PRINCIPLES AND PRACTICE OF GYNECOLOGIC ONCOLOGY

PRINCIPLES AND PRACTICE OF GYNECOLOGIC ONCOLOGY

FIFTH EDITION

Edited by

Richard R. Barakat, MD, FACOG, FACS
Chief, Gynecology Service, Department of Surgery
Ronald O. Perelman Chair in Gynecologic Surgery
Vice Chairman, Clinical Affairs, Department of Surgery
Memorial Sloan-Kettering Cancer Center
New York, New York

Maurie Markman, MD
Vice President for Clinical Research
The University of Texas M. D. Anderson Cancer Center
Houston, Texas

Marcus E. Randall, MD, FACR
Chairman, Department of Radiation Medicine
University of Kentucky
Lexington, Kentucky

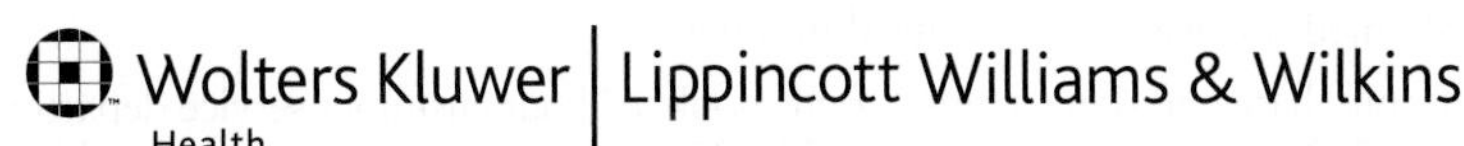

Philadelphia • Baltimore • New York • London
Buenos Aires • Hong Kong • Sydney • Tokyo

Acquisitions Editor: Jonathan W. Pine, Jr.
Managing Editor: Joyce Murphy
Marketing Manager: Angela Panetta
Project Manager: Paula C. Williams
Designer: Stephen Druding
Production Services: International Typesetting and Composition

Fifth Edition

351 West Camden Street
Baltimore, MD 21201

530 Walnut Street
Philadelphia, PA 19106

Printed in China

9 8 7 6 5 4 3 2 1

Library of Congress Cataloging-in-Publication Data

Principles and practice of gynecologic oncology.—5th ed. / [edited by]
Richard R. Barakat, Maurie Markman, Marcus Randall.
p. ; cm.
Includes bibliographical references and index.
ISBN-13: 978-0-7817-7845-9
ISBN-10: 0-7817-7845-X
1. Generative organs, Female—Cancer. I. Barakat, Richard R. II. Markman, Maurie. III. Randall, Marcus, 1956-
[DNLM: 1. Genital Neoplasms, Female. 2. Breast Neoplasms. WP 145 P957 2009]
RC280.G5P75 2009
616.99'465—dc22

2008045509

DISCLAIMER

Care has been taken to confirm the accuracy of the information present and to describe generally accepted practices. However, the authors, editors, and publisher are not responsible for errors or omissions or for any consequences from application of the information in this book and make no warranty, expressed or implied, with respect to the currency, completeness, or accuracy of the contents of the publication. Application of this information in a particular situation remains the professional responsibility of the practitioner; the clinical treatments described and recommended may not be considered absolute and universal recommendations.

The authors, editors, and publisher have exerted every effort to ensure that drug selection and dosage set forth in this text are in accordance with the current recommendations and practice at the time of publication. However, in view of ongoing research, changes in government regulations, and the constant flow of information relating to drug therapy and drug reactions, the reader is urged to check the package insert for each drug for any change in indications and dosage and for added warnings and precautions. This is particularly important when the recommended agent is a new or infrequently employed drug.

Some drugs and medical devices presented in this publication have Food and Drug Administration (FDA) clearance for limited use in restricted research settings. It is the responsibility of the health care provider to ascertain the FDA status of each drug or device planned for use in their clinical practice.

To purchase additional copies of this book, call our customer service department at (800) 638-3030 or fax orders to (301) 223-2320. International customers should call (301) 223-2300.

Visit Lippincott Williams & Wilkins on the Internet: http://www.lww.com. Lippincott Williams & Wilkins customer service representatives are available from 8:30 am to 6:00 pm, EST.

CCS0409

This book is dedicated to our families—Catherine Barakat and children Joanna, Richard Jr., and Christian Barakat; Brabham Morgan Randall and children Ken, Morgan, and Marycobb Randall; and Tomes Markman and children Margaret, Jonathan, Timothy, and Elisabeth Markman. By virtue of their patience, good humor, encouragement, and tolerance of our long hours at work, they have each made significant contributions to this book.

FOREWORD

Stuart Freeman, in charge of production of oncology textbooks at Lippincott Publishers (now Lippincott Williams & Wilkins) approached the three of us—Carlos Perez, Robert Young, and me—in the early 1990s to collaborate in editing a textbook on gynecologic cancer. We met to plan the text in 1992, and 2 years later, in 1994, the first edition was published. With the able guidance of Stuart, we developed several basic principles: (a) The textbook would be multidisciplinary, with the disease chapters authored by a surgeon, a medical oncologist, a radiation oncologist, and a pathologist; (b) the editors would strive to make the textbook a definitive reference that would be written at the level of an expert in surgery, medical oncology, and radiation oncology; (c) the text would be divided into three sections: basic science, modalities of therapy, and the disease chapters, which cover current principles of treatment; (d) we would edit the book in two sessions, each lasting 2 to 3 days, with all the editors sitting at one table reading the same chapter; (e) we would strive to publish an updated edition every 3 years.

Over the next 12 years, we published four editions of the text, the first three under the guidance of Stuart Freeman and the last edition under the guidance of Jonathan Pine. We appreciate the assistance and support that we received from Lippincott Williams & Wilkins throughout. We were, and remain, grateful for the opportunity to develop a close friendship and, most important, we were satisfied that our book was a definitive and valuable text for those physicians who treat gynecologic cancer.

In the planning for the fourth edition, the three editors agreed that it would be our last edition and that we should select new editors to continue the publication of the text. As a group, we chose Richard Barakat, MD, Maurie Markman, MD, and Marcus Randall, MD, and they worked with us on the preparation of the fourth edition. In this fifth edition of *Principles and Practice of Gynecologic Oncology,* our only involvement is to write the Foreword. This edition and the ones to come are the work of Rich, Maurie, and Marc. We are grateful that the current editors have agreed to carry on the text, and we anticipate that this text will be outstanding and uphold the tradition of presenting the state of the art in gynecologic oncology.

The landscape in the management of patients with gynecologic cancer has rapidly evolved in recent years. A vaccine for human papillomavirus (HPV) is being administered worldwide, with the expectation that it will substantially decrease the incidence and mortality of carcinoma of the uterine cervix. All aspects of the diagnosis and treatment of gynecologic cancer have become more complex. Surgical procedures are more radical, and there are many new chemotherapeutic and targeted agents (both cytotoxic and biologic) and new equipment and techniques in radiation oncology. Survival rates for ovarian and cervical cancer have improved, and survival for corpus cancer is stable. In 2007, the 5-year survival for all stages and all races was 45% for ovary, 72% for cervix, and 83% for corpus cancers.

This text continues to be the most comprehensive and up-to-date book for the physicians who treat women with gynecologic cancer, and with its multidisciplinary approach still addresses the most important aspects of basic biology, pathology, modalities of therapy, and therapeutic options by disease site.

As the original editors of this text, we are very pleased with this fifth edition of *Principles and Practice of Gynecologic Oncology* and congratulate the new editors, Drs. Richard Barakat, Maurie Markman, and Marcus Randall, for their achievement. We are confident they will continue to produce timely and up-to-date editions in the future.

William J Hoskins, MD
Carlos A Perez, MD
Robert C Young, MD

CONTENTS

SECTION I: EPIDEMIOLOGY OF GYNECOLOGIC CANCER

SECTION II: THERAPEUTIC MODALITIES AND RELATED SUBJECTS

SECTION III: DISEASE SITES

SECTION IV: SPECIAL MANAGEMENT TOPICS

CONTRIBUTING AUTHORS

Nadeem R. Abu-Rustum, MD
Associate Attending Director
Minimally Invasive Surgery Program
Gynecology Service, Department of Surgery
Memorial Sloan-Kettering Cancer Center
New York, New York

David S. Alberts, MD
Professor of Medicine, Pharmacology, Nutritional Sciences, and Public Health
Director, Arizona Cancer Center
University of Arizona
Tucson, Arizona

Kaled M. Alektiar, MD
Attending Radiation Oncologist
Department of Radiation Oncology
Memorial Sloan-Kettering Cancer Center
New York, New York

Christina M. Annunziata, MD, PhD
Associate Clinical Investigator
Molecular Signaling Section
Medical Oncology Branch
Center for Cancer Research
National Cancer Institute
Bethesda, Maryland

Susan M. Ascher, MD
Professor
Department of Radiology
Director, Division of Abdominal Imaging
Georgetown University Hospital
Washington, DC

Nilofer S. Azad, MD
Medical Oncology Fellow
Molecular Signaling Section
Medical Oncology Branch
Center for Cancer Research
National Cancer Institute
Bethesda, Maryland

Andrew Berchuck, MD
Professor and Director
Division of Gynecologic Oncology
Duke University Medical Center
Durham, North Carolina

Ross S. Berkowitz, MD
William H. Baker Professor of Gynecology
Harvard Medical School
Director
Gynecologic Oncology and Gynecology
Co-director, New England Trophoblastic Disease Center
Brigham and Women's Hospital
Dana Farber Cancer Center
Boston, Massachusetts

Michael J. Birrer, MD, PhD
Director
Gynecologic Cancer Research Program
Diana Farber/Harvard Cancer Center
Professor of Medicine, Harvard Medical School
Director, Gillette Center for Gynecologic Oncology
Massachusetts General Hospital Cancer Center
Boston, Massachusetts

Michael A. Bookman, MD
Member
Division of Medical Science
Fox Chase Cancer Center
Philadelphia, Pennsylvania

Jeff Boyd, PhD
Vice President for Laboratory Science
Memorial Health University Medical Center
Associate Director for Laboratory Science
Anderson Cancer Institute
Savannah, Georgia

Mark F. Brady, PhD
Director of Statistics
Gynecological Oncology Group (GOG) Statistical Office and Data Center
Roswell Park Cancer Institute
Buffalo, New York

Louise A. Brinton, PhD
Chief
Hormonal and Reproductive Epidemiology Branch
National Cancer Institute
Rockville, Maryland

Robert E. Bristow, MD
Professor and Director
The Kelly Gynecologic Oncology Service
Department of Gynecology and Obstetrics
The Johns Hopkins Medical Institutions
Baltimore, Maryland

James J. Burke II, MD
Associate Professor
Department of Obstetrics and Gynecology
Division of Gynecologic Oncology
Mercer University School of Medicine
Memorial University Medical Center
Savannah, Georgia

Joanna M. Cain, M.D.
Chace/Joukowsky Professor and Chair
Surgeon-in-Chief
Department of Gynecology and Obstetrics
Rhode Island Hospital
Obstetrician and Gynecologist-in-Chief
Women & Infants Hospital
Providence, Rhode Island

Higinia Cárdenes, MD, PhD
Professor
Radiation Oncology Department
Indiana University School of Medicine
Indianapolis, Indiana

Jeanne Carter, PhD
Assistant Attending Psychologist
Department of Psychiatry
Memorial Sloan-Kettering Cancer Center
New York, New York

David Cella, PhD
Professor and Executive Director
Center on Outcomes Research and Education
Evanston Northwestern Healthcare
Robert H. Lurie Comprehensive Cancer Center of Northwestern University
Evanston, Illinois

David Z. Chang, MD, PhD
Assistant Professor of Medicine
Department of Gastrointestinal Medical Oncology and Immunology
The University of Texas M. D. Anderson Cancer Center
Houston, Texas

Dana Chase, M.D.
Clinical Instructor
Division of Gynecologic Oncology
Department of Obstetrics and Gynecology
University of California Irvine
Irvine, California

Dennis S. Chi, MD
Associate Member
Gynecology Service, Department of Surgery
Memorial Sloan-Kettering Cancer Center
New York, New York

Cirrelda Cooper, MD
Professor
Department of Radiology
Division of Abdominal Imaging
Georgetown University Hospital
Washington, DC

Mary B. Daly, MD, PhD
Senior Vice President for Population Science
Fox Chase Cancer Center
Philadelphia, Pennsylvania

Chaitanya R. Divgi, MD
Professor of Radiology and Radiation Oncology
Professor
Wistar Institute
Member, Abramson Cancer Center
University of Pennsylvania
Chief, Division of Nuclear Medicine
and Clinical Molecular Imaging
Hospital of the University of Pennsylvania
Philadelphia, Pennsylvania

Don S. Dizon, MD
Director of Medical Oncology and Integrative Care
Co-Director, Center for Sexuality, Intimacy, and Fertility
Program in Women's Oncology
Women and Infants Hospital of Rhode Island
Assistant Professor, Obstetrics-Gynecology and Medicine
The Warren Alpert Medical School of Brown University
Providence, Rhode Island

Robert T. Dorr, Ph.D.
Professor of Pharmacology
Arizona Cancer Center
Cancer Center Division
University of Arizona
Tucson, Arizona

Beth A. Erickson-Wittmann, MD, FACR
Professor of Radiation Oncology
Radiation Oncology Clinic
Medical College of Wisconsin
Milwaukee, Wisconsin

John H. Farley, MD, COL, FACOG, FACS
Associate Professor
Senior Medical Coordinator Advisor
Department of Obstetrics and Gynecology
Uniformed Services University of the Health Sciences
Bethesda, Maryland

Gwenael Ferron, MD
Department of Surgery
Institut Claudius Regaud Cancer Center
Toulouse, France

Gini F. Fleming, MD
Professor of Medicine
University of Chicago Medical Center
Chicago, Illinois

Damean Freas, MD
Fellow
Department of Pain Medicine and Palliative Care
Beth Israel Medical Center
New York, New York

Daniel P. Gaile, PhD
Assistant Professor
Department of Biostatistics
School of Public Health and Health Professions
Roswell Park Cancer Institute
New York State Center of Excellence in Bioinformatics
and Life Sciences
Buffalo, New York

Donald G. Gallup, MD
Professor, Chair, and Program Director
Department of Obstetrics and Gynecology
Mercer University School of Medicine
Savannah, Georgia

Ginger J. Gardner, MD
Assistant Attending Surgeon
Gynecology Service, Department of Surgery
Memorial Sloan-Kettering Cancer Center
New York, New York

Jennifer S. Gass, MD, FACS
Chief of Surgery
Director of the Breast Fellowship
Women and Infants Hospital of Rhode Island
Assistant Professor (Clinical)
The Warren Alpert Medical School of Brown University
Providence, Rhode Island

Aleksandra Gentry-Maharaj, PhD
Research Fellow
Gynaecological Cancer Research Centre
EGA Institute for Women's Health
University College London
London, United Kingdom

David M. Gershenson, MD
Professor and Chairman
Department of Gynecologic Oncology
University of Texas M.D. Anderson Cancer Center
Houston, Texas

Donald P. Goldstein, MD
Professor of Obstetrics, Gynecology, and Reproductive Biology
Harvard Medical School
Co-director
New England Trophoblastic Disease Center
Department of Obstetrics and Gynecology
Brigham and Women's Hospital
Dana Farber Cancer Institute
Boston, Massachusetts

Lynn C. Hartmann, MD
Professor of Oncology
Co-leader, Mayo Women's Cancer Program
Mayo Clinic Cancer Center
Rochester, Minnesota

Lisa M. Hess, MD, PhD
Science Officer
Cancer Center Division
Leon-Levy Cancer Center
University of Arizona
Tucson, Arizona

Ebony R. Hoskins, MD
Cancer Research Training Award Fellow
Molecular Signaling Section
Medical Oncology Branch
Center for Cancer Research
National Cancer Institute
Bethesda, Maryland

Alan N. Houghton, MD
Virginia and Daniel K. Ludwig Clinical Chair
Member, Attending Physician, and Chief, Clinical Immunology Service
Vice-Chair
Department of Medicine
Head, Swim Across America Laboratory of Tumor Immunology
Memorial Sloan-Kettering Cancer Center
Professor of Medicine and Immunology
Weill Medical School
Graduate School of Medical Sciences of Cornell University
New York, New York

Hedvig Hricak, MD, PhD, Dr hc
Professor of Radiology
Weill Medical College of Cornell University
Chairman, Department of Radiology
Memorial Sloan-Kettering Cancer Center
New York, New York

Alan D. Hutson, PhD
Chair and Professor
Department of Biostatistics
School of Public Health and Health Professions
The University of Buffalo, SUNY
Buffalo, New York

Ian Jacobs, MD, FRCOG
Professor of Women's Health
Dean, UCL and Partners Health Sciences Research
Gynaecological Cancer Research Centre
EGA Institute for Women's Health
University College London
London, United Kingdom

Amir A. Jazaeri, MD
Assistant Professor
Department of Obstetrics and Gynecology
Division of Gynecologic Oncology
Charlottesville, Virginia

John Kavanagh, MD
Professor and Associate Director of Therapeutic Development
Department of Gynecologic Oncology
The University of Texas M. D. Anderson Cancer Center
Houston, Texas

Hanan I. Khalil, MD
Women's Imaging
Women and Infants Hospital of Rhode Island
Assistant Professor of Diagnostic Imaging (Clinical)
The Warren Alpert Medical School of Brown University
Providence, Rhode Island

Kevin Khater, MD, PhD
Medical Director
Radiation Oncology of Northern Illinois
Ottawa, Illinois

Susan L. Koelliker, MD
Women's Imaging, Body Imaging
Women and Infants Hospital of Rhode Island
Assistant Professor of Diagnostic Imaging (Clinical)
The Warren Alpert Medical School of Brown University
Providence, Rhode Island

Wui-Jin Koh, MD
Associate Professor
Department of Radiation Oncology
University of Washington Medical Center
Seattle, Washington

Elise C. Kohn, MD
Head
Molecular Signaling Section
Medical Oncology Branch
National Cancer Institute
Bethesda, Maryland

Eric Leblanc, MD
Département de Cancérologie Gynécologique
Centre Oscar Lambret
Lille, France

Robert D. Legare, MD
Director
Breast Health Center
Director
Cancer Risk and Prevention Program
Women and Infants Hospital of Rhode Island
Assistant Professor of Medicine and Obstetrics-Gynecology
The Warren Alpert Medical School of Brown University
Providence, Rhode Island

Pauline Lesage, MD
Director of the Palliative Care
Division, Department of Pain Medicine and Palliative Care
Medical Director, Continuum Hospice Care/
Jacob Perlow Hospice
Beth Israel Hospital
New York, New York

Philip O. Livingston, MD
Member and Attending Physician
Memorial Sloan-Kettering Cancer Center
Head, Laboratory of Tumor Vaccinology
Professor of Medicine
Weill Medical School
Graduate School of Medical Sciences of Cornell University
New York, New York

Harry Long III, MD
Professor of Oncology
Division of Medical Oncology
Mayo Clinic College of Medicine
Rochester, Minnesota

Stephanie MacAusland, MD
Assistant Professor of Radiation Oncology
The Warren Alpert Medical School of Brown University
Providence, Rhode Island

Maurie Markman, MD
Vice President for Clinical Research
Chairman, Department of Gynecologic Medical Oncology
Professor of Cancer Medicine
The University of Texas M. D Anderson Cancer Center
Houston, Texas

Daniela E. Matei, MD
Associate Professor
Melvin and Bren Simon Cancer Center
Indiana University
Indianapolis, Indiana

G. Larry Maxwell, MD
Director
Gynecologic Disease Center
Chief, Division of Gynecologic Oncology
Walter Reed Army Medical Center
Professor, Uniformed Services University
Washington, DC

William P. McGuire, MD
Director
Harry and Jeanette Weinberg Cancer Institute
Baltimore, Maryland

D. Scott McMeekin, MD
Virginia Kerley Cade Chair in Cancer
Developmental Therapeutics
Section Chief
Gynecologic Oncology
University of Oklahoma
Oklahoma City, Oklahoma

Usha Menon, MD, FRCOG
Senior Lecturer/Consultant Gynaecologist
Gynaecological Cancer Research Centre
EGA Institute for Women's Health
University College London
London, United Kingdom

Helen Michael, MD
Professor
Department of Pathology
Indiana University School of Medicine
Chief, Pathology and Laboratory Medicine
Clarian North Medical Center
Indianapolis, Indiana

David Moore, MD
Mary Fendrich Hulman Professor of Gynecologic Oncology
Indiana University
Indianapolis, Indiana

Arno J. Mundt, MD
Professor and Chair
Department of Radiation Oncology
Moores UCSD Cancer Center
La Jolla, California

David G. Mutch, MD
Judith and Ira Gall Professor of Gynecologic Oncology
Director, Division of Gynecologic Oncology
Washington University School of Medicine
St. Louis, Missouri

Steven A. Narod, MD, FRCP
Canada Research Chair in Breast Cancer
Professor, Public Health Sciences
Women's College Research Institute
Toronto, Ontario, Canada

Brigid O'Connor, MD
Assistant Professor of Radiation Oncology
The Warren Alpert Medical School of Brown University
Providence, Rhode Island

Janet L. Osborne, MD
Assistant Professor
Department of Obstetrics and Gynecology
Division of Gynecologic Oncology
Froedtert Memorial Lutheran Hospital
Milwaukee, Wisconsin

Richard Penson, MD, MRCP
Clinical Director
Medical Gynecologic Oncology
Massachusetts General Hospital
Assistant Professor, Harvard Medical School
Boston, Massachusetts

Marie Plante, MD
Associate Professor
Department of Obstetrics and Gynecology
Laval University
Quebec, Canada

Russell K. Portenoy, MD
Chairman, Department of Pain Medicine and Palliative Care
Beth Israel Medical Center
New York, New York

Denis Querleu, MD
Professor and Head
Department of Surgery
Institut Claudius Regaud
Toulouse, France

Issam I. Raad, MD, FACP, FIDSA
Professor of Medicine
Chairman, Department of Infectious Diseases, Infection Control, and Employee Health
The University of Texas M. D. Anderson Cancer Center
Houston, Texas

Marcus E. Randall, MD, FACR
Markey Foundation Chair and Professor
Department of Radiation Medicine
University of Kentucky
Lexington, Kentucky

Laurel W. Rice, MD
Professor and Chair
Department of Obstetrics and Gynecology
University of Wisconsin School of Medicine and Public Health
Madison, Wisconsin

John I. Risinger, PhD
Associate Member
Memorial University Medical Center
Anderson Cancer Institute
Savannah, Georgia

Brigitte M. Ronnett, MD
Professor
Departments of Pathology and Gynecology and Obstetrics
The Johns Hopkins University School of Medicine and Hospital
Baltimore, Maryland

Lawrence M. Roth, MD
Professor Emeritus of Pathology
Indiana University School of Medicine
Indianapolis, Indiana

Eric K. Rowinsky, MD
Chief Medical Officer, Senior Vice President
ImClone Systems Incorporated
Branchburg, New Jersey
Adjunct Professor of Medicine
New York University School of Medicine
New York, New York

Jason Rownd, MS, DABMP
Senior Medical Physicist
Radiation Oncology Clinic
Medical College of Wisconsin
Milwaukee, Wisconsin

Stephen C. Rubin, MD
Director
Division of GYN Oncology
University of Pennsylvania Medical Center
Philadelphia, Pennsylvania

Anthony H. Russell, MD
Associate Professor of Radiation Oncology
Harvard Medical School
Chief
Gynecologic Radiation Oncology Service
Department of Radiation Oncology
Massachusetts General Hospital
Boston, Massachusetts

Paul J. Sabbatini, MD
Associate Attending Physician
Gynecologic Medical Oncology Service
Department of Medicine
Memorial Sloan-Kettering Cancer Center
New York, New York

Amar Safdar, MD, FACP, FIDSA
Associate Professor of Medicine
Director
Clinical Mycobacterial Research
Department of Infectious Diseases, Infection Control, and Employee Health
The University of Texas M. D. Anderson Cancer Center
Houston, Texas

Mark Schattner, MD
Attending Gastroenterologist
Department of Medicine, GI/Nutrition
Memorial Sloan-Kettering Cancer Center
New York, New York

Mark Schiffman, MD, MPH
Deputy Chief, Hormonal and Reproductive Epidemiology Branch
National Cancer Institute
Rockville, Maryland

Jeanne M. Schilder, MD
Associate Professor
Department of Obstetrics and Gynecology
Division of Gynecologic Oncology
Indiana University School of Medicine
Indianapolis, Indiana

Leslie Scoutt, MD
Professor of Diagnostic Radiology
Chief of Ultrasound Service
Department of Diagnostic Radiology
Yale University School of Medicine
New Haven, Connecticut

Jeffrey Seidman, MD
Director of Gynecological Pathology
Department of Pathology
Washington Hospital Center
Washington, DC

Christopher K. Senkowski, MD, FACS
Associate Professor of Surgery
Mercer University School of Medicine
Savannah Campus Memorial University Medical Center
Savannah, Georgia

Moshe Shike, MD
Director
Memorial Sloan-Kettering Cancer Prevention and Wellness Program
Department of Medicine, GI/Nutrition
Memorial Sloan-Kettering Cancer Center
New York, New York

Yukio Sonoda, MD
Assistant Attending Surgeon
Gynecology Service, Department of Surgery
Memorial Sloan-Kettering Cancer Center
New York, New York

Margaret M. Steinhoff, MD
Director
Division of Gynecologic Pathology
Women and Infants Hospital of Rhode Island
Professor of Pathology and Laboratory Medicine
The Warren Alpert Medical School of Brown University
Providence, Rhode Island

C. James Sung, MD
Director of Clinical Pathology
Women and Infants Hospital of Rhode Island
Professor of Pathology and Laboratory Medicine
The Warren Alpert Medical School of Brown University
Providence, Rhode Island

Gregory Sutton, MD
Medical Director
Gynecologic Oncology
St. Vincent Hospitals and Health Services
Indianapolis, Indiana

Charu Taneja, MD
Director
Breast Health Program
Roger Williams Medical Center
Providence, Rhode Island
Clinical Assistant Professor
Department of Surgery
Boston University Medical Center
Boston, Massachusetts

Sean Tedjarati, MD, MPH
Associate Professor
Division of Gynecologic Oncology
Texas Tech University Health Sciences Center
Amarillo, Texas

Trevor Tejada-Berges, MD
Gynecologic Oncologist and Breast Surgeon
Program in Women's Oncology
Women and Infants Hospital of Rhode Island
Assistant Professor, Obstetrics-Gynecology
The Warren Alpert Medical School of Brown University
Providence, Rhode Island

Susan Tolle, MD
Cornelia Hayes Stevens Chair
Director
Center for Ethics in Health Care
Professor of Medicine
Oregon Health and Science University
Portland, Oregon

Carmen Tornos, MD
Professor of Pathology
Stony Brook University Medical Center
Stony Brook, New York

Daniel D. Von Hoff, MD, FACP
Physician in Chief, Senior Investigator
Translational Genomics Research Institute (TGen)
Clinical Professor of Medicine
University of Arizona
Phoenix, Arizona

Lari Wenzel, PhD
Professor
College of Health Sciences
University of California, Irvine
Irvine, California

Edward J. Wilkinson, MD, FACOG, FCAP
Professor and Vice Chairman
Department of Pathology and Laboratory Medicine
University of Florida College of Medicine
Gainesville, Florida

Darcy J. Wolfman, MD
Assistant Professor
Department of Radiology
Division of Abdominal Imaging
Georgetown University Hospital
Washington, DC

Aaron Wolfson, MD
Professor and Vice Chair
Department of Radiation Oncology
Sylvester Cancer Center
University of Miami School of Medicine
Miami, Florida

Thomas C. Wright Jr, MD
Professor of Pathology
Department of Pathology
College of Physicians and Surgeons of Columbia University
New York, New York

Catheryn Yashar, MD
Assistant Professor of Radiation Oncology
Chief
Breast and Gynecologic Services
University of California, San Diego Moores Cancer Center
La Jolla, California

Robert H. Young, MD
Robert E. Scully Professor of Pathology
Harvard Medical School
Director, Surgical Pathology
Massachusetts General Hospital
Boston Massachusetts

Richard J. Zaino, MD
Professor of Pathology
Milton S. Hershey Medical Center
Pennsylvania State University
Hershey, Pennsylvania

Kristin K. Zorn, MD
Assistant Professor
Department of Obstetrics, Gynecology, and Women's Health
Magee–Women's Hospital of the University of Pittsburgh Medical Center
Pittsburgh, Pennsylvania

PREFACE

The publication of the fifth edition of *Principles and Practice of Gynecologic Oncology* marks the completion of the transition to three new editors, Richard Barakat, Maurie Markman, and Marcus Randall. As editors and cancer specialists, we are excited about the fifth edition and are honored to follow in the tradition of excellence established by our three predecessors, William J. Hoskins, MD, Carlos A. Perez, MD, and Robert C. Young, MD, who had worked together on this textbook for over 15 years. Without their guidance and friendship, this seamless transition wouldn't have been possible. We look forward to building on their important contribution to the medical literature.

We remain committed to the multidisciplinary theme of the textbook, with chapters authored by teams consisting of a surgeon, a medical oncologist, a radiation oncologist, and a pathologist. The increasing complexity of all aspects of gynecologic cancer treatment requires this type of approach. As in previous editions, we have rotated approximately 30% of the authors, and all chapters have been either completely rewritten or extensively updated, including the chapters on the three major disease sites—ovarian, uterine, and cervical cancer—as well as breast cancer. We are certain that this edition contains the most up-to-date information available about the treatment of gynecologic cancers. This textbook was designed for specialists who care for women afflicted with gynecologic cancer, including surgeons, medical oncologists, radiation oncologists, pathologists, and nurses. It also serves as a valuable resource for residents and fellows in training for a career in cancer care.

Finally, we wish to thank the readers for their support in the past and look forward to their continued support and advice in the future. We will continually strive to improve the content and quality of this comprehensive textbook. It is our hope that this textbook will play a significant role in developing future treatments to benefit women afflicted with gynecologic cancer.

Richard Barakat, MD
Maurie Markman, MD
Marcus Randall, MD

ACKNOWLEDGMENTS

The editors acknowledge the contributions of numerous individuals without whom this book would not have been possible. The talented staff of the publisher, Lippincott Williams & Wilkins, especially Jonathan Pine, senior executive editor; Joyce Murphy, associate director of content; Anne Jacobs, senior managing editor; and Paula Williams, senior project editor, provided invaluable encouragement, direction, and guidance during the creative process and in technical execution. Charu Dutt, senior project manager for International Typesetting and Composition, provided outstanding production services.

From the Gynecology & Breast Services Academic Office, Department of Surgery, Memorial Sloan-Kettering Cancer Center (MSKCC), we acknowledge the invaluable contributions of K. Alexandra MacDonald, senior editor; Jennifer Grady, assistant editor; and Shan-san Wu, assistant editor. Their attention to detail, patience, and communication skills were of the utmost importance throughout the publication process. Our appreciation for all their efforts cannot be adequately expressed, but we hope they know how much we value their contributions.

miRNA genes
Pol II
NUCLEUS
CYTOPLASM
Pol II Trans-cription
m7Gpp
Pri-miRNA
AAA
Pol II
Drasha
RISC
ORF
3′ UTR
Translation
Mature miRNA
Mature siRNA
Pre-miRNA
RISC
ORF
ORF
3′ UTR
RNA-GTP
Exporin 5
miRNA:miRNA* duplex
Helicase
Pre-miRNA
Dicer
Dicer
Helicase
Degradation
Cell membrane
Foreign dsRNA
*siRNA
*miRNA

COLOR PLATE 3.10.

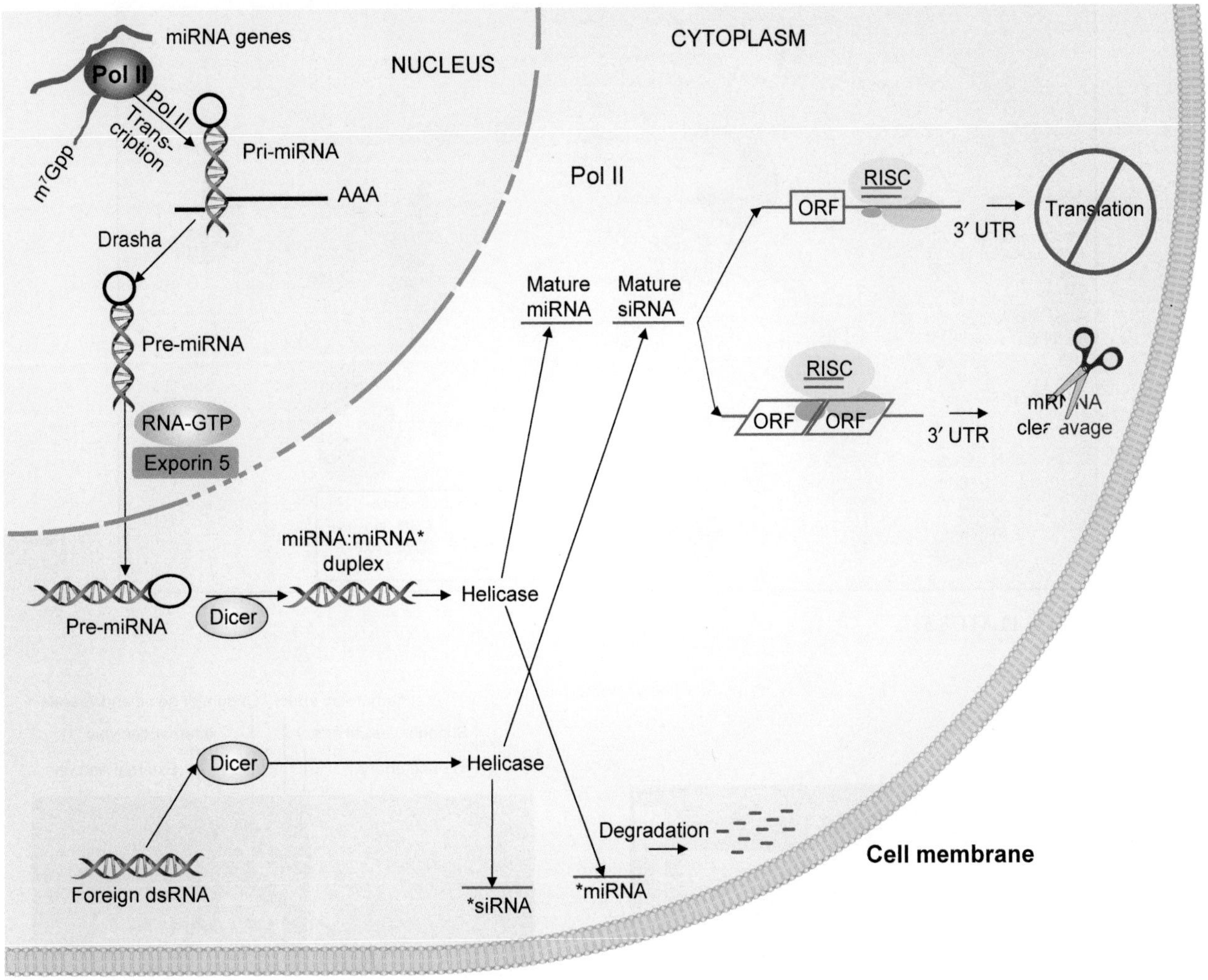

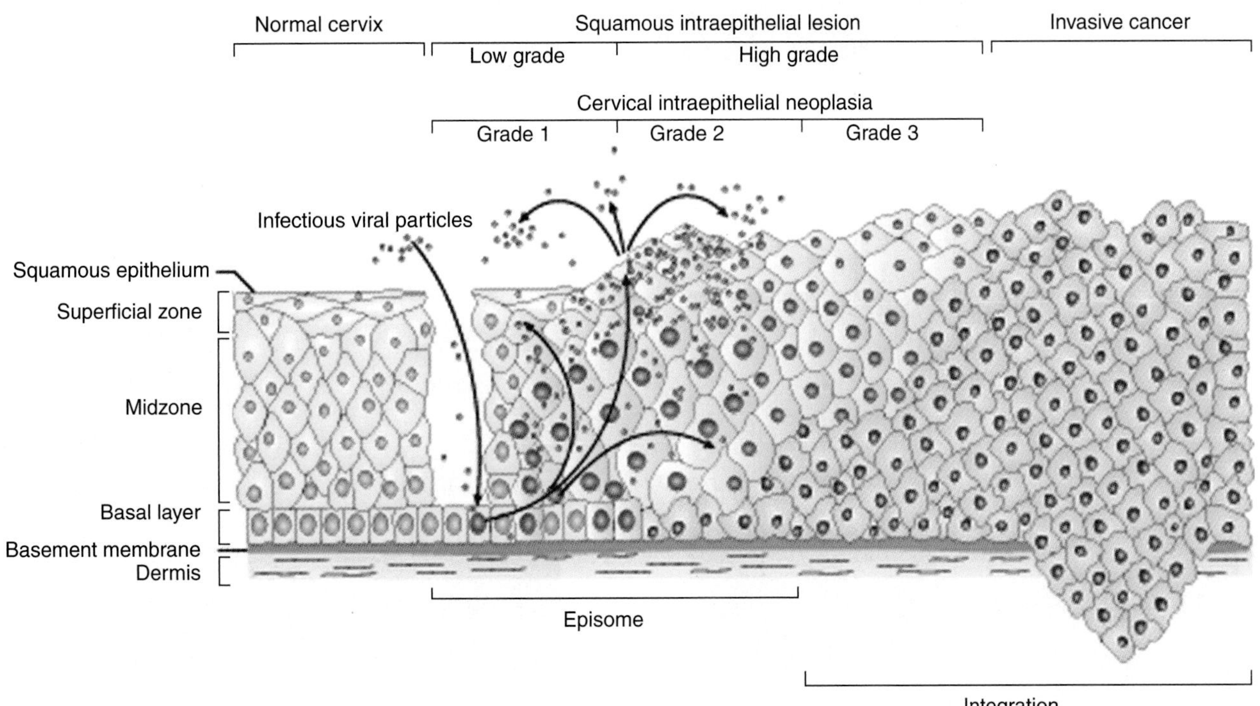
Normal cervix
Squamous intraepithelial lesion
Invasive cancer
Low grade
High grade
Cervical intraepithelial neoplasia
Grade 1
Grade 2
Grade 3
Infectious viral particles
Squamous epithelium
Superficial zone
Midzone
Basal layer
Basement membrane
Dermis
Episome
Integration

COLOR PLATE 8.4.

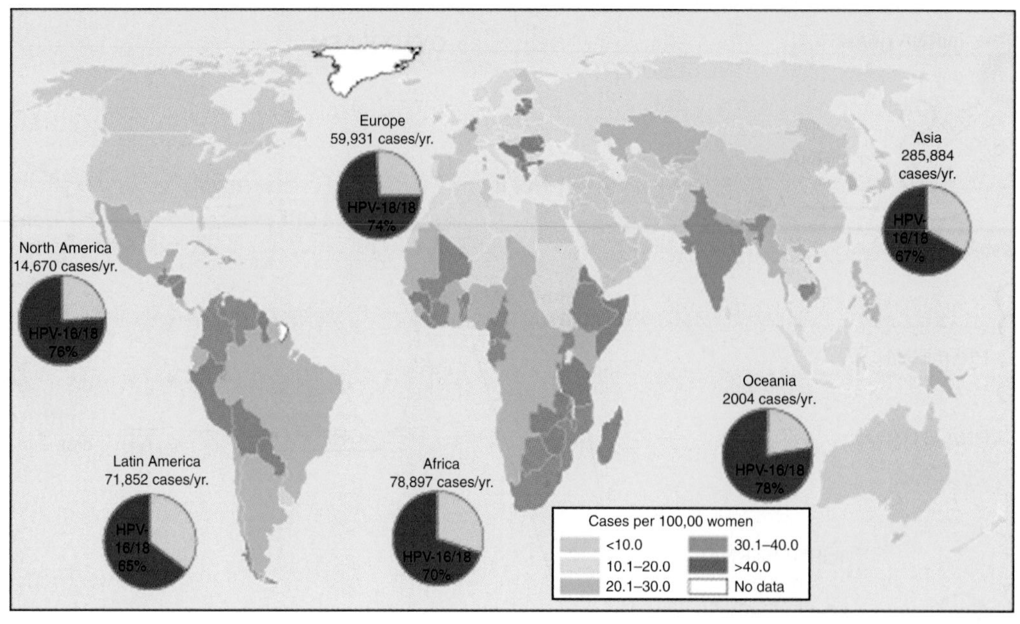

COLOR PLATE 8.5.

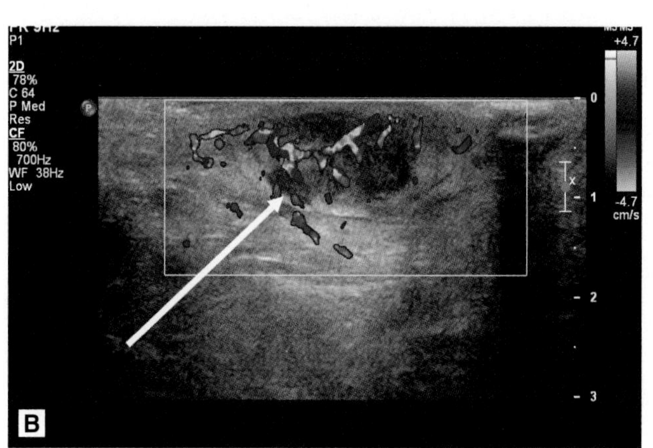

COLOR PLATE 10.39B.

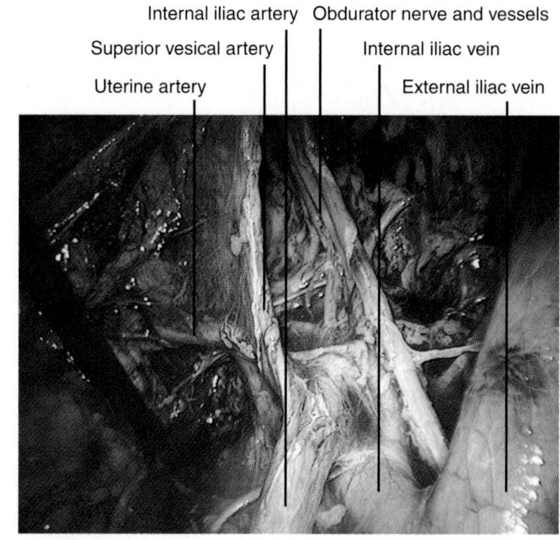

COLOR PLATE 13.3.

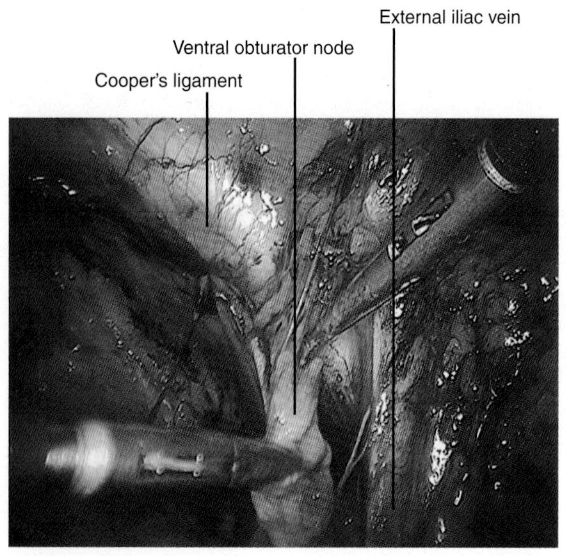

COLOR PLATE 13.2.

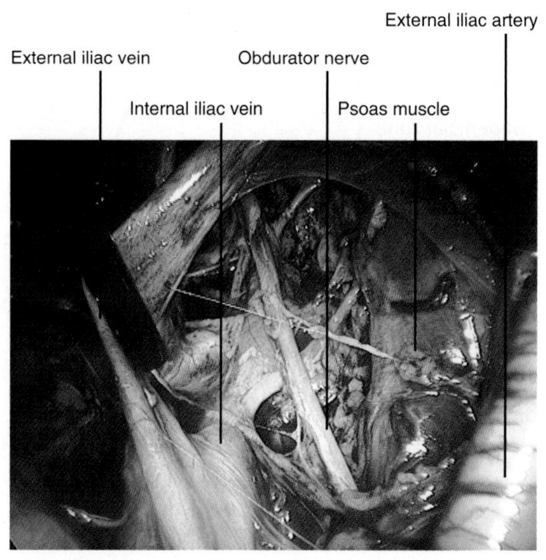

COLOR PLATE 13.4.

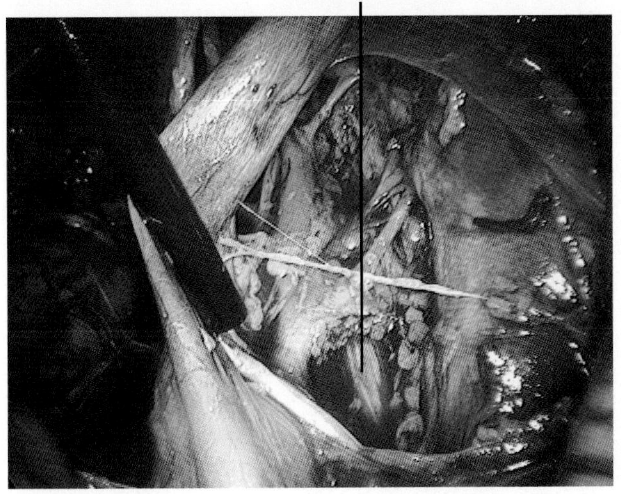

COLOR PLATE 13.5.

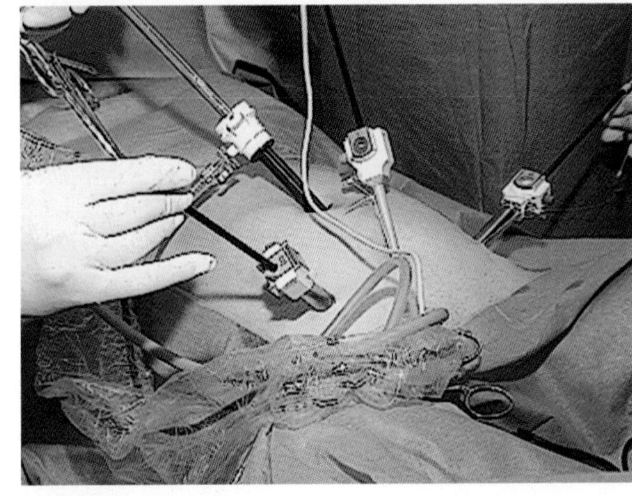

COLOR PLATE 13.8.

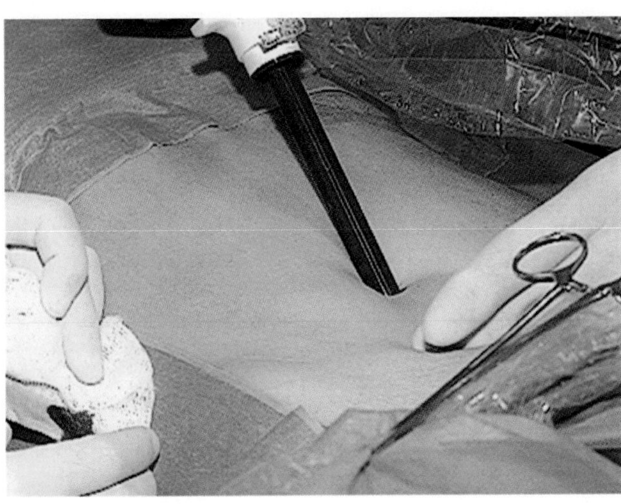

COLOR PLATE 13.6.

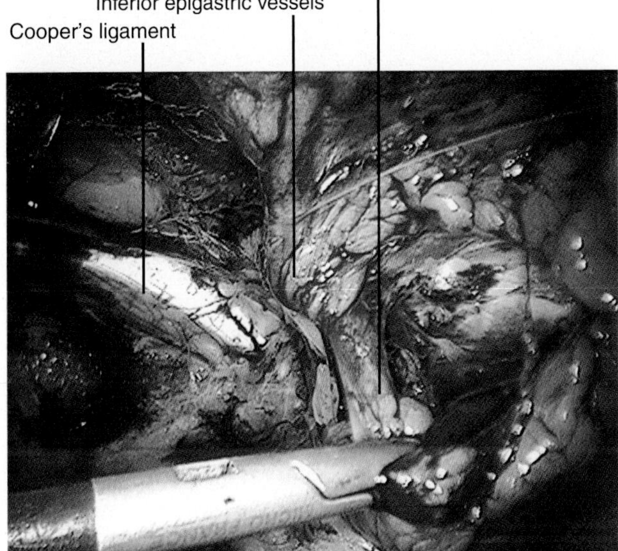

COLOR PLATE 13.9.

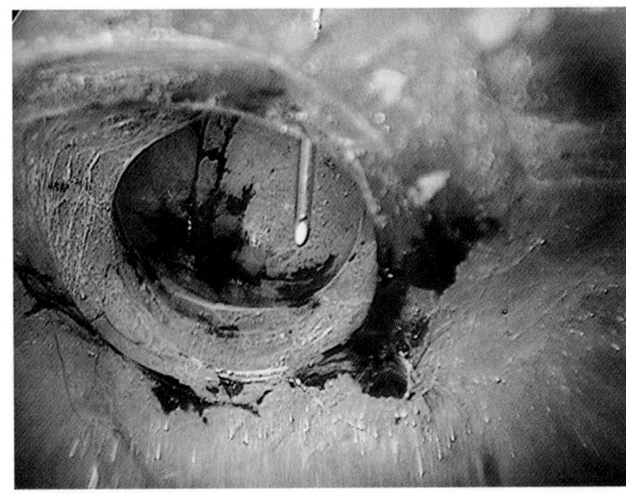

COLOR PLATE 13.7.

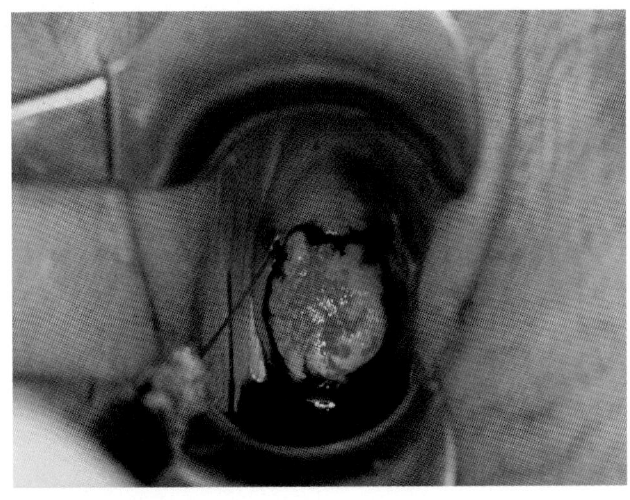

COLOR PLATE 13.10.

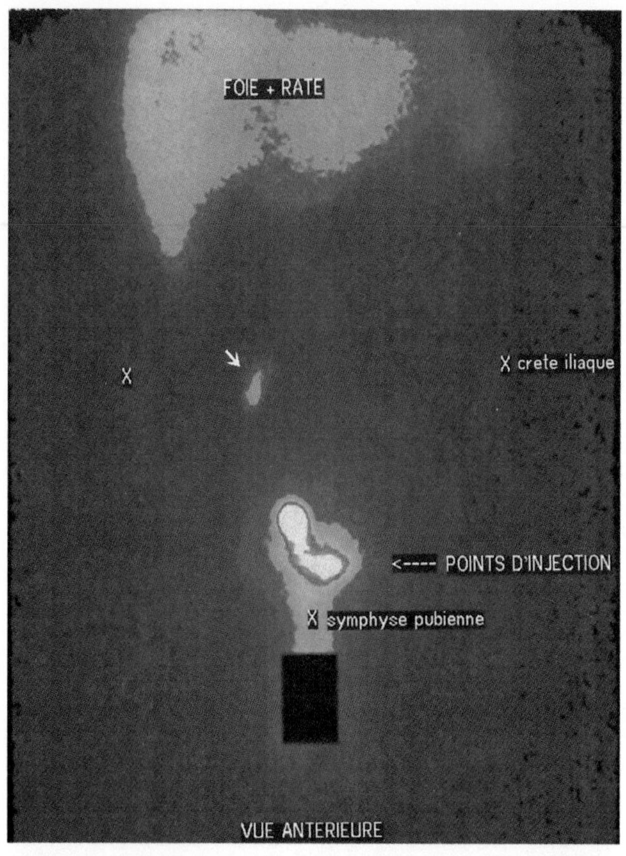

COLOR PLATE 13.11.

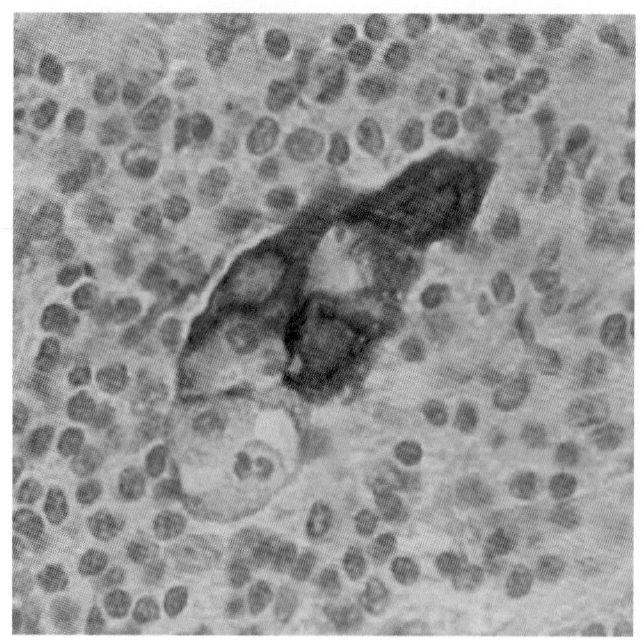

COLOR PLATE 13.14.

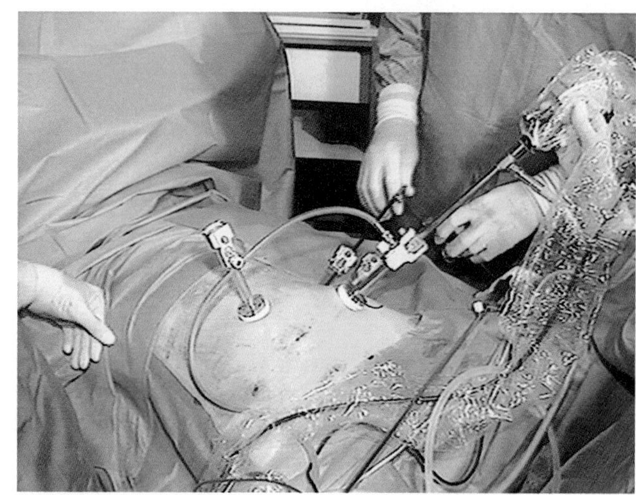

COLOR PLATE 13.15.

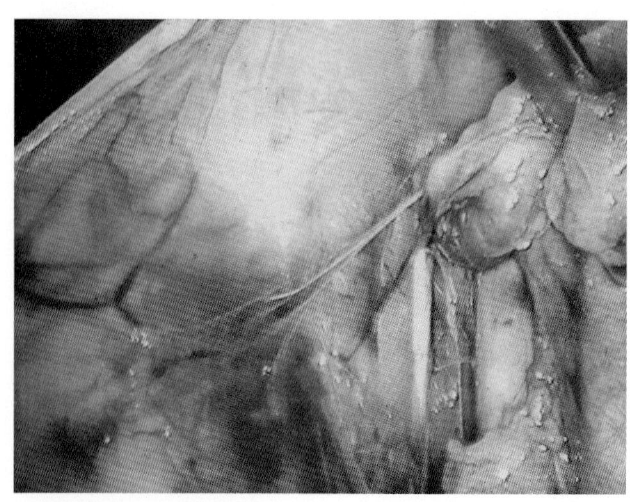

COLOR PLATE 13.12.

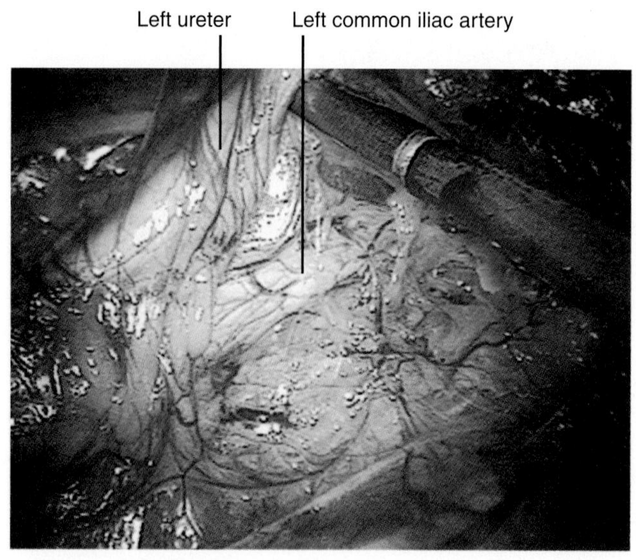

COLOR PLATE 13.16.

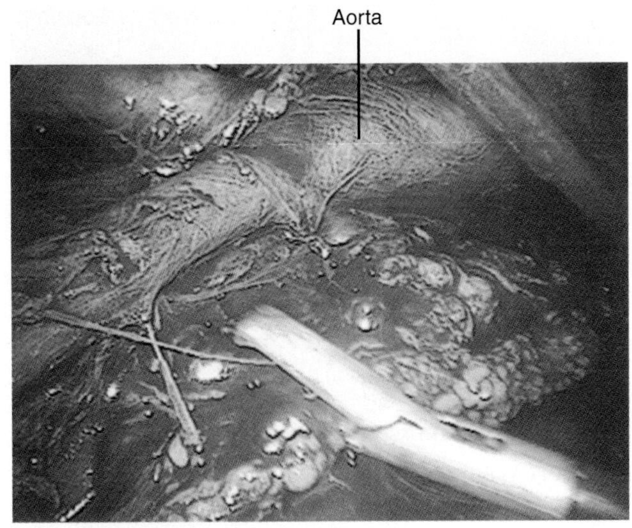

COLOR PLATE 13.17.

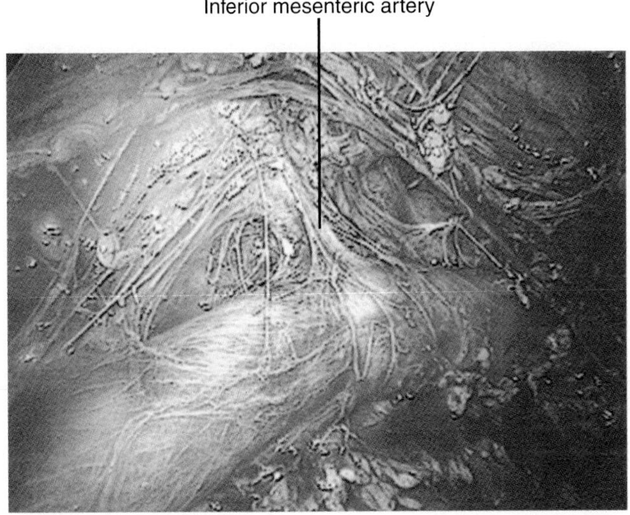

COLOR PLATE 13.18.

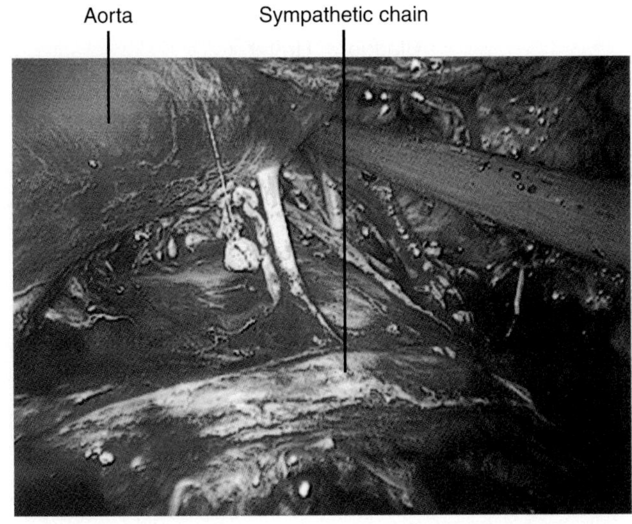

COLOR PLATE 13.19.

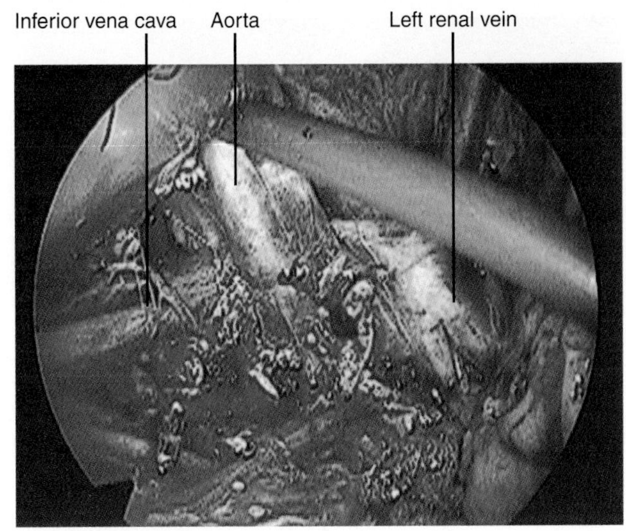

COLOR PLATE 13.20.

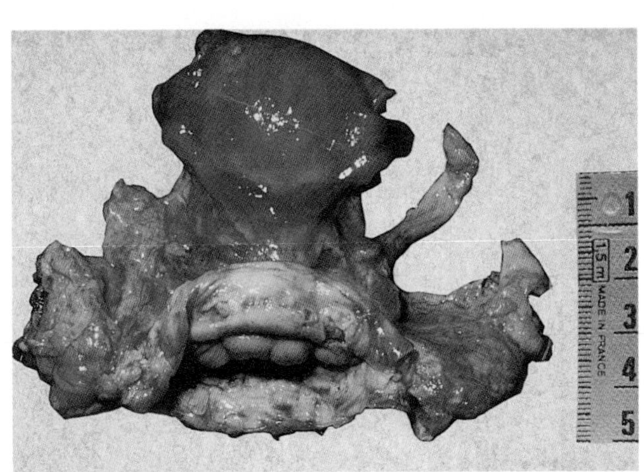

COLOR PLATE 13.21.

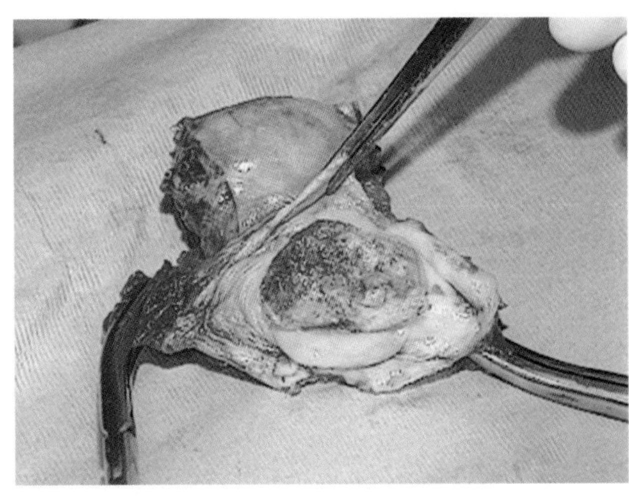

COLOR PLATE 13.22.

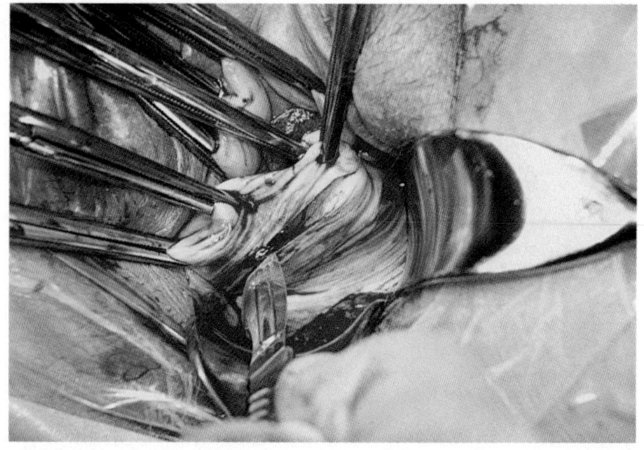

COLOR PLATE 13.23.

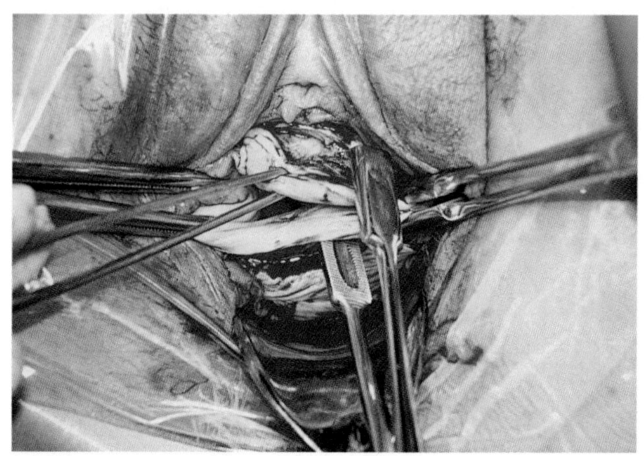

COLOR PLATE 13.24.

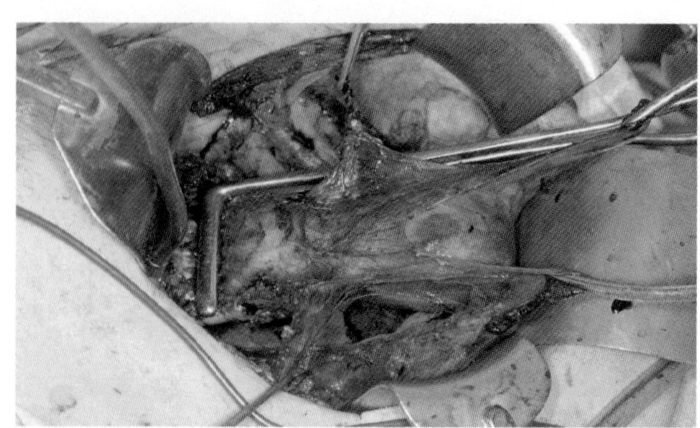

COLOR PLATE 13.25.

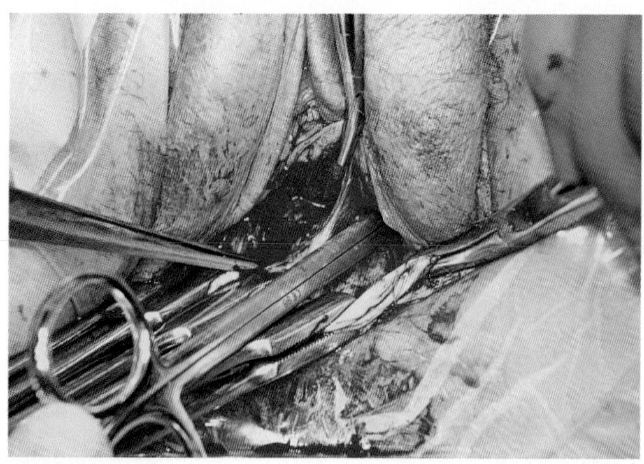

COLOR PLATE 13.26.

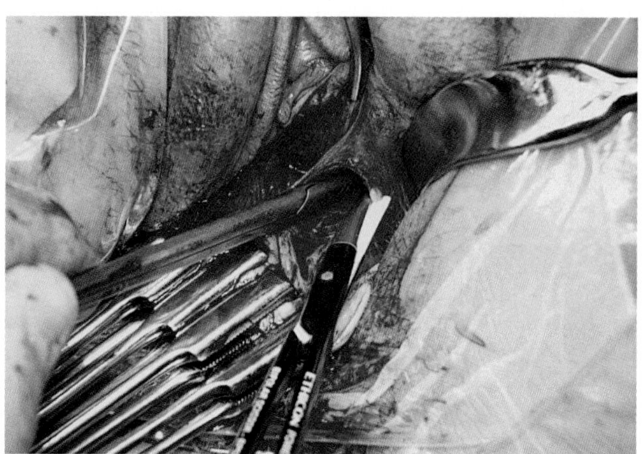

COLOR PLATE 13.27.

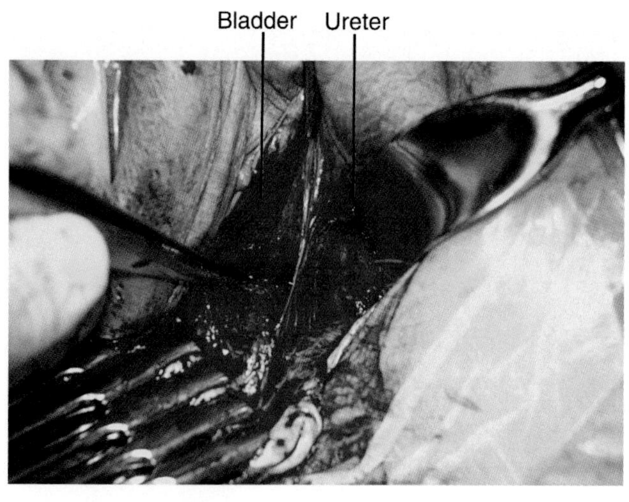

COLOR PLATE 13.28.

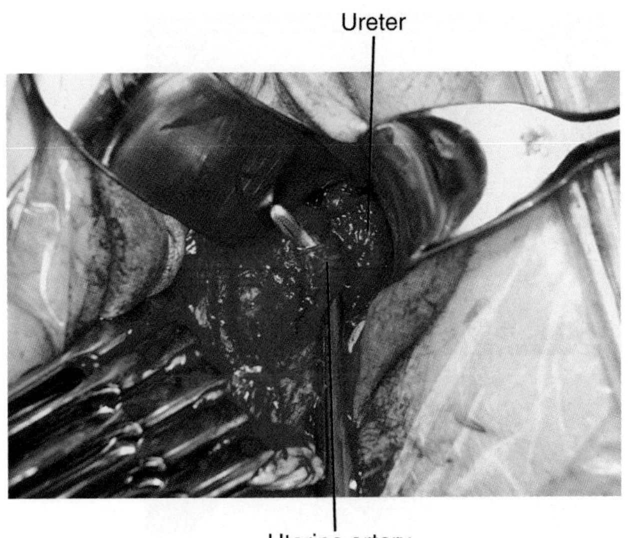

COLOR PLATE 13.29.

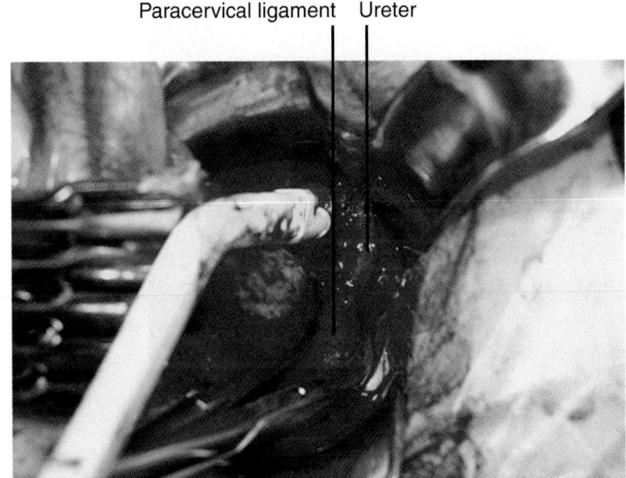

COLOR PLATE 13.30.

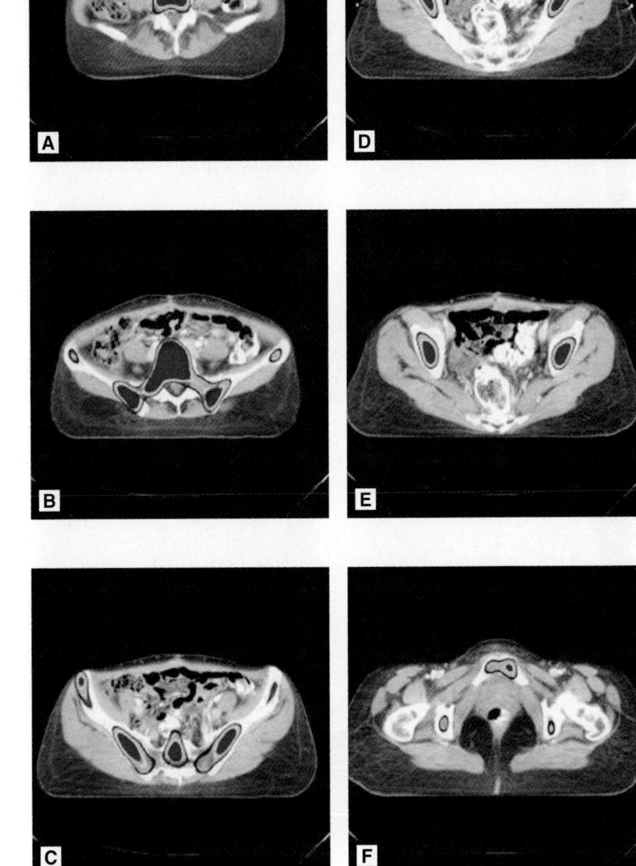

COLOR PLATE 18.9 A–F.

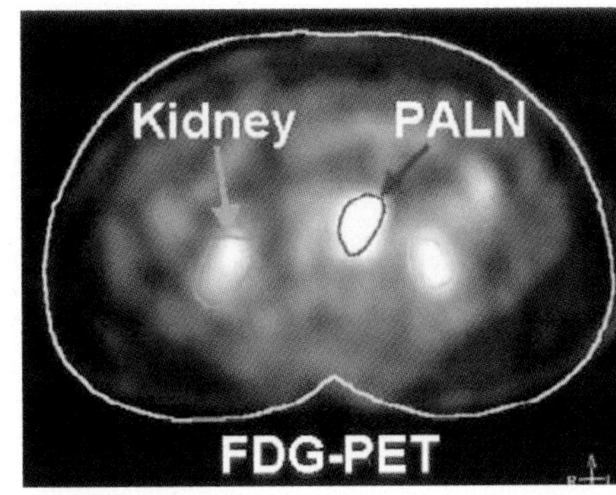

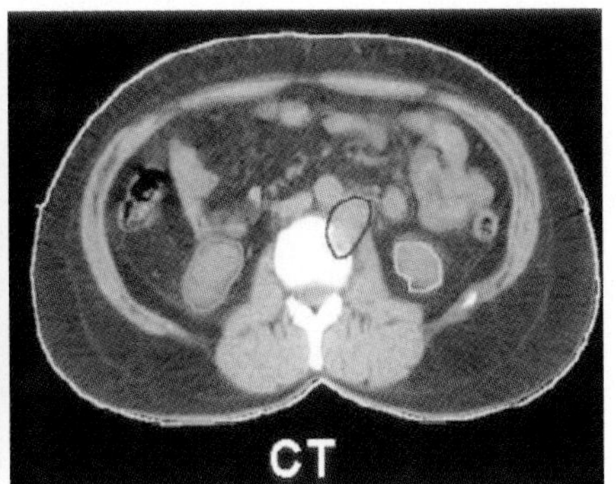

COLOR PLATE 18.8.

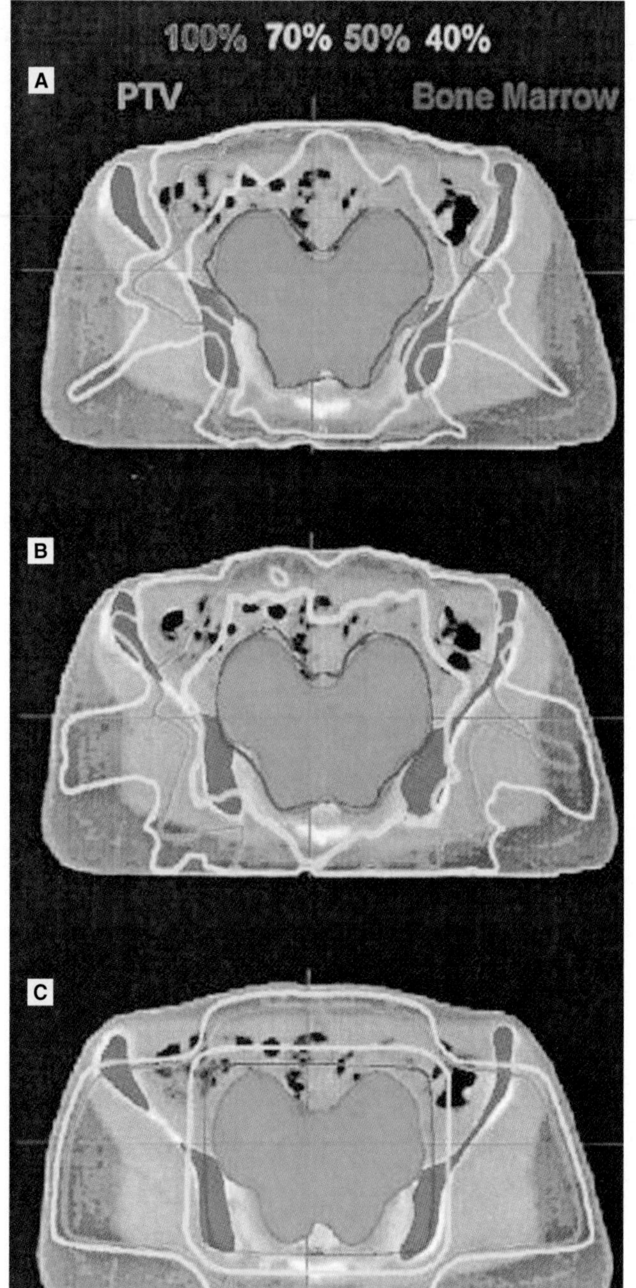

COLOR PLATE 18.10.

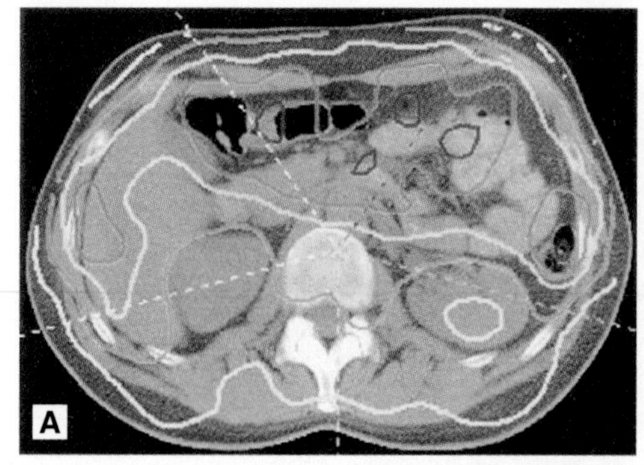

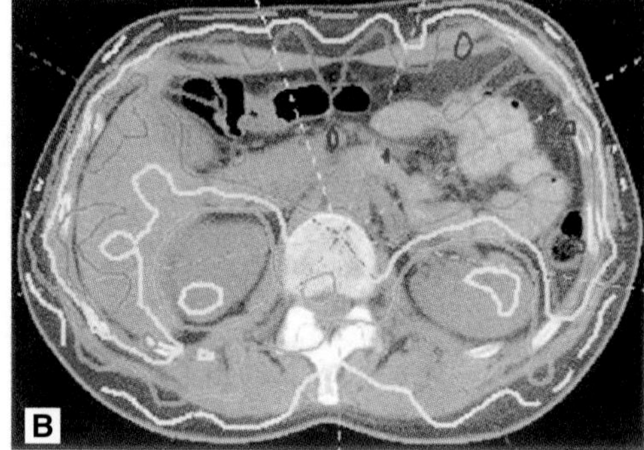

110%

100%

90%

70%

50%

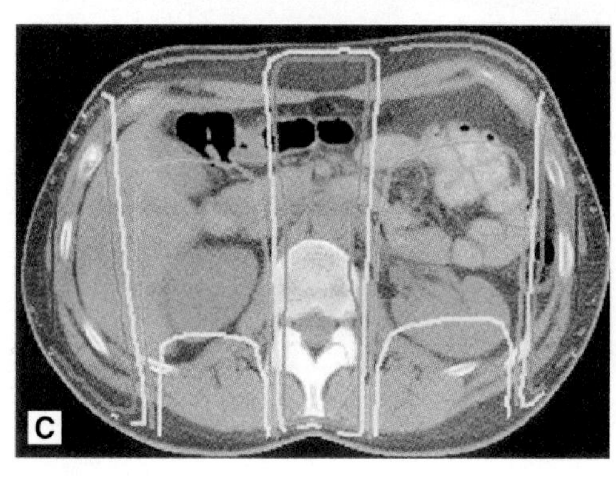

COLOR PLATE 18.11.

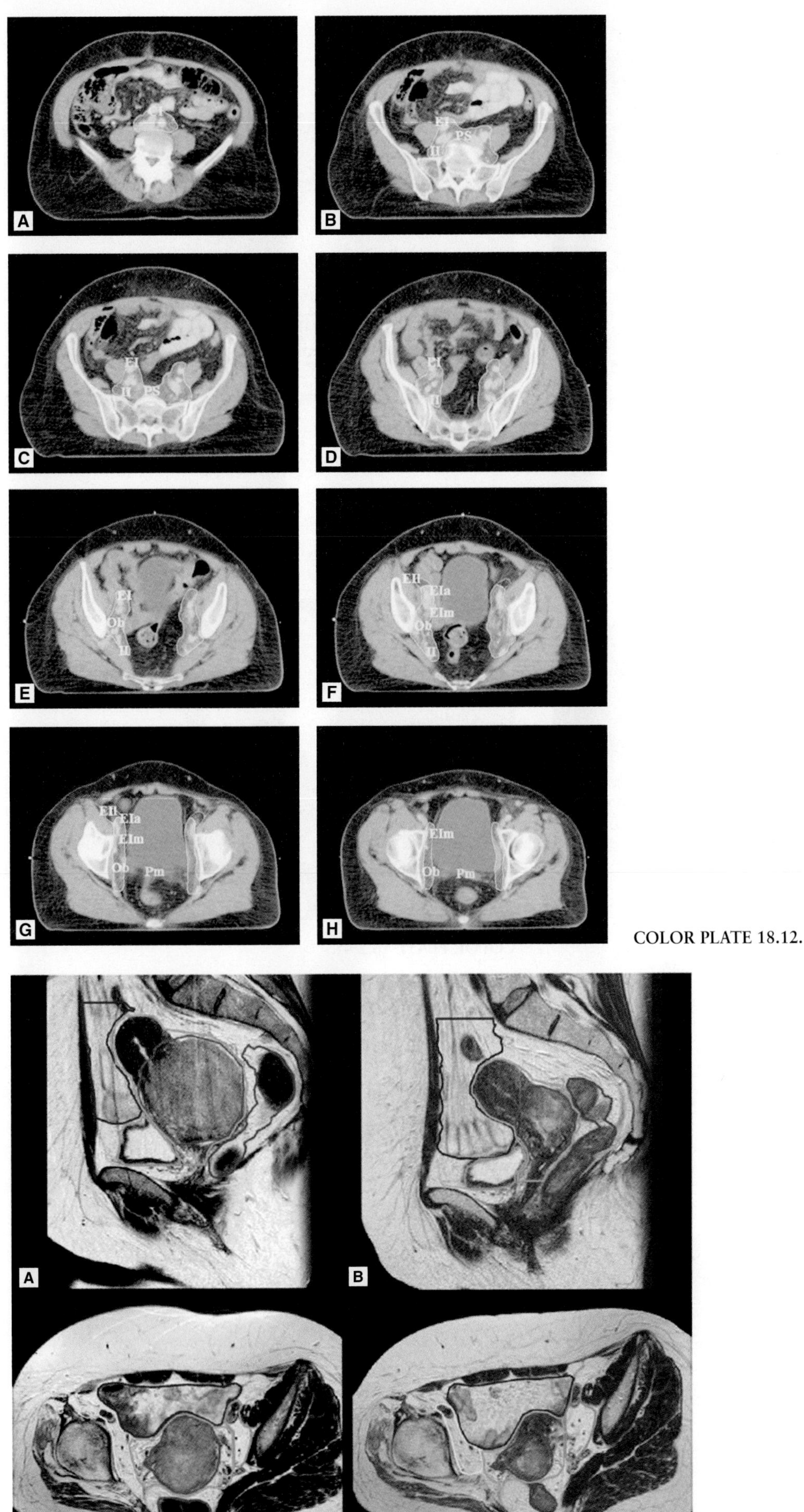

COLOR PLATE 18.12.

COLOR PLATE 18.14.

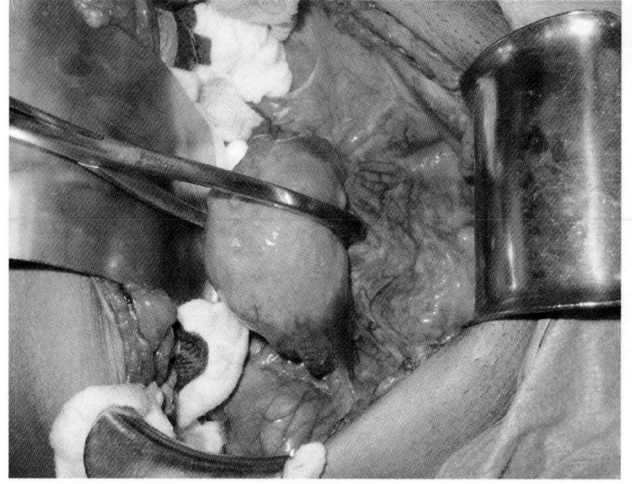

COLOR PLATE 18.23.

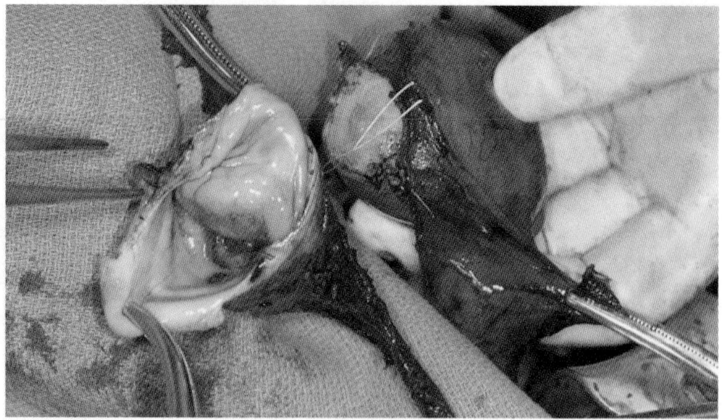

COLOR PLATE 18.28.

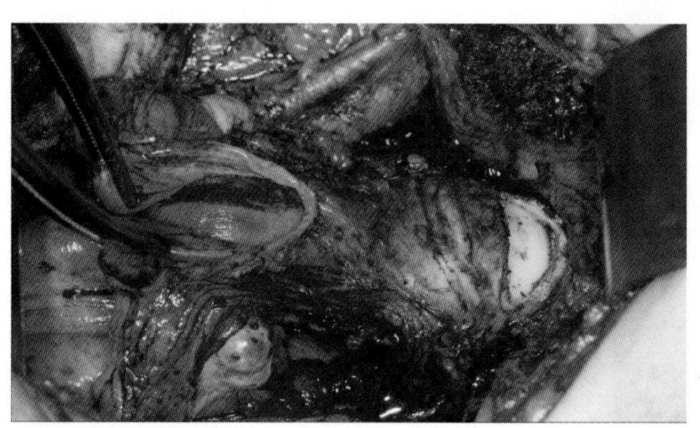

COLOR PLATE 18.24.

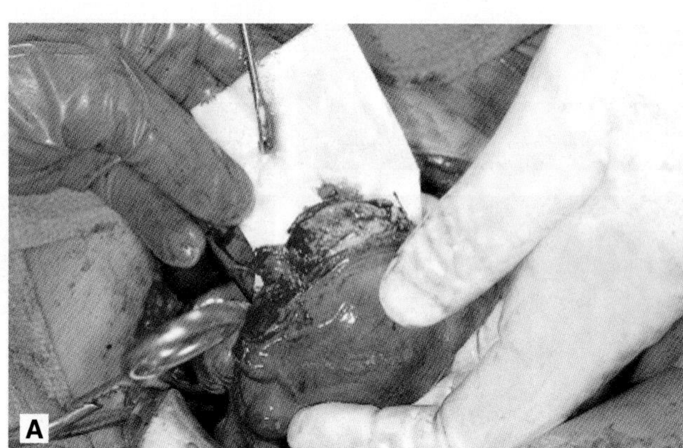

COLOR PLATE 18.29A.

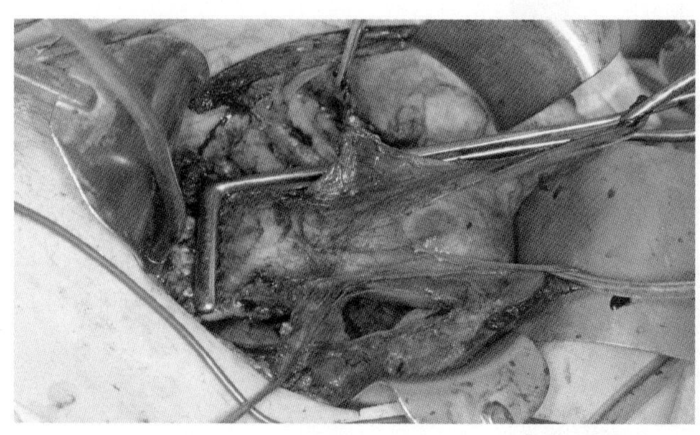

COLOR PLATE 18.25.

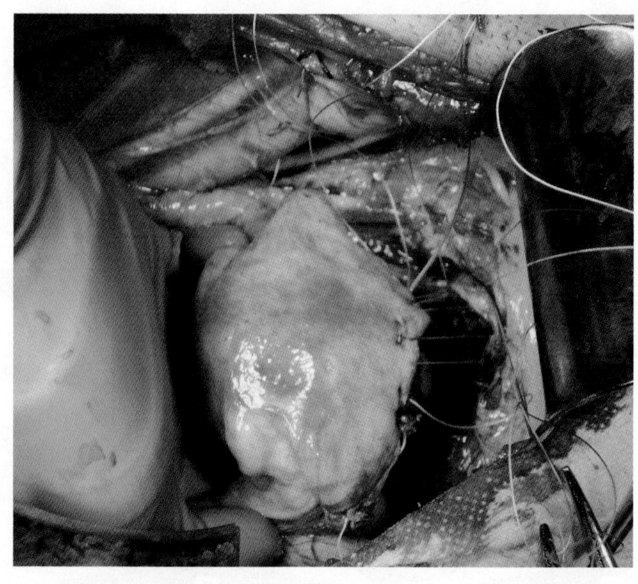

COLOR PLATE 18.33.

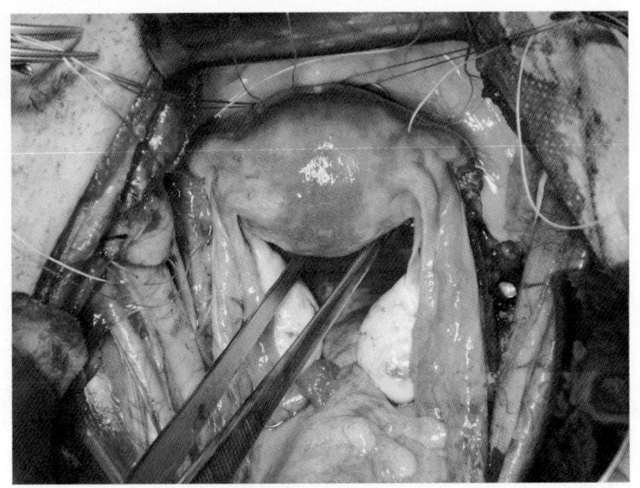

COLOR PLATE 18.34.

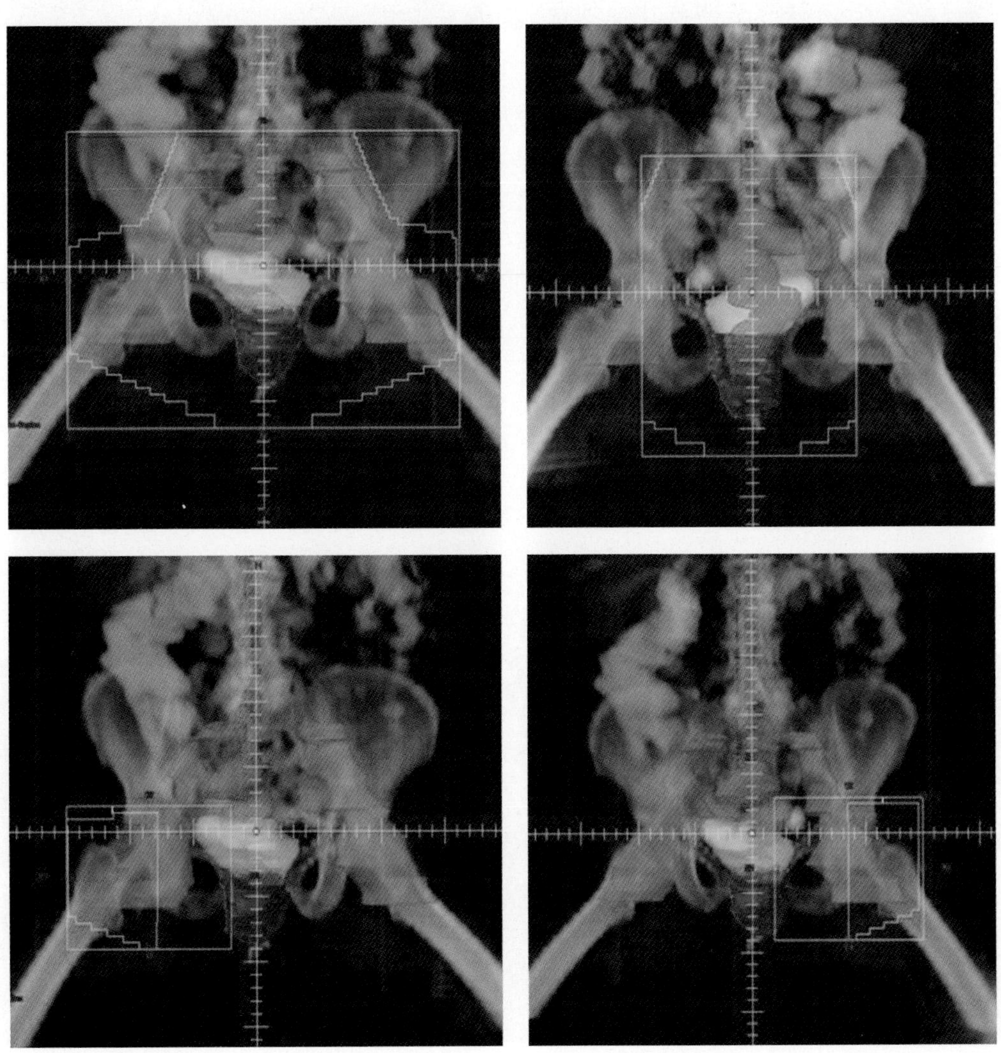

A

COLOR PLATE 21.5A.

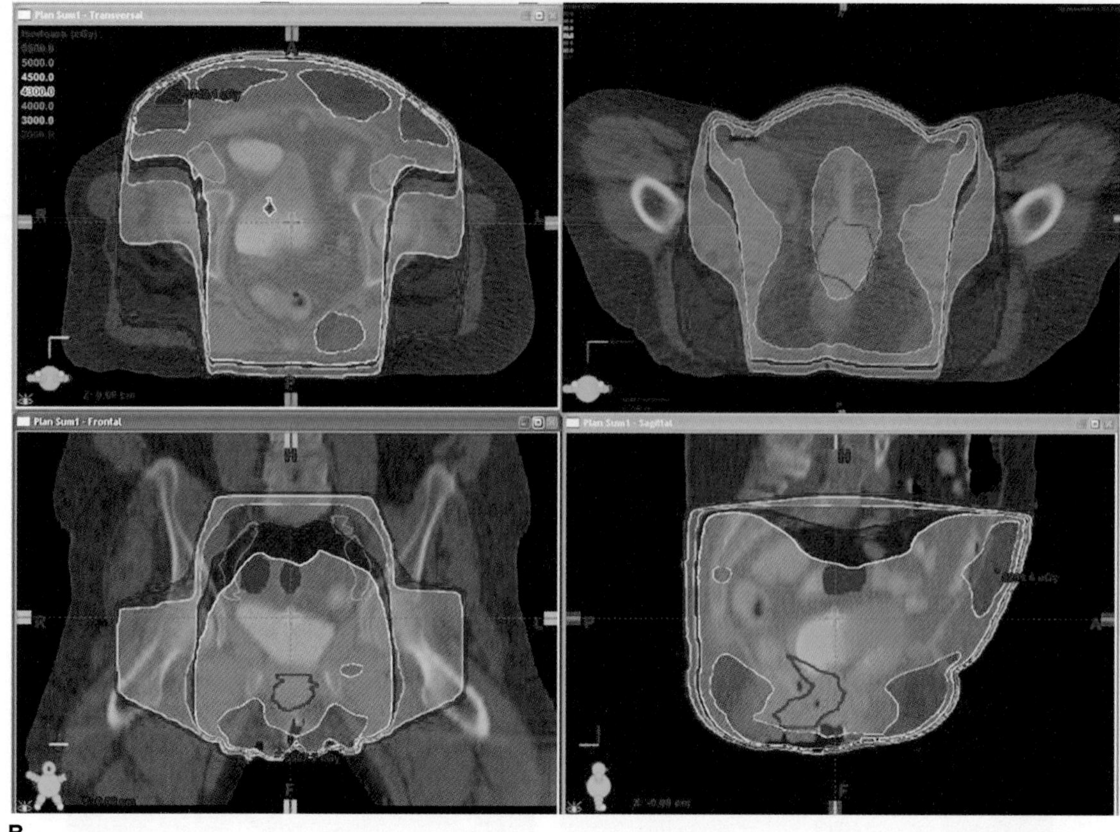

B

COLOR PLATE 21.5B.

A

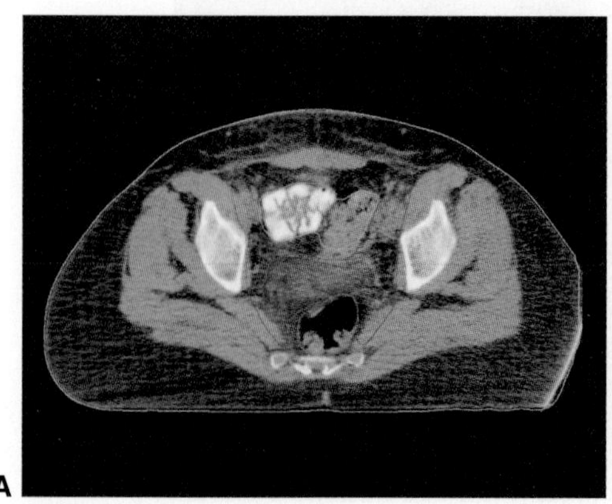

Axial

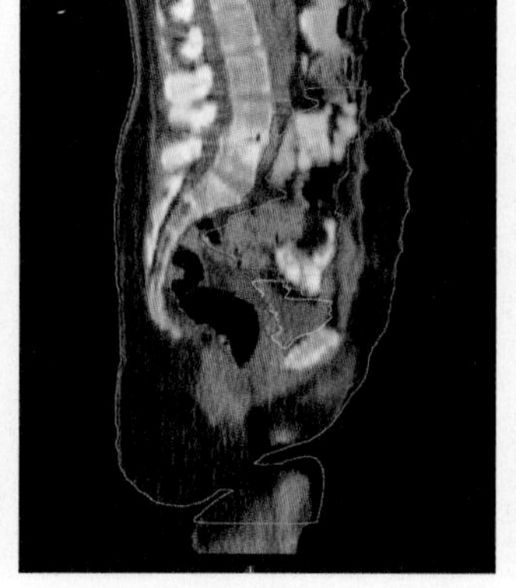

Sagittal

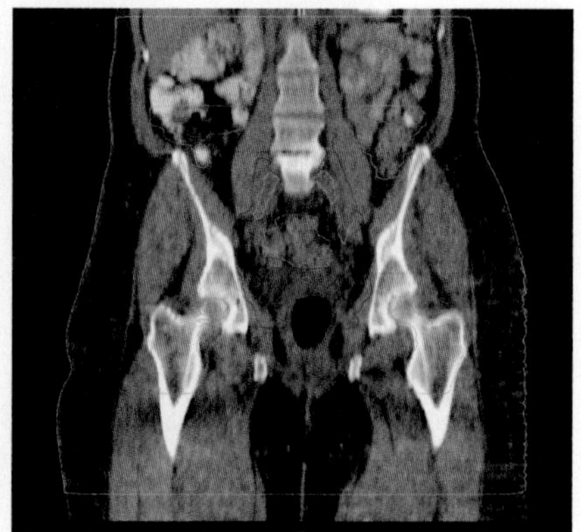

Coronal

COLOR PLATE 21.6A.

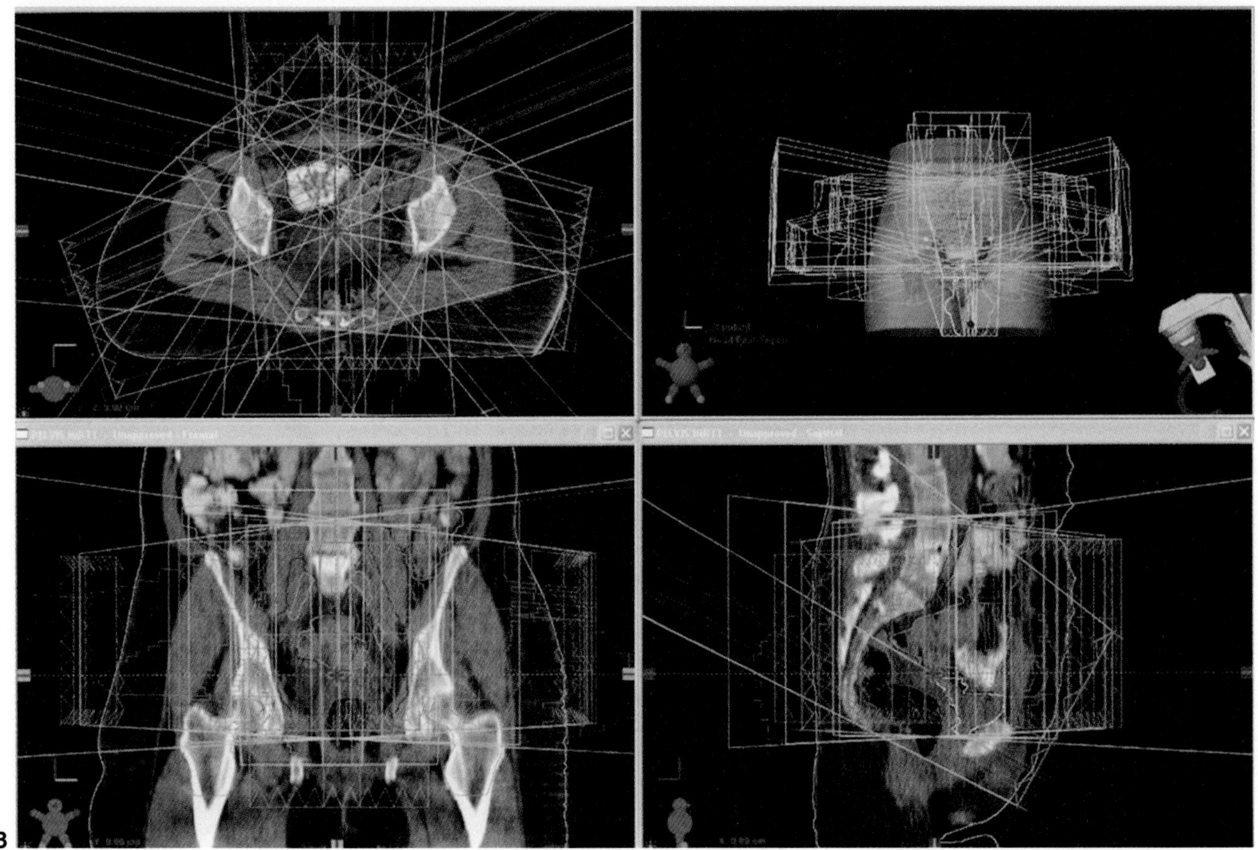

COLOR PLATE 21.6B.

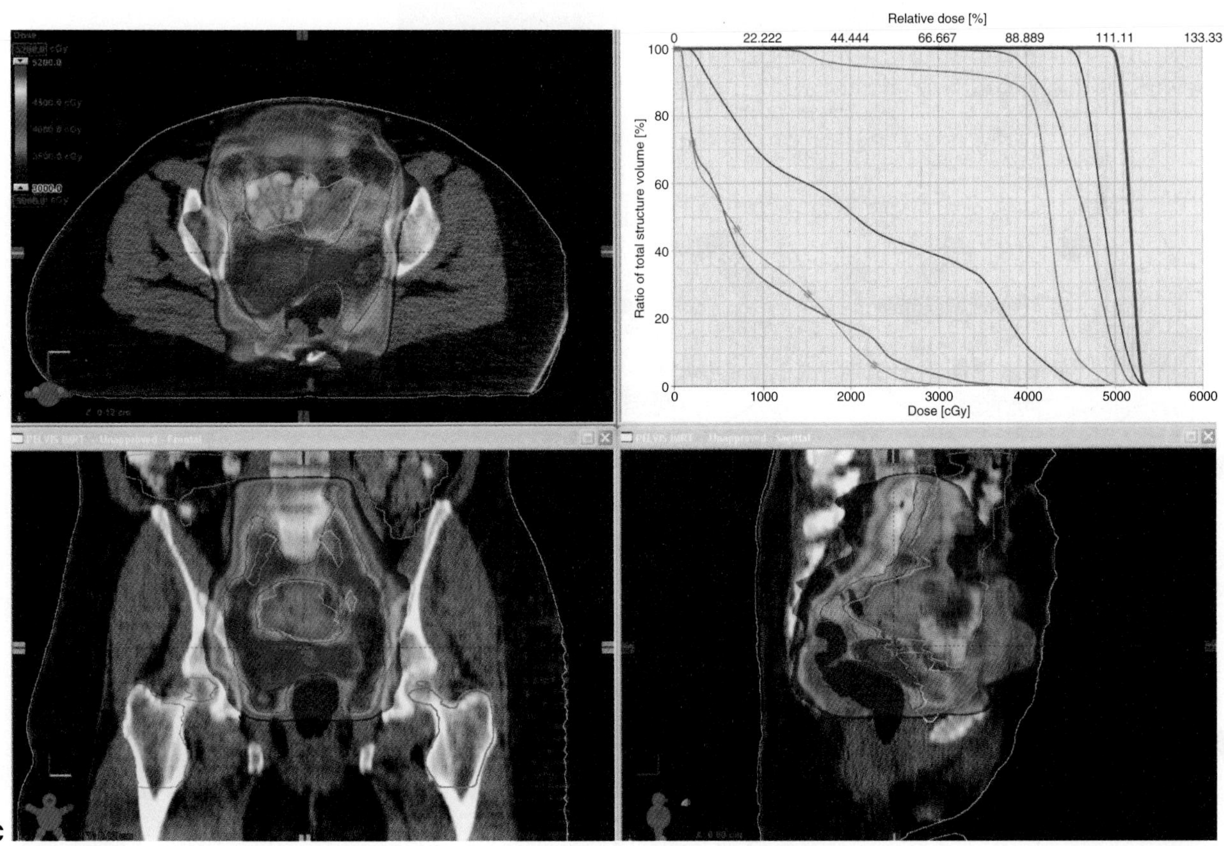

COLOR PLATE 21.6C.

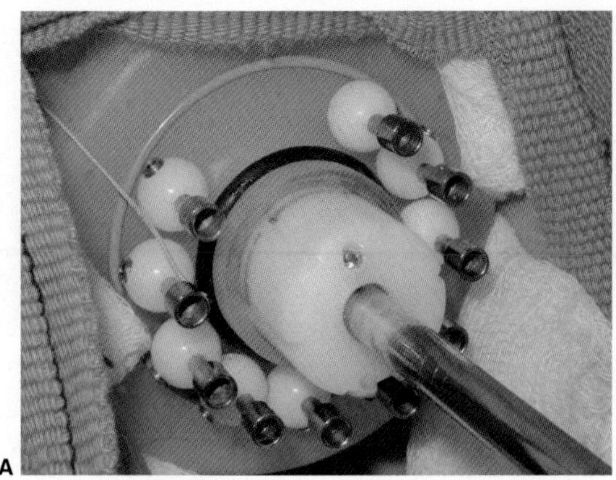

A

COLOR PLATE 21.7A.

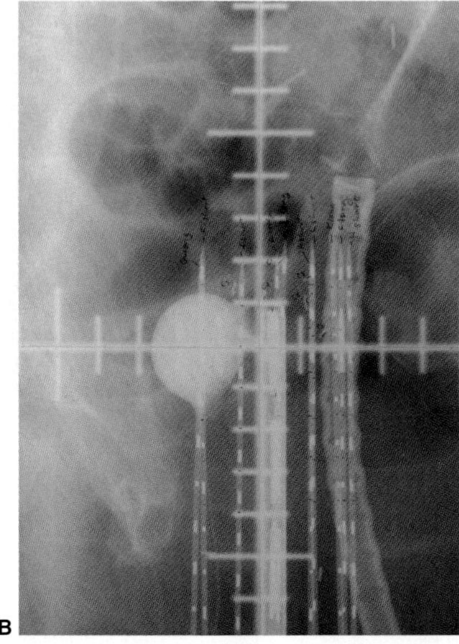

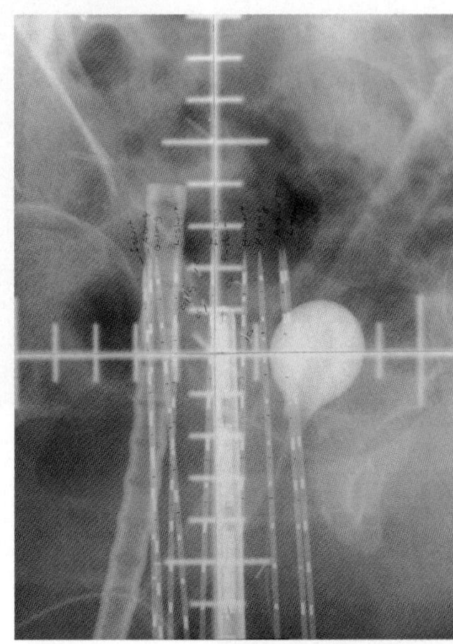

B

LAO

RAO

COLOR PLATE 21.7B.

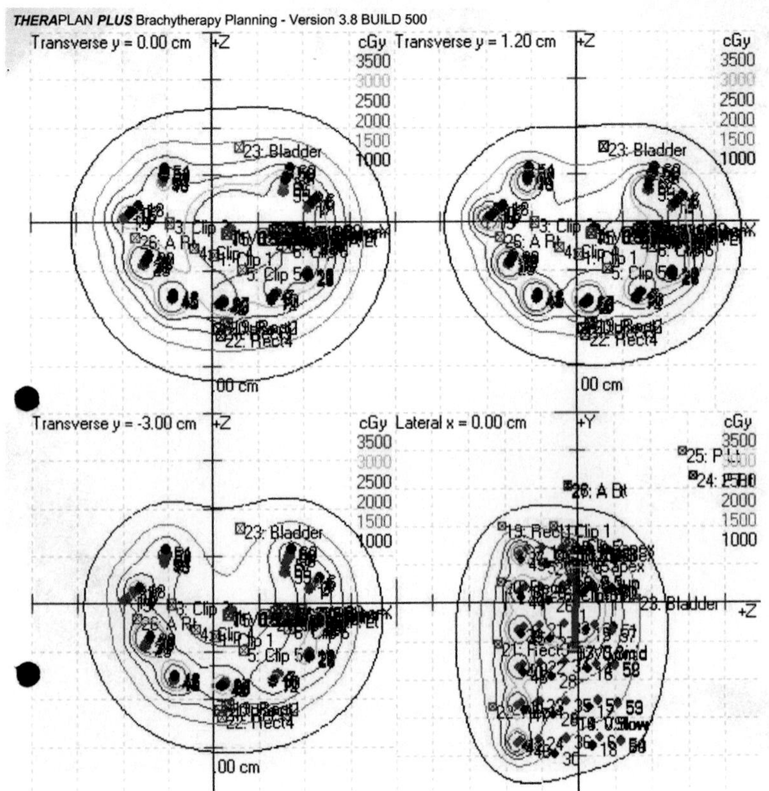

C

COLOR PLATE 21.7C.

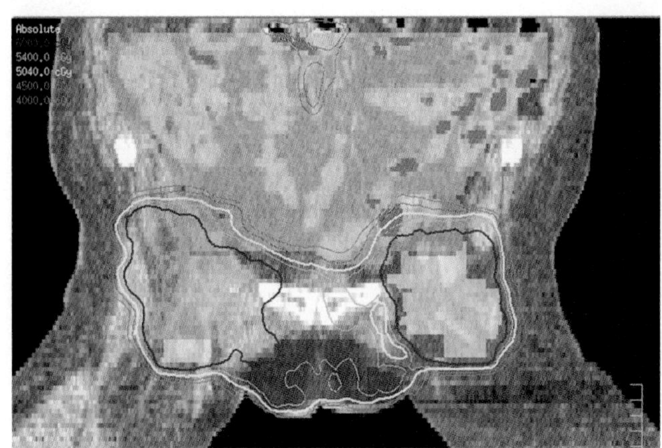

COLOR PLATE 22.14.

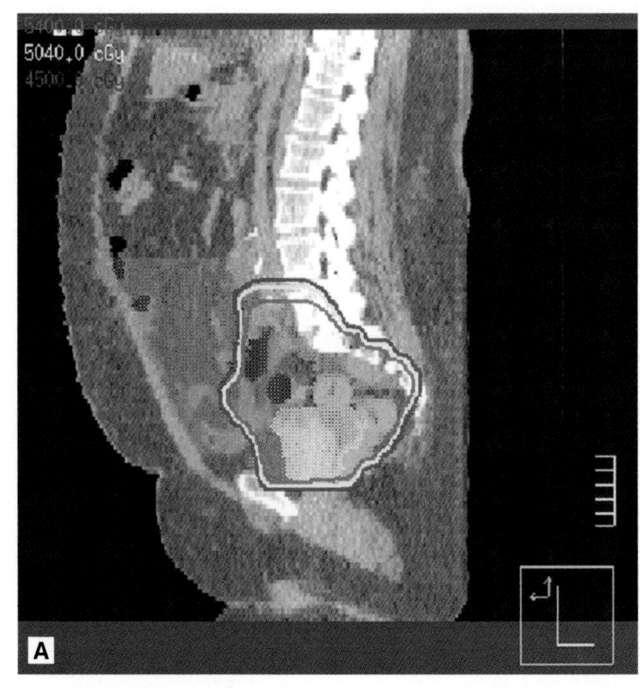

COLOR PLATE 22.16A.

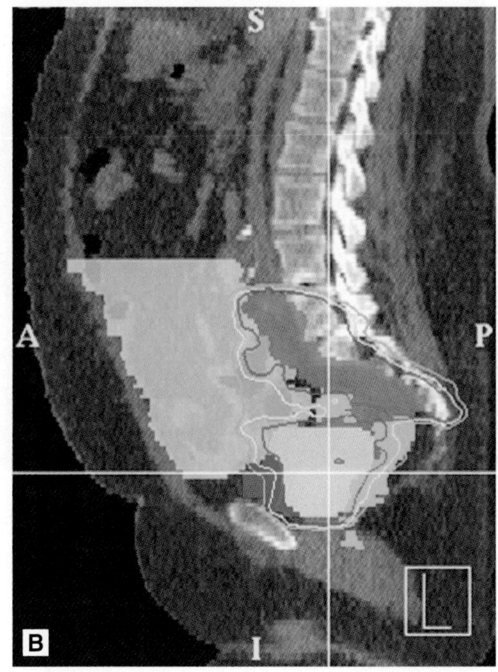

COLOR PLATE 22.16B.

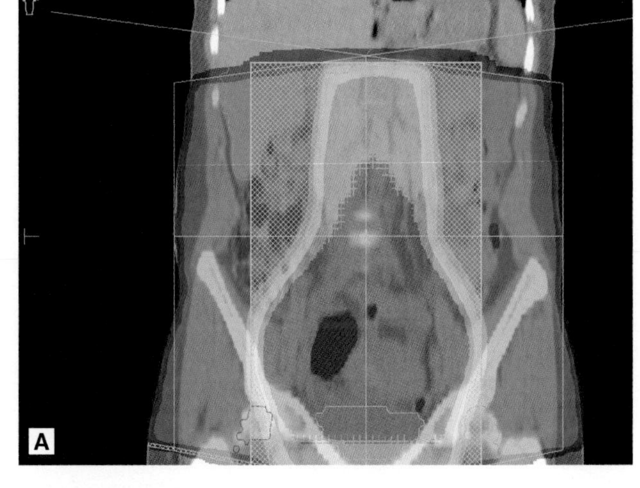

COLOR PLATE 22.18A.

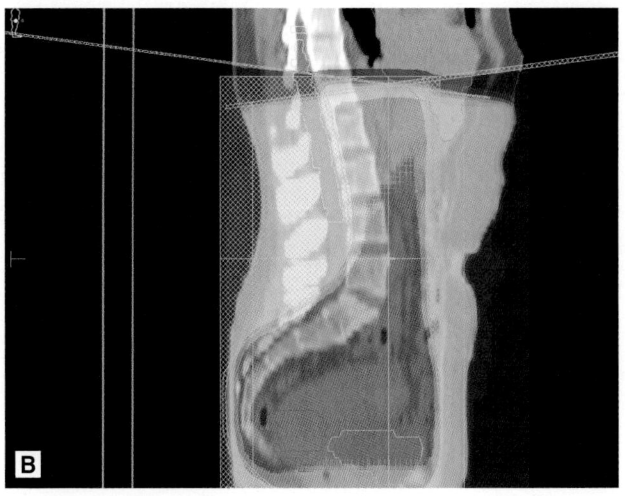

COLOR PLATE 22.18B.

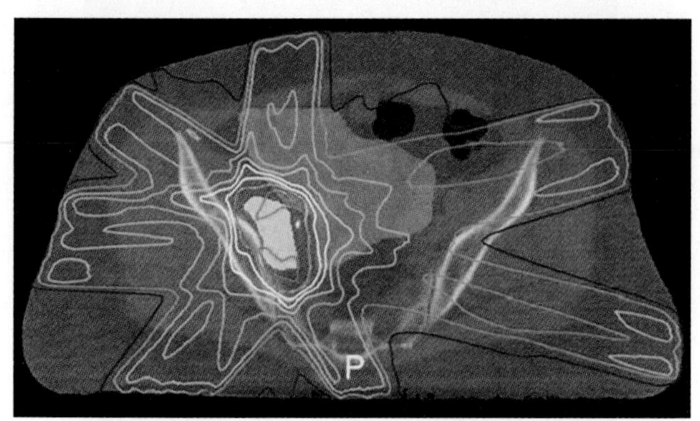

COLOR PLATE 22.20.

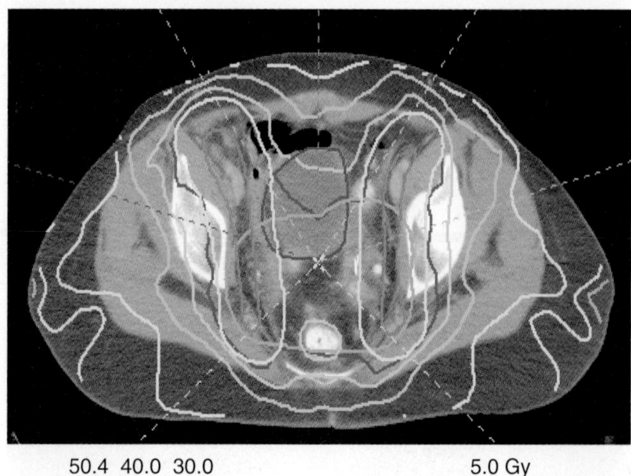

COLOR PLATE 23.13.

SECTION I:

EPIDEMIOLOGY OF GYNECOLOGIC CANCER

CHAPTER 1 ■ EPIDEMIOLOGY OF GYNECOLOGIC CANCERS

LOUISE A. BRINTON AND MARK SCHIFFMAN

Disease-oriented texts often include a chapter on epidemiology or etiology, which is considered perfunctory if the book is used by therapists whose daily practice is rarely influenced by these considerations. This is not the case for physicians who treat patients with gynecologic cancers, because these clinicians have frequent opportunities to interpret epidemiologic findings and make observations of etiologic importance. Moreover, public health measures based on epidemiologic findings influence gynecologic practice perhaps more than any other clinical discipline. In particular, epidemiologic data are critical for the prevention and treatment of cervical and uterine cancers.

From the observation 150 years ago of the rarity of cervical cancer in nuns to the most recent follow-up studies of type-specific human papillomavirus infection, determining the cause, natural history, and prevention of this disease has focused on sexual practices and suspect infectious agents. Screening interventions based on natural history studies have fundamentally altered the usual presentation of this disease, and as more information about preceding infectious processes becomes available, even more radical changes in presentation and management are likely.

The probable estrogenic cause of endometrial cancer was proposed by etiologically oriented gynecologists decades before its demonstration by epidemiologists. Unfortunately, this did not prevent the largest epidemic of iatrogenic cancer in recorded history (i.e., endometrial cancer caused by estrogen replacement therapy). The resurgent interest in hormone replacement therapy, effects of progestins added to this regimen, and associated risk-benefit questions are certain to link the epidemiologist and the gynecologist for the foreseeable future. The iatrogenic chemoprevention of endometrial and ovarian cancer through oral contraception has similarly thrust the two disciplines together around issues ranging from basic biology to risk-benefit assessments.

The rich tradition of the mingling of epidemiology and gynecologic oncology has led to better opportunities for prevention, screening, and insights into basic mechanisms of disease than for any other subspecialty concerned with cancer. This chapter is written with the aim of clarifying how epidemiology is an integral part of the effort to reduce the morbidity and mortality from gynecologic cancers in women.

UTERINE CORPUS CANCER

Demographic Patterns

Cancer of the uterine corpus (hereafter referred to as uterine cancer) is the most common invasive gynecologic cancer and the fourth most frequently diagnosed cancer among American women today. One in 40 American women will develop uterine cancer during their lives, and it is estimated that there will be approximately 40,100 diagnoses during 2008 (1). The average annual age-adjusted (2000 U.S. standard) incidence from the Surveillance, Epidemiology, and End Results (SEER) program, a cancer reporting system involving approximately 26% of U.S. residents, was 22.7 per 100,000 women for 2000 to 2004; the corresponding age-adjusted mortality rate was 2.0 per 100,000 women, reflecting the relatively good prognosis for this cancer (2). The 5-year survival rate is approximately 84%. It is estimated that approximately 7,470 women will die from uterine cancer during 2008 (1).

Uterine cancer rates are highest in North America, intermediate in Europe and temperate South America, and low in Southern and Eastern Asia (including Japan) and in most of Africa (except southern Africa) (3). The disease is rare before the age of 45 years, but the risk rises sharply among women in their late 40s to middle 60s. The age-adjusted incidence for whites is approximately twice the incidence for nonwhites (Fig. 1.1). Reasons for the discrepancy remain largely undefined. Within the last several decades in the United States, a dramatic change in the incidence pattern for uterine cancer has occurred, characterized by a marked increase that peaked about 1975 (Fig. 1.2) (4). Considerable evidence has linked this rise and fall with the widespread use of estrogen replacement therapy in the late 1960s and early 1970s. Mortality rates, albeit considerably lower, have generally mirrored incidence rates.

Reproductive Risk Factors

Nulliparity is a recognized risk factor for uterine cancer. Most studies demonstrate a two- to threefold higher risk for nulliparous than parous women. The association of uterine cancer with nulliparity has been suggested to reflect prolonged periods of infertility. The hypothesis that infertility is a risk factor for uterine cancer is supported by studies showing higher risks for married nulliparous women than for unmarried women. Several studies have found that infertile women experience a three- to eightfold increase in risk (5–7). Mechanisms that may mediate the risk associated with infertility include anovulatory menstrual cycles (i.e., prolonged exposure to estrogens without sufficient progesterone); high serum levels of androstenedione (i.e., excess androstenedione is available for conversion to estrone); and the absence of monthly sloughing of the endometrial lining (i.e., residual tissue may become hyperplastic). In addition, nulliparity has been associated with lower levels of serum sex hormone–binding globulin (SHBG), leading to increased bioavailable estrogen (8).

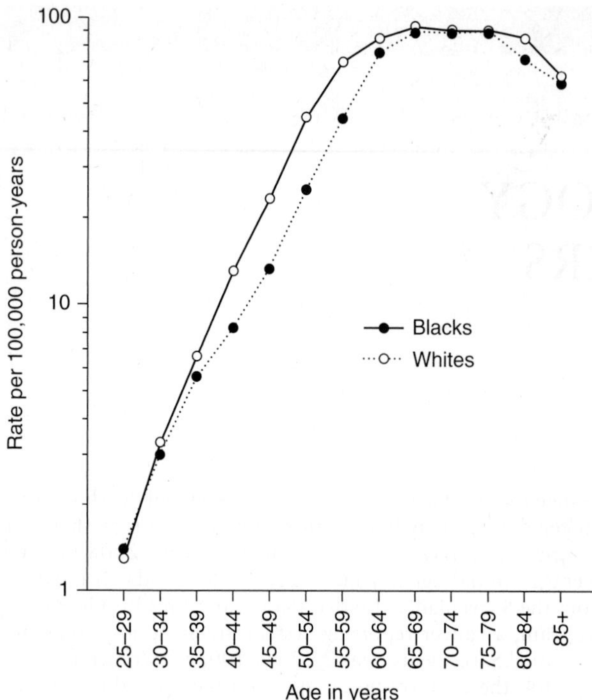

FIGURE 1.1. Age-specific incidence of cancer of the corpus uteri by race. *Source:* Data from the Surveillance, Epidemiology, and End Results Program, 2000–2004.

It has been established for many years that the risk of uterine cancer decreases with increasing parity, especially among premenopausal women (6,9,10). More recent attention has focused on characteristics of ages at which these births occurred. Several investigators have found decreased risks with either older ages at or shorter intervals since a last birth, and have suggested that this might reflect a protective effect of mechanical clearance of initiated cells (11,12). However, a recent analysis, which accounted for the correlation of multiple reproductive parameters, concluded that protection appeared to derive more from a late age at a first birth, suggesting an adverse effect of infertility among women who are unable to conceive at older ages (10). Additional studies are needed to confirm these latest findings and to shed further light on endogenous hormonal alterations that might underlie reproductive associations with uterine cancer risk.

An understanding of the effects of infertility on cancer risk must also consider relationships according to different methods of birth control, including oral contraceptives (discussed later in this chapter). However, it is also of interest that a number of investigations have noted reductions in risk among users of intrauterine devices (13–16). The mechanisms involved with this apparent protective effect have not been elaborated, although it is possible that the devices may affect risk by causing structural or biochemical changes that alter the sensitivity of the endometrium to circulating hormones.

An additional area of interest is the effect of exposure to fertility drugs, given a recent study showing that users of clomiphene citrate are at an increased risk of developing uterine cancers (17). Although this finding requires replication, it is of interest given the structural similarity of clomiphene and tamoxifen, which has been extensively linked with the occurrence of uterine cancers (discussed in more detail below).

The relationship of risk to breast-feeding remains controversial. Although some recent studies suggest that prolonged lactation may offer protection (18,19), in one of these investigations

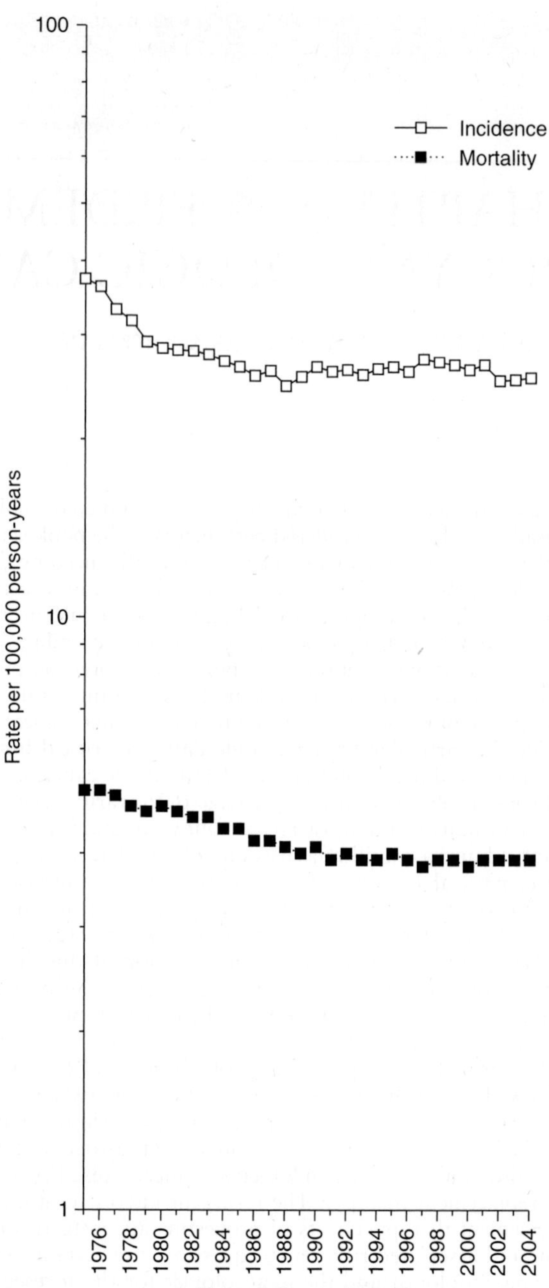

FIGURE 1.2. Incidence and mortality trends among U.S. white females for cancer of the corpus uteri. *Source:* Data from the Surveillance, Epidemiology, and End Results Program, 1975–2004.

the reduced risk did not persist into the age range when uterine cancer becomes common (19).

Menstrual Risk Factors

Early ages at menarche have been related to an elevated risk for uterine cancer in several studies, although associations have generally been rather weak and trends inconsistent (5,6). Several studies have found stronger effects of ages at menarche among younger women, although this has not been consistently demonstrated (6). The extent to which these relationships reflect increased exposure to ovarian hormones or other correlates of early menarche (e.g., increased body weight) is unresolved.

Most studies have indicated that age at menopause is directly related to the risk of developing uterine cancer. About 70% of all women diagnosed with uterine cancer are postmenopausal. Most studies support the estimate that there is about a twofold risk associated with natural menopause after the age of 52 years as compared to before age 49 years (20). It has been hypothesized that the effect of late age at menopause on risk may reflect prolonged exposure of the uterus to estrogen stimulation in the presence of anovulatory (progesterone-deficient) cycles. The interrelationships among menstrual factors, age, and weight are complex, and the biologic mechanisms of these variables operating in the pathogenesis of uterine cancer are subject to substantial speculation.

Exogenous Hormones

Oral Contraceptives

Studies have demonstrated significantly higher risks in users of sequential oral contraceptives (i.e., containing a high dose of estrogen and a weak dose of progestin) as compared to users of estrogen-progestin combination pills. Studies have shown that women who used Oracon, a sequential preparation that employed dimethisterone (weak progestogen) with a large dose of a potent estrogen (ethinyl estradiol), had substantially elevated risks of uterine cancer (6,21). The risk associated with the use of other sequential oral contraceptives remains unclear, mainly because these drugs are no longer marketed.

In contrast, the use of combination oral contraceptives may reduce the risk of uterine cancer by 50% compared to nonuse, and long-term use may decrease risk further (21–24). Kaufman et al. (23) showed that the reduced risk persisted for at least 5 years after discontinuation, but Weiss and Sayvetz (21) found that the protective effect waned within 3 years. In several studies, the greatest reduction in risk was associated with high-progestin-dose pills, although recent findings indicate that this may be true only among obese women (25). A number of studies indicate that the protective effect of the pill appears greatest among nulliparous women (6,22). In other studies, the protection has been limited to nonobese women or those who have not been exposed to menopausal estrogens (6,21).

Menopausal Hormones

It is well established that unopposed estrogens are associated with a 2- to 12-fold elevation in uterine cancer risk (26–29). In most investigations, the increased risk does not become apparent until the drugs have been used for at least 2 to 3 years, and longer use of estrogens is generally associated with higher risk (26,30,31). The highest relative risks (RRs) have been observed after 10 years of use (up to 20-fold), although it is unclear whether risk increases after 15 years. Most but not all studies have found that cessation of use is associated with a relatively rapid decrease in risk, although a number of studies have found significantly elevated risks to persist 10 or more years after last usage (26,30–33). Although higher doses of estrogen are associated with the greatest elevations in risk, one study showed that even 0.3 mg of unopposed equine estrogen can result in a significant increase in risk (34).

This large body of evidence linking estrogen use to increases in the risk of uterine cancers has led to estrogens being prescribed in conjunction with progestins among women who have not had a hysterectomy. Progesterone has been shown to cause regression of endometrial hyperplasia, the presumed precursor of uterine cancers (35). The large Women's Health Initiative (WHI) clinical trial showed that women assigned to 0.625 mg of conjugated equine estrogen plus 2.5 mg of medroxyprogesterone acetate daily had a lower hazard ratio (0.81, 95% confidence interval [CI] 0.48 to 1.36) than those assigned to placebo, but this risk was based on relatively small numbers of endometrial cancers and short follow-up (36). Similar observational results derive from the Million Women Study in the United Kingdom, where usage of continuous combined therapy resulted in a relative risk of 0.71 (95% CI 0.56 to 0.90) (37).

It is unresolved whether protection from estrogens can be achieved when progestins are prescribed sequentially (usually defined as less than 10 to 15 days per month) as opposed to continuously. Although a number of studies indicate that the excess risk of uterine cancer can be significantly reduced if progestins are given for at least 10 days each month (27,38–40), several studies have shown that subjects prescribed progestins for less than 10 days per month experience some increase in risk, with only a slight reduction compared to estrogen-only users (27,38,40,41). The sharp contrast between the effects of <10 and ≥ 10 days of progestin use has led to the suggestion that the extent of uterine sloughing or of "terminal" differentiation at the completion of the progestin phase may play a critical role in determining risk (27). It remains questionable whether <10 days of progestin administration per month is sufficient for complete protection, particularly for long-term users (42). Few studies have had large numbers of long-term sequential users, and in two studies there has been evidence that this pattern of usage may result in some persistence of risk (27,41). Other studies, however, have not confirmed this (43).

Studies have shown that the effects of hormonal therapy (both unopposed estrogens as well as combination therapy) may vary by user characteristics, most notably by a woman's body mass. The Million Women Study showed that the adverse effects of unopposed estrogens were greatest in nonobese women and that the beneficial effects of combined therapy were greatest in obese women (37). Studies have also suggested that effects of unopposed estrogens are strongest in nondiabetic, normotensive, and nonsmoking women (26,31,44), but less information is available on how these other risk factors modify the effects of combination therapy. These findings suggest either that estrogen metabolism differs among certain women, or that risk is already high enough in women who are obese, diabetic, hypertensive, or smokers that exposure to exogenous estrogens has only a small additional effect.

Most data regarding effects of hormones derive from studies of users of pills. Unresolved is whether the use of estrogen patches, creams, or injections can affect risk; given relationships of risk with even low dose estrogens, it is plausible that these regimens may confer some increase in risk.

Tumors associated with estrogen use generally demonstrate favorable characteristics, including earlier stage at diagnosis, lower grade, and less frequent myometrial invasion (26,33). Estrogen users tend to be younger at diagnosis than nonusers, and the tumors are more frequently accompanied by hyperplasia or adenomyosis (45,46). The fact that estrogen remains linked to risk in studies limited to pathologically confirmed cases and that risk is increased for both early- and late-stage cancers (32,47) suggests that the increased risk is not related to pathologic overdiagnosis.

Tamoxifen

A number of clinical trials and one population-based case-control study have demonstrated an increased risk of uterine cancer among tamoxifen-treated breast cancer patients (48–50). This is consistent with tamoxifen's estrogenic effects on the endometrium. Elevated risks have been observed primarily among women receiving high cumulative doses of therapy, usually in the range of 15 g or greater. According to a recent investigation, the risk for malignant mixed müllerian tumors may be especially high (51). One study documented a poor prognosis among long-term tamoxifen users who developed uterine cancer, presumably reflecting less favorable histologies and higher stages of disease at diagnosis (52). Whether this finding is generalizable to other populations remains unclear.

Anthropometry and Physical Activity

Obesity

Obesity is a well-recognized risk factor for uterine cancer and may account for up to 25% of cases (53–55). Very heavy women appear to have exceptionally high risks (55,56). Although studies have demonstrated significant positive trends of uterine cancer with both weight and various measures of obesity, including the Quetelet's index (weight/height^2), height has not been consistently associated with risk. Obesity appears to affect both premenopausal and postmenopausal uterine cancer (55).

Although initial studies hypothesized that adolescent and long-standing obesity may be more important than adult weight, recent studies support that contemporary weight and weight gain during adulthood are the most important predictors of uterine cancer risk (55,56). Relationships with obesity appear stronger for postmenopausal disease and among women not exposed to exogenous hormones (56,57).

Recent interest has focused on determining whether the distribution of body fat predicts uterine cancer risk. A number of studies have shown that central obesity may have an effect independent of overall body size (56,58), although not all studies confirm this relationship.

Physical Activity

Recent investigations have focused on the role of physical activity in the etiology of uterine cancer. A potential relationship is biologically appealing given that physical activity can result in changes in the menstrual cycle, body fat distribution, and levels of endogenous hormones. Although several recent studies suggest a protective effect of physical activity on uterine cancer risk that appears independent of relationships with body weight (59–64), the apparent relationships are not as convincing as have been observed for breast cancer risk. For instance, recent results from the large European Prospective Investigation into Cancer and Nutrition (EPIC) indicate that the protective effect of physical activity may be restricted to premenopausal women (65). Further, other studies have not shown dose-response relationships, and the types of activities associated with risk reductions have varied across studies. Two recent reviews on the topic emphasize the need for further investigation to determine the types, characteristics, or time periods of physical activity that could optimally impact risk (66,67).

Dietary Factors

Despite the fact that obesity has been consistently related to uterine cancer, the role of dietary factors remains controversial. Geographic differences in disease rates (i.e., high rates in Western and low rates in Eastern societies) suggest that nutrition has a role, especially the high content of animal fat in Western diets. Armstrong and Doll (68) demonstrated a strong correlation between a country's total fat intake and uterine cancer incidence.

Dietary Fat

Although a number of studies have assessed uterine cancer risk in relation to consumption of dietary fat, the association remains unclear. A clear assessment of risk depends on careful control for effects of both body size and caloric intake (energy). Several case-control studies have found a relationship with dietary fat intake (particularly animal fat) that appeared independent of other dietary factors (69–71). Another case-control study (53) found that the risk associated with fat calories was partially explained by body size. Several other case-control studies did not confirm a relationship with fat intake (72,73). In addition, a recent cohort study found an opposite trend; namely, some decrease in risk with relatively high intakes of saturated or animal fat (54).

Fruits, Vegetables, and Associated Micronutrients

A somewhat more consistent observation has been the reduction of uterine cancer related to high intakes of fruits and vegetables (53,69,73–75). There is some support for this relating to consumption of fruits and vegetables that are high in either beta-carotene (74) or lutein (53). Various other micronutrients have been implicated in the etiology of uterine cancer, although their independence from each other and from other risk factors has not been fully resolved (71–73). Further, not all studies support relationships with micronutrients, including a large Canadian prospective study (54).

Other Dietary Factors

Given the recognized role of diabetes in the etiology of uterine cancers, a number of studies have assessed risk in relation to carbohydrate intake, glycemic intake, and glycemic load, which are known to increase insulin and estrogen levels. There are suggestions that all three factors may relate to risk (76–79), although further studies are needed to sort out their independence from other risk factors, including obesity, diabetes, and physical activity levels.

Several studies have found that consumption of phytoestrogens and omega-3 fatty acids (found in fatty fish) may be protective (53,80,81), but confirmatory studies are needed. In addition, future studies are needed to assess whether risk reductions associated with certain dietary patterns reflect modified hormone metabolism, as suggested in both observational and intervention studies (82–85).

Alcohol Consumption

In several studies, regular consumption of alcoholic beverages has been linked to substantial reductions in uterine cancer risk (86–88). Several studies suggest more pronounced effects among premenopausal or overweight women, indicating that an attenuation in endogenous estrogen levels may be responsible for the reduced risk (86,88). However, other studies have failed to find a relationship between alcohol consumption and uterine cancer risk (89–91).

Cigarette Smoking

A reduced risk of uterine cancer among smokers has been reported, with current smokers having approximately half the risk of nonsmokers (90,92–94). Cigarette smoking has been linked to an earlier age at natural menopause in some populations and to reduced levels of endogenous estrogens. Reduced risk associated with long-term smoking is more pronounced in postmenopausal than premenopausal women (92). In addition, reduced risk associated with smoking may be most apparent in parous or obese patients (92,95).

At present, biologic mechanisms underlying the inverse relationship of smoking to uterine cancer risk remain elusive. Alterations in endogenous hormones or metabolites are likely involved. In one report, the inverse association of smoking with uterine cancer risk appeared to be more strongly related to higher serum androstenedione levels than to lower serum estrogen levels, except perhaps among overweight women (96).

Medical Conditions

Numerous clinical reports link polycystic ovarian syndrome (PCOS) with an increase in the risk of uterine cancer, particularly among younger women (97–99); however, it is uncertain whether this risk is independent of obesity. In a follow-up study at the Mayo Clinic, women with chronic anovulation were found to be at a threefold increased risk of developing uterine cancer (100). Assessing histories of PCOS is challenging in case-control studies, but it is of interest that uterine cancer has been associated with histories of either hirsutism or acne (5,101), which are conditions often associated with hyperandrogenism.

A number of studies have noted a high risk of uterine cancer among diabetics, but again the issue is whether the association is independent of weight. Various cohort studies (102–105) and a number of case-control studies (5,106–108) suggest that the relationship persists when analyses are restricted to nonobese women or are adjusted for weight. However, in several other studies (109,110), the effect of diabetes on uterine cancer risk was apparent only among obese women, suggesting the possible involvement of selected metabolic abnormalities, including hyperinsulinemia. Further studies are needed to resolve the association, as well as to elaborate on how specific types of diabetes may be involved.

A variety of other conditions have been suggested as possibly predisposing to uterine cancer risk, including hypertension, arthritis, thyroid conditions, and cholecystectomy. In a number of studies, positive findings may be partially explained by the correlation of the diseases with other factors. Similar to relationships with breast cancer, patients with previous fractures have been found to have a reduced risk of uterine cancer (111,112), presumably reflecting the association of lowered bone density with altered endogenous hormone levels.

Host Factors

Although studies have shown that a family history of uterine cancer is a risk factor for the disease, particularly among younger subjects (113), this appears to explain only a small proportion of disease occurrence (114). In addition, subjects with a family history of colon cancer are at increased risk, an association that is now recognized as reflective of hereditary nonpolyposis colorectal cancer, a dominantly inherited syndrome associated with mutations in the DNA mismatch repair genes *MSH2, MLH1,* and *MSH6.*

A number of recent studies have focused on relationships of uterine cancer risk with common genetic polymorphisms, including those involved with hormone biosynthesis and metabolism (115–119), DNA repair (120), and folate metabolism (121). Additional studies are needed to resolve effects of these genes as well as their interactions with environmental factors.

Environmental and Occupational Risk Factors

Geographic variation in rates of uterine cancer, with high rates in certain industrial areas, has led to the suggestion that certain environmental agents may affect risk. Given the well-recognized influence of hormones on the disease, there has been particular concern about a potential role for certain endocrine disruptors, including dichlorodiphenyltrichloroethane (DDT). Several studies have addressed this issue by comparing dichlorodiphenyldichloroethylene (DDE) levels (the active metabolite of DDT) in the sera of cases and controls, finding no significant differences (122,123).

Studies assessing the relationship of uterine cancer risk to exposure to electromagnetic radiation (electric blanket or mattress covers) have been negative (124). Data for occupational exposures are limited. Elevated endometrial cancer rates have been found among teachers in California (125) and individuals exposed to animal dust and sedentary work in Finland (126). The extent to which these relationships reflect the influence of social class is unknown.

Biologic Mechanisms Underlying Risk Factor Associations

Many of the identified risk factors are thought to operate through alterations in various endogenous hormones. The majority of studies have found increased risks associated with higher levels of circulating estrogens among postmenopausal women that persisted after adjustment for the effects of body mass (127–130), although in one study associations were considerably reduced after adjustment for body mass (129). In this same investigation, estrogens appeared to be less predictive of premenopausal disease, suggesting that anovulation or progesterone deficiency might be more predictive of risk.

Less well investigated is whether other endogenous hormones are related to uterine cancer risk. Key and Pike (131) suggested that uterine carcinogenesis is dependent on uterine mitosis, which is increased by estrogens and reduced by progesterone, but risk associated with progesterone levels has not been well explored. Several studies have shown positive associations of uterine cancer risk with serum androstenedione and testosterone levels (128,129). It has been hypothesized that this may reflect a role of chronic anovulation and progesterone deficiency in premenopausal women, whereas after menopause, aromatase and local conversion of estrone from androstenedione may be involved (132).

Obesity, which is hypothesized to reflect elevated estrogen levels (131), seems to represent a key risk factor for both uterine carcinoma and endometrial hyperplasias, but the mechanisms mediating this are unclear. One case-control analysis of serum estrogen levels (129) reported that the risk associated with obesity was not entirely mediated by estrogen, especially among premenopausal women. In another cohort study of postmenopausal women, elevated serum estrogen levels appeared to account for the majority of the risk associated with obesity (130). A potential role for insulin and insulin-like growth factors (IGF) has been suggested, although studies generally have not found support for a role of either c-peptide (133) or IGF (134) levels.

Conclusions

A unified theory of how risk factors for uterine cancer might operate through one common hormonal pathway has been suggested. Estrogen promotes proliferation in the endometrium, which is opposed by progesterone. Therefore, exposure to estrogen, particularly bioavailable estrogen that is weakly bound or unbound to plasma protein, is viewed as carcinogenic. Functional ovarian tumors, PCOS, late menopause, and administration of exogenous estrogens and sequential oral contraceptives produce higher levels of estrogen exposure without the antiproliferative effects of progesterone. Obesity could also contribute in a variety of ways (135). Adipose tissue is the primary site for conversion of androstenedione to estrone, which is the primary source for estrogen after menopause. Obesity is associated with higher conversion rates and/or elevated plasma levels of estrogen. In addition, obesity is related to lower levels of SHBG and more frequent anovulatory menstrual cycles

TABLE 1.1

RISK FACTORS FOR UTERINE CANCER

Factors influencing risk	Estimated relative risk[a]
Older ages	2–3
Residency in North America, Northern Europe	3–18
Higher levels of education or income	1.5–2.0
White race	2
Nulliparity	3
History of infertility	2–3
Menstrual irregularities	1.5
Early ages at menarche	1.5–2.0
Late ages at natural menopause	2–3
Long-term use or high dosages of menopausal estrogens	10–20
Use of oral contraceptives	0.3–0.5
High cumulative doses of tamoxifen	3–7
Obesity	2–5
Stein-Leventhal disease or estrogen-producing tumors	>5
Histories of diabetes, hypertension, gallbladder disease or thyroid disease	1.3–3.0
Cigarette smoking	0.5

[a]Relative risks depend on the study and referent group employed.

(i.e., less progesterone). Vegetarianism is associated with lower plasma estrogen levels, presumably on the basis of the relationship of diet composition to estrogen metabolism. The beneficial effects of combination oral contraceptives and cyclic progestins added to hormone replacement therapy presumably operate through the antiestrogenic effects of progesterone. The peculiar age incidence patterns for uterine cancer (i.e., extremely rare under age 45 years, followed by a rapid and progressive rise from ages 45 to 60 years) could also reflect the waning influence of progesterone. Nulliparity, hypertension, diabetes, the absence of smoking, and race may yet be added to the unifying scheme as knowledge of endocrinologic mechanisms in endometrial tissue increases.

Although there are a number of identified risk factors for uterine cancer (Table 1.1), important gaps in knowledge currently limit a full understanding of the proposed carcinogenic process. We need to understand when in a woman's life obesity matters most and how risk is influenced by weight loss; whether the number of adipocytes, their fat composition, or other factors determine peripheral conversion of androstenedione; and the precise hormonal mechanisms associated with vegetarianism. Perhaps the most important gap is in understanding the basic mechanism of estrogen carcinogenesis. It is unclear whether estrogens are complete carcinogens, classic "promoters" that affect initiated cells, or growth stimulants that act on vulnerable genetic material. The epidemiologic data are consistent with estrogens acting at a relatively late stage of carcinogenesis. If this reflects their position as tumor promoters, then the need to identify initiators of the process becomes even more crucial.

OVARIAN CANCER

Demographic Patterns

Ovarian cancer accounts for 3% of all incident cancers in U.S. women (1). Approximately 1 in 70 American women develops ovarian cancer during her lifetime. The average annual age-adjusted incidence for all SEER areas between 2000 and 2004 was 13.5 per 100,000 women (2). An estimated 21,650 new cases will be diagnosed in the United States in 2008 (1).

Diagnosis usually occurs at advanced stages; the overall 5-year survival between 2000 and 2004 was only 45%. The average annual age-adjusted mortality rate is 8.9 per 100,000 women (2). The estimated 15,520 deaths due to ovarian cancer in 2008 will make it the fifth leading cause of cancer death among U.S. women (1).

After rising during the mid-20th century, age-adjusted mortality rates have since remained relatively constant (1). Incidence rates show little variation over the past 30 years, but both incidence and mortality rates may be declining for U.S. women under age 40 years (136). U.S. blacks and whites have nearly identical mortality rates, but incidence rates remain higher for U.S. white women (137) (Fig. 1.3).

The highest incidence occurs in North American, Scandinavian, and Northern European countries, whereas the lowest rates occur in African nations and some eastern countries, such as China (3). Age-standardized rates vary 4.5-fold across countries. Mortality data show a similar but slightly less dramatic pattern. The estimated age-standardized mortality rates are 6.2 in developed countries and 2.8 in developing countries (138).

Reproductive Risk Factors

Gravidity is consistently associated with a decreased risk of ovarian cancer (139–142). Compared with nulligravidous women, women with a single pregnancy have an RR of 0.6 to 0.8. Each additional pregnancy decreases risk another 10% to 15%. The number of full-term births seems most influential, but several studies have also found decreased risks associated with an increasing number of incomplete pregnancies (143,144). Most studies that adjusted for parity report no residual association with age at first or last birth (145), but some investigators argue that both number of births and timing matter (146,147).

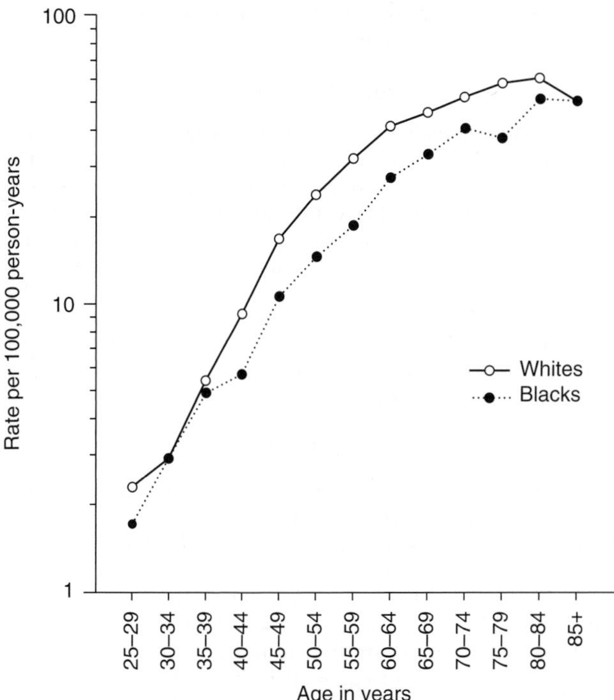

FIGURE 1.3. Age-specific incidence of cancer of the ovary by race. *Source:* Data from the Surveillance, Epidemiology, and End Results Program, 2000–2004.

Whether these risk relationships reflect a hazardous role for infertility or merely the protective role of pregnancy is unclear. Comparing subfertile women with ovarian abnormalities to subfertile women with normal ovarian function has thus far shown no increased risk for the former, but the data are not definitive (148). Studies with higher risks among infertile women support some role for abnormal endocrine factors (149). In one study (139), sexually active women who were not using contraceptives and had not conceived for 10 or more years were at a sixfold excess risk compared with other women. Another large study similarly found a high risk associated with nulliparity despite unprotected intercourse, especially in women with long periods of ovulatory experience (149).

Although several early studies showed substantial increases in ovarian cancer risk linked to use of fertility drugs (142,150), subsequent studies have generally not confirmed an association (151). The prospect that the causes of subfertility and infertility, not the associated treatments, are the causative factors appears to be gaining support (148,151,152).

A number of studies have found a reduced risk of ovarian cancer associated with breast-feeding, although the association has not always been shown to be independent of parity or to relate to risk in a dose-response relation (141,153–157). A recent pooling of two large cohort studies showed significant trends of risk with extended breast-feeding that were independent of parity effects (158). Notably, each month of breast-feeding decreased the relative risk of ovarian cancer by 2%. Suppression of ovulation and decreased gonadotropin levels were proposed as explanatory to the reduced risks, but further studies are needed to confirm this.

Menstrual Factors and Gynecologic Surgery

Numerous studies have noted reduced risks among women who have had a hysterectomy or tubal ligation (139,159–162). These patients' risks were 30% to 40% lower than the risks among women who had not undergone surgery. Surgery offers an opportunity to remove abnormal-appearing ovaries, but this alone is unlikely to explain the protective effect (163). Partial devascularization and reduced ovarian function represent a possible alternative mechanism (164).

A number of studies have linked late age at natural menopause with an increased risk of ovarian cancer (139,165), although not all studies have confirmed this relationship (166). The marked flattening in the age-specific incidence curves shortly after menopausal ages is consistent with the conclusion that early or late menopause has little effect on ovarian cancer risk. Most studies have not found earlier ages at menarche to increase risk, but some have reported weak positive associations (139,165).

Hormonal Risk Factors

Oral Contraceptives

Almost all epidemiologic studies show a reduced risk of ovarian cancer among women who use oral contraceptives. Their use for only a few months introduces lasting protection, but long-term use generates the largest risk reduction (141,167). In one study, the protective effect of long-term use (≥10 years) reached 80% (168). The protection appears to persist for many years after their last use (167–170). The lower-dose formulations now in use seem to reduce risk at least as effectively as their higher dose predecessors (171–174). In addition, the androgenicity of the progestins used does not appear to differentiate risks (175).

Menopausal Hormones

Accumulating evidence links use of menopausal hormones to an increased risk of ovarian cancer (176–182). In most of these studies, risk has been highest among long-term users. Although most of the earlier studies focused on effects of unopposed estrogens, more recent studies have addressed effects of combined estrogen plus progestin therapy. There are inconsistent results regarding how risk is affected by regimen and mode of administration of hormones (177–179,181), which may reflect small numbers involved in many of the analyses. In the WHI clinical trial, women exposed to estrogen plus progestin therapy had a 58% nonsignificantly increased risk of ovarian cancer compared to those receiving a placebo (36). The recently published Million Women Study found no variation in risk according to type of preparation used, its constituents, or mode of administration (176). The study did note a higher risk of serous tumors related to use of exogenous hormones, a finding requiring further replication.

Endogenous Hormones

Recent interest has focused on the role of endogenous hormones in the etiology of ovarian cancer. Although one nested case-control study found higher levels of androgens and lower levels of gonadotropins among cases compared to controls (183), this was not confirmed in a more recent investigation (184). This latter study, however, found some suggestion that free testosterone might play a role in early onset ovarian cancers. Another investigation, which pooled data from three studies, reported null associations with estrogens, androgens, SHBG, IGF-1, and associated binding proteins (IGFBPs) (185,186). Despite these initial null results, the strong biologic rationale for these hormones in ovarian carcinogenesis warrants further investigation.

Medical Conditions and Medications

Several studies surveyed whether certain medical conditions predispose to ovarian cancer. Diabetes, hypertension, and thyroid diseases seem unrelated to risk (102,187). In line with a number of clinical studies showing simultaneous occurrences of endometriosis and ovarian cancer, several epidemiologic studies have found that women with a diagnosis of endometriosis have elevated risks for developing ovarian cancer (152,188,189). In one of these studies, the relationship was shown to be specific to clear cell and endometrioid ovarian cancers (189). As reviewed by Ness (190), the two conditions share a number of pathophysiologic processes, including estrogen excesses and progesterone deficits, immunologic responses, and inflammatory reactions. Pelvic inflammatory disease has also been found in several studies to be a possible risk factor for ovarian cancer (191,192). This finding supports a role for inflammation in ovarian carcinogenesis.

Medications recently surfaced both as potential risk and protective factors. Several studies showed increased risks among users of psychotropic medications, particularly those operating through dopaminergic mechanisms (193). However, subsequent studies that employed cohort designs or improved exposure assessment reported null associations (194–197). Other data suggested a reduced risk among women who used anti-inflammatory or other analgesic medications (198–201). However, as with the psychotropic medication data, subsequent studies showed, at most, a weak or inconsistent association. Chemoprevention via the use of these medications remains a premature concept.

Anthropometry and Physical Activity

Obesity has recently received increased scrutiny as a possible risk factor. Most studies fail to show a generalized effect (202), although some studies have shown possible inverse relationships (203). In those studies that do show positive relationships, it has usually been restricted to certain subgroups, including premenopausal women (204,205), nulliparous women (206), women who never used menopausal estrogens (207), or those who are physically inactive (208). Further, some studies have suggested that obesity is a risk factor only for certain types of tumors. However, the histologic subgroups identified as being increased among obese women have varied across studies (209,210). Further complicating assessment of effects are suggestions that increased risks may be restricted to women who are clinically obese (211) or who became obese when they were teenagers (212). These diverse results regarding the effects of obesity on ovarian cancer risk could reflect statistical chance or other systematic biases.

Studies have also examined effects of physical activity levels on ovarian cancer risk, although results are inconclusive. Case-control studies in China (213), Canada (214), and the United States (215) have reported inverse associations with increasing activity, but the cohort analyses published to date (216,217) suggest that increasing activity might put women at increased, rather than decreased, risk.

Dietary Factors

Correlations between ovarian cancer incidence and per capita fat availability and noted increased incidence rates among migrants who moved to areas with higher per capita fat availability have stimulated interest in dietary risk factors (68). Initial studies in unique populations, such as ovolactovegetarians (218) or meat abstainers (219), provided conflicting results. Since then, studies have targeted a few classes of foods: lactose and dairy foods, fats, vitamins, fiber, fruits, and vegetables.

Lactose Consumption

Findings linking higher consumption of yogurt, cottage cheese, and other lactose-rich dairy products with an increased risk of ovarian cancer (220) were viewed with interest given that galactose-related enzymes can influence gonadotropin levels, which are hypothesized to be crucial ovarian cancer risk determinants. The majority of subsequent studies failed to show increases in risk with lactose consumption or galactose metabolism (221–225), although a few studies have provided some support for the hypothesis (226,227). Recent results from the Nurses' Health Study suggest that further attention may be warranted regarding effects for serous tumors (228).

Fat Intake

Although some case-control studies have reported higher risks of ovarian cancer associated with intake of fatty foods (e.g., butter and meats) as well as types of fat, the data on this are not entirely consistent (229–233). In contrast, most cohort studies have failed to find relationships with dietary fat consumption (226,229). The most recent analysis (234), a meta-analysis of 12 cohort studies, found no overall association with fat, cholesterol, or egg intakes, but some suggestion that very high levels of saturated fat intake might increase risk, a finding that merits further investigation.

Fruits, Vegetables, and Micronutrient Intake

Although some studies have suggested that ovarian cancer risk might be reduced by higher consumption of fruits and vegetables (221,226,235) or fiber (236,237), other studies, including a recent pooling project of 12 cohorts, fail to support these relations (238–241). Some studies showed inverse associations with particular vitamins, such as vitamins A, C, E, or beta-carotene (232,242–246), although results have not been consistent across studies. Further clarification of effects may require considering effects according to other risk factors and within histologic subgroups.

Alcohol and Coffee Consumption

A number of studies have examined effects on ovarian cancer risk related to alcohol consumption. Most have not found any convincing relationships (210,247–251), including a recent pooled analysis of ten cohort studies (252). Coffee consumption was linked to an elevated risk of ovarian cancer in early studies (253,254), but more recent studies have not replicated that association (210,248). One study actually suggested an inverse association with coffee consumption, but concluded that this was not due to caffeine intake since no relationship was observed with tea consumption (255).

Host Factors

A family history of ovarian cancer is the strongest risk factor identified to date. Which family member was affected is less important than the total number of affected relatives or their age at diagnosis (256). Women with two or more affected relatives or whose relative was diagnosed before 50 years of age experience the highest risks (257). Approximately 5% to 10% of ovarian cancer patients have a first-degree relative with ovarian cancer (256).

Inherited mutations in two autosomal dominant genes—*BRCA1* and *BRCA2*—are strongly linked to familial ovarian cancer (and breast and other cancers) (258). Whereas the lifetime probability of developing ovarian cancer in most women is 2%, the probabilities in women with a family history or women with a *BRCA1/2* mutation are 9.4% (259) and 15% to 40% (260,261), respectively. Despite these increases, *BRCA1/2* mutations explain less than one third of the elevated risk in women with familial ovarian cancer (257). Other candidate high-risk genes have not been identified but are almost certain to exist (256).

In addition to assessing the role of high-penetrance genes, studies have begun to evaluate relationships of ovarian cancer risk with the more common genetic polymorphisms, including various genes involved in hormone metabolism. To date, no markers have been conclusively linked with risk increases (262,263).

Talc

Over-the-counter talc chemically resembles asbestos, a known cause of mesothelioma, and mesothelioma histologically resembles ovarian cancer. The published case-control studies generally report positive associations between ovarian cancer and perineal talc exposure. However, a lack of consistent statistical significance and inconsistent associations with different patterns of talc use raise questions about the validity of this association (264–268).

Cigarette Smoking

In general, cigarette smoking is not considered a major risk factor for ovarian cancer. However, a number of studies have found evidence that there may be an increased risk of mucinous tumors associated with smoking. In a recent systematic review, smoking was found to lead to a significant doubling in risk for mucinous tumors, but no increased risk for endometrioid or clear cell tumors (269). The risk of mucinous cancers increased with amount smoked but returned to that of never smokers within 20 to 30 years of stopping smoking. Fewer studies have evaluated effects of passive smoking on ovarian cancer risk, with no consensus as to whether this might alter risk or have histologic specificity (270,271).

Environmental and Occupational Risk Factors

Certain occupations came under scrutiny when studies linked hair dyes and triazine herbicides to ovarian cancer (272,273). Record linkage studies in Finland (274), Norway (275), Sweden (276), Canada (277), and the United States· (125,278) have suggested a pattern of increased risks among certain professions (e.g., teachers, health care workers) or with particular occupational exposures (e.g., solvents, asbestos). Until additional data address the potential for inconsistent or chance findings and the challenge of finding large populations with sufficient data on other potential confounding variables, occupation will likely not be considered a major risk factor for ovarian cancer (279).

Conclusions

Much of the clinical and epidemiologic evidence concerning risk factors for ovarian cancer implicates ovulatory activity (Table 1.2). Conditions associated with reduced ovulation, for example, pregnancy and oral contraceptives, consistently reduce risk. Combining these and other menstrual factors into single "ovulatory age" or "lifetime ovulatory cycles" indexes has generally produced the expected associations with ovarian cancer risk; that is, older ovulatory ages (280) or higher cycle counts (281) increase risk. However, the misclassification inherent in these indexes is sufficient to generate different risk estimates (282), and the magnitude of risk reduction for short-term oral contraceptive use or a single pregnancy exceeds the proportional decrease in ovulatory cycles that would be expected to be associated with these exposures.

TABLE 1.2

RISK FACTORS FOR OVARIAN CANCER

Factors influencing risk	Estimated relative risk[a]
Older ages	3
Residency in North America, Northern Europe	2–5
Higher levels of education or income	1.5–2.0
White race	1.5
Nulligravity	2–3
History of infertility	2–5
Early ages at menarche	1.5
Late ages at natural menopause	1.5–2.0
History of a hysterectomy	0.5–0.7
Use of oral contraceptives	0.3–0.5
Long-term use of menopausal estrogens	10–20
Perineal talc exposure	1.5–2.0
Female relative with ovarian cancer	3–4

[a]Relative risks depend on the study and referent group employed.

The putative mechanisms behind ovulatory inhibition and the risk associated with "increased ovulation" (283) raise additional questions. An early report suggested, based on the associations with parity and infertility, that an unidentified endocrine abnormality predisposed women to relative or absolute infertility and ovarian cancer. The protection associated with oral contraceptives seems unlikely to fit this hypothesis unless, in some improbable manner, use induces an endocrine milieu similar to that underlying fertility.

A second popular unifying hypothesis is that ovarian cancer is the result of accumulated exposure to circulating pituitary gonadotropins (284). Although this is consistent with the parity, menopause, and oral contraceptive associations, a study that directly measured gonadotropin levels failed to find a relationship with subsequent development of ovarian cancer (183). This theory also fails to account for the risks associated with clinical infertility, and it predicts that menopausal hormone therapy use would decrease risk, because both exposures are associated with reduced gonadotropin levels.

A third explanation points to a biologic effect of ovulation on ovarian surface epithelium. Ovulation prompts a cascade of epithelial events, including minor trauma, increased local concentrations of estrogen-rich follicular fluid, and increased epithelial proliferation. Such proliferation, particularly near the point of ovulation, can recruit inclusions into the ovarian parenchyma. Some or all of these "incessant ovulation" events may lie on the causal path to ovarian cancer (285,286). This is consistent with most of the endocrine-related risk factors except for the risks associated with clinical infertility.

No single theory adequately incorporates the available data. A unifying hypothesis may lie in a combination of ovulation, hormones, and local effects. Additional factors, such as genetic alterations; androgens, progestogens, and other hormones

(283); inflammation (191); and endometriosis (190), also appear to be important.

Each hypothesis identifies testable possibilities. Discriminating between the roles of voluntary versus involuntary infertility could identify the mechanisms underlying the role of parity. Characterizing the specific reproductive abnormalities associated with clinical infertility could reveal new biologic mechanisms involved in ovarian carcinogenesis. Determining why hysterectomy and tubal ligation reduce risk could generate insights into the role of gynecologic conditions and ovarian carcinogenesis. Exploring the interactive contributions of the hormones along the hypothalamic-pituitary-gonadal axis could explain how specific hormones seem to influence risk at different time periods. In addition, verifying that inflammation or related conditions and pathways play an etiologic role in ovarian carcinogenesis could open new lines of inquiry.

Ovarian cancer epidemiology presents both simple and complex patterns. Rates have largely remain unchanged over the last 40 years, and virtually all studies show consistent associations with some exposures, such as oral contraceptives, parity, and family history. But where some uncertainty exists, it is substantial. Other reproductive or lifestyle factors that are consistently associated with other reproductive cancers—smoking, obesity, menopausal hormone therapy—have been published with such diversity that traditional attempts to quantitatively summarize the divergent data likely will not prove to be useful. Although it is tempting to attribute the differences to histology-specific associations, such hypotheses will require substantially more epidemiologic, clinical, genetic, and transitional data before their acceptance is certain. Careful a priori attempts to systematically assess the mechanisms of histologic differences may yet prove fruitful.

So where can epidemiology contribute to increasing the opportunities to reduce ovarian cancer's toll? The highly penetrant genes account for only a small proportion (10%) of women who develop ovarian cancer, but a better understanding of the mechanisms behind those risks could introduce immediate benefits for high-risk women. Continued close collaboration between geneticists and epidemiologists should pay dividends. A clear picture has emerged for some protective factors, such as oral contraceptives and parity, but risk associated with other important public health issues, such as smoking, obesity, and physical activity, remains uncertain. Continued attempts to account for the differences between studies should help delineate the spurious associations from the etiologically relevant risk factors. Doing so should help identify targets for improving detection, treatment, and prevention of this deadly tumor.

CERVICAL CANCER

It is now known that virtually all cases of cervical cancer and precancerous changes can be attributed to persistent infection with carcinogenic genotypes of human papillomaviruses (HPV) (287). Cervical cancer has a remarkably uniform etiology and pathogenesis worldwide. Consequently, the last two decades have witnessed the transformation of human HPV epidemiology from a narrow field of research to essential knowledge for gynecologists. Of the more than 100 genotypes of HPV, several dozen can infect the anogenital epithelium and approximately 15 to 20 (including types 16, 18, 26, 31, 33, 35, 39, 45, 51, 52, 56, 58, 59, 66, 68, 73, 82) can cause anogenital cancer, although the types differ greatly in carcinogenic risk (287). HPV-16 is by far the most carcinogenic type, and accounts for half of cervical cancer cases. However, cervical infection with carcinogenic types of HPV, even HPV-16, is extremely common compared to the relatively rare development of cervical cancer. Thus, additional etiologic factors are involved, in particular, variability in the human host immunologic response. Other possible causal cofactors might act by affecting immunity or via genotoxic mechanisms. These include smoking, high parity, oral contraceptive use, and coinfection with other infectious agents (287, 288).

Key Aspects of HPV Natural History Related to Cervical Cancer Epidemiology

It is possible to define new prevention strategies using HPV-based technologies that are even more effective than cervical cytologic screening and colposcopy. These topics, including the pathogenesis, diagnosis, and prevention of cervical cancer precursors, are detailed by Wright in Chapter 19. Although the current chapter concentrates mainly on the descriptive epidemiology of invasive cervical cancer, and broad relationships with major demographic and behavioral risk factors, the epidemiology of cervical cancer is most coherently understood in terms of the effects that factors exert on the natural history of HPV infection, including (a) exposure/acquisition of infection, (b) persistence of HPV infection and progression to precancer (cervical intraepithelial neoplasia 3 [CIN 3]), and (c) development of invasion (Fig. 1.4) (289).

Cervical HPV transmission, which is primarily sexual, is studied best at the molecular level, because types must be distinguished for natural history studies and because most infections (more than two thirds) are not microscopically or

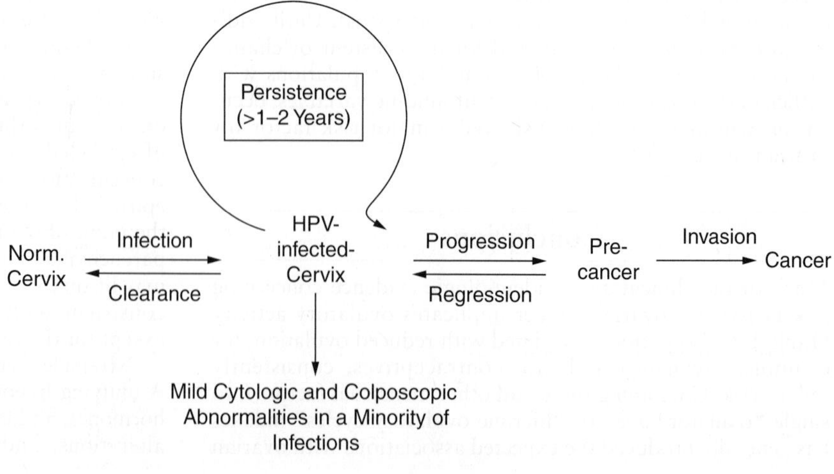

FIGURE 1.4. An epidemiologic model of the natural history of cervical carcinogenesis. The major steps in cervical carcinogenesis are human papillomavirus (HPV) infection (balanced by viral clearance), progression to precancer (partly offset by regression of precancer), and invasion. The persistence of oncogenic HPV types is necessary for progression and invasion. HPV infection is frequently, but not necessarily, associated with cytologic and histologic abnormalities. *Source:* From Schiffman M, Kjaer SK. Natural history of anogenital papillomavirus infection and neoplasia. *J Natl Cancer Inst Monogr* 2003;(31):14–19, with permission.

macroscopically evident (290). Each HPV type is a separate genetic entity and should be considered a separate sexually transmitted infection. Because all carcinogenic types are transmitted by the same sexual route, concurrent multiple-type infections are common. The available data, which are limited, seem to indicate that HPV types influence each other minimally (291, 292). The typical age of cervical HPV infection is similar to other sexually transmitted infections, with a large peak following sexual initiation.

Cervical HPV infections tend to clear after 6 to 24 months, as do warts anywhere on the body (291,293,294). Acquisition (293–296) and clearance dynamically oppose each other in each cohort of women to produce the characteristic age distributions as infections are transmitted sexually when women have new partners and are then cleared (297).

The immune response to HPV is an important determinant of viral clearance versus persistence and, by extension, a major determinant of cervical cancer risk. The key immune responses involved in the clearance of HPV infections are known to be cell mediated, but the specific immunological markers of immune protection are difficult to measure and poorly understood.

A major unresolved question of HPV natural history relates to viral latency. In follow-up studies lasting up to 10 years, virtually all HPV infections become nondetectable by sensitive HPV DNA tests, usually within 2 years, except for those that lead to precancer. Little else is known about latency, including what might cause re-emergence like that seen in renal transplant patients and HIV-immunosuppressed women, and what fraction of cancers (apparently small) arises following a period of latency. Answers to these questions will greatly affect prevention strategies reliant on HPV DNA detection.

It is the *overt persistence* of one of the carcinogenic types that is strongly linked to precancer, which histologically corresponds to CIN 3, including carcinoma in situ (298–302). Persistence of carcinogenic types of HPV and development of precancer are not identical, but thus far they are so closely linked that epidemiologists are only beginning to disentangle them. Part of the problem is that precancers begin as extremely small clonal lesions that may be below the limits of detection of microscopy. HPV type greatly affects both the absolute risk of viral persistence, and of progression to precancer associated with viral persistence (295,296,303). The most common carcinogenic type, HPV-16, is also the most common type in the general population, linked to its greater propensity to persist. However, even noncarcinogenic types like HPV-61 can also be persistent and common, although they do not cause malignant transformation (304).

The average time of viral persistence that leads to diagnosable precancer is not clear. Virgins who begin sexual activity can develop apparent precancers within a few years of initial HPV infection as detected by DNA. This short time period represents the leading edge of what is typically a longer incidence curve of precancer in persistently HPV infected women. The average age at microscopic diagnosis of precancer is approximately 25 to 30 years (305), approximately 5 to 10 years after the average peak ages of carcinogenic HPV prevalence and associated minor cytologic abnormalities in screening populations.

Noncarcinogenic HPV infections are capable of producing lesions falsely diagnosed as precancer, especially CIN2, showing that this level of abnormality is not a perfect surrogate for cancer risk (306). Still, because of the U.S. emphasis on safety and concern over loss to follow-up, treating precancer (except as appropriate in very young women, etc.) is a valid clinical strategy to provide a margin of safety, given that it is not yet possible to know which lesions pose a threat. Eventually, better accuracy based on molecular profiling is the goal.

Precancerous lesions (CIN 3, in particular) tend not to regress over short-term follow-up; however, even among precancerous lesions, risk and timing of invasion versus eventual regression are matters of probability. The absolute risk of untreated precancer developing into invasive disease is argued, with estimates averaging about 30% but ranging from 10% to 90%.

The high ratio of precancerous lesions to cancers supports the belief that many cases of precancer, particularly CIN2, would not invade but rather would regress if followed for many years. In any case, the epidemiologic risk factors for invasive cervical cancer among HPV-infected women are the same as mentioned above for precancer, except for age. Screened detected cases of invasive cancer, on average, occur approximately 15 to 20 years or more later than for precancer, suggesting a long sojourn time in the precancerous state. The median age moves toward even older ages as the quality of screening decreases, and the average stage of cancer at diagnosis also worsens due to this diagnostic delay.

Demographic Patterns

Cervical cancer is the second most common cancer of women worldwide, with 471,000 incident cases estimated in 2000 (307), and a 5-year prevalence of more than 1.4 million cases. Cervical cancer accounted for approximately 233,000 deaths worldwide in the year 2000, or about one tenth of the total number of female cancer deaths (307). The cancer burden (incidence and mortality) is disproportionately high (~80%) in the developing world.

The incidence rate per 100,000 women-years for invasive cervical cancer in various geographic areas is highly variable, linked to HPV infection and screening practices (287). The highest age-standardized rates, more than five times the rates in the United States and Canada, were reported from East Africa, Central America, and the Pacific Islands. Comparing regions without extensive effective screening, geographic studies using sensitive polymerase chain reaction (PCR) DNA testing methods to detect the carcinogenic HPV types have observed HPV prevalence rates to correlate with the population risks of cervical cancer.

An examination of age-specific cervical cancer incidence in countries prior to introduction of screening has demonstrated that rates begin to increase around age 25 (when cases are still quite rare), with an unusually early plateau or peak starting at age 40 to 50 (308). It is unusual for incidence rates of a cancer to plateau or fall with increasing age, and this age structure reflects that cervical cancers originate from HPV infections transmitted mainly in late adolescence and early adulthood.

It is estimated that 11,070 women will be diagnosed with and 3,870 will die from cervical cancer during 2008 in the United States (1). The corresponding average annual age-adjusted incidence for invasive cervical cancer in all SEER areas was 8.7 per 100,000 women for the period 2000 to 2004 (2). Previously striking regional differences in incidence, with excesses particularly in Appalachia, are now less visible, although high-incidence areas such as the Mexican-U.S. border still exist.

Cervical cancer rates began to fall during the early 20th century, before the advent of cytologic screening. Reduced parity may have contributed to this pattern, given that multiparity appears to be a cofactor for progression of HPV infection to cervical neoplasia. In the latter half of the last century, effective screening contributed to a further reduction in cancer incidence and mortality, particularly among women of 30 to 74 years because of targeting of this age group in many countries (309,310).

In the United States and many other developed nations, rates of squamous cell carcinomas, accounting for approximately

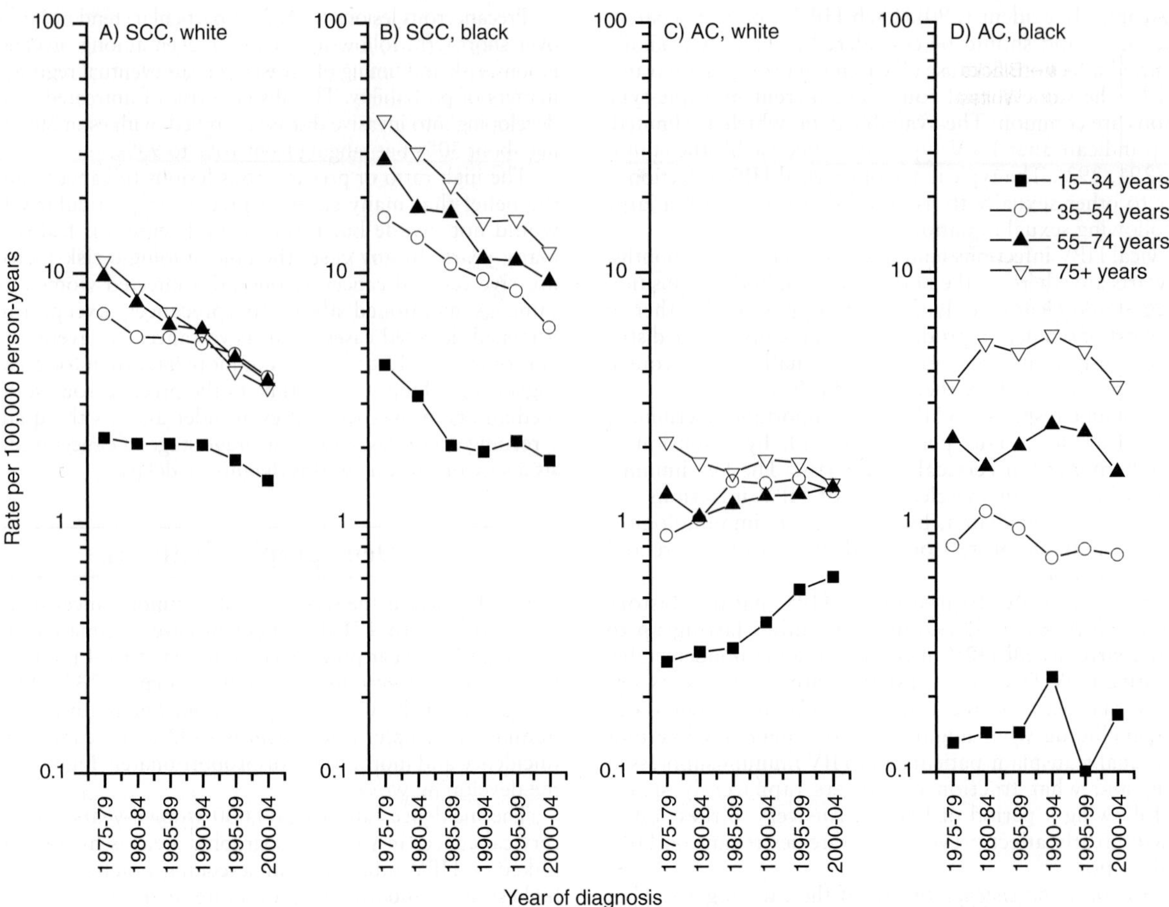

FIGURE 1.5. Incidence trends for cervical squamous cell carcinoma and adenocarcinoma by race. *Source:* Data from the Surveillance, Epidemiology, and End Results Program, 1976–1995, and from Wang SS, Sherman ME, Hildesheim A, Lacey JV, Devesa S. Cervical adenocarcinoma and squamous cell carcinoma incidence trends among white women and black women in the United States for 1976–2000. *Cancer* 2004;100;(5):1035–1044, with permission.

80% of invasive cervical cancers (310), have declined steadily since the introduction of Pap smear screening, while adenocarcinomas (accounting for approximately 15%) have not (311–318). In fact, rates of cervical adenocarcinomas have risen in the past two to three decades in various countries including the United States, both relative to rates of squamous cell carcinoma and in absolute numbers (Fig. 1.5).

The overall incidence and stage of invasive squamous cell cancer has declined substantially over the past 25 years, with the pace of decline having been more pronounced in black than white women (Fig. 1.6). Although rates for invasive carcinoma remain higher for blacks than whites, the difference has narrowed over time, with major differences now being observed only among older women.

The 5-year survival rate for cervical cancer is greater than 70%, with survival being highly dependent on stage at diagnosis. Younger women and white women are more likely than older women and black women, respectively, to be diagnosed with localized cancer that carries a good prognosis.

HPV Infection

For more than a century, epidemiologic studies have suggested an association between sexual activity and cervical cancer, but proof that HPV is the sexually transmitted agent responsible for this association was not achieved until sensitive methods for detecting HPV DNA were developed. The epidemiologic association between HPV infection and cervical cancer fulfills all of the established epidemiologic criteria for causality. As a result, HPV is now accepted to be the central, necessary causal factor for virtually all cases of cervical cancer in the world. The recognition of the key etiologic role of HPV infection has profoundly altered the epidemiologic study of cervical cancer. It is increasingly clear which previously "established" epidemiologic risk factors for cervical cancer are correlates of HPV infection, which lead to infection, and which are HPV cofactors operating only in the presence of infection (319, 320). For example, because HPV is transmitted by direct physical contact, virgins (women without any sexual contact at all) almost invariably test negative for HPV (321,322) explaining their virtually negligible risk of cervical cancer regardless of other behaviors.

Numerous case-control and cohort studies have now shown that sexual behavior, specifically numbers of partners, is the main determinant of incident HPV detection and subsequent risk of cervical precancer and cancer (323–326). HPV infections are easily transmitted with few acts of sexual intercourse and, therefore, sexual frequency is not a major risk factor for cervical neoplasia. The variable "age at first intercourse" tends to weaken as a risk factor once HPV infection is taken into account (325,327) and remains an

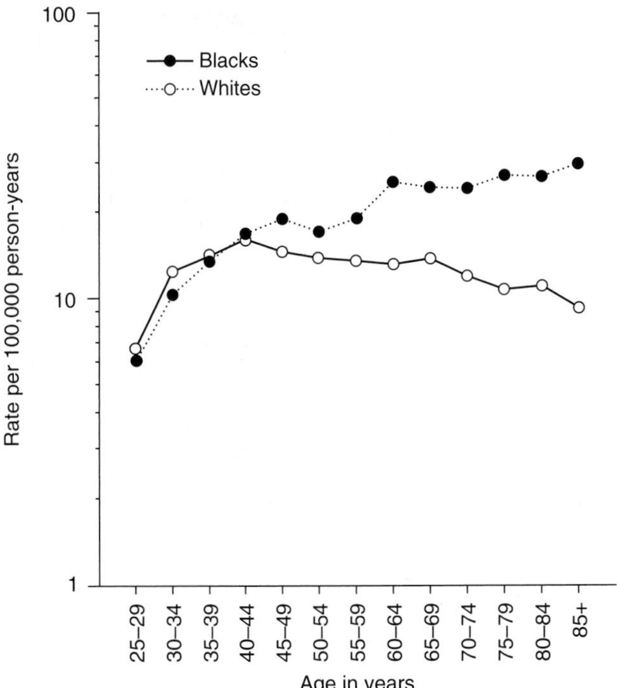

FIGURE 1.6. Age-specific incidence of invasive cancer of the cervix uteri by race. *Source:* Data from the Surveillance, Epidemiology, and End Results Program, 2000–2004.

apparent proxy for time of HPV infection (328), i.e., the start of viral "latency" (327).

A protective effect against cervical cancer risk has been noted for careful, consistent condom use. Condom use affords modest protection against HPV infection and resultant external warts (HPV-6 and HPV-11) and cervical lesions caused by carcinogenic HPV types (329). Given that users of condoms may not report sporadic unprotected contacts, and that the entire skin and mucosal genital area at risk for infection is not protected with this contraceptive method, only modest protection against transmission would be expected (330).

Historically, and still in many regions of the world, female monogamy has been valued more than male monogamy. Thus, cervical cancer risk from HPV infection transmitted from a male partner to his monogamous partner can properly be seen as "the male factor." Confirmed associations supporting this view include the geographic clustering of cervical and penile cancer, the increased risk of cervical cancer among wives of men who have penile cancer, the increased risk among partners of men who have had a previous partner who died of cervical cancer, and the increased risk among women whose partners travel (331). Circumcision is associated with a reduced risk of HPV detection in penile samples, and the wives of men with a history of multiple partners were at lower risk of cervical cancer if the men had been circumcised (331). Circumcision appears to reduce male HPV infection, but studies to understand details of HPV transmission between sexual partners have proved challenging. Contact between women and multiple partners at different times, clearance of infection in one partner but not the other, and difficulties in collecting satisfactory specimens for HPV testing from men all complicate the demonstration of concordant infection among partners (332).

Transient HPV infections are ubiquitous among sexually active young women, but progression to a cervical cancer precursor requires persistence of carcinogenic types (296,299, 300,333,334). This has prompted epidemiologic studies to investigate "cofactors" that influence persistence and progression to precancer. Persistence and progression to CIN 3 occur concurrently, complicating the independent examination of these two processes.

Viral Factors Associated with Persistence and Progression

HPV type is by far the strongest predictor of risk of precancer (see Wright, chapter 19). Persistent HPV-16 infection is an extremely strong risk factor for subsequent diagnosis of CIN 3 and invasive cancer. HPV types, are more predictive of risk than subtleties of minor and equivocal cytopathic effects, colposcopic findings, or behavioral cofactors like smoking. However the existence of many HPV types prevents easy-to-follow clinical protocols. Furthermore, intratypic sequence variants of HPV-16 and possibly other types have been associated with altered risk, although these risk modifications are weaker than the intertypic variation. The role of elevated viral load (i.e., HPV content in samples obtained from infected women) in predicting persistence and progression of infection is complicated and varies by HPV type. A clear trend of increasing prospective risk with increasing viral load has been demonstrated only for HPV-16. Viral load assessment is not useful clinically. Although studies suggest that women with prevalent infections may be more likely to acquire additional infections, infection with one HPV type does not seem to influence the risk of persistence and development of precancer from another concurrent infection (291,335). Finally, while the state of the virus (integrated into human host DNA vs. episomal), methylation status, and transcript levels for the oncogenes E6 and E7 may be associated with risk of persistence and subsequent neoplasia, clinically useful assays and protocols are not yet available.

Host Factors Associated with Persistence and Progression

Immunity

Whereas humoral (antibody-mediated) immunity appears to play a central role in preventing HPV infection (leading to the prophylactic vaccines), elimination of HPV seems more closely related to mounting an effective cellular immune response (336–338). Impaired cellular immunity, attributable to human immunodeficiency virus (HIV) infection, transplantation, or immunosuppressive drugs, has been shown to increase HPV prevalence, persistence, warts, CIN, and cancer (339,340). In contrast, deficiencies in humoral immunity appear unrelated to these conditions. The U.S. Centers for Disease Control and Prevention (CDC) has identified cervical cancer as an acquired immune deficiency syndrome (AIDS)–defining illness among women infected with HIV. Compared to the general population, women with AIDS have a fivefold excess risk of carcinoma in situ of the cervix, with risk increasing over time (341). Although risk was similarly elevated for invasive cancers, rates did not increase over time, suggesting that HIV infection probably has a limited impact on the transition from in situ to invasive disease. Although highly active antiretroviral therapy (HAART) improves CD4 levels, this has not been associated with regression of cervical cancer precursors (339).

Human Leukocyte Antigens

Human leukocyte antingens (HLAs) are important determinants of the efficiency of antigen presentation to immune effector cells and, therefore, may influence the outcome of HPV infections. Both class I HLA genes (those that encode

HLA molecules that are present in all nucleated cells) and class II HLA genes (those that encode HLA molecules that are present in lymphocytes and other immune-related cells) are involved in immune presentation. To date, HLA class II genes have been more extensively studied than HLA class I genes for their association with cervical cancer. A protective association with HLA DRB1*13 and/or DQB1*603 has been found consistently among studies, whereas specific HLA class II markers of increased risk have not been identified. Data for risk associations with polymorphic variants of HLA class I antigens are sparse; a protective association with HLA C*0202 was reported in an analysis combining data from three diverse populations (342). Since the C*0202 allele is involved not only in acquired immune response to viruses (i.e., the antigen-specific, memory immune responses associated with T cells of the immune system) but also in the innate immune response to foreign pathogens (i.e., nonspecific, inflammatory immune responses), this finding has prompted the speculation that not only the HPV-type specific T-cell mediated immune responses but also nonspecific innate immune responses might be important in the immune response to HPV infections and in cervical cancer pathogenesis. Results regarding other genes involved in the immune response are still inconclusive.

Familial Factors

Whatever the mechanism, studies conducted largely in Scandinavian countries with established nationwide tumor, twin, and other family registries clearly indicate that cervical cancer aggregates in families (343–349). In general, an approximate twofold increase in risk of precancer or invasive cervical cancer relative to general population risk is observed in family members of cervical cancer patients. It is not settled how much of this elevation in risk among relatives of individuals affected with cervical cancer can be attributed to shared environment versus genetic effects (343,347).

Behavioral Factors Associated with Persistence and Progression

Socioeconomic Status

Internationally, women defined as low social class were found in a recent meta-analysis to have twice the risk of cervical cancer compared to women defined as belonging to a high social class (350). In the United States, the inverse relationships of risk with income and education prevail among both whites and blacks, and among HPV-infected women (351). In one analysis, when adjustment was made for socioeconomic variables, the relative risk of cervical cancer among blacks compared to whites was substantially reduced (352). On the other hand, controlling for race or ethnicity, or exposure to HPV infection does not account for the socioeconomic status (SES) association entirely (351). The correlates of low socioeconomic level that are HPV cofactors for cervical cancer are not known. Of note, another socioeconomic variable formerly linked to cervical cancer risk, religion, has not been reassessed in studies incorporating accurate HPV testing.

Cigarette Smoking

Case-control and cohort studies among groups of women infected with carcinogenic HPV have shown that smokers are at increased risk compared with infected women who do not smoke (288,327,353–355). Current smoking is the main risk factor, not past smoking, with no clear trend with time since stopping smoking. Among current smokers, evidence of increasing risk has been found with increasing intensity and duration (or early start) of smoking. Several investigations have attempted to define possible mechanisms by which smoking might alter cervical epithelium. Tobacco-derived carcinogens are secreted into the cervix at levels higher than in serum (356–359), suggesting possible genotoxicity. The immunosuppressive effects of smoking (360) might enhance the persistence of HPV infection (361). In a randomized clinical trial, quitting smoking was associated with increased regression rates of microscopically identified HPV infections, possibly due to an effect on cell-mediated immunity (362).

Parity and Other Obstetrical and Gynecologic Events

HPV-infected women who have many live births are at increased risk of cervical cancer and precancer. There is a dose-dependent increase in risk with numbers of live births, most evident among women with many live births (288,363–367). Although this epidemiologic association is firmly established, the explanatory mechanism is not clear. Mechanisms underlying the association between parity and cervical neoplasia include trauma during parturition, hormonal changes associated with pregnancy, immunosuppression, and possibly altered anatomy of the transformation zone, specifically eversion. Other menstrual and reproductive factors, including miscarriages, abortions, stillbirths, ectopic pregnancies, cesarean sections, age at first pregnancy, age at menarche, and age at menopause, are not independently associated with risk (365,368).

Oral Contraceptives

Studies examining the relationship of oral contraceptive use to cervical cancer risk among HPV infected women are especially complex, with questions arising about the potential for confounding, particularly by the duration of HPV infection and screening behavior (288,369–373). Use of oral contraceptives could plausibly potentiate the carcinogenicity of HPV infection, because transcriptional regulatory regions of HPV DNA contain hormone-recognition elements and transformation of cells in vitro with viral DNA is enhanced by hormones (374). A recent large multi-center case-control study and meta-analysis found an elevated risk of invasive cervical cancer among HPV-positive women who used oral contraceptives for more than 10 years (288, 373). Shorter durations of use were not associated with elevated risk. There is not yet prospective confirmation of the risk of precancer among HPV-infected women taking oral contraceptives. Evidence linking oral contraceptives to cervical abnormalities has raised concern about long-acting steroid preparations, notably depot-medroxyprogesterone acetate (DMPA). Although these agents are widely used in many countries, studies evaluating their effects, particularly among HPV-infected women, are limited (328,375).

In sum, Bosch et al. (376) concluded that HPV infection associated with one or more leading candidate cofactors (pregnancy, smoking, and oral contraceptive use) might account for about 75% of cervical cancer. This interesting analysis has not been replicated sufficiently; thus, the search for other cofactors continues.

Infectious Agents Other than HPV

In the 1970s, herpes simplex virus (HSV-2) was hypothesized to be the sexually transmitted cause of cervical cancer (377). Now, HPV infection is known to be the central, necessary cause of cervical cancer, but other sexually transmitted agents could increase the risk of cervical cancer among HPV-infected women. Of the other agents examined, there is still some interest in HSV-2, but most attention now is focused on *Chlamydia trachomatis*. Although residual confounding by some aspect of HPV infection has not been completely ruled out, despite adjusting for HPV exposure using DNA tests and/or serology, *C. trachomatis* seropositive women are sometimes observed to be at increased risk compared to seronegative women (377–380) No consistent association with cervical cancer risk has been observed for other sexually transmitted agents (except for HIV, related to immunosuppression). It is interesting that the mildly immunosuppressive retrovirus HTLV-1 has not been linked to an increased risk of precancer and cancer among HPV-infected women (381). One investigation (382) but not another (383) noted a rise in risk of cervical cancer with multiple, concurrent infections, consistent with the hypothesis and some epidemiologic evidence (384) that long-term cervicovaginal inflammation (dominated by neutrophils), regardless of causal agent, might increase the carcinogenicity of HPV infection.

Nutrients

The influence of nutrient status on risk of cervical neoplasia has received substantial research attention (385,386). Although epidemiologists continue to suspect that diet, e.g., antioxidant micronutrient intake, is important in cervical carcinogenesis, no firm associations between a specific aspect of nutritional status and HPV infection or cervical cancer risk has been established or completely discarded, perhaps due to methodologic difficulties. Low folate levels or high homocysteine levels have been linked to risk of cervical cancer, leading to interest in markers of one-carbon metabolism and DNA repair (384,387). Unfortunately, seven phase 3 chemoprevention trials giving folic acid or beta-carotene failed to significantly ameliorate HPV lesions and precancers, although topical administration of retinoic acid did lead to lesion regression, similar to its therapeutic utility on facial warts (384).

Risk Factors for Cervical Adenocarcinoma

While infection with a carcinogenic HPV is a necessary cause of both squamous cell carcinomas and adenocarcinomas, the distribution of carcinogenic HPV types and variants detected in these two tumor types vary, with HPV-18 accounting for a relatively higher percentage of adenocarcinomas as compared to squamous cell carcinomas (388).

Interpreting increasing rates of cervical adenocarcinomas over time poses challenges because of gradual improvements in clinical practices (including the use of devices to obtain better endocervical sampling), stricter criteria for adequate Pap tests, development of cytologic criteria for recognizing adenocarcinoma in situ (AIS), and recently, formal inclusion of the AIS category in the new Bethesda System (314,315,389). In addition, proposed but unsubstantiated explanations for these upward trends include increased rates of HPV infection without improved cytologic detection of AIS, a specific increase in rates of HPV-18 infection, and increased exposure to HPV cofactors specific to adenocarcinoma.

Although our understanding of the etiology of cervical adenocarcinoma is incomplete, a picture is emerging in which adenocarcinoma seems to share some risk factors with cervical squamous carcinomas (acquisition of HPV through sexual contact) and others with uterine carcinoma (a tumor etiologically related to hormones). Two strongly linked factors for squamous carcinoma, parity and smoking, have not been shown to increase the risk for adenocarcinoma (390–392); in fact, there is some evidence that both factors might be associated with decreases in risk. In contrast, increased weight (or related measures) appears to be related to increases in the risk of cervical adenocarcinomas (391,393,394). Oral contraceptives have been linked to an increased risk for AIS or adenocarcinoma in a number of studies (391,395–398). The increased risk of cervical adenocarcinoma associated with obesity and reduced risk with parity and smoking resemble the epidemiology of endometrial adenocarcinoma. However, the relationship between cervical adenocarcinoma and oral contraceptives is more similar to reported results for squamous carcinomas of the cervix. The association between estrogen replacement therapy and increased risk for adenocarcinoma has been inconsistent (399,400).

Conclusions

Knowledge of the epidemiology of HPV and its causal role in cervical carcinogenesis has been successfully translated into clinical practice (401–405), particularly to reduce rates of squamous lesions. In many developed countries, women with equivocal cytology are tested for HPV DNA; a negative result provides strong reassurance that immediate follow-up is not required and can reduce patient anxiety and health costs (406). Comparison of HPV test results with cytologic interpretations provides important quality assurance for both tests (407,408). Repeated HPV testing is also finding application in following women without intervention and in determining the risk of recurrence among those treated for CIN. HPV testing as an adjunct to primary screening has been adopted in the United States, and screening studies are under way to develop new optimized approaches that focus resources on at-risk women (409). Finally, encouraging early results from vaccine trials suggest that primary prevention of HPV infection may be possible, potentially allowing eradication of cervical cancer in even the poorest nations of the world (410,411). Following these accomplishments, the epidemiologic study of HPV and cervical cancer will continue in order to target public health strategies, improve patient management, and monitor success in prevention.

VULVAR CANCER

Demographic Patterns and the Importance of Pathologic Classifications

Carcinoma of the vulva is a rare genital neoplasm with an average annual age-adjusted incidence in all SEER areas during 2000 to 2004 of 2.2 per 100,000 women (2). During 2008, an estimated 3,460 women will develop the disease and 870 will die as a consequence of it.

Vulvar cancer is etiologically heterogeneous, and pathologic subtypes have distinct epidemiologic features. The great majority of cases are squamous, but two subclassifications of squamous cancers, basaloid and warty, are more linked to HPV than keratinizing squamous tumors (412). Most vulvar intraepithelial neoplasias, similar to CIN, show risk factors that resemble basaloid and warty carcinomas. The HPV-associated subtypes are associated with younger age and black race (413). The non-HPV-associated types are associated with chronic inflammatory states such as lichen sclerosus.

Because vulvar cancer is heterogeneous, and because epidemiologic data usually do not separate the subtypes, compiled summary data must be interpreted very cautiously. Although vulvar cancer has been noted in clinical series to occur frequently among blacks, recent incidence data do not support any substantial differences in *overall* incidence by race (2.3 per 100,000 for white women and 1.9 per 100,000 for black women). Although the disease occurs primarily among older women (a mixture of HPV- and non-HPV-related pathologies), recent analyses of SEER data indicate substantial increases in the incidence of in situ vulvar carcinomas (mainly HPV related), which generally occur at much younger ages than invasive diseases (414).

Cancer of the vulva occurs significantly more frequently among women with primary cancers of the cervix, and the two diseases often occur simultaneously (415,416). Approximately 15% to 20% of women with vulvar cancer have a second primary cancer occurring simultaneously or nonsimultaneously in the cervix, vagina, or anogenital area. As many as 10% to 15% of women with cancer of the vulva have a second primary lesion of the cervix. This association probably reflects multifocal HPV infection. When multiple primaries are not diagnosed simultaneously, cancer of the cervix usually precedes cancer of the vulva. Many patients with vulvar cancer have multifocal genital lesions, commonly including a mixture of condyloma acuminatum planum and intraepithelial neoplasia. They may also have similar changes at other anogenital sites, including the vagina, cervix, and perianal region (417).

SEER incidence data indicate nearly a doubling in the rate of vulvar cancer between 1973 and 1976 and between 1985 and 1987 (418). This is in contrast to rates of invasive squamous cell carcinomas, which have remained relatively stable. Given that *in situ* cancers develop on average significantly earlier than invasive vulvar cancers, it may be that changes in certain risk factors (e.g., increased sexual activity and HPV infection) may have been too recent in order for effects to be seen for invasive cancers. Alternatively, successful treatment of *in situ* tumors may have prevented the occurrence of invasive disease. Again, the most likely explanation for the patterns observed is etiologic differences, with HPV being important for a larger proportion of *in situ* cancers (412).

HPV and Smoking

Early case-control studies reported higher risks among women reporting multiple sexual partners (419,420). Subsequent studies postulated a role for HPV in the etiology of the tumors, finding high rates of detection of the virus in vulvar tumor tissue and high subsequent disease risks among patients with seropositive tests to HPV-16 (421–423). HPV-16 appears to be the most predominant type detected among vulvar cancer patients (376).

Findings of elevated risks of vulvar cancer associated with cigarette smoking (419,423–425) have prompted several studies to examine interactions with HPV infection status. Two studies have found particularly high risks associated with HPV seropositivity among cigarette smokers, suggesting that the effect of HPV may depend on smoking as a cofactor (422,423).

Social Class

Although the incidence of vulvar cancer has been discussed in relation to social class, results from one case-control study indicated that control for sexual factors eliminated this effect (419). Suggestions that the risk of vulvar cancer is elevated among nulliparous women and those with late ages at first birth were also not confirmed in this study.

Medical Conditions

Vulvar carcinomas often arise within genital warts, but more specific temporal associations between the two remain unclear. Several studies have suggested that a history of vulvar warts is associated with an elevated risk of vulvar cancer, with RRs ranging from 15 to 23 (419,426). In one study, a particularly high risk was associated with multiple episodes of genital warts, possibly reflecting poor immunologic response to HPV infection among these women (419). However, the HPV types that cause vulvar warts, HPV-6 and HPV-11, are not genetically close to the major types in vulvar cancers and preceding vulvar intra-epithelial neoplasia (predominantly HPV-16), so the exact relationship between warts and cancer is somewhat obscure.

Several clinical studies have suggested that vulvar cancer may be elevated among women with diabetes, obesity, or hypertension, but this has not been confirmed in the one epidemiologic study assessing these factors (419). An excess risk of vulvar cancer among users of oral contraceptives was found in one study but not in another (419,425).

Host Factors

Recent attention has focused on the possible etiologic role of genetic factors. Although it has been hypothesized that some carcinogen-metabolizing genes might be involved, particularly those involved in the metabolism of cigarette smoke, studies have failed to find relationships of risk with either glutathione S-transferase (GST) or debrisoquine 4-hydroxylase (CYP2D6) genetic polymorphisms (427,428).

Conclusions

The cervix and vulva are covered by squamous-cell epithelium with a common embryologic origin from the cloacogenic membrane. These similarities have led to the theory that the entire lower genital tract responds to various carcinogens as a single tissue field, resulting in a relatively high proportion of multicentric squamous carcinomas (429). The multicentric nature of the disease; its association with cervical, vaginal, and perianal malignancies; and several risk factors common to it and cervical cancer suggest that the etiologic mechanisms for a fraction of vulvar cancer and cervical cancer may be similar, linked to HPV infection.

VAGINAL CANCER

Demographic Patterns

Cancer of the vagina is also rare, with an average annual age-adjusted incidence of 0.7 per 100,000 women in the SEER areas for the period from 2000 to 2004 (2). The incidence is higher for blacks (1.1 per 100,000 for blacks vs. 0.7 per 100,000 for whites), but the reasons for the discrepancy are unknown. During 2008 it is estimated that 2,210 women will develop the disease and 760 will die from it (1). The average 5-year survival rate is 52% for whites (50% for all races). The majority of vaginal cancers are squamous-cell carcinomas and occur in the upper part of the vagina.

Vaginal cancer is primarily a disease of older women (430), with almost 60% occurring among women 60 years of age or older. In the past, carcinoma of the vagina was only rarely reported in infants and children but, beginning in the late 1960s, cases of clear-cell adenocarcinoma of the vagina, an uncommon cancer in any age group, began to be observed with much greater frequency than expected among women between 15 and 22 years of age. Most of these cases have been related to prenatal exposure to diethylstilbestrol (DES).

Medical and Sexual Risk Factors

The rarity of vaginal cancer has limited the conduct of definitive epidemiologic investigations. One case-control study of vaginal cancer, based on relatively few cases, found associations of risk with low socioeconomic status, histories of genital warts or other genital irritations, and previous abnormal Pap smears (431). A more recent and larger study linked risk with histories of multiple sexual partners, early ages at first intercourse, and current cigarette smoking (432). Epidemiologic studies have also shown high risks associated with prior hysterectomies, although this apparently is due to the predisposition of women with anogenital cancers (particularly those with cervical cancer) to subsequently develop vaginal cancers (432).

HPV Infection

Findings that vaginal cancer is frequently found as a synchronous or a metachronous neoplasm with cervical cancer have led to the suggestion that there may be shared etiologic features between vaginal and cervical cancers. HPV has been related to disease through findings of HPV antigens or DNA in vaginal cancer tissue. In the largest study of this issue, HPV DNA was found in tumor blocks in over 80% of patients with in situ and over 60% of patients with invasive cancers (432). In addition, serologic antibodies to HPV have been linked to subsequent disease risk (421).

Diethylstilbestrol and Clear-Cell Adenocarcinomas

In 1971, seven clear-cell carcinomas of the vagina and one closely related endometrioid carcinoma developed in young women (ages 15 to 22 years) (433). An epidemiologic study found that the mothers of seven of the eight women had taken DES during the first trimester of pregnancy as opposed to none of the mothers of 32 matched controls. The relationship between DES exposure in utero and adenocarcinoma of the vagina was soon confirmed in New York State and at the Mayo Clinic (434,435). Since then, a registry of clear-cell cancer of the vagina and cervix has been established, and many more cases have been reported (436). Among these patients, about twice as many have clear-cell adenocarcinoma of the vagina as have clear-cell adenocarcinoma of the cervix.

Recent data from an assembly of all established DES cohorts indicate that the majority of patients with vaginal or cervical adenocarcinomas are diagnosed prior to age 25, with the incidence after this age decreasing by 80% (437). The estimated attack rate for clear-cell adenocarcinoma of the vagina and cervix through 39 years of age was estimated to be 1.6 per 1,000 DES-exposed daughters. Thus, DES exposure leads to a large relative increase in risk, but it affects only a small proportion of all exposed women. It remains to be seen what risk will be encountered by DES daughters when they reach their 50s and 60s, the peak ages of adenocarcinomas of the vagina in women unexposed to DES.

Conclusions

Even less is known about risk factors for vaginal cancer than is known for vulvar cancer. It has recently been suggested that there may be two types of vaginal cancers with age-related etiology (438). In young patients, the etiology may be similar to cervical cancer and relate to HPV, smoking, and low socioeconomic status, while the most common occurrences in older women may be due to hormonal factors or trauma to the vagina. Further attention should focus on the relative contributions of these factors.

The rare occurrence of vaginal adenocarcinoma in young women is distinctive in being essentially an iatrogenic disease related to in utero exposure to DES and other estrogens. A proposed mechanism involves nests of abnormal cells of müllerian duct origin, which are stimulated by endogenous hormones during puberty and promoted into adenocarcinomas.

GESTATIONAL TROPHOBLASTIC DISEASES

Gestational trophoblastic diseases (GTDs) (which include hydatidiform moles, invasive moles, and choriocarcinoma) encompass a range of interrelated conditions characterized by abnormal growth of chorionic tissues with various propensities for local invasion and metastasis (439). Hydatidiform moles can be either complete or partial and have distinctive pathologies and etiologies. Complete moles have paternally derived nuclear DNA but maternally derived cytoplasmic DNA. In contrast, partial moles generally have a triploid karyotype, with the extra haploid set of chromosomes being of paternal origin.

Demographic Patterns

Choriocarcinoma is a rare malignancy in the United States, with a reported incidence in all SEER areas of 0.1 per 100,000 women, or approximately 1 per 25,674 live births (440). Hydatidiform moles occur about once in every 1,000 pregnancies, and approximately one of six occurrences results in invasive complications (either invasive mole or choriocarcinoma). Trophoblastic diseases have been reported to be more common in certain parts of the world, although some of the differences may be due to a variety of selection, detection, and reporting biases (441), including whether risk is expressed in relation to women at risk, conceptions, or live births. In the United States, incidence rates have declined over time, and survival improved, but blacks continue to have higher incidence and lower survival than women of other ethnicities (442).

The epidemiologic study of choriocarcinoma has been complicated by its relative infrequency. Most studies have, therefore, focused on defining risk factors for hydatidiform moles, but it is uncertain the extent to which these findings can be extrapolated to malignant trophoblastic disease.

Host Factors

Trophoblastic disease rates are considerably higher in Asian and African countries, but the true extent of difference from Western rates is difficult to decipher because of variations in reporting practices (443). A survey in Britain showed that the incidence of gestational trophoblastic diseases in Asians was nearly twice as high as among non-Asians (444). One incidence survey in the United States showed that, even after adjustment for age and birth distribution effects, blacks had a 2.1-fold greater risk and other nonwhite races had a 1.8-fold greater risk than whites (445). American Indians and Alaskan natives have also recently been shown to have high rates of GTDs (446).

One clearly established risk factor for choriocarcinoma and hydatidiform moles is maternal age. A recent study showed women at extreme maternal ages (either very early or late) to have nearly twofold elevated rates, with even further age differences noted for the occurrence of complete moles (444).

A history of hydatidiform moles is also a strong risk factor. The risk of another molar pregnancy in a subsequent conception is about 1% and the risk appears to increase to about 25% in women who have had more than one previous hydatidiform mole (447). Although two studies have reported a higher risk of hydatidiform moles associated with a history of a complete mole (448,449), other studies have not confirmed this. Hydatidiform moles are associated with a 1,000 to 2,000 times increase for development of subsequent choriocarcinoma, with an even further enhancement after a complete molar pregnancy (2,500 times higher than after a live birth). One study suggested that some women might have multiple episodes of hydatidiform moles despite different male partners, suggesting either a role for oocyte defects or environmental factors (450).

Two studies have found an association between blood group A and choriocarcinoma (451,452). The combination of mother's group A and father's group O generated over a 10-fold increased risk. Blood groups A and AB were associated with elevated risks of hydatidiform moles in one study but not in another (453,454). These findings may support a role for genetic factors or immunologic factors related to the histocompatibility of maternal and trophoblastic tissues.

Menstrual, Reproductive, and Anthropometric Risk Factors

In several studies that have adjusted for the effects of late maternal age, parous women have remained at a substantially reduced risk of GTDs compared with nulliparous women, with some evidence of further reductions in risk with multiple births (453,455,456). Several studies have found an increased risk associated with a prior spontaneous abortion, although this has not been consistently observed (453,455–457). An increased risk of GTDs has been found related to a history of induced abortions in a number of studies, although information was not available on reasons for the terminations (455). A history of infertility has also been suggested as a risk factor for gestational trophoblastic disease, although not confirmed in all studies (453,455,457). In one study, Chinese patients reporting the use of herbal medicines during the first trimester of a previous pregnancy were at elevated risk (455).

Low body mass, unrelated to dieting or exercise, has been reported as a risk factor for choriocarcinoma in one study (458). Patients also had later onset of menarche and lighter menstrual periods than controls, possibly reflecting lower estrogen levels.

Exogenous Hormones

Several studies have found an increased risk of trophoblastic diseases associated with long-term use of oral contraceptives (455,459,460). Two other case-control studies, however, found no influence of oral contraceptives on risk (453,457). In one study, the association was considerably stronger for partial than complete moles (461). Others have suggested that oral contraceptives may increase the risk of malignant sequelae after mole evacuation through a tumor-stimulating effect (462,463). In one study, this effect was restricted to users of high-dose estrogens, although in others there were no effects of the pill on postmolar complications (459,464,465).

Other Risk Factors

Late paternal age was suggested in one study to increase the risk of trophoblastic diseases, but other investigations failed to confirm this (453,455,466). Cigarette smoking has also been linked with the occurrence of trophoblastic disease (457). One study suggested that low carotene intake affected the risk of hydatidiform mole, but no specific dietary associations were observed in another study (455,459).

Conclusions

Although a genetic role in the development of hydatidiform moles is now certain, little is known about genotypes that predispose to hydatidiform moles or environmental factors that may increase the risk of defective ova. Except for the possible role of oral contraceptives, few potential environmental promoters have been identified.

The trophoblast plays an active role in pregnancy, including metabolizing and detoxifying xenobiotic substances, regulating nutrient and waste product transfer, synthesizing steroid and protein hormones, and controlling the immune response of the maternofetal unit. Injury to the trophoblast can occur in pregnancy as a result of environmental exposure (e.g., heavy metals and polycyclic hydrocarbons), resulting in the breakdown of trophoblastic processes. When the trophoblast malfunctions, mutagenic, teratogenic, lethotoxic, and carcinogenic compounds may gain access to the developing embryo, causing injury and death. The genotype of hydatidiform moles results in a trophoblast that malfunctions, and exposure to certain environmental agents during the molar pregnancy may promote choriocarcinoma. Before implantation, the trophoblast forms most of the embryonic tissue, which already metabolizes environmental agents. Even preimplanted moles, with their impaired metabolic capabilities, may increase the toxicity of environmental agents and promote carcinogenesis.

Recent advances in identifying genetic and molecular markers involved with partial versus complete moles (439) open a number of avenues for assessing the interaction of these markers with a variety of proposed environmental risk factors. This could include a focus on early stages in the disease process or on factors involved in the progression of molar pregnancies to more invasive complications.

SUMMARY

The goal of both medical practice and epidemiology is to reduce morbidity and mortality. For many diseases, the focus has turned to the ultimate aim of prevention. The link between identification of etiologic factors and possibilities for prevention is well illustrated for tobacco- and alcohol-related tumors and for those associated with specific pharmaceutical, radiogenic, and occupational exposures. Fortunately, for gynecologic cancers, there are a number of identified etiologic factors that are also amenable to preventive approaches.

Undoubtedly, the prospects for prevention are best for cervical cancer. For some time, secondary prevention in the form of screening for pathologic precursors of invasive disease has been the hallmark of the public health approach to this malignancy. The establishment of HPV as a central etiologic agent for the disease presents other avenues for prevention, including application of recently developed vaccines against the virus (410). Knowledge of when and how infection and other factors operate in the natural history of the disease has revolutionized screening strategies and shifted treatment from cell ablation to antiviral therapies. As always, combined laboratory, clinical, and epidemiologic research is needed to realize these propositions.

Many believe that more is known about the cause of endometrial carcinoma than for almost any other tumor. A unified theory of how all risk factors may operate through a final common estrogenic pathway is popular and well supported. A woman's hormonal milieu may prove to be favorable to modification at a practical level. There is substantial evidence that elimination of obesity an intervention actively promoted for other reasons—should also reduce endometrial cancer risk. After the epidemic of endometrial cancer due to estrogen replacement therapy, changes in the management of menopause occurred, resulting in a marked decline in the rates of endometrial cancer.

More care is devoted to identifying women who truly need estrogen therapy, treatment of menopausal symptoms is for a much shorter period of time, the use of cyclic progestin in combination with estrogen is advised if indicated, and regular endometrial sampling is frequently practiced for long-term estrogen users.

Although past alterations in patient management led to a decline in endometrial cancer, current events make future patterns less clear. Previous enthusiasm for 1ong-term treatment of large segments of the population of menopausal women with hormones to control symptoms and prevent osteoporosis and heart disease may have implications for endometrial cancer in the future. On the other hand, current patterns of use of oral contraceptives could lead to reductions in endometrial cancer rates in the general population. The impact of widespread oral contraceptive use at young ages on endometrial cancer risk at older ages is not well studied. However, if it is anywhere near the reduced risk seen at young ages, the resulting reduction in endometrial cancer overall could be substantial.

With further research, it is also possible that pharmacologic interventions aimed specifically at groups at high risk for endometrial cancer due to endogenous hormonal factors could be justified. More must be learned about the associations of risk for endometrial cancer and the quantitative levels of estrogens and other hormones and their relative proportions. Once these factors are known, women with PCOS, diabetes, morbid obesity, or other predisposing conditions could be evaluated for unfavorable hormone profiles and appropriately targeted for treatment.

Although a substantial amount has been learned about ovarian cancer risks, the prospects for meaningful preventive measures aimed at this tumor are probably worse than for the other gynecologic malignancies. Although several ovarian cancer risk factors seem to indict ovulatory activity as a common pathway to increased risk, the mechanism by which this occurs is unknown. Even if some of the hypothesized mechanisms prove to be correct (e.g., levels of circulating gonadotropins), it is unclear how reasonable any interventions may be. However, if the long-term effect of oral contraceptive use on ovarian cancer risk is similar to its short-term effect, a substantial decline in ovarian cancer rates should result from pill use patterns of the past 40 years. Another reason for the limited prospects for prevention is that for several risk factors (e.g., protection associated with hysterectomy), no credible mechanism has been suggested. The associations promising the greatest opportunities for preventive actions are several recently suggested dietary relationships, specifically, decreased risks with consumption of diets high in fruit and vegetable and certain micronutrients. However, these observations need to be replicated in additional studies. Because of the preventive implications, attempts at confirmation should have high priority.

For cervical cancer, endometrial cancer, and ovarian cancer, much is known about the risk factors. Less is known about the precise biologic mechanisms through which the known risk factors operate. There is substantial enthusiasm for current interdisciplinary studies that incorporate state-of-the-art laboratory assays into robust epidemiologic research designs focused on answering these mechanistic questions. Even among some of the more conservative etiologists, there is a belief that the gynecologic oncologist may soon be able to intervene much earlier in the natural history of these diseases and, in some instances, engage in primary prevention.

References

1. Jemal A, Siegel R, Ward E, et al. Cancer statistics, 2008. *CA Cancer J Clin* 2008;58(2):71–96.
2. Ries LAG, Melbert D, Krapcho M, et al., eds. *SEER Cancer Statistics Review, 1975–2004, National Cancer Institute*. Bethesda, MD: http://Seer.Cancer.Gov/Csr/1975_2004/, Based on November 2006 SEER Data Submission, Posted to the SEER Web Site; 2007.
3. Parkin DM, Pisani P, Ferlay J. Global cancer statistics. *CA Cancer J Clin* 1999;49(1):33–64.
4. Weiss NS, Szekely DR, Austin DF. Increasing incidence of endometrial cancer in the United States. *N Engl J Med* 1976;294(23):1259–1262.
5. Brinton LA, Berman ML, Mortel R, et al. Reproductive, menstrual, and medical risk factors for endometrial cancer: results from a case-control study. *Am J Obstet Gynecol* 1992;167(5):1317–1325.
6. Henderson BE, Casagrande JT, Pike MC, et al. The epidemiology of endometrial cancer in young women. *Br J Cancer* 1983;47(6):749–756.
7. Modan B, Ron E, Lerner-Geva L, et al. Cancer incidence in a cohort of infertile women. *Am J Epidemiol* 1998;147(11):1038–1042.
8. Bernstein L, Pike MC, Ross RK, et al. Estrogen and sex hormone-binding globulin levels in nulliparous and parous women. *J Natl Cancer Inst* 1985;74(4):741–745.
9. La Vecchia C, Franceschi S, Decarli A, et al. Risk factors for endometrial cancer at different ages. *J Natl Cancer Inst* 1984;73(3):667–671.
10. Brinton LA, Sakoda LC, Lissowska J, et al. Reproductive risk factors for endometrial cancer among Polish women. *Br J Cancer* 2007;96(9): 1450–1456.
11. Albrektsen G, Heuch I, Tretli S, et al. Is the risk of cancer of the corpus uteri reduced by a recent pregnancy? A prospective study of 765,756 Norwegian women. *Int J Cancer* 1995;61(4):485–490.
12. Lambe M, Wuu J, Weiderpass E, et al. Childbearing at older age and endometrial cancer risk (Sweden). *Cancer Causes Control* 1999;10(1):43–49.
13. Castellsague X, Thompson WD, Dubrow R. Intra-uterine contraception and the risk of endometrial cancer. *Int J Cancer* 1993;54(6):911–916.
14. Hill DA, Weiss NS, Voigt LF, et al. Endometrial cancer in relation to intrauterine device use. *Int J Cancer* 1997;70(3):278–281.
15. Sturgeon SR, Brinton LA, Berman ML, et al. Intrauterine device use and endometrial cancer risk. *Int J Epidemiol* 1997;26(3):496–500.
16. Tao MH, Xu WH, Zheng W, et al. Oral contraceptive and IUD use and endometrial cancer: a population-based case-control study in Shanghai, China. *Int J Cancer* 2006;119(9):2142–2147.
17. Althuis MD, Moghissi KS, Westhoff CL, et al. Uterine cancer after use of clomiphene citrate to induce ovulation. *Am J Epidemiol* 2005;161(7): 607–615.
18. Newcomb PA, Trentham-Dietz A. Breast feeding practices in relation to endometrial cancer risk, USA. *Cancer Causes Control* 2000;11(7):663–667.
19. Rosenblatt KA, Thomas DB. Prolonged lactation and endometrial cancer. WHO Collaborative Study of Neoplasia and Steroid Contraceptives. *Int J Epidemiol* 1995;24(3):499–503.
20. MacMahon B. Risk factors for endometrial cancer. *Gynecol Oncol* 1974;2(2-3):122–129.
21. Weiss NS, Sayvetz TA. Incidence of endometrial cancer in relation to the use of oral contraceptives. *N Engl J Med* 1980;302(10):551–554.
22. The Cancer and Steroid Hormone Study of the Centers for Disease Control and the National Institute of Child Health and Human Development. Combination oral contraceptive use and the risk of endometrial cancer. *JAMA* 1987;257(6):796–800.
23. Kaufman DW, Shapiro S, Slone D, et al. Decreased risk of endometrial cancer among oral-contraceptive users. *N Engl J Med* 1980;303(18): 1045–1047.
24. Voigt LF, Deng Q, Weiss NS. Recency, duration, and progestin content of oral contraceptives in relation to the incidence of endometrial cancer (Washington, USA). *Cancer Causes Control* 1994;5(3):227–233.
25. Maxwell GL, Schildkraut JM, Calingaert B, et al. Progestin and estrogen potency of combination oral contraceptives and endometrial cancer risk. *Gynecol Oncol* 2006;103(2):535–540.
26. Brinton LA, Hoover RN. Estrogen replacement therapy and endometrial cancer risk: unresolved issues. The Endometrial Cancer Collaborative Group. *Obstet Gynecol* 1993;81(2):265–271.
27. Pike MC, Peters RK, Cozen W, et al. Estrogen-progestin replacement therapy and endometrial cancer. *J Natl Cancer Inst* 1997;89(15):1110–1116.
28. Shapiro S, Kelly JP, Rosenberg L, et al. Risk of localized and widespread endometrial cancer in relation to recent and discontinued use of conjugated estrogens. *N Engl J Med* 1985;313(16):969–972.
29. Strom BL, Schinnar R, Weber AL, et al. Case-control study of postmenopausal hormone replacement therapy and endometrial cancer. *Am J Epidemiol* 2006;164(8):775–786.
30. Green PK, Weiss NS, McKnight B, et al. Risk of endometrial cancer following cessation of menopausal hormone use (Washington, United States). *Cancer Causes Control* 1996;7(6):575–580.
31. Levi F, La Vecchia C, Gulie C, et al. Oestrogen replacement treatment and the risk of endometrial cancer: an assessment of the role of covariates. *Eur J Cancer* 1993;29A(10):1445–1449.
32. Rubin GL, Peterson HB, Lee NC, et al. Estrogen replacement therapy and the risk of endometrial cancer: remaining controversies. *Am J Obstet Gynecol* 1990;162(1):148–154.
33. Shapiro JA, Weiss NS, Beresford SA, et al. Menopausal hormone use and endometrial cancer, by tumor grade and invasion. *Epidemiology* 1998; 9(1):99–101.
34. Cushing KL, Weiss NS, Voigt LF, et al. Risk of endometrial cancer in relation to use of low-dose, unopposed estrogens. *Obstet Gynecol* 1998;91(1): 35–39.

35. Randall TC, Kurman RJ. Progestin treatment of atypical hyperplasia and well-differentiated carcinoma of the endometrium in women under age 40. *Obstet Gynecol* 1997;90(3):434–440.
36. Anderson GL, Judd HL, Kaunitz AM, et al. Effects of estrogen plus progestin on gynecologic cancers and associated diagnostic procedures: the Women's Health Initiative randomized trial. *JAMA* 2003;290(13): 1739–1748.
37. Beral V, Bull D, Reeves G. Endometrial cancer and hormone-replacement therapy in the Million Women Study. *Lancet* 2005;365(9470):1543–1551.
38. Newcomb PA, Trentham-Dietz A. Patterns of postmenopausal progestin use with estrogen in relation to endometrial cancer (United States). *Cancer Causes Control* 2003;14(2):195–201.
39. Persson I, Adami HO, Bergkvist L, et al. Risk of endometrial cancer after treatment with oestrogens alone or in conjunction with progestogens: results of a prospective study. *BMJ* 1989;298(6667):147–151.
40. Weiderpass E, Adami HO, Baron JA, et al. Risk of endometrial cancer following estrogen replacement with and without progestins. *J Natl Cancer Inst* 1999;91(13):1131–1137.
41. Beresford SA, Weiss NS, Voigt LF, et al. Risk of endometrial cancer in relation to use of oestrogen combined with cyclic progestagen therapy in postmenopausal women. *Lancet* 1997;349(9050):458–461.
42. Archer DF. The effect of the duration of progestin use on the occurrence of endometrial cancer in postmenopausal women. *Menopause* 2001;8(4): 245–251.
43. Lacey JV, Jr., Leitzmann MF, Chang SC, et al. Endometrial cancer and menopausal hormone therapy in the National Institutes of Health-AARP Diet and Health Study cohort. *Cancer* 2007;109(7):1303–1311.
44. Newcomer LM, Newcomb PA, Trentham-Dietz A, et al. Hormonal risk factors for endometrial cancer: modification by cigarette smoking (United States). *Cancer Causes Control* 2001;12(9):829–835.
45. Elwood JM, Boyes DA. Clinical and pathological features and survival of endometrial cancer patients in relation to prior use of estrogens. *Gynecol Oncol* 1980;10(2):173–187.
46. Silverberg SG, Mullen D, Faraci JA, et al. Endometrial carcinoma: clinical-pathologic comparison of cases in postmenopausal women receiving and not receiving exogenous estrogens. *Cancer* 1980;45(12):3018–3026.
47. Weiss JM, Saltzman BS, Doherty JA, et al. Risk factors for the incidence of endometrial cancer according to the aggressiveness of disease. *Am J Epidemiol* 2006;164(1):56–62.
48. Andersson M, Storm HH, Mouridsen HT. Incidence of new primary cancers after adjuvant tamoxifen therapy and radiotherapy for early breast cancer. *J Natl Cancer Inst* 1991;83(14):1013–1017.
49. Fisher B, Costantino JP, Wickerham DL, et al. Tamoxifen for the prevention of breast cancer: current status of the National Surgical Adjuvant Breast and Bowel Project P-1 study. *J Natl Cancer Inst* 2005;97(22): 1652–1662.
50. van Leeuwen FE, Benraadt J, Coebergh JW, et al. Risk of endometrial cancer after tamoxifen treatment of breast cancer. *Lancet* 1994;343(8895): 448–452.
51. Curtis RE, Freedman DM, Sherman ME, et al. Risk of malignant mixed müllerian tumors after tamoxifen therapy for breast cancer. *J Natl Cancer Inst* 2004;96(1):70–74.
52. Bergman L, Beelen ML, Gallee MP, et al. Risk and prognosis of endometrial cancer after tamoxifen for breast cancer. Comprehensive Cancer Centres' ALERT Group. Assessment of liver and endometrial cancer risk following tamoxifen. *Lancet* 2000;356(9233):881–887.
53. Goodman MT, Hankin JH, Wilkens LR, et al. Diet, body size, physical activity, and the risk of endometrial cancer. *Cancer Res* 1997;57(22): 5077–5085.
54. Jain MG, Rohan TE, Howe GR, et al. A cohort study of nutritional factors and endometrial cancer. *Eur J Epidemiol* 2000;16(10):899–905.
55. Swanson CA, Potischman N, Wilbanks GD, et al. Relation of endometrial cancer risk to past and contemporary body size and body fat distribution. *Cancer Epidemiol Biomarkers Prev* 1993;2(4):321–327.
56. Friedenreich C, Cust A, Lahmann PH, et al. Anthropometric factors and risk of endometrial cancer: the European prospective investigation into cancer and nutrition. *Cancer Causes Control* 2007;18(4):399–413.
57. Chang SC, Lacey JV, Jr., Brinton LA, et al. Lifetime weight history and endometrial cancer risk by type of menopausal hormone use in the NIH-AARP diet and health study. *Cancer Epidemiol Biomarkers Prev* 2007;16(4):723–730.
58. Shu XO, Brinton LA, Zheng W, et al. Relation of obesity and body fat distribution to endometrial cancer in Shanghai, China. *Cancer Res* 1992;52(14):3865–3870.
59. Colbert LH, Lacey JV, Jr., Schairer C, et al. Physical activity and risk of endometrial cancer in a prospective cohort study (United States). *Cancer Causes Control* 2003;14(6):559–567.
60. Friberg E, Mantzoros CS, Wolk A. Physical activity and risk of endometrial cancer: a population-based prospective cohort study. *Cancer Epidemiol Biomarkers Prev.* 2006;15(11):2136–2140.
61. Littman AJ, Voigt LF, Beresford SA, et al. Recreational physical activity and endometrial cancer risk. *Am J Epidemiol* 2001;154(10):924–933.
62. Matthews CE, Xu WH, Zheng W, et al. Physical activity and risk of endometrial cancer: a report from the Shanghai endometrial cancer study. *Cancer Epidemiol Biomarkers Prev* 2005;14(4):779–785.
63. Moradi T, Weiderpass E, Signorello LB, et al. Physical activity and postmenopausal endometrial cancer risk (Sweden). *Cancer Causes Control* 2000;11(9):829–837.
64. Schouten LJ, Goldbohm RA, van den Brandt PA. Anthropometry, physical activity, and endometrial cancer risk: results from the Netherlands Cohort Study. *J Natl Cancer Inst* 2004;96(21):1635–1638.
65. Friedenreich C, Cust A, Lahmann PH, et al. Physical activity and risk of endometrial cancer: the European prospective investigation into cancer and nutrition. *Int J Cancer* 2007;121(2):347–355.
66. Cust AE, Armstrong BK, Friedenreich CM, et al. Physical activity and endometrial cancer risk: a review of the current evidence, biologic mechanisms and the quality of physical activity assessment methods. *Cancer Causes Control* 2007;18(3):243–258.
67. Voskuil DW, Monninkhof EM, Elias SG, et al. Physical activity and endometrial cancer risk, a systematic review of current evidence. *Cancer Epidemiol Biomarkers Prev* 2007;16(4):639–648.
68. Armstrong B, Doll R. Environmental factors and cancer incidence and mortality in different countries, with special reference to dietary practices. *Int J Cancer* 1975;15(4):617–631.
69. Littman AJ, Beresford SA, White E. The association of dietary fat and plant foods with endometrial cancer (United States). *Cancer Causes Control* 2001;12(8):691–702.
70. Potischman N, Swanson CA, Brinton LA, et al. Dietary associations in a case-control study of endometrial cancer. *Cancer Causes Control* 1993;4(3):239–250.
71. Xu WH, Dai Q, Xiang YB, et al. Nutritional factors in relation to endometrial cancer: a report from a population-based case-control study in Shanghai, China. *Int J Cancer* 2007;120(8):1776–1781.
72. Barbone F, Austin H, Partridge EE. Diet and endometrial cancer: a case-control study. *Am J Epidemiol* 1993;137(4):393–403.
73. McCann SE, Freudenheim JL, Marshall JR, et al. Diet in the epidemiology of endometrial cancer in western New York (United States). *Cancer Causes Control* 2000;11(10):965–974.
74. Negri E, La Vecchia C, Franceschi S, et al. Intake of selected micronutrients and the risk of endometrial carcinoma. *Cancer* 1996;77(5):917–923.
75. Tao MH, Xu WH, Zheng W, et al. A case-control study in Shanghai of fruit and vegetable intake and endometrial cancer. *Br J Cancer* 2005;92(11):2059–2064.
76. Augustin LS, Polesel J, Bosetti C, et al. Dietary glycemic index, glycemic load and ovarian cancer risk: a case-control study in Italy. *Ann Oncol* 2003;14(1):78–84.
77. Folsom AR, Demissie Z, Harnack L. Glycemic index, glycemic load, and incidence of endometrial cancer: the Iowa women's health study. *Nutr Cancer* 2003;46(2):119–124.
78. Larsson SC, Friberg E, Wolk A. Carbohydrate intake, glycemic index and glycemic load in relation to risk of endometrial cancer: a prospective study of Swedish women. *Int J Cancer* 2007;120(5):1103–1107.
79. Silvera SA, Rohan TE, Jain M, et al. Glycaemic index, glycaemic load and risk of endometrial cancer: a prospective cohort study. *Public Health Nutr* 2005;8(7):912–919.
80. Horn-Ross PL, John EM, Canchola AJ, et al. Phytoestrogen intake and endometrial cancer risk. *J Natl Cancer Inst* 2003;95(15):1158–1164.
81. Terry P, Wolk A, Vainio H, et al. Fatty fish consumption lowers the risk of endometrial cancer: a nationwide case-control study in Sweden. *Cancer Epidemiol Biomarkers Prev* 2002;11(1):143–145.
82. Armstrong BK, Brown JB, Clarke HT, et al. Diet and reproductive hormones: a study of vegetarian and nonvegetarian postmenopausal women. *J Natl Cancer Inst* 1981;67(4):761–767.
83. Barbosa JC, Shultz TD, Filley SJ, et al. The relationship among adiposity, diet, and hormone concentrations in vegetarian and nonvegetarian postmenopausal women. *Am J Clin Nutr* 1990;51(5):798–803.
84. Goldin BR, Adlercreutz H, Gorbach SL, et al. The relationship between estrogen levels and diets of Caucasian American and Oriental immigrant women. *Am J Clin Nutr* 1986;44(6):945–953.
85. Prentice R, Thompson D, Clifford C, et al. Dietary fat reduction and plasma estradiol concentration in healthy postmenopausal women. The Women's Health Trial Study Group. *J Natl Cancer Inst* 1990;82(2): 129–134.
86. Newcomb PA, Trentham-Dietz A, Storer BE. Alcohol consumption in relation to endometrial cancer risk. *Cancer Epidemiol Biomarkers Prev* 1997; 6(10):775–778.
87. Swanson CA, Wilbanks GD, Twiggs LB, et al. Moderate alcohol consumption and the risk of endometrial cancer. *Epidemiology* 1993;4(6): 530–536.
88. Webster LA, Weiss NS. Alcoholic beverage consumption and the risk of endometrial cancer. Cancer and Steroid Hormone Study Group. *Int J Epidemiol* 1989;18(4):786–791.
89. Gapstur SM, Potter JD, Sellers TA, et al. Alcohol consumption and postmenopausal endometrial cancer: results from the Iowa Women's Health Study. *Cancer Causes Control* 1993;4(4):323–329.
90. Loerbroks A, Schouten LJ, Goldbohm RA, et al. Alcohol consumption, cigarette smoking, and endometrial cancer risk: results from the Netherlands Cohort Study. *Cancer Causes Control* 2007;18(5):551–560.
91. Weiderpass E, Baron JA. Cigarette smoking, alcohol consumption, and endometrial cancer risk: a population-based study in Sweden. *Cancer Causes Control* 2001;12(3):239–247.

92. Brinton LA, Barrett RJ, Berman ML, et al. Cigarette smoking and the risk of endometrial cancer. *Am J Epidemiol* 1993;137(3):281–291.
93. Terry PD, Miller AB, Jones JG, et al. Cigarette smoking and the risk of invasive epithelial ovarian cancer in a prospective cohort study. *Eur J Cancer* 2003;39(8):1157–1164.
94. Viswanathan AN, Feskanich D, De V, I, et al. Smoking and the risk of endometrial cancer: results from the Nurses' Health Study. *Int J Cancer* 2005;114(6):996–1001.
95. Terry PD, Miller AB, Rohan TE. A prospective cohort study of cigarette smoking and the risk of endometrial cancer. *Br J Cancer* 2002;86(9): 1430–1435.
96. Austin H, Drews C, Partridge EE. A case-control study of endometrial cancer in relation to cigarette smoking, serum estrogen levels, and alcohol use. *Am J Obstet Gynecol* 1993;169(5):1086–1091.
97. Jafari K, Javaheri G, Ruiz G. Endometrial adenocarcinoma and the Stein-Leventhal syndrome. *Obstet Gynecol* 1978;51(1):97–100.
98. Wild S, Pierpoint T, Jacobs H, et al. Long-term consequences of polycystic ovary syndrome: results of a 31 year follow-up study. *Hum Fertil (Camb)* 2000;3(2):101–105.
99. Wood GP, Boronow RC. Endometrial adenocarcinoma and the polycystic ovary syndrome. *Am J Obstet Gynecol* 1976;124(2):140–142.
100. Coulam CB, Annegers JF, Kranz JS. Chronic anovulation syndrome and associated neoplasia. *Obstet Gynecol* 1983;61(4):403–407.
101. Dahlgren E, Friberg LG, Johansson S, et al. Endometrial carcinoma: ovarian dysfunction—a risk factor in young women. *Eur J Obstet Gynecol Reprod Biol* 1991;41(2):143–150.
102. Weiderpass E, Ye W, Vainio H, et al. Diabetes mellitus and ovarian cancer (Sweden). *Cancer Causes Control* 2002;13(8):759–764.
103. Wideroff L, Gridley G, Mellemkjaer L, et al. Cancer incidence in a population-based cohort of patients hospitalized with diabetes mellitus in Denmark. *J Natl Cancer Inst* 1997;89(18):1360–1365.
104. Friberg E, Mantzoros CS, Wolk A. Diabetes and risk of endometrial cancer: a population-based prospective cohort study. *Cancer Epidemiol Biomarkers Prev* 2007;16(2):276–280.
105. Zendehdel K, Nyren O, Ostenson CG, et al. Cancer incidence in patients with type 1 diabetes mellitus: a population-based cohort study in Sweden. *J Natl Cancer Inst* 2003;95(23):1797–1800.
106. Inoue M, Okayama A, Fujita M, et al. A case-control study on risk factors for uterine endometrial cancer in Japan. *Jpn J Cancer Res* 1994;85(4): 346–350.
107. Parazzini F, La Vecchia C, Negri E, et al. Diabetes and endometrial cancer: an Italian case-control study. *Int J Cancer* 1999;81(4):539–542.
108. Weiderpass E, Persson I, Adami HO, et al. Body size in different periods of life, diabetes mellitus, hypertension, and risk of postmenopausal endometrial cancer (Sweden). *Cancer Causes Control* 2000;11(2):185–192.
109. Anderson KE, Anderson E, Mink PJ, et al. Diabetes and endometrial cancer in the Iowa women's health study. *Cancer Epidemiol Biomarkers Prev* 2001;10(6):611–616.
110. Shoff SM, Newcomb PA. Diabetes, body size, and risk of endometrial cancer. *Am J Epidemiol* 1998;148(3):234–240.
111. Newcomb PA, Trentham-Dietz A, Egan KM, et al. Fracture history and risk of breast and endometrial cancer. *Am J Epidemiol* 2001;153(11): 1071–1078.
112. Persson I, Adami HO, McLaughlin JK, et al. Reduced risk of breast and endometrial cancer among women with hip fractures (Sweden). *Cancer Causes Control* 1994;5(6):523–528.
113. Hemminki K, Vaittinen P, Dong C. Endometrial cancer in the family-cancer database. *Cancer Epidemiol Biomarkers Prev* 1999;8(11):1005–1010.
114. Hemminki K, Bermejo JL, Granstrom C. Endometrial cancer: population attributable risks from reproductive, familial and socioeconomic factors. *Eur J Cancer* 2005;41(14):2155–2159.
115. Doherty JA, Weiss NS, Freeman RJ, et al. Genetic factors in catechol estrogen metabolism in relation to the risk of endometrial cancer. *Cancer Epidemiol Biomarkers Prev* 2005;14(2):357–366.
116. McGrath M, Lee IM, Hankinson SE, et al. Androgen receptor polymorphisms and endometrial cancer risk. *Int J Cancer* 2006;118(5):1261–1268.
117. Olson SH, Bandera EV, Orlow I. Variants in estrogen biosynthesis genes, sex steroid hormone levels, and endometrial cancer: a HuGE review. *Am J Epidemiol* 2007;165(3):235–245.
118. Rebbeck TR, Troxel AB, Wang Y, et al. Estrogen sulfation genes, hormone replacement therapy, and endometrial cancer risk. *J Natl Cancer Inst* 2006;98(18):1311–1320.
119. Tao MH, Cai Q, Zhang ZF, et al. Polymorphisms in the CYP19A1 (aromatase) gene and endometrial cancer risk in Chinese women. *Cancer Epidemiol Biomarkers Prev* 2007;16(5):943–949.
120. Weiss JM, Weiss NS, Ulrich CM, et al. Nucleotide excision repair genotype and the incidence of endometrial cancer: effect of other risk factors on the association. *Gynecol Oncol* 2006;103(3):891–896.
121. Xu WH, Shrubsole MJ, Xiang YB, et al. Dietary folate intake, MTHFR genetic polymorphisms, and the risk of endometrial cancer among Chinese women. *Cancer Epidemiol Biomarkers Prev* 2007;16(2):281–287.
122. Sturgeon SR, Brock JW, Potischman N, et al. Serum concentrations of organochlorine compounds and endometrial cancer risk (United States). *Cancer Causes Control* 1998;9(4):417–424.
123. Weiderpass E, Adami HO, Baron JA, et al. Organochlorines and endometrial cancer risk. *Cancer Epidemiol Biomarkers Prev* 2000;9(5):487–493.
124. McElroy JA, Newcomb PA, Trentham-Dietz A, et al. Endometrial cancer incidence in relation to electric blanket use. *Am J Epidemiol* 2002; 156(3):262–267.
125. Bernstein L, Allen M, Anton-Culver H, et al. High breast cancer incidence rates among California teachers: results from the California Teachers Study (United States). *Cancer Causes Control* 2002;13(7):625–635.
126. Weiderpass E, Pukkala E, Vasama-Neuvonen K, et al. Occupational exposures and cancers of the endometrium and cervix uteri in Finland. *Am J Ind Med* 2001;39(6):572–580.
127. Austin H, Austin JM, Jr., Partridge EE, et al. Endometrial cancer, obesity, and body fat distribution. *Cancer Res* 1991;51(2):568–572.
128. Lukanova A, Lundin E, Micheli A, et al. Circulating levels of sex steroid hormones and risk of endometrial cancer in postmenopausal women. *Int J Cancer* 2004;108(3):425–432.
129. Potischman N, Hoover RN, Brinton LA, et al. Case-control study of endogenous steroid hormones and endometrial cancer. *J Natl Cancer Inst* 1996;88(16):1127–1135.
130. Zeleniuch-Jacquotte A, Akhmedkhanov A, Kato I, et al. Postmenopausal endogenous oestrogens and risk of endometrial cancer: results of a prospective study. *Br J Cancer* 2001;84(7):975–981.
131. Key TJ, Pike MC. The dose-effect relationship between 'unopposed' oestrogens and endometrial mitotic rate: its central role in explaining and predicting endometrial cancer risk. *Br J Cancer* 1988;57(2):205–212.
132. Kaaks R, Lukanova A, Kurzer MS. Obesity, endogenous hormones, and endometrial cancer risk: a synthetic review. *Cancer Epidemiol Biomarkers Prev* 2002;11(12):1531–1543.
133. Troisi R, Potischman N, Hoover RN, et al. Insulin and endometrial cancer. *Am J Epidemiol* 1997;146(6):476–482.
134. Weiderpass E, Brismar K, Bellocco R, et al. Serum levels of insulin-like growth factor-I, IGF-binding protein 1 and 3, and insulin and endometrial cancer risk. *Br J Cancer* 2003;89(9):1697–1704.
135. Siiteri PK. Steroid hormones and endometrial cancer. *Cancer Res* 1978;38(11 Pt 2):4360–4366.
136. Gnagy S, Ming EE, Devesa SS, et al. Declining ovarian cancer rates in U.S. women in relation to parity and oral contraceptive use. *Epidemiology* 2000;11(2):102–105.
137. Mink PJ, Sherman ME, Devesa SS. Incidence patterns of invasive and borderline ovarian tumors among white women and black women in the United States. Results from the SEER Program, 1978-1998. *Cancer* 2002;95(11):2380–2389.
138. Pisani P, Parkin DM, Bray F, et al. Estimates of the worldwide mortality from 25 cancers in 1990. *Int J Cancer* 1999;83(1):18–29.
139. Booth M, Beral V, Smith P. Risk factors for ovarian cancer: a case-control study. *Br J Cancer* 1989;60(4):592–598.
140. Hankinson SE, Colditz GA, Hunter DJ, et al. A prospective study of reproductive factors and risk of epithelial ovarian cancer. *Cancer* 1995;76(2):284–290.
141. Risch HA, Marrett LD, Howe GR. Parity, contraception, infertility, and the risk of epithelial ovarian cancer. *Am J Epidemiol* 1994;140(7):585–597.
142. Whittemore AS, Harris R, Itnyre J. Characteristics relating to ovarian cancer risk: collaborative analysis of 12 US case-control studies. II. Invasive epithelial ovarian cancers in white women. Collaborative Ovarian Cancer Group. *Am J Epidemiol* 1992;136(10):1184–1203.
143. Chen MT, Cook LS, Daling JR, et al. Incomplete pregnancies and risk of ovarian cancer (Washington, United States). *Cancer Causes Control* 1996;7(4):415–420.
144. Greggi S, Parazzini F, Paratore MP, et al. Risk factors for ovarian cancer in central Italy. *Gynecol Oncol* 2000;79(1):50–54.
145. Voigt LF, Harlow BL, Weiss NS. The influence of age at first birth and parity on ovarian cancer risk. *Am J Epidemiol* 1986;124(3):490–491.
146. Cooper GS, Schildkraut JM, Whittemore AS, et al. Pregnancy recency and risk of ovarian cancer. *Cancer Causes Control* 1999;10(5):397–402.
147. Negri E, Franceschi S, Tzonou A, et al. Pooled analysis of 3 European case-control studies: I. Reproductive factors and risk of epithelial ovarian cancer. *Int J Cancer* 1991;49(1):50–56.
148. Klip H, Burger CW, Kenemans P, et al. Cancer risk associated with subfertility and ovulation induction: a review. *Cancer Causes Control* 2000;11(4):319–344.
149. Whittemore AS, Wu ML, Paffenbarger RS, Jr., et al. Epithelial ovarian cancer and the ability to conceive. *Cancer Res* 1989;49(14):4047–4052.
150. Rossing MA, Daling JR, Weiss NS, et al. Ovarian tumors in a cohort of infertile women. *N Engl J Med* 1994;331(12):771–776.
151. Brinton LA, Moghissi KS, Scoccia B, et al. Ovulation induction and cancer risk. *Fertil Steril* 2005;83(2):261–274.
152. Ness RB, Cramer DW, Goodman MT, et al. Infertility, fertility drugs, and ovarian cancer: a pooled analysis of case-control studies. *Am J Epidemiol* 2002;155(3):217–224.
153. Chiaffarino F, Pelucchi C, Negri E, et al. Breastfeeding and the risk of epithelial ovarian cancer in an Italian population. *Gynecol Oncol* 2005;98(2):304–308.
154. Rosenblatt KA, Thomas DB. Lactation and the risk of epithelial ovarian cancer. The WHO Collaborative Study of Neoplasia and Steroid Contraceptives. *Int J Epidemiol* 1993;22(2):192–197.

155. Siskind V, Green A, Bain C, et al. Breastfeeding, menopause, and epithelial ovarian cancer. *Epidemiology* 1997;8(2):188–191.
156. Titus-Ernstoff L, Perez K, Cramer DW, et al. Menstrual and reproductive factors in relation to ovarian cancer risk. *Br J Cancer* 2001;84(5):714–721.
157. Zhang M, Xie X, Lee AH, et al. Prolonged lactation reduces ovarian cancer risk in Chinese women. *Eur J Cancer Prev* 2004;13(6):499–502.
158. Danforth KN, Tworoger SS, Hecht JL, et al. Breastfeeding and risk of ovarian cancer in two prospective cohorts. *Cancer Causes Control* 2007;18(5):517–523.
159. Green A, Purdie D, Bain C, et al. Tubal sterilisation, hysterectomy and decreased risk of ovarian cancer. Survey of Women's Health Study Group. *Int J Cancer* 1997;71(6):948–951.
160. Hankinson SE, Hunter DJ, Colditz GA, et al. Tubal ligation, hysterectomy, and risk of ovarian cancer. A prospective study. *JAMA* 1993;270(23):2813–2818.
161. Kreiger N, Sloan M, Cotterchio M, et al. Surgical procedures associated with risk of ovarian cancer. *Int J Epidemiol* 1997;26(4):710–715.
162. Rosenblatt KA, Thomas DB. Reduced risk of ovarian cancer in women with a tubal ligation or hysterectomy. The World Health Organization Collaborative Study of Neoplasia and Steroid Contraceptives. *Cancer Epidemiol Biomarkers Prev* 1996;5(11):933–935.
163. Weiss NS, Harlow BL. Why does hysterectomy without bilateral oophorectomy influence the subsequent incidence of ovarian cancer? *Am J Epidemiol* 1986;124(5):856–858.
164. Ellsworth LR, Allen HH, Nisker JA. Ovarian function after radical hysterectomy for stage IB carcinoma of cervix. *Am J Obstet Gynecol* 1983;145(2):185–188.
165. Franceschi S, La Vecchia C, Booth M, et al. Pooled analysis of 3 European case-control studies of ovarian cancer: II. Age at menarche and at menopause. *Int J Cancer* 1991;49(1):57–60.
166. Schildkraut JM, Bastos E, Berchuck A. Relationship between lifetime ovulatory cycles and overexpression of mutant p53 in epithelial ovarian cancer. *J Natl Cancer Inst* 1997;89(13):932–938.
167. Rosenberg L, Palmer JR, Zauber AG, et al. A case-control study of oral contraceptive use and invasive epithelial ovarian cancer. *Am J Epidemiol* 1994;139(7):654–661.
168. The Cancer and Steroid Hormone Study of the Centers for Disease Control and the National Institute of Child Health and Human Development. The reduction in risk of ovarian cancer associated with oral-contraceptive use. *N Engl J Med* 1987;316(11):650–655.
169. Bosetti C, Negri E, Trichopoulos D, et al. Long-term effects of oral contraceptives on ovarian cancer risk. *Int J Cancer* 2002;102(3):262–265.
170. Franceschi S, Parazzini F, Negri E, et al. Pooled analysis of 3 European case-control studies of epithelial ovarian cancer: III. Oral contraceptive use. *Int J Cancer* 1991;49(1):61–65.
171. Lurie G, Thompson P, McDuffie KE, et al. Association of estrogen and progestin potency of oral contraceptives with ovarian carcinoma risk. *Obstet Gynecol* 2007;109(3):597–607.
172. Ness RB, Grisso JA, Klapper J, et al. Risk of ovarian cancer in relation to estrogen and progestin dose and use characteristics of oral contraceptives. SHARE Study Group. Steroid Hormones and Reproductions. *Am J Epidemiol* 2000;152(3):233–241.
173. Royar J, Becher H, Chang-Claude J. Low-dose oral contraceptives: protective effect on ovarian cancer risk. *Int J Cancer* 2001;95(6):370–374.
174. Schildkraut JM, Calingaert B, Marchbanks PA, et al. Impact of progestin and estrogen potency in oral contraceptives on ovarian cancer risk. *J Natl Cancer Inst* 2002;94(1):32–38.
175. Greer JB, Modugno F, Allen GO, et al. Androgenic progestins in oral contraceptives and the risk of epithelial ovarian cancer. *Obstet Gynecol* 2005;105(4):731–740.
176. Beral V, Bull D, Green J, et al. Ovarian cancer and hormone replacement therapy in the Million Women Study. *Lancet* 2007;369(9574):1703–1710.
177. Danforth KN, Tworoger SS, Hecht JL, et al. A prospective study of postmenopausal hormone use and ovarian cancer risk. *Br J Cancer* 2007;96(1):151–156.
178. Lacey JV, Jr., Mink PJ, Lubin JH, et al. Menopausal hormone replacement therapy and risk of ovarian cancer. *JAMA* 2002;288(3):334–341.
179. Lacey JV, Jr., Brinton LA, Leitzmann MF, et al. Menopausal hormone therapy and ovarian cancer risk in the National Institutes of Health-AARP Diet and Health Study Cohort. *J Natl Cancer. Inst* 2006;98(19):1397–1405.
180. Negri E, Tzonou A, Beral V, et al. Hormonal therapy for menopause and ovarian cancer in a collaborative re-analysis of European studies. *Int J Cancer* 1999;80(6):848–851.
181. Riman T, Dickman PW, Nilsson S, et al. Hormone replacement therapy and the risk of invasive epithelial ovarian cancer in Swedish women. *J Natl Cancer Inst* 2002;94(7):497–504.
182. Rodriguez C, Patel AV, Calle EE, et al. Estrogen replacement therapy and ovarian cancer mortality in a large prospective study of U.S. women. *JAMA* 2001;285(11):1460–1465.
183. Helzlsouer KJ, Alberg AJ, Gordon GB, et al. Serum gonadotropins and steroid hormones and the development of ovarian cancer. *JAMA* 1995;274(24):1926–1930.
184. Rinaldi S, Dossus L, Lukanova A, et al. Endogenous androgens and risk of epithelial ovarian cancer: results from the European Prospective Investigation into Cancer and Nutrition (EPIC). *Cancer Epidemiol Biomarkers Prev* 2007;16(1):23–29.
185. Lukanova A, Lundin E, Micheli A, et al. Risk of ovarian cancer in relation to prediagnostic levels of C-peptide, insulin-like growth factor binding proteins-1 and -2 (USA, Sweden, Italy). *Cancer Causes Control* 2003;14(3):285–292.
186. Lukanova A, Lundin E, Akhmedkhanov A, et al. Circulating levels of sex steroid hormones and risk of ovarian cancer. *Int J Cancer* 2003;104(5):636–642.
187. Parazzini F, Moroni S, La Vecchia C, et al. Ovarian cancer risk and history of selected medical conditions linked with female hormones. *Eur J Cancer* 1997;33(10):1634–1637.
188. Brinton LA, Gridley G, Persson I, et al. Cancer risk after a hospital discharge diagnosis of endometriosis. *Am J Obstet Gynecol* 1997;176(3):572–579.
189. Brinton LA, Sakoda LC, Sherman ME, et al. Relationship of benign gynecologic diseases to subsequent risk of ovarian and uterine tumors. *Cancer Epidemiol Biomarkers Prev* 2005;14(12):2929–2935.
190. Ness RB. Endometriosis and ovarian cancer: thoughts on shared pathophysiology. *Am J Obstet Gynecol* 2003;189(1):280–294.
191. Ness RB, Cottreau C. Possible role of ovarian epithelial inflammation in ovarian cancer. *J Natl Cancer Inst* 1999;91(17):1459–1467.
192. Risch HA, Howe GR. Pelvic inflammatory disease and the risk of epithelial ovarian cancer. *Cancer Epidemiol Biomarkers Prev* 1995;4(5):447–451.
193. Harlow BL, Cramer DW, Baron JA, et al. Psychotropic medication use and risk of epithelial ovarian cancer. *Cancer Epidemiol Biomarkers Prev* 1998;7(8):697–702.
194. Dalton SO, Johansen C, Mellemkjaer L, et al. Antidepressant medications and risk for cancer. *Epidemiology* 2000;11(2):171–176.
195. Dublin S, Rossing MA, Heckbert SR, et al. Risk of epithelial ovarian cancer in relation to use of antidepressants, benzodiazepines, and other centrally acting medications. *Cancer Causes Control* 2002;13(1):35–45.
196. Kato I, Zeleniuch-Jacquotte A, Toniolo PG, et al. Psychotropic medication use and risk of hormone-related cancers: the New York University Women's Health Study. *J Public Health Med* 2000;22(2):155–160.
197. Lacey JV, Jr., Sherman ME, Hartge P, et al. Medication use and risk of ovarian carcinoma: a prospective study. *Int J Cancer* 2004;108(2):281–286.
198. Cramer DW, Harlow BL, Titus-Ernstoff L, et al. Over-the-counter analgesics and risk of ovarian cancer. *Lancet* 1998;351(9096):104–107.
199. Rodriguez C, Henley SJ, Calle EE, et al. Paracetamol and risk of ovarian cancer mortality in a prospective study of women in the USA. *Lancet* 1998;352(9137):1354–1355.
200. Tzonou A, Polychronopoulou A, Hsieh CC, et al. Hair dyes, analgesics, tranquilizers and perineal talc application as risk factors for ovarian cancer. *Int J Cancer* 1993;55(3):408–410.
201. Schildkraut JM, Moorman PG, Halabi S, et al. Analgesic drug use and risk of ovarian cancer. *Epidemiology* 2006;17(1):104–107.
202. Lacey JV, Jr., Leitzmann M, Brinton LA, et al. Weight, height, and body mass index and risk for ovarian cancer in a cohort study. *Ann Epidemiol* 2006;16(12):869–876.
203. Lukanova A, Toniolo P, Lundin E, et al. Body mass index in relation to ovarian cancer: a multi-centre nested case-control study. *Int J Cancer* 2002;99(4):603–608.
204. Beehler GP, Sekhon M, Baker JA, et al. Risk of ovarian cancer associated with BMI varies by menopausal status. *J Nutr* 2006;136(11):2881–2886.
205. Fairfield KM, Willett WC, Rosner BA, et al. Obesity, weight gain, and ovarian cancer. *Obstet Gynecol* 2002;100(2):288–296.
206. Greer JB, Modugno F, Ness RB, et al. Anthropometry and the risk of epithelial ovarian cancer. *Cancer* 2006;106(10):2247–2257.
207. Rodriguez C, Calle EE, Fakhrabadi-Shokoohi D, et al. Body mass index, height, and the risk of ovarian cancer mortality in a prospective cohort of postmenopausal women. *Cancer Epidemiol Biomarkers Prev* 2002;11(9):822–828.
208. Purdie DM, Bain CJ, Webb PM, et al. Body size and ovarian cancer: case-control study and systematic review (Australia). *Cancer Causes Control* 2001;12(9):855–863.
209. Farrow DC, Weiss NS, Lyon JL, et al. Association of obesity and ovarian cancer in a case-control study. *Am J Epidemiol* 1989;129(6):1300–1304.
210. Riman T, Dickman PW, Nilsson S, et al. Some life-style factors and the risk of invasive epithelial ovarian cancer in Swedish women. *Eur J Epidemiol* 2004;19(11):1011–1019.
211. Schouten LJ, Goldbohm RA, van den Brandt PA. Height, weight, weight change, and ovarian cancer risk in the Netherlands cohort study on diet and cancer. *Am J Epidemiol* 2003;157(5):424–433.
212. Lubin F, Chetrit A, Freedman LS, et al. Body mass index at age 18 years and during adult life and ovarian cancer risk. *Am J Epidemiol* 2003;157(2):113–120.
213. Zhang M, Lee AH, Binns CW. Physical activity and epithelial ovarian cancer risk: a case-control study in China. *Int J Cancer* 2003;105(6):838–843.
214. Pan SY, Ugnat AM, Mao Y. Physical activity and the risk of ovarian cancer: a case-control study in Canada. *Int J Cancer* 2005;117(2):300–307.
215. Cottreau CM, Ness RB, Kriska AM. Physical activity and reduced risk of ovarian cancer. *Obstet Gynecol* 2000;96(4):609–614.

216. Bertone ER, Willett WC, Rosner BA, et al. Prospective study of recreational physical activity and ovarian cancer. *J Natl Cancer Inst* 2001;93(12):942–948.
217. Mink PJ, Folsom AR, Sellers TA, et al. Physical activity, waist-to-hip ratio, and other risk factors for ovarian cancer: a follow-up study of older women. *Epidemiology* 1996;7(1):38–45.
218. Phillips RL, Garfinkel L, Kuzma JW, et al. Mortality among California Seventh-Day Adventists for selected cancer sites. *J Natl Cancer Inst* 1980;65(5):1097–1107.
219. Kinlen LJ. Meat and fat consumption and cancer mortality: a study of strict religious orders in Britain. *Lancet* 1982;1(8278):946–949.
220. Cramer DW, Harlow BL, Willett WC, et al. Galactose consumption and metabolism in relation to the risk of ovarian cancer. *Lancet* 1989;2(8654):66–71.
221. Bosetti C, Negri E, Franceschi S, et al. Diet and ovarian cancer risk: a case-control study in Italy. *Int J Cancer* 2001;93(6):911–915.
222. Goodman MT, Wu AH, Tung KH, et al. Association of dairy products, lactose, and calcium with the risk of ovarian cancer. *Am J Epidemiol* 2002;156(2):148–157.
223. Herrinton LJ, Weiss NS, Beresford SA, et al. Lactose and galactose intake and metabolism in relation to the risk of epithelial ovarian cancer. *Am J Epidemiol* 1995;141(5):407–416.
224. Risch HA, Jain M, Marrett LD, et al. Dietary lactose intake, lactose intolerance, and the risk of epithelial ovarian cancer in southern Ontario (Canada). *Cancer Causes Control* 1994;5(6):540–548.
225. Webb PM, Bain CJ, Purdie DM, et al. Milk consumption, galactose metabolism and ovarian cancer (Australia). *Cancer Causes Control* 1998;9(6):637–644.
226. Kushi LH, Mink PJ, Folsom AR, et al. Prospective study of diet and ovarian cancer. *Am J Epidemiol* 1999;149(1):21–31.
227. Larsson SC, Bergkvist L, Wolk A. Milk and lactose intakes and ovarian cancer risk in the Swedish Mammography Cohort. *Am J Clin Nutr* 2004;80(5):1353–1357.
228. Fairfield KM, Hunter DJ, Colditz GA, et al. A prospective study of dietary lactose and ovarian cancer. *Int J Cancer* 2004;110(2):271–277.
229. Bertone ER, Rosner BA, Hunter DJ, et al. Dietary fat intake and ovarian cancer in a cohort of US women. *Am J Epidemiol* 2002;156(1):22–31.
230. Cramer DW, Welch WR, Hutchison GB, et al. Dietary animal fat in relation to ovarian cancer risk. *Obstet Gynecol* 1984;63(6):833–838.
231. Lubin F, Chetrit A, Modan B, et al. Dietary intake changes and their association with ovarian cancer risk. *J Nutr* 2006;136(9):2362–2367.
232. McCann SE, Moysich KB, Mettlin C. Intakes of selected nutrients and food groups and risk of ovarian cancer. *Nutr Cancer* 2001;39(1):19–28.
233. Risch HA, Jain M, Marrett LD, et al. Dietary fat intake and risk of epithelial ovarian cancer. *J Natl Cancer Inst* 1994;86(18):1409–1415.
234. Genkinger JM, Hunter DJ, Spiegelman D, et al. A pooled analysis of 12 cohort studies of dietary fat, cholesterol and egg intake and ovarian cancer. *Cancer Causes Control* 2006;17(3):273–285.
235. Larsson SC, Holmberg L, Wolk A. Fruit and vegetable consumption in relation to ovarian cancer incidence: the Swedish Mammography Cohort. *Br J Cancer* 2004;90(11):2167–2170.
236. McCann SE, Freudenheim JL, Marshall JR, et al. Risk of human ovarian cancer is related to dietary intake of selected nutrients, phytochemicals and food groups. *J Nutr* 2003;133(6):1937–1942.
237. Pelucchi C, La Vecchia C, Chatenoud L, et al. Dietary fibres and ovarian cancer risk. *Eur J Cancer* 2001;37(17):2235–2239.
238. Fairfield KM, Hankinson SE, Rosner BA, et al. Risk of ovarian carcinoma and consumption of vitamins A, C, and E and specific carotenoids: a prospective analysis. *Cancer* 2001;92(9):2318–2326.
239. Koushik A, Hunter DJ, Spiegelman D, et al. Fruits and vegetables and ovarian cancer risk in a pooled analysis of 12 cohort studies. *Cancer Epidemiol Biomarkers Prev* 2005;14(9):2160–2167.
240. Mommers M, Schouten LJ, Goldbohm RA, et al. Consumption of vegetables and fruits and risk of ovarian carcinoma. *Cancer* 2005;104(7):1512–1519.
241. Schulz M, Lahmann PH, Boeing H, et al. Fruit and vegetable consumption and risk of epithelial ovarian cancer: the European Prospective Investigation into Cancer and Nutrition. *Cancer Epidemiol Biomarkers Prev* 2005;4(11 Pt 1):2531–2535.
242. Byers T, Marshall J, Graham S, et al. A case-control study of dietary and nondietary factors in ovarian cancer. *J Natl Cancer Inst* 1983;71(4):681–686.
243. Fleischauer AT, Olson SH, Mignone L, et al. Dietary antioxidants, supplements, and risk of epithelial ovarian cancer. *Nutr Cancer* 2001;40(2):92–98.
244. Pan SY, Ugnat AM, Mao Y, et al. A case-control study of diet and the risk of ovarian cancer. *Cancer Epidemiol Biomarkers Prev* 2004;13(9):1521–1527.
245. Slattery ML, Schuman KL, West DW, et al. Nutrient intake and ovarian cancer. *Am J Epidemiol* 1989;130(3):497–502.
246. Tung KH, Wilkens LR, Wu AH, et al. Association of dietary vitamin A, carotenoids, and other antioxidants with the risk of ovarian cancer. *Cancer Epidemiol Biomarkers Prev* 2005;14(3):669–676.
247. Chang ET, Canchola AJ, Lee VS, et al. Wine and other alcohol consumption and risk of ovarian cancer in the California Teachers Study cohort. *Cancer Causes Control* 2007;18(1):91–103.
248. Kuper H, Titus-Ernstoff L, Harlow BL, et al. Population based study of coffee, alcohol and tobacco use and risk of ovarian cancer. *Int J Cancer* 2000;88(2):313–318.
249. Peterson NB, Trentham-Dietz A, Newcomb PA, et al. Alcohol consumption and ovarian cancer risk in a population-based case-control study. *Int J Cancer* 2006;119(10):2423–2427.
250. Schouten LJ, Zeegers MP, Goldbohm RA, et al. Alcohol and ovarian cancer risk: results from the Netherlands Cohort Study. *Cancer Causes Control* 2004;15(2):201–209.
251. Webb PM, Purdie DM, Bain CJ, et al. Alcohol, wine, and risk of epithelial ovarian cancer. *Cancer Epidemiol Biomarkers Prev* 2004;13(4):592–599.
252. Genkinger JM, Hunter DJ, Spiegelman D, et al. Alcohol intake and ovarian cancer risk: a pooled analysis of 10 cohort studies. *Br J Cancer* 2006;94(5):757–762.
253. La Vecchia C, Franceschi S, Decarli A, et al. Coffee drinking and the risk of epithelial ovarian cancer. *Int J Cancer* 1984;33(5):559–562.
254. Whittemore AS, Wu ML, Paffenbarger RS, Jr., et al. Personal and environmental characteristics related to epithelial ovarian cancer. II. Exposures to talcum powder, tobacco, alcohol, and coffee. *Am J Epidemiol* 1988;128(6):1228–1240.
255. Jordan SJ, Purdie DM, Green AC, et al. Coffee, tea and caffeine and risk of epithelial ovarian cancer. *Cancer Causes Control* 2004;15(4):359–365.
256. Hemminki K, Granstrom C. Familial invasive and borderline ovarian tumors by proband status, age and histology. *Int J Cancer* 2003;105(5):701–705.
257. Pharoah PD, Ponder BA. The genetics of ovarian cancer. *Best Pract Res Clin Obstet Gynaecol* 2002;16(4):449–468.
258. Venkitaraman AR. Cancer susceptibility and the functions of *BRCA1* and *BRCA2*. *Cell* 2002;108(2):171–182.
259. Hartge P, Whittemore AS, Itnyre J, et al. Rates and risks of ovarian cancer in subgroups of white women in the United States. The Collaborative Ovarian Cancer Group. *Obstet Gynecol* 1994;84(5):760–764.
260. Struewing JP, Hartge P, Wacholder S, et al. The risk of cancer associated with specific mutations of *BRCA1* and *BRCA2* among Ashkenazi Jews. *N Engl J Med* 1997;336(20):1401–1408.
261. Wooster R, Weber BL. Breast and ovarian cancer. *N Engl J Med* 2003;348(23):2339–2347.
262. Garcia-Closas M, Brinton LA, Lissowska J, et al. Ovarian cancer risk and common variation in the sex hormone-binding globulin gene: a population-based case-control study. *BMC Cancer* 2007;7:60.
263. Holt SK, Rossing MA, Malone KE, et al. Ovarian cancer risk and polymorphisms involved in estrogen catabolism. *Cancer Epidemiol Biomarkers Prev* 2007;16(3):481–489.
264. Cook LS, Kamb ML, Weiss NS. Perineal powder exposure and the risk of ovarian cancer. *Am J Epidemiol* 1997;145(5):459–465.
265. Cramer DW, Welch WR, Scully RE, et al. Ovarian cancer and talc: a case-control study. *Cancer* 1982;50(2):372–376.
266. Gertig DM, Hunter DJ, Cramer DW, et al. Prospective study of talc use and ovarian cancer. *J Natl Cancer Inst* 2000;92(3):249–252.
267. Harlow BL, Weiss NS. A case-control study of borderline ovarian tumors: the influence of perineal exposure to talc. *Am J Epidemiol* 1989;130(2):390–394.
268. Mills PK, Riordan DG, Cress RD, et al. Perineal talc exposure and epithelial ovarian cancer risk in the Central Valley of California. *Int J Cancer* 2004;112(3):458–464.
269. Jordan SJ, Whiteman DC, Purdie DM, et al. Does smoking increase risk of ovarian cancer? A systematic review. *Gynecol Oncol* 2006;103(3):1122–1129.
270. Baker JA, Odunuga OO, Rodabaugh KJ, et al. Active and passive smoking and risk of ovarian cancer. *Int J Gynecol Cancer* 2006;16(Suppl 1):211–218.
271. Goodman MT, Tung KH. Active and passive tobacco smoking and the risk of borderline and invasive ovarian cancer (United States). *Cancer Causes Control* 2003;14(6):569–577.
272. Boffetta P, Andersen A, Lynge E, et al. Employment as hairdresser and risk of ovarian cancer and non-Hodgkin's lymphomas among women. *J Occup Med* 1994;36(1):61–65.
273. Donna A, Crosignani P, Robutti F, et al. Triazine herbicides and ovarian epithelial neoplasms. *Scand J Work Environ Health* 1989;15(1):47–53.
274. Vasama-Neuvonen K, Pukkala E, Paakkulainen H, et al. Ovarian cancer and occupational exposures in Finland. *Am J Ind Med* 1999;36(1):83–89.
275. Langseth H, Kjaerheim K. Ovarian cancer and occupational exposure among pulp and paper employees in Norway. *Scand J Work Environ Health* 2004;30(5):356–361.
276. Shields T, Gridley G, Moradi T, et al. Occupational exposures and the risk of ovarian cancer in Sweden. *Am J Ind Med* 2002;42(3):200–213.
277. Macarthur AC, Le ND, Abanto ZU, et al. Occupational female breast and reproductive cancer mortality in British Columbia, Canada, 1950-94. *Occup Med (Lond)* 2007;57(4):246–253.
278. Sala M, Dosemeci M, Zahm SH. A death certificate-based study of occupation and mortality from reproductive cancers among women in 24 U.S. states. *J Occup Environ Med* 1998;40(7):632–639.
279. Shen N, Weiderpass E, Antilla A, et al. Epidemiology of occupational and environmental risk factors related to ovarian cancer. *Scand J Work Environ Health* 1998;24(3):175–182.

280. Franceschi S, La Vecchia C, Helmrich SP, et al. Risk factors for epithelial ovarian cancer in Italy. *Am J Epidemiol* 1982;115(5):714–719.
281. Purdie DM, Bain CJ, Siskind V, et al. Ovulation and risk of epithelial ovarian cancer. *Int J Cancer* 2003;104(2):228–232.
282. Moorman PG, Schildkraut JM, Calingaert B, et al. Ovulation and ovarian cancer: a comparison of two methods for calculating lifetime ovulatory cycles (United States). *Cancer Causes Control* 2002;13(9):807–811.
283. Risch HA. Hormonal etiology of epithelial ovarian cancer, with a hypothesis concerning the role of androgens and progesterone. *J Natl Cancer Inst* 1998;90(23):1774–1786.
284. Cramer DW, Welch WR. Determinants of ovarian cancer risk. II. Inferences regarding pathogenesis. *J Natl Cancer Inst* 1983;71(4):717–721.
285. Fathalla MF. Incessant ovulation—a factor in ovarian neoplasia? *Lancet* 1971;2(7716):163.
286. Zajicek J. Ovarian cystomas and ovulation, a histogenetic concept. *Tumori* 1977;63(5):429–435.
287. Bosch FX, de Sanjose S. Chapter 1: human papillomavirus and cervical cancer—burden and assessment of causality. *J Natl Cancer Inst Monogr* 2003;(31):3–13.
288. Castellsague X, Munoz N. Chapter 3: cofactors in human papillomavirus carcinogenesis—role of parity, oral contraceptives, and tobacco smoking. *J Natl Cancer Inst Monogr* 2003;(31):20–28.
289. Schiffman M, Kjaer SK. Chapter 2: natural history of anogenital human papillomavirus infection and neoplasia. *J Natl Cancer Inst Monogr* 2003;(31):14–19.
290. Kovacic MB, Castle PE, Herrero R, et al. Relationships of human papillomavirus type, qualitative viral load, and age with cytologic abnormality. *Cancer Res* 2006;66(20):10112–10119.
291. Plummer M, Schiffman M, Castle PE, et al. A 2-year prospective study of human papillomavirus persistence among women with a cytological diagnosis of atypical squamous cells of undetermined significance or low-grade squamous intraepithelial lesion. *J Infect Dis* 2007;195(11):1582–1589.
292. Thomas KK, Hughes JP, Kuypers JM, et al. Concurrent and sequential acquisition of different genital human papillomavirus types. *J Infect Dis* 2000;182(4):1097–1102.
293. Burk RD. Pernicious papillomavirus infection. *N Engl J Med* 1999; 341(22):1687–1688.
294. Richardson H, Kelsall G, Tellier P, et al. The natural history of type-specific human papillomavirus infections in female university students. *Cancer Epidemiol Biomarkers Prev* 2003;12(6):485–490.
295. Hildesheim A, Schiffman MH, Gravitt PE, et al. Persistence of type-specific human papillomavirus infection among cytologically normal women. *J Infect Dis* 1994;169(2):235–240.
296. Ho GY, Bierman R, Beardsley L, et al. Natural history of cervicovaginal papillomavirus infection in young women. *N Engl J Med* 1998;338 (7):423–428.
297. Castle PE, Schiffman M, Herrero R, et al. A prospective study of age trends in cervical human papillomavirus acquisition and persistence in Guanacaste, Costa Rica. *J Infect Dis* 2005;191(11):1808–1816.
298. Ho GY, Burk RD, Klein S, et al. Persistent genital human papillomavirus infection as a risk factor for persistent cervical dysplasia. *J Natl Cancer Inst* 1995;87(18):1365–1371.
299. Kjaer SK, van den Brule AJ, Paull G, et al. Type specific persistence of high risk human papillomavirus (HPV) as indicator of high grade cervical squamous intraepithelial lesions in young women: population based prospective follow up study. *BMJ* 2002;325(7364):572.
300. Nobbenhuis MA, Walboomers JM, Helmerhorst TJ, et al. Relation of human papillomavirus status to cervical lesions and consequences for cervical-cancer screening: a prospective study. *Lancet* 1999;354(9172):20–25.
301. Schlecht NF, Kulaga S, Robitaille J, et al. Persistent human papillomavirus infection as a predictor of cervical intraepithelial neoplasia. *JAMA* 2001;286(24):3106–3114.
302. Nobbenhuis MA, Walboomers JM, Helmerhorst TJ, et al. Relation of human papillomavirus status to cervical lesions and consequences for cervical-cancer screening: a prospective study. *Lancet* 1999;354(9172):20–25.
303. Molano M, van den BA, Plummer M, et al. Determinants of clearance of human papillomavirus infections in Colombian women with normal cytology: a population-based, 5-year follow-up study. *Am J Epidemiol* 2003;158(5):486–494.
304. Schiffman M, Herrero R, Desalle R, et al. The carcinogenicity of human papillomavirus types reflects viral evolution. *Virology* 2005;337(1):76–84.
305. Schiffman MH. Recent progress in defining the epidemiology of human papillomavirus infection and cervical neoplasia. *J Natl Cancer Inst* 1992;84(6):394–398.
306. Clifford GM, Rana RK, Franceschi S, et al. Human papillomavirus genotype distribution in low-grade cervical lesions: comparison by geographic region and with cervical cancer. *Cancer Epidemiol Biomarkers Prev* 2005;14(5):1157–1164.
307. Parkin DM, Bray F, Ferlay J, et al. Estimating the world cancer burden: Globocan 2000. *Int J Cancer* 2001;94(2):153–156.
308. Gustafsson L, Ponten J, Bergstrom R, et al. International incidence rates of invasive cervical cancer before cytological screening. *Int J Cancer* 1997;71(2):159–165.
309. Gustafsson L, Ponten J, Zack M, et al. International incidence rates of invasive cervical cancer after introduction of cytological screening. *Cancer Causes Control* 1997;8(5):755–763.
310. Wang SS, Sherman ME, Hildesheim A, et al. Cervical adenocarcinoma and squamous cell carcinoma incidence trends among white women and black women in the United States for 1976-2000. *Cancer* 2004;100(5): 1035–1044.
311. Alfsen GC, Thoresen SO, Kristensen GB, et al. Histopathologic subtyping of cervical adenocarcinoma reveals increasing incidence rates of endometrioid tumors in all age groups: a population based study with review of all nonsquamous cervical carcinomas in Norway from 1966 to 1970, 1976 to 1980, and 1986 to 1990. *Cancer* 2000;89(6):1291–1299.
312. Beral V, Hermon C, Munoz N, et al. Cervical cancer. *Cancer Surv* 1994;19-20:265–285.
313. Peters RK, Chao A, Mack TM, et al. Increased frequency of adenocarcinoma of the uterine cervix in young women in Los Angeles County. *J Natl Cancer Inst* 1986;76(3):423–428.
314. Vizcaino AP, Moreno V, Bosch FX, et al. International trends in the incidence of cervical cancer: I. Adenocarcinoma and adenosquamous cell carcinomas. *Int J Cancer* 1998;75(4):536–545.
315. Smith HO, Tiffany MF, Qualls CR, et al. The rising incidence of adenocarcinoma relative to squamous cell carcinoma of the uterine cervix in the United States—a 24-year population-based study. *Gynecol Oncol* 2000;78(2):97–105.
316. Vizcaino AP, Moreno V, Bosch FX, et al. International trends in incidence of cervical cancer: II. Squamous-cell carcinoma. *Int J Cancer* 2000; 86(3):429–435.
317. Sasieni P, Adams J. Changing rates of adenocarcinoma and adenosquamous carcinoma of the cervix in England. *Lancet* 2001;357(9267):1490–1493.
318. Herbert A, Singh N, Smith JA. Adenocarcinoma of the uterine cervix compared with squamous cell carcinoma: a 12-year study in Southampton and South-west Hampshire. *Cytopathology* 2001;12(1):26–36.
319. Schiffman MH, Schatzkin A. Test reliability is critically important to molecular epidemiology: an example from studies of human papillomavirus infection and cervical neoplasia. *Cancer Res* 1994;54(7 Suppl):1944s–1947s.
320. Wacholder S. Chapter 18: statistical issues in the design and analysis of studies of human papillomavirus and cervical neoplasia. *J Natl Cancer Inst Monogr* 2003;(31):125–130.
321. Andersson-Ellstrom A, Hagmar BM, Johansson B, et al. Human papillomavirus deoxyribonucleic acid in cervix only detected in girls after coitus. *Int J STD AIDS* 1996;7(5):333–336.
322. Kjaer SK, Chackerian B, van den Brule AJ, et al. High-risk human papillomavirus is sexually transmitted: evidence from a follow-up study of virgins starting sexual activity (intercourse). *Cancer Epidemiol Biomarkers Prev* 2001;10(2):101–106.
323. Franco EL, Villa LL, Sobrinho JP, et al. Epidemiology of acquisition and clearance of cervical human papillomavirus infection in women from a high-risk area for cervical cancer. *J Infect Dis* 1999;180(5):1415–1423.
324. Moscicki AB, Hills N, Shiboski S, et al. Risks for incident human papillomavirus infection and low-grade squamous intraepithelial lesion development in young females. *JAMA* 2001;285(23):2995–3002.
325. Schiffman MH, Bauer HM, Hoover RN, et al. Epidemiologic evidence showing that human papillomavirus infection causes most cervical intraepithelial neoplasia. *J Natl Cancer Inst* 1993;85(12):958–964.
326. Winer RL, Lee SK, Hughes JP, et al. Genital human papillomavirus infection: incidence and risk factors in a cohort of female university students. *Am J Epidemiol* 2003;157(3):218–226.
327. Deacon JM, Evans CD, Yule R, et al. Sexual behaviour and smoking as determinants of cervical HPV infection and of CIN3 among those infected: a case-control study nested within the Manchester cohort. *Br J Cancer* 2000;83(11):1565–1572.
328. Hildesheim A, Herrero R, Castle PE, et al. HPV co-factors related to the development of cervical cancer: results from a population-based study in Costa Rica. *Br J Cancer* 2001;84(9):1219–1226.
329. Winer RL, Hughes JP, Feng Q, et al. Condom use and the risk of genital human papillomavirus infection in young women. *N Engl J Med* 2006;354(25):2645–2654.
330. Manhart LE, Koutsky LA. Do condoms prevent genital HPV infection, external genital warts, or cervical neoplasia? A meta-analysis. *Sex Transm Dis* 2002;29(11):725–735.
331. Castellsague X, Bosch FX, Munoz N, et al. Male circumcision, penile human papillomavirus infection, and cervical cancer in female partners. *N Engl J Med* 2002;346(15):1105–1112.
332. Franceschi S, Castellsague X, Dal Maso L, et al. Prevalence and determinants of human papillomavirus genital infection in men. *Br J Cancer* 2002;86(5):705–711.
333. Ylitalo N, Josefsson A, Melbye M, et al. A prospective study showing long-term infection with human papillomavirus 16 before the development of cervical carcinoma in situ. *Cancer Res* 2000;60(21): 6027–6032.
334. Moscicki AB, Shiboski S, Broering J, et al. The natural history of human papillomavirus infection as measured by repeated DNA testing in adolescent and young women. *J Pediatr* 1998;132(2):277–284.
335. Liaw KL, Hildesheim A, Burk RD, et al. A prospective study of human papillomavirus (HPV) type 16 DNA detection by polymerase chain reaction and its association with acquisition and persistence of other HPV types. *J Infect Dis* 2001;183(1):8–15.
336. Konya J, Dillner J. Immunity to oncogenic human papillomaviruses. *Adv Cancer Res* 2001;82:205–238.

337. Man S, Fiander A. Immunology of human papillomavirus infection in lower genital tract neoplasia. *Best Pract Res Clin Obstet Gynaecol* 2001; 15(5):701–714.
338. Woodworth CD. HPV innate immunity. *Front Biosci* 2002;7:d2058–d2071.
339. Palefsky JM, Holly EA. Chapter 6: immunosuppression and co-infection with HIV. *J Natl Cancer Inst Monogr* 2003;(31):41–46.
340. Moscicki AB, Ellenberg JH, Farhat S, et al. Persistence of human papillomavirus infection in HIV-infected and -uninfected adolescent girls: risk factors and differences, by phylogenetic type. *J Infect Dis* 2004;190(1):37–45.
341. Frisch M, Biggar RJ, Goedert JJ. Human papillomavirus-associated cancers in patients with human immunodeficiency virus infection and acquired immunodeficiency syndrome. *J Natl Cancer Inst* 2000;92(18):1500–1510.
342. Wang SS, Hildesheim A, Gao X, et al. Human leukocyte antigen class I alleles and cervical neoplasia: no heterozygote advantage. *Cancer Epidemiol Biomarkers Prev* 2002;11(4):419–420.
343. Ahlbom A, Lichtenstein P, Malmstrom H, et al. Cancer in twins: genetic and nongenetic familial risk factors. *J Natl Cancer Inst* 1997;89(4):287–293.
344. Goldgar DE, Easton DF, Cannon-Albright LA, et al. Systematic population-based assessment of cancer risk in first-degree relatives of cancer probands. *J Natl Cancer Inst* 1994;86(21):1600–1608.
345. Hemminki K, Dong C, Vaittinen P. Familial risks in cervical cancer: is there a hereditary component? *Int J Cancer* 1999;82(6):775–781.
346. Hemminki K, Li X, Mutanen P. Familial risks in invasive and in situ cervical cancer by histological type. *Eur J Cancer Prev* 2001;10(1):83–89.
347. Lichtenstein P, Holm NV, Verkasalo PK, et al. Environmental and heritable factors in the causation of cancer—analyses of cohorts of twins from Sweden, Denmark, and Finland. *N Engl J Med* 2000;343(2):78–85.
348. Magnusson PK, Sparen P, Gyllensten UB. Genetic link to cervical tumours. *Nature* 1999;400(6739):29–30.
349. Hemminki K, Vaittinen P. Familial cancers in a nationwide family cancer database: age distribution and prevalence. *Eur J Cancer* 1999;35(7):1109–1117.
350. Parikh S, Brennan P, Boffetta P. Meta-analysis of social inequality and the risk of cervical cancer. *Int J Cancer* 2003;105(5):687–691.
351. Khan MJ, Partridge EE, Wang SS, et al. Socioeconomic status and the risk of cervical intraepithelial neoplasia grade 3 among oncogenic human papillomavirus DNA-positive women with equivocal or mildly abnormal cytology. *Cancer* 2005;104(1):61–70.
352. Devesa SS, Diamond EL. Association of breast cancer and cervical cancer incidence with income and education among whites and blacks. *J Natl Cancer Inst* 1980;65(3):515–528.
353. Appleby P, Beral V, Berrington de GA, et al. Carcinoma of the cervix and tobacco smoking: collaborative reanalysis of individual data on 13,541 women with carcinoma of the cervix and 23,017 women without carcinoma of the cervix from 23 epidemiological studies. *Int J Cancer* 2006;118(6):1481–1495.
354. Castle PE, Wacholder S, Lorincz AT, et al. A prospective study of high-grade cervical neoplasia risk among human papillomavirus-infected women. *J Natl Cancer Inst* 2002;94(18):1406–1414.
355. Castle PE, Wacholder S, Sherman ME, et al. Absolute risk of a subsequent abnormal pap among oncogenic human papillomavirus DNA-positive, cytologically negative women. *Cancer* 2002;95(10):2145–2151.
356. McCann MF, Irwin DE, Walton LA, et al. Nicotine and cotinine in the cervical mucus of smokers, passive smokers, and nonsmokers. *Cancer Epidemiol Biomarkers Prev* 1992;1(2):125–129.
357. Prokopczyk B, Cox JE, Hoffmann D, et al. Identification of tobacco-specific carcinogen in the cervical mucus of smokers and nonsmokers. *J Natl Cancer Inst* 1997;89(12):868–873.
358. Schiffman M, Brinton L, Holly E, et al. Regarding mutagenic mucus in the cervix of smokers. *J Natl Cancer Inst* 1987;78(3):590–591.
359. Schiffman MH, Haley NJ, Felton JS, et al. Biochemical epidemiology of cervical neoplasia: measuring cigarette smoke constituents in the cervix. *Cancer Res* 1987;47(14):3886–3888.
360. Barton SE, Maddox PH, Jenkins D, et al. Effect of cigarette smoking on cervical epithelial immunity: a mechanism for neoplastic change? *Lancet* 1988;2(8612):652–654.
361. Burger MP, Hollema H, Gouw AS, et al. Cigarette smoking and human papillomavirus in patients with reported cervical cytological abnormality. *BMJ* 1993;306(6880):749–752.
362. Szarewski A, Maddox P, Royston P, et al. The effect of stopping smoking on cervical Langerhans' cells and lymphocytes. *BJOG* 2001;108(3):295–303.
363. Brinton LA, Hamman RF, Huggins GR, et al. Sexual and reproductive risk factors for invasive squamous cell cervical cancer. *J Natl Cancer Inst* 1987;79(1):23–30.
364. Brinton LA, Reeves WC, Brenes MM, et al. Parity as a risk factor for cervical cancer. *Am J Epidemiol* 1989;130(3):486–496.
365. Munoz N, Franceschi S, Bosetti C, et al. Role of parity and human papillomavirus in cervical cancer: the IARC multicentric case-control study. *Lancet* 2002;359(9312):1093–1101.
366. International Collaboration of Epidemiological Studies of Cervical Cancer. Cervical carcinoma and reproductive factors: collaborative reanalysis of individual data on 16,563 women with cervical carcinoma and 33,542 women without cervical carcinoma from 25 epidemiological studies. *Int J Cancer* 2006;119(5):1108–1124.
367. Kjaer SK, Dahl C, Engholm G, et al. Case-control study of risk factors for cervical neoplasia in Denmark. II. Role of sexual activity, reproductive factors, and venereal infections. *Cancer Causes Control* 1992;3(4):339–348.
368. Hildesheim A, Wang SS. Host and viral genetics and risk of cervical cancer: a review. *Virus Res* 2002;89(2):229–240.
369. Beral V, Hannaford P, Kay C. Oral contraceptive use and malignancies of the genital tract. Results from the Royal College of General Practitioners' Oral Contraception Study. *Lancet* 1988;2(8624):1331–1335.
370. Brinton LA, Huggins GR, Lehman HF, et al. Long-term use of oral contraceptives and risk of invasive cervical cancer. *Int J Cancer* 1986;38(3): 339–344.
371. Brinton LA, Reeves WC, Brenes MM, et al. Oral contraceptive use and risk of invasive cervical cancer. *Int J Epidemiol* 1990;19(1):4–11.
372. Moreno V, Bosch FX, Munoz N, et al. Effect of oral contraceptives on risk of cervical cancer in women with human papillomavirus infection: the IARC multicentric case-control study. *Lancet* 2002;359(9312): 1085–1092.
373. Smith JS, Green J, Berrington dG, et al. Cervical cancer and use of hormonal contraceptives: a systematic review. *Lancet* 2003;361(9364):1159–1167.
374. de Villiers EM. Relationship between steroid hormone contraceptives and HPV, cervical intraepithelial neoplasia and cervical carcinoma. *Int J Cancer* 2003;103(6):705–708.
375. Herrero R, Brinton LA, Reeves WC, et al. Injectable contraceptives and risk of invasive cervical cancer: evidence of an association. *Int J Cancer* 1990;46(1):5–7.
376. Bosch FX, Lorincz A, Munoz N, et al. The causal relation between human papillomavirus and cervical cancer. *J Clin Pathol* 2002;55(4):244–265.
377. Aurelian L. Viruses and carcinoma of the cervix. *Contrib Gynecol Obstet* 1991;18:54–70.
378. Smith JS, Munoz N, Franceschi S, et al. Chlamydia trachomatis and cervical squamous cell carcinoma. *JAMA* 2001;285(13):1704–1706.
379. Smith JS, Munoz N, Herrero R, et al. Evidence for *Chlamydia trachomatis* as a human papillomavirus cofactor in the etiology of invasive cervical cancer in Brazil and the Philippines. *J Infect Dis* 2002;185(3): 324–331.
380. Smith JS, Bosetti C, Munoz N, et al. *Chlamydia trachomatis* and invasive cervical cancer: a pooled analysis of the IARC multicentric case-control study. *Int J Cancer* 2004;111(3):431–439.
381. Castle PE, Escoffery C, Schachter J, et al. *Chlamydia trachomatis*, herpes simplex virus 2, and human T-cell lymphotrophic virus type 1 are not associated with grade of cervical neoplasia in Jamaican colposcopy patients. *Sex Transm Dis* 2003;30(7):575–580.
382. Schmauz R, Okong P, de Villiers EM, et al. Multiple infections in cases of cervical cancer from a high-incidence area in tropical Africa. *Int J Cancer* 1989;43(5):805–809.
383. de Sanjose S, Munoz N, Bosch FX, et al. Sexually transmitted agents and cervical neoplasia in Colombia and Spain. *Int J Cancer* 1994;56(3): 358–363.
384. Castle PE, Giuliano AR. Chapter 4: genital tract infections, cervical inflammation, and antioxidant nutrients—assessing their roles as human papillomavirus cofactors. *J Natl Cancer Inst Monogr* 2003;(31):29–34.
385. Giuliano AR. The role of nutrients in the prevention of cervical dysplasia and cancer. *Nutrition* 2000;16(7-8):570–573.
386. Potischman N, Brinton LA. Nutrition and cervical neoplasia. *Cancer Causes Control* 1996;7(1):113–126.
387. Weinstein SJ, Ziegler RG, Selhub J, et al. Elevated serum homocysteine levels and increased risk of invasive cervical cancer in U.S. women. *Cancer Causes Control* 2001;12(4):317–324.
388. Comparison of risk factors for invasive squamous cell carcinoma and adenocarcinoma of the cervix: collaborative reanalysis of individual data on 8,097 women with squamous cell carcinoma and 1,374 women with adenocarcinoma from 12 epidemiological studies. *Int J Cancer* 2007; 120(4):885–891.
389. Solomon D, Davey D, Kurman R, et al. The 2001 Bethesda System: terminology for reporting results of cervical cytology. *JAMA* 2002;287(16): 2114–2119.
390. Altekruse SF, Lacey JV, Jr., Brinton LA, et al. Comparison of human papillomavirus genotypes, sexual, and reproductive risk factors of cervical adenocarcinoma and squamous cell carcinoma: Northeastern United States. *Am J Obstet Gynecol* 2003;188(3):657–663.
391. Ursin G, Pike MC, Preston-Martin S, et al. Sexual, reproductive, and other risk factors for adenocarcinoma of the cervix: results from a population-based case-control study (California, United States). *Cancer Causes Control* 1996;7(3):391–401.
392. Lacey JV, Jr., Frisch M, Brinton LA, et al. Associations between smoking and adenocarcinomas and squamous cell carcinomas of the uterine cervix (United States). *Cancer Causes Control* 2001;12(2):153–161.
393. Lacey JV, Jr., Swanson CA, Brinton LA, et al. Obesity as a potential risk factor for adenocarcinomas and squamous cell carcinomas of the uterine cervix. *Cancer* 2003;98(4):814–821.
394. Parazzini F, La Vecchia C, Negri E, et al. Risk factors for adenocarcinoma of the cervix: a case-control study. *Br J Cancer* 1988;57(2):201–204.
395. Lacey JV, Jr., Brinton LA, Abbas FM, et al. Oral contraceptives as risk factors for cervical adenocarcinomas and squamous cell carcinomas. *Cancer Epidemiol Biomarkers Prev* 1999;8(12):1079–1085.
396. Madeleine MM, Daling JR, Schwartz SM, et al. Human papillomavirus and long-term oral contraceptive use increase the risk of adenocarcinoma in situ of the cervix. *Cancer Epidemiol Biomarkers Prev* 2001;10(3): 171–177.

397. Thomas DB, Ray RM. Oral contraceptives and invasive adenocarcinomas and adenosquamous carcinomas of the uterine cervix. The World Health Organization Collaborative Study of Neoplasia and Steroid Contraceptives. *Am J Epidemiol* 1996;144(3):281–289.
398. Ursin G, Peters RK, Henderson BE, et al. Oral contraceptive use and adenocarcinoma of cervix. *Lancet* 1994;344(8934):1390–1394.
399. Parazzini F, Negri E, La Vecchia C, et al. Treatment for infertility and risk of invasive epithelial ovarian cancer. *Hum Reprod* 1997;12(10): 2159–2161.
400. Lacey JV, Jr., Brinton LA, Barnes WA, et al. Use of hormone replacement therapy and adenocarcinomas and squamous cell carcinomas of the uterine cervix. *Gynecol Oncol* 2000;77(1):149–154.
401. Cuzick J. Role of HPV testing in clinical practice. *Virus Res* 2002;89(2): 263–269.
402. Saslow D, Runowicz CD, Solomon D, et al. American Cancer Society guideline for the early detection of cervical neoplasia and cancer. *CA Cancer J Clin* 2002;52(6):342–362.
403. Wright TC, Jr., Cox JT, Massad LS, et al 2001 Consensus guidelines for the management of women with cervical cytological abnormalities. *JAMA* 2002;287(16):2120–2129.
404. Wright TC, Jr., Cox JT, Massad LS, et al 2001 consensus guidelines for the management of women with cervical intraepithelial neoplasia. *Am J Obstet Gynecol* 2003;189(1):295–304.
405. Wright TC, Jr., Schiffman M, Solomon D, et al. Interim guidance for the use of human papillomavirus DNA testing as an adjunct to cervical cytology for screening. *Obstet Gynecol* 2004;103(2):304–309.
406. Kim JJ, Wright TC, Goldie SJ. Cost-effectiveness of alternative triage strategies for atypical squamous cells of undetermined significance. *JAMA* 2002;287(18):2382–2390.
407. Sherman ME, Schiffman MH, Lorincz AT, et al. Toward objective quality assurance in cervical cytopathology. Correlation of cytopathologic diagnoses with detection of high-risk human papillomavirus types. *Am J Clin Pathol* 1994;102(2):182–187.
408. Zuna RE, Moore W, Dunn ST. HPV DNA testing of the residual sample of liquid-based Pap test: utility as a quality assurance monitor. *Mod Pathol* 2001;14(3):147–151.
409. Franco EL. Chapter 13: primary screening of cervical cancer with human papillomavirus tests. *J Natl Cancer Inst Monogr* 2003;(31):89–96.
410. Koutsky LA, Ault KA, Wheeler CM, et al. A controlled trial of a human papillomavirus type 16 vaccine. *N Engl J Med* 2002;347(21):1645–1651.
411. Schiffman M, Castle PE. The promise of global cervical-cancer prevention. *N Engl J Med* 2005;353(20):2101–2104.
412. Trimble CL, Hildesheim A, Brinton LA, et al. Heterogeneous etiology of squamous carcinoma of the vulva. *Obstet Gynecol* 1996;87(1):59–64.
413. Kurman RJ, Toki T, Schiffman MH. Basaloid and warty carcinomas of the vulva. Distinctive types of squamous cell carcinoma frequently associated with human papillomaviruses. *Am J Surg Pathol* 1993;17(2):133–145.
414. Judson PL, Habermann EB, Baxter NN, et al. Trends in the incidence of invasive and in situ vulvar carcinoma. *Obstet Gynecol* 2006;107(5): 1018–1022.
415. Sherman KJ, Daling JR, Chu J, et al. Multiple primary tumours in women with vulvar neoplasms: a case-control study. *Br J Cancer* 1988;57(4): 423–427.
416. Rose PG, Herterick EE, Boutselis JG, et al. Multiple primary gynecologic neoplasms. *Am J Obstet Gynecol* 1987;157(2):261–267.
417. Beckmann AM, Kiviat NB, Daling JR, et al. Human papillomavirus type 16 in multifocal neoplasia of the female genital tract. *Int J Gynecol Pathol* 1988;7(1):39–47.
418. Sturgeon SR, Brinton LA, Devesa SS, et al. In situ and invasive vulvar cancer incidence trends (1973 to 1987). *Am J Obstet Gynecol* 1992;166(5): 1482–1485.
419. Brinton LA, Nasca PC, Mallin K, et al. Case-control study of cancer of the vulva. *Obstet Gynecol* 1990;75(5):859–866.
420. Sherman KJ, Daling JR, Chu J, et al. Genital warts, other sexually transmitted diseases, and vulvar cancer. *Epidemiology* 1991;2(4):257–262.
421. Bjorge T, Dillner J, Anttila T, et al. Prospective seroepidemiological study of role of human papillomavirus in non-cervical anogenital cancers. *BMJ* 1997;315(7109):646–649.
422. Hildesheim A, Han CL, Brinton LA, et al. Human papillomavirus type 16 and risk of preinvasive and invasive vulvar cancer: results from a seroepidemiological case-control study. *Obstet Gynecol* 1997;90(5): 748–754.
423. Madeleine MM, Daling JR, Carter JJ, et al. Cofactors with human papillomavirus in a population-based study of vulvar cancer. *J Natl Cancer Inst* 1997;89(20):1516–1523.
424. Daling JR, Sherman KJ, Hislop TG, et al. Cigarette smoking and the risk of anogenital cancer. *Am J Epidemiol* 1992;135(2):180–189.
425. Newcomb PA, Weiss NS, Daling JR. Incidence of vulvar carcinoma in relation to menstrual, reproductive, and medical factors. *J Natl Cancer Inst* 1984;73(2):391–396.
426. Daling JR, Chu J, Weiss NS, et al. The association of condylomata acuminata and squamous carcinoma of the vulva. *Br J Cancer* 1984;50(4): 533–535.
427. Chen C, Madeleine MM, Weiss NS, et al. Glutathione S-transferase M1 genotypes and the risk of vulvar cancer: a population-based case-control study. *Am J Epidemiol* 1999;150(5):437–442.
428. Chen C, Cook LS, Li XY, et al. CYP2D6 genotype and the incidence of anal and vulvar cancer. *Cancer Epidemiol Biomarkers Prev* 1999;8(4 Pt 1): 317–321.
429. Okagaki T. Female genital tumors associated with human papillomavirus infection, and the concept of genital neoplasm-papilloma syndrome (GENPS). *Pathol Annu* 1984;19(Pt 2):31–62.
430. Creasman WT. Vaginal cancers. *Curr Opin Obstet Gynecol* 2005;17(1): 71–76.
431. Brinton LA, Nasca PC, Mallin K, et al. Case-control study of in situ and invasive carcinoma of the vagina. *Gynecol Oncol* 1990;38(1):49–54.
432. Daling JR, Madeleine MM, Schwartz SM, et al. A population-based study of squamous cell vaginal cancer: HPV and cofactors. *Gynecol Oncol* 2002;84(2):263–270.
433. Herbst AL, Ulfelder H, Poskanzer DC. Adenocarcinoma of the vagina. Association of maternal stilbestrol therapy with tumor appearance in young women. *N Engl J Med* 1971;284(15):878–881.
434. Greenwald P, Barlow JJ, Nasca PC, et al. Vaginal cancer after maternal treatment with synthetic estrogens. *N Engl J Med* 1971;285(7):390–392.
435. Noller KL, Decker DG, Lanier AP, et al. Clear-cell adenocarcinoma of the cervix after maternal treatment with synthetic estrogens. *Mayo Clin Proc* 1972;47(9):629–630.
436. Herbst AL, Anderson S, Hubby MM, et al. Risk factors for the development of diethylstilbestrol-associated clear cell adenocarcinoma: a case-control study. *Am J Obstet Gynecol* 1986;154(4):814–822.
437. Troisi R, Hatch EE, Titus-Ernstoff L, et al. Cancer risk in women prenatally exposed to diethylstilbestrol. *Int J Cancer* 2007;121(2):356–360.
438. Hellman K, Silfversward C, Nilsson B, et al. Primary carcinoma of the vagina: factors influencing the age at diagnosis. The Radiumhemmet series 1956-96. *Int J Gynecol Cancer* 2004;14(3):491–501.
439. Fulop V, Mok SC, Gati I, et al. Recent advances in molecular biology of gestational trophoblastic diseases. A review. *J Reprod Med* 2002;47(5): 369–379.
440. Smith HO, Qualls CR, Prairie BA, et al. Trends in gestational choriocarcinoma: a 27-year perspective. *Obstet Gynecol* 2003;102(5 Pt 1): 978–987.
441. Bracken MB, Brinton LA, Hayashi K. Epidemiology of hydatidiform mole and choriocarcinoma. *Epidemiol Rev* 1984;6:52–75.
442. Smith HO, Wiggins C, Verschraegen CF, et al. Changing trends in gestational trophoblastic disease. *J Reprod Med* 2006;51(10):777–784.
443. Steigrad SJ. Epidemiology of gestational trophoblastic diseases. *Best Pract Res Clin Obstet Gynecol* 2003;17(6):837–847.
444. Tham BW, Everard JE, Tidy JA, et al. Gestational trophoblastic disease in the Asian population of Northern England and North Wales. *BJOG* 2003;110(6):555–559.
445. Brinton LA, Bracken MB, Connelly RR. Choriocarcinoma incidence in the United States. *Am J Epidemiol* 1986;123(6):1094–1100.
446. Smith HO, Hilgers RD, Bedrick EJ, et al. Ethnic differences at risk for gestational trophoblastic disease in New Mexico: a 25-year population-based study. *Am J Obstet Gynecol* 2003;188(2):357–366.
447. Altieri A, Franceschi S, Ferlay J, et al. Epidemiology and aetiology of gestational trophoblastic diseases. *Lancet Oncol* 2003;4(11):670–678.
448. Goto S, Yamada A, Ishizuka T, et al. Development of postmolar trophoblastic disease after partial molar pregnancy. *Gynecol Oncol* 1993; 48(2):165–170.
449. Kodama A, Kanazawa K, Honma S, et al. Epidemiologic and clinicopathologic studies of partial hydatidiform mole. *Nippon Sanka Fujinka Gakkai Zasshi* 1991;43(9):1219–1225.
450. Tuncer ZS, Bernstein MR, Wang J, et al. Repetitive hydatidiform mole with different male partners. *Gynecol Oncol* 1999;75(2):224–226.
451. Bagshawe KD, Rawlins G, Pike MC, et al. ABO blood-groups in trophoblastic neoplasia. *Lancet* 1971;1(7699):553–556.
452. Dawood MY, Teoh ES, Ratnam SS. ABO blood group in trophoblastic disease. *J Obstet Gynaecol Br Commonw* 1971;78(10):918–923.
453. Messerli ML, Lilienfeld AM, Parmley T, et al. Risk factors for gestational trophoblastic neoplasia. *Am J Obstet Gynecol* 1985;153(3):294–300.
454. Parazzini F, La Vecchia C, Franceschi S, et al. ABO blood-groups and the risk of gestational trophoblastic disease. *Tumori* 1985;71(2): 123–126.
455. Brinton LA, Wu BZ, Wang W, et al. Gestational trophoblastic disease: a case-control study from the People's Republic of China. *Am J Obstet Gynecol* 1989;161(1):121–127.
456. Parazzini F, La Vecchia C, Pampallona S, et al. Reproductive patterns and the risk of gestational trophoblastic disease. *Am J Obstet Gynecol* 1985;152(7 Pt 1):866–870.
457. La Vecchia C, Franceschi S, Parazzini F, et al. Risk factors for gestational trophoblastic disease in Italy. *Am J Epidemiol* 1985;121(3):457–464.
458. Buckley JD, Henderson BE, Morrow CP, et al. Case-control study of gestational choriocarcinoma. *Cancer Res* 1988;48(4):1004–1010.
459. Berkowitz RS, Cramer DW, Bernstein MR, et al. Risk factors for complete molar pregnancy from a case-control study. *Am J Obstet Gynecol* 1985;152(8):1016–1020.

460. Palmer JR, Driscoll SG, Rosenberg L, et al. Oral contraceptive use and risk of gestational trophoblastic tumors. *J Natl Cancer Inst* 1999;91(7): 635–640.
461. Parazzini F, Cipriani S, Mangili G, et al. Oral contraceptives and risk of gestational trophoblastic disease. *Contraception* 2002;65(6): 425–427.
462. Ho YB, Burch P. Relationship of oral contraceptives and the intrauterine contraceptive devices to the regression of concentrations of the beta subunit of human chorionic gonadotropin and invasive complications after molar pregnancy. *Am J Obstet Gynecol* 1983;145(2): 214–217.
463. Stone M, Dent J, Kardana A, et al. Relationship of oral contraception to development of trophoblastic tumour after evacuation of a hydatidiform mole. *Br J Obstet Gynaecol* 1976;83(12):913–916.
464. Curry SL, Schlaerth JB, Kohorn EI, et al. Hormonal contraception and trophoblastic sequelae after hydatidiform mole (a Gynecologic Oncology Group Study). *Am J Obstet Gynecol* 1989;160(4):805–809.
465. Morrow P, Nakamura R, Schlaerth J, et al. The influence of oral contraceptives on the postmolar human chorionic gonadotropin regression curve. *Am J Obstet Gynecol* 1985;151(7):906–914.
466. La Vecchia C, Parazzini F, Decarli A, et al. Age of parents and risk of gestational trophoblastic disease. *J Natl Cancer Inst* 1984;73(3):639–642.

CHAPTER 2 ■ CLINICAL GENETICS OF GYNECOLOGIC CANCER

STEVEN A. NAROD

GENETICS IN CLINICAL PRACTICE OF GYNECOLOGIC ONCOLOGY

The identification of *BRCA1* in 1994 and *BRCA2* in 1995 has introduced a new component to the practice of gynecologic oncology. Genetic testing for predisposition to ovarian cancer became available by 1996 and is now well established. There are five genes for ovarian cancer susceptibility that are now in clinical use (*BRCA1, BRCA2, MLH1, MSH2,* and *MSH6*). *BRCA1* and *BRCA2* are responsible for the hereditary breast-ovarian cancer syndrome (13% of all ovarian cancers) and *MLH1, MSH2,* and *MSH6* are responsible for the hereditary nonpolyposis colon cancer syndrome (2% of ovarian cancers). Our ability to use laboratory testing to predict the later development of ovarian cancer requires that clinicians have a clear understanding of the role of genetic testing in risk assessment and in patient care. Advances in preventive oncology have had the effect of increasing the number of healthy women who seek advice from a gynecologic oncologist. Increasing numbers of prophylactic salpingo-oophorectomies are performed on healthy women by surgeons who, for the most part, had previously treated patients for cancer. Information is now available to support the practice of genetic testing for *BRCA* mutations as a means to prevent ovarian cancer in high-risk women. Current strategies for prevention include prophylactic surgery and chemoprevention with oral contraceptives. Screening for ovarian cancer is widespread, but its utility has not been proven.

OVARIAN CANCER

Genetic Epidemiology

Approximately 13% of all women with invasive ovarian cancer carry a *BRCA1* or *BRCA2* mutation (1–3) and it is reasonable to offer genetic testing to all women diagnosed with invasive epithelial ovarian cancer (women with mucinous cancer may be exempted). In the event of a positive genetic test, testing is extended to unaffected female relatives. However, if there is no living affected relative, then testing may begin with an unaffected woman.

The frequency of *BRCA* mutations among ovarian cancer patients is not the same for all ethnic groups. In some populations, there are recurrent (founder) mutations. In these populations, the overall frequency of *BRCA1* mutations tends to be high and a large proportion of mutations will be accounted for by one, or a small number, of specific mutations. For example, approximately 30% to 40% of Jewish women with ovarian cancer carry one of three founder mutations (two in *BRCA1* and one in *BRCA2*) (4,5). Moslehi et al. (4) found that 41% of Jewish women with ovarian cancer from North America carried a mutation, including the majority of those diagnosed between the ages of 40 and 60. Modan et al. (5) found one of the three mutations in 29% of 840 Jewish women with ovarian cancer in Israel. In Poland, 13.5% of unselected patients with ovarian cancer carry one of three common *BRCA1* mutations (6) (one of these [5382insC] is also one of the Jewish founder mutations). Three mutations account for 86% of all *BRCA* mutations found in Poland (7). The frequency of *BRCA* mutations has been estimated at 1 in 12 cases of ovarian cancer in French-Canadians (8) and one in six cases in Pakistan (9). In these populations, it may be possible to offer testing for a limited number of mutations.

The excess risk of ovarian cancer in Jewish families with multiple cases of breast or ovarian cancer appears to be almost entirely due to the three Jewish founder mutations. Liede et al. studied a cohort of 290 Jewish women undergoing surveillance for ovarian cancer because of a family history of breast or ovarian cancer (10). Among women with a *BRCA* mutation, the ovarian cancer incidence was 32 times greater than expected. However, among women who did not carry a mutation, no excess risk of ovarian cancer was observed. Kauff et al. followed 199 women from site-specific *BRCA*-negative breast cancer families (11). They observed an elevated risk for breast cancer (standardized incidence ratio [SIR] = 3.1; $p < 0.001$), but not for ovarian cancer (SIR = 1.5; $p = 0.5$) (11). Phelan et al. screened 160 Jewish families with site-specific breast cancer or the breast-ovarian cancer syndrome (12). These families had previously been found to be negative for the three Jewish founder mutations. Only a single nonfounder mutation was identified. Together, these studies indicate that if a founder mutation is not identified through screening of a Jewish family, it is exceedingly unlikely that a different mutation will be found. This also implies that a Jewish woman without one of the three mutations should not be considered to be at increased risk for ovarian cancer (although she may be at higher than average risk for breast cancer). Testing for mutations other than these three in Jewish women should be conducted in exceptional circumstances—an example would be a family with four or more cases of early-onset breast cancer or invasive ovarian cancer.

In the ethnically mixed populations of North America, approximately 13% of all patients with invasive ovarian cancer carry a mutation in *BRCA1* or *BRCA2* (1–3). However, the range of mutations is wide and genetic testing must be comprehensive (full genomic screening). In Ontario, Canada, a mutation was found in 129 of 977 (13.2%) unselected cases of ovarian cancer (2). There were 75 *BRCA1* mutations and 54 *BRCA2*

TABLE 2.1

LIFETIME RISKS OF CANCERS ASSOCIATED WITH SPECIFIC GENES

	BRCA1	*BRCA2*	MMR[a]
Breast	50%–85%	50%–85%	NI
Ovarian	30%–40%	15%–25%	5%–10%
Endometrial	NI	NI	40%–60%

NI, not increased.
[a]Mismatch repair genes *MSH2*, *MLH1*, and *MSH6*.

mutations. Women with *BRCA1* mutations were diagnosed with ovarian cancer at an average age of 52.6 years, compared to 58.8 years for carriers of *BRCA2* mutations and 57.3 years for the nonhereditary cases. *BRCA1* mutations represented 71% of the mutations found in women diagnosed under age 50 and *BRCA2* mutations represented 62% of those diagnosed after age 60.

Among *BRCA1* carriers, the risk of ovarian cancer is significant in women above the age of 35 (13) (approximately 1% per year) and preventive measures must be initiated early. Women who carry a pathogenic mutation in the *BRCA1* gene have a lifetime risk of approximately 40% for developing invasive ovarian cancer (14–18) (Table 2.1). Among *BRCA2* carriers, the risk is much lower and ovarian cancer rarely occurs below age 50. Antoniou et al. estimated the lifetime risk for *BRCA2* carriers to be 11% (15); Satagopan et al. estimated the risk of ovarian cancer to be 21% (17). A recent meta-analysis (which included these two studies) estimated the risk of ovarian cancer to be 16% (18). Also, among *BRCA2* carriers, the risk of ovarian cancer varies with the position of the mutation. Thompson et al. (16) estimated that the risk of ovarian cancer to age 70 was 20% for carriers of *BRCA2* mutations within the Ovarian Cancer Cluster Region (OCCR: nucleotides 4075–6503) and was 11% for mutations outside of this region. This assignment was confirmed by Lubinski et al. in 2004 (19). These investigators studied 440 families with a *BRCA2* mutation. They found that families with a mutation in the OCCR (nucleotides 3035–6629) were twice as likely to contain one or more cases of ovarian cancer than were families with a *BRCA2* mutation located outside of this region (odds ratio [OR] = 2.2; $p = 0.0002$).

Metcalfe et al. followed a cohort of women with breast cancer and a *BRCA1* or *BRCA2* mutation (20). In the ten-year period following the cancer diagnosis, the risk of ovarian cancer was 13% for *BRCA1* carriers and 7% for *BRCA2* mutation carriers. In this study, 25% of the deaths in women with stage I breast cancer were due to subsequent ovarian cancer.

Pathology and Surgical Presentation of Hereditary Ovarian Cancer

Ovarian cancers that occur in women with a *BRCA* mutation appear to be similar to their sporadic counterparts (1,2,21,22), with the exception that mucinous tumors and tumors of low malignant potential (or "borderline" tumors) are rarely observed in women with a *BRCA* mutation. The great majority of *BRCA*-linked ovarian cancers show moderate to poor differentiation. Most hereditary ovarian tumors present at an advanced surgical stage (4,21), but stage I or II tumors are now being discovered in the context of high-risk screening programs, or as an incidental finding associated with a prophylactic oophorectomy in an asymptomatic woman. Several studies have reported on the presence of early ovarian cancers among pathology specimens obtained at the time of prophylactic surgery (23–30). In one study (23), 4 of 33 women (12%) at high risk were found to have clinically unsuspected ovarian cancer at the time of prophylactic oophorectomy. In a second study (24), two of eight women with germ-line *BRCA1* mutations had ovarian cancer at the time of prophylactic oophorectomy. Salazar et al. (25) reviewed the ovaries of 20 women who had a prophylactic oophorectomy and found two cases of microscopic cancer. Finch et al. described a series of 159 female *BRCA1* or *BRCA2* carriers who underwent prophylactic oophorectomy (26). Six of 94 *BRCA1* carriers were found to have an occult cancer (6.4%). In contrast, only one of the 65 *BRCA2* carriers was found to have an occult cancer (1.5%). Three of the seven cases of occult malignancy involved the fallopian tube and not the ovaries.

In a study from Boston, 122 of *BRCA1* and *BRCA2* carriers underwent preventive ovarian surgery (27). Seven cancers were found (6% of total). All cancers were found in the distal portion of the fallopian tube. Powell et al. found seven cancers among 67 women who underwent a prophylactic oophorectomy (28). Seven cancers were found: four in the fallopian tubes and three in the ovaries. These studies support the theory that the distal fallopian tube is the site of origin of the majority of ovarian/fallopian cancers in high-risk women (30–32). Carcinoma of the fallopian tube has also been noted in several *BRCA*-linked breast and ovarian cancer kindreds. In a population-based study of unselected cases of carcinoma of the fallopian tube, 7 of 44 (16%) tested patients were found to harbor a germ-line *BRCA* mutation: five in *BRCA1* (11%) and two in *BRCA2* (5%) (33). It is necessary that the fallopian tube be completely removed and serially sectioned when a prophylactic oophorectomy is performed.

Several study groups have asked whether morphologic alterations of the ovarian surface epithelium are prevalent in women with ovarian cancer (34–37) or who are at high genetic risk for ovarian cancer (38). Alterations of these types are common and it has not yet been proven that they are present at a higher frequency than expected in cancer-prone ovaries.

Clinical Outcome and Treatment Effects

Several studies have reported that the survival of patients with *BRCA*-associated ovarian cancer is improved, compared to women with sporadic ovarian cancer (21,39–43). A study of consecutive cases of ovarian cancers, which compared *BRCA*-associated to sporadic ovarian cancers from the same institution, found that *BRCA* mutation status was a favorable and independent predictor of survival for women with advanced disease (21). It is not yet clear if the improved survival rate is the result of a difference in the natural history of ovarian cancer in the two subgroups or a better response of *BRCA*-associated tumors to current therapies. Cass et al. reported that *BRCA1* carriers with ovarian cancer had a higher response rate to primary therapy than did matched noncarriers, and carrier patients with advanced disease had improved survival (91 months for *BRCA1* carriers vs. 54 months for noncarriers; $p = 0.05$) (41).

Prophylactic Oophorectomy

In 1995, a consensus panel of the National Institutes of Health (NIH) recommended prophylactic oophorectomy for high-risk women at age 35 years, or after childbearing is complete (44). It seems logical that prophylactic oophorectomy should eliminate the incidence of ovarian cancer, but there are two reasons for potential failure of prophylactic oophorectomy. First, it is possible that the removed ovaries or fallopian tubes contain foci of occult carcinoma and that the cancer has spread locally to the peritoneum at the time of the resection. In this case, the peritoneal cancer is not, in fact, a primary cancer, but a metastatic ovarian cancer. Second, it is possible that *de novo* cancer arises in the peritoneum after oophorectomy. The peritoneum is derived from coelomic epithelium, of the same embryologic origin as the surface epithelium of the ovary.

Liede et al. (10) followed a cohort of 33 Jewish women with *BRCA* mutations for a mean of eight years. Five cases of primary peritoneal cancer were diagnosed. The ten-year risk of peritoneal cancer was 16%. However, the women in this study had both ovaries intact and the peritoneal origin of the tumors was not definite. It is difficult to measure the risk of peritoneal cancer in women with intact ovaries. Peritoneal, fallopian, and serous ovarian cancers are histologically indistinguishable, and symptomatic women often present with multiple foci of cancer involving the peritoneum, tubes, omentum, and ovary. Tubal cancer is difficult to discriminate from ovarian cancer and is often misclassified as ovarian cancer (45). It is easier to make the diagnosis of primary peritoneal cancer in women without ovaries. New serous cancers that arise in the abdominal peritoneum, following an oophorectomy, and with normal ovaries on pathological examination are generally considered to be primary peritoneal cancers.

Piver et al. (46) reported that 6 of 324 women who underwent prophylactic oophorectomy experienced primary peritoneal cancer. The mutation status of these women was unknown and there was no standard period of follow-up. Struewing et al. (47) reported that the cancer risk in women after prophylactic oophorectomy was 13 times greater than that expected from population-based rates, but this was based on only two observed cases of peritoneal cancer. Kauff et al. (48) followed 170 *BRCA* carriers for an average of two years. They observed one peritoneal cancer among 98 women who chose salpingo-oophorectomy, versus five ovarian/peritoneal cancers in 72 women with intact ovaries. In a historical cohort study of 551 *BRCA1* and *BRCA2* carriers, Rebbeck et al. (49) reported that the incidence of ovarian or peritoneal cancer was diminished by 96% (95% confidence interval [CI], 84% to 99%) in women who underwent prophylactic oophorectomy, compared to those with intact ovaries.

Finch et al. followed 1,045 women with a mutation who underwent a bilateral prophylactic salpingo-oophorectomy and compared the cancer risk with 783 women who did not undergo the procedure (13). After a mean follow-up of 3.5 years, 50 incident ovarian, fallopian tube, or peritoneal cancer cases were reported in the cohort. There were 32 incident cancers diagnosed in women with intact ovaries. Eleven cancer cases were identified at the time of prophylactic oophorectomy, and seven were diagnosed following prophylactic oophorectomy. The overall reduction in cancer risk associated with bilateral oophorectomy was 80% (hazard ratio = 0.20; 95% CI, 0.07 to 0.58; p = 0.003). The estimated cumulative incidence of peritoneal cancer was 4.3% at 20 years after oophorectomy.

An additional benefit of prophylactic oophorectomy is a marked reduction in the risk of breast cancer (48–50). Oophorectomy performed at a relatively early age (<40) is associated with a greater degree of protection than surgery performed near the age of menopause. In the largest study to date, Eisen et al. found that oophorectomy was associated with a significant reduction in breast cancer risk of 56% for *BRCA1* carriers and 46% for *BRCA2* carriers (50). The risk reduction was greater if the oophorectomy was performed before age 40 (OR = 0.36) than after age 40 (OR = 0.53) and the protective effect was evident for 15 years postoophorectomy. Reductions of similar magnitude have been reported in other studies (48,49).

Hormone Replacement Therapy

Premenopausal oophorectomy is associated with the induction of acute menopause. There is concern that the use of hormone replacement therapy in these women may be associated with an increased risk of breast cancer, or may offset the protective effect of the oophorectomy itself. There is one study of hormone replacement therapy in *BRCA1* and *BRCA2* carriers. Rebbeck et al. estimated the effect of oophorectomy on breast cancer risk in a study of 462 *BRCA1* and *BRCA2* carriers (51). They found that the odds ratio for breast cancer associated with oophorectomy in the entire study group was 0.40 (95% CI, 0.18 to 0.92) and was 0.37 (95% CI, 0.14 to 0.96) in the subgroup of women with oophorectomies who used hormone replacement therapy. This single study suggests that it is safe to offer hormone replacement therapy, but this is a relatively small sample and additional studies are required.

Oral Contraceptives and Tubal Ligation

A protective effect of oral contraceptives against ovarian cancer has been reported in *BRCA* carriers (52–54). In a recent matched case-control study of 799 ovarian cancer cases and 2,424 controls, three to five years of oral contraceptive use was associated with a 64% reduction in the risk of ovarian cancer (p = 0.0001) (53). In a second, smaller study (54), six or more years of use of oral contraceptives was associated with a decrease in risk of 38% (OR = 0.62; 95% CI, 0.35 to 1.09). Tubal ligation has been found to be protective against ovarian cancer in the general population. There is some evidence that it is also effective among *BRCA1* carriers (53). McLaughlin et al. reported an adjusted relative risk of 0.78 (95% CI, 0.61 to 1.0) for tubal ligation and subsequent ovarian cancer (a risk reduction of 22%) (53).

Screening for Hereditary Ovarian Cancer

Screening for ovarian cancer using serial CA-125 levels and abdominal ultrasound has been proposed as a method of reducing mortality through early detection. There have been no randomized trials of screening in *BRCA1* carriers, but observational cohort studies have been disappointing. Liede et al. (10) identified seven incident ovarian/peritoneal cancers in a historical cohort of 33 *BRCA* carriers who underwent regular screening examinations. Six of the seven cases were stage III at the time of diagnosis. For the majority of cases, the ultrasound findings were normal prior to diagnosis and the women presented with pain or abdominal distension. In a randomized trial of CA-125 and ultrasound in women at average risk, Jacobs et al. (55) identified 16 ovarian cancers in the screened group. Eleven of the 16 tumors were diagnosed at stage III or IV. Neither CA-125 nor ultrasound has proven to be a sensitive means of detecting stage I and stage II ovarian cancers.

ENDOMETRIAL CANCER

The most important factor in the etiology of endometrial cancer is prolonged estrogen exposure, but inherited factors are important for a small proportion of cases as well. Susceptibility genes for endometrial cancer include *BRCA1, PTEN,* and the three mismatch repair genes *MSH2, MLH1,* and *MSH6* (Table 2.2). These genes are responsible for the hereditary breast-ovarian cancer syndrome, Cowden syndrome, and hereditary nonpolyposis colon cancer, respectively (discussed later).

TABLE 2.2

GENES ASSOCIATED WITH COMMON CANCERS

Breast	Ovary	Colon	Endometrial
BRCA1	*BRCA1*		
BRCA2	*BRCA2*	*APC*	
ATM	*MSH2*	*MSH2*	*MSH2*
CHEK2	*MLH1*	*MLH1*	*MLH1*
NBS1	*MSH6*	*MSH6*	*MSH6*
TP53			*PTEN*

The Breast Cancer Linkage Consortium reported that some endometrial cancers were due to mutations in *BRCA1* (56) but none were due to mutations in *BRCA2* (57). Among *BRCA1* carriers the risk for endometrial cancer was reported to be 2.6 times higher than expected (95% CI, 1.7 to 4.2). However, two smaller studies (one of patients with papillary serous endometrial tumors [58] and one on patients with endometrial carcinomas in general [59]) concluded that the risk of endometrial carcinoma in women with a germ-line *BRCA1* mutation was not increased. These findings suggest that it is likely that some cases of endometrial carcinoma are due to an inherited *BRCA1* mutation, but the penetrance of *BRCA1* mutations for endometrial carcinoma is low and the hereditary fraction is small.

Beiner et al. prospectively followed a cohort of *BRCA1* and *BRCA2* carriers who had an intact uterus (60). After an average follow-up period of 3.3 years, six women were diagnosed with endometrial cancer, compared to 1.1 cancers expected (SIR = 5.3, $p = 0.001$). Four of the six patients had used tamoxifen in the past. Among the 226 participants who had used tamoxifen (220 as treatment and six for the primary prevention of breast cancer) the relative risk for endometrial cancer was 12 ($p = 0.0004$). The risk among women who were never exposed to tamoxifen treatment was not significantly elevated. These data suggest that the excess risk of endometrial cancer among *BRCA* carriers can be attributed to past tamoxifen use, and not to the effect of the gene.

Somatic mutations in *PTEN* are common in endometrial cancers (61) and, rarely, inherited constitutional mutations in *PTEN* are present in women with endometrial cancer. In the latter case, endometrial cancer is seen in the context of Cowden syndrome—a rare dominant disease of the skin that is associated with increased risks of cancer of the breast, thyroid, and endometrium (62).

Women in families with the syndrome of hereditary familial nonpolyposis colon cancer (HNPCC) are also at elevated risk for endometrial and ovarian cancer (63). This syndrome is characterized by an autosomal dominant inherited tendency to develop colon and other cancers. The colon cancers tend to be of young onset, are right-sided, and are often multicentric. Adenomatous polyps are seen, but florid polyposis is rare. Individuals in families with HNPCC are at risk for a range of cancer types, and endometrial cancer is the second most frequent site of cancer among women (63,64). Genes that are responsible for the repair of mismatched DNA (mismatch repair) are defective in families with this syndrome. *MSH2, MLH1,* and *MSH6* are the three major genes responsible. The risk of colon cancer is high in families with a mutation in any of these genes, and the lifetime risk for endometrial cancer in women from these families is reported to be from 40% to 60% (63,64). The risk of endometrial cancer also depends on which gene carries the mutation. Mutations in *MSH2* and *MSH6* have been implicated in most HNPCC families with endometrial cancer, but families with *MSH1* mutations have been reported as well. Germ-line mutations in *MSH6* are relatively rare in HNPCC but are overrepresented in families with multiple cases of endometrial cancer (65). Goodfellow et al. reported that an inactivating germ-line *MSH6* mutation was present in 7 of 441 women with unselected ovarian cancer (1.6%) (66). Cancers were diagnosed in women with mutations on average ten years earlier than in women without mutations. Malander et al. studied 128 women with ovarian cancer, unselected for age of diagnosis or family history (67). They found one mutation in *MLH1* and one mutation in *MSH2*. This small study suggests that about 2% of unselected cases of ovarian cancer are due to mutations in the mismatch repair genes.

It is possible that other genetic variants in the genes in the mismatch repair pathway may also contribute to ovarian cancer. This may be due to the effect of common variants associated with lower penetrance. To test this hypothesis, Beiner et al. studied 672 unselected cases of endometrial cancer for a variant in the *MLH1* gene (nt-93 A) (68). They found that women who carried this variant were at 1.5-fold increased risk of endometrial cancer (OR = 1.5; 95% CI, 1.2 to 2.0). A positive association was also seen for ovarian cancer (OR = 1.5; 95% CI, 1.3 to 3.9) (69). A similar association has been seen for colon cancer with microsatellite instability (70).

The majority of tumors in individuals from HNPCC families demonstrate microsatellite instability. Microsatellite instability is a feature of tumors that are genetically unstable, i.e., that are associated with error-prone DNA replication during cell division. Microsatellite instability is limited to tumor DNA and the phenotype is visualized in the laboratory by comparison of tumor and lymphocyte DNA from the same individual. Microsatellite instability is highly predictive of colon and endometrial cancers that are attributable to mutations in one of three mismatch repair genes *(MSH2, MLH1,* and *MSH6)*. These mutations may be germ-line (inherited), but are more often somatic (restricted to tumor tissue only). Approximately one quarter of women with nonhereditary endometrial cancer (sporadic cancer) have tumors that demonstrate microsatellite instability (71). If the mutation is present in the germ line, it may be transmitted from the carrier parent to child. In this case, genetic counseling is warranted. Counseling should include a full pedigree review, and may involve predictive genetic testing for unaffected individuals. Other individuals found to carry the family mutation should be apprised of the risks and the range of tumor types involved. It is not necessary that genetic counseling be undertaken when the mutation is limited to the tumor tissue only, as this situation does not pose a risk to relatives. The gene may also be silenced by methylation of the gene regulatory regions. The *MLH1* gene is usually silenced through methylation in the tumor tissues (72).

Individuals with an inherited mutation in one of the mismatch repair genes are also at risk for additional cancers, including ovarian, gastric, urologic tract, and small bowel cancers, but the risk for these is much less than the risk for colon or endometrial cancer. Members of the International Collaborative Group on HNPCC collected information on 80 women with ovarian cancer who were members of HNPCC families (64). The mean age of diagnosis was 43 years. The majority of cancers were moderately or well differentiated and 85% were stage I or II. Synchronous endometrial cancer was reported in 22% of cases.

There is currently no consensus on the screening and management of women with inherited mutations in the mismatch repair genes. Annual endometrial ultrasound surveillance has been recommended by the International Collaborative Group on HNPCC, but the effectiveness of this screening regimen has not been established. Although there are no data on the effectiveness of hysterectomy as a preventive measure for hereditary endometrial cancer, there have been no reports of failures of hysterectomy to prevent endometrial cancer. Because of the high lifetime risk of endometrial cancer in women with mutations in the mismatch repair genes, preventive hysterectomy may be warranted.

References

1. Risch HA, McLaughlin JR, Cole DEC, et al. Prevalence and penetrance of germline *BRCA1* and *BRCA2* mutations in a population series of 649 women with ovarian cancer. *Am J Hum Genet* 2001;68:700–710.
2. Risch HA, McLaughlin J, Cole DE, et al. Population *BRCA1* and *BRCA2* mutation frequencies and cancer penetrances: a kin-cohort study in Ontario, Canada. *J Natl Cancer Inst* 2006;98:1694–1706.
3. Pal T, Permuth-Wey J, Betts J, et al. *BRCA1* and *BRCA2* mutations account for a large proportion of ovarian carcinoma cases. *Cancer* 2005;104: 2807–2816.
4. Moslehi R, Chu W, Karlan B, et al. *BRCA1* and *BRCA2* mutation analysis of 208 Ashkenazi Jewish women with ovarian cancer. *Am J Hum Genet* 2000;66:1259–1272.
5. Modan B, Hartge P, Hirsh-Yechezkel G, et al. Parity, oral contraceptives, and the risk of ovarian cancer among carriers and non-carriers of a *BRCA1* or *BRCA2* mutation. *N Engl J Med* 2001;345(4):235–240.
6. Menkiszak J, Gronwald J, Gorski B, et al. Hereditary ovarian cancer in Poland. *Int J Cancer* 2003;106:942–945.
7. Gorski B, Jakubowska A, Huzarski T, et al. A high proportion of founder *BRCA1* mutations in Polish breast cancer families. *Int J Cancer* 2004;110: 683–686.
8. Tonin MP, Mes-Masson AM, Narod SA, et al. Founder *BRCA1* and *BRCA2* mutations in French-Canadian ovarian cancer cases unselected for family history. *Clin Genet* 1999;55:318–324.
9. Liede A, Malik IA, Aziz Z, et al. Contribution of *BRCA1* and *BRCA2* mutations to breast and ovarian cancer in Pakistan. *Am J Hum Genet* 2002;71(3):595–606.
10. Liede A, Karlan BY, Baldwin RL, et al. Cancer incidence in a population of Jewish women at risk of ovarian cancer. *J Clin Oncol* 2002;20:1570–1577.
11. Kauff ND, Mitra N, Robson ME, et al. Risk of ovarian cancer in *BRCA1* and *BRCA2* mutation-negative hereditary breast cancer families. *J Natl Cancer Inst* 2005;97:1382–1384.
12. Phelan CM, Kwan E, Jack E, et al. A low frequency of non-founder mutations in Ashkenazi Jewish breast-ovarian cancer families. *Hum Mutat* 2002;20:352–357.
13. Finch A, Beiner M, Lubinski J, et al. Salpingo-oophorectomy and the risk of ovarian, fallopian tube and peritoneal cancers in women with a *BRCA1* or *BRCA2* mutation. *JAMA* 2006;296:185–192.
14. Ford D, Easton DF, Stratton M, et al. Genetic heterogeneity and penetrance analysis of the *BRCA1* and *BRCA2* genes in breast cancer families. *Am J Hum Genet* 1998;62:676–689.
15. Antoniou A, Pharaoh PD, Narod SA, et al. Average risks of breast and ovarian cancer associated with *BRCA1* or *BRCA2* mutations detected in case series unselected for ovarian cancer: a combined analysis of 22 studies. *Am J Hum Genet* 2003;72:1117–1130.
16. Thompson D, Easton D, Breast Cancer Linkage Consortium. Variation in cancer risks, by mutation position, in *BRCA2* mutation carriers. *Am J Hum Genet* 2001;68:410–419.
17. Satagopan JM, Boyd J, Kauff ND, et al. Ovarian cancer risk in Ashkenzi Jewish carriers of *BRCA1* and *BRCA2* mutations. *Clin Cancer Res* 2002;8:3776–3781.
18. Chen S, Parmigiani G. Meta-analysis of *BRCA1* and *BRCA2* penetrance. *J Clin Oncol* 2007;25:1320–1333.
19. Lubinski J, Phelan CM, Ghadirian P, et al. Cancer variation associated with the position of the mutation in the *BRCA* gene. *Fam Cancer* 2004;3:1–10.
20. Metcalfe KA, Lynch HT, Ghadirian P, et al. The risk of ovarian cancer after breast cancer in *BRCA1* and *BRCA2* carriers. *Gynecol Oncol* 2005;96: 222–226.
21. Boyd J, Sonoda Y, Federici MG, et al. Clinicopathologic features of *BRCA*-linked and sporadic ovarian cancer. *JAMA* 2000;283:2260–2265.
22. Werness BA, Ramus SJ, Whittemore AS, et al. Histopathology of familial ovarian tumors in women from families with and without germline *BRCA1* mutations. *Hum Pathol* 2000;31:1420–1424.
23. Lu KH, Garber JE, Cramer DE, et al. Occult ovarian tumours in women with *BRCA1* or *BRCA2* mutations undergoing prophylactic oophorectomy. *J Clin Oncol* 2000;18:2728–2732.
24. Johannsson OT, Ranstam J, Borg A, et al. Survival of *BRCA1* breast and ovarian cancer patients: a population-based study from southern Sweden. *J Clin Oncol* 1998;16:397–404.
25. Salazar H, Godwin AK, Daly MB, et al. Microscopic benign and invasive malignant neoplasms and a cancer-prone phenotype in prophylactic oophorectomies. *J Natl Cancer Inst* 1996;88:1810–1820.
26. Finch A, Shaw P, Rosen B, et al. Clinical and pathologic findings of prophylactic salpingo-oophorectomies in 159 *BRCA1* and *BRCA2* carriers. *Gynecol Oncol* 2006;100:58–64.
27. Callahan MJ, Crum CP, Medeiros F, et al. Primary fallopian tube malignancies in *BRCA*-positive women undergoing surgery for ovarian cancer risk reduction. *J Clin Oncol* 2007;25:3985–3990.
28. Powell CB, Kenley E, Chen LM, et al. Risk-reducing salpingo-oophorectomy in *BRCA* mutation carriers: role of serial sectioning in the detection of occult disease. *J Clin Oncol* 2005;23:127–132.
29. Medeiros F, Muto MG, Lee Y, et al. The tubal fimbria is a preferred site for early adenocarcinoma in women with familial ovarian cancer syndrome. *Am J Surg Pathol* 2006;30:230–236.
30. Narod SA, Sun P, Ghadirian P, et al. Tubal ligation and risk of ovarian cancer in carriers of *BRCA1* or *BRCA2* mutations: a case-control study. *Lancet* 2001;357:1467–1470.
31. Piek JM, van Diest PJ, Zweemer RP, et al. Tubal ligation and risk of ovarian cancer. *Lancet* 2001;358:844.
32. Crum CP, Drapkin R, Kindelberger D, et al. Lessons from *BRCA*: the tubal fimbria emerges as an origin for pelvic serous cancer. *Clin Med Res* 2007;5:35–44.
33. Aziz S, Kuperstein G, Rosen B, et al. A genetic epidemiological study of carcinoma of the fallopian tube. *Gynecol Oncol* 2001;80:341–345.
34. Westhoff C, Murphy P, Heller D, et al. Is ovarian cancer associated with an increased frequency of germinal inclusion cysts? *Am J Epidemiol* 1993;138: 90–93.
35. Stratton JF, Buckley CH, Lowe D, et al. Comparison of prophylactic oophorectomy specimens from carriers and noncarriers of a *BRCA1* or *BRCA2* gene mutation. *J Natl Cancer Inst* 1999;91:626–628.
36. Deligdisch L, Gil J, Kerner H, et al. Ovarian dysplasia in prophylactic oophorectomy specimens. *Cancer* 1999;86:1544–1550.
37. Barakat RR, Federici MG, Saigo PE, et al. Absence of premalignant histologic, molecular, or cell biological alterations in prophylactic oophorectomy specimens from *BRCA1* heterozygotes. *Cancer* 2000;89: 383–390.
38. Casey MJ, Bewtra C, Hoehne LL, et al. Histology of prophylactically removed ovaries from *BRCA1* and *BRCA2* mutation carriers compared with noncarriers in hereditary breast ovarian cancer syndrome kindreds. *Gynecol Oncol* 2000;78:278–287.
39. Pharoah PDP, Easton DF, Stockton DL, et al. Survival in familial, *BRCA1*-associated, and *BRCA2*-associated epithelial ovarian cancer. *Cancer Res* 1999;59:868–871.
40. McGuire V, Whittemore AS, Norris R, et al. Survival in epithelial ovarian cancer patients with prior breast cancer. *Am J Epidemiol* 2000;152:528–532.
41. Cass I, Baldwin RL, Varkey T, et al. Improved survival in women with *BRCA*-associated ovarian carcinoma. *Cancer* 2003;97:2127–2129.
42. Ben David Y, Chetrit A, Hirsch-Yechezkel G, et al. Effect of *BRCA* mutations on the length of survival in ovarian epithelial tumours. *J Clin Oncol* 2002;20:463–466.
43. Pal T, Permuth Wey J, Kapoor R, et al. Improved survival in *BRCA2* carriers with ovarian cancer. *Fam Cancer* 2007;6:113–119.
44. NIH Consensus Development Panel on Ovarian Cancer. Ovarian cancer: screening, treatment and follow-up. *JAMA* 1995;273:491–497.
45. Woolas R, Smith J, Paterson JM, et al. Fallopian tube carcinoma: an under-reported primary neoplasm. *Int J Gynecol Oncol* 1997;7:284–288.
46. Piver MS, Jishi MF, Tsukada Y, et al. Primary peritoneal carcinoma after prophylactic oophorectomy in women with a family history of ovarian cancer. A report from the Gilda Radner Family Ovarian Cancer Registry. *Cancer* 1993;71:2751–2755.
47. Struewing JP, Watson P, Easton DF, et al. Prophylactic oophorectomy in inherited breast/ovarian cancer families. *J Natl Cancer Inst Monogr* 1995;33–35.
48. Kauff ND, Satagopan JM, Robson ME, et al. Risk-reducing salpingo-oophorectomy in women with a *BRCA1* mutation. *N Engl J Med* 2002; 346:1609–1615.
49. Rebbeck TR, Lynch HT, Neuhausen SL, et al. Prophylactic oophorectomy in carriers of *BRCA1* and *BRCA2* mutations. *N Engl J Med* 2002;346: 1616–1622.
50. Eisen A, Lubinski J, Klijn J, et al. Breast cancer risk following bilateral oophorectomy in *BRCA1* and *BRCA2* mutation carriers: an international case-control study. *J Clin Oncol* 2005;23:7491–7496.
51. Rebbeck HRT, Rebbeck TR, Friebel T, et al. Effect of short-term hormone replacement therapy on breast cancer risk reduction after bilateral prophylactic oophorectomy in *BRCA1* and *BRCA2* mutation carriers: the PROSE Study Group. *J Clin Oncol* 2005;23:7804–7810.
52. Narod SA, Risch H, Mosleh R, et al. Oral contraceptives and the risk of hereditary ovarian cancer. *N Engl J Med* 1998;339:424–428.
53. McLaughlin JR, Risch HA, Lubinski J, et al. Reproductive risk factors for ovarian cancer in carriers of *BRCA1* or *BRCA2* mutations: a case-control study. *Lancet Oncol* 2007;8:26–34.
54. Whittemore AS, Balise RR, Pharoah PD, et al. Oral contraceptive use and ovarian cancer risk among carriers of *BRCA1* or *BRCA2* mutations. *Br J Cancer* 2004;91:1911–1915.
55. Jacobs I, Skates SJ, MacDonald N, et al. Screening for ovarian cancer: a pilot randomized control trial. *Lancet* 1999;353(9160):1207–1210.
56. Thompson D, Easton DF, Breast Cancer Linkage Consortium. Cancer incidence in *BRCA1* mutation carriers. *J Natl Cancer Inst* 2002;94L: 1358–1365.

57. Breast Cancer Linkage Consortium. Cancer risks in *BRCA2* mutations carriers. *J Natl Cancer Inst* 1999;91:1310–1316.
58. Goshen R, Chu W, Elit L, et al. Is uterine papillary serous adenocarcinoma a manifestation of the hereditary breast-ovarian cancer syndrome? *Gynecol Oncol* 2000;79:477–481.
59. Levine DA, Lin O, Barakat RR, et al. Risk of endometrial carcinoma associated with *BRCA* mutation. *Gynecol Oncol* 2001;80:395–398.
60. Beiner ME, Finch A, Rosen B, et al. The risk of endometrial cancer in women with *BRCA1* or *BRCA2* mutations. A prospective study. *Gynecol Oncol* 2007;104(1):7–10.
61. Zhou XP, Kusismanen S, Nystrom-Lahti M, et al. Distinct *PTEN* mutational spectrum in hereditary non-polyposis cancer syndrome-related endometrial carcinomas compared to sporadic microsatellite unstable tumors. *Hum Molec Genet* 2002;11:445–450.
62. Eng C. *PTEN:* one gene, many syndromes. *Hum Mutat* 2003;22:183–198.
63. Watson P, Lynch HT. Cancer risk in mismatch repair gene carriers. *Fam Cancer* 2001;1:57–60.
64. Watson P, Butzow R, Lynch HT, et al. The clinical features of ovarian cancer in hereditary non-polyposis colorectal cancer. *Gynecol Oncol* 2001;82:223–228.
65. Wijnen J, de Leeuw W, Vasen H, et al. Familial endometrial cancer in female carriers of *MSH6* germline mutations. *Nat Genet* 1999;23:142–144.
66. Goodfellow PJ, Buttin BM, Herzog TJ, et al. Prevalence of defective DNA mismatch repair and *MSH6* mutation in an unselected series of endometrial cancers. *Proc Natl Acad Sci USA* 2003;100:5908–5913.
67. Malander S, Rambech E, Kristoffersson U, et al. The contribution of the hereditary non-polyposis colorectal cancer syndrome to the development of ovarian cancer. *Gynecol Oncol* 2006;101:238–243.
68. Beiner ME, Rosen B, Fyles A, et al. Endometrial cancer risk is associated with variants of the mismatch repair genes *MLH1* and *MSH2*. *Cancer Epidemiol Biomarkers Prev* 2006;15:1636–1640.
69. Harley I, Rosen B, Risch HA, et al. Ovarian cancer risk is associated with a common variant in the promoter sequence of the mismatch repair gene *MLH1*. *Gynecol Oncol* 2008;109(3):384–387.
70. Raptis S, Mrkonjic M, Green RC, et al. *MLH1* –93G>A promoter polymorphism and the risk of microsatellite-unstable colorectal cancer. *J Natl Cancer Inst* 2007;99:463–474.
71. Gurin CC, Federci MG, Kang L, et al. Causes and consequences of microsatellite instability in endometrial carcinoma. *Cancer Res* 1999;59: 462–466.
72. Simpkins SB, Bocker T, Swisher EM, et al. *MLH1* promoter methylation and gene silencing is the primary cause of microsatellite instability in sporadic endometrial cancers. *Hum Mol Genet* 1999;8:661–666.

CHAPTER 3 ■ THE BIOLOGY OF GYNECOLOGIC CANCER

KRISTIN K. ZORN, GINGER J. GARDNER, JOHN H. FARLEY, AND MICHAEL J. BIRRER

INTRODUCTION TO THE BIOLOGY OF GYNECOLOGIC NEOPLASIA

A neoplasm represents new growth and may be defined as an abnormal mass of tissue, the growth of which exceeds and is uncoordinated with that of the normal tissues. Growth persists in the same excessive manner after cessation of the stimuli that evoked the change (1). Neoplasia traditionally has been classified as benign or malignant on the basis of structural and growth characteristics. Most benign tumors mimic their tissue of origin in both cellular form and function. Cancerous tumors exhibit a spectrum from well differentiated to anaplastic (undifferentiated, characterized by both cytologic pleomorphism and architectural disorganization). Benign masses are typically well demarcated, with a broad, expansive front, and do not invade local normal tissues. Although some malignancies grossly appear to be encapsulated, they may infiltrate adjacent noncancerous tissue. In addition, malignancies tend to have a faster growth rate that is, in general, inversely related to the degree of differentiation. Finally, the ability to metastasize, a behavior that many malignant tumors exhibit, is a feature that benign tumors uniformly lack (2).

Nonneoplastic processes can alter the structure and/or function of a tissue, but are usually reversible. These conditions represent an adaptation to stress, such as an injury or infection, or a physiologic response to biochemical (e.g., hormonal) stimulation. *Hypertrophy* refers to an increase in cell size within a tissue, whereas *hyperplasia* is an increase in cell number. *Metaplasia* describes the process by which one differentiated cell type is replaced with another. *Dysplasia* is disordered cellular proliferation characterized by structural variability and disorganization of tissue architecture. When the full thickness of an epithelium is involved through this process, it is termed carcinoma *in situ*, and is considered to be a preinvasive process (2).

Biologic Properties of Transformed Cells and Tumors

Our understanding of the biologic behavior of malignant cells has been derived from *in vitro* comparisons of normal and transformed cells, the study of cell lines established by culturing human cancer cells, and the evaluation of tumors transplanted or induced in animals. Normal human cells display a finite ability to proliferate in cell culture, stopping after about 50 generations of cell division. These cells have specific requirements for growth, including the availability of nutrients and growth factors, attachment to a substratum, and lack of contact with other cells. In the event of temporary nutritional deprivation, they will arrest in a nonproliferative state but retain the capacity to resume replication with replenishment of growth-promoting substances.

Malignant cells, in contrast, demonstrate decreased reliance on exogenous growth factors, anchorage independence, and a lack of contact inhibition. As a result, transformed cells generally require less serum and supplements to grow, demonstrate nonadherent growth (such as growth in suspension or in a semisolid medium), and exhibit greater cell-population density. Cellular transformation produces disorganization of actin filaments, which results in more rounded, refractile cells.

Depending on location and accessibility to physical examination or imaging techniques, most tumors become clinically detectable at a mass of 1 to 10 g (10^9 to 10^{10} cells). A tumor mass of 1 kg (10^{12} cells) represents approximately 40 doublings and is generally lethal to the host in animal models. The time it takes for a given human malignancy to double in volume is usually constant, consistent with an exponential growth pattern (Fig. 3.1). Tumors frequently demonstrate a growth deceleration generally attributed to inadequate nutrition as they enlarge. Extrapolation into the preclinical phase reveals a slower rate of growth during this portion of the tumor's life span as well, which may be related to the early growth requirements of establishing a supporting vascular network and overcoming the host's immune surveillance.

Doubling times for human malignancies range from a few days for certain lymphomas and leukemias to up to several months for epithelial tumors such as lung and colorectal carcinomas. The growth rates for tumors of identical origin and histology may also be quite variable. A formula that includes the growth fraction and duration of DNA synthesis may be used to estimate the theoretical doubling time for a given tumor. This potential tumor doubling time is often considerably shorter than the actual doubling time seen clinically (3). Reasons for this discrepancy include tumor cell death (apoptosis or necrosis) or lowered growth fraction due to cellular senescence, in part due to the lack of an adequate vascular supply.

Cell Cycle, Senescence, Apoptosis, and Necrosis

Cell Cycle

During the process of replication, a cell passes through a series of phases beginning with DNA synthesis (S phase) and culminating in mitosis (M phase), the process by which the cell actually divides (Fig. 3.2). These two periods are separated by the presynthetic (G_1) and premitotic (G_2) phases. Cells that

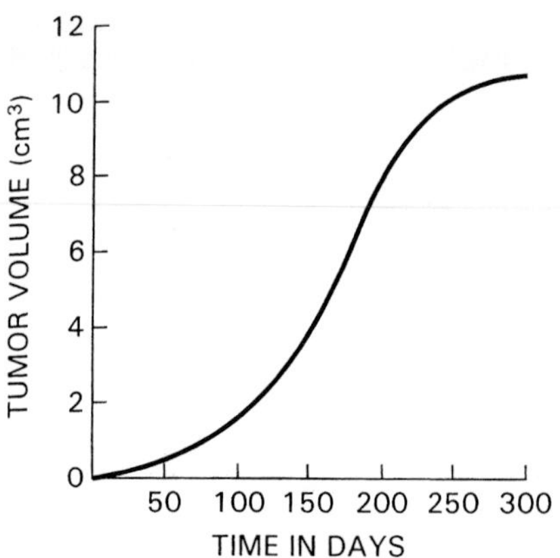

FIGURE 3.1. An exponential growth curve with preclinical lag and terminal growth deceleration. The abscissa represents time of tumor growth in days. The ordinate displays tumor volume in square centimeters. A slower rate of tumor growth is shown during the tumor's preclinical phase as well as when it attains a large volume.

are not actively proliferating are in the G_0 phase. Some of these nonproliferating cells retain the ability to progress through the cell cycle given the appropriate stimulus and environmental conditions. Others have lost the capacity for replication, which occurs secondary to terminal differentiation or damage sufficient to result in eventual cell death. The proportion of cells in a tumor that are actively proliferating is known as the tumor's growth fraction (3).

Entry into and transit through the cell cycle appear to be controlled by a number of regulatory proteins (3). Events necessary for G_0/G_1 cells to enter the S phase include the transduction of growth factor signals to the nucleus and the activation of "early response" genes, whose products bind to DNA and regulate the expression of other genes necessary for progression through the cell cycle (Fig. 3.3). The proteins necessary for this progression include the cyclins, cyclin-dependent kinases (CDKs), and the CDK inhibitors (4,5). It is now abundantly clear that progression through the cell cycle requires the interaction of these proteins in a coordinated fashion.

The cyclins are a group of proteins that are synthesized and degraded during the cell cycle. They can be divided into two major classes depending on where in the cell cycle they are active: the G_1 cyclins include cyclins D, A, and E, whereas the mitotic cyclins include cyclins A and B. The cyclins bind to and activate the CDKs. The cyclin/CDK complex is critical for the phosphorylation and activation of proteins and enzymes involved in DNA replication. For instance, the cyclin D/CDK4, cyclin D/CDK6, cyclin E/CDK2, and cyclin A/CDK2 complexes phosphorylate the retinoblastoma gene product (pRb) (6). pRb is a protein with tumor-suppressor function. The Rb protein and a structurally related protein, p107, are modified by a variety of different cyclins and CDKs (7). Their phosphorylation results in the release of transcription factor E2F, which then drives the transcription of "growth genes" (8–10). Another example is the activation of the protein kinase $p34^{cdc\text{-}2}$ by dephosphorylation and binding to a regulatory cofactor, which appears important for cell cycle transit. Kinase activity is maximal during mitosis, when $p34^{cdc\text{-}2}$ is bound to the protein cyclin B.

The stimulatory activity of cyclin/CDK complexes is opposed by CDK inhibitors (4). The CDK inhibitors are a group of small proteins that are able to directly inhibit the activity of the cyclin/CDK complex. The G_1 cyclin/CDK complexes are inhibited by p15, p16, and p27.

The interaction of cyclins, CDKs, and CDK inhibitors provides for a regulated progression through the cell cycle (5). The cell passes through a number of checkpoints where assurance of proper completion of prior phases is required (11,12). If this assurance is not achieved, the cell arrests. The p53 protein mediates two of these checkpoints (13). Overexpression of wild-type (nonmutated) p53 arrests cell cycle progression in G_1 at or near a restriction point regulating the G_1/S transition, in part by transcriptionally activating the expression of the CDK inhibitor p21 Waf1/Cip1 (13). Although routine cellular functions may not require the presence of p53, conditions such as DNA damage and cellular stress stimulate the expression of p53 and produce a G_1 arrest (5). If the DNA damage is minor, it is repaired during this arrest; extensive damage causes the cell to undergo apoptosis (discussed below) (14). Elevated levels of p53 can also produce a G_2/M arrest, providing another period of rest for the cell during which it can repair damaged chromosomes. Although the mechanism for G_2 arrest is less clear than that involved in the G_1 checkpoint, it appears to involve the inactivation of mitotic cyclins A and B (15–17). The formation of a functional mitotic spindle is critical for successful cell division. It is not surprising, therefore, that a checkpoint exists during mitotic spindle formation (18). The genes involved in this process have only recently been characterized, but some appear to be involved in human cancers (19).

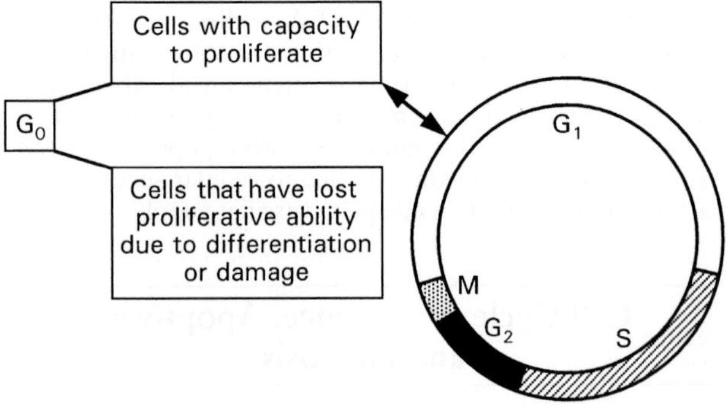

FIGURE 3.2. The cell cycle. The normal cell cycle, with relative time spent in each phase, is illustrated. G_0 cells are "resting," with an ability to replicate given the appropriate conditions and stimulus, or they have lost the ability to proliferate secondary to damage, death, or differentiation. G_1 represents the presynthetic phase; DNA synthesis occurs during the S phase; G_2 is the premitotic phase; and M represents mitosis, the briefest portion of the cycle.

Senescence

Cell growth slows as the finite number of cell doublings, known as the Hayflick limit, approaches (20). This process is governed by the loss of telomeres on chromosomal ends. Telomeres are protective DNA sequences rich in TTAGGG repeats that are shortened with successive replications. When the ends become critically shortened, the cell enters replicative senescence or mortality stage 1. In epithelial cells, the first barrier appears to be mediated by stress-induced cyclin-dependent kinase inhibitors (CKIs) (p16, p21) inhibiting Rb inactivation (21). Some cells escape senescence and continue to divide until they undergo crisis, which is also known as mortality stage 2. The rare cell that emerges from this stage still able to replicate is considered to be immortalized because it has acquired the ability to proliferate indefinitely. Continued telomere erosion in cells that overcame the first barrier eventually leads to unprotected telomeric ends generating widespread genomic instability. Immortalized cells are able to continue dividing because they maintain telomere length, usually through reactivation of telomerase (21,22). Telomerase is an RNA-dependent DNA polymerase that synthesizes the telomeric DNA sequences. It consists of an RNA template, which is universally

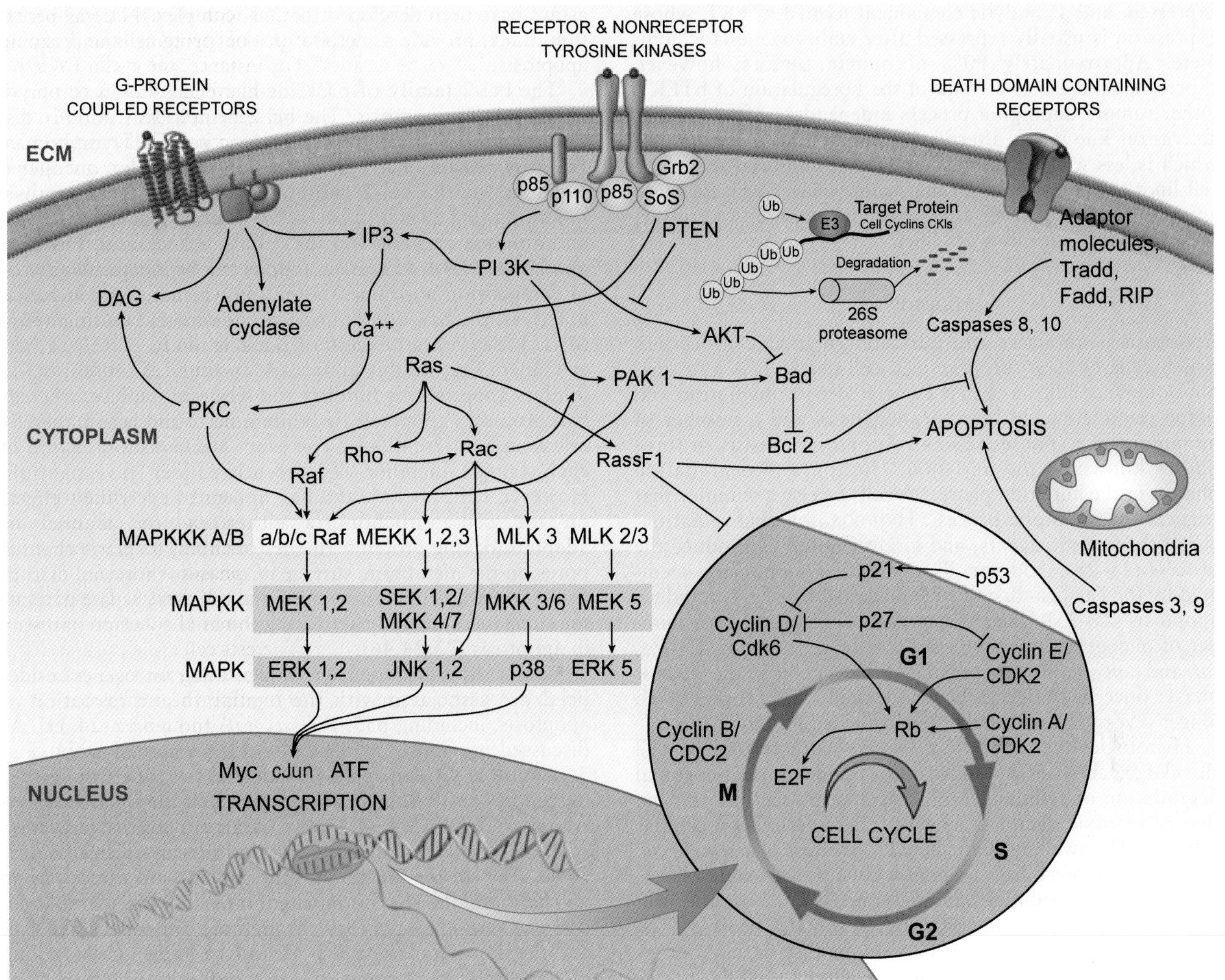

FIGURE 3.3. Signal transduction, regulation of the cell cycle, ubiquitin proteasome protein degradation, and apoptotic pathways. The covalent modification of intracellular constituents is illustrated by receptor and nonreceptor protein tyrosine kinases. Input from tyrosine kinases results in increased generation of activated ras bound to GTP, which in turn associates with ras effectors: raf, Rho, Rac, and RassF1. Raf (MAPKKK) propagates the signal to microtubule-associated protein kinase kinase (MAPKK), which activates MAPK. MAPK phosphorylates a host of substrates, including cytoplasmic phospholipase A_2, cytoskeletal components, protein synthesis machinery, and, most importantly, transcription factors such as myc, cJun, and ATF. Parallel pathways exist that use different MAPKKKs, MAPKKs, and MAPKs. Different MAPKs, such as ERK, JNK, and p38, phosphorylate and activate downstream targets that ultimately drive the cell cycle. The upstream activators of the MAPKKK are not as well characterized as other portions of the cascade; as such, only ras, PAK 1, and rac have been listed for simplicity. Although the MAP kinase cascades are parallel in nature, there is extensive cross talk between these pathways. The generation of "secondary messengers" that act upon intracellular receptor sites is exemplified by G-protein-coupled receptors. G-proteins interact with adenylate cyclase and certain phospholipases. Consequent hydrolysis of membrane phosphatidylinositol 4,5-bis-phosphate yields inositol 1,4,5-tris-phosphate (IP 3), which releases Ca^2, from internal stores, and diacylglycerol (DAG), which activates protein kinase C (PKC). Activation of PI3K by tyrosine kinases increases IP 3 levels, allowing cross talk between growth factor and G-protein-coupled receptors. The ultimate effect of growth factors is to trigger the enzymatic cascade involving cyclins and cyclin-dependent kinases (CDKs) that play critical roles in stimulating cells to enter and transit through the cell cycle. The protein levels of cyclins and CDKs are controlled by ubiquitylating enzymes. Ubiquitin (Ub) is a small 8-kDa protein, which is covalently attached to the target protein by E3 ubiquitin ligase, leading to the formation of a polyubiquitin chain. The polyubiquitylated protein is recognized by the 26S proteosome, and is destroyed in an ATP-dependent manner. Extrinsic apoptotic pathways are triggered by activation of a variety of receptors (Fas, TNF-R) containing death domains, which leads to the activation of caspases and programmed cell death (apoptosis). Intrinsic apoptotic pathways are activated by a wide range of stress stimuli and result in an up-regulation of proapoptotic mediators (BCL-2 members) on the outer mitochondrial membrane, with subsequent apoptosome assembly and activation of caspases and apoptosis. These pathways have extensive cross talk with other cellular pathways, including the one depicted here. Elevated activity of PI3K leads to activation of AKT, which in turn phosphorylates Bad, leaving its protein partner Bcl-2 available to inhibit apoptosis.

expressed, and a catalytic component termed hTERT, whose expression is usually repressed after embryogenesis is complete. Approximately 90% of human tumors, however, express telomerase as a result of the upregulation of hTERT. Other tumors undergo a process independent of telomerase activation known as alternative lengthening of telomeres, which is less well understood. Although immortalized, these cell lines are generally not tumorigenic when implanted into animals. Further genetic alterations are required to convert these into tumor-forming cell lines.

Apoptosis

Apoptosis is an active and intricately regulated process in which cells undergo programmed cell death. It is a normal physiologic condition that is associated with involution and tissue remodeling during morphogenesis and a number of immunologic responses (23,24). Apoptosis consists of three phases known as the initiation, effector, and degradation phases. In the initiation phase, the cells receive a stimulus that triggers the apoptotic process. Hypoxia, ionizing radiation, chemotherapeutic agents, and viral infection can induce the process (25–28). Additionally, cytotoxic lymphocytes, mediated by the Fas ligand, and p53, mediated by *bax*, can induce apoptosis (29–33). The entire process is regulated by a number of oncogenes and tumor-suppressor genes (p53, *Rb*, *ras*, *raf*, and c-*myc*) (34). Apoptosis is still reversible in the effector phase; once degradation begins, though, the process is no longer reversible and cellular death ensues (24, 28).

Histologically, apoptotic cells are characterized by cell shrinkage, chromatin condensation, and internucleosomal degradation of cellular DNA. This appearance differs from that of hypoxic necrosis, which is characterized by cellular swelling. The swelling is attributed to the loss of selective cell membrane permeability and to mitochondrial swelling, resulting in plasma membrane rupture with DNA, RNA, and protein degradation from the release of lysosomal hydrolases. The enzymatic degradation leads to an intense inflammatory response in the surrounding tissue, resulting in cellular necrosis (23,24,35). In contrast, this inflammatory response does not occur with apoptosis. During the final stages of apoptosis, the cell becomes convoluted and breaks into several membrane-bound vesicles containing intact organelles and nuclear fragments. Typically 180 to 200 base pairs in length, DNA fragments are the biochemical hallmark of apoptosis and can be used for morphologic analysis (24,35). Although apoptotic cells can be visualized and quantified with routine staining of tumor material, techniques using labeling of the 3′ free ends of the DNA fragments by radioactive or nonradioactive means allow for accurate identification of single apoptotic cells and quantification of the extent of apoptosis in tumor material via an apoptotic index (24,36,37). The index commonly measures either the number of apoptotic cells per 1,000 tumor cells or per ten high-power fields (24,38,39).

Apoptosis can be induced by cytotoxic lymphocytes ($CD8^+$ T lymphocytes) via the Fas ligand/receptor pathway (30,31). Fas (or Apo-1) is a glycosylated transmembrane receptor belonging to the tumor necrosis factor (TNF) receptor family. The binding of Fas receptor to Fas ligand (FasL), a transmembrane protein present on cytotoxic T lymphocytes, activates a pathway eventually leading to apoptotic cellular death (30,31). Downstream of the Fas receptor is FADD (Fas-associated death domain), which binds to a conserved amino acid sequence known as the "death domain" of the cytoplasmic end of the Fas receptor. Together, these two proteins form an apoptotic signaling complex with FLICE (FADD-like interleukin-2 converting enzyme [ICE], also known as caspase-8). Recently, caspases have been identified as the "common final pathway" in the execution of apoptosis in highly divergent systems (31). Caspase assays have been developed that, as with the DNA fragmentation index, provide a method of identifying cells undergoing apoptosis.

The bcl-2 family of proteins has been shown to play a major role in apoptosis. The bcl-2 protein was initially discovered as an overexpressed protein in B-cell lymphomas. For this reason, bcl-2 is considered to be an oncogene. Members of the bcl-2 protein family are both apoptosis inhibiting (bcl-2, bcl-xl, bcl-w, bfl-1, brag-1, mcl-1, and A1) and apoptosis promoting (bax, bak, bcl-xS, bad, bid, bik, and Hrk) (24,40–45). Their actions can be independent of or in competition with one another. For instance, when bax is in excess, the bax homodimers predominate, favoring apoptosis. However, an excess of bcl-2 leads to bcl-2/bax heterodimers that inhibit apoptosis. In other examples, bcl-xl inhibits apoptosis by binding and sequestering bax, whereas bad promotes apoptosis by binding bcl-2 and bcl-xl, thereby releasing bax (24,43,44). The exact mechanism of action of each family member is currently under investigation. However, bcl-2, bcl-xl, and bax appear to exert their effects on the cell mitochondria either as ion channel or adapter/docking proteins. As these proteins form ion channel pores on the membrane surface of the mitochondria, disruption of the transmembrane potential releases caspase-activating substances, thereby activating the final common pathway in apoptosis (23,24,46).

Tumor-suppressor genes as well as other oncogenes besides bcl-2 are associated with the regulation and execution of apoptosis, including p53, *Rb*, *ras*, *raf*, and c-*myc* (24,34). As discussed previously, p53 monitors the status of DNA (Fig. 3.3). With DNA damage, p53 stalls the cell cycle through the induction of CIP/WAF/p21, a protein that prevents phosphorylation of CDKs (24,34,47,48). CDKs are positive regulators of the cell cycle. In the absence of this phosphorylated (active) CDK, Rb will remain unphosphorylated, and the cell cycle will halt until the DNA is repaired. If the DNA is not repaired, p53 can promote apoptosis through the upregulation of bax and the downregulation of bcl-2 (24,34,49,50). Cells lacking p53 are resistant to some apoptotic induction events, such as ionizing radiation, chemotherapeutic agents, loss of Rb, and expression of c-myc. The effect of c-myc on the apoptotic process is growth-factor dependent. It induces proliferation in the presence of growth factors, but in their absence has apoptotic effects (24,51). Overexpression of ras may lead to increased or decreased apoptosis (24,52–54). Additionally, ras-induced apoptosis is inhibited by bcl-2. However, phosphorylation of bcl-2 negates its capacity to protect cells from ras-induced apoptosis (24,55).

Several investigators have examined differing aspects of apoptotic mechanisms in gynecologic malignancies (56–61). In general, overexpression of the oncogenes *bcl-2* and *bcl-xl* protects many cell types against inducers of apoptosis (hypoxia, ionizing radiation, chemotherapeutic agents, and viral infection), and therefore promotes tumorigenesis. Additionally, downregulation of the p53 tumor-suppressor gene or of the proapoptotic *bax* gene also promotes tumorigenesis. In gynecologic malignancies, bcl-2 is strongly expressed in normal endometrial epithelium and is downregulated in atypical hyperplasia and endometrial adenocarcinoma. However, the use of bcl-2 expression as a prognostic factor is not well established (59). With respect to p53, immunohistochemical detection of p53 in tissue correlates closely with the presence of mutations in the gene, which is attributable to a much longer half-life of the mutated protein. Mutations of p53 are absent in normal endometrium but present in endometrial cancer, particularly the endometrioid subtype; p53 expression in endometrial cancer has been shown to correlate with tumor type, stage, and grade but not significantly with prognosis (57,60,62–66).

Necrosis

Historically, three types of cell death have been distinguished in mammalian cells by morphological criteria. Type I cell death, better known as apoptosis, is defined by characteristic changes in the nuclear morphology, including chromatin condensation (pyknosis) and fragmentation (karyorrhexis) (67). All of these changes occur before plasma membrane integrity is lost. Type II cell death is characterized by a massive accumulation of two-membrane autophagic vacuoles in the cytoplasm. Type III cell death, better known as necrosis, is often defined in a negative manner as death lacking the characteristics of the type I and type II processes, and is usually considered to be uncontrolled (67). Necrosis can include signs of controlled processes such as mitochondrial dysfunction, enhanced generation of reactive oxygen species, adenosine 5′-triphosphate (ATP) depletion, proteolysis by calpains and cathepsins, and early plasma membrane rupture (67). Recent research suggests, however, that the process of necrosis might be tightly regulated. Specific processes thought to be involved in the regulation of necrosis include receptor-induced necrotic cell death through receptor interacting protein RIP1 and cyclophilin D. RIP kinases constitute a family of seven members and are crucial regulators of cell survival and death (68). RIP kinases are classified as serine/threonine kinases and are closely related to members of the interleukin-1 receptor-associated kinase (IRAK) family. RIP1 and RIP2 (CARDIAK/RICK) also bear a C-terminal domain belonging to the death domain, allowing recruitment to large protein complexes initiating different signaling pathways (68). Cyclophilin D is a mitochondrial matrix protein that can interact with inner membrane proteins and participate in the opening of nonspecific channels, causing dissipation of the inner mitochondrial transmembrane potential (67). Knockout of the cyclophilin D gene induces resistance to necrotic cell death.

In Vivo Biology

Proliferation Indices

Various methods have been developed to measure the percentage of cells actively proliferating, the percentage of cells in specific phases of the cell cycle, the duration of different phases, and the total cell-cycle time. The labeling index (LI) is a crude estimate of the percentage of proliferating cells within a tumor. The LI identifies the proportion of cells that have completed S phase during the assay by using autoradiography to detect ^{3}H-thymidine that has been incorporated into cellular DNA. Another crude estimate of proliferation is given by the mitotic index (MI), which relies on enumeration of mitotic figures. This measure is limited by the relatively short duration of mitosis and the ability to correctly identify cells in mitosis. The percent labeled mitosis (PLM) method is used to estimate the duration of the cell cycle and its component phases. Serial biopsies are obtained after thymidine injection to follow the labeled cohort of cells as it passes through the cell cycle. Ideally, waves of labeled mitoses of width T_S (S-phase duration) are separated by T_C (cell-cycle duration). Phase duration variability, however, causes dampening of these waves. Computer models are required to generate approximations of the phase and cycle times. Drawbacks of the PLM method include the preferential collection of data from the cells with shorter cycle times and the inability to distinguish nonproliferating from slowly proliferating cells (3).

Flow cytometry has been used to analyze the cell cycle and growth fraction. The histogram generated by fluorescent emission allows estimation of the proportion of cells with DNA content that is diploid (G_1 and G_0 cells), tetraploid (G_2 and M cells), or intermediate (S-phase cells). The S-phase fraction (SPF) provides an approximation of the growth fraction. Phase determination may be complicated by background contamination due to cellular debris and by the imprecision involved in interpreting DNA distribution, especially in the presence of aneuploidy. A more specific method for estimating the SPF involves the administration of a nonradioactive DNA precursor, such as 5-bromodeoxyuridine or 5-iododeoxyuridine, followed by treatment with a DNA-intercalating fluorescent dye. The precursor may be recognized in denatured DNA by a fluorescent-labeled monoclonal antibody. Two-parameter flow cytometry is used to follow the labeled cohort of cells as it traverses the cell cycle. This method can generate estimates for T_S and LI from a single biopsy performed at a known interval after administration of the precursor. Similar to the PLM method, however, these flow cytometric measurements favor data collection from the most rapidly dividing cells. Another application of flow cytometry is the estimation of growth fraction via fluorescent-labeled antibody recognition of cellular antigens expressed only by actively proliferating cells (proliferation-dependent antigens) (3).

Estimates for the LI or SPF of solid human malignancies are generally in the range of 3% to 15%, a proliferation rate lower than that of normal bone marrow and intestinal epithelium, but higher than that of other normal tissues such as liver and lung (31). Typical values for tumor T_S and T_C are 12 to 24 hours and 2 to 3 days, respectively. These values are somewhat longer than comparable estimates for nonmalignant, rapidly proliferating tissues. Many studies have addressed indices of proliferation for gynecologic malignancies. The PI (proliferation index, generally defined as %S + G_2 cells) and SPF are the measures that are commonly used. SPF and PI have been used as both discrete and continuous variables when establishing levels of significance.

Some retrospective investigations of epithelial ovarian cancer have found the SPF or PI to be prognostic indicators, while others have not (69–72). A prospective evaluation of 47 cases of ovarian carcinoma of all stages assessed SPF and expression of Ki-67, a proliferation-dependent nuclear antigen. Expression of Ki-67 and elevated SPF were both found to confer an adverse prognosis. When the cases were stratified by disease dissemination, stage I/II versus stage III/IV, the SPF retained its significance within both groups (73).

Increasing SPF and PI have been noted to accompany increasing severity of endometrial hyperplasia (74); several investigators have also found a correlation between advanced grade and elevated indices in endometrial carcinoma (75–77). Two prospective studies, including 304 evaluable clinical stage I/II patients and 101 patients of all stages of endometrial cancer, reported SPF to be of independent prognostic significance in multivariate analyses (75,77). Another prospective study of 209 clinical stage I/II cases, however, found a high PI not to have adverse implications (78).

Increasing proliferative activity, as measured by mitotic index, has been reported to correlate with increasing degree of cervical dysplasia (79). One prospective evaluation of 242 squamous cell carcinoma patients of all stages found SPF to be significantly related to survival in both univariate and multivariate analyses, whereas another prospective study of 195 similar cases determined that SPF alone did not predict survival (80,81). A few investigators have noted the subset of diploid cases with high proliferative indices to have a significantly worsened prognosis (81–83).

Some studies of proliferation have assessed the less commonly occurring gynecologic malignancies. Retrospective analyses of uterine sarcomas have revealed the mitotic index or SPF to be useful for predicting clinical outcome (84–86). For discriminating molar versus nonmolar hydropic gestations, elevated SPF was found to be useful in one study, but not in another (87,88). In an evaluation of 51 complete mole patients with available follow-up, no significant difference was noted in the SPF for those with persistent disease versus those without (88). A retrospective evaluation of 42 cases with all stages of squamous cell carcinoma of the vulva failed to show a significant association between SPF and recurrence or overall survival (89).

Precursor Lesions

A wide range of neoplasia is encountered in gynecology. Squamous cell carcinoma of the cervix has the most well-defined precursor lesion among the gynecologic malignancies in the form of cervical dysplasia. High-grade cervical dysplasia has a known high propensity for eventual infiltration into the subepithelial tissue, whereas most low-grade dysplasia will spontaneously regress (90). Endometrial cancer has two forms of precursor lesions: endometrioid endometrial cancer is associated with atypical hyperplasia arising in a setting of estrogen excess, whereas serous and some clear cell endometrial cancer arises from endometrial intraepithelial neoplasia (EIN) in a setting of atrophy (91). A precursor lesion for epithelial ovarian cancer has not been identified consistently, although some researchers have found dysplasia of the ovarian surface epithelium, particularly in ovarian inclusion cysts, to be associated with ovarian cancer (92). Atypical endometriosis appears to be a preinvasive lesion for 28% of endometrioid and 49% of clear cell ovarian cancers (92). Further evaluation of all of these precursor lesions is under way to define the critical events that cause a small fraction of them to progress to overt cancer while the rest remain premalignant or even regress.

Gynecologic neoplasms range from noninvasive benign tumors, such as uterine leiomyomata, to aggressive malignancies, such as high-grade epithelial ovarian carcinoma. Ovarian tumors of low malignant potential (LMP, also called borderline tumors) are relatively unique with respect to the criteria distinguishing benign from malignant neoplasia. Although originally thought to represent a preinvasive stage in ovarian malignancy, recent molecular evidence suggests a more complicated relationship between LMP and invasive tumors. Serous LMP tumors do not have p53 mutations and display loss of heterogeneity (LOH) on the long arm of the inactivated X chromosome, whereas invasive serous ovarian cancer frequently displays p53 mutations and has a different pattern of LOH involving multiple chromosomes (93). Mucinous LMP tumors, on the other hand, have similar patterns of K-*ras* mutation and LOH as invasive mucinous ovarian cancer (92). These results suggest that, whereas mucinous LMP tumors may progress to invasive cancer, serous LMP tumors do not and, in fact, likely represent a distinct disease process. Other gynecologic neoplasms such as advanced endometriosis, with its ability to invade structures such as the bowel and ureter despite being a benign lesion, and pseudomyxoma peritonei, with an indolent but nevertheless potentially lethal course, also blur the boundaries between the behavior of benign and malignant tumors.

Stem Cells

Stem cells are a recent focus of intense research that ultimately may contribute to our understanding of the pathogenesis of ovarian cancer, as well as strategies for its prevention and treatment. Somatic stem cells divide asymmetrically, giving rise to a cell that can replace normal differentiated tissue cells and another stem cell. Somatic stem cells are thought to play a role in the normal function of organs and in normal tissue repair. Because of these repeated cycles of division, the stem cells are prone to accumulating genetic mutations over time. Cellular transformation may occur, creating a population of cancer stem cells (reviewed in Ref. 94). The properties of stem cells may explain some of the clinical features of tumors; their ability to differentiate may explain the heterogeneous nature of many tumors, while their ability to remain quiescent in a niche until stimulated to undergo potentially limitless self-renewal may help explain the process of recurrence.

Cancer stem cells, also referred to as "side population" cells, were described first in leukemia and breast cancer. Goodell et al. first identified a subset of cells in murine bone marrow on the basis of their ability to efflux the Hoechst 33342 vital dye with dual-wavelength flow cytometry. These side population cells were found to have the features of hematopoietic stem cells (95). Recent work has identified side population cells in epithelial ovarian cancer animal models, cell lines, and patients. Animal models for ovarian cancer have progressed significantly with the identification of the müllerian inhibiting substance type II promoter in a mouse model of serous ovarian cancer as well as the *Kras/PTEN* Cre recombinase mouse model for endometrioid ovarian cancer (96,97).

Szotek et al. utilized these two models to identify side population cells. One cell line derived from each model was found to have side population cells based on a sort using Hoechst 33342. These cells, in turn, were capable of forming tumors when injected into the dorsal fat pad of nude mice. In addition, side population cells were identified in three of four human ovarian cancer cell lines and the ascites from four of six patients with ovarian cancer (98).

Bapat et al. also examined the tumor cells in ascites from a patient with advanced ovarian cancer for evidence of cancer stem cells. Initially, one tumorigenic clone was identified, but another spontaneously transformed in culture. Both clones were capable of producing anchorage-independent spheroids that self-renewed. They also induced serous tumors when injected subcutaneously or intraperitoneally into nude mice. These features suggest that the clones represent true cancer stem cells (99).

Genetic Alterations

Chromosomal Abnormalities

Karyotypic and molecular biologic analyses have provided evidence that most cancers arise in association with clonal genetic changes. Multiple genetic alterations appear necessary for conversion from the normal to the cancerous state, with primary events that are responsible for tumor initiation and secondary changes that account for tumor progression and heterogeneity. Gross chromosomal abnormalities include translocations, deletions, inversions, and amplifications affecting entire sections of a chromosome (100). Most forms of malignant neoplasia demonstrate both intertumoral and intratumoral heterogeneity with respect to chromosomal aberrations. Molecular chromosomal abnormalities in cancer consist of point mutations affecting a specific locus on the chromosome, frequently involving dominant (e.g., *ras*) or recessive (e.g., p53) oncogenes (101).

Classic examples of chromosomal abnormalities found in cancer are the reciprocal translocations that occur in chronic myelogenous leukemia (CML) [t(9;22)] and Burkitt's lymphoma [t(8;14)] and the inherited deletions of 13q14 in retinoblastoma (102). In CML, the protooncogene *abl* is translocated from chromosome 9 to 22. This results in the formation of a new protein that represents a fusion of the *abl* and *bcr* gene products. Experimental infection of mice with retroviruses carrying the gene encoding this fusion protein has produced a CML-like condition in these animals. In Burkitt's lymphoma, the *myc* protooncogene is repositioned near genes encoding the immunoglobulin heavy or light chains and is constitutively activated. Deregulated expression of the *myc* gene results in cellular proliferation. Characterization of chromosomal abnormalities at 13q14 in hereditary retinoblastoma resulted in the identification of the retinoblastoma gene (*Rb*). The identification of allelic loss in tumors from patients heterozygous at this locus (loss of heterozygosity or LOH analysis) has provided evidence that similar molecular mutations appear to be operating in the hereditary and sporadic forms of the disease. The Rb protein appears to have a major role in regulating cell division; the consequences of alterations at the Rb locus have led to its characterization as a tumor-suppressor gene.

Gross chromosomal alterations have been described in both benign and malignant gynecologic neoplasia, but are more frequent and generally more extensive in the latter. In uterine leiomyomata, clonal chromosomal aberrations have been reported in 15% to 54% of tumors studied, with abnormalities involving chromosomes 12 and 14 being most frequently detected (103,104). In uterine sarcomas, up to 71% of tumors have demonstrable and often multiple abnormalities, with chromosomes 1, 7, and 11 most commonly involved, especially 11q22 (105,106). Cervical carcinoma is characterized by chromosome 1 alterations in greater than 90% of tumors, as well as by frequent deletions involving 3p, 11q, and 17p (107–110), while karyotypic analysis of epithelial ovarian cancers reveals frequent abnormalities of chromsomes 1, 3, 7, 11, and 12 (111–113).

In general, less aggressive malignancies are associated with less complex karyotypic changes. Simple chromosomal abnormalities have been reported for some granulosa cell tumors, tumors of low malignant potential, low-grade epithelial ovarian cancer, and early-stage endometrial and ovarian carcinomas, whereas advanced epithelial ovarian carcinoma frequently demonstrates complex chromosomal changes (112–118). In addition, specific changes for certain tumors may represent a later event in tumorigenesis or may confer a worse prognosis. The frequency of polysomy for chromosome 1 increases as the severity of cervical intraepithelial neoplasia increases (109). Gallion et al. detected LOH on 17p in benign, borderline, and invasive epithelial ovarian tumors, but found allelic loss on 11p in the invasive cancer cases only (119). LOH on 13q was noted in 58% of informative cases overall, including 80% of stage I tumors. Worsham et al. analyzed six squamous cell carcinomas of the vulva, each containing multiple chromosomal rearrangements (120). Two specific deletions, 10q23–25 and 18q22–23, were present in all four of the patients who died of disease but in neither of the long-term survivors.

Somatic Versus Germ-Line Mutations

In addition to the above classification, genetic changes may be characterized as germ-line versus somatic. Whereas all of the cells in an individual with a germ-line mutation will manifest the genetic alteration, somatic mutations occur in a single cell and are detectable in tumors secondary to clonal proliferation. Germ-line genetic changes have been shown to be the basis of the hereditary cancers seen in syndromes such as *BRCA1, BRCA2,* and hereditary nonpolyposis colon cancer (HNPCC). In general, these hereditary syndromes are thought to account for only a minority of gynecologic cancers. Somatic mutations, on the other hand, occur in the majority of cancers.

Clonality

Many human tumors exhibit extensive heterogeneity with respect to cellular properties such as morphology, surface markers, and chromosomal abnormalities. This diversity has raised the question of whether tumors originate from a monoclonal or polyclonal origin. One method of assessing clonality evaluates X-linked gene products such as the isozymic expression of glucose-6-phosphate dehydrogenase (G6PD) (121). Another technique utilizes restriction fragment length polymorphism (RFLP) analysis, exploiting the differential methylation patterns of X-linked genes such as hypoxanthine phosphoribosyl transferase (HPRT), phosphoglycerate kinase (PGK), and the human androgen receptor (HUMARA assay) (122). The use of proliferation-independent X chromosome–linked markers is based on lyonization, the phenomenon of random inactivation of one X chromosome in the embryonic cells of mammalian females. The somatic cells of heterozygous women will be mosaics, with approximately equal numbers of cells expressing either the maternal or paternal allele, but no cells expressing both. A tumor arising in a woman heterozygous for an X-linked gene would be expected to express only one allele if it originated from a single antecedent cell, but to express both alleles if its origin were polyclonal (121). Although the studies utilizing these techniques have generally suggested a monoclonal origin for tumors, the interpretation of the results is complicated by technical issues with the assays, particularly the presence of monoclonal patches in many of the surrounding normal tissues, raising the possibility that the monoclonal tumor simply reflects the clonal composition of the normal tissue.

Genetic markers acquired secondary to somatic events have also been studied to assess clonality. Examples include the rearrangement of immunoglobulin and T-cell receptor genes in lymphoid malignancies (120), the allelic loss on autosomes described for a number of different cancers (123), and point mutations. Immunohistochemistry or molecular probes are used to determine if the same gene product or gene arrangement is present in all of the cells within the tumor, suggesting their origin from a common precursor cell. LOH analysis is employed to discern whether the pattern of allelic loss is identical in all of the cells in a given tumor. Point mutations may be assessed by techniques such as RFLP analysis using restriction endonuclease digestion. Studies using these techniques have been performed on acute myelogenous leukemia, Burkitt's lymphoma, and many epithelial tumors. The results have provided overwhelming evidence for a monoclonal origin of most human malignancies.

Many studies have analyzed the clonal nature of gynecologic malignancies. Fialkow reported the use of G6PD analysis for a variety of tumors, including cervical carcinoma, but this method was thought to be inconclusive, owing in part to its inability to reliably exclude the presence of contaminating normal tissue in the assay (120,124,125). Other problems noted with this method included the requirement for a relatively large amount of tissue and the low frequency of G6PD polymorphism in the female population. In contrast, Vogelstein et al. demonstrated that RFLP analysis of the *HPRT* and *PGK* genes could be used to assess the clonality of tumors in greater than 50% of American women. Of 92 tumors tested with the *HPRT* and *PGK* probes, the X-inactivation patterns seen reflected clonality accurately in greater than 95% (122). Sawada et al. evaluated the clonality of 25 gynecologic malignancies (4 cervical, 11 uterine, 7 ovarian, and 3 tubal) in women heterozygous for the BstXI polymorphism of the *PGK* gene. All 25 tumors were determined to be monoclonal, whereas adjacent normal tissue was polyclonal. DNA preparations from separate areas of the same primary tumor and from corresponding metastatic lesions again revealed identical allelic inactivation (125). The differential methylation patterns of the *PGK* gene on which this RFLP analysis is based could potentially limit the utility of this approach, however, since DNA methylation patterns are sometimes altered in malignancy.

Several investigators have employed a strategy of combined X-chromosome inactivation and autosomal LOH analysis to assess the clonality of metastatic epithelial ovarian cancer.

Jacobs et al. investigated the primary tumor and metastatic implants for LOH at five loci on chromosomes 5, 11, 13, and 17 and sequenced exons 5–8 of the p53 gene in 17 cases. X-chromosome inactivation of the *PGK* gene could be assessed in five of these patients. Strong evidence for a single precursor cell was presented for 15 of 17 cases. In two cases, data were thought to be compatible with either a monoclonal origin or origin from two primary ovarian carcinomas (126). Tsao et al. tested for LOH at 12 loci on chromosome 17 in 16 patients and were able to evaluate allelic inactivation of the *HPRT* gene in four of these 16. In all cases, the X-chromosome inactivations and LOH patterns were identical for all tumor deposits tested in each individual patient (127). Li et al. examined eight cases of invasive and one case of borderline ovarian carcinoma. Analysis of LOH at 86 polymorphic autosomal loci and X-chromosome inactivation patterns of the RFLP DXS255 in five informative patients strongly suggested a monoclonal origin for all of the tumors tested (128).

In contrast, Muto et al. have provided evidence for a polyclonal origin in four of six cases of papillary serous carcinoma of the peritoneum. Eight loci on chromosomes 1, 3, 4, and 17 were assessed for LOH at five or more different tumor sites within each patient. Screening for p53 mutations was also performed. Four of the six patients demonstrated selective allelic loss at all sites tested. One of these four patients also had a p53 mutation detected by single-strand conformational polymorphism (SSCP) analysis and confirmed by DNA sequencing at only half of the distinct anatomic sites tested (129). Recent analysis of borderline tumors has also determined that a small subset of these malignancies is multiclonal in origin (130). Additional studies of primary peritoneal serous carcinoma and borderline tumors are needed to clarify their clonal origin and their relationship to, or distinction from, primary ovarian serous carcinoma (131).

Ploidy

The cells in a tumor may be described in terms of their overall DNA content as compared to that of normal tissue. Normal tissue primarily contains cells that have a diploid (2n) complement of chromosomes, a subset of cells that have undergone DNA synthesis (4n) but have not yet divided, and a smaller number of cells with an intermediate amount of DNA. Deviation from this distribution is termed aneuploidy and occurs in approximately 70% of human tumors (132). Tumor ploidy status is frequently described by a ratio known as the DNA index. The numerator is the DNA content in tumor cells that are either not actively proliferating or are in the process of replicating but have not yet undergone DNA synthesis, whereas the denominator is the DNA content of normal diploid cells. Index values deviant from 1 are used to define aneuploidy (3).

Flow cytometry and, more recently, image cytometry are methods that have been used to assess the ploidy status of tumors. In flow cytometry, a DNA intercalating fluorescent dye, such as propidium iodide, is applied to a single-cell suspension. Laser excitation of the stained nuclei, which have been isolated from the cell, generates a fluorescent emission proportional to the amount of DNA in each cell. A histogram is generated, which is analyzed for evidence of tumor aneuploidy (Fig. 3.4) (3). Flow cytometry may be applied to paraffin-embedded as well as fresh-frozen tissue. In addition, because of the large number of cells evaluated, it may be used to describe other cellular parameters, such as the cell-cycle composition of the tumor cell population. Potential confounding factors associated with this method include cellular debris and normal cells contained in the suspension. In image cytometry, touch imprints of the tumor are stained with a stoichiometric nuclear dye, such as feulgen. To quantify DNA staining, a computer measures the optical density in intact cells that have been prescreened by light microscopy to exclude nontumorous cells. The number of cells analyzed is usually 100 to 200, which is in contrast to the 20,000 to 50,000 required by flow cytometry. Both paraffin-embedded and fresh-frozen tissue may be used for image cytometry. Other applications of image cytometry include the description of nuclear architecture and the quantification of hormone receptors (133–135). Although flow cytometry and image cytometry have provided comparable estimates of aneuploidy between series of cancer cases, the classification within series of cases evaluated by both methods may differ by as much as 15% (135).

Several important caveats regarding the use of ploidy status should be noted. Normal ploidy status should not be equated with a normal karyotype. Because ploidy determination provides an estimate of overall DNA content only, tumors with structural chromosomal abnormalities may still manifest a normal DNA content. Also, different areas of the same tumor may manifest heterogeneity with respect to ploidy status (71,136,137). Thus, differences in sampling techniques such as obtaining single versus multiple tissue specimens may partially explain the discrepant results of various investigators examining the same tumor type.

Ploidy studies of epithelial ovarian cancer have detected aneuploidy in 0% to 34% of LMP tumors and in 50% to 80% of invasive carcinomas (70–73,113,134–143). The three largest published series of LMP tumors are case-control studies that reached conflicting conclusions regarding the significance of aneuploidy and prognosis (139–141). In invasive disease, studies have suggested that ploidy status may be of prognostic importance. Several studies have found ploidy status to be of independent prognostic significance in early-stage invasive disease (70,73,142,144,145). Many investigations that have included advanced-stage invasive disease have also reported a significant adverse association between aneuploidy and

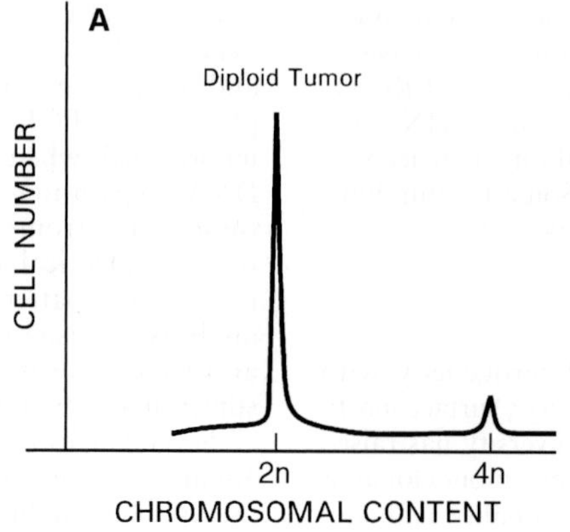

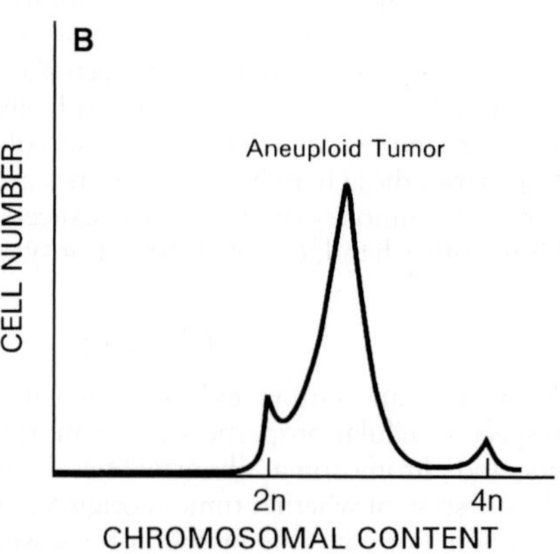

FIGURE 3.4. DNA histograms for (A) diploid and (B) aneuploid tumors. A: The normal distribution of cells in somatic tissue is shown, with the majority possessing a 2n DNA content, and a smaller fraction having a 4n or intermediate amount of DNA. B: In contrast, a tumor-cell population is shown that contains a prominent population of cells with an intermediate DNA content.

median time to recurrence or long-term survival (70–73,144, 146,147). Subset analysis by stage in some of these studies, however, has shown the association to be significant only in patients with early-stage tumors (73,144). Suboptimal tumor debulking at the primary surgery, a higher frequency of positive second-look laparotomies, and a greater likelihood of recurrence after a negative reassessment procedure have all been associated with aneuploidy, although the relationships have not always been statistically significant (69–73,77,78,80–83,133, 135,136,138–150). Overall, it appears that cytometric analysis of tumor DNA content is an important prognostic indicator in ovarian cancer and is associated with a shortened median time to recurrence and long-term survival. This association appears particularly true in early-stage tumors.

The clinical value of DNA ploidy status has also been analyzed in both endometrial hyperplasia and carcinoma (74,78,151–153). Norris et al. defined a set of combined morphometric and DNA content criteria to help distinguish between various forms of endometrial hyperplasia and carcinoma (154). Lindahl and Alm prospectively evaluated 156 patients with endometrial hyperplasia (109 cystic glandular, 35 adenomatous, and 12 atypical). The frequency of aneuploidy was 21%, 20%, and 33%, respectively. Follow-up at 24 months for a subset of patients treated with dilatation and curettage only revealed nonhyperplastic endometria in 64% of those whose hyperplasias were initially diploid compared to 36% of those whose lesions were nondiploid. The difference was not statistically significant, but they noted that this may have resulted from the small number of cases analyzed because a number of patients were lost to follow-up (74). Whereas earlier studies produced conflicting results with respect to the clinical value of DNA ploidy status on prognosis in endometrial carcinoma, more recent studies have shown DNA ploidy status to be an important prognostic indicator with respect to survival (78,151–153). In a subgroup of 293 women with early-stage disease from a Gynecologic Oncology Group protocol, Zaino et al. found a significant increased risk of disease-related death for patients with aneuploid tumor type as compared to patients with diploid tumor type (151). Although this study examined early-stage disease, Nordstrom et al. recently examined DNA ploidy status in 266 patients with advanced-stage or early-stage grade 3 tumors. In this study, World Health Organization (WHO), International Federation of Gynecology and Obstetrics (FIGO), and nuclear grading were evaluated for prognostic impact in relation to clinical variables and DNA ploidy. Patients with clinical stage I (grades 1–2) tumors were excluded. In univariate Cox analyses, WHO, FIGO, and especially nuclear grading ($p < 0.001$), as well as age, stage, and ploidy, were prognostic regarding survival. In the multivariate Cox analyses, WHO and FIGO grades yielded little further independent information beyond nuclear grade. When DNA ploidy was added to the analyses, nuclear grade lost most of its impact because aneuploidy was a powerful factor ($p < 0.001$) that covaried with nuclear grade (152). Thus, it appears that recent data would suggest aneuploidy as being an independent indicator of poor prognosis with respect to endometrial carcinomas.

Preinvasive and invasive cervical diseases have also been evaluated for the prognostic significance of aneuploidy (155–164). A good correlation has been demonstrated between normal or dysplastic Papanicolaou smears and normal or aneuploid DNA histograms, respectively (158,159). An increasing DNA index and a higher frequency of aneuploidy have been reported for increasing degrees of cervical intraepithelial neoplasia (CIN) (158,160–162). Some investigators have suggested defining a subset of CIN at high risk for progression by quantitating the degree of aneuploidy (161,163). Bibbo et al. (164) found that polyploid CIN was more likely to revert to normal histology than aneuploid, nonpolyploid CIN. Additionally, in a prospective study examining the natural history of CIN, Kashyap et al. (162) noted that aneuploid CIN 1 and CIN 2 lesions were more likely to progress to CIN 3 than euploid lesions. Retrospective and prospective studies of invasive cancer, however, have not demonstrated a consistent relationship between aneuploidy and prognosis (81–83, 154–156). Other gynecologic malignancies such as uterine sarcoma, gestational trophoblastic disease, granulosa cell tumors, vulvar cancer, and fallopian tube cancer have not shown a consistent relationship between ploidy status and prognosis (84–86,88–89,165–169).

Genomic and Proteomic Analysis Techniques

Recent advances in molecular techniques have provided new genomic and proteomic approaches that allow for a more precise analysis and definition of the genetic lesions within cancer cells (170). Loss of genetic material may reflect the presence of tumor-suppressor genes, whereas gain of chromosomal regions identifies the presence of dominant oncogenes.

Fluorescent *In Situ* Hybridization. Gross chromosomal abnormalities are detected by the examination of cultured tumor cells arrested in mitosis by spindle poisons using standard cytogentic techniques. Fluorescent *in situ* hybridization (FISH) is an excellent technique for identifying the copy number and location of specific genes (or chromosomal regions) within a tumor. A nucleic acid probe that recognizes a specific gene (chromosomal region) is labeled with a fluorescent dye and hybridized to chromosomal spreads. A control for chromosome number is accomplished by using a centromeric probe labeled with a different fluorescent dye (Fig. 3.5). Using these probes, total and relative (per chromosome) gene copy number can be derived. Loss of genetic material may reflect the presence of tumor-suppressor genes, whereas gain of chromosomal regions identifies the presence of dominant oncogenes.

A related technique known as comparative genomic hybridization (CGH) allows a much broader assessment of chromosomal imbalances (171). CGH represents the first approach to scanning the entire genome for DNA copy number abnormalities. The technique utilizes total genomic DNA from control and test samples, which are then labeled with different fluorescent dyes, mixed, and hybridized to normal metaphase spreads. A region that is deleted in the test sample will not hybridize to its chromosomal location, causing the control sample's dye to be in excess. Conversely, the test sample's dye will be in excess if a region is amplified. Thus, a global assessment of chromosomal imbalances can be determined. A more recently developed version of CGH utilizes microarrays (see below) that contain genomic DNA probes. Hybridization of the above-described labeled probes to microarrays containing genomic DNA from a variety of chromosomal regions can provide a quantitative evaluation of chromosomal imbalances.

Whereas FISH allows a specific locus of interest to be identified, CGH represents an advance in its ability to assess the whole genome for gene copy number alterations. FISH has demonstrated that 3q26 has increased copy number in 40% of ovarian cancers (172). Various studies utilizing CGH have consistently revealed aberrant gains in 3q26-qer, 7q32-qter, 8q24-qter, 17q32-qter, and 20q13.2-qter and losses in 4, 13q, 16qter, 18qter, and Xq12 in the genome of fallopian tube and ovarian cancers (173–175). CGH analysis has also been used to evaluate for copy number abnormalities in *BRCA1* and *BRCA2* mutation carriers compared to sporadic ovarian cancer cases (176–178). Inconsistent results have been obtained so far, likely due to small sample sizes and varying inclusion of specific mutations. However, two studies have shown increased copy numbers on 2q (176,178), while two have shown losses on chromosomes 9 and 19, particularly in the *BRCA1* group (177,178), and merit further evaluation.

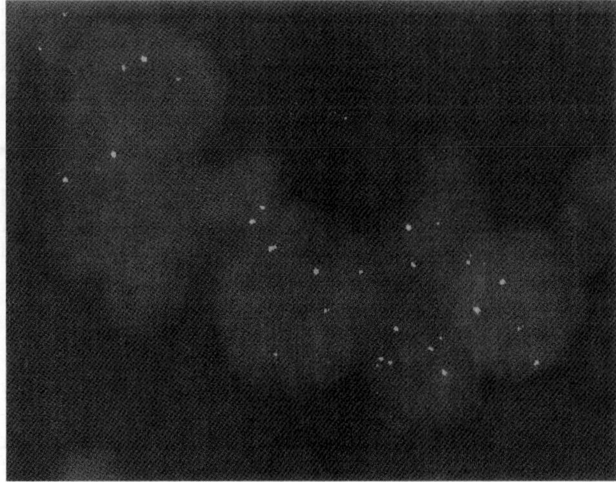

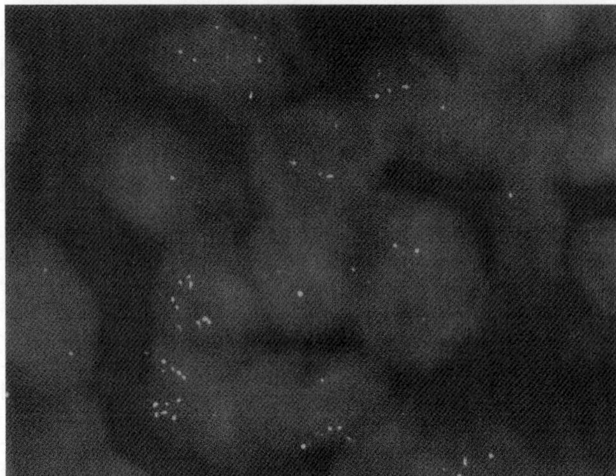

FIGURE 3.5. FISH analysis of advanced ovarian cancers for cyclin E. The BAC clone containing the CCNE1 (cyclin E) gene was labled with spectrum orange, whereas the BAC clone containing the INSR gene (to control for aneusomy) was labeled with spectrum green.

Microarrays. Subsequent advances in technique have allowed genomic segments spotted onto arrays to be substituted for the metaphase spreads used in the CGH technique. Microarrays allow for increased resolution, and the potential to improve efficiency and reproducibility. The first array platforms utilized bacterial artificial chromosomes (BAC) as large inserts. Investigators then developed cDNA microarrays. Currently, commercially produced oligonucleotide arrays or single nucleotide polymorphism (SNP) arrays are widely used. Arrays can be designed to focus on a specific area, such as a particular chromosome or region of a chromosome, or can include a large number of genomic segments to assess across the entire genome.

Using microarrays, expression profiles can be established for tumors of different histology, stage, and grade and compared to those of normal tissues. These comparisons can identify genes whose aberrant expression is present in the malignant cell compared to that of its normal counterpart. The selection of the appropriate control sample is critical as it serves as the basis for this analysis. For ovarian tumors, the control sample can be selected to include RNA harvested from the whole ovary or RNA isolated solely from the ovarian surface epithelium. Since the majority of ovarian cancers are thought to be of epithelial origin, the surface epithelium may provide a more specific normal counterpart. Alternatively, there is the potential loss of genetic alterations in the ovarian stroma, the local host microenvironment, which may be important to the adjacent tumor cell growth. This question was evaluated by profiling the five tissues typically selected as a normal ovarian control in ovarian cancer microarray studies (179). Each normal tissue's comparison to the same set of ovarian cancer samples generated a unique set of differentially expressed genes, emphasizing the importance of the normal control when assessing the list of genes found to be up- or down-regulated in a comparison to cancer. Although there is no broadly accepted standard for the optimal normal ovarian control, this data indicates the potential hazards in cross-comparison between microarray studies if different normal controls are used.

Ovarian cancers of different histologic subtypes have been profiled (180–185). The expression of genes unique to a particular histologic subtype may help explain clinical and biologic characteristics of these subtypes and generate the basis for additional study. For example, clear cell carcinoma of the ovary has traditionally been associated with chemoresistance and an overall poor clinical outcome. Using oligonucleotide arrays, Schwartz et al. analyzed the four major histologic types of ovarian cancer among 113 separate tumors. A unique expression profile of 73 genes was demonstrated in the clear cell ovarian cancers (180). Similarly, other investigators have also noted a distinct profile among clear cell ovarian cancers compared to ovarian cancers of other histologic subtype (181). One study compared the expression profiles of ovarian cancers of different histologies to the analogous subtypes of endometrial cancer. This analysis showed a strong influence of the organ of origin for papillary serous and endometrioid histologies. In contrast, tumors of clear cell histology demonstrated a striking similarity despite different organs of origin, even when renal clear cell carcinomas were included in the analysis, which implies a unique cell of origin and/or biology for all clear cell cancers (182). Collectively, this data suggests that there may be a benefit to subtype-specific diagnostic and therapeutic strategies for ovarian cancer. Subsequent validation studies with clinical correlation have identified up-regulation of the *ABCF2* gene in clear cell ovarian cancers (183). *ABCF2* belongs to the ATP-binding cassette gene superfamily. Currently this gene requires further characterization as it may represent a useful prognostic marker or a potential therapeutic target in clear cell ovarian malignancy.

Other investigators have focused on the molecular signature identified in mucinous ovarian tumors. Microdissection of mucinous cystadenomas, mucinous tumors of low malignant potential, and mucinous adenocarcinomas was performed. The tumors were compared to normal ovarian surface epithelium and a series of microdissected serous ovarian tumors. Hierarchical clustering showed a close association of mucinous tumors. Analysis of the gene expression profiles in mucinous tumors demonstrated an up-regulation of genes involved in cytoskeletal function, which was confirmed with reverse transcriptase polymerase chain reaction (RT-PCR) (184). Other investigators have utilized whole tissue samples to demonstrate a distinct pattern of gene expression among mucinous tumors (185). One gene highly overexpressed in mucinous ovarian cancers is *LGALS4*, an intestinal cell surface molecule. Interestingly, *LGALS4* is located at 19q13.3, a region previously identified to harbor a high frequency of loss of heterozygosity in mucinous ovarian cancers (186).

Other research has focused on clarifying whether a continuum from normal to premalignant to malignant tissue exists for ovarian cancer as it does for other malignancies such as colorectal and cervical cancer. For instance, tumors of low malignant potential (LMPs), also known as borderline tumors of the ovary, have metastatic potential and some histologic features similar to invasive ovarian cancers; however, LMPs generally demonstrate a slow growth rate and an indolent clinical course. Recently, gene expression profiling was applied to

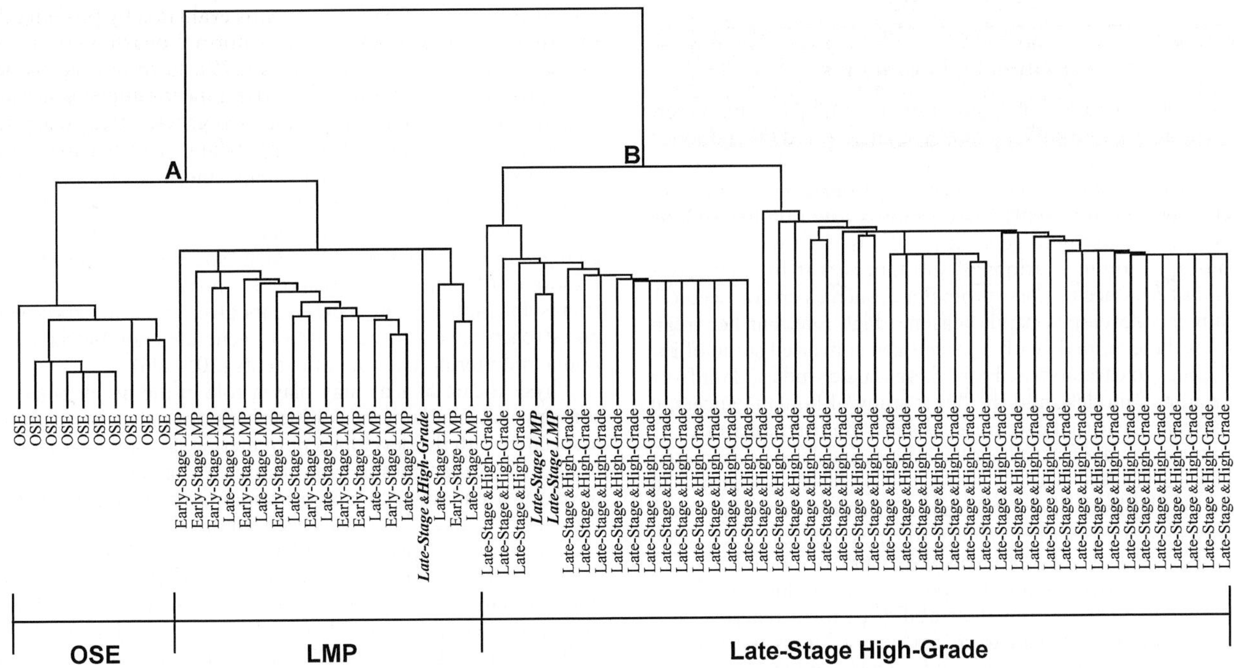

FIGURE 3.6. Hierarchical clustering analysis of the 14,119 probe sets passing the filtering criteria for LMP, low-grade, high-grade, and OSE specimens and binary tree validation. Clustering analysis was completed using the 1 – correlation metric with centroid linkage. Overall tree structure was retained despite the association of low-grade tumors with LMP tumors and the grouping of early-stage and late-stage high-grade lesions. Low-grade and early-stage high-grade samples are indicated in bold. Misclassified specimens are bold and italicized.

define the relationship between LMPs and invasive ovarian cancers (Fig. 3.6). Microdissected LMPs and invasive ovarian cancer of both serous and mucinous histology were compared to normal ovarian surface epithelium. Unsupervised clustering of the expression profiles demonstrated that the serous LMPs cluster separately from high-grade tumors and closer to normal epithelial cells. Interestingly, the majority of low-grade serous invasive tumors clustered with serous LMP tumors, with p53-dependent genes prominently represented on the gene lists. The high-grade invasive tumors showed enhanced expression of genes linked to proliferation, chromosomal instability, and epigenetic silencing compared to the low-grade tumors and LMPs (187). These findings strongly support the concept that serous LMP tumors develop via a pathway that includes the low-grade tumors, whereas high-grade tumors develop along an independent route. In contrast, analysis of mucinous tumors revealed a much closer relationship between LMP tumors and their invasive counterparts. In fact, a molecular continuum from benign mucinous cystadenoma to mucinous LMPs to invasive cancer seems to exist. This supports the idea that a benign mucinous cyst can progress via a borderline lesion to invasive tumor, whereas a serous cyst typically will not undergo transformation to a high-grade ovarian cancer. Additional insights from profiling research such as these may identify the specific molecular events involved in the etiology of each type of ovarian tumor. Understanding these molecular events can then be utilized as targets for screening strategies or for therapeutic intervention.

Gene expression profiling has also been used to identify expression gene patterns in ovarian cancer that correlate with important clinical outcomes. One study employed an oligonucleotide array with over 40,000 features to achieve a whole-genome assessment in which 1,191 genes demonstrated differential expression when compared to normal ovarian surface epithelium. RT-PCR was utilized as a confirmatory analysis on 14 randomly selected genes. The differentially expressed genes include those associated with cell growth, differentiation, adhesion, apoptosis, and migration (188). With regard to other known clinical prognostic markers, unique gene expression profiles have been demonstrated for early- versus late-stage disease, tumor grade, and surgical resectability (189–191).

Recently, correlation of gene expression profiles with ovarian cancer chemoresistance has been defined (192–194). Unique profiles are associated with primary ovarian cancers that subsequently demonstrate either sensitivity or resistance to chemotherapy. Intrinsic and acquired chemoresistance yield different patterns of gene expression. Further, gene expression profiles have been used to predict early recurrence and positive second-look surgical findings, clinical markers of chemoresistant disease (195,196).

Serial Analysis of Gene Expression. Serial analysis of gene expression (SAGE) is one of several new techniques that allow determination of the expression patterns of thousands of genes simultaneously. SAGE was developed on the basic principles that a short sequence tag (10 base pairs) contains sufficient information to uniquely identify a transcript and that the concatenation of tags in a serial fashion allows for increased efficiency in a sequence-based analysis. The procedure involves the synthesis of cDNA, which is then cleaved. The fragments eventually are amplified via polymerase chain reaction (PCR), concatenated, and sequenced. The identity and abundance for individual transcripts in a tissue can thus be determined (197). The advantage of SAGE is that it is an "open" technique that does not require prior knowledge of the sequences to be analyzed. Microarray technology requires the knowledge of the target sequences (cDNAs or oligonucleotides printed on the microarrays). However, microarrays tend to be easier to utilize.

Carcinogenesis

Initiation and Promotion

The biologic processes of tumor initiation and promotion were first characterized from experiments that involved the induction of skin tumors in mice (198). Animals given high doses of an agent such as a polycyclic aromatic hydrocarbon (initiator or carcinogen) would eventually develop a low number of skin papillomas. If subtumorigenic doses of this agent were followed by multiple administrations of substances that by themselves could not produce tumors (promoters), such as croton seed oil, the animals developed papillomas at a high rate. Further treatment of these animals with a carcinogen converted some of the papillomas to carcinomas. From these classic studies, data from other animal models, and the direct study of human cancers, it has become clear that carcinogenesis is a multistep process.

Initiation is the first stage of carcinogenesis and is characterized by irreversible changes in the cellular DNA. Initiators can be chemical, physical, or viral agents. Chemical carcinogens are usually identified by their ability to cause malignancies when given as a single agent to animals or by epidemiologic studies of environmental/occupational exposures. Their mechanism of action stems in part from their ability to form reactive electrophilic species that can form covalent adducts with nucleophilic sites found in nucleic acids. These adducts can cause DNA structural distortions and, if not repaired prior to subsequent DNA synthesis, heritable mutations. The activity of a chemical carcinogen may vary depending on the dose received and host factors, such as age, sex, species, and target organ specificity. Examples of chemical carcinogens are aromatic amines, nitrosamines, hydrazines, chlorocarbons, reactive alkylating agents, and some natural products, including heavy metals such as cobalt, chromium, and nickel (198). Physical carcinogens include ionizing and ultraviolet radiation, which produce DNA mutations and chromosomal abnormalities through the formation of intermediates such as free radicals and pyrimidine dimers, respectively. Agents such as ultraviolet light, x-rays, certain viruses and chemicals, and tumor-cell DNA can be used to produce cell lines that are not only immortalized but capable of forming tumors in immunocompromised animals (199).

Promotion, the second stage of carcinogenesis, involves a series of generally reversible cellular and tissue changes that inevitably involve cellular proliferation. This proliferation results in the clonal expansion of initiated cells, which then accumulate more mutations, resulting eventually in a transformed cell. Most tumor promoters do not form electrophilic species. Activities associated with tumor promoters include changes in phospholipid, polyamine, and nucleic acid synthesis; enzyme induction; and release of prostaglandins, with concomitant alterations in cell morphology, differentiation, and mitotic rate. Some promoters bind to protein kinase C, a known second messenger in signal transduction pathways (198). Examples of substances classified as promoters include phorbol esters, phenobarbital, saccharin, and hormones such as estrogen (198,200).

The molecular mechanisms of tumor promotion involve proliferative stimuli from growth factors and hormones, the activation of second messenger cascades, stimulation of transcription factor activities, and ultimately changes in the expression of effector genes involved in the biologic processes of cellular growth and/or differentiation. The net effect is to alter cell division, produce clonal expansion of initiated cells, and allow for the continued accumulation of key mutations necessary for the development of the fully transformed phenotype (201).

Potential tumor promoters have been identified for gynecologic malignancies. For example, monocyte products interleukin (IL)-1, IL-6, and TNF-α have all been demonstrated to stimulate the growth of ovarian cancer cells (202). The role of these and other growth factors in the development of gynecologic cancer is more fully described above. In addition, another example is provided by the well-known growth stimulatory effect of estrogen on endometrial glands.

Occupational/environmental exposure to chemicals has not been identified as an important risk factor for the development of gynecologic malignancies, unlike other cancers such as those of the lung and bladder. The limited data that exist have been derived primarily from animal studies. Multiple chemicals have been shown to have the potential for causing ovarian granulosa cell tumors, benign mixed neoplasms, or nonneoplastic toxic changes in some, but not all, rodent species tested (203,204). Examples of such agents include 1,3-butadiene, benzene, and tricresylphosphate. Chemical agents given in conjunction with an estrogen have also been used to generate endometrial carcinoma and uterine sarcoma in rodents (205,206).

Physical carcinogens may play a role in the development of some gynecologic tumors. A history of prior pelvic irradiation is associated with the development of uterine sarcoma, particularly malignant mixed mesodermal tumor. Case series of patients developing endometrial adenocarcinoma following irradiation for cervical cancer have also been reported, with a disproportionate number of cases of papillary serous histology (207).

Agents that function as tumor promoters in the development of female genital cancers have been better characterized. Unopposed estrogen, whether exogenous or endogenous, is a well-known risk factor for endometrial carcinoma. More recently, concern has been raised over the partial agonist activity of the antiestrogenic agent tamoxifen, which is used most often in the prevention and treatment of breast cancer. Also, sequential oral contraceptives (OCPs) have been associated with an elevated risk of endometrial cancer, but have been replaced by combination preparations, which, in contrast, impart protection against both uterine and ovarian epithelial carcinoma.

Exposure to some hormonal agents has been associated with an increased risk for the development of other gynecologic malignancies as well, although their precise role (initiator vs. promoter) in the pathogenesis remains unclear. For example, several studies have reported an increased rate of cervical cancer among long-time users of OCPs. Also, intrauterine exposure to diethylstilbestrol is associated with an increased risk of developing clear cell adenocarcinoma of the vagina and cervix.

Viral Carcinogenesis

Experiments in the early 1900s in which inoculations of filtered, cell-free extracts from the cancer cells of one animal could induce a tumor in a healthy recipient provided evidence for the role of a transmissible agent in some forms of animal carcinogenesis (208). This phenomenon was initially demonstrated for chicken leukemia and sarcoma, with the responsible infectious agents isolated known as avian leukemia viruses (ALVs) and avian or Rous sarcoma viruses (ASV or RSV), respectively. Subsequently, the mouse mammary tumor viruses (MMTVs) were shown to transmit mammary carcinomas from nursing mothers to newborn mice via breast milk, and murine leukemia viruses (MuLV) were found to spread horizontally by means of cell-free extracts. These viruses are all examples of RNA-containing retroviruses.

The general structure and life cycle of a retrovirus are depicted in Figure 3.7. A retrovirus consists of an outer envelope and an inner core, within which resides the viral genome. The envelope is a lipid bilayer containing viral glycoproteins encoded by the *env* gene. The core contains capsid proteins specified by the *gag* gene, and two identical single viral RNA strands with bound reverse transcriptase enzyme encoded by the *pol* gene (208). A retrovirus enters a host cell by absorption and endocytosis via specific cell-surface receptors. For example, the human immunodeficiency virus (HIV) is a retrovirus with a known specificity for $CD4^+$ cells. Inside the host cell cytoplasm, the viral RNA is released from the envelope

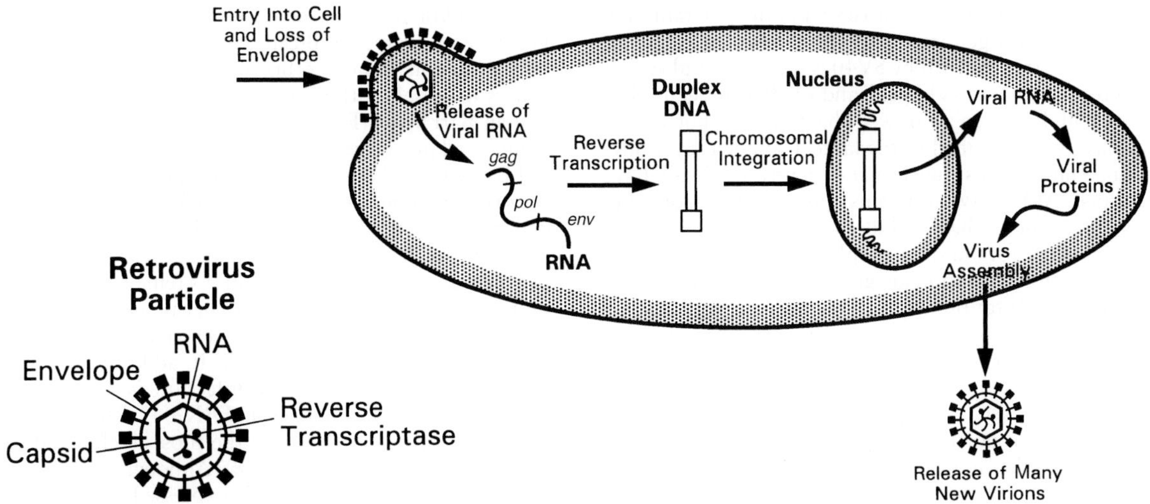

FIGURE 3.7. The structure and life cycle of a retrovirus. The outer envelope of a retrovirus is a lipid bilayer containing viral glycoproteins encoded by the *env* gene. The inner core consists of capsid proteins, specified by the *gag* gene, and two identical single viral RNA strands with bound reverse transcriptase enzyme encoded by the *pol* gene. After entry into the host cell cytoplasm via absorption and endocytosis, the viral RNA is released from the viral particle and reverse transcribed into DNA. An extension of a nucleotide repeat sequence of the ends of the viral RNA is also synthesized, forming a long terminal repeat (LTR) on the DNA that contains sequences necessary for viral RNA synthesis. The DNA then localizes to the nucleus and is randomly integrated into the host genome. The viral genome is replicated and mRNA encoding viral proteins are produced and translated. New virions are assembled from their component parts and released from the cell.

and capsid proteins are then reverse transcribed into DNA. An extension of a nucleotide repeat sequence on the ends of the viral RNA is also synthesized, forming a long terminal repeat (LTR) on the DNA that contains promoter, enhancer, and polyadenylation sequences required for viral RNA synthesis. Between the LTRs are located the *env*, *gag*, *pol*, and various other genes, depending on the type of retrovirus. This DNA localizes to the nucleus and is randomly integrated into the host genome by means of sequences at the ends of the LTR. The integrated DNA serves as a transcription template to replicate the viral genome or produce mRNA for structural and functional viral proteins. Virions are assembled from the viral RNA and processed proteins and are then released (208).

Transforming retroviruses may be classified into two basic types based on their mechanism of action (209). The first group consists of the acute transforming viruses, which can transform cells in culture within several days. These viruses contain viral oncogenes (v-*onc*) derived from normal host cell sequences called protooncogenes (c-*onc*) through the process of transduction, which involves recombination of viral and host genomes during viral integration. In the process of transduction, viral sequences necessary for reproduction are replaced by cellular DNA (c-*onc*), rendering the retrovirus replication defective and dependent on competent "helper viruses" to complete the replication process. In fact, oncogenes were first identified by the study of tumor-causing viruses. V-*oncs* frequently differ from c-*oncs* by containing mutations and no intervening/noncoding sequences (introns). Protooncogene products include a wide range of proteins that are critical for the control of cell growth. They include growth factors and their receptors, nuclear transcription factors, and signal transduction proteins. Because retroviruses carrying these genes will express high levels of these products upon infection, the effects of these retroviruses on cell function are seen acutely.

Chronic or slow-acting retroviruses constitute the other major class of transforming retroviruses. They contain no oncogenes, are replication competent, and are associated with a long latency period. The mechanism of transformation by these viruses is via insertional mutagenesis (209). Random and rare viral genomic integration near a protooncogene or growth-effector gene (e.g., c-*erb*B, c-K-*ras*, or *IL-2*) results in abnormal transcriptional activation of the cellular gene. If the integration is upstream of the gene and in the same orientation for transcription as the gene, it is considered functionally a promoter insertion. When the integration occurs downstream from the target or upstream but in an opposite transcriptional orientation, the viral LTRs are thought to operate through enhancer insertion. An example of insertional mutagenesis is demonstrated by ALV, which can induce bursal lymphoma in chickens following integration of viral LTRs near the c-*myc* protooncogene by either promoter or enhancer insertion.

Viruses containing linear or circular double-stranded DNA have also been implicated in carcinogenesis. The Shope papillomaviruses, extracted from the warts of cottontail rabbits and transmitted horizontally to tumor-free animals, were the first such viruses isolated. Another early isolate was the polyoma virus, capable of causing murine salivary gland adenocarcinoma (208). The structures and activities of the DNA tumor viruses are more complex than those of the retroviruses. In general, the mechanisms of transformation may be direct or indirect (210). Direct methods include activation of cellular or viral oncogenes, alteration of host cell protein expression at the site of viral integration, and the interaction of viral oncoproteins with cellular proteins, such as the products of tumor-suppressor genes (210,211). Indirect actions include altering the host cell genome without persistence of the viral DNA or induction of host immunosuppression.

One example of a DNA tumor virus is simian virus 40 (SV40), a member of the papovavirus family (208). Although nonpathogenic in its natural adult monkey host, it can cause tumors when inoculated into newborn hamsters and certain strains of neonatal mice. Cell culture studies have shown that papovaviruses can cause either a lytic infection, in which the virus undergoes replication and subsequent release from the host cell via lysis and cell death, or an abortive infection, characterized by cell survival but with a subset undergoing transformation with viral DNA integrated in the host cell genome. Permissive cells that can support viral replication, like adult monkey cells, are subject to lytic infection. Nonpermissive or semipermissive cells, such as hamster cells, will typically be transformed.

Cells transformed by papovaviruses will often contain only a portion of the viral genome. The only consistent segment integrated in cells transformed by SV40 is the early viral region encoding proteins known as large-T and small-T antigens. The role of the small-T antigen is not well characterized, but several functions have been ascribed to the large-T antigen. By studying experimental mutants, functional domains of large-T have been identified. At least two domains appear to be involved in transformation. One of these includes amino acids 105–114, a segment necessary for binding to pRb (the product of the retinoblastoma tumor-suppressor gene) and p107 (a 107-kD cellular protein). Mutations within this domain will destroy the ability of SV40 to transform cells. Another domain includes that of amino acids 272–625, which contains binding sites for the p53 protein, DNA polymerase-α, and ATP, and is involved with helicase and self-oligomerization activities. Mutations within this portion of the SV40 genome will abolish its transforming ability in some, but not all, cell lines. Large-T antigen is also instrumental in the initiation and regulation of viral DNA replication and transcription.

The adenoviruses constitute another group of DNA tumor viruses studied in animal models and cell culture (208). In humans, they can cause acute infections of the eye and upper respiratory and intestinal tracts, whereas in rodents, they can cause tumors in neonates or transform cultured rodent cells. Similar to SV40, only a portion of the viral genome is consistently integrated. For the adenoviruses, this is represented by the *E1A* (early region 1A) and *E1B* gene sequences. Multiple gene products can be produced from both *E1A* and *E1B* as a result of differential splicing of transcripts. *E1A* products can immortalize cells but require the presence of *E1B* or an activated ras in cell culture to cause transformation. *E1A* can also regulate cellular and viral transcription. There are three conserved amino acid sequence domains for *E1A*. The first two are required for transformation and contain the binding sites for *pRb*. In addition, *E1A* can bind p107 and a 300-kD cellular protein, whereas *E1B* binds p53.

Despite extensive investigations of the role of transforming viruses in animal models and in *in vitro* cell culture, their role in human cancer remains speculative. Human T-cell leukemia virus (HTLV-1) is a retrovirus that confers risk for human adult T-cell leukemia (ATL) (211). Infection is specific for $CD4^+$ lymphocytes, and can be transmitted vertically through breast milk or horizontally via sexual intercourse or blood transfusions. After random integration into the host genome, polyclonal expansion of T cells occurs during a latency period, which can last several years. Only a subgroup of infected patients actually develops leukemia, which is manifested by a clonal cell population that has the same viral site of insertion within all of the malignant cells of a given patient. In addition to the *env*, *gag*, and *pol* genes typical of retroviruses, the HTLV-1 genome encodes proteins known as Tax and Rex (212). The mechanism of transformation by HTLV-1 appears to involve Tax protein transcriptional activation of cellular genes. Genes whose expression is altered include *IL-2*, c-*sis*, c-*fos*, granulocyte-macrophage colony-stimulating factor, and a subunit of the IL-2 receptor.

Acquired immune deficiency syndrome (AIDS) patients are known to be at increased risk for developing certain malignancies, such as lymphoma and Kaposi's sarcoma (KS). HIV is a $CD4^+$ tropic retrovirus that causes AIDS, but its relationship to the above cancers remains unclear. For instance, although KS is commonly found in AIDS patients, its tumor cells lack evidence of viral genomic integration. However, supernatants from HIV-infected cells have been shown to be growth enhancing for the KS cells of AIDS patients secondary to the presence of the *tat* gene product encoded by the virus. In addition, germline insertion of the *tat* gene into mice precipitates skin tumors resembling KS (61). HIV, therefore, may act indirectly to induce and/or promote the development of KS. An increasing incidence of aggressive B-cell lymphomas has also been noted in HIV patients. Whether this is a result of reactivation of other viruses or an alteration in immune surveillance is unknown. Epstein-Barr virus (EBV) and c-myc overexpression appear to be involved in a large number of these cases (213).

EBV is a member of the DNA herpesvirus family. In addition to causing mononucleosis by acute infection, it has been associated with Burkitt's lymphoma (BL), lymphoma of the immunocompromised host, and nasopharyngeal carcinoma (214,215). The mechanisms of these associations remain to be defined. It is known that B cells and nasopharyngeal epithelium contain the cell-surface receptor CR2, which serves as a receptor for both C3d serum complement and EBV. In addition, B lymphocytes can be immortalized by EBV infection *in vitro*. Viral genes encoding EBV nuclear antigen 1 (*EBNA-1*), *EBNA-2*, and latent membrane protein (*LMP*) are the most likely candidates for effectors of immortalization (208). Although *EBNA-1* has been the only latent gene consistently expressed in BL, experiments with *LMP* mutants have suggested that *LMP* is required for the transformation of B lymphocytes, but which domain is necessary is currently unclear (216,217). BL characteristically contains chromosomal translocations, primarily t(8;14) but also t(2;8) and t(8;22), which reposition the protooncogene c-*myc* near immunoglobulin (Ig) genes. The resulting deregulation of c-*myc* favors cellular proliferation. Magrath et al. have proposed a theory regarding the development of BL in African children (217). Infectious diseases such as malaria may alter the relative and absolute numbers of B-cell precursors in the bone marrow and perhaps mesentery, which are cells that are susceptible to the translocations found in BL. Ig enhancers may increase the frequency of translocations, and therefore play a role in c-*myc* deregulation. Magrath et al. believe that EBV probably increases Ig enhancer activity. BL is seen as a consequence of collaboration between EBV infection and these chromosoml aberrations. EBV may also cooperate with HIV in the development of some other B-cell lymphomas. When B lymphocytes from EBV-seropositive donors are infected with HIV, a subset of these cells is subsequently transformed. These transformed cells show marked elevations of c-*myc* transcripts and protein, as well as EBV DNA and RNA (213).

Another DNA virus associated with a human cancer is the hepatitis B virus (HBV). Chronic HBV infection is strongly associated with the development of hepatocellular carcinoma. HBV is hepatotropic secondary to the presence of HBV receptors on liver cells that recognize the viral coat protein. Acute infection is frequently hepatotoxic, resulting in destruction of liver cells. Chronic infection is associated with viral integration. The precise mechanism by which HBV increases the risk of developing hepatocellular carcinoma remains unknown. Although HBV is not an acutely transforming virus, two viral genes can be consistently demonstrated after integration. They are *ORF* (open reading frame) *X*, and *preS2/S*, which encode proteins that can function as transcriptional activators (208). Insertional events may be important in the role of HBV in the pathogenesis of liver cancer. Modification of cyclin A has been reported secondary to HBV viral genomic integration into an intron of the cyclin-A gene in cancerous liver cells. The resultant hybrid HBV-cyclin A transcript encodes a stabilized cyclin A resistant to degradation. This may play a role in the process of carcinogenesis, as cyclin A is intimately involved with cell-cycle control through its association with protein kinases such as $p34^{cdc-2}$ and is a component of protein complexes involving E2F transcription factor and p107 (218,219). Insertional mutagenesis involving the retinoic acid receptor-β gene and the mevalonate kinase gene owing to EBV integration has also been reported (220).

Historically, herpes simplex virus 2 (HSV-2) was the first viral agent suspected of playing a role in the pathogenesis of gynecologic malignancies. It is a member of the herpes family of DNA viruses. Epidemiologic studies showing a higher frequency of HSV-2 antibodies in women with cervical cancer than in healthy women suggested a possible link between HSV-2 infection and cervical cancer. Fragments of the HSV-2 genome have been identified in some cases of cervical and vulvar carcinoma, but are usually not integrated into the host genome (221,222). Genital keratinocytes previously immortalized by integration of human papillomavirus 16 have been transformed in cell culture by transfection with a subgenomic region of HSV-2 known as BglII N (223). However, with subsequent cell passages, the transformed phenotype was maintained despite loss of the HSV-2 genetic material. In addition, normal epithelial cells transfected with HSV-2/BglII N were not transformed. These data support the hypothesis that if HSV-2 plays a role in the development of cervical cancer, it most likely functions indirectly as a cofactor.

The study of viral infections as possible contributors to the process of gynecologic carcinogenesis is now focused primarily on human papillomavirus (HPV). HPVs are epitheliotropic DNA viruses and members of the papovavirus family (224). The HPV viral particle consists of an approximately 8,000-base pair (bp) circular double-stranded DNA molecule surrounded by an icosahedral capsid structure (225). The viral DNA contains seven early (E1–*E7*) and two late (L1 and L2) open reading frames (ORFs), plus a noncoding region (NCR) of about 1,000 bp involved in the control of replication and transcription (Fig. 3.8). E1 contains the DNA sequences for at least two proteins involved in DNA replication. Genes encoding activator and repressor proteins, which regulate viral mRNA synthesis, are located in E2. E4 may play a role in the maturation of viral particles. The E5 and *E6*/*E7* ORFs were originally identified by their participation in the *in vitro* transformation of rodent cells by fragments of the bovine papillomavirus genome. L1 and L2 contain genes that encode the viral capsid proteins.

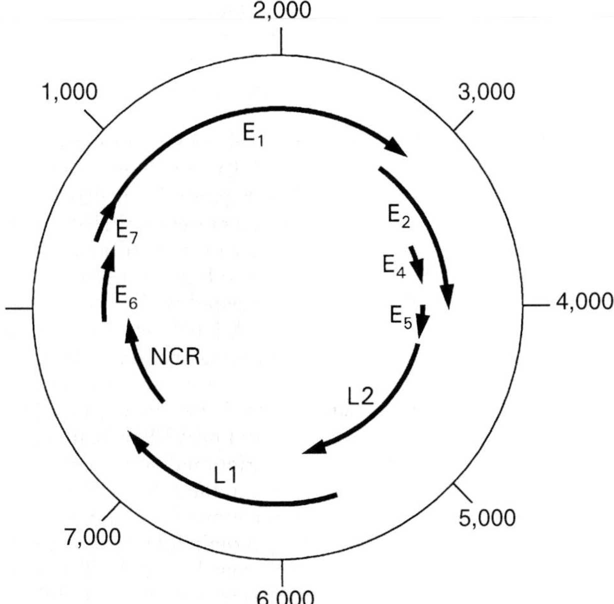

FIGURE 3.8. The HPV genome. The HPV genome is an approximately 8,000-bp circular double-stranded DNA molecule containing seven early (E_1–E_7) and two late (L1 and L2) open reading frames (ORFs), plus a noncoding region (NCR) involved in the control of replication and transcription. E_1 contains sequences for proteins involved in DNA replication. E_2 encodes activator and repressor proteins that regulate viral mRNA synthesis. E_4 is thought to be involved in the maturation of viral particles. *E6* and E_7 can immortalize human keratinocytes and cooperate with oncogenes in the process of malignant transformation. L1 and L2 encode viral capsid proteins.

Over 60 HPV types have been identified by cross-hybridization procedures demonstrating less than 50% DNA sequence homology between any two types (224). Approximately 20 of these have been isolated from the anogenital tract. The lesions associated with HPV infections vary depending on the viral type involved. Lorincz et al. analyzed the relationship between 15 common anogenital types of HPV and cervical dysplasia in 2,627 women (226). Evidence of HPV viral DNA was found in 84% of the 153 invasive carcinoma cases, predominantly HPV-16, -18, -45, or -56, with about 10% containing HPV-31, -33, -35, -51, -52, or -58. They referred to the former group of HPV types as "high risk" and to the latter group as "intermediate risk." Of the 261 cases of high-grade intraepithelial lesions (HGSILs), 54% contained high-risk HPV, 24% had intermediate-risk types, and 4% included viral DNA from their designated "low-risk" group, which included HPV-6, -11, -42, -43, and -44. The 377 low-grade intraepithelial lesions (LGSILs) contained high-risk types in 23%, intermediate-risk HPV in 17%, low-risk types in 20%, and no evidence of HPV in 30%. Nine percent of the LGSIL cases could not be classified. Multiple other investigators have also demonstrated the frequent association of HPV-16 and -18 with HGSILs and invasive carcinoma, while HPV-6 and -11 are more often found in condylomas and low-grade dysplasia. Squamous cell histology has been studied more extensively than that of adenocarcinoma and adenosquamous carcinoma. The prevalence of HPV DNA in these less common types of cervical cancer has varied from 20% to 80%, depending on the method of detection used (226). The vast majority of vulvar condylomata acuminata are also associated with the low-risk HPV types, whereas high-risk types have been demonstrated in invasive vulvar carcinoma.

HPV DNA has been detected in host cells in both integrated and nonintegrated (episomal or extrachromosomal) states (225,226). Episomal viral DNA is characteristic of benign cervical precursor lesions, although integrated HPV is sometimes found in HGSILs. Invasive carcinoma almost always contains integrated viral DNA, but episomal forms of the viral genome have also been detected. Although integration has occurred near cellular protooncogenes, in general the site of viral integration appears to be random with respect to the host genome. However, there is a consistent pattern with respect to the site of disruption of the circular viral genome in the process of integration. The viral DNA is usually interrupted in the E1/E2 region, which is the viral transcriptional regulatory system. Upon integration into the host genome, two ORFs, *E6* and *E7*, are consistently retained (224).

Human keratinocyte cell cultures and tumor cell lines have illustrated the participation of the HPV *E6* and *E7* proteins in the processes of immortalization and transformation. Transfection of human foreskin keratinocytes with high-risk HPV DNA, but not with low-risk HPV DNA, has been demonstrated to immortalize these cells (227). Integration and expression of both *E6* and *E7* are usually required for efficient immortalization, since *E7* alone has weak activity and *E6* alone has none (227). The role of HPV in the multistage process of cervical/vulvar carcinogenesis would appear to be early in the course of the disease since the effect of HPV has generally been limited to immortalization. Progression to the fully transformed phenotype has been described in an HPV-18–immortalized keratinocyte cell line after multiple passages, but in general, this phenomenon is quite rare (228). The transfection of an activated *Ha-ras* oncogene into HPV-16–immortalized cervical cells can render them tumorigenic, demonstrating the ability of HPV to cooperate with another cellular insult to effect carcinogenesis (229). Persistent expression of *E6* and *E7* appears to be necessary to maintain the transformed phenotype. The application of synthetic anti-*E6* and anti-*E7* oligonucleotides to cervical and oral cancer cell lines containing HPV-18 significantly inhibits cell growth (230). Treatment of the cells with both antisense oligonucleotides inhibits growth more effectively than either one applied alone.

An important property of the *E6* and *E7* oncoproteins is their biochemical interaction with tumor-suppressor gene products. Similar to adenovirus E1A and the SV40 large-T antigen, HPV *E7* can bind pRb. The *E7* proteins from HPV-16, -18, -6, and -11 have all been demonstrated to bind pRb *in vitro,* although the binding affinities of the high-risk HPV types are higher (231). The *E6* proteins of HPV-16 and -18 have been shown to bind p53 *in vitro,* which is analogous to adenovirus E1B and SV40 large-T (231). Inactivation of p53 and pRb, secondary to protein binding or mutation, may disrupt control of cellular proliferation. The small proportion of cervical cancer that is HPV-negative frequently harbors a demonstrable p53 mutation. By use of p53-responsive reporter plasmids and a HeLa cervical cancer cell line, Hoppe-Seyler and Butz have shown that HPV-16 *E6*, as well as mutant p53, can disrupt p53-mediated transactivation (232). Additional investigation is needed to further define the specific role of HPV in cellular transformation.

Molecular Basis of Carcinogenesis

Early epidemiologic studies suggested that the development of human epithelial cancers is a complex multistage process. The study of tumors that rise in frequency with age has revealed that cancer incidence is proportional to the *n*th power of age (233). This relationship may be interpreted to suggest that some *n* events, each time dependent but independent of each other, must occur before a tumor can develop. Two models have been proposed to explain how these events might take place. One proposal is that a single cell accumulates multiple genetic lesions (single target, multihit). The other suggests that multiple cells receive a single insult (multiple targets, single hit). Because of evidence suggesting that most human tumors have a monoclonal origin, the former theory has received the most support. Whether or not the *n* events need to occur in a certain order for a given malignancy to develop is unclear.

These epidemiologic data, combined with results from the aforementioned animal models of carcinogenesis, strongly suggest that human cancer results from a complex, multistage process. The application of modern molecular biologic techniques to the biologic mysteries of cancer has supplied additional critical evidence for the multistage hypothesis. The identification and characterization of oncogenes as cancer-causing genes has provided the structural link between the carcinogen/promoter model of malignancy and the biochemical pathways known to be activated in the process of cellular transformation. A recent review proposed that despite the enormous variety of human cancers, five basic rules exist for making human tumor cells (234). According to these rules, malignant cells must have the ability to generate their own mitogenic signals, to resist exogenous growth-inhibitory controls, to evade apoptosis, to proliferate without limits, and to acquire vasculature. In addition, advanced tumors acquire the ability to invade and metastasize.

Oncogenes have been described by (a) identification as transforming sequences found within retroviruses; (b) gene transfer experiments in which DNA sequences from tumor cells were shown to transform normal recipient cells; (c) characterization of fusion genes at chromosomal breakpoints; and (d) identification by nucleic acid sequence homology. Protooncogenes are cellular genes that play important roles in cellular proliferation. Activation of protooncogenes occurs secondary to point mutation, gene amplification, or loss of normal control mechanisms regulating gene expression. Overexpression or overactivity of the protein product results in the transformation of normal cells (235). Protooncogenes that have been well characterized include growth factors and their receptors, nuclear transcription factors, and components of signal transduction pathways (235).

Multiple activated oncogenes have been detected within gynecologic malignancies, some of which have been previously described in this chapter (236). For example, overexpression of c-*erb*B2, which encodes a transmembrane tyrosine kinase with 40% sequence homology to the epidermal growth factor (EGF) receptor, occurs in approximately 30% of epithelial ovarian carcinomas. The *ras* family of oncogenes encodes a protein with GTPase activity and is activated by point mutation. Activation of *ras* genes has been detected in endometrial carcinomas and ovarian LMP tumors. Overexpression of the nuclear transcription factor c-*myc* has been described in a large number of female genital cancers.

Another type of oncogene known to be important in carcinogenesis is the tumor-suppressor gene. Historically, two independent lines of evidence supported its existence (235). Somatic cell hybrids, formed by the fusion of tumor cells with normal cells, frequently display a normal, rather than transformed, phenotype. This suggests that the normal cells harbor factors with tumor-suppressive activity. In addition, epidemiologic studies of the pediatric malignancy retinoblastoma strongly support the existence of recessive oncogenes. Retinoblastoma occurs in two forms. The inherited form occurs early in life, with tumors that are frequently bilateral and multifocal. The sporadic form occurs later in life and is unilateral. Hethcote and Knudson hypothesized that this tumor results from the loss of function of a key regulatory gene (236). In the hereditary form, a mutated allele is inherited; a tumor results when the second allele undergoes a somatic mutation. The sporadic form of the disease occurs as a result of two independent somatic events occurring in the same cell. Careful cytogenetic evaluation of retinoblastoma tumors revealed gross chromosomal abnormalities at 13q14. Molecular analysis of this area led to the identification and characterization of the retinoblastoma gene. Subsequently, other tumor-suppressor genes have been identified and shown to have dramatic effects on cellular proliferation. Mutational inactivation of these genes leads to deregulation of cell growth.

Mutation of the tumor-suppressor gene p53 is the most common genetic alteration in human cancer. Mutation of this gene, which frequently leads to overexpression of the p53 protein, is associated with a large number of human malignancies, including tumors of the female genital tract. In advanced-stage ovarian carcinoma, for example, p53 mutations occur in about 50% of cases. Multiple other tumor-suppressor genes have been proposed by the identification of other nonrandom allelic losses occurring within certain tumors.

Multistage Carcinogenesis Model

Careful analysis of human epithelial cancers has provided substantial evidence for the general model of multistage carcinogenesis. For instance, the study of colorectal carcinoma has identified a series of histologic and molecular correlates in the progression from normal epithelium to hyperplasia, adenoma, and, ultimately, carcinoma. Some of the molecular events in this sequence are now known and include inactivation of the *APC* and p53 tumor-suppressor genes and activation of the *ras* protooncogene (237). In other human cancers, such as lung cancer, activated *ras* genes, p53 mutations, and 3p deletions are frequently found, whereas p53 mutations, overexpression of EGF receptors, and gene amplifications of c-*myc* and *neu* are common genetic alterations in breast cancer (238,239).

Although our knowledge about the molecular biology of gynecologic malignancies has been steadily expanding, much remains unclear. Current research is directed at defining which molecular events are critical to tumor development and when these events occur. These efforts have allowed the construction

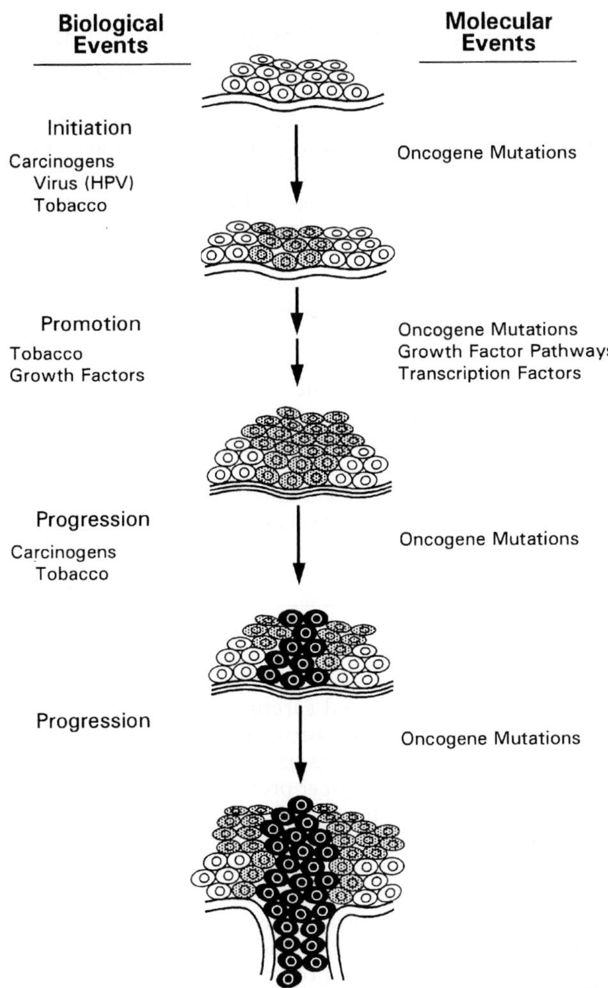

FIGURE 3.9. Multistage model for the development of cervical carcinoma. The transition from normal to dysplastic to malignant cervical epithelium is shown in association with known risk factors, such as HPV infection, tobacco use, and growth-factor stimulation. Molecular mechanisms accompanying these changes include the binding of tumor-suppressor gene products by HPV oncoproteins, activation of growth-factor pathways, and genetic alterations such as c-*myc* amplification and LOH at 3p. Tumor promoters stimulate the division of initiated, partially transformed cells. Accumulation of additional oncogene/tumor-suppressor gene mutations effects full transformation and invasion of the basement membrane.

of hypothetical models of the development of gynecologic cancers, such as that for cervical carcinoma seen in Figure 3.9. The transition from normal to dysplastic to malignant cervical epithelium is shown in association with known risk factors for this process, such as HPV infection, tobacco use, and growth factor stimulation. Molecular mechanisms accompanying these histologic changes include the binding of tumor-suppressor gene products by HPV oncoproteins, activation of growth factor pathways, and genetic alterations such as c-*myc* amplification and LOH at 3p (235). Initiated cells are stimulated to divide under the influence of tumor promoters, producing clonal expansion of partially transformed cells. As more oncogene/tumor-suppressor gene mutations occur, cells become fully transformed and invade the basement membrane.

The multistage model of carcinogenesis provides multiple opportunities for intervention. Primary prevention involves risk factor modification. Smoking cessation, avoidance of unopposed estrogen, prophylactic salpingo-oophorectomy, and dietary modification are activities aimed at preventing the initiation and/or promotion of gynecologic cancers. Secondary prevention implies intervening once the early events in tumor formation have occurred. This involves identification of the histologic stages of early carcinogenesis and treatment of the affected tissue. Traditionally, this has meant addressing preinvasive disease by surgery, topical applications, and hormonal manipulation. More recently, laser ablation and immunotherapy have been used. Identification of the molecular events occurring early in the development of gynecologic cancers may provide new, more sensitive, and more specific markers for the early detection of these tumors.

Improved understanding of the molecular basis of the multistage process of human carcinogenesis has also provided novel approaches to cancer prevention and therapy. For initiation and progression events, compounds that inhibit the activity of activated *ras* genes, antisense oligonucleotides that can reverse the transformed phenotype of HPV-associated cancer cells, and the potential to replace the lost functions of mutated tumor-suppressor genes by gene therapy exist (230). Better understanding of the role of tumor promotion in the development of epithelial cancers has provided other excellent targets for intervention. The development of growth-factor antagonists might inhibit or reverse growth-factor-induced cellular proliferation, which is critical for tumor promotion.

Another approach aimed at inhibiting tumor-promoter-induced cellular proliferation has been suggested by the work of Brown et al., who have created a dominant-negative mutant of the nuclear transcription factor c-jun (240). This mutant protein can block the activities of wild-type transcription factors in the c-jun and c-fos families and block cellular transformation by a wide range of oncogenes. Blocking transcriptional activity may be a potent method of inhibiting cellular proliferation associated with tumor promotion. A similar but more pharmacologic approach is the use of antioxidants for chemoprevention. Epidemiologic studies have found an association between decreased serum levels of the micronutrient beta-carotene and either a diagnosis of cervical dysplasia and carcinoma or a future risk of such disease (241,242). Research regarding the potential effect of beta-carotene therapy is ongoing.

Retinoids have been shown to retard the growth and differentiation of HPV-16–immortalized human cervical cells (243,244). These agents may trigger transcriptional factor pathways that either directly or indirectly interact with other proteins to redirect cellular programming. Meyskens et al. have published the results of a randomized phase III trial in which patients with moderate or severe cervical intraepithelial neoplasia (CIN) received either topical all-*trans* retinoic acid or a placebo (245). A significant increase in the complete regression rate of CIN 2 was achieved, but no significant treatment effect was seen for the CIN 3 group. More data regarding the clinical usefulness of retinoic acid are needed.

BIOCHEMISTRY OF NEOPLASTIC CELLS

Cell Structure

Malignant cells differ from normal cells by dramatic changes in their overall size and shape, as well as changes involving their intracellular components. The nuclei of malignant cells are often enlarged and irregular, containing coarse, clumped chromatin. The nucleus:cytoplasm ratio, normally in the range of 1:4 to 1:6, frequently approaches 1:1 (2). Nucleoli are often more prominent in cancerous cells than in normal cells. These differences can be quantitated and exploited as a measure of cellular transformation. For example, the technique of silver staining and counting nucleolar organizer regions (AgNORs) has been applied to cervical dysplasia and ovarian tumors. Wistuba et al.

demonstrated an increasing number of AgNORs with increasing severity of cervical dysplasia (246). In another study involving 24 mucinous and 28 serous epithelial ovarian tumors, a higher number of AgNORs were found in invasive carcinomas than in borderline or benign tumors. The differences were not significant for mucinous tumors, but a significant difference was demonstrated for the invasive serous versus noninvasive serous neoplasms (72).

Cellular fibrils appear to have important structural and functional roles in both normal and neoplastic cells. As presented in the description of the transformed cell, disorganization of actin microfilaments is thought to underlie some of the morphologic changes and random orientation manifested by these cells (246). Experimental evidence suggests that increased actin organization is associated with *in vitro* growth suppression (247). The distribution of intermediate filaments, such as desmin, vimentin, and the keratins, varies among different types of tumors. Monoclonal antibodies that recognize these filaments can aid in the diagnosis of poorly differentiated neoplasms. In addition to their traditionally ascribed functions, such as maintenance of cell structure and assistance with cell movement, intermediate filaments have been shown to play a role in cell division and nuclear function. They are demonstrated substrates for protein kinases involved with regulation of cellular proliferation, such as $p34^{cdc-2}$ and C-kinase. Phosphorylation of intermediate filaments is associated with their depolymerization during mitosis (248,249). Also, data suggest that lamin B, a component of the nuclear laminin complex, may be involved with the organization of chromatin during DNA replication (250).

Significant alterations in the structure and function of the cell membrane accompany malignant transformation. Modification of membrane glycoproteins, glycolipids, and cell surface adhesive properties are associated with the ability to invade and metastasize. An increased degree of branching in the glycan chains of glycoproteins has been noted as well as abnormal fucosylation and sialylation of membrane carbohydrate moieties (251,252). In some cases, new gangliosides or other novel structures are produced. These aberrantly glycosylated membrane components are recognized by monoclonal antibodies as tumor-associated carbohydrate antigens.

Tumor Metabolism

The process of malignant transformation produces profound changes in cellular metabolism. Tumor cells demonstrate a higher rate of both glycolysis and glutaminolysis, providing intermediary phosphometabolites for the biosynthesis of nucleotides, lipids, and complex carbohydrates. Alterations in the concentrations and activities of certain isoenzymes, such as the greatly increased activity of pyruvate kinase type M2, underlie these changes. Phosphometabolite levels are also higher secondary to lowered levels of their degradative enzymes (253–255). Other metabolic aberrations described in tumor cells include alterations in cholesterol biosynthesis and intramitochondrial aldehyde catabolism (255).

One consequence of altered tumor metabolism is the higher level of fucoproteins seen in the sera of cancer patients as compared to healthy individuals. Elevated serum levels of α-1,3 fucosyltransferase and fucosylated forms of α_1-antitrypsin and haptoglobin have been detected in patients with ovarian cancer, and these levels appeared to correlate with disease status (256). Another secondary effect of the abnormal metabolism of cancer cells is its effect on the host metabolism. When cancer strips its host of nutrients, the host metabolism adapts by processes such as increasing gluconeogenesis. Eventually, anorexia and depletion of energy stores are manifested in the clinical condition known as cachexia.

Tumor-Associated Antigens, Oncofetal Proteins, Hormones, and Enzymes

Tumor cells may produce substances unique to the tissue cell of origin, such as prostate-specific antigen and human chorionic gonadotropin (2). Other substances that are secreted by tumors are infrequently or never elaborated by their normal cellular counterparts. These include ectopic hormones responsible for the paraneoplastic syndromes, tumor-associated antigens such as CA-125, and oncofetal antigens such as α-fetoprotein (2). Oncofetal antigens, although absent from normal adult tissues, can be found in developmental precursor cells. Many of these tumor products are particularly useful as tumor markers that can assist with cancer diagnosis and surveillance. In addition, cancer cells frequently demonstrate an imbalance between the activities of proteolytic enzymes, such as plasminogen activator, metalloproteinases, and cathepsins, and their inhibitors. These deregulated enzyme activities are thought to play a role in the processes of tumor invasion and metastasis (257).

Protein Processing and Degradation

For proteins to serve their roles in cellular function, they require proper structure and carefully regulated levels that reflect a steady-state balance between synthesis, folding, and degradation. Recent discoveries have shown that protein folding, which is required for proper protein function, is mediated through a group of proteins called chaperones. Heat shock protein 90 (Hsp-90) is a typical chaperone that binds to a large number of client proteins and assists in their appropriate folding (258). Once appropriately folded, these proteins are fully functional until they become denatured and then targeted for degradation. Proteins are degraded in part by ubiquitination and targeting to the proteosome. Ubiquitination is accomplished by a family of ubiquitin ligases whose substrate specificity depends upon protein sequence and phosphorylation status. The proteosome is a complex of proteins including proteases that degrades a wide range of proteins. This complex process accounts for the tissue-specific and cell-cycle regulation of expression of many critical proteins.

The ubiquitination/proteosome process has received a great deal of attention in relation to its contribution to cancer development. Mutations and alterations in the phosphorylation state have been shown to change ubiquitination status and turnover of critical proteins including those involved in the cell cycle. Based in part upon these observations, the proteosome has been targeted for the development of novel small molecule inhibtors. It is hypothesized that these inhibtors would potentially be effective chemotherapeutic agents (258).

Signal Transduction Pathways

Neoplasia may be viewed fundamentally as a disorder of cell proliferation in both space and time. Central to the orderly occurrence of normal cell proliferation is the response to environmental cues. Growth factors, originally defined as peptides or proteins extractable from living tissues that promote cell proliferation in artificial (e.g., cell and organ cultures) systems, have come to be viewed as the means by which these signals are conveyed. In this way, neoplasia can also be viewed as a disorder of cellular communication.

"Signal transduction" refers to the biochemical mechanisms by which small molecules alter the state or activities of the intracellular milieu. Two broad mechanisms for signal transduction have emerged. The first involves the covalent modification in intracellular constituents consequent to the action, with the "signal" lasting as long as the modification is present. A common covalent modification is phosphorylation accomplished by protein kinases, enzymes that transfer the gamma phosphate of ATP to substrate molecules whose function is altered because of the attached phosphate. Two types of protein kinases of greatest importance in the regulation of cell growth are those that phosphorylate proteins on tyrosine residues and those that phosphorylate proteins on serine or threonine residues (16). Protein phosphatases function in an opposing manner to protein kinases, providing a regulatory mechanism for the previously described signaling cascades.

The second general mechanism for signal transduction is found in the generation of "second messenger" molecules produced consequent to the action of a growth factor, acting upon intracellular receptor sites to effect functional changes, usually by allosteric mechanisms. The second messengers whose role in growth control is most clearly defined include, but are not limited to, calcium, cyclic AMP (cAMP), and phospholipid metabolites. This section gives a broad overview of the growth-regulating pathways modified by growth factors employing these effector mechanisms.

Ras Pathway

Nowhere in signal transduction research has more progress been achieved than in characterizing the downstream pathways from *ras*. Multiple protein kinases have been identified and their mode of interaction characterized (259). The view of growth-factor-induced cellular activation that emerges from this train of recent investigation is represented in Figure 3.3, where input from either receptor-associated or nonreceptor-associated TKs is reflected in increased generation of activated *ras* bound to guanosine 5′-triphosphate (GTP). Three *ras* protooncogenes have been identified: the H-*ras* gene (homologous to the oncogene of the Harvey murine sarcoma virus), the K-*ras* gene (homologous oncogene of the Kirsten murine sarcoma virus), and the N-*ras* gene (which does not have a retroviral homologue and was first isolated from a neuroblastoma cell line) (260). The *ras* oncogenes encode four 21-kd proteins called $p21^{ras}$ that are localized to the inner surface of the cell membrane (260). Ras proteins are members of the family of GTPases. Ras functions as a molecular switch that cycles between an inactive guanosine 5′-diphosphate (GDP)-bound form and an active GTP-bound state. Ras, synthesized as a biologically inactive cytosolic propeptide, is localized to the inner surface of cell membranes only after it has undergone a series of posttranslational modifications, the first and most critical of which is farnesylation, which adds a farnesyl isoprenoid group to Ras and is catalyzed by farnesyltransferase (260). Activated *ras* in turn associates with *raf* and increases the catalytic activity of the latter protein, which propagates the signal to microtubule-associated protein (MAP) kinase (261).

The c-*raf* protooncogene was originally defined as the cellular homologue of the transforming oncogene v-*raf*. However, accumulating evidence from genetic approaches, summarized by Van Aelst et al., indicates that *raf* functions downstream of *ras*. Specifically, activated *raf* abrogates the need for *ras* to transform cells. Mutations of *raf* can block *ras* transformation. Growth-factor agonists that activate *ras* have hyperphosphorylated *raf*. Most importantly, a family of serine threonine kinases, the MAP kinases, were themselves activated by MAP kinase kinases (MAPKK), which are substrates for *raf* (262). These genetic results led to a concerted effort to identify a biochemical association between *ras* or *ras*-associated molecules and *raf*. Indeed, several groups using recombinant-expressed protein or fusion proteins produced in yeast have clearly demonstrated a noncovalent association between ras and raf proteins (262,263). This association has been confirmed by precipitation of raf using ras affinity reagents (264). However, although it is clear that inactive raf is brought to the cell membrane by GTP-ras, the precise mechanism by which ras activates raf still remains unknown. Activated raf in turn phosphorylates MAPKK (MEK), which activates MAP kinases (261).

One question regarding *ras* signaling is how a single protein can mediate such diverse biologic effects as apoptosis, proliferation, and differentiation. In the GTP-bound state, *ras* can activate several downstream effector pathways. These effector pathways include *raf*, GTP-binding proteins Rac and Rho, PI3K, and MEKK. Some of these *ras* effectors may play a role in the development of gynecologic cancer (265). For instance, Noey2 was originally described as a down-regulated ras effector in ovarian cancer (266). This protein mediates growth inhibition and may function as a tumor-suppressor gene. The ras effectors ERK and PI3K have been implicated in the growth control of ovarian cancer cell lines (267).

Although activated ras proteins are usually associated with driving growth and transformation, they may also induce senescence, apoptosis, and terminal differentiation. Ras association domain in the tumor suppressor, RASSF1, which binds ras in a GTP-dependent manner, is an example. Moreover, activated ras enhances and dominant negative ras inhibits the cell death induced by transient transfection of RASSF1. This cell death appears to be apoptotic in nature. Hypermethylation of the RASSF1A promoter region is common in 45% of adenocarcinomas of the uterine cervix and 40% of ovarian tumors, and is rare in squamous carcinoma of the uterine cervix (268,269). Thus, the RASSF1 tumor suppressor may serve as a novel ras effector that mediates the apoptotic effects of oncogenic ras.

Consequently, *ras*-like genes may also be important for the development of gynecologic cancers. Ras is mutationally activated in 30% of all cancers, with pancreas (90%), colon (50%), thyroid (50%), lung (30%), and melanoma (25%) having the highest prevalence (270). The mutant *ras* genes in human cancers encode mutated proteins that harbor single amino-acid substitutions primarily at residues G12 or Q61. The *K-ras* gene is mutationally activated in only 5% of invasive epithelial ovarian cancers (271). In borderline ovarian malignancies, however, *K-ras* is mutationally activated in 22% of serous and 46% of mucinous borderline ovarian tumors (272). The precise role for these effectors is not yet clear, but presumably they will serve important functions in a variety of biologic processes.

Growth Factor Receptor–Associated Tyrosine Kinases

The importance of tyrosine kinases as mediators of carcinogenic stimuli was discovered due to the identification of their capture by acutely transforming RNA tumor viruses. Characterization of the structure of these captured genes identified them as kinases, while examination of the mass of phosphorylated amino acids in virally transformed cells demonstrated an increase in tyrosine phosphate, normally a minor phosphoamino acid constituent. Antisera specific for the transforming proteins precipitated proteins that have the ability to phosphorylate themselves and, in some cases, the precipitating antibody. Characterization of the proteins demonstrated the presence of phosphorylated tyrosine moieties. Subsequently, it was demonstrated that receptors for certain growth factors also possessed kinase activity for tyrosine. Truncated or mutated versions of the receptors had oncogenic potential in certain instances. Conceptually, this links tyrosine kinase activity to the action of growth-regulatory substances.

As outlined in detail by Cadena and Gill, receptor–tyrosine kinases have at least four structural domains: (a) an extracellular domain that binds ligand; (b) a transmembrane helix domain that links the external portion with the rest of the molecule; (c) an intracellular catalytic domain that contains the core ATP binding and phosphoryl transfer elements; and (d) regulatory domains that regulate the endogenous activity of the kinases by allosteric or intrachain "pseudosubstrate"-like mechanisms or mediate association of the receptor–tyrosine kinase with either substrates or regulatory molecules involved in the propagation of signals (273). Receptor-associated tyrosine kinases are divided into groups according to the structure of their extracellular domains, including the presence of a variable number of immunoglobulin-like domains, the number of cysteine-rich motifs, leucine-rich regions, cadherin domains, fibronectin type III repeats, discoid I–like domains, and epidermal growth factor (EGF)-like domains. These various structures result in at least 14 different families of receptor-associated tyrosine kinases.

In addition to causing dimerization and autophosphorylation of the receptor, activation of growth-factor-receptor tyrosine kinases results in phosphorylation of key substrate molecules thought to be important in propagating the growth-promoting stimulus. Both of these reactions create tyrosine phosphates, which can then form complexes with Src homology region 2 (SH2) domains. SH2 domains are approximately 100 amino acid regulatory motifs originally defined by similarity to a portion of pp60$^{c\text{-}src}$. Importantly, SH2 domains are found in a number of signaling molecules, including phospholipase-C-gamma, phosphatidylinositol 3′-kinase (PI 3′K), the GTPase activator for ras proteins, protein phosphatase-1C, and many nonreceptor–tyrosine kinases, including pp60$^{c\text{-}src}$. This important family of "adapter" molecules, represented prototypically by grb2, contains small molecules devoid of catalytic functions that consist of two SH2 domains centered around the SH3 domain and are capable of mediating protein–protein interactions. Through their SH2 domains, these adapter molecules function to physically associate proteins phosphorylated on tyrosine.

The important result of growth-factor-receptor–kinase activation is the assembly of multimeric complexes through SH2 domains of molecules with distinct signaling capabilities. Phospholipase-C-gamma (PLC-gamma) hydrolyzes membrane phosphatidylinositol bisphosphate (PIP_2), producing inositol triphosphate and increases in intracellular diacylglycerol (DAG). Inositol triphosphate interacts with the cell membrane and releases calcium. The increased DAG and calcium maximally activates protein kinase C (PKC). PI 3′K phosphorylates phosphatidylinositols at the 3′ position, creating new substrates for PLC-gamma. In addition, a substrate for PI 3′K is protein kinase B (AKT), which has been demonstrated to be important in suppressing apoptosis. Finally, ras GTP hydrolysis is stimulated by ras GAP (GTPase-activating protein).

In this way, a large signaling complex is rapidly assembled around activated receptors, from which a variety of signal transduction cascades emanate. The multiple components activated through ligand binding exemplifies the profound effect that growth factors have on target cells, because each signaling pathway activated can initiate or amplify multiple functional responses. Additionally, many growth factor ligands induce receptor heterodimerization with multiple receptors and signaling pathways, providing a mechanism that generates a large number of different cellular responses from a limited number of receptors (274). Once activated, growth factor receptors are rapidly internalized by the endocytotic pathway and degraded by lysosomes (274). Ligand binding can also act as a signal for ubiquitinoylation and subsequent proteasome degradation. Thus, ligand binding not only activates a myriad of signaling pathways, but also causes complementary down-regulation of cell surface receptors and attenuation of signaling transduction cascades.

In addition to the associations described above with receptor tyrosine–protein kinases, the adapter protein grb2 can form complexes with the mammalian homolog of the son of sevenless (Sos) protein originally described in the sevenless *Drosophila* mutant. The importance of this observation is that the Sos protein has GDP-exchange activity for mammalian ras proteins. Thus, receptor–tyrosine kinase activation can both accelerate ras protein activation (through exchange of GDP for GTP) as well as lead to ras inactivation (through GAP). These findings provide a biochemical basis for the original observations that neoplastic transformation by receptor–tyrosine or nonreceptor–tyrosine kinases could be blocked by genetic maneuvers that inhibited ras function.

Nonreceptor-Associated Tyrosine Kinases

Tyrosine kinases (TKs) are enzymes that transfer the γ-phosphate groups from ATP to the hydroxyl group of tyrosine residues (275). They can be characterized as either nonreceptor type or, more commonly, transmembrane receptor type. The nonreceptor TKs are found in the cytoplasm, lack a transmembrane segment, and generally function downstream of the transmembrane receptor tyrosine kinases (RTKs). The prototype for oncogenic, nonreceptor TKs is *pp60*$^{c\text{-}src}$, the cellular homologue of the transforming oncogene of Rous sarcoma virus, *pp60*$^{v\text{-}src}$. It is representative of at least eight families of molecules with distinct domain structures. In addition to the Src family, these include the Abl, Fes/Fps, focal adhesion (FAK), c-Src kinase (CSK), Janus kinase (JAK), spleen tyrosine kinase (syk), and interleukin-2–inducible kinase (ITK) families. These kinases can have either relatively ubiquitous expression (e.g., abl, src) or tissue-restricted distribution (e.g., fyn, lyn). Although they are anatomically distinct from RTKs, they have functional similarities in that the kinase-specific activity of the nonreceptor-tyrosine kinases increases following ligand stimulation of cells in which they are found. For example, thrombin activation of platelets and platelet-derived growth factor (PDGF) activation of fibroblasts results in increased pp60$^{c\text{-}src}$ activity, while activation of T lymphocytes through the CD4 or CD8 determinants activates pp56$^{c\text{-}lck}$, a pp60$^{c\text{-}src}$ family member (276).

Another example of a nonreceptor TK with clinical relevance is Abl. The Philadelphia (Ph) chromosome found in some forms of leukemia is a result of a chromosomal translocation that juxtaposes the c-*abl* nonreceptor TK gene on chromosome 9 with a breakpoint cluster region *(bcr)* gene on chromosome 22 (275). The resulting fusion protein Bcr-Abl, is a constitutively activated form of Abl TK that drives uncontrolled growth of Ph cells. Normally, Abl can translocate into the nucleus, where it has a role in DNA-damage-induced apoptosis. However, truncated fusion protein Bcr-Abl is retained in the cytoplasm in association with the cytoskeleton, where its lack of proapoptotic activity contributes to its oncogenic properties (275).

The consequences of the activation of the nonreceptor TKs include the phosphorylation of many of the same substrates described above for the receptor-linked TKs. In particular, the activation of *ras* through grb2/Sos underscores that activation can proceed through input from a number of different sources and points to the importance of the molecules downstream of *ras* as representing a "final common pathway" of cellular activation.

Epidermal Growth Factor and Receptor

Epidermal growth factor (EGF) is so named because of growth-promoting activity originally recognized by its promotion of the normal formation of facial structures in neonatal mice. It is now recognized as the prototype for a family of growth factors widely distributed in a number of anatomic sites, including EGF, transforming growth factor-β (TGF-β), amphiregulin, neu differentiation factor, and neu/*erb*B2 ligand growth factor (277,278). The growth factors share several structural motifs and bind to receptors that possess intrinsic tyrosine kinase activity. These receptors include the classic EGF receptor (EGFR, also known as c-*erb*B1), which also binds to TGF-β, and the related receptor c-*erb*B2 (also known as p185*neu*), originally defined by its similar structure but distinct pattern of amplification and expression in tumors (279).

The clinical significance of EGFR protein expression in the development and progression of human ovarian carcinoma was studied in seven ovarian cystadenomas, six mucinous LMP tumors, and 25 invasive adenocarcinomas by immunohistochemistry. EGF and EGFR expression were found to be significantly higher in mucinous cystadenocarcinomas than in mucinous cystadenomas or mucinous LMP tumors (280). In a series of 226 patients with early-stage epithelial ovarian carcinomas, EGFR status was a significant independent prognostic factor with regard to disease-free survival (DFS). A prognostic model based on the presence of grade 3, p53-positive, and EGFR-positive disease found the poorest DFS for patients with all three clinical factors (281).

As outlined by Bast et al., autocrine stimulation by TGF-β and overexpression of c-*erb*B2 appear to be of clear importance in ovarian carcinoma, where the level of c-*erb*B2 expression appears to correlate adversely with prognosis in some series (282–284). The conflicting results regarding c-*erb*B2 protein expression and survival in the literature could be explained by discrepancies between c-*erb*B2 protein overexpression and the frequency of c-*erb*B2 gene amplification.

Since the advent of tissue microarray (TMA) technology, researchers are able to evaluate large numbers of specimens by FISH analysis. For example, FISH analysis of 79 FIGO stage I and II epithelial ovarian cancers found a 6.7% rate of c-*erb*B2 amplification. No clinical correlation of survival was attempted in this study due to the limited number of informative cases in the sample set (285). FISH analysis of 103 advanced stage ovarian cancer specimens found c-*erb*B2 amplification rates of 10.7% and 33.3%, depending on the fluorescence ratio cutoff (286). No correlation between c-*erb*B2 protein expression by immunohistochemistry and c-*erb*B2 amplification by FISH analysis was seen. In addition, no correlation between c-*erb*B2 amplification and DFS was seen (286).

Another comprehensive FISH analysis of 173 invasive ovarian cancers of all stages revealed good correlation between FISH analysis and immunohistochemistry, but no correlation between c-*erb*B2 amplification and histological type, stage, grade, or prognosis (287). In this study, 79% of the invasive epithelial ovarian cancer specimens analyzed was of serous histology. The treatment period spanned from 1985 to 2002, including a variety of adjuvant chemotherapy regimens. Although the authors concluded that c-*erb*B2 amplification did not correlate with FIGO stage, the percentages of early- and advanced-stage cancers analyzed were not provided. The inclusion of borderline or germ cell tumors also was not clarified (287).

Thus, the strong correlation between c-*erb*B2 immunostaining and amplification seen in breast carcinoma might not be present in ovarian carcinoma. In addition, the expression of c-*erb*B2 and potential relation to tumor cell growth have been outlined in endometrial and cervical carcinomas (65). Although receptors for EGF have been proposed as targets for antibodies that create a negative growth regulatory signal, initial trials have been disappointing (288–289).

Insulin-Like Growth Factors

Insulin-like growth factors (IGFs) have metabolic effects and an amino acid sequence analogous to insulin. IGF-I and IGF-II have been described. The IGF-1 receptor (IGF-1R) belongs to a family that includes the insulin receptor (IR) and IGF-2R (290). IGF-1R is expressed on the cell surface membrane as preformed dimers. Upon binding of IGF-I or IGF-II, IGF-1R undergoes autophosphorylation and conformational change (290). Signaling then depends on phosphorylation of intracellular substrates, leading to activation of the MAPK and PI3K/Akt pathways. IGF-1R signaling can be regulated on several levels, including receptor expression, ligand production, and ligand binding to proteins. Transcription of the IGF-1R gene is up-regulated by growth factors including PDGF, EGFR, hormones, and oncogenes. Transcription of IGF-1R is down-regulated by the tumor suppressor genes *Wt1* and p53. Production of IGFs occurs primarily in the liver and is regulated by growth hormone. Only 2% of IGFs circulate in their free form, while the vast majority are bound to a series of six IGF binding proteins (IGF-BPs) (290,291).

Expression of IGF-1R is observed in most solid tumors examined to date, while overexpression of IGF-II has been demonstrated in cancer cells (292). High circulating levels of IGF-1 in serum have been associated with increased risk of breast, prostate, and colon cancer (291,292). Recent studies have implicated these receptors and their cognate growth factors in the promotion of ovarian carcinoma (293). Relative expression of IGF-II was measured in 109 epithelial ovarian cancers and eight normal ovarian surface epithelial samples using quantitative real-time polymerase chain reaction. Expression of the IGF-II gene was more than 300-fold higher in ovarian cancers compared with normal ovarian surface epithelium samples (294). High IGF-II expression was associated with advanced-stage disease at diagnosis, high-grade cancers, and suboptimal surgical cytoreduction. In multivariate analysis, relative IGF-2 expression was an independent predictor of poor survival. As such, IGF-II is a molecular marker and might be a potential therapeutic target for the most aggressive epithelial ovarian cancers (294).

IGF-II, IGF binding protein 3 (IGFBP-3), and estrogen-receptor-α expressions were evaluated in 215 patients with primary epithelial ovarian cancer. Survival analysis was done to examine the associations of IGF-II with disease progression. IGF-II expression was found to be higher in tumors with poor prognosis, including tumors with advanced stage, poor differentiation, serous histology, and large residual lesions. This study found evidence that IGF-II expression is associated with disease progression, suggesting that IGF-II and IGF signaling are potential targets for ovarian cancer treatment (295).

Platelet-Derived Growth Factor

The platelet-derived growth factor (PDGF) is of historic significance owing to its structural and functional homology to the v-*sis* viral oncogene. PDGFs are a growth factor family, each member of which contains one of four different polypeptide chains: PDGF-A, PDGF-B, PDGF-C, or PDGF-D (296). Each chain is encoded by an individual gene located on chromosomes 7, 22, 4, and 11, respectively. The polypeptide chains are linked with an amino acid disulfide bond forming homo- or heterodimers, of which five have so far been described: PDGF-AA, PDGF-AB, PDGF-BB, PDGF-CC, and PDGF-DD. These factors exert their cellular effects through PDGF-α and PDGF-β protein tyrosine kinase receptors. The platelet-derived growth factor receptor (PDGFR) system, located primarily on mesenchymal cells, transduces signals for cell survival, growth, and chemotaxis. As reviewed in detail by Fantl et al., the PDGFR is a receptor-linked tyrosine kinase with distinctive features, including an extracellular domain with five regions with homology to immunoglobulins and an intracellular domain that interrupts the kinase region and is thought to serve as a "dock" for presentation of phosphotyrosines to molecules that can bind to phosphotyrosine through SH2 domains (298). PDGFR-α can be activated by PDGF-AA, PDGF-AB, PDGF-BB, and PDGF-CC, while PDGF-BB and PDGF-DD bind and activate PDGF-β. Ligand binding induces receptor dimerization, activation, and autophosphorylation of the tyrosine kinase domain. This in turn recruits SH2-domain-containing signal transduction proteins and activates signaling enzymes including Src, PI3K. This precipitates a complex network of downstream signaling events, which have yet to be fully characterized. Activation of the receptors ultimately promotes cell migration, proliferation, and survival (299).

Ovarian and choriocarcinoma cells have been reported to express PDGF and PDGF receptors (299,300). A number of ovarian and cervical carcinomas express either c-kit and/or steel ligand, and have receptors for M-CSF (301,302). High levels of PDGF and PDGFR-α have been reported in advanced epithelial ovarian cancer, while overexpression of PDGFR-α has been shown to be associated with a reduced overall survival (299). Tissue arrays containing 84 epithelial ovarian tumors were studied by immunohistochemistry with antibodies specific for c-kit, PDGFR-α, and PDGFR-β (298). PDGFR-α was expressed in the largest percentage of ovarian tumors (58%), whereas 29% expressed PDGFR-β. No mutations were detected in six ovarian tumors with elevated immunoreactivity for each of the RTKs (c-kit, PDGFR-α, and PDGFR-β). This study demonstrates that PDGFR-α, PDGFR-β, and c-kit are expressed in a high percentage of epithelial ovarian cancers, suggesting that tyrosine kinase inhibitors may be useful in the treatment of these tumors (298).

In a mouse model of human ovarian cancer, the tyrosine kinase inhibitor SU6668 exhibited antitumor effects, both as a single agent and with paclitaxel (296,303). Reduction in tumor growth, ascites production, and metastatic spread were observed. Improvement in overall survival has also been demonstrated in mouse models of peritoneally disseminated ovarian cancer after treatment with SU6668 (303). Although the functional importance of these receptors has not been established, their presence raises the possibility that gynecologic neoplasms will depend, at some point in their pathogenesis, on the action of members of this growth-factor-receptor family. The initial clinical data in ovarian cancer, however, has been disappointing. A phase-II study of patients with relapsed ovarian cancer expressing c-KIT (CD117) or PDGFR was conducted with imatinib mesylate (304). Patients were treated daily with 400 mg of imatinib mesylate orally. Of the 19 evaluable patients, 2 (11%) had tumors expressing c-Kit, while 17 (89%) had tumors expressing PDGFR. There were no objective responders. Thirteen patients (68%) had increasing disease or symptomatic deterioration, and six (32%) went off protocol during the first month due to adverse events.

Vascular Endothelial Growth Factor and Other Angiogenic Factors

Angiogenesis, the formation of new blood vessels, is a process required by many biologic processes including the development of cancer (305). Maturation is usually incomplete in neoplastic growth. Endothelial cells of immature blood vessels require growth signals for survival to avoid apoptosis. Autocrine and paracrine loops exist between the tumor cells and stromal and/or endothelial cells (306). Autocrine stimulation by the tumor cell consists of growth factors such as vascular endothelial growth factor (VEGF), fibroblast growth factor (FGF), and PDGF, all of which stimulate the host cells in a paracrine fashion, to trigger the neovasculature that will irrigate the tumor cells. The VEGF family of glycoproteins consists of six related growth factors, VEGF-A (known as VEGF) through VEGF-E, as well as placental growth factor (PIGF)-1 and -2 (307). The VEGF gene, located on the short arm of chromosome 6, is composed of eight exons and is differentially spliced to yield four mature isoforms (308). VEGF mediates angiogenic signals to the vascular endothelium through high affinity receptor tyrosine kinases (RTKs) that are thought to activate the MAPK pathway. The VEGF family members bind their related receptors. The receptors identified so far include VEGFR-1, VEGFR-2, VEGFR-3, and the neuropilins (NP-1 and NP-2). These receptors are transmembrane tyrosine kinases that, upon ligand binding, activate a cascade of downstream proteins. These downstream pathways include PI3 kinase/AKT, ERK-1/2, and Raf-MEK-ERK pathways (308).

Although many stimulators and inhibitors of angiogenesis have been identified, the trigger that causes a dormant tumor to transform into a proangiogenic tumor remains elusive. Expression of VEGF in ovarian carcinomas was evaluated by immunohistochemistry and revealed focal or diffuse strong immunostaining in 48% to 51% of carcinomas (309). Significant associations between the VEGF expression and FIGO stage and histologic grade were observed (309,310). The survival of patients with high VEGF expression was significantly worse than that of patients with low or no VEGF expression. Multivariate analysis revealed that disease stage and VEGF expression were significant independent prognostic indicators of overall survival.

The family of FGFs comprises several members distinguished originally by binding to heparin and elution at a spectrum of pH, thus allowing their characterization as basic or acidic FGFs (311). These entities have been proposed to mediate not only the direct promotion of tumor cell growth but also the stimulation of stroma formation and blood vessel growth to sustain tumors beyond the microscopic stage. Additional angiogenic factors include platelet-derived endothelial growth factor and vascular permeability factor. Basic FGF and its receptor are expressed in human ovarian carcinomas (312). Ovarian and endometrial neoplasms have recently been demonstrated to secrete both PDGF and VEGF (313,314).

Bevacizumab (BEV) is a humanized monoclonal antibody against vascular endothelial growth factor. In a phase-II trial, 32 patients not participating in an ongoing clinical trial were treated with BEV (15 mg/kg every 3 weeks IV) (315). All patients had failed multiple prior cytotoxic chemotherapies prior to BEV. A median of six cycles (range 1 to 20) with 196 total doses of BEV was administered. A 16% response rate was seen with 62.5% of patients demonstrating stable disease. Median overall survival (OS) was 6.9 months, with median progression-free survival (PFS) of 5.5 months. BEV was generally well tolerated after multiple prior cytotoxic regimens and resulted in significant clinical benefit among women with recurrent ovarian cancer (315).

Transforming Growth Factor-β

TGF-β was originally recognized as a mediator of natural killer cell transformation. TGF-β binds directly to a receptor that is a constitutively active transmembrane serine/threonine kinase (316). Ligand binding of TGF-β results in heterodimerization with both TGF-β receptors, TβR1 and TβR2, and the ensuing phosphorylation of TβR1 (317). Phosphorylated TβR1 phosphorylates a SMAD protein that forms a heterodimer with SMAD4, travels into the nucleus, binds to DNA, and (with other factors) initiates transcription. TβR1 can also interact with a subunit of farnesyl transferase, which is involved in the farnesylation of the ras gene product. Also, H-ras has been shown to up-regulate expression of TβR1 and down-regulate expression of TβR2 (317). The importance of TGF-β to gynecologic neoplasia extends in part from the recognition that müllerian inhibitor substance (MIS), important in the embryogenesis of the normal genitourinary tract, is a member of the TGF-β family (318). TGF-β itself is recognized as a negative growth regulator of a variety of cell types, including ovarian tumor cells (252).

Ovarian cancer is resistant to the antiproliferative effects of TGF-β; however, the mechanism of this resistance remains unclear. Investigators used oligonucleotide arrays to profile 37 undissected, 68 microdissected advanced-stage, and 14 microdissected early-stage papillary serous cancers to identify TGF-β signaling pathways involved in ovarian cancer (319). A total of seven genes involved in TGF-β signaling were identified that had altered expression >1.5-fold in the ovarian cancer specimens, compared with normal ovarian surface epithelium. Genes that inhibit TGF-β signaling (DACH1, BMP7, and EVI1) were up-regulated in advanced-stage ovarian cancers while, conversely, genes that enhance TGF-β signaling (PCAF, TFE3, TGFBRII, and SMAD4) were down-regulated compared with the normal samples (319). These results suggest that altered expression of these genes is responsible for disrupted TGF-β signaling in ovarian cancer, potentially making them useful as novel therapeutic targets for ovarian cancer.

Tumor Necrosis Factor, TNF-Related Apoptosis-Inducing Ligand, and Interleukin-1

The tumor necrosis factor (TNF) superfamily consists of proteins involved in proliferation, differentiation, and apoptosis (320). Members of this superfamily such as TNF-α, Fas ligand (FasL), and TNF-related apoptosis-inducing ligand (TRAIL) have been shown to directly induce apoptosis. The cytokines bind TNF-family receptors that contain a conserved cytosolic structure known as the death domain; this is a protein interaction module that allows the TNF receptors to communicate with adapter proteins, which in turn bind to specific caspases (in humans, caspase-8 and caspase-10), thereby triggering apoptosis. TRAIL specifically induces apoptosis of transformed cells through the action of death domain receptors DR-4 and DR-5. It also directly induces apoptosis through an extrinsic pathway, which involves the activation of caspases. Unlike TNF and FasL, TRAIL appears to have a unique selectivity for triggering apoptosis in tumor cells while leaving normal tissues intact (320). Activation of caspase-8 by TRAIL can lead to a mitochondrial-independent signal that activates caspases downstream of caspase-8 and a mitochondrial-dependent caspase activation following caspase-8 activation and BID cleavage. It has been proposed that TNF and interleukin-1 (IL-1), cytokines originally defined as hematopoietic growth factors, operate via yet another distinct signaling mechanism. This involves the hydrolysis of membrane sphingomyelin, with the resulting ceramide acting as a second messenger to activate a ceramide-dependent protein kinase (321). Recent evidence has been accumulating that IL-1 can directly inhibit the growth of ovarian carcinoma cells and is expressed by this cell type and endometrial carcinoma cells in culture (322,323). IL-1 has also been found to regulate the secretion of collagenase, which is important in mediating invasiveness in choriocarcinoma cells (324). TNF can act as an autocrine and paracrine growth factor for ovarian carcinoma cells (325,326).

Calcium-Mobilizing Growth Factors

The importance of the G-protein–linked calcium-mobilizing growth factors and their receptors to the growth of gynecologic neoplasms has been less completely characterized than the entities described above. However, it has recently been demonstrated that the peptide bombesin can modulate sensitivity of ovarian carcinoma cells to TNF and platinum, perhaps by modulating calcium levels (327). In addition, pharmacologic treatments that seek to interfere with the increase in calcium in response to growth factors of this class are under clinical evaluation in patients with gynecologic neoplasms (328).

MAP Kinases

MAP kinase was originally defined as a distinctive protein whose phosphorylation on both tyrosine and threonine residues increased shortly after addition of growth factors to cells. It is now appreciated that there are multiple different MAP kinases and isoforms (329,330). Each family of MAP kinases has unique (although overlapping) downstream substrates and upstream activators (MAPKKs). MAP kinase families include the extracellular-signal-regulated kinase (ERK), c-Jun N-terminal kinase (JNK), and p38 families. The ERKs are phosphorylated and activated by MEK 1,2, while the JNKs are activated by JNKK1 (SAPKK1), and the p38s are activated by MKK 3 and 6. These MAPKKs are in turn activated by specific MAPKKKs. Thus, raf signals through MEK 1,2 to the ERK family members, whereas JNK and p38 receive their activation signals from other upstream kinases. These kinase cascades allow for rapid transduction and amplification of signals from the cell membrane. Recent work has demonstrated that activation of one MAPK pathway can suppress the activity of the others (331). Thus, although these are primarily vertical pathways, there is ample lateral cross talk between them, providing integration of multiple unique cell membrane signals.

As reviewed by Garrington and Johnson, MAP kinases in turn phosphorylate a diverse series of substrates, including cytoplasmic phospholipase A_2, cytoskeletal components, protein synthesis machinery, and, perhaps most importantly, transcription factors (332). The substrate specificities of different MAP kinase families, although overlapping, are unique (333). Thus, a unique combination of proteins is activated by each MAP kinase. It is proposed that activation of transcription of new genes in response to growth-factor action extends in part from these actions of MAP kinases. Included among the transcription factors affected are those that govern the synthesis of cyclins, which allow entry into the cell cycle (334,335).

The role of the MAPK pathway in ovarian cancer has been investigated. Activation of MAPK family members was detected following stimulation of ovarian cancer cells with transforming growth factor, as well as through epidermal growth factor receptor activation (336). Treatment of ovarian carcinoma cell lines *in vitro* with paclitaxel or cisplatin resulted in measurable changes in MAPK levels, with resulting effects toward proliferation or apoptosis (337). In another analysis, ERK expression was associated with clinical parameters related to better outcome, such as lower volume of residual disease (336). Moreover, it correlated significantly with improved survival. Thus, there is evidence of a beneficial prognostic role for ERK in human ovarian cancer patients.

Phosphatidylinositol 3′-Kinase

Phosphatidylinositol 3′-kinase (PI3K) is a lipid kinase that appears to play an important role in mediating a wide variety of signals involved in diverse processes including proliferation, apoptosis, and vesicular trafficking (338). PI3K is a heterodimeric protein that is activated by a wide variety of receptor–TKs such as the insulin, PDGF, and EGF receptors. It has been well established that phosphorylation of a tyrosine residue on the receptor will serve as a docking site for a component of PI3K (p85) that in turn recruits the catalytic subunit of PI3K (p110). Alternatively, PI3K can be activated through a *ras*-dependent mechanism. The PI3K/AKT pathway has been implicated as a major determinant of oncogenic transformation in ovarian cancer. Amplification of PI3K renders ovarian cancer cells resistant to the effects of paclitaxel (339). This process can subsequently be reversed by inhibitors of PI3K. PI3K inhibitors decrease cell proliferation, increase sensitivity to paclitaxel, increase apoptosis, and decrease vascularization *in vivo* (339). PI3K is up-regulated in 30% to 45% of ovarian cancers (340,341). Only 2.3% of serous carcinomas had PI3K mutations compared with 20.0% of endometrioid and clear cell cancers. In contrast, PI3K gene amplification (>sevenfold) was common among all histologic subtypes (24.5%) and was inversely associated with the presence of mutations. Overall, PI3K mutation or gene amplification was detected in 30.5% of all ovarian cancers. Intriguingly, multiple other components of the PI3K signaling cascade, including AKT1, AKT2, P70S6 kinase, TCL1, and GSK3α, are located at sites of copy number abnormalities in ovarian cancer, providing further evidence that this pathway is potentially important in the development of ovarian cancer (339).

As mentioned above, PI3K has been widely recognized as being able to phosphorylate phosphatidylinositols at the 3′ position, which in turn activates protein kinase C (PKC). However, it is appreciated that there are other substrates of PI3K including p70, S6K, and, most importantly, PKB/AKT. AKT is a protein kinase that has been demonstrated to mediate multiple biologic processes. Of particular importance, PI3K has been identified as amplified in breast and ovarian cancers. Increased PI3K activity has been detected in a large subset of ovarian cancers, while inhibition of this pathway leads to inhibition of cellular proliferation (342).

AKT

AKT, a member of the protein kinase B family, represents a subfamily of the serine/threonine protein kinases, and the primary mediator of the effects of PI3K (338). Three members of this family, AKT1, AKT2, and AKT3, have been identified. A broad spectrum of substrates is phosphorylated by AKT, including transcription factors (Creb, Forkhead), proteins critical for apoptosis (caspase-9, BAD, IKK), and cell-cycle proteins (p21, p27) and other kinases (GSK-3). These substrates in turn activate multiple other pathways, including cross talk with the MAPK pathway. The downstream effects of AKT activation include suppression of apoptosis, induction of cell-cycle progression, and induced resistance to cytotoxic drugs. Given these effects, it is not surprising to note evidence linking AKT to the development of cancer. AKT has been found to be activated and amplified in ovarian cancer (343). It has also been shown to play a major role in drug resistance in a variety of human malignancies. Approximately 36% of primary ovarian tumors show elevated AKT2 activity (340,344). The majority of these tumors were of high grade and late stage, implicating the kinase in tumor progression. AKT3 has been shown to be highly expressed in 21% of primary ovarian tumors (340). Strikingly, purified AKT3 exhibited up to tenfold higher specific activity than AKT1. Consistent with this finding, AKT3 levels in a range of ovarian cancer cell lines correlated with total AKT activity and proliferation rates, implicating AKT3 as a key mediator of ovarian oncogenesis. Specific silencing of AKT3 using short hairpin RNA markedly inhibited proliferation of the two cell lines with the highest AKT3 expression and total AKT activity by slowing G(2)-M phase transition (340). These findings are consistent with AKT3 playing a key role in the genesis of at least one subset of ovarian cancers.

Protein Kinase C

PKC was originally described as a calcium (hence the C) and phospholipid-dependent kinase distinct from the cAMP-dependent protein kinase A. It is now recognized that the term *protein kinase C* can refer to at least eight distinct molecular isoforms that, in some cases, may actually be independent of calcium, but are related to other members of the family because of structural similarities.

The importance of PKC in tumorigenesis was suggested by the finding that PKC isoforms are receptors for the tumor-promoting phorbol esters, one of the first demonstrations of a discrete molecular effector of a carcinogenetic stimulus (345). The addition of growth factors was recognized to increase the enzymatic activity of diacylglycerols, which are normal activators of PKC that can be produced by phospholipase-C. Thus, tyrosine kinase–linked growth factors could be shown to phosphorylate and activate the phospholipase-C-gamma isoform, whereas calcium-linked growth factors (see discussion of G-protein and calcium-related signals below) activate phospholipase-C-gamma. PKC, once activated, can directly influence the activity of the MAP kinase pathway by phosphorylating raf (346). Additional pathways leading to activation of transcription from PKC-sensitive promoter elements exist.

Cyclin-Dependent Kinases

The ultimate consequence of growth factor action is the entry of quiescent cells into the cell cycle. The molecular events responsible for this process are currently being elucidated. Classic biochemical experiments showed that, at the onset of mitosis, there was an increase in protein kinase activity directed at histones. It was hypothesized that altered phosphorylation of nuclear proteins allows or promotes the morphologically apparent changes in chromosomal condensation. It was therefore of great interest when a protein with histone H1-kinase activity was found to complement a yeast mutant defective in cell-cycle progression. The responsible protein, $p34^{cdc\text{-}2}$, was found to be a serine/threonine kinase whose activity was cyclically regulated by the appearance during the normal yeast cell cycle of a family of molecules called cyclins, with the active H1-kinase enzyme consisting of a complex of cyclin and an appropriately phosphorylated $p34^{cdc2}$ catalytic subunit (347–351).

Subsequently, through the use of homology cloning and complementation of function in yeast, it became apparent that progression through G_1 is also regulated by a family of analogous molecules now collectively referred to as cyclin-dependent kinases (cdk). There are at least nine cdks (cdk1 through cdk9) and 15 cyclins (cyclin A through cyclin T) (352). Cdk4 and cdk6, along with their D-type cyclins, are responsible for progression through G_1 phase. Cdk2 and cyclin E complex are responsible for progression from G_1 to S phase. Cdk2 and cyclin A are responsible for progression through S phase, while cdk1 and cyclin B are required for mitosis. These complexes in turn are inhibited by a combination of small proteins called cdk inhibitors (CKIs this is the same acronym as used earlier). The INK4 (inhibitor of cdk4) family consists of $p16^{ink4a}$, $p15^{ink4b}$, $p18^{ink4c}$, and $p19^{ink4d}$ and specifically inhibits cyclin D–associated kinases. The protein kinase inhibitor family of $p21^{waf1}$, $p27^{Kip1}$, and $p57^{kip2}$ inhibits the cyclin E/cdk2 and cyclin A/cdk2 complexes. Loss of expression of CKIs confers a poor prognosis in a variety of cancers (352). Of great current interest is how growth factors regulate the enzymatic cascade that is directly responsible for entry into the cell cycle. Of fundamental importance is the observation that the tumor-suppressor gene product of the retinoblastoma-related locus (pRb) is a substrate for cdk2 and that phosphorylation of Rb correlates with entry into the S phase (353,354).

It is now well documented that cyclin D-cdk4/6 and cyclin E-cdk2 complexes phosphorylate Rb, causing it to release the transcription factor E2F. E2F in turn regulates the expression of S-phase genes, which are required for DNA replication. Thus, the G_1–S-phase transition is critically dependent on sufficient cdk activity and, as expected, is a frequent target for alteration in cancer cells. For instance, recent analysis has demonstrated that cyclin E is frequently amplified and overexpressed in ovarian cancer (355). Genetic abnormalities such as these may provide important enzymatic targets for novel therapeutic agents.

G-Protein and Calcium-Related Signals

Second-messenger control of intracellular events was first demonstrated convincingly in the case of cAMP and glycolysis in liver treated with α-adrenergic agonists. Paramount to establishing the mechanism of this process was the observation that guanine nucleotides were necessary for the efficient generation of cAMP. This led to the purification of proteins that, in the GTP-bound state, stimulated adenylate cyclase, and thus were called G-proteins (356). G-protein-coupled receptors (GPCR), the prototype of which is the adrenergic receptor, are structurally very distinct in comparison to receptor-linked tyrosine kinases. The GPCR superfamily, now with over 200 members, has an external ligand-binding portion, seven transmembrane segments, and a carboxyl-terminal tail. These serpentine receptors couple to G-proteins, which are now understood to interact not only with adenylate cyclase, but also with certain phospholipases including phospholipase-C-β (325). The membrane lipid phosphatidylinositol-4,5-bisphosphate then is hydrolyzed to yield the soluble metabolite inositol 1,4,5-tris-phosphate, which releases calcium from internal stores as well as diacylglycerol, described above as the endogenous regulator of PKC (Fig. 3.3) (357).

Recent work has demonstrated that a subfamily of GPCRs that bind lysophospholipids appear to play a role in the development of ovarian cancer (358). These receptors include PSP24 and the EDG receptors. These receptors do not bind all lysophospholipids, but are activated by lysophatidic acid (LPA) and sphingosine-1-phosphate (325,359,360). The combination of multiple receptor family members, different ligands, and the available intracellular G-proteins produces a wide range of biologic effects including proliferation, invasion, and cellular survival.

Protein Phosphatases

Protein phosphatases are a relatively newly described group of proteins that function in an opposing manner to protein kinases, providing important regulatory mechanisms to the above-described signal cascades. In fact, it has been proposed that phosphatases play as critical a role in cellular functions, such as proliferation, differentiation, and apoptosis, as protein kinases (361,362).

Protein phosphatases are divided into groups by different criteria, but the most commonly used is that of substrate specificity: protein tyrosine phosphatases (PTPs), protein serine/threonine phosphatases (PSPs), and dual-specificity phosphatases (DSPs). PTPs are further classified according to whether they contain a transmembrane (TM) domain or not. TM-domain-containing PTPs called receptor PTPs (RPTPs) have extracellular domains and a catalytic domain in their intracellular portion. Many RPTPs (such as CD45, LAR, and PTP-β) possess structural features that suggest a role in cellular adhesion (363). Indeed, studies have revealed that several RPTPs are important regulators of neuronal adhesion (364).

Non-TM PTPs are also important regulators of tyrosine phosphorylation. Some appear to associate with tyrosine kinases through the SH2 domains found within their structures (SHP-1, SHP-2). SHP-1 and SHP-2 play critical roles in regulating tyrosine kinase signals within hematopoietic cells (349,365). *PTEN* is a tyrosine phosphatase that has been demonstrated to have an inhibitory effect on cellular proliferation (366). This inhibitory activity has been traced to a negative regulation of PI3K and AKT activity (367,368). Whether this is a direct effect of *PTEN's* ability to dephosphorylate phosphotyrosine residues or its additional activity as a lipid phosphatase remains unclear. However, mutations in *PTEN* have been identified in a wide variety of tumors as well as in the germ line of patients with Cowden's syndrome (369). Based upon these observations, it is widely concluded that *PTEN* is a tumor-suppressor gene. Recent work has identified mutations within this gene in endometrial cancers and endometrioid ovarian cancers (370,371). In a wider number of ovarian cancers, *PTEN* activity is suppressed, leading to an overactivity of the PI3K pathway.

PSPs comprise a group of protein phosphatases containing three subunits: regulatory, variable, and catalytic (372). Previously, four major families had been identified (PP1, PP2A, PP2B, and PP2C), although a fifth family has recently been added. Multiple members exist within each family with some evidence for substrate specificity differences between families. Type 2A PSPs have selective substrate specificity for PKC phosphorylated proteins and the ribosomal S6 protein. Type 2A PSPs are of particular interest because they have been found to associate with complexes formed by DNA tumor virus proteins and cellular proteins. The presence of PP2A in these complexes suggests it may play a role in the alteration of cellular proliferation mediated by DNA tumor viruses (373,374).

Dual-specificity phosphatases are frequently grouped with PTPs owing to their ability to dephosphorylate phosphotyrosine moieties. However, they are also able to use phosphoserine and phosphothreonine as substrates. DSPs such as MKP-1 and Cdi1 localize to the nucleus, where they have been shown to dephosphorylate MAP kinases (375). Thus, this represents an important family of proteins that may serve to regulate the incoming proliferative signals from various MAP kinase cascades. For instance, MKP-1/CL100 has been found to be differentially expressed between normal and malignant ovarian epithelium (376). Reexpression of this gene in ovarian cancer cells decreases the malignant phenotype.

Wnt/β-Catenin Pathway

The Wnt/β-catenin pathway is an important signal transduction pathway frequently disrupted in cancer cells (377). In the absence of Wnt signaling, β-catenin expression is controlled by the formation of a degradation complex that includes GSK3B, APC, and Axin (378). This complex produces ubiquitination of β-catenin and its subsequent degradation by the proteosome. When the Wnt ligand binds to its receptor Frizzled, the degradation complex is destabilized, resulting in higher levels of nonphosphorylated β-catenin. High levels of β-catenin translocate to the nucleus, where it acts as a cofactor for TCF/LEF transcription factor.

This pathway has been studied extensively in human cancers (377). Mutations in this pathway are very common in colorectal cancers. Germ-line mutations within the APC gene form the molecular basis for familial adenomatous polyposis (FAP). Somatic mutations of APC (and to a lesser extent β-catenin) are common in sporadic colorectal cancers. Activating mutations of the Wnt pathway are found in a wide variety of other cancers, including gynecologic cancers. This is especially true for the endometrioid histologic subtype of ovarian and endometrial cancers.

The expression of β-catenin in uterine serous carcinoma (USC) and endometrioid endometrial carcinoma (EEC) was investigated in tissue microarrays created from 20 cases of grade 3 EEC and 73 cases of USC (379). β-catenin was present in both tumor types. Expression of β-catenin was also examined by immunohistochemistry in 253 ovarian carcinomas (380). Membrane-associated staining of β-catenin was detected in nearly all cases with no correlation to clinical parameters. Most of the samples (84%) also had cytoplasmic localization, while only 13% had nuclear β-catenin localization. Nuclear β-catenin was almost exclusively present in endometrioid carcinomas. Fifty-three percent of all endometrioid tumors were positive for nuclear β-catenin expression. Better prognostic outcome was found for patients with nuclear β-catenin localization compared to the cases without it. Although the study showed no correlation between β-catenin expression, FIGO stage, and genomic instability, as determined by DNA ploidy status in ovarian carcinoma, nuclear β-catenin expression again was strongly associated with the endometrioid histologic subtype (380).

RNA Interference

Small RNAs. The most familiar role for RNA is as a relatively passive intermediary in the translation of information from genes into proteins, but other functions for this versatile molecule have been emerging (381). Although the first hints about silencing were seen decades ago, the real breakthrough in mechanistic understanding came in 1998. A landmark paper by Fire et al. showed that the trigger for gene silencing is double-stranded RNA (dsRNA) (382). RNA interference (RNAi) was identified as a potent and highly specific gene-silencing phenomenon that is initiated or triggered by dsRNA (383). Since then, other components of the RNAi machinery have been identified at a startling rate, although the picture is still incomplete. RNAi was first observed in plants in the guise of a mysterious immune response to viral pathogens. Based on their origin or function, three types of naturally occurring small RNA have been described. The first is endogenous or artificial micro RNAs (miRNAs), which are expressed from Pol II promoters as primary miRNA transcripts subsequently processed into mature miRNAs in a regulated multistep process. The second is exogenous, short, synthetic, double-stranded, small interfering RNAs (siRNAs), while the third is endogenous siRNAs (381,384).

Micro RNAs. miRNAs are a subset of small (typically 21 to 23 nucleotides) noncoding RNAs evolutionarily conserved in many organisms including yeast, fruit flies, humans, and plants (384). miRNAs have important roles in many functions including development, proliferation, hematopoiesis, and apoptosis (383). Unlike siRNAs, miRNAs usually do not cleave the messenger RNA (mRNA) of a target gene, but instead suppress mRNA translation (384,385). RNA Pol II transcribes miRNA genes in the cell nucleus and gives rise to a large primary miRNA (Fig. 3.10). These initial primary miRNAs are then processed by RNase III, Drasha, to form pre-miRNAs in the nucleus. The pre-miRNAs are exported into the cytoplasm by the transporter exportin 5 and undergo processing by another RNase III, Dicer, to produce a miRNA duplex (384). The RNA duplex is unwound by helicase. The

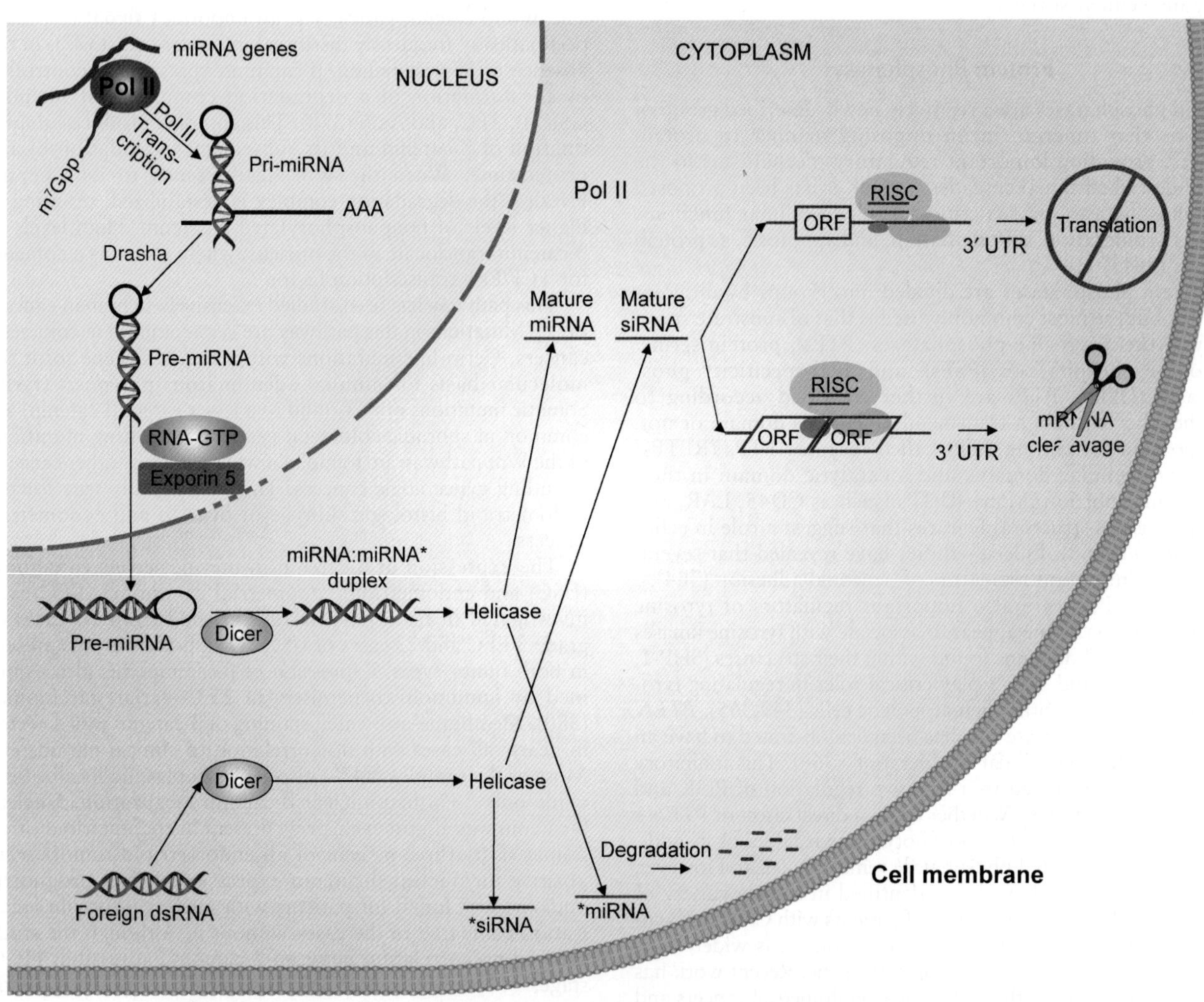

FIGURE 3.10. (*See color plate section.*) This figure depicts distinct roles for dsRNA in a network of interacting silencing pathways. In some cases dsRNA functions as the initial stimulus (or trigger), for example, when foreign dsRNA (blue) is introduced experimentally. In other cases transcription can produce dsRNA (red) by read through from adjacent transcripts. miRNA genes often cluster on the chromosome and are transcribed by RNA Pol II to form pri-miRNAs in the nucleus. The primary miRNAs then undergo procession by RNase III, Drasha, and are exported to the cytoplasm by exportin 5. Another RNase III, Dicer, further processes the small RNA products of the Dicer, pre-miRNA or pre-siRNA, to generate a ~22nt mi/siRNA:mi/siRNA* duplex, where mi/siRNA* is complementary to mi/siRNA. Helicase can divide the duplex into two separate ones. Whereas *mi/*siRNA is degraded, mature mi/siRNA can enter the RNA-induced silence complex (RISC). The RISC complex blocks protein synthesis by imperfectly binding to the 3′UTR of the mRNA (**upper right**), causing inhibition of translation; the other one is to endonucleolytically cleave the target mRNA by perfect or nearly perfect base pairing (**lower right**).

mature miRNA enters the miRNA-induced silencing complex, which then blocks protein synthesis by binding to the 3′ untranslated region (UTR) of the mRNA.

miRNAs can influence the signaling pathway by repressing several secreted signaling proteins (384). For example, the 3′UTR of ras genes contains multiple *let-7* complementary sites allowing *let-7* to regulate ras expression. Conversely, miRNA expression can be regulated by protooncogenes. c-Myc directly binds to the locus of six miRNAs and stimulates their expression (384).

Small-Interfering RNAs. Small-interfering RNAs (siRNAs) are similar to their cousin miRNAs. The initial processing of dsRNA in the nucleus by Dicer is similar. The small RNA products of the Dicer-mediated dsRNA processing reaction guide distinct protein complexes to their targets, including the RNA-induced silencing complex, which is implicated in mRNA destruction and translational repression, and the RNA-induced transcriptional silencing complex, which is implicated in chromatin silencing (381). The single-stranded siRNA in the RNA-induced silencing complex then guides sequence-specific degradation of complementary or near-complementary target mRNA. In summary, these small interfering siRNAs trigger gene silencing by binding to their target RNA sequences and cleaving them.

Endogenous siRNAs. In addition to the endogenous miRNAs and exogenous siRNAs, endogenous siRNAs have been discovered in various organisms and fall into at least four classes: trans-acting siRNAs (tasiRNAs), repeat-associated siRNAs (rasiRNAs), small-scan RNAs (scnRNAs), and Piwi-interacting RNAs (piRNAs) (383). tasiRNAs are small (approximately 21 nucleotides) RNAs that have been reported in plants that are encoded in intergenic regions that correspond to both the sense and antisense strands (386). In *Arabidopsis thaliana*, tasiRNAs require components of the miRNA machinery and cleave their target mRNAs in transcription. It has been postulated that rasiRNAs that match sense and antisense sequences could be involved in transcriptional gene silencing in *Schizosaccharomyces pombe* and *A. thaliana* (387). scnRNAs are approximately 28-nucleotide RNAs that have been found in *Tetrahymena thermophila* and are thought to be involved in scanning DNA sequences in order to induce genome rearrangement (388). piRNAs are possibly important in mammalian gametogenesis (389). Whereas miRNA and siRNA range between 21 and 26 nucleotides, piRNAs are larger (between 26 and 31 nucleotides) and lack 20 and/or 30 OH termini (390). They tend to cluster and are diversely distributed among exonic, intronic, intergenic, and repeat sequences in the mouse genome, suggesting their potentially diverse roles in regulating gene expression. A fraction of piRNAs are associated with polysomes. Interestingly, piRNAs associate with MIWI, a murine PIWI Argonaute protein expressed exclusively in spermatogenic cells and required for initiating the spermiogenic program (389). As a result these piRNAs can control gene expression involved in sperm development.

RNAi Clinical Potential. The rationale for RNAi-based therapeutic agents is that new siRNAs could be designed to treat diseases by lowering the concentrations of disease-causing gene products. However, the development of such siRNA-based therapies faces two major challenges: the identification of chemically stable and effective siRNA sequences, and the efficient delivery of these sequences to tissue-specific targets *in vivo* with siRNA amounts that are not too toxic to humans (383). Recent advances in understanding the rules for chemically modifying siRNA sequences without compromising gene-silencing efficiencies have allowed the design and synthesis of therapeutically effective siRNA molecules that can silence target genes *in vivo* (383). Based on this rapid progress in understanding the structure and function of siRNAs and their applications in disease models, it is likely that RNAi-based therapeutics will become a reality in the near future.

As our knowledge about tumor biology and the molecular mechanisms underlying the process of carcinogenesis continues to expand, so too will the potential for intervention. In this respect, basic science and clinical research will continue to complement each other in increasingly important ways.

References

1. Willis R. *The Spread of Tumors in the Human Body*. London: Butterworth; 1952.
2. Cotran R, Robbins SL, Kumar V. *Pathologic Basis of Disease*. 5th ed. Philadelphia: Harcourt Brace Jovanovich; 1994.
3. Tannock I. *Cell Proliferation*. Toronto: McGraw-Hill; 1992.
4. Roberts JM, Koff A, Polyak K, et al. Cyclins, CDKs, and cyclin kinase inhibitors. *Cold Spring Harb Symp Quant Biol* 1994;59:31–38.
5. Sherr CJ. Cancer cell cycles. *Science* 1996;274:1672–1677.
6. Knudsen ES, Buckmaster C, Chen TT, et al. Inhibition of DNA synthesis by RB: effects on G1/S transition and S-phase progression. *Genes Dev* 1998;12:2278–2292.
7. Ewen ME. The cell cycle and the retinoblastoma protein family. *Cancer Metastasis Rev* 1994;13:45–66.
8. Shirodkar S, Ewen M, DeCaprio JA, et al. The transcription factor E2F interacts with the retinoblastoma product and a p107–cyclin A complex in a cell cycle–regulated manner. *Cell* 1992;68:157–166.
9. Ludlow JW, Shon J, Pipas JM, et al. The retinoblastoma susceptibility gene product undergoes cell cycle–dependent dephosphorylation and binding to and release from SV40 large T. *Cell* 1990;60:387–396.
10. Weintraub SJ, Prater CA, Dean DC. Retinoblastoma protein switches the E2F site from positive to negative element. *Nature* 1992;358:259–261.
11. Elledge SJ. Cell cycle checkpoints: preventing an identity crisis. *Science* 1996;274:1664–1672.
12. Planas-Silva MD, Weinberg RA. The restriction point and control of cell proliferation. *Curr Opin Cell Biol* 1997;9:768–772.
13. el-Deiry WS, Tokino T, Velculescu VE, et al. WAF1: a potential mediator of p53 tumor suppression. *Cell* 1993;75:817–825.
14. Polyak K, Xia Y, Collins JL. A model for p53-induced apoptosis (see comments). *Nature* 1993;389:300.
15. Fiscella M, Ullrich SJ, Zambrano N, et al. Mutation of the serine 15 phosphorylation site of human p53 reduces the ability of p53 to inhibit cell cycle progression. *Oncogene* 1993;8:1519–1528.
16. Peng CY, Graves PR, Thoma RS, et al. Mitotic and G2 checkpoint control: regulation of 14–3–3 protein binding by phosphorylation of Cdc25C on serine–216. *Science* 1997;277:1501–1505.
17. Sanchez Y, Wong C, Thoma RS, et al. Conservation of the Chk1 checkpoint pathway in mammals: linkage of DNA damage to CDK regulation through Cdc25. *Science* 1997;277:1497–1501.
18. Hardwick KG. The spindle checkpoint. *Trends Genet* 1998;14:1–4.
19. Cahill DP, Lengauer C, Yu J, et al. Mutations of mitotic checkpoint genes in human cancers. *Nature* 1998;392:300–303.
20. Schmitt CA. Senescence: apoptosis and therapy—cutting the lifelines of cancer. *Nat Rev Cancer* 2003;3:286–295.
21. Stampfer MR, Yaswen P. Human epithelial cell immortalization as a step in carcinogenesis. *Cancer Lett* 2003;194:199–208.
22. Newbold RF. The significance of telomerase activation and cellular immortalization in human cancer. *Mutagenesis* 2002;17:539–550.
23. Granville DJ, Carthy CM, Hunt DW, et al. Apoptosis: molecular aspects of cell death and disease. *Lab Invest* 1998;78:893–913.
24. Soini Y, Paakko P, Lehto VP. Histopathological evaluation of apoptosis in cancer. *Am J Pathol* 1998;153:1041–1053.
25. Kamesaki H. Mechanisms involved in chemotherapy-induced apoptosis and their implications in cancer chemotherapy. *Int J Hematol* 1998;68: 29–43.
26. Mesner PW Jr., Budihardjo II, Kaufmann SH. Chemotherapy-induced apoptosis. *Adv Pharmacol* 1997;41:461–499.
27. Milas L, Gregoire V, Hunter N, et al. Radiation-induced apoptosis in tumors: effect of radiation modulating agents. *Adv Exp Med Biol* 1997;400B:559–564.
28. Susin SA, Zamzami N, Castedo M, et al. The central executioner of apoptosis: multiple connections between protease activation and mitochondria in Fas/APO–1/CD95– and ceramide-induced apoptosis. *J Exp Med* 1997;186:25–37.
29. Berke G. The CTL's kiss of death. *Cell* 1995;81:9–12.
30. Nagata S. Fas-mediated apoptosis. *Adv Exp Med Biol* 1996;406:119–124.
31. Nagata S. Apoptosis by death factor. *Cell* 1997;88:355–365.
32. Miyashita T, Reed JC. Tumor suppressor p53 is a direct transcriptional activator of the human bax gene. *Cell* 1995;80:293–299.
33. Wu GS, Burns TF, McDonald ER 3rd, et al. KILLER/DR5 is a DNA damage–inducible p5-regulated death receptor gene. *Nat Genet* 1997;17: 141–143.
34. Lane DP. Cancer. p53, guardian of the genome. *Nature* 1992;358:15–16.

35. Kerr JF, Winterford CM, Harmon BV. Apoptosis. Its significance in cancer and cancer therapy. *Cancer* 1994;73:2013–2026.
36. Gavrieli Y, Sherman Y, Ben-Sasson SA. Identification of programmed cell death *in situ* via specific labeling of nuclear DNA fragmentation. *J Cell Biol* 1992;119:493–501.
37. Wijsman JH, Jonker RR, Keijzer R, et al. A new method to detect apoptosis in paraffin sections: *in situ* end-labeling of fragmented DNA. *J Histochem Cytochem* 1993;41:7–12.
38. Lipponen P, Aaltomaa S, Kosma VM, et al. Apoptosis in breast cancer as related to histopathological characteristics and prognosis. *Eur J Cancer* 1994;30A:2068–2073.
39. Shinohara T, Ohshima K, Murayama H, et al. Apoptosis and proliferation in gastric carcinoma: the association with histological type. *Histopathology* 1996;29:123–129.
40. Hockenbery DM. Bcl-2 in cancer: development and apoptosis. *J Cell Sci Suppl* 1994;18:51–55.
41. Krueger NX, Van Vactor D, Wan HI, et al. The transmembrane tyrosine phosphatase DLAR controls motor axon guidance in *Drosophila*. *Cell* 1996;84:611–622.
42. Reed JC. Bcl-2 and the regulation of programmed cell death. *J Cell Biol* 1994;124:1–6.
43. White E. Life, death, and the pursuit of apoptosis. *Genes Dev* 1996;10:1.
44. Yang E, Korsmeyer SJ. Molecular thanatopsis: a discourse on the BCL2 family and cell death. *Blood* 1996;88:386–401.
45. Yin XM, Oltvai ZN, Korsmeyer SJ. BH1 and BH2 domains of Bcl-2 are required for inhibition of apoptosis and heterodimerization with bax. *Nature* 1994;369:321–323.
46. Kroemer G. The proto-oncogene Bcl-2 and its role in regulating apoptosis. *Nat Med* 1997;3:614–620.
47. Martinez J, Georgoff I, Levine AJ. Cellular localization and cell cycle regulation by a temperature-sensitive p53 protein. *Genes Dev* 1991;5:151–159.
48. Michalovitz D, Halevy O, Oren M. Conditional inhibition of transformation and of cell proliferation by a temperature-sensitive mutant of p53. *Cell* 1990;62:671–680.
49. Miyashita T, Krajewski S, Krajewska M, et al. Tumor suppressor p53 is a regulator of bcl-2 and bax gene expression *in vitro* and *in vivo*. *Oncogene* 1994;9:1799–1805.
50. Yonish-Rouach E, Resnitzky D, Lotem J, et al. Wild-type p53 induces apoptosis of myeloid leukaemic cells that is inhibited by interleukin-6. *Nature* 1991;352:345–347.
51. Evan GI, Wyllie AH, Gilbert CS, et al. Induction of apoptosis in fibroblasts by c-myc protein. *Cell* 1992;69:119–128.
52. Kauffmann-Zeh A, Rodriguez-Viciana P, Ulrich E, et al. Suppression of c-Myc–induced apoptosis by Ras signalling through PI(3)K and PKB. *Nature* 1997;385:544–548.
53. Trent JC 2nd, McConkey DJ, Loughlin SM, et al. Ras signaling in tumor necrosis factor–induced apoptosis. *EMBO J* 1996;15:4497–4505.
54. Ward R, Todd AV, Santiago F, et al. Activation of the K-ras oncogene in colorectal neoplasms is associated with decreased apoptosis. *Cancer* 1997;79:1106.
55. Chen CY, Faller DV. Phosphorylation of Bcl-2 protein and association with p21Ras in ras-induced apoptosis. *J Biol Chem* 1996;271:2376–2379.
56. Chieng D, Ross JS, Ambros, RA. Bcl-2 expression and the development of endometrial carcinoma. *Mod Pathol* 1996;9:402.
57. Giatromanolaki A, Sivridis E, Koukourakis MI, et al. Bcl-2 and p53 expression in stage I endometrial carcinoma. *Anticancer Res* 1998;18:3689–3693.
58. Heatley MK. Association between the apoptotic index and established prognostic parameters in endometrial adenocarcinoma. *Histopathology* 1995;27:469–472.
59. Henderson GS, Brown KA, Perkins SL, et al. Bcl-2 is down-regulated in atypical endometrial hyperplasia and adenocarcinoma. *Mod Pathol* 1996;9:430–438.
60. Ioffe OB, Papadimitriou JC, Drachenberg CB. Correlation of proliferation indices, apoptosis, and related oncogene expression (bcl-2 and c-erbB-2) and p53 in proliferative, hyperplastic, and malignant endometrium. *Hum Pathol* 1998;29:1150–1159.
61. Saegusa M, Kamata Y, Isono M, et al. Bcl-2 expression is correlated with a low apoptotic index and associated with progesterone receptor immunoreactivity in endometrial carcinomas. *J Pathol* 1996;180:275–282.
62. Bur ME, Perlman C, Edelmann L, et al. p53 expression in neoplasms of the uterine corpus. *Am J Clin Pathol* 1992;98:81–87.
63. Kohler MF, Berchuck A, Davidoff AM, et al. Overexpression and mutation of p53 in endometrial carcinoma. *Cancer Res* 1992;52:1622–1627.
64. Koshiyama M, Konishi I, Wang DP, et al. Immunohistochemical analysis of p53 protein over-expression in endometrial carcinomas: inverse correlation with sex steroid receptor status. *Virchows Arch A Pathol Anat Histopathol* 1993;423:265–271.
65. Nielsen AL, Nyholm HC. p53 protein and c-erbB-2 protein (p185) expression in endometrial adenocarcinoma of endometrioid type. An immunohistochemical examination on paraffin sections. *Am J Clin Pathol* 1994;102:76–79.
66. Reinartz JJ, George E, Lindgren BR, et al. Expression of p53, transforming growth factor alpha, epidermal growth factor receptor, and c-erbB-2 in endometrial carcinoma and correlation with survival and known predictors of survival. *Hum Pathol* 1994;25:1075–1083.
67. Golstein P, Kroemer G. Cell death by necrosis: towards a molecular definition. *Trends Biochem Sci* 2007;32:37–43.
68. Festjens N, Vanden Berghe T, Cornelis S, et al. RIP1, a kinase on the crossroads of a cell's decision to live or die. *Cell Death Differ* 2007;14:400–10.
69. Barnabei VM, Miller DS, Bauer KD, et al. Flow cytometric evaluation of epithelial ovarian cancer. *Am J Obstet Gynecol* 1990;162:1584–1592.
70. Kallioniemi OP, Punnonen R, Mattila J, et al. Prognostic significance of DNA index, multiploidy, and S-phase fraction in ovarian cancer. *Cancer* 1988;61:334–339.
71. Brescia RJ, Barakat RA, Beller U, et al. The prognostic significance of nuclear DNA content in malignant epithelial tumors of the ovary. *Cancer* 1990;65:141–147.
72. Griffiths AP, Cross D, Kingston RE, et al. Flow cytometry and AgNORs in benign, borderline, and malignant mucinous and serous tumours of the ovary. *Int J Gynecol Pathol* 1993;12:307–314.
73. Henriksen R, Strang P, Backstrom T, et al. Ki-67 immunostaining and DNA flow cytometry as prognostic factors in epithelial ovarian cancers. *Anticancer Res* 1994;14:603–608.
74. Lindahl B, Alm P. Flow cytometrical DNA measurements in endometrial hyperplasias. A prospective follow-up study after abrasio only or additional high-dose gestagen treatment. *Anticancer Res* 1991;11:391–395.
75. Strang P, Stendahl U, Tribukait B. Prognostic significance of S-phase fraction as measured by DNA flow cytometry in gynecologic malignancies. *Ann NY Acad Sci* 1993;677:354–363.
76. Takahashi Y, Matsumoto H, Wakuda K, et al. Analysis of cell cycle kinetics using flow cytometry from paraffin-embedded tissues in endometrial adenocarcinoma. *Asia Oceania J Obstet Gynaecol* 1991;17:73–81.
77. Wagenius G, Bergstrom R, Strang P, et al. Prognostic significance of flow cytometric and clinical variables in endometrial adenocarcinoma stages I and II. *Anticancer Res* 1992;12:725–732.
78. Lindahl B, Gullberg B. Flow cytometrical DNA and clinical parameters in the prediction of prognosis in stage I-II endometrial carcinoma. *Anticancer Res* 1991;11:397–401.
79. Mariuzzi G, Sisti S, Santinelli A, et al. Evolutionary somatic cell changes in cervical tumour progression quantitatively evaluated with morphological, histochemical and kinetic parameters. *Pathol Res Pract* 1992;188:454–460.
80. Strang P, Stendahl U, Bergstrom R, et al. Prognostic flow cytometric information in cervical squamous cell carcinoma: a multivariate analysis of 307 patients. *Gynecol Oncol* 1991;43:3–8.
81. Willen R, Himmelmann A, Langstrom-Einarsson E, et al. Prospective malignancy grading: flow cytometry DNA-measurements and adjuvant chemotherapy for invasive squamous cell carcinoma of the uterine cervix. *Anticancer Res* 1993;13:1187–1196.
82. Naus GJ, Zimmerman RL. Prognostic value of flow cytophotometric DNA content analysis in single treatment stage IB-IIA squamous cell carcinoma of the cervix. *Gynecol Oncol* 1991;43:149–153.
83. Zanetta GM, Katzmann JA, Keeney GL, et al. Flow-cytometric DNA analysis of stages IB and IIA cervical carcinoma. *Gynecol Oncol* 1992;46:13–19.
84. Malmstrom H, Schmidt H, Persson PG, et al. Flow cytometric analysis of uterine sarcoma: ploidy and S-phase rate as prognostic indicators. *Gynecol Oncol* 1992;44:172–177.
85. Peters WA 3rd, Howard DR, Andersen WA, et al. Deoxyribonucleic acid analysis by flow cytometry of uterine leiomyosarcomas and smooth muscle tumors of uncertain malignant potential. *Am J Obstet Gynecol* 1992;166:1646–1653; discussion 1653–1654.
86. Wolfson AH, Wolfson DJ, Sittler SY, et al. A multivariate analysis of clinicopathologic factors for predicting outcome in uterine sarcomas. *Gynecol Oncol* 1994;52:56–62.
87. Bocklage TJ, Smith HO, Bartow SA. Distinctive flow histogram pattern in molar pregnancies with elevated maternal serum human chorionic gonadotropin levels. *Cancer* 1994;73:2782–2790.
88. Fukunaga M, Ushigome S, Sugishita M. Application of flow cytometry in diagnosis of hydatidiform moles. *Mod Pathol* 1993;6:353–359.
89. Dolan JR, McCall AR, Gooneratne S, et al. DNA ploidy, proliferation index, grade, and stage as prognostic factors for vulvar squamous cell carcinomas. *Gynecol Oncol* 1993;48:232–235.
90. Hatch KD. Preinvasive cervical neoplasia. *Semin Oncol* 1994;21:12–16.
91. Sherman ME. Theories of endometrial carcinogenesis: a multidisciplinary approach. *Mod Pathol* 2000;13:295–308.
92. Feeley KM, Wells M. Precursor lesions of ovarian epithelial malignancy. *Histopathology* 2001;38:87–95.
93. Teneriello MG, Ebina M, Linnoila RI, et al. p53 and Ki-ras gene mutations in epithelial ovarian neoplasms. *Cancer Res* 1993;53:3103–3108.
94. Sell S. Stem cell origin of cancer and differentiation therapy. *Crit Rev Oncol Hemat* 2004;51:1–28.
95. Goodell MA, Brose K, Pradis G, et al. Isolation and functional properties of murine hematopoietic stem cells that are replicating *in vivo*. *J Exp Med* 1996;183:1797–1806.
96. Connolly DC, Bao R, Nikitin AY, et al. Female mice chimeric for expression of the simian virus 40 Tag under control of the *MISIIR* promoter develop epithelial ovarian cancer. *Cancer Res* 2003;63:1389–1397.
97. Dinulescu DM, Ince TA, Quade BJ, et al. Role of *K-ras* and *Pten* in the development of mouse models of endometriosis and endometrioid ovarian cancer. *Nat Med* 2005;11:63–70.

98. Szotek PP, Pieretti-Vanmarcke R, Masiakos PT, et al. Ovarian cancer side population defines cells with stem cell-like characteristics and müllerian inhibiting substance responsiveness. *Proc Natl Acad Sci USA* 2006;103: 11154–11159.
99. Bapat SA, Mali AM, Koppikar CB, et al. Stem and progenitor-like cells contribute to the aggressive behavior of human epithelial ovarian cancer. *Cancer Res* 2005;65:3025–3029.
100. Squire J, Phillips RA. *Genetic Basis of Cancer*. 2nd ed. Toronto: McGraw-Hill; 1992.
101. Kurzrock R, Talpaz, M. *Molecular Biology in Cancer Medicine*. London: Martin Dunitz; 1995.
102. Sandberg A, Chen, Z. *Cancer Cytogenetics: Nomenclature and Clinical Applications*. London: Martin Dunitz; 1995.
103. Hu J, Surti U. Subgroups of uterine leiomyomas based on cytogenetic analysis. *Hum Pathol* 1991;22:1009–1016.
104. Rein MS, Friedman AJ, Barbieri RL, et al. Cytogenetic abnormalities in uterine leiomyomata. *Obstet Gynecol* 1991;77:923–926.
105. Emoto M, Iwasaki H, Kikuchi M, et al. Characteristics of cloned cells of mixed müllerian tumor of the human uterus. Carcinoma cells showing myogenic differentiation *in vitro*. *Cancer* 1993;71:3065–3075.
106. Laxman R, Currie JL, Kurman RJ, et al. Cytogenetic profile of uterine sarcomas. *Cancer* 1993;71:1283–1288.
107. Hampton GM, Penny LA, Baergen RN, et al. Loss of heterozygosity in cervical carcinoma: subchromosomal localization of a putative tumor-suppressor gene to chromosome 11q22-q24. *Proc Natl Acad Sci USA* 1994;91: 6953–6957.
108. Kohno T, Takayama H, Hamaguchi M, et al. Deletion mapping of chromosome 3p in human uterine cervical cancer. *Oncogene* 1993;8:1825–1832.
109. Segers P, Haesen S, Amy JJ, et al. Detection of premalignant stages in cervical smears with a biotinylated probe for chromosome 1. *Cancer Genet Cytogenet* 1994;75:120–129.
110. Sreekantaiah C, De Braekeleer M, Haas O. Cytogenetic findings in cervical carcinoma. A statistical approach. *Cancer Genet Cytogenet* 1991;53:75–81.
111. Gallion HH, Powell DE, Smith LW, et al. Chromosome abnormalities in human epithelial ovarian malignancies. *Gynecol Oncol* 1990;38:473–477.
112. Kohlberger PD, Kieback DG, Mian C, et al. Numerical chromosomal aberrations in borderline, benign, and malignant epithelial tumors of the ovary: correlation with p53 protein overexpression and Ki-67. *J Soc Gynecol Investig* 1997;4:262–264.
113. Persons DL, Hartmann LC, Herath JF, et al. Fluorescence *in situ* hybridization analysis of trisomy 12 in ovarian tumors. *Am J Clin Pathol* 1994;102:775–779.
114. Gorski GK, McMorrow LE, Blumstein L, et al. Trisomy 14 in two cases of granulosa cell tumor of the ovary. *Cancer Genet Cytogenet* 1992;60: 202–205.
115. Crickard K, Marinello MJ, Crickard U, et al. Borderline malignant serous tumors of the ovary maintained on extracellular matrix: evidence for clonal evolution and invasive potential. *Cancer Genet Cytogenet* 1986;23:135–143.
116. Pejovic T, Heim S, Mandahl N, et al. Chromosome aberrations in 35 primary ovarian carcinomas. *Genes Chromosomes Cancer* 1992;4:58–68.
117. Milatovich A, Heerema NA, Palmer CG. Cytogenetic studies of endometrial malignancies. *Cancer Genet Cytogenet* 1990;46:41–53.
118. Tharapel SA, Qumsiyeh MB, Photopulos G. Numerical chromosome abnormalities associated with early clinical stages of gynecologic tumors. *Cancer Genet Cytogenet* 1991;55:89–96.
119. Gallion HH, Powell DE, Morrow JK, et al. Molecular genetic changes in human epithelial ovarian malignancies. *Gynecol Oncol* 1992;47:137–142.
120. Worsham MJ, Van Dyke DL, Grenman SE, et al. Consistent chromosome abnormalities in squamous cell carcinoma of the vulva. *Genes Chromosomes Cancer* 1991;3:420–432.
121. Williams GT, Wynford-Thomas D. How may clonality be assessed in human tumours? *Histopathology* 1994;24:287–292.
122. Vogelstein B, Fearon ER, Hamilton SR, et al. Clonal analysis using recombinant DNA probes from the X-chromosome. *Cancer Res* 1987;47:4806–4813.
123. Fearon ER, Hamilton SR, Vogelstein B. Clonal analysis of human colorectal tumors. *Science* 1987;238:193–197.
124. Fialkow PJ. Clonal origin of human tumors. *Biochim Biophys Acta* 1976;458:283–321.
125. Sawada M, Azuma C, Hashimoto K, et al. Clonal analysis of human gynecologic cancers by means of the polymerase chain reaction. *Int J Cancer* 1994;58:492–496.
126. Jacobs IJ, Kohler MF, Wiseman RW, et al. Clonal origin of epithelial ovarian carcinoma: analysis by loss of heterozygosity, p53 mutation, and X-chromosome inactivation. *J Natl Cancer Inst* 1992;84:1793–1798.
127. Tsao SW, Mok CH, Knapp RC, et al. Molecular genetic evidence of a unifocal origin for human serous ovarian carcinomas. *Gynecol Oncol* 1993;48:5–10.
128. Li S, Han H, Resnik E, et al. Advanced ovarian carcinoma: molecular evidence of unifocal origin. *Gynecol Oncol* 1993;51:21–25.
129. Muto MG, Welch WR, Mok SC, et al. Evidence for a multifocal origin of papillary serous carcinoma of the peritoneum. *Cancer Res* 1995;55: 490–492.
130. Lu KH, Bell DA, Welch WR, et al. Evidence for the multifocal origin of bilateral and advanced human serous borderline ovarian tumors. *Cancer Res* 1998;58:2328–2330.
131. Gardner GJ, Birrer MJ. Ovarian tumors of low malignant potential: can molecular biology solve this enigma? *J Natl Cancer Inst* 2001;93:1122–1123.
132. Barlogie B, Raber MN, Schumann J, et al. Flow cytometry in clinical cancer research. *Cancer Res* 1983;43:3982–3997.
133. Berchuck A, Boente MP, Kerns BJ, et al. Ploidy analysis of epithelial ovarian cancers using image cytometry. *Gynecol Oncol* 1992;44:61–65.
134. Russack V. Image cytometry: current applications and future trends. *Crit Rev Clin Lab Sci* 1994;31:1–34.
135. Strang P, Stenkvist B, Bergstrom R, et al. Flow cytometry and interactive image cytometry in endometrial carcinoma. A comparative and prognostic study. *Anticancer Res* 1991;11:783–788.
136. Hamaguchi K, Nishimura H, Miyoshi T, et al. Flow cytometric analysis of cellular DNA content in ovarian cancer. *Gynecol Oncol* 1990;37:219–223.
137. Kaern J, Trope CG, Kristensen GB, et al. Flow cytometric DNA ploidy and S-phase heterogeneity in advanced ovarian carcinoma. *Cancer* 1994;73:1870–1877.
138. Demirel D, Laucirica R, Fishman A, et al. Ovarian tumors of low malignant potential. Correlation of DNA index and S-phase fraction with histopathologic grade and clinical outcome. *Cancer* 1996;77:1494–1500.
139. Guerrieri C, Hogberg T, Wingren S, et al. Mucinous borderline and malignant tumors of the ovary. A clinicopathologic and DNA ploidy study of 92 cases. *Cancer* 1994;74:2329–2340.
140. Harlow BL, Fuhr JE, McDonald TW, et al. Flow cytometry as a prognostic indicator in women with borderline epithelial ovarian tumors. *Gynecol Oncol* 1993;50:305–309.
141. Lai CH, Hsueh S, Chang TC, et al. The role of DNA flow cytometry in borderline malignant ovarian tumors. *Cancer* 1996;78:794–802.
142. Eissa S, Khalifa A, Laban M, et al. Comparison of flow cytometric DNA content analysis in fresh and paraffin-embedded ovarian neoplasms: a prospective study. *Br J Cancer* 1998;77:421–425.
143. Bakshi N, Rajwanshi A, Patel F, et al. Prognostic significance of DNA ploidy and S-phase fraction in malignant serous cystadenocarcinoma of the ovary. *Anal Quant Cytol Histol* 1998;20:215–220.
144. Gajewski WH, Fuller AF Jr, Pastel-Ley C, et al. Prognostic significance of DNA content in epithelial ovarian cancer. *Gynecol Oncol* 1994,53:5–12.
145. Pietrzak K, Olszewski W. DNA ploidy as a prognostic factor in patients with ovarian carcinoma. *Pol J Pathol* 1998;49:141–144.
146. Friedlander ML, Hedley DW, Swanson C, et al. Prediction of long-term survival by flow cytometric analysis of cellular DNA content in patients with advanced ovarian cancer. *J Clin Oncol* 1988;6:282–290.
147. Iversen OE. Prognostic value of the flow cytometric DNA index in human ovarian carcinoma. *Cancer* 1988;61:971–975.
148. Resnik E, Trujillo YP, Taxy JB. Long-term survival and DNA ploidy in advanced epithelial ovarian cancer. *J Surg Oncol* 1997;64:299–303.
149. Kaern J, Trope C, Kjorstad KE, et al. Cellular DNA content as a new prognostic tool in patients with borderline tumors of the ovary. *Gynecol Oncol* 1990;38:452–457.
150. Wagner TM, Adler A, Sevelda P, et al. Prognostic significance of cell DNA content in early-stage ovarian cancer (FIGO stages I and II/A) by means of automatic image cytometry. *Int J Cancer* 1994;56:167–172.
151. Zaino RJ, Davis AT, Ohlsson-Wilhelm BM, et al. DNA content is an independent prognostic indicator in endometrial adenocarcinoma. A Gynecologic Oncology Group study. *Int J Gynecol Pathol* 1998;17:312–319.
152. Nordstrom B, Strang P, Lindgren A, et al. Carcinoma of the endometrium: do the nuclear grade and DNA ploidy provide more prognostic information than do the FIGO and WHO classifications? *Int J Gynecol Pathol* 1996;15:191–201.
153. Xue F, Jiao S, Zhao F. A study on DNA content and cell cycle phase analysis in endometrial carcinoma. *Zhonghua Fu Chan Ke Za Zhi* 1996;31: 216–219.
154. Norris HJ, Becker RL, Mikel UV. A comparative morphometric and cytophotometric study of endometrial hyperplasia, atypical hyperplasia, and endometrial carcinoma. *Hum Pathol* 1989;20:219–223.
155. Connor JP, Miller DS, Bauer KD, et al. Flow cytometric evaluation of early invasive cervical cancer. *Obstet Gynecol* 1993;81:367–371.
156. Jarrell MA, Heintz N, Howard P, et al. Squamous cell carcinoma of the cervix: HPV 16 and DNA ploidy as predictors of survival. *Gynecol Oncol* 1992;46:361–366.
157. Anton M, Nenutil R, Rejthar A, et al. DNA flow cytometry: a predictor of a high-risk group in cervical cancer. *Cancer Detect Prev* 1997;21:242–246.
158. Monsonego J, Valensi P, Zerat L, et al. Simultaneous effects of aneuploidy and oncogenic human papillomavirus on histological grade of cervical intraepithelial neoplasia. *Br J Obstet Gynaecol* 1997;104:723–727.
159. Multhaupt H, Bruder E, Elit L, et al. Combined analysis of cervical smears. Cytopathology, image cytometry and *in situ* hybridization. *Acta Cytol* 1993;37:373–378.
160. Clavel C, Zerat L, Binninger I, et al. DNA content measurement and *in situ* hybridization in condylomatous cervical lesions. *Diagn Mol Pathol* 1992;1:180–184.
161. Hanselaar AG, Vooijs GP, Mayall BH, et al. DNA changes in progressive cervical intraepithelial neoplasia. *Anal Cell Pathol* 1992;4:315–324.
162. Kashyap V, Das BC. DNA aneuploidy and infection of human papillomavirus type 16 in preneoplastic lesions of the uterine cervix: correlation with progression to malignancy. *Cancer Lett* 1998;123:47–52.

163. Bocking A, Hilgarth M, Auffermann W, et al. DNA-cytometric diagnosis of prospective malignancy in borderline lesions of the uterine cervix. *Acta Cytol* 1986;30:608–615.
164. Bibbo M, Dytch HE, Alenghat E, et al. DNA ploidy profiles as prognostic indicators in CIN lesions. *Am J Clin Pathol* 1989;92:261–265.
165. Lage JM, Mark SD, Roberts DJ, et al. A flow cytometric study of 137 fresh hydropic placentas: correlation between types of hydatidiform moles and nuclear DNA ploidy. *Obstet Gynecol* 1992;79:403–410.
166. Martin DA, Sutton GP, Ulbright TM, et al. DNA content as a prognostic index in gestational trophoblastic neoplasia. *Gynecol Oncol* 1989;34:383–388.
167. Haba R, Miki H, Kobayashi S, et al. Combined analysis of flow cytometry and morphometry of ovarian granulosa cell tumor. *Cancer* 1993;72:3258.
168. Jacoby AF, Young RH, Colvin RB, et al. DNA content in juvenile granulosa cell tumors of the ovary: a study of early- and advanced-stage disease. *Gynecol Oncol* 1992;46:97–103.
169. Rosen AC, Graf AH, Klein M, et al. DNA ploidy in primary fallopian-tube carcinoma using image cytometry. *Int J Cancer* 1994;58:362–365.
170. Baak JP, Path FR, Hermsen MA, et al. Genomics and proteomics in cancer. *Eur J Cancer* 2003;39:1199–1215.
171. Lichter P, Joos S, Bentz M, et al. Comparative genomic hybridization: uses and limitations. *Semin Hematol* 2000;37:348–357.
172. Shayesteh L, Lu Y, Kuo WL, et al. *PIK3CA* is implicated as an oncogene in ovarian cancer. *Nature Genet* 1999;21:99–102.
173. Snijders A, Nowee M, Fridlyand J, et al. Genome-wide-array-based comparative genomic hybridization reveals genetic homogeneity and frequent copy number increases encompassing *CCNE1* in fallopian tube carcinoma. *Oncogene* 2003;22:4281–4286.
174. Pere H, Tapper J, Seppala M, et al. Genomic alterations in fallopian tube carcinoma: comparison to serous uterine and ovarian carcinomas reveals similarity suggesting likeness in molecular pathogenesis. *Cancer Res* 1998;58:4274–4276.
175. Heselmeyer K, Hellstrom AC, Blegen H, et al. Primary carcinoma of the fallopian tube: comparative genomic hybridization reveals high genetic instability and a specific, recurring pattern of chromosomal aberrations. *Int J Gynecol Pathol* 1998;17:245–254.
176. Tapper J, Sarantaus L, Vahteristo P, et al. Genetic changes in inherited and sporadic ovarian carcinomas by comparative genomic hybridization: extensive similarity except for a difference at chromosome 2q24-q32. *Cancer Res* 1998;58:2715–2719.
177. Patael-Karasik Y, Daniely M, Gotlieb WH, et al. Comparative genomic hybridization in inherited and sporadic ovarian tumors in Israel. *Cancer Genet Cytogenet* 2000;121:26–32.
178. Israeli O, Gotlieb WH, Friedman E, et al. Familial vs. sporadic ovarian tumors: characteristic genomic alterations analyzed by CGH. *Gynecol Oncol* 2003;90:629–636.
179. Zorn K, Jazaeri AA, Awtrey CS, et al. Choice of normal ovarian control influences determination of differentially expressed genes in ovarian cancer expression profiling studies. *Clin Cancer Res* 2003;9(13):4811–4818.
180. Schwartz DR, Kardia SL, Shedden KA, et al. Gene expression in ovarian cancer reflects both morphology and biological behavior, distinguishing clear cell from other poor-prognosis ovarian carcinomas. *Cancer Res* 2002;62(16):4722–4729.
181. Schaner ME, Ross DT, Ciaravino G, et al. Gene expression patterns in ovarian carcinomas. *Mol Biol Cell* 2003;14(11):4376–4386.
182. Zorn K, Bonome T, Gangi L, et al. Gene expression profiles of serous, endometrioid, and clear cell subtypes of ovarian and endometrial cancer. *Clin Cancer Res* 2005;11(18):6422–6430.
183. Tsuda H, Ito YM, Ohashi Y, et al. Identification of overexpression and amplification of ABCF2 in clear cell ovarian adenocarcinomas by cDNA microarray analyses. *Clin Cancer Res* 2005;11(19 Pt 1):6880–6888.
184. Wammuyokoli FW, Bonome T, Lee JY, et al. Exression profiling of mucinous tumor of the ovary identifies genes of clinicopathologic importance. *Clin Cancer Res* 2006;12(3 Pt1):690–700.
185. Heinzelmann-Schwartz VA, Gardiner-Garden M, Henshall SM. A distinct molecular profile associated with mucinous epithelial ovarian cancer. *Br Cancer* 2006;94:904–913.
186. Felmate CM, Lee KR, Johnson M, et al. Whole-genome allelotyping identified distinct loss-of-heterozygosity patterns in mucinous ovarian and appendiceal carcinomas. *Clin Cancer Res* 2005;11:7651–7657.
187. Bonome T, Lee JY, Park DC, et al. Expression profiling of serous low malignant potential, low grade, and high grade tumors of the ovary. *Cancer Res* 2005;65(22):10602–10612.
188. Donninger H, Bonome T, Radonovich M, et al. Whole genome expression profiling of advanced stage papillary serous ovarian cancer reveals activated pathways. *Oncogene* 2004;23(49):8065–8077.
189. Berchuck A, Iversen ES, Lancaster JM, et al. Patterns of gene expression that characterize long-term survival in advanced stage serous ovarian cancers. *Clin Cancer Res* 2005;11(10):3686–3696.
190. Shridhar V, Lee J, Pandita A, et al. Genetic analysis of early- versus late-stage ovarian tumors. *Cancer Res* 2001;61(15):5895–5904.
191. Berchuck A, Iversen ES, Lancaster JM, et al. Prediction of optimal versus suboptimal cytoreduction of advanced-stage serous ovarian cancer with the use of microarrays. *Am J Obstet Gynecol* 2004;190(4):910–925.
192. Jazaeri AA, Lu K, Schmandt R, et al. Molecular determinants of tumor differentiation in papillary serous ovarian carcinoma. *Mol Carcinog* 2003;36(2):53–59.
193. Jazaeri AA, Awtrey CS, Chandramouli GV, et al. Gene expression profiles associated with response to chemotherapy in epithelial ovarian cancers. *Clin Cancer Res* 2005;11(17):6300–6310.
194. Hellman J, Jansen MP, Span PN, et al. Molecular profiling of platinum resistant ovarian cancer. *Int J Cancer* 2006;118(8):1963–1971.
195. Hartmann LC, Lu KH, Linette GP, et al. Gene expression profiles predict early relapse in ovarian cancer after platinum-paclitaxel chemotherapy. *Clin Cancer Res* 2005;11(6):2149–2155.
196. Spentzos D, Levine DA, Kolia S, et al. Unique gene expression profile based on pathologic response in epithelial ovarian cancer. *J Clin Oncol* 2005;23(31):7911–7918.
197. Velculescu VE, Zhang L, Vogelstein B, et al. Serial analysis of gene expression. *Science* 1995;270:484–487.
198. Archer M. The basic science of oncology. In: Tannock IHR, ed. *Chemical Carcinogenesis*. 2nd ed. Toronto: McGraw-Hill; 1992:102.
199. Buick R, Tannock, I. Properties of malignant cells. In: Tannock IHR, ed. *The Basic Science of Oncology*. Toronto: McGraw-Hill; 1992:139.
200. Sutherland D. *Hormones and Cancer*. Toronto: McGraw-Hill; 1992.
201. Ames BN, Shigenaga MK, Gold LS. DNA lesions, inducible DNA repair, and cell division: three key factors in mutagenesis and carcinogenesis. *Environ Health Perspect* 1993;101(Suppl)5:35–44.
202. Wu S, Rodabaugh K, Martinez-Maza O, et al. Stimulation of ovarian tumor cell proliferation with monocyte products including interleukin-1, interleukin-6, and tumor necrosis factor-alpha. *Am J Obstet Gynecol* 1992;166:997–1007.
203. Maronpot RR. Ovarian toxicity and carcinogenicity in eight recent National Toxicology Program studies. *Environ Health Perspect* 1987;73:125–130.
204. Smith BJ, Mattison DR, Sipes IG. The role of epoxidation in 4-vinylcyclohexene–induced ovarian toxicity. *Toxicol Appl Pharmacol* 1990;105:372–381.
205. Nagaoka T, Takeuchi M, Onodera H, et al. Experimental induction of uterine adenocarcinoma in rats by estrogen and N-methyl-N-nitrosourea. *In Vivo* 1993;7:525–530.
206. Turusov VS, Raikhlin NT, Smirnova EA, et al. Uterine sarcomas in CBA mice induced by combined treatment with 1,2-dimethylhydrazine and estradiol dipropionate. Light and electron microscopy. *Exp Toxicol Pathol* 1993;45:161–166.
207. Parkash V, Carcangiu ML. Uterine papillary serous carcinoma after radiation therapy for carcinoma of the cervix. *Cancer* 1992;69:496–501.
208. Benchimol S. Viruses and cancer. In: Tannock IHR, ed. *The Basic Science of Oncology*. Toronto: McGraw-Hill; 1992:88.
209. Varmus H. Retroviruses. *Science* 1988;240:1427–1435.
210. zur Hausen H. Viruses in human cancer. *Science* 1991;254:1167.
211. Van Dyke T. Analysis of viral–host protein interactions and tumorigenesis in transgenic mice. *Semin Cancer Biol* 1994;5:47.
212. Green PL, Chen IS. Regulation of human T cell leukemia virus expression. *FASEB J* 1990;4:169–175.
213. Laurence J, Astrin SM. Human immunodeficiency virus induction of malignant transformation in human B lymphocytes. *Proc Natl Acad Sci USA* 1991;88:7635.
214. Stewart JP, Arrand JR. Expression of the Epstein-Barr virus latent membrane protein in nasopharyngeal carcinoma biopsy specimens. *Hum Pathol* 1993;24:239–242.
215. Young LS, Rowe M. Epstein-Barr virus, lymphomas and Hodgkin's disease. *Semin Cancer Biol* 1992;3:273–284.
216. Izumi KM, Kaye KM, Kieff ED. Epstein-Barr virus recombinant molecular genetic analysis of the LMP1 amino-terminal cytoplasmic domain reveals a probable structural role, with no component essential for primary B-lymphocyte growth transformation. *J Virol* 1994;68:4369–4376.
217. Magrath I, Jain V, Bhatia K. Epstein-Barr virus and Burkitt's lymphoma. *Semin Cancer Biol* 1992;3:285–295.
218. Brechot C. Oncogenic activation of cyclin A. *Curr Opin Genet Dev* 1993;3:11–18.
219. Wang J, Zindy F, Chenivesse X, et al. Modification of cyclin A expression by hepatitis B virus DNA integration in a hepatocellular carcinoma. *Oncogene* 1992;7:1653–1656.
220. Graef E, Caselmann WH, Wells J, et al. Insertional activation of mevalonate kinase by hepatitis B virus DNA in a human hepatoma cell line. *Oncogene* 1994;9:81–87.
221. Di Luca D, Costa S, Monini P, et al. Search for human papillomavirus, herpes simplex virus and c-myc oncogene in human genital tumors. *Int J Cancer* 1989;43:570–577.
222. Manservigi R, Cassai E, Deiss LP, et al. Sequences homologous to two separate transforming regions of herpes simplex virus DNA are linked in two human genital tumors. *Virology* 1986;155:192–201.
223. DiPaolo JA, Woodworth CD, Popescu NC, et al. HSV-2–induced tumorigenicity in HPV16-immortalized human genital keratinocytes. *Virology* 1990;177:777–779.
224. Lancaster WD. Viral role in cervical and liver cancer. *Cancer* 1992;70:1794–1798.
225. Gissmann L. Human papillomaviruses and genital cancer. *Semin Cancer Biol* 1992;3:253–261.

226. Lorincz AT, Reid R, Jenson AB, et al. Human papillomavirus infection of the cervix: relative risk associations of 15 common anogenital types. *Obstet Gynecol* 1992;79:328–337.
227. Woodworth CD, Doniger J, DiPaolo JA. Immortalization of human foreskin keratinocytes by various human papillomavirus DNAs corresponds to their association with cervical carcinoma. *J Virol* 1989;63: 159–164.
228. Hurlin PJ, Kaur P, Smith PP, et al. Progression of human papillomavirus type 18-immortalized human keratinocytes to a malignant phenotype. *Proc Natl Acad Sci USA* 1991;88:570–574.
229. DiPaolo JA, Woodworth CD, Popescu NC, et al. J. Induction of human cervical squamous cell carcinoma by sequential transfection with human papillomavirus 16 DNA and viral Harvey ras. *Oncogene* 1989;4: 395–399.
230. Steele C, Cowsert LM, Shillitoe EJ. Effects of human papillomavirus type 18–specific antisense oligonucleotides on the transformed phenotype of human carcinoma cell lines. *Cancer Res* 1993;53:2330–2337.
231. Werness BA, Levine AJ, Howley PM. Association of human papillomavirus types 16 and 18 *E6* proteins with p53. *Science* 1990;248:76–79.
232. Hoppe-Seyler F, Butz K. Repression of endogenous p53 transactivation function in HeLa cervical carcinoma cells by human papillomavirus type 16 *E6*, human mdm-2, and mutant p53. *J Virol* 1993;67:3111–3117.
233. Stein WD. Analysis of cancer incidence data on the basis of multistage and clonal growth models. *Adv Cancer Res* 1991;56:161–213.
234. Hahn WC, Weinberg RA. Rules for making human tumor cells. *N Engl J Med* 2002,347:1593–1603.
235. Taylor RR, Teneriello MG, Nash JD, et al. The molecular genetics of gyn malignancies. *Oncology (Huntingt)* 1994;8:63–70, 73; discussion 73, 78–82.
236. Hethcote HW, Knudson AG Jr. Model for the incidence of embryonal cancers: application to retinoblastoma. *Proc Natl Acad Sci USA* 1978;75:2453–2457.
237. Fearon ER, Vogelstein B. A genetic model for colorectal tumorigenesis. *Cell* 1990;61:759–767.
238. Perera F, Santella R, Brandt-Rauf, P. *Molecular Epidemiology of Lung Cancer*. New York: Cold Spring Harbor Laboratory Press; 1991.
239. Harris A. *Breast Cancer, Molecular Oncology and Cancer Therapy*. New York: Cold Spring Harbor Laboratory Press; 1991.
240. Brown PH, Alani R, Preis LH, et al. Suppression of oncogene-induced transformation by a deletion mutant of c-jun. *Oncogene* 1993;8:877–886.
241. Batieha AM, Armenian HK, Norkus EP, et al. Serum micronutrients and the subsequent risk of cervical cancer in a population-based nested case-control study. *Cancer Epidemiol Biomarkers Prev* 1993;2:335–339.
242. Palan PR, Mikhail MS, Basu J, et al. Beta-carotene levels in exfoliated cervicovaginal epithelial cells in cervical intraepithelial neoplasia and cervical cancer. *Am J Obstet Gynecol* 1992;167:1899–1903.
243. Agarwal C, Hembree JR, Rorke EA, et al. Interferon and retinoic acid suppress the growth of human papillomavirus type 16 immortalized cervical epithelial cells, but only interferon suppresses the level of the human papillomavirus transforming oncogenes. *Cancer Res* 1994;54:2108–2112.
244. Agarwal C, Rorke EA, Irwin JC, et al. Immortalization by human papillomavirus type 16 alters retinoid regulation of human ectocervical epithelial cell differentiation. *Cancer Res* 1991;51:3982–3989.
245. Meyskens FL Jr, Surwit E, Moon TE, et al. Enhancement of regression of cervical intraepithelial neoplasia II (moderate dysplasia) with topically applied all-trans-retinoic acid: a randomized trial. *J Natl Cancer Inst* 1994;86:539–543.
246. Wistuba I, Roa I, Araya JC, et al. Nucleolar organizer regions in uterine cervical cancer and its precursor epithelial lesions. *Rev Med Chil* 1993;121:1110–1117.
247. Miyamoto S, Nishida M, Miwa K, et al. Increased actin cable organization after single chromosome introduction: association with suppression of *in vitro* cell growth rather than tumorigenic suppression. *Mol Carcinog* 1994;10:88–96.
248. Ando S, Tsujimura K, Matsuoka Y, et al. Phosphorylation of synthetic vimentin peptides by cdc2 kinase. *Biochem Biophys Res Commun* 1993;195:837–843.
249. Kusubata M, Matsuoka Y, Tsujimura K, et al. cdc2 kinase phosphorylation of desmin at three serine/threonine residues in the amino-terminal head domain. *Biochem Biophys Res Commun* 1993;190:927–934.
250. Moir RD, Montag-Lowy M, Goldman RD. Dynamic properties of nuclear lamins: lamin B is associated with sites of DNA replication. *J Cell Biol* 1994;125:1201–1212.
251. Dohi T, Nemoto T, Ohta S, et al. Different binding properties of three monoclonal antibodies to sialyl Le(x) glycolipids in a gastric cancer cell line and normal stomach tissue. *Anticancer Res* 1993;13:1277–1282.
252. Hakomori S, Nudelman E, Levery SB, et al. Novel fucolipids accumulating in human adenocarcinoma. I. Glycolipids with di- or trifucosylated type 2 chain. *J Biol Chem* 1984;259:4672–4680.
253. Eigenbrodt E, Reinacher M, Scheefers-Borchel U, et al. Double role for pyruvate kinase type M2 in the expansion of phosphometabolite pools found in tumor cells. *Crit Rev Oncog* 1992;3:91–115.
254. Newsholme EA, Board M. Application of metabolic-control logic to fuel utilization and its significance in tumor cells. *Adv Enzyme Regul* 1991;31:225–246.
255. Baggetto LG. Deviant energetic metabolism of glycolytic cancer cells. *Biochimie* 1992;74:959–974.
256. Thompson S, Cantwell BM, Matta KL, et al. Parallel changes in the blood levels of abnormally-fucosylated haptoglobin and alpha 1,3 fucosyltransferase in relationship to tumour burden: more evidence for a disturbance of fucose metabolism in cancer. *Cancer Lett* 1992;65:115–121.
257. Hill R. *Metastasis*. 2nd ed. Toronto: McGraw-Hill; 1992.
258. Maloney A, Workman P. HSP90 as a new therapeutic target for cancer therapy: the story unfolds. *Expert Opin Biol Ther* 2002;2:3–24.
259. Widmann C, Gibson S, Jarpe MB, et al. Mitogen-activated protein kinase: conservation of a three-kinase module from yeast to human. *Physiol Rev* 1999;79:143–180.
260. Rowinsky EK, Windle JJ, Von Hoff DD. Ras protein farnesyltransferase: a strategic target for anticancer therapeutic development. *J Clin Oncol* 1999;17:(11)3631–3652.
261. Morrison DK, Cutler RE. The complexity of Raf-1 regulation. *Curr Opin Cell Biol* 1997;9:174–179.
262. Van Aelst L, Barr M, Marcus S, et al. Complex formation between RAS and RAF and other protien kinases. *Proc Natl Acad Sci USA* 1993;90:6213.
263. Warne PH, Viciana PR, Downward J. Direct interaction of Ras and the amino-terminal region of Raf-1 *in vitro*. *Nature* 1993;364:352–355.
264. Moodie SA, Willumsen BM, Weber MJ, et al. Complexes of Ras.GTP with Raf-1 and mitogen-activated protein kinase kinase. *Science* 1993;260: 1658–1661.
265. Vos MD, Ellis CA, Bell A, et al. Ras uses the novel tumor suppressor RASSF1 as an effector to mediate apoptosis. *J Biol Chem* 2000;275:35669–35672.
266. Yu Y, Xu F, Peng H, et al. NOEY2 (ARHI), an imprinted putative tumor suppressor gene in ovarian and breast carcinomas. *Proc Natl Acad Sci USA* 1999;96:214–219.
267. Sewell JM, Smyth JF, Langdon SP. Role of TGF alpha stimulation of the ERK, PI3 kinase and PLC gamma pathways in ovarian cancer growth and migration. *Exp Cell Res*. 2005;304:305–316.
268. Cohen Y, Singer G, Lavie O, et al. The RASSF1A tumor suppressor gene is commonly inactivated in adenocarcinoma of the uterine cervix. *Clin Cancer Res* 2003;9:2981–2984.
269. Yoon JH, Dammann R, Pfeifer GP. Hypermethylation of the CpG island of the RASSF1A gene in ovarian and renal cell carcinomas. *Int J Cancer* 2001;94:212–217.
270. Roberts PJ, Der CJ. Targeting the Raf-MEK-ERK mitogen-activated protein kinase cascade for the treatment of cancer. *Oncogene* 2007;26:3291–3310.
271. Teneriello MG, Ebina M, Linnoila RI, et al. p53 and Ki-ras gene mutations in epithelial ovarian neoplasms. *Cancer Res* 1993;53:3103–3108.
272. Mayr D, Hirschmann A, Lohrs U, et al. KRAS and BRAF mutations in ovarian tumors: a comprehensive study of invasive carcinomas, borderline tumors and extraovarian implants. *Gynecol Oncol* 2006;103: 883–887.
273. Cadena DL, Gill GN. Receptor tyrosine kinases. *Faseb J* 1992;6:2332–2337.
274. Uings IJ, Farrow SN. Cell receptors and cell signalling. *Mol Pathol* 2000;53:(6)295–299.
275. Vlahovic G, Crawford J. Activation of tyrosine kinases in cancer. *Oncologist* 2003;8:(6)531–538.
276. Cantley LC, Auger KR, Carpenter C, et al. Oncogenes and signal transduction. *Cell* 1991;64:281–302.
277. Derynck R. The physiology of transforming growth factor-alpha. *Adv Cancer Res* 1992,58:27–52.
278. Wen D, Peles E, Cupples R, et al. Neu differentiation factor: a transmembrane glycoprotein containing an EGF domain and an immunoglobulin homology unit. *Cell* 1992;69:559–572.
279. Yamamoto T, Ikawa S, Akiyama T, et al. Similarity of protein encoded by the human c-erb-B-2 gene to epidermal growth factor receptor. *Nature* 1986;319:230–234.
280. Niikura H, Sasano H, Sato S, et al. Expression of epidermal growth factor-related proteins and epidermal growth factor receptor in common epithelial ovarian tumors. *Int J Gynecol Pathol* 1997;16:60–68.
281. Skirnisdottir I, Seidal T, Sorbe B. A new prognostic model comprising p53, EGFR, and tumor grade in early stage epithelial ovarian carcinoma and avoiding the problem of inaccurate surgical staging. *Int J Gynecol Cancer* 2004;14:259–270.
282. Bast RC Jr., Boyer CM, Jacobs I, et al. Cell growth regulation in epithelial ovarian cancer. *Cancer* 1993;71:1597–1601.
283. Meden H, Marx D, Rath W, et al. Overexpression of the oncogene c-erb B2 in primary ovarian cancer: evaluation of the prognostic value in a Cox proportional hazards multiple regression. *Int J Gynecol Pathol* 1994;13:45–53.
284. Slamon DJ, Godolphin W, Jones LA, et al. Studies of the HER-2/neu proto-oncogene in human breast and ovarian cancer. *Science* 1989;244: 707–712.
285. Wu Y, Soslow RA, Marshall DS, et al. Her-2/neu expression and amplification in early stage ovarian surface epithelial neoplasms. *Gynecol Oncol* 2004;95(3):570–575.
286. Lee CH, Huntsman DG, Cheang MC, et al. Assessment of Her-1, Her-2, and Her-3 expression and Her-2 amplification in advanced stage ovarian carcinoma. *Int J Gynecol Pathol* 2005;24:147–152.
287. Mayr D, Kanitz V, Amann G, et al. HER-2/neu gene amplification in ovarian tumours: a comprehensive immunohistochemical and FISH analysis on tissue microarrays. *Histopathology* 2006;48(2):149–156.
288. Harwerth IM, Wels W, Schlegel J, et al. Monoclonal antibodies directed to the erbB-2 receptor inhibit *in vivo* tumour cell growth. *Br J Cancer* 1993;68:1140–1145.

289. Bookman MA, Darcy KM, Clarke-Pearson D, et al. Evaluation of monoclonal humanized anti–HER2 antibody, trastuzumab, in patients with recurrent or refractory ovarian or primary peritoneal carcinoma with overexpression of HER2: a phase II trial of the Gynecologic Oncology Group. *J Clin Oncol* 2003;21:283–290.
290. Pollak MN, Schernhammer ES, Hankinson SE. Insulin-like growth factors and neoplasia. *Nat Rev Cancer* 2004;4(7):505–518.
291. Pollak M. Insulin-like growth factor-related signaling and cancer development. *Recent Results Cancer Res* 2007;174:49–53.
292. LeRoith D, Roberts CT Jr. The insulin-like growth factor system and cancer. *Cancer Lett* 2003;195(2):127–137.
293. Resnicoff M, Ambrose D, Coppola D, et al. Insulin-like growth factor-1 and its receptor mediate the autocrine proliferation of human ovarian carcinoma cell lines. *Lab Invest* 1993;69:756–760.
294. Sayer RA, Lancaster JM, Pittman J, et al. High insulin-like growth factor-2 (IGF-2) gene expression is an independent predictor of poor survival for patients with advanced stage serous epithelial ovarian cancer. *Gynecol Oncol* 2005;96:355–361.
295. Lu L, Katsaros D, Wiley A, et al. The relationship of insulin-like growth factor-II, insulin-like growth factor binding protein-3, and estrogen receptor-alpha expression to disease progression in epithelial ovarian cancer. *Clin Cancer Res* 2006;12:1208–1214.
296. Board R, Jayson GC. Platelet-derived growth factor receptor (PDGFR): a target for anticancer therapeutics. *Drug Resist Updat* 2005;8(1-2):75–83.
297. Fantl WJ, Johnson DE, Williams LT. Signalling by receptor tyrosine kinases. *Annu Rev Biochem* 1993;62:453–481.
298. Wilczynski SP, Chen YY, Chen W, et al. Expression and mutational analysis of tyrosine kinase receptors c-kit, PDGFRalpha, and PDGFRbeta in ovarian cancers. *Hum Pathol* 2005;36:242–249.
299. Henriksen R, Funa K, Wilander E, et al. Expression and prognostic significance of platelet-derived growth factor and its receptors in epithelial ovarian neoplasms. *Cancer Res* 1993;53:4550–4554.
300. Versnel MA, Haarbrink M, Langerak AW, et al. Human ovarian tumors of epithelial origin express PDGF *in vitro* and *in vivo*. *Cancer Genet Cytogenet* 1994;73:60–64.
301. Inoue M, Kyo S, Fujita M, et al. Coexpression of the c-kit receptor and the stem cell factor in gynecologic tumors. *Cancer Res* 1994;54:3049–3053.
302. Baiocchi G, Kavanagh JJ, Talpaz M, et al. Expression of the macrophage colony–stimulating factor and its receptor in gynecologic malignancies. *Cancer* 1991;67:990–996.
303. Garofalo A, Naumova E, Manenti L, et al. The combination of the tyrosine kinase receptor inhibitor SU6668 with paclitaxel affects ascites formation and tumor spread in ovarian carcinoma xenografts growing orthotopically. *Clin Cancer Res* 2003;9(9):3476–3485.
304. Alberts DS, Liu PY, Wilczynski SP, et al. Phase II trial of imatinib mesylate in recurrent, biomarker positive, ovarian cancer (Southwest Oncology Group Protocol S0211). *Int J Gynecol Cancer* 2007;17(4):784–788.
305. Paley PJ. Angiogenesis in ovarian cancer: molecular pathology and therapeutic strategies. *Curr Oncol Rep* 2002;4:165–174.
306. Rasila KK, Burger RA, Smith H, et al. Angiogenesis in gynecologic oncology-mechanism of tumor progression and therapeutic targets. *Int J Gynecol Cancer* 2005;15(5):710–726.
307. Starling N, Cunningham D. Monoclonal antibodies against vascular endothelial growth factor and epidermal growth factor receptor in advanced colorectal cancers: present and future directions. *Curr Opin Oncol* 2004;16:385–390.
308. Otrock ZK, Makarem JA, Shamseddine AI. Vascular endothelial growth factor family of ligands and receptors: Review. *Blood Cells Mol Dis* 2007;38(3):258–268.
309. Shen GH, Ghazizadeh M, Kawanami O, et al. Prognostic significance of vascular endothelial growth factor expression in human ovarian carcinoma. *Br J Cancer* 2000;83:196–203.
310. Paley PJ, Staskus KA, Gebhard K, et al. Vascular endothelial growth factor expression in early stage ovarian carcinoma. *Cancer* 1997;80:98–106.
311. Baird A, Bohlen P. Peptide growth factors and their receptors I. In: Sporn MRA, ed. *Handbook of Experimental Pharmacology*. Berlin: Springer-Verlag; 1990:369.
312. Di Blasio AM, Cremonesi L, Vigano P, et al. Basic fibroblast growth factor and its receptor messenger ribonucleic acids are expressed in human ovarian epithelial neoplasms. *Am J Obstet Gynecol* 1993;169:1517–1523.
313. Olson TA, Mohanraj D, Carson LF, et al. Vascular permeability factor gene expression in normal and neoplastic human ovaries. *Cancer Res* 1994;54:276–280.
314. Reynolds K, Farzaneh F, Collins WP, et al. Association of ovarian malignancy with expression of platelet-derived endothelial cell growth factor. *J Natl Cancer Inst* 1994;86:1234–1238.
315. Monk BJ, Han E, Josephs-Cowan CA, et al. Salvage bevacizumab (rhuMAB VEGF)-based therapy after multiple prior cytotoxic regimens in advanced refractory epithelial ovarian cancer. *Gynecol Oncol* 2006;102:140–144.
316. Wrana JL, Attisano L, Wieser R, et al. Mechanism of activation of the TGF-beta receptor. *Nature* 1994;370:341–347.
317. Nash MA, Ferrandina G, Gordinier M, et al. The role of cytokines in both the normal and malignant ovary. *Endocr Relat Cancer* 1999;6(1):93–107.
318. Cate R, Donohoe P, MacLaughlin D. Mullerian inhibting substance. In: Sporn MRA, ed. *Peptide Growth Factors and Their Receptors I. Handbook of Experimental Pharmacology*. Berlin: Springer-Verlag; 1990:179.
319. Sunde JS, Donninger H, Wu K, et al. Expression profiling identifies altered expression of genes that contribute to the inhibition of transforming growth factor-β signaling in ovarian cancer. *Cancer Res* 2006;66:8404–8412.
320. Suliman A, Lam A, Datta R, et al. Intracellular mechanisms of TRAIL: apoptosis through mitochondrial-dependent and -independent pathways. *Oncogene* 2001;20(17):2122–2133.
321. Kolesnick R, Golde DW. The sphingomyelin pathway in tumor necrosis factor and interleukin-1 signaling. *Cell* 1994;77:325–328.
322. Kilian PL, Kaffka KL, Biondi DA, et al. Antiproliferative effect of interleukin-1 on human ovarian carcinoma cell line (NIH:OVCAR-3). *Cancer Res* 1991;51:1823–1828.
323. Li BY, Mohanraj D, Olson MC, et al. Human ovarian epithelial cancer cells cultures *in vitro* express both interleukin 1 alpha and beta genes. *Cancer Res* 1992;52:2248–2252.
324. Lewis MP, Sullivan MH, Elder MG. Regulation by interleukin-1 beta of growth and collagenase production by choriocarcinoma cells. *Placenta* 1994;15:13–20.
325. Savarese TM, Fraser CM. *In vitro* mutagenesis and the search for structure-function relationships among G protein–coupled receptors. *Biochem J* 1992;283(Pt 1):1–19.
326. Wu S, Meeker WA, Wiener JR, et al. Transfection of ovarian cancer cells with tumor necrosis factor-alpha (TNF-alpha) antisense mRNA abolishes the proliferative response to interleukin-1 (IL-1) but not TNF-alpha. *Gynecol Oncol* 1994;53:59–63.
327. Isonishi S, Jekunen AP, Hom DK, et al. Modulation of cisplatin sensitivity and growth rate of an ovarian carcinoma cell line by bombesin and tumor necrosis factor-alpha. *J Clin Invest* 1992;90:1436–1442.
328. Kohn EC, Sandeen MA, Liotta LA. *In vivo* efficacy of a novel inhibitor of selected signal transduction pathways including calcium, arachidonate, and inositol phosphates. *Cancer Res* 1992;52:3208–3212.
329. Gutkind JS. The pathways connecting G protein–coupled receptors to the nucleus through divergent mitogen-activated protein kinase cascades. *J Biol Chem* 1998;273:1839–1842.
330. Su B, Karin, M. Mitogen-activated protein kinase cascades and regulation of gene expression. *Curr Opin Immunol* 1996;8:402.
331. Shen YH, Godlewski J, Zhu J, et al. Cross-talk between JNK/SAPK and ERK/MAPK pathways: sustained activation of JNK blocks ERK activation by mitogenic factors. *J Biol Chem* 2003;278:26715–26721.
332. Garrington TP, Johnson GL. Organization and regulation of mitogen-activated protein kinase signaling pathways. *Curr Opin Cell Biol* 1999;11:211–218.
333. Cobb MH. MAP kinase pathways. *Prog Biophys Mol Biol* 1999;71:479–500.
334. Davis RJ. The mitogen-activated protein kinase signal transduction pathway. *J Biol Chem* 1993;268:14553–14556.
335. Nevins JR. E2F: a link between the Rb tumor suppressor protein and viral oncoproteins. *Science* 1992;258:424–429.
336. Givant-Horwitz V, Davidson B, Lazarovici P, et al. Mitogen-activated protein kinases (MAPK) as predictors of clinical outcome in serous ovarian carcinoma in effusions. *Gynecol Oncol* 2003;91:160–172.
337. Persons DL, Yazlovitskaya EM, Cui W, et al. Cisplatin-induced activation of mitogen-activated protein kinases in ovarian carcinoma cells: inhibition of extracellular signal-regulated kinase activity increases sensitivity to cisplatin. *Clin Cancer Res* 1999;5:1007–1014.
338. Chang F, Lee JT, Navolanic PM, et al. Involvement of PI3K/Akt pathway in cell cycle progression, apoptosis, and neoplastic transformation: a target for cancer chemotherapy. *Leukemia* 2003;17:590–603.
339. Mills GB, Fang X, Lu Y, et al. Specific keynote: molecular therapeutics in ovarian cancer. *Gynecol Oncol* 2003;88:S88–S92; discussion S93–S96.
340. Cristiano BE, Chan JC, Hannan KM, et al. A specific role for AKT3 in the genesis of ovarian cancer through modulation of G(2)-M phase transition. *Cancer Res* 2006;66:11718–11725.
341. Campbell IG, Russell SE, Choong DY, et al. Mutation of the PIK3CA gene in ovarian and breast cancer. *Cancer Res* 2004;64:7678–7681.
342. Shayesteh L, Lu Y, Kuo WL, et al. PIK3CA is implicated as an oncogene in ovarian cancer. *Nat Genet* 1999;21:99–102.
343. Cheng JQ, Godwin AK, Bellacosa A, et al. AKT2, a putative oncogene encoding a member of a subfamily of protein-serine/threonine kinases, is amplified in human ovarian carcinomas. *Proc Natl Acad Sci USA* 1992;89:9267–9271.
344. Yuan ZQ, Sun M, Feldman RI, et al. Frequent activation of AKT2 and induction of apoptosis by inhibition of phosphoinositide-3-OH kinase/Akt pathway in human ovarian cancer. *Oncogene* 2000;19:2324–2330.
345. Azzi A, Boscoboinik D, Hensey C. The protein kinase C family. *Eur J Biochem* 1992;208:547–557.
346. Rossomando A, Wu J, Weber MJ, et al. The phorbol ester–dependent activator of the mitogen-activated protein kinase p42mapk is a kinase with specificity for the threonine and tyrosine regulatory sites. *Proc Natl Acad Sci USA* 1992;89:5221–5225.
347. Heichman KA, Roberts JM. Rules to replicate by. *Cell* 1994;79:557–562.
348. Hunter T, Pines J. Cyclins and cancer. II: Cyclin D and CDK inhibitors come of age. *Cell* 1994;79:573–582.
349. Klingmuller U, Lorenz U, Cantley LC, et al. Specific recruitment of SH-PTP1 to the erythropoietin receptor causes inactivation of JAK2 and termination of proliferative signals. *Cell* 1995;80:729–738.

350. Nurse P. Ordering S phase and M phase in the cell cycle. *Cell* 1994;79:547–550.
351. Sherr CJ. G1 phase progression: cycling on cue. *Cell* 1994;79:551–555.
352. Farley JH, Birrer MJ. Biologic directed therapies in gynecologic oncology. *Curr Oncol Rep* 2003;5:459–467.
353. Akiyama T, Ohuchi T, Sumida S, et al. Phosphorylation of the retinoblastoma protein by CDK2. *Proc Natl Acad Sci USA* 1992;89:7900–7904.
354. DeCaprio JA, Furukawa Y, Ajchenbaum F, et al. The retinoblastoma-susceptibility gene product becomes phosphorylated in multiple stages during cell cycle entry and progression. *Proc Natl Acad Sci USA* 1992;89:1795–1798.
355. Farley J, Smith LM, Darcy KM, et al. Cyclin E expression is a significant predictor of survival in advanced, suboptimally debulked ovarian epithelial cancers: a Gynecologic Oncology Group study. *Cancer Res* 2003;63:1235–1241.
356. Casey PJ, Gilman AG. G protein involvement in receptor-effector coupling. *J Biol Chem* 1988;263:2577–2580.
357. Cockcroft S, Thomas GM. Inositol-lipid–specific phospholipase C isoenzymes and their differential regulation by receptors. *Biochem J* 1992;288(Pt 1):1–14.
358. Fang X, Gaudette D, Furui T, et al. Lysophospholipid growth factors in the initiation, progression, metastases, and management of ovarian cancer. *Ann NY Acad Sci* 2000;905:188–208.
359. Guo Z, Liliom K, Fischer DJ, et al. Molecular cloning of a high-affinity receptor for the growth factor-like lipid mediator lysophosphatidic acid from *Xenopus* oocytes. *Proc Natl Acad Sci USA* 1996;93:14367–14372.
360. Kelvin DJ, Michiel DF, Johnston JA, et al. Chemokines and serpentines: the molecular biology of chemokine receptors. *J Leukoc Biol* 1993;54:604–612.
361. Neel BG, Tonks NK. Protein tyrosine phosphatases in signal transduction. *Curr Opin Cell Biol* 1997;9:193–204.
362. Tonks NK, Neel BG. From form to function: signaling by protein tyrosine phosphatases. *Cell* 1996;87:365–368.
363. Brady-Kalnay SM, Tonks NK. Protein tyrosine phosphatases as adhesion receptors. *Curr Opin Cell Biol* 1995;7:650–657.
364. Peles E, Nativ M, Campbell PL, et al. The carbonic anhydrase domain of receptor tyrosine phosphatase beta is a functional ligand for the axonal cell recognition molecule contactin. *Cell* 1995;82:251–260.
365. Lorenz U, Bergemann AD, Steinberg HN, et al. Genetic analysis reveals cell type–specific regulation of receptor tyrosine kinase c-Kit by the protein tyrosine phosphatase SHP1. *J Exp Med* 1996;184:1111–1126.
366. Li DM, Sun H. *PTEN*/MMAC1/TEP1 suppresses the tumorigenicity and induces G1 cell cycle arrest in human glioblastoma cells. *Proc Natl Acad Sci USA* 1998;95:15406–15411.
367. Haas-Kogan D, Shalev N, Wong M, et al. Protein kinase B (PKB/Akt) activity is elevated in glioblastoma cells due to mutation of the tumor suppressor *PTEN*/MMAC. *Curr Biol* 1998;8:1195–1198.
368. Ramaswamy S, Nakamura N, Vazquez F, et al. Regulation of G1 progression by the *PTEN* tumor suppressor protein is linked to inhibition of the phosphatidylinositol 3-kinase/Akt pathway. *Proc Natl Acad Sci USA* 1999;96:2110.
369. Eng C. Genetics of Coden syndrome: through the looking glass of oncology. *Int J Oncol* 1998;12:701.
370. Obata K, Morland SJ, Watson RH, et al. Frequent *PTEN*/MMAC mutations in endometrioid but not serous or mucinous epithelial ovarian tumors. *Cancer Res* 1998;58:2095–2097.
371. Risinger JI, Hayes AK, Berchuck A, Barrett JC. *PTEN*/MMAC1 mutations in endometrial cancers. *Cancer Res* 1997;57:4736–4738.
372. Villafranca JE, Kissinger CR, Parge HE. Protein serine/threonine phosphatases. *Curr Opin Biotechnol* 1996;7:397–402.
373. Goldberg Y. Protein phosphatase 2A: who shall regulate the regulator? *Biochem Pharmacol* 1999;57:321–328.
374. Schonthal AH. Role of PP2A in intracellular signal transduction pathways. *Front Biosci* 1998;3:D1262–D1273.
375. Tonks NK. Protein tyrosine phosphatases and the control of cellular signaling responses. *Adv Pharmacol* 1996;36:91–119.
376. Manzano RG, Montuenga LM, Dayton M, et al. CL100 expression is down-regulated in advanced epithelial ovarian cancer and its re-expression decreases its malignant potential. *Oncogene* 2002;21:4435–4447.
377. Giles RH, van Es JH, Clevers H. Caught up in a Wnt storm: Wnt signaling in cancer. *Biochim Biophys Acta* 2003;1653:1–24.
378. Orford K, Crockett C, Jensen JP, et al. Serine phosphorylation-regulated ubiquitination and degradation of beta-catenin. *J Biol Chem* 1997;272:24735–24738.
379. Monaghan H, MacWhinnie N, Williams AR. The role of matrix metalloproteinases-2, -7 and -9 and beta-catenin in high grade endometrial carcinoma. *Histopathology* 2007;50:348–357.
380. Kildal W, Risberg B, Abeler VM, et al. Beta-catenin expression, DNA ploidy and clinicopathological features in ovarian cancer: a study in 253 patients. *Eur J Cancer* 2005;41:1127–1134.
381. Mello CC, Conte D Jr. Revealing the world of RNA interference. *Nature* 2004;431:338–342.
382. Fire A, Xu S, Montgomery MK, et al. Potent and specific genetic interference by double-stranded RNA in *Caenorhabditis elegans. Nature.* 998;391:806–811.
383. Rana TM. Illuminating the silence: understanding the structure and function of small RNAs. *Nat Rev Mol Cell Biol* 2007;8:(1)23–36.
384. Liu W, Mao SY, Zhu WY. Impact of tiny miRNAs on cancers. *World J Gastroenterol* 2007;13:497–502.
385. Bartel DP. MicroRNAs: genomics, biogenesis, mechanism, and function. *Cell* 2004;116:281–297.
386. Vazquez F, Vaucheret H, Rajagopalan R, et al. Endogenous trans-acting siRNAs regulate the accumulation of Arabidopsis mRNAs. *Mol Cell* 2004;16(1):69–79.
387. Volpe TA, Kidner C, Hall IM, et al. Regulation of heterochromatic silencing and histone H3 lysine-9 methylation by RNAi. *Science* 2002;297(5588):1833–1837.
388. Mochizuki K, Gorovsky MA. Small RNAs in genome rearrangement in Tetrahymena. *Curr Opin Genet Dev* 2004;14(2):181–187.
389. Grivna ST, Pyhtila B, Lin H. MIWI associates with translational machinery and PIWI- interacting RNAs (piRNAs) in regulating spermatogenesis. *Proc Natl Acad Sci USA* 2006;103:13415–13420.
390. Zaratiegui M, Irvine DV, Martienssen RA. Noncoding RNAs and gene silencing. *Cell* 2007;128(4):763–776.

CHAPTER 4 ■ TUMOR INVASION, ANGIOGENESIS, AND METASTASIS: BIOLOGY AND CLINICAL APPLICATION

CHRISTINA M. ANNUNZIATA, NILOFER S. AZAD,
EBONY R. HOSKINS, AND ELISE C. KOHN

Genetic instability is at the heart of malignant transformation. This is manifest in part by the activation of signaling events triggering malignant cells to stimulate their local microenvironment, invade locally, and then metastasize to distant sites (Fig. 4.1). Invasive and metastatic disease is responsible for much of the morbidity and mortality associated with cancer. The search for factors affecting this process began as far back as 1889 when Sir James Paget noted that women who died of breast cancer tended to have a higher frequency of metastases to bone and ovaries. He further commented that the process was not random and, even more importantly, represented a relationship between the "seed," tumor cells of a given type, and "soil," the microenvironment providing the growth advantage to the cells (1). Scientists have turned much attention toward dissecting the sequence of events that comprises these key steps in the disease process and translating that understanding to development of targeted therapeutics (2). Signals in the cancers that stimulate and maintain the invasive and angiogenic phenotype can also drive survival. Recognition of the regulation and roles of angiogenesis, invasion, and tumor survival in the dissemination of gynecologic cancers has and will continue to lead to improved patient care and outcome.

CLINICAL IMPLICATIONS OF INVASION, ANGIOGENESIS, AND METASTASIS

Invasion

Survival, recurrence, and response to treatment strongly correlate with tumor invasion that leads to nodal and distant metastases (3). Epithelial ovarian tumors of low malignant potential (LMP/borderline) are characterized by their lack of penetration into the ovarian stroma (4). These tumors rarely metastasize, recur late, and have an overall survival at 5 years in excess of 95% (4). The importance of invasion depth is reflected in the International Federation of Gynecology and Obstetrics (FIGO) staging systems for both cervical and endometrial cancer (5). The stage and frequency of cervical cancer metastasis increases as the depth of invasion exceeds 5 mm (6,7). Extent of invasion significantly contributed to a model predicting disease-free survival in multivariate analyses of early cervical cancer and other cancers (8). Clinical outcome in endometrial cancer is also affected by depth of invasion. As myometrial invasion proceeds beyond the depth of 50%, the risks of nodal metastases and treatment failure escalate (9). In addition to FIGO stage and tumor type, depth of invasion has independent prognostic value in endometrial cancer (10). Invasion has been used as a discriminating clinical feature in the application of therapeutic modalities, especially for local therapies such as radiation and intraperitoneal chemotherapy. Invasion is thus an important behavior contributing to the clinical outcome of gynecologic malignancies.

Angiogenesis

Angiogenesis is the process of forming new blood vessels from a preexisting vascular network. Its role in cancer was first detailed by Folkman (11,12) and Liotta (13) in the 1970s. Angiogenesis is now considered to be an invasive process itself, and is prognostically important in tumor survival and progression. Several points in the process of angiogenesis have been successfully targeted in cancer therapy (11).

Endothelial cells from tumor samples can be identified and quantified by immunohistochemistry analysis of angiogenic markers such as von Willebrand's factor, factor VIII, CD31, or CD34 (14). Microvessel density has been correlated with disease relapse in cervical cancer (15), ovarian cancer (16,17), and endometrial cancer (18). High microvessel counts occurred in cervical cancer patients of all stages who developed early disease recurrence (19). Increased microvessel number in endometrial carcinomas has been associated with recurrent disease, progression-free survival, and overall survival (18,20). The extent of angiogenesis correlated with progression-free survival and overall survival in ovarian cancers. CD34 was the most useful discriminator of microvessels in advanced-stage ovarian cancers (21); counts and stage of disease were associated with overall survival and disease-free survival, respectively.

The expression of vascular endothelial growth factor (VEGF), a potent angiogenesis stimulator, can complement microvessel density (MVD) in the clinical assessment of angiogenesis. VEGF correlated with poor outcome in early-stage and LMP ovarian tumors; a statistically significantly worse median disease-free survival was found in patients with VEGF-positive tumors (22). Raspollini et al. (16) demonstrated that increased MVD and higher expression of VEGF were independent predictors of disease survival in serous ovarian cancer. Thus, neoangiogenesis is a consistent clinical predictor of poor progression-free survival in gynecologic malignancies.

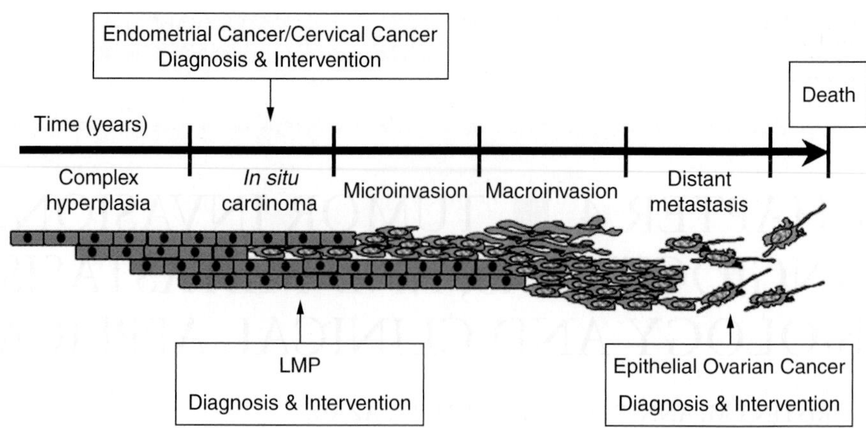

FIGURE 4.1. Paradigm of cancer progression. The average age at diagnosis of cervical intraepithelial neoplasia III and/or carcinoma *in situ* (CIS) is approximately 42 years. Progression from CIS to invasive carcinoma occurs over 8 to 10 years. The majority of patients with invasive cervical cancer die within 10 to 15 years of their diagnosis. In comparison, a precursor or early detectable lesion for invasive ovarian cancer has not yet been found. Low malignant potential tumors are diagnosed between the fourth and fifth decade. Invasive ovarian cancer is diagnosed approximately 15 years later, with the majority of patients diagnosed dying of the disease within 5 years.

Metastasis

Both autocrine and paracrine signaling by growth factors and cytokines activate programs for invasion and angiogenesis in the progression toward metastasis. Once activated, these events set the stage for dissemination. Activation and modulation of the local microenvironment induces further permissive events supporting tumor metastasis.

Metastatic activity and pattern of spread is important in the diagnosis, prognosis, and treatment of all malignancies. Patterns of spread vary between and within tumors and follow the biology and location of the primary tumor. Consider distinct patterns of spread of gynecologic cancers. Cervical and endometrial cancers tend to follow the general adenocarcinoma pattern of early local extension with nodal involvement predicted by locally invasive behavior, followed by distant dissemination (23,24). The presence of nodal metastases is a poor prognostic sign for gynecologic malignancies, a manifestation of invasion that results in upstaging and high risk of relapse. A study of fallopian tube cancer revealed a 76-month median survival in patients without lymph node metastases. This was in contrast to a 33-month median survival in patients with documented nodal disease (25).

Unlike other invasive adenocarcinomas, however, epithelial ovarian tumors disseminate broadly within the abdominal cavity prior to nodal and hematogenous dissemination (26–28). This occurs from tumor cell shedding, followed by adhesion to the serosal and peritoneal surfaces and migration of the malignant epithelium. Common sites of early extension are bowel and bladder serosal surfaces and the abdominal and pelvic peritoneum. Surface shedding, a nurturing milieu within the ascites, and the supportive local microenvironment of the serosa and peritoneum can result in extensive microscopic tumor burden. The microscopic and insidious nature of the surface extension of ovarian cancer limits the success of complete surgical resection. Disease can be found on the abdominal peritoneum of the diaphragm in patients before microscopic nodal involvement (FIGO stage IIIA vs. IIIC). This is in sharp contrast to other gynecologic malignancies; Matsumoto et al. compared the process of lymphatic invasion of ovarian, cervical, and endometrial cancers (29) and showed that cervical and endometrial cancers tended to involve pelvic nodes earlier in the metastatic process than ovarian malignancies.

BIOLOGY OF INVASION

Invasion is the active translocation of a cell across tissue boundaries and through host cellular and extracellular matrix barriers (Figure 4.2). It is tightly regulated in the physiologic settings of wound healing, embryogenesis, and trophoblast implantation.

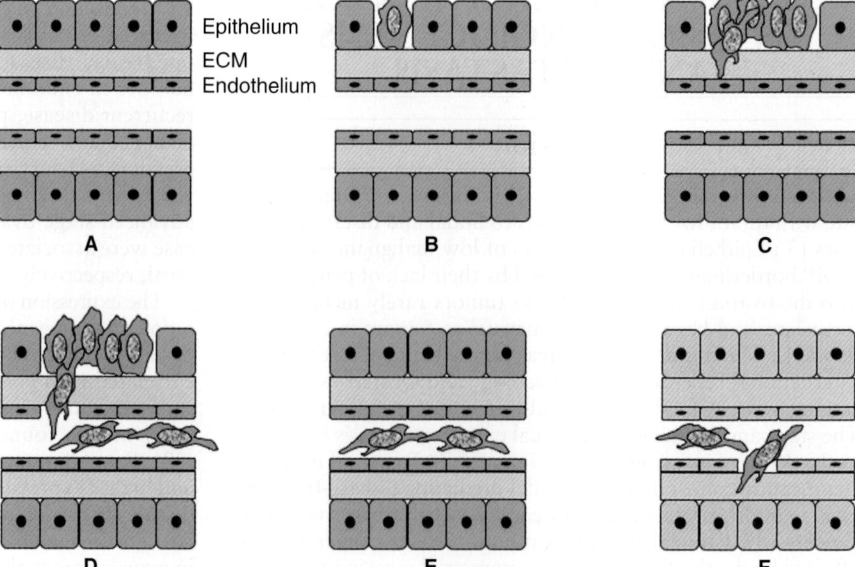

FIGURE 4.2. Schema of invasion and metastasis. (**A**) Normal epithelium, extracellular matrix (ECM), and endothelium. (**B**) Early transformation and carcinoma *in situ*. (**C**) Stromal invasion requiring proteolysis and ECM degradation. (**D**) Intravasation requiring further proteolysis. (**E**) Migration. (**F**) Extravasation into distant sites.

The components and events of physiological invasion and malignant invasion are similar. Invasion requires cellular adhesion and proteolysis, coupled with activation of migration and survival pathways (30). Quantity, activation, and regulation are what set the two forms of invasion apart. These checkpoints are disrupted or altered in the setting of malignancy.

Adhesion

Both cell-cell and cell-stroma interactions are involved in physiologic and malignant invasion. Connections through cell adhesion molecules, integrins, and cadherins stabilize tissue integrity and provide survival and activation signals (31). Loss of these connections is associated with increased metastatic potential (32,33). Cell polarity and organization during spreading and migration are regulated by cell interaction with extracellular matrix (ECM) proteins through the integrin family, and with other cells through the transmembrane glycoproteins, cadherins. Activation of these cell surface receptors passes signals from the microenvironment to the intracellular environment, thereby affecting cellular behavior. Differential expression and activation of adhesion molecules has been described as differentiating normal from malignant cells (32).

Cadherins

Cadherins are transmembrane glycoproteins that mediate cell-cell interactions in a fashion dependent upon extracellular calcium. The intracellular domain of the cadherins form complexes with the catenin family of cytoplasmic proteins (34). Cadherin-catenin complexes are linked to the cytoskeleton through direct interactions between α-catenin and α-actinin (35). Interaction with the ECM thus transmits signals intracellularly via cadherin/catenin complexes, thereby affecting both structural morphology and functional differentiation.

E-cadherin is the most extensively studied member of the family. E-cadherin functions as a metastasis-suppressor molecule in several types of carcinomas (36). Loss of E-cadherin expression is associated with an invasive phenotype. A transgenic mouse model of pancreatic islet cell carcinoma demonstrated that loss of E-cadherin was associated with early invasion and metastasis (37). The role of E-cadherin is less defined in ovarian cancer, based on its variable patterns of expression. In contrast to other normal epithelial cells, normal ovarian surface epithelium (OSE) rarely expresses E-cadherin (38,39), whereas activated metaplastic OSE cells and primary ovarian cancers often express this protein. E-cadherin protein expression is then lost as tumors become more poorly differentiated or increase their metastatic potential (37). E-cadherin expression becomes scant or absent in metastases, consistent with its description as a metastatic suppressor (36,40–42). Exogenous expression of E-cadherin in OSE cells induced expression of markers associated with preneoplastic and metaplastic OSE (43). Hence, alterations associated with control of E-cadherin could facilitate invasion in malignancy.

Integrins

The integrins are transmembrane glycoproteins composed of noncovalently linked α- and β-subunit heterodimers. Integrins serve both as cell adhesion molecules and as signaling molecules regulating apoptosis, proliferation, invasion, metastasis, angiogenesis, and survival. A variety of extracellular matrix proteins interact as ligands, including collagens, laminin, tenascin, fibronectin, vitronectin, von Willebrand's factor, and thrombospondin (44). Matrix engagement is an important stimulus of invasive behavior, signaling through integrins to activate focal adhesion kinase (FAK), phosphatidylinositol 3′-kinase (PI3K) and the AKT/protein kinase B pathway. Feedback interdependence between these proteins was demonstrated experimentally when overexpression of AKT2 in ovarian cancer led to up-regulation of β1 integrins and resulted in increased invasion and metastasis (45).

Integrins also exhibit the capability of serving as mechanoreceptors, allowing for the translation of mechanical external signals into biochemical messages such as during collagen matrix contraction (46). The αvβ3 integrin plays a fundamental role in angiogenesis, invasion, and survival. Its activation initiates a calcium-dependent signaling pathway, leading to an increase in cell motility and survival signals. This integrin is expressed on epithelial, endothelial, and uterine smooth muscle cells, as well as leukocytes. αvβ3 integrin is expressed minimally in normal or resting blood vessels and is up-regulated both on activated vascular endothelium and tumor epithelium, suggesting a role in tumor proliferation as well as angiogenesis (47–51). There is elevated expression of αvβ3 in cervical cancers (52) and ovarian cancers (53), that shows an increasing gradient of expression as cells progress from LMP tumors to invasive epithelial cancers (54). Cross talk may occur between the αvβ3 integrin and the tyrosine kinase domains of angiogenic growth factor receptors, amplifying downstream activation of survival and proliferation cascade (55,56). Agents directed against integrins have been tested in a variety of models, with clinical results still forthcoming. Examples of these agents can be found in Table 4.1.

Proteolysis

Local proteolysis occurs in both the tumor and stromal compartments. The process of intravasation and extravasation depends upon the ability to secrete proteolytic enzymes required to degrade the barriers within the extracellular matrix. Overexpression of such enzymes occurs in almost all cells within the tumor-host microenvironment (30). Degradation of the basement membrane is affected by net proteolytic activity that is determined by the balance of activated proteolytic enzymes and their inhibitors. A positive correlation with tumor aggressiveness has been shown for a variety of degradative enzymes, including heparanases and seryl-, thiol-, and metal-dependent enzymes (57–59). Proteolytic behavior may therefore be a logical molecular target to interrupt the invasive and metastatic process in malignancy.

Matrix Metalloproteases

Matrix metalloproteases (MMPs) are a family of neutral metalloenzymes secreted as latent proenzymes. They require cleavage of the amino-terminal domain, and their activity depends on the presence of Zn^{2+} and/or Ca^{2+} (60). There are five subclasses grouped according to substrate specificity: interstitial collagenases, gelatinases, stromelysins, membrane-type MMPs, and elastases. Increased MMP activity has been detected in and shown to correlate with invasive and metastatic potential in a wide rage of cancers, including gynecologic, lung, prostate, breast, and pancreatic cancers (30,61–63). Epithelial ovarian carcinoma cells derived from primary ovarian tumors, metastatic lesions, or ascites overexpressed MMP-2 (gelatinase A) and MMP-9 (gelatinase B) (64). Increased MMP-2 expression was observed in cervices with high-grade cervical intraepithelial neoplasia (CIN) and invasive cervical carcinoma when compared to normal and low-grade CIN cervices (65). Expression of MMP-13 (collagenase-3) is abundant in vulvar carcinomas metastatic to lymph nodes. MMP-13 was associated with tumor-cell expression of MTI-MMP and stromal-cell expression of MMP-2 (66). Therefore, MMPs may serve as useful markers for detection of disease and/or as targets for therapeutic intervention to prevent tumor progression.

The activity of MMPs is regulated by a family of five proteins known as the tissue inhibitors of metalloproteases (TIMPs).

TABLE 4.1

MOLECULAR THERAPEUTICS OF INVASION, ANGIOGENESIS, AND METASTASIS

Target	Drug
AKT	Perifosine PX-316 A-443654
c-Kit	Imatinib
Epidermal growth factor receptor (EGFR1)	Cetuximab Panitumumab Matuzumab Gefitinib Erlotinib Lapatinib Vandetanib Canertinib Leflunomide
Heparanase	PI-88
ERBB2 (HER2/neu)	Trastuzumab Lapatinib Canertinib
Integrins	Volociximab Cilengitide Vitaxin Endostatin Angiostatin
Matrix metal oproteases (MMPs)	Marimastat COL-3 BAY 12-9566 MMI 270 ABT-518
mTOR/FRAP	Temsirolimus Rapamycin RAD001
p53	ONYX-015
PI3K	PX-866
Platelet-derived growth factor receptor (PDGFR)	Imatinib Sunitinib Leflunomide
Protein kinase C-a (PKC-a)	Bryostatin-1 UCN 01
Raf-kinase	Sorafenib ISIS 5132 ISIS 2503
Ras	Tipifarnib Lonafarnib L-778123
Vascular endothelial growth factor (VEGF)	Bevacizumab VEGF trap
Vascular endothelial growth factor receptor-1/2 (VEGFR-1/2)	Sorafenib Vandetanib Sunitinib
Angiogenesis (unknown targets)	Thalidomide Lenalidomide IL-12

In concert with MT1-MMP, TIMP-2 can regulate activation of MMP-2, whereas it can also directly inhibit MMP-2 function (67). The balance between levels of activated MMPs and free TIMPs determines the balance between matrix degradation and matrix formation. Altering this equilibrium affects the progression of the invasive phenotype. Immunohistochemistry of MMP-2 and TIMP-2 in endometrial tumors showed that the quantity of MMP-2 increased with histologic grade, while TIMP-2 decreased (68). This pattern of MMP and TIMP expression correlated clinically, serving as indicator of local and distant metastasis. Similar data for MMPs and their inhibitors were found in ovarian cancer (69).

TIMPs have independent activities as well. TIMP-2 inhibits basic fibroblast growth factor-induced stimulation of endothelial-cell proliferation independent of its ability to inhibit MMP activity (70). TIMP-1 and TIMP-2 have been shown to inhibit tumor-induced angiogenesis in experimental systems (71) and to have antiapoptotic activity in lymphomas (72). Such information has led to development of novel agents affecting the expression or activity of MMPs and TIMPs. Multiple synthetic inhibitors of MMPs have been studied in preclinical and clinical trials (73,74) demonstrating a variety of antineoplastic effects that have not translated successfully to the clinic. Clinical response to the MMP inhibitor class has been disappointing either from lack of activity and/or unexpected toxicity. A new generation of inhibitors has been developed and is reaching clinical testing (see Table 4.1 for examples) (75).

Serine Proteases

Plasminogen activators (PAs) are serine-specific proteases that convert inactive plasminogen to active plasmin, a trypsin-like enzyme that degrades a variety of proteins, including fibrin, fibronectin, type IV collagen, vitronectin, and laminin. Plasminogen activator exists in two forms: tissue-type plasminogen activator (tPA), the primary plasminogen activator in plasma, and urokinase plasminogen activator (uPA). uPA is involved primarily in cell-mediated proteolysis during macrophage invasion, wound healing, embryogenesis, and metastasis (76). Production of uPA in ovarian carcinoma cells is reported as 17- to 38-fold higher than that found in normal ovarian epithelial cells (77,78). The role of uPA in ovarian cancer has been shown in preclinical models. Its production is stimulated by multiple ovarian-cancer-derived growth factors, such as lysophosphatidic acid (79). Approaches to molecular targeting of uPA and its related family of regulatory molecules are undergoing preclinical evaluation. New inhibitory agents directed to uPA include bikunin and soybean kunitz inhibitor, which block messenger RNA (mRNA) and protein expression of uPA, and down-regulate uPA through Src-dependent signaling pathways, respectively (80–82).

Cellular Events Promoting Invasion

ras Family

The ras family of oncoproteins is a group of integral modulators of signal transduction pathways and its members are potent inducers of mitogenesis and invasion (83). K-ras mutations have been found in 50% of mucinous ovarian cancers and 40% of LMP tumors, but are generally uncommon in serous ovarian cancers (84). Approximately 10% to 30% of endometrial cancers show K-ras mutations (85,86). H-ras mutations have been associated with the progression of papillomavirus-induced lesions in the uterine cervix (87). Mutated or overexpressed, ras functions in invasion and angiogenesis in multiple ways.

Several ras family members have been shown to regulate angiogenesis. Colorectal carcinoma cell lines constitutively expressing K-ras- and H-ras-mutant cell lines had increased VEGF expression (88). H-ras induction of VEGF expression was mediated by TGF-β and basic fibroblast growth factor (bFGF), both of which are potent proangiogenic growth factors produced in tumor autocrine and paracrine loops (89). Therapeutics inhibiting farnesyltransferase (FTase) proteins such as RAS can decrease VEGF expression *in vitro* and *in vivo* (90), suggesting that farnesyltransferase inhibitors (FTIs) may have a multifunctional role in cancer treatment (Table 4.1). FTIs are an evolving family of agents under investigation.

BIOLOGY OF ANGIOGENESIS

New Vessel Formation

Blood Vessels

Angiogenesis is a rate-limiting step in the growth of tumors and in the development of metastases (91,92). Tumor growth is limited by nutrient requirements and waste removal, and metastasis depends on tumor cells' access to the vasculature for dissemination (92–95). Net tumor volume represents a balance between cellular proliferation and cell death. Lack of angiogenesis limits growth, creating a balance between proliferation and death rates (Fig. 4.3) (93). A tumor mass larger than 0.125 mm^2 exceeds its capacity to acquire nutrients by simple diffusion. Further expansion of the tumor mass requires new blood vessel formation (11).

The formation of tumor neovasculature consists of multiple, interdependent steps similar to the process of invasion (96). Activation of endothelial cells by stimuli such as injury or inflammation, and tumor secretion of proangiogenic cytokines and growth factors, induces expression of a pro-invasive phenotype in the endothelial cells. This is manifest by local degradation of the capillary basement membrane, followed by endothelial-cell invasion into the surrounding stroma and migration of endothelial cells in the direction of the angiogenic stimulus. Proliferation of endothelial cells occurs at the leading edge of the migrating column, and the endothelial cells begin to organize into three-dimensional structures to form new capillary tubes (3,97). The switch of endothelial cells from quiescent to activated is regulated by angiostimulatory and angiostatic signals (91). These include cytokines, fibrin, and integrins (98–101). These different angioregulatory processes have been targeted for therapeutic inhibition in cancer and inflammatory diseases. The results of these efforts are promising, as some cancers are highly responsive to antiangiogenic therapy. Investigators are characterizing a number of new molecular pathways that may be involved in the process of angiogenesis. Examples of these pathways include the ephrin (102), notch (103), hedgehog (104), sprouty (105), roundabouts (106), and slits pathways (106). These may prove to be novel sites for molecular targeting (Table 4.1 and Fig. 4.3).

Lymphangiogenesis

Tumors frequently metastasize to lymph nodes. The lymphatic system is composed of ducts ending in lymphatic capillaries analogous to the blood circulatory system. Lymphangiogenesis is the process of forming new lymphatic vessels. It is similarly a dynamic system and undergoes remodeling. A tumor, therefore, may prompt formation of its own lymphatic drainage by secreting factors stimulating lymphangiogenesis (107). The cytokines and receptors for lymphangiogenesis, described in the next section, are analogous to, yet distinct from, those involved in new blood vessel formation. Our understanding of this process is in its infancy, but the identification of lymphatic-specific markers has provided initial structural insights (108).

Angio-Immunology (Vascular Leukocytes)

An alternative model of neoangiogenesis proposes that tumor-infiltrating leukocytes can be stimulated to differentiate into endothelial cell precursors (109). Typically, leukocytes express CD45 but not VE-cadherin, while endothelial cells have VE-cadherin but not CD45 (110). A distinct population of cells was isolated from primary cases of stage III ovarian cancer

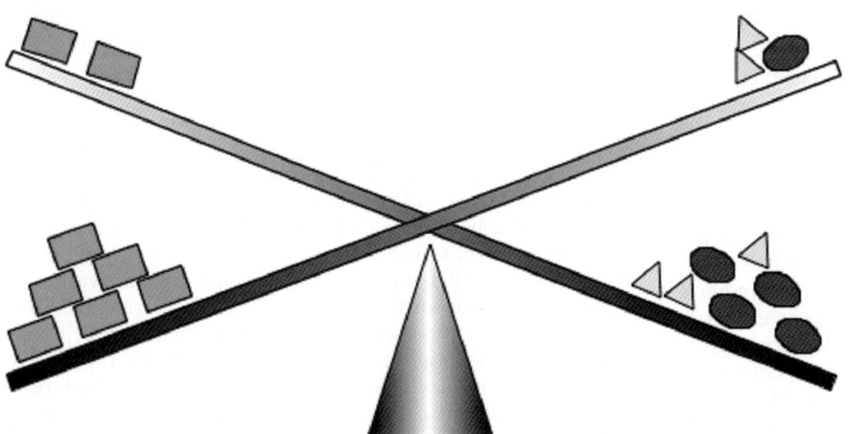

FIGURE 4.3. Schematic representation of angiogenesis. Vascular homeostasis represents a balance between physiologic activators and inhibitors of vessel formation. This balance is disrupted in cancer. Pharmacologic agents have been targeted at various elements of the angiogenic cascade in attempts to shift the balance away from an environment favorable to cancer.

based on their expression of these two markers: those that expressed markers of both leukocytes (CD45) and endothelial cells (VE-cadherin) (110). Such cells also expressed vascular endothelial growth factor receptor-2 (VEGFR2) and formed vessel-like structures when stimulated *in vitro* with VEGF (110). New blood vessels, therefore, may be derived from two distinct yet interrelated pathways, each under the influence of VEGF. The proposed vascular leukocytes may provide additional targets for therapeutic intervention based on their unique pattern of cell surface markers.

Growth Factors Promoting Angiogenesis

Vascular Endothelial Growth Factor

VEGF, described initially as vascular permeability factor, was purified from ovarian cancer xenograft ascites (98,111). Five isoforms of VEGF have been identified (A through E). VEGF-A, -B, and -E stimulate angiogenesis by binding VEGFR1 (VEGF-A and -B) or VEGFR2 (VEGF-A and -E); isoforms -C and -D signal through VEGFR3 to stimulate lymphangiogenesis (108). VEGFs are mitogens for vascular endothelial cells, induce capillary tube formation, cause increased vascular permeability and protein extravasation, stimulate endothelial-cell migration, and promote endothelial-cell survival (112). They have critical roles in normal gynecologic function, including endometrial cycling, ovarian follicle maturation, and corpus luteum formation and regression (113). VEGF-A also functions in gynecologic pathologies, including endometriosis (114) and polycystic ovarian disease (115). VEGFs are products of known tumor-growth-factor signaling cascades, such as the lysophosphatidic acid (LPA), NF-kB, and PI3K pathways in ovarian cancer (116–118). Expression is up-regulated in a variety of tumors, including most gynecologic malignancies, and correlates with poor outcome (119,120). Tumor cells, stromal support cells, and endothelial cells express VEGFs, indicating that they are paracrine mediators of angiogenesis in cancer. Both primary and metastatic ovarian carcinoma cells can coexpress VEGFs and VEGF receptors 1 (Flt) and 2 (KDR), thus providing autocrine stimulation (121). This was the first example of localization of VEGFR2 expression in nonendothelial cells.

A strong correlation exists between the degree of vascularization of a tumor and VEGF expression (122). Circulating VEGF concentrations may be influenced by numerous factors including hormones, cytokines, and hypoxia that affect the expression of VEGF protein and mRNA (123–125). Plasma and urine concentrations of VEGF increase during tumor progression. In a study of advanced epithelial ovarian carcinomas, patients with tumors expressing higher levels of VEGF had shorter survival (126) and concordant results were found with serum levels of VEGF (120). This growth factor accumulates in malignant ascites and contributes to increasing the ascites burden through its effects on vascular permeability (127,128). The role of VEGF in malignant ascites of ovarian cancer has been exploited therapeutically in several studies, which noted decreases in ascites volume after treatment with bevacizumab, the anti-VEGF monoclonal antibody (129–132). Thus, VEGF is a prognostic factor and molecular target for gynecologic malignancies.

Epidermal Growth Factor

Epidermal growth factor (EGF) is a potent mitogen and chemoattractant for many tumor types, stromal cells, and endothelial cells (133). It is a prototype for successful targeting of growth-factor pathways in the era of molecularly targeted therapeutics. EGF expression has been correlated with malignant invasion and angiogenesis in a variety of tumors (133–136). This is a pathway subject to positive feedback, since tumors that produce and secrete EGF can up-regulate expression of EGF receptor (EGFR) in the local vasculature. This phenomenon was associated with an antivascular and antitumor response to EGFR inhibition (137). This may be an important site of intervention, but can also lead to a mechanism for escape from single molecular targeted therapies, for example, by tumor production of bFGF when VEGF is down-regulated (138,139).

The EGFR pathway may be important in gynecologic cancers. Ovarian cancer patients with circulating EGF concentrations below 1 ng/mL had significantly better survival than those with higher EGF concentrations (140). Increased expression of EGF receptors ErBB1/HER1(EGFR) and ErBB2/HER2/neu was associated with increased metastasis and reduced survival in ovarian carcinoma (140–142). Concurrent expression of EGF-related proteins such as EGFR and cripto ligand correlated with stage of serous and clear cell ovarian cancers at surgery (143).

EGFR antagonists have putative antiangiogenic activity. ERBB2 (HER2/neu) is expressed at a lower level in gynecologic malignancies as compared to breast cancer, but is nonetheless a poor prognostic factor (141). Overexpression of ERBB2 in cultured cells has been shown to overcome therapeutic inhibition of EGFR kinase owing to shifting the balance from EGFR homodimers to ERBB2 heterodimers that retain signaling capacity (144). Laboratory investigation and clinical targeting of this class of agents is complicated by the potential of members of the EGFR (HER) family of receptors to heterodimerize. Gefitinib is an oral EGFR inhibitor that was studied in phase 2 trials in ovarian cancer, but was ineffective in achieving objective responses or stabilization of disease (145,146). Thus, it may be important to evaluate the expression of the family of receptors and/or to identify expression of the family of ligands to optimize therapeutic intervention of this pathway. Optimal intervention may require combinations of inhibitors that target multiple family members or multiple approaches to inhibition such as simultaneous inhibition of both ligand binding and kinase signaling.

Platelet-Derived Growth Factor

Platelet-derived growth factor (PDGF) expression has been demonstrated in epithelial ovarian carcinomas but not borderline ovarian tumors (147). PDGF is a dimeric protein composed of two closely related A- and B-chain polypeptides encoded by independent genes (148). The dimer is a multifunctional cytokine that acts in an autocrine and paracrine fashion in ovarian cancer and angiogenesis. Three isoforms of PDGF (AA, AB, and BB) bind to two distinct receptors, PDGFRβ and -α (149). PDGF and its receptors promote tumor angiogenesis (123,150,151). PDGF stimulates migration of endothelial cells by increasing transcription and secretion of VEGF by PDGFRβ-expressing endothelial cells; activation of PI3K is important for this response (123). Similarly, PDGF-BB induced VEGF expression in vascular smooth muscle cells and support cells through activation of the PI3K-AKT pathway (152). In addition, PDGF-mediated secretion of VEGF protected endothelial cells *in vitro* from apoptosis caused by serum starvation, indicating an indirect role of PDGF in supporting tumor angiogenesis through activation of survival pathways (152). There is a greater expression of PDGF and PDGFRβ and -α genes in ovarian cancer than in normal epithelial ovarian cells and borderline tumors (149,153). PDGF and PDGFRβ were detected by immunohistochemistry in 73% and 36% of malignant tumor samples, respectively, but no staining occurred in normal ovarian surface epithelial (OSE) cells or benign tumors (149). Furthermore, those patients without detectable PDGFRβ had a 76% chance of survival at 40 months, equivalent to that of patients with early-stage ovarian cancer. Stromal expression of PDGFRβ supports its role in angiogenesis (31,149). Imatinib is an oral inhibitor of PDGFR in addition to bcr-abl and c-KIT, and has been approved for treatment of chronic myelogenous leukemia and gastrointestinal stromal tumors (154). Preclinical studies demonstrating that imatinib inhibited the PDGFR kinase led to the hypothesis that it could have antiangiogenic activity and potentially direct anticancer activity (155). This hypothesis was not borne out in phase 2 trials, which showed no clinical benefit of single-agent imatinib in ovarian cancer (156,157).

Intracellular Signals Promoting Angiogenesis

p53

p53 regulates multiple cellular functions including gene transcription, DNA synthesis and repair, apoptosis, angiogenesis, invasion, and metastasis (158,159). p53 is mutated in over half of all human cancers (160), including ovarian (161,162), endometrial (163), and cervical cancers (164). p53 has been linked to angiogenesis through several intermediates. Loss of wild-type p53 can down-regulate thrombospondin-1, an ECM protein and potent inhibitor of angiogenesis. Higher levels of thrombospondin-1 expression were demonstrated in fibroblasts with wild-type p53, whereas loss of p53 was associated with a decrease in thrombospondin-1 (165). An inverse relationship between thombospondin-1 expression and angiogenic activity was also found. The migration of endothelial cells and cancer cell lines grown in media from wild-type p53 fibroblasts was abrogated by antibody against thrombospondin-1. Thus, one mechanism of p53-mediated angiogenesis is its regulation of thrombospondin-1.

VEGF is downstream of p53 regulation through several mechanisms. First, hypoxia induces VEGF expression via multiple intermediates, such as hypoxia-inducible factor-1α (HIF-1α) and src (166–168). Hypoxia-induced src-mediated overexpression of VEGF may be augmented by mutant p53 (167). Cell lines containing mutant p53 expressed 80% less VEGF than those with wild-type p53. Overexpression of *src* increased VEGF in cells with p53 mutations, but wild-type p53 had a dominant effect, causing a net decrease in VEGF expression (167). Secondly, coexpression of MDM-2 with p53 correlates with increased VEGF expression in angiosarcomas (169). Eighty percent of the angiosarcomas showed elevated expression of both MDM-2 and p53 and had increased VEGF expression. Mutant p53 also has been shown to act through the protein kinase C pathway to increase VEGF expression (170,171). Thus, several mechanisms for p53-regulated VEGF expression exist, suggesting a key role for p53 in the modulation of angiogenesis.

Biology of Metastasis

Intravasation occurs first in the progression toward metastasis. The tumor cell must migrate toward and adhere to the stromal side of the vascular basement membrane, degrade the matrix at that local site, migrate through the damaged basement membrane, and interpolate between endothelial cells in order to enter the vasculature (Fig. 4.2). Circulating tumor cells cannot complete the process of metastatic dissemination without reversing the process, extravasating at a favorable secondary site. That, coupled with stimulation of local angiogenesis and tumor cell proliferation, leads to a metastatic focus. All these events are programmed into the cell. However, the metastatic cascade is a very inefficient process. Although millions of tumor cells are shed into the circulation system daily, less than 0.01% of the shed cells successfully lead to metastases (172). Such heterogeneity in metastatic competence implies that not all patients with circulating tumor cells will develop detectable metastatic disease. Thus, insight into these biological mechanisms may lead to new and better therapeutic targets and interventions.

Migration

Neoplastic cells migrate from the primary tumor mass and successfully traverse tissue barriers to induce metastasis to a site distant from the primary tumor (Fig. 4.1). This may involve simple cell locomotion from the primary into the interstitial stroma and subsequent shedding as seen in early ovarian cancer spread. Alternatively, it may require penetration and proteolysis of tissue obstacles, as occurs in active invasion. Furthermore, tumor cells have to survive the stage of vascular transport and arrest in the capillary bed of distant organs to engage in a second round of invasion and extravasation, whereby neoplastic cells exit from the vessel lumen into the surrounding stromal tissue (173). This key step in the cascade of events composing the invasive process of angiogenesis and metastasis is endothelial-cell and tumor-cell migration.

Chemokines and Growth Factors Promoting Metastasis

In order to achieve locomotion, cancer cells must initiate and maintain a complicated dynamic consisting of coordinated pseudopodal extension and attachment coupled with cell translocation and detachment. Tumor cells respond to a number of stimuli including host-derived motility and growth factors, extracellular matrix components, and tumor-secreted autocrine factors. Examples of these include the insulin-like growth factors (IGF-I, IGF-II), hepatocyte growth factor (HGF, also known as scatter factor) (174), fibroblast growth factors (FGFs), and PDGFs (175). ECM proteins or fragments may also stimulate chemotaxis (176–178). Some of these ECM fragments, such as endostatin and angiostatin, can have inhibitory activity (179,180). Thus, the dynamic process of migration is the balance of positive and negative regulatory influences in the local environment. This process stops in physiologic migration when sufficient events have occurred. Regulation of migration is aberrant in malignancy, allowing for progression of the metastatic phenotype. Advancements in our understanding of autocrine and paracrine stimulation of migration have uncovered new molecular targets for therapeutic interruption.

Autotaxin

The concept and role of autocrine growth factors is a longstanding and well-accepted biologic event. Some growth factors support motility and survival. Autotaxin (ATX) is a potent motility-stimulating glycoprotein that acts on both the tumor and the extracellular environment (181,182). ATX has been shown to stimulate tumor-cell migration, endothelial-cell migration and tube formation, and angiogenesis (183). ATX is linked to the production of lysophosphatidic acid (LPA) in the cellular microenvironment, cleaving lysophosphatidylcholine (LPC) to release LPA. It is thus an important component of the LPA regulatory pathway and a novel extracellular molecular target.

Lysophosphatidic Acid

LPA is a lipid that was initially characterized as a factor propagating ovarian cancer cells in ascites (184,185). It has been proposed as both a biomarker for diagnosis and a potential target for therapy of ovarian cancer (186). LPA is known to induce tumor and endothelial cell proliferation, migration, and survival through its stimulation of the PI3K pathway in ovarian cancer (185,187). Interestingly, one study with ovarian cancer cells *in vitro* showed that LPA-induced migration could be inhibited by alendronate, a commercially available bisphosphonate (188). The receptor for LPA is a G-protein-coupled receptor; since G-protein-coupled receptors are the most successfully druggable targets (189), agents inhibiting the LPA receptor are in development (190).

Intracellular Signals Promoting Metastasis

Anoikis, or homelessness, is defined as apoptosis that occurs from loss of adhesion-linked survival signals (191). Malignant cells surviving in effusions or ascites have developed mechanisms to overcome anoikis. Ovarian cancer cells must develop such survival mechanisms early in their progression since malignant ascites and effusions occur before parenchymal metastases, in contrast to most other solid tumors. A molecular pattern of this process has been detected in ovarian cancer cells harvested from malignant effusions (192). Anoikis can be overcome by constitutive activation of the survival signals through genomic, transcriptional, and protein activation events that no longer depend on the "home" extracellular environment. These signals allow metastasis to occur. Malignant tumors consist of phenotypically heterogeneous populations that differ in their capacity to invade surrounding tissue, induce angiogenesis, and travel to distant sites (92,95,193). As with cellular transformation, loss of function and gain of function events have been demonstrated in the regulation of metastatic suppression and promotion.

PIK3CA

PIK3CA encodes the p110α catalytic subunit of PI3K. It has been implicated in ovarian carcinogenesis and may act synergistically with RAS-mediated pathways to increase cell motility and metastasis (194). The PI3K p110 catalytic subunit shows increased gene copy number that results in increased transcription and translation of *PIK3CA* in ovarian cancer cell lines and patient samples, and that signal is transmitted through overactivation of the PI3K p85 regulatory subunit. This in turn activates the AKT pro-survival pathway and provides protection from anoikis in the absence of integrin engagement (46,194–196). Further, PI3K has lipid kinase activity wherein it phosphorylates phosphatidylinositol 4,5-phosphate (PIP2) to generate PIP3, a regulatory molecule for several other pathways involved in adhesion and motility such as phospholipase C-δ (PLC-δ), which is involved in the detachment process required for motility (197).

PTEN

PTEN (phosphate and tensin homolog) has been identified as a tumor- and metastasis-suppressor gene. Loss-of-function mutations of *PTEN* that result in the loss of the catalytic domain have been found in multiple human tumors including endometrial and ovarian cancers (196,198,199). It encodes a tyrosine and lipid phosphatase (200) that inhibits cell migration, spreading, and focal adhesion, in part by dephosphorylating focal adhesion kinase (FAK). A significant decrease in integrin-mediated cell spreading and focal adhesion formation *in vitro* was associated with a 60% decrease in tyrosine phosphorylation of FAK in *PTEN*-overexpressing cells (201). Cell invasion, migration, and growth were down-regulated by expressing *PTEN* in an ovarian cancer cell line, confirming the metastatic suppressor phenotype (201). *PTEN* is also important as a regulator of survival pathways. Loss of *PTEN* function leaves PI3K and AKT in their activated states, driving the pro-invasive, pro-angiogenic, and pro-survival pathways. Thus, *PTEN* activity is a critical step in metastasis regulation.

NOVEL TECHNOLOGIES TO STUDY MOLECULAR MECHANISMS OF METASTASIS

Advances in technology are yielding new genes and new directions for studying the molecular mechanism of invasion, angiogenesis, and metastasis. To date, this information has been gained through examination of cultured cells and through animal models. Analysis from metastatic cell populations as they exist in their native environment may provide new insight into additional genes, proteins, and signal transduction pathways critical to oncogenic events. Several technologies have been developed that may aid in the direct evaluation of cancer cells.

Microdissection

Laser capture microdissection has provided more control in microdissection and markedly advanced our ability to evaluate events ongoing in human gynecologic and other tumors (202). Captured cells isolated from the appropriately fixed tissues can be used for genomic, expression, and protein studies. In one instance of the use of microdissected ovarian cancer cells from fixed tissues, a 50% loss of heterozygosity at chromosomal locus 8p21 was identified. This high rate of allelic loss, suggesting the presence of a tumor-suppressor gene at that locus, was missed by prior studies in which hand microdissection or no cell selection was performed and has led to further studies to identify the putative suppressor gene (203). Advances in the field of microdissection use immunohistochemistry guidance for identification of target cells (204) and have led to more precise interrogation of ovarian tumor vasculature (205).

High-Throughput cDNA Screening

The use of frozen or ethanol-fixed tissues is optimal for gene expression studies, and these products have been applied to investigative and high-throughput screening techniques. cDNA libraries from microdissected tissues have the advantage of representing the genes expressed from a specific cell population and can be compared to local stroma to discern differential gene regulation in the microenvironment. A novel growth factor, granulin-epithelin precursor (GEP), was identified as a possible ovarian cancer invasion gene from differential analysis of cDNA libraries from microdissected ovarian tumor epithelium (206–208). This finding would have been missed using nonmicrodissected cells since this gene is expressed ubiquitously in stromal cells. Microdissected samples can be adapted to high-throughput gene expression profiling by microarray analysis (209).

Proteomic Technology

New proteomic technologies applied to gynecologic cancer tumors and serum samples can identify proteins and protein pathways involved in the development and progression of these cancers. High-throughput approaches for global unbiased searches can uncover protein family associations or signatures (210). Application of surface-enhanced or matrix-associated mass spectrometry with higher order bioinformatics and mass sequencing is now being used to generate large volumes of information related to the malignant process. This will advance development of databases of proteomic information from which target validation and therapeutic application can proceed in a directed fashion.

We recently completed clinical trials applying tissue proteomics to evaluate effects of targeted agents (145). The clinical trials assessed the targeted activity of the EGFR-inhibitor gefitinib and the c-kit/PDGFR inhibitor imatinib in patients with recurrent ovarian cancer. Percutaneous 16- to 18-gauge core needle tumor biopsies were obtained prior to beginning therapy and after 4 weeks of treatment. Tumor and stromal cells were separated using laser capture microdissection and analyzed separately by tissue lysate arrays (TLA). Arrayed samples were analyzed for the levels of EGFR and its activated (phosphorylated) forms, as well as downstream signaling molecules AKT and extracellular-signal-regulated kinase (ERK), and their activated forms. No clinical benefit was seen with either agent, but the TLAs confirmed the targeted activity of each drug. TLA results from both trials suggested that target inhibition was present but that the blocked signal was not essential for tumor growth, the level of inhibition was insufficient to completely prevent receptor signaling, and/or the receptor function was unrelated to the malignancy at this advanced and recurrent state of disease. Statistics did show, however, a relationship for signaling parameter and clinical toxicity by grade and by trend of toxicity. Increasing EGFR, AKT, p-ERK, and p-EGFR moieties in tumor after treatment were statistically significantly associated with increasing overall toxicity ($p \leq 0.05$), gastrointestinal toxicity ($p < 0.05$), and skin toxicity ($p = 0.029$) (157). This illustrates the strength of the tissue lysate array. These clinical trials demonstrated the ability to incorporate invasive sample collection and detailed biochemical analysis to confirm target modulation and to correlate the biochemical proteomic events with clinical and toxicity events.

CLINICAL APPLICATION: THERAPY DIRECTED AGAINST INVASION, ANGIOGENESIS, AND METASTASIS

Molecular Targeted Agents: Monoclonal Antibodies

Bevacizumab is a recombinant humanized version of the murine antihuman VEGF monoclonal antibody. The VEGF-neutralizing antibody inhibits VEGF-induced signaling, resulting in reduced angiogenesis and tumor growth. It has been FDA-approved based on prolonging survival when given in combination with chemotherapy in metastatic colon cancer, and has activity in breast and lung cancer as well (211,212). As a single agent, bevacizumab has been shown to prolong progression-free survival compared to placebo in a phase 2 trial in renal cell cancer (213). Moreover, a phase 2 study (GOG 170D) of bevacizumab in ovarian cancer demonstrated a 17% response rate with an added 40% of patients having stable disease in women treated with two or fewer prior therapies (214). The addition of bevacizumab to front-line chemotherapy and to maintenance therapy in epithelial ovarian cancer is now being evaluated in a large phase 3 trial (GOG 218). Recent results from the GOG phase II trial of bevacizumab in cervical cancer are promising. NB not publised yet.

Cetuximab is a recombinant chimeric antibody to EGFR1 that is presently approved for treatment of metastatic colon cancer and unresectable head and neck cancer, with activity in breast and non-small-cell lung cancer as well. As monotherapy, cetuximab produced a 9% response rate in irinotecan refractory colon cancer (215) and showed responses in head and neck cancer (216). Cetuximab has also been effective as a radiation sensitizer, prolonging survival (49 vs. 29 months) in unresectable head and neck cancer treated with concomitant radiation (217). It is being evaluated in advanced cervical cancer in combination with cisplatin (GOG 76DD) and with radiation (GOG 9918). Panitumumab is a second-generation human antibody to the extracellular domain of EGFR1 and has been approved as last-line therapy in metastatic colon cancer (218,219). Preclinical and early-phase clinical work is pending for multiple other monoclonal antibodies that target pro-angiogenic receptors and pathways.

ERBB2 (HER2/neu) is expressed in less than 10% of epethelial ovarian cancer (EOC) and approximately 18% of uterine papillary serous carcinoma (220,221). Trastuzumab is a monoclonal antibody to ERBB2 and prolongs survival significantly in ERBB2 positive breast cancer in both the adjuvant and metastatic settings (222,223). A phase 2 trial of trastuzumab in recurrent ovarian cancer (GOG-160) showed only a 7.3% response rate in 41 patients with ERBB2 overexpression (2+ or 3+ by immunohistochemistry) (224). It is presently under study in a phase 2 trial in advanced endometrial cancer.

Molecular Targeted Agents: Kinase Inhibitors

In addition to direct targeting of VEGF with bevacizumab, a number of small-molecule inhibitors of the VEGF receptors have been developed and have reached clinical trials. VEGFR2 is the most commonly targeted. Preclinical data have shown this approach to be active in reducing endothelial-cell proliferation, migration, and vascular development, and xenograft models have confirmed activity in a number of solid tumors (225).

Sorafenib is an oral Raf and VEGFR2 kinase inhibitor that has been approved for treatment of metastatic renal cell cancer (226); it is presently being studied in a GOG phase 2 study in ovarian cancer (GOG-170F). Gefitinib, an oral EGFR inhibitor, was studied in phase 2 trials in ovarian cancer but did not produce objective responses or stabilization of disease (145,146). Imatinib, an oral inhibitor of bcr-abl, c-KIT, and PDGFR, has been approved for treatment of chronic myelogenous leukemia and gastrointestinal stromal tumors; it had no activity in phase 2 trials of relapsed/refractory ovarian and endometrial cancer (154,156,157). Lapatinib is an oral EGFR and ERBB2 inhibitor that has activity in breast cancer (227,228) and is being studied in a phase 2 trial in ovarian cancer, among other malignancies. Sunitinib, a VEGFR and PDGFR inhibitor, is approved for treatment of metastatic renal cell cancer (229), while erlotinib, another EGFR inhibitor, is approved as a single agent for treatment of metastatic lung cancer (230) and in combination with gemcitabine for pancreatic cancer (231). Vandetanib, a dual EGFR and VEGFR inhibitor, has been shown in preclinical work to have activity in EOC (232) and is currently in a phase 2 trial for recurrent ovarian cancer. Numerous other small molecules targeting these pathways are presently under development.

Combination Therapy

Further refinement of targeted therapy is focused on the hypothesis that inhibiting angiogenesis signals in combination with each other or with chemotherapy may be more effective

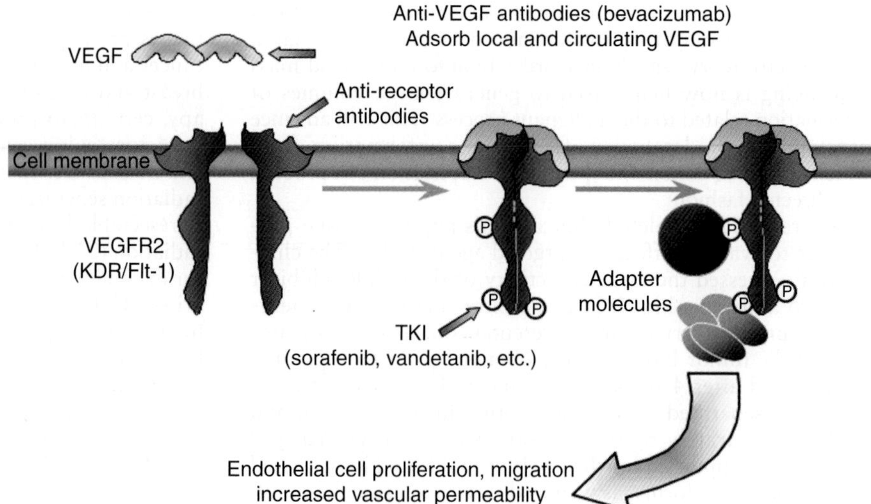

FIGURE 4.4. Example of combined targeted therapy against angiogenesis. Bevacizumab blocks VEGF from binding to its receptor, VEGFR2. Sorafenib inhibits downstream signaling from the receptor by blocking its tyrosine kinase activity, as well as that of other signal transduction molecules such as Raf.

than when used as single agents. In an attempt to target the VEGF pathway in vertical series, bevacizumab was combined with sorafenib, as Raf-kinase is a downstream effector of VEGFR2 (Fig. 4.4). A phase 1 trial of sorafenib and bevacizumab in combination has demonstrated a partial response rate of 47% (7 out of 15 patients) in heavily pretreated EOC (233). A phase 2 trial of bevacizumab combined with sorafenib for ovarian cancer is accruing at the National Cancer Institute as of this writing. Many other ongoing phase 2 clinical trials are testing targeted agents combined with chemotherapy in gynecologic malignancies (234). Trials are widely varied and range from paclitaxel and carboplatin in combination with an EGFR tyrosine kinase inhibitor or an anti-EGFR monoclonal antibody, to proteasome inhibitor with irinotecan.

CONCLUSIONS

Continued scientific, epidemiologic, and clinical advances are critically needed until successful, reproducible, and accurate early detection of gynecologic tumors becomes routine. Understanding the biology, regulation, and implications of the process of invasion and angiogenesis will continue to drive new biomarker and therapeutic target identification and intervention. Similarity between dysregulated invasion of angiogenesis and unregulated motility of metastasis allows the potential for duality of intervention. The tumor's interaction with its microenvironment becomes the focus for scientific dissection and therapeutic application (31). Here, the process of autocrine and paracrine regulation, signal pathway activation, and cell-cell conversation are critical. The use of the newer and high-throughput technologies to identify collections of biologic targets rather than one gene or protein at a time can make the process more streamlined and provide a broader view of the interaction of events. Together, improved understanding, study of events in the patient populations, and cooperative and collaborative progress will allow us to overcome invasion and metastasis, the major causes of morbidity and mortality associated with gynecologic cancers.

References

1. Paget J. The distribution of secondary growths in cancer of the breast. *Lancet.* 1889;1:571–573.
2. Norton L, Massague J. Is cancer a disease of self-seeding? *Nat Med* 2006;12(8):875–878.
3. Fidler IJ. Critical determinants of metastasis. *Semin Cancer Biol* 2002;12(2):89–96.
4. Taylor H. Malignant and semimalignant tumors of the ovary. *Surg Gynecol Obstet* 1929;48:204.
5. Benedet JL, Bender H, Jones H 3rd, et al. FIGO staging classifications and clinical practice guidelines in the management of gynecologic cancers. FIGO Committee on Gynecologic Oncology. *Int J Gynaecol Obstet* 2000;70(2):209–262.
6. Silva-Filho AL, Reis FM, Traiman P, et al. Clinicopathological features influencing pelvic lymph node metastasis and vaginal and parametrial involvement in patients with carcinoma of the cervix. *Gynecol Obstet Invest* 2005;59(2):92–96.
7. Hirai Y, Takeshima N, Tate S, et al. Early invasive cervical adenocarcinoma: its potential for nodal metastasis or recurrence. *BJOG* 2003;110(3):241–246.
8. Grisaru DA, Covens A, Franssen E, et al. Histopathologic score predicts recurrence free survival after radical surgery in patients with stage IA2-IB1-2 cervical carcinoma. *Cancer* 2003;97(8):1904–1908.
9. Bucy GS, Mendenhall WM, Morgan LS, et al. Clinical stage I and II endometrial carcinoma treated with surgery and/or radiation therapy: analysis of prognostic and treatment-related factors. *Gynecol Oncol* 1989;33(3):290–295.
10. Steiner E, Eicher O, Sagemuller J, et al. Multivariate independent prognostic factors in endometrial carcinoma: a clinicopathologic study in 181 patients: 10 years experience at the Department of Obstetrics and Gynecology of the Mainz University. *Int J Gynecol Cancer* 2003;13(2):197–203.
11. Folkman J. Tumor angiogenesis: therapeutic implications. *N Engl J Med* 1971;285(21):1182–1186.
12. Folkman J, Merler E, Abernathy C, et al. Isolation of a tumor factor responsible for angiogenesis. *J Exp Med* 1971;133(2):275–288.
13. Liotta LA, Saidel GM, Kleinerman J. Diffusion model of tumor vascularization and growth. *Bull Math Biol* 1977;39(1):117–128.
14. Hlatky L, Hahnfeldt P, Folkman J, et al. Clinical application of antiangiogenic therapy: microvessel density, what it does and doesn't tell us. *J Natl Cancer Inst* 2002;94(12):883–893.
15. Cantu De Leon D, Lopez-Graniel C, Frias Mendivil M, et al. Significance of microvascular density (MVD) in cervical cancer recurrence. *Int J Gynecol Cancer* 2003;13(6):856–862.
16. Raspollini MR, Amunni G, Villanucci A, et al. Prognostic significance of microvessel density and vascular endothelial growth factor expression in advanced ovarian serous carcinoma. *Int J Gynecol Cancer* 2004;14(5):815–823.
17. Taskiran C, Erdem O, Onan A, et al. The prognostic value of endoglin (CD105) expression in ovarian carcinoma. *Int J Gynecol Cancer* 2006;16(5):1789–1793.
18. Ozalp S, Yalcin OT, Acikalin M, et al. Microvessel density as a prognosticator in endometrial carcinoma. *Eur J Gynaecol Oncol* 2003;24(3-4):305–308.
19. Schlenger K, Hockel M, Mitze M, et al. Tumor vascularity—a novel prognostic factor in advanced cervical carcinoma. *Gynecol Oncol* 1995;59(1):57–66.
20. Kaku T, Kamura T, Kinukawa N, et al. Angiogenesis in endometrial carcinoma. *Cancer* 1997;80(4):741–747.
21. Hollingsworth HC, Kohn EC, Steinberg SM, et al. Tumor angiogenesis in advanced stage ovarian carcinoma. *Am J Pathol* 1995;147(1):33–41.
22. Paley PJ, Staskus KA, Gebhard K, et al. Vascular endothelial growth factor expression in early stage ovarian carcinoma. *Cancer* 1997;80(1):98–106.
23. Beyer FD Jr., Murphy A. Patterns of spread of invasive cancer of the uterine cervix. *Cancer* 1965;18:34–40.

24. Creasman WT, Morrow CP, Bundy BN, et al. Surgical pathologic spread patterns of endometrial cancer. A Gynecologic Oncology Group Study. *Cancer* 1987;60(8 Suppl):2035–2041.
25. di Re E, Grosso G, Raspagliesi F, et al. Fallopian tube cancer: incidence and role of lymphatic spread. *Gynecol Oncol* 1996;62(2):199–202.
26. Ahmed N, Pansino F, Clyde R, et al. Overexpression of $\alpha v\beta 6$ integrin in serous epithelial ovarian cancer regulates extracellular matrix degradation via the plasminogen activation cascade. *Carcinogenesis* 2002;23(2):237–244.
27. Jacobs A. Ovarian cancer. *Clin Symp* 1996;48(2):2–32.
28. Knapp RC, Friedman EA. Aortic lymph node metastases in early ovarian cancer. *Am J Obstet Gynecol* 1974;119(8):1013–1017.
29. Matsumoto K, Yoshikawa H, Yasugi T, et al. Distinct lymphatic spread of endometrial carcinoma in comparison with cervical and ovarian carcinomas. *Cancer Lett* 2002;180(1):83–89.
30. Liotta LA, Stetler-Stevenson WG. Tumor invasion and metastasis: an imbalance of positive and negative regulation. *Cancer Res* 1991;51(18 Suppl): 5054s–5059s.
31. Liotta LA, Kohn EC. The microenvironment of the tumour-host interface. *Nature* 2001;411(6835):375–379.
32. Davies BR, Worsley SD, Ponder BA. Expression of E-cadherin, α-catenin and β-catenin in normal ovarian surface epithelium and epithelial ovarian cancers. *Histopathology* 1998;32(1):69–80.
33. Stupack DG, Cho SY, Klemke RL. Molecular signaling mechanisms of cell migration and invasion. *Immunol Res* 2000;21(2-3):83–88.
34. Chen YT, Stewart DB, Nelson WJ. Coupling assembly of the E-cadherin/β-catenin complex to efficient endoplasmic reticulum exit and basal-lateral membrane targeting of E-cadherin in polarized MDCK cells. *J Cell Biol* 1994;144:687–699.
35. Klingelhofer J, Troyanovsky RB, Laur OY, et al. Exchange of catenins in cadherin-catenin complex. *Oncogene* 2003;22(8):1181–1188.
36. Christofori G, Semb H. The role of the cell-adhesion molecule E-cadherin as a tumour-supressor gene. *Trends Biochem Sci* 1999;24:73–76.
37. Perl AK, Wilgenbus P, Dahl U, et al. A causal role for E-cadherin in the transition from adenoma to carcinoma. *Nature* 1998;392(6672):190–193.
38. Sundfeldt K, Piontkewitz Y, Ivarsson K, et al. E-cadherin expression in human epithelial ovarian cancer and normal ovary. *Int J Cancer* 1997;74(3): 275–280.
39. Maines-Bandiera SL, Auersperg N. Increased E-cadherin expression in ovarian surface epithelium: an early step in metaplasia and dysplasia? *Int J Gynecol Pathol* 1997;16(3):250–255.
40. Berx G, Van Roy F. The E-cadherin/catenin complex: an important gatekeeper in breast cancer tumorigenesis and malignant progression. *Breast Cancer Res* 2001;3(5):289–293.
41. Fujimoto J, Ichigo S, Hirose R, et al. Expression of E-cadherin and α- and β-catenin mRNAs in ovarian cancers. *Cancer Lett* 1997;115(2):207–212.
42. Risinger JI, Berchuck A, Kohler MF, et al. Mutations of the E-cadherin gene in human gynecologic cancers. *Nat Genet* 1994;7(1):98–102.
43. Auersperg N, Pan J, Grove BD, et al. E-cadherin induces mesenchymal-to-epithelial transition in human ovarian surface epithelium. *Proc Natl Acad Sci USA* 1999;96(11):6249–6254.
44. Giancotti FG, Ruoslahti E. Integrin signaling. *Science* 1999;285(5430): 1028–1032.
45. Arboleda MJ, Lyons JF, Kabbinavar FF, et al. Overexpression of AKT2/protein kinase Bβ leads to up-regulation of β1 integrins, increased invasion, and metastasis of human breast and ovarian cancer cells. *Cancer Res* 2003;63(1):196–206.
46. Tian B, Lessan K, Kahm J, et al. β1 integrin regulates fibroblast viability during collagen matrix contraction through a phosphatidylinositol 3-kinase/Akt/protein kinase B signaling pathway. *J Biol Chem* 2002; 277(27):24667–24675.
47. Eliceiri BP, Cheresh DA. Role of alpha v integrins during angiogenesis. *Cancer J* 2000;6(Suppl 3):S245–S249.
48. Kerr JS, Slee AM, Mousa SA. The αv integrin antagonists as novel anti-cancer agents: an update. *Expert Opin Investig Drugs* 2002;11(12): 1765–1774.
49. Naik MU, Mousa SA, Parkos CA, et al. Signaling through JAM-1 and (vβ3 is required for the angiogenic action of bFGF: dissociation of the JAM-1 and (vβ3 complex. *Blood* 2003;102(6):2108–2114.
50. Nam JO, Kim JE, Jeong HW, et al. Identification of the $\alpha v\beta 3$ integrin-interacting motif of βig-h3 and its anti-angiogenic effect. *J Biol Chem* 2003;278(28):25902–25909.
51. Sudhakar A, Sugimoto H, Yang C, et al. Human tumstatin and human endostatin exhibit distinct antiangiogenic activities mediated by $\alpha v\beta 3$ and $\alpha 5\beta 1$ integrins. *Proc Natl Acad Sci USA* 2003;100(8):4766–4771.
52. Chattopadhyay N, Chatterjee A. Studies on the expression of $\alpha v\beta 3$ integrin receptors in non-malignant and malignant human cervical tumor tissues. *J Exp Clin Cancer Res* 2001;20(2):269–275.
53. Ahmed N, Riley C, Rice G, et al. Role of integrin receptors for fibronectin, collagen and laminin in the regulation of ovarian carcinoma functions in response to a matrix microenvironment. *Clin Exp Metastasis* 2005;22(5):391–402.
54. Liapis H, Adler LM, Wick MR, et al. Expression of $\alpha v\beta 3$ integrin is less frequent in ovarian epithelial tumors of low malignant potential in contrast to ovarian carcinomas. *Hum Pathol* 1997;28(4):443–449.
55. Vacca A, Ria R, Presta M, et al. $\alpha v\beta 3$ integrin engagement modulates cell adhesion, proliferation, and protease secretion in human lymphoid tumor cells. *Exp Hematol* 2001;29(8):993–1003.
56. Ria R, Vacca A, Ribatti D, et al. (vβ3 integrin engagement enhances cell invasiveness in human multiple myeloma. *Haematologica* 2002;87(8):836–845.
57. Fundyler O, Khanna M, Smoller BR. Metalloproteinase-2 expression correlates with aggressiveness of cutaneous squamous cell carcinomas. *Mod Pathol* 2004;17(5):496–502.
58. Nuttall RK, Pennington CJ, Taplin J, et al. Elevated membrane-type matrix metalloproteinases in gliomas revealed by profiling proteases and inhibitors in human cancer cells. *Mol Cancer Res* 2003;1(5):333–345.
59. Riethdorf L, Riethdorf S, Petersen S, et al. Urokinase gene expression indicates early invasive growth in squamous cell lesions of the uterine cervix. *J Pathol* 1999;189(2):245–250.
60. Verma RP, Hansch C. Matrix metalloproteinases (MMPs): chemical-biological functions and (Q)SARs. *Bioorg Med Chem* 2007;15(6):2223–2268.
61. Di Nezza LA, Misajon A, Zhang J, et al. Presence of active gelatinases in endometrial carcinoma and correlation of matrix metalloproteinase expression with increasing tumor grade and invasion. *Cancer* 2002;94(5): 1466–1475.
62. Iwata H, Kobayashi S, Iwase H, et al. Production of matrix metalloproteinases and tissue inhibitors of metalloproteinases in human breast carcinomas. *Jpn J Cancer Res* 1996;87(6):602–611.
63. Rosenthal EL, Matrisian LM. Matrix metalloproteases in head and neck cancer. *Head Neck* 2006;28(7):639–648.
64. Fishman DA, Bafetti LM, Banionis S, et al. Production of extracellular matrix-degrading proteinases by primary cultures of human epithelial ovarian carcinoma cells. *Cancer* 1997;80(8):1457–1463.
65. Nasr M, Ayyad SB, El-Lamie IK, et al. Expression of matrix metalloproteinase-2 in preinvasive and invasive carcinoma of the uterine cervix. *Eur J Gynaecol Oncol* 2005;26(2):199–202.
66. Johansson N, Vaalamo M, Grenman S, et al. Collagenase-3 (MMP-13) is expressed by tumor cells in invasive vulvar squamous cell carcinomas. *Am J Pathol* 1999;154(2):469–480.
67. Bernardo MM, Fridman R. TIMP-2 (tissue inhibitor of metalloproteinase-2) regulates MMP-2 (matrix metalloproteinase-2) activity in the extracellular environment after pro-MMP-2 activation by MT1 (membrane type 1)-MMP. *Biochem J* 2003;374(Pt 3):739–745.
68. Graesslin O, Cortez A, Uzan C, et al. Endometrial tumor invasiveness is related to metalloproteinase 2 and tissue inhibitor of metalloproteinase 2 expressions. *Int J Gynecol Cancer* 2006;16(5):1911–1917.
69. Sakata K, Shigemasa K, Nagai N, et al. Expression of matrix metalloproteinases (MMP-2, MMP-9, MT1-MMP) and their inhibitors (TIMP-1, TIMP-2) in common epithelial tumors of the ovary. *Int J Oncol* 2000;17(4):673–681.
70. Murphy AN, Unsworth EJ, Stetler-Stevenson WG. Tissue inhibitor of metalloproteinases-2 inhibits bFGF-induced human microvascular endothelial cell proliferation. *J Cell Physiol* 1993;157(2):351–358.
71. Ikenaka Y, Yoshiji H, Kuriyama S, et al. Tissue inhibitor of metalloproteinases-1 (TIMP-1) inhibits tumor growth and angiogenesis in the TIMP-1 transgenic mouse model. *Int J Cancer* 2003;105(3):340–346.
72. Guedez L, Stetler-Stevenson WG, Wolff L, et al. *In vitro* suppression of programmed cell death of B cells by tissue inhibitor of metalloproteinases-1. *J Clin Invest* 1998;102(11):2002–2010.
73. Crul M, Beerepoot LV, Stokvis E, et al. Clinical pharmacokinetics, pharmacodynamics and metabolism of the novel matrix metalloproteinase inhibitor ABT-518. *Cancer Chemother Pharmacol* 2002;50(6):473–478.
74. Nyormoi O, Mills L, Bar-Eli M. An MMP-2/MMP-9 inhibitor, 5a, enhances apoptosis induced by ligands of the TNF receptor superfamily in cancer cells. *Cell Death Differ* 2003;10(5):558–569.
75. Mannello F, Tonti G, Papa S. Matrix metalloproteinase inhibitors as anti-cancer therapeutics. *Curr Cancer Drug Targets* 2005;5(4):285–298.
76. Conese M, Nykjaer A, Petersen CM, et al. α-2 Macroglobulin receptor/Ldl receptor-related protein(Lrp)-dependent internalization of the urokinase receptor. *J Cell Biol* 1995;131(6 Pt 1):1609–1622.
77. Kiziridou AD, Toliou T, Stefanou D, et al. u-PA expression in benign, borderline and malignant ovarian tumors. *Anticancer Res* 2002;22(2A): 985–990.
78. Kobayashi H, Moniwa N, Sugimura M, et al. Increased cell-surface urokinase in advanced ovarian cancer. *Jpn J Cancer Res* 1993;84(6):633–640.
79. Pustilnik TB, Estrella V, Wiener JR, et al. Lysophosphatidic acid induces urokinase secretion by ovarian cancer cells. *Clin Cancer Res* 1999;5(11): 3704–3710.
80. Inagaki K, Kobayashi H, Yoshida R, et al. Suppression of urokinase expression and invasion by a soybean Kunitz trypsin inhibitor are mediated through inhibition of Src-dependent signaling pathways. *J Biol Chem* 2005;280(36):31428–31437.
81. Kobayashi H, Suzuki M, Kanayama N, et al. Genetic down-regulation of phosphoinositide 3-kinase by bikunin correlates with suppression of invasion and metastasis in human ovarian cancer HRA cells. *J Biol Chem* 2004;279(8):6371–6379.
82. Kobayashi H, Suzuki M, Tanaka Y, et al. A Kunitz-type protease inhibitor, bikunin, inhibits ovarian cancer cell invasion by blocking the calcium-dependent transforming growth factor-β1 signaling cascade. *J Biol Chem* 2003;278(10):7790–7799.
83. Bourne HR, Sanders DA, McCormick F. The GTPase superfamily: conserved structure and molecular mechanism. *Nature* 1991;349(6305):117–127.
84. Teneriello MG, Ebina M, Linnoila RI, et al. p53 and Ki-ras gene mutations in epithelial ovarian neoplasms. *Cancer Res* 1993;53(13):3103–3108.

85. Lax SF, Kendall B, Tashiro H, et al. The frequency of p53, K-ras mutations, and microsatellite instability differs in uterine endometrioid and serous carcinoma: evidence of distinct molecular genetic pathways. *Cancer* 2000; 88(4):814–824.
86. Swisher EM, Peiffer-Schneider S, Mutch DG, et al. Differences in patterns of TP53 and KRAS2 mutations in a large series of endometrial carcinomas with or without microsatellite instability. *Cancer* 1999;85(1):119–126.
87. Alonio LV, Picconi MA, Dalbert D, et al. Ha-ras oncogene mutation associated to progression of papillomavirus induced lesions of uterine cervix. *J Clin Virol* 2003;27(3):263–269.
88. Okada F, Rak JW, Croix BS, et al. Impact of oncogenes in tumor angiogenesis: mutant K-ras up-regulation of vascular endothelial growth factor/vascular permeability factor is necessary, but not sufficient for tumorigenicity of human colorectal carcinoma cells. *Proc Natl Acad Sci USA* 1998;95(7):3609–3614.
89. Breier G, Blum S, Peli J, et al. Transforming growth factor-beta and Ras regulate the VEGF/VEGF-receptor system during tumor angiogenesis. *Int J Cancer* 2002;97(2):142–148.
90. Gu WZ, Joseph I, Wang YC, et al. A highly potent and selective farnesyltransferase inhibitor ABT-100 in preclinical studies. *Anticancer Drugs* 2005;16(10):1059–1069.
91. Hanahan D, Folkman J. Patterns and emerging mechanisms of the angiogenic switch during tumorigenesis. *Cell* 1996;86(3):353–364.
92. Liotta LA, Kleinerman J, Saidel GM. Quantitative relationships of intravascular tumor cells, tumor vessels, and pulmonary metastases following tumor implantation. *Cancer Res* 1974;34(5):997–1004.
93. Holmgren L, O'Reilly MS, Folkman J. Dormancy of micrometastases: balanced proliferation and apoptosis in the presence of angiogenesis suppression. *Nat Med* 1995;1(2):149–153.
94. Klauber N, Parangi S, Flynn E, et al. Inhibition of angiogenesis and breast cancer in mice by the microtubule inhibitors 2-methoxyestradiol and taxol. *Cancer Res* 1997;57(1):81–86.
95. Parangi S, O'Reilly M, Christofori G, et al. Antiangiogenic therapy of transgenic mice impairs *de novo* tumor growth. *Proc Natl Acad Sci USA* 1996;93(5):2002–2007.
96. Kohn EC, Liotta LA. Molecular insights into cancer invasion: strategies for prevention and intervention. *Cancer Res* 1995;55(9):1856–1862.
97. Auerbach W, Auerbach R. Angiogenesis inhibition: a review. *Pharmacol Ther* 1994;63(3):265–311.
98. Ferrara N, Gerber HP, LeCouter J. The biology of VEGF and its receptors. *Nat Med* 2003;9(6):669–676.
99. Folkman J, Klagsbrun M. Angiogenic factors. *Science* 1987;235(4787): 442–447.
100. Joseph-Silverstein J, Silverstein RL. Cell adhesion molecules: an overview. *Cancer Invest* 1998;16(3):176–182.
101. Yancopoulos GD, Davis S, Gale NW, et al. Vascular-specific growth factors and blood vessel formation. *Nature* 2000;407(6801):242–248.
102. Ogawa K, Pasqualini R, Lindberg RA, et al. The ephrin-A1 ligand and its receptor, EphA2, are expressed during tumor neovascularization. *Oncogene* 2000;19(52):6043–6052.
103. Liu ZJ, Shirakawa T, Li Y, et al. Regulation of Notch1 and Dll4 by vascular endothelial growth factor in arterial endothelial cells: implications for modulating arteriogenesis and angiogenesis. *Mol Cell Biol* 2003;23(1): 14–25.
104. Pola R, Ling LE, Silver M, et al. The morphogen Sonic hedgehog is an indirect angiogenic agent upregulating two families of angiogenic growth factors. *Nat Med* 2001;7(6):706–711.
105. Lee SH, Schloss DJ, Jarvis L, et al. Inhibition of angiogenesis by a mouse sprouty protein. *J Biol Chem* 2001;276(6):4128–4133.
106. Huminiecki L, Gorn M, Suchting S, et al. Magic roundabout is a new member of the roundabout receptor family that is endothelial specific and expressed at sites of active angiogenesis. *Genomics* 2002;79(4):547–552.
107. Achen MG, Stacker SA. Tumor lymphangiogenesis and metastatic spread—new players begin to emerge. *Int J Cancer* 2006;119:1755–1760.
108. Al-Rawi MAA, Mansel RE, Jiang WG. Molecular and cellular mechanisms of lymphangiogenesis. *Eur J Surg Oncol* 2005;31:117–121.
109. Conejo-Garcia JR, Buckanovich RJ, Benencia F, et al. Vascular leukocytes contribute to tumor vascularization. *Blood* 2005;105(2):679–681.
110. Conejo-Garcia JR, Benencia F, Courreges MC, et al. Tumor-infiltrating dendritic cell precursors recruited by a beta-defensin contribute to vasculogenesis under the influence of Vegf-A. *Nat Med* 2004;10(9):950–958.
111. Senger DR, Galli SJ, Dvorak AM, et al. Tumor cells secrete a vascular permeability factor that promotes accumulation of ascites fluid. *Science* 1983;219(4587):983–985.
112. Ferrara N, Houck K, Jakeman L, et al. Molecular and biological properties of the vascular endothelial growth factor family of proteins. *Endocr Rev* 1992;13(1):18–32.
113. Ferrara N, Chen H, Davis-Smyth T, et al. Vascular endothelial growth factor is essential for corpus luteum angiogenesis. *Nat Med* 1998;4(3):336–340.
114. Mahnke JL, Dawood MY, Huang JC. Vascular endothelial growth factor and interleukin-6 in peritoneal fluid of women with endometriosis. *Fertil Steril* 2000;73(1):166–170.
115. Ferrara N, Frantz G, LeCouter J, et al. Differential expression of the angiogenic factor genes vascular endothelial growth factor (VEGF) and endocrine gland-derived VEGF in normal and polycystic human ovaries. *Am J Pathol* 2003;162(6):1881–1893.
116. Hu YL, Tee MK, Goetzl EJ, et al. Lysophosphatidic acid induction of vascular endothelial growth factor expression in human ovarian cancer cells. *J Natl Cancer Inst* 2001;93(10):762–768.
117. Hsieh CY, Chen CA, Chou CH, et al. Overexpression of Her-2/NEU in epithelial ovarian carcinoma induces vascular endothelial growth factor C by activating NF-kappa B: implications for malignant ascites formation and tumor lymphangiogenesis. *J Biomed Sci* 2004;11(2):249–259.
118. Hu L, Hofmann J, Jaffe RB. Phosphatidylinositol 3-kinase mediates angiogenesis and vascular permeability associated with ovarian carcinoma. *Clin Cancer Res* 2005;11(22):8208–8212.
119. Gombos Z, Xu X, Chu CS, et al. Peritumoral lymphatic vessel density and vascular endothelial growth factor C expression in early-stage squamous cell carcinoma of the uterine cervix. *Clin Cancer Res* 2005;11(23):8364–8371.
120. Li L, Wang L, Zhang W, et al. Correlation of serum VEGF levels with clinical stage, therapy efficacy, tumor metastasis and patient survival in ovarian cancer. *Anticancer Res* 2004;24(3b):1973–1979.
121. Boocock CA, Charnock-Jones DS, Sharkey AM, et al. Expression of vascular endothelial growth factor and its receptors flt and KDR in ovarian carcinoma. *J Natl Cancer Inst* 1995;87(7):506–516.
122. Bamberger ES, Perrett CW. Angiogenesis in epithelian ovarian cancer. *Mol Pathol* 2002;55(6):348–359.
123. Wang D, Huang HJ, Kazlauskas A, et al. Induction of vascular endothelial growth factor expression in endothelial cells by platelet-derived growth factor through the activation of phosphatidylinositol 3-kinase. *Cancer Res* 1999;59(7):1464–1472.
124. Sivridis E, Giatromanolaki A, Gatter KC, et al. Association of hypoxia-inducible factors 1α and 2α with activated angiogenic pathways and prognosis in patients with endometrial carcinoma. *Cancer* 2002;95(5): 1055–1063.
125. Hyder SM, Chiappetta C, Stancel GM. Pharmacological and endogenous progestins induce vascular endothelial growth factor expression in human breast cancer cells. *Int J Cancer* 2001;92(4):469–473.
126. Hartenbach EM, Olson TA, Goswitz JJ, et al. Vascular endothelial growth factor (VEGF) expression and survival in human epithelial ovarian carcinomas. *Cancer Lett* 1997;121(2):169–175.
127. Zebrowski BK, Liu W, Ramirez K, et al. Markedly elevated levels of vascular endothelial growth factor in malignant ascites. *Ann Surg Oncol* 1999;6(4):373–378.
128. Kraft A, Weindel K, Ochs A, et al. Vascular endothelial growth factor in the sera and effusions of patients with malignant and nonmalignant disease. *Cancer* 1999;85(1):178–187.
129. Cohn DE, Valmadre S, Resnick KE, et al. Bevacizumab and weekly taxane chemotherapy demonstrates activity in refractory ovarian cancer. *Gynecol Oncol* 2006;102(2):134–139.
130. Gerber HP, Ferrara N. Pharmacology and pharmacodynamics of bevacizumab as monotherapy or in combination with cytotoxic therapy in preclinical studies. *Cancer Res* 2005;65(3):671–680.
131. Numnum TM, Rocconi RP, Whitworth J, et al. The use of bevacizumab to palliate symptomatic ascites in patients with refractory ovarian carcinoma. *Gynecol Oncol* 2006;102(3):425–428.
132. Wright JD, Hagemann A, Rader JS, et al. Bevacizumab combination therapy in recurrent, platinum-refractory, epithelial ovarian carcinoma: A retrospective analysis. *Cancer* 2006;107(1):83–89.
133. Boonstra J, Rijken P, Humbel B, et al. The epidermal growth factor. *Cell Biol Int* 1995;19(5):413–430.
134. Brabender J, Danenberg KD, Metzger R, et al. Epidermal growth factor receptor and HER2-neu mRNA expression in non-small cell lung cancer Is correlated with survival. *Clin Cancer Res* 2001;7(7):1850–1855.
135. Salomon DS, Brandt R, Ciardiello F, et al. Epidermal growth factor-related peptides and their receptors in human malignancies. *Crit Rev Oncol Hematol* 1995;19(3):183–232.
136. van Cruijsen H, Giaccone G, Hoekman K. Epidermal growth factor receptor and angiogenesis: opportunities for combined anticancer strategies. *Int J Cancer* 2005;117(6):883–888.
137. Mathur RS, Mathur SP, Young RC. Up-regulation of epidermal growth factor-receptors (EGF-R) by nicotine in cervical cancer cell lines: this effect may be mediated by EGF. *Am J Reprod Immunol* 2000;44(2):114–120.
138. Jain RK, Carmeliet PF. Vessels of death or life. *Sci Am* 2001;285(6):38–45.
139. Izumi Y, Xu L, di Tomaso E, et al. Tumour biology: herceptin acts as an anti-angiogenic cocktail. *Nature* 2002;416(6878):279–280.
140. Shah NG, Bhatavdekar JM, Doctor SS, et al. Circulating epidermal growth factor (EGF) and insulin-like growth factor-I (IGF-I) in patients with epithelial ovarian carcinoma. *Neoplasma* 1994;41(5):241–243.
141. Hogdall EV, Christensen L, Kjaer SK, et al. Distribution of HER-2 overexpression in ovarian carcinoma tissue and its prognostic value in patients with ovarian carcinoma: from the Danish MALOVA Ovarian Cancer Study. *Cancer* 2003;98(1):66–73.
142. Khalifa MA, Mannel RS, Haraway SD, et al. Expression of EGFR, HER-2/neu, P53, and PCNA in endometrioid, serous papillary, and clear cell endometrial adenocarcinomas. *Gynecol Oncol* 1994;53(1):84–92.
143. Niikura H, Sasano H, Sato S, et al. Expression of epidermal growth factor-related proteins and epidermal growth factor receptor in common epithelial ovarian tumors. *Int J Gynecol Pathol* 1997;16(1):60–68.
144. Shankaran H, Wiley HS, Resat H. Modeling the effects of HER/ErbB1-3 coexpression on receptor dimerization and biological response. *Biophys J* 2006;90(11):3993–4009.

145. Posadas EM, Liel MS, Kwitkowski V, et al. A phase II and pharmacodynamic study of gefitinib in patients with refractory or recurrent epithelial ovarian cancer. *Cancer* 2007;109(7):1323–1330.
146. Schilder RJ, Sill MW, Chen X, et al. Phase II study of gefitinib in patients with relapsed or persistent ovarian or primary peritoneal carcinoma and evaluation of epidermal growth factor receptor mutations and immunohistochemical expression: a Gynecologic Oncology Group Study. *Clin Cancer Res* 2005;11(15):5539–5548.
147. Link CJ, Jr., Kohn E, Reed E. The relationship between borderline ovarian tumors and epithelial ovarian carcinoma: epidemiologic, pathologic, and molecular aspects. *Gynecol Oncol* 1996;60(3):347–354.
148. Heldin CH, Westermark B. Mechanism of action and *in vivo* role of platelet-derived growth factor. *Physiol Rev* 1999;79(4):1283–1316.
149. Henriksen R, Funa K, Wilander E, et al. Expression and prognostic significance of platelet-derived growth factor and its receptors in epithelial ovarian neoplasms. *Cancer Res* 1993;53(19):4550–4554.
150. Hellstrom M, Kalen M, Lindahl P, et al. Role of PDGF-B and PDGFR-β in recruitment of vascular smooth muscle cells and pericytes during embryonic blood vessel formation in the mouse. *Development* 1999;126(14): 3047–3055.
151. Sundberg C, Ljungstrom M, Lindmark G, et al. Microvascular pericytes express platelet-derived growth factor-beta receptors in human healing wounds and colorectal adenocarcinoma. *Am J Pathol* 1993;143(5): 1377–1388.
152. Reinmuth N, Liu W, Jung YD, et al. Induction of VEGF in perivascular cells defines a potential paracrine mechanism for endothelial cell survival. *Faseb J* 2001;15(7):1239–1241.
153. Versnel MA, Haarbrink M, Langerak AW, et al. Human ovarian tumors of epithelial origin express PDGF *in vitro* and *in vivo*. *Cancer Genet Cytogenet* 1994;73(1):60–64.
154. Dushkin H, Schilder RJ. Imatinib mesylate and its potential implications for gynecologic cancers. *Curr Treat Options Oncol* 2005;6(2):115–120.
155. Matei D, Chang DD, Jeng MH. Imatinib mesylate (Gleevec) inhibits ovarian cancer cell growth through a mechanism dependent on platelet-derived growth factor receptor alpha and Akt inactivation. *Clin Cancer Res* 2004;10(2):681–690.
156. Coleman RL, Broaddus RR, Bodurka DC, et al. Phase II trial of imatinib mesylate in patients with recurrent platinum- and taxane-resistant epithelial ovarian and primary peritoneal cancers. *Gynecol Oncol* 2006;101(1): 126–131.
157. Posadas EM, Kwitkowski V, Kotz HL, et al. A prospective analysis of imatinib-induced c-kit modulation in ovarian cancer: a phase II clinical study with proteomic profiling. *Cancer* 2007;110(2):309–317.
158. Levine AJ, Momand J, Finlay CA. The p53 tumour suppressor gene. *Nature* 1991;351(6326):453–456.
159. Greenblatt MS, Bennett WP, Hollstein M, et al. Mutations in the p53 tumor suppressor gene: clues to cancer etiology and molecular pathogenesis. *Cancer Res* 1994;54(18):4855–4878.
160. Chang F, Syrjanen S, Syrjanen K. Implications of the p53 tumor-suppressor gene in clinical oncology. *J Clin Oncol* 1995;13(4):1009–1022.
161. Skilling JS, Sood A, Niemann T, et al. An abundance of p53 null mutations in ovarian carcinoma. *Oncogene* 1996;13(1):117–123.
162. Kohler MF, Marks JR, Wiseman RW, et al. Spectrum of mutation and frequency of allelic deletion of the p53 gene in ovarian cancer. *J Natl Cancer Inst* 1993;85(18):1513–1519.
163. Tsuda H, Hirohashi S. Frequent occurrence of p53 gene mutations in uterine cancers at advanced clinical stage and with aggressive histological phenotypes. *Jpn J Cancer Res* 1992;83(11):1184–1191.
164. Borresen AL, Helland A, Nesland J, et al. Papillomaviruses, p53, and cervical cancer. *Lancet* 1992;339(8805):1350–1351.
165. Dameron KM, Volpert OV, Tainsky MA, et al. Control of angiogenesis in fibroblasts by p53 regulation of thrombospondin-1. *Science* 1994; 265(5178):1582–1584.
166. Carmeliet P, Dor Y, Herbert JM, et al. Role of HIF-1(in hypoxia-mediated apoptosis, cell proliferation and tumour angiogenesis. *Nature* 1998; 394(6692):485–490.
167. Mukhopadhyay D, Tsiokas L, Sukhatme VP. Wild-type p53 and v-Src exert opposing influences on human vascular endothelial growth factor gene expression. *Cancer Res* 1995;55(24):6161–6165.
168. Tsuzuki Y, Fukumura D, Oosthuyse B, et al. Vascular endothelial growth factor (VEGF) modulation by targeting hypoxia-inducible factor-1α—> hypoxia response element—> VEGF cascade differentially regulates vascular response and growth rate in tumors. *Cancer Res* 2000;60(22):6248–6252.
169. Zietz C, Rossle M, Haas C, et al. MDM-2 oncoprotein overexpression, p53 gene mutation, and VEGF up-regulation in angiosarcomas. *Am J Pathol* 1998;153(5):1425–1433.
170. Khwaja A, Rodriguez-Viciana P, Wennstrom S, et al. Matrix adhesion and Ras transformation both activate a phosphoinositide 3-OH kinase and protein kinase B/Akt cellular survival pathway. *Embo J* 1997;16(10):2783–2793.
171. Kieser A, Weich HA, Brandner G, et al. Mutant p53 potentiates protein kinase C induction of vascular endothelial growth factor expression. *Oncogene* 1994;9(3):963–969.
172. Price JT, Bonovich MT, Kohn EC. The biochemistry of cancer dissemination. *Crit Rev Biochem Mol Biol* 1997;32(3):175–253.
173. Quigley JP, Armstrong PB. Tumor cell intravasation elucidated: the chick embryo opens the window. *Cell* 1998;94(3):281–284.
174. Stoker M, Gherardi E, Perryman M, et al. Scatter factor is a fibroblast-derived modulator of epithelial cell mobility. *Nature* 1987;327(6119): 239–242.
175. Kohn EC, Francis EA, Liotta LA, et al. Heterogeneity of the motility responses in malignant tumor cells: a biological basis for the diversity and homing of metastatic cells. *Int J Cancer* 1990;46(2):287–292.
176. Shibayama H, Tagawa S, Hattori H, et al. Laminin and fibronectin promote the chemotaxis of human malignant plasma cell lines. *Blood* 1995;86(2):719–725.
177. Nelson PR, Yamamura S, Kent KC. Extracellular matrix proteins are potent agonists of human smooth muscle cell migration. *J Vasc Surg* 1996;24(1):25–32; discussion, 33.
178. Doerr ME, Jones JI. The roles of integrins and extracellular matrix proteins in the insulin-like growth factor I-stimulated chemotaxis of human breast cancer cells. *J Biol Chem* 1996;271(5):2443–2447.
179. Shichiri M, Hirata Y. Antiangiogenesis signals by endostatin. *Faseb J* 2001;15(6):1044–1053.
180. Dell'Eva R, Pfeffer U, Indraccolo S, et al. Inhibition of tumor angiogenesis by angiostatin: from recombinant protein to gene therapy. *Endothelium* 2002;9(1):3–10.
181. Brindley DN. Lipid phosphate phosphatases and related proteins: signaling functions in development, cell division, and cancer. *J Cell Biochem* 2004;92(5):900–912.
182. Xie Y, Meier KE. Lysophospholipase D and its role in LPA production. *Cell Signal* 2004;16(9):975–981.
183. Nam SW, Clair T, Campo CK, et al. Autotaxin (ATX), a potent tumor motogen, augments invasive and metastatic potential of ras-transformed cells. *Oncogene* 2000;19(2):241–247.
184. Xu Y, Gaudette DC, Boynton JD, et al. Characterization of an ovarian cancer activating factor in ascites from ovarian cancer patients. *Clin Cancer Res* 1995;1(10):1223–1232.
185. Ren J, Xiao YJ, Singh LS, et al. Lysophosphatidic acid is constitutively produced by human peritoneal mesothelial cells and enhances adhesion, migration, and invasion of ovarian cancer cells. *Cancer Res* 2006;66(6): 3006–3014.
186. Mills GB, Eder A, Fang X, et al. Critical role of lysophospholipids in the pathophysiology, diagnosis, and management of ovarian cancer. *Cancer Treat Res* 2002;107:259–283.
187. Mills GB, Moolenaar WH. The emerging role of lysophosphatidic acid in cancer. *Nat Rev Cancer* 2003;3(8):582–591.
188. Sawada K, Morishige K, Tahara M, et al. Alendronate inhibits lysophosphatidic acid-induced migration of human ovarian cancer cells by attenuating the activation of rho. *Cancer Res* 2002;62(21):6015–6020.
189. Nassar N, Cancelas J, Zheng J, et al. Structure-function based design of small molecule inhibitors targeting Rho family GTPases. *Curr Top Med Chem* 2006;6(11):1109–1116.
190. Sengupta S, Kim KS, Berk MP, et al. Lysophosphatidic acid downregulates tissue inhibitor of metalloproteinases, which are negatively involved in lysophosphatidic acid-induced cell invasion. *Oncogene* 2007;26(20): 2894–2901.
191. Frisch SM, Francis H. Disruption of epithelial cell-matrix interactions induces apoptosis. *J Cell Biol* 1994;124(4):619–626.
192. Davidson B, Zhang Z, Kleinberg L, et al. Gene expression signatures differentiate ovarian/peritoneal serous carcinoma from diffuse malignant periitoneal mesothelioma. *Clin Cancer Res* 2006;12(20 Pt 1):5944–5950.
193. Woodhouse EC, Chuaqui RF, Liotta LA. General mechanisms of metastasis. *Cancer* 1997;80(8 Suppl):1529–1537.
194. Shayesteh L, Lu Y, Kuo WL, et al. PIK3CA is implicated as an oncogene in ovarian cancer. *Nat Genet* 1999;21(1):99–102.
195. Bretland AJ, Lawry J, Sharrard RM. A study of death by anoikis in cultured epithelial cells. *Cell Prolif* 2001;34(4):199–210.
196. Tokunaga E, Kimura Y, Mashino K, et al. Activation of PI3K/Akt signaling and hormone resistance in breast cancer. *Breast Cancer* 2006;13(2): 137–144.
197. Bondeva T, Pirola L, Bulgarelli-Leva G, et al. Bifurcation of lipid and protein kinase signals of PI3Kgamma to the protein kinases PKB and MAPK. *Science* 1998;282(5387):293–296.
198. Hayes MP, Wang H, Espinal-Witter R, et al. PIK3CA and *PTEN* mutations in uterine endometrioid carcinoma and complex atypical hyperplasia. *Clin Cancer Res* 2006;12(20 Pt 1):5932–5935.
199. Sato N, Tsunoda H, Nishida M, et al. Loss of heterozygosity on 10q23.3 and mutation of the tumor suppressor gene *PTEN* in benign endometrial cyst of the ovary: possible sequence progression from benign endometrial cyst to endometrioid carcinoma and clear cell carcinoma of the ovary. *Cancer Res* 2000;60(24):7052–7056.
200. Steck PA, Pershouse MA, Jasser SA, et al. Identification of a candidate tumour suppressor gene, MMAC1, at chromosome 10q23.3 that is mutated in multiple advanced cancers. *Nat Genet* 1997;15(4):356–362.
201. Tamura M, Gu J, Matsumoto K, et al. Inhibition of cell migration, spreading, and focal adhesions by tumor suppressor *PTEN*. *Science* 1998;280(5369):1614–1617.
202. Bonner RF, Emmert-Buck M, Cole K, et al. Laser capture microdissection: molecular analysis of tissue. *Science* 1997;278(5342):1481–1483.
203. Jones MB, Krutzsch H, Shu H, et al. Proteomic analysis and identification of new biomarkers and therapeutic targets for invasive ovarian cancer. *Proteomics* 2002;2(1):76–84.

204. Tangrea MA, Chuaqui RF, Gillespie JW, et al. Expression microdissection: operator-independent retrieval of cells for molecular profiling. *Diagn Mol Pathol* 2004;13(4):207–212.
205. Buckanovich RJ, Sasaroli D, O'Brien-Jenkins A, et al. Tumor vascular proteins as biomarkers in ovarian cancer. *J Clin Oncol* 2007;25(7):852–861.
206. Jones MB, Michener CM, Blanchette JO, et al. The granulin-epithelin precursor/PC-cell-derived growth factor is a growth factor for epithelial ovarian cancer. *Clin Cancer Res* 2003;9(1):44–51.
207. Jones MB, Spooner M, Kohn EC. The granulin-epithelin precursor: a putative new growth factor for ovarian cancer. *Gynecol Oncol* 2003;88(1 Pt 2):S136–S139.
208. He Z, Ong CH, Halper J, Bateman A. Progranulin is a mediator of the wound response. *Nat Med* 2003;9(2):225–229.
209. Caretti E, Devarajan K, Coudry R, et al. Comparison of RNA amplification methods and chip platforms for microarray analysis of samples processed by laser capture microdissection. *J Cell Biochem* 2008;103(2):556–563.
210. Petricoin EF, Zoon KC, Kohn EC, et al. Clinical proteomics: translating benchside promise into bedside reality. *Nat Rev Drug Discov* 2002;1(9): 683–695.
211. Johnson DH, Fehrenbacher L, Novotny WF, et al. Randomized phase II trial comparing bevacizumab plus carboplatin and paclitaxel with carboplatin and paclitaxel alone in previously untreated locally advanced or metastatic non-small-cell lung cancer. *J Clin Oncol* 2004;22(11):2184–2191.
212. Miller KD. E2100: a phase III trial of paclitaxel versus paclitaxel/bevacizumab for metastatic breast cancer. *Clin Breast Cancer* 2003;3(6): 421–422.
213. Yang JC, Haworth L, Sherry RM, et al. A randomized trial of bevacizumab, an anti-vascular endothelial growth factor antibody, for metastatic renal cancer. *N Engl J Med* 2003;349(5):427–434.
214. Burger RA, Sill M, Monk BJ, et al. Phase II trial of bevacizumab in persistent or recurrent epithelial ovarian cancer (EOC) or primary peritoneal cancer (PPC): A Gynecologic Oncology Group (GOG) study. *J Clin Oncol* 2007;25(33):5165–5171.
215. Saltz LB, Meropol NJ, Loehrer PJ Sr., et al. Phase II trial of cetuximab in patients with refractory colorectal cancer that expresses the epidermal growth factor receptor. *J Clin Oncol* 2004;22(7):1201–1208.
216. Cohen EE. Role of epidermal growth factor receptor pathway-targeted therapy in patients with recurrent and/or metastatic squamous cell carcinoma of the head and neck. *J Clin Oncol* 2006;24(17):2659–2665.
217. Bonner JA, Harari PM, Giralt J, et al. Radiotherapy plus cetuximab for squamous-cell carcinoma of the head and neck. *N Engl J Med* 2006;354(6):567–578.
218. Wainberg Z, Hecht JR. Panitumumab in colon cancer: a review and summary of ongoing trials. *Expert Opin Biol Ther* 2006;6(11):1229–1235.
219. Wainberg Z, Hecht JR. A phase III randomized, open-label, controlled trial of chemotherapy and bevacizumab with or without panitumumab in the first-line treatment of patients with metastatic colorectal cancer. *Clin Colorectal Cancer* 2006;5(5):363–367.
220. Riener EK, Arnold N, Kommoss F, et al. The prognostic and predictive value of immunohistochemically detected HER-2/neu overexpression in 361 patients with ovarian cancer: a multicenter study. *Gynecol Oncol* 2004;95(1):89–94.
221. Slomovitz BM, Broaddus RR, Burke TW, et al. Her-2/neu overexpression and amplification in uterine papillary serous carcinoma. *J Clin Oncol* 2004;22(15):3126–3132.
222. Piccart-Gebhart MJ, Procter M, Leyland-Jones B, et al. Trastuzumab after adjuvant chemotherapy in HER2-positive breast cancer. *N Engl J Med* 2005;353(16):1659–1672.
223. Romond EH, Perez EA, Bryant J, et al. Trastuzumab plus adjuvant chemotherapy for operable HER2-positive breast cancer. *N Engl J Med* 2005;353(16):1673–1684.
224. Bookman MA, Darcy KM, Clarke-Pearson D, et al. Evaluation of monoclonal humanized anti-HER2 antibody, trastuzumab, in patients with recurrent or refractory ovarian or primary peritoneal carcinoma with overexpression of HER2: a phase II trial of the Gynecologic Oncology Group. *J Clin Oncol* 2003;21(2):283–290.
225. Adjei AA. Novel small-molecule inhibitors of the vascular endothelial growth factor receptor. *Clin Lung Cancer* 2007;8(Suppl 2):S74–S78.
226. Escudier B, Eisen T, Stadler WM, et al. Sorafenib in advanced clear-cell renal-cell carcinoma. *N Engl J Med* 2007;356(2):125–134.
227. Gomez HL, Chavez MA, Doval DC, et al. A phase II, randomized trial using the small molecule tyrosine kinase inhibitor lapatinib as a first-line treatment in patients with FISH positive advanced or metastatic breast cancer. *ASCO Meeting Abstracts* 2005;23(16 Suppl):3046.
228. Spector NL, Blackwell K, Hurley J, et al. EGF103009, a phase II trial of lapatinib monotherapy in patients with relapsed/refractory inflammatory breast cancer (IBC): clinical activity and biologic predictors of response. *J Clin Oncol.* (Meeting Abstracts) 2006;24(18 Suppl):502.
229. Figlin RA. Newly approved therapies for RCC and their effect on the standard of care. *Clin Adv Hematol Oncol* 2007;5(1):35–36, 66.
230. Shepherd FA, Rodrigues Pereira J, Ciuleanu T, et al. Erlotinib in previously treated non-small-cell lung cancer. *N Engl J Med* 2005;353(2):123–132.
231. Moore MJ, Goldstein D, Hamm J, et al. Erlotinib plus gemcitabine compared with gemcitabine alone in patients with advanced pancreatic cancer: a phase III trial of the National Cancer Institute of Canada Clinical Trials Group. *J Clin Oncol* 2007;25(27):4320–4321.
232. Ryan AJ, Wedge SR. ZD6474—a novel inhibitor of VEGFR and EGFR tyrosine kinase activity. *Br J Cancer* 2005;92(Suppl 1):S6–S13.
233. Azad N, Posadas EM, Kwitkowski VE, et al. Combination targeted therapy with sorafenib and bevacizumab results in enhanced anti-tumor activity and toxicity. *J Clin Oncol* 2008:26:3709–3714.
234. Chon HS, Hu W, Kavanagh JJ. Targeted therapies in gynecologic cancers. *Curr Cancer Drug Targets* 2006;6(4):333–363.

CHAPTER 5 ■ ONCOGENES AND TUMOR SUPPRESSOR GENES

JEFF BOYD, JOHN I. RISINGER, AND ANDREW BERCHUCK

HISTORICAL PERSPECTIVE

Discoveries over the past three decades have brought us to a new frontier in cancer research that is founded upon the identification and understanding of the basic cellular processes that become disrupted during cancer development. Historically, numerous empirical models have been proposed to explain the etiology of cancers. Attention has focused on viruses, environmental agents, chemical carcinogens, and congenital predisposition. We now know that all of these factors may contribute to carcinogenesis by disrupting genes whose products are involved in regulating cell proliferation, senescence, death, and the ability to invade and survive in ectopic locations. Most cancers are believed to arise from a single progenitor cell that has sustained mutations in several of these critical genes (1).

The genetic basis of human cancer development was implied by the work of some of the earliest cell biologists and is now considered among the most robust of biologic paradigms. In the mid-19th century, the great German pathologist Rudolph Virchow recognized that metastatic cancer cells resemble those of the corresponding primary tumor, and in the course of developing his cell theory, postulated that all cells of a cancer may arise from a single progenitor (2). Thus, the neoplastic phenotype is heritable from one tumor cell generation to the next, prompting the famous aphorism widely attributed to him, "*omnis cellulae cellula*" (every cell from a cell). In the early 1900s, Theodor Boveri extended this concept to the cytogenetic level, suggesting that gains and losses of specific chromosomes might lead to abnormal cell division and other aspects of the cancer phenotype. In his remarkable landmark treatise, *Zur Frage der Entstehung Maligner Tumoren* (*On the Origin of Malignant Tumors*), Boveri initiated the age of cancer genetics, presaging the existence of tumor-suppressor genes, oncogenes, cell cycle checkpoints, multistep tumor progression, cancer predisposition through tumor-suppressor genes, the clonal origin of tumors, and other aspects of the neoplastic phenotype (3).

It required another half century, however, for Boveri's predictions to begin to be realized, with the discovery by Nowell and Hungerford in 1960 of a specific chromosomal translocation (the Philadelphia chromosome), which is characteristic of chronic myeloid leukemia (4). Nowell later provided a detailed and modernized version of the earlier notion of Virchow and Boveri that tumors are monoclonal with his theory on the clonal evolution of tumor cell populations (5). At this time in the mid-1970s, the stage was now set for the discovery by Bishop and Varmus that genetic sequences homologous to the transforming gene (v-*src*) of an avian cancer retrovirus exist in the host chicken genome (6), and indeed in the genomes of vertebrates including humans (7). This was the first direct evidence for the existence of cellular "oncogenes," which laid the groundwork for the field of cancer molecular genetics, and was a discovery of sufficient magnitude to warrant awarding of the Nobel Prize to Bishop and Varmus in 1989.

This brief history of cancer genetics comes full circle with discoveries in 1973 that the Philadelphia chromosome represents a reciprocal translocation involving chromosomes 9 and 22 (8), in 1983 that this translocation results in the constitutive activation of the cellular oncogene c-*abl* (9), and in 2001 that a specific inhibitor of the ABL tyrosine kinase (Gleevec) is associated with extraordinary efficacy in the treatment of a subset of patients with leukemias harboring the Philadelphia chromosome (10). Although this "bench to bedside" success story is so far the exception rather than the rule, the molecular genetic basis of cancer has been defined in sufficient detail to allow an unprecedented optimism that we will eventually attain a thorough understanding of the molecular etiology of cancer. Although the number of genes that may be mutated and contribute to the development of the various cancer types is large, perhaps in the hundreds, the problem is clearly not intractable. Recent successes in elucidating the sequence of the human genome and in using comprehensive gene expression profiles to classify human malignancies in clinically relevant contexts contribute to this optimism. As our understanding of the molecular pathogenesis of cancer evolves, it is reasonable to assume that this knowledge will facilitate the development of new approaches to prevention, early diagnosis, and treatment.

GENETIC PARADIGM OF TUMORIGENESIS

All cancers are genetic in origin in the sense that the driving force of tumor development is genetic mutation. A given tumor may arise through the accumulation of acquired (somatic) mutations or through the inheritance of a mutation(s) through the germ line followed by the acquisition of additional somatic mutations. These two genetic scenarios distinguish what are colloquially referred to as "sporadic" and "hereditary" cancers, respectively (Fig. 5.1).

Although alterations in gene expression also contribute to the malignant phenotype, the sequential mutation of cancer-related genes leading to outgrowth of a clonal population of cells is the major determinant of whether a cancer develops as well as the time required for its development and progression. The data supporting this multistep genetic paradigm are extensive (11,12), but perhaps the most compelling evidence is that the age-specific incidence rates for most epithelial tumors increase at roughly the fourth to eighth power of elapsed time, suggesting that a series of four to eight genetic alterations are

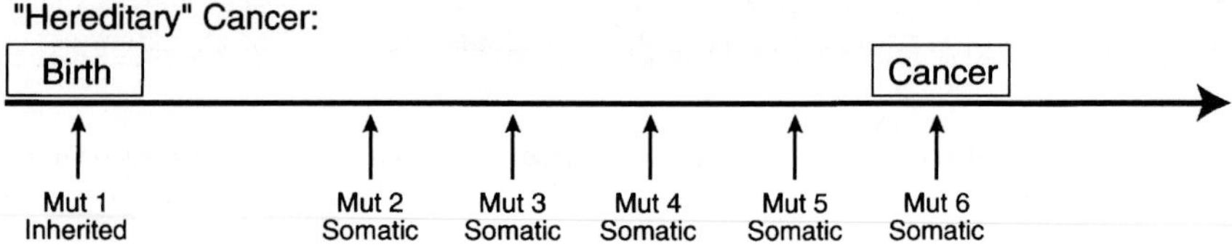

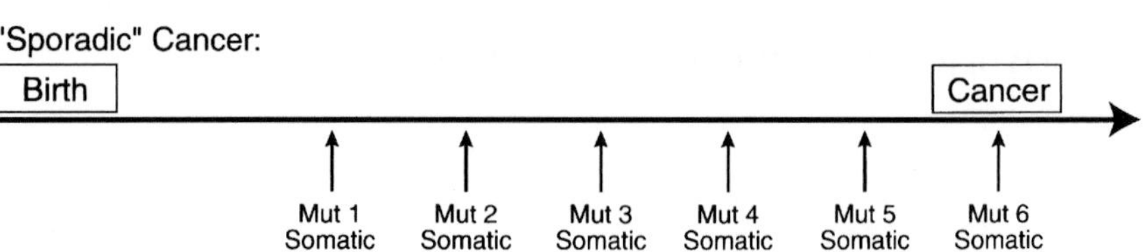

FIGURE 5.1. All cancers are genetic. "Hereditary" cancers differ from "sporadic" cancers by virtue of association with a predisposing mutation inherited through the germ line. In contrast, all of the mutations associated with sporadic tumorigenesis are acquired somatically.

rate limiting for cancer development (12). Additionally, it would seem rather self-evident that the well-characterized histopathologic progression of several common tumor types, for example, through hyperplasia, dysplasia, carcinoma *in situ,* and invasive carcinoma, reflects this multistep, multigenic model at the morphologic level.

Genetic alterations in cancer cells occur in two major families of genes: oncogenes and tumor-suppressor genes. Proteins encoded by oncogenes may generally be viewed as stimulatory and those encoded by tumor-suppressor genes as inhibitory to the neoplastic phenotype. Gain-of-function mutations resulting in the activation of "protooncogenes" to oncogenes and loss-of-function mutations resulting in the inactivation of tumor-suppressor genes both are requisite for cancer development. Protooncogene mutations are nearly always somatic, presumably because such cellular dominant mutations in the germ line are incompatible with normal development. Two known exceptions involve the *RET* and *MET* protooncogenes, mutations of which may be inherited through the germ line, predisposing to multiple endocrine neoplasia type II (13) and papillary renal carcinoma (14), respectively. Tumor-suppressor gene mutations may be inherited or acquired somatically, and nearly all hereditary cancer syndromes for which predisposing genes have been identified are linked to mutant tumor-suppressor genes. Genes encoding proteins involved in various pathways of DNA repair have been proposed to represent a third class of genes involved in cancer development (15), but, as will be discussed below, these genes possess many of the features of tumor-suppressor genes and are considered as such in this chapter.

A human cancer represents the endpoint of a long and complex process involving multiple cellular changes in genotype and phenotype. Human solid tumors generally are monoclonal, with every cell in a given cancer having arisen from a single progenitor cell. This does imply that all cells of a tumor are genetically identical, as the genetic instability characteristic of most malignancies results in substantial genetic heterogeneity as clonal evolution occurs (16). Clonal evolution, or clonal expansion (Fig. 5.2), is the process through which a cell and its offspring sustain and accumulate multiple mutations with the stepwise selection of variant sublines (5,17). A long-term goal of studying the molecular genetics of a particular tumor type is to catalogue the specific genes that are affected by mutations and the relative order in which they are affected and, ultimately, to use this molecular genetic blueprint to improve methods of diagnosis, prognostication, and treatment. This task will undoubtedly prove to be difficult, however, because of the aforementioned genetic instability characteristic of cancers. There are multiple types of such instability that are operative at both the chromosomal and molecular levels (18). Distinguishing the genetic mutations that are simply the by-product of genetic instability from those that are critical to the neoplastic phenotype or, indeed, responsible for increasing genetic instability of one form or another is among the most formidable challenges to be faced in human cancer research.

The greatest progress in this context perhaps has been achieved for colorectal carcinoma, and a rudimentary model has been proposed that applies molecular detail to the general paradigm of multistep tumorigenesis and clonal evolution. In addition, most colon cancers are affected by one of two distinct types of genetic instability (18), and specific molecular genetic alterations have been shown to occur at discrete histologic stages of neoplastic progression in the colon: for example, mutation of the *APC* tumor-suppressor gene at a very early stage of hyperproliferation, mutation of the *KRAS* oncogene in the transition of early to intermediate adenoma, and mutation of the *TP53* tumor-suppressor gene in the transition of late adenoma to carcinoma (19). Several features of colorectal

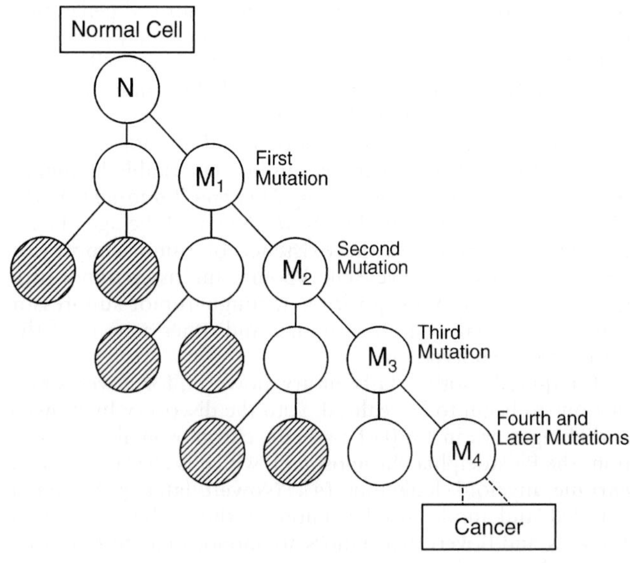

FIGURE 5.2. Model of clonal evolution in neoplasia. Following the initiating mutation in a normal cell, stepwise genetic mutations and selective pressures result in a cancer consisting of a clonal population of cells all derived from the original progenitor cell. Each critical mutation in the evolving tumor may be viewed as having provided a selective advantage leading to clonal expansion.

cancers facilitate this type of characterization, including the well-defined histopathologic progression of normal colonic epithelium to cancer and the accessibility of the various premalignant lesions for molecular analyses, as well as the occurrence of some of these genetic mutations in large fractions of colorectal tumors. This type of model is more difficult to apply to other cancer types, however, as premalignant precursor lesions for many solid tumor types (e.g., ovarian carcinoma) are not readily detectable, and few genetic alterations have been described that occur in major fractions of other cancer types.

TUMOR-SUPPRESSOR GENES

The protein products of tumor-suppressor genes normally function to inhibit various aspects of the neoplastic phenotype, such as cell proliferation, and are inactivated through loss-of-function mutations. Tumor-suppressor genes (having formerly been referred to variously as "recessive oncogenes" or "antioncogenes") are, by definition, recessive at the cellular level insofar as inactivation of both alleles (the copies present on both chromosomes) must occur for a phenotypic effect on tumorigenesis to be manifest. This is in contrast to the concept of mendelian recessivity, which refers to the necessity of germ-line transmission of two mutant alleles for a phenotype to be manifest. Most tumor-suppressor genes responsible for hereditary cancer syndromes are dominant at the mendelian level, which means that inheritance of a single mutant allele is sufficient to confer a high probability of developing the phenotype (cancer in this case); cellular recessivity must then occur through somatic inactivation of the second allele, and mechanisms through which this may occur are discussed below.

Several lines of evidence led to the discovery of tumor-suppressor genes. In addition to Boveri's predictions, a statistical analysis of carcinogen-induced mouse papillomas in 1942 led to the conclusion that a cellular recessive gene must be involved in carcinogenesis (20). Nearly 30 years later, Harris et al. demonstrated that somatic cell hybrids created from tumor cells and normal cells invariably expressed a nonmalignant phenotype, again implicating a cellular recessive class of cancer genes (21). Application of this notion of a recessive cancer gene was first applied to cancer predisposition by Knudson, who in 1971 published a statistical analysis of pediatric retinoblastoma and concluded that inactivation of both alleles of a single gene, one through the germ line and one somatically, was necessary for tumor development (22). This concept became widely known as the "two-hit hypothesis" (a term not coined by Knudson), and is now inextricably linked to the more general concept of cellular recessivity of tumor-suppressor genes, the first of which to be discovered was the gene responsible for retinoblastoma, *RB1* (23).

This two-hit model for pediatric retinoblastoma is frequently misunderstood and misapplied, especially in the context of hereditary cancers generally, having become synonymous with the notion that inactivation of both alleles of a single gene is necessary *and* sufficient for tumorigenesis. It is important to recognize that this theory estimates only the number of events that are rate limiting for hereditary pediatric cancer development (22,24). As implied by Figure 5.1, most adult solid tumors, hereditary and sporadic, are likely to require mutations in multiple genes, most of which may occur at a relatively high frequency approaching zero-order kinetics, thus not appearing in the type of kinetic analysis performed by Knudson. This is especially true in cases where the inherited mutation affects a tumor-suppressor gene involved in DNA repair, with the result being increased genetic instability of one form or another.

The location and type of inactivating mutations in tumor-suppressor genes vary among genes and cancer types (Fig. 5.3). In some cases, most notably *TP53*, missense mutations occur that change a single amino acid in the encoded protein (25). More often, however, mutations in tumor-suppressor genes alter the base sequence such that the encoded protein product is truncated owing to generation of a premature stop codon. Truncated protein products may result from several types of mutational events. Included in this category are nonsense mutations in which a single base substitution changes the sequence from a specific amino acid to a stop codon (e.g., AAG to TAG). In addition, microdeletions or insertions of one or several nucleotides that disrupt the reading frame of the DNA (frameshifts) also lead to the generation of stop codons downstream in the gene. Less commonly, large genomic deletions are known sometimes to include portions of tumor-suppressor genes. Any of these types of mutations in one allele, whether germ line or somatic, is then "revealed" following somatic inactivation of the homologous wild-type allele, as discussed earlier. In theory, the same spectrum of mutational events could contribute to inactivation of the second allele, but what is typically observed in tumors is homozygosity or hemizygosity for the first mutation, indicating "loss" of the wild-type allele. As originally demonstrated for the retinoblastoma gene, loss of the second allele may occur through mitotic nondisjunction or recombination mechanisms or large deletions (Fig. 5.3) (26). This so-called "loss of heterozygosity" (LOH) has become recognized as the hallmark of tumor-suppressor gene inactivation. Table 5.1 lists some of the most well-characterized tumor-suppressor genes and the cancer syndromes and sporadic cancers with which they are associated.

Although some tumor-suppressor gene products reside outside the nucleus, many are nuclear proteins that prevent proliferation by arresting molecular pathways directly involved in cell cycle progression. The retinoblastoma gene (*RB1*) is a prototypical tumor-suppressor gene that encodes a nuclear protein involved in G_1 cell cycle arrest (27). Mutations in *RB1* have been noted primarily in retinoblastomas and sarcomas, but also occasionally in other types of cancers. In G_1, phosphorylated RB protein binds to the E2F transcription factor and prevents it from activating transcription of other genes involved in cell cycle progression (Fig. 5.4).

When RB is dephosphorylated, E2F is released and stimulates entry into the DNA synthetic (S) phase of the cell cycle. The phosphorylation of RB is regulated by a complex series of events that involves cyclins and cyclin-dependent kinases (CDKs). Cyclin-CDK complexes implicated in G_1 progression include cyclin D-CDK4/6, cyclin E-CDK2, and cyclin A-CDK2. Conversely, G_1 progression is restrained by CDK inhibitors such as p21, p16, and p27 (28, 29). CDK inhibitors are classified as tumor-suppressor genes because of their ability to inhibit G_1 progression, and inactivation of CDK inhibitors, particularly the gene encoding p16 (*CDKN2A*), is a frequent event in human cancers (30). In contrast to the classic "two-hit" model of tumor-suppressor inactivation in which there is a mutation in one allele and deletion of the other, loss of p16 function usually involves deletion of both alleles or silencing of gene transcription due to promoter methylation. After DNA synthesis occurs in S phase, other classes of cyclins and genes such as *CHK1* and *CHK2* are involved in regulating progression from G_2 to mitosis (M phase). Germ-line mutations in the *CHK2* (*CHEK2*) gene have been implicated in Li-Fraumeni syndrome (30) and breast cancer predisposition (31).

Several tumor-suppressor genes involved in hereditary predisposition to cancer have been shown to function in the recognition and/or repair of various forms of DNA damage. The mutational inactivation of DNA repair genes contributes to tumorigenesis indirectly by promoting one or another type of genetic instability, which leads to the mutation of additional cancer-related genes. This unique mechanism of tumor suppression has led some to suggest that the DNA repair genes should represent a third cancer gene family. In all cases

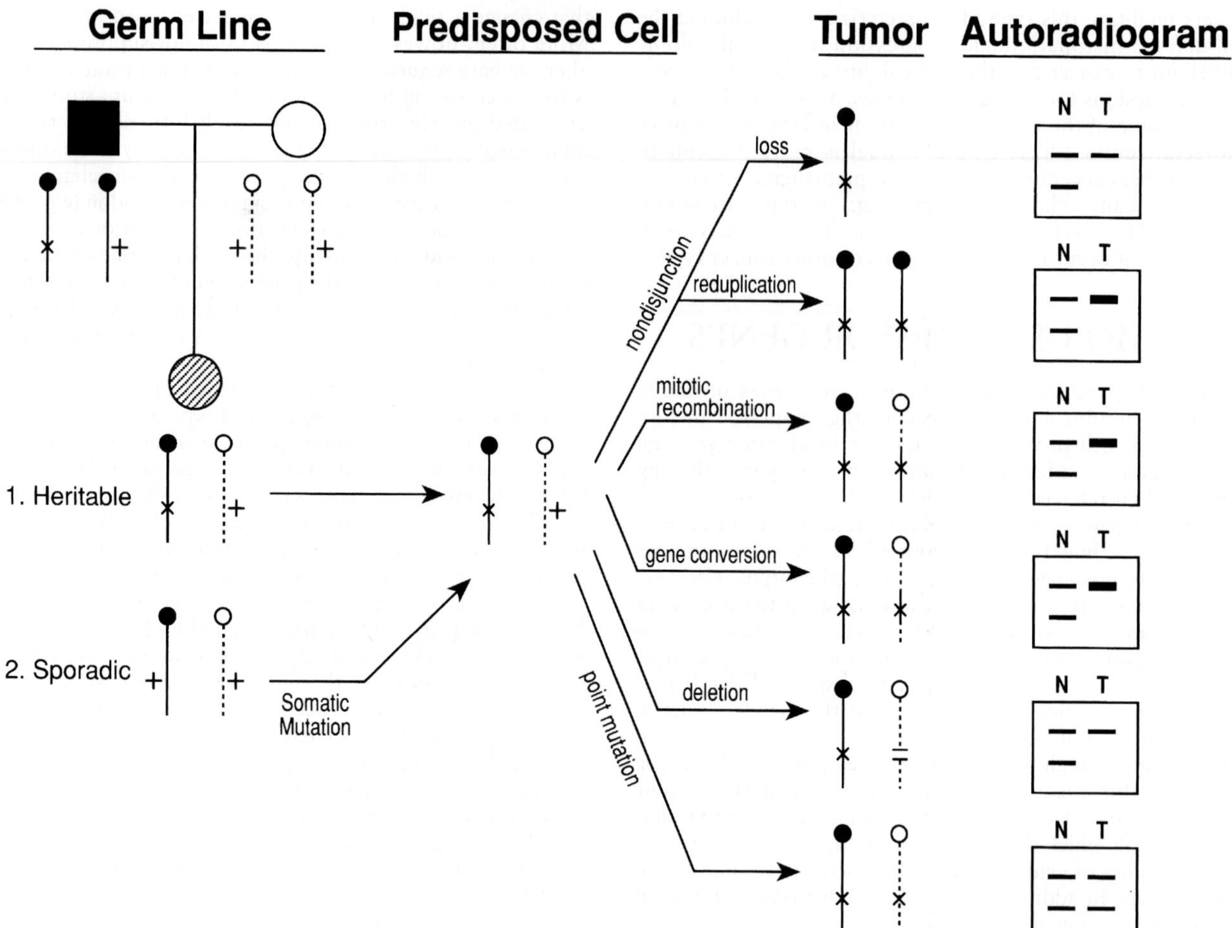

FIGURE 5.3. Model for loss of tumor-suppressor gene function and recessivity at the cellular level. In hereditary tumorigenesis, one mutant allele is inherited from either parent, in which case the "predisposed cell" is, in effect, every cell in the body. In sporadic tumorigenesis, one allele is mutated somatically, in which case there is one predisposed cell in, for example, the ovarian surface epithelium. Loss of inactivation of the remaining wild-type allele may occur through any number of somatic chromosomal mechanisms, most commonly through nondisjunction or recombination. This so-called loss of heterozygosity is manifest through Southern blotting or PCR-based procedures that allow visualization of loss of one or another polymorphic allele at or near the tumor-suppressor locus, in tumor (T) DNA compared to nontumor (N) DNA from the same individual.

described to date, however, the genetic mechanism appears to involve a cellular recessive mechanism involving loss of function, which is consistent with the tumor-suppressor categorization. Perhaps more appropriate is the classification scheme proposed by Kinzler and Vogelstein in which tumor-suppressor genes are subdivided into the categories of "gatekeepers" and "caretakers" (15). The former category includes those genes that function directly to inhibit cell proliferation or promote cell death (e.g., *RB1*, *TP53*, and *APC*), whereas the latter category consists of those genes that function to maintain genomic integrity (e.g., the mismatch repair genes involved in HNPCC, the nucleotide excision repair genes involved in xeroderma pigmentosum, the *ATM* gene, and the *BRCA1* and *BRCA2* genes). It should be noted that some of these genes do not readily adhere to this distinction; *BRCA1* and *BRCA2*, for example, may function as both gatekeepers and caretakers.

Although numerous tumor-suppressor genes are mutated in various human cancers, only a limited number have been shown to play a significant role in gynecologic malignancies. Somatic mutations of *TP53* are observed at variable frequencies in gynecologic sarcomas and in ovarian and endometrial carcinomas, wherease viral inactivation of the p53 protein is a central mechanism in cervical tumorigenesis. Germ-line mutations in DNA mismatch repair genes, primarily *MSH2* or *MLH1*, lead to endometrial and ovarian carcinomas in association with the Lynch syndrome, also known as hereditary nonpolyposis colorectal cancer (HNPCC) syndrome, whereas epigenetic silencing of *MLH1* is associated with some cases of sporadic endometrial carcinoma. Most cases of hereditary ovarian carcinoma are associated with inherited mutation of *BRCA1* or *BRCA2*, whereas somatic mutations in these genes are occasionally observed in sporadic ovarian carcinomas. Finally, the *PTEN* gene is somatically mutated in many endometrial carcinomas. The role of these tumor suppressors in specific cancer types will be discussed in greater detail in a later section of this chapter following a discussion of the molecular function of these genes.

TP53

The *TP53* tumor-suppressor gene is the most frequently inactivated gene described thus far in both human cancers in general as well as specifically in gynecologic cancers. Originally

TABLE 5.1

REPRESENTATIVE EXAMPLES OF TUMOR-SUPPRESSOR GENES MUTATED IN HUMAN CANCERS

Gene	Chromosomal location	Function	Hereditary cancers	Sporadic cancers
RB1	13q14	Cell cycle regulator	Retinoblastoma, osteosarcoma	Retinoblastoma, sarcomas, and others
WT1	11p13	Transcription factor	Wilms tumor	Wilms tumor
TP53	17p13	Transcription factor; regulator of cell cycle, apoptosis	Li-Fraumeni syndrome	Many
APC	5q21-q22	Signal transduction	Familial adenomatous polyposis	Colorectal, gastric
VHL	3p26-p25	Transcriptional elongation	von Hippel-Lindau syndrome	Renal
MSH2, MLH1, PMS2, MSH6	2p21, 3p21, 7p22, 2p21	DNA mismatch repair	Hereditary nonpolyposis colorectal cancer	Colorectal, endometrial
BRCA1	17q12-21	DNA repair; transcription factor	Breast, ovary	Ovary (rare)
BRCA2	13q12	DNA repair; transcription factor	Breast, ovary	Ovary (rare)
NF1	17q11	Negative regulator of RAS	Neurofibromatosis	None
DPC4	18q21	TGF-β signaling	None	Pancreatic
CDKN2A (p16)	9p21	Negative regulator of cyclin D	Melanoma	Many
PTEN (MMAC1)	10q24	Phosphatase	Cowden's syndrome	Many

TGF-β, transforming growth factor-β.

identified through the physical interaction of its protein product with the SV40 large T antigen (32,33), *TP53* has been an intensely studied gene over the last 30 years. The gene was first classified as a cellular oncogene because of its apparent dominant transforming potential when transfected into rodent cells; subsequent studies confirmed, however, that the original cDNA clones used in the original studies all contained inactivating mutations, and that wild-type p53 is actually a tumor suppressor (34). Subsequently, several convergent lines of research provided unequivocal evidence that *TP53* functions as a tumor-suppressor gene. Overexpression of exogenous wild-type p53 dramatically inhibits the growth of human colorectal carcinoma and osteosarcoma cell lines with endogenous p53 mutations (35,36), and loss of heterozygosity at chromosome 17p, seen frequently in a variety of human tumors, correlates with mutational inactivation of p53 in

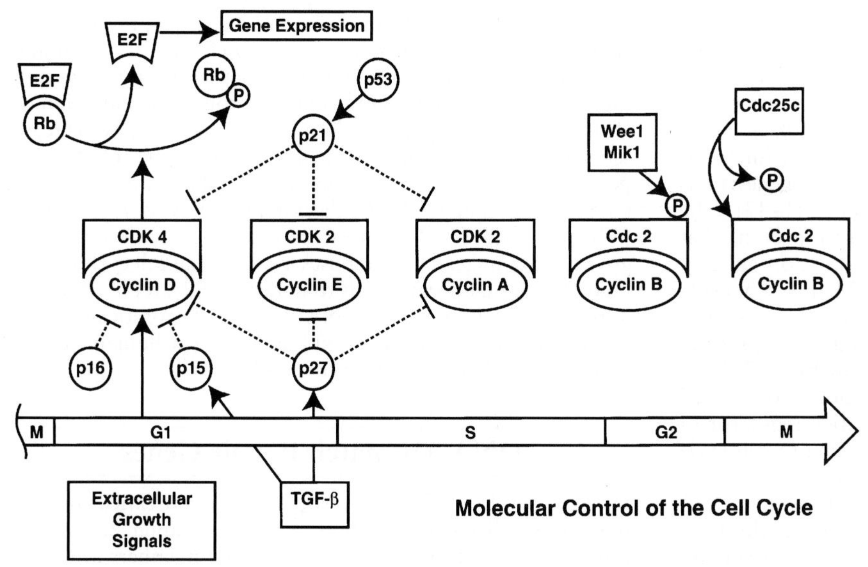

FIGURE 5.4. Molecular control of cell-cycle progression. A linear version of the various stages of the cell cycle is shown with the various cyclin/cyclin-dependent kinase complexes corresponding to the stages that they control.

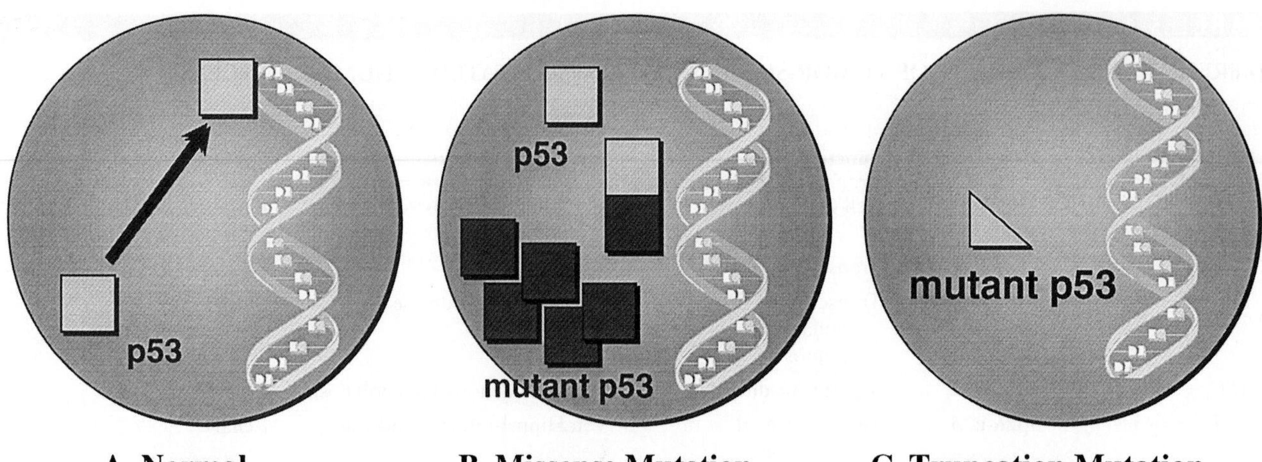

FIGURE 5.5. Inactivation of the p53 gene. **A:** Normal p53 protein binds to transcriptional regulatory elements in DNA. **B:** p53 missense mutations encode proteins that no longer bind to DNA and the mutant protein complexes with and inactivates any remaining normal p53 in the nucleus. **C:** p53 mutations that encode truncated protein products result in proteins that no longer bind to DNA, and these mutations usually are accompanied by deletion of the wild-type p53 allele.

human colorectal carcinomas (37). Mutant p53 protein inactivates wild-type p53 protein by formation of inactive oligomeric complexes, reconciling the earlier observations of cellular transformation by the expression of exogenous mutant p53 constructs.

The most common class of mutation observed in *TP53* is the single nucleotide substitution that results in a missense alteration (change in one amino acid) (Fig. 5.5). Mutations that lead to truncated protein products are less common and include nonsense alterations, which directly encode premature stop codons, and frameshift mutations, which consist of small deletions or insertions. The vast majority (greater than 80%) of missense mutations occur within highly conserved regions in the middle third of p53 encoded by exons 5 through 8 (38). Structural studies reveal that these regions are involved in a physical interaction between the p53 protein and DNA (39), consistent with the known role of p53 as a transcription factor. Disruption of the ability of p53 to interact with DNA appears to be a critical mechanism of p53 inactivation. Because p53 missense mutants are relatively resistant to degradation within the cell, mutant proteins accumulate within the nucleus, leading to apparent "overexpression," which can be detected immunohistochemically. As a result, immunostaining of p53 has been used as a rapid method of screening cancers for *TP53* mutations. However, positive immunostaining usually is not observed in cancers with protein truncating (nonsense and frameshift) mutations, so immunohistochemical analysis is relatively imprecise when used as a surrogate for mutational analysis (40).

The mechanism through which the p53 protein functions as a central element in the suppression of tumorigenesis has now been revealed in great molecular detail (41–43). The *TP53* gene encodes a 53-kD nuclear phosphoprotein that exists at low levels in all normal cells. Functioning as a homotetrameric complex, p53 binds to DNA in a sequence-specific fashion to regulate gene transcription, and oncogenic forms of p53 inhibit this transcriptional activation. Expression of p53 can be down-regulated when appropriate by the *MDM2* gene product, which targets it for degradation. Conversely, under other circumstances, p14^{ARF} , a negative regulator of *MDM2*, can increase expression of p53, leading to cell cycle arrest. It has become abundantly clear that the primary function of p53 is to activate the expression of genes involved in a DNA damage response pathway(s). Cell cycle arrest at the G_1-S checkpoint prior to DNA replication and at the G_2-M checkpoint prior to mitosis facilitates DNA damage repair and prevents mutations and aneuploidy, respectively. Additionally, the induction of apoptosis (programmed cell death) may be considered to be a fail-safe mechanism in cases where irreparable DNA damage has occurred. The accumulation of p53 in response to DNA damage leads to an enhanced transcriptional activation of genes involved in apoptosis, such as *BAX, FAS,* and *BCL2*, as well as genes involved in cell cycle arrest, such as *CDKN1A* (encoding p21), which encodes a potent inhibitor of most CDKs. The molecular pathway linking DNA damage to p53 protein accumulation is still obscure. The carboxyl-terminal of p53 can bind nonspecifically to the ends of DNA molecules to catalyze renaturation and strand transfer, and can also bind to extrahelical regions of DNA affected by insertion or deletion mismatches. Double-strand breaks in DNA are especially efficient in causing p53 accumulation, probably through reduced ubiquitin-mediated proteolysis.

By activating transcription of these other genes, p53 induces cell cycle arrest in late G_1 phase or may induce apoptosis in response to DNA damage. Cells expressing mutant p53 do not pause in G_1 or undergo apoptosis, but continue directly into S phase before DNA repair is complete. *TP53* has therefore been referred to as the "guardian of the genome," as it prevents entry into S phase until the genome has been cleared of potentially carcinogenic mutations. As many chemotherapeutic drugs and radiation exert their cytotoxic effects through the induction of DNA damage and apoptosis, loss of p53 function may decrease sensitivity to these agents, enhancing the emergence of resistant populations of cancer cells. Indeed, p53 and p21 are also essential in maintaining the G_2-M checkpoint following γ irradiation (44). Although *TP53* mutation provides cells with a selective growth advantage, it also imposes a substantial cell cycle checkpoint deficit that permits cells to undergo DNA replication and mitosis in the presence of DNA damage. Theoretically, such checkpoint defects might be exploited to treat human cancers with abnormalities of p53 function (45).

DNA Mismatch Repair Genes

HNPCC syndrome is an autosomal dominant cancer-predisposition syndrome described in detail in Chapter 2. In addition to colorectal cancers, HNPCC family members are at an increased risk for cancers of the endometrium, ovary, gastrointestinal sites, and upper urologic tract (46). This syndrome is believed to account for essentially all cases of hereditary endometrial carcinoma and up to 5% of cases of hereditary ovarian carcinoma. The estimated lifetime risk for endometrial cancer in female HNPCC gene carriers is 40% to 60%, corresponding to a relative risk of 13 to 20, whereas that of ovarian cancer is 6% to 20%, corresponding to a relative risk of 4 to 8 (47–52). Cloning and characterization of the genes responsible has provided substantial insight into the molecular etiology of HNPCC-associated malignancies, as well as that of some sporadic gynecologic cancers.

Clues to the genetic basis of HNPCC first emerged in 1993 with several independent observations of somatic hypermutability of a class of DNA repetitive elements, known as "microsatellites," in sporadic and familial colorectal tumors (53–55). This observation was accompanied by reports of the genetic linkage of HNPCC kindreds to two loci: one on chromosome 2p (56) and another on chromosome 3p (57). Identification and cloning of the responsible genes at these loci, *MSH2* on chromosome 2 (58,59) and *MLH1* on chromosome 3 (60,61), quickly followed, together with the realization that these genes encoded human orthologs of yeast DNA mismatch repair proteins. Thus, the microsatellite instability phenotype previously observed in colorectal and other cancer types associated with the HNPCC syndrome could be explained by loss of function of these DNA mismatch repair (MMR) genes. In HNPCC, one of these genes is inherited in a mutant form through the germ line followed by somatic loss of the wild-type allele, whereas in sporadic colorectal, endometrial, and gastric carcinomas affected by microsatellite instability, somatic silencing of *MLH1* through promoter hypermethylation appears to be the primary pathogenic mechanism (62).

Although most HNPCC kindreds appear to be linked to either *MSH2* or *MLH1*, a small fraction are linked to a third MMR gene, *MSH6*. There is some evidence that this gene may account for a substantial number of atypical or low-penetrance HNPCC kindreds, as well as those affected by a disproportionately high number of gynecologic cancers (63–66). A recent report indicates that about 2% of all newly diagnosed endometrial cancers have germ-line defects in *MSH6* and that most of these cases are not known to be associated with classic HNPCC syndrome criteria (67). Early evidence suggested that the MMR genes *PMS1* and *PMS2* may also play a role in HNPCC (68), but these observations were not widely confirmed, and a recent report involving investigators originally linking these genes to HNPCC kindreds indicates that these genes are less likely to be involved in the syndrome (69).

The genetic instability phenotype associated with defective MMR genes is most readily observed through somatic length alterations in simple repeat sequences, for example, (CA)*n*, located throughout the genome and known as "microsatellites." Replication errors in these repeat sequences are probably common, and their inefficient repair results in the "microsatellite instability" phenotype. Since the discovery of mutant MMR genes and the corresponding microsatellite instability, a large number of studies have documented microsatellite instability in many sporadic tumor types, including those not associated with the HNPCC syndrome. Although mutations of the MMR genes have been readily identified in many HNPCC kindreds, somatic MMR gene mutations in sporadic tumors with the microsatellite instability phenotype are not commonly detected. It appears to be likely that hypermethylation of the *MLH1* promoter, resulting in down-regulation of its expression, is the causative mechanism in most sporadic colorectal, gastric, and endometrial carcinomas with microsatellite instability (70–72).

It is not clear how microsatellite instability contributes to tumorigenesis in the endometrium, ovary, or other organs affected by the HNPCC syndrome. Microsatellites exist throughout the genome in predominantly noncoding regions of DNA. Simple repeat sequences are known to occur in the coding regions of genes, however, and their somatic mutation may result in loss of function for genes critical to the regulation of proliferation, invasion, or metastasis. Examples include genes encoding the transforming growth factor-β (TGF-β) receptor type II, the regulator of apoptosis BAX, and the insulin-like growth factor II receptor, all of which contain homopolymeric microsatellite repeats (e.g., A_8) that are mutated in some cancers with microsatellite instability (73). Frequently overlooked is the fact that the DNA mismatch repair system also functions in the repair of single nucleotide mismatches, so that defective mismatch repair would also lead to point mutations. Although the assay for this type of DNA damage is less straightforward than that for microsatellite instability, these single base-pair substitution mutations may play a more important role in tumorigenesis than microsatellite mutations.

BRCA1 and *BRCA2*

Approximately 10% of all epithelial ovarian carcinomas are associated with an autosomal dominant genetic predisposition. The great majority of these cases is attributable to the *BRCA1* or *BRCA2* tumor-suppressor genes and arises in the context of the hereditary breast and ovarian cancer syndrome, with a small fraction occurring in the HNPCC syndrome. (Clinical genetics aspects of this topic are discussed in Chapter 2.) Following the original reports of genetic linkage of early-onset breast cancer families (74) and some breast and ovarian cancer families (75) to the *BRCA1* locus on chromosome 17q, the *BRCA1* gene was cloned and characterized in 1994 (76). Shortly thereafter, the *BRCA2* locus on chromosome 13q was defined (77), and the gene was identified in 1995 (78). It is now clear that 60% to 90% of breast and ovarian cancer families are linked to *BRCA1*, with most of the remainder being linked to *BRCA2*, especially those with cases of male breast cancer.

The *BRCA1* and *BRCA2* genes share remarkable similarities in both structure and function, and will be discussed together. Both genes are unusually large, *BRCA1* consisting of 22 coding exons and a 7.8-kb mRNA transcript, and *BRCA2* consisting of 26 coding exons and a transcript exceeding 10 kb. Both genes contain a very large 11th exon that encodes nearly half of the transcript, a start codon located in exon 2, and a high A/T to G/C content. Mutations occur throughout both genes, with no evidence of hotspots or clustering. Over 80% of detected mutations are nonsense or frameshift alterations that are predicted to lead to a truncated protein product, with the remainder representing missense and other miscellaneous "variants of uncertain significance" (79). Somatic LOH at the *BRCA* loci in breast and ovarian cancers invariably affects the wild-type allele, which is consistent with their function as classic tumor-suppressor genes (80,81). In the search for genotype/phenotype correlations in the *BRCA* genes, it has become clear that no strong association is likely to exist for *BRCA1*, but that *BRCA2* contains an "ovarian cancer cluster region" (OCCR) in exon 11; the ratio of ovarian to breast cancers is significantly higher in families segregating a *BRCA2* OCCR mutation (82) for reasons that remain obscure.

Prior to discovery of the *BRCA* genes, it was well documented that LOH affecting the relevant regions of chromosomes 17q and 13q was common in sporadic breast and ovarian cancers, and thus it came as a surprise that somatic mutations in *BRCA1* and *BRCA2* are virtually nonexistent in sporadic breast cancers and rare in sporadic ovarian cancers. Gene silencing of *BRCA1* through promoter hypermethylation appears to play a role in the pathogenesis of a small fraction of sporadic ovarian cancers (83,84), whereas methylation of *BRCA2* has not been reported. Attempts to explain this paradox have centered on the argument that inactivation of *BRCA* genes early in development (i.e., through the germ line) may be important for tumorigenesis, but not somatic inactivation in adult tissues. Recently, several lines of evidence suggest that inactivation of the *BRCA* pathway may play an important role in ovarian tumorigenesis through mechanisms other than inactivation of the *BRCA* genes themselves. Microarray-based gene expression profiling experiments indicate that rather than clustering as a third group, sporadic ovarian cancers all cluster as either *BRCA1*-like or *BRCA2*-like, implying the existence of a BRCA-deficient gene expression fingerprint in all ovarian cancers (85). Additionally, the novel EMSY protein was recently identified as a suppressor of *BRCA2* activity, and the *EMSY* gene is amplified in 17% of ovarian cancers, providing a genetic mechanism for inactivation of *BRCA2* in some sporadic cancers (86).

Over the past 10 years, a large body of data has been generated with respect to BRCA function, which appears to be related for the two genes, but a coherent picture of precisely how these proteins function to suppress tumorigenicity remains elusive. Generally, there is substantial evidence for a role of *BRCA1* and *BRCA2* in cellular processes related to the prevention of genomic instability, including DNA damage recognition and repair, transcriptional regulation, and control of cell cycle checkpoints (87,88). A seminal research finding in this area was that *BRCA1* colocalizes *in vivo* and physically associates *in vitro* with the RAD51 protein, known to function in the repair of double-strand DNA breaks, implying a role for *BRCA1* in the control of recombination and genomic integrity (89). Other early work on the role of *Brca2* in mouse development indicated that loss of the protein confers radiation hypersensitivity and also that *Brca2* physically interacts with Rad51 in repair of double-strand DNA breaks (90). Remarkably, *BRCA1* and *BRCA2* proteins appear to be involved in the same biochemical pathway, mediated by RAD51, regulating genomic integrity.

Data derived from the study of embryonic cells and tissues from mice rendered nullizygous for *Brca1* or *Brca2* provide strong evidence for the role of these proteins in the response to DNA damage. An embryonic lethal phenotype is observed in mice with a homozygous null mutation in *Brca1* (91) or *Brca2* (90,92), suggesting their requirement for embryonic cellular proliferation prior to gastrulation. Partial rescue of this developmental lethality is achieved by simultaneous knockout of the *TP53* gene (93,94), implying that the accumulation of DNA damage in *Brca* knockout mice leads to the arrest of cell division by p53, and that their concomitant knockout allows additional cell division to take place before eventual lethality. In cells from these Brca-deficient animals, gross chromosomal rearrangements are evident, and considerable data suggest that this chromosomal instability results from the inappropriate repair of DNA double-strand breaks during the S and G_2 phases of the cell cycle. Specifically, homology-directed repair of double-strand breaks, an error-free pathway, is defective in *Brca1*-deficient mouse cells (95–97) and in *BRCA2*-deficient human and mouse cells (98–100). The error-prone pathway of nonhomologous end joining remains intact in Brca-deficient cells, however, and the attempted repair of spontaneous and induced double-strand breaks because of inappropriate routing through this mechanism probably contributes to chromosomal instability observed in Brca-deficient cells. The precise roles of BRCA proteins in homology-directed repair remain to be determined, but evidence suggests that *BRCA1* performs the general function of linking DNA damage sensing or signaling to effector components of the cellular response to DNA damage (88), whereas *BRCA2* physically interacts with and controls the RAD51 recombinase (101), a catalytic activity essential for homologous recombination.

In contrast to *BRCA2*, there are considerable data linking the *BRCA1* protein to other functions possibly involved in tumor suppression, especially the transcriptional regulation of gene expression. Fragments of *BRCA1* are capable of transcriptional transactivation *in vitro* (102,103), and *BRCA1* is a component of the RNA polymerase II holoenzyme (104) through its interaction with RNA helicase A (105). In response to DNA damage, *BRCA1* functions as a p53-independent transactivator of the CDK inhibitor p21 (106,107). Ectopic expression of *BRCA1* results in the p53-independent induction of GADD45 expression (108), as well as the selective coactivation of p53-dependent transcription (109), one target of which appears to be the gene encoding the G_2/M checkpoint control protein 14–3-3σ (110). Microarray-based expression profiling experiments indicate that the selective expression of *BRCA1* in mouse and human cells leads to alterations in expression of numerous additional genes involved in cell cycle control and DNA repair (108,110,111).

BRCA1 is a large protein that, in addition to its role in the DNA damage and transcriptional pathways mentioned above, has been found to associate with a variety of other cellular components. Of these proteins BARD1 (*BRCA1* associated ring domain 1) appears to enhance some other cellular functions of *BRCA1* not associated with DNA interaction. Through its interaction with BARD1, *BRCA1* has been identified as an E3 ubiquitin ligase (112,113). E3 ubiquitin ligases function by attaching the ubiquitin monomer to specific target proteins, making them subject to degradation. Ubiquitin-directed degradation is a key process in regulating the levels of proteins post-transcriptionally. Defects in this process have been implicated in carcinogenesis previously. Specifically, the Von Hippel Lindau (*VHL*) tumor suppressor is a well known E3 ubiquitin ligase. VHL predominantly targets the hypoxia inducible factor (HIF1A) transcription factor for degradation in normoxic conditions. Loss of VHL leads to increased HIF1 and its subsequent transcription targets that are involved in cell survival, blood vessel development, and mitogenesis. The *VHL* mutation ultimately promotes kidney and other cancers. The role of *BRCA1's* E3 ubiquitin ligase activity and cancer formation is much less clear. Specifically, the protein(s) targeted by *BRCA1* for ubiquitination are largely unknown (114). Recently, however, estrogen receptor alpha (ER) was found to be a specific target of *BRCA1*-mediated ubiquitination (115). The implications of this finding are not yet clarified, but may in part explain the tissue specificity of tumor formation in *BRCA1*-defective kindreds. It is conceptually difficult to understand how a protein involved in DNA repair that is expressed in a wide variety of tissues could protect only breast and ovary cells from tumor formation. However, it is more tractable to understand how an enzyme that acts on a variety of targets, some of which are tissue specific, could. Indeed the role of the *ER/BRCA1* genes in promoter transactivation has been suggested as a factor in determining the tumor spectrum of *BRCA1* mutation carriers. Tissue specific modulatin of ER levels by *BRCA1* could effect diverse transcriptional targets, and the importance of ER has been demonstrated in the murine BRCA knockout mouse (116). Interestingly, most *BRCA1* mutant breast cancers are ER negative, which is counterintuitive if *BRCA1* normally functions to target the receptor for degradation. The significance of these recent findings remains intriguing, and the role of BRCA ubiquitination in carcinogenesis of the breast and ovary remains unclear.

Thus, the emerging model of BRCA function implies a dual role for the BRCA-deficient state in the initiation of tumorigenesis as well as targeted cancer therapy. In BRCA-deficient cells, the defective maintenance of genomic integrity may accelerate cancer initiation and progression, yet also render the resultant cancer more susceptible to therapeutic agents whose cytotoxic potential is mediated through the induction of the specific type of DNA damage that BRCA normally functions to repair. A number of commonly used cancer therapies are believed to cause DNA interstrand cross links, a lesion that appears to be repaired through creation of an intermediate double-strand break followed by homologous recombination. Prototypical agents from this mechanistic category include cisplatin, mitomycin C, and γ radiation (117). That BRCA-deficient cancers may respond favorably to this class of DNA-damaging agents is suggested by studies in which modulation of *BRCA1* expression in various isogenic cell clones is shown to affect sensitivity to cisplatin (118–120), mitomycin C (97), and γ radiation (121–124). This mechanism likely represents the underlying biologic basis for improved outcome in *BRCA*-linked hereditary ovarian cancer patients compared to matched sporadic cases (125–127). Further, this suggests a rational basis for trials investigating the efficacy of platinum-based chemotherapy in breast cancer patients with germ-line BRCA mutations.

PTEN

A novel tumor-suppressor gene responsible for the very rare, autosomal dominant hereditary cancer syndrome Cowden's syndrome was cloned and characterized in 1997 (128,129). Cowden's syndrome, also known as multiple hamartoma syndrome, is characterized by benign hamartomas of multiple organs, including skin, intestine, breast, and thyroid. In addition to benign lesions, breast cancers develop in 30% to 50% of affected women and thyroid cancers occur in 10% of affected individuals. Bannayan-Zonana syndrome, a closely related condition, was also subsequently found to be caused by mutations in the same gene (130). Named *PTEN*, this gene was originally noted to encode a likely tyrosine phosphatase with additional significant homologies to the cytoskeletal proteins tensin and auxilin. Early studies aimed at uncovering *PTEN* function indicated that its phosphatase activity may function to suppress tumorigenesis by negatively regulating cell interactions with the extracellular matrix, specifically the inhibition of integrin-mediated cell spreading and cell migration through dephosphorylation of focal adhesion kinase (FAK) (131). Additionally, expression of *PTEN* selectively inhibits activation of the extracellular signal-regulated kinase (ERK) mitogen-activated protein kinase (MAPK) pathway (132). Other cellular targets for the phosphatase activity of *PTEN* include elements of the phosphoinositide 3-kinase/AKT pathway (133). Specifically, the *PTEN* gene functions as a lipid phosphatase negatively regulating the lipid second messenger phoshatidylinositol 3, 4, 5,-triphosphate (134). Because constitutive activation of either PI3-kinase or AKT is known to induce cellular transformation, an increase in the activity of this pathway caused by mutations in *PTEN* provided additional support for its complex role in tumor suppression. It is now well established that *PTEN's* lipid phosphatase activity, acting through the PI3K/AKT and MAPK pathways, plays a critical role in the regulation of growth arrest, apoptosis, and other important cellular functions (135).

Although endometrial carcinoma has been suggested to represent a component tumor of Cowden's syndrome according to revised diagnostic criteria (136), germ-line mutations in *PTEN* are not associated with a significant proportion of unselected endometrial carcinomas. Remarkably, however, sporadic endometrial carcinomas frequently exhibit loss of heterozygosity in a region of chromosome 10q that includes the *PTEN* gene (137,138). Mutation analyses of *PTEN* in endometrial carcinomas indicate that this gene is somatically inactivated in 30% to 50% of all such tumors (139-141), representing the most frequent molecular genetic alteration in endometrial cancers yet defined. Inactivation of *PTEN* may represent an early event in a subset of endometrial cancers, as mutations are detected at a significant frequency in premalignant endometrial hyperplasia specimens (142). Interestingly, *PTEN* mutations are also seen in a fraction of ovarian carcinomas of endometrioid histology (143), but not in those of serous or other histologic subtypes (141–144). More recent findings on the role of *PTEN* in specific gynecologic cancers are discussed later in this chapter.

ONCOGENES

It has been convincingly demonstrated that alterations in genes whose products normally act to stimulate cell proliferation or other aspects of the neoplastic phenotype (oncogenes) can cause malignant transformation (Fig. 5.6) (145,146). Oncogenes can be activated via several mechanisms. In solid tumors, the most common mechanism of oncogene activation appears to be gene amplification with resultant overexpression of the corresponding protein. Instead of two copies of one of these genes, there may be many copies. The *ERBB2* (HER2/neu) oncogene is activated in this fashion. Some oncogenes may become resistant to inactivation when affected by specific point mutations in regulatory domains, resulting in constitutive signaling. The *RAS* family of oncogenes is prototypical in this regard. Finally, oncogenes may be translocated from one chromosomal location to another and then come under the influence of promoter sequences that cause overexpression of the gene. This mechanism frequently occurs in leukemias and lymphomas (e.g., the Philadelphia chromosome), but appears to be less common in solid tumors.

In addition to gene amplification and other mechanisms mentioned above, expression of some genes can be increased due to loss of imprinted transcriptional control. Loss of imprinting (LOI) remains poorly understood in carcinogenesis. A small subset of genes in the genome is expressed solely from either the maternal or paternal inherited copy. During the carcinogenic process the maintenance of allele-specific silencing is often lost, resulting in increased expression. For example, the mitogenic peptide insulin-like growth factor 2 (IGF2) is commonly up-regulated in a variety of cancers where it functions to promote cell division by signaling through the insulin receptor and the IGFI receptor. Loss of imprinting of this

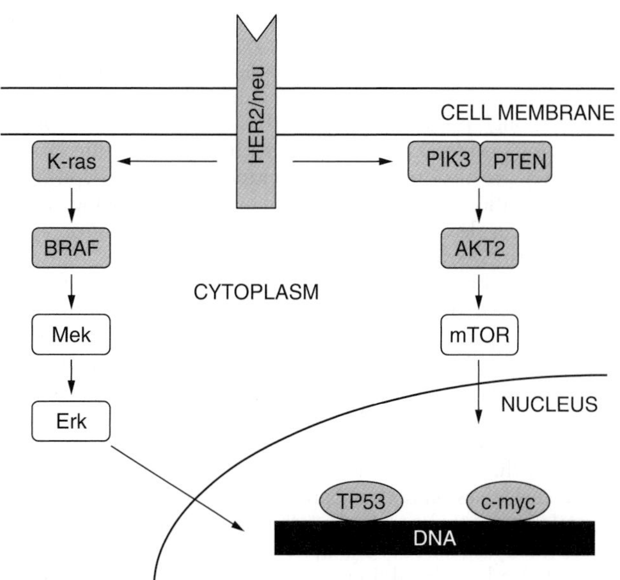

FIGURE 5.6. Cellular localization of representative oncogenes and tumor-suppressor genes that are altered in gynecologic cancers.

growth factor is common in some cancers, including some ovarian malignancies, and increases the susceptibility of tumor formation (147). However, the up-regulation of IGF2 is more common in cancers than the frequency of LOI, indicating that LOI alone is not responsible for all observed IGF2 increases. The increased levels of IGF2 are likely due to LOI in some cases and other epigenetic events in most cases at this complex genomic locus (148,149). Thus, LOI is just one of several epigenetic mechanisms that can disregulate the expression of genes with oncogenic potential.

In various model systems and *in vitro,* many genes that are involved in normal pathways of cell proliferation, signal transduction, and transcriptional regulation can elicit neoplastic transformation when altered to overactive forms via amplification, mutation, translocation, or simple overexpression. On this basis, a large number of genes have been classified as "oncogenic." However, the actual spectrum of such genes that have been shown to be altered mutationally in human cancers (the formal criterion for classification as an oncogene) is much more limited. Presently, it appears that inactivation of tumor-suppressor genes is significantly more common than activation of oncogenes. With the advent of large gene-sequencing efforts directed at identifying activating mutations in protein kinases, it is likely that the number of genes satisfying the classic oncogene definition will increase. This may reflect the fact that mutations are more apt to disrupt the function of a gene than to create a product that is hyperactive. Alternatively, it is possible that the involvement of tumor-suppressor genes in malignant transformation has been more easily identifiable because of their association with hereditary cancer syndromes. In this section, the various classes of oncogenes are summarized, with particular attention being paid to those that are altered in gynecologic cancers.

Peptide Growth Factors and Their Receptors

Peptide growth factors in the extracellular space can stimulate a cascade of molecular events that leads to proliferation by binding to cell membrane receptors. Unlike endocrine hormones, which are secreted into the bloodstream to act in distant target organs, peptide growth factors usually act in the local environment. The concept that autocrine growth stimulation might be a key strategy by which cancer cell proliferation becomes autonomous has received considerable attention. In this model, it is postulated that cancers secrete stimulatory growth factors that then interact with receptors on the same cell. Although production of growth factors may play a role in enhancing proliferation associated with malignant transformation, they are also involved in development, stromal-epithelial communication, tissue regeneration, and wound healing. Thus, it remains unclear whether autocrine growth stimulation actually is a critical event in cancer development.

Cell membrane receptors that bind peptide growth factors are composed of an extracellular ligand-binding domain, a membrane-spanning region, and a cytoplasmic tyrosine kinase domain (150). More than a dozen receptor tyrosine kinases have been identified thus far that bind peptide growth factors. Binding of a growth factor to the extracellular domain results in aggregation and conformational shifts in the receptor and activation of the inner tyrosine kinase. This kinase phosphorylates tyrosine residues on both the growth factor receptor (autophosphorylation) and targets in the cell interior, leading to activation of secondary signals. For example, phosphorylation of phospholipase C leads to breakdown of cell membrane phospholipids and generation of diacylglycerol and inositol-triphosphate (IP3), both of which play a role in propagation of the mitogenic signal.

Epidermal Growth Factor Receptor Family

The role of the epidermal growth factor (EGF) receptor family of transmembrane receptors and their ligands in growth regulation and transformation has been a prominent focus in cancer research over the past three decades (151). The salient findings are summarized in this section. EGF is a peptide growth factor of 53 amino acids that maintains its secondary structure by virtue of disulfide bonds between cysteine residues. At least 10 other peptide growth factors, including TGF-α, also interact with and activate the EGF receptor(s) (152). TGF-α was so named because of its ability to act in concert with TGF-β to transform some types of cells in culture. EFG, TGF-α, and other EGF receptor ligands are produced as proforms that are inserted into the cell membrane. The membrane-anchored growth factor can interact with receptors on adjacent cells, a phenomenon known as juxtacrine growth regulation. Alternatively, the active peptide then can be cleaved and released into the extracellular space. The free peptide may interact with receptors on the same (autocrine) or nearby (paracrine) cells to stimulate growth.

The EGF family of receptors has been extensively characterized from both a genetic and biochemical standpoint. Similar to other growth factor receptors, the EGF family members are composed of an extracellular ligand-binding domain, a hydrophobic membrane-spanning region, and an intracellular tyrosine kinase domain (153,154). A truncated form of the EGF receptor that lacks the outer ligand-binding domain is the viral oncogene (v-*erb*B) responsible for avian erythroblastosis. The v-*erb*B gene encodes a receptor that is constantly activated and sending growth stimulatory signals to the nucleus. The EGF receptor is ubiquitously expressed in both epithelial and stromal cells and plays a role in growth stimulation of most cell types

The EGF receptor has been shown to be massively amplified in the A431 human vulvar squamous cell carcinoma cell line, and these cells have been widely used as a model for studying the biochemical functions of the EGF receptor. In some head and neck and lung cancers, the EGF receptor also appears to be significantly amplified, and amplification may be associated with virulent behavior. In these cancers, the EGF receptor can be targeted therapeutically with monoclonal antibodies (155). In normal squamous epithelium, expression of EGF receptor is high in the basal proliferative layer and decreases as cells migrate toward the surface and differentiate. Although levels of EGF receptor vary between different primary squamous cancers of the lower genital tract in women, gene amplification rarely occurs, and EGF receptor levels do not appear to correlate closely with clinical behavior of these cancers (156). Similarly, EGF receptor is expressed in normal ovarian epithelium and endometrium, and although the level of expression varies between cancers, this is not a strong predictor of clinical behavior.

In some human cancers, such as non-small-cell lung cancer, specific inhibitors of the EGF receptor, such as gefitinib (Iressa) or erlotnib (Tarceva), have recently been proven to be effective in their treatment, and multiple clinical trials are now under way to test the efficacy of these agents alone or in combination with traditional chemotherapeutic agents (157). Efficacy of these inhibitors is largely predictable based on whether the cancer has specific mutations within the EGF receptor. Patients with certain mutations that constitutively activate the receptor tend to preferentially respond to anti-EGFR treatment. About half of these mutations are an in-frame deletion of amino acids 747-750; most of the other mutants occur at amino acid 858 (158). The occurrence of tumors with a strong dependence on one oncogene has led to the so-called oncogene addiction theory (159). Many genetic and epigenetic alterations may have occurred in these cancers, yet they are vulnerable to a single targeted treatment directed to a dependence on a particular oncogene. It is theorized that the anti-EGFR therapy causes an "oncogenic shock," leading to high levels of apoptosis and significant clinical response when pro-growth stimulations are replaced by apoptotic signals. Unfortunately, many of these cancers will recover from this treatment by acquiring drug resistance.

As mentioned, the EGF receptor family of receptors is also often referred to as the *ERBB* family because the first member identified was the v-*erb*B oncogene. The second member of the family (*ERBB2*) initially was called *neu* because it was found to be the transforming gene responsible for the generation of neuroblastomas in rats treated with a chemical carcinogen. It subsequently was discovered that the *neu* gene encoded a 185-kD transmembrane receptor that is highly homologous with the EGF receptor (160). This human EGF receptor–like molecule was named both HER2/neu and *erb*B2 by investigators working in the field. The transforming activity of *neu* in the animal model was due to the presence of a mutation in the transmembrane portion of the molecule that results in constitutive activation of the inner tyrosine kinase domain. Biochemical studies of HER2/neu (formally designated *ERBB2*) have shown that activation of this receptor is not driven by ligand binding, but rather is dependent on activation of other members of the *ERBB* family (161). Two members of the *ERBB* receptor family are nonautonomous and require dimerization with other family members for function. Specifically, *ERBB2* lacks ligand-binding capability, while *ERBB3* lacks the kinase activity. These two receptors develop potency of growth factor signal transmission via heterodimerization. Whereas *ERBB2* and *ERBB3* require heterodimerization for function, *ERBB1* (EGFR) and *ERBB4* can function autonomously or as heterodimers. *ERBB2* is the preferential partner for *ERBB3* and *ERBB4*. Recent attempts to characterize the complex signaling via these receptors and their ligands at systems biology level imply that *ERBB2* functions as the system amplifier (152).

In contrast to EGF receptor, which normally is expressed in both stromal and epithelial cells, ERBB2 is expressed primarily in epithelial cells. As originally shown for breast and ovarian cancers (162), the expression of ERBB2 is increased in several human cancer types as a result of gene amplification. In addition, artificial overexpression of this gene in some cell types in culture leads to acquisition of a malignant phenotype. In human cancers, *ERBB2* may also be overexpressed owing to alterations in regulation of transcription in the absence of gene amplification. Regardless of the underlying mechanism, it has been shown that overexpression correlates strongly with aggressive features in breast, ovarian, and endometrial cancers.

As noted above, activation of the ERBB3 and ERBB4 transmembrane receptors is requisite for ERBB2 kinase activity. At least four families of ligands, collectively called neuregulins (e.g., heregulin, *neu* differentiating factor), bind to ERBB3 and ERBB4 (161). Interestingly, there is considerable promiscuity between ERBB ligands and receptors. For example, amphiregulin can activate both the EGF receptor (ERBB1) and ERBB3. And one of the more recently described ligands (epiregulin) can activate heterodimers of any of the ERBB family members; these heterodimers are more potent growth stimulators than homodimers of any individual ERBB receptor. Finally, although their molecular signaling mechanisms have not yet been fully elucidated, the ERBB family of receptors has also been exploited as therapeutic targets. Success has been achieved with the anti-ERBB2 monoclonal antibody trastuzumab (Herceptin), which is approved for treatment of ERBB2-positive metastatic breast cancer. In combination with chemotherapy, trastuzumab provides significant clinical benefit in terms of increased response rate and extended survival compared with chemotherapy alone in patients with ERBB2-positive advanced breast cancer. Trastuzumab also has therapeutic activity as monotherapy in the front-line management of ERBB2-overexpressed or ERBB2-amplified metastatic breast cancer. Given its proven efficacy in the metastatic setting, the combination and sequential use of trastuzumab with adjuvant and neoadjuvant chemotherapy are the focus of several ongoing clinical studies (163). In ovarian cancers with *ERBB2* amplification and/or overexpression, however, trastuzumab has been proven to be disappointing in terms of efficacy compared to that observed in breast cancer (164).

Extranuclear Signal Transduction

Following interaction of peptide growth factors and their receptors, secondary molecular signals are generated to transmit the mitogenic stimulus toward the nucleus. This function is served by a multitude of complex and overlapping signal transduction pathways that occur in the inner cell membrane and cytoplasm. Many of these signals involve phosphorylation of proteins by enzymes known as kinases. Cellular processes other than growth are also regulated by kinases, but one family of kinases appears to have evolved specifically for the purpose of transmitting growth stimulatory signals. These tyrosine kinases transfer a phosphate group from ATP to tyrosine residues of target proteins. Some kinases that phosphorylate proteins on serine and/or threonine residues (e.g., protein kinase C, AKT2) also are involved in stimulating proliferation. The activity of kinases is regulated by phosphatases, which act in opposition to the kinases by removing phosphates from the target proteins. Although several families of intracellular kinases have been identified that can elicit transformation when activated *in vitro* (e.g., *SRC*), structural alterations in these molecules appear to play a role in the development of human cancers only rarely. Recently, sequencing of kinase genes in common human cancers identified a low frequency of mutations (165). The frequency of these alterations and their significance will need to be validated in future studies; however, it appears clear that widespread mutation of specific kinases is not common. Rather, cancer is typified by a low frequency of mutations in multiple kinases.

RAS

G-proteins represent another class of molecules involved in transmission of growth stimulatory signals from the cell membrane to the nucleus (166). The RAS family of G-proteins functions as a relay switch that is positioned downstream of cell surface receptor tyrosine kinases and upstream of a cytoplasmic cascade of kinases that include the mitogen-activated protein (MAP) kinases (167,168). Activated MAP kinases in turn regulate the activities of nuclear transcription factors. RAS proteins are 21-kD molecules that localize to the inner aspect of the cell membrane. They have intrinsic GTPase activity that catalyzes the exchange of guanosine 5′-triphosphate (GTP) for guanosine 5′-diphosphate (GDP). In their active GTP-bound form, G-proteins interact with MAP kinases. Conversely, hydrolysis of GTP to GDP, which is stimulated by GTPase-activating proteins (GAPs), leads to inactivation of G-proteins.

It is estimated that point mutations in *RAS* genes are present in about one third of cancers (11). Mutations in this family of G-proteins (*KRAS*, *HRAS*, and *NRAS*) are among the most frequently observed genetic alterations in human cancers (e.g., gastrointestinal and endometrial cancers). In human cancers and in a wide range of chemically induced rodent tumors, activating mutations in *RAS* are observed at codon 12, 13, or 61 (169). The encoded amino acids at these three locations appear to play a critical structural role in the active site of ras, such that missense mutations at one of these codons destroy the ability of RAS to convert GTP to GDP. The end result of such an activating mutation is accumulation of GTP-RAS protein that chronically transmits its growth stimulatory signal. In human epithelial malignancies, the most frequently observed mutation is that of *KRAS* codon 12; such is the case for gynecologic cancers, as is discussed later in this chapter.

To be biologically active, RAS must move from the cytoplasm to the inner plasma membrane. A posttranslational modification, specifically addition of a farnesyl group to the C-terminal cysteine, is requisite for membrane localization. Farnesylation of RAS is catalyzed by the enzyme farnesyltransferase. Recently, several compounds have been developed that can inhibit farnesylation. Preclinical studies indicate that these molecules can suppress transformation and tumor growth *in vitro* and in animal models with little toxicity to normal cells (170).

Nuclear Factors

If proliferation is to occur in response to signals generated in the cytoplasm, these events must lead to activation of nuclear factors responsible for DNA replication and cell division. Expression of several genes that encode nuclear proteins increases dramatically within minutes of treatment of normal cells with peptide growth factors. Once induced, the products of these genes (e.g., FOS, JUN, MYC) bind to specific DNA regulatory elements and induce transcription of genes involved in DNA synthesis and cell division. When inappropriately amplified and/or overexpressed, however, these transcription factors can act as oncogenes.

Among the nuclear transcription factors involved in stimulating proliferation, amplification and/or overexpression of members of the *MYC* family has most often been implicated in the development of human cancers (161). MYC proteins are key regulators of mammalian cell proliferation, and treatment of cells with MYC antisense oligonucleotides inhibits proliferation. It has been shown that MYC acts as part of a heterodimeric complex with the protein MAX to initiate transcription of other genes involved in cell cycle progression (171). Ironically, in some instances in which MYC expression is low, its inappropriate reexpression can elicit apoptosis (172).

The T-cell–like transcription factor 4, *TCF4/LEF1*, and the *TCF3* (now known as *TCF7L1* and *TCF7L2*) transcription factors are implicated in carcinogenesis. These factors are thought to be the chief effectors of constitutive alteration of the Wnt signal transduction pathway. As discussed elsewhere in this chapter, inactivating mutation of the APC tumor suppressor, activating mutation of *CTNNB1*, or multiple epigenetic inactivation events in secreted Frizzled receptors all lead to increases of β-catenin (173). β-catenin associates with the TCF4 factor and activates or represses gene transcription from certain promoters. The exact targets of transcription remain poorly known in most cancer types. However, the c-*myc* gene contains canonical TCF/Lef binding sites within its promoter and may be one key target gene. Whether alterations in this pathway are relevant in the transformation of gynecologic cancers largely remains to be elucidated.

GYNECOLOGIC MALIGNANCIES

Considerable evidence has accumulated to suggest that the clinical heterogeneity of gynecologic cancers with respect to behavior (borderline vs. invasive), histologic type, stage, and outcome is attributable, to a great extent, to differences in underlying molecular alterations between cancers. The spectrum of oncogene and tumor-suppressor gene defects clearly varies both between cancer types and within a given type of cancer. A comprehensive understanding of the molecular pathogenesis of gynecologic cancers has not yet been achieved, but new genomic technologies that allow global assessment of molecular alterations are accelerating the pace of discovery. Elucidation of the molecular pathology of gynecologic cancers promises not only to illuminate their origins, but also to facilitate the development of new approaches to diagnosis, treatment, and prevention.

Although expression of many genes and molecular pathways is dysregulated in gynecologic cancers, most of these are secondary changes that contribute to evolution of the malignant phenotype. The main focus of this chapter is on the primary mutational alterations in oncogenes and tumor-suppressor genes that lead to the initial development of gynecologic cancers.

ENDOMETRIAL CANCER

Epidemiologic and clinical studies of endometrial cancer have suggested that there are two distinct types of endometrial cancer (174). Type I cases are associated with unopposed estrogen stimulation and often develop in a background of endometrial hyperplasia. These cancers are characterized by well-differentiated, endometrioid histology, early stage, and favorable outcome. In contrast, type II cancers are poorly differentiated and/or nonendometrioid and are more virulent. They often present at an advanced stage and survival is relatively poor. In practice, not all cases can be neatly characterized as either type I or II lesions, and endometrial cancers can also be viewed as a spectrum with respect to etiology and clinical behavior. However, as the genetic events involved in the development of endometrial cancer have been elucidated, it has been found that specific alterations often, but not always, are seen primarily in either type I or II cases (Table 5.2, Fig. 5.7).

The molecular basis for the relationship between unopposed estrogenic stimulation of the endometrium and endometrial cancer remains uncertain. It has long been thought that estrogens contribute to the development of endometrial cancer by virtue of their mitogenic effect on the endometrium. A higher rate of proliferation in response to estrogens may lead to an increased frequency of spontaneous mutations. In addition, when genetic damage occurs, regardless of the cause, the presence of estrogens may facilitate clonal expansion. It has also been postulated that estrogens may act as "complete carcinogens" that both promote proliferation and act as initiating agents due to free-radical generation and production of carcinogenic metabolites. In contrast, progestins oppose the action of estrogens both by down-regulating estrogen receptor levels and by decreasing proliferation and increasing apoptosis.

The initial evidence of genetic alterations in endometrial cancers came from cytogenetic studies that revealed changes in the number of copies of specific chromosomes as well as deletions and translocations (175). Subsequently, comparative genomic hybridization (CGH) studies have demonstrated specific areas of chromosomal loss and gain in both endometrial cancers and atypical hyperplasias (176,177). The most common sites of chromosomal gain are 1q, 8q, 10p, and 10q (178–180). Chromosomal losses also are frequently observed both using CGH and in loss of heterozygosity studies (181). A correlation has been noted between higher numbers of chromosomal alterations on CGH and more virulent clinical features (182). The overall number of chromosomal alterations detected using CGH is lower in endometrial cancers relative to other cancer types.

Ploidy analysis simply measures total nuclear DNA content. About 80% of endometrial cancers have a normal diploid DNA content as measured by ploidy analysis. Aneuploidy occurs in 20% and is associated with advanced stage, poor grade, nonendometrioid histology, and poor survival (183).

TABLE 5.2

GENETIC ALTERATIONS IN SPORADIC ENDOMETRIAL CARCINOMAS

	Class	Mechanism	Approximate frequency	Type I/II[a]
Hereditary				
MSH2, MLH1, PMS1, PMS2, MSH6	DNA repair	Mutation	5%	I
Sporadic				
Oncogenes				
HER2/neu	Tyrosine kinase	Amplification/overexpression	10%	II
K-*ras*	G-protein	Mutation	10%–30%	I/II
β-catenin	Transcription factor	Mutation	10%	I
c-*myc*	Transcription factor	Amplification/overexpression	20%–30%	?
FGFR2	Tyrosine kinase	Mutation	10%	I
PI3KCA	Tyrosine kinase	Amplification	20%–30%	I/II
Tumor-suppressor genes				
TP53	Transcription factor	Mutation/overexpression	20%	II
PTEN	Phosphatase	Mutation/deletion	40%	I
MLH1	Mismatch repair	Promoter methylation	10%–20%	I
CDC4	Cell cycle	Mutation/deletion	15%	II

[a]Type I = well-differentiated, endometrioid, estrogen-associated cancers; Type II = poorly differentiated, nonendometrioid cancers.

The frequency of aneuploidy is relatively low in endometrial cancers relative to ovarian cancers (80%). The differences in frequency of aneuploidy between endometrial and ovarian cancers correlate well with the disparate outcomes of these two diseases.

More recently, microarrays that measure the expression of all the genes in a cancer have been used to identify patterns that distinguish between normal and malignant endometrium and between various histologic types of endometrial cancer (181,184,185). This approach has the potential to complement studies of the individual oncogenes and tumor-suppressor genes reviewed below and to enhance understanding of the biology of endometrial cancer.

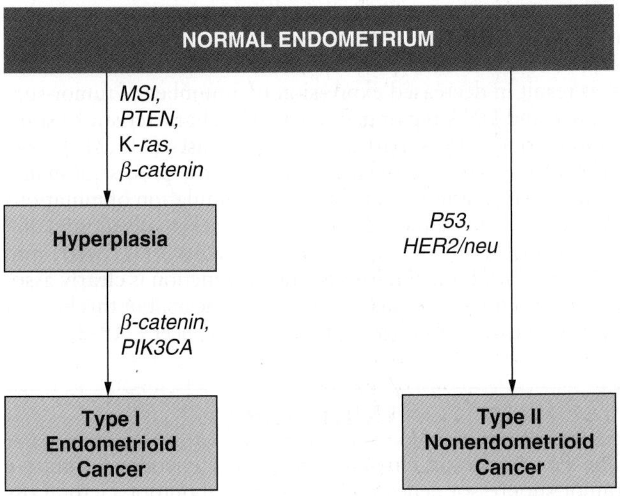

NORMAL ENDOMETRIUM

MSI,
PTEN,
K-*ras,*
β-catenin

Hyperplasia

β-catenin,
PIK3CA

Type I Endometrioid Cancer

P53,
HER2/neu

Type II Nonendometrioid Cancer

FIGURE 5.7. Molecular pathogenesis of type I and type II endometrial cancers.

Tumor-Suppressor Genes

TP53

Inactivation of the *TP53* tumor-suppressor gene is among the most frequent genetic events in endometrial cancers (186). The mechanisms of *TP53* inactivation were discussed in detail earlier in this chapter. Overexpression of mutant TPTP53 protein occurs in about 20% of endometrial adenocarcinomas and is associated with several known prognostic factors, including advanced stage, poor grade, and nonendometrioid histology (Fig. 5.8) (183,187). Overexpression occurs in about

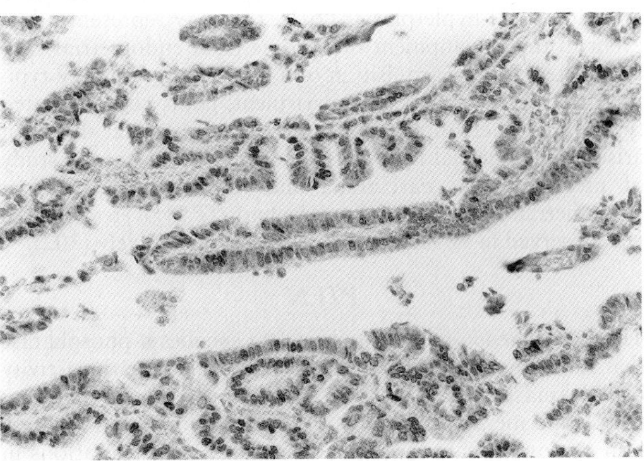

FIGURE 5.8. Overexpression of p53. About 50% of ovarian cancers and 20% of endometrial cancers have missense mutations in the p53 tumor-suppressor gene that result in protein products that are resistant to degradation. As is demonstrated in this endometrial cancer these mutant p53 proteins overaccumulate in the nucleus of the cell and can be visualized using immunohistochemistry.

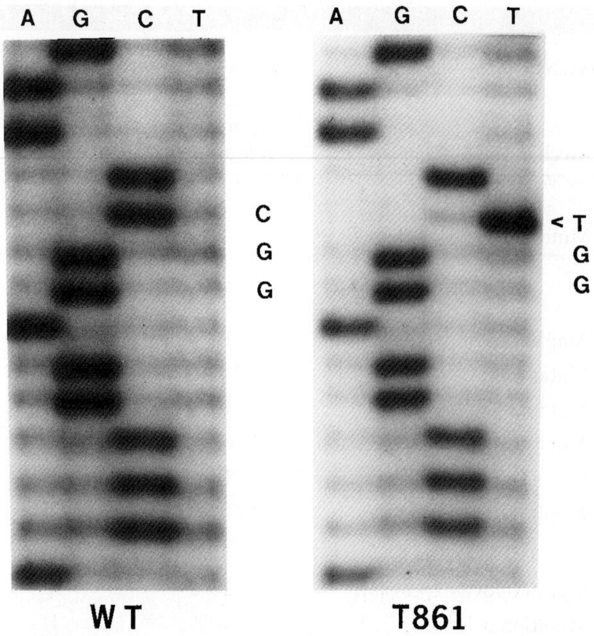

FIGURE 5.9. Mutation of the p53 gene. Endometrial cancer T861 has a missense mutation in codon 248 of the p53 gene that changes the sequence from CGG to TGG and results in the substitution of tryptophan for arginine. On the left is the normal wild-type (WT) sequence.

10% of stage I/II and 40% of stage III/IV cancers (187). Numerous studies have confirmed the strong association between *TP53* overexpression and other poor prognostic factors and decreased survival (188–194). In some of these studies, *TP53* overexpression has been associated with worse survival even after controlling for stage (195,196). This suggests that loss of *TP53* tumor-suppressor function confers a particularly virulent phenotype. Although little is known regarding molecular alterations in uterine sarcomas, overexpression of mutant *TP53* occurs in a majority of mixed mesodermal sarcomas of the uterus (74%) and in some leiomyosarcomas (197,198).

Endometrial cancers that overexpress *TP53* protein usually harbor missense mutations in exons 5 through 8 of the gene that result in amino acid substitutions in the protein (Fig. 5.9) (187,199,200). Most of these mutations lead to loss of DNA-binding activity. Because *TP53* mutations rarely, if ever, occur in endometrial hylperplasias (201), this may represent a late event in the development of endometrioid endometrial cancers. Alternatively, acquisition of a *TP53* mutation may typically lead to development of a virulent, poorly differentiated type II endometrioid cancer or serous cancer that does not arise in endometrial hyperplasia. In this regard, in one study of uterine serous carcinoma and its putative precursor (endometrial intraepithelial carcinoma), *TP53* overexpression was observed in 90% and 78% of cases, respectively (202).

PTEN

The *PTEN* gene on chromosome 10q encodes a phosphatase that functions as a tumor suppressor by opposing the activity of PI3 kinase, which is a lipid kinase involved in generating the second messenger PIP3 that in turn contributes to activation of downstream targets such as Akt (203). Mutations in the *PTEN* tumor-suppressor gene occur in about half of endometrial cancers (139–141), and this represents the most frequent genetic alteration described thus far in these cancers. Most of these mutations are deletions, insertions, and nonsense mutations that lead to truncated protein products, whereas only about 15% are missense mutations that change a single amino acid in the critical phosphatase domain. Loss of *PTEN* tumor-suppressor function generally also involves deletion of the second non-mutated copy of the gene.

Mutations in the *PTEN* gene are associated with endometrioid histology, early stage, and favorable clinical behavior (204). Well-differentiated, noninvasive cases have the highest frequency of mutations. In addition, *PTEN* mutations have been observed in 20% of endometrial hyperplasias, suggesting that this is an early event in the development of some type I endometrial cancers (205). It has been reported that loss of *PTEN* protein may occur in normal-appearing endometrial glands even before the emergence of hyperplasia, suggesting that this may be a critical initiating event in endometrial carcinogenesis (206,207).

Synchronous endometrioid cancers are sometimes encountered in the endometrium and ovary that are indistinguishable microscopically. In some of these cases, identical *PTEN* mutations have been identified, suggesting that the ovarian tumor represents a metastasis from the endometrium (208). In other cases, the *PTEN* mutation seen in the endometrial cancer was not found in the ovarian tumor, suggesting that these represent two distinct primary cancers. *PTEN* mutations have also been observed in about 20% of endometrioid ovarian cancers that arise in the absence of endometrial cancers (143).

DNA Mismatch Repair Genes

As noted in Chapter 2, about 3% to 5% of endometrial cancers occur in women with a strong hereditary predisposition due to germ-line mutations in DNA repair genes in the context of the HNPCC syndrome. Endometrial cancer is the second most common malignancy observed in women with HNPCC. Cancers that arise in these individuals are characterized by mutations in multiple microsatellite repeat sequences throughout the genome. Microsatellite instability also occurs in about 20% of sporadic endometrial cancers (209,210). Endometrial cancers that exhibit microsatellite instability tend to be type I cancers. Because microsatellite instability has been noted in some sporadic endometrial cancers in women who do not carry germ-line DNA repair gene mutations that cause HNPCC syndrome (209), several groups have attempted to identify acquired somatic mutations in these genes. DNA repair gene mutations have been identified in only a minority of endometrial cancers with microsatellite instability (70,211). Loss of mismatch repair in these cases appears to be most often due to silencing of the *MLH1* gene by way of promoter methylation (212,213). Methylation of the *MLH1* promoter has also been noted in endometrial hyperplasias (210,214) and normal endometrium adjacent to cancers, suggesting that this is an early event in the development of some of these cancers (215). It is thought that global changes in methylation that result in decreased expression of a number of tumor-suppressor and DNA repair genes may be a characteristic of some endometrial cancers, particularly type I cases (216,217). Loss of DNA mismatch repair may accelerate the process of malignant transformation by facilitating accumulation of mutations in microsatellite sequences present in genes involved in malignant transformation such as *PTEN, BAX, TGFβRII,* and *CASP5* (218). Loss of mismatch repair function is clearly associated with favorable survival in colon cancers, but this has not been a consistent finding in endometrial cancer (219–222).

Other Genes

The *Par-4* gene on chromosome 12q21 encodes a putative tumor-suppressor gene that acts as a proapoptotic factor. Loss of expression of this gene has been demonstrated in some human cancers, and mice in which Par-4 has been inactivated develop endometrial cancer. *Par-4* expression is lower in secretory than in proliferative endometrium. Reduced expression occurs in about 40% of endometrial cancers and may be attributable to methylation of the promoter region of the gene (223). Expression of *Par-4* was correlated with ER expression and microsatellite instability (MSI), but not with mutations in *PTEN*, *K-ras*, or β-*catenin*.

The *Cables* gene on chromosome 18q11–12 is a putative tumor suppressor involved in regulating phosphorylation of cyclin-dependent kinase 2 in a manner that restrains cell cycle progression. *Cables* mutant mice develop endometrial hyperplasia at an early age, and exposure to low levels of estrogen causes endometrial cancer (224). *Cables* expression is up-regulated by estrogen and decreases following progestin treatment. Loss of *Cables* expression also occurs in human endometrial hyperplasias and cancers.

Finally, mutations in the *CDC4* gene, which is involved in regulating cyclin E expression during cell cycle progression, have been noted in 16% of endometrial cancers (225). Mutations were accompanied by loss of the wild-type allele and were more common in cancers with poor prognostic factors such as high-grade and lymph-node metastases. It is postulated that *CDC4* may act as a tumor suppressor by restraining the activity of cyclin E in promoting progression from G_1 to S phase. An additional study failed to reproduce this finding. This study evaluated 73 endometrial cancers for hCDC4 mutation and was able to detect only a single case with a variant of uncertain significance (226). The frequency and significance of hCDC4 alterations in endometrial cancer are uncertain.

Oncogenes

HER2/neu/ERBB2

Alterations in oncogenes have been demonstrated in endometrial cancers, but these occur less frequently than inactivation of tumor-suppressor genes (Table 5.2). Increased expression of the *HER2/neu* receptor tyrosine kinase has been noted in about 10% of endometrial cancers (192,227–229) and is associated with advanced stage and poor outcome. In some studies, multivariate analysis revealed that high expression was an independent variable associated with poor survival (228,230). Serous endometrial cancers most frequently overexpress *HER2/neu* (231). In one study of 27 serous endometrial cancers, overexpression was seen in 70% of African American cases compared to 24% of Caucasian cases, and it was suggested that this may have contributed to an observed racial disparity in outcome (232). The levels of *HER2/neu* overexpression in endometrial cancers are much less striking than in breast cancers, but there have been isolated reports that Herceptin (anti-*HER2/neu* antibody) treatment is of therapeutic benefit in some endometrial cancers (233).

K-*ras* and *BRAF*

The *RAS* family of genes encodes cell-membrane-associated GTPases that frequently undergo point mutations in codons 12, 13, or 61 in many human cancers. These mutations produce constitutively activated oncogenic molecules. Initially, these codons of the K-*ras*, H-*ras*, and N-*ras* genes were examined in 11 immortalized endometrial cancer cell lines (234). Mutations in codon 12 of K-*ras* were seen in four cell lines, whereas three had mutations in codon 61 of H-*ras*. Subsequent studies of primary endometrial adenocarcinomas have confirmed that codon 12 of K-*ras* is mutated in about 10% of American cases and 20% of Japanese cases (235–242). These mutations occur more often, but not exclusively, in type I endometrial cancers. K-*ras* mutations have also been identified in some endometrial hyperplasias (236,242,243), which suggests that this may be a relatively early event in the development of some type I cancers.

The *BRAF* gene product acts downstream of K-*ras*, and also is frequently mutated in several types of cancers. Most reports have suggested that *BRAF* mutations are not a feature of endometrial hyperplasias or cancers (244,245). However, one paper from Japan found *BRAF* mutations in 21% of endometrial cancers and 11% of hyperplasias (246). These alterations were not found at locations proven to constitutively activate the BRAF protein. Furthermore, many were found in tumors with mismatch repair deficiency, suggesting that they may be passenger alterations. Evaluation of these "mutants" requires further study. It is also possible that these disparate findings may be due to differences between American and Japanese endometrial cancers, as has been noted with K-*ras* mutation frequency between these populations.

PI3KCA

As noted above, the *PTEN* tumor-suppressor gene, which normally acts to restrain PI3K activity, is frequently inactivated in type I endometrial cancers. Conversely, the *PI3KCA* gene is oncogenically activated in some cases. The catalytic subunit of *PI3K* (*PI3KCA*) is located on chromosome 3q26.3 and activating mutations in this gene have been described in several types of cancers. In an initial study, *PI3KCA* mutations were seen in 36% of endometrial cancers, and 24% of cases had mutations in both *PTEN* and *PI3KCA* (247). This suggested that there is an additive effect of two mutations in the same pathway. In a subsequent study, 39% of endometrial cancers and 7% of atypical endometrial hyperplasias were found to harbor mutations in *PI3KCA* (248). This study also implied that *PI3KCA* mutation occurred at the time of tumor invasion and could serve as a marker for invasion. As in the initial study, a high fraction of cases had mutations in both *PTEN* and *PI3KCA*. These and other studies confirm that PI3KCA activating mutations are common in endometrial cancers.

β-catenin

Alterations in a molecular pathway involving E-*cadherin*, *APC*, and β-*catenin*, the product of the *CTNNB1* gene, have been noted in some endometrial cancers. E-*cadherin* is a transmembrane glycoprotein involved in cell-cell adhesion, and its decreased expression in cancer cells is associated with increased invasiveness and metastatic potential. E-*cadherin* mutations occur only rarely in endometrial cancers (249), but cadherin expression may also be down-regulated in the absence of mutations (250,251). The cytoplasmic tail of E-*cadherin* exists as a macromolecular complex with the β-*catenin* and *APC* gene products, which link it to the cytoskeleton. It appears that a critical function of the *APC* tumor-suppressor gene is to regulate phosphorylation of serine and threonine residues (codons 33, 37, 41, 45) in exon 3 of β-*catenin*, which results in degradation of β-*catenin*. Mutational inactivation of *APC* allows accumulation of β-*catenin*, which translocates to the nucleus and acts as a transcription factor to induce expression of cyclin D1 and perhaps other genes involved in cell cycle progression (251). Germ-line *APC* mutations are responsible for the adenomatous polyposis coli syndrome, and somatic mutations are common in sporadic colon cancers, but *APC* mutations have not been described in endometrial cancers. The *APC* gene may be inactivated in some endometrial cancers owing to promoter methylation (252). In addition, it has been shown that missense mutations in exon 3 of *β-catenin* lead to the same end result—namely, abrogation of the ability of *APC* to induce β-*catenin* degradation, which results in abnormal transcriptional activity. In view of this, the β-*catenin* gene is considered an oncogene (253).

β-catenin can function as an oncogene in some endometrial cancers and is a key regulatory protein involved in canonical Wnt signaling. Disruptions in Wnt signaling have been implicated in numerous cancer types (254). In addition to the defects present in the gene itself, which lead to constitutive activity, epigenetic silencing of other negative regulators of this pathway has been observed. The complexities of Wnt signaling remain poorly understood; however, it appears that these additional defects in the pathway are related to an increased signaling cascade in the absence of key proteins that normally dampen the Wnt signal. Mutations in exon 3 of *β-catenin* have been observed in several types of cancers, including hepatocellular, prostatic, and endometrial cancers. Mutation of *β-catenin* occurs in about 10% to 15% of endometrial cancers, but abnormal accumulation of *β*-catenin protein occurs in about one third of cases, suggesting that mechanisms other than mutation might be involved in some cases (255,256). Mutation of *β-catenin* tends to be associated with type I endometrial cancers, and mutations have been noted in some endometrial hyperplasias (257).

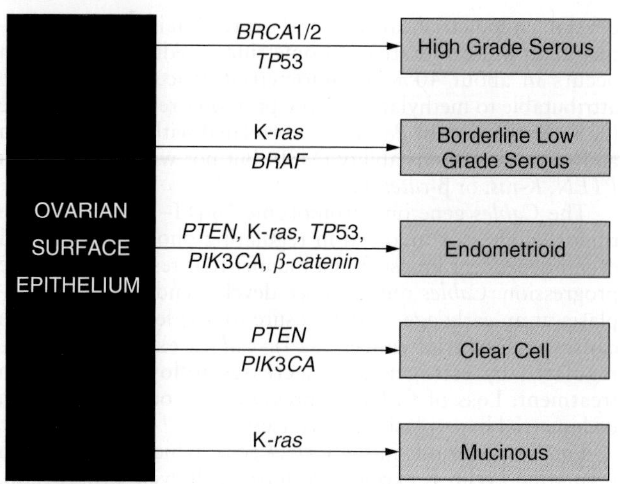

FIGURE 5.10. Molecular pathogenesis of different histological types of ovarian cancer.

FGFR2

Efforts designed to sequence kinase genes in human cancers identified mutations of fibroblast growth factor receptors (FGFRs) in some common epithelial cancers including ovarian cancer (258). The *FGFR2* gene encodes one of a family of tyrosine kinase growth factor receptors that receive signals from a large family of ligands. Recently, one study evaluated the *FGFR2* gene for activating mutations in a series of endometrial cancers (259). The study was initiated after the unbiased sequencing approach identified mutations in two endometrial cancer cell lines and one endometrial stromal sarcoma cell line. *FGFR2* mutations were subsequently identified in about 10% of endometrioid cancers. Mutations were found almost exclusively in cancers with endometrioid histology. There was no association with clinical outcome. Further studies will be needed to evaluate the significance of the identified mutations and other mechanisms of increased FGF signaling in endometrial cancer as well as any potential clinical utility by drug targeting of the receptor.

c-*myc*

Among nuclear transcription factors involved in stimulating proliferation, amplification of members of the *myc* family has most often been implicated in the development of human cancers. It has been shown that c-*myc* is expressed in normal endometrium (260) with higher expression in the proliferative phase. Several studies have suggested that *myc* may be amplified in a fraction of endometrial cancers (261–263).

OVARIAN CANCER

About 10% of ovarian cancers arise in women who carry germ-line mutations in cancer susceptibility genes—predominantly *BRCA1* or *BRCA2*, which are involved in repair of double-stranded DNA breakage. The vast majority of ovarian cancers is sporadic and arises due to accumulation of genetic alterations. The etiology of the molecular alterations involved in malignant transformation of the ovarian epithelium remains uncertain, and with the possible exception of talc, exogenous carcinogens have not been strongly implicated. Some mutations may arise spontaneously due to increased epithelial proliferation required to repair ovulatory defects. Oxidative stress and free-radical formation due to inflammation and repair at the ovulatory site may also contribute to accumulation of damage in cancer-causing genes.

Regardless of the mechanisms involved in causing genetic alterations, reproductive events that decrease lifetime ovulatory cycles (e.g., pregnancy and birth control pills) are strongly protective against ovarian cancer (264). The protective effect of these factors is greater in magnitude than one would predict based on the extent that ovulation is interrupted. Five years of oral contraceptive use provides a 50% risk reduction while only decreasing total years of ovulation by less than 20%. There is evidence to suggest that the progestagenic milieu of pregnancy and the pill might also protect against ovarian cancer by increasing apoptosis of ovarian epithelial cells, thereby cleansing the ovary of cells that have acquired genetic damage (265). The action of other reproductive hormones such as estrogens, androgens, and gonadotropins also may contribute to the development of ovarian cancers.

Epithelial ovarian cancers are heterogeneous with respect to behavior (borderline vs. invasive), histologic type (serous, mucinous, endometrioid, clear cell), stage, and outcome. These clinical and pathologic differences are reflected in diverse patterns of underlying genetic alterations (Fig 5.10). As our understanding of the molecular pathogenesis of ovarian cancer continues to mature, it is likely that the various disease subsets will increasingly be thought of as distinct entities that are defined by characteristic patterns of underlying epidemiologic risk factors, clinical features, and molecular signatures.

Global Genomic Changes

Invasive epithelial ovarian carcinoma is generally a monoclonal disease that develops as a clonal expansion of a single transformed cell in the ovary (266). There is evidence that some serous borderline tumors (229) as well as cancers that arise in the peritoneum of patients with *BRCA1* mutations may be polyclonal, however (267). Most ovarian cancers are characterized by a high degree of genetic damage that is manifest at the genomic and molecular levels. Gains and losses of various segments of the genome have been demonstrated using comparative genomic hybridization (CGH) (268). Likewise, loss of heterozygosity (LOH), indicative of deletion of specific genetic loci, also has been demonstrated to occur at a high frequency on many chromosomal arms (269). It is unclear whether the wide range of genetic alterations in ovarian cancers reflects the need to alter several genes in the process of malignant transformation or is the result of generalized genomic instability.

Both CGH and LOH studies have shown that advanced-stage, poorly differentiated cancers have a higher number of genetic changes than early-stage, low-grade cases (270–272). This finding could be interpreted as reflective of the fact that the number of genetic changes accumulates with progression from an early to an advanced cancer. Alternatively, advanced stage cancers may be intrinsically more virulent even at their early stages by virtue of their specific mutations and/or increased genomic instability. If this latter theory is correct, then early- and advanced-stage ovarian cancers could be thought of as different diseases rather than as steps in a progressive pathway. This could have significant implications for early diagnosis, treatment, and prevention of ovarian cancer.

It is estimated that the human genome contains about 25,000 genes. Recently, microarray chips that contain sequences complementary to the messenger RNAs of thousands of genes have been created that allow global assessment of gene expression. It is likely that levels of gene expression ascertained using microarrays are reflective of all the mechanisms that can affect expression, including amplification, deletion, and mutation, as well as changes in promoter methylation. Expression arrays have proven useful in predicting clinical phenotypes of various types of cancers. Several groups have applied expression array technology to the analysis of ovarian cancers. Many of these studies have compared gene expression between normal ovarian epithelial cells and ovarian cancers. Numerous genes have been identified that appear to be up- or down-regulated in the process of malignant transformation (273–275). In addition, microarrays have demonstrated patterns of gene expression that distinguish between invasive and borderline cases (276), histologic types (277), and early- and advanced-stage cases (275,278) and that predict survival (279,280). Although most of the changes in gene expression observed using microarrays are not reflective of oncogene or tumor-suppressor gene mutations, it has been shown that complex expression signatures reflective of specific oncogene alterations can be reliably ascertained (281).

Tumor-Suppressor Genes

TP53

Alteration of the *TP53* tumor-suppressor gene is the most frequent genetic event described thus far in ovarian cancers (Table 5.3) (40,282–287). The frequency of overexpression of mutant *TP53* is significantly higher in advanced-stage (40% to 60%) relative to early-stage cases (20%), but differences in frequencies of histologic types likely account for this difference. In this regard, about two thirds of early-stage serous ovarian cancers were found to have *TP53* mutations compared to only 21% of nonserous cases (288). The higher frequency of *TP53* alterations in advanced-stage cases may indicate that this is a "late event" in ovarian carcinogenesis. Alternatively, it is possible that loss of *TP53* confers an aggressive phenotype associated with more rapid progression. There

TABLE 5.3

GENETIC ALTERATIONS IN EPITHELIAL OVARIAN CANCERS

	Class	Mechanism	Approximate frequency	Comments
Hereditary				
BRCA1	Double-stranded DNA repair	Mutation/deletion	6%	Breast/ovarian syndrome
BRCA2	Double-stranded DNA repair	Mutation/deletion	3%	Breast/ovarian syndrome
MSH2/MLH1	DNA mismatch repair	Mutation/deletion	1%	HNPCC syndrome
Sporadic				
Oncogenes				
HER2/neu	Tyrosine kinase	Amplification/overexpression	5%–10%	Gene amplification rare
K-*ras*	G-protein	Mutation	20%–30%	Mostly serous borderline
BRAF	Serine/threonine kinase	Mutation	10%–20%	Serous borderline only
AKT2	Serine/threonine kinase	Amplification	5%–10%	
PI3KCA	Tyrosine kinase	Amplification	5%–10%	
c-myc	Transcription factor	Amplification/overexpression	20%–30%	
β-catenin	Transcription factor	Mutation	30%	Endometrioid only Type I
Tumor-suppressor genes				
TP53	Transcription factor	Mutation/deletion	50%–70%	Most common in invasive
p16	CDK inhibitor	Deletion, promoter methylation	15%	
p21, p27	CDK inhibitor	Promoter methylation	10%–40%	
BRCA1	Double-stranded DNA repair	Promoter methylation	10%	
CCNE (cyclin E)	Cyclin-dependent kinase	Overexpression	40%	

CDK, cyclin-dependent kinase; HNPCC, hereditary nonpolyposis colorectal cancer.

is a suggestion that overexpression of mutant TP53 protein may be associated with slightly worse survival in advanced-stage ovarian cancers (282–284,286,287,289–291). Finally, although there is a high concordance between *TP53* missense mutations in exons 5 through 8 and protein overexpression, about 20% of advanced ovarian cancers contain mutations that result in truncated protein products, which usually are not overexpressed (40,291). Some of these mutations may lie outside of exons 5 through 8. Overall, about 70% of advanced ovarian cancers have either missense or truncation mutations in the *TP53* gene. Most *TP53* missense mutations are transitions rather than transversions (292,293), which suggests that these mutations occur spontaneously, rather than due to exogenous carcinogens.

It has been postulated that loss of functional *TP53* might confer a chemoresistant phenotype because of its role in chemotherapy-induced apoptosis. In this regard, several studies have examined the correlation between chemosensitivity and *TP53* mutation in ovarian cancers *in vitro* (294–299). Some have suggested a relationship between *TP53* mutation and loss of chemosensitivity, but in other equally valid studies such a relationship has not been observed. It is likely that the status of the *TP53* gene is just one of a multitude of factors that determines chemosensitivity.

Overexpression of *TP53* is rare in stage I serous borderline tumors, but occurs in as many as 20% of advanced-stage borderline cases (300,301). In a study of advanced serous borderline tumors, *TP53* overexpression was associated with a sixfold higher risk of death (301). In some cases, invasive serous cancers may arise following an earlier diagnosis of borderline tumor. It has been shown that *TP53* mutational status was not concordant between the original borderline tumor and the subsequent invasive cancer (302). This suggests that the invasive cancer either arises independently or as a clonal outgrowth within the original tumor.

Rb Gene

Although mutations in the *Rb* tumor-suppressor gene are not a common feature of ovarian cancers, evidence suggests that inactivation of *Rb* greatly enhances tumor formation in ovarian cells with p53 mutations (303). In a mouse model in which these genes were inactivated in the ovarian epithelium, few cancers developed in response to loss of either p53 or *Rb* alone. When both genes were inactivated, epithelial ovarian cancers with serous features developed in almost all cases. Given that *Rb* mutations are rare in ovarian cancers, it is possible that inactivation of one of a number of genes in the *Rb* pathway can initiate transformation cooperatively with *TP53*. Inactivation of *Rb* itself may not be requisite. This mouse model of ovarian cancer has the potential to add greatly to our understanding of epithelial ovarian carcinogenesis. A notable feature of this model is the development of dysplastic premalignant epithelium. Although ovarian dysplasia has long been thought to represent the precursor of serous ovarian cancers (304) and is an appealing target for early detection and prevention (305), the inaccessibility of the ovaries has presented a significant obstacle to studying its natural history. The ability to track the development of preinvasive and invasive lesions in this new mouse model presents the opportunity to develop chemoprevention approaches in a setting that appears similar to human ovarian carcinogenesis.

Cyclin-Dependent Kinase Inhibitors

The cyclin-dependent kinase (CDK) inhibitors act as tumor suppressors by virtue of their inhibition of cell cycle progression from G_1 to S phase. Expression of several CDK inhibitors appears to be decreased in some ovarian cancers. The *CDKN2A* (p16) gene undergoes homozygous deletions in about 15% of ovarian cancers (306). There is evidence to suggest that p16 (307), *CDKN2B* (p15) (308), and some other tumor-suppressor genes such as *BRCA1* (83,84,309) may be inactivated via transcriptional silencing due to promoter methylation rather than mutation and/or deletion. Likewise, decreased expression of the CDK inhibitor *CDKN1A* (p21) has been noted in a significant fraction of ovarian cancers despite the absence of inactivating mutations (310,311), and in some studies has been associated with poor survival (312). Loss of *CDKN1B* (p27) also may occur and correlates with poor survival in some studies (313–316). It has been suggested that abberant expression of p27 in the cytoplasm may be most associated with poor outcome (317).

Other Genes

The TGF-β pathway is believed to play an important role in suppression of proliferation and malignant transformation. Normal ovarian epithelial cells are inhibited by the growth inhibitory peptide TGF-β, whereas some ovarian cancers are unresponsive (318,319). There is some evidence that mutations may occur in cell surface TGF-β receptors or in the *Smad* family of genes that are involved in downstream signaling (320), but in other studies these signaling pathways have been found to be intact (319).

A number of other genes involved in inhibiting proliferation that are not inactivated by mutation and/or deletion may be silenced due to methylation of their promoters. Examples include the *ARHI* gene on chromosome 1p31 and the *ARLTS1* gene on 13q14 (321,322).

Oncogenes

HER2/neu

Normal and malignant ovarian epithelial cells produce and respond to various peptide growth factors such as epidermal growth factor (323), insulin-like growth factors (324), platelet-derived growth factor (325), and fibroblast growth factors (326–328). Production of these growth-accelerating peptides appears to be increased during carcinogenesis. These growth factors interact with membrane-spanning tyrosine kinase receptors. The only one of these receptor tyrosine kinases convincingly shown to be activated in some ovarian cancers is HER2/neu.

About 30% of breast cancers express increased levels of HER2/neu (162), often as a result of gene amplification. Overexpression of HER2/neu in breast cancer has been associated with poor survival. Expression of HER2/neu is increased in a fraction of ovarian cancers (Fig. 5.11) and overexpression has been associated with poor survival in some studies (162,329), but ovarian cancers that exhibit HER2/neu overexpression rarely have high-level gene amplification. Monoclonal antibodies that bind to HER2/neu can decrease growth of ovarian cancer cell lines that overexpress this receptor (330). Anti-HER2/neu antibody therapy (Herceptin) has demonstrated efficacy in the treatment of breast cancer and is often administered in concert with paclitaxel (331). In a Gynecologic Oncology Group (GOG) study, only 11% of ovarian cancers exhibited significant HER2/neu overexpression (332). The response rate to single-agent Herceptin therapy was disappointingly low (7.3%), but perhaps some benefit may be found in the future using combination regimens that also include taxanes or other cytotoxics.

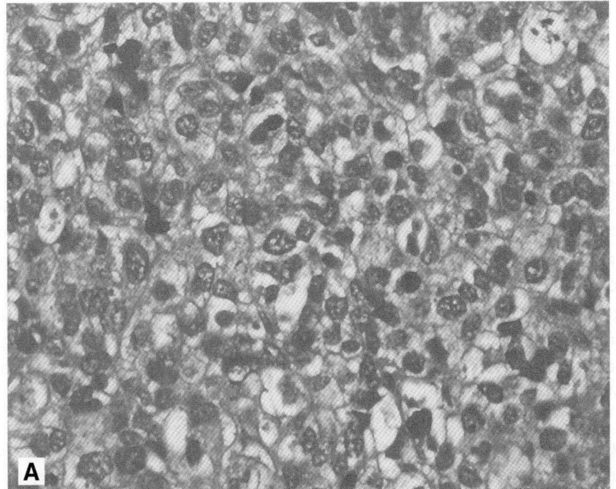

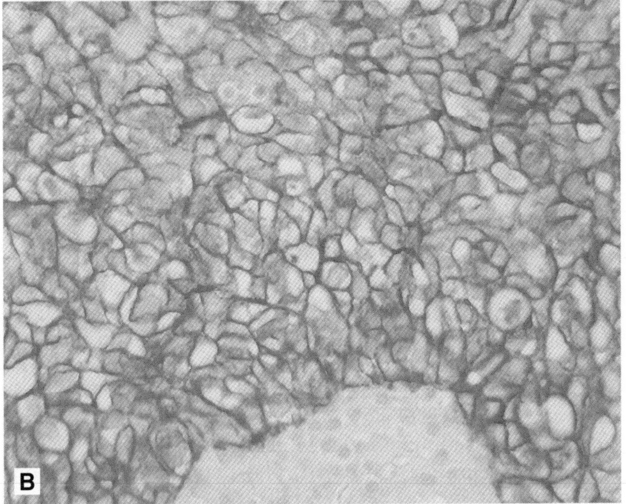

FIGURE 5.11. Overexpression of HER2/neu in ovarian cancer. **A:** Serous ovarian cancer. **B:** Immunostaining for HER2/neu demonstrates intense cell membrane staining indicative of overexpression.

K-*ras* and *BRAF*

Activating mutations in codons 12 and 13 of the K-*ras* gene are rare in invasive serous ovarian cancers (333–335). Some types of cancers that lack K-*ras* mutations have activating mutations in codon 599 of the downstream *BRAF* gene, but this is not the case in serous ovarian cancers. In contrast, K-*ras* mutations are common in borderline serous ovarian tumors, occurring in about 25% to 50% of cases (336,337). In addition, mutations in *BRAF* occur in about 20% of serous borderline cases lacking K-*ras* mutations (338). Mutations in K-*ras* and *BRAF* have also been noted in cystadenoma epithelium adjacent to serous borderline tumors, suggesting that this is an early event in their development (339). K-*ras* mutations have been noted in about 50% of mucinous ovarian cancers, but *BRAF* mutations have not been found (340). These findings highlight the distinct differences in the molecular pathology between various histologic types and between borderline tumors and invasive ovarian cancers.

PI3KCA and *AKT2*

Similar to endometrial cancers, activation of the *PI3KCA* and *AKT2* oncogenes occurs in some ovarian cancers. The region of chromosome 3p26 that includes the phosphatidylinositol 3-kinase (*PI3KCA*) is amplified in some ovarian cancers (341). In addition, activating mutations in *PI3KCA* occur in about 10% of ovarian cancers, and are much more common in endometrioid and clear cell cancers (20%) compared to serous cancers (2%) (342). Likewise, the *AKT2* serine/threonine kinase that is downstream of *PI3KCA* also has been shown to be amplified and overexpressed in some ovarian cancers (343). *PI3KCA* and *AKT2* kinase activity is opposed by the *PTEN* phosphatase, and this tumor-suppressor gene also is inactivated in about 20% of endometrioid ovarian cancers (344).

β-catenin

As noted previously, mutations in the *β-catenin* gene are a feature of some endometrial cancers. Similarly, *β-catenin* mutations are present in about 30% of endometrioid ovarian cancers (345), but not other histologic types. This provides further evidence of the molecular heterogeneity of the various histologic types of ovarian cancer. In some endometrioid ovarian cancers with abnormal nuclear accumulation of β-catenin that lack mutations, the *APC*, *AXIN1*, or *AXIN2* genes that regulate β-catenin activity were found to be mutated (345). This suggests that alterations in this wnt signaling pathway are a feature of endometrioid ovarian cancers. Mouse models in which the wnt and the PIK3/*PTEN* pathways are inactivated in the ovarian epithelium lead to the development of endometrioid cancer and endometriosis (346,347).

c-*myc*

Increased activity of nuclear transcription factors also may enhance malignant transformation. In this regard, amplification of the c-*myc* oncogene has been reported to occur in some ovarian cancers. Several studies have suggested that the c-*myc* gene is amplified in about 30% of cases, although high-level amplification is rare (348–350). Despite these reports of gene amplification, evidence of c-*myc* protein overexpression has been less convincing.

CCNE (Cyclin E)

Cell cycle progression factors may also exert an oncogenic effect when overactive. In this regard, some ovarian cancers have been reported to show increased expression of cyclin E, which is involved in cell cycle progression from G_1 to S phase. In a study of advanced-stage suboptimally debulked ovarian cancers treated on GOG protocols, high cyclin E expression was associated with a 6-month decrease in median survival (351). In some, but not all, cases, amplification of the cyclin *E* gene was found to be the underlying cause of overexpression. In a large study using a tissue microarray, cyclin E overexpression has been shown to be associated with serous/clear cell histology, advanced stage, and poor outcome (352).

Other Genes

Global genomic approaches such as CGH have also suggested the presence of amplified genes in other chromosomal regions in some ovarian cancers. An amplicon on chromosome 11q13 results in amplification of *Cyclin D1* and/or the *BRCA2* interacting protein *EMSY* in some cases (353). Likewise, the Notch3 gene on chromosome 19p13, the Aurora-A kinase on 20q13, and eIF-5A2 on 3q26 also may be targets for amplification (354–356).

Large-scale sequencing of 518 protein kinases was performed on a panel of human cancers, including 25 ovarian cancers (258). Although the analysis did not detect a gene or genes with high prevalence of mutation, several genes were mutated infrequently in ovarian cancers including *CDKL2*, *CDKL5*, *STK36*, and *TRRAP*. The investigators performed more sequencing on additional ovarian cancers and did not find widespread alteration in these genes. Interestingly, this screen identified a single *FGFR2* mutation in 25 ovarian cancers. There were only two endometrioid histology ovarian cancers among the 25 sequenced. Given the high similarity of mutation and histologic appearance of endometrioid ovarian cancer and endometrioid endometrial cancer, it seems possible that a low frequency of *FGFR2* mutations will be found in endometrioid ovarian cancers.

Ovarian cancer ascites also contain lipid factors such as lysophosphatidic acid (LPA) that stimulate proliferation and invasiveness of ovarian cancer cells (357). The edg-2 G-protein–coupled receptors act as functional receptors for LPA. It also has been shown that LPA induces the *Groα* gene that acts to stimulate proliferation (358). The finding that neutralization of LPA activity decreases growth and increases apoptosis of ovarian cancers suggests that manipulation of this pathway may be therapeutically beneficial (359).

CERVICAL CANCER

Cervical cancer is the most common gynecologic malignancy worldwide and accounts for over 400,000 cases annually. Molecular and epidemiologic studies have demonstrated that sexually transmitted human papillomavirus (HPV) infections play a role in almost all cervical dysplasias and cancers (360). HPV infection is also involved in the development of dysplasias and cancers of the vagina and vulva. The peak incidence of HPV infection is in the 20s and 30s and the incidence of cervical cancer increases from the 20s to a plateau between age 40 and 50. Although HPV plays a major role in the development of most cervical cancers, only a small minority of women who are infected develop invasive cervical cancer. This suggests that other genetic alterations and/or environmental factors also are involved in cervical carcinogenesis. For example, individuals who are immunosuppressed, either due to HIV infection (361) or immunosuppressive drugs, are more likely to develop dysplasia and invasive cervical cancer following HPV infection.

Cervical screening programs in developed nations dramatically reduced both the incidence of invasive cervical cancer and disease-related mortality in the 20th century. The recent development of vaccines against oncogenic HPV subtypes promises to further decrease the incidence of cervical dysplasia and cancer. Although cervical cancer mortality is now low in the United States and Western Europe, it remains among the leading causes of cancer deaths in women in underdeveloped nations. Complete eradication of cervical cancer through screening and prevention strategies that are based on an understanding of HPV biology may be within reach in the 21st century.

Human Papillomavirus Infection

There are over 80 HPV subtypes, but not all infect the lower genital tract. HPV-16 and -18 are the most common types associated with cervical cancer, and are found in over 80% of cases. Types 31, 33, 35, 39, 45, 51, 52, 56, 58, 59, 68, 73, and 82 should be considered high-risk types, and types 26, 53, and 66 should be considered probably carcinogenic (360). Low-risk types that may cause dysplasias or condyloma in the lower genital tract, but rarely cause cancers, include types 6, 11, 40, 42, 43, 44, 54, 61, 70, 72, and 81. The advent of HPV typing now allows assessment of whether patients carry high-risk or low-risk HPV types and this has proven to be clinically useful in the management of patients with low-grade Pap smear abnormalities.

The HPV DNA sequence consists of 7,800 nucleotides divided into "early" and "late" open reading frames (ORFs). Early ORFs are within the first 4,200 nucleotides of the genome and encode proteins (E1–E8) important in viral replication and cellular transformation. Late ORFs (L1 and L2) are found within the latter half of the sequence and encode structural proteins of the virion. In oncogenic subtypes like HPV-16 and -18, transformation may be accompanied by integration of episomal HPV DNA into the host genome. Opening of the episomal viral genome usually occurs in the E1/E2 region, resulting in a linear fragment for insertion. The location of the opening may be significant since E2 acts as a repressor of the E6/E7 promotor, and disruption of E2 can lead to unregulated expression of the E6/E7 transforming genes. HPV-16 DNA may be found in its episomal form in some cervical cancers, however, and unregulated E6/E7 transcription may occur independent of viral DNA integration into the cellular genome.

Examination of the biological effects of HPV-encoded proteins has shed light on the mechanisms of HPV-associated transformation. Expression of the E4 transcript results in the production of intermediate filaments that colocalize with cytokeratins. E4 proteins of oncogenic subtypes disrupt the cytoplasmic cytokeratin matrix, whereas those of nononcogenic strains do not. It has been suggested that this may facilitate the release of HPV particles in oncogenic subtypes such as HPV-16. The E5 oncogene encodes a 44 amino acid protein that usually forms dimmers within the cellular membrane. The transforming properties of E5 appear to involve potentiation of membrane-bound epidermal growth factor receptors or platelet-derived growth factor receptors. HPV E2 proteins are thought to cause a mitotic block that leads to genomic instability.

The E6 and E7 oncoproteins are the main transforming genes of oncogenic strains of HPV (Fig. 5.12) (362). Transfection of these genes *in vitro* results in immortalization and transformation of some cell lines. The HPV E7 protein acts primarily by binding to and inactivating the retinoblastoma (Rb) tumor-suppressor gene product. E7 contains two domains, one of which mediates binding to Rb while the other serves as a substrate for casein kinase II (CKII) phosphorylation. Variations in oncogenic potential between HPV subtypes may be related to differences in the binding efficacy of E7 to Rb. High-risk HPV types contain E7 oncoproteins that bind Rb with more affinity than E7 from low-risk types. The transforming activity of E7 may be increased by CKII mutation, implying a role for this binding site in the development of HPV-mediated neoplasias. The E6 proteins of oncogenic HPV subtypes bind to and inactivate the *TP53* tumor-suppressor gene product (363,364). There is also a correlation between oncogenicity of various HPV strains and the ability of their E6 oncoproteins to inactivate *TP53*. Inactivation of Rb and *TP53* by E6/E7

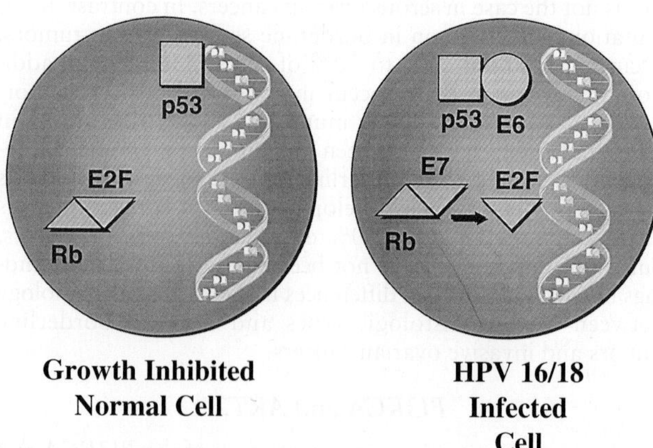

FIGURE 5.12. Role of p53 and Rb genes in cervical carcinogenesis. The HPV-16/18 E6 and E7 proteins inactivate the p53 and Rb genes, respectively.

circumvents the need for mutational inactivation of these key growth regulatory genes. HPV-negative cervical cancers are uncommon, but have been reported to exhibit overexpression of mutant *TP53* protein (365). This suggests that inactivation of the *TP53* tumor-suppressor gene either by HPV E6 or by mutation is a requisite event in cervical carcinogenesis. In some studies, the levels of E6 and E7 in invasive cervical cancers have been found to predict outcome, whereas HPV viral load does not (366).

Genomic Changes

Comparative genomic hybridization techniques have been used to identify chromosomal loci that are either increased or decreased in copy number in cervical cancers. A strikingly consistent finding of various studies is the high frequency of gains on chromosome 3q in both squamous cell cancers (367–370) and adenocarcinomas (371). Other chromosomes that exhibit frequent gains include 1q and 11q. The most common areas of chromosomal loss include chromosomes 3p and 2q. For the most part, with the exception of the *FHIT* gene on chromosome 3p, it has not been proven that these genomic gains and losses result in the recruitment of specific oncogenes and tumor-suppressor genes in the process of malignant transformation. It is conceivable that these chromosomal alterations may be frequent sequelae of infection with oncogenic HPVs while playing no significant role in the pathogenesis of cervical cancers. Abnormalities seen in invasive cancers using comparative genomic hybridization also have been identified in high-grade dysplasias, however, suggesting that these are early events in cervical carcinogenesis (368,369,372).

Oncogenes and Tumor-Suppressor Genes

Only a small fraction of HPV-infected women develop cervical cancer. This suggests that additional genetic alterations are requisite for progression to high-grade dysplasia and cancer, but little is known regarding these events. Allele loss suggestive of involvement of tumor-suppressor genes has been noted at loci on chromosomes 3p, 11p, and others, but alterations in specific genes remain elusive. Interestingly, the cyclin-dependent kinase inhibitor p16 is strikingly up-regulated in almost all cervical dysplasias and cancers (373). Clinical trials are ongoing to determine whether this will represent a useful adjunct to improve the positive predictive value of high-risk HPV testing for detection of cervical dysplasia.

The role of several oncogenes has been examined in cervical carcinomas. Although the epidermal growth factor receptor gene is amplified and overexpressed in some squamous cell cancers that arise in the aerodigestive tract, this is not observed in cervical cancers (374). Mutant *ras* genes are capable of cooperating with HPV in transforming cells *in vitro*. There is some evidence that mutations in either K-*ras* or H-*ras* may play a role in a subset of cervical cancers (365,375–378). Alterations in *ras* genes have not been seen in cervical intraepithelial neoplasia, suggesting that mutation of *ras* is a late event in the pathogenesis of some cervical cancers. In contrast, c-*myc* amplification and overexpression may be an early event in the development of some cervical cancers (379). Overexpression of c-*myc* has been demonstrated in one third of early invasive carcinomas and some CIN 3 lesions, but not in normal cervical epithelium or lower grade dysplasia. It has been reported that overexpression of c-*myc* gene may be due to amplification of the gene (4- to 20-fold) in some cases. In some studies, amplification correlated with poor prognosis in early-stage cases (380). Other studies have not confirmed the finding of amplification of c-*myc* in cervical cancers, however. Integration of the HPV genome near c-*myc* on chromosome 8q may lead to increased expression due to enhanced transcription of the gene rather than amplification. Further studies are needed to clarify the role of *ras* genes, c-*myc*, and other oncogenes in cervical carcinogenesis.

The fragile histidine triad (*FHIT*) gene localized within human chromosomal band 3p14.2 is frequently deleted in many different cancers, including cervical cancer (381–383). Decreased expression of this putative tumor-suppressor gene is an early event in some cervical cancers (383,384). In one study, FHIT protein expression was markedly reduced or absent in 71% of invasive cancers, 52% of high-grade squamous intraepithelial lesions (HSILs) associated with invasive cancer, and 21% of HSILs without associated invasive cancer (383). In addition, reduced expression is associated with poor prognosis in advanced cervical cancers (385).

As is the case in endometrial and ovarian cancers, it is thought that gene silencing due to promoter hypermethylation also may play a role in cervical carcinogenesis (386,387). In this regard, the *RASSF1A* gene is located on chromosome 3p21.3 in an area that is frequently the site of deletions in cervical cancer. The function of this gene is not completely understood, but is thought to be involved in *ras*-mediated signal transduction pathways. Although mutations in *RASSF1A* do not occur in cervical cancers, inactivation of the gene due to promoter methylation occurs in a fraction of cases, particularly adenocarcinomas (388,389).

Molecular analyses can readily be performed using cell pellets obtained from liquid-based Pap smears. This promises to facilitate future investigation of the role of promoter methylation and other alterations in the molecular pathogenesis of cervical cancer (390,391).

GESTATIONAL TROPHOBLASTIC DISEASE

The genetic alterations that underlie gestational trophoblastic disease have been elucidated to a great extent. The most prominent feature of these tumors is an imbalance of parental chromosomes. In the case of partial moles this involves an extra haploid copy of one set of paternal chromosomes, while complete moles generally are characterized by two complete haploid sets of paternal chromosomes and an absence of maternal chromosomes. Although the risk of repeat molar pregnancy is only about 1%, women who have had two molar pregnancies have about a 25% risk of developing another mole. Although this suggests a hereditary defect that affects gametogenesis, this remains speculative. Thus far there is no convincing evidence that damage to specific tumor-suppressor genes or oncogenes contributes to the development of gestational trophoblastic disease.

References

1. Bishop JM. Cancer: the rise of the genetic paradigm. *Genes Dev* 1995;9:1309–1315.
2. Virchow R. *Die Cellularpathologie in Ihrer Begrundung auf Physiologiche and Pathologiche Gewebslehre*; 1858.
3. Boveri T. *Zur Frage der Entstehung Maligner Tumoren*. Jena: Verlag von Gustav Fischer; 1914.
4. Nowell PC, Hungerford DA. A minute chromosome in human chronic granulocytic leukemia. *Science* 1960;132:1497.
5. Nowell PC. The clonal evolution of tumor cell populations. *Science* 1976;194:23–28.
6. Stehelin D, Varmus HE, Bishop JM, et al. DNA related to the transforming gene(s) of avian sarcoma viruses is present in normal avian DNA. *Nature* 1976;260:170–173.
7. Spector DH, Varmus HE, Bishop JM. Nucleotide sequences related to the transforming gene of avian sarcoma virus are present in DNA of uninfected vertebrates. *Proc Natl Acad Sci USA* 1978;75:4102–4106.

8. Rowley JD. Letter: a new consistent chromosomal abnormality in chronic myelogenous leukaemia identified by quinacrine fluorescence and Giemsa staining. *Nature* 1973;243:290–293.
9. Heisterkamp N, Stephenson JR, Groffen J, et al. Localization of the c-ab1 oncogene adjacent to a translocation break point in chronic myelocytic leukaemia. *Nature* 1983;306:239–242.
10. Druker BJ, Talpaz M, Resta DJ, et al. Efficacy and safety of a specific inhibitor of the BCR-ABL tyrosine kinase in chronic myeloid leukemia. *N Engl J Med* 2001;344:1031–1037.
11. Vogelstein B, Kinzler KW. The multistep nature of cancer. *Trends Genet* 1993;9:138–141.
12. Hanahan D, Weinberg RA. The hallmarks of cancer. *Cell* 2000;100: 57–70.
13. Hofstra RM, Landsvater RM, Ceccherini I, et al. A mutation in the RET proto-oncogene associated with multiple endocrine neoplasia type 2B and sporadic medullary thyroid carcinoma. *Nature* 1994;367:375–376.
14. Schmidt L, Duh FM, Chen F, et al. Germline and somatic mutations in the tyrosine kinase domain of the MET proto-oncogene in papillary renal carcinomas. *Nat Genet* 1997;16:68–73.
15. Kinzler KW, Vogelstein B. Cancer-susceptibility genes. Gatekeepers and caretakers. *Nature* 1997;386:761.
16. Loeb LA. A mutator phenotype in cancer. *Cancer Res* 2001;61:3230–3239.
17. Foulds L. *Neoplastic Development.* London: Academic Press; 1969.
18. Lengauer C, Kinzler KW, Vogelstein B. Genetic instabilities in human cancers. *Nature* 1998;396:643–649.
19. Fearon ER, Vogelstein B. A genetic model for colorectal tumorigenesis. *Cell* 1990;61:759–767.
20. Charles DR, Luce-Clausen EM. The kinetics of papilloma formation in benzpyrene-treated mice. *Cancer Res* 1942;2:261–263.
21. Harris H, Miller OJ, Klein G, et al. Suppression of malignancy by cell fusion. *Nature* 1969;223:363–368.
22. Knudson AG. Two genetic hits (more or less) to cancer. *Nat Rev Cancer* 2001;1:157–162.
23. Friend SH, Bernards R, Rogelj S, et al. A human DNA segment with properties of the gene that predisposes to retinoblastoma and osteosarcoma. *Nature* 1986;323:643–646.
24. Haber DA, Housman DE. Rate-limiting steps: the genetics of pediatric cancers. *Cell* 1991;64:5–8.
25. Greenblatt MS, Bennett WP, Hollstein M, et al. Mutations in the p53 tumor suppressor gene: clues to cancer etiology and molecular pathogenesis. *Cancer Res* 1994;54:4855–4878.
26. Cavenee WK, Dryja TP, Phillips RA, et al. Expression of recessive alleles by chromosomal mechanisms in retinoblastoma. *Nature* 1983;305:779–784.
27. Bartek J, Bartkova J, Lukas J. The retinoblastoma protein pathway in cell cycle control and cancer. *Exp Cell Res* 1997;237:1–6.
28. Fischer PM, Endicott J, Meijer L. Cyclin-dependent kinase inhibitors. *Prog Cell Cycle Res* 2003;5:235–248.
29. Milde-Langosch K, Riethdorf S. Role of cell-cycle regulatory proteins in gynecologic cancer. *J Cell Physiol* 2003;196:224–244.
30. Bell DW, Varley JM, Szydlo TE, et al. Heterozygous germ line hCHK2 mutations in Li-Fraumeni syndrome. *Science* 1999;286:2528–2531.
31. Meijers-Heijboer H, van den OA, Klijn J, et al. Low-penetrance susceptibility to breast cancer due to CHEK2(*)1100delC in noncarriers of *BRCA1* or *BRCA2* mutations. *Nat Genet* 2002;31:55–59.
32. Lane DP, Crawford LV. T antigen is bound to a host protein in SV40-transformed cells. *Nature* 1979;278:261–263.
33. Linzer DI, Levine AJ. Characterization of a 54K dalton cellular SV40 tumor antigen present in SV40-transformed cells and uninfected embryonal carcinoma cells. *Cell* 1979;17:43–52.
34. Finlay CA, Hinds PW, Levine AJ. The p53 proto-oncogene can act as a suppressor of transformation. *Cell* 1989;57:1083–1093.
35. Baker SJ, Markowitz S, Fearon ER, et al. Suppression of human colorectal carcinoma cell growth by wild- type p53. *Science* 1990;249:912–915.
36. Chen PL, Chen YM, Bookstein R, et al. Genetic mechanisms of tumor suppression by the human p53 gene. *Science* 1990;250:1576–1580.
37. Baker SJ, Fearon ER, Nigro JM, et al. Chromosome 17 deletions and p53 gene mutations in colorectal carcinomas. *Science* 1989;244:217–221.
38. Hollstein M, Sidransky D, Vogelstein B, Harris CC. p53 mutations in human cancers. *Science* 1991;253:49–53.
39. Cho Y, Gorina S, Jeffrey PD, et al. Crystal structure of a p53 tumor suppressor-DNA complex: understanding tumorigenic mutations. *Science* 1994;265:346–355.
40. Casey G, Lopez ME, Ramos JC, et al. DNA sequence analysis of exons 2 through 11 and immunohistochemical staining are required to detect all known p53 alterations in human malignancies. *Oncogene* 1996;13:1971–1981.
41. Levine AJ. p53, the cellular gatekeeper for growth and division. *Cell* 1997;88: 323–331.
42. Oren M. Regulation of the p53 tumor suppressor protein. *J Biol Chem* 1999;274:36031–36034.
43. Vogelstein B, Lane D, Levine AJ. Surfing the p53 network. *Nature* 2000;408: 307–310.
44. Bunz F, Dutriaux A, Lengauer C, et al. Requirement for p53 and p21 to sustain G2 arrest after DNA damage. *Science* 1998;282:1497–1501.
45. Sherr CJ, McCormick F. The RB and p53 pathways in cancer. *Cancer Cell* 2002;2:103–112.
46. Lynch HT, Smyrk T. Hereditary nonpolyposis colorectal cancer (Lynch syndrome). An updated review. *Cancer* 1996;78:1149–1167.
47. Watson P, Lynch HT. Extracolonic cancer in hereditary nonpolyposis colorectal cancer. *Cancer* 1993;71:677–685.
48. Watson P, Vasen HF, Mecklin JP, et al. The risk of endometrial cancer in hereditary nonpolyposis colorectal. *Cancer Am J Med* 1994;96: 516–520.
49. Aarnio M, Mecklin JP, Aaltonen LA, et al. Life-time risk of different cancers in hereditary non-polyposis colorectal cancer (HNPCC) syndrome. *Int J Cancer* 1995;64:430–433.
50. Vasen HF, Wijnen JT, Menko FH, et al. Cancer risk in families with hereditary nonpolyposis colorectal cancer diagnosed by mutation analysis. *Gastroenterology* 1996;110:1020–1027.
51. Dunlop MG, Farrington SM, Carothers AD, et al. Cancer risk associated with germline DNA mismatch repair gene mutations. *Hum Mol Genet* 1997;6:105–110.
52. Aarnio M, Sankila R, Pukkala E, et al. Cancer risk in mutation carriers of DNA-mismatch-repair genes. *Int J Cancer* 1999;81:214–218.
53. Ionov Y, Peinado MA, Malkhosyan S, et al. Ubiquitous somatic mutations in simple repeated sequences reveal a new mechanism for colonic carcinogenesis. *Nature* 1993;363:558–561.
54. Aaltonen LA, Peltomaki P, Leach FS, et al. Clues to the pathogenesis of familial colorectal cancer. *Science* 1993;260:812–816.
55. Thibodeau SN, Bren G, Schaid D. Microsatellite instability in cancer of the proximal colon. *Science* 1993;260:816–819.
56. Peltomaki P, Aaltonen LA, Sistonen P, et al. Genetic mapping of a locus predisposing to human colorectal cancer. *Science* 1993;260:810–812.
57. Lindblom A, Tannergard P, Werelius B, et al. Genetic mapping of a second locus predisposing to hereditary non-polyposis colon cancer. *Nat Genet* 1993;5:279–282.
58. Fishel R, Lescoe MK, Rao MR, et al. The human mutator gene homolog *MSH2* and its association with hereditary nonpolyposis colon cancer. *Cell* 1994;77:167.
59. Leach FS, Nicolaides NC, Papadopoulos N, et al. Mutations of a mutS homolog in hereditary nonpolyposis colorectal cancer. *Cell* 1993;75: 1215–1225.
60. Bronner CE, Baker SM, Morrison PT, et al. Mutation in the DNA mismatch repair gene homologue hMLH1 is associated with hereditary nonpolyposis colon cancer. *Nature* 1994;368:258–261.
61. Papadopoulos N, Nicolaides NC, Wei YF, et al. Mutation of a mutL homolog in hereditary colon cancer. *Science* 1994;263:1625–1629.
62. Peltomaki P. Deficient DNA mismatch repair: a common etiologic factor for colon cancer. *Hum Mol Genet* 2001;10:735–740.
63. Wijnen J, de Leeuw W, Vasen H, et al. Familial endometrial cancer in female carriers of *MSH6* germline mutations. *Nat Genet* 1999;23:142–144.
64. Miyaki M, Konishi M, Tanaka K, et al. Germline mutation of *MSH6* as the cause of hereditary nonpolyposis colorectal cancer. *Nat Genet* 1997;17: 271–272.
65. Akiyama Y, Sato H, Yamada T, et al. Germ-line mutation of the hMSH6/GTBP gene in an atypical hereditary nonpolyposis colorectal cancer kindred. *Cancer Res* 1997;57:3920–3923.
66. Kolodner RD, Tytell JD, Schmeits JL, et al. Germ-line msh6 mutations in colorectal cancer families. *Cancer Res* 1999;59:5068–5074.
67. Hampel H, Frankel W, Panescu J, et al. Screening for Lynch syndrome (hereditary nonpolyposis colorectal cancer) among endometrial cancer patients. *Cancer Res* 2006;66:7810–7817.
68. Nicolaides NC, Papadopoulos N, Liu B, et al. Mutations of two PMS homologues in hereditary nonpolyposis colon cancer. *Nature* 1994;371:75–80.
69. Liu T, Yan H, Kuismanen S, et al. The role of hPMS1 and hPMS2 in predisposing to colorectal cancer. *Cancer Res* 2001;61:7798–7802.
70. Gurin CC, Federici MG, Kang L, et al. Causes and consequences of microsatellite instability in endometrial carcinoma. *Cancer Res* 1999;59: 462–466.
71. Herman JG, Umar A, Polyak K, et al. Incidence and functional consequences of hMLH1 promoter hypermethylation in colorectal carcinoma. *Proc Natl Acad Sci USA* 1998;95:6870–6875.
72. Leung SY, Yuen ST, Chung LP, et al. hMLH1 promoter methylation and lack of hMLH1 expression in sporadic gastric carcinomas with high-frequency microsatellite instability. *Cancer Res* 1999;59:159–164.
73. Duval A, Hamelin R. Mutations at coding repeat sequences in mismatch repair-deficient human cancers: toward a new concept of target genes for instability. *Cancer Res* 2002;62:2447–2454.
74. Hall J, Lee M, Newman B, et al. Linkage of early onset familial breast cancer to chromosome 17q21. *Science* 1990;250:1684–1689.
75. Narod SA, Feunteun J, Lynch HT, et al. Familial breast-ovarian cancer locus on chromosome 17q12-q23. *Lancet* 1991;338:82–83.
76. Miki Y, Swensen J, Shattuck-Eidens D, et al. A strong candidate for the breast and ovarian cancer susceptibility gene *BRCA1*. *Science* 1994;266: 66–71.
77. Wooster R, Neuhausen SL, Mangion J, et al. Localization of a breast cancer susceptibility gene, *BRCA2*, to chromosome 13q12-13. *Science* 1994;265:2088–2090.
78. Wooster R, Bignell G, Lancaster J, et al. Identification of the breast cancer susceptibility gene *BRCA2*. *Nature* 1995;378:789–791.
79. Breast Cancer Information Core Database. http://research.nhgri.nik.gov/bic/.

80. Gudmundsson J, Johannesdottir G, Bergthorsson JT, et al. Different tumor types from *BRCA2* carriers show wild-type chromosome deletions on 13q12-q13. *Cancer Res* 1995;55:4830–4832.
81. Smith SA, Easton DF, Evans DG, et al. Allele losses in the region 17q12-21 in familial breast and ovarian cancer involve the wild-type chromosome. *Nat Genet* 1992;2:128–131.
82. Thompson D, Easton D. Variation in cancer risks, by mutation position, in *BRCA2* mutation carriers. *Am J Hum Genet* 2001;68:410–419.
83. Esteller M, Silva JM, Dominguez G, et al. Promoter hypermethylation and *BRCA1* inactivation in sporadic breast and ovarian tumors. *J Natl Cancer Inst* 2000;92:564–569.
84. Baldwin RL, Nemeth E, Tran H, et al. *BRCA1* promoter region hypermethylation in ovarian carcinoma: a population-based study. *Cancer Res* 2000;60:5329–5333.
85. Jazaeri AA, Yee CJ, Sotiriou C, et al. Gene expression profiles of *BRCA1*-linked, *BRCA2*-linked, and sporadic ovarian cancers. *J Natl Cancer Inst* 2002;94:990–1000.
86. Hughes-Davies L, Huntsman D, Ruas M, et al. EMSY links the *BRCA2* pathway to sporadic breast and ovarian cancer. *Cell* 2003;115:523–535.
87. Scully R, Livingston DM. In search of the tumour-suppressor functions of *BRCA1* and *BRCA2*. *Nature* 2000;408:429–432.
88. Venkitaraman AR. Cancer susceptibility and the functions of *BRCA1* and *BRCA2*. *Cell* 2002;108:171–182.
89. Scully R, Chen J, Plug A, et al. Association of *BRCA1* with Rad51 in mitotic and meiotic cells. *Cell* 1997;88:265–275.
90. Sharan SK, Morimatsu M, Albrecht U, et al. Embryonic lethality and radiation hypersensitivity mediated by Rad51 in mice lacking *BRCA2*. *Nature* 1997;386:804–810.
91. Hakem R, de la Pompa JL, Sirard C, et al. The tumor suppressor gene *BRCA1* is required for embryonic cellular proliferation in the mouse. *Cell* 1996;85:1009–1023.
92. Suzuki A, de la Pompa JL, Hakem R, et al. *BRCA2* is required for embryonic cellular proliferation in the mouse. *Genes Dev* 1997;11:1242–1252.
93. Hakem R, de la Pompa JL, Elia A, et al. Partial rescue of *BRCA1* (5–6) early embryonic lethality by p53 or p21 null mutation. *Nat Genet* 1997;16: 298–302.
94. Ludwig T, Chapman DL, Papaioannou VE, et al. Targeted mutations of breast cancer susceptibility gene homologs in mice: lethal phenotypes of *BRCA1, BRCA2, BRCA1/BRCA2, BRCA1*/p53, and *BRCA2*/p53 nullizygous embryos. *Genes Dev* 1997;11:1226–1241.
95. Moynahan ME, Chiu JW, Koller BH, et al. *BRCA1* controls homology-directed DNA repair. *Mol Cell* 1999;4:511–518.
96. Snouwaert JN, Gowen LC, Latour AM, et al. *BRCA1* deficient embryonic stem cells display a decreased homologous recombination frequency and an increased frequency of non-homologous recombination that is corrected by expression of a *BRCA1* transgene. *Oncogene* 1999;18:7900–7907.
97. Moynahan ME, Cui TY, Jasin M. Homology-directed DNA repair, mitomycin-c resistance, and chromosome stability is restored with correction of a *BRCA1* mutation. *Cancer Res* 2001;61:4842–4850.
98. Moynahan ME, Pierce AJ, Jasin M. *BRCA2* is required for homology-directed repair of chromosomal breaks. *Mol Cell* 2001;7:263–272.
99. Tutt A, Bertwistle D, Valentine J, et al. Mutation in *BRCA2* stimulates error-prone homology-directed repair of DNA double-strand breaks occurring between repeated sequences. *EMBO J* 2001;20:4704–4716.
100. Xia F, Taghian DG, DeFrank JS, et al. Deficiency of human *BRCA2* leads to impaired homologous recombination but maintains normal nonhomologous end joining. *Proc Natl Acad Sci USA* 2001;98:8644–8649.
101. Yang H, Jeffrey PD, Miller J, et al. *BRCA2* function in DNA binding and recombination from a *BRCA2*-DSS1-ssDNA structure. *Science* 2002;297: 1837–1848.
102. Chapman MS, Verma IM. Transcriptional activation by *BRCA1*. *Nature* 1996;382:678–679.
103. Monteiro AN, August A, Hanafusa H. Evidence for a transcriptional activation function of *BRCA1* C-terminal region. *Proc Natl Acad Sci USA* 1996;93:13595–13599.
104. Scully R, Anderson SF, Chao DM, et al. *BRCA1* is a component of the RNA polymerase II holoenzyme. *Proc Natl Acad Sci USA* 1997;94: 5605–5610.
105. Anderson SF, Schlegel BP, Nakajima T, et al. *BRCA1* protein is linked to the RNA polymerase II holoenzyme complex via RNA helicase A. *Nat Genet* 1998;19:254–256.
106. Somasundaram K, Zhang H, Zeng YX, et al. Arrest of the cell cycle by the tumour-suppressor *BRCA1* requires the CDK-inhibitor p21WAF1/CiP1. *Nature* 1997;389:187–190.
107. Li S, Chen PL, Subramanian T, et al. Binding of CtIP to the BRCT repeats of *BRCA1* involved in the transcription regulation of p21 is disrupted upon DNA damage. *J Biol Chem* 1999;274:11334–11338.
108. Harkin DP, Bean JM, Miklos D, et al. Induction of GADD45 and JNK/SAPK-dependent apoptosis following inducible expression of *BRCA1*. *Cell* 1999;97:575–586.
109. Ouchi T, Monteiro AN, August A, et al. *BRCA1* regulates p53-dependent gene expression. *Proc Natl Acad Sci USA* 1998;95:2302–2306.
110. Aprelikova O, Pace AJ, Fang B, et al. *BRCA1* is a selective co-activator of 14-3-3 sigma gene transcription in mouse embryonic stem cells. *J Biol Chem* 276:25647–25650.
111. MacLachlan TK, Somasundaram K, Sgagias M, et al. *BRCA1* effects on the cell cycle and the DNA damage response are linked to altered gene expression. *J Biol Chem* 2000;275:2777–2785.
112. Hashizume R, Fukuda M, Maeda I, et al. The RING heterodimer *BRCA1*-BARD1 is a ubiquitin ligase inactivated by a breast cancer-derived mutation. *J Biol Chem* 2001;276:14537–14540.
113. Baer R, Ludwig T. The *BRCA1*/BARD1 heterodimer, a tumor suppressor complex with ubiquitin E3 ligase activity. *Curr Opin Genet Dev* 2002;12:86–91.
114. Starita LM, Parvin JD. Substrates of the *BRCA1*-dependent ubiquitin ligase. *Cancer Biol Ther* 2006;5:137–141.
115. Eakin CM, Maccoss MJ, Finney GL, et al. Estrogen receptor alpha is a putative substrate for the *BRCA1* ubiquitin ligase. *Proc Natl Acad Sci USA* 2007;104:5794–5799.
116. Li W, Xiao C, Vonderhaar BK, et al. A role of estrogen/ERalpha signaling in *BRCA1*-associated tissue-specific tumor formation. *Oncogene* 2007;26: 7204–7212.
117. Hoeijmakers JH. Genome maintenance mechanisms for preventing cancer. *Nature* 2001;411:366–374.
118. Husain A, He G, Venkatraman ES, et al. *BRCA1* up-regulation is associated with repair-mediated resistance to cis-diamminedichloroplatinum(II). *Cancer Res* 1998;58:1120–1123.
119. Bhattacharyya A, Ear US, Koller BH, et al. The breast cancer susceptibility gene *BRCA1* is required for subnuclear assembly of Rad51 and survival following treatment with the DNA cross-linking agent cisplatin. *J Biol Chem* 2000;275:23899–23903.
120. Lafarge S, Sylvain V, Ferrara M, et al. Inhibition of *BRCA1* leads to increased chemoresistance to microtubule-interfering agents, an effect that involves the JNK pathway. *Oncogene* 2001;20:6597–6606.
121. Abbott DW, Thompson ME, Robinson-Benion C, et al. *BRCA1* expression restores radiation resistance in *BRCA1*-defective cancer cells through enhancement of transcription-coupled DNA repair. *J Biol Chem* 1999;274: 18808–18812.
122. Scully R, Ganesan S, Vlasakova K, et al. Genetic analysis of *BRCA1* function in a defined tumor cell line. *Mol Cell* 1999;4:1093–1099.
123. Cortez D, Wang Y, Qin J, et al. Requirement of ATM-dependent phosphorylation of *BRCA1* in the DNA damage response to double-strand breaks. *Science* 1999;286:1162–1166.
124. Lee JS, Collins KM, Brown AL, et al. hCds1-mediated phosphorylation of *BRCA1* regulates the DNA damage response. *Nature* 2000;404:201–204.
125. Rubin SC, Benjamin I, Behbakht K, et al. Clinical and pathological features of ovarian cancer in women with germ-line mutations of *BRCA1*. *N Engl J Med* 1996;335:1413–1416.
126. Boyd J, Sonoda Y, Federici MG, et al. Clinicopathologic features of BRCA-linked and sporadic ovarian cancer. *JAMA* 2000;283:2260–2265.
127. Ben DY, Chetrit A, Hirsh-Yechezkel G, et al. Effect of BRCA mutations on the length of survival in epithelial ovarian tumors. *J Clin Oncol* 2002;20:463–466.
128. Li J, Yen C, Liaw D, et al. *PTEN*, a putative protein tyrosine phosphatase gene mutated in human brain, breast, and prostate cancer [see comments]. *Science* 1997;275:1943–1947.
129. Steck PA, Pershouse MA, Jasser SA, et al. Identification of a candidate tumour suppressor gene, MMAC1, at chromosome 10q23.3 that is mutated in multiple advanced cancers. *Nat Genet* 1997;15:356–362.
130. Marsh DJ, Dahia PL, Zheng Z, et al. Germline mutations in *PTEN* are present in Bannayan-Zonana syndrome. *Nat Genet* 1997;16:333–334.
131. Tamura M, Gu J, Matsumoto K, et al. Inhibition of cell migration, spreading, and focal adhesions by tumor suppressor *PTEN*. *Science* 1998;280:1614–1617.
132. Gu J, Tamura M, Yamada KM. Tumor suppressor *PTEN* inhibits integrin- and growth factor-mediated mitogen-activated protein (MAP) kinase signaling pathways. *J Cell Biol* 1998;143:1375–1383.
133. Wu X, Senechal K, Neshat MS, et al. The *PTEN*/MMAC1 tumor suppressor phosphatase functions as a negative regulator of the phosphoinositide 3-kinase/Akt pathway. *Proc Natl Acad Sci USA* 1998;95: 15587–15591.
134. Maehama T, Dixon JE. The tumor suppressor, *PTEN*/MMAC1, dephosphorylates the lipid second messenger, phosphatidylinositol 3,4,5-trisphosphate. *J Biol Chem* 1998;273:13375–13378.
135. Waite KA, Eng C. Protean *PTEN*: form and function. *Am J Hum Genet* 2002;70:829–844.
136. Eng C. Will the real Cowden syndrome please stand up: revised diagnostic criteria. *J Med Genet* 2000;37:828–830.
137. Nagase S, Yamakawa H, Sato S, et al. Identification of a 790-kilobase region of common allelic loss in chromosome 10q25-q26 in human endometrial cancer. *Cancer Res* 1997;57:1630–1633.
138. Peiffer SL, Herzog TJ, Tribune DJ, et al. Allelic loss of sequences from the long arm of chromosome 10 and replication errors in endometrial cancers. *Cancer Res* 1995;55:1922–1926.
139. Kong D, Suzuki A, Zou TT, et al. *PTEN1* is frequently mutated in primary endometrial carcinomas. *Nat Genet* 1997;17:143–144.
140. Risinger JI, Hayes AK, Berchuck A, et al. *PTEN*/MMAC1 mutations in endometrial cancers. *Cancer Res* 1997;57:4736–4738.
141. Tashiro H, Blazes MS, Wu R, et al. Mutations in *PTEN* are frequent in endometrial carcinoma but rare in other common gynecologic malignancies. *Cancer Res* 1997;57:3935–3940.

142. Maxwell GL, Risinger JI, Gumbs C, et al. Mutation of the *PTEN* tumor suppressor gene in endometrial hyperplasias. *Cancer Res* 1998;58: 2500–2503.
143. Obata K, Morland SJ, Watson RH, et al. Frequent *PTEN*/MMAC mutations in endometrioid but not serous or mucinous epithelial ovarian tumors. *Cancer Res* 1998;58:2095–2097.
144. Maxwell GL, Risinger JI, Tong B, et al. Mutation of the *PTEN* tumor suppressor gene is not a feature of ovarian cancers. *Cancer Res* 1998;70: 13–16.
145. Bishop JM. Molecular themes in oncogenesis. *Cell* 1991;64:235–248.
146. Weinberg RA. Oncogenes, antioncogenes, and the molecular bases of multistep carcinogenesis. *Cancer Res* 1989;49:3713–3721.
147. Kim HT, Choi BH, Niikawa N, et al. Frequent loss of imprinting of the H19 and IGF-II genes in ovarian tumors. *Am J Med Genet* 1998;80: 391–395.
148. Kaneda A, Feinberg AP. Loss of imprinting of IGF2: a common epigenetic modifier of intestinal tumor risk. *Cancer Res* 2005;65:11236–11240.
149. Murphy SK, Huang Z, Wen Y, et al. Frequent IGF2/H19 domain epigenetic alterations and elevated IGF2 expression in epithelial ovarian cancer. *Mol Cancer Res* 2006;4:283–292.
150. Madhani HD. Accounting for specificity in receptor tyrosine kinase signaling. *Cell* 2001;106:9–11.
151. Boerner JL, Danielsen A, Maihle NJ. Ligand-independent oncogenic signaling by the epidermal growth factor receptor: v-ErbB as a paradigm. *Exp Cell Res* 2003;284:111–121.
152. Citri A, Yarden Y. EGF-ERBB signalling: towards the systems level. *Nat Rev Mol Cell Biol* 2006;7:505–516.
153. Cantley LC, Auger KR, Carpenter C, et al. Oncogenes and signal transduction. *Cell* 1991;64:281–302.
154. Pinkas-Kramarski R, Shelly M, Guarino BC, et al. ErbB tyrosine kinases and the two neuregulin families constitute a ligand-receptor network. *Mol Cell Biol* 1998;18:6090–6101.
155. Fan Z, Mendelsohn J. Therapeutic application of anti-growth factor receptor antibodies. *Curr Opin Oncol* 1998;10:67–73.
156. Berchuck A, Rodriguez G, Kamel A, et al. Expression of epidermal growth factor receptor and HER-2/neu in normal and neoplastic cervix, vulva, and vagina. *Obstet Gynecol* 1990;76:381–387.
157. Sridhar SS, Seymour L, Shepherd FA. Inhibitors of epidermal-growth-factor receptors: a review of clinical research with a focus on non-small-cell lung cancer. *Lancet Oncol* 2003;4:397–406.
158. Sharma SV, Bell DW, Settleman J, et al. Epidermal growth factor receptor mutations in lung cancer. *Nat Rev Cancer* 2007;7:169–181.
159. Weinstein IB. Cancer. Addiction to oncogenes—the Achilles heal of cancer. *Science* 2002;297:63–64.
160. Bargmann CI, Hung MC, Weinberg RA. The neu oncogene encodes an epidermal growth factor receptor-related protein. *Nature* 1986;319: 226–230.
161. Penuel E, Schaefer G, Akita RW, et al. Structural requirements for ErbB2 transactivation. *Semin Oncol* 2001;28:36–42.
162. Slamon DJ, Godolphin W, Jones LA, et al. Studies of HER-2/neu protooncogene in human breast and ovarian cancer. *Science* 1989;244:707–712.
163. Tan AR, Swain SM. Ongoing adjuvant trials with trastuzumab in breast cancer. *Semin Oncol* 2003;30(5 Suppl 16):54–64.
164. Bookman MA, Darcy KM, Clarke-Pearson D, et al. Evaluation of monoclonal humanized anti-HER2 antibody, trastuzumab, in patients with recurrent or refractory ovarian or primary peritoneal carcinoma with overexpression of HER2: a phase II trial of the Gynecologic Oncology Group. *J Clin Oncol* 2003;21:283–290.
165. Futreal PA, Wooster R, Stratton MR. Somatic mutations in human cancer: insights from resequencing the protein kinase gene family. *Cold Spring Harb Symp Quant Biol* 2005;70:43–49.
166. Neves SR, Ram PT, Iyengar R. G protein pathways. *Science* 2002;296: 1636–1639.
167. Campbell SL, Khosravi-Far R, Rossman KL, et al. Increasing complexity of Ras signaling. *Oncogene* 1998;17:1395–1413.
168. Gutkind JS. Cell growth control by G protein-coupled receptors: from signal transduction to signal integration. *Oncogene* 1998;17:1331–1342.
169. Bos JL. ras oncogenes in human cancer: a review. *Cancer Res* 1989;49: 4682–4689.
170. Baum C, Kirschmeier P. Preclinical and clinical evaluation of farnesyltransferase inhibitors. *Curr Oncol Rep* 2003;5:99–107.
171. Grandori C, Cowley SM, James LP, et al. The Myc/Max/Mad network and the transcriptional control of cell behavior. *Annu Rev Cell Dev Biol* 2000;16:653–699.
172. Nilsson JA, Cleveland JL. Myc pathways provoking cell suicide and cancer. *Oncogene* 2003;22:9007–9021.
173. Morin PJ, Sparks AB, KorinekV, et al. Activation of beta-catenin-Tcf signaling in colon cancer by mutations in beta-catenin or APC. *Science* 1997;275:1787–1790.
174. Deligdisch L, Holinka CF. Endometrial carcinoma: two diseases? *Cancer Detect Prev* 1987;10:237–246.
175. Shah NK, Currie JL, Rosenshein N, et al. Cytogenetic and FISH analysis of endometrial carcinoma. *Cancer Genet Cytogenet* 1994;73:142–146.
176. Baloglu H, Cannizzaro LA, Jones J, et al. Atypical endometrial hyperplasia shares genomic abnormalities with endometrioid carcinoma by comparative genomic hybridization. *Hum Pathol* 2001;32:615–622.
177. Kiechle M, Hinrichs M, Jacobsen A, et al. Genetic imbalances in precursor lesions of endometrial cancer detected by comparative genomic hybridization. *Am J Pathol* 2000;156:1827–1833.
178. Suzuki A, Fukushige S, Nagase S, et al. Frequent gains on chromosome arms 1q and/or 8q in human endometrial cancer. *Hum Genet* 1997;100:629–636.
179. Sonoda G, du MS, Godwin AK, et al. Detection of DNA gains and losses in primary endometrial carcinomas by comparative genomic hybridization. *Genes Chromosomes Cancer* 1997;18:115–125.
180. Hirasawa A, Aoki D, Inoue J, et al. Unfavorable prognostic factors associated with high frequency of microsatellite instability and comparative genomic hybridization analysis in endometrial cancer. *Clin Cancer Res* 2003;9:5675–5682.
181. Risinger JI, Maxwell GL, Chandramouli GV, et al. Microarray analysis reveals distinct gene expression profiles among different histologic types of endometrial cancer. *Cancer Res* 2003;63:6–11.
182. Suehiro Y, Umayahara K, Ogata H, et al. Genetic aberrations detected by comparative genomic hybridization predict outcome in patients with endometrioid carcinoma. *Genes Chromosomes Cancer* 2000;29:75–82.
183. Lukes AS, Kohler MF, Pieper CF, et al. Multivariable analysis of DNA ploidy, p53, and HER-2/neu as prognostic factors in endometrial cancer. *Cancer* 1994;73:2380–2385.
184. Moreno-Bueno G, Sanchez-Estevez C, Cassia R, et al. Differential gene expression profile in endometrioid and nonendometrioid endometrial carcinoma: STK15 is frequently overexpressed and amplified in nonendometrioid carcinomas. *Cancer Res* 2003;63:5697–5702.
185. Maxwell GL, Chandramouli GV, Dainty L, et al. Microarray analysis of endometrial carcinomas and mixed mullerian tumors reveals distinct gene expression profiles associated with different histologic types of uterine cancer. *Clin Cancer Res* 2005;11:4056–4066.
186. Berchuck A, Kohler MF, Marks JR, et al. The p53 tumor suppressor gene frequently is altered in gynecologic cancers. *Am J Obstet Gynecol* 1994;170:246–252.
187. Kohler MF, Berchuck A, Davidoff AM, et al. Overexpression and mutation of p53 in endometrial carcinoma. *Cancer Res* 1992;52:1622–1627.
188. Hachisuga T, Fukuda K, Uchiyama M, et al. Immunohistochemical study of p53 expression in endometrial carcinomas: correlation with markers of proliferating cells and clinicopathologic features. *Int J Gynecol Cancer* 1993;3:363–368.
189. Hamel NW, Sebo TJ, Wilson TO, et al. Prognostic value of p53 and proliferating cell nuclear antigen expression in endometrial carcinoma. *Cancer Res* 1996;62:192–198.
190. Inoue M, Okayama A, Fujita M, et al. Clinicopathological characteristics of p53 overexpression in endometrial cancers. *Int J Cancer* 1994;58: 14–19.
191. Ito K, Watanabe K, Nasim S, et al. Prognostic significance of p53 overexpression in endometrial cancer. *Cancer Res* 1994;54:4667–4670.
192. Khalifa MA, Mannel RS, Haraway SD, et al. Expression of EGFR, HER2/neu, p53, and PCNA in endometrioid, serous papillary, and clear cell endometrial adenocarcinomas. *Cancer Res* 1994;53:84–92.
193. Kohlberger P, Gitsch G, Loesch A, et al. p53 protein overexpression in early stage endometrial cancer. *Cancer Res* 1996;62:213–217.
194. Service RF. Research news: stalking the start of colon cancer. *Science* 1994;263:1559–1560.
195. Clifford SL, Kaminetsky CP, Cirisano FD, et al. Racial disparity in overexpression of the p53 tumor suppressor gene in stage I endometrial cancer. *Am J Obstet Gynecol* 1997;176:S229–S232.
196. Kohler MF, Carney P, Dodge R, et al. p53 overexpression in advanced-stage endometrial adenocarcinoma. *Am J Obstet Gynecol* 1996;175: 1246–1252.
197. Liu FS, Kohler MF, Marks JR, et al. Mutation and overexpression of the p53 tumor suppressor gene frequently occurs in uterine and ovarian sarcomas. *Obstet Gynecol* 1994;83:118–124.
198. Hall KL, Teneriello MG, Taylor RR, et al. Analysis of Ki-ras, p53, and MDM2 genes in uterine leiomyomas and leiomyosarcomas. *Cancer Res* 1997;65:330–335.
199. Risinger JI, Dent GA, Ignar-Trowbridge D, et al. Mutations of the p53 gene in human endometrial carcinoma. *Molec Carcinog* 1992;5:250–253.
200. Yaginuma Y, Westphal H. Analysis of the p53 gene in human uterine carcinoma cell lines. *Cancer Res* 1991;51:6506–6509.
201. Kohler MF, Nishii H, Humphrey PA, et al. Mutation of the p53 tumor-suppressor gene is not a feature of endometrial hyperplasias. *Am J Obstet Gynecol* 1993;169:690–694.
202. Tashiro H, Isacson C, Levine R, et al. p53 gene mutations are common in uterine serous carcinoma and occur early in their pathogenesis. *Am J Pathol* 1997;150:177–185.
203. Kanamori Y, Kigawa J, Itamochi H, et al. Correlation between loss of *PTEN* expression and Akt phosphorylation in endometrial carcinoma. *Clin Cancer Res* 2001;7:892–895.
204. Risinger JI, Hayes K, Maxwell GL, et al. *PTEN* mutation in endometrial cancers is associated with favorable clinical and pathologic characteristics. *Clin Cancer Res* 1998;4:3005–3010.
205. Milner J, Ponder B, Hu. Transcriptional activation functions in *BRCA2*. *Nature* 1997;386:772–773.
206. Mutter GL, Ince TA, Baak JP, et al. Molecular identification of latent precancers in histologically normal endometrium. *Cancer Res* 2001;61: 4311–4314.

207. Mutter GL, Lin MC, Fitzgerald JT, et al. Altered *PTEN* expression as a diagnostic marker for the earliest endometrial precancers. *J Natl Cancer Inst* 2000;92:924–930.
208. Lin WM, Forgacs E, Warshal DP, et al. Loss of heterozygosity and mutational analysis of the *PTEN*/MMAC1 gene in synchronous endometrial and ovarian carcinomas. *Clin Cancer Res* 1998;4:2577–2583.
209. Risinger JI, Berchuck A, Kohler MF, et al. Genetic instability of microsatellites in endometrial carcinoma. *Cancer Res* 1993;53:5100–5103.
210. Faquin WC, Fitzgerald JT, Lin MC, et al. Sporadic microsatellite instability is specific to neoplastic and preneoplastic endometrial tissues. *Am J Clin Pathol* 2000;113:576–582.
211. Kowalski LD, Mutch DG, Herzog TJ, et al. Mutational analysis of *MLH1* and *MSH2* in 25 prospectively-acquired RER+ endometrial cancers. *Genes Chromosomes Cancer* 1997;18:219–227.
212. Simpkins SB, Bocker T, Swisher EM, et al. *MLH1* promoter methylation and gene silencing is the primary cause of microsatellite instability in sporadic endometrial cancers. *Hum Mol Genet* 1999;8:661–666.
213. Salvesen HB, MacDonald N, Ryan A, et al. Methylation of hMLH1 in a population-based series of endometrial carcinomas. *Clin Cancer Res* 2000;6:3607–3613.
214. Esteller M, Catasus L, Matias-Guiu X, et al. hMLH1 promoter hypermethylation is an early event in human endometrial tumorigenesis. *Am J Pathol* 1999;155:1767–1772.
215. Kanaya T, Kyo S, Maida Y, et al. Frequent hypermethylation of *MLH1* promoter in normal endometrium of patients with endometrial cancers. *Oncogene* 2003;22:2352–2360.
216. Risinger JI, Maxwell GL, Berchuck A, et al. Promoter hypermethylation as an epigenetic component in type I and type II endometrial cancers. *Ann NY Acad Sci* 2003;983:208–212.
217. Momparler RL. Cancer epigenetics. *Oncogene* 2003;22:6479–6483.
218. Vassileva V, Millar A, Briollais L, et al. Apoptotic and growth regulatory genes as mutational targets in mismatch repair deficient endometrioid adenocarcinomas of young patients. *Oncol Rep* 2004;11:931–937.
219. Maxwell GL, Risinger JI, Alvarez AA, et al. Favorable survival associated with microsatellite instability in endometrioid endometrial cancers. *Obstet Gynecol* 2001;97:417–422.
220. Black D, Soslow RA, Levine DA, et al. Clinicopathologic significance of defective DNA mismatch repair in endometrial carcinoma. *J Clin Oncol* 2006;24:1745–1753.
221. Cohn DE, Frankel WL, Resnick KE, et al. Improved survival with an intact DNA mismatch repair system in endometrial cancer. *Obstet Gynecol* 2006;108:1208–1215.
222. Zighelboim I, Goodfellow PJ, Gao F, et al. Microsatellite instability and epigenetic inactivation of *MLH1* and outcome of patients with endometrial carcinomas of the endometrioid type. *J Clin Oncol* 2007;25:2042–2048.
223. Moreno-Bueno G, Fernandez-Marcos PJ, Collado M, et al. Inactivation of the candidate tumor suppressor par-4 in endometrial cancer. *Cancer Res* 2007;67:1927–1934.
224. Zukerberg LR, DeBernardo RL, Kirley SD, et al. Loss of cables, a cyclin-dependent kinase regulatory protein, is associated with the development of endometrial hyperplasia and endometrial cancer. *Cancer Res* 2004;64:202–208.
225. Spruck CH, Strohmaier H, Sangfelt O, et al. hCDC4 gene mutations in endometrial cancer. *Cancer Res* 2002;62:4535–4539.
226. Cassia R, Moreno-Bueno G, Rodriguez-Perales S, et al. Cyclin E gene (CCNE) amplification and hCDC4 mutations in endometrial carcinoma. *J Pathol* 2003;201:589–595.
227. Berchuck A, Rodriguez G, Kinney RB, et al. Overexpression of HER-2/neu in endometrial cancer is associated with advanced stage disease. *Am J Obstet Gynecol* 1991;164(1 Pt 1):15–21.
228. Hetzel DJ, Wilson TO, Keeney GL, et al. HER-2/neu expression: a major prognostic factor in endometrial cancer. *Cancer Res* 1992;47:179–185.
229. Lu KH, Bell DA, Welch WR, et al. Evidence for the multifocal origin of bilateral and advanced human serous borderline ovarian tumors. *Cancer Res* 1998;58:2328–2330.
230. Morrison C, Zanagnolo V, Ramirez N, et al. HER-2 is an independent prognostic factor in endometrial cancer: association with outcome in a large cohort of surgically staged patients. *J Clin Oncol* 2006;24:2376–2385.
231. Santin AD, Bellone S, Gokden M, et al. Overexpression of HER-2/neu in uterine serous papillary cancer. *Clin Cancer Res* 2002;8:1271–1279.
232. Santin AD, Bellone S, Siegel ER, et al. Racial differences in the overexpression of epidermal growth factor type II receptor (HER2/neu): a major prognostic indicator in uterine serous papillary cancer. *Am J Obstet Gynecol* 2005;192:813–818.
233. Jewell E, Secord AA, Berchuck A, et al. Use of trastuzumab in the treatment of metastatic endometrial cancer. *Int J Gynecol Cancer* 2006;16:1370–1373.
234. Boyd J, Risinger JI. Analysis of oncogene alterations in human endometrial carcinoma: prevalence of ras mutations. *Mol Carcinog* 1991;4:189–195.
235. Ignar-Trowbridge D, Risinger JI, Dent GA, et al. Mutations of the Ki-ras oncogene in endometrial carcinoma. *Am J Obstet Gynecol* 1992;167:227–232.
236. Duggan BD, Felix JC, Muderspach LI, et al. Early mutational activation of the c-Ki-ras oncogene in endometrial carcinoma. *Cancer Res* 1994;54:1604–1607.
237. Enomoto T, Inoue M, Perantoni AO, et al. K-ras activation in neoplasms of the human female reproductive tract. *Cancer Res* 1990;50:6139–6145.
238. Enomoto T, Inoue M, Perantoni AO, et al. K-ras activation in premalignant and malignant epithelial lesions of the human uterus. *Cancer Res* 1991;51:5308–5314.
239. Enomoto T, Fujita M, Inoue M, et al. Alterations of the p53 tumor suppressor gene and its association with activation of the c-K-ras-2 protooncogene in premalignant and malignant lesions of the human uterine endometrium. *Cancer Res* 1993;53:1883–1888.
240. Fujimoto I, Shimizu Y, Hirai Y, et al. Studies on ras oncogene activation in endometrial carcinoma. *Cancer Res* 1993;48:196–202.
241. Mizuuchi H, Nasim S, Kudo R, et al. Clinical implications of K-ras mutations in malignant epithelial tumors of the endometrium. *Cancer Res* 1992;52:2777–2781.
242. Sasaki H, Nishii H, Tada A, et al. Mutation of the Ki-ras protooncogene in human endometrial hyperplasia and carcinoma. *Cancer Res* 1993;53:1906–1910.
243. Mutter GL, Wada H, Faquin WC, et al. K-ras mutations appear in the premalignant phase of both microsatellite stable and unstable endometrial carcinogenesis. *Mol Pathol* 1999;52:257–262.
244. Mutch DG, Powell MA, Mallon MA, et al. RAS/RAF mutation and defective DNA mismatch repair in endometrial cancers. *Am J Obstet Gynecol* 2004;190:935–942.
245. Pappa KI, Choleza M, Markaki S, et al. Consistent absence of BRAF mutations in cervical and endometrial cancer despite KRAS mutation status. *Gynecol Oncol* 2006;100:596–600.
246. Feng YZ, Shiozawa T, Miyamoto T, et al. BRAF mutation in endometrial carcinoma and hyperplasia: correlation with KRAS and p53 mutations and mismatch repair protein expression. *Clin Cancer Res* 2005;11:6133–6138.
247. Oda K, Stokoe D, Taketani Y, et al. High frequency of coexistent mutations of PI3KCA and *PTEN* genes in endometrial carcinoma. *Cancer Res* 2005;65:10669–10673.
248. Hayes MP, Wang H, Espinal-Witter R, et al. PI3KCA and *PTEN* mutations in uterine endometrioid carcinoma and complex atypical hyperplasia. *Clin Cancer Res* 2006;12:5932–5935.
249. Risinger JI, Berchuck A, Kohler MF, et al. Mutations of the E-cadherin gene in human gynecologic cancers. *Nat Genet* 1994;7:98–102.
250. Fujimoto J, Ichigo S, Hori M, et al. Expressions of E-cadherin and alpha- and beta-catenin mRNAs in uterine endometrial cancers. *Eur J Gynaecol Oncol* 1998;19:78–81.
251. Hirohashi S. Inactivation of the E-cadherin-mediated cell adhesion system in human cancers. *Am J Pathol* 1998;153:333–339.
252. Zysman M, Saka A, Millar A, et al. Methylation of adenomatous polyposis coli in endometrial cancer occurs more frequently in tumors with microsatellite instability phenotype. *Cancer Res* 2002;62:3663–3666.
253. Mitra AB, Murty VV, Pratap M, et al. ERBB2 (HER2/neu) oncogene is frequently amplified in squamous cell carcinoma of the uterine cervix. *Cancer Res* 1994;54:637–639.
254. Polakis P. The many ways of Wnt in cancer. *Curr Opin Genet Dev* 2007;17:45–51.
255. Fukuchi T, Sakamoto M, Tsuda H, et al. Beta-catenin mutation in carcinoma of the uterine endometrium. *Cancer Res* 1998;58:3526–3528.
256. Moreno-Bueno G, Hardisson D, Sanchez C, et al. Abnormalities of the APC/beta-catenin pathway in endometrial cancer. *Oncogene* 2002;21:7981–7990.
257. Brachtel EF, Sanchez-Estevez C, Moreno-Bueno G, et al. Distinct molecular alterations in complex endometrial hyperplasia (CEH) with and without immature squamous metaplasia (squamous morules). *Am J Surg Pathol* 2005;29:1322–1329.
258. Greenman C, Stephens P, Smith R, et al. Patterns of somatic mutation in human cancer genomes. *Nature* 2007;446:153–158.
259. Pollock PM, Gartside MG, Dejeza LC, et al. Frequent activating FGFR2 mutations in endometrial carcinomas parallel germline mutations associated with craniosynostosis and skeletal dysplasia syndromes. *Oncogene* 2007 Nov 1;26(50):7158–7162.
260. Odom LD, Barrett JM, Pantazis CG, et al. Immunocytochemical study of ras and myc proto-oncogene polypeptide expression in the human menstrual cycle. *Am J Obstet Gynecol* 1989;161:1663–1668.
261. Borst MP, Baker VV, Dixon D, et al. Oncogene alterations in endometrial carcinoma. *Cancer Res* 1990;38:s364–366.
262. Monk BJ, Chapman JA, Johnson GA, et al. Correlation of c-myc and HER-2/neu amplification and expression with histopathologic variables in uterine corpus cancer. *Am J Obstet Gynecol* 1994;171:1193–1198.
263. Williams JA Jr, Wang ZR, Parrish RS, et al. Fluorescence in situ hybridization analysis of HER-2/neu, c-myc, and p53 in endometrial cancer. *Exp Mol Pathol* 1999;67:135–143.
264. Whittemore AS, Harris R, Itnyre J. Characteristics relating to ovarian cancer risk. Collaborative analysis of twelve US case-control studies: IV. The pathogenesis of epithelial ovarian cancer. *Am J Epidemiol* 1992;136:1212–1220.
265. Rodriguez GC, Walmer DK, Cline M, et al. Effect of progestin on the ovarian epithelium of macaques: cancer prevention through apoptosis? *J Soc Gynecol Investig* 1998;5:271–276.
266. Jacobs IJ, Kohler MF, Wiseman RW, et al. Clonal origin of epithelial ovarian carcinoma: analysis by loss of heterozygosity, p53 mutation, and X-chromosome inactivation. *J Natl Cancer Inst* 1992;84:1793–1798.

267. Schorge JO, Muto MG, Welch WR, et al. Molecular evidence for multifocal papillary serous carcinoma of the peritoneum in patients with germline *BRCA1* mutations. *J Natl Cancer Inst* 1998;90:841–845.
268. Kallioniemi A, Kallioniemi OP, Sudar D, et al. Comparative genomic hybridization for molecular cytogenetic analysis of solid tumors. *Science* 1992;258:818–821.
269. Cliby W, Ritland S, Hartmann L, et al. Human epithelial ovarian cancer allelotype. *Cancer Res* 1993;53(10 Suppl):2393–2398.
270. Dodson MK, Hartmann LC, Cliby WA, et al. Comparison of loss of heterozygosity patterns in invasive low-grade and high-grade epithelial ovarian carcinomas. *Cancer Res* 1993;53:4456–4460.
271. Iwabuchi H, Sakamoto M, Sakunaga H, et al. Genetic analysis of benign, low-grade, and high-grade ovarian tumors. *Cancer Res* 1995;55:6172–6180.
272. Suzuki S, Moore DH, Ginzinger DG, et al. An approach to analysis of large-scale correlations between genome changes and clinical endpoints in ovarian cancer. *Cancer Res* 2000;60:5382–5385.
273. Welsh JB, Zarrinkar PP, Sapinoso LM, et al. Analysis of gene expression profiles in normal and neoplastic ovarian tissue samples identifies candidate molecular markers of epithelial ovarian cancer. *Proc Natl Acad Sci USA* 2001;98:1176–1181.
274. Ono K, Tanaka T, Tsunoda T, et al. Identification by cDNA microarray of genes involved in ovarian carcinogenesis. *Cancer Res* 2000;60:5007–5011.
275. Schummer M, Ng WV, Bumgarner RE, et al. Comparative hybridization of an array of 21,500 ovarian cDNAs for the discovery of genes overexpressed in ovarian carcinomas. *Gene* 1999;238:375–385.
276. Bonome T, Lee JY, Park DC, et al. Expression profiling of serous low malignant potential, low-grade, and high-grade tumors of the ovary. *Cancer Res* 2005;65:10602–10612.
277. Schwartz DR, Kardia SL, Shedden KA, et al. Gene expression in ovarian cancer reflects both morphology and biological behavior, distinguishing clear cell from other poor-prognosis ovarian carcinomas. *Cancer Res* 2002;62:4722–4729.
278. Shridhar V, Lee J, Pandita A, et al. Genetic analysis of early- versus late-stage ovarian tumors. *Cancer Res* 2001;61:5895–5904.
279. Berchuck A, Iversen ES, Lancaster JM, et al. Patterns of gene expression that characterize long-term survival in advanced stage serous ovarian cancers. *Clin Cancer Res* 2005;11:3686–3696.
280. Spentzos D, Levine DA, Ramoni MF, et al. Gene expression signature with independent prognostic significance in epithelial ovarian cancer. *J Clin Oncol* 2004;22:4648–4658.
281. Dressman HK, Berchuck A, Chan G, et al. An integrated genomic-based approach to individualized treatment of patients with advanced-stage ovarian cancer. *J Clin Oncol* 2007;25:517–525.
282. Bennett M, Macdonald K, Chan SW, et al. Cell surface trafficking of Fas: a rapid mechanism of p53-mediated apoptosis. *Science* 1998;282:290–293.
283. Eltabbakh GH, Belinson JL, Kennedy AW, et al. p53 overexpression is not an independent prognostic factor for patients with primary ovarian epithelial cancer. *Cancer* 1997;80:892–898.
284. Hartmann L, Podratz K, Keeney G, et al. Prognostic significance of p53 immunostaining in epithelial ovarian cancer. *J Clin Oncol* 1994;12:64–69.
285. Kohler MF, Kerns BJ, Humphrey PA, et al. Mutation and overexpression of p53 in early-stage epithelial ovarian cancer. *Obstet Gynecol* 1993;81:643–650.
286. Marks JR, Davidoff AM, Kerns B, et al. Overexpression and mutation of p53 in epithelial ovarian cancer. *Cancer Res* 1991;51:2979–2984.
287. van dZAG, Hollema H, Suurmeijer AJ, et al. Value of P-glycoprotein, glutathione S-transferase pi, c-erbB-2, and p53 as prognostic factors in ovarian carcinomas. *J Clin Oncol* 1995;13:70–78.
288. Leitao MM, Soslow RA, Baergen RN, et al. Mutation and expression of the *TP53* gene in early stage epithelial ovarian carcinoma. *Gynecol Oncol* 2004;93:301–306.
289. Henriksen R, Strang P, Backstrom T, et al. Ki-67 immunostaining and DNA flow cytometry as prognostic factors in epithelial ovarian cancers. *Anticancer Res* 1994;14:603–608.
290. Berns EM, Klijn JG, van PWL, et al. p53 protein accumulation predicts poor response to tamoxifen therapy of patients with recurrent breast cancer. *J Clin Oncol* 1998;16:121–127.
291. Havrilesky L, Hamdan H, Darcy K, et al. Relationship between p53 mutation, p53 overexpression and survival in advanced ovarian cancers treated on Gynecologic Oncology Group studies #114 and #132. *J Clin Oncol* 2003;21:3814–3825.
292. Kohler MF, Marks JR, Wiseman RW, et al. Spectrum of mutation and frequency of allelic deletion of the p53 gene in ovarian cancer. *J Natl Cancer Inst* 1993;85:1513–1519.
293. Kupryjanczyk J, Thor AD, Beauchamp R, et al. p53 mutations and protein accumulation in human ovarian cancer. *Proc Natl Acad Sci USA* 1993;90:4961–4965.
294. Brown R, Clugston C, Burns P, et al. Increased accumulation of p53 protein in cisplatin-resistant ovarian cell lines. *Int J Cancer* 1993;55:678–684.
295. Eliopoulos AG, Kerr DJ, Herod J, et al. The control of apoptosis and drug resistance in ovarian cancer: influence of p53 and Bcl-2. *Oncogene* 1995;11:1217–1228.
296. Herod JJ, Eliopoulos AG, Warwick J, et al. The prognostic significance of Bcl-2 and p53 expression in ovarian carcinoma. *Cancer Res* 1996;56:2178–2184.
297. Perego P, Giarola M, Righetti SC, et al. Association between cisplatin resistance and mutation of p53 gene and reduced bax expression in ovarian carcinoma cell systems.*Cancer Res* 1996;56:556–562.
298. Righetti SC, Della TG, Pilotti S, et al. A comparative study of p53 gene mutations, protein accumulation, and response to cisplatin-based chemotherapy in advanced ovarian carcinoma. *Cancer Res* 1996;56:689–693.
299. Havrilesky LJ, Elbendary A, Hurteau JA, et al. Chemotherapy-induced apoptosis in epithelial ovarian cancers. *Obstet Gynecol* 1995;85:1007–1010.
300. Berchuck A, Kohler MF, Hopkins MP, et al. Overexpression of p53 is not a feature of benign and early-stage borderline epithelial ovarian tumors. *Cancer Res* 1994;52:232–236.
301. Gershenson DM, Deavers M, Diaz S, et al. Prognostic significance of p53 expression in advanced-stage ovarian serous borderline tumors. *Clin Cancer Res* 1999;5:4053–4058.
302. Ortiz BH, Ailawadi M, Colitti C, et al. Second primary or recurrence? Comparative patterns of p53 and K-ras mutations suggest that serous borderline ovarian tumors and subsequent serous carcinomas are unrelated tumors. *Cancer Res* 2001;61:7264–7267.
303. Flesken-Nikitin A, Choi KC, Eng JP, et al. Induction of carcinogenesis by concurrent inactivation of p53 and Rb1 in the mouse ovarian surface epithelium. *Cancer Res* 2003;63:3459–3463.
304. Plaxe SC, Deligdisch L, Dottino PR, et al. Ovarian intraepithelial neoplasia demonstrated in patients with stage I ovarian carcinoma. *Cancer Res* 1990;38:367–372.
305. Brewer MA, Johnson K, Follen M, et al. Prevention of ovarian cancer: intraepithelial neoplasia. *Clin Cancer Res* 2003;9:20–30.
306. Schultz DC, Vanderveer L, Buetow KH, et al. Characterization of chromosome 9 in human ovarian neoplasia identifies frequent genetic imbalance on 9q and rare alterations involving 9p, including CDKN2. *Cancer Res* 1995;55:2150–2157.
307. McCluskey LL, Chen C, Delgadillo E, et al. Differences in p16 gene methylation and expression in benign and malignant ovarian tumors. *Cancer Res* 1999;72:87–92.
308. Liu Z, Wang LE, Wang L, et al. Methylation and messenger RNA expression of p15INK4b but not p16INK4a are independent risk factors for ovarian cancer. *Clin Cancer Res* 2005;11:4968–4976.
309. Catteau A, Harris WH, Xu CF, et al. Methylation of the *BRCA1* promoter region in sporadic breast and ovarian cancer: correlation with disease characteristics. *Oncogene* 1999;18:1957–1965.
310. Schmider A, Gee C, Friedmann W, et al. p21 (WAF1/CIP1) protein expression is associated with prolonged survival but not with p53 expression in epithelial ovarian carcinoma. *Cancer Res* 2000;77:237–242.
311. Levesque MA, Katsaros D, Massobrio M, et al. Evidence for a dose-response effect between p53 (but not p21WAF1/Cip1) protein concentrations, survival, and responsiveness in patients with epithelial ovarian cancer treated with platinum-based chemotherapy. *Clin Cancer Res* 2000;6:3260–3270.
312. Bali A, O'Brien PM, Edwards LS, et al. Cyclin D1, p53, and p21Waf1/Cip1 expression is predictive of poor clinical outcome in serous epithelial ovarian cancer. *Clin Cancer Res* 2004;10:5168–5177.
313. Masciullo V, Ferrandina G, Pucci B, et al. p27Kip1 expression is associated with clinical outcome in advanced epithelial ovarian cancer: multivariate analysis. *Clin Cancer Res* 2000;6:4816–4822.
314. Sui L, Dong Y, Ohno M, et al. Implication of malignancy and prognosis of p27(kip1), cyclin E, and CDK2 expression in epithelial ovarian tumors. *Cancer Res* 2001;83:56–63.
315. Hurteau JA, Allison BM, Brutkiewicz SA, et al. Expression and subcellular localization of the cyclin-dependent kinase inhibitor p27(Kip1) in epithelial ovarian cancer. *Cancer Res* 2001;83:292–298.
316. Korkolopoulou P, Vassilopoulos I, Konstantinidou AE, et al. The combined evaluation of p27Kip1 and Ki-67 expression provides independent information on overall survival of ovarian carcinoma patients. *Cancer Res* 2002;85:404–414.
317. Rosen DG, Yang G, Cai KQ, et al. Subcellular localization of p27kip1 expression predicts poor prognosis in human ovarian cancer. *Clin Cancer Res* 2005;11:632–637.
318. Hurteau J, Whitaker RS, Rodriguez GC, et al. Effect of transforming growth factor-β on proliferation of human ovarian cancer cells obtained from ascites. *Soc Gynecol Invest* 1993;40:128.
319. Baldwin RL, Tran H, Karlan BY. Loss of c-myc repression coincides with ovarian cancer resistance to transforming growth factor beta growth arrest independent of transforming growth factor beta/Smad signaling. *Cancer Res* 2003;63:1413–1419.
320. Wang D, Kanuma T, Mizunuma H, et al. Analysis of specific gene mutations in the transforming growth factor-beta signal transduction pathway in human ovarian cancer. *Cancer Res* 2000;60:4507–4512.
321. Rosen DG, Wang L, Jain AN, et al. Expression of the tumor suppressor gene ARHI in epithelial ovarian cancer is associated with increased expression of p21WAF1/CIP1 and prolonged progression-free survival. *Clin Cancer Res* 2004;10:6559–6566.
322. Petrocca F, Iliopoulos D, Qin HR, et al. Alterations of the tumor suppressor gene ARLTS1 in ovarian cancer. *Cancer Res* 2006;66:10287–10291.
323. Rodriguez GC, Berchuck A, Whitaker RS, et al. Epidermal growth factor receptor expression in normal ovarian epithelium and ovarian cancer. II.

Relationship between receptor expression and response to epidermal growth factor. *Am J Obstet Gynecol* 1991;164:745–750.
324. Yee D, Morales FR, Hamilton TC, et al. Expression of insulin-like growth factor I, its binding proteins, and its receptor in ovarian cancer. *Cancer Res* 1991;51:5107–5112.
325. Henrikson R, Funa K, Wilander E, et al. Expression and prognostic significance of platelet-derived growth factor and its receptors in epithelial ovarian neoplasms. *Cancer Res* 1993;53:4550–4554.
326. Di Blasio AM, Cremonesi L, Vigano P, et al. Basic fibroblast growth factor and its receptor messenger ribonucleic acids are expressed in human ovarian epithelial neoplasms. *Am J Obstet Gynecol* 1993;169:1517–1523.
327. Siemans CH, Auersperg N. Serial propagation of human ovarian surface epithelium in culture. *J Cell Physiol* 1991;134:347–356.
328. Ziltener HJ, Maines-Bandiera S, Schrader JW, et al. Secretion of bioactive interleukin-1, interleukin-6 aand colony-stimulating factors by human ovarian surface epithelium. *Biol Reprod* 1993;49:635–641.
329. Berchuck A, Kamel A, Whitaker R, et al. Overexpression of HER-2/neu is associated with poor survival in advanced epithelial ovarian cancer. *Cancer Res* 1990;50:4087–4091.
330. Rodriguez GC, Boente MP, Berchuck A, et al. The effect of antibodies and immunotoxins reactive with HER- 2/neu on growth of ovarian and breast cancer cell lines. *Am J Obstet Gynecol* 1993;168:228–232.
331. Pegram MD, Lipton A, Hayes DF, et al. Phase II study of receptor-enhanced chemosensitivity using recombinant humanized anti-p185 HER2/neu monoclonal antibody plus cisplatin in patients with HER2/neu-overexpressing metastatic breast cancer refractory to chemotherapy treatment. *J Clin Oncol* 1998;16:2659–2671.
332. Bookman MA, Darcy KM, Clarke-Pearson D, et al. Evaluation of monoclonal humanized anti-HER2 antibody, trastuzumab, in patients with recurrent or refractory ovarian or primary peritoneal carcinoma with overexpression of HER2: a phase II trial of the Gynecologic Oncology Group. *J Clin Oncol* 2003;21:283–290.
333. Baker SJ, Fearon ER, Nigro JM, et al. Chromosome 17 deletions and p53 gene mutations in colorectal carcinomas. *Science* 1989;244:217–221.
334. Haas M, Isakov J, Howell SB. Evidence against ras activation in human ovarian carcinomas. *Mol Biol Med* 1987;4:265–275.
335. Feig LA, Bast RC Jr, Knapp RC, et al. Somatic activation of rasK gene in a human ovarian carcinoma. *Science* 1984;223:698–701.
336. Teneriello MG, Ebina M, Linnoila RI, et al. p53 and ki-ras gene mutations in epithelial ovarian neoplasms. *Cancer Res* 1993;53:3103–3108.
337. Mok SCH, Bell DA, Knapp RC, et al. Mutation of K-ras protooncogene in human ovarian epithelial tumors of borderline malignancy. *Cancer Res* 1993;53:1489–1492.
338. Singer G, Oldt R III, Cohen Y, et al. Mutations in BRAF and KRAS characterize the development of low-grade ovarian serous carcinoma. *J Natl Cancer Inst* 2003;95:484–486.
339. Ho CL, Kurman RJ, Dehari R, et al. Mutations of BRAF and KRAS precede the development of ovarian serous borderline tumors. *Cancer Res* 2004;64:6915–6918.
340. Gemignani ML, Schlaerth AC, Bogomolniy F, et al. Role of KRAS and BRAF gene mutations in mucinous ovarian carcinoma. *Cancer Res* 2003;90:378–381.
341. Shayesteh L, Lu Y, Kuo WL, et al. PI3KCA is implicated as an oncogene in ovarian cancer. *Nat Genet* 1999;21:99–102.
342. Campbell IG, Russell SE, Choong DY, et al. Mutation of the PI3KCA gene in ovarian and breast cancer. *Cancer Res* 2004;64:7678–7681.
343. Cheng JQ, Godwin AK, Bellacosa A, et al. AKT2, a putative oncogene encoding a member of a subfamily of protein-serine/threonine kinases, is amplified in human ovarian carcinomas. *Proc Natl Acad Sci USA* 1992;89: 9267–9271.
344. Obata K, Morland SJ, Watson RH, et al. Frequent *PTEN*/MMAC mutations in endometrioid but not serous or mucinous epithelial ovarian tumors. *Cancer Res* 1998;58:2095–2097.
345. Wu R, Zhai Y, Fearon ER, et al. Diverse mechanisms of beta-catenin deregulation in ovarian endometrioid adenocarcinomas. *Cancer Res* 2001;61:8247–8255.
346. Wu R, Hendrix-Lucas N, Kuick R, et al. Mouse model of human ovarian endometrioid adenocarcinoma based on somatic defects in the Wnt/beta-catenin and PI3K/*Pten* signaling pathways. *Cancer Cell* 2007;11: 321–333.
347. Dinulescu DM, Ince TA, Quade BJ, et al. Role of K-ras and *Pten* in the development of mouse models of endometriosis and endometrioid ovarian cancer. *Nat Med* 2005;11:63–70.
348. Berns EMJJ, Klijn JGM, Henzen-Logmans SC, et al. Receptors for hormones and growth factors (onco)-gene amplification in human ovarian cancer. *Int J Cancer* 1992;52:218–224.
349. Sasano H, Garrett C, Wilkinson D, et al. Protoocogene amplification and tumor ploidy in human ovarian neoplasms. *Hum Pathol* 1990;21: 382–391.
350. Tashiro H, Niyazaki K, Okamura H, et al. c-myc overexpression in human primary ovarian tumors: its relevance to tumor progression. *Int J Cancer* 1992;50:828–833.
351. Farley J, Smith LM, Darcy KM, et al. Cyclin E expression is a significant predictor of survival in advanced, suboptimally debulked ovarian epithelial cancers: a Gynecologic Oncology Group study. *Cancer Res* 2003;63: 1235–1241.
352. Rosen DG, Yang G, Deavers MT, et al. Cyclin E expression is correlated with tumor progression and predicts a poor prognosis in patients with ovarian carcinoma. *Cancer* 2006;106:1925–1932.
353. Brown LA, Irving J, Parker R, et al. Amplification of EMSY, a novel oncogene on 11q13, in high grade ovarian surface epithelial carcinomas. *Gynecol Oncol* 2006;100:264–270.
354. Park JT, Li M, Nakayama K, et al. Notch3 gene amplification in ovarian cancer. *Cancer Res* 2006;66:6312–6318.
355. Yang H, Ou CC, Feldman RI, et al. Aurora-A kinase regulates telomerase activity through c-Myc in human ovarian and breast epithelial cells. *Cancer Res* 2004;64:463–467.
356. Guan XY, Fung JM, Ma NF, et al. Oncogenic role of eIF-5A2 in the development of ovarian cancer. *Cancer Res* 2004;64:4197–4200.
357. Furui T, LaPushin R, Mao M, et al. Overexpression of edg-2/vzg-1 induces apoptosis and anoikis in ovarian cancer cells in a lysophosphatidic acid-independent manner. *Clin Cancer Res* 1999;5:4308–4318.
358. Lee Z, Swaby RF, Liang Y, et al. Lysophosphatidic acid is a major regulator of growth-regulated oncogene alpha in ovarian cancer. *Cancer Res* 2006;66:2740–2748.
359. Tanyi JL, Morris AJ, Wolf JK, et al. The human lipid phosphate phosphatase-3 decreases the growth, survival, and tumorigenesis of ovarian cancer cells: validation of the lysophosphatidic acid signaling cascade as a target for therapy in ovarian cancer. *Cancer Res* 2003;63: 1073–1082.
360. Munoz N, Bosch FX, de Sanjose S, et al. Epidemiologic classification of human papillomavirus types associated with cervical cancer. *N Engl J Med* 2003;348:518-527.
361. Sun XW, Kuhn L, Ellerbrock TV, et al. Human papillomavirus infection in women infected with the human immunodeficiency virus. *N Engl J Med* 1997;337:1343–1349.
362. Scheffner M, Werness BA, Huibregtse JM, et al. The E6 oncoprotein encoded by human papillomavirus types 16 and 18 promotes the degradation of p53. *Cell* 1990;63:1129–1136.
363. Scheffner M, Munger K, Byrne JC, et al. The state of the p53 and retinoblastoma gene in human cervical carcinoma cell lines. *Proc Natl Acad Sci USA* 1991;88:5523–5527.
364. Werness BA, Levine AJ, Howley PM. Association of human papillomavirus types 16 and 18 E6 proteins with p53. *Science* 1990;248:76–79.
365. Parker MF, Arroyo GF, Geradts J, et al. Molecular characterization of adenocarcinoma of the cervix. *Cancer Res* 1997;64:242–251.
366. de Boer MA, Jordanova ES, Kenter GG, et al. High human papillomavirus oncogene mRNA expression and not viral DNA load is associated with poor prognosis in cervical cancer patients. *Clin Cancer Res* 2007;13: 132–138.
367. Narayan G, Pulido HA, Koul S, et al. Genetic analysis identifies putative tumor suppressor sites at 2q35-q36.1 and 2q36.3-q37.1 involved in cervical cancer progression. *Oncogene* 2003;22:3489–3499.
368. Umayahara K, Numa F, Suehiro Y, et al. Comparative genomic hybridization detects genetic alterations during early stages of cervical cancer progression. *Genes Chromosomes Cancer* 2002;33:98–102.
369. Kirchhoff M, Rose H, Petersen BL, et al. Comparative genomic hybridization reveals a recurrent pattern of chromosomal aberrations in severe dysplasia/carcinoma in situ of the cervix and in advanced-stage cervical carcinoma. *Genes Chromosomes Cancer* 1999;24:144–150.
370. Heselmeyer K, Macville M, Schrock E, et al. Advanced-stage cervical carcinomas are defined by a recurrent pattern of chromosomal aberrations revealing high genetic instability and a consistent gain of chromosome arm 3q. *Genes Chromosomes Cancer* 1997;19:233–240.
371. Yang YC, Shyong WY, Chang MS, et al. Frequent gain of copy number on the long arm of chromosome 3 in human cervical adenocarcinoma. *Cancer Genet Cytogenet* 2001;131:48–53.
372. Lin WM, Michalopulos EA, Dhurander N, et al. Allelic loss and microsatellite alterations of chromosome 3p14.2 are more frequent in recurrent cervical dysplasias. *Clin Cancer Res* 2000;6:1410–1414.
373. Wang SS, Trunk M, Schiffman M, et al. Validation of p16INK4a as a marker of oncogenic human papillomavirus infection in cervical biopsies from a population-based cohort in Costa Rica. *Cancer Epidemiol Biomarkers Prev* 2004;13:1355–1360.
374. Berchuck A, Rodriguez G, Kamel A, et al. Expression of epidermal growth factor receptor and HER-2/neu in normal and neoplastic cervix, vulva, and vagina. *Obstet Gynecol* 1990;76:381–387.
375. Grendys ECJ, Barnes WA, Weitzel J, et al. Identification of H, K, and N-ras point mutations in stage IB cervical carcinoma. *Cancer Res* 1997;65:343–347.
376. Koulos JP, Wright TC, Mitchell MF, et al. Relationships between c-Ki-ras mutations, HPV types, and prognostic indicators in invasive endocervical adenocarcinomas. *Cancer Res* 48:364–369.
377. Riou G, Barrois M, Sheng ZM, et al. Somatic deletions and mutations of c-Ha-ras gene in human cervical cancers. *Oncogene* 1998;3:329–333.
378. Van Le L, Stoerker J, Rinehart CA, et al. H-ras condon 12 mutation in cervical dysplasia. *Cancer Res* 1993;49:181–184.
379. Riou G, Le MG, Favre M, et al. Human papillomavirus-negative status and c-myc gene overexpression: independent prognostic indicators of distant metastasis for early-stage invasive cervical cancers. *J Natl Cancer Inst* 1992;84:1525–1526.

380. Bourhis J, Le MG, Barrois M, et al. Prognostic value of c-myc proto-oncogene overexpression in early invasive carcinoma of the cervix. *J Clin Oncol* 1990;8:1789–1796.
381. Birrer MJ, Hendricks D, Farley J, et al. Abnormal FHIT expression in malignant and premalignant lesions of the cervix. *Cancer Res* 1999;59:5270–5274.
382. Huang LW, Chao SL, Chen TJ. Reduced FHIT expression in cervical carcinoma: correlation with tumor progression and poor prognosis. *Cancer Res* 2003;90:331–337.
383. Connolly DC, Greenspan DL, Wu R, et al. Loss of FHIT expression in invasive cervical carcinomas and intraepithelial lesions associated with invasive disease. *Clin Cancer Res* 2000;6:3505–3510.
384. Liu FS, Hsieh YT, Chen JT, et al. FHIT (fragile histidine triad) gene analysis in cervical intraepithelial neoplasia. *Cancer Res* 2001;82:283–290.
385. Krivak TC, McBroom JW, Seidman J, et al. Abnormal fragile histidine triad (FHIT) expression in advanced cervical carcinoma: a poor prognostic factor. *Cancer Res* 2001;61:4382–4385.
386. Dong SM, Kim HS, Rha SH, et al. Promoter hypermethylation of multiple genes in carcinoma of the uterine cervix. *Clin Cancer Res* 2001;7:1982–1986.
387. Virmani AK, Muller C, Rathi A, et al. Aberrant methylation during cervical carcinogenesis. *Clin Cancer Res* 2001;7:584–589.
388. Wong YF, Selvanayagam ZE, Wei N, et al. Expression genomics of cervical cancer: molecular classification and prediction of radiotherapy response by DNA microarray. *Clin Cancer Res* 2003;9:5486–5492.
389. Kuzmin I, Liu L, Dammann R, et al. Inactivation of RAS association domain family 1A gene in cervical carcinomas and the role of human papillomavirus infection. *Cancer Res* 2003;63:1888–1893.
390. Lin WM, Ashfaq R, Michalopulos EA, et al. Molecular Papanicolaou tests in the twenty-first century: molecular analyses with fluid-based Papanicolaou technology. *Am J Obstet Gynecol* 2000;183:39–45.
391. Manavi M, Hudelist G, Fink-Retter A, et al. Gene profiling in Pap-cell smears of high-risk human papillomavirus-positive squamous cervical carcinoma. *Gynecol Oncol* 2007;105:418–426.

CHAPTER 6 ■ IMMUNOTHERAPY OF GYNECOLOGIC MALIGNANCIES

PAUL J. SABBATINI, DAVID Z. CHANG, CHAITANYA R. DIVGI, PHILIP O. LIVINGSTON, AND ALAN N. HOUGHTON

The natural clinical history of ovarian cancer makes it ideally suited for the evaluation of immune-based strategies. Although the majority of patients are diagnosed with advanced disease, 70% are in a complete clinical remission following initial cytoreductive surgery and platinum and taxane–based primary chemotherapy (1). However, data from second-look surgical assessments show that more than 60% of patients actually have persistent disease, which is supported by the fact that only 30% of optimally debulked stage III patients will remain disease-free with a median progression-free interval of approximately 24 months (2). Despite the high relapse rate, many patients return to a complete or partial clinical remission following additional chemotherapy. With this chronic course of relapse and response, the median survival of optimally debulked patients exceeded 60 months in a study evaluating intraperitoneal (IP) therapy as part of primary treatment (3). Neither higher doses and protracted schedules nor non-cross-resistant consolidation chemotherapy has provided additional benefit. These ovarian cancer patients with minimal disease burdens are therefore appropriate candidates for the evaluation of immune-based strategies, which typically have excellent side effect profiles.

With regard to other gynecologic malignancies, the outcome of both early-stage and locally advanced cervical cancer has been improved with the addition of chemotherapy to radiation therapy, yet for those patients who relapse, survival in the metastatic setting is short (4,5). The bulk of immune strategies being evaluated in patients with cervical cancer target human papillomavirus, and this important subject is covered separately in chapters 19 and 22 (6,7). The treatment of patients with metastatic recurrent endometrial cancer is also characterized by limited chemotherapy responses of short duration (8). There is a need in each of these gynecologic cancers for more effective therapy, especially in the adjuvant setting, when the target is circulating cancer cells and micrometastases or peritoneal implants. A variety of approaches utilizing the specificity and potency of the immune system are under evaluation including cytokines or other immunologic modulators, monoclonal antibodies, and vaccines.

CANCER IMMUNOLOGY: OVERVIEW

The immune system evolved to fight foreign invaders such as bacteria, viruses, and parasites. However, strong evidence suggests that the immune system also plays a crucial role in controlling or even rejecting incipient cancers. Mice that have major defects in immunologic molecules develop cancer more frequently, including carcinomas, supporting the hypothesis that the immune system detects and destroys incipient cancers, the theory of *immune surveillance of cancer*. This theory has been modified to propose that the immune system not only destroys incipient cancers, but that cancer cells are able to escape this early immunity through changes in gene expression, leading to outgrowth of tumors with the capacity to escape recognition by the immune system. The process of tumor cells escaping from immunity is termed *immune editing*.

Innate Immunity

The immune system is broadly divided into two arms. *Innate immunity* is present at birth and does not require adaptation to react against microorganisms or tumors. Examples of cells that are part of innate immunity include natural killer (NK) cells, macrophages, and dendritic cells. NK cells are lymphocytes that are programmed to recognize and destroy tissues that have been altered or stressed, e.g., by viruses or by malignant transformation. Macrophages play many roles in immunity and inflammation, including production of a multitude of soluble secreted proinflammatory proteins, which are growth factors for other cells of the immune system, for neovasculature, and for cancer cells. These growth factors include *cytokines* and *chemokines*, and they support the growth, movement, and survival of immune and inflammatory cells. Macrophages play important roles in tissue remodeling during wound healing, mediating inflammatory responses, sampling molecules from the environment through internalization, and presenting antigens to stimulate T cells. Macrophages can also play a counterproductive role through production of molecules that promote tumor growth and angiogenesis (e.g., vascular endothelial growth factor [VEGF] and basic fibroblast growth factor [FGF]). Macrophages can also inhibit immune responses through production of cytokines and other molecules that down-regulate immunity, such as prostaglandins E2, arginase I, and transforming growth factor-β. Thus, the role of macrophages in tumors is complex. Dendritic cells have some properties that are similar to macrophages, including production of cytokines and sampling of molecules from the environment. Most importantly, dendritic cells are a primary link between the innate immune system and the adaptive or acquired immune system through presentation of antigens to initiate T-cell activation. For this reason, dendritic cells are professional antigen-presenting cells.

Adaptive Immunity

Adaptive immunity is characterized by adaptation to antigens, e.g., antigens of infectious pathogens (or potentially by cancer).

This arm of the immune system is not mature or activated at birth, but rather adapts through maturation in response to antigens of pathogens. It is characterized by receptors encoded by the immunoglobulin (Ig) gene family. These receptors have the capacity to rearrange, creating enormous diversity ($>10^{11-12}$ different receptors). This provides a system to generate enormous specificity that recognizes and responds to a wide range of antigens that have not previously been encountered.

The two major cell types of acquired immunity are *T lymphocytes* (T cells) and *B lymphocytes* (B cells). T cells have the capacity to recognize antigens sequestered in different compartments within cells, for instance, antigens generated in the cytoplasm or nucleus by viral infections. T cells recognize antigens as short peptides, 8 to 16 amino acids in length. These peptides must be complexed with and presented by specialized antigen-presenting molecules, the major histocompatibility complex (MHC) molecules, to T-cell receptors. In humans, MHC molecules are the human leukocyte antigens (HLAs) expressed on virtually every cell in the body. On the other hand, B cells produce secreted *antibodies* that can recognize soluble and cell surface molecules. Both T cells and B cells initially develop with a limited range of receptors for immune recognition. However, in response to antigen (e.g., from a virus or cancer cell) presented by a professional antigen-presenting cell, T cells or B cells that have receptors with the best "fit" to the antigen itself (for B cells) or antigen/MHC complex (for T cells) are stimulated to proliferate and this subpopulation is quickly expanded.

Humoral Immunity

B cells recognize antigens usually in their natural configuration (9). An individual host has a repertoire of B cells that are capable of generating antibodies against the full range of pathogens encountered in the environment. To do this, the total population of B lymphocytes expresses a diverse repertoire of immunoglobulins. Each B cell expresses immunoglobulin against a single antigenic determinant, with the immunoglobulin expressed at the cell surface of the B cell where it acts as a specific receptor to transduce signals in response to that antigen. Once activated, the B cell is to create an individual monoclonal antibody (mAb). The diversity of specificities in different B cells is generated by rearrangements of the immunoglobulin genes, and new antibody specificities continue to be generated in response to new antigens. During development, B cells with high avidity immunoglobulins against ubiquitous self-antigens are eliminated. This elimination of B cells reactive with autoantigens is not absolute, however, as a broad array of antibodies against autoantigens is found in the blood of humans. Peripheral blood B cells consist of naïve and relatively short-lived B cells, long-lived memory B cells resulting from maturation in response to antigenic stimulation, and a small population of B cells expressing germ-line immunoglobulins that have not undergone rearrangement (which are found in the CD5+ B-cell population) (10).

B cells are very mobile, and after development in the bone marrow they migrate through the peripheral blood to B-cell-rich areas in lymphoid organs, e.g., the follicles of lymph nodes, spleen, and gastrointestinal tract. Many B cells continue recirculating in the blood. If cognate antigen is encountered in lymphoid organs, the B lymphocyte migrates to the T-cell-rich areas where appropriate T-cell help can be provided to promote increased antibody diversity and increased affinity through immunoglobulin gene rearrangements. This T-cell help does not have to be induced by the same antigen. Chemical conjugation of the antibody-recognized antigen to highly immunogenic bacterial or xenogeneic proteins or, alternatively, expression of the antigen in bacterial or viral vectors, are widely used approaches to ensure adequate T-cell help in vaccines. The result of T-cell help is generation of plasma cells, the most mature form of B cell with the highest capacity for antibody production. In addition, T-cell help promotes formation of germinal centers in lymphoid organs where hypermutation in immunoglobulin genes and class and subclass switching occur to generate antibodies with higher affinities for antigen. Class switching refers to changes in antibody class during an immune response, with the IgM class of antibodies appearing first, generally followed by antibodies of the IgG class (different subclasses of IgG antibodies have different blood half-lives and different capacities for effector functions, such as fixation of complement or binding to Fc receptors). The consequence is plasma cells secreting increasingly higher affinity IgG antibodies as the immune response matures over time. In addition, some B cells that generally recognize non-protein antigens, e.g., carbohydrate or glycolipid antigens, can be stimulated to proliferate in the absence of T-cell help. Class switching, affinity maturation, and memory B cells do not occur "without cell help;" rather, low-affinity IgM antibodies of shorter duration result.

The immunoglobulin variable region (called the Fv region) determines antibody specificity and is located in the Fab domain of immunoglobulins. This region mediates effective binding to antigens. However, the constant region (Fc), where antibody class and subclass are determined, is equally critical. Binding of antibody to antigen results in a conformational change in the Fc portion, leading to activation of several effector mechanisms, including complement activation (discussed below). IgM antibodies are synthesized early in the response, but if T-cell help is available, antibody responses mature through immunoglobulin gene rearrangements into the higher affinity IgG classes, which are capable of improved binding to antigen as well as receptors on the bone marrow-derived cells for the Fc domain, expanding potential effector functions. The responses to most non-protein antigens are IgM class and generally do not mature to IgG responses. The IgM pentamer structure is specialized to increase avidity of binding to multimeric antigens and to efficiently activate one type of effector function: complement. Activation of complement, which includes blood components with different enzymatic properties, results in opsonization (coating of pathogens by complement components), recognition by complement receptors on macrophages, monocytes, neutrophils, and dendritic cells, with subsequent activation of these cells leading to phagocytosis and/or killing. In addition, complement can form a membrane attack complex, which creates holes in membranes of target pathogens and cancer cells, producing complement-dependent cytotoxicity (CDC). IgG antibodies are synthesized following immunoglobulin gene rearrangements, with switches in Fc domains, as the B cell matures in response to T-cell help. IgG antibodies usually have higher affinity, and can be found in the extracellular space as well as in the blood. IgG1 and IgG3 antibodies in humans are especially effective at activating complement and also at sensitization of pathogens for killing by NK cells, macrophages, and other cells with complement receptors and immunoglobulin Fc receptors.

Opsonization for ingestion and destruction by phagocytes can occur through complement activation, but also occurs directly as a consequence of engagement of Fc receptors on phagocytic cells. Antibodies complexed to antigen bind to Fc receptors, which can lead to activation signals through activating Fc receptors (e.g., FcRIII), but activation can be countered by IgG binding to the inhibitory Fc receptor, FcRIIB. Fc receptors, which are bound effectively by IgG1 and IgG3 subclasses of human antibodies, are expressed on monocytes, macrophages, NK cells, neutrophils, mast cells, and other cells. Cross-linking of Fc receptors leads to activation of the cells, in some cases leading to antibody-dependent cell-mediated cytotoxicity (ADCC) of tumor cells through production of cytotoxic molecules, e.g., perforin and granzymes by NK cells and reactive molecular species by macrophages. Monoclonal antibodies are commonly used for cancer therapy. Antitumor effects can be in part mediated by antibody binding to critical molecules on the surface of tumor cells, for example by inhibiting tumor cell attachment or growth receptors. However, generally interactions of antibody with cell antigen are not very effective unless Fc receptor–mediated effector mechanisms are also activated.

Cellular Immunity

T lymphocytes recognize processed (digested) molecules that complex with MHC molecules within antigen-presenting cells. The antigen/MHC molecules are then trafficked to the cell surface for recognition by T-cell receptors, which are encoded by genes of the immunoglobulin family. Similar to generation of antibodies, great diversity of T-cell receptors is generated by rearrangements of these immunoglobulin family genes. Each monoclonal T-cell receptor must bind to its cognate antigen/MHC complex presented on the surface of antigen-presenting cells. Signaling from the T-cell receptor following engagement of antigen/MHC complex is insufficient to activate the T cell. Additional signals are required (co-stimulatory signals or "signal 2"). The most important co-stimulatory signal in T cells comes from the T-cell surface molecule CD28, which engages B7 molecules (CD80 and CD86) on antigen-presenting cells. Engagement of T-cell receptor by antigen/MHC in conjunction with CD28 engagement of B7 is sufficient to activate naïve T cells. Interestingly, within several days following T-cell activation, a second molecule, CTLA-4, appears on the T-cell surface to provide a brake to the T-cell response. CTLA-4 also binds B7 molecules, but with much higher affinity, therefore displacing CD28 activation signals. CTLA-4 signaling leads to down-regulation of the T-cell response. A variety of other co-stimulatory molecules are up-regulated on the surface of activated T cells, including OX40 and 4-1BB, which promote survival of T cells and help generate long-lived T-cell memory responses. Once T cells are activated by professional antigen-presenting cells (primarily dendritic cells), they gain a variety of effector functions, including the production of cytokines and cytotoxic molecules, which lead to death of target cells. Recently, a cell type combining properties of NK cells and T cells, called NKT cells, has been characterized. NKT cells can rapidly produce cytokines and also cytotoxic effector molecules in response to cognate antigen, and remarkably recognize lipid antigens presented by MHC-related molecules on antigen-presenting cells.

Antigen-Presenting Cells

Dendritic cells, the prototype professional antigen-presenting cells, sit at the crossroads of innate immunity and acquired immunity. These are phagocytic cells that sit on epidermal surfaces, including skin and mucosal membranes, constantly sampling their environment to search for infectious organisms. Although dendritic cells continuously ingest molecules from their environment, uptake of antigen is insufficient to activate dendritic cells. Rather, dendritic cells have a set of receptors, most notably the toll-like receptors (TLRs), which can recognize lipid-containing molecules and CpG-rich DNA and poly-U RNA sequences produced specifically by microbial organisms. Engagement of TLR signals for activation of the dendritic cell, with increased expression of MHC and B7 molecules, and movement of cells with captured antigen to draining lymph nodes. It is in draining lymph nodes that dendritic cells activate appropriate T cells that recognize that particular antigen presented by MHC molecules. Subsequently, activated T cells can then travel from the draining lymph node to distant sites of infection or tumor to carry out the effector functions. One of the central problems for cancer immunology is that dendritic cells may ingest and process cancer antigens, but without activation through TLRs or other receptors, the dendritic cells remain incapable of activating T cells (because of insufficient expression of co-stimulatory molecules, such as B7) and do not move to draining lymph nodes. In fact, insufficiently activated dendritic cells presenting antigens can induce anergy, a form of immune tolerance where T cells become paralyzed and incapable of responding to cognate antigens. This is one of the mechanisms used to maintain immune tolerance to self to prevent autoimmunity, but also presents a major hurdle for cancer immunity. Cancer cells do not have any readily apparent mechanism to activate dendritic cells, although several self molecules, including heat shock protein, hyaluronate, and uric acid crystals, have been suggested to activate dendritic cells.

Helper and Regulatory T Cells

Several types of T cells are activated by dendritic cells, and which type is influenced by whether antigens are presented by MHC class I or MHC class II molecules on antigen-presenting cells. MHC class I molecules complexed with antigen stimulate CD8+ T cells that are cytotoxic and kill target cells (infected cells or tumor cells). Antigens presented by class II MHC molecules stimulate CD4+ helper T cells. Helper T cells produce chemokines and cytokines to help recruit and orchestrate other components of the immune system. Helper T cells come in several "flavors," and different cytokines in the milieu determine what type of T cell is generated. Each type of helper T cell mediates different types of immune responses with different characteristics. Th1 T cells produce interferon (IFN)-γ to activate cytotoxic T cells and macrophages for *cellular immune responses*. On the other hand, Th2 helper T cells produce interleukin (IL)-4 and other cytokines that favor antibody responses, or *humoral immunity*. The newly discovered Th17 CD4+ T cell produces IL-17 to mediate inflammatory autoimmune diseases, such as arthritis, colitis, and encephalitis, and may play a role in cancer pathogenesis, either by promoting cancer progression or by destroying tumors. Another type of CD4+ T cell restricted by MHC II presentation negatively regulates immune responses. These are regulatory T cells, or Tregs. Tregs recognize self antigens, are dependent on IL-2, and produce inhibitory molecules such as IL-10 and transforming growth factor-β. Th1 cellular immunity may be particularly effective at attacking tumors in tissues, while humoral immunity may be better at controlling circulating metastatic tumor cells. Infiltration of ovarian cancers and other cancers by Treg cells is associated with a poorer prognosis (11–13).

Cancer Immunity and Immunotherapy

The notion that both the innate and acquired immune arms of the immune system can recognize and reject cancer had been controversial over the last hundred years. Careful studies over the past 3 decades have shown that the immune system can recognize and destroy cancers, usually involving interactions between multiple arms of the immune system. For instance, simple recognition by T cells, antibodies, or NK cells is usually not sufficient to reject cancers. Cytotoxic T cells and NK cells produce soluble and cell surface molecules that induce death of target tumor cells. Helper T cells can produce cytokines and chemokines that not only recruit cytotoxic T cells or B cells to make antibodies, but also inflammatory cells which mediate tissue destruction. Antibodies can activate NK cells, macrophages, or other cells that have receptors for the antibodies' Fc domain, leading to activation of the recruited cells, a mechanism implicated in the antitumor effects of monoclonal antibody therapies. Antibodies can also activate complement proteins in the blood that can directly kill tumor cells and activate inflammatory cells at the tumor site.

Thus, based on solid evidence that the immune system can recognize antigens on tumor cells and that immunity is sufficient to destroy tumors, strategies are being developed for *immunotherapy*. These approaches can be broadly divided into three groups. First, *immune modulation* uses nonspecific approaches to treat cancer. Examples include cytokines such as IL-2, IL-12, interferons, BCG (*Bacillus* Calmette-Guérin, an attenuated *Mycobacterium* strain used successfully for treatment of early recurrent bladder cancer), and other microbial products. This approach tends to rely on components from the innate immune arm. *Passive therapy* refers to the transfer of specific components from the acquired immune system to the host with cancer. The best examples are monoclonal antibodies directed against antigens expressed on the surface of cancer cells. Rituximab against the CD20 antigen expressed by normal B cells is an effective part of the armamentarium for treatment of B-cell lymphomas, and trastuzumab (Herceptin) has been approved for treatment of breast cancer in combination with chemotherapy. Although the antitumor effects of trastuzumab in part probably involve inhibition of signaling by the HER2 tyrosine kinase oncogene, evidence strongly supports a major role for immune activation of Fc receptor–positive cells by both rituximab and trastuzumab (14).

A second example of passive immunotherapy is adoptive cellular therapy, where cells from the blood or bone marrow donor are purified, cultured, and/or manipulated outside the body and reinfused into the same patient (autologous) or a different patient (allogeneic). Cellular therapy has particularly focused on T cells and more recently on NK cells. Recent strategies have used genetic approaches to transduce T cells with receptors against tumor antigens (using either cloned T-cell receptors or antibody Fv regions to determine antigen specificity linked to intracellular signaling domains). In addition, genetic approaches are exploring transduction of T cells with genes encoding co-stimulatory molecules such as CD28 or 4-1BB.

Finally, active immunization refers to vaccines that trigger the patient to make her own immune response. Both passive and active immunotherapy must be directed against specific antigens on cancer cells.

Immunotherapy is already a routine part of cancer treatment (e.g., interferons, IL-2, BCG, monoclonal antibodies, and adoptive cellular therapy as part of allogeneic bone marrow transplantation). Potential difficulties remain in developing new immunotherapies, including insufficient activation of dendritic cells by cancer cells, inhibition of responses by Treg cells, and both intrinsic and extrinsic mechanisms that down-regulate T-cell responses, e.g., signaling through CTLA-4. These checkpoints all participate to dampen immune responses against cancer. On the other hand, identification of these checkpoints is leading to development of strategies with the potential of overcoming these barriers. Vaccines need to incorporate immune adjuvants that can sufficiently activate dendritic cells, often using microbial products. Therapeutic strategies to target Tregs are being assessed preclinically and clinically, including chemotherapy and new drugs targeting the CD25 molecule expressed by Tregs. Blockade of CTLA-4 by monoclonal antibodies has led to responses in patients with ovarian cancer, melanoma, and other cancers. Passive therapy with monoclonal antibodies or with adoptive cellular treatments may be able to bypass some of these checkpoints.

Five groups of antigens have been defined on cancer cells that are recognized by the immune system: (a) Differentiation antigens, expressed by cancer cells and their normal cell counterparts; for instance, antigens expressed by ovarian carcinomas and normal ovarian epithelium are differentiation antigens. (b) Germ cell antigens, expressed by germ cells, particularly sperm, and silenced in normal adult somatic tissues, but re-expressed by certain tumors, commonly called cancer-testis antigens. (c) Genetic mutations and other alterations, such as translocations. (d) Over-expressed antigens, such as Her2 or the alpha isoform of the folate receptor. (e) Viral antigens, such as antigens encoded by oncogenic human papillomavirus.

In summary, cancer immunology has begun to create a firm scientific footing over the last few decades. In particular, identification of molecules on cancer cells that are recognized by the immune system provides new strategies for passive immunotherapy and vaccination. A number of clinical trials are in various stages of development to explore these strategies.

IMMUNOMODULATION AND CYTOKINE THERAPY

Cytokines play important roles in immune modulation. Many cytokines, including IL-2, IL-3, IL-4, IL-6, IL-10, IL-12, tumor necrosis factor-α (TNF-α), macrophage colony-stimulating final factor, and IFNs, have been studied for their roles in tumor treatment. Some of these cytokines (IL-2 and IFN-α) have been approved by the U.S. Food and Drug Administration (FDA) specifically for the treatment of melanoma and renal-cell carcinoma.

Gynecologic cancers, particularly ovarian cancer, provide a unique environment for cytokine therapy in that the peritoneal cavity is a rich milieu for the elaboration of cytokines (15). The bulk of ovarian cancer occurs in the peritoneal cavity, making the regional administration of biologic therapy theoretically attractive. Distinct patterns of cytokine expression have been observed between the tumor and peritoneal compartments. Some of these cytokines may be counter-regulatory components of T-lymphocyte networks that have the potential to either augment or inhibit host antitumor responses (16). The successful outcome of cytokine treatment in ovarian cancer may be the result of a number of mechanisms. Whereas some cytokines may inhibit tumor cell growth, down-regulating the production of growth and survival factors, other cytokines may stimulate adaptive immunity or modulate angiogenesis. It is also possible that an individual cytokine has more than one role (17). The major cytokines that have been tested in gynecologic cancers are IFN-α, IL-2, and IL-12.

Interferons

Cytokine therapy in gynecologic cancers has been studied most extensively with IFN-α. There has been no head-to-head comparison between IFN-α and IFN-γ; nonetheless, they appear to have similar antitumor efficacy in ovarian cancer (18–20), and most studies have focused on IFN-α. Although the exact mode of action of IFN in patients with ovarian cancer is unknown, several mechanisms have been proposed: (a) stimulation of NK cells and macrophages, both of which are known to have antitumor properties (21); (b) anti-angiogenic effects; and (c) inhibition of expression of dysregulated oncogenes (such as *HER2/neu*) and thereby improving the responsiveness of cisplatin-resistant cells (22).

Initial trials with IFN evaluated administration of systemic IFN-α to patients with advanced ovarian cancer. The objective response rate was generally low at about 10% in a Gynecologic Oncology Group (GOG) study, where patients with measurable disease in whom higher priority treatment methods had failed were treated with IFN intramuscularly (23). The role of IFN-α as a maintenance treatment after initial surgical resection and chemotherapy was also evaluated by a randomized phase 3 study and was recently reported to be negative (24). The systemic IFN-α was also associated with frequent dose-limiting toxicity, including fatigue and flu-like symptoms, and moderate toxicity, such as leukopenia and thrombocytopenia. Because of the poor response rate and frequent toxicity of systemic administration, further studies were focused on IP administration of IFN-α. Multiple clinical trials with IP IFN therapy were carried out in women with persistent ovarian cancer (21,25–33). The surgically documented response rates from these studies ranged from 30% to 50%. An important finding was that the response rate was inversely correlated with tumor bulk and was not observed in patients with tumors >5 mm. For example, in a study where an overall response rate was 44%, patients with minimal residual disease (defined as <5 mm) had a response rate of 71%, whereas none of the four patients whose tumors were ≥5 mm responded (25). Systemic IFN toxicity developed following peritoneal absorption, and the maximal tolerable dose (MTD) was defined as 50 MU IP once per week (15). A randomized, placebo-controlled GOG phase 3 trial attempted to address the value of IP recombinant IFN-α as an adjuvant therapy in stage III ovarian patients with no evidence of disease at second-look surgery. Unfortunately, the study was prematurely terminated owing to slow accrual secondary to a decline of frequency of second-look surgery nationwide.

Some *in vitro* studies had suggested that IFN (both IFN-α and IFN-γ) could increase the sensitivity of cytotoxic drugs, such as cisplatin and doxorubicin, in cancer cells (19,34). It was found that IFN produced no significant change in the uptake of cisplatin. Studies indicated that the mechanism of IFN-induced sensitization in human ovarian cancer cell lines is multifactorial. Several phase 1 studies have been carried out to define the optimal dosing schedule of IP IFN-α in combination with cis-platinum–based chemotherapy (30,35,36). The MTDs were generally 20 to 30 MU/m^2 of IFN-α with 60 to 75 mg/m^2 cis-platinum. The most common toxicities were myelosuppression, flu-like symptoms, abdominal pain, and fatigue. In general, the combination of IP IFN-α with cis-platinum was less tolerated than IFN-α alone. Several phase 2 studies have evaluated the efficacy of this combination with response rates in the range of 20% to 50% (28,30,37). IP carboplatin with or without IFN-α was also evaluated in a randomized trial in 111 patients with advanced ovarian cancer and minimal residual disease who had previously had platinum-based front-line chemotherapy (38,39,40). Median survival was 22 and 29 months in the carboplatin arm and in the carboplatin plus IFN-α arm, respectively (p = 0.9). The IP IFN-α did not add benefit to the results achievable with IP carboplatin alone, while the toxicity and the costs of the combination were consistently higher. Based on data suggesting that cyclosporine A could potentiate the cytotoxic activity of platinum, a phase 2 trial was conducted with subcutaneous injection of IFN-α added to a continuous infusion of cyclosporine A combined with carboplatin in patients with recurrent ovarian cancer. Thirty patients with both platinum-sensitive and -resistant disease were included. Only three partial responses were seen, and toxicities included myelosuppression, nausea, vomiting, and headache. Insufficient clinical resistance reversal was observed to warrant further investigation of this combination (39). Taking together all of these studies, there is no evidence to date showing that those combinations of IP IFN-α with cytotoxic chemotherapy provide any benefit over single agents. A more recent study with IP IFN-α chemotherapy in ovarian cancer patients with minimal residual disease reported a total complete remission rate of 49% (40). This somewhat higher response rate remains to be confirmed by prospective controlled trials.

The combination of IFN-γ with chemotherapy has also been evaluated. A randomized phase 3 trial evaluating cyclophosphamide and cisplatin for first-line therapy in 148 patients of a planned 200 with or without IFN-γ demonstrated a progression-free survival advantage of 17 versus 48 months (p = 0.031) in favor of the IFN-γ–containing arm. Accrual was halted early when taxane and platinum-based combination therapy became standard and power in the study was compromised. No statistically significant survival benefit was seen (41). A follow-up phase 1/2 study combining IFN-γ with the newer standard chemotherapy paclitaxel and carboplatin showed that the combination was safe and had a response rate of 71% as first-line treatment for ovarian cancer (42). Randomized trial results will be required to determine if a benefit exists for the addition of IFN-γ to standard therapy.

In cervical cancer, monotherapy with IFN-α had minimal activity (43,44). In a multi-institutional, prospective phase-2 clinical trial by the Eastern Cooperative Oncology Group (ECOG) evaluating the activity of IFN-α2b in women with metastatic or locally recurrent cervical cancer, only 10% achieved a clinical response. Further studies had been focused on the combination of IFN-α and retinoids because of observed synergistic antiproliferative, differentiating, and anti-angiogenic activities in some human hematologic and solid-tumor systems (45,46,47,48). The proposed mechanisms include (a) the additive activation of transcription of a retinoic reporter gene (45); (b) the induction of higher levels of IFN-α–stimulated genes than the levels induced by either agent alone (46); (c) the up-regulation of HLA class I and intracellular adhesion molecule-1 (ICAM-1) molecules, inducing an additive effect on the expression of immunologically important surface antigens on human cervical cancer cells (47). An initial phase 2 study with this combination for untreated locally advanced cervical or uterine cancer patients yielded response rates of 50% to 58% (45). However, in pretreated recurrent cervical cancers, this combination appears to be less active, with response rates of 0% to 31% (49–52). Another study for patients with locally advanced cervical cancer showed a response rate of 47% with mild fever being the major toxicity (53). In addition, the combination of IFN-α with cytotoxic agents, namely, cisplatin plus 5-fluorouracil (5-FU), has also been evaluated in the treatment of cervical cancer (54). It was relatively well tolerated, as toxicity was comparable to that of cisplatin plus 5-FU alone with a major response rate of 31%. Recent studies have shown that concurrent cisplatin-based radiotherapy and chemotherapy have significantly improved survival in both early- and locally advanced-stage cervical cancer (4,5,55), and has now become the standard of care. Future studies may test whether addition of IFN-α and/or retinoic acid will provide additional benefit.

Regional therapy with IFN-α gel for vulvar intraepithelial neoplasia was also evaluated in a prospective, randomized, double-armed crossover study comparing IFN-α with and without 1% nonoxynol-9. An overall response rate of 67% was achieved, and the toxicity was lower than previously reported for topical 5-FU. These data support the hypothesis that IFN-α is an active agent in the treatment of vulvar intraepithelial neoplasia III (56). Intralesional IFN-α was also evaluated for cervical intraepithelial neoplasia (57). However, with the good surgical success rate, this approach has received less enthusiasm.

In summary, IP IFN-α is well tolerated, and while it has produced clinical responses in ovarian cancer patients with minimal residual disease, no randomized data has supported a survival benefit to date. The combination of IFN-α with standard cytotoxic agents adds toxicity without adding significant antitumor activity. The improved progression-free survival with IFN-γ in conjunction with platinum-based primary chemotherapy is intriguing, and the evaluation of IFN-γ in combination with current standard regimens in appropriately randomized and controlled trials is reasonable. Combinations of IFN and retinoic acid or chemotherapy may have clinical benefit in cervical cancer, and appropriate controlled trials could be considered.

Interleukin-2

IL-2 is a T-cell growth factor that plays a central role in the immune system. Initial studies of IL-2 in the treatment of ovarian cancer involved continuous intravenous infusion therapy for patients with minimal residual disease at second-look surgery. The toxicity was significant and about 86% required dose reduction (58). Subsequent studies had been focused on IP administration of IL-2. A phase 1-2 study (59) of IP IL-2 in patients with laparotomy-confirmed persistent or recurrent ovarian cancer after ≥6 courses of prior platinum-based chemotherapy had shown an overall response rate of 25.7%, with an overall 5-year survival probability of 13.9%. For the patients who responded to therapy, the median survival time had not been reached (range 27 to 90+ months) at the time of the report. This study also showed that IP IL-2 is better tolerated as a weekly infusion compared with a 7-day infusion. In the follow-up phase 2 study of outpatient weekly infusion of IP IL-2 in patients with persistent ovarian cancer after primary paclitaxel (Taxol) and platinum therapy in patients with minimal residual disease (<2 cm), 17.6% had a surgically documented response and 41% of patients had stable disease. This study suggests that IP IL-2 may have activity in persistent epithelial ovarian cancer and is well tolerated as an outpatient regimen (60). The combination of IL-2 and cytotoxic agents, for example, cisplatin, has been studied in mouse ovarian tumor models. In tumors that were minimally responsive to treatment with either of the drugs alone, combined local treatment with low doses of cisplatin and IL-2 resulted in an effective antitumor response with a complete response of 60%. Analysis of tumor-associated leukocytes showed that the combination of cisplatin and IL-2 resulted in enhanced nonspecific cytolytic activity of peritoneal leukocytes. Therefore, in the mouse model, combined local treatment with low doses of cis-platinum and IL-2 was more effective than cisplatin alone. Randomized data would be required to determine if similar efficacy exists in human ovarian cancer (61).

A disadvantage of frequent administration of high-dose IL-2 is the occurrence of dose-limiting side effects. Therefore, delivery of IL-2-from an expression plasmid has been evaluated for the treatment of ovarian cancer. IP treatment of ovarian tumors with an IL-2–expressing plasmid resulted in an increase in local IL-2 levels, a change in the cytokine profile of the tumor ascites, and a significant antitumor effect in a mouse model (62). A phase 1 trial with an IL-2 gene–modified tumor in refractory ovarian cancer patients was proposed and the result is not yet available (63).

In summary, IL-2–based therapy has been reported to be associated with long-term remissions in selected ovarian cancer patients as with other solid tumors. The treatment, however, is hindered by significant toxicity. Approaches to minimize toxicity and optimize efficacy are being tested. The combination of low doses of cis-platinum with IL-2 seems to be a promising strategy in mouse models and warrants clinical trials to assess efficacy in humans.

Interleukin-12

IL-12 is a cytokine mainly produced by activated monocytes, tissue macrophages, and B cells. It can induce IFN-γ and together with IL-2 becomes a potent activator of cytotoxic T lymphocytes and NK cells (64,65). Whereas IL-4 and IL-10 mediate the development of Th2-type immunity, IL-12 initiates the differentiation to the Th1 phenotype. In addition, IL-12 production can be negatively or positively regulated by cytokines. For example, IL-10 and IL-4 have been shown to inhibit the production of IL-12 (16,66), whereas IL-2 and IFN-α enhance its production. In addition, IL-12 has potent anti-metastatic and antitumor effects in several murine tumor models, as well as in human tumor cells *in vitro* and *in vivo* (65,67). IL-12 was better than IL-2 in enhancing the cytotoxicity against ovarian cancer cells of lymphocytes from ascites or peripheral blood from patients (68). IL-12 and IL-2 have a synergistic effect on the lymphokine-activated killer activity in peripheral blood mononuclear cells cultured in ovarian cancer ascitic fluid (69). It has been suggested that the antitumor effects of IL-12 involve enhanced IFN-γ production by antitumor T cells, their accumulation to tumor sites, and *in situ* IFN-γ production (70). In addition, IL-12 promotes IFN-γ–mediated up-regulation of adhesion molecules (vascular cell adhesion molecule [VCAM-1] and ICAM-1) on tumor-associated blood vessels, providing access for circulating lymphocytes (68). However, ascitic IL-12 has also been shown to be an independent prognostic factor for adverse outcome in ovarian cancer (71).

A phase 2 GOG clinical trial (72) evaluated intravenously administered recombinant human IL-12 in patients with recurrent or refractory ovarian cancer. The study showed that, as a single agent, IL-12 could be tolerated, and myelotoxicity and capillary leak syndrome were the major adverse events. However, the response rate was low, with no complete responders, and a partial response rate of 3.8%. IP administration of human recombinant IL-12 was also evaluated in patients with refractory ovarian and gastrointestinal malignancies after primary standard therapy (73). Among the 29 patients, two patients (one with ovarian cancer and one with mesothelioma) had no remaining disease at laparoscopy, eight patients had stable disease, and 19 had progressive disease. In this study, the dose-limiting toxicity was elevated transaminases. More frequent toxicities included fever, fatigue, abdominal pain, nausea, and catheter-related infections. Preclinical data had suggested that IL-12 may potentiate the activity of the HER2 monoclonal antibody trastuzumab. A phase 1 trial with this combination in HER2-positive malignancies in 15 patients showed no clinical evidence of increased activity with the combination with one complete response and otherwise disease stabilization as best response (74).

BASIS FOR ANTIBODY-MEDIATED THERAPY OF CANCER

Antibodies are the primary mechanism for eliminating infectious pathogens from the bloodstream. The effect of all commonly used vaccines against infectious agents is thought to be primarily a consequence of antibody induction. Antibodies are also ideally suited for elimination of circulating tumor cells and micrometastases. The importance of antibodies in mediating protection from tumor recurrence is well documented in experimental animals (75,76). Experiments involving administration of monoclonal antibody 3F8 against GD2 or induction of GD2 antibodies by vaccination after challenge with EL4 lymphoma (which expresses GD2) are two examples. Administration of 3F8 prior to intravenous tumor challenge or as late as 4 days after tumor challenge results in complete protection of a majority of mice (76). Comparable protection from EL4 challenge was induced by immunization with a GD2-KLH conjugate vaccine. This timing may be comparable to antibody induction, or administration, in patients in the adjuvant setting after surgical resection of the primary or lymph node or peritoneal metastases, or after response to chemotherapy. In both cases, the targets may be circulating tumor cells and micrometastases.

There is also evidence in cancer patients that natural or passively administered antibodies in the adjuvant setting are associated with clinical benefit:

1. Natural antibodies (antibodies present in patient sera prior to vaccination) and vaccine-induced antibodies have been correlated with an improved prognosis. This is true for patients with paraneoplastic syndromes where high titers of antibodies against onconeural antigens expressed on particular cells in the nervous system and certain types of tumors have been associated both with debilitating autoimmune neurologic disorders and with delayed tumor progression and prolonged survival. Also patients with American Joint Commission for Cancer (AJCC) stage III melanoma and natural antibodies against GM2 ganglioside treated at two different medical centers have had an 80% to 100% 5-year survival compared to the expected 40% rate (77–79). Tumor vaccine–induced antibodies in the adjuvant setting against GM2 and several other melanoma antigens at four different medical centers, and against sialyl Tn (sTn) antigen in adenocarcinoma patients, have been correlated with prolonged disease-free interval and survival (reviewed in Ref. 80).
2. A series of monoclonal antibodies against antigens expressed at the cell surface of cancer cells has now been shown to has clinical efficacy in the advanced disease setting and has been approved by the FDA. These include rituximab, ibritumomab, and tositumomab for B-cell lymphomas; gemtuzumab for acute myelocytic leukemias; alemtuzumab for chronic lymphocytic leukemias; cetuximab for colorectal and head and neck squamous cell carcinomas; and trastuzumab for breast cancer. It is likely that all of these mAbs would be more effective if administered in the adjuvant setting. This appears to be the case for trastuzumab. Treatment of patients with advanced *HER2/neu* positive breast cancers resulted in an overall response rate of 19% to 26% and response duration of 9 to 15 months, while treatment with trastuzumab in the adjuvant setting has resulted in a 50% decrease in the recurrence rate at 1-year median follow-up and at 3 years (81).

Hence, passively administered and vaccine-induced antibodies have been shown to correlate with clinical responses or improved disease-free and overall survival in the mouse and human. Preclinical studies strongly suggest that the optimal setting for antibody therapy is the adjuvant setting. Since the great majority of gynecologic cancer patients are initially rendered free of detectable disease by surgery and/or chemotherapy after initial diagnosis, administration of mAbs or vaccines inducing antibodies may have broad applicability. There are advantages to each approach. Titers of anticancer antibodies are generally acutely higher after administration of mAbs, and mAbs can be generated against virtually any antigen. On the other hand, human antimouse and anti-idiotype antibodies may limit the usefulness of continued administration of mAbs, and maintenance of antibody titers with vaccines is more practical and less expensive than with mAbs.

Target Antigens for Antibodies

We have screened a variety of malignancies and normal tissues with a series of 40 mAbs against 25 antigens that were potential target antigens for immunotherapy of cancer (82–84). Since recognition of antigens on living cancer cells by antibodies is largely restricted to the cancer cell surface, the focus was on cell surface antigens. Antigen expression on ovarian and endometrial cancers and several other malignancies for the seven defined antigens expressed strongly in at least three of five biopsy specimens are shown in Table 6.1 (82–86). The antigens expressed by ovarian and endometrial cancers are similar, and quite different from those expressed by melanomas, and similar to, although not the same as, those expressed by prostatic cancers. The 18 excluded antigens (including CEA and *HER2/neu*) were expressed in one or zero of five specimens. With the possible exception of GM2 (for which there are no previous reports), our results are consistent with the separate studies describing the expression of these individual ovarian cancer antigens from other centers. Our studies identify ganglioside GM2 as an antigen present on many malignancies, which is a conclusion supported by an increasing number of recent reports (87,88).

TABLE 6.1

NUMBER OF TUMOR BIOPSY SPECIMENS WITH 50% OR MORE OF TUMOR CELLS POSITIVE BY IMMUNOHISTOLOGY

	Antigen (mAb)[a]									
Tumor	sTn (CC49)	sTn (B72.3)	TF (49H.8)	Le^y (3S193)	Le^y (BR96)	GM2 (696)	Globo H (Mbr1)	MUC-1 (HMFG2)	KSA (GA7333)	MUC-16/ (CA-125)
Ovarian	4/5	3/5	5/5	4/5	99/133[b]	5/5	18/19	5/5	5/5	53/62[c]
Endometrial	4/5	2/5	4/5	3/5	2/5	5/5	4/5	3/5	5/5	—
Melanoma	0/5	0/5	0/5	0/5	0/5	10/10	0/10	0/5	0/5	0/4
Small-cell Lung	0/5	0/5	0/5	2/5	1/5	6/6	4/6	2/5	4/5	0/2
Prostate	4/5	3/5	1/5	3/5	3/5	5/5	2/5	1/5	5/5	0/5

[a]All the tumor tissues were stained by avidin-biotin complex immunoperoxidase methods (82–84).
[b](85)
[c](86)

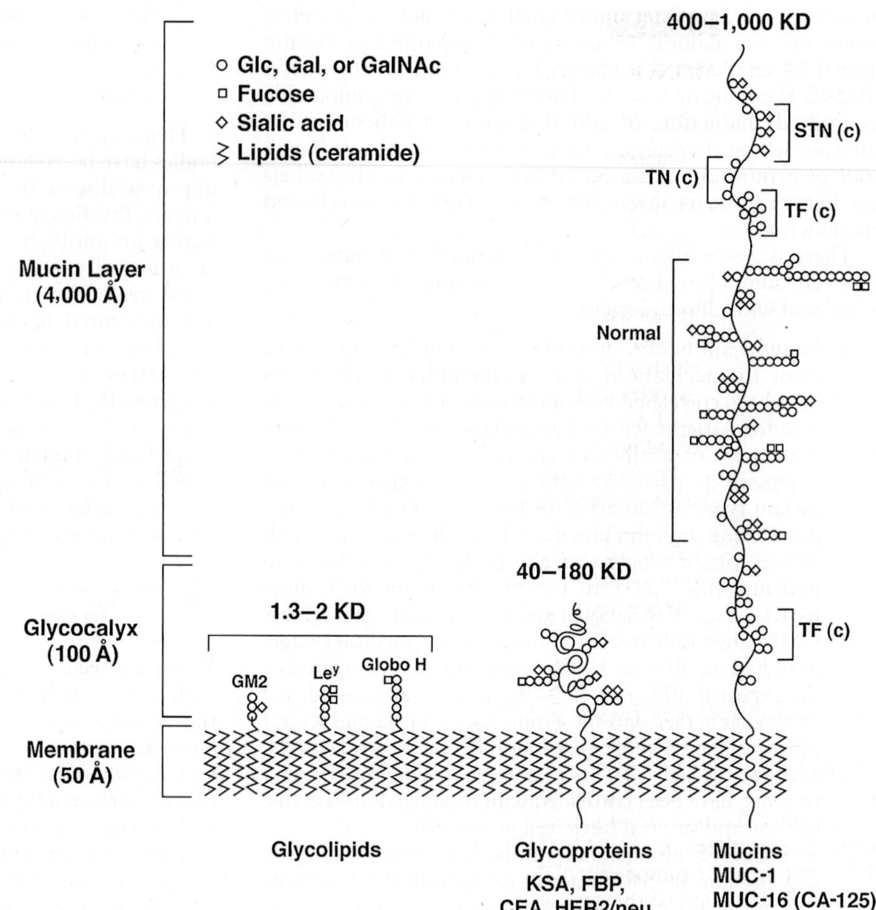

FIGURE 6.1. Glycolipid and glycoprotein antigens expressed at the cell surface of gynecologic cancers. *Symbols:* ◇ = sialic acid; □ = fucose; ○ = glucose, galactose, N-acetylgalactosamine, or N-acetylgl cosamine.

The expression of these eight antigens on normal tissues is essentially restricted to apical epithelial cells at luminal borders, a site that appears not to be accessible to the immune system. Administered mAbs to several of these antigens have induced clinical responses but have not induced autoimmunity, indicating that antigen in these locations may not be accessible to antibodies. The exception is GM2, which is also expressed in the brain, although far less than the related ganglioside GD3, where the blood-brain barrier prevents autoimmune toxicity (infusions of monoclonal antibodies against GD3 have been associated with many clinical responses and no incidents of central nervous system [CNS] toxicity). BR96 recognizes a broader specificity than Lewis-y (Le^y) (89,90), also including Lewis-X (Le^x), which explains the reactivity with polymorphonucleocytes (which express Le^x but do not express Le^y). Hemorrhagic gastritis has been reported after high doses of BR96 (against Le^y), possibly related to a broader specificity of BR96, since treatment with another mAb, 3S193, against Le^y has not been associated with these toxicities. The extensive expression of CA-125 in over 80% of serous and endometrioid ovarian cancers has been well documented since the early 1980s (91). Following the successful cloning of CA-125 and identifying it as a complex mucin, it has been termed MUC-16 (92–94). Contributing to tumor mucin specificity is the less intense glycosylation of tumor mucins than normal mucins, involving shorter carbohydrate chains. The simplified structures of these antigens in relation to the cancer cell surface lipid bilayer are shown in Figure 6.1.

There is now sufficient experience from clinical trials with vaccine-induced antibody responses against GM2, TF, sTn, MUC-1, and KSA antigens, and passive administration of mAbs against sTn, MUC-16 (CA-125), and KSA to draw conclusions about the consequences of antigen distribution on various normal tissues. GM2 exposure on cells in the brain and GM2, sTn, TF, MUC-1, and KSA antigen expression in cells at the secretory borders of epithelial tissues induce neither immunologic tolerance nor autoimmunity once antibodies are present, suggesting that they are sequestered from the immune system. Against this background, GM2, T, Tn, sTn, Globo H, MUC-1, MUC-16 (CA-125), and KSA all appear to be good cell surface targets for active immunotherapy with vaccines that induce antibodies, or for passive immunotherapy with monoclonal antibodies.

Antibody Selection

Tumor cells have defined antigens and receptors on the cell surface that may differ from those present on normal cells. mAbs directed against these targets have potential diagnostic and therapeutic applications. The selection of the optimal antigen-antibody system for clinical development depends on a number of biologic and technical factors, including antigen density, pathways of catabolism, tumor specificity, heterogeneity of expression, effector mechanisms, and binding affinity. Antigens that have been used for immune targeting of gynecologic malignancies with mAbs for antibody development include (a) over-expressed tumor antigens (e.g., CA-125, TAG-72 [sTn], MUC-1, polymorphic epithelial mucin [PEM], folate-binding protein [FBP], and Lewis-Y); (b) over-expressed growth-factor receptors (e.g., *HER2/neu* [erbB2], epidermal

TABLE 6.2

MONOCLONAL ANTIBODIES TARGETING GYNECOLOGIC MALIGNANCIES

Targeted antigens	Antibody examples	Therapeutic considerations
Mucins		
CA-125 (MUC-16)	OVAREX (B43.13), OC125 ACA125 (anti-id OC125)	Ovarian cancer
MUC-1	HMFG1, HMFG2	
Tumor-associated glycoprotein		
TAG-72 (sTn)	B72.3, CC49	Ovarian cancer
Human folate-binding protein (FBP)	MOv18, MOv19	Ovarian cancer
Markers of epithelial differentiation		
CEA	MN-14	Ovarian cancer
Blood type substance		
Lewis-Y-related cell surface antigens	BR55, BR96, B3, 3S193	Ovarian cancer
Oncogene-associated growth factor receptor		
HER2/neu receptor	Trastuzumab	Ovarian cancer
CAIX (MN antigen)	M75	Endo/cervix

CEA, carcinoembryonic antigen.

growth-factor receptor [EGFR], and vascular endothelial growth factor [VEGF]); and (c) mutated tumor-suppressor genes (e.g., p53 and *BRCA-1*). Binding of mAb to these antigens may have antitumor effect generated through these possible mechanisms: (a) antibody-mediated recruitment of human effector mechanisms *in situ*, ADCC against the tumor cells; (b) development of tumor-specific cytotoxic T lymphocytes (CTLs); (c) activation of the complement system; (d) stimulation of granulocytes cytotoxic to the cancer cells; and (e) induction of an anti-idiotypic antibody that can elicit active immunity. The available antibodies and their targeting antigens that have been tested in gynecologic malignancies are summarized in Table 6.2.

Obstacles in Antibody Therapy and Engineering Strategies

Despite decades of efforts, there are currently few nonimmunogenic antibodies against cell-surface antigens that are of therapeutic significance in gynecologic cancers. The major obstacles have been (a) development of human anti-murine antibodies (HAMA) that form immune complexes with subsequent antibody administration, which results in altered patterns of catabolism and host toxicity; (b) limited immunobiologic activity of nonconjugated antibody; (c) expression of antigens (e.g., growth-factor receptors on a wide range of normal host tissue); and (d) heterogeneity of antigen expression among different histologies and patients. Various engineering strategies have been tested to overcome these obstacles.

Overcoming HAMA

Because murine mAbs are xenotypic proteins, the immunocompetent human will recognize them as foreign and generate antibody responses (HAMA) against them. Although the resultant immune complexes may potentially boost the immune response to the antigen epitope, leading to enhanced recognition by the immune system and an increased processing by dendritic and antigen-presenting cells, the more likely outcome is increased blood clearance and less effective tumor targeting, precluding repeat administration. This has been one of the major obstacles in the application of murine mAbs to the treatment of human cancers. To minimize the effect of HAMA, various strategies have been explored, including construction of smaller antibody fragments, design of recombinant antibodies with substitution of human for murine sequences, and direct cloning of human variable regions with the desired binding specificity. Chimeric or fully humanized antibodies have been developed to reduce HAMA responses associated with the administration of murine mAbs, with the concomitant possibility of manipulating the effector function (95). The reduced immunogenicity of humanized antibodies allows their repeated administration in many cases. Initial efforts involved development of a mouse-human chimeric mAb by replacing the murine immunoglobulin heavy- and light-chain constant regions with those of the human Ig (chimerization).

A widely used procedure for the humanization of xenogeneic antibodies is based on grafting the hypervariable or complementarity-determining regions (CDRs) of a xenogeneic antibody onto the human Ig framework. With this approach, a minimally immunogenic variant of humanized anti-CC49 mAb has been developed (96). Construction of smaller molecules has also been explored to decrease HAMA. Immunoglobulins have been engineered to retain only the domains that are required for antigen binding and/or effector functions and have also been rebuilt into multivalent, high-affinity reagents to achieve the desired efficacy (97). Studies with different forms of mAbs have shown that antibody fragments of lower molecular weight can penetrate tumor faster than whole IgG molecules (98,99). A humanized CC49 single-chain (scFv) construct (hu/muCC49 scFv) has been prepared, where the murine CC49 variable light chain was entirely replaced by a homologous human light chain. Pharmacokinetic studies in mice showed rapid blood and whole-body clearance with a half-life of 6 minutes, and biodistribution studies demonstrated equivalent tumor targeting to human colon carcinoma xenografts for muCC49 and hu/muCC49 scFv (100), indicating that it has potential diagnostic and therapeutic applications for TAG72-positive tumors. mAb constructs that have a deletion of the CH_2 portion of the constant region have been created: h-ΔCH_2CC49 is a humanized CC49 with its CH_2 region deleted, with identical affinity for TAG-72 (101). The clinical characteristics of these constructs and conjugates are being tested. Conjugates of these constructs with radionuclides, for example, ^{225}Ac, have also been made (102). A more recent technology uses immunization of transgenic mice with human immunoglobulin genes (and deleted mouse immunoglobulin genes) to generate fully human monoclonal antibodies.

Antibody Conjugates

In view of the limited efficacy of unconjugated antibody, efforts have been made to optimize the antitumor activity by conjugating with radionuclides, toxins, cytotoxic drugs, or second antibodies (Table 6.3) (15). Combinations of multiple antibodies to

TABLE 6.3

RADIONUCLIDES, TOXINS, AND CYTOTOXIC AGENTS USED AS mAb CONJUGATES

Reagents	Mechanistic considerations	Therapeutic considerations
RADIONUCLIDES		
^{125}I	Auger electron antitumor effects	Standard iodination chemistry, subject to dehalogenation. Auger effects limited to 15 Å radius. β penetrates ~1 mm and can kill adjacent antigen-negative cells. γ associated with wider penetration and dose-limiting marrow suppression.
^{131}I	$T_{1/2}$ 60 d 364 KeVγ (imaging) 606 Kevβ (therapy) $T_{1/2}$ 8 d	
^{90}Y	2.27 Mev β $T_{1/2}$ 2.7 d	Requires chelation. Almost pure β penetrates ~3 mm. Free ^{90}Y localizes to bone, associated with dose-limiting marrow suppression.
^{212}Bi	High LET 6.2 MeVα $T_{1/2}$ 1 h	α penetrates only several cell diameters (~20–100 μm). Toxicity not oxygen dependent, increased energy deposition compared to β.
^{211}At	High LET 6.0 Me11Vα $T_{1/2}$ 7.2 h	^{212}Bi has very short $T_{1/2}$ (demanding rapid localization), requires chelation, and can be generated in laboratory. ^{211}At requires a cyclotron for generation, and can be directly conjugated.
^{186}Re	137 KeVγ (imaging) 1.1 Mevβ (therapy) $T_{1/2}$ 3.7 d	Techniques available for direct conjugation or chelation. Low abundance γ suitable for imaging.
^{177}Lu	208 KeVγ (imaging) 0.5 Mevβ (therapy) $T_{1/2}$ 6.7 d	Evaluated as chelate. Low abundance γ suitable for imaging.
TOXINS		
PE	Bacterial *Pseudomonas* exotoxin A. Enzymatic inactivation of protein synthesis by ADP ribosylation of elongation factor 2.	Both PE and RA require internalization and cytoplasmic translocation for protein synthesis inhibition. PE requires acid hydrolysis. No mechanisms for killing adjacent antigen-negative or non-targeted cells. Recombinant PE and RA fragments available for chemical conjugation or construction of single-chain chimeric proteins.
RA	Ricin A-chain from castor beans. N-glycosidase-mediated inactivation of 28S ribosomal RNA.	
CYTOTOXIC AGENTS		
DOX	Doxorubicin-associated free-radical formation, DNA intercalation, inhibition of topoisomerase-II	Toxicity requires internalization and acid hydrolysis to release free DOX.
Anti-CD	Effector activation via the T-cell receptor complex	Requires simultaneous presence of activated effector cells, antibody, and antigen-positive tumor. Indirect cytokine effects, recruitment of inflammatory cells, and enhancement of immunity can occur.
Anti-FcR	Effector activation via NK/LGL FcγRIII complex	
Biotin	Multistep amplification using biotin-streptavidin system	Permits adding second- and third-step reagents with high affinity for the primary antibody. Allows for systemic clearing with increased tumor localization and tumor-to-normal-tissue ratios.

Source: Modified from Bookman MA, Boente MP, Bast R. Immunology and immunotherapy of gynecologic cancer. In: *Principles and Practice of Gynecologic Oncology.* 3rd ed. Philadelphia: Lippincott Williams & Wilkins, 2000:129–163.

compensate for antigen heterogeneity in ovarian carcinomas have been evaluated. The choice of conjugates and specific antibodies is influenced by features such as antigen internalization, lysosomal degradation, shedding, and heterogeneity of expression. Although internalization is a prerequisite for cellular toxicity of some drug and toxin conjugates, it may result in reduced efficacy and increased host toxicity due to intracellular catabolism (15).

Radionuclides

A variety of radionuclides have been conjugated with antibodies for imaging and treatment. The optimal radionuclide for cancer therapy is not easy to define (15). Radioconjugates with β (i.e., ^{131}I and ^{90}Y) and α (i.e., ^{211}At and ^{212}Bi) emitters have been proposed for regional therapy of peritoneal implants. Estimates of dosimetry suggest that adequate therapy (i.e., 20 Gy) could be delivered to tumors with a depth <300 μg using ^{211}At, <0.1 cm using ^{131}I, and <1 cm using ^{90}Y when conjugated to antibodies. Delivery of effective radiation dose is greatly influenced by the extent of tumor binding, depth of tumor penetration, catabolism, and relative distribution between tumor and normal tissues. Although internalization is usually detrimental owing to enhanced catabolism, internalization is required for maximal Auger electron chromosomal toxicity from ^{131}I owing to an extremely limited sphere of penetration (15). At the present time, β emitters are considered to be the optimal candidates for radiotherapy, as they avoid excessive systemic exposure associated with γ radiation. Conjugates with ^{131}I have been most extensively studied because of isotope availability, ease of chemical conjugation, and ability to perform γ imaging and β therapeutic studies with the same reagent. There has been an interest in finding alternatives to ^{131}I due to the nonspecific γ irradiation, bone marrow toxicity, and the tendency for rapid dehalogenation, which limits tumor retention. ^{90}Y provides 100% decay suitable for therapy over several millimeters (15), although it has no γ emission useful for imaging. Lutetium-177 (^{177}Lu) is a rare earth metal with a physical half-life of 6.7 days and β emissions that penetrate 0.2 to 0.3 mm in soft tissue. ^{177}Lu also emits two relatively low-abundance, low-energy rays (113 to 208 keV) that allow imaging with a gamma camera, but pose less radiation hazard to health care personnel compared with ^{131}I (103).

Immunotoxins, Drugs, and Cytokines

An important factor limiting the treatment of cancer is the low therapeutic index, which may be improved by targeted delivery of cytotoxic agents (Table 6.3) (15) to tumor sites. mAbs have been attractive carriers for tumor-directed therapy by increasing the intratumoral concentration of targeted agent, and to minimize toxicity by reducing systemic exposure (104). Drugs, toxins, and cytokines conjugated to mAb have been evaluated in gynecologic cancers. Immunotoxins incorporate an antibody-binding domain and a toxin joined by a chemical cross-linker, peptide, or disulfide bond. The specific targeting afforded by mAbs and the relative potency of the toxin moiety present potential therapeutic advantages. The two most studied toxins have been *Pseudomonas* exotoxin A (PE), originally isolated from bacteria, and ricin, initially extracted from castor beans (15). In general, there has been less enthusiasm for antibodies conjugated with conventional cytotoxic drugs owing to concerns about quantitative drug delivery compared to treatment with maximally tolerated doses of the drug alone (15). The major drug conjugate that has been investigated in ovarian cancer is BR96-DOX, an immunoconjugate of doxorubicin (DOX) and an anti–Lewis-Y mAb. Studies utilizing these antibody conjugates are discussed in respective sections below and summarized in Table 6.4. Ref. (103, 105–130).

CLINICAL TRIALS WITH MONOCLONAL ANTIBODIES

Antibodies Targeting CA-125: OvaRex (mAb B43.13) and OC125 Conjugates

CA-125, a tumor-specific antigen that is found in 97% of patients with late-stage ovarian cancer, was first described by Bast et al. as an antigen that is elevated in the serum of patients with epithelial ovarian cancer (131). CA-125 has been cloned and identified as a mucin MUC-16 (89); its function is not clear. *In vitro* studies suggested that CA-125 can produce a dose-dependent increase in invasiveness in a collagen gel invasion assay (132). It has also been shown that CA-125 can be induced by IL-1β, TNF-α, and TGF-α, whereas glucocorticoids and TGF-β can suppress the release of CA-125 from ovarian cancer cells (133). These findings may have a clinical implication on the measurement of CA-125 levels as an indicator of response to cytokine therapy (134). Two mAbs against CA-125 have been used in a series of clinical trials: mAb B43.13 (OvaRex) and OC125 (Table 6.4) (103, 105–130).

mAb B43.13 (OvaRex)

mAb B43.13, a murine anti–CA-125 mAb, was radiolabeled with ^{99m}Tc for detection of recurrent ovarian cancer. The therapeutic potential was serendipitously discovered when a retrospective study noted that patients who received radiolabeled mAb B43.13 for immunoscintigraphy exhibited unexpected prolonged survival times (95,135). It has been speculated that mAb B43.13 binds to circulating CA-125 antigens to form complexes that are recognized as foreign because they contain the foreign antibody. Several *in vitro* and *in vivo* studies have been carried out to explore the robustness of this finding. A series of prospective placebo-controlled and open-label studies in patients with ovarian cancer was carried out to assess therapeutic efficacy of naked mAb B43.13 or in combination with cytokines (e.g., IFN) or chemotherapy. Immunologic parameters in 100 patients with ovarian cancer who had been injected with mAb B43.13 were studied to explain the serendipitous observation of prolonged survival after such treatment (136). In addition to CA-125–specific humoral and cellular responses, IFN-γ was also found to be induced in those patients receiving the antibody. *In vitro* studies indicated that the expression of MHC I, MHC II, and ICAM-1 in ovarian tumor cells was up-regulated in response to IFN-γ. Such tumor cells were also found to be more sensitive to CA-125–specific cytotoxic T cells compared with cells that were not incubated with IFN-γ. It was further noted that the clinical outcome was attributed to the induction of an anti-idiotypic network by this antibody (135). In addition, these anti–CA-125 antibodies were able to conduct Fc-mediated tumor-cell killing (ADCC). In a multivariate analysis of clinical and immunologic profiles of 60 patients exposed to labeled mAb B43.13 compared to a contemporaneous historical cohort of 247 patients, the patients in the mAb B43.13 group were 2.7 times less likely to die from ovarian caner than were control patients managed with chemotherapy alone ($p < 0.001$) (137). The mAb B43.13 group had a twofold higher median survival time compared with the control group. The 5-year survival rate was 40.7% in the mAb B43.13 group compared with 11.4% in the control group. Survival correlated with changes in three humoral immune parameters, including nonspecific HAMA responses,

TABLE 6.4

CLINICAL TRIALS WITH mABS IN GYNECOLOGIC MALIGNANCIES

Antibody	Phase	Disease	Antibody dose or combination	N	Responses	Toxicity	Remarks	References
B43.13	I	Recurrent ovarian cancer	2 mg, IV	13	HAMA: 92%; Ab2: 66%; anti–CA-125: 33% Six survived at least 50 weeks Three experienced a prolonged period of disease stability with survival approaching 2 years	Well tolerated	Administration of the antibody was well tolerated without infusion-related adverse events	105
B43.13	I	Recurrent ovarian cancer	IV B43.13/Chemo, sequential	—	HAMA: 50%; Ab2: 75%, Patients remained progression-free for 50 weeks, 39 weeks, 18 weeks, and 36 weeks	Well tolerated	Subsequent chemotherapy did not abrogate the induced immune responses Patients with a T-cell response to CA-125 showed a highly significant benefit in time to progression and survival compared with non-responders (p <0.01)	106, 107
B43.13	I	Recurrent ovarian cancer	IV B43.13/Chemo, concurrent	19	HAMA/Ab2: 75% Functional T cells: 62.5%	Well tolerated	—	108
B43.13	II	Recurrent ovarian cancer	IV B43.13/Chemo, concurrent	16	2 CR TTP: 10.9 months	Side effects not additive between chemotherapy and B43.13	Chemotherapy did not abrogate the ability to generate an immune response	109
ACA-125	—	Recurrent ovarian cancer	IV ACA-125	42	Ab2: 66.7% Overall survival: 14.9 ± 12.9 months	Well tolerated	Patient survival with a positive immune response was 19.9 ± 13.1 months, in contrast with 5.3 ± 4.3 months in those patients without detectable anti–CA-125 immunity	110
B43.13	III	Consolidation in CA-125 elevation patients	IV B43.13	55	DFS at 6 months: 75% (vs. 35% in placebo group)	Well tolerated	Limited by early relapse	111
B43.13	III	Consolidation in CA-125 elevation patients	IV B43.13	345	55% generated Ab2 or HAMA responses Twofold prolongation of survival compared with placebo control group	Well tolerated	Limited by early relapse	105
B43.13	III	Consolidation in CA-125 elevation patients	IV B43.13	345	HAMA: 51%; Ab2 63% DFS: 24.0 months in the mAb B43.13 group and 10.8 months in the placebo group (hazard ratio 0.53; $p = 0.06$)	Well tolerated	Limited by early relapse	112

B43.13	III	Consolidation	IV B43.13	102	Awaits long-term follow-up	Well tolerated	—	113
^{131}I-OC125	I	Recurrent ovarian cancer	IV versus IP	10	IP ^{131}I-OC125 resulted in a higher uptake of antibody in the tumor and a lower uptake of antibody in normal tissues	Well tolerated	IP is preferable route to IV	114
^{131}I-OC125	I	Recurrent ovarian cancer	IP	20	12 of 20 patients were alive 3 to 17 months following therapy Tumor progression was noted in the majority of patients, although three patients had documented decreases in tumor burden of short duration	Rare nausea and mild diarrhea. No dose-limiting toxicity has been observed for doses ≤120 mCi of ^{131}I	At doses ≤120 mCi, ^{131}I-OC125 could be safely administered intraperitoneally and may have antitumor effects	115
^{131}I-OC125	II	Minimal residual disease ovarian cancer	IP ^{131}I-OC125, 120 mCi	6	All six developed HAMA response Two patients without change, three with POD on biopsy at 3 months, one not biopsied	Grade III neutropenia and thrombocytopenia in two patients	Little therapeutic benefit from IP radioimmunotherapy in patients with residual ovarian carcinoma	116
^{131}I-HMFG1	I	Chemo-resistant ovarian cancer	IP	24	Nine of the 16 patients with small-volume disease at the time of treatment with radiolabeled antibody responded	Mild abdominal pain, pyrexia, diarrhea, and moderate reversible pancytopenia	IP of ≥ 140 mCi ^{131}I-HMFG1 is more effective than lower doses	117
^{90}Y-HMFG1	I/II	Adjuvant ovarian	IP	30 and 52	Two of 21 patients with minimal residual disease have died of their disease with a median follow-up 35 months	The treatment was well tolerated and the only significant toxicity observed was reversible myelosuppression	With IV chelating agent, EDTA, allowed dose increase from 18 to 30 mCi without causing severe myelotoxicity Suggests that patients with advanced ovarian cancer who achieve a CR following conventional therapy may benefit from further treatment with intraperitoneal radioactive monoclonal Ab	118, 119
^{90}Y-HMFG1	III	Adjuvant ovarian	IP	447	No differences in time to relapse between Ab versus placebo	Reversible myelosuppression	Largest randomized consolidation study evaluation of a monoclonal antibody to date	120

(continued)

TABLE 6.4

CLINICAL TRIALS WITH mABS IN GYNECOLOGIC MALIGNANCIES (CONTINUED)

Antibody	Phase	Disease	Antibody dose or combination	N	Responses	Toxicity	Remarks	References
^{177}Lu-CC49	I	Chemo-resistant ovarian cancer	IP ^{177}Lu-CC49	12	Localization of ^{177}Lu-CC49 in 11 of 12 patients One of eight patients with gross disease had >50% tumor reduction, while six progressed and one went off study with stable disease Of the patients with microscopic or occult disease, one relapsed at 10 months and three remained free of disease after 18 months	Mild discomfort with administration, delayed transient arthralgia, and mild marrow suppression	The MTD had not been reached with levels ≤30 mCi/m^2	121
^{177}Lu-CC49	I/II	Chemo-resistant ovarian cancer	IP ^{177}Lu-CC49	27	Antitumor effects were noted even at lower dose levels and resulted in prolonged disease-free survival of most patients with microscopic disease	Dose-limiting toxicity was bone marrow suppression	MTD: 45 mCi/m^2	103
^{177}Lu-CC49	I	Chemo-resistant ovarian cancer	IP ^{177}Lu-CC49 + IFN + Taxol	44	Four of the 17 patients with CT-measurable disease had a PR	Well tolerated with the expected reversible hematologic toxicity	MTD: 40 mCi/m^2 ^{177}Lu-CC49, when given with IFN-α in combination with 100 mg/m^2 Taxol did not have a significant effect on pharmacokinetic or dosimetry parameters	121
^{177}Lu-CC49	I	Chemo-resistant ovarian cancer	SC IFN-α2b, IP Taxol, and IP ^{90}Y-CC49	20	Of nine patients with measurable disease, two had PR Of the 11 patients with non-measurable disease, seven patients recurred	Primarily hematologic toxicity	MTD: 24.2 mCi/m^2 of ^{90}Y-CC49 ^{90}Y -CC49-based radioimmunotherapy in combination with IFN-α 2b and IP Taxol is feasible and well tolerated at a dose of ≤24.2 mCi/m^2	122
^{131}I-MOv18	Pilot	Chemo-resistant ovarian cancer	A single dose of IP ^{131}I-MOv18 (mean dose 14 mg) with 3,700 GBq ^{131}I	16	The majority of patients (15/16, 94%) produced HAMA responses CR: 5; SD: 6; POD: 5	The toxicity was negligible, with only mild and transient bone marrow suppression in one patient	—	123
cMOv18	Pilot	Chemo-resistant ovarian cancer	A single IV dose of c-MOv18 (5 mg to 75 mg)	15	No HACA response was found up to 12 weeks post-injection	Only minor side effects at doses of ≥50 mg	—	124

cMOv18	Pilot	Recurrent ovarian cancer	IV injections of cMOv18 for 4 weeks	5	No HACA response was found Increased ADCC levels Three patients had stable disease for up to 4 months, 9 months, and 14 months, respectively	Toxicity was mild and transient	Immunotherapy has minor effects in patients with ovarian cancer that have been heavily pretreated with chemotherapy Such strategies should be evaluated in patients who are more immunocompetent	125
^{131}I-cMOv18	Pilot	Recurrent ovarian cancer	IV 3 GBq ^{131}I-cMOv18	3	No HACA responses All patients achieved a stable disease state	Only mild myelosuppression	Tumor-absorbed doses ranged from 600 to 3,800 cGy	126
^{111}In-mAb B3	I	Advanced ovarian cancer with Lewis-Y antigen	IV ^{90}Y-mAb B3 (5 to 25 mCi)	26	Definite tumor imaging was observed in 20 of 26 patients	DLT: myelosuppression	The MTD of ^{90}Y-mAb B3 was 20 mCi	127
LMB-1	I	Patients with solid tumors who failed conventional therapy and whose tumors expressed the Lewis-Y antigen	IV LMB-1	38	Objective antitumor activity was observed in five patients, 18 had stable disease, and 15 progressed	The major toxicity reported at this dose was vascular leak syndrome	The MTD of LMB-1 was 75 μg/kg given intravenously three times every other day	128
^{131}I-MN-14	I	Ovarian cancer	Escalating IV doses of ^{131}I-MN-14 mAb	14	The mAb scan was positive in all 14 treated patients 1 CR	Myelosuppression was the only observed treatment-related toxicity	MTD: 50 mCi/m^2	129
^{125}I- or ^{131}I-MX35	I	Ovarian cancer	Escalation doses, 2, 10, or 20 mg, administered by IV or IP injection	25	Specific localization of mAb in tumor was demonstrated by tumor:normal tissue ratios ranging from 2.3:1 to 34:1	Mild	mAb MX35 localizes well to tumor in selected patients with ovarian cancer	130

Note: ADCC, antibody-dependent cell-mediated cytotoxicity; CR, complete response; DFS, disease free survival; DLT, dose limiting toxicity; EDTA, ethylenediamine tetraacetic acid; HACA, human anti-chimeric antibodies; HAMA, human anti-murine antibodies; IP, intraperitoneal; IV, intravenous; MTD, maximal tolerable dose; POD, progression of disease; PR, partial response; SC, subcutaneous; SD, stale disease; TTP, time to progression.

Ab2, and anti–CA-125 antibody development. This study suggested that mAb B43.13 exerts its therapeutic effects via stimulation of specific and nonspecific immune responses.

mAb B43.13 (OvaRex) in Recurrent Disease

Ehlen et al. reported a single-center, open-label trial to assess the induction of tumor protective immunity utilizing mAb B43.13 in a cohort of 13 patients with advanced chemorefractory recurrent ovarian cancer (105). It was noted that HAMA induction occurred in 12 of 13 patients, Ab2 was found in approximately two thirds of the patients, and anti–CA-125–specific antibodies were elicited in one third of the patients. These immunologic data demonstrate that the injection of a murine antibody to CA-125 can induce CA-125–specific antibody and T-cell responses even in late-stage cancer patients with substantial tumor burden. Administration of the antibody was well tolerated without infusion-related adverse events. Notably, six patients survived at least 50 weeks and three patients experienced a prolonged period of disease stability with survival approaching 2 years. The use of mAb B43.13 in combination with second-line chemotherapy in patients with recurrent ovarian cancer has been evaluated (106–109). The treatment has been well tolerated without significant added toxicities. Immune responses in this disease setting included HAMA and Ab2, as well as T-cell responses to CA-125 and autologous tumor cells. CA-125 measured prior to dosing of the antibody was noted to decline prior to additional chemotherapy. Patients remained progression-free for prolonged periods of time. Subsequent or concurrent chemotherapy did not abrogate the induced immune responses, and T-cell responses to autologous tumor actually increased. Patients with a T-cell response to CA-125 on the autologous tumor showed a highly significant benefit in time to progression (TTP) and survival compared with non-responders ($p < 0.01$). Furthermore, the T-cell responses were MHC class I and II restricted, indicating the activation of CTLs and T helper cells. Chemotherapy did not ablate the immune response as traditionally thought. A long-term follow-up study of 49 of the 218 patients who received injections of mAb B43.13 demonstrated periods of disease stabilization and showed that the magnitude of immunologic responses to mAb B43.13 assessed by serial evaluation of HAMA levels, anti–CA-125 antibody levels, and T-cell responses appeared to correlate with the clinical impact of treatment. A significant survival benefit post–antibody treatment was observed in patients with HAMA responses >2,000 ng/mL ($p = 0.001$). Long-term survival was noted in 7 of these 49 patients who remained alive with disease 3 to 6 years after receiving mAb B43.13. These results suggest that treatment with mAb B43.13 can stimulate immune responses even in patients with relapsed ovarian cancer, and activity is associated with disease stabilization in some patients (138).

mAb B43.13 (OvaRex) in Consolidation

One of the first randomized, double-blind, placebo-controlled studies of mAb B43.13 for adjuvant consolidation in epithelial ovarian cancer was reported by Bookman et al. (111). In this study, 55 patients who had no clinical or radiographic evidence of disease after surgery and first-line chemotherapy, but presented elevated CA-125 levels (>35 U/mL), were randomized to receive either mAb B43.13 or placebo. Immune responses were induced at a frequency similar to that reported by other studies. However, the limitation here was that the study population relapsed rapidly, and treatment was discontinued upon clinical relapse. Nevertheless, the subpopulation of patients who had time to mount an immune response had a trend of improved survival, with a 6-month progression-free survival of 75% for the mAb B43.13–treated group and 35% for the placebo cohort. The impact of different schedules on immune responses and clinical outcomes has been evaluated in a study of 102 patients with stage III-IV epithelial ovarian cancer treated with surgery and chemotherapy. Patients were randomized to adjuvant mAb B43.13 in three different schedules. Antibody responses specific for the constant (HAMA) and variable (Ab2) regions of mAb B43.13 were analyzed serially by enzyme-linked immunosorbent assay (ELISA) and T-cell responses by IFN-γ enzyme-linked immunosorbent spot (ELISPOT). It was noted that mAb B43.13 dosing can be increased without adversely affecting safety, and more than two doses were needed for optimal immune responses (108,109). A randomized, placebo-controlled trial with 145 patients with stage III or IV epithelial ovarian cancer (EOC) received intravenous oregovomab in their first clinical remission (109,112,113). No significant toxicity was seen. The median TTP from randomization post front-line therapy for patients receiving oregovomab versus placebo was 13.3 months versus 10.3 months ($p = 0.71$). In a subgroup of patients (≤2 cm residual at debulking, CA-125 ≤65 U/mL before third cycle, and CA-125 ≤35 U/mL at entry), TTP for patients receiving oregovomab versus placebo was 24 months versus 10.8 months (hazard ratio [HR] 0.543; 95% CI, 0.287 to 1.025). Using the eligibility criteria of the subgroup, the investigators have completed prospective enrollment of phase 3 Immunotherapy Pivotal ovarian Cancer Trials I and II (IMPACT) with 354 patients. Efficacy results from these studies are expected to be available when sufficient events have occurred for analysis.

mAb B43.13 (OvaRex) in First-Line Chemo-immunotherapy

The use of anti–CA-125 antibodies in chemo-immunotherapy as first-line therapy remains controversial. Traditionally, it has been thought that the combination of immunotherapy and chemotherapy was not desirable because of the immunosuppressive nature of cytotoxic agents. However, several reports have suggested that chemotherapy may selectively eliminate immunosuppressive lymphocyte populations, and thereby may beneficially alter the characteristics of an immune response (139). The study with concurrent mAb B43.13 and chemotherapy in recurrent epithelial ovarian cancer reported above also supports the idea that favorable specific immune responses could be generated despite concurrent chemotherapy (108). This observation, coupled with benign toxicity profiles and the association between antibody response and survival prolongation, suggests that concurrent chemo-immunotherapy should be evaluated as a first-line therapy for this and other vaccine approaches.

mAb B43.13 (OvaRex) with Conjugates

A drug-antibody conjugate was tested in human ovarian serous adenocarcinomas after it showed selective toxicity *in vitro* against dividing cell populations of the human ovarian cancer cell lines expressing CA-125 (140). Daunorubicin (DNR)-OC125 was made from a new analog (PIPP-DNR) of daunorubicin that chemically links the drug to monoclonal antibodies. The immunofluorescence data show that the DNR-OC125 conjugate had high affinity and specificity for proliferating malignant cells from human ovarian tumors and indicated that the OC125 monoclonal antibody can indeed serve as a cancer-targeting carrier for daunorubicin and its analogs. The clinical efficacy has not been tested.

Immunoconjugated antibodies have been tested in the treatment of ovarian cancer. A distribution and pharmacokinetics study of ^{131}I-OC125 in patients with gynecologic tumors revealed that IP versus IV administration of the radiolabeled antibody resulted in a higher uptake of antibody in the tumor and a lower uptake of antibody in normal tissues (114). Therefore, this study suggested that for radioimmunotherapy of ovarian cancer, IP administration of radiolabeled antibodies is preferable to intravenous administration. This was also consistent with a study in nude mice with ovarian cancer xenografts (141). In a phase 1 study, 20 patients with recurrent or persistent epithelial ovarian cancer failing conventional therapies were treated with a single IP injection of ^{131}I-OC125 mAb (115). Rare acute side effects were nausea and mild diarrhea, and no dose-limiting toxicity has been observed for doses $\leq$120 mCi of ^{131}I. Only three patients had partial responses of short duration. A phase 2 study with IP radioimmunotherapy in patients with minimal residual ovarian adenocarcinoma after primary treatment with surgery and chemotherapy showed little therapeutic benefit (116). Toxicity was mainly hematologic, with grade III neutropenia and thrombocytopenia in two patients. In a retrospective study of patients with ovarian carcinoma who received 1 mg of ^{131}I-OC125 mAb one to five times after radical surgery and polychemotherapy, patients who developed high titers of Ab2 responses had a significantly higher survival rate than the ones with weak or no immunologic response to ^{131}I-OC125 mAb treatment ($p < 0.05$) (142). The diagnostic value of ^{131}I-OC125 to localize ovarian tumors was tested prospectively. Scintigraphy revealed the presence of active disease, which was confirmed by laparotomy/laparoscopy in the majority of patients considered to be in clinical remission. Therefore, the sensitivity of scintigraphy with ^{131}I-OC125 was high enough and may have diagnostic value (143). The assessment of clinical efficacy will require randomized, prospective clinical trials.

Antibodies Targeting MUC-1: HMFG1 and HMFG2

A murine immunoglobulin G1 mAb raised against human milk fat globules (HMFG1) reacts with an epitope in the protein core of polymorphic epithelial mucin (PEM) antigen (MUC-1) that is expressed by >90% of epithelial ovarian cancers and many other carcinomas. The therapeutic potential of HMFG1 has mainly been assessed in the form of conjugates with radionuclide. In one study, 24 patients with persistent epithelial ovarian cancer were treated with IP ^{131}I-labeled mAbs directed against tumor-associated antigens, including HMFG1 (117). Acute side effects were mild abdominal pain, pyrexia, diarrhea, and moderate reversible pancytopenia. Of the 16 patients with small-volume disease (<2 cm) at the time of treatment with radiolabeled antibody, 9 responded. Analysis of the data on relapse indicated that doses >140 mCi were more effective than lower doses. This study suggested that the IP administration of $\geq$140 mCi ^{131}I-labeled tumor-associated monoclonal antibodies had activity in patients with small-volume stage III ovarian cancer. In a phase 1-2 trial of IP ^{90}Y-HMFG1 in patients with ovarian cancer, the dose was limited by myelotoxicity as described by bone deposition of free ^{90}Y carcinoma (118). The intravenous use of a chelating agent, ethylenediamine tetraacetic acid (EDTA) (Ledclair), allowed the dose to be increased from 18 to 30 mCi without causing severe myelotoxicity. An additional 52 patients with epithelial ovarian cancer were treated with IP ^{90}Y-HMFG1 following conventional surgery and chemotherapy, results showed that patients with advanced ovarian cancer who receive conventional therapy and achieve a complete remission may benefit from further treatment with IP radioactive mAbs (119). Another adjuvant study with one dose of 25 mg of HMFG1 labeled with 18 mCi/m^2 ^{90}Y given intraperitoneally yielded a 5-year survival of 80% compared to 55% in control cases selected from the database ($p = 0.0035$). All patients developed serologic evidence of HAMA. This study was hypothesis generating and suggested a survival benefit for patients with ovarian cancer who receive IP radioimmunotherapy in the adjuvant setting (144). To overcome the myelosuppression toxicity from bone deposition of ^{90}Y, stable chelating agents, such as the benzyl analog of diethylene triamine pentaacetic acid (DTPA), 6-p-isothiocyanatobenzyl diethylene triamine penta-acetic acid (CITCDTPA), was conjugated with ^{90}Y-HMFG1. However, anti-chelate antibody responses developed against the macrocycle benzyl-DOTA, resulting in clinical side effects with hypersensitivity syndrome (145). Despite the provocative activity suggested in the phase 2 trials with ^{90}Y-HMFG1, a large randomized, placebo-controlled study failed to show benefit. In the study by Verheijen et al., a total of 844 stage IC to IV patients were initially screened, of whom 447 patients with a negative second-look laparoscopy after primary surgery and chemotherapy were randomly assigned to receive either a single IP dose of ^{90}Y-muHMFG1 followed by observation or observation alone. The study had an 80% power to detect a 15% improvement in survival. After a median follow-up of 3.5 years, 70 patients had died in the active treatment arm compared with 61 patients in the control arm. Cox proportional hazards analysis of survival demonstrated no difference between treatment arms. It was concluded that a single IP administration of ^{90}Y-muHMFG1 given to patients having a negative second-look laparoscopy after primary therapy did not extend survival or time to relapse. Several factors have been suggested as contributing to the negative results such as inadequate dose or dosing frequency. A follow-up analysis of this study further characterized the negative result, showing that treatment was associated with improved control of intraperitoneal disease ($p < 0.05$) but a shorter time to disease recurrence in extraperitoneal sites ($p < 0.05$) (146). Nonetheless, this represents the largest randomized consolidation study to date in patients with ovarian cancer utilizing radionuclides with unfortunately disappointing results.

Antibodies Targeting Tumor-Associated Glycoprotein-72: CC49, B72.3

Human mammary and other carcinoma cells secrete and express on their cell surfaces complex, mucin-like glycoproteins that are recognized as tumor-associated antigens by a variety of mAbs. One such mAb, B72.3, was initially developed using a membrane-enriched fraction of human metastatic mammary carcinoma tissue as an immunogen (147). This mAb has been extensively studied with respect to the range of reactivity for a variety of carcinomas versus normal tissues. Tumor-associated glycoprotein-72 (TAG-72) is a tumor-associated glycoprotein recognized by mAb B72.3, which has more recently been shown to be specific for clusters of sTn (148). This high-molecular-weight mucin is expressed by the majority of common epithelial tumors. In an effort to improve the parental mAb B72.3, a series of second-generation mAbs has been developed that also recognize TAG-72 (149,150). Among the members of the initial library of antibodies produced, murine mAb CC49 was selected for further clinical studies because of its higher affinity and more rapid plasma clearance compared with mAb B72.3. mAb CC49 recognizes a different epitope than mAb B72.3 (although still sTn related) and exhibits higher reactivity to several carcinomas (151,152). The potential value of this mAb in immunotherapy has been tested for conjugates with various radionuclides in different cancers, including that of the breast (153,154), colon (155–159), and prostate (160–162). The studies in ovarian cancers are summarized below.

Animal model studies have shown considerable antitumor activity for ^{177}Lu-CC49 in TAG-72–positive human tumor xenograft models (103,163). Several phase 1 trials (121) showed that treatment with ^{177}Lu-CC49 was well tolerated. Side effects included mild discomfort with administration, delayed transient arthralgia, and marrow suppression. The dose-limiting toxicity was bone marrow suppression with an MTD of 45 mCi/m^2. Antitumor effects were noted against chemotherapy-resistant ovarian cancer, even at lower dose levels, and resulted in prolonged disease-free survival of most patients with microscopic disease. The combination of IFN and paclitaxel (Taxol) with IP ^{177}Lu-CC49 was also evaluated in persistent ovarian cancer (164). Human recombinant IFN-α was administered to increase the expression of the tumor-associated antigen TAG-72. Paclitaxel, which has radiosensitizing effects and antitumor activity against ovarian cancer, was given intraperitoneally 48 hours before radioimmunotherapy. The therapy was well tolerated with the expected reversible hematologic toxicity, and addition of IFN-α increased hematologic toxicity. The MTD was 40 mCi/m^2 ^{177}Lu-CC49 when given with IFN-α in combination with 100 mg/m^2 paclitaxel. A different radionuclide isotope, ^{90}Y, was also evaluated with mAb CC49. Treatment of patients with persistent ovarian cancer with a combination of subcutaneous IFN-α2b, IP paclitaxel, and IP ^{90}Y-CC49 was associated with primarily hematologic toxicity (122). The MTD of IP ^{90}Y-CC49 was established at 24.2 mCi/m^2 in this combined regimen. Partial responses were observed in some of the patients with measurable disease.

The CC49 mAb was also evaluated as a drug conjugate with doxorubicin in mouse models. The immunoconjugate, designated CC49-BAMME-CH-DOX, was approximately a log less potent than unconjugated doxorubicin in an *in vitro* cytotoxicity assay (165). Immunoreactivity of the antibody was fully retained. When evaluated in a nude (*nu/nu*) mouse xenograft model with the antigen-positive human colorectal tumor target, CC49-BAMME-CH-DOX and free doxorubicin had similar tumor-suppressive activities. However, the immunoconjugate was clearly less toxic, as measured by weight loss and deaths. When evaluated in an NIH:OVCAR-3 human ovarian carcinoma xenograft model, CC49-BAMME-CH-DOX was superior at prolonging survival in comparison to free doxorubicin, unmodified CC49, and a non–tumor-binding doxorubicin immunoconjugate (165). These results indicate that targeting of doxorubicin with the CC49 antibody may improve the toxicity and/or the potency of the drug depending on the tumor target being evaluated.

In summary, these phase 1-2 studies have shown that IP treatment with radiolabeled antibodies is well tolerated. Although these studies were not designed to estimate response rate or survival, they do provide evidence of antitumor activities with this approach. One advantage of administering isotopes conjugated to antibodies intraperitoneally is to ameliorate bowel complications associated with IP administration of unconjugated radioisotopes. Various forms of mAb CC49 have been engineered to improve delivery of radiation doses to tumors and minimize undesirable pharmacokinetics that lead to significant radiation exposure of normal tissues. The clinical efficacy of these different constructs will be tested.

Antibodies Targeting Folate-Binding Proteins: MOv18 and MOv19

The mAbs MOv18 and MOv19 were raised against a membrane preparation from an ovarian carcinoma surgical specimen. They reacted with a surface antigen present on the majority of non-mucinous ovarian malignant tumors tested but not with normal adult tissue (166). This antigen was subsequently identified to be folate-binding protein (FBP) (167), which is over-expressed in ovarian adenocarcinoma. The therapeutic potentials of these mAbs in ovarian cancer have been assessed in several pilot and phase 1 studies. A pilot study in 16 patients with minimal residual ovarian cancer with a single dose of ^{131}I-MOv18 (mean dose 14 mg) with 3,700 GBq ^{131}I showed complete response in 5 of 16 patients, and the majority of patients produced HAMA responses (123). The toxicity of radioimmunotherapy was negligible, with only mild and transient bone marrow suppression in one patient. A chimeric form of MOv18 (c-MOv18) was evaluated in several clinical trials with single or repeated injections of c-MOv18 (124,125,168). Toxicity was generally mild and transient. No human anti-chimeric antibody (HACA) response was found. Increased ADCC levels corresponding to a slight increase in CD4$^+$ and CD8$^+$ fractions were observed, whereas the CD4/CD8 ratio and the levels of CD25 remained unchanged. The radionuclide-labeled MOv18 (^{131}I-cMOv18) was also demonstrated to be safe with only mild myelosuppression, again without significant HACA response (126). These studies showed that immunotherapy aimed at boosting the patient's immunologic capacity has minor effects in patients with ovarian cancer who have been heavily pretreated with chemotherapy and suggested that such strategies should be evaluated in patients who are more immunocompetent.

A bispecific OC/TR mAb that cross-links the CD3 molecule on T cells with human FBP was also generated and produced some complete and partial responses in clinical trials of patients with ovarian carcinoma (169). Most patients developed HAMA, which can inhibit OC/TR mAb-mediated lysis. An antibody-cytokine conjugate was constructed as a fusion protein between IL-2 and the scFv of MOv19 (170). This small molecule combines the specificity of MOv19 with the immunostimulatory activity of IL-2. The newly designed molecule may have improved tissue penetration and distribution within the tumor and reduced immunogenicity, and it may lack the toxicity related to the systemic administration of IL-2. In a syngeneic mouse model, IL-2/MOv19 scFv specifically targeted α-folate receptor gene–transduced metastatic tumor cells without accumulating in normal tissues owing to its fast clearance from the body. Treatment with IL-2/MOv19 scFv, but not with recombinant IL-2, significantly reduced the volume of subcutaneous venographic tumors. The pharmacokinetics and biologic characteristics of IL-2/NMOV19 scFv may allow the combination of systemically administered IL-2/NMOV19 scFv and adoptive transfer of *in vitro* retargeted T lymphocytes for the treatment of ovarian cancer, thereby providing local delivery of IL-2 without toxicity.

It is worth noting that unlike other cancer-associated antigens, for example, CA-125 and TAG-72, whose expression may be enhanced by IFN, expression of MOv18 and MOv19 was not modulated by IFN-α, INF-β, or IFN-γ (125,171). Addition of IL-2 *in vitro* also did not change any immunologic parameters (125).

Antibodies Targeting the Lewis-Y Antigen: BR5, BR96, B3, 3S193

The Lewis-Y (Le^y) antigen is a type 2 blood group–related glycoprotein that is expressed by 60% to 90% of human carcinomas of epithelial cell origin, including breast, pancreas, ovary, colon, gastric, and lung cancer (83,90,172–175). A total of 75% of the analyzed ovarian cancer specimens expressed Lewis-Y (175). Because of its high frequency in tumors, high density and altered expression on the surface of tumor cells, and relatively homogeneous expression in primary and metastatic lesions, Lewis-Y has been an antigenic target for solid tumor immunotherapy (176). Several mAbs have been developed, including BR55 (177), BR64, and BR96 (178), B1 and B3 (179), and 3S193 (180). Some of these mAbs have been evaluated for their potential therapeutic use in gynecologic malignancies.

mAb B3 radiolabeled with ^{111}In demonstrated good tumor localization in patients with advanced epithelial tumors (127).

The MTD of ^{90}Y-mAb B3 was 20 mCi, with myelosuppression as the dose-limiting toxicity. An immune toxin conjugate of B3 and *Pseudomonas* exotoxin, designated LMB-1, had excellent antitumor activity in nude mice bearing Lewis-Y–positive tumors (181). In a phase 1 study of 38 patients with solid tumors who failed conventional therapy and whose tumors expressed the Lewis-Y antigen, LMB-1 produced objective antitumor activity. The MTD of LMB-1 was 75 μg/kg given intravenously three times every other day. The major toxicity reported at this dose was vascular leak syndrome.

A drug conjugate consisting of chimeric mAb BR96 and doxorubicin, BR96-Dox has been shown to cure 94% of athymic rats with subcutaneous human lung cancer (182). BR96-Dox conjugate was generally well tolerated with mild gastrointestinal toxicities, and did not show significant clinical antitumor activity in metastatic breast cancer (183–185). Another humanized anti–Lewis-Y mAb (hu3S193) was evaluated using a radionuclide conjugate of the ^{131}I isotope alone or in combination with paclitaxel in an MCF-7 xenografted BALB/c nude mouse, which is a breast cancer model (186). It has been noted that the combination of paclitaxel and ^{131}I-hu3S193 had a synergistic effect with significant tumor inhibition in 80% of the analyzed mice. Its value in the treatment of ovarian or other gynecologic cancers has not been well studied and remains to be tested in the future.

Antibodies Targeting Carcinoembryonic Antigen: MN-14

Carcinoembryonic antigen (CEA) belongs to the class of tumor-associated antigens and has been most extensively studied in gastrointestinal cancers. The diagnostic and therapeutic value of CEA has also been evaluated in ovarian cancers. An anti-CEA mAb radiolabeled with ^{99}Tc was shown to be a promising radioimmunoimaging method for the detection of malignant ovarian tumors with excellent sensitivity and specificity (187). Complete clinical remission was observed in a patient with advanced ovarian cancer, refractory to paclitaxel therapy, treated with two cycles of ^{131}I-labeled murine MN-14 anti-CEA mAb (188). A follow-up phase 1 therapy trial with intravenously administered ^{131}I-MN-14 anti-CEA mAb in patients with epithelial ovarian cancer showed that myelosuppression was the only observed treatment-related toxicity, and dose-limiting toxicity was seen at 50 mCi/m^2. It seems that MN-14 anti-CEA mAb is a suitable agent for tumor targeting, and it may have a therapeutic potential in patients with chemotherapy-refractive epithelial ovarian cancer, especially those with minimal disease (129).

Antibodies Targeting MX35 Antigen

mAb MX35 is a murine IgG1 that was initially developed at Memorial Sloan-Kettering Cancer Center (189,190). It detects an antigen expressed strongly and homogeneously on approximately 90% of human epithelial ovarian cancers (130), and was subsequently identified to be a 95-kD glycoprotein (191). The exact function of this antigen is yet to be defined; however, given its strong expression in ovarian cancers but not in normal peritoneum, mAb MX35 in the form of immune radionuclide conjugate has been tested for its therapeutic potential in ovarian cancer. In one study, 25 patients with advanced ovarian cancer were entered into a clinical trial using ^{125}I- or ^{131}I-labeled MX35 in escalation doses administered by intravenous or IP injection (130). Specific localization of mAb in tumor was demonstrated by tumor:normal tissue ratios ranging from 2.3:1 to 34:1 (mean 10.18:1), demonstrating that mAb MX35 localizes well to tumor in selected patients with ovarian cancer. Another study to quantify the targeting of the mAb MX35 to micrometastatic epithelial ovarian cancer demonstrated that mAb MX35 localizes to the micrometastatic ovarian carcinoma deposits within the peritoneal cavity (192). These two dosimetry results suggest a therapeutic potential for this antibody in patients with minimal residual disease (<5 mm).

Antibodies Targeting ERBB1 (EGF), ERBB2 (HER2/neu), and VEGF

The epidermal growth factor receptor (EGFR) has been a frequent target for cancer treatment development in the past decade. Several EGFR antibodies have been approved by the FDA for cancer treatment such as cetuximab and panitumumab for colorectal cancer. These encouraging data have prompted their evaluation in other malignancies. In ovarian cancer, the EGF tyrosine kinase inhibitor gefitinib had a minimal objective single agent response rate of 4% in unscreened patients (9% in EGF + patients). The patient with the only objective response had a mutation in the catalytic domain of EGFR, and the frequency of mutation in this study was 1/32 or 3% (193). The anti-EGFR antibody, matuzumab, was then tested in patients with recurrent, EGFR-positive ovarian or primary peritoneal cancer in a multi-institutional single-arm phase 2 trial of 75 patients, and showed no significant clinical activity as a monotherapy in this population of very heavily pretreated patients. Taken together, these data suggest that anti-EGF targeted therapy as a single agent in ovarian cancer is relatively inactive, but combination studies with chemotherapy are ongoing (178).

Original data had suggested that approximately 30% of ovarian cancer patients overexpress HER2, providing a rationale for investigation (194). Furthermore, HER2 overexpression appears inversely correlated with overall survival when considered in univariate and multivariate analysis among other usual prognostic factors (195). However, the most significant treatment experience in patients with recurrent or refractory ovarian or primary peritoneal cancer comes from the GOG study that screened 837 tumor samples for HER2 expression, and showed the required 2+/3+ expression in only 95 (11.4%) of patients (196). Forty-five patients were entered into the study with an overall response rate of 7.3% with a median progression-free interval of 2.0 months. Based on infrequent HER2 expression, and the low rate of objective responses, the clinical value of single-agent trastuzumab appears limited in these patients. It is unknown whether a clinical benefit could be seen by combining chemotherapy with trastuzumab in those patients with appropriate HER2 expression, but this benefit would be limited by the frequency of expression.

Recent intriguing results have been published from a small series evaluating HER2 overexpression in the aggressive papillary serous variant of endometrial cancer. In 10 consecutive specimens, eight patients showed 2+/3+ expression, and this series is currently being expanded (197). The need for better treatment for patients with uterine papillary serous cancer is apparent, and if this degree of overexpression is confirmed, clinical studies will be warranted.

The growth and metastasis of malignant neoplasms require the presence of an adequate blood supply, and recent data have confirmed the therapeutic potential of antivascular strategies. Bevacizumab, a humanized recombinant antibody against VEGF that prevents its binding to VEGFR, inhibits angiogenesis and tumor growth. Randomized trials have shown statistically significant improvements in progression-free and overall survival when bevacizumab is combined with chemotherapy in several solid tumors, including colorectal cancer (198), non-small-cell lung cancer (199), and breast cancer (200). In these particular tumor types, significant single-agent activity was not observed despite the improvements when used in combination. By contrast, single-agent bevacizumab did improve progression-free survival in renal cell cancer (201). Interestingly, single-agent activity of bevacizumab has also been clearly established in recurrent ovarian cancer by two prospective trials with a response rate of 16% to 18% (202,203). A combination of bevacizumab with metronomic oral cyclophosphamide in recurrent ovarian cancer patients with up to two prior regimens showed a response rate of 28% (204). It should be noted that in the trial by Cannistra et al., a gastrointestinal perforation rate of 11.4% was seen resulting in the death of one patient. This prompted a National Cancer Institute Investigational New Drug (IND) action letter dated October 4, 2005, which alerted investigators to the risk of gastrointestinal perforation in patients with advanced ovarian cancer treated with bevacizumab. A recent analysis has combined data from all available studies in ovarian cancer, resulting in an estimated risk of gastrointestinal perforation of 5.4% (95% CI, 2.2 to 9.4), which appears to exceed the published risk in colorectal cancer of 2.4% (205,206). Randomized phase 3 trials evaluating the addition of bevacizumab to the adjuvant treatment of patients with ovarian cancer after surgical debulking are ongoing and will provide awaited estimates of clinical efficacy and toxicity when used in this patient population.

Antibodies Targeting MN/CAIX Antigens: M75

The MN antigen is a tumor-associated antigen initially identified from a cervical carcinoma cell line HeLa (207), and was later identified to be CAIX, a carbonic anhydrase (208). It was found to be expressed in cervical intraepithelial neoplasia and 90% of invasive cervical cancer but not in normal cervical tissue (207–209). Although the exact role of MN/CAIX antigen in carcinogenesis is not known, it has been suggested that it may facilitate acidification of the extracellular milieu surrounding cancer cells and in this way may promote tumor growth and spread (210). A retrospective study of 130 squamous cell cervical carcinomas demonstrated that a semiquantitative immunohistochemical analysis of CAIX expression in tumor biopsies is a significant and independent prognostic indicator of overall survival and metastasis-free survival after radiation therapy. Prospective studies have shown that MN/CAIX expression is up-regulated in hypoxic human cervical tumors and is a significant and independent poor prognostic indicator (211). Therefore, CAIX may act as an intrinsic marker of tumor hypoxia and poor outcome after radiation therapy. The level of CAIX expression may be used to aid in the selection of patients who would benefit most from hypoxia-modification therapies or bioreductive drugs. Mouse mAb M75 has been used in immunohistochemical staining in the above studies.

Summary of mAb Trials

In summary, progress has been made in the application of mAb to treatment of B-cell malignancies, breast cancer, and colorectal cancer. Bevacizumab has shown promise in ovarian cancers. Additional human or humanized antibodies against cell surface antigens that are of therapeutic significance needed to be studied in gynecologic cancers. A panel discussion of mAb in the treatment of ovarian cancers was held at the Helene Harris Memorial Trust 9th Biennial Forum on Ovarian Cancer in Stratford, England (17). It was concluded that future trials should aim to develop humanized monoclonal antibodies to surface antigens that can be internalized. More effective radionuclide conjugates and chelates should be developed. Work should be encouraged with isotopes that are primarily α or possibly β emitters. The priorities in the development of effective mAb therapy, as summarized by the panel, are (a) development of human/humanized mAbs to surface antigens that are internalized; (b) development of more effective radionuclides, chelates; (c) definition of suitable surrogate markers; (d) development of xenotypic antibodies that can induce immunity to autologous antigens; and (e) exploration of combinations with chemotherapy.

ADOPTIVE CELLULAR THERAPY

The goal of most immunotherapeutic approaches is to generate large numbers of highly reactive specific antitumor lymphocytes. Adoptive cellular therapy seeks to overcome tolerance hurdles by selecting and activating large numbers of lymphocytes *in vitro*, and manipulating the host environment to which they are introduced for maximum effect (139). Recent provocative data correlated progression-free and overall survival in patients with epithelial ovarian cancer to the presence or absence of tumor-infiltrating T cells. The 5-year overall survival rate was 38% among ovarian cancer patients whose tumor cells contained T cells and 4.5% among patients whose tumors did not contain T cells ($p < 0.001$). This finding could represent a prognostic phenomenon, and the addition of T cells via the adoptive transfer approach or via vaccination may or may not be beneficial, but it warrants further exploration (212). The adoptive immunotherapeutic approach has resulted in striking clinical responses in melanoma patients after pretreatment with myeloablative chemotherapy (139). In the study by Dudley et al., 13 HLA-A2+ patients with metastatic melanoma received immuno-depleting chemotherapy with cyclophosphamide and fludarabine followed by the transfer of highly selected *in vitro* expanded MART-1 (melanocyte differentiation antigen) reactive T cells and high-dose IL-2. Six of 13 patients had clinical responses, and four had a mixed response. Immunohistochemical studies of tumor deposits revealed predominant infiltrates of CD8+ cells, and both MHC class I and II antigens were highly expressed. The first phase 1 study in patients with EOC using gene-modified autologous T cells with reactivity against the ovarian cancer–associated antigen α-folate receptor (FR) was reported (213). Cohort 1 received T cells with IL-2, and cohort 2 received dual specific T cells followed by allogeneic peripheral blood mononuclear cells. Five patients in cohort 1 experienced toxicity likely due to the cytokine. No reduction in tumor burden was seen in any patient. Polymerase chain reaction (PCR) analysis showed that gene-modified T cells were present in the circulation the first 2 days after transfer, but declined. An inhibitory factor developed in the serum of three of six patients tested over the period of treatment, which significantly reduced the ability of gene-modified T cells to respond against FR+ tumor cells. Future studies need to employ strategies to extend T-cell persistence. There is much interest in further exploring adoptive T-cell approaches in patients with epithelial ovarian cancer.

CANCER VACCINES DESIGNED TO AUGMENT ANTIBODY RESPONSES

Selection of KLH Conjugation Plus QS-21 for Vaccine Construction

A variety of approaches have been explored to induce the antibody responses against carbohydrate and peptide cancer antigens, including the use of autologous and allogeneic tumor cells modified in various ways, or not (reviewed in Ref. 17), different immunologic adjuvants (214–217), anti-idiotype

TABLE 6.5

ROLE OF CONJUGATE VACCINE COMPONENTS IN ANTIBODY INDUCTION AGAINST CANCER ANTIGENS

Antigen	Carrier (KLH)	Adjuvant (QS-21)
1) Antigen configuration mimics expression on tumor cell. Conjugation site and tertiary structure are key.	1) Highly immunogenic carrier molecule is key for optimal cytokine release and overcoming tolerance.	The mechanism of action for most adjuvants includes:
2) High density of antigen per carrier molecule optimal.	2) Sequence of cytokine release may be important, so an immunogenic carrier may be better than a cytokine, cytokine mixture, or cytokine inducer.	1) Activation of APCs 2) B-cell activation 3) T-cell activation 4) Depot effect

vaccines (218,219), chemical modification of antigens to make them more immunogenic (220–222), and conjugation to various immunogenic carrier proteins (223,224). The conclusion from these studies is that the use of a carrier protein plus an immunologic adjuvant is the optimal approach. The optimal immunologic adjuvant in each case was one of two saponins (QS-21 or GPI-0100) obtained from the bark of *Quillaja saponaria* (225,226). The optimal carrier protein was in each case KLH (227–230). Each component of this approach is absolutely required; conjugate without adjuvant, antigen plus adjuvant, antigen plus KLH not conjugated plus adjuvant, all result in greatly diminished antibody responses. The rationale for this approach is reviewed above and in Table 6.5.

Conjugate Vaccines Against Cell Surface Antigens

Based on this background, GM2-KLH plus QS-21 (termed GMK) was tested in patients. It induced eight times higher titers of IgM antibody that lasted twice as long compared to our previous GM2/BCG vaccine, and for the first time GMK induced consistent IgG antibodies as well (231). Antibodies were induced in >95% of patients vaccinated with GMK instead of <85% as seen with the GM2/BCG vaccine. Previous trials comparing high-dose IFN-α to no treatment (232) and GM2/BCG to BCG (79) resulted in comparable benefit for IFN and GM2/BCG. However, the time in follow-up needed to detect the benefit was different, which may be important to consider as future trials are designed to ensure adequate follow-up periods. The beneficial effect of IFN was evident during the initial 6 to 8 months of follow-up, whereas the effect of GMK vaccine was not clearly evident until after 2 years. Consequently, a randomized multicenter intergroup trial comparing GMK to high-dose IFN-α was conducted by ECOG in stage III and high-risk stage II melanoma patients. An assessment after 18 months median follow-up demonstrated a significantly prolonged disease-free survival for the patients receiving IFN (233), and the trial was discontinued. It remains possible that one explanation for the lack of benefit for vaccine is the low or heterogeneous expression of GM2 in most melanomas. The presence of tumor cell heterogeneity, heterogeneity of the human immune response, and the correlation between overall antibody titer against tumor cells and antibody effector mechanisms (234) provide a rationale for favoring the evaluation of polyvalent vaccines in future studies.

A randomized adjuvant multicenter trial with a vaccine against sTn has recently been conducted by Biomira, Inc. (Edmonton, Alberta, Canada). The vaccine contained sTn disaccharide (also referred to as TAG-72) covalently linked to KLH and mixed with immunologic adjuvant Detox. Biomira conducted the trial in patients with high-risk breast cancer at multiple centers in Canada, the United States, and Europe. This trial was based on the high titer antibodies induced by this vaccine in this patient population, the correlation between expression of sTn on tumors and a more aggressive phenotype, and the correlation between antibody induction against sTn and longer disease-free and overall survival in previous studies (80). This trial did not meet its predetermined statistical endpoints of time to disease progression or survival (235), again possibly because of the low or heterogeneous expression of sTn on most breast cancers. While the study failed to reach its primary endpoint, a subgroup analysis showed prolonged survival in patients who were treated with concomitant hormonal therapy compared with patients who received a control vaccine with KLH (median survival for theratope 36.5 months and for KLH 30.7 months, $p = 0.0360$) (236,237).

The strategy to use KLH conjugate plus QS21 has been applied to the development of vaccines against gynecologic malignancies. Vaccines have been tested against seven antigens expressed by gynecologic malignancies, in a series of monovalent vaccine trials. These vaccines have induced antibodies against GM2, MUC-1, and sTn in 80% to 90% of patients, and against Globo H, TF, and Tn in 50% to 80% of patients (223,238–240). Le^y has proved less immunogenic than the other antigens with only 20% to 30% of patients receiving Le^y-KLH vaccines producing significant antibody responses (241). With each of these antigens, the antibodies induced by the antigen-KLH conjugate plus QS21 vaccines reacted by flow cytometry with tumor cells expressing these antigens. The IgG subclasses in all trials have been restricted to IgG1 and IgG3, the two subclasses known to mediate CDC and ADCC.

Preclinical models have shown that a heptavalent KLH conjugate plus QS21 vaccine induced antibody titers comparable to those induced by monovalent vaccines containing Tn, sTn, TF, MUC-1, and Globo-H. Lower titers were produced against Lewis-Y and GM2 than when evaluated as monovalent antigens (242). Recently, a pilot study was performed to test a heptavalent vaccine in ovarian cancer patients in second or greater complete clinical remission (241). The objectives of this phase 1 study were to characterize safety and immunogenicity in preparation for an adequately powered randomized efficacy trial. Eleven patients in this study received a heptavalent vaccine subcutaneously containing GM2 (10 μg), Globo-H (10 μg), Le^y (10 μg), Tn(c) (3 μg), sTn(c) (3 μg), TF(c) (3 μg), and Tn-MUC-1 (3 μg) individually conjugated to KLH and mixed with adjuvant QS21 (100 μg). Vaccinations were administered at weeks 1, 2, 3, 7, and 15. No systemic toxicity was seen. After immunization, median IgM titers were as follows: Tn–MUC-1, 1:640 (IgG 1:80); Tn, 1:160; TF, 1:640; Globo-H, 1:40; and sTn, 1:80. Only one response was seen against Lewis-Y, two against GM2. Eight of nine patients developed responses against at least three antigens. Fluorescent-activated cell sorting (FACS) and CDC analysis showed substantially increased reactivity against MCF7 cells in seven of nine patients, with some increase seen in all patients (241).

As exemplified in the case of the GM2 and sTn vaccines discussed above, where signals suggesting activity in phase 2 trials did not translate into clinical benefit in the phase 3 setting, a randomized phase 3 trial of a multivalent-KLH construct with QS21 as the adjuvant is the next step to follow the phase 1 study. This study is planned to randomize patients in second or greater clinical remission to a multivalent-KLH construct + QS21 versus QS21. The endpoint will be an improvement in the proportion of patients remaining in remission at 12 months.

CANCER VACCINES DESIGNED TO AUGMENT T-LYMPHOCYTE RESPONSES

Options Available

There is a wide range of options for augmenting the immunogenicity of the antigenic targets for T-cell immunity (242,243, 244). For these antigens, the options include (a) the full proteins or MHC-restricted peptides modified by amino acid substitutions to increase immunogenicity; (b) genes or mini-genes for these proteins or peptides used as DNA vaccines; or (c) genes expressed in viral or bacterial vectors. Co-stimulatory molecules, cytokines, or molecules targeting antigens to particular processing compartments can be incorporated into these vaccines. DNA vaccines are especially appealing in this regard because of ease of production, versatility, and adaptability to such combinations. Most of these approaches can also be applied to expressing these antigens in antigen-presenting cells, such as dendritic cells, that are then used to vaccinate the patient. Furthermore, since many tumor-rejection antigens detected by T cells in experimental animals are individually unique (mutated), a variety of individualized vaccines are being tested. Whole-cell vaccines can be prepared from a specific patient (if accessible tumor is available) and immunogenicity may be increased by the use of an immunologic adjuvant and transduction with genes for cytokines or co-stimulatory molecules, or treatment with haptens such as dinitrophenyl (DNP). Other approaches to increasing the immunogenicity of unique and shared antigens include the use of heat shock proteins that may carry the full range of cancer peptides, anti-idiotype vaccines, and DNA or messenger RNA vaccines that may be obtained from smaller biopsy specimens. The range of options for augmenting T-cell immunity against cancer is daunting. Clinical trials with each of these approaches to augmenting T-cell immunity have been recently completed, are ongoing, or have been planned. There is no basis for selecting one over the other at this time.

Target Antigens to T Lymphocytes: Selecting a Strategy

Antigens shared by ovarian or endometrial cancers from different patients are KSA, MUC-16, WT1, CEA, MUC-1, HER2/neu, and cancer-testis antigens (including the MAGE family) and NY-ESO-1. None of these cancer antigens defined as targets for T cells to date is a perfect candidate for the majority of patients due to (a) over-expression on less than 50% of ovarian or endometrial cancers (HER2/neu, CEA, and the cancer-testis antigens) and (b) wide expression (though at lower levels) on normal tissues (KSA, CEA, HER2/neu, MUC-1). The highly polar extensive expression of KSA and some other antigens on cells apically at mucosal borders (lumens) in many normal epithelial tissues does not exclude them as a target for antibodies because IgG1, IgG3, and IgM antibodies are present in much lower concentrations in these lumens, or not at all, and there is little or no complement and no antibody-dependent cell-mediated cytotoxicity (ADCC) effector cells. Since antigen presentation to T cells in the context of HLA antigens is not known to have the same polar distribution, KSA would be a worrisome target for T cells. MUC-16 for ovarian cancers and human papillomavirus (HPV)-related antigens for cervical cancer are especially strong candidates at this time because of their widespread expression on the respective cancers and restricted expression on normal tissues.

Molecular analysis of endometrial carcinomas has identified a variety of proteins that may serve as target antigens for vaccine-based therapy. For example, over-expression of HER2/neu has been correlated with advanced disease and poor outcome in both adenocarcinoma and uterine papillary serous carcinoma (245,246). More recent reports have implicated alterations in the hMLH1, p16(ink4a) (p16), and *PTEN* genes as promoters of carcinogenesis, as well as over-expression of the *SART-1* gene, which encodes the SART-1 (247) tumor antigen that is recognized by HLA-A26–restricted cytotoxic T lymphocytes (32% of tested specimens) (248,249).

CLINICAL TRIALS WITH SELECTED VACCINES DESIGNED PRIMARILY TO INDUCE T-CELL RESPONSES

NY-ESO-1 Vaccine

The NY-ESO-1 antigen belongs to the cancer-testis antigen family that includes the MAGE-1 protein (first human gene product recognized by $CD8^+$ T cells identified in a patient with cancer), and the GAGE and BAGE families (250,251). NY-ESO-1 has shown consistent immunogenicity, and the existence of overlapping $CD8^+$ and $CD4^+$ T-cell epitopes within these antigens has provided the opportunity of using one short peptide, ESO 157–170, to generate both $CD4^+$ and CD 8^+ T cells (252). Immunoscreening studies have found NY-ESO-1 expression in ovarian cancers, and interestingly the cancer-testis family antigens are represented by the MAGE series (with the exception of MAGE-10), LAGE-1, and PRAME genes, but NY-ESO-1 expression is absent in patients with cervical cancer (253,254). The represented antigens would be appropriate targets for vaccines, and studies with a peptide vaccine targeted at NY-ESO-1 are ongoing in patients with ovarian cancer at the Memorial Sloan-Kettering and Roswell Park Cancer Centers. An existing phase 1 clinical trial immunized 12 patients with metastatic NY-ESO-1–expressing tumors (seven were NY-ESO-1 serum antibody negative and five patients were NY-ESO-1 positive at the start of the study) using intradermal administration of three HLA A2–restricted peptides. Primary peptide-specific $CD8^+$ T-cell reactions were generated in four of seven NY-ESO-1 antibody-negative patients. Although there were no complete or partial clinical responses, induction of a specific $CD8^+$ T-cell response to NY-ESO-1 in immunized antibody-negative patients was associated with disease stabilization and objective regression of single metastases. Stabilization of disease was observed overall in four of the seven seronegative patients who developed $CD8^+$ T-cell responses by ELISPOT and delayed-type hypersensitivity (DTH) reactions after vaccination (one of the two ovarian cancer patients had decreasing ascites and stable peritoneal carcinomatosis lasting 20 weeks) (255).

Granulocyte-Macrophage Colony-Stimulating Factor–Secreting Tumor-Cell Vaccines

Granulocyte-macrophage colony-stimulating factor (GM-CSF) has a variety of properties desirable for vaccine production including enhancing immune responses by inducing the proliferation, maturation, and migration of dendritic cells and the expansion of both T- and B-cell lymphocytes (256). A recent characterization of its adjuvant response has shown the early elevation of inflammatory molecules such as IL-6, TNF-α, and monocyte chemotactic protein-1 (MCP-1) followed later by IL-12 and IFN-δ production, among others (257). *In vitro* characterization of a GM-CSF–secreting vaccine was performed by genetically engineering UCI-107 (ovarian cancer cell line) to secrete GM-CSF by retrovirus-mediated gene transduction with the LXSN retroviral vector containing the human GM-CSF gene and the neomycin resistance selection marker. A clone (UCI-107 GM-SF-MPS) was extensively characterized and shown to secrete high levels of GM-CSF over 6 months of study (258). In human trials, a variety of studies have shown that vaccination with irradiated tumor cells engineered to secrete GM-CSF stimulates long-lasting immunity in murine models and in patients with metastatic melanoma. A phase 1 study evaluated patients with metastatic non-small-cell lung carcinoma. A metastatic site was resected, processed to single-cell suspension, infected with a replication-defective adenoviral vector encoding GM-CSF, irradiated, cryopreserved, and then given intradermally at weekly and biweekly intervals. Vaccines were made successfully for 34 of 35 patients. Dendritic cell, macrophage, granulocyte, and lymphocyte infiltrates were elicited in 18 of 25 assessable patients. Two patients rendered disease-free by surgical removal of metastatic disease prior to trial enrollment were disease-free at 43 and 42 months; five patients had stable disease ranging from 3 to 33 months; and one patient had a mixed response (259). Additional trials in other solid tumor types, including gynecologic malignancies, are warranted.

Folate Receptor–Targeted Vaccines

Previous studies have identified the alpha isoform of the folate receptor (FR), which is a 38-kD GPI-anchored protein constitutively expressed at high levels in 90% of non-mucinous ovarian cancer and at low levels in normal tissues (247). The reason for over-expression is unknown, but one hypothesis is that over-expression provides an alternate folate-processing pathway to compensate for deletion of the tetrahydrofolate reductase gene that is deleted frequently in cancer cells (167). FR expression has been shown in preclinical models to confer a growth advantage in FR-transfected cells, which suggests a role for the receptor in the control of cell proliferation (260). Growth regulation may be related to an inverse relationship between folate receptor expression and Cav-1, a 21- to 24-kD protein that may negatively regulate the activity of several cytoplasmic signaling proteins and tyrosine kinase inhibitors (258).

The preferential over-expression of the folate receptor in malignant tissue has prompted the investigation of this antigen in several preclinical immunization studies. Neglia et al. (261) evaluated FR alpha cDNA after ligation into the VR1012 (Vical) expression vector under transcriptional control of the cytomegalovirus promoter. Purified plasma DNA was injected into BALB/c mice three times at 14-day intervals. At 10 days after the second injection, sera (100%) showed antibody titers against syngeneic C26 cells transduced with FR alpha, but not against unmodified C26 cells. Specific cytotoxic T-lymphocyte activity against FR alpha–transduced C26 cells could be seen in splenocytes from all immunized animals. Challenge by subcutaneous injection with FR alpha–transduced C26 cells (administered 10 days after third injection) showed a statistically significant delay in tumor growth (261). Further studies by Peoples et al. showed that both immunodominant E39 (folate-binding protein [FBP], 194–202) and subdominant E41 (FBP, 246, 248–255) epitopes of human high-affinity FBP are presented by HLA-A2 in both ovarian and breast cancers (262). Tumor-associated lymphocytes stimulated with FBP peptides exhibit cytotoxicity not only against peptide-loaded targets but also against FBP-expressing epithelial tumors of different histologies. Finally, FBP peptides induced E39-specific cytotoxic T lymphocytes (CTLs) and E39- and E41-specific IFN-δ and IP-10 secretion in a proportion of healthy donors. These studies provide motivation for proceeding to clinical trials with DNA and peptide FR vaccines in ovarian cancer patients.

Dendritic-Cell Approaches

Dendritic cells (DC) are phenotypically distinct, potent antigen-presenting cells well suited for vaccine strategies (263). They are found throughout the body, particularly at the portals of entry for infectious organisms, such as in the epidermis and other epithelial surfaces. Cancers may be ineffective at attracting DCs, may attract the wrong type of DCs, or may attract immature DCs that induce tolerance. Zou et al. observed that ovarian carcinoma cells express high levels of the chemokine SDF-1 that attracts a subset of DC precursors with capacity to differentiate into plasmacytoid DCs, which are implicated in immune suppression through induction of IL-10 by T cells. Myeloid DCs, which are more effective at inducing immune responses, were not detected (264). Also, plasmacytoid DCs have been implicated in inducing a set of CD8+ regulatory T cells in ovarian carcinoma (265). DCs from patients with ovarian cancer can be matured *ex vivo* to activate T cells producing IFN-γ in response to autologous tumor cell lysates, but not cytotoxic T cells (266). Ovarian carcinoma cell lines can directly inhibit maturation of DCs (267). These results and many others suggest that DCs from cancer patients can be defective at fully activating T cells. Curiel et al. showed that myeloid DCs from tumor or draining lymph nodes of ovarian carcinoma expressed B7-H1, a molecule in the B7 family implicated in inhibiting immune responses (268). Blockade of B7-H1 led to marked increases in T-cell responses. Multiple animal studies have demonstrated CTL-mediated protective immunity and even regression of established tumors with the administration of antigen pulsed dendritic cells (269,270). A variety of approaches have been considered with regard to antigen type and loading techniques to include recombinant or fusion proteins (271), peptides as tumor antigen-derived CTL epitopes (272), DC-tumor cell hybrids (273), HLA-restricted antigens (274), and autologous antigens from tumor cell lysates and apoptotic tumor cells (275,276). A number of antigen sources are possible for DC-based treatment of ovarian cancer, including germ cells/cancer testis antigens, HER2, and MUC-16 (CA-125) (92).

Both the clinical relevance and presence of the target are obviously essential when using this tumor antigen approach. For example, several studies have demonstrated the effectiveness of using *in vitro*-generated DCs loaded with HLA-A2 restricted peptide fragments from either HER2 (E75) or the HER2 intracellular domain (ICD) in terms of immune response. Brossart et al. vaccinated patients with advanced breast cancer or ovarian cancer with DCs pulsed with peptides from HER2 or MUC-1, detecting peptide-specific cytotoxic T-cell responses in T cells from peripheral blood of 5 of 10 patients (277). However, recent data from a GOG study showed that only 11.4% of 837 screened ovarian cancer tumor samples showed 2+ or 3+ over-expression of HER2. Furthermore, using the monoclonal humanized anti-HER2 antibody trastuzumab, an overall response rate of 7.3% was seen, showing that even with appropriate over-expression, minimal single-agent activity is seen (278).

Santin et al. showed that DCs loaded with lysates of autologous ovarian cancer cells from three patients were able to induce specific cytotoxic T-cell responses *in vitro*, suggesting feasibility of this approach (279). Using the autologous tumor antigen pulsed DC approach in patients with ovarian cancer (n = 8) and uterine sarcoma (n = 2), Hernando et al. harvested DCs, and pulsed them with KLH and autologous tumor cell lysate in the presence of GM-CSF (270). Significant tumor antigen-specific lymphoproliferative responses were seen in two ovarian cancer patients. Progression-free intervals of 25 to 45 weeks were seen in three patients (two with demonstrable immune responses), suggesting an effect of disease stabilization. Homma et al. treated 21 patients, including patients with ovarian cancer, with DCs fused to tumor cells using polyethylene glycol, with or without systemic treatment with IL-12 (280). They observed antibody responses against autologous tumor cells in one patient and resolution of malignant ascites in a patient with gastric carcinoma. These data combined with DCs pulsed with lysates from other solid tumors such as melanoma, renal cell carcinoma, and selected pediatric tumors showing specific T-cell immunity, and some objective responses further support evaluation of this approach in patients with gynecologic cancers (275,281,282).

Dendritic cell approaches are potent at inducing T-cell responses. A variety of variables require further study to optimize the approach including choice of DC subtype, maturational status at immunization, adjuvant cytokines, antigen loading method, and route and frequency of administration.

ANTI-IDIOTYPE VACCINES

Anti-idiotype vaccines strive to augment both antibody and T-cell responses by using antibody facsimiles of the native antigens to overcome their poor immunogenicity and availability. Tumor-associated antigens are traditionally weakly immunogenic as the large majority of them in humans are non-mutated self-antigens. One approach has been to present the desired epitope to the now tolerant host in a different molecular environment, but the problem with many tumor antigens is that they are ill-defined chemically and difficult to purify and produce (110).

The "immune network hypothesis" attempts to transform epitope structures into idiotypic determinants expressed on the surface of antibodies, and was originally proposed in the 1970s (283,284). This approach assumes that immunization with a given antigen will generate the production of antibodies against this antigen (termed Ab1). Ab1 can generate anti-idiotypic antibodies against Ab1, termed Ab2. Some of the anti-idiotypic antibodies (Ab2β) express the internal image of the antigen recognized by the Ab1 antibody and can be used as surrogate antigens. Immunization with Ab2β can cause the production of anti–anti-Id antibodies (termed Ab3) that recognize the corresponding original antigen identified by Ab1 (285,286). (Since Ab3 can have Ab1-like reactivity, it is also called Ab1′ to distinguish it from the original Ab1.)

ACA-125 (Abagovomab)

The generation and production of the murine anti-idiotypic antibody ACA-125 (abagovomab) for clinical use has been described in detail (287). Briefly, BALB/c mice were immunized with murine monoclonal antibody OC125 (CIS; Bio International, Gif-Sur-Yvette, France) directed against the tumor-associated antigen CA-125. Splenic cells of immunized mice were fused with myeloma cells yielding an ACA-125–producing hybridoma that was adapted to serum-free medium. Large-scale production of mAb ACA-125 was performed in a hollow fiber system with yields of 10 to 15 mg of antibody per day. mAb ACA-125 was purified from culture supernatant by affinity chromatography with protein G-sepharose and the preparation was checked by SDS-PAGE analysis (PHAST-System; Pharmacia Biotech, Uppsala, Sweden) to give >95% purity. The final product for vaccination in previous phase 1-2 trials contained 2 mg of Ab2 IgG1 in sterile, pyrogen-free, polynucleotide-free, mycoplasma virus–free, and retrovirus-free phosphate-buffered saline (PBS) solution.

The anti-idiotype approach has been used in a variety of clinical studies including patients with colon cancer, melanoma, small-cell lung cancer, and neuroblastoma. Immune responses have been demonstrated, and some have suggested a benefit in those patients in whom antibody develops (288–292). Problems with interpreting such phase 2 studies have been appropriately recognized, and prospective phase 3 studies are in development in several tumor types directed toward a variety of antigens.

A two-step study with ACA-125 has been conducted in Germany in patients with ovarian cancer and reported by Wagner et al. (293). Initially, 18 patients were enrolled in the phase 1 portion, which was extended into a phase 2 study with a total of 42 patients being treated. The objective of the phase 1 portion was to confirm safety. The objectives of the phase 2 portion were to (a) further characterize the effect of ACA-125 vaccination on the Ab3 titer as a marker of a specific anti–ACA-125 immune response, and (b) to evaluate overall survival comparing those patients in whom antibody was generated with those in whom it was not. Other immunologic parameters evaluated to better characterize the humoral response included assays of Ab1 and ADCC. The cytolytic activity of immunized patients' peripheral blood lymphocytes against human ovarian cancer cells (CA-125 expressing = OAW-42 and non-expressing = SK-OV3) was also evaluated using a standard europium-release cytotoxicity assay.

Forty-two patients with advanced/recurrent epithelial ovarian carcinoma were enrolled with an average number of 2.1 prior regimens (range 1 to 5). All patients had tumors that strongly expressed CA-125 and received an intramuscular injection of 2 mg of alum-precipitated ACA-125 for four injections at 2-week intervals followed by monthly administration. A mean number of 16.6 + 10.8 vaccinations were delivered (range 2 to 46). Minimal pain at the injection site was seen but no other systemic adverse effects. Hyperimmune sera of 27 of 42 patients (64.2%)

showed an increase in HAMAs (>100 ng/mL). Ab3 responses were negative in all patients before ACA-125 administration, and 28 of 42 patients (66.7%) developed specific anti–anti-idiotype antibodies (Ab3) during ACA-125 administration. The IgG subclass was evaluated in 10 patients: predominantly IgG1 and IgG2. No correlation could be shown between number of doses, serologic CA-125 concentration, and maximum Ab3 reactivity. The specificity of the immune responses induced after vaccination was demonstrated by a series of competition experiments showing that binding of Ab3 to the anti-idiotype ACA-125 could be inhibited by the idiotypic mAb OC125 and the CA-125 antigen (293). Cell-mediated cytotoxicity from peripheral blood lymphocytes (PBLs) against CA-125–expressing and CA-125–non-expressing human ovarian cancer cell lines in 18 patients was evaluated with measured cell kill increasing in 9 of 18 patients from 19.6% ± 11.7% to 52.7% ± 13.6% at the effector:target cell ratio of 100:1 (259). Cell-mediated lysis was accompanied by the induction of Ab3 in eight of nine patients, prompting only humoral response evaluation in the remaining patients. Overall survival of all patients vaccinated with ACA-125: 14.9 ± 12.9 months; of all patients with a positive response to ACA-125: 19.9 ± 13.1 months; and of all patients with no detectable response to ACA-125: 5.3 ± 4.3 months; $p < 0.0001$.

Two additional studies have explored different doses (2.0 mg vs. 0.2 mg), routes (subcutaneous vs. intramuscular), and number of immunizations (nine vs. six) of abagovomab. A phase 1 trial with 42 patients showed that neither route ($p = 0.628$) nor dose ($p = 0.4602$) was statistically significant in terms of effect on maximum post-baseline Ab3 titer (294). Induction of Ab3 was observed in all evaluable patients. A second phase 1 study in 36 patients evaluated two subcutaneous vaccination schedules (nine vs. six injections) (295). No treatment-limiting toxicities occurred in either group and induction of Ab3 was observed in all evaluable patients. IFN-γ–expressing CA-125 specific CD8+ T cells were significantly more frequent in those receiving nine vaccinations, while there was no significant difference between CD4+ T cells in the two groups.

Therefore, vaccination with a suitable anti-idiotypic antibody may offer a way to induce immunity against undefined antigens or poorly immunogenic tumor antigen, such as CA-125. As seen in other immune approaches, phase 1/1 data show an association between the desired immune response and longer survival, but a randomized, appropriately powered trial is required to confirm benefit. Side effects have been minimal. More recently, a study in mice has suggested that injection of the ACA-125 antibody fused to IL-6 may increase the specific humoral response against CA-125, although the clinical relevance has not been studied (296).

Based on the sum of the phase 1 data, an international, multicenter, randomized phase 3 trial of abagovomab versus placebo for stage III or IV epithelial ovarian cancer patients, with an accrual goal of 870 patients, began accruing patients in 2007 under the direction of the Arbeitsgemeinschaft Gynäkologische Onkologie (AGO) group and the Cooperative Ovarian Cancer Group for Immunotherapy (COGI). Eligible patients have completed standard debulking and platinum with taxane-based chemotherapy (intravenous or intraperitoneal) and are in complete remission. The primary endpoint of this study is progression-free survival with a secondary endpoint of overall survival.

CONCLUSIONS

Most patients with cervical, endometrial, or ovarian cancer who will eventually die of disease can be initially rendered free of detectable disease by surgery, radiation therapy, and/or chemotherapy for varying periods. This adjuvant setting where the targets are circulating tumor cells or micrometastasis is ideal for treatment with immune interventions such as cytokines administered intraperitoneally, adoptive immunotherapy with monoclonal antibodies or cellular therapy, and vaccines that induce T cells or antibodies. This is especially true for cervical and ovarian cancers where HPV-related antigens and MUC-16 (CA-125), respectively, are uniquely specific target antigens. HPV-related interventions against cervical cancer are discussed in chapter 19 by Dr. Thomas Wright. Initial studies in ovarian cancer patients using IFN or IL-2 administered IP have resulted in occasional partial or complete regressions of metastatic disease, especially of tumors less than 5 mm in diameter, but the impact on overall survival has yet to be demonstrated in randomized trials. Administration of mAbs against MUC-16, MUC-1, and sTn have resulted in occasional clinical responses and evidence of prolonged survival compared to historical controls, but results of randomized trials in ovarian cancer evaluating the benefit of these approaches are not yet available. A well-conducted randomized trial of the radionuclide ^{90}Y-HMFG1 showed no benefit, but many other conjugates using other doses and schedules remain to be tested (120). Vaccines have augmented T-cell or B-cell immunity, and these responses have been associated with stabilization of disease in some patients with advanced disease and prolongation of disease-free and overall survival compared to historical controls. Again, randomized trials confirming the benefit of vaccines remain to be accomplished but several are now ongoing. The suggestion of clinical efficacy to date in trials with IP cytokines, monoclonal antibodies, and vaccines is encouraging but not definitive. As awareness of the unique features of the peritoneal cavity, radiolabeled mAb technologies, and vaccine design for augmentation of antibodies and T cells continues to evolve, further progress is likely (128). However, over the next several years, the focus will need to be on testing the clinical impact of these immunologic interventions in appropriately controlled randomized trials in the adjuvant setting. Only in this way can a firm foundation be built on which to explore combinations of these treatments with each other and with surgery, radiation, and chemotherapy.

References

1. McGuire WP, Hoskins WJ, Brady MF, et al. Cyclophosphamide and cisplatin compared with paclitaxel and cisplatin in patients with stage III and stage IV ovarian cancer. *N Engl J Med* 1996;334:1–6.
2. Muggia FM, Braly PS, Brady MF, et al. Phase III randomized study of cisplatin versus paclitaxel versus cisplatin and paclitaxel in patients with suboptimal stage III or IV ovarian cancer: a Gynecologic Oncology Group study. *J Clin Oncol* 2000;18:106–115.
3. Armstrong DK, Bundy B, Wenzel L, et al. Intraperitoneal cisplatin and paclitaxel in ovarian cancer. *N Engl J Med* 2006;354:34–43.
4. Morris M, Eifel PJ, Lu J, et al. Pelvic radiation with concurrent chemotherapy compared with pelvic and para-aortic radiation for high-risk cervical cancer. *N Engl J Med* 1999;340:1137–1143.
5. Keys HM, Bundy BN, Stehman FB, et al. Cisplatin, radiation, and adjuvant hysterectomy compared with radiation and adjuvant hysterectomy for bulky stage IB cervical carcinoma. *N Engl J Med* 1999;340:1154–1161.
6. Koutsky LA, Ault KA, Wheeler CM, et al. A controlled trial of a human papillomavirus type 16 vaccine. *N Engl J Med* 2002;347:1645–1651.
7. FUTURE II Study Group. Quadrivalent vaccine against human papillomavirus to prevent high-grade cervical lesions. *N Engl J Med* 2007;356:1915–1927.
8. Fleming GF, Brunetto VL, Cella D, et al. Phase III trial of doxorubicin plus cisplatin with or without paclitaxel plus filgrastim in advanced endometrial carcinoma: a Gynecologic Oncology Group study. *J Clin Oncol* 2004;22:2159–2166.
9. Curiel TJ, Coukos G, Zou L, et al. Specific recruitment of regulatory T cells in ovarian carcinoma fosters immune privilege and predicts reduced survival. *Nat Med* 2004;10(9):942–949.

10. Sato E, Olson SH, Ahn J, et al. Intraepithelial CD8+ tumor-infiltrating lymphocytes and a high CD8+/regulatory T cell ration are associated with favorable prognosis in ovarian cancer. *Proc Natl Acad Sci USA* 2005;105(51):18538–18543.
11. Zhang L, Conejo-Garcia JR, Katsaros D, et al. Intratumoral T cells, recurrence, and survival in epithelial ovarian cancer. *N Engl J Med* 2003;348(3):203–213.
12. Wolf D, Wolf AM, Rumpold H, et al. The expression of the regulatory T cell-specific forkhead box transcription factor FoxP3 is associated with poor prognosis in ovarian cancer. *Clin Cancer Res* 2005;11(23): 8326–8331.
13. Verheijen RH, Massuger LF, Benigno BB, et al. Phase III trial of intraperitoneal therapy with yttrium-90-labeled HMFG1 murine monoclonal antibody in patients with epithelial ovarian cancer after a surgically defined complete remission. *J Clin Oncol* 2006;24:571–579.
14. Clynes RA, Towers TL, Presta LG, et al. Inhibitory Fc receptors modulate *in vivo* cytotoxicity against tumor targerts. *Nat Med* 2000;6(4):443–446.
15. Bookman MA, Boente MP, Bast R. Immunology and immunotherapy of gynecologic cancer. In: *Principles and Practice of Gynecologic Oncology.* 3rd ed. Philadelphia: Lippincott Williams & Wilkins, 2000:129–163.
16. Nash MA, Lenzi R, Edwards CL, et al. Differential expression of cytokine transcripts in human epithelial ovarian carcinoma by solid tumour specimens, peritoneal exudate cells containing tumour, tumour-infiltrating lymphocyte (TIL)–derived T cell lines and established tumour cell lines. *Clin Exp Immunol* 1998;112:172–180.
17. Balkwill F, Schlom J, Berek J, et al. Discussion: immunological therapeutics in ovarian cancer. *Gynecol Oncol* 2003;88:S110–S113.
18. Allavena P, Peccatori F, Maggioni D, et al. Intraperitoneal recombinant gamma-interferon in patients with recurrent ascitic ovarian carcinoma: modulation of cytotoxicity and cytokine production in tumor-associated effectors and of major histocompatibility antigen expression on tumor cells. *Cancer Res* 1990;50:7318–7323.
19. Nehme A, Julia AM, Jozan S, et al. Modulation of cisplatin cytotoxicity by human recombinant interferon-gamma in human ovarian cancer cell lines. *Eur J Cancer* 1994;30A:520–525.
20. Saito T, Berens ME, Welander CE. Direct and indirect effects of human recombinant gamma-interferon on tumor cells in a clonogenic assay. *Cancer Res* 1986;46:1142–1147.
21. Berek JS. Intraperitoneal immunotherapy for ovarian cancer with alpha interferon. *Eur J Cancer* 1992;28A:719–721.
22. Windbichler GH, Hausmaninger H, Stummvoll W, et al. Interferon-gamma in the first-line therapy of ovarian cancer: a randomized phase III trial. *Br J Cancer* 2000;82:1138–1144.
23. Abdulhay G, DiSaia PJ, Blessing JA, et al. Human lymphoblastoid interferon in the treatment of advanced epithelial ovarian malignancies: a Gynecologic Oncology Group study. *Am J Obstet Gynecol* 1985;152: 418–423.
24. Hall GD, Brown JM, Coleman RE, et al. Maintenance treatment with interferon for advanced ovarian cancer: results of the Northern and Yorkshire Gynecology Group randomized phase III study. *Br J Cancer* 2004;91(4):621–626.
25. Berek JS, Hacker NF, Lichtenstein A, et al. Intraperitoneal recombinant alpha 2-interferon for "salvage" immunotherapy in persistent epithelial ovarian cancer. *Cancer Treat Rev* 1985;12(Suppl B):23–32.
26. Berek JS, Hacker NF, Lichtenstein A, et al. Intraperitoneal recombinant alpha-interferon for "salvage" immunotherapy in stage III epithelial ovarian cancer: a Gynecologic Oncology Group study. *Cancer Res* 1985;45: 4447–4453.
27. Berek JS. Intraperitoneal adoptive immunotherapy for peritoneal cancer. *J Clin Oncol* 1990;8:1610–1612.
28. Nardi M, Cognetti F, Pollera CF, et al. Intraperitoneal recombinant alpha-2-interferon alternating with cisplatin as salvage therapy for minimal residual-disease ovarian cancer: a phase II study. *J Clin Oncol* 1990;8:1036–1041.
29. Willemse PH, de Vries EG, Mulder NH, et al. Intraperitoneal human recombinant interferon alpha-2b in minimal residual ovarian cancer. *Eur J Cancer* 1990;26:353–358.
30. Berek JS, Welander C, Schink JC, et al. A phase I-II trial of intraperitoneal cisplatin and alpha-interferon in patients with persistent epithelial ovarian cancer. *Gynecol Oncol* 1991;40:237–243.
31. Pujade-Lauraine E, Guastella J, Colombo N, et al. Intraperitoneal administration of interferon gamma. An efficient adjuvant to the chemotherapy of ovarian cancers. Apropos of an European study of 108 patients. *Bull Cancer* 1993;80(2):163–170.
32. Pujade-Lauraine E, Guastalla JP, Colombo N, et al. Intraperitoneal recombinant interferon gamma in ovarian cancer patients with residual disease at second-look laparotomy. *J Clin Oncol* 1996;14:343–350.
33. Berek JS, Markman M, Stonebraker B, et al. Intraperitoneal interferon-alpha in residual ovarian carcinoma: a phase II gynecologic oncology group study. *Gynecol Oncol* 1999;75:10–14.
34. Welander CE, Morgan TM, Homesley HD, et al. Combined recombinant human interferon alpha 2 and cytotoxic agents studied in a clonogenic assay. *Int J Cancer* 1985;35:721–729.
35. Moore DH, Valea F, Walton LA, et al. A phase I study of intraperitoneal interferon-alpha 2b and intravenous cis-platinum plus cyclophosphamide chemotherapy in patients with untreated stage III epithelial ovarian cancer: a Gynecologic Oncology Group pilot study. *Gynecol Oncol* 1995;59:267–272.
36. Frasci G, Tortoriello A, Facchini G, et al. Intraperitoneal (ip) cisplatin-mitoxantrone-interferon-alpha 2b in ovarian cancer patients with minimal residual disease. *Gynecol Oncol* 1993;50:60–67.
37. Berek JS, Markman M, Blessing JA, et al. Intraperitoneal alpha-interferon alternating with cisplatin in residual ovarian carcinoma: a phase II Gynecologic Oncology Group study. *Gynecol Oncol* 1999;74:48–52.
38. Bruzzone M, Rubagotti A, Gadducci A, et al. Intraperitoneal carboplatin with or without interferon-alpha in advanced ovarian cancer patients with minimal residual disease at second look: a prospective randomized trial of 111 patients. G.O.N.O. Gruppo Oncologic Nord Ovest. *Gynecol Oncol* 1997;65:499–505.
39. Morgan RJ Jr, Synold TW, Gandara D, et al. Phase II trial of carboplatin and infusional cyclosporine with alpha-interferon in recurrent ovarian cancer: a California Cancer Consortium trial. *Int J Gynecol Cancer* 2007;17(2):373–378.
40. Ambrosio D, Piscopo L, Lauro C, et al. Trattamento del carcinoma ovarico con interferone alpha 2b somministrato per via intraperitoneale. *Minerva Ginecol* 2001;53:67–71.
41. Windbichler GH, Hausmaninger H, Stummvoll W, et al. Interferon-gamma in the first-line therapy of ovarian cancer: a randomized phase III trial. *Br J Cancer* 2000;82(6):1138–1144.
42. Marth C, Windbichler GH, Hausmaninger H, et al. Interferon-gamma in combination with carboplatin and paclitaxel as a safe and effective first-line treatment option for advanced ovarian cancer: results of a phase I/II study. *Int J Gynecol Cancer* 2006;16(4):1522–1528.
43. Vasilyev RV, Bokhman Ja V, Smorodintsev AA, et al. An experience with application of human leucocyte interferon for cervical cancer treatment. *Eur J Gynaecol Oncol* 1990;11:313–317.
44. Wadler S, Burk RD, Neuberg D, et al. Lack of efficacy of interferon-alpha therapy in recurrent, advanced cervical cancer. *J Interferon Cytokine Res* 1995;15:1011–1016.
45. Lotan R, Dawson MI, Zou CC, et al. Enhanced efficacy of combinations of retinoic acid- and retinoid X receptor–selective retinoids and alpha-interferon in inhibition of cervical carcinoma cell proliferation. *Cancer Res* 1995;55:232–236.
46. Moore DM, Kalvakolanu DV, Lippman SM, et al. Retinoic acid and interferon in human cancer: mechanistic and clinical studies. *Semin Hematol* 1994;31:31–37.
47. Santin AD, Hermonat P, Ravaggi A, et al. Effects of retinoic acid combined with interferon-gamma on the expression of major-histocompatibility-complex molecules and intercellular adhesion molecule-1 in human cervical cancer. *Int J Cancer* 1998;75:254–258.
48. Lippman SM, Parkinson DR, Itri LM, et al. 13-Cis-retinoic acid and interferon alpha-2a: effective combination therapy for advanced squamous cell carcinoma of the skin [Comment]. *J Natl Cancer Inst* 1992; 84:235–241.
49. Paredes Espinoza M, Lippman SM, Kavanagh JJ, et al. Treatment of 32 cervico-uterine cancer patients with 13-cis-retinoic acid and interferon alpha. *Rev Invest Clin* 1994;46:105–111.
50. Hallum AV 3rd, Alberts DS, Lippman SM, et al. Phase II study of 13-cis-retinoic acid plus interferon-alpha 2a in heavily pretreated squamous carcinoma of the cervix. *Gynecol Oncol* 1995;56:382–386.
51. Wadler S, Schwartz EL, Haynes H, et al. All-trans retinoic acid and interferon-alpha-2a in patients with metastatic or recurrent carcinoma of the uterine cervix: clinical and pharmacokinetic studies. New York Gynecologic Oncology Group. *Cancer* 1997;79:1574–1580.
52. Weiss GR, Liu PY, Alberts DS, et al. 13-cis-retinoic acid or all-trans-retinoic acid plus interferon-alpha in recurrent cervical cancer: a Southwest Oncology Group phase II randomized trial. *Gynecol Oncol* 1998;71:386–390.
53. Park TK, Lee JP, Kim SN, et al. Interferon-alpha 2a, 13-cis-retinoic acid and radiotherapy for locally advanced carcinoma of the cervix: a pilot study. *Eur J Gynaecol Oncol* 1998;19:35–38.
54. Gonzales-de Leon C, Lippman SM, Kudelka AP, et al. Phase II study of cisplatin, 5-fluorouracil and interferon-alpha in recurrent carcinoma of the cervix. *Invest New Drugs* 1995;13:73–76.
55. Rose PG, Bundy BN, Watkins EB, et al. Concurrent cisplatin-based radiotherapy and chemotherapy for locally advanced cervical cancer. *N Engl J Med* 1999;340:1144–1153.
56. Spirtos NM, Smith LH, Teng NN. Prospective randomized trial of topical alpha-interferon (alpha-interferon gels) for the treatment of vulvar intraepithelial neoplasia III. *Gynecol Oncol* 1990;37:34–38.
57. Bornstein J, Ben-David Y, Atad J, et al. Treatment of cervical intraepithelial neoplasia and invasive squamous cell carcinoma by interferon. *Obstet Gynecol Surv* 1993;48:251–260.
58. Benedetti Panici P, Scambia G, Greggi S, et al. Recombinant interleukin-2 continuous infusion in ovarian cancer patients with minimal residual disease at second-look. *Cancer Treat Rev* 1989;16(Suppl A):123–127.
59. Edwards RP, Gooding W, Lembersky BC, et al. Comparison of toxicity and survival following intraperitoneal recombinant interleukin-2 for persistent ovarian cancer after platinum: twenty-four-hour versus 7-day infusion. *J Clin Oncol* 1997;15:3399–3407.
60. Edwards RP, Gooding W, Lembersky BC, et al. Comparison of toxicity and survival following intraperitoneal recombinant interleukin-2 for

persistent ovarian cancer after platinum: twenty-four-hour versus 7-day infusion. *J Clin Oncol* 1997;15(11):3399–3407.
61. Bernsen MR, Van Der Velden AW, Everse LA, et al. Interleukin-2: hope in cases of cisplatin-resistant tumours. *Cancer Immunol Immunother* 1998;46:41–47.
62. Horton HM, Dorigo O, Hernandez P, et al. IL-2 plasmid therapy of murine ovarian carcinoma inhibits the growth of tumor ascites and alters its cytokine profile. *J Immunol* 1999;163:6378–6385.
63. Berchuck A, Lyerly H. A phase I study of autologous human interleukin-2 (IL-2) gene modified tumor cells in patients with refractory metastatic ovarian cancer. *Human Gene Transfer Protocols, Office of Recombinant DNA Activities*. Bethesda, MD: National Institutes of Health, 1995.
64. Gately MK. Interleukin-12: a recently discovered cytokine with potential for enhancing cell-mediated immune responses to tumors. *Cancer Invest* 1993;11:500–506.
65. Brunda MJ, Luistro L, Warrier RR, et al. Antitumor and antimetastatic activity of interleukin 12 against murine tumors. *J Exp Med* 1993;178:1223–1230.
66. Coffman RL, Varkila K, Scott P, et al. Role of cytokines in the differentiation of CD4+ T-cell subsets *in vivo*. *Immunol Rev* 1991;123:189–207.
67. Nastala CL, Edington HD, McKinney TG, et al. Recombinant IL-12 administration induces tumor regression in association with IFN-gamma production. *J Immunol* 1994;153:1697–1706.
68. DeCesare SL, Michelini-Norris B, Blanchard DK, et al. Interleukin-12–mediated tumoricidal activity of patient lymphocytes in an autologous *in vitro* ovarian cancer assay system. *Gynecol Oncol* 1995;57:86–95.
69. Barton DP, Blanchard DK, Duan C, et al. Interleukin-12 synergizes with interleukin-2 to generate lymphokine-activated killer activity in peripheral blood mononuclear cells cultured in ovarian cancer ascitic fluid. *J Soc Gynecol Invest* 1995;2:762–771.
70. Fujiwara H, Hamaoka T. The anti-tumor effects of IL-12 involve enhanced IFN-gamma production by anti-tumor T cells, their accumulation to tumor sites and *in situ* IFN-gamma production. *Leukemia* 1997;11(Suppl 3):570–571.
71. Zeimet AG, Widschwendter M, Knabbe C, et al. Ascitic interleukin-12 is an independent prognostic factor in ovarian cancer [Comment]. *J Clin Oncol* 1998;16:1861–1868.
72. Hurteau JA, Blessing JA, DeCesare SL, et al. Evaluation of recombinant human interleukin-12 in patients with recurrent or refractory ovarian cancer: a Gynecologic Oncology Group study. *Gynecol Oncol* 2001;82:7–10.
73. Lenzi R, Rosenblum M, Verschraegen C, et al. Phase I study of intraperitoneal recombinant human interleukin 12 in patients with müllerian carcinoma, gastrointestinal primary malignancies, and mesothelioma. *Clin Cancer Res* 2002;8:3686–3695.
74. Parihar R, Nadella P, Lewis A, et al. A phase I study of interleukin 12 with trastuzumab in patients with human epidermal growth factor receptor-2-over-expressing malignancies: analysis of sustained interferon gamma production in a subset of patients. *Clin Cancer Res* 2004;10(15):5027–5037.
75. Zhang H, Zhang S, Cheung NK, et al. Antibodies can eradicate cancer micrometastases. *Cancer Res* 1998;58:2844–2849.
76. Livingston PO. The case for melanoma vaccines that induce antibodies. In: Kirkwood, JM, ed. *Molecular Diagnosis and Treatment of Melanoma*. New York: Marcel Dekker; 1998.
77. Jones PC, Sze LL, Liu PY, et al. Prolonged survival for melanoma patients with elevated IgM antibody to oncofetal antigen. *J Natl Cancer Inst* 1981;66:249–254.
78. Livingston PO, Ritter G, Srivastava P, et al. Characterization of IgG and IgM antibodies induced in melanoma patients by immunization with purified GM2 gangliosic. *Cancer Res* 1989;49:7045–7050.
79. Livingston PO, Wong GYC, Adluri S, et al. Improved survival in AJCC stage III melanoma patients with GM2 antibodies: a randomized trial of adjuvant vaccination with GM2 ganglioside. *J Clin Oncol* 1994;12:1036–1044.
80. MacLean GD, Reddish MA, Koganty RR, et al. Antibodies against mucin-associated sialyl-Tn epitopes correlate with survival of metastatic adenocarcinoma patients undergoing active specific immunotherapy with synthetic STn vaccine. *J Immunother* 1996;19:59–68.
81. Piccart-Gebhart MJ, Procter M, Leyland-Jones B, et al. Trastuzumab after adjuvant chemotherapy in HER2-positive breast cancer. *N Engl J Med* 2005;353(16):1659–1672.
82. Zhang S, Cordon-Cardo C, Zhang HS, et al. Selection of carbohydrate tumor antigens as targets for immune attack using immunohistochemistry. I. Focus on gangliosides. *Int J Cancer* 1997;73:42–49.
83. Zhang S, Zhang HS, Cordon-Cardo C, et al. Selection of tumor antigens as targets for immune attack using immunohistochemistry. II. Blood group–related antigens. *Int J Cancer* 1997;73:50–56.
84. Zhang S, Zhang HS, Cordon-Cardo C, et al. Selection of tumor antigens as targets for immune attack using immunohistochemistry. III. Protein antigens. *Clin Cancer Res* 1998;4:2669–2676.
85. Mark FF, Kudryashov V, Saigo PE, et al. Selection of carbohydrate antigens in human epithelial ovarian cancers as targets for immunotherapy: serous and mucinous tumors exhibit distinctive patterns of expression. *Int J Cancer* 1999;81:193–198.
86. Kabawat SE, Bast RC Jr, Welch WR, et al. Immunopathologic characterization of a monoclonal antibody that recognizes common surface antigens of human ovarian tumors of serous, endometrioid, and clear cell types. *Am J Clin Pathol* 1983;79(1):98–104.
87. Nakamura K, Koike M, Shitara K, et al. Chimeric anti-ganglioside GM2 antibody with antitumor activity. *Cancer Res* 1994;54:1511–1516.
88. Nishinaka Y, Ravindranath MNH, Ire RF. Development of a human monoclonal antibody to ganglioside GM2 with potential for cancer treatment. *Cancer Res* 1996;56:5666–5671.
89. Lloyd KO. Blood group antigens as markers for normal differentiation and malignant change in human tissues. *Am J Clin Pathol* 1987;87:129–139.
90. Hellström I, Garrigues HJ, Garrigues U, et al. Highly tumor-reactive, internalizing, mouse monoclonal antibodies to Ley-related cell surface antigens. *Cancer Res* 1990;50:2183–2190.
91. Bast RC, Feeney M, Lazarus H, et al. Reactivity of a monoclonal antibody with human ovarian carcinoma. *J Clin Invest* 1981;68:1331–1337.
92. Yin BWT, Dnistrian A, Lloyd KO. Ovarian cancer antigen CA125 is encoded by the MUC16 mucin gene. *Int J Cancer* 2002;98:737–740.
93. Yin BWT, Lloyd, KO. Molecular cloning of the CA125 ovarian cancer antigen. *J Biol Chem* 2001;276:27371–27375.
94. O'Brien TJ, Beard JB, Underwood LJ, et al. The CA 125 gene: an extracellular superstructure dominated by repeat sequences. *Tumor Biol* 2001;22:348–366.
95. Baum RP, Noujaim AA, Nanci A, et al. Clinical course of ovarian cancer patients under repeated stimulation of HAMA using MAb OC125 and B43.13. *Hybridoma* 1993;12:583–589.
96. Kashmiri SV, Iwahashi M, Tamura M, et al. Development of a minimally immunogenic variant of humanized anti-carcinoma monoclonal antibody CC49. *Crit Rev Oncol Hematol* 2001;38:3–16.
97. Goel A, Colcher D, Baranowska-Kortylewicz J, et al. Genetically engineered tetravalent single-chain Fv of the pancarcinoma monoclonal antibody CC49: improved biodistribution and potential for therapeutic application. *Cancer Res* 2000;60:6964–6971.
98. Kennel SJ, Chappell LL, Dadachova K, et al. Evaluation of 225Ac for vascular targeted radioimmunotherapy of lung tumors [Comment]. *Cancer Biother Radiopharmaceut* 2000;15:235–244.
99. Yokota T, Milenic DE, Whitlow M, et al. Rapid tumor penetration of a single-chain Fv and comparison with other immunoglobulin forms. *Cancer Res* 1992;52:3402–3408.
100. Pavlinkova G, Colcher D, Booth BJ, et al. Pharmacokinetics and biodistribution of a light-chain-shuffled CC49 single-chain Fv antibody construct. *Cancer Immunol Immunother* 2000;49:267–275.
101. Kashmiri SV, Shu L, Padlan EA, et al. Generation, characterization, and *in vivo* studies of humanized anticarcinoma antibody CC49. *Hybridoma* 1995;14:461–473.
102. Kennel SJ, Brechbiel MW, Milenic DE, et al. Actinium-225 conjugates of MAb CC49 and humanized delta CH2CC49. *Cancer Biother Radiopharmaceut* 2002;17:219–231.
103. Alvarez RD, Partridge EE, Khazaeli MB, et al. Intraperitoneal radioimmunotherapy of ovarian cancer with 177Lu-CC49: a phase I/II study. *Gynecol Oncol* 1997;65:94–101.
104. Trail PA, Bianchi AB. Monoclonal antibody drug conjugates in the treatment of cancer. *Curr Opin Immunol* 1999;11:584–588.
105. Ehlen TG, Gordon AG, Fingert HJ, et al. Adjuvant treatment with monoclonal antibody, OvaRex MAb-B43.13 (OV) targeting CA125, induces robust immune responses associated with prolonged time to relapse (TTR) in a randomized, placebo-controlled study in patients with advanced epithelial ovarian cancer (EOC). *Proc Am Soc Clin Oncol* 2002(abst 31).
106. Gordon A, Whiteside T, Nicodemus C, et al. An interim assessment of OvaRex® MAb-B43.13 in the management of recurrent ovarian cancer. *Proc Am Soc Clin Oncol* 2001;20:187b.
107. Schultes B, Gordon A, Ehlen T. Induction of tumor- and CA125-specific T cell responses in patients with epithelial ovarian cancer treated with OvaRex MAb B43.13. *Proc Am Assoc Cancer Res* 2002;43:144.
108. Gordon A, Stringer A, Edwards RP, et al. Clinical and immunologic outcomes of patients with recurrent epithelial ovarian cancer treated with OvaRex MAb and chemotherapy. *Gynecol Oncol* 2002;84:501 (abst 74).
109. Gordon AN, Schultes BC, Gallion H, et al. CA125- and tumor-specific T-cell responses correlate with prolonged survival in oregovomab-treated recurrent ovarian cancer patients. *Gynecol Oncol* 2004;94(2):340–351.
110. Foon KA, Bhattacharya-Chatterjee M. Are solid tumor anti-idiotype vaccines ready for prime time? Commentary re: Wagner U, et al. Immunological consolidation of ovarian carcinoma recurrences with monoclonal anti-idiotype antibody ACA-125: immune responses and survival in palliative treatment. *Clin Cancer Res* 2001;7:1154–1162; 1112–1115.
111. Bookman MA, Rettenmaier M, Gordon A. Monoclonal antibody (Oregovomab) targeting of CA125 in patients (pts) with advanced epithelial ovarian cancer (EOC) and elevated CA125 after response to initial therapy. *Clin Cancer Res* 2001;7:3756s (abst 510).
112. Berek JS, Taylor PT, Gordon A, et al. Randomized, placebo-controlled study of oregovomab for consolidation of clinical remission in patients with advanced ovarian cancer. *J Clin Oncol* 2004;22(17):3507–3516.
113. Method MW, Gordon A, Finkler F, et al. Randomized evaluation of 3 treatment schedules to optimize clinical activity of OvaRex® MAb-B43.13 (OV) in patients (pts) with epithelial ovarian cancer (EOC). *Proc Am Soc Clin Oncol* 2002;(abst 80).
114. Haisma HJ, Moseley KR, Battaile A, et al. Distribution and pharmacokinetics of radiolabeled monoclonal antibody OC 125 after intravenous and intraperitoneal administration in gynecologic tumors. *Am J Obstet Gynecol* 1988;159:843–848.

115. Finkler NJ, Muto MG, Kassis AI, et al. Intraperitoneal radiolabeled OC 125 in patients with advanced ovarian cancer. *Gynecol Oncol* 1989;34:339–344.
116. Mahe MA, Fumoleau P, Fabbro M, et al. A phase II study of intraperitoneal radioimmunotherapy with iodine-131–labeled monoclonal antibody OC-125 in patients with residual ovarian carcinoma. *Clin Cancer Res* 1999;5:3249s–3253s.
117. Epenetos AA, Munro AJ, Stewart S, et al. Antibody-guided irradiation of advanced ovarian cancer with intraperitoneally administered radiolabeled monoclonal antibodies. *J Clin Oncol* 1987;5:1890–1899.
118. Hird V, Stewart JS, Snook D, et al. Intraperitoneally administered ^{90}Y-labelled monoclonal antibodies as a third line of treatment in ovarian cancer. A phase 1–2 trial: problems encountered and possible solutions. *Br J Cancer* 1990;10(Suppl):48–51.
119. Hird V, Maraveyas A, Snook D, et al. Adjuvant therapy of ovarian cancer with radioactive monoclonal antibody. *Br J Cancer* 1993;68:403–406.
120. Verheijen RH, Massuger LF, Benigno BB, et al. Phase III trial of intraperitoneal therapy with yttrium-90-labeled HMFG1 murine monoclonal antibody in patients with epithelieal ovarian cancer after a surgically defined complete remission. *J Clin Oncol* 2006;24:571–579.
121. Meredith RF, Partridge EE, Alvarez RD, et al. Intraperitoneal radioimmunotherapy of ovarian cancer with lutetium-177-CC49. *J Nucl Med* 1996;37:1491–1496.
122. Alvarez RD, Huh WK, Khazaeli MB, et al. A phase I study of combined modality (90)yttrium-CC49 intraperitoneal radioimmunotherapy for ovarian cancer. *Clin Cancer Res* 2002;8:2806–2811.
123. Crippa F, Bolis G, Seregni E, et al. Single-dose intraperitoneal radioimmunotherapy with the murine monoclonal antibody I-131 MOv18: clinical results in patients with minimal residual disease of ovarian cancer. *Eur J Cancer* 1995;31A:686–690.
124. Molthoff CF, Prinssen HM, Kenemans P, et al. Escalating protein doses of chimeric monoclonal antibody MOv18 immunoglobulin G in ovarian carcinoma patients: a phase I study. *Cancer* 1997;80:2712–2720.
125. van Zanten-Przybysz I, Molthoff C, Gebbinck JK, et al. Cellular and humoral responses after multiple injections of unconjugated chimeric monoclonal antibody MOv18 in ovarian cancer patients: a pilot study. *J Cancer Res Clin Oncol* 2002;128:484–492.
126. van Zanten-Przybysz I, Molthoff CF, Roos JC, et al. Radioimmunotherapy with intravenously administered ^{131}I-labeled chimeric monoclonal antibody MOv18 in patients with ovarian cancer. *J Nucl Med* 2000;41: 1168–1176.
127. Pai-Scherf LH, Carrasquillo JA, Paik C, et al. Imaging and phase I study of ^{111}In- and ^{90}Y-labeled anti-LewisY monoclonal antibody B3. *Clin Cancer Res* 2000;6:1720–1730.
128. Pai LH, Wittes R, Setser A, et al. Treatment of advanced solid tumors with immunotoxin LMB-1: an antibody linked to *Pseudomonas* exotoxin. *Nat Med* 1996;2:350–353.
129. Juweid M, Swayne LC, Sharkey RM, et al. Prospects of radioimmunotherapy in epithelial ovarian cancer: results with iodine-131-labeled murine and humanized MN-14 anti-carcinoembryonic antigen monoclonal antibodies. *Gynecol Oncol* 1997;67:259–271.
130. Rubin SC, Kostakoglu L, Divgi C, et al. Biodistribution and intraoperative evaluation of radiolabeled monoclonal antibody MX35 in patients with epithelial ovarian cancer. *Gynecol Oncol* 1993;51:61–66.
131. Bast RC Jr, Klug TL, St John E, et al. A radioimmunoassay using a monoclonal antibody to monitor the course of epithelial ovarian cancer. *N Engl J Med* 1983;309:883–887.
132. Gaetje R, Winnekendonk DW, Scharl A, et al. Ovarian cancer antigen CA 125 enhances the invasiveness of the endometriotic cell line EEC 145. *J Soc Gynecol Invest* 1999;6:278–281.
133. Marth C, Zeimet AG, Widschwendter M, et al. Regulation of CA 125 expression in cultured human carcinoma cells. *Int J Biol Markers* 1998;13:207–209.
134. Balkwill FR. Tumour necrosis factor and cancer. *Prog Growth Factor Res* 1992;4:121–137.
135. Schultes BC, Baum RP, Niesen A, et al. Anti-idiotype induction therapy: anti-CA125 antibodies (Ab3) mediated tumor killing in patients treated with Ovarex mAb B43.13 (Ab1). *Cancer Immunol Immunother* 1998;46:201–212.
136. Madiyalakan R, Yang R, Schultes BC, et al. OVAREX MAb-B43.13:IFN-gamma could improve the ovarian tumor cell sensitivity to CA125-specific allogenic cytotoxic T cells. *Hybridoma* 1997;16:41–45.
137. Berek JS, Dorigo O, Schultes B, et al. Specific keynote: immunological therapy for ovarian cancer. *Gynecol Oncol* 2003;88:S105–S109; discussion, S110–S113.
138. Bolle M, Niesen A, Korz W, et al. Possible role of anti-CA125 monoclonal antibody B43.13 (OvaRex) administration in long-term survival of relapsed ovarian cancer patients. *Proc Am Soc Clin Oncol* 2000;19:476a.
139. Dudley ME, Wunderlich JR, Robbins PF, et al. Cancer regression and autoimmunity in patients after clonal repopulation with antitumor lymphocytes. *Science* 2002;298:850–854.
140. Dezso B, Torok I, Rosik LO, et al. Human ovarian cancers specifically bind daunorubicin–OC-125 conjugate: an immunofluorescence study. *Gynecol Oncol* 1990;39:60–64.
141. Thedrez P, Saccavini JC, Nolibe D, et al. Biodistribution of indium-111–labeled OC 125 monoclonal antibody after intraperitoneal injection in nude mice intraperitoneally grafted with ovarian carcinoma. *Cancer Res* 1989;49:3081–3086.
142. Schmolling J, Wagner U, Reinsberg J, et al. Immune reactions and survival of patients with ovarian carcinomas after administration of 131I-F(Ab)2 fragments of the OC 125 monoclonal antibody. *Geburtshilfe Frauenheilkd* 1995;55:200–203.
143. Kalofonos HP, Karamouzis MV, Epenetos AA. Radioimmunoscintigraphy in patients with ovarian cancer. *Acta Oncol* 2001;40:549–557.
144. Nicholson S, Gooden CS, Hird V, et al. Radioimmunotherapy after chemotherapy compared to chemotherapy alone in the treatment of advanced ovarian cancer: a matched analysis. *Oncol Rep* 1998;5:223–226.
145. Maraveyas A, Snook D, Hird V, et al. Pharmacokinetics and toxicity of an yttrium-90-CITC-DTPA-HMFG1 radioimmunoconjugate for intraperitoneal radioimmunotherapy of ovarian cancer. *Cancer* 1994;73:1067–1075.
146. Verheijen RH, Massuger LF, Benigno BB, et al. Phase III trial of intraperitoneal therapy with yttrium-90-labeled HMFG1 murine monoclonal antibody in patients with epithelial ovarian cancer after a surgically defined complete remission. *J Clin Oncol* 2006;24:571–578.
147. Colcher D, Hand PH, Nuti M, et al. Differential binding to human mammary and nonmammary tumors of monoclonal antibodies reactive with carcinoembryonic antigen. *Cancer Invest* 1983;1(2):127–138.
148. Zhang S, Walberg LA, Ogata S, et al. Immune sera and monoclonal antibodies define two configurations for the sialyl Tn tumor antigen. *Cancer Res* 1995;55:3364–3368.
149. Colcher D, Minelli MF, Roselli M, et al. Radioimmunolocalization of human carcinoma xenografts with B72.3 second generation monoclonal antibodies. *Cancer Res* 1988;48:4597–4603.
150. Muraro R, Kuroki M, Wunderlich D, et al. Generation and characterization of B72.3 second generation monoclonal antibodies reactive with the tumor-associated glycoprotein 72 antigen. *Cancer Res* 1988;48:4588–4596.
151. Sheer DG, Schlom J, Cooper HL. Purification and composition of the human tumor-associated glycoprotein (TAG-72) defined by monoclonal antibodies CC49 and B72.3. *Cancer Res* 1988;48:6811–6818.
152. Molinolo A, Simpson JF, Thor A, et al. Enhanced tumor binding using immunohistochemical analyses by second generation anti-tumor-associated glycoprotein 72 monoclonal antibodies versus monoclonal antibody B72.3 in human tissue. *Cancer Res* 1990;50:1291–1298.
153. Macey DJ, Grant EJ, Kasi L, et al. Effect of recombinant alpha-interferon on pharmacokinetics, biodistribution, toxicity, and efficacy of ^{131}I-labeled monoclonal antibody CC49 in breast cancer: a phase II trial. *Clin Cancer Res* 1997;3:1547–1555.
154. Murray JL, Macey DJ, Grant EJ, et al. Enhanced TAG-72 expression and tumor uptake of radiolabeled monoclonal antibody CC49 in metastatic breast cancer patients following alpha-interferon treatment. *Cancer Res* 1995;55:5925s–5928s.
155. Rucker R, Bresler HS, Heffelfinger M, et al. Low-dose monoclonal antibody CC49 administered sequentially with granulocyte-macrophage colony-stimulating factor in patients with metastatic colorectal cancer. *J Immunol* 1999;22:80–84.
156. Triozzi PL, Kim JA, Martin EW Jr, et al. Clinical and immunologic effects of monoclonal antibody CC49 and interleukin-2 in patients with metastatic colorectal cancer. *Hybridoma* 1997;16:147–151.
157. Divgi CR, Scott AM, Gulec S, et al. Pilot radioimmunotherapy trial with 131I-labeled murine monoclonal antibody CC49 and deoxyspergualin in metastatic colon carcinoma. *Clin Cancer Res* 1995;1:1503–1510.
158. Divgi CR, Scott AM, Dantis L, et al. Phase I radioimmunotherapy trial with iodine-131-CC49 in metastatic colon carcinoma. *J Nucl Med* 1995;36:586–592.
159. Murray JL, Macey DJ, Kasi LP, et al. Phase II radioimmunotherapy trial with 131I-CC49 in colorectal cancer. *Cancer* 1994;73:1057–1066.
160. Meredith RF, Khazaeli MB, Macey DJ, et al. Phase II study of interferon-enhanced ^{131}I-labeled high affinity CC49 monoclonal antibody therapy in patients with metastatic prostate cancer. *Clin Cancer Res* 1999;5:3254s–3258s.
161. Meredith RF, Bueschen AJ, Khazaeli MB, et al. Treatment of metastatic prostate carcinoma with radiolabeled antibody CC49. *J Nucl Med* 1994;35:1017–1022.
162. Slovin SF, Scher HI, Divgi CR, et al. Interferon-gamma and monoclonal antibody ^{131}I-labeled CC49: outcomes in patients with androgen-independent prostate cancer. *Clin Cancer Res* 1998;4:643–651.
163. Schlom J, Siler K, Milenic DE, et al. Monoclonal antibody-based therapy of a human tumor xenograft with a 177-lutetium-labeled immunoconjugate. *Cancer Res* 1991;51:2889–2896.
164. Meredith RF, Alvarez RD, Partridge EE, et al. Intraperitoneal radioimmunochemotherapy of ovarian cancer: a phase I study. *Cancer Biother Radiopharmaceut* 2001;16:305–315.
165. Johnson DA, Briggs SL, Gutowski MC, et al. Anti-tumor activity of CC49-doxorubicin immunoconjugates. *Anticancer Res* 1995;15:1387–1393.
166. Miotti S, Canevari S, Menard S, et al. Characterization of human ovarian carcinoma-associated antigens defined by novel monoclonal antibodies with tumor-restricted specificity. *Int J Cancer* 1987;39:297–303.
167. Coney LR, Tomassetti A, Carayannopoulos L, et al. Cloning of a tumor-associated antigen: MOv18 and MOv19 antibodies recognize a folate-binding protein. *Cancer Res* 1991;51:6125–6132.
168. Buist MR, Molthoff CF, Kenemans P, et al. Distribution of OV-TL 3 and MOv18 in normal and malignant ovarian tissue. *J Clin Pathol* 1995;48: 631–636.

169. Luiten RM, Warnaar SO, Sanborn D, et al. Chimeric bispecific OC/TR monoclonal antibody mediates lysis of tumor cells expressing the folate-binding protein (MOv18) and displays decreased immunogenicity in patients. *J Immunol* 1997;20:496–504.
170. Melani C, Figini M, Nicosia D, et al. Targeting of interleukin 2 to human ovarian carcinoma by fusion with a single-chain Fv of antifolate receptor antibody. *Cancer Res* 1998;58:4146–4154.
171. Greiner JW, Guadagni F, Goldstein D, et al. Intraperitoneal administration of interferon-gamma to carcinoma patients enhances expression of tumor-associated glycoprotein-72 and carcinoembryonic antigen on malignant ascites cells. *J Clin Oncol* 1992;10:735–746.
172. Sakamoto J, Furukawa K, Cordon-Cardo C, et al. Expression of Lewis-a, Lewis-b, X, and Y blood group antigens in human colonic tumors and normal tissue and in human tumor-derived cell lines. *Cancer Res* 1986;46:1553–1561.
173. Hakomori S. General concept of tumor-associated carbohydrate antigens: their chemical, physical and enzymatic basis. In: Oettgen HF, ed. *Gangliosides and Cancer*. Weiheim, Germany: VHC Publishers; 1989: 93–102.
174. Miyake M, Taki T, Hitomi S, et al. Correlation of expression of H/Le(y)/Le(b) antigens with survival in patients with carcinoma of the lung [Comment]. *N Engl J Med* 1992;327:14–18.
175. Yin BW, Finstad CL, Kitamura K, et al. Serological and immunochemical analysis of Lewis y (Ley) blood group antigen expression in epithelial ovarian cancer. *Int J Cancer* 1996;65:406–412.
176. Scott AM, Geleick D, Rubira M, et al. Construction, production, and characterization of humanized anti-Lewis Y monoclonal antibody 3S193 for targeted immunotherapy of solid tumors. *Cancer Res* 2000;60:3254–3261.
177. Masucci G, Lindemalm C, Frodin JE, et al. Effect of human blood mononuclear cell populations in antibody dependent cellular cytotoxicity (ADCC) using two murine (CO17–1A and Br55–2) and one chimeric (17–1A) monoclonal antibodies against a human colorectal carcinoma cell line (SW948). *Hybridoma* 1988;7:429–440.
178. Seiden MV, Burris HA, Matulonis U, et al. A phase II trial of EMD72000 (matuzumab), a humanized anti-EGFR monoclonal antibody, in patients with platinum-resistant ovarian and primary peritoneal malignancies. *Gynecol Oncol* 2007;104(3):727–731.
179. Pastan I, Lovelace E, Gallo M, et al. Characterization of monoclonal antibodies B1 and B3 that react with mucinous adenocarcinomas. *Cancer Res* 1991;51:3781–3787.
180. Kitamura K, Stockert E, Garin-Chesa P, et al. Specificity analysis of blood group Lewis-y (Le(y)) antibodies generated against synthetic and natural Le(y) determinants. *Proc Natl Acad Sci USA* 1994;91:12957–12961.
181. Pai LH, Batra JK, FitzGerald DJ, et al. Anti-tumor activities of immunotoxins made of monoclonal antibody B3 and various forms of Pseudomonas exotoxin. *Proc Natl Acad Sci USA* 1991;88:3358–3362. [Erratum appears in *Proc Natl Acad Sci USA* 1991;88:5066.]
182. Trail PA, Willner D, Lasch SJ, et al. Cure of xenografted human carcinomas by BR96-doxorubicin immunoconjugates. *Science* 1993;261:212–215. [Erratum appears in *Science* 1994;263:1076.]
183. Tolcher AW, Sugarman S, Gelmon KA, et al. Randomized phase II study of BR96-doxorubicin conjugate in patients with metastatic breast cancer [Comment]. *J Clin Oncol* 1999;17:478–484.
184. Tolcher AW: BR96-doxorubicin: been there, done that! [Comment]. *J Clin Oncol* 2000;18:4000.
185. Saleh MN, Sugarman S, Murray J, et al. Phase I trial of the anti–Lewis Y drug immunoconjugate BR96-doxorubicin in patients with Lewis Y–expressing epithelial tumors [Comment]. *J Clin Oncol* 2000;18:2282–2292.
186. Clarke K, Lee FT, Brechbiel MW, et al. Therapeutic efficacy of anti-Lewis(y) humanized 3S193 radioimmunotherapy in a breast cancer model: enhanced activity when combined with Taxol chemotherapy. *Clin Cancer Res* 2000;6:3621–3628.
187. Juweid M, Sharkey RM, Alavi A, et al. Regression of advanced refractory ovarian cancer treated with iodine-131-labeled anti-CEA monoclonal antibody. *J Nucl Med* 1997;38:257–260.
188. Wu LY, Wu AR, Zhan J. Radioimmunoimaging assay of ovarian tumor with 99mTc labeled anti-carcinoembryonic antigen monoclonal antibody. *Chin J Obstet Gynecol* 1994;29:340–342, 381–382.
189. Mattes MJ, Lloyd KO, Lewis JL Jr. Binding parameters of monoclonal antibodies reacting with ovarian carcinoma ascites cells. *Cancer Immunol Immunother* 1989;28:199–207.
190. Mattes MJ, Look K, Furukawa K, et al. Mouse monoclonal antibodies to human epithelial differentiation antigens expressed on the surface of ovarian carcinoma ascites cells. *Cancer Res* 1987;47:6741–6750.
191. Welshinger M, Yin BW, Lloyd KO. Initial immunochemical characterization of MX35 ovarian cancer antigen. *Gynecol Oncol* 1997;67:188–192.
192. Finstad CL, Lloyd KO, Federici MG, et al. Distribution of radiolabeled monoclonal antibody MX35 F(ab′)2 in tissue samples by storage phosphor screen image analysis: evaluation of antibody localization to micrometastatic disease in epithelial ovarian cancer. *Clin Cancer Res* 1997;3:1433–1442.
193. Schilder RJ, Sill MW, Chen X, et al. Phase II study of gefitinib in patients with relapsed or persistent ovarian or primary peritoneal carcinoma and evaluation of epidermal growth factor receptor mutations and immunohistochemical expression: a Gynecologic Oncology Group study. *Clin Cancer Res* 2005;11(15):5539–5548.
194. Slamon DJ, Godephin W, Jones LA, et al. Studies of the HER-2/neu proto-oncogene in human breast and ovarian cancer. *Science* 1989;244:707–712.
195. Hogdall EV, Christensen L, Kjaer SK, et al. Distribution of HER-2 overexpression in ovarian carcinoma tissue and its prognostic value in patients with ovarian carcinoma: from the Danish MALOVA Ovarian Cancer Study. *Cancer* 2003;98:66–73.
196. Bookman M, Darcy K, Clarke-Pearson D, et al. Evaluation of monoclonal humanized anti–HER-2 antibody, trastuzumab, in patients with recurrent or refractory ovarian or primary peritoneal carcinoma with over expression of HER-2: a phase II trial of the Gynecologic Oncology Group. *J Clin Oncol* 2003;21:283–290.
197. Santin AD, Bellone S, Gokden M, et al. Overexpression of HER-2/neu in uterine serous papillary cancer. *Clin Cancer Res* 2002;8:1271–1279.
198. Hurwitz H, Fehrenbacher L, Novotny W, et al. Bevacizumab plus irinotecan, fluorouracil, and leucovorin for metastatic colorectal cancer. *N Engl J Med* 2004;350(23):2335–2342.
199. Sandler A, Gray R, Perry MC, et al. Paclitaxel-carboplatin alone or with bevacizumab for non-small-cell lung cancer. *N Engl J Med* 2006;355(24): 2542–2550.
200. Miller KD, Chap LI, Holmes FA, et al. Randomized phase III trial of capecitabine compared with bevacizumab plus capecitabine in patients with previously treated metastatic breast cancer. *J Clin Oncol* 2005;23(4): 792–799.
201. Yang JC, Haworth L, Sherry RM, et al. A randomized trial of bevacizumab, an anti-vascular endothelial growth factor antibody, for metastatic renal cancer. *N Engl J Med* 2003;349(5):427–434.
202. Burger R, Sill MW, Monk BJ, et al. Phase II trial of bevacizumab in persistent or recurrent epithelial ovarian cancer (EOC) or primary peritoneal cancer (PPC): a Gynecologic Oncology Group (GOG) study. 2005 PROC ASCO: Abs #5009.
203. Cannistra SA, Matulonis U, et al. Bevacizumab in patients with advanced platinum-resistant ovarian cancer. 2006 PROC ASCO 24: Abs #5006.
204. Garcia AA, Oza AM, et al. Interim report of a phase II clinical trial of bevacizumab (Bev) and low dose metronomic oral cyclophosphamide (mCtx) in recurrent and primary peritoneal carcinoma: A California Cancer Consortium trial. 2005 PROC ASCO: Abs #5000.
205. Gordon MS, Cunningham D. Managing patients treated with bevacizumab combination therapy. *Oncology* 2005;69(Suppl 3):25–33.
206. Han ES, Monk BJ. What is the risk of bowel perforation associated with bevacizumab therapy in ovarian cancer? *Gynecol Oncol* 2007;105(1):3–6.
207. Liao SY, Brewer C, Zavada J, et al. Identification of the MN antigen as a diagnostic biomarker of cervical intraepithelial squamous and glandular neoplasia and cervical carcinomas. *Am J Pathol* 1994;145:598–609.
208. Pastorek J, Pastorekova S, Callebaut I, et al. Cloning and characterization of MN, a human tumor-associated protein with a domain homologous to carbonic anhydrase and a putative helix-loop-helix DNA binding segment. *Oncogene* 1994;9:2877–2888.
209. Zavada J, Zavadova Z, Pastorekova S, et al. Expression of MaTu-MN protein in human tumor cultures and in clinical specimens. *Int J Cancer* 1993;54:268–274.
210. Ivanov S, Liao SY, Ivanova A, et al. Expression of hypoxia-inducible cell-surface transmembrane carbonic anhydrases in human cancer. *Am J Pathol* 2001;158:905–919.
211. Loncaster JA, Harris AL, Davidson SE, et al. Carbonic anhydrase (CA IX) expression, a potential new intrinsic marker of hypoxia: correlations with tumor oxygen measurements and prognosis in locally advanced carcinoma of the cervix. *Cancer Res* 2001;61:6394–6399.
212. Zhang L, Conejo-Garcia JR, Katsaros D, et al. Intratumoral T cells, recurrence, and survival in epithelial ovarian cancer. *N Engl J Med* 2003;348:203–213.
213. Kershaw MH, Westwood JA, Parker LL, et al. A phase I study on adoptive immunotherapy using gene-modified T cells for ovarian cancer. *Clin Cancer Res* 2006;12(20 Pt 1):6106–6115.
214. Kim S-K, Ragupathi G, Cappello S, et al. Effect of immunological adjuvant combinations on the antibody and T-cell response to vaccination with MUC-1-KLH and GD3-K conjugates. *Vaccine* 2000;19:530–537.
215. Kim S-K, Ragupathi G, Musselli C, et al. Comparison of the effect of different immunological adjuvants on the antibody and T cell response to immunization with MUC1-KLH and GD3-KLH conjugate vaccines. *Vaccine* 1999;18:597–603.
216. Livingston PO, Adluri S, Raychaudhuri S, et al. A phase I trial of the immunological adjuvant SAF-m in melanoma patients vaccinated with the anti-idiotype antibody MELIMMUNE-1. *Vaccine Res* 1994;3:71–81.
217. Livingston PO, Adluri S, Helling F, et al. Phase I trial of immunological adjuvant QS-21 with a GM2 ganglioside-KLH conjugate vaccine in patients with malignant melanoma. *Vaccine* 1994;12:1275–1280.
218. Livingston PO, Adluri S, Zhang S, et al. Impact of immunological adjuvants and administration route on HAMA response after immunization with murine monoclonal antibody MELIMMUNE-1 in melanoma patients. *Vaccine Res* 1995;4:87–94.
219. Chapman PB, Livingston PO, Morrison ME, et al. Immunization of melanoma patients with anti-idiotypic monoclonal antibody BEC2 (which mimics GD3 ganglioside): pilot trials using no immunological adjuvant. *Vaccine Res* 1994;3:59.
220. Ritter G, Boosfeld E, Calves MJ, et al. Antibody response after immunization with gangliosides GD3, GD3 lactones, GD3 amide and GD3 gangliosidol

in the mouse. GD3 lactone I induces antibodies reactive with human melanoma. *Immunobiology* 1990;182:32–43.
221. Ritter G, Boosfeld E, Adluri R, et al. Antibody response to immunization with ganglioside GD3 and GD3 congeners (lactones, amide and gangliosidol) in patients with malignant melanoma. *Int J Cancer* 1991;48: 379–385.
222. Ritter G, Ritter-Boosfeld E, Adluri R, et al. Analysis of the antibody response to immunization with purified O-acetyl GD3 gangliosides in patients with malignant melanoma. *Int J Cancer* 1995;62:1–5.
223. Slovin SF, Ragupathi G, Musselli C, et al. Thomsen-Friedenreich (TF) antigen as a target for prostate cancer vaccine: clinical trial results with TF cluster (c)-KLH plus QS21 conjugate vaccine in patients with biochemically relapsed prostate cancer. *Cancer Immunol Immunother* 2005;54(7) 694–702.
224. Helling F, Shang A, Calves M, et al. GD3 vaccines for melanoma: superior immunogenicity of keyhole limpet hemocyanin conjugate vaccines. *Cancer Res* 1994;54:197–203.
225. Kensil CR, Patel U, Lennick M, et al. Separation and characterization of saponins with adjuvant activity from *Quillaja saponaria molina* cortex. *J Immunol* 1982;12:91–96.
226. Marciani DJ, Press JB, Reynolds RC, et al. Development of semisynthetic triterpenoid saponin derivatives with immune stimulating activity. *Vaccine* 2000;18:3141–3151.
227. Ragupathi G, Park TK, Zhang S, et al. Immunization of mice with the synthetic hexasaccharide Globo H results in antibodies against human cancer cells. *Angewandte Chem Int Engl* 1997;125–128.
228. Zhang S, Walberg LA, Helling F, et al. Augmenting the immunogenicity of synthetic MUC-1 vaccines in mice. *Cancer Res* 1996;55:3364–3368.
229. Livingston PO. Approaches to augmenting the immunogenicity of melanoma gangliosides: from whole melanoma cells to ganglioside-KLH conjugate vaccines. *Immunol Rev* 1995;145:147–166.
230. Chapman PB, Morissey DM, Pangeas KS, et al. Induction of antibodies against GM2 ganglioside by immunizing melanoma patients using GM2-keyhole limpet hemocyanin + QS21 vaccine: a dose response study. *Clin Cancer Res* 2000;6:874–879.
231. Helling F, Zhang A, Shang A, et al. GM2-KLH conjugate vaccine: increased immunogenicity in melanoma patients after administration with immunological adjuvant QS-21. *Cancer Res* 1995;55:2783–2788.
232. Kirkwood JM, Strawderman MH, Ernstoff MS, et al. Interferon alfa-2b adjuvant therapy of high-risk resected cutaneous melanoma: the Eastern Co-operative Oncology Group trial EST 1684. *J Clin Oncol* 1996; 14:7–17.
233. Kirkwood JM, Ibrahim JG, Sosman JA, et al. High-dose interferon alfa-2b significantly prolongs relapse-free and overall survival compared with the GM2-KLH/QS-21 vaccine in patients with resected stage IIB-III melanoma: results of Intergroup Trial E1694/S9512/C509801. *J Clin Oncol* 2001;19:2370–2380.
234. Ragupathi G, Gathuru J, Livingston P. Antibody inducing polyvalent cancer vaccines. *Cancer Treat Res* 2005;123:157–180.
235. Biomira and M. KGaA 2003. Biomira and Merck KGaA announce phase III Theratope vaccine trial does not meet primary endpoints. http://biomira.com/new/detailNewsRelease/166/%3E. Accessed on June 9, 2007.
236. Biomira and Braun DP, Crist KA, et al. Aromatase inhibitors increase the sensitivity of human tumor cells to monocyte-mediated, antibody-dependent cellular cytotoxicity. *Am J Surg* 2005;190(4):570–571.
237. Exploratory analysis shows statistically significant survival advantage for women in hormonal therapy subset receiving Theratope vaccine in phase III study. June 7, 2004. http://www.biomira.com/news/detailNewsRelease/189. Accessed on July 29, 2007.
238. Helling F, Zhang S, Shang A, et al. GM2-KLH conjugate vaccine: increased immunogenicity in melanoma patients after administration with immunological adjuvant QS-21. *Cancer Res* 1995;55(13):2783–2788.
239. Gilewski T, Adluri S, Ragupathi G, et al. Vaccination of high-risk breast cancer patients with mucin-1 (MUC1) keyhole limpet hemocyanin conjugate plus QS 21. *Clin Cancer Res* 2000;6(5):1693–1701.
240. Gilewski T, Ragupathi G, Bhuta S, et al. Immunization of metastatic breast cancer patients with a fully synthetic globo H conjugate: a phase I trial. *Proc Natl Acad Sci USA* 2001;98(6):3270–3275.
241. Sabbatini PJ, Ragupathi G, Hood C, et al. Pilot study of a heptavalent vaccine-KLH conjugate plus QS-21 in patients with epithelial ovarian, fallopian tube, or peritoneal cancer. *Clin Cancer Res* 2007;13(14):4170–4177.
242. Ragupathi G, Koide F, Sathyan N, et al. A preclinical study comparing approaches for augmenting the immunogenicity of a heptavalent KLH-conjugate vaccine against epithelial cancers. *Cancer Immunol Immunother* 2003;52(10):608–616.
243. Rosenberg SA. The identification of cancer antigens impact on the development of cancer vaccines. *Cancer J* 2000;6(Suppl 2):S142–S149.
244. Moingeon P. Review: cancer vaccines. *Vaccine* 2001;19:1305–1326.
245. Santin AD, Bellone S, Gokden M, et al. Over expression of HER-2/neu in uterine serous papillary cancer. *Clin Cancer Res* 2002;8:1271–1279.
246. Khalifa MA, Mannel RS, Haraway SD, et al. Expression of EGFR, HER-2/neu, P53, and PCNA in endometrioid, serous papillary, and clear cell endometrial adenocarcinomas. *Gynecol Oncol* 1994;53:84–92.
247. Miotti S, Facheris P, Tomassetti A, et al. Growth of ovarian-carcinoma cell lines at physiological folate concentration: effect on folate-binding protein expression *in vitro* and *in vivo*. *Int J Cancer* 1995;63:395–401.
248. Martini M, Ciccarone M, Garganese G, et al. Possible involvement of hMLH1, p16(INK4a) and *PTEN* in the malignant transformation of endometriosis. *Int J Cancer* 2002;102:398–406.
249. Matsumoto H, Shichijo S, Kawano K, et al. Expression of the SART-1 antigens in uterine cancers. *Jpn J Cancer Res* 1998;89:1292–1295.
250. van der Bruggen P, Traversari C, Chomez P, et al. A gene encoding an antigen recognized by cytolytic T lymphocytes on a human melanoma. *Science* 1991;254:1643–1647.
251. Chen YT, Scanlan MJ, Sahin U, et al. A testicular antigen aberrantly expressed in human cancers detected by autologous antibody screening. *Proc Natl Acad Sci USA* 1997;94:1914–1918.
252. Zeng G, Li Y, El-Gamil M, et al. Generation of NY-ESO-1–specific CD4+ and CD8+ T cells by a single peptide with dual MHC class I and class II specificities: a new strategy for vaccine design. *Cancer Res* 2002; 62:3630–3635.
253. Sarcevic B, Spagnoli GC, Terracciano L, et al. Expression of cancer/testis tumor associated antigens in cervical squamous cell carcinoma. *Oncology* 2003;64:443–449.
254. Stone B, Schummer M, Paley PJ, et al. Serologic analysis of ovarian tumor antigens reveals a bias toward antigens encoded on 17q. *Int J Cancer* 2003;104:73–84.
255. Jager E, Gnjatic S, Nagata Y, et al. Induction of primary NY-ESO-1 immunity: CD8+ T lymphocyte and antibody responses in peptide-vaccinated patients with NY-ESO-1+ cancers. *Proc Natl Acad Sci USA* 2000; 97:12198–12203.
256. Nasi ML, Lieberman P, Busam KJ, et al. Intradermal injection of granulocyte-macrophage colony-stimulating factor (GM-CSF) in patients with metastatic melanoma recruits dendritic cells. *Cytokines Cell Mol Ther* 1999;5:139–144.
257. Perales MA, Fantuzzi G, Goldberg SM, et al. GM-CSF DNA induces specific patterns of cytokines and chemokines in the skin: implications for DNA vaccines. *Cytokines Cell Mol Ther* 2003;7:125–133.
258. Santin AD, Ioli GR, Hiserodt JC, et al. Development and in vitro characterization of a GM-CSF secreting human ovarian carcinoma tumor vaccine. *Int J Gynecol Cancer* 1995;5:401–410.
259. Salgia R, Lynch T, Skarin A, et al. Vaccination with irradiated autologous tumor cells engineered to secrete granulocyte-macrophage colony-stimulating factor augments antitumor immunity in some patients with metastatic non–small-cell lung carcinoma. *J Clin Oncol* 2003;21:624–630.
260. Bagnoli M, Canevari S, Figini M, et al. A step further in understanding the biology of the folate receptor in ovarian carcinoma. *Gynecol Oncol* 2003;88:S140–S144.
261. Neglia F, Orengo AM, Cilli M, et al. DNA vaccination against the ovarian carcinoma-associated antigen folate receptor alpha (FR alpha) induces cytotoxic T lymphocyte and antibody responses in mice. *Cancer Gene Ther* 1999;6:349–357.
262. Peoples GE, Anderson BW, Lee TV, et al. Vaccine implications of folate binding protein, a novel cytotoxic T lymphocyte-recognized antigen system in epithelial cancers. *Clin Cancer Res* 1999;5:4214–4223.
263. Santini SM, Belardelli F. Advances in the use of dendritic cells and new adjuvants for the development of therapeutic vaccines. *Stem Cells* 2003;21:495–505.
264. Zou W, Machelon V, Coulomb-L'Hermin A, et al. Stromal-derived factor-1 in human tumors recruits and alters the function of plasmacytoid precursor dendritic cells. *Nat Med* 2001;7(12):1339–1346.
265. Wei S, Kryczek I, Zou L, et al. Plasmacytoid dendritic cells induce CD8+regulatory T cells in human ovarian carcinoma. *Cancer Res* 2005;65(12):5020–5026.
266. Schlienger K, Chu CS, Woo EY, et al. TRANCE and CD40 ligand-matured dendritic cells reveal MHC class I-restricted T cells specific for autologous tumor in late-stage ovarian cancer patients. *Clin Cancer Res* 2003;9(4): 1517–1527.
267. Ye F, Chen HZ, Xie X, et al. Ovarian carcinoma cells effectively inhibit differentiation and maturation of dendritic cells derived from hematopoietic progenitor cell *in vitro*. *Cancer Invest* 2005;23(5):379–385.
268. Curiel TJ, Wei S, Don H, et al. Blockade of B7-H1 improves myeloid dendritic cell-mediated antitumor immunity. *Nat Med* 2003;9(5):562–567.
269. Mayordomo JI, Zorina T, Storkus WJ, et al. Bone marrow-derived dendritic cells serve as potent adjuvants for peptide-based antitumor vaccines. *Stem Cells* 1997;15:94–103.
270. Hernando JJ, Park TW, Kubler K, et al. Vaccination with autologous tumour antigen-pulsed dendritic cells in advanced gynecologic malignancies: clinical and immunological evaluation of a phase I trial. *Cancer Immunol Immunother* 2002;51:45–52.
271. Hsu FJ, Benike C, Fagnoni F, et al. Vaccination of patients with B-cell lymphoma using autologous antigen-pulsed dendritic cells. *Nat Med* 1996;2:52–58.
272. Brossart P, Wirths S, Stuhler G, et al. Induction of cytotoxic T-lymphocyte responses in vivo after vaccinations with peptide-pulsed dendritic cells. *Blood* 2000;96:3102–3108.
273. Kugler A, Stuhler G, Walden P, et al. Regression of human metastatic renal cell carcinoma after vaccination with tumor cell-dendritic cell hybrids. *Nat Med* 2000;6:332–336.
274. Engleman EG, Fong L. Induction of immunity to tumor-associated antigens following dendritic cell vaccination of cancer patients. *Clin Immunol* 2003;106:10–15.

275. Geiger JD, Hutchinson RJ, Hohenkirk LF, et al. Vaccination of pediatric solid tumor patients with tumor lysate-pulsed dendritic cells can expand specific T cells and mediate tumor regression. *Cancer Res* 2001;61:8513–8519.
276. Nestle FO, Alijagic S, Gilliet M, et al. Vaccination of melanoma patients with peptide- or tumor lysate-pulsed dendritic cells. *Nat Med* 1998;4:328–332.
277. Brossart P, Wirths S, Stuhler G, et al. Induction of cytotoxic T-lymphocyte responses in vivo after vaccinations with peptide-pulsed dendritic cells. *Blood* 2000;96(9):3102–3108.
278. Bookman MA, Darcy KM, Clarke-Pearson D, et al. Evaluation of monoclonal humanized anti-HER2 antibody, trastuzumab, in patients with recurrent or refractory ovarian or primary peritoneal carcinoma with overexpression of HER2: a phase II trial of the Gynecologic Oncology Group. *J Clin Oncol* 2003;21:283–290.
279. Santin AD, Hermonat PL, Ravaggi A, et al. *In vitro* induction of tumor-specific human lymphocyte antigen class I-restricted CD8 cytotoxic T lymphocytes by ovarian tumor antigen-pulsed autologous dendritic cells from patients with advanced ovarian cancer. *Am J Obstet Gynecol* 2000;183(3):601–609.
280. Homma S, Sagawa Y, Ito M, et al. Cancer immunotherapy using dendritic/tumor-fusion vaccine induces elevation of serum anti-nuclear antibody with better clinical responses. *Clin Exp Immunol* 2006;144(1):41–47.
281. Lodge PA, Jones LA, Bader RA, et al. Dendritic cell-based immunotherapy of prostate cancer: immune monitoring of a phase II clinical trial. *Cancer Res* 2000;60:829–833.
282. Chakraborty NG, Sporn JR, Tortora AF, et al. Immunization with a tumor-cell-lysate-loaded autologous-antigen-presenting-cell-based vaccine in melanoma. *Cancer Immunol Immunother* 1998;47:58–64.
283. Lindemann J. Speculations on idiotypes of homobodies. *Ann Immunol* 1973;124:171–184.
284. Jerne NK. Towards a network theory of the immune system. *Ann Immunol* 1974;125:373–389.
285. Birebent B, Somasundaram R, Purev E, et al. Anti-idiotypic antibody and recombinant antigen vaccines in colorectal cancer patients. *Crit Rev Oncol Hematol* 2001;9:107–113.
286. Herlyn D, Harris D, Zaloudik J, et al. Immunomodulatory activity of monoclonal anti-idiotypic antibody to anti-colorectal carcinoma antibody CO17-1A in animals and patients. *J Immunother Emphasis Tumor Immunol* 1994;15:303–311.
287. Saleh MN, Lalisan DY, Pride MW, et al. Immunologic response to the dual murine anti-Id vaccine Melimmune-1 and Melimmune-2 in patients with high risk melanoma without evidence of systemic disease. *J Immunother* 1998;21:379–388.
288. Wang X, Luo W, Foon KA, et al. Tumor associated antigen (TAA) mimicry and immunotherapy of malignant diseases from anti-idiotypic antibodies to peptide mimics. *Cancer Chemother Biol Response Modif* 2001;19:309–326.
289. Baral R, Sherrat A, Das R, et al. Murine monoclonal anti-idiotypic antibody as a surrogate antigen for human Her-2/neu. *Int J Cancer* 2001;92:88–95.
290. Safa MM, Foon KA. Adjuvant immunotherapy for melanoma and colorectal cancers. *Semin Oncol* 2001;28:68–92.
291. Foon KA, John WJ, Chakraborty M, et al. Clinical and immune responses in resected colon cancer patients treated with anti-idiotype monoclonal antibody vaccine that mimics the carcinoembryonic antigen. *J Clin Oncol* 1999;17:2889–2895.
292. Grant SC, Kris MG, Houghton AN, et al. Long survival of patients with small cell lung cancer after adjuvant treatment with the anti-idiotypic antibody BEC2 plus *Bacillus* Calmette-Guerin. *Clin Cancer Res* 1999;5:1319–1323.
293. Wagner U, Kohler S, Reinartz S, et al. Immunological consolidation of ovarian carcinoma recurrences with monoclonal anti-idiotype antibody ACA-125: immune responses and survival in palliative treatment. See the biology behind: Foon KA, Bhattacharya-Chatterjee M. Are solid tumor anti-idiotype vaccines ready for prime time? *Clin Cancer Res* 2001;7: 1112–1115; 1154–1162.
294. Sabbatini P, Dupont J, Aghajanian C, et al. Phase I study of abagovomab in patients with epithelial ovarian, fallopian tube, or primary peritoneal cancer. *Clin Cancer Res* 2006;12(18):5503–5510.
295. Pfisterer J, du Bois A, Sehouli J, et al. The anti-idiotypic antibody abagovomab in patients with recurrent ovarian cancer. A phase I trial of the AGO-OVAR. *Ann Oncol* 2006;17(10):1568–1577.
296. Reinartz S, Hombach A, Kohler S, et al. Interleukin-6 fused to an anti-idiotype antibody in a vaccine increases the specific humoral immune response against CA125(+) (MUC-16) ovarian cancer. *Cancer Res* 2003;63:3234–3240.

CHAPTER 7 ■ DEVELOPMENT AND IDENTIFICATION OF TUMOR MARKERS

ALEKSANDRA GENTRY-MAHARAJ, IAN JACOBS, AND USHA MENON

Tumor markers are biological substances that are produced by malignant tumors and enter the circulation in detectable amounts. In the management of cancer, the most useful biochemical markers are the macromolecular tumor antigens, including enzymes, hormones, receptors, growth factors, biological response modifiers, and glycoconjugates. Global nondirected screening strategies looking at DNA, RNA, and protein levels are constantly identifying novel tumor markers that could complement those previously identified by candidate gene or antibody-based techniques.

Tumor markers are used for screening, diagnosis, monitoring therapeutic response, and detecting recurrence. An ideal tumor marker would need to have 100% sensitivity, specificity, and positive predictive value (PPV). The calculation of each of these attributes is outlined in Table 7.1. *Sensitivity* refers to the percentage of patients with tumor correctly identified as a result of a positive test, whereas *specificity* refers to the percentage of the population without tumor correctly identified as a result of a negative test. PPV refers to the percentage of patients with positive test that have tumor (true positives). In addition, it would need to be tumor-specific and produced in sufficient amounts to allow detection of minimal disease so that it quantitatively reflects the tumor burden. There are few, if any, markers that satisfy these criteria. The most limiting factor is *lack of specificity* as the majority of markers are tumor associated rather than tumor specific, and such markers are elevated in multiple cancers, in benign and physiological conditions, and in the fetal circulation. This restricts their use, with few exceptions, to monitoring therapeutic response and follow-up. This chapter focuses on those markers that are clinically relevant to female genital tract malignancies.

OVARIAN AND FALLOPIAN TUBE CANCERS

Epithelial ovarian cancers represent the majority of ovarian malignancies. A great number of markers have been investigated for use in screening, prognosis, monitoring of response, and recurrence, with CA125 being the best-known marker.

CA125

CA125 was first described by Bast et al. in 1981 as an antigenic determinant on a high-molecular-weight glycoprotein recognized by the murine monoclonal antibody OC-125 (1). It carries two major antigenic domains, classified as A, the domain binding monoclonal antibody OC-125, and B, the domain binding monoclonal antibody M11 (2). During fetal development, CA125 is expressed by amniotic and coelomic epithelium. In the adult, the determinant is found in structures derived from the coelomic epithelium (the mesothelial cells of the pleura, pericardium, and peritoneum) and in tubal, endometrial, and endocervical epithelium. Surprisingly, CA125 is not expressed by the surface epithelium of normal fetal and adult ovaries with the exception of inclusion cysts, areas of metaplasia, and papillary excrescences (3).

Serum CA125 was originally quantified using a homologous assay based on the monoclonal antibody OC-125 alone. This assay has been replaced by a heterologous assay that uses OC-125 as the capture antibody and M11 as the detection antibody. There are a number of CA125 assays available, most of which correlate well with each other and are clinically reliable. For some samples, however, differences between methods exist, suggesting a need for parallel testing when introducing a new method (4,5).

A CA125 serum value of 35 U/mL, representing 1% of female healthy donors, is often accepted as the upper limit of normal in clinical practice (6). It should be noted that this is an arbitrary cutoff and may not be suitable for all applications of CA125. In postmenopausal women or in patients who have undergone hysterectomy, for example, CA125 levels tend to be lower than in the general population and lower cutoffs may be more suitable: levels of 20 U/mL and 26 U/mL have been suggested (7–9). Approximately 85% of patients with epithelial ovarian cancer have CA125 levels of >35 U/mL (6,10). Elevated levels of >35 U/mL are found in 50% of patients with stage I disease, but raised levels are found in over 90% of patients with advanced disease (11). CA125 levels are less frequently elevated in mucinous, clear cell, and borderline tumors compared to serous tumors (11–13). CA125 can be elevated in other malignancies (pancreas, breast, colon, and lung cancer) and in benign conditions and physiological states such as pregnancy, endometriosis, and menstruation (11). Many of these nonmalignant conditions are not found in postmenopausal women, thus improving the diagnostic accuracy of elevated CA125 in this population.

Screening

The role of CA125 in screening for ovarian cancer is still under investigation. Elevation of CA125 in apparently healthy postmenopausal women is a powerful predictor of increased risk of ovarian cancer (14,15). However, if used alone, it is not a suitable screening test as it lacks sufficient specificity (16). When combined with abnormal ovarian imaging, the risk of ovarian cancer is increased (15). A multimodal screening strategy combining CA125 with pelvic ultrasound achieves high specificity (99.9%) and PPV (26.8%) in postmenopausal

TABLE 7.1

PARAMETERS OF TUMOR MARKER ASSAYS

Tumor marker result	True tumor status	
	Positive	Negative
Positive	a (True positives)	b (False positives)
Negative	c (False negatives)	d (True negatives)

Sensitivity = True positives/All with tumor = a/a + c
Specificity = True negatives/All tumor free = d/d + b
Positive predictive value (PPV) = True positives/All with positive tumor-marker result = a/a + b

women (17). Preliminary data has shown that this may impact on survival. In a randomized controlled trial (RCT) of ovarian cancer screening (OCS) involving 22,000 postmenopausal women, median survival of those diagnosed with ovarian cancer in the screened group (72.9 months) was significantly better than that of women in the control group (41.8 months) (18).

CA125 was initially interpreted using a fixed cutoff. Sensitivity and specificity has been improved by the development of a statistical algorithm (Risk of Ovarian Cancer [ROC] algorithm) based on the age-specific risk of the disease and the behavior of CA125 with time in women with ovarian cancer versus normal controls (19). When the ROC algorithm was applied retrospectively to serial samples from an OCS trial of postmenopausal women, the area under the curve was significantly improved in comparison to a fixed CA125 cutoff (93% vs. 84%). For a target specificity of 98%, the ROC calculation achieved a sensitivity of 86% for preclinical detection of ovarian cancer, whereas CA125 cutoff achieved a lower sensitivity of 62% (20). The performance of the ROC algorithm has been evaluated prospectively in an RCT of 13,582 postmenopausal women aged over 50. Women with normal ROC results were returned to annual screening; those with intermediate values had repeat CA125 testing, while those with elevated values underwent transvaginal ultrasound (TVS). Women with abnormal or persistently equivocal findings on TVS were referred for a gynecologic opinion. High specificity (99.8%; 95% CI, 99.7 to 99.9) and PPV (19%; 95% CI, 4.1 to 45.6) for primary invasive epithelial ovarian cancer was achieved by using the ROC algorithm strategy in the prevalence screen involving 6,532 women (21).

There is controversy as to whether a raised CA125 in asymptomatic postmenopausal women is a predictor of nongynecologic cancer. An initial nested case control study of 1,542 women with elevated (≥30 U/mL) and normal (<30 U/mL) CA125 levels using data from an RCT of 22,000 postmenopausal women (18) reported that elevated serum CA125 was not a predictor of a nongynecologic malignancy on mean follow-up of 2,269 days (22). However, it was associated with significantly increased risk of death from all causes in the next 5 years (23). In contrast, data from the Norwegian OCS trial of 5,500 women showed that breast and lung cancer were overrepresented among women with elevated CA125 (24). The two reports, although discrepant in their findings, agree that elevated CA125 is a risk factor for death from malignant disease. It is probably best to rule out other malignancies such as breast, lung, and pancreas in asymptomatic postmenopausal women with rising CA125 levels with no evidence of gynecologic malignancy.

One of the limitations of CA125 is that 15% to 20% of ovarian cancers do not express the antigen. Rosen et al. explored 10 potential serum markers that could complement CA125 in 65 ovarian cancers with weak or absent CA125 tissue expression. All specimens lacking CA125 expressed human kallikrein 10 (HK10), human kallikrein 6 (HK6), osteopontin, and claudin 3. A small proportion of CA125-negative ovarian cancers expressed DF3 (95%), vascular endothelial growth factor (VEGF) (81%), MUC1 (62%), mesothelin (MES) (34%), HE4 (32%), and CA-19-9 (29%). MES and HE4 showed the greatest specificity when reactivity with normal tissues was considered. Differential expression was also found for HK10, osteopontin, DF3, and MUC1 (25). Several of these markers are currently being assessed in nested case control studies using serum samples from ovarian cancer screening trials.

There are currently two large RCTs of OCS in postmenopausal women that incorporate CA125 measurement. Both seek to address the key issue of whether OCS will impact disease mortality in the general population. The U.K. Collaborative Trial of Ovarian Cancer Screening (UKCTOCS) involves 202,638 postmenopausal women aged 50 to 74, randomized to annual screening until the end of 2011 with serum CA125 using the ROC algorithm (50,640), TVS (50,639), or no screening (101,359) (www.ukctocs.org.uk) (Menon U, Gentry-Maharaj A, Ryan A, et al. Recruitment to multicentre trials–lessons from UKCTOCS: descriptive study. *Bmj* 2008;337:a2079.) The ovarian cancer screening arm of the National Institutes of Health Prostate Lung Colorectal and Ovarian Cancer Screening trial (PLCO) has randomized 78,237 women aged 55 to 74 (26,27). A proportion of women are not eligible for the ovarian screening as they have undergone bilateral oophorectomy. A total of 28,816 women had a serum CA125 (interpreted using a cutoff) and a TVS as part of the ovarian cancer prevalence screen. Of these, 1,338 (4.7%) had abnormal TVS and 402 (1.4%) had abnormal CA125 and 29 neoplasms; 26 ovarian, 2 fallopian, and 1 primary peritoneal neoplasm were identified (9 were tumors of low malignant potential and 20 were invasive). The positive predictive value for invasive cancer was 3.7% for an abnormal CA125, 1.0% for an abnormal TVS, and 23.5% if both tests were abnormal (27). Both trials are ongoing and will report in 2012–2014.

Women at increased risk of ovarian cancer due to hereditary predisposition often seek screening. It needs to be highlighted that in this population, the current recommendation is that women consider risk-reducing bilateral salpingo-oophorectomy once they have completed their families. The sensitivity and effectiveness of screening is still not established. Studies so far have not been of sufficient size or rigor to be able to draw any definitive conclusions with regard to the effectiveness of ovarian cancer screening in the high-risk group (28). In addition, multifocal primary peritoneal cancer is probably a phenotypic variant of familial ovarian cancer, and both CA125 and ultrasound are not reliable in detecting early-stage disease (29). False positive rates for CA125 and ultrasound are also higher in this population as most women are premenopausal (30,31). Table 7.2 gives details of studies involving 1,000 or more women. A more detailed review of all studies in this area is available elsewhere (37). One of the most promising trials to report so far is the U.S.-based Cancer Genetics Network (CGN) (38). Unlike previous studies, which used annual CA125 with a fixed cutoff and TVS, this trial used the ROC algorithm to screen 2,343 high-risk women at 3 monthly intervals. Thirty-eight women underwent surgery following 6,284 screens. Five ovarian cancers were detected, two prevalent (one early, one late stage) and three incident (three early) cases resulting in a PPV of 13%. Three further occult cancers were detected at risk-reducing salpingo-oophorectomy and one woman developed an interval (late-stage) cancer (36). Currently, there are two ongoing ovarian cancer screening trials in the high-risk population: the U.K. Familial Ovarian Cancer Screening Study

TABLE 7.2

STUDIES OF OVARIAN CANCER SCREENING IN WOMEN AT HIGH RISK (ONLY THOSE WITH OVER 1,000 PARTICIPANTS ARE LISTED)

Study	No.	Inclusion criteria	Screening tests	No. of invasive detected (LMP Tumors)	Cancers in screen-negative women (months from last screen)
Karlan et al. 1999 (29)	1,261	OC diagnosis since enrollment in the Gilda Radner OC Detection Program (women with *BRCA1/2* gene mutation)	TVS, CD, and CA125	One EOC, three PP (two), one stage I	Four PP (5, 6, 15, 16 mo); one EOC (2 mo)
van Nagell et al. 2000 (32)	3,299	Women over 50 and women over 25 with documented family history of OC in at least one first- or second-degree relative	TVS, CD, and CA125	Three (one), two stage I	Two (12, 14 mo)
Tailor et al. 2003 (33)	2,500	Prospective study of symptom-free women with at least one close relative who had developed ovarian cancer	TVS and CD	Six (four), four stage I	Two PP (20–40 mo); seven EOC (9–46 mo)
Stirling et al. 2005 (34)	1,110	First-degree relative with either one OC and one BC (age <50); one OC and two BC (age >60); hMLH1, hMSH2 mutation carrier; two or more OC; individual with BC and OC; three or more individuals with BC or OC over three generations; known *BRCA1*, *BRCA2* mutation carrier	TVS and CA125	Nine (one), two stage I	Three (2, 4, 12 mo)
Jacobs et al. 2005[a] (35) (data as presented at the meeting)	2,005	Two first-degree relatives with OC; first-degree relatives with one OC and one BC (age <50); first-degree relatives with one OC and two BC (age >60); HNPCC (first-degree relatives with one OC and three colorectal cancers—1 <50); mutation positive families (*BRCA1*, *BRCA2*, *MLH1*, *MSH2*, *MSH6*, PMS1, PMS2)	CA125 (ROCA) and TVS	Nine, five early stage, four late stage	Not reported
Skates et al. 2007[a] (36)	2,343	First- or second-degree relative with either *BRCA1/2* mutation; two of OC or early onset BC (age = 50); Ashkenazi ethnicity and one of OC or BC	CA125 (ROCA) and TVS	Six early stage, three late stage	Not reported

Note: BC, breast cancer; CD, Color Doppler; EOC, epithelial ovarian cancer; HNPCC, hereditary nonpolyposis colorectal cancer; OC, ovarian cancer; PP, primary peritoneal cancer; ROCA, Risk of Ovarian Cancer algorithm; TVS, transvaginal ultrasound; MO, months.
[a]Abstract only.

(UK FOCSS) with 3,300 of the target of 5,000 women recruited, and gynecologic Oncology Group 199 trial (39) which aims to recruit 2,332 women. Both trials are using the ROC algorithm with a screening interval of 3 to 4 months. It is likely that they will report in 2012 at the same time as the general population trials.

Differential Diagnosis of an Adnexal Mass

Serum CA125 is of value in differential diagnosis of benign and malignant adnexal masses, especially in postmenopausal women. Using an upper limit of 35 U/mL, sensitivity of 78%, specificity of 95%, and PPV of 82% was achieved for malignant disease in women with palpable adnexal masses (40). This has since been confirmed by numerous studies (41–43). Further improvements in specificity were achieved by using a panel of markers (CA125 II, CA-72-4, CA-15-3, and lipid-associated sialic acid) and an artificial neural network approach to differentiate malignant from benign pelvic masses (44).

The most valuable clinical tool has been combining serum CA125 values with ultrasound findings and menopausal status to calculate a Risk of Malignancy Index (RMI). It yielded a sensitivity of 85% and a specificity of 97%. Patients with an elevated RMI score had, on average, a 42-fold increase in the background risk of ovarian cancer (45). The RMI has since been validated both retrospectively and prospectively in gynecologic oncology and general gynecologic units (46–55) with prospective studies reporting lower sensitivity, specificity, and PPV (46,53). Higher sensitivity can be achieved by increasing the RMI cutoff (49,52,54), using artificial neural networks or altering the RMI calculation (46,50,51).

Recently the performance of RMI values of 25 to 1,000 in combination with specialist ultrasound (US), magnetic resonance imaging (MRI), and radioimmunoscintigraphy (RS) in a prospective cohort study of 180 women with an adnexal mass referred to a teaching hospital has been assessed. In women with an RMI cutoff of ≥25 and <1,000, addition of US and MRI provided a sensitivity of 94% and a specificity of 90%. The authors concluded that utilizing this approach in contrast to an RMI cutoff value of 250 can improve the correct referral of cancer patients to a cancer center, without change in the proportion of patients with benign disease being managed locally (55,57). It has also been suggested that the use of an RMI over 200 and the absence of an ovarian crescent sign (an ultrasound feature that depends on the fact that healthy ovarian tissue can be seen adjacent to the cyst within an ipsilateral ovary) used sequentially may improve the accuracy of ovarian cancer diagnosis (56). Despite limited value in borderline, stage I invasive, and nonepithelial ovarian cancers, the RMI is a simple, easily applicable method in the primary evaluation of patients with adnexal masses that identifies ovarian cancers more accurately than any other criterion used in diagnosis of this disease (47).

Prognosis

In ovarian malignancy, preoperative serum CA125 levels are related to tumor stage, tumor volume, and histological grade. Although initial studies did not find preoperative CA125 to be an independent prognostic factor (58–60), more recent work has confirmed it to be of value in localized/early-stage disease (61). A recent study of 118 patients with FIGO stage I epithelial ovarian cancer demonstrated that patients with stage I epithelial ovarian cancer and preoperative serum CA125 levels <65 U/mL had a significantly longer survival compared to stage I patients with preoperative serum CA125 ≥65 U/mL (62). This was confirmed in a study of 600 patients from gynecologic cancer centers in Australia, the United States, and Europe with stage I epithelial ovarian cancer. On multivariate analysis, preoperative serum CA125 >30 U/mL and age >70 years at diagnosis were the only independent predictors for overall survival. Levels of CA125 of ≤30 U/mL dominated over histological cell type, substage, and grade and were able to identify a subgroup of FIGO stage I patients with a genuinely good prognosis and extremely good survival who could possibly be spared of adjuvant chemotherapy (63). Additional parameters such as cyclooxygenase-2 overexpression in combination with preoperative CA125 level of under 30 U/mL have recently been found to be independent predictors of survival in univariate and multivariate analyses (64). In advanced ovarian cancer, CA125 does not seem to be an independent prognostic factor (61).

Postoperative CA125 levels have been found to be significant prognostic factors (58) with patients with a low CA125 prognostic score composed of two CA125 values, one taken preoperatively and the other taken 1 month after surgery, having significantly better prognosis than patients with high scores (65). It should be noted that CA125 levels can be elevated in the immediate postoperative period as a result of the abdominal surgery, and therefore measurements are best postponed for at least 4 weeks (66).

During primary chemotherapy, serum CA125 half-life is an independent prognostic factor in patients with advanced epithelial ovarian cancer, for both complete remission and survival (67–69). The most commonly used cutoff is a CA125 half-life of 20 days (69–71). In patients with CA125-positive tumors, other useful prognostic indicators of survival are the serum CA125 levels prior to a third course of chemotherapy (67,72,73) and the slope of the CA125 exponential regression curve. A recent retrospective analysis of patients treated in maintenance chemotherapy trials suggests that, in women achieving a clinically defined complete response to primary chemotherapy with a baseline CA125 level of ≤35 U/mL, the baseline CA125 level before initiation of maintenance chemotherapy strongly predicts the risk of subsequent relapse. Patients with premaintenance baseline CA125 values ≤10 U/mL have a superior progression-free survival compared to those with higher levels in the normal CA125 range (74).

Serum CA125 continues to be of prognostic significance when ovarian cancer recurs, with patients with normal serum CA125 levels (≤35 U/mL) at relapse having a better prognosis than patients with elevated levels (75).

Monitoring Response to Treatment

Serum CA125 levels reflect progression or regression of disease in over 90% of ovarian cancer patients with elevated preoperative levels (6,76) (Fig. 7.1). These findings have resulted in the widespread use of serum CA125 levels to monitor the clinical course of ovarian cancer and its response to chemotherapy (77). It is to be noted that CA125 should not be used as the sole criterion to determine clinical response (78) as studies involving second-look laparotomy have confirmed that CA125 values of <35 U/mL do not exclude active disease (79). The pattern of CA125 over time is a more useful parameter than using an arbitrary cutoff level (71,72,80,81). Precise mathematical definitions to evaluate response to treatment have been suggested, with 50% response corresponding to a 50% decrease in CA125 after two samples, confirmed by a third sample collected at least 28 days later, and a 75% response defined as a serial decrease over three samples of greater than 75% (82,83). A recent French multicenter study on the kinetics of CA125 under induction chemotherapy has again confirmed that prechemotherapy CA125, its half-life, nadir concentration, and time to nadir, all had a univariate prognostic value for disease-free and overall survival (84).

Detecting Recurrence

Among patients with elevated CA125 levels at diagnosis, serial monitoring following initial chemotherapy can lead to the early detection of recurrent disease. Median lead time prior to clinical progression of 63 to 99 days has been demonstrated between marker detection of disease progression and clinically apparent progressive disease (85,86). The value of marker lead time depends ultimately on a patient's remaining therapeutic options, and the clinical value of this approach is unclear (87).

In a study of 39 patients with elevated serum CA125 at time of diagnosis and complete clinical and radiographic response to initial treatment with normalization of serum CA125, Santillan et al. reported that a relative increase in CA125 of 100% (odds ratio [OR] = 23.7; 95% CI, 2.9 to 192.5) was significantly predictive of recurrence. From baseline CA125 nadir

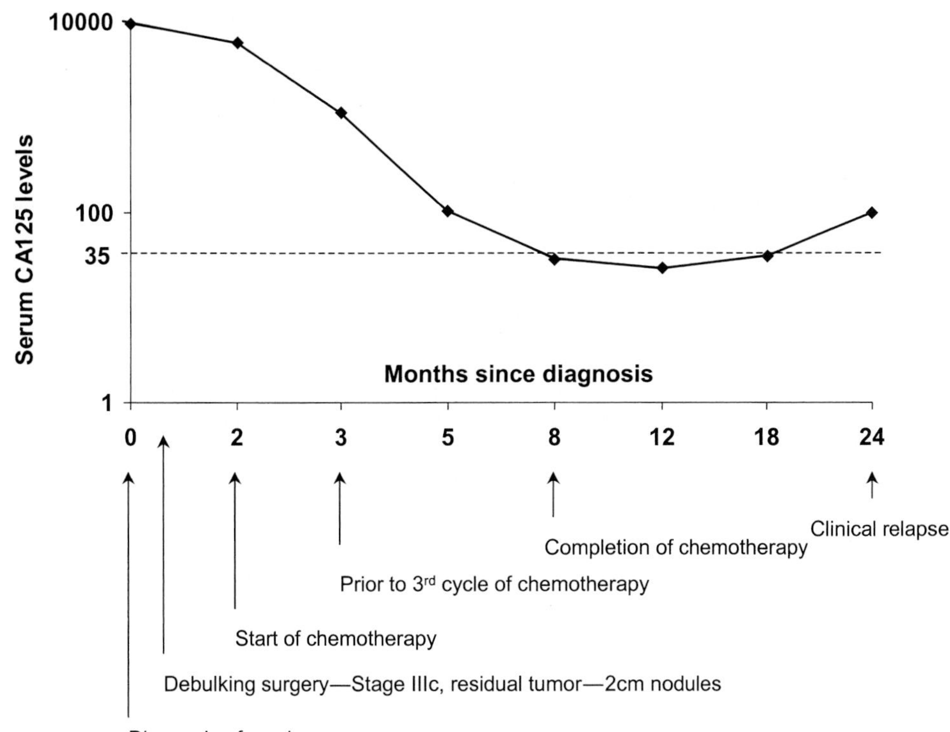

FIGURE 7.1. Correlation between serum CA125 and clinical course in ovarian cancer.

levels, an absolute increase in CA125 of 5 U/mL (OR = 8.4; 95% CI, 2.2 to 32.6) and 10 U/mL (OR = 71.2; 95% CI, 4.8 to >999.9) were also significantly associated with the likelihood of concurrent disease recurrence. These data suggest that for patients in complete clinical remission, a progressive low-level increase in serum CA125 levels is strongly predictive of disease recurrence (88).

CA125 measurements together with thin-section computed tomography (CT) and careful review of the clinical history are recommended in follow-up of patients with ovarian carcinomas (89). However, a study of 58 patients with recurrent ovarian cancer revealed that 98% of recurrences were identified by physical examination and CA125, with ultrasound and CT not providing additional clinically relevant information during follow-up (90).

Combination With Other Markers

Tumour-associated trypsin inhibitor (TATI), CA-19-9, CA-72-4, and carcinoembryonic antigen (CEA) in addition to CA125 may be useful in mucinous ovarian cancer (91). Increased preoperative sensitivity for early-stage disease has been reported by combining CA125 with CA-72-4, CA-15-3, and M-CSF (92). The majority of studies, however, report limited ability to improve diagnostic sensitivity by addition of other serum markers for patients with nonmucinous tumors (81,93–96). In clinical situations when CA125 is inconclusive or negative, Cancer-associated serum antigen (CASA) may be useful in the follow-up of patients with advanced disease (97). A more recent immunohistochemical study of CA125-negative ovarian cancers showed that all specimens expressed human kallikrein 10, human kallikrein 6, osteopontin, and claudin 3 with a smaller proportion expressing DF3 (95%), VEGF (81%), MUC1 (62%), MES (34%), HE4 (32%), and CA-19-9 (29%). From all the markers assayed, MES and HE4 exhibited greatest specificity (25). Further investigation of these markers in serum is underway.

Carcinoembryonic Antigen

Carcinoembryonic antigen (CEA) was first identified in 1965 in serum of rabbits immunized with colon carcinoma (98). It is an oncofetal antigen that is found in small amounts in the adult colon. Elevated levels are associated with colon and pancreatic cancer. CEA levels are also raised in benign diseases of the liver, gastrointestinal tract, and lung, and in smokers. In ovarian cancer, CEA is expressed by most endometrioid and Brenner tumors, and in areas of intestinal differentiation in mucinous tumors. In contrast to CA125, this marker is not expressed in normal and inflammatory conditions of the adnexa. Around 25% to 50% of ovarian cancer patients have elevated levels of CEA, and the correlation with ovarian cancer is not as well established as with the other markers (99,100).

Alpha-Fetoprotein

Alpha-fetoprotein (AFP) is an oncofetal protein produced by the fetal yolk sac, liver, and upper gastrointestinal tract. Elevated levels of AFP occur in pregnancy and benign liver disease. Serum levels are raised in most patients with liver tumors, and some patients with gastric, pancreatic, colon, and bronchogenic malignancies have elevated AFP levels (99). AFP levels were investigated in 135 patients with germ-cell tumors, and elevated levels were found in all patients with endodermal sinus tumors, 62% with immature teratomas and 12% with dysgerminoma (101). AFP also accurately predicts the presence of yolk sac elements in mixed germ-cell tumors (102). Although AFP production in epithelial ovarian cancers is extremely rare, a case of ectopic production of AFP by an ovarian endometrioid tumor has been described in the literature (103).

In women with endodermal sinus tumors, AFP is a reliable marker for monitoring therapeutic response and detecting recurrence (104,105). On univariate analysis, AFP levels of over 1,000 ng/mL, age over 22, and histology were found to be major prognostic factors in 43 patients with ovarian and extragonadal germ-cell tumors (106).

Human Chorionic Gonadotropin

Human chorionic gonadotropin (hCG) is synthesized in pregnancy by the syncytiotrophoblast. It is a glycoprotein hormone made up of two dissimilar covalently linked subunits α and β. Production of hCG by the tumor is accompanied by varying degrees of release of the free subunits into circulation. Recent advances in our understanding of hCG/hCG-β synthesis by trophoblastic and nontrophoblastic tissues alongside an improvement in techniques measuring hCG have helped define its role in clinical practice. hCG is elevated in virtually all cases of gestational trophoblastic disease (hydatidiform mole, invasive mole, and choriocarcinoma) and serves as an ideal tumor marker. There is a close correlation between hCG levels and tumor burden, and hCG levels are used in staging and clinical management. Serum hCG can also be detected in patients with nontrophoblastic cancers. Although gynecologic cancers are prominent in this group, the sensitivity of using hCG is lower than for other markers in current use except in germ-cell tumors with a chorionic component (107).

In a retrospective analysis of 113 patients with stage IC to IV malignant ovarian germ-cell tumors, both on univariate and multivariate analyses, stage of disease and elevation of serum hCG-β and AFP were significant predictors of overall survival, whereas age at diagnosis was of no prognostic value (108). It is worth noting that this is the first study to demonstrate stage and tumor markers as prognostic parameters in patients with malignant ovarian germ-cell tumors and may help in deciding on a therapeutic regimen.

Inhibin and Related Peptides

Inhibins and activins are structurally related dimeric proteins, first isolated from ovarian follicular fluid on the basis of their ability to modulate pituitary follicle-stimulating hormone secretion. They are members of a larger group of diverse proteins, the transforming growth factor-β (TGF-β) superfamily, which are involved in cell growth and differentiation. Inhibin is a heterodimeric glycoprotein composed of a common α-subunit and one of two β-subunits, resulting in either inhibin A (αβA) or inhibin B (αβB), for which specific immunoassays are now available. The serum also contains immunoreactive forms of the alpha subunit not attached to the beta subunit, the most abundant of which is pro-αC and pro-αN-αC. The pro-αC assay measures these precursor forms of inhibin. The original Monash assay detected immunoreactive inhibin that included a range of inhibin-related peptides in addition to biologically active inhibin dimers.

In 1989, Lappohn et al. (109) reported elevated serum immunoreactive inhibin concentrations in women with granulosa-cell tumors. Numerous studies have since confirmed serum inhibin elevation in ovarian sex cord/stromal tumors and established its role in differential diagnosis and surveillance of these malignancies (110–112). The major molecular forms detected are bioactive dimeric inhibins A and B (113,114). Antimüllerian hormone, or müllerian inhibitory factor, is another member of the TGF-β superfamily that is being investigated as a marker for granulosa-cell tumor (113,115,116).

In epithelial ovarian cancer, the role of the inhibin peptides remains to be determined. Using the initial nonspecific Monash assay, elevated serum inhibin levels were reported in 25% to 90% of women with epithelial ovarian cancer (117–119). In 2004, an ELISA assay for total inhibin was developed (120). Tsigkou et al. investigated the sensitivity/specificity of serum total inhibin for epithelial ovarian cancer in 89 postmenopausal women with stage II to III epithelial ovarian cancer and found that patients with serous or mucinous tumors showed the highest total inhibin levels. At 95% specificity, the total inhibin assay detected 93% of serous and 94% of mucinous tumors (121). Mucinous ovarian cancers are most likely to be associated with increased inhibin levels (111,122). In contrast, using specific assays that measure bioactive dimeric inhibin A, elevated serum levels were only found in 5% to 31% of women with epithelial ovarian cancer (116,122,123). Overall, the picture is emerging that dimeric inhibin A and B levels are not informative in epithelial ovarian cancer, and total inhibin/pro-αC immunoreactive forms are the most commonly elevated of the inhibin-related peptides (121,123,124). Furthermore, although there is preferential secretion of precursor forms of the alpha subunit rather than dimeric inhibin A by epithelial ovarian cancer, pro-αC is unlikely to be a useful marker if used alone (125). Combining pro-αC with CA125 may improve the sensitivity for detection of epithelial ovarian cancer (123). More recently, when total inhibin was combined with CA125, all cases of serous and mucinous tumors were detected and the overall sensitivity for epithelial ovarian cancers was 99% at 95% specificity, respectively. On further follow-up, it became clear that an increase of total inhibin levels was associated with recurrence. These recent data suggest that total inhibin is a sensitive and specific marker of epithelial ovarian cancer in postmenopausal women and may therefore be combined with CA125 for noninvasive diagnosis of epithelial ovarian cancer. Furthermore, it may also be a useful serum marker to monitor disease-free intervals (121).

In conclusion, the data suggest that functional inhibin is secreted by most ovarian granulosa-cell tumors and may be superior to estradiol in assessing therapeutic response and predicting recurrence. For epithelial ovarian cancer, dimeric inhibin A and B levels are probably not informative. While the role of total inhibin/pro-αC needs further investigation, most recent data suggest that total inhibin displays high sensitivity and specificity for serous and mucinous cancer, which is improved when total inhibin is combined with CA125.

Activin is a dimer of the two-beta subunits of inhibin and exists as activin A (βA βA), activin B (βB βB), and activin AB (βA βB). Serum activin A has been shown to be significantly elevated in epithelial ovarian cancer (113,125,126), with highest levels detected in undifferentiated tumors. More recently, high concentrations of activin A in the peritoneal fluid of women with serous ovarian carcinoma have been shown to be useful in distinguishing serous ovarian cancer from cystadenoma (128). Preliminary data suggest a poor correlation of activin levels and the clinical course of the disease (113). It is possible that activin A could play a role in ovarian cancer but further investigation is needed.

Estrogen/Androgen

Estrogen secretion is associated with granulosa-cell tumors. Serial estradiol levels are of significant value in monitoring these patients after surgery, in view of the difficulty in assessing the malignant potential of these tumors on histological grounds. Androgen levels are elevated in women with Sertoli-Leydig–cell tumors.

Kallikreins

The human kallikrein gene family currently consists of 15 members. There is accumulating evidence that in addition to prostate-specific antigen (PSA, hK3) and human glandular kallikrein (hK2) (both prostate cancer biomarkers), many other members of the human kallikrein gene family are differentially regulated in breast, ovarian, and testicular cancers. Recently it has been shown that the malignant phenotype of ovarian cancer cells can be enhanced by overexpression of the human tissue kallikrein genes 4, 5, 6, and 7 (129). Potential biomarkers for ovarian cancer include kallikreins 5, 6, 7, 8, 10, 11, and 14 (130,132,133) . Kallikrein 4 is up-regulated in epithelial ovarian carcinoma cells in effusions (132) and kallikrein expression may have some value in differentiating ascites resulting from ovarian cancer from other malignant and nonmalignant causes (134). Human kallikrein 8 seems to be an independent marker of favorable prognosis in ovarian cancer (135), while kallikrein 7, although not an independent prognosticator for ovarian cancer, has been found to be associated with unfavorable characteristics of the disease (136).

Mesothelin

Mesothelin is a marker that was initially identified in mesotheliomas and ovarian cancers in 1996 (137). Serum levels are higher in ovarian cancer patients when compared to women with benign ovarian tumors or from the normal population. The levels increase significantly from early to advanced stages. Elevated mesothelin levels before therapy are associated with poor overall survival both in patients with optimal debulking surgery and in those with advanced disease (138). It is possible that mesothelin may prove to be a useful tumor marker for differential diagnosis of epithelial ovarian cancer as well as for prognosis.

Prostasin

Prostasin, a serine protease secreted by the prostate gland, was identified following use of cDNA microarray technology on RNA pooled from ovarian cancer and normal human ovarian surface epithelial cell lines to detect overexpressed genes for secretory proteins that might be potential serum biomarkers (139). The initial study reported higher levels of prostasin in ovarian cancer patients compared to controls, with levels decreasing following surgery. For a fixed specificity of 94%, sensitivity for detection of ovarian cancer for CA125 was 64.9% (95% CI, 47.5 to 78.9), for prostasin 51.4% (95% CI, 34.4 to 68.1), and for the combination 92% (95% CI, 78.1 to 98.3) (139). Prostasin may have clinical potential but it needs further investigation and validation.

Osteopontin

Osteopontin is another biomarker that has been identified using gene-expression profiling techniques. The initial investigation showed osteopontin tissue expression to be weak or absent in 93% of ovarian adenocarcinomas, compared to positive expression in 81.5% in borderline tumors and 50% in omental and lymph node implants. Its expression did not correlate with histological type, grade, or clinical stage (140). In 2002, Kim et al. showed an increased expression of this marker in ovarian cancer cell lines, microdissected tissues, and plasma of epithelial ovarian cancer patients (141). Preoperative plasma osteopontin and CA125 levels were investigated in patients with ovarian cancer, benign ovarian tumor, other gynecologic cancers, and healthy women and showed significantly higher levels in patients with ovarian cancer than the other groups. Higher plasma osteopontin levels were detected in late-stage ovarian cancer patients (stage IV) and ovarian cancer patients with ascites with no correlation with histological type. Sensitivity of preoperative plasma osteopontin in detecting ovarian cancer was 81.3%, which increased to 93.8% when combined with CA125, suggesting that preoperative osteopontin may be a useful biomarker for differential diagnosis of ovarian cancer, particularly when combined with CA125 (25,142). Osteopontin levels have been shown to correlate with the presence of ascites, bulky disease, and recurrence (143). In predicting clinical response to therapy, osteopontin is inferior to CA125. However, levels increase earlier in 90% of patients developing recurrent disease, leading the authors to suggest that it may be useful as a complementary marker in detecting recurrent ovarian cancer (144).

Cytokines

Cytokines are soluble mediator substances produced by cells that exercise a specific effect on other target cells. Their importance in tumor biology has increased since the demonstration that many cytokines are produced by cancer cells and can influence the malignant process in a positive and a negative manner (127). However, cytokines do not fulfil the classic criteria for tumor markers, as they may be elevated in a number of pathological conditions, are invariably produced by nonmalignant surrounding tissue rather than the tumor itself, and are not specific for one cell type. Despite this, their measurement in malignant conditions may provide valuable clinical information regarding prognosis and response to treatment.

Details of some of the cytokines and their roles as tumor markers in ovarian malignancy are shown in Table 7.3. The majority are at an early stage of evaluation, with conflicting reports associated with some. The most studied cytokine in the context of ovarian cancer is serum M-CSF (or CSF-1). It appears to be a marker with high specificity for ovarian malignancy with elevation being related to stage (163,167). When combined with other markers, it may have a role in ovarian cancer screening (165,167). Combination of CA125II, CA-72-4, and M-CSF significantly increased sensitivity for detecting early-stage disease compared to CA125II alone (70% vs. 45%) while maintaining 98% specificity (92). M-CSF may be highly sensitive and specific for malignant germ-cell tumors of the ovary, especially dysgerminoma (166). It has been shown that elevated serum levels are associated with poor outcome after adjusting for stage, grade, and degree of surgical clearance (59). In patients with advanced disease, low ascitic fluid M-CSF was associated with longer overall survival and was a better indicator in comparison to other prognostic factors except for zero residual disease (164). Serum M-CSF does not seem to be useful in follow-up of women with advanced disease (168).

Interleukins have also been studied in ovarian cancer. Preliminary reports demonstrated IL-6 elevation in 50% of ovarian cancers (145,146). However, the combination of IL-6 and CA125 did not improve the sensitivity of CA125 alone (146). A more recent report investigating the role of CA125, IL-6, IL-7, and IL-10 in 187 ovarian cancer patients, 45 patients with benign ovarian tumors, and 50 healthy controls found that a combination of IL-7 and CA125 could accurately predict 69% of the ovarian cancer patients, without falsely classifying patients with benign pelvic mass (152).

Cytokeratins

Cytokeratins are intermediate filaments that are part of the cytoskeleton of all epithelial cells. They are specific markers of epithelial differentiation and continue to be expressed by epithelial cells following malignant transformation. Fragments of cytokeratins, in contrast to cytokeratins themselves, are soluble in serum and can be detected and measured using monoclonal

TABLE 7.3

STUDIES REPORTED ON THE ROLE OF CYTOKINES AS TUMOR MARKERS IN OVARIAN CANCER

Cytokines	Description
Interleukin-6 (IL-6)	High levels of IL-6 in 50% of patients with primary ovarian cancer (145,146). Serum levels correlate with stage of disease (147). IL-6 sensitivity lower than that of CA125, and the combination of both assays did not increase the sensitivity of CA125 alone (146). Conflicting reports on the role of elevated IL-6 serum levels in predicting prognosis (146,148–150). It has been shown that *IL6-174* promoter polymorphism impacts serum cytokine levels through transcriptional regulation. Recent data has shown that the *IL6-174* GG genotype has a strong, independent, and favorable impact on survival for women with ovarian and peritoneal carcinoma (151).
Interleukin-7 (IL-7)	Serum levels of CA125, IL-6, IL-7, and IL-10 were determined in 187 ovarian cancer patients with complete clinicopathologic data and follow-up, 45 patients with benign ovarian tumors, and 50 healthy controls and were found to be elevated in ovarian cancer patients compared to patients with benign ovarian tumors. A combination of IL-7 and CA125 serum levels accurately predicted 69% of the ovarian cancer patients, without falsely classifying patients with benign pelvic mass. IL-7 was not an independent predictor of overall survival when clinicopathologic parameters were included (152).
Soluble interleukin-2 receptor (sIL-2R)	Elevated in numerous malignancies and in liver, renal, and autoimmune diseases. Only patients with advanced epithelial ovarian cancer had elevated preoperative serum sIL-2R alpha levels (153). Conflicting reports on the usefulness of sIL-2R as an adjunctive tool for the differential diagnosis of ovarian masses (154, 155). Limited benefit for monitoring response to chemotherapy and follow-up of patients with epithelial ovarian cancer (153,156–158).
Tumor necrosis factor (TNF)	Raised levels documented in various malignancies and several benign conditions. Significantly higher levels were reported in patients with epithelial ovarian cancer than in those with benign ovarian disease (159). A more recent study has shown that serum TNF-α levels differed between benign tumors and endometriomas ($p < 0.01$), but not between endometriomas and malignant tumors (160). No correlation has been shown between preoperative TNF values and common prognostic variables or the clinical outcome of patients (159).
Soluble receptors of TNF (sTNF-R)	Initial studies suggested that preoperative serum levels might have a potential role for detection, prognosis, and monitoring disease (159,161). The ratio of preoperative serum TNF-α receptor 1 (p55) and 2 (p75) may be of value in differential diagnosis of ovarian cancer (162).
Macrophage colony-stimulating factor (M-CSF)	Levels significantly elevated in 61% to 64% of patients with ovarian cancer compared with 6% to 7% of patients with benign ovarian tumors. Elevation related to stage of disease and independent of histologic type (163,164). Serum M-CSF, but not CA125, significantly associated with outcome following adjustment for stage, grade, and degree of surgical clearance (54). May have a role in ovarian cancer screening (163,165). Combination of CA125II, CA-72-4, and M-CSF significantly increased sensitivity for detecting early-stage disease compared to CA125II alone (70% versus 45%) while maintaining 98% specificity (92). M-CSF may be highly sensitive and specific for malignant germ-cell tumors of the ovary, especially dysgerminoma (166).

antibodies. Their role as tumor markers in various malignancies is currently being investigated.

Tissue Polypeptide-Specific Antigen

Tissue polypeptide-specific antigen (TPS) is a proliferation marker closely related to the tumor marker TPA. It is recognized by a monoclonal antibody raised against the M3 epitope on cytokeratin 18. TPS is elevated in 50% to 77% of ovarian cancers studied with a specificity of 84% to 85% (169–172). Preoperatively, serum levels of TPS and CA125 were significantly higher in patients with cancer rather than benign disease and in those with advanced compared to early-stage disease. Similarly, levels of TPS and CA125 were higher in malignant and benign tumor cysts and ascitic fluids than in corresponding sera with levels in cyst fluid from cancer patients being the highest (173). However, no correlation between TPS levels and survival have been shown (172). Its serial measurement may be of value in the follow-up of patients (169,170). When combined with CA125, sensitivity for predicting recurrence of 81% was achieved with a specificity and PPV of 82% and 58%, respectively (171,172).

CYFRA 21-1

CYFRA 21-1 is a fragment of cytokeratin 19. The assay was first developed in 1993 by Stieber et al. (174). It was initially found to be elevated in cervical and endometrial cancers (175). It does not seem to be very useful in the differential diagnosis of adnexal masses, with most studies reporting sensitivities of 40% to 45% (176,177). It may have a role as a prognostic factor but there are conflicting reports. Elevated CYFRA 21-1 levels prior to therapy were reported to be associated with poor overall and disease-free survival in ovarian cancer (177). However, preoperative levels of CYFRA 21-1 were higher in patients with advanced disease, but Cox regression analysis failed to detect a significant association between preoperative CYFRA 21-1 values and survival. For patients with advanced ovarian cancer, preoperative CYFRA 21-1 levels appear to be predictive of response to chemotherapy but not of survival (178). In a recent case report, elevated levels of CYFRA 21-1 together with neuron-specific enolase, estradiol, and CA125 were described in a patient with Sertoli-Leydig–cell tumor of the ovary, and it was suggested that it may be useful to further investigate the role of these tumor markers in individualized monitoring (179).

Proteomics

Proteomics is the study of the expression, structure, and function of all proteins as a function of state, time, age, and environment (180–182). It complements the genomics-based approaches and has become very popular in the past few years. While two-dimensional gel electrophoresis continues to be the cornerstone of protein separation, mass spectrometry is increasingly being used for diagnostics, tissue imaging, and biomarker discovery as it is a high-throughput technique requiring small amounts of sample (183). Surface-enhanced laser desorption ionization time-of-flight (SELDI-TOF) analysis and matrix-associated laser desorption ionization time-of-flight (MALDI-TOF) technology have the potential to identify patterns or changes in thousands of proteins in the mass range under 20 kDa. When combined with matrices that selectively absorb certain serum proteins, these approaches can globally analyze almost all small proteins in complex solutions, such as serum or plasma (184,185). Two proteomic approaches have been used: one examines the pattern of peaks on mass spectometry, and the other uses proteomic analysis to identify a limited number of critical markers that are then assayed by more conventional methods. Both approaches are promising but require further development.

In a preliminary study, SELDI-TOF in combination with powerful computer algorithms identified a pattern of protein changes in serum with sensitivity of 100%, specificity of 95%, and PPV of 94% for both early and late ovarian cancer in a limited set of samples from 50 patients with ovarian cancer and 50 unaffected women (186). There were numerous issues with the study design (131,187–189) and the results are still to be validated. In a multicenter case-control study that followed, three potential serum biomarkers for ovarian cancer were identified: lower levels of apolipoprotein A1, lower levels of a truncated form of transthyretin, and elevated levels of a cleavage fragment of inter-alpha-trypsin inhibitor heavy chain H4 (ITIH4) (190). These findings were confirmed in an independently conducted blinded study of 42 women with ovarian cancer, 65 with benign tumors, and 76 with digestive diseases. The mean levels of five of the six forms of transthyretin were significantly lower in cases than in controls (191). The specificity of a model including transthyretin and apolipoprotein A1 alone was high (96.5%; 95% CI, 91.9 to 98.8) but sensitivity was low (52.4%; 95% CI, 36.4 to 68.0). A class prediction algorithm using all seven markers, CA125, and age maintained high specificity (94.3%) but had higher sensitivity (78.6%) (191). Proteomic analysis of plasma samples has also yielded informative protein spots that may be complementary to those identified in the serum. Using four specific protein peaks in plasma, a sensitivity of 90% to 96.3% and specificity of 100% for the studied cases and controls were reached (192). However encouraging these results are, further validation studies with due consideration to the influences of sample handling, subject characteristics, and other covariates on biomarker levels need to be undertaken. A recent report has confirmed that sample processing after venipuncture affects serum protein profile with the largest effect related to room temperature prior to sample separation. Certain proteins (transthyretin, apolipoprotein C1, and transferrin) were unaffected by handling, while others (ITIH4 and hemoglobin β) displayed significant variability (193). This further highlights the need for biomarker discovery to be carried out on samples collected in a standardized fashion. More recent efforts have involved exploring antibodies raised to 35 of 217 protein spots obtained by proteomic profiling of ovarian cancer and normal tissue (194) and subtype-specific biomarker candidates obtained by differential protein expression of tissue specimens from clear cell and mucinous ovarian cancers (195,196). In contrast to the biomarker studies described above, where proteomic profile is assessed in differing numbers of specimens from cases and controls, another proposed approach is the creation and use of standard serum sets developed from pooled healthy donors and pooled sera from ovarian cancer cases. Preliminary data show that CA125 remains the best single marker for nonmucinous ovarian cancer, complemented by CA-15-3 or soluble mesothelin-related protein (36).

The high volume of data obtained from proteomic analyses is difficult to handle. Various algorithms are being developed to analyze the preprocessed mass-spectrometry data and identify the most informative "common" peaks, but these approaches still need fine tuning (197–199). It is critical that once the technology is standardized, large, prospective, multicenter trials are carried out to ensure validation (200).

Metabolite Profiling

Metabolites are the end products of cellular regulatory processes. Alterations in their levels can be regarded as response to genetic or environmental changes. Analysis of 66 invasive ovarian carcinomas and nine borderline ovarian tumors by gas chromatography/time-of-flight mass spectrometry (GC-TOF MS) using a novel contamination-free injector was undertaken to assess if quantitative signatures of primary metabolites can be used to characterize molecular changes in ovarian tumor tissues. A total of 291 metabolites were detected and 114 were already annotated compounds. Principal component analysis as well as additional supervised predictive models allowed a separation of 88% of the borderline tumors from the carcinomas. The data suggest that metabolomics is a promising high-throughput, automated approach in addition to functional genomics and proteomics for analyses of molecular changes in malignant tumors (201).

Other Serum Markers

Table 7.4 details other serum markers that have been assessed in isolation and as part of panels in women with ovarian cancer, both in the context of screening and differential diagnosis, as well as in assessing prognosis, monitoring response to treatment, and detecting recurrence. Table 7.5 details their current role in ovarian cancer. It is important to note that in women with ovarian cancer, no single marker or combination of markers has emerged with a clear clinical advantage over CA125, except in specific tumor subtypes such as germ-cell tumors with yolk sac and chorionic elements, and granulosa-cell tumors. The results of the proteomic and genomics studies are therefore eagerly awaited. The consensus is that these new approaches are most likely to identify novel markers or marker panels that in combination with CA125 will improve biomarker accuracy in ovarian cancer.

ENDOMETRIAL CANCERS

There are no serum markers with an established role in the clinical management of endometrial cancer. Serum CA125 is elevated in 10% to 31% of patients (265–268) with elevated

TABLE 7.4

OTHER TUMOR MARKERS FOR OVARIAN CARCINOMA THAT ARE NOT REFERRED TO IN DETAIL IN THE TEXT

Tumor marker	Description
CA-15-3	Tumor-associated antigen in human milk fat globule membrane. Most used in breast carcinoma. Elevated levels in 57% to 71% of ovarian cancer patients and 2% to 6% of patients with benign tumors (202,203). Not useful on its own (204), but in combination with CA125 increases the specificity of the CA125 assay in the differential diagnosis of adnexal masses (203). Preoperative sensitivity for early-stage disease was 45% for CA125II; 67% for CA125II and CA-72-4; 70% for CA125II, CA-72-4, and M-CSF; and 68% for CA125II, CA-72-4, M-CSF, and CA-15-3. CA-15-3 in combination with the other three markers performed second in comparison to using the other markers alone (92).
CA-72-4 or TAG-72	Defines a glycoprotein surface antigen found in colon, gastric, and ovarian cancer. Levels elevated in 67% of ovarian cancers (205) with a better sensitivity than CA125 for mucinous tumors (206,207). The specificity of CA-72-4 for ovarian malignancy was >95%, and combination with CA125 increased sensitivity without substantial change in specificity (208). Combination of CA125II, CA-72-4, and M-CSF significantly increased preoperative sensitivity for early-stage disease from 45% with CA125II alone to 70%, while maintaining 98% first-line specificity (92). The addition of serum CA-72-4 to the combination of pelvic examination, ultrasound, and serum CA125 improved discrimination between malignant and benign pelvic masses (209).
CA-19-9	Defines an antigen that is part of the Lewis blood group antigens. Elevated in gastrointestinal, lung, ovarian, and endometrial carcinoma. Most useful in pancreatic carcinoma. Mucinous ovarian cancers express the antigen more frequently (76%) than serous tumors (27%). Unlike CA125, not affected by pregnancy (210). Together with CA125, was the most useful marker in patients with borderline ovarian tumors (12). In patients with mature cystic teratomas of the ovary, elevated levels were found in 38.8%, whereas serum CA125 was elevated in 25% of the patients. Patients with an elevated serum CA-19-9 level showed significantly higher rates of bilateral tumors (51.6% versus 12.2%) than the patients with low levels (211). In a recent study of 28 stage I ovarian cancers, preoperative serum CA125 and CA-19-9 levels in stage IA patients were much lower than in patients with stage IC disease (212).
OVX1	Antigenic determinant on a high-molecular-weight mucin-like glycoprotein present in ovarian and breast cancer cells. Recognized by murine monoclonal antibody OVX1 (213). Elevated serum levels (>7.2 U/mL) reported in 5% of 184 normal individuals and in 70% of 93 epithelial ovarian cancer patients (214). OVX1 as a part of a panel of markers improved the sensitivity for discriminating malignant from benign pelvic masses (165,215). However, although the combination of serum OVX1, CA125II, and M-CSF markers had greater sensitivity than CA125 alone for all stages of ovarian cancer, only CA125 was able to distinguish invasive stage I tumors from apparently healthy women (216). A preliminary report found that serial measurement of OVX1 in combination with CA125 improved the sensitivity, specificity, and PPV of CA125 alone in primary screening for epithelial ovarian cancer (217). However, the OVX1 radioimmunoassay is highly dependent on sample handling (96) and therefore is not widely used.
CASA/OSA	Tumor-associated antigens assayed by dual epitope ELISAs using the same capture monoclonal antibody (BC2) and different second antibodies (OM-1 and BC3, respectively). Elevated levels reported in 38% to 58% of ovarian cancers (94,218) with CASA showing higher specificity (94). In addition, CASA was elevated in patients with breast, lung, prostate, and bladder cancer (218). CASA may have a role in prognosis and monitoring disease—postoperative OSA and CASA assays were superior to CA125 for detection of small-volume occult ovarian carcinoma (219); on multivariate analysis of survival rates postoperative CASA levels ranked above all prognostic factors except age (220); postoperative CASA levels supplemented the prognostic value of CA125 measurements in monitoring disease (221,222); in patients with recurrent ovarian carcinoma, elevated level of CASA before treatment was an adverse prognostic factor for survival (223); high serum levels of CASA were associated with increased risk of second-line chemoresistance (224).
Growth factors	Insulin-like growth factors (IGFs) and IGF-binding proteins (IGFBPs) have been shown to play a physiologic role in the female genital system, including the ovarian follicular system. Expression of the insulin-like growth factor binding protein-2 (*IGFBP-2*) gene is elevated in advanced epithelial ovarian cancers in comparison to normal ovarian epithelium. This is also reflected in the serum with elevated serum *IGFBP-2* levels detected in epithelial ovarian cancers compared to both normal controls and patients with benign gynecologic disease (225,226). The relationship between circulating levels of IGF-I and its major binding protein (IGFBP-3) in relation to ovarian cancer risk was investigated in a case-control study nested within the European Prospective Investigation into Cancer and Nutrition involving prediagnostic serum samples of 214 women who subsequently

	developed ovarian cancer and 388 matched control subjects. No association was found between the circulating IGF-I or IGFBP-3 levels and the risk of ovarian cancer in the cohort. However, for women diagnosed with ovarian cancer aged 55 or younger, the relative risk was higher in the middle or top tertiles of serum IGF-I, when compared with women in the lowest tertile. In premenopausal women with ovarian cancer relative risks for ovarian cancer diagnosed before age 55 were higher for second and third tertiles. The results suggest that IGF-I circulating levels may play a role in the development of ovarian cancer in women of a pre- or perimenopausal age (227).
Tetranectin	A tetrameric, plasminogen-binding plasma protein first discovered in 1986. Blood levels reduced in patients with a variety of cancers. At a false-positive rate of 1%, the sensitivity for ovarian cancer stages I and II was 33% for serum tetranectin against 76% for CA125. Combining tetranectin with CA125 increases sensitivity without causing a concomitant increase in the rate of false-positive results. However, neither marker rose to levels that would allow use in the discrimination of localized cancer and benign tumors (228). Preoperative tetranectin leves correlated with survival and were a strong prognostic variable in patients with advanced ovarian cancer (61,229). Chemotherapy induced significant increases in serum tetranectin levels with a decrease in serum tetranectin during chemotherapy being highly indicative of recurrence and poor outcome (230). Hogdall et al. (231) measured serum tetranectin, CA125, and CASA prior to 63 second-look and five third-look operations for ovarian cancer. Patients with residual tumor had significantly lower levels of tetranectin and higher levels of CASA and CA125 compared with tumor-free patients. Using multivariate Cox analyses, it was found that all three markers were independent prognostic predictors of survival.
Tumor-associated trypsin inhibitor (TATI)	In ovarian cancer patients, a 6 kD polypeptide, TATI, can occur in elevated concentrations in both urine and serum (232). When used as a single marker, serum TATI has lower sensitivity and specificity than CA125. However, it is more sensitive than CA125 in diagnosing mucinous and poorly differentiated carcinomas (233,234). TATI may also be useful in differentiation of primary and metastatic ovarian tumors. In a recent report of 38 patients with secondary ovarian malignancies and 76 control patients with primary epithelial ovarian cancer, although the preoperative serum CA125 was not different between the two groups, patients with secondary malignancies displayed higher levels of serum TATI and CEA. The study demonstrated that tumors less than 9 cm with solid structure, absence of ascites, and elevated serum CEA and TATI levels are typical of secondary ovarian malignancies (235). Unlike CA125, TATI levels seem to correlate with tumor grade (234). It may have a prognostic role as elevated preoperative levels have been associated with a twofold increase in risk of death (60) and a 5-year cumulative survival in advanced ovarian cancer of 8% as opposed to 45% in patients with normal preoperative values (236). In patients with stage III and IV disease on multivariate analysis, TATI tissue expression along with tumor grade has been reported to be an independent prognostic factor for adverse cancer-specific and progression-free survival (237).
GAT (galactosyltransferase associated with tumor)	Elevated in 4.5% to 6.0% of women with endometriosis and 46% to 48% of women with ovarian cancer. GAT may be useful in discriminating ovarian malignancy from endometriosis (238,239). GAT has been shown to be a marker of ovarian cancer with a high specificity. Human serum contains certain factors that decrease the GAT level, but these factors seem to be inhibited in ovarian cancer patients so that a high GAT level persists. (240).
LASA (lipid-associated sialic acid)	The assay predominantly determines glycogen-bound sialic acid and has high positivity rate in leukemia, Hodgkin's disease, melanoma, sarcoma, advanced ovarian carcinoma, and oropharyngeal tumors (241). The value of determination of LASA in addition to CA125 in invasive epithelial ovarian cancer is due to lack of specificity (242,243). When used as part of a panel of serum markers, it may be useful in women with a pelvic mass (215). It was investigated as part of a panel of multiple markers (CA125, HER2/neu, urinary gonadotropin peptide, lipid-associated sialic acid, and Dianon marker 70/K) in serial samples obtained during 6 years of follow-up of 1,257 healthy women at high risk of ovarian cancer. The findings suggested that individual-specific screening rules may be developed with the potential to improve early detection of ovarian cancer (244) using these markers.
VEGF (vascular endothelial growth factor)	A promoter of angiogenesis, VEGF is believed to play a pivotal role in tumor growth and metastasis. In a preliminary study, serum VEGF had a sensitivity of 54% for ovarian cancer and was not useful in the differential diagnosis of adnexal mass (245). A more recent study has shown that higher serum VEGF, higher FIGO stage, and presence of residual tumor mass after primary surgery were independently associated with a shortened overall survival and that serum VEGF is an independent prognostic parameter regardless of the stage (246).
IAP (immunosuppressive acid protein)	Increased levels detected in 70% of patients with ovarian cancer, 25% with benign tumors, and in 4.5% of normal women. The simultaneous determination of IAP and CA125 allowed an overall sensitivity of 84% without any significant reduction of specificity (247). On multivariate analysis, there was significant association with survival (248). Since then, the performance of IAP in combination with IL-6 and M-CSF was examined in 61 serum samples of previously untreated ovarian cancer patients. Whereas a direct correlation between IL-6 and M-CSF was found, IAP serum levels failed to correlate with M-CSF and IL-6 levels (249).

(*continued*)

TABLE 7.4

OTHER TUMOR MARKERS FOR OVARIAN CARCINOMA THAT ARE NOT REFERRED TO IN DETAIL IN THE TEXT (CONTINUED)

Tumor marker	Description
Lysophosphatidic acid (LPA)	LPA is a bioactive phospholipid with mitogenic and growth-factor-like activities that stimulates the proliferation of cancer cells (250,251). It has been shown to increase cell proliferation, cell survival, resistance to cisplatin, and production of VEGF in ovarian cancer cells, but not in normal ovarian surface epithelial cells (252), and accounts for the ability of ascites to activate ovarian cancer cells (253). LPA levels were significantly higher in ascites from ovarian cancer patients than in malignant effusions from other cancer patients, suggesting a role for LPA-like lipids in the peritoneal spread of ovarian cancer (254). In an initial study, elevated plasma LPA levels were detected in 9 out of 10 patients with stage I ovarian cancer; all 24 patients with stage II, III, and IV ovarian cancer; and 14 patients with recurrent ovarian cancer. In contrast, raised plasma LPA levels were detected in 5 of 48 controls, 4 out of 17 women with benign disease, and in no women with breast cancer or leukemia (255). Using a new highly specific, sensitive, and reproducible assay, Bast et al. demonstrated elevated levels of LPA in more than 90% of stage I or II ovarian cancer patients, less than 50% of whom had elevated CA125 levels (256). There have, however, been no further studies validating the potential of plasma LPA as a potential biomarker for ovarian cancer.
DNA methylation	Circulating methylated DNA may represent a new generation of tumor marker (257), as changes in DNA methylation are one of the most common alterations in human neoplasia (258). Hypermethylation of tumor-derived DNA can be found in serum and plasma of cancer patients (259,260). Recently, in colorectal cancer the pattern of methylation of serum DNA has been shown to be a prognostic factor (261). In the next decade it is possible that this approach may identify novel tumor markers for ovarian cancer.
Cadherin	Cadherin expression has been explored as a potential tool to differentiate ovarian cancer from malignant mesothelioma cell effusions. However, it turned out that different cadherins are co-expressed and P-cadherin, E-cadherin, and N-cadherin are not useful for differentiation between ovarian/primary peritoneal and malignant mesothelioma cell in effusions (262).
Shed glycans	Shed glycans can be used as possible markers for ovarian cancer (263). Glycoproteins shed by cancer cells are found in the supernatant (or conditioned media) of cultured cells. They can be profiled for their oligosaccharide content using beta-elimination conditions, and any changes in glycosylation can be monitored by matrix-assisted laser desorption/ionization Fourier transform ion cyclotron resonance mass spectrometry (MALDI-FTICR-MS). As glycoproteins can be detected in the serum, oligosaccharide profiling data can be applied to ovarian cancer patients and normal sera to determine at least 15 unique serum glycan markers in ovarian cancer patients that were absent in normal individuals (264).

Note: There were initial studies in the early 1990s exploring the role of sialyl SSEA-1 antigen, TPA, and serum CA-130 in ovarian cancer but none since 1995. Hence, these markers have been omitted from the above table. CASA, Cancer-associated serum antigen; CEA, carcinoembryonic antigen; OSA, Ovarian serum antigen; PPV, positive predictive value.

levels detected in 63% to 67% of patients with advanced-stage and 10% to 19% of those with early-stage disease (269,276). Preoperative assessment of serum CA125 may be of use in predicting the presence of extra-uterine and metastatic disease and, to a lesser extent, myometrial invasion (270, 271). It was suggested that serum CA125 may be useful in follow-up of patients with early-stage endometrial cancer but has not been shown to add to clinical examination and imaging (272). While distant metastases may raise CA125 levels, isolated recurrences in the vagina do not. Levels can be falsely elevated in the presence of severe radiation injury (266). In an analysis of 97 patients with endometrial cancer, elevations of CA125 and CA-15-3 were significantly associated with poor prognostic clinical factors. On multivariate analysis, CA-15-3 was highly significant and had a larger hazard ratio than CA125 (268).

In the 1990s, the role of a number of serum markers was explored in endometrial cancer— CYFRA 21-1 (175), urinary beta-core or UGF levels (273,274), SCC and CA-15-3 (275), CA-19-9 (267), amino-terminal propeptide of type III procollagen (276), placental protein 4 (277), CA-72-4 (278), OVX1 antigen (253), soluble interleukin-2 receptor (279), and M-CSF (265,280). However, none proved to be very useful and this is confirmed by the lack of further publications.

Recent publications indicate significantly higher levels of serum and plasma human kallikrein 6 in women with uterine serous papillary endometrial cancer compared to those with endometrioid carcinoma and controls without cancer (281), increased expression of inhibin βB in grade 3 compared to grade 2 endometrial cancer (282), and an association of matrix metalloproteinase 2 (MMP-2) expression with CA125 and clinical course in endometrial carcinoma. Expression of the MMP-2 and MMP-9 proteins was found in 88% and 70% of the primary endometrial cancers with positive MMP-2 immunostaining associated with a shortened recurrence-free and cancer-specific survival. MMP-2 negativity seemed linked to favorable prognosis. Preoperative serum levels of CA125 were higher in the patients presenting with tumors positive for MMP-2 than in those with negative immunostaining (283). However, the value of such observations still remains to be determined.

CERVICAL CANCERS

Screening for cervical cancer is based on exfoliative cytology and high-risk HPV DNA detection in cervical specimens. Currently, no serological markers are being explored.

TABLE 7.5

STATUS OF CURRENT TUMOR MARKERS IN OVARIAN CANCER

	Screening	Differential diagnosis of an adnexal mass	Prognostic indicator	Monitoring response to therapy	Monitoring disease and recurrence
EPITHELIAL CANCERS					
Clinical practice		CA125 is the main marker—when combined with menopausal status and ultrasound features in the risk of malignancy index (RMI), a sensitivity of 71% to 85% and specificity of 96% to 97% are achieved. CEA	CA125 levels post surgery and during chemotherapy are independent prognostic indicators. Various criteria are used based on CA125 half-life.	Serial CA125 levels reflect clinical course in 90% of positive tumors and are used routinely for monitoring patients.	CA125 detects recurrence with a sensitivity of 84% to 94% and a false-positive rate of <2%. Median lead time compared with clinical diagnosis of recurrence is 60 to 99 days.
Research	Serum CA125 being assessed in screening trials in the general (UKCTOCS and PLCO) and high-risk (UKFOCSS and trials by GOG and CGN in the United States) populations. Results expected in 2012 to 2014. Main emphasis on algorithms to interpret serial CA125 and transvaginal ultrasound, as a second-line test. M-CSF free serum DNA methylation	Inhibin pro-α C/total inhibin, kallikreins, mesothelin, prostasin, osteopontin, M-CSF, TPS, proteomic markers (profile, transthyretin, apolipoprotein A). CA-15-3, CA-72-4, CA-19-9, TATI, GAT, free serum DNA methylation, free glycans, IL-7, TNF-α receptors	Kallikrein 8, mesothelin, CYFRA 21-1, M-CSF, TATI, VEGF, CASA, tetranectin	CASA	Osteopontin, TPS CASA
GERM-CELL TUMORS					
Clinical practice		Serum AFP in tumors with endodermal sinus/yolk sac elements, serum β hCG in tumors with chorionic elements			
Research		M-CSF especially in dysgerminomas			
SEX CORD STROMAL TUMORS					
Clinical practice		Inhibin, estradiol in granulosa-cell tumors		Inhibin, anti–müllerian hormone (AMH) in granulosa-cell tumors CYFRA 21-1 in Sertoli Leydig tumors	

Note: Further discussion and references are in the appropriate section in the accompanying text or in Table 7.4. CASA, Cancer-associated serum antigen; CEA, carcinoembryonic antigen; CGN, Cancer Genetics Network; GAT, galactosyltransferase associated with tumor; GOG, Gynecologic Oncology Group; TATI, tumor-associated trypsin inhibitor; TNF, tumor necrosis factor; TPS, tissue polypeptide-specific antigen; VEGF, vascular endothelial growth factor.

However, a variety of serum markers have been investigated in assessing prognosis, monitoring response to treatment, and detecting recurrence.

Squamous-Cell Carcinoma Antigen

In 1977, Kato and Torigoe (283) isolated the tumor antigen TA-4 from a cervical squamous-cell carcinoma antigen (SCC). SCC is one of 14 subfractions of tumor antigen TA-4. Elevated levels of SCC are found in 57% to 70% of women with primary squamous-cell carcinoma of the cervix (284–286). The release of SCC into the circulation is independent of local tissue content, as high antigen concentrations are found in the cytosol of normal cervical squamous epithelia, but in these cases serum levels are always in the normal range (287). The antigen is not specific for cervical squamous-cell carcinoma with elevated levels found in other squamous-cell carcinomas of the head and neck, esophagus, and lung, and in adenocarcinoma of the uterus, ovary, and lung. SCC levels can also be raised in skin diseases such as psoriasis and eczema (288). SCC is probably a marker of cellular differentiation of squamous cells, as the incidence of elevated serum levels is higher in women with well-differentiated (78%) and moderately differentiated carcinoma (67%) than in those with poorly differentiated tumors (38%) (287). Its levels before treatment correlate with stage, tumor volume, lymph node status, and blood vessel invasion (289–293).

In the past, there have been conflicting reports on the prognostic significance of pretreatment SCC levels (285,289,290, 292,294–296), but increasingly it seems that a combination of pre- and post-treatment values may be useful both for predicting prognosis and for estimating clinical response in women, especially in those undergoing neoadjuvant chemotherapy (296–299). On multivariate analysis of 352 patients with stage IIB to IVA squamous-cell carcinoma of the cervix managed with both external irradiation and high-dose-rate intracavitary brachytherapy, pretreatment SCC antigen level and lymph node metastases were found to have a significant independent effect on absolute survival and disease-free survival (300). Elevated post-treatment serum SCC levels have been shown to be indicators of treatment failure (295,299,301) and be associated with poor survival rates (296). In a recent study involving 211 patients treated with concurrent chemoradiotherapy, SCC levels normalized in 93% of patients at 1 month after completing treatment. In patients with complete remission who had previously elevated pretreatment SCC antigen, the values were normalized in 96% (134 out of 139) at 1 month (286). Various authors have suggested the need for further treatment in patients with elevated SCC levels at completion of treatment. Nonetheless, the evidence is preliminary and further studies are needed before any definitive conclusions can be drawn.

In serum SCC-positive patients, serial measurements correlated with clinical course of the disease in 72% of women (302). Raised SCC levels were found in 50% to 71% of patients with recurrent carcinoma, with a lead time ranging from 0 to 12 months (284,303).

Preliminary studies suggest that SCC antigen (SCCA) isoforms may provide additional clinical information when compared to total SCCA. In early-stage cervical cancer, it has been shown that 2-year disease-free survival is significantly lower in patients with high SCCA2/SCCA1 mRNA ratios (50%) compared to those with low SCCA2/SCCA1 mRNA ratios (92%) (304). More recently, Roijer et al. have developed and evaluated specific serum immunoassays for the different forms of SCC antigen (free SCCA2, total SCCA2, total SCCA1, and total SCCA). Both SCCA1 and SCCA2 levels were elevated in serum from cervical cancer patients and followed the clinical course of the disease during monitoring of treatment. Patients with recurrence or progressive disease had rising levels of SCCA1 and SCCA2, with elevations in SCCA2 being more prominent than those in SCCA1. SCCA2 did not show improved tumor specificity as compared to SCCA1 (305). These results need to be confirmed in a larger study in order to make firm conclusions.

CYFRA 21-1

Following detection of elevated levels of CYFRA 21-1 in patients with squamous-cell carcinoma of the lung, various groups started investigating its role in cervical carcinoma. Tsai et al. detected elevated CYFRA 21-1 levels in 14% of controls, 35% of patients with stage IB to IIA squamous-cell carcinoma of the cervix, and 64% of patients with stage IIB to IV disease (306). Although CYFRA 21-1 was related to tumor stage and size in patients with cervical cancer (307) and there was a positive correlation with SCC, its sensitivity and specificity for detection of squamous-cell carcinoma of the cervix were lower than SCC (306). In cervical adenocarcinoma, it was elevated in 63% of patients (308). CYFRA 21-1 may have a role in follow-up of women with cervical cancer (309). In the study by Pras et al. (299) elevated CYFRA 21-1 levels after chemoradiation for cervical cancer indicated residual tumor in 70% of patients. Nonetheless, the evidence available so far does not justify the routine measurements of these markers.

CA125/CEA

Serum CA125 is only elevated in 13% to 21% of women with squamous-cell carcinoma (275,302). It is a better marker than SCC for cervical adenocarcinoma (275,302,310). In combination with CA-19-9, a sensitivity of 60% for cervical adenocarcinoma was reported, with the addition of CEA to this combination increasing sensitivity to 70% (311). Elevated CA125 levels have been found to contribute to prognosis (312,313) with levels falling in women who respond to chemotherapy (314). In adenosquamous cervical cancer, serum CA125, SCC, and CEA were found to be elevated in patients with progressive disease, whereas only CA125 was elevated in women with adenocarcinoma (310). Serum CEA alone is less useful in cervical cancers, with an overall sensitivity of 15% and specificity of 90%. Patients with cervical adenocarcinoma have significantly higher levels of CEA than those with squamous-cell cancers (315).

VULVAR AND VAGINAL CANCERS

Tumors of the vulva and the vagina are rare and there are relatively few studies on circulating markers in these conditions. TPS has been shown to be elevated in 80% of patients with vulvar or vaginal cancer (169), whereas SCC levels were elevated in 43% (316). Carter et al. (317) studied the urinary core fragment of the β-subunit of hCG in these cancers. Although the sensitivity of beta-core was only 38%, a highly significant difference was observed in the survival curve between those with elevated beta-core levels compared to those with normal levels. Ninety percent of patients with elevated levels died within 24 months in contrast to 32% of those with normal levels. It might also be useful in detecting recurrence, as rising urinary gonadotropin fragment (UGF) levels at an earlier clinic visit predicted recurrence in four of seven patients. These data, albeit limited, suggest that for lower genital tract malignancies, the measurement of urinary beta-core may be valuable as a prognostic indicator, allowing a more informed approach to treatment and in follow-up.

CONCLUSIONS

The potential role of serum tumor markers is hampered by the fact that these markers are neither confined to the malignant tumor cell nor limited to the malignant phenotype. Of all the markers available in gynecologic malignancies, serum hCG in gestational trophoblastic disease remains closest to the ideal tumor marker. Serum CA125 continues to be the most useful clinical marker, with an established role in diagnosis and monitoring of epithelial ovarian cancer.

Biomarkers are increasingly being used in the differential diagnosis of adnexal masses. Numerous tumor markers have been recognized as promising prognostic factors, and this will aid the development of novel treatment strategies in the future. The role of markers in monitoring therapeutic response and detecting recurrence is yet to be fully explored. In screening trials, serial serum CA125 in combination with ultrasonography is currently being investigated in ovarian cancer screening trials in the general and high-risk populations.

Promising novel biomarkers, especially for ovarian cancer, identified through proteomics and genomics are undergoing validation studies and continuing developments in these two fields, metabolomics and DNA methylation, will probably lead to further candidates that can be used either alone or in combination with existing tumor markers.

References

1. Bast RC Jr, Feeney M, Lazarus H, et al. Reactivity of a monoclonal antibody with human ovarian carcinoma. *J Clin Invest* 1981;68(5):1331–1337.
2. Nustad K, Bast RC Jr, Brien TJ, et al. Specificity and affinity of 26 monoclonal antibodies against the CA 125 antigen: first report from the ISOBM TD-1 workshop. International Society for Oncodevelopmental Biology and Medicine. *Tumour Biol* 1996;17(4):196–219.
3. Kabawat SE, Bast RC Jr, Bhan AK, et al. Tissue distribution of a coelomic-epithelium-related antigen recognized by the monoclonal antibody OC125. *Int J Gynecol Pathol* 1983;2(3):275–285.
4. Davelaar EM, van Kamp GJ, Verstraeten RA, et al. Comparison of seven immunoassays for the quantification of CA 125 antigen in serum. *Clin Chem* 1998;44(7):1417–1422.
5. Mongia SK, Rawlins ML, Owen WE, et al. Performance characteristics of seven automated CA 125 assays. *Am J Clin Pathol* 2006;125(6):921–927.
6. Bast RC Jr, Klug TL, St John E, et al. A radioimmunoassay using a monoclonal antibody to monitor the course of epithelial ovarian cancer. *N Engl J Med* 1983;309(15):883–887.
7. Alagoz T, Buller RE, Berman M, et al. What is a normal CA125 level? *Gynecol Oncol* 1994;53(1):93–97.
8. Bon GG, Kenemans P, Verstraeten R, et al. Serum tumor marker immunoassays in gynecologic oncology: establishment of reference values. *Am J Obstet Gynecol* 1996;174(1 Pt 1):107–114.
9. Zurawski VR Jr, Orjaseter H, Andersen A, et al. Elevated serum CA 125 levels prior to diagnosis of ovarian neoplasia: relevance for early detection of ovarian cancer. *Int J Cancer* 1988;42(5):677–680.
10. Canney PA, Moore M, Wilkinson PM, et al. Ovarian cancer antigen CA125: a prospective clinical assessment of its role as a tumour marker. *Br J Cancer* 1984;50(6):765–769.
11. Jacobs I, Bast RC Jr. The CA 125 tumour-associated antigen: a review of the literature. *Hum Reprod* 1989;4(1):1–12.
12. Tamakoshi K, Kikkawa F, Shibata K, et al. Clinical value of CA125, CA19-9, CEA, CA72-4, and TPA in borderline ovarian tumor. *Gynecol Oncol* 1996;62(1):67–72.
13. Vergote IB, Bormer OP, Abeler VM. Evaluation of serum CA 125 levels in the monitoring of ovarian cancer. *Am J Obstet Gynecol* 1987;157(1):88–92.
14. Jacobs IJ, Skates S, Davies AP, et al. Risk of diagnosis of ovarian cancer after raised serum CA 125 concentration: a prospective cohort study. *BMJ* 1996;313(7069):1355–1358.
15. Menon U, Talaat A, Jeyarajah AR, et al. Ultrasound assessment of ovarian cancer risk in postmenopausal women with CA125 elevation. *Br J Cancer* 1999;80(10):1644–1647.
16. Bell R, Petticrew M, Luengo S, et al. Screening for ovarian cancer: a systematic review. *Health Technol Assess* 1998;2(2):i–iv, 1–84.
17. Jacobs I, Davies AP, Bridges J, et al. Prevalence screening for ovarian cancer in postmenopausal women by CA 125 measurement and ultrasonography. *BMJ* 1993;306(6884):1030–1034.
18. Jacobs IJ, Skates SJ, MacDonald N, et al. Screening for ovarian cancer: a pilot randomised controlled trial. *Lancet* 1999;353(9160):1207–1210.
19. Skates SJ, Xu FJ, Yu YH, et al. Toward an optimal algorithm for ovarian cancer screening with longitudinal tumor markers. *Cancer* 1995;76(10 Suppl):2004–2010.
20. Skates SJ, Menon U, MacDonald N, et al. Calculation of the risk of ovarian cancer from serial CA-125 values for preclinical detection in postmenopausal women. *J Clin Oncol* 2003;21(10 Suppl):206–210.
21. Menon U, Skates SJ, Lewis S, et al. Prospective study using the risk of ovarian cancer algorithm to screen for ovarian cancer. *J Clin Oncol* 2005; 23(31):7919–7926.
22. Jeyarajah AR, Ind TE, Skates S, et al. Serum CA125 elevation and risk of clinical detection of cancer in asymptomatic postmenopausal women. *Cancer* 1999;85(9):2068–2072.
23. Jeyarajah AR, Ind TE, MacDonald N, et al. Increased mortality in postmenopausal women with serum CA125 elevation. *Gynecol Oncol* 1999;73(2): 242–246.
24. Sjovall K, Nilsson B, Einhorn N. The significance of serum CA 125 elevation in malignant and nonmalignant diseases. *Gynecol Oncol* 2002;85(1):175–178.
25. Rosen DG, Wang L, Atkinson JN, et al. Potential markers that complement expression of CA125 in epithelial ovarian cancer. *Gynecol Oncol* 2005;99(2):267–277.
26. Prorok PC, Andriole GL, Bresalier RS, et al. Design of the Prostate, Lung, Colorectal and Ovarian (PLCO) cancer screening trial. *Control Clin Trials* 2000;21(6 Suppl):273S–309S.
27. Buys SS, Partridge E, Greene MH, et al. Ovarian cancer screening in the Prostate, Lung, Colorectal and Ovarian (PLCO) cancer screening trial: findings from the initial screen of a randomized trial. *Am J Obstet Gynecol* 2005;193(5):1630–1639.
28. Jacobs I. Screening for familial ovarian cancer: the need for well-designed prospective studies. *J Clin Oncol* 2005;23(24):5443–5445.
29. Karlan BY, Baldwin RL, Lopez-Luevanos E, et al. Peritoneal serous papillary carcinoma, a phenotypic variant of familial ovarian cancer: implications for ovarian cancer screening. *Am J Obstet Gynecol* 1999;180(4):917–928.
30. Karlan BY, Raffel LJ, Crvenkovic G, et al. A multidisciplinary approach to the early detection of ovarian carcinoma: rationale, protocol design, and early results. *Am J Obstet Gynecol* 1993;169(3):494–501.
31. Muto MG, Cramer DW, Brown DL, et al. Screening for ovarian cancer: the preliminary experience of a familial ovarian cancer center. *Gynecol Oncol* 1993;51(1):12–20.
32. van Nagell JR Jr, DePriest PD, Reedy MB, et al. The efficacy of transvaginal sonographic screening in asymptomatic women at risk for ovarian cancer. *Gynecol Oncol* 2000;77(3):350–356.
33. Tailor A, Bourne TH, Campbell S, et al. Results from an ultrasound-based familial ovarian cancer screening clinic: a 10-year observational study. *Ultrasound Obstet Gynecol* 2003;21(4):378–385.
34. Stirling D, Evans DG, Pichert G, et al. Screening for familial ovarian cancer: failure of current protocols to detect ovarian cancer at an early stage according to the International Federation of Gynecology and Obstetrics system. *J Clin Oncol* 2005;23(24):5588–5596.
35. Jacobs IJ MJ, Rosenthal AN, Fraser L, et al. *Progress in the UK Familial Ovarian Cancer Screening Study (UKFOCSS) in European Society of Gynaecological Oncology.* Istanbul, Turkey: International Gynaecological Cancer Society; 2005.
36. Skates SJ, DCW, Isaacs C, Schildcraut JM, et al. A prospective multi-center ovarian cancer screening study in women at increased risk. Abstract #5510, Journal of Clinical Oncology, 2007 ASCO Annual Meeting Proceedings Part I. Vol 25, No. 18S, 2007:5510.
37. Rosenthal A, Jacobs I. Familial ovarian cancer screening. *Best Pract Res Clin Obstet Gynaecol* 2006;20(2):321–338.
38. www.clinicaltrials.gov. http://clinicaltrials.gov/ct/gui/show/NCT00039559?order=5. Accessed May 25, 2007. Available from: http://clinicaltrials.gov/ct/gui/show/NCT00039559?order=5.
39. www.clinicaltrials.gov. http://clinicaltrials.gov/ct/show/NCT00049049?order=5. Accessed March 22, 2007. Available from: http://clinicaltrials.gov/ct/show/NCT00049049?order=5.
40. Einhorn N, Bast RC Jr, Knapp RC, et al. Preoperative evaluation of serum CA 125 levels in patients with primary epithelial ovarian cancer. *Obstet Gynecol* 1986;67(3):414–416.
41. Curtin JP. Management of the adnexal mass. *Gynecol Oncol* 1994;55(3 Pt 2): S42–S46.
42. Maggino T, Gadducci A, D'Addario V, et al. Prospective multicenter study on CA 125 in postmenopausal pelvic masses. *Gynecol Oncol* 1994;54(2): 117–123.
43. Parker WH, Levine RL, Howard FM, et al. A multicenter study of laparoscopic management of selected cystic adnexal masses in postmenopausal women. *J Am Coll Surg* 1994;179(6):733–737.
44. Zhang Z, Barnhill SD, Zhang H, et al. Combination of multiple serum markers using an artificial neural network to improve specificity in discriminating malignant from benign pelvic masses. *Gynecol Oncol* 1999;73(1):56–61.
45. Jacobs I, Oram D, Fairbanks J, et al. A risk of malignancy index incorporating CA 125, ultrasound and menopausal status for the accurate preoperative diagnosis of ovarian cancer. *Br J Obstet Gynaecol* 1990;97(10):922–929.
46. Tingulstad S, Hagen B, Skjeldestad FE, et al. Evaluation of a risk of malignancy index based on serum CA125, ultrasound findings and menopausal status in the pre-operative diagnosis of pelvic masses. *Br J Obstet Gynaecol* 1996;103(8):826–831.

47. Andersen ES, Knudsen A, Rix P, et al. Risk of malignancy index in the preoperative evaluation of patients with adnexal masses. *Gynecol Oncol* 2003;90(1):109–112.
48. Aslam N, Tailor A, Lawton F, et al. Prospective evaluation of three different models for the pre-operative diagnosis of ovarian cancer. *Bjog* 2000;107(11):1347–1353.
49. Ma S, Shen K, Lang J. A risk of malignancy index in preoperative diagnosis of ovarian cancer. *Chin Med J (Engl)* 2003;116(3):396–399.
50. Manjunath AP, Pratapkumar, Sujatha K, et al. Comparison of three risk of malignancy indices in evaluation of pelvic masses. *Gynecol Oncol* 2001;81(2):225–229.
51. Morgante G, la Marca A, Ditto A, et al. Comparison of two malignancy risk indices based on serum CA125, ultrasound score and menopausal status in the diagnosis of ovarian masses. *Br J Obstet Gynaecol* 1999;106(6):524–527.
52. Davies AP, Jacobs I, Woolas R, et al. The adnexal mass: benign or malignant? Evaluation of a risk of malignancy index. *Br J Obstet Gynaecol* 1993;100(10):927–931.
53. Ulusoy S, Akbayir O, Numanoglu C, et al. The risk of malignancy index in discrimination of adnexal masses. *Int J Gynaecol Obstet* 2007;96(3):186–191.
54. Bailey J, Tailor A, Naik R, et al. Risk of malignancy index for referral of ovarian cancer cases to a tertiary center: does it identify the correct cases? *Int J Gynecol Cancer* 2006;16(Suppl 1):30–34.
55. van Trappen PO, Rufford BD, Mills TD, et al. Differential diagnosis of adnexal masses: risk of malignancy index, ultrasonography, magnetic resonance imaging, and radioimmunoscintigraphy. *Int J Gynecol Cancer* 2007;17(1):61–67.
56. Yazbek J, Aslam N, Tailor A, et al. A comparative study of the risk of malignancy index and the ovarian crescent sign for the diagnosis of invasive ovarian cancer. *Ultrasound Obstet Gynecol* 2006;28(3):320–324.
57. Tingulstad S, Hagen B, Skjeldestad FE, et al. The risk-of-malignancy index to evaluate potential ovarian cancers in local hospitals. *Obstet Gynecol* 1999;93(3):448–452.
58. Makar AP, Kristensen GB, Kaern J, et al. Prognostic value of pre- and postoperative serum CA 125 levels in ovarian cancer: new aspects and multivariate analysis. *Obstet Gynecol* 1992;79(6):1002–1010.
59. Scholl SM, Bascou CH, Mosseri V, et al. Circulating levels of colony-stimulating factor 1 as a prognostic indicator in 82 patients with epithelial ovarian cancer. *Br J Cancer* 1994;69(2):342–346.
60. Venesmaa P, Lehtovirta P, Stenman UH, et al. Tumour-associated trypsin inhibitor (TATI): comparison with CA125 as a preoperative prognostic indicator in advanced ovarian cancer. *Br J Cancer* 1994;70(6):1188–1190.
61. Hogdall CK, Norgaard-Pedersen B, Mogensen O. The prognostic value of pre-operative serum tetranectin, CA-125 and a combined index in women with primary ovarian cancer. *Anticancer Res* 2002;22(3):1765–1768.
62. Petri AL, Hogdall E, Christensen IJ, et al. Preoperative CA125 as a prognostic factor in stage I epithelial ovarian cancer. *APMIS* 2006;114(5):359–363.
63. Obermair A, Fuller A, Lopez-Varela E, et al. A new prognostic model for FIGO stage 1 epithelial ovarian cancer. *Gynecol Oncol* 2007;104(3):607–611.
64. Raspollini MR, Amunni G, Villanucci A, et al. COX-2 and preoperative CA-125 level are strongly correlated with survival and clinical responsiveness to chemotherapy in ovarian cancer. *Acta Obstet Gynecol Scand* 2006;85(4):493–498.
65. Rosen A, Sevelda P, Klein M, et al. A CA125 score as a prognostic index in patients with ovarian cancer. *Arch Gynecol Obstet* 1990;247(3):125–129.
66. Yedema CA, Kenemans P, Thomas CM, et al. CA 125 serum levels in the early post-operative period do not reflect tumour reduction obtained by cytoreductive surgery. *Eur J Cancer* 1993;29A(7):966–971.
67. Gadducci A, Zola P, Landoni F, et al. Serum half-life of CA 125 during early chemotherapy as an independent prognostic variable for patients with advanced epithelial ovarian cancer: results of a multicentric Italian study. *Gynecol Oncol* 1995;58(1):42–47.
68. Rosman M, Hayden CL, Thiel RP, et al. Prognostic indicators for poor risk epithelial ovarian carcinoma. *Cancer* 1994;74(4):1323–1328.
69. Yedema CA, Kenemans P, Voorhorst F, et al. CA 125 half-life in ovarian cancer: a multivariate survival analysis. *Br J Cancer* 1993;67(6):1361–1367.
70. van der Burg ME, Lammes FB, van Putten WL, et al. Ovarian cancer: the prognostic value of the serum half-life of CA125 during induction chemotherapy. *Gynecol Oncol* 1988;30(3):307–312.
71. Hawkins RE, Roberts K, Wiltshaw E, et al. The prognostic significance of the half-life of serum CA 125 in patients responding to chemotherapy for epithelial ovarian carcinoma. *Br J Obstet Gynaecol* 1989;96(12):1395–1399.
72. Makar AP, Kristensen GB, Bormer OP, et al. Serum CA 125 level allows early identification of nonresponders during induction chemotherapy. *Gynecol Oncol* 1993;49(1):73–79.
73. Redman CW, Blackledge GR, Kelly K, et al. Early serum CA125 response and outcome in epithelial ovarian cancer. *Eur J Cancer* 1990;26(5):593–596.
74. Markman M, Liu PY, Rothenberg ML, et al. Pretreatment CA-125 and risk of relapse in advanced ovarian cancer. *J Clin Oncol* 2006;24(9):1454–1458.
75. Makar AP, Kristensen GB, Bormer OP, et al. Is serum CA 125 at the time of relapse a prognostic indicator for further survival prognosis in patients with ovarian cancer? *Gynecol Oncol* 1993;49(1):3–7.
76. Hawkins RE, Roberts K, Wiltshaw E, et al. The clinical correlates of serum CA125 in 169 patients with epithelial ovarian carcinoma. *Br J Cancer* 1989;60(4):634–637.
77. Hempling RE, Piver MS, Natarajan N, et al. Predictive value of serum CA125 following optimal cytoreductive surgery during weekly cisplatin induction therapy for advanced ovarian cancer. *J Surg Oncol* 1993;54(1):38–44.
78. Morgan RJ Jr, Speyer J, Doroshow JH, et al. Modulation of 5-fluorouracil with high-dose leucovorin calcium: activity in ovarian cancer and correlation with CA-125 levels. *Gynecol Oncol* 1995;58(1):79–85.
79. Gallion HH, Hunter JE, van Nagell JR, et al. The prognostic implications of low serum CA 125 levels prior to the second-look operation for stage III and IV epithelial ovarian cancer. *Gynecol Oncol* 1992;46(1):29–32.
80. Buller RE, Berman ML, Bloss JD, et al. Serum CA125 regression in epithelial ovarian cancer: correlation with reassessment findings and survival. *Gynecol Oncol* 1992;47(1):87–92.
81. de Bruijn HW, van der Zee AG, Aalders JG. The value of cancer antigen 125 (CA 125) during treatment and follow-up of patients with ovarian cancer. *Curr Opin Obstet Gynecol* 1997;9(1):8–13.
82. Rustin GJ, Nelstrop AE, McClean P, et al. Defining response of ovarian carcinoma to initial chemotherapy according to serum CA 125. *J Clin Oncol* 1996;14(5):1545–1551.
83. Rustin GJ, Nelstrop AE, Crawford M, et al. Phase II trial of oral altretamine for relapsed ovarian carcinoma: evaluation of defining response by serum CA125. *J Clin Oncol* 1997;15(1):172–176.
84. Riedinger JM, Wafflart J, Ricolleau G, et al. CA 125 half-life and CA 125 nadir during induction chemotherapy are independent predictors of epithelial ovarian cancer outcome: results of a French multicentric study. *Ann Oncol* 2006;17(8):1234–1238.
85. Rustin GJ, Nelstrop AE, Tuxen MK, et al. Defining progression of ovarian carcinoma during follow-up according to CA 125: a North Thames Ovary Group study. *Ann Oncol* 1996;7(4):361–364.
86. Cruickshank DJ, Terry PB, Fullerton WT. The potential value of CA125 as a tumour marker in small volume, non-evaluable epithelial ovarian cancer. *Int J Biol Markers* 1991;6(4):247–252.
87. Duffy MJ, Bonfrer JM, Kulpa J, et al. CA125 in ovarian cancer: European Group on Tumor Markers guidelines for clinical use. *Int J Gynecol Cancer* 2005;15(5):679–691.
88. Santillan A, Garg R, Zahurak ML, et al. Risk of epithelial ovarian cancer recurrence in patients with rising serum CA-125 levels within the normal range. *J Clin Oncol* 2005;23(36):9338–9343.
89. Ferrozzi F, Bova D, De Chiara F, et al. Thin-section CT follow-up of metastatic ovarian carcinoma correlation with levels of CA-125 marker and clinical history. *Clin Imaging* 1998;22(5):364–370.
90. Fehm T, Heller F, Kramer S, et al. Evaluation of CA125, physical and radiological findings in follow-up of ovarian cancer patients. *Anticancer Res* 2005;25(3A):1551–1554.
91. Stenman UH, Alfthan H, Vartiainen J, et al. Markers supplementing CA 125 in ovarian cancer. *Ann Med* 1995;27(1):115–120.
92. Skates SJ, Horick N, Yu Y, et al. Preoperative sensitivity and specificity for early-stage ovarian cancer when combining cancer antigen CA-125II, CA 15-3, CA 72-4, and macrophage colony-stimulating factor using mixtures of multivariate normal distributions. *J Clin Oncol* 2004;22(20):4059–4066.
93. Padungsutt P, Thirapagawong C, Senapad S, et al. Accuracy of tissue polypeptide specific antigen (TPS) in the diagnosis of ovarian malignancy. *Anticancer Res* 2000;20(2B):1291–1295.
94. Sehouli J, Akdogan Z, Heinze T, et al. Preoperative determination of CASA (cancer associated serum antigen) and CA-125 for the discrimination between benign and malignant pelvic tumor mass: a prospective study. *Anticancer Res* 2003;23(2A):1115–1118.
95. Senapad S, Neungton S, Thirapakawong C, et al. Predictive value of the combined serum CA 125 and TPS during chemotherapy and before second-look laparotomy in epithelial ovarian cancer. *Anticancer Res* 2000;20(2B):1297–1300.
96. Hogdall EV, Hogdall CK, Kjaer SK, et al. OVX1 radioimmunoassay results are dependent on the method of sample collection and storage. *Clin Chem* 1999;45(5):692–694.
97. Oehler MK, Sutterlin M, Caffier H. CASA and Ca 125 in diagnosis and follow-up of advanced ovarian cancer. *Anticancer Res* 1999;19(4A):2513–2518.
98. Gold P, Freedman SO. Specific carcinoembryonic antigens of the human digestive system. *J Exp Med* 1965;122(3):467–481.
99. Onsrud M. Tumour markers in gynaecologic oncology. *Scand J Clin Lab Invest Suppl* 1991;206:60–70.
100. Roman LD, Muderspach LI, Burnett AF, et al. Carcinoembryonic antigen in women with isolated pelvic masses. Clinical utility? *J Reprod Med* 1998;43(5):403–407.
101. Kawai M, Kano T, Kikkawa F, et al. Seven tumor markers in benign and malignant germ cell tumors of the ovary. *Gynecol Oncol* 1992;45(3):248–253.
102. Olt G, Berchuck A, Bast RC Jr. The role of tumor markers in gynecologic oncology. *Obstet Gynecol Surv* 1990;45(9):570–577.
103. Maida Y, Kyo S, Takakura M, et al. Ovarian endometrioid adenocarcinoma with ectopic production of alpha-fetoprotein. *Gynecol Oncol* 1998;71(1):133–136.

104. Chow SN, Yang JH, Lin YH, et al. Malignant ovarian germ cell tumors. *Int J Gynaecol Obstet* 1996;53(2):151–158.
105. Zalel Y, Piura B, Elchalal U, et al. Diagnosis and management of malignant germ cell ovarian tumors in young females. *Int J Gynaecol Obstet* 1996;55(1):1–10.
106. Mayordomo JI, Paz-Ares L, Rivera F, et al. Ovarian and extragonadal malignant germ-cell tumors in females: a single-institution experience with 43 patients. *Ann Oncol* 1994;5(3):225–231.
107. Mann K, Saller B, Hoermann R. Clinical use of HCG and hCG beta determinations. *Scand J Clin Lab Invest Suppl* 1993;216:97–104.
108. Murugaesu N, Schmid P, Dancey G, et al. Malignant ovarian germ cell tumors: identification of novel prognostic markers and long-term outcome after multimodality treatment. *J Clin Oncol* 2006;24(30):4862–4866.
109. Lappohn RE, Burger HG, Bouma J, et al. Inhibin as a marker for granulosa-cell tumors. *N Engl J Med* 1989;321(12):790–793.
110. Boggess JF, Soules MR, Goff BA, et al. Serum inhibin and disease status in women with ovarian granulosa cell tumors. *Gynecol Oncol* 1997;64(1): 64–69.
111. Cooke I, O'Brien M, Charnock FM, et al. Inhibin as a marker for ovarian cancer. *Br J Cancer* 1995;71(5):1046–1050.
112. Jobling T, Mamers P, Healy DL, et al. A prospective study of inhibin in granulosa cell tumors of the ovary. *Gynecol Oncol* 1994;55(2):285–289.
113. Petraglia F, Luisi S, Pautier P, et al. Inhibin B is the major form of inhibin/activin family secreted by granulosa cell tumors. *J Clin Endocrinol Metab* 1998;83(3):1029–1032.
114. Yamashita K, Yamoto M, Shikone T, et al. Production of inhibin A and inhibin B in human ovarian sex cord stromal tumors. *Am J Obstet Gynecol* 1997;177(6):1450–1457.
115. Rey RA, Lhomme C, Marcillac I, et al. Antimullerian hormone as a serum marker of granulosa cell tumors of the ovary: comparative study with serum alpha-inhibin and estradiol. *Am J Obstet Gynecol* 1996;174(3): 958–965.
116. Silverman LA, Gitelman SE. Immunoreactive inhibin, mullerian inhibitory substance, and activin as biochemical markers for juvenile granulosa cell tumors. *J Pediatr* 1996;29(6):918–921.
117. Blaakaer J, Micic S, Morris ID, et al. Immunoreactive inhibin-production in post-menopausal women with malignant epithelial ovarian tumors. *Eur J Obstet Gynecol Reprod Biol* 1993;52(2):105–110.
118. Healy DL, Burger HG, Mamers P, et al. Elevated serum inhibin concentrations in postmenopausal women with ovarian tumors. *N Engl J Med* 1993;329(21):1539–1542.
119. Phocas I, Sarandakou A, Sikiotis K, et al. A comparative study of serum alpha-beta A immunoreactive inhibin and tumor-associated antigens CA125 and CEA in ovarian cancer. *Anticancer Res* 1996;16(6B): 3827–3831.
120. Khosravi J, Krishna RG, Khaja N, et al. Enzyme-linked immunosorbent assay of total inhibin: direct determination based on inhibin alpha subunit-specific monoclonal antibodies. *Clin Biochem* 2004;37(5):370–376.
121. Tsigkou A, Marrelli D, Reis FM, et al. Total inhibin is a potential serum marker for epithelial ovarian cancer. *J Clin Endocrinol Metab* 2007;92(7): 2526–2531.
122. Burger HG, Robertson DM, Cahir N, et al. Characterization of inhibin immunoreactivity in post-menopausal women with ovarian tumours. *Clin Endocrinol (Oxf)* 1996;44(4):413–418.
123. Lambert-Messerlian GM, Steinhoff M, Zheng W, et al. Multiple immunoreactive inhibin proteins in serum from postmenopausal women with epithelial ovarian cancer. *Gynecol Oncol* 1997;65(3):512–516.
124. Burger HG, Baillie A, Drummond AE, et al. Inhibin and ovarian cancer. *J Reprod Immunol* 1998;39(1-2):77–87.
125. Menon U, Riley SC, Thomas J, et al. Serum inhibin, activin and follistatin in postmenopausal women with epithelial ovarian carcinoma. BJOG 2000;107(9):1069–1074.
126. Welt CK, Lambert-Messerlian G, Zheng W, et al. Presence of activin, inhibin, and follistatin in epithelial ovarian carcinoma. *J Clin Endocrinol Metab* 1997;82(11):3720–3727.
127. Michiel DF, Oppenheim JJ. Cytokines as positive and negative regulators of tumor promotion and progression. *Semin Cancer Biol* 1992;3(1):3–15.
128. Cobellis L, Reis FM, Luisi S, et al. High concentrations of activin A in the peritoneal fluid of women with epithelial ovarian cancer. *J Soc Gynecol Investig* 2004;11(4):203–206.
129. Prezas P, Arlt MJ, Viktorov P, et al. Overexpression of the human tissue kallikrein genes KLK4, 5, 6, and 7 increases the malignant phenotype of ovarian cancer cells. *Biol Chem* 2006;387(6):807–811.
130. Diamandis EP, Yousef GM, Soosaipillai AR, et al. Human kallikrein 6 (zyme/protease M/neurosin): a new serum biomarker of ovarian carcinoma. *Clin Biochem* 2000;33(7):579–583.
131. Diamandis EP. Proteomic patterns in serum and identification of ovarian cancer. *Lancet* 2002;360(9327):170; author reply 170–171.
132. Davidson B, Xi Z, Klokk TI, et al. Kallikrein 4 expression is up-regulated in epithelial ovarian carcinoma cells in effusions. *Am J Clin Pathol* 2005;123(3):360–368.
133. Paliouras M, Borgono C, Diamandis EP. Human tissue kallikreins: the cancer biomarker family. *Cancer Lett* 2007;249(1):61–79.
134. Oikonomopoulou K, Scorilas A, Michael IP, et al. Kallikreins as markers of disseminated tumour cells in ovarian cancer—a pilot study. *Tumour Biol* 2006;27(2):104–114.
135. Borgono CA, Kishi T, Scorilas A, et al. Human kallikrein 8 protein is a favorable prognostic marker in ovarian cancer. *Clin Cancer Res* 2006;12(5): 1487–1493.
136. Shan SJ, Scorilas A, Katsaros D, et al. Unfavorable prognostic value of human kallikrein 7 quantified by ELISA in ovarian cancer cytosols. *Clin Chem* 2006;52(10):1879–1886.
137. Chang K, Pastan I. Molecular cloning of mesothelin, a differentiation antigen present on mesothelium, mesotheliomas, and ovarian cancers. *Proc Natl Acad Sci USA* 1996;93(1):136–140.
138. Huang CY, Cheng WF, Lee CN, et al. Serum mesothelin in epithelial ovarian carcinoma: a new screening marker and prognostic factor. *Anticancer Res* 2006;26(6C):4721–4728.
139. Mok SC, Chao J, Skates S, et al. Prostasin, a potential serum marker for ovarian cancer: identification through microarray technology. *J Natl Cancer Inst* 2001;93(19):1458–1464.
140. Tiniakos DG, Yu H, Liapis H. Osteopontin expression in ovarian carcinomas and tumors of low malignant potential (LMP). *Hum Pathol* 1998;29(11): 1250–1254.
141. Kim JH, Skates SJ, Uede T, et al. Osteopontin as a potential diagnostic biomarker for ovarian cancer. *JAMA* 2002;287(13):1671–1679.
142. Nakae M, Iwamoto I, Fujino T, et al. Preoperative plasma osteopontin level as a biomarker complementary to carbohydrate antigen 125 in predicting ovarian cancer. *J Obstet Gynaecol Res* 2006;32(3):309–314.
143. Brakora KA, Lee H, Yusuf R, et al. Utility of osteopontin as a biomarker in recurrent epithelial ovarian cancer. *Gynecol Oncol* 2004;93(2):361–365.
144. Schorge JO, Drake RD, Lee H, et al. Osteopontin as an adjunct to CA125 in detecting recurrent ovarian cancer. *Clin Cancer Res* 2004;10(10):3474–3478.
145. Scambia G, Testa U, Panici PB, et al. Interleukin-6 serum levels in patients with gynecologic tumors. *Int J Cancer* 1994;57(3):318–323.
146. Scambia G, Testa U, Benedetti Panici P, et al. Prognostic significance of interleukin 6 serum levels in patients with ovarian cancer. *Br J Cancer* 1995;71(2):354–356.
147. Schroder W, Ruppert C, Bender HG. Concomitant measurements of interleukin-6 (IL-6) in serum and peritoneal fluid of patients with benign and malignant ovarian tumors. *Eur J Obstet Gynecol Reprod Biol* 1994;56(1): 43–46.
148. Plante M, Rubin SC, Wong GY, et al. Interleukin-6 level in serum and ascites as a prognostic factor in patients with epithelial ovarian cancer. *Cancer* 1994;73(7):1882–1888.
149. Tempfer C, Zeisler H, Sliutz G, et al. Serum evaluation of interleukin 6 in ovarian cancer patients. *Gynecol Oncol* 1997;66(1):27–30.
150. Maccio A, Lai P, Santona MC, et al. High serum levels of soluble IL-2 receptor, cytokines, and C reactive protein correlate with impairment of T cell response in patients with advanced epithelial ovarian cancer. *Gynecol Oncol* 1998;69(3):248–252.
151. Garg R, Wollan M, Galic V, et al. Common polymorphism in interleukin 6 influences survival of women with ovarian and peritoneal carcinoma. *Gynecol Oncol* 2006;103(3):793–796.
152. Lambeck AJ, Crijns AP, Leffers N, et al. Serum cytokine profiling as a diagnostic and prognostic tool in ovarian cancer: a potential role for interleukin 7. *Clin Cancer Res* 2007;13(8):2385–2391.
153. Barton DP, Blanchard DK, Michelini-Norris B, et al. Serum soluble interleukin-2 receptor alpha levels in patients with gynecologic cancers: early effect of surgery. *Am J Reprod Immunol* 1993;30(2-3):202–206.
154. Ferdeghini M, Gadducci A, Prontera C, et al. Serum soluble interleukin-2 receptor assay in epithelial ovarian cancer. *Tumour Biol* 1993;14(5): 303–309.
155. Hurteau JA, Woolas RP, Jacobs IJ, et al. Soluble interleukin-2 receptor alpha is elevated in sera of patients with benign ovarian neoplasms and epithelial ovarian cancer. *Cancer* 1995;76(9):1615–1620.
156. Gadducci A, Ferdeghini M, Malagnino G, et al. Elevated serum levels of neopterin and soluble interleukin-2 receptor in patients with ovarian cancer. *Gynecol Oncol* 1994;52(3):386–391.
157. Pavlidis NA, Bairaktari E, Kalef-Ezra J, et al. Serum soluble interleukin-2 receptors in epithelial ovarian cancer patients. *Int J Biol Markers* 1995;10(2):75–80.
158. de Bruijn HW, ten Hoor KA, van der Zee AG. Serum and cystic fluid levels of soluble interleukin-2 receptor-alpha in patients with epithelial ovarian tumors are correlated. *Tumour Biol* 1998;19(3):160–166.
159. Gadducci A, Ferdeghini M, Castellani C, et al. Serum levels of tumor necrosis factor (TNF), soluble receptors for TNF (55- and 75-kDa sTNFr), and soluble CD14 (sCD14) in epithelial ovarian cancer. *Gynecol Oncol* 1995;58(2):184–188.
160. Darai E, Detchev R, Hugol D, et al. Serum and cyst fluid levels of interleukin (IL) -6, IL-8 and tumour necrosis factor-alpha in women with endometriomas and benign and malignant cystic ovarian tumours. *Hum Reprod* 2003;18(8):1681–1685.
161. Grosen EA, Granger GA, Gatanaga M, et al. Measurement of the soluble membrane receptors for tumor necrosis factor and lymphotoxin in the sera of patients with gynecologic malignancy. *Gynecol Oncol* 1993;50(1):68–77.
162. Rzymski P, Opala T, Wilczak M, et al. Serum tumor necrosis factor alpha receptors p55/p75 ratio and ovarian cancer detection. *Int J Gynaecol Obstet* 2005;88(3):292–298.
163. Suzuki M, Ohwada M, Sato I, et al. Serum level of macrophage colony-stimulating factor as a marker for gynecologic malignancies. *Oncology* 1995;52(2):128–133.

164. Price FV, Chambers SK, Chambers JT, et al. Colony-stimulating factor-1 in primary ascites of ovarian cancer is a significant predictor of survival. *Am J Obstet Gynecol* 1993;168(2):520–527.
165. Woolas RP, Xu FJ, Jacobs IJ, et al. Elevation of multiple serum markers in patients with stage I ovarian cancer. *J Natl Cancer Inst* 1993;85(21): 1748–1751.
166. Suzuki M, Kobayashi H, Ohwada M, et al. Macrophage colony-stimulating factor as a marker for malignant germ cell tumors of the ovary. *Gynecol Oncol* 1998;68(1):35–37.
167. Suzuki M, Ohwada M, Aida I, et al. Macrophage colony-stimulating factor as a tumor marker for epithelial ovarian cancer. *Obstet Gynecol* 1993;82(6):946–950.
168. Gadducci A, Ferdeghini M, Castellani C, et al. Serum macrophage colony-stimulating factor (M-CSF) levels in patients with epithelial ovarian cancer. *Gynecol Oncol* 1998;70(1):111–114.
169. Salman T, el-Ahmady O, Sawsan MR, et al. The clinical value of serum TPS in gynecologic malignancies. *Int J Biol Markers* 1995;10(2):81–86.
170. Shabana A, Onsrud M. Tissue polypeptide-specific antigen and CA 125 as serum tumor markers in ovarian carcinoma. *Tumour Biol* 1994;15(6): 361–367.
171. Sliutz G, Tempfer C, Kainz C, et al. Tissue polypeptide specific antigen and cancer associated serum antigen in the follow-up of ovarian cancer. *Anticancer Res* 1995;15(3):1127–1129.
172. Tempfer C, Hefler L, Haeusler G, et al. Tissue polypeptide specific antigen in the follow-up of ovarian and cervical cancer patients. *Int J Cancer* 1998;79(3):241–244.
173. Harlozinska A, Sedlaczek P, Van Dalen A, et al. TPS and CA 125 levels in serum, cyst fluid and ascites of patients with epithelial ovarian neoplasms. *Anticancer Res* 1997;17(6D):4473–4478.
174. Stieber P, Bodenmuller H, Banauch D, et al. Cytokeratin 19 fragments: a new marker for non-small-cell lung cancer. *Clin Biochem* 1993;26(4): 301–304.
175. Inaba N, Negishi Y, Fukasawa I, et al. Cytokeratin fragment 21-1 in gynecologic malignancy: comparison with cancer antigen 125 and squamous cell carcinoma-related antigen. *Tumour Biol* 1995;16(6):345–352.
176. Hasholzner U, Baumgartner L, Stieber P, et al. Significance of the tumour markers CA 125 II, CA 72-4, CASA and CYFRA 21-1 in ovarian carcinoma. *Anticancer Res* 1994;14(6B):2743–2746.
177. Tempfer C, Hefler L, Heinzl H, et al. CYFRA 21-1 serum levels in women with adnexal masses and inflammatory diseases. *Br J Cancer* 1998;78(8): 1108–1112.
178. Gadducci A, Ferdeghini M, Cosio S, et al. The clinical relevance of serum CYFRA 21-1 assay in patients with ovarian cancer. *Int J Gynecol Cancer* 2001;11(4):277–282.
179. Lenhard M, Kuemper C, Ditsch N, et al. Use of novel serum markers in clinical follow-up of Sertoli-Leydig cell tumours. *Clin Chem Lab Med* 2007;45(5):657–661.
180. Wilkins MR, Sanchez JC, Gooley AA, et al. Progress with proteome projects: why all proteins expressed by a genome should be identified and how to do it. *Biotechnol Genet Eng Rev* 1996;13:19–50.
181. Reynolds T. For proteomics research, a new race has begun. *J Natl Cancer Inst* 2002;94(8):552–554.
182. Wilkins MR, Sanchez JC, Williams KL, et al. Current challenges and future applications for protein maps and post-translational vector maps in proteome projects. *Electrophoresis* 1996;17(5):830–838.
183. Plebani M. Proteomics: the next revolution in laboratory medicine? *Clin Chim Acta* 2005;357(2):113–122.
184. Baak JP, Path FR, Hermsen MA, et al. Genomics and proteomics in cancer. *Eur J Cancer* 2003;39(9):1199–1215.
185. Mills GB, Bast RC Jr, Srivastava S. Future for ovarian cancer screening: novel markers from emerging technologies of transcriptional profiling and proteomics. *J Natl Cancer Inst* 2001;93(19):1437–1439.
186. Petricoin EF, Ardekani AM, Hitt BA, et al. Use of proteomic patterns in serum to identify ovarian cancer. *Lancet* 2002;359(9306):572–577.
187. Rockhill B. Proteomic patterns in serum and identification of ovarian cancer. *Lancet* 2002;360(9327):169; author reply 170–171.
188. Pearl DC. Proteomic patterns in serum and identification of ovarian cancer. *Lancet* 2002;360(9327):169–70; author reply 170–171.
189. Elwood M. Proteomic patterns in serum and identification of ovarian cancer. *Lancet* 2002;360(9327):170; author reply 170–171.
190. Zhang Z, Bast RC Jr, Yu Y, et al. Three biomarkers identified from serum proteomic analysis for the detection of early stage ovarian cancer. *Cancer Res* 2004;64(16):5882–5890.
191. Moore LE, Fung ET, McGuire M, et al. Evaluation of apolipoprotein A1 and posttranslationally modified forms of transthyretin as biomarkers for ovarian cancer detection in an independent study population. *Cancer Epidemiol Biomarkers Prev* 2006;15(9):1641–1646.
192. Lin YW, Lin CY, Lai HC, et al. Plasma proteomic pattern as biomarkers for ovarian cancer. *Int J Gynecol Cancer* 2006;16(Suppl 1):139–146.
193. Timms JF, Arslan-Low E, Gentry-Maharaj A, et al. Preanalytic influence of sample handling on SELDI-TOF serum protein profiles. *Clin Chem* 2007;53(4):645–656.
194. Bengtsson S, Krogh M, Szigyarto CA, et al. Large-scale proteomics analysis of human ovarian cancer for biomarkers. *J Proteome Res* 2007;6(4): 1440–1450.
195. Zhu Y, Wu R, Sangha N, et al. Classifications of ovarian cancer tissues by proteomic patterns. *Proteomics* 2006;6(21):5846–5856.
196. Morita A, Miyagi E, Yasumitsu H, et al. Proteomic search for potential diagnostic markers and therapeutic targets for ovarian clear cell adenocarcinoma. *Proteomics* 2006;6(21):5880–5890.
197. Fushiki T, Fujisawa H, and Eguchi S. Identification of biomarkers from mass spectrometry data using a "common" peak approach. *BMC Bioinformatics* 2006;7:358.
198. Oh JH, Gao J, Nandi A, et al. Diagnosis of early relapse in ovarian cancer using serum proteomic profiling. *Genome Inform* 2005;16(2):195–204.
199. Bast RC Jr, Badgwell D, Lu Z, et al. New tumor markers: CA125 and beyond. *Int J Gynecol Cancer* 2005;15(Suppl 3):274–281.
200. van der Merwe DE, Oikonomopoulou K, Marshall J, et al. Mass spectrometry: uncovering the cancer proteome for diagnostics. *Adv Cancer Res* 2007;96:23–50.
201. Denkert C, Budczies J, Kind T, et al. Mass spectrometry-based metabolic profiling reveals different metabolite patterns in invasive ovarian carcinomas and ovarian borderline tumors. *Cancer Res* 2006;66(22):10795–10804.
202. Scambia G, Benedetti Panici P, Baiocchi G, et al. CA 15-3 serum levels in ovarian cancer. *Oncology* 1988;45(3):263–267.
203. Bast RC Jr, Knauf S, Epenetos A, et al. Coordinate elevation of serum markers in ovarian cancer but not in benign disease. *Cancer* 1991;68(8):1758–1763.
204. Soper JT, Hunter VJ, Daly L, et al. Preoperative serum tumor-associated antigen levels in women with pelvic masses. *Obstet Gynecol* 1990;75(2): 249–254.
205. Scambia G, Benedetti Panici P, Perrone L, et al. Serum levels of tumour associated glycoprotein (TAG 72) in patients with gynaecological malignancies. *Br J Cancer* 1990;62(1):147–151.
206. Negishi Y, Iwabuchi H, Sakunaga H, et al. Serum and tissue measurements of CA72-4 in ovarian cancer patients. *Gynecol Oncol* 1993;48(2):148–154.
207. Hasholzner U, Baumgartner L, Stieber P, et al. Clinical significance of the tumour markers CA 125 II and CA 72-4 in ovarian carcinoma. *Int J Cancer* 1996;69(4):329–334.
208. Guadagni F, Roselli M, Cosimelli M, et al. CA 72-4 serum marker—a new tool in the management of carcinoma patients. *Cancer Invest* 1995;13(2): 227–238.
209. Schutter EM, Sohn C, Kristen P, et al. Estimation of probability of malignancy using a logistic model combining physical examination, ultrasound, serum CA 125, and serum CA 72-4 in postmenopausal women with a pelvic mass: an international multicenter study. *Gynecol Oncol* 1998;69(1): 56–63.
210. Gocze PM, Szabo DG, Than GN, et al. Occurrence of CA 125 and CA 19-9 tumor-associated antigens in sera of patients with gynecologic, trophoblastic, and colorectal tumors. *Gynecol Obstet Invest* 1988;25(4):268–272.
211. Dede M, Gungor S, Yenen MC, et al. CA19-9 may have clinical significance in mature cystic teratomas of the ovary. *Int J Gynecol Cancer* 2006;16(1): 189–193.
212. Muramatsu T, Mukai M, Sato S, et al. Clinical usefulness of serum and immunohistochemical markers in patients with stage Ia and Ic ovarian cancer. *Oncol Rep* 2005;14(4):861–865.
213. Xu FJ, Yu YH, Li BY, et al. Development of two new monoclonal antibodies reactive to a surface antigen present on human ovarian epithelial cancer cells. *Cancer Res* 1991;51(15):4012–4019.
214. Xu FJ, Yu YH, Daly L, et al. OVX1 radioimmunoassay complements CA-125 for predicting the presence of residual ovarian carcinoma at second-look surgical surveillance procedures. *J Clin Oncol* 1993;11(8):1506–1510.
215. Woolas RP, Conaway MR, Xu F, et al. Combinations of multiple serum markers are superior to individual assays for discriminating malignant from benign pelvic masses. *Gynecol Oncol* 1995;59(1):111–116.
216. van Haaften-Day C, Shen Y, Xu F, et al. OVX1, macrophage-colony stimulating factor, and CA-125-II as tumor markers for epithelial ovarian carcinoma: a critical appraisal. *Cancer* 2001;92(11):2837–2844.
217. Berek JS, Bast RC Jr. Ovarian cancer screening. The use of serial complementary tumor markers to improve sensitivity and specificity for early detection. *Cancer* 1995;76(10 Suppl):2092–2096.
218. Devine PL, McGuckin MA, Ramm LE, et al. Serum mucin antigens CASA and MSA in tumors of the breast, ovary, lung, pancreas, bladder, colon, and prostate. A blind trial with 420 patients. *Cancer* 1993;72(6):2007–2015.
219. McGuckin MA, Layton GT, Bailey MJ, et al. Evaluation of two new assays for tumor-associated antigens, CASA and OSA, found in the serum of patients with epithelial ovarian carcinoma—comparison with CA125. *Gynecol Oncol* 1990;37(2):165–171.
220. Ward BG, McGuckin MA, Ramm LE, et al. The management of ovarian carcinoma is improved by the use of cancer-associated serum antigen and CA 125 assays. *Cancer* 1993;71(2):430–438.
221. Kierkegaard O, Mogensen O, Mogensen B, et al. Predictive and prognostic values of cancer-associated serum antigen (CASA) and cancer antigen 125 (CA 125) levels prior to second-look laparotomy for ovarian cancer. *Gynecol Oncol* 1995;59(2):251–254.
222. Meisel M, Straube W, Weise J, et al. A study of serum CASA and CA 125 levels in patients with ovarian carcinoma. *Arch Gynecol Obstet* 1995; 256(1):9–15.
223. Gronlund B, Dehn H, Hogdall CK, et al. Cancer-associated serum antigen level: a novel prognostic indicator for survival in patients with recurrent ovarian carcinoma. *Int J Gynecol Cancer* 2005;15(5):836–843.

224. Gronlund B, Hogdall EV, Christensen IJ, et al. Pre-treatment prediction of chemoresistance in second-line chemotherapy of ovarian carcinoma: value of serological tumor marker determination (tetranectin, YKL-40, CASA, CA 125). *Int J Biol Markers* 2006;21(3):141–148.
225. Lancaster JM, Sayer RA, Blanchette C, et al. High expression of insulin-like growth factor binding protein-2 messenger RNA in epithelial ovarian cancers produces elevated preoperative serum levels. *Int J Gynecol Cancer* 2006;16(4):1529–1535.
226. Flyvbjerg A, Mogensen O, Mogensen B, et al. Elevated serum insulin-like growth factor-binding protein 2 (*IGFBP-2*) and decreased IGFBP-3 in epithelial ovarian cancer: correlation with cancer antigen 125 and tumor-associated trypsin inhibitor. *J Clin Endocrinol Metab* 1997;82(7):2308–2313.
227. Peeters PH, Lukanova A, Allen N, et al. Serum IGF-I, its major binding protein (IGFBP-3) and epithelial ovarian cancer risk: the European Prospective Investigation into Cancer and Nutrition (EPIC). *Endocr Relat Cancer* 2007;14(1):81–90.
228. Hogdall CK, Mogensen O, Tabor A, et al. The role of serum tetranectin, CA 125, and a combined index as tumor markers in women with pelvic tumors. *Gynecol Oncol* 1995;56(1):22–28.
229. Hogdall CK, Hogdall EV, Hording U, et al. Pre-operative plasma tetranectin as a prognostic marker in ovarian cancer patients. *Scand J Clin Lab Invest* 1993;53(7):741–746.
230. Hogdall CK, Hording U, Norgaard-Pedersen B, et al. Serum tetranectin and CA-125 used to monitor the course of treatment in ovarian cancer patients. *Eur J Obstet Gynecol Reprod Biol* 1994;57(3):175–178.
231. Hogdall CK, Hogdall EV, Hording U, et al. Use of tetranectin, CA-125 and CASA to predict residual tumor and survival at second- and third-look operations for ovarian cancer. *Acta Oncol* 1996;35(1):63–69.
232. Halila H, Huhtala ML, Haglund C, et al. Tumour-associated trypsin inhibitor (TATI) in human ovarian cyst fluid. Comparison with CA 125 and CEA. *Br J Cancer* 1987;56(2):153–156.
233. Medl M, Ogris E, Peters-Engl C, et al. TATI (tumour-associated trypsin inhibitor) as a marker of ovarian cancer. *Br J Cancer* 1995;71(5): 1051–1504.
234. Peters-Engl C, Medl M, Ogris E, et al. Tumor-associated trypsin inhibitor (TATI) and cancer antigen 125 (CA125) in patients with epithelial ovarian cancer. *Anticancer Res* 1995;15(6B):2727–2730.
235. Antila R, Jalkanen J, Heikinheimo O. Comparison of secondary and primary ovarian malignancies reveals differences in their pre- and perioperative characteristics. *Gynecol Oncol* 2006;101(1):97–101.
236. Venesmaa P, Stenman UH, Forss M, et al. Pre-operative serum level of tumour-associated trypsin inhibitor and residual tumour size as prognostic indicators in Stage III epithelial ovarian cancer. *Br J Obstet Gynaecol* 1998;105(5):508–511.
237. Paju A, Vartiainen J, Haglund C, et al. Expression of trypsinogen-1, trypsinogen-2, and tumor-associated trypsin inhibitor in ovarian cancer: prognostic study on tissue and serum. *Clin Cancer Res* 2004;10(14): 4761–4768.
238. Udagawa Y, Aoki D, Ito K, et al. Clinical characteristics of a newly developed ovarian tumour marker, galactosyltransferase associated with tumour (GAT). *Eur J Cancer* 1998;34(4):489–495.
239. Nozawa S, Udagawa Y, Ito K, et al. Clinical significance of galactosyltransferase associated with tumor (GAT), a new tumor marker for ovarian cancer—with special reference to the discrimination between ovarian cancer and endometriosis. *Gan To Kagaku Ryoho* 1994;21(4):507–516.
240. Saitoh E, Aoki D, Susumu N, et al. Galactosyltransferase associated with tumor in patients with ovarian cancer: factors involved in elevation of serum galactosyltransferase. *Int J Oncol* 2003;23(2):303–310.
241. Schutter EM, Visser JJ, van Kamp GJ, et al. The utility of lipid-associated sialic acid (LASA or LSA) as a serum marker for malignancy. A review of the literature. *Tumour Biol* 1992;13(3):121–132.
242. Petru E, Sevin BU, Averette HE, et al. Comparison of three tumor markers—CA-125, lipid-associated sialic acid (LSA), and NB/70K—in monitoring ovarian cancer. *Gynecol Oncol* 1990;38(2):181–186.
243. Schwartz PE, Chambers JT, Taylor KJ, et al. Early detection of ovarian cancer: preliminary results of the Yale Early Detection Program. *Yale J Biol Med* 1991;64(6):573–582.
244. Crump C, McIntosh MW, Urban N, et al. Ovarian cancer tumor marker behavior in asymptomatic healthy women: implications for screening. *Cancer Epidemiol Biomarkers Prev* 2000;9(10):1107–1111.
245. Obermair A, Tempfer C, Hefler L, et al. Concentration of vascular endothelial growth factor (VEGF) in the serum of patients with suspected ovarian cancer. *Br J Cancer* 1998;77(11):1870–1874.
246. Hefler LA, Zeillinger R, Grimm C, et al. Preoperative serum vascular endothelial growth factor as a prognostic parameter in ovarian cancer. *Gynecol Oncol* 2006;103(2):512–517.
247. Castelli M, Battaglia F, Scambia G, et al. Immunosuppressive acidic protein and CA 125 levels in patients with ovarian cancer. *Oncology* 1991;48(1):13–17.
248. Scambia G, Foti E, Ferrandina G, et al. Prognostic role of immunosuppressive acidic protein in advanced ovarian cancer. *Am J Obstet Gynecol* 1996;175(6):1606–1610.
249. Foti E, Ferrandina G, Martucci R, et al. IL-6, M-CSF and IAP cytokines in ovarian cancer: simultaneous assessment of serum levels. *Oncology* 1999;57(3):211–215.
250. Mills GB, May C, McGill M, et al. A putative new growth factor in ascitic fluid from ovarian cancer patients: identification, characterization, and mechanism of action. *Cancer Res* 1988;48(5):1066–1071.
251. Mills GB, May C, Hill M, et al. Ascitic fluid from human ovarian cancer patients contains growth factors necessary for intraperitoneal growth of human ovarian adenocarcinoma cells. *J Clin Invest* 1990;86(3):851–855.
252. Fang X, Gaudette D, Furui T, et al. Lysophospholipid growth factors in the initiation, progression, metastases, and management of ovarian cancer. *Ann N Y Acad Sci* 2000;905:188–208.
253. Xu FJ, Yu YH , Daly L, et al. *OVX1 as a marker for early stage endometrial carcinoma.* Cancer, 1994;73(7):p.1855–1858.
254. Westermann AM, Havik E, Postma FR, et al. Malignant effusions contain lysophosphatidic acid (LPA)-like activity. *Ann Oncol* 1998;9(4): 437–442.
255. Xu Y, Shen Z, Wiper DW, et al. Lysophosphatidic acid as a potential biomarker for ovarian and other gynecologic cancers. *JAMA* 1998;280(8): 719–723.
256. Bast RC Jr, Xu FJ, Yu YH, et al. CA 125: the past and the future. *Int J Biol Markers* 1998;13(4):179–187.
257. Widschwendter M, Menon U. Circulating methylated DNA: a new generation of tumor markers. *Clin Cancer Res* 2006;12(24):7205–7208.
258. Jones PA, Baylin SB. The fundamental role of epigenetic events in cancer. *Nat Rev Genet* 2002;3(6):415–428.
259. Jen J, Wu L, Sidransky D. An overview on the isolation and analysis of circulating tumor DNA in plasma and serum. *Ann N Y Acad Sci* 2000; 906:8–12.
260. Laird PW. The power and the promise of DNA methylation markers. *Nat Rev Cancer* 2003;3(4):253–266.
261. Wallner M, Herbst A, Behrens A, et al. Methylation of serum DNA is an independent prognostic marker in colorectal cancer. *Clin Cancer Res* 2006;12(24):7347–7352.
262. Sivertsen S, Berner A, Michael CW, et al. Cadherin expression in ovarian carcinoma and malignant mesothelioma cell effusions. *Acta Cytol* 2006;50(6):603–607.
263. Cottingham K. Shed glycans as possible markers for ovarian cancer. *J Proteome Res* 2006;5(7):1525.
264. An HJ, Miyamoto S, Lancaster KS, et al. Profiling of glycans in serum for the discovery of potential biomarkers for ovarian cancer. *J Proteome Res* 2006;5(7):1626–1635.
265. Hakala A, Kacinski BM, Stanley ER, et al. Macrophage colony-stimulating factor 1, a clinically useful tumor marker in endometrial adenocarcinoma: comparison with CA 125 and the aminoterminal propeptide of type III procollagen. *Am J Obstet Gynecol* 1995;173(1):112–119.
266. Patsner B, Orr JW Jr, Mann WJ Jr. Use of serum CA 125 measurement in posttreatment surveillance of early-stage endometrial carcinoma. *Am J Obstet Gynecol* 1990;162(2):427–429.
267. Takeshima N, Shimizu Y, Umezawa S, et al. Combined assay of serum levels of CA125 and CA19-9 in endometrial carcinoma. *Gynecol Oncol* 1994;54(3):321–326.
268. Lo SS, Cheng DK, Ng TY, et al. Prognostic significance of tumour markers in endometrial cancer. *Tumour Biol* 1997;18(4):241–249.
269. Gadducci A, Ferdeghini M, Prontera C, et al. A comparison of pretreatment serum levels of four tumor markers in patients with endometrial and cervical carcinoma. *Eur J Gynaecol Oncol* 1990;11(4):283–288.
270. Takami M, Sakamoto H, Ohtani K, et al. An evaluation of CA125 levels in 291 normal postmenopausal and 20 endometrial adenocarcinoma-bearing women before and after surgery. *Cancer Lett* 1997;121:69–72.
271. Kurihara T, Mizunuma H, Obara M, et al. Determination of a normal level of serum CA125 in postmenopausal women as a tool for preoperative evaluation and postoperative surveillance of endometrial carcinoma. *Gynecol Oncol* 1998;69(3):192–196.
272. Price FV, Chambers SK, Carcangiu ML, et al. CA 125 may not reflect disease status in patients with uterine serous carcinoma. *Cancer* 1998;82(9): 1720–1725.
273. Cole LA, Tanaka A, Kim GS, et al. Beta-core fragment (beta-core/UGF/UGP), a tumor marker: a 7-year report. *Gynecol Oncol* 1996;60(2):264–270.
274. Kinugasa M, Nishimura R, Koizumi T, et al. Combination assay of urinary beta-core fragment of human chorionic gonadotropin with serum tumor markers in gynecologic cancers. *Jpn J Cancer Res* 1995;86(8):783–789.
275. Matorras R, Rodriguez-Escuderoi FJ, Diez J, et al. Monitoring endometrial adenocarcinoma with a four tumor marker combination. CA 125, squamous cell carcinoma antigen, CA 19.9 and CA 15.3. *Acta Obstet Gynecol Scand* 1992;71(6):458–464.
276. Tomas C, Penttinen J, Risteli J, et al. Serum concentrations of CA 125 and aminoterminal propeptide of type III procollagen (PIIINP) in patients with endometrial carcinoma. *Cancer* 1990;66(11):2399–2406.
277. Ota Y, Inaba N, Shirotake S, et al. Enzyme immunoassay for placental protein 4 (PP4) and its possible diagnostic significance in patients with genital tract cancer. *Arch Gynecol Obstet* 1990;247(3):139–147.
278. Hareyama H, Sakuragi N, Makinoda S, et al. Serum and tissue measurements of CA72-4 in patients with endometrial carcinoma. *J Clin Pathol* 1996;49(12):967–970.
279. Ferdeghini M, Gadducci A, Prontera C, et al. Serum soluble interleukin-2 receptor (sIL-2R) assay in cervical and endometrial cancer. Preliminary data. *Anticancer Res* 1993;13(3):709–713.

280. Santin AD, Diamandis EP, Bellone S, et al. Human kallikrein 6: a new potential serum biomarker for uterine serous papillary cancer. *Clin Cancer Res* 2005;11(9):3320–3325.
281. Worbs S, Shabani N, Mayr D, et al. Expression of the inhibin/activin subunits (-alpha, -betaA and -betaB) in normal and carcinogenic endometrial tissue: possible immunohistochemical differentiation markers. *Oncol Rep* 2007;17(1):97–104.
282. Honkavuori M, Talvensaari-Mattila A, Soini Y, et al. MMP-2 expression associates with CA 125 and clinical course in endometrial carcinoma. *Gynecol Oncol* 2007;104(1):217–221.
283. Kato H, Torigoe T. Radioimmunoassay for tumor antigen of human cervical squamous cell carcinoma. *Cancer* 1977;40(4):1621–1628.
284. Lozza L, Merola M, Fontanelli R, et al. Cancer of the uterine cervix: clinical value of squamous cell carcinoma antigen (SCC) measurements. *Anticancer Res* 1997;17(1B):525–529.
285. Ngan HY, Cheung AN, Lauder IJ, et al. Prognostic significance of serum tumour markers in carcinoma of the cervix. *Eur J Gynaecol Oncol* 1996;17(6):512–517.
286. Yoon SM, Shin KH, Kim JY, et al. The clinical values of squamous cell carcinoma antigen and carcinoembryonic antigen in patients with cervical cancer treated with concurrent chemoradiotherapy. *Int J Gynecol Cancer* 2007;17(4):872–878.
287. Crombach G, Scharl A, Vierbuchen M, et al. Detection of squamous cell carcinoma antigen in normal squamous epithelia and in squamous cell carcinomas of the uterine cervix. *Cancer* 1989;63(7):1337–1342.
288. Duk JM, van Voorst Vader PC, ten Hoor KA, et al. Elevated levels of squamous cell carcinoma antigen in patients with a benign disease of the skin. *Cancer* 1989;64(8):1652–1656.
289. Bolger BS, Dabbas M, Lopes A, et al. Prognostic value of preoperative squamous cell carcinoma antigen level in patients surgically treated for cervical carcinoma. *Gynecol Oncol* 1997;65(2):309–313.
290. Duk JM, Groenier KH, de Bruijn HW, et al. Pretreatment serum squamous cell carcinoma antigen: a newly identified prognostic factor in early-stage cervical carcinoma. *J Clin Oncol* 1996;14(1):111–118.
291. Massuger LF, Koper NP, Thomas CM, et al. Improvement of clinical staging in cervical cancer with serum squamous cell carcinoma antigen and CA 125 determinations. *Gynecol Oncol* 1997;64(3):473–476.
292. Scambia G, Benedetti Panici P, Foti E, et al. Squamous cell carcinoma antigen: prognostic significance and role in the monitoring of neoadjuvant chemotherapy response in cervical cancer. *J Clin Oncol* 1994;12(11): 2309–2316.
293. Takeshima N, Hirai Y, Katase K, et al. The value of squamous cell carcinoma antigen as a predictor of nodal metastasis in cervical cancer. *Gynecol Oncol* 1998;68(3):263–266.
294. Gaarenstroom KN, Bonfrer JM, Kenter GG, et al. Clinical value of pretreatment serum Cyfra 21-1, tissue polypeptide antigen, and squamous cell carcinoma antigen levels in patients with cervical cancer. *Cancer* 1995;76(5):807–813.
295. Hong JH, Tsai CS, Chang JT, et al. The prognostic significance of pre- and posttreatment SCC levels in patients with squamous cell carcinoma of the cervix treated by radiotherapy. *Int J Radiat Oncol Biol Phys* 1998;41(4): 823–830.
296. Bonfrer JM, Gaarenstroom KN, Korse CM, et al. Cyfra 21-1 in monitoring cervical cancer: a comparison with tissue polypeptide antigen and squamous cell carcinoma antigen. *Anticancer Res* 1997;17(3C):2329–2334.
297. Scambia G, Benedetti P, Foti E, et al. Multiple tumour marker assays in advanced cervical cancer: relationship to chemotherapy response and clinical outcome. *Eur J Cancer* 1996;32A(2):259–263.
298. Bae SN, Namkoong SE, Jung JK, et al. Prognostic significance of pretreatment squamous cell carcinoma antigen and carcinoembryonic antigen in squamous cell carcinoma of the uterine cervix. *Gynecol Oncol* 1997;64(3): 418–424.
299. Pras E, Willemse PH, Canrinus AA, et al. Serum squamous cell carcinoma antigen and CYFRA 21-1 in cervical cancer treatment. *Int J Radiat Oncol Biol Phys* 2002;52(1):23–32.
300. Ogino I, Nakayama H, Okamoto N, et al. The role of pretreatment squamous cell carcinoma antigen level in locally advanced squamous cell carcinoma of the uterine cervix treated by radiotherapy. *Int J Gynecol Cancer* 2006;16(3):1094–1100.
301. Hung YC, Shiau YC, Chang WC, et al. Early predicting recurrent cervical cancer with combination of tissue polypeptide specific antigen (TPS) and squamous cell carcinoma antigen (SCC). *Neoplasma* 2002;49(6):415–417.
302. Gocze PM, Vahrson HW, Freeman DA. Serum levels of squamous cell carcinoma antigen and ovarian carcinoma antigen (CA 125) in patients with benign and malignant diseases of the uterine cervix. *Oncology* 1994; 51(5):430–434.
303. Rose PG, Baker S, Fournier L, et al. Serum squamous cell carcinoma antigen levels in invasive cervical cancer: prediction of response and recurrence. *Am J Obstet Gynecol* 1993;168(3 Pt 1):942–946.
304. Hsu KF, Huang SC, Shiau AL, et al. Increased expression level of squamous cell carcinoma antigen 2 and 1 ratio is associated with poor prognosis in early-stage uterine cervical cancer. *Int J Gynecol Cancer*, 2007. 17(1):p.174–81.
305. Roijer E, de Bruijn HW, Dahlen U, et al. Squamous cell carcinoma antigen isoforms in serum from cervical cancer patients. *Tumour Biol* 2006;27(3): 142–152.
306. Tsai SC, Kao CH, Wang SJ. Study of a new tumor marker, CYFRA 21-1, in squamous cell carcinoma of the cervix, and comparison with squamous cell carcinoma antigen. *Neoplasma* 1996;43(1):27–29.
307. Bonfrer JM, Gaarenstroom KN, Kenter GG, et al. Prognostic significance of serum fragments of cytokeratin 19 measured by Cyfra 21-1 in cervical cancer. *Gynecol Oncol* 1994;55(3 Pt 1):371–375.
308. Ferdeghini M, Gadducci A, Annicchiarico C, et al. Serum CYFRA 21-1 assay in squamous cell carcinoma of the cervix. *Anticancer Res* 1993; 13(5C):1841–1844.
309. Callet N, Cohen-Solal Le Nir CC, Berthelot E, et al. Cancer of the uterine cervix: sensitivity and specificity of serum Cyfra 21.1 determinations. *Eur J Gynaecol Oncol* 1998;19(1):50–56.
310. Duk JM, Aalders JG, Fleuren GJ, et al. Tumor markers CA 125, squamous cell carcinoma antigen, and carcinoembryonic antigen in patients with adenocarcinoma of the uterine cervix. *Obstet Gynecol* 1989;73(4):661–668.
311. Borras G, Molina R, Xercavins J, et al. Tumor antigens CA 19.9, CA 125, and CEA in carcinoma of the uterine cervix. *Gynecol Oncol* 1995;57(2): 205–211.
312. Avall-Lundqvist EH, Sjovall K, Nilsson BR, et al. Prognostic significance of pretreatment serum levels of squamous cell carcinoma antigen and CA 125 in cervical carcinoma. *Eur J Cancer* 1992;28A(10):1695–1702.
313. Duk JM, De Bruijn HW, Groenier KH, et al. Adenocarcinoma of the uterine cervix. Prognostic significance of pretreatment serum CA 125, squamous cell carcinoma antigen, and carcinoembryonic antigen levels in relation to clinical and histopathologic tumor characteristics. *Cancer* 1990;65(8):1830–1837.
314. Leminen A, Alftan H, Stenman UH, et al. Chemotherapy as initial treatment for cervical carcinoma: clinical and tumor marker response. *Acta Obstet Gynecol Scand* 1992;71(4):293–297.
315. Lam CP, Yuan CC, Jeng FS, et al. Evaluation of carcinoembryonic antigen, tissue polypeptide antigen, and squamous cell carcinoma antigen in the detection of cervical cancers. *Zhonghua Yi Xue Za Zhi (Taipei)* 1992;50(1):7–13.
316. Nam JH, Chang KC, Chambers JT, et al. Urinary gonadotropin fragment, a new tumor marker. III. Use in cervical and vulvar cancers. *Gynecol Oncol* 1990;38(1):66–70.
317. Carter PG, Iles RK, Neven P, et al. Measurement of urinary beta core fragment of human chorionic gonadotrophin in women with vulvovaginal malignancy and its prognostic significance. *Br J Cancer* 1995;71(2):350–353.

CHAPTER 8 ■ CANCER PREVENTION STRATEGIES

MARY B. DALY

INTRODUCTION

The prevention of gynecologic cancer is becoming a reality due to the recognition that cancer initiation and progression is a multistep process characterized by distinct molecular genetic events that provide opportunities to intervene in the carcinogenic process at several steps and reverse its early stages. The concept of preventing gynecologic cancer is based on an understanding of causally related risk factors, their role in carcinogenesis, and opportunities for their avoidance and/or reversal of their effect. There are three distinct models that can be applied to gynecologic cancer prevention: (a) *risk avoidance and adoption of protective practices* includes the identification of key risk factors and the development of strategies for their avoidance. Included in risk avoidance are the avoidance of exogenous and endogenous exposures (chemical, hormonal, infectious, etc.) and the avoidance of risky health behaviors. The adoption of protective practices, such as vaccination with the human papillomavirus (HPV) vaccine, a healthy diet, and exercise, may forestall early premalignant events; (b) the use of *chemopreventive agents*, both natural and synthetic, to reverse early, premalignant changes; and (c) *surgical prophylaxis* to remove either healthy at-risk organs or tissues with premalignant changes.

In addition to establishing valid interventions for cancer prevention, it is important to identify optimal target populations for their application, and to tailor the interventions to the level of risk. Interventions for use in the general population at average risk must be highly effective, safe, inexpensive, and socially acceptable. Population groups with high risks may tolerate interventions that confer more risk and higher costs. All prevention efforts are greatly enhanced by public and professional education about their use and by a health care system that values, promotes, and invests in prevention activities.

The avoidance of environmental, occupational, and lifestyle risk factors through public education and social policies has the potential to prevent a large proportion of human cancer. The epidemiological literature has provided a wealth of information about the risks associated with cancers of the cervix, uterus, and ovary, which allows us to devise risk avoidance and risk reduction strategies. This chapter focuses on the opportunities for primary prevention of these three cancers and directions for the future.

CERVIX CANCER

Risk Factors

There are approximately 14,000 new cases of cervical cancer per year in the United States, and 5,000 women die of the disease. The disease burden is not distributed equally but is overrepresented among African American, Mexican American, American Indian, Vietnamese American, and rural poor women (1). The burden of cervical cancer is worldwide (Fig. 8.1), where 470,000 new cases are diagnosed each year, and 250,000 women die of the disease (2). Traditionally, the most significant factor associated with the risk of cervical cancer has been number of sexual partners and the early onset of sexual activity. This observation has led to the discovery that the primary cause of cervical cancer, and its precursor, intraepithelial lesions, is persistent infection with HPV, which is sexually transmitted. The HPVs are a large (over 100 types, Fig. 8.2) family of viruses that infect skin and mucosa. Of the approximately 40 HPV types that infect the genital tract, about one half are associated with anogenital warts and are considered low risk for malignancy, or non-oncogenic. The other half may give rise to a range of anogenital cancers, including cervix, vulva, and anus in women, and penis and anus in men, and are referred to as high-risk or oncogenic (3). HPV types 16 and 18 alone account for >70% (Fig. 8.3) of all cervical cancers. Similarly, HPV types 6 and 11 account for >90% of all anogenital warts. In the United States, close to 20% of girls are sexually active by age 15 years, and close to 60% are sexually active at age 18 years. As a result, the infection rate of HPV among the general population is high, peaking in the second and third decades of life when infection rates range from 27% to 46% (1). The median length of infection is 8 to 12 months and most individuals have cleared the virus by two years. A small proportion, 10% to 13%, however, develop chronic persistent HPV infection, which can lead to genital warts, cervical dysplasia, carcinoma *in situ,* and invasive cancer (Fig. 8.4). Persistence of HPV infection is likely to be related to modifying factors, including immune status, the use of oral contraceptives (OCP), and smoking. Prolonged duration of OCP use is thought to function as a promoter of HPV-related carcinogenesis, not as a facilitator of HPV infection, although the mechanisms are uncertain (4). Tobacco carcinogens have been found in cervical secretions, and it is postulated that smoking constituents may interact with HPV to induce immunologic changes leading to cervical dysplasia, or may produce genomic damage via genotoxins (5,6).

The HPVs are nonenveloped, double-stranded DNA viruses whose circular DNA encodes eight genes, six early genes, which encode nonstructural proteins (E1, E2, E3, E4, E5, and E6) responsible for viral replication and transcription, and two late genes (L1 and L2), which encode the structural components of the viral capsid. HPV can infect the basal cells of the cervical epithelium and replicate in an extrachromosomal form. In HPV-related malignancy, the virus can integrate into cellular DNA and interact with p53 and RB (retinoblastoma), which prolongs the cell cycle, inhibits apoptosis, and can result in malignant transformation (2,7). Another potential mechanism for carcinogenesis that has been observed in HPV-16–infected

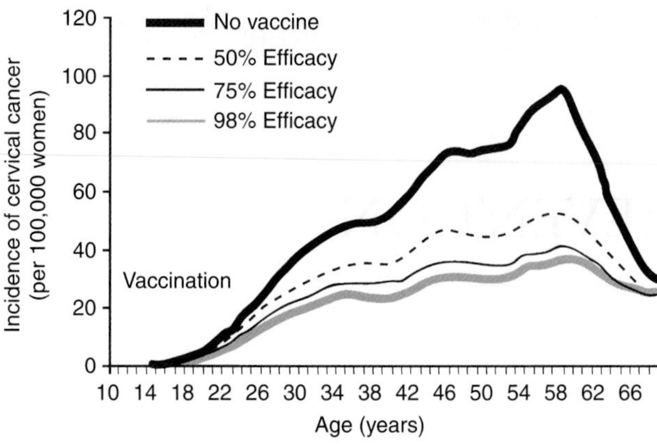

FIGURE 8.1. Age-standardized rates of new cases of cervical cancer per 100,000 women, 2002.

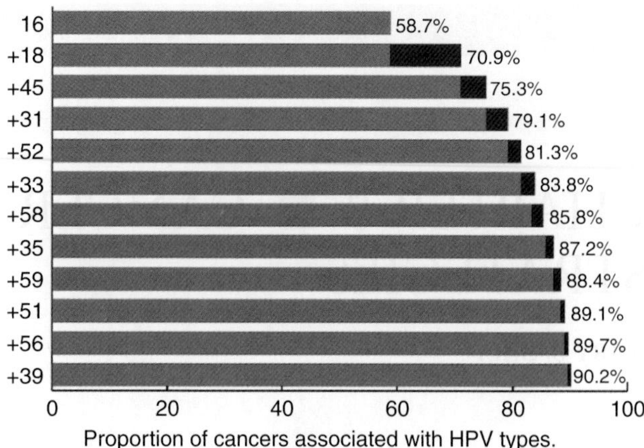

FIGURE 8.3. HPV types in cervical cancer.

cells is aberrant mitotic spindle pole formation resulting in genetic instability (8). The recent production of prophylactic vaccines that induce the generation of neutralizing antibodies to certain oncogenic types of HPV, therefore, represents a major breakthrough in the prevention of cervical cancer.

Prevention

Risk Reduction and/or Adoption of Healthy Practices

Cervical cancer prevention requires decreasing the risk of infection with oncogenic strains of HPV. Having few sexual partners and the use of condoms have been associated with a reduced risk for cervical cancer (9). Avoidance of those factors that enhance the persistence of HPV infection, viz. smoking and OCP use, has the potential to reduce the rate of malignant change. OCPs, however, are the most effective means of contraception, and their avoidance overall is not a wise public health strategy. Safe and effective vaccines now offer the best option for cervical cancer prevention. Early studies in animal models provided the proof of principle that neutralizing antibodies, directed to determinants on the major viral capsid protein, were generated by infection with HPV and could be detected in the serum. In the early 1990s it was found that the L1 protein, when expressed in recombinant vectors, self-assembled into virus-like particles (VLPs), which closely resemble the antigenic characteristics of the wild-type virions (10). VLPs formulated on aluminum adjuvants were shown to induce a strong virus-neutralizing antibody response in nonhuman primates (11,12), leading to their development for human populations. A series of phase 1 trials in humans tested the immunogenicity and safety of monovalent VLP-based vaccines and found that they generated levels of neutralizing antibodies that far exceeded those seen in natural infections, and were well tolerated. The predominant antibody responses are of the immunoglobulin GI (IgG1) subclass (3). Prevention of persistent HPV-16 and HPV-18 was also demonstrated, although only short-term follow-up was available (13).

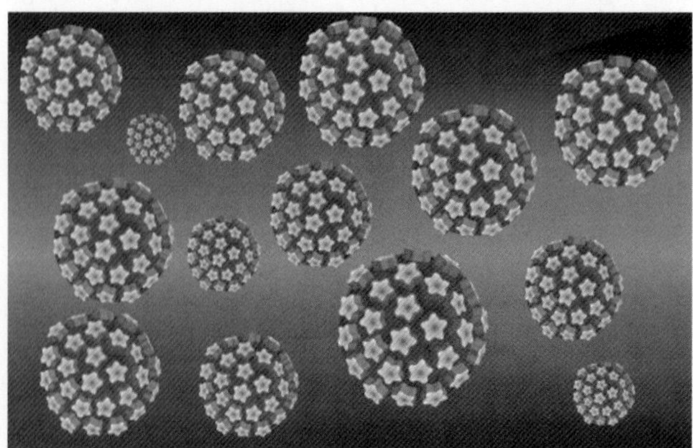

FIGURE 8.2. Human papillomavirus.

Subsequently, two vaccines have been developed for use in humans, Gardisal (Merck), a quadrivalent vaccine that includes HPV-16, -18, -6, and -11 and is formulated with aluminum adjuvant, and a bivalent vaccine Cervarix (GlaxoSmithKline), which includes HPV-16 and -18 and is formulated with a proprietary adjuvant, AS04, which contains aluminum and a bacterial lipid. Gardasil has undergone four randomized, placebo-controlled trials among a total of 20,583 women. In a U.S. multicenter proof of principle study, 2,391 young women aged 16 to 25 were assigned to a monovalent yeast-derived HPV-16L1 VLP, formulated on aluminum adjuvant, by intramuscular injection at day 0, month 2, and month 6 or placebo. The primary outcomes were persistent HPV-16 infection and HPV-16–related carcinoma *in situ* (CIN) 2 and 3. At a follow-up of 48 months, administration of the three-dose regimen of HPV-16 vaccine resulted in a 94% reduction in persistent HPV infection in those treated according to protocol. The vaccine was 100% effective in protecting against HPV-16–related CIN 2 and 3 (14).

A phase 2 dose-ranging assessment of immunogenicity and efficacy was conducted in the United States, Brazil, and Europe among 552 women aged 16 to 23 years. Women were randomized to one of three vaccine doses versus placebo given at day 1, month 2, and month 6. At close to 3 years of follow-up, vaccine efficacy for persistent HPV infection was 90% and for clinical disease (cytologic abnormalities, CIN, cervical cancer, or external genital lesions) was 100%. Vaccine efficacy was similar for each of the three doses. All women who received the vaccine developed high antibody titers by month 7 (15).

The two pivotal phase 3 trials enrolled >18,000 women and included both precancerous lesions, CIN 2, CIN 3, adenocarcinoma *in situ* (AIS), or invasive cervical cancer with documented HPV-16 or -18 in DNA from the involved tissue, vulvar and vaginal lesions, and genital warts as outcomes.

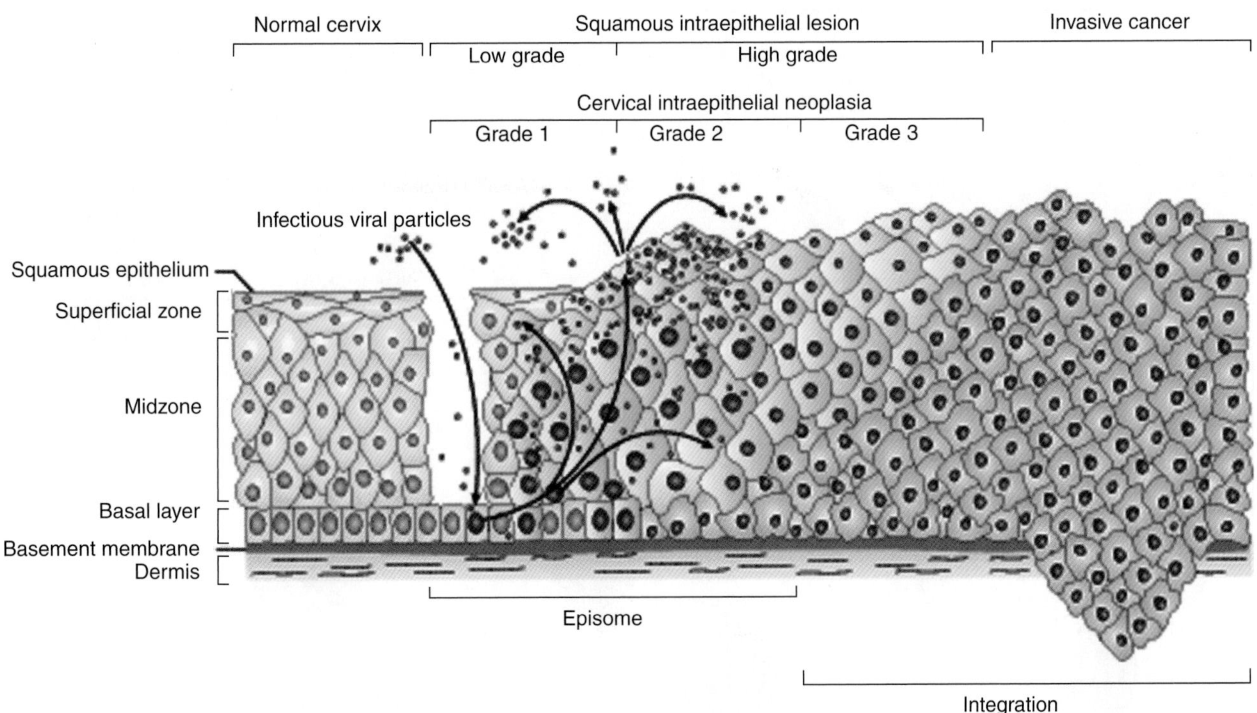

FIGURE 8.4. (*See color plate section.*) HPV-mediated progression to cervical cancer.

Women with evidence of previous infection with HPV, or with cytologic abnormalities, were not excluded. At 3 years, vaccine efficacy in those women treated according to protocol was 99%, with only one case of CIN 3 occurring among the vaccine recipients. In the intent to treat population, which included women with prevalent HPV-16/18 infection and women who did not complete the vaccination schedule, CIN 2/3 and AIS were reduced by 44% (16,17). The vaccine was also efficacious against high-grade vulval and vaginal lesions (18). Side effects in all of the studies were minimal and included discomfort at the injection site and occasional mild fever. Anti-HPV antibody titers remain high 5 years after administration. In June 2006, Gardasil received FDA approval for the vaccination of women aged 9 to 26, followed closely by approval for its use in children and adults aged 9 to 26 years by the European Commission.

The initial trial of Cervarix randomized 1,113 women aged 15 to 25 years to receive a bivalent HPV-16, -18 vaccine versus placebo. No cases of persistent HPV-16 or HPV-18 were seen in the women vaccinated according to protocol, whereas there were seven cases of infection in the control group. The vaccine was 95% effective against persistent infection and 93% effective against cytologic abnormalities even when including those women who did not complete the vaccine regimen. In an extended follow-up of 776 women, the vaccine continued to demonstrate 98% efficacy at close to 4 years. The bivalent vaccine also showed significant efficacy against two additional oncogenic strains, HPV-45 and -31 (13,19). A second study randomized 18,644 women to three doses of Cervarix versus hepatitis A vaccine. HPV vaccine efficacy, assessed in women who were seronegative DNA for HPV-16/18 at baseline, against CIN 2+ lesions was 90% at 14.8 months (20).

Overall, achieving close to 100% effective vaccination of a cohort of 12-year-old girls is estimated to result (Fig. 8.5) in a 76% reduction in the incidence of cervical cancer (21). Markov modeling has been used to estimate the clinical benefits and cost-effectiveness of a population-based HPV-16/18 vaccination program. Parameters considered were the natural history of HPV and cervical cancer, age at vaccination, vaccine cost, vaccine efficacy (Fig. 8.1), waning immunity, the risk of replacement with other oncogenic strains of HPV, age at onset of screening, and screening intervals. One model that combined vaccination at age 12 with triennial cytologic screening beginning at age 25 years resulted in a cost-effectiveness ratio of less than $60,000 per quality-adjusted life year (QALY) and a 94% reduction in a woman's lifetime risk of cervical cancer (22,23). Another model found that vaccination plus biennial cytologic screening beginning at age 24 years had the most attractive cost-effectiveness ratio ($44,889) (24). In both models, the combination of a highly effective vaccine, a delay in the onset of cytologic screening, and a decrease in colposcopy rates result in a cost-effective use of health care resources. The Advisory Committee on Immunization Practices (ACIP) of the Centers for Disease Control and Prevention (CDC) recommends routine vaccination for HPV of girls age 11 to 12 (range, 9 to 26 years) and has added Gardasil to its Vaccines for Children program (25,26). Similarly, the American Cancer Society recommends that all girls should be vaccinated against HPV at age 11 to 12 years.

There are several questions remaining regarding the use of HPV vaccines. The duration of protection afforded by HPV vaccines is not known, although data from animal models report long-lasting protection even with low levels of circulating antibody. Evidence from recent clinical trials in humans suggests persistence of immunity beyond 4 years. The need for a booster dose is at this time unknown. Because the neutralizing antibodies generated by the current vaccines appear to be type specific, it is not clear if there is cross-reactivity with other HPV types. It is also unclear whether vaccinating an adolescent population will be socially acceptable in all cultures. Most of the randomized trials performed to date focused on young women in their late teens and early 20s, an age when sexual activity has likely already begun. Because HPV vaccines are ineffective after infection with HPV, vaccination should

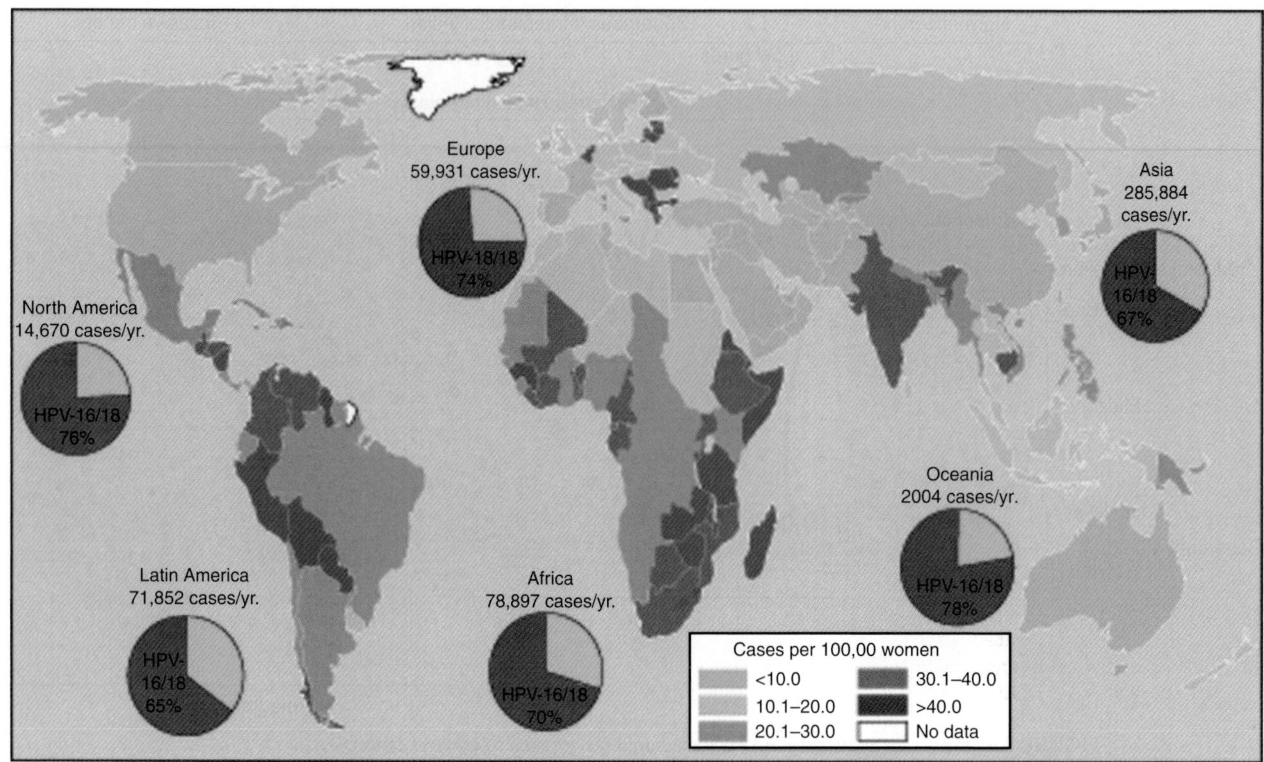

FIGURE 8.5. (*See color plate section.*) Impact of HPV-16/18 vaccines on incidence of cervical cancer.

occur prior to the onset of sexual activity, or at a younger age. The majority of females will become infected with HPV within 2 to 3 years of the onset of sexual activity. Depending on sociocultural variations in sexual debut, the target age for vaccination would ideally be girls aged 9 to 12. There is currently no systematic vaccination program beyond infancy and preschool in the United States. Although vaccinating older women who are uninfected with HPV is likely to induce an effective immune response, studies have shown that antibody response is higher among 10 to 15 year olds than among 16 to 23 year olds (14,27).

Another unanswered question is the added benefit of vaccinating males. Although the majority of morbidity associated with HPV is seen in females, males remain the major vector for the disease. Furthermore, both males and females would need to be vaccinated to achieve herd immunity. Information on the natural history of HPV in males is lacking, and vaccination studies to date have focused predominantly on females. A study is currently under way to evaluate the safety and effectiveness of Gardasil in males.

Among women, the impact of effective vaccination on subsequent screening practices is not known. There is concern that women who receive the HPV vaccine might be less likely to adhere to screening guidelines because they feel protected from cervical cancer. Women who have been vaccinated will, however, need to continue cytologic screening since the current vaccines do not protect against all oncogenic types, and since some women will have already been infected at the time of vaccination. It is likely, however, that the onset of screening could safely be delayed. Concerns about the impact of HPV vaccination on subsequent accuracy of cytologic screening have also been raised.

Much work remains to be done to educate the public about HPV and cervical cancer. Recent studies have shown that the majority of women are unaware of the link between HPV and cervical cancer. Awareness of HPV is increased among young women, more educated women, and those with more access to the health care system (28,29). Public health efforts to introduce the vaccine will clearly need to be accompanied by vigorous educational programs directed at both young women and their parents to increase acceptability and the success of the HPV vaccine program. One concern that parent and other groups have expressed is the fear that vaccination against HPV may lead to a sense of invulnerability, would undermine abstinence-based messages, and may increase high-risk sexual behavior. There is no data, however, to suggest that fear of HPV is an important deterrent from sexual activity in young men or women. Several states have considered legislation to mandate HPV vaccination, although few have actually enacted such laws. All of the proposed laws have opt-out provisions for parents who object. However, they do not address the potential financial burdens imposed by the mandate. Mandating HPV vaccination would certainly boost vaccine coverage rates, but at a price of loss of parental autonomy.

These and other vaccine-related concerns will need to be addressed by primary care providers as well as public health officials. Surveys of physicians indicate a relatively high rate of acceptance of HPV vaccination, although many are reluctant to vaccinate the youngest age groups (10 to 12 years) for whom the vaccination is likely to offer the most benefit (30). Providers cite safety, durability, and affordability of the vaccine as important determinants of their acceptance, and indicated that they would be influenced by the recommendations of their professional organizations (23,31,32).

The most significant unresolved issue pertains to the application of HPV vaccines to underdeveloped nations, where the greatest burden of disease attributable to HPV is found (Fig. 8.5). The highest rates of cervical cancer occur in Africa, Central and South America, and Micronesia (1). Contributing to this burden is a lack of understanding of the dimensions of the disease, weak infrastructures and insufficient funds for population-wide vaccination programs, and a lack of the political

TABLE 8.1

CERVIX CANCER—MAJOR POINTS

Virtually all cervix cancer is related to persistent infection with HPV.
HPV infection is common, affects up to 50% of women, and peaks in the second and third decades of life.
Altered immune status, smoking, and the use of OCPs affect the rate of persistent HPV infection.
Rates of cervical cancer are highest in the underdeveloped countries of the world.
Two HPV vaccines have shown high efficacy in eliminating persistent HPV infection and cervical lesions in previously uninfected women.

HPV, human papillomavirus; OCPs, oral contraceptives.

will to address a sexually transmitted disease. The delivery of a new vaccine to a non-pediatric population is particularly problematic in countries with limited public health resources. Yet it is precisely in these countries that the potential benefit for a widespread vaccination program is greatest. Administering the vaccine in infancy along with other basic childhood vaccines may be the best choice, even though the duration of protection is at this time unknown. Clearly, the contribution of the international community will be required to make HPV vaccination a reality in the third world.

Chemoprevention

Several promising targets for the chemoprevention of cervical cancer have been identified, including topical retinoids, carotenoids, prostaglandins, indole-3-carbinol, and immune modulators (33). In phase 1 and 2 trials topical retinoids applied directly to the cervix resulted in significant complete histologic regression of CIN 2 lesions compared to placebo (34). None of the proposed agents, however, have been subject to definitive phase 3 randomized trials.

Surgical Prophylaxis

The introduction of widespread cervical cancer screening using the Papaniculaou (Pap) smear has dramatically reduced the incidence of invasive cervical cancer through the detection of treatable, premalignant lesions, referred to as cervical intraepithelial neoplasia (CIN). Because of the high rate of spontaneous regression, management of women with CIN 1 and satisfactory colposcopy (visualization of the entire squamocolumnar junction) is repeat cytology at 6 and 12 months or DNA testing for oncogenic types of HPV at 12 months. Alternatively, ablative (cryotherapy, electrocoagulation, or laser vaporization) or excisional (cold-knife conization or loop electrosurgical excision procedure [LEEP]) treatment may be offered. If the entire squamocolumnar junction cannot be visualized, an excisional procedure is the preferred approach. Treatment of CIN 2,3 lesions with satisfactory colposcopy involves excision or ablation of the entire transformation zone rather than just the colposcopically identified lesion (35). Cryotherapy, laser vaporization, and LEEP all appear to be effective modalities, although over time LEEP has become the procedure most widely chosen. When colposcopy is not satisfactory, a diagnostic excisional procedure is recommended. A variety of posttreatment surveillance protocols utilizing cervical cytology with or without colposcopy and HPV testing at frequent intervals have been proposed. Hysterectomy is reserved for recurrent or persistent biopsy-confirmed CIN 2,3 or for positive margins when repeat diagnostic excision is not possible (36). This approach to cervical cancer prevention based on large-scale cytologic screening programs is not feasible, however, in countries in the developing world, due to lack of infrastructure, funding, and public health education (Tables 8.1 and 8.2).

OVARIAN CANCER

Risk Factors

Ovarian cancer is the most common cause of death from a gynecologic cancer in the United States and accounts for approximately 14,000 deaths per year. Worldwide there are 192,000 new cases per year (37). Due to a lack of effective screening tools to identify ovarian cancer at early, highly curable stages, the majority of ovarian cancers are diagnosed at

TABLE 8.2

CERVIX CANCER—REMAINING QUESTIONS

What is the duration of protection of HPV vaccines?
What is the extent of cross-vaccination with the current HPV vaccines?
What is the sociocultural acceptability of vaccinating adolescent girls?
What is the added benefit of vaccinating males?
What is the impact of effective vaccination on subsequent screening practices and screening performance?
Which methods will best educate the public about HPV vaccines?
How should HPV vaccines be made available to underdeveloped nations?

HPV, human papillomavirus.

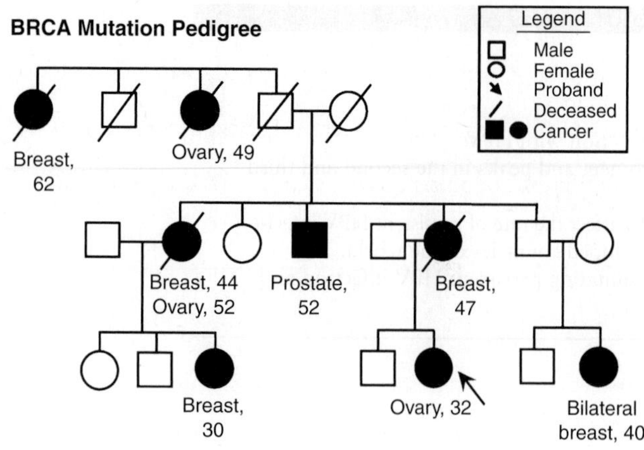

FIGURE 8.6. Family pedigree illustrating BRCA mutation.

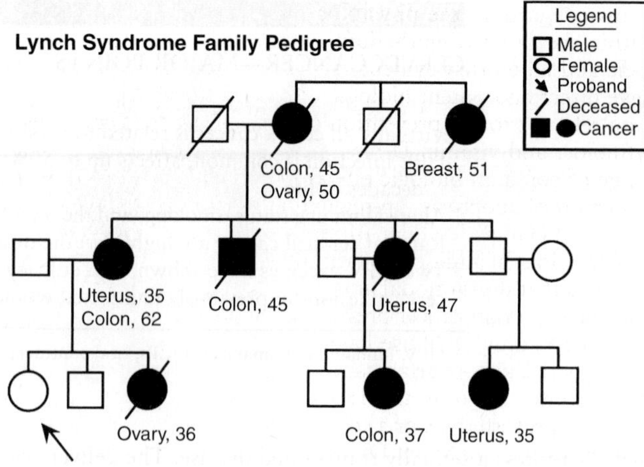

FIGURE 8.7. Family pedigree illustrating Lynch syndrome.

advanced stages when survival is poor. While our understanding of the biology of epithelial ovarian cancer is slowly advancing, most of our current knowledge regarding risks for ovarian cancer has emerged from the epidemiologic literature. Advancing age, reproductive factors (specifically, nulliparity), and heredity are established risk factors for the disease. The majority of ovarian cancers are diagnosed after menopause. Rates are higher in nulliparous women, while parity has been found to offer protection. The risk of ovarian cancer is increased twofold in women who are infertile, and the risk appears to be independent of fertility drug treatment (37). Although the majority of cases of ovarian cancer are sporadic, approximately 5% to 10% are thought to fit a hereditary pattern of autosomal dominant inheritance. Epidemiologic studies have estimated a two- to fourfold increase in risk among first-degree relatives of women with ovarian cancer. Recently, a number of genes have been identified that account for a large percentage of hereditary ovarian cancer and that allow more precise estimates of risk. Since the identification of *BRCA1* on chromosome 17q in 1994, and *BRCA2* on chromosome 13q in 1995, several hundred mutations in these genes have been characterized, many of which lead to premature truncation of protein transcription and, therefore, presumably defective gene products. Ovarian cancer in these families is characterized by multiple cases of ovarian and breast cancer in successive generations, earlier age of onset, and evidence of both maternal and paternal transmission (Fig. 8.6). The penetrance of *BRCA1/2*, i.e., the likelihood that a mutation will actually result in ovarian cancer, is estimated to range anywhere from 16% to 39% for *BRCA1* mutation carriers, and from 11% to 16% for *BRCA2* mutation carriers (37). Some mutations may be more specifically related to ovarian cancer risk than others. An ovarian cancer cluster region has been identified, for example, in exon 11 of *BRCA2*, which is associated with a higher rate of ovarian cancer than other mutations in the gene. The wide variation observed may also reflect the interaction of the genetic mutation with other genetic and/or environmental factors, and suggests that these genes may function as "gatekeepers" and, when lost, allow other genetic alterations to accumulate. Ovarian cancer is also included in the phenotype of the recently described mismatch repair genes associated with the hereditary nonpolyposis colon cancer (HNPCC), or Lynch syndrome, in which the lifetime risk for ovarian cancer is estimated to be approximately 12% (38) (Fig. 8.7). The identification of hereditary syndromes of ovarian cancer provides new opportunities to understand the biology of the disease and to devise novel preventive strategies.

Prevention

Risk Avoidance and/or Adoption of Protective Practices

The available evidence regarding factors that lower ovarian cancer risk has been based primarily on the results of case-control studies retrospectively comparing the reproductive, hormonal, or behavioral characteristics of ovarian cancer cases with matched controls, not on prospective randomized trials. These studies have consistently shown an inverse association of ovarian cancer with increasing parity, with the first birth conferring significantly more protection (35%) than subsequent births (15%). The protective effect of pregnancy occurs regardless of fertility history and is not age dependent (39). Pregnancy is characterized by a prolonged period of anovulation as well as high levels of circulating progesterone, which may cause terminal differentiation of premalignant cells on the surface of the ovary (40,41).

The evidence supporting a protective effect of breast-feeding against epithelial ovarian cancer risk is weak and inconsistent. Some studies suggest a 10% to 20% decrease in ovarian cancer risk associated with breast-feeding. In those studies that are positive, the impact of breast-feeding on ovarian cancer risk appears to be greatest for the first 6 months of lactation with no apparent increase in ovarian cancer protection with longer-term lactation (42,43).

Several studies have examined the association of hormone replacement therapy (HRT) with ovarian cancer risk. While the majority finds a modest increase in risk, most lack statistical significance. The strongest association is seen in endometrioid histologies, where relative risks range from 1.2 to 5.5 (44).

Several retrospective and prospective studies have examined associations between dietary factors and ovarian cancer risk. Modest levels of protection have been reported for fruits and vegetables in general, and for vitamin A and beta-carotene in particular, although findings are inconsistent (45–50). Nor is there a consistent relationship between physical activity or obesity and ovarian cancer risk (37,51,52).

Chemoprevention

The ovarian epithelium is a hormonally responsive target organ that expresses receptors for most members of the steroid hormone superfamily, including receptors for progestins, retinoids, androgens, and vitamin D. Although little is known regarding the physiologic role of steroid hormones within the ovarian epithelium, there is mounting epidemiologic and laboratory evidence suggesting that these hormones have direct and potent biologic effects on the ovarian epithelium relevant to the prevention of ovarian cancer. Progestins, retinoids, and vitamin D have been shown to exert a broad range of common biologic effects in epithelial cells, including induction of apoptosis, up-regulation of transforming growth factor-β (TGF-β), cellular differentiation, and inhibition of proliferation. In addition to hormonal agents, there is growing evidence that nonsteriodal anti-inflammatory drugs (NSAIDs) may have ovarian cancer preventive effects (53).

To date, only OCP use has been consistently shown to be protective against ovarian cancer. OCPs were first introduced in the United States in the 1960s. Most formulations include estrogen, progesterone, or a combination of the two. In addition to suppressing ovulation, OCPs also reduce pituitary secretion of gonadotropins. In addition to these potential mechanisms, a 3-year study in primates demonstrated that the progestin component of an OCP has a potent effect on apoptotic and TGF-β signaling pathways in the ovarian epithelium, raising the possibility that progestin-mediated biologic effects may underlie the ovarian cancer protective effects of OCPs (54,55). The use of OCPs appears to decrease a woman's risk for ovarian cancer by 30% to 60%. Risk reduction is apparent with as little as 3 months of use, increases in magnitude with increased duration of use, and persists for as long as 10 years after discontinuation of use. The risk reduction applies to nulliparous as well as parous women, to all histologic subtypes, including tumors of low malignant potential, to women with a hereditary risk for ovarian cancer, is consistent across races, and is independent of age at use or menopausal status (41,56,57). Although there has never been a randomized clinical trial to demonstrate the protective effect of OCPs on ovarian cancer risk, it is often recommended empirically to women with a family history of ovarian cancer to reduce their risk.

Epidemiologic and laboratory evidence suggest a potential role for retinoids as preventive agents for ovarian cancer (58). Retinoids are natural and synthetic derivatives of vitamin A. They have great potential for cancer prevention, due to a broad range of important biologic effects on epithelial cells, including inhibition of cellular proliferation, induction of cellular differentiation, induction of apoptosis, cytostatic activity, and induction of TGF-β. *In vitro,* it has been reported that the growth of human ovarian carcinoma cell lines and normal human ovarian epithelium is inhibited by retinoids. The mechanism underlying this effect may involve induction of TGF-β and/or apoptosis in ovarian epithelial cells. The most significant evidence supporting a rationale for retinoids as chemopreventive agents for ovarian cancer is that of a recently published Italian study suggesting an ovarian cancer preventive effect from the retinoid 4-HPR. Among women randomized to receive either 4-HPR or placebo in a trial designed to evaluate 4-HPR as a chemopreventive for breast carcinoma, significantly fewer ovarian cancer cases were noted in the 4-HPR group as compared to controls (59).

Vitamin D is a fat-soluble vitamin that is essential as a positive regulator of calcium homeostasis. The vitamin D receptor and the retinoic acid receptors share strong homology and readily dimerize, making it likely that vitamin D and retinoids have common signaling pathways in the cell (60). Vitamin D has been shown to have diverse biologic effects in epithelial cells relevant to cancer prevention, including retardation of growth, induction of cellular differentiation, induction of apoptosis and up-regulation of TGF-β (61). With regard to ovarian cancer, a recent study has correlated population-based data regarding ovarian cancer mortality in large cities across the United States with geographically based long-term sunlight data reported by the National Oceanic and Atmospheric Administration. The study demonstrated a statistically significant inverse correlation between regional sunlight exposure and ovarian mortality risk (62). Given that sunlight induces production of native vitamin D in the skin, it might confer protection against ovarian cancer via direct biologic effects on nonmalignant ovarian epithelium, for example, through induction of apoptosis and/or TGF-β in the ovarian epithelium, leading to selective removal of nonmalignant but genetically damaged epithelial cells.

Epidemiologic studies have suggested that use of NSAIDs may lower ovarian cancer risk (63). Several biologic mechanisms have been proposed to account for the chemopreventive effects of NSAIDs, including inhibition of ovulation, inhibition of COX and down-regulation of prostaglandins, enhancement of the immune response, and induction of apoptosis (41,64,65). Despite a growing body of preclinical data indicating chemopreventive effects of several agents, clinical research exploring their efficacy to reduce rates of ovarian cancer is hindered by the relatively low incidence of the disease, insufficient understanding of the preclinical course of ovarian cancer, the lack of validated preclinical biomarkers, and inadequate screening strategies.

Surgical Prophylaxis

For women with a family history of ovarian cancer, or a hereditary pattern of breast cancer, bilateral salpingo-oophorectomy (BSO) has been shown to lower the risk of subsequent epithelial ovarian cancer by 80% to 95% (66–68). There is also a 50% reduction in rates of breast cancer in women who undergo prophylactic BSO (69). Occult ovarian and fallopian tube tumors have been found at the time of BSO in 3% to 4% of *BRCA1/2* mutation carriers (70), emphasizing the need for both deliberate removal of the fallopian tubes at the time of prophylactic surgery, and of careful pathologic examination of the surgical specimen. The incidence of primary peritoneal cancer following BSO is reported to be approximately 2% to 5% (68). Because the median age of diagnosis of ovarian cancer among women with a hereditary risk is 50 years, the recommended age for prophylactic surgery is at the completion of childbearing, or at age 35 years.

In addition to the significant reduction in ovarian cancer incidence associated with BSO, several studies have found a significant decline in ovarian cancer worry and anxiety following the procedure (71–73). These potential benefits of prophylactic oophorectomy must, however, be weighed against its adverse consequences, including the short- and long-term surgical risks, the physical and psychological impact of early menopause, and the potential subsequent risks of cardiovascular disease and osteoporosis related to early estrogen/progesterone depletion. Although the use of combined estrogen/progesterone HRT has been associated with an increased risk for breast cancer among postmenopausal women in the general population, one study with short follow-up found no increased risk of breast cancer among *BRCA1/2* mutation carriers who took HRT following BSO (74). And data from the Mayo Clinic showed that there was no increase in breast cancer among women under the age of 50 years undergoing BSO (75). Women seeking information regarding prophylactic oophorectomy should be counseled about the practical short- and long-term sequelae of the surgery, the risks and benefits of postoperative HRT, and the small potential for primary peritoneal cancer (76).

Tubal ligation has been associated with lower ovarian cancer risk in both case-control and cohort studies. A strong inverse association was observed between tubal ligation and ovarian cancer risk in the Nurses Health Study, with a relative risk of 0.33 (CI, 0.16 to 0.64) after controlling for age, OCP use, and parity (77). A Danish population-based study also supports a significant association between tubal sterilization

TABLE 8.3

OVARIAN CANCER—MAJOR POINTS

Several risk factors, including age, nulliparity, and family history, have been identified for ovarian cancer.
Germ-line mutations in the *BRCA1/2* genes and the DNA mismatch repair genes associated with Lynch syndrome significantly increase the risk of ovarian cancer.
Primary cancer of the fallopian tube is considered a component of the hereditary ovarian cancer syndromes.
OCPs confer significant protection from ovarian cancer and the level of protection is related to the duration of use.
Tubal ligation also confers a significant protection from ovarian cancer, although the physiologic mechanism is unknown.
Prophylactic bilateral salpingo-oophorectomy is the most effective method of preventing ovarian cancer in women with a hereditary pattern of ovarian cancer.
No effective method of screening for ovarian cancer has been identified.

OCPs, oral contraceptives.

and ovarian cancer (78). A case-control study among *BRCA1/2* carriers found an odds ratio of 0.39 for ovarian cancer among women with *BRCA1* mutations who had undergone tubal ligation. No effect was seen in *BRCA2* carriers (79). Proposed mechanisms include changes in local or circulating hormones, reduced access of carcinogens to the ovary, or a reduction in inflammatory processes on the ovarian surface. Although the protective effect of tubal ligation appears to be substantial, the ability to perform BSO using a laparoscopic approach would seem to make this procedure a preferable choice among women with an increased risk of ovarian cancer (Tables 8.3 and 8.4).

ENDOMETRIAL CANCER

Risk Factors

Endometrial cancer is the most common gynecologic cancer in the United States, but the least common cause of gynecologic cancer death. Close to 40,000 new cases are diagnosed each year, and there are 7,400 deaths annually (80). Worldwide, there are close to 200,000 new cases and over 50,000 deaths (81). The relatively low case fatality rate is due to early detection and treatment at early-stage disease. The majority of risk factors associated with type 1 (endometrioid) endometrial cancer, viz. increased age, nulliparity, early age at menarche, late age at menopause, obesity, the long-term use of unopposed estrogen replacement therapy, and the use of tamoxifen, are all thought to exert their effect through estrogen-induced endometrial proliferation leading to hyperplasia and malignant transformation. The increased risk associated with diabetes, hypertension, and thyroid disease suggests a role for altered growth hormone pathways in addition to the steroid hormone pathways. There are also genetic syndromes associated with endometrial cancer. Women with mutations in the DNA repair genes associated with the HNPCC or Lynch syndrome have a 40% to 60% risk of endometrial cancer (82). Endometrial cancer is also a component of Cowden syndrome (Fig. 8.8), in which it is estimated that mutations in the PTEN gene confer a lifetime risk for endometrial cancer of approximately 5% (83). Type 2 serous endometrial cancer is uncommon and is not related to unopposed estrogen exposure.

TABLE 8.4

OVARIAN CANCER—REMAINING QUESTIONS

What is the duration of latent, preclinical ovarian cancer?
Can effective screening strategies, using biomarkers and/or imaging studies, be identified?
Are there effective chemopreventive agents that will reduce the risk of ovarian cancer?

Prevention

Risk Avoidance and Uptake of Protective Behaviors

It has been estimated that approximately 40% of endometrial cancers are attributable to excess body weight in developed countries (84). Maintenance of ideal body weight, regular physical activity, and control of diseases associated with endometrial cancer (diabetes, hypertension, and thyroid

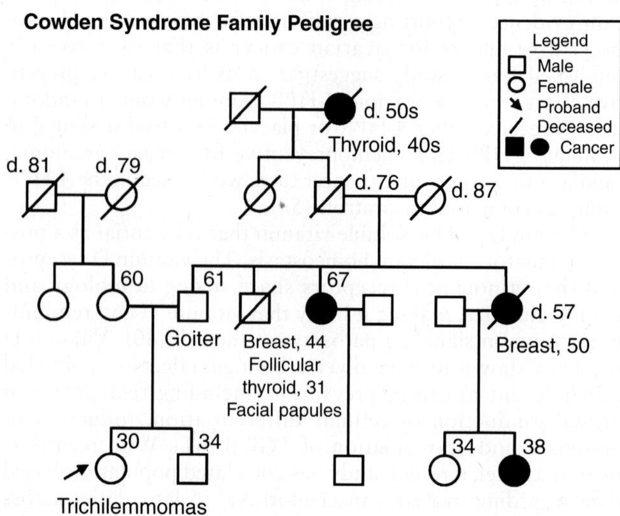

FIGURE 8.8. Family pedigree illustrating Cowden syndrome.

TABLE 8.5

ENDOMETRIAL CANCER—MAJOR POINTS

The major risk factors for type 1 endometrial cancer exert their effect through estrogen stimulation of the endometrial surface epithelium.
Altered growth hormone pathways may also be involved in endometrial carcinogenesis.
Hereditary forms of endometrial cancer have been associated with the Lynch syndrome and with Cowden syndrome.
The majority of endometrial cancers present at an early stage with abnormal uterine bleeding.
Endometrial cancer screening is not recommended for the general population, although women with a hereditary risk are recommended to undergo annual endometrial biopsy.
Prophylactic hysterectomy in high-risk women has been shown to protect women from subsequent endometrial cancer.

disease) are all prudent approaches to reduce disease risk. Women considering the use of tamoxifen or raloxifene for breast cancer risk reduction should carefully weigh the risk of endometrial cancer with the benefits as they make their decision.

Chemoprevention

The addition of a progestin to the estrogen component of HRT has been shown to eliminate the increased risk of endometrial cancer. Progesterone reverses the estrogen effect on the endometrium and prevents the development of hyperplasia. Women with an intact uterus who elect HRT are routinely prescribed a combined estrogen-progestin preparation. Long-term use of combination OCPs also reduces the risk of endometrial cancer by approximately 10% per year of use (40). The reduction in risk associated with OCP use is attributed to the suppression of endometrial hyperplasia by the progestin component (85).

Surgical Prophylaxis

It is thought that the majority of invasive endometrial cancers progress through a series of premalignant stages, simple hyperplasia, complex hyperplasia, simple atypical hyperplasia, and complex atypical hyperplasia, all of which may present with abnormal vaginal bleeding (86). Conservative management of these conditions involves the use of progestational agents, which results in a complete regression of atypical hyperplasia in 50% to 94% of cases. Even in complete responders, however, there is a high rate of recurrence, and definitive therapy of atypical hyperplasia is hysterectomy (33). Among women with documented germ-line mutations associated with the Lynch syndrome, a retrospective study found that prophylactic hysterectomy conferred 100% protection from subsequent endometrial cancer (87). Because of the high success rate for endometrial cancer treatment, however, it is not clear if this protection would translate into a significant survival benefit. This study also found 100% protection from ovarian cancer, which may warrant the consideration of prophylactic total abdominal hysterectomy–bilateral salpingo-oophorectomy (TAH-BSO) in this population. Alternatively, annual endometrial biopsy starting at age 30 to 35 is recommended in women with Lynch syndrome to detect early, premalignant endometrial lesions (82) (Tables 8.5 and 8.6).

TABLE 8.6

ENDOMETRIAL CANCER—REMAINING QUESTIONS

Can interventions targeting weight control and physical activity impact the incidence of endometrial cancer?
Does prophylactic hysterectomy translate into a survival benefit?

FUTURE DIRECTIONS

The prevention of gynecologic malignancies involves many disciplines and requires the collaboration of basic scientists, clinicians, behavioral scientists, and policy makers. The successful development of the HPV vaccines is a major breakthrough in the prevention of cervical cancer and will likely undergo further improvements and refinements. Advances in molecular genetics, molecular pathology, and molecular imaging will contribute to the early identification of specific markers of premalignant change associated with gynecologic malignancies. The identification of safe and effective chemopreventive agents will provide additional strategies for prevention. Accompanying this progress will be the need to address the psychosocial and cultural barriers to the adoption of preventive strategies.

References

1. Saslow D, Castle PE, Cox JT, et al. American Cancer Society Guideline for human papillomavirus (HPV) vaccine use to prevent cervical cancer and its precursors. *CA Cancer J Clin* 2007;57(1):7–28.
2. Jansen KU, Shaw AR. Human papillomavirus vaccines and prevention of cervical cancer. *Annu Rev Med* 2004;55:319–331.
3. Stanley M. HPV vaccines. *Best Pract Res Clin Obstet Gynaecol* 2006;20(2): 279–293.
4. Moreno V, Bosch FX, Munoz N, et al. Effect of oral contraceptives on risk of cervical cancer in women with human papillomavirus infection: the IARC multicentric case-control study. *Lancet* 2002;359(9312):1085–1092.
5. McCann MF, Irwin DE, Walton LA, et al. Nicotine and cotinine in the cervical mucus of smokers, passive smokers, and nonsmokers. *Cancer Epidemiol Biomarkers Prev* 1992;1(2):125–129.
6. McIntyre-Seltman K, Castle PE, Guido R, et al. Smoking is a risk factor for cervical intraepithelial neoplasia grade 3 among oncogenic human papillomavirus DNA-positive women with equivocal or mildly abnormal cytology. *Cancer Epidemiol Biomarkers Prev* 2005;14(5):1165–1170.
7. Tomson TT, Roden RB, Wu TC. Human papillomavirus vaccines for the prevention and treatment of cervical cancer. *Curr Opin Investig Drugs* 2004;5(12):1247–1261.
8. Duensing S, Lee LY, Duensing A, et al. The human papillomavirus type 16 E6 and E7 oncoproteins cooperate to induce mitotic defects and genomic instability by uncoupling centrosome duplication from the cell division cycle. *Proc Natl Acad Sci USA* 2000;97(18):10002–10007.
9. Bailey J, Cymet TC. Planning for the HPV vaccine and its impact on cervical cancer prevention. *Compr Ther* 2006;32(2):102–105.
10. Zhou J, Doorbar J, Sun XY, et al. Identification of the nuclear localization signal of human papillomavirus type 16 L1 protein. *Virology* 1991;185(2): 625–632.
11. Lowe RS, Brown DR, Bryan JT, et al. Human papillomavirus type 11 (HPV-11) neutralizing antibodies in the serum and genital mucosal secretions of African green monkeys immunized with HPV-11 virus-like particles expressed in yeast. *J Infect Dis* 1997;176(5):1141–1145.
12. Palker TJ, Monteiro JM, Martin MM, et al. Antibody, cytokine and cytotoxic T lymphocyte responses in chimpanzees immunized with human papillomavirus virus-like particles. *Vaccine* 2001;19(27):3733–3743.
13. Harper DM, Franco EL, Wheeler C, et al. Efficacy of a bivalent L1 virus-like particle vaccine in prevention of infection with human papillomavirus types 16 and 18 in young women: a randomised controlled trial. *Lancet* 2004;364(9447):1757–1765.
14. Mao C, Koutsky LA, Ault KA, et al. Efficacy of human papillomavirus-16 vaccine to prevent cervical intraepithelial neoplasia: a randomized controlled trial. *Obstet Gynecol* 2006;107(1):18–27.

15. Villa LL, Costa RL, Petta CA, et al. Prophylactic quadrivalent human papillomavirus (types 6, 11, 16, and 18) L1 virus-like particle vaccine in young women: a randomised double-blind placebo-controlled multicentre phase II efficacy trial. *Lancet Oncol* 2005;6(5):271–278.
16. Shi L, Sings HL, Bryan JT, et al. Gardasil: prophylactic human papillomavirus vaccine development—from bench top to bed-side. *Clin Pharmacol Ther* 2007;81(2):259–264.
17. FUTURE II Study Group. Quadrivalent vaccine against human papillomavirus to prevent high-grade cervical lesions. *N Engl J Med* 2007;356(19): 1915–1927.
18. Joura EA, Leodolter S, Hernandez-Avila M, et al. Efficacy of a quadrivalent prophylactic human papillomavirus (types 6, 11, 16, and 18) L1 virus-like-particle vaccine against high-grade vulval and vaginal lesions: a combined analysis of three randomised clinical trials. *Lancet* 2007;369(9574): 1693–1702.
19. Harper DM, Franco EL, Wheeler CM, et al. Sustained efficacy up to 4.5 years of a bivalent L1 virus-like particle vaccine against human papillomavirus types 16 and 18: follow-up from a randomised control trial. *Lancet* 2006;367(9518):1247–1255.
20. Paavonen J, Jenkins D, Bosch FX, et al. Efficacy of a prophylactic adjuvanted bivalent L1 virus-like-particle vaccine against infection with human papillomavirus types 16 and 18 in young women: an interim analysis of a phase III double-blind, randomised controlled trial. *Lancet* 2007;369(9580): 2161–2170.
21. Kohli M, Ferko N, Martin A, et al. Estimating the long-term impact of a prophylactic human papillomavirus 16/18 vaccine on the burden of cervical cancer in the UK. *Br J Cancer* 2007;96(1):143–150.
22. Goldie SJ, Kohli M, Grima D, et al. Projected clinical benefits and cost-effectiveness of a human papillomavirus 16/18 vaccine. *J Natl Cancer Inst* 2004;96(8):604–615.
23. Dinh TA, Benoit MF. Human papillomavirus vaccine: progress and the future. *Expert Opin Biol Ther* 2007;7(4):479–485.
24. Kulasingam SL, Kim JJ, Lawrence WF, et al. Cost-effectiveness analysis based on the atypical squamous cells of undetermined significance/low-grade squamous intraepithelial lesion Triage Study (ALTS). *J Natl Cancer Inst* 2006;98(2):92–100.
25. Markowitz LE, Dunne EF, Saraiya M, et al. Quadrivalent human papillomavirus vaccine: recommendations of the Advisory Committee on Immunization Practices (ACIP). *MMWR Recomm Rep* 2007;56(RR-2): 1–24.
26. Charo RA. Politics, parents, and prophylaxis—mandating HPV vaccination in the United States. *N Engl J Med* 2007;356(19):1905–1908.
27. Block SL, Nolan T, Sattler C, et al. Comparison of the immunogenicity and reactogenicity of a prophylactic quadrivalent human papillomavirus (types 6, 11, 16, and 18) L1 virus-like particle vaccine in male and female adolescents and young adult women. *Pediatrics* 2006;118(5):2135–2145.
28. Moreira ED Jr, de Oliveira BG, Neves RC, et al. Assessment of knowledge and attitudes of young uninsured women toward human papillomavirus vaccination and clinical trials. *J Pediatr Adolesc Gynecol* 2006;19(2): 81–87.
29. Tiro JA, Meissner HI, Kobrin S, et al. What do women in the U.S. know about human papillomavirus and cervical cancer? *Cancer Epidemiol Biomarkers Prev* 2007;16(2):288–294.
30. Daley MF, Liddon N, Crane LA, et al. A national survey of pediatrician knowledge and attitudes regarding human papillomavirus vaccination. *Pediatrics* 2006;118(6):2280–2289.
31. Kahn JA, Zimet GD, Bernstein DI, et al. Pediatricians' intention to administer human papillomavirus vaccine: the role of practice characteristics, knowledge, and attitudes. *J Adolesc Health* 2005;37(6):502–510.
32. Widdice LE, Kahn JA. Using the new HPV vaccines in clinical practice. *Cleve Clin J Med* 2006;73(10):929–935.
33. Alberts DS, Barakat RR, Daly M, et al. Prevention of gynecologic malignancies. In: Gershenson DM, McGuire WP, Gore M, et al., eds. *Gynecologic Cancer Controversies in Management.* Philadelphia: Elsevier Ltd.; 2004:883–919.
34. Meyskens FL Jr, Surwit E, Moon TE, et al. Enhancement of regression of cervical intraepithelial neoplasia II (moderate dysplasia) with topically applied all-trans-retinoic acid: a randomized trial. *J Natl Cancer Inst* 1994;86(7):539–543.
35. Spitzer M, Apgar BS, Brotzman GL. Management of histologic abnormalities of the cervix. *Am Fam Physician* 2006;73(1):105–112.
36. Wright TC Jr, Cox JT, Massad LS, et al. 2001 Consensus Guidelines for the Management of Women with Cervical Intraepithelial Neoplasia. *J Low Genit Tract Dis* 2003;7(3):154–167.
37. Hanna L, Adams M. Prevention of ovarian cancer. *Best Pract Res Clin Obstet Gynaecol* 2006;20(2):339–362.
38. Lu KH, Dinh M, Kohlmann W, et al. Gynecologic cancer as a "sentinel cancer" for women with hereditary nonpolyposis colorectal cancer syndrome. *Obstet Gynecol* 2005;105(3):569–574.
39. Whiteman DC, Murphy MF, Cook LS, et al. Multiple births and risk of epithelial ovarian cancer. *J Natl Cancer Inst* 2000;92(14):1172–1177.
40. Pike MC, Pearce CL, Wu AH. Prevention of cancers of the breast, endometrium and ovary. *Oncogene* 2004;23(38):6379–6391.
41. Barnes MN, Grizzle WE, Grubbs CJ, et al. Paradigms for primary prevention of ovarian carcinoma. *CA Cancer J Clin* 2002;52(4):216–225.
42. Risch HA, Marrett LD, Howe GR. Parity, contraception, infertility, and the risk of epithelial ovarian cancer. *Am J Epidemiol* 1994;140(7): 585–597.
43. Rosenblatt KA, Thomas DB. Lactation and the risk of epithelial ovarian cancer. The WHO Collaborative Study of Neoplasia and Steroid Contraceptives. *Int J Epidemiol* 1993;22(2):192–197.
44. Auranen A, Hietanen S, Salmi T, et al. Hormonal treatments and epithelial ovarian cancer risk. *Int J Gynecol Cancer* 2005;15(5):692–700.
45. Tung KH, Wilkens LR, Wu AH, et al. Association of dietary vitamin A, carotenoids, and other antioxidants with the risk of ovarian cancer. *Cancer Epidemiol Biomarkers Prev* 2005;14(3):669–676.
46. Larsson SC, Holmberg L, Wolk A. Fruit and vegetable consumption in relation to ovarian cancer incidence: the Swedish Mammography Cohort. *Br J Cancer* 2004;90(11):2167–2170.
47. Koushik A, Hunter DJ, Spiegelman D, et al. Intake of the major carotenoids and the risk of epithelial ovarian cancer in a pooled analysis of 10 cohort studies. *Int J Cancer* 2006;119(9):2148–2154.
48. Schulz M, Lahmann PH, Boeing H, et al. Fruit and vegetable consumption and risk of epithelial ovarian cancer: the European Prospective Investigation into Cancer and Nutrition. *Cancer Epidemiol Biomarkers Prev* 2005;14(11 Pt 1): 2531–2535.
49. Fairfield KM, Hankinson SE, Rosner BA, et al. Risk of ovarian carcinoma and consumption of vitamins A, C, and E and specific carotenoids: a prospective analysis. *Cancer* 2001;92(9):2318–2326.
50. Cramer DW, Kuper H, Harlow BL, et al. Carotenoids, antioxidants and ovarian cancer risk in pre- and postmenopausal women. *Int J Cancer* 2001;94(1):128–134.
51. Weiderpass E, Margolis KL, Sandin S, et al. Prospective study of physical activity in different periods of life and the risk of ovarian cancer. *Int J Cancer* 2006;118(12):3153–3160.
52. Cottreau CM, Ness RB, Kriska AM. Physical activity and reduced risk of ovarian cancer. *Obstet Gynecol* 2000;96(4):609–614.
53. Rodriguez-Burford C, Barnes MN, Oelschlager DK, et al. Effects of nonsteroidal anti-inflammatory agents (NSAIDs) on ovarian carcinoma cell lines: preclinical evaluation of NSAIDs as chemopreventive agents. *Clin Cancer Res* 2002;8(1):202–209.
54. Rodriguez GC, Walmer DK, Cline M, et al. Effect of progestin on the ovarian epithelium of macaques: cancer prevention through apoptosis? *J Soc Gynecol Investig* 1998;5(5):271–276.
55. Rodriguez GC, Nagarsheth NP, Lee KL, et al. Progestin-induced apoptosis in the Macaque ovarian epithelium: differential regulation of transforming growth factor-beta. *J Natl Cancer Inst* 2002;94(1):50–60.
56. Whittemore AS, Balise RR, Pharoah PD, et al. Oral contraceptive use and ovarian cancer risk among carriers of *BRCA1* or *BRCA2* mutations. *Br J Cancer* 2004;91(11):1911–1915.
57. Whittemore AS. Personal characteristics relating to risk of invasive epithelial ovarian cancer in older women in the United States. *Cancer* 1993;71(2 Suppl):558–565.
58. Brewer MA, Johnson K, Follen M, et al. Prevention of ovarian cancer: intraepithelial neoplasia. *Clin Cancer Res* 2003;9(1):20–30.
59. De Palo G, Veronesi U, Camerini T, et al. Can fenretinide protect women against ovarian cancer? *J Natl Cancer Inst* 1995;87(2):146–147.
60. Campbell MJ, Park S, Uskokovic MR, et al. Expression of retinoic acid receptor-beta sensitizes prostate cancer cells to growth inhibition mediated by combinations of retinoids and a 19-nor hexafluoride vitamin D3 analog. *Endocrinology* 1998;139(4):1972–1980.
61. Studzinski GP, Moore DC. Sunlight—can it prevent as well as cause cancer? *Cancer Res* 1995;55(18):4014–4022.
62. Lefkowitz ES, Garland CF. Sunlight, vitamin D, and ovarian cancer mortality rates in US women. *Int J Epidemiol* 1994;23(6):1133–1136.
63. Moysich KB, Mettlin C, Piver MS, et al. Regular use of analgesic drugs and ovarian cancer risk. *Cancer Epidemiol Biomarkers Prev* 2001;10(8): 903–906.
64. Rodriguez C, Patel AV, Calle EE, et al. Estrogen replacement therapy and ovarian cancer mortality in a large prospective study of US women. *JAMA* 2001;285(11):1460–1465.
65. Akhmedkhanov A, Toniolo P, Zeleniuch-Jacquotte A, et al. Aspirin and epithelial ovarian cancer. *Prev Med* 2001;33(6):682–687.
66. Kauff ND, Satagopan JM, Robson ME, et al. Risk-reducing salpingo-oophorectomy in women with a *BRCA1* or *BRCA2* mutation. *N Engl J Med* 2002;346(21):1609–1615.
67. Rebbeck TR. Prophylactic oophorectomy in *BRCA1* and *BRCA2* mutation carriers. *Eur J Cancer* 2002;38(Suppl 6):S15–S17.
68. Finch A, Beiner M, Lubinski J, et al. Salpingo-oophorectomy and the risk of ovarian, fallopian tube, and peritoneal cancers in women with a *BRCA1* or *BRCA2* Mutation. *JAMA* 2006;296(2):185–192.
69. Rebbeck TR, Lynch HT, Neuhausen SL, et al. Prophylactic oophorectomy in carriers of *BRCA1* or *BRCA2* mutations. *N Engl J Med* 2002;346(21): 1616–1622.
70. Dowdy SC, Stefanek M, Hartmann LC. Surgical risk reduction: prophylactic salpingo-oophorectomy and prophylactic mastectomy. *Am J Obstet Gynecol* 2004;191(4):1113–1123.
71. Tiller K, Meiser B, Butow P, et al. Psychological impact of prophylactic oophorectomy in women at increased risk of developing ovarian cancer: a prospective study. *Gynecol Oncol* 2002;86(2):212–219.

72. Meiser B, Tiller K, Gleeson MA, et al. Psychological impact of prophylactic oophorectomy in women at increased risk for ovarian cancer. *Psychooncology* 2000;9(6):496–503.
73. Madalinska JB, Hollenstein J, Bleiker E, et al. Quality-of-life effects of prophylactic salpingo-oophorectomy versus gynecologic screening among women at increased risk of hereditary ovarian cancer. *J Clin Oncol* 2005;23(28):6890–6898.
74. Rebbeck TR, Friebel T, Wagner T, et al. Effect of short-term hormone replacement therapy on breast cancer risk reduction after bilateral prophylactic oophorectomy in *BRCA1* and *BRCA2* mutation carriers: the PROSE Study Group. *J Clin Oncol* 2005;23(31):7804–7810.
75. Olson JE, Sellers TA, Iturria SJ, et al. Bilateral oophorectomy and breast cancer risk reduction among women with a family history. *Cancer Detect Prev* 2004;28(5):357–360.
76. Conner KM, Daly MB, Cherry C, et al. *Ovarian Cancer Risk-Reducing Surgery: A Decision-Making Resource.* Philadelphia: Fox Chase Cancer Center; 2006:140.
77. Hankinson SE, Hunter DJ, Colditz GA, et al. Tubal ligation, hysterectomy, and risk of ovarian cancer. A prospective study. *JAMA* 1993;270(23):2813–2818.
78. Kjaer SK, Mellemkjaer L, Brinton LA, et al. Tubal sterilization and risk of ovarian, endometrial and cervical cancer. A Danish population-based follow-up study of more than 65,000 sterilized women. *Int J Epidemiol* 2004;33(3): 596–602.
79. Narod SA, Sun P, Ghadirian P, et al. Tubal ligation and risk of ovarian cancer in carriers of *BRCA1* or *BRCA2* mutations: a case-control study. *Lancet* 2001;357(9267):1467–1470.
80. Jemal A, Siegel R, Ward E, et al. Cancer statistics, 2007. *CA Cancer J Clin* 2007;57(1):43–66.
81. Parkin DM, Bray F, Ferlay J, et al. Global cancer statistics, 2002. *CA Cancer J Clin* 2005;55(2):74–108.
82. Lindor NM, Petersen GM, Hadley DW, et al. Recommendations for the care of individuals with an inherited predisposition to Lynch syndrome: a systematic review. *JAMA* 2006;296(12):1507–1517.
83. Eng C. Will the real Cowden syndrome please stand up: revised diagnostic criteria. *J Med Genet* 2000;37(11):828–830.
84. Bergstrom A, Pisani P, Tenet V, et al. Overweight as an avoidable cause of cancer in Europe. *Int J Cancer* 2001;91(3):421–430.
85. Sonoda Y, Barakat RR. Screening and the prevention of gynecologic cancer: endometrial cancer. *Best Pract Res Clin Obstet Gynaecol* 2006;20(2): 363–377.
86. Sherman ME, Sturgeon S, Brinton L, et al. Endometrial cancer chemoprevention: implications of diverse pathways of carcinogenesis. *J Cell Biochem Suppl* 1995;23:160–164.
87. Schmeler KM, Sun CC, Bodurka DC, et al. Prophylactic bilateral salpingo-oophorectomy compared with surveillance in women with BRCA mutations. *Obstet Gynecol* 2006;108(3 Pt 1):515–520.

CHAPTER 9 ■ CLINICAL TRIALS METHODOLOGY AND BIOSTATISTICS

MARK F. BRADY, ALAN D. HUTSON, AND DANIEL P. GAILE

Issues involved in the design, conduct, and analyses of clinical trials are presented in this chapter. Phase 1, 2, and 3 trials are presented, as well as screening trials. Since translational research objectives are often integrated into modern clinical trials, this topic is also described. Statistical jargon and mathematical notation is avoided wherever possible. Studies from the field of gynecologic oncology are used as examples in order to illustrate specific points. This chapter is an overview of these very expansive topics. Details can be found in books dedicated to the subject of clinical trials, like Piantadosi, 2005 (1), Green et al., 2003 (2), or Everett and Pickles, 1999 (3).

This chapter begins with general systems for classifying interventions and study designs. Then, some historical highlights from medical research are described. This synopsis of history is intended to provide a sense of how the concepts of clinical trials matured from an intuition-based practice of medicine to the more sophisticated evidence-based medicine used today. The procedures for designing, conducting, and analyzing clinical trials continue to mature as the demand for evidence-based medicine increases. The following sections in this chapter describe the components of a clinical trial and some essential considerations for each of these components. Since translational research objectives are incorporated into many modern clinical trials, some issues related to design and analyses of these components are also considered.

CLASSIFICATION OF INTERVENTIONS AND STUDY DESIGNS

In general, a clinical trial is any experiment involving human subjects that evaluates an intervention that attempts to reduce the impact of a specific disease in a particular population. When an intervention is applied in order to prevent the onset of a particular disease, the trial is classified as a primary prevention trial. For example, a primary prevention trial may evaluate healthy lifestyles or a vitamin supplement in a population of individuals who are considered to be at risk of a particular disease. Secondary prevention trials evaluate interventions that are applied to individuals with early stages of a disease in order to reduce their risk of progressing to more advanced stages of the disease. Tertiary intervention trials are aimed at evaluating interventions that reduce the risk of morbidity or mortality due to a particular disease.

Clinical trials that evaluate methods for detecting a disease in a preclinical state are called screening trials. Early detection may mean diagnosing a malignancy in an early stage (e.g., the use of mammography in the detection of breast cancer) or in a premalignant state (e.g., the use of Papanicolaou smear in the detection of cervical intraepithelial neoplasia). There are typically two interventions in a screening trial. The first intervention is the screening program (e.g., annual mammograms), which involves individuals who appear to be free of the disease. However, once the disease is detected in an individual, a secondary intervention (e.g., surgery) is performed in hopes of stopping the disease from progressing to more advanced stages. Consequentially, screening trials require *both* interventions to be effective. An effective screening procedure is useless if the secondary intervention does not alter the course of the disease. On the other hand, an ineffective screening procedure would cause the secondary intervention to be applied indiscriminately.

Nonexperimental studies (or observational studies) can be classified into three broad design categories: cohort (or prospective), case-control (or retrospective), and cross-sectional. In a cohort study individuals are initially identified according to their exposure status, which can include environmental, genetic, or lifestyle factors. These individuals are then followed in order to determine who develops the disease. The aim of these studies is to assess whether the exposure is associated with the incidence of the disease under study. This design is in contrast to the case-control study, which identifies individuals on the basis of whether they have the disease and then measures and compares their exposure histories. Measuring exposure may be as simple as questioning the individuals about their personal or employment history, or it may involve a more sophisticated assessment such as analyzing the individual's blood for markers of exposure. Though the case-control study is susceptible to several methodological flaws, it has the advantage of often being less expensive, and easier and quicker to perform than a cohort study, especially when the disease is rare. The power of the case-control design is apparent from a review of the case-control studies published between 1975 and 1983 (4), which demonstrated the deleterious effects of exogenous estrogens in perimenopausal women. Finally, the goal of the cross-sectional study is to describe the prevalence of a disease and an exposure in a population during a specific period of time. These studies can often be conducted more quickly than either the cohort or case-control study, but they are frequently not used when the time between exposures and the disease onset is long, as it is for cancer.

HISTORICAL PERSPECTIVE

Clinicians make treatment recommendations daily. These recommendations arise from culling information from standardized clinical guidelines, published reports, expert opinion, or

Brian N. Bundy, PhD, contributed to prior editions of this chapter.

personal experiences. The synthesis of information from these sources into a particular recommendation for an individual patient is based on a clinician's personal judgment. But what constitutes reliable and valid information worthy of consideration? Clinicians have long recognized that properly planned and conducted clinical trials are important sources of empirical evidence for shaping clinical judgment.

The Greek physician Hippocrates in the 5th century BCE had a profound influence in freeing medicine from superstitions. He rejected the notion that the cause of an individual's disease had a divine origin. Rather, he postulated that diseases originated from natural causes that could be determined from observing environmental factors like diet, drinking water, or local weather. He also proposed the revolutionary concept that a physician could anticipate the course of a disease after carefully observing a sufficient number of cases. Despite these insights, medicine continued to frequently consist of a mixture of herbal concoctions, purging, bloodletting, and astrology.

In the Middle Ages, Avicenna (980–1037 CE) wrote *The Canon of Medicine*, a work considered to be the preeminent source of medical and pharmaceutical knowledge of its time. In his writings Avicenna proposed some rules for testing clinical interventions. First, he pointed to the need to experiment in humans since "testing a drug on a lion or horse might not prove anything about its effect on man." Also, he described the basic experiment as observing pairs of individuals with uncomplicated but similar forms of the disease. Finally, he emphasized the need for careful observation of the times of an intervention and then reporting the reproducibility of its effects (5). Despite these insights, *The Canon of Medicine* does not include any specific reports of clinical experimentation.

Early trials frequently lacked concurrent comparison groups. For example, Lady Mary Wortley-Montague in 1721 urged King George I to commute the sentences of six inmates from the Newgate prison if they agreed to participate in a smallpox inoculation trial (5). The prisoners were inoculated with smallpox matter from a patient with a naturally occurring form of the disease. Since these individuals remained free of smallpox, this was considered evidence supporting treatment by inoculation. Later, however, the results of this trial were considered less compelling, when it was discovered that some of these inmates might have been exposed to smallpox prior to the trial (6). Without a proper control group, it can be difficult to interpret the efficacy of an intervention. There are frequently many factors, both known and unknown, that influence an individual's outcome.

Subjective assessments from either the subject or the practitioner may also influence the interpretability of a trial. In the late 18th century the King of France selected Benjamin Franklin to head a royal commission to investigate the physician Franz Mesmer's claims that he could promote good health by manipulating a force he called "animal magnetism" (7). Franklin devised several ingenious experiments in which the subjects were blindfolded and not told whether or not they were receiving Mesmer's treatment. These trials led Franklin to conclude that the therapeutic effects of mesmerism were due to imagination or illusion. Several years later John Haygarth demonstrated the importance of controlling for assessment biases. At that time magnetic healing rods were commonly used to relieve pain due to chronic rheumatism (6). He treated five patients on two consecutive days once with sham wooden rods and once with genuine magnetic rods. He noted that four individuals reported pain relief and one experienced no relief, regardless of which rods were used. Franklin's and Haygarth's trials established the importance of implementing experimental procedures aimed at removing all sources of subjectivity from the assessment of treatment effects.

It had long been appreciated that there is a potential for misguided inference about the effectiveness of a treatment when the comparison involves a group with a dissimilar prognosis. The apparent benefits attributed to a new treatment might in fact be biases due to prognostic differences in patients between treatment groups. One of the earliest clinical trials to attempt to address this bias was reported in 1898 by Johannes Fibiger (8). Four hundred and eighty-four patients admitted to his clinic with diphtheria were given either standard care or diphtheria serum twice daily. In order to disassociate the mode of treatment from the individual's prognosis, the patient's treatment was to be determined by the day of clinic admission, and it alternated from day to day (9). Using this type of procedure to disassociate prognosis from treatment is only partially effective, since the practitioner or the subject knew which treatment would be applied and this knowledge may have influenced the individual's decision to participate in the study. Therefore, masking the treatment assignment so that it cannot be part of the decision to participate in the trial is important for controlling this source of selection bias.

Treatment randomization in clinical trials was performed as early as 1926 (10). However, it was not until the 1940s when Corwin Hinshaw (11), using a coin toss, and later Bradford Hill (12), using random numbers in sealed envelopes, established the methodologic importance of randomizing treatments in clinical trials. Balancing the unpredictable and spontaneous remissions exhibited by some patients with pulmonary tuberculosis motivated Amberson (10) and later Hinshaw (11). While methodological principles motivated Hill, the short supply of streptomycin after World War II provided the opportunity to use randomization as an equitable way to distribute the drug (13).

One of the first randomized clinical trials in the study of gynecologic malignancies was initiated in 1948 (14). This trial compared ovarian irradiation to standard treatment for breast cancer. Initially, shuffled sealed envelopes were used to designate treatment. However, this procedure was later changed due to administrative difficulties so that treatment depended on the woman's date of birth. This latter procedure is susceptible to the same selection bias mentioned in Fibiger's trials since the treatments were not masked.

Despite these methodological advances, the inadequate justification for selecting one medical procedure over another led one contemporary physician to express his frustration: "Early in my medical career I was appalled at the 'willy-nilly' fashion by which treatment regimens slipped in and out of popularity. How many operations that I was trained to do or medicines that I was instructed to give because of somebody's conviction they were beneficial passed into oblivion for no apparent reason, only to be replaced by others of equally dubious worth?" (15).

The first randomized clinical trial at the National Cancer Institute (NCI) was begun in 1955 (16). This trial involved 65 evaluable patients with acute leukemia from four different institutions. The trial incorporated many elements that should be part of most modern clinical trials: uniform criteria for response assessment, a randomized comparison of at least two treatment regimens, and a complete accounting of all patients entered. The published report included considerations for such issues as patient selection bias and the study's impact on the patient's welfare (17). The first NCI randomized clinical trial in solid tumors followed shortly thereafter and was organized by the Eastern Group for Solid Tumor Chemotherapy (18). By 2007, there were 12 NCI-sponsored cooperative groups conducting clinical trials, and the annual funding for these groups was $155 million (19).

In the late 1950s most patients with gynecologic cancers were included incidentally in small trials to screen new agents for broad-range activity. The first NCI-sponsored group to organize trials specifically for gynecologic malignancies was the Surgical Ovarian Adjuvant Group. This group was formed in the late 1950s, initiated a few trials, and then disbanded in 1964. Starting in 1963 the Surgical Endometrial Adjuvant Group was one of the earliest efforts toward a multidisciplinary group. This multidisciplinary cooperative group included gynecologic surgeons, medical oncologists, pathologists, radiation oncologists, and biostatisticians. It was from this group that the Gynecologic Oncology Group (GOG) was eventually formed in 1970 to deal with a broader range of gynecologic malignancies (20). Over the following 10 years, the field of gynecologic oncology matured. Board certification procedures for gynecologic oncologists were developed, fellowship programs were initiated in the comprehensive cancer centers, and a professional Society of Gynecologic Oncologists was organized in 1969.

COMPONENTS OF A CLINICAL TRIAL

Objectives

In clinical oncology research, where the disease is often fatal, the ultimate purpose of a research program is to develop a treatment plan that puts patients into a disease-free state, reduces the risk of cancer recurrence, and allows patients to return to their normal lifestyle within a reasonable period of time. The objectives of a particular clinical trial are often more specific and less grandiose. A clinical trial attempts to answer a precisely defined set of questions with respect to the effects of a particular treatment(s) (21). These questions (objectives) form the foundation upon which the rest of the trial is built. The study objective typically incorporates three elements: the interventions to be evaluated, the "yardstick" to be used to measure treatment benefit (see the Endpoints section), and a brief description of the target population (see the Eligibility Criteria section). These three elements (i.e., "what," "how," and "who") should be stated in the most precise, clear, and concise terms possible.

The choice of experimental therapy to be evaluated in a randomized clinical trial is not always easy. Both a plethora of new therapies and the absence of innovative concepts make for difficult choices. The former is problematic since many malignancies in gynecologic oncology are relatively uncommon. Definitive clinical trials may require 4 to 5 years to accrue a sufficient number of patients even in a cooperative group setting. This time frame limits the number of new therapies that can be evaluated. The absence of new therapies is a problem since substantial increases in patient benefit are less likely to be observed in trials that merely alter doses or schedules of already acceptable therapies. An open dialogue among expert investigators remains the most effective approach for establishing the objectives of any clinical trial.

Endpoints

The endpoint of a trial is some measurable entity in the patient's disease process that can be used to assess the effectiveness of an intervention. A study may assess more than one endpoint, but in these instances the endpoint of primary interest should be clearly specified or else the study design should carefully reflect the complexity of interpreting multiple outcomes. Endpoints can be a composite measure of multiple outcomes. For instance, some studies assessing quality of life aggregate patient-reported scores from several related items that are all considered components of a larger concept called quality of life.

Selecting endpoints that will reflect the effectiveness of an experimental therapy is not always obvious. First, endpoints should be a valid (unbiased) measure of the treatment effect on the disease process. Endpoints that are susceptible to a systematic error that favors one treatment lead to biased treatment effects. For instance, trials assessing time to disease progression, in which the schedule for computed tomography (CT) scans is different for each treatment group, are susceptible to this assessment bias. This problem is not uncommon in studies comparing two different modalities such as chemotherapy and radiation therapy. Second, the measurement of an endpoint should be reliable and not susceptible to subjective interpretation. In some cases clinical response can be considered unreliable, since it is not uncommon for experts to disagree when interpreting the same radiograms (22). Third, endpoints that are directly relevant to the patient are preferable, although valid surrogate endpoints are considered indirectly relevant to the patient. Finally, endpoints that are not too expensive or inconvenient for the patient are preferred. It is not always possible for a single endpoint to exhibit all of these characteristics simultaneously. For example, avoiding death is extremely relevant to a patient with a lethal disease like advanced gynecologic cancer. Also, survival can be measured very reliably. However, most cancer patients will not only receive the treatments prescribed by the study, but after exhibiting signs of disease progression, they may also receive other anticancer therapies. In this case, the validity of overall survival comparisons is suspect since they not only reflect the effects of the study treatment, but also the effects of other therapies that are external to the study. For example, a meta-analysis of those trials comparing the survival of patients who were randomized to non-platinum versus platinum regimens for the treatment of advanced ovarian cancer concluded that these trials appear to have underestimated the true effect of platinum on survival. The reason is that many patients who were not randomized to the platinum regimen eventually received platinum treatment (23). For this reason, progression-free survival (PFS) may be considered a more appropriate endpoint in those trials, since it is unaffected by subsequent therapies. Survival may remain a reasonable endpoint in trials that explicitly compare a strategy of immediate treatment versus delayed treatment.

Endpoints may be classified as categorical (e.g., clinical response), continuous (e.g., serum CA125 values), or time-to-event (e.g., survival time). A time-to-event endpoint includes both time (a continuous measure) and censoring status (categorical measure). The data type influences the methods of analysis.

Measurement Errors

The susceptibility of an outcome to measurement errors is an important consideration when choosing an endpoint. Both random and systematic errors are components of measurement error. Random error refers to that part of the variation that occurs among measurements that is not predictable, and appears to be due to chance alone. For example, a serum sample could be divided into 10 aliquots and submitted to the laboratory for CA125 determinations. If the laboratory returns nearly the same value for each aliquot, then the associated random error is low and the measurement may be deemed reproducible. On the other hand, if the CA125 values vary considerably among aliquots, perhaps due to inconsistent laboratory procedures, then individual values may be considered unreliable. In this case, taking the average CA125 measurement across all 10 aliquots is expected to be a better estimate of the patient's true CA125 value than any single measurement.

Concern for reliability is one of the reasons for incorporating several items into a quality of life questionnaire. Quality of life is a complex entity and no single question can be expected to reliably measure it. A measurement of an individual's quality of life is therefore typically composed from an individual's responses to several items that are all considered to be associated with quality of life. Indeed, one step toward demonstrating the usefulness of any quality of life instrument is to show that it provides reproducible results when assessing individuals under the same conditions (24).

Systematic error, also called bias, refers to deviations from the true values that occur in a systematic fashion. For example, suppose an investigator initiates a randomized clinical trial comparing two treatments with time to disease progression being the primary endpoint. The protocol indicates that the patient should be assessed after each cycle of therapy. However, suppose that a cycle duration is 2 weeks for one treatment group and 4 weeks for the second treatment group. Using a more intense assessment schedule for one treatment group would tend to detect failures earlier in that group. Therefore, the time to failure comparison between treatments would systematically favor the second treatment group.

When there are recognized sources of error, it is important that the study design implement procedures to avoid or minimize their effect. For example, random error in many cases can be accommodated by either increasing the number of individuals in the study, or in some cases by increasing the number of assessments performed on each individual. Systematic measurement error cannot be addressed by increasing the sample size. In fact, increasing the sample size may exacerbate the problem since small systematic errors in large comparative trials can erroneously contribute to a "significant" treatment effect. The approaches to controlling sources of systematic error tend to be procedural. For example, treatment randomization is used to control selection bias, placebos are used to control observer bias, standardized assessment procedures and schedules are used to control measurement bias, and stratified analyses are used to control biases due to confounding. For an extensive description of biases that can occur in analytic research see Sackett, 1979 (25).

Surrogate Endpoints

Surrogate endpoints do not necessarily have direct clinical relevance to the patient. Instead, surrogate endpoints are intermediate events in the etiologic pathway to other events that are directly relevant to the patient (26). The degree to which a treatment's effect on a surrogate endpoint predicts the treatment's effect on a clinically relevant endpoint is a measure of the surrogate's validity. The ideal surrogate endpoint is an observable event that is a necessary and sufficient precursor in the causal pathway to a clinically relevant event. Additionally, the treatment's ability to alter the surrogate endpoint must be directly related to its impact on the true endpoint. It is important that the validity and reliability of an endpoint be established with appropriate evidence and not presupposed (27,28). Surrogate endpoints are sometimes justified on the basis of an analysis that demonstrates a statistical correlation between the surrogate event and a true endpoint. However, while such a correlation is a necessary condition, it is not a sufficient condition to justify using a particular surrogate as an endpoint in a clinical trial. For example, CA125 levels following first-line treatment of ovarian cancer have been shown to be associated with subsequent overall survival. Those patients with normal CA125 levels at the end of treatment tend to survive longer than those who have abnormal levels. However, it has not (yet) been demonstrated that the degree to which treatments reduce CA125 levels reliably predicts their effects on clinically relevant endpoints like overall survival.

The most frequently cited reasons for incorporating surrogate endpoints into a study include reduction in study size and duration, decreased expense, and convenience.

Primary Endpoints in Gynecologic Oncology Treatment Trials

The Food and Drug Administration (FDA) recently held a conference to consider endpoints for trials involving women diagnosed with advanced ovarian cancer (29). Meta-analyses were presented which indicate that PFS can be considered a valid endpoint for trials involving women with advanced ovarian cancer. It is important to recognize that although the general validity of PFS for predicting overall survival in this patient population has been established, PFS comparisons in a particular study can be biased. One source of bias arises from using different disease assessment schedules for each treatment group either intentionally or unintentionally. Delaying assessments for one treatment group artificially increases the apparent time to progression. Survival time is generally not susceptible to this source of bias.

Progression-free interval (PFI) may be a more reasonable endpoint in trials involving patients with early or locally advanced ovarian cancer. PFI should be distinguished from PFS. The difference resides in how patients who die without any evidence of disease progression are handled in the analysis. Patients who die without evidence of progression are censored at the time of their death in a PFI analysis, but considered an uncensored event in a PFS analysis.

Response (disease status) assessed via reassessment laparotomy following treatment has been proposed for use as a study endpoint in ovarian cancer trials (30). The justification is that those patients with no pathologic evidence of disease are more likely to experience longer survival than those with evidence of disease. The principal drawback to this endpoint is that reassessment laparotomy is a very onerous procedure for the patient, and many patients refuse reassessment surgery or the surgery may become medically contraindicated. Even among highly motivated and very persuasive investigators the percentage of patients not reassessed is typically greater than 15%. These missing evaluations can significantly undermine the interpretability of the study.

To date PFS has not been formally validated for use in trials involving patients with advanced cervical, endometrial, or vulvar cancers. In the absence of a formally validated endpoint, overall survival or symptom relief are reasonable endpoints. Since relief from symptoms is susceptible to assessment bias, trials utilizing these endpoints should consider blinding the study treatments when possible.

The endpoint selection for trials involving patients with recurrent cervical cancer has been controversial. Historically, some trials have been designed with clinical response as the primary endpoint. However, in recent GOG trials involving these patients, such as GOG Protocol 179 (A Randomized Phase III Study of Cisplatin Versus Cisplatin Plus Topotecan Versus MVAC [methotrexate, vinblastine, adriablastine, and cisplatin] in Stage IVB, Recurrent, or Persistent Squamous Cell Carcinoma of the Cervix), overall survival is considered the primary endpoint. The rationale for this choice arises from the observation that treatments that have demonstrated an improvement in the frequency of response have not consistently prolonged survival (31–33). Although subsequent therapies may have distorted the cause-effect relationship, the effect is probably at best minimal since there are currently no known treatments that have consistently demonstrated an ability to influence the survival time of patients with advanced or recurrent cervical cancer (i.e., median survival: 8.5 months).

In summary, the ideal endpoint provides reasonable assurance that inference about the causal relationship between the intervention and the endpoint is valid. The ideal endpoint can be measured reliably. It is convenient and cost-effective to measure. Unfortunately, in some trials these features are not available simultaneously. If a surrogate endpoint is used then its validity should be established, not presumed.

Eligibility Criteria

The eligibility criteria serve two purposes in a clinical trial. The immediate purpose is to define those patients with a particular disease, clinical history, and personal and medical characteristics that may be considered for enrollment into the clinical trial. The subsequent purpose of eligibility criteria comes after the clinical trial is completed and the results are available. Physicians must then decide whether the trial results are applicable to their particular patient. A physician may consider the trial results to be applicable when the patient meets the eligibility criteria of the published study. Unfortunately, this principle is problematic. The necessary sampling procedure for selecting patients for the study (i.e., a random sample of all patients) is never actually applied in clinical trials. Moreover, the principle ignores the fact that extrapolation is an inherent part of medical practice.

Within the general population there is a target population that includes those patients to whom the results of the trial are intended to apply (e.g., women with advanced endometrial cancer having had no prior systemic cytotoxic therapies). While an investigator can typically specify an idealized definition for the target population, additional practical issues also frequently need to be considered. For example, there are varying opinions about whether patients diagnosed with an adenocarcinoma of the fallopian tube should be included in studies that target the treatment of patients with adenocarcinomas of the ovary. Some clinical investigators will argue for the need to study a "pure" study population and ignore the fact that their treatment decisions for patients with cancers of the fallopian tube frequently come from the results of trials involving only patients with advanced ovarian cancer. Ideally, the size of a subgroup represented in a study should be in proportion to their presence in the target population (see the Ethics section). The degree to which a study sample reflects the target population determines the generalizability or external validity of the study results. Eligibility criteria should reflect a concern for the generalizability of the trial results. When clinicians frequently resort to extrapolating the results of a trial to patient groups that were not eligible for the trial, this may be considered a serious indictment of the study's eligibility criteria.

The ideal situation is when each patient who meets the eligibility criteria of a clinical trial is asked to participate. This is seldom possible since not all physicians who treat such patients participate in the study. Also, not all patients wish to be involved in a clinical trial. Impediments in traveling to a participating treatment center further reduce the target population. The source population is the subset of patients in the target population who have access to the study. Figure 9.1 displays common restrictions that can limit the entry of patients to a clinical trial.

Restricted access to the study may contribute a biased sample from the target population, referred to as selection bias. For example, participating investigators at university hospitals might tend to enroll disproportionately more patients with ovarian cancer who have undergone very aggressive initial debulking surgeries than their counterparts at community hospitals.

A potentially useful approach for determining the necessity of a particular eligibility criterion is to clearly identify its function. There are four distinct functions that an eligibility criterion may serve: benefit-morbidity equipoise (safety), homogeneity of benefit (scientific), logistic, and regulatory (34).

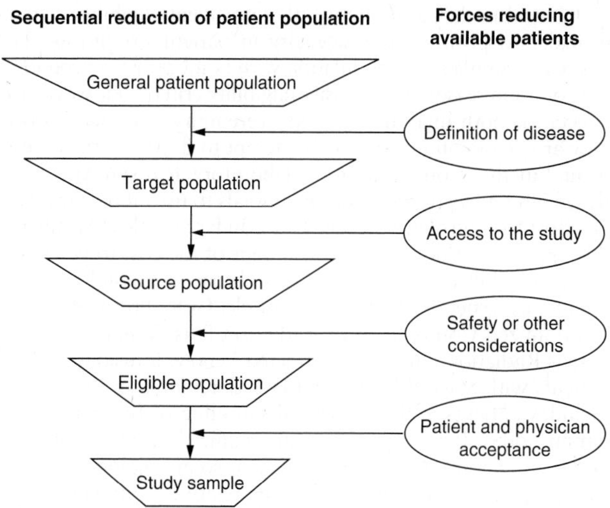

FIGURE 9.1. Sequential reduction of patient population.

Criteria for benefit-morbidity equipoise or safety are frequently imposed to eliminate patients for whom the risk of adverse effects from treatment is not commensurate with the potential for benefit (see the Ethics section). This concern can manifest in two ways. First, in oncology trials there is often some concern that study treatments may be too toxic for those with compromised bone-marrow reserves or kidney function. These patients are frequently excluded from trials when the potential benefits of treatment are not consistent with the risk associated with treatment. Second, even otherwise healthy cancer patients may be eliminated from the study when the risks from treatment are considered too great. For example, chemoradiation after hysterectomy is normally considered excessive treatment for a patient with stage IA cervix cancer since even without this treatment the risk of relapse is relatively small, but the morbidity of this combined modality following hysterectomy may be substantial. Therefore, eligibility criteria that eliminate these patients may be justified.

Eligibility criteria may be warranted when there is a scientific or biologic rationale for a variation in treatment benefit across patient subgroups. There is no scientific reason to expect that the effect of treatment is entirely homogeneous across all subgroups of patients included in the study. The effect of a new therapy may be expected to have such dramatic inconsistencies across the entire spectrum of the target population that statistical power is compromised (34). One example of this type of exclusion criterion is found in GOG Protocol 152 (A Phase III Randomized Study of Cisplatin [NSC #119875] and Taxol [Paclitaxel] [NSC #125973] with Interval Secondary Cytoreduction Versus Cisplatin and Paclitaxel in Patients with Suboptimal Stage III and IV Epithelial Ovarian Carcinoma). This study was designed to assess the value of secondary cytoreductive surgery in patients with stage III ovarian cancer. All patients entered into this study were to receive three courses of cisplatin and paclitaxel. After completing this therapy they are then randomized to either three additional courses of chemotherapy or interval secondary cytoreductive surgery followed by three additional courses of chemotherapy. The eligibility criteria excluded patients with only microscopic residual disease since there is no scientific reason to expect interval debulking would be of any value to patients with no gross residual disease.

Clinical investigators frequently implement eligibility criteria in order to promote homogeneity in patient prognoses. The desire to attain a study population with homogeneous prognoses is a common reason for excessive eligibility criteria. However, the concept is both unattainable and overemphasized. This notion may arise from an investigator's attempt to duplicate the experimental method conducted in the laboratory. It is standard practice in laboratory experiments on animals to use inbred strains in an effort to control genetic variability. In large-scale clinical trials this approach seldom has merit in light of the cost to generalizability. Eligibility criteria should be as broad as possible in order to enhance generalizability. For example, GOG Protocol 165 (A Randomized Comparison of Radiation Plus Weekly Cisplatin Versus Radiation Plus PVI [Protracted Venous Infusion] 5-FU in Patients with Stage IIB, IIIB, and IVA Carcinoma of the Cervix) includes patients with no surgical sampling of the para-aortic lymph nodes. Previous GOG trials required sampling of these nodes. However, there is no evidence or sound biological justification to support the notion that the relative treatment benefit depends on the extent of surgical staging. This is not to say whether or not surgical staging is itself beneficial.

Eligibility criteria can be justified on the basis of logistic considerations. For example, a study that requires frequent clinic visits for proper evaluation or toxicity monitoring may restrict patients who are unable to arrange reliable transportation. The potential problem with such a restriction is how it is structured. A criterion requiring that the patient have a car at her disposal is probably too restrictive in a trial of women with advanced cervical cancer, since patients from this target population tend toward poorer socioeconomic status (SES) and may not have access to private transportation. Such a restriction erodes the generalizability of the trial by over sampling those with higher SES and may prolong study accrual. Moreover, complicated eligibility criteria are more likely to function ineffectively. In general, complicated eligibility restrictions should be avoided.

Eligibility criteria based on regulatory considerations include those institutional and governmental regulations that require a signed and witnessed informed consent and study approval by the local Institutional Review Board. These restrictions are required in most research settings and are not subject to the investigator's discretion.

Currently many biostatisticians believe that eligibility criteria in oncology trials tend to be too restrictive and complicated (34,35). Overly restrictive or complex eligibility criteria hamper accrual, prolong the study's duration, and delay the reporting of results. The Medical Research Council has demonstrated that it is possible to conduct trials with simple and few eligibility criteria (36). The ICON3 (International Collaborative Ovarian Neoplasms) trial compared standard carboplatin or cisplatin-adriamycin-cyclophosphamide regimen to paclitaxel plus carboplatin in women with newly diagnosed ovarian cancer. This trial had six eligibility criteria, three of which were for safety: (a) fit to receive, and no clear contraindication to, chemotherapy, (b) absence of sepsis, and (c) bilirubin less than twice the normal level for the center. This is in sharp contrast to GOG Protocol 162 (A Phase III Randomized Trial of Cisplatin [NSC #119875] with Paclitaxel [NSC #125973] Administered by Either 24-Hour Infusion or 96-Hour Infusion in Patients with Selected Stage III and Stage IV Epithelial Ovarian Cancer), which compared two different paclitaxel infusion durations in patients with advanced ovarian cancer and had 34 eligibility criteria.

PHASES OF DRUG DEVELOPMENT TRIALS

The traditional approach to identifying and evaluating new drugs has relied on sequential evidence from phase 1, 2, and 3 clinical trials. Each of these study designs stems from very distinct study objectives. Phase 2 trials build on the evidence gathered from phase 1 trial results, and similarly phase 3 trials build on phase 2 and phase 1 trial results. The investigation of a given treatment may be halted at any phase, either due to safety and/or efficacy issues. Depending upon the underlying investigation, the time from the initiation of a phase 1 trial for a given treatment to the completion of a phase 3 trial often spans several years.

Phase 1 Trials

The purpose of a phase 1 therapeutic trial in cancer-related research is to determine an acceptable dose or schedule for a new therapy as determined by toxicity and/or pharmacokinetics. A phase 1 trial marks the first use of a new experimental agent in humans. Most phase 1 trials escalate the dose or schedule of the new agent after either a prespecified number of consecutive patients have been successfully treated or within an individual as each dose is determined to be tolerable. The usual phase 1 trial of a cytotoxic agent attempts to balance the delivery of the greatest dose intensity against an acceptable risk of dose-limiting toxicity (DLT). The conventional approach increases the dose after demonstrating that a small cohort of consecutive patients (three to six) is able to tolerate the regimen. However, once an unacceptable level of toxicity occurs (e.g., two or three patients experiencing DLT), the previously acceptable dose level is used to treat a few additional patients in order to provide additional evidence that the current dose has an acceptably low risk of DLT. If this dose is still regarded as acceptable, it becomes the dose and schedule studied in subsequent trials and it is referred to as the recommended dose level (RDL). The RDL should not be confused with the maximum tolerated dose (MTD). The MTD is a theoretical concept used to design phase 1 trials, while the RDL is an estimate of the MTD, which may or may not be close to it. Due to the limited number of patients involved in phase 1 trials, outcome measures such as response and survival are not the primary interest in these studies. When these outcomes are reported, they are considered anecdotal evidence of treatment activity. Eligibility criteria for phase 1 trials in oncology typically limit accrual to patients in whom conventional treatments have failed.

Early phase 1 trial designs were often ad hoc. Alternative strategies for estimating the MTD have recently been proposed. The primary motivation for these newer strategies is to reduce the number of patients treated at therapeutically inferior doses and to reduce the overall size of the study. One of these alternatives implements a Bayesian approach and is referred to as the continual reassessment method (CRM) (37). It has the attractive feature of determining the dose level for the next patient based on the toxicity experience from all of the previously treated patients. While the traditional approach has been criticized for treating too many patients at sub-therapeutic doses and providing unreliable estimates of the MTD, CRM has been criticized for tending to treat too many patients at doses higher than the MTD (38). Refinements to CRM have been proposed (39) and found to have good properties when compared to alternative dose-seeking strategies (40). Another family of designs termed the accelerated titration design (ATD) allows doses to be escalated within each patient and incorporates toxicity or pharmacologic information from each course of therapy into the decision of whether to further escalate or not (41). Both the modified-CRM and ATD designs can provide significant advantages over the conventional phase 1 design.

Even though the majority of phase 1 trials in cancer research follow what was described above, it should be noted that alternative phase 1 trials may arise in other settings such as medical device trials, prevention trials, education intervention trials, behavior modification trials, and where the first phase of investigation may actually utilize healthy subjects, like studies interested in determining the utility of a new educational intervention on smoking cessation. The phase 1 trial may simply be utilized as an approach toward gaining some experience with the intervention prior to moving forward to the next phase of investigation.

Phase 2 Trials

Once a dose and schedule for a new regimen have been deemed acceptable, a reasonable next step is to seek evidence that the new regimen is worthy of further evaluation in a particular patient population. The principle goal of a phase 2 trial is to prospectively quantify the potential efficacy of the new therapy. Since a phase 2 trial treats more patients at the RDL than in a phase 1 trial, it also provides an opportunity to more reliably assess toxicities. A phase 2 trial is often referred to as a drug-screening trial because it attempts to judiciously identify active agents worthy of further study in much the same way a clinician screens a patient for further evaluation. The study should have adequate sensitivity to detect active treatments and adequate specificity for rejecting inactive treatments. A phase 2 trial may evaluate a single new regimen, or incorporate randomization to evaluate several new therapies or treatment schedules simultaneously. However, in oncology a concurrent control arm is often not included in randomized phase 2 trials since these trials are too small to draw a reliable inference about relative therapeutic efficacy of the experimental treatments.

Phase 2 trials can have a single-stage or multi-stage design. In a single-stage design, a fixed number of patients are treated with the new therapy. The goal of the single-stage design is to achieve a predetermined level of precision in estimating the endpoint. While precision is one important goal in cancer trials, there is also a concern for reducing the number of patients treated with inferior regimens. For this reason many phase 2 cancer trials use multi-stage designs. Multi-stage designs implement interim analyses of the data and apply predetermined rules to assess whether there is sufficient evidence to warrant continuing the trial. These rules, which are established prior to initiating the study, tend to terminate those trials with regimens having less than the desired activity, and tend to continue to full accrual those trials with regimens having at least a minimally acceptable level of activity. Two-stage designs, which minimize the expected sample size when the new treatment has a clinically uninteresting level of activity, have been proposed (42). These designs are often appropriate for trials involving a small number of clinics. However, phase 2 trials in the cooperative group setting demand more flexibility in specifying when the interim analysis will occur. This is due to the significant administrative and logistic overhead of coordinating the study in several clinics. Modifications to the optimal design, which do not require that the interim analyses occur after a precise number of patients are entered, are useful in the cooperative group setting (43).

Regardless of the measure of treatment efficacy, most designs treat toxicity as merely a secondary observation. This approach is not likely to be appropriate in phase 2 trials of very aggressive treatments, such as high-dose chemotherapy with bone marrow support. In these trials, stopping rules that explicitly consider both response and the cumulative incidence of certain toxicities may be more appropriate (44–46). Bayesian designs, which permit continuous monitoring of both toxicity and response, have also been proposed (47).

The procession from phase 1 to phase 3 is a typical research path for evaluating a new therapy in humans. However, this research paradigm may not always be appropriate, and all three elements (i.e., "what," "how," and "who") of a phase 2 trial (see the Objectives section) have been challenged. It may be justifiable to eliminate strict phase 2 testing of a new combination of known active agents, if the combination is known to be safe and there is no antagonism anticipated between the agents, especially if the phase 3 trial includes provisions for futility analyses (see the Data Monitoring section). Another challenge to the paradigm is directed at whether patients whose disease is no longer responsive to standard treatments represent a fair test of a promising treatment plan. If the subsequent phase 3 trial of the therapy will involve newly diagnosed patients, it is debatable whether patients with treatment-refractory disease represent the proper phase 2 study population. Finally, clinical response has been a classic measure of activity in phase 2 oncology clinical trials. However, response may be considered a surrogate endpoint and is frequently not an ideal one, especially in trials of patients with cervical cancer. Additionally, new treatments that exhibit a different mode of action from the traditional cytotoxic drugs (e.g., antiangiogenesis drugs) may render response an unsuitable endpoint. In this case, PFI and survival time may be preferable endpoints for evaluating treatment efficacy in phase 2 trials (48). There are many issues that come to bear on whether the conventional research paradigm is appropriate. A thoughtful discussion among experts should precede all clinical research endeavors.

Phase 3 Trials

The goal of a phase 3 trial is to prospectively and definitively determine the effects of a new therapy relative to a standard therapy in a well-defined patient population. Phase 3 trials are also used to determine an acceptable standard therapy when there is no prior consensus on the appropriate standard therapy. Some phase 3 trial methodologies, such as randomization and blocking, have origins in comparative laboratory experiments. However, in clinical trials the experimental unit is a human being and, consequently, there are two very important distinctions. First, each individual must be informed of the potential benefits as well as the risks and must freely consent to participate before enrollment into the study (see the Ethics section). Second, an investigator has very limited control over the patient's environment during the observation period. This latter distinction can have a profound statistical implication, which will be discussed later.

Trials With Historical Controls

The strict definition of a phase 3 trial does not necessitate concurrent controls (i.e., prospectively enrolled patients assigned the standard treatment) or randomization (i.e., random treatment allocation). However, these two features are almost synonymous with phase 3 trials today. The basic phase 3 design is what is termed a two-arm randomized parallel design, i.e., given an appropriately executed randomization, the only potential difference (from a statistical perspective) between the two experimental groups in terms of an outcome variable is the experimental factor. In contrast, the principal drawback from inferring treatment differences from a historically controlled trial is that the treatment groups may differ in a variety of characteristics that are not apparent. Differences in outcome, which are in fact due to differences in characteristics between the groups, may be erroneously attributed to the treatment. While statistical models are often used to adjust for some potential biases, adjustments are possible only for factors that have been recorded accurately and consistently from both samples. Shifts in medical practice over time, differences in the definition of the disease, eligibility criteria, follow-up procedures, or recording methods can all contribute to a differential bias (see the Endpoints section). Unlike random error, this type of error cannot be reduced by increasing the sample size. Moreover, the undesirable consequences of moderate biases may be exacerbated with larger sample sizes. When a trial includes concurrent controls, the definition of disease and the eligibility criteria can be applied consistently to both treatment groups. Also, the standard procedures for measuring the endpoint can be uniformly applied to all patients. Inclusion of prospectively treated controls within the clinical trial requires a method of assigning the treatments to patients. Randomization and its benefits are discussed in the next section (see the Other Design Considerations section).

It is useful to distinguish phase 3 objectives as having an efficacy, equivalency, or non-inferiority design consideration. An efficacy design is characterized by the search for an intervention strategy that provides a therapeutic advantage over the current standard of care. An equivalency trial seeks to demonstrate that two interventions can be considered sufficiently similar on the basis of outcome that one can be reasonably substituted for the other. Non-inferiority trials seek to identify new treatments that reduce toxicity, patient inconvenience, or treatment costs without significantly compromising efficacy.

Efficacy Trials

Efficacy designs are very common in oncology trials. Examples include trials that assess the benefit of adding chemotherapy to radiation for the treatment of early-stage cervical cancer or trials that compare standard versus dose-intense platinum regimens for treating ovarian cancer. In each of these cases, the trial seeks to augment the standard of care in order to attain a better treatment response. From the outset of these trials it is recognized that the treatment benefit may be accompanied by an increased risk of toxicity, inconvenience, or financial cost. However, it is hoped that the benefits will be sufficiently large to offset these drawbacks. Suppose treatment A is the standard of care for a particular target disease population. The quantitative difference between treatments with respect to a particular outcome (B-A) can be described on a horizontal axis as in Figure 9.2. If we are reasonably certain that the difference between treatments is less than zero (left of 0) then we would consider treatment A to be better. On the other hand, if the treatment difference is greater than zero (right of 0) then we would conclude that the new treatment, B, is better. Furthermore, we can use dotted lines to demarcate on this graphic a region in which the difference between A and B is small enough to warrant no clinical preference for A or B. Consider the results from a trial expressed as the estimated difference between treatments and the corresponding 95% or 99% confidence interval superimposed on this graph. The confidence interval depicts those values of the treatment difference that can reasonably be considered consistent with the data from the trial. An inconclusive trial is characterized by having such broad confidence intervals that the data cannot distinguish between A being preferred or B being preferred (Fig. 9.2). This is a typical consequence of a small trial. On the other hand, if the confidence interval entirely excludes the region where A is better than B, then we can conclude that B is significantly better than A (Fig. 9.2). Note that in this case the lower bound of the confidence interval may extend into the region of clinical indifference, but the confidence interval must exclude the region below (left of) 0 difference.

Equivalency Trials

The equivalency study design is perhaps a misnomer, since it is actually impossible to generate enough data from any trial to definitively claim that the two treatments are equivalent. Instead, an investigator typically defines the limits for treatment differences that can be interpreted as clinically irrelevant. If it is a matter of opinion what differences in effect sizes can be considered clinically irrelevant, this issue can become a major source for controversy in the final interpretation of the trial results. Survival or progression-free survival endpoints are seldom used in equivalency trials; however, bio-equivalency designs are sometimes used for drug development. For example, if one agent is known to influence a particular biologic marker, then it may be desirable to design a trial to determine whether a new agent is as effective at modifying the expression of this biomarker. In this case, an investigator has some notion about the acceptable range of activity that can be considered clinically biologically equivalent. These studies are designed so that within tolerable limits, the treatments can be considered equivalent.

Notice that the results from the inconclusive trial in Figure 9.2 cannot be interpreted as demonstrating equivalency. Even when the estimated difference between the treatments is nearly zero, the confidence interval cannot rule out treatment differences that would lead to preferring A or B. Caution should be exercised in interpreting the results from studies that conclude

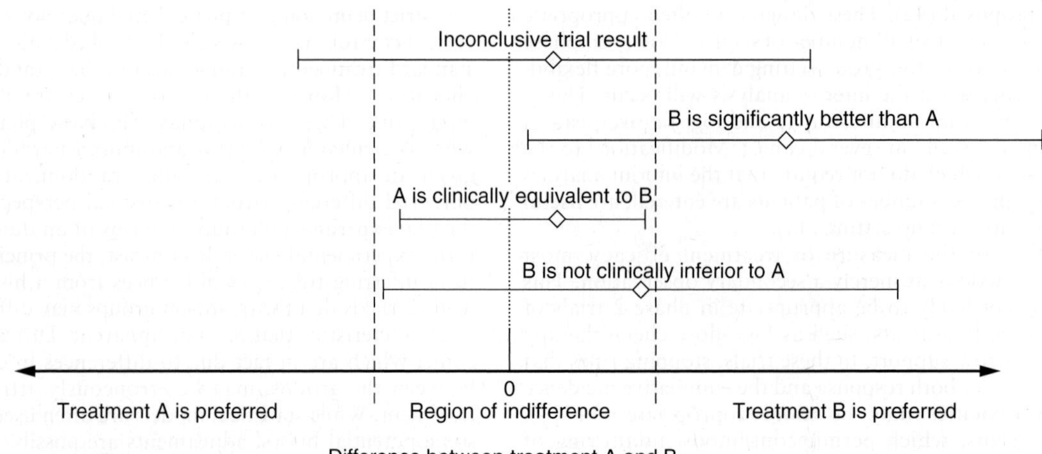

FIGURE 9.2. Graphical representation of the point estimates and confidence intervals describing the results from four hypothetical trials.

"therapeutic equivalency" when only a small difference between treatments with regard to the outcome is observed and it is declared to be not statistically significant. Even results from moderately large trials, which suggest therapeutic equivalence, may in fact be due to inadequate statistical power to detect clinically relevant differences.

Non-inferiority Trials

A non-inferiority study design may be considered when the currently accepted standard treatment is associated with significant toxicity and a new and less toxic treatment becomes available. The goal of this type of study is to demonstrate that substituting the new treatment for the current standard treatment does not appreciably compromise efficacy (49–52). Referring to Figure 9.2, the trial seeks to provide sufficient evidence to be reasonably certain that the difference between A and B lies above the lower boundary of the indifference region. This lower boundary is often called the "non-inferiority margin." Notice that if an investigator wishes to be reasonably certain that the new treatment does not sacrifice *any* activity of the standard treatment (treatment A) then the non-inferiority margin is set to zero. However, this would be equivalent to an efficacy design (described above).

The justification for the non-inferiority margin selected in a particular study is often controversial. If this margin is set too low, then the study has an unacceptably high probability of recommending an inferior treatment. If it is too high, then the trial utilizes too many clinical and financial resources. In order to select an appropriate margin of non-inferiority it is important to recognize that even though a non-inferiority trial may explicitly compare only two treatments, implicitly there is a third treatment to be considered. Suppose that several historical studies indicate that treatment A is better than a placebo for treating a specific disease. In this case, the goal of a non-inferiority study is to demonstrate that a new experimental treatment, B, does not significantly compromise efficacy when compared to currently accepted active standard treatment, A. However, it should also demonstrate that B would have been better than a placebo, if a placebo had been included in the current trial. In other words, the current trial will directly estimate the effectiveness of B relative to A, but it must also indirectly consider the effectiveness of B relative to the previous control treatment (placebo in this case). This indirect comparison relies on obtaining a reliable and unbiased estimate of the effectiveness of the current active control to the previous control from previous trials. Sometimes the margin of non-inferiority is expressed as a proportion of the effectiveness of A relative to the previous standard treatment. For example, a non-inferiority study could be designed to have a high probability of concluding that a new treatment retains at least 50% of the activity of the standard regimen, A. Note that an investigator may decide that she is unwilling to give up any of the benefit attributed to the current standard treatment. In this case, the margin of non-inferiority is set at zero (Fig. 9.2) and the design is the same as the efficacy trial. Indeed, an efficacy trial can be considered a study in which the investigator is willing to accept the new treatment B, only if the trial results indicate that B is superior to A.

Obtaining reliable estimates for the activity of the currently accepted active standard treatment can be a very troublesome aspect of non-inferiority oncology trials. For example, cisplatin 75 mg/m^2 and paclitaxel 135 mg/m^2 infused over 24 hours was the first platinum-taxane combination to demonstrate activity in the treatment of advanced ovarian cancer (53). Subsequently, several trials were conducted to assess whether carboplatinum could be safely substituted for cisplatinum (54–56) or whether taxotere could be substituted for paclitaxel (57). However, there has been some controversy about the size of the benefit provided by paclitaxel (58). An investigator can reasonably ask, "What is the effect size of paclitaxel and how much of this effect can I reasonably be certain is preserved by taxotere?"

Randomized Phase 3 Trials

There are several design features that may be considered for phase 3 trials. Some are more pertinent than others to gynecologic oncology trials. The most important feature to be considered is treatment randomization. A study with this feature, a randomized clinical trial (RCT), has several scientific advantages. First, both the known and unknown prognostic factors tend to be distributed similarly across the treatment groups when a trial implements randomized treatments. Second, a potential source of differential selection bias is eliminated. This bias could occur when there is an association between treatment choice and prognosis. It need not be intentional. When a physician's interest in a trial or a patient's decision to participate in the trial depends on the assigned treatment, a nonrandom association between treatment and prognosis can be introduced. Finally, randomization provides the theoretical underpinning for the significance test (59). In other words, the probability of a false-positive trial as stated in the study design is justified with randomization. It is important to recognize that these advantages, which are provided by randomizing the study treatments, are forfeited when all of the randomized patients are not included in the final analyses. All randomized patients registered on the trial should be included in the final analysis in order to promote the validity of the conclusions.

It is sometimes argued that since many factors that influence prognosis are known, perhaps other approaches to allocating treatments can be considered and statistical models should be used to adjust for any imbalances in prognosis. However, the conclusions from this type of trial must be conditioned on the completeness of knowledge about the disease and acceptability of the modeling assumptions. If the disease is moderately unpredictable with regard to the outcome, or the statistical model is inappropriate, then the conclusions are suspect. Results from nonrandomized studies can polarize the medical community. They frequently provide enough evidence for those who already support the conclusions but insufficient evidence for those who are skeptical.

Kunz and Oxman (60) have compared the results from overviews of randomized and nonrandomized clinical trials that evaluated the same intervention. They reported that the nonrandomized studies tended to overestimate the treatment effect from the randomized trials by 76% to 160%. Schulz et al. (61) compared 33 randomized, controlled trials that had inadequate concealment of the random treatment assignments to those studies that had adequate concealment. They found that those with inadequate concealment tended to overestimate the treatment effect (relative odds) by 40%. Some investigators do not appreciate the importance of concealment and will go to considerable lengths to subvert it (62). When the randomization technique requires pregenerated random treatment assignments, one must guarantee that the investigators who are enrolling patients do not have access to the assignment lists.

The patient-physician relationship can occasionally be challenged by introducing the concept of treatment randomization (63). Patients may prefer a sense of confidence from their physician regarding the "best" therapy for them. However, physicians involved in an RCT must honestly acknowledge that the best therapy is unknown and that an RCT is preferred to continued ignorance. One survey of 600 women seen in a breast clinic suggested that 90% of women prefer their doctor to admit uncertainty about the best treatment option rather than give them false hope (64).

Randomization Techniques

The simplest approach to randomization is to assign treatments based on a coin flip, sequential digits from random number tables, or computerized pseudo-random number generators. On average, each individual has a defined probability of being allocated to a particular study treatment when they enter the study. Although this approach is simple, the statistical efficiency of the analyses can be enhanced by constraining the randomization so that each treatment is allocated an equal number of times. Permuted block randomization is sometimes used in order to promote equal treatment-group sizes. A block can be created by shuffling a fixed number of cards for each treatment and then assigning the patients according to the random order of the deck. After completing each block there are an equal number of patients assigned to the treatment groups. For example, consider a trial comparing treatments A and B. There are six possible ways the deck will be ordered when the block size is four: AABB, ABBA, BBAA, BABA, ABAB, and BAAB. A sufficient number of assignments for an RCT can be created by randomly selecting a series of blocks from the six distinct possibilities. There are three features of blocked randomization that may be problematic. First, the probability of a particular treatment being allocated is not the same throughout the study, as in simple randomization. Taking the example above, every fourth treatment is predetermined by the previous three allocations. Second, the use of small blocks in a single-institution study may undermine concealment and allow an investigator to deduce the next treatment. This potential problem can be corrected by continually changing the block size throughout the assignment list. Third, large block sizes can subvert the benefits of blocking. As block sizes increase, the procedure resembles simple randomization.

The statistical efficiency of the study can be further enhanced by stratifying patients into groups with similar prognoses and using separate lists of blocked treatments for each stratum. This procedure is called stratified block randomization. It is worth noting that using simple randomization within strata would defeat the purpose of stratification, since this is equivalent to using simple randomization for all patients. Likewise, trials that stratify on too many prognostic factors are likely to have many uncompleted treatment blocks at the end of the study, which also defeats the intent of blocking (65).

When it is desirable to balance on more than a few prognostic factors, an alternative is dynamic randomization, a particular type being minimization. Whereas stratified block randomization will balance treatment assignments within each combination of the various factor levels, minimization tends to balance treatments within each level of the factor separately. Each time a new patient is entered into the study, the number of individuals who share any of the prognostic characteristics of the new patient is tabulated. A metric that measures the imbalance of these factors among the study treatments is computed as if the new patient were allocated to each of the study treatments in turn. The patient is then allocated to the treatment that would favor the greatest degree of balance. In the event that the procedure indicates equal preference for two or more possible treatment allocations, simple randomization can be used to determine the individual's treatment assignment.

Masking Treatment

Concealment. Concealment refers to the procedure in which the assigned study treatment is not revealed to the patient or the investigator until after the subject has successfully enrolled into the study. The purpose of concealment is to eliminate a bias that can arise from an individual's decision to participate in the study depending on the treatment assignment (66). Concealment is an essential component of randomized clinical trials.

Blinding. Blinding is a procedure that prevents the patient or physician from knowing which treatment is being used. In a single-blinded study patients are unaware of which study treatments they are receiving. A double-blinded study results in a situation in which neither the patients nor the healthcare providers are aware of that information. One purpose of blinding is to avoid measurement bias, particularly differential measurement bias (see the Endpoints section). This type of bias occurs when the value of a measurement is influenced by the knowledge of which treatment is being received (see the Historical Perspective section). It can occur when the measurement of an endpoint is subjective. Most methods for assessing pain are subjective and require treatment blinding in order to promote the validity of the study.

Oncology trials frequently do not implement blinding for several reasons. It is rather difficult to blind treatments when various treatment modalities are used (e.g., surgery versus radiation therapy, or intravenous versus oral administrations), when good medical practice is jeopardized (e.g., special tests are required to monitor toxicity), or when it is logistically difficult (e.g., the evaluating physician must be kept isolated from the treatment of the patient). In the absence of blinding, care should be taken that the method of measuring the endpoint is precisely stated in the protocol and consistently applied to each patient uniformly. Trials that assess quality of life or relief from symptoms should give serious consideration to treatment blinding.

Schulz et al. (67) reviewed 110 randomized clinical trials published between 1990 and 1991 in four journals of obstetrics and gynecology. Thirty-one of these trials reported being double-blinded. However, blinding seemed to be compromised in at least three of the trials. Schultz et al. concluded that blinding should have been used more often, despite frequent impediments.

Placebo. A placebo is an inert treatment, usually in a self-administered form (e.g., tablet). Placebos blind patients and also, usually, physicians to the knowledge of whether they are receiving the active or inert treatment. Placebos are frequently used in trials where there is no accepted standard treatment and the endpoint is susceptible to measurement bias. The use of a placebo is also important when the endpoint can be affected by the patient's psychological response to the knowledge of receiving therapy combined with a belief that the therapy is effective. This phenomenon is aptly named the "placebo effect." In such circumstances, the use of a placebo provides a treatment-to-control comparison that measures only the therapeutic effect. Note that the placebo effect is a distinctly different type of measurement bias from those that have been previously discussed.

GOG Protocol 137 (A Randomized Double-Blinded Trial of Estrogen Replacement Therapy Versus Placebo in Women With Stage I or II Endometrial Adenocarcinoma [IND #43,226]) is a randomized, double-blinded comparison of estrogen replacement therapy versus a placebo in women who have had a total abdominal hysterectomy and bilateral salpingo-oophorectomy for early-stage endometrial cancer. One primary reason for the use of a placebo in this trial was the potential for differential measurement bias being introduced by the physician monitoring patients on estrogens much more closely.

Sham procedures are similar to placebos in their function. The sham procedure is one that mimics the experimental procedure under study (excluding the therapeutic portion) to the extent that patients are blinded to whether they received the experimental component of the intervention. Careful ethical considerations must precede the use of a placebo or sham procedure in any clinical trial (68).

Factorial Designs

Factorial designs enable several interventions to be studied simultaneously. For example, each patient enrolled onto a study may be randomly assigned to receive one of two different chemotherapy regimens in addition to two being randomized to receive one of two different radiation regimens. The key assumption necessary for a factorial design is that all treatments can be given simultaneously without interaction or interference.

The term *factorial* arises from historical terminology in which the treatments were referred to as factors. Each factor has corresponding levels; for example, an investigator may wish to compare a study agent administered at three dose levels: high dose, medium dose, and none. The total number of factor combinations being studied is the product of the number of levels for each factor or treatment. For example, a trial that evaluates treatment A at three levels and treatment B at two levels is called a 3-by-2 (denoted 3 × 2) factorial design. If the relative effects due to the various levels of treatment A are independent of the levels of B, the two treatments (A and B) can be evaluated simultaneously. The factorial design provides a significant reduction in the required sample size when compared to trials that study A and B separately.

The most commonly utilized factorial design is the 2 × 2 factorial design, which includes two distinct treatment regimens at each of two factor levels. For example, suppose individuals entering a cancer prevention trial are randomly assigned to receive vitamin E (placebo-A or 50 mg/day) and beta-carotene (placebo-B or 20 mg/day) in a 2 × 2 factorial design. In this case, the factors are vitamin E and beta-carotene, while the respective factor levels are placebo-A or 50 mg/day for vitamin E, and placebo-B or 20 mg/day for beta-carotene. There are four treatment combinations. In a standard 2 × 2 design the main effect of vitamin E can be ascertained by utilizing information from each of the four treatment groups. In some studies, however, the main effects may be of secondary importance as compared to the "interaction" between each factor. An interaction exists when the effect due to one of the factors (i.e., treatment A) depends on the level of the other factor (treatment B). In drug discovery, a "positive" interaction may imply a synergistic effect of two drugs in combination, i.e., the effect of the combination therapy is greater than the sum of the individual additive effects. Reliable tests of an interaction require a relatively large number of patients in each of the four treatment groups. This testing, in turn, reduces the advantage of the factorial design over a standard four-arm study. Attention to the statistical power of such tests is an important part of interpreting the study results (69–71).

DIAGNOSTIC STUDIES

In a diagnostic study the objective is to develop a model that accurately predicts a particular disease state based upon other clinical information. In cancer-related diagnostic models this predictive information typically consists of some combination of demographic risk factors, medical history information, imaging data, and biomarker data, and can consist of a combination of qualitative and quantitative information. The simplest diagnostic model consists of a single binary marker of disease, e.g., whether a biomarker has positive expression (yes/no).

In order to determine the utility of a given diagnostic model several global measures of accuracy have been defined. These are described below. However, it must first be noted that a critical feature of these models is the actual *true* diagnosis of disease, oftentimes referred to as the "gold standard." If the gold standard diagnosis is not easily ascertained, this can in turn influence the empirical estimates of accuracy of a given diagnostic model in terms of biasing the results in either the positive or negative direction. In certain instances, the gold standard determination is clear cut, such as death or no death. However, in other instances the absolute determination is made by a committee of experts; for example, a panel of radiologists who may come to a consensus regarding a cancer/no cancer diagnosis would be referred to as the "gold standard committee." When designing a study to develop a diagnostic test, the accuracy of the gold standard determination is a vitally important consideration.

Under the assumption that the gold standard diagnosis is correct, the accuracy of a binary disease marker can be simplified. The quantities most often used for assessing overall accuracy include prevalence, sensitivity, specificity, accuracy, and positive predictive value (PPV). If we let *Pr* denote the probability of an event, *T* represent the test result being positive (+) or negative (−), and *D* represent the disease diagnosis as it is determined by the gold standard being present (+) or absent (−), then the following definitions apply:

Prevalence = $Pr(D+)$ = Probability of having the disease determined by the gold standard.

Sensitivity = $Pr(D+|T+)$ = Probability of having the disease among those who test positive.

Specificity = $Pr(D-|T-)$ = Probability of not having disease among those who test negative.

Accuracy = $Pr(D+|T+) \times Pr(D+) + Pr(D-|T-) \times Pr(D-)$ = Probability of the test correctly classifying an individual.

PPV = $Pr(D+|T+) \times Pr(D+)/\text{Accuracy}$ = Probability of correctly diagnosing positive disease proportional to all correct diagnoses.

Empirical estimates of these quantities are merely estimates of simple proportions or a combination of proportions conditional on the disease and test state.

Consider two separate tests (generically Test A and Test B) evaluated in two hypothetical studies involving 1,200 individuals and summarized in Table 9.1a. The calculations for the empirical estimates are demonstrated in Table 9.1b. Test A and Test B are equally accurate, with an estimated accuracy of 0.87. Specifically, each test is expected to correctly classify 87% of those tested in the population consisting of individuals with or without disease. Note, however, that in both instances the probability of the test being positive among those individuals with disease is quite low with PPVs of 14% and 8% for Test A and Test B, respectively. This is particularly noteworthy given the relatively high sensitivity and specificity

TABLE 9.1A

RESULTS FROM TWO HYPOTHETICAL SCREENING TRIALS

TEST A	T−	T+	
D+	140	60	200
D−	100	900	1000
	240	960	1200

TEST B	T−	T+	
D+	80	120	200
D−	40	960	1000
	120	1080	1200

TABLE 9.1B

RELATIVE ACCURACY COMPARISONS OF TEST A VERSUS TEST B

Estimates	Test A	Test B
Prevalence	200/1200 = 0.17	200/1200 = 0.17
Sensitivity	140/200 = 0.70	80/200 = 0.40
Specificity	900/1,000 = 0.90	960/1,000 = 0.96
Accuracy	0.70 × 0.17 + 0.90 × 0.83 = 0.87	0.40 × 0.17 + 0.96 = 0.83 = 0.87
PPV	0.70 × 0.17/0.87 = 0.14	0.40 × 0.17/0.87 = 0.08

Note: PPV, positive predictive value.

values for Test A (70%) as compared to Test B (40%). In general, the lower the prevalence is for a given test with fixed accuracy, the lower the PPV. In other words, for very rare diseases it is nearly impossible to obtain high PPV values even for tests with good sensitivity and specificity. This concept is extremely important when considering screening studies across large groups of subjects when the diagnosis of interest has very low prevalence, yet the accuracy measure appears relatively high.

What happens in the setting where a researcher is interested in a marker of disease that is measured on a continuous or discrete scale and/or would like to combine information from several variables in order to construct a diagnostic model? In the instance of a single continuous marker of disease, the problem is often framed in terms of determining an optimal cut point so that the continuous marker is transformed into a simple binary value. In the case where we are combining several pieces of information, the problem statistically reduces to a data dimension reduction problem that ultimately transforms a multivariate set of measurements into a single measure. One such technique is to utilize a logistic regression model, regressing the gold standard on the diagnostic variables of interest and then using the predicting probability of disease as the single univariate measure, which in turn then needs to be transformed to a single dichotomized measure. Other popular approaches to this aspect of data reduction in diagnostic testing problems include neural networks and classification trees.

Once the problem has been reduced down to a single continuous measure the next step is to examine the various potential threshold values from which a positive or negative diagnosis will be arrived at. One approach toward examining all possible thresholds is through the use of receiver operating characteristic (ROC) curves. An ROC curve is a plot of the estimated probability of a positive test result among individuals with disease (sensitivity) on the y-axis versus the estimated probability of a positive test result among individuals without disease (1-specificity) on the x-axis across all possible threshold values or cut points. (See Figure 9.3 for an example of an empirical ROC curve.) In essence, each point on the ROC curve represents one possible threshold value. The nature of the step function feature of the plot represents the empirical nature of the estimate, that is, for real data there are only a finite number of potential cut points. The area under the ROC curve provides a global measure of accuracy and ranges from 0.5 (worst case) to 1.0 (perfect diagnostic accuracy). This measure is sometimes denoted as the C statistic. For our example plot the estimated area under the ROC curve is C = 0.83. The area under the ROC curve has a similar interpretation as the measure of accuracy defined above. Specifically, the model is expected to accurately predict approximately 83% of the cases correctly over all possible decision rules. Once the ROC curve has been generated and the diagnostic model appears to have good relative accuracy, how does one determine the "best" decision threshold? In essence, the best threshold value determination comes down to putting more or less weight on sensitivity relative to specificity as it pertains to the specific clinical setting. There is not a one-size-fits-all approach in determining the best sensitivity-to-specificity tradeoff. Oftentimes, however, if sensitivity and specificity are given equal weight, a good rule of thumb is to utilize the threshold value that corresponds to the point on the ROC curve that is closest to the upper left-hand corner. In our example plot given in Figure 9.3 this point is marked approximately above with "*". Once an acceptable cut point has been defined, additional estimates for the diagnostic test of interest, such as the PPV, may be calculated as they were in the previous example.

The next issue of concern with respect to diagnostic model building is whether or not the model that has been fit based on a given diagnostic study will perform as well on a *future* sample of patients. As a general rule of thumb, when we optimize the fit of a model involving limited available data, there is a tendency to overestimate the accuracy of a diagnostic test relative to future performance. One commonly used strategy for assessing this bias is to divide the study sample into two distinctly separate sets: a training set and a validation set. The training set is used to develop a statistical model that provides the desired accuracy for classifying individuals into diseased and nondiseased categories. This modeling process is often called a supervised analysis, since it involves knowing the true disease state of each individual. In the validation phase the exact same classification

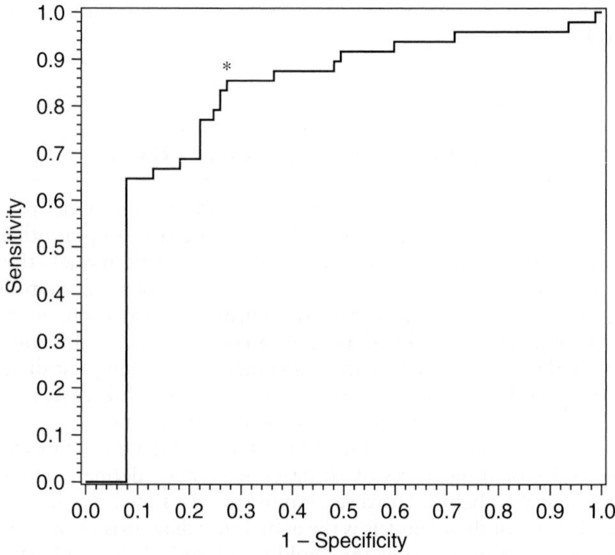

FIGURE 9.3. Empirical receiver operator characteristic curve.

procedure that was developed using the training set is applied to individuals in the validation set. The predicted disease state is compared to the actual disease state. The validation phase provides more realistic estimates of the accuracy of the classification procedure with respect to its performance in practice. Modifying the classifier in order to improve accuracy in the validation phase would introduce biases due to overfitting and therefore defeat the purpose of a validation phase. When designing a study to develop a new diagnostic test, one needs to consider not only the sample size needed for the training phase, but also the sample size needed for the validation phase. For smaller pilot studies where a validation phase is not feasible, there are statistical methods that can be employed in order to reduce biases from overfitting. However, the most meaningful diagnostic studies contain a true validation component.

STUDIES INVOLVING ADVANCED EXPERIMENTAL BIOTECHNOLOGIES

Many modern day experimental and study designs now involve data generated from advanced biotechnologies such as expression microarrays, comparative genomic hybridization microarrays, single nucleotide polymorphism platforms, and proteiomic platforms. These biotechnologies are typically designed for simultaneously performing a large number of assays (e.g., possibly greater than 1,000,000) on a given sample or pair of samples. The quantification of the assay results can involve multiple layers of data processing, and methods for inference utilizing such quantified values can be quite complex. *It is important to note that the naïve analyses of such datasets can have profound negative consequences* (72) and that *the development of optimal experimental/study designs and optimal data analytic methodologies are open and active areas of research* (73,74). There is currently a pressing need for the development of improved methodologies for the analysis of data generated by advanced biotechnologies. The complexity of the problems being addressed by research efforts involving advanced experimental biotechnologies, coupled with the complexities of the technologies (both physical and methodological) being brought to bear on problems, often can only be managed by research teams composed of diverse collections of investigators. Often such teams must not only include bench scientists and clinicians, but also scientists with expertise in biostatistics, computational sciences (e.g., high-performance computing) and bioinformatics. Indeed, the development and proliferation of collaborative research efforts involving advanced biotechnologies are part of a larger trend in which the practice of "team science" is becoming much more prevalent. For example, the National Institutes of Health (NIH) has recently implemented a multiple principal investigators (PI) model (http://grants.nih.gov/grants/multi%5Fpi/) to accommodate "projects or activities that clearly require a 'team science' approach."

Although advanced biotechnologies present new and important avenues to conduct research, it is important to approach the utilization of such technologies with reasonable expectations. Such technologies are not as automated as a naïve researcher might expect. The analysis of such datasets often requires the investment of significant sweat equity. For example, such datasets often require meticulous inspection to eliminate samples and spot assays of poor quality. "Garbage in, garbage out" is a common expression in data analytic circles (75) and reflects the belief that even when the best of data analytic methodologies is applied to data of poor quality, the results can also be expected to be poor. This is true for data analyses in general, but the expression is particularly relevant to analyses involving advanced biotechnologies given the size and nature of the datasets that they generate. Once the data is cleaned and incorporated into an appropriate analysis plan, researchers must also contend with the time-consuming task of inspecting the possibly high-dimensioned results of their experiment/study. Researchers new to such experiments/studies should understand that high-dimensioned data are not guaranteed to provide low-dimension result (e.g., a single highly significant gene), especially for exploratory studies, which are typically underpowered.

Researchers wishing to conduct research involving advanced biotechnologies such as microarrays are strongly encouraged to review the materials presented in Dupuy and Simon (2007) (72). The manuscript provides a review of 90 published outcome-related microarray studies as well as an invaluable set of guidelines for the statistical analysis and reporting of such studies. Several general concepts related to the analysis of such datasets are presented below.

Multi-stage Analyses

The analysis of advanced biotechnical data often involves the implementation of multiple data analytic steps that form a composite analysis. Multiple assays are performed and quantification of their outcomes is stored in a raw data set, which is typically a matrix with dimensions equal to the number of samples crossed with the number of assays performed on each sample. For example, for the 244K Agilent array comparative genomic hybridization (aCGH) arrays, the number of assays is ~244K where each assay corresponds to a two-color competitive hybridization. Typically, tumor and control samples are labeled with different fluorescent dyes (i.e., cy3 and cy5) and the relative fluorescence of the dyes at each spot on the array is used to measure the outcomes of the competitive hybridizations. The quantification of this relative fluorescence is rather complicated as it involves spot identification and determining a summary intensity value for each spot, since spots may not have a uniform intensity. There are many competing heuristics that provide such measures and it is an open area of research. Once assay values have been obtained (usually from imaging heuristics), the data is often subjected to a first stage of analyses, which involves the application of algorithms designed to correct and normalize/standardize the raw dataset. The second major stage of the composite analysis often involves inference on the population from which the assayed samples can be considered a representative sample; inference that is conducted via the application of statistical methodologies to the processed dataset.

It is commonly assumed that the application of algorithms designed to correct and normalize/standardize a raw biotechnical dataset will provide processed data that is devoid of meaningful systematic biases and spurious correlations. Whenever possible, the results from any analysis involving advanced biotechnologies should be interrogated to ascertain whether such an assumption is warranted. It should also be noted that proper experimental/study design can minimize the extent to which biotechnical data must be normalized/standardized and corrected, and that improper design can provide data that may be impossible to correct (76–78).

Multiple Hypothesis Testing

Dupuy and Simon (2007) (72) noted that the analyses of microarray experiments can usually be assigned to general classes such as outcome-related gene finding, class discovery, and supervised prediction. The authors defined outcome-related gene finding as "generally involving statistical methods to identify genes that were differentially expressed according to two categories." Such concepts extend to the analysis of other advanced biotechnologies and usually involve a large number of univariate tests (e.g., tests for differential expression in the case of expression arrays).

Certain complications present themselves when the number of univariate tests greatly exceeds the number of samples that were assayed—complications that are often ascribed to the "curse of dimensionality" (79). In the context of multiple testing the large number of tests presents challenges with respect to error control—challenges that can be particularly difficult to manage if the number of samples is relatively small and the univariate tests are under powered. Table 9.2 provides a summary of the possible outcomes of a set of m univariate tests where m_0 of the tests are true null hypotheses and m-m_0 of the tests are not true null hypotheses. The table entries U, V, T, S, and R depend upon the application of a given test function (i.e., a function that applies a test statistic to the data and determines whether the test result is "significant"). Note that V and T denote the total number of type I and type II errors, respectively. The expected value (i.e., the average or "expected" outcome that would be observed if the experiment were replicated many times) of both of these counts is of particular importance. For example, if univariate t-tests for differential expression were conducted for each of 10,000 genes and each test was conducted at a significance level of 0.05, then the expected value of V would be $0.05 \times 10{,}000 = 500$. Hence, such an analysis can be expected to produce, by random chance alone, approximately 500 spuriously significant findings. Conducting each test with a type I error rate of 0.05 controls the comparison-wise type I error rate but this control does not extend to the complete family (e.g., the set of 10,000 tests in the present example) of tests. The probability of committing at least one type I error across a family of tests is referred to as the family-wise error rate (FWER) and equals 1 – (probability of committing no type I errors) $= 1 - 0.95^{10{,}000} \approx 1$ for the given example. Therefore, if the goal of the analysis is to identify a set of significant genes that is unlikely to contain spuriously significant results, then conducting each univariate test at a level of 0.05 would be ill advised.

Statistical methods exist for the control of the FWER and are well described by Dudoit et al. (2003) (80). The most common of these include the Bonferroni, Sidak, and minP methods, with the Bonferroni correction being the most conservative but easiest to implement. To control the FWER at 0.05 the Bonferroni correction specifies that the comparison-wise error rate be controlled at $0.05/m$. For the given example, this would correspond to a comparison-wise error rate of $0.05/10{,}000 = 0.000005$ and would provide an FWER of $1 - (0.999995)^{10{,}000} = 0.0488 < 0.05$. Controlling the FWER is considered to be a conservative method of error control because it often requires that the univariate tests be conducted at comparison-wise error rates that are quite small.

A popular alternative to the control of the FWER is the control of the false discovery rate (FDR). The false discovery rate corresponds to the expected value of the ratio of false discoveries to the total number of discoveries (i.e., the expected value of $\frac{V}{R}$). Control of the FDR is appropriate in cases where researchers are willing to accept a certain percentage of spurious findings within their final list of significant findings. Development of methodologies for the control of the false discovery rate is an open and active area of research and the reader is referred to Cheng and Pounds (2007) (81) for a useful review of this topic.

Developing and Validating Classifiers

The development of classifiers of prognostic value (e.g., a gene expression signature that can predict clinical outcome) is an important and very active area of research. As with the multiple testing procedures, the development of classifiers is also complicated by the curse of dimensionality. Namely, when the number of features (e.g., a subset of assays) is much larger than the number of samples, it is often possible to overfit the data and identify perfect (with respect to the observed data) but spurious (with respect to the clinical population from which the samples were obtained) classification rules. Classifiers are commonly developed using either split sample or cross-validation procedures. In the former case, the assayed samples are split into training and test sets whereby the data in the training set is used to develop the classifier and the data in the test set is used to validate it. In the latter case, the data is partitioned into training and test sets multiple times and the validation results are, in essence, averaged over all such partitionings. Cross-validation procedures are mathematically more attractive, but a split sample approach with an independent and blinded test set provides the greatest protection against intentional or unintentional reporting biases (e.g., it prevents researchers from running multiple classifiers under multiple settings and only reporting the classifier that achieved the highest level of performance with respect to the test set). Hastie et al. (2001) (82) provide an overview of many of the basic methodologies for building classifiers. Dupuy and Simon (2007) (72) provide useful guidelines for their implementation.

HYPOTHESIS TEST

A hypothesis is a conjecture based on prior experiences that leads to refutable predictions (83). A hypothesis is frequently framed in the context of either a null or an alternative hypothesis. A null hypothesis may postulate that a treatment does not influence patients' outcomes. The alternative hypothesis is that a particular, well-defined treatment approach will influence the patients' outcomes to a prespecified degree. These hypotheses cast the purpose of the trial into a clear framework. A type I error is committed when the null hypothesis is in fact true, but the results of the study lead the investigator to incorrectly conclude it to be false. Committing a type I error would be disastrous if it means discontinuing the use of an active control treatment that is well tolerated and substituting an experimental therapy that is more toxic but, in reality, no better. A type II error is committed when the null hypothesis is

TABLE 9.2

CATEGORIZATION OF THE OUTCOMES OF m UNIVARIATE TESTS

	Number declared not significant	Number declared significant	Total
Number of true null hypotheses	U	V	m_0
Number of not true null hypotheses	T	S	$m-m_0$
Total	m−R	R	m

not true, but the study results lead the investigator to conclude that it is true. Prospectively quantifying the acceptable probabilities of these errors provides the underpinning for determining the appropriate design and sample size of a particular trial.

p VALUE

Some researchers are overly fond of reporting *p* values. At times statisticians play the role of the conservative physician, cautiously prescribing a significance test only when it is appropriate. There is a general concern that the *p* value is overused, even abused, and overemphasized. A common misconception is that the *p* value is the probability that the null hypothesis is true. The null hypothesis is either true or false, and so it is therefore not subject to a probability statement. It is the inference that an investigator makes, based on his data, that is susceptible to error.

Misconceptions about the *p* value (or significance level) may arise in part from a poor distinction between the *p* value and the α level (the type I error) of a study (84). The α level is the probability of the test statistic rejecting the null hypothesis when it is true. It is specified during the design phase of the study and is unaltered by the results obtained. The *p* value results from a statistical test on the observed data. It is the probability of the observed result or a more extreme result, given that the null hypothesis is true. R. A. Fisher, who is credited with developing the concept of the *p* value, suggested that it be used as a measure of credibility for the null hypothesis. Neymann and Pearson developed the notion of acceptance and rejection regions for the null hypothesis based on a critical value. Consequently, the concepts of type I and II errors were spawned. Fisher was very much against this "black and white" approach to measuring the evidence of the true state of reality.

The *p* value is not without problems. First, it confounds the relative treatment benefit and the amount of data (sample size) (85). Suppose two trials studying the same disease and the same treatments yield the same *p* value but one study is four times larger than the other. Assuming both were well-designed studies, one should have much more confidence in the estimate of the benefit from the larger trial. In short, the *p* value tells us little about the size of the treatment effect.

Second, important clinical differences and statistically significant differences do not correspond as frequently as they should. A large meta-analysis, which combines the results from several clinical trials, may yield a statistically significant difference that is not considered important clinically. Conversely, the literature contains many small trials with non-significant results that are statistically underpowered and cannot rule out clinically important differences (86).

Third, a *p* value of 0.05 is not necessarily a compelling result. Suppose a trial is properly designed to limit the probability of type I error to 5% (a two-tail test) and type II error to 10% for a treatment difference, D, which is considered the smallest clinically relevant difference. Also, suppose the trial is properly executed and the final *p* value equals precisely 0.05. In this case, the relative benefit between treatment groups would only be approximately 60% of the specified difference, D (84). Ironically, this statistically significant estimate of the treatment benefit is not within the range of clinically relevant differences specified by the study investigators. Furthermore, suppose that after reviewing this study result, the investigators agree that the benefit is clinically important and they wish to repeat the study exactly in order to confirm the original study result. These investigators will be surprised to learn that the size of their second trial is wholly inadequate to detect the treatment difference that was observed in the first trial. In fact, if the second trial is only as large as the first trial, then the probability of the second trial committing a type II error is 50%. That is, the probability of obtaining a statistically significant result from the second trial is no better than obtaining tails with the flip of a coin (84). These results are perhaps counterintuitive, but they emphasize the shortcomings of overinterpreting *p* values.

DATA MONITORING

Data monitoring can be classified into three categories: administrative, quality control, and endpoint monitoring. Observing extremely poor accrual in a trial that questions the feasibility of completing the trial is an example of administrative monitoring. Any evaluation of an actively accruing trial that addresses whether the study will produce valid results is quality control monitoring. Endpoint monitoring is when comparisons are made of the endpoints between treatment groups. This last category is the only one that attempts to test the hypothesis earlier than the formal end of the trial. Although much of the statistical methodology for data monitoring was published 20 or more years ago, formal plans for data monitoring have only become routine and expected in RCT designs in the last several years. The most uncomplicated situation is when an ongoing trial provides incontrovertible evidence that one of the treatments is inferior. In this situation the need to close the trial (or the arm using the inferior treatment) becomes essential. The challenge in a data monitoring plan is the definition of "incontrovertible evidence." The sophistication of data monitoring statistical methods and the formality associated with a data monitoring committee stem from a simple premise that knowledge of benefit (or harm) of an experimental treatment accumulates slowly over time. Many trials can be monitored because patients are enrolled over a period of years and differences in patient outcome may emerge between treatment groups before other patients are even enrolled. Endpoint monitoring was initially driven by the ethics of do no harm (see the Ethics section). However, endpoint monitoring has expanded to include terminating a trial due to the lack of improvement among those in the experimental group. Continuing the trial in this situation is not as much an ethical dilemma as a poor use of clinical resources. This type of data monitoring is referred to as futility analysis. The term is ideal in that it conveys the thought that continuing the trial is futile in the hopes of seeing a significant improvement in the experimental group when compared to the control group. Unless futility analysis is specially mentioned, the remaining discussion involves the more common data monitoring for dramatic differences.

The cost in monitoring endpoints (for the purpose of stopping the trial) is subtle and influences the characteristics of the hypothesis tests. Most physicians' understanding of statistics comes from frequentist theory and fixed sample size designs. Fixed sample size designs evaluate a hypothesis using a test statistic once at the end of the study (see the Hypothesis Test section). Data monitoring for the purpose of stopping the trial early, and thus varying the sample size, is in direct conflict with fixed sample size methods. The specific problem is that the rule that was established to declare significance (i.e., rejecting the null hypothesis) for a one-time test at the end of the trial is no longer appropriate when conducting the test multiple times throughout the study. Figure 9.4 is a theoretical illustration of how defining statistical significance is a by-product of how often the emerging data is to be analyzed. The lines in the graph display the evolving *p* values for 20 fictitious RCTs in which there were no differences in the effect of treatment (i.e., the null hypothesis is true). The thick horizontal line demarcates the conventional boundary for declaring statistical significance

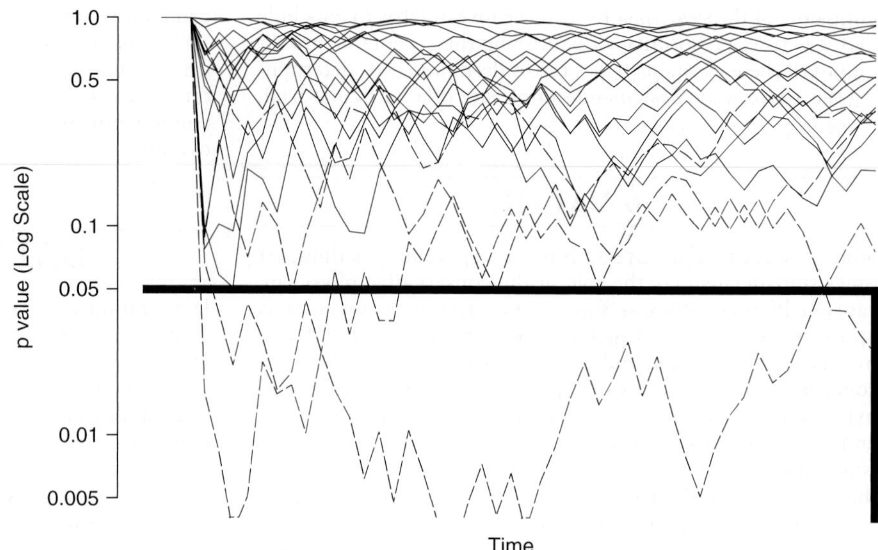

FIGURE 9.4. Continual monitoring of 20 trials. Conventional significance level under null hypothesis.

for a statistical test performed once at the end of the study. Note that if the data were analyzed only once at the end of these trials, only one trial in 20 (1/20 or 5% error) would be considered "significant." However, if the data are monitored throughout the trials, then four additional trials reach or exceed the critical boundary, and therefore ([1+ 4]/20) 25% of these trials would be erroneously considered "significant." This represents a fivefold increase in the type I error since all 20 trials were simulated under the null hypothesis. This figure illustrates why interim monitoring rules must be structured appropriately in order to properly control the experimental errors. Notice that the four additional lines that attained p values ≤ 0.05 eventually return to a nonsignificant p value. This illustrates that it is not the act of monitoring data that causes the increase in the type I error but rather premature study closure and declaring "significance."

Data monitoring has a much greater impact than changing the rules for declaring "significance"; it also changes the meaning of the p value and confidence interval estimates. Reporting fixed sample size p value in a trial that achieves the entire sample size but had data monitoring procedures is technically incorrect. However, some authors ignore this fact to avoid the complexity that would result by providing adjusted p values. Also, data monitoring affects the estimation of the statistical parameters. The parameter associated with the hypothesis being tested is biased when interim stopping rules are in use. For example, a trial that is stopped early due to extreme improvement in the survival rate among the experimental group will likely provide overly optimistic estimates of the reduction in the mortality rate. Another cost to data monitoring is that the decision to stop a trial early may preclude the study from properly addressing all of the research objectives. For example, the Women's Health Initiative (the component that evaluated estrogen plus progestin in healthy postmenopausal women with an intact uterus) was terminated early in the follow-up phase due to the alarming increase in breast cancer risk in the treated group and the lack of any evidence of reducing coronary heart disease events (87). The study's Data Monitoring Committee voted to unblind the study treatments and release results early. All study participants were made aware of the deleterious effects so that they could consider the consequences of continuing treatment. Any endpoints that depended on long-term follow-up may no longer be feasible due to the fact that so many women stopped their study treatments.

Ideally, investigators should have a thorough understanding of the options and the consequences of monitoring clinical trials. It is only then that they will be able to provide guidance to the statistician in order to implement the optimal monitoring plan for the trial under design that is ethical, efficient, and valid.

ETHICS IN CLINICAL TRIALS

Historically, there have been many personal views expressed regarding the appropriateness of clinical studies involving human beings. Specifically, Claude Bernard in 1865 wrote, "Medicine by its nature is an experimental science, but it must apply the experimental method systematically." Prior to World War II, clinical trials tended to be small and, therefore, they did not attract significant debate. However, at the Nuremberg Trials following World War II, it became apparent that Nazi physicians and military officials had performed strange and cruel experiments on war prisoners. These egregious violations of ethical conduct horrified the world and led to the development of the first international codes of ethics for human experimentation. Most notable of these is the Nuremberg Code, which was adopted in 1947. These ethical standards were intended to apply not only to war crimes, but to human experimentation in general (88). The Nuremberg Code advanced 10 principles (89):

1. The subjects of a trial should provide voluntary consent.
2. Consent to participate is an ongoing process, which an individual can revoke at any time.
3. The study should provide worthwhile results unavailable by other means.
4. The design should reflect the current state of knowledge from animal studies or other empirical studies.
5. The study procedures should be conducted so as to avoid unnecessary injury or suffering.
6. The risk to the subject should be consistent with the study benefits.
7. No deaths or disabling injury can be expected to result from the study procedures.
8. Appropriate precautions must be taken to protect subjects from any harm.
9. The assessment of risk and benefit is a continuous process. An investigator is obliged to terminate the trial when the risk of injury is imminent.
10. The study should be planned, executed, and reported by qualified individuals.

Unfortunately, at the time these codes were adopted they had very little practical influence on the practices of human experimentation within the U.S. medical community. Many investigators considered them unrelated to clinical trials (90). Also, some important issues were not addressed in these guidelines, such as the inclusion of individuals who are mentally or physically unable to provide an informed consent.

Based on the standards set forth at the Nuremberg Trials, the World Medical Association (WMA), at its 18th Assembly held in Helsinki, Finland, in 1964, adopted recommendations to guide physicians who participate in medical research involving human subjects. This document has become known as the Helsinki Declaration (91). It has been subsequently amended several times and most recently at the 52nd General Assembly, in Edinburgh, Scotland, in 2000. The current guidelines concede that "medical progress is based on research that ultimately must rest in part on experimentation involving human subjects." It stresses that the risks to an individual incurred through participation in a research trial must be balanced against the potential benefits. While all subjects must be adequately informed of the goals, procedures, anticipated benefits, and potential hazards, ultimately, responsibility for the human subject must always rest with a medically qualified person and never with the research subject him- or herself. Finally, in research involving human beings, "the interests of science and society should never take precedence over considerations related to the well-being of the subject" (91).

A few years after the Helsinki Declaration was adopted, Henry Beecher published an article that identified 22 clinical trials with serious deficiencies in clinical ethics (92). Each trial violated one or more of the principles advanced in the Helsinki Declaration and endangered the health or the life of the subjects. Many of these studies were conducted at prominent U.S. university medical schools, and many were either federally funded or funded by well-known pharmaceutical companies. In order to explain why an investigator would participate in these studies, Beecher suggested that the pressures for career advancement and promotion might have influenced ambitious physicians. Shortly afterwards, the Tuskegee and Willowbrook incidents also captured national attention. In the first incident the U.S. Public Health Service monitored 201 men in Tuskegee, Alabama, with advanced syphilis to determine the natural history of this disease. This study continued despite the availability of an effective treatment. In the second incident mentally handicapped children at the Willowbrook Hospital in New York State were intentionally infected with viral hepatitis.

In reaction to these incidents the U.S. Congress established the National Commission for the Protection of Human Subjects of Biomedical and Behavioral Research by passing the National Research Act of 1974. The purpose of this commission was to investigate the ethical problems in clinical research. This act also mandated that all research studies funded entirely or in part by the federal government be reviewed by Institutional Review Boards (IRBs). The commission described the role of the IRBs and provided ethical guidelines for research involving human subjects. These guidelines are presented in the Commission's 1978 Belmont Report. There are three important ethical principles for clinical research articulated in this report: respect for persons, beneficence, and justice.

The principle of respect for persons acknowledges that autonomous individuals, who are properly informed, should be free to exercise self-determination. At the same time, it recognizes that not all individuals are capable of self-determination and these persons must be protected (93,94). The informed-consent process arises from this principle. The principle of beneficence acknowledges that there is often a potential for both benefit and harm to the subjects of clinical research. This principle not only requires that there be a favorable balance toward benefit, but that the potential for harm be minimized and justified. The principle of justice requires that the burdens and benefits of research be distributed fairly. An injustice occurs when one group bears a disproportionate burden of research while another reaps a disproportionate share of its benefits. Therefore, those obstacles that tend to limit access to clinical trials, such as study eligibility criteria, must be appropriately justified or else eliminated (see the Eligibility Criteria section).

The actualization of these principles can be controversial. For example, some authors have noted that there is a natural tension between the science and practice of medicine. On one hand, physicians have an uncompromisable covenant of loyalty and fidelity with their patients. This obliges the physician to exercise his or her best judgment in making treatment recommendations for each individual. The "randomized clinical trial routinely asks physicians to sacrifice the interests of their patients for the sake of the study" (95). On the other hand, there are many diseases in which the best available treatment is not known, or worse, the recommended treatment is based on limited scientific data and hunches that may be ineffective or even harmful. Historical examples include bezoar stone as a general antidote, bloodletting or purging for dysentery (5), thalidomide for sedation of pregnant women, and antiarrythmic drugs following a myocardial infarction (96).

Dichotomizing the role of a physician as either caregiver or scientist is problematic. These roles should be viewed as part of a continuum that requires balance. "The tension between the interdependent responsibilities for providing personal and compassionate care, as well as scientifically sound and valid treatment, is intrinsic to the practice of medicine today. This tension is structurally part of the medical profession's covenant with the human community, not merely the expression of an individual physician-investigator's disordered intentions" (97). Not every medical issue is amenable to an experimental study. The efficacy of penicillin and the hazards of smoking were recognized without subjecting them to the rigors of a randomized clinical trial. Even among those issues that can be studied, it is not always clear that they should be. There certainly are many instances when clinical trials have been initiated in the absence of an ethical consensus (98,99).

This dichotomized view of the physician's role arises from the physician's responsibility to both the individual patient and the community. However, clinical trials are not the only instance when ethical consideration of the individual and the collective ethics can conflict. For example, it may be in the best interest of an individual to always be operated on by the most experienced surgeon, but society needs inexperienced surgeons to gain experience for future patients (100). The rising cost of health care also makes it necessary to frequently weigh the needs of the individual against the community's resources. This dichotomy in the physician's role leads to an artificial double standard, one for the practitioner and another for the investigator. Physicians who are not involved in clinical trials are no less obligated to inform their patients of treatment alternatives, as well as of the potential risks and benefits of each alternative. Also, respect for a patient's right to self-determination is appropriate regardless of whether the patient is involved in a clinical trial (89).

Another controversial area in clinical trials occurs when a new therapeutic approach consists of the standard therapy augmented with a promising new experimental drug. The experimental therapy is frequently associated with more risks than the standard approach. The justification for the randomized trial arises from the uncertainty over whether the additional risks may be offset by the benefits of new treatment. However, when given a choice between standard therapy and randomization, some patients with a generally fatal disease prefer to refuse randomization and "take their chances" with the experimental treatment outside the study. In this case, some investigators are reluctant to expose a patient to the risks of an unproven therapy, *outside* of a clinical trial. It has been suggested that this provides another example of when clinical trials "violate the physician-patient relationship, forcing investigators to use patients instead of treating them as individuals" (63). Markman (101) has proposed another twist on this same issue. When paclitaxel was first being evaluated in ovarian cancer trials (in 1990), the supply of the drug was limited and it was not generally available outside of a clinical trial. The only chance a patient had to receive paclitaxel in front-line therapy was to accept randomization with a clinical trial. In this case the patient's choice was to receive standard therapy or consent to a randomized trial in return for a 50-50 chance of getting the experimental therapy.

There are ethical considerations that must be addressed at every point throughout a study, beginning with its design. "An experiment is ethical or not at its inception; it does not become ethical *post hoc*" (92). The study must begin with clear and meaningful objectives that are worthy of investigation. Studies that address unimportant issues cannot be ethically justified. The study methods and design follow directly from these objectives. Since a study needs to be both scientifically and ethically justified, the investigators involved in the study must be both technically and humanely competent (89). Technical competence implies an appropriate level of education, knowledge, certification, and experience, while humanistic competence implies both compassion and empathy. The execution of the study must be devoid of scientific misconduct. Scientific misconduct includes any behavior that compromises the validity of the findings or violates the rights of the subjects who participate in the study (102). Since misconduct can arise from either fraud or incompetence, constant vigilance is the only countermeasure.

Finally, since those physicians not involved in the study base their judgments about the internal and external validity of the study on summaries, all publications must be prepared accurately, completely, and objectively.

References

1. Piantadosi S. *Clinical Trials: A Methodologic Perspective.* 2nd ed. Hoboken, NJ: John Wiley and Sons, Inc.; 2005.
2. Green S, Benedetti J, Crowley J. *Clinical Trials in Oncology.* Boca Raton, FL: Chapman and Hall/CRC; 2003.
3. Everett BS, Pickles A. *Statistical Aspects of the Design and Analysis of Clinical Trials.* London, UK: Imperial College Press; 1999.
4. Kelsey JL, Hildreth NG. *Breast and Gynecologic Cancer Epidemiology.* Boca Raton, FL: CRC Press, Inc.; 1983.
5. Bull JP. The historical development of clinical therapeutic trials. *J Chronic Dis* 1959;10(3):218–248.
6. Meinert CL, Tonascia S. *Clinical Trials: Design, Conduct and Analysis.* New York: Oxford University Press; 1986.
7. Kaptchik TJ. Intentional ignorance: a history of blind assessment and placebo controls in medicine. *Bull Hist Med* 1998;72(3):389–433.
8. Fibiger J. Om Serumbehandling af difteri. *Hospitalstidende* 1898;6: 765–769.
9. Hrobjartsson A, Gotzsche PC, Gluud C. The controlled clinical trial turns 100 years: Fibiger's trial of serum treatment of diphtheria. *BMJ* 1998;317:1243–1245.
10. Neuhauser D, Diaz M. Shuffle the deck, flip that coin: randomization comes to medicine. *Qual Saf Health Care* 2004;13(4):315–316.
11. Hinshaw H, Feldman W. Evaluation of chemotherapeutic agents in clinical tuberculosis: a suggested procedure. *Am Rev Tuberc* 1944;50:202–213.
12. Medical Research Council Streptomycin in Tuberculosis Trials Committee. Streptomycin treatment for pulmonary tuberculosis. *BMJ* 1948;ii:769–782.
13. Yoshioka A. Use of randomisation in the Medical Research Council's clinical trial of streptomycin in pulmonary tuberculosis in the 1940's. *BMJ* 1998;317:1220–1223.
14. Paterson R, Russell M. Clinical trials in malignant disease. Breast cancer: value of radiation of the ovaries. *J Faculty Radiologists* 1959;10:130–133.
15. Fisher B. Winds of change in clinical trials—from Daniel to Charlie Brown. *Control Clin Trials* 1982;4:65–73.
16. Frei III E, Holland JF, Schneiderman MA, et al. A comparative study of two regimens of combination chemotherapy in acute leukemia. *Blood* 1958;13:1126–1148.
17. Gehan EA, Schneiderman MA. Historical and methodolgic developments in clinical trials at the National Cancer Institute. *Stat Med* 1990;9:871–880.
18. Zubrod CG, Schneiderman M, Frei III E, et al. Appraisal of methods for the study of chemotherapy of cancer in man: comparative therapeutic trial of nitrogen mustard and thiophophoramide. *J Chronic Dis* 1960;11:7–33.
19. Goldberg K. Cooperative groups get reprieve from cut as budget is flatlined at fiscal 2006 level. *Cancer Lett* 2007;33(22):1–6.
20. Lewis GC, Blessing J, Kellner JR. *Clinical Trials in Gynecology Oncology: Cooperative Group Research.* Boston: Martinus Nijhoff Publishers; 1983.
21. Buyse ME, Staquet MJ, Sylvester RJ, eds. *Cancer Clinical Trials, Methods and Practice.* New York: Oxford University Press; 1984.
22. Therasse P. Measuring the clinical response. What does it mean? *Eur J Cancer* 2002;38(14):1817–1823.
23. Group AOCT. Chemotherapy in advanced ovarian cancer: an overview of randomised clinical trials. *BMJ* 1991;303(6807):884–893.
24. Guyatt G, Walter S, Norman G. Measuring change over time: assessing the usefulness of evaluative instruments. *J Chronic Dis* 1987;40(2):171–178.
25. Sackett DL. Bias in analytic research. *J Chronic Dis* 1979;32(1-2):51--63.
26. Fleming TR, DeMets DL. Surrogate end points in clinical trials: are we being misled? *Ann Intern Med* 1996;125(7):605–613.
27. Lesko LJ, Atkinson AJ Jr. Use of biomarkers and surrogate endpoints in drug development and regulatory decision making: criteria, validation, strategies. *Annu Rev Pharmacol Toxicol* 2001;41:347–366.
28. Buyse M, Molenberghs G, Burzykowski T, et al. The validation of surrogate endpoints in meta-analyses of randomized experiments. *Biostatistics* 2000;1(1): 49–67.
29. Public Workshop on Endpoints for Ovarian Cancer. 2006. http://www.fda.gov/cder/drug/cancer_endpoints/#ovarian. Accessed June 10, 2007.
30. Creasman WT. Second-look laparotomy in ovarian cancer. *Gynecol Oncol* 1994;55(3 Pt 2):S122–S127.
31. Omura GA, Blessing JA, Vaccarello L, et al. Randomized trial of cisplatin versus cisplatin plus mitolactol versus cisplatin plus ifosfamide in advanced squamous carcinoma of the cervix: a Gynecologic Oncology Group Study. *J Clin Oncol* 1997;15(1):165–171.
32. Moore DH, Blessing JA, McQuellon RP, et al. Phase III study of cisplatin with or without paclitaxel in stage IVB, recurrent, or persistent squamous cell carcinoma of the cervix: a gynecologic oncology group study. *J Clin Oncol* 2004;22(15):3113–3119.
33. Moore KN, Herzog TJ, Lewin S, et al. A comparison of cisplatin/paclitaxel and carboplatin/paclitaxel in stage IVB, recurrent or persistent cervical cancer. *Gynecol Oncol* 2007;105(2):299–303.
34. George SL. Reducing patient eligibility criteria in cancer clinical trials. *J Clin Oncol* 1996;14(4):1364–1370.
35. Begg CB, Engstrom PF. Eligibility and extrapolation in cancer clinical trials. *J Clin Oncol* 1987;5(6):962--968.
36. ICON Group T. Paclitaxel plus carboplatin versus standard chemotherapy with either single-agent carboplatin or cyclophosphamide, doxorubicin, and cisplatin in women with ovarian cancer: the ICON3 randomised trial. *Lancet* 2002;360(9332):505–515.
37. O'Quigley J, Pepe M, Fisher L. Continual reassessment method: a practical design for phase I clinical trials in caner. *Biometrics* 1990;46:33–48.
38. Korn EL, Midthune D, Chen TT, et al. A comparison of two phase I trial designs. *Stat Med* 1994;13:1799–1806.
39. Goodman SN, Zahurak ML, Piantadosi S. Some practical improvements in the continual reassessment method for phase I studies. *Stat Med* 1995;14: 1149–1161.
40. Ahn C. An evaluation of phase I cancer clinical trial designs. *Stat Med* 1998;17:1537–1549.
41. Simon R, Freidlin B, Rubinstein L, et al. Accelerated titration designs for phase I clinical trials in oncology. *J Natl Cancer Inst* 1997;89:1138–1147.
42. Simon R. Optimal two-stage designs for phase II clinical trials. *Control Clin Trials* 1989;10:1–10.
43. Chen TT, Ng TH. Optimal flexible designs in phase II clinical trials. *Stat Med* 1998;17:2301–2312.
44. Conaway MR, Petroni GR. Designs for the phase II trials allowing for a trade-off between response and toxicity. *Biometrics* 1996;52:1375–1386.
45. Bryant J, Day R. Incorporating toxicity considerations into the design of two-stage phase II clinical trials. *Biometrics* 1995;51:1372–1383.
46. Jennison C, Turnbull BW. Group sequential tests for bivariate response: interim analyses of clinical trials with both efficacy and safety endpoints. *Biometrics* 1993;49:741–752.
47. Thall P, Simon R, Estey E. New statistical strategy for monitoring safety and efficacy in single-arm clinical trials. *J Clin Oncol* 1996;14(1):296–303.
48. Korn EL, Arbuck SG, Pluda JM, et al. Clinical trial designs for cytostatic agents: are new approaches needed? *J Clin Oncol* 2001;19(1):265–272.
49. Wiens B. Choosing an equivalence limit for noninferiority or equivalence studies. *Control Clin Trials* 2002;23:2–14.
50. Rothmann M, Li N, Chen G, et al. Design and analysis of non-inferiority mortality trials in oncology. *Stat Med* 2003;22(2):239–264.
51. Senn S. Inherent difficulties with active control equivalence studies. *Stat Med* 1993;12:2367–2375.
52. Durrleman S, Simon R. Planning and monitoring of equivalence studies. *Biometrics* 1990;46:329–336.

53. McGuire WP, Hoskins WJ, Brady MF, et al. Cyclophosphamide and cisplatin versus paclitaxel and cisplatin: a phase III randomized trial in patients with suboptimal stage III/IV ovarian cancer (from the Gynecologic Oncology Group). *Semin Oncol* 1996;23:40-47.
54. du Bois A, Luck HJ, Meier W, et al. A randomized clinical trial of cisplatin/paclitaxel versus carboplatin/paclitaxel as first-line treatment of ovarian cancer. *J Natl Cancer Inst* 2003;95(17):1320–1329.
55. Neijt JP, Engelholm SA, Tuxen MK, et al. Exploratory phase III study of paclitaxel and cisplatin versus paclitaxel and carboplatin in advanced ovarian cancer. *J Clin Oncol* 2000;18(17):3084–3092.
56. Ozols RF, Bundy BN, Greer BE, et al. Phase III trial of carboplatin and paclitaxel compared with cisplatin and paclitaxel in patients with optimally resected stage III ovarian cancer: a Gynecologic Oncology Group study. *J Clin Oncol* 2003;21(17):3194–3200.
57. Vasey PA. Role of docetaxel in the treatment of newly diagnosed advanced ovarian cancer. *J Clin Oncol* 2003;21(10 Suppl):136–144.
58. Sandercock J, Parmar MK, Torri V, et al. First-line treatment for advanced ovarian cancer: paclitaxel, platinum and the evidence. *Br J Cancer* 2002;87(8):815–824.
59. Byar DP, Simon RM, Friedewald WT, et al. Randomized clinical trials. Perspectives on some recent ideas. *N Engl J Med* 1976;295:74–80.
60. Kunz R, Oxman A. The unpredictability paradox: review of empirical comparisons of randomised and non-randomised clinical trials. *BMJ* 1998;317: 1185–1190.
61. Schulz KF, Chalmers I, Hayes RJ, et al. Empirical evidence of bias. Dimensions of methodological quality associated with estimates of treatment effects in controlled trials. *JAMA* 1995;273(5):408–412.
62. Schulz KF. Subverting randomization in controlled trials. *JAMA* 1995; 274(18):1456–1458.
63. Emanuel EJ, Patterson WB. Ethics of randomized clinical trials. *J Clin Oncol* 1998;16(1):365–371.
64. Ellis PM, Coates AS. Ethics of randomized clinical trials. *J Clin Oncol* 1998;16(7):2570.
65. Therneau TM. How many stratification factors are "too many" to use in a randomization plan? *Control Clin Trials* 1993;14(2):98–108.
66. Schulz KF, Altman DG, Moher D. Allocation concealment in clinical trials. *JAMA* 2002;288(19):2406–2407; author reply 8–9.
67. Schulz KF, Grimes DA, Altman DG, et al. Blinding and exclusions after allocation in randomized contolled trials: survery of published parallel group trials in obstetrics and gynaecology. *BMJ* 1996;312:742–744.
68. Rothman KJ, Michels KB. The continuing unethical use of placebo controls. *N Engl J Med* 1994;331(6):394–398.
69. Xiang AH, Sather HN, Azen SP. Power considerations for testing an interaction in a 2xk factorial design with failure time outcome. *Control Clin Trials* 1994;15:489–502.
70. Peterson B, George SL. Sample size requirements and length of study for testing interactions in a 2xk factorial design when time-to-failure is the outcome. *Control Clin Trials* 1993;14:511–522.
71. Green S, Liu PY, O'Sullivan J. Factorial design considerations. *J Clin Oncol* 2002;20(16):3424–3430.
72. Dupuy A, Simon RM. Critical review of published microarray studies for cancer outcome and guidelines on statistical analysis and reporting. *J Natl Cancer Inst* 2007;99(2):147–157.
73. Rosa GJ, de Leon N, Rosa AJ. Review of microarray experimental design strategies for genetical genomics studies. *Physiol Genomics* 2006;28(1): 15–23.
74. Johnson WE, Li C, Rabinovic A. Adjusting batch effects in microarray expression data using empirical Bayes methods. *Biostatistics* 2007;8(1): 118–127.
75. Wikipedia. Garbage in, garbage out. http://en.wikipedia.org/w/index.php?title=Garbage_In%2C_Garbage_Out&oldid=137752376. Accessed June 24, 2007.
76. Hu J, Coombes KR, Morris JS, et al. The importance of experimental design in proteomic mass spectrometry experiments: some cautionary tales. *Brief Funct Genomic Proteomic* 2005;3(4):322–331.
77. Dabney AR, Storey JD. A reanalysis of a published Affymetrix GeneChip control dataset. *Genome Biol* 2006;7(3):401.
78. Gaile DP, Miecznikowski JC. Putative null distributions corresponding to tests of differential expression in the Golden Spike dataset are intensity dependent. *BMC Genomics* 2007;8:105.
79. Bellman RE. *Dynamic Programming.* Princeton, NJ: Princeton University Press; 1957.
80. Dudoit S, Shaffer JP, Boldrick JC. Multiple hypothesis testing in microarray experiments. *Stat Sci* 2003;18:71–103.
81. Cheng C, Pounds S. False discovery rate paradigms for statistical analyses of microarray gene expression data. *Bioinformation* 2007;1(10): 436–446.
82. Hastie T, Tibshirani R, Friedman J. The elements of statistical learning: data mining, inference and prediction. New York. Springer; 2001.
83. Last, JM, ed. *A Dictionary of Epidemiology.* 3rd ed. New York: Oxford University Press; 1995.
84. Goodman SN. p values, hypothesis tests, and likelihood: implications for epidemiology of a neglected historical debate. *Am J Epidemiol* 1993;137(5): 485–499.
85. Lang JM, Rothman KJ, Cann CI. That confounded p-value. *Epidemiology* 1998;9(1):7–8.
86. Machin D, Stenning SP, Parmar MKB, et al. Thirty years of Medical Research Council randomized trials in solid tumors. *Clin Oncol* 1997;9:100–114.
87. Rossouw JE, Anderson GL, Prentice RL, et al. Risks and benefits of estrogen plus progestin in healthy postmenopausal women: principal results from the Women's Health Initiative randomized controlled trial. *JAMA* 2002;288(3):321–333.
88. Katz J. The Nuremberg Code and the Nuremberg Trial: a reappraisal. *JAMA* 1996;276:1662–1666.
89. Piantadosi S. Clinical trials: a methodologic perspective. New York: John Wiley and Sons; 1997.
90. Faden RR, Lederer SE, Moreno JD. US medical researchers, the Nuremberg Doctors Trial, and the Nuremberg Code. *JAMA* 1996;276: 1667–1671.
91. World Medical Association General Assembly. World Medical Association's Declaration of Helsinki: ethical principles for medical research involving human subjects. *J International Bioethics* 2004;15:124–129. research involving human subjects (revised: 1975, 1983, 1989, 1996, 2000, 2002, 2004). In; 1964.
92. Beecher HK. Ethics and clinical research. *N Engl J Med* 1966;274(24): 1354–1360.
93. Michels R. Are research ethics bad for our mental health? *N Engl J Med* 1999;340(18):1427–1430.
94. Capron AM. Ethical and human-rights issues in research on mental disorders that may effect decision-making capacity. *N Engl J Med* 1999;340(18):1430–1434.
95. Hellman S, Hellman DS. Of mice but not men: problems of the randomized clinical trial. *N Engl J Med* 1991;324(22):1585–1589.
96. Epstein AE, Hallstrom AP, Rogers WJ, et al. Mortality following ventricular arrhythmia suppression by encainide, flecainide and moricizine after myocardial infarcation: the original design concept of the Cardiac Arrhthmia Suppression Trial (CAST). *JAMA* 1993;270:2451–2455.
97. Roy DJ. Controlled clinical trials: an ethical imperative. *J Chronic Dis* 1986;39(3):159–162.
98. Adami H, Baron J, Rothman K. Ethics of a prostate cancer screening trial. *Lancet* 1994;343(8903):958–960.
99. Noonan E. Ethicists fault mental health researchers over use of 'date-rape drug' on test subjects. *Buffalo News* January 1, 1999:A8.
100. Armitage P. Attitudes in clinical trials. *Stat Med* 1998;17:2675–2683.
101. Markman M. Ethical difficulties with randomized clinical trials involving cancer patients: examples from the field of gynecologic oncology. *J Clin Ethics* 1992;3(3):193–195.
102. Shapiro MF, Charrow RP. Scientific misconduct in investigational drug trials. *N Engl J Med* 1985;312(11):731–736.

CHAPTER 10 ■ DIAGNOSTIC IMAGING TECHNIQUES IN GYNECOLOGIC ONCOLOGY

DARCY J. WOLFMAN, SUSAN M. ASCHER, HEDVIG HRICAK,
CIRRELDA COOPER, AND LESLIE SCOUTT

INTRODUCTION

This chapter addresses the role of diagnostic imaging in evaluating gynecologic malignancy. Comprehensive imaging of the female pelvis can be achieved using a combination of ultrasound (US), computed tomography (CT), magnetic resonance imaging (MRI), and 2-[^{18}F]-fluoro-2-deoxy-D-glucose positron emission tomography (FDG-PET). The objectives of imaging in gynecologic oncology are straightforward: primary tumor detection and characterization, image-guided percutaneous biopsy, staging, monitoring treatment response, and detecting tumor recurrence. Each imaging modality listed above is appropriate only in certain clinical situations and this chapter discusses not only what is possible in imaging of the female pelvis, but also what is appropriate for a given clinical situation. In some instances, more than one modality may be appropriate, and it is best to discuss the clinical question with the radiologist to determine which modality will be most useful. As with any changing technologic arena, imaging strategies are not static and require continuous updating and reevaluation.

IMAGING MODALITIES

Ultrasound

US is considered the initial imaging modality of choice in the workup of most pelvic disorders. Currently, the accepted roles of US in women with suspected gynecologic malignancy include characterization of adnexal masses to help differentiate benign from malignant ovarian masses, identification of endometrial abnormalities in women with intermenstrual or postmenopausal bleeding, and detection of primary or recurrent gestational trophoblastic disease in women with elevated serum beta human chorionic gonadotropin (β-hCG) levels. US is also used to guide biopsy of primary pelvic tumors and/or metastases and to guide drainage of postoperative fluid collections such as lymphoceles, seromas, or abscesses. The role of US in screening high-risk patient populations for ovarian or endometrial carcinoma remains controversial.

US offers many advantages: it is relatively inexpensive, is widely available, provides multiplanar imaging, and is without known risk. However, US has many limitations as well: it is operator dependent; it is a limited, targeted exam; and image quality may be significantly degraded by patient body habitus and/or bowel gas. Transvaginal ultrasound (TVS) provides the best spatial and soft-tissue resolution, but it comes at the cost of a significant decrease in the size of the field of view. Sonohysterosalpingogram (SHg), which utilizes TVS while distending the endometrial cavity with fluid, can be useful in evaluating the endometrium.

Computed Tomography

CT is the primary imaging modality for evaluating the overall extent of a known gynecologic malignancy and for detecting residual and recurrent pelvic tumors. CT staging is more accurate than clinical staging in locally advanced disease and in cancers with a high propensity for lymphatic or peritoneal metastases. CT can also survey the brain, chest, and upper abdomen to provide information about extrapelvic disease. CT-guided biopsy can confirm metastatic spread of disease. Small and difficult to access masses are sometimes more readily biopsied using CT fluoroscopy (1).

Advantages of CT include ready availability, short scanning times, large field of view, and high spatial resolution. The advent of multidetector CT (MDCT) using continuous spiral (helical) acquisitions and multirow detector arrays (4-, 16-, 32-, and 64-slice systems) allows for faster scanning with higher image quality. Rapid technologic advances in MDCT include the ability to obtain submillimeter slice thickness, multiphasic contrast studies (such as arterial and venous phase enhancement after a single injection), CT angiography, endoluminal "fly-through" techniques (as used in CT colonoscopy), and rapid three-dimensional (3-D) reconstructions.

Disadvantages of CT include the use of ionizing radiation, degradation of image quality by patient body habitus or metallic implants, such as a hip prosthesis, and the morbidity and mortality associated with iodinated contrast agents. Despite technical improvements, CT remains of limited utility in the detection of primary gynecologic malignancies and the characterization of early-stage disease.

Magnetic Resonance Imaging

There is substantial evidence supporting the usefulness of MRI in staging gynecologic malignancies. MRI has been shown to be superior to CT in the staging of endometrial and cervical cancers (2,3). MRI may also be useful in the staging of ovarian cancer and gestational trophoblastic disease (GTD). In addition, MRI can often differentiate radiation fibrosis from recurrent tumor (4) and is useful in the detection of recurrent cervical cancer. The accuracy of MRI assessment of lymph node invasion is similar to that of CT; both rely on size criteria to detect adenopathy (5). In addition, MRI-guided biopsies are gaining wider clinical acceptance.

Although MRI is still relatively expensive, it minimizes costs in some clinical settings by limiting or eliminating the need for more expensive and/or more invasive diagnostic or surgical procedures (6,7). There are at least three cost-minimizing indications for MRI in the evaluation of women with gynecologic malignancy: (a) the staging of invasive cervical carcinoma as an adjunct to clinical examination; (b) the preoperative management of women with endometrial cancer (8); and (c) the characterization of adnexal lesions when US and clinical examination are indeterminate (6,7). In addition, a meta-analysis of imaging endometrial cancer found that MRI was the best modality for multifactorial assessment (8).

Advantages of MRI include superior soft-tissue contrast, absence of ionizing radiation, multiplanar capability, and relatively fast (i.e., breath-hold and breathing-independent) techniques. MRI is the modality of choice for patients with allergies to iodinated intravenous contrast media or renal impairment. However, clinicians should be aware that gadolinium contrast agents used in MRI have recently been associated with the development of nephrogenic systemic fibrosis (NSF), a rare progressive connective tissue disease, in patients with end-stage renal disease and/or acute renal failure. Current recommendations from the American College of Radiology (9) include immediate dialysis after administration of a gadolinium contrast agent and a risk-benefit assessment on the use of gadolinium contrast in this patient population.

One disadvantage of MRI is the longer scan times when compared to CT. In addition, MRI is contraindicated in patients with pacemakers, cochlear implants, certain vascular clips, metallic objects in the eye, and neural stimulators. Furthermore, some patients may experience claustrophobia and may require sedation in order to complete a diagnostic examination.

Positron Emission Tomography

PET with the glucose analog FDG images tumors by showing areas of increased glucose uptake (10). FDG-PET thus takes advantage of a biochemical change (the accelerated rate of glycolysis) associated with malignancy that often precedes, and can be more specific than, the structural changes visualized by more conventional imaging means. This capability is the biggest advantage FDG-PET has over other modalities. FDG-PET does not have the same spatial resolution or soft tissue contrast as US, CT, or MRI, but image fusion techniques that overlay FDG-PET images onto anatomic images are available. PET-CT scanners, which are equipped with both PET and CT detectors, allow both modalities to be performed at once and have gained wide clinical acceptance.

In recent years, research has shown that FDG-PET is useful for the detection of recurrent ovarian, cervical, and endometrial cancer and for the staging of cervical cancer. As further research is done, more applications of FDG-PET in evaluation of gynecologic malignancies will become known.

There are several disadvantages of FDG-PET. False negatives can occur with lesions smaller then 1.0 cm and with certain tumor types that demonstrate low metabolic activity. False-positive results can be seen with several inflammatory disorders such as tuberculosis and granulomatous disease.

Excretory Urography

The use of excretory urography in the evaluation of gynecologic malignancies has been on the decline for several years; it is neither sensitive nor accurate in delineating tumor extent and bladder invasion (11). Today, cross-sectional examinations provide similar and, in most instances, additional information.

Barium Enema

Barium enema (BE) in the workup of gynecologic pelvic cancers is also on the decline. If BE is used, signs of bowel involvement include fixation and tethering of the bowel wall, irregular serrations at the mass–colon interface, an annular defect from circumferential involvement, and mucosal ulceration and fistulization from complete transmural invasion. Unfortunately, these signs are not specific for involvement from gynecologic cancer (12). In fact, BE has a low positive yield when used in the routine evaluation of women with gynecologic malignancy—it is useful only in the workup of women with advanced disease for the detection of specific complications (13). Cross-sectional imaging has the advantage of providing information about structures surrounding the bowel and, thus, eliminates the need to infer this information indirectly from findings on BE.

EXAMINATION TECHNIQUES AND NORMAL ANATOMY

Ultrasound

Techniques

Adequate ultrasound evaluation of the female pelvis requires a transvaginal approach. By placing the transducer closer to the organs of interest, less penetration of the US beam is necessary and a higher frequency probe can be used. The use of a higher frequency transducer, typically 5.0 to 7.5 MHz, results in significantly improved spatial resolution and fewer imaging artifacts in comparison to transabdominal imaging but at the cost of a smaller field of view. Hence, transabdominal imaging must be considered an important complementary imaging technique if the mass is larger than the TVS field of view, the ovaries are displaced out of the pelvis, the ovaries are not visualized because of the presence of bowel gas, or to evaluate important ancillary findings such as hydronephrosis, ascites, peritoneal and/or hepatic implants, and liver metastases. Transabdominal imaging also provides a better overall view of the pelvis and the relationship of female pelvic organs to the pelvic sidewall and bladder.

Patients undergoing TVS are examined with an empty bladder in the supine position with the knees flexed and the hips slightly elevated and externally rotated. A gel-filled condom is placed over the 5.0- to 7.5-MHz probe, which is inserted into the vagina following application of an external lubricant. Transabdominal pelvic imaging is performed with a 3.5- to 5.0-MHz curved array transducer using a distended urinary bladder as an acoustic window to view the female pelvic organs.

Three-dimensional ultrasound is a new ultrasound technique that has been shown to decrease scanning time and possibly improve diagnostic confidence in pelvic imaging (14,15).

Sonohysterography (SHG) is a technique that is increasingly performed to better evaluate the endometrium (Fig. 10.1). With this technique, sterile saline is infused into the endometrial cavity under continuous TVS guidance. The sterile saline distends the endometrial cavity, separating the anterior and posterior endometrial layers and outlining the endometrial surface.

To perform a SHg, a baseline TVS examination is initially done. After insertion of a single-hinged speculum, the cervix is cleansed with Betadine and a 5F to 7F catheter is threaded through the cervical os. The catheter should be flushed with saline prior to insertion to remove the air from the lumen of

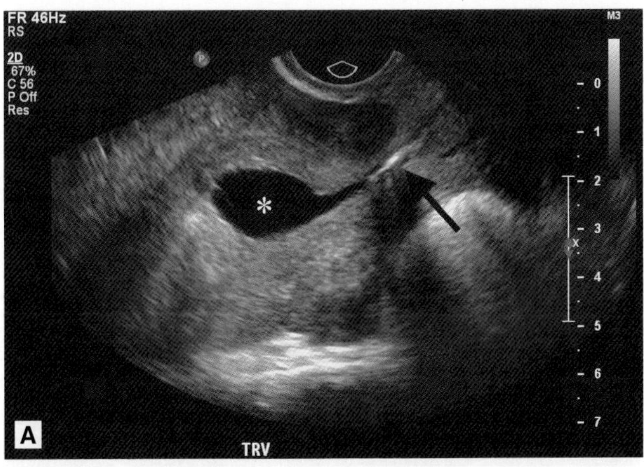

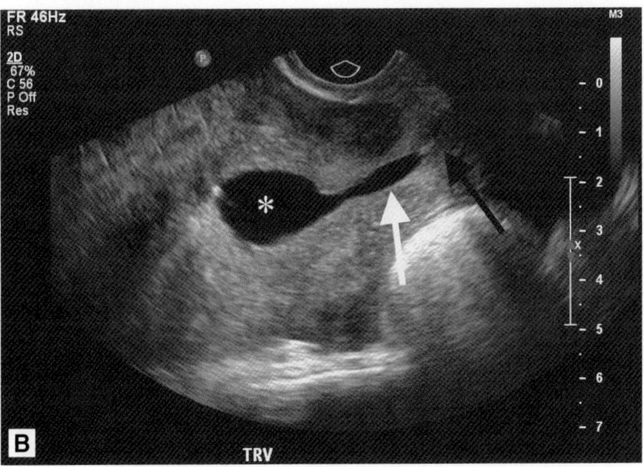

FIGURE 10.1. Normal sonohysterosalpingogram. Endometrial cavity is distended with fluid (white asterisk). Catheter (black arrow) is within the lower uterine segment (**A**) and then is pulled back (**B**) to allow visualization of the endometrial cavity within the lower uterine segment (white arrow).

the catheter. A balloon catheter may be used, but care should be taken to remove the air from the balloon before insertion. The speculum is removed and the endovaginal probe reinserted. Under continuous ultrasound imaging, 10 to 60 mL of sterile saline is slowly infused and images are obtained in both sagittal (long axis) and transverse (short axis) planes (16,17). If a balloon catheter is utilized, it should be deflated at the end of the procedure to allow complete visualization of the lower uterine segment. Antibiotic prophylaxis can be considered in patients who normally take prophylactic antibiotics prior to dental work. Premedication with nonsteroidal anti-inflammatory agents will minimize uterine cramping. Contraindications to SHG include hematometria and acute pelvic inflammatory disease.

Three-dimensional SHG is becoming more commonly used. This technique reduces operator dependence and length of examination time and has been reported to provide significant additional information in a majority of patients (18).

Normal Uterus

The normal myometrium (Fig. 10.2) is homogeneous in echotexture and intermediate in echogenicity. Anechoic tubular structures separating the outer one third from the inner two thirds of the myometrium represent the arcuate vessels, which are best seen on color flow imaging. The internal os can be recognized as a slight constriction of the uterine contour. Uterine volume is calculated using the formula 1/2 (L × W × D).

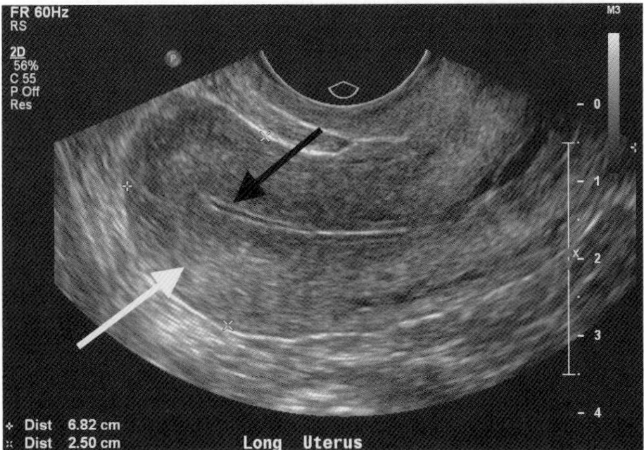

FIGURE 10.2. Normal uterus on ultrasound. Uterine myometrium demonstrates a homogeneous echotexture (white arrow). The endometrium is a highly echogenic thin line (black arrow). Note the trace amount of anechoic fluid in the endometrial canal.

The endometrium should be measured at the thickest part of the endometrial stripe in the uterine fundus on a midline sagittal image, and by convention is always reported as a double-layer measurement. The normal endometrium is highly echogenic. However, the thickness and echotexture of the endometrium vary with the hormonal status of the patient. At the end of the menses, the endometrial stripe is highly echogenic and measures approximately 2 to 3 mm. During the proliferative stage, the endometrium becomes less echogenic and thickens, reaching a maximum of 8 mm. Before ovulation, a trilaminar appearance of the endometrium has been described. The central thin echogenic line represents a reflective artifact and/or mucus and secretions between the anterior and posterior layers of the endometrium. Subjacent is the second layer, which is the relatively hypoechoic functionalis layer. The third layer is the surrounding deeper basalis layer, which remains echogenic. Following ovulation, the functionalis layer becomes thicker and more echogenic then during the secretory phase such that the entire stripe may reach 15 mm in thickness and is more uniformly echogenic just prior to menstruation (19). In some patients, the innermost layer of myometrium is relatively hypoechoic compared to the immediately subjacent endometrium and is termed the subendometrial halo. The subendometrial halo is less commonly visualized in postmenopausal women. Neither the subendometrial halo nor fluid or debris within the endometrial cavity should be included in measurements of the endometrial stripe. At SHG, the endometrium should be homogeneous, symmetric, and regular without mass effect. The sum of the width of the two layers should not exceed the maximum acceptable width for the patient's hormonal status.

The uterine artery originates from the internal iliac artery. Pulse Doppler examination will demonstrate a high impedance waveform characterized by an early diastolic notch and relatively little diastolic flow. Only minor changes occur in the uterine artery waveform during the menstrual cycle.

In postmenopausal women, the uterine corpus shrinks until it approximates the length of the cervix. The endometrium atrophies and should appear as a thin, regular echogenic line <5 mm in width (20). In women taking hormonal replacement therapy (HRT) less uterine and endometrial atrophy occurs (21). Women taking sequential HRT are best examined following withdrawal bleeding and the progesterone phase of their cycle when the endometrium is expected to be at the thinnest.

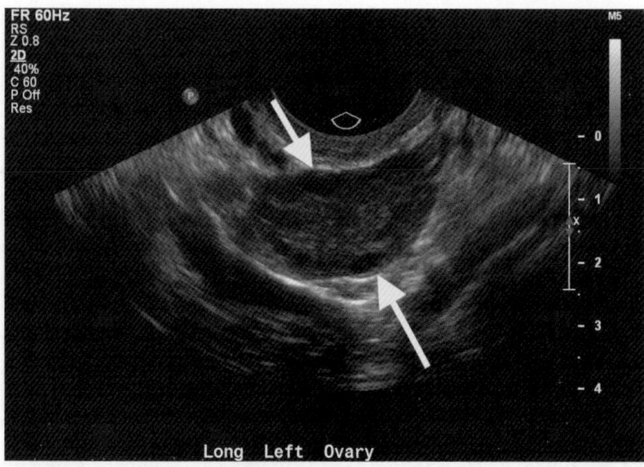

FIGURE 10.3. Normal ovary on ultrasound. Ovarian parenchyma demonstrates a homogeneous echotexture with multiple anechoic follicles (arrows).

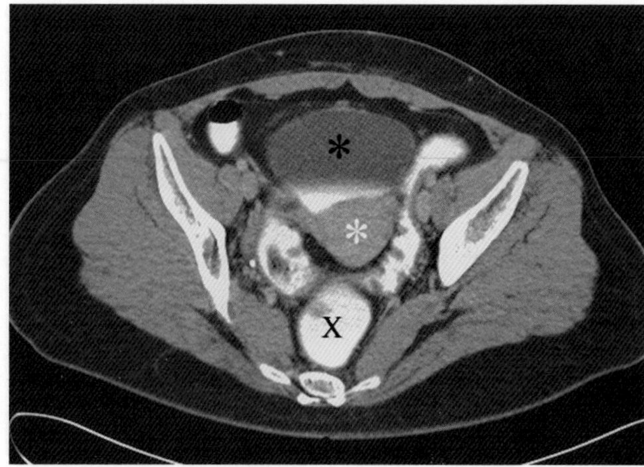

FIGURE 10.4. Normal uterus on CT. Uterus (white asterisk) is a triangular-shaped soft-tissue density posterior to the bladder (black asterisk) and anterior to the bowel (black X).

Normal Ovaries

The US appearance of the ovaries (Fig. 10.3) also changes with the patient's hormonal status. The premenopausal ovary has a relatively homogeneous outer cortex with a more echogenic central medulla. Small anechoic follicles are common. At ovulation, one follicle becomes dominant, reaching a maximum diameter of 2.0 to 2.5 cm. Following ovulation, the corpus luteum develops. The corpus luteum may contain debris and/or hemorrhage and often involutes, appearing to be crenelated just prior to menstruation. The ovaries atrophy with menopause and contain fewer follicles. Therefore, postmenopausal ovaries are more difficult to visualize with ultrasound. In women taking HRT, less ovarian atrophy will occur and follicles will continue to develop.

Doppler evaluation of ovarian blood flow is best performed during days 3 to 7 of the menstrual cycle. The ovary undergoing ovulation in a given cycle demonstrates a relatively high-velocity, low-resistance arterial waveform with continuous forward diastolic flow. The contralateral ovary will typically demonstrate a higher-resistance low-velocity arterial waveform with either very low or no diastolic flow.

Computed Tomography

Techniques

CT studies of the pelvis require contrast opacification of the distal small bowel and colon. In some centers, patients receive 500 mL of a 2% barium solution the evening preceding the examination and an additional 500 mL 45 minutes before the CT scan. In other protocols, the patient receives 600 to 1,000 mL of dilute oral contrast at least 1 hour before the examination, coupled with a 200-mL dilute contrast enema. Iodinated intravenous (IV) contrast is used in pelvic CT imaging to opacify the bladder and ureters, to differentiate contrast-filled blood vessels from adjacent lymph nodes, to enhance the myometrium, to visualize the endometrial cavity, and to delineate hypodense tumor boundaries from contiguous normal organ parenchyma.

MDCT is the standard of care in most hospital and outpatient settings. Optimal IV contrast enhancement for these faster scanners requires a mechanical power injector to administer 100 to 120 mL of IV contrast at a rate of 2 mL/s or more. Scan parameters including injection rates, scan delays, and collimation vary based on the specific protocol used and imaging objective. With MDCT, it is easy to obtain multiphasic contrast examinations with arterial and venous phase images. Increased radiation exposure for multiple passes must be balanced with the likelihood of increased clinical yield. The enormous data sets generated by MDCT studies require sophisticated software and computer workstations to fully exploit the technology (1).

Normal Uterus and Pelvic Structures

On CT, the vagina, cervix, and uterine corpus can be differentiated based on both morphologic and enhancement characteristics. The uterine corpus appears as a triangular or ovoid soft-tissue mass posterior to the urinary bladder (Fig. 10.4). The cervix is a more rounded structure. At the level of the fornix, the vagina has a flat rectangular or crescentic shape. Following bolus intravenous contrast administration, the myometrium in the uterine corpus enhances to a greater degree than that of the cervix. The endometrium can often be delineated from the enhancing myometrium. The broad and round ligaments can be seen coursing laterally and anteriorly, respectively. Occasionally, the uterosacral ligaments are depicted as arc-like structures extending from the cervix to the sacrum.

Normal Ovaries

In the premenopausal patient, the normal ovaries are routinely seen, usually posterolateral to the uterine corpus. Their uniform soft-tissue density is punctuated by small cystic regions representing follicles (Fig. 10.5). In the postmenopausal patient, the ovaries are small and less readily detected.

Magnetic Resonance Imaging

Techniques

It is recommended that patients fast for 4 to 6 hours before an MRI examination or be given an antiperistaltic (e.g., 1.0 mg glucagon intramuscularly). The routine use of bowel contrast agents is controversial, but some investigators advocate the administration of varying amounts (typically 400 to 600 mL) of oral contrast 10 to 40 minutes prior to an MRI examination (22). When an oral contrast agent is used, the antiperistaltic is given just before scanning to optimize image quality (23). Gadolinium contrast (0.1 µmol/kg) is administered intravenously to opacify vessels, to highlight tumor interfaces, to

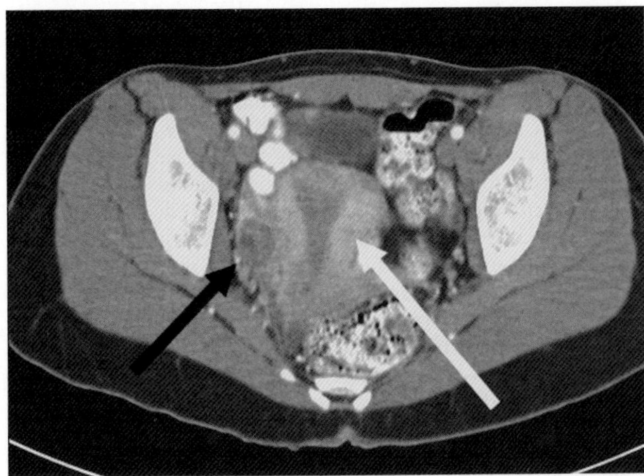

FIGURE 10.5. Normal ovary on CT. Ovary (black arrow) is a soft-tissue density with small cystic spaces corresponding to follicles. Note the uterus (white arrow) adjacent to the right ovary.

assess lymph nodes, to detect fistulas, and to identify local, regional, and distant metastases. Patients are usually scanned in the supine position, with the bladder empty at the beginning of the study.

Using a high field strength (≥1 tesla) MRI system and a phased-array body surface coil, high-resolution T2-weighted (T2W) images are obtained in under 5 minutes using fast-spin echo technique (FSE) (24). Recently, parallel imaging has been gaining momentum. Parallel imaging allows for faster acquisition of T2W-FSE sequences by a factor of two or provides twice the spatial resolution for a given acquisition time. Although there are even faster imaging techniques (e.g., breath-hold FSE and breathing-independent half Fourier acquisition single-shot turbo spin echo [HASTE]), they do not have the same spatial resolution as FSE and therefore cannot replace T2W-FSE for evaluating the primary tumor and extent of disease (24,25). These other T2W sequences (e.g., rapid acquisition relaxation enhanced [RARE], HASTE), however, are particularly attractive for performing MRI urography (MRIU) as an adjunct to T2W-FSE images (26).

Normal Uterus and Pelvic Structures

Pelvic anatomy is exquisitely demonstrated on MRI scans. On T1-weighted (T1W) sequences, the normal pelvic musculature and viscera demonstrate homogeneous low to medium signal intensity. Cortical bone demonstrates low signal intensity and fatty marrow is high in signal intensity. Similarly, intrapelvic fat demonstrates high signal intensity.

It is the soft-tissue contrast afforded by T2W sequences, however, that is the basis for the strength of MRI in pelvic imaging. On these sequences, the uterus, cervix, and vagina all exhibit distinct layers of different signal intensity—the so-called zonal architecture (Figs. 10.6 and 10.7). The endometrium shows high signal intensity, usually higher than the signal intensity of subcutaneous fat. The peripheral myometrium is intermediate in signal intensity, being higher in signal intensity than striated muscle. Interposed between these two layers is a narrow band of decreased signal intensity, the junctional zone, which corresponds to the innermost myometrium (Fig. 10.6). The signal properties of the junctional zone reflect its lower water content, compared with the rest of the myometrium, which may be a function of its decrease in extracellular matrix per unit volume (27,28). The three zones seen on MRI images are not comparable to the different zones seen on US (29). The endometrium is well visualized with MRI, including the varying width of the endometrium (both leaflets) seen with the menstrual cycle (30). In postmenopausal women not receiving exogenous hormones, uterine zonal anatomy is indistinct, and the endometrium typically measures less than 3 mm (30).

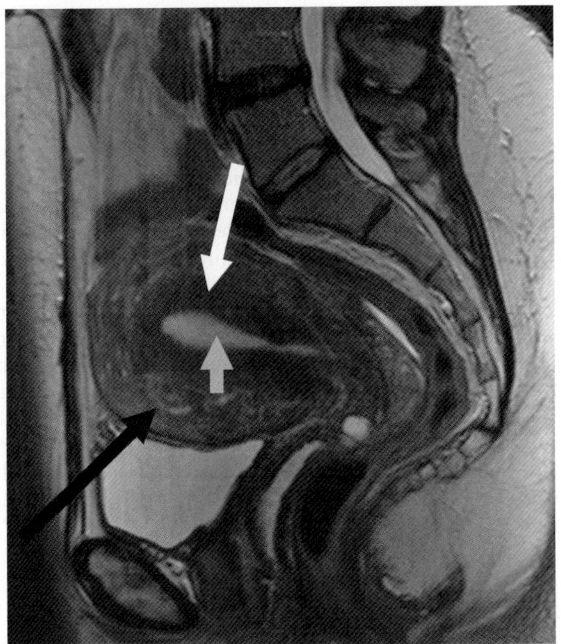

FIGURE 10.6. Normal uterus on MRI. Sagittal T2W image through the uterine midline. The uterine zonal anatomy is seen with the intermediate-T2W-signal myometrium (long black arrow), low-T2W-signal junctional zone (white arrow), and high-T2W-signal endometrium (short grey arrow).

The cervix also demonstrates zonal architecture on T2W sequences (Fig. 10.7). There is an inner area of high signal intensity, which is believed to represent epithelium and mucus; a middle area of predominantly low signal intensity, which is believed to represent fibrous stroma with a higher cell count or more nuclei; and an outer area of medium signal intensity,

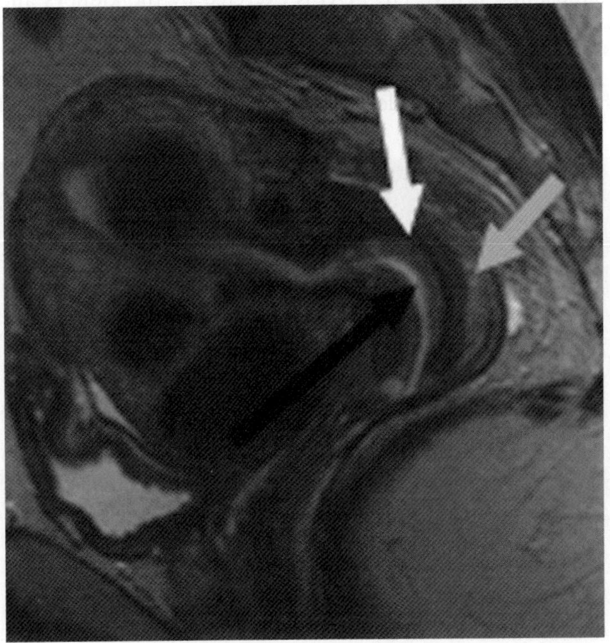

FIGURE 10.7. Normal cervix on MRI. Sagittal T2W image through the cervix. The cervical zonal anatomy is apparent with an innermost high signal layer (long black arrow), outermost intermediate signal layer (short grey arrow), and a low signal layer in between (white arrow).

which is believed to represent fibrous stroma with a lower cell count or fewer nuclei and a high degree of vascularity (31,32). The use of pelvic surface coils has revealed yet another cervical layer: interposed between the high-signal-intensity endocervical canal and the low-signal-intensity fibrocervical stroma is a feathery layer of intermediate signal intensity, which is thought to represent the mucosal folds or plicae palmatae.

T2W images of the vagina reveal two zones, the bright vaginal mucosa and the intermediate-signal-intensity vaginal wall. The low-signal-intensity ligamentous structures are identified by their anatomic location.

Following the administration of gadolinium contrast, the zonal anatomy of the uterus is demonstrated on fat-saturated T1W images. The endometrium and outer myometrium enhance to a greater extent than the junctional zone. Similarly, in the cervix, the inner cervical mucosa and outer smooth muscle enhance more than the fibrocervical stroma. The parametrial tissues, vaginal wall, and submucosa also enhance after gadolinium contrast administration.

Normal Ovaries

On T1W images, the ovaries display homogeneous low to medium signal intensity, whereas on T2W images (Fig. 10.8), the follicles become brighter than the surrounding stroma. The normal fallopian tubes are not routinely imaged because of their small size and tortuous course.

Positron Emission Tomography

Techniques

Patient preparation is crucial to high-quality FDG-PET imaging. Physiologic uptake of tracer needs to be limited in order to achieve the best signal-to-noise ratio. After intravenous injection, FDG is distributed by the bloodstream and taken up by glycolytically active tissues including the brain, myocardium, liver, spleen, bone marrow, gastrointestinal tract, testes, and skeletal muscle. Other less common sites of FDG uptake include the endometrium, breast, major and minor salivary glands, and brown fat. FDG is excreted by the kidneys and therefore intense uptake can be seen in the renal collecting systems, ureters, and bladder.

The patient is asked to fast for at least 4 hours prior to the FDG-PET scan in order to keep insulin levels low. Elevated insulin levels drive FDG into skeletal muscle, often leading to a nondiagnostic examination. Blood glucose is checked prior to FDG injection. Blood glucose levels less than 200 mg/dL are acceptable at most institutions. If blood glucose levels are found to be above this level, most institutions will not perform the study or will evaluate the situation on a case-by-case basis. Specific protocols are used for diabetic patients.

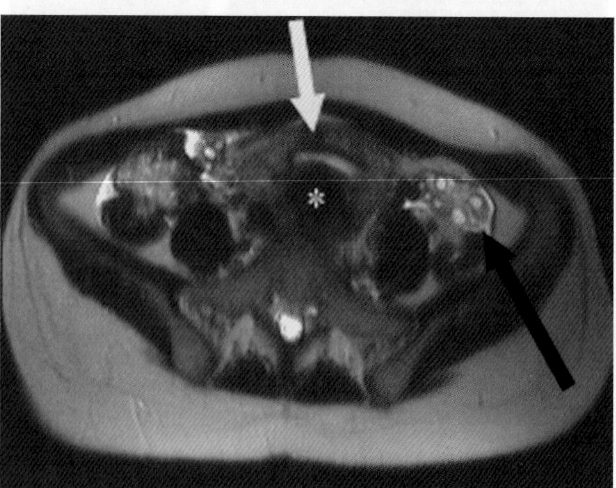

FIGURE 10.8. Normal ovary on MRI. Axial T2W image showing the normal ovary (black arrow) with intermediate-T2W-signal stroma and high-T2W-signal follicles. Note the uterus in the midline (white arrow) with a posterior fibroid (white asterisk).

Bladder/urine activity cannot be removed, but steps are taken to reduce the amount of activity. Adequate hydration and frequent urination, including voiding immediately prior to imaging, are used to help reduce this activity. Some centers use IV hydration. However, care should be taken to ensure that no dextrose is in the IV fluid.

Patients are asked to not engage in any heavy activity or gum chewing the day before the FDG-PET exam. After the injection of 5 to 10 mCi FDG intravenously, the patient is asked to lie quietly in the supine position without talking in order to limit skeletal muscle FDG uptake. Imaging occurs 60 to 90 minutes after FDG injection and lasts 30 to 45 minutes, depending on the specific protocol.

Normal Pelvic Structures

In premenopausal patients, uterine and ovarian FDG uptake is related to the menstrual cycle. Ovarian FDG uptake occurs in the late follicular to early luteal phase of the menstrual cycle. The most intense endometrial FDG uptake occurs during the first 3 days of the menstrual cycle (33). Therefore, premenopausal patients should be imaged a week before to a few days after menstruation.

There is no physiologic uptake of FDG in the uterus or ovaries of postmenopausal patients (33). No studies to date have evaluated physiologic uptake of FDG in the uterus and ovaries in women on tamoxifen or HRT.

CERVICAL CANCER

Introduction

Cervical cancer is typically detected clinically (Pap smear and/or physical exam), with imaging being most often reserved for staging, monitoring treatment, and detecting recurrence in patients with advanced disease. US, CT, MRI, and FDG-PET all play a role in the management of patients with known cervical cancer.

Primary Detection and Characterization of Cervical Cancer

Cervical cancer is usually detected by physical exam or from results of a Pap smear. Imaging rarely plays a role in the primary detection and characterization of cervical cancer.

Ultrasound

Early cervical carcinoma is difficult to detect with either transabdominal or transvaginal sonography. Transrectal ultrasound (TRUS) can sometimes allow better visualization of the uterine cervix (34). High-frequency 20-MHz miniature intracervical US probes are a promising technique in the evaluation of cervical cancer. These probes are able to detect early cancers (invasion >5 mm) (35,36). However, more research is needed before this technique is useful clinically.

On US, cervical tumors are hypoechoic or isoechoic masses with ill-defined margins. Occasionally, a hypoechoic cervical tumor can mimic a cervical myoma. If the tumor obstructs the endocervical canal, hydrometra and/or hematometra will be present, which is readily detectable with US.

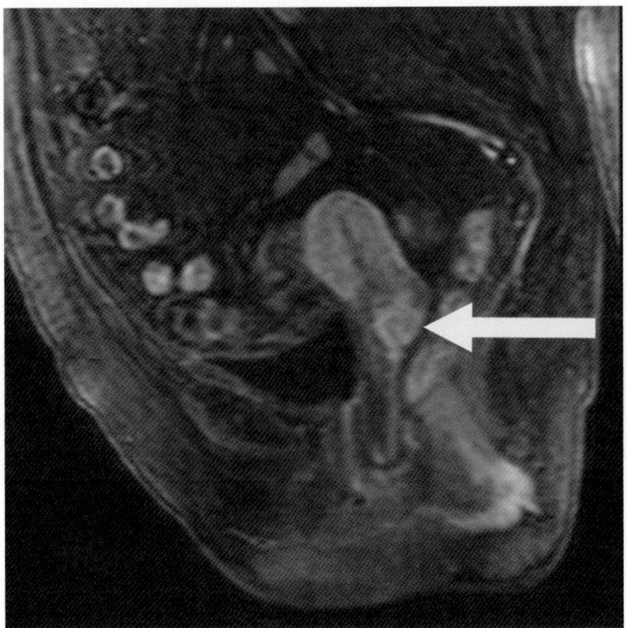

FIGURE 10.9. Cervical mass on MRI. Sagittal T1W post-contrast fat-saturated image demonstrating an enhancing cervical mass (arrow).

Magnetic Resonance Imaging

The ever-increasing body of literature on MRI and cervical cancer suggests that MRI is superior to US for delineating the primary tumor site and size. These MRI advantages are primarily due to the superior soft-tissue contrast of MRI and the ability to define the tumor in the orthogonal plane (37,38). On T2W images, the characteristic feature of cervical cancer is an intermediate-signal-intensity mass. The T2W signal intensity of the tumor is usually greater than the normal low T2W signal intensity of the fibrocervical stroma.

On T1W images, cervical tumors are usually isointense compared to the normal cervix and may not be visible. Gadolinium contrast highlights tumor heterogeneity and aids in the differentiation of viable tumor from debris and necrosis (39). Primary cervical tumors demonstrate increased early enhancement relative to the normal adjacent cervical stroma (Fig. 10.9). On later postcontrast T1W images the tumor enhancement becomes less marked, and on delayed images the tumor may be isointense or hypointense compared to the adjacent normal cervical stroma (40). Dynamic imaging may improve the detection of small lesions and assessment of stromal invasion (40,41). Signal-intensity-versus-time curves, however, do not appear to make a significant contribution to the evaluation of tumor aggressiveness (42).

In contrast to squamous-cell cervical carcinoma, adenoma malignum, a rare form of cervical adenocarcinoma, is depicted as a high-signal-intensity multicystic lesion on T2W sequences. The tumor extends from the endocervical glands to the deep cervical stroma and may mimic nabothian cysts. On postcontrast T1W images, solid portions within the tumor enhance, which is a feature that helps distinguish adenoma malignum from nabothian cysts (43).

Primary Detection and Characterization of Cervical Cancer Recommendations

Cervical carcinoma is most commonly detected by physical exam or from the results of a Pap smear. MRI is the current study of choice if imaging is necessary in this situation.

Staging Cervical Cancer

Recommendations for diagnostic evaluation of tumor staging derive from the International Federation of Gynecology and Obstetrics (FIGO) clinical staging system and are based on findings from physical examination, colposcopy, lesion biopsies, chest radiography, cystoscopy, sigmoidoscopy, intravenous urography (IVU), and BE. When compared with surgical staging, clinical FIGO staging is flawed, with a reported error rate of 17% to 67%. These sobering statistics primarily reflect failure to identify parametrial extension (38,44,45). The detection of parametrial invasion is crucial in the treatment decision process. The staging accuracy for both BE and IVU are dismal, with both tests being positive only in advanced disease. Whereas hydronephrosis or a nonfunctioning kidney can be detected with IVU, it is insensitive to tumor extent (46,47). Furthermore, clinical FIGO staging does not include evaluation of lymph node metastases. Although cross-sectional imaging is not mandated by FIGO, many women are referred for cross-sectional imaging to stage cervical cancer when advanced-stage disease is suspected.

Ultrasound

Transabdominal sonography plays a limited role in the staging of cervical cancer and is inferior to other cross-sectional modalities in this role. Although the improved spatial resolution achieved with TVS and TRUS is helpful in the evaluation of tumor size and locoregional extent, poor soft-tissue contrast impedes differentiation between tumor and normal adjacent cervical, uterine, parametrial, and vaginal tissue (48,49). Sonographic findings in parametrial invasion include irregularity or loss of the normal cervical contour (50). Pelvic sidewall involvement is diagnosed on US by a parametrial soft-tissue mass or tumor extension to the sidewall and/or encasement of the iliac vessels (50). Bladder invasion is suggested by loss of the fat plane between cervix and bladder or direct extension of the tumor mass through the bladder wall. Enlarged pelvic lymph nodes may also be detected.

One study reports an overall accuracy of 83% for TRUS in the staging of cervical cancer (50). The accuracy increases to 87% for parametrial involvement, with a sensitivity of 78% and a specificity of 89%. Unfortunately, these results have not been reproduced, limiting enthusiasm for this modality. Most agree that both the soft-tissue contrast and field of view with US are too limited to allow adequate evaluation of the parametria. Therefore, US is significantly limited in its usefulness in the staging of patients with cervical cancer.

Computed Tomography

CT has been used extensively for staging cervical cancer, and its strengths and limitations are well known. Intravenous contrast is essential to delineate the interfaces of tumor, normal cervical stroma, and myometrium and to differentiate normal parauterine fat margins from irregular hypodense borders caused by tumor infiltration.

CT staging criteria are derived from FIGO staging (Table 10.1). Stage I cervical cancer is confined to the cervix. Tumor confined to the cervix does not alter the normal, smooth, well-defined cervical contour; periureteral fat planes are preserved; and there is neither stranding of the parametria nor a parametrial soft-tissue mass. The primary tumor may appear as diffuse cervical enlargement or as a discrete low-attenuation cervical mass. The regions of decreased attenuation are a function of tumor necrosis/ulceration and/or inherent differences in the attenuation between tumor and normal cervical tissue. Distinguishing tumor from the normal cervix is often problematic, as half of cervical tumors show isoattenuation to normal

TABLE 10.1

CORRESPONDING CT FINDINGS FOR STAGING CERVICAL CANCER

Stage	Substage	CT findings
Stage 0		No tumor present
Stage I	IA	No tumor present
	IB	No tumor present or tumor does not alter cervical contour
Stage II	IIA	Thickening of vaginal wall (upper two thirds)
	IIB	Irregular lateral cervical margin parametrial mass or strands Obliteration of periureteral fat
Stage III	IIIA	Thickening of vaginal wall (lower one third)
	IIIB	Tumor extends to obturator internus, piriformis, or levator ani muscles Dilated ureter
Stage IV	IVA	Thickening, nodularity, or serration of bladder or rectal wall Obliteration of perivesical or perirectal fat
	IVB	Tumor in distant organs

cervical stroma on CT (2). Obstruction of the endocervical canal by cervical tumor can result in uterine enlargement with a fluid-filled endometrial cavity (51).

Stage II cervical cancer extends beyond the cervix to involve the upper two thirds of the vagina (stage IIA) or the parametria, but not the pelvic sidewall (stage IIB). Intravaginal tumor (stage IIA) is best staged by clinical examination (Fig. 10.10) (52). CT criteria for parametrial invasion (stage IIB) include irregularity or effacement of the lateral cervical margins, thick parametrial soft-tissue stranding, an eccentric soft-tissue mass, and/or obliteration of the normal periureteral fat planes. Diagnosis of early parametrial invasion is problematic on CT as irregular cervical margins and prominent parametrial soft tissue can be simulated by parametritis associated with previous uterine curettage or cervical conization. Loss of the periureteral fat plane around the pelvic ureter is the only reliable finding of parametrial tumor extension but indicates advanced disease (47,53).

Stage III cervical carcinoma involves either the lower third of the vagina (stage IIIA) or the pelvic sidewall (stage IIIB). Stage IIIA cervical cancer is best staged clinically. Stage IIIB tumors appear as irregular soft-tissue strands extending to the piriformis, levator ani, and/or obturator internus muscles. Alternatively, confluent soft-tissue masses may envelop the pelvic sidewall musculature and iliac vessels. A fat plane of 3 mm or less between a parametrial mass and the pelvic sidewall indicates stage IIIB disease, since clinicians consider tumor to involve the sidewall if they are unable to interpose their fingers between the tumor and pelvic sidewall during pelvic examination under anesthesia (51). Detection of hydronephrosis also indicates stage IIIB disease. CT is more accurate than IVU in demonstrating the exact site of ureteral obstruction and the entire course of a hydroureter even in the absence of renal function (47,54).

Stage IVA cervical carcinoma indicates spread of tumor to adjacent pelvic organs, while stage IVB indicates spread of disease to distant organs. CT criteria for urinary bladder or rectal invasion (stage IVA) include focal loss of the normal perivesical/perirectal fat plane accompanied by asymmetric wall thickening, nodular indentations or serrations along the bladder or rectal wall, an intraluminal tumor mass, and/or a vesicovaginal or rectovaginal fistula (Fig. 10.11) (52). Early invasion of the bladder or rectum is not reliably detected by CT. Distant disease (stage IVB) is detected in the usual manner.

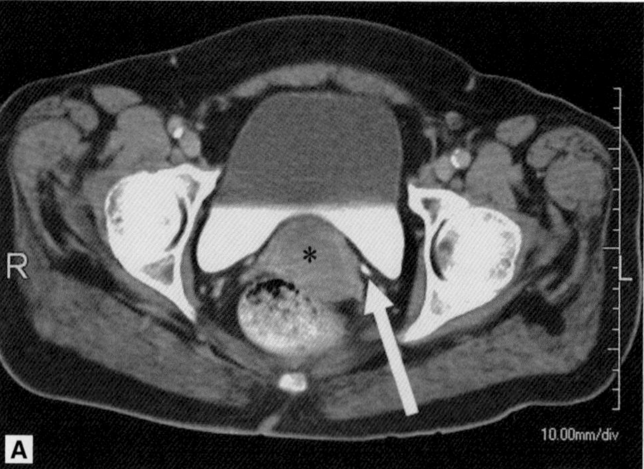

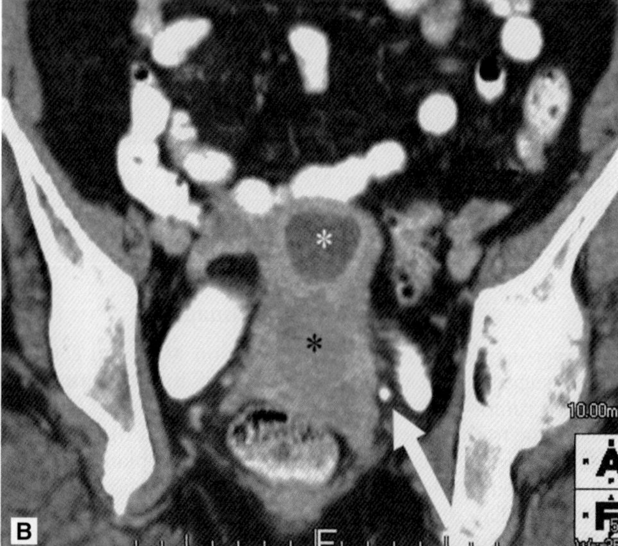

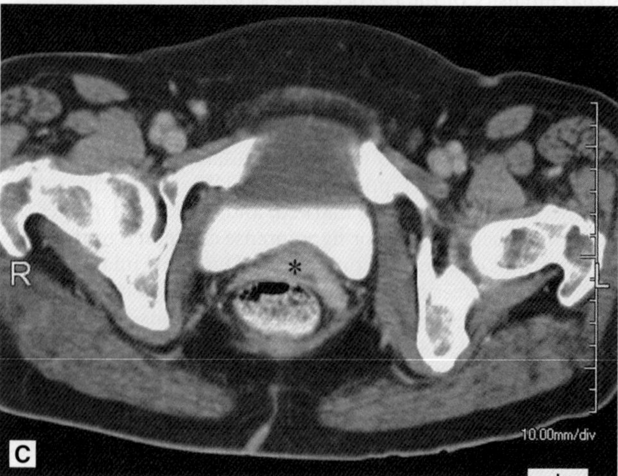

FIGURE 10.10. Stage IIA cervical cancer on CT. Axial (**A and C**) and coronal (**B**) contrast-enhanced CT images. Cervical enlargement secondary to a low attenuation cervical mass (black asterisk in **A** and **B**). Cervical mass extends into the vagina (black asterisk in **C**). Note fluid-filled endometrial canal (white asterisk in **B**) secondary obstruction of the endocervical canal. Note the well-opacified left ureter (white arrow in **A** and **B**) with a preserved periureteral fat plane.

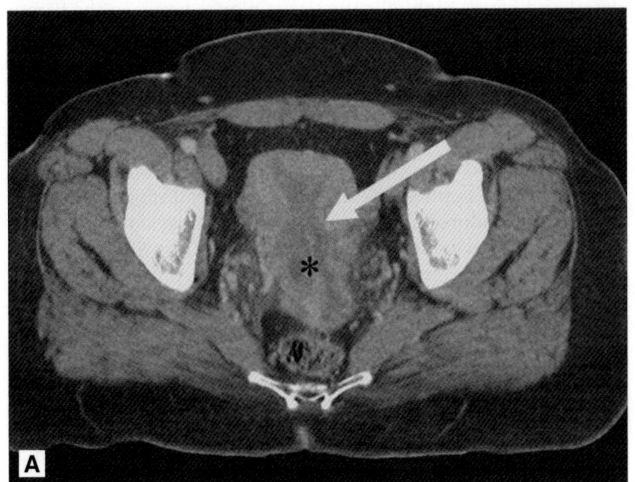

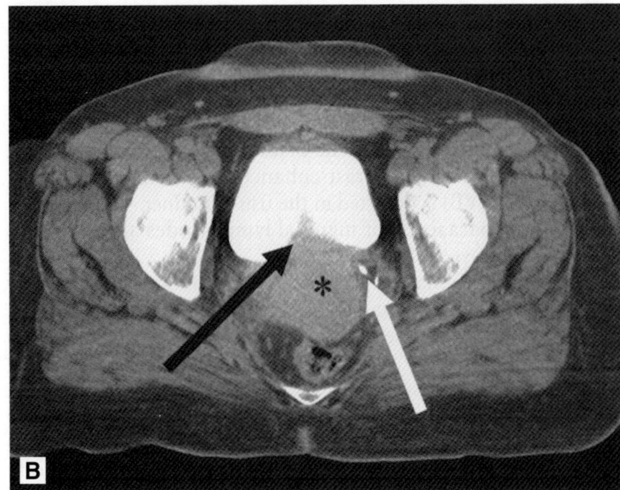

FIGURE 10.11. Stage IVA cervical cancer on CT. Contrast-enhanced CT images at two levels (**A and B**). Images demonstrate a heterogeneous mass arising in the cervix (black asterisk) with extension into the uterus (white arrow in **A**) and bladder (black arrow in **B**). Note the loss of the normal periureteral fat plane around the left ureter (white arrow in **B**).

Although the FIGO system does not include lymph node status, the presence of adenopathy affects prognosis. Detection of pathologically enlarged paraaortic or inguinal lymph nodes by CT is considered to be extrapelvic tumor extension and correlates with stage IVB disease. Lymph nodes greater than 1 cm in the short axis are considered to be pathologically enlarged. Adenopathy with central necrosis is associated with a high likelihood of metastatic disease (55). However, lymph node enlargement may also be secondary to benign inflammatory or reactive hyperplasia and, conversely, normal-sized lymph nodes may contain microscopic tumor foci. CT-guided biopsy can be useful to further assess patients with suspected nodal disease.

CT is often used for the staging of advanced cervical carcinoma because of the large field of view, widespread availability, and large numbers of experienced readers. However, CT has many limitations including poor detection of small primary tumors, parametrial invasion, and early invasion of the rectum and bladder. The diagnosis of stage IIB disease may be crucial to determine which patients are candidates for surgical resection. In the largest study to date the sensitivity, specificity, and negative predictive value (NPV) of CT in staging cervical carcinoma of stage IIB or greater were 42%, 82%, and 84%, respectively (56). Recent studies have shown that the staging accuracy of CT (53%) is better than that of clinical examination (47%) (57). Despite its limitations, CT is a valuable complement to clinical staging because of its accuracy in detecting advanced disease. In fact, 92% of stage IIIB through IVB lesions are accurately staged with CT (47).

The use of MDCT may help improve the accuracy of CT in cervical cancer staging by imaging thinner tissue slices, improving spatial resolution, and utilizing multiplanar reformatted images (58). However, more research is needed in this area.

Magnetic Resonance Imaging

The most recent literature suggests that MRI is superior to CT and clinical examination in the staging of cervical cancer (56,57). For this reason, MRI is becoming more frequently used in the staging of cervical cancer. MRI staging criteria are derived from FIGO staging conventions (Table 10.2).

An intact area of low T2W signal intensity, representing normal peripheral fibrous cervical stroma, is a reliable indication that the tumor is confined to the cervix (stage IB) (37,38,59).

Vaginal tumor involvement (stage IIA or IIIA) is recognized by segmental disruption of the intermediate- to low-signal-intensity vaginal wall on T2W images (37,60). However, vaginal tumor involvement is best staged by clinical examination. MRI determination of parametrial tumor extension (stage IIB) includes both morphologic and tissue signal alterations. Criteria include an irregular lateral cervical margin, prominent parametrial strands, eccentric parametrial enlargement, loss of parametrial fat planes on T1W images, and/or abnormal high-signal tumor extending through the low-signal-intensity ring of fibrocervical stroma into the parametria or cardinal-uterosacral ligaments on T2W images (37,38,59).

MRI criteria for pelvic sidewall extension (stage IIIB) are tumor extending beyond the lateral margins of the cardinal

TABLE 10.2

CORRESPONDING MRI FINDINGS FOR STAGING OF CERVICAL CANCER (T2W OR CONTRAST-ENHANCED T1W IMAGES)

Stage 0		No tumor present
Stage I	IA	No tumor present
	IB	Partial or complete disruption of low-signal-intensity stromal ring with intact tissue surrounding tumor
Stage II	IIA	Segmental disruption of low-signal-intensity vaginal wall (upper two thirds)
	IIB	Complete disruption of low signal intensity stromal ring with tumor extending into parametrium
Stage III	IIIA	Segmental disruption of low-signal-intensity vaginal wall (lower one third)
	IIIB	Tumor extends to obturator internus, piriformis, or levator ani muscles Dilated ureter
Stage IV	IVA	Signal loss of low-signal-intensity bladder or rectal wall
	IVB	Tumor in distant organs

ligaments and loss of the normal low signal intensity of the piriformis, levator ani, and/or obturator internus muscles on T2W images (Fig. 10.12) (37). The presence of hydronephrosis also indicates stage IIIB disease.

In stage IVA disease, there is segmental loss of the normal low-signal-intensity wall of the bladder or rectum. This is best seen on T2W and/or contrast-enhanced T1W images. Distant disease (stage IVB) is detected in the usual manner. The presence of abnormal paraaortic or inguinal lymph nodes also indicates stage IVB disease.

Recent studies have shown the overall staging accuracy of MRI in cervical carcinoma to be high at 77% to 93% (57,61). The accuracy for the detection of parametrial invasion is also high, ranging from 94% to 95% (61). However, the sensitivity for parametrial invasion on MRI was low, 38% (61).

Surface coil imaging (e.g., endovaginal, endorectal, or phased-array coil) results in higher spatial resolution than conventional body coil imaging. When compared with body coil images, endorectal coil images provide greater anatomic detail and better highlight the tissue planes between the tumor and normal structures (62). Whether these imaging improvements change patient management, however, is controversial. Results from one study indicated that the use of an endorectal coil improved accuracy in detecting parametrial invasion. Accuracy was 95% with the endorectal coil as opposed to 79% with a body coil (62). Other studies, however, have found no statistically significant difference in overall staging accuracy between the endorectal coil and the phased-array coil or between the phased-array coil and the body coil (89% vs. 89% and 91% vs. 89%, respectively). Nor was it possible to prove a significant difference in accuracy for detecting parametrial invasion (93% vs. 96% and 95% vs. 94%, respectively) (63).

Positron Emission Tomography

FDG-PET has been shown to be useful in the staging of advanced cervical cancer, especially the detection of pathologic lymph nodes. Although adenopathy is not part of the

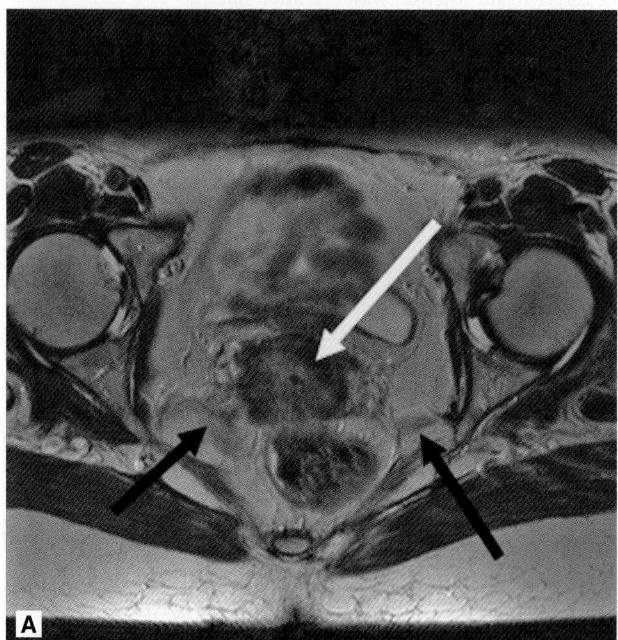

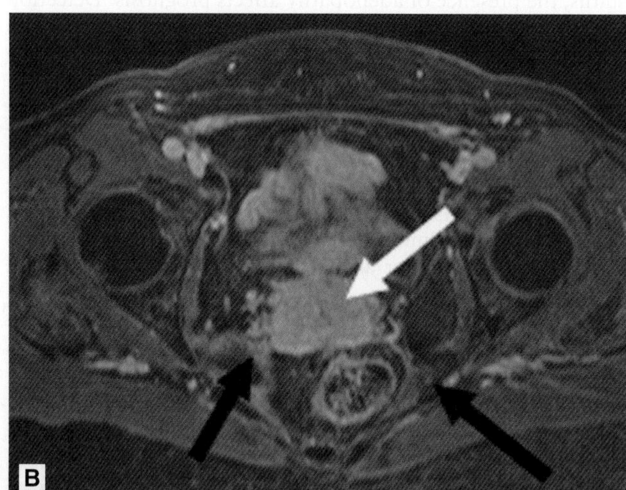

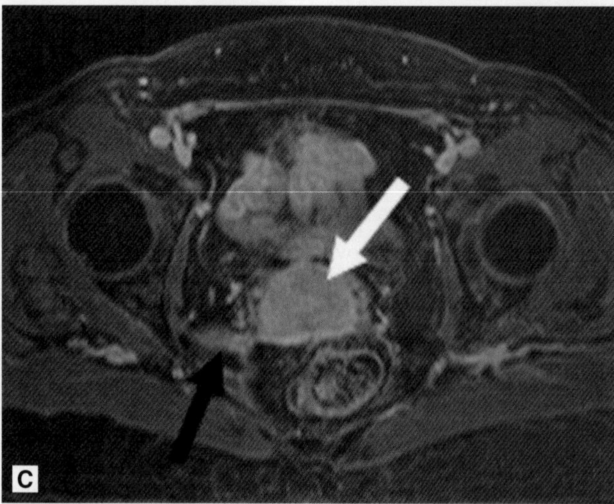

FIGURE 10.12. Stage IIIB cervical cancer on MRI. Axial T2W (A) and T1W post-contrast fat-saturated images at the same level (B) and slightly cranial (C). Images demonstrate a cervical mass (white arrow) with adjacent intermediate T2W signal and post-contrast enhancement (black arrows) extending to the pelvic sidewall bilaterally.

FIGO staging system, it is considered stage IVB disease and is therefore crucial information when developing a treatment plan (Fig. 10.13). Conventional cross-sectional imaging modalities rely on size criteria for the diagnosis of adenopathy and, as such, microscopic disease is often not detected.

FDG-PET is better than the conventional imaging modalities in the detection of adenopathy in patients with cervical cancer. Reinhardt et al. (64) found that in the detection of involved lymph nodes, sensitivity, specificity, and positive predictive value (PPV) were 91%, 100%, and 100%, respectively, for FDG-PET, as compared to 73%, 83%, and 67%, respectively, for MRI. Another study demonstrated that the accuracy of FDG-PET in the detection of lymph node metastasis was 88%, compared to 75% with MRI (48). A recent study concluded that pretreatment FDG-PET compatible with abnormal lymph node uptake predicted disease recurrence and altered treatment management decisions in some patients (49).

Staging Cervical Cancer Recommendations

MRI outperforms clinical and CT staging for cervical cancer. In the largest study to date, Hricak et al. (56) determined that MRI performs significantly better in the detection of cervical tumors. Further, the sensitivity in detecting stage IIB disease or greater was 29% for clinical staging, 42% for CT, and 53% for MRI. Another study found that for staging, MRI had significantly higher accuracy (86%) than clinical staging (47%) or CT (53%) (57). Another recent study showed that MRI is superior to both CT and clinical examination for evaluating uterine body involvement and measuring tumor size (65). Moreover, when pretreatment MRI is used to guide clinical management decisions, it has been shown to help minimize costs. In a study by Hricak et al. (6), the use of MRI findings to guide treatment decisions in women with cervical cancer greater than 2 cm in diameter resulted in a decrease in the number of diagnostic tests ordered and a decrease in the number of invasive procedures performed. In fact, therapy based on MRI findings led to a net cost savings of $401 for all patients and $449 for patients with stage IB disease.

Recent work has shown that FDG-PET is superior to both CT and MRI for the evaluation of adenopathy in patients with cervical cancer (48,64). However, more research is needed in the use of FDG-PET in the primary staging of cervical cancer before widespread clinical use.

In the meantime, MRI appears to be the modality of choice for the preoperative evaluation of women with cervical cancer, with FDG-PET being used in certain situations. MRI should be performed in women with primary tumor with a transverse diameter greater than 2 cm on clinical examination, women with primary tumor that is endocervical or predominantly infiltrative and cannot be accurately assessed clinically, and women who are pregnant or have concomitant uterine lesions, making it difficult to assess the primary tumor by other means (6,53,66).

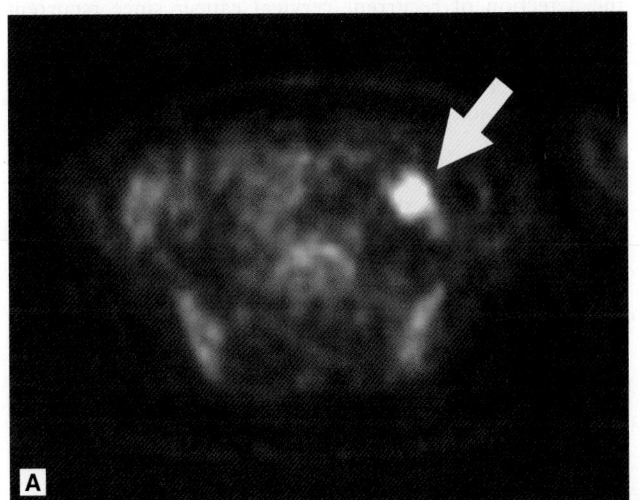

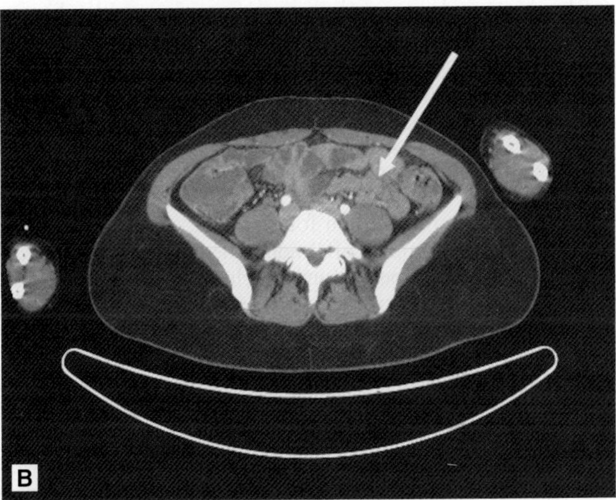

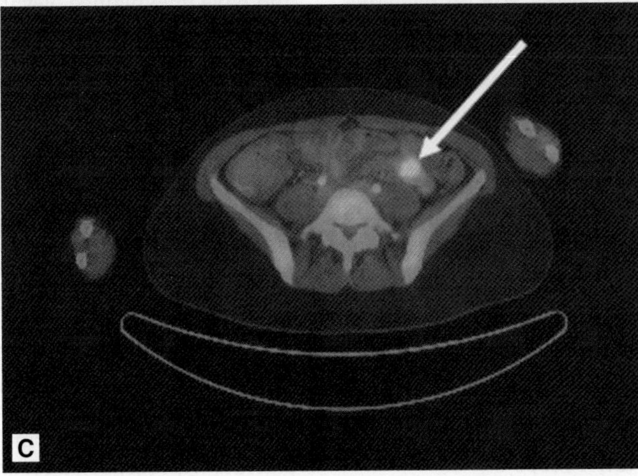

FIGURE 10.13. Stage IVB cervical cancer on FDG-PET. FDG-PET (**A**), CT (**B**), and fused PET-CT (**C**) images show increased FDG uptake (arrow in **A**). PET-CT image demonstrates that the increased FDG uptake corresponds to the pelvic lymph node (arrow in **C**). Pelvic lymph node on CT alone (arrow in **B**) does not meet criteria for an abnormal lymph node.

Monitoring Treatment Response and Detecting Recurrent Cervical Cancer

Ultrasound

TRUS has a role, albeit small, in the evaluation of recurrent cervical cancer and for biopsy guidance in selected patients (67). Reports from one study indicate that in approximately 25% of cases, TRUS provides information that is complementary to that obtained from CT. TRUS is most likely to be helpful in patients with small-volume recurrence in areas of previous irradiation (67). Unfortunately, differentiation between radiation fibrosis and recurrent disease cannot be made on the basis of US soft-tissue appearance or Doppler vascularity. However, TRUS can be used to guide biopsy of these areas. Furthermore, because of its limited field of view, TRUS is not useful in the assessment of the cephalic extent of tumor, abnormalities of the upper urinary tract, or the presence of extrapelvic metastases (67). However, hydronephrosis is easily detected by transabdominal imaging, which can also serve to guide stent placement. Both TRUS and TVS also have an important role, complementary to CT and MRI, in detecting complications of therapy or advanced disease such as lymphoceles, fistulae, or abscesses.

Computed Tomography

CT has been used extensively to monitor patients with a history of cervical cancer and plan subsequent therapy (47,68,69). Serial CT scans provide an objective measure of tumor response to radiation therapy or chemotherapy in nonsurgical candidates. Compared with its use for initial staging of cervical cancer, CT has higher sensitivity and specificity and a lower false-negative rate when used for the detection of recurrent disease (68).

Recurrent tumor is often found in the central pelvis, the surgical bed, the vaginal cuff, and/or the preserved cervix. CT features of recurrent pelvic tumor include soft-tissue asymmetry, soft-tissue mass with hypoattenuation tumor foci, compression and invasion of adjacent organs, and/or tumor extension to the pelvic sidewall, the iliopsoas muscle, and/or the innominate bone. Pelvic and paraaortic nodal metastases are also often present in patients with recurrent disease and are well depicted by CT (69).

Complications of therapy and/or advanced disease are well delineated on CT. Fistula formation, to the bladder and/or rectum, is well evaluated with CT. CT is also useful for detecting and defining the site of ureteral obstruction, which is common in patients with recurrent cervical cancer (70).

Radiation therapy changes of the intact uterus are characterized by bilateral parametrial "whiskers" or poor definition and irregularity of the parametria without pelvic sidewall extension. Other classic radiation-induced changes on CT are thickening of the perirectal fascia, widening of the presacral space, a thick-walled bladder and rectum, a diffuse increase in the density of fat in the posterior pelvis, and thickening of small bowel loops in the pelvic inlet (71). A major limitation of CT is the inability to reliably differentiate postradiation or postsurgical fibrosis from recurrent tumor (47,68).

In patients with equivocal findings, CT-guided fine-needle aspiration or core biopsy is an accurate way to differentiate recurrent tumor from posttreatment changes (71). In some cases, however, dense fibrous tissue surrounding nests of tumor cells may lead to a false-negative biopsy.

Because of the extensive use of pelvic radiation therapy as well as improved CT imaging techniques, detection of recurrent disease outside the pelvis is increasing (72). CT is useful for the assessment of metastases to solid organs (particularly the liver, lungs, and adrenal glands), the peritoneum and omentum, and the osseous structures.

Magnetic Resonance Imaging

Residual or recurrent cervical cancer demonstrates intermediate signal intensity on T1W images and heterogeneous high signal intensity on T2W images, whereas uninvolved cervical stroma retains its low signal intensity (73–75). Lesions larger than 1 cm are accurately depicted, but smaller lesions are more difficult to assess because of partial volume averaging and limits in spatial resolution with MRI. On T2W images, tumor extension into the rectum and/or bladder is seen as disruption of the low-signal-intensity walls of these structures. The appearance of pelvic sidewall involvement is similar to that described earlier for the extension of a primary tumor.

MRI is the most utilized modality for differentiating recurrent tumor from posttreatment fibrosis secondary to irradiation, chemotherapy, and/or surgery (75). In a patient with a history of remote radiation therapy (>1 year), radiation-induced changes tend to be of low signal intensity on both T1W and T2W images, whereas recurrent tumor tends to be of moderate to high signal intensity on T2W sequences. In this situation (remote radiation treatment), the difference in signal intensity between posttreatment fibrosis and recurrent tumor is statistically significant, and a sensitivity of 86% and a specificity of 94% have been reported for detection of recurrent cervical cancer (76). Contrast enhancement may further aid in the detection of recurrent cervical cancer since recurrent tumor shows early enhancement compared with benign conditions. The accuracy of dynamic contrast-enhanced MRI for identifying recurrent disease approaches 85% compared to 64% to 68% for unenhanced T2W images (4,77).

Positron Emission Tomography

FDG-PET has been shown to be useful in the restaging of potentially curable recurrent cervical cancer (Fig. 10.14) and in the evaluation of patients with previously treated cervical cancer and unexplained tumor marker elevation. In a recent study, FDG-PET was shown to have a sensitivity of 96%, specificity of 84%, and accuracy of 92% in the detection of recurrent cervical cancer (78). In this study, 40% of patients diagnosed with recurrence received therapy with curative intent. Although more research needs to be done, there is hope that FDG-PET imaging will have a favorable impact on prognosis and survival.

In patients who have received treatment for cervical cancer and have unexplained elevations in tumor markers, FDG-PET is an excellent imaging choice. In one study, FDG-PET was performed on patients previously treated for cervical cancer with unexplained elevated serum squamous cell carcinoma antigen (SCC-Ag) and no evidence of recurrent disease on conventional imaging. The FDG-PET scans were positive in 94% of patients with documented recurrence (79).

Monitoring Treatment Response and Detecting Recurrent Cervical Cancer Recommendations

For the routine surveillance of patients with a history of cervical cancer and to diagnose complications from advanced cervical cancer or treatment, CT is the study of choice. In order to differentiate recurrent tumor from posttreatment fibrosis, MRI is the study of choice. Both MRI and CT have been used, with limited success, in monitoring response to therapy. In patients with suspected recurrence because of unexplained elevated tumor markers, and in patients with potentially curable recurrent cervical cancer, FDG-PET is the study of choice. More research is needed in the use of FDG-PET in monitoring cervical cancer treatment and detecting recurrent disease.

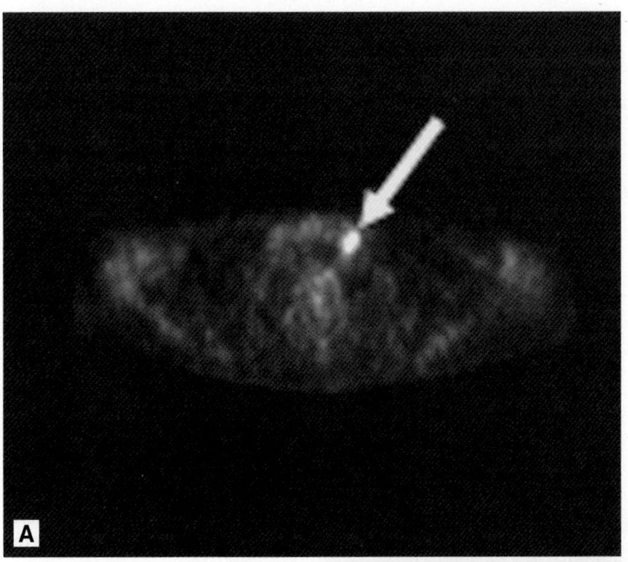

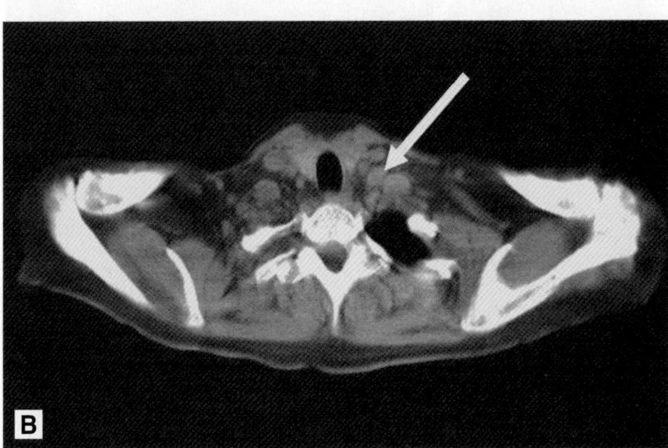

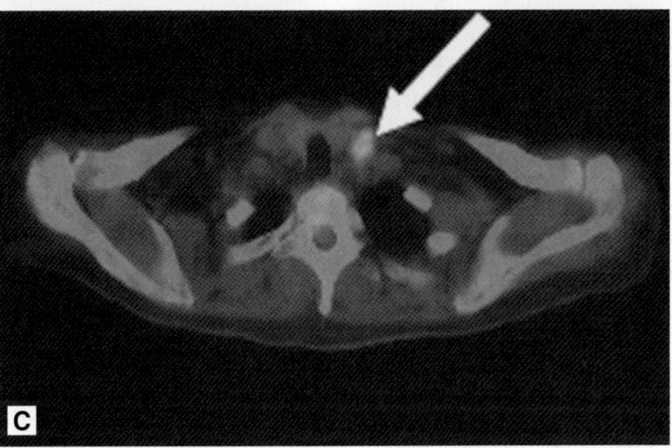

FIGURE 10.14. Recurrent cervical cancer on FDG-PET. FDG-PET (**A**), noncontrast CT (**B**), and fused PET-CT (**C**) images. Increased FDG-PET uptake in the left supraclavicular region (arrow in **A**) corresponds to a left supraclavicular lymph node on CT (arrow in **B**). Fused image demonstrates that the increased FDG uptake corresponds to the left supraclavicular lymph node (arrow in **C**).

Summary

Cervical cancer is most often diagnosed clinically with imaging reserved for staging, monitoring treatment response, and detecting recurrence. Cervical cancer staging is most accurately done with MRI; however, recent research suggests that FDG-PET may be the best staging technique for cervical cancer. More research is needed before staging with FDG-PET is routinely used. Both CT and MRI have utility in monitoring treatment response and detecting recurrent cervical cancer. In certain clinical scenarios, FDG-PET is useful for monitoring treatment response and detecting recurrence.

ENDOMETRIAL CANCER

Introduction

Endometrial carcinomas are typically diagnosed by endometrial biopsy or dilation and curettage (D&C). US remains the primary imaging modality to evaluate the endometrium, especially in patients with postmenopausal bleeding. Most other cross-sectional imaging studies are reserved for the evaluation of the extent of disease (3,39,80–83). Imaging criteria for staging of endometrial cancer is surgical–pathological and based on the FIGO classification. CT and MRI are the most useful modalities to stage endometrial carcinoma. Evaluation for recurrent disease does not often require imaging as most recurrences occur at the vaginal cuff, which is well evaluated by physical exam. However, in cases of recurrent metastatic disease or for problem solving, CT, MRI, and PET may all be useful depending on the clinical question.

Primary Diagnosis of Endometrial Cancer

Endometrial biopsy and/or D&C has traditionally been the gold standard for histologic diagnosis of endometrial pathology. However, if routine endometrial sampling were performed in all women with postmenopausal bleeding, only one of every ten samples would be expected to be positive. In addition, significant sampling error has been reported with false-negative rates ranging from 2% to 6% (84,85). In order to decrease unnecessary endometrial biopsies, screening patients with postmenopausal bleeding with TVS and/or SHG has been advocated (86–91).

Double layer endometrial thickness greater than 4 or 5 mm on TVS is used as the sole ultrasound criterion for determining whether endometrial sampling is warranted in postmenopausal patients (Fig. 10.15) (86,87). This endometrial thickness is based on numerous trials that looked to establish a threshold

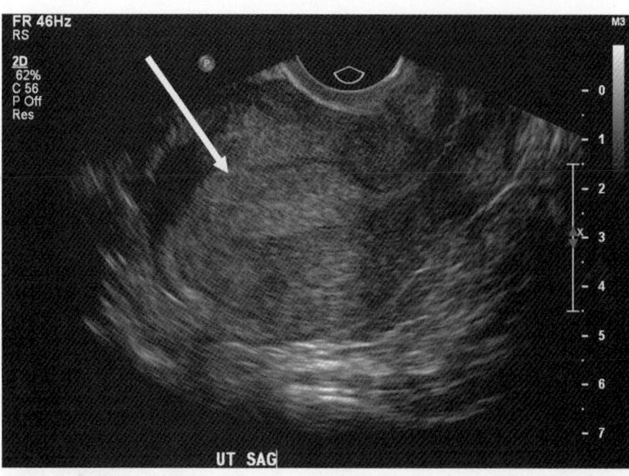

FIGURE 10.15. Thickened endometrium on ultrasound. Gray-scale ultrasound image through the sagittal midline of the endometrial canal demonstrating marked thickening of the hyperechoic endometrium (arrow).

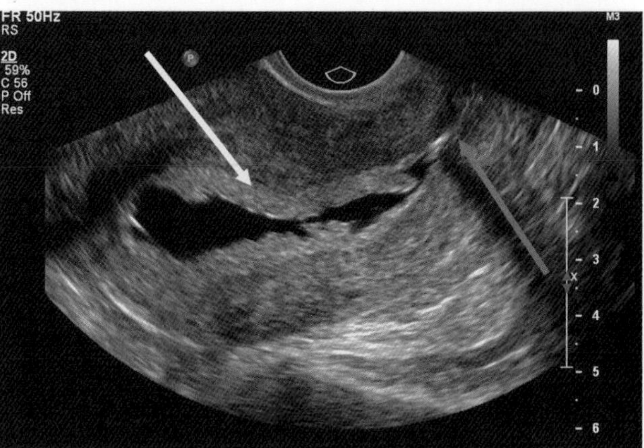

FIGURE 10.16. Thickened endometrium on sonohysterosalpingogram. Sagittal midline gray-scale image from a sonohysterosalpingogram. Note the thickened, irregular endometrium (white arrow). Catheter with deflated balloon can be seen in the lower uterine segment (gray arrow).

endometrial thickness in postmenopausal patients below which endometrial pathology is unlikely. However, the specificity of this criterion is low, ranging from 59% to 63% (87,92).

When endometrial thickness is greater then 5 mm, endometrial sampling is suggested not only because of increased posttest probability of endometrial carcinoma, but also because of the inability of TVS and/or SHG to differentiate accurately between benign and malignant causes of endometrial thickening (88,93–95). In a meta-analysis of 35 articles including 5,892 women, Smith-Bindman et al. (87) reported that using a cut-off of 5 mm for endometrial thickness, 96% of women with endometrial cancer had an abnormal TVS. In this series, a woman with a 10% pretest probability of endometrial carcinoma and a negative TVS had a posttest probability of endometrial carcinoma of only 1%. They concluded that TVS is highly accurate in identifying a subgroup of patients at extremely low risk, obviating the need for endometrial sampling in these patients.

In women taking HRT, the specificity of the 5 mm cut-off is even lower, as HRT increases endometrial thickness. However, since the pretest probability of endometrial carcinoma is also likely increased in these patients, the same cut-off value of 4 or 5 mm is generally used. In women on sequential HRT regimens, scanning should be performed after the progesterone part of the cycle when the endometrium is expected to be at its thinnest.

Investigators have attempted to correlate the morphology of the endometrium on US with histology in order to increase specificity. Endometrial cancer tends to be an irregular, heterogeneous mass, whereas endometrial hyperplasia tends to be more homogenous and echogenic. Cystic areas within the endometrium are more often associated with polyps, cystic endometrial hyperplasia, or tamoxifen use (96–98), rather than with endometrial carcinoma. However, there is considerable overlap of these morphologic features. The most specific and only reliable US finding for endometrial carcinoma is invasion of the myometrium or disruption of the subendometrial halo by an endometrial mass.

On SHG, endometrial carcinoma is most commonly depicted as a broad-based, irregular mass (Fig. 10.16) (99). Difficulty in distending the endometrial cavity has also been described (100). Three-dimensional SHG has been reported to be more accurate than either TVS or two-dimensional (2-D) SHG for the diagnosis of endometrial carcinoma. Endometrial volume and thickness are reported to be higher in patients with postmenopausal bleeding and endometrial carcinoma than in patients without endometrial carcinoma (101).

Doppler US has not been shown to be useful in distinguishing benign from malignant endometrial pathology as a wide range of peak systolic velocities and resistive indices is reported for benign and malignant endometrial pathology (102). However, benign endometrial polyps are more likely to have a single feeding vessel, whereas cancers more often have numerous feeding vessels and generalized increased vascularity (103).

Staging Endometrial Cancer

Staging in endometrial carcinoma is surgical–pathological and based on the FIGO classification. US, CT, and MRI all have utility in the staging of endometrial carcinoma.

Ultrasound

The role of ultrasound in staging endometrial carcinoma is limited to evaluating stage I disease by assessing the depth of myometrial invasion. According to the FIGO classification, stage IA indicates tumor confined to the endometrium; stage IB indicates tumor invading less than one half of the myometrium; and stage IC indicates tumor invading more than one half of the myometrium. For endometrial carcinoma to be considered stage IA by ultrasound criteria the myometrial/endometrial interface should be smooth and regular and the hypoechoic subendometrial halo, if present, should be regular, symmetric, and uninterrupted. Myometrial invasion is documented when the tumor mass disrupts the subendometrial halo and/or extends into the subjacent myometrium. TVS has been reported to have a sensitivity of 77% to 100%, a specificity of 65% to 93%, and an overall accuracy of 60% to 76% in assessing the degree of myometrial invasion (104–106). Understaging can occur with microscopic or minimal myometrial invasion. In addition, assessment of myometrial invasion is more difficult when the myometrium is thinned or distorted by fibroids (104). Three-dimensional SHG has been reported to be more accurate in detecting myometrial and cervical invasion by endometrial carcinoma (107).

Computed Tomography

CT is widely used for the staging of endometrial cancer (68,108,109). CT staging criteria, based on the FIGO classification, for endometrial carcinoma have been well described (Table 10.3). IV contrast, as well as good bowel opacification with oral and/or rectal contrast, is necessary for adequate CT

TABLE 10.3

CORRESPONDING CT FINDINGS FOR STAGING ENDOMETRIAL CARCINOMA

Stage I	
IA	Normal myometrium enveloping central low-attenuation tumor
IB	Normal myometrium enveloping central low-attenuation tumor <50% myometrial invasion
IC	Normal myometrium enveloping central low-attenuation tumor 50% myometrial invasion
Stage II	Central low-attenuation tumor extends into cervix
Stage III	
IIIA	Irregular uterine configuration Parametrial or pelvic sidewall extension Adnexal mass
IIIB	Thickening of vaginal wall
IIIC	Regional lymph nodes >1 cm in diameter in short axis
Stage IV	
IVA	Thickening or serration of bladder or rectal wall Obliteration of perivesical or perirectal fat
IVB	Tumor in distant organs or anatomic sites

evaluation. On noncontrast CT, endometrial carcinoma is the same attenuation as the normal surrounding myometrium, making evaluation difficult. On contrast-enhanced CT, endometrial carcinoma appears as a hypodense mass relative to the normal myometrium.

In stage I disease, the tumor may reside solely within the endometrial cavity as a diffuse, circumscribed, vegetative, or polypoid mass, or it may invade the adjacent myometrium (Fig. 10.17). If myometrial invasion is detected on CT, this usually corresponds to invasion of greater than one third to one half of the myometrium (109). Tumor may also occlude the cervical os or vagina, resulting in uterine obstruction. In these instances, CT demonstrates an enlarged uterus with a distended, fluid-density endometrial cavity surrounded by contrast-enhanced myometrium of varying thickness. Demonstration of intrauterine gas usually indicates a necrotic neoplasm, gas introduced by curettage or endometrial biopsy, or a fistula secondary to tumor invasion (110). Rarely, in this circumstance, does gas represent pyometria.

In stage II disease, there is endometrial tumor involvement of the cervix, which is characterized on CT as cervical enlargement greater than 3.5 cm in diameter and heterogeneous low-attenuation areas within the fibromuscular cervical stroma (Fig. 10.18).

Stage III disease, parametrial extension, is depicted by a loss of the normal periureteral fat. Pelvic sidewall involvement is indicated by the depiction of less than 3 mm of intervening fat between the soft-tissue mass and the pelvic sidewall (45). Fallopian tube and/or ovarian involvement are also consistent with stage III disease.

Stage IV disease, pathologically enlarged lymph nodes and distant metastases, are detected in the usual manner on CT.

The utility of CT in patients with stage I and II disease is limited. CT accuracy in these cases is variable, ranging from 58% to 92% (69). Detection of stage I disease had an accuracy of 76% in one study (108). In another study, CT had a specificity of 42% for detection of deep myometrial invasion (stage IC) and a sensitivity of only 25% for cervical involvement (stage II) (111).

The greatest clinical impact of CT use is in confirming parametrial and sidewall extension in stage III tumors and in detecting pelvic adenopathy and metastatic disease. Stage III tumors may be upstaged if extrapelvic metastases are depicted on CT studies (69). The accuracy of CT in patients with stage III or IV disease is 83% to 86% (69).

Limitations of CT include a tendency to understage endometrial carcinoma because of a failure to detect microscopic parametrial, lymph node, bowel, or bladder invasion (69). CT is also particularly unreliable in the determination of myometrial invasion in elderly women with atrophic myometrium and a polypoid tumor in the endometrial cavity (69,108,109).

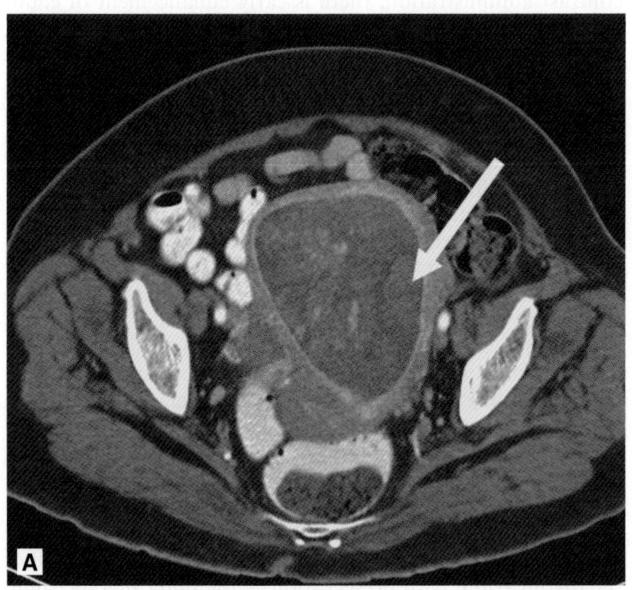

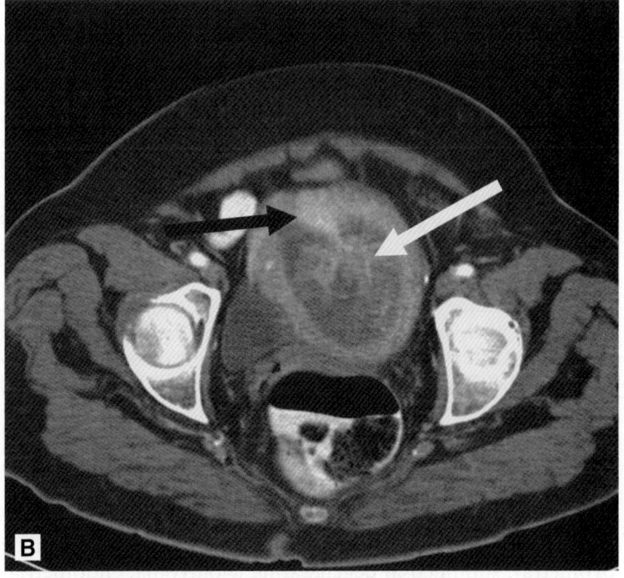

FIGURE 10.17. Stage I endometrial cancer on CT. Contrast-enhanced CT images (**A and B**) demonstrate enhancing tumor (white arrows in **A** and **B**) within an enlarged endometrial canal. Note the myometrial invasion (black arrow in **B**).

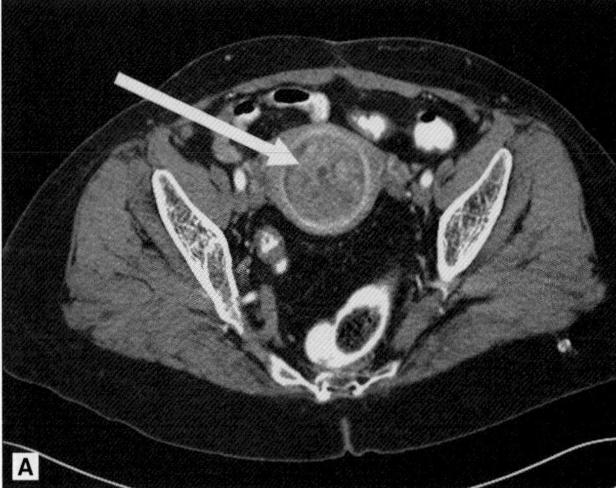

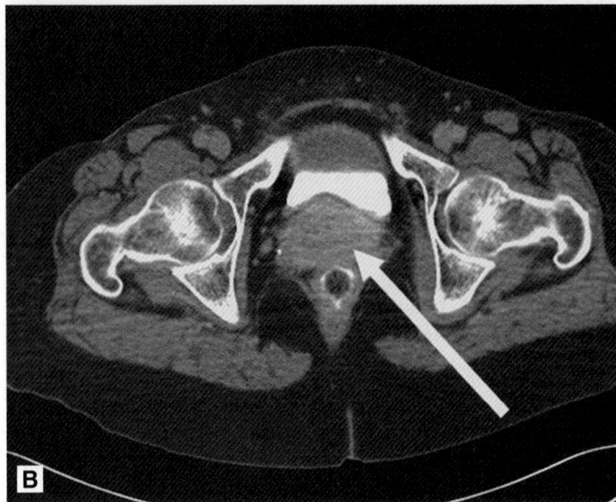

FIGURE 10.18. Stage II endometrial cancer on CT. Contrast-enhanced CT images (**A** and **B**) demonstrate enhancing tumor within the endometrial canal (white arrow in **A**) with associated low attenuation enlargement of the cervix (white arrow in **B**) indicating cervical involvement of tumor.

TABLE 10.4

CORRESPONDING MRI FINDINGS (T2W OR CONTRAST-ENHANCED T1W IMAGES) FOR STAGING ENDOMETRIAL CARCINOMA

Stage	Findings
Stage 0	Normal or thickened endometrial stripe
Stage I	
IA	Thickened endometrial stripe with diffuse or focal abnormal signal intensity Endometrial stripe may be normal Intact junctional zone with smooth endometrial–myometrial interface
IB	Signal intensity of tumor extends into myometrium <50% Partial or full-thickness disruption of junctional zone with irregular endometrial–myometrial interface
IC	Signal intensity of tumor extends into myometrium >50% Full-thickness disruption of junctional zone Intact stripe of normal outer myometrium
Stage II	
IIA	Internal os and endocervical canal are widened Low signal of fibrous stroma remains intact
IIB	Disruption of fibrous stroma
Stage III	
IIIA	Disruption of continuity of outer myometrium Irregular uterine configuration Adnexal mass
IIIB	Segmental loss of hypointense vaginal wall
IIIC	Regional lymph nodes >1 cm in diameter in short axis
Stage IV	
IVA	Tumor signal disrupts normal tissue planes with loss of low signal intensity of bladder or rectal wall
IVB	Tumor in distant organs or anatomic sites

Magnetic Resonance Imaging

Contrast-enhanced MRI is considered the most accurate imaging method for staging endometrial carcinoma (106). MRI staging criteria based on the FIGO classification have been well described (Table 10.4). Most MRI scans in women with endometrial cancer are performed after diagnostic D&C, and it is important to recognize post-D&C hemorrhage on MRI, which can be seen as a linear focal signal void. The results of at least one study indicate that this finding does not interfere with MRI staging evaluation of the uterus (112).

On unenhanced T1W images, endometrial carcinoma is isointense with the normal endometrium, and small tumors do not expand the canal. Therefore, these cancers usually go undetected on unenhanced T1W images. With larger tumors, the endometrium is thickened and may be lobulated or irregular on T1W images. Although endometrial cancer may demonstrate homogeneous high signal intensity on T2W sequences, it is more typically heterogeneous and may even be low in signal intensity. The MRI appearance of endometrial carcinoma is not specific and can also be seen with uterine fluid (hematometra or pyometra), submucosal degenerating leiomyoma, endometrial hyperplasia, endometrial polyps, and blood clots (80).

Routine use of gadolinium contrast is necessary for MRI evaluation of endometrial carcinoma. Following gadolinium contrast administration, there is early enhancement of endometrial cancer relative to the normal endometrium, allowing the identification of small tumors, even those contained by the endometrium. Contrast-enhanced images also differentiate viable tumor from necrosis, providing a more accurate assessment of tumor volume. Similarly, the distinction between tumor and endometrial fluid is obvious after gadolinium contrast administration; the former enhances, whereas the latter does not. The dynamic contrast-enhanced appearance of endometrial cancer has been described in a number of reports. Tumor conspicuity was more pronounced on dynamic enhanced images than on standard postcontrast T1W images, although the tumors themselves enhanced heterogeneously (109,113).

The MRI correlates of surgical FIGO subdivisions for stage I tumors have been described. Tumors are considered to be confined to the endometrium (stage IA) when the junctional zone is preserved. Alternatively, in cases without a visualized junctional zone, as is common in postmenopausal women, stage IA disease is characterized by a sharp tumor–myometrium interface. In stage IB disease, there is disruption of the junctional zone with an irregular myometrial–endometrial interface, and/or there is tumor of high T2W signal intensity in the inner half of the myometrium with preservation of the outer myometrium. In contradistinction, stage IC disease is characterized by high-T2W-signal-intensity tumor that extends into the outer myometrium with a thin, intact outer rim of normal myometrium.

Stage II tumors are characterized by widening and expansion of the cervical canal, with associated heterogeneity of the cervical stroma. Assessment of cervical involvement is facilitated by the multiplanar capabilities of MRI and dynamic contrast-enhanced sequences (Fig. 10.19) (82).

Extraserosal invasion (stage III) is depicted on T2W images as high-signal-intensity tumor extending beyond the outer uterine borders (80). Focal disruption of the normally low-signal-intensity wall of the bladder or rectum signifies stage IVA disease (66). Pathologically enlarged lymph nodes and metastatic disease are diagnosed in the usual fashion on MRI.

Reports of the overall MRI accuracy in staging of endometrial carcinoma range from 70% to 94% (39,80,81,114). Reports of accuracy in evaluation of myometrial invasion (stage I) on T2W images vary from 58% to 88% (80,81,113–117). Limitations of nonenhanced T2W-MRI staging of endometrial carcinoma include difficulty in differentiating tumor from some benign entities, difficulty in determining myometrial invasion in postmenopausal women with poorly defined or absent junctional zones, and difficulty in detecting extrauterine spread. High-resolution T2W images increase the conspicuity of the tumor–myometrial interface and the high soft-tissue contrast allows accurate determination of cervical involvement. And although there are single-institution studies of high-resolution T2W staging with a phased-array coil that report accuracy rates equal to those of dynamic contrast-enhanced imaging for the evaluation of myometrial and cervical invasion (118), to date these have not been reproduced in multi-institutional trials. Accuracy rates for the determination of cervical invasion using high-resolution T2W images are 82% to 91% (118,119).

These limitations have been at least partially overcome by the routine use of gadolinium contrast. Static contrast-enhanced MRI increases the accuracy of determining myometrial invasion to 68% to 78% (39,83,113,117,119). However, dynamic contrast-enhanced MRI is the best MRI technique for detection of myometrial invasion, with an accuracy of 85% to 93%, compared with 68% to 78% for static contrast-enhanced images and 58% to 88% for T2W images (72,113).

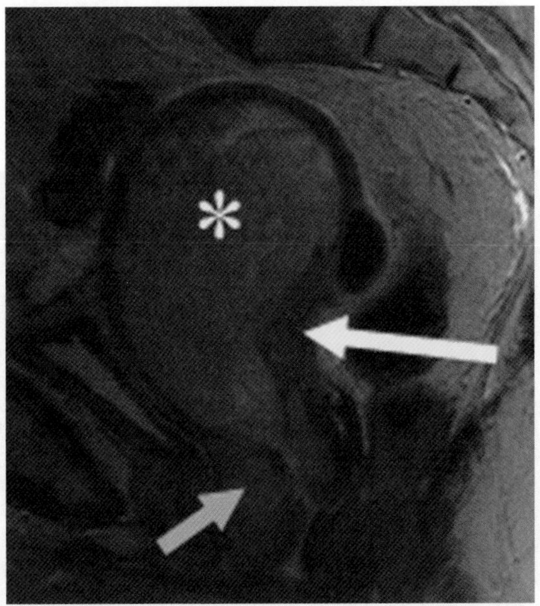

FIGURE 10.19. Stage II endometrial cancer on MRI. Sagittal T2W MRI image. The endometrial canal is expanded and contains heterogeneous signal (white asterisk). There is loss of the normal junctional zone along the posterior aspect of the uterus (white arrow); furthermore, the cervix is heterogeneous (grey arrow), compatible with tumor involvement.

Staging Endometrial Cancer Recommendations

Several studies suggest that MRI outperforms conventional CT in the assessment of depth of myometrial invasion (3). Two studies have reported that TVS is equivalent to T2W-MRI in evaluating myometrial invasion (68% to 69% vs. 68% to 74%) (116,117), but contrast-enhanced MRI is superior to TVS (85% vs. 68%) (117). A meta-analysis of studies showed significant differences in the accuracy of assessment of myometrial invasion among CT, TVS, and MRI. Contrast-enhanced MRI was significantly better than TVS and showed a trend toward better performance than CT (82). A follow-up meta-analysis and Bayesian analysis limited to detecting deep myometrial invasion also found contrast-enhanced MRI to be superior to other modalities (72).

Detecting Recurrent Endometrial Cancer

Endometrial cancer tends to recur locally in women treated with surgery alone. The most common site of local recurrence is the vaginal cuff. Because the vaginal cuff is amenable to physical examination in the majority of patients, imaging is usually reserved for problem solving in this group of patients. For patients who fail radiation therapy, either alone or in combination with surgery, recurrences tend to be distant disease. In these cases, CT or MRI is usually performed (Figs. 10.20 and 10.21). Detection of distant metastases by CT or MRI is performed in the usual fashion for these modalities.

FDG-PET has recently been evaluated for use in detecting recurrent endometrial carcinoma. In patients who are evaluated with FDG-PET after therapy, the sensitivity and specificity in detecting recurrent disease have been found to be 96% to 100% and 78% to 88%, respectively (120,121). Also, several studies have shown that FDG-PET in combination with anatomic imaging (CT and/or MRI) is more sensitive, specific, and accurate than anatomic imaging alone in detecting recurrent endometrial carcinoma (121,122).

Summary

In patients without a diagnosis of endometrial carcinoma, but with a clinical concern (e.g., postmenopausal bleeding), TVS is the study of choice. SHG, 3-D TVS, and 3-D SHg can also be helpful for primary detection of endometrial carcinoma.

The imaging evaluation of patients with known endometrial cancer is a function of physical examination, tumor type, and tumor stage. A chest radiograph is the only imaging study necessary in the majority of patients diagnosed with low-grade, clinical stage I tumor—that is, tumors that have a low pretest probability of extrauterine disease. However, TVS is also reasonable for estimating myometrial invasion in patients with a low pretest probability of myometrial involvement.

In patients with a high pretest probability of extrauterine disease (e.g., high tumor grade, aggressive cell type, suspicious physical examination, positive endocervical curettage, or elevated serum CA125), more extensive imaging is indicated. There is a growing body of evidence that dynamic contrast-enhanced MRI is more sensitive, specific, and accurate than CT and TVS in the staging of endometrial carcinoma. CT, however, remains an acceptable alternative. No studies to date have evaluated the utility of FDG-PET imaging in the staging of endometrial carcinoma. However, this is an area where FDG-PET may prove useful in the future.

For the detection of recurrent disease, FDG-PET combined with CT and/or MRI has preliminarily been shown to be superior to CT and/or MRI alone (120,121). However, because these studies involved only a small number of patients, more work in this area is needed and CT and/or MRI alone remains an acceptable alternative.

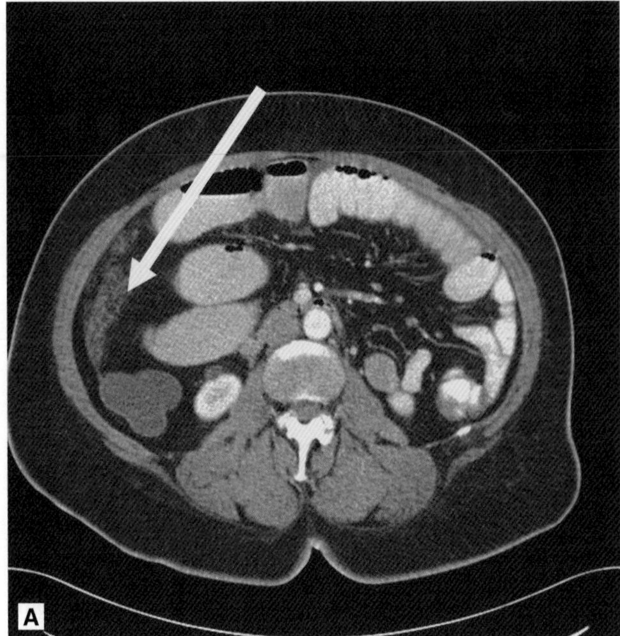

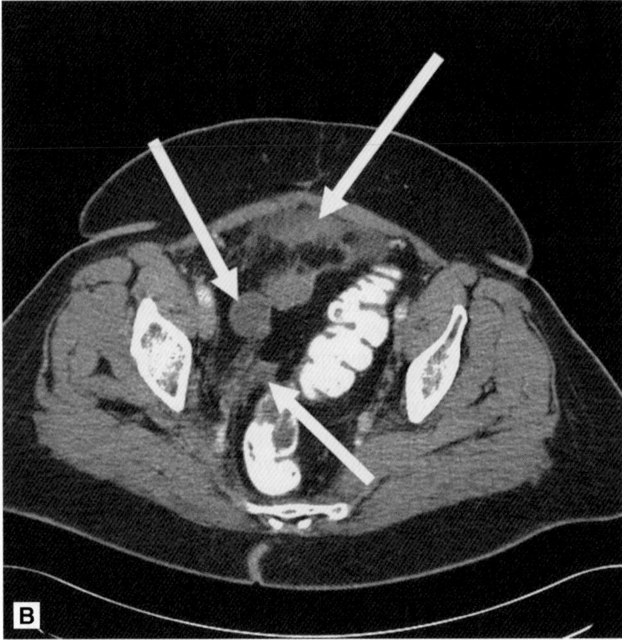

FIGURE 10.20. Endometrial cancer recurrence on CT. Axial contrast-enhanced CT images. Images demonstrate peritoneal and omental spread of tumor (white arrows in A and B).

GESTATIONAL TROPHOBLASTIC DISEASE

Introduction

Gestational trophoblastic disease (GTD) encompasses a spectrum of placental lesions including hydatidiform mole, invasive mole, choriocarcinoma, and placental site trophoblastic tumor. The role of imaging in GTD is primarily to document metastatic disease or to evaluate for persistent disease. No specific imaging findings allow differentiation between the different GTD lesions (123–125).

Primary Detection, Characterization, Staging, and Monitoring for Recurrence of Gestational Trophoblastic Disease

Ultrasound

TVS is considered the study of choice in the evaluation of suspected GTD. In patients with GTD, TVS examination most commonly demonstrates a soft-tissue mass distending the endometrial cavity. Typically, the mass is echogenic and heterogeneous, containing numerous cystic spaces (Fig. 10.22A) (126–128). In the case of complete hydatidiform mole, the

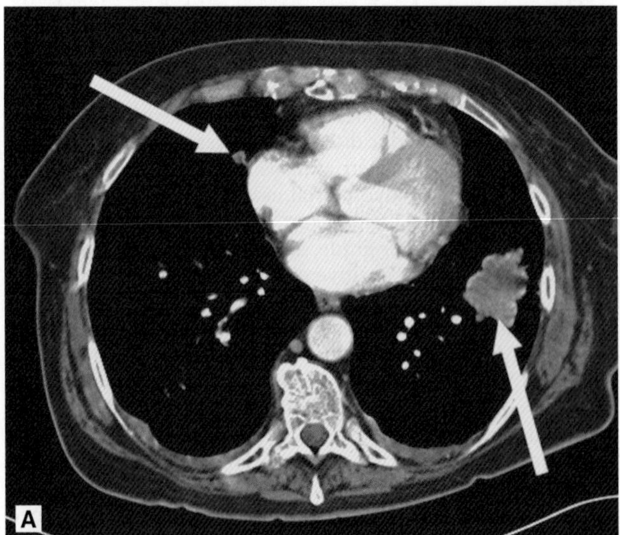

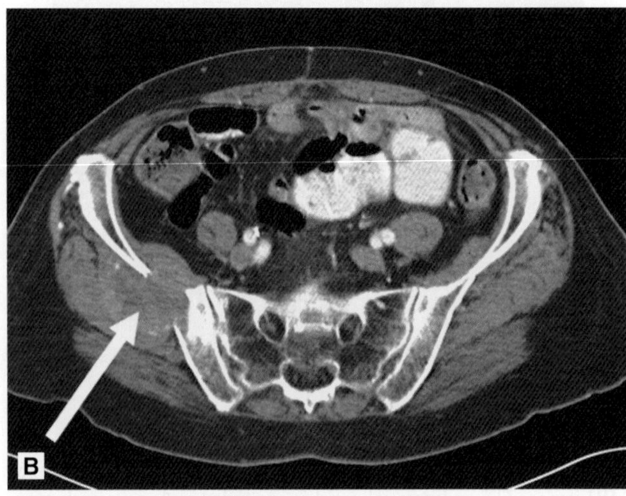

FIGURE 10.21. Endometrial cancer recurrence on CT. Axial contrast-enhanced CT images through the lower chest (A) and pelvis (B) of the same patient. Images demonstrate lung nodules (white arrows in A) and a soft-tissue mass with osseous destruction (white arrow in B) both proven to be recurrent endometrial cancer.

small cystic spaces correspond to the hydropic villi (126). Hydropic degeneration of the placenta may have a similar US appearance. The mass is usually extremely vascular, demonstrating increased vessel density and an abnormal uterine arterial waveform characterized by high peak systolic velocity and high diastolic blood flow (low resistance index [RI]) compared to the normal uterine arterial waveform (129). Irregularity of the border of the mass or asymmetric extension of the mass into the myometrium suggests myometrial invasion.

The ovaries may become enlarged with numerous theca lutein cysts (Fig. 10.22C and D). This ovarian enlargement can result in symptomatic ovarian torsion or hemorrhage (130). However, theca lutein cysts may not be detected in the early stages of the disease (127).

US can be helpful in assessing for persistent or recurrent disease by documenting an endometrial mass. Persistent GTD can be treated with US-guided direct injection of methotrexate (131).

GTD is the most common cause of uterine vascular malformations. These vascular malformations usually present after treatment is complete and can be easily diagnosed with US. Recently, it has been shown that these vascular malformations can be treated with uterine artery embolization (132).

Computed Tomography

The role of CT in the evaluation of GTD is primarily limited to the detection of metastatic disease. Uterine enlargement is the most common CT feature of GTD. Following administration of intravenous contrast, uterine enhancement is typically heterogeneous with focal enlargement or irregular hypodense regions within the myometrium (Fig. 10.22B) (130,133). These low-attenuation areas correspond to foci of hemorrhage and/or necrosis (133). Contrast-enhanced CT often demonstrates vascular uterine lesions and dilated uterine vessels in the broad ligaments (130).

Locoregional spread is characterized by avidly enhancing soft-tissue nodules in the parametria and/or obliteration of the pelvic fat and/or muscle planes.

GTD spreads hematogenously, with the lungs being the most common site of metastatic disease. Metastases to the lung, liver, and brain are vascular and prone to hemorrhage (130). CT detects these metastatic lesions in the usual manner. Trophoblastic emboli to the lungs may produce symptoms of acute pulmonary embolism and occasionally result in large intravascular masses (130).

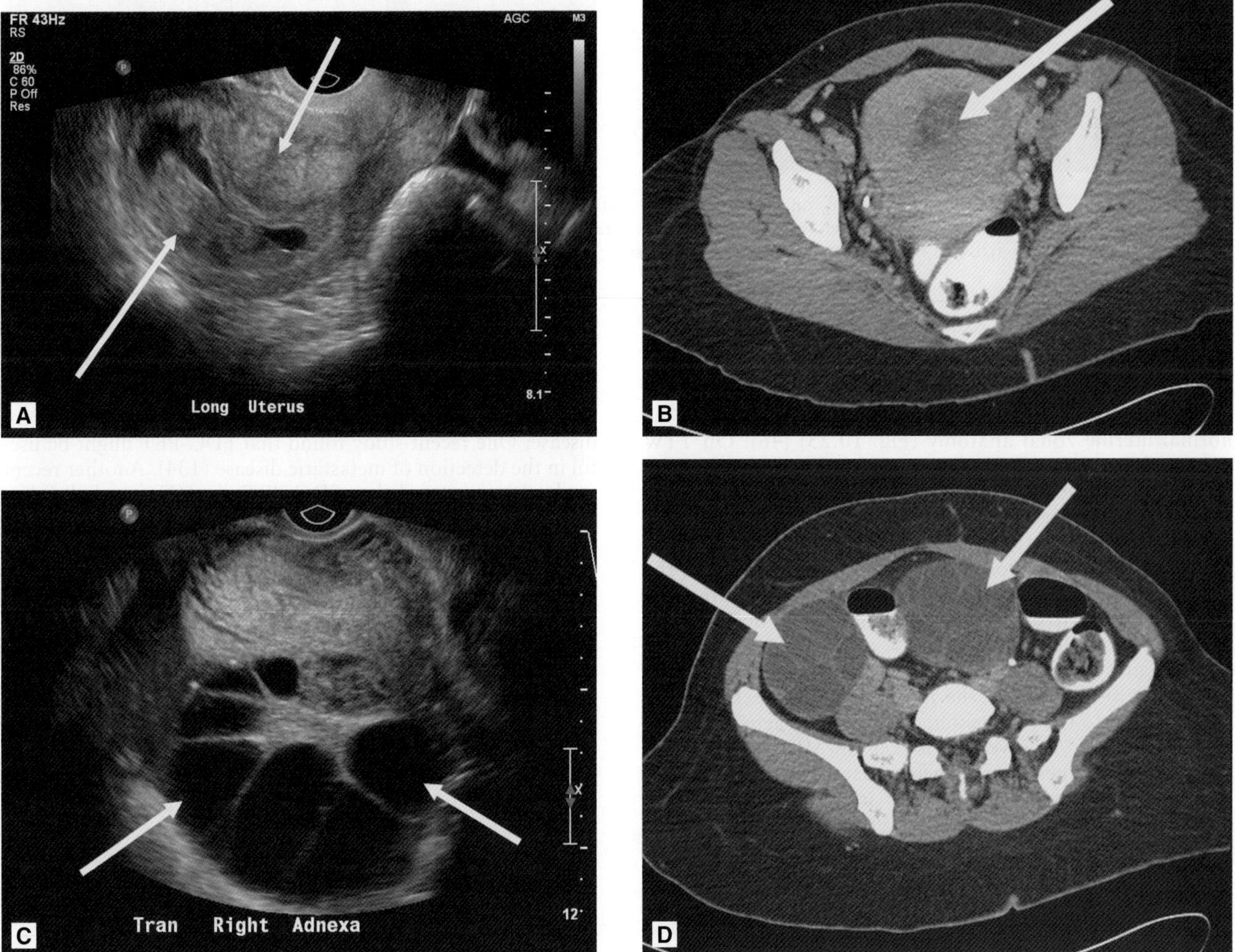

FIGURE 10.22. Hydatidiform mole on ultrasound and CT. Gray-scale sagittal ultrasound image of the uterus (A) demonstrating an echogenic, heterogeneous mass within the endometrial canal (white arrows in A). Axial contrast-enhanced CT image (B) in the same patient demonstrates enhancing soft-tissue distending the endometrial canal (white arrow in B). Gray-scale ultrasound image (C) of the right ovary and contrast-enhanced CT image (D) through the pelvis in the same patient demonstrating bilateral enlarged ovaries with innumerable theca lutein cysts (white arrows in C and D).

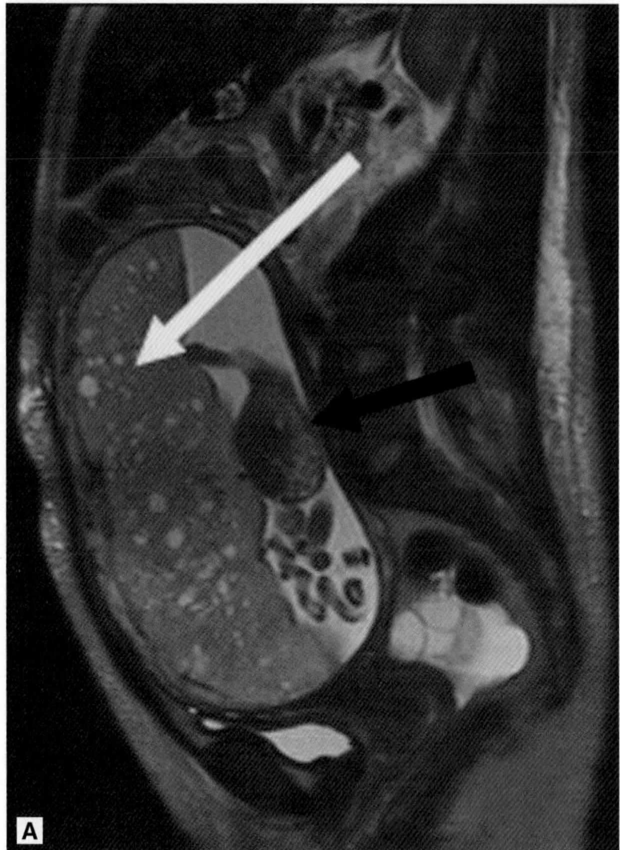

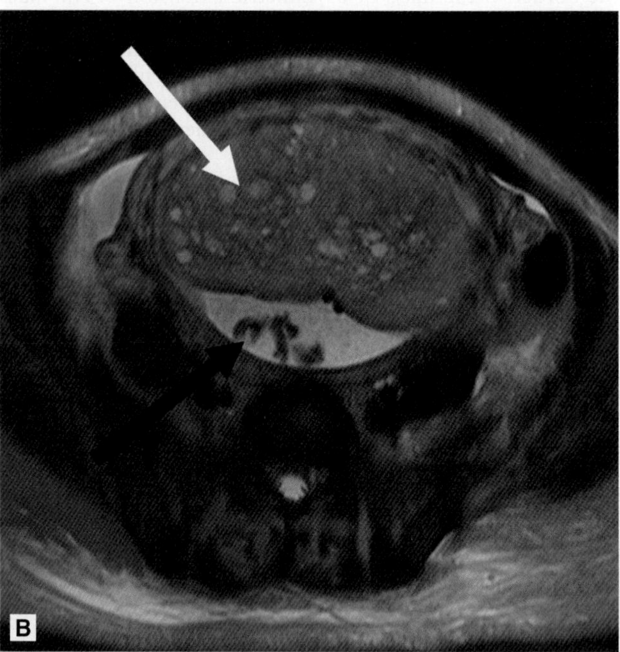

FIGURE 10.23. Partial mole on MR. Sagittal (A) and axial (B) T2W MRI images demonstrating a heterogeneous mass within the uterus (white arrows). Fetal abdomen (black arrow in A) and umbilical cord (black arrow in B) can be seen adjacent to the mass.

Magnetic Resonance Imaging

MRI is primarily used for staging and detecting recurrent disease. On T2W images, GTD is seen as a heterogeneous, predominantly high-signal-intensity mass that obliterates the normal uterine zonal anatomy (Fig. 10.23) (46). On T1W images, the mass may be isointense or hyperintense compared to the adjacent normal myometrium. The tumors are hypervascular, and enlarged vessels in the broad ligament and the uterus are depicted as signal voids on both T1W and T2W images. Following gadolinium contrast administration, the tumors avidly enhance and multiple enlarged vessels are often seen. MRI is able to depict tumors that invade the myometrium but spare the endometrium, a cause of nondiagnostic and/or false-negative D&Cs.

MRI is also useful in the identification of extrauterine pelvic spread to the parametria, adnexa, and vaginal fornices (46). Parametrial involvement is seen on MRI as high T2W signal masses within the parametria that avidly enhance after gadolinium contrast. MRI is better at detecting parametrial involvement than US. MRI is the preferred method for determining vaginal spread of tumor. Vaginal involvement is identified on MRI as a high-2W-signal-intensity mass within the vagina with associated gadolinium contrast enhancement. Metastatic disease is usually hypervascular and is detected in the usual manner.

Another role of MRI is to monitor patients' response to therapy. MRI findings of regression of vascular abnormalities, development of intralesional hemorrhage, and return of normal uterine zonal anatomy parallel a favorable response to chemotherapy (46). Normal uterine zonal anatomy should be seen 6 to 9 months after treatment (46).

Positron Emission Tomography

Very little data is available in the use of FDG-PET with GTD. The little data that is available has shown that FDG-PET may be helpful in the detection of metastatic disease and recurrent disease. One recent study found that FDG-PET might be useful in the detection of metastatic disease (134). Another recent study demonstrated that FDG-PET plus CT was helpful in 43.8% of patients when compared with CT alone (135). More research into the use of FDG-PET is needed before the clinical utility of this modality is established.

Summary

Imaging plays an important, albeit limited, role in the evaluation of GTD. US, CT, and MRI all play a role in the evaluation of suspected and documented GTD. The limited data available on the use of FDG-PET in the setting of GTD suggest that this modality may be useful for the detection of metastatic disease and the evaluation of recurrent GTD.

OVARIAN CANCER

Introduction

The detection of early ovarian cancer is difficult for a variety of reasons and currently involves a combination of physical examination, CA125 levels, and TVS. At present, there is no screening strategy that reliably detects early ovarian cancer.

Because of this, ovarian cancer is often not diagnosed until it has spread to other organs. Two staging systems for ovarian cancer exist, the TNM (tumor, node, metastasis) system and the FIGO staging system. US, CT, MRI, and FDG-PET all have a role to play in the accurate staging of ovarian cancer. These modalities also play a role in the monitoring of therapy and detection of recurrent disease.

Primary Detection and Characterization of Ovarian Cancer

The 5-year survival rates for stage I and stage II ovarian cancer are 80% to 90% and 70%, respectively (136); however, the 5-year survival rate for stages III and IV ranges from 5% to 50%. Therefore, if more ovarian cancers were detected as stage I disease rather than stage III or IV disease, 5-year survival would dramatically improve. Unfortunately, there are no good screening methods for ovarian cancer at present; most use a combination of physical exam, CA125 levels, and TVS.

Ultrasound

US plays a crucial role in the detection and characterization of adnexal masses and is an important component of screening programs for women at high risk for ovarian carcinoma. US is the initial imaging modality of choice for characterizing an ovarian mass as benign or malignant.

The early diagnosis of ovarian carcinoma when cure is possible but tumors are clinically asymptomatic (silent) is made difficult by the low prevalence of ovarian carcinoma in the general population. Therefore, efforts at screening patients for ovarian carcinoma have focused on high-risk populations. Risk factors include older age, high socioeconomic status, factors that increase the number of ovulatory cycles such as early menarche, nulliparity, late-onset menopause, and having a first-degree relative with ovarian carcinoma (137,138). Approximately 10% of ovarian carcinomas are believed to be due to an inherited susceptibility. Three syndromes have been described: the breast/ovarian cancer syndrome; the Lynch 2 syndrome, or the hereditary nonpolyposis colorectal cancer syndrome; and hereditary site-specific ovarian cancer. In 1994, a National Institutes of Health (NIH) consensus conference (139) recommended that screening be offered to women with two or more first-degree relatives with ovarian carcinoma. It is also recommended that women with an inherited predisposition to ovarian cancer be screened (139,140). In practice, many women with a single first-degree relative are enrolled in screening programs.

Most screening programs for ovarian cancer rely on a combination of physical examination, serologic markers, and TVS. The results of these screening trials have consistently demonstrated that US detects more stage I ovarian carcinomas than CA125 levels and physical examination (141). Nonetheless, very few stage I carcinomas have been found in such screening programs (142). The most recent data from the Prostate, Lung, Colorectal, and Ovarian (PLCO) Cancer Screening Trial (143) demonstrated that the PPV value for invasive cancer was 1.0% for an abnormal TVS, 3.7% for an abnormal CA125, and 23.5% if both tests (CA125 and TVS) were abnormal. Only one study has demonstrated ovarian cancer screening trials to have a survival benefit. Van Nagell et al. (144) reported a decrease in case-specific ovarian cancer mortality with 89.9% 2-year and 77.2% 5-year survival in women with US-detected ovarian carcinoma.

Ultrasound is considered the initial imaging modality of choice to differentiate a benign from a malignant clinically suspected ovarian mass. Although a likely benign mass can be followed or removed by a general gynecologist, suspicion of a malignant ovarian mass initiates referral to a gynecologic oncologist who can better perform the more complex therapeutic and staging cytoreduction surgery for ovarian carcinoma. Morphologic features remain the primary criteria for differentiating complex ovarian masses as benign or malignant on US. Hence, TVS is the critical US imaging approach because of the improved spatial and soft-tissue resolution afforded by the higher frequency endovaginal probe. Nonetheless, transabdominal ultrasound remains an important, complementary component of the US examination when a larger field of view is required—for example, if a mass is displaced out of the pelvis or is so large that it is incompletely visualized by TVS. In addition, transabdominal imaging is required for evaluation of secondary findings in ovarian cancer, such as ascites, peritoneal implants, or hydronephrosis. Such findings can be important not only to confirm the impression of malignancy but also for staging.

Numerous studies have reported that when strict US criteria and a pattern recognition approach for identification of benign ovarian masses are used, US examination has a near 95% to 99% NPV in excluding malignancy (145–147). US features consistent with benign etiology include smooth, thin walls; few, thin septations; absence of solid components or mural nodularity; as well as pattern recognition for certain benign diagnoses. Simple cysts will be anechoic with a smooth, thin wall and posterior acoustic enhancement. Hemorrhagic cysts or endometriomas (Fig. 10.24) may contain uniform low-level echoes but should still demonstrate a smooth, thin wall and increased through transmission. Hemorrhagic cysts may contain complex internal echoes; however, the appearance of the internal echoes should change over time and should never demonstrate internal vascularity. Several US patterns associated with dermoid cysts have been described including uniform increased echogenicity with posterior acoustic attenuation, echogenic shadowing mural nodules, and layering with or without floating debris.

Conversely, mural nodules, mural thickening or irregularity, solid components, thick septations (>3 mm) (Fig. 10.25), and associated findings such as ascites, peritoneal implants, and/or hydronephrosis suggest malignancy. Such US descriptors have been reported to have a high sensitivity but lower specificity for malignancy (144,146,147). The lower specificity reflects overlap in the imaging appearance of benign, borderline, and malignant lesions. For example, benign lesions such as hemorrhagic cysts, cystadenomas, or cystadenofibromas may have thick septations and apparent mural nodules; borderline

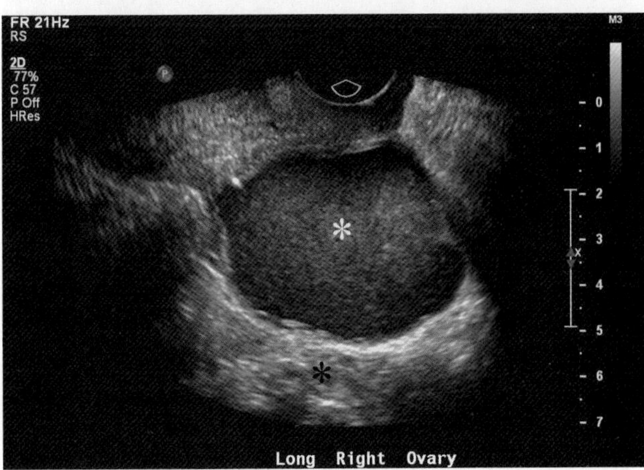

FIGURE 10.24. Endometrioma. Gray-scale ultrasound image demonstrating uniform low-level internal echoes (white asterisk) and increased through transmission (black asterisk).

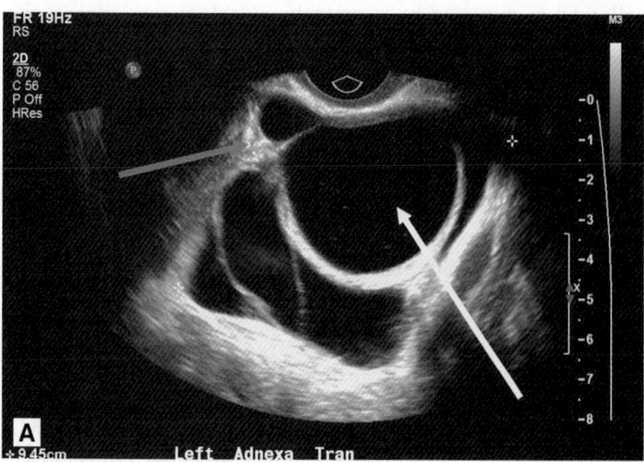

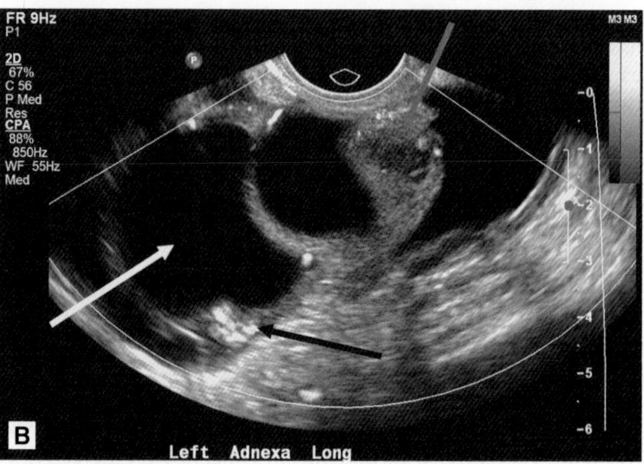

FIGURE 10.25. Solid and cystic ovarian mass on ultrasound. Gray-scale (**A**) and color Doppler (**B**) images demonstrate a mostly cystic mass (white arrows) with an associated solid component (grey arrows). Note the internal flow within the solid components (black arrow in **B**).

tumors may have minimal findings; and Brenner's tumors, fibromas, and fibrothecomas are solid but benign (Fig. 10.26). Furthermore, pedunculated fibroids, dermoids, and endometriomas can masquerade as solid ovarian lesions.

The use of color and pulse Doppler in the evaluation of ovarian masses is controversial, with some investigators considering blood flow characteristics to be merely confirmatory but others considering the Doppler examination to be a helpful discriminator (148–150). Tumor neovascularity is known to be characterized by an increased number of often tortuous vessels with arteriovenous shunts. Malignant neovascularity lacks the normal amount of smooth muscle cells in the vessel walls. Researchers had hoped that Doppler evaluation, which could potentially assess vascular compliance or resistance as well as vessel morphology, density, and distribution, would be helpful in characterizing ovarian masses. Malignant lesions more often demonstrate increased vessel density and tortuosity than benign lesions, but significant overlap exists. Malignant ovarian lesions also tend to demonstrate higher peak systolic velocities and lower resistive indices than benign masses, but again, considerable overlap exists and no discriminatory cut-off values are accepted (148–150).

Three-dimensional US is a new imaging technique that may improve characterization of adnexal masses. In one early study of 71 pelvic masses, 3-D power Doppler US improved the specificity and PPV compared to conventional 2-D US from 54% to 75% and from 35% to 50%, respectively (151). Further research is needed with this technique to better define its role in the characterization of adnexal masses.

Scoring systems have been proposed to standardize evaluation of ovarian masses in an attempt to improve specificity (152,153). Using a stepwise logistic regression analysis to determine the most discriminating gray-scale and Doppler sonographic features of malignancy, Brown et al. (153) reported that a multiparameter approach, which assessed for nonhyperechoic solid components, central blood flow on color Doppler, ascites, and thick septations, had a 93% sensitivity and specificity for malignancy. To achieve 100% sensitivity, specificity dropped to 86% in this study (153). However, Timmerman et al. (154) have reported similar findings and interobserver variability when readers used subjective criteria for evaluating ovarian masses.

Computed Tomography

CT is not the study of choice to evaluate a suspected ovarian lesion; however, ovarian lesions are detected incidentally on CT and can be characterized. In studies of adnexal lesions, the

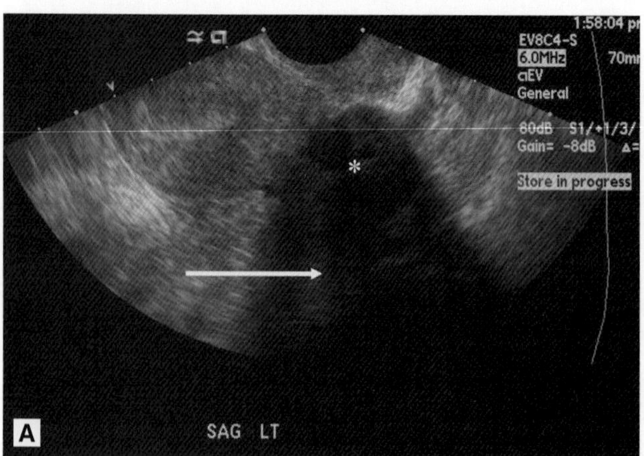

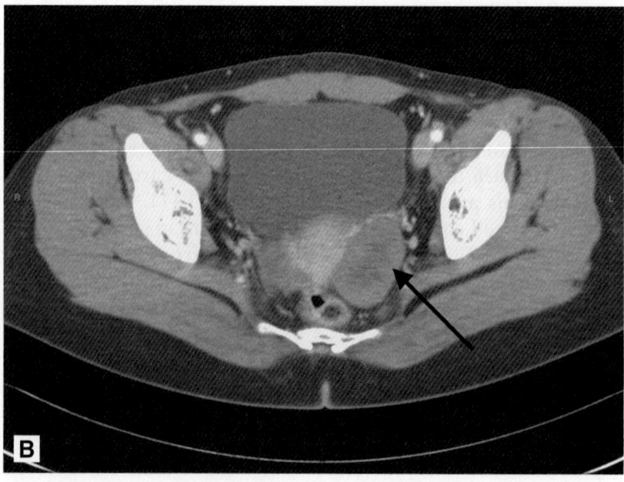

FIGURE 10.26. Ovarian fibroma. Gray-scale ultrasound (**A**) and axial CT (**B**) images. On ultrasound (**A**), the lesion is a solid mass (white asterisk) with homogeneous decreased echogenicity with associated dark shadowing (white arrow). A CT scan (**B**) of the same patient demonstrates a solid homogeneous left adnexal mass (black arrow).

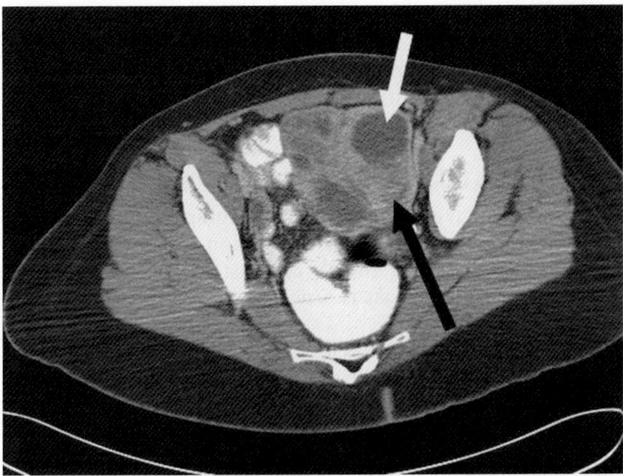

FIGURE 10.27. Poorly differentiated ovarian carcinoma on CT. Axial contrast-enhanced CT image demonstrating an adnexal mass with both solid (black arrow) and cystic (white arrow) components.

sensitivity, specificity, and accuracy of CT for characterizing benign versus malignant lesions are reported to be 89%, 96% to 99%, and 92% to 94%, respectively (155,156).

On CT, ovarian cancer demonstrates varied morphologic patterns, including a multilocular cyst with thick internal septations and solid mural or septal components, a partially cystic and solid mass, and a lobulated, papillary solid mass (Fig. 10.27). The outer border of the mass may be irregular and poorly defined, and amorphous, coarse calcifications and contrast enhancement may be seen in the cyst wall or soft-tissue components. Since the CT appearance of ovarian metastases is indistinguishable from a primary ovarian neoplasm, the stomach and colon should be carefully examined as potential primary tumor sites when an ovarian mass is detected on CT (157).

Magnetic Resonance Imaging

MRI functions as a complementary exam to US in the evaluation of a suspected ovarian lesion. To optimize MRI detection and characterization of an adnexal mass, contrast-enhanced protocols and attention to eliminating, or at least limiting, bowel motion are needed. Additionally, imaging should be performed with a phased-array surface coil to maximize spatial resolution.

Primary and ancillary criteria have been proposed for the characterization of an adnexal mass as being malignant. In a study of 60 lesions (158), statistical analyses yielded the following five significant primary criteria for malignancy: size greater than 4 cm, solid mass or large solid component, wall thickness greater than 3 mm, septal thickness greater than 3 mm, and/or the presence of vegetations or nodularity and necrosis (Fig. 10.28). Four ancillary criteria of malignancy were also statistically formulated: involvement of pelvic organs or pelvic sidewall; peritoneal, mesenteric, or omental disease; ascites; and adenopathy. When gadolinium contrast-enhanced T1W and unenhanced T1W and T2W images were analyzed collectively, the presence of one or more of the five primary criteria, coupled with a single criterion from the ancillary group, correctly characterized 95% of malignant lesions (158). These rates reflect improvements in lesion characterization produced by the addition of gadolinium contrast to the protocol and have been reproduced in other studies (159,160).

As with CT, disease metastatic to the ovary is often indistinguishable from primary ovarian cancer on MRI scans and both the colon and the stomach should be examined as potential primary tumor sites if an ovarian mass is detected on MRI (157,161).

Ovarian masses at times can grow large and it can be difficult to determine the organ of origin on US and/or CT. Uterine fibroids and other pelvic masses can also grow to a large size and mimic an ovarian tumor. The multiplanar capabilities of MRI are helpful in this situation and often help to delineate the organ of origin of a large pelvic mass.

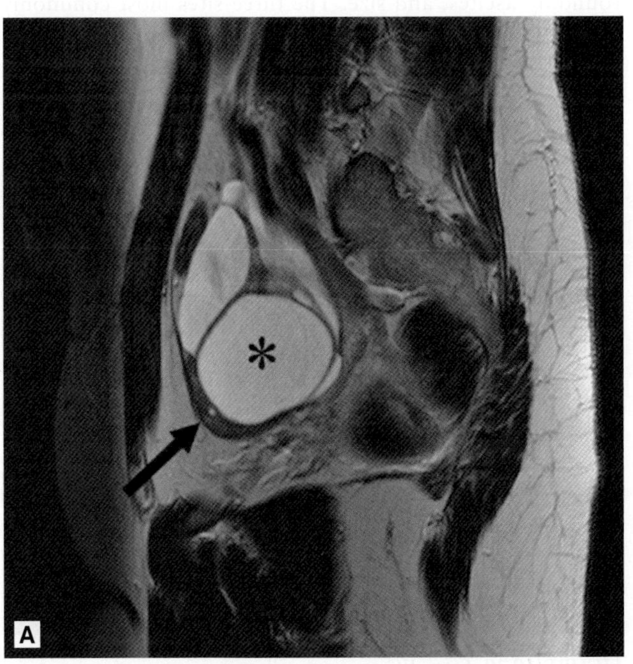

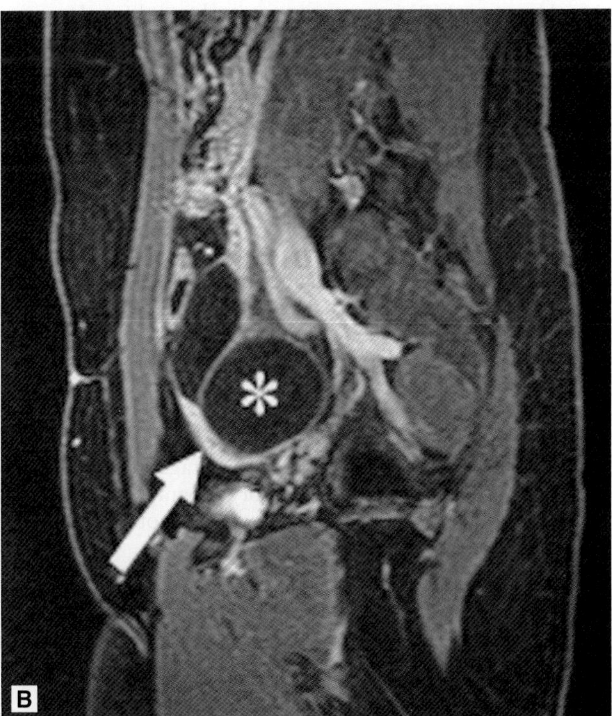

FIGURE 10.28. Solid and cystic ovarian mass on MR. Sagittal T2W (A) and T1W contrast-enhanced fat-saturated (B) images. The cystic components are high signal on the T2W image (black asterisk) and do not enhance on the T1W post-contrast fat-saturated image (white asterisk). Abnormally thickened wall is intermediate signal on the T2W image (black arrow) and enhances post contrast (white arrow).

Positron Emission Tomography

FDG-PET has little clinical role in the primary detection of a pelvic mass. However, FDG-PET appears to be promising for the characterization of ovarian masses because of its potential to detect tumor prior to significant morphologic changes. This is important, as currently most patients with ovarian cancer present late in their disease owing to a lack of early clinical or imaging manifestations. A study by Hubner et al. (162) found good correlation between FDG-PET and histologic findings in women with suspected ovarian cancer imaged prior to laparotomy. Specifically, the sensitivity, specificity, accuracy, PPV, and NPV of FDG-PET were 83%, 80%, 82%, 86%, and 76%, respectively. A recent study found that PET-CT imaging had a sensitivity of 100% and a specificity of 92.5% for the detection of a malignant mass (163).

Recommendations for Primary Detection and Characterization of Ovarian Cancer

Several studies have compared MRI to CT and US for characterizing adnexal masses, with mixed results (159,164,165). One study found that low-field-strength MRI was equivalent to CT for this determination, with accuracies of 86% and 92%, respectively (156). Another study suggested that TVS was superior to unenhanced MRI for lesion characterization (166), and yet another study found that the specificity of MRI with intravenous contrast was higher than that of TVS (97% vs. 69%) (164). Both TVS and MRI with gadolinium contrast have high sensitivity (97% and 100%, respectively) in the identification of solid components within an adnexal mass. MRI, however, shows higher specificity (98% vs. 46%) (165). Furthermore, MRI was shown to be the most efficient second test when an indeterminate ovarian mass was detected at gray-scale US and provides the greatest change in posttest probability when compared to combined color and gray-scale US and CT (167).

At present, the relatively high cost of MRI precludes its use as a screening modality, and US should be used for this indication. However, MRI is most appropriately used for characterization of an adnexal lesion in cases where US and clinical examination are indeterminate (7,167). Further research is necessary to determine the role of FDG-PET and/or PET-CT in the primary detection and characterization of adnexal masses.

Staging Ovarian Cancer

Cross-sectional imaging is widely accepted and more commonly used in the evaluation and staging of ovarian carcinoma than for other gynecologic malignancies. Two staging systems exist for ovarian cancer: the TNM system and the FIGO system. The FIGO system is surgically based and is the more frequently used of the two systems, and it will be the staging system referred to in the remainder of this chapter. Imaging is an adjunct to surgical staging. It is useful in the detection of pathologic adenopathy, the presence of which may alter staging and therapy. Although barium enema and excretory urography are still performed at some institutions, these studies are not recommended as routine staging procedures (168).

Ultrasound

US has a limited role in the staging of ovarian cancer except for detecting the presence of ascites. Transabdominal US is an excellent modality not only for identifying ascites, but for guiding paracentesis as well. However, the detection of stage II and III disease by US is limited. Peritoneal implants can sometimes be documented on careful US examination. The specificity of US examination in documenting abdominal spread of disease has been reported to be slightly higher than that of CT or MRI (169). However, the sensitivity of US for the detection of implants less than 2 cm (stage IIIB) is lower than that of CT or MRI owing to a limited field of view and decreased spatial and soft-tissue resolution (169,170). US, therefore, should only be used for specific indications.

Computed Tomography

CT is the primary cross-sectional imaging modality used to stage ovarian cancer. For this indication, CT should be performed with both oral and IV contrast. Opacification of the bowel with oral contrast is crucial for the detection of peritoneal implants on CT.

Stage I ovarian cancer is limited to either one (stage IA) or both (stage IB) ovaries. The presence of malignant ascites with tumor confined to one or both ovaries is stage IC disease. Ascites on CT is easily identified; however, the distinction between stage IC and stage III, or peritoneal, disease is often difficult to make and has significant clinical implications. In one series of patients, the presence of ascites on CT had a PPV of 72% to 80% as a sign of peritoneal metastasis (171).

Stage II disease occurs when there is direct extension into or implants on the uterus and/or fallopian tubes (stage IIA) or the rectum, bladder, and/or peritoneum (stage IIB). The presence of stage IIA or IIB disease with malignant ascites is stage IIC disease (Fig. 10.29). Irregularity or obliteration of the fat plane between the uterus and the ovarian mass indicates stage IIA disease. Loss of the normal fat plane around the rectum or bladder, less than 3 mm between the tumor and the pelvic sidewall, and/or displacement or encasement of the iliac vessels indicates stage IIB disease (172).

Stage III disease is defined as the presence of extra-pelvic peritoneal and/or lymph node metastasis. Microscopic extra-pelvic peritoneal implants are stage IIIA disease and are not detectable with CT. Stage IIIB, extra-pelvic peritoneal implants less than 2 cm and stage IIIC (Fig. 10.30), extra-pelvic peritoneal implants larger than 2 cm or lymph node metastasis are sometimes detectable with CT.

CT detection of peritoneal implants depends on several factors including location, the presence or absence of surrounding ascites, and size. The three sites most commonly involved are the right subphrenic space, the greater omentum,

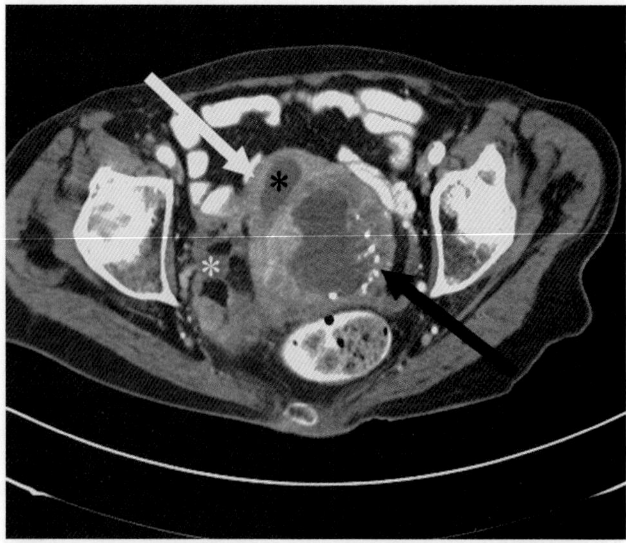

FIGURE 10.29. Stage IIC serous papillary ovarian carcinoma. Axial CT image with oral and intravenous contrast. Obliteration of the fat plane between the solid and cystic ovarian mass (black arrow) and uterus (white arrow). Note fluid in the endometrial canal (black asterisk) secondary to obstruction. Ascites (white asterisk) is also present.

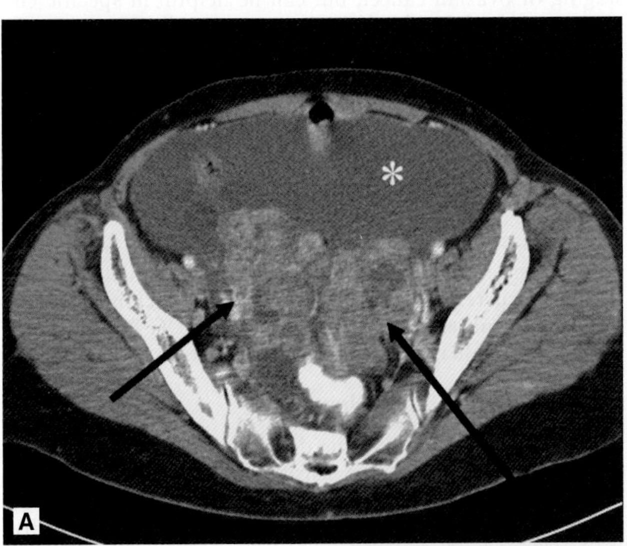

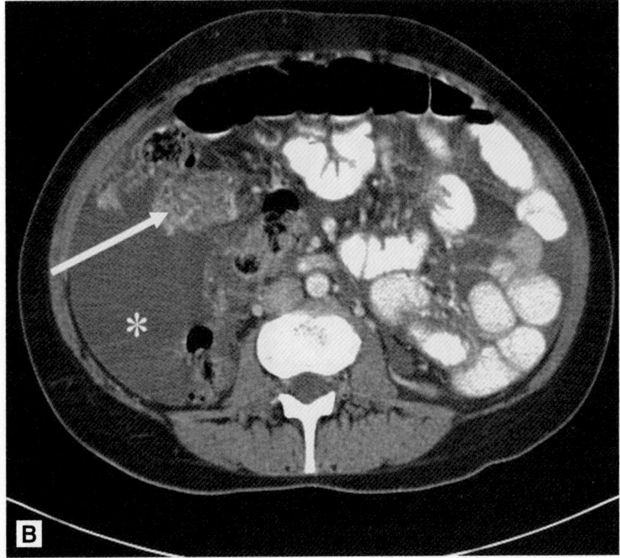

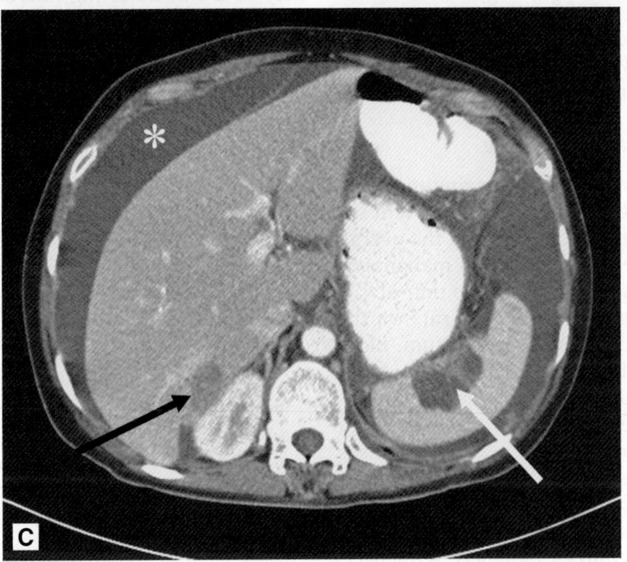

FIGURE 10.30. Stage IIIC serous papillary ovarian carcinoma. Axial CT images with oral and IV contrast (A–C). Images demonstrate bilateral ovarian solid and cystic masses (black arrows in **A**), omental (white arrow in **B**), subcapsular liver (black arrow in **C**) and splenic (white arrow in **C**) implants, and ascites (white asterisk in **A–C**).

and the pouch of Douglas (173). The presence of surrounding ascites aids in the detection of small peritoneal implants by increasing their conspicuity. In addition, the presence of ascites on CT is suggestive of peritoneal spread, as previously discussed. Size plays an important role in the reliable detection of peritoneal implants. Peritoneal implants smaller than 1 cm are not consistently detected on CT, especially in the absence of ascites, with a sensitivity of only 14% to 27% in this situation (172,174). However, the use of coronal and sagittal reformatted images allows for better detection of smaller lesions and has the potential to improve the sensitivity of CT (175).

Mesenteric metastases appear on CT scans as either round or ill-defined soft-tissue masses surrounded by small-bowel loops and mesenteric fat, or as thickened leaves of the mesentery caused by tumor coating the peritoneal surfaces. Omental metastases are characterized as stranding or soft tissue nodules embedded in omental fat or the replacement of the omental fat with thick, nodular tumor ("omental cake") along the greater curvature of the stomach, in the gastrosplenic ligament, or anterior to the transverse colon and small bowel in the lower abdomen (Fig. 10.31) (176). The sensitivity of CT for detection of omental metastasis is reported to be 80% to 86% (172,174). Capsular implants on the surface of the liver are seen as soft-tissue nodules studded along the peritoneal surface of the liver. Prominent hematogenous spread to the liver can occur in ovarian cancer and is considered stage IV disease, but it is unusual and should raise the suspicion for a gastrointestinal primary tumor.

Lymph node metastases are defined by a size criterion on CT as having a short axis greater than 1 cm. As with other malignancies, this criterion is flawed, as it does not take into account microspread of tumor.

Stage IV disease is defined as liver parenchymal metastasis and/or disease outside the peritoneal cavity (lung, bone, brain, etc.). These findings are diagnosed on CT in the usual manner.

The sensitivity of CT for the detection of extrapelvic disease is approximately 95% to 100% for liver involvement and 50% to 60% for nodal involvement (172,174). Overall staging

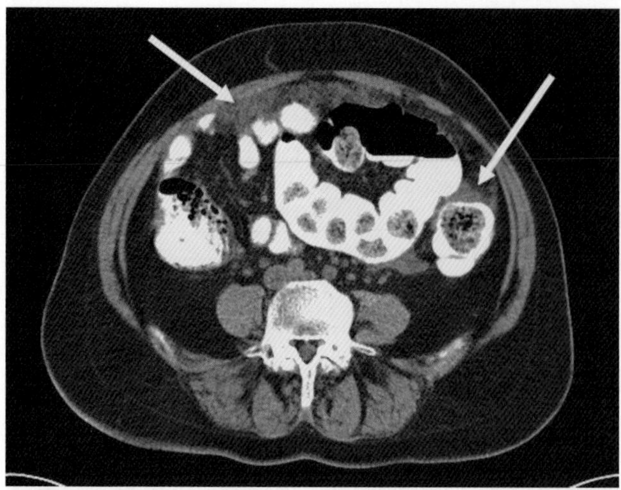

FIGURE 10.31. Omental implants on CT. Axial CT image through the lower abdomen demonstrating omental caking (arrows).

accuracy for CT has been reported to be 77% (172). CT also has a high PPV for imaging bulky disease and is therefore useful for identifying patients with inoperable disease (172,174).

Magnetic Resonance Imaging

Although CT is the primary cross-sectional imaging modality used to stage ovarian cancer, MRI can be useful in certain situations (contrast allergy, renal failure, etc.). In fact, the overall staging accuracy of MRI in patients with ovarian malignancy is 75% to 78% (158,172), which is comparable to that of CT.

Stage II disease, direct extension into or implants on the uterus and/or fallopian tubes (stage IIA) or the rectum, bladder, and/or peritoneum (stage IIB), is well depicted on MRI. Invasion is characterized by a tumor/normal structure interface of greater than 90% or direct soft-tissue extension with irregular margins into the adjacent structure. Accuracy ranges from 70% to 94% for the assessment of spread of ovarian tumor to the uterus, bladder, rectum, and pelvic sidewall (172).

Depiction of stage III disease on MRI is aided by the use of T1W fat-suppressed gadolinium contrast-enhanced sequences. T1W fat-suppressed contrast-enhanced sequences are used to depict intra-abdominal disease (i.e., omental, peritoneal, and mesenteric metastases), which enhance and have high-signal intensity contrasting with the low signal intensity of intra-abdominal fat. This technique makes lesions as small as 1 cm conspicuous (159).

Stage IV disease is diagnosed in the usual manner on MRI.

Positron Emission Tomography

The role of FDG-PET in the initial staging of ovarian cancer is controversial. However, at least one study has demonstrated FDG-PET to be a useful adjunct in the initial staging of ovarian cancer. In this recent study, the addition of FDG-PET imaging to CT alone increased staging accuracy from 79% to 81% within the pelvis and from 85% to 93% outside the pelvis (177).

Staging Recommendations

CT is the primary modality for staging ovarian cancer. The few prospective studies comparing CT and MRI found that MRI was at least equivalent and, in some cases, superior to CT for showing the relationship between tumor and adjacent pelvic structures and delineating the intra-abdominal extent of disease (159). The use of MRI, however, is limited by longer exam time, limited availability, expense, and lack of widespread reader experience. US has limited usefulness in the staging of ovarian cancer, but can be helpful in specific circumstances such as identifying ascites or guiding paracentesis. The use of FDG-PET for the initial staging of ovarian cancer is controversial. Further research is needed to determine the appropriate role for FDG-PET in this situation.

Detecting Persistent or Recurrent Ovarian Cancer

Imaging, especially US and CT, has been used to detect persistent or recurrent ovarian cancer and to document tumor response to subsequent therapy. Recently, FDG-PET has been shown to be valuable for the detection of recurrent disease.

Ultrasound

US plays a limited role in the detection of recurrent ovarian cancer. US has the greatest sensitivity in detecting recurrent tumor in the pelvis or around the liver and right hemidiaphragm in the setting of ascites (178). However, the sensitivity of US in detecting microscopic disease, miliary peritoneal seeding, and macroscopic disease less than 2 cm of the peritoneum and/or omentum is poor (178,179). Additionally, small, plaque-like lesions on the pelvic peritoneum or lesions high in the false pelvis are often missed on US (179). Therefore, US is not sufficient to replace second-look laparotomy (which is still performed in some centers) in making patient-management decisions (178). Despite these limitations, US can reliably confirm a clinical suspicion of gross macroscopic recurrent disease (Figs. 10.32 and 10.33) and is more accurate than clinical examination (178,179). US can also be used to guide biopsy of areas of suspected recurrence.

Computed Tomography

CT is the most commonly used cross-sectional imaging modality for the detection of recurrent ovarian cancer (Figs. 10.34 and 10.35). Although the use of CT allows assessment of more potential sites of tumor recurrence than US, it too has significant limitations. In the detection of persistent or recurrent ovarian cancer, the sensitivity of conventional CT is 51% to 84% and its specificity is 81% to 93% (180–183). False-positive results are usually caused by misdiagnosis of adherent bowel loops as a tumor mass. The sensitivity of CT for disease detection is proportional to lesion size (180). Many studies report limitations in the detection of small (1- to 3-cm) tumor nodules in the mesentery and omentum, and along peritoneal surfaces (180,181). However, the use of sagittal and coronal reformatted images improves the detection of peritoneal implants (175). Nevertheless, a negative CT does not exclude microscopic disease or small tumor implants and thus cannot substitute for second-look laparotomy in some patient populations (180,181,183). Serum levels of the tumor-specific antigen CA125 and FDG–PET can help to differentiate patients with small-volume disease and a false-negative CT from those with a true negative CT (181).

If recurrent ovarian cancer is detected by CT, determination of nonresectability is an important next step. Currently, there is no consensus on CT criteria that determine nonresectability. However, in a recent study, Funt et al. (184) determined that hydronephrosis and invasion of the pelvic sidewall were most indicative of tumor nonresectability. CT-guided biopsy can be used to confirm suspected recurrence (181).

Magnetic Resonance Imaging

MRI can be useful for the detection of recurrent disease, especially in patients unable to undergo CT (due to contrast allergy, renal failure, etc.) (Figs. 10.36 and 10.37). Few studies

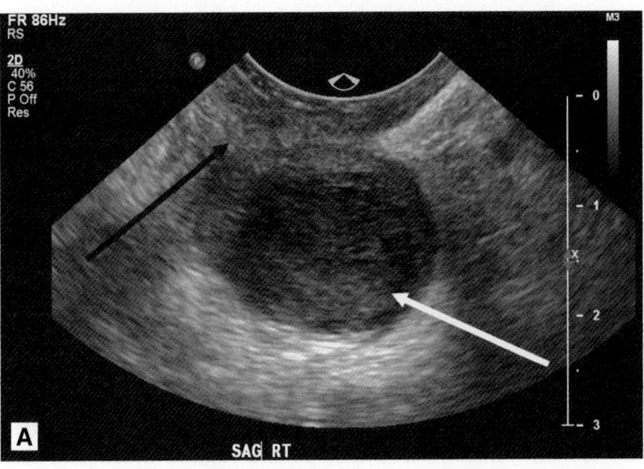

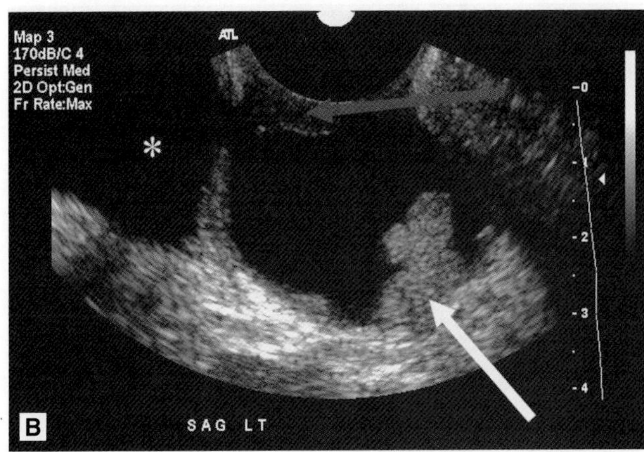

FIGURE 10.32. Ovarian cancer recurrence on ultrasound. Gray-scale images from two different patients demonstrating recurrence at the vaginal cuff. Image (A) shows a solid mass (white arrow) arising from the right side of the vaginal cuff (black arrow). Image (B) shows a solid and cystic mass (white arrow) arising from the left side of the vaginal cuff (grey arrow). Note the full bladder in image (B) (asterisk).

have compared MRI to second-look laparotomy. In the largest series to date, gadolinium contrast-enhanced MRI detected residual tumor in women treated for ovarian cancer with accuracy, PPV, and NPV that were comparable to those of laparotomy (185). Reports from another study, using recurrent tumor size greater than 2 cm as a criterion for inoperability, suggest that the accuracy of MRI is 82% for identification of patients who would not benefit from second-look surgery. The accuracy rate decreased to 38%, however, for lesions less than 2 cm in size (186).

Positron Emission Tomography

Although CT and MRI are the most commonly used imaging modalities for the detection of recurrence, they are both limited in the detection of disease smaller than 2 cm, as discussed above. FDG-PET has been shown to be an extremely useful adjunct in the evaluation of recurrent ovarian cancer (Fig. 10.38). A recent study by Torizuka et al. (187) concluded that FDG-PET is more accurate than conventional imaging (i.e., CT/MRI) with sensitivity, specificity, and accuracy of 80%, 100%, and 84%, respectively, compared to 55%, 100%, and 64% for conventional imaging alone. Studies have also demonstrated that the sensitivity, specificity, and accuracy of conventional imaging increase from 73%–76% to 83%–92%, 75%–83% to 92%–100%, and 73%–74% to 86%–94%, respectively, with the addition of FDG-PET (188,189).

Recommendations for Detecting Persistent or Recurrent Ovarian Cancer

When disease recurrence is suspected, complete abdominal-pelvic evaluation with conventional imaging is advised. Both contrast-enhanced CT and MRI offer a comprehensive examination, albeit one that is limited in its detection of small tumor nodules. Both have comparable sensitivity, specificity, and accuracy (183). The additional use of FDG-PET has been shown to be extremely useful in this situation and should be considered as an adjunct to, rather then a replacement for, conventional imaging.

Summary

A large number of factors make the early detection of ovarian cancer difficult. Furthermore, results from screening trials have been disappointing with few early ovarian cancers

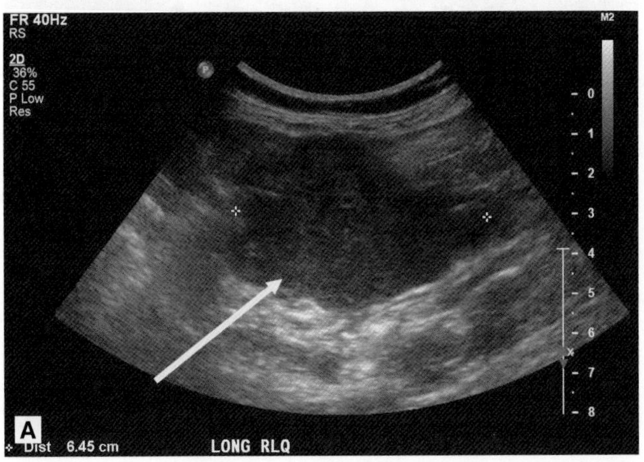

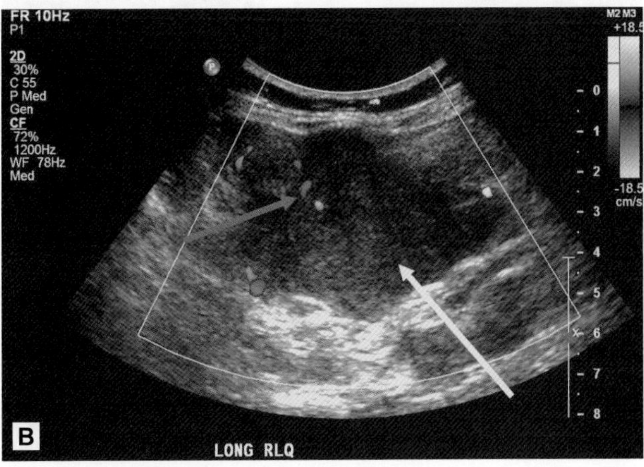

FIGURE 10.33. Ovarian cancer recurrence on ultrasound. Patient presented with a palpable right lower quadrant lesion and a history of ovarian cancer. Gray-scale (A) and color Doppler (B) images demonstrate a solid mass (white arrow) with internal flow (grey arrow) that proved to be recurrent ovarian cancer.

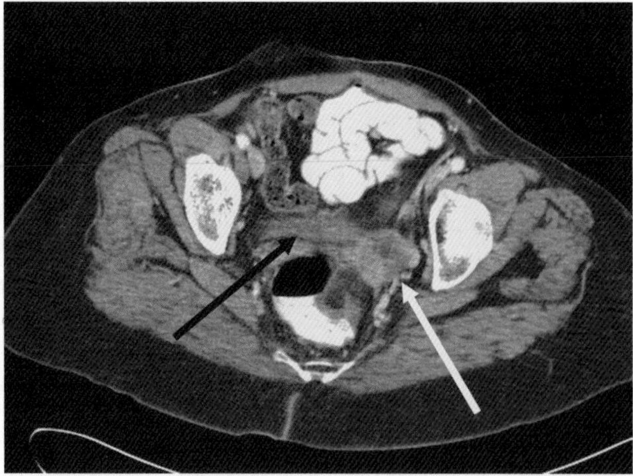

FIGURE 10.34. Ovarian cancer recurrence on CT. Solid and cystic mass (white arrow) along the left side of the vaginal cuff (black arrow).

detected. Therefore, most ovarian cancers are not detected until they are at an advanced stage. US is the study of choice for the primary detection and characterization of a suspected ovarian mass. Contrast-enhanced MRI is valuable in cases where an adnexal mass is suspected but US is indeterminate (167). CT and MRI are both useful for the initial staging of ovarian cancer. Initial research into the use of FDG-PET for the initial staging of ovarian cancer is promising, but more work in this area is needed. For the detection of recurrent ovarian cancer, a combination of conventional imaging, CT or MRI, and FDG-PET appears to be the most beneficial. New techniques, such as dual time point FDG-PET imaging, are currently being investigated. Preliminary data indicate that this technique may help to distinguish benign processes, especially inflammatory ones, from malignant lesions (190), but further research is required.

VAGINAL CANCER

Vaginal cancer is most often diagnosed and staged clinically. Diagnostic imaging is often performed only for the detection of pelvic adenopathy or metastatic disease.

There is virtually no role for diagnostic imaging in the primary detection and characterization of vaginal cancer. On MRI, vaginal tumors appear isointense on T1W sequences and may only be apparent if they alter the vaginal contour (66). On T2W sequences, a vaginal tumor appears as an intermediate- to high-signal-intensity soft-tissue mass.

Staging of vaginal cancer is most often clinical; however, MRI has a limited role in the staging of vaginal cancer. MRI criteria that correlate to the FIGO staging scheme have been developed. Stage I disease is defined as tumor that has invaded the epithelium but is confined to the vaginal mucosa. These lesions may be occult on MRI, or there may be abnormal high T2W signal penetrating the vaginal wall. The surrounding perivaginal fat is preserved.

Vaginal tumor that has invaded the paravaginal tissues but does not involve the pelvic sidewall is considered stage II disease. With stage II disease, the normally high-T2W-signal perivaginal fat is invaded by intermediate-signal tumor.

Tumor that extends to involve the pelvic sidewall and/or pelvic adenopathy defines stage III disease. Tumor contiguous with the levator ani, obturator internus, or the piriformis muscle is diagnostic of pelvic sidewall invasion. Pelvic adenopathy is diagnosed in the usual manner on MRI.

Stage IV is defined as tumor invading the bladder and/or rectum and/or extrapelvic spread of disease. MRI is particularly well suited for imaging stage IV disease because of its multiplanar capabilities. Invasion of the bladder and/or rectum is diagnosed by identifying disruption of the normal high-T2W-signal mucosa of the bladder and/or rectum. Extrapelvic metastases are diagnosed in the usual manner.

Although these staging criteria have been developed, care must be taken when using MRI for the evaluation of vaginal cancer. It has been shown that inflammatory changes and/or congestion of the vagina may appear similar to carcinoma (60).

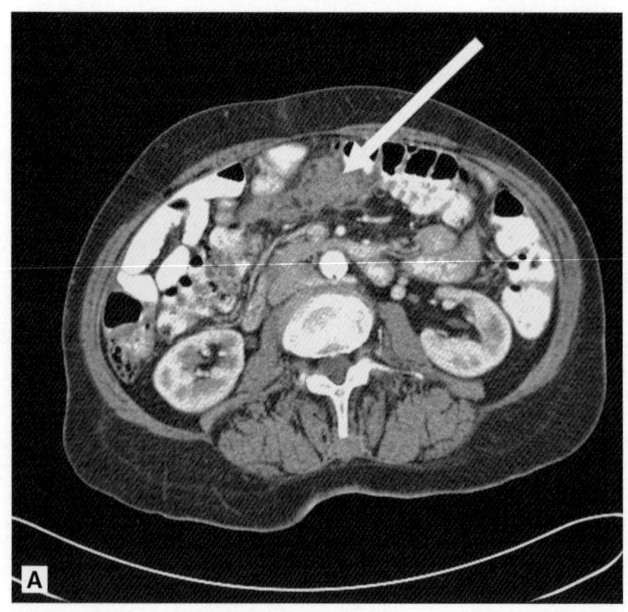

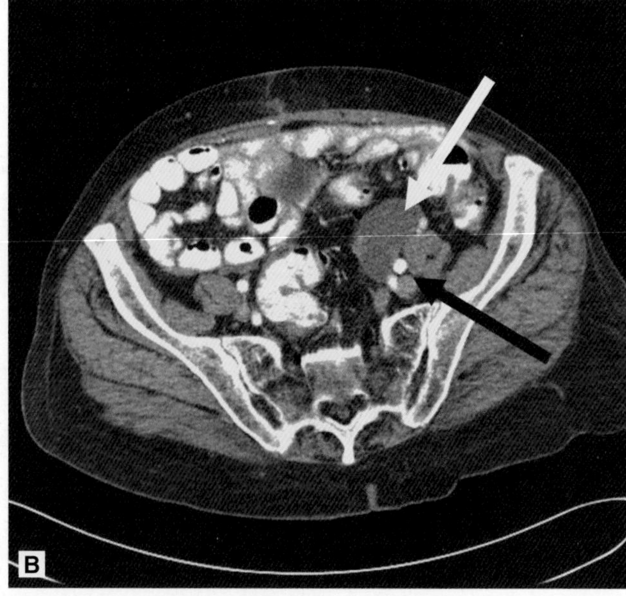

FIGURE 10.35. Recurrent ovarian cancer on CT. Contrast-enhanced CT images in a patient with a remote history of ovarian cancer. Soft-tissue nodularity within the mesentery (white arrow in **A**) and cystic mass (white arrow in **B**) adjacent to the iliac vessels (black arrow in **B**) are recurrent ovarian cancer.

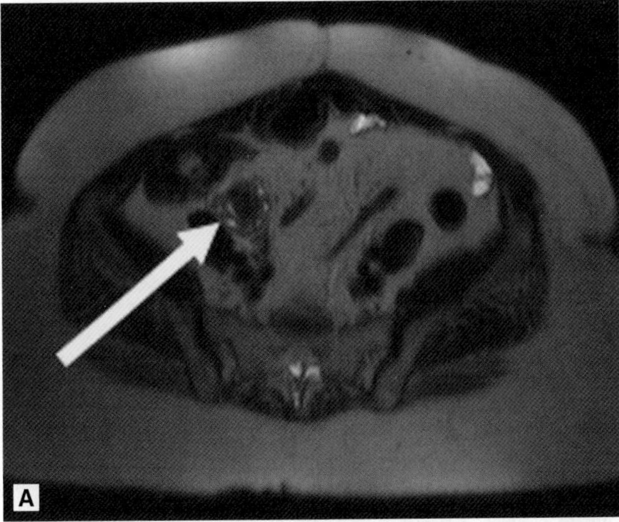

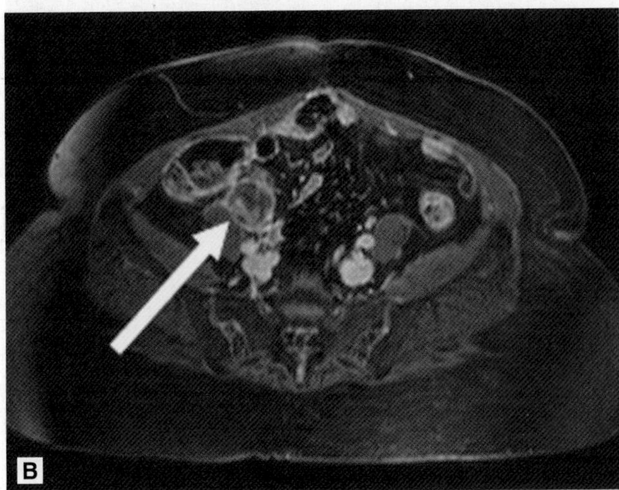

FIGURE 10.36. Ovarian cancer recurrence on MRI. Axial T2W (**A**) and T1W post-contrast fat-saturated (**B**) images. Images demonstrate a solid and cystic enhancing mass in the right pelvis (arrows).

CT and US have little role in the staging of vaginal cancer, although CT can be used for the detection of pelvic adenopathy.

Complications from vaginal cancer and/or vaginal cancer treatment can be imaged with US, CT, and/or MRI depending on the clinical concern. Known complications include fistulae, fluid collections, and post-radiation therapy colitis. Fistulae are best diagnosed with contrast-enhanced CT or MRI.

Very little data is available on the utility of FDG-PET with vaginal cancer. However, a recent study demonstrated that FDG-PET was superior to CT in the detection of the primary tumor and pelvic adenopathy in patients with vaginal cancer (191). While more research is needed in this area, this research is promising.

Summary

Overall, diagnostic imaging plays a limited and directed role in the evaluation of vaginal cancer. Although preliminary results of FDG-PET and vaginal cancer are promising, more research is needed before this modality is used clinically.

VULVAR CANCER

Vulvar cancer is diagnosed and staged clinically. Diagnostic imaging is limited to searching for deep pelvic adenopathy in patients with known inguinal lymph node metastasis. Lymph node status plays an important role in the staging, treatment, and prognosis of patients with vulvar cancer. However, to date no imaging modality has been shown to be adequate in the evaluation of deep pelvic adenopathy in patients with vulvar cancer.

There is no role for diagnostic imaging in the primary detection and characterization of vulvar cancer. Vulvar cancer appears on US as a soft-tissue mass with internal vascularity (Fig. 10.39). On CT, vulvar cancer appears as a nonspecific soft-tissue mass. On MRI, this type of cancer demonstrates intermediate signal intensity on T1W sequences and high signal intensity on T2W sequences.

In select cases, CT and MRI may be used to evaluate for tumor extension into adjacent structures (i.e., urethra) (85). MRI may also be used to differentiate recurrence from post-therapy

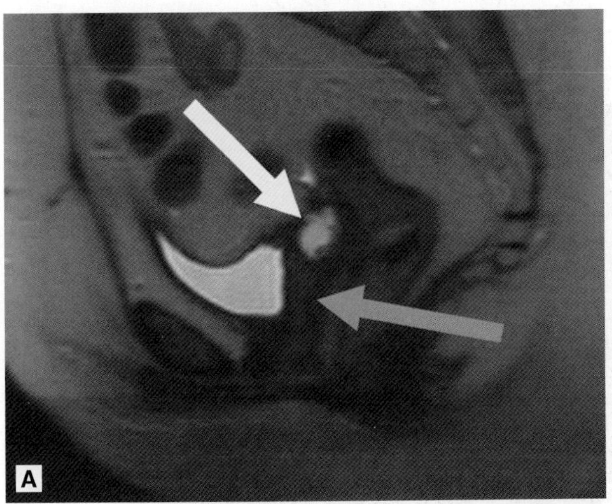

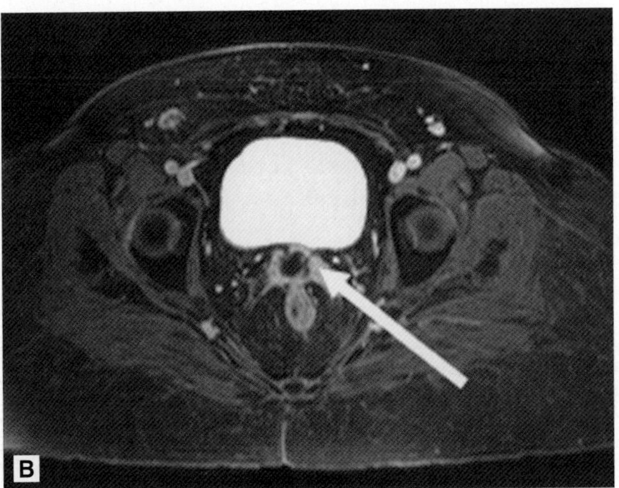

FIGURE 10.37. Recurrent papillary ovarian carcinoma at the vaginal cuff on MRI. Sagittal T2W (**A**) and axial T1W post-contrast fat-saturated (**B**) images. Images demonstrate a solid and cystic enhancing mass (white arrow) at the vaginal cuff (grey arrow).

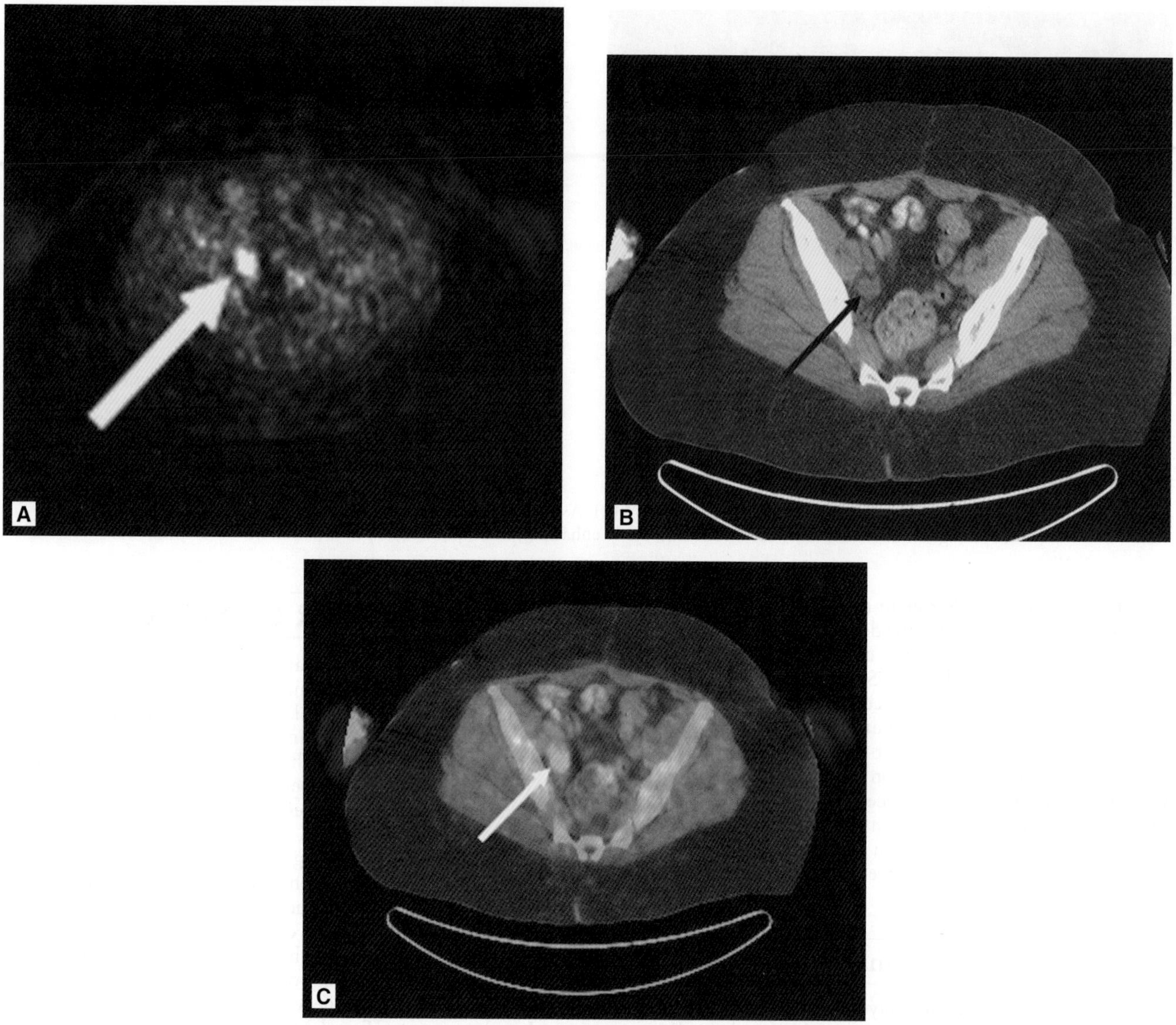

FIGURE 10.38. Recurrent ovarian carcinoma on FDG-PET. FDG-PET image (**A**), noncontrast CT image (**B**), and fused PET-CT images demonstrating an area of focal increased activity in the right pelvis (arrow in **A**) corresponding to soft-tissue density on CT (arrow in **B**). Fused PET-CT image demonstrates that the focal increased activity definitely corresponds to the focal soft-tissue density (arrow in **C**).

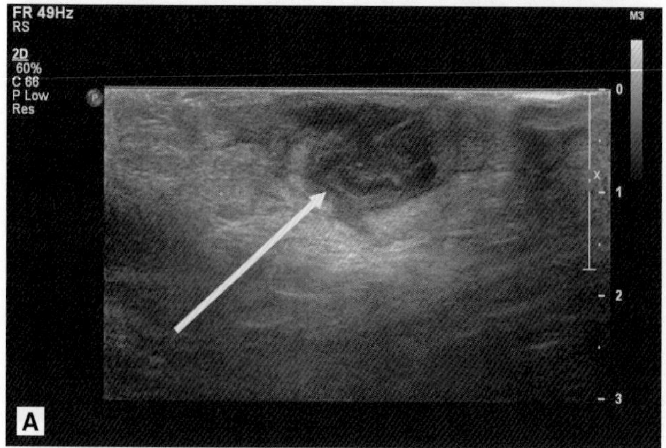

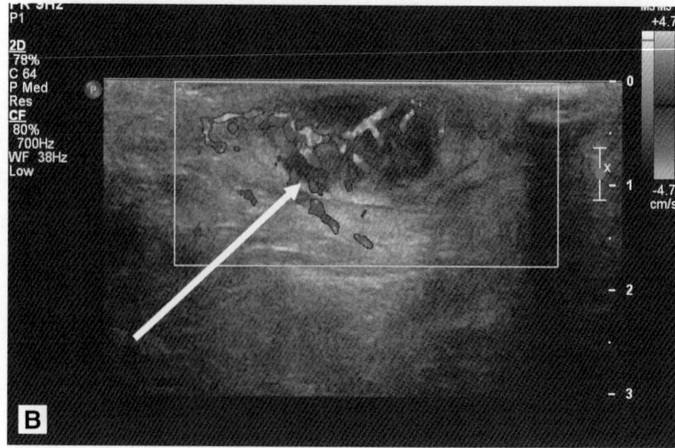

FIGURE 10.39. Vulvar mass on ultrasound. Gray-scale (**A**) and color Doppler (**B**, *See color plate section*) images demonstrating a hypoechoic solid vulvar mass with internal flow (arrow).

changes, with the former demonstrating high signal intensity on T2W images and the latter demonstrating intermediate signal intensity on T2W sequences.

Pelvic adenopathy in vulvar cancer is usually diagnosed by surgical lymph node dissection. US combined with fine-needle aspiration biopsy (FNA) has recently been shown to influence surgical management with sensitivity, specificity, NPV, and PPV of 80%, 100%, 93%, and 100%, respectively (192).

Very little research has been done on the use of FDG-PET for vulvar cancer. In one recent study, the detection of pelvic adenopathy with FDG-PET was evaluated. FDG-PET had a sensitivity of 80%, specificity of 90%, PPV of 80%, and NPV of 90% in the detection of pelvic adenopathy (193). Although these results are promising, more research in this area is needed.

Summary

Diagnostic imaging is not routinely used in the management of patients with vulvar cancer. Recent research, however, has shown that US combined with FNA may be useful for evaluating pelvic adenopathy (192). The utility of FDG-PET for vulvar cancer appears promising.

CONCLUSION

Increased use of CT and MRI for staging gynecologic pelvic malignancies has led to a significant decline in the use of conventional and invasive radiologic studies such as intravenous urography and barium enema. In addition, transabdominal US is no longer used for primary gynecologic cancer staging. TVS, however, in conjunction with Doppler US, is helpful in characterizing ovarian and endometrial masses, with TRUS being reserved for evaluating cervical cancer.

CT maintains a high-profile role in pelvic imaging because of its lower cost, high spatial resolution, fast examination time, and wide availability. It ably detects adenopathy and guides percutaneous biopsy of metastases and recurrent tumor. CT has been proven useful for the staging of ovarian cancer, cervical cancer, endometrial cancer, and GTD, and for the evaluation of recurrent pelvic malignancies.

MRI has been gaining favor for gynecologic pelvic cancer staging because of its superb soft-tissue contrast and multiplanar imaging capabilities. It also has advantages over CT for patients allergic to iodinated intravenous contrast or with impaired renal function. Early reservations about MRI, vis-à-vis long scanning times and lack of oral contrast, no longer apply. MRI shows excellent soft-tissue contrast between tumor, cervical stroma, endometrium, myometrium, uterine ligaments, parametrial fat, and blood vessels. Most comparative studies show MRI to have advantages over CT and US in the local staging of cervical and endometrial cancers. MRI is also useful for the detection of recurrent cervical cancer and the staging of GTD.

FDG-PET and PET-CT are increasingly being used to evaluate gynecologic malignancies. Studies have shown the utility of FDG-PET in the detection of recurrent ovarian, cervical, and endometrial cancer. Also, FDG-PET may be useful in the staging of cervical cancer. Further research in this area will help define the clinical role of FDG-PET in the evaluation of gynecologic malignancies.

FUTURE DIRECTIONS

Future innovations in gynecologic oncology imaging will go beyond anatomy to focus on function. Specifically, functional imaging aims to provide *in vivo* cellular characterization and, ultimately, biologic signatures for both premalignant and malignant conditions. Functional technologies range in maturity: (a) reasonably established (e.g., MRI spectroscopy), (b) less well developed (e.g., MRI with ultrasmall superparamagnetic iron oxide [USPIO] particles), and (c) nascent technologies (e.g., electron paramagnetic resonance imaging [EPRI]). These technologies will likely have a twofold impact on cancer incidence and mortality by allowing (a) improvements in existing methods (e.g., use of USPIO particles as a supplement to routine MRI imaging) and (b) development of new approaches to detect early or preinvasive cancers that traditionally have low survival rates and no proven early-detection algorithms (e.g., optical coherence tomography for surface epithelial ovarian cancer) (194).

Advances in functional imaging raise issues in data management and display. Image fusion, which marries anatomic and functional data, coupled with soft-copy display, will provide roadmaps for gynecologic cancer prevention and treatment.

References

1. Ros PR, Ji H. Multisection (multi-detector) CT: applications in the abdomen. *Radiographics* 2002;22:697–700.
2. Kim SH, Choi BI, Han JK, et al. Preoperative staging of uterine cervical carcinoma: comparison of CT and MRI in 99 patients. *J Comput Assist Tomogr* 1993;17:633–640.
3. Kim SH, Kim HD, Song YS, et al. Detection of deep myometrial invasion in endometrial carcinoma: comparison of transvaginal ultrasound, CT, and MRI. *J Comput Assist Tomogr* 1995;19:766–772.
4. Kinkel K, Ariche M, Tardivon AA, et al. Differentiation between recurrent tumor and benign conditions after treatment of gynecologic pelvic carcinoma: value of dynamic contrast-enhanced subtraction MR imaging. *Radiology* 1997;204:55–63.
5. Dooms GC, Hricak H, Crooks LE, et al. Magnetic resonance imaging of the lymph nodes: comparison with CT. *Radiology* 1984;153:719–728.
6. Hricak H, Powell B, Yu KK, et al. Invasive cervical carcinoma: role of MR imaging in pretreatment work-up—cost minimization and diagnostic efficacy analysis. *Radiology* 1996;198:403–409.
7. Yu KK, Hricak H. Can MRI of the pelvis be cost effective? *Abdom Imaging* 1997;22:597–601.
8. Hardesty LA, Sumkin JH, Nath ME, et al. Use of preoperative MR imaging in the management of endometrial carcinoma: cost analysis. *Radiology* 2000;215:45–49.
9. Kanal E, Barkovich AJ, Bell C, et al. ACR guidance document for safe MR practices: 2007. *Am J Roentgenol* 2007;188(6):1447–1474.
10. Strauss LG, Conti PS. The application of PET in clinical oncology. *J Nucl Med* 1991;32:623–648.
11. Hillman BJ, Clark RL, Babbitt G. Efficacy of the excretory urogram in the staging of gynecologic malignancies. *AJR Am J Roentgenol* 1984;143: 997–999.
12. Gedgaudas RK, Kelvin FM, Thompson WM, et al. The value of the preoperative barium-enema examination in the assessment of pelvic masses. *Radiology* 1983;146:609–613.
13. Pearl ML, Griffen T, Valea FA, et al. The utility of pretreatment barium enema in women with endometrial carcinoma. *Gynecol Oncol* 1997;64: 442–445.
14. Andreotti RF, Fleischer AC, Mason LE Jr. Three-dimensional sonography of the endometrium and adjacent myometrium: preliminary observations. *J Ultrasound Med* 2006;25(10):1313–1319.
15. Hagel J, Bicknell SG. Impact of 3D sonography on workroom time efficiency. *Am J Roentgenol* 2007;188(4):966–969.
16. Lev-Toaff AS. Sonohysterography: evaluation of endometrial and myometrial abnormalities. *Semin Roentgenol* 1996;31:288–298.
17. Sohaey R, Woodward P. Sonohysterography: technique, endometrial findings, and clinical applications. *Semin Ultrasound CT MR* 1999;20:250–258.
18. Lev-Toaff AS, Pinheiro LW, Bega, G, et al. Three-dimensional multiplanar sonohysterography. Comparison with conventional two-dimensional sonohysterography and X-ray hysterosalpingography. *J Ultrasound Med* 2001;20:295–306.
19. Lyons EA, Gratton D, Harrington C. Transvaginal sonography of normal pelvic anatomy. *Radiol Clin North Am* 1992;30:663–676.
20. Arger PH. Transvaginal ultrasonography in postmenopausal patients. *Radiol Clin North Am* 1992;30:759–767.
21. Levine D, Gosink BB, Johnson LA. Change in endometrial thickness in postmenopausal women undergoing hormone replacement therapy. *Radiology* 1995;197:603–608.
22. Pels Rijcken TH, Davis MA, Ros PR. Intraluminal contrast agents for MR imaging of the abdomen and pelvis. *J Magn Reson Imaging* 1994;4: 291–300.

23. Brown JJ, Duncan JR, Heiken JP, et al. Perfluoroctylbromide as a gastrointestinal contrast agent for MR imaging: use with and without glucagon. *Radiology* 1991;81:455–460.
24. Ascher SM. MR imaging of the female pelvis: the time has come. *Radiographics* 1998;18:931–945.
25. Ascher SM, O'Malley J, Semelka RC, et al. T2-weighted MRI of the uterus: fast spin echo vs. breath-hold fast spin echo. *J Magn Reson Imaging* 1999;9:384–390.
26. Nolte-Ernsting CCA, Bücker A, Adam GB, et al. Gadolinium-enhanced excretory MR urography after low-dose diuretic injection: comparison with conventional excretory urography. *Radiology* 1998;209:147–157.
27. McCarthy S, Scott G, Majumdar S, et al. Uterine junctional zone: MR study of water content and relaxation properties. *Radiology* 1989;171: 241–243.
28. Scoutt LM, Flynn SD, Luthringer DJ, et al. Junctional zone of the uterus: correlation of MR imaging and histologic examination of hysterectomy specimens. *Radiology* 1991;179:403–407.
29. Mitchell DG, Schonholz L, Hilpert PL, et al. Zones of the uterus: discrepancy between US and MR images. *Radiology* 1990;174:827.
30. Demas BE, Hricak H, Jaffe RB. Uterine MR imaging effects of hormonal stimulation. *Radiology* 1986;159:123–126.
31. deSouza NM, Hawley IC, Schwieso JE, et al. The uterine cervix on *in vitro* and *in vivo* MR images: a study of zonal anatomy and vascularity using an enveloping cervical coil. *AJR Am J Roentgenol* 1994;163:607–612.
32. Scoutt LM, McCauley TR, Flynn SD, et al. Zonal anatomy of the cervix: correlation of MR imaging and histologic examination of hysterectomy specimens. *Radiology* 1993;186:159–162.
33. Nishizawa S, Inubushi M, Okada H. Physiological 18F-FDG uptake in the ovaries and uterus of healthy female volunteers. *Eur J Nucl Med Mol Imaging* 2005;32(5):549–556.
34. Hawnaur JM, Johnson RJ, Carrington BM, et al. Predictive value of clinical examination, transrectal ultrasound and magnetic resonance imaging prior to radiotherapy in carcinoma of cervix. *Br J Radiol* 1998;71: 819–827.
35. Kikuchi A, Okai T, Kobayashi K, et al. Intracervcial US with a high-frequency miniature probe: a method for diagnosing early invasive cervical cancer. *Radiology* 1996;198:411–413.
36. Dubinsky TJ, Reed SD, Grieco V, et al. Intracervical sonographic-pathologic correlation: preliminary results. *J Ultrasound Med.* 2003;22:61–67.
37. Hricak H, Lacey CG, Sandles LG, et al. Invasive cervical carcinoma: comparison of MR imaging and surgical findings. *Radiology* 1988;166:623–631.
38. Togashi K, Nishimura D, Sagoh T, et al. Carcinoma of the cervix: staging with MR imaging. *Radiology* 1989;171:245–251.
39. Hricak H, Hamm B, Semelka RC, et al. Carcinoma of the uterus: use of gadopentetate dimeglumine in MR imaging. *Radiology* 1991;181:95–106.
40. Yamashita Y, Takahashi M, Sawada T, et al. Carcinoma of the cervix: dynamic MR imaging. *Radiology* 1992;182:643–648.
41. Seki H, Azumi R, Kimura M, et al. Stromal invasion by carcinoma of the cervix: assessment with dynamic MR imaging. *AJR Am J Roentgenol* 1997;168:1579–1585.
42. Postema S, Pattynama PMT, Van Rijswijk CSP, et al. Cervical carcinoma: can dynamic contrast-enhanced MR imaging help predict tumor aggressiveness? *Radiology* 1999;210:217–220.
43. Doi T, Yamashita Y, Yasunaga T, et al. Adenoma malignum: MR imaging and pathologic study. *Radiology* 1997;204:39–42.
44. Villasanta U, Whitley NO, Haney PJ, et al. Computed tomography in invasive carcinoma of the cervix: an appraisal. *Obstet Gynecol* 1983;62: 218–224.
45. Walsh JW, Vick CW. Staging of female genital tract cancer. In: Walsh JW, ed. *Computed Tomography of the Pelvis*. New York: Churchill Livingstone; 1985:163.
46. Hricak H, Demas BE, Braga CA, et al. Gestational trophoblastic neoplasm of the uterus: MR assessment. *Radiology* 1986;161:11–16.
47. Kilcheski TS, Arger PH, Mulhern CB Jr, et al. Role of computed tomography in the presurgical evaluation of carcinoma of the cervix. *J Comput Assist Tomogr* 1981;5:378–383.
48. Narayan K, Hicks RJ, Jobling T, et al. A comparison of MRI and PET scanning in surgically staged locoregionally advanced cervical cancer: potential impact in treatment. *Int J Gynecol Cancer* 2001;11:263–271.
49. Unger JB, Lilien DL, Caldito G, et al. The prognostic value of pretreatment 2-[F]-fluoro-2-deoxy-d-glucose positron emission tomography scan in women with cervical cancer. *Int J Gynecol Cancer* 2007;17: 1062–1067.
50. Innocenti P, Pulli F, Savino L, et al. Staging of cervical cancer: reliability of transrectal US. *Radiology* 1992;185:201–205.
51. Ascher SM, Silverman PM. Applications of computed tomography in gynecologic diseases. *Urol Radiol* 1991;13:16–28.
52. Walsh JW, Goplerud DR. Prospective comparison between clinical and CT staging in primary cervical carcinoma. *AJR Am J Roentgenol* 1981;137: 997–1003.
53. Hricak H, Yu KK. Radiology in invasive cervical cancer. *AJR Am Roentgenol* 1996:167:1101–1108.
54. Goldman SM, Fishman EK, Rosenshein NB, et al. Excretory urography and computed tomography in the initial evaluation of patients with cervical cancer: Are both examinations necessary? *AJR Am J Roentgenol* 1984;143:991–996.
55. Yang WT, Lam WWM, Yu MY, et al. Comparison of dynamic helical CT and dynamic MR imaging in the evaluation of pelvic lymph nodes in cervical carcinoma. *AJR Am J Roentgenol* 2000;175:759–766.
56. Hricak H, Gatsonis C, Chi DS, et al. Role of imaging in pretreatment evaluation of early invasive cervical cancer: results of the intergroup study American College of Radiology Imaging Network 6651-Gynecologic Oncology Group 183. *J Clin Oncol* 2005;23(36):9329–9337.
57. Ozsarlako O, Tjalma W, Schepens E, et al. The correlation of preoperative CT, MR imaging, and clinical (FIGO) staging with histopathology findings in primary cervical carcinoma. *Eur Radiol* 2003;13(10): 2338–2345.
58. Pannu HK, Fishman EK. Evaluation of cervical cancer by computed tomography: current status. *Cancer* 2003;98(9 suppl):2039–2043.
59. Sironi S, Belloni C, Taccagni GL, et al. Carcinoma of the cervix: value of MR in detecting parametrial involvement. *AJR Am J Roentgenol* 1991;156:753–756.
60. Chang YCF, Hricak H, Thurnher S, et al. Vagina: evaluation with MR imaging. Part II. neoplasms. *Radiology* 1988;169:175–179.
61. Choi SH, Kim SH, Choi HJ, et al. Preoperative magnetic resonance imaging staging of uterine cervical carcinoma: results of prospective study. *J Comput Assist Tomogr* 2004;28(5):620–627.
62. Kaji Y, Sugimura K, Kitao M, et al. Histopathology of uterine cervical carcinoma: diagnostic comparison of endorectal surface coil and standard body coil MRI. *J Comput Assist Tomogr* 1994;18:785–792.
63. Yu KK, Hricak H, Subak LL, et al. Preoperative staging of cervical carcinoma: phased array coil fast spin-echo versus body coil spin-echo T2-weighted MR imaging. *AJR Am J Roentgenol* 1998;171:707–711.
64. Reinhardt MJ, Ehritt-Braun C, Vogelgesang D, et al. Metastatic lymph nodes in patients with cervical cancer: detection with MR imaging and FDG PET. *Radiology* 2001;218:776–782.
65. Mitchell DG, Snyder B, Coakley F, et al. Early invasive cervical cancer: Tumor delineation by magnetic resonance imaging, computed tomography, and clinical exam, verified by pathologic results, in the ACRIN 6651/GOG 183 intergroup study. *J Clin Oncol* 2006;24(36):5687–5694.
66. Carrington B, Hricak H. The uterus and vagina. In: Hricak H, Carrington BM, eds. *MRI of the Pelvis: A Text Atlas*. London: Appleton & Lange; 1991:93.
67. Meanwell CA, Rolfe EB, Blackledge G, et al. Recurrent female pelvic cancer: assessment with transrectal ultrasonography. *Radiology* 1987;162:278–281.
68. Franchi M, La Fianza A, Babilonti L, et al. Clinical value of computerized tomography (CT) in assessment of recurrent uterine cancers. *Gynecol Oncol* 1989;35:31–37.
69. Walsh JW, Goplerud DR. Computed tomography of primary, persistent, and recurrent endometrial malignancy. *AJR Am J Roentgenol* 1982;139: 1149–1154.
70. Fulcher AS, O'Sullivan SG, Segreti EM, et al. Recurrent cervical carcinoma: typical and atypical manifestations. *Radiographics* 1999;19: S103–S116.
71. Doubleday LC, Bernadino ME. CT findings in the perirectal area following radiation therapy. *J Comput Assist Tomogr* 1980;4:634–638.
72. Frei KA, Kinkel K, Bonel HM, et al. Prediction of deep myometrial invasion in patients with endometrial cancer: clinical utility of contrast-enhanced MR imaging—a meta-analysis and Bayesian analysis. *Radiology* 2000;216:444–449.
73. Flueckiger F, Ebner F, Poschauko H, et al. Cervical cancer: serial MR imaging before and after primary radiation therapy—a 2-year follow-up study. *Radiology* 1992;184:89–93.
74. Manfredi R, Maresca G, Smaniotto D, et al. Cervical cancer response to neoadjuvant therapy: MR imaging assessment. *Radiology* 1998;209: 819–824.
75. Sugimura K, Carrington BM, Quivey JM, et al. Postirradiation changes in the pelvis: assessment with MR imaging. *Radiology* 1990;175:805–813.
76. Weber TM, Sostman DH, Spritzer CE, et al. Cervical carcinoma: determination of recurrent tumor extent versus radiation changes with MR imaging. *Radiology* 1995;194:135–139.
77. Yamashita Y, Harada M, Torashima M, et al. Dynamic MR imaging of recurrent postoperative cervical cancer. *J Magn Reson Imaging* 1996;1: 167–171.
78. Chung HH, Kim SK, Kim TH, et al. Clinical impact of FDG PET imaging in post-therapy surveillance of uterine cervical cancer: from diagnosis to prognosis. *Gynecol Oncol* 2006;103(1):165–170.
79. Chang TC, Law KS, Hong JH, et al. Positron emission tomography for unexplained serum SCC-Ag elevation in cervical cancer patients—a phase II study. *Cancer* 2004;101:164–171.
80. Hricak H, Stern JL, Fisher MR, et al. Endometrial carcinoma staging by MR imaging. *Radiology* 1987;162:297–305.
81. Hricak H, Rubinstein LV, Gherman GM, et al. MR imaging evaluation of endometrial carcinoma: results of an NCI cooperative study. *Radiology* 1991;179:829–832.
82. Kinkel K, Yu KK, Kaji Y, et al. Radiological staging in patients with endometrial cancer: a meta-analysis. *Radiology* 1999:212:711–718.
83. Sironi S, Colombo E, Villa G, et al. Myometrial invasion by endometrial carcinoma: assessment with plain and gadolinium-enhanced MR imaging. *Radiology* 1992;185:207–212.
84. Grimes DA. Diagnostic dilatation and curettage: a reappraisal. *Am J Obstet Gynecol* 1982;142:1–6.

85. Guido RS, Kanbour-Shakir A, Rulin MC, et al. Pipelle endometrial sampling. Sensitivity in the detection of endometrial cancer. *J Reprod Med* 1995;40:553–555.
86. Karlsson B, Granberg S, Wikland M, et al. Transvaginal ultrasonography of the endometrium in women with postmenopausal bleeding—a Nordic multicenter study. *Am J Obstet Gynecol* 1995;172:1488–1494.
87. Smith-Bindman R, Kerlikowske K, Feldstein VA, et al. Endovaginal ultrasound to exclude endometrial cancer and other endometrial abnormalities. *JAMA* 1998;280:1510–1517.
88. Goldstein RB, Bree RL, Benson CB, et al. Evaluation of the woman with postmenopausal bleeding. Society of Radiologist in Ultrasound-Sponsored Consensus Conference Statement. *J Ultrasound Med* 2001;20:1025–1036.
89. Medverd JR, Dubinsky TJ. Cost analysis model: US versus endometrial biopsy in evaluation of peri- and postmenopausal abnormal vaginal bleeding. *Radiology* 2002;222:619–627.
90. Lev-Toaff AS, Toaff ME, Liu J-B, et al. Value of sonohysterography in the diagnosis and management of abnormal uterine bleeding. *Radiology* 1996;201:179–184.
91. Laifer-Narin S, Ragavendra N, Parmenter EK, et al. False-normal appearance of the endometrium on conventional transvaginal sonography: comparison with saline hysterosonography. *AJR Am J Roentgenol* 2002;178: 129–133.
92. Langer RD, Pierce JJ, O'Hanlan KA, et al. Transvaginal ultrasonography compared with endometrial biopsy for the detection of endometrial disease. *N Engl J Med* 1997;337:1792–1798.
93. Laifer-Narin SL, Ragavendra N, Lu DSK, et al. Transvaginal saline hysterosonography: characteristics distinguishing malignant and various benign conditions. *AJR Am J Roentgenol* 1999;172:1513–1520.
94. Dubinsky TJ, Stroehlein K, Abu-Ghazzeh Y, et al. Prediction of benign and malignant endometrial disease: hysterosonographic-pathologic correlation. *Radiology* 1999;210:393–397.
95. Williams PL, Laifer-Narin SL, Ragavendra N. US of abnormal uterine bleeding. *Radiographics* 2003;23:703–718.
96. Sheth S, Hamper UM, Kurman RJ. Thickened endometrium in the postmenopausal woman: sonographic-pathologic correlation. *Radiology* 1993;187:135–139.
97. Hann LE, Giess CS, Bach AM, et al. Endometrial thickness in tamoxifen-treated patients: correlation with clinical and pathological findings. *AJR Am J Roentgenol* 1997;168:657–661.
98. Hulka CA, Hall DA. Endometrial abnormalities associated with tamoxifen therapy for breast cancer: sonographic and pathologic correlation. *AJR Am J Roentgenol* 1993;160:809–812.
99. Dubinsky TJ, Stroehlein K, Abu-Ghazzeh Y, et al. Prediction of benign and malignant endometrial disease: hysterosonographic-pathologic correlation. *Radiology* 1999;210:393–397.
100. Affinito P, Palomba S, Pellicano M, et al. Ultrasonographic measurement of endometrial thickness during hormonal replacement therapy in postmenopausal women. *Ultrasound Obstet Gynecol* 1998;11:343–346.
101. Bonilla-Musoles F, Raga R, Osborne NG, et al. Three dimensional hysterosonography for the study of endometrial tumors: comparison with conventional transvaginal sonography, hysterosalpingography, and hysteroscopy. *Gynecol Oncol* 1997;65:245–252.
102. Sheth S, Hamper UM, McCollum ME, et al. Endometrial blood flow analysis in postmenopausal women: can it help differentiate benign from malignant causes of endometrial thickening? *Radiology* 1995;195:661–665.
103. Sladkevicius P, Valentin L, Marsal K. Endometrial thickness and Doppler velocimetry of the uterine arteries as discriminators of endometrial status in women with postmenopausal bleeding: a comparative study. *Am J Obstet Gynecol* 1994;171:722–728.
104. DelMaschio A, Vanzulli A, Sironi S, et al. Estimating the depth of myometrial involvement by endometrial carcinoma: efficacy of transvaginal sonography vs. MR imaging. *AJR Am J Roentgenol* 1993;160:533–538.
105. Teefey SA, Stahl JA, Middleton WD, et al. Local staging of endometrial carcinoma: comparison of transvaginal and intraoperative sonography and gross visual inspection. *AJR Am J Roentgenol* 1996;166:547–552.
106. Kinkel K, Kaji Y, Yu KK, et al. Radiologic staging in patients with endometrial cancer: a meta-analysis. *Radiology* 1999;212:711–718.
107. Gruboeck K, Jurkovic D, Lawton F, et al. The diagnostic value of endometrial thickness and volume measurements by three-dimensional ultrasound in patients with postmenopausal bleeding. *Ultrasound Obstet Gynecol* 1996;8:272–276.
108. Dore R, Moro B, D'Andrea F, et al. CT evaluation of myometrium invasion in endometrial carcinoma. *J Comput Assist Tomogr* 1987;11:282–289.
109. Hamlin DJ, Burgener FA, Beecham JB. CT of intramural endometrial carcinoma: contrast enhancement is essential. *AJR Am J Roentgenol* 1981;137: 551–554.
110. Gross BH, Jafri SZH, Glazer GM. Significance of intrauterine gas demonstrated by computed tomography. *J Comput Assist Tomogr* 1983;7:842–845.
111. Hardesty LA, Sumkin JH, Hakim C, et al. The ability of helical CT to preoperatively stage endometrial carcinoma. *AJR Am J Roentgenol* 2001;176: 603–606.
112. Ascher SM, Scoutt LM, McCarthy SM, et al. Uterine changes after dilation and curettage: MR imaging findings. *Radiology* 1991;80:433–435.
113. Seki H, Kimura M, Sakai K. Myometrial invasion of endometrial carcinoma: assessment with dynamic MR and contrast-enhanced T1-weighted images. *Clin Radiol* 1997;52:18–23.
114. Seki H, Takano T, Sakai K. Value of dynamic MR imaging in assessing endometrial carcinoma involvement of the cervix. *AJR Am J Roentgenol* 2000;175:171–176.
115. Ito K, Matsutomo T, Nakada T, et al. Assessing myometrial invasion by endometrial carcinoma with dynamic MRI. *J Comput Assist Tomogr* 1994;18:77–86.
116. DelMaschio A, Vanzulli A, Sironi S, et al. Estimating the depth of myometrial involvement by endometrial carcinoma: efficacy of transvaginal sonography vs. MR imaging. *AJR Am J Roentgenol* 1993;160:533–538.
117. Minderhoud-Bassie W, Treurniet FEE, Koops W, et al. Magnetic resonance imaging (MRI) in endometrial carcinoma: preoperative estimation of depth of myometrial invasion. *Acta Obstet Gynecol Scand* 1995;74:827–831.
118. Takahashi S, Murakami T, Narumi Y, et al. Preoperative staging of endometrial carcinoma: diagnostic effect of T2-weighted fast spin-echo MR imaging. *Radiology* 1998;206:539–547.
119. Yamashita Y, Mizutani H, Torashima M, et al. Assessment of myometrial invasion by endometrial carcinoma: transvaginal sonography vs. contrast-enhanced MR imaging. *AJR Am J Roentgenol* 1993;161:595–599.
120. Belhocine T, DeBarsy C, Hustinx R, et al. Usefulness of (18)F-FDG PET in the post-therapy surveillance of endometrial carcinoma. *Eur J Nucl Med Mol Imaging* 2002;29(9):1132–1139.
121. Saga T, Higashi T, Ishimari T, et al. Clinical value of FDG-PET in the follow up of post-operative patients with endometrial cancer. *Ann Nucl Med* 2003;17:197–203.
122. Chao A, Chang TC, Ng KK, et al. 18F-FDG PET in the management of endometrial cancer. *Eur J Nucl Med Mol Imaging* 2006;33(1):36–44.
123. Green CL, Angtuaco TL, Shah HR, et al. Gestational trophoblastic disease: a spectrum of radiologic diagnosis. *Radiographics* 1996;16: 1371–1384.
124. Preidler KW, Luschin G, Tamussino K, et al. Magnetic resonance imaging in patients with gestational trophoblastic disease. *Invest Radiol* 1996;31: 492–496.
125. Wagner BJ, Woodward PJ, Dickey GE. From the archives of the AFIP. Gestational trophoblastic disease: radiologic–pathologic correlation. *Radiographics* 1996:16:131–148.
126. Green CL, Angtuaco TL, Shah HR, et al. Gestational trophoblastic disease: a spectrum of radiologic diagnosis. *Radiographics* 1996;16: 1371–1384.
127. Lazarus E, Hulka C, Siewert B, et al. Sonographic appearance of early complete molar pregnancies. *J Ultrasound Med* 1999;18:589–594.
128. Benson CB, Enest DR, Bernstein MR, et al. Sonographic appearance of first trimester complete hydatidiform moles. *Ultrasound Obstet Gynecol* 2000;16:188–191.
129. Dobkin GR, Berkowitz RS, Goldstein DP, et al. Duplex ultrasonography for persistent gestational trophoblastic tumor. *J Reprod Med* 1991;36:14–16.
130. Miyasaka M, Hachiya J, Furuya Y, et al. CT evaluation of invasive trophoblastic disease. *J Comput Assist Tomogr* 1984;9:459–462.
131. Su WH, Wang PH, Chang SP. Successful treatment of a persistent mole with myometrial invasion by direct injection of methotrexate. *Eur J Gynaecol Oncol* 2001;22:283–286.
132. Lim AK, Agarwal R, Seckl MJ, et al. Embolization of bleeding residual uterine vascular malformations in patients with treated gestational trophoblastic tumors. *Radiology* 2002;222:640–644.
133. Rose PG. Hydatidiform mole: diagnosis and management. In: Yarbro JW, Bornstein RS, Mastrangelo MJ, MacFeem, eds. *Gestational Trophoblastic Neoplasia*. Philadelphia: WB Saunders; 1995:149–154.
134. Sironi S, Picchio M, Mangili G, et al. [18F]fluorodeoxyglucose positron emission tomography as a useful indicator of metastatic gestational trophoblastic tumor: preliminary results in three patients. *Gynecol Oncol* 2003;91:226–230.
135. Chang TC, Yen TC, Li YT, et al. The role of 18F-fluorodeoxyglucose positron emission tomography in gestational trophoblastic tumors: a pilot study. *Eur J Nucl Med Mol Imaging* 2006;33(2):156–163.
136. Cannistra SA. Cancer of the ovary. *N Engl J Med* 1993;329:1550–1559.
137. Taylor KJW, Schwartz PE. Screening for early ovarian cancer. *Radiology* 1994;192:1–10.
138. Schwartz PE. Nongenetic screening of ovarian malignancies. *Obstet Gynecol Clin* 2001;28:1–13.
139. National Institutes of Health Consensus Development Conference Statement: Ovarian cancer: Screening, treatment, and follow-up. *Gynecol Oncol* 1994;55:S4–S14.
140. Burke W, Daly M, Garber J, et al. Recommendations for follow-up care of individuals with an inherited predisposition to cancer: II. *BRCA1* and *BRCA2*. *JAMA* 1997;277:997–1003.
141. Troiano RN, Quedans-Case C, Taylor KJW. Correlation of findings on transvaginal sonography with serum CA125 levels. *AJR Am J Roentgenol* 1997;168:1587–1590.
142. Olivier RI, Lubsen-Brandsma MA, Verhoef S, et al. CA125 and transvaginal ultrasound monitoring in high-risk women cannot prevent the diagnosis of advanced ovarian cancer. *Gynecol Oncol* 2006;100(1):20–26.
143. Buys SS, Partridge E, Greene MH, et al. Ovarian cancer screening in the Prostate, Lung, Colorectal and Ovarian cancer screening trial: findings from the initial screen of a randomized trial. *Am J Obstet Gynecol* 2005;193(5):1630–1639.
144. Van Nagell JR Jr, Depriest PD, Ueland FR, et al. Ovarian cancer screening with annual transvaginal sonography: findings of 25,000 women screened. *Cancer* 2007;109(9):1887–1896.

145. Buy JN, Ghossain MA, Hugol D, et al. Characterization of adnexal masses: combination of color Doppler and conventional sonography compared with spectral Doppler analysis alone and conventional sonography alone. *AJR Am J Roentgenol* 1996;166:385–393.
146. Jain KA. Prospective evaluation of adnexal masses with endovaginal grayscale and duplex and color Doppler US: correlation with pathologic findings. *Radiology* 1994;191:63–67.
147. Stein SM, Laifer-Narin S, Johnson MB, et al. Differentiation of benign and malignant adnexal masses: relative value of gray-scale, color Doppler, and spectral Doppler sonography. *AJR Am J Roentgenol* 1995;164:381–386.
148. Hamper UM, Sheth S, Abbas FM, et al. Transvaginal color Doppler sonography of adnexal masses: differences in blood flow impedance in benign and malignant lesions. *AJR Am J Roentgenol* 1993;160:1225–1228.
149. Levine D, Feldstein VA, Babcock CJ, et al. Sonography of ovarian masses: poor sensitivity of resistive index for identifying malignant lesions. *AJR Am J Roentgenol* 1994;162:1355–1359.
150. Fleischer AC, Brader KR. Sonographic depiction of ovarian vascularity and flow: current improvements and future applications. *J Ultrasound Med* 2001;20:241–250.
151. Cohen LS, Escobar PF, Scharm C, et al. Three-dimensional power Doppler ultrasound improves the diagnostic accuracy for ovarian cancer prediction. *Gynecol Oncol* 2001;82(1):40–48.
152. DePriest PD, Varner E, Powell J, et al. The efficacy of a sonographic morphology index in identifying ovarian cancer: a multi-institutional investigation. *Gynecol Oncol* 1994;55:174–178.
153. Brown DL, Doubilet PM, Miller FH, et al. Benign and malignant ovarian masses; selection of the most discriminating gray-scale and Doppler sonographic features. *Radiology* 1998;208:103–110.
154. Timmerman D, Schwarzler P, Collins WP, et al. Subjective assessment of adnexal masses with the use of ultrasonography: an analysis of interobserver variability and experience. *Ultrasound Obstet Gynecol* 1999;13:8–10.
155. Buy JN, Ghossain MA, Sciot C, et al. Epithelial tumors of the ovary: CT findings and correlation with US. *Radiology* 1991;1178:811–818.
156. Ghossain MA, Buy JN, Ligneres C, et al. Epithelial tumors of the ovary: comparison of MR and CT findings. *Radiology* 1991;181:863–870.
157. Kim SH, Kim WH, Park KJ, et al. CT and MR findings of Krukenberg tumors: comparison with primary ovarian tumors. *Comput Assist Tomogr* 1996;20:393–398.
158. Stevens SK, Hricak H, Stern JL. Ovarian lesions: detection and characterization with gadolinium-enhanced MR imaging at 1.5 T. *Radiology* 1991;181: 481–488.
159. Semelka RC, Lawrence PH, Shoenut JP, et al. Primary ovarian cancer: prospective comparison of contrast-enhanced CT and pre- and post-contrast, fat-suppressed MR imaging with histologic correlation. *J Magn Reson Imaging* 1993;3:99–106.
160. Thurnher SA. MR imaging of pelvic masses in women: contrast-enhanced vs. unenhanced images. *AJR Am J Roentgenol* 1992;159:1243–1250.
161. Ha HK, Baek SY, Kim SH, et al. Krukenberg's tumor of the ovary: MR imaging features. *AJR Am J Roentgenol* 1995;164;1435–1439.
162. Hubner KF, McDonald TW, Niethammer JG, et al. Assessment of primary and metastatic ovarian cancer by positron emission tomography (PET) using 2-[18-F]deoxyglucose(2-[18F]FDG). *Gynecol Oncol* 1993;51:197–204.
163. Risum S, Hogdall C, Loft A, et al. The diagnostic value of PET/CT for primary ovarian cancer: a prospective study. *Gynecol Oncol* 2007;105(1):145–149.
164. Hata K, Hata T, Manabe A, et al. A critical evaluation of transvaginal Doppler studies, transvaginal sonography, magnetic resonance imaging and CA 125 in detecting ovarian cancer. *Obstet Gynecol* 1992;80;922–926.
165. Komatsu T, Konishi I, Mandai M, et al. Adnexal masses: transvaginal US and gadolinium-enhanced MR imaging assessment of intratumoral structure. *Radiology* 1996;198:109–115.
166. Jain KA, Friedman DL, Pettinger TW, et al. Adnexal masses: comparison of specificity of endovaginal US and pelvic MR imaging. *Radiology* 1993;186: 697–704.
167. Kinkel K, Ying L, Mehdizade A, et al. Indeterminate ovarian mass at US: Incremental value of second imaging test for characterization-meta-analysis and Bayesian analysis. *Radiology* 2005;236:85–94.
168. Buchsbaum HJ, Lifshitz S. Staging and surgical evaluation of ovarian cancer. *Semin Oncol* 1984;11:227–237.
169. Kurtz AB, Tsimikas JV, Tempany CMC, et al. Diagnosis and staging of ovarian cancer: comparative values of Doppler and conventional US, CT, and MR imaging correlated with surgery and histopathologic analysis—report of the Radiology Diagnostic Oncology Group. *Radiology* 1999;212:19–27.
170. Tempany CMC, Zou KH, Silverman SG, et al. Staging of advanced ovarian cancer: comparison of imaging modalities—report from the Radiological Diagnostic Oncology Group. *Radiology* 2000;215:761–767.
171. Coakley FV, Choi PH, Gougoutas CA, et al. Peritoneal metastasis: detection with spiral CT in patients with ovarian cancer. *Radiology* 2002;223: 495–499.
172. Forstner R, Hricak H, Occhipinti KA, et al. Ovarian cancer: staging with CT and MR imaging. *Radiology* 1995;197:619–626.
173. Buy JN, Moss AA, Ghossain MA, et al. Peritoneal implants from ovarian tumors: CT findings. *Radiology* 1988;169:691–694.
174. Meyer JI, Kennedy AW, Friedman R, et al. Ovarian carcinoma: value of CT in predicting success of debulking surgery. *AJR Am J Roentgenol* 1995;165:875–878.
175. Pannu HK, Bristow RE, Montz, FJ, et al. Multidetector CT of peritoneal carcinomatosis from ovarian cancer. *Radiographics* 2003;23:687–701.
176. Cooper CR, Jeffrey RB, Silverman PM, et al. Computed tomography of omental pathology. *J Assist Tomogr* 1986;10:62–66.
177. Yoshida Y, Kurokawa T, Kawahara K, et al. Incremental benefits of FDG positron emission tomography over CT alone for the preoperative staging of ovarian cancer. *Am J Roentgenol* 2004;182(1):227–233.
178. Murolo C, Constantini S, Foglia G, et al. Ultrasound examination in ovarian cancer patients. A comparison with second look laparotomy. *J Ultrasound Med* 1989;8:441–443.
179. Khan O, Cosgrove DO, Fried AM, et al. Ovarian carcinoma follow-up: US versus laparotomy. *Radiology* 1986;159:111–113.
180. Goldhirsch A, Triller JK, Greiner R, et al. Computed tomography prior to second-look operation in advanced ovarian cancer. *Obstet Gynecol* 1983;62:630–634.
181. Megibow AJ, Bosniak MA, Ho AG, et al. Accuracy of CT in detection of persistent or recurrent ovarian carcinoma: correlation with second-look laparotomy. *Radiology* 1988;166:341–345.
182. Prayer L, Kainz C, Kramer J, et al. CT and MR accuracy in the detection of tumor recurrence in patients treated for ovarian cancer. *J Comput Assist Tomogr* 1993;17:626–632.
183. Reuter KL, Griffin T, Hunter RE. Comparison of abdominopelvic computed tomography results and findings at second-look laparotomy in ovarian carcinoma patients. *Cancer* 1989;63:1123–1128.
184. Funt SA, Hricak H, Abu-Rustum N, et al. Role of CT in the management of recurrent ovarian cancer. *AJR Am J Roentgenol* 2004;182:393–398.
185. Low RN, Duggan B, Barone RM, et al. Treated ovarian cancer: MR imaging, laparotomy reassessment, and serum CA-125 values compared with clinical outcome at 1 year. *Radiology* 2005;235:918–926.
186. Forstner R, Hricak H, Powell CB, et al. Ovarian cancer recurrence: value of MR imaging. *Radiology* 1995;196:715–720.
187. Torizuka T, Nobezawa S, Kanno T, et al. Ovarian cancer recurrence: role of whole-body positron emission tomography using 2-[fluorine-18]-fluoro-2-deoxy-D-glucose. *Eur J Nucl Med Mol Imaging* 2002;29(6):797–803.
188. Nakamoto Y, Saga T, Ishimori T, et al. Clinical value of positron emission tomography with FDG for recurrent ovarian cancer. *Am J Roentgenol* 2001;176(6):1449–1454.
189. Picchio M, Sironi S, Messa C, et al. Advanced ovarian carcinoma: usefulness of [(18)F]FDG-PET in combination with CT for lesion detection after primary treatment. *Q J Nucl Med* 2003;47(2):77–84.
190. Zhuang H, Pourdehnad M, Lambright ES, et al. Dual time point 18F-FDG PET imaging for differentiating malignant from inflammatory processes. *J Nucl Med* 2001;42(9):1412–1417.
191. Lamoreaux WT, Grigsby PW, Dehdashti F, et al. FDG-PET evaluation of vaginal carcinoma. *Int J Radiation Oncology Biol Phys* 2005;62(3):733–737.
192. Land R, Herod J, Moskovic E, et al. Routine computerized tomography scanning, groin ultrasound with or without fine needle aspiration cytology in the surgical management of primary squamous cell carcinoma of the vulva. *Int J Gynecol Cancer* 2006;16:312–317.
193. Cohn DE, Dehdashti F, Gibb RK, et al. Prospective evaluation of positron emission tomography for the detection of groin node metastases from vulvar cancer. *Gynecol Oncol* 2002;85:179–184.
194. Report of the Joint Working Group on Quantitative *In Vivo* Functional Imaging in Oncology. Washington DC, USA. January 6–8, 1999. *Acad Radiol* 1999;6(Suppl 6):S259–S300.

SECTION II:

THERAPEUTIC MODALITIES AND RELATED SUBJECTS

CHAPTER 11 ■ PERIOPERATIVE AND CRITICAL CARE

JAMES J. BURKE II, JANET L. OSBORNE, AND CHRISTOPHER K. SENKOWSKI

Surgery remains the mainstay of treatment for women with gynecologic malignancies. Ultimately, outcomes of the surgical intervention rest with the gynecologic oncologist in concert with anesthesiologists, nursing staff, stomal therapists, physical therapists, pharmacists, social workers, and the social network/support of the patient as well as others. Careful assessment of the patient prior to surgery can lead to improved outcomes and minimize surprises in the postoperative period. Should the need arise, prudent consultation with other medical specialists prior to or following surgery can further enhance patient care, and result in better outcomes.

The chapter has been divided into two sections: preoperative care/risk recognition and postoperative care/critical care. Within each section, clinical information has been arranged by organ system and recommendations are based upon evidence (when available). The critical care section provides basic yet practical information for the reader so that comanagement of the critically ill gynecologic oncology patient with an intensivist may be seamless.

PREOPERATIVE RISK ASSESSMENT

Initial Preoperative Evaluation

When patients are found to have a gynecologic malignancy (or suspicion is high as in the case of an adnexal mass), hopefully they are referred to a gynecologic oncologist for consultation and ultimate treatment. During this meeting, the gynecologic oncologist should take a thorough history, assessing for comorbid conditions, which may impact perioperative risk (1). Similarly, a thorough physical examination, looking for signs of diseases of which the patient is unaware, will aid in finding diseases that can impact surgical outcome. Review of accompanying medical records and radiographs is important. Ultimately, those patients who will benefit from surgery will be identified and will be deemed operative candidates, operative candidates who need further evaluation from specialists prior to surgery, or inoperable candidates. Subsequent discussions should focus on the course of treatment. If surgical, the planned operative procedure should be described to the patient in nonmedical terminology. Attendant risks of the procedure should be described to the patient as well as alternatives for therapy (if they exist). The length of time for the operation and length of anticipated hospital stay should be estimated for the patient and her family. These elements of the treatment plan constitute *informed consent,* and should be documented in the medical record by the physician at the initial consultation. Preferably, this "consenting" should be done before the patient is in the preoperative holding area on the day of her surgery. Should further evaluation be needed from a specialist (e.g., a cardiologist or a pulmonologist), a letter outlining the proposed surgical intervention should be sent to the consultant.

Ideally, laboratory data will be dictated by findings from the history and physical examination. However, most institutions have a battery of required laboratory testing prior to surgical intervention. A logical review of laboratory testing is available and we refer the reader to this review (2). Table 11.1 shows recommendations for laboratory testing prior to surgery, the incidences of abnormalities that influence changes in surgical management, and the indications for each test. Further, minimal evaluation for specific comorbid disease states will be presented in the following sections of this chapter.

If the patient's condition requires the possibility of a stoma(s) (colostomy or urostomy), consultation with an enterostomal therapist for marking of the planned stoma(s) should be considered. During this visit, the therapist will take into account the location of the patient's "waist," how she wears her clothing, the types of clothing she wears, and the location of the future stoma when she stands or sits. In addition, the therapist can initiate education on the function and care of the stoma(s).

Should the proposed surgery result in a marked change of body image or possible sexual dysfunction (e.g., exenteration, radical vulvectomy, or vaginal reconstruction), consultation with prior patients who have successfully recovered from similar operations may be warranted. In addition, these patients may benefit from psychologic counseling prior to their surgery.

Assessment of Cardiac Risk

Any gynecologic oncologist must be aware of the underestimation of cardiac disease in women when evaluating cardiac risk preoperatively. In the last decade, a great deal of literature has been published on this subject. In 2001, the National Heart, Lung, and Blood Institute (NHLBI) launched the Heart Truth Project to promote education about heart disease among women (3). Statistics have shown that only one of three primary physicians correctly cited coronary artery disease as a leading cause of death in women. Similarly, studies have demonstrated that women are less often counseled on cardiac risk factors, less often prescribed lipid-lowering medications, less often offered invasive procedures, and less often prescribed cardiac rehabilitation. Further, compared to men, women who had a myocardial infarction (MI) had a greater interval from onset of pain until arrival at hospital, were less likely to be treated with thrombolytics and beta-blocking agents, were less often evaluated with invasive methods, had higher rates of reinfarction, and had greater mortality (3).

TABLE 11.1

RECOMMENDED PREOPERATIVE LABORATORY ASSESSMENTS WITH INDICATIONS FOR TESTING

Test	Incidence of abnormalities that influence management (%)	Indications
Hemoglobin	0.1	Anticipated major blood loss or symptoms of anemia
White blood cell count	0.0	Symptoms that suggest infection, myeloproliferative disorder, or myelotoxic medications
Platelet count	0.0	History of bleeding diathesis, myeloproliferative disorder, or myelotoxic medications
Prothrombin time	0.0	History of bleeding diathesis, chronic liver disease, malnutrition, recent or long-term antibiotic use
Partial thromboplastin time	0.1	History of bleeding diathesis
Electrolytes	1.8	Known renal insufficiency, CHF, medications that affect electrolytes
Renal function	2.6	Age >50 years, hypertension, cardiac disease, major surgery, diabetes, medications that affect renal function
Glucose	0.5	Obesity or known diabetes
Liver function tests	0.1	No indication. Consider albumin measurement for major surgery or chronic illness
Urinalysis	1.4	No indication
Electrocardiogram	2.6	Age >50 years; known CAD, diabetes, or hypertension
Chest radiograph	3.0	Age >50 years; known cardiac or pulmonary disease; symptoms or exam suggesting cardiac or pulmonary disease.

Note: CAD, coronary artery disease; CHF, congestive heart failure.
Source: Adapted from Smetana GW, Macpherson DS. The case against routine preoperative laboratory testing. *Med Clin N Am* 2003;87:7–40, with permission.

In the assessment of perioperative risk, cardiac risk factors are certainly one of the top concerns for clinicians. There have been a number of reviews and different systems created for the purposes of assessing cardiac risk for patients undergoing noncardiac surgery (4–7). Realize that approximately 1 in 12 patients (>65 years old) will have significant coronary artery disease (8). It is estimated that over 30% of patients undergoing major elective surgery have at least one cardiac risk factor (9).

Cardiac risk indices have been published by at least 10 different investigators (10). Goldman et al. published the Multifactorial Index of Cardiac Risk (MICR) in 1977 (11). This risk index was the first large, prospective, multivariate analysis of patients undergoing noncardiac surgery. They used definite endpoints of cardiac death, ventricular tachycardia, pulmonary edema, and myocardial infarction. The MICR involves nine independent risk factors to create a point risk index and predict morbidity and mortality (Tables 11.2 and 11.3). One weakness of this index is underestimating risk in vascular surgery patients. Nonetheless, these criteria have been validated and have stood the test of time. In response to a shift in the literature from calculation of risk with indices to clinical decision making, especially in regard to the need for preoperative evaluation, the American College of Cardiology/American Heart Association (ACC-AHA) guidelines were developed (12). Recently, the AHA updated guidelines for cardiovascular disease prevention in women (13). This document provides risk classification of coronary vascular disease (CVD), based upon clinical criteria and/or the Framingham 10-year global risk score (14) (Table 11.4). This CVD risk stratification has not been assessed specifically for preoperative risk assessment, but provides classification of women who may need further (noninvasive or invasive) evaluation.

Clearly, the approach to the patient must include a careful history and physical examination. Initially, age greater than 70 years was thought to be a risk factor for cardiac morbidity, but a recent clinical trial showed no increased independent risk for cardiac complications (15). Any prior history of cardiac disease such as angina, MI, arrhythmia, pulmonary edema, or valvular disease must be elaborated. Patients with unstable angina, recent myocardial infarction, class III-IV heart failure,

TABLE 11.2

MULTIFACTORIAL INDEX OF CARDIAC RISK (MICR)

Risk factor	Points
S3 gallop or increased jugular venous pressure	11
Myocardial infarction in previous 6 months	10
More than five premature ventricular ectopic beats per minute	7
Rhythm other than sinus or premature atrial contractions	7
Age >70 years	5
Emergency noncardiac operative procedure	4
Significant aortic stenosis	3
Poor general health status	3
Abdominal or thoracic surgery	3
Possible total	53

Source: Adapted from Goldman L, Caldera DL, Nussbaum SR, et al. Multifactorial index of cardiac risk in noncardiac surgical procedures. *N Engl J Med* 1977;297:845–880.

decompensated congestive failure, or aortic stenosis present the highest risk. These patients will likely require further invasive testing.

In patients without overt cardiac risks, other factors are considered to be helpful for uncovering subclinical disease. Classically, these risk factors are smoking, hyperlipidemia, hypertension, and diabetes mellitus.

In 2002, the ACC-AHA published guidelines to direct invasive, interventional evaluations (12). The classification defines clinical predictors as major, intermediate, and minor. In addition, the guidelines now utilize functional capacity in terms of metabolic equivalents (METs), with a level <4 being considered poor. The ability to climb one flight of stairs or walk up a hill would classify the patient in the >4 group (12).

Testing available for further evaluation includes both invasive and noninvasive methods. Echocardiography can predict postoperative congestive heart failure (CHF) in patients with ejection fractions (EFs) less than 35% (16). Unfortunately, echocardiography cannot reliably predict ischemia. However, echocardiography is quite useful in the evaluation of valvular diseases and for follow-up of patients with known left ventricular (LV) dysfunction.

Exercise or pharmacological stress testing provides valuable information for perioperative ischemic risk. Nuclear scintigraphy with evaluation of perfusion defects has shown a positive predictive value of 12% to 16% and a negative predictive value of 99% (17). Dobutamine stress echocardiography has shown similar predictive values.

The ACC-AHA recommendations provide a way to segregate patients who should have their surgery delayed for further cardiac evaluation because of a recent MI; who should have their CHF optimized; or who should optimize control of dysrhythmias. In selected patients, it may be that coronary revascularization, angioplasty, stent placement, or valve replacement is prudent before the planned noncardiac surgery (12).

TABLE 11.4

CLASSIFICATION OF CVD RISK IN WOMEN

Risk status	Criteria
High risk	Established coronary heart disease Cerebrovascular disease Peripheral arterial disease Abdominal aortic aneurysm End-stage or chronic renal disease Diabetes mellitus 10-year Framingham global risk >20%[a]
At risk	≥1 major risk factors for CVD, including: Cigarette smoking Poor diet Physical inactivity Obesity, especially central adiposity Family history of premature CVD (CVD at <55 years of age in male relative and <65 years of age in female relative) Evidence of subclinical vascular disease (e.g., coronary calcification) Metabolic syndrome Poor exercise capacity on treadmill test and/or abnormal heart rate recovery after stopping exercise
Optimal risk	Framingham global risk <10% and a healthy lifestyle, with no risk factors

Note: CVD, coronary vascular disease.
[a]Or at high risk on the basis of another population-adapted tool used to assess global risk.
Source: Adapted from Mosca L, Banka CL, Benjamin EJ, et al. Evidence-based guidelines for cardiovascular disease prevention in women: 2007 update. *Circulation* 2007;115:1481–1501.

The risks of reinfarction after a recent MI are clearly related to the timing of an event, which could precipitate an MI. However, these rates have been declining secondary to improved perioperative care. Reported reinfarction rates have dropped from 37% in patients undergoing surgery within 3 months following MI to more recent figures of 5% to 10%. The rates fall even further the longer the interval from the original MI, with rates of reinfarction being 2% to 3% in the 4 to 6 months following and 1% to 2% after 6 months (18).

TABLE 11.3

MULTIFACTORIAL INDEX OF CARDIAC RISK (MICR), CARDIAC RISK CLASS, MORBIDITY, AND MORTALITY

Cardiac risk (%)	Total points	Morbidity (%)	Mortality (%)
Class I	0–5	0.7	0.2
Class II	6–12	5.0	1.6
Class III	12–25	11.5	2.3
Class IV	>26	22.2	55.6

Source: Adapted from Goldman L, Caldera DL, Nussbaum SR, et al. Multifactorial index of cardiac risk in noncardiac surgical procedures. *N Engl J Med* 1977;297:845–850.

Perioperative Beta Blockade

In 1996, a multicenter, randomized, placebo-controlled trial was published that evaluated the use of beta blockade with atenolol versus placebo in patients undergoing noncardiac surgery (19). Although no differences in perioperative mortality or MI were seen, the atenolol group had significantly fewer ischemic episodes (24% vs. 39%). Furthermore, in a 2-year follow-up, the atenolol group had a decreased mortality (9 vs. 21 deaths) and decreased number of cardiac events (16 vs. 32). Based on the findings of this study, patients with or at risk for coronary artery disease should receive preoperative and postoperative beta blockade.

Pulmonary Risk Assessment

Postoperative pulmonary complications represent a significant cause for morbidity and mortality in patients undergoing elective surgery. Approximately 25% of deaths within the early postoperative period (first week) are related to pulmonary issues. Pulmonary complications after major abdominal surgery range from 20% to 30% (20). Laparotomy results in a 45% decrease in vital capacity and a 20% reduction in functional residual capacity (FRC) (21). When the patient is in the supine position, FRC is reduced below alveolar closing volume (i.e., the volume at which point alveoli start closing), which results in atelectasis (22).

When examining risk factors for postoperative pulmonary problems, a number of issues surface. General medical status (e.g., functional status, obesity, nutrition) is related to postoperative pulmonary complications (PPCs) (23). A history of congestive failure, renal failure, poor mental status, and immunosuppression are all associated with a higher PPC rate (24). Surgical issues such as the type of incision (thoracic and upper abdominal being worse than midline or lower abdominal), duration of anesthetic (>2 hours), the use of a nasogastric tube (increased risk), and the use of parenteral (increased risk) versus epidural (decreased risk) analgesics are all correlated with PPC incidence (25).

In terms of direct pulmonary risk factors, the most common preexisting pulmonary disease is chronic obstructive pulmonary disease (COPD) (26). These patients retain carbon dioxide, have poor gas exchange, and have an increased residual volume. Smoking, history of dyspnea, pneumonia, and sleep apnea are other risk categories. Patients with asthma and other restrictive lung diseases (low forced vital capacity [FVC] with normal forced expiratory volume in the first second of expiration [FEV_1]/FVC ratio) have minimal increased risk for PPCs (27).

When interpreting the usual preoperative radiographic and laboratory values, several caveats must be kept in mind. A preoperative chest radiograph in normal adults has no predictive value other than providing essential baseline data for an at-risk patient. Arterial blood gas analysis in prospective trials has been shown not to be useful in providing risk stratification. However, it is useful in providing baseline data for patients with preexisting disease, that is, COPD (28). Preoperative pulmonary function tests (PFTs) have few supporting clinical trials other than in preparation for lung resection, where they are clearly beneficial (29). A consensus statement was forwarded from the American College of Physicians in 1990 that recommended preoperative PFTs in the following settings: in patients with a history of smoking or dyspnea scheduled to undergo upper abdominal operations, coronary bypass, or lung resection; in patients with unexplained pulmonary disease; and in patients with planned extensive lower abdominal, head and neck, or orthopedic operations (30). It would appear from the data that PFTs are overutilized. In the case of major abdominal surgery in a patient with moderate to severe COPD, however, they may aid greatly in risk stratification and in providing baseline data.

Preoperative and perioperative strategies for reducing risk of PPCs include pulmonary expansion, smoking cessation, and optimization of gas exchange. Although preoperative and postoperative incentive spirometery has shown mixed results in reducing the rate of pulmonary complications, it continues to be widely recommended (31), and it should be considered as a preventive strategy for any patient undergoing laparotomy. In order to maximize patient compliance, preoperative counseling and education is necessary. Clearly, COPD must be optimized with control of infection and maximizing medical regimens. Reactive airway disease should be prevented with the use of perioperative inhalation therapy such as beta agonists. Steroid therapy is generally reserved for patients already utilizing them as part of their medical regimen. These steroid-dependent patients will need stress-dose steroids to prevent insufficiency (see "Adrenal Suppression" section). Prophylactic antibiotics are not indicated in COPD patients to prevent pulmonary infections.

Smoking-cessation programs have had an unclear effect on postoperative pulmonary complications (32). Although the data consist of poorly controlled trials, it appears that short-term abstinence (<8 weeks from the time of surgery) may actually increase the complication rate (33). Abstinence for greater than 10 weeks showed complication rates similar to nonsmokers (34). Unfortunately, the long-term success rate of smoking-cessation programs is low, and in the case of malignancy, the gynecologic oncologist rarely has the opportunity to delay the operation for 8 to 10 weeks.

Endocrinologic Risk Assessment

Diabetes

The incidence of diabetes is rising because of the obesity pandemic, the sedentary lifestyle of Americans, and the rapidly aging population (35). Interestingly, one third to one half of these patients are unaware that they have diabetes and are currently receiving no treatment. It is only during preoperative evaluation for elective surgery or acute hospitalization that most of those patients will be diagnosed (36). Understanding the basic physiology of diabetes and how it impacts perioperative risk is crucial for the surgeon.

There are two types of diabetes of concern for the surgeon. Type 1 diabetes occurs as a result of insulinopenia, with all type 1 diabetics being insulin dependent. In the absence of sufficient insulin, these patients are prone to ketosis. Type 1 diabetics account for approximately 10% of all diabetics. Type 2 diabetes occurs as a result of insulin resistance and impaired insulin secretion. Type 2 diabetics may be treated with diet alone, oral hypoglycemic agents, or insulin. These patients account for approximately 90% of all diabetics (37). Intraoperative as well as postoperative glycemic control is dictated by the type of diabetes a patient has.

When evaluating patients with diabetes for surgery, attention should be directed toward the long-term complications of diabetes, as these can impact perioperative risk. Most complications of diabetes are related to microvascular changes, such as diabetic retinopathy, neuropathy, nephropathy, and cardiovascular disease (38). In addition to a thorough history and physical examination, preoperative studies should include an electrocardiogram to rule out a prior "silent" MI (especially in patients with diabetes for more than 10 years); serum creatinine, blood urea nitrogen, and urinary analyses to assess renal function; and a hemoglobin A_{1c} to evaluate recent glycemic control. Should abnormalities be found, consultation with an appropriate specialist should be entertained (39). Ultimately, the type of diabetes, preoperative glycemic control, the extent and magnitude of the intended surgery, the elective or emergent nature of that surgery, and other comorbid medical conditions will affect the metabolic changes these patients face intraoperatively and postoperatively.

The physiologic changes that diabetic patients encounter during surgery all result in a hyperglycemic state. The stress of surgery increases secretion of epinephrine, norepinephrine, cortisol, and growth hormone, all of which directly antagonize insulin action (40,41). In addition, gluconeogenesis and lipolysis are increased with mobilization of glucose precursors, and a net protein catabolism ensues. All of these factors affect ketosis and acidosis and require intraoperative glucose measurement, especially if the surgery lasts longer than 2 hours.

Although diabetic patients with vascular disease are at risk of silent postoperative MI and acute renal failure, postoperative infections (respiratory, urinary, and wound infections) account for about two thirds of all postoperative complications and 20% of all postoperative deaths among diabetics undergoing surgery (42,43). Hyperglycemia has been shown to impair phagocytic function and chemotaxis of granulocytes when glucose levels are higher than 250 mg/dL (44). Other wound complications such as superficial wound dehiscence or fascial dehiscence are common among diabetic patients because of suppressed collagen synthesis by glucose levels higher than 200 mg/dL (45).

Although no prospective studies demonstrating better perioperative outcome from tight glycemic control in diabetics undergoing surgery have been done, several retrospective studies of diabetics undergoing cardiac surgery suggest a lower incidence of postoperative wound infections and complications (46–48). Similarly, a randomized prospective study of intensive insulin therapy (maintaining glucose levels between 80 and 110 mg/dL) versus conventional insulin therapy (glucose levels between 180 and 200 mg/dL) in critically ill postoperative patients demonstrated a 46% reduction in episodes of septicemia and a 34% reduction of in-hospital mortality (49).

Glycemic control during surgery will depend upon the type of diabetes the patient has, the medications currently being utilized for treatment, the expected length of time that the patient will be nil per os (npo), and the type of surgery the patient is having. Patients who are taking oral hypoglycemic agents for control should not take their morning dose on the day of surgery (because of the longer half-life of metformin and chlorpropamide, patients should be instructed to stop these medications 24 to 48 hours prior to surgery) (39). Table 11.5 shows recommendations for management of diabetic patients undergoing surgery (39).

Thyroid Disorders

When patients give history of hypothyroidism or hyperthyroidism during evaluation for surgery, thyroid-stimulating hormone (TSH) and thyroxine (T4) levels should be obtained. The primary objective is to determine if the patient is euthyroid or mildly abnormal prior to surgical intervention so as to avoid the complications of myxedema or thyroid storm in the postoperative period.

Decisions to operate on patients with hypothyroidism will depend upon the level of hypothyroidism and the urgency of the surgery. Hypothyroidism can influence many physiologic functions such as myocardial function, respiration, gastrointestinal motility, hemostasis, and free water balance (39). Although there have been no prospective, randomized studies looking at the surgical outcome of hypothyroid patients versus controls, several retrospective case-matched control studies have evaluated hypothyroid patients undergoing surgery. A study by Weinberg et al. demonstrated no differences between hypothyroid and euthyroid controls for perioperative complications. In addition, no differences in outcome were seen when hypothyroidism was stratified by thyroxine levels. The investigators concluded that patients with mild to moderate hypothyroidism should not be denied needed surgery in order to correct the metabolic problem. They further stated that insufficient numbers of patients with severe hypothyroidism precluded recommendations for perioperative care of these patients (50). In another retrospective study, Ladenson et al. reviewed perioperative complications among hypothyroid patients undergoing surgery, finding more intraoperative hypotension in noncardiac surgery, more heart failure in cardiac surgery, and more gastrointestinal and neuropsychiatric complications. They also noted that patients were unable to mount fever in the face of infection, although infection rates were not different. Further, no differences were found in the

TABLE 11.5

MANAGEMENT OF DIABETES MELLITUS DURING SURGERY

Type	Minor surgery	Major surgery
TYPE I		
DM on insulin therapy	1/2–2/3 of usual AM insulin dose SC	IV insulin infusion during surgery—frequent blood glucose monitoring necessary
TYPE II		
DM controlled with diet alone	No insulin during surgery	No insulin during surgery
DM controlled with oral medications	No insulin during surgery	Insulin may be required during surgery—frequent blood glucose monitoring may be required
DM poorly controlled with oral medications	Insulin may be required during surgery—frequent blood glucose monitoring may be required	IV insulin infusion during surgery—frequent blood glucose monitoring necessary

Note: DM, diabetes mellitus; IV, intravenous; SC, subcutaneous.
Source: Adapted from Schiff RL, Welsh GA. Perioperative evaluation and management of the patient with endocrine dysfunction. *Med Clin N Am* 2003;87(1):175–192, with permission.

duration of hospitalization, perioperative arrhythmias, delayed anesthesia recovery, pulmonary complications, or mortality (51).

Patients with mild to moderate hypothyroidism requiring urgent surgery may have it without delay. These patients may have more minor complications of ileus, postoperative delirium, or infection without fever. Patients with severe hypothyroidism (myxedema coma, decreased mentation, pericardial effusions, heart failure, or very low levels of thyroxine) who are to undergo urgent/emergent surgery will need intravenous thyroxine and stress-dose glucocorticoids (see "Adrenal Suppression" section) started prior to, during, and continued after surgery (52). Patients who develop seizures, coma, unexplained heart failure, hypothermia, prolonged ileus, or postoperative delirium should be evaluated for undiagnosed hypothyroidism or myxedematous coma (53–55).

Patients using thyroid replacement preparations can have their doses withheld during the immediate postoperative period until they are able to tolerate oral intake, as the half-life of these drugs is 5 to 9 days (39).

Most complications occurring in hyperthyroid patients undergoing surgery involve cardiac function, as T4 and T3 have a direct inotropic and chronotropic effect on the heart. Atrial fibrillation occurs in 10% to 20% of patients (56–59). The greatest perioperative risk for patients who have undiagnosed hyperthyroidism or who are inadequately treated is a rare, yet life-threatening, condition known as thyroid storm. Thyroid storm should be considered in any postoperative patient with fever, tachycardia, confusion, cardiovascular collapse, and death (60, 61).

Patients with mild hyperthyroidism may have surgery with preoperative beta blockade. However, patients with moderate or severe disease should have surgery canceled until a euthyroid state is attained.

Thyrotoxic patients who require emergent/urgent surgery need premedication with antithyroid agents, beta blockade, and corticosteroids. Antithyroid medications include thionamides, propythiouracil (PTU), and iodine. Methimazole is a thionamide drug that blocks thyroid hormone synthesis, and iodine blocks thyroid hormone release (62,63). Because adrenal reserve may be low in these patients, stress-dose steroids (see "Adrenal Suppression" section) should be administered prior to and following surgery (64). Should thyroid storm occur, treatment with beta blockade, thionamides, iodine, and corticosteroids should be instituted. It is important to give the thionamides at least 1 hour prior to iodine administration to prevent uptake of iodine and synthesis of further hormone. Occasionally, supportive care in the intensive care unit (ICU) with correction of cardiac dysfunction and electrolyte abnormalities may be necessary (39).

Adrenal Suppression

Corticosteroids are used to treat a myriad of diseases, and it is not unusual to obtain a history from patients revealing steroid usage. It is important to ascertain the type of steroid used, the dosage prescribed, the duration of treatment, and whether or not a tapering schedule was used in stopping the medication.

Although some case series demonstrate biochemical evidence of hypothalamic-pituitary axis (HPA) suppression after exogenous steroid usage, none has demonstrated frank adrenal insufficiency, hypotension, and shock in surgical patients (65). However, recommendations for stress-dose steroids perioperatively have been made to prevent the occurrence of this life-threatening situation in patients with either "presumed" or documented HPA suppression. Giving stress-dose glucocorticoids needs to be weighed against the potential side effects of the drug (such as poor wound healing, fluid retention, and increased risk of infection) versus the benefits of supporting the HPA axis in a surgically stressed patient.

Three tiers of chronic glucocorticoid usage and subsequent HPA axis suppression have emerged. Several studies have shown that steroid equivalent to 5 mg of prednisone as a single morning dose, alternate-day short-acting steroids given as a morning dose, and any dose of steroid given for less than 3 weeks seldom results in clinical suppression of the HPA and requires no stress-dose steroids perioperatively (66–68). However, patients who are chronically taking 20 mg prednisone (or equivalent) per day for more than 3 weeks or who appear clinically cushingoid require stress-dose steroids based upon the type of surgical stress (69) (Fig. 11.1). Patients whose steroid usage falls in between the first two tiers are more controversial and may require HPA testing to ascertain the functionality of the adrenal gland (70).

Renal Risk Assessment

Chronic kidney disease affects 8 million Americans, with most having a glomerular filtration rate (GFR) of less than 60 mL/min/1.73 m^2 (71). The most common form of renal failure facing the surgeon is acute renal failure (ARF) occurring during the postoperative period. This condition will be discussed below in the section on postoperative/critical care. However, with the aging population, increasing prevalence of diabetes and hypertension, and the advances in dialytic therapy, the number of patients living with end-stage renal disease (ESRD) is increasing. Therefore, surgeons must be cognizant of the potential perioperative risks associated with these patients.

The causes of ESRD are predominantly diabetes and hypertension, which account for 68% of patients with ESRD (72). As such, patients with these underlying diseases tend to have other comorbid conditions such as coronary artery disease and peripheral vascular disease. Obviously, patients with ESRD have problems with fluid balance, electrolyte levels, and acid-base management. Furthermore, with reduced or absent renal function, these patients metabolize drugs such as antibiotics, anesthetics, and analgesics poorly. Finally, patients with ESRD are immunocompromised and are more susceptible to infections postoperatively. Taking this complex picture into consideration, the morbidity rate among ESRD patients undergoing surgery is 54% (range, 12% to 64%) and the mortality rate is 4% (range, 0% to 47%) (73).

Evaluation of ESRD patients undergoing surgery should focus on three areas: cardiac evaluation, fluid and electrolyte management and anemia, and bleeding diatheses. Of course, glycemic control for diabetics and blood pressure control for hypertensives are obvious. Cardiac disease is the leading cause of death among ESRD patients (72,74). Unfortunately, a large proportion of these patients have asymptomatic coronary artery disease (23% to 40%) (75,76), with 75% of diabetics being asymptomatic (77,78). Therefore, these patients need formal cardiac clearance from a cardiologist prior to surgical intervention.

ESRD patients who are dependent upon dialysis will need to be euvolemic prior to surgery. Thus, communication with the patient's nephrologist is paramount. Details about the operation should be discussed, with planned preoperative dialysis (without heparin 24 hours prior to surgery) and postoperative dialysis on the day of surgery for large intraoperative fluid loads. Electrolytes should be monitored in the immediate postoperative period, with hyperkalemia being aggressively managed with dialysis or medically if necessary. Hyperkalemia may be treated with glucose and insulin, which will drive the NaK-ATPase pump resulting in an increase of intracellular potassium and a lowering of extracellular potassium. Ten milliliters of calcium gluconate can afford cardioprotection and membrane stabilization in patients with abnormal electrocardiograms (ECGs). Finally, 40 g of sodium

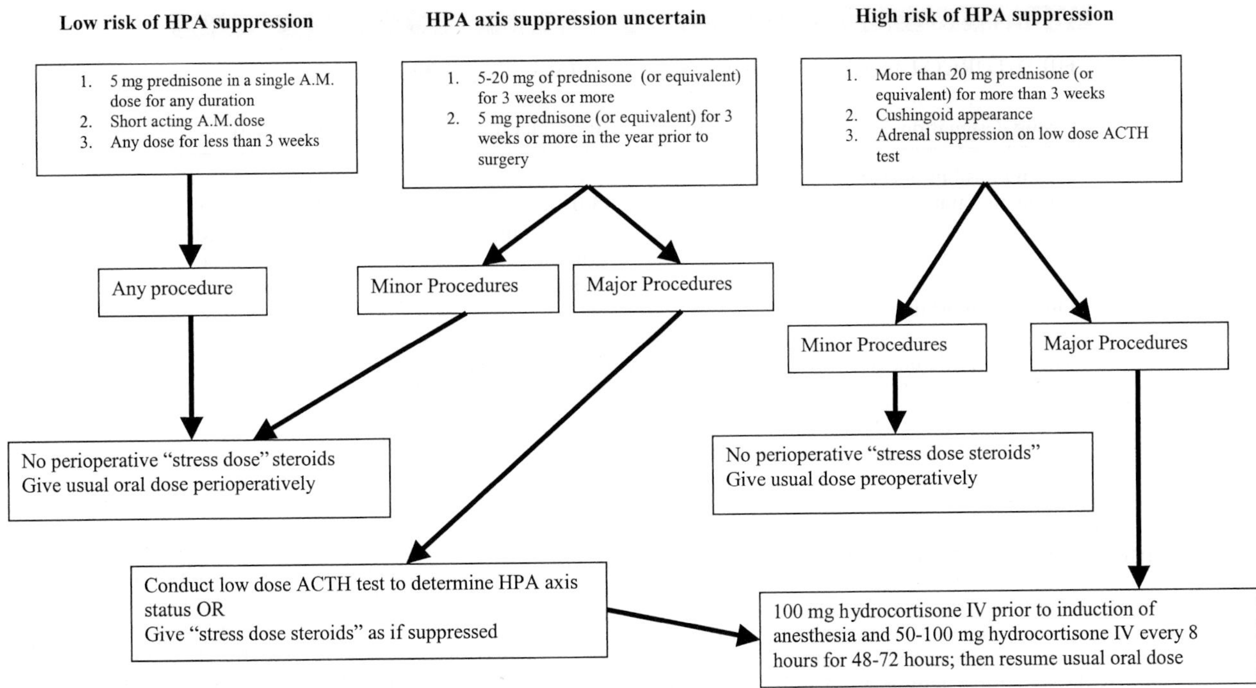

Low risk of HPA suppression
HPA axis suppression uncertain
High risk of HPA suppression
1. 5 mg prednisone in a single A.M. dose for any duration
2. Short acting A.M. dose
3. Any dose for less than 3 weeks
1. 5-20 mg of prednisone (or equivalent) for 3 weeks or more
2. 5 mg prednisone (or equivalent) for 3 weeks or more in the year prior to surgery
1. More than 20 mg prednisone (or equivalent) for more than 3 weeks
2. Cushingoid appearance
3. Adrenal suppression on low dose ACTH test
Any procedure
Minor Procedures
Major Procedures
Minor Procedures
Major Procedures
No perioperative "stress dose" steroids
Give usual oral dose perioperatively
No perioperative "stress dose steroids"
Give usual dose preoperatively
Conduct low dose ACTH test to determine HPA axis status OR
Give "stress dose steroids" as if suppressed
100 mg hydrocortisone IV prior to induction of anesthesia and 50-100 mg hydrocortisone IV every 8 hours for 48-72 hours; then resume usual oral dose

FIGURE 11.1. Algorithm for stress-dose steroids. ACTH, adrenal corticotropin hormone; HPA, hypothalmus-pituitary-adrenal axis; IV, intravenous. *Source:* Adapted from Schiff RL, Welsh GA. Perioperative evaluation and management of the patient with endocrine dysfunction. *Med Clin North Am* 2003;87(1):175–192, with permission.

polystyrene sulfonate (Kionex, Kayexalate) dissolved in 80 mL of sorbitol may be given orally, or alternatively 50 to 100 g in 200 mL of water may be given rectally as a retention enema by inserting a Foley catheter into the rectum and filling the balloon. These administrations should be repeated every 2 to 4 hours until the potassium level is in a normal range (see section below on potassium derangements). Caution with the use of this resin in postoperative patients is urged as intestinal necrosis can occur (79).

Patients with ESRD usually receive erythropoietin to maintain hemoglobin levels. In urgent situations, transfusion of blood is necessary to maintain hemoglobin prior to and during surgery. Uremic patients may have platelet dysfunction resulting in bleeding (80). If a patient has demonstrated prior bleeding because of uremic platelet dysfunction, these patients must be treated with 1-deamino-8-D-arginine vasopressin (dDAVP) intravenously or intranasally and with cryoprecipitate to prevent bleeding during surgery (81). In addition, patients may be treated with intravenous conjugated estrogens (0.6 mg/kg) if they are given 4 to 5 days prior to surgery (82).

Drug administration in ESRD must be done judiciously with careful attention to the pharmacokinetics of particular drugs. Multiple guidelines exist that can direct drug dose reductions for patients with ESRD (83).

Hepatic Risk Assessment

The incidence of liver disease in gynecologic oncology is not known. However, patients may present with a history of cirrhosis or acute or chronic hepatitis in conjunction with a gynecologic malignancy. Awareness of liver disorders and how they impact the perioperative risk is necessary to avoid unnecessary morbidity and mortality.

As mentioned earlier, thorough preoperative evaluation of patients includes a comprehensive history and physical examination, with further laboratory testing based upon historical and physical findings. Routine testing of liver function in asymptomatic patients rarely yields abnormal levels or changes in perioperative management (2). However, patients with histories of jaundice, blood transfusions, the use of alcohol or other recreational drugs, hepatitis, or physical findings of icterus, hepatosplenomegaly, palmar erythema, or spider nevi should be tested to rule out occult or active liver diseases (84).

Patients with acute hepatitis (viral or alcohol induced) should have surgery delayed until the acute phase of the disease process has passed and liver function tests have returned to normal. The older literature has demonstrated mortality rates of 0% to 58% in this patient group (84). Contrarily, patients with chronic hepatitis tolerate surgery well with no mortality (85,86).

Surgical risk in patients with cirrhosis of the liver is significant and correlates directly with the Child-Turcotte classification (Table 11.6). This system takes into consideration five components, three of which are subjective. Nonetheless, for predicting operative outcome, this system is quite reproducible and has been validated in a number of studies (87–90). Postoperative mortality rates have been shown to be 10% in Child class A and 30% and 80%, respectively, for Child classes B and C (87,89). Patients with cirrhosis of the liver also have coagulopathies, which need to be corrected prior to surgery. Vitamin K administration, fresh frozen plasma, or cryoprecipitate may be administered to correct the prothrombin time to within 3 seconds of normal. Figure 11.2 presents an algorithm for patients with liver disease facing surgery (84).

Finally, selection of medications in patients with hepatic dysfunction needs to be done judiciously. Patients with liver dysfunction are particularly susceptible to anesthetic effects such as changes in hepatic metabolism of medications and changes in hepatic blood flow. Alterations in the type and the dose of an agent are necessary to avoid postoperative hepatic dysfunction and hepatitis. Postoperative pain management with narcotic agents needs to be reduced by as much as 50% to account for the altered hepatic metabolism in these patients (91).

TABLE 11.6

CHILD-TURCOTTE CLASSIFICATION AND OPERATIVE MORTALITY

Group designation	A (minimal)	B (moderate)	C (advanced)
Serum bilirubin (mg/dL)	<2.0	2.0–3.0	>3.0
Serum albumin (g/dL)	>3.5	3.0–3.5	<3.0
Ascites	None	Easily controlled	Poorly controlled
Neurologic disorder	None	Minimal	Advanced, coma
Nutrition	Excellent	Good	Poor, wasting
Operative mortality	10%	30%	80%

Source: Adapted from Child CG, Turcotte JG. Surgery and portal hypertension. In: Child CG, ed. *The Liver and Portal Hypertension*. Philadelphia: WB Saunders; 1964:50, with permission.

Preoperative Nutritional Assessment

Clearly, the status of nourishment plays an important role in the way patients respond to the various stresses of their cancer care. The broader consideration of nutrition in gynecologic cancer patients is discussed in Chapter 33. The intent of this section is to present the concepts of preoperative nutritional evaluation and nutritional support of the gynecologic oncology patient. Early refeeding in the postoperative patient as well as enteral and parenteral nutritional support in the critically ill gynecologic patient are discussed later.

The prevalence of malnutrition among cancer patients has been shown to be quite high (92,93). In addition, a direct correlation between the level of malnutrition and surgical outcome has been demonstrated (94,95). Specific rates of malnutrition among gynecologic oncology patients have been described. Tunca showed a high prevalence of severe protein malnutrition among ovarian cancer patients without gastrointestinal involvement. However, he was unable to demonstrate malnutrition among other gynecologic cancer sites (96). Orr et al. have shown increased rates of malnutrition with increasing stages of cervical cancer among patients (97). Recently, Santoso et al.

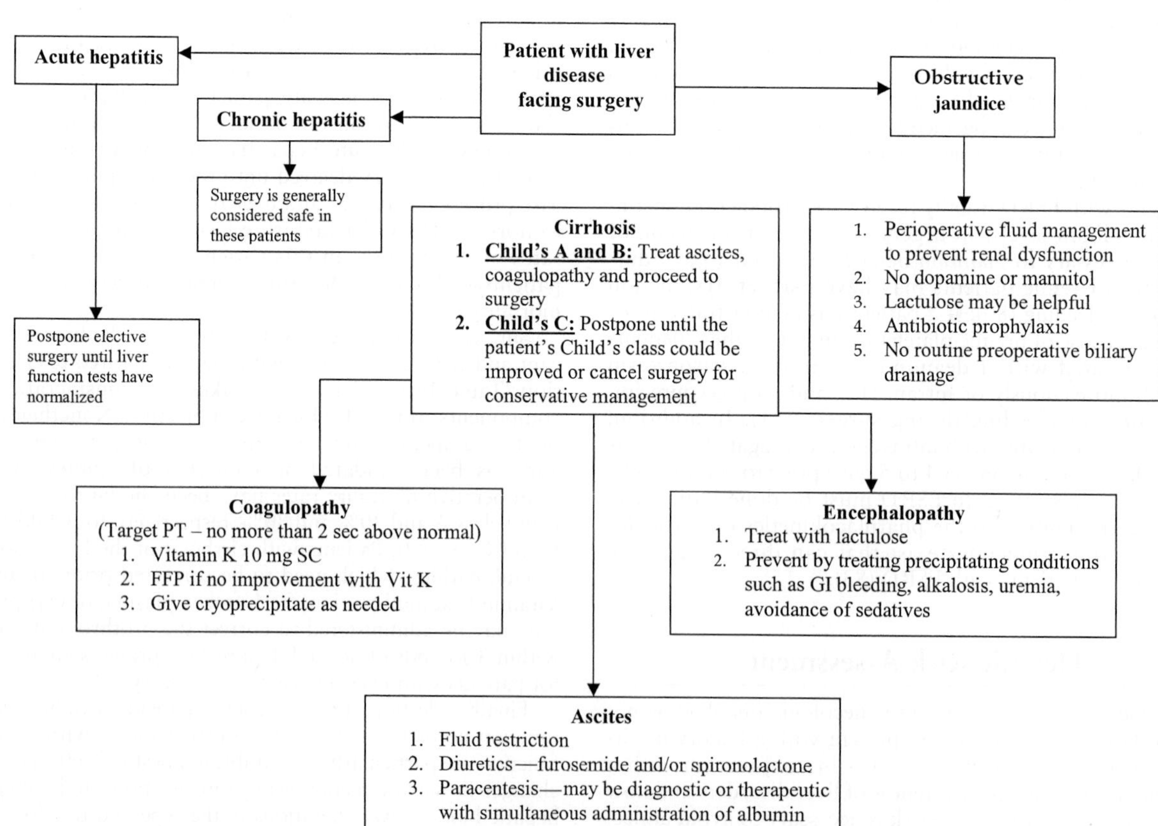

FIGURE 11.2. Perioperative assessment of the patient with liver disease. FFP, fresh frozen plasma; GI, gastrointestinal; SC, subcutaneously. *Source:* From Rizvon MK, Chou CL. Surgery in the patient with liver disease. *Med Clin North Am* 2003;87:211–227, with permission.

demonstrated that 54% of their patients admitted to the gynecologic oncology ward (medical and surgical admissions) demonstrated malnutrition. Most of their patients had cervical or uterine carcinomas, were obese, and were admitted for major abdominal surgeries (98). The question remains, how best to assess patients for nutritional status and what intervention(s) can correct deficiencies, producing improved postoperative outcomes?

Simply attaining a history of weight loss (amount and over what duration) can identify patients who may be malnourished, especially if the weight loss is greater than 10% of the patient's normal weight (99). However, recalled weights may be inaccurate and require corroboration of family members or comparison to prior recorded weights (100). Other important historical elements that may identify patients who are at risk are the type and/or duration of any "diets," recent surgical interventions, radiation or chemotherapy treatment, nausea or vomiting, and a history of alcohol or drug abuse (101).

Other methods for assessing nutritional status include body measurements and laboratory values. Table 11.7 lists these measures of nutritional depletion. The anthropometric measurements assess fat stores (the triceps skin fold) and protein stores (mid-arm circumference). The resulting measurements are compared to standard tables of these measurements and a percentage is calculated to arrive at the level of depletion (or nourishment). Although the measurements are quite easy to obtain, there is a lack of standardization of measurement techniques, which can introduce error and produce inaccurate assessments of nutritional status. Total lymphocyte count is calculated by multiplying the percentage of lymphocytes, determined in the differential by the total white blood cell count. Several conditions can affect the percentage of lymphocytes, such as infection or recent chemotherapy or radiation administration, producing artificially low levels of lymphocytes and inaccurate nutritional assessments. A serum albumin level is usually included in most complete metabolic profiles. Because the half-life of serum albumin is 20 days, levels can give a picture of the patient's visceral protein stores over longer periods of time. However, the plasma level of serum albumin can be affected by the patient's volume status and events that increase catabolism, all of which may interfere with the clinical usefulness of this assessment method (102).

Several schemes have been developed to combine several of the measures in Table 11.7 and correlate them to surgical outcomes. The prognostic nutritional index (PNI) has been studied the most (98,103). This index combines the triceps skin fold, the serum albumin and transferrin levels, and delayed hypersensitivity response to mumps, tuberculin, and *Candida* antigens. Because it requires measurements of immune response, it is a cumbersome index to complete and probably has little clinically utility. Serum albumin emerges as the single test with the most predictive value of poor operative outcome due to malnutrition. Santoso et al. found that albumin levels correlated with the PNI and predicted longer lengths of stay for hospitalized, malnourished patients (98). Gibbs et al., through the National Veterans Affairs Surgical Risk Study, found that albumin levels less than 2.1 mg/dL were associated with an increased surgical morbidity from 10% to 65% (especially in predicting sepsis and major infections), as well as an increased 30-day mortality from 1% to 29% (104). Further, Delgado-Rodriguez et al. showed that lower levels of serum albumin were predictive of longer lengths of stay, increased rates of nosocomial infections, and in-hospital deaths among a general surgical population. This group of investigators also correlated their outcome measures to lower levels of high-density lipoprotein-cholesterol fractions (105).

Finally, studies have shown that experienced clinicians are able to assess nutritional status subjectively, as well as through objective laboratory or anthropometric measures, merely by obtaining a history and examining the patient (106,107).

Since the mid 1980s several trials of total parenteral nutrition (TPN) to correct deficiencies preoperatively in order to improve operative outcomes were done. This controversial practice was called into question and ultimately answered with several prospective, randomized trials, which defined patients who would benefit from such repletion. The largest trial, the Veterans Affairs Cooperative Study, randomized 395 mostly male, surgical (abdominal or noncardiac thoracic surgeries) patients to receive at least 7 days of preoperative and 3 days of postoperative TPN or to receive no perioperative nutritional supplementation. The TPN group had a greater number of infectious complications, mostly among patients classified as borderline or mildly malnourished compared to the unfed patients (14.1% vs. 6.4%). However, a subset of severely malnourished patients derived benefit from lower operative complication rates (5% vs. 43%, $p = 0.03$) without incurring an increase in infectious complications. The overall 30- and 90-day mortality rates were not different between the groups (108). A similar study by Bozzetti et al. randomized severely malnourished patients undergoing resection of gastric or colonic malignancies to 10 days of preoperative TPN and 9 days of postoperative TPN or no supplementation. His group showed that noninfectious postoperative complication rates were lower among the TPN group versus the unfed control group (12% vs. 34%, $p = 0.02$) (109). Although the method of nutritional assessment was different in these two studies, it is clear that patients assessed to be severely malnourished should be considered for preoperative TPN prior to abdominal surgery.

TABLE 11.7

MEASUREMENT OF NUTRITIONAL DEPLETION

Parameters	Mild	Moderate	Severe
Triceps skin fold (TSF), % standard	50–90	30–50	<30
Mid-arm muscle circumference (MAMC), % standard	80–90	70–80	<70
Albumin g/dL	3.0–3.4	2.1–3.0	<2.1
Total lymphocyte count (TLC) Cmm	1,200–1,500	800–1,200	<800
Weight loss, % initial			
In 1 week	<1	1–2	>2
In 1 month	<2	2–5	>5
In 3 months	<5	5.0–7.5	>7.5
In 6 months	<7.5	7.5–10.0	>10.0

PREPARATION FOR SURGERY

Infection Prophylaxis

Surgical site infections (SSIs) account for nearly 40% of nosocomial infections in surgical patients and occur in up to 20% of patients undergoing abdominal surgery (110,111). They are a significant source of postoperative morbidity resulting in longer hospital stays, increased rates of intensive care unit admissions, hospital readmissions, and subsequently increased costs. Patients who develop an SSI have a mortality rate two to three times that of uninfected patients (112,113). Patient and operative environmental factors influence surgical infection rates. The goal of preoperative skin preparation is to reduce the risk of SSI by reducing the microbial count to a subpathogenic level in a time-efficient and atraumatic manner. A meta-analysis of six trials concluded that although whole-body scrubs or showers with antiseptic agents such as chlorhexidine or povidone-iodine prior to surgery reduce bacterial counts on the skin, this practice did not reduce wound infection rates (114). Patients undergoing surgery should simply be instructed to bathe or shower normally the night or morning prior to surgery, removing any debris from the skin surface.

Inappropriate hair removal techniques can traumatize the skin and provide an opportunity for colonization of microorganisms. There is no evidence that hair removal prior to surgery will prevent or reduce SSI. To the contrary, meta-analysis evaluating hair removal techniques demonstrated a twofold increase in SSI when patients underwent hair removal by shaving versus clipping (115). Hair is generally sterile and therefore does not need to be removed unless the hair around the incision will interfere with the operation. When hair removal is necessary the simplest and least irritating method of hair removal is an electric or battery-powered clipper with a disposable head (110,115). Some infection control experts advocate removing all razors from hospitals and operating rooms (116).

The use of prophylactic antimicrobials plays a large role in reducing the rates of SSI and should be used in clean or clean-contaminated operations, which include most procedures performed by gynecologic oncologists. Factors that increase the risk of postoperative infection in women undergoing radical pelvic surgery include longer duration of surgery, extremes of age, increased blood loss, anemia, potential hypothermia, poor nutritional status, the presence of tumor, prior pelvic irradiation, diabetes, obesity, peripheral vascular disease, and a history of post-surgical infection (110,117). Prophylactic antibiotics should provide coverage consistent with the microbial milieu most likely to be encountered. In gynecologic oncology surgery, potential infecting organisms are coliforms, enterococci, streptococci, clostridia, and bacteroides.

Several guidelines for antibiotic prophylaxis in surgery have been published (110,111,118–120). Most recommend cefazolin for gynecologic procedures. Because of its longer half-life and broad spectrum coverage, cefotetan had been the preferred antibiotic for prophylaxis in longer radical gynecologic operations and was also recommended for prophylaxis prior to colorectal surgery (118); however, it is no longer available. An appropriate alternative for surgical procedures with a higher chance of bowel resection or injury is cefazolin plus metronidazole or ampicillin-sulbactam (120). Cefoxitin is another option, but availability has been limited. Most patients with a penicillin allergy can be treated with cefazolin; however, when allergy prohibits the administration of a cephalosporin, alternative regimens are clindamycin with gentamicin, a fluoroquinolone, or aztreonam (111). Itani et al. reported on a randomized, double-blinded trial in patients undergoing elective colorectal surgery that suggested ertapenem as an effective alternative to cefotetan (121). Ertapenem has received FDA approval for prophylaxis for elective colon resection; however, the 2006 Medical Letter guidelines caution against the routine use of ertapenem for surgical prophylaxis due to cost and concerns that this practice may result in increased rates of antibiotic resistance (120).

In order to achieve and maintain effective tissue levels, parenteral antibiotics should be given within 1 hour (between 1 and 2 hours for fluoroquinolones and vancomycin) prior to skin incision as a loading dose (111). For patients weighing >70 kg, the dosage should be doubled (i.e., cefazolin 2 g intravenously [IV]) or weight-based dosing should be used. Repeat doses should be given intraoperatively for surgeries lasting longer than 3 to 4 hours or when blood loss exceeds 1,000 mL (118,120). Guidelines from the National Surgical Site Infection Project recommend that prophylactic antibiotic use for abdominal or vaginal procedures end within 24 hours of the operation (111). The majority of the published evidence supports the use of an appropriately timed administration of a single dose of antibiotic and that repeat doses postoperatively are unnecessary and subject the patient to the potential emergence of resistant organisms (110,111,118,120).

Bowel Preparation

It is generally accepted that full mechanical bowel preparation is indicated when intestinal injury or bowel resection is anticipated. Mechanical bowel cleansing is considered to be a crucial factor in preventing postoperative infectious complications and disruption of bowel anastomosis. Mechanical bowel preparation has several advantages unrelated to the risk of infection. It facilitates palpation of the entire colon during laparotomy. It may decrease operative time by enabling the surgeon to work with a clean bowel and improve handling during bowel anastomosis or repair. Furthermore, removal of solid material from the gastrointestinal tract prior to laparoscopy may improve exposure and lessen the chance of injury from manipulation of a heavy and distended feces-laden colon with the relatively traumatic laparoscopic grasping instruments.

Historically, clearing the colon in preparation for surgery was a complicated procedure requiring several days of clear liquid diet, cathartics, enemas, and preoperative hospitalization. The introduction of polyethylene glycol (PEG) electrolyte solution in the early 1980s revolutionized bowel preparation (122). PEG is an isoosmotic solution with especially designed electrolyte concentrations that result in virtually no net absorption of ions or water, and large volumes can be administered without significant fluid or electrolyte alterations. Several randomized studies have demonstrated that bowel cleansing with PEG can be performed safely as an outpatient preparation prior to colorectal surgery without increasing complication rates (123). Bowel preparation with PEG has some disadvantages. It requires oral intake of 4 L of a salty-tasting solution over a relatively short period of time. Many patients experience nausea, vomiting, and abdominal bloating and discomfort, and are unable to drink the required volume.

Sodium phosphate is an osmotic cathartic that provides quality bowel cleansing while avoiding the need to ingest a large volume of solution (124,125). Generally, a 45-mL dose (or two doses taken 4 hours apart) is taken with at least four glasses of clear liquid with each dose. Colonic cleansing with this method may cause intravascular volume contraction in some patients. A randomized, blinded study showed that rehydration with a carbohydrate-electrolyte "sport" drink resulted in significantly less intravascular volume contraction as compared to rehydration with water (126). A meta-analysis of eight blinded studies that compared sodium phosphate to PEG for colonoscopy preparation suggests that sodium phosphate is an effective, better tolerated, and less costly regimen (127).

Comparisons between these two preparations have also been studied in patients undergoing colorectal surgery with similar results (125,128). The use of sodium phosphate is not recommended for patients with renal insufficiency, symptomatic CHF, and liver failure with ascites (129). Hyperphosphatemia, hypernatremia, hypocalcemia, and hypokalemia have been reported after bowel preparation with sodium phosphate, but generally without clinical significance (124,125,127,130). However, serious and fatal metabolic derangements have been reported, and caution should be used in elderly patients or when prescribing multiple dose regimens (129–132). The FDA suggests obtaining post-treatment laboratory evaluation (basic metabolic panel, calcium, phosphate), especially if more than 45 mL is taken in a 24-hour period (129).

Although regarded as being essential in preventing complications of colorectal surgery, the necessity of mechanical bowel cleansing has been strongly disputed for the past 15 years. The claims that preoperative mechanical bowel preparation reduces anastomotic leakage and SSI are based on observational studies and expert clinical experience. Since 1992 several prospective randomized trials reported that elective colon and rectal surgery may be performed safely without mechanical bowel preparation. All patients in these trials received systemic antibiotics. However, the majority of these trials were greatly underpowered with a 60% or greater chance that a type II error occurred (133,134). In 2004, Bucher et al. published a meta-analysis of 1,297 patients from seven randomized, controlled trials and concluded that mechanical bowel preparation does not reduce the incidence of infectious complications and may be harmful with respect to leakage at the anastomosis (135). Another meta-analysis of 1,592 patients (nine trials) came to the same conclusions and stated that the dogma that mechanical bowel preparation is necessary before elective colorectal surgery should be reconsidered (136). In a survey of members of the American Society of Colon and Rectal Surgeons, essentially all routinely used mechanical bowel preparation, although 10% questioned its importance. Of the 515 surgeons who responded to the questionnaire, 47% routinely used sodium phosphate, 32% routinely used PEG, and 14% alternated between the two agents (137).

The importance of appropriate intravenous antimicrobial prophylaxis in patients undergoing colorectal surgery is well established and was discussed earlier in this chapter. There are conflicting opinions and data regarding whether preoperative oral antibiotics as part of a bowel preparation add any additional benefit for reduction of SSI (138,139). Although there are still strong proponents of this practice (140), oral antibiotic usage with preoperative mechanical bowel cleansing is declining (137).

Blood Transfusion Prophylaxis

Medications associated with increased bleeding risks need to be stopped prior to surgery. Elderly patients are more likely to be taking daily aspirin, nonsteroidal anti-inflammatory medications, platelet aggregation inhibitors, and anticoagulants. It will take approximately 4 days after warfarin therapy is discontinued for the international normalized ratio (INR) to reach 1.5 for those patients with INR levels between 2.0 and 3.0. Many patients on warfarin do not need to be covered with heparin therapy preoperatively. Administration of treatment-dose intravenous heparin or low-molecular-weight heparin (LMWH) while the INR is subtherapeutic is recommended for patients with a history of mechanical mitral valve, ball and cage valve, acute venous, or arterial thromboembolism within 3 months of surgery, or atrial fibrillation with a history of thromboembolic stroke (141). Patients also need to be asked about over-the-counter drug and dietary supplement usage. *Ginkgo biloba*, garlic supplements, ginseng, and vitamin E have antiplatelet activity and may enhance bleeding risk (142). If possible, anemia should be corrected preoperatively. The use of recombinant human erythropoietin with concurrent iron and folic acid supplementation 2 to 3 weeks preoperatively has been shown to reduce allogeneic blood transfusions in patients undergoing elective surgery (143). It has been estimated that 60% of all blood transfused in the United States is given to surgical patients. Transfusion rates of approximately 5% have been reported for patients undergoing abdominal hysterectomy for benign disease (144). Radical procedures performed for the treatment of gynecologic malignancies are associated with an estimated blood loss of 1,000 mL or greater. Transfusion rates for patients undergoing radical hysterectomy have been reported as high as 80% (145), but rates of 10% to 20% are more typical in the recent literature. There is a growing demand by patients for better information about their care, risks involved, and alternatives available. Transfusion-associated risks should be explained to the patient as part of routine preoperative counseling. The risk of transfusion-transmitted infection of human immunodeficiency virus, hepatitis B virus, and hepatitis C virus from red blood cell transfusion is estimated at 1:2.1 million units, 1:250,000 units, and 1:1.9 million units, respectively (146). Although these rates have significantly decreased in the last decade with the introduction of new screening technologies, transmission of other agents, bacterial contamination, transfusion reactions, increased infection complications, and immunosuppression remain risks of allogeneic blood transfusion (147,148). Increasing awareness of these adverse effects has prompted both physicians and patients to search for alternatives to the use of donor blood in the perioperative period.

Since the mid 1980s preoperative autologous blood donation (PABD) has been utilized in order to avoid allogeneic blood transfusion in patients undergoing elective surgery where excessive blood loss is anticipated. Although this practice decreases homologous blood use, 15% of autologous donors will still receive allogeneic transfusions, and 50% of units collected are not used and must be discarded (149). Furthermore, PABD greatly increases the likelihood of any transfusion being necessary and is not without medical risks. Severe reactions during autologous donation occurred at a rate of 0.32% per unit collected and 0.75% per donor. Serious incidents during blood collection that required hospitalization were 12 times more likely in PABD compared to allogeneic donors (150). Transfusion to the wrong recipient, bacterial contamination, febrile nonhemolytic reactions, and allergic reactions have also been reported with autologous transfusion. The cost-effectiveness of PABD has been found to be extremely poor and has steadily deteriorated over the decade (149,151,152).

Acute normovolemic hemodilution (ANH) is an autologous blood-procurement strategy that is equivalent to PABD in reducing allogeneic transfusion needs. Its clinical utility has been extensively studied in patients undergoing radical prostatectomy, total joint replacement, and, more recently, major colorectal surgery. During ANH, blood is procured in the holding or operating room and replaced simultaneously with colloid and crystalloid until a target hematocrit level of 28% is reached or blood volume of 1,500 mL is removed (153). The patient's blood becomes diluted and the amount of actual red cell mass lost during surgery is reduced. ANH obviates the costs of blood testing, storage, or wastage because all blood collected during ANH is kept in the operating room and returned to the patient before the end of surgery. It is simple to perform and more convenient for the patient. Since the blood is collected at point-of-care there is no possibility for clerical error or contamination. ANH has been shown to be a cost-effective yet underutilized strategy to reduce allogeneic blood transfusions (153–155). ANH in which the blood is kept in a continuous circuit with the patient is often a workable alternative for a Jehovah's Witness patient (153,156).

Special Considerations for Obese Patients

Coexisting medical disorders, including coronary artery disease, hypertension, obesity-hypoventilation syndrome, obstructive sleep apnea, adult-onset diabetes mellitus, pulmonary hypertension, gastroesophageal reflux, impaired cardiac function, and hypercoagulability are common in morbidly obese patients and contribute to increased perioperative morbidity and mortality. These comorbidities may not have been previously diagnosed and symptoms may not manifest themselves until the patient undergoes physiologic stress related to surgery. For example, baseline pulmonary function studies of markedly obese patients demonstrate mild hypoxemia; decreased vital capacity, tidal volume, and expiratory reserve volume; increased resistance; and ventilation-perfusion inequalities (157). During the postoperative period, severe hypoxemia may occur secondary to sedation, pain, immobility, atelectasis, and anemia, leading to cardiac arrhythmia or ischemia. A thorough preoperative medical evaluation is necessary to detect coexisting disease and minimize surgical risk. A comprehensive review of the pathophysiology associated with morbid obesity is beyond the scope of this chapter, and we direct the reader elsewhere for a thorough review (158).

Surgery in morbidly obese patients poses many challenges for teams on both sides of the surgical drape. The primary concern of the anesthesiologist is gaining adequate control of the airway. The combined problems of increased aspiration risk, rapid oxygen desaturation caused by decreased functional residual capacity, baseline hypoxemia, and increased oxygen demand, in addition to technical difficulties due to anatomic fat deposits, make intubation a high-risk procedure. An awake, fiberoptic-assisted intubation is often the technique of choice for obtaining an airway. Extubation should be delayed until the patient is fully awake and ideally sitting upright (159). There are technical operating room and instrumentation issues, which need to be addressed as well. Standard operating tables, stretchers, and hospital beds have weight limits, which have prompted specifically designed wider and sturdier models for the obese patient. Staff and patient safety during transfer of the patient from the operating table to the bed or gurney is also a concern in the extremely obese patient and must be taken into consideration. Proper retractors and extra long instruments are essential and may not be available in all hospitals. Although these practical considerations are ostensibly mundane, failure to prepare will obviate a successful outcome, add frustration to all involved, and possibly put the patient at risk.

Recent reports in the gynecologic oncology literature suggest performing panniculectomy to improve exposure of the peritoneal cavity and pelvic structures (160–162). Although this is a relatively straightforward procedure, it does require some experience and planning for optimal results. Hospital credentialing of surgical privileges may require the involvement of a plastic surgeon or proctoring until proficiency is demonstrated. In addition, since panniculectomy is considered a cosmetic procedure, many insurers may require prior authorization with documentation of medical necessity or may deny any reimbursement.

CRITICAL CARE AND POSTOPERATIVE MANAGEMENT

Cardiovascular Issues

Monitoring Issues

There are many tools at the hands of the modern-day clinician when it comes to monitoring the cardiovascular function of the patient. Clinical examination, heart rate, blood pressure, and ECG are a few. In the critical care setting, the addition of the arterial catheter, central venous pressure, and pulmonary artery catheter increases sophistication. Most patients in the ICU can be managed with simple clinical parameters. Fluid status can be assessed by daily weights, pulse rate, blood pressure, and urine output. Continuous ECG monitoring is helpful for detecting arrhythmias and ischemia. Central venous pressure (CVP) is often used for assessment of volume status and a crude estimation of cardiac function. If a patient has a central line then a port can be continuously transduced for CVP. It is a common mistake among novices to evaluate a single reading of CVP rather than reviewing the trend. When the CVP is correlated with volume status, the resulting graph is a scatter graph (i.e., no correlation). There is only correlation over time and in response to, for example, fluid challenges, transfusion, or therapy. One must remember that the CVP is a pressure measurement and not the desired measurement of volume (preload). Therefore, only crude estimations of fluid status can be made. When the status of a patient's cardiac output or fluid state is unclear, a pulmonary artery (PA) catheter (e.g., Swan-Ganz catheter) may be helpful.

These catheters are placed via a central vein (subclavian or jugular) as a central line. The catheter has a balloon-tipped transducer and is "floated" into the pulmonary artery. Waveforms of the right ventricle, pulmonary artery, and pulmonary capillary wedge pressure (PCWP) are directly visualized as the catheter progresses through the heart (Fig. 11.3), and confirmed placement is verified by chest radiograph (Fig. 11.4). Complications of placement include pneumothorax, arrhythmia, line sepsis (2%), and, rarely, pulmonary artery rupture. The PA catheter allows the measurement of cardiac output and oxygen delivery and estimation of preload by obtaining the pulmonary artery occlusive pressure (PAOP) or PCWP, the "wedge."

A number of formulas for calculation of hemodynamic parameters are crucial in utilizing the PA catheter for the care of the critically ill patient (Table 11.8). Assessment of preload is desirable for determining fluid administration or diuretic requirements for patients. The ideal measure of preload would be left ventricular end-diastolic volume; however, since this is unobtainable with current technology, intensivists settle for "the wedge" as an estimation. By inflating the balloon placed in the pulmonary artery, a direct column of standing fluid exists between the left atrium, through the pulmonary vasculature, and back to the balloon (transducer). The PAOP can be measured and is a crude reflection of left atrial pressure. If the PAOP is elevated, the preload is adequate (or excessive), and if it is low, the patient may be volume depleted. These measurements, as previously mentioned with CVP, are dynamic and trend is important. For example, if the PAOP is low and a fluid bolus is given, the PAOP should increase if the diagnosis of volume depletion was correct.

Thermodilution techniques are used to calculate cardiac output by injecting saline via a proximal port in the PA catheter and measuring the thermal changes at the distal tip of the PA catheter. By combining the preload assessment provided by the PAOP and the calculated cardiac output, differentiation between volume depletion and cardiogenic disease states can be made (see section on shock). Newer PA catheters have been developed that can calculate right ventricular ejection fraction.

By taking a blood sample from the tip of the PA catheter, the most desaturated blood in the body is retrieved. In normal circulation, the blood from the superior vena cava and the inferior vena cava mix and the blood from the coronary sinus is added to give a sample known as the mixed venous blood. By evaluating the oxygen saturation of this blood, oxygen delivery can be calculated (Table 11.8). This measurement is perhaps the most important function of the PA catheter, and current technology allows this function to be continuous via

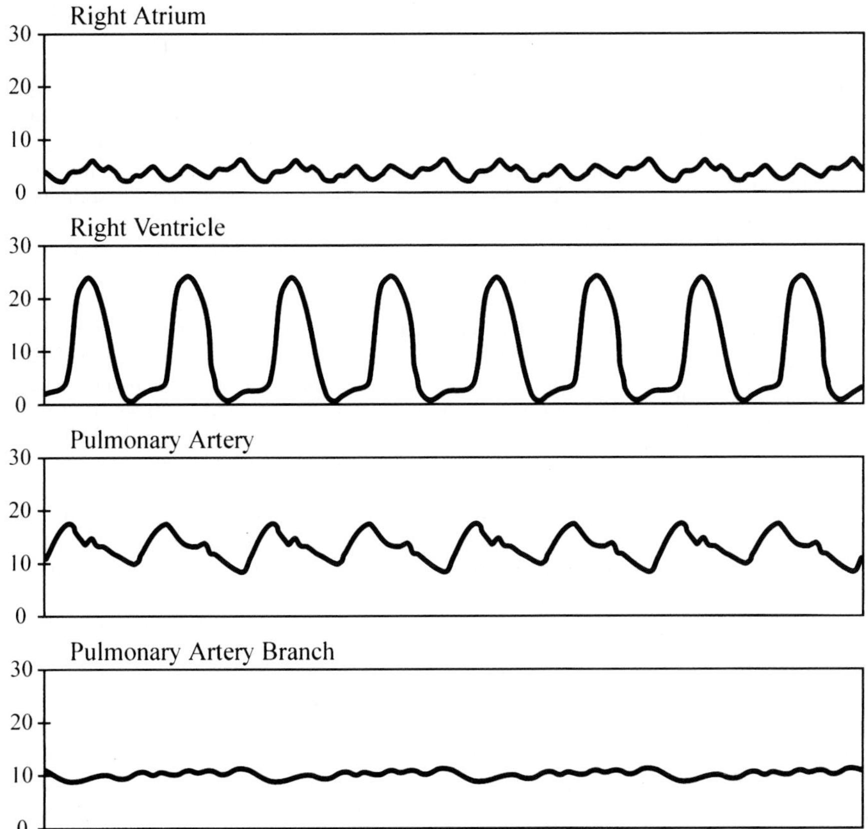

FIGURE 11.3. Pulmonary artery catheter wave form readings as the catheter passes through the heart into the pulmonary artery. Y-axis is reading in millimeters of mercury (mm Hg).

an infrared sensor at the tip of the PA catheter. For example, if oxygen delivery is determined to be low, there are only three situations that can be influenced by the clinician: increase cardiac output (with fluid, chronotropes, or inotropes), increase the hemoglobin, or increase the oxygen saturation. In a patient with a major operation and medical comorbidities, the measurement of a normal oxygen delivery provides reassurance to the clinician that end organs are being perfused.

Calculation of the systemic vascular resistance (SVR) is also possible with a PA catheter. Because the SVR is a calculated value and not directly measured, inaccuracies are inherent and overinterpretation of this value is cautioned. Rather than relying on the calculated SVR, the clinician should have complete understanding of the measured blood pressure and cardiac output and the ramifications therein to make therapeutic decisions (the SVR combines the two previously mentioned measured variables).

In one study of ovarian cancer patients undergoing cytoreductive surgery, 18% of patients had indications for PA catheter use (163). Because of the issues of volume status in

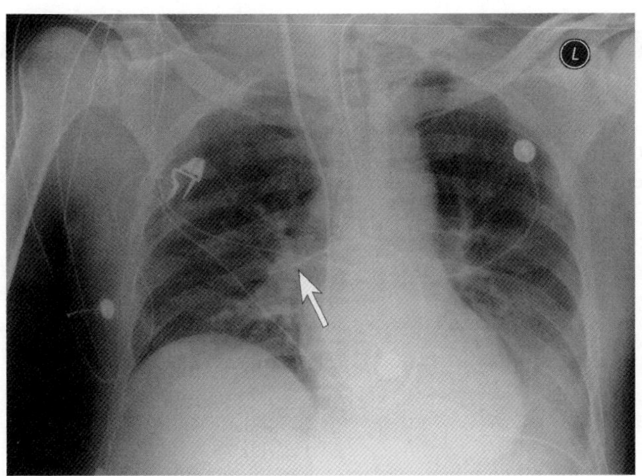

FIGURE 11.4. Chest radiograph showing proper placement of pulmonary artery catheter in the pulmonary artery (*arrow* shows tip of pulmonary catheter).

TABLE 11.8

HEMODYNAMIC FORMULAS

Cardiac output (CO) = stroke volume (SV) × heart rate (HR) [4–8 L/min]
Cardiac index (CI) = CO/body surface area (BSA)
Systemic vascular resistance (SVR) = mean arterial pressure (MAP) − central venous pressure (CVP) × 80/CO [800−1,200 dyne/s/cm^{-5}/m^2]
Arterial O_2 content (CaO_2) = (1.36) (hemoglobin) (oxygen saturation) + 0.003 (partial pressure of oxygen) [20 mL O_2/dL]
O_2 delivery ($\dot{D}O_2$) = CO × CaO_2 × 10 [600–1,000 mL O_2/min]
O_2 availability (O_2AVI) = CI × CaO_2 × 10 [500–600 mL/min/m^2]
O_2 extraction ratio = (CaO_2 − CvO_2)/CaO_2 [25%]

Note: Values in brackets are normal values.

these patients, PA catheter placement for postoperative fluid management may be especially helpful.

Acute Postoperative Myocardial Infarction

MI usually manifests with acute chest discomfort, elevated cardiac enzymes, and ECG changes. Dyspnea, diaphoresis, nausea, and anxiety may also be associated. Risk factors that increase mortality from postoperative MI include female gender, advanced age, tachycardia, hypotension, and CHF (164). Treatment includes ICU monitoring with continuous ECG monitoring and supplemental oxygen, aspirin 325 mg immediately, sublingual nitroglycerin, and morphine sulfate as needed until pain resolves. Beta-blockers have been shown to decrease mortality by decreasing fatal arrhythmias and are also part of the early treatment regimen. An evaluation for heparin therapy or thrombolytics can be made in consultation with a cardiologist.

Congestive Heart Failure

Patients with known CHF will be risk stratified, as previously mentioned, before major elective surgery. However, in the postoperative setting, CHF will present in a number of ways (165). Patients with CHF are in a continuous hypervolemic state, and issues of fluid balance (strict "ins" and "outs") will be paramount during the perioperative period. In difficult cases, insertion of a PA catheter can be very helpful. Judicious fluid administration guided by the PAOP as well as selective use of inotropic support for augmentation of the cardiac output will aid the clinician in a successful outcome in these difficult patients (166).

Inotropes and Vasopressors

A variety of hemodynamically active drugs are available to support the cardiovascular function of patients in the perioperative period (167). In the broadest sense, they can be categorized as vasopressors, which elevate blood pressure, and inotropes, which enhance cardiac output (Table 11.9) (168). When faced with a patient in whom oxygen delivery is low and an increase in cardiac output is desired, inotropes such as dopamine or dobutamine should be used. Dopamine, at lower doses, activates dopaminergic receptors and increases circulation in mesenteric, cerebral, and renal vascular beds. At intermediate doses, dopamine stimulates beta-receptors in the heart and peripheral circulation. This activation causes tachycardia, increasing stroke volume and cardiac output. Increasing cardiac output in this fashion also increases demands for myocardial oxygen and could precipitate angina or an MI (169). At high doses, dopamine acts as an alpha agonist, causing vasoconstriction. Dobutamine is a β_1 agonist with much greater inotropic effect than dopamine and causes peripheral arterial vasodilation, decreasing afterload (this dilation is abrupt and can cause hypotension in some patients). It is the drug of choice for severe heart failure.

Epinephrine is a potent sympathomimetic with varying effects based on the dose. The drug has beta-mimetic effects at lower doses and alpha-mimetic effects at higher doses. Epinephrine causes an acute increase in myocardial oxygen demand and is mainly reserved for cardiac arrest or severe circulatory failure. Norepinephrine and phenylephrine are pure alpha-mimetic agents, utilized for vasoconstriction (neurogenic shock). In most situations of shock, fluid resuscitation is preferred to administration of alpha agents. Although these agents will give a false sense of security that the blood pressure is normal, one must remember that the vasoconstriction underperfuses capillary beds, leading to an increased incidence of renal hypoperfusion (renal failure), splanchnic hypoperfusion (resulting in translocation of gut flora), and a myriad of other problems.

Vasopressin has emerged as an option similar to epinephrine with some important differences. This antidiuretic hormone in high doses provides potent vasoconstriction and leads to improved cerebral and coronary blood flow in shock states. Unlike epinephrine, there is less increase in myocardial oxygen demand and less propensity for inducing arrhythmias.

Amrinone (or inamrinone) is a phosphoesterase inhibitor that provides a positive inotropic effect on cardiac musculature while causing vasodilation. It is used in refractory cardiac failure.

Valvular Disease

In a recent study, approximately 4% of patients undergoing elective, noncardiac surgery were found to have clinically significant valvular disease. Important considerations in perioperative management are directed at patients with aortic stenosis (AS) and the level of associated ventricular failure. In addition, these patients need endocarditis antibiotic prophylaxis (Table 11.10). AS is an independent risk factor for poor

TABLE 11.9

VASOPRESSORS: EFFECTS AND DOSAGE

Drug	Systemic vasodilation	Systemic vasoconstriction	Inotropic effect	Chronotropic effect	Dysrhythmias	Dosing
Dopamine	+	0 to +++	++	+++	++	0.5–5 μg/kg/min for low range 5–10 mid range 10–20 high range
Dobutamine	++	0 to +	++++	++	+	2.5–20 μg/kg/min
Epinephrine	++	+++	++++	+++	+++	0.5–10 μg/min
Norepinephrine	0	++++	++	0	+	0.5–20 μg/min
Phenylephrine	0	+++	0	0	0	20–200 μg/min
Vasopressin	0	+++	0	0	0	0.04–0.12 U/min
Amrinone	++	0	++++	+	+	Load 0.75 mg/kg Maintenance 5–15 μg/kg/min

Note: 0, no effect; +, slight effect, to ++++, strong effect.

TABLE 11.10

ANTIBIOTIC REGIMENS FOR ENDOCARDITIS PROPHYLAXIS IN HIGH- AND MODERATE-RISK PATIENTS UNDERGOING GENITOURINARY/GASTROINTESTINAL PROCEDURES

Patient type	Antibiotic	Regimen
High-risk patients[a]	Ampicillin plus gentamicin	Ampicillin 2.0 g IM/IV plus 1.5 mg/kg (not to exceed 120 mg) within 30 minutes of starting procedure; 6 hours later, ampicillin 1.0 g IM/IV or amoxicillin 1.0 g orally
High-risk patients[a] allergic to ampicillin/amoxicillin	Vancomycin plus gentamicin	Vancomycin 1.0 g IV over 1–2 hours plus gentamicin 1.5 mg/kg IM/IV (not to exceed 120 mg); complete injection/infusion within within of starting procedure
Moderate-risk patients[b]	Ampicillin or amoxicillin	Ampicillin 2.0 g IM/IV within 30 minutes of starting procedure or amoxicillin 2.0 g orally 1 hour 30 minutes before procedure
Moderate-risk patients[b] allergic to ampicillin/amoxicillin	Vancomycin	Vancomycin 1.0 g IV over 1–2 hours; complete infusion within 30 minutes of starting procedure

Note: IM, intramuscular; IV, intravenous.
[a]High-risk patients: prosthetic cardiac valves; previous history of bacterial endocarditis; complex cyanotic heart disease (e.g., tetralogy of Fallot); surgically constructed systemic pulmonary shunts or conduits.
[b]Moderate-risk patients: other congenital cardiac malformations; acquired valvar dysfunction; hypertrophic cardiomyopathy; mitral valve prolapse with valvar regurgitation and/or thickened leaflets.

operative outcome, as previously mentioned (170). Patients with severe AS need valve replacement before elective surgery, whereas patients with mild to moderate AS need careful anesthetic control of blood pressure. Some patients may need intraoperative, continuous transesophageal echocardiography (171). The presence of aortic regurgitation, mitral stenosis, and mitral regurgitation require assessment of left ventricular function for the presence of congestive heart failure. Treatment and support will be related to support of ventricular function. Recently, the American Heart Association revised their recommendations for antibiotic prophylaxis for endocarditis (172). The common antibiotic regimens for endocarditis prophylaxis are presented in Table 11.10 for patients with anatomic cardiac defects and for whom risk is highest for the development of endocarditis after extended gastrointestinal or genitourinary operations.

Arrhythmias

Whenever an arrhythmia occurs in the postoperative setting, myocardial ischemia must first be ruled out (173). If ECG and cardiac enzyme measurement are normal, an electrolyte or metabolic derangement or drug toxicity exists. Fortunately, most arrhythmias in the postoperative period are transient and self-resolving. Asymptomatic arrhythmias, except in the preoperative period (Table 11.2), are generally of little clinical signi-ficance. Hypercapnia, hypoxemia, hypokalemia, acidosis, inadequate analgesia, and anemia can all promote cardiac arrhythmias. Supraventricular tachycardia is the most common rhythm disturbance seen in the postoperative period (174). Treatment with cardizem or a beta-blocker is usually effective after correction of the underlying etiology. One significant new development has been the use of amiodarone as first-line treatment of acute-onset atrial fibrillation. Its usage has been associated with a lower incidence of recurrent atrial fibrillation (175).

Pulmonary Issues

Ventilator Management

The ability to provide ventilatory support to the surgical patient has been a tremendous advance in postoperative care. Mechanical ventilators have enabled oncologic surgeons to perform major operations for aggressive control of lesions that were once considered to be unresectable. Although preemptive preoperative therapies attempt to avoid postoperative mechanical ventilation, some patients will require this therapy. Mechanical ventilation must be thought of as providing two functions: ventilation and oxygenation. However, these two functions must be separated and applied independently to each particular situation. A more difficult concept for residents and fellows to understand is that ventilation has nothing to do with oxygenation. Many patients decompensate on the ward despite supplemental oxygen and 100% oxygen saturation because tidal volumes were low and the patient was not ventilating.

When contemplating mechanical ventilation, one must ask two questions: is the patient able to oxygenate her tissues adequately and can she ventilate adequately to maintain normal partial pressure of carbon dioxide (PCO_2) and acid-base function? Adequate oxygenation can be determined by measurement of oxygen saturation and arterial partial pressure of oxygen (PO_2). Targets are generally an O_2 saturation >92% or PO_2 greater than 65 mm Hg. Poor oxygenation may be caused by fluid overload, depressed mental status, underlying pulmonary disease, or shunt. Evaluation of the arterial blood gas will also give a pH and PCO_2 measurement. Patients may hypoventilate for a number of reasons. Postoperative pain may prohibit deep inspiration. Conversely, overuse of pain medication may depress the level of consciousness, leading to fewer and poorer respirations. Atelectasis, pneumonia, and poor pulmonary compliance all lead to difficulties in ventilation. Finally, a bronchial mucous plug or a pneumothorax will lead life-threatening ventilatory compromise. A respiratory rate greater than 35 per minute or a PCO_2 greater than 55 mm Hg are accepted indications for intubation and mechanical ventilation.

When intubating patients, the size of the endotracheal tube must be considered, as this may impact removal of mechanical ventilation. The larger the tube, the less resistance and the easier it will be for the patient to participate in "weaning" trials to discontinue ventilatory support (176). Typical recommendations are an 8.5-mm tube for women and a 9.0-mm tube for men.

Traditionally, there are pressure-cycled ventilators and volume-cycled ventilators. Pressure-cycled ventilators are used routinely in neonatal ICU patients because overinflation can be dangerous to neonates. In the adult ICU, most ventilators are volume cycled, meaning that the clinician sets the tidal volume, and regardless of the pressures necessary to give the volume, the volume will be delivered. In patients in whom pulmonary compliance is reduced (i.e., due to a stiff lung or acute respiratory distress syndrome [ARDS]), efforts at controlling pressure are important. When setting the ventilator, a number of decisions must be made. The mode of delivery, tidal volume, and rate will determine ventilation, whereas the fraction of inspired oxygen (FIO_2) and positive end-expiratory pressure (PEEP) will determine oxygenation.

Mode

There are a number of ventilator modes. The first developed was controlled mechanical ventilation (CMV), where the tidal volume and rate are set and that is exactly what the patient receives—no more and no less. This mode is very good for patients under general anesthesia or who are paralyzed. However, this mode is very disturbing to the patient who wishes to participate, however slightly, in her own ventilation. This mode has evolved into the current assist/control mode (A/C), whereby the patient is guaranteed the fixed rate and tidal volume but can also trigger breaths in between with a similar tidal volume. In addition, the machine will synchronize the breath when the patient triggers such a breath. This mode provides complete rest for the patient by performing all the work of breathing and is generally used for patients in the immediate postoperative period or for patients whose organ failure or ongoing sepsis is a more pressing concern.

Intermittent mandatory ventilation (IMV) is a mode whereby the clinician sets a rate and a tidal volume, which the machine delivers. Any breath initiated by the patient is delivered in relation to the amount of effort the patient puts forth, meaning a strong effort gives the patient a large breath and a meager effort a smaller one. This is sometimes called a weaning mode. The patient is given full support with rate and tidal volume until she is stronger. The rate is slowly turned down, allowing the patient more frequent, spontaneous breaths until extubation. Synchronized IMV (SIMV) ensures that a machine-delivered breath does not stack onto a patient-initiated breath.

Pressure support ventilation (PSV) is a mode where patient-initiated breaths are given support from the ventilator only during the beginning of ventilation (inspiratory phase). The support is meant to help the patient overcome the large amount of resistance present in the valves of the machine, the ventilator circuit, and the endotracheal tube. By titrating PSV to the spontaneous tidal volume produced by the patient, one can fully or partially support patient breathing and overcome the work of breathing. This mode of ventilation is important during the "weaning" process.

Work of Breathing

When conceptualizing the job of the ventilator, the different types of work must be defined (177). In addition to the physiologic work of breathing that all humans do on a daily basis, huge workloads are imposed from the resistance of the ventilator equipment (e.g., breathing through a straw analogy). Finally, there is the pathologic work of breathing from the pneumonia, the incision, etc. The intent of mechanical ventilation during disease states is to assume the last two types of "work" so that the patient may convalesce. As a patient improves and the pathologic work has been removed, then the patient should be able to resume normal, physiologic work.

More Advanced Modes of Ventilation

With advanced circuitry and computer microprocessors, newer ventilator modes have been developed. Pressure-regulated volume control (PRVC) has largely replaced AC ventilation (ACV). PRVC provides the same function as AC while preventing overinflation. Recent data have shown that preventing overinflation (or stretch) of alveoli prevents trauma and has a decreased incidence of ARDS (178). PRVC delivers the same tidal volume but changes the flow rate to prevent high pressures by measuring the pressure on a breath-to-breath basis. Volume control (VC ventilation) is a mode whereby a tidal volume target is set and the ventilator continually titrates the amount of PSV to provide this volume. This mode has been termed "autowean" or "weekend" mode because as the patient gets stronger, he or she will be able to meet the tidal volume setting. In situations where difficulties in ventilation are encountered, such as ARDS, hypercarbia, and acidosis, pressure control (PC) is used. This mode is similar to the neonatal pressure-cycled ventilator where the maximum pressure is set and the flow rate is decreased but the inspiratory time is lengthened to achieve proper ventilation. Airway pressure release ventilation (APRV), high-frequency jet ventilation, and inverse ratio ventilation are other advanced modes beyond the scope of this chapter.

Setting the Ventilator

Initial ventilator settings require a rate of 12 to 14 breaths per minute with a tidal volume of 6 to 8 cc/kg. This is a departure from the traditional 12 cc/kg, which has been determined to result in greater alveolar trauma and increased risk for the development of ARDS (179). After initial setting of the ventilator, measurements of pH, PO_2, and PCO_2 from arterial blood gas are used to make further ventilator adjustments.

Oxygenation

Oxygenation is controlled by two settings: FIO_2 and PEEP. The inspired oxygen content can easily be controlled on the ventilator, keeping oxygen saturation greater than 92%. Inspired oxygen levels greater than 60% are considered to be potentially toxic, with such levels leading to pathologic changes similar to ARDS with acute inflammation and fibroproliferative changes. Human studies are few and have only examined effects on normal lungs, whereas no studies have clearly delineated the toxic effects of high oxygen levels in patients with underlying pulmonary disease (180). If it is necessary to have oxygen concentrations above 60%, the recommendation is to wean these levels as soon as possible. PEEP is another mechanism for improving oxygenation. In normal physiology, the glottis closes before full expiration, creating a PEEP of approximately 4 cm H_2O, and is termed physiologic PEEP. When ventilating patients, the addition of 5 cm H_2O PEEP is used as a baseline and is increased if added oxygen delivery is required. Increasing PEEP is the preferred method for improving oxygenation in postsurgical patients as opposed to increasing the FIO_2. Postsurgical patients have atelectasis and shunting secondary to operative pain and anesthesia. The addition of PEEP recruits collapsed alveoli, improving oxygenation and lung compliance. However, the use of PEEP must be balanced by potential adverse effects, which include decreased cardiac output and the risk for barotrauma. Kirby et al. have shown that PEEP levels of 30 to 40 mm H_2O are easily tolerable in most patients; however, few clinical situations present in which patients need levels of PEEP this high (181).

Weaning From Ventilator

Multiple opinions exist on the techniques of weaning patients from mechanical ventilation, and no prospective randomized trial has proven one method to be superior to another (182). T-piece trials, spontaneous breathing trials, SIMV, and PSV are just a few. The best method of weaning is a treatment pathway agreed upon by clinicians, nurses, and respiratory therapists. Before discontinuing mechanical ventilation, the disease process that required ventilation should have resolved and patients should have proper mental status and the ability to generate a cough. Copious secretions are often an initial reason not to consider weaning or extubation. Criteria for extubation, whether on T-piece or minimal PSV, have traditionally included a respiratory rate less than 35, a PCO_2 less than 50 mm Hg, and a negative inspiratory force (NIF) greater than –20 cm H_2O.

Acute Respiratory Distress Syndrome

ARDS is a condition that has been well recognized and extensively studied (183). It is a form of refractory hypoxemia that can be elicited by a number of insults. In 1994, a consensus of American and European intensivists defined the criteria for ARDS and a lesser form deemed acute lung injury (ALI) (184). Criteria include (a) acute onset after defined insult; (b) bilateral diffuse infiltrates on chest radiograph; (c) no evidence of left atrial hypertension, CHF, or a PAOP less than or equal to 18 mm Hg; and, most importantly, (d) impaired oxygenation. Impaired oxygenation was classified as ALI if the partial pressure of arterial oxygen (PaO_2)/FIO_2 ratio was ≥300 mm Hg and ARDS if the PaO_2/FIO_2 ratio was ≥200 mm Hg. Postmortem examination of lungs with ARDS shows atelectasis, edema, inflammation, hyaline membrane deposition, and fibrosis. The mortality of ARDS is 30% to 40%. Treatment of these severely hypoxemic patients consists of mechanical ventilatory support with FIO_2 and PEEP. Because of alveolar damage, ventilation/perfusion mismatch occurs, resulting in a worsening shunt fraction and increasing dead space. As the pathologic process continues, not only does oxygenation become difficult, but so also does ventilation as a result of decreased pulmonary compliance. The end result is a hypercapneic state and respiratory acidosis.

The recent ARDS NET trial comparing high tidal volume to achieve normocapnia with low tidal volumes to prevent barotrauma has shown significantly improved survival with the low-volume protective strategy (178). Current strategies employ tidal volumes of 6 cc/kg and accept elevated PCO_2 levels (permissive hypercapnea).

The last 15 years have seen the elucidation of a number of systemic factors that are released upon physiologic insult (185). For example, cytokines, leukotrienes, endothelial adhesion molecules, and interleukins are useful in the defense of the organism, but are systemically detrimental when activated by certain disease states. Investigations of the multiple organ dysfunction syndrome (MODS) where sequential organ failure leads to patient death have given significant credibility to the hypothesis that the lung may be the first organ system susceptible to these circulating inflammatory mediators (186). The pulmonary endothelium is acutely sensitive to circulating cytokines and is the first to manifest damage. In addition to supportive treatment for ARDS, operative injuries or postoperative complications (e.g., intra-abdominal abscess, anastomotic leak) must be sought and ruled out aggressively. ARDS is the result of some inciting cause and does not arise *de novo* as a primary problem.

Pneumonia

Pneumonia is a significant complication in postsurgical patients. Patients requiring mechanical ventilation are particularly susceptible to pneumonia (ventilator acquired pneumonia [VAP]) with rates as high as 30% after 72 hours of ventilation. The mortality rate from VAP ranges from 25% to 50%. The pathogens are often gram negative and resistant to multiple antibiotics. High clinical suspicion and aggressive treatment of VAP is crucial. An exhaustive review of this complicated and serious topic by Chastre and Fagon is recommended for further reading (187).

Pulmonary Embolism and Deep Venous Thrombosis Prophylaxis

The prevention of venous thromboembolism is an important component of perioperative management of the gynecologic oncology patient. The American College of Chest Physicians consensus statement published in 1998 reviews the data exhaustively and provides recommendations (188). Risk factors include age greater than 40 years, prolonged immobility, prior deep venous thrombosis (DVT), cancer diagnosis, major surgery, obesity, CHF, MI, stroke, indwelling femoral catheter, inflammatory bowel disease, estrogen use, nephrotic syndrome, and hypercoagulable states. The incidence of DVT in large groups of general surgical patients is around 20% and increases to 30% in patients with cancer diagnoses. The incidence of pulmonary embolism (PE) is 1.6% with a fatal PE rate of 0.9%. In trials comparing low-dose unfractionated heparin (LDUH) with no therapy in general surgical patients, the DVT rate was decreased from 25% to 8%. These studies also produced a 50% decrease in rate of fatal PE (188). Comparisons of low-molecular-weight heparin (LMWH) versus unfractionated heparin have shown equal efficacy. LMWH may have less bleeding complication (mostly wound hematomas) and greater ease of use with once daily dosing.

Sequential pneumatic compression devices (PCDs) are attractive for patients at risk for bleeding complications. In trials comparing PCD with LDUH, both have shown efficacy. Elastic stockings (Ted's hose) and aspirin usage are not currently recommended as DVT prophylaxis. Recently, studies have shown D-dimer positivity with DVT and PE, but the presence of any released blood or hematoma (i.e., any postoperative patient) makes the D-dimer positivity nonspecific. In the surgical patient, a negative D-dimer makes DVT or PE highly unlikely; however, a positive test is essentially useless.

Patients at low risk (age less than 40 years, no risk factors, and minor surgery) need no prophylaxis, but early ambulation is encouraged. Moderate-risk patients (minor surgery in a patient with risk factors, major surgery with no risk factors) should receive PCD, LMWH, or LDUH, with equal results. High-risk patients require LWMH in addition to PCD.

Diagnosis of DVT is performed by duplex ultrasonography, and treatment is with either heparinization to 1.5 times control prothrombin time or therapeutic doses of LMWH. Diagnosis of PE was traditionally made by pulmonary arteriogram. This practice has recently been abandoned because dynamic contrast-enhanced computerized tomography has better sensitivity. Once diagnosis is confirmed, the patient is anticoagulated with IV heparin or LMWH. Ultimately, the patient is converted to warfarin (Coumadin) therapy for at least 3 months in the case of DVT and 6 months in the case of PE.

Fluid and Electrolyte Issues

Understanding fluid and electrolyte physiology in gynecologic oncology is paramount because of the underlying disease processes that face the gynecologic oncologist and the ultimate,

TABLE 11.11

BODY FLUID COMPARTMENTS

Total body water	Body weight (%)	Total body water (%)
Total	60	100
Intracellular	40	67
Extracellular	20	33
Intravascular	5	8
Interstitial	15	25

Source: From Wait RB, Kahng KU, Dresner LS. Fluid and electrolytes and acid-base balance. In: Greenfield LJ, Mulholland M, Oldham KT, et al. eds. *Surgery: Scientific Principles and Practice.* 2nd ed. Philadelphia: Lippincott–Raven Publishers, 1997:242–266, with permission.

radical surgical interventions that are needed to treat them. These treatments result in great fluid shifts perioperatively, requiring careful attention to input of fluids (volume and content/type) as well as output from renal and gastrointestinal sources, insensible sources, and drains. Since extensive discussions of these topics can be found elsewhere, this section presents a brief review of normal fluid and electrolyte physiology and discusses strategies for fluid resuscitation and correction of electrolyte deficiencies.

Total body water (TBW) can be calculated by various methods and varies directly with the amount of adipose or lean tissue present in an individual patient. TBW estimates, therefore, must be adjusted based on the adiposity of the patients. In women, TBW accounts for approximately 60% of a patient's weight. TBW is distributed into extracellular fluid (ECF) and intracellular fluid (ICF), with the ECF being further divided into intravascular (one quarter of the ECF) and interstitial (three quarters of the ECF) compartments. The ECF accounts for approximately one third of the TBW, whereas ICF accounts for two thirds (189,190). Direct measurement of the ECF and TBW are possible with the resulting difference being an estimated ICF. Table 11.11 describes the body fluid compartments and their contributions to body weight. Despite these arbitrary compartments (and electrolyte concentration differences between compartments, which are discussed in the paragraph below), water flows freely across all compartments. Thus, a derangement in one compartment will result in a compensatory change in another (191).

The electrolyte composition of the various compartments is different. Sodium is the predominant cation in the ECF and potassium is the predominant cation of the ICF. Table 11.12 describes the various concentrations of electrolytes in the various fluid compartments. Because of the Donnan principle of equilibration, the content of cations and anions in the interstitial compartment is slightly higher than the intravascular compartment. This principle describes the unique relation between solutions of permeable and impermeable complex anions when these anions are unevenly distributed across a semipermeable membrane. Water, on the other hand, as mentioned earlier, freely equilibrates between the compartments (191).

Effective circulating volume (ECV) is a term used to describe the portion of the ECF that perfuses the organs of the body and affects baroreceptors (see next paragraph). In healthy patients, the ECV equates to the intravascular volume/compartment. But in disease states that increase "third spacing" such as sepsis (leaky capillaries), ascites due to intra-abdominal metastasis, or bowel obstruction with resulting edema and transudation, the interstitial compartment increases at the expense of the intravascular compartment, decreasing the ECV (189).

The osmotic activity of a fluid compartment is affected by the component ions and is described in milliosmoles (mOsm). Normal serum osmolality (in the ECF, of course) averages 290 mOsm/kg of H_2O. Osmoreceptors in the hypothalamus respond to small changes in serum osmolality, increasing or decreasing secretion of antidiuretic hormone (ADH) and modifying the thirst response. These receptors are responsible for the day-to-day fine tuning of fluid balance. Baroreceptors, on the other hand, in the intrathoracic vena cava, the atria, the aortic arch, the carotid arteries, and the renal parenchyma, sense volume changes by changes in pressure. These receptors begin a cascade of mediators such as aldosterone, atrial natriuretic peptide (ANP), prostaglandins, and the renin-angiotensin system, which ultimately result in changes of water and sodium

TABLE 11.12

ELECTROLYTE CONCENTRATIONS IN THE VARIOUS FLUID COMPARTMENTS

	Extracellular fluid		
	Plasma	Interstitial fluid	Intracellular fluid
CATIONS			
Na^+	140	146	12
K^+	4	4	150
Ca^{2+}	5	3	10^{-7}
Mg^{2+}	2	1	7
ANIONS			
Cl^-	103	114	3
HCO_3^-	24	27	10
SO_4^{2-}	1	1	—
HPO_4^{3-}	2	2	116
Protein	16	5	40
Organic anions	5	5	—

Source: From Wait RB, Kahng KU, Dresner LS. Fluid and electrolytes and acid-base balance. In: Greenfield LJ, Mulholland M, Oldham KT, et al. eds. *Surgery: Scientific Principles and Practice.* 2nd ed. Philadelphia: Lippincott–Raven Publishers, 1997:242–266, with permission.

balance mediated through the kidneys. These baroreceptors have little to do with the day-to-day fluid management and require intravascular losses of 10% to 20% to initiate activity (191).

The goal of fluid resuscitation is to maintain the ECV and return the patient to a homeopathic state. Many gynecologic oncology procedures are lengthy and can result in large blood losses requiring immediate intraoperative replacement. In addition, following procedures where evacuation of large amounts of ascites has occurred and/or "peritoneal stripping" has left denuded surfaces, these patients may have large fluid shifts into the interstitial compartment requiring large volumes of fluid to maintain the ECV. Finally, losses are not water alone and include electrolytes and clotting factors, which may need repletion. Selecting fluids to administer to a given patient is akin to selecting the correct intravenous medication to give; not *all* fluids are for *all* patients. The physician should understand the amount of daily maintenance fluid and electrolytes required by patients, calculate losses (fluid and electrolytes), determine ongoing fluid and electrolyte losses, and replace them with the appropriate fluid and electrolyte combinations. It is easy to fall into the trap of giving all patients an 8-hour rate (125 mL/h) of maintenance fluid. However, an octogenarian, even with normal cardiac and renal function, weighing 50 kg does not need that much maintenance fluid. "Formulas" for calculating appropriate maintenance fluid requirements exist (191), but calculating 30 to 40 mL/kg/day, depending upon body frame size, is a much simpler and quicker estimate of maintenance fluid requirements for patients.

In general, the normal maintenance requirement of sodium is 1 to 2 mEq/kg/day and for potassium 0.5 to 1.0 mEq/kg/day. Table 11.13 lists the various IV fluid preparations available for fluid resuscitation. Which fluid to be used is controversial and driven, in more instances, by "dogma," varying from physician to physician and institution to institution rather than by evidence. Controversy over which fluid type to use in fluid resuscitation continues to this day. Several meta-analyses have shown no advantage of colloid over crystalloid for resuscitation in surgical patients (192–199). Almost all studies have shown that administered colloid leaks from the intravascular compartment to the interstitial compartment in several hours, decreasing the ECV and requiring further administration of colloid (192–199). The use of colloid has been shown to be advantageous in conditions of hypoproteinemia or malnourished states where patients require plasma volume expansion and cannot tolerate large amounts of fluid (199).

Most of the time patients are given isotonic solutions, such as lactated Ringer's solution, to cover perioperative losses. In the immediate postoperative course, patients are given their maintenance fluid requirements in addition to the immediate intraoperative losses. It is helpful to convert all losses to equivalents of crystalloid to determine fluid rates. For example, to replace 500 mL of blood loss, one would give 1,500 mL of isotonic fluid, a ratio of 3 mL of crystalloid to 1 mL of blood loss. It is traditional to replace one half of the intraoperative losses in the first 24 hours, with the rest being replaced during the ensuing several days. Other intraoperative losses, which need to be accounted for, are the insensible losses that occur through evaporation from the incision (5 to 10 mL/kg/h of operation) and from the anesthesia circuit and ascites.

Sodium Derangements

Hyponatremia is the most common electrolyte abnormality seen in postoperative patients and is caused by excess free water rather than a depletion of sodium. Increases in free water absorption are mediated by a self-limited, physiologic increase in the secretion of ADH in response to the stress of surgery. Serum sodium levels rarely fall below 130 mEq/L, but may be further exacerbated by intravenous administration of large volumes of hypotonic solutions (i.e., 0.2%, 0.33%, 0.45% sodium solutions). Other disease states can result in a hyperosmolar condition, resulting in a hyperosmolar ECF, causing fluid to shift from the ICF and lowering the sodium levels. These conditions include hyperglycemia, mannitol ethylene glycol or ethanol ingestion, and uremia. For each increase of 180 mg/dL of glucose above 100 mg/dL, there is a concomitant decrease in the serum sodium of 5 mEq/L (198). In addition, during situations where potassium is low, there is a compensatory exchange of sodium for potassium, resulting in hyponatremia. In either of these prior cases, total body sodium does not change. Finally, patients with hyperproteinemia or hyperlipidemia may have falsely low sodium values, which result from errors in the laboratory measurement of sodium. This *pseudohyponatremia* does not result in any symptoms of hyponatremia (191).

The symptoms of hyponatremia are driven by cellular water intoxication and are related to the central nervous system (CNS) (e.g., lethargy, headaches, confusion, delirium, weakness, muscle cramps). The rate at which hyponatremia occurs also determines the symptoms. Chronic hyponatremia tends to be asymptomatic, whereas acute drops in the serum sodium (levels 120 to 130) result in the symptoms listed

TABLE 11.13

ELECTROLYTE CONTENT OF COMMONLY USED INTRAVENOUS ELECTROLYTE SOLUTIONS

	Electrolyte concentration (mEq/L)					
Solution	Na^+	K^+	Ca^{2+}	Mg^{2+}	Cl^-	HCO^{3-}
Lactated Ringer's solution	130	4	4	—	109	28
0.2% NaCl	34	—	—	—	34	—
0.33% NaCl	56	—	—	—	56	—
0.45% NaCl	77	—	—	—	77	—
0.9% NaCl	154	—	—	—	154	—
3.0% NaCl	513	—	—	—	513	—
5.0% NaCl	855	—	—	—	855	—

Source: Adapted from Wait RB, Kahng KU, Dresner LS. Fluid and electrolytes and acid-base balance. In: Greenfield LJ, Mulholland M, Oldham KT, et al. eds. *Surgery: Scientific Principles and Practice.* 2nd ed. Philadelphia: Lippincott–Raven Publishers, 1997:242–266, with permission.

above. Correction of hyponatremia must be done carefully to avoid central pontine myelinolysis, which results in the "locked-in syndrome."

Because most hyponatremia is related to dehydration (low ECV) simple correction of this state will increase the sodium plasma level. If the patient has a high ECV (such as the syndrome of inappropriate antidiuretic hormone [SIADH] secretion) or is in an edematous state, free water restriction should normalize the sodium level. However, if patients have symptoms of hyponatremia, aggressive replacement of sodium is prudent should the duration of the hyponatremia be determined to be no longer than 48 hours. Hyponatremic states longer than 48 hours increase the risk of central pontine myelinolysis. Chronic cases need replacement at rates not to exceed 0.5 mEq/L/h. Acute cases may be replaced at rates of 5 mEq/L/h.

Hypernatremia is an uncommon finding and is related to large volumes of free water loss (through insensible routes such as breathing, sweating, and ventilation), diabetes insipidus, adrenal hyperfunction, or ingestion or administration of increased sodium solutions. Again, the symptoms are predominantly CNS oriented because of brain cell dehydration. Symptoms rarely occur until serum sodium levels exceed 160 mEq/L. In addition, the rapidity at which the derangement occurs determines the symptoms manifested. Treatment is carefully done with replacement of free water. Replacement too rapidly can cause cerebral edema and herniation. Patients with chronic hypernatremia need free water administration, which decreases the serum sodium no faster than 0.7 mEq/L.

Potassium Derangements

Whereas sodium is the major extracellular cation, potassium is the major intracellular cation by a ratio of 30:1. The intracellular potassium concentrations tend to be relatively constant, whereas the extracellular concentrations vary depending upon renal function/excretion. The majority of potassium secretion occurs in the distal tubule and the collecting duct of the nephron. Secretion is stimulated by increased urine flow, increased sodium delivery, high potassium levels, alkalosis, aldosterone, vasopressin, and β-adrenergic agonists. Insulin causes potassium to move into cells (as previously mentioned), reducing the extracellular concentration of potassium. Serum potassium levels are further affected by the acid-base status of patients. In alkalotic states, the potassium shifts into cells in exchange for hydrogen ions, whereas in acidotic states the exchange is opposite.

The predominant reason for hyperkalemia in a postoperative patient is renal dysfunction or failure. When these patients become critically ill, serum potassium concentrations can increase by 0.3 to 0.5 mEq/L/day in noncatabolic patients and 0.7 mEq/L/day in catabolic patients. It is important to rule out a spuriously elevated level secondary to hemolysis at the time of the blood draw either from too small a gauge of needle or simply from the application of the tourniquet and squeezing (191).

Hyperkalemia changes the membrane potential established by differences between the intracellular and extracellular milieu. This increased concentration has deleterious effects on cardiac muscle function, causing peaked T waves, flattened P waves, prolonged QRS complexes, and deep S waves on the ECG and possibly resulting in ventricular fibrillation and cardiac arrest. Skeletal musculature is also affected with paresthesias and weakness, which can progress to a flaccid paralysis.

Treatment for hyperkalemia has been outlined in the section on renal risk factors. The mainstay is saline diuresis unless ECG changes are present, then infusion of calcium gluconate can be lifesaving. Utilization of 25 to 50 g of glucose and 10 to 20 units of regular insulin can drive potassium intracellularly and transiently lower plasma levels. Ultimately, definitive therapy relies upon increased excretion of potassium. For each gram of sodium polystyrene sulfonate (Kayexalate, given in the doses previously mentioned) used either orally or rectally, 0.5 mEq of potassium will be removed. Finally, in patients not responding to these therapies or patients with renal failure, hemodialysis may be indicated.

Hypokalemia is caused by decreased intake, increased gastrointestinal losses (vomiting, diarrhea, fistulae), excessive renal losses (metabolic alkalosis, magnesium deficiency, hyperaldosteronism), a shift of potassium into the intracellular space (acute or uncompensated metabolic alkalosis, glucose and insulin administration, catecholamines), or any combination thereof. A reduction of serum potassium by 1 mEq/L represents a total body deficiency of about 100 to 200 mEq. (Remember that total exchangeable potassium is approximately 3,000 mEq with the majority being intracellular and thus the majority of the loss [191].) Symptoms of hypokalemia cause ECG changes with flattening of the T waves, depression of S-T segments, prominent U waves, and prolongation of the Q-T interval. Treatment is accomplished by replacement of potassium either orally or intravenously, depending upon the severity of symptoms and whether or not the patient is able to take oral preparations. Intravenous replacement of potassium can be done at approximately 10 mEq/h and should not be more concentrated than 40 mEq/L. If less fluid is desired, 20 mEq can be placed in 100 mL, but administration should not exceed 40 mEq/h (191).

Magnesium Derangements

Most magnesium in the body is confined to the intracellular space and bone. Less than 1% of total body magnesium is in the serum. Of the magnesium in the serum, 60% is ionized, 25% is protein bound, and 15% is complexed with nonprotein anionic species (191). Magnesium is absorbed in the small intestine, directed by levels of vitamin D, and filtered by the kidney for excretion. Approximately 40% of renally excreted magnesium is reabsorbed in the ascending loop of Henle. Loop diuretics, hypermagnesemia, hypercalcemia, acidosis, and phosphate depletion result in increased excretion of magnesium.

Patients with renal failure and receiving magnesium-containing antacids or laxatives can become hypermagnesemic. In addition, patients with acidosis and dehydration may become hypermagnesemic. Patients present with CNS depression, loss of deep tendon reflexes, and ECG changes (prolonged P-R interval and QRS complex) in the face of elevated magnesium levels (greater than 8 mg/dL). As levels rise, patients will develop coma, respiratory failure, and/or cardiac arrest. Acute treatment of hypermagnesemia is slow IV infusion of 5 to 10 mEq of calcium. Because the etiology of this condition is usually renal failure, withholding magnesium-containing preparations may be all that is necessary. In severe instances, hemodialysis is required.

In gynecologic oncology patients, the overwhelming reason for hypomagnesemia is a history of cisplatin administration. However, other conditions such as hypoparathyroidism, malabsorptive states, chronic loop diuretic use, and the diuretic phase of acute renal failure can cause hypomagnesemia. Symptoms are similar to hypocalcemia with muscle weakness, fasciculations, tetany, hypokalemia, and ECG changes (Q-T prolongation, torsade de pointes). Treatment can be accomplished with oral preparations in less acute situations. However, large doses may produce diarrhea, worsening the situation. Intravenous boluses of 2 to 3 g followed by infusions of 1 to 2 mEq/kg/day can be utilized for patients with severe symptoms.

Calcium Derangements

Almost all the calcium in the body is in bone, stored as hydroxyapatite crystals, and provides a supply that can be exchanged to the serum. Calcium homeostasis is controlled by parathyroid hormone (PTH), controlling intestinal absorption of calcium, renal excretion of calcium, and exchange of calcium from the bone. In the serum, calcium exists in three phases: 45% as an ionized form, which is responsible for most of the physiologic function of calcium; 40% in a protein bound form, bound mostly to albumin; and 15% in a nonionized form, complexed with nonprotein anions that do not easily dissociate. A serum total calcium level is usually obtained when assessing calcium homeostasis, as measurement of ionized calcium is cumbersome. The total calcium levels change by 0.8 g/dL for each 1 g/dL change of albumin (up or down) (191).

In gynecologic oncology patients with hypercalcemia, the underlying malignancy is usually the etiologic agent. Hypercalcemia may be caused by direct bony involvement or, more commonly, secretion of PTH-like peptides and/or other humoral factors, which increase serum calcium levels. Other reasons for hypercalcemia include primary, secondary, or tertiary hyperparathyroidism, thiazide diuretic use, or lithium usage (191,200). Patients present with muscle fatigue, weakness, confusion, coma, ECG changes (shortening of the Q-T interval), nausea, and vomiting. The goal of treatment is to increase calcium excretion and stop bone turnover in order to decrease serum total calcium. Initial measures include vigorous hydration (200 mL/h) with 0.9% or 0.45% saline solutions. Furosemide or other loop diuretics may be helpful in patients with borderline cardiac function or in patients with fluid overload. If the underlying malignancy is a breast carcinoma, patients may respond to high doses of steroids to reduce calcium levels. Other pharmacologic agents have been developed to stop bone resorption and reduce serum calcium levels. Calcitonin (4 IU/kg every 12 hours via subcutaneous or intramuscular injection) has a rapid onset of action and works by interfering with osteoclast maturation at several points (200). However, the duration of response is usually about 48 hours because of down-regulation of calcitonin receptors by osteoclasts. Bisphosphonates have emerged as the drug of choice for treatment of hypercalcemia in malignancy. These agents work by inhibiting osteoclast activity and survival. The nitrogen-containing bisphosphonates are the most potent. Pamidronate (approved in 1991) and zoledronic acid (approved in 2001) are utilized in the United States. Another agent, ibandronate, is utilized in Europe but has not been approved for use in the United States. Zoledronic acid is the current drug of choice because of its proven superiority over pamidronate (201). The effective dose of zoledronic acid is 4 mg infused over 15 minutes and dosed every 3 to 4 weeks. Serum calcium levels return to normal in approximately 10 days and duration of response lasts approximately 40 days (202). Surgical resection is the treatment of choice for primary, secondary, or tertiary hyperparathyroidism (191,200).

Hypocalcemia is caused by hypoparathyroidism, hypomagnesemia, pancreatitis, and malnutrition. Patients present with tetany, hyperactive deep tendon reflexes, a positive Chvostek sign, positive Trousseau sign, and ECG changes (prolonged Q-T interval, prolonged S-T segment). Low levels of calcium may be present because of low albumin levels, but these levels do not affect the ionized portion of calcium and usually do not cause symptoms. Symptomatic hypocalcemia can be treated with intravenous infusion of either calcium gluconate or calcium chloride at a rate not to exceed 50 mg/min. Calcium chloride dissociates into the ionized form of calcium more readily and is the treatment of choice to raise serum ionized calcium level.

Acid-Base Disturbances

Optimum cellular function requires a very narrow range of pH for chemical reactions to occur normally. Several buffering systems exist within the body to maintain this optimum pH. The predominant buffering system is the carbonic acid-bicarbonate buffering system. Derangements in the concentration of bicarbonate (HCO_3^-) or in concentrations of carbon dioxide (CO_2) result in acid-base disorders. Because the kidneys control excretion/generation of bicarbonate and the lungs exchange CO_2, these organs play a central role in the compensation of any acid-base disorder. Therefore, four situations arise in acid-base balance: metabolic acidosis and alkalosis, and respiratory acidosis and alkalosis. Compensatory mechanisms exist in each situation in order to blunt the effect on pH (Table 11.14).

Metabolic Acidosis

Most clinically significant metabolic acidosis occurs with a net loss of bicarbonate either due to direct loss or when consumption is greater than generation. Situations where extra renal losses of bicarbonate occur include diarrhea, gastrointestinal fistulae, and urinary diversions (ureterosigmoidostomy or ureteroileostomy, which result in reabsorption of NH_4Cl from urine). Certain disease states result in the production of organic acids (ketoacidosis and lactic acidosis), which consume bicarbonate and outpace the renal compensatory mechanisms. Similarly, overdoses of certain drugs (e.g., aspirin) or ingestion of toxins (e.g., ethylene glycol, methanol) consume bicarbonate and outpace the renal compensatory mechanisms. Renal acidosis occurs when the intrinsic acid-excreting function of the kidney malfunctions, resulting in retention of acid and consumption of bicarbonate without concomitant regeneration of bicarbonate. These are classified as renal tubular acidosis (RTA I, distal tubule dysfunction; or RTA-II, proximal tubule dysfunction). Cardiac effects are the major findings in metabolic acidosis (peripheral arteriolar dilation, decreased

TABLE 11.14

CONCENTRATIONS OF HCO_3^- AND PCO_2 IN PRIMARY ACID-BASE DERANGEMENTS AND THE COMPENSATORY RESPONSE

	Primary		Compensatory response		
Disorder	pH	HCO_3^-	PCO_2	HCO_3^-	PCO_2
Metabolic acidosis	↓	↓			↓
Metabolic alkalosis	→	→			→
Respiratory acidosis	↓		→	→	
Respiratory alkalosis	→		↓	↓	

Source: Adapted from Wait RB, Kahng KU, Dresner LS. Fluid and electrolytes and acid-base balance. In: Greenfield LJ, Mulholland M, Oldham KT, et al. eds. *Surgery: Scientific Principles and Practice.* 2nd ed. Philadelphia: Lippincott–Raven Publishers, 1997:242–266, with permission.

cardiac contractility, and central venous constriction). Other manifestations of metabolic acidosis include gastric distention, abdominal pain, nausea, and vomiting. In surgical patients, lactic acidosis is the primary cause of metabolic acidosis and results from tissue hypoperfusion. Therefore, treatment should be aimed at increasing tissue perfusion with fluid and blood administration. The use of bicarbonate is best reserved for patients with other, not easily reversible causes of metabolic acidosis. Older patients and patients with cardiovascular disease may benefit from administration of bicarbonate. Administration should be instituted when the pH is 7.1 to 7.2. One or two ampules of bicarbonate (approximately 55 mEq/amp) can be administered intravenously, with further administrations being dictated by the pH obtained from an arterial blood gas measurement. In diabetic ketoacidosis, treatment with insulin and glucose infusion should not only reverse the acidosis but also treat the hyperglycemia.

Metabolic Alkalosis

Sustained metabolic alkalosis is an uncommon clinical entity and is related to renal dysfunction. Loss of HCl is the most common reason for an increase in extracellular bicarbonate. This situation occurs with prolonged nausea and vomiting or prolonged nasogastric suctioning of gastric contents. As acid is removed from the gastrointestinal tract, a net gain of bicarbonate occurs. Other situations that can result in metabolic alkalosis include volume contraction, exogenous administration of bicarbonate or bicarbonate precursors (citrate, lactate, or calcium carbonate), hypokalemia, hypercalcemia, hypochloremia, excess mineralocorticoid usage, and high PCO_2. Patients rarely present with symptoms, as metabolic alkalosis occurs gradually. However, in patients who develop this situation acutely, most symptoms are CNS oriented (e.g., confusion, stupor, coma, muscle fasiculations, tetany). Correction of the underlying disease state usually corrects the metabolic alkalosis. Repletion of electrolyte abnormalities and infusion of appropriate fluids (chloride containing) restore volume and result in normal renal excretion of excess bicarbonate.

Respiratory Acidosis

A depression of the pH occurs when there is hypoventilation. This occurs secondary to airway obstruction, COPD, depression of the respiratory center, impaired excursion of the thorax, or inappropriate ventilatory management in the mechanically ventilated patient. Development of symptoms depends upon the chronicity or acute nature of the event. If chronic, most patients have no symptoms. If it is an acute change, drowsiness, restlessness, headache, or development of a flapping tremor may occur. Treatment of this condition is aimed at the underlying cause of the hypoventilation. In chronic conditions, the hypoxemia, and subsequent hypercapnia, resulting from the hypoventilation may be the sole drive for the patient's respirations. Correction of the hypoxemia may further worsen the respiratory acidosis and must be considered. In general, correction of the PCO_2 must be done slowly because re-equilibration of cerebral bicarbonate concentration lags behind systemic changes (191).

Respiratory Alkalosis

Respiratory alkalosis occurs when the PCO_2 decreases with hyperventilation. Hyperventilation may occur because of hypoxia, drugs, decreased lung compliance, and mechanical ventilation. With drops in the arterial PO_2, the peripheral chemoreceptors (in the carotid and aortic body) sense this change and result in hyperventilation to increase arterial PO_2 with a resulting decrease in PCO_2. Because of renal compensatory mechanisms, this condition is usually asymptomatic. However, in acute situations, patients may have a sensation of breathlessness, dizziness, nervousness with altered levels of consciousness, and tetany. Treatment of underlying hypoxia should address the hyperventilation. If acute symptoms are present, having the patient re-breathe expired air should temporarily relieve the symptoms.

Postoperative Nutritional Issues

As mentioned earlier, the full consideration of nutrition in the gynecologic oncology patient is presented in Chapter 33. In this section, we will discuss early refeeding in the postoperative gynecologic oncology patient, indications for enteral nutrition, and total parenteral nutrition (TPN).

Although malnutrition has been shown to be prevalent among gynecologic oncology patients (98), many patients are adequately nourished, undergo surgery uneventfully, and have return of bowel function in 2 to 5 days while simultaneously resuming oral intake. Recently, several prospective randomized trials have been conducted that demonstrate the utility of early refeeding in the postoperative period. In these studies, patients in the early feeding group were fed on the first postoperative day, with 90% or more tolerating diets. The underlying malignancies, types of operations, and complications occurred at similar rates between the early refeeding and the "traditionally fed" patients in all the studies. The placement of nasogastric tubes (NGTs) for intolerance of diet was low among the studies (less than 10% incidence). Finally, length of hospital stay was shorter among the earlier fed patients (203–208).

The use of the enteral route is preferred in sustaining or repleting patients in the postoperative period after extensive procedures. Enteral nutrition utilizes normal physiologic absorptive mechanisms, maintains gut epithelial integrity, and reduces infectious morbidity (209,210). Studies on nutrition have found that the splanchnic circulation and support of the mucosal integrity of the small bowel may prevent progression to MODS (see Section on Multi-Organ Dysfunction Syndrome). Specifically, the intestinal mucosa will atrophy secondary to lack of luminal nutrients and intermittent activation of the destructive cytokine pathways, and/or intermittent translocation of bacteria into the blood stream will occur. These events result in "priming" neutrophils, which ultimately leads to a full-blown systemic inflammatory response, causing organ damage. A number of well-designed randomized trails have compared early enteral feeds to TPN in patients with pancreatitis, major elective surgery, and trauma (209,210). All of these studies have shown a clear benefit for early enteral feeding, with a decrease in infectious complications (210).

Although considered a nonessential amino acid in nourished, healthy patients, glutamine has emerged as an essential amino acid in patients who are stressed and critically ill. This amino acid has been shown to be an important component in maintaining enterocyte integrity and has now been added to most enteral preparations (101,209,210).

Enteral feeds may be given in a variety of fashions and each is associated with its own type and number of complications. Intragastric feeds may be accomplished with NGTs, oral-gastric tubes, or percutaneous endoscopic gastrostomy tubes (PEGs). Intragastric feeding has the advantage of utilizing the stomach as a reservoir for bolus feeding. In addition, stretching of the stomach stimulates the biliary-pancreatic axis, which may be trophic to the small bowel. Finally, the gastric secretions mix with the feeding material and decrease the osmolarity, thus reducing the incidence of diarrhea. The main disadvantage of this route of enteral feeding is the increased risk of gastric overdistention with high residual amounts of feeding material and the increased risk of aspiration pneumonia (209). Enteral feeds may also be accomplished through the placement of nasal tubes, which are positioned into the pylorus, duodenum, or jejunum (such as Dobhoff tubes). These tubes have the advantage of being placed (or migrating) more distal in the upper gastrointestinal tract, greatly reducing the risk of aspiration. These types of tubes are preferred in patients who require long-term ventilation. Because of advances in endoscopic instrumentation, many of the tubes can be placed via this method. At the time of laparotomy, gastrostomy, or jejunostomy, tubes (such as a Stamm or Witzel tube) may be placed. These have the advantage of being placed at the time of major abdominal surgery under direct visualization/palpation. The techniques are described in other texts (209,211). Several enteral feeding preparations are available, but vary from hospital to hospital depending upon formulary makeup. The use of the enteral route is contraindicated in patients with mechanical intestinal obstructions, and for these patients nutritional support can be accomplished through the parenteral route.

TPN took the forefront in nutritional sustenance and replacement in the 1980s. The basic premise of TPN is to provide dietary precursors to maintain anabolic function. TPN can be broken into three components of replacement: glucose and lipid preparations for normal or increased energy expenditures, and amino acid preparations for protein synthesis. Because of the higher osmolar load presented by these preparations, central venous access is necessary for administration. Subclavian, internal jugular, or peripherally inserted central catheters (PICCs) will need to be placed, and they present the first of several potential complications associated with TPN administration. At the time of placement, pneumothorax, intubation of arterial structures, air embolism, or cardiac arrhythmias may occur. Later complications include the possibility of infection at the skin entrance site or line sepsis. Should these infectious complications occur, removal of the catheter and antibiotic administration will be necessary (101).

The Harris-Benedict equation is utilized to calculate basal energy expenditure (BEE) for patients and approximates the BEE of a sedentary, fasting, nonstressed individual (212).

$$\text{BEE} = 666 + (9.6 \times \text{weight [kg]}) + (1.7 \times \text{height [cm]}) - (4.7 \times \text{age [yr]})$$

Because stress of disease and surgical intervention need to be considered, "stress factors" have been developed and are multiplied by the BEE to arrive at kilocalories per day. Stress level multipliers are 1.2 for a resting individual, 1.3 for an ambulatory individual or moderate stress (e.g., systemic inflammatory response syndrome [SIRS], sepsis), and 1.5 for severe stress/burn patients.

After calculation of caloric requirements, the composition of the TPN solution to be administered should be determined. Because there are many different types of TPN preparations available, consultation with the nutrition team or pharmacists in an individual hospital is necessary to arrive at the desired solution.

In aerobic situations, glucose is the primary substrate for energy expenditure. It provides 3.4 kcal/g and is usually given in a concentrated form in order to provide 70% of the calculated calories. The remaining 30% of calories is provided by lipid preparations. Not only does this component have denser caloric content (it provides 9 kcal/g), but administration precludes the development of a fatty acid deficiency. Adjustment of the composition of TPN may be necessary depending upon the disease state (e.g., more contribution of kilocalories from fat vs. carbohydrate in a ventilated patient because of the respiratory quotient of fat vs. glucose).

Protein requirements are provided by amino acid solutions and are determined by the patient's age, sex, nutritional status, ongoing stress, and comorbid conditions. In general, 25% of protein requirements are obtained by normal oral intake. The remaining protein comes from breakdown of serum and organic proteins. Thus, periods of prolonged malnutrition, with decreased protein intake, and increased stress of disease will lead to breakdown of visceral protein. An estimate of maintenance protein requirements is 1 g nitrogen per kilogram of body weight. In situations of increased stress, the patient may need 1.2 to 1.5 g/kg in order to maintain and/or replace protein losses. Table 11.15 shows serum protein measurements and their respective half-lives, which are useful for determining anabolic versus catabolic response to TPN treatment. Another method to assess nitrogen balance (positive or negative) is (192):

$$\text{Nitrogen balance} = \text{protein intake}/6.25 - (\text{urinary urea nitrogen} + 4)$$

The amount of protein intake is divided by 6.25 to give the grams of nitrogen taken in. The urinary urea nitrogen is expressed in grams based upon a 24-hour collection. The correction factor of 4 is meant to adjust for the grams of nitrogen lost in the stool or non–urea nitrogen losses.

In addition to these three main components of TPN, daily requirements of vitamins, trace elements, and insulin are necessary to maintain/regain nourishment. Again, these preparations vary by hospital formulary and need consultation with resident pharmacists.

The rate of infusion of TPN needs to be titrated upward to take into account the large glucose load that the patient will be receiving. This lower rate allows the pancreas time to increase insulin secretion in order to meet the glucose load being presented. Similarly, the rate of infusion needs to be decreased when TPN is being stopped to prevent hypoglycemia. During TPN administration, blood glucose measurements by finger stick are required so that hyperglycemia is avoided. For the first several days, measurement of serum electrolytes, with adjustments being made daily, is necessary.

TABLE 11.15

VISCERAL PROTEINS UTILIZED AS INDICATORS FOR NUTRITIONAL STATUS DURING NUTRITIONAL REPLETION

Protein	Normal range	Half-life (days)	Levels low in	Levels high in
Albumin	3.5–5.4 g/dL	18	Liver disease, pregnancy, overhydration, nephrotic syndrome	Dehydration
Transferrin	200–400 mg/dL	8	Chronic infection, chronic inflammation, liver disease, iron overload, nephrotic syndrome	Iron deficiency, pregnancy
Prealbumin	20–40 mg/dL	2	Liver disease, inflammation, surgery, nephrotic syndrome	
Retinol-binding protein (RBP)	3–6 mg/dL	0.5	Liver disease, hyperthyroidism, zinc deficiency, nephrotic syndrome	Renal insufficiency

As previously mentioned, complications from venous access are some of the drawbacks of TPN administration. Other complications include metabolic derangements, which most often are mild but need correcting as soon as they are identified, abnormalities of liver function tests, the clinical significance of which is unclear (101), and cholelithiasis/cholecystitis secondary to gallbladder sludge.

Renal Issues

Acute renal failure (ARF) or hospital-acquired renal insufficiency (HARI) continues to be a common problem among postsurgical patients. Although the incidence of HARI is 1.5 patients per 1,000 admitted, the impact of HARI on morbidity and mortality is quite high (mortality averages 45% but may exceed 80% if dialysis is required). The best methods for preventing HARI are reducing risk factors and reversing the condition by early detection and intervention (213).

When HARI presents in the postoperative patient, causes can be divided into three parts: prerenal, renal, or postrenal (inflow, parenchymal, and outflow). The function of glomeruli to create the urinary filtrate depends upon adequate renal perfusion and represents the prerenal component. If the renal mean arterial pressure (MAP) falls below 80 mm Hg, perfusion of the glomeruli decreases (some disease states require the renal MAP to be higher for adequate perfusion). Many situations can decrease renal MAP and include anesthetics, atherosclerotic emboli, decreased vascular resistance, hypotension, intravascular volume contraction, mechanical ventilation, sepsis, and any form of shock. Autoregulation of the glomeruli can be disrupted by nonsteroidal anti-inflammatory drugs (NSAIDs), angiotensin-converting enzyme (ACE) inhibitors, calcium channel blockers (diltiazem or verapamil), and endotoxins produced by gram-negative sepsis.

Renal parenchymal damage occurs most commonly in the postoperative patient because of prolonged hypotension or direct injury from inflammatory responses initiated by sepsis. In general, if the hypoperfusion is corrected quickly, reversible azotemia, creatinine elevation, and decreased urine output may be the only manifestations. However, prolonged hypoperfusion can cause acute tubular necrosis (ATN), which results in sloughing of renal tubular cells into the tubular lumen and obstruction. In addition, the production of Tamm-Horsfall proteins forms coarse granular casts, inciting an intense inflammatory response, further injuring the renal parenchyma (214,215). Other agents that can induce ATN include aminoglycoside antibiotics and iodinated contrast media. Approximately 15% of patients who receive aminoglycosides will have nephrotoxicity, and serum levels of these antibiotics need to be carefully monitored (216). Iodinated contrast media, used in multiple radiographic procedures, induces ATN by impairing nitric oxide production and increasing free radical formation (217,218). Diabetic patients with creatinine clearance rates less than 50 mL/min are at particularly high risk (219).

The final reason for ARF in the postoperative gynecologic oncology patient is outflow obstruction. Because of the radical pelvic procedures performed by gynecologic oncologists, ureteral injury is possible and needs to be excluded early in the evaluation of patients with ARF. Prompt reversal of the obstruction can further limit renal damage.

In general, expected postoperative urinary output should be maintained at 0.5 mL/kg of weight per hour. Most oliguria can be treated with intravascular expansion in the first 24 to 48 hours postsurgery. Hypoperfusion of the renal parenchyma must be avoided to prevent ATN from occurring. The definition of ARF is not standardized, but includes rising serial creatinine measurements, urine output less than 400 mL/24 hours, or, in drastic situations, the initiation of dialysis (213). Once diagnosed, calculating the fractional excretion of sodium (FENa) or chloride can help to discern between prerenal causes or renal causes (hypoperfusions versus ATN). The formula is presented below (213):

$$\text{FENa} = (\text{urine Na level} \times \text{serum Cr level})/(\text{serum Na level} \times \text{urine Cr level}) \times 100\%$$

If the FENa is less than 1% and the urine specific gravity is greater than 1.025, the diagnosis is hypoperfusion. However, if ischemia has occurred, the FENa will be greater than 4% and the urine specific gravity will fall to 1.01 because of tubular damage and loss of renal concentrating mechanisms. One cannot calculate FENa in patients who have received diuretics or hyperosmotic agents (e.g., mannitol or contrast media). If prerenal and renal causes of low urine output have been excluded, ultrasonography may be useful in evaluating for outflow obstruction.

Once the underlying causes for HARI have been eliminated (e.g., hypoperfusion, obstruction, sepsis), only time can be offered as treatment. Therapies such as low-dose dopamine, furosemide, or mannitol administration, or atrial natriuretic peptide use have not demonstrated prevention of or improved recovery from HARI (220–225). Dialysis remains the only intervention that can support patients until return of renal function. Indications for dialysis include (a) hyperkalemia, metabolic acidosis, or volume expansion that cannot be controlled; (b) symptoms of uremia or encephalopathy; or (c) platelet dysfunction inducing a bleeding diasthesis (213).

Shock

Definition

Shock is defined in its simplest terms as a decrease in tissue perfusion—a decrease below the lowest metabolic needs of the tissue bed. This usually results in a depletion of stored energy and an increase in anaerobic metabolism with a buildup of lactic acid in addition to other toxic waste products. Hypotension is incorrectly thought of as a defining component of shock. Hypotension often leads to hypoperfusion, but the hypotensive patient is not in shock until evidence of hypoperfusion occurs. Various types of shock exist.

Hemorrhagic Shock

The first thought for a surgeon managing a postoperative patient who manifests signs and symptoms of shock is hemorrhage. Hypovolemic shock secondary to inadequate preload can be the result of excessive or ongoing blood loss or inadequate replacement or both. Certainly after radical debulking procedures or major extirpative procedures, the potential for postoperative hemorrhage exists. Tachycardia, hypotension, and oliguria are typical clinical signs. In the face of these clinical signs, the surgeon should have high suspicion for active bleeding and be preparing to return the patient to the operating room for correction. Measurement of hemoglobin or hematocrit can be normal in the setting of acute blood loss since a decrease in red cells is accompanied by a decrease in mass. Once fluid is given for resuscitation, dilution will occur and the hemoglobin/hematocrit will fall. With invasive monitoring, the CVP will be low, as will cardiac output and the PAOP. As the stroke volume decreases to inadequate amounts, the heart compensates by increasing the heart rate in order to maintain cardiac output. The treatment in these cases is aggressive volume resuscitation and control of ongoing blood loss. The controversy between resuscitation with colloid (albumin, plasma) or crystalloid (normal saline or lactated Ringer's solution) was mentioned earlier in the chapter. However, The Cochrane evidence-based review on this subject has proclaimed no benefit for colloid and perhaps an increased mortality with colloid (as well as cost). Recently, a large multicenter Australian study began in an attempt to shed more light on this subject, and its results are anticipated. As mentioned earlier, the ratio of crystalloid replacement to blood loss is 3 to 1 (3 cc crystalloid for each estimated 1-cc loss of blood). Blood products including packed red blood cells and fresh frozen plasma (in the case of a coagulopathy) are also indicated.

Endpoints of resuscitation include normalization of serum lactic acid and base deficit. Measurement of the base deficit via an arterial blood gas analysis has become an effective means for following response to resuscitation. Following large operations where patients are admitted to the ICU and where large, expected fluid shifts occur, the base deficit should be monitored serially until it has returned to normal. If a patient has a worsening base deficit (i.e., becomes more negative), then a search for other problems, such as ongoing hemorrhage, subacute anastamotic leak(s), or tissue ischemia, must be made and be addressed before the base deficit will normalize. The base deficit should normalize within the first 24 hours after surgery.

In the case of continued or rapid bleeding, the obvious course of treatment is reoperation. A number of options are now available intraoperatively in these situations. Obvious bleeders are controlled and ligated. Raw surfaces can be coagulated or treated with fibrin sealants. Damage-control packing has been shown to increase survival in the direst situations. Massive transfusion, defined as greater than 1.5 blood volumes, presents a number of additional problems. These patients will have a dilutional coagulopathy, hypocalcemia, and hyperkalemia. After six to eight red blood cell transfusions have been given in rapid fashion for massive bleeding, some would advocate empiric fresh frozen plasma and platelets. Platelet transfusion is indicated for a platelet count <50,000 in the actively bleeding patient. Attention to delivery of warm transfusions is critical as hypothermia and acidosis will promote coagulopathy and worsening in bleeding. Once any of the "lethal triad" is manifested then the operation needs to be quickly terminated even if this means damage-control packing and transport to an ICU setting.

Cardiogenic Shock

A patient with adequate preload who shows signs of poor perfusion secondary to poor cardiac output is categorized as being in cardiogenic shock. The etiology may be a decrease in contractility (secondary to myocardial infarction) or an increase in afterload (severe hypertension). Typically, "pump failure" results in decreased stroke volume and backup of fluid into the pulmonary circulation. This leads to pulmonary edema and decreased oxygen delivery. The most common provocation for pump failure is the overadministration of fluid in a patient with compromised ventricular function. Treatment consists of diuresis and optimization of cardiac output without increasing myocardial oxygen demand (a difficult task). In the case where significant failure has led to hypotension, dopamine and dobutamine are usually the drugs of choice. The usage of these drugs was discussed previously. Digoxin is commonly used for increasing contractility, but its effects are minor in the acute setting. In addition to inotropic support, correction of electrolyte disturbances (particularly potassium, calcium, and magnesium), maintenance of proper systemic oxygen saturation, and analgesia are important factors in decreasing myocardial stress.

Septic Shock

Septic shock has commonly been defined as hypotension related to infection with eventual organ failure secondary to hypoperfusion despite adequate fluid resuscitation. This definition has changed with that of SIRS and is discussed in the section on "Sepsis and Systemic Inflammatory Response Syndrome" below. Sepsis is defined as a subset of patients with SIRS who have a documented infectious process.

Infectious Disease Issues

Infections in the critically ill patient population are a significant cause of morbidity and mortality. Approximately 45% of ICU patients will have an infection and approximately half of those will have acquired the infection while in the ICU (226). Nosocomial infections are commonly associated with complications of medical or surgical therapy. Patients in the ICU are particularly vulnerable to infection because of decreased host defenses and the high incidence of resistant bacterial isolates found in ICUs. In addition, the presence of indwelling catheters and lines lowers the inoculum needed to cause infection and provides portals of entry (226). Initial therapy involves identifying and eradicating the source of infection and promptly initiating empirical antibiotic therapy aimed at multidrug-resistant gram-negative and gram-positive organisms. If an intra-abdominal or pelvic source is suspected, empiric antibiotic therapy should include anaerobic coverage. Appropriate antibiotic classes include carbapenems, extended-spectrum penicillins, fluoroquinolone-metronidazole, aminoglycoside-metronidazole, or clindamycin combinations (227). In Chapter 30 the management of infections in the gynecologic cancer patient is discussed; therefore, information here is limited to infections pertaining to the critically ill patient.

Fungal Infections

Systemic fungal infections are a significant cause of morbidity and mortality in patients admitted to the ICU. A nonspecific and variable presentation makes the diagnosis of systemic candidal infection difficult. Risk factors that have been associated with candidemia and invasive candidiasis include treatment with multiple antibiotics for extended periods, the presence of central venous catheters, the use of TPN, abdominal surgery, prolonged ICU stay, and compromised immune status (228). Although a positive blood culture is the gold standard for diagnosis, blood culture techniques are relatively insensitive and clinicians frequently must rely on clinical judgment about the probability that candidemia is responsible for a patient's symptoms. ICU patients who have persistent fever, hypothermia, or unexplained hypotension, despite broad spectrum antibiotic coverage, may have candidemia. The initial choice of therapeutic agents depends on the epidemiologic characteristics of the particular ICU and host factors such as the severity of illness, infection site(s), neutropenia, and organ dysfunction. Fluconazole has excellent activity against *Candida albicans*, but infections caused by *Candida glabrata* or *Candida krusei* must be treated with amphotericin B or caspofungin. Amphotericin B should not be used in patients with renal failure, and azoles and echinocandins (caspofungin) should be used with caution in patients with hepatic dysfunction. Antifungal therapy should be continued for 14 days past the first negative blood culture for candidemia or until clinical microbiological or radiographical resolution of the infection (229). In addition to antifungal therapy, it is generally recommended that all patients with candidemia have a dilated eye exam by an ophthalmologist and that all catheters be removed if possible (although tunneled catheters are at less risk) (228).

Abdominal Infections

The diagnosis of an intra-abdominal source of infection can be difficult in critically ill patients. Symptoms such as abdominal pain and peritoneal signs may not be apparent in patients who are obtunded or sedated and on a ventilator. Fever and leukocytosis may be absent in 35% and 55% of peritoneal infections, respectively (230). Ultrasonography is a useful diagnostic test that can be performed in the ICU and may assist with therapeutic intervention as well. It is extremely sensitive for evaluations of the pelvis and right upper quadrant, but evaluation of the entire abdomen can be limited by bowel gas, surgical dressings, and operator experience. For many of these reasons, a computed tomographic (CT) scan is the preferred study for the evaluation of patients with suspected intra-abdominal infection. To avoid misdiagnosing fluid-filled bowel as a possible abnormal fluid collection, it is essential that contrast agents be used when performing these studies. CT also has limitations, especially when used in the critically ill population. The presence of renal insufficiency precludes the use of intravenous contrast, and ileus or bowel obstruction may prevent complete opacification of the gastrointestinal tract. Diagnostic laparoscopy can be performed in the ICU with minimal anesthesia and is a safe, accurate, and cost-effective alternative to laparotomy when managing suspected intra-abdominal processes (231).

Once identified, an intra-abdominal abscess must be fully evacuated and the source controlled. Radiologically assisted percutaneous drainage has become the preferred method for treating most abscesses located in the abdomen and pelvis. For well-delineated unilocular fluid collections, percutaneous drainage has a success rate better than 80% (232). Percutaneous drainage of complex abscesses or those with an enteric communication has a lower success rate, but remains a reasonable alternative treatment for the high-risk patient (233).

In some cases, surgery may be the only appropriate lifesaving intervention. Timely laparotomy in the critically ill patient with diffuse peritonitis allows for peritoneal toilet, debridement of infected and necrotic tissue, and control or repair of the source. Laparoscopic drainage of complex intra-abdominal abscess has also been reported with good success rates (234). Complex intra-abdominal infections that cannot be effectively controlled by a single laparotomy may be managed best with an open-abdomen approach with temporary wound closure utilizing a composite, negative pressure (vacuum-pack) dressing (235). Potential advantages of the open-abdomen approach include facilitation of repeated debridement, effective drainage, repeat exploration of the peritoneal cavity (at the ICU bedside if necessary), and reduction in intra-abdominal pressure. In general, the intervention that accomplishes the source control objective with the least physiologic upset should be employed (236).

Sepsis and Systemic Inflammatory Response Syndrome

Inflammation is the body's initial response to tissue injury produced by chemical, mechanical, or microbial stimuli. Inflammation is an exceedingly complex cellular and humoral response involving interaction between the complement, kinin, coagulation, and fibrolytic cascades. The goal of inflammation is to enhance the movement of nutrients and phagocytic cells to the injury site in order to prevent invasion of microbes and limit the extension of injury. As a local response, this is beneficial, but appropriate regulation is necessary to prevent a pathologic, exaggerated systemic response, which is clinically identified as SIRS. Sepsis is the clinical syndrome of SIRS that is due to severe infection. The mediator response in SIRS can be divided into four phases based on the cytokine/cellular response: induction, triggering of cytokine synthesis, evolution of cytokine and coagulation cascade, and elaboration of secondary mediators leading to cellular injury. The three most important mediators operating in SIRS appear to be tumor necrosis factor-α (TNF-α), interleukin-1 (IL-1), and interleukin-6 (IL-6). The microcirculation endothelium is the key target for injury in the sepsis syndrome (237).

TABLE 11.16

DEFINITIONS FOR SYSTEMIC INFLAMMATORY RESPONSE AND SEPSIS (SIRS)

SIRS	Two or more of the following in the setting of a known cause of inflammation: Temperature >38°C or <36°C Pulse >90 Respirations >20/min or $PaCO_2$ <32 mm Hg WBC count >12,000 or <4,000 cells/mm³ or >10% band forms
Sepsis	SIRS due to known infection
Severe sepsis	Sepsis with evidence of organ dysfunction, hypoperfusion, or hypotension
Septic shock	Sepsis with hypotension despite adequate fluid resuscitation

Source: Adapted from 1991 American College of Chest Physicians/ Society of Critical Care Medicine Consensus Conference definitions.

In 1992, the American College of Chest Physicians and the Society of Critical Care Medicine published definitions for SIRS and sepsis (Table 11.16) with the goal of standardizing terminology to aid clinicians in the diagnosis and treatment and to aid in the interpretation of research in this field (238). Many have criticized the 1992 consensus definitions as too nonspecific to be of use. In 2001, a group of experts reconvened and expanded the list of signs and symptoms of sepsis to reflect clinical bedside experience. In addition to the original criteria, altered mental status, oliguria, skin mottling, coagulopathy, hypoxemia, hyperglycemia in the absence of diabetes, thrombocytopenia, and altered liver function tests can also be used to establish the diagnosis of sepsis (239).

The host response, more than the pathogen, is the primary determinant of patient outcome. Failure to develop a fever, leukopenia, and hypothermia are associated with increased fatality rates in patients with sepsis and are thought to represent abnormalities in the host's inflammatory response. Other risk factors for mortality from sepsis include age greater than 40, underlying medical conditions, malnutrition, immune suppression, and cancer. The presence or absence of a positive blood culture does not influence outcomes; however, sepsis due to a nosocomial infection has a higher mortality than community-acquired infection (240).

Sepsis with acute organ dysfunction (severe sepsis) is a complex condition that represents a major challenge to the critical care team and carries a crude mortality rate of 28% to 50% (241). Gram-negative and gram-positive organisms as well as fungi cause systemic sepsis and septic shock. Early recognition is crucial to patient survival because mortality rates are exceedingly high if the full clinical picture of shock and organ dysfunction develops. Septic shock is divided into an early hyperdynamic state and a late hypodynamic state.

Low systemic vascular resistance, splanchnic vasoconstriction, and increased cardiac output characterize the hyperdynamic phase of shock. Venous capacitance is increased and results in diminished effectiveness of the circulating blood volume. Aggressive volume resuscitation must be provided to restore cardiac preload and ventricular filling. These patients are best managed in an ICU with the placement of an arterial line, a PA catheter, and a bladder catheter. Appropriate cultures should be obtained and intravenous broad-spectrum antibiotics should be started within the first hour of recognition of severe sepsis. Laboratory tests of immediate concern include arterial blood gas determinations, creatinine, electrolytes, lactate, coagulation panel, and a complete blood count. Oxygenation and ventilation should be optimized with mechanical ventilation if indicated. If hypotension persists after optimization of the PCWP, the use of norepinephrine or dopamine may be necessary. Surgical debridement or manipulation of infected material should not be performed until the patient has been stabilized.

Early goal-directed therapy of the septic patient has been shown to improve survival. During the first 6 hours of resuscitation, the goals of therapy as outlined by the Surviving Sepsis Campaign guidelines include CVP of 8 to 12 mm Hg, mean arterial pressure ≥65 mm Hg, urine output ≥0.5 mL/kg/h, and central venous or mixed venous oxygen saturation ≥70%. If during the first 6 hours oxygen saturation goals are not achieved despite appropriate CVP, then transfusion of red blood cells to achieve a Hct >30% and/or initiation of a dobutamine infusion is the next step (242).

In the hypodynamic phase of septic shock, hypotension results from cardiac output deterioration. The patient is often cool, mottled, oliguric, diaphoretic, and confused. The etiology of the hypodynamic cardiovascular response to sepsis may be inadequate volume resuscitation, underlying cardiac disease, or myocardial dysfunction associated with sepsis. This is a state of gross decompensation with global tissue hypoxia and is associated with greater mortality.

Numerous clinical trials have attempted to find specific agents that could modulate the underlying disease process in sepsis. Candidate therapies included agents that target mediators of inflammatory response, agents that boost the immune system, and prostaglandin inhibitors, but none was shown to be beneficial until recently. The Recombinant Human Activated Protein C Worldwide Evaluation in Severe Sepsis (PROWESS) study is the first clinical trial to show a clinically significant reduction in the 28-day all-cause mortality rate due to severe sepsis (243). This multicenter, prospective, double-blind, placebo-controlled study enrolled 1,690 patients who were randomized to treatment with a continuous infusion of drotrecogin alfa (activated) at a dose of 24 μg/kg/h for a total of 96 hours or placebo. Drotrecogin alfa (activated) is a recombinant form of human activated protein C, an endogenous protein with antithrombotic, pro-fibrinolytic, and anti-inflammatory properties that is frequently deficient in sepsis. Eligible patients were 18 years of age or older with a documented or a highly suspicious source of infection, at least three of the SIRS criteria, and evidence of acute end-organ dysfunction, including shock, severe hypoxia, oliguria, or acidosis for less than 24 hours. Patients began treatment within 24 hours of meeting study criteria. Drotrecogin alfa (activated) has significant anticoagulant properties; therefore, patients at high risk of or from bleeding were excluded, as well as those who were pregnant or breast-feeding, had human immunodeficiency virus infection with CD4 cell count ≤50/mm^3, weighed >35 kg, had a transplanted organ other than a kidney, or were expected to die from non-sepsis-related disease within 1 month. The mortality rate was 30.8% in the placebo group and 24.7% in the treatment arm, with a reduction in relative risk of death of 19.4% and an absolute reduction in risk of death of 6.1% ($p = 0.005$). Although patients considered to be at higher risk of bleeding were excluded, serious bleeding conditions were higher in the drotrecogin alfa (activated) group (3.5% vs. 2.0%, $p = 0.06$). The FDA has approved drotrecogin alfa (activated) for the treatment of patients with sepsis who have a high risk of death. In light of the increased bleeding risk, appropriate patient selection for treatment with drotrecogin alfa (activated) should be an important consideration (242).

In addition to early goal-directed therapy with hemodynamic interventions that balance systemic oxygen delivery with oxygen demand and the use of drotrecogin alfa (activated), other management strategies have also been shown in randomized, controlled trials to reduce mortality associated with severe sepsis. These include limiting the tidal volume to 6 to 7 mL/kg ideal body weight for patients requiring mechanical ventilation for ARDS, the use of moderate-dose corticosteroids (hydrocortisone 200 to 300 mg and fludrocortisone 50 μg daily) for 7 days in patients with refractory septic shock, and maintaining serum glucose levels <150 mg/dL (242). These therapies are not mutually exclusive and optimal patient management may require a combination of approaches. Some of these strategies vary dramatically from traditional approaches and will require education and established protocols to safely incorporate them into practice.

Multiple Organ Dysfunction Syndrome

Multiple organ dysfunction syndrome (MODS) can be defined as the development of progressive physiologic dysfunction of two or more organ systems after an acute threat to systemic homeostasis (238). Inciting factors are diverse and include SIRS, sepsis, massive trauma, burns, ischemia, and reperfusion injury. Consensus has not been reached as to the criteria used to define this clinical syndrome, that is, which organ systems are important or the degree of physiologic derangement necessary to constitute dysfunction. Pulmonary dysfunction is common and typically develops early in the course of SIRS or sepsis. Renal dysfunction initially is a prerenal azotemia unless the initial insult promoted a sudden oliguric acute tubular necrosis. Hyperbilirubinemia is the earliest marker of hepatic dysfunction. Gastrointestinal abnormalities include ileus, stress ulcers, diarrhea, and mucosal atrophy. The platelet count has been used as a surrogate marker of the hematologic system. Cardiac function is often measured by the degree of hypotension or the need for vasopressors. Deterioration of the nervous system is manifested by encephalopathy and peripheral neuropathies. The treatment of MODS is support of individual organ function and aggressive therapies aimed at correcting the underlying process. Mortality is related to the number of dysfunctional systems and is greater than 80% once four organ systems fail (244).

The Acute Physiology and Chronic Health Evaluation (APACHE) provided population-based estimates of mortality for the day of ICU admission (245). Several versions of the APACHE scoring system have been utilized, most recently APACHE IV. Organ failure scores, such as the Sequential Organ Failure Assessment (SOFA), can help assess organ dysfunction over time and are useful to evaluate morbidity. Independent of the initial value, an increase of the SOFA score (Table 11.17) during the first 48 hours of an ICU admission predicts a mortality rate of 50% or greater, and improvement of cardiovascular, renal, or respiratory SOFA score from baseline through day 1 of ICU admission is significantly related to greater survival (246). It is important to note that these and other outcome prediction models were designed as tools to be used in critical care research in order to stratify patients by severity of illness. They have not been validated for making decisions relating to individual patients.

Abdominal Compartment Syndrome

Abdominal compartment syndrome (ACS) is an important but often unrecognized cause of acute deterioration of a patient after massive fluid resuscitation for septic or hypovolemic shock. Although most commonly associated with trauma patients, it has also been observed in patients with massive ascites, bowel obstruction or ileus, peritonitis, pancreatitis, and intraperitoneal blood. Intra-abdominal pressure (IAP) is usually measured indirectly by a balloon-tipped catheter in the bladder. Intra-abdominal hypertension is defined as an IAP of

TABLE 11.17

THE SEQUENTIAL ORGAN FAILURE ASSESSMENT (SOFA) SCORE

	SOFA score				
Variables	0	1	2	3	4
Respiratory: PaO_2/FIO_2, mm Hg	>400	≤400	≤300	≤200[a]	≤100[a]
Coagulation: platelets × $10^3/\mu L$[b]	>150	150	100	50	20
Liver bilirubin, mg/dL[b]	<1.2	1.2–1.9	2.0–5.9	6.0–11.9	>12.0
Cardiovascular hypotension	No hypotension	Mean arterial pressure <70 mm Hg	Dop ≤5 or Dob (any dose)[c]	Dop >5, Epi 0.1, or Norepi 0.1[c]	Dop >15, Epi >0.1, or Norepi >0.1[c]
Central nervous system, Glasgow Coma Scale score	15	13–14	10–12	6–9	<6
Renal creatinine, mg/dL or urine output, mL/d	<1.2	1.2–1.9	2.0–3.4	3.5–4.9 or <500	>5.0 or <200

Note: Dob, dobutamine; Dop, dopamine; Epi, epinephrine; FIO_2, fraction of inspired oxygen; Norepi, norephinephrine; PaO_2, partial pressure oxygen.
[a]Values are with respiratory support.
[b]To convert bilirubin from mg/dL to μmol/L, multiply by 17.1.
[c]Adrenergic agents administered for at least 1 hour (doses given are in μg/kg per minute).
Source: From Ferreira FL, Bota DP, Bross A, et al. Serial evaluation of the SOFA score to predict outcome in critically ill patients. *JAMA* 2001;286:1754–1758, with permission.

12 mm Hg or greater recorded by a minimum of three standard measurements conducted 4 to 6 hours apart (247). ACS is defined by an IAP of 20 mm Hg or greater and single or multiple organ failure that was not previously present. Although ACS can impair the function of every organ system, it is generally manifested as hypotension, reduced urine output, and decreased pulmonary compliance. Operative decompression of the abdominal cavity with maintenance of an open abdomen via use of temporary closure techniques such as a vacuum pack is the only treatment that reverses the physiological abnormalities resulting from ACS.

Withdrawal of Life-Sustaining Treatment

The decision to withdraw or withhold life-sustaining treatment is most difficult for patients, families, and health professionals. The ethical aspect of foregoing treatment resides in the legal and ethical right of the patient to self-determination. Unfortunately, the majority of critically ill patients are unable to speak for themselves when decisions to limit treatment are considered. Therefore, careful attention must be paid to previously expressed wishes and the input of surrogate decision makers. If a medical power of attorney is not in place, some states stipulate who the surrogate will be by a legal hierarchy. The ethical basis for identification of an appropriate surrogate is primary if none of the preceding legal bases apply. In this situation, the physician and other health care providers have the responsibility to help identify the person or persons who have knowledge of the patient's values and preferences in order to assist with medical decisions on the patient's behalf. This process can become difficult in circumstances when family members or others close to the patient are in disagreement as to who should be the surrogate or what the patient would prefer. In these cases, health care providers should be knowledgeable of applicable legal directives and their ethical responsibility to act in their patient's best interest. Consultation with the institution's ethics committee may be helpful in trying to reach consensus (248). Although not responsible for the patient's death, those close to the patient often are left with feelings of guilt and anxiety in addition to their bereavement. It is important that the health care providers support the family both before and after the decision to withhold or withdraw life-sustaining treatment has been made.

End of life care of patients in the ICU requires a dramatic paradigm shift in attitude and interventions from intensive rescue-type care to intensive palliative care. When considering the array of interventions that may be discontinued or held, physicians and surrogates should focus on clearly articulating the goals of care. For example, a goal for survival until the patient's important loved ones can gather to say their good-byes may justify short-term continuation of ventilator support. If the only goal is patient comfort, then such treatment should be stopped. The withdrawal of life-sustaining treatment is a clinical procedure that deserves the same preparation and expectation of quality as other medical procedures. Honest, caring, and culturally sensitive communication with the patient's loved ones and the patient, if competent, should include explanations of how therapies will be withdrawn, what symptoms are expected, strategies to assess and ensure the patient's comfort, and information about the expected survival after interventions are withdrawn. Informed consent should be documented along with a formulated plan for withdrawing care (249). Adequate analgesia and sedation should be prescribed to relieve symptoms of pain, dyspnea, and anxiety during the dying process. Intravenous opioids and shorter acting benzodiazepines are the drugs of choice. The clinician's primary goal should be to prevent suffering and ensure the patient's comfort even if doing so unintentionally hastens the patient's death.

Neurologic Issues

The critically ill patient is invariably anxious, stressed, confused, uncomfortable, or in pain from immobility, wounds, preexisting disease, infection, invasive medical interventions, and routine nursing care such as airway suctioning, repositioning, or dressing changes. The restlessness and distress often associated with critical illness must be quelled with analgesia, sedation, and neuromuscular blockade as a last resort. The Society of Critical Care Medicine and American Society of Health-System Pharmacists (ASHP) clinical practice guidelines for sedation, analgesia, and neuromuscular blockade of the critically ill adult were revised in 2002. This comprehensive document is available online at www.ashp.org (250,251).

Analgesia

Maintaining an optimal level of comfort and safety for critically ill patients is a universal goal for all involved in their care. Unrelieved pain contributes to inadequate sleep and agitation. Pain may contribute to pulmonary dysfunction through localized guarding and generalized muscle rigidity that restricts movement of the chest wall and diaphragm. Unrelieved pain also evokes a stress response characterized by tachycardia, increased myocardial oxygen consumption, hypercoagulability, immunosuppression, and persistent catabolism (252). The combined use of effective analgesia and sedation may ameliorate the stress response and diminish pulmonary complications in postoperative critically ill patients. A comprehensive overview of pain management is covered in Chapter 32; therefore, only key aspects of pain management applicable to patients in the ICU will be addressed.

Pharmacologic therapies include opioids, NSAIDs, and acetaminophen. ASHP guidelines recommend fentanyl, hydromorphone, and morphine given as a continuous infusion or scheduled doses rather than "as needed." Fentanyl has the most rapid onset and shortest duration, but repeated dosing may cause accumulation and prolonged effects. Fentanyl may also be administered via a transdermal patch to hemodynamically stable patients with more chronic analgesic needs, but it is not recommended for the management of acute pain. Morphine has a quick onset but longer duration of action, so intermittent doses may be given. However, morphine causes histamine release, which contributes to hypotension, especially in a hemodynamically unstable patient. Hydromorphone's duration of action is similar to morphine but lacks an active metabolite or histamine release, making it an ideal drug for continuous infusion and for use in patients who cannot tolerate hypotension. Meperidine has an active metabolite that causes neuroexcitation including apprehension, tremors, delirium, and seizures, so its use is not recommended in critically ill patients who may need repeated doses. The characteristics of analgesics and sedatives commonly used in ICU patients are summarized in Table 11.18.

Sedation

Sedatives are commonly used adjuncts for the treatment of anxiety and agitation. The physical environment of the ICU, limited ability to communicate, sleep deprivation, and medical circumstances precipitating the ICU admission are contributing factors creating anxiety in critically ill patients. Efforts to reduce anxiety, including frequent reorientation, provision of adequate analgesia, and optimization of the environment, may be supplemented with sedatives. Agitation is also common in ICU patients; however, not all patients with anxiety will exhibit agitation. Sedatives reduce the stress response and improve tolerance to routine ICU procedures. They may be necessary to facilitate mechanical ventilation. Generally, sedatives should be administered intermittently to determine the dose needed to achieve the sedation goal, but they may be given as a continuous infusion if necessary. Daily interruption of sedative infusion is associated with shorter duration of mechanical ventilation, shorter ICU stays, and fewer instances of posttraumatic stress disorder (253,254). Benzodiazepines are sedatives and hypnotics that cause anterograde amnesia but lack analgesic properties. Midazolam has a rapid onset and short duration of effect with single doses, making it ideal for treating acutely agitated patients or for brief sedation with invasive procedures. Lorazepam has a slower onset but fewer potential drug interactions because of its metabolism via glucuronidation (Table 11.18).

TABLE 11.18

CHARACTERISTICS OF SELECTED ANALGESICS AND SEDATIVES FREQUENTLY USED IN CRITICALLY ILL PATIENTS

Agent	Indication	Active metabolites (effect)	Adverse effects	Intermittent dose (IV)[a]	Infusion dose range
Fentanyl	Pain	No metabolite, patient accumulates	Rigidity with high doses	0.35–1.5 µg/kg q 0.5–1 h	0.7–10 µg/kg/h
Hydromorphone	Pain	None	—	10–30 µg/kg q 1–2 h	7–15 µg/kg/h
Morphine	Pain	Yes (sedation)	Histamine release	0.01–0.15 mg/kg q 1–2 h	0.07–0.5 mg/kg/h
Ketorolac	Pain	None	GI bleeding, renal	15–30 mg q 6 h; decrease if >65 yr; avoid >5 day use	—
Midazolam	Acute agitation	Yes (prolonged sedation)	—	0.02–0.08 mg/kg q 0.5–2 h	0.04–0.2 mg/kg/h
Lorazepam	Sedation	None	Solvent-related acidosis/renal failure in high doses	0.02–0.06 mg/kg q 2–6 h	0.01–0.1 mg/kg/h
Propofol	Sedation	None	Elevated triglycerides	—	5–80 µg/kg/min
Haloperidol	Delirium	Yes (EPS)	QT interval prolongation	0.03–0.15 mg/kg q 0.5–6 h	0.04–0.15 mg/kg/h

Note: EPS, extrapyramidal symptoms; GI, gastrointestinal; IV, intravenous.
[a]More frequent doses may be needed for acute management in mechanically ventilated patients.

Propofol is an intravenous general anesthetic that has sedative and hypnotic properties at lower doses. Like the benzodiazepines, propofol has no analgesic properties. Propofol has a rapid onset and short duration of sedation once discontinued. Propofol is a phospholipid emulsion that provides 1.1 kcal/mL from fat and should be counted as a caloric source. Long-term infusions may result in hypertriglyceridemia and monitoring is recommended after 2 days of use (250). Physiologic dependence and potential withdrawal symptoms have been described in ICU patients who have been exposed to more than 1 week of sedative or narcotic therapy, including the use of propofol (255).

Neuromuscular Blockade

Neuromuscular blocking agents (NMBAs) can be used to facilitate mechanical ventilation, to manage intracranial pressure in head trauma, to ablate muscle spasms, and to decrease oxygen consumption only when all other means to accomplish these aims have failed (251). Pancuronium is a long-acting NMBA that is effective for up to 90 minutes after intravenous bolus dose of 0.06 to 0.1 mg/kg. It can be used as a continuous infusion by adjusting the dose to the degree of neuromuscular blockade that is desired. Since pancuronium is vagolytic, 90% of patients will have an increase in heart rate of greater than 10 beats per minute. For patients who cannot tolerate an increase in heart rate, vecuronium can be used. If neuromuscular blockade is necessary for patients with significant hepatic or renal failure, cisatracurium or atracurium should be used. Patients receiving any NMBA should be assessed using electronic twitch monitoring with a goal of adjusting the blockade to achieve one or two twitches. Before initiating neuromuscular blockade, patients should be adequately medicated with sedative and analgesic drugs as it is difficult to assess pain and anxiety after NMBAs are given. Furthermore, neuromuscular paralysis without sedation is an extremely frightening and unpleasant experience.

Acute quadriplegic myopathy syndrome, also referred to as postparalytic quadriparesis, is a clinical triad of acute paresis, myonecrosis with increased creatine phosphokinase concentration, and abnormal electromyography that is related to prolonged exposure to NMBAs. This is a devastating complication of NMBA therapy and one of the reasons that indiscriminate use of these agents is discouraged. Increased risk of acute quadriplegic myopathy is associated with the concurrent use of corticosteroids; drug "holidays" may decrease the risk (256).

ICU Syndrome/Delirium

The ICU syndrome, first reported in the 1960s, describes a range of psychological disturbances exhibited by many critically ill patients (257). Other designations commonly used are ICU psychosis and postoperative delirium. The ICU syndrome has been defined as an altered emotional state occurring in a highly stressful environment that may manifest itself in a variety of psychological reactions including fear, memory disturbance, anxiety, confusion, withdrawal, despair, agitation, and disorientation. Sleep deprivation, noise, constant light exposure, restriction of movement, limited ability to communicate, as well as the patient's preadmission mental state and coping ability have all been reported as causative factors of ICU syndrome. Current medical literature challenges this concept and argues that what is being called ICU syndrome or psychosis is diagnostic of delirium and not due to the ICU environment per se. Concerns have been raised that using the term *ICU syndrome* implies that confusion can be expected in the ICU setting and may reduce the vigilance necessary to recognize delirium and identify and treat the physiologic disturbances leading to it (258). Delirium is found in as many as 80% of critically ill patients and is associated with longer ICU admissions and increased mortality (259,260).

Delirium in the ICU setting is commonly caused by metabolic disturbances, hypoxia, electrolyte imbalances, alcohol or drug withdrawal, acute infection, and medications (Table 11.19) (258,260). Many drugs have anticholinergic properties that can exert an additive effect causing neurotoxicity, especially in elderly patients. Anticholinergic-related delirium can be differentiated from other causes of delirium if the mental status clears after administration of the cholinesterase inhibitor physostigmin. Delirium presents in both a hypoactive and hyperactive form. Hypoactive delirium, which is associated with the worst prognosis, is characterized by psychomotor retardation, represents more global cerebral dysfunction, and is manifested by a calm appearance, inattention, and obtundation in extreme cases. Hyperactive delirium is more easily recognized by agitation and combative behaviors. Elderly patients may pose a particular diagnostic challenge when delirium is superimposed on baseline dementia.

TABLE 11.19

COMMONLY USED ICU DRUGS ASSOCIATED WITH DELIRIUM[a]

Anesthetics	Anticonvulsants	Atropine[b]
Lidocaine	Carbamazepine	Cimetidine[b]
Propofol	Phenobarbital	Corticosteroids[b]
	Phenytoin	Digoxin[b]
Antibiotics		
Amphotericin B	Antihypertensives	Narcotic analgesics
Aztreonam	Diltiazem	Fentanyl
Cephalosporins	Enalapril	Meperidine[b]
Ciprofloxacin	Hydralazine	Morphine
Doxycycline	Methyldopa	
Imipenem	Propranolol	Nitroprusside
Metronidazole	Verapamil	Phenylephrine
Penicillins		Procainamide[b]
Tobramycin		Scopolamine[b]
		Tricyclic antidepressants[b]

[a]Listing is not intended to be all-inclusive.
[b]Drugs known to have significant anticholinergic properties.

The medical management of delirium consists of finding and treating underlying medical conditions and then controlling any behavioral disturbances if necessary. Neuroleptic drugs are the first-line agents for the treatment of delirium due to causes other than alcohol withdrawal syndrome, which is managed with benzodiazepines. Haloperidol is the neuroleptic of choice because it has minimal anticholinergic or hypotensive effects. A dose of 2 to 10 mg intravenously can be given every 20 to 30 minutes until agitation resolves. Once the delirium is controlled, scheduled doses every 4 to 6 hours consisting of 25% of necessary loading doses can be used and tapered off over several days. A continuous infusion can also be used (Table 11.18). Patients receiving repeat doses of haloperidol should be monitored for electrocardiographic changes. Extrapyramidal side effects such as rigidity, tremor, or facial tics can be managed with diphenhydramine hydrochloride (250).

References

1. Dean MM, Finan MA, Kline RC. Predictors of complications and hospital stay in gynecologic cancer surgery. *Obstet Gynecol* 2001;97(5 Pt 1):721–724.
2. Smetana GW, Macpherson DS. The case against routine preoperative laboratory testing. *Med Clin North Am* 2003;87:7–40.
3. National Institutes of Health, National Heart, Lung, and Blood Institute. *Women's Heart Health: Developing a National Health Education Action Plan.* NIH Publication No. 01–2963, Sep 2001.
4. Hollenberg SM. Preoperative cardiac risk assessment. *Chest* 1999;115 (5 Suppl):51–57.
5. Freeman WK, Gibbons RJ, Shub C. Preoperative assessment of cardiac patients undergoing noncardiac surgical procedures. *Mayo Clin Proc* 1989;64:1105–1117.
6. Romero L, de Virgillo C. Preoperative cardiac risk assessment: an updated approach. *Arch Surg* 2001;136:1370–1376.
7. Cerino M, Nattel S, Boucher Y, et al. Preoperative and long-term cardiac risk assessment. Predictive value of 23 clinical descriptors, 7 multivariate scoring systems and quantitative dipyridamole imaging in 360 patients. *Ann Surg* 1992;216:192–204.
8. Eagle KA, Boucher CA. Cardiac risk of noncardiac surgery. *N Engl J Med* 1989;321:1330–1332.
9. Blaustein AS. Preoperative and perioperative management of cardiac patients undergoing noncardiac surgery. *Cardiol Clin* 1995;13:149–161.
10. Cohn SL, Goldman L. Preoperative risk evaluation and perioperative management of patients with coronary artery disease. *Med Clin North Am* 2003;87(1):111–136.
11. Goldman L, Caldera DL, Nussbaum SR, et al. Multifactorial index of cardiac risk in noncardiac surgical procedures. *N Engl J Med* 1977;297:845–850.
12. Eagle KA, Berger PB, Calkins H, et al. ACC/AHA guideline update for perioperative cardiovascular evaluation for noncardiac surgery: a report of the American College of Cardiology/American Heart Association Task Force on Practice Guidelines (Committee to Update the 1996 Guidelines on Perioperative Cardiovascular Evaluation for Noncardiac Surgery). American College of Cardiology Web site. www.acc.org/clinical/guidelines/perio/ update/periupdate_sendindex.htm. Accessed November 15, 2002.
13. Mosca L, Banka CL, Benjamin EJ, et al. Evidence-based guidelines for cardiovascular disease prevention in women: 2007 update. *Circulation* 2007;115:1481–1501.
14. National Cholesterol Education Program. Detection, evaluation and treatment of high blood cholesterol. www.nhlbi.nih.gov/guidelines/cholesterol/index.htm. Accessed September 15, 2004.
15. Shammash JB, Ghali WA. Preoperative assessment and perioperative management of the patient with nonischemic heart disease. *Med Clin North Am* 2003;87:137–152.
16. Halm EA, Browner WS, Tubau JF, et al. Echocardiography for assessing cardiac risk in patients having noncardiac surgery. *Ann Intern Med* 1996;125:433–441.
17. Ferreira MJ. The role of nuclear cardiology for preoperative risk assessment prior to noncardiac surgery. *Rev Port Cardiol* 2001;19(Suppl 1):163–169.
18. Ashton CM, Petersen NJ, Wray, NP, et al. The incidence of perioperative myocardial infarction in men undergoing noncardiac surgery. *Ann Intern Med* 1993;188:504–510.
19. Mangano DT, Layug EL, Wallace A, et al. Effect of atenolol on mortality and cardiovascular morbidity after noncardiac surgery. *N Engl J Med* 1996;335:1713–1720.
20. Fisher BW, Majumdar SR, McAlistar FA. Predicting pulmonary complications after nonthoracic surgery: a systematic review of blinded studies. *Am J Med* 2002;112:219–225.
21. Mitchell CK, Smoger SH, Pfeifer MP, et al. Multivariate analysis of factors associated with postoperative pulmonary complications following general elective surgery. *Arch Surg* 1998;133:194–198.
22. Beecher HK. Effect of laparotomy on lung volumes: demonstration of a new type of pulmonary collapse. *J Clin Invest* 1933;12:651–666.
23. The VA Total Parenteral Nutrition Cooperative Study Group. Perioperative total parenteral nutrition in surgical patients. *N Engl J Med* 1991;325: 525–532.
24. Arozullah AM, Khuri SF, Henderson WG, et al. Development and validation of a multifactorial risk index for predicting postoperative pneumonia after major noncardiac surgery. *Ann Intern Med* 2001;135:847–857.
25. Smetana GW. Preoperative pulmonary evaluation. *N Engl J Med* 1999; 340:937–944.
26. Wong DH, Weber EC, Shell MJ, et al. Factors associated with postoperative pulmonary complications in patients with severe chronic obstructive pulmonary disease. *Anesth Analg* 1995;80:276–284.
27. Arozullah AM, Conde MV, Lawrence VA. Preoperative evaluation of postoperative pulmonary complications. *Med Clin North Am* 2003;87: 153–173.
28. Latimer RG, Dickman M, Day WC, et al. Ventilatory patterns and pulmonary complications after upper abdominal surgery determined by preoperative and postoperative computerized spirometry and blood gas analysis. *Am J Surg* 1971;122:622–632.
29. Celli BR, Rodriguez KS, Snider GL. A controlled trial of intermittent positive pressure breathing, incentive spirometry, and deep breathing exercises in preventing pulmonary complications after abdominal surgery. *Am Rev Respir Dis* 1984;130:12–15.
30. Ferguson GT, Enright PL, Buist AS, et al. Office spirometry for lung health assessment in adults: a consensus statement from the National Lung Health Education Program. *Respir Care* 2000;45:513–530.
31. De Nino LA, Lawrence VA, Averyt EC, et al. Preoperative spirometry and laparotomy: blowing away dollars. *Chest* 1997:111:1536–1541.
32. Bluman LG, Mosca L, Newman N, et al. Preoperative smoking habits and postoperative pulmonary complications. *Chest* 1998;113:883–889.
33. Moller AM, Villebro N, Pedersen P, et al. Effect of preoperative smoking intervention on postoperative complications: a randomized clinical trial. *Lancet* 2002;359:114–117.
34. Nakagawa M, Tanaka H, Tsukuma H, et al. Relationship between the duration of the preoperative smoke-free period and the incidence of postoperative pulmonary complications after pulmonary surgery. *Chest* 2001;120:705–710.
35. Harris MI, Flega KM, Cowie CC, et al. Prevalence of diabetes, impaired fasting glucose, and impaired glucose tolerance in U.S. adults. *Diabetes Care* 1998;21:518–524.
36. Guyuron B, Raszewskie R. Undetected diabetes and the plastic surgeon. *Plast Reconstr Surg* 1990;86:471–474.
37. Hoogwerf BJ. Postoperative management of the diabetic patient. *Med Clin North Am* 2001;85(5):1213–1228.
38. Walter DP, Gatling W, Houston AC, et al. Mortality in diabetic subjects: an eleven year follow-up of a community-based population. *Diabet Med* 1994;11:968–973.
39. Schiff Rl, Welsh GA. Perioperative evaluation and management of the patient with endocrine dysfunction. *Med Clin North Am* 2003;87: 175–192.
40. Hirsch IB, McGill JB. Role of insulin in management of surgical patients with diabetes mellitus. *Diabetes Care* 1990;13:980–981.
41. Hirsch IB, McGill JB, Cryer PE. Perioperative management of surgical patients with diabetes mellitus. *Anesthesiology* 1991;74:346–359.
42. DiPalo S, Ferrari G, Castoldi R, et al. Surgical septic complications in diabetic patients. *Acta Diabetol Latina* 1988;25:49–54.
43. Schiff RL, Emanuele MA. The surgical patient with diabetes mellitus: guidelines for management. *J Gen Intern Med* 1995;10:154–161.
44. Gallacher SJ, Thomason F, Fraser WD, et al. Neutrophil bactericidal function in diabetes mellitus: evidence for association with blood glucose control. *Diabet Med* 1995;12:916–920.
45. Scherpereel PA, Travernier B. Perioperative care of diabetic patients. *Eur J Anesthesiol* 2001;18:277–294.
46. Furnary AP, Zerr KJ, Grunkemeier GL. Continuous intravenous insulin infusion reduces the incidence of deep sternal wound infection in diabetic patients after cardiac surgical procedures. *Ann Thorac Surg* 1999;67: 352–362.
47. Golden SH, Peart-Vigilance C, Kao WHL. Perioperative glycemic control and the risk of infectious complications in a cohort of adults with diabetes. *Diabetes Care* 1999;22:1408–1414.
48. Pompocelli JJ, Baxter JK, Babineau TJ, et al. Early postoperative glucose control predicts nosocomial infection rate in diabetic patients. *JPEN J Parenter Enter Nutr* 1998;22:77–81.
49. Van Den Berghe G, Wouters P, Weekers F, et al. Intensive insulin therapy in critically ill patients. *N Engl J Med* 2001;345:1359–1367.
50. Weinberg AD, Brennan MD, Gorman CA. Outcome of anesthesia and surgery in hypothyroid patients. *Arch Intern Med* 1983;143:893–897.
51. Ladenson PW, Levin AA, Ridgway EC, et al. Complications of surgery in hypothyroid patients. *Am J Med* 1984;77(2):261–266.
52. Bennett-Guerrero E, Kramer DC, Schwinn DA. Effect of chronic and acute thyroid reduction on perioperative outcome. *Anesth Analg* 1997;85: 30–36.
53. Appoo JJ, Morin JF. Severe cerebral and cardiac dysfunction associated with thyroid decompensation after cardiac operations. *J Thorac Cardiovasc Surg* 1997;114:496.

54. Catz B, Russell S. Myxedema, shock and coma. *Arch Intern Med* 1961;108: 407–417.
55. Holvey DN, Goodner CJ, Nicoloff JT, el al. Treatment of myxedema coma with intravenous thyroxine. *Arch Intern Med* 1964;113:89–96.
56. Forfar JC, Muir AL, Sawrers SA, et al. Abnormal left ventricular function in hyperthyroidism. *N Engl J Med* 1982;307:1165–1170.
57. Klein I, Ojamaa K. Mechanisms of disease: thyroid hormone and the cardiovascular system. *N Engl J Med* 2001;344:501–509.
58. Sawin CT, Geller A, Wolf PA. Low serum thyrotropin concentration as a risk factor for atrial fibrillation in older patients. *N Engl J Med* 1994;331: 1249–1252.
59. Woeber KA. Thyrotoxicosis and the heart. *N Engl J Med* 1992;327: 94–97.
60. Strube PJ. Thyroid storm during beta-blockade. *Anaesthesia* 1984;39: 343–346.
61. McArthur JW, Rawson RW, Means JH, et al. Thyrotoxic crisis. *JAMA* 1947;132:868.
62. Baez A, Aguayo J, Varrie M, et al. Rapid preoperative preparation in hyperthyroidism. *Clin Endocrinol* 1991;35:439–442.
63. Roti E, Robuschi G, Gardini E, et al. Comparison of methimazole and saturated solution of potassium iodide in early treatment of hyperthyroidism in Graves' disease. *Clin Endocrinol* 1988;28:305–314.
64. Mazzaferri EL, Skillman TG. Thyroid storm: a review of 22 episodes with special emphasis on the use of guanethidine. *Arch Intern Med* 1969;124: 684–690.
65. Salem M, Rainsh RE, Bromberg J, et al. Perioperative glucocorticoid coverage: a reassessment 42 years after the emergence of a problem. *Ann Surg* 1994;219:416–425.
66. Ackerman GL, Nolan CM. Adrenocortical responsiveness after alternate-day corticosteroid therapy. *N Engl J Med* 1968;278:405–409.
67. Fauci AS. Alternate-day corticosteroid therapy. *Am J Med* 1978;64: 729–731.
68. LaRochelle GE, LaRochelle AG, Ratner RE, et al. Recovery of the hypothalamic-pituitary-adrenal (HPA) axis in patients with rheumatic disease receiving low-dose prednisone. *Am J Med* 1993;95:258–264.
69. Christy NP. Corticosteroid withdrawal. In: Bardin CW, ed. *Current Therapy in Endocrinology and Metabolism.* 3rd ed. New York: BC Decker; 1988:113.
70. Tordjman R, Jaffe A, Grazas N, et al. The role of the low dose (1 microgram) adrenocorticotropin test in the evaluation of patients with pituitary diseases. *J Clin Endocrinol Metab* 1995;80:1301–1305.
71. NKF-K/DOQI clinical practice guidelines for chronic kidney disease: evaluation, classification and stratification. *Am J Kidney Dis* 2000;37(Suppl 1): S1–S266.
72. United States Renal Data System. USRDS 2001 annual data report: atlas of end-stage renal disease in the United States. Bethesda, MD: National Institutes of Health, National Institute of Diabetes and Kidney Diseases; 2001.
73. Kellerman PS. Perioperative care of the renal patient. *Arch Intern Med* 1994;154(15):1674–1688.
74. Foley RN, Parfrey PS, Sarnack MJ. Clinical epidemiology of cardiovascular disease in chronic renal disease. *Am J Kidney Dis* 1998;32(5 Suppl 3): S112–S119.
75. Conlon PJ, Krucoff MW, Minda S, et al. Incidence and long-term significance of transient S-T segment deviation in hemodialysis patients. *Clin Nephrol* 1998;49(4):236–239.
76. Pochmalicki G, Jan F, Fouchard I. Frequency of painless myocardial ischemia during hemodialysis in 50 patients with chronic kidney failure. *Arch Mal Coeur Vaiss* 1990;83:1671–1675.
77. Braun WE, Phillips DF, Vidt DG. Coronary artery disease in 100 diabetics with end-stage renal failure. *Transplant Proc* 1984;16:603–607.
78. Koch M, Gradaus F, Schoebel DC, et al. Relevance of conventional cardiovascular risk factors for the prediction of coronary artery disease in diabetic patients on renal replacement therapy. *Nephrol Dial Transplant* 1997;12:1187–1191.
79. Joseph AJ, Cohn SL. Perioperative care of the patient with renal failure. *Med Clin North Am* 2003;87:193–210.
80. Remuzzi G, Livio M, Marchiaro G, et al. Bleeding in renal failure: altered platelet function in chronic uraemia only partially corrected by haemodialysis. *Nephron* 1978;22(4–6):347–353.
81. Mannucci PM, Remuzzi G, Pusineri F, et al. Deamino-8-arginine vasopressin shortens the bleeding time in uremia. *N Engl J Med* 1983;308:8–12.
82. Livio M, Mannucci PM, Vigano G, et al. Conjugated estrogens for the management of bleeding associated with renal failure. *N Engl J Med* 1986;315:731–735.
83. Benett WM, Aronoff GR, Golper TA, et al. *Drug Prescribing in Renal Failure: Dosing Guidelines for Adults.* 4th ed. Philadelphia: American College of Physicians; 2000.
84. Rizvon MK, Chou CL. Surgery in the patient with liver disease. *Med Clin North Am* 2003;87:211–227.
85. Runyon BA. Surgical procedures are well tolerated by patients with asymptomatic chronic hepatitis. *J Clin Gastroenterol* 1986;8:542–544.
86. O'Sullivan MJ, Envoy D, O'Donnell C, et al. Gallstones and laparoscopic cholecystectomy in hepatitis C patients. *Ir Med J* 2001;94:114–117.
87. Garrison RN, Cryer HM, Howard DA, et al. Clarification of risk factors for abdominal operations in patients with hepatic cirrhosis. *Ann Surg* 1984;199:648–655.
88. Isozaki H, Okajima K, Morita S, et al. Surgery for cholelithiasis in cirrhotic patients. *Surg Today* 1993;23:504–508.
89. Mansour A, Wateson W, Shayani V, et al. Abdominal operations in patients with cirrhosis: still a major surgical challenge. *Surgery* 1997;122:730–735; discussion 735–736.
90. Ziser A, Plevak DJ, Wiesner RH, et al. Morbidity and mortality in cirrhotic patients undergoing anesthesia and surgery. *Anesthesiology* 1999;90:42–53.
91. Gholson CF, Provenza JM, Bacon BR. Hepatologic considerations in patients with parenchymal liver disease undergoing surgery. *Am J Gastroenterol* 1990;85:487–496.
92. Bozetti F. Is enteral nutrition a primary therapy in cancer patients? *Gut* 1994;35:S65.
93. Daly JM, Redmond HP, Gallagher H. Perioperative nutrition in cancer patients. *JPEN J Parenter Enteral Nutr* 1992;16:S100.
94. Smale BF, Mullen JL, Buzby GP, et al. The efficacy of nutritional assessment and support in cancer patients. *Cancer* 1981;47:2375.
95. Hickman DM, Miller RA, Rombeau JL, et al. Serum albumin and body weight as predictors of postoperative course in colorectal cancer. *Cancer* 1980;4:314.
96. Tunca JC. Nutritional evaluation of gynecologic cancer patients during initial diagnosis of their disease. *Am J Obstet Gynecol* 1983;8:893–896.
97. Orr JW, Wilson K, Bodiford C, et al. Nutritional status of patients with untreated cervical cancer. I. Biochemical and immunology assessment. *Am J Obstet Gynecol* 1985;151:625.
98. Santoso JT, Canada T, Latson B, et al. Prognostic nutritional index in relation to hospital stay in women with gynecologic cancer. *Obstet Gynecol* 2000;95:844–846.
99. Dempsey DT, Mullen JL, Buzby GP. The link between nutritional status and clinical outcome: can nutritional intervention modify it? *Arch Surg* 1985;120:721–727.
100. Morgon DB, Hill GL, Burkinshow L. The assessment of weight loss from a single measurement of body weight: the problem and limitations. *Am J Clin Nutr* 1980;33:2102–2105.
101. Mann WJ. Nutritional complications. In: Orr JW, Shingleton HM, eds. *Complications in Gynecologic Surgery: Prevention, Recognition and Management.* Philadelphia: J.B. Lippincott; 1994:260–277.
102. Smith LC, Mullen JL. Nutritional assessment and indications for nutritional support. *Surg Clin North Am* 1991;71:449–457.
103. Buzby GP, Mullen JL, Matthews DC, et al. Prognostic nutritional index in gastrointestinal surgery. *Am J Surg* 1980;139:160–167.
104. Gibbs J, Cull W, Henderson W, et al. Preoperative serum albumin level as a predictor of operative mortality and morbidity: results from the National VA Surgical Risk Study. *Arch Surg* 1999;134:36–42.
105. Delgado-Rodriguez M, Medina-Cuadros M, Gomez-Ortega A, et al. Cholesterol and serum albumin levels as predictors of cross infection, death, and length of hospital stay. *Arch Surg* 2002;137:805–812.
106. Baker JP, Detsky AS, Wesson DE, et al. Nutritional assessment: a comparison of clinical judgment and objective measurements. *N Engl J Med* 1991;325:525–532.
107. Detsky AS, Baker JP, O'Rourke K, et al. Predicting nutrition-associated complications for patients undergoing gastrointestinal surgery. *JPEN J Parenter Enter Nutr* 1987;11:440–446.
108. Anonymous. Perioperative total parenteral nutrition in surgical patients. The Veterans Affairs Total Parenteral Nutrition Cooperative Study Group. *N Engl J Med* 1991;325:525–532.
109. Bozzetti F, Gavazzi C, Miceli R, et al. Perioperative total parenteral nutrition in malnourished, gastrointestinal cancer patients: a randomized, clinical trial. *JPEN J Parenter Enter Nutr* 2000;24:7–14.
110. Mangram AJ, Horan TC, Pearson ML, et al. Guideline for prevention of surgical site infection, 1999. Centers for Disease Control and Prevention (CDC) Hospital Infection Control Practices Advisory Committee. *Am J Infect Control* 1999;27:97–132.
111. Bratzler DW, Houck PM. Antimicrobial prophylaxis for surgery: an advisory statement from the National Surgical Infection Prevention Project. *Am J Surg* 2005;189:395–404.
112. Kirkland KB, Briggs JP, Trivette L, et al. The impact of surgical-site infections in the 1990s: attributable mortality, excess length of hospitalization, and extra costs. *Infect Control Hosp Epidemiol* 1999;20:725-730.
113. Perencevich EN, Sands KE, Cosgrove SE, et al. Health and economic impact of surgical site infections diagnosed after hospital discharge. *Emerg Infect Dis* 2003;9:196–203.
114. Webster J, Osborne S. Preoperative bathing or showering with skin antiseptics to prevent surgical site infection. *Cochrane Database of Systematic Reviews.* 2007, Issue 2. Art. No.: CD004985. DOI: 10.1002/14651858. CD004985.pub3.
115. Tanner J, Woodings D, Moncaster K. Preoperative hair removal to reduce surgical site infection. *Cochrane Database of Systematic Reviews.* 2006, Issue 3. Art. No.: CD004122. DOI: 10.1002/14651858.CD004122.pub3.
116. Bratzler DW, Hunt DR. The Surgical Infection Prevention and Surgical Care Improvement projects: national initiatives to improve outcomes of patients having surgery. *Clin Infect Dis* 2006;43:322–330.
117. Malone DL, Genuit T, Tracy JK, et al. Surgical site infections: reanalysis of risk factors. *J Surg Res* 2002;103:89–95.
118. ASHP therapeutic guidelines on antimicrobial prophylaxis in surgery. *Am J Health Syst Pharm* 1999;56:1839–1888.
119. ACOG Practice Bulletin No. 74: antibiotic prophylaxis for gynecologic procedures. *Obstet Gynecol* 2006;108:225–234.

120. Antimicrobial prophylaxis for surgery. *Treat Guidel Med Lett* 2006;4:83–88.
121. Itani K, Wilson S, Awad S, et al. Ertapenem versus cefotetan prophylaxis in elective colorectal surgery. *N Engl J Med* 2006;355:2640–2651.
122. Bowden TA Jr, DiPiro JT, Michael KA. Polyethylene glycol electrolyte lavage solution (PEG-ELS). A rapid, safe mechanical bowel preparation for colorectal surgery. *Am Surg* 1987;53:34–36.
123. Frazee RC, Roberts J, Symmonds R, et al. Prospective, randomized trial of inpatient vs. outpatient bowel preparation for elective colorectal surgery. *Dis Colon Rectum* 1992;35:223–226.
124. Curran MP, Plosker GL. Oral sodium phosphate solution: a review of its use as a colorectal cleanser. *Drugs* 2004;64:1697–1714.
125. Oliveira L, Wexner SD, Daniel N, et al. Mechanical bowel preparation for elective colorectal surgery. A prospective, randomized, surgeon-blinded trial comparing sodium phosphate and polyethylene glycol-based oral lavage solutions. *Dis Colon Rectum* 1997;40:585–591.
126. Barclay RL, Depew WT, Vanner SJ. Carbohydrate-electrolyte rehydration protects against intravascular volume contraction during colonic cleansing with orally administered sodium phosphate. *Gastrointest Endosc* 2002;56:633–638.
127. Hsu CW, Imperiale TF. Meta-analysis and cost comparison of polyethylene glycol lavage versus sodium phosphate for colonoscopy preparation. *Gastrointest Endosc* 1998;48:276–282.
128. Itani K, Wilson S, Awad S. Polyethyleneglycol versus sodium phosphate mechnical bowel preparation in elective colorectal surgery. *Am J Surg* 2007;193:190–194.
129. Valantas M, Beck D, DiPalma J. Mechanical bowel preparation in the older surgical patient. *Curr Surg* 2004;61:320–324.
130. Beloosesky Y, Grinblat J, Weiss A, et al. Electrolyte disorders following oral sodium phosphate administration for bowel cleansing in elderly patients. *Arch Intern Med* 2003;163:803–808.
131. Tan HL, Liew QY, Loo S, et al. Severe hyperphosphataemia and associated electrolyte and metabolic derangement following the administration of sodium phosphate for bowel preparation. *Anaesthesia* 2002;57:478–483.
132. Pitcher DE, Ford RS, Nelson MT, et al. Fatal hypocalcemic, hyperphosphatemic, metabolic acidosis following sequential sodium phosphate-based enema administration. *Gastrointest Endosc* 1997;46:266–268.
133. Platell C, Hall J. What is the role of mechanical bowel preparation in patients undergoing colorectal surgery? *Dis Colon Rectum* 1998;41:875–882; discussion 882–883.
134. Zmora O, Pikarsky AJ, Wexner SD. Bowel preparation for colorectal surgery. *Dis Colon Rectum* 2001;44:1537–1549.
135. Bucher P, Mermillod B, Gervas P, et al. Mechanical bowel preparation for elective colorectal surgery, a meta-analysis. *Arch Surg* 2004;139:1359–1364.
136. Guenaga K, Atallah AN, Castro AA, et al. Mechanical bowel preparation for elective colorectal surgery. *Cochrane Database of Systemic Reviews* 2005, Issue 1. Art No.: CD001544. DOI: 10.1002114651858.CD001544.pub2.
137. Zmora O, Wexner SD, Hajjar L, et al. Trends in preparation for colorectal surgery: survey of the members of the American Society of Colon and Rectal Surgeons. *Am Surg* 2003;69:150–154.
138. Lewis RT. Oral versus systemic antibiotic prophylaxis in elective colon surgery: a randomized study and meta-analysis send a message from the 1990s. *Can J Surg* 2002;45:173–180.
139. Espin-Basany E, Sanchez-Garcia JL, Lopez-Cano M, et al. Prospective, randomized study on antibiotic prophylaxis in colorectal surgery. Is it really necessary to use oral antibiotics? *Int J Colorectal Dis* 2005;20:542–546.
140. Nichols R, Choe EU, Weldon CB. Mechanical and antibiotic bowel preparation in colon and rectal surgery. *Chemotherapy* 2005;51(Suppl 1):115–121.
141. Ansell J, Hirsch J, Poller L, et al. The pharmocology and management of vitamen K antagonists: the Seventh ACCP Conference on Antithrombolic and Thrombolytic Therapy. *Chest* 2004;126:204S–233S.
142. Ang-Lee MK, Moss J, Yuan CS. Herbal medicines and perioperative care. *JAMA* 2001;286:208–216.
143. Crosby E. Perioperative use of erythropoietin. *Am J Ther* 2002;9:371–376.
144. Ng SP. Blood transfusion requirements for abdominal hysterectomy: 3-year experience in a district hospital (1993–1995). *Aust N Z J Obstet Gynaecol* 1997;37:452–457.
145. Lentz SS, Shelton BJ, Toy NJ. Effects of perioperative blood transfusion on prognosis in early-stage cervical cancer. *Ann Surg Oncol* 1998;5:216–219.
146. Dodd RY, Notari EP, Stramer SL. Current prevalence and incidence of infectious disease markers and estimated window-period risk in the American Red Cross blood donor population. *Transfusion* 2002;42:975–979.
147. Dunne JR, Malone D, Tracy JK, et al. Perioperative anemia: an independent risk factor for infection, mortality, and resource utilization in surgery. *J Surg Res* 2002;102:237–244.
148. Taylor RW, Manganaro L, O'Brien J, et al. Impact of allogenic packed red blood cell transfusion on nosocomial infection rates in the critically ill patient. *Crit Care Med* 2002;30:2249–2254.
149. Vanderlinde ES, Heal JM, Blumberg N. Autologous transfusion. *BMJ* 2002;324:772–775.
150. Popovsky MA, Whitaker B, Arnold NL. Severe outcomes of allogeneic and autologous blood donation: frequency and characterization. *Transfusion* 1995;35:734–737.
151. Goldman M, Savard R, Long A, et al. Declining value of preoperative autologous donation. *Transfusion* 2002;42:819–823.
152. Horowitz NS, Gibb RK, Menegakis NE, et al. Utility and cost effectiveness of preoperative autologous blood donation in gynecologic and gynecologic oncology patients. *Obstet Gynecol* 2002;5:771–776.
153. Shander A, Rijhwani TS. Acute normovolemic hemodilution. *Transfusion* 2004;44:26S–34S.
154. Monk TG, Goodnough LT, Brecher ME, et al. A prospective randomized comparison of three blood conservation strategies for radical prostatectomy. *Anesthesiology* 1999;91:24–33.
155. Goodnough LT, Despotis GJ, Merkel K, et al. A randomized trial comparing acute normovolemic hemodilution and preoperative autologous blood donation in total hip arthroplasty. *Transfusion* 2000;40:1054–1057.
156. Jabbour N, Gagandeep S, Maeteo R, et al. Live donor liver transplantation without blood products: strategies developed for Jehovah's Witnesses offer broad application. *Ann Surg* 2004;240:350–357.
157. Koenig SM. Pulmonary complications of obesity. *Am J Med Sci* 2001;321: 249–279.
158. Haslam DW, James WP. Obesity. *Lancet* 2005;366:1197–1209.
159. Gaszynski T. Anesthetic complications of gross obesity. *Curr Opin Anaesthesiol* 2004;17:271–276.
160. Hopkins MP, Shriner AM, Parker MG, et al. Panniculectomy at the time of gynecologic surgery in morbidly obese patients. *Am J Obstet Gynecol* 2000;182:1502–1505.
161. Pearl ML, Valea FA, Disilvestro PA, et al. Panniculectomy in morbidly obese gynecologic oncology patients. *Int J Surg Invest* 2000;2:59–64.
162. Tillmanns TD, Kamelle SA, Abudayyeh I, et al. Panniculectomy with simultaneous gynecologic oncology surgery. *Gynecol Oncol* 2001;83:518–522.
163. Eisner RF, Montz FJ, Berek JS. Cytoreductive surgery for advanced ovarian cancer: cardiovascular evaluation with pulmonary artery catheter. *Gynecol Oncol* 1990;37:11.
164. Weitz HH. Perioperative cardiac complications. *Med Clin North Am* 2001;85:1151–1169.
165. Ho K, Pinsky JL, Kannel WB, et al. The epidemiology of heart failure: the Framingham Study. *J Am Coll Cardiol* 1993;22:6A–13A.
166. American Heart Association. Heart and stroke statistical update. http://www.americanheart.org/downloadable/heart/10148328094661013190990123HS_State_send02.pdf. Accessed November 15, 2002.
167. Zaloga GP, Prielipp RC, Butterworth JF, et al. Pharmacologic cardiovascular support. *Crit Care Clin* 1993;9:335–362.
168. Guidelines for cardiopulmonary resuscitation and emergency cardiac care. Emergency Cardiac Care Committee and Subcommittees, American Heart Association. Part III. Adult advanced cardiac life support. *JAMA* 1992; 268:2199–2241.
169. Chiolero R, Flatt J-P, Revelly J-P, et al. Effects of catecholamines on oxygen consumption and oxygen delivery in critically ill patients. *Chest* 1991;100: 1676–1684.
170. Raymer K, Yang H. Patients with aortic stenosis: cardiac complications in non-cardiac surgery. *Can J Anaesth* 1998;45:855–859.
171. Torsher LC, Shub C, Rettke SR, et al. Risk of patients with severe aortic stenosis undergoing noncardiac surgery. *Am J Cardiol* 1998;81:448–452.
172. Dajani AS, Taubert KA, Wilson W, et al. Prevention of bacterial endocarditis. *Circulation* 1997;96:358–366.
173. Christians KK, Wu B, Quebbeman EJ, et al. Postoperative atrial fibrillation in noncardiothoracic surgical patients. *Am J Surg* 2001;182:713–715.
174. Balser JR, Martinez EA, Winters BD, et al. Beta-adrenergic blockade accelerates conversion of postoperative supraventricular tachyarrhythmias. *Anesthesiology* 1998;89:1052–1059.
175. Roy D, Talajic M, Dorian P, et al. Amiodarone to prevent recurrrence of atrial fibrillation. *N Engl J Med* 2000;342:913–920.
176. Bersten AD, Rutten AJ, Vedig AE. Additional work of breathing imposed by endotracheal tubes, breathing circuits, and intensive care ventilators. *Crit Care Med* 1989;21:1333–1337.
177. Banner MJ, Jaeger MJ, Kirby RR. Components of the work of breathing and implications for monitoring ventilator-dependent patients. *Crit Care Med* 1994;22:515–518.
178. Stewart T, Meade M, Cook D, et al. The Pressure and Volume-Limited Ventilation Strategy Group (1998). Evaluation of a ventilation strategy to prevent barotrauma in patients at high risk for acute respiratory distress syndrome. *N Engl J Med* 1998;338:356–361.
179. Amoto M, Barbas C, Medeiros D, et al. Effect of a protective-ventilation strategy on mortality in the acute respiratory distress syndrome. *N Engl J Med* 1998;338:347–354.
180. Lodat, R. Oxygen toxicity. *Crit Care Clin* 1990;6:749–765.
181. Kirby R, Downs J, Civetta J, et al. High level positive end expiratory pressure (PEEP) in acute respiratory insufficiency. *Chest* 1975;67:156–163.
182. Dries D. Weaning from mechanical ventilation. *J Trauma* 1997;43:372–384.
183. Bulger E, Jurkovich G, Gentilello L, et al. Current clinical options for the treatment and management of acute respiratory distress syndrome. *Crit Care Rev* 2000;48:562–572.
184. Bernard G, Artigas A, Brigham, KL, et al. Report of the American-European Consensus Conference on Acute Respiratory Distress Syndrome: definitions, mechanisms, relevant outcomes, and clinical trial coordination. Consensus Committee. *J Crit Care* 1994;9:72–81.
185. Luce J. Acute lung injury and the acute respiratory distress syndrome. *Crit Care Med* 1998;26:369–376.
186. Marshall J, Cook D, Christou N, et al. Multiple organ dysfunction score: a reliable descriptor of a complex clinical outcome. *Crit Care Med* 1995;23: 1638–1652.
187. Chastre J, Fagon JY. Ventilator-associated pneumonia. *Am J Respir Crit Care Med* 2002;165:867–903.

188. Clagett P, Anderson F, Geerts W, et al. Prevention of venous thromboembolism. *Chest* 1998;(114):531S–560S.
189. Pestana C. *Fluids and Electrolytes in the Surgical Patient*. 4th ed. Baltimore: Williams & Wilkins; 1989.
190. Vanatta JC, Fogelman MJ, eds. *Moyer's Fluid Balance: A Clinical Manual*. 2nd ed. Chicago: Year Book; 1976.
191. Wait RB, Kahng KU, Dresner LS. Fluids and electrolytes and acid-base balance. In: Greenfield LJ, Mulholland M, Oldham KT, et al., eds. *Surgery: Scientific Principles and Practice*. 2nd ed. Philadelphia: Lippincott–Raven Publishers; 1997:242–266.
192. Lowe RJ, Moss GS, Jilek J, et al. Crystalloid versus colloid in the etiology of pulmonary failure after trauma. A randomized trial in man. *Surgery* 1977;81:676–683.
193. Virgilio RW, Rice CL, Smith DE, et al. Crystalloid versus colloid resuscitation: is one better? A randomized clinical study. *Surgery* 1979;85:129–139.
194. Weinstein PD, Doerfler ME. Systemic complications of fluid resuscitation. *Crit Care Clin* 1992;8:439–448.
195. Metildi LA, Shackford SR, Virgilio RW, et al. Crystalloid versus colloid in fluid resuscitation of patients with severe pulmonary insufficiency. *Surg Gynecol Obstet* 1984;158:207–212.
196. Rizoli SB. Crystalloids and colloids in trauma resuscitation: a brief overview of the current debate. *J Trauma* 2003;54(5 Suppl):S82–S88.
197. Alderson P, Schierhout G, Roberts I, et al. Colloids versus crystalloids for fluid resuscitation in critically ill patients. *Cochrane Database Syst Rev* 2000;(2):CD000567.
198. Choi PT, Yip G, Quinonez LG, et al. Crystalloids vs. colloids in fluid resuscitation: a systematic review. *Crit Care Med* 1999;27:200–210.
199. Roberts JS, Bratton SL. Colloid volume expanders. Problems, pitfalls and possibilities. *Drugs* 1998;55:621–630.
200. Berenson JR. Treatment of hypercalcemia of malignancy with bisphosphonates. *Semin Oncol* 2002;29(Suppl 21):12–18.
201. Mundy GR. Hypercalcemia. In: *Bone Remodeling and Its Disorders*. 2nd ed. London: Martin Dunitz; 1999:107–122.
202. Major P, Lortholary A, Hon J, et al. Zolendronic acid is superior to pamidronate in the treatment of hypercalcemia of malignancy: a pooled analysis of two randomized, controlled clinical trials. *J Clin Oncol* 2001;19:558–567.
203. Pearl ML, Frandina M, Mahler L, et al. A randomized controlled trial of a regular diet as the first meal in gynecologic oncology patients undergoing intraabdominal surgery. *Obstet Gynecol* 2002;100:230–234.
204. Pearl ML, Valea FA, Fischer M, et al. A randomized controlled trial of early postoperative feeding in gynecologic oncology patients undergoing intra-abdominal surgery. *Obstet Gynecol* 1998;92:94–97.
205. Cutillo G, Maneschi F, Franchi M, et al. Early feeding compared with nasogastric decompression after major oncologic gynecologic surgery: a randomized study. *Obstet Gynecol* 1999;93:41–45.
206. MacMillan SL, Kammerer-Doak D, Rogers RG, et al. Early feeding and the incidence of gastrointestinal symptoms after major gynecologic surgery. *Obstet Gynecol* 2000;96:604–608.
207. Steed HL, Capstick V, Flood C, et al. A randomized controlled trial of early versus "traditional" postoperative oral intake after major abdominal gynecologic surgery. *Am J Obstet Gynecol* 2002;186:861–865.
208. Schilder JM, Hurteau JA, Look KY, et al. A prospective controlled trial of early postoperative oral intake following major abdominal gynecologic surgery. *Gynecol Oncol* 1997;67:235–240.
209. Souba WW, Austen WG Jr. Nutrition and metabolism. In: Greenfield LJ, Mulholland M, Oldham KT, et al., eds. *Surgery: Scientific Principles and Practice*. 2nd ed. Philadelphia: Lippincott–Raven Publishers; 1997:42–67.
210. Marik PE, Zaloga GP. Early enteral nutrition in acutely ill patients: a systematic review. *Crit Care Med* 2001;29;2264–2270.
211. Morrow CP, Curtin JP. *Gynecologic Cancer Surgery*. New York: Churchill Livingstone; 1996:194–205.
212. Blackburn GL, Bistrian BR, Moini BS, et al. Nutritional and metabolic assessment of the hospitalized patient. *JPEN J Parenter Enter Nutr* 1977;1:11–22.
213. Edwards BF. Postoperative renal insufficiency. *Med Clin North Am* 2001;85:1241–1254.
214. Klausner JM, Paterson IS, Goldman G, et al. Postischemic renal injury is mediated by neutrophils and leukotrienes. *Am J Physiol* 1989;256(5 Pt 2): F794–F802.
215. Kribben A, Edelstein CL, Schrier RW. Pathophysiology of acute renal failure. *J Nephrol* 1999;12(Suppl 2):S142–S151.
216. Prins JM, Buller HR, Kuijper EJ, et al. Once versus thrice daily gentamicin in patients with serious infections. *Lancet* 1993;341:335–339.
217. Murphy SW, Barrett BJ, Parfrey PS. Contrast nephropathy. *J Am Soc Nephrol* 2000;11:177–182.
218. Rudnick MR, Berns JS, Cohen RM, et al. Contrast media-associated nephrotoxicity. *Semin Nephrol* 1997;17:15–26.
219. McCullough PA, Wolyn R, Rocher LL, et al. Acute renal failure after coronary intervention: incidence, risk factors and relationship to mortality. *Am J Med* 1997;103:368–375.
220. Baldwin L, Henderson A, Hickman P. Effect of postoperative low-dose dopamine on renal function after elective major vascular surgery. *Ann Intern Med* 1994;120:744–747.
221. Dishart MK, Kellum JA. An evaluation of pharmacological strategies for the prevention and treatment of acute renal failure. *Drugs* 2000;59:79–91.
222. Lassnigg A, Donner E, Grubhofer G, et al. Lack of renoprotective effects of dopamine and furosemide during cardiac surgery. *J Am Soc Nephrol* 2000;11:97–104.
223. Marik PE, Iglesias J. Low-dose dopamine does not prevent acute renal failure in patients with septic shock and oliguria. NORASEPT II Study Investigators. *Am J Med* 1999;107:387–390.
224. Sirivella S, Gielchinsky I, Parsonnet V. Mannitol, furosemide and dopamine infusion in postoperative renal failure complicating cardiac surgery. *Ann Thorac Surg* 2000;69:501–506.
225. Allgren RL, Marbury TC, Rahman SM, et al. Anaritide in acute tubular necrosis. Auriculin Anaritide Acute Renal Failure Study Group. *N Engl J Med* 1997;336:828–834.
226. National Nosocomial Infections Surveillance (NNIS) system report, data summary from January 1992 through June 2004, issued October 2004. *Am J Infect Control* 2004;32:470–485.
227. Stafford RE, Weigelt JA. Surgical infections in the critically ill. *Curr Opin Crit Care* 2002;8:449–452.
228. Ostrosky-Zeichner L, Pappas PG. Invasive candidiasis in the intensive care unit. *Crit Care Med* 2006;34:857–863.
229. Pappas PG, Rex JH, Sobel JD, et al. Guidelines for treatment of candidiasis. *Clin Infect Dis* 2004;38:161–189.
230. Crabtree TD, Pelletier SJ, Antevil JL, et al. Cohort study of fever and leukocytosis as diagnostic and prognostic indicators in infected surgical patients. *World J Surg* 2001;25:739–744.
231. Jaramillo EJ, Trevino JM, Berghoff KR, et al. Bedside diagnostic laparoscopy in the intensive care unit: a 13-year experience. *JSLS* 2006;10:155–159.
232. Cinat ME, Wilson SE, Din AM. Determinants of successful percutaneous image-guided drainage of intra-abdominal abscess. *Arch Surg* 2002;137: 845–849.
233. Garvais DA, Ho CH, O'Neill MJ, et al. Recurrent abdominal and pelvic abscesses: incidence, results of repeated percutaneous drainage, and underlying causes in 956 drainages. *Am J Roentgenol* 2004;182: 463–466.
234. Kok KY, Yapp SK. Laparoscopic drainage of postoperative complicated intra-abdominal abscess. *Surg Laparosc Endosc Percutan Tech* 2000;10:311–313.
235. Schecter WP, Ivatury RR, Rotondo MF, et al. Open abdomen after trauma and abdominal sepsis: a strategy for management. *J Am Coll Surg* 2006;203: 390–396.
236. Marshall JC, Maier RV, Jimenez M, et al. Source control in the management of severe sepsis and septic shock: an evidence-based review. *Crit Care Med* 2004;32(11 Suppl):S513–S526.
237. Aird WC. The role of endothelium in severe sepsis and multiple organ dysfunction syndrome. *Blood* 2003;101:3765–3777.
238. American College of Chest Physicians/Society of Critical Care Medicine Consensus Conference. Definitions for sepsis and organ failure and guidelines for the use of innovative therapies in sepsis. *Crit Care Med* 1992;20:864–874.
239. Levy MM, Fink MP, Marshall JC, et al. 2001 SCCM/ESICM/ACCP/ ATS/SIS International Sepsis Definitions Conference. *Crit Care Med* 2003;31:1250–1256.
240. Shorr AF, Tabak YP, Killian AD, et al. Healthcare-associated bloodstream infection: a distinct entity? Insights from a large U.S. database. *Crit Care Med* 2006;34:2588–2595.
241. Angus DC, Linde-Zwirble WT, Lidicker J, et al. Epidemiology of severe sepsis in the United States: analysis of incidence, outcome, and associated costs of care. *Crit Care Med* 2001;29:1303–1310.
242. Dellinger RP, Carlet JM, Masur H, et al. Surviving Sepsis Campaign guidelines for management of severe sepsis and septic shock. *Crit Care Med* 2004;32:858–873.
243. Bernard GR, Vincent JL, Laterre PF, et al. Efficacy and safety of recombinant human activated protein C for severe sepsis. *N Engl J Med* 2001;344: 699–709.
244. Vincent JL, de Mendonca A, Cantraine F, et al. Use of the SOFA score to assess the incidence of organ dysfunction/failure in intensive care units: results of a multicenter, prospective study. Working group on "sepsis-related problems" of the European Society of Intensive Care Medicine. *Crit Care Med* 1998;26:1793–1800.
245. Zimmerman JE, Kramer AA, McNair DS, et al. Acute Physiology and Chronic Health Evaluation (APACHE) IV: Hospital mortality assessment for today's critically ill patients. *Crit Care Med* 2006;34:1297–1310.
246. Levy MM, Macias WL, Vincent JL, et al. Early changes in organ function predict eventual survival in severe sepsis. *Crit Care Med* 2005;33: 2194–2201.
247. Sugrue M. Abdominal compartment syndrome. *Curr Opin Crit Care* 2005;11:333–338.
248. Way J, Back AL, Curtis JR. Withdrawing life support and resolution of conflict with families. *BMJ* 2002;325:1342–1345.
249. Luce JM, Alpers A. Legal aspects of withholding and withdrawing life support from critically ill patients in the United States and providing palliative care to them. *Am J Respir Crit Care Med* 2000;162:2029–2032.
250. Society of Critical Care Medicine and American Society of Health-System Pharmacists. Clinical practice guidelines for the sustained use of sedatives and analgesics in the critically ill adult. *Am J Health Syst Pharm* 2002;59:150–178.
251. Society of Critical Care Medicine and American Society of Health-System Pharmacists. Clinical practice guidelines for sustained neuromuscular

blockade in the adult critically ill patient. *Am J Health Syst Pharm* 2002;59:179–195.
252. Epstein J, Breslow MJ. The stress response of critical illness. *Crit Care Clin* 1999;15:17–33.
253. Kress JP, Gehlbach B, Lacy M, et al. The long-term psychological effects of daily sedative interruption on critically ill patients. *Am J Respir Crit Care Med* 2003;168:1457–1461.
254. Kress JP, Pohlman AS, O'Connor MF, et al. Daily interruption of sedative infusions in critically ill patients undergoing mechanical ventilation. *N Engl J Med* 2000;342:1471–1477.
255. Cammarano WB, Pittet JF, Weitz S, et al. Acute withdrawal syndrome related to the administration of analgesic and sedative medications in adult intensive care unit patients. *Crit Care Med* 1998;26:676–684.
256. Bird SJ. Diagnosis and management of critical illness polyneuropathy and critical illness myopathy. *Curr Treat Options Neurol* 2007;9:85–92.
257. McKegney FP. The intensive care syndrome. The definition, treatment and prevention of a new "disease of medical progress." *Conn Med* 1966;30: 633–636.
258. McGuire BE, Basten CJ, Ryan CJ, et al. Intensive care unit syndrome: a dangerous misnomer. *Arch Intern Med* 2000;160:906–909.
259. Ely EW, Inouye SK, Bernard GR, et al. Delirium in mechanically ventilated patients: validity and reliability of the confusion assessment method for the intensive care unit (CAM-ICU). *JAMA* 2001;286:2703–2710.
260. Thomason J, Shintani A, Peterson J, et al. Intensive care unit delirium is an independent predictor of longer hospital stay: a prospective study of 261 nonventilated patients. *Crit Care* 2005;94:R375–R381.

CHAPTER 12 ■ SURGICAL PRINCIPLES IN GYNECOLOGIC ONCOLOGY

DENNIS S. CHI, ROBERT E. BRISTOW, AND DONALD G. GALLUP

The management of most human cancers involves multimodal therapy, and this is especially true for female genital malignancies. Although some early gynecologic cancers can be eradicated by surgery alone, and chemotherapy as a single modality can often cure gestational trophoblastic malignancies, the optimal treatment for the majority of gynecologic malignancies requires surgery combined with chemotherapy and/or irradiation.

In this chapter, surgery is discussed both as a separate discipline and as an integral part of multimodal therapeutic planning. Although specific operations and relatively new surgical techniques are described for some disease sites, many procedures are addressed more completely in surgical texts and atlases to which the reader is referred (1–3). The role of surgical intervention in the treatment of gynecologic cancers is addressed herein with a more philosophic approach than would be taken in a surgical atlas. However, select illustrations and tips are included that have enabled us to approach various radical procedures more rapidly and safely. The major goal of this chapter is to give the reader an appreciation and understanding of the surgical principles of the subspecialty of gynecologic oncology.

TECHNICAL ASPECTS OF SURGERY

Many physicians who practice the art and science of surgery tend to focus on the technical craft of the specialty only when teaching young surgeons. At other times, we are acutely aware that the most difficult part of our practice is the decision of whether or not to utilize surgical therapy. Preoperative and postoperative management is also demanding since therapy must be tailored for individual patients depending not only on their specific disease but also on their overall medical status. Owing to the significance of these pressing issues, we often take for granted the many years of preparation and experience in the craft of surgery.

Mastering the skills of surgery involves a thorough understanding of proper technique. It also requires frequent and consistent practice to keep surgical maneuvers well honed. For the student, this means actual practice in tying knots, manipulating instruments, and suturing. For the accomplished surgeon, it means that a sufficient case load must be maintained to ensure adequate practice of the technical art of the specialty. The surgeon should also keep abreast of new suture materials, instruments, and technical developments.

Anatomy

There is no substitute for a detailed knowledge of the anatomy of the pelvis and abdomen. The physician who pursues gynecologic oncology as a career must be completely familiar with the pelvis, abdomen, retroperitoneum, and the lymphatic drainage of the female genital tract. No amount of surgical skill or knowledge of cancer therapy can compensate for the lack of this knowledge.

Lymphatic drainage from the cervix follows the uterine arteries and cardinal ligaments to the pelvic lymph nodes that include the external iliac, internal iliac (hypogastric), and obturator node groups (Fig. 12.1). From these pelvic lymph nodes, the drainage proceeds superiorly through the common iliac lymph nodes and then up to the paraaortic nodes.

The lymphatic drainage from both the uterine corpus and the ovaries follows one of three routes (Fig. 12.1): (a) along the uterine arteries in the broad ligaments to the pelvic nodes, (b) in channels following the round ligaments to the inguinal lymph nodes, or (c) along the ovarian lymphatics in the infundibulopelvic ligaments directly up to the paraaortic nodes.

The anatomy of the paraaortic lymph nodes has been well described by Fowler and Johnson (4). The paraaortic lymph nodes are part of the lumbar lymph node group. There are three subgroups: preaortic, retroaortic, and lateral aortic (right and left). The preaortic group drains the abdominal part of the gastrointestinal tract down to the mid rectum, whereas the retroaortic group has no special area of drainage. The lateral group receives lymphatic drainage from the iliac lymph nodes, ovaries, and other pelvic viscera (apart from the alimentary tract), and therefore it is this group of nodes that is sampled in the surgical staging of gynecologic malignancies.

There are typically 15 to 20 lateral aortic nodes per side. They are located adjacent to the aorta, anterior to the lumbar spine, extending bilaterally to the medial margins of the psoas major muscles, and up to the diaphragmatic crura (4). The lateral nodes usually dissected in gynecologic oncology span the region from the aortic bifurcation up to either the inferior mesenteric artery (IMA) or the renal veins.

The first major blood vessel encountered during a caudad-to-cephalad paraaortic node dissection is the IMA (Fig. 12.1). The IMA originates from the anterior surface of the aorta approximately 3 to 4 cm above the aortic bifurcation. Next, the right and left ovarian arteries arise from their respective sides of the aorta about 5 to 6 cm above the bifurcation (Fig. 12.1). The right ovarian vein inserts into the right side of the inferior vena cava (IVC) approximately 1 cm below the right renal vein. The left ovarian vein does not insert directly into the IVC, but rather follows a path close to the left ureter inserting into the left renal vein lateral to the left border of the aorta. Three to four pairs of lumbar arteries and veins arise from the posterior surfaces of the aorta and IVC, respectively.

The gynecologic oncologist who operates on patients with advanced ovarian carcinoma often encounters disease spread involving upper abdominal structures such as the diaphragm, liver, pancreas, and spleen. Debulking of tumor from these

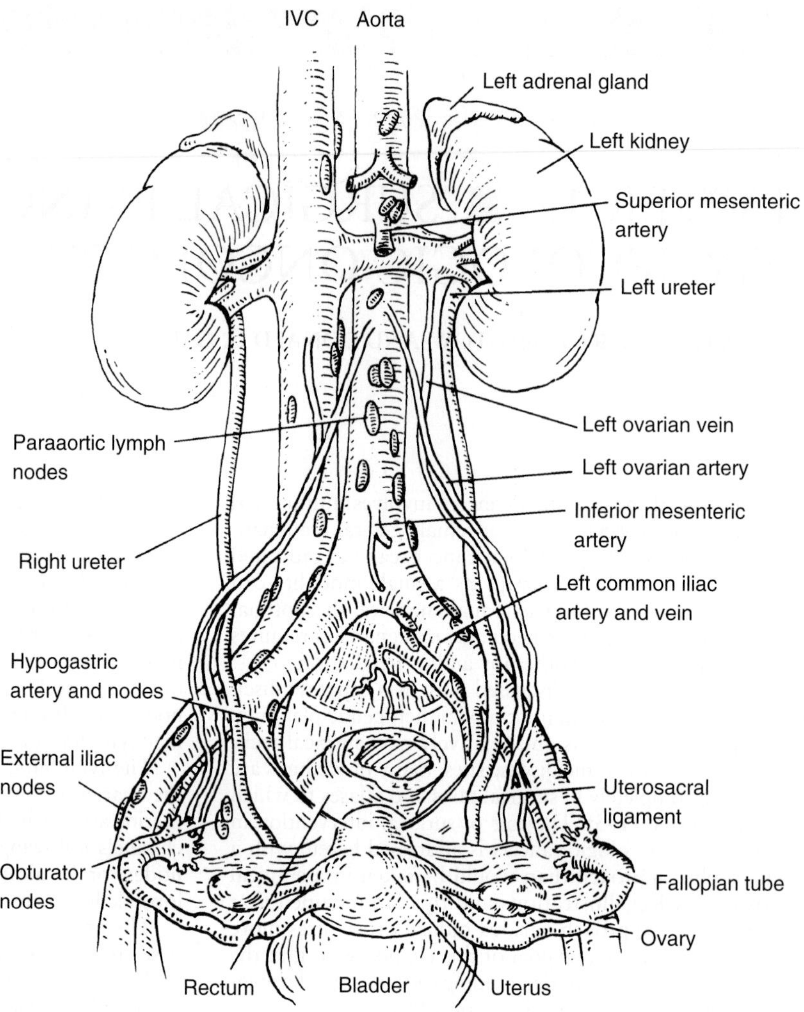

FIGURE 12.1. The pelvic and paraaortic lymph nodes and their relationship to the major retroperitoneal vessels.

areas has been demonstrated to improve the rate of optimal cytoreduction and subsequent survival (5,6). Anatomic considerations for diaphragm surgery include the relevant hepatic attachments and the underlying central vasculature (7,8) (Fig. 12.2). The anterior hepatic attachment is the falciform ligament, which contains the ligamentum teres in its infrahepatic portion, and attaches the liver to the anterior abdominal wall in its membranous hepatic portion. As the falciform ligament continues superiorly, its peritoneal surface divides laterally on each side to form the anterior right and left coronary ligaments. These coronary ligaments reflect off the liver capsule and delineate the posterior extent of peritoneum covering the superior diaphragm. The IVC lies to the right side of this falciform ligament division. The right and left hepatic veins drain into the anterior surface of the IVC at the level of this peritoneal reflection. The anterior coronary ligaments continue laterally and inferiorly along the posterior liver edge, where they join the posterior right and left coronary ligaments to form the right and left triangular ligaments, respectively. The right triangular ligament reflects from the liver to the diaphragm, right kidney, and right adrenal gland. The left triangular ligament reflects primarily to the diaphragm; the posterior left coronary ligament lies higher than the esophageal hiatus and the esophagus is generally not encountered. The coronary ligaments on each side delineate the larger "bare area" of the liver on the right and a smaller "bare area" on the left, which underlie the central tendon of the diaphragm. The right phrenic nerve penetrates this central tendon lateral to the vena caval foramen on the right and is usually not encountered until the "bare area" is exposed. The left phrenic nerve may penetrate the left diaphragm muscle above the central tendon and is a consideration during left-sided anterior diaphragm surgery.

In the left upper quadrant of the abdomen, the spleen lies under the 9th, 10th, and 11th ribs. It is situated adjacent and slightly deep to the stomach and colon, lateral to the pancreas, and sits on the superior aspect of the left kidney. The posterior aspect of the spleen is in contact with the adrenal gland as well as Gerota's fascia of the kidney. The tail of the pancreas often approaches the splenic hilum and sometimes contacts the spleen. The spleen varies in size between individuals, but in general measures 12 cm in length, 7 cm in width, and 3 to 4 cm in width. The peritoneum creates folds that form the suspensory ligaments of the spleen. The four main "suspensory" ligaments are gastrosplenic, splenorenal, splenophrenic, and splenocolic ligaments. The splenophrenic and splenocolic ligaments are avascular. The gastrosplenic ligament contains the short gastric vessels. The splenorenal ligament has an anterior and posterior aspect and surrounds the splenic hilum. The splenic hilum contains the splenic artery, splenic vein, and sometimes the tail of the pancreas. The splenic vessels sometimes branch before entering the spleen. The splenic artery is tortuous and is one of the three branches of the celiac trunk. It runs along the superior aspect of the pancreas and gives rise to the short gastric arteries prior to entering the spleen, which course in the gastrosplenic ligament and supply the portion of the greater curvature of the stomach superior to the splenic artery (Fig. 12.3) (9). The splenic artery also gives rise to the left gastroepiploic

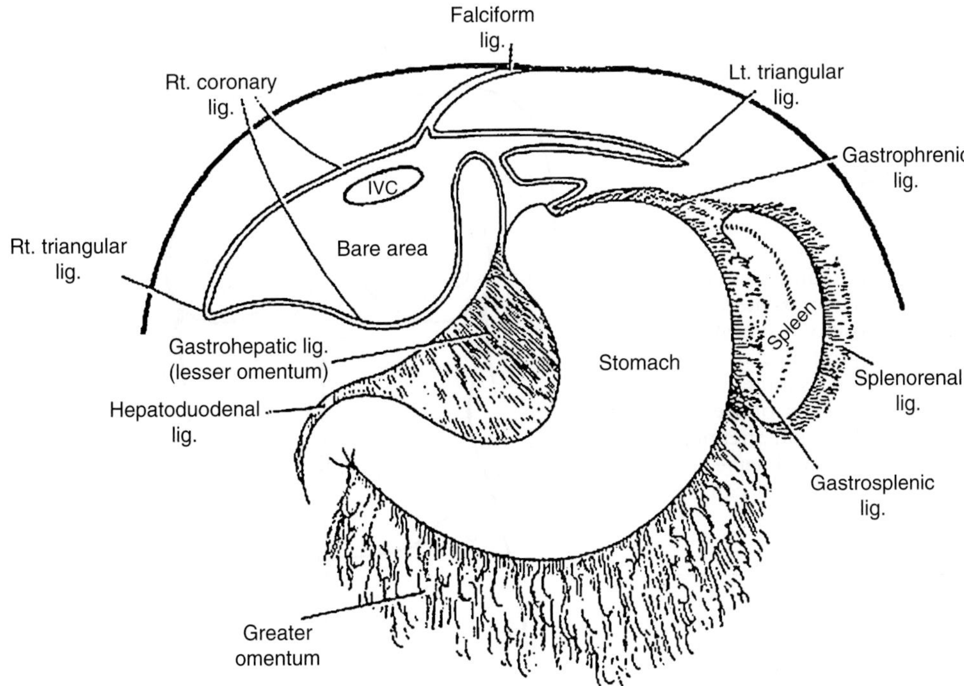

FIGURE 12.2. Peritoneal reflections of the liver: the lesser omentum (hepatogastric and hepatoduodenal ligaments) and its relation to the coronary ligament of the liver and diaphragm. *Source:* Reprinted with permission from Skandalakis JE, Gray SW, Rowe JR, eds. *Anatomical Complications in General Surgery.* New York: McGraw-Hill; 1983.

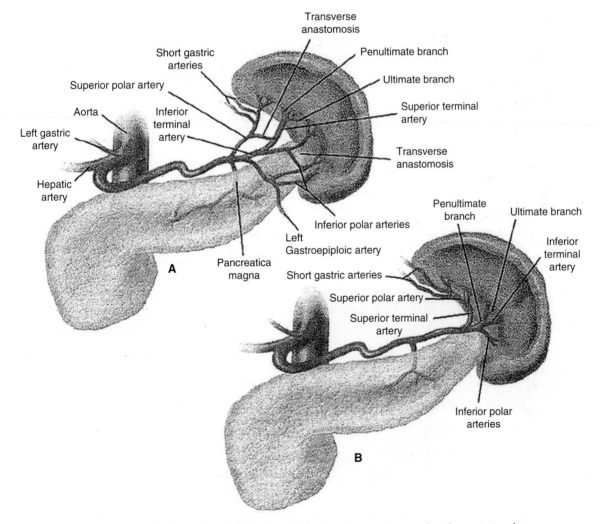

FIGURE 12.3. A,B. Variations of splenic vascularization. *Source:* Reprinted with permission from Poulin EC, Schlachta DM, Maazza J. Splenectomy. Gastroinestinal tract and abdomen. In: Souba WW, Fink MJ, Jurkovich GJ, et al., eds. *ACS Surgery*. New York: WebMd; 2005.

artery, which supplies the remainder of the greater curvature of the stomach and the gastrocolic omentum. The splenic vein is slightly inferior and follows the course and branching of the artery.

Patient Positioning

Patient positioning for radical gynecologic oncology procedures is often critical in improving exposure, particularly in obese patients. For most women undergoing radical hysterectomy, ovarian cancer cytoreduction, or pelvic exenterative procedures, we prefer the low lithotomy position using Allen stirrups (Fig. 12.4) (1). The buttocks should protrude 2 to 3 cm over the end of the table. This position allows simultaneous access to the perineum and abdomen. The weight of the leg should be on the foot with the legs well padded and attention paid to prevent pressure on the calf and the peroneal nerve. To further improve pelvic exposure, a blanket or pad can be placed under the small of the back.

Abdominal Incisions

Abdominal incisions in gynecologic oncology vary with the indication for the procedure, associated preoperative conditions (such as the presence of ascites or bowel obstruction), suspicion of upper abdominal pathology, and the presence of a previous abdominal scar. Incisions for surgery for gynecologic oncology patients should be highly individualized. Three basic incisions are used for intraperitoneal exposure (Fig. 12.5) (2). Additionally, extraperitoneal access to the pelvic and paraaortic nodes can be achieved through a J-shaped incision (10) or a "sunrise" incision (11).

Transverse incisions offer the advantages of being the best cosmetic incisions for pelvic surgery while also being the least painful, resulting in less interference with postoperative pulmonary function. In addition, compared to vertical incisions, transverse incisions are allegedly stronger and allow better exposure to the pelvic sidewalls. Many gynecologic oncologists use transverse incisions when performing a radical hysterectomy or pelvic exenteration.

In performing the Maylard incision, it is recommended that the deep inferior epigastric vessels be isolated, sectioned, and ligated prior to dividing the rectus muscle (Fig. 12.6) (2). Occasionally, the pelvic surgeon will make a Pfannenstiel incision and find it inadequate. When more exposure is needed, the appropriate maneuver is to convert the Pfannenstiel to a Cherney-type incision. This conversion can be accomplished by dissecting the rectus muscles from the pyramidalis muscles and the anterior rectus sheath and then transecting the rectus tendons at their insertion into the pubic bone.

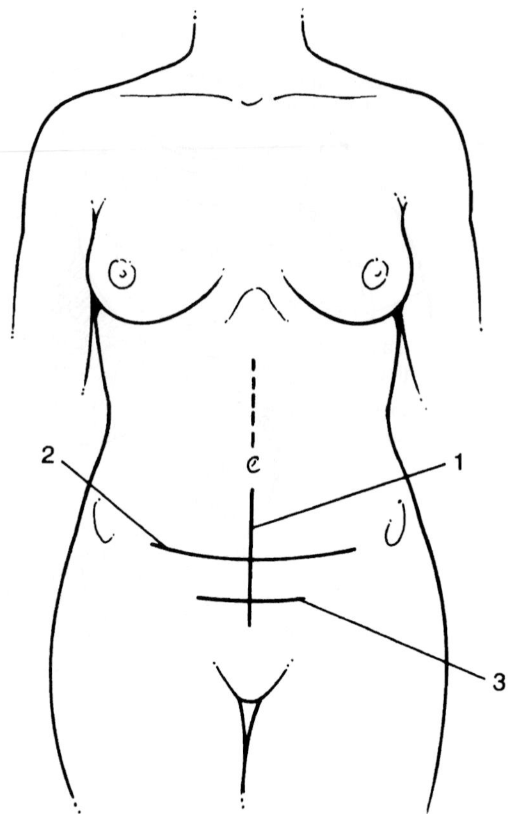

FIGURE 12.5. Entry into the abdominal cavity can be made by three basic incisions: (1) the midline incision; (2) the transverse Maylard-type incision from anterior-superior iliac spine to anterior-superior iliac spine; and (3) the Pfannenstiel incision. The latter is not an incision for radical pelvic surgery, but it can be converted to a Cherney-type incision for improved exposure. For the patient who has some type of transverse incision, and for whom later exposure of the upper abdominal cavity is necessary, a midline upper abdominal incision can be separately used. *Source:* Reprinted with permission from Gallup DG, Talledo OE. *Surgical Atlas of Gynecologic Oncology.* Philadelphia: WB Saunders Co.; 1994:44.

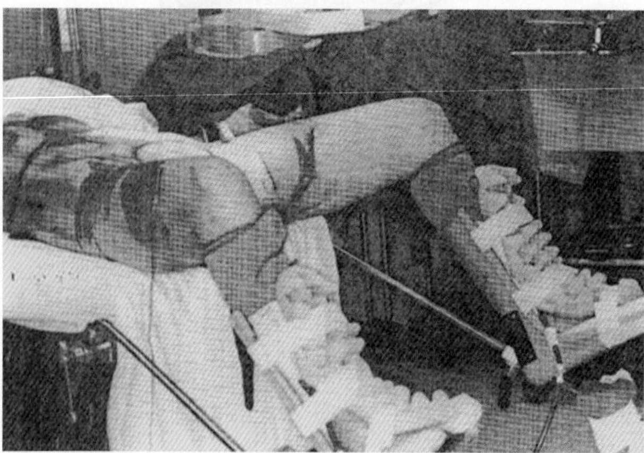

FIGURE 12.4. Low lithotomy position using Allen stirrups. *Source:* Reprinted with permission from Morrow CP, Curtin JP, eds. *Gynecologic Cancer Surgery.* New York: Churchill Livingstone; 1996.

Lymph Node Dissection

The surgical technique used to dissect the pelvic and paraaortic lymph nodes involves either a transperitoneal or extraperitoneal approach. The approach utilized is generally dictated by the primary site of disease and the planned accompanying procedure. In cases of endometrial and ovarian carcinoma where the anticipated procedure includes a hysterectomy and/or surgical debulking, the approach is invariably transperitoneal. However, in the pretreatment surgical staging of patients with advanced-stage cervical cancer, the transperitoneal approach has been associated with significant radiation-induced intestinal morbidity due to postoperative adhesion formation (12). Therefore, current clinical trials that require pretreatment surgical staging recommend that the lymph node sampling be performed via the extraperitoneal approach or by operative laparoscopy (13).

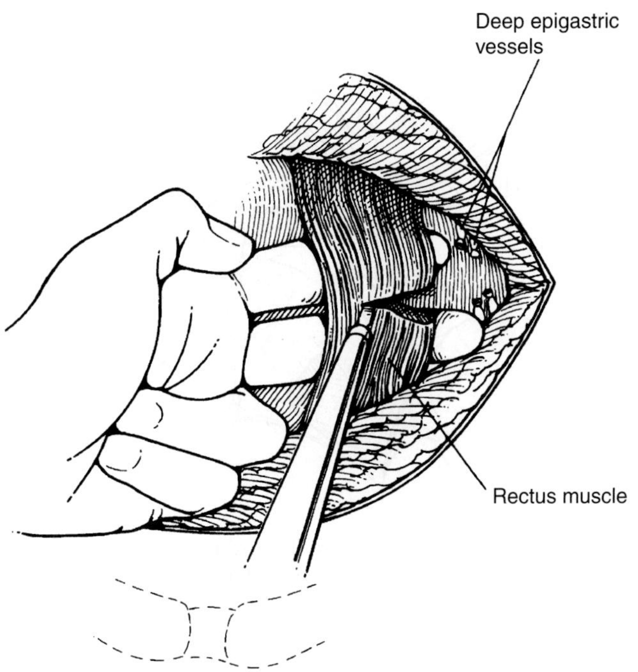

FIGURE 12.6. The Maylard incision. A transverse incision has been made from the anterior-superior iliac spine to the opposite anterior-superior iliac spine. The fascia has been incised transversely. The deep inferior epigastric vessels are located on the lateral and posterior borders of the rectus muscle. They are bluntly dissected from this position by the finger of the operator, isolated, clamped, sectioned, and tied. Only after they are tied should the rectus muscle be incised. This can be done with the Bovie. *Source:* Reprinted with permission from Gallup DG, Talledo OE. *Surgical Atlas of Gynecologic Oncology.* Philadelphia: WB Saunders Co.; 1994:45.

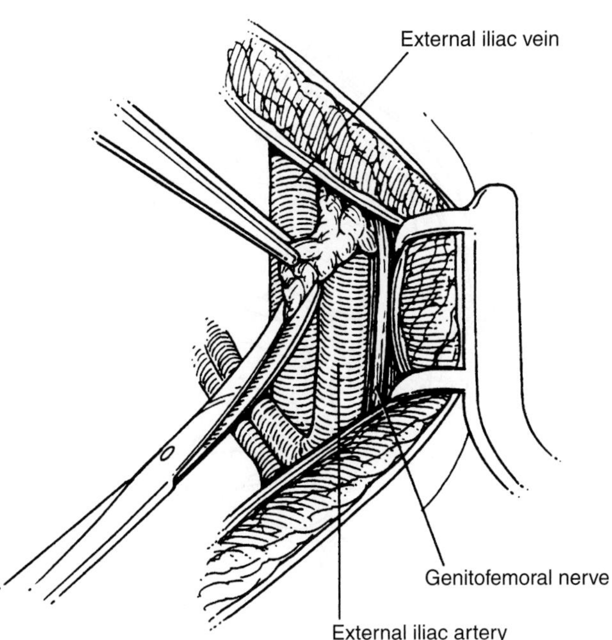

FIGURE 12.7. Starting at the bifurcation of the common iliac vessels, the loose areolar tissue over the vein is excised from cephalad to caudad. Clips should be used at the bifurcation of the common iliac to avoid troublesome bleeding. *Source:* Reprinted with permission from Gallup DG, Talledo OE. *Surgical Atlas of Gynecologic Oncology.* Philadelphia: WB Saunders Co.; 1994:57.

Pelvic Lymph Node Dissection

Whether a transperitoneal or extraperitoneal approach is used, most surgeons initially remove pelvic nodes by excising the loose areolar tissue over the external iliac vessels (Fig. 12.7) (2). The genitofemoral nerve courses laterally to the external iliac artery and should be identified and preserved prior to excising the lymphatic tissue. Mobilization and retraction of the external iliac vessels allows access to the obturator space. The obturator nodes are most easily teased away from the nerve and vessels if one begins the dissection caudad (Fig. 12.8) (2).

Transperitoneal Approach to the Paraaortic Nodes

The transperitoneal approach to the paraaortic lymph nodes can be accomplished by either the direct or the lateral approach. With the direct approach, the dissection begins with an incision in the peritoneum directly over the common iliac arteries and aorta. The lateral approach starts with an incision in the lateral paracolic gutters with subsequent medial reflection of the right and/or left colon. The advantage of the direct approach is that it involves less dissection of the intestine and ureter, whereas one of its main disadvantages is that it is associated with a greater degree of difficulty in exposing the left paraaortic nodes. Consequently, many surgeons sample the right paraaortic lymph nodes via the direct approach and use the lateral approach for the left-sided nodes.

With the direct approach to the right paraaortic nodes, an incision is made in the peritoneum overlying the right common iliac artery (Fig. 12.9). The incision is carried up over the aorta to the level of the duodenum. If the nodal dissection is to be carried out only to the level of the IMA, the duodenum may not need to be mobilized. Using blunt dissection, the ureter and

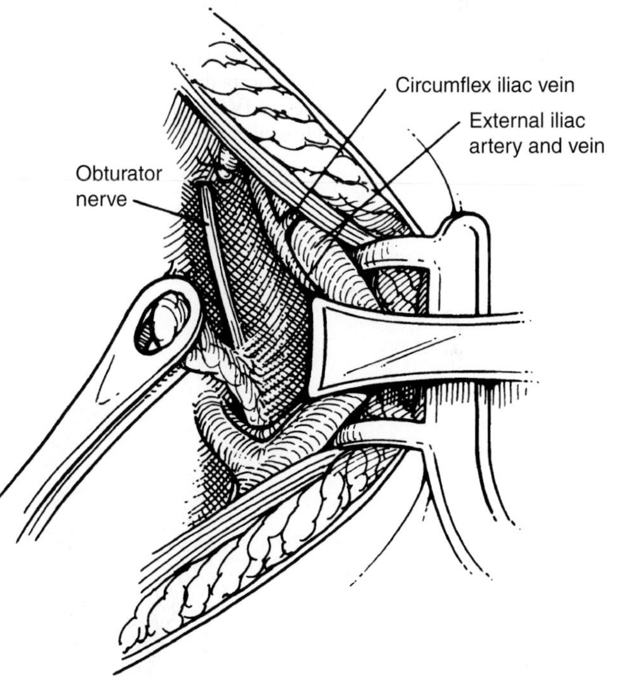

FIGURE 12.8. A vein retractor is used to retract the external iliac veins anterior and lateral to expose the obturator space. Lymphatic tissue is gently teased from the psoas muscle. The entire lymphatic bundle is clamped, sectioned at its caudal end, and ligated at the pelvic sidewall. With the use of the Singley forceps, the lymphatic bundle is bluntly dissected from the obturator nerve and mobilized superiorly. Often, the obturator vein and artery must be sacrificed to obtain access to tissue posterior and lateral to the nerve. Once the tissue is mobilized superiorly, all areolar tissue is cleaned off the hypogastric vessels to the level of the bifurcation of the common iliac artery. The large tissue bundle is clamped and removed en bloc. A tie or clips may be used at the level of the bifurcation. *Source:* Reprinted with permission from Gallup DG, Talledo OE. *Surgical Atlas of Gynecologic Oncology.* Philadelphia: WB Saunders Co.; 1994:58.

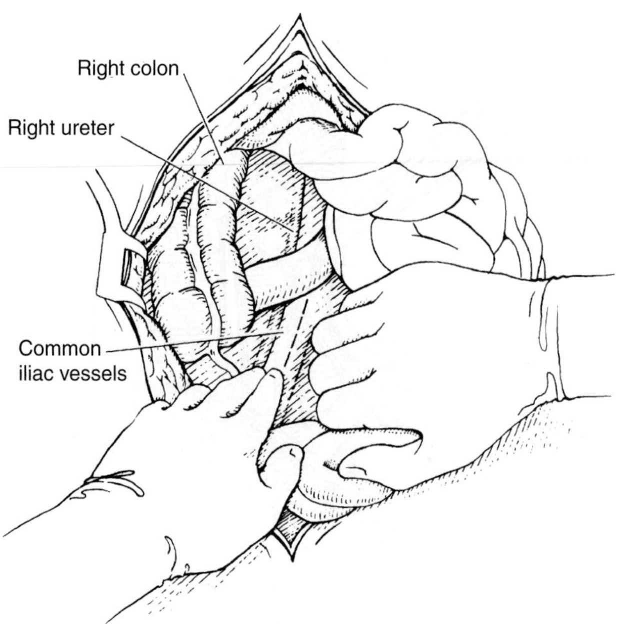

FIGURE 12.9. The small bowel is elevated out of the pelvis placing the mesentery on gentle traction. The right ureter and common iliac artery are identified and the peritoneum overlying the artery is incised.

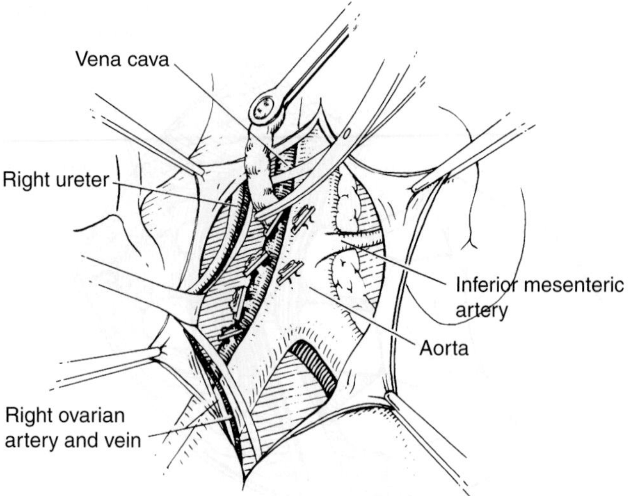

FIGURE 12.10. The specimen is dissected in a cephalad direction. Hemostatic clips are used on either side of the developing pedicle as it is mobilized and divided, and also at the most cephalad extent of the dissection before the specimen is removed.

ovarian vessels are identified and mobilized laterally. The lymphatic tissue lateral to the right common iliac artery is elevated and the caudal end is clipped and divided. The dissection then proceeds in a caudad-to-cephalad direction. A plane is created between the IVC and the lymphatic pedicle. The majority of the right paraaortic nodes overlie the IVC and they are generally easily dissected off the vessel. However, there is a fairly constant small vein within the lymphatics anterior to the IVC that inserts just above its bifurcation. If care is not taken to identify and ligate this so-called "fellow's" vein early in the dissection, it can easily be torn with resultant heavy bleeding (1). When the most cephalad extent of the dissection is reached, the pedicle is clipped and divided (Fig. 12.10).

If the nodes above the IMA need to be sampled, the third portion of the duodenum is mobilized by bilaterally incising the peritoneum around it and then sharply dissecting the areolar

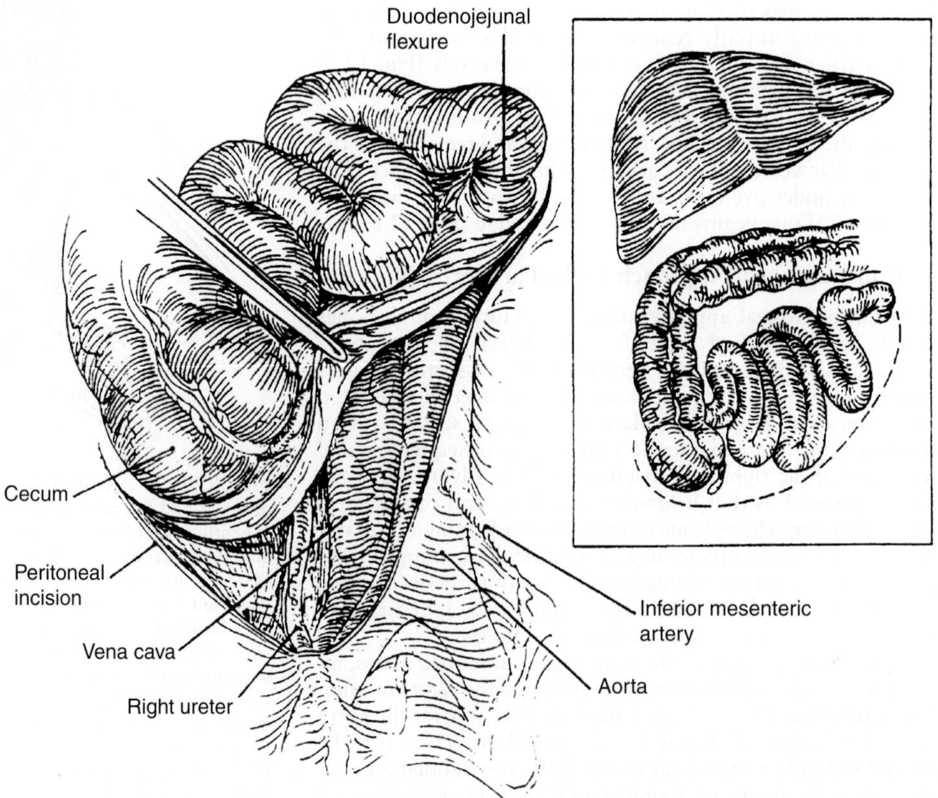

FIGURE 12.11. Extended peritoneal incision. The peritoneal incision is extended over the right ureter around the cecum and the cephalad along the right paracolic gutter. This allows for mobilization of the small bowel mesentery as well as the ascending colon. *Source:* Reprinted with permission from Fowler JM, Johnson PR. Transperitoneal para-aortic lymphadenectomy. *Oper Tech Gynecol Surg* 1996;1:9.

tissue underneath (4). The superior portion of the peritoneal incision can be carried up as high as the ligament of Treitz, which can also be divided if needed. Inferiorly, the peritoneal incision is extended over the right ureter around the cecum and up along the right paracolic gutter to mobilize the small bowel mesentery and part of the right colon (Fig. 12.11) (4). The small bowel can then be packed into the upper abdomen or completely removed from the peritoneal cavity and stabilized outside of the abdominal cavity or put into a bowel bag outside the abdomen. The duodenum is retracted superiorly, allowing identification and ligation of the right ovarian artery and vein. The lymphatic tissue can then be safely dissected off of the right side of the aorta and the anterior surface of the IVC up to the level of the renal veins.

The left paraaortic lymph nodes may be removed through the same peritoneal incision. Sharp dissection is used to identify the left common iliac artery, left side of the aorta, IMA, left ureter, and left psoas muscle (Fig. 12.12). The ureter is again mobilized laterally. The lymphatic tissue lateral to the left common iliac artery and aorta is then removed in a caudad-to-cephalad direction. The left paraaortic lymph nodes lie lateral and partially behind the aorta. In dissecting these nodes, judicious use of vascular clips will help prevent troublesome bleeding from the lumbar vessels. Safe removal of the lymph nodes above the IMA frequently requires identification and division of the left ovarian artery and vein, and occasionally ligation of the inferior mesenteric artery.

To remove right-sided paraaortic nodes via the lateral approach, the right paracolic gutter is incised along the line of Toldt (Fig. 12.13). The peritoneum is elevated off the psoas muscle and the incision is extended up to the hepatic flexure of the colon. Using sharp and blunt dissection, the right colon is reflected medially. The ureter and ovarian vessels can be identified attached to the undersurface of the reflected peritoneum. They may be left attached or mobilized laterally for better exposure. Further medial mobilization of the colon exposes the IVC and aorta. With the essential structures identified, the lymphatic tissue can then be dissected as previously described in a caudad-to-cephalad direction up to the third portion of the duodenum (Fig. 12.14).

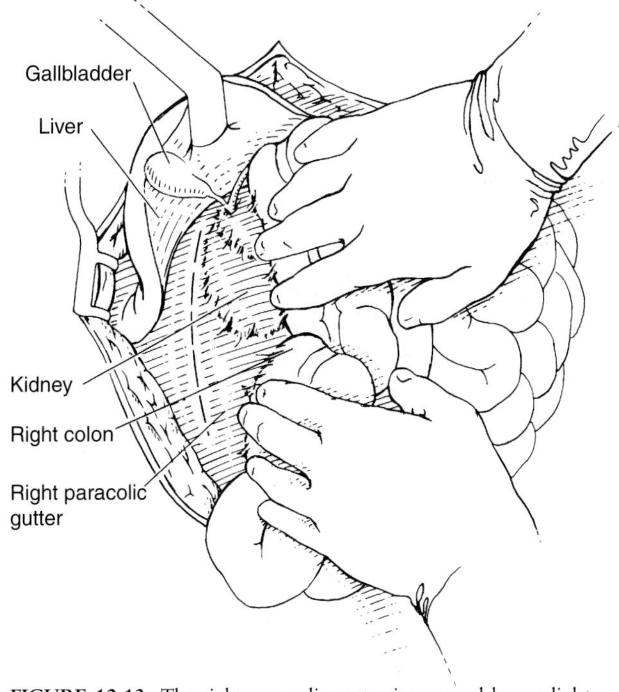

FIGURE 12.13. The right paracolic gutter is exposed by medial traction on the ascending colon. The gutter is incised along the line of Toldt.

If the lymph nodes above the IMA need to be sampled, the Kocher maneuver is used to reflect the duodenum medially. The peritoneum lateral to the convexity of the C-curve of the duodenum is incised and the second portion of the duodenum is then dissected off of the IVC. For further exposure, the peritoneal incision along the line of Toldt may need to be extended cephalad to mobilize completely the hepatic flexure of the colon (Fig. 12.15). The right ovarian artery and vein are identified and divided. The right-sided paraaortic lymph

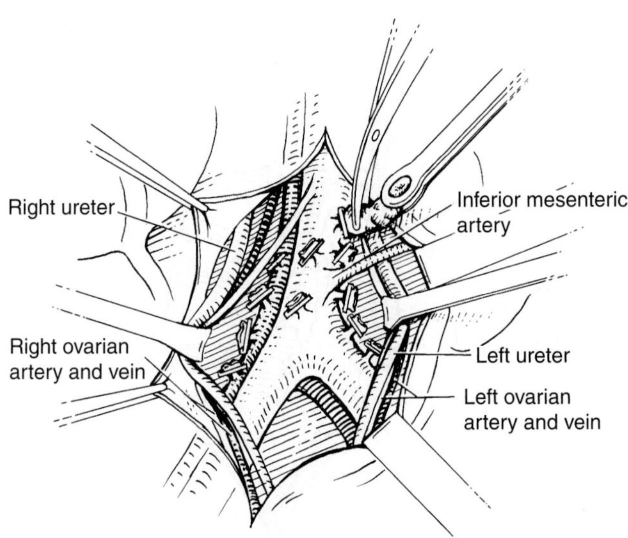

FIGURE 12.12. Removal of the left paraaortic nodes through the same peritoneal incision. The dissection also proceeds in a cephalad direction, again using hemostatic clips on the lateral and medial margins. Care should be taken to avoid injury to the inferior mesenteric artery that arises approximately 3 to 4 cm above the aortic bifurcation.

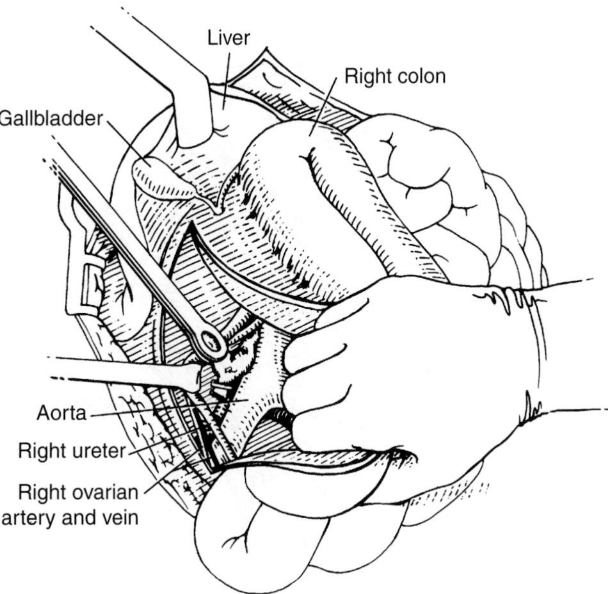

FIGURE 12.14. With the ureter and ovarian vessels identified, the dissection begins at the right common iliac artery and proceeds cephalad up to the third portion of the duodenum.

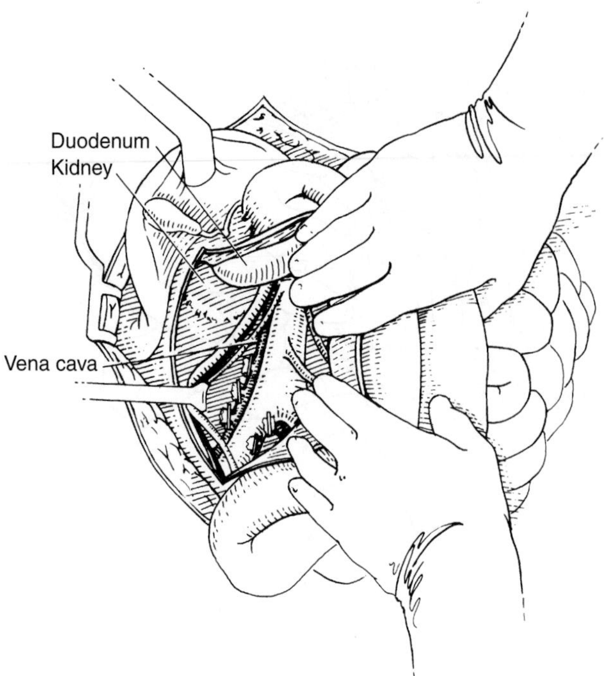

FIGURE 12.15. The Kocher maneuver can be used to gain access to the lymph nodes above the IMA. The peritoneum lateral to the convexity of the C-curve of the duodenum is incised and the second portion of the duodenum is then dissected off of the IVC. The common bile duct and pancreatic duct enter the second portion of the duodenum posteromedially. For further exposure, the incision along the line of Toldt can be extended cephalad to mobilize completely the hepatic flexure of the colon.

nodes are then able to be dissected off of the IVC and right aorta up to the level of the renal vessels.

The lateral approach to the left paraaortic lymph nodes is accomplished in a similar fashion by incising along the line of Toldt and mobilization of the left colon medially (Fig. 12.16). Again, the ureter and ovarian vessels are identified on the undersurface of the reflected peritoneum, and they may be left attached or mobilized laterally for better exposure (Fig. 12.17). After further mobilization of the left colon and identification of the aorta and the IMA, the left-sided nodes are removed in a caudad-to-cephalad direction (Fig. 12.18). Dissection of the nodes above the IMA requires mobilization of the splenic flexure of the colon, division of the left ovarian artery and vein, and occasionally ligation of the inferior mesenteric artery.

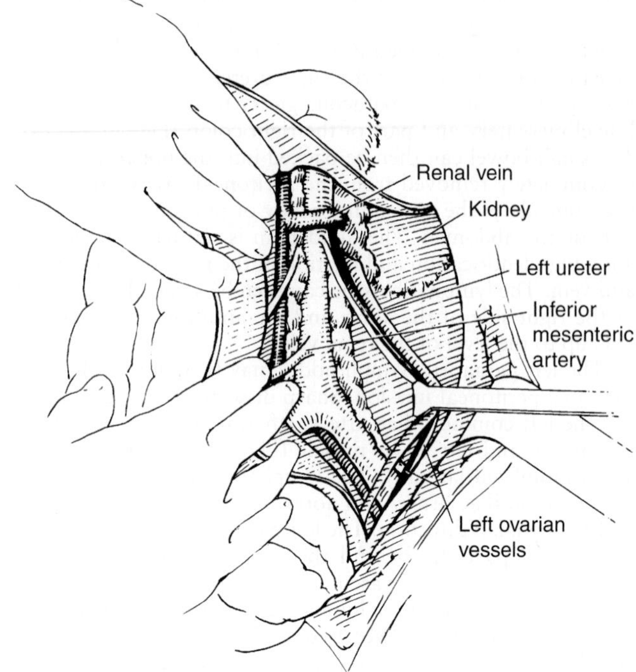

FIGURE 12.17. Using sharp and blunt dissection, the left colon can be mobilized medially, exposing the left ureter, ovarian vessels, and aorta.

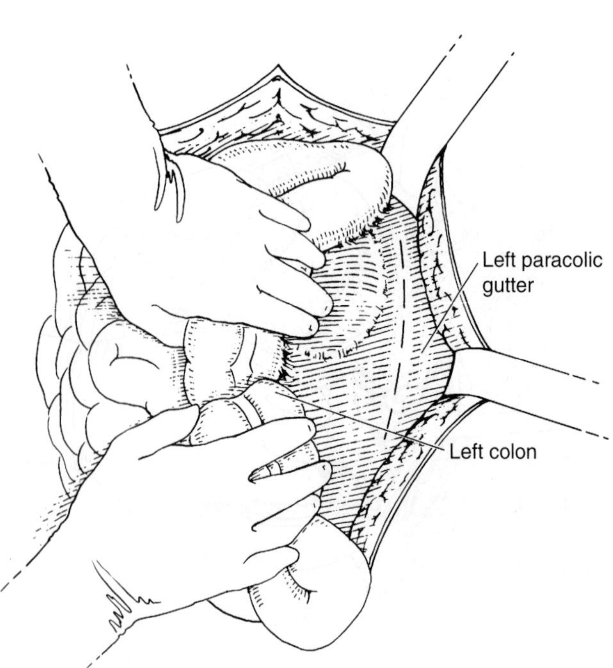

FIGURE 12.16. The lateral approach to the left paraaortic nodes is accomplished by retracting the descending colon medially and incising along the line of Toldt.

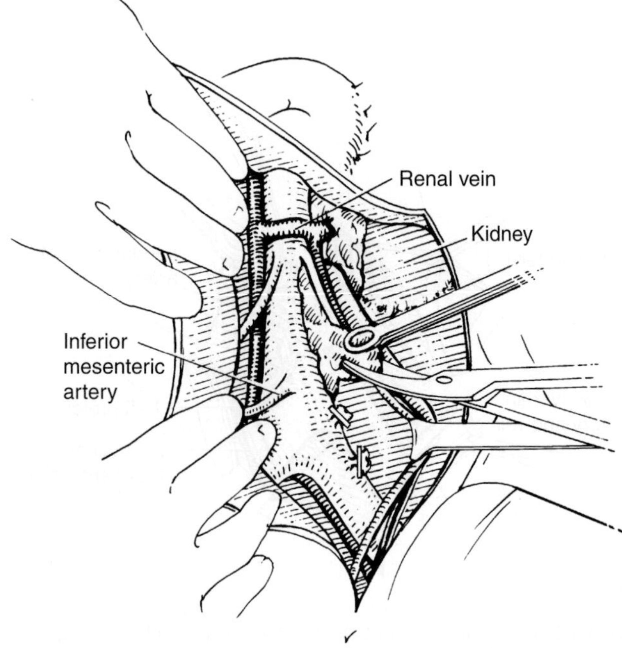

FIGURE 12.18. Dissection begins at the left common iliac artery and proceeds cephalad using hemostatic clips. Care should be taken to avoid injury to the inferior mesenteric artery that arises approximately 3 to 4 cm above the aortic bifurcation.

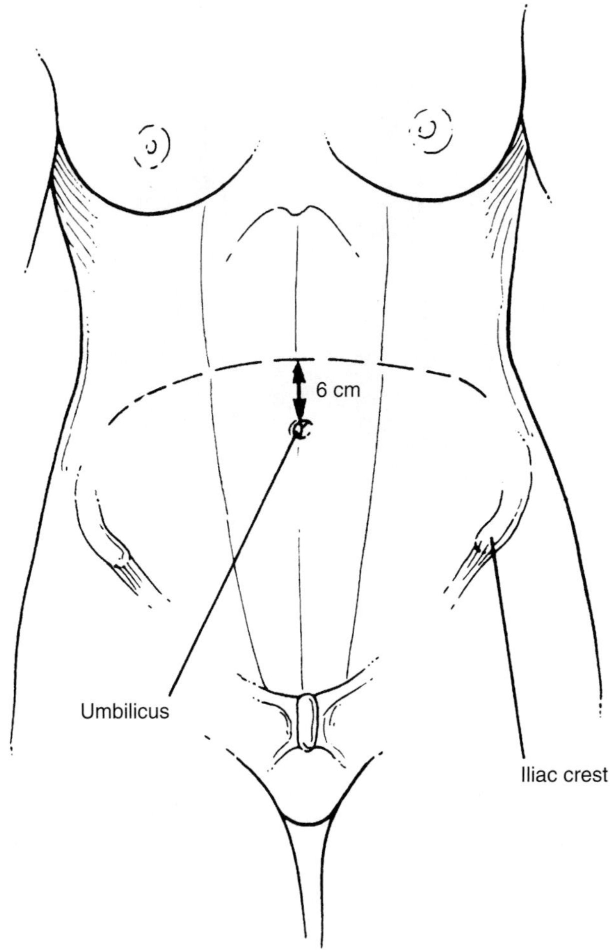

FIGURE 12.19. The "sunrise" incision. In the center, the incision is approximately 6 cm above the umbilicus. The incision is carried laterally in a downward fashion to the level of the iliac crests. *Source:* Reprinted with permission from Gallup DG, Talledo OE. *Surgical Atlas of Gynecologic Oncology.* Philadelphia: WB Saunders Co.; 1994:118.

Extraperitoneal Approach to the Paraaortic Nodes

The extraperitoneal approach to the paraaortic lymph nodes by means of a supraumbilical transverse sunrise incision was initially described by Gallup et al. (11). The skin incision is made 6 cm above the umbilicus in the midline and is carried laterally and caudad to the level of the iliac crests bilaterally (Fig. 12.19) (2).

The fascia is incised transversely. The rectus muscles are dissected off of the anterior-lying fascia cephalad and caudad. The right rectus muscle is transected. The right transversus muscle is then identified and transected caudally and laterally. The hand of the operator is inserted deep into the incision until the right psoas muscle and external iliac vessels are palpated. The peritoneum is then bluntly dissected from caudad and lateral to cephalad and medial, separating it from the underlying common iliac vessels until the great vessels are exposed (Fig. 12.20) (2). If the peritoneum is inadvertently entered, it must be closed immediately.

After identification of the right ureter and ovarian vessels, the right paraaortic nodes can be removed. In thin patients, the left paraaortic nodes may be able to be removed through a right abdominal approach. However, if exposure is difficult, the left rectus and transversus muscles can be transected and the peritoneum mobilized medially in a similar fashion to gain access to the left paraaortic nodes.

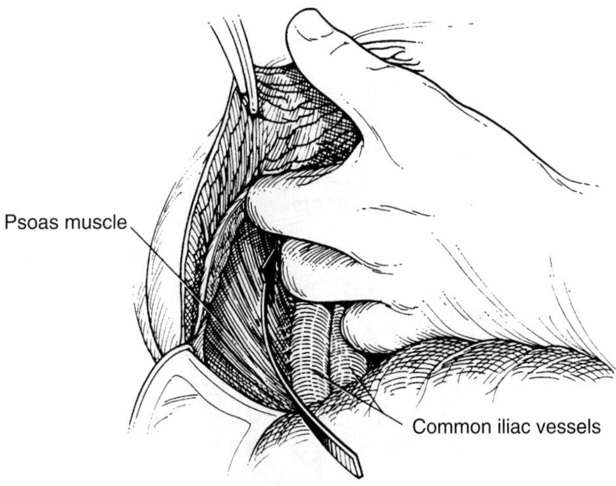

FIGURE 12.20. With the rectus and transversus muscles transected, the operator's hand is inserted caudad until the psoas muscle and external iliac vessels are palpated. The peritoneum is then bluntly dissected from caudad and lateral to cephalad and medial, separating it from the underlying common iliac vessels until the aorta and vena cava are exposed. *Source:* Reprinted with permission from Gallup DG, Talledo OE. *Surgical Atlas of Gynecologic Oncology.* Philadelphia: WB Saunders Co.; 1994:121.

Radical Hysterectomy

In performing a radical hysterectomy, one of the most troublesome areas is intraoperative bleeding from the lateral cardinal ligament, which is also known as the "web." In order to have better access and exposure in this area, the surgeon can release the uterus posteriorly in the earlier steps of the procedure. The six classic spaces are developed prior to sectioning the uterosacral ligaments. With maximal mobility of the uterus achieved, the ureter is unroofed from the tunnel of tissue that contains the uterine vessels and its branches (Fig. 12.21).

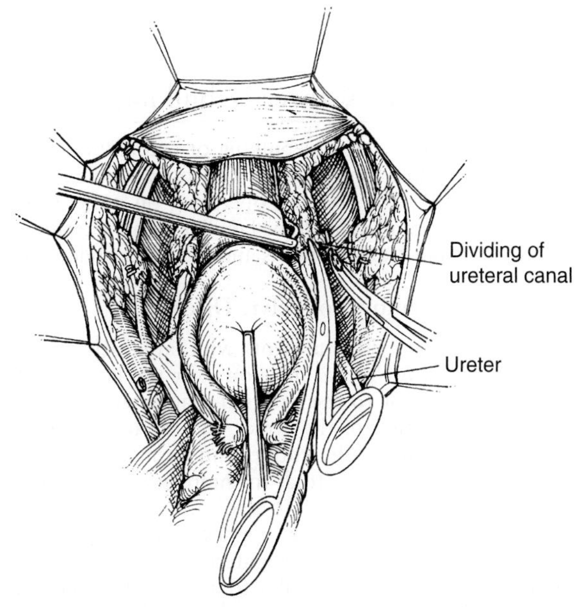

FIGURE 12.21. Dissection of the ureter from the parametrium is begun. The ureteral canal is unroofed by placing traction on the medial stump of the uterine vessels. Because of the rich blood supply from anastomosis of vessels in this area, a clamp-cut technique is often used. *Source:* Reprinted with permission from Gallup DG, Talledo OE. *Surgical Atlas of Gynecologic Oncology.* Philadelphia: WB Saunders Co.; 1994:79.

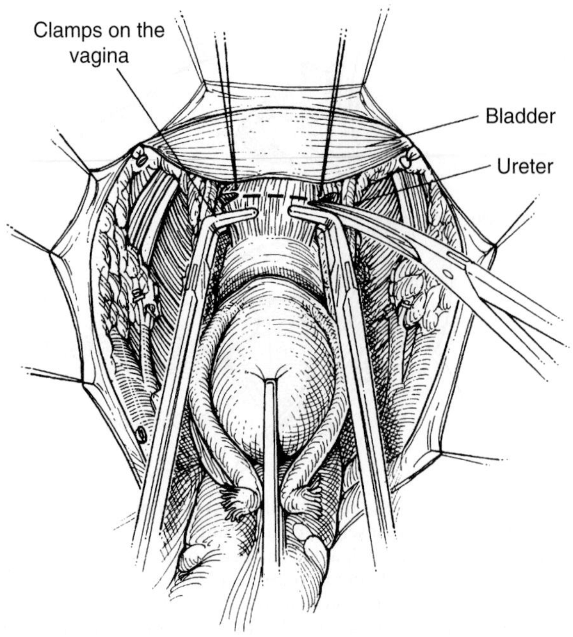

FIGURE 12.22. The vaginal angles are clamped and sectioned after placing right-angle clamps across the proximal vagina. Note the vaginal incision is made caudad to these clamps. *Source:* Reprinted with permission from Gallup DG, Talledo OE. *Surgical Atlas of Gynecologic Oncology.* Philadelphia: WB Saunders Co.; 1994:81.

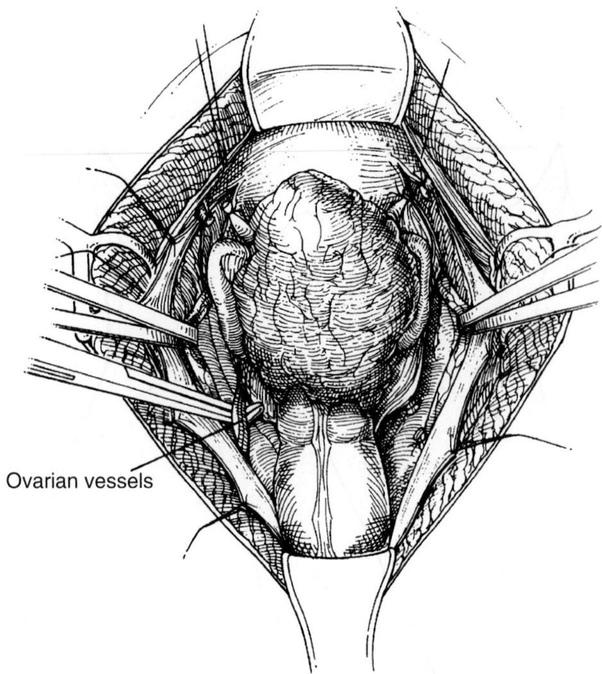

FIGURE 12.23. The ovarian vessels are skeletonized and divided at the pelvic brim. Early control of these vessels will help reduce blood loss during the later dissection. The ureter can be mobilized off the medial leaf of the broad ligament and retracted laterally on a Penrose drain or vessel loop. *Source:* Reprinted with permission from Gallup DG, Talledo OE. *Surgical Atlas of Gynecologic Oncology.* Philadelphia: WB Saunders Co.; 1994:92.

Once the ureter is unroofed, removal of any remaining cardinal ligament is accomplished with the ureter pulled laterally. To ensure that adequate vaginal margins are obtained, right-angle clamps are placed proximal to the level of resection of the specimen (Fig. 12.22). The pelvic lymphadenectomy can be done prior to or following the radical hysterectomy. The use of closed suction drains is advocated by many, although some avoid their use.

Ovarian Cancer Debulking

The goal of ovarian cancer debulking or cytoreduction is to remove all or as close as possible to all grossly visible and palpable tumor (14). The surgeon operating on patients with advanced ovarian cancer should be familiar with the techniques used to clear tumor from the pelvis and the upper abdomen.

Removal of Pelvic Disease

Ovarian malignancy often presents with large pelvic masses filling the pelvis. An initial incision over the lateral pelvic sidewall just anterior to the external iliac artery will allow adequate visualization of the ureter and the ovarian vessels (Fig. 12.23). The paracolic gutters can be incised cephalad along the avascular line of Toldt for more adequate exposure of the retroperitoneal space. To avoid further troublesome hemorrhage with large adnexal masses, if a hysterectomy is part of the planned procedure, the uterine vessels can be separately isolated and divided similar to a modified radical hysterectomy. When the anatomy is distorted by peritoneal implants, the ureters may need to be followed down to the tunnel and retracted laterally prior to removal of the uterus.

In cases where ovarian tumors are densely adherent to or involve the rectosigmoid, a reverse hysterectomy can often help identify the rectovaginal plane. Once the uterine vessels are ligated bilaterally, the vagina is incised anteriorly below the level of the cervix. The posterior vagina is incised after elevating the anterior vaginal flap. The vaginal angles are ligated and the posterior vaginal wall is grasped with Kocher clamps and retracted cephalad (Fig. 12.24). The cardinal and uterosacral ligaments are then clamped and sectioned. Resection of the rectosigmoid with tumor is frequently required to clear all pelvic tumor. Low rectal anastomosis in this setting is generally performed and associated with a low rate of complications in well-trained hands (15,16).

Upper Abdominal Disease

A recent meta-analysis by Bristow et al. demonstrated that expert centers with primary optimal cytoreduction rates of 75% or greater provided their patients with a 50% improvement in overall survival when compared to less experienced centers with primary optimal cytoreduction rates of 25% or less (17). A subsequent study by Chi et al. illustrated that in order to achieve primary optimal cytoreduction rates of 75% or more in advanced-stage ovarian cancer patients, the surgeon's armamentarium should include the ability to remove disease involving upper abdominal structures such as the liver, diaphragm, spleen, and pancreas (5).

Adequate exposure is the most important factor in determining whether resection of diaphragm disease can be performed safely (7). Once an exploratory laparotomy has been performed and the presence of bulky diaphragm disease confirmed on one or both hemidiaphragms, the midline incision is extended to the xiphoid process. For maximum exposure, it can be extended to the sternum to the right of the xiphoid, or in some cases the xiphoid can be divided or removed. The procedure can almost always be performed through this midline incision, and although extending a subcostal incision 2 to 3 cm below the costal margin has been described, we have not generally found this to be necessary.

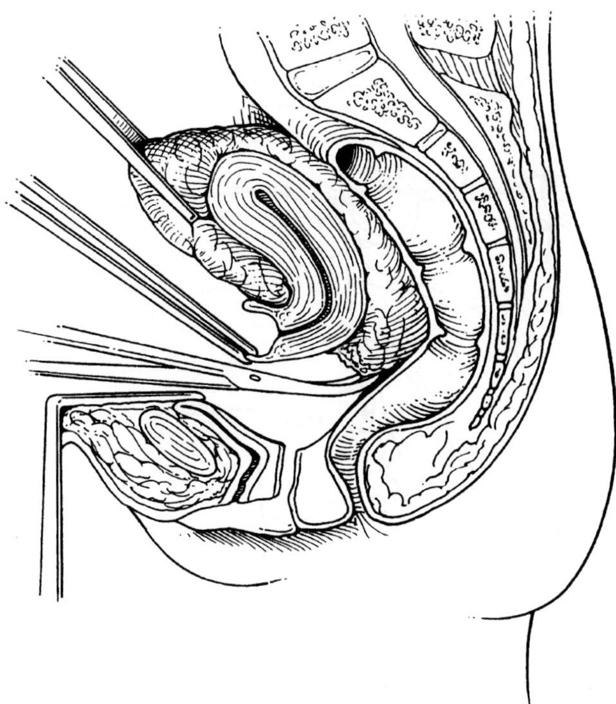

FIGURE 12.24. The posterior vaginal wall is grasped and retracted cephalad. The uterus can now be sharply dissected off of the rectosigmoid. *Source:* Reprinted with permission from Gallup DG, Talledo OE. *Surgical Atlas of Gynecologic Oncology.* Philadelphia: WB Saunders Co.; 1994:103.

The extent of liver mobilization required depends on the distribution of tumor involving the hemidiaphragm. Large volume disease is common on the right side, and a greater proportion of the right hemidiaphragm is obscured by the liver. A right-sided liver mobilization will be described primarily. Tumor involvement on the left diaphragm is more easily resected without fully mobilizing the liver, although in certain cases splenectomy may be necessary to clear the metastatic deposits on the left diaphragm.

The infrahepatic edge of the falciform ligament containing the ligamentum teres is grasped between two Kelly clamps, and is divided and ligated. The suture on the lower edge is left long to aid with downward traction of the liver and remaining falciform ligament. The falciform ligament should be transected all the way to the coronary ligament. This can be used for traction of the liver. The coronary ligament is incised from the falciform to the right triangular ligament. Care must taken in the area of the hepatic notch. The hepatic notch contains the right hepatic vein as it enters the inferior vena cava and is found lateral to the union of the falciform and coronary ligaments. If further mobilization of the liver is necessary, the lateral attachments may be incised and the liver bluntly lifted off Gerota's fascia of the right kidney and diaphragm.

The extent of diaphragm peritonectomy is determined by the distribution of the tumor implants and the method can be modified accordingly. When a full right diaphragm peritonectomy is performed, the peritoneum on the anterior edge of the diaphragm is incised along the costal margin using either cautery or Metzenbaum scissors. This anterior free edge is grasped with several Allis or Mixter clamps, which are then retracted inferiorly to visualize the line of attachment between the diaphragm and its overlying peritoneum. The plane between is developed with a combination of blunt and sharp dissection as determined by the patient's tissue laxity and/or peritoneal adherence. This may not be possible if the tumor has extended through the peritoneum and diaphragm.

If tumor implants are securely fixed to the diaphragm muscle and/or are suspicious for full thickness diaphragm involvement, diaphragm resection should be considered. The technique for diaphragm resection depends largely on the size of the lesion to be resected. Small penetrating lesions can be resected using the EndoGIA stapler alone without entering the pleural cavity. The lesion is grasped with a long Allis clamp, the diaphragm tented downward away from the lung, and the EndoGIA used to staple and divide the tented diaphragm and invasive lesion. Larger lesions require entry into the pleural space and this is generally performed sharply with a Metzenbaum scissors to avoid an inadvertent cautery burn to the lung. Once entered and the lung visualized/retracted, cautery can be used to circumscribe the lesion and resect it en bloc with the peritoneal, muscular, and pleural layers. The defect can almost always be closed primarily with limited tension, using interrupted horizontal mattress or figure-of-eight permanent sutures. Larger defects that cannot be closed primarily without significant tension should be closed with a permanent mesh secured to the peritoneal diaphragm surface with interrupted permanent sutures (18). The majority of patients undergoing diaphragm resection can have their pleural cavity closed and the air from the thorax evacuated using the red Robinson catheter. A purse-string suture is placed widely around the hole and a #14 French red Robinson catheter is passed through the hole into the pleural cavity. The anesthesiologist is asked to give the patient a maximal inspiration, suction may be applied to the catheter, and the catheter is pulled as the purse-string suture is tied down. For patients undergoing more extensive resections or with other reasons to benefit from prolonged pleural drainage, such as pleurodesis, a chest tube can be placed in the operating room and removed postoperatively as required.

To remove tumor from the left upper quadrant, occasionally a splenectomy with or without distal pancreatectomy is required. Usually, the initial step is to enter the lesser sac to evaluate the posterior aspect of the stomach and pancreas. The gastrosplenic ligament and then the short gastrics are carefully divided. The spleen is mobilized medially and out of the left upper quadrant by dividing the splenophrenic and splenocolic ligaments and the other attachments to the adrenal gland and Gerota's fascia of the left kidney. The spleen can now be elevated out of the splenic bed and into the incision. The splenic hilum is now grasped between the fingers. Palpation of the pancreas is attempted. Identification of the pancreas may be facilitated by viewing the hilum posteriorly. The anterior splenorenal ligament is entered sharply. The splenic artery and vein can then be identified. These vessels should be ligated and divided separately. The splenic vessels may also be ligated prior to elevating the spleen in cases where lateral mobilization is not possible secondary to tumor and/or dense adhesions. A linear stapler may be placed across the tail of the pancreas if necessary to remove tumor involving the distal pancreas and/or splenic hilum. Reinforcement of this staple line with 3-0 delayed absorbable suture, either continuously or interrupted, is optional.

Continent Urinary Diversion

Over the past decade, interest in performing continent urinary diversions for patients with gynecologic malignancies has emerged. Most gynecologic oncologists will use a modification of the Indiana (19) or Miami (20) pouch. Poor candidates for continent urinary diversion include those with crippling arthritis or those psychologically unable to tolerate frequent self-catheterization of the pouch.

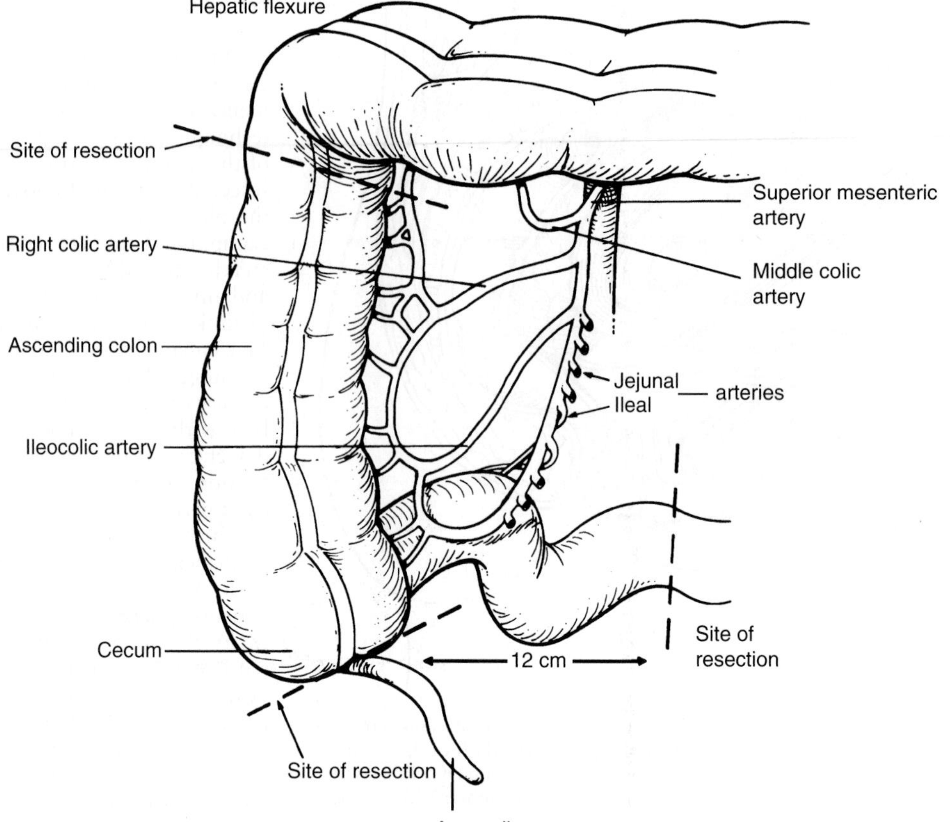

FIGURE 12.25. The anatomic location and vascularity of the right colon segment utilized for formation of the continent urinary pouch. Illustrated are the anatomic sites of division for creation of the continent pouch. The ascending colon is divided distal to the right colic artery. The terminal ileum is divided approximately 12 cm from the ileocecal valve. The resection can be accomplished with the use of surgical staplers or by intestinal clamps. If the appendix is present, it should be removed. The ileocecal segment has a rich blood supply derived from the right colic artery and the ileocolic artery. If one is performing the Miami pouch type of urinary diversion, the transverse colon would be divided distal to the middle colic artery. *Source:* Reprinted with permission from Gallup DG, Talledo OE. *Surgical Atlas of Gynecologic Oncology.* Philadelphia: WB Saunders Co.; 1994:186.

A modification of these pouches is shown (2). The colon is transected just proximal to the hepatic flexure (Fig. 12.25). The colon is then detubularized by a longitudinal incision along the tinea. The continent mechanism is created by two maneuvers. First, the terminal ileal segment is tapered down over a #14 French Foley catheter by using a gastrointestinal anastomosis (GIA) stapling device along the antimesenteric border of the ileum. The second maneuver is to plicate the ileocecal valve by placing concentric purse-string sutures of 0 silk or polypropylene around it. The ureters are then implanted under direct vision (Fig. 12.26) (2). After closing the pouch, the ileal stoma can be brought out in several areas of the abdominal wall (Fig. 12.27) (2). Some use the umbilicus as the exit site. The ureteral stents can exit the abdomen via the ileal stoma or through separate incisions in the pouch and abdominal wall. The use of a Penrose drain and a cecostomy tube for irrigation to remove mucus is optional.

Abdominal Closure

With the advent of more recently published closure methods and newer suture materials, the vertical, allegedly stronger paramedian incision is unnecessary. A midline incision is preferable in modern-day gynecologic oncology. It is the least hemorrhagic of all incisions, and rapid entry is feasible. Exposure is excellent, and minimal nerve damage occurs.

In the past, many surgeons have advocated the relatively time-consuming Smead-Jones closure (21). However, in the 1980s it was noted that midline incisions could be safely closed with a running, mass closure. In 1989, Gallup et al. (22) reported on 210 patients, most of whom were at high risk for evisceration, who had midline incisions closed with a running, mass closure using #2 monofilament polypropylene suture. No eviscerations occurred. Since that publication, several gynecologic oncology services have published excellent results using monofilament absorbable or monofilament permanent sutures in a running, mass closure method (23–26). Figure 12.28 illustrates a popular technique utilizing an absorbable suture (2). Eviscerations using this technique almost never occur.

SURGICAL MANAGEMENT OF GYNECOLOGIC CANCER

The gynecologic oncologist must be able to evaluate the woman with a genital tract malignancy, direct her management, perform the necessary surgical procedures, and supervise her postoperative care and surveillance. A patient who is managed by a surgeon who is not a gynecologic oncologist may receive an operative procedure that is inappropriate or inadequate. Over 20 years ago, McGowan et al. (27) reviewed the intraoperative evaluation of 291 women with primary ovarian cancer. Ninety-seven percent of the patients who underwent surgery by a gynecologic oncologist received complete staging operations, but only 52% and 35% had adequate operations by an obstetrician-gynecologist or a general surgeon, respectively.

Two more recent British studies retrospectively analyzed the outcomes of over 1,800 patients with ovarian cancer (28,29). Both studies found on multivariate analysis that patients' survival was adversely impacted when their initial operation was performed by a general surgeon as opposed to a gynecologic surgeon. These results are similar to those obtained by Nguyen et al. in a national survey of ovarian carcinoma (30). Eisenkop et al. analyzed the outcomes of 263 patients with stages IIIC and IV ovarian carcinoma (31). When

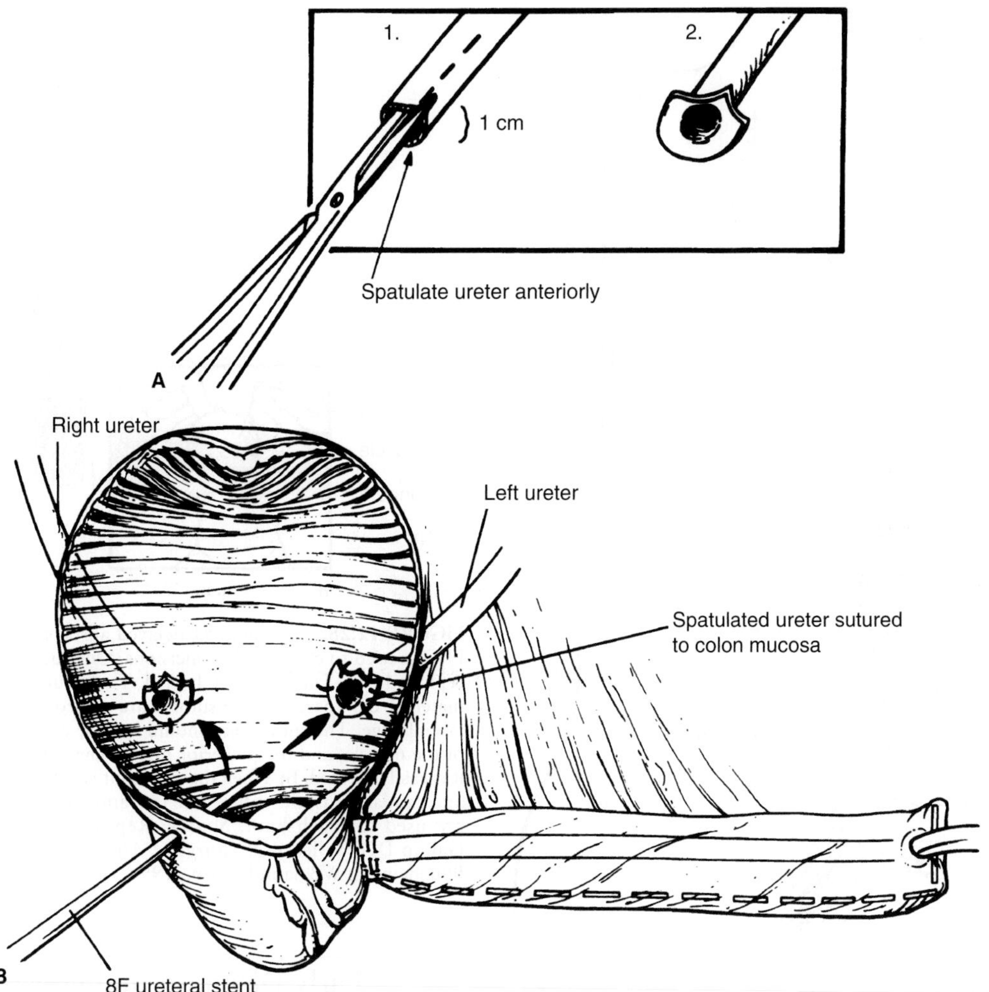

FIGURE 12.26. A, B: Prior to beginning the continent diversion, the ureters have been transected (usually at the pelvic brim) and mobilized so that they are able to be brought to the area where the continent pouch will be located without tension. If necessary, the left ureter can be brought through or under the mesentery of the colon to facilitate its placement into the urinary pouch. An appropriate site is selected on what will be the posterior wall of the pouch, and a long thin clamp is used to perforate the colon and pull the ureter through. An approximately 1-cm segment of ureter is brought into the pouch. For ease of ureterointestinal anastomosis, the ureter should be secured posteriorly to the pouch by suturing the adventitial tissue of the ureter to the seromuscular layers of the pouch with three or four permanent 3-0 sutures. The ureter is spatulated to increase the lumen diameter. The ureter is sutured directly to the colon and is not tunneled. We use 4-0 polyglycolic suture. This is a full-thickness approximation of the colon and ureter. Once both ureters have been sutured into the pouch, two #8 French ureterointestinal stents or long pediatric feeding tubes are placed retrograde into the renal pelvis. If a feeding tube is used, it should be sutured to the ureter with 4-0 chromic to ensure against displacement due to ureteral peristalsis. Note the three concentric sutures at the ileocecal valve. *Source:* Reprinted with permission from Gallup DG, Talledo OE. *Surgical Atlas of Gynecologic Oncology.* Philadelphia: WB Saunders Co.; 1994:191.

the primary surgery was performed by gynecologic oncologists, as compared to general obstetricians-gynecologists and general surgeons, the rate of optimal cytoreduction was significantly higher, the operative mortality substantially lower, and the median survival significantly longer.

Accordingly, other countries have attempted to centralize the care of patients with ovarian cancer so that they are primarily operated on by gynecologic oncologists (32,33). However, patterns of care studies in the United States have demonstrated that a significant percentage of women with ovarian cancer are not receiving their primary treatment from gynecologic oncologists (34,35). Consequently, in this country, many women with ovarian cancer are still not receiving the recommended comprehensive primary surgery (36,37).

In the three decades since the establishment of gynecologic oncology as a subspecialty, cancer therapy has become increasingly sophisticated and complex, and it is difficult for any one physician to master all the skills necessary for treating gynecologic malignancies. More often, we must use multimodal therapy and be involved in multidisciplinary care. There are many medical and radiation oncologists who have specialized in gynecologic cancer, and they are integral members of the multidisciplinary team. The Gynecologic Oncology Group (GOG), with its emphasis on multidisciplinary research, has demonstrated the effectiveness of such an approach.

Another important factor in providing optimal patient care is the environment in which gynecologic oncology is practiced. The facilities used by the gynecologic oncologist should offer

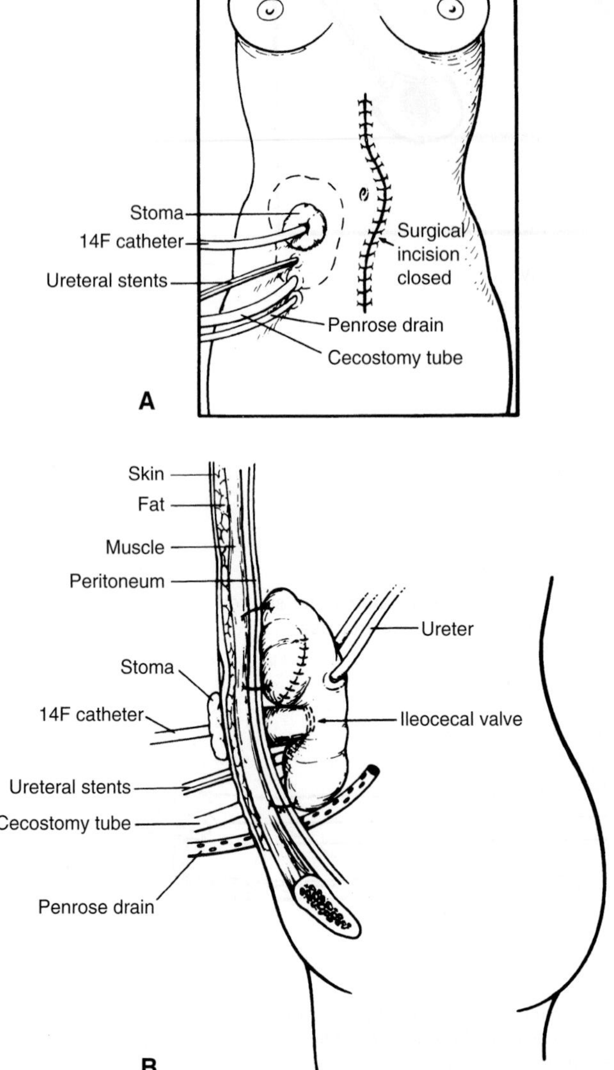

FIGURE 12.27. A, B: The site for the ileal stoma is selected on the anterior abdominal wall and then incised through all abdominal tissue layers. The stoma is created for catheterization and the #14 French catheter should exit the pouch through this stoma. It is critical that the ileal segment be at a 90° angle with the abdominal wall so that catheterization is a "straight shot." The pouch may be sutured to the abdominal wall to accomplish this. All stents and drainage tubes are brought out through the anterior abdominal wall and secured. The pouch may also be anchored posteriorly (i.e., to the sacrum). *Source:* Reprinted with permission from Gallup DG, Talledo OE. *Surgical Atlas of Gynecologic Oncology.* Philadelphia: WB Saunders Co.; 1994:193.

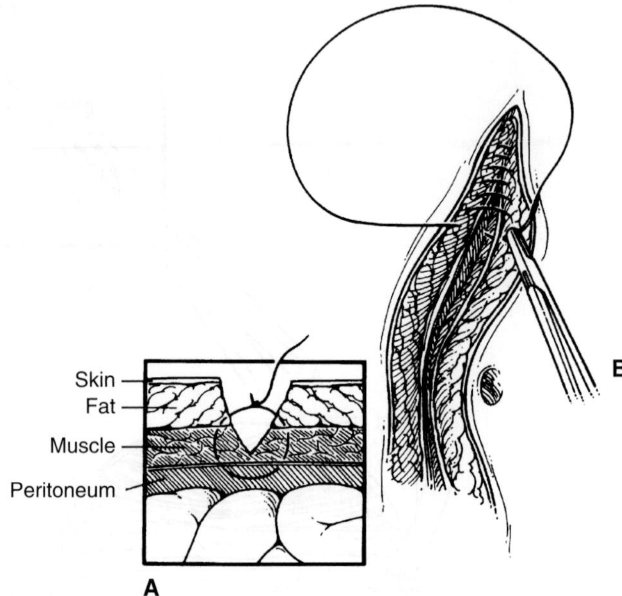

FIGURE 12.28. A running #1 delayed absorbable suture (Maxon or PDS) is used to close midline incisions. One suture is started from the cephalad end. The knots are buried. The sutures are placed approximately 1 cm apart. A: The sutures are placed at least 2 cm from the fascial edge. The suture bite should include anterior fascia, a portion of the muscle, and the posterior fascia. The peritoneum is included if it is easily located. B: When the midpoint is reached from the cephalad and caudad ends, the sutures are tied and the knot buried. Six throws are used for each knot. *Source:* Reprinted with permission from Gallup DG, Talledo OE. *Surgical Atlas of Gynecologic Oncology.* Philadelphia: WB Saunders Co.; 1994:51.

state-of-the-art radiation therapy and chemotherapy. Patients should receive care tailored to the type and extent of their disease and not be determined by the limitations of the available facilities. Mortality rates for complex oncologic procedures, such as pelvic exenteration, have been demonstrated to be significantly lower in hospitals where the procedures are performed with a relatively high volume as compared to those in which the procedures are performed infrequently (38). The recent meta-analysis performed by Bristow et al. evaluated 81 studies involving 6,885 patients with advanced ovarian cancer (17). This study demonstrated a 50% increase in median survival if patients' primary surgery was performed at an "expert" center compared to less experienced centers.

Early Diagnosis and Prevention

There is a role for early diagnosis and prevention in virtually all female genital cancers. The management of a patient with an abnormal Papanicolaou (Pap) smear allows the gynecologic oncologist to use limited surgery to prevent the development of an invasive malignancy of the cervix or vagina. Guided by colposcopy, the surgeon can employ traditional surgical excision, laser surgery, cryotherapy, or a loop electrosurgical excision procedure (LEEP) to preserve function and prevent cancer. Preinvasive lesions of the vulva can be diagnosed and managed by laser or local excision, thereby potentially avoiding progression to invasive disease and its associated extensive surgical therapy.

The proper management of endometrial hyperplasia can prevent the subsequent development of endometrial cancer. Optimal management requires individualization of treatment. Complex hyperplasia without atypia in a premenopausal patient indicates the need for medical therapy with progesterone, but a similar problem in a postmenopausal patient may indicate the need for a hysterectomy. Atypia in either case requires consideration of hysterectomy to prevent the development of endometrial cancer. It is essential that the gynecologic oncologist recognize the significance of these cancer precursors.

No diagnostic test or early symptoms reliably herald the onset of ovarian or tubal cancer, and no preinvasive lesion has been identified. The only method of prevention for these cancers is surgical removal of the tubes or ovaries before cancer develops. Although quite rare, women can be identified who may have as high as a 40% lifetime risk of developing ovarian cancer. These are women who have a family history of ovarian cancer, who have a family history of breast and ovarian cancer, or who are members of hereditary nonpolyposis colorectal cancer (HNPCC) families. These cancer-prone families are described elsewhere in this book. These syndromes are seen infrequently, and certain criteria must be fulfilled before the diagnosis can be made. For women who fall into one of these high-risk categories, surgical removal of the tubes and ovaries (and the uterus in HNPCC) should be considered after child-bearing is complete (39,40). Before that time, close monitoring is essential.

The decision to remove the ovaries and fallopian tubes to prevent ovarian cancer is generally accepted for the post-menopausal patient who undergoes an exploratory pelvic operation or a hysterectomy for benign disease. The removal of the fallopian tubes and ovaries represents little additional surgery, and although the chance of the disease in any woman is quite low, prevention is worthwhile because of the lack of an effective screening modality combined with the devastating effects of ovarian and fallopian tube cancer. However, removal of the ovaries and fallopian tubes in premenopausal women is controversial. For a patient younger than 40 years of age, it seems advisable not to recommend removal of the fallopian tubes and ovaries unless she has a familial risk of ovarian cancer. Between the ages of 40 and 50 years, the pros and cons should be carefully discussed with the patient, and her wishes must be taken into account.

Diagnosis and Staging

The diagnosis of any gynecologic cancer requires a surgical biopsy. The manner in which the histologic diagnosis is obtained varies with the disease and the clinical situation. A punch biopsy or an instrument biopsy may be sufficient for the diagnosis of an invasive cancer of the vulva, vagina, or cervix, but an excisional biopsy is necessary for the diagnosis of microinvasive or preinvasive cancer. A fine-needle aspiration biopsy for cytologic analysis may be adequate for establishing the extent of spread of a cancer, but not for providing histologic cell type and grade for the primary diagnosis. The histologic diagnosis of ovarian or fallopian tube carcinoma requires surgical exploration.

The current International Federation of Gynecology and Obstetrics (FIGO) staging system of gynecologic cancers requires surgical staging for vulvar, endometrial, and ovarian cancer. Cervical cancer remains a clinically staged disease, although many centers use surgical staging (by laparotomy or laparoscopy) for treatment planning. No official FIGO staging exists for fallopian tube cancer or uterine sarcomas, but fallopian tube cancers are usually staged on the basis of surgical and pathologic findings similar to ovarian carcinoma. Table 12.1 lists the current methods of staging for the various gynecologic malignancies.

The initial surgical procedure in a patient with known or suspected gynecologic cancer should be performed by a trained gynecologic oncologist because the accuracy of diagnosis and staging significantly influences subsequent therapy. As stated earlier, numerous studies have demonstrated that ovarian cancer staging operations performed by general obstetricians-gynecologists or general surgeons are inadequate much more frequently than if the operation is performed by a gynecologic oncologist. Young et al. (41) reported excellent survival in patients with early ovarian cancer, but stressed that these data were applicable only to patients with adequate surgical staging.

In addition to the anatomic site and stage of disease, the plan of therapy for most gynecologic malignancies is also influenced by the histologic cell type and histologic grade (differentiation) of the cancer. The cooperation of the surgeon, pathologist, and cytologist cannot be overemphasized in the diagnosis and staging of cancer. It is the surgeon's responsibility to provide the pathologist or cytologist with a complete clinical history and an indication of what he or she hopes to learn from the anatomic specimen. Without this communication, the pathologist and cytologist will be unable to provide the information needed to direct the clinical care of the patient. Both the pathologist and the cytologist must be sure that the surgeon is aware of any special handling that is necessary for a particular specimen. There is no excuse for misinterpretation of a tissue or cytologic specimen because of a failure in communication.

TABLE 12.1

FIGO STAGING OF GYNECOLOGIC CANCERS

Site	Staging
Vulva	Surgical and pathologic staging
Vagina	Clinical staging
Cervix	Clinical staging
Corpus (endometrium)	Surgical and pathologic staging
Corpus (sarcoma)	None (most use modified clinical endometrial cancer staging)
Fallopian tube	None (most use modified surgical and pathology staging)
Ovary	Surgical and pathologic staging
Gestational trophoblastic disease	FIGO staging (clinical) NIH classification WHO classification (risk-oriented)

Note: FIGO, International Federation of Gynecology and Obstetrics; NIH, National Institutes of Health; WHO, World Health Organization.

Surgery as Primary Therapy

Surgery is usually the treatment method of choice for preinvasive diseases of the vulva, vagina, and cervix, for which local excision is both diagnostic and curative. Surgical margins should clear only gross and microscopic disease; removal of large areas of normal tissue is not required. For microinvasive lesions of these organs, wide local excision with a 1- to 2-cm normal tissue margin is appropriate.

Localized disease, such as stage I through stage III vulvar cancer, stage I vaginal cancer, and stages IB1 and IIA cervical cancer, are usually managed by an en bloc radical resection of the primary tumor and regional lymphadenectomy. In these surgical procedures, the operations themselves are designed to be curative without adjunctive therapy unless high-risk conditions are identified. As described in the chapter on vulvar cancer, there is a trend toward more conservative therapy for vulvar malignancies. This allows preservation of normal tissues and prevents some of the disfigurement usually associated with this surgery. Surgery may be curative without adjuvant therapy for other cancers as well, including early-stage endometrial cancer, stage IA ovarian cancer, and early sarcomas of the uterus.

Findings at surgery may indicate the need for additional treatment. This therapy is usually called adjuvant therapy. It is administered because of the potential for occult spread of disease based on a surgical finding (e.g., positive lymph nodes). The use of adjuvant therapy requires that information be available to allow the selection of patients with a high risk of recurrence. These risk groups are defined for each disease site in the appropriate chapters of this book.

Surgery Combined With Other Therapies

In some cancers of the female genital system, surgery is the cornerstone of treatment but is not curative when used alone. Primary cytoreduction of gross disease is vital in advanced ovarian and fallopian tube cancer, but it is of little benefit without adjunctive therapy. Chemotherapy after surgery is a vital and necessary part of the treatment regimen for these cancers. For patients with clinical stage I or II endometrial cancer who have high-grade cancer or deep myometrial penetration, surgical removal of the uterus is an extremely important part of therapy. However, depending on the histopathologic findings of the surgical specimens, additional regional radiotherapy and/or chemotherapy may be indicated. It is the responsibility of the gynecologic oncologist to coordinate surgical therapy with chemotherapy and/or radiation therapy to ensure that the patient receives optimal care.

Surgery as Salvage Therapy

Occasionally, surgical resection can be curative in patients who have failed other therapies. These surgical procedures are almost always extensive and produce some limitation of function. After the failure of other therapies, radical surgery may be the patient's last chance of survival. The classic examples of this situation are vulvar, vaginal, cervical, or uterine cancers that have failed primary surgery and irradiation or irradiation alone. In such cases, pelvic exenteration with removal of virtually all pelvic tissues may offer the only possibility for a cure. Five-year survival rates of 23% to 61% have been reported after pelvic exenteration (42–44).

The possibility of cure with pelvic exenteration is not without cost. The loss of the bladder and the rectum often requires permanent stomas, and sexual function is impaired or lost in many patients. For some patients, reconstructive techniques can prevent the need for stomas and may also restore sexual function. These procedures are described in detail in other chapters in this book. During the last three decades, improvements in initial surgery and radiation therapy along with refinements in selection criteria have made operations like pelvic exenteration infrequent (45). Today, most patients experience distant failure rather than regional failure, and they are therefore not candidates for attempts at curative pelvic exenteration.

Surgery as salvage therapy may also play an important role in the management of ovarian, fallopian tube, and some endometrial cancers. For patients who have failed initial therapy and chemotherapy, second attempts at cytoreduction may be beneficial, provided that reasonable salvage therapy is available (46–48).

Surgery for Metastatic Disease

In selected cases, distant metastases from gynecologic tumors may be curable by surgical resection, or the resection may produce a prolonged disease-free interval. Fuller et al. (49) reported on 15 patients who underwent pulmonary resection of distant metastases from a variety of gynecologic malignancies. They reported a 5-year survival rate of 36% and a 10-year survival rate of 26%. Patients with solitary metastases had a median survival of 64 months, with a median survival of 48 months for those with multiple metastases. Levenback et al. (50) reported their experience with 45 patients who underwent pulmonary resection of metastases from uterine sarcomas. From the date of the pulmonary resection, the 5-year survival rate was 41%, with a 10-year survival rate of 35%. They found a statistically improved chance of survival for patients who developed pulmonary metastases 1 year or longer from their original therapy and for those with unilateral metastases. There was no statistical difference in survival based on the number of nodules (in one lung), the size of the lesion, the age of the patient, or the use of postresection adjunctive therapy. However, the small numbers of patients in this study precluded adequate evaluation of these factors.

Resection of intra-abdominal or pelvic disease may offer palliation by removal of tumor bulk or may allow chemotherapy or irradiation a greater chance of eradicating disease. Resection of tumors that have a poor blood supply often leaves behind smaller tumors with a better blood supply that are more amenable to treatment with chemotherapy or irradiation. Resection of bulk disease also increases the number of residual tumor cells that enter the active cell cycle, in which they may be more responsive to these adjunctive therapies. The availability of new techniques for intraoperative electron beam irradiation or intraoperative brachytherapy may result in more utility for resection of distant and regional metastatic disease.

There is increasing evidence that salvage therapy in ovarian and fallopian tube cancers is likely to be effective only in patients with minimal residual disease. Secondary cytoreduction or resection of regional and distant metastases may play an important role in the treatment of these patients. Recent reports have demonstrated promising results with surgical resection of isolated metastases to the parenchyma of the liver and spleen (51,52).

Surgical Procedures for Specialized Care

Surgical placement of indwelling intravenous access systems allows patients to receive chemotherapy and nutritional supplements and to have necessary blood samples drawn with relative ease and comfort. Placement of these devices, usually semipermanent subcutaneous systems, is safe, contributes to the patient's well-being, and allows for more effective therapy.

The use of intracavitary therapy requires the temporary or semipermanent placement of chest tubes or intraperitoneal access devices. Results of many studies confirm that peritoneal access or vascular access devices placed totally beneath the skin have a low infection rate and a low rate of malfunction (53,54). Implanted arterial infusion devices are being evaluated in research studies to allow direct infusion of therapeutic agents into a tumor mass by means of the arterial system. This therapy often requires intra-abdominal surgery to place the device into the appropriate portion of the vascular system.

Surgery for Reconstruction

Reconstructive surgery may be performed at the time of resection of the cancer, as a delayed procedure, or as required therapy to correct a complication of treatment. Vulvar reconstruction is usually done at the time of initial resection and may involve the use of free skin grafts, rotational flaps of adjacent skin and fat tissue, or myocutaneous grafts from the thigh, buttocks, or anterior abdominal wall. Vaginal reconstruction may also be performed, usually as a planned, delayed phase of reconstruction. Vaginal reconstruction requires free skin grafts or myocutaneous flaps depending on the size of the defect and whether or not there has been previous irradiation of the vaginal bed. The techniques of vulvar and vaginal reconstruction are explained in detail in other chapters of the book.

Reconstruction as therapy for complications of treatment may be required for the closure of defects from improper wound healing, radiation necrosis, or tissue loss after extravasation of chemotherapeutic agents. Although free skin grafts may be used to reconstruct surgical wound disruption or tissue loss due to chemotherapy extravasation, radiation necrosis usually requires the use of myocutaneous flaps because of a lack of adequate blood supply in the area of the injury.

Surgery for Palliation

Surgery for palliation may involve resection of tumor to relieve symptoms, or it may involve diversion or bypass of portions of the gastrointestinal or urinary tract to prolong life and provide comfort. Surgical procedures may also be used to provide pain relief by interrupting sensory nerve transmissions. Surgical removal of tumor bulk to provide palliation has been discouraged by many authorities. They point out that without effective adjunctive therapy, tumor regrowth occurs quickly and the surgical procedure proves to be futile. Although this may be true in most cases, the gynecologic oncologist should not uniformly dismiss the concept of surgical palliation. A surgical procedure to provide relief of symptoms is usually considered a failure if the tumor regrows in 6 to 12 months. However, palliative administration of a chemotherapeutic agent for 6 to 12 months is considered to be successful if there is minor tumor shrinkage or stabilization of disease despite the side effects of the chemotherapy. As a surgeon, the gynecologic oncologist must remember that a surgical procedure with limited risk and a reasonable recovery period may provide as much relief as 6 to 12 months of palliative chemotherapy or a course of palliative irradiation. The difficult decision about when to employ surgical palliation requires astute surgical judgment and a realistic assessment of the patient's condition and wishes.

Palliative surgery is more frequently used to relieve specific dysfunctions, such as obstruction of the urinary or intestinal tract. Relief of urinary tract obstruction may be accomplished by ureteroneocystostomy or by urinary conduit depending on the location of the obstruction and the location or extent of disease. A urinary conduit can provide immediate and permanent relief to the patient who has a ureterovaginal, vesicovaginal, or urethrovaginal fistula. It may also provide relief of urinary obstruction, which will prolong life and allow for the administration of additional chemotherapy or irradiation. The judgment of the surgeon and the desires of the patient become essential factors in this decision process. For the patient who is miserable because of constant urinary leakage or who may benefit from additional therapy, the decision to perform a urinary diversion is quite simple. If diversion is done to prolong life, however, the decision must be weighed carefully. For a patient who has a limited life expectancy or is in uncontrollable pain, performing a urinary diversion may do more harm than good.

The gynecologic oncologist must also consider the relative benefits of nonsurgical urinary diversion, such as placement of a ureteral stent or a percutaneous nephrostomy. For many patients, percutaneous nephrostomy is a better choice than surgical intervention. This is particularly true if the aim is to employ adjunctive chemotherapy or irradiation, or if a surgical procedure is not feasible because of medical conditions or other surgical considerations. Unfortunately, a percutaneous nephrostomy cannot help the patient with a fistula because the nephrostomy will not totally divert the urine.

Placement of a ureteral stent, by cystoscopy or antegrade through a percutaneous nephrostomy, is usually better and safer than urinary diversion for the relief of obstruction. Current technology allows the placement of stents that can be left in place for months and can be changed easily over a guide wire by means of the cystoscope.

Intestinal obstruction threatens the patient's quality of life, and the decision of whether to perform an intestinal diversion is usually easy. Deciding whether the operation is feasible can be more difficult. For the patient with localized disease, a diverting colostomy or an intestinal bypass is usually possible and is not very difficult. For the patient with intra-abdominal carcinomatosis, the decision is more complex. The surgeon may not be able to determine the extent of intestinal involvement preoperatively and may have difficulty deciding whether the surgical procedure will benefit the patient.

Pothuri et al. (55) recently evaluated 68 palliative operations performed on 64 patients with recurrent ovarian cancer and intestinal obstruction. In 84% of cases, a corrective surgical procedure was able to be performed, whereas no corrective surgical procedure was possible for the remaining 16%. Of the 57 cases where corrective surgery was possible, 71% were successfully palliated ("successful palliation" is defined as the ability to tolerate a regular or low-residue diet at least 60 days postoperatively). If surgery resulted in successful palliation, median survival was 11.6 months compared to 3.9 months for all other patients.

THE FUTURE OF GYNECOLOGIC ONCOLOGY

As of 2008, the subspecialty of gynecologic oncology is over 30 years old. From a cadre of farsighted individuals with a variety of training backgrounds, a cohesive subspecialty has developed with consistent standards of training, a system of certification, and recognition in the medical community. None of this has come easily, and we owe a great deal to that first generation of gynecologic oncologists.

Several current issues are affecting the future role of gynecologic oncology within the medical community. Our relationship with our parent specialty of obstetrics and gynecology is being reexamined, as well as our ties with general surgery and urology, specialties with which we often seem even more closely allied. As technologic advances occur, we are becoming more integrated with the specialties of medical oncology and radiation oncology. Although we remain primarily surgeons, and surgery remains our principal mode of therapy, it is critical to emphasize the integrated multidisciplinary management of the patient with gynecologic cancer.

The benefits of multidisciplinary care were recently highlighted in a clinical announcement by the National Cancer Institute (NCI) concerning concurrent chemoradiation for cervical cancer (56). In each of five randomized phase 3 trials of women with various stages of cervical cancer, the addition of chemotherapy to radiotherapy was found to provide a significant survival benefit (13,57–60). The risk of death from cervical cancer was decreased by 30% to 50% with the multimodality approach.

Changes in Surgical Therapy

If the past decade is any indication of the future, significant changes in the technology of surgery can be expected to occur as we proceed through the new millennium. New materials, new surgical instruments, and new devices will be invented, and many of these will make surgical treatment better. Certainly, laparoscopic surgery appears to have made a significant impact on our specialty, as well as on the other surgical specialties.

Innovative methods of supportive care will be developed to further the technical capabilities that we now possess, such as computerized anesthesia machines and transesophageal ultrasound. Anesthetic agents will become better and safer, and will be joined by a new generation of antibiotics and cardiovascular medications. We will be able to treat the older patient surgically with relative safety, which is especially important because of the increased incidence of cancer in the elderly and because of the advancing age of our population. Our responsibilities include staying abreast of these advances and judiciously integrating them into our practices.

Changes in the Indications for Surgery

Early diagnosis will change the indications for surgery and the types of procedures that should be done. We will be able to treat more patients with less disfigurement and with greater preservation of function. A larger proportion of patients will present with early disease, allowing surgery to be used more frequently for definitive cure.

Better adjunctive therapies will increase the importance of initial surgical therapy. More patients will benefit from surgical cytoreduction to minimize disease. The availability of effective irradiation and chemotherapeutic regimens will make adjuvant therapy feasible in more cases, and it will become more important for us to identify risk groups who are likely to develop recurrent disease after surgery.

Multidisciplinary Therapy and Primary Care

In outlining the extent of surgical training required for the gynecologic oncologist, the founders of this discipline were careful to include adequate training that would enable the gynecologic oncologist to become an accomplished abdominopelvic surgeon. The gynecologic oncologist must be trained to perform the gynecologic, gastrointestinal, and urologic surgery necessary to manage gynecologic cancer and its potential complications. As stated by John L. Lewis Jr. (61), in reference to pelvic exenteration by a team of gynecologists, general surgeons, and urologists, "Even when the surgery was successful, the postoperative care required committee meetings and its outcome was often less than successful."

These same founders realized that, although training can produce a qualified surgical oncologist, the complete care of the cancer patient requires knowledge of the basic biologic, physical, and pharmacologic principles of radiation therapy and chemotherapy. This does not mean that the gynecologic oncologist must be a radiation oncologist or a medical oncologist, but it does demand that he or she know enough to ensure proper integration of all therapeutic modalities. Throughout the United States, this collaboration in the care of patients with gynecologic cancer has produced multidisciplinary teams of gynecologic oncologists, radiation oncologists, medical oncologists, and pathologists who provide state-of-the-art cancer care. The GOG, a national cooperative research group, has demonstrated how this multidisciplinary approach to gynecologic oncology research can be achieved.

Despite the emphasis on multidisciplinary care, the gynecologic oncologist should maintain active involvement during all aspects of a patient's care. The principle of being the patient's physician until she is either cured or dies of her disease has been an integral part of our subspecialty and must be maintained. The constant involvement of the gynecologic oncologist through all phases of cancer treatment ensures optimal integration of surgery, irradiation, and chemotherapy. The patient receives continuity of care and the reassurance of a physician who is involved at each stage of her therapy and follow-up.

CONCLUSION

After three decades, the gynecologic oncologist has emerged as a surgical oncologist for women. The specialist has sufficient familiarity with radiation oncology and medical oncology to ensure the proper integration of all modalities of treatment, and he or she is able to apply surgical skills for primary therapy, secondary therapy, reconstruction, and palliation. The gynecologic oncologist stands in the obstetrics and gynecology community but has one foot in the community of surgeons.

The emergence of cooperative research groups, particularly the GOG, has allowed a generation of gynecologic oncologists to develop superior clinical research skills. These skills must be continually stressed in the training of young oncologists and as an integral part of the practice of our subspecialty. A growing number of young oncologists are receiving additional training in basic research. This is vital for the continued development of the subspecialty and for progress toward the prevention and care of gynecologic cancers. Our position in the arena of clinical practice is well established, and we must now establish ourselves equally well as scientists and surgical researchers.

References

1. Morrow CP, Curtin JP, eds. *Gynecologic Cancer Surgery*. New York: Churchill Livingstone; 1996.
2. Gallup DG, Talledo OE, eds. *Surgical Atlas of Gynecologic Oncology*. Philadelphia: WB Saunders; 1994.
3. Levine DA, Barakat RR, Hoskins WJ. *Atlas of Procedures in Gynecologic Oncology*. London: Inform Healthcare; 2008.
4. Fowler JM, Johnson PR. Transperitoneal para-aortic lymphadenectomy. *Oper Tech Gynecol Surg* 1996;1:8–12.
5. Chi DS, Franklin CC, Levine DA, et al. Improved optimal cytoreduction rates for stage IIIC and IV epithelial ovarian, fallopian tube, and primary peritoneal carcinoma: a change in surgical approach. *Gynecol Oncol* 2004;94:650–654.
6. Eisenhauer EL, Abu-Rustum NR, Sonoda Y, et al. The addition of extensive upper abdominal surgery to achieve optimal cytoreduction improves survival in patients with stage IIIC-IV epithelial ovarian cancer. *Gynecol Oncol* 2006;103:1083–1090.
7. Eisenhauer EL, Chi DS. Liver mobilization and diaphragm peritonectomy/resection. *Gynecol Oncol* 2007;104(2):S25–S28.
8. Skandalakis JE, Gray SW, Rowe JR, eds. *Anatomical Complications in General Surgery*. New York: McGraw-Hill; 1983.
9. Poulin EC, Schlachta DM, Maazza J. Splenectomy. Gastroinestinal tract and abdomen. In: Souba WW, Fink MJ, Jurkovich GJ, et al., eds. *ACS Surgery*. New York: WebMd; 2005.
10. Berman ML, Lagasse LD, Watring WG, et al. The operative evaluation of patients with cervical cancer by an extraperitoneal approach. *Obstet Gynecol* 1977;50:658–664.
11. Gallup DG, King LA, Messing MJ, et al. Paraaortic lymph node sampling by means of an extraperitoneal approach with a supraumbilical transverse "sunrise" incision. *Am J Obstet Gynecol* 1993;169:307–312.
12. Weiser EB, Bundy BN, Hoskins WJ, et al. Extraperitoneal versus transperitoneal selective paraaortic lymphadenectomy in the pretreatment surgical staging of advanced cervical carcinoma: a Gynecologic Oncology Group study. *Gynecol Oncol* 1989;33:283–289.
13. Rose PG, Bundy BN, Watkins EB, et al. Concurrent cisplatin-based chemoradiation for locally advanced cervical cancer: *New Engl J Med* 1999;340:1144–1153.
14. Chi DS, Eisenhauer EL, Lang J, et al. What is the optimal goal of primary cytoreductive surgery for bulky stage IIIC epithelial ovarian carcinoma? *Gynecol Oncol* 2006;103:559–564.
15. Bristow RE, del Carmen MG, Kaufman JS, et al. Radical oophorectomy with primary stapled colorectal anastomosis for resection of locally advanced epithelial ovarian cancer. *J Am Coll Surg* 2003;197(4):565–574.
16. Mourton SM, Temple LK, Abu-Rustum NR, et al. Morbidity of rectosigmoid resection and anastomosis in high risk patients undergoing primary cytoreductive surgery for advanced epithelial ovarian cancer. *Gynecol Oncol* 2005;99:608–614.
17. Bristow RE, Tomacruz RS, Armstrong DK, et al. Survival effect of maximal cytoreductive surgery for advanced ovarian carcinoma during the platinum era: a meta-analysis. *J Clin Oncol* 2002;20:1248–1259.
18. Juretzka M, Abu-Rustum NR, Sonoda Y, et al. Full thickness diaphragmatic resection for stage IV ovarian carcinoma using the EndoGIA stapling device with diaphragmatic reconstruction using a gortex graft: a case report and review of the literature. *Gynecol Oncol* 2006;100:618–620.
19. Rowland RG, Mitchell ME, Bihrle R, et al. Indiana continent urinary reservoir. *J Urol* 1987;137:1136–1139.
20. Penalver MA, Benjany DE, Averette HE, et al. Continent urinary diversion in gynecologic oncology. *Gynecol Oncol* 1989;34:274–288.
21. Wallace D, Hernandez W, Schlaerth JB, et al. Prevention of abdominal wound disruption utilizing the Smead-Jones closure technique. *Obstet Gynecol* 1980;56:226–230.
22. Gallup DG, Talledo OE, King LA. Primary mass closure of midline incisions with a continuous running monofilament suture in gynecologic patients. *Obstet Gynecol* 1989;675–677.
23. Gallup DG, Nolan TE, Smith RP. Primary mass closure of midline incisions with a continuous polyglyconate monofilament absorbable suture. *Obstet Gynecol* 1990;76:872–875.
24. Montz FJ, Creasman WT, Eddy G, et al. Running mass closure of abdominal wounds using absorbable looped suture. *J Gynecol Surg* 1991;7:107–110.

25. Orr JW, Orr PF, Barrett JM, et al. Continuous or interrupted fascial closure: a prospective evaluation of no. 1 Maxon suture on 402 gynecologic procedures. *Am J Obstet Gynecol* 1990;163:1485–1489.
26. Sutton G, Morgan S. Abdominal wound closure using a running, looped monofilament polybutester suture: comparison to Smead-Jones closure in historic controls. *Obstet Gynecol* 1992;80:650–654.
27. McGowan L, Lesher LP, Norris HJ, et al. Misstaging of ovarian cancer. *Obstet Gynecol* 1985;65:568–572.
28. Kehoe S, Powell J, Wilson S, et al. The influence of the operating surgeon's specialisation on patient survival in ovarian cancer. *Br J Cancer* 1994;70:1014–1017.
29. Woodman C, Baghdady A, Collins S, et al. What changes in the organisation of cancer services will improve the outcome for women with ovarian cancer? *Br J Obstet Gynecol* 1997;104:135–139.
30. Nguyen HN, Averette HE, Hoskins W, et al. National survey of ovarian carcinoma, part V. The impact of physician's specialty on patient's survival. *Cancer* 1993;72:3663–3670.
31. Eisenkop SM, Spirtos NM, Montag TW, et al. The impact of subspecialty training on the management of advanced ovarian cancer. *Gynecol Oncol* 1992;47:203.
32. Tingsulstad S, Skjeldestad FE, Hagen B. The effect of centralization of primary surgery on survival in ovarian cancer patients. *Obset Gynecol* 2003;102:499–505.
33. Andersen ES, Knudsen A, Svarrer T, et al. The results of treatment of epithelial ovarian cancer after centralisation of primary surgery. Results from North Jutland, Denmark. *Gynecol Oncol* 2005;99:552–556.
34. Harlan LC, Clegg LX, Trimble EL. Trends in surgery and chemotherapy for women diagnosed with ovarian cancer in the United States. *J Clin Oncol* 2003;21:3488–3494.
35. Goff BA, Matthews BJ, Wynn M, et al. Ovarian cancer: patterns of surgical care across the United States. *Gynecol Oncol* 2006;103:383–390.
36. Chan JK, Kapp DS, Shin JY, et al. Influence of the gynecologic oncologist on the survival of ovarian cancer patients. *Obstet Gynecol* 2007;109: 1342–1350.
37. Goff BA, Matthews BJ, Larson EH, et al. Predictors of comprehensive surgical treatment in patients with ovarian cancer. *Cancer* 2007;109(10): 2031–2042.
38. Begg CB, Cramer LD, Hoskins WJ, et al. Impact of hospital volume on operative mortality for major cancer surgery. *JAMA* 1998;280:1747–1751.
39. Kauff ND, Satagopan JY, Robson ME, et al. Risk reducing salpingo-oophorectomy in women with a *BRCA1* or *BRCA2* mutation. *N Engl J Med* 2002;346:1609–1615.
40. Rebbeck TR, Lynch HT, Neuhausen SL, et al. Prophylactic oophorectomy in carriers of *BRCA1* or *BRCA2* mutations. *N Engl J Med* 2002;346:1616–1622.
41. Young RC, Walton LA, Ellenberg SS, et al. Adjuvant therapy in stage I and stage II epithelial ovarian cancer: results of two prospective randomized trials. *N Engl J Med* 1990;332:1021–1027.
42. Lawhead RA, Clark GC, Smith DH, et al. Pelvic exenteration for recurrent or persistent gynecologic malignancies: a 10-year review of the Memorial Sloan-Kettering Cancer Center Experience (1972–1981). *Gynecol Oncol* 1989;33:279–282.
43. Morley GW, Hopkins MP, Lindenauer SM, et al. Pelvic exenteration, University of Michigan: 100 patients at 5 years. *Obstet Gynecol* 1989;74:934–943.
44. Matthews CM, Morris M, Burke TW, et al. Pelvic exenteration in the elderly patient. *Obstet Gynecol* 1992;79:773–777.
45. Chi DS, Gemignani ML, Curtin JP, et al. Long-term experience in the surgical management of cancer of the uterine cervix. *Semin Surg Oncol* 1999;17:161–167.
46. Eisenkop SM, Friedman RL, Spirtos NM. The role of secondary cytoreductive surgery in the treatment of patients with recurrent epithelial ovarian carcinoma. *Cancer* 2000;88:144–153.
47. Scarabelli C, Gallo A, Carbone A. Secondary cytoreductive surgery for patients with recurrent epithelial ovarian carcinoma. *Gynecol Oncol* 2001;83:504–512.
48. Chi DS, McCaughty K, Schwabenbauer S, et al. Guidelines and selection criteria for secondary cytoreductive surgery in patients with recurrent platinum sensitive epithelial ovarian carcinoma. *Cancer* 2006;106(9): 1933–1939.
49. Fuller AF, Scannell JG, Wilkins W Jr. Pulmonary resection for metastases from gynecologic cancers: MGH experience, 1943–1982. *Gynecol Oncol* 1985;22:174–180.
50. Levenback C, Rubin SC, McCormack PM, et al. Resection of pulmonary metastases from uterine sarcomas. *Gynecol Oncol* 1992;45:202–205.
51. Yoon SS, Jarnagin WR, DeMatteo RP, et al. Resection of recurrent ovarian or fallopian tube carcinoma involving the liver. *Gynecol Oncol* 2003;91(2): 383–388.
52. Gemignani ML, Chi DS, Gurin CC, et al. Splenectomy in recurrent epithelial ovarian cancer. *Gynecol Oncol* 1999;72:407–410.
53. Davidson SA, Hoskins WJ, Rubin SC, et al. Intraperitoneal chemotherapy: analysis of complications with an implanted subcutaneous port and catheter system. *Gynecol Oncol* 1991;41:101–106.
54. Makhija S, Leitao M, Sabbatini P, et al. Complications associated with intraperitoneal chemotherapy catheters. *Gynecol Oncol* 2001;81:77–81.
55. Pothuri B, Vaidya A, Aghajanian C, et al. Palliative surgery for bowel obstruction in recurrent ovarian cancer: an updated series. *Gynecol Oncol* 2003;89:306–313.
56. National Cancer Institute. Clinical announcement regarding concurrent chemoradiation for cervical cancer. February 22, 1999.
57. Whitney CW, Sause W, Bundy BN, et al. Randomized comparison of fluorouracil plus cisplatin versus hydroxyurea as an adjunct to radiation therapy is stage IIB-IVA carcinoma of the cervix with negative para-aortic lymph nodes: a Gynecologic Oncology Group and Southwest Oncology Group study. *J Clin Oncol* 1999;17:1339–1348.
58. Morris M, Eifel PJ, Lu J, et al. Pelvic radiation with concurrent chemotherapy compared with pelvic and para-aortic radiation for high risk cervical cancer. *N Engl J Med* 1999;340:1137–1143.
59. Keys HM, Bundy BN, Stehman FB, et al. Cisplatin, radiation, and adjuvant hysterectomy compared with radiation and adjuvant hysterectomy for bulky stage IB cervical carcinoma. *N Engl J Med* 1999;340:1154–1161.
60. Peters WA, Liu PY, Barrett R, et al. Concurrent chemotherapy and pelvic radiation therapy compared with pelvic radiation therapy alone as adjuvant therapy after radical surgery in high-risk early-stage cancer of the cervix. *J Clin Oncol* 2000;18:1606–1613.
61. Lewis JL Jr. Training of the gynecologic oncologist. In: Coppleson M, ed. *Gynecologic Oncology: Fundamental Principles and Clinical Practice.* Edinburgh: Churchill Livingstone; 1981:4–20.

CHAPTER 13 ■ LAPAROSCOPIC SURGERY IN GYNECOLOGIC CANCER

DENIS QUERLEU, MARIE PLANTE, YUKIO SONODA AND ERIC LEBLANC

Laparoscopy became a regular feature in the practice of gynecology during the 1960s. Although it played a role in the early detection of pelvic, mainly ovarian, malignancies (1), the concept of using it in the management of gynecologic cancer did not emerge until the late 1980s. A special mention must be given to Daniel Dargent, who pioneered the concept of laparoscopy in the field of gynecologic oncology. Daniel Dargent, trained as a vaginal surgeon, was dedicated to maintaining the tradition of the Schauta operation, which explains his original design of the radical vaginal trachelectomy. His vast surgical culture extended beyond the field of gynecologic oncology, which explains his adaptation of the urologic concept of selecting for radical surgery only those patients with negative nodes, and for the same reason his dedication to the typically "urologic" extraperitoneal approach. Finally, he was aware of the early development of advanced laparoscopic techniques in Clermont-Ferrand, France. All these combined factors led him to pioneer the developments of extraperitoneal lymph node dissection in the staging of cervical cancer. This chapter is an update, not a complete revision, of the same chapter of the previous edition of this book with Daniel Dargent as the first author. The general style of writing and argumentation of concept have been preserved throughout the previous contribution of Daniel Dargent.

Urologists were the first to consider whether endoscopy could play a role in the management of pelvic tumors. The first report was published in 1980 by Hald and Rasmussen (2). These Danish urologists used an instrument derived from the Carlens mediastinoscope for assessing the iliac nodes in patients affected by urinary bladder or prostatic cancer. The tip of the instrument was placed in direct contact with the iliac vessels after digital preparation was made through a short inguinal incision. Small samples were taken from the tissues surrounding the vessels using forceps introduced through the instrument. The decision to perform radical surgery, which is only of benefit for node-negative patients, was made according to the result of the endoscopic assessment.

When laparoscopic surgery was pioneered in patients affected by gynecologic cancer, the rationale was similar: By assessing the pelvic lymph nodes in patients affected by cervical cancer, candidates for vaginal radical hysterectomy (VRH) could be determined (3). The technique was also similar except that the laparoscope was used instead of direct endoscopy.

THE EARLY YEARS (1987–1992): RETROPERITONEAL LAPAROSCOPIC PELVIC LYMPHADENECTOMY

The first laparoscopic pelvic assessments were performed through two separate inguinal incisions. The view obtained of the pelvic sidewall was much wider than the view obtained with the mediastinoscope, and node sampling was easier with an instrument introduced through a separate port. After a dozen attempts, the technique was refined and required only a suprapubic midline incision. This approach, panoramic retroperitoneal pelviscopy, was first described in a monograph published in 1989 by Dargent and Salvat (4), who reported the data of 107 procedures. Thereafter, the data for 200 patients' operations performed between December 1986 and February 1991 were detailed in the classic textbook edited by Nichols and published in 1993 (5).

There was some criticism during the 5 years following the initial description of laparoscopic lymphadenectomy. Critics were concerned about operative risks, the limited area of dissection, and oncologic risks (two abdominal implants occurred among the first 200 operations), but the main obstacle was cultural in nature. The surgical anatomy of the retroperitoneal space was unfamiliar to the gynecologic surgeon, especially when viewed through a laparoscope. It was only after Querleu (6) devised the transumbilical transperitoneal laparoscopic approach that the concept of the "oncolaparoscopy" began to emerge.

THE MATURATION PERIOD: 1992–2003

In June 1989, Querleu (6) presented his first report on laparoscopic transumbilical transperitoneal lymphadenectomy as a staging procedure for patients affected by cervical cancer. The technique used was the routine laparoscopic technique: Both broad ligaments were opened using a peritoneal incision made alongside the axis of the iliac vessels, allowing dissection and retrieval of the pelvic nodes under laparoscopic guidance. The data on the first 39 operations were published in 1991 in the *American Journal of Obstetrics and Gynecology* (7).

Months after Querleu's publication, Childers and Surwit (8) published the first two American cases—both patients with endometrial cancer. They added a low para-aortic sampling to the pelvic lymphadenectomy. The operation was completed with a transvaginal hysterectomy.

After these early publications, the concept of laparoscopically assisted surgical staging emerged. That same year, the use of the laparoscope in the management of cervical cancer was reported (9). The "oncolaparoscopic" movement began by (a) applying this new concept to malignancies other than endometrial cancer, (b) increasing the thoroughness of the staging dissection, and (c) combining staging with the preparation for radical vaginal surgery with a progressive move to purely laparoscopic radical surgery.

The transition of laparoscopy-assisted surgical staging from endometrial cancer to cervical cancer was not unexpected. The first reports did not clearly indicate the rationale for the laparoscopic staging, but only demonstrated that the staging was feasible and probably safe (9,10). Subsequently, surgeons began to distinguish the different roles of laparoscopy between early- and advanced-stage disease (11,12). The use of laparoscopic surgery in the management of ovarian cancer was first reported in 1973 (13); however, it was not until 1990 that laparoscopic management of ovarian cancer was first reported (14). Except for the concept of laparoscopic restaging for incidental adnexal cancers, which was accepted after the first reported cases of laparoscopic infrarenal aortic dissection (15), this application remains the most questionable. Endoscopy, specifically inguinoscopy, was also introduced into the management of vaginal and vulvar cancers (16) but never gained acceptance, probably because of the development of the sentinel node technique. With time, laparoscopy found a place in the management of the majority of gynecologic malignancies.

The extent of laparoscopic staging has gone through a pendular development. In its earliest form, laparoscopic lymphadenectomy was limited to the interiliac area (4). The laparoscopic pelvic lymphadenectomy described by Querleu et al. (7) soon progressed to the common iliac area and then to the inframesenteric aortic area (8,17,18). Beginning in 1994 (15), the infrarenal para-aortic nodes were included in laparoscopic dissection, and thereafter Possover et al. (19) described laparoscopic suprarenal retrocrural dissection. It was around this time that the concept of sentinel node biopsy emerged as a procedure that could potentially eliminate the need for systemic dissection. This concept has been combined with laparoscopy to produce a convenient method for carrying out this type of biopsy (20).

Laparoscopy-assisted radical surgery and purely laparoscopic radical surgery were foreseeable developments from the concept of laparoscopic staging. Laparoscopically assisted surgical staging was being established during a period when the use of laparoscopically assisted vaginal hysterectomy was commonplace for benign conditions (21). Thus, it was a natural extension of laparoscopically assisted vaginal hysterectomy to apply it to the treatment of endometrial cancer (8). The use of laparoscopy in the management of cervical cancer was initiated by combining laparoscopically assisted surgical staging with the Schauta radical vaginal hysterectomy (3). Descriptions of the laparoscopically assisted vaginal radical hysterectomy, or coelio-Schauta, began appearing in the early 1990s (22–24), and soon after, series using this new procedure began to appear in the literature (25,26). In spite of this, the use of the laparoscopically assisted vaginal radical hysterectomy remains limited because of the lack of training of most gynecologic surgeons in the field of advanced vaginal surgery. As more surgeons became familiar with the abdominal approach to radical hysterectomy, the use of laparoscopy resulted in the development of laparoscopic radical hysterectomy, which was also initially described in the early 1990s by Canis et al. (27) and Nezhat et al. (10). Conceptually, this approach is easier to grasp by those more familiar with the abdominal approach, as witnessed by the growing number of publications demonstrating its feasibility and safety (28–30). Laparoscopy has recently also been used to perform pelvic exenteration (31).

OTHER DEVELOPMENTS AND THE QUESTIONS THEY RAISE

The next technical development in the field of laparoscopy may come from robotics. The biggest drawbacks of these robots are the cost and size. For the experienced laparoscopic surgeon, these "heavy" robots have yet to demonstrate an obvious benefit except for fine suturing in which the robot excels. Thus, these robots may eventually be employed when laparoscopic suturing is required, that is, during reconstruction operations following exenterative surgery. As the use of robots grows, these procedures will undoubtedly be further developed.

The future of laparoscopic extirpative surgery is a second point of discussion. The data available on total laparoscopic or laparoscopically assisted radical surgery seem to be comparable to those of open surgery. The radical nature of the surgeries can be preserved with laparoscopy. In general, the operative time is increased, but the blood loss is generally diminished and the postoperative morbidity is improved. However, good level-one evidence regarding the use of laparoscopy is not yet available in the field of gynecologic cancer surgery. During the emergence of laparoscopy, improvements in open abdominal surgery have also occurred. Newer technologies (i.e., Ligasure, Tyco; Biclamp, Erbe, Tubingen, Germany) and better analgesics decrease blood loss, operative time, and postoperative pain for open surgery. Only through well-designed randomized trials will the better surgical approach be determined.

The future of laparoscopically assisted surgical staging is the third point open to discussion. There are no doubts about its feasibility and safety. One can, in spite of the absence of direct manual sensation, assess the peritoneal cavity and the retroperitoneal spaces with the same accuracy as through an open incision. One may also argue that the visual assessment is better thanks to the optical magnification. On the other hand, if doubts exist about the benefits of laparoscopy in extirpative surgery, they do not exist in the specific field of surgical staging. Laparoscopy paralleled with xiphopubic laparotomy or J-shaped large side incisions that were the standard in the past, and is a more acceptable surgical staging procedure. However, in spite of its obvious benefits, laparoscopic staging has been challenged. A recent randomized trial has demonstrated that surgically staged patients with cervical cancer had a worse survival irrespective of the surgical approach used (open surgery or laparoscopy) (32). The results of this trial are largely biased (see below), but one has to recognize that surgical staging has an excellent potential to separate the good and the poor prognostic cases without necessarily improving life expectancy. In the future, prognostic information obtained from newer procedures, such as the sentinel node biopsy, or from the molecular analysis of the tumor itself could replace the information obtained from imaging and surgical staging.

BASIC ELEMENTS OF LAPAROSCOPIC SURGERY

Laparoscopic surgery is usually performed via CO_2 insufflation to create a pneumoperitoneum. There are several techniques used to enter the abdomen for laparoscopic procedures.

"Closed" laparoscopy, employing a Veress needle followed by blind insertion of the first trocar, is favored by many laparoscopic surgeons. Others prefer direct "blind" trocar insertion. The use of disposable trocars with retractable blades for direct trocar insertion does not appear to significantly reduce the risk of bowel or vascular injuries. This is of particular concern since the majority of complications following laparoscopic surgery are related to trocar insertion (33). Conversely, the "open" technique where the fascia and the peritoneum are surgically opened and the trocar inserted under direct visualization is considered by many to be the safest access technique, although this is likely not to be true in patients with a history of laparotomy.

CO_2 Laparoscopy: Closed Versus Open Technique

Bonjer et al. (34) reviewed the literature and compared data between 12,444 open laparoscopic and 489,335 closed laparoscopic cases. Rates of visceral and vascular injury were 0.083% and 0.075%, respectively, after closed laparoscopy and 0.048% and 0.0%, respectively, after open laparoscopy ($p = 0.002$). Mortality rates were 0.003% for the closed and 0.0% for the open laparoscopy technique (p = NS). In another randomized trial of blind versus open laparoscopy for laparoscopic cholecystectomy, the major complication rate was 4% in the blind group and 1.3% in the open group, respectively ($p < 0.05$). Minor complications occurred in 6.7% of patients in both groups (35). In a large series of 2,000 cases performed for general surgery procedures, there was no vascular injury and only one bowel injury with the open laparoscopy technique (36). Perone (37) published a series of 585 cases of laparoscopy using a simplified open technique. There were no technical failures or major complications, despite the fact that nearly 30% of the patients had undergone previous laparoscopy or laparotomy.

Decloedt et al. (38) performed laparoscopic surgery in patients with gynecologic malignancies and reported only a 1% complication rate for the open laparoscopy technique, despite the fact that a high proportion of the patients had previous major surgery and/or radiation therapy. In another study of patients who underwent operations for pelvic masses, it was noted that all the vascular injuries occurred during direct trocar insertion in patients without prior abdominal surgery, and the authors now routinely use an open technique in all their cases (39). Altogether, the data seem to indicate that the open laparoscopy technique is safer than closed laparoscopy. A recent large series, however, comparing 8,324 cases of direct laparoscopic entry versus 1,562 cases of open laparoscopy for gynecologic procedures did not show a difference in the rate of major complications. In fact, there were more conversions to laparotomy in the open technique group (40). A recent review on laparoscopic entry concludes that there is no evidence that the open entry technique is superior or inferior to other entry techniques currently available (level II-2C evidence) (41). Authors also conclude that direct entry with shielded trocars may decrease entry injuries. The visual entry cannula system may represent an advantage over traditional trocars, as it allows a clear optical entry; however, that does not necessarily avoid all visceral or vascular injuries (41).

In patients with prior abdominal surgery, using midline incisions, Childers et al. (42) proposed the use of the Veress needle in the left upper quadrant to first insufflate the abdomen prior to the trocar entry. Also, in cases where the risk of injury appears high because of prior abdominal surgery, smaller 5- or 7-mm trocars may be used to enter the abdomen, as opposed to the traditional 10- to 12-mm trocars. Choosing the lateral flank, rather than the midline subumbilical area, as an entry site may also be useful. This can potentially decrease the risk of damaging bowel loops that could be adherent under the anterior abdominal wall from prior surgeries.

Gasless Laparoscopy

With hopes of decreasing tumor cell spillage, gasless laparoscopy was developed in the early 1990s (43). The gasless system involves lifting the abdominal wall using an abdominal wall-lifting device. Valveless ports and conventional instruments or laparoscopic instruments can be used without gas leak (44,45). Several devices have been developed that avoid the use of CO_2 to distend the abdomen. Two devices frequently used are the Laparolift retraction system (Origin Medsystems, Menlo Park, California, USA) and the Abdo-lift (Karl Storz, Tuttlingen, Germany).

Theoretically, gasless laparoscopy has numerous advantages over the traditional CO_2 laparoscopy: It avoids the problem of CO_2 leakage as well as difficulties associated with creating and maintaining adequate CO_2 pressure. Indeed, high-pressure irrigation and large-volume suction devices can be used without losing the CO_2 gas, which, when lost, can seriously impair adequate visibility. Gasless laparoscopy can also avoid the potential for infectious particles contaminating the CO_2 insufflation gas and the problem of lowering the body temperature (46), thus avoiding potential risks of metabolic and hemodynamic instability from CO_2 insufflation (47). In patients for whom general anesthesia and CO_2 pneumoperitoneum are contraindicated, gasless laparoscopy can be used, as it does not significantly increase the intra-abdominal pressures. The procedure can also be performed under epidural anesthesia and has been successfully performed during pregnancy (48–53).

Galen et al. (45) performed 80 gynecologic procedures using gasless laparoscopy. They compared their gasless laparoscopically assisted vaginal hysterectomy with 150 laparoscopically assisted vaginal hysterectomies performed with CO_2 pneumoperitoneum. They concluded that the Laparolift retraction system satisfactorily maintained visualization during the entire procedure, including the vaginal portion of the surgery. In another series of 49 laparoscopic gynecologic surgeries performed with gasless laparoscopy, the success rate was 90%. It allowed the surgical team to use the vaginal and laparoscopic approaches simultaneously (54). Tintara et al. from Thailand performed 40 gynecologic procedures using gasless laparoscopy and reported no surgical complications. They considered the operative field virtually the same as that of the CO_2 pneumoperitoneum, except in morbidly obese patients (55).

Tintara et al. also recently published a series comparing 31 gasless laparoscopic hysterectomies (GLHs) with 31 total abdominal hysterectomies (56). The operating time was longer by almost 1 hour, but blood loss, hospital stay, and convalescence were lower in the GLH group (56). Comparable results were also reported by others (57). Conversely, a clinical trial of 30 cases looking at the measure of visualization as primary outcome concluded that exposure with conventional laparoscopy using pneumoperitoneum is superior to that offered by gasless laparoscopy (58).

Data in gynecologic oncology are limited. A gasless pelvic lymphadenectomy has been reported by one team (44); the authors retrieved 45 lymph nodes and found this approach satisfactory. On the other hand, Johnson and Sibert (59) reported a randomized comparison of gasless versus CO_2 laparoscopy for tubal ligation and reported markedly increased technical difficulty with the gasless approach. Another group conducted a randomized comparison of gasless and CO_2 laparoscopy in 57 patients undergoing infertility surgery (60). Six patients in the gasless group had to be converted to CO_2 pneumoperitoneum because of inadequate exposure. The authors concluded that times to achieve exposure and close incisions were longer, and exposure and ease of surgery were worse in the gasless group. They found no advantages to this procedure over the conventional CO_2 approach (60). In a randomized prospective study, postoperative pain appeared to be similar for both techniques in patients undergoing laparoscopic tubal ligation (61).

Currently, gasless laparoscopy is not as widely used as CO_2 laparoscopy and the data on the procedure are more limited. However, the technique does merit further evaluation in oncology patients, particularly because of the concerns that CO_2 pneumoperitoneum may increase tumor spread (see next section on port-site metastasis).

Port-Site Metastasis

There has been increasing concern among surgical oncologists about the apparent increased rate of port-site metastases following laparoscopic procedures. The reported rate of abdominal-wall recurrences from two large studies following traditional abdominal surgery was 1% to 1.5% (62,63). In the last few years, as laparoscopic procedures have become more popular in oncology patients, there have been several reports in the literature of port-site metastases following laparoscopic surgery for a variety of cancers.

Schaeff et al. (64) conducted a literature review of port-site metastasis and found 164 reported cases from 90 publications, including 29 cases in gynecologic procedures. Wang et al. (65) recently conducted a similar MEDLINE search and found that the rate of port-site metastasis in ovarian cancer varies between 1.1% and 13.5%. A recent series of 83 patients who underwent laparoscopy for diagnosis, treatment, or staging of gynecologic cancers shows an overall incidence of port-site metastasis of 2.3%. As expected, the risk was highest in patients with recurrence of ovarian and peritoneal malignancies in the presence of ascites (66). Vergote et al. also observed a high rate of port-site metastasis after laparoscopic surgery in patients with advanced ovarian cancer, but concluded that the prognosis was not worse in those patients and that laparoscopy remains a convenient technique to diagnose advanced ovarian cancer or rule out other primary tumors (67).

Initial reports in gynecologic oncology surgery suggested that patients with adenocarcinomas of the ovaries with ascites and peritoneal seeding were at highest risk for port-site metastasis. Although most reports suggest that port-site metastases occur in advanced-stage cancer and poorly differentiated tumors, thus being an indicator of tumor virulence, there have been worrisome reports of low-stage and well-differentiated tumors causing postlaparoscopy tumor seeding (64). Borderline tumors (65), squamous cell cancers of the cervix (68,70), and adenocarcinomas of the endometrium have also been reported to metastasize to port sites (71). In a recent literature review of 58 reported port-site metastases, Ramirez et al. confirmed that port-site metastases are a potential complication of laparoscopic surgery in patients with gynecologic malignancies, even in patients with early-stage disease (69).

The time period between the laparoscopic surgery and the appearance of port-site metastasis varies between 1 week and 3 years (71). Of concern, a number of port-site metastases have been documented to develop very rapidly after laparoscopic procedures, as early as 1 to 2 weeks. Timely referral for staging and definitive treatment becomes very important, as delays in referral have been shown to increase the rate of port-site metastasis and worsen prognosis. Several measures have been recommended to decrease the risk of port-site metastasis. These include thorough irrigation of the port sites (72), use of large volumes of saline for lavage of the abdominal cavity (73) and of the port sites (65), slow abdominal-wall deflation, use of a wound protector, and use of a specimen bag to retrieve the specimen (74).

Clearly, morcellation of suspicious solid tumors should be avoided at all cost, and according to Canis et al., if the abdominal wall is protected with a bag and the tumor is not morcellated, the incidence of trocar site metastasis is approximately 1% (75). To further reduce the risk of trocar-site metastasis, some authors recommend the resection of the laparoscopic ports in a full-thickness fashion at the time of the staging laparotomy, ideally within 1 week of the laparoscopic surgery (76–78). Van Dam et al. also recommend closing all the layers of the trocar sites at the end of the laparoscopic procedure, i.e., the peritoneum, the rectus sheath, and the skin. Indeed, in their study, they noted that trocar site metastasis developed in 58% of their patients with only the skin closure of the trocar site compared to 2% of patients with closure of all layers (78).

The causes of port-site metastasis seem to be multifactorial: gas used, local trauma, tumor manipulation, biologic properties of the tumor, and individual surgical skills (64). Wang et al. (65) have identified a number of risk factors associated with port-site metastasis: ovarian cancer, adenocarcinoma histology, peritoneal carcinomatosis, presence of ascites, and diagnostic or palliative procedures performed for malignancy. Based on a review of experimental data, Canis et al. concluded that the risk of dissemination following laparoscopic surgery is increased when a large number of malignant cells are present. For that reason, they suggested that adnexal tumors with external vegetations and bulky lymph nodes should be considered as contraindications to CO_2 laparoscopy (79). Other reported etiologies of port-site recurrence include trauma to the port site from frequent removal of instruments, tumor seeding from removal of the specimen through the port, and potential leakage of ascites (64,65). Trocar-site hematomas seem to also favor the rapid growth of tumor implants.

In an animal model, it was demonstrated that pneumoperitoneum itself may play an important role in the etiology of port-site metastasis (80). Others are concerned about the use of CO_2, as it may increase tumor cell spillage and implantation (81). Local immune suppression and growth-factor secretion may also be involved (82). Recent data from animal studies suggest that the underlying immune or metabolic status of the host has a marked independent effect on tumor spread and implantation (83).

Due to concerns regarding the potential increased risk of tumor dissemination associated with CO_2 laparoscopy, some experts advocate the use of gasless laparoscopy. An animal model comparing gasless laparoscopy, CO_2 laparoscopy, and laparotomy was performed to study peritoneal tumor growth and abdominal-wall metastasis. The study concluded that CO_2 insufflation promotes tumor growth in the peritoneum and is associated with greater abdominal-wall metastasis than gasless laparoscopy. They also found that direct contact between a solid tumor and the port site enhances local tumor growth (81). Other studies in rats have also shown that CO_2 may have an effect on growth stimulation on tumor cells (84), and CO_2 insufflation results in tumor dissemination during laparoscopy, leading to port-site metastasis (85). In these rat models, it appears that gasless laparoscopy may reduce the risk of wound metastasis following laparoscopic surgery for cancer (86). Conversely, using an ovarian cancer xenograft animal model, two recent studies from the same authors seem to indicate that CO_2 laparoscopy has a minor impact on visceral metastasis and survival and has no deleterious effect on tumor growth compared to gasless laparoscopy (87,88). Similar results have been shown in humans. Abu-Rustum et al. retrospectively reviewed patients with persistent metastatic intra-abdominal peritoneal or ovarian cancer at time of second-look surgery. There was no difference in overall survival between patients who underwent laparoscopy or laparotomy; thus, the authors concluded that CO_2 pneumoperitoneum did not appear to reduce overall survival (89). In fact, a higher rate of port-site metastasis with gasless laparoscopy has been reported in some series (90). In a large review of 2,593 laparoscopic procedures on 1,288 women, all with malignant disease, Abu-Rustum et al. identified seven patients who developed a trocar-related subcutaneous implant. However, there were no "isolated" trocar-related implants noted, and all seven patients had synchronous metastasis or carcinomatosis. The authors argued that subcutaneous implantation should not be routinely used as an argument against laparoscopy (91).

Despite the above data, it is still controversial as to whether the use of gasless laparoscopy will reduce the risk of port-site metastasis. Some argue that the risk of tumor dissemination is just as great with gasless laparoscopy (65,85,92). Others argue that the surgical technique and the thorough lavage of the port site are probably more important than the use of CO_2 (93). Reymond et al. (93) claim that gasless laparoscopy is not the solution to the problem, since numerous port-site metastases have been reported after thoracoscopy where CO_2 insufflation was not used. In their opinion, the surgeon's role in seeding tumor cells is important and can be decreased by avoiding excessive tumor manipulation and frequent replacement of trocars. Variation in surgeons' techniques may explain the large differences in the reported incidence of port-site metastasis (0% to 21%). Meticulous surgical technique and the use of preventive measures will keep the incidence of port-site metastasis to about 1%, comparable to that seen with open laparotomy (93).

Laparoscopic Management of Pelvic Masses

A growing body of literature indicates that the laparoscopic management of pelvic masses is safe and effective. It significantly reduces the length of hospital stay, operative morbidity, and overall postoperative recuperation time. Despite careful preoperative evaluation, it appears inevitable that some of those masses will turn out to be malignant. Proper management and following strict surgical guidelines is very important in achieving optimal results.

Large series reported that among all patients approached laparoscopically for pelvic masses, the overall rate of malignancy is low (Table 13.1) (39,94–110). The rate varies greatly among the studies according to the preoperative selection criteria used and the study design. It is also interesting that the rate of malignancy reported since 1997 seems to be higher. This may be explained by the fact that more surgeons are becoming comfortable with invasive laparoscopic techniques and are thus more likely to approach high-risk pelvic masses laparoscopically.

Preoperative Selection

In 1994, Canis et al. (96) published an extensive, retrospective 12-year analysis with long-term follow-up of 757 patients from 1980 to 1991. All patients had ovarian masses and were managed by laparoscopy. The authors followed a strict set of criteria to select cases for laparoscopic management. The complete preoperative investigation included a pelvic sonogram, CA-125 measurement, and pelvic examination. Obviously

TABLE 13.1

LITERATURE CONCERNING LAPAROSCOPIC MANAGEMENT OF PELVIC MASSES

Authors	No. of ovarian malignancies/no. of laparoscopies for pelvic masses	%
Nezhat et al., 1992 (94)	4/1,011	0.40
Hulka et al.,1992 (95)	55/13,739	0.40
Canis et al., 1994 (96)	1 9/757	2.5
Blanc et al., 1994 (97)	78/5,307	1.4
Marana et al.,1995 (98)	2/949	0.21
Wenzl et al., 1996 (99)	108/16,601	0.65
Yuen et al., 1997 (100)	0/102	0
Hidlebaugh et al., 1997 (101)	8/405 ~	2.0
Guglielmina et al., 1997 (102)	34/803	4.2
Malik et al., 1998 (103)	11/292	3.7
Dottino et al., 1999 (39)	17/160	10.6
Sadik et al., 1999 (104)	2/220	1.0
Ulrich et al., 2000 (105)	10/211	4.7
Serur et al., 2001 (106)	7/100	7.0
Mettler et al., 2001 (107)	6/493	1.2
Mendilcioglu et al., 2002 (108)	2/61	3.3
Havrileski et al., 2003 (109)	8/396	2.0
Leng et al., 2006 (110)	16/2083	0.77

Source: Leng JH, Lang JH, Zhang JJ, et al. Role of laparoscopy in the diagnosis and treatment of adnexal masses. *Chin Med J (Engl)* 2006;119(3):202–206.

malignant or suspicious masses were managed with laparotomy. The others underwent a laparoscopic evaluation, which included a peritoneal cytology, cyst puncture, and endocystic evaluation also referred to as "cystoscopy." At laparoscopy, if a malignant mass was encountered or was considered highly suspicious, an immediate midline laparotomy was performed. Following this algorithm, their rate of inadvertent malignancy was 2.5% (19 of 757), including 12 borderline and 7 invasive cancers. Additionally, 27 masses were falsely diagnosed as malignant (3.6%), which means that these patients had an unnecessary laparotomy. Based on that experience, Canis et al. consider laparoscopic management of pelvic masses to be safe and reliable (96).

Although it is generally agreed that by careful preoperative and intraoperative assessment most cancers can be adequately diagnosed and properly managed, the preoperative evaluation is frequently of limited value and cannot discriminate a benign mass from a malignant mass. Benacerraf et al. (111) used sonography to study 100 women undergoing laparotomy for ovarian masses; in their study, sonography was misleading in 15% of cases. Guglielmina et al. (102) reviewed their experience with laparoscopic management of over 800 ovarian cysts and concluded that neither ultrasound nor laparoscopic evaluation can accurately predict the exact nature of an adnexal mass. Even when carefully conducted, preoperative investigation cannot accurately detect all ovarian cancers (103). Maiman et al. (112) noted that four of the so-called "benign" characteristics were present in 31% of the pelvic masses found to be malignant. According to Nezhat et al. (94), neither the CA-125 level, pelvic ultrasound, nor peritoneal cytologic testing had sufficient specificity to predict malignancy.

Laparoscopic Approach

In general, laparoscopic management for pelvic masses is considered safe and effective. There are several reported advantages to this approach: shorter hospital stay, decreased postoperative pain and recovery time, less adhesion formation, decreased hospital cost, and lower complication rate. The failure rate of laparoscopy in removing pelvic masses is low (less than 5%) (10,112,113).

In a randomized trial, Yuen et al. (100) compared laparoscopy with laparotomy in the management of ovarian masses in 102 patients. Exclusion criteria included masses suspicious for malignancy and lesion diameter greater than 10 cm. Their data showed that inadvertent cyst rupture was frequent in both groups and operative time was comparable. The laparoscopic approach was associated with significant reductions in operative morbidity, postoperative pain, required analgesia, hospital stay, and recovery period. Those findings were confirmed by others (14,113–115). Recently, Jennings et al. (116) reported a significantly decreased length of hospital stay without adverse effect on the surgical complication rate in patients undergoing operations in a gynecologic oncology unit.

Concerns Regarding Laparoscopic Management of Pelvic Masses

There are several concerns regarding the laparoscopic management of benign-appearing pelvic masses. These include failure to diagnose malignancy; underestimation of the extent of disease; tumor spillage from rupture of the masses; inability to perform complete staging, implying another surgery for the patient; and, most important, long delays before a staging procedure or definitive treatment that can adversely affect the ultimate prognosis of the patient (39,117). The risk of port-site metastasis has been discussed extensively above.

Intraoperative Frozen Section

The management of any pelvic mass, either by laparoscopy or by laparotomy, should include access to accurate frozen section, so the necessary procedure can be performed immediately. In one large series, the overall accuracy of frozen section was 92.7% (118). However, in a collected series of over 11,000 laparoscopies for ovarian cysts, Lehner et al. (117) reported that frozen section was obtained at the time of laparoscopy in only 34% of cases. Frozen section was obtained in 40% of cases in the survey of Society of Gynecologic Oncologists (SGO) members by Maiman et al. (112). Also of interest in the latter study is that the average age of patients with invasive cancers was 44 years, and 29% of these tumors were borderline. Ovarian cancer is thus not uncommon in perimenopausal women, and surgeons should always keep a high index of suspicion. A recent series of 141 patients undergoing laparoscopic surgery for a pelvic mass looked at the accuracy of frozen section to guide the surgical management. This study showed that the frozen section diagnosis was accurate in 95.5% of benign tumors, 77.8% of borderline tumors, and in only 75% of cancers (119). These results confirm that frozen section is a useful tool to guide the intraoperative management but also that pelvic masses should always be handled as though they could be malignant (119). The accuracy of the frozen section (FS) is also size dependent: for masses larger than 10 cm, FS becomes less reliable (120). The recent use of magnetic resonance imaging does not appear to be superior to the intraoperative frozen section analysis with regard to the diagnosis of pelvic masses (120). Most authors agree that availability of frozen section at the time of laparoscopy is mandatory, even in younger women, so that a staging procedure can be performed without delay when indicated (39,94,117,121,122).

Tumor Spillage

It remains controversial as to whether intraoperative tumor spillage carries a poorer prognosis. Some authors have noted that preoperative tumor rupture or the presence of ascites may worsen the prognosis (43), while others did not find any difference in survival among stage I patients with intraoperative spillage (121). Mettler et al. (123) found that tumor propagation does not occur in ruptured stage I cases if definitive surgery is performed within 1 week. According to others, the grade of the tumor and the presence of ascites in stage I cancer of the ovary is more important in relation to survival than is rupture of the ovarian capsule at surgery (124,125). Nevertheless, all pelvic masses should be considered potentially malignant, and consequently, all efforts should be made to avoid rupture.

Delayed Staging

Maiman et al. (112) surveyed SGO members with regard to their management of ovarian neoplasms later found to be malignant. The response rate from members was 42% and 42 cases of ovarian malignancy were reported. In that survey, immediate staging had been performed in 17% of cases, delayed in 71% (median, 36 days), and not performed in 12%. The authors raised significant concerns with regard to the negative outcome of some laparoscopically managed ovarian cancers, particularly as it related to the significant number of patients who were not restaged and to the delay between the initial procedure and the definitive treatment. They concluded that delays of more than 4 weeks had a negative impact on patient outcome.

Blanc et al. (126) conducted a similar multi-institutional French survey and recorded 5,307 ovarian lesions treated laparoscopically, of which 1.4% were malignant. Staging of cancer cases was performed immediately in 25% of the cases, delayed in 58% (median, 78 days), and not performed in 16%. In those who had delayed staging, 22.4% were upstaged.

Kindermann et al. (122) also sent a questionnaire to 273 German departments of obstetrics and gynecology with a response rate of 46%. They collected a total of 192 ovarian cases managed laparoscopically. Overall, 16% of borderline stage IA and 39% of malignant stage IA tumors (based on laparoscopy) had spread of disease identified at staging laparotomy. In 92% of cases, capsule rupture and tumor morcellation with intra-abdominal spillage occurred at laparoscopy. Endoscopy bags were used in only 7.4% of ovarian cancer cases. In patients staged more than 8 days after initial laparoscopy, nearly 75% of cases were upstaged (20% to stage IC and 53% to stages II-III). Most disturbing, trocar-site metastasis was identified in 52% of patients with stages IC-III at initial laparoscopy if definitive surgery was delayed more than 8 days.

Leminen and Lehtovirta (127) reported on eight patients who had their staging laparotomy after laparoscopic surgery within a mean of 17 days (range, 7 to 29). In four patients, the disease had spread from a localized to an advanced stage during the delay. The authors concluded that laparoscopic surgery of ovarian masses later found to be malignant can cause considerable and rapid spread of the disease. Hopkins et al. reported a similar experience with three young women who had laparoscopic removal of what appeared to be benign lesions. All three underwent re-exploration within 3 weeks, yet trocar site metastasis and intra-abdominal tumor spread had already occurred (77).

Lastly, Lehner et al. (117) sent a questionnaire to all gynecology departments in Austria regarding laparoscopic management of ovarian masses later found to be malignant. Of the 70 cancers identified, 48 patients underwent an immediate laparotomy to complete surgery, 24 had a laparotomy within 17 days (median, 9.9 days), and 24 patients had delays of more than 17 days (median, 47.7 days). The cutoff of 17 days was chosen arbitrarily. Only 10% of malignant tumors were reported using an endoscopy bag. They found that patients in whom definitive surgery was delayed more than 17 days were more likely to be upstaged (odds ratio of 5.3 for borderline tumors and 9.2 for invasive cancers). In a multivariate analysis, delay of more than 17 days was an independent prognostic factor for stage of disease in borderline cases. This was not statistically significant in the cases of invasive ovarian cancer. The study does not provide data as to whether survival was subsequently affected by the upstaging.

The above studies emphasize that poor surgical technique and delayed definitive surgery when managing ovarian masses by laparoscopy can have a very serious impact on patients' survival. It also underscores the fact that, because of the subsequent upstaging, a number of patients will likely be subjected to adjuvant chemotherapy, which they may not have otherwise needed.

Comprehensive Management of Suspicious Pelvic Masses

Recently, Dottino et al. (39) challenged the concept that patients with a suspicious pelvic mass should necessarily undergo laparotomy. In their study, they purposely approached all the pelvic masses referred to their oncology unit by laparoscopy regardless of the suspicion of malignancy, except when there was evidence of gross metastatic disease (i.e., omental cake) or masses extending above the umbilicus. All masses were sent for immediate frozen-section analysis. Despite the fact that the majority of the masses were considered suspicious for malignancy preoperatively, 87% of the masses were in fact benign, and 88% were successfully managed by laparoscopy. Not surprisingly, compared with other series (Table 13.1) (39,94–109), a higher proportion of the masses turned out to be malignant (10.6%), but most of them were managed laparoscopically following oncologic standards. If debulking was deemed to be best performed by laparotomy, the laparoscopy was converted to an open case. In many instances, adequate surgery could be completed by laparoscopy. Long-term data on overall outcome and survival following laparoscopic surgery for ovarian cancer are not available. Canis et al. (121) also suggest performing a diagnostic laparoscopy regardless of the ultrasonographic appearance of the pelvic mass, although they recommend an immediate laparotomy for staging of cancer cases. They also reiterate the importance of frozen-section analysis to appropriately decide definitive treatment. When indicated, they consider restaging of cancers as an "oncologic emergency." Quinlan et al. (115) included complex masses and septated cysts in their selection criteria. Laparoscopy by trained laparoscopists can be used to evaluate adnexal masses in women with risk factors for ovarian cancer with a low complication rate and reduced hospital stay (128). A recent study of 313 patients comparing the performance of ultrasound findings, laparoscopy findings, and frozen-section analysis showed that laparoscopy correctly identified ovarian cancer and borderline tumors with a sensitivity and a specificity of 100% and 99%, respectively (129).

It would thus appear that even though suspicious masses have traditionally been managed by laparotomy, laparoscopic management of high-risk pelvic masses can be successfully performed in an oncology referral population if there is expertise in operative laparoscopy, availability of immediate and accurate pathologic evaluation, and appropriate further treatment where indicated. In many cases, having an oncologist skilled in advanced laparoscopic procedures allows laparoscopic completion of the staging procedure. However, when skilled assistance is unavailable, it is best to terminate the laparoscopic procedure after a cancer diagnosis and to promptly refer the patient for definitive surgery. As stated by Alvarez et al. (130), "accuracy is more important than immediacy."

According to the literature, laparoscopy for the management of pelvic masses can eliminate the need for unnecessary laparotomy in most cases. Statistically, the majority of them will be benign and can be adequately managed laparoscopically, and most of the recent publications conclude that laparoscopy is a safe approach for the treatment of adnexal masses (Table 13.1) (39,94–109). However, the above data clearly demonstrate that delayed staging and definitive treatment can have a negative impact on patient outcome more than the laparoscopic procedure itself. When appropriate referral for a staging operation is made in a timely fashion, ideally within 2 weeks, it is unlikely that disease progression will occur (122,130). Moreover, until proven otherwise, ovarian masses should always be considered potentially malignant. Thus, surgeons should be technically meticulous in order to minimize the risk of ovarian cyst rupture and spillage, and specimens should always be retrieved intact through an endobag to reduce the risk of trocar-site metastasis. With advances in laparoscopic surgical technique, suspicious ovarian masses can be approached laparoscopically as long as a plan is in place for appropriate staging and treatment by laparotomy or laparoscopy (39).

Borderline Tumors

Borderline tumors often present as multilocular lesions on sonogram and may have elevated CA-125 levels. Darai et al. (131) reported a series of 43 borderline tumors of which 34 were approached by laparoscopy. Of those, 27 were completely managed by laparoscopy. There were four recurrences, three of which occurred in patients who had ovarian cystectomies only. The authors concluded that laparoscopic management of borderline tumors is feasible, but ovarian cystectomies are associated with a higher risk of recurrence. Two other recent French studies showed that the initial laparoscopic surgery in the management of borderline tumors is associated with a lower rate of complete staging, a higher rate of cyst rupture, and a higher recurrence rate following conservative treatment (132,133). However, despite an incomplete staging, there does not appear to be a detrimental effect on outcome in patients with apparent early borderline tumors (134). A Scandinavian group also retrospectively compared the short-term outcome of 107 patients with borderline tumors operated on by laparoscopy or laparotomy. The authors concluded that laparoscopic treatment of borderline tumors is feasible in moderate size tumors (<10 cm) and is associated with fewer complications and shorter hospital stay. However, in larger size tumors, cyst rupture was significantly more frequent in the laparoscopy group (135).

LAPAROSCOPIC RETROPERITONEAL STAGING: PELVIC AND AORTIC LYMPH NODE DISSECTIONS

Laparoscopy enables visual assessment, sampling, and systematic dissection of the lymph nodes located in the extraperitoneal space along the pelvic sidewall and in the para-aortic area. Both direct and indirect transumbilical approaches are discussed.

Transumbilical Transperitoneal Laparoscopic Lymphadenectomies

The transumbilical transperitoneal technique for laparoscopic lymphadenectomy remains the most popular approach employed by gynecologists. This in part has to do with the familiarity of gynecologists with this indirect approach. The setup is essentially the same as for routine laparoscopy. The ports are placed in a similar configuration as that used for traditional pelvic laparoscopy (Fig. 13.1). The size of the ports will depend on the instruments that are to be employed. When para-aortic lymphadenectomy is to be performed, it is helpful to place the lateral ports slightly more cephalad, avoiding the abdominal wall vasculature, and an additional port in the left upper quadrant may be required to assist with retraction of the intestines.

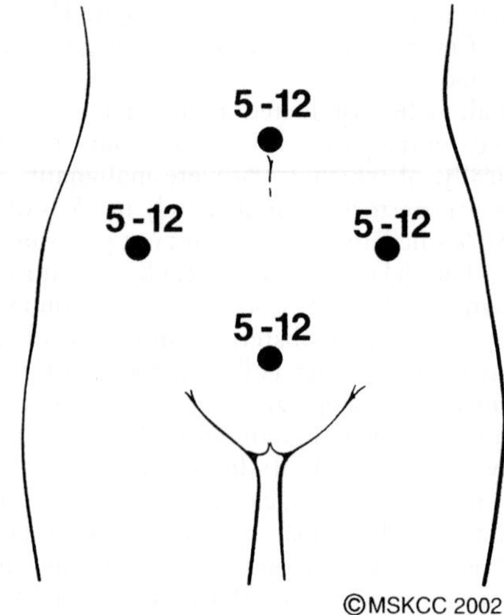

FIGURE 13.1. Transperitoneal trocar placement for laparoscopic lymphadenectomy.

Pelvic Dissection

The surgeon intending to perform a pelvic dissection stands on the patient's left side. The video monitor is placed at the foot of the operating table. The peritoneum is divided along the pelvic brim between the round ligament and the infundibulopelvic (IP) ligament, which are best left undivided until the dissection is finished. Prior to opening the peritoneum, the umbilical ligament is located, which is seen as an oblique peritoneal fold on the posterior surface of the abdominal wall. By following this "Ariadne's thread" from front to back, once the broad ligament is opened, it is easy to identify the superior vesical artery and its ventral continuation, the umbilical ligament. The superior vesical artery is the first surgical landmark in the pelvic dissection. Retracting it medially enables one to open the paravesical space and free the pelvic sidewall. This exposes the external iliac vessels at the point where they cross Cooper's ligament. In obese patients whose anatomic structures are covered with fatty tissue, it is recommended to locate Cooper's ligament first. This can be identified by palpation with a blunt instrument on the posterior surface of the pubis, lateral to the umbilical ligament—much the same way a blind person seeks the edge of the pavement with a cane.

Prior to dissection, one must identify the major vascular landmarks including the common, external, and internal iliac vessels. The dissection starts with grasping the tissues located anterior to the external iliac vessels and gently placing them on traction. A second instrument can then be used to dissect the connective fibers and lymphatic channels joining the node-bearing tissues to the surrounding structures (Fig. 13.2). In 20% of cases, an accessory obturator vein will be found in the obturator nodal tissue and inserted on the inferior surface of the external iliac vein; blunt dissection is generally enough to free the nodal tissue from this structure. Once the nodes are freed from beneath the vein and the obturator nerve is exposed, the external iliac vein is traced back to the bifurcation of the common iliac vessels.

The next step is to dissect the node-bearing tissues located between the external iliac vessels and the psoas muscle. One starts ventrally at the level of the origin of the circumflex artery and continues dorsally to the level of the common iliac artery. At that point, it is often necessary to make a lateral peritoneal incision in order to reflect the ileocecal junction upward on the right side and the sigmoid colon on the left side. The ureter is identified at the level at which it crosses the iliac vessels. If the IP ligament has not been divided and the posterior sheet of the broad ligament is intact, the ureter remains attached to its natural support. Both are pushed medially. The pararectal space is then opened. The node-bearing tissues alongside the inferior aspect of the common iliac artery and posterior aspect of the internal iliac artery are exposed.

Dissection techniques and the sequence in which the landmarks are identified vary from surgeon to surgeon. The most basic technique of dissection is recommended, that is, grasping

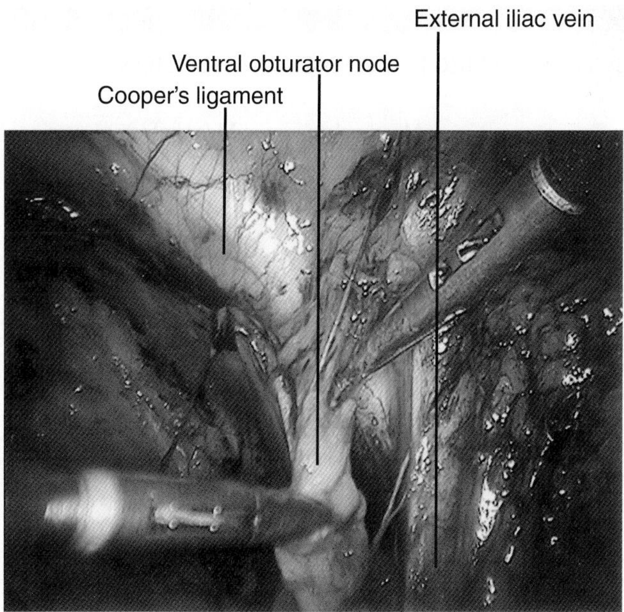

FIGURE 13.2. (*See color plate section.*) Pelvic laparoscopic lymphadenectomy. The pelvic lymphadenectomy is initiated. Picture of the ventral part of the right pelvic sidewall.

the nodes with grasping forceps and employing blunt dissection to separate the node-bearing tissue from the underlying structures. Such a technique (Fig. 13.2) requires skill, but once this skill is acquired, less blood loss is involved. Only the resistant structures, that is, the blood vessels, must be controlled before being divided, and these are few if the dissection is performed in the correct tissue planes. Needless to say, other techniques exist that can yield comparable results.

Removal of the nodes can be accomplished by (a) gathering them (e.g., in the uterovesical space) and extracting them at the end of the procedure using an extracting bag, or (b) using a specialized nodal extractor such as the Coelio-Extractor (Groupe Lepine, Lyon, France) to deliver the nodes without contaminating the abdominal wall.

Querleu et al. (7) were the first to provide data describing the feasibility and safety of transumbilical transperitoneal laparoscopic pelvic dissection. There were 39 procedures performed on patients with cancer of the cervix, stage IB to IIB, and the mean duration of the procedure was 80 minutes. No conversion to laparotomy was required. The mean node count was 8.7 (range, 3 to 22). Positive nodes were found in 5 patients who were subsequently treated with radiotherapy, and the remaining 34 patients underwent either an abdominal radical hysterectomy or a VRH. All patients were followed for 5 years (136), and the 5-year survival rate was similar to the survival of a historical group of patients who underwent standard abdominal radical hysterectomy. Patients were matched for age, stage, and therapy. Childers et al. (9) reported the experience from 18 patients with cervical cancer who were initially managed with laparoscopy. Five patients had immediate abdominal radical hysterectomy and 13 were subsequently treated with radiotherapy. No complications were observed. The duration of the staging procedure was 75 to 175 minutes for the patients assessed prior to radiotherapy. The mean number of lymph nodes was 31.4 (range, 17 to 37) for patients submitted to abdominal radical hysterectomy. One year later, Childers et al. (137) provided data for 53 patients with endometrial cancer. All the patients underwent laparoscopic assessment, and 29 underwent pelvic lymphadenectomy plus aortic sampling. Three intraoperative complications occurred (one pneumothorax, one transection of the ureter, and one bladder injury) and three postoperative complications (two patients had a postoperative ileus and one patient had significant atelectasis). The issue was addressed again 5 years later (138) in 125 patients. The rate of complications did not vary. However, the rate of conversion to laparotomy dropped from 8% (2 of 25) to 0% (0 of 100), whereas the operative time decreased from 196 minutes to 128 minutes ($p < 0.02$) and the hospital stay from 3.2 days to 1.8 days ($p < 0.0001$).

Aortic Dissection

Two techniques have been described for performing an aortic dissection with the laparoscope. In the first (9), the setup is the same as the one used for the pelvic dissection. Two details differ: The video monitor is put on the side of the patient opposite the side where the surgeon stands, and the video camera is turned clockwise 90 degrees, so that the axis of the aorta appears to be horizontal. The intestines are pushed under the diaphragmatic areas. The dorsal peritoneum is opened longitudinally alongside the axis of the aorta. The upper peritoneal flap is developed upward. The right ovarian vessels and the right ureter are identified and pushed laterally. The nodal tissue on the ventral aspect of the vena cava is removed followed by that in the interaorticocaval space. Finally, the nodes from the anterior aspect of the aorta are removed. The origin of the inferior mesenteric artery is identified, and the nodes lying on the left side of the aorta are mobilized and delivered.

In the second technique (18), the surgeon stands between the patient's legs with the monitor at the head of the bed. The dorsal peritoneum is opened transversely alongside the axis of the right common iliac vessels. The upper peritoneal flap is pushed cranially at the same time as the last ileal loop. The right gonadal vessels are identified at the level of the third portion of the duodenum. After having mobilized and divided the ovarian vessels, one finds the left renal vein and begins the dissection that is performed alongside the anterior aspect of the vena cava and then continued in the interaorticocaval space, alongside the ventral aspect of the aorta, and, finally, alongside the left aspect of the aorta. Gaining access to the retroaortic and retrocaval spaces necessitates mobilizing the vessels laterally and medially in order to clear out each of the spaces in two steps. The lumbar arteries and veins represent major danger during this final part of the dissection.

Since 1993, many series have appeared in the literature describing laparoscopic lymphadenectomy (11,12,17,127–136). Most have included data from an inframesenteric dissection as well. Summarizing the larger series (Table 13.2) (7,11,12,17,27, 139–149), one can assume that the mean number of pelvic nodes retrieved laparoscopically was 21 and the mean number of aortic nodes was eight. This number is close to the number of nodes retrieved by laparotomy (150). Comparative studies confirm that the numbers are approximately the same (29,151). Fowler et al. (152) addressed the fact that 25% of the pelvic nodes were still present at laparotomy after the patient underwent a laparoscopic lymphadenectomy; however, no patients with negative nodes at laparoscopy had positive nodes at laparotomy.

The thoroughness of laparoscopic lymphadenectomy has been demonstrated by the recent Gynecologic Oncology Group (GOG) study (149). In this series in which laparoscopic pelvic and para-aortic lymphadenectomy was immediately followed by laparotomy, the mean number of retrieved pelvic nodes was 32.1 (16.6 on the left side and 15.5 on the right side). In spite of this large number, the results were judged to be incomplete in 6 of the 40 patients who subsequently underwent laparotomy after laparoscopic lymphadenectomy. The objective

TABLE 13.2

SELECTED SERIES OF LAPAROSCOPIC PELVIC AND/OR INFRAMESENTERIC LYMPH NODE DISSECTION

Author (ref.)	Year	No. of patients	Disease site	Mean pelvic nodes	Mean inframesenteric nodes
Querleu et al. (7)	1991	39	Cervix	8.7	—
Childers et al. (17)	1993	61	Gyn	—	6.3
Spirtos et al. (140)	1995	40	Endometrium	20.8	7.9
Su et al. (143)	1995	38	Cervix	15	—
Hatch et al. (12)	1996	37	Cervix	35	11
Chu et al. (11)	1997	67	Cervix	26.7	8
Possover et al. (139)	1998	150	Gyn	26.8	7.3
Vidaurreta et al. (144)	1999	84	Cervix	18.5	—
Dottino et al. (141)	1999	94	Gyn	11.9	3.7
Renaud et al. (145)	2000	57	Cervix	27	3
Altgassen et al. (146)	2000	108	Cervix	21.0–24.3	5.1–10.6
Scribner et al. (142)	2001	103	Endometrium	18.1	11.9
Vergote et al. (147)	2002	41	Cervix	—	6
Spirtos et al. (148)	2002	78	Cervix	23.8	10.3
Schlaerth et al. (148)	2002	69	Cervix	32.1	12.1
Abu-Rustum et al. (149)	2003	114	Gyn	10.7	5.7

Note: Gyn: cervical, endometrial, and ovarian tumors.

of laparoscopic lymphadenectomy should be to remove the nodes at risk for spread of disease. The rarity of pelvic sidewall recurrences in node-negative patients managed without a complete lymphadenectomy suggests that laparoscopy enables us to remove the significant nodes. If a criterion to judge the adequacy of the procedure had to be selected, photographic records taken at the end of the laparoscopic procedure would provide the best means to this end. In the GOG study, the result was judged to be inadequate in three of the patients whose photographic records were reviewed by two independent observers. If clearly identifying the dorsal part of the obturator nerve and lumbosacral nerve is required (Figs. 13.3 to 13.5), the risk of missing positive pelvic nodes is very low, at least in cases of cervical and endometrial cancer.

Lymphadenectomy is one of the cornerstone procedures in gynecologic oncology. The development of the laparoscopic

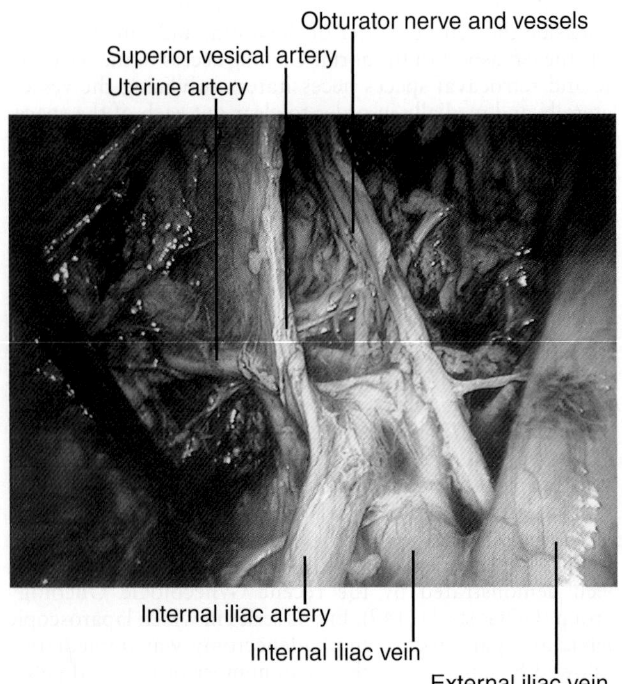

FIGURE 13.3. (*See color plate section.*) Pelvic laparoscopic lymphadenectomy. The pelvic lymphadenectomy is complete. Picture of the dorsal part of the right pelvic sidewall.

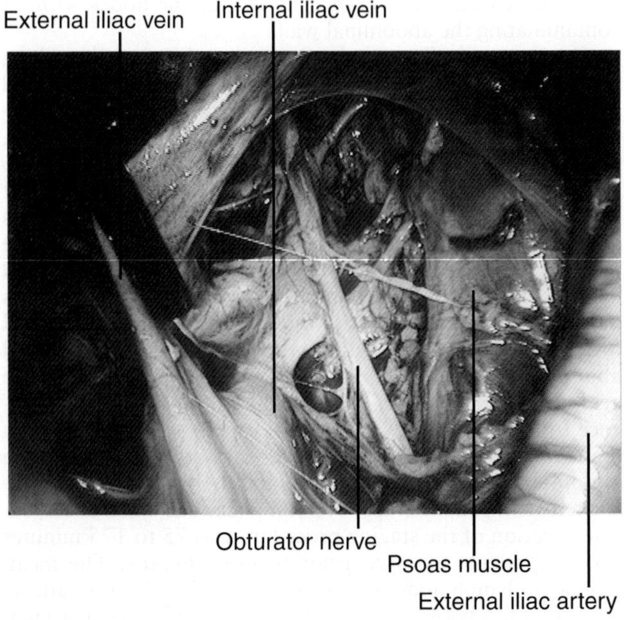

FIGURE 13.4. (*See color plate section.*) Pelvic laparoscopic lymphadenectomy. The pelvic lymphadenectomy is complete. Same view as Figure 13.2, but the external iliac vein has been pushed medially.

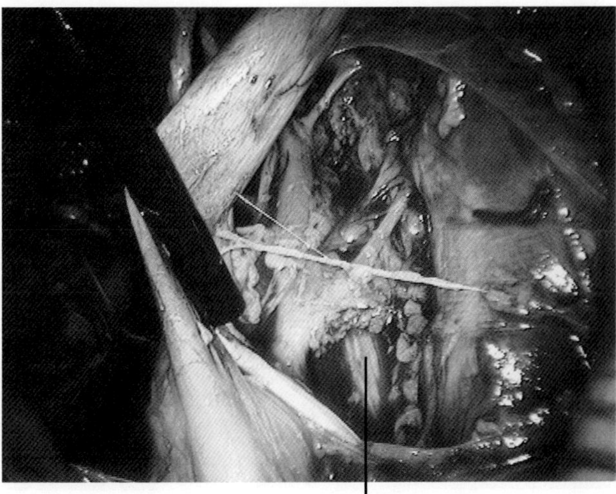

FIGURE 13.5. (*See color plate section.*) Pelvic laparoscopic lymphadenectomy. The pelvic lymphadenectomy is complete. Same view as Figure 13.3, but the external iliac vein and the obturator nerve have been pushed medially. The lumbosacral nerve is visible; this, more than the lymph node count, is proof that the pelvic lymphadenectomy has been done thoroughly.

lymphadenectomy has opened the door for the use of minimally invasive surgery in the management of gynecologic malignancies. The benefits of the procedure alone are difficult to assess since in most of the reported series the procedure is combined with additional operations. This makes it difficult to assess the role of laparoscopic lymphadenectomy either in duration of surgery, appraising intraoperative or postoperative complications, and duration of hospital stay. In the inaugural series by Querleu et al. (7), the procedure was discontinued in 1 of 14 patients owing to an anesthetic problem. One case of intraoperative bleeding was controlled laparoscopically, and all patients except one were discharged the day after the procedure. Possover et al. (138) reported that ten major vessel injuries were registered among 150 procedures (four vena cava, two right renal vein, two external iliac vein, one internal iliac vein, and one internal iliac artery). A conversion to laparotomy was necessary in four of these cases. The mean hospital stay for the 26 patients submitted to lymphadenectomy for pure staging was 3.2 days. Dottino et al. (140) reviewed 94 cases of laparoscopic lymphadenectomies of which 3 required conversion. There was one vascular injury, one case of densely adherent nodal tissue that was felt to be laparoscopically unresectable, and one case of a bulky cervical tumor making laparoscopy difficult. Thirty patients had laparoscopic lymphadenectomy alone and the mean hospital stay was 3.6 days; however, this number included a group of patients who received postoperative chemotherapy. Patients who did not receive chemotherapy were discharged in 1.7 days. Scribner et al. (141) reviewed their first 103 laparoscopic lymphadenectomies. Laparoscopy was completed in 70.9% of patients, with obesity, adhesions, and intraperitoneal disease being the main reasons for not being able to complete the laparoscopic procedure. Three procedural complications included a bladder laceration, a ureteral injury, and one vessel injury at trocar insertion. Other operative procedures were performed and direct correlation with the lymphadenectomy was not mentioned. These studies provided evidence that laparoscopic lymphadenectomy is feasible with an acceptable complication rate.

Childers initially limited the surgical effort to the right inframesenteric area. Consequently, the mean lymph node yield was about eight (Table 13.2) (7,11,12,17,27,139–149). This number is not much different from the number reported for the same dissection at laparotomy (150). It is now known from studies like those published by Benedetti-Panici et al. (153) that the actual number of nodes is around 20 if the dissection is continued to the level of the left renal vein. Michel et al. (154) report that, in cervical cancer involving aortic nodes, the involvement on the left side of the aorta is 72% (23 of 32) and involves the supramesenteric level in 25% of cases (8 of 32). Because of these findings, the aortic dissection must be extended to the left side and to the level of the left renal vein. The feasibility of such an extensive dissection has been demonstrated since the early report by Querleu and Leblanc in 1992 (15), and the yield of 20 nodes, with acceptable morbidity, has been reached in a large series of patients (155).

As the need to perform a systematic infrarenal dissection became more evident, data regarding this procedure under transumbilical transperitoneal laparoscopic guidance began to appear for adnexal cancers (15). Possover et al. (139) also performed such operations in selected cases (ovarian cancer and uterine cancer with high risk of metastasis). When comparing the infrarenal lymphadenectomy to the inframesenteric lymphadenectomy, Kohler et al. (156) confirmed that this could be performed safely. This extended para-aortic lymphadenectomy only took an additional 31 minutes on average and significantly increased the mean node counts from 9.0 to 19.6. A report from the same group (157) indicates that the greatest dangers are not in the higher part of the dissection, but they are lower where tributaries to the anterior aspect of the vena cava are found in the area of the bifurcation of the vena cava in 58.0% of cases, versus 19.6% in the area between the bifurcation and the inferior mesenteric artery, and 0.9% of cases in the area between the inferior mesenteric artery and the right ovarian vein. Furthermore, it appears that if need be, dissection higher than the left renal vein is feasible. Possover et al. (19) attempted this in patients with stage IIIB cervical cancer, transecting at first the left paracolic peritoneum and the left phrenicocolic ligament and mobilizing medially the colonic flexure, left kidney and adrenal gland, tail of pancreas, and spleen. The median number of retrieved nodes was ten. No intraoperative or postoperative complications occurred.

Extraperitoneal Laparoscopic Pelvic Lymphadenectomy

Laparoscopic pelvic lymphadenectomy can be performed using the direct extraperitoneal approach. Historically, this approach was the first method described. Although it is no longer routinely used, one remaining application may be laparoscopic preparation for vaginal radical trachelectomy. The direct extraperitoneal approach had the advantage of completely avoiding the "other surface" of the peritoneum and thus minimizing the risk of postoperative adhesions potentially impairing fertility. This risk, however, appears to be low with the indirect transumbilical approach, and the direct approach does have two drawbacks: (a) loss of time (approximately 15 minutes) and (b) potential for postoperative collections, that is, hematomas, abscesses, lymphoceles (which may be preventable by creating a peritoneotomy at the end of the dissection).

In spite of the above disadvantages to the direct approach to the pelvic extraperitoneal spaces, this approach may be useful in cases where the pelvic cavity is not accessible or not easily accessible such as in pregnancy more than 16 weeks or when severe postoperative adhesions are present. This approach starts with a blind digital preparation of the preperitoneal space. It is also possible to obtain access to the correct space under direct optical guidance through a 10-mm incision thanks to the new laparoscopic trocars that have a cutting tip (Endotip, Storz, Tuttingen, Germany) or accommodate a cutting and transparent punch (Visiport, Tyco; Optiview, Ethicon, Cincinnati, Ohio, USA).

Midline Suprapubic Access

Midline suprapubic access is obtained through an incision made 3 to 4 cm above the pubis. The surgeon stands across from the pelvic sidewall to be dissected and handles the trocar obliquely in order to get access directly to the iliopubic bone at an equal distance from the midline and the external iliac vessels. Once the bone is located, the extraperitoneal space is insufflated and the ancillary trocars can be placed (at 5 to 6 cm from each other on a vertical line running perpendicular to the pubis at 3 to 4 cm lateral to the midline). Cooper's ligament leads to the external iliac vessels that can be traced in ideal conditions from the femoral ring to the bifurcation of the common iliac artery.

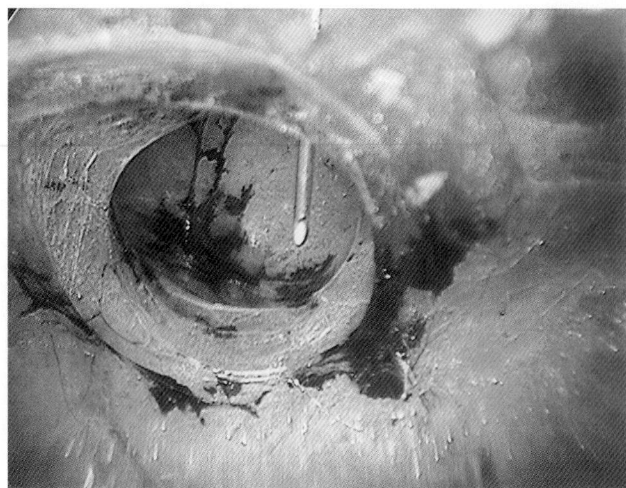

FIGURE 13.7. (*See color plate section.*) Umbilical extraperitoneal laparoscopic approach. A spinal needle is introduced in the midline in the extraperitoneal space before the ancillary instruments are put in place.

Transumbilical Access

Direct access to the extraperitoneal spaces while using a transumbilical microincision (Fig. 13.6) can be obtained using the same technique one uses for routine transumbilical laparoscopy. One only has to use the previously mentioned dissecting trocars (see above) and stop the sharp dissection once the fascia parietalis is opened, that is, before entering the peritoneal serosa. Once the fascia is opened, the CO_2 insufflation begins, and one proceeds to use the laparoscope as a blunt dissector until the symphysis pubis is reached. After using a fine-needle puncture to check the retroperitoneal channel one has created on the midline (Fig. 13.7), a 10- to 20-mm trocar is introduced in the midline that will accommodate the laparoscopic scissors that are used to prepare the posterior surface of the abdominal wall up to the level of McBurney's point. Care must be taken not to dissect too close to the muscle (staying posterior to the inferior epigastric vessels) and not too close to the serosa (accidental peritoneotomy makes the continuation of the surgery very difficult if not impossible). Having prepared the posterior surface of the abdominal wall on both sides, the setup is exactly the same as that used for routine laparoscopy (Fig. 13.8). The access to the retropubic space is ideal, but access to the iliac vessels is limited by the adherent nature of the peritoneum to the abdominal wall, particularly at the level of the inguinal canals. In order to mobilize this, division of the round ligaments is required at the most distal point where they disappear into the inguinal canals (Fig. 13.9). Once the ligaments are divided and the peritoneum developed dorsally, the view obtained of the pelvic sidewall is similar to that seen in the transumbilical transperitoneal approach. The only difference is the superior vesical arteries and umbilical ligaments now run dorsally since the bladder has been detached from the abdominal wall and reflected dorsally.

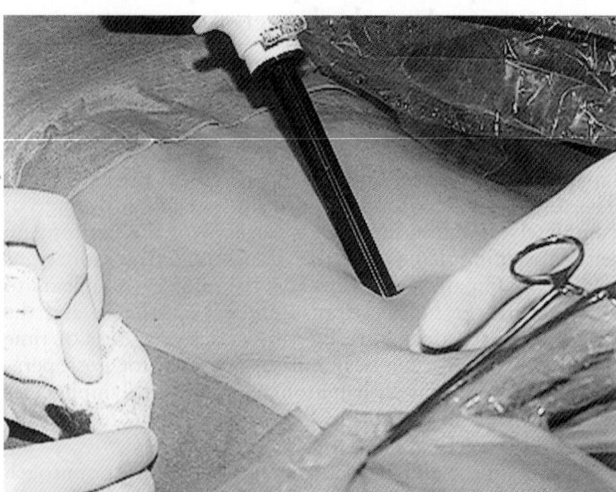

FIGURE 13.6. (*See color plate section.*) Umbilical extraperitoneal laparoscopic approach. The instrument used is the Visiport (U.S. Surgical Corporation Norwalk, Connecticut, USA).

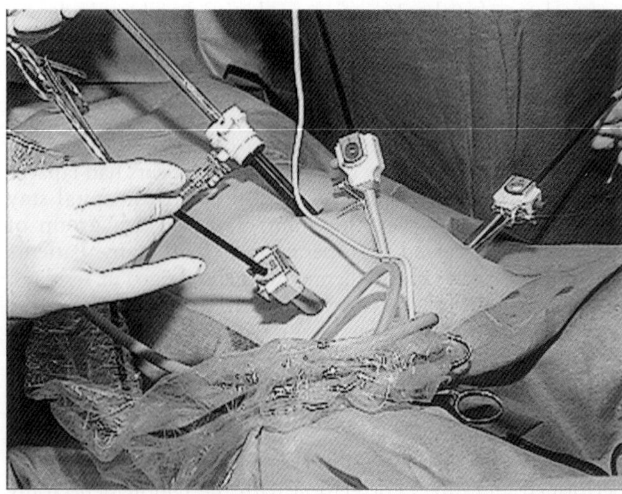

FIGURE 13.8. (*See color plate section.*) Umbilical extraperitoneal laparoscopic approach. Position of laparoscopic trocar and ancillary trocars.

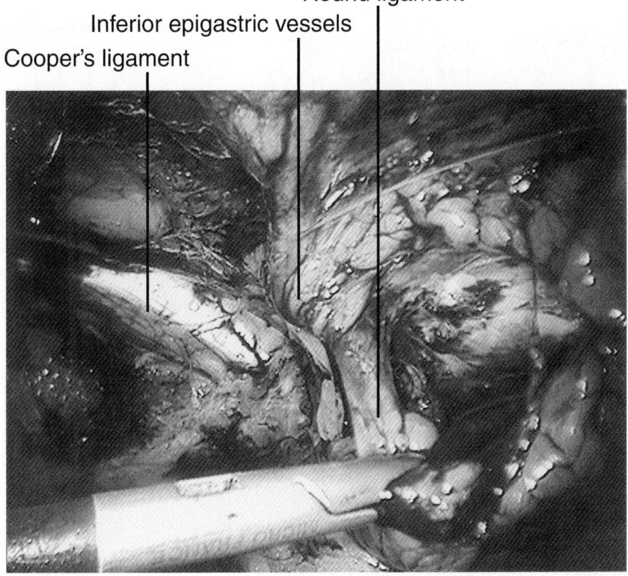

FIGURE 13.9. (*See color plate section.*) Umbilical extraperitoneal laparoscopic approach. The round ligament on the right side is freed before being divided.

Sentinel Node Biopsy

The use of the sentinel node (SN) concept in the clinical management of epithelial malignancies started in the 1970s. The urologist Cabanas (158) proposed replacement of full inguinofemoral dissection that was traditionally combined with radical surgery for penile cancer with only a biopsy of the so-called sentinel node. The use of the new technique spread rapidly beginning in the early 1990s. In gynecologic oncology, the first application was in vulvar cancer (159), but this was soon followed by its application in cervical cancer (20,160–175) and endometrial cancer (175,175). Numerous opinions about techniques of injection, methods of dissection, modality of pathologic assessment, and, even more, the practical use of the end results have been put forth. The only point that gives rise to quasiunanimity is that the laparoscope is a tool perfectly suitable for SN biopsy technique in the field of cervical cancer. Table 13.3 (20,160–166,167–171,173,176,177) summarizes the early literature concerning the use of SN biopsy in early cervical carcinoma. The data should be interpreted carefully because of the different techniques employed among the teams. A recent systematic review by van de Lande et al. (178) reported on a pooling of carefully selected publications. Only 23 out of 98 articles met the selection criteria. Ultimately, 12 studies used the combined technique with a sensitivity of 92% (95% CI, 84% to 98%). Five studies used (99m)Tc-colloid, with a pooled sensitivity of 92% (95% CI, 79% to 98%; $p = 0.71$ vs. combined technique), and four used blue dye with a pooled sensitivity of 81% (95% CI, 67% to 92%, $p = 0.17$ vs. combined technique). The SN detection rate was highest for the combined technique: 97% (95% CI, 95% to 98%) vs. 84% for blue dye (95% CI, 79% to 89%; $p < 0.0001$), and 88% (95% CI, 82% to 92%; $p = 0.0018$) for (99m)Tc colloid. The authors concluded that SN biopsy has the highest SN detection rate when (99m)Tc is used in combination with blue dye (97%), and a sensitivity of 92%.

The SN injection is started by injecting the normal tissues surrounding the tumor. The size of the needle is ideally 21 gauge. The injection must not be too deep and not too superficial (Fig. 13.10). A "learning curve effect" does exist with this technique. Many factors may contribute to the discrepancies in the literature such as the nature of the injected medium: either a blue dye (Lymphazurin or Patent Blue Violet) or radioisotopic colloidal particles. The blue dyes have to be used at an appropriate dilution and in appropriate quantity. The isotope used for the radioisotopic technique is generally technetium 99m, but the colloidal particles vary in nature and size (2 to 80 nm), which contributes to variability in the transit time and number of detected nodes. No matter what the radioisotopic colloid used, the detection rate is generally higher and the number of detected nodes greater with the radioisotopic technique. It appears that the combination of blue dye and isotopes is the most accurate. The result of the radioisotopic injection can be assessed 3 hours after a lymphoscintigraphy (Fig. 13.11). The result of the blue dye injection is assessed at the time of surgery, which is performed soon after injection.

The surgery is performed in the usual fashion for laparoscopic pelvic surgery, usually within 12 hours of injection of the colloidal radioisotope and immediately after the injection of the blue dye. The procedure starts with the transperitoneal assessment. If the injection has been done correctly, the blue channels are located through the dorsal leaf of the broad ligament and traced from the center of the pelvis to the pelvic sidewall. The isotopic detection probe demonstrates where the injected nodes are situated (level of radioactivity ten or more times higher than the basic level). In order to dissect the nodes, the pelvic peritoneum is opened alongside the external iliac vessel axis, and the broad ligament is opened. Some surgeons, in particular those who use an isotope, immediately search for the SNs, whereas others first identify the blue channels and trace them to the SNs. Technique plays a major role in the chances for success, and may explain the variations in the "SN detection rate." It also may explain the great variations in the number and the topography of the detected nodes.

The use of blue dye will demarcate one or more lymphatic channels at the base of broad ligament. They run parallel to the uterine artery, cross the obliterated obturator artery, and end in a node situated in the so-called interiliac area, that is, at the bifurcation to the common iliac artery either medial or dorsal to the external iliac vein (Fig. 13.12) or between it and the external iliac artery. One node is usually found (or two or three juxtaposed micronodes). However, in 5% of the cases, injected nodes are found in two distant basins. At least one node should be found on each pelvic sidewall. In approximately 15% of cases (Fig. 13.13), the SN is located either in the region of the internal iliac artery or in the common iliac and/or low aortic area. Such results are usually observed when the dissection is performed by first identifying the blue lymphatic channels.

The results may be different when isotopes are used. Detected nodes are found in distant basins. This means that the sensitivity of the isotopic technique is higher than the sensitivity of the blue dye technique. But this questions the specificity and even challenges the concept itself. Since SN dissection with a radioisotope may include multiple anatomic areas, it may tend to resemble a systematic dissection more than a true "sentinel node" biopsy.

Pathologic assessment of the SN can be performed by various techniques. Frozen section has been criticized because of the higher rate of false negatives. It does have the advantage of immediate answers in patients with metastasis to the SN (no false positive). The classic unilevel sectioning after paraffin embedment and the hematoxylin and eosin (H&E) staining are the most widely used techniques. Micrometastasis, however, can be missed. Multilevel sectioning may help minimize this problem. The literature concerning the topic is very

TABLE 13.3

EARLY REPORTS IN THE LITERATURE CONCERNING SENTINEL NODE BIOPSY IN EARLY CERVICAL CANCER

Author (ref.)	No. of patients	FIGO stage	Injection technique	Surgical technique	SN detection/ no. of patients (%)	Average no. of SNs	Pathologic assessment	No. of SN-positive patients (%)	No. of SN false-negative patients (%)
Echt et al., 1999 (160)	13	IB	B	Laparotomy	2 (15)	1.5	H&E	2 (100)	0
Medl et al., 2000 (161)	3	NS	B	Laparotomy	3 (100)	—	NS	3 (100)	0
O'Boyle et al., 2000 (162)	20	IB-IIA	B	Laparotomy	12 (60)	1.9	H&E	4 (33)	0[a]
Dargent et al., 2000 (20)	69[b]	IA2-IB1	B	Laparoscopy	59 (85)[b]	1.1 b	H&E	6 (10)[b]	0
Verheijen et al., 2000 (164)	10	IB	B and R	Laparotomy	8 (80)	1.8	IHC	1 (12)	0
Kamprathet al., 2000 (163)	18	I-II	R	Laparoscopy	16 (88)	—	—	1 (6)	0
Lantzsch et al., 2001 (170)	14	IB1	R	Laparotomy	13 (93)	2	IHC	1 (8)	0
Malur et al., 2001 (168)	50	I-IV	B and R	Laparoscopy	39 (78)[c]	2	H&E	5 (13)	1 (3)[d]
Levenback, 2002 (176)	39	I-IIA	B and R	Laparotomy	39 (100)	4.7	IHC	8 (20)	1 (3)
Barranger et al., 2003 (166)	13	IA-IIA	B and R	Laparoscopy	12 (92)	1.7	IHC	2 (15)	0
Lambaudie et al., 2003 (165)	12	IA2-IB1	B and R	Laparoscopy	11 (92)	1.7	IHC	2 (18)	1 (9)[e]
Buist et al., 2003 (169)	25	I-IIA	B and R	Laparoscopy	25 (100)	2.3	IHC	9 (36)	1 (4)
Plante et al., 2003 (171)	70	IA-IIA	B and R	Laparoscopy	61 (87)[f]	1.9	IHC	8 (11)	0
Dargent and Enria, 2003 (171)	139[g]	IA2-IB1	B	Laparoscopy	125 (90)[g]	1.1[g]	H&E	18 (14)	0
Dargent et al., 2004 (177)	29	IA2-IB1	B	Laparoscopy	29 (100)	2	IHC	5 (17)	3 (10)

Note: B, blue dye; FIGO, International Federation of Gynecology and Obstetrics; H&E, hematoxylin and eosin; IHC, immunohistochemistry; NS, not significant; R, radioactive isotope; SN, sentinel node.
[a]One pN1 patient among the eight patients with no SN detected (149).
[b]Sixty-nine pelvic sidewalls assessed in 35 patients.
[c]Detection rate: 55.5% with B alone, 76% with R alone, and 90% with B and R.
[d]Four pN1 patients among the eleven patients with no SN detected (155).
[e]One metastasis in one node of the only patient with no SN detected.
[f]Detection rate: 79% with B alone, 93% with R alone, and 93% with B and R.
[g]One hundred and thirty-nine pelvic sidewalls assessed in 70 patients.

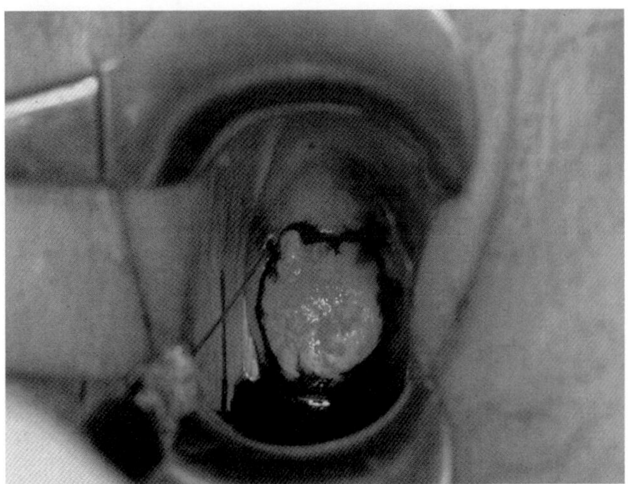

FIGURE 13.10. (*See color plate section.*) Injection of the dye. The dye is injected into the tissue surrounding the tumor. The sentinel lymph node procedure should only be used for early-stage cancers.

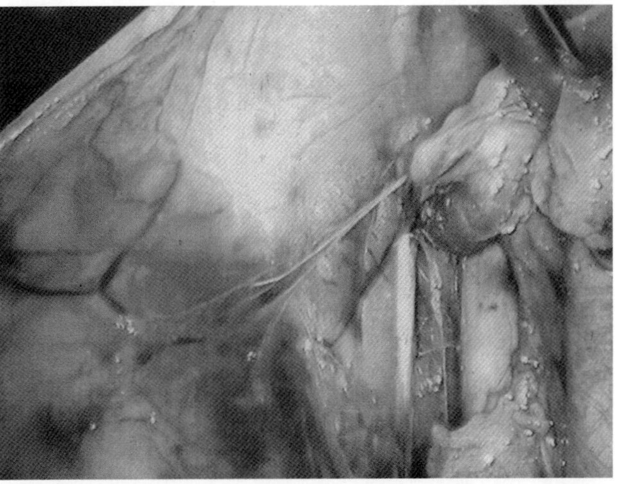

FIGURE 13.12. (*See color plate section.*) Dissection of the sentinel node. The main lymphatic channel crosses the umbilical ligament and ends in a node situated between the external iliac vein and the obturator nerve.

confusing. Ideally, the best technique is serial sectioning of the entire node with all slides being stained and assessed, but this is unrealistic. The semiserial sectioning entails examining slides at 40- to 200-μm (depending on institutional protocol) intervals. Even the so-called micromicrometastasis can thus be identified. Using immunostains can improve the sensitivity. The most common antibodies used in current practice are those directed toward the cytokeratins. Very small clusters of epithelial cells (Fig. 13.14) and isolated epithelial cells can be identified that were previously impossible to identify after the standard H&E staining. However, if true serial sectioning is not employed, these epithelial cells can be missed as well. Molecular biology analysis for cytokeratins or human papillomavirus (HPV) may provide the highest sensitivity. Each group has its own personal technique, and this explains the great variability of the rate of positive and false-negative SNs reported in the literature. With the unilevel sectioning and classic H&E staining, the rate of SN positives is, in cervical cancer stage IB1, approximately 15%, and the rate of false negatives varies between 0% and 17%. Both rates are much

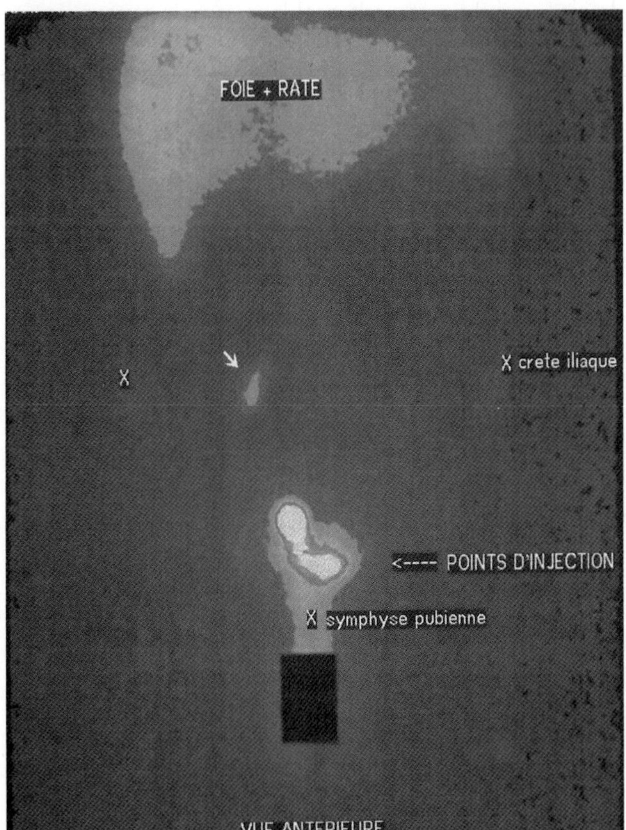

FIGURE 13.11. (*See color plate section.*) Lymphoscintigraphy. One hot spot only is visible. No sentinel lymph node was detected on the left side. The sentinel lymph node on the right side was a common iliac node.

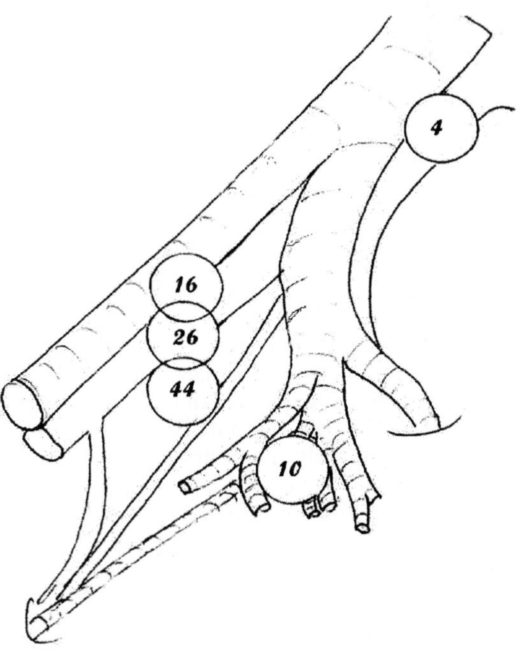

FIGURE 13.13. Topography of sentinel node location. The most common place where the sentinel node is situated is at the contact of the external iliac vein, ventral to the origin of the uterine artery.

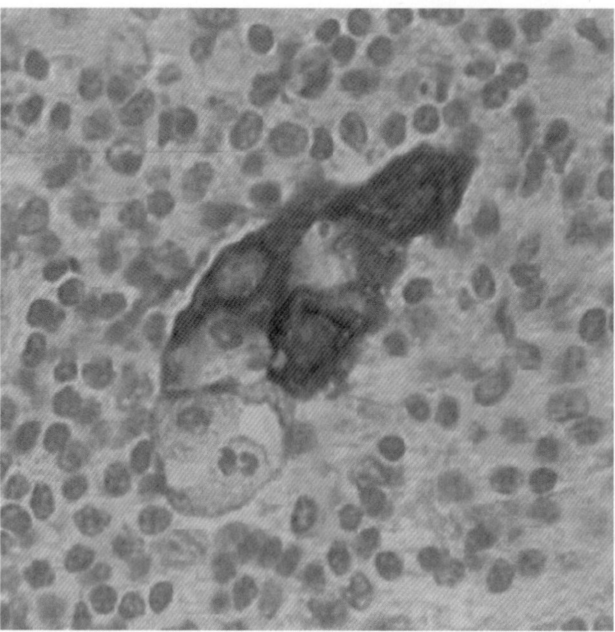

FIGURE 13.14. (*See color plate section.*) Micrometastasis. Immunohistochemistry can be used to identify micrometastasis in the sentinel lymph node.

higher if semiserial sectioning and immunostaining are used both for the assessment of the SN and the non-SN. In the series by Marchiole et al. (179), the rate of SN positivity increased from 10.3% (3 of 29) to 27.5% (5 of 29) using semiserial sectioning and cytokeratin AE1 and AE3 immunostaining. However, the rate of false negatives was also increased to 37% as three of the five micrometastases were discovered in non-SNs with the SNs being uninvolved. This questions the role of SN biopsy in the clinical management of early cervical cancer.

The goal of the SN concept is avoiding systematic dissection in patients who do not have node metastasis. This goal is reached if one does not consider micrometastasis as being clinically relevant. However, in spite of the fact that the clinical significance of micrometastasis is not clearly established, it seems oncologically safer to remove nodes that could be involved. On the other hand, laparoscopy makes systematic dissection a relatively safe and acceptable procedure that may be no more morbid than a laparoscopic SN biopsy. A reasonable strategy may include (a) laparoscopy with SN biopsy, (b) frozen sections of the SN, and (c) systematic dissection if the frozen section is negative. In the cases where either the SN biopsy or other nodes have metastasis, chemoradiation can be given. The risk for radiation enteritis is minimized by the decreased adhesion formation after laparoscopy.

The concept of SN biopsy has been tested in advanced cervical carcinoma. The detection rate is low, and the clinical value is only theoretical. In endometrial cancer, several publications (175,180,181) demonstrate similarities with the early cervical cancer model. Injections of the cervix give better results than injections of the fundus (180), which give rise to a larger amount of diffusion and result in a higher false-negative rate (50% in one of the published series) (175). Laparoscopy can also be used with SN biopsy in endometrial cancer. However, SN biopsy may not have the impact on the current management of endometrial cancer as it does with cervical cancer. In ovarian, tubal, and peritoneal cancers, the application of the SN concept is not likely to be applicable.

Extraperitoneal Laparoscopic Aortic Lymphadenectomy

Unlike pelvic lymphadenectomy, the use of the extraperitoneal approach to laparoscopically remove the aortic nodes followed the introduction of the transperitoneal technique. Transperitoneal laparoscopic aortic lymphadenectomy still remains the more common approach employed by the majority of gynecologic oncologists. However, this innovative extraperitoneal approach does have several advantages when compared to the transperitoneal technique and has gained increasing popularity.

An extraperitoneal approach to the aorta is begun by using a 3-cm incision made at McBurney's point (or at the point exactly opposite on the left side of the patient). The contralateral nodes can be removed using a one-sided approach. The left-sided approach is preferred for several reasons, which will be illustrated below. The successive layers of the abdominal wall are transected, including the parietal fascia, leaving the parietal peritoneum intact. Insertion of a transperitoneal laparoscopic trocar is recommended so that the area where the extraperitoneal dissection starts can be visualized to prevent entry into the peritoneal cavity. Once the parietal fascia is opened, the surgeon's forefinger is introduced into the extraperitoneal space and develops the retroperitoneal space along the psoas muscle and common iliac artery. With gentle blunt dissection, the peritoneal sac is elevated off the underlying structures. The second landmark is the iliac crest, which is followed laterally in order to open the inferior part of the side. At this time, a laparoscopic trocar with a pneumostatic tool (Blunt Tip Auto Suture, Norwalk, Connecticut, USA) is introduced.

Once the extraperitoneal space has been adequately developed, insufflation begins, the gas from the peritoneal cavity is drained, and the extraperitoneal laparoscopic assessment can begin. This trocar accommodates one laparoscopic forceps, which is used to develop the extraperitoneal spaces to the level of the lower ribs. A second ancillary trocar is introduced in the infracostal area in the midaxillary line.

The video monitor is placed on the opposite side of the table from the surgeon as he or she seeks the first landmark (Fig. 13.15): the fascia of the psoas muscle. Detaching the

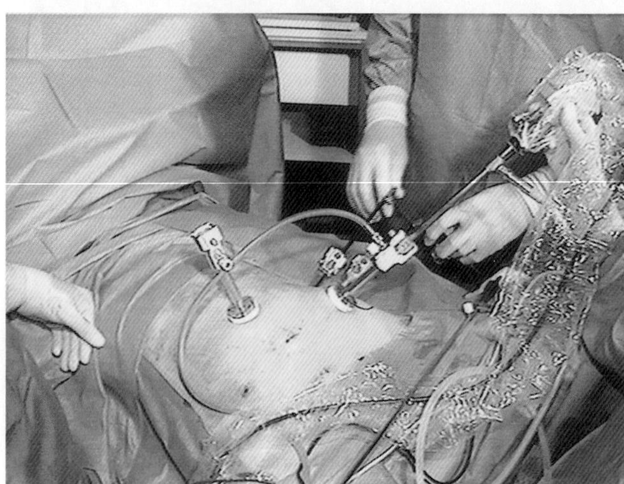

FIGURE 13.15. (*See color plate section.*) Left-sided extraperitoneal laparoscopic approach. Position of laparoscopic trocar and ancillary trocars (the extraperitoneal approach is preceded by a transumbilical transperitoneal approach; the umbilical trocar is left in place after exsufflation).

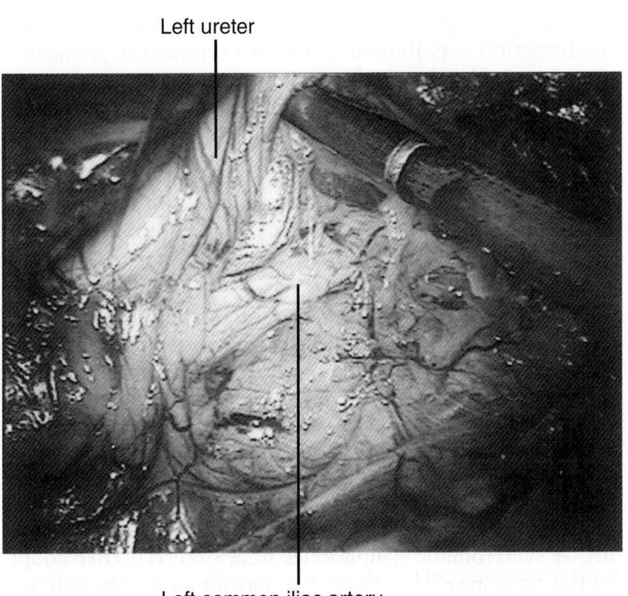

FIGURE 13.16. (*See color plate section.*) Left-sided extraperitoneal laparoscopic approach. The left ureter is pushed ventrally. The left common iliac artery is visible.

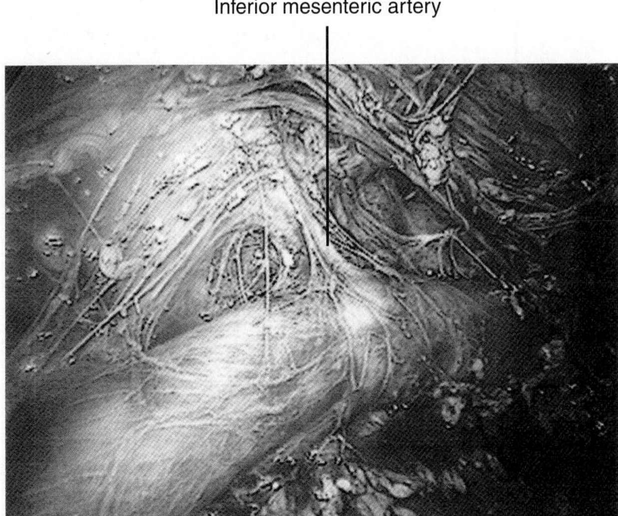

FIGURE 13.18. (*See color plate section.*) Left-sided extraperitoneal laparoscopic approach. Picture taken at the end of the aortic dissection.

peritoneum from the muscle reveals the second landmark, the ureter (Fig. 13.16), and then the third landmark, the ovarian vein, a fragile structure that must be handled carefully. After pushing the peritoneum medially, the common iliac vessels can be identified and the aortic dissection can begin. The lower aspect of the dissection is shown in Figure 13.17.

The lateral aspect of the aorta is approached in a caudal-to-cranial direction. At the level of the origin of the inferior mesenteric artery, the dissection becomes more difficult owing to the presence of the lower mesenteric autonomic nervous plexus. There are no drawbacks in dividing this plexus in a woman. Once the nervous plexus is divided and the ventrolateral aspect of the aorta is freed up, the dissection is continued cranially up to the level of the left renal vein. This is the superior limit of the dissection of the left para-aortic lymph nodes. The anterior aspect of the completed dissection is shown in Figure 13.18.

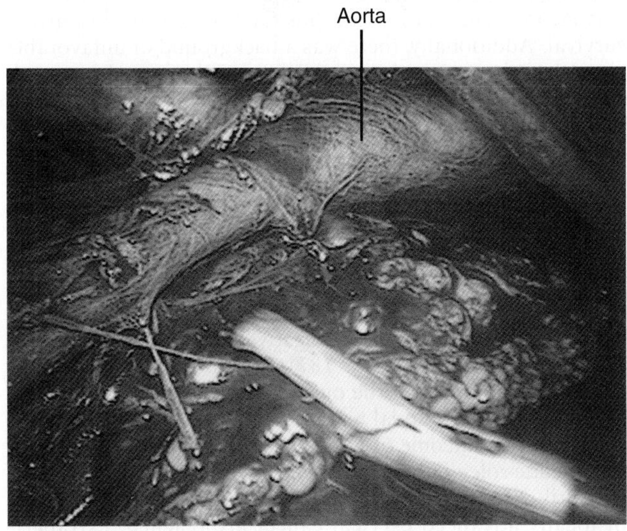

FIGURE 13.17. (*See color plate section.*) Left-sided extraperitoneal laparoscopic approach. Picture taken at the end of the common iliac and lower aortic dissection.

If one starts with the right-sided dissection, it is easy to remove the nodal tissue on the anterior aspect of the vena cava and the interaorticocaval space where the right lateroaortic nodes lie. However, the difficulty lies in reaching the left lateral aspect of the aorta. This is largely due to the noncompressible nature of the aorta. Conversely, if dissection is started on the left side, exposing the right lateral aspect of the aorta can be simplified by dissecting from beneath the aorta. Hence, it is recommended to start with the left side and move to the right side only if difficulties arise. When comparing the unilateral to the bilateral approach, the total node counts of a unilateral left-sided approach have been shown to be comparable to those from a bilateral extraperitoneal approach and a transperitoneal approach; however, the right-sided node counts are significantly decreased compared to the bilateral approach (182).

During the unilateral left-sided technique, the separation of the left aortic nodes is performed either cranially to caudally or vice versa. The nodes are located between the artery and the psoas muscle. Separating these structures reveals the lumbar sympathetic chain and the vertebral vessels. Once the left aortic lymph nodes have been retrieved, attention now moves to the retroaortic space. The aorta is separated from the common ventral vertebral ligament. The aim of this maneuver is to remove the few nodes lying in the retroaortic space while exposing the nodes on the right side of the aorta and the interaorticocaval space. This dissection can be made in the spaces located between the successive lumbar arteries (Fig. 13.19) but access to the interaorticocaval space is limited. It is better to divide the collaterals of the aorta: the fifth lumbar arteries in all cases and the fourth if needed. Division of these lumbar vessels opens the retroaortic space and simplifies the removal of the right aortic nodes (Fig. 13.20). The additional exposure allows the right laterocaval nodes to be removed via the retrocaval or

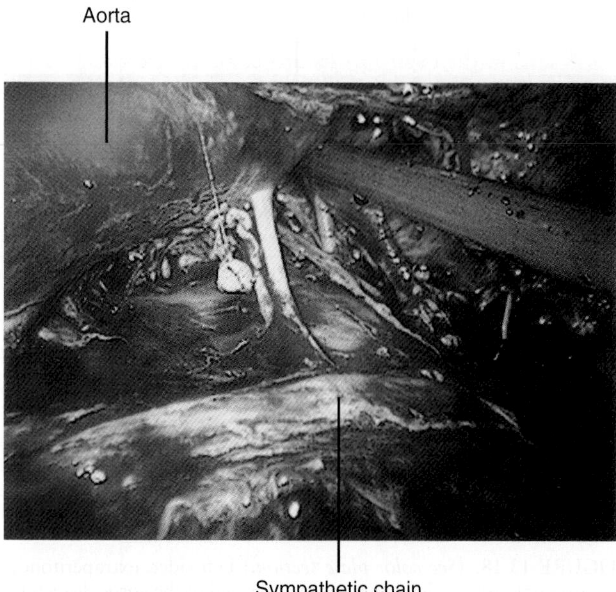

FIGURE 13.19. (*See color plate section.*) Left-sided extraperitoneal laparoscopic approach. Picture taken at the beginning of the retroaortic dissection: the lumbar arteries and veins are visible.

the precaval route. Dissection of these nodes is usually only performed for a right ovarian tumor. Thus, except for cases of ovarian cancer, there is no need to proceed this far if the caval dissection appears from the left side to be dangerous (owing to the distribution of the vertebral veins).

Reports on this particular approach are relatively sparse in the gynecologic oncology literature and have been limited to patients with cervical cancer. Vasilev and McGonigle (183) were the first to publish data on laparoscopic extraperitoneal para-aortic lymphadenectomy using a left-sided approach in humans. They reported an average of five nodes in four cases; the dissection was limited to the inframesenteric area. In a larger series, Querleu et al. used this technique to perform an infrarenal aortic dissection, and by doing such, the mean node count rose to 20.7 (184).

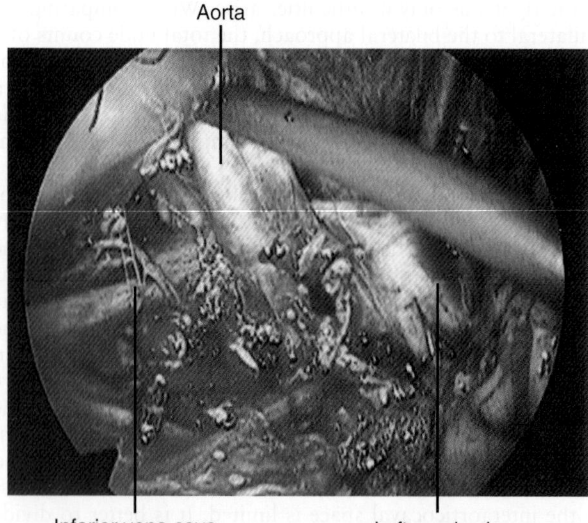

FIGURE 13.20. (*See color plate section.*) Left-sided extraperitoneal laparoscopic approach. Picture taken after the lumbar arteries and veins have been divided and the interaorticocaval space appeared: the junction of the left renal vein and inferior vena cava is visible.

Sonoda et al. (185) reported on 111 patients with locally advanced cervical cancer who underwent surgical staging. This comprises the largest series to date using this novel approach for the management of locally advanced cervical cancer. In this study, 30 patients were found to have positive nodes. The mean duration of the procedure was 157 ± 46 minutes and the average number of nodes was 19. The mean postoperative stay was 2 days. Perioperative complications occurred in 14 patients. The majority of these complications were symptomatic lymphoceles that occurred in 11 patients: Eight of these lymphoceles were drained under radiologic guidance, two required a catheter placed under anesthesia, and one required laparoscopic drainage. In the final 37 patients, marsupialization of the peritoneum was performed to drain the retroperitoneal fluid into the peritoneal cavity. No further symptomatic lymphoceles were observed after adopting this maneuver. There were two retroperitoneal hematomas and one bowel obstruction from a trocar-site hernia. Only two patients in the series required a reoperation for a complication. Of the 30 patients with positive nodes, only the patient who had a trocar-site hernia that required small bowel resection developed radiation enteritis. This is consistent with the finding that the laparoscopic extraperitoneal approach is associated with less adhesion formation in the radiation field (186). The benefits of surgical staging of locally advanced cervical cancer remain controversial, and procedure-related morbidity must be taken into consideration. Thirty (27%) of 111 patients in this series were found to have positive lymph nodes in spite of negative imaging studies and received extended field radiation with or without chemotherapy. However, the overall survival was still significantly worse in this group of patients with positive aortic nodes.

The subject of surgical staging for locally advanced cervical cancer remains controversial and has been prospectively studied in only one small, randomized trial (32). The primary objective of this study was to determine percentage of improvement in detection of para-aortic node metastasis with survival being secondary. Unfortunately, the study was closed prematurely because both a significantly worse progression-free and overall survival were identified in the group undergoing surgical staging. Treatment after the staging procedure was inconsistent and biased, thus tainting the conclusions on survival. Additionally, there was a background of unfavorable characteristics facing the surgically staged group. In general, the surgically staged patients were of higher stage, had larger tumor size, and fewer received concurrent chemoradiation as compared to the patients who were clinically staged. These differences in variables did not reach statistical significance, but this was most likely due to the small sample size.

In spite of this randomized prospective trial, the option on surgical staging for locally advanced cervical cancer is still adopted in a growing number of centers, on the basis of acceptable morbidity and the evidence of an acceptable oncologic outcome in aortic node–negative patients managed without aortic radiation therapy (187). In addition, the same study from France found that the outcome for patients with laparoscopically removed nodal micrometastases in the aortic area is similar to the outcome of node-negative patients, suggesting a therapeutic role of aortic node dissection.

Until definitive conclusions on the optimal management of locally advanced cervical cancer are reached, extraperitoneal laparoscopic aortic lymphadenectomy appears to be a reasonable approach for these patients when surgical staging is employed.

LAPAROSCOPIC ASSISTANCE TO RADICAL SURGERY AND LAPAROSCOPIC RADICAL SURGERY

Laparoscopy can be used to assist extirpative transvaginal surgery or it can be used to perform the entire operation, after which the specimen is removed transvaginally.

Laparoscopically Assisted Vaginal Hysterectomy and Laparoscopic Hysterectomy

The concept of laparoscopic assistance to vaginal hysterectomy emerged in 1984 (21) as a procedure for the management of benign conditions. Its use for the management of endometrial cancer was naturally foreseeable. The main contraindication to the vaginal approach in endometrial cancer was the inability to assess the ovaries and tubes, the peritoneal serosa, and the retroperitoneal spaces. This was made possible by using laparoscopic assessment of the pelvis before undertaking the hysterectomy. Laparoscopically assisted vaginal hysterectomy (LAVH) includes five types, which are listed here, and whose descriptions can be found elsewhere (188):

Type 0: Laparoscopy is only used to assess the pelvic cavity and the organs it includes.

Type 1: Laparoscopic management of inflammatory peritoneal adhesions and control of the round ligaments and infundibulopelvic ligaments.

Type 2: Laparoscopic preparation and division of the uterine arteries.

Type 3: Laparoscopic management of the paracervical ligaments.

Type 4: Laparoscopic transection of the vagina, transvaginal extraction of the specimen, and laparoscopic closure of the vagina.

Type 4 LAVH corresponds to the total laparoscopic hysterectomy first described by Reich et al. (189). This technique as well as others has been used in the field of endometrial cancer. Childers and Surwit (8) were the first to report on the combined use of laparoscopy with vaginal hysterectomy for the treatment of early-stage endometrial cancer. This group later reported on a series of 59 patients with clinical stage I endometrial cancer who were staged by this new procedure (136). Their technique included an inspection of the intraperitoneal cavity, intraperitoneal washings, and LAVH. Patients with preoperative grade 2 or 3 tumors or grade 1 tumors with greater than 50% myometrial invasion underwent laparoscopic pelvic and para-aortic lymphadenectomy. Six patients had intraperitoneal disease. Two patients could not undergo laparoscopic lymphadenectomy secondary to obesity, and two patients required conversion to laparotomy for intraoperative complications. These reports stimulated the interest in laparoscopic management of endometrial cancer.

Laparoscopically Assisted Vaginal Radical Hysterectomy

The introduction of laparoscopy into the realm of gynecologic oncology was first proposed as a means of expanding the use of VRH for the management of cervical cancer. The laparoscope was to perform the lymphadenectomy before the radical hysterectomy, which was entirely done through the vaginal approach. Subsequently, the concept of laparoscopically assisted vaginal radical hysterectomy (LAVRH) appeared with variations in the degree of laparoscopic preparation for the vaginal part of the surgery with the ultimate development being the total laparoscopic radical hysterectomy.

Vaginal Radical Hysterectomy After Laparoscopic Staging

Type 0 LAVRH, although not discussed here, combines pelvic lymphadenectomy as previously described and a VRH whose description can be found elsewhere (190).

The first large series of LAVRH (5) reported on type 0 LAVRH. The technique was used until June 1992. At that time (unpublished data), the series included 95 cases. The mean duration of the laparoscopic staging was 60.4 ± 25.8 minutes. The Schauta-Stoeckel technique (less radical) was used in 28 cases and the Schauta-Amreich technique (more radical) was used in 67 cases. The mean duration of the surgery was 74 ± 31 minutes and 89 ± 26 minutes, respectively. No perioperative complication was observed with the Schauta-Stoeckel technique, whereas six complications were observed with the Schauta-Amreich technique: one cystotomy, four ureterotomies, and one proctotomy (all repaired immediately with no postoperative complications). Only one patient required reoperation for postoperative bleeding after a Schauta-Amreich procedure. Only 14 patients received transfusions. Among the 28 patients who underwent the Schauta-Stoeckel operation, 8 suffered from urinary bladder problems but only 1 had persistent dysuria after 6 months. Among the 67 patients who underwent the Schauta-Amreich procedure, 27 suffered the same bladder problems and 10 had persistent dysuria after 6 months.

Laparoscopic Vaginal Radical Hysterectomy

As with LAVH, there are different techniques between the two extremes of the spectrum, that is, laparoscopy for staging purposes only and laparoscopy for the entire procedure. The techniques first described were highly radical comparable to types 3 and 4 abdominal radical hysterectomy (ARH). A less radical approach appears to be possible leading to surgery like type 2 ARH. Laparoscopically assisted vaginal radical trachelectomy (LVRT) is a conservative modification of this less radical LAVRH.

Supraradical Laparoscopically Assisted Vaginal Radical Hysterectomy. Since 1992 a series (12,22,25,26,176) of reports have been published describing a variety of techniques of LAVRH that could be designated as type 3, and that involved preparation of the parametrium during the laparoscopic step. The common feature of these techniques was the quest for radicalness that was made possible by the laparoscope. In fact, one of the technical difficulties of the radical vaginal approach is the clamping of the parametrium close to the pelvic sidewall due to the obliquity of the latter to the former; this is in contrast to the oblique angle along which the "vaginal" surgeon naturally works. Alternatively, using an ipsilateral iliac laparoscopic port, one can operate in the plane of the pelvic sidewall, and using endoscopic staplers, bipolar cauterization, the argon-beam coagulator, or other devices, the surgeon can divide the parametrium at its lateral insertion. As a consequence, the operative specimen (Fig. 13.21) is very large, that is, identical to type 3 ARH. It can even be extended (26) by the addition of a piece of the "posterior parametrium," that is, uterosacral ligaments, which are easily divided during laparoscopy.

In 1993, Kadar and Reich (191) reported an operative time of 10 hours. However, the postoperative course was uneventful and the patient went back to work after 3 weeks. The operative time for the second patient was 8 hours. The blood loss was 2 L, and the postoperative pyelogram revealed a transection of the

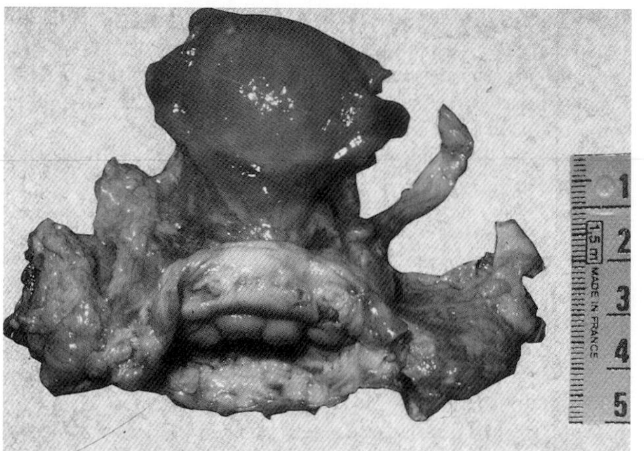

FIGURE 13.21. (*See color plate section.*) Specimen of supraradical LAVRH (distal celio-Schauta).

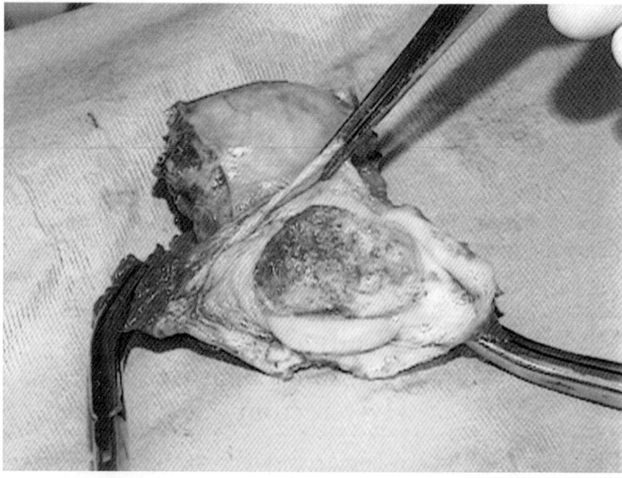

FIGURE 13.22. (*See color plate section.*) Specimen of modified LAVRH (proximal celio-Schauta).

left ureter, which was reimplanted by laparotomy. Pulmonary embolism and vesicovaginal fistula occurred after the reoperation. Roy et al. (25) reported on 25 cases with a mean duration of the operation of 270 minutes. Two conversions to laparotomy occurred, one for an external iliac vein injury and the second for a cystotomy. One other cystotomy was repaired transvaginally. Five patients received a transfusion. These data were similar to those collected in a comparative group of 27 patients who underwent ARH. In the series of 37 cases reported by Hatch et al. (12), the mean operative time was 225 minutes. Two intraoperative bladder injuries and one large bowel injury occurred. Two postoperative ureterovaginal fistulas developed. Four patients required blood transfusion. When compared to a matched series of 30 patients treated by ARH, the mean operative time was significantly longer for LAVRH, but blood loss, rate of transfusion, and mean hospital stay were significantly lower for LAVRH. Martin (192) reported on Dargent's experience in 28 patients from June 1992 to June 1994. The mean duration of the operation was 204 minutes. Four complications occurred during the transvaginal portion of the surgery: one bladder injury, two ureteral injuries, and one internal iliac vein collateral injury. The first three injuries were repaired transvaginally. The bleeding complication was managed by laparoscopic re-exploration, and eight patients received blood transfusions. During the postoperative course, a surgical re-exploration was necessary in three instances: one for bleeding, one for incisional dehiscence, and one for intestinal obstruction. Fourteen patients suffered from bladder problems, and one had persistent dysuria after 6 months. Schneider et al. (26) reported a series of 33 patients. The mean operative time was 295 minutes. Three patients sustained injury to the bladder, one patient had injury to the left ureter, and another patient had an injury to the left internal iliac vein. Blood transfusions were necessary in four women.

Since 1999 a larger series has been compiled demonstrating that the oncologic outcomes are at an acceptable level. Operative complications are less frequent, which may be due to the "learning curve effect" as well as the trend toward less radical surgery. The standard operation of today ends up with an operative specimen that is similar to type 2 ARH (Fig. 13.22), but this is combined with laparoscopic paracervical lymphadenectomy to preserve the radical nature.

Modified Laparoscopically Assisted Vaginal Radical Hysterectomy.

Laparoscopic Step. The route used for introducing the laparoscope can be either transperitoneal or extraperitoneal. Pelvic lymphadenectomy is performed first and then "paracervical cellulolymphadenectomy." Paracervical cellulolymphadenectomy consists of removing all the lymph node–bearing tissues located in the vasculonervous web making up the lateral part of the paracervical ligament. It is a multistep procedure.

First, the "deep obturator nodes" (nodes located underneath the obturator nerve) are removed, which completely opens up the paravesical space, reveals the origin of the obturator vessels, and exposes the ventral surface of the paracervical ligament.

The dorsal aspect of the paracervix is exposed in the second step. The pararectal space opens when pushing the posterior sheet of the broad ligament, to which the ureter is attached, medially. Following the ureter ventrally, one arrives at the point where the ureter crosses the uterine artery. Starting from this point, the pararectal space is developed as far as the sacrospinous muscle. The fatty tissues lying between the ventral aspect of the sacrum, the lateral aspect of the rectum, and the medial aspect of the pelvic sidewall are removed. During this part of the procedure, one must proceed carefully owing to the confined nature of the pararectal space, especially on the left side where the presence of the left common iliac vein poses an added obstacle.

Once the two aspects of the paracervical ligament are exposed, the fatty tissue among the paracervical vascular network must be removed. This can be done by using the grasping and dissecting forceps similar to the technique that is recommended for pelvic dissection. This technique is better suited to paracervical dissection for which the use of scissors is dangerous. Another solution could be using a vacuum curette as recommended by Hockel et al. (193) for open dissection. It is perfectly possible to adapt this technique to laparoscopic dissection, but with the disadvantage of working in a gasless environment.

The last step of the paracervical dissection is cleaning out the retrovascular area (i.e., the space located lateral to the common iliac vessels and medial to the psoas muscle). The lymph node–bearing tissues located in this space are quite abundant. One must take care not to injure the collateral vasculature from the common iliac vessels to the psoas muscle. Once the deepest part of the obturator nerve and the lumbosacral nerve crossing the sacroiliac joint have been identified, the procedure is completed (Figs. 13.2 to 13.4).

Since paracervical cellulolymphadenectomy has been performed, there is no need to divide the cardinal ligament at the level of its origin. The division can be performed in the mid part and is easiest when performed transvaginally. This is the rationale of the technique of LVRH recommended by Dargent and Querleu.

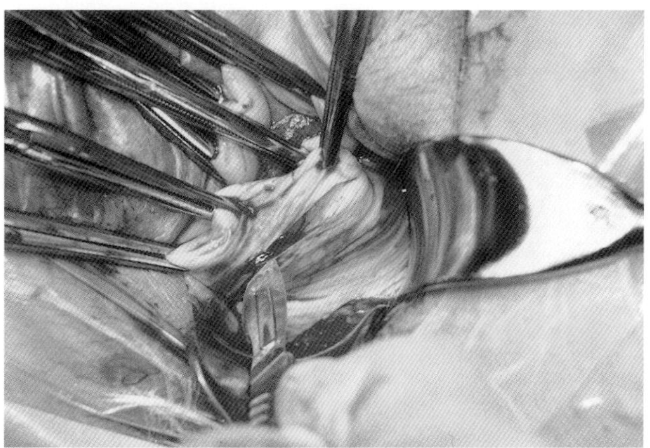

FIGURE 13.23. (*See color plate section.*) Technique of modified LAVRH (proximal celio-Schauta). Incision of the vagina.

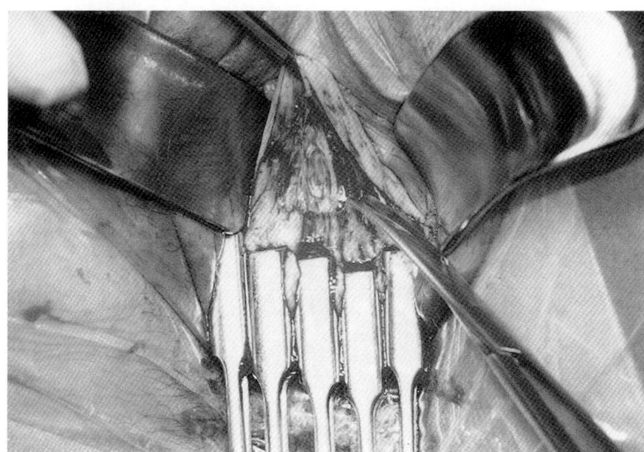

FIGURE 13.25. (*See color plate section.*) Technique of modified LAVRH. Opening the vesicovaginal space.

Transvaginal Step. The transvaginal portion of the Dargent and Querleu LAVRH simulates the modified VRH described by Stoeckel. In both, the paracervical ligaments are divided at an intermediate level. However, the technique differs in that no paravaginal incisions are used in the Dargent and Querleu LAVRH. Stoeckel made two incisions: one on each side of the patient.

The first step of the transvaginal operation is the formation of the vaginal cuff. A series of Kocher forceps is put onto the vaginal mucosa following a circular line located at the level of the junction between the upper and the middle thirds. Traction is exerted on the forceps, creating an internal vaginal prolapse. The two sheets of the vaginal fold raised by the traction are separated from each other by injection with saline midway between each traction forceps. The outside sheet of the fold is then divided. The division is gradually made outside a line drawn by exerting appropriate traction on each pair of forceps. The pressure on the scalpel blade must be released as soon as the saline drop appears, so as not to enter the opposite sheet of the fold. This full-thickness incision (incision of the three layers of the vaginal wall) is made only on the anterior and posterior aspects of the developed vaginal cuff (Fig. 13.23). Only the skin is incised on the dorsolateral aspects (between three and four o'clock and between eight and nine o'clock), so that the relationship between the vaginal cuff and the paracervical ligaments is maintained.

Once separated from the remainder of the vagina, the cuff is taken into strong grasping forceps that are aligned in a frontal plane (Fig. 13.24). It is retracted dorsally in order to free the ventral aspect of the vaginal cuff at the same time as the ventral aspect of the uterus and surrounding tissues (i.e., paracervical and parametrial ligaments). The bladder floor and terminal ureter are attached to these structures and must be separated from them. The vesicovaginal space is carefully developed in the midline so as not to injure the bladder, which is very close to the tips of the grasping forceps. Caution must be taken because of the condensation of the cellular tissue joining the bladder floor to the vagina. This condensation raises a pseudoaponeurotic coronal structure named the supravaginal septum, which must be perforated (Fig. 13.25) to reach the appropriate space. Once the midline intervisceral space has been opened, the bladder pillars can be approached.

The bladder pillars are divided in two steps. Initially, the pillar is separated into the lateral and medial parts by opening the caudal brim of the pillar at an equal distance from its two sides and two extremities. After opening, the scissors are pushed laterally (Fig. 13.26). One ensures that the instrument is placed lateral to the ureter by palpating and feeling the "plop." These fibers are divided after stapling or bipolar cauterization (Fig. 13.27), making the paravesical space wider. A bigger retractor is put in place and the knee of the ureter appears in the deepest part. Once the knee of the ureter has

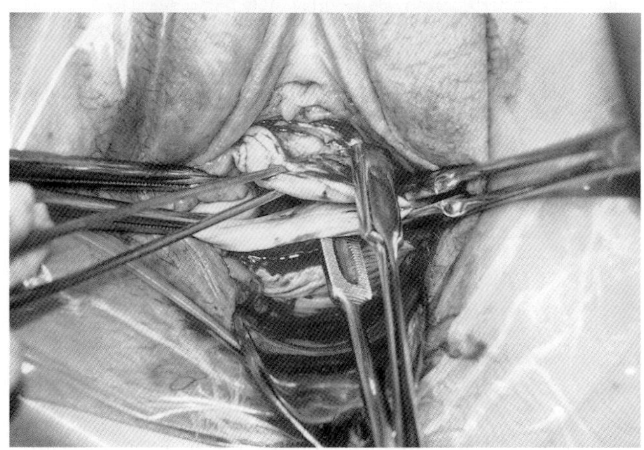

FIGURE 13.24. (*See color plate section.*) Technique of modified LAVRH. Closing the vaginal cuff with Chroback forceps.

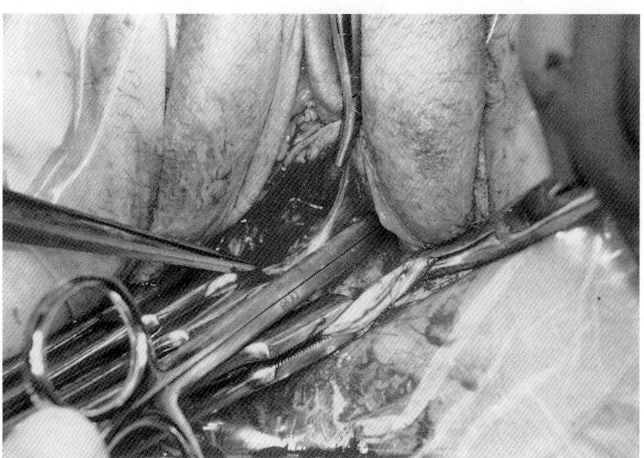

FIGURE 13.26. (*See color plate section.*) Technique of modified LAVRH. Opening the paravesical space on the left side of the patient.

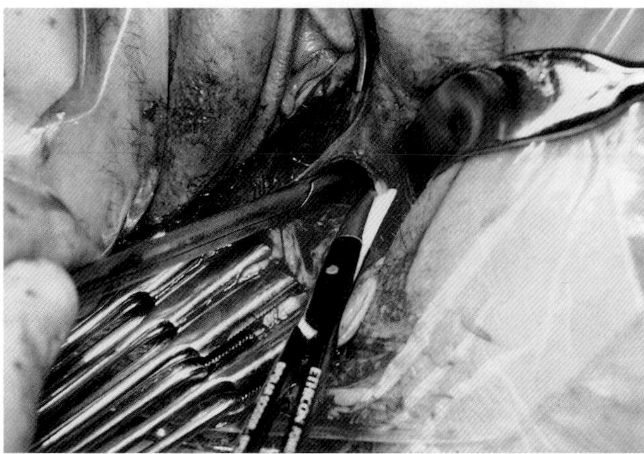

FIGURE 13.27. (*See color plate section.*) Technique of modified LAVRH. Dividing the lateral fibers of the bladder pillar on the left side of the patient.

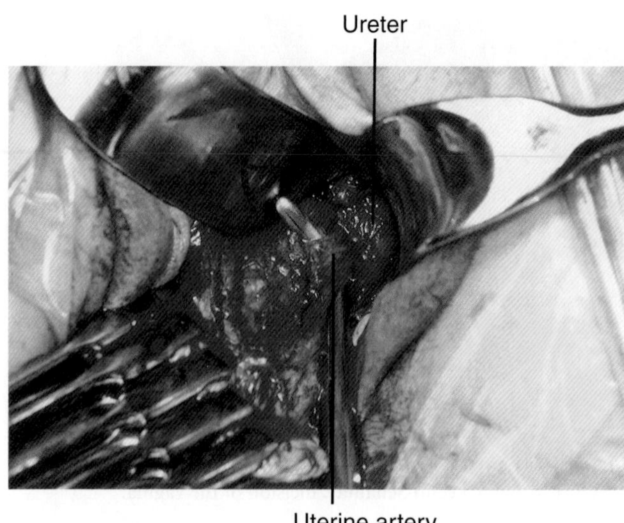

FIGURE 13.29. (*See color plate section.*) Technique of modified LAVRH. The medial fibers of the bladder pillar have been divided; the arch of the uterine artery is demonstrated.

been identified, the medial fibers (Fig. 13.28) of the pillar can be divided. This division exposes the ventral aspect of the juxtauterine part of the paracervical ligament. The paraisthmic window (the inferior brim of which is the superior brim of the paracervical ligament) is identified by palpation. The arch of the uterine artery is located inside it. The afferent branch of the arch is isolated (Fig. 13.29) and dissected upward as far as the level of the knee of the ureter. Then the dissection is pushed further laterally inside the knee of the ureter and the artery is cut close to its origin.

Freeing the dorsal aspect of the vaginal cuff is easier than freeing its ventral aspect. The grasping forceps are retracted ventrally. The pouch of Douglas is opened in the midline and the rectal pillars are divided, that is, the sacrouterine ligaments or, more precisely, the medial part of them (i.e., the rectouterine peritoneal folds). Once these ligaments have been divided, the dorsal aspect of the paraisthmic windows is palpated. Their inferior brim corresponds to the superior brim of the paracervical ligaments.

A right-angle dissector is pushed from back to front through the parauterine ligament. Opening the dissector frees the upper brim of the paracervical ligament. This is done while dividing the paracolpos, that is, the expansion that the paracervix sends to the vagina. This division is done by deepening the dorsolateral incision in the vagina and pushing it laterally while controlling the bleeders encountered during this action.

Now that the dorsal and ventral aspects of the paracervical ligaments are both exposed with the superior and inferior brims, they can be divided. Two clamps are placed on each ligament, the most lateral being just at the contact of the tip of the knee of the ureter (Fig. 13.30).

Once the two paracervical ligaments have been divided, the operation can be completed without difficulty.

Sardi et al. (194) reported on 47 patients who underwent a procedure closer to type 0 LAVRH than to type 3. After 4 years, the overall survival was 100% for stage IA, 88% for stage IB1, and 85% for stage IB2. Sardi et al. suggested that 20 cases were needed to obtain the minimum skill to perform

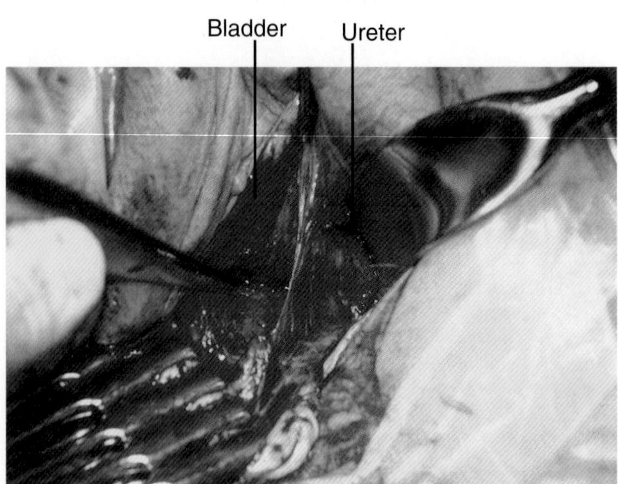

FIGURE 13.28. (*See color plate section.*) Technique of modified LAVRH. The location where the ureter enters the bladder floor is visible. The medial fibers of the bladder pillar can be cut.

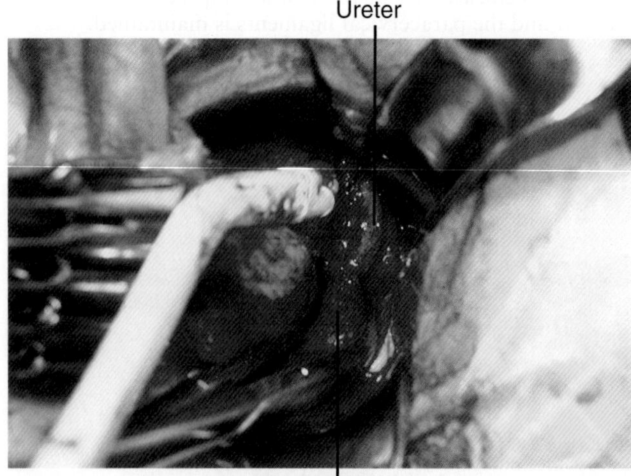

FIGURE 13.30. (*See color plate section.*) Technique of modified LAVRH. Two clamps are put on the paracervical ligament, the distal one being just underneath the tip of the knee of the ureter.

LAVRH. Renaud et al. (145) reviewed the charts of 102 patients affected by cervical cancer who had laparoscopic lymphadenectomy followed by VRH or trachelectomy in 91 of them (stage IA in 77%, IB1 in 17%, and IIA in 6%). There were two intraoperative complications due to laparoscopy and four due to VRH; however, only one postoperative complication was considered to be major (an abscess which required surgical drainage). With a median follow-up of 36 months, there were four recurrences in 91 patients. Three of the intraoperative and postoperative complications occurred in the first 25 cases compared to four in the following 77 cases. Querleu et al. (195) used personal interview and a standardized questionnaire in 60 of 95 patients who underwent LAVRH in order to assess the impact of the paracervical lymphadenectomy on late urinary bladder dysfunction. No difference was found between the patients operated before and after introduction of the new procedure. However, the paracervical dissection apparently failed to prevent the pelvic recurrences observed in the patients who had cancers 2 cm or greater. Six of 14 patients with tumors 2 cm or greater recurred with no difference being observed between those who underwent paracervical lymphadenectomy and those who did not. Conversely, only one recurrence was observed in the group of 81 patients affected by a tumor less than 2 cm. The uselessness of a very large surgery in small tumors is demonstrated in Dargent's series (unpublished data). Among 216 patients affected by cervical cancer stages pIA2 and pIB1 who underwent LAVRH between December 1986 and May 2002, the actuarial 5-year disease-free survival was 94.2%. No recurrence was observed in the 144 patients with stage pIA and stage pIB1 <2 cm large cancers. Conversely, among the 72 patients affected by stage pIB1 ≥2 cm, the addition of a paracervical dissection was likely to decrease the risk of recurrence, which was as high as 18.9% during the first 3 years. Among the 53 patients followed during 3 years or more, the number of early recurrences was 3 of 11 after a proximal radical hysterectomy, 4 of 23 with a distal radical hysterectomy, and 3 of 19 with a proximal radical hysterectomy combined with a laparoscopic paracervical dissection. Hertel et al. (196) reported on 200 patients with cervical cancer stages IA to IIIA treated in Jena using LAVRH, and confirmed that the incidence of complications decreased significantly when comparing the first half with the second half of the series (65% of the complications in the first half vs. 35% in the second). This decrease could be linked to improvement in the technique (197,198). It could also be due to a change in the surgical radicality. In the reported series, the VRH was either performed according to the Schauta-Stoeckel technique that is similar to type 2 radical hysterectomy (102 cases) or according to a more extensive original technique (98 cases) described by Possover et al. (199). At the time of the report, no change in the indications was formally introduced, but after having identified three independent risk factors for recurrence (tumor node metastasis (TNM) stage IB2 or greater, lymph node metastasis, and lymphovascular space involvement), the investigators decided not to use LAVRH for high-risk cases and to reserve it only for low-risk cases. This resulted in a projected 98% 5-year overall survival rate, even when the more patient-friendly Schauta-Stoeckel technique was used (average duration of the surgery 298 minutes vs. 371; $p = 0.0001$).

Laparoscopic Vaginal Radical Trachelectomy

Radical trachelectomy is a conservative variant of radical hysterectomy for young patients affected by early invasive cancer on the superficial aspect of the cervix. This operation was devised by the Romanian gynecologist Aburel using a laparotomy. None of his patients ever became pregnant. Postoperative adhesions, excessive tissue removal, and inaccurate isthmovaginal suturing were the probable causes for the lack of pregnancies in his patients. Using the laparoscopic vaginal approach allows successful outcomes.

The operation proceeds the same way as LAVRH. The arch of the uterine artery is identified, and the uterine artery must be preserved. Once the arch is identified, the afferent branch is followed laterally, ensuring that no lymph node is located along its course (if so, this node is removed). Once this dissection has been completed, the dorsal aspect of the paracervical ligament and its superior and inferior brims are cleared. The paracervical ligament is then divided at the same level that it is divided in LAVRH. The clamps are put in place taking care not to compromise the uterine artery. The uterine artery collaterals going to the lateral fornix and to the cervix (cervicovaginal arteries) are controlled and divided. At this stage, the most important difference from LAVRH occurs: The uterus is divided 5 mm below the isthmus (Fig. 13.31), which is generally easy to locate owing to the previous dissections that have freed its anterior, posterior, and lateral aspects. The specimen is sent to the laboratory for assessment of its superior margin by frozen section. The cavity is sounded and a dilator is inserted to widen the canal and facilitate the reconstruction.

Once the results of the frozen section determine negative margins, the reconstruction is undertaken. Initially, the pouch of Douglas is closed with a circular running suture, including the posterior aspect of the supraisthmic part of the uterus and taking the stumps of the paracervical ligaments that reattach the uterus to its natural support. Isthmic cerclage, using the same suture used for the conventional prophylaxis of miscarriage, is then performed. Finally, the isthmovaginal suturing is performed using two Sturmdorf stitches approximating the vaginal mucosa and the isthmic mucosa with great care—the previous dilation facilitates this crucial step of the operation. The reconstruction is completed by three interrupted stitches in each lateral part and eventually results in a new os (Fig. 13.32).

The data on laparoscopic vaginal radical trachelectomy are sparse. After the first presentation made by Dargent et al. (200) in 1996, Schneider et al. (201) published two cases and then Shepherd et al. (202) reported ten cases. The patients all had invasive cancer stage IB1 <2 cm in diameter. No complications were reported. Six pregnancies occurred after surgery and three live infants were delivered. One septic abortion occurred at 18 weeks and there were no recurrences. Roy and Plante (203) reviewed their first 31 cases in 1998. Most of the

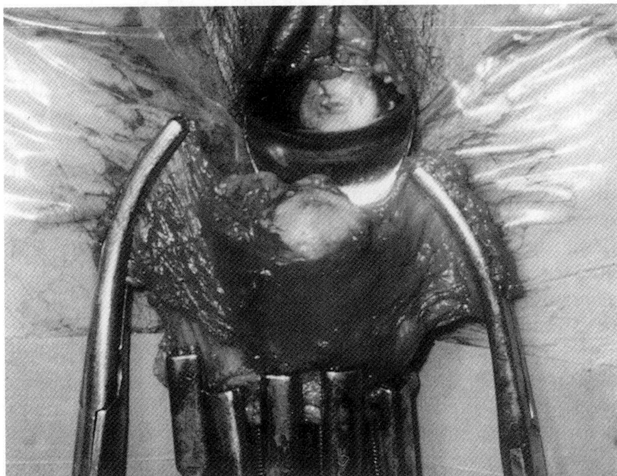

FIGURE 13.31. Specimen of LVRT. The radicality is the same as in the modified LAVRH. The transected uterine isthmus is visible.

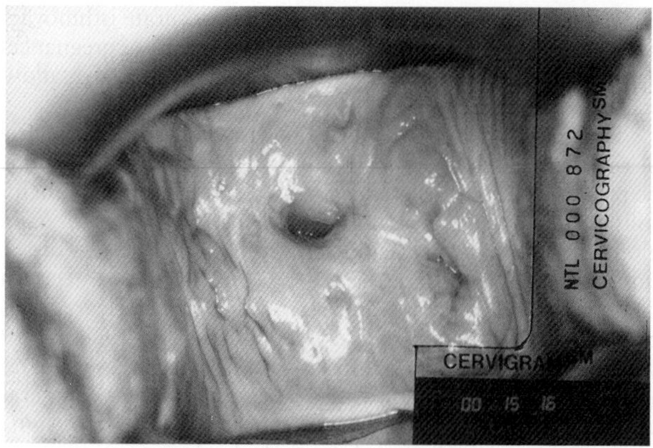

FIGURE 13.32. Postoperative picture after LVRT. The contour of the cervix has disappeared but the uterine orifice remains patent.

patients were stage IA and stage IB1 <2 cm in diameter. Only two patients had lesions >2 cm. Four complications required laparotomy: two external iliac vessel injuries during the laparoscopic step of the operation, one episode of intraoperative bleeding, and one bladder injury during the transvaginal step. Seven pregnancies occurred and four births were registered, one of them at 25 weeks of gestation. One recurrence was observed among the 26 patients followed for more than 6 months (median follow-up 25 months). The patient had a stage IIA 3-cm squamous cancer. Covens et al. (204) compared 31 patients treated with laparoscopic vaginal radical trachelectomy for stage IB1 cervical cancer <2 cm with two control groups, one matched and the other one unmatched (541 patients). The 2-year actuarial recurrence-free survival rates were 95%, 100%, and 98%, respectively. The cumulative actuarial conception rate at 12 months was 40%.

Dargent's experience was reviewed in May 2002 (205). Of the 96 patients with a follow-up of 1 to 15 years, one secondary cancer was observed (bilateral suprarenal gland cancer in a patient treated for neuroendocrine cancer of the cervix) as well as four recurrences. The retrospective univariate analysis demonstrated that the maximal tumor diameter (≥2 cm) and the depth of infiltration (≥1 cm) were the only two significant factors of risk. The chance of recurrence was zero for the small tumors, 19% for the tumors ≥2 cm (n = 21), and 25% for the tumors ≥2 cm with a depth of infiltration ≥1 cm (n = 19). The obstetric outcomes (unpublished data) were assessed at the same time. Forty-seven patients attempted to become pregnant, of which 36 succeeded and 11 did not (3 because of male factors). The 55 pregnancies ended with 11 early miscarriages, eight late miscarriages, and 36 live births. No recurrences were reported in the 61 patients from Shepherd et al. (206), Schlaerth et al. (207), and Burnett et al. (208). However, Picone et al. (209) reported the first central pelvic recurrence after radical trachelectomy. The tumor was 21 mm large, and the proximal tumor-free margin was only 4 mm. The recurrence developed on the isthmus 26 months after the surgery. Bernardini et al. (210) reported on the obstetric outcomes of 30 patients attempting to become pregnant after radical trachelectomy, of which 18 succeeded and 12 did not. Among the 22 registered pregnancies, 3 resulted in first-trimester abortion and 1 in an induced 17-week abortion after rupture of the membranes. Of the 18 pregnancies lasting past the seventeenth week, all resulted in a viable birth, but six occurred at or before 36 weeks of gestation.

One might assume, from summarized data, that laparoscopic vaginal radical trachelectomy provides the same chances for survival as either VRH or ARH. The question remains, however, as to whether the operation is acceptable for tumors >2 cm in which the risk of recurrence is significant. There is no question about the absolute contraindication when the proximal tumor-free margin is too short (less than 10 mm). With regard to reproductive outcome, the main problem is miscarriage. Dargent's early experience suggests that cervical closure performed by the Saling method (211) at the end of the first trimester of pregnancy could improve the efficacy of the cerclage placed at the time of the initial procedure.

Laparoscopic Radical Hysterectomy

Laparoscopic radical hysterectomy was first introduced by Canis et al. (27) and shortly thereafter by Nezhat et al. (1992) (10). These two early cases were limited to stage IA2 tumors; however, as experience grew, the procedure was applied to larger tumors (212).

Spirtos et al. described a standardized technique to perform what was termed a laparoscopic type 3 radical hysterectomy (213). He separated this operation into eight components: (a) right and left aortic lymphadenectomy, (b) right and left pelvic lymphadenectomy, (c) development of the paravesical and pararectal spaces, (d) ureteral dissection, (e) ligation and dissection of the uterine artery, (f) development of the vesicouterine and rectovaginal spaces, (g) resection of the parametria, and (h) resection of the upper vagina. All the steps are carried out with the laparoscope, including the vaginal closure. Spirtos et al. use staplers for transecting the parametria and an argon-beam coagulator for dissection of the uterine artery, ureter, and paravaginal tissue and to open the vagina. Other American surgeons have found this technique to be successful (29). However, the procedure can be performed with basic bipolar coagulation (214) as well as ultrasonic energy (215).

As more surgeons began mastering the techniques of advanced laparoscopy, additional reports demonstrating the feasibility of this procedure began to appear in the literature. Ramirez et al. (216) reported the M. D. Anderson experience on 20 patients who underwent the laparoscopic radical hysterectomy. The procedure was completed laparoscopically in all patients with a median operative time of 332.5 minutes (range, 275 to 442) despite nine of the patients having additional procedures performed. The median hospital stay was only 1 day (range, 1 to 5). There were three perioperative and two long-term complications in this series. Others have reported a high level of success with the procedures. Gil-Moreno et al. (217) were able to complete the procedure laparoscopically in 26 of the 27 patients with no reported intraoperative complications. The one conversion reported was due to technical considerations. In a large series of over 300 patients, Xu et al. (218) reported an intraoperative complication rate of 4.4%. Vascular injury was the most common intraoperative complication. However, the majority of intraoperative complications were managed laparoscopically and the conversion rate was only 1.3%. There was a 5.1% postoperative complication rate with fistula being the most common complication.

When compared to abdominal radical hysterectomy, total laparoscopic radical hysterectomy has been shown to be feasible, safe, and associated with low morbidity. Abu-Rustum et al. (29) compared a group of patients who underwent a laparoscopic radical hysterectomy with pelvic lymphadenectomy to a group of patients managed with laparotomy. Patient age, body mass index, stage, histology, and mean pelvic lymph node counts were similar in both groups. Although the median operative time for the laparoscopic procedure was significantly longer (360 vs. 285, $p < 0.01$), the estimated blood loss and hospital stay were significantly less. Similarly, Frumovitz et al. (219) reported on a comparison between 35 patients who underwent total laparoscopic radical hysterectomy and 54 patients who underwent an abdominal radical hysterectomy. Patient demographics and tumor factors were comparable in both groups. Although operative time was longer for the laparoscopic group, hospital stay, mean blood loss, and infectious morbidity were significantly less. Mean pelvic lymph node counts of patients undergoing laparoscopic procedure were less in this report; however, other larger comparative series have demonstrated that pelvic node counts are the same irrespective of the approach (219). Such a technically demanding procedure can be taught to trainees without compromising adequacy. In a recent case-controlled study specifically examining the use of total laparoscopic radical hysterectomy in a fellowship program, Zakashansky et al. (220) demonstrated that greater node counts, decreased hospital stay, and less blood loss are possible without increased morbidity in a training program.

Recently, follow-up data on the oncologic outcomes have been reported. In the largest series to date, Spirtos et al. (221) reported on 78 consecutive patients who underwent laparoscopic radical hysterectomy with aortic and pelvic lymphadenectomy. The average operative time was 205 minutes (150 to 430 minutes) and the average blood loss was 225 mL (range, 50 to 700 mL). With a mean follow-up of 66.8 months (± 1.78 months), the estimated 5-year disease-free survival was 89.7% and the estimated 5-year overall survival was 93.6%. Similar survival data have been reported by other groups performing laparoscopic radical hysterectomy (222). Pomel et al. reported a 5-year survival rate of 96% in 50 patients with stages IA2 and IB1 cervical cancers treated with laparoscopic radical hysterectomy (222). Several groups have compared the oncologic outcomes of laparoscopic radical hysterectomy with those of abdominal radical hysterectomy. In one of the larger series published to date, Li et al. (223) compared 90 patients treated with laparoscopic radical hysterectomy to 35 patients treated with traditional open surgery. Although the median follow-up was only 26 months, the recurrence rates for the laparoscopic and laparotomy groups were similar.

Since laparoscopic radical hysterectomy is a technically demanding procedure, some have implemented robotic-assisted surgery to perform the surgery. Sert and Abeler (224) recently published a case report on robotic-assisted radical hysterectomy with bilateral pelvic node dissection for a stage IB1 cervical cancer. In a larger series, Boggess et al. (225) reported on seven type III radical hysterectomies with pelvic node dissection for stage IB1 cervical cancers. The mean blood loss was 143 mL (range, 25 to 300) and mean operative time was 252 minutes (range, 187 to 290). The mean node count was 35 (range, 25to 55) and all patients were discharged on postoperative day 1. The authors recently compared their experience in obese patients using a robotically assisted approach to an open approach. Those obese patients undergoing a robotically assisted approach had a superior node count, shorter hospital stay, and lower blood loss, which the authors reasoned may all contribute to reduced morbidity in this group of patients (226).

Laparoscopic radical hysterectomy appears to be a reasonable option for patients with early-stage cervical cancer. It can be performed with an acceptable morbidity and outcomes appear comparable to patients who undergo traditional open surgery. The application of robotic assistance may allow a greater number of surgeons to perform the laparoscopic radical hysterectomy without requiring them to acquire advanced laparoscopic skills.

Laparoscopic Pelvic Exenteration

Using the laparoscope to assess the feasibility of pelvic exenteration was addressed for the first time by Plante and Roy (227) and subsequently reported by Köhler et al. (228). Pomel et al. (31) extended the procedure by actually performing a total laparoscopic pelvic exenteration with a small incision to create an ileal conduit and the diverting ileostomy. The operative time was 9 hours, and the postoperative course was uneventful. One can imagine that the complementary reconstruction will eventually be performed with a closed abdomen as well!

LAPAROSCOPY AND CANCER OF THE CERVIX

Although more than a century has passed since the first radical hysterectomy was performed by Clark (229), the role of surgery in the management of cervical cancer still remains a matter for debate. It is generally accepted that early cases can be managed using surgery or radiotherapy. Advanced cases must be treated using radiotherapy. The controversy arises from the many discrepancies existing among the definition of early and advanced cases. For some experts, the concept of ruling out surgery in the management of bulky but resectable tumors appears to be inappropriate considering that these tumors are less likely to be cured by radiotherapy. What should be the place of laparoscopic surgery in this controversial area of management? For simplification, the question will be addressed separating tumors <4 cm from tumors ≥4 cm.

Early Stages

Surgery and radiotherapy produce comparable survival in the treatment of early cervical cancer (230). Even if the question of cost-effectiveness is not clearly settled, the majority of gynecologic oncologists have a preference for surgery, especially in young patients whose ovarian function can be preserved. Data obtained from the extensive use of radical surgery have demonstrated that the chances for cure depend in large part on the state of regional lymph nodes (231,232). For tumors <4 cm in diameter, the 5-year disease-free survival is approximately 90% as long as the nodes are negative, and approximately 60% if one or two nodes are involved. Disease-free survival drops to 15% if three or more nodes are involved. The opportunity to identify nodal spread is one of the advantages of a surgical versus a radiotherapeutic approach. However, when nodal spread is discovered after surgery is completed, it only serves to help adjust adjuvant therapy that has a low efficacy (63,233–235). Knowledge of lymph node status before the onset of radiotherapy is obviously better. Here lies the first indication for laparoscopy—the assessment of the regional lymph nodes to help decide on treatment modalities.

Staging

If accepted, the concept of pretherapeutic laparoscopic staging raises a series of practical questions, which we will try to answer in the order in which they appear in daily practice.

Prelaparoscopic Imaging

The sensitivity and specificity of computed tomographic (CT) scanning are approximately 60% and 85%, respectively (236). Lymphangiography has a slightly better accuracy, but it cannot be easily obtained in many centers. CT scanning (and/or magnetic resonance imaging [MRI]) must be performed in every case, and if enlarged nodes are detected, they must be assessed by guided biopsy. If the biopsy reveals metastatic involvement, there is no point in performing a laparoscopy. If the biopsy is negative, laparoscopy should be undertaken.

Sentinel Node Biopsy. Although SN biopsy does not replace systematic lymphadenectomy, it deserves to be implemented in all cases. The first reason is that there are no false positives. Since involved lymph nodes can lead to altered therapy, the information is priceless. For the pathologist, identification of the node(s) at greatest risk for metastasis may help minimize the false-negative rate. The final (and possibly the best) reason for performing SN biopsy is that the scientific community needs more data and should encourage surgicopathologic studies regarding this matter.

Management of Bulky Nodes. Even if prelaparoscopic imaging does not suggest suspicious lymph nodes, it is still possible to encounter an obviously metastatic node. Freeing such a node laparoscopically is technically possible (139) even if vascular adhesions exist. One should, however, refrain from undertaking this dissection because of the hazard of tumor dissemination from nodal rupture. Two options for management are suggested: (a) referring the patient to the radiotherapist after having documented the metastatic involvement by fine-needle aspiration, or (b) opening the abdomen and performing nodal debulking.

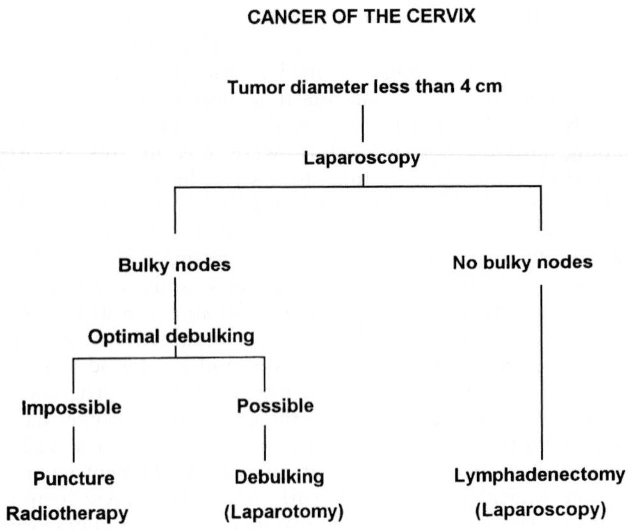

FIGURE 13.33. Algorithm for laparoscopy in early cervical cancer (1).

Pelvic Versus Pelvic and Aortic Lymphadenectomy

In cases where the pelvic lymph nodes appear to be uninvolved whether at prelaparoscopic imaging, laparoscopic assessment, or at frozen section (frozen sections done on the SN and on the other pelvic nodes), the question is whether an aortic dissection has to be added. The risk of involvement of the aortic nodes is small if the pelvic nodes are negative (237). Therefore, we assume that aortic dissection is not indicated. If pelvic node involvement is found at the time of the initial laparoscopic staging, one should perform a para-aortic dissection using the same approach—the transumbilical transperitoneal one. If the pelvic node involvement is discovered at final pathology (no frozen sections during the initial procedure or a false negative of the frozen section: 20% to 40% of the cases), aortic dissection is performed at a second surgery. We recommend using the left-side extraperitoneal approach to do this. The dissection has to be extended up to the level of the left renal vein because isolated supramesenteric metastasis can exist (154).

Proposed Algorithms

Many opinions exist as to the exact role of lymphadenectomy in the management of early cervical cancers. The lymphadenectomy itself clearly plays a role in prognosis as nodes are found to be apparently free of disease. Radiotherapy given as adjuvant treatment to pN1 patients decreases the chance of recurrence; however, it can produce iatrogenic complications such as radiation enteritis, which is increased if radiation follows surgical dissection (230). Taking these facts into account, some oncologists abort surgery as soon as they know that lymph node involvement exists. Others may proceed with radical surgery in spite of nodal disease, and in such cases, these surgeons deny any value to laparoscopic staging. The former group may have interest in laparoscopic staging, but the question remains of how to adopt this in the pN1 cases. The proposed algorithms (Figs. 13.33 and 13.34) represent a compromise taking into account the truth in surgical dissection for patients with limited nodal involvement and the necessity of radiotherapy in all pN1 cases. If bulky nodes are noted at laparoscopy, debulking probably is useful (238,239), but it appears to be safer to do such by laparotomy.

If the nodes appear to be endoscopically normal but are involved on frozen section, the decision depends essentially on the number of involved nodes. If this number is less than three, radical surgery is a reasonable choice. We prefer performing it by laparotomy for safety (and rapidity) reasons. If the number of positive lymph nodes exceeds two, primary chemoradiotherapy is the best option, and we recommend aborting the radical hysterectomy.

If the nodes are normal, radical surgery is the treatment of choice. The laparoscopically assisted and the purely laparoscopic radical hysterectomies are offered as alternatives to classic ARH.

Laparoscopic Assistance to Radical Surgery

After deciding to use the laparoscopic approach for performing radical hysterectomy, one must decide between the various forms of laparoscopic assistance to VRH and purely laparoscopic radical hysterectomy. The data concerning both types of approaches have been addressed in the previous sections of this chapter. We favor the combined approach for three reasons. The first is that the purely laparoscopic approach requires a large degree of manipulation of the tumor, whereas in the laparoscopically assisted operation there is no tumor

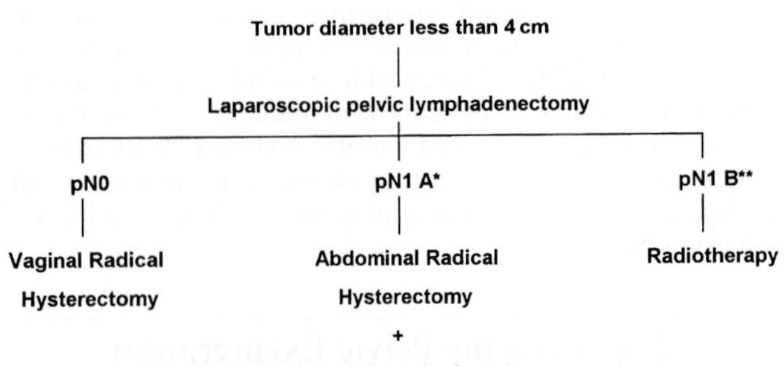

FIGURE 13.34. Algorithm for laparoscopy in early cervical cancer (2).

manipulation during the laparoscopic step and the tumor is protected inside the vaginal cuff at the beginning of the vaginal step. The second reason is that the vaginal approach allows easy management of the juxtauterine tissues, especially the vesicovaginal spaces, bladder pillars, and parametrium. Additionally, delineation of the vaginal cuff is much more precise using the vaginal route. The third and most important reason favoring the mixed approach is that this is good training for performing radical vaginal trachelectomy.

Advanced Cases and Recurrences

Radiotherapy given for advanced cervical cancers fails in two of three cases because of extrapelvic recurrences. These recurrences arise mostly in the abdominal cavity either extraperitoneally (aortic nodes) or intraperitoneally. One way of tackling this problem could be to give systematic extended-field radiotherapy. However, a prospective study (240) in which extended-field radiotherapy was given either routinely or after lymphangiographic selection did not yield the expected results. Moreover, extended-field radiotherapy includes a risk of severe complications close to 20% (241). Thus, the indications for its use must be limited to appropriately selected cases.

Staging laparotomy was devised as an answer to the question of selection of the indications for extended-field radiotherapy. It has some success in spite of its drawbacks, which include intraoperative and postoperative complications and enhanced risk of radiation enteritis because of peritoneal adhesions resulting from surgery. A GOG study (242) demonstrated that an extraperitoneal approach decreases these drawbacks, and laparoscopy may produce an even better result.

Laparoscopic staging of advanced cervical cancer can be performed using the classic transumbilical transperitoneal approach, which enables the surgeon to assess the peritoneal cavity and perform pelvic and aortic dissections. A more conservative approach could be limiting dissection to the pelvic area and going further only in the cases where the pelvic nodes are involved. Another approach entails using transumbilical laparoscopy only for assessing the peritoneal cavity and guiding digital preparation preceding extraperitoneal aortic dissection (discussed above). Most important in the selection of extended-field radiotherapy are (a) peritoneal cytology and (b) the status of the aortic nodes. The status of the pelvic lymph nodes does not alter pelvic radiation fields. This highlights the benefits of the combination of transumbilical laparoscopy and extraperitoneal dissection. It is the ideal way to perform laparoscopic staging in the management of advanced cervical cancer (Fig. 13.35). The benefits of this staging should not be overestimated since using laparoscopy in place of laparotomy avoids the deleterious effects of operative adhesions but does not increase survival.

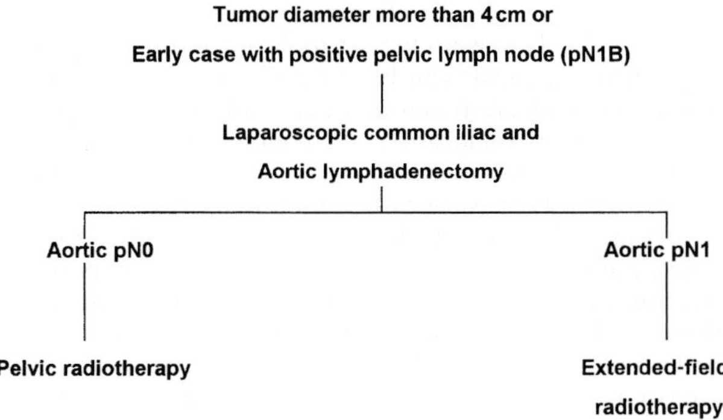

FIGURE 13.35. Algorithm for laparoscopy in advanced cervical cancer.

An additional benefit of pretherapeutic laparoscopy is the possibility of performing ovarian transposition for patients less than 40 or 45 years of age. Studies demonstrate that laparoscopic transposition is both feasible and effective (243).

An additional indication for combined laparoscopic assessment is selection for pelvic exenteration in patients diagnosed with pelvic recurrence of cervical cancer (227,228). Both positive peritoneal cytology and positive aortic nodes are contraindications to exenteration. As previously mentioned, it is advantageous to identify these findings without having to perform a laparotomy.

Laparoscopic Surgery and Endometrial Cancer

Surgery remains the cornerstone for the treatment of endometrial cancer. Hysterectomy and bilateral salpingo-oophorectomy are part of all traditional treatment protocols. Total hysterectomy has been traditionally performed through an open approach to completely assess the peritoneal cavity and perform lymph-node sampling or lymphadenectomy. Vaginal hysterectomy has been used in the management of endometrial cancers in certain situations (244). However, the vaginal route does not allow for the evaluation of the peritoneal cavity or the retroperitoneal lymph nodes. Since the introduction of laparoscopic lymphadenectomy, minimally invasive surgery has become increasingly popular in the management of gynecologic malignancies. With the development of improved instruments and surgeons' skills, laparoscopic surgeons began to perform more complicated procedures for the management of gynecologic malignancies. Case series began to appear in the literature, and recently, more prospective studies have been reported, with the largest one being the GOG LAP-2 study.

Using a combined laparoscopic and vaginal approach, all the procedures required for endometrial cancer surgery can be accomplished. Complete assessment of the peritoneal surfaces and retroperitoneal dissection are possible. Thus, the addition of laparoscopy transforms the basic transvaginal hysterectomy into an oncologic complete operation. Minimally invasive management of endometrial cancer is appealing, and does not require long training. This explains why the use of LAVH in the treatment of endometrial cancer gained popularity long before LAVRH in the treatment of cervical cancer.

Feasibility studies concerning minimally invasive surgery in endometrial cancer are becoming more numerous. In addition to the two early publications regarding laparoscopic management (81,137), there have been many additional reports (244,245) that confirm the feasibility. Recently, the GOG completed the largest prospective, randomized trial to date (LAP-2) in patients with clinical early-stage uterine cancer comparing a traditional open surgical approach to laparoscopic management (246). Although survival data are not available, the study did demonstrate that laparoscopic staging can be completed in 76.3% of patients. The patients undergoing laparoscopic staging were less likely to have their para-aortic nodes sampled but the node positivity rate and International Federation of Obstetrics and Gynecology (FIGO) stage were the same in both arms.

The advantages of laparoscopically assisted vaginal hysterectomy (LAVH) have been illustrated when compared to abdominal hysterectomy for the management of early-stage endometrial cancer in several retrospective studies. In a retrospective review of 320 patients, Gemignani et al. (247) demonstrated that LAVH was associated with a decreased hospital stay, fewer complications, and resulted in lower overall hospital charges. Others have also demonstrated significantly lower hospital costs when patients with early endometrial cancer are managed by laparoscopy (151), but total costs may be higher when surgeons' fees are added (248). Cost savings are most likely a direct result of the significantly shorter hospital stay and have been consistently reported in both single institutional retrospective and prospective series (249,250). The multi-institutional GOG LAP-2 study also demonstrated a shorter hospitalization with a median hospital stay of 3 days for patients treated with laparoscopy versus a median of 4 days in those patients treated with open surgery (246).

Patients who undergo laparoscopic surgery seem to report a higher level of satisfaction with laparoscopy when compared to patients treated with total abdominal hysterectomy. They benefit from a shorter recovery time and are able to return to work and full activity more quickly (248). In a recent prospective, randomized study comparing laparoscopy to laparotomy in the management of endometrial cancer, Zullo et al. (250) prospectively demonstrated that patients treated with laparoscopy did indeed have improved quality of life for the first 6 months after surgery. Improved short-term quality of life was also demonstrated in the GOG LAP-2 study, which employed the Functional Assessment of Cancer Therapy-General (FACT-G) tool. At the 1-, 3-, and 6-week postoperative intervals, scores were higher for the patients treated with laparoscopic surgery, illustrating that quality of life was better. However, at the 6-month postoperative interval, scores were the same, signifying that improved quality of life was generally seen within the first 6 weeks after surgery (251).

When evaluating the two techniques in regard to their oncologic adequacy, both appear to be comparable. In a prospective comparison of the two techniques, Malur et al. (252) demonstrated that there was no significant difference in the number of pelvic or para-aortic lymph nodes obtained. Oncologic outcomes also appear comparable in small prospective and retrospective studies of women with early-stage endometrial cancer treated by either laparoscopy or laparotomy (250,253). Tozzi et al. reported on the survival of 122 women prospectively randomized to either laparoscopy or laparotomy. With a median follow-up of 44 months (range, 5 to 96), cause-specific survival was similar in the two groups: laparoscopy, 90.5% versus laparotomy, 94.9% ($p = 0.47$) (253).

Prospective comparisons between the combined laparoscopic and vaginal approach and the abdominal approach are available in the literature. Malur et al. (252) compared 37 patients treated by a laparoscopic and vaginal approach to 33 patients treated by laparotomy. All patients underwent pelvic and aortic lymph node dissection except for patients with well-differentiated tumors that invaded to less than the inner third of the myometrium. There was no difference in the mean Quetelet index (QI), mean number of lymph nodes, and mean operation time. The laparoscopic group did have less blood loss, fewer transfusions, and shorter hospital stay. With a mean follow up of 16.5 (range, 2 to 43) and 21.6 (range, 2 to 48) months for the laparoscopic and laparotomy groups, respectively, the recurrence-free and overall survivals were not significantly different (97.3% vs. 93.3% and 83.9% vs. 90.9%, respectively). Other small prospective trials have demonstrated the association of laparoscopy with less blood loss and shorter hospital stay in the management of endometrial cancer (254,255).

Since obesity is a major risk factor for the development of endometrial cancer, many patients will present with a high QI. Performing a staging procedure in an obese patient can be difficult, but may not be an absolute contraindication. Scribner et al. (256) reported on their experience of laparoscopic pelvic and para-aortic lymphadenectomy in the obese patient. In 55 patients, laparoscopic staging was completed in 44% of patients with a QI ≥ 35 compared to a completion rate of 82% in patients with a QI < 35 ($p = 0.004$). In spite of this difference, the authors concluded that obesity is not an absolute contraindication to laparoscopic staging. Similarly, the same authors studied the surgical management of a group of patients 65 years or older with endometrial cancer. Although the operating room time and transfusion rate were significantly higher in the patients managed by laparoscopy compared to laparotomy, laparoscopy was associated with decreased hospital stay, less postoperative ileus, and fewer infectious complications with comparable blood loss and node counts. The authors concluded that older age was not an absolute contraindication to laparoscopic staging (257).

One potential drawback to laparoscopic management was the potential for retrograde seeding with the use of a uterine manipulator, which was suggested in a retrospective study of 377 patients undergoing either LAVH or total abdominal hysterectomy (TAH) for early-stage endometrial cancer (258). The authors found that patients in the LAVH group had a significantly higher incidence of positive peritoneal washings (10.3% vs. 2.8%, $p = 0.002$). A subsequent report by Vergote et al. (259) similarly reviewed the experience with endometrial cancer patients treated with either TAH or LAVH without the use of a uterine manipulator, and no difference in positive peritoneal cytology was observed. In a prospective study of patients with clinical stage I endometrial cancer undergoing laparoscopic surgery, Eltabbakh et al. demonstrated that routine use of a uterine manipulator does not result in an increased incidence of positive peritoneal cytology (260).

Laparoscopic surgery for the management of endometrial cancer undoubtedly has its limitations. Large fibroid uteri that cannot be removed without morcellation should not be operated on using laparoscopic surgery if endometrial cancer is present. Placing such unusual situations aside, the preliminary results from the GOG LAP-2 trial are encouraging and support many of the benefits of laparoscopic surgery identified in the studies to date. If equivalency in cancer outcomes is demonstrated, it is likely that laparoscopy will become a mainstay in the surgical management of early-stage endometrial cancer.

LAPAROSCOPY IN OVARIAN CANCER

Laparoscopy can be used in several different ways in the management of ovarian cancer depending on the stage of the disease and the anticipated goals of the procedures.

Advanced Ovarian Cancer

In patients with advanced ovarian cancer characterized by ascites, carcinomatosis, and omental cake, optimal surgical debulking may not be feasible even by laparotomy. Unfortunately, there is no perfect tool to determine preoperatively whether patients can be optimally debulked surgically. CT scan often underestimates the extent of the disease, in particular the extent and location of carcinomatosis. Nelson et al. have proposed a set of criteria that appear to accurately predict the inability to surgically debulk patients (261). They found that CT scan was highly sensitive for detection of ascites, mesenteric, and omental disease, but was poor for detection of liver involvement, omental attachment to the spleen, gallbladder fossa disease, and peritoneal nodules smaller than 2 cm (262). In the early 1990s, Schwartz et al. pioneered the concept of neoadjuvant chemotherapy in patients with advanced disease with the goals of chemoreducing the tumor bulk then using surgical debulking for those who show a good response to the chemotherapy (262,263). Recent studies suggest that quality of life is improved with this approach (264). However, other malignancies, particularly of gastrointestinal (GI) origin (such as colon, pancreas, stomach, and others) can mimic ovarian cancer. In some series, up to 20% of patients with presumed advanced ovarian cancer had a GI primary (265) due in part to inconclusive cytologic examination of ascitic fluid. Some, however, have argued that it is extremely accurate and helpful (266).

In cases where the diagnosis remains unclear, histologic confirmation of an ovarian primary is critical before initiation of chemotherapy. However, an adequate biopsy specimen cannot always be safely obtained under radiologic guidance. This is where laparoscopy becomes a valuable diagnostic tool. Indeed, the laparoscopic exploration of the abdominal cavity allows the surgeon to determine whether the disease can be optimally surgically debulked or not. If so, then a laparotomy can be performed to complete the surgery. If not, an adequate tissue specimen can be obtained for histologic confirmation. In a recent series of 18 patients with ovarian cancer explored laparoscopically, 7 (40%) were found to have unresectable disease and were spared a laparotomy. In the remaining patients, a laparotomy was performed and complete debulking was accomplished (267). In patients with advanced disease, diagnostic laparoscopy is an accurate diagnostic tool that may obviate the need for unnecessary laparotomies and thus contribute to a better quality of life in patients found to have unresectable disease (268).

In a recent series, 87 patients with advanced ovarian cancer underwent first a diagnostic open laparoscopy (269). In 61% of patients, optimal cytoreductive surgery was deemed possible and those patients underwent a laparotomy and debulking surgery. The goal was correctly achieved in 96% of cases. Conversely, in 39% of cases, optimal debulking appeared impossible. These patients then underwent neoadjuvant chemotherapy followed by interval debulking and adjuvant chemotherapy. Of note, the first cycle of chemotherapy was quickly initiated the day following the laparoscopic surgery. Overall, 80% of patients could be optimally debulked following three cycles of chemotherapy. The authors concluded that diagnostic open laparoscopy is a valid diagnostic tool to evaluate the extent of disease and avoids unnecessary laparotomies in patients where optimal debulking cannot be accomplished (269). To that extent, Fagotti et al. proposed a simple laparoscopy-based scoring system to estimate the chances of achieving optimal cytoreduction based on the presence of an omental cake, diaphragmatic carcinomatosis, mesenteric retraction, etc. A score of >8 predicted a suboptimal surgery with a specificity of 100%, a positive predictive value of 100%, and a negative predictive value of 70% (270).

However, the diagnostic laparoscopic procedure can have some pitfalls: first, the presence of a large amount of ascites may lead to a reduced visibility; second, the GI anatomy can be distorted, or the colon and/or small bowel may be adherent to the anterior abdominal wall or omentum, which may increase the risk of bowel injury. An open laparoscopic approach may be preferable in such cases, although a recent large trial does not seem to indicate that open laparoscopy reduces the risk of major complications (40). Lastly, the issue of trocar-site implantation remains controversial, particularly in patients with adenocarcinoma, ascites, and carcinomatosis (see section on port-site metastasis). However, when trocar sites are carefully closed after the procedure and the chemotherapy is initiated within 1 week, the risk of trocar-site metastasis can be reduced substantially (271,272). In cases of advanced ovarian cancer, laparoscopy appears to be a good triage method to select out patients who would not benefit from a laparotomy and can thus be spared the associated morbidity.

Second-Look Surgery

For those who perform second-look evaluation following first-line chemotherapy, laparoscopy may be a valuable approach to reduce the morbidity of the procedure. The magnification of the view allows a good evaluation of the peritoneal surfaces, in particular the costodiaphragmatic recessus and pelvic cul-de-sac. However, laparoscopy may be less accurate in the prerenal and porta hepatis regions, as well as in the root of the mesentery where small implants may go unnoticed. It is reassuring that the rate of negative evaluations and the rate of recurrences in patients with negative laparoscopic second looks are equivalent to those described in studies of second-look assessment by laparotomy (273). Conversely, in a prospective comparative study, a French group found the laparoscopic second-look evaluation to be suboptimal when compared to the abdominal approach, mainly because of the presence of adhesions which appeared to limit the thoroughness of the evaluation (274). In that study, the positive predictive value was 100%, but the negative predictive value was 86% (two false-negative cases) (274). Clearly, if residual tumor implants are readily confirmed at laparoscopy, then a laparotomy can be avoided in those patients. In patients with negative laparoscopic evaluation, it remains uncertain if laparotomy is more accurate, particularly in patients with diffuse adhesions. Large randomized trials are not available to answer this important question.

However, in a recent study 99 patients who had achieved a complete clinical response following first-line chemotherapy underwent second-look surgery. Nearly 70% had a negative second-look laparoscopy and were converted to a planned laparotomy, whereas 32% had positive findings at laparoscopy and thus were spared a laparotomy. In that study, the negative second-look laparoscopy predicted a negative laparotomy in 91% of the cases and was associated with a lower complication rate. The authors concluded that the small increase in sensitivity offered by laparotomy does not warrant the increased morbidity (275).

In terms of morbidity, a pilot study from Memorial Sloan-Kettering demonstrated that the laparoscopic approach results in less morbidity, shorter operating time, shorter hospital stay, less blood loss, and lower total hospital charges (276). In a series of 150 cases, Husain et al. also concluded that the complication rate of the laparoscopic approach is low and that it is a safe approach even in patients who had a prior abdominal surgery (273). Clough et al. have also reported similar findings (274). Concerns about the effect of CO_2 pneumoperitoneum on the risk of tumor dissemination have been raised (see section on gasless laparoscopy). However, a recent study including 131 patients operated on by laparoscopy does not seem to indicate that laparoscopic surgical procedures with CO_2 pneumoperitoneum reduce overall survival of patients with metastatic intra-abdominal carcinoma of ovarian/peritoneal origin (89). Lastly, in the context of second-look surgery, laparoscopy may be used to place intraperitoneal catheters under direct laparoscopic guidance in patients found to have residual disease at the time of the second-look operation (277).

Staging Procedure in Early-Stage Disease

On occasion, despite thorough preoperative investigation, patients are operated on for a presumed benign ovarian mass, yet an unexpected diagnosis of ovarian cancer occurs on final pathology, or the operating surgeon does not feel comfortable completing the staging procedure. In such situations, a complete surgical staging at a second surgery should be performed to determine the true stage. This information is critical for recommendations of adjuvant chemotherapy. Roughly, in presumed stage I disease, the chances of finding more advanced disease is in the range of 20% to 30% and the most frequent sites of metastasis are the lymph nodes (278,279). Laparoscopy may be an excellent alternative to complete the staging in such cases since a complete pelvic and para-aortic node sampling, an infracolic omentectomy, and a complete peritoneal assessment (+/− contralateral bilateral salpingo oophorectomy [BSO] and vaginal hysterectomy in older women), can be safely performed laparoscopically (280–283). Early studies showed that the morbidity of the laparoscopic procedure is low and the results are accurate (280–283). In the early 1990s, Querleu and Leblanc even demonstrated that a complete laparoscopic infrarenal lymph node dissection could be accomplished in the context of restaging ovarian or fallopian tube cancers (15). In a more recent study including 46 cases, infrarenal lymphadenectomies were performed laparoscopically (156). The morbidity was low and the authors noted that the number of lymph nodes obtained was doubled compared to the number of lymph nodes obtained by the more frequently performed inframesenteric lymphadenectomy (156).

Over a 10-year experience, Leblanc et al. laparoscopically restaged 42 patients with apparent early ovarian cancer and 7 with fallopian tube cancers. Only one patient had to be converted to a laparotomy because of adhesions and 19% were upstaged as a result of the staging procedure. They concluded that laparoscopic surgery meets the standards of a complete staging procedure, spares the patients the inconvenience of a laparotomy, and accurately identifies patients with more advanced disease who require adjuvant chemotherapy (284). In a recent GOG trial, Spirtos et al. completed the staging of incompletely staged gynecologic malignancies including ovarian and fallopian tube cancers. They noted a conversion rate of 20% to laparotomy, most often due to the presence of adhesions. Nevertheless, nearly 70% of patients had a successful complete laparoscopic staging and 11% were found to have more advanced disease (285).

Although there are no randomized trials comparing both approaches, it would appear that a comprehensive laparoscopic restaging of patients with early-stage ovarian cancer is feasible, accurate, and the morbidity is lower compared to the same procedure done by laparotomy. However, this procedure should only be performed by experienced and skilled laparoscopists capable of performing advanced and complex oncologic laparoscopic procedures.

With regard to borderline tumors, the value of a restaging procedure is controversial since the prognosis of patients with presumed stage I disease is excellent, and the value of adjuvant treatment is questionable even in more advanced disease. In a series of 56 patients referred with a suspected stage IA disease, only 4 (7%) were upstaged (286). Conversely, in a recent series of 30 patients who underwent complete laparoscopic staging for presumed ovarian cancer, 26.6% of patients were upstaged as a result of the staging procedure (287). However, all the patients are alive with the exception of only one patient who developed a recurrence (287). The authors concluded that whenever staging of a patient with a borderline tumor is considered, laparoscopy appears to be the method of choice since the procedure is accurate, the complication rate and the morbidity are low, and, very importantly, the incidence of infertility in young patients is minimized (287). It would appear, however, that laparoscopic ovarian cystectomy only for borderline tumor is associated with a higher risk of recurrence compared to a complete oophorectomy (131). Indeed, Darai et al. recently published their results regarding the laparoscopic restaging of borderline tumors and confirmed the feasibility of that surgical approach. In their series, there were no conversions and no intraoperative or postoperative complications. As expected, they noted that ovarian cystectomies were associated with a higher risk of persistent lesions, and the risk of upstaging was higher in cases of serous borderline tumors (288).

Laparoscopic Surgical Management of Early-Stage Ovarian Cancer

It is uncommon for gynecologic oncologists to knowingly operate on women with ovarian cancer laparoscopically unless it is to determine the resectability of patients with advanced disease (see section above). Thus, in most instances the ovarian cancer is diagnosed inadvertently at the time of surgery for a presumed benign ovarian mass. There are two options: (a) complete the surgery laparoscopically or (b) convert to a laparotomy.

In experienced hands, the surgery can technically be completed laparoscopically, particularly when the cancer appears to be limited to the ovary and when there is no evidence of gross metastatic disease (39). In a recent series reported by Havrilesky et al., the ovarian malignancies discovered at the time of laparoscopy for pelvic masses were managed laparoscopically and this was not associated with an adverse outcome (109). A recent study comparing 15 cases of early ovarian cancer managed by laparoscopy to 19 cases managed by laparotomy shows no difference in outcome between the two groups. Complication rate and shorter hospital stay were in favor of the laparoscopy group (289). Lecuru et al. found no deleterious influence of laparoscopy as first surgical access on outcome of patients with early-stage cervical cancer (290). However, in a recent survey, Leblanc et al. concluded that complete laparoscopic management of early-stage ovarian cancer is feasible in selected cases, but should be reserved to surgeons with advanced skills in laparoscopic surgery (291). Obviously, when faced with the discovery of an ovarian malignancy, another option is to convert the laparoscopy to a laparotomy to complete the surgery if surgeons do not feel comfortable performing the whole staging laparoscopically (106,292).

Whether or not laparoscopy compromises outcome in patients managed laparoscopically for a pelvic mass compared with patients managed by laparotomy is not clear (293). Unfortunately, there are no prospective, randomized trials with a large number of patients and long-term follow-up to answer this very important question. There are several uncertainties that are still not well answered with regard to the safety and efficacy of minimally invasive surgery in early-stage ovarian cancer (294). Until such solid data are available, oncologists should remain very cautious with regard to the use of laparoscopy in the management of suspicious complex adnexal masses and early-stage ovarian cancer. Caution should be used when counseling such patients. First and foremost, minimal access surgery should not compromise outcome, particularly for patients with early-stage disease who have an excellent prognosis.

There are a few concerning reports of trocar-site recurrences following laparoscopic surgery. For instance, an isolated abdominal wall metastasis has been reported in a woman operated on for early-stage ovarian cancer 10 years earlier (295). Port-site metastasis at the trocar site of a previous endocholecystectomy performed 7 months prior to abdominal surgery for advanced ovarian cancer has also been reported; the metastasis appeared after completion of platinum-based chemotherapy (296). These two reports suggest that cancer cells can probably be trapped at the level of trocar sites and remain dormant for several years. Trocar-site metastasis may also be only the tip of the iceberg. Indeed, CT scan may show more extensive spread either within the abdominal wall tracking or associated with intra-abdominal carcinomatosis (297). Huang et al. also recently reported that port-site metastasis that appears during chemotherapy or after adequate chemotherapy is associated with a very poor prognosis (298). Trocar-site metastasis associated with laparoscopic surgery is a very serious condition and all efforts should be made to reduce its occurrence.

Despite the above, the risk of malignancy in patients operated on for presumed benign pelvic masses is relatively low (Table 13.1) (39,94–109) but will always be present despite adequate and thorough preoperative evaluation. The majority of women will benefit from the minimally invasive laparoscopic approach, which is clearly associated with lower morbidity and cost. In the event of a malignancy discovered at the time of surgery, clear mechanisms have to be in place to minimize the risk of tumor dissemination, particularly at the level of trocar sites: appropriate surgical technique to prevent tumor spillage (avoid cyst puncture or morcellation, use of endobag, proper closure of trocar sites, etc.), conversion to immediate laparotomy if satisfactory surgery cannot be adequately completed laparoscopically, and rapid referral to proper centers to either complete surgery or for adjuvant chemotherapy. Proper teaching following strict oncologic and surgical principles is thus essential to promote safe laparoscopic surgery (299). If strict guidelines are followed, in the end, women will benefit from the minimally invasive laparoscopic surgery for the management of benign masses, and outcome should not be jeopardized for those found to have a malignancy discovered inadvertently.

Hand-Assisted Laparoscopy

Hand-assisted laparoscopy (HAL) has been introduced as an adjunct to conventional laparoscopic surgery to facilitate the surgery and reduce the rate of conversion to laparotomy. It is used more frequently by GI and genitourinary (GU) surgeons, and procedures such as splenectomy, pancreatectomy, hepatectomy, nephrectomy, prostatectomy, and colectomy have been successfully performed by HAL. The HAL approach implies a 6 to 8 cm skin incision in order to place the gel port through which the surgeon's hand and the laparoscopic instruments can be introduced while maintaining the pneumoperitoneum. HAL confers several advantages over laparoscopy alone: return of tactile sensation, improved spatial relationships, rapid exploration of the abdomen, palpation of intra-abdominal organs and masses, retraction and reflection of tissue planes, atraumatic blunt dissection, rapid control of bleeding, and lysing of dense adhesions. Even though a longer incision has to be made, HAL appears to maintain all the benefits of conventional laparoscopic surgery, i.e., less postoperative ileus and pain, less blood loss, and shorter hospital stay. In addition, HAL frequently reduces the operating time and shortens the learning curve.

HAL seems underused in gynecologic oncology surgery, and only a few groups have reported their experience so far. Spannuth et al. recently reported their experience with the management of 29 patients with a pelvic mass by HAL versus 41 managed by conventional laparotomy. The two groups were comparable in terms of age, body mass index (BMI), and size of the mass, and they found that HAL was associated with statistically lower blood loss, shorter hospital stay, and fewer postoperative complications (300). Krivak et al. approached 25 patients with ovarian cancer by HAL. Of the 19 with apparent early-stage disease, 10 (53%) were up-staged as a result of the full staging procedure done by HAL, and 88% of the cases were successfully completed by HAL (301). HAL has also recently been used to manage recurrent disease. The ideal situation is one where the recurrence appears to be an isolated mass. Chi et al. recently described the technique for HAL splenectomy in five patients with an isolated recurrence in the spleen. The procedure was safely performed without complications (302).

VIDEOENDOSCOPIC SURGERY AND CANCER OF THE VULVA AND VAGINA

Surgery for the management of cancers of the vagina and/or vulva includes lymph node dissection. For cancers of the upper half of the vagina, the management is similar to that of patients with cervical cancers. Open surgery is the standard, but laparoscopically assisted vaginal radical surgery can be used as well (303). The best indication for laparoscopy may be for the reoperation of patients with incidental cervical cancer discovered at simple hysterectomy. This "Schauta *sine utero*" (304) seems to be safer than the classic open restaging. In a series of 17 patients managed between 1987 and 2003, no recurrence was observed among the 4 patients considered as being free of disease after laparoscopic vaginal restaging versus 1 of 4 patients who underwent only laparoscopic restaging and 1 of 3 patients who underwent abdominal restaging and were considered to be disease-free (DFD, unpublished data).

CONCLUSIONS

The most difficult question to answer is the actual benefit both the patient and the surgeon garner from the use of laparoscopic surgery rather than classic open surgery. For extirpative surgery, this benefit remains purely hypothetical as there is a paucity of level one evidence on this subject. The GOG has launched a trial to assess the advantages of laparoscopic surgery in the management of endometrial cancer. A French group has done the same for the management of early cervical cancer. Both organizations have met similar difficulties in enrolling patients owing to the public awareness that laparoscopic surgery is more patient friendly. This concept may deter patients from participating in randomized trials that could result in patients foregoing laparoscopy for laparotomy. However, without such randomized trials, the questions surrounding the laparoscopic approach, which include quality of life, will never be answered. The only truly recognized improvement is radical trachelectomy. Although no births were reported after the initial attempts of the pioneers using an abdominal approach, one birth was reported by the new supporters of the older method (305). This one success is in contrast to the numerous births reported after the laparoscopic vaginal operation. In regard to staging surgery, laparoscopically assisted staging surgery greatly reduces morbidity without sacrificing accurate assessment of disease spread. A brief operative procedure and hospitalization can now provide definitive information upon which appropriate treatment can be prescribed. Here may be the future of laparoscopic oncosurgery. However, even with this indication where the superiority to open surgery looks clear, we still require prospective evidence upon which it can be justified.

References

1. De Brux JA, Dupre-Froment J, Mintz M. Cytology of the peritoneal fluids sampled by coelioscopy or by cul de sac puncture, its value in gynecology. *Acta Cytol* 1968;12:395–405.
2. Hald T, Rasmussen F. Extraperitoneal pelvioscopy: a new aid in staging of lower urinary tract tumors. A preliminary report. *J Urol* 1980;124: 245–248.

3. Dargent D. A new future for Schauta's operation through pre-surgical retroperitoneal pelviscopy. *Eur J Gynecol Oncol* 1987;8:292–296.
4. Dargent D, Salvat J. Envahissement ganglionnaire pelvien: place de la pelviscopie rétropéritonéale. In: Dargent D, Salvat J, eds. *L'Envahissement Ganglionnaire Pelvien.* Paris: Medsi McGraw-Hill; 1989.
5. Dargent D, Arnould P. Percutaneous pelvic lymphadenectomy under laparoscopic guidance. In: Nichols D, ed. *Gynecologic and Obstetrics Surgery.* St. Louis: Mosby; 1993:583.
6. Querleu D. Laparoscopic lymphadenectomy. Presented at the Second World Congress of Gynecologic Endoscopy, Clermont-Ferrand, France, June 5–8, 1989.
7. Querleu D, Leblanc E, Castelain B. Laparoscopic pelvic lymphadenectomy in the staging of early carcinoma of the cervix. *Am J Obstet Gynecol* 1991;164:579–583.
8. Childers JM, Surwit EA. Combined laparoscopic and vaginal surgery for the management of two cases of stage I endometrial cancer. *Gynecol Oncol* 1992;45:46–48.
9. Childers JM, Hatch K, et al. The role of laparoscopic lymphadenectomy in the management of cervical carcinoma. *Gynecol Oncol* 1992;47:38–41.
10. Nezhat CR, Burrell MO, Nezhat FR, et al. Laparoscopic radical hysterectomy with paraaortic and pelvic node dissection. *Am J Obstet Gynecol* 1992;166:864–866.
11. Chu KK, Chang SD, Chen FP, et al. Laparoscopic surgical staging in cervical cancer—preliminary experience among Chinese. *Gynecol Oncol* 1997;64:49–53.
12. Hatch KD, Hallum AV III, Nour M. New surgical approaches to treatment of cervical cancer. *J Natl Cancer Inst Monogr* 1996;21:71–75.
13. Bagley CM Jr, Young RC, Schein PS, et al. Ovarian carcinoma metastatic to the diaphragm—frequently undiagnosed at laparotomy. A preliminary report. *Am J Obstet Gynecol* 1973;116:397–400.
14. Reich H, McGlynn F, Wilkie W. Laparoscopic management of stage I ovarian cancer. *J Reprod Med* 1990;35:601–604.
15. Querleu D, Leblanc E. Laparoscopic infrarenal paraaortic lymph node dissection for restaging of carcinoma of the ovary or fallopian tube. *Cancer* 1994;73:1467–1471.
16. Mathevet P. Laparoscopic surgery in the management of gynecologic cancer: vulvar and vaginal cancers. In: Querleu D, Childers J, Dargent D, eds. *Laparoscopic Surgery in Gynecologic Oncology.* Oxford, UK: Blackwell Science; 1999:170–175.
17. Childers JM, Hatch KD, Tran AN, et al. Laparoscopic para-aortic lymphadenectomy in gynecologic malignancies. *Obstet Gynecol* 1993;82: 741–747.
18. Querleu D. Laparoscopic paraaortic node sampling in gynecologic oncology: a preliminary experience. *Gynecol Oncol* 1993;49:24–29.
19. Possover M, Krause N, Drahonovsky J, et al. Left-sided suprarenal retrocrural para-aortic lymphadenectomy in advanced cervical cancer by laparoscopy. *Gynecol Oncol* 1998;71:219–222.
20. Dargent D, Martin X, Mathevet P. Laparoscopic assessment of the sentinel lymph node in early stage cervical cancer. *Gynecol Oncol* 2000;79:411–415.
21. Semm K. *Operationslehre für Endoskopische Abdominal Chirurgie—Operativ Pelviscopie.* Stuttgart: Schattauerpub; 1984.
22. Querleu D. Radical hysterectomies by the Schauta-Amreich and Schauta-Stoeckel techniques assisted by coelioscopy. *J Gynecol Obstet Biol Reprod (Paris)* 1991;20:747–748.
23. Dargent D, Mathevet P. Radical laparoscopic vaginal hysterectomy. *J Gynecol Obstet Biol Reprod (Paris)* 1992;21:709–710.
24. Querleu D. Laparoscopically assisted radical vaginal hysterectomy. *Gynecol Oncol* 1993;51:248–254.
25. Roy M, Plante M, Renaud MC, et al. Vaginal radical hysterectomy versus abdominal radical hysterectomy in the treatment of early-stage cervical cancer. *Gynecol Oncol* 1996;62:336–339.
26. Schneider A, Possover M, Kamprath S, et al. Laparoscopy-assisted radical vaginal hysterectomy modified according to Schauta-Stoeckel. *Obstet Gynecol* 1996;88:1057–1060.
27. Canis M, Mage G, Wattiez A, et al. Does endoscopic surgery have a role in radical surgery of cancer of the cervix uteri? *J Gynecol Obstet Biol Reprod (Paris)* 1990;19:921.
28. Spirtos NM, Eisenkop SM, Schlaerth JB, et al. Laparoscopic radical hysterectomy (type III) with aortic and pelvic lymphadenectomy in patients with stage I cervical cancer: surgical morbidity and intermediate follow-up. *Am J Obstet Gynecol* 2002;187:340–348.
29. Abu-Rustum NR, Gemignani ML, Moore K, et al. Total laparoscopic radical hysterectomy with pelvic lymphadenectomy using the argon-beam coagulator: pilot data and comparison to laparotomy. *Gynecol Oncol* 2003;91:402–409.
30. Pomel C, Atallah D, Le Bouedec G, et al. Laparoscopic radical hysterectomy for invasive cervical cancer: 8-year experience of a pilot study. *Gynecol Oncol* 2003;91:534–539.
31. Pomel C, Rouzier R, Pocard M, et al. Laparoscopic total pelvic exenteration for cervical cancer relapse. *Gynecol Oncol* 2003;91:616–618.
32. Lai CH, Huang KG, Hong JH, et al. Randomized trial of surgical staging (extraperitoneal or laparoscopic) versus clinical staging in locally advanced cervical cancer. *Gynecol Oncol* 2003;89:160–167.
33. Bateman BG, Kolp LA, Hoeger K. Complications of laparoscopy—operative and diagnostic. *Fertil Steril* 1996;66:30–35.
34. Bonjer HJ, Hazebroek EJ, Kazemier G, et al. Open versus closed establishment of pneumoperitoneum in laparoscopic surgery. *Br J Surg* 1997;84:599–602.
35. Cogliandolo A, Manganaro T, Saitta FP, et al. Blind versus open approach to laparoscopic cholecystectomy: a randomized study. *Surg Laparosc Endosc* 1998;8:353–355.
36. Rice JG, McCall JG, Wattchow DA. Improving the ease and safety of laparoscopy: a technique for open insertion of the umbilical trocar. *Aust N Z J Surg* 1998;68:664–665.
37. Perone N. Laparoscopy using a simplified open technique. A review of 585 cases. *J Reprod Med* 1992;37:921–924.
38. Decloedt J, Berteloot P, Vergote I. The feasibility of open laparoscopy in gynecologic-oncologic patients. *Gynecol Oncol* 1997;66:138–140.
39. Dottino PR, Levine DA, Ripley DL, et al. Laparoscopic management of adnexal masses in premenopausal and postmenopausal women. *Obstet Gynecol* 1999;93:223–228.
40. Chapron C, Cravello L, Chopin N, et al. Complications during set-up procedures for laparoscopy in gynecology: open laparoscopy does not reduce the risk of major complications. *Acta Obstet Gynecol Scand* 2003;82: 1125–1129.
41. Vilos GA, Ternamian A, Dempster J, et al. Laparoscopic entry: a review of techniques, technologies, and complications. *J Obstet Gynaecol Can* 2007;9(5):433–465.
42. Childers JM, Brzechffa PR, Surwit EA, et al. Laparoscopy using the left upper quadrant as the primary trocar site. *Gynecol Oncol* 1992;50:221–225.
43. Sjovall K, Nilsson B, Einhorn N. Different types of rupture of the tumor capsule and the impact on survival in early ovarian carcinoma. *Int J Gynecol Cancer* 1994;4:333–336.
44. Bojahr B, Lober R, Straube W, et al. Gasless laparoscopic-assisted radical vaginal hysterectomy with lymphadenectomy for cervical carcinoma. *J Am Assoc Gynecol Laparosc* 1996;3:S4.
45. Galen DI, Jacobson A, Weckstein LN, et al. Gasless laparoscopy for gynecology. *J Am Assoc Gynecol Laparosc* 1995;2:S68.
46. Hill DJ, Maher PJ, Wood EC. Gasless laparoscopy—useless or useful? *J Am Assoc Gynecol Laparosc* 1994;1:265–268.
47. Chang FH, Soon YK, Lee CL, et al. Laparoscopic removal of a large leiomyoma using airlift gasless laparoscopy. *J Am Assoc Gynecol Laparosc* 1996;3:S7.
48. Akira S, Yamanaka A, Ishihara T, et al. Gasless laparoscopic ovarian cystectomy during pregnancy: comparison with laparotomy. *Am J Obstet Gynecol* 1999;180:554–557.
49. Pelosi MA. Gasless laparoscopy under epidural anesthesia during pregnancy. *J Am Assoc Gynecol Laparosc* 1995;2:S75.
50. Tanaka H, Futamura N, Takubo S, et al. Gasless laparoscopy under epidural anesthesia for adnexal cysts during pregnancy. *J Reprod Med* 1999;44:929–932.
51. Schmidt T, Nawroth F, Foth D, et al. Gasless laparoscopy as an option for conservative therapy of adnexal pedical torsion with twin pregnancy. *J Am Assoc Gynecol Laparosc* 2001;8:621–622.
52. Romer T, Bojahr B, Schwesinger G. Treatment of a torqued hematosalpinx in the thirteenth week of pregnancy using gasless laparoscopy. *J Am Assoc Gynecol Laparosc* 2002;9:89–92.
53. Stepp KJ, Tulikangas PK, Goldberg JM, et al. Laparoscopy for adnexal masses in the second trimester of pregnancy. *J Am Assoc Gynecol Laparosc* 2003;10:55–59.
54. D'Ercole C, Cravello L, Guyon F, et al. Gasless laparoscopic gynecologic surgery. *Eur J Obstet Gynecol Reprod Biol* 1996;66:137–139.
55. Tintara H, Leetanaporn R, Getpook C, et al. Simplified abdominal wall-lifting device for gasless laparoscopy. *Int J Gynaecol Obstet* 1998;61: 165–170.
56. Tintara H, Choobun T, Geater A. Gasless laparoscopic hysterectomy: a comparative study with total abdominal hysterectomy. *J Obstet Gynaecol Res* 2003;29:38–44.
57. Li B, Hao J, Gao X, et al. Gynecologic procedures under gasless laparoscopy. *Chin Med J* 2001;114:514–516.
58. Lukban JC, Jaeger J, Hammond KC, et al. Gasless versus conventional laparoscopy. *N J Med* 2000;97:29–34.
59. Johnson PL, Sibert KS. Laparoscopy. Gasless vs. CO_2 pneumoperitoneum. *J Reprod Med* 1997;42:255–259.
60. Goldberg JM, Maurer WG. A randomized comparison of gasless laparoscopy and CO_2 pneumoperitoneum. *Obstet Gynecol* 1997;90:416–420.
61. Guido RS, Brooks K, McKenzie R, et al. A randomized, prospective comparison of pain after gasless laparoscopy and traditional laparoscopy. *J Am Assoc Gynecol Laparosc* 1998;5:149–153.
62. Hughes ES, McDermott FT, Polglase AL, et al. Tumor recurrence in the abdominal wall scar tissue after large-bowel cancer surgery. *Dis Colon Rectum* 1983;26:571–572.
63. Reilly WT, Nelson H, Schroeder G, et al. Wound recurrence following conventional treatment of colorectal cancer. A rare but perhaps underestimated problem. *Dis Colon Rectum* 1996;39:200–207.
64. Schaeff B, Paolucci V, Thomopoulos J. Port site recurrences after laparoscopic surgery. A review. *Dig Surg* 1998;15:124–134.
65. Wang PH, Yuan CC, Lin G, et al. Risk factors contributing to early occurrence of port site metastases of laparoscopic surgery for malignancy. *Gynecol Oncol* 1999;72:38–44.
66. Nagarsheth NP, Rahaman J, Cohen CJ, et al. The incidence of port-site metastases in gynecologic cancers. *JSLS* 2004;8(2):133–139.

67. Vergote I, Marquette S, Amant F, et al. Port-site metastases after open laparoscopy: a study in 173 patients with advanced ovarian carcinoma. *Int J Gynecol Cancer* 2005;15(5):776–779.
68. Pastner B, Damien M. Umbilical metastasis from a stage IB cervical cancer after laparoscopy: a case report. *Fertil Steril* 1992;58:1248–1249.
69. Ramirez PT, Frumovitz M, Wolf JK, et al. Laparoscopic port-site metastases in patients with gynecologic malignancies. *Int J Gynecol Cancer* 2004;14(6): 1070–1077.
70. Wang PH, Yuan CC, Chao KC, et al. Squamous cell carcinoma of the cervix after laparoscopic surgery. A case report. *J Reprod Med* 1997;42:801–804.
71. Wang PH, Yen MS, Yuan CC, et al. Port site metastasis after laparoscopic-assisted vaginal hysterectomy for endometrial cancer: possible mechanisms and prevention. *Gynecol Oncol* 1997;66:151–155.
72. Childers JM, Aqua KA, Surwit EA, et al. Abdominal-wall tumor implantation after laparoscopy for malignant conditions. *Obstet Gynecol* 1994;84: 765–769.
73. Umpleby HC, Fermor B, Symes MO, et al. Viability of exfoliated colorectal carcinoma cells. *Br J Surg* 1984;71:659–663.
74. Jeon HM, Kim JS, Lee CD, et al. Late development of umbilical metastasis after laparoscopic cholecystectomy for a gallbladder carcinoma. *Oncol Rep* 1999;6:283–287.
75. Canis M, Mage G, Botchorishvili R, et al. Laparoscopy and gynecologic cancer: is it still necessary to debate or only convince the incredulous? *Gynecol Obstet Fertil* 2001;29:913–918.
76. Morice P, Viala J, Pautier P, et al. Port-site metastasis after laparoscopic surgery for gynecologic cancer. A report of six cases. *J Reprod Med* 2000;45:837–840.
77. Hopkins MP, von Gruenigen V, Gaich S. Laparoscopic port site implantation with ovarian cancer. *Am J Obstet Gynecol* 2000;182:735–736.
78. van Dam PA, DeCloedt J, Tjalma WA, et al. Trocar implantation metastasis after laparoscopy in patients with advanced ovarian cancer: can the risk be reduced? *Am J Obstet Gynecol* 1999;181:536–541.
79. Canis M, Botchorishvili R, Wattiez A, et al. Cancer and laparoscopy, experimental studies: a review. *Eur J Obstet Gynecol Reprod Biol* 2000;91:1–9.
80. Cavina E, Goletti O, Molea N, et al. Trocar site tumor recurrences. May pneumoperitoneum be responsible? *Surg Endosc* 1998;12:1294–1296.
81. Bouvy ND, Giuffrida MC, Tseng LN, et al. Effects of carbon dioxide pneumoperitoneum, air pneumoperitoneum, and gasless laparoscopy on body weight and tumor growth. *Arch Surg* 1998;133:652–656.
82. Neuhaus SJ, Texler M, Hewett PJ, et al. Port-site metastases following laparoscopic surgery. *Br J Surg* 1998;85:735–741.
83. Mathew G, Watson DI, Ellis TS, et al. The role of peritoneal immunity and the tumour-bearing state on the development of wound and peritoneal metastases after laparoscopy. *Aust N Z J Surg* 1999;69:14–18.
84. Jacobi CA, Sabat R, Bohm B, et al. Pneumoperitoneum with carbon dioxide stimulates growth of malignant colonic cells. *Surgery* 1997;121:72–78.
85. Mathew G, Watson DI, Ellis T, et al. The effect of laparoscopy on the movement of tumor cells and metastasis to surgical wounds. *Surg Endosc* 1997;11:1163–1166.
86. Watson DI, Mathew G, Ellis T, et al. Gasless laparoscopy may reduce the risk of port site metastasis following laparoscopic tumor surgery. *Arch Chir* 1997;132:166–168.
87. Lecuru F, Agostini A, Camatte S, et al. Impact of pneumoperitoneum on visceral metastasis rate and survival. Results in two ovarian cancer models in rats. *Br J Obstet Gynaecol* 2001;108:733–737.
88. Lecuru F, Agostini A, Camatte S, et al. Impact of pneumoperitoneum on tumor growth. *Surg Endosc* 2002;16:1170–1174.
89. Abu-Rustum NR, Sonoda Y, Chi DS, et al. The effects of CO_2 pneumoperitoneum on the survival of women with persistent metastatic ovarian cancer. *Gynecol Oncol* 2003;90:431–434.
90. Agostini A, Robin F, Aggerbeck M, et al. Influence of peritoneal factors on port-site metastases in a xenograft ovarian cancer model. *Br J Obstet Gynaecol* 2001;108:809–812.
91. Abu-Rustum NR, Rhee EH, Chi DS, et al. Subcutaneous tumor implantation after laparoscopic procedures in women with malignant disease. *Obstet Gynecol* 2004;103:480–487.
92. Bouvy ND, Marquet RL, Jeekel H, et al. Impact of gas(less) laparoscopy and laparotomy on peritoneal tumor growth and abdominal wall metastases. *Ann Surg* 1996;224:694–700.
93. Reymond MA, Schneider C, Kastl S, et al. The pathogenesis of port-site recurrences. *J Gastrointest Surg* 1998;2:406–414.
94. Nezhat F, Nezhat C, Welander CE, et al. Four ovarian cancers diagnosed during laparoscopic management of 1011 women with adnexal masses. *Am J Obstet Gynecol* 1992;167:790–796.
95. Hulka JF, Parker WH, Surrey MW, et al. Management of ovarian masses. AAGL 1990 survey. *J Reprod Med* 1992;37:599–602.
96. Canis M, Mage G, Pouly JL, et al. Laparoscopic diagnosis of adnexal cystic masses: a 12-year experience with long-term follow-up. *Obstet Gynecol* 1994;83:707–712.
97. Blanc B, Boubli L, D'Ercole C, et al. Laparoscopic management of malignant ovarian cysts: a 78 case national survey. Part 1: preoperative and laparoscopic evaluation. *Eur J Obstet Gynecol Reprod Biol* 1994;56:177–180.
98. Marana R, Vittori G, Porpora MG, et al. Laparoscopic treatment of ovarian cysts in women under 40 years of age. *J Am Assoc Gynecol Laparosc* 1995;2:S20.
99. Wenzl R, Lehner R, Husslein P, et al. Laparoscopic surgery in cases of ovarian malignancies: an Austria-wide survey. *Gynecol Oncol* 1996;63:57–61.
100. Yuen PM, Yu KM, Yip SK, et al. A randomized prospective study of laparoscopy and laparotomy in the management of benign ovarian masses. *Am J Obstet Gynecol* 1997;177:109–114.
101. Hidlebaugh DA, Vulgaropulos S, Orr RK. Treating adnexal masses. Operative laparoscopy vs. laparotomy. *J Reprod Med* 1997;42:551–558.
102. Guglielmina JN, Pennehouat G, Deval B, et al. Treatment of ovarian cysts by laparoscopy. *Contracept Fertil Sex* 1997;25:218–229.
103. Malik E, Bohm W, Stoz F, et al. Laparoscopic management of ovarian tumors. *Surg Endosc* 1998;12:1326–1333.
104. Sadik S, Onoglu AS, Gokdeniz R, et al. Laparoscopic management of selected adnexal masses. *J Am Assoc Gynecol Laparosc* 1999;6:313–316.
105. Ulrich U, Paulus W, Schneider A, et al. Laparoscopic surgery for complex ovarian masses. *J Am Assoc Gynecol Laparosc* 2000;7(3):373–380.
106. Serur E, Emeney PL, Byrne DW. Laparoscopic management of adnexal masses. *JSLS* 2001;5:143–151.
107. Mettler L, Jacobs V, Brandenburg K, et al. Laparoscopic management of 641 adnexal tumors in Kiel, Germany. *J Am Assoc Gynecol Laparosc* 2001;8:74–82.
108. Mendilcioglu I, Zorlu CG, Trak B, et al. Laparoscopic management of adnexal masses. Safety and effectiveness. *J Reprod Med.* 2002;47:36–40.
109. Havrilesky LJ, Peterson BL, Dryden DK, et al. Predictors of clinical outcomes in the laparoscopic management of adnexal masses. *Obstet Gynecol* 2003;102:243–251.
110. Leng JH, Lang JH, Zhang JJ, et al. Role of laparoscopy in the diagnosis and treatment of adnexal masses. *Chin Med J (Engl)* 2006;119(3):202–206.
111. Benacerraf BR, Finkler NJ, Wojciechowski C, et al. Sonographic accuracy in the diagnosis of ovarian masses. *J Reprod Med* 1990;35:491–495.
112. Maiman M, Seltzer V, Boyce J. Laparoscopic excision of ovarian neoplasms subsequently found to be malignant. *Obstet Gynecol* 1991;77:563–565.
113. Hidlebaugh DA, Vulgaropulos S, Orr R. Trends in oophorectomy by laparoscopic versus open techniques. *J Am Assoc Gynecol Laparosc* 1996;3:S17–S18.
114. Parker WH, Levine RL, Howard FM, et al. A multicenter study of laparoscopic management of selected cystic adnexal masses in postmenopausal women. *J Am Coll Surg* 1994;179:733–737.
115. Quinlan DJ, Townsend DE, Johnson GH. Laparoscopic removal of adnexal masses. *Mt Sinai J Med* 1999;66:31.
116. Jennings TS, Dottino P, Rahaman J, et al. Results of selective use of operative laparoscopy in gynecologic oncology. *Gynecol Oncol* 1998;70:323–328.
117. Lehner R, Wenzl R, Heinzl H, et al. Influence of delayed staging laparotomy after laparoscopic removal of ovarian masses later found malignant. *Obstet Gynecol* 1998;92:967–971.
118. Rose PG, Rubin RB, Nelson BE, et al. Accuracy of frozen-section (intraoperative consultation) diagnosis of ovarian tumors. *Am J Obstet Gynecol* 1994;171:823–826.
119. Canis M, Mashiach R, Wattiez A, et al. Frozen section in laparoscopic management of macroscopically suspicious ovarian masses. *J Am Assoc Gynecol Laparosc* 2004;11(3):365–369.
120. Geomini PM, Zuurendonk LD, Bremer GL, et al. The impact of size of the adnexal mass on the accuracy of frozen section diagnosis. *Gynecol Oncol* 2005;99(2):362–366.
121. Canis M, Botchorishvili R, Kouyate S, et al. Surgical management of adnexal tumors. *Ann Chir* 1998;52:234–248.
122. Kindermann G, Maassen V, Kuhn W. Laparoscopic preliminary surgery of ovarian malignancies. Experiences from 127 German gynecologic clinics. *Geburtshilfe Frauenheilk* 1995;55:687–694.
123. Mettler L, Semm K, Shive K. Endoscopic management of adnexal masses. *J Soc Laparoendosc Surg* 1997;1:103–112.
124. Dembo AJ, Davy M, Stenwig AE, et al. Prognostic factors in patients with stage I epithelial ovarian cancer. *Obstet Gynecol* 1990;75:263–273.
125. Sevelda P, Dittrich C, Salzer H. Prognostic value of the rupture of the capsule in stage I epithelial ovarian carcinoma. *Gynecol Oncol* 1989;35:321–322.
126. Blanc B, D'Ercole C, Nicoloso E, et al. Laparoscopic management of malignant ovarian cysts: a 78 case national survey. Part 2: follow-up and final treatment. *Eur J Obstet Gynecol Reprod Biol* 1995;61:147–150.
127. Leminen A, Lehtovirta P. Spread of ovarian cancer after laparoscopic surgery: report of eight cases. *Gynecol Oncol* 1999;75:387–390.
128. Ripley D, Golden A, Fahs MC, et al. The impact of laparoscopic surgery in the management of adnexal masses. *Mt Sinai J Med* 1999;66:31–34.
129. Bensaid C, Le Frere Belda MA, Metzger U, et al. Performance of laparoscopy in identifying malignant ovarian cysts. *Surg Endosc* 2006;20(9): 1410–1414.
130. Alvarez RD, Kilgore LC, Partridge EE, et al. Staging ovarian cancer diagnosed during laparoscopy: accuracy rather than immediacy. *South Med J* 1993;86:1256–1258.
131. Darai E, Teboul J, Walker-Combrouze F, et al. Borderline ovarian tumors: a series of 43 patients. *Contracept Fertil Sex* 1997;25:933–938.
132. Fauvet R, Boccara J, Dufournet C, et al. Laparoscopic management of borderline ovarian tumors: results of a French multicenter study. *Ann Oncol* 2005;16(3):403–410.
133. Desfeux P, Chatellier G, Bats AS, et al. Impact of surgical access on staging of early borderline and invasive tumors of the ovary. *Bull Cancer* 2006; 93(7):723–730.

134. Desfeux P, Bats AS, Bensaid C, et al. Impact of the surgical route on staging and outcome of early borderline ovarian tumors. *Gynecol Obstet Fertil* 2007;35(3):193–198.
135. Odegaard E, Staff AC, Langebrekke A, et al. Surgery of borderline tumors of the ovary: retrospective comparison of short-term outcome after laparoscopy or laparotomy. *Acta Obstet Gynecol Scand* 2007;86(5):620–626.
136. Querleu D, Leblanc E. Laparoscopic modified radical hysterectomy in laparoscopic surgery. In: Querleu D, Childers J, Dargent D, eds. *Laparoscopic Surgery in Gynaecological Oncology*. Oxford, UK: Blackwell Science; 1999:49–52.
137. Childers JM, Brzechffa PR, Hatch KD, et al. Laparoscopically assisted surgical staging (LASS) of endometrial cancer. *Gynecol Oncol* 1993;51:33–38.
138. Melendez TD, Childers JM, Nour M, et al. Laparoscopic staging of endometrial cancer: the learning experience. *J Soc Laparoendosc Surg* 1997;1:45–49.
139. Possover M, Krause N, Plaul K, et al. Laparoscopic para-aortic and pelvic lymphadenectomy: experience with 150 patients and review of the literature. *Gynecol Oncol* 1998;71:19–28.
140. Spirtos NM, Schlaerth JB, Spirtos TW, et al. Laparoscopic bilateral pelvic and paraaortic lymph node sampling: an evolving technique. *Am J Obstet Gynecol* 1995;173:105–111.
141. Dottino PR, Tobias DH, Beddoe A, et al. Laparoscopic lymphadenectomy for gynecologic malignancies. *Gynecol Oncol* 1999;73:383–388.
142. Scribner DR Jr, Walker JL, Johnson GA, et al. Laparoscopic pelvic and paraaortic lymph node dissection: analysis of the first 100 cases. *Gynecol Oncol* 2001;82:498–503.
143. Su TH, Wang KG, Yang YC, et al. Laparoscopic para-aortic lymph node sampling in the staging of invasive cervical carcinoma: including a comparative study of 21 laparotomy cases. *Int J Gynaecol Obstet* 1995;49:311–318.
144. Vidaurreta J, Bermudez A, di Paola G, et al. Laparoscopic staging in locally advanced cervical carcinoma: a new possible philosophy? *Gynecol Oncol* 1999;75:366–371.
145. Renaud MC, Plante M, Roy M. Combined laparoscopic and vaginal radical surgery in cervical cancer. *Gynecol Oncol* 2000;79:59–63.
146. Altgassen C, Possover M, Krause N, et al. Establishing a new technique of laparoscopic pelvic and para-aortic lymphadenectomy. *Obstet Gynecol* 2000;95:348–352.
147. Vergote I, Amant F, Berteloot P, et al. Laparoscopic lower para-aortic staging lymphadenectomy in stage IB2, II, and III cervical cancer. *Int J Gynecol Cancer* 2002;12:22–26.
148. Schlaerth JB, Spirtos NM, Carson LF, et al. Laparoscopic retroperitoneal lymphadenectomy followed by immediate laparotomy in women with cervical cancer: a Gynecologic Oncology Group study. *Gynecol Oncol* 2002;85: 81–88.
149. Abu-Rustum NR, Chi DS, Sonoda Y, et al. Transperitoneal laparoscopic pelvic and para-aortic lymph node dissection using the argon-beam coagulator and monopolar instruments: an 8-year study and description of technique. *Gynecol Oncol* 2003;89:504–513.
150. Gallup DG, King LA, Messing MJ, et al. Paraaortic lymph node sampling by means of an extraperitoneal approach with a supraumbilical transverse "sunrise" incision. *Am J Obstet Gynecol* 1993;169:307–311.
151. Spirtos NM, Schlaerth JB, Gross GM, et al. Cost and quality-of-life analyses of surgery for early endometrial cancer: laparotomy versus laparoscopy. *Am J Obstet Gynecol* 1996;174:1795–1799.
152. Fowler JM, Carter JR, Carlson JW, et al. Lymph node yield from laparoscopic lymphadenectomy in cervical cancer: a comparative study. *Gynecol Oncol* 1993;51:187–192.
153. Benedetti-Panici P, Maneschi F, Scambia G, et al. Lymphatic spread of cervical cancer: an anatomical and pathological study based on 225 radical hysterectomies with systematic pelvic and aortic lymphadenectomy. *Gynecol Oncol* 1996;62:19–24.
154. Michel G, Morice P, Castaigne D, et al. Lymphatic spread in stage Ib and II cervical carcinoma: anatomy and surgical implications. *Obstet Gynecol* 1998;91:360–363.
155. Querleu D, Leblanc E, Cartron G, et al. Audit of preoperative and early complications of laparoscopic lymph node dissection in 1000 gynecologic cancer patients. *Amer J Obstet Gynecol* 2006;195:1287–1292.
156. Kohler C, Tozzi R, Klemm P, et al. Laparoscopic paraaortic left-sided transperitoneal infrarenal lymphadenectomy in patients with gynecologic malignancies: technique and results. *Gynecol Oncol* 2003;91:139–148.
157. Possover M, Plaul K, Krause N, et al. Left-sided laparoscopic para-aortic lymphadenectomy: anatomy of the ventral tributaries of the infrarenal vena cava. *Am J Obstet Gynecol* 1998;179:1295–1297.
158. Cabanas RM. An approach for the treatment of penile carcinoma. *Cancer* 1977;39:456–466.
159. Levenback C, Burke TW, Gershenson DM, et al. Intraoperative lymphatic mapping for vulvar cancer. *Obstet Gynecol* 1994;84:163–167.
160. Echt ML, Finan MA, Hoffman MS, et al. Detection of sentinel lymph nodes with lymphazurin in cervical, uterine, and vulvar malignancies. *South Med J* 1999;92:204–208.
161. Medl M, Peters-Engl C, Schutz P, et al. First report of lymphatic mapping with isosulfan blue dye and sentinel node biopsy in cervical cancer. *Anticancer Res* 2000;20:1133–1134.
162. O'Boyle JD, Coleman RL, Bernstein SG, et al. Intraoperative lymphatic mapping in cervix cancer patients undergoing radical hysterectomy: a pilot study. *Gynecol Oncol* 2000;79:238–243.
163. Kamprath S, Possover M, Schneider A. Laparoscopic sentinel lymph node detection in patients with cervical cancer. *Am J Obstet Gynecol* 2000;182: 1648.
164. Verheijen RH, Pijpers R, van Diest PJ, et al. Sentinel node detection in cervical cancer. *Obstet Gynecol* 2000;96:135–138.
165. Lambaudie E, Collinet P, Narducci F, et al. Laparoscopic identification of sentinel lymph nodes in early stage cervical cancer: prospective study using a combination of patent blue dye injection and technetium radiocolloid injection. *Gynecol Oncol* 2003;89:84–87.
166. Barranger E, Grahek D, Cortez A, et al. Laparoscopic sentinel lymph node procedure using a combination of patent blue and radioisotope in women with cervical carcinoma. *Cancer* 2003;97:3003–3009.
167. Rhim CC, Park JS, Bae SN, et al. Sentinel node biopsy as an indicator for pelvic nodes dissection in early stage cervical cancer. *J Korean Med Sci* 2002;17:507–511.
168. Malur S, Krause N, Kohler C, et al. Sentinel lymph node detection in patients with cervical cancer. *Gynecol Oncol* 2001;80:254–257.
169. Buist MR, Pijpers RJ, van Lingen A, et al. Laparoscopic detection of sentinel lymph nodes followed by lymph node dissection in patients with early stage cervical cancer. *Gynecol Oncol* 2003;90:290–296.
170. Lantzsch T, Wolters M, Grimm J, et al. Sentinel node procedure in Ib cervical cancer: a preliminary series. *Br J Cancer* 2001;85:791–794.
171. Plante M, Renaud MC, Tetu B, et al. Laparoscopic sentinel node mapping in early-stage cervical cancer. *Gynecol Oncol* 2003;91:494–503.
172. van Dam PA, Hauspy J, Vanderheyden T, et al. Intraoperative sentinel node identification with technetium-99m–labeled nanocolloid in patients with cancer of the uterine cervix: a feasibility study. *Int J Gynecol Cancer* 2003;13:182–186.
173. Dargent D, Enria R. Laparoscopic assessment of the sentinel lymph nodes in early cervical cancer. Technique—preliminary results and future developments. *Crit Rev Oncol Hematol* 2003;48:305–310.
174. Gargiulo T, Giusti M, Bottero A, et al. Sentinel lymph node (SLN) laparoscopic assessment early stage in endometrial cancer. *Minerva Ginecol* 2003;55:259–262.
175. Burke TW, Levenback C, Tornos C, et al. Intraabdominal lymphatic mapping to direct selective pelvic and paraaortic lymphadenectomy in women with high-risk endometrial cancer: results of a pilot study. *Gynecol Oncol* 1996;62:169–173.
176. Levenback C. Lymphatic mapping and sentinel node identification in patients with cervix cancer undergoing radical hysterectomy and pelvic lymphadenectomy. *J Clin Oncol* 2002;20:688–893.
177. Dargent D, Marchiole P, Buenerd A, et al. Is the absence of metastases, including micrometastases, in the sentinel nodes predictive of the absence of metastases in the other regional nodes in early stage cervical cancer patients? Society of Gynecologic Oncologists, San Diego, February 7–11, 2004. Abstract #58.
178. van de Lande J, Torrenga B, Raijmakers PG, et al. Sentinel lymph node detection in early stage uterine cervix carcinoma: a systematic review. *Gynecol Oncol* 2007;106(3):604–613.
179. Marchiole P, Buenerd A, Scoazec JY, et al. Sentinel lymph node biopsy is not accurate in predicting lymph node status for patients with cervical carcinoma. *Cancer* 2004;100:2154–2159.
180. Holub Z, Jabor A, Kliment L. Comparison of two procedures for sentinel lymph node detection in patients with endometrial cancer: a pilot study. *Eur J Gynaecol Oncol* 2002;23:53–57.
181. Pelosi E, Arena V, Baudino B, et al. Pre-operative lymphatic mapping and intra-operative sentinel lymph node detection in early stage endometrial cancer. *Nucl Med Commun* 2003;24:971–975.
182. Dargent D, Ansquer Y, Mathevet P. Technical development and results of left extraperitoneal laparoscopic paraaortic lymphadenectomy for cervical cancer. *Gynecol Oncol* 2000;77:87–92.
183. Vasilev SA, McGonigle KF. Extraperitoneal laparoscopic para-aortic lymph node dissection. *Gynecol Oncol* 1996;61:315–320.
184. Querleu D, Dargent D, Ansquer Y, et al. Extraperitoneal endosurgical aortic and common iliac dissection in the staging of bulky or advanced cervical carcinomas. *Cancer* 2000;88:883–891.
185. Sonoda Y, Leblanc E, Querleu D, et al. Prospective evaluation of surgical staging of advanced cervical cancer via a laparoscopic extraperitoneal approach. *Gynecol Oncol* 2003;91:326–331.
186. Occelli B, Narducci F, Lanvin D, et al. *De novo* adhesions with extraperitoneal endosurgical para-aortic lymphadenectomy versus transperitoneal laparoscopic para-aortic lymphadenectomy: a randomized experimental study. *Am J Obstet Gynecol* 2000;183:529–533.
187. Leblanc E, Narducci F, Frumovitz M, et al. Therapeutic value of pretherapeutic extraperitoneal laparoscopic staging of locally advanced cervical carcinoma. *Gynecol Oncol* 2007;105:304–311.
188. Donnez J, Nisolle M. *An Atlas of Operative Laparoscopy and Hysteroscopy*. 2nd ed. Boca Raton, FL: CRC Press–Parthenon; 2001.
189. Reich HJ, De Caprio J, McGlynn F. Laparoscopic hysterectomy. *J Gynecol Surg* 1989;5:213.
190. Dargent D, Mathevet P. Radical vaginal hysterectomy in the primary management of invasive cervical cancer. In: Rubin S, Hoskins W, eds. *Cervical Cancer and Preinvasive Neoplasia*. New York: Raven Press; 1996:207.
191. Kadar N, Reich H. Laparoscopically assisted radical Schauta hysterectomy and bilateral laparoscopic pelvic lymphadenectomy for the treatment of bulky stage IB carcinoma of the cervix. *Gynaecol Endosc* 1993;2:135.

192. Martin X. Hysterectomie elargie laparoscopico-vaginale dans le traitement des cancers du col uterin. *These Medecine Lyon* 1997;191.
193. Hockel M, Konerding MA, Heussel CP. Liposuction-assisted nerve-sparing extended radical hysterectomy: oncologic rationale, surgical anatomy, and feasibility study. *Am J Obstet Gynecol* 1998;178:971–976.
194. Sardi J, Vidaurreta J, Bermudez A, et al. Laparoscopically assisted Schauta operation: learning experience at the Gynecologic Oncology Unit, Buenos Aires University Hospital. *Gynecol Oncol* 1999;75:361–365.
195. Querleu D, Narducci F, Poulard V, et al. Modified radical vaginal hysterectomy with or without laparoscopic nerve-sparing dissection: a comparative study. *Gynecol Oncol* 2002;85:154–158.
196. Hertel H, Kohler C, Michels W, et al. Laparoscopic-assisted radical vaginal hysterectomy (LARVH): prospective evaluation of 200 patients with cervical cancer. *Gynecol Oncol* 2003;90:505–511.
197. Possover M, Stober S, Plaul K, et al. Identification and preservation of the motoric innervation of the bladder in radical hysterectomy type III. *Gynecol Oncol* 2000;79:154–157.
198. Possover M. Technical modification of the nerve-sparing laparoscopy-assisted VRH type 3 for better reproducibility of this procedure. *Gynecol Oncol* 2003;90:245–247.
199. Possover M, Krause N, Kuhne-Heid R, et al. Laparoscopic assistance for extended radicality of radical vaginal hysterectomy: description of a technique. *Gynecol Oncol* 1998;70:94–99.
200. Dargent D, Brun JL, Remy I. Pregnancies following radical trachelectomy for invasive cervical cancer. *Gynecol Oncol* 1994;52:105(abst).
201. Schneider A, Krause N, Kuhne-Heid R, et al. Laparoscopic paraaortic and pelvic lymph node excision—initial experiences and development of a technique. *Zentralbl Gynakol* 1996;118:498–504.
202. Shepherd JH, Crawford RA, Oram DH. Radical trachelectomy: a way to preserve fertility in the treatment of early cervical cancer. *Br J Obstet Gynaecol* 1998;105:912–916.
203. Roy M, Plante M. Pregnancies after radical vaginal trachelectomy for early-stage cervical cancer. *Am J Obstet Gynecol* 1998;179:1491–1496.
204. Covens A, Shaw P. Is radical trachelectomy a safe radical hysterectomy for early-stage IB carcinoma of the cervix. *Cancer* 1999;86:2273–2279.
205. Dargent D, Franzosi F, Ansquer Y, et al. Extended trachelectomy relapse: plea for patient involvement in the medical decision. *Bull Cancer* 2002;89: 1027–1030.
206. Shepherd JH, Mould T, Oram DH. Radical trachelectomy in early stage carcinoma of the cervix: outcome as judged by recurrence and fertility rates. *Br J Obstet Gynaecol* 2001;108:882–885.
207. Schlaerth JB, Spirtos NM, Schlaerth AC. Radical trachelectomy and pelvic lymphadenectomy with uterine preservation in the treatment of cervical cancer. *Am J Obstet Gynecol* 2003;188:29–34.
208. Burnett AF, Roman LD, O'Meara AT, et al. Radical vaginal trachelectomy and pelvic lymphadenectomy for preservation of fertility in early cervical carcinoma. *Gynecol Oncol* 2003;88:419–423.
209. Picone O, L'homme C, Tournaire M, et al. Preservation of pregnancy in a patient with a stage IIIB ovarian epithelial carcinoma diagnosed at 22 weeks of gestation and treated with initial chemotherapy. *Gynecol Oncol* 2004;94(2):600–604.
210. Bernardini M, Barrett J, Seaward G, et al. Pregnancy outcomes in patients after radical trachelectomy. *Am J Obstet Gynecol* 2003;189:1378–1382.
211. Saling E. Early total occlusion of os uteri prevents habitual abortion and premature deliveries. *Z Geburtshilfe Perinatol* 1981;185:259–261.
212. Nezhat CR, Nezhat FR, Burrell MO, et al. Laparoscopic radical hysterectomy and laparoscopically assisted vaginal radical hysterectomy with pelvic and paraaortic node dissection. *J Gynecol Surg* 1993;9:105–120.
213. Spirtos NM, Schlaerth JB, Kimball RE, et al. Laparoscopic radical hysterectomy (type III) with aortic and pelvic lymphadenectomy. *Am J Obstet Gynecol* 1996;174:1763–1767.
214. Canis M, Wattiez A, Mage G, et al. Laparoscopic radical hysterectomy for cervical cancer. In: Querleu D, Childers J, Dargent D, eds. *Laparoscopic Surgery in Gynaecological Oncology.* Paris: Blackwell Science;1999: 70–77.
215. Nezhat F, Mahdavi A, Nagarsheth NP. Total laparoscopic radical hysterectomy and pelvic lymphadenectomy using harmonic shears. *J Minim Invasive Gynecol* 2006;13(1):20–25.
216. Ramirez PT, Slomovitz BM, Soliman PT, et al. Total laparoscopic radical hysterectomy and lymphadenectomy: the M. D. Anderson Cancer Center experience. *Gynecol Oncol* 2006;102(2):252–255.
217. Gil-Moreno A, Puig O, Pérez-Benavente MA, et al. Total laparoscopic radical hysterectomy (type II-III) with pelvic lymphadenectomy in early invasive cervical cancer. *J Minim Invasive Gynecol* 2005;12(2):113–120.
218. Xu H, Chen Y, Li Y, et al. Complications of laparoscopic radical hysterectomy and lymphadenectomy for invasive cervical cancer: experience based on 317 procedures. *Surg Endosc* 2007;21(6):960–964.
219. Frumovitz M, Dos Reis R, Sun CC, et al. Comparison of total laparoscopic and abdominal radical hysterectomy for patients with early-stage cervical cancer. *Obstet Gynecol* 2007;110(1):96–102.
220. Zakashansky K, Chuang L, Gretz H, et al. A case-controlled study of total laparoscopic radical hysterectomy with pelvic lymphadenectomy versus radical abdominal hysterectomy in a fellowship training program. *Int J Gynecol Cancer* 2007:17(5):1075–1082.
221. Spirtos NM, Eisenkop SM, Schlaerth JB, et al. Laparoscopic radical hysterectomy (type III) with aortic and pelvic lymphadenectomy in patients with stage I cervical cancer: surgical morbidity and intermediate follow-up. *Am J Obstet Gynecol* 2002;187(2):340–348.
222. Pomel C, Atallah D, Bouedec GL, et al. Laparoscopic radical hysterectomy for invasive cervical cancer: 8-year experience of a pilot study. *Gynecol Oncol* 2003;91:534–539.
223. Li G, Yan X, Shang H, et al. A comparison of laparoscopic radical hysterectomy and pelvic lymphadenectomy and laparotomy in the treatment of Ib-IIa cervical cancer. *Gynecol Oncol* 2007;105(1):176–180.
224. Sert BM, Abeler VM. Robotic-assisted laparoscopic radical hysterectomy (Piver type III) with pelvic node dissection—case report. *Eur J Gynaecol Oncol* 2006;27(5):531–533.
225. Boggess J, Gehrig P, Rutledge T, et al. Robotic type III radical hysterectomy with pelvic lymph-node dissection: description of a novel technique for treating stage IB1 cervical cancer. Annual Meeting of the Society of Gynecologic Oncologists, 2006.
226. Shafer A, Boggess JF, Gehrig P, et al. Type III radical hysterectomy for obese women with cervical carcinoma: robotic versus open. Annual Meeting of the Society of Gynecologic Oncologists, 2007.
227. Plante M, Roy M. Operative laparoscopy prior to a pelvic exenteration in patients with recurrent cervical cancer. *Gynecol Oncol* 1998;69:94–99.
228. Köhler C, Tozzi R, Possover M, et al. Explorative laparoscopy prior to exenterative surgery. *Gynecol Oncol* 2002;86:311–315.
229. Clark VG. A more radical method of performing hysterectomy for cancer of the uterus. *Bull Johns Hopkins Hosp* 1895:120–124.
230. Landoni F, Maneo A, Colombo A, et al. Randomised study of radical surgery versus radiotherapy for stage IB-IIA cervical cancer. *Lancet* 1997;350:535–540.
231. Alvarez RD, Potter ME, Soong SJ, et al. Rationale for using pathologic tumor dimensions and nodal status to subclassify surgically treated stage IB cervical cancer patients. *Gynecol Oncol* 1991;43:108–112.
232. Delgado G, Bundy B, Zaino R, et al. Prospective surgical-pathological study of disease-free interval in patients with stage IB squamous cell carcinoma of the cervix: a Gynecologic Oncology Group study. *Gynecol Oncol* 1990;38:352–357.
233. Fiorica JV, Roberts WS, Greenberg H, et al. Morbidity and survival patterns in patients after radical hysterectomy and postoperative adjuvant pelvic radiotherapy. *Gynecol Oncol* 1990;36:343–347.
234. Soisson AP, Soper JT, Clarke-Pearson DL, et al. Adjuvant radiotherapy following radical hysterectomy for patients with stage IB and IIA cervical cancer. *Gynecol Oncol* 1990;37:390–395.
235. Thomas GM, Dembo AJ. Is there a role for adjuvant pelvic radiotherapy after radical hysterectomy in early stage cervical cancer? *Int J Gynecol Cancer* 1993;3:193.
236. Dargent D, Salvat J. Valeur des méthodes non invasives dans l'appréciation de l'état des ganglions ilio-pelviens et lombo-aorticques. In: Dargent D, Salvat J, eds. *L'Envahissement Ganglionnaire Pelvien.* Paris: Medsi McGraw-Hill; 1989:55.
237. Berman ML, Bergen S, Salazar H. Influence of histological features and treatment on the prognosis of patients with cervical cancer metastatic to pelvic lymph nodes. *Gynecol Oncol* 1990;39:127–131.
238. Hacker NF, Wain GV, Nicklin JL. Resection of bulky positive lymph nodes in patients with cervical carcinoma. *Int J Gynecol Cancer* 1995;5:250–256.
239. Cosin JA, Fowler JM, Chen MD, et al. Pretreatment surgical staging of patients with cervical carcinoma: the case for lymph node debulking. *Cancer* 1998;82:2241–2248.
240. Haie C, Pejovic MH, Gerbaulet A, et al. Is prophylactic para-aortic irradiation worthwhile in the treatment of advanced cervical carcinoma? Results of a controlled clinical trial of the EORTC radiotherapy group. *Radiother Oncol* 1988;11:101–112.
241. Cunningham MJ, Dunton CJ, Corn B, et al. Extended-field radiation therapy in early-stage cervical carcinoma: survival and complications. *Gynecol Oncol* 1991;43:51–54.
242. Weiser EB, Bundy BN, Hoskins WJ, et al. Extraperitoneal versus transperitoneal selective paraaortic lymphadenectomy in the pretreatment surgical staging of advanced cervical carcinoma (a Gynecologic Oncology Group study). *Gynecol Oncol* 1989;33:283–289.
243. Johnson PL, Sibert KS. Laparoscopy. Gasless vs. CO_2 pneumoperitoneum. *J Reprod Med* 1997;42:255–259.
244. Chan JK, Lin YG, Monk BJ, et al. Vaginal hysterectomy as primary treatment of endometrial cancer in medically compromised women. *Obstet Gynecol* 2001;97(5 Pt 1):707–711.
245. Holub Z, Voracek J, Shomani A. A comparison of laparoscopic surgery with open procedure in endometrial cancer. *Eur J Gynaecol Oncol* 1998;19:294.
246. Walker JL. Surgical staging of uterine cancer: Randomized phase III trial of laparoscopy vs laparotomy—A Gynecologic Oncology Group Study (GOG): Preliminary results. Abstract - No. 5010 Annual meeting of the American Society of Clinical Oncology, 2006.
247. Gemignani ML, Curtin JP, Zelmanovich J, et al. Laparoscopic-assisted vaginal hysterectomy for endometrial cancer: clinical outcomes and hospital charges. *Gynecol Oncol* 1999;73(1):5–11.
248. Eltabbakh GH, Shamonki MI, Moody JM, et al. Laparoscopy as the primary modality for the treatment of women with endometrial carcinoma. *Cancer* 2001;91(2):378–387.
249. Zapico A, Fuentes P, Grassa A, et al. Laparoscopic-assisted vaginal hysterectomy versus abdominal hysterectomy in stages I and II endometrial cancer. Operating data, follow up and survival. *Gynecol Oncol* 2005;98(2): 222–227.
250. Zullo F, Palomba S, Russo T, et al. A prospective randomized comparison between laparoscopic and laparotomic approaches in women with early

stage endometrial cancer: a focus on the quality of life. *Am J Obstet Gynecol* 2005;193(4):1344–1352.

251. Kornblith A, Walker J, Huang H, et al. Quality of life (QOL) of patients in a randomized clinical trial of laparoscopy (scope) vs. open laparotomy (open) for the surgical resection and staging of uterine cancer: a Gynecologic Oncology Group (GOG) study. SGO 2006.
252. Malur S, Possover M, Michels W, et al. Laparoscopic-assisted vaginal versus abdominal surgery in patients with endometrial cancer—a prospective randomized trial. *Gynecol Oncol* 2001;80(2):239–244.
253. Tozzi R, Malur S, Koehler C, et al. Laparoscopy versus laparotomy in endometrial cancer: first analysis of survival of a randomized prospective study. *J Minim Invasive Gynecol* 2005;12(2):130–136.
254. Fram KM. Laparoscopically assisted vaginal hysterectomy versus abdominal hysterectomy in stage I endometrial cancer. *Int J Gynecol Cancer* 2002;12(1):57–61.
255. Kalogiannidis I, Lambrechts S, Amant F, et al. Laparoscopy-assisted vaginal hysterectomy compared with abdominal hysterectomy in clinical stage I endometrial cancer: safety, recurrence, and long-term outcome. *Am J Obstet Gynecol* 2007;196(3):248(e1–e8).
256. Scribner DR Jr, Walker JL, Johnson GA, et al. Laparoscopic pelvic and paraaortic lymph node dissection in the obese. *Gynecol Oncol* 2002;84(3): 426–430.
257. Scribner DR Jr, Walker JL, Johnson GA, et al. Surgical management of early-stage endometrial cancer in the elderly: is laparoscopy feasible? *Gynecol Oncol* 2001;83(3):563.
258. Sonoda Y, Zerbe M, Smith A, et al. High incidence of positive peritoneal cytology in low-risk endometrial cancer treated by laparoscopically assisted vaginal hysterectomy. *Gynecol Oncol* 2001;80(3):378–382.
259. Vergote I, De Smet I, Amant F. Incidence of positive peritoneal cytology in low-risk endometrial cancer treated by laparoscopically assisted vaginal hysterectomy. *Gynecol Oncol* 2002;84(3):537–538.
260. Eltabbakh GH, Mount SL. Laparoscopic surgery does not increase the positive peritoneal cytology among women with endometrial carcinoma. *Gynecol Oncol* 2006;100(2):361–364.
261. Nelson BE, Rosenfield AT, Schwartz PE. Preoperative abdominopelvic computed tomographic prediction of optimal cytoreduction in epithelial ovarian carcinoma. *J Clin Oncol* 1993;11:166–172.
262. Schwartz PE, Chambers JT, Makuch R. Neoadjuvant chemotherapy for advanced ovarian cancer. *Gynecol Oncol* 1994;53:33–37.
263. Schwartz PE, Rutherford TJ, Chambers JT, et al. Neoadjuvant chemotherapy for advanced ovarian cancer: long-term survival. *Gynecol Oncol* 1999;72:93–99.
264. Chan YM, Ng TY, Ngan HY, et al. Quality of life in women treated with neoadjuvant chemotherapy for advanced ovarian cancer: a prospective longitudinal study. *Gynecol Oncol* 2003;88:9–16.
265. Plante M, Renaud MC, Roy M. Flaws in the use of neoadjuvant chemotherapy in advanced ovarian cancer. In: 8th Biennial Meeting of the International Gynecologic Cancer Society, Bologna: Monduzzi Editore; 2001:197.
266. Schwartz PE, Zheng W. Neoadjuvant chemotherapy for advanced ovarian cancer: the role of cytology in pretreatment diagnosis. *Gynecol Oncol* 2003;90:644–650.
267. Ben David Y, Bustan M, Shalev E. Laparoscopy as part of the evaluation and management of ovarian and cervix neoplasms. *Harefuah* 2001;140:464–467.
268. Deffieux X, Castaigne D, Pomel C. Role of laparoscopy to evaluate candidates for complete cytoreduction in advanced stages of epithelial ovarian cancer. *Int J Gynecol Cancer* 2006;16(Suppl 1):35–40.
269. Angioli R, Palaia I, Zullo MA, et al. Diagnostic open laparoscopy in the management of advanced ovarian cancer. *Gynecol Oncol* 2006;100(3): 455–461.
270. Fagotti A, Ferrandina G, Fanfani F, et al. A laparoscopy-based score to predict surgical outcome in patients with advanced ovarian carcinoma: a pilot study. *Ann Surg Oncol* 2006;13(8):1156–1161.
271. van Dam PA, DeCloedt J, Tjalma WA, et al. Trocar implantation metastasis after laparoscopy in patients with advanced ovarian cancer: can the risk be reduced? *Am J Obstet Gynecol* 1999;181(3):536–541.
272. Ansquer Y, Leblanc E, Clough K, et al. Neoadjuvant chemotherapy for unresectable ovarian carcinoma: a French multicenter study. *Cancer* 2001;15:91:2329–2334.
273. Husain A, Chi DS, Prasad M, et al. The role of laparoscopy in second-look evaluations for ovarian cancer. *Gynecol Oncol* 2001;80:44–47.
274. Clough KB, Ladonne JM, Nos C, et al. Second look for ovarian cancer: laparoscopy or laparotomy? A prospective comparative study. *Gynecol Oncol* 1999;72:411–417.
275. Little RD, Hallonquist H, Matulonis U, et al. Negative laparoscopy is highly predictive of negative second-look laparotomy following chemotherapy for ovarian, tubal, and primary peritoneal carcinoma. *Gynecol Oncol* 2006; 103(2):570–574.
276. Abu-Rustum NR, Barakat RR, Siegel PL, et al. Second-look operation for epithelial ovarian cancer: laparoscopy or laparotomy? *Obstet Gynecol* 1996;88(4 Pt 1):549–553.
277. Anaf V, Gangji D, Simon P, et al. Laparoscopical insertion of intraperitoneal catheters for intraperitoneal chemotherapy. *Acta Obstet Gynecol Scand* 2003;82:1140–1145.
278. Soper JT, Johnson P, Johnson V, et al. Comprehensive restaging laparotomy in women with apparent early ovarian carcinoma. *Obstet Gynecol* 1992;80:949–953.
279. Faught W, Le T, Fung Kee Fung M, et al. Early ovarian cancer: what is the staging impact of retroperitoneal node sampling? *J Obstet Gynaecol Can* 2003;25:18–21.
280. Chu KK, Chen FP, Chang SD. Laparoscopic surgical procedures for early ovarian cancer. *Acta Obstet Gynecol Scand* 1995;74:391–392.
281. Amara DP, Nezhat C, Teng NN, et al. Operative laparoscopy in the management of ovarian cancer. *Surg Laparosc Endosc* 1996;6:38–45.
282. Childers JM, Lang J, Surwit EA, et al. Laparoscopic surgical staging of ovarian cancer. *Gynecol Oncol* 1995;59:25–33.
283. Pomel C, Provencher D, Dauplat J, et al. Laparoscopic staging of early ovarian cancer. *Gynecol Oncol* 1995;58:301–306.
284. Leblanc E, Querleu D, Narducci F, et al. Laparoscopic restaging of early stage invasive adnexal tumors: a 10-year experience. *Gynecol Oncol* 2004; 94(3):624–629.
285. Spirtos NM, Eisekop SM, Boike G, et al. Laparoscopic staging in patients with incompletely staged cancers of the uterus, ovary, fallopian tube, and primary peritoneum: a Gynecologic Oncology Group (GOG) study. *Am J Obstet Gynecol* 2005;193(5):1645–1649.
286. Land R, Perrin L, Nicklin J. Evaluation of restaging in clinical stage 1A low malignant potential ovarian tumours. *Aust N Z J Obstet Gynaecol* 2002;42:379–382.
287. Querleu D, Papageorgiou T, Lambaudie E, et al. Laparoscopic restaging of borderline ovarian tumours: results of 30 cases initially presumed as stage IA borderline ovarian tumours. *Br J Obstet Gynaecol* 2003;110: 201–204.
288. Darai E, Tulpin L, Prugnolle H, et al. Laparoscopic restaging of borderline ovarian tumors. *Surg Endosc* 2007 May 19 [Epub ahead of print].
289. Ghezzi F, Cromi A, Uccella S, et al. Laparoscopy versus laparotomy for the surgical management of apparent early stage ovarian cancer. *Gynecol Oncol* 2007;105(2):409–413.
290. Lecuru F, Desfaux P, Camatte S, et al. Impact of initial surgical access on staging and survival of patients with stage I ovarian cancer. *Int J Gynecol Cancer* 2006;16(1):87–94.
291. Leblanc E, Sonoda Y, Narducci F, et al. Laparoscopic staging of early ovarian carcinoma. *Curr Opin Obstet Gynecol* 2006;18(4):407–412.
292. Biran G, Golan A, Sagiv R, et al. Conversion of laparoscopy to laparotomy due to adnexal malignancy. *Eur J Gynaecol Oncol* 2002;23:157–160.
293. Canis M, Botchorishvili R, Manhes H, et al. Management of adnexal masses: role and risk of laparoscopy. *Semin Surg Oncol* 2000;19:28–35.
294. Theodoridis TD, Bontis JN. Laparoscopy and oncology: where do we stand today? *Ann N Y Acad Sci* 2003;997:282–291.
295. Haughney RV, Slade RJ, Brain AN. An isolated abdominal wall metastasis of ovarian carcinoma ten years after primary surgery. *Eur J Gynaecol Oncol* 2001;22:102.
296. Carlson NL, Krivak TC, Winter WE 3rd, et al. Port site metastasis of ovarian carcinoma remote from laparoscopic surgery for benign disease. *Gynecol Oncol* 2002;85:529–531.
297. Viala J, Morice P, Pautier P, et al. CT findings in two cases of port-site metastasis after laparoscopy for ovarian cancer. *Eur J Gynaecol Oncol* 2002;23:293–294.
298. Huang KG, Wang CJ, Chang TC, et al. Management of port-site metastasis after laparoscopic surgery for ovarian cancer. *Am J Obstet Gynecol* 2003;189:16–21.
299. Canis M, Rabischong B, Houlle C, et al. Laparoscopic management of adnexal masses: a gold standard? *Curr Opin Obstet Gynecol* 2002;14: 423–428.
300. Spannuth WA, Rocconi RP, Huh WK, et al. A comparison of hand-assisted laparoscopy and conventional laparotomy for the surgical evaluation of pelvic masses. *Gynecol Oncol* 2005;99(2):443–446.
301. Krivak TC, Elkas JC, Rose GS, et al. The utility of hand-assisted laparoscopy in ovarian cancer. *Gynecol Oncol* 2005;96(1):72–76.
302. Chi DS, Abu-Rustum NR, Sonoda Y, et al. Laparoscopic and hand-assisted laparoscopic splenectomy for recurrent and persistent ovarian cancer. *Gynecol Oncol* 2006;101(2):224–227.
303. Magrina JF, Walter AJ, Schild SE. Laparoscopic radical parametrectomy and pelvic and aortic lymphadenectomy for vaginal carcinoma: a case report. *Gynecol Oncol* 1999;75:514–516.
304. Kohler C, Tozzi R, Klemm P, et al. "Schauta *sine utero*": technique and results of laparoscopic-vaginal radical parametrectomy. *Gynecol Oncol* 2003;91:359–368.
305. Rodriguez M, Guimares O, Rose PG. Radical abdominal trachelectomy and pelvic lymphadenectomy with uterine conservation and subsequent pregnancy in the treatment of early invasive cervical cancer. *Am J Obstet Gynecol* 2001;185:370–374.

CHAPTER 14 ■ BIOLOGIC AND PHYSICAL ASPECTS OF RADIATION ONCOLOGY

BETH A. ERICKSON-WITTMANN, JASON ROWND, AND KEVIN KHATER

RADIATION ONCOLOGY AS A SPECIALTY

Radiation oncology is a specialty focused primarily on the treatment of malignancies, although there are a number of benign diseases for which radiation can be used. Training in radiation oncology begins with internship followed by 4 years of residency. Board certification follows, requiring successful completion of both written and oral exams. Residency training includes an in-depth understanding of the natural history and treatment of all malignancies including the roles of surgery and systemic therapy in this era of multimodality therapies. An in-depth understanding of surgical procedures, pathology, and radiologic anatomy, as well as the efficacies and toxicities of systemic therapy, are required. Formal instruction in physics and radiobiology is also part of the residency training. Subspecialization can follow with a specific practice focus on gynecologic or other cancers. Only a few centers sponsor fellowships, which are usually focused on brachytherapy or other special procedures. Brachytherapy skills are especially important in the curative treatment of patients with gynecologic cancer. In addition, contemporary treatment of gynecologic malignances requires mastery of rapidly evolving technology for delivering external beam irradiation with techniques such as intensity-modulated radiation therapy (IMRT) and image-guided radiation therapy (IGRT). Radiation oncologists are important contributors in the management of individual patients and in multidisciplinary tumor boards. Having a knowledgeable and subspecialized radiation oncologist and gynecologic oncologist paired is a great benefit to all. In addition to radiation oncologists, other allied health professionals are integral to the radiation oncology department and treatment delivery. Radiation therapists are the individuals who actually operate the radiation equipment and deliver the radiation treatments. Some of them will obtain a Bachelor of Science degree followed by a 13-month training program in radiation therapy. Alternatively, a 2-year associate degree in diagnostic radiology can be obtained followed by 1 to 2 years in radiation therapy training. Dosimetrists are primarily responsible for doing the radiation therapy planning or dosimetry prior to treatment delivery. Most of these individuals are former radiation therapists. An additional 1 to 2 years of training under a physicist and board certified dosimetrist, as well as additional years of practice, are required to be eligible for board certification. Radiation physicists supervise and review the work of dosimetrists. Physicists are also integral to the introduction and maintenance of the rapidly evolving technology in radiation oncology departments. They are very involved with quality assurance and radiation safety. They can be Master's level or PhD level physicists and should be board certified.

INTRODUCTION TO RADIOBIOLOGY

Radiobiology is the study of the action of ionizing radiations on living things (1). It is important for radiation oncologists to know the most appropriate dose to potentially irradicate the tumor and the normal tissue tolerance doses for those organs in the radiation field. The published literature includes clinical and laboratory data to support various dose/fractionation schemes as well as acceptable dose ranges to the normal tissues. The size and histology of the tumor as well as the relationship of the tumor to the normal organs within the radiation field will help to determine the total dose and the dose per fraction. Almost every radiation oncologist approaches treatment planning by considering whether the therapy is curative verses palliative. If curative, then the focus becomes identifying the location of the disease and how best to irradicate it. Typically, radiation and chemotherapy treatments take place over many months, and upon completion of treatment, if there is still a clonogenically viable cell that remains, then the tumor will ultimately recur. Clinical radiobiology focuses on steps that maximize the chance for cure and decrease the chance for side effects.

As in pharmacology, radiation effects exhibit a sigmoidal dose-response curve. In the case of radiation, the interpretation of the curve becomes far more complex because multiple independent processes govern responses to radiation. Pharmacology, on the other hand, tends to be simpler because classic examples can be described by a ligand binding to a group of receptors initiating subsequent events. Keeping this in mind, consider the following theoretical dose-response curve for tumor control probability and normal tissue complications in the presence and absence of chemotherapy (Fig. 14.1). Ideally, there is a great deal of separation between the curve on the left, representing chances of tumor control, and the curve on the right, representing the chance for toxicity. An intolerable situation is where the curves are close together since, as they approach one another, the chances of control and toxicity become equal and the therapeutic range (TR) narrows. Therefore, the most important goal of radiobiology is to understand the basic science behind the interaction of radiation and cells with the hope of maximizing the risk-benefit ratio for patients.

Models for Cell Kill

Tumor Control Probability

The simplest model one can envision for the sterilization of cancer cells by radiation in a given volume is the log cell kill model. A typical course of radiation therapy is given in 10 to

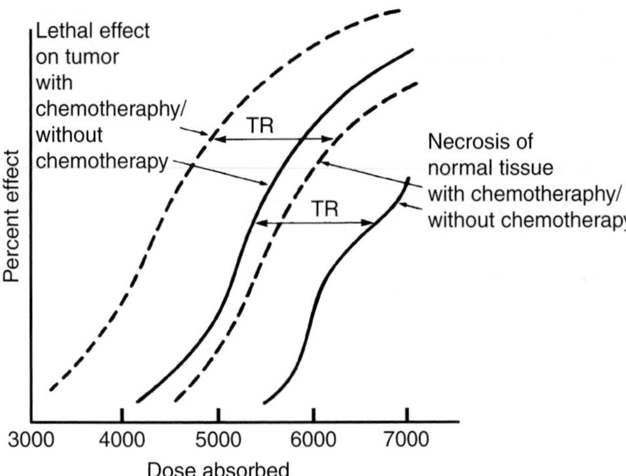

FIGURE 14.1. Theoretic curves for tumor control and complications as a function of radiation dose both with and without chemotherapy. TR, therapeutic range, or the difference between tumor control and complication frequency. *Source:* Reprinted from Perez CA, Thomas PRM. Radiation therapy: basic concepts and clinical implications. In: Sutow WW, Fernbach DJ, Vietti TJ, eds. *Clinical Pediatric Oncology*. 3rd ed. St. Louis: Mosby; 1984:167, with permission from Elsevier.

40 fractions administered over 2 to 8 weeks. Each fraction kills a fixed percentage of cells. We are trained at a young age to mathematically think in base 10, and therefore a convenient number to consider is the D_{10} or the dose which kills 90% of the cells. If there are 100 cells and a D_{10} dose is administered, 10 viable cells remain. D_0, a commonly used term, is the dose of radiation that kills 63% of cells. D_0 is related to the more convenient parameter D_{10} by the following formula: $D_{10} = 2.3 \times D_0$. Consider a tumor 1 g in size, which has 10^9 cells. If the D_{10} for this tumor is 3 Gy, how many fractions are required for a 90% chance of sterilization? The log cell kill model gets slightly more complicated when dealing in fractions since 1/10 of a viable cell does not exist. Instead, 0.1 cells represent a 10% chance that a viable cell will exist at the end of therapy. Therefore, a tumor with 10^9 cells requires 10 decades of cell kill for a 90% chance of tumor control. Three Gy × 10 fractions = 30 Gy total dose. This model makes a number of invalid assumptions such as D_{10} remaining constant throughout the course of radiation. As discussed later, there are data that support D_{10} both increasing and decreasing throughout treatment.

When it comes to actually treating patients, physicians do not actively engage in the above mental exercise. However, the basic concepts of the log kill model are reflected in the administered treatments. Consider, for example, curative therapy for cervical cancer. Radiation oncologists begin treatment planning by first identifying the targets GTV (gross target volume) and CTV (clinical target volume) (Fig. 14.2). The CTV is any region that has a high likelihood of harboring malignancy, but otherwise appears normal. For cervical cancer, this could be normal-sized pelvic and possibly paraaortic lymph nodes or an area of positive margin. The CTV typically requires a lower dose of radiation for control, ranging from 45 to 54 Gy. The GTV is defined as any disease that is identified either radiographically or by physical exam and requires a higher dose of radiation, such as 80 to 90 Gy in cervical cancer patients. Attaining these doses of radiation while respecting normal tissue tolerance is not feasible with external beam radiation therapy alone and brachytherapy is required. If a patient undergoes a hysterectomy where bulk tumor is removed, then there is not a GTV and brachytherapy is often not needed. So, while the cell kill model is of little practical importance, it is used nonquantitatively for almost every patient receiving radiation treatments.

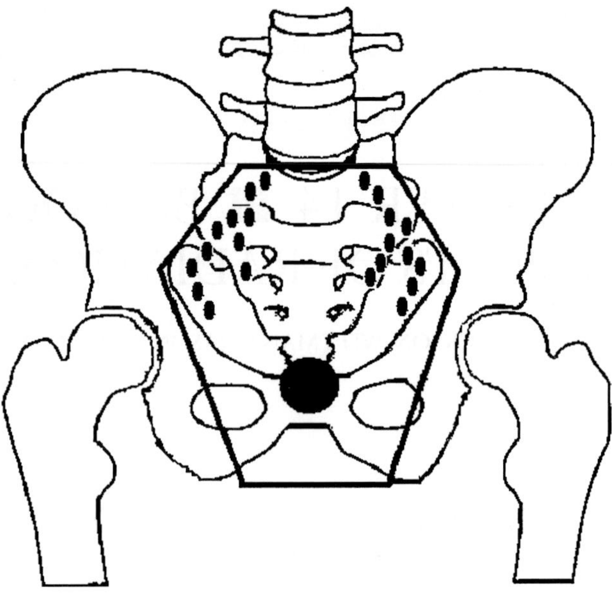

FIGURE 14.2. Target definition in radiation treatment planning for cervical cancer. The solid circle represents the gross target volume (GTV), which is the cervical primary defined both clinically and radiographically. The clinical target volume (CTV) is the pelvic lymph nodes, which have a high probability of at least microscopic involvement. The planning target volume (PTV) is shown as the outer solid line and represents the margin added to the CTV to account for organ motion and daily setup error.

Cell Survival Curves

The log cell kill model describes cell kill in very simplistic terms such that a given radiation dose will kill a certain percentage of cells and that a tumor receiving a fractionated course of radiation gets progressively smaller with time. This approach looks at behavior in a population of cells, which is practical, but gains very little insight into events at the molecular level. The reason is that measuring the diameter of the tumor is not a very accurate way of estimating cell kill. Additionally, tumor cells may have undergone clonogenic cell death, wherein they are still present but unable to reproduce. Therefore, one does not necessarily have to kill all cancer cells in order to achieve cure if the remaining ones are unable to reproduce.

In order to understand events at the molecular level, one needs to accurately measure cell kill. The technique used most commonly first involves creating a suspension containing the target population of cells at a known concentration (Fig. 14.3). An aliquot with a known number of cells is plated on agarose growth media and allowed to incubate. As one would expect, not all the cells successfully form a colony, and so plating efficiency must be calculated by dividing the number of formed colonies by the starting number of cells. The experiment is repeated, but after plating and before incubation, the petri dish is irradiated. The number of colonies formed is divided by the starting number of cells, which is then divided by plating efficiency to yield the ratio of surviving cells. This experiment is repeated over a range of doses of radiation and under various conditions to yield a cell survival curve. The first feature to notice about a cell survival curve is that it uses a logarithmic scale on the y-axis such that as survival approaches 0, the curve goes to negative infinity. The benefit of plotting the data on a logarithmic scale is that, visually speaking, we are able to interpret whether the events driving cell kill are simple or complex. Consider the analogy of a completely different process, such as the decay of a pure radioisotope over time.

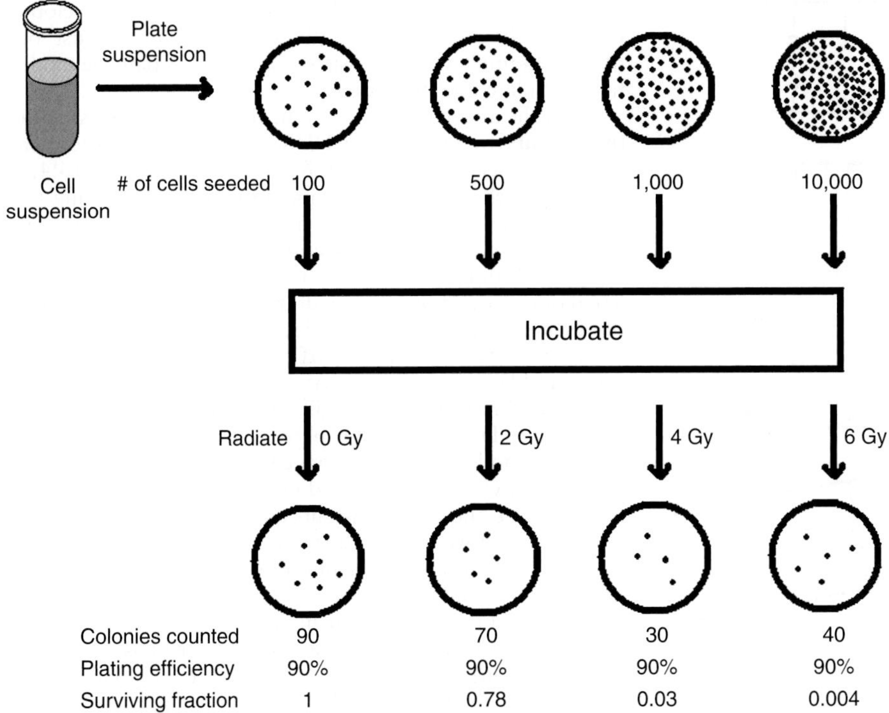

FIGURE 14.3. Cell culture technique used to generate a cell survival curve. A cell suspension is used to plate Petri dishes with a known number of cells, which are subsequently irradiated. Viable cells will form colonies after incubation. The number of viable cells divided by the plating efficiency is used to calculate the surviving fraction. The experiment is repeated over a wide range of doses to produce the cell survival curve.

Plotting this on a linear scale over time would yield an exponential curve, which is difficult to interpret. However, plotting this on a logarithmic scale would yield a perfect straight line indicating that a single isotope is involved. Consider a slightly more complex situation where the decay is represented by two radioactive isotopes with similar half-lives. Plotting this on a linear scale would also reveal an exponential curve, which is unrevealing by inspection. However, creating a plot on a logarithmic scale would yield two lines superimposed on one another, clearly indicating that two radioisotopes are involved.

Two theoretical experimental cell survival curves are shown in Figure 14.4 under LDR (low dose rate) and HDR (high dose rate) radiation conditions. The curve for LDR is best fit by a straight line, while the HDR curve is shown to have two components, an earlier linear component mirroring

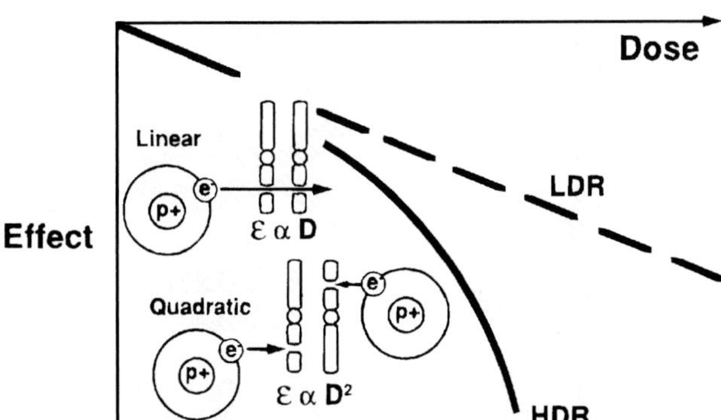

FIGURE 14.4. Cell killing by radiation is largely due to aberrations caused by breaks in two chromosomes. The dose-response curve for high dose rate (HDR) irradiation is linear-quadratic: the two breaks may be caused by the same electron (dominant at low doses) or by two different electrons (dominant at higher doses). For low dose rate (LDR) irradiation, where radiation is delivered over a protracted period, the principal mechanism of cell killing is by the single electron. Consequently, the LDR survival curve is an extension of the low-dose region of the HDR survival curve.

the LDR curve followed by a quadratic component. At higher doses of radiation, the HDR curve always has a higher proportion of cell kill than the LDR curve for any given dose.

The rate at which radiation is delivered causes dramatic differences in the shape of the cell survival curve. This is best described by considering the linear-quadratic model with DNA as the lethal target. The evidence for DNA as one of the targets for radiation is substantial: (a) incorporation of radioactive tritium into DNA causes cell death at greater rates than cytoplasmic tritium (2); (b) halogenated pyrimidines, when present in DNA, increase the cell's inherent radiosensitivity in an amount proportionate to the degree of incorporation; (c) a correlation between radiation, DNA double-stranded break repair, and clonogenic survival has also been observed; (d) the concentration of DNA in the nucleus correlates positively with radiosensitivity (3); (e) microirradiation techniques have shown the nucleus to be the most radiosensitive organelle (4).

In most instances, radiation must cause DNA damage that results in a net loss of genetic material, thereby causing a lethal outcome. Radiation exerts most of its deleterious effects by causing breaks in the DNA backbone. Figure 14.5 shows possible outcomes of photon interaction with the DNA backbone. Because DNA is composed of a double helix with multiple local base pairs acting cooperatively, a single-strand nick is thought to be inconsequential and is repaired by the cellular machinery (Fig. 14.5b). In fact, multiple single-strand nicks can occur, and if they are remote from one another, a normal cell can repair the damage with little chance of a deleterious outcome (Fig. 14.5c). However, two opposing single-strand breaks locally disrupt cooperativity, and a double-stranded break (DSB) develops.

Once a DSB develops, the cell attempts repair by rejoining the cut ends, as shown in Figure 14.6. There are two possible outcomes with repair of the DSBs: the lethal outcomes are shown at the top of Figure 14.6, wherein the chromosomes rearrange such that a portion lacks a centromere, an acentric fragment. When the cell undergoes mitosis, these acentric fragments are eventually lost and may be identified in micronuclei, a smaller "sub-nucleus" found in the cytoplasm in a separate compartment from the chromosomes (5–7). The nonlethal

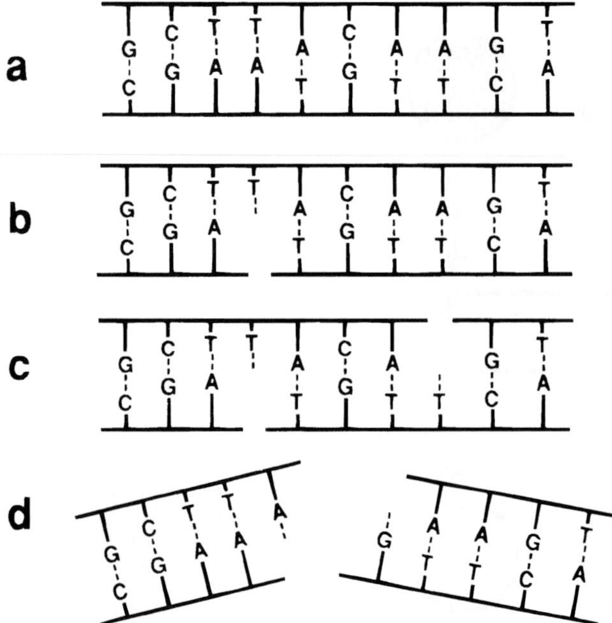

FIGURE 14.5. Diagrams of single- and double-strand DNA breaks caused by radiation. **a:** two-dimensional representation of the normal DNA double helix. The base pairs carrying the genetic code are complementary (i.e., adenine pairs with thymine, guanine pairs with cytosine). **b:** a break in one strand is of little significance because it is readily repaired, using the opposite strand as a template. **c:** breaks in both strands, if well separated, are repaired as independent breaks. **d:** if breaks occur in both strands and are directly opposite or separated by only a few base pairs, this may lead to a double-strand break, where the chromatin snaps into two pieces. *Source:* Courtesy of Dr. John Ward. From Hall EJ. *Radiobiology for the Radiologist.* 4th ed. Philadelphia: JB Lippincott Co.; 1994.

outcomes are shown at the bottom of Figure 14.6, where repair results in a reciprocal translocation and preservation of the genetic information. In some instances, the reciprocal translocation results in activation of an oncogene, which may manifest as a malignancy. It is worth noting that a "bystander effect" has been described using microbeam irradiation techniques (8). In this approach, a nanoscale α-particle beam is directed at the nucleus of a single cell. DSBs can be seen to develop in immediately adjacent unirradiated cells. This is just one notable example where classic radiation DNA damage models fail to explain an observation.

With the above information, the differences in the shape of the cell survival curve under HDR verses LDR conditions can be more easily understood. Referring back to Figure 14.4, in the inset is shown the linear-quadratic model depicting two DSBs that develop as result of a photon ejecting an electron, which interacts with DNA. Recall from Figure 14.6 that two separate chromosomal breaks are necessary for a potentially lethal outcome. Above the quadratic model is the linear model represented as a single ejected electron causing both DSBs and described mathematically by $\varepsilon\alpha D$ where ε and α are both constants and D is dose. The important point is that the degree of the linear component of cell kill, also known as α kill, is proportional to D since only one photon/electron is involved. The quadratic model also shows two chromosomal breaks. This is caused by two separate ejected electrons and is described by $\varepsilon\beta D^2$ where ε and β are constants and D is again dose. Cell kill accounted for by the quadratic model, or β kill, is proportional to D^2 because two photons/electrons are involved. Looking at the HDR curve at low doses of radiation, there is very little β kill; however, at higher doses the β component increases exponentially because of D^2. Under LDR conditions, the β component is absent, leaving only α kill. This is best explained by the idea that β kill involves damage to one chromosome and so is more easily repaired provided that the radiation dose rate and rate of DSB formation is not significantly greater than the cell's repair capacity.

DNA Damage Repair and the Shape of Cell Survival Curves

The concept that DNA damage repair drives the shapes of cell survival curves is well illustrated by experiments showing the effectiveness of oxygen as a sensitizer. Oxygen is known to chemically modify radiation-induced DNA damage making it irreparable (8). This is known as the oxygen fixation hypothesis. Therefore, under anoxic conditions, DNA damage repair would be expected to increase considerably. Figure 14.7 shows an experiment on cultured human embryo liver cells irradiated under 100% oxygen and nitrogen conditions. Hypoxia causes the cell survival curve to shift to the right and change shape.

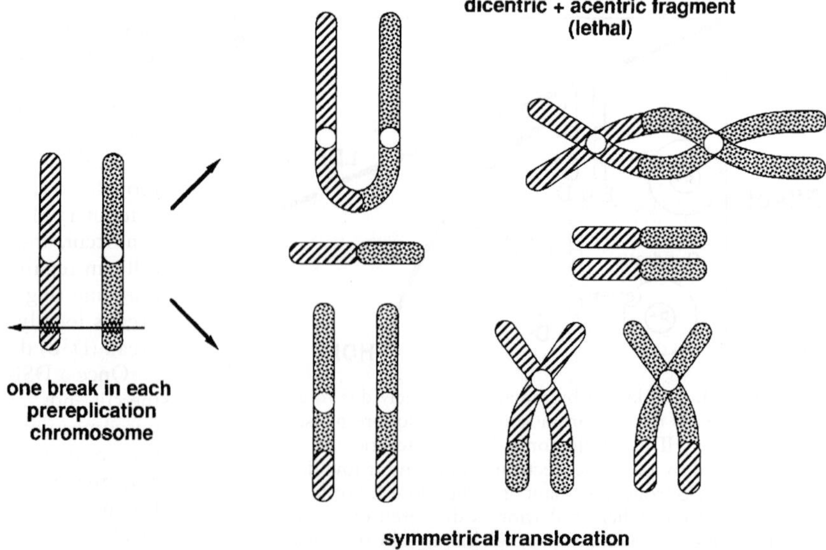

FIGURE 14.6. Most biologic effects of radiation are due to the incorrect joining of breaks in two chromosomes. For example, the two broken chromosomes may recombine to form a dicentric (a chromosome with two centromeres) and an acentric fragment (a fragment with no centromere). This is a lethal lesion resulting in cell death. Alternatively, the two broken chromosomes may exchange broken ends, called symmetrical translocation, which does not lead to death of the cell, but in a few special cases activates an oncogene by moving it from a quiescent to an active site.

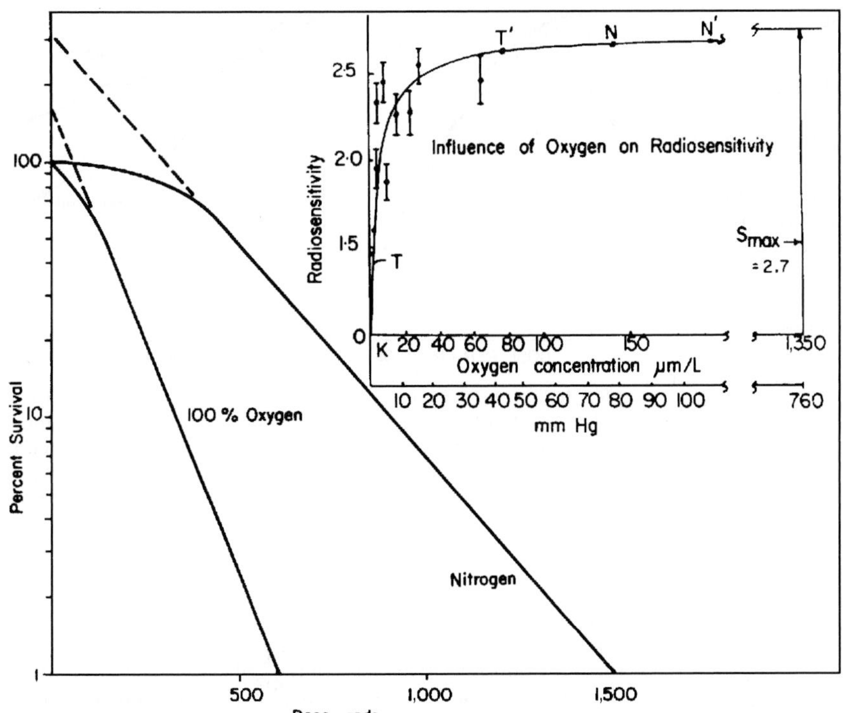

FIGURE 14.7. Influence of oxygen tension on radiosensitivity. Survival curve for human embryo liver cells in tissue culture irradiated with and without oxygen. *Source:* From Johns HE, Cunningham JR. *The Physics of Radiology.* 3rd ed. Springfield, IL: Charles C Thomas; 1972, with permission.

Up to this point, the linear-quadratic model has been used to describe cell survival curve experiments. Another way to describe the observations is using the multi-target single hit model, which simply states that multiple targets within a cell must be damaged for a lethal outcome. Therefore, at very low doses of radiation there will be nearly 100% survival. The model is described mathematically by Survival $= 1-(1-e^{-D/Do})^n$, where D is dose delivered, D is the amount of radiation to achieve approximately 63% cell kill. The parameter n is the extrapolation coefficient or the number of targets in each cell, and is identified by where an imaginary straight line drawn back from the linear portion of the cell survival curve crosses the y-intercept. It is important to note that this model makes no statement about what the targets actually are. Since we already know that the primary target is DNA, which can trigger multiple complicated events such as repair and apoptosis, the single hit multi-target model falls short of perfection. Nevertheless, it is a good model for understanding the general shapes of survival curves. Contrast this model to the single-target single hit model, which states that a cell needs only to sustain a single hit for lethality, and is described mathematically by Survival $= e^{-D/Do}$. Therefore, even at very low doses of radiation, there will be cell kill. Note that this model does not have an extrapolation coefficient.

Referring back to Figure 14.7, the cell survival curve under anoxic conditions can be interpreted as having a higher extrapolation coefficient when compared to 100% oxygen. The extrapolation coefficient is shown diagrammatically by following the dotted lines of the survival curves back to the y-intercept. n is where the dotted line crosses the y-intercept.

The inset shows a dose-response relationship between oxygen and radiosensitivity. The typical sigmoidal relationship is lost because oxygen is extremely effective at fixing DNA damage even at low pressures. In fact, only approximately 20 mm Hg or 2% to 3% oxygen is required to achieve the maximum oxygen effect. The half-maximum sensitization is typically observed at 3 mm Hg or 0.5% of oxygen.

The linear-quadratic model is stated more explicitly by the following equation:

$$-\ln S = \alpha D + \beta D^2$$

where S is the surviving fraction and the remaining parameters α, β, and D are the same definitions as above. The formula was used to generate Figure 14.8. The dashed line represents the α component and is generated by extrapolating the initial slope of the curve to higher doses of radiation. The point at which the α and β kill are equal is shown, and the dose at which this occurs is called the α/β ratio. It is worth noting that the α/β ratio is a bit of a misnomer since ratios typically are unitless values. However, α/β has the units of Gy^{-1}. The α/β ratio for early side effects is thought to be higher, around 10 Gy^{-1}, than for tumor control and late side effects, which is around 3 Gy^{-1}.

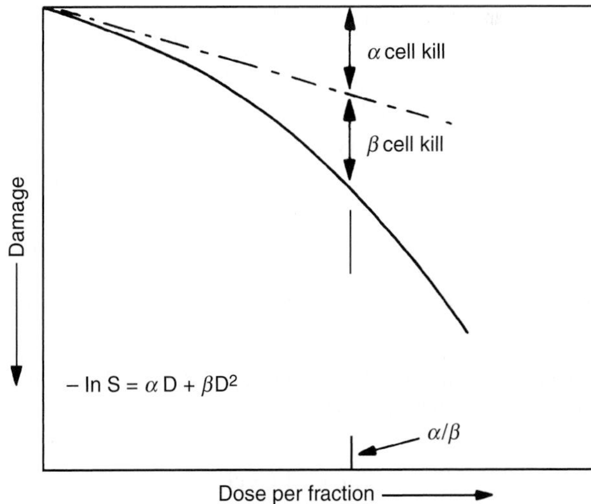

FIGURE 14.8. At a dose equal to the α/β ratio, the log cell kill due to the α process (nonreparable) is equal to that due to the β process (reparable injury): α/β is thus a measure of how soon the survival curve begins to bend over significantly. *Source:* Reprinted from Fowler JR. Fractionation and therapeutic gain. In: Steel GG, Adams GE, Peckham MJ, eds. *Biologic Basis of Radiotherapy*. Amsterdam: Elsevier Science; 1983:181–194, with permission from Elsevier.

Biologically Equivalent Dose

It is clear from Figure 14.4 that both the total dose of radiation and how fast it is delivered can produce very different outcomes. The same holds true for fractionated courses of radiation. For example, 16 Gy delivered in a single treatment, as is the case for radiosurgery, can sterilize a small tumor of cancer cells. However, the same treatment delivered over 8 days would be clinically insignificant. Figure 14.9 shows theoretical cell survival curves for early and late reactions under two separate experimental conditions, single fraction and multi-fraction regimens. Note that by breaking up the radiotherapy in fractions, the shoulder of the cell survival curve is repeated. A formula that would normalize a biologic endpoint under various dose fractionation schemes is necessary. The linear-quadratic equation can be used to derive an equation to be used as a guide to predict various biologic endpoints and is given by the following equation:

$$BED = D[1 + d/(\alpha/\beta)]$$

Where:

BED = biologically equivalent dose
D = total dose
d = dose per fraction
α/β = dose where the α component of cell kill equals the β component

A good example where the formula aided the design of a randomized trial, RTOG 8305, is shown below (9). This trial investigated two different fractionation schemes in the treatment of metastatic melanoma.

Early Side Effects (assumes an α/β of 10)
Arm 1 (32 Gy at 8 Gy/fxn):

$$\begin{aligned} BED &= D[1 + d/(\alpha/\beta)] \\ &= 32\text{ Gy } (1 + 8\text{ Gy}/10\text{ Gy}) \\ &= 57.6\text{ Gy} \end{aligned}$$

Arm 2 (50 Gy at 2.5 Gy/fxn):

$$\begin{aligned} BED &= D[1 + d/(\alpha/\beta)] \\ &= 50\text{ Gy } (1 + 2.5\text{Gy}/10\text{ Gy}) \\ &= 62.5\text{ Gy} \end{aligned}$$

Late Side Effects/Tumor Control (assumes an α/β of 3)
Arm 1 (32 Gy at 8 Gy/fxn):

$$\begin{aligned} BED &= D[1 + d/(\alpha/\beta)] \\ &= 32\text{ Gy } (1 + 8\text{ Gy}/3\text{ Gy}) \\ &= 117\text{ Gy} \end{aligned}$$

Arm 2 (50 Gy at 2.5 Gy/fxn):

$$\begin{aligned} BED &= D[1 + d/(\alpha/\beta)] \\ &= 50\text{ Gy } (1 + 2.5\text{Gy}/3\text{ Gy}) \\ &= 92\text{ Gy} \end{aligned}$$

In this instance, the BED calculations predict that arm 1 will have slightly more early and late side effects but better tumor control. BED calculations are used as a guide for determining doses. Oftentimes the calculations do not translate directly into the clinical setting outcomes. For example, RTOG 8305 was not able to detect a difference between the two dose fractionation schemes.

The Cell Cycle

The cell cycle is an ordered set of events, resulting in cell growth and division into two daughter cells. The steps, pictured in the middle of Figure 14.10, are G_1-S-G_2-M. The G_1 stands for "gap 1," and S phase stands for "synthesis" and is the point at which DNA replication occurs. Late S phase is the most radioresistant phase of the cell cycle since the DNA repair machinery for replication can also repair radiation damage.

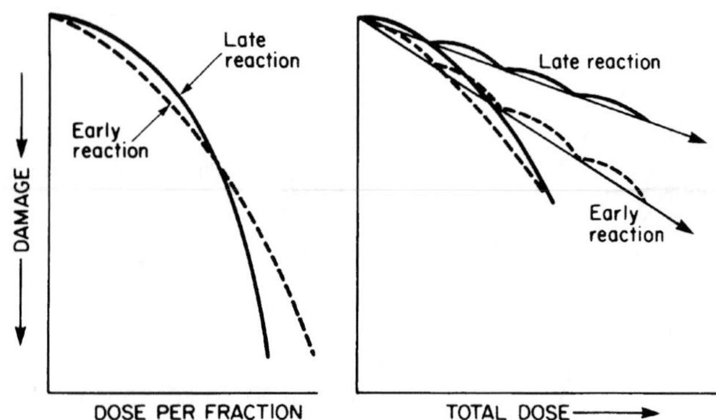

FIGURE 14.9. Difference in cell survival curves for acute and late radiation effects with single or multifractionated doses of irradiation. *Source:* Reprinted from Fowler JF. Fractionation and therapeutic gain. In: Steel GG, Adams GE, Peckham MT, eds. *Biologic Basis of Radiotherapy.* Amsterdam: Elsevier Science; 1983:181, with permission from Elsevier.

The G_2 stage stands for "gap 2," and M phase stands for "mitosis" and is when nuclear division occurs. M phase is also the most radiosensitive phase of the cell cycle since this is an all or nothing event. In other words, once the cell enters into M phase, it will attempt to complete this phase of the cycle without arresting. Therefore, any DNA damage caused generally will be passed along to the daughter cells and may be fatal. This is one important reason why rapidly dividing cells such as cancers are radiosensitive. Not shown in Figure 14.10 is G_0, which is a stable state of the cell and is typically observed with well-differentiated cells that have reached end stage of development and are no longer dividing (i.e., neuron).

There are three major classes of proteins that orchestrate the cell cycle in mammalian cells: (a) cyclins, (b) cyclin-dependent kinases (cdk in mammals, cdc in yeast), (c) proteins that regulate (a) and (b). Cyclins are generally synthesized and degraded for each phase of the cell cycle. Alone they have no intrinsic enzymatic activity; rather, they bind to and activate cdks. Monomeric cdks are protein kinases that are inactive and require association with a specific cyclin and phosphorylation of a series of conserved threonine residues to become active. Cyclin D/cdk4 is involved with G_1 phase of the cell cycle, cyclin E/cdk2 with G_1 to S phase, cyclin A/cdk2 with S to G_2, and cyclin B/cdk1 with M.

Cellular Response to Radiation

When a cell is irradiated, there are, in general, four possible outcomes. The cell can survive, undergo apoptosis, undergo a mitotic death, or senesce. Survival requires cell cycle arrest and repair of damaged DNA. Apoptosis requires intact molecular biologic pathways that favor an ordered process of programmed cell death within hours of exposure to radiation. Unfortunately, most tumors have mutations in these pathways, but in malignancies such as lymphoma where these pathways are intact, the tumors can respond after only a couple of radiation treatments. Cells that die a mitotic death undergo a catastrophic event when trying to replicate and so responses may take days. Tumors that die via this mechanism are more radioresistant and result in necrotic masses on imaging after completing a course of radiation. Senescence is a state in which proliferation is irreversibly arrested and the cell may eventually die. Note that senescence is a metabolically active state, which is different from G_0, which is typically metabolically inactive.

Inherent to the cell is a type of thermostat, which influences the radiation responses to favor any of the above processes. Protooncogenes are regulator proteins that, due to

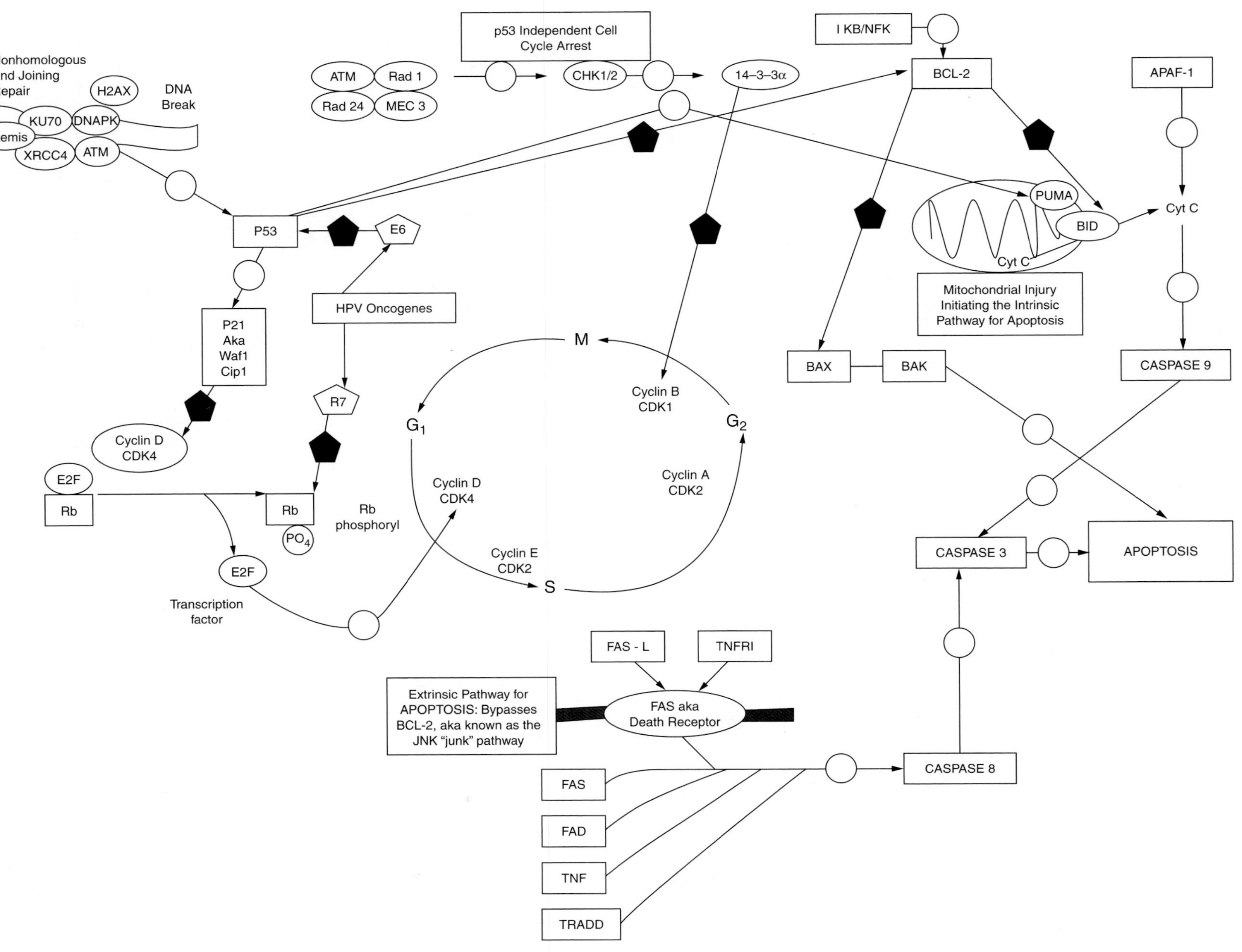

FIGURE 14.10. The cell cycle and important molecular biologic pathways driving cell cycle arrest, aptoptosis, and survival are shown. The solid pentagon denotes a net inhibitory step and the open circle indicates a downstream step.

either overexpression or mutation, have a higher activity level, thereby promoting unregulated division. Because this mechanism is a net gain of function, only one allele need be affected in order to see phenotypic expression. Tumor suppressor genes keep the cell cycle in check, and so loss of function of both alleles is typically required for dysregulation to be observed.

Cell Cycle Arrest

As previously mentioned, when a cell is irradiated, repair of the DNA backbone is attempted, and in order for this process to occur the cell cycle must typically arrest. There are two prototypical points in the cell cycle during which arrest occurs: G_1 and G_2 (10,11). A major regulator of the cell cycle is the transcription factor p53, which is a tumor suppressor gene that has many pathways both upstream and downstream and is important for G_1 arrest (Fig. 14.10) (12). For example, breaks in the DNA backbone are rejoined via the nonhomologous end-joining (NHEJ) repair mechanisms (top left of Fig. 14.10) (13). One critical gene, the ataxia telangiectasia gene (ATM) has a net positive regulatory effect on p53, which, via p21 (CCDKN1A), has a net inhibitory effect on cyclin D/cdk4, thereby favoring arrest. This is the p53-dependent pathway of cell-cycle arrest. An alternative pathway, independent of p53, operates via chk1/2 and 14-3-3α gene products and has a net inhibitory effect on cyclin B/cdk1, which promotes arrest during G_2 (14).

Retinoblastoma Gene, E2F, and Human Papillomavirus

Retinoblastoma protein (Rb) is another critical regulator of the G_1 phase of the cell cycle (15). This gene is located on chromosome 13 and mutations can cause a number of tumors, the earliest of which to manifest is retinoblastoma. Knudson et al. developed the two-hit hypothesis for the inheritance pattern of this disease (16). He recognized that there were two forms: (a) sporadic, which compromises 60% of the cases of retinoblastoma, whereby mutations occur as random events in both alleles. Patients typically have unilateral disease and a marginal risk for developing second malignancies in response to radiation. (b) Inherited, where a germ-line mutation results when an abnormal allele is inherited from a parent. Patients with this form of retinoblastoma are more likely to develop bilateral disease and have a profound sensitivity toward developing radiation-induced second malignancies. Rb acts by binding and inhibiting E2F, a transcription factor essential for G_1. Phosphorylation of Rb results in release of inhibition of E2F and subsequent cell cycle progression. Human papillomavirus gene product produces an oncogene, E7, which binds to Rb and releases inhibition of E2F, thereby promoting cell division (17).

Apoptosis

Apoptosis can begin in two distinct manners: (a) extrinsic pathway, where the apoptotic stimulus occurs extracellularly, or (b) intrinsic pathway, where the cascade of events is contained intracellularly. Figure 14.10 shows both pathways converging on caspase 8 (cysteine aspartic acid-specific proteases). Caspases are expressed as inactive precursors (procaspases), which are proteolytically cleaved to an active state following an apoptotic stimulus. Upstream from caspase 8, the pathways diverge. The extrinsic pathway begins by binding of a specific ligand such as Fas-L or tumor necrosis factor (TNF) to a membrane bound death receptor. The intrinsic pathway, on the other hand, requires disruption of the mitochondrial membrane, release of mitochondrial cytochrome to the cytoplasm. Cyt c then combines with two other cytosolic protein factors, Apaf-1 (apoptotic protease activating factor-1) and procaspase-9, to promote the assembly of a caspase-activating complex termed the apoptosome, thereby promoting the apoptotic caspase cascade. Bcl-2 and its family member proteins are important regulators of apoptosis. Bcl-2 is anti-apoptotic by inhibiting proapoptotic factor bax and inhibiting the release of cyt c into the cytoplasm. p53 is an important inhibitor of bcl-2. All of these pathways interact to determine whether a cell will survive or apoptose in response to an insulting stimulus such as radiation.

Radiation Effects on Embryo and Fetus

In Utero Exposure to Ionizing Radiation

There are two models that describe the negative clinical sequelae of exposure to radiation to a developing fetus or embryo. (a) Deterministic effects describe how radiation affects a large population of cells resulting in end organ damage. A large number of cells must die in order to induce organ failure. As such, deterministic effects tend to have a sigmoidal dose-response relationship with a threshold dose. As long as the threshold dose is respected, there is very little chance of a given toxicity. (b) Stochastic effects describe events at the cellular level and how radiation induces malignancies. Stochastic effects have more of a constant, steep dose-response relationship. As such, there is no threshold dose, i.e., exposure to even miniscule amounts of additional radiation theoretically increases the chance of inducing a malignancy.

Deterministic Effects—End Organ Damage and Failure

The most sensitive phase of the cell cycle to ionizing radiation is M phase because little repair to the DNA backbone occurs during this period. Most of the cell molecular machinery is geared toward completing mitosis and any DNA double-stranded breaks are passed along to the daughter cells and are typically fatal. Since embryos and fetuses are composed of rapidly dividing cells, they are exquisitely sensitive to radiation and exhibit an extremely low threshold dose. Gestational age is also a key determinant when predicting outcomes of radiation exposure. As Figure 14.11 shows, exposure of several gray during the first 1 to 2 weeks of gestation (peri-implantation stage) results in loss of the embryo. However, if the embryo survives the insult, it will go on to develop without obvious abnormalities. This phenomenon is termed the "all or nothing effect." During weeks 2 to 6, the period of organogenesis is occurring and exposure at this point results in congenital anomalies, neonatal death, and temporary growth retardation. Doses as low as 2 Gy have a 70% mortality. The fetal period occurs beyond 6 weeks and exposure results in permanent growth retardation. Irradiation during weeks 4 through 16 may produce severe eye, skeletal, and genital organ abnormalities as well as microcephaly and mental retardation. According to the Japanese survival data, the risk is approximately 40% per gray. Exposure during weeks 16 through 20 may cause a less severe form of stunting of growth, microcephaly, and mental retardation. After 30 weeks, low doses of radiation do not typically result in gross abnormalities.

Stochastic Effects—Cancer Induction

The Oxford Survey by Kneale and Stewart suggested that there was an association between leukemia risk and *in utero* exposure to diagnostic x-rays (18). Doll and Wakeford summarized the data with the following general conclusions: Low-dose irradiation increases the risk of childhood malignancies, particularly in the third trimester (19). An x-ray exam increases the risk by approximately 40% above the spontaneous rate. Doses as low as approximately 10 mGy increase the risk, and the excess absolute risk is around 6% per gray.

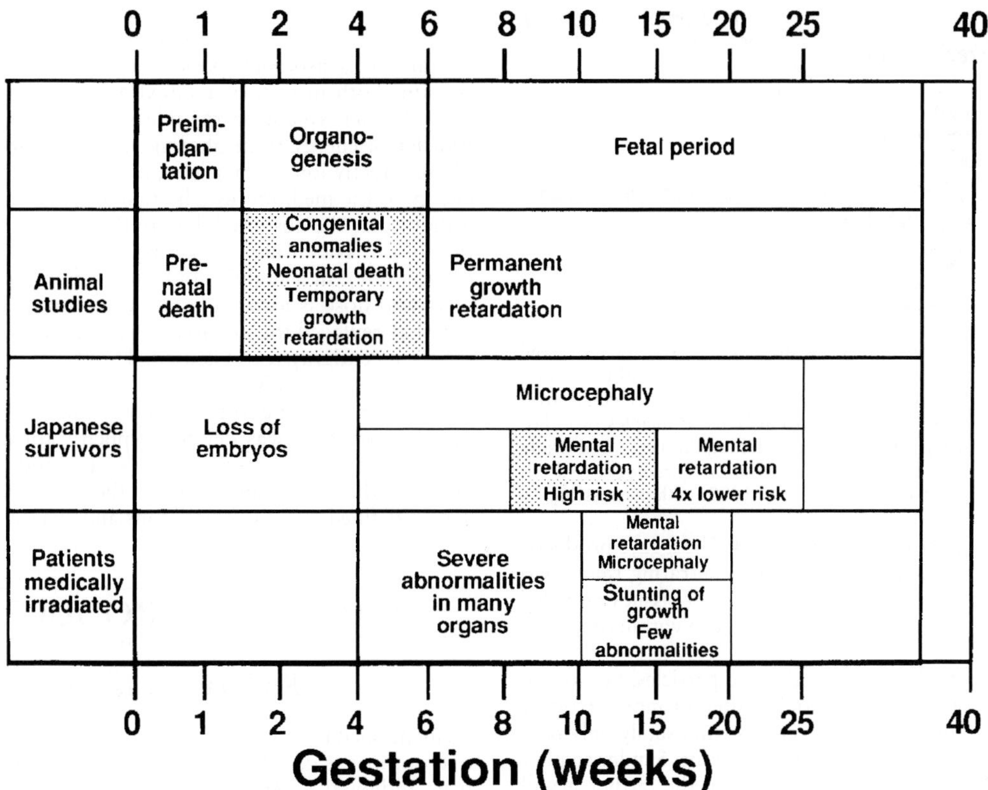

FIGURE 14.11. Summary of the effects of radiation on the developing embryo and fetus from three principal sources: medical radiation, laboratory animal studies, and survivors of the atomic bomb attacks on Nagasaki and Hiroshima. The animal studies indicate a wide range of structural abnormalities during organogenesis, whereas the principal effect observed in humans is reduced head diameter with or without severe mental retardation. *Source:* Modified from Hall EJ. *Radiobiology for the Radiologist.* 4th ed. Philadelphia: JB Lippincott Co.; 1994.

Solid tumors have a longer latency period of approximately 20 to 40 years, whereas leukemias have an average latency of around 7 years. When counseling the pregnant patient or worker, it is important to let them know the magnitude of and potential for side effects. According to the International Council of Radiation Protection (ICRP) Publication 84, doses less than 1 mGy may be considered negligible, which is the approximate dose of normal background radiation (20). Exposures above 1 mGy require a more in-depth discussion with the patient. ICRP Publication 84 provides detailed risk assessments and counseling guidelines for *in utero* exposure.

Occupational Exposure

Once a pregnancy has been declared, the employee is encouraged to formally inform her employer. Further, the radiation safety officer should interview her, her employment should be evaluated for exposure history, and steps should be taken to minimize exposure. The National Council on Radiological Protection recommends that the embryo/fetus have limited exposure to less than 0.5 Sv/month (21).

INTRODUCTION TO RADIATION PHYSICS

Radiation physics is the study of the interaction of radiation with matter. In the treatment of patients with radiation, this matter is either tumor tissue or normal tissues such as the skin, the internal organs, or the supporting tissues and structures.

Units Used in Radiation and Radiation Therapy

Radiation is an abbreviation for electromagnetic radiation. It can occur in numerous forms. The most common forms used in radiation therapy are x-rays, γ-rays, and electrons. X-rays and γ-rays are also known as photons or packets of energy and are used to treat most body sites where radiation is deemed efficacious. Other particles or forms of radiation, such as protons, neutrons, and heavier alpha particles, are less commonly used in radiation therapy except in select clinical situations. Protons are used increasingly in the treatment of prostate cancers, choroidal melanomas, skull base and paraspinal tumors, and pediatric tumors. Neutrons have been used for salivary gland tumors, sarcomas, and prostate cancers.

X-rays and γ-rays are forms of electromagnetic radiation, similar to visible light, but with a much smaller wavelength, i.e., greater energy. The difference between x-rays and γ-rays is only their respective origins. X-rays are derived from interactions in the atom that are outside the nucleus, typically by bombardment of the atom or target with high-speed electrons. This is the source of radiation produced by most modern radiotherapy treatment machines termed linear accelerators or linacs. Their name derives from acceleration of these electrons. γ-rays arise from a process within the nucleus of the atom called radioactive decay, which occurs in brachytherapy sources and cobalt (^{60}Co) teletherapy treatment machines. This type of electromagnetic radiation can penetrate several millimeters to centimeters of normal tissue, in close proximity to tumors or tissues at risk. There is increased penetration as

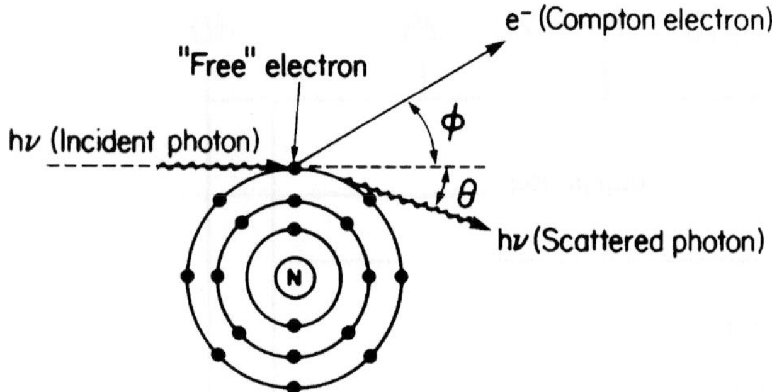

FIGURE 14.12. Schematic drawing illustrating the process of the Compton effect. The incident photon interacts with one of the atom's outer electrons, and the energy is shared between the ejected electron and a scattered photon. *Source:* From Purdy JA. Principles of radiologic physics, dosimetry, and treatment planning. In: Perez CA, Brady LW, eds. *Principles and Practice of Radiation Oncology*. 3rd ed. Philadelphia: Lippincott-Raven Publishers; 1998, with permission.

the energy of the gamma rays is increased. The x-rays produced by linear accelerators are much more penetrating than ^{60}Co gamma rays and are used to treat tumors or tissues at a distance from the linear accelerator such as deep within the pelvis or abdomen.

Electrons are small, negatively charged particles. Because of their inherent charge, these particles interact more strongly with the atoms found in tissue. Electrons will usually only penetrate a few millimeters to centimeters in tissue. Similar to photons, the higher the energy of the electron, the farther it will penetrate into the tissue. Electrons are used to treat tumors or tissues close to the skin surface such as superficial inguinal nodes and tumors of the skin, including vulvar cancers.

Regarding photon interactions with tissue, the dominant process at energies used in radiation therapy is termed the Compton effect (Fig. 14.12). The probability that a photon will interact with a target atom is inversely proportional to the energy of the incident photon and nearly independent of the atomic number of the target material. As a result, at the energies used in radiation therapy, termed megavoltage (MV), the absorbed dose in normal tissues is comparable to that in nearby bone. At much lower energies, termed kilovoltage (kV), the absorbed dose would scale with the atomic number of the target with higher absorbed dose in bone compared to normal soft tissues.

At the second International Congress of Radiology in 1928, the basic unit of exposure, the roentgen (R) was defined (22). Although the original definition evolved over time, the fundamental idea remained the same. The roentgen is the amount of photon radiation that causes 0.001293 g of air to produce one electrostatic unit of positive or negative charge (esu). The value of 0.001293 g is the mass of 1 cc of air at a temperature of 0°C and a pressure of 760 mm Hg. The definition of the roentgen can also be expressed in other equivalent terms:

$$1 \text{ R} = 2.58 \times 10^{-4} \text{ C/kg air}$$

or, conversely, expressed in SI units, the unit of exposure is defined by

$$1 \text{ C/kg} = 3{,}876 \text{ R}$$

Table 14.1 lists some basic units of radiation and radiation therapy, both in historic context and in terms of modern SI units. Kerma (kinetic energy release per unit mass) defines the transfer of energy from photons to directly ionized particles. These directly ionized particles, in turn, transfer some of their energy to the medium (usually tissue). This transfer of energy is defined as the absorbed dose to the medium from the radiation beam. The SI unit for kerma is joule per kilogram (J/kg) or gray (Gy). In a slightly confusing definition, the SI unit for absorbed dose is also joule per kilogram or gray. The term gray has replaced the previously used term "rad". Oftentimes the term centigray (cGy) is used. The cGy is equivalent to the rad and 1 gray equals 100 cGy.

Another rationale to think and communicate in SI units is that the roentgen was defined explicitly for photon interactions and not charged particles. Kerma and absorbed dose, although they have equivalence to the roentgen and exposure, can be defined equally for photons and charged particles.

RADIATION PRODUCTION

Radioactive Isotopes

As mentioned before, γ-rays are typically derived from radioactive isotopes, e.g., ^{60}Co. Electrons or beta particles also come from radioactive isotopes. In fact, most radioactive material produces a combination of photons (gamma rays) and electrons during the decay process. Radioactivity is the result of an atom changing its "energy" state, usually to a lower "energy" state, by the emission/absorption/internal conversion of photons or electrons in the atom. These processes result in disintegrations or radioactive decay whereby the atom releases photons or electrons or both during the change in "energy" states. The release of these particles is a form of radiation (or energy) that can be used to irradiate tissues. The absorbed dose resulting from this radiation depends on the energy and particle type as mentioned above, as well as the tissue in which it interacts.

Radioactivity, or activity, is denoted by the symbol A and is defined as the number of disintegrations per unit of time. The following relationship defines activity, the decay constant, and ultimately the half-life for a radioactive material:

$$A = N/t = \gamma N$$

This equation is solved using an exponential solution:

$$A = A_o e^{-\lambda t}$$

where A is the initial activity, λ is the decay constant, and t is some unit of time later. Other important units for radioactivity and radioactive decay are the half-life, $T_{1/2}$, and the average life, T_a. The half-life is the amount of time necessary to reduce the original amount of material by half. This is also equivalent to reducing the original activity by half. $T_{1/2}$ is related to the decay constant by $T_{1/2} = 0.693/\lambda$. The average life represents

TABLE 14.1

SI UNITS FOR RADIATION THERAPY

Quantity	SI unit (special name)	Non-SI unit	Conversion factor
Exposure	C kg^{-1}	roentgen (R)	1 C $kg^{-1} \approx$ 3876 R
Absorbed dose, kerma	J kg^{-1} (gray [Gy])	rad	1 Gy = 100 rad
Dose equivalent	J kg^{-1} (sievert [Sv])	rem	1 Sv = 100 rem
Activity	s^{-1} (becquerel [Bq])	curie	1 Bq = 2.7×10^{-11} Ci

the period of time that a hypothetical source would need, if it retained its original activity for a fixed period of time (T_a) before suddenly decaying to zero activity, to produce the same number of disintegrations over an infinite amount time by the same source if it decayed exponentially. T_a is related to the decay constant and the half-life by $T_a = 1/\lambda = 1.44\ T_{1/2}$.

Radioactive isotopes can occur naturally or be created artificially. Artificially created isotopes are usually created by neutron bombardment of otherwise stable isotopes. The resulting interactions produce atoms that are inherently unstable and will decay to a more stable form with a predictable half-life, releasing energy or radiation through this decay. Naturally occurring radioactive isotopes originally come from one of three standard series—the uranium series, the actinium series, and the thorium series—so named because of a dominant radioactive isotope in each series. In general, the higher the atomic number, the more likely an isotope will be radioactive. Table 14.2 lists many of the more common radioactive isotopes and their physical properties. For gynecologic cancers, use of radium 226 (^{226}Ra) sources is now historic. Though cost-effective because of its long half-life (1,622 years), radium releases a by-product, radon gas, if the integrity of the source capsule is compromised. This could require closure of hospital wards due to radon gas contamination. Cesium 137 (^{137}Cs) has replaced radium as a safer yet effective radioisotope. Less shielding is required for cesium than radium, and there is no

TABLE 14.2

PHYSICAL PROPERTIES AND USES OF BRACHYTHERAPY RADIONUCLIDES

Element	Isotope	Energy (MeV)	Half-life	HVL-lead (mm)	Source form	Clinical application
OBSOLETE SEALED SOURCES OF HISTORIC SIGNIFICANCE						
Radium	^{226}Ra	0.83 (avg)	1,626 years	16	Radium salt encapsulated in tubes and needles	LDR intracavitary and interstitial
Radon	^{222}Rn	0.83 (avg)	3.83 days	16	Radon	Permanent interstitial; temporary molds
CURRENTLY USED SEALED SOURCES						
Cesium	^{137}Cs	0.662	30 years	6.5	Cesium salt encapsulated in tubes and needles	LDR intracavitary and interstitial
Iridium	^{192}Ir	0.397 (avg)	74 days	6	Seeds in nylon ribbon; encapsulated source on steel cable	LDR temporary interstitial; HDR interstitial and intracavitary
Cobalt	^{60}Co	1.25	5.26 years	11	Encapsulated spheres	HDR intracavitary
Iodine	^{125}I	0.028	59.6 days	0.025	Seeds	Permanent interstitial
Palladium	^{103}Pd	0.020	17 days	0.013	Seeds	Permanent interstitial
Gold	^{198}Au	0.412	2.7 days	6	Seeds	Permanent interstitial
Strontium	^{90}Sr-^{90}Y	2.24 MeV β_{max}	28.9 years	—	Plaque	Superficial ocular lesions
DEVELOPMENTAL SEALED SOURCES						
Americium	^{241}Am	0.060	432 years	0.12	Tubes	LDR intracavitary
Ytterbium	^{169}Yb	0.093	32 days	0.48	Seeds	LDR temporary interstitial
Californium	^{252}Cf	2.4 (avg) neutrons	2.65 years	—	—	—
Samarium	^{145}Sm	0.043	340 days	0.060	Seeds	LDR temporary interstitial
UNSEALED RADIOISOTOPES USED FOR RADIOPHARMACEUTICAL THERAPY						
Strontium	^{89}Sr	1.4 MeV β_{max}	51 days	—	SrCl2 IV solution	Diffuse bone metastases
Iodine	^{131}I	0.61 MeV β_{max} 0.364 MeV *g*	8.06 days	—	Capsule NaI oral solution	Thyroid cancer
Phosphorus	^{32}P	1.71 MeV β_{max}	14.3 days	—	Chromic phosphate colloid instillation; Na^2PO^3 solution	Ovarian cancer seeding: peritoneal surface; polycythemia vera, chronic leukemia

Note: LDR, low dose rate; HDR, high dose rate.

risk of radon gas leakage. With a half-life of 30 years it is also cost-effective due to the infrequent need for replacement. Cesium can be used clinically for years without replacement, but the treatment duration must be adjusted to allow for radioactive decay (23). It is typically used for low dose rate gynecologic brachytherapy in tandem and ovoid and cylinder applicators. Iridium 192 (^{192}Ir) comes in various activities and can be used for interstitial and intracavitary gynecologic implants. Its half-life of 74.2 days requires frequent replacement and, typically, this is custom ordered individually for each implant rather than stored in the radiation oncology department like ^{137}Cs sources. High activity ^{192}Ir (^{10}Ci) sources are used for high dose rate brachytherapy and are replaced every 3 months, and lower activity ^{192}Ir sources are used for low dose rate brachytherapy.

Linear Accelerators

Linacs are another method of producing radiation for treatment of malignancies. Linacs can produce both photon and electron beams of different energies depending on their construction. The principles behind a linac involve accelerating an initial beam of electrons across a variable electric field. The greater the strength of the electric field, the more energetic the electron beam. This electron beam can be adjusted to control its shape and intensity before delivery to the patient. Alternatively, the electron beam can be directed to a tungsten target. The electron-target interaction creates a forward scattered photon beam or x-ray. The resulting photon beam can then be modified by the machine using filters and collimators to produce the desired radiation field shape.

Photon beams of different energies have a different absorbed dose pattern within tissues. This pattern is normally characterized as a percent depth dose or variation of dose as a function of depth within tissue, as shown in Figure 14.13 and Figure 14.14, and by dose profiles, or variation of dose as a function of lateral distance at a given depth (Fig. 14.15). The key feature in all of the figures is that higher energy photons deposit dose at greater depths. Because of the way dose is deposited and absorbed in tissue, the higher the photon energy, the less dose is deposited at shallow depths toward the surface of the patient. This is called "skin sparing" and is a characteristic of high-energy photons. In fact, the higher the photon energy, the deeper the point at which the maximum absorbed dose is deposited. After this D_{max}, the absorbed dose decreases because the photon beam is attenuated by the tissues through which it passes.

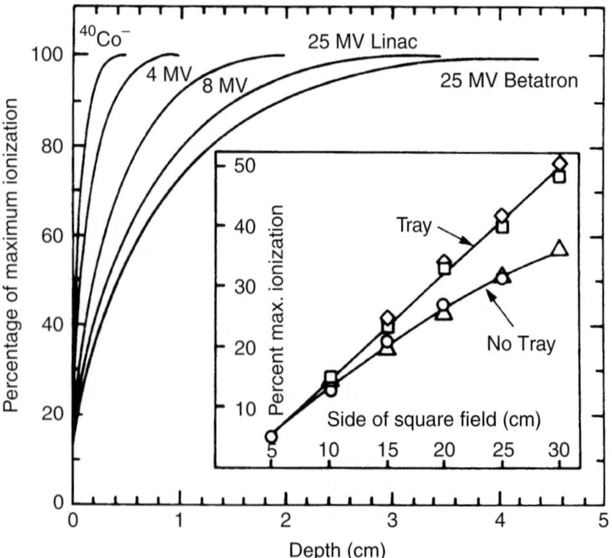

FIGURE 14.13. ^{60}Co to 25-MV x-rays. *Source:* From Velkley DE, Manson DJ, Purdy JA, et al. Build-up region of megavoltage photon radiation sources. *Med Phys* 1975;2:14–19, with permission.

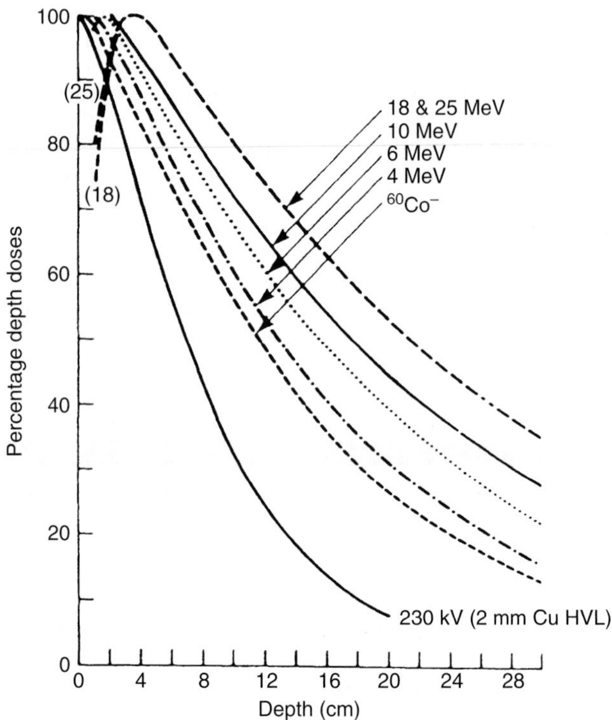

FIGURE 14.14. Typical x-ray or photon beam central-axis percentage depth-dose curves for a 10 × 10 cm beam for 230 kV (2 mm Cu HVL) at 50 cm SSD, ^{60}Co and 4 MV at 80 cm SSD, and 6 MV, 10 MV, 18 MV, and 25 MV at 100 cm SSD. The last two beams coincide at most depths but do not coincide in the first few millimeters of the build-up region. The 4-MV, 6-MV, 18-MV, and 25-MV data are for the Varian Clinic 4, 6, 20, and 35 units, respectively, at the Department of Radiation Oncology, Washington University in St. Louis. *Source:* From Cohen M, Jones DEA, Greene D. Central axis depth dose data for use in radiotherapy. *Br J Radiol* 1972;11:21, with permission.

Figure 14.16 shows a simplified drawing of a linac. The gantry (or part of the linac where radiation exits the machine) can rotate 360° around the patient on the treatment table. The table can also be rotated about the vertical axis of the radiation beam. This combination of angles allows the radiation to be directed to almost any part of a patient's body.

Modern linacs come equipped with mulitleaf collimators (MLCs) and asymmetric jaws to control the shape of the radiation beam directed before it reaches the patient (Fig. 14.17). Prior to asymmetric jaws and MLCs, photon beam shaping was achieved using poured blocks mounted below the lowest machine jaws. The composition and thickness of the poured block material are sufficient to block more than 97% of the radiation, allowing less than 3% of the radiation to penetrate the block and reach the patient. MLCs have mostly replaced poured blocks, but in some cases poured blocks are still necessary for detailed field shaping.

MLCs are small (projected size at the patient ~1 cm), adjustable collimators built into the linac gantry that work together to create a shaped opening mimicking the effects of a poured block. Because each MLC is adjustable, a new field shape can be "programmed" into the gantry without the necessity of pouring a different block for every treatment field. With the advent of computer-controlled motion of the MLCs,

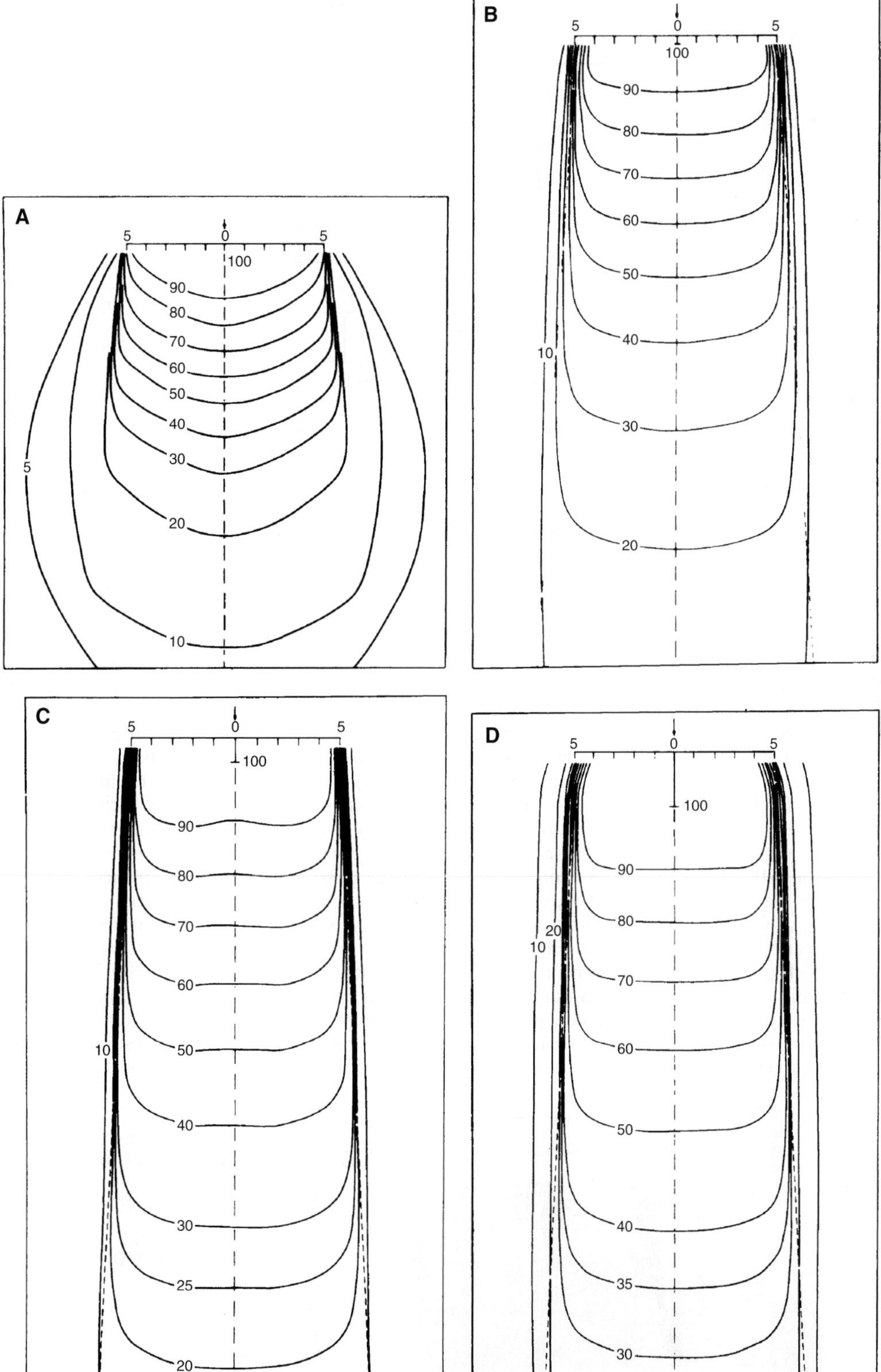

FIGURE 14.15. Isodose distributions for different quality radiation. **A:** 200 kVp, SSD = 50 cm, HVL = 1 mm Cu, field size = 10 × 10 cm. **B:** ^{60}Co, SSD = 80 cm, field size = 10 × 10 cm. **C:** 4-MV x-rays, SSD = 100 cm, field size = 10 × 10 cm. **D:** 10-MV x-rays, SSD = 100 cm, field size = 10 × 10 cm. *Source:* From Khan FM. *The Physics of Radiation Therapy*. 2nd ed. Baltimore: Williams & Wilkins; 1994, with permission.

the radiation field can be further controlled to produce an intensity modulated radiation therapy (IMRT) treatment. In IMRT treatments, the MLCs are used to create many small fields of radiation within a larger treatment field. By opening and closing these small fields, the intensity at any point within the large field can be modulated to give more or less dose to the tissues directly exposed to the radiation. At one gantry angle, the IMRT field may need to spare a critical normal structure but still treat the target to a lower dose, while in another gantry angle, that same critical structure may be out

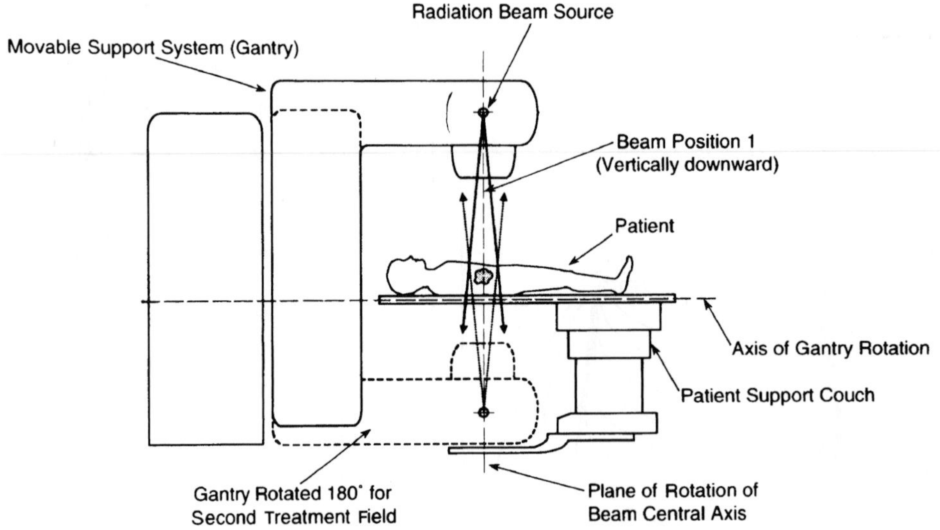

FIGURE 14.16. Example of multifield radiation therapy using parallel opposite beams with an isocentrically mounted radiation source.

of the field and the target can get a higher intensity to compensate for the lowered intensity in the first field. This adaptability allows the radiation treatment planner to create and deliver very complex treatment fields that improve target coverage while attempting to spare normal tissues. In practical terms, IMRT treatment plans are an improvement of the more conventional three-dimensional (3D) conformal treatment plans. 3D conformal treatment plans use fewer fields to achieve nominal coverage of the treatment target. At each gantry angle, the radiation is either hitting the target/normal tissue or not with a simple shaped treatment field. Normal tissues may be impossible to spare relative to adjacent targets. IMRT treatment plans may use similar gantry angle setups, but with the additional intensity modulation, the IMRT fields can create a complicated dose distribution within the patient. In some cases, where the normal tissues are relatively far from the target tissues, there may be no benefit or rationale for the more complex IMRT treatment plan compared to 3D conformal treatment plans. In cases where the proximity of normal tissues and target vary across a field and between gantry angles, IMRT may prove the more efficient treatment plan to protect normal tissues while focusing dose onto the target (Fig. 14.18).

IMRT is being explored for the treatment of gynecologic cancers. The setting where it may be the most helpful is in the postoperative setting for select endometrial and cervical cancer presentations. In this setting, there is often a significant amount of small bowel in the pelvis that can be avoided to a greater degree with IMRT than 3D conformal radiation techniques (24–27) (Fig. 14.19). Bone marrow sparing can also be improved over a 3D conformal approach (24). Bladder and rectosigmoid doses can also be reduced. Margin size around the target and bladder and rectal filling are important considerations as are immobilization techniques when using IMRT. RTOG 0418 has defined parameters for contouring of targets and normal organs, margin size, and dose volume constraints in the postoperative setting in early cervical or endometrial cancers. An online atlas has been developed to improve consistency between multiple contouring physicians (28). Other atlases are available to guide radiation oncologists in defining these structures of interest (29–30). When using IMRT to treat the intact uterus, bladder filling can have even more influence on the position of the uterus, and the vagina and uterus can move several centimeters as a result. Stool in the rectosigmoid can also cause movement of the adjacent pelvic organs and

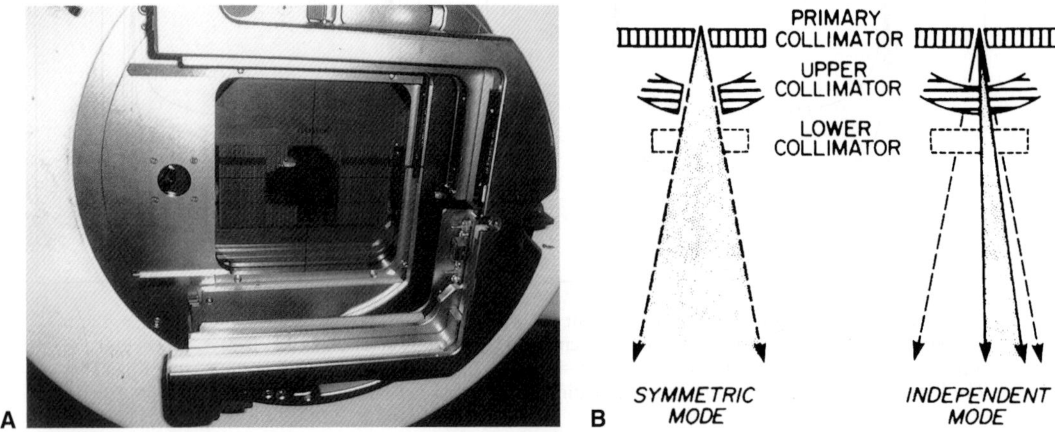

FIGURE 14.17. **A:** Multileaf collimator. *Source:* Courtesy of Varian Associates, Palo Alto, California, USA. **B:** Treatment technique for breast cancer using independent collimators. *Source:* From Purday JA, Klein EE. External photon beam dosimetry and treatment planning. In: Perez CA, Brady LW, eds. *Principles and Practice of Radiation Oncology*. 3rd ed. Philadelphia: Lippincott-Raven Publishers; 1998:281, with permission.

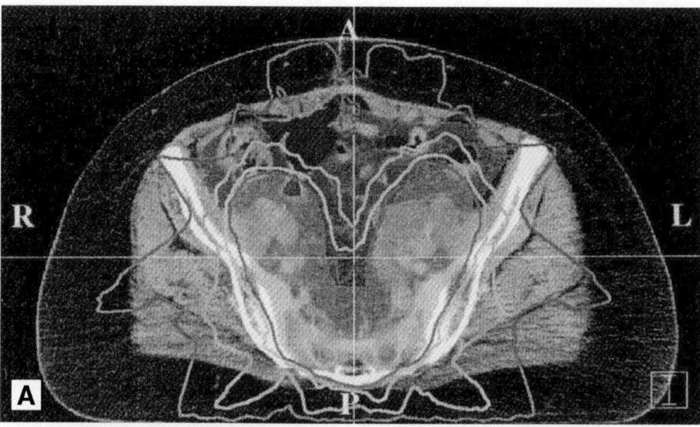

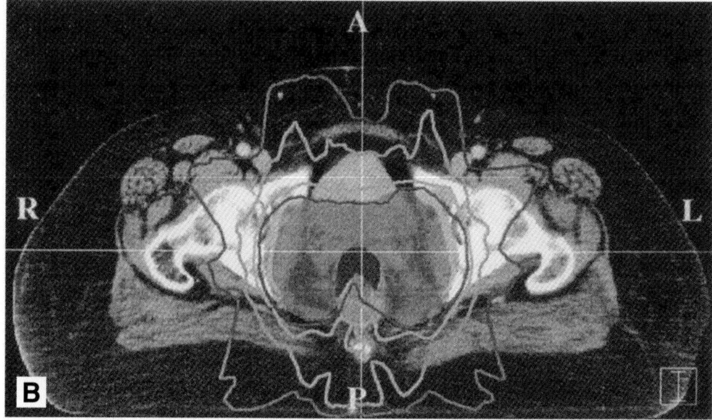

FIGURE 14.18. **A:** Isodose curves from a whole pelvic intensity-modulated radiation therapy plan superimposed on an axial CT slide through the upper pelvis. Highlighted are the 100%, 90%, 70%, and 50% isodose curves. **B:** Isodose curves from a whole pelvic intensity-modulated radiation therapy plan superimposed on an axial CT slide through the lower pelvis. Highlighted are the 100%, 90%, 70%, and 50% isodose curves. *Source:* Reprinted from Mundt AJ, Lujan AE, Rotmensch J, et al. Intensity-modulated whole pelvic radiotherapy in women with gynecologic malignancies. *Int J Radiat Oncol Biol Phys* 2002;52:1330, with permission from Elsevier.

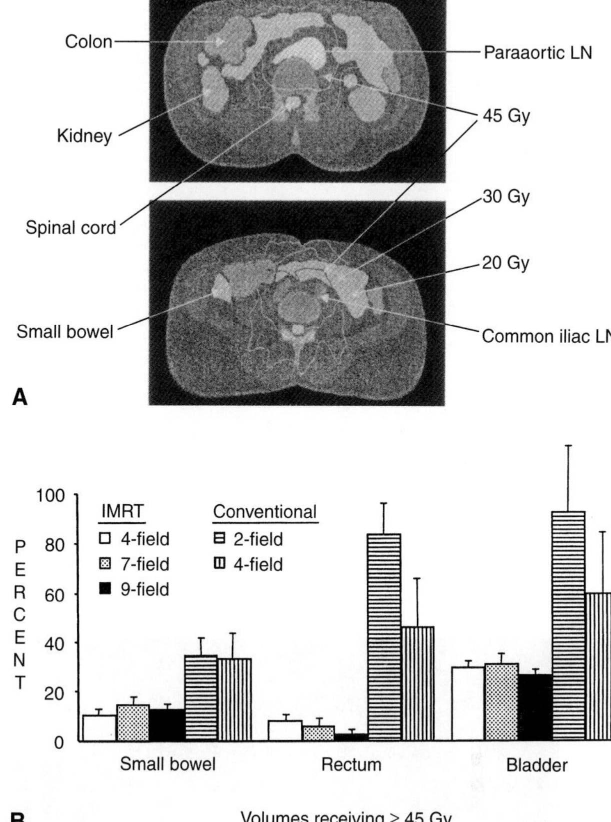

FIGURE 14.19. **A:** Axial views of intensity-modulated radiation therapy dose distribution. **B:** The functional volume of the small bowel, rectum, and bladder receiving ≥45 Gy with intensity-modulated radiation therapy and conventional techniques when 100% of the target volume (uterus) receives ≥95% of the prescription dose (45 Gy). *Source:* Reprinted from Portelance L, Chao KSCC, Grigsby PW, et al. Intensity-modulated radiation therapy (IMRT) reduces small bowel and bladder doses in patients with cervical cancer receiving pelvic and para-aortic irradiation. *Int J Radiat Oncol Biol Phys* 2001;51:261–266, with permission from Elsevier.

alter the dose distribution in the rectosigmoid. Use of IMRT in the definitive management of cervical cancer has been piloted at the University of Chicago (31–33). In their series, IMRT has reduced both acute and late gastrointestinal (GI) toxicities (34–35). The University of Chicago experience also revealed that IMRT in the setting of concurrent chemotherapy and radiation can also spare bone marrow during treatment (36). Use of IMRT for extended field irradiation, used for treating the pelvic and paraaortic regions, is also being explored to decrease dose to the small bowel, kidneys, liver, spinal cord, and bone marrow (Fig. 14.20). Selective boosting of gross nodal disease may allow for safer dose escalation (37–40). IMRT techniques are also being explored for whole abdominal irradiation to reduce doses to the gastrointestinal tract, liver, kidneys, and bone marrow and increase dose to the peritoneal surfaces and lymph nodes (41–42).

A relatively new feature for radiotherapy treatments is image-guided radiation therapy (IGRT). Historically, treatment setups were verified by orthogonal radiographs and treatment fields by port films or x-rays of the treatment fields superimposed on the patient. Modern linacs have added on-board imaging (OBI) that allows the treatment fields to be recorded electronically at every treatment setup using an electronic portal imaging device (EPID). By comparing computer generated radiographs (DRRs, or digitally reconstructed radiographs) with the actual patient images, discrepancies in field shape and patient setup can be corrected before the delivered treatment. This type of corrective behavior before treatment is the foundation of IGRT. The latest variation on IGRT is the addition of computed tomography (CT) scanners within the linear accelerator to verify more completely the correct alignment of the patient on the treatment table prior to treatment. CT scans are obtained prior to each treatment. In some cases, the CT scans are constructed based on the photon beams (MV) that will be used for treatment. In other cases, a different photon source (kV) is used to reconstruct the CT scan. Because cone beam CT (CBCT) or megavoltage CT (MVCT) uses a high-energy photon beam to gather the information for reconstruction, the image quality suffers because of poor soft-tissue contrast. kVCT or normal CT images, because they use a lower energy photon beam to reconstruct the patient image, have better soft-tissue contrast but are prone to distorting artifacts from high density objects within the patient, i.e., hip prostheses. In either case, the CT image at the time of treatment and its corresponding isocenter location are compared to the treatment planning CT and isocenter for agreement. Adjustments for rotation, lateral, vertical, and longitudinal discrepancies are made prior to treatment. The intent of these

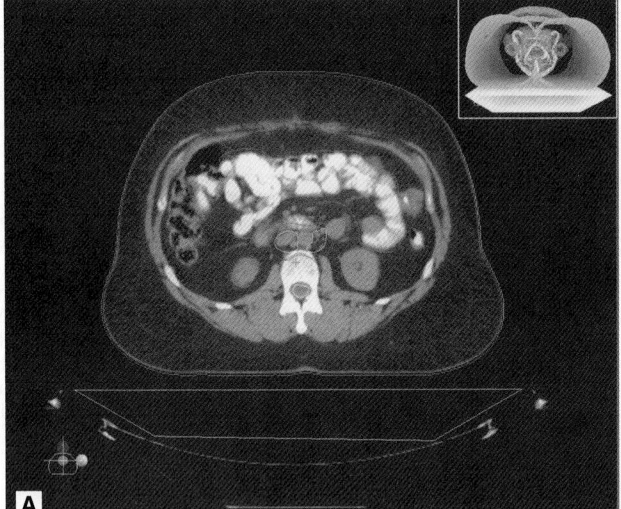

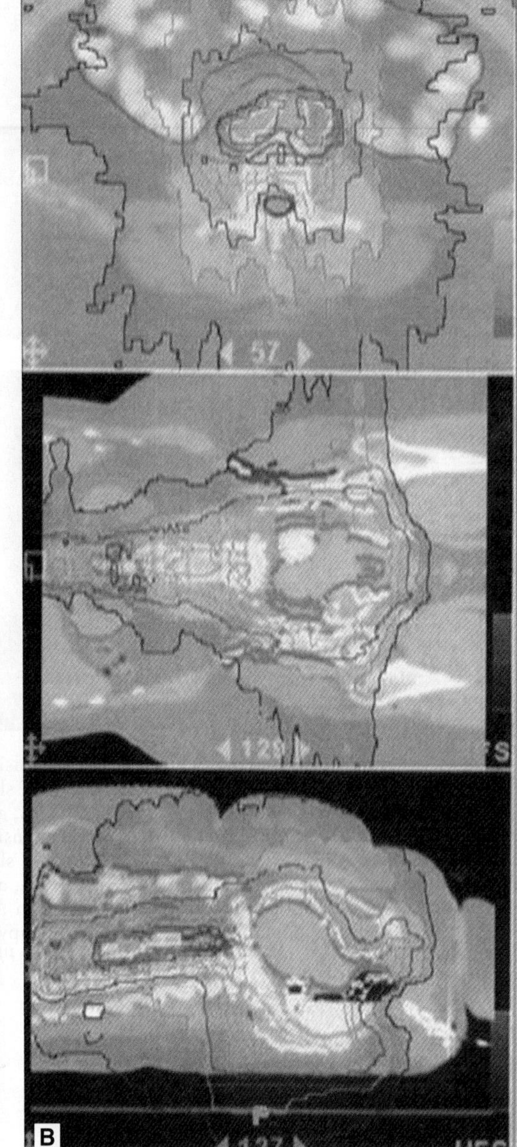

FIGURE 14.20. A: Contours of enlarged paraaortic nodes with margin are shown in close proximity to small bowel. **B:** IMRT plan for extended field irradiation in axial, coronal, and sagittal projections.

IGRT treatments is to improve the accuracy of the treatment setup on a daily basis relative to the original treatment plan. This enables decreasing the size of the radiation fields, as there is not as much need for a large margin on the target, which can decrease normal tissue irradiation and even allow for dose escalation to the target.

TomoTherapy (Fig. 14.21) is special type of linac/CT combination. TomoTherapy units were the first commercially available treatment machines that directly combined CT (MVCT in this case) with highly complex MLCs to deliver IMRT using IGRT. Each day, the patient receives an MVCT, a comparison using 3D fusion to the original treatment plan is made, adjustments to the patient position are made, and IMRT treatment is delivered without the patient needing to change machines. Corrections to the delivered dose can even be modeled based on the patient's current anatomy as visualized by the MVCT built into the TomoTherapy machine.

In addition to photon beams, many linacs also provide the option to treat patients with electron beams of various energies (e.g., 4 to 21 millionelecton volts [MeV]). Compared to photon beams, electron beams have different depth dose and dose profiles (Fig. 14.22), when electrons, even at the same energy as photons, do not penetrate as far as photons do within tissues. While electron depth doses have a D_{max} that increases with increasing energy, unlike photons, the higher the electron energy, the higher the surface dose to tissue, i.e., loss of "skin sparing."

Simulation

The conventional simulator used in radiation oncology departments reproduces all the gantry, collimator, and table rotations used in a linac treatment, and therefore "simulates" the actual treatment. Instead of a therapy (MV) photon beam, the conventional simulator uses a diagnostic (kV) photon beam to simulate the treatment beam. Previously, the conventional simulator (Fig. 14.23) allowed the radiation oncologist to determine beam direction and treatment fields that would be needed for a radiotherapy treatment based on x-ray fluoroscopy. The radiographic visualization of internal structures allowed special

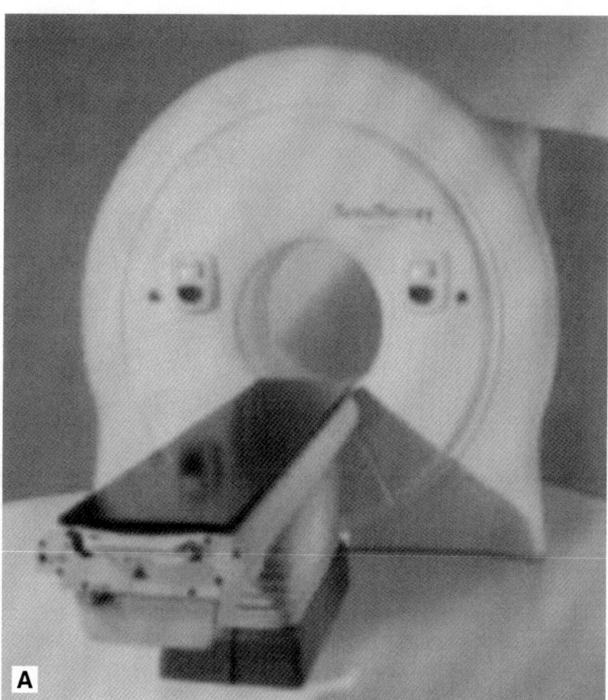

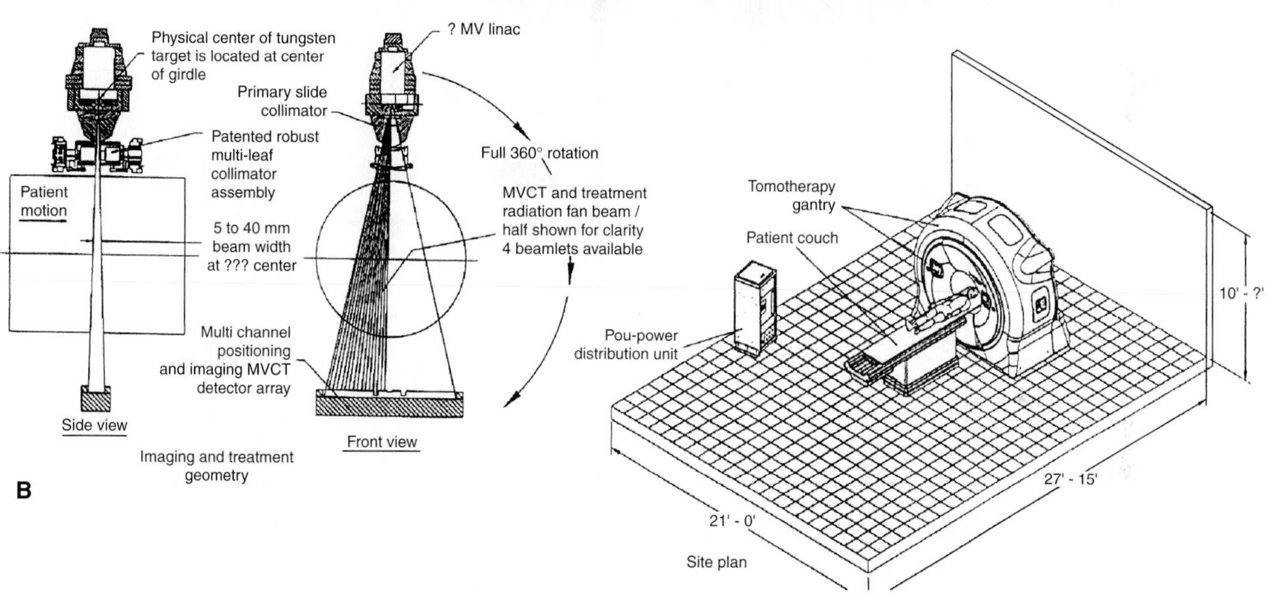

FIGURE 14.21. **A:** Helical TomoTherapy device commercially available for IMRT. **B:** Diagrammatic representation of the device. *Source:* Courtesy of TomoTherapy Inc., Madison, Wisconsin, USA.

shielding (poured blocks) to be constructed. All the geometric parameters of the conventional simulator are nearly identical to the actual treatment linacs. The intersections of the gantry rotation axis, collimator rotation axis (the machine isocenter), and patient location are identified and marked on the patient's skin with removable ink or a permanent series of tattoos. These marks facilitate the reproduction of the same clinical setup for the patient each day of treatment. Hard copy radiographs can also be used to document the expected treatment fields for comparison with port films obtained on the treatment linac.

CT-based simulators ("CTSims") have largely replaced conventional simulators in most radiation oncology departments. CTSims (Fig. 14.23) combine a diagnostic CT scanner with a software package that allows for the simulation of the patient setup in the virtual world of the computer. All of the necessary gantry angles and table angles are modeled in the computer. Computer controlled room lasers tied into the CTSim software allow the simulator therapist to identify the treatment isocenter in a fashion similar to the conventional simulator. DRRs are created for later comparison to actual treatment images. The treatment isocenter and the full CT images can then be transferred to the computer planning system for further treatment planning.

Computerized Dosimetry

In a modern radiotherapy department, computers are necessary to accurately calculate the absorbed doses to tissues. These absorbed doses within tissues are termed isodoses, or lines of the same dose. To initiate this process, CT images are acquired of the area of interest at a pretreatment planning

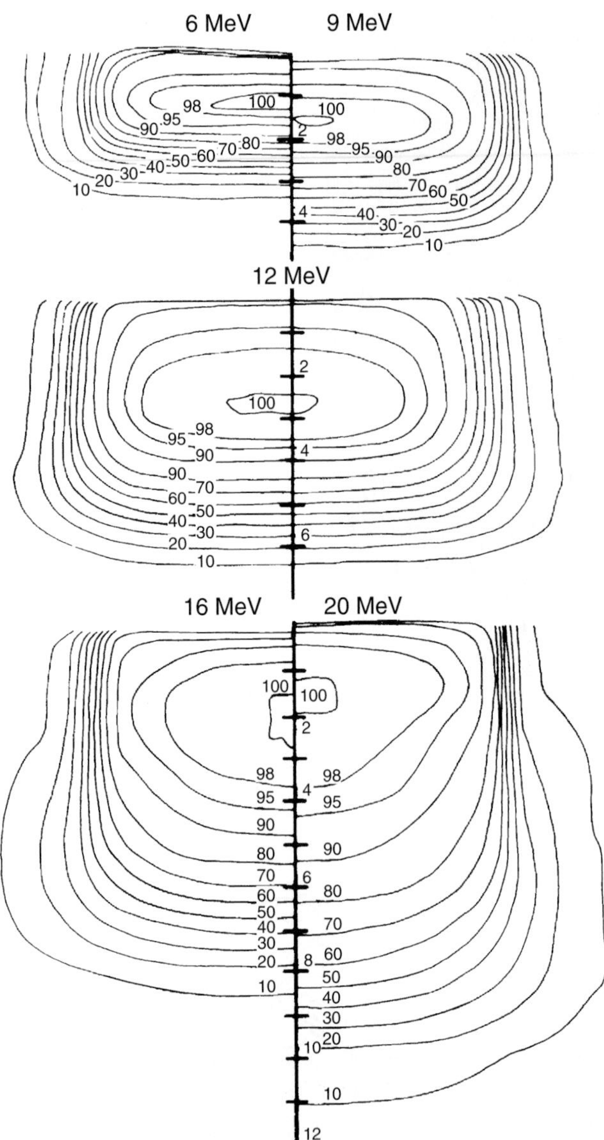

FIGURE 14.22. Electron beam central axis isodose curves for a 10 × 10 cm field at 100 cm SSD. These data are for the Varian Clinac 20 at the Department of Radiation Oncology, Washington University in St. Louis, MO. *Source:* From Glasgow GP, Purdy JA. External beam dosimetry and treatment planning. In: Perez CA, Brady LW, eds. *Principles and Practice of Radiation Oncology*. 2nd ed. Philadelphia: JB Lippincott Co.; 1992:208–245.

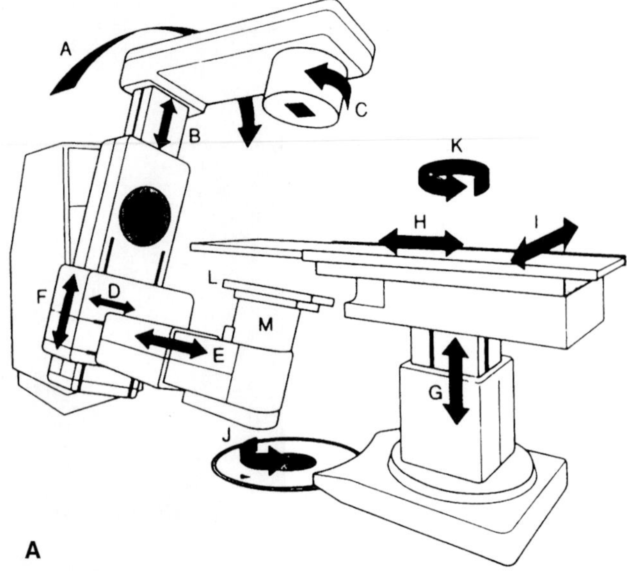

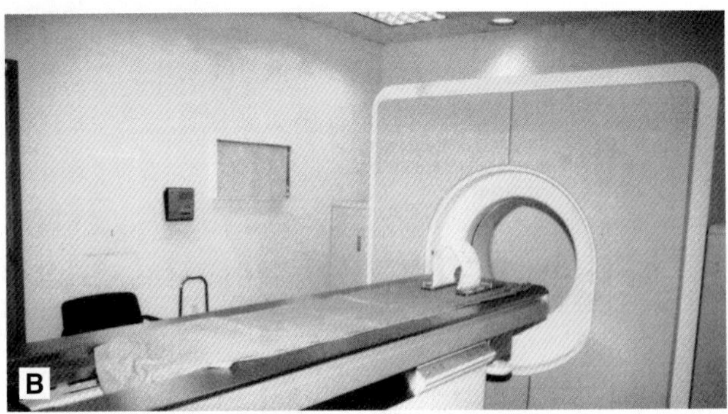

FIGURE 14.23. **A:** The basic components and motions of a radiation therapy simulator. A, gantry rotation; B, source-axis distance; C, collimator rotation; D, image intensifier (lateral); E, image intensifier (longitudinal); F, image intensifier (radial); G, patient table (vertical); H, patient table (longitudinal); I, patient table (lateral); J, patient table rotation about isocenter; K, patient table rotation about pedestal; L, film cassette; M, image intensifier. Motions not shown include field size delineation, radiation beam diaphragms, and source-tray distance. *Source:* From Van Dyk J, Mah K. Simulators and CT scanners. In: Williams JR, Thwaites DI, eds. *Radiotherapy Physics*. New York: Oxford Medical Publications; 1993:118 (Fig. 7.3). Reprinted by permission of Oxford University Press. **B:** Three-dimensional simulator that is basically a modified CT scanner with a flat couch suite for treatment planning.

session or simulation. These scans are typically obtained on the CT simulator. Treatment targets such as pelvic lymph nodes, the uterus, or vagina are identified through contouring on these images, as are normal tissues such as the rectosigmoid, bladder, and small bowel. Dose goals are identified for the targets and normal tissues. A dosimetrist uses this information to design the radiation treatment plan. Treatment beams are planned and the resulting dosimetry is reviewed by the treating physician and a physicist and altered as needed to best address the tumor and avoid the normal organs and tissues. In order for a computer treatment planning system to do all this, the depth dose and dose profiles for all the treatment beams (photons and electrons) must be accurately entered into the planning system.

There are varying complexities of treatment plans that might be used. For simple targets, e.g., metastatic cancer to the spine, a simple single field or parallel opposed, two-dimensional (2D) plan might be all that is required. Complexities of internal anatomy and external surface contours can be ignored while still successfully delivering a palliative treatment plan to the patient. More complicated target definitions might require specific and accurate knowledge of adjacent internal anatomy and the details of the patient's surface in order to accurately deliver a successful treatment plan. In these cases, a 3D conformal treatment plan is developed. In still more complicated target/normal tissue regions, IMRT treatment planning might be required in order to give sufficient dose to the target while minimizing the dose to an adjacent normal tissue. The goal for most treatment plans is to treat the target to a specified dose while minimizing dose to adjacent normal tissues.

In all of these examples, the word "target" is used. The goal is to encompass the target with the desired dose. Targets are more formally defined in ICRU 50 (43). Figure 14.24 illustrates the gross target volume (GTV), the clinical target volume (CTV),

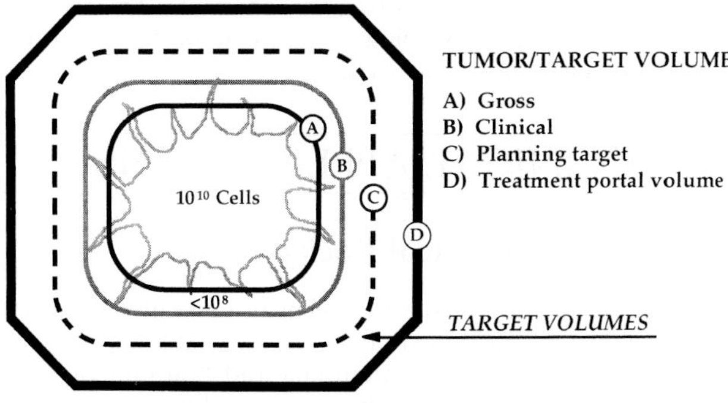

FIGURE 14.24. Schematic representation of "volumes" in radiation therapy. The treatment portal volume includes the gross target volume, potential areas of local and regional microscopic disease around the tumor (clinical), and a margin of surrounding normal tissue (planning). *Source:* From Perez CA, Purdy, JA. Rationale for treatment planning in radiation therapy. In: Levitt SH, Khan FM, Potish RA, eds. *Levitt and Tapley's Technological Basis of Radiation Therapy: Practical and Clinical Applications.* 2nd ed. Philadelphia: Lea & Febiger; 1992. Modified in Perez CA, Brady LW, Roti JL. Overview. In: Perez CA, Brady LW, eds. *Principles and Practice of Radiation Oncology.* 3rd ed. Philadelphia: Lippincott-Raven Publishers; 1998:1, with permission.

the planning target volume (PTV), and the treated volume. Each of the target or tumor volumes is larger than the previous target volume by some margin. The CTV includes all of the GTV plus possible microscopic extensions. The PTV includes all of the CTV plus a margin to account for possible geometric uncertainties of the patient or treatment margin. The irradiated volume includes all of the PTV plus any margins that might be included in the treatment plan to provide minimum dose coverage to the PTV.

Brachytherapy Principles

Brachytherapy is a term with Greek roots where "brachy" means "short distance." With brachytherapy, a highly concentrated dose of radiation is delivered to immediately surrounding tissues within millimeters to several centimeters of the applicators that carry the radioactive sources. This allows for a high dose of radiation to be delivered to closely approximated tumor and to relatively spare surrounding normal tissues such as the rectosigmoid, bladder, and small bowel. This is in comparison to teletherapy, where "tele" means "far distance" and refers to external beam irradiation where the radiation source is at a greater distance from the patient (~100 cm) than with brachytherapy. With external beam irradiation, the tumor and/or tumor bed are typically irradiated along with adjacent tissues at risk such as lymph nodes. External beam irradiation typically is much more penentrating than brachytherapy unless electron beam external irradiation is used. With electron beam therapy, superficial structures such as the skin and or superficial lymph nodes are optimally treated unlike the deep abdominopelvic tissues, which are best irradiated with the penetrating photons produced by a linear accelerator.

There are different types of brachytherapy or radioactive implants. Temporary implants are used most frequently and are categorized as interstitial or intracavitary. With interstitial brachytherapy, the radioactive sources are transiently inserted into tumor-bearing tissues directly through placement in hollow needles or tubes. With intracavitary brachytherapy, radioactive sources are placed into naturally occurring body cavities or orifices such as the vagina or uterus using commercially available hollow applicators such as a vaginal cylinder or tandem and ovoids. Temporary surface applications or plesiotherapy for ophthalmic or skin tumors and intraluminal applications in the esophagus, bronchus, and bile duct are other possible approaches. Permanent interstitial implants entail insertion of radioactive seeds (iodine 125 [^{125}I]; gold 198 [^{198}Au]; palladium 103 [^{103}Pd]) directly into tumor-bearing tissues to emit radiation continuously as they decay to a nonradioactive form (44). Radioactive sources are also sealed or unsealed, referring to whether they are solid (^{137}Cs; ^{192}Ir) or liquid radioisotopes (phosphorus 32 [^{32}P]). The most common sealed radioactive sources used for gynecologic brachytherapy are ^{192}Ir and ^{137}Cs. Historically, unsealed radioactive sources such as ^{32}P have been used to treat the entire peritoneal cavity in ovarian cancer. The limitation of this source was that the beta rays emitted only penetrated a distance of 3 mm, making it useful only for patients with microscopic or very thin residual tumor deposits following debulking.

Dose rate is also an important variable in brachytherapy. Traditional low dose rate (LDR) irradiation has been used for decades in gynecologic cancers using ^{226}Ra and ^{137}Cs sources for intracavitary insertions and low activity ^{192}Ir sources for interstitial insertions. High dose rate (HDR) brachytherapy has gradually been introduced over the last several decades and entails the use of a highly radioactive (^{10}Ci) ^{192}Ir source. There are several definitions for the dose rates used in brachytherapy. The ICRU 38 classifies LDR as 0.4 to 2 Gy/hr, MDR (medium dose rate) as 2 to 12 Gy/hr, and HDR as >12 Gy/hr (45). More standard ranges for LDR are 40 to 100 cGy/hr, and for HDR 20 to 250 cGy/min, which is 1,200 to 15,000 cGy/hr. Pulsed dose rate (PDR) is increasingly popular with the scarcity of available new ^{137}Cs sources. Rather than using a high activity ^{10}Ci ^{192}Ir source with short dwell times as in HDR, PDR uses a medium strength ^{192}Ir source of 0.5 to 1.0 Ci with dose rates of up to 3 Gy/hr. The radiation with PDR is typically delivered in a "pulsed" method over only 10 to 30 minutes of each hour as opposed to LDR techniques, which deliver 30 to 100 cGy/hr continuously over several days (46). PDR delivers the same total dose over the same total time at the same hourly rate as LDR, but with an instantaneous dose rate higher than LDR. PDR brachytherapy was developed to combine the isodose optimization of HDR brachytherapy with the biologic advantages of LDR.

The term "afterloading," whereby an unloaded applicator is inserted first and the radioactive sources introduced later, was popularized by Henschke (47–49). Nearly all modern brachytherapy exploits afterloading. An ideal implant is established with the appropriate applicator before being loaded with the radioactive sources. This sequence allows for more careful and accurate applicator placement than inherent to earlier "hot loaded" applicators, which were placed in the operating room preloaded with radium. Radiation exposure to medical personnel is reduced and exposure of operating room personnel is totally eliminated. Remote afterloading, which eliminates all personnel exposure, entails the use of a computer-driven machine to insert and retract the source(s), which are attached to a cable. During treatment, the source is transported from its shielded safe to the patient's applicators via a transfer tube. Sources are retracted automatically whenever visitors or hospital personnel enter the room. With modern remote afterloading techniques, a single cable-driven radioactive source is propelled through an array of dwell positions in needles, plastic tubes, or intracavitary applicators within an implanted volume. Through computerized dosimetry, the source stops for a specified duration at a preselected number of locations during its transit, delivering a specified dose to a defined volume of tissue. This dose may be delivered rapidly in a large fraction, as in the case of HDR brachytherapy, or a series of small "pulsed doses" delivered at a given frequency over a period of days, as in PDR brachytherapy (46). Typically, these treatment units are housed in shielded rooms in the hospital (LDR or PDR) or the radiation oncology department (HDR) to further eliminate radiation exposure (44).

Radiation Protection

The amount of radiation that a person other than patients under treatment can receive is governed by state and federal regulations. The actual values depend on whether the person is considered part of the general public or an occupationally exposed worker. These values can change with different regulations. The National Council on Radiation Protection and Measurements (21) set the following reccomendations for limits on exposure to ionizing radiation:

Public exposures <1 mSv or 0.1 rem annually
Occupational exposures <50 mSv or 5 rem annually

Additionally, NCRP Report #91 placed limits on embryo-fetus exposures:

Total dose limit <5 mSv or 0.5 rem
Dose equivalent limit in 1 month <0.5 mSv or 0.05 rem

These recommended limits were adopted by the Nuclear Regulatory Commission (10 CFR 20, Standards for Protection Against Radiation).

Linacs produce radiation using electrical power. Once the linac is turned "off," there is little, if any, radiation exposure risk to staff. Radioactive isotopes, used most often for brachytherapy, however, do not have an "off" switch. They are always undergoing radioactive decay with the resultant radiation production of x-rays, γ-rays, electrons, and other particles.

Radiation safety is an important focus for patient and health care workers. All hospitals that house radioactive sources or linear accelerators will have a special department termed radiation safety. Radiation personnel are responsible for monitoring radiation exposure in hospitals and clinics. All health care workers exposed to radiation must wear badges that track radiation exposure. There are three words that encompass all of the important aspects of radiation safety and protection: time, distance, and shielding. All three can be used to reduce radiation exposure. The dose delivered to a target from a radioactive source is directly proportional to the amount of time the target is exposed to the radioactive source (50). The dose delivered to a target is inversely proportional to the square of the distance from the radioactive source double the distance and the dose is reduced by a factor of four.

$$\text{Dose} \sim \text{time}$$
$$\text{Dose} \sim 1/r^2$$

This is the inverse square rule. The relationship between shielding and absorbed dose is more complicated. The simplest explanation is that the absorbed dose is reduced in an exponential relationship to the physical amount of shielding. The exact relationship (μ) depends on the energy of radiation and the specific material, e.g., concrete or lead, used to provide the protection. More material (x) means more protection. Less energy means more protection for the same thickness (x) of material.

$$\text{Dose} \sim e^{-\mu x}$$

Minimizing time, maximizing distance, and maximizing shielding will reduce one's absorbed radiation dose. Fortunately, there is relatively little exposure to radiation for most health care providers. The linear accelerators in radiation oncology are strategically located and shielded to minimize radiation to anyone other than the treated patient. Many brachytherapy insertions are typically performed with remote afterloading to minimize exposure, and often outpatient brachytherapy can be realized because of high dose rate techniques. This takes the patient off the hospital ward and thereby avoids exposure to the health professional caring for inpatients. The shielded rooms in the radiation oncology department protect the attendant staff from exposure as well.

CLINICAL APPLICATIONS

Historical Background

The use of radiation in the treatment of gynecologic cancers has a rich history. Roentgen rays were used externally as early as 1902 to treat cervical carcinoma and "radium rays" in 1906. In Europe, the use of intracavitary radium was reported in 1903 for the treatment of inoperable uterine cancers (51). Dr. Margaret Cleaves reported one of the first uses of intracavitary radium along with roentgen rays for the treatment of cervical carcinoma in New York in 1903 (52). In October of 1903, Dr. James Morton reported the use of a radium applicator "to be introduced within cavities where it had been heretofore impossible to practically introduce the X-ray" (53,54). In 1913, Robert Abbe was the first to report a true cure with a patient alive and well after 8 years of follow-up (54,55). In these early years, there was little knowledge of the biologic effects of radiation on the normal and tumor tissues. Typically, a uterine tandem was used alone without vaginal colpostats. There was little understanding of the dose distribution in the tumor and surrounding normal tissues, and implant duration, and thereby dose, was entirely empirical. Complications and failures were common.

Brachytherapy Systems for the Treatment of Cervical Cancer

Intracavitary brachytherapy for cervical carcinoma was profoundly impacted by the development of various "systems" that attempted to combine empiricism with a more scientific and systematic approach. A dosimetric system refers to a set of rules concerning a specific applicator type, radioactive isotope, and distribution of the sources in the applicator to deliver a defined dose to a designated treatment region (45,56). Within any system, specification of treatment in terms of dose, timing, and administration is necessary to implement the prescription in a consistent manner. Three systems were developed in Europe, including the Paris system, the Stockholm system, and the Manchester system (57,58). The Manchester system principles are an integral part of modern brachytherapy.

The Manchester System

The Manchester system was developed in 1932 by Tod and Meredith (59–61), and was later modified in 1953 (62) at the Holt Radium Institute. It standardized treatment with predetermined doses and dose rates directed to fixed points in the pelvis. The fixed points A and B were selected on the theory that the dose in the paracervical triangle impacted normal tissue tolerance rather than the actual doses to the bladder, rectum, and vagina. The paracervical triangle was described as a pyramidal-shaped area with its base resting on the lateral vaginal fornices and its apex curving around with the anteverted uterus. "Point A" was defined as 2 cm lateral to the central canal of the uterus and 2 cm from the mucous membrane of the lateral fornix in the axis of the uterus (Fig. 14.25). It often correlates anatomically with the point of crossage of the

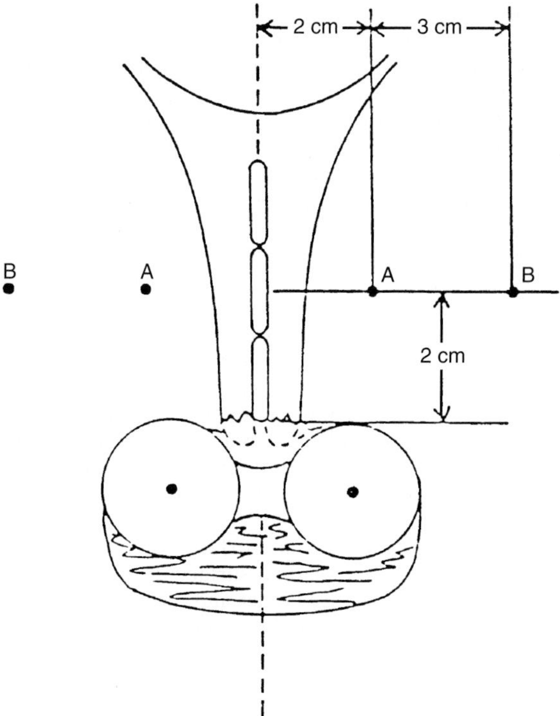

FIGURE 14.25. The Manchester system. Definitions of points A and B in the classical Manchester system are found in the text. In a typical application, the loading of intrauterine applicators varied between 20 and 35 mg of radium and between 15 and 25 mg of radium for each vaginal ovoid. The resultant treatment time to get 8,000 R at point A was 140 hours. Source: From Meredith WJ. *Radium Dosage: The Manchester System*. Edinburgh: Livingstone, 1967, with permission.

ureter and uterine artery and was taken as an average point from which to assess dose in the paracervical region. "Point B" was located 5 cm from midline at the level of point A and was thought to correspond to the location of the obturator lymph nodes. To achieve consistent dose rates, a set of strict rules dictating the relationship, position, and activity of radium sources in the uterine and vaginal applicators was devised. The amount of radium would vary based on ovoid size and uterine length such that the same dose in roentgen would be delivered to point A regardless of the size of the patient or the size and shape of the tumor, uterus, and vagina. The vaginal ovoids were available in three sizes: small (2.0-cm diameter), medium (2.5-cm diameter), and large (3.0-cm diameter) and were preloaded or "hot loaded" with radium. The amount of radium per ovoid varied by size to get a uniform dose rate at the ovoid surface. It was recommended to use the largest ovoid size possible and place the ovoids as far laterally as possible in the fornices to carry the radium closer to point B and increase the depth dose. Vaginal packing was used to limit the dose to the bladder and rectum to <80% of point A. Two intracavitary applications of 72 hours with a 4- to 7-day interval between them were given to deliver a dose of 8,000 R at 55.5 R/hr to point A and 3,000 R to point B. External beam irradiation with a midline block in place was later used to deliver a total cumulative dose of 6,000 R to point B.

The Manchester system underlies contemporary intracavitary techniques and dose specification (59–62). With current LDR applications using cesium rather than radium, it is considered standard to have a point A dose rate of 50 to 60 cGy/hr and to deliver a total dose of 85 Gy to point A and 60 Gy to point B when combined with external beam therapy.

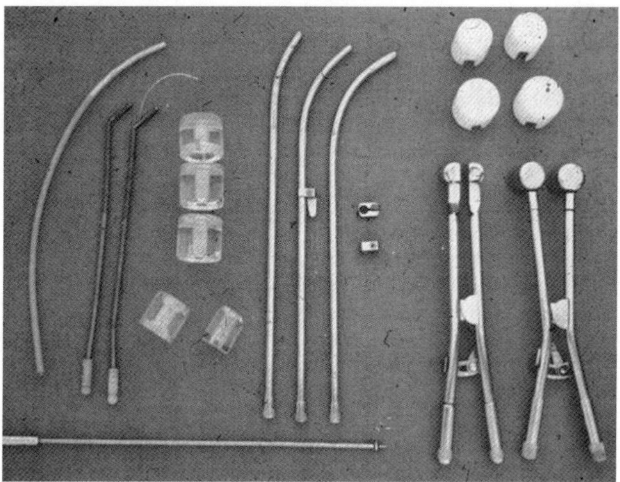

FIGURE 14.26. Fletcher Suit Delclos low dose rate applicators. **Left to right:** Afterloading colpostats, mini ovoids, tandems, cylinders, and source inserters. *Source:* Reprinted with permission from Fletcher, Gilbert H, eds. *Textbook of Radiotherapy*. 3rd ed. Philadelphia: Lea & Febiger; 1980:741 (Fig. 18A).

The Fletcher (M.D. Anderson) System

The Fletcher system was established at M.D. Anderson Hospital in the 1940s (63). The Fletcher applicator was subsequently developed and remains an integral part of gynecologic brachytherapy (Fig. 14.26) (64). The initial dosimetric work at M.D. Anderson was done prior to the development of computerized dosimetry in the 1960s (65–69). As in the Paris system, milligram-hours (mg-hrs) were used for dose prescription with the premise that with any geometric arrangement of specified sources, dose at any point is proportional to the amount of radioactivity and the implant duration. Though previous systems (Paris and Stockholm) had used mg-hrs, clinical experience alone determined the amount of radium tolerable to the tissues. Fletcher predicted that better results and less morbidity could be obtained if knowledge of the energy absorbed at various points in the pelvis ("measured data") such as the bladder and rectum and pelvic lymph nodes could be determined (70). According to Fletcher, a dosimetric approach should meet the following requirements: (a) ensure that the primary disease in the cervix and fornices and immediate extensions into the paracervical triangle are adequately treated; (b) guide treatments in such a way that the bladder and rectum are not overdosed (respect mucosal tolerance); and (c) determine the dose received by the various lymph node groups. Individualization to fit the anatomical situation was an essential aspect of this system (71).

The primary prescription parameter in the Fletcher system was tumor volume and prescription rules were based on maximum mg-hrs and maximum time, taking into account the total external beam dose and the calculated sigmoid dose. An application was left in place until either of these two maximums was reached. Large mg-hr implants were halted by the mg-hr prescription while smaller mg-hr implants were terminated by time. A set of maxima of mg-hrs was established for combinations with external irradiation, which were published in tables (72,73). Standardized source arrangements and limits on the vaginal surface dose and mg-hrs were all used to help specify treatment.

Despite a more elaborate dosimetry system, the Fletcher system combined many elements of the Paris and Manchester systems, including using the largest size ovoid possible positioned as far laterally and cephalad as possible to give the highest tumor dose at depth for a given mucosal dose. By using a larger ovoid, the radium-mucous membrane distance was increased, allowing a greater increase in the total number of mg-hrs and a greater volume of adequate irradiation (63). The Fletcher colpostats were actually a further evolution of the Manchester ovoids and were made with the same diameters of 2, 2.5, and 3 cm but were more cylindrical than Manchester "ovoids" and were attached to handles, with shielding in the direction of the bladder and rectum. Initially these were preloaded with radium, but later an afterloading model was developed and loaded instead with ^{137}Cs (74–77). Recommended loadings were 15, 20, and 25 mg of radium for the 2, 2.5, and 3 cm colpostats, respectively, and 5 to 10 mg for the mini-ovoids (74). Like the earlier systems, it was also recommended to use the longest tandem available and load the tandem so that sources reached the uterine fundus to give an adequate distribution in the lower uterine segment and paracervical areas and to increase the dose to the obturator lymph nodes. Additionally, a high position of the applicator in the pelvis and a wide separation of the ovoids were thought to increase the dose to the pelvic wall (63,78). Tight packing was also recommended to displace the system upward and centrally and to decrease the dose to the bladder and rectum (63). Recommended tandem loadings were usually 15-10-10 mg of radium with the amount of radium in the tandem usually greater than that in the ovoids (71). The distal source in the tandem was to be positioned to produce an even pear-shaped dose distribution with no drop in dose rate between the tandem and ovoids, without excessive overlap that would cause a hot spot on the adjacent bladder or rectal mucosa. With the ovoids well positioned, this was usually accomplished by placing the physical end of the distal source at or a few millimeters beyond the external os of the cervix. A 10-mg protruding source was recommended if the vaginal ovoids were separated by more than 5 cm or displaced caudally, with each ovoid then decreased by 5 mg.

A careful review of implant films was outlined (Figure 14.27). It was recommended to keep the tandem in the axis of the pelvis, equidistant from the sacral promontory and pubis and the lateral pelvic walls to avoid overdosage to the bladder, sigmoid, or one ureter. The tandem was recommended to bisect the ovoids on the AP films and bisect their height on the lateral films (79). The flange of the tandem was to be flush against the cervix and the ovoids surrounding it, verified by confirming the proximity of the applicators to radio-opaque cervical seeds. Radio-opaque vaginal packing was used to hold the system in place and displace the bladder and rectum. Scrutiny of implant films prior to treatment remains an important tenant of brachytherapy. Two or more intracavitary insertions were thought to make more efficient use of the inverse square law such that the second and third implants would deliver intense radiation to the tumor periphery because of interval tumor regression. A recent retrospective review of implant geometry has confirmed the consistency of the M.D. Anderson approach and the good outcomes achieved when attention is paid to applicator position in the pelvis (80).

The current M.D. Anderson approach to treatment specification reflects a policy of treating advanced cervical carcinoma to normal tissue tolerance (81). This includes integrating standard loadings and mg-hrs with calculated doses to the bladder, rectum, sigmoid, and vaginal surface. The activity in the ovoids is limited by the vaginal surface dose, which is kept below 140 Gy. Calculated bladder and rectal doses are noted and are sometimes used to limit the duration of the intracavitary system, with the combined external beam and implant doses for the bladder kept at <75 to 80 Gy and for the rectum at <70 to 75 Gy. Mg-Ra-eq-hrs are usually limited to 6,000 to 6,500 after 40 to 45 Gy external beam. Though mg-hrs have usually been used to guide and report doses at M.D. Anderson, recent retrospective reviews have also reported point doses, though these have not been used to plan or prescribe treatment. With the implant loadings and durations outlined by Fletcher, typical dose rates at point A are approximately 57 cGy per hour and vaginal surface dose rates are 100 cGy/hr (80,82). The median doses to point B and to the International Commission on Radiation Units & Measurements (ICRU) rectal and bladder reference points averaged 28%, 59%, and 60% of the point A doses, respectively (80). The median total dose to point A from external beam and intracavitary irradiation

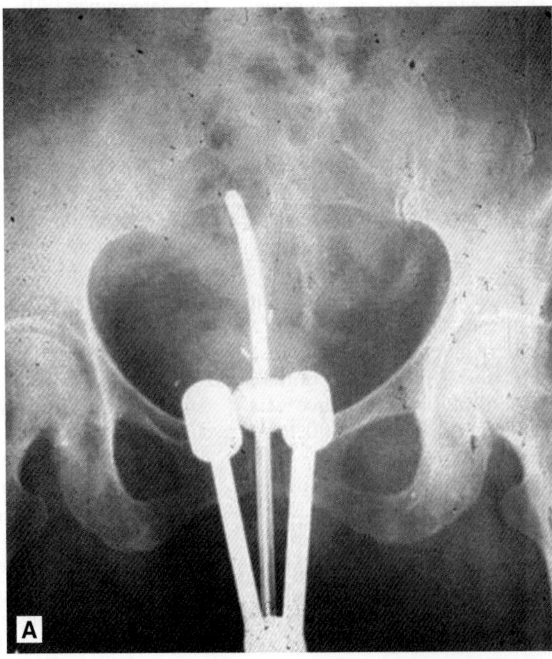

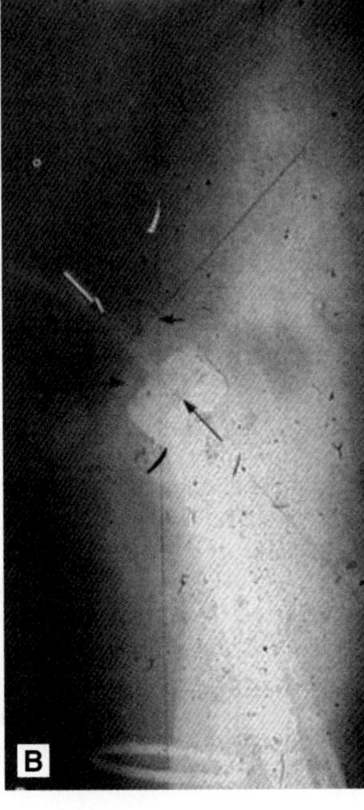

FIGURE 14.27. Ideal position of tandem and ovoid applicator on an AP radiograph (A) and a lateral radiograph (B). Note the metallic seeds inserted into the cervix. *Source:* Reprinted with permission from Fletcher, Gilbert H, eds. *Textbook of Radiotherapy*. 3rd ed. Philadelphia: Lea & Febiger; 1980:745 (Fig. 11–24).

was 87 Gy, and the median doses to the bladder and rectum were 68 and 70 Gy. The total dose delivered to the vaginal surface was limited to 120 to 140 Gy or 1.4 to 2.0 times the point A dose (80). These total doses to point A and the vagina, bladder, and rectum are used as contemporary guidelines for determining implant duration and therefore dose.

Point A Redefined

The failure of localization radiographs to show the surfaces of the ovoids made implementation of the initial definition of point A difficult. The definition of point A was modified in 1953 to be "2 cm up from the lower end of the intrauterine source and 2 cm laterally in the plane of the uterus, as the external os was assumed to be at the level of the vaginal fornices" (Fig. 14.28) (62). This definition of point A is currently used at many institutions (83,84). A seed or marker ball placed near the exocervix and coincident with the tandem flange is used to identify the exocervix on the localization films. This definition, however, becomes problematic when the cervix protrudes between the ovoids (Fig. 14.29). This causes a resultant increase in dose rate at point A because point A lies in the higher dose "bulge" around the ovoids (78). The variation of point A often occurs in a high-gradient region of the isodose distribution. A consistent location for dose specification should fall sufficiently superior to the ovoids where the dose distribution runs parallel to the tandem (Fig. 14.30) (85,86). In patients with deep vaginal fornices, reverting to use of the ovoid surface rather than the exocervix can help to solve this problem (85,87).

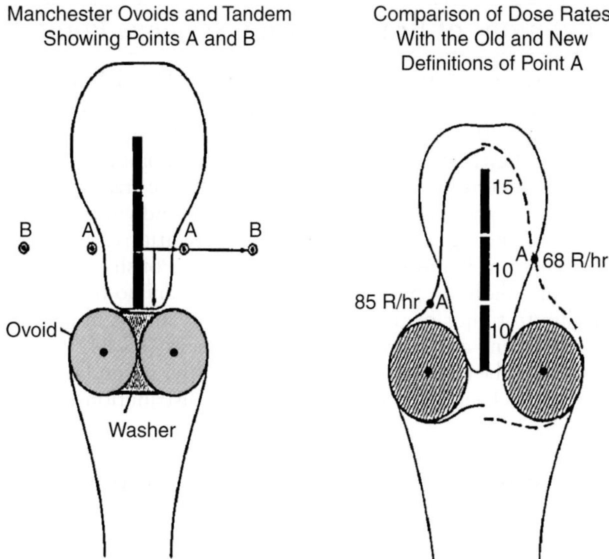

FIGURE 14.29. The definition of point A using the revised Manchester definition becomes problematic when the cervix protrudes between the ovoids, causing an increase in dose rate at point A. Use of the classical Manchester definition of point A (point A defined from the level of the upper vaginal fornices rather than the location of the exocervix) may be helpful. *Source:* Reprinted with permission from Batley F, Constable WC. The use of the Manchester system for treatment of cancer of the uterine cervix with modern afterloading radium applicators. *Am J Roentgenol Rad Ther* 1967;18:397 (Figs. 1 and 2).

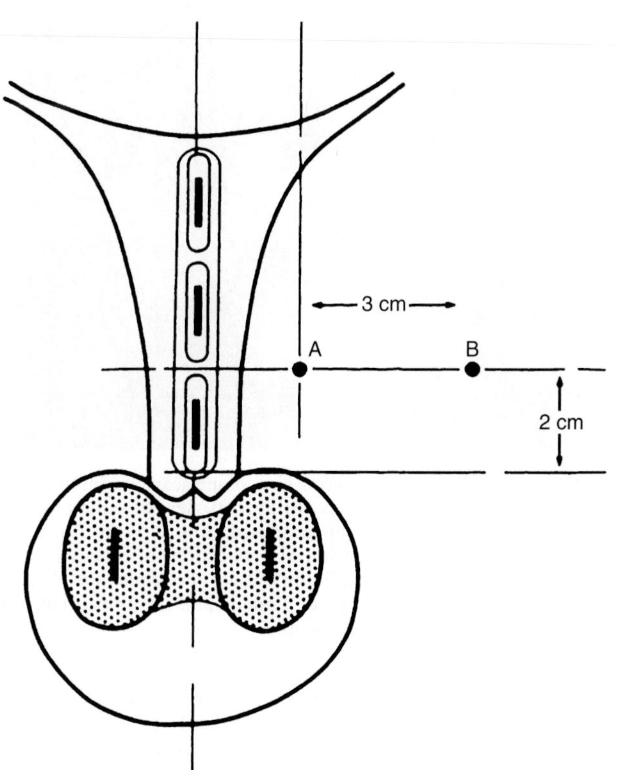

FIGURE 14.28. Revised Manchester system definition of point A. *Source:* From Morita K. Cancer of the cervix. In: Vahrson HW, ed. *Radiation Oncology of Gynecologic Cancers.* 1st ed. Berlin, Heidelburg, New York: Springer-Verlag; 1997:185.

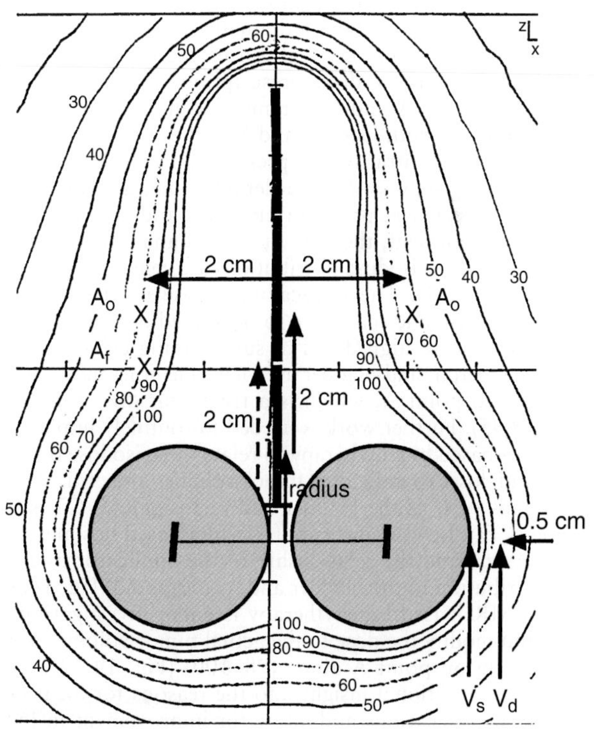

FIGURE 14.30. Variations of point A based on definition. A consistent location for dose specification should fall superior to the ovoids where the dose distribution runs parallel to the tandem and not close to bulge of the pear. *Source:* Reprinted with permission from Nag S, Chao C, Erickson B, et al. American Brachytherapy Society recommendations for low-dose rate brachytherapy for carcinoma of the cervix. *Int J Radiat Oncol Biol Phys* 2002;52(1):38 (Fig. 2).

Limitations of Brachytherapy Systems: Point A

It has become clear over time that points A and B are not anatomic sites. The actual specification is related to the position of the intracavitary sources rather than to an anatomical structure. Lewis et al. also demonstrated that point A does not maintain a constant relationship to any specific structure and its position varies with the type of applicator, individual tumor anatomy, and age of the patient. No correlation was found between point B and the pelvic wall (88,89). Potish also questions the validity of point A as its position bears no fixed relationship to tumor or normal tissue anatomy and is in a steep dose gradient and sensitive to displacement (83,84,90,91). Point A can be identical for implants that differ in fundamental ways and deliver different overall 3D dose distributions.

Limitations of Brachytherapy Systems: Mg-Hr Systems

The use of mg-hr systems also continues at many institutions to guide the choice of source strength and duration of the implant, estimate the risk of complications, compare treatment between patients and institutions, and estimate efficacy (92,93). In the past, little attempt was made to obtain dose information to anatomical structures, and mg-hr prescriptions were not necessarily accompanied by isodose distributions so that the dose prescription was not related to patient anatomy.

Contemporary Dose Specification for Cervical Cancer

The advent of afterloading applicators and computerized dosimetry has brought about a dramatic change in dosimetric analysis (65,66,94). For cervical cancer, there continue to be two basic systems of dose prescription, mg-hrs and the Manchester point A and B systems, and many prescription systems combine both Fletcher and Manchester elements. The basic principle of intracavitary prescription is to leave a specific loading of sources in for a definite time, determined by empirical experience, prescription rules, and computerized dosimetry. At present, the dose at several anatomic points is evaluated, and the isodose distributions are generated by computer (Fig. 14.31). The intracavitary dose is based on the extent of disease and may have to be altered if computer calculations indicate high doses to surrounding critical structures. The rectum and bladder are viewed as tolerance points, compared to point A, which is a treatment dose reference point (78,95). Further work is needed to routinely implement 3D-image–based brachytherapy to relate these isodose distributions and doses to individual tumor volumes and critical normal organs such as the bladder and rectosigmoid. CT-based dosimetry can be used instead of 2D film-based dosimetry to better understand the relationship of the applicator and the dose distribution to the bladder and rectosigmoid (Fig. 14.32) (96,97). MRI-based brachytherapy is under investigation to assess and modify the dose to the actual tumor volume rather than relying on point A alone (98–100) (Fig. 14.33). This should give additional insight into the reasons for local failures and complications and allow for improvement in local control and late toxicities.

Dose Specification Points for Cervical Cancer

At institutions using a derivation of the Manchester system, dose is typically specified at various points such as A and B.

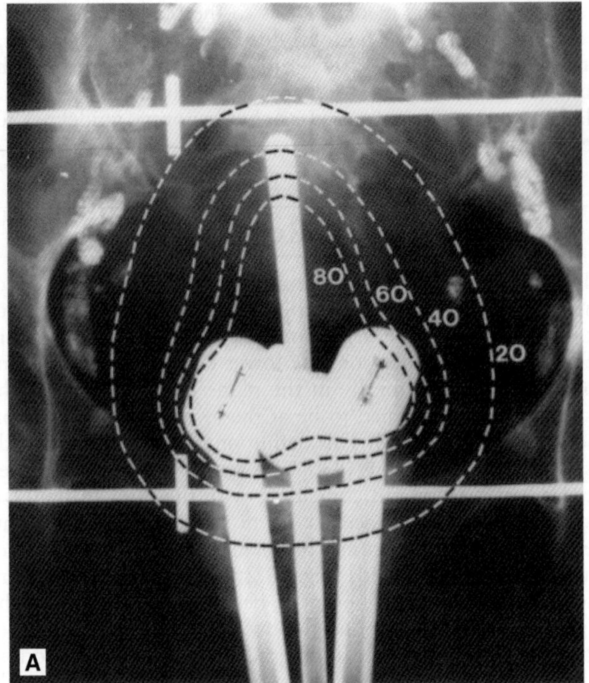

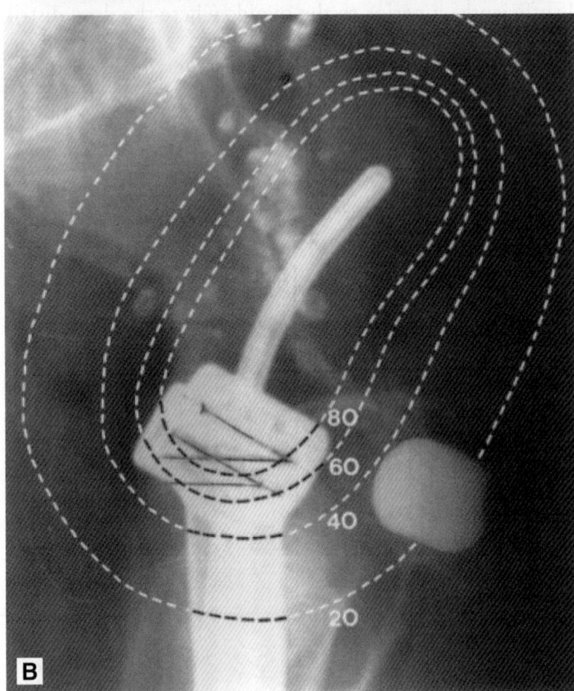

FIGURE 14.31. A: Anteroposterior view of intracavitary insertion for carcinoma of the uterine cervix. **B:** Lateral view of same implant. Isodose curves (cGy/hr) are superimposed. *Source:* From Perez CA, Grigsby PW, Williamson JF. Clinical applications of brachytherapy. I: low dose-rate. In: Perez CA, Brady LW, eds. *Principles and Practice of Radiation Oncology*. 3rd ed. Philadelphia: Lippincott-Raven Publishers; 1998:487, with permission.

A combination of both mg-hrs and point doses is used at some institutions to guide implant duration (81,101). Though these definitions vary from institution to institution, most will attempt to quantify doses in the paracervical region (point A), and at either point B or the pelvic wall (C or E), and the rectum and bladder (83,84). Unfortunately, intracavitary point dose calculations are not recorded as often for the sigmoid, vaginal mucosa, or cervix. Dose evaluation at these points is

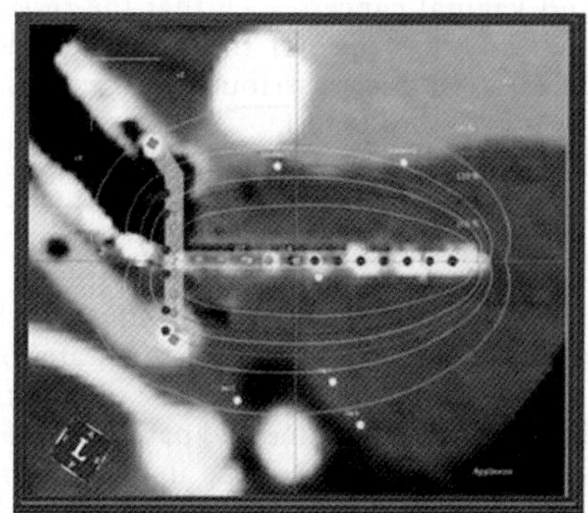

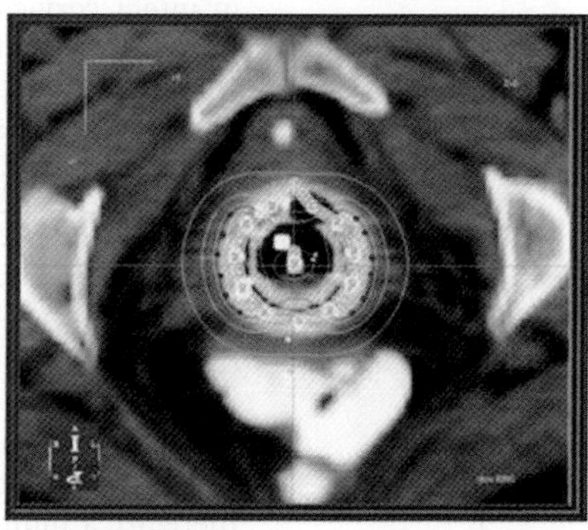

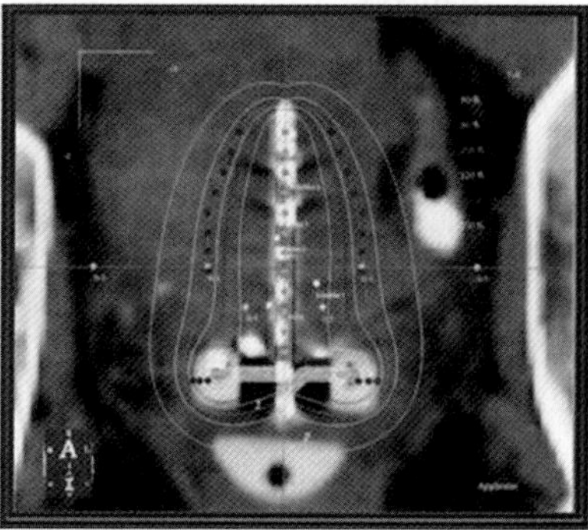

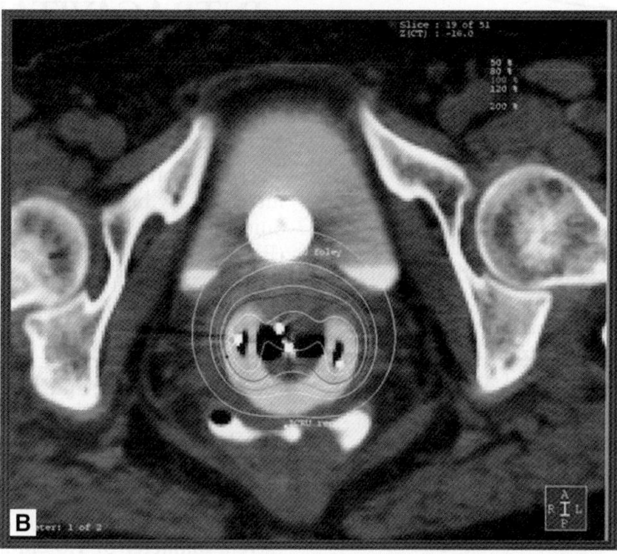

FIGURE 14.32. A: Sagittal, coronal, and axial CT images with MRI/CT compatible applicator in place showing the isodose distribution around the applicator and within the surrounding tissues. B: Axial CT at the level of the Foley catheter bulb near the traditional ICRU 38 bladder and rectal points. Contrast is present within the bladder and rectum as well as the bladder catheter bulb.

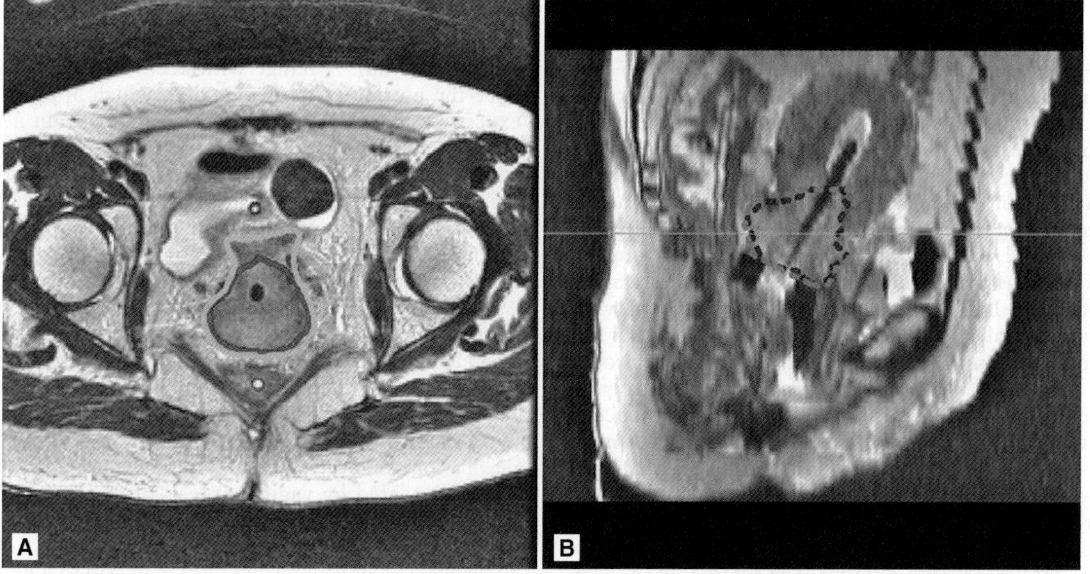

FIGURE 14.33. Axial (A) and sagittal (B) MRI images with MRI compatible applicator in place with contours of the gross target volume (GTV) and high risk clinical target volume (HRCTV).

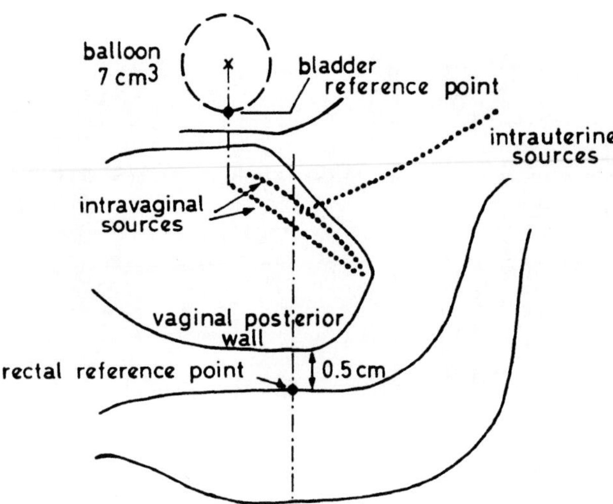

FIGURE 14.34. Reference points for bladder and rectal brachytherapy doses proposed by ICRU. *Source:* From International Commission on Radiation Units and Measurements. *Report 38: Dose and Volume Specification for Reporting Intracavitary Therapy in Gynecology.* Bethesda, MD: International Commission on Radiation Units; 1985:11, with permission.

also recommended. Maruyama et al. defined a point T (tumor dose) located 1 cm above the cervical marker and 1 cm lateral to the tandem, which is usually 2 to 3 times the dose at point A (102) and has been used at other institutions (103,104). Vaginal surface dose rates, defined at the lateral ovoid surface, will vary based on applicator diameter and available source strengths and should be in the range of 1.4 to 2.0 (the point A dose) (80,105).

Though frequently confused, the ICRU 38 system (Dose and Volume Specification for Reporting Intracavitary Therapy in Gynecology) is a dose reporting system, not a dose specification system (Fig. 14.34) (45). This was developed so that comparisons could be made between centers using different brachytherapy systems. It provides definitions for determining dose to the bladder and rectum in addition to other characteristics of the implant.

Importance of Brachytherapy in Cervical Cancer

When curative treatment is planned, patients with cervical carcinoma treated with definitive irradiation should receive a combination of external beam irradiation and brachytherapy. As revealed in the Patterns of Care Studies (PCS) and the retrospective series of Perez et al., recurrences and complications are decreased when brachytherapy is used in addition to external beam (82,101,106–108). Use of an intracavitary implant was the single most important treatment factor in multivariate analysis for stage IIIB cervical cancer with respect to survival and pelvic control in the 1973 and 1978 PCS (109,110). Retrospective series with external beam alone have proven marginal outcomes with this approach. The efficacy of brachytherapy is attributable to the ability of radioactive implants to deliver a higher concentrated radiation dose more precisely to tissues than external beam alone, which contributes to improved local control and survival. At the same time, surrounding healthy tissues such as the bladder and rectosigmoid are relatively spared due to the rapid fall-off of dose around the applicators with distance. The external beam component of treatment is also very important as it addresses tissues at a distance from the applicator such as the pelvic lymph nodes. The external beam also brings about tumor regression in intact cervical and vaginal cancers such that the residual tissue is brought within the range of the pear-shaped or cylindrical-shaped radiation dose distribution around standard applicators (44).

Brachytherapy Applicators

Given the importance of brachytherapy, it is important to select the appropriate applicator to accommodate patient anatomy and the disease and shape the associated isodose distribution to encompass the disease. Tumor volume and patient anatomy are key in this decision. Tumor size and shape are variable, and there are a multitude of applicators available to address these diverse presentations.

INTRACAVITARY APPLICATORS: CERVICAL CANCER

Low Dose Rate

There are varieties of low dose rate applicators available for intracavitary brachytherapy. The best known are the Fletcher-Suit and Henschke tandem and ovoid (colpostat) applicators (Fig. 14.26). In 1953, Fletcher published an article introducing his preloaded radium applicator, which was designed to produce the largest possible volume of adequate radiation in each of the common directions of spread of disease—the uterine body, parametria, and perivaginal tissues—with relative sparing of the bladder trigone and anterior rectum due to the addition of shielding (63,64). The applicator was modified in the 1960s for afterloading (Fletcher-Suit applicator) (74,76,77,111) and in the 1970s to accommodate ^{137}Cs sources (75,76). In the 1970s, the Delclos mini-ovoid was developed for use in narrow vaginal vaults (Fig. 14.26) (74, 6,112,113). The mini-colpostats have a diameter of 1.6 cm and a flat inner surface. The mini-ovoids do not have shielding added inside the colpostat, and this together with their smaller diameter produces a higher surface dose than regular ovoids with resultant higher doses to the rectum and bladder. Appropriate source strength and treatment duration adjustment are important considerations to prevent complications. Fletcher tandems are available in four curvatures, with the greatest curvature used in cavities measuring >6 cm and lesser curvatures used for smaller cavities (Fig. 14.26). A flange with keel is added to the tandem once the uterine canal is sounded, which approximates the exocervix and defines the length of source train needed. The keel prevents rotation of the tandem after packing. The distal end of the tandem near the cap is marked so that rotation of the tandem after insertion can be assessed.

The Henschke tandem and ovoid applicator was initially unshielded (111,114) but later modified with rectal and bladder shielding (103,104). It consists of hemispheroidal ovoids with the ovoids and tandem fixed together. Sources in the ovoids are parallel to the sources in the uterine tandem (103). The Henschke applicator may be easier to insert into shallow vaginal fornices in comparison to Fletcher ovoids.

The Fletcher-Suit-Delclos tandem and cylinder applicator was designed to accommodate narrow vaginas where ovoids may be contraindicated and to treat varying lengths of the vagina when mandated by vaginal spread of disease. The cylinders vary in size from 2 to 5 cm to accommodate varying vaginal sizes (Fig. 14.26) (112). A narrow vagina poses a therapeutic challenge. Use of vaginal cylinders may lead to a higher rate of local failure as the dose to the lateral cervix and pelvic sidewall is reduced in the absence of ovoids, which produce the optimum

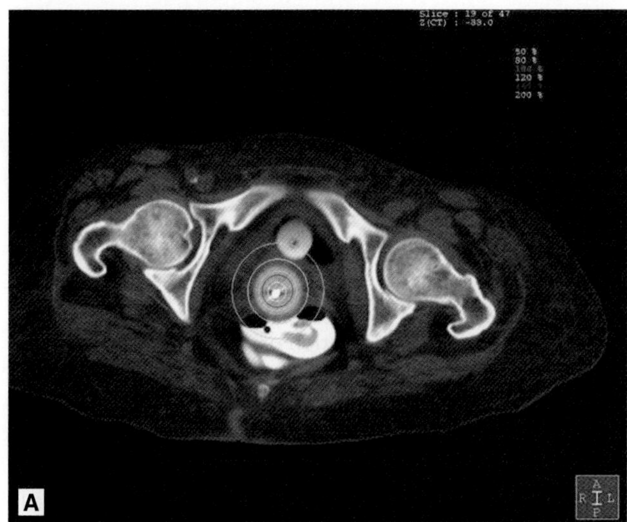

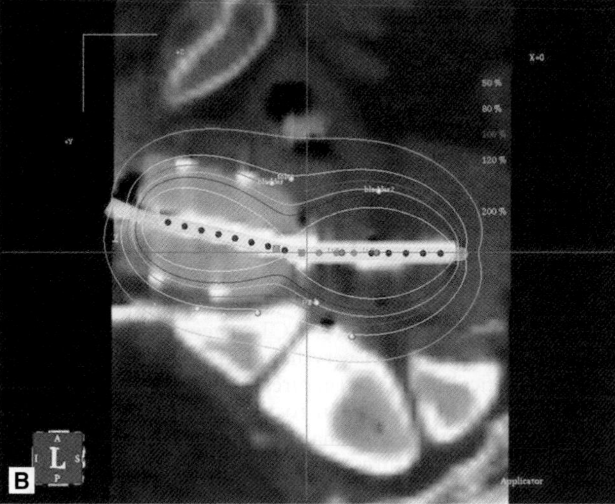

FIGURE 14.35. MRI/CT compatible tandem and cylinder applicator with associated isodose distribution in (A) axial and (B) sagittal views, demonstrating the close proximity to the rectum due to the absence of packing or rectal retraction.

pear-shaped distribution. These patients also tend to receive lower total doses due to the proximity of the rectum and bladder (Fig. 14.35) (81). There is less of a dose gradient between the vaginal mucosa and the bladder and rectum than in a patient with a wider vagina (115). Additionally, packing cannot be used with cylinders to decrease the rectal and bladder doses (116–119). Vaginal cylinders increase the length of vagina and rectum treated, with an associated increase in complications (120,121). Vaginal fistulae, rectal ulcers, and strictures are reported with increased frequency when vaginal cylinders are used (122–124). Pourquier et al. indicated that doses should be reduced with the use of vaginal cylinders and mini-ovoids to reduce complications as these applicators have no shielding (125,126). Interstitial implantation should also be a consideration for patients with a narrow vagina or with distal vaginal disease.

The Importance of Optimal Applicator Placement

Geometrically optimal intracavitary implants improve outcome over suboptimal implants. Corn et al. reported an analysis of the 1978 and 1983 PCSs, which attempted to analyze the outcome of cervical cancer patients by the technical quality of the implant. A technically good implant correlated significantly with improved local control, with a trend toward improved survival (127). Perez et al. observed that "inadequate" insertions increased the incidence of pelvic failures (101) and that the quality of the intracavitary insertion had a measurable impact on the incidence of complications (128). Attention to the details of implant geometry has been linked to improved outcome in the series of Katz and Eifel at M.D. Anderson (80). Prior to afterloading, it was much more difficult to obtain adequate applicator placement due to the need to complete the insertion quickly to avoid excessive exposure to the sources in the preloaded applicators. In the era of afterloading, applicator placement can be more methodical. Orthogonal films or other imaging (CT, magnetic resonance imaging [MRI]) should always be obtained following applicator placement to assess applicator geometry and the need for adjustment to ensure optimum placement. It is imperative that geometrically favorable applicator placement, as described in detail previously by Fletcher, be achieved in as many patients as possible.

Optimum applicator placement is pivotal in maximizing local control. Placement of the brachytherapy applicators in direct proximity to the cervix is necessary to avoid underdosage. There will be a cold spot if the ovoids or other vaginal applicators are displaced away from the cervix (Fig. 14.36). Proper applicator selection is important in avoiding malpositioning. It is extremely important to place metallic markers on the cervix so that the flange of the tandem and the ovoids/cylinder dome are positioned in close proximity to these markers as confirmed on orthogonal check films (80).

Likewise, suboptimal applicator placement can increase the risk of complications. Applicators that are too close to the bladder and rectum can increase rectal and bladder complications. Sources in the tandem can give very high doses of radiation to the small bowel (ileum), sigmoid, and upper bladder, often not

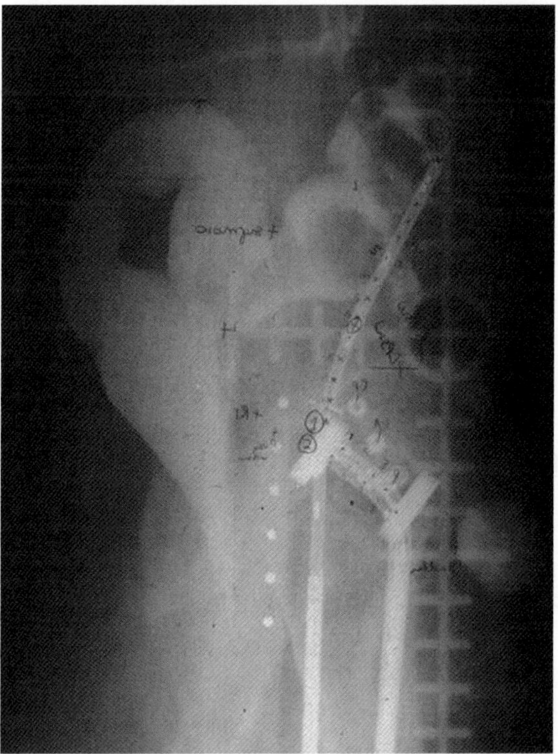

FIGURE 14.36. Lateral radiograph of a poorly positioned HDR tandem and ovoid applicator. Note that the tandem does not bisect the ovoids and that the ovoid appears to be displaced inferiorly from the cervical marker balls.

revealed by orthogonal x-rays. Tandems that have perforated through the uterus can cause tremendous hot spots in the nearby normal organs (79).

Interstitial Applicators: Cervical and Vaginal Cancers—LDR and HDR

The size of the reference pear-shaped isodose achieved with tandem and ovoids is not variable except by increasing the duration (dose) of the implant. The shape of the reference pear-shaped isodose can be altered to some degree by varying the source strengths and applicator type, but it may not be able to encompass a bulky tumor, particularly when there is bulky parametrial or vaginal disease. In these settings, the disease may be better accommodated by an interstitial application (Fig. 14.37). Patients with large, bulky lesions will have a higher rate of local failure because of a decrease in dose to the periphery of the tumor due to the rapid fall-off of dose beyond the relevant pear-shaped distribution. The use of higher doses of external beam prior to implantation and interstitial techniques are important considerations. These patients should not be treated with external beam alone, as achieving the curative radiation doses required may be impossible because of the limited tolerance of the interposed small bowel, rectum, and bladder. Standard intracavitary applications may be suboptimal or prohibited either by tumor bulk or distorted normal anatomy, and these patients should not be treated with geometrically unfavorable intracavitary implants.

The limitations of intracavitary techniques contrast with the strengths of interstitial techniques in certain settings. Determine which approach is best on a patient-by-patient basis. Interstitial implantation is appropriate in select patients with bulky tumors, anatomical distortion such as an obliterated endocervical canal or narrow vagina, or recurrent disease (129).

The development of prefabricated perineal templates, through which stainless steel needles were inserted and afterloaded with ^{192}Ir or ^{125}I, was pivotal in advancing interstitial techniques for the treatment of cervical and vaginal cancers. With these interstitial techniques, rather that doing a freehand implant, the template concept allows for a predictable distribution of needles inserted across the entire perinum through a perforated template according to an optimum pattern. Commercially available and institution-specific templates are used in these patients to accommodate varying disease presentations. Stainless steel and plastic needles are used, which are

Indications for Transperineal Interstitial Implantation of Gynecologic Malignancies
1 Bulky Disease
• IB Barrel
• IIB, III, IVA
2 Anatomical Distortion
• Narrow/obliterated vagina
• Obliterated fornices
• Stenotic/obliterated endocervical canal
3 Recurrent Disease

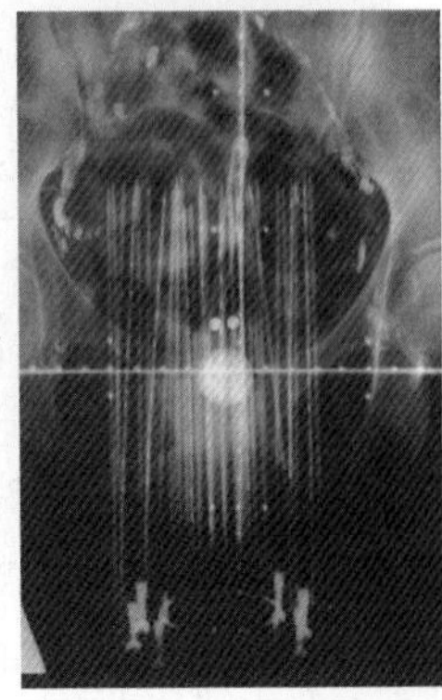

FIGURE 14.37. Indications for interstitial implantation and associated AP radiograph of the implanted needles.

afterloaded with low- or high-activity ^{192}Ir sources. The MUPIT (Martinez Universal Perineal Interstitial Template, Beaumont Hospital, Royal Oak, Michigan, USA) template (Fig. 14.38) accommodates implantation of multiple pelvic-perineal malignancies (prostate, anorectal, gynecologic) (129–133). In this system, one template accommodates many different disease presentations. Recent modifications of this template and needle system enabling HDR implants have become available (134). The Syed-Neblett (Best Industries, Springfield, Virginia, USA) is the other well-known commercially available template system (129,135–139). Currently, there are three LDR Syed-Neblett templates of varying size and shape for use in implantation of gynecologic malignances (GYN 1-36 needles, GYN 2-44 needles, GYN 3-53 needles), as well as templates for implantation of the anus, prostate, and urethra (Fig. 14.39). There is also a disposable template for gynecologic presentations that accommodates HDR needles (140,141).

The Syed-Neblett and MUPIT templates are particularly suited for treatment of vaginal disease as the vaginal obturator needles can be strategically loaded to encompass disease from the fornices to the introitus. Additionally, the obturator needles can be advanced directly into the cervix, along with a uterine tandem, and may be essential to deliver tumorcidal radiation doses to the cervix by preventing a central "cold spot," especially if an intrauterine tandem is not used. The more peripheral needles are used for implantation of the parametria, which is often underdosed in intracavitary approaches. Modifications of these standard templates have evolved and other innovative templates have been developed for vulvar, vaginal, and cervical carcinomas (129).

Individualized computer-generated dosimetry is an integral part of interstitial dose delivery. CT imaging following needle implantation has proven very helpful to identify tumor volume and critical normal structures, confirm the adequacy of needle placement in relation to these structures or needed adjustments, analyze and manipulate the dose distribution related to these structures, and assist with dose specification and the integration of external beam irradiation (129,142). Post-procedure epidural anesthesia provides optimal pain control and allows the needles and tandem to be manipulated outside the operating room if necessary. Modification of the planned source placement based upon the location of specific needles and critical structures can therefore be made before or after source loading.

With LDR techniques, traditional low dose rates are the goal (142), achieved through differential loading (core sources $\leq$½ activity of peripheral sources) of low-activity sources. "Reference" dose rates of 60 to 80 cGy/hr are optimal. The implant dose rates as well as the dose homogeneity and distribution can be manipulated by selectively changing the activity associated with a particular needle or needles or by selectively unloading, either immediately or during the implant, strategic needles in the pattern. With HDR techniques, optimization of the dose distribution with predetermined parameters for the reference dose, normal organ doses, and dose homogeneity can produce even more ideal implant dosimetry (Fig. 14.40). Typically, total LDR doses to the tumor volume or reference isodose from the implant range from 23 to 40 Gy over 2 to 4 days (142). The total HDR dose will be approximately 60% of the total LDR dose and will be given in divided fractions. With either approach, careful attention to significant hot spots within the implant and doses to the bladder, rectosigmoid, and vaginal surface are requisite to obtaining the best outcome.

External whole pelvic irradiation (39.6 to 45.0 Gy) generally precedes implantation. For either LDR or HDR, one or two template implants can be done 1 to 2 weeks following external beam. With HDR, one to two fractions can be delivered per day over a period of 2 to 5 days, whereas with LDR, continuous hourly

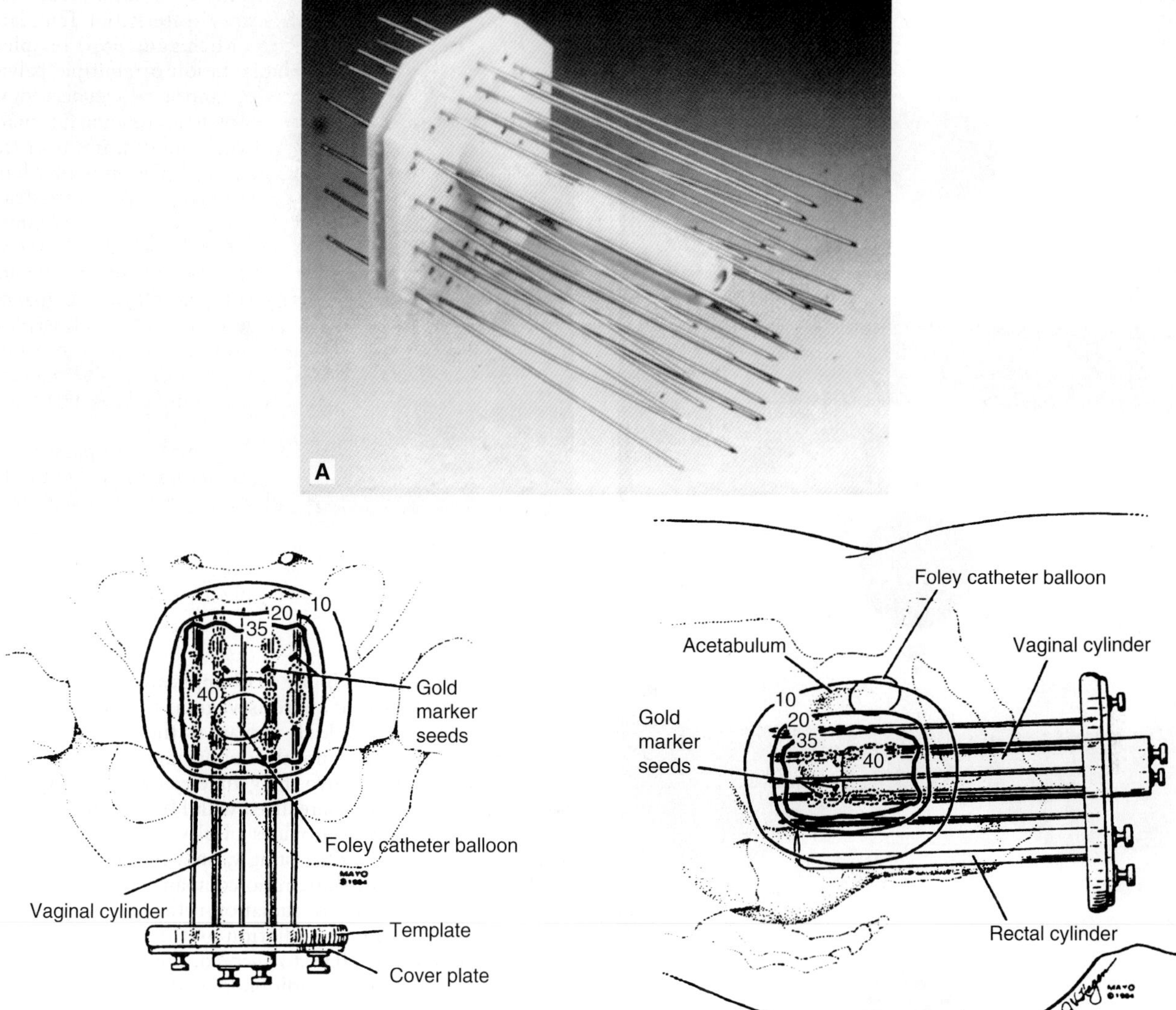

FIGURE 14.38. **A:** Martinez Universal Perineal Interstitial Template (MUPIT). *Source:* Courtesy of Dr. Alvaro Martinez, William Beaumont Hospital, Detroit, Michigan, USA. **B:** Diagrammatic representation in coronal and sagittal planes of the same template. *Source:* Reprinted from Martinez A, Edmundson GK, Cox RS, et al. Combination of external beam irradiation and multiple-site perineal applicator (MUPIT) for treatment of locally advanced or recurrent prostatic, anorectal, and gynecologic malignancies. *Int J Radiat Oncol Biol Phys* 1985;11:391–398, with permission from Elsevier.

radiation is delivered. After the implant, selective external irradiation boosting can be done as needed. The total LDR dose to the reference volume from the combined implant and external beam approximates 70 to 85 Gy over 8 weeks.

High Dose Rate Brachytherapy for Cervical Cancer

Though LDR techniques have been the traditional standard for decades for gynecologic brachytherapy, there appear to be some inherent advantages with the implementation of HDR techniques (143). Because the treatment time is very short, treatment is performed on an outpatient basis without the need for several days of bed rest, with greater patient acceptance and comfort. This allows treatment of some patients with medical comorbidities, which would prohibit LDR techniques because of the prolonged bed rest. With the shorter treatment time, the implant reproducibility is superior to traditional LDR approaches as more stable positioning of applicators is possible. The shortened treatment time provides a greater degree of certainty that the sources will remain in the 3D positions documented in the isodose distributions, and that applicator displacement as a function of time will be decreased (56). The use of external applicator fixation devices allows more constant and reproducible geometry of source positioning (56,144–146). The newer systems, which allow a single source to "dwell" at a site for a calculated period of time, combined with dose optimization software programs, provide a significant further improvement in the ability to shape the dose distribution. The small source size allows for finer increments in source location and relative weighting for each source location than with the fixed source sizes and activities inherent to the LDR ^{137}Cs sources (86,146,147). This allows for greater precision coupled with greater flexibility and perhaps a reduction in normal tissues doses. Additionally, the

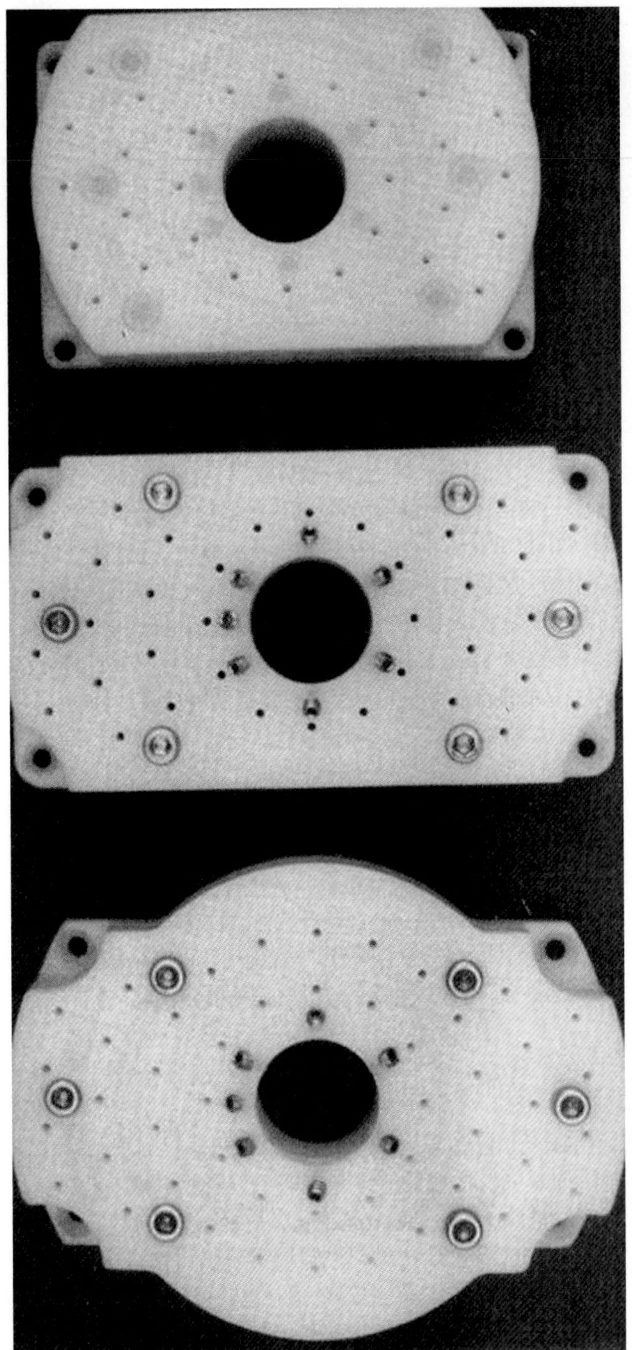

FIGURE 14.39. LDR Syed-Neblett templates (**top to bottom**) Gyn 1, Gyn 2, Gyn 3. *Source:* Reprinted with permission from Erickson B, Gillin M. Interstitial implantation of gynecologic malignancies. In: Nag S, ed. Principles and Practice of Brachytherapy. New York: Futura; 1997:518 (Fig. 1).

rectal retraction devices available with the HDR applicators maximize displacement of the rectum for short periods of time and may give superior and more predictable displacement than traditional vaginal gauze packing (56,144–146). These two factors lead to improved dose delivery to the tumor relative to surrounding normal tissues (148). There is also increased integration of external beam with HDR as external beam irradiation can be given three to four times per week and HDR one to two times per week. This can lead to a shorter overall treatment duration, which may be pivotal in maximizing cure (149,150). Additionally, due to the small physical size of the ^{192}Ir source, the HDR applicators are lighter and smaller than bulky LDR applicators and are easier to insert, particularly if there is vaginal narrowing. Many institutions use only one LDR implant so that if the applicator geometry is poor, there is not the opportunity to perform multiple implants and improve the geometry or change applicators in future insertions as realized with HDR techniques. The remote afterloading also provides a lack of radiation exposure to health-care givers. Contrastingly, on a radiobiologic basis, HDR lowers the therapeutic ratio compared to LDR as there may be more late effects of radiation if the rectosigmoid and bladder receive as much radiation as the tumor than with LDR techniques. For HDR to succeed, the geometric advantages must overcome the radiobiologic disadvantages (146). Himmelmann et al. concluded that with HDR regimens, reoxygenation of hypoxic cells can take place between fractions, and this may in fact be a radiobiologic advantage of HDR (151). Disadvantages of HDR may include loss of the radiobiologic advantage of LDR, a potential increase in late tissue effects with large fraction sizes, and an increase in the number of implants per patient from 1–3 to 3–6 (range: 2–16), which is labor intensive for all involved. The need for sedation may still exclude high-risk patients even though bed rest is not required.

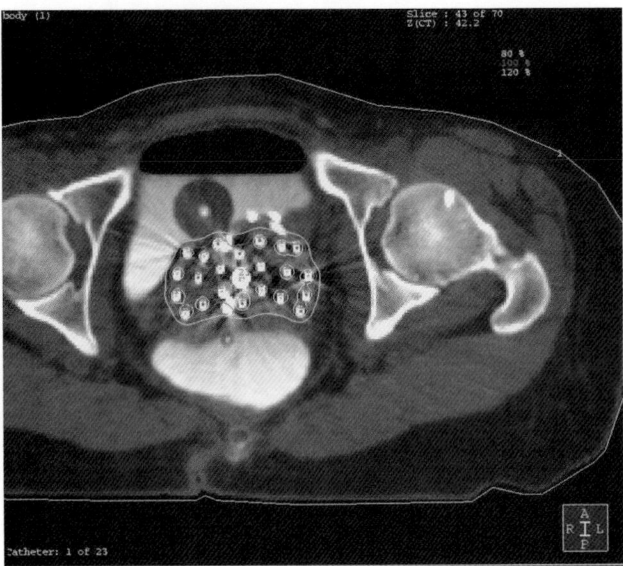

FIGURE 14.40. Axial CT scan with needles inserted into the cervical and paracervical tissues between the bladder and rectum. Isodose curves shown are 80%, 100%, and 120% of the prescription dose.

Conversion from LDR to HDR

There have been numerous suggestions regarding how to convert total LDR doses to HDR doses in order to implement reasonable dose-fractionation schemes. Efforts have been made by many investigators to compare the biologic effects of LDR with HDR regimens using various dose conversion models. The linear-quadratic model has typically been used, but this does not address the optimal number of fractions. A basic concept is that the total dose with HDR must be less than with LDR and the number of fractions must increase (151–155). This concept comes from early radiobiologic studies. The Equivalent Radiation Dose (ERD) mathematical model can be used to determine the HDR dose per fraction (156,157). The ERD is a biologic dose unit, which utilizes the linear-quadratic model. To determine an appropriate dose for high dose rate

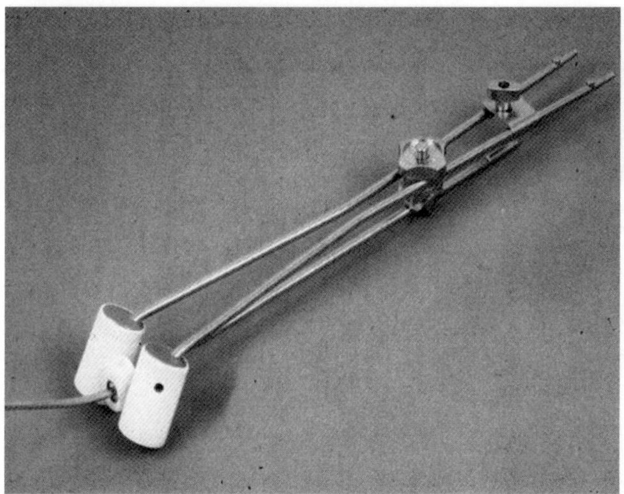

FIGURE 14.41. HDR tandem and ovoids. *Source:* Courtesy of Nucletron.

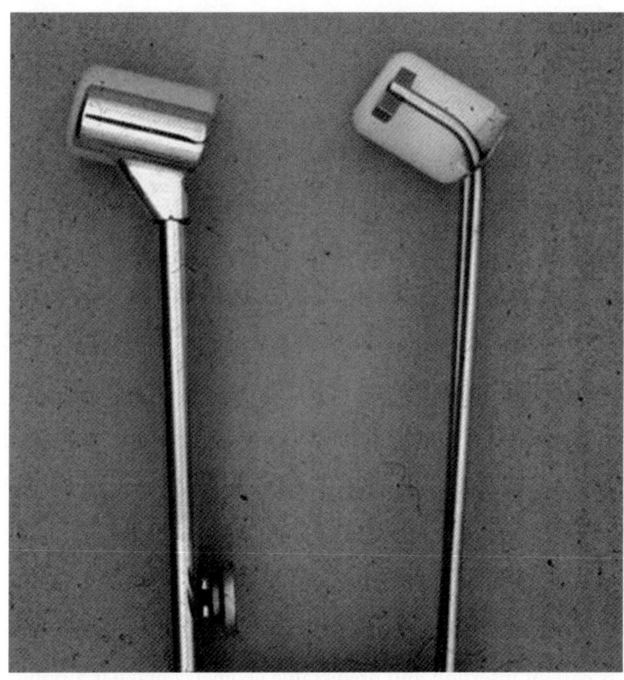

FIGURE 14.42. LDR versus HDR ovoid angles. The low dose rate ovoids are positioned at a 15° or 30° angle to the vaginal axis versus 60° in the HDR ovoids. *Source:* Courtesy of Nucletron.

treatments based upon low dose rate techniques, the ERDs are assumed to be equal. The alpha/beta for tumor is assumed to be 10, while u is assumed to be 1.4 hours^{-1}. For this calculation, the LDR total dose, LDR dose rate, and desired number of HDR fractions are required to calculate an HDR fraction size. These calculations have shown that one must give approximately 60% of the LDR dose with HDR (143,156,157).

High Dose Rate Applicators

The tandems and ovoids used with HDR are variations of the traditional Fletcher and Henschke LDR applicators but are lighter, narrower, and smaller (Fig 14.41). The ovoids are 2.0, 2.5, and 3.0 cm in diameter with and without shielding. The relationship of the colpostat to the handle is different between HDR and LDR colpostats so that the cable-driven HDR source can negotiate the angle between the handle and the colpostat. The Selectron colpostats are angled at 60° to the applicator handles. Standard Fletcher-Suit LDR colpostats are angled most often at 15° and sometimes at 30° with respect to the colpostat handles (Fig 14.42). This can lead to a different relationship between the tandem and the colpostats and between the colpostats and the cervix, best seen on the lateral orthogonal x-rays taken for dosimetry after applicator insertion.

The ring applicator, which is an adaptation of the Stockholm technique, has become a popular applicator (147,158–161) (Fig. 14.43). The plastic caps that come with the ring applicator place the vaginal mucosa 0.6 cm from the source path, compared to the caps for the ovoids, which distance the vaginal mucosa from the source path by 1 to 1.5 cm. The short distance from the ring to vaginal mucosa can result in very high surface doses if fixed weighting, nonoptimized techniques are used (144,145,160). The bladder and rectum may also receive higher doses with fixed weighting nonoptimized dosimetry (159). It is important not to activate all the positions in the ring, as this will increase the dose to the rectum, bladder, and vaginal

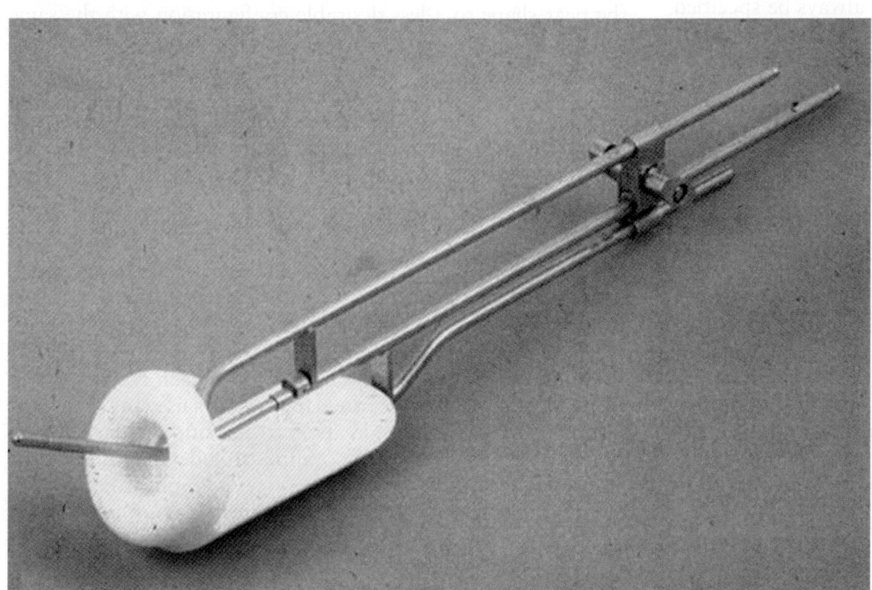

FIGURE 14.43. Tandem and ring applicator with associated rectal retractor. *Source:* Courtsey of Nucletron.

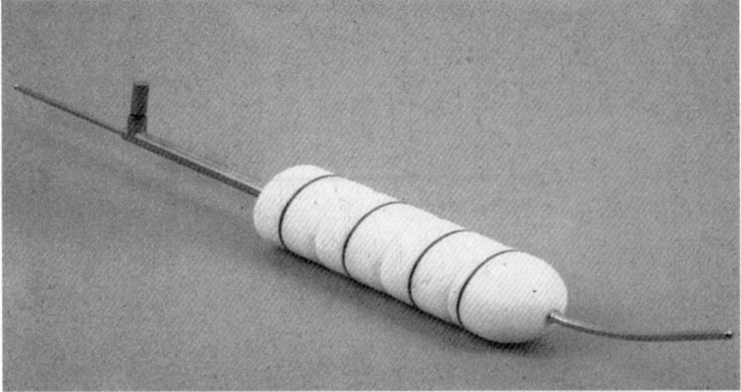

FIGURE 14.44. Tandem and cylinder applicator. *Source:* Courtesy of Nucletron.

mucosa (159). Typically, four dwells are activated on each side of the smallest ring (36 mm), five on each side of the medium ring (40 mm), and six on each side of the large ring (44 mm). The tandems are available in lengths of 2 to 8 cm. Four ring-tandem angles are available including 30°, 45°, 60°, and 90°. The shape of the isodose curves comparing the ring with tandem and ovoids will also have a different shape and the volume of tissue irradiated will also differ (159,160). The ring applicator is ideal for patients without lateral vaginal fornices. Its ease of insertion and predictable geometry make it a popular alternative to tandem and ovoids.

Tandem and cylinder applicators are used in the setting of a narrow vagina or vaginal extension of disease and are available in diameters of 2.0 to 4.0 cm (Fig. 14.44). In most cases, rectal and bladder displacement are not possible with this applicator, although some of the cylinders have built-in shielding. A posterior speculum blade to displace the rectum can be used if there is not posterior vaginal disease. As with LDR tandem and cylinder applicators, the bladder and rectal doses may increase with this applicator, and the dose distribution will be more cylindrical than pear-shaped, which can underdose bulky tumors (Fig. 14.35). Careful attention to normal tissue doses and target coverage is necessary in this setting.

HDR Treatment Planning

The dose distribution with HDR tandem and ovoids and tandem and ring applicators model the LDR pear-shaped isodose distribution. Most HDR regimens use a paracervical dose specification point (A) rather than mg-hrs. Rectal, bladder, sigmoid, and vaginal surface doses should always be specified or documented, and some assessment of dose to the pelvic lymph nodes and lateral parametria should be documented.

The HDR system utilizes special vocabulary to describe certain functions and applications. A "dwell position" is a position at which the source is driven to stop or dwell. Dwell positions can be 2.5 and 5 mm apart. Up to 48 dwell positions can be specified per channel. The physicists will ask for the active length and convert the active length into a number of dwell positions. "Patient points" are points of interest at which the dose is calculated; they are defined on the orthogonal implant films. Examples include bladder, rectum, and sigmoid. "Applicator points" are points of interest at which the dose is calculated; they are defined by manually inputting the coordinates. Typically, applicator points include point A and points on the lateral surface of a ring, ovoid, or cylinder. "Dose points" are points at which the dose is optimized. In general, doses are specified using dose points. The optimization program then attempts to give the prescription dose at each of these points. With the tandem and ring, a similar system is used. The entire ring should never be activated, as this will cause high rectal, bladder, and vaginal doses. For the tandem and cylinder, again, a similar system is used with the

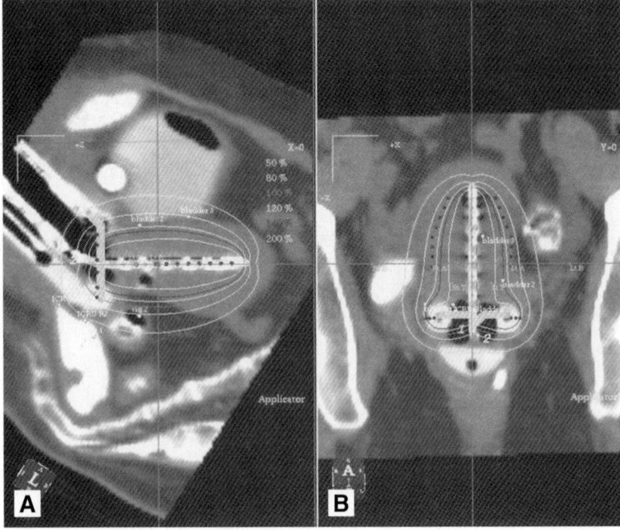

FIGURE 14.45. Dose distribution around a tandem and ring applicator in (**A**) sagittal and (**B**) coronal projections with dose specified at the ring surface and at the level of point A.

exception that at the cylinder interface, dose points are entered laterally from the dwell positions at the distances representing the cylinder surface. Due to the close proximity of the bladder and rectum in women requiring vaginal cylinders because of a narrow vagina, it may be wise to decrease the vaginal surface dose to 100% to 120% of the point A dose rather than 140% to 200% of the point A dose, as recommended with tandem and ovoid or ring applications.

Dose specification at point A alone can result in underdosing of target tissue and overdosing of dose-limiting tissues (162). In addition to point A, specifying dose at the vaginal applicator surface and use of optimization may allow for design of an optimal dose distribution (Fig. 14.45). Optimization is a term used in HDR dosimetry planning. With optimized plans, dose points are defined relative to the applicators and are used by the planning system to determine the dwell times necessary to deliver the specified dose to the points. With nonoptimized plans, fixed relative dwell weights are input into the planning system and are used to calculate the dose distribution. By altering the dwell times and dwell weights, it is possible to alter the dose distribution, and thereby optimize tumor volume coverage, and minimize normal tissue exposure. Excessive optimization can alter the pear shape to a less desirable configuration with the same point A dose (163,164). When altering the standard dwell times and weights, it is important to also monitor point T (defined at 1 cm superior to the cervical os and 1 cm lateral to the tandem with a dose two to three times the point A dose), and the vaginal surface (defined at the lateral radius of the ovoid and ring applicator with a dose 1.4 to 2.0 times the point A dose) (80,102,105). In addition, doses to the rectum, sigmoid, and bladder should be carefully monitored and adjusted if they are above the threshold tolerance.

HDR Dosimetry Generation

It is important to perform dosimetry for each fraction of an HDR regimen even if the same applicator is used, as there may be quite a bit of variation in applicator position with each fraction (165–173). There is also applicator deformation of the adjacent structures, which varies with applicator position (168). Variables that impact applicator position are vaginal packing, the presence and effectiveness of sedation/anesthesia, as well as use of the dorsal lithotomy versus legs down position. The bladder and rectosigmoid may also change configuration

Variation in Anatomy by Fraction

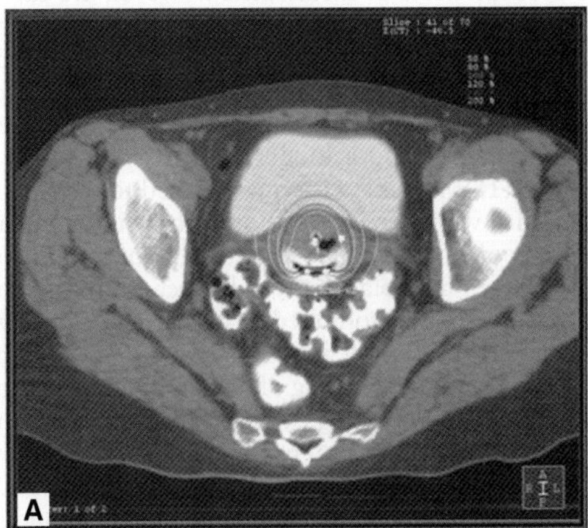

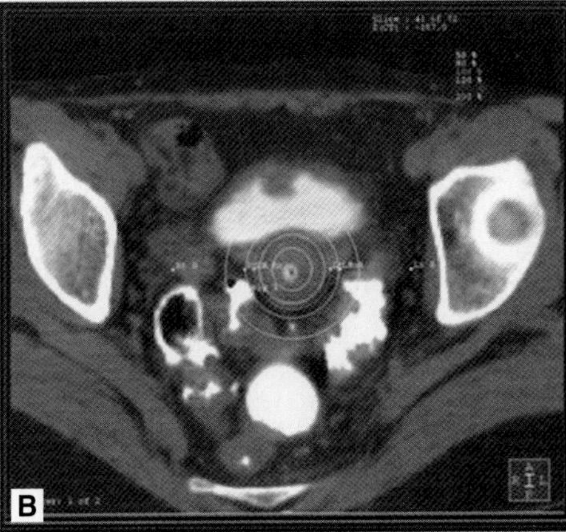

FIGURE 14.46. Variation in anatomy between fraction 2 (**A**) and fraction 3 (**B**) of a 5 fraction high dose rate (HDR) course. Note the difference in the position of normal organs at the level of point A between fractions 2 and 3.

due to changes in filling and position, and doses to these organs will vary from fraction to fraction. Uterine and sigmoid mobility may also impact the dose distribution in these organs. Additionally, disease regression and vaginal narrowing will vary from fraction to fraction and can also result in changes in dose distribution. A change in applicator can also result in changes in dose distribution as can changing the ovoid or ring size, ovoid separation, and tandem curvature. The ovoids may also change in separation and their relative position to the tandem over time if there is not a fixed relationship between the tandem and ovoids (167,169–172). Jones et al. found that when treatment planning was not performed for each fraction and only the initial dosimetry was used, there was increased dose to at-risk normal organs (172). This is also true when using a tandem and ring, even though it has a fixed geometry. The applicator position relative to the pelvic organs is the important factor rather than the relationship of the tandem to the ring (Fig. 14.46).

Dose-Fractionation Schemes

In the 1990 literature review by Fu and Phillips of the randomized and nonrandomized studies of HDR, multiple dose-fractionation schemes were tabulated. Most centers used point A as a reference point, although the definition of point A varied. The dose per fraction at point A varied from 3 to 10.5 Gy, the number of fractions varied from 2 to 13, and the number of fractions per week varied from one to three. At that time, most centers used a schedule of 7 to 8 Gy/fx for three to six fractions. The external beam dose was variable and in most centers was carried out concurrently with or after intracavitary brachytherapy (174). The 1991 Orton et al. survey of 56 institutions reported treatment of over 17,000 cervix patients with HDR and found that the average fractionation scheme was five fractions of 7.5 Gy to point A. Fractionation of the HDR treatments significantly influenced toxicity as morbidity rates were significantly lower for point A doses per fraction of ≤7 Gy compared with >7 Gy (175,176). Fraction sizes <7.5 Gy are recommended by the American Brachytherapy Society (86). In a literature analysis by Petereit and Pearcey of the HDR fractionation schedules, a dose-response relationship could not be identified for tumor control or complications (177). There is no consensus as to the optimal number of fractions and dose per fraction except that the choice will depend on the external beam dose and on whether central shielding is used, normal tissue doses, medical comorbidities, and the stage of disease. The linear-quadratic model was suggested as a guide to formulate the regimens chosen at each institution (86,178). Currently, Gynecologic Oncology Group (GOG) protocols define a dose/fractionation scheme of 6 Gy × 5 to point A (87). Radiation Therapy Oncology Group (RTOG) protocols allow more variation depending on the external beam dose with fraction sizes of 5.3 to 7.4 Gy when using four to seven fractions. Tables for combining various external beam doses with varying HDR fractions using the linear-quadratic formula and normal-tissue-modifying factor have been provided with these protocols (179). Currently, the most common approach in the United States is to use five fractions of 5 to 6 Gy in combination with whole pelvis irradiation of 45 to 50 Gy (180).

Sequencing with External Beam

In nonbulky disease presentations, HDR insertions are often integrated early in the treatment course after approximately 20 Gy of external beam RT. Alternatively, some institutions choose to take the whole pelvis to 40 to 45 Gy initially, preceding the five HDR insertions, unless the patient has very early disease or evidence of early vaginal stenosis. When delivering 40 to 45 Gy to the whole pelvis before initiation of HDR, it is important to avoid treatment prolongation by giving two HDR fractions per week to complete the radiation within 50 to 56 days (86,87). Compressing the duration of treatment to <60 days may be desirable (149,181–183).

Midline blocks are used at variable points in time at many institutions (Fig. 14.47). It is important to understand when the midline block is placed as this will influence the HDR fraction size. Higher whole pelvis doses can be utilized without a midline block (56,145,146), but the HDR doses have to be appropriately reduced. HDR and external beam fractions should not be given on the same day.

Brachytherapy for Endometrial Cancer

Hysterectomy is the cornerstone of treatment for endometrial carcinoma. Selective use of vaginal brachytherapy, external beam irradiation, or both in the postoperative setting is based

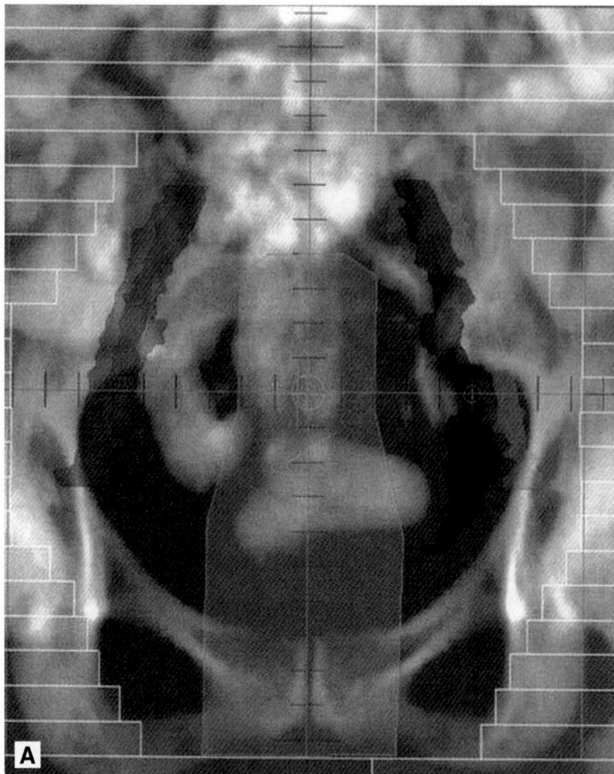

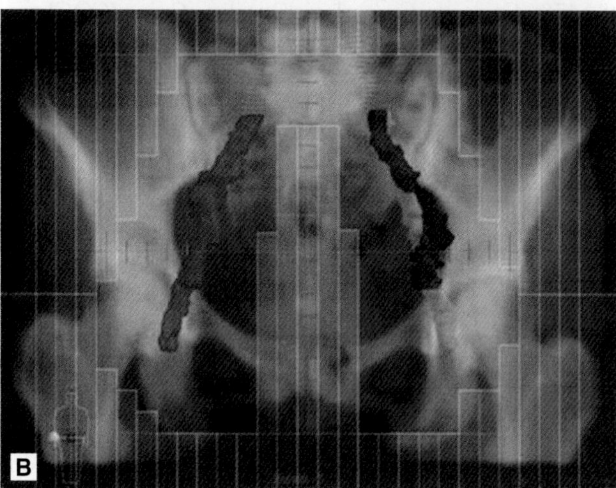

FIGURE 14.47. Midline blocks. (A) A custom cerrobend block protecting the area previously treated by the tandem and ring implant. (B) A midline block defined by the leaves of the multileaf collimator.

on the histopathologic risk factors identified in the tissues removed at the time of surgical staging. Vaginal brachytherapy is typically performed using Fletcher colpostats, or a variety of vaginal cylinders (Delclos, Burnette). Both LDR and HDR techniques are used (Fig. 14.48). The choice of ovoids versus cylinders is individual and both have relative advantages and disadvantages (184). Vaginal ovoids are available in diameters of 2 to 3 cm with associated caps and shielding. Vaginal cylinders are available in diameters of 2 to 5 cm, with or without shielding. Vaginal ovoids generally require sedation for insertion, whereas cylinders do not. The length of the vagina treated with vaginal ovoids is approximately the upper third, whereas vaginal cylinders can treat a portion of or the entire vagina. Though rare, when present, distal vaginal metastases tend to be located in the periurethral area (185,186). Poorly differentiated tumors may recur earlier and present in the distal vagina or distant disease sites, whereas well-differentiated lesions tend to recur later and are often in the upper vagina (187). Distal vaginal recurrences or metastases, however, are rare after radiation and occurred in 0.5% to 1% of patients when the upper vagina was treated (188). It is therefore not suggested to treat more than the upper half of the vagina routinely. Typically, the length of vagina treated with vaginal cylinders is between 4 and 5 cm, perhaps favoring a longer length when using brachytherapy alone (189). Packing is typically used to displace the rectum and bladder with ovoids and not with cylinders. Due to the longer length of vagina treated and the lack of packing, a larger volume of rectum and bladder will be treated with cylinders. Vaginal ovoids may be prohibited in a narrow vagina, whereas vaginal cylinders may not be in close approximation with all of the vaginal mucosa in the setting of a wide vaginal apex or if the cuff has been closed with "dog ears" rather than in a cylindrical shape.

Most vaginal brachytherapy for endometrial cancer is performed with vaginal cylinders using HDR techniques (Fig. 14.48) (189). The dose distribution should ideally conform to the shape of the cylinder (190). Dose is typically specified either at the vaginal applicator surface (mucosal surface) or at a depth of 0.5 cm from the applicator or vaginal mucosal surface. Dose prescription at 0.5 cm can lead to excessively high mucosal doses and surface doses should also be tracked (191,192). Additionally, careful assessment of dose to the rectum and bladder through use of computerized dosimetry should also be performed for the first fraction of radiation delivered (Fig. 14.48). Choo et al. have revealed that 95% of the vaginal lymphatic channels are located within 3 mm of the vaginal surface and that dose prescription to a depth of less than 5 mm may be adequate (193). For LDR insertions, dose rates at the surface of the applicator should be in the range of 80 to 100 cGy/hr, and perhaps 50 to 70 cGy/hr if the prescription is at 0.5 cm (190). Total vaginal surface doses of 50 to 80 Gy are reported most frequently in the literature. When used with external beam, cumulative doses of 60 to 100 Gy at the vaginal surface are reported in the literature. Doses in excess of 80 Gy to the vaginal mucosa are not necessary in the setting of adjuvant therapy and can be associated with increased morbidity. For a vaginal recurrence of endometrial cancer, doses of 80 Gy and higher may be needed when combining external beam and brachytherapy (194).

Vaginal brachytherapy alone is generally considered an option for patients treated with hysterectomy, with either no or selective lymph node sampling, who are thought to be at low risk for lymph node metastases. These patients typically have grade 1 or 2 disease without significant myometrial invasion (<1/3) (195,196). Additionally, vaginal brachytherapy alone is considered an option at some institutions in the setting of a negative pelvic lymph node dissection, even when high-risk factors such as high grade or deep myometrial invasion are present (196–198).

There is great debate if a vaginal cuff boost is routinely necessary in addition to external beam irradiation for early-stage endometrial cancer and little data to support it (199,200). Practice patterns are based more on institutional tradition and individual preference rather than prospective randomized trials. The rationale for use of a vaginal boost is the supposition that there may be a critical dose needed at the vaginal apex to optimally decrease the likelihood of a vaginal apex recurrence. Doses in excess of the 45 to 50 Gy typically delivered with external beam may be necessary if there are microscopic tumor cells embedded in the hypoxic vaginal cuff.

There are some clinical situations in which more complex brachytherapy procedures are required in the treatment of endometrial cancer. Patients with bulky stage II endometrial cancers may benefit from preoperative radiation with external beam alone, brachytherapy alone, or a combination of the

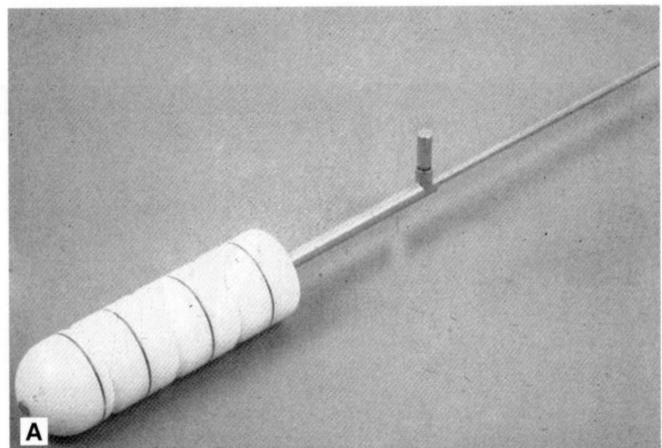

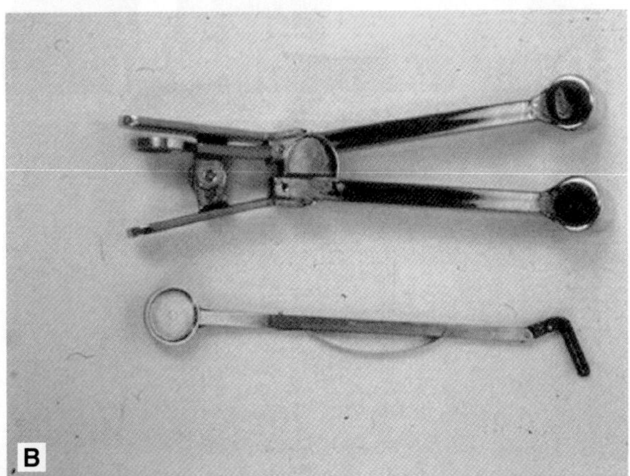

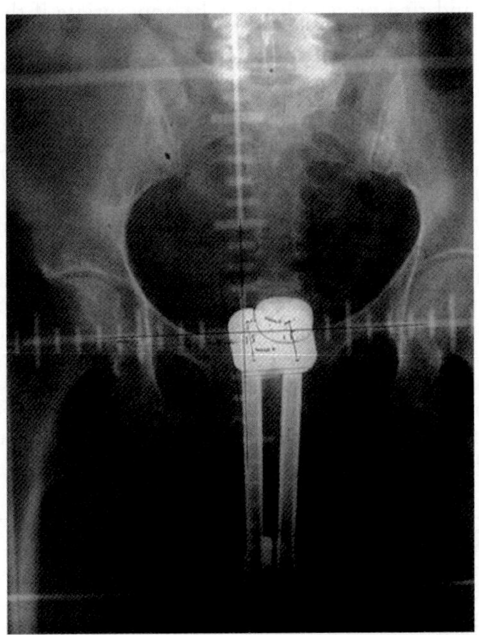

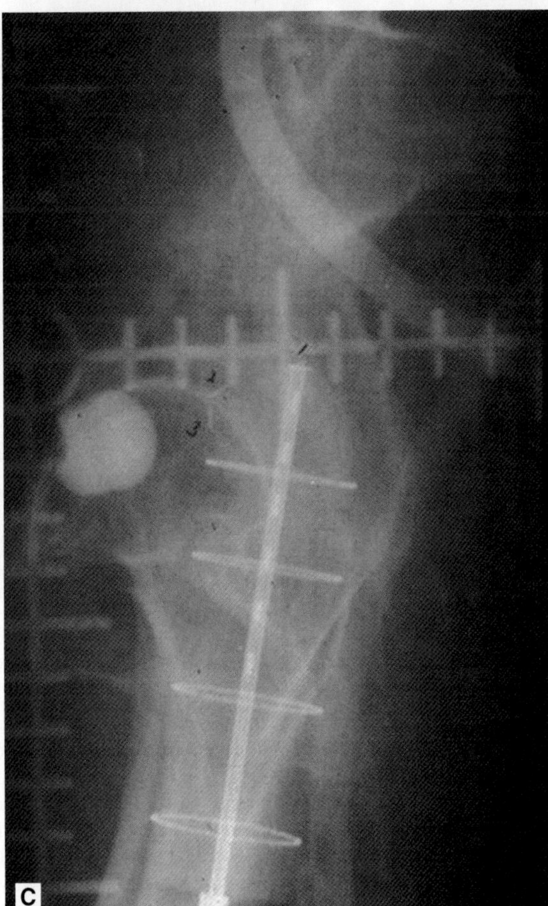

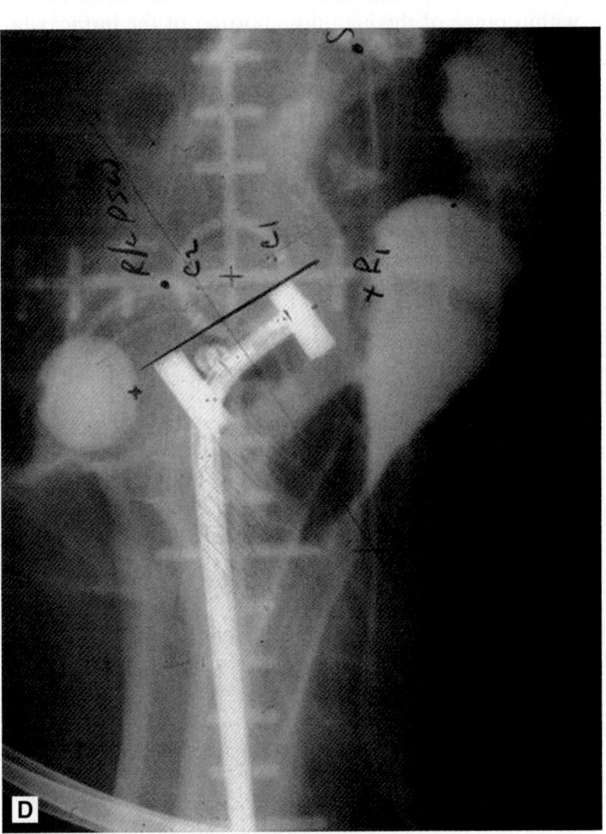

FIGURE 14.48. (A) High dose rate domed vaginal applicator. *Source:* Courtesy of Nucletron. (B) Low dose rate (LDR) Fletcher ovoids with associated radiograph. Lateral radiographs are shown of cylinder (C) and ovoids (D) with bladder bulb contrast in both and rectal contrast in (C).

two. Tandem and ovoids or tandem and ring or cylinder applicators are used in this setting. Medically inoperable endometrial cancer is a rare phenomenon in the current era of aggressive surgical staging. When encountered, it can require the use of sophisticated radiation techniques. Either external beam alone or brachytherapy alone or a combination of the two may be appropriate for some patients. Tandem and ovoids or a tandem and ring or cylinder may be appropriate if the uterine cavity is small. If the uterus is large or if there is more extensive disease, special uterine applicators such as dual and triple tandems or Heyman-Simons capsules may be helpful (Fig. 14.49). There is better coverage of the entire endometrial cavity with these applicators, and dose can be delivered through the uterine wall to the serosa of the uterus (201–203). HDR and LDR techniques can be used.

Patients with recurrent endometrial cancer usually benefit from both external beam and brachytherapy. Doses in excess of 80 Gy may lead to better local control in these patients (194). In patients with residual vaginal disease less than 0.5 cm in maximum thickness, vaginal cylinders or ovoids can be used, whereas in patients with thicker lesions following external beam, interstitial techniques are needed. For apical lesions, laparotomy or laparoscopy may be required for optimum needle placement and to avoid small bowel tethered to the pelvic floor (129,204–206).

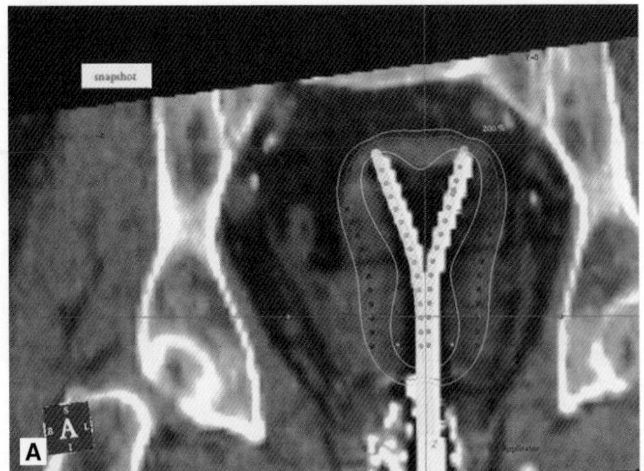

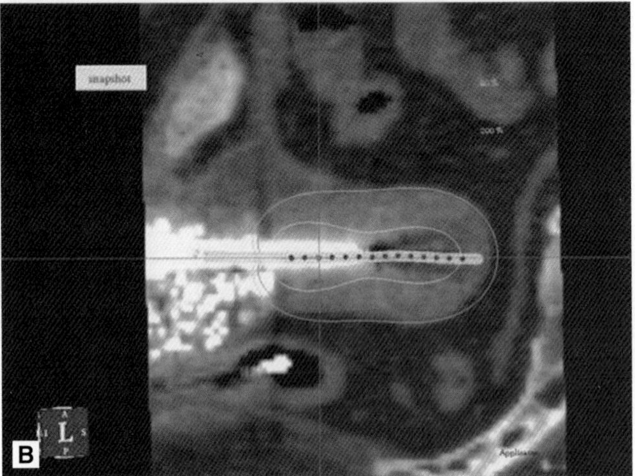

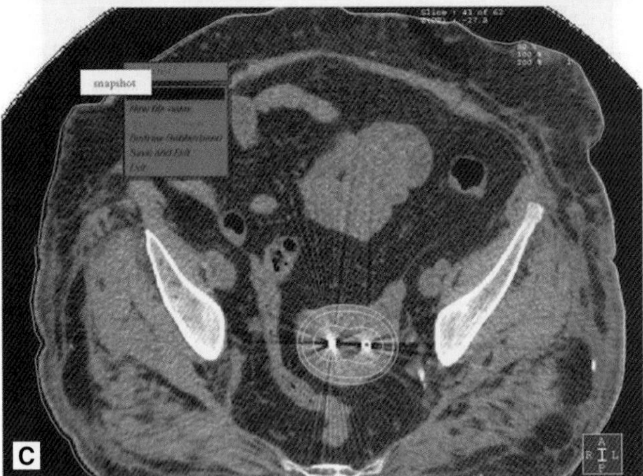

FIGURE 14.49. Brachytherapy plan for a patient with medically inoperable endometrial cancer in (A) coronal, (B) sagittal, and (C) axial dimensions. Note dual tandems on the coronal image (A).

EXTERNAL BEAM IRRADIATION FOR GYNECOLOGIC CANCERS

Cervical and Vaginal Cancers

In cervical and vaginal cancers, the role of external beam irradiation is to shrink bulky tumor prior to implantation to bring it within range of the high-dose portion of the intracavitary dose distribution, improve tumor geometry by shrinking tumor that may distort anatomy and prevent optimal brachytherapy, and sterilize paracentral and nodal disease that lies beyond reach of the intracavitary system (72,85). Some institutions maximize the brachytherapy component of the treatment regimen and perform the first intracavitary insertion after 10 to 20 Gy with subsequent external beam delivered with a central block (207). Other institutions treat the whole pelvis to 40 to 50 Gy and perform brachytherapy once the external beam is completed. The total dose at point A or to the vaginal dose specification point(s), however, should remain the same, stage for stage. Implementing brachytherapy early with subsequent reliance on only the implant to treat the central disease may be considered an advantage as a greater portion of the central dose is delivered with the implant, with relative sparing of the bladder and rectum, perhaps permitting delivery of a higher central dose over a shorter period of time. More reliance, however, is placed on the extremely complex match between the intracavitary system and the edge of the midline block, making good implant geometry imperative when brachytherapy contributes a large portion of the central dose. Those who prefer to deliver an initial 40 to 45 Gy of external beam first believe that the ability to deliver a homogeneous distribution to the entire region at risk for microscopic disease and the ability to have more shrinkage of central disease prior to intracavitary irradiation outweigh other considerations. The brachytherapy dose is accordingly decreased to respect normal tissue tolerance. In addition to causing regression of central disease, the external beam fields are also directed at the regional lymph nodes at risk. In cervical and vaginal cancer, the risk of pelvic lymph node involvement is related to the stage of disease, tumor size, and lymphatic vascular space invasion. Other histomorphologic factors influencing lymph node involvement in cervical cancer include pathologic tumor diameter, depth of stromal invasion, uterine body involvement, parametrial spread, and the number of cervical quadrants involved by tumor (208). Early necropsy studies reported the lymphatic pathways for patients with cervical cancer (209). The primary lymphatic pathway is to the parametrial and paracervical nodes, and the obturator and internal and external iliac nodes. Secondary spread can occur to the sacral and common iliac nodes, with subsequent spread to the paraaortic nodes. Unlike in endometrial cancer, paraaortic lymph node involvement in the absence of pelvic lymph node involvement is rare. Inguinal lymph node involvement occurs with distal vaginal spread of disease or via the round ligament if there is extensive involvement of the corpus. The cervical lymphatics are located in three plexuses in the mucosa, muscularis, and serosa of the cervix and anastamose extensively with the lymphatics of the uterine isthmus. This interconnected lymphatic supply is one of the reasons why the entire uterus should be within the external beam fields when treating cervical cancer. Additionally, there may also be lower uterine segment and endometrial extension of tumor. There are lymph vessels running posteriorly in the uterosacral ligaments to lymph nodes located in the sacrum between the rectum and internal iliac vessels. These posterior nodes may terminate in the common iliac, subaortic, or paraaortic lymph nodes (208,210,211). Recent CT studies have added further information on the location of these lymph nodes and variants of spread (212).

For all gynecologic cancers, these patterns of lymphatic spread influence the external beam field borders. Traditionally, design of "standard" pelvic fields, as shown in many radiation oncology textbooks, has been thought to be quite simple and straightforward and based primarily on skeletal landmarks. The skeletal landmarks are not sufficient for field design (213–215). Traditionally, many institutions have used the "four-field box" technique to treat the pelvis with typical AP-PA field sizes of 15 × 15 cm and lateral field widths of 8 to 9 cm (Fig. 14.50) (79). The intent of the four fields is to use rather narrow lateral beams to avoid some of the small bowel anteriorly and a portion of the rectum posteriorly. As radiation technique must be "predicated on knowing where things are as opposed to where they ought to be," there exist no such entities as "standard" radiation treatment volumes, "standard" portal design, or "standard" field sizes. Surgical and imaging series using CT, MRI, and Lymphangiogram (LAG) have revealed that fields of these sizes can easily miss the primary tumor and its extensions and the regional lymphatics at risk, and design of the pelvic fields needs to be done with care and use of confirmatory imaging (214,216–222). Plain films do not visualize the important soft tissues such as the cervical tumor and its extensions, the uterus, or the lymph nodes at risk. Additionally, bladder and rectal contrast and a vaginal obturator or cervical markers have been used to guide field design but are not sufficient (218,223). As with the brachytherapy component of treatment, the adequacy of the external beam fields and margins has a direct relationship with local and regional control (217). What may be considered a mysterious failure following definitive irradiation, perhaps caused by "radiation resistance," may actually be the result of a marginal miss due to external beam field design. Placement of radiation fields must take into account the alteration of the spatial relationship between the tumor and normal anatomy due to individual anatomic, tumor-induced, or treatment-related positional variations of the uterus and cervix, as well as a knowledge of the location of the regional lymphatics (218,220). Radiation oncologists must be aware of these patterns of disease spread as well as have an in-depth understanding of CT anatomy when designing radiation fields following CT simulation. Identification and contouring of enlarged nodes in nodal regions at risk as well as identification of the iliac vessels, which serve as surrogates for the location of unenlarged lymph nodes, are important in subsequently defining radiation field borders (Fig 14.51). Additionally, contouring of the entire uterus and portions of the vagina will also ensure that these tissues are included in the radiation fields (Fig. 14.51).

Generally, the superior border of the pelvic fields is at the S1-L5 interspace for early-stage disease (i.e., nonbulky IB or IIA) or at the L4-5 interspace for more advanced disease. The latter is used if one wants to cover the common iliac lymph nodes. Interestingly, Greer et al. evaluated "standard" pelvic fields

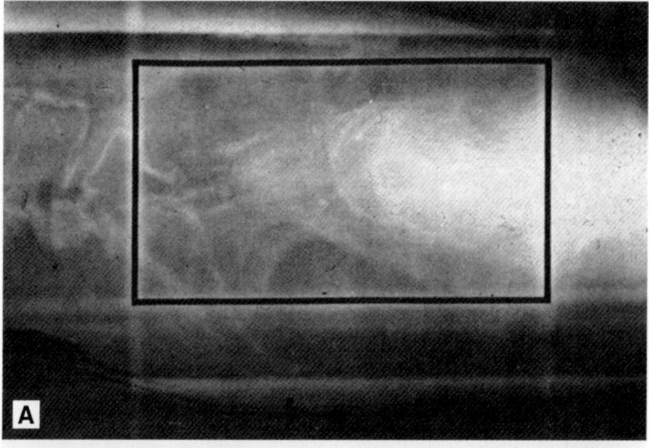

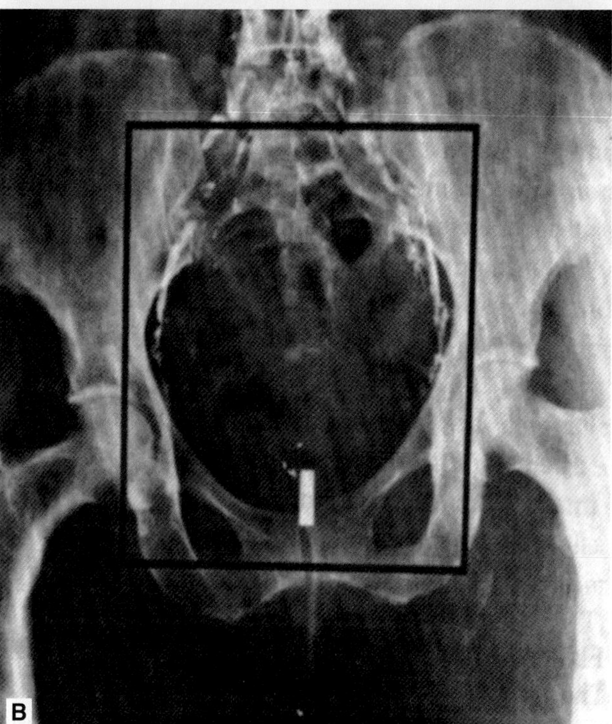

FIGURE 14.50. Traditional four field pelvic box technique with short and narrow fields with the potential to miss the uterine fundus and the pelvic lymph nodes. *Source:* Reprinted with permission from Fletcher, Gilbert H, eds. *Textbook of Radiotherapy*. 3rd ed. Philadelphia: Lea & Febiger; 1980:761–762 (Fig. 37B and D).

(Anterior-Posterior [AP] - Posterior-Anterior [PA], 15 × 15 cm; lateral, 8 to 9 cm wide) for the treatment of cervical cancer in relationship to intraoperative findings. Based on intraoperative measurements of the location of the aortic bifurcation and the bifurcation of the common iliac arteries relative to the lumbosacral prominence (the anterior caudal border of L5), Greer et al. concluded that anterior and posterior treatment fields with a superior border at the L4-5 interspace are required to cover the internal iliac, external iliac, and obturator nodes as the bifurcations of the common iliac arteries were above the lumbosacral prominence in 87% of the patients studied. Coverage of the common iliacs could require extending the upper field border to the L3-4 interspace or even the L2-3 interspace in some patients (224). In a later series, Greer et al. treated 38 patients with cervical carcinoma with these expanded fields (AP-PA fields: median length and width of 20 and 17.5 cm; lateral fields: median width of 16.5 cm, posterior border including the entire sacrum), with an acceptable late

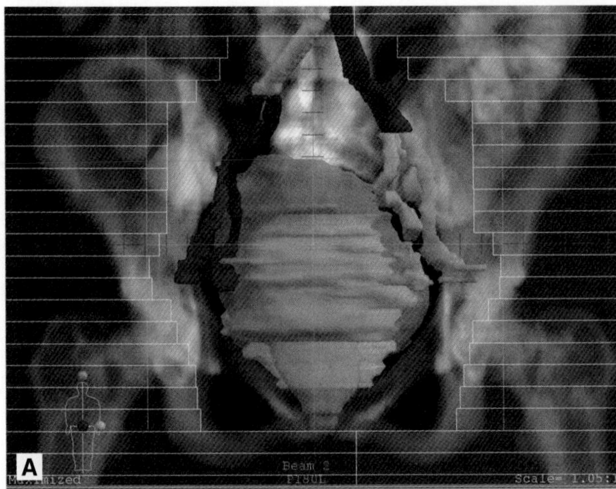

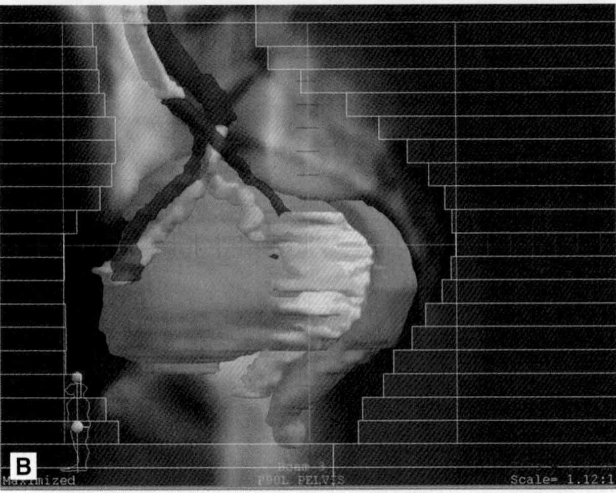

FIGURE 14.51. Digitally reconstructed AP (A) and lateral (B) radiographs with associated contoured targets including the pelvic lymph nodes and uterus. Note the multileaf collimator leaves defining the field shape in accordance with coverage of the targets of interest.

actuarial severe complication rate of 14.8% (223). Obviously, with CT-based dosimetry, it is imperative to outline the vessels and/or nodes in these areas to determine the appropriate field borders as unnecessary irradiation of bowel could occur if all patients were treated to the L2-3 interspace based on this assumption (Fig. 14.51). CT is an excellent tool to either identify pathologically enlarged nodes, multiple small lymph nodes that by increased number rather than size are suspicious, or in the absence of nodes, the aortic and iliac bifurcations and the iliac vessels (212,214). Finlay et al., using CT-based planning, found that 79% of patients treated with conventional fields had inadequate coverage. For adequate coverage, the superior border may need to be as high as L3-4 to cover the common iliac nodes. Using CT-based planning, Finlay et al. reported that 95.4% of the patients who had "conventional" pelvic fields had inadequate coverage of nodes when these were contoured on treatment planning CT scans (225). The inferior border of the pelvic field is usually at the bottom of the ischial tuberosities or 3 to 4 cm below the most distal vaginal component of disease. Inguinal nodes are included if there is distal vaginal spread, in which case treatment of the vaginal introitus with margin would also be required. MRI is especially helpful in imaging vaginal tumor extension (218). The lateral borders of the AP-PA fields are important to design carefully as the 1.5- to 2.0-cm margin from the pelvic brim standardly recommended may be too narrow. Using lymphangiography, Pendlebury et al. found that in order to cover the lymphatic channels in the pelvis in 90% of cases, the lateral margins of the AP-PA fields would need to be 2.5 cm lateral to the pelvic brim (range of medial margins to cover lymph nodes: 0.5 to 3.0 cm) (215), and Bonin et al. found a margin of 2.6 cm (213). Intraoperative measurements have confirmed these findings (224). The lateral fields are even more prone to marginal misses than the AP-PA fields, as demonstrated in multiple series that have compared the standard textbook lateral fields (8 to 12 cm wide) to fields designed based on CT and MRI images (Fig. 14.52) (214,216,217, 219–221,226). For the lateral fields, a commonly employed guideline is to place the posterior border in a horizontal line, parallel to the treatment couch that divides the mid-rectum and intersects the sacrum between the second and third sacral segments (S2-3 interspace), and the anterior border by a horizontal line, parallel to the treatment couch from the anteroinferior lip of L5 to the anterior aspect of the pubic symphysis (219). These "standard" lateral fields are too narrow. For the lateral fields, careful consideration needs to be given to the anterior border to include the external iliac nodes. Based on lymphangiography, Pendlebury et al. found that to cover the external iliac nodes, the anterior border of the lateral field was sometimes as much as 2 cm anterior to the pubic symphysis (215), which was later confirmed by Bonin et al. (213). Chun et al. found that based on CT definition of the external iliac lymph nodes, when using standard lateral fields, only 50% of the patients studied had adequate coverage of these nodes (214). Additionally, the anterior border must also be drawn to include the entire uterus, given the interconnecting lymphatics of the uterus and cervix and the possibility of lower uterine segment/endometrial extension (Fig. 14.52) (211,216,220). Enlargement of the uterine fundus by the presence of hematometra or massive fundal extension of cancer can displace the fundus anteriorly and cephalad, as can an anteverted or retroverted uterus (216, 221,227). The prone position may accentuate this displacement (218,220). The anterior field border should be based on CT or MRI delineation of the tumor and/or normal anatomical variants to avoid underdosing of these structures (214,216,218, 219,221,226,227). The posterior border of the lateral fields must be designed carefully. Based on intraoperative findings, Greer et al. showed that the cardinal and uterosacral ligaments extend posterior to the rectum and sigmoid in their attachments to the sacrum. As part of the parametria, these tissues often contain nodes, even in early disease (IB and II, 22.5%) or are involved by direct extension and need to be covered in most patients by including the entire sacrum in the lateral fields (223). If there is uterosacral ligament involvement, it is especially important to include the entire sacrum in the lateral fields, although some institutions will use this as a criterion for AP-PA fields alone (210). The internal iliac lymph nodes can also lie very close to the rectum and splitting of the rectum can result in a marginal miss of these nodes (Fig. 14.53) (212). For posterior cervical lesions, there can also be direct extension to the superior rectal nodes or sacral lymph nodes (208). Tumor can also extend directly around the rectum. Kim et al. found that the most common site of an inadequate margin was near the portion of the lateral field blocking the rectum. On CT, it was found that tumor often fell along the lateral aspect of the rectum. The second most common site of inadequate margin was the posterior border at the S2-3 interspace (216). Zunino et al. also found inadequate posterior border margins when the uterus was both retroverted and anteverted (Fig. 14.52) (221). The reason for narrow lateral fields is typically concern over the rectum and the small bowel. Russell et al. have included the entire sacrum in the lateral fields of all patients with cervical cancer treated at their institution, and they have reported no increase in acute or late morbidity. When present, all rectal injuries observed have been on the anterior rectal wall due to the proximity of the implants used in the definitive management

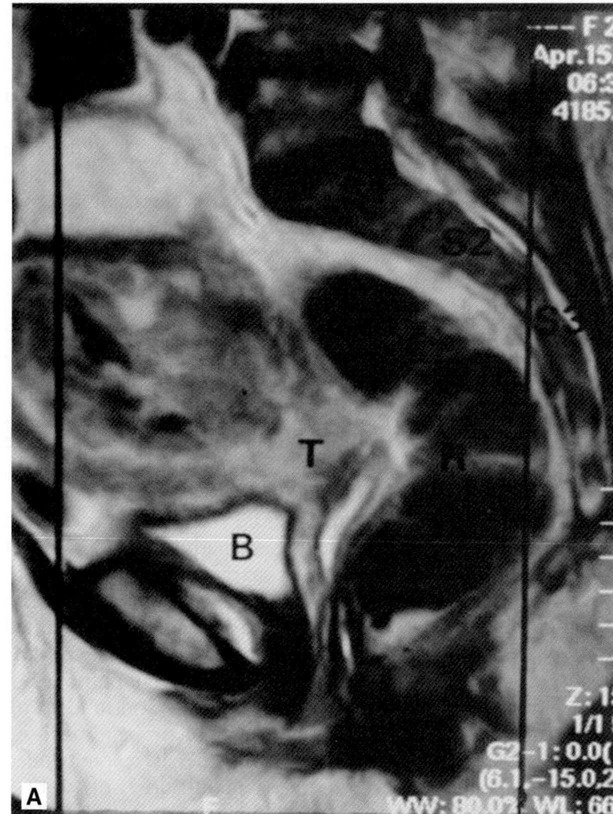

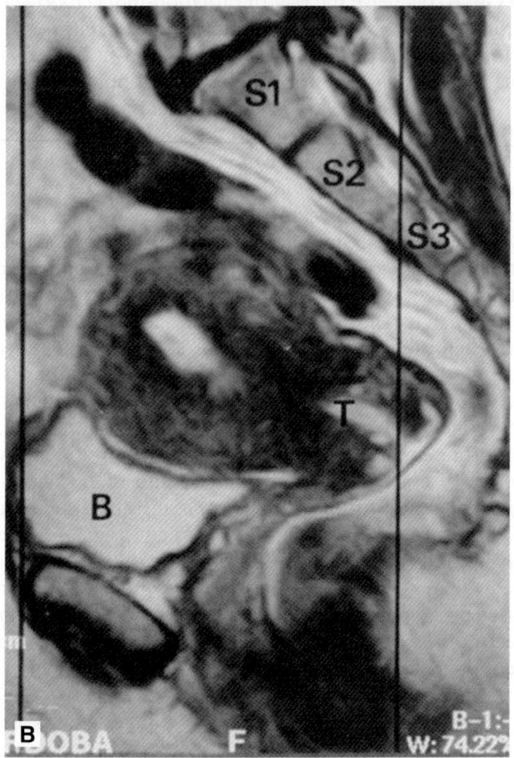

FIGURE 14.52. (A–B): Traditional lateral fields are superimposed on sagittal MRI scans to evaluate target coverage with traditional fields. Note in (A) that the traditional lateral fields would not completely cover the uterine fundus, and that in (B) the traditional lateral field would cut through cervical tumor within the anteverted uterus. *Source:* Reprinted with permission from Zunino S, Rosato O, Lucino S, et al. Anatomic study of the pelvis and carcinoma of the uterine cervix as related to the box technique. *Int J Radiat Oncol Biol Phys* 1999;44(1):56–57 (Figs. 2 and 3).

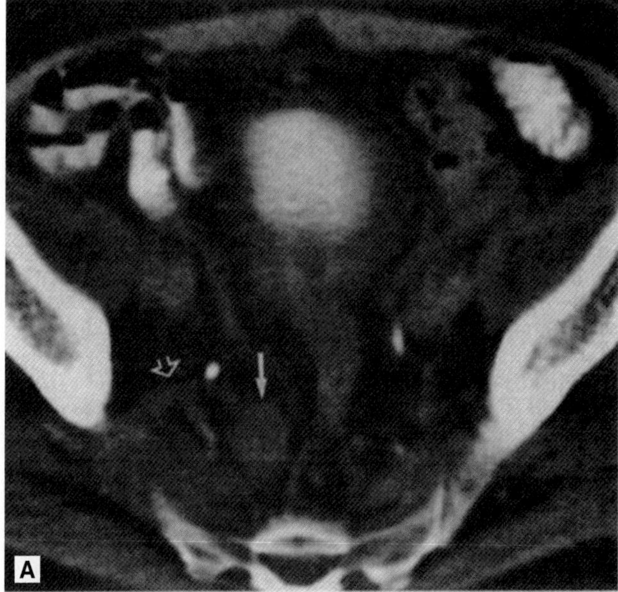

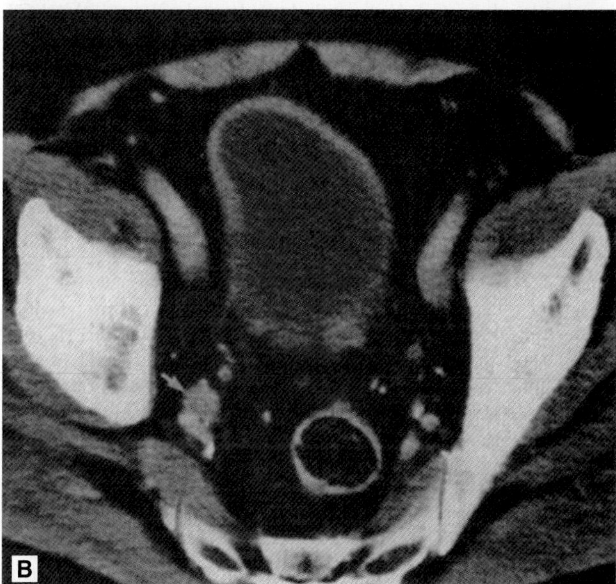

FIGURE 14.53. **A:** The location of the presacral lymph nodes mandates including the entire sacrum to cover disease in the uterosacral and cardinal ligaments and superior rectal (pre-sacral) nodes. The right lateral sacral node (solid arrow) is medial to the hypogastric vessels (open arrow). **B:** Note the proximity of the internal iliac lymph node (solid arrow) to the rectum. This spatial relationship would exclude partial blocking of the rectum on the lateral fields. Source: Reprinted with permission from Park J, Charnsangavej C, Yoshimitsu K, et al. Pathways of nodal metastases from pelvic tumors: CT demonstration. *Radiographics* 1994;14(6):1311 (Figs. 2 and 3).

of these patients (219). Greer et al. also reported no increase in late rectal complications when including the entire sacrum in the field (223). It may also be a mistake to avoid the chance of a marginal miss by treating just with anterior and posterior fields, as in most cases some of the small bowel can be omitted from the lateral fields when using imaged-based planning (219). Gerstner et al. found that by using beam's eye view–based 3D treatment planning, though the rectal volume treated increased to avoid a marginal miss, there was an overall reduction in the lateral field treatment volume as compared to standard treatment fields due to beam shaping to exclude portions of the bladder and small bowel and bladder distention (226). MRI has been found to be an invaluable tool for delineating normal anatomy and the extent of cervical tumor involvement because of its superior soft-tissue contrast when compared to CT. MRI also allows direct imaging in sagittal, coronal, and transverse plains (221). Sagittal MRI images are exceedingly helpful in designing radiation fields (Fig. 14.52). Design of the anterior and posterior borders of the lateral fields can be especially influenced by these images (218–221,227). Thomas et al. performed MRI rather than CT in the treatment position, and found better delineation of the tumor volume due to the superior contrast resolution (220). Lymphangiograms are very helpful in defining the location and architecture of lymph nodes when designing radiation fields, and are especially helpful in designing the lateral fields and subsequent nodal boost fields (213,215, 221,228). They do not routinely image the internal iliac lymph nodes, although sometimes these will fill in a retrograde manner. Unfortunately, lymphangiography is available at only a few institutions due to the fact that it is time consuming for both the radiologist and patient, and fewer radiologists are trained in such procedures (213). Positron emission tomography (PET)/CT scans have largely replaced lymphangiograms at most institutions with Medicare approval in 2005 and can detect involved pelvic and paraaortic lymph nodes better than CT alone (229–232). PET does not rely on lymph node size alone, unlike CT, but rather metabolic alterations for detection of disease. PET has better accuracy than can be achieved with CT or MRI with a sensitivity of 85% to 90%, a specificity of 95% to 100%, and overall accuracy of 90% to 95%. Nodes as small as 6 mm can be imaged with PET, providing information to guide therapy and predict outcome.

Midline Blocks

A midline block is used during external beam to avoid regions of excessive dose adjacent to the implant and to deliver an adequate dose to potential tumor-bearing regions outside of the implant. When using a midline block early in the treatment course, more reliance is placed on the extremely complex match between the intracavitary system and the edge of the midline block. Some institutions customize the midline shield for each patient by defining the Cerrobend block edges as the contour of the isodose line passing through point A (233), or the 50% isodose line. Other institutions further customize this by stepping or altering the block thickness at specific isodose level intervals to achieve a dose "feathering" effect between the external beam and brachytherapy doses. The step-wedge or variable thickness transmission block used at Mallinckrodt (MIR) was initially designed to correspond to the various isodoses of the intracavitary insertions with various tandem and ovoid configurations (128,234,235). Over time, a customized step-wedge was not fabricated for each patient, but a number of standard prefabricated sizes were made available for repeated use. Several other institutions have published use of customized step-wedge midline blocks based on individual implants (236). Most institutions use rectangular blocks 4 to 5 cm in width rather than production of blocks based on the isodose distributions (Fig. 14.47) (233,237).

There are some important safety issues when using midline blocks. The midline block position should be based on films with similar isocenters. If patients receive external beam irradiation in the prone position, it may be wise to simulate them in the supine position for their parametrial boosts so that they are in the same position as they are for their implants. Midline blocks can be positioned to account for applicator deviation. Wolfson et al. found that most institutions using the standard rectangular midline blocks align the superior-inferior central axis of the block along the midplane of the patient's pelvis, while those using customized midline blocks usually align the midline block along the axis of the tandem (233). The step-wedge corrects for the lateral gradient of the intracavitary system and not the rapid dose gradient anterior and posterior to the plane of the implant or for variations in the positions of the implants. The contribution of scattered radiation may increase the dose under narrow midline blocks, which may exceed the anticipated 5% of the primary pelvic dose when using a 5 to 6 half-value layer (HVL) midline block. Midline blocks that are too narrow may not adequately shield the bladder and rectosigmoid given their ability to move in and out of the blocked field. Filling and emptying of these organs may also alter their position relative to the block. Eifel et al. point out that the distance between the distal ureters is usually 4 to 5 cm. A narrow block may fail to shield a portion of the ureters during external beam (238). Reviewing the M.D. Anderson experience, Eifel et al. detected an increase in complications in patients with midline blocks (4 cm) used throughout the course of external beam. Since the ureters are typically 2 to 3 cm from midline, the explanation for the ureteral stenosis could have been an overlap between the external beam fields and the high dose region of the intracavitary implants (238). A margin of 0.5 cm lateral to the lateral ovoid surface is recommended in designing the width of the midline block for each patient to protect the implanted volume. If the intracavitary system is broad, a wide midline block may potentially shield the external iliac lymph nodes. If tissues immediately adjacent to the colpostats and tandem tip are not shielded, portions of the ileocecal junction and rectosigmoid may be overdosed (239,240). Huang et al. recommended avoiding a combination of parametrial boost doses of ≥54 Gy and a cumulative rectal biologically effective dose (CRBED) $\geq 100\ Gy_3$ to decrease the risk of radiation-induced bowel complications (240). Chun et al. also found increasing rectal complications with parametrial boosts >55 Gy (241). When a midline block is inserted prior to 40 Gy, it should not extend to the top of the field since it will shield the common iliac and presacral lymph nodes, which will be underdosed (228,233). Kuipers notes that the uterus can be displaced cranially toward the sigmoid during intracavitary irradiation because of vaginal packing. It may be important to make the midline block high enough to protect the sigmoid so that it does not receive further radiation during external beam (242). The inferior edge of the midline block should be coincident with the caudal aspect of the whole pelvis fields to avoid overdosage of the distal vagina (233). When there is suspicion of uterosacral ligament involvement, it is safer to avoid early placement of the midline block, which will shield disease lying posterior to the implant (210). Due to concern over rectal tolerance, the rectum is shielded after a certain amount of external beam radiation therapy, which can block tumor in the perirectal area and uterosacral space. The geometric configuration of the intracavitary implant emphasizes lateral rather than posterior coverage and does not effectively treat the perirectal and uterosacral space effectively. This can lead to underdosing of tissues in this area and an increased risk of central recurrence. Higher whole pelvis external beam doses, interstitial implantation, or addition of a supplemental posterior oblique external beam boost may offer ways to compensate dose in this area (210). As there may be some disparity in implant position if multiple fractions are used over time, such as with HDR, it is necessary to reassess the midline block configuration after each implant (243).

Parametrial/Nodal Boosting in Cervical Cancer

Parametrial boosting is often recommended for patients with bulky parametrial or sidewall disease, after completion of the whole pelvis field and midline block fields, as the parametria are a common site of failure. The need for boosting is usually based on the status of disease regression following whole pelvis irradiation. MRI may be helpful in making this assessment both before and during radiation. Mayr et al. found MRI imaging useful in the localization of parametrial tumor extension and enlarged their parametrial boost fields based on these MRI images to include the disease and exclude small bowel (218). Logsdson and Eifel suggest boosting residual lateral pelvic wall disease after 40 to 45 Gy whole pelvis to 60 to 62 Gy to small volumes (82). Perez et al. found a trend toward increased pelvic control with point B doses (defined at 6 cm lateral to the central axis) >45 Gy (101,244). In the 1973 and 1978 PCS, there was no relationship between lateral dose >60 Gy and either infield pelvic control or survival, but the lateral dose did impact complications with an increase above 50 Gy (107,109,110). There was a trend toward decreased failure with increasing parametrial doses in stage III disease (108). Perez et al. found that the incidence of pelvic recurrence was correlated with tumor size and dose of irradiation delivered to the lateral parametrium. There was an increase in the incidence of pelvic recurrence in patients receiving less than 50 Gy, but no correlation with increasing doses of irradiation (245). Doses needed to eradicate parametrial disease in the literature are typically around 60 Gy, combining the external beam doses with the implant doses. The proximity of small bowel can make this a risky proposition. Perez et al. noted that with doses below 50 Gy to the lateral pelvic wall, the risk of small bowel complications was about 1% and somewhat higher with larger doses (128). In a later series, grade 3 small bowel sequelae were 1% with doses of 50 Gy and 2% to 4% with doses over 60 Gy ($p = 0.04$) (246). At present, Perez et al. recommend limiting the small bowel doses to less than 60 Gy (246). Ferrigno et al. found an increase in small bowel complications when parametrial boosts were above 59 Gy. They recommended dropping the superior border of the parametrial fields to the S2-3 level and limiting the total dose to 54 Gy (181). The use of concurrent chemoradiation may allow a decrease in these doses, but data is too preliminary to conclude what this dose should be. When there is uterosacral space involvement, thought should be given to the use of a supplemental posterior oblique external beam boost (210). Grigsby et al. used PET/CT scans to evaluate lymph node size, irradiation dose, and patterns of failure. The parametrial and lymph node boost doses used were in the range of 9.0 to 14.4 Gy following large field doses of 50.4 Gy. Radiation dose and lymph node size were not significant predicators of lymph node failure. The risk of an isolated lymph node failure was <2% (247). A reoperation series following definitive irradiation and chemotherapy was reported by Houvenaegel et al. After 45 Gy and whole pelvis and selective parametrial or nodal boosting to 55 to 60 Gy, 15.9% of patients had biopsy-proven residual disease in the pelvic nodes and 11.7% of paraaortic nodes (248). Use of IMRT may be a method to increase dose to bulky nodes or residual parametrial disease while sparing adjacent normal structures (37,40,249).

EXTERNAL BEAM IRRADIATION FOR GYNECOLOGIC CANCERS

Endometrial Cancer

For endometrial cancer, many of the same nodes are at risk as in cervical cancer, but the spread of disease is not as predictable with the paraaortic nodes independently at risk. The presacral nodes are also not at risk unless there is cervical involvement. Both the pelvic and paraaortic nodes are at risk in all sites of uterine involvement, and grade, myometrial invasion, and lymphatic vascular space invasion are more predictive of risk than location (250–254). Cervical and lower uterine segment involvement also increases the likelihood of pelvic and paraaortic lymph node metastases compared to fundal location, as do increasing histologic grade and myometrial invasion. In the surgical staging series of Boronow et al., 18 of 222 patients had lower uterine segment involvement and six (33%) had pelvic lymph node metastases (253,255). In the final GOG surgical staging series report, by location, patients with fundal lesions had a 4% risk of paraaortic and 8% risk of pelvic lymph node involvement, whereas patients with lower uterine segment involvement had a 16% risk of pelvic and 14% risk of paraaortic lymph node involvement (254).

In endometrial cancer, external beam irradiation is generally recommended for patients thought to be at significant risk for lymph node metastases and/or a vaginal cuff recurrence. This has traditionally been recommended in the absence of a lymph node dissection or a limited lymph node sampling. External beam irradiation is also still delivered at many institutions in the setting of a negative lymph node dissection when high risk features such as deep myometrial invasion, high grade, lymphatic vascular space invasion, lower uterine segment involvement, or cervical invasion are present (256,257).

External beam irradition typically covers the upper one half to two thirds of the vagina, the pelvic lymph node regions, and the surgical bed (Fig. 14.54). External beam field design must necessarily include the pelvic lymphatics with exclusion of as

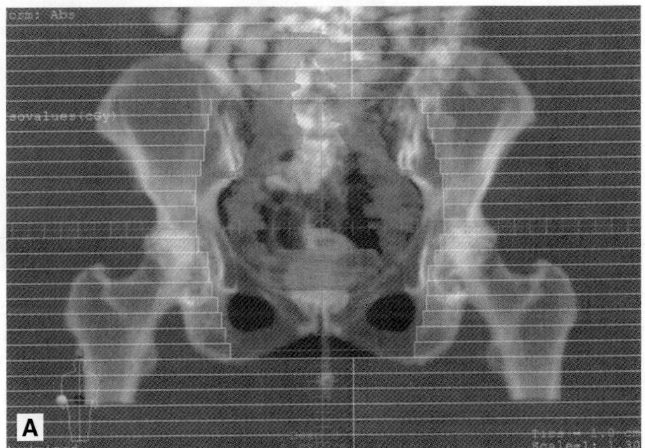

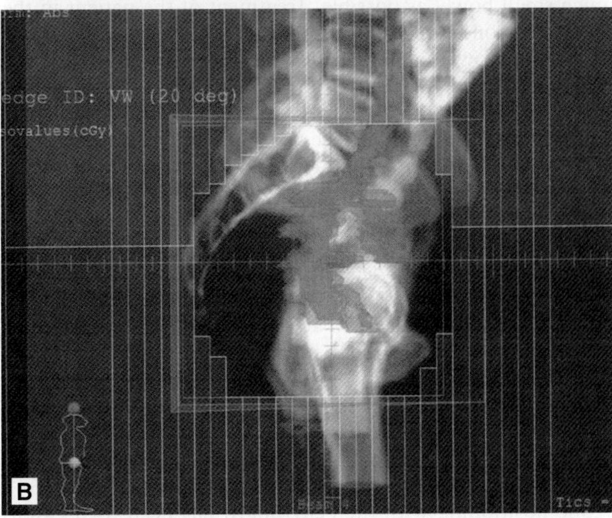

FIGURE 14.54. Digitally reconstructed AP (A) and lateral (B) radiographs with nodal volumes contoured as well as the vaginal apex and the fields defined by the leaves of multileaf collimator. This is a standard field design for patients with endometrial cancer.

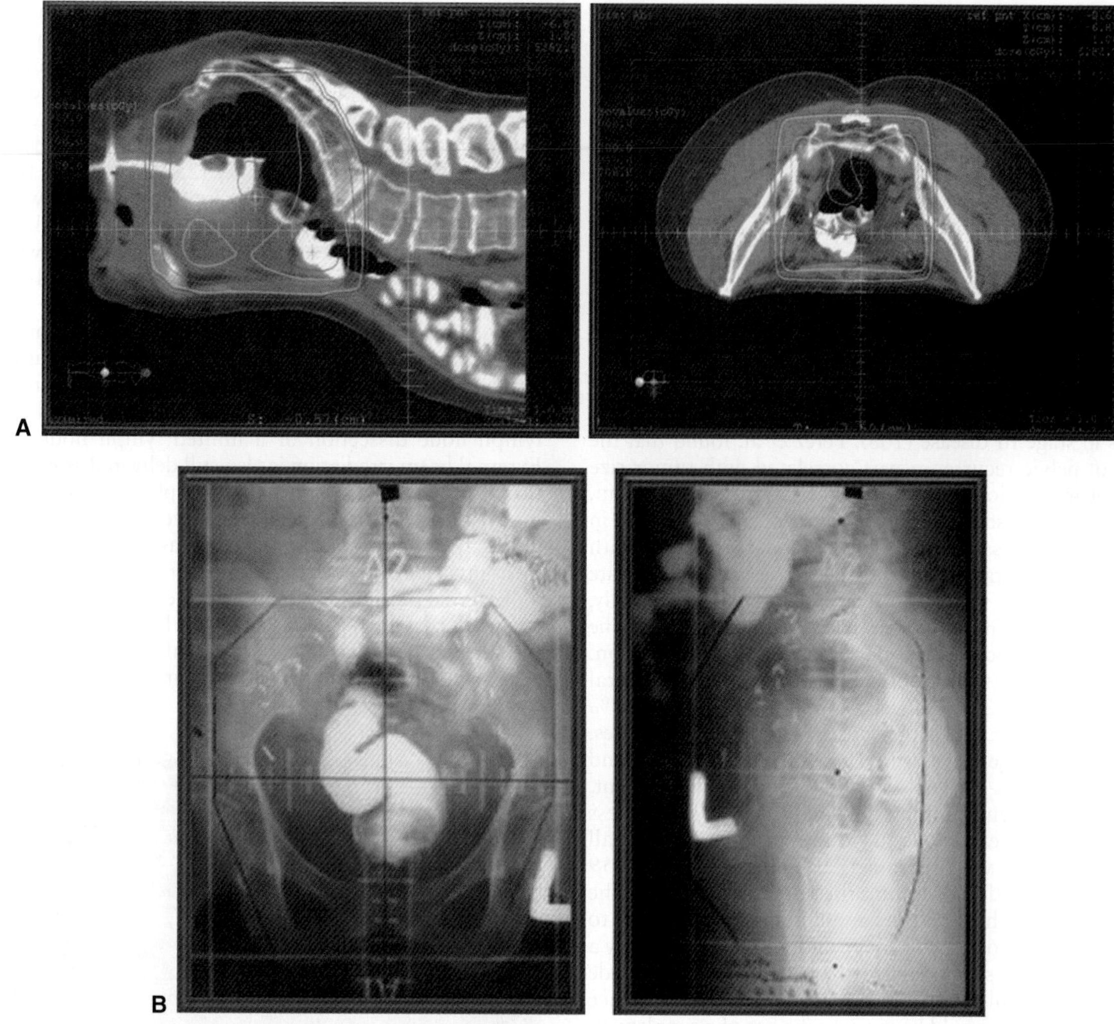

FIGURE 14.55. **A:** Utility of the prone technique for small bowel displacement as shown on a sagittal and axial CT scan of a patient with endometrial cancer planned in the prone position. **B:** Radiographs of the pelvis showing significant amount of small bowel in the radiation fields.

much small bowel as possible. Treatment of the patient in the prone position with a full bladder will help to exclude at least some small bowel in most patients unless these loops are fixed in the pelvis (Fig. 14.55). It is important, however, for the lateral fields to also cover the course of the external iliac nodes, which are quite anterior in the pelvis and require inclusion of some small bowel in the lateral fields to be adequately covered. Doses of 45 to 50.4 Gy are typical with some institutions treating to 40 Gy and as high as 60 Gy to reduced fields in the setting of nodal disease. Whole pelvic fields are generally reduced or a midline block is added after variable doses.

Prone techniques have been used in the treatment of many other pelvic malignancies to attempt to exclude small bowel from the field. Use of a belly board device to further enhance small bowel displacement has become standard practice for many pelvic malignancies (258–260). Use of prone position with or without a belly board for the treatment of patients with cervical cancer has been reported in a few series, in the postoperative (258,259,261–263) and definitive settings (258–260,263,264). Prone positioning with the belly board has been used extensively for patients with rectal cancers when using a PA and two lateral fields. Concern over use of this technique for patients with gynecologic malignancies when adding a fourth field (AP) to cover the external iliac nodes has been raised by Ghosh et al. due to the uncertainty in source to skin distance (SSD) and variation in tissue thickness from the anterior field. In patients who underwent postoperative irradiation for cervical cancer, they observed that the small bowel was best excluded from the AP-PA fields when the patient was positioned prone without the belly board, thereby compressing the small bowel laterally out of the AP-PA fields. They recommended an alternating routine (261). Bladder distention can also help to optimally displace bowel when using the belly board (258,260). Concern over use of the belly board in patients treated with definitive versus postoperative irradiation for cervical cancer is also raised due to the potential change in position of the uterus when prone, the impact and variability of bladder filling, and the potential daily variation in the setup (261,263,264). There is also some concern that, in patients with intact uteri, the prone position may increase the volume of the rectum treated (263). CT- based dosimetry has documented that the prone position, particularly with bladder filling, can alter the position of the uterus within the radiation field (218,220,264). Hence, if patients are simulated prone, it is even more imperative to use CT- or MRI-based dosimetry in the prone position to make sure that the entire uterus is in the pelvic fields, and it is also imperative to consistently fill or empty the bladder (264,265). IGRT may also be helpful in ensuring that the daily setup is reproducible and reliable.

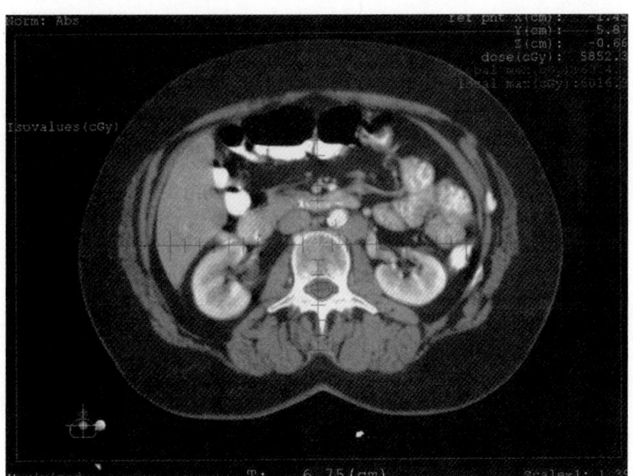

FIGURE 14.56. Axial CT scan demonstrating an enlarged periaortic lymph node near the left renal hilum.

Extended Field Irradiation

Extended field irradiation refers to inclusion of both the pelvic and paraaortic nodes in the radiation fields. Common indications for extended field irradiation in gynecologic cancers include patients with positive paraaortic nodes or those with positive pelvic nodes or bulky primary lesions feared to be at risk for microscopic paraaortic disease (Fig. 14.56). Extended fields include more normal organs than pelvic fields alone. Limitation of dose to the small bowel, kidneys, liver, stomach, and spinal cord are essential. Three-dimensional conformal techniques are helpful in achieving an acceptable therapeutic ratio. Use of IMRT has recently been piloted in this setting with further attempts to decrease acute and late toxicity (Fig. 14.20). Selective boosting of gross nodal disease may allow for safer dose escalation (37–39,249).

Whole Abdominal Irradiation

Whole abdominal irradiation is used to cover the entire abdominopelvic cavity in ovarian cancers or high-risk uterine cancers such as those with positive peritoneal washings or adnexal involvement (IIIA disease). This requires limiting the radiation dose to a maximum of 30 Gy to the entire abdomen and using lower fraction sizes of 150 to 170 cGy. This will reduce both acute and late toxicities. Careful attention to and limitation of the dose of radiation delivered to the liver and kidneys requires selective blocking of these structures at different doses (266,267). IMRT techniques are also being explored for whole abdominal irradiation to reduce doses to the GI tract, liver, kidneys, and bone marrow and increase dose to the peritoneal surfaces and lymph nodes (41,42).

Radiation-Induced Tissue Effects

Side effects that develop during the course of radiation and persist for 3 months or less following completion of radiation are termed acute side effects. Those toxicities that develop later than 3 months after the completion of radiation are termed late or chronic effects. The late effects of radiation are due to damage at the capillary level where there is endothelial cell proliferation resulting in less diffusion of oxygen into the tissues with resulting fibrosis. There is less resistance to infection, trauma, or functional stress due to this change in vasculature and circulation (268,269). When treating gynecologic cancers, the normal tissues most often incidentally irradiated in the pelvis are the rectosigmoid, small bowel, bladder, vagina, and pelvic bones and bone marrow. In the upper abdomen, the kidneys, liver, stomach, small bowel, and spinal cord may be in the radiation field. The response of a tissue or organ to radiation depends on two factors: (a) the inherent sensitivity of the individual cells, and (b) the kinetics of the population as a whole of which the cells are a part. These factors combine to account for the substantial variation in response to radiation characteristic of different tissues (1). Additionally, the volume of tissue irradiated as well as the dose, dose rate, and fractionation scheme will affect both acute and late toxicities. The addition of chemotherapy or other systemic agents may impact toxicity, as may other medical comorbidites such as diabetes, hypertension, collagen vascular diseases, Crohn's disease, and ulcerative colitis, as well as social risk factors such as smoking. The most comprehensive data describing the effects of radiation on the normal tissues was published by Rubin and Casarett and later updated by Emani et al. (269,270). Rubin and Casarett defined tolerance doses (TD) for almost all of the tissues. The TD 5/5 is defined as the probability of a 5% risk of complications within 5 years of the completion of radiation, and TD 5/50 as the probability of a 50% risk of complications within 5 years (269).

Skin

When treating abdominopelvic tumors with radiation, often there will be minimal skin reactions due to the skin-sparing quality of the high-energy radiation beams used to treat these sites deep within the body. Contrastingly, when treating the vulvar and inguinal regions, where electrons or lower energy x-rays are more often used, there can be marked skin reactions. Skin reactions are also more likely to develop in skin folds such as the inguinal creases or intergluteal fold. The cells in the basal layer of the skin are very sensitive to radiation, but because of the time required for these differentiating cells to move from the basal layer to the keratinized layer of skin, there is a 2 to 3 week delay between the start of radiation and the appearance of skin reactions. Erythema is the first visible skin reaction due to dilation of the small capillaries and is usually seen about the 3rd week of radiation. Other skin reactions include dry desquamation and moist desquamation occurring after the 4th week of radiation. Moist desquamation occurs with transient loss of the epidermis and exposure of the dermis. Serous fluid often oozes from the exposed and inflamed dermis (269,271). These effects may be enhanced by the combination of irradiation and some chemotherapeutic agents, particularly actinomycin D and doxorubicin (Adriamycin) (272). It is also well known that chemotherapy agents such as Adriamycin or gemcitabine can "recall" radiation reactions after the original reaction has subsided. Radiation-induced skin reactions are treated with various topical ointments and creams as well as with sitz baths and special emphasis on cleansing all stool and urine gently from the perineum. Additionally, if the distal vagina or vulva is in the radiation field, patients may also complain of dysuria or painful defecation, which is due to the caustic effects of the urine and stool on the denuded epithelium of the distal vagina, perianal area, and vulva. Diarrhea control and use of barrier creams to protect the irritated skin from stool and urine will help to minimize discomfort and hasten skin healing. Sulfa-based creams and Domeboro soaks can be used to expedite healing. Return of the epidermis can take 10 to 14 days. Residual surviving basal cells form islands of regeneration, which proliferate to re-epithelize the area. Islands of skin forming in the desquamated skin herald skin renewal. The new skin is thin and pink with gradual return to normal in 2 to 3 weeks (269). Late manifestations of radiation on the skin include depigmentation, subcutaneous fibrosis, dryness and thinning with loss of apocrine and sebaceous glands, thinning or loss of hair, and telangiectases. Necrosis of the skin is rare and generally occurs only with very high doses of radiation in excess of 60 Gy (269,272).

Vagina

There are few noticeable acute reactions when treating the upper two thirds of the vagina with radiation. Some patients may notice a white-yellow vaginal discharge, which is due to mucositis of the vaginal mucosa. This can be evident during radiation and continue for several months after radiation (269). The lower third of the vagina, however, will become quite irritated when irradiated, in part due to irradiation of the vulva and urethra as described above. The distal vagina is less tolerant of radiation than the proximal and the tolerance doses are in the range of 80 to 90 Gy versus 120 to 150 Gy, respectively (273). Vaginal narrowing and shortening is a late sequela of radiation, which can alter and impede sexual function. Combined brachytherapy and external beam irradiation will cause more late effects than either modality alone. Use of a vaginal dilator or intercourse 2 to 3 times/week can help to keep the vagina open. Use of lubrication with intercourse as well as estrogen creams to build up the vaginal mucosa can also make intercourse more comfortable (272,274). Rarely, with excessive doses of radiation, patients can develop vaginal necrosis. This is due to a change in blood supply to the vaginal tissues and is much more common at the introitus than at the vaginal apex, perhaps due to the vascular supply of the vagina. The posterior vaginal wall is most frequently involved (273). Interstitial implants are more likely to cause necrosis than intracavitary implants. Hydrogen peroxide douches, antibiotics, and hyperbaric oxygen therapy can help the vaginal tissues to heal (275,276). Narcotics are often necessary to control the associated pain until healing has occurred. Trental (pentoxifylline) can also help soft-tissue necrosis to heal (277). The uterus is very resistant to high doses of radiation as is evident in patients treated with external beam and brachytherapy for cervical cancer. Rare cervical necrosis can occur and will respond readily to hyperbaric oxygen treatments and pentoxifylline (269,276,278). Necrosis can also be caused by recurrent tumor, and distinguishing recurrent disease from necrosis can be very difficult and sometimes will mandate surgical intervention (269).

Bladder/Ureters/Urethra

The bladder and ureters have a rapidly renewing transitional epithelium. The effect of radiation is early denudation similar to the skin due to injury to the rapidly dividing basal cells. Epithelial desquamation leads to focal ulcerations, hyperemia, and edema of the bladder wall, which is visible at cystoscopy (269,271,279). Acute and transient radiation cystitis may be observed with moderate doses of irradiation (>30 Gy) and usually requires no specific treatment. Patients will report urinary frequency and urgency as well as mild dysuria, as well as decreased bladder capacity. However, with higher radiation doses, more severe symptoms of cystitis develop, such as severe dysuria and hematuria, which may require treatment. Agents such as Pyridium may help lessen these symptoms. Significant spasms of the bladder musculature, which may be improved with administration of smooth muscle relaxants, may also occur. It is important to rule out the presence of a concomitant bacterial infection, which may exacerbate the symptoms. Infections are seen at an increased rate in irradiated patients, perhaps in part due to radiation-induced diarrhea and contamination of the perineum. Urinalysis and urine cultures obtained under sterile conditions, when indicated, should be obtained before institution of antibiotic therapy. Radiation cystitis is characterized by the presence of white cells and red cells without bacteria on urinalysis.

With doses above 60 Gy, chronic cystitis and hematuria may be observed due to telangiectasias, which can develop in the bladder lining. With higher doses, more severe chronic cystitis, fibrosis, and decreased bladder capacity can occur. Rarely, bladder neck contractures as well as fistulas may occur, which can necessitate surgical intervention. Fistulas are more likely to occur if there is invasion of the bladder wall by tumor or in the setting of interstitial implants. Surgery may be required to deal with some of these complications (269). Hyperbaric oxygen therapy can be very helpful with hemorrhagic cystits as can the drug pentosan polysulfate (Elmiron), which has been used for interstitial cystitis (276,280,281). Studies have demonstrated that with doses below 75 to 80 Gy to limited volumes of the bladder, the incidence of grade 3 or 4 complications is 5% or less, whereas with higher doses, a greater incidence of sequelae is noted (238,246). The ureters are quite resistant to radiation and rare ureteral stenosis is reported in some series (238,269,279,282). This can require stenting or rarely diversion. Interstitial implants are more likely to cause this than intracavitary implants, as can early placement of a narrow midline block (238). Urethral stenosis is also rare and is also more likely to occur with interstitial than intracavitary approaches. Careful dilation can be helpful in sustaining bladder outflow (279).

Small and Large Intestine, Stomach

The acute effects of radiation on the small intestine are due to the inherent radiation sensitivity of the rapidly dividing undifferentiated crypt of Lieberkuhn cells. The normal lining of the GI tract is a self-renewing tissue. These undifferentiated stem cells normally migrate and differentiate upward from the lower half of the crypts to the tips of the intestinal villi as they mature, providing a continuous supply of surface cells as they divide. Their function is to primarily form absorbtive cells but also mucous-secreting goblet cells and endocrine cells (268,269,271). The mature cells at the surface of the villi are repeatedly sloughed and replaced by the cells, which originate in the crypts. These undifferentiated crypt cells are the most sensitive to radiation and are preferentially depleted, leading to loss of mature replacement cells at the surface of the villi. When these mature mucosal cells cannot be replaced, the villi shorten and the loss of absorbtive function of the small intestine occurs. This loss of function results in fluid and nutrient wasting, diarrhea, and dehydration. This constellation of symptoms is termed acute radiation enteritis. Fortunately, re-epithelialization occurs within several days due to recovery of the rapidly dividing crypt cells (271). Mucosal healing will occur within 10 to 14 days if radiation is terminated, and symptoms will accordingly improve and resolve in most patients. It is common to observe watery diarrhea with intermittent abdominal cramping starting in the 2nd or 3rd week of abdominal or pelvic irradiation. Increased peristalsis, disturbance of the absorption mechanisms, and a decreased transit time also occur. Patients will report increased flatulence and noisy bowel sounds. Rarely patients will report nausea. Implementation of a low residue diet, hydration, and use of antimotility agents can be very helpful. Some patients may be lactose and fat intolerant as well. Judicious use of narcotics to calm the bowel can also be helpful. Concurrent 5-FU or gemcitabine can worsen small bowel toxicity with diarrhea from the 5-FU often appearing before the radiation enteritis has had time to evolve. The late effects of radiation on the small bowel can be a continuation of the acute effects. Some patients will experience chronic diarrhea that will require a permanent change in diet. Certain foods may trigger diarrhea such as those high in fiber or fat. Spicy foods and MSG may also trigger diarrhea. Areas of narrowing corresponding to regions of high dose or adhesions can occur in the small bowel loops and lead to partial obstruction of the small bowel. Patients may report abdominal pain and distention followed by diarrhea and relief of these symptoms. A complete bowel obstruction would also be characterized by abdominal pain and distention in addition to vomiting and lack of bowel movements. Small bowel obstructions occur in approximately 5% of irradiated patients and surgical intervention is required in some to relieve these obstructions. Prior surgeries or a history of a perforated appendix or pelvic abscess as well as inflammatory bowel disease can increase the risk of small bowel toxicity. Hypertension and diabetes can also be risk factors as can thin body habitus. Radiation to large volumes of bowel or high doses to even small volumes of bowel can lead to bowel obstructions. The ileum is the most common loop of bowel involved (269). Malabsorbtion of fats, carbohydrates, protein, B12, and lactose can occur in some patients. Excessive bile salts can reach the colon and act as a cathartic, and medications such as cholestyramine can be helpful in controlling the resultant loose stools.

The rectosigmoid mucosa is also a rapid renewal system similar to the small bowel. When the rectum is included in the irradiated volume, there is rectal discomfort with tenesmus and mucous production, sometimes mixed with blood in the stools. Patients may report frequent and sometimes painful evacuations of only small amounts of stool mixed with mucus. Hemorrhoids may worsen during radiation. This constellation of symptoms is termed "proctitis." Medications to decrease the number of stools as well as antispasmodic agents can be helpful. Suppositories or foams with steroids can be helpful, as can topical perianal skin ointments and lotions. Uncontrolled radiation enteritis can worsen radiation proctitis due to frequent stooling through the irritated rectum. For late effects, if the dose of radiation is large enough, it may cause temporary or permanent ulceration and bleeding due to telangiectasias (Fig. 14.57). Cortisone-containing rectal suppositories and foams or sulfasalazine instillations can also help to heal the

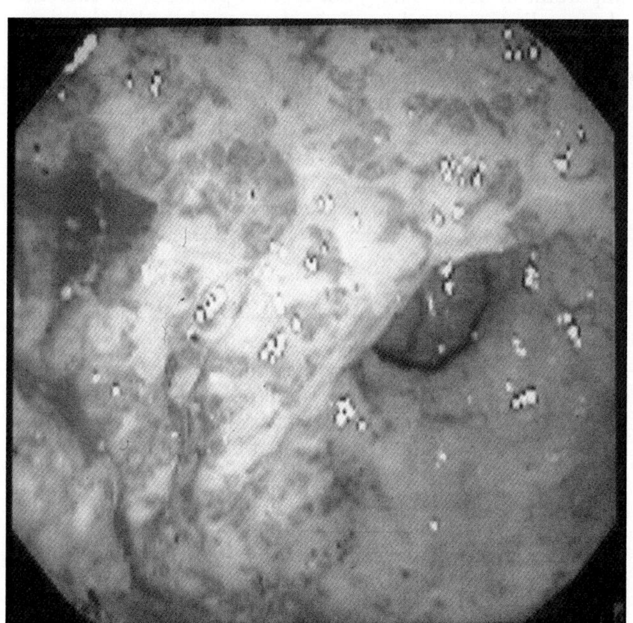

FIGURE 14.57. Radiation-induced telangiectasias of the rectum consistent with radiation proctitis.

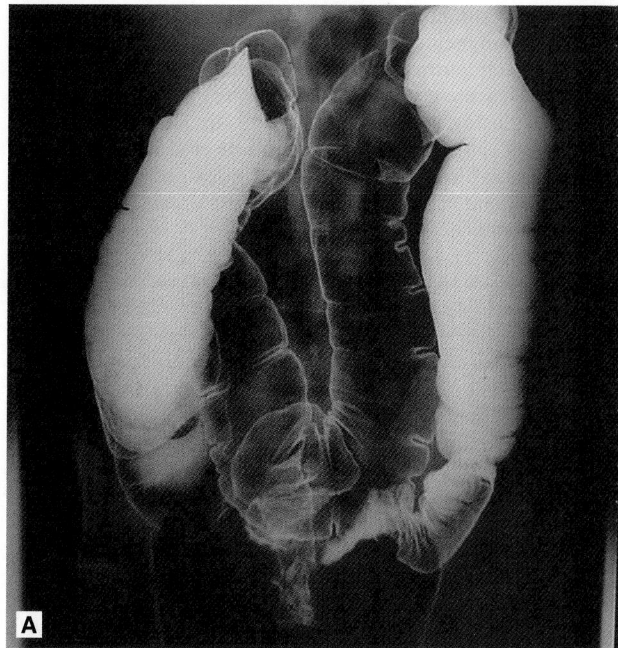

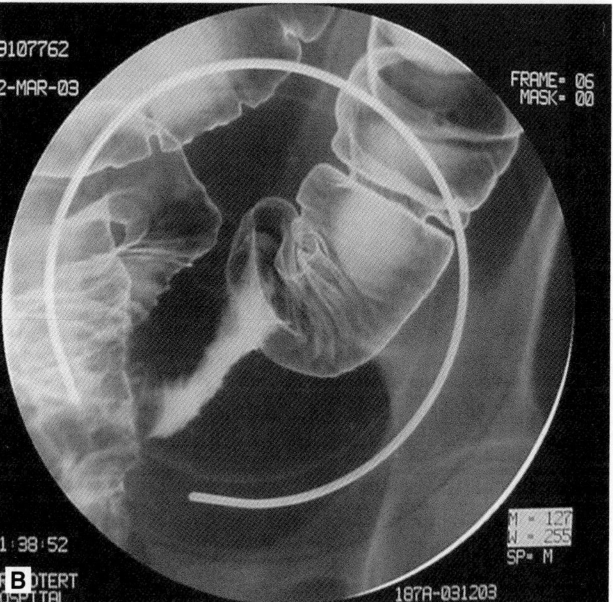

FIGURE 14.58. Radiation-induced sigmoid stricture noted on a contrast study ([A] full view, [B] magnified view) following definitive chemoradiation.

bleeding and ulcerated rectal mucosa as can argon laser ablation of the telangiectasias.

Hyperbaric oxygen therapy can be helpful in controlling bleeding when severe (276,280,283,284). Fibrosis, stenosis, perforation, and fistula formation are more rare (Fig. 14.58). In general, doses in excess of 60 Gy are necessary to produce this more advanced radiation damage to the small bowel and rectosigmoid. Fecal diversion may be necessary in the setting of stenosis, necrosis, or fistula formation. Retrospective analyses have shown that limited volumes of the rectum can tolerate about 75 Gy (external beam and brachytherapy) with acceptable morbidity (238,246).

The stomach is also lined with a mucous membrane, which is columnar epithelium and sensitive to radiation. Like the small and large bowel reactions, the stomach lining develops erosions and thinning and subsequent edema and ulceration. Symptoms can include nausea, vomiting, reflux, and pain. Use of prophylactic antiemetics and proton pump inhibitors can decrease the acute effects of radiation. Acid production can be decreased during radiation and for up to 1 to 2 years after. Late effects can include gastritis and ulceration with associated bleeding. Progressive fibrosis can lead to gastric outlet obstruction and rarely perforation, all of which are dose and volume dependent (269).

Ovaries

In premenopausal patients treated with definitive irradiation, the ovaries will be irradiated incidentally and ovarian failure will occur. Hot flashes and other menopausal symptoms can begin to develop during radiation. Hormone replacement therapy is an important consideration in women younger than 50. Alternatively, midline oophoropexy has been used in young women requiring irradiation for Hodgkin's disease in an effort to spare the ovaries. The ovaries can also be elevated out of the radiation field and placed above the true pelvis to attempt to avoid them when treating cervical cancer. The radiosensitivity of the ovarian cells varies considerably with age. The dose necessary to castrate a woman depends on her age. A larger dose is required during the period of more active follicular proliferation. A single dose of 4.0 to 8.0 Gy or fractionated doses of 12 to 20 Gy (depending on age) are known to produce permanent castration and sterility in most patients (268,269,272).

Bone Marrow/Pelvic Bones

The lymphocytes are the most radiosensitive cells in the bone marrow. The rate of fall of the various components of the marrow is a function of the half-lives of the mature cells. These half-lives are as follows: erythrocytes, 120 days; granulocytes, 6.6 hours; platelets, 8 to 10 days (269). Pelvic irradiation may cause transient lymphopenia. This is even more of an issue when whole abdominal or extended field irradiation is used due to the increased bone marrow in the radiation fields. This decrease in lymphocytes is thought to be the result of irradiation of the lymphocytes circulating through the vascular bed and may not be indicative of bone marrow reserve depletion. Prior or concurrent chemotherapy will also lead to increased bone marrow toxicity. Frequent monitoring of the CBC is considered standard of care with pelvic or abdominal irradiation. Permanent chronic changes are noted even when small segments of the bone marrow are irradiated to doses over 30 Gy, and recovery may take up to 18 months or longer in a proportion of patients with good reparative capacity.

Insufficiency fractures can also develop in irradiated pelvic bones (285–287). These most commonly involve the sacrum and ileum, followed by the pubic bones, and rarely the acetabulum. Patients may complain of sudden onset of back or groin pain, which worsens with weight bearing and changes in position. MRI is the best imaging modality to detect them and also rule out recurrent disease. Sometimes edema will be reported in the absence of actual fractures, and in other cases actual fractures will be seen. It is important not to confuse these changes with metastatic disease, as further palliative irradiation would worsen the integrity of the bone. Symptoms from these changes in the pelvic bones will often improve over time, but patients may also suffer future symptoms from exacerbation of these fractures or development of new fractures over time. Sacroplasty can be used if patients remain symptomatic. Narcotics and changes in activity are often required. Femoral neck complications can include avascular necrosis as well as fracture. This is a rare complication following irradiation of the inguinal nodes. Hip replacement surgery is required to resolve this problem (278).

Liver

During whole abdominal irradiation or paraaortic irradiation, the liver is in the radiation field and dose must be limited to this critical organ. Clinical and pathologic studies have shown that the liver is not a radioresistant organ. Venoocclusive disease is the pathologic entity caused by radiation. Necrosis and atrophy of the hepatic cells result from this change in blood supply. CT scanning following radiation can show changes in perfusion of the liver corresponding to the radiation fields. These changes are not always associated with toxicity. The clinical course and liver changes depend on the dose and volume of irradiation as well as the presence of chemotherapy and preexisting liver disease. During radiation, the liver enzymes may be elevated. This can continue following completion of radiation. Signs of radiation hepatitis can include a marked elevation of alkaline phosphatase (3 to 10 times normal) with much less elevation of the transaminases (normal to 2 times normal) (269,288). Liver enlargement and varying amount of ascites can also evolve. If the doses and volumes are high enough liver failure can occur. The TD 5/5 for whole liver is 30 Gy. Small portions of the liver can receive up to 70 Gy (269).

Kidney

The kidneys are very sensitive to small doses of radiation, and a common goal is to avoid greater than 18 to 20 Gy whole kidney dose. When delivering whole abdominal irradiation the kidneys are at risk and must be blocked at acceptable doses to prevent renal failure. When delivering paraaortic irradiation, the kidneys are also at risk and treatment planning CT scans can help to define which beam angles are best to irradiate the nodal regions yet miss, in part, the kidneys. When planning radiation fields, sometimes one kidney will need to be irradiated more than the other and the equivalent of one kidney must be spared. Functional renal studies prior to radiation are important in documenting unexpected perfusion or excretion abnormalities and in determining how much each kidney contributes to total renal function. Functional changes have been described after exposure of the kidney to more than 20 Gy, and signs and symptoms of renal dysfunction can follow including hypertension, leg edema, and a urinalysis showing albuminuria and low specific gravity. A normocytic, normochromic anemia may also appear. Renal function studies will ultimately show decreased blood flow and filtration rates. CT scans may reveal a small kidney if one kidney has been preferentially irradiated to protect the other (269).

Bladder and Rectosigmoid—LDR

The bladder and rectosigmoid are the organs of concern in the setting of combined external beam irradiation and brachytherapy. Dose and volume are considered two important variables related to complications. Dose has been thought to be an important determinant of normal tissue complications. Attempts have been made to determine the maximum tolerable normal tissue dose with an acceptable risk of complications. There is no consensus as to what these values should be. Point doses may or may not coincide with complication risk, as they do not account for the volume of organ irradiated. They are also not defined consistently. Maximum bladder doses of 75 to 80 Gy and rectal doses of 70 to 75 Gy are guidelines (79,246). Small bowel doses should be limited to 45 to 50 Gy with 60 Gy maximum (246). Additionally, the ratio of dose to the rectum and bladder and dose to point A is also important with a low incidence of rectal (0.3% vs. 5%) and bladder (2% vs. 2% to 5%) complications when this ratio was less than 80% (246). Other factors such as external beam dose and intracavitary dose rate are also important in the etiology of complications. The volume of rectum and bladder irradiated is an important variable in the development of complications in addition to the cumulative dose (289). Both external beam and use of tandem and cylinder applicators can increase the volume of bladder and rectum treated (116,290). Stage, patient age, and medical comorbidities such as hypertension, diabetes, diverticulitis, or inflammatory bowel disease may also increase the risk of complications. Individual radiosensitivity may also impact complication risk (291).

Bladder and Rectosigmoid—HDR

Acceptable normal tissue doses are even more debatable in HDR than LDR (177). Using HDR techniques, the therapeutic range is narrower and the risk of complications seems to rise faster than the rate of improved tumor control. Available clinical data also suggests that in addition to total HDR dose, the most important factor in late complication development is the dose per fraction and the number of fractions (56,291,292). The organ most at risk for complications is the rectosigmoid, whereas the bladder complication risk is comparatively low (150,174,293,294). Rectal and sigmoid complications occur earlier than bladder complications (291,292). Rectal bleeding is the most frequent rectal morbidity occurring in approximately 30% of patients (241,293–295). To avoid excessive morbidity, better physical dose distributions must be achieved with HDR to reduce doses to critical normal structures. This implies the use of rectal and bladder displacement. Fowler has speculated that if only 80% of the tumor dose is received by the critical normal tissues, then 4 to 6 HDR fractions can be used safely, whereas 12 to 16 fractions would be required if the normal structures receive 90% of the point A dose, and 30 fractions if the normal structures received 100% of the HDR dose (56,296).

Various disparate recommendations concerning normal tissue fraction size and total dose exist in the literature. Sakata et al. found that the probability of rectal complications increased dramatically above a maximal rectal dose (Deq) of 60 Gy (297). Cheng et al. found that patients with >62 Gy of summed external beam and intracavitary doses to the proximal rectum and >110 Gy maximal proximal rectal BED had significant increase in complications (298). Takeshi et al. noted that radiation dose significantly impacted rectal dose complication rate with an increase above 65 Gy (299). Teshima et al. noted a marked increase in rectal reactions beyond a rectal time-dose fractionation (TDF) factor value of 80 (300,301), and Ogino et al. noted no grade 4 rectal complications below a TDF of 130 and a BED below 147. The calculated incidence of complications ranged from 5% to 10% at TDF values from 104 to 124 and BED values from 119 to 146 (294). Sood et al. found that a rectal or bladder BED_3 <100 Gy_3 was associated with negligible late toxicity (302). Chun et al. noted increasing complications with an ICRU 38 CRBED >100 Gy (241). Chen et al. found the risk of rectal complications to increase with cumulative rectal doses >65 Gy and a CRBED >110 Gy (303). When using 45 Gy to the whole pelvis, Chen et al. found that complications were increased with cumulative ICRU 38 HDR rectal doses >16 Gy and cumulative ICRU 38 HDR bladder doses >24 Gy (304). Ferrigno et al. found that patients treated with a cumulative BED at rectum points above 110 Gy_3 and at bladder points above 125 Gy_3 had a higher risk of complications (181). Correlation of bladder BED with radiation complications has been unreliable (225,304). Toita et al. suggested that the cumulative BED at the rectal point should be kept below 100 to 120 Gy_3 (305). In the series of Lee et al., late rectal complications increased with cumulative rectal BED $\geq$131 (306). Huang et al. recommended cumulative rectal BED $\leq$100 Gy_3 when using parametrial boosting, and recommended boost doses of <54 Gy to the parametria (240). Van Lancker and Storme have not found point A or normal tissue dose points helpful as predictors of complications, but rather that volume calculations were extremely helpful in predicting complications, and they found a significant correlation between rectal complications and the ICRU reference 60 Gy isodose volumes (307).

Rectal retractors have become an integral component of insertion techniques and perhaps improve the effectiveness and reproducibility of rectal displacement over gauze vaginal packing (56,144–146). Whatever the case, a rectal retractor, vaginal speculum blade, or gauze packing should be used to displace the rectum (157,175).

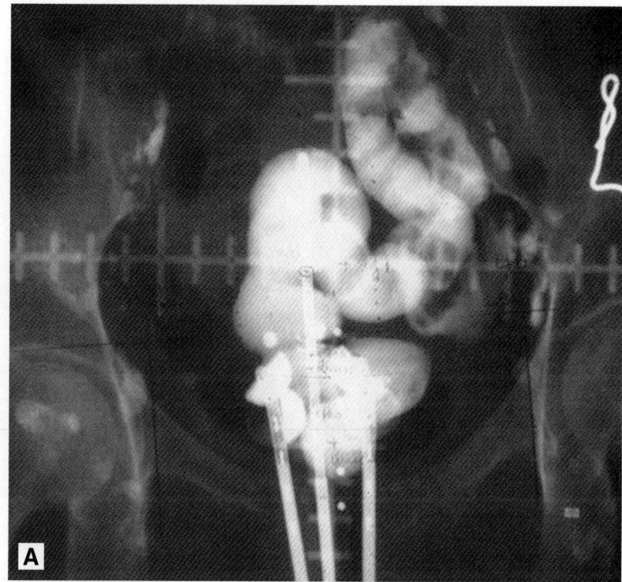

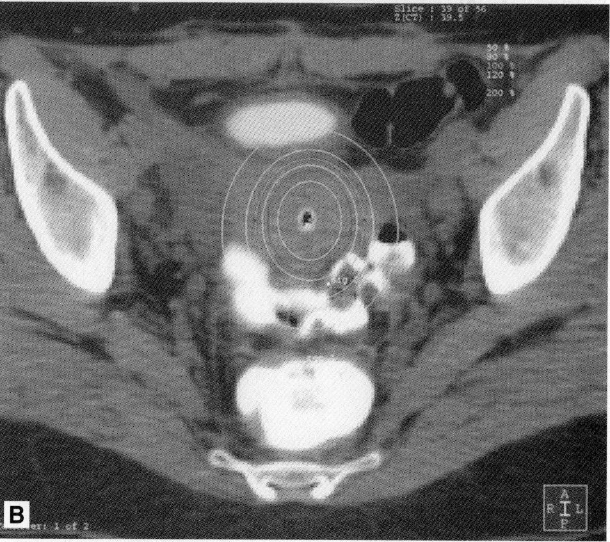

FIGURE 14.59. Radiograph of the pelvis with a tandem and ovoid applicator in place demonstrates the circuitous course of the sigmoid (**A**). The axial CT scan (**B**) demonstrates a more accurate relationship of the sigmoid to the uterine tandem and the need to limit dose to this loop of sigmoid positioned very close to the high dose region of the implant.

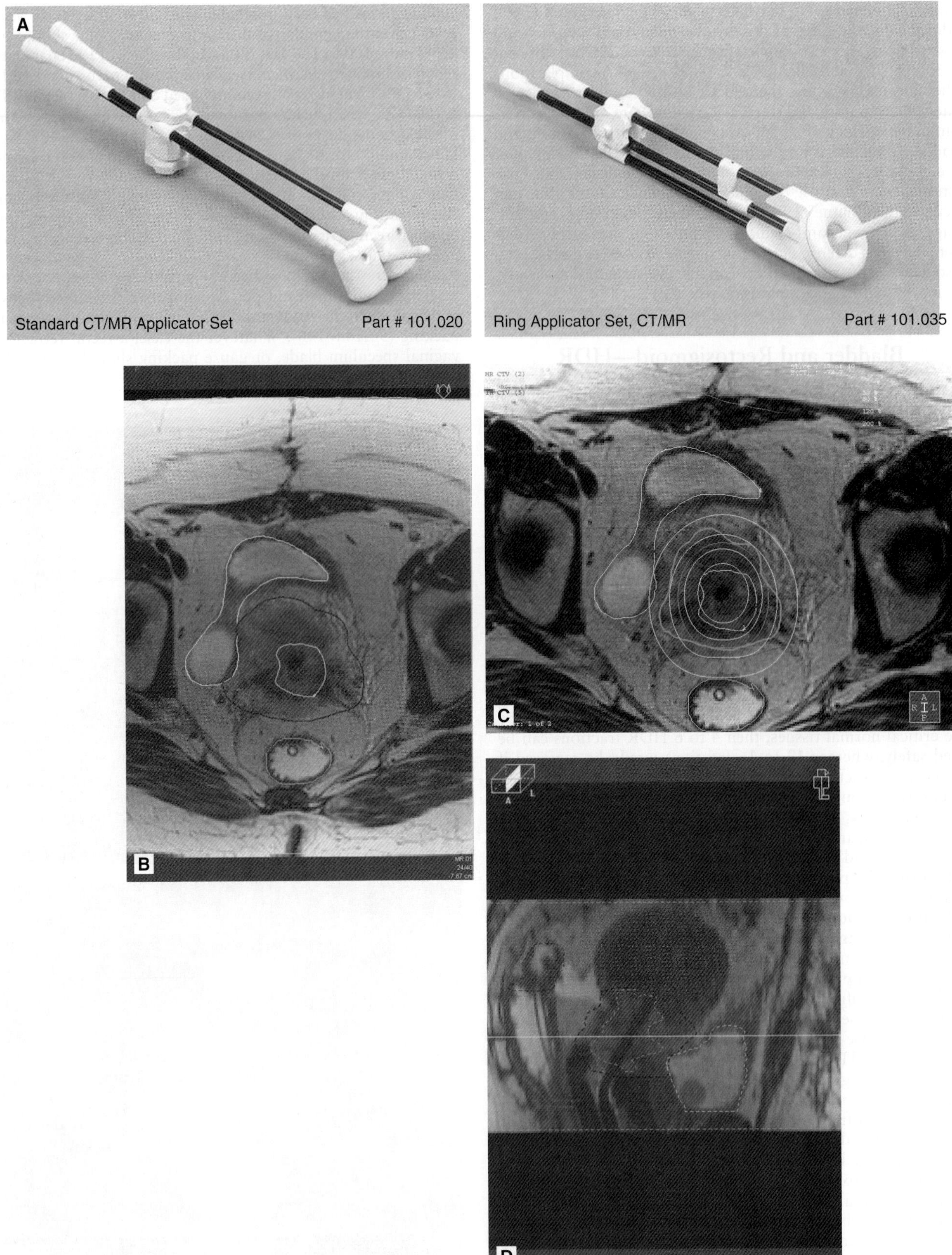

FIGURE 14.60. **A:** MRI compatible applicators. *Source:* Courtesy of Nucletron. **B:** MRI of the pelvis with an MRI/CT compatible applicator in place. Note the associated dose distribution relative to visible tumor within the cervix, in axial (B,C) and sagittal (D) orientations.

It is very important to choose points related to critical structures very carefully on the orthogonal films. Rectum above the level of the vaginal applicators and rectal retractor should be identified and sigmoid in addition to rectal points should be evaluated, as should bladder and vaginal points. Various methods for determining normal tissue doses have been described. When possible, the doses to the normal critical structures should be less than the dose at point A, perhaps in the range of 50% to 80%. The portions of the rectum and sigmoid that are above the range of the rectal retractor are most often the hot spots, and every effort must be made to decrease the dose to the rectosigmoid relative to the point A dose. Consideration to decreasing the dwell times or turning off dwell positions in the tandem should be given. To avoid underdosing endometrial extension of tumor, at least treating 4 cm above the exocervix so that point A is not in a region of dose constriction may be wise. Tandem lengths of 6 to 8 cm are typical. If there is endometrial extension, a longer tandem may be needed. Additionally, use of a tapered tandem will decrease sigmoid, bladder, and small bowel doses (162). Contrast in the sigmoid is helpful in making these decisions. CT scanning after applicator placement is exceedingly helpful and much more reliable in assessing the proximity of the sigmoid to the tandem and in manipulating the dose distribution (Fig. 14.59). Assessment of the anterior and posterior uterine wall thickness measured on CT with the applicator in place, along the course of the tandem, as well as the measured distances from the tandem to the rectosigmoid, small bowel, and bladder, can help to guide dose prescription and potentially decrease toxicity if the distribution is altered appropriately (308). Sigmoid doses can often be higher than the rectal ICRU doses (298).

FUTURE FOCUS

Reduction of morbidity and improvement in local control and cure is a common goal in the treatment of patients with gynecologic cancers. Use of 3D and functional imaging will be increasingly important to define tumor and normal tissues. This can perhaps allow escalation of dose to the tumor and reduction of dose to the critical normal tissues. There has been, however, a reluctance to vary from traditional dose specification as good outcomes have been published at institutions skilled in the care of gynecologic patients. It is potentially dangerous to optimize therapy to such an extent that the dose distribution looks dramatically different from the traditional "pear shape," which effectively encompasses the primary tumor and parametria in cervical cancer presentations. Making this pear too narrow to avoid critical structures may lead to a higher rate of local recurrence. Yet it is important to treat the disease and not just strive for an ideal dose distribution. Preliminary studies using CT indicate that we underestimate normal tissue doses with the present 2D dosimetric analysis used at most institutions (96,291,309). Whether this information should change the way we prescribe doses remains debatable. Directly relating the intracavitary system to the anatomy through use of CT and MRI seems to be the next step in the lineage of dosimetric systems (Fig. 14.60) (96,97,309–312). The GEC ESTRO Gyn Working Group has developed guidelines for defining and contouring tumor volumes and normal tissues on MRI scans with the brachytherapy applicators in place (99–100). The excellent soft-tissue resolution of MRI allows visualization of residual tumor in relation to the isodose distribution around the MRI compatible brachytherapy applicators (Figs. 14.33 and 14.60) (98,313). Data from Potter et al. has shown a decrease in complications and an increase in local control with the use of MRI-guided brachytherapy for cervical cancer (314). Additionally, the use of dose-volume histogram analysis may add new insight into optimizing local control and decreasing morbidity with a better understanding of the importance of dose/volume relationships (311,312,315). This may be a powerful tool to help improve the therapeutic ratio in patients with gynecologic cancer and will best be achieved through collaboration of radiation oncologists, gynecologic oncologists, and diagnostic radiologists.

References

1. Hall EJ, Giaccia AJ. *Radiobiology for the Radiologist*. 6th ed. Philadelphia: Lippincott Williams & Wilkins; 2006.
2. Warters RL, Hofer KG, Harris CR, et al. Radionuclide toxicity in cultured mammalian cells: elucidation of the primary site of radiation damage. *Curr Top Radiat Res Q* 1978;12(1–4):389–407.
3. Hawkins RB. The influence of concentration of DNA on the radiosensitivity of mammalian cells. *Int J Radiat Oncol Biol Phys* 2005;63(2):529–535.
4. Cremer C, Cremer T, Zorn C, et al. Induction of chromosome shattering by ultraviolet irradiation and caffeine: comparison of whole-cell and partial-cell irradiation. *Mutat Res* 1981;84(2):331–348.
5. Hatayoglu SE, Orta T. Relationship between radiation induced dicentric chromosome aberrations and micronucleus formation in human lymphocytes. *J Exp Clin Cancer Res* 2007;26(2):229–234.
6. Garaj-Vrhovac V, Fucic A, Horvat D. The correlation between the frequency of micronuclei and specific chromosome aberrations in human lymphocytes exposed to microwave radiation in vitro. *Mutat Res* 1992;281(3):181–186.
7. Silva MJ, Carothers A, Dias A, et al. Dose dependence of radiation-induced micronuclei in cytokinesis-blocked human lymphocytes. *Mutat Res* 1994;322(2):117–128.
8. Ewing D. The oxygen fixation hypothesis: a reevaluation. *Am J Clin Oncol* 1998;21(4):355–361.
9. Sause WT, Cooper JS, Rush S, et al. Fraction size in external beam radiation therapy in the treatment of melanoma. *Int J Radiat Oncol Biol Phys* 1991;20(3):429–432.
10. Li CY, Nagasawa H, Dahlberg WK, et al. Diminished capacity for p53 in mediating a radiation-induced G1 arrest in established human tumor cell lines. *Oncogene* 1995;11(9):1885–1892.
11. Davis TW, Wilson-Van Patten C, Meyers M, et al. Defective expression of the DNA mismatch repair protein, MLH1, alters G2-M cell cycle checkpoint arrest following ionizing radiation. *Cancer Res* 1998;58(4):767–778.
12. Kachnic LA, Wu B, Wunsch H, et al. The ability of p53 to activate downstream genes p21(WAF1/cip1) and MDM2, and cell cycle arrest following DNA damage is delayed and attenuated in scid cells deficient in the DNA-dependent protein kinase. *J Biol Chem* 1999;274(19):13111–13117.
13. Canman CE, Lim DS, Cimprich KA, et al. Activation of the ATM kinase by ionizing radiation and phosphorylation of p53. *Science* 1998;281(5383):1677–1679.
14. Wang X, Khadpe J, Hu B, et al. An overactivated ATR/CHK1 pathway is responsible for the prolonged G2 accumulation in irradiated AT cells. *J Biol Chem* 2003;278(33):30869–30874.
15. McCabe MT, Azih OJ, Day ML. pRb-Independent growth arrest and transcriptional regulation of E2F target genes. *Neoplasia* 2005;7(2):141–151.
16. Knudson AG, Hethcote HW, Brown BW. Mutation and childhood cancer: a probabilistic model for the incidence of retinoblastoma. *Proc Natl Acad Sci USA* 1975;72(12):5116–5020.
17. Huang PS, Patrick DR, Edwards G, et al. Protein domains governing interactions between E2F, the retinoblastoma gene product, and human papillomavirus type 16 E7 protein. *Mol Cell Biol* 1993;13(2):953–960.
18. Kneale GW, Stewart AM. Mantel-Haenszel analysis of Oxford data. I. Independent effects of several birth factors including fetal irradiation. *J Natl Cancer Inst* 1976;56(5):879–883.
19. Doll R, Wakeford R. Risk of childhood cancer from fetal irradiation. *Br J Radiol* 1997;70:130–139.
20. International Commission on Radiological Protection. http://www.icrp.org/. Accessed October 1, 2007.
21. *Recommendation on Limits for Exposure to Ionizing Radiation*. Report no. 91. Bethesda, MD: National Council on Radiation Protection and Measurements; 1987.
22. Johns HE, Cunningham JR. *The Physics of Radiology*. 4th ed. Springfield, IL: Charles C. Thomas; 1983.
23. Khan FM. *The Physics of Radiation Therapy*. 3rd ed. Philadelphia: Lippincott Williams & Wilkins; 2003.
24. Wong E, D'Souza D, Chen J, et al. Intensity-modulated ARC therapy for treatment of high-risk endometrial malignancies. *Int J Radiat Oncol Biol Phys* 2005;61(3):830–841.
25. D'Souza W, Ahamad A, Iyer R, et al. Feasibility of dose escalation using intensity-modulated radiotherapy in posthysterectomy cervical carcinoma. *Int J Radiat Oncol Biol Phys* 2005;61(4):1062–1070.

26. Ahamad A, D'Souza W, Salehpour M, et al. Intensity-modulated radiation therapy after hysterectomy: comparison with conventional treatment and sensitivity of the normal-tissue-sparing effect to margin size. *Int J Radiat Oncol Biol Phys* 2005;62(4):1117–1124.
27. Heron D, Gerszten K, Selvaraj G, et al. Conventional 3D conformal versus intensity-modulated radiotherapy for the adjuvant treatment of gynecologic malignancies: a comparative dosimetric study of dose-volume histograms. *Gynecol Oncol* 2003;91:39–45.
28. Small W, Mundt A. *Gynecologic Pelvis Atlas.* RTOG Radiation Therapy Oncology Group. http://www.rtog.org/gynatlas/main.html, 2007. Accessed January 9, 2009.
29. Taylor A, Rockall A, Reznek R, et al. Mapping pelvic lymph nodes: guidelines for delineation in intensity-modulated radiotherapy. *Int J Radiat Oncol Biol Phys* 2005;63(5):1604–1612.
30. Martinez-Monge R, Fernandes P, Gupta N, et al. Cross-sectional nodal atlas: a tool for the definition of clinical target volumes in three-dimensional radiation therapy planning. *Radiology* 1999;211:815–828.
31. Roeske J, Lujan A, Rotmensch J, et al. Intensity-modulated whole pelvic radiation therapy in patients with gynecologic malignances. *Int J Radiat Oncol Biol Phys* 2000;48(5):1613–1621.
32. Mundt A, Roeske J, Lujan A, et al. Initial clinical experience with intensity-modulated whole-pelvis radiation therapy in women with gynecologic malignancies. *Gynecol Oncol* 2001;82:456–463.
33. Mundt A, Lujan A, Rotmensch J, et al. Intensity-modulated whole pelvic radiotherapy in women with gynecologic malignancies. *Int J Radiat Oncol Biol Phys* 2002;52(5):1330–1337.
34. Roeske J, Bonta D, Mell L, et al. A dosimetric analysis of acute gastrointestinal toxicity in women receiving intensity-modulated whole-pelvic radiation therapy. *Radiother. Oncol.* 2003;69:201–207.
35. Mundt A, Mell L, Roeske J. Preliminary analysis of chronic gastrointestinal toxicity in gynecology patients treated with intensity-modulated whole pelvic radiation therapy. *Int J Radiat Oncol Biol Phys* 2003;56(5):1354–1360.
36. Lujan A, Mundt A, Yamada SD, et al. Intensity-modulated radiotherapy as a means of reducing dose to bone marrow in gynecologic patients receiving whole pelvic radiotherapy. *Int J Radiat Oncol Biol Phys* 2003;57(2):516–521.
37. Kochanski J, Mell L, Roeske J, et al. Intensity-modulated radiation therapy in gynecologic malignancies: current status and future directions. *Clin Adv Hematol Oncol* 2006;4(5):379–386.
38. Portlance L, Chao C, Grigsby P, et al. Intensity-modulated radiation therapy (IMRT) reduces small bowel, rectum, and bladder doses in patients with cervical cancer receiving pelvic and para-aortoc irradiation. *Int J Radiat Oncol Biol Phys* 2001;51(1):261–266.
39. Ahmed R, Kim R, Duan J, et al. IMRT dose escalation for positive para-aortic lymph nodes in patients with locally advanced cervical cancer while reducing dose to bone marrow and other organs at risk. *Int J Radiat Oncol Biol Phys* 2004;60(2):505–512.
40. Kavanagh B, Schefter T, Wu Q, et al. Clinical application of intensity-modulated radiotherapy for locally advanced cervical cancer. *Semin Radiat Oncol* 2002;12(3):260–271.
41. Hong L, Alektiar K, Chui C, et al. IMRT of large fields: whole-abdomen irradiation. *Int J Radiat Oncol Biol Phys* 2002;54(1):278–289.
42. Duthoy W, Gersem W, Vergote K, et al. Whole abdominopelvic radiotherapy (WAPRT) using intensity-modulated ARC therapy (IMAT): first clinical experience. *Int J Radiat Oncol Biol Phys* 2003;57(4):1019–1032.
43. *International Commission on Radiation Units and Measurements, Prescribing, Recording, and Reporting Photon Beam Therapy.* ICRU Report 50. Bethesda, MD: International Commission on Radiation Units and Measurements; 1993.
44. Erickson B, Wilson JF. Clinical indications for brachytherapy. *J Surg Oncol* 1997;65:218–227.
45. *Dose and Volume Specification for Reporting Intracavitary Therapy in Gynecology.* ICRU Report 38. Bethesda, MD: International Commission on Radiation Units and Measurements; 1985.
46. Swift P, Purser P, Roberts L, et al. Pulsed low dose rate brachytherapy for pelvic malignancies. *Int J Radiat Oncol Biol Phys* 1997;37(4):811–817.
47. Henschke UK, Hilaris BS, Mahan GD. Afterloading in interstitial and intracavitary radiation therapy. *Am J Roentgenol* 1963;90:386–395.
48. Henschke UK, Hilaris BS, Mahan GD. Remote afterloading with intracavitary applicators. *Radiology* 1964;83:344–345.
49. Henschke UK, Hilaris BS, Mahan GD. Intracavitary radiation therapy of cancer of the uterine cervix by remote afterloading with cycling sources. *Am J Roentgenol* 1966;96:45–51.
50. Nath R, Anderson L, Luxton G, et al. Dosimetry of interstitial brachytherapy sources: recommendations of AAPM Radiation Therapy Committee Task Group No. 43. *Med Phys* 1995;22:209–234.
51. Vahrson H, Glaser FH. History of HDR afterloading in brachytherapy. *Strahlenther Onkol* 1988;82(Suppl):2–6.
52. Cleaves MA. Radium: with a preliminary note on radium rays in the treatment of cancer. *Med Rec* 1903;64:601–606.
53. Morton WJ. Treatment of cancer by the x-ray, with remarks on the use of radium. *Int J Surg* 1903;14:289–300.
54. Abbe R. The use of radium in malignant disease. *Lancet* 1913;2:524–527.
55. O'Brien F. The radium treatment of cancer of the cervix. *Am J Roent & Rad Therapy* 1947;57:281–297.
56. Stitt JA, Fowler JF, Thomadsen BR, et al. High dose rate intracavitary brachytherapy for carcinoma of the cervix: the Madison system: I. Clinical and radiobiological considerations. *Int J Radiat Oncol Biol Phys* 1992;24: 335–348.
57. Heyman J. The so-called Stockholm method and the results of treatment of uterine cancer at the Radiumhemmet. *Acta Radiol* 1935;16:129–147.
58. Lenz M. Radiotherapy of cancer of the cervix at the Radium Institute, Paris, France. *Am J Roentgenol Rad Ther Nucl Med* 1927;17:335–342.
59. Tod MC, Meredith WJ. A dosage system for use in the treatment of cancer of the uterine cervix. *Br J Radiol* 1938;11:809–824.
60. Tod MC. The optimum dosage in the treatment of carcinoma of the uterine cervix by radiation. *Br J Radiol* 1941;14:23–29.
61. Tod MC. Optimum dosage in the treatment of cancer of the cervix by radiation. *Acta Radiol* 1947;28:565–575.
62. Tod M, Meredith WJ. Treatment of cancer of the cervix uteri—a revised "Manchester method." *Br J Radiol* 1953;26:252–257.
63. Fletcher GH, Shalek RJ, Wall JA, et al. A physical approach to the design of applicators in radium therapy of cancer of the cervix uteri. *Am J Roentgenol* 1952;68:935–949.
64. Fletcher GH. Cervical radium applicators with screening the direction of bladder and rectum. *Radiology* 1953;60:77–84.
65. Adams GD, Meurk ML. The use of a computer to calculate isodose information surrounding distributed gynaecological radium sources. *Phys Med Biol* 1964;9:533–540.
66. Adams RM, Peterson M, Collins VP, et al. Clinically useful calculations of the dose distribution from multiple radiation sources. *Radiology* 1965;85: 361–364.
67. Batten GW. The M.D. Anderson method for the computation of isodose curves around interstitial and intracavitary radiation sources II. Mathematical and computational aspects. *Am J Roentgenol* 1968;102: 673–676.
68. Shalek RJ, Stoval M. The M.D. Anderson method for the computation of isodose curves around interstitial and intracavitary radiation sources I. Dose from linear sources. *Am J Roentgenol* 1968;102:662–672.
69. Stovall M, Shalek RJ. The M.D. Anderson method for the computation of isodose curves around interstitial and intracavitary radiation sources. III. Roentgenograms for input data and the relation of isodose calculations to the Paterson-Parker system. *Am J Roentgenol* 1968;102:677–687.
70. Fletcher GH, Brown TC, Rutledge FN. Clinical significance of rectal and bladder dose measurements in radium therapy of cancer of the uterine cervix. *Am J Roentgenol Rad Ther Nucl Med* 1958;79:421–450.
71. Fletcher GH, Wall JA, Bloedorn FG, et al. Direct measurements and isodose calculations in radium therapy of carcinoma of the cervix. *Radiology* 1953;61:885–902.
72. Fletcher GH, Rutledge FN, Chau PM. Policies of treatment in cancer of the cervix uteri. *Am J Roentgenol* 1962;87:6–21.
73. Fletcher GH. Cancer of the uterine cervix: Janeway lecture, 1970. *Am J Roentgenol Rad Ther Nucl Med* 1971;3:225–242.
74. Delclos L, Fletcher GH, Sampiere V, et al. Can the Fletcher gamma ray colpostat system be extrapolated to other systems? *Cancer* 1978;41: 970–979.
75. Haas JS, Dean RD, Mansfield CM. Evaluation of a new Fletcher applicator using cesium-137. *Int J Radiat Oncol Biol Phys* 1980;6:1589–1595.
76. Haas JS, Dean RD, Mansfield CM. Dosimetric comparison of the Fletcher family of gynecologic colpostats 1950-1980. *Int J Radiat Oncol Biol Phys* 1985;11:1317–1321.
77. Suit HD, Moore EB, Fletcher GH, et al. Modification of Fletcher ovoid system for afterloading, using standard-sized radium tubes (milligram and microgram). *Radiology* 1963;81:126–131.
78. Batley F, Constable WC. The use of the Manchester system for treatment of cancer of the uterine cervix with modern after-loading radium applicators. *Am J Roentgenol Rad Ther Nucl Med* 1967;18:396–400.
79. Fletcher, Gilbert H., eds. *Textbook of Radiotherapy.* 3rd ed. Philadelphia: Lea & Febiger; 1980:720–772.
80. Katz A, Eifel P. Quantification of intracavitary brachytherapy parameters and correlation with outcome in patients with carcinoma of the cervix. *Int J Radiat Oncol Biol Phys* 2000;48(5):1417–1425.
81. Eifel PJ, Morris M, Wharton JT, et al. The influence of tumor size and morphology on the outcome of patients with FIGO stage IB squamous cell carcinoma of the uterine cervix. *Int J Radiat Oncol Biol Phys* 1994;29:9–16.
82. Logsdson M, Eifel P. FIGO IIIB squamous cell carcinoma of the cervix: an analysis of prognostic factors emphasizing the balance between external beam and intracavitary radiation therapy. *Int J Radiat Oncol Biol Phys* 1999;43(4):763–775.
83. Potish RA, Gerbi BJ. Cervical cancer: intracavitary dose specification and prescription. *Radiology* 1987;165:555–560.
84. Potish RA. The effect of applicator geometry on dose specification in cervical cancer. *Int J Radiat Oncol Biol Phys* 1990;18:1513–1520.
85. Nag S, Chao C, Erickson B, et al. The American Brachytherapy Society recommendations for low dose-rate brachytherapy for carcinoma of the cervix. *Int J Radiat Oncol Biol Phys* 2002;52(1):33–48.
86. Nag S, Erickson B, Thomadsen B, et al. The American Brachytherapy Society recommendations for high-dose-rate brachytherapy for carcinoma of the cervix. *Int J Radiat Oncol Biol Phys* 2000;48(1):201–211.

87. Petereit D, Sakaria J, Potter D, et al. High dose rate vs. low dose rate brachytherapy in the treatment of cervical cancer: analysis of tumor recurrence—The University of Wisconsin experience. *Int J Radiat Oncol Biol Phys* 1999;45(5):1267–1274.
88. Lewis GC, Raaventos A, Half J. Space dose relationships for points A and B in the radium therapy of cancer of the uterine cervix. *Am J Roentgenol Rad Ther Nucl Med* 1960;83:432–446.
89. Gebara W, Weeks K, Jones E, et al. Carcinoma of the uterine cervix: a 3D-CT analysis of dose to the internal, external and common iliac nodes in tandem and ovoid applications. *Radiother Oncol* 2000;56:43–48.
90. Potish RA, Gerbi BJ. Role of point A in the era of computerized dosimetry. *Radiology* 1986;158:827–831.
91. Potish RA. Cervix cancer. In: Levitt SH, Khan FM, Potish RA, eds. *Technological Basis of Radiation Therapy*. Philadelphia: Lea & Febiger; 1992:289–299.
92. Cunningham DE, Stryker JA, Velkley DE, et al. Intracavitary dosimetry: a comparison of mg-hr prescription to doses at points A and B in cervical cancer. *Int J Radiat Oncol Biol Phys* 1981;7:121–123.
93. Potish RA, Deibel FC, Khan FM. The relationship between milligram-hours and dose to point A in carcinoma of the cervix. *Radiology* 1982;145:479–483.
94. Durrance FY, Fletcher GH. Computer calculation of dose contribution to regional lymphatics from gynecologic radium insertions. *Radiology* 1968;91:140–147.
95. Krishnan L, Cytacki EP, Wolf CD, et al. Dosimetric analysis in brachytherapy of carcinoma of the cervix. *Int J Radiat Oncol Biol Phys* 1990;18: 965–970.
96. Stuecklschweiger GF, Arian-Schad KS, Poier E, et al. Bladder and rectal dose of gynecologic high-dose-rate implants: comparison of orthogonal radiographic measurements with in vivo and CT-assisted measurements. *Radiology* 1991;181:889–894.
97. Potter R, Knocke T, Fellner C, et al. Definitive radiotherapy based on HDR brachytherapy with iridium 192 in uterine cervix carcinoma: report on the Vienna University Hospital findings (1993–1997) compared to the preceding period in the context of ICRU 38 recommendations. *Cancer Radiother* 2000;4:159–172.
98. Dimopoulos J, Schard G, Berger D, et al. Systematic evaluation of MRI findings in different stages of treatment of cervical cancer: potential of MRI on delineation of target, pathoanatomic structures, and organs at risk. *Int J Radiat Oncol Biol Phys* 2006;64(5):1380–1388.
99. Haie-Meder C, Potter R, Van Limbergen E, et al. Recommendations for Gynecological (GYN) GEC-ESTRO Working Group (I): concepts and terms in 3D image-based 3D treatment planning in cervix cancer brachytherapy with emphasis on MRI assessment of GTV and CTV. *Radiother Oncol* 2005;74:235–245.
100. Potter R, Haie-Meder C, Van Limbergen E, et al. Recommendations for Gynecological (GYN) GEC ESTRO Working Group (II): concepts and terms in 3D image-based treatment planning in cervix cancer brachytherapy 3D volume parameters and aspects of 3D image-based anatomy, radiation physics radiobiology. *Radiother Oncol* 2006;78:67–77.
101. Perez CA, Breaux S, Madoc-Jones H, et al. Radiation therapy alone in the treatment of carcinoma of the uterine cervix I. Analysis of tumor recurrence. *Cancer* 1983;51:1393–1402.
102. Maruyama Y, Van Nagell JR, Wrede DE, et al. Approaches to optimization of dose in radiation therapy of cervix carcinoma. *Radiology* 1976;120:389–398.
103. Hilaris BS, Nori D, Anderson LL. Brachytherapy in cancer of the cervix. In: Hilaris BS, Nori D, Anderson LL, eds. *Atlas of Brachytherapy*. New York: Macmillan Publishing Co.; 1988:244–256.
104. Mohan R, Ding IY, Toraskar J, et al. Computation of radiation dose distributions for shielded cervical applicators. *Int J Radiat Oncol Biol Phys* 1985;11:823–830.
105. Decker W, Erickson B, Albano K, et al. Comparison of traditional low dose rate to optimized and nonoptimized high dose rate tandem and ovoid dosimetry. *Int J Radiat Oncol Biol Phys* 2001;50(2):561–567.
106. Coia L, Won M, Lanciano R, et al. The patterns of care outcome study for cancer of the uterine cervix. *Cancer* 1990;66:2451–2456.
107. Lanciano RM, Won M, Coia LR, et al. Pretreatment and treatment factors associated with improved outcome in squamous cell carcinoma of the uterine cervix: a final report of the 1973 and 1978 Patterns of Care Studies. *Int J Radiat Oncol Biol Phys* 1991;20:667–676.
108. Montana GS, Martz KL, Hanks GE. Patterns and sites of failure in cervix cancer treated in the USA in 1978. *Int J Radiat Oncol Biol Phys* 1991;20:87–93.
109. Hanks GE, Herring DF, Kramer S. Patterns of Care outcome studies results of the National Practice in Cancer of the Cervix. *Cancer* 1983;51:959–967.
110. Lanciano R, Martz K, Coia L, et al. Tumor and treatment factors improving outcome in stage IIIb cervix cancer. *Int J Radiat Oncol Biol Phys* 1991;20(1):95–100.
111. Perez CA, Kuske R, Glasgow GP. Review of brachytherapy techniques for gynecologic tumors. *Endocuriether Hyperthermia Oncol* 1985;1: 153–175.
112. Delclos L, Fletcher GH, Moore EB, et al. Minicolpostats, dome cylinders, other additions and improvements of the Fletcher-Suit afterloadable system: indications and limitations of their use. *Int J Radiat Oncol Biol Phys* 1980;6:1195–1206.
113. Haas JS, Dean RD, Mansfield CM. Fletcher-Suit-Delclos gynecologic applicator: evaluation of a new instrument. *Int J Radiat Oncol Biol Phys* 1983;9:763–768.
114. Henschke UK. Afterloading applicator for radiation therapy of carcinoma of the uterus. *Radiology* 1960;74:834.
115. Kagan AR, DiSaia PJ, Wollin M, et al. The narrow vagina, the antecedent for irradiation injury. *Gynecol Oncol* 1976;4:291–298.
116. Crook JM, Esche BA, Chaplain G, et al. Dose-volume analysis and the prevention of radiation sequelae in cervical cancer. *Radiother Oncol* 1987;8:321–332.
117. Cunningham DE, Stryker JA, Velkley DE, et al. Routine clinical estimation of rectal, rectosigmoidal, and bladder doses from intracavitary brachytherapy in the treatment of carcinoma of the cervix. *Int J Radiat Oncol Biol Phys* 1981;7:653–660.
118. Villasanta U. Complications of radiotherapy for carcinoma of the uterine cervix. *Am J Obstet Gynecol* 1972;6:717–726.
119. Barillot I, Horiot J, Maingon P, et al. Impact on treatment outcome and late effects of customized treatment planning in cervix carcinomas: baseline results to compare new strategies. *Int J Radiat Oncol Biol Phys* 2000;48(1):189–200.
120. Esche BA, Crook JM, Horiot JC. Dosimetric methods in the optimization of radiotherapy for carcinoma of the uterine cervix. *Int J Radiat Oncol Biol Phys* 1987;13:1183–1192.
121. Esche BA, Crook JM, Isturiz J, et al. Reference volume, milligram-hours and external irradiation for the Fletcher applicator. *Radiother Oncol* 1987;9:255–261.
122. Hamberger AD, Unal A, Gershenson DM, et al. Analysis of the severe complications of irradiation of carcinoma of the cervix: whole pelvis irradiation and intracavitary radium. *Int J Radiat Oncol Biol Phys* 1983;9: 367–371.
123. Strockbine MF, Hancock JE, Fletcher GH. Complications in 831 patients with squamous cell carcinoma of the intact uterine cervix treated with 3,000 rads or more whole pelvis irradiation. *Am J Roentgenol* 1970;108: 293–304.
124. Unal A, Hamberger AD, Seski JC, et al. An analysis of the severe complications of irradiation of carcinoma of the uterine cervix: treatment with intracavitary radium and parametrial irradiation. *Int J Radiat Oncol Biol Phys* 1981;7:999–1004.
125. Paris KJ, Spanos WJ, Day TG, et al. Incidence of complications with mini vaginal culpostats in carcinoma of the uterine cervix. *Int J Radiat Oncol Biol Phys* 1991;21:911–917.
126. Pourquier H, Dubois JB, Delard R. Exclusive use of radiotherapy in cancer of the cervix prevention of late pelvic complications. *Cervix* 1990;8: 61–74.
127. Corn BW, Hanlon AL, Pajak TF, et al. Technically accurate intracavitary insertions improve pelvic control and survival among patients with locally advanced carcinoma of the uterine cervix. *Gynecol Oncol* 1994;53:294–300.
128. Perez CA, Breaux S, Bedwinek JM, et al. Radiation therapy alone in the treatment of carcinoma of the uterine cervix. II. Analysis of complications. *Cancer* 1984;54:235–246.
129. Erickson B, Gillin M. Interstitial implantation of gynecologic malignancies. *J Surg Oncol* 1997;66:285–295.
130. Gupta A, Vicini F, Frazier A, et al. Iridium-192 transperineal interstitial brachytherapy for locally advanced or recurrent gynecologic malignancies. *Int J Radiat Oncol Biol Phys* 1999;43(5):1055–1060.
131. Martinez A, Herstein P, Portnuff J. Interstitial therapy of perineal and gynecologic malignancies. *Int J Radiat Oncol Biol Phys* 1983;9: 409–416.
132. Martinez A, Cox RS, Edmundson GK. A multiple site perineal applicator (MUPIT) for treatment of prostatice, anorectal, and gynecologic malignancies. *Int J Radiat Oncol Biol Phys* 1984;10:297–305.
133. Martinez A, Edmundson GK, Clarke D. The role of transperineal template implants in gynecologic malignancies. *Brachther J* 1991;5:107–113.
134. Inoue T, Inoue T, Tanaka E, et al. High dose rate fractionated interstitial brachytherapy as the sole treatment for recurrent carcinoma of the uterus. *J Brachyther Internat* 1999;15:161–167.
135. Feder BH, Syed AMN, Neblett D. Treatment of extensive carcinoma of the cervix with the "transperineal parametrial butterfly." *Int J Radiat Oncol Biol Phys* 1978;4:735–472.
136. Fleming P, Syed AMN, Neblett D, et al. Description of an afterloading ^{192}Ir interstitial-intracavitary technique in the treatment of carcinoma of the vagina. *Obstet Gynecol* 1980;55:525–530.
137. Gaddis O, Morrow CP, Klement V, et al. Treatment of cervical carcinoma employing a template for transperineal interstitial ^{192}Ir brachytherapy. *Int J Radiat Oncol Biol Phys* 1983;9:819–827.
138. Syed AMN, Puthawala AA, Neblett D et al. Transperineal interstitial-intracavitary "Syed-Neblett" applicator in the treatment of carcinoma of the uterine cervix. *Endocuriether Hypertherm Oncol* 1986;2:1–13.
139. Syed A, Puthawala A, Abdelaziz N, et al. Long-term results of low-dose-rate interstitial-intracavitary brachytherapy in the treatment of carcinoma of the cervix. *Int J Radiat Oncol Biol Phys* 2002;54(1):67–78.
140. Demanes D, Rodriguez R, Bendre D, et al. High dose rate transperineal interstitial brachytherapy for cervical cancer: high pelvic control and low complication rates. *Int J Radiat Oncol Biol Phys* 1999;45(1):105–112.

141. Beriwal S, Bhatnagar A, Heron D, et al. High dose rate interstitial brachytherapy for gynecologic malignancies. *Brachytherapy* 2006;5: 218–222.
142. Erickson B, Albano K, Gillin M. CT-guided interstitial implantation of gynecologic malignancies. *Int J Radiat Oncol Biol Phys* 1996;36(3): 699–709.
143. Orton C. High and low dose rate brachytherapy for cervical carcinoma. *Acta Oncol* 1998;37(2):117–125.
144. Sarkaria JN, Petereit DG, Stitt JA, et al. A comparison of the efficacy and complication rates of low dose-rate versus high dose-rate brachytherapy in the treatment of uterine cervical carcinoma. *Int J Radiat Oncol Biol Phys* 1994;30:75–82.
145. Stitt JA. High-dose-rate intracavitary brachytherapy in gynecologic malignancies. *Oncology* 1992;6:59–70.
146. Thomadsen BR, Shahabi S, Stitt JA, et al. High dose rate intracavitary brachytherapy for carcinoma of the cervix: the Madison system: II. Procedural and physical considerations. *Int J Radiat Oncol Biol Phys* 1992;24:349–357.
147. Houdek PV, Schwade JG, Abitbol AA, et al. Optimization of high dose-rate cervix brachytherapy: Part I: Dose distribution. *Int J Radiat Oncol Biol Phys* 1991;21:1621–1625.
148. Speiser B. Advantages of high dose rate remote afterloading systems: physics or biology. *Int J Radiat Oncol Biol Phys* 1991;20:1133–1135.
149. Delaloye JF, Coucke PA, Pampallona S, et al. Effect of total treatment time on event-free survival in carcinoma of the cervix. *Gynecol Oncol* 1996;60: 42–48.
150. Le Pechoux C, Akine Y, Sumi M, et al. High dose rate brachytherapy for carcinoma of the uterine cervix: comparison of two different fractionation regimens. *Int J Radiat Oncol Biol Phys* 1995;31:735–741.
151. Himmelmann A, Holmberg E, Oden A, et al. Intracavitary irradiation of carcinoma of the cervix stage IB and IIA. *Acta Radiol Oncol* 1985;24: 139–144.
152. Brenner DJ, Huang Y, Hall EJ. Fractionated high dose-rate versus low dose-rate regimens for intracavitary brachytherapy of the cervix: equivalent regimens for combined brachytherapy and external irradiation. *Int J Radiat Oncol Biol Phys* 1991;21:1415–1423.
153. Brenner D. HDR brachytherapy for carcinoma of the cervix: fractionation considerations. *Int J Radiat Oncol Biol Phys* 1991;22:221–222.
154. Joslin CAF. High-activity source afterloading in gynecologic cancer and its future prospects. *Endocuriether Hyperther Oncol* 1989;5:69–81.
155. Newman G. Increased morbidity following the introduction of remote afterloading, with increased dose rate for cancer of the cervix. *Radiother Oncol* 1996;39:97–103.
156. Orton CG. Biologic treatment planning. In: Martinez AA, Orton CG, Mould RF, eds. *Brachytherapy HDR and LDR*. Columbia: Nucletron; 1990:205–215.
157. Orton CG. Application of the linear quadratic model to radiotherapy for gynaecological cancers. *Selectron Brachytherapy J* 1991;2(Suppl):15–18.
158. Abitbol AA, Houdek P, Schwade JG, et al. Ring applicator with rectal retractor: applicability to high dose rate brachytherapy of cervical cancer. *Selectron Brachytherapy J* 1990;4:6869.
159. Wollin M, Kagan AR, Olch A, et al. Comparison of the ring applicator and the Fletcher applicator for HDR gynaecological brachytherapy. *Selectron Brachytherapy J* 1991;2(Suppl)2:25–27.
160. Erickson B, Jones R, Rownd J, et al. Is the tandem and ring applicator a suitable alternative to the high dose rate Selectron tandem and ovoid applicator? *J Brachytherapy Int* 2000;16:31–144.
161. Brooks S, Bownes P, Lowe G, et al. Cervical brachytherapy utilizing ring applicator: comparison of standard and conformal loading. *Int J Radiat Oncol Biol Phys* 2005;63(3):934–939.
162. Mai J, Erickson B, Rownd J, et al. Comparison of four different dose specification methods for high dose rate intracavitary radiation for treatment of cervical cancer. *Int J Radiat Oncol Biol Phys* 2001;51(4):1131–1141.
163. Kim R, Caranto J, Pareek P, et al. Dynamics of pear-shaped dimensions and volume of intracavitary brachytherapy in cancer of the cervix: a desirable pear shape in the era of three-dimensional treatment planning. *Int J Radiat Oncol Biol Phys* 1997;37(5):1193–1199.
164. Cetingoz R, Ataman O, Tuncel N, et al. Optimization in high dose rate brachytherapy for utero-vaginal applications. *Radiother Oncol* 2001;58: 31–36.
165. Hoskin PJ, Cook M, Bouscale D, et al. Changes in applicator position with fractionated high dose rate gynaecological brachytherapy. *Radiother Oncol* 1996;40:59–62.
166. Grigsby PW, Georgiou A, Williamson JF, et al. Anatomic variation of gynecologic brachytherapy prescription points. *Int J Radiat Oncol Biol Phys* 1993;27:725–729.
167. Kim RY, Meyer JT, Plott WE, et al. Major geometric variations between multiple high-dose-rate applications of brachytherapy in cancer of the cervix: frequency and types of variation. *Radiology* 1995;195:419–422.
168. Christensen G, Carlson B, Chao C, et al. Imaged-based dose planning of intracavitary brachytherapy: registration of serial-imaging studies using deformable anatomic templates. *Int J Radiat Oncol Biol Phys* 2001;51(1): 227–243.
169. Kim R, Meyer J, Spencer S, et al. Major geometric variation between intracavitary applications in carcinoma of the cervix: high dose rate vs. low dose rate. *Int J Radiat Oncol Biol Phys* 1996;35(5):1035–1038.
170. Kim R, Meyer J, Plott W, et al. Major geometric variation between multiple high dose rate applications of brachytherapy in cancer of the cervix: frequency and types of variation. *Radiology* 1995;195:419–422.
171. Elhanafy O, Das R, Paliwal B, et al. Anatomic variation of prescription points and treatment volume with fractionated high-dose-rate gynecologic brachytherapy. *J Appl Clin Med Phys* 2002;3(1):1–5.
172. Jones N, Rankin J, Gaffney D. Is simulation necessary for each high-dose-rate tandem and ovoid insertion in carcinoma of the cervix? *Brachytherapy* 2004;3:120–124.
173. Pham H, Chen Y, Rouby E, et al. Changes in high-dose-rate tandem and ovoid applicator position during treatment in an unfixed brachytherapy system. *Radiology* 1998;206:525–531.
174. Fu KK, Phillips TL. High-dose-rate versus low-dose-rate intracavitary brachytherapy for carcinoma of the cervix. *Int J Radiat Oncol Biol Phys* 1990;19:791–796.
175. Orton CG. HDR: forget not "time" and "distance." *Int J Radiat Oncol Biol Phys* 1991;20:1131–1132.
176. Orton CG, Seyedsadr M, Somnay A. Comparison of high and low dose rate remote afterloading for cervix cancer and the importance of fractionation. *Int J Radiat Oncol Biol Phys* 1991;21:1425–1434.
177. Petereit D, Pearcey R. Literature analysis of high dose rate brachytherapy fractionation schedules in the treatment of cervical cancer: Is there an optimal fractionation schedule? *Int J Radiat Oncol Biol Phys* 1999;43(2): 359–366.
178. Nag S, Abitbol AA, Anderson LL, et al. Consenus guidelines for high dose rate remote brachytherapy in cervical, endometrial, and endobronchial tumors. *Int J Radiat Oncol Biol Phys* 1993;27:1241–1244.
179. Nag S, Gupta N. A simple method of obtaining equivalent doses for use in HDR brachytherapy. *Int J Radiat Oncol Biol Phys* 2000;46(2): 507–513.
180. Erickson B, Eifel P, Moughan J, et al. Patterns of brachytherapy practice for patients with carcinoma of the cervix (1996-1999): a Patterns of Care study. *Int J Radiat Oncol Biol Phys* 2005;63(4):1083–1092.
181. Ferrigno R, Novaes P, Pellizzon A, et al. High dose rate brachytherapy in the treatment of uterine cervix cancer. Analysis of dose effectiveness and late complications. *Int J Radiat Oncol Biol Phys* 2001;50(5):1123–1135.
182. Chen SW, Liang JA, Yang SN, et al. The adverse effect of treatment prolongation in cervical cancer by high-dose-rate intracavitary brachytherapy. *Radiother Oncol* 2003;67:69–76.
183. Ferrigno R, Nishimoto IN, Dos Santos Novaes PER, et al. Comparison of low and high dose rate brachytherapy in the treatment of uterine cervix cancer. Retrospective analysis of two sequential series. *Int J Radiat Oncol Biol Phys* 2005;62(4):1108–1116.
184. Kim R, Pareek K, Duan J, et al. Postoperative intravaginal brachytherapy for endometrial cancer: dosimetric analysis of vaginal colpostats and cylinder applicators. *Brachytherapy* 2002;1:138–144.
185. Dobbie BMW. Vaginal recurrences in carcinoma of the body of the uterus and their prevention. *J Obstet Gynaecol Brit Emp* 1953;60:702–705.
186. Greven KM, Randall M, Fanning J, et al. Patterns of failure in patients with stage I, grade 3 carcinoma of the endometrium. *Int J Radiat Oncol Biol Phys* 1990;19:529–534.
187. Price JJ, Hahn GA, Rominger CJ. Vaginal involvement in endometrial carcinoma. *Am J Obstet Gynecol* 1965;91(8):1060–1065.
188. Grigsby PW, Perez CA, Kuten A, et al. Clinical stage I endometrial cancer: results of adjuvant irradiation and patterns of failure. *Int J Radiat Oncol Biol Phys* 1991;21(2):379–385.
189. Small W, Erickson B, Kwakwa F. American Brachytherapy Society survey regarding practice patterns of post-operative irradiation for endometrial cancer: current status of vaginal brachytherapy. *Int J Radiat Oncol Biol Phys* 2005;63(5):1502–1507.
190. Gore E, Gillin M, Albano K, et al. Comparison of high dose rate and low dose rate dose distributions for vaginal cancers. *Int J Radiat Oncol Biol Phys* 1995;31(1):165–170.
191. Li Z, Liu C, Palta J. Optimized dose distribution of a high dose rate vaginal cylinder. *Int J Radiat Oncol Biol Phys* 1998;41(1):239–244.
192. Li S, Aref I, Walker E, et al. Effects of prescription depth, cylinder size, treatment length, tip space, and curved end on doses in high-dose-rate vaginal brachytherapy. *Int J Radiat Oncol Biol Phys* 2007;67(4): 1268–1277.
193. Choo J, Scudiere J, Bitterman P, et al. Vaginal lymphatic channel location and its implication for intracavitary brachytherapy radiation treatment. *Brachytherapy* 2005;4:236–240.
194. Jhingran A, Burke T, Eifel, P. Definitive radiotherapy for patients with isolated vaginal recurrence of endometrial carcinoma after hysterectomy. *Int J Radiat Oncol Biol Phys* 2003;56(5):1366–1372.
195. Alektiar K, McKee A, Venkatraman E, et al. Intravaginal high dose rate brachytherapy for stage IB (FIGO Grade 1, 2) endometrial cancer. *Int J Radiat Oncol Biol Phys* 2002;53(3):707–713.
196. Chadha M. Gynecologic brachytherapy. II: Intravaginal brachytherapy for carcinoma of the endometrium. *Semin Radiat Oncol* 2002;12(1):53–61.
197. Alektiar K, Venkatramam E, Chi D, et al. Intravaginal brachytherapy alone for intermediate risk endometrial cancer. *Int J Radiat Oncol Biol Phys* 2005;62(1):111–117.
198. Chada M, Nanavati PJ, Liu P, et al. Patterns of failure in endometrial carcinoma stage IB grade 3 and IC patients treated with postoperative vaginal vault brachytherapy. *Gynecol Oncol* 1999;75:103–107.

199. Greven MKM, D'Agostino RB Jr, Lanciano RM, et al. Is there a role for a brachytherapy vaginal cuff boost in the adjuvant management of patients with uterine-confined endometrial cancer? *Int J Radiat Oncol Biol Phys* 1998;42(1):101–104.
200. Randall ME, Wilder J, Greven K, et al. Role of intracavitary cuff boost after adjuvant external irradiation in early endometrial carcinoma. *Int J Radiat Oncol Biol Phys* 1990;19:49–54.
201. Naizi T Souhami L, Portlance L, et al. Long-term results of high-dose-rate brachytherapy in the primary treatment of medically inoperable stage I-II endometrial carcinoma. *Int J Radiat Oncol Biol Phys* 2005;63(4): 1108–1113.
202. Taghian A, Pernot M, Hoffstetter S, et al. Radiation therapy alone for medically inoperable patients with adenocarcinoma of the endometrium. *Int J Radiat Oncol Biol Phys* 1988;15(4):1135–1140.
203. Knocke T, Kucera H, Weidinger B, et al. Primary treatment of endometrial carcinoma with high-dose-rate brachytherapy: results of 12 years of experience with 280 patients. *Int J Radiat Oncol Biol Phys* 1997;37(2): 359–365.
204. Disaia PJ, Syed AMN, Puthawala AA. Malignant neoplasia of the upper vagina. *Endocureither Hypertherm Oncol* 1994;10:83–86.
205. Puthawala AA, Syed AMN, Fleming, et al. Reirradiation with interstitial implant for recurrent pelvic malignancies. *Cancer* 1982;50: 2810–2814.
206. Monk BJ, Walker JL, Tewari K, et al. Open interstitial brachytherapy for the treatment of local-regional recurrences of uterine corpus and cervix cancer after primary surgery. *Gynecol Oncol* 1994;52:222–228.
207. Perez C, Brady L, eds. *Principles and Practice of Radiation Oncology*. 2nd ed. Philadelphia: Lippincott Co.; 1992:1143–1202.
208. Rotman M, Aziz H, Eifel P. Irradiation of pelvic and para-aortic nodes in carcinoma of the cervix. *Semin Radiat Oncol* 1994;4(1):23–29.
209. Hendriksen E. The lymphatic spread of carcinoma of the cervix and of the body of the uterus. A study of 420 necropsies. *Am J Obstet Gynecol* 1949;58(5):924–942.
210. Chao C, Williamson J, Grigsby P, et al. Uterosacral space involvement in locally advanced carcinoma of the uterine cervix. *Int J Radiat Oncol Biol Phys* 1998;40(2):397–403.
211. Netter, F. *The CIBA Collection of Medical Illustrations, Vol 2. Reproductive System*. Summitt, NJ, CIBA Pharmaceutical; 1988.
212. Park J, Charnsangavej C, Yoshimitsu K, et al. Pathways of nodal metastasis from pelvic tumors: CT demonstration. *RadioGraphics* 1994;14(6): 1309–1321.
213. Bonin S, Lanciano R, Corn B, et al. Bony landmarks are not an adequate substitute for lymphangiography in defining pelvic lymph node location for the treatment of cervical cancer with radiotherapy. *Int J Radiat Oncol Biol Phys* 1996;34(1):167–172.
214. Chun M, Timmerman R, Mayer R, et al. Radiation therapy of external iliac lymph nodes with lateral pelvic portals: identification of patients at risk for inadequate regional coverage. *Radiology* 1995;194:147–150.
215. Pendlebury S, Cahill S, Crandon A, et al. Role of bipedal lymphangiogram in radiation treatment planning for cervical cancer. *Int J Radiat Oncol Biol Phys* 1993;27(4):959–962.
216. Kim R, McGinnis S, Spencer S, et al. Conventional four-field pelvic radiotherapy technique without CT treatment planning in cancer of the cervix: potential geographic miss. *Radiother Oncol* 1994;30:140–145.
217. Kim R, McGinnis S, Spencer S, et al. Conventional four-field pelvic radiotherapy technique without computed tomography treatment planning in cancer of the cervix: potential geographic miss and its impact on pelvic control. *Int J Radiat Oncol Biol Phys* 1995;31(1):109–112.
218. Mayr N, Tali E, Yuh W, et al. Cervical cancer: application of MR imaging in radiation therapy. *Radiology* 1993;189:601–608.
219. Russell A, Walter J, Anderson M, et al. Sagittal magnetic resonance imaging in the design of lateral radiation treatment portals for patients with locally advanced squamous cancer of the cervix. *Int J Radiat Oncol Biol Phys* 1992;23(2):449–455.
220. Thomas L, Chacon B, Kind M, et al. Magnetic resonance imaging in the treatment planning of radiation therapy in carcinoma of the cervix treated with the four-field pelvic technique. *Int J Radiat Oncol Biol Phys* 1997;37(4):827–832.
221. Zunino S, Rosato O, Lucino S, et al. Anatomic study of the pelvis in carcinoma of the uterine cervix as related to the box technique. *Int J Radiat Oncol Biol Phys* 1999;44(1):53–59.
222. McAlpine J, Schlaerth JB, Lim P, et al. Radiation fields in gynecologic oncology: correlation of soft tissue (surgical) to radiologic landmarks. *Gynecol Oncol* 2004;92:25–30.
223. Greer B, Koh W, Stelzer K, et al. Expanded pelvic radiotherapy fields for treatment of local-regionally advanced carcinoma of the cervix: outcome and complications. *Am J Obstet Gynecol* 1996;174(4):1141–1150.
224. Greer B, Koh WJ, Figge D, et al. Gynecologic radiotherapy fields defined by intraoperative measurements. *Gynecol Oncol* 1990;38:421–424.
225. Finlay M, Ackerman I, Tirona R, et al. Use of CT simulation for treatment of cervical cancer to assess the adequacy of lymph node coverage of conventional pelvic fields based on bony landmarks. *Int J Radiat Oncol Biol Phys* 2006;64(1):205–209.
226. Gerstner N, Wachter S, Knocke T, et al. The benefit of beam's eye view based 3D treatment planning for cervical cancer. *Radiother Oncol* 1999;51:71–78.
227. Russell A. Contemporary radiation treatment planning for patients with cancer of the uterine cervix. *Semin Oncol* 1994;21(1):30–41.
228. Terry L, Piver S, Hanks G. The value of lymphangiography in malignant disease of the uterine cervix. *Radiology* 1972;103:175–177.
229. Grigsby P, Siegel B, Dehdashti F, et al. Lymph node staging by positron emission tomography in patients with carcinoma of the cervix. *J Clin Oncol* 2001;19(17):3745–3749.
230. Rose P, Adler L, Rodriguez M, et al. Positron emission tomography for evaluating para-aortic nodal metastasis in locally advanced cervical cancer before surgical staging: a surgicopathologic study. *J Clin Oncol* 1999;17(1):41-45.
231. Lin W, Hung Y, Yeh L, et al. Usefulness of ^{18}F-fluorodeoxyglucose positron emission tomography to detect para-aortic lymph nodal metastasis in advanced cervical cancer with negative computed tomography findings. *Gynecol Oncol* 2003;89:73–76.
232. Tsai CS, Chang TC, Lai CH, et al. Preliminary report of using FDG-PET to detect extrapelvic lesions in cervical cancer patients with enlarged pelvic lymph nodes on MRI/CT. *Int J Radiat Oncol Biol Phys* 2004;58(5): 1506–1512.
233. Wolfson A, Abdel-Wahab M, Markoe A, et al. A quantitative assessment of standard vs. customized midline shield construction for invasive cervical carcinoma. *Int J Radiat Oncol Biol Phys* 1997;37(1):237–242.
234. Perez CA, Camel HM, Kuske RR, et al. Radiation therapy alone in the treatment of carcinoma of the uterine cervix: a 20-year experience. *Gynecol Oncol* 1986;23:127–140.
235. Walz B, Perez C, Feldman A, et al. Individualized compensating filter and dose optimization in pelvic irradiation. *Radiology* 1973;107: 611–614.
236. Han I, Malviya V, Chuba P, et al. Multifractionated high dose rate brachytherapy with concomitant daily teletherapy for cervical cancer. *Gynecol Oncol* 1996;63:71–77.
237. Ling C, Smith A, Hanlon A, et al. Treatment planning for carcinoma of the cervix: a Patterns of Care Study report. *Int J Radiat Oncol Biol Phys* 1998;34(1):13–19.
238. Eifel PJ, Levenback C, Wharton JT, et al. Time course and incidence of late complications in patients treated with radiation therapy for FIGO stage IB carcinoma of the uterine cervix. *Int J Radiat Oncol Biol Phys* 1995;32:1289–1300.
239. Huang E, Lin H, Hsu H, et al. High external parametrial dose can increase the probability of radiation proctitis in patients with uterine cervix cancer. *Gynecol Oncol* 2000;79:406–410.
240. Huang EY, Wang CJ, Hsu HC, et al. Dosimetric factors predicting severe radiation-induced bowel complications in patients with cervical cancer: combined effect of external parametrial dose and cumulative rectal dose. *Gynecol Oncol* 2004;95:101–108.
241. Chun M, Kang S, Kil HJ, et al. Rectal bleeding and its management after irradiation for uterine cervical cancer. *Int J Radiat Oncol Biol Phys* 2004;58(1):98–105.
242. Kuipers TJ. Stereo x-ray photogrammetry applied for prevention of sigmoid-colon damage caused by radiation from intrauterine sources. *Int J Radiat Oncol Biol Phys* 1982;8:1011–1017.
243. Bahena J, Martinez A, Yan D, et al. Spatial reproducibility of the ring and tandem high dose rate cervix applicator. *Int J Radiat Oncol Biol Phys* 1998;41(1):13–19.
244. Perez CA, Fox S, Lockett MA, et al. Impact of dose in outcome of irradiation alone in carcinoma of the uterine cervix: analysis of two different methods. *Int J Radiat Oncol Biol Phys* 1991;21:885–898.
245. Perez C, Grigsby P, Chao C, et al. Tumor size, irradiation dose, and long-term outcome of carcinoma of uterine cervix. *Int J Radiat Oncol Biol Phys* 1998;41(2):307–317.
246. Perez C, Grigsby P, Lockett M, et al. Radiation therapy morbidity in carcinoma of the uterine cervix: dosimetric and clinical correlation. *Int J Radiat Oncol Biol Phys* 1999;44(4):855–866.
247. Grigsby P, Singh A, Siegel B, et al. Lymph node control in cervical cancer. *Int J Radiat Oncol Biol Phys* 2004;59(3):706–712.
248. Houvenaegel G, Lelievre L, Rigouard A, et al. Residual pelvic lymph node involvement after concomitant chemoradiation for locally advanced cervical cancer. *Gynecol Oncol* 2006;102:74–79.
249. Brixey C, Roeske J, Lujan A, et al. Impact of intenstity-modulated radiotherapy on acute hematologic toxicity in women with gynecologic maliganies. *Int J Radiat Oncol Biol Phys* 2002;54(5):1388–1396.
250. Johnsson JE. Recurrences and metastases in carcinoma of the uterine body correlated to the size and localization of the primary tumor. *Acta Obstet Gynecol Scand* 1979;58:405–408.
251. Creasman WT, Boronow RC, Morrow CP, et al. Adenocarcinoma of the endometrium: Its metastatic lymph node potential. *Gynecol Oncol* 1976;4:239–243.
252. Creasman WT, Morrow P, Bundy BN, et al. Surgical pathologic spread patterns of endometrial cancer. *Cancer* 1987;60:2035–2041.
253. Boronow RC, Morrow CP, Creasman WT, et al. Surgical staging in endometrial cancer: clinical–pathologic findings of a prospective study. *Obstet Gynecol* 1984;63(6):825–832.
254. Morrow PC, Bundy BN, Kurman RJ, et al. Relationship between surgical-pathological risk factors and outcome in clinical stage I and II carcinoma of the endometrium: a Gynecologic Oncology Group study. *Gynecol Oncol* 1991;40:55–65.

255. DiSaia PJ, Creasman WT, Boronow RC, et al. Risk factors and recurrent patterns in stage I endometrial cancer. *Am J Obstet Gynceol* 1985;151: 1009–1015.
256. Greven KM, Corn BW, Case D, et al. Which prognostic factors influence the outcome of patients with surgically staged endometrial cancer treated with adjuvant radiation? *Int J Radiat Oncol Biol Phys* 1997;39(2): 413–418.
257. Morrow CP, Di Saia J, Townsend DE. The role of postoperative irradiation in the management of stage I adenocarcinoma of the endometrium. *Am J Roentgenol* 1976;127:325–329.
258. Gallagher M, Brereton H, Rostock R, et al. A prospective study of treatment techniques to minimize the volume of pelvic small bowel with reduction of acute and late effects associated with pelvic irradiation. *Int J Radiat Oncol Biol Phys* 1986;12(9):1565–1573.
259. Huh S, Lim D, Ahn Y, et al. Effect of customized small bowel displacement system in pelvic irradiation. *Int J Radiat Oncol Biol Phys* 1998; 40(3):623–627.
260. Shanahan T, Mehta M, Bertelrud K, et al. Minimization of small bowel volume within treatment fields utilizing customized "belly boards." *Int J Radiat Oncol Biol Phys* 1990;19(2):469–476.
261. Ghosh K, Padilla L, Murray K, et al. Using a belly board device to reduce the small bowel volume within pelvic radiation fields in women with postoperatively treated cervical carcinoma. *Gynecol Oncol* 2001;83: 271–275.
262. Olofsen-van Acht M, van den Berg H, Quint S, et al. Reduction of irradiated small bowel volume and accurate patient positioning by use of a belly board device in pelvic radiotherapy of gynecologic cancer patients. *Radiother Oncol* 2001;59:87–93.
263. Pinkawa M, Gagel B, Demirel C, et al. Dose-volume histogram for prone and supine patient position in external beam radiotherapy for cervical and endometrial cancer. *Radiother Oncol* 2003;69:99–105.
264. Weiss E, Eberlein K, Pradier O, et al. The impact of patient positioning on the adequate coverage of the uterus in the primary irradiation of cervical carcinoma: a prospective analysis using magnetic resonance imaging. *Radiother Oncol* 2002;63:83–87.
265. Buchali A, Koswig S, Dinges S, et al. Impact of the filling status of the bladder and rectum on their integral dose distribution and movement of the uterus in the treatment planning of gynaecological cancer. *Radiother Oncol* 1999;52:29–34.
266. Martinez A, Weiner S, Podratz K, et al. Improved outcome at 10 years for serous-papillary/clear cell or high-risk endometrial cancer patients treated by adjuvant high-dose-whole abdomino-pelvic irradiation. *Gynecol Oncol* 2003;90:537–546.
267. Small W, Mayadevan A, Roland P, et al. Whole-abdominal radiation in endometrial carcinoma: an analysis of toxicity, patterns of recurrence, and survival. *Cancer J* 2000;6(6):394–400.
268. Rotman M, Aziz H, Choi K. Radiation damage of normal tissues in the treatment of gynecologic cancers. *Front Radiat Ther Oncol* 1989;23: 349–366.
269. Rubin P, Casarett G. *Clinical Radiation Pathology*. Vol. 1–2. Philadelpha: WB Saunders Co.; 1968.
270. Emani B, Lyman J, Brown, A, et al. Tolerance to therapeutic irradiation. *Int J Radiat Oncol Biol Phys* 1991;21:109–122.
271. Cox J, Ang K, eds. *Radiation Oncology: Rationale, Technique, Results*. 8th ed. St. Louis, MO: Mosby; 2003.
272. Grigsby P, Russell A, Bruner D, et al. Late injury of cancer therapy on the female reproductive tract. *Int J Radiat Oncol Biol Phys* 1995;31(5): 1289–1299.
273. Hintz BL, Kagan AR, Chan P, et al. Radiation tolerance of the vaginal mucosa. *Int J Radiat Oncol Biol Phys* 1980;6:711–716.
274. Au S, Grigsby P. The irradiation tolerance dose of the proximal vagina. *Radiother Oncol* 2003;67:77–85.
275. Williams J, Clarke D, Dennis W, et al. The treatment of pelvic soft tissue radiation necrosis with hyperbaric oxygen. *Am J Obstet Gynecol* 1992;167(2):412–416.
276. Pasquier D, Hoelscher T, Schmutz J, et al. Hyperbaric oxygen therapy in the treatment of radio-induced lesions in normal tissues: a literature review. *Radiother Oncol* 2004;72:1–13.
277. Okunieff P, Augustine E, Hicks J, et al. Pentoxifylline in the treatment of radiation-induced fibrosis. *J Clin Oncol* 2004;22(11):2207–2213.
278. Grigsby P, Roberts H, Perez C. Femoral head fracture following groin irradiation. *Int J Radiat Oncol Biol Phys* 1995;32(1):63–67.
279. Marks L, Carroll P, Dugan T, et al. The response of the urinary bladder, urethra, and ureter to radiation and chemotherapy. *Int J Radiat Oncol Biol Phys* 1995;31(5):1257–1280.
280. Mayer R, Klemen H, Quehenberger F, et al. Hyperbaric oxygen—an effective tool to treat radiation morbidity in prostate cancer. *Radiother Oncol* 2001;61:151–156.
281. Bevers RFM, Bakker D, Kurth KH. Hyperbaric oxygen treatment for haemorrhagic radiation cystitis. *Lancet* 1995;346:803–804.
282. McIntyre J, Eifel P, Levenback C, et al. Ureteral stricture as a late complication of radiotherapy for stage IB carcinoma of the uterine cervix. *Cancer* 1995;75(3):836–843.
283. Carl U, Peusch-Dreyer D, Frieling T, et al. Treatment of radiation proctitis with hyperbaric oxygen: what is the optimal number of HBO treatments? *Strahlenther Onkol* 1998;174(9):482–483.
284. Woo TCS, Joseph D, Oxer H, et al. Hyperbaric oxygen treatment for radiation proctitis. *Int J Radiat Oncol Biol Phys* 1997;38(3):619–622.
285. Ikushima H, Osaki K, Furutani S, et al. Pelvic bone complications following radiation therapy of gynecologic malignancies: clinical evaluation of radiation-induced pelvic insufficiency fractures. *Gynecol Oncol* 2006;103:1100–1104.
286. Tai P, Hammond A, Van Dyk J, et al. Pelvic fractures following irradiation of endometrial and vaginal cancer—a case series and review of lecture. *Radiother Oncol* 2000;56:23–28.
287. Huh S, Kim B, Kang M, et al. Pelvic insufficiency fracture after pelvic irradiation in uterine cervix cancer. *Gynecol Oncol* 2002;86:264–268.
288. Lawrence T, Robertson J, Anscher M, et al. Hepatic toxicity resulting from cancer treatment. *Int J Radiat Oncol Biol Phys* 1995;31(5): 1237–1248.
289. Roeske J, Mundt A, Halpern H, et al. Late rectal sequelae following definitive radiation therapy for carcinoma of the uterine cervix: a dosimetric analysis. *Int J Radiat Oncol Biol Phys* 1997;37(2):351–358.
290. Stryker J, Bartholomew M, Velkley D, et al. Bladder and rectal complications following radiotherapy for cervix cancer. *Gynecol Oncol* 1988; 29:1–11.
291. Kapp K, Stueckschweiger G, Kapp D, et al. Carcinoma of the cervix: analysis of complications after primary external beam radiation and Ir-192 HDR brachytherapy. *Radiother Oncol* 1997;42:143–153.
292. Wang C, Leung S, Chen H, et al. High-dose rate intracavitary brachytherapy (HDR-IC) in treatment of cervical carcinoma: 5-year results and implication of increased low-grade rectal complication on initiation of an HDR-IC fractionation scheme. *Int J Radiat Oncol Biol Phys* 1997;38(2): 391–398.
293. Ito H, Kutuki S, Nishiguchi I, et al. Radiotherapy for cervical cancer with high-dose rate brachytherapy correlation between tumor size, dose and failure. *Radiother Oncol* 1994;31:240–247.
294. Ogino I, Kitamura T, Okamoto N, et al. Late rectal complication following high dose rate intracavitary brachytherapy in cancer of the cervix. *Int J Radiat Oncol Biol Phys* 1995;31:725–734.
295. Chen MS, Lin FJ, Hong CH, et al. High-dose-rate afterloading technique in the radiation treatment of uterine cervical cancer: 399 cases and 9 years experience in Taiwan. *Int J Radiat Oncol Biol Phys* 1991;20:915–919.
296. Fowler JF. The radiobiology of brachytherapy. In: Martinez AA, Orton CG, Mould RF, eds. *Brachytherapy HDR and LDR*. Columbia: Nucletron; 1990:121–137.
297. Sakata KI, Nagakura H, Oouchi A, et al. High-dose-rate intracavitary brachytherapy: results of analyses of late rectal complications. *Int J Radiat Oncol Biol Phys* 2002;54(5):1369–1376.
298. Cheng JCH, Peng LC, Chen YH, et al. Unique role of proximal rectal dose in late rectal complications for patients with cervical cancer undergoing high-dose-rate intracavitary brachytherapy. *Int J Radiat Oncol Biol Phys* 2003;57(4):1010–1018.
299. Takeshi K, Katsuyuki K, Yoshiaki T, et al. Definitive radiotherapy combined with high dose rate brachytherapy for stage III carcinoma of the uterine cervix: retrospective analysis of prognostic factors concerning patient characteristics and treatment parameters. *Int J Radiat Oncol Biol Phys* 1998;41(2):319–327.
300. Teshima T, Chatani M, Hata K, et al. Rectal complication after remote afterloading intracavitary therapy for carcinoma of the uterine cervix. *Strahlenther* 1985;161:343–347.
301. Teshima T, Chatani M, Hata K, et al. High-dose rate intracavitary therapy for carcinoma of the uterine cervix: II. Risk factors for rectal complication. *Int J Radiat Oncol Biol Phys* 1988;14:281–286.
302. Sood B, Garg M, Avadhani J, et al. Predictive value of linear-quadratic model in the treatment of cervical cancer using high-dose-rate brachytherapy. *Int J Radiat Oncol Biol Phys* 2002;54(5):1377–1387.
303. Chen S, Liang J, Yang S, et al. The prediction of late rectal complications following the treatment of uterine cervical cancer by high dose rate brachytherapy. *Int J Radiat Oncol Biol Phys* 2000;47(4):955–961.
304. Chen SW, Liang JA, Yeh LS, et al. Comparative study of reference points by dosimetric analyses for late complications after uniform external radiotherapy and high-dose-rate brachytherapy for cervical cancer. *Int J Radiat Oncol Biol Phys* 2004;60(2):663–671.
305. Toita T, Kakinohana Y, Ogawa K, et al. Combination external beam radiotherapy and high-dose-rate intracavitary brachytherapy for uterine cervical cancer: analysis of dose and fractionation schedule. *Int J Radiat Oncol Biol Phys* 2003;56(5):1344–1353.
306. Lee SW, Suh CO, Chung EJ, et al. Dose optimization of fractionated external radiation and high-dose-rate intracavitary brachytherapy for FIGO stage IB uterine cervical carcinoma. *Int J Radiat Oncol Biol Phys* 2002;52(5):1338–1344.
307. Van Lancker M, Storme G. Prediction of severe late complications in fractionated, high dose-rate brachytherapy in gynecologic applications. *Int J Radiat Oncol Biol Phys* 1991;20:1125–1129.
308. Mai J, Rownd J, Erickson B. CT-guided high dose rate prescription for cervical carcinoma: the importance of uterine wall thickness. *Brachytherapy* 2002;1:27–35.
309. Kapp KS, Stuecklschweiger GF, Kapp DS, et al. Dosimetry of intracavitary placements for uterine and cervical carcinoma: results of orthogonal film, TLD, and CT-assisted techniques. *Radiother Oncol* 1992;24: 137–146.

310. Mishra S, Chadha M, Panigrahi N, et al. Computed tomography-assisted three-dimensional dosimetry in high dose rate brachytherapy. *Endocurie Hypertherap Oncol* 1994;10:71–77.
311. Schoeppel SL, Fraass BA, Hopkins MP, et al. A CT-compatible version of the Fletcher system intracavitary applicator: clinical application and 3-dimensional treatment planning. *Int J Radiat Oncol Biol Phys* 1989;17:1103–1109.
312. Schoeppel SL, Ellis JH, LaVigne ML, et al. Magnetic resonance imaging during intracavitary gynecologic brachytherapy. *Int J Radiat Oncol Biol Phys* 1992;23:169–174.
313. Viswanathan A, Cormack R, Holloway C, et al. Magnetic resonance-guided interstitial therapy for vaginal recurrence of endometrial cancer. *Int J Radiat Oncol Biol Phys* 2006;66(1):91–99.
314. Potter R, Dimopoulos J, Georg P, et al. Clinical impact of MRI assisted dose volume adaptation and dose escalation in brachytherapy of locally advanced cervix cancer. *Radiother Oncol* 2007;83:148–155.
315. Terahara A, Nakano T, Ishikawa A, et al. Dose-volume histogram analysis of high dose rate intracavitary brachytherapy for uterine cervix cancer. *Int J Radiat Oncol Biol Phys* 1996;35:549–554.

CHAPTER 15 ■ PRINCIPLES OF CHEMOTHERAPY IN GYNECOLOGIC CANCER

MICHAEL A. BOOKMAN

HISTORICAL OVERVIEW OF CANCER CHEMOTHERAPY

The first report of a drug-mediated tumor response was noted over 125 years ago using Fowler's solution (arsenic trioxide in potassium bicarbonate) in patients with Hodgkin's disease and leukemia (1). Arsenic compounds had been used for various medicinal purposes for over 2,000 years, and it was not surprising that they were tested in patients with cancer. Cyclic hematologic toxicity was observed following arsenic administration in normal individuals and patients with leukemia (2), establishing a close association between tumor response and host toxicity that still exists today. Cumulative dose-limiting toxicity (arsenic poisoning) was also described following expanded utilization of arsenic in chronic myelogenous leukemia (3), coinciding with a transition toward radiation therapy for the management of leukemia and lymphoma around 1940.

The term *chemotherapy* has been attributed to Paul Ehrlich, a Nobel laureate physician and bacteriologist, who developed *in vivo* rodent models of infection, including the introduction in 1910 of Salvarsan, an organic arsenical originally used to cure syphilis and still used in the management of trypanosomiasis. His early *in vivo* modeling also encouraged the development of inbred transplantable rodent tumors, thereby establishing a paradigm that has been widely adopted for screening new antitumor agents.

Although the topical vesicant properties of sulfur mustard received much attention during World War I, multiple systemic effects, including leukopenia, bone marrow aplasia, and mucosal ulceration, emerged with further study, and would ultimately have greater importance. Cancer chemotherapy, in the traditional sense, began with the demonstration that nitrogen mustard had reproducible activity against transplanted lymphoma in mice, prompting clinical trials as early as 1942 (4). However, owing to World War II, much of the research remained classified until 1946. Following the demonstration by Farber in 1948 that aminopterin, an antifolate, could induce temporary remission in childhood leukemia (5), antimetabolites became the next major category of agents to be developed, and were ultimately associated with cures in women with choriocarcinoma (6). Research during the 1940s also included the Nobel Prize–winning observations of Huggins and others (7) regarding the antitumor effect of estrogens in prostatic cancer.

Between 1945 and 1965, many important chemotherapeutic agents, such as actinomycin D, cyclophosphamide, 5-fluorouracil, Vinca alkaloids, and progestogens, were developed and demonstrated to have antitumor activity in clinical trials. Between 1965 and 1975, the pace of new drug discovery and development continued. During this period, cisplatin was shown to have activity in testicular and ovarian tumors, and doxorubicin, bleomycin, etoposide, and tamoxifen entered our clinical arsenal. This was followed by identification of analogs, such as carboplatin, idarubicin, and vinorelbine, with antitumor activity similar to the parent compound but with a reduction in nonhematologic toxicity. The 1990s and beyond have brought important new agents into clinical practice, including the taxanes (paclitaxel and docetaxel), non-taxane microtubule binding agents (epothilones), camptothecins (topotecan and irinotecan), nucleoside analogs (gemcitabine and capecitabine), alternative organoplatinums (oxaliplatin, satraplatin), an inhibitor of the proteasome complex (bortezomib), and an agent that binds to the minor groove of DNA, distinct from other alkylating agents (ecteinascidin).

Attention has also been directed at alternative formulations of standard agents, including liposomal or polymer-based encapsulation, protein conjugation, nanoparticles, or lipid solubilization, to modify drug disposition, tumor targeting, and the potential for host toxicity. In addition, conventional agents have been utilized for regional (intraperitoneal) administration, prolonged intravenous infusion, continuous oral administration, high-dose therapy with hematopoietic progenitor cell support, and weekly low-dose therapy, each with the goal of improving the therapeutic ratio, but with a variable impact on host toxicity and clinical outcomes.

With the availability of multiple agents, each with a different molecular target, mechanism of action, pattern of resistance, and spectrum of host toxicity, we have also seen frequent utilization of multidrug combinations, particularly as primary therapy for advanced disease. The use of adjuvant therapy, including concurrent chemoradiation for early-stage disease, has been greatly expanded in selected clinical situations, with the result that a larger proportion of patients is exposed to chemotherapy at an earlier point in the natural history of their disease. Based on a combination of intrinsic and acquired factors, the majority of advanced tumors eventually demonstrate broad resistance to conventional cytotoxic chemotherapy, and there has been renewed interest in novel biologic and immunologic approaches with non–cross-resistant mechanisms. In addition, with improved understanding of the mechanisms associated with drug resistance, newer agents have been developed that may partially reverse the resistant phenotype through blockade of specific pathways or promotion of cellular apoptosis.

Exploration of the biologic mechanisms associated with tumor invasion, metastasis, and angiogenesis has led to the development of inhibitors directed against metalloproteinases, adhesion molecules, and growth factors important for angiogenesis. As basic research in molecular biology uncovers specific genetic and growth-regulatory factors associated with tumorigenesis, targeted small molecules have been developed that modulate a number of intracellular pathways. These include inhibition of protein tyrosine kinases associated with specific growth-factor receptors and downstream components of signal transduction pathways, cyclin-dependent kinases associated with cell cycle progression, as well as interference with posttranslational protein modifications, such as farnesylation of the *ras* oncogene and other intracellular targets (8).

TUMOR BIOLOGY IN RELATION TO CHEMOTHERAPY

Tumor Growth and Cellular Kinetics

Many of the principles of modern chemotherapy are derived from knowledge of the growth characteristics of normal and tumor tissues. Each tissue has an innate capacity for growth that is regulated by internal and external factors. The growth characteristics of tumors differ from normal tissues, and the exploitation of these differences has provided the historical basis for utilization of radiation and chemotherapy. The cellular kinetics of normal tissues also explains many of the toxicities associated with chemotherapy. All normal tissues, particularly during fetal development and variably during adult life, possess the capacity for cellular division and growth.

The *static* population includes well-differentiated cells that arise from pluripotential fetal stem cells and rarely undergo cell division during adult life. Typical of this group are striated muscle, neurons, and nephrons, with oocytes representing a specialized subcategory. Damage to these cells can have long-term consequences, and has prompted interest in stem cell biology.

The *expanding* population of normal tissues retains the capacity to grow, but in their adult state, they are normally quiescent. Under stress, especially after injury, a proliferative burst is followed by return to quiescence. Typical of this pattern of growth are the components of liver parenchymal tissue, including hepatocytes, bile duct epithelium, and vascular endothelium.

The *renewing* cell population is in a continuous proliferative state with ongoing cell division balanced by cell loss and terminal differentiation. Typical renewing populations include the bone marrow, epidermis, gastrointestinal epithelium, and spermatocytes.

The patterns of normal cell growth partially explain some of the toxic effects of cytotoxic therapy and why some tissues are commonly spared (9). Renewing cell populations with constant turnover are most sensitive to acute injury from conventional chemotherapy or irradiation. This is reflected by the frequent occurrence of dose-limiting bone marrow suppression, mucositis, and azoospermia during cytotoxic drug treatment, with relative sparing of nonproliferative compartments, such as brain, muscle, kidney, bone, and oocytes. However, even nondividing tissues can experience late chronic effects related to DNA damage.

Dysregulated growth of cancer cells occurs because of altered growth-factor signaling and/or disruption of checkpoint mechanisms that exist in normal cells. Despite a capacity for continuous growth, the actual process of cancer cell division is not more rapid than division in normal cells.

Programmed cell death, or apoptosis, has emerged as a major mechanism for regulating growth and development of tissues. Furthermore, certain oncogenes, like c-*myc* and *bcl-2*, and tumor-suppressor genes (antioncogenes), including *Rb* and *TP53*, are central to the regulation of apoptosis. Expression of these genes can alter the sensitivity of cancer cells to treatment with chemotherapy and radiation. For instance, overexpression of functional *bcl-2* and nonfunctional p53 genes can render tumor cells resistant to a number of chemotherapeutic agents (10), suggesting that efforts to restore apoptotic signaling may improve chemosensitivity.

Antioncogenes, such as *Rb* or *TP53*, contribute to growth restraint in normal cells. Within the spectrum of gynecologic malignancies, their role is best illustrated in the setting of cervical cancer, where the papillomavirus E7 protein directly inhibits *Rb*, allowing cell cycle release (11). In addition, the papillomavirus E6 protein increases *TP53* degradation, promoting cellular proliferation.

Gompertzian Tumor Growth

During initial cell divisions, tumor growth seems to follow an exponential pattern. As the tumor grows larger, the rate of growth slows. This pattern of exponential growth with exponential growth retardation and is known as gompertzian growth (Fig. 15.1). As the tumor mass increases, the time required to double the tumor volume also increases. The kinetic explanation for this apparent paradox is illustrated in Figure 15.2, showing the effect of exponential growth by comparing the number of cells in the tumor mass with the number of doublings (12). In accordance with gompertzian kinetics, exponential growth is not strictly maintained throughout the entire growth history. For example, if a skilled radiologist recognized a 0.5-cm tumor on a chest radiograph, or a clinician palpated a 1-cm tumor mass, we might assume that the tumor had been detected quite early. In reality, the tumor has already

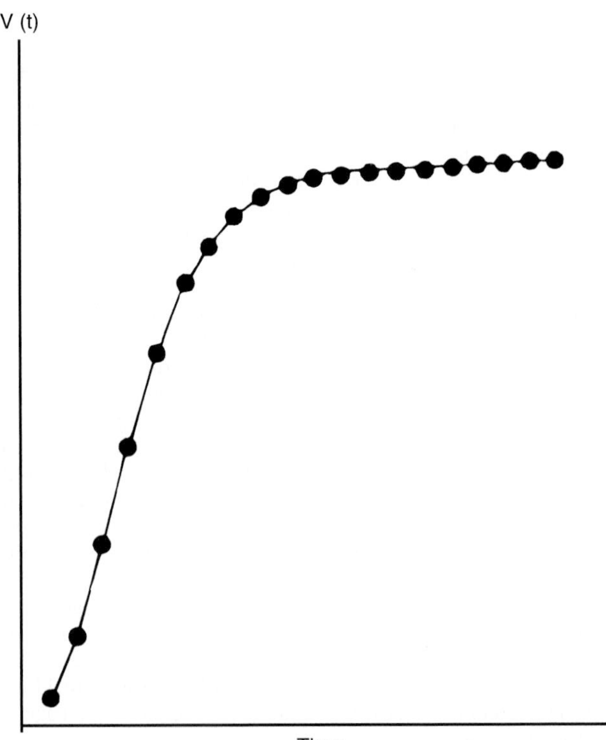

FIGURE 15.1. Hypothetical gompertzian tumor growth curve. Exponential tumor growth with exponential growth retardation. The vertical axis is tumor volume, and the horizontal axis is time.

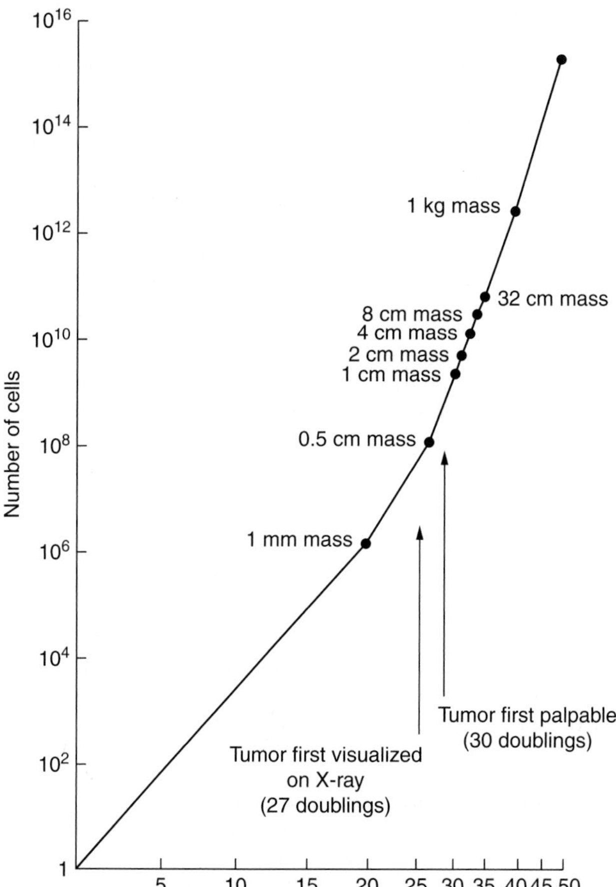

FIGURE 15.2. Theoretical tumor doubling curve assumes exponential tumor growth. The vertical axis is the number of cells, and the horizontal axis is the number of doublings.

undergone at least 30 doublings prior to detection (Fig. 15.2). If we adjust for ongoing cell loss, the number of actual cell doublings would be much greater.

Limited information exists regarding the actual doubling times of human tumors *in vivo* (13,14), as summarized in Table 15.1. For this analysis, tumors were relatively circumscribed and serially measurable by radiographic imaging, often as pulmonary metastases, representing a selective sample. It is clear that embryonal tumors, lymphomas, and mesenchymal tumors have shorter doubling times than adenocarcinomas or squamous-cell carcinomas. In addition, metastases generally have faster doubling times than their corresponding primary lesions. The average doubling time observed in human tumors is approximately 50 days, with a broad range.

The model also suggests other conclusions of clinical relevance. First, metastatic spread may occur well before obvious evidence of the primary lesion. Second, at later stages of tumor growth, a small number of doublings can produce a marked change in tumor size with an increased potential for adverse clinical consequences. For instance, a 1-cm mass (at least 30 prior doublings) becomes a 4-cm mass after just two more doublings.

TABLE 15.1

DOUBLING TIMES OF HUMAN TUMORS

Tumor histology	Patients (n)	Doubling time (Mean ± 2 SD, days)
Embryonal tumors (lung metastases)	76	27 ± 5
Lymphomas	51	29 ± 6
Malignant mesenchymal tumors	87	41 ± 7
Squamous-cell carcinomas (lung metastases)	51	58 ± 9
Squamous-cell carcinomas (primary tumors)	97	82 ± 14
Adenocarcinomas (lung metastases)	134	83 ± 12
Adenocarcinomas (primary tumors)	34	166 ± 48

Host-Tumor Interactions

Ultimately, dysregulated growth exceeds local resources, and the tumor becomes dependent on the manipulation of host angiogenic pathways for delivery of oxygen, access to nutrients, and removal of waste products. In contrast, tumors generally grow without induction of host lymphatics, and are characterized by increased interstitial pressures as a consequence of disordered capillary proliferation with leaky vessels and accumulation of extracellular fluid. Together, these factors result in regional hypoxia, acidosis, and necrosis that can limit the effective delivery of chemotherapy and may protect viable tumor cells that are more distant from functional capillaries. One of the potential benefits observed with antiangiogenic therapy has been normalization of tumor vessels with reduced interstitial pressures and improved drug delivery (15).

Cell Cycle Kinetics

The kinetic behavior of individual tumor cells is also important in understanding tumor growth. Figure 15.3 is a schematic view of the cell cycle. Cells can remain in a noncycling postmitotic

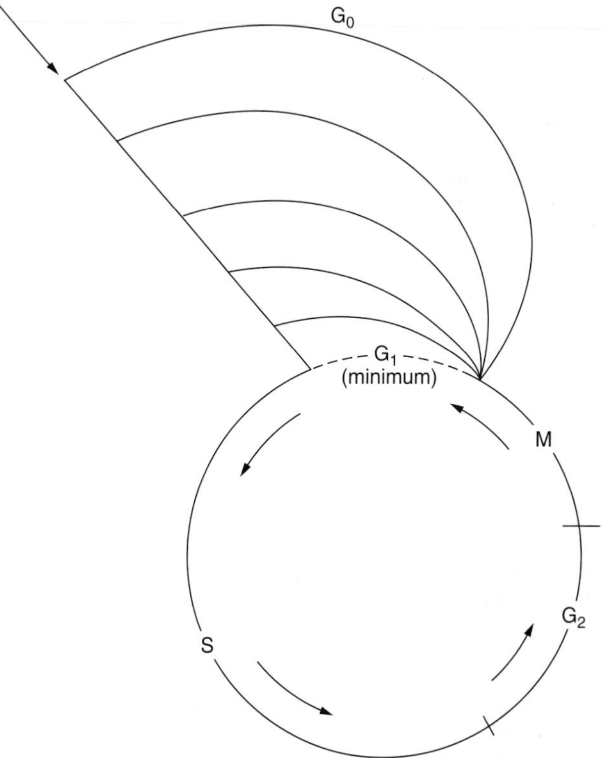

FIGURE 15.3. Phases of the cell cycle, beginning with M (mitosis) and proceeding through G_1 (postmitotic phase), S (DNA synthetic phase), and G_2 (premitotic phase). As G_1 becomes progressively longer, it is known as G_0.

compartment (G_0) for extended periods of time, but retain the ability to reenter active cycling when triggered by growth factors or other local signals. The point of entry, or first gap phase (G_1), can be of variable length and associated with diverse cellular activities, including protein and RNA synthesis, DNA repair, and cell growth. After passing the first checkpoint in G_1, the cell enters the DNA synthetic phase (S), during which a complete copy of the cellular DNA is created through replication. The second gap phase (G_2) provides another opportunity for checkpoint control before entering active mitosis (M), during which the nuclear membrane disappears and the chromosomes condense (prophase) and align (metaphase) in conjunction with the appearance of the mitotic apparatus, consisting of microtubules, centrioles, and the kinetochore. Mitotic alignment is associated with one final checkpoint prior to actual separation (anaphase), followed by dissolution of the mitotic apparatus (telophase) and creation of daughter cells through cytokinesis. The postmitotic period (G_1) is variable, and cells can further differentiate, enter a noncycling state (G_0), or initiate another cycle.

Cell cycle events have important implications for the patient, tumor, and cancer therapist. Most chemotherapeutic agents disrupt DNA, RNA, or protein synthesis. Rapidly proliferating cells (i.e., short G_1) are most sensitive to chemotherapy, whereas cells that slowly proliferate (i.e., G_0 or long G_1) are generally less sensitive. Nondividing cells, such as the differentiated elements of a mature teratoma, may occupy space and contribute to tumor bulk and symptoms, but are relatively insensitive to chemotherapy.

Cell cycle times may be estimated by performing labeled mitotic curves *in vivo* or *in vitro,* and appear to be relatively similar for many solid tumors, with cycle times ranging from 10 to 31 hours (16). Compared with the tremendous variation in human tumor doubling times, this is a relatively narrow range, suggesting that the primary reason for variations in clinical tumor growth cannot be ascribed to variations in the cell cycle.

Growth fraction and programmed cell death also influence the overall tumor growth rate and response to therapy. The growth fraction is the proportion of tumor cells that are actively cycling. In a typical solid tumor, only a fraction of the cells are rapidly proliferating, primarily those that are most proximal to small blood vessels. With the marked heterogeneity of human tumors at a microscopic level, growth fractions are quite variable, ranging from 25% to 95%. Although it may seem paradoxical, cell loss is very high in human tumors, ranging from 70% to more than 95%, and small changes in cell loss could produce major changes in overall tumor growth (17).

Log Cell Kill

In principle, the rational use of chemotherapy relies on basic concepts of cellular kinetics, but the translation from preclinical models to solid tumors has been challenging. In animals, the curability of transplanted tumors is inversely proportional to the tumor cell number, size, and timing of treatment initiation. In part, this is the result of important tumor-host interactions, such as the time required to establish a blood supply. However, this is also an illustration of first-order cell-kill kinetics, whereby a constant fraction of exposed cells is killed, rather than a constant number. Using first-order kinetics, a single treatment for a tumor weighing 1 g (approximately 10^9 cells) might yield 90% cell kill and would only decrease the tumor population by one log, leaving 10^8 viable cells. Without further treatment, the tumor would grow back at a constant rate, with only a modest delay in lethality. Only when the log cell kill is very large (>99%) and the therapies are repetitive can chemotherapy be curative. Although certain unusual cancers, such as choriocarcinoma, can be cured with a single application of a single drug, most human cancers are intrinsically less sensitive, and more sophisticated therapeutic techniques are needed to achieve adequate tumor response. This is one reason why multidrug combinations have been developed. In addition, chemotherapy is usually distributed over multiple cycles to allow for host recovery and achieve the cumulative cell kill required for tumor regression and cure.

It is thought that prolonged survival or cure can be achieved only when the cell population is reduced to between 10^1 and 10^4 cells. In most circumstances, cell burdens of this size are not clinically detectable. This realization has led to the use of adjuvant chemotherapy in the early stages of cancer, where microscopic residual disease is suspected. It has also been used to rationalize the continuation of active chemotherapy for several cycles beyond clinical evidence of tumor remission.

Cell Cycle Specificity

Chemotherapeutic agents have complex mechanisms of action and can affect tumor cells through multiple pathways. Nevertheless, certain anticancer drugs are known to be proliferation dependent and cell cycle specific. Other drugs are cycle nonspecific, and are capable of killing in all phases of the cell cycle, generally without dependence on the proliferative rate. Examples of cycle-nonspecific drugs include alkylating agents, particularly nitrogen mustard, which are effective against a variety of solid tumors, including those with low growth fractions. Cell cycle–specific agents depend on the proliferative fraction of the tumor and phase of the cell cycle. A typical example is hydroxyurea, which inhibits ribonucleotide reductase. Not surprisingly, cell cycle–specific drugs tend to be more effective against tumors with a high proliferative rate and growth fractions. The interaction of specific cytotoxic agents with the cell cycle is summarized in Table 15.2.

PHARMACOLOGIC PRINCIPLES OF CHEMOTHERAPY

General pharmacologic principles should be considered by the physician in selecting individual drugs and managing their administration according to standards of dose and schedule. Many factors may influence the effectiveness and/or toxicity of chemotherapy, including absorption, distribution, metabolism, and excretion, as well as clinical complications, such as renal impairment, malnutrition, or drug-drug interactions.

Absorbtion, Distribution, and Transport

Drugs may be given orally, intravenously, intramuscularly, intraarterially, or intraperitoneally. Selection of the route of administration depends on solubility, requirements for drug activation, local tissue tolerance, feasibility for an individual patient, and optimal tumor drug exposure, which is estimated as the area under the concentration-time curve (AUC) for the drug and active metabolites. The ultimate effectiveness of any chemotherapeutic agent depends on optimizing the AUC at critical tumor sites. However, there are no established techniques for noninvasive measurement of active drug concentration at these critical sites, and we are forced to extrapolate tumor drug exposure from preclinical models and plasma concentrations over time. Promising research in magnetic resonance spectroscopy and positron emission tomography may soon provide clinically relevant information on drug distribution and tumor metabolism using selected agents.

TABLE 15.2

RELATIONSHIP OF CHEMOTHERAPY AGENTS TO INTRACELLULAR TARGETS AND CELL CYCLE PROGRESSION

Classification	Cell-cycle arrest	Cellular targets and mechanisms	Examples
Inhibition of DNA synthesis and repair	G_1, S	Inhibition of nucleotide synthesis and metabolism. Inhibition of thymidylate synthase, thymidylate phosphorylase, dihydrofolate reductase, ribonucleotide reductase	Antifolates (methotrexate, pemetrexed), nucleoside analogues (6-mercaptopurine, 5-fluorouracil, cytarabine, fludarabine, gemcitabine), hydroxyurea
	S	Stabilization of DNA-topoisomerase II cleavable complex, DNA intercalation, +/− free radical formation	Anthracyclines (doxorubicin, daunomycin, idarubicin, epirubicin), anthracenediones (mitoxantrone), epipodophyllotoxins (etoposide), actinomycin-D
		Stabilization of DNA-topoisomerase I cleavable complex	Camptothecins (topotecan, irinotecan)
Alkylating agents and related compounds	G_1, G_2, S	Direct DNA damage, DNA adduct formation, free radical production, strand breakage	Radiation, platinum compounds (cisplatin, carboplatin, oxaliplatin); bleomycin, mitomycin C, nitrogen mustard, nitrosoureas, ecteinascidin
Antimicrotubule reagents	M	Inhibition of tubulin polymerization	Vinca alkaloids (vinristine, vinblastine, vinorelbine), colchicine
		Promotion of tubulin polymerization	Taxanes (paclitaxel, docetaxel), epothilones
		Kinesin spindle proteins	Investigational agents
Cell cycle agents	G_1, S, G_2, M	Mitotic checkpoint control, cyclin-dependent kinases (CDK), aurora kinases	Flavopiridol, investigational agents
Signal transduction modulators	G_0, G_1, S, G_2	Growth factor sequestration, receptor blockade	Trastuzumab, cetuximab, pertuzumab, VEGF-trap, bevacizumab
		Inhibition of tyrosine kinase mediated signal transduction	Erlotinib, gefitinib, desatinib, imatinib, sorafenib, sunitinib, lapatinib
		Modulation of protein kinase C	Bryostatin, enzastaurin
		Inhibition of hormonal pathways	Tamoxifen, raloxifene, anastrazole, letrozole, fulvestrant, megestrol, mifepristone, flutamide, leuprolide
Gene regulation	NA	Gene regulation by inhibition of methylation, DNA methyltransferase, inhibition of histone deacetylase	Azacytidine, suberoylanilide hydroxamic acid (vorinostat)
Protein modifications	NA	Post-translational protein modifications, inhibition of farnesylation	Tipifarnib, bisphosphonates
		Inhibition of the proteasome complex and clearance of ubiquinated proteins	Bortezomib

The increasing utilization of oral chemotherapy and development of oral molecular targeted agents has renewed interest in bioavailability in the setting of meals and other factors that can modulate local intestinal transport. Most often, dose and schedule information from Food and Drug Administration (FDA)-approved package inserts reflects data from large phase 3 trials, rather than smaller studies that might examine dietary or drug interactions. For example, the bioavailability of one tyrosine kinase inhibitor could be increased over threefold in the setting of a high-fat meal (18), but the package insert recommends taking the drug on an empty stomach, at least 1 hour before or after meals. With the high cost of chronic medication, it is apparent that there could also be substantial economic implications to these pharmacokinetic observations (19).

Another interesting association concerns ingestion of grapefruit juice, which contains compounds that can inhibit local compounds within the intestinal mucosa, particularly the cytochrome P450 isozyme, CYP3A4 (20), and possibly the drug efflux pump, p-glycoprotein. Drugs that are substrates for either of these compounds can be more efficiently absorbed after ingestion of grapefruit juice, due to reduced local metabolism, leading to increased serum levels that may have clinical consequences, including cyclosporine, erythromycin, calcium channel blockers, and benzodiazepines.

The extent of drug binding to serum proteins, as well as physical properties, such as lipid solubility, diffusion, or molecular weight, may have an impact on tumor drug exposure. In addition, some areas of the body, particularly the brain, are actively protected from drug exposure and can serve as pharmacologic tumor sanctuaries, where sequestered cancer cells may survive otherwise curative systemic therapy. Although uncommon with solid tumors that disrupt the blood-brain barrier, this was a common problem in acute leukemia until effectively managed with intrathecal drug delivery and/or high peak plasma levels. In addition to achieving local delivery, most drugs must be internalized within tumor cells to achieve cytotoxicity. Internalization can be accomplished by passive diffusion, active transport, pinocytosis, or receptor-mediated endocytosis.

Many chemotherapeutic agents are lipophilic and highly protein bound in plasma, particularly to albumin. Commonly used agents with greater than 95% protein binding include cisplatin, paclitaxel, docetaxel, etoposide, and the active metabolite of irinotecan (SN-38). Agents with less protein binding include doxorubicin (75%), topotecan (35%), gemcitabine (10%), carboplatin (<5%), and ifosfamide (<5%). It is generally the unbound "free" drug that mediates toxicity, and any condition associated with variability in protein binding can have an impact on cumulative drug exposure. For example, the toxicity of chemotherapy is frequently accentuated in patients with poor nutritional status, which is associated with reduced protein levels and other metabolic changes (21). Docetaxel offers an interesting example for potential interactions, due to extensive binding to albumin, lipoproteins, and α-acidic glycoprotein (AAG), which has been correlated with changes in drug clearance, prompting further evaluation of optimized dosing (22).

Intraperitoneal Chemotherapy

Although most chemotherapy is administered by the systemic route, there are unique situations in which the regional use of chemotherapy has been studied, with intraperitonal administration a specific example. If primary tumors or their metastases are anatomically confined to specific organs or particular regions of the body, or if unique pharmacokinetic circumstances exist that favor regional clearance, there is a theoretical rationale for regional chemotherapy. For example, intraarterial drug administration has been studied in cervical cancer, localized recurrence of rectal carcinoma, and head and neck cancer. Local complications are potentially serious, including arterial thrombosis, wound slough, lymphedema, and osteonecrosis caused by the shared arterial blood supply between the tumor and neighboring normal tissues. While high response rates can be achieved in selected patients, larger randomized trials are needed to evaluate overall risks and long-term outcomes.

Intracavitary chemotherapy has been used for tumors confined to the peritoneum, pleura, or pericardium. The rationale for this approach is based on the fact that clearance from a body cavity is delayed compared to the systemic circulation, achieving more prolonged exposure to higher regional concentrations of active agents. This technique has been most extensively studied in ovarian cancer, with evaluation of many agents, including 5-fluorouracil, doxorubicin, cisplatin, carboplatin, cytarabine, melphalan, etoposide, and paclitaxel (23,24). Phase 1-2 studies have uniformly demonstrated a pharmacologic advantage favoring the intraperitoneal compartment, but have not documented enhanced drug delivery to actual sites of disease. Of key importance, penetration of peritoneal tumor nodules by passive diffusion is limited by fibrotic adhesions, tumor encapsulation, and high interstitial pressures as a consequence of intratumoral capillary leak without functional lymphatic drainage. In addition, both cisplatin and carboplatin are rapidly cleared from the peritoneal compartment and recirculate through the blood, limiting the window for direct tumor penetration, exposing the host to systemic toxicity, and raising questions about the clinical importance of the local pharmacokinetic advantage. Based on these observations, it has been postulated that the major role for intracavitary therapy would be in patients with minimal residual disease.

Cisplatin has received the greatest attention for intraperitoneal delivery in ovarian cancer, achieving a laparotomy-confirmed response rate of greater than 32% at doses between 50 and 150 mg/m^2, using systemic thiosulfate rescue at the higher dose levels (25). One long-term analysis reported an actuarial 2-year survival rate of 74% for patients with minimal residual disease treated with a variety of intraperitoneal therapies (26), although this may partially reflect the biology of small-volume disease, which can also be managed effectively with observation followed by systemic therapy. In view of the risk of systemic toxicity from cisplatin, there has been renewed interest in the substitution of carboplatin, which differs in terms of protein binding and overall time required for activation (via aquation), suggesting that biologic and clinical properties could be different from intraperitoneal cisplatin.

In contrast to cisplatin, paclitaxel was poorly absorbed from the peritoneal compartment, suggesting that patients might benefit from combined intravenous and intraperitoneal administration to optimize tumor drug exposure. As a single agent, intraperitoneal paclitaxel demonstrated a 61% pathology-confirmed complete response rate among 28 assessable patients with initial microscopic disease (27). However, only 1 of 31 patients (3%) with greater than microscopic disease achieved a complete response, emphasizing the limitations of drug access and penetration by diffusion from the peritoneal space.

Intraperitoneal therapy could also have an impact on the tumor-host relationship through alterations in local cytokine production, angiogenic potential, or immunoregulation. Hopefully, future studies will evaluate some of these biologic parameters to assist with optimization of therapy.

Biotransformation

Some agents, such as cyclophosphamide, ifosfamide, and capecitabine, are administered as true prodrugs and must undergo irreversible metabolism to the active form, most commonly in the liver, but also in tumor or other host tissues. For many of these agents, intraperitoneal or intraarterial administration would be ineffective, as it would achieve high local concentrations of the native compound, but without an opportunity for bioconversion. Other agents are in reversible equilibrium with reactive intermediates, such as irinotecan and SN-38 (7-ethyl-10-hydroxycamptothecin), with dependencies on local pH and presence of specific enzymes, such as carboxyesterase. Cisplatin and carboplatin require activation through irreversible aquation to a reactive intermediary before they can initiate DNA adduct formation. Although the final reactive compounds are identical, the rate of aquation and adduct formation is much slower with carboplatin (28), but can be accelerated in the presence of activating nucleophiles, such as glutathione (29), even though the same nucleophiles can partially block cisplatin adduct formation at higher concentrations.

Renal Excretion and Physiologic Age

Drug inactivation, elimination, or excretion can dramatically influence cumulative exposure, which significantly affects antitumor activity and host toxicity. Inactivation and excretion of chemotherapeutic agents occurs primarily through the liver, kidneys, and body tissues, with lesser elimination through the stool. While any impairment of normal liver or kidney function can disturb drug metabolism and excretion, the most common problem encountered in the setting of gynecologic cancer is acute or chronic renal insufficiency due to tumor-mediated obstruction, drug-induced toxicity, advanced age, or preexisting comorbidities.

The use of combination chemotherapy in the elderly patient can pose a number of challenges related to bone marrow reserve and vital organ function (30). Although the risk of hematologic toxicity is generally increased, overall benefits from active chemotherapy regimens can still be demonstrated, as illustrated by the analysis of data from several breast cancer trials (31). Studies in ovarian cancer have indicated that age is an adverse prognostic factor, but it seems reasonable to expect that delivery of effective treatments can still have an incremental benefit regardless of age. From that perspective, it is important to define tolerable and effective treatment regimens that can be safely administered in elderly patients, incorporating adjustments for age-related changes in vital organ function.

In surveying the general nondiabetic female population, the incidence of moderate renal insufficiency dramatically increases with advancing age, which is of particular relevance to the care of women with gynecologic cancer (32). For example, in the 60 to 69 year age group, over one third of women have an estimated glomerular filtration rate (GFR) of less than 60 mL/min/1.73 m^2 (Fig. 15.4). In addition, serum creatinine levels can be inappropriately low in women with gynecologic cancer, as a consequence of reduced muscle mass, malnutrition, or alterations in fluid balance, and any of the standard formulae will overestimate GFR, with potential clinical consequences. Clearly, universal caution in dosing drugs with high renal clearance, especially carboplatin, is required.

Several methods are available to estimate GFR and classify the extent of renal injury based on age, sex, serum creatinine, and other factors. In general, serum creatinine is the dominant factor, and it remains unclear if minor differences between formulae might have meaningful and/or consistent clinical consequences with regard to drug dosing. In most cases, it is sufficient to estimate the magnitude of renal injury rather than obtain a precise measure of GFR. However, all of these formulae are based on stable normalized biologic parameters, and are less useful in the setting of dynamic changes following acute renal injury, or nonrenal fluctuations in serum creatinine and fluid status, such as might occur in the postoperative setting or in the presence of large-volume ascites or in patients with abnormal muscle mass. While urine collection for measurement of creatinine clearance may provide a better estimate of GFR, it is also subject to variability, and the use of ^{51}Cr-ethylenediamine tetraacetic acid (EDTA) clearance remains the standard for measurement of GFR, but is rarely used in clinical practice due to the cost and complexity associated with radioisotopes. A nonradioactive alternative is the measurement of iodine in blood after administration of iohexol (a nonionic contrast agent), but this has not yet gained wide clinical acceptance (33).

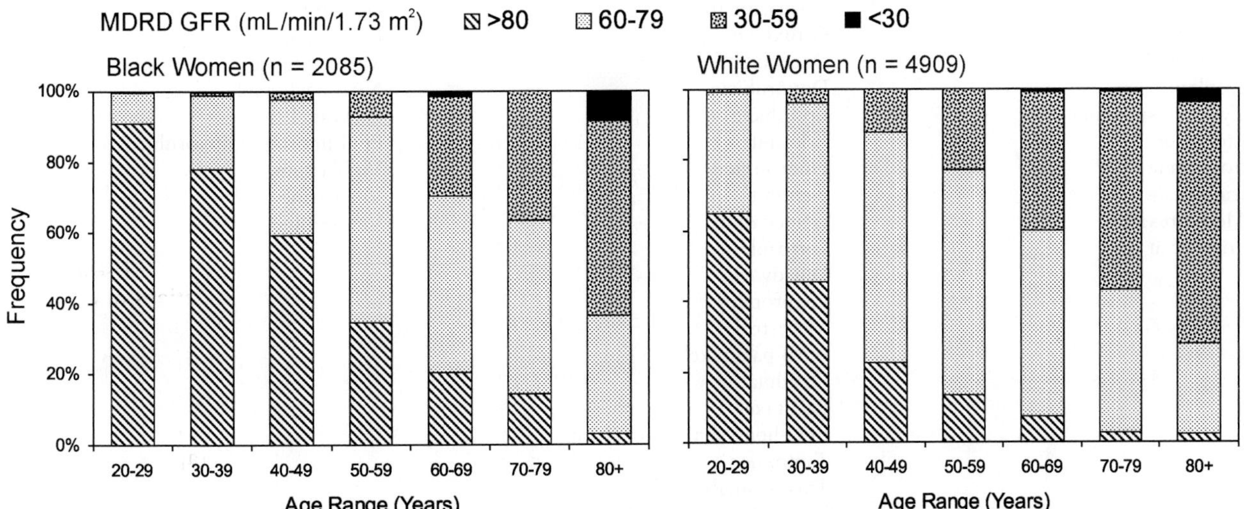

FIGURE 15.4. Distribution of renal function in nondiabetic adults. Weighted distribution of predicted GFR (mL/min/1.73 m^2) based on the MDRD formula from the Third National Health and Nutrition Examination Survey (NHANES III). *Source:* From Clase CM, Garg AX, Kiberd BA. Prevalence of low glomerular filtration rate in nondiabetic Americans: Third National Health and Nutrition Examination Survey (NHANES III). *J Am Soc Nephrol* 2002;13:1338–1349.

TABLE 15.3

COMMONLY UTILIZED FORMULAE TO ESTIMATE CREATININE CLEARANCE

Formula name	Estimation of creatinine clearance (CrCl)
Cockcroft–Gault formula (35)	CrCl (mL/min) = (140 − age) × weight (kg) × (0.85 if female)/serum Cr (mg/dL) × 72
Jelliffe formula (36)	CrCl (mL/min) = {98 − [0.8 × (age − 20)]} × (0.9 if female)/serum Cr (mg/dL)
MDRD formula (34)	GFR (mL/min/1.73 m^2) = 170 × [serum Cr (mg/dL)]$^{-0.999}$ × (age)$^{-0.176}$ × (0.762 if female) × (1.180 if African American) × [SUN (mg/dL)]$^{-0.170}$ × [Alb (g/dL)]$^{+0.318}$

Note: Alb, serum albumin concentration; Cr, creatinine; GFR, glomerular filtration rate; MDRD formula, the Modification of Diet in Renal Disease study equation; SUN, serum urea nitrogen concentration.

For characterization of chronic renal dysfunction, there is emerging support for the formula derived from the Modification of Diet in Renal Disease (MDRD) study, which has also been incorporated in standardized laboratory reports (34). The Cockroft–Gault (35) and Jelliffe (36) formulae are also commonly used (Table 15.3). Staging of chronic renal disease has been used to reflect overall severity and guide management decisions, including dose modifications. The most commonly used staging system is from the National Kidney Foundation (http://www.kidney.org/professionals/kdoqi/guidelines_ckd/toc.htm) (37).

Specific guidelines exist for modifying drug doses for patients with renal impairment (38), with special attention to a growing list of agents with renal-dominant clearance (Table 15.4). Dosing parameters for patients on dialysis receiving individual drugs, such as cisplatin (39) and carboplatin (40), are also available. However, owing to the rapid introduction of new agents, clinicians are urged to consult updated prescribing information and online database resources.

Metabolism and Pharmacogenomics

Modifications of drug doses may also be required for patients with liver disease (41), particularly for paclitaxel, docetaxel, nanoparticle albumin-bound paclitaxel (42), doxorubicin, and the Vinca alkaloids (vincristine, vinblastine, and vinorelbine), which are primarily metabolized in the liver and/or excreted in the bile. Excessive toxicity may occur with doses that would ordinarily be acceptable, and guidelines for treating patients with impaired liver function should be consulted. However, variability in nonhepatic clearance and compensatory host adaptations, such as increased renal clearance, make these recommendations less rigid than those provided for patients with

TABLE 15.4

MODIFICATIONS IN THE SETTING OF RENAL AND HEPATIC DYSFUNCTION

Agents that should be considered for modification in the presence of moderate to severe renal dysfunction	Agents that generally do not require modification in the presence of moderate renal dysfunction	Agents that should be considered for modification in the presence of hepatic dysfunction
Actinomycin D	Anastrozole	Docetaxel
Bleomycin	Bevacizumab	Doxorubicin
Capecitabine	Cetuximab	Epirubicin
Carboplatin	Docetaxel	Mitoxantrone
Cisplatin[a]	Doxorubicin	NAB-paclitaxel
Cyclophosphamide	Epirubicin	Paclitaxel
Etoposide	Erlotinib	PEG-liposomal doxorubicin
Ifosfamide	Fluorouracil	Vinblastine
Irinotecan	Gefitinib	Vincristine
Methotrexate	Gemcitabine	Vinorelbine
Topotecan	Letrozole	
	Leucovorin	
	Leuprorelin	
	Megestrol	
	NAB-paclitaxel	
	Oxaliplatin	
	Paclitaxel	
	PEG-liposomal doxorubicin	
	Tamoxifen	
	Trastuzumab	
	Vinblastine	
	Vincristine	
	Vinorelbine	

[a]Can be administered at full doses in anephric patients receiving hemodialysis.

renal dysfunction. For example, dose reduction of etoposide in the setting of biliary obstruction remains controversial and may not be required (43).

With expanded knowledge of metabolic pathways and awareness of polymorphisms in key enzymes, it has also been possible to identify individuals with a dramatic increased risk of toxicity. For example, dihydropyrimidine dehydrogenase (DPD) controls the rate-limiting step in fluoropyrimidine metabolism, and approximately 10 variant DPD alleles can occur with sufficient frequency to merit consideration of screening, as patients can be at risk for life-threatening mucosal injury and bone marrow suppression after receiving a single standard dose of 5-fluorouracil. While methods are available for screening, current assays can be expensive, and the potential reduction in risk needs to be balanced against the costs of a widespread screening program (44). The use of 5-fluorouracil during primary treatment of gynecologic cancer has declined, with the exception of some chemoradiation strategies and occasional palliative management of recurrent disease.

Uridine diphospho-glucuronosyl-transferase 1A1 (UGT1A1) is responsible for glucuronidation of bilirubin and a number of drug metabolites, most notably SN-38, the major active metabolite of irinotecan. As such, patients with a deficiency in UGT1A1 are at increased risk for life-threatening diarrhea and bone marrow suppression after receiving irinotecan, and potentially other camptothecin derivatives with SN-38 metabolites (45). While the UGT1A1*28 promotor mutation has been studied most extensively, mutations in the coding region can also occur, particularly in Asian populations, and may predict for efficacy in addition to toxicity (46). Gilbert's syndrome is associated with a mild unconjugated hyperbilirubinemia and reduced activity of UGT1A1 that is also associated with an increased risk of toxicity in both homozygous and heterozygous patients (47). The family of adenosine triphosphate-binding cassette (ABC) proteins is involved in biliary transport and conjugation of camptothecins. Polymorphisms of ABCB1, also known as p-glycoprotein or multidrug resistance protein 1 (MDR1) as well as ABCC2, also known as canalicular multispecific organic anion transporter (cMOAT)

TABLE 15.5

PHYSIOLOGIC AND PHARMACOLOGIC INTERACTIONS IN CANCER CHEMOTHERAPY

Interaction		Cause and/or agent	Impact
Renal dysfunction		Obstruction, renal dysfunction, hypovolemia, hypotension, nonsteroidals, nephrotoxins (aminoglycosides, cisplatin)	Decreased clearance of methotrexate, carboplatin, and other agents
Hepatobiliary dysfunction		Biliary obstruction, hepatic dysfunction	Decreased clearance of doxorubicin, mitoxantrone, vincristine, vinblastine, etoposide, paclitaxel, docetaxel
		Gilbert's syndrome, glucuronidation polymorphisms (UGTA1A)	Increased exposure to SN-38 (irinotecan)
Microsomal activation		Hepatic dysfunction	Impaired activation of cyclophosphamide and ifosfamide
Altered protein binding		Carrier displacement (sulfonamide, salicylates, phenytoin)	Increased toxicity, higher free drug levels (methotrexate)
		Reduced carrier proteins (malnutrition)	Increased toxicity, higher free drug levels (cisplatin, paclitaxel, docetaxel, etoposide, SN-38)
Altered intestinal absorption		Oral antibiotics (neomycin)	Decreased absorption of methotrexate
		High-fat meal	Increased bioavailability (lapatinib) Decreased bioavailability (capecitabine)
		Grapefruit juice (intestinal CYP3A4 inhibition)	Increased bioavailability (cyclosporine, erythromycin, benzodiazepines)
Decreased metabolism		Allopurinol	Delayed clearance (6-mercaptopurine)
		Dihydropyrimidine dehydrogenase (DPD) deficiency	Lethal toxicity (5-fluorouracil)
Cholinesterase inhibition		Cyclophosphamide, glucocorticoids	Decreased clearance (succinylcholine)
Monoamine oxidase inhibition		Procarbazine	Neurotoxicity and seizures (tricyclic antidepressants and phenothiazines)
MDR-1 competition		Natural products and other substrates, including verapamil, cyclosporine, tamoxifen	Decreased efflux and increased toxicity from natural products (doxorubicin, vincristine, paclitaxel, docetaxel)
CYP2C9	Inhibition	Capecitabine	Increased AUC (warfarin)
CYP3A4	Induction	Glucocorticoids, barbiturates, rifampin	Increased activation (cyclophosphamide)
	Inhibition	Ketoconazole, itraconazole, fluconazole, erythromycin	Decreased metabolism of substrates (potentially significant)
	Substrate competition	Cyclophosphamide, ifosfamide, paclitaxel, docetaxel, etoposide, vincristine, vinblastine, tamoxifen, gefitinib	Decreased metabolism of other substrates (usually not clinically significant)

or MRP2, also appear to have an impact on the clinical efficacy and toxicity (neutropenia and diarrhea) associated with irinotecan therapy in Asian patients (48).

Other gene polymorphisms have been described with an impact on DNA repair or detection of DNA damage, as described in subsequent sections. Techniques for screening and identification of pharmacogenomic elements are expanding, with potential implications for individualized drug selection, dosing, prediction of efficacy, and risk of toxicity.

Drug Interactions

During routine care, patients may receive a variety of drugs, including antiemetics, antihistamines (H_1 and H_2), steroids, nonsteroidal anti-inflammatory agents, anticoagulants, narcotics, and anti-infective agents. In addition, adult patients are frequently receiving medication to manage underlying comorbidities, such as diabetes, hypertension, and elevated cholesterol. In view of the number and diversity of medications in common use, it is somewhat surprising that most drug interactions with cytotoxic chemotherapy appear to be of little consequence. However, prospective studies of chemotherapy administration in noncancer volunteers are impractical, and many potential interactions have not been fully explored. Although recent clinical trials acknowledge that these interactions may exist, patients are likely to be excluded from enrollment on the basis of concomitant medications, rather than prospectively collecting valuable data to document safety or the need for treatment modifications. In clinical practice, the occurrence of excessive hematologic and/or nonhematologic toxicity in an individual patient treated with chemotherapy is usually attributed directly to the chemotherapy and managed with treatment modifications, rather than ascribed to a potential drug interaction.

In some instances, interactions may be critical, and some of the more important drug interactions are listed in Table 15.5. Particular attention should be placed on drugs that could alter renal function, such as aminoglycoside antibiotics, nonsteroidal anti-inflammatory agents, and diuretics, in patients with reduced fluid intake. Typical of *in vivo* interactions relevant in gynecologic cancer chemotherapy are the displacement of methotrexate from its transport protein by aspirin or sulfonamides, suppression of pseudocholinesterase by alkylating agents with increased apnea duration during succinylcholine-assisted general anesthesia, impairment of doxorubicin clearance by preadministration of paclitaxel, and impairment of paclitaxel clearance by preadministration of cisplatin.

Increased attention has been focused on drug metabolism and potential interactions at the level of cytochrome P450 (CYP) isozymes, particularly CYP3A4, which is potentially linked to the metabolism of nearly half of all pharmaceutical agents (49). These interactions are guided by several common principles. Drugs that are *substrates* for the same isozyme may competitively inhibit metabolism, but these interactions are usually not of clinical consequence. Drugs that *directly inhibit* CYP isozymes without being a substrate for that isozyme are more likely to have clinical consequences. In this regard, itraconazole, ketoconazole, and fluconazole can inhibit CYP3A4 at low concentrations, and erythromycin can inhibit CYP3A4 via covalent binding and inactivation. Other drugs act as *inducers* of CYP isozymes by increasing gene expression or protein levels, such as glucocorticoids, barbiturates, and rifampin, which can increase the net activity of CYP3A4, resulting in decreased concentrations of susceptible compounds. In addition, many drugs that interact with CYP3A4 are natural products and may also interact with the MDR-1 multidrug resistance transporter P 170 (see mechanisms of multidrug resistance). Among the anticancer agents that are substrates for CYP3A4 are cyclophosphamide, ifosfamide, docetaxel, etoposide, paclitaxel (also CYP2C8), docetaxel, vincristine, vinblastine, tamoxifen, and gefitinib (50). CYP2C9 and CYP2D6 are inhibited by imatinib, and doxorubicin can inhibit CYP2D6. Cyclosporine and verapamil can increase concentrations of doxorubicin and etoposide, probably through blockade of the P-170 drug efflux pump (Table 15.6).

Owing to the diversity and rapid adoption of new chemotherapy and nonchemotherapy compounds, information regarding drug interactions is best obtained from online

TABLE 15.6

SPECIFIC MECHANISMS OF TUMOR DRUG RESISTANCE

Mechanism	Examples	Specific target or effects
Impaired activation	5-Fluorouracil	Reduced levels of thymidylate synthase, thymidylate phosphorylase, or dihydropyrimidine dehydrogenase
	Methotrexate	Reduced intracellular polyglutamation
	Doxorubicin	Low P450 enzymes
	Cyclophosphamide, ifosfamide	Decreased microsomal function
	Gemcitabine	Decreased deoxycytidine kinase
Increased drug efflux	Natural products	Increased *MDR 1* (P 170)
	Topotecan, mitoxantrone	Increased *BCRP* (ABCG2)
Increased drug inactivation	Alkylating agents, platinum	Elevated glutathione and other cellular thiols
Accelerated DNA repair	Alkylating agents, platinum, radiation	Induction of DNA repair enzymes
Increased damage tolerance	Alkylating agents, platinum, radiation	Loss of DNA mismatch repair
Transport defects	Melphalan	Reduced carrier-mediated uptake
	Gemcitabine	Decreased nucleoside transporter
	Platinum	Decreased copper transporter-1
Target alterations	Methotrexate	*DHFR* gene amplification
	Vincristine, paclitaxel	Altered beta-tubulin binding
	Hydroxyurea, gemcitabine	Decreased ribonucleotide reductase
	Glucocorticoids	Decreased receptor binding
	Camptothecins	Decreased topoisomerase-I
	Anthracyclines, etoposide	Decreased topoisomerase-II

databases (e.g., http://www.medicalletter.com or http://www.micromedex.com or http://www.druginteractioninfo.org/Home.aspx), or the drug manufacturer.

DRUG RESISTANCE AND TUMOR CELL HETEROGENEITY

The curative potential of chemotherapy is limited by the emergence of drug resistance, which can be either intrinsic or acquired, and may involve one drug or multiple agents (pleiotropic resistance). Of interest, tumors with intrinsic or primary drug resistance to natural products often arise from duct cells or cells lining excretory organs (51). These cells, which normally detoxify, transport, and excrete a wide variety of toxic compounds, may retain these normal functions after transformation, manifesting as chemoresistance. With few exceptions, attempts to differentiate prospectively drug-responsive tumors from their resistant counterparts using morphologic, cytogenetic, immunologic, or molecular biologic techniques have not yet been successful. However, within the next few years, high-throughput molecular profiling by gene expression or proteomic array is expected to identify patterns that are predictive of tumor resistance or response to specific chemotherapeutic agents.

The presence of intrinsic drug resistance is inferred based on clonal survival of tumor populations after initial chemotherapy exposure. Solid tumors are thought to consist of a mixture of clonal variants with different mutations and patterns of resistance. Following repetitive cycles of chemotherapy, a process of clonal selection can occur, enriching for resistant populations, even while there could be a reduction in clinical tumor volume associated with elimination of more sensitive tumor elements. From a clinical perspective, the end result of this process is indistinguishable from acquired resistance, which develops from cumulative mutations, or phenotypic alterations, over a period of time. However, acquired resistance is more likely to have a reversible component that could influence the timing and selection of subsequent chemotherapy. The most well-documented specific example is amplification of the dihydrofolate reductase (*DHFR*) gene, which is associated with acquired resistance to methotrexate (52). *DHFR* gene amplification is not generally observed prior to methotrexate exposure and can be reversed in the absence of drug exposure.

From the perspective of gynecologic oncology, there are two major patterns of drug resistance that emerge with continued treatment. The first is broad-based multidrug, or pleiotropic, drug resistance that has been associated with overexpression of *MDR 1* (P 170 glycoprotein) and/or other membrane-associated transport proteins (53,54). This multidrug resistance phenotype has maximal impact on natural products and their analogs, including the anthracyclines, Vinca alkaloids, and taxanes. The second is resistance to alkylating agents, especially platinum compounds, mediated through a completely different set of cellular mechanisms, including reduced cellular uptake due to loss of membrane transport proteins, increased detoxification of reactive intermediates by glutathione production, increased damage tolerance due to defective detection and/or apoptotic signaling, and expanded capacity for DNA repair (55).

Mechanisms of Multidrug Resistance

After exposure to a potential *MDR 1* substrate, tumor cells will develop cross resistance to a variety of structurally and functionally unrelated agents derived from natural products. This pleiotropic resistance is associated with increased drug efflux and a net lowering of intracellular drug concentration. Although relatively uncommon in ovarian cancer (56,57), with increased utilization of natural products, including taxanes, etoposide, and liposomal doxorubicin, this pattern of resistance may become more prevalent. Mutations in the β-tubulin subunit have been associated with paclitaxel resistance in preclinical models, but this does not appear to be a common mechanism in the clinical setting (58), and expression of *MDR 1* has been more frequently observed as a potential marker of resistance (59).

Other chemotherapeutic agents are not substrates for *MDR 1* and remain unaffected by increased expression. For example, several cell lines with multidrug resistance mediated by *MDR 1* demonstrated increased uptake, phosphorylation, and sensitivity to gemcitabine, a nucleoside analog, which could be reversed by verapamil, an inhibitor of *MDR 1* (60). This has potential implications for optimal timing, sequence, and combination of agents in the clinical setting.

Other energy-dependent transporter proteins have been identified in drug-resistant cell lines that do not overexpress *MDR 1*. These include the multidrug resistance–associated protein (MRP), which is representative of a family of cMOAT proteins (61). Similar to *MDR 1*, these proteins include multiple transmembrane domains, but appear to have more broad tissue distribution and greater association with intracellular membrane–bound compartments. Another member of the family with relevance to gynecologic cancer is the breast cancer resistance protein (BCRP) or adenosine triphosphate–binding cassette protein G2 (ABCG2) that dimerizes to form a membrane-associated energy-dependent drug efflux pump responsible for atypical multidrug resistance following exposure to mitoxantrone or camptothecins, including topotecan. Overexpression of BCRP has been documented in ovarian cancer cells resistant to topotecan (62).

Platinum Resistance and DNA Repair

Although a number of DNA alkylating agents and radiation are used in the treatment of gynecologic cancer, platinum derivatives are the most important compounds utilized in clinical practice. The dramatic success of platinum-based therapy is nearly overshadowed by the emergence of platinum resistance, and this observation has stimulated a substantial body of research over the last 30 years.

As a highly polar compound, cisplatin enters cells relatively slowly, and uptake can be influenced by local cation concentrations, pH, and the presence of reducing agents, prompting a search for membrane transporter proteins that could supplement passive diffusion. The major transporter involved in copper homeostasis, copper transporter-1 (CTR1), has now been shown to have a substantial role in cisplatin influx (63). Down-regulation of CTR1 expression can reduce cisplatin uptake, leading to one mechanism of resistance. Targeted methods to safely and selectively increase platinum uptake in tumors are not yet available. However, it has been observed that ovarian cancer cell lines can rapidly down-regulate membrane CTR1 after cisplatin exposure, followed by proteasomal-mediated degradation (64), suggesting that sequence and schedule of drug administration could have an impact on platinum uptake. An orally active analogue of carboplatin, satraplatin or bis-acetato-ammine-dichloro-cyclohexylamine platinum (IV), has shown promising activity in the treatment of prostate cancer (65) and undergoes biotransformation to JM118 or cis-ammine-dichloro-cyclohexylamine-platinum (II), which retains activity in tumor cells that have lost CTR1 (66), suggesting another avenue for clinical development.

Human ovarian cell lines resistant to alkylating agents, cisplatin, and irradiation contain elevated levels of cellular glutathione (GSH). Using resistant cell lines, it has been possible to demonstrate a restoration of drug sensitivity by exposure to the synthetic amino acid buthionine sulfoximine (BSO), which inhibits gamma-glutamylcysteine synthetase, causing GSH depletion (67). The exact mechanism by which GSH and other thiol compounds modulate cytotoxicity is unknown, although they can interfere with the formation of DNA-platinum adducts (68). There is also evidence of increased drug metabolism through GSH-linked transferases, which can vary for specific platinum compounds (69), and which may also contribute to cisplatin-mediated nephrotoxicity (70). Although clinical trials of BSO with melphalan have documented an 80% to greater than 90% reduction in tumor-associated GSH levels (71,72), this approach has not yet been demonstrated to improve the outcomes of platinum-based therapy.

In view of the prominent role of thiols in mediating a subset of platinum resistance, a sterically hindered platinum complex, picoplatin (JM473, ZD0473), was developed with the expectation that it would favor interacting with DNA rather than glutathione or metallothioneins (73). A phase 2 trial in recurrent ovarian cancer documented response rates of 8.4% in platinum-resistant disease and 32.4% in platinum-sensitive disease, similar to expectations with cisplatin or carboplatin (74). Of interest, there was no documented peripheral neuropathy or nephrotoxicity even in this group of patients with prior platinum therapy, implicating thiol reactions in the generation of these nonhematologic toxicities.

Enhanced capacity for DNA repair can play a role in drug resistance to alkylating agents and cisplatin. Human ovarian cancer cell lines resistant to melphalan demonstrate increased ability to repair melphalan damage, and this phenotype can be reversed by aphidicolin, a potent inhibitor of alpha and beta DNA polymerase (75). Increased damage tolerance is another mechanism that contributes to resistance, and is perhaps best illustrated by the mismatch repair system. Errors in DNA replication following platinum adduct formation can be detected by the postreplicative DNA mismatch repair system, which contains several well-characterized genes, including *MLH1* and *MSH2*. Of note, cellular attempts to repair platinum alkylation by this mechanism are not successful as the repair is directed at the nascent daughter DNA strand rather than the platinated parental strand. Eventually, abortive attempts at repair are associated with apoptotic cell death. Thus, loss of mismatch repair can actually promote cell survival by ignoring DNA damage in noncritical areas of the genome and has emerged as another mechanism of drug resistance.

Loss of *MLH1* or other mismatch repair genes is not uncommon in ovarian cancer and appears to increase after exposure to carboplatin or cisplatin (76). In addition, functional loss of *MLH1* activity in patients with ovarian cancer can also occur through hypermethylation-mediated silencing of the *MLH1* gene following exposure to platinum, and has been correlated with poor survival (77). Preclinical models with platinum-resistant cell lines have shown improved treatment outcomes following exposure to 2′-deoxy-5-azacytidine (decitabine), which blocks DNA methylation, unmasking expression of *MLH1* (78), providing a basis for exploratory clinical trials.

Oxaliplatin is one of several diaminocyclohexane (DACH) platinum derivatives that forms platinum adducts that differ in three-dimensional structure from the more established diamine compounds, such as cisplatin and carboplatin (79). As a consequence of these structural differences, oxaliplatin adducts are not detected by the mismatch repair system (80), and there was hope that oxaliplatin would retain clinical activity in patients with platinum-resistant tumors. However, in phase 2 studies, the response rate among ovarian cancer patients with less than a 6-month platinum-free interval was less than 7% (81,82).

Nucleotide excision repair (NER) is the primary mechanism to remove platinum-DNA adducts from genomic DNA. Excision repair cross-complementing 1 (*ERCC1*) is a critical gene on the NER pathway. Platinum resistance has been linked to *ERCC1* mRNA levels in tumors, including ovarian cancer (83). In lung cancer, immunohistochemical evaluation of *ERCC1* levels was also predictive for survival following cisplatin-based adjuvant therapy, with improved survival in patients with *ERCC1*-negative tumors (84). However, *ERCC1* may also have prognostic significance independent of chemotherapy, as lung cancer patients assigned to observation with *ERCC1*-positive tumors had better survival compared with those with *ERCC1*-negative tumors (85). These observations have prompted randomized trials to prospectively assign chemotherapy for lung cancer based on *ERCC1* status, with the suggestion of higher response rates among patients receiving customized therapy, but without a difference in progression-free or overall survival (86). The role of *ERCC1* in selecting treatment for women with ovarian cancer remains to be established, but optimal selection will probably require information from additional cellular pathways.

Other Mechanisms of Agent-Specific Resistance

A number of specific alterations have been identified in the setting of individual drugs (Table 15.6). For example, *DHFR* gene amplification was demonstrated in a patient with methotrexate-resistant ovarian cancer who had localized *DHFR* gene copies on an abnormally staining region of chromosome 4q (87). Methotrexate resistance has also been associated with defects in polyglutamation, limiting intracellular methotrexate accumulation (88).

The action of nucleoside analogs, such as gemcitabine (2,2-difluorodideoxycytidine), is dependent on active membrane transport for uptake, which is followed by double phosphorylation and potential incorporation in DNA. This complex process offers several opportunities for development of resistance, such as decreased activity of specific nucleoside transport proteins or reduced phosphorylation by depletion of deoxycytidine kinase (89). In addition, the main enzymatic target of phosphorylated gemcitabine, the M2 subunit of ribonucleotide reductase, can undergo gene amplification in resistant cell lines (90) similar to the primary mechanism of resistance to hydroxyurea, an inhibitor of ribonucleotide reductase. Of interest, sensitivity to gemcitabine can actually be increased severalfold by prior exposure to flavopiridol, an inhibitor of cyclin-dependent kinase activity, which has been shown to accelerate catabolism of the M2 subunit protein through the proteasome complex (91). Increased levels of target gene expression or protein, including thymidylate synthase, thymidylate phosphorylase, and dihydropyrimidine dehydrogenase, have also been associated with resistance to 5-fluorouracil in colon cancer, and have been correlated with clinical outcomes following 5-fluorouracil treatment (92,93). Even a superficial analysis of these specific examples would suggest potential strategies for screening of tumor tissue to guide the selection of optimal chemotherapy regimens, providing a basis for the application of tissue, gene, and protein arrays.

Tumor Heterogeneity and Assays of Chemotherapy Response

Solid tumors have traditionally been considered to be a homogeneous collection of clonally derived cells with similar features, but it is now clear that tumors are composed of subpopulations with diverse biologic characteristics. Through genetic instability and regulatory processes, such as gene methylation, these subpopulations may exhibit different kinetic properties, angiogenic potential, receptor content, immunogenicity, and susceptibility to chemotherapy. In addition, there can be variability in the potential for metastatic spread among cells that appear to be similar at a morphologic and genetic level (94). Recognition of tumor heterogeneity has altered our understanding of tumor behavior with implications for multiagent and multimodality treatment programs.

Following the development of model systems for screening new anticancer compounds, it is not surprising that attention was focused on the process of screening actual human tumor cells for sensitivity and resistance to chemotherapy agents (95). A variety of methods have been developed utilizing clonogenic survival, ^{3}H-thymidine incorporation, vital dye exclusion, treatment of transplanted tumor xenografts, and colorimetric analysis of adenosine triphosphate levels. Although there is relatively good correlation between high-level resistance to individual agents demonstrated in vitro and lack of a clinical response in vivo, it is more difficult to predict sensitivity to specific agents, or to guide the utilization of drug combinations (96), reflecting tumor cell heterogeneity, assay complexity, and inability to evaluate the tumor-host relationship, including angiogenesis. A nonrandomized phase 2 trial in recurrent epithelial ovarian cancer has suggested good correlation between ex vivo assay sensitivity and clinical response (97). Wider adoption of these approaches will need to address the lack of prospective randomized data, as well as the complexities of obtaining and shipping fresh tumor tissue, delay in receiving assay results, and substantial costs. In addition, with the rapid development of gene expression and proteomic arrays, it is possible that adequate predictions can be obtained from profiling existing frozen tumor specimens, as opposed to assays on fresh tumor biopsies.

Dose Intensity and Density

The dose and frequency of drug administration can contribute to the overall effectiveness of a treatment regimen, as well as the spectrum and severity of host toxicity. Dose intensity is a standardized measure of the amount of drug administered over time, most commonly expressed as mg/m^2 per week.

Preclinical studies demonstrate a sigmoidal relationship between dose and tumor response. This is characterized by a *lag phase* and a lower-limit *threshold* for observing benefit; a *linear phase*, where increases in dose are matched by improved efficacy; and a *plateau*, where toxicity continues to increase but there is no incremental improvement in response. In highly responsive tumors (e.g., choriocarcinoma, dysgerminoma), the entire dose-response curve is shifted to the left, with the result that standard chemotherapy doses are already situated near the upper plateau, and further dose increases are unlikely to achieve any improvement in clinical outcomes. In resistant tumors (e.g., previously treated cervical cancer), the curve is shifted to the right, and is also flattened, reducing the maximal potential benefit. For heterogeneous tumors with sensitive and resistant populations, such as epithelial ovarian cancer, it is unlikely that increased dose intensity would achieve long-term clinical benefit. However, lower than standard doses are potentially suboptimal, and arbitrary dose reductions or delays for nonphysiologic factors should be avoided. True dose-intense regimens have not been demonstrated to improve long-term clinical outcomes in women with gynecologic cancer, with the possible exception of recurrent germ-cell tumors.

The dose intensity hypothesis has been extensively evaluated in the setting of advanced ovarian cancer, beginning with a series of retrospective studies (98) suggesting a correlation between actual delivered dose intensity and clinical outcomes. However, within practical dose ranges that can be achieved in the clinical setting, prospective randomized trials have not demonstrated significant improvements in either disease-free or overall survival (99). While front-line studies focused on platinum dose intensity, the question of paclitaxel dose intensity was also addressed in the setting of recurrent disease, again without evidence of improved outcomes.

Dose intensity is limited by acute (single-cycle) and cumulative (multi-cycle) non-hematologic and hematologic toxicity. Although multiple cycles of high-dose carboplatin and paclitaxel (with or without topotecan or gemcitabine) can be safely administered with hematopoietic progenitor and growth factor support, it is more difficult to overcome serious non-hematologic toxicities. Thus far, there is no evidence that a two- to threefold increase in carboplatin dose intensity and cumulative dose delivery is associated with a substantial improvement in clinical outcomes (100–102), and it is unlikely that this approach will be further evaluated.

In contrast, there is renewed interest in "dose-dense" therapy, in which a series of two or three individual single agents are sequentially administered at maximal tolerated doses using short cycle intervals. This approach has been favorably evaluated in the adjuvant therapy of breast cancer (103), although it has not been clearly established if the clinical benefit is secondary to dose density or weekly scheduling of specific components. Short cycle intervals may offer a safer approach for intensification by reinforcing normal biologic rhythms that can accelerate repair and minimize host toxicity.

GENERAL PRINCIPLES OF CHEMOTHERAPY

Treatment Objectives

Although certain general principles guide the clinician in choosing the appropriate classes of drugs or combinations, the decision to use these agents *at all* must be considered carefully. The critical factors involved in formulating a recommendation are reviewed in Table 15.5.

Natural History

Antineoplastic agents should be used only in patients whose malignancy has been established histologically, with consideration of the expected natural history, based on the primary tumor site, extent of disease, and rate of progression. Individual factors that could have an impact on tolerance for therapy must be evaluated in the context of treatment goals, including physiologic age (as reflected by vital organ function), general health, performance status, desire for treatment, and the presence of underlying illness. Prior history, including any previous cancer treatment and residual functional impairment, as well as patterns of recurrence, should also be considered. Finally, the emotional, social, and financial concerns of the patient and family must be respected (Table 15.7). Recommendations and goals should be presented to the patient and family in conjunction with a reasonable analysis of potential risks and benefits, which contributes to the process of informed consent, and which should be followed by sharing of written information for future reference.

Clinical Assessment

Chemotherapy should not be instituted unless the physician is prepared to monitor tumor response (if applicable) carefully while managing expected and unexpected toxicities. If proper

TABLE 15.7

IMPORTANT CONSIDERATIONS BEFORE USING ANTINEOPLASTIC DRUGS

Natural history of the malignancy
- Biopsy proof of malignancy
- Identification of primary site
- Rate of progression or grade
- Stage of disease, patterns of spread

Patient characteristics
- Physiologic age, nutritional status, performance status
- Vital organ function; bone marrow reserve
- Comorbid conditions
- Extent of previous treatment

Supportive care
- Adequate facilities to evaluate, monitor, and treat potential drug toxicities
- Emotional, social, and financial status; support from family
- Collaboration with referring physician

Treatment goals
- Parameters to monitor objective response to treatment
- Potential benefits
  - Curative intent
  - Improved or sustained quality of life
  - Control of disease
  - Palliation of symptoms

facilities are not readily available, and the decision is made to begin therapy, the patient should be referred to a physician or facility that can provide integrated care.

In view of the potential for serious toxicity, it is desirable to have some objective means of measuring tumor response by physical examination, radiographic imaging, and/or analysis of serum tumor markers. However, it is not uncommon to administer multiple cycles of adjuvant or postoperative chemotherapy without any direct means of documenting tumor response. In these circumstances, the physician should be alert for any clinical evidence of tumor recurrence or progression during treatment. In patients with evaluable disease, continued administration of chemotherapy requires verification of ongoing benefit.

Expectations

The likelihood of achieving long-term benefit influences the choice of treatment and the acceptance of potential toxicity. Primary tumors (and recurrence after surgical resection or radiation without prior chemotherapy) can generally be grouped according to the likelihood of achieving a durable response. However, chemotherapy is also being utilized more frequently in the setting of early-stage disease, including postoperative adjuvant therapy of ovarian cancer, concurrent chemoradiation in cervical cancer, and postoperative treatment (with or without sequential radiation) in endometrial cancer. While the use of chemotherapy in each of these scenarios is supported by data from phase 3 clinical trials, it is also apparent that more patients are being exposed to platinum-based therapy at earlier points in their natural history, with an increased risk of treatment-resistant disease at the time of recurrence.

Most importantly, there is a group of tumors for which primary chemotherapy has been curative in the majority of patients, including choriocarcinoma and ovarian germ cell tumors. These patients should be treated aggressively with curative intent. Toxicity in this setting is acceptable, assuming that it is reversible, as the probability of long-term survival is high.

A second group, including advanced epithelial ovarian carcinoma, has high response rates to primary therapy (exceeding 75%), with prolongation of disease-free and median overall survival, but with only a modest improvement in overall mortality. Patients with these tumors usually benefit from therapy in terms of extended survival or quality-adjusted survival, and they should receive primary treatment at full doses unless contraindicated.

A third group of cancers, including advanced (or recurrent) endometrial cancer, cervical cancer, and uterine mixed müllerian tumors, have intermediate or lower response rates to primary chemotherapy, with shorter duration of remission and limited improvement in overall survival. Treatment with an initial course of therapy is reasonable, with careful monitoring of toxicity and response.

Other tumors, including uterine leiomyosarcoma, are more resistant to primary therapy, achieving a low frequency of objective response without prolongation of survival. In this setting, the use of chemotherapy should be restricted and particular emphasis placed on including these patients in well-structured clinical trials to evaluate innovative treatments.

In patients with recurrent or progressive disease after prior chemotherapy, the expectations of response are reduced due to the emergence of drug resistance and the impact of prior therapy and/or disease on performance status and vital organ function. As such, treatment goals are usually palliative, with attention to quality of life and control of symptoms. In this population, the frequency of stable disease usually exceeds the objective response rate. With appropriate chemotherapy regimens that avoid cumulative toxicity, patients without further disease progression may remain on therapy for prolonged periods of time with an acceptable quality of life. Most patients are best managed with single-agent chemotherapy with regular assessment of ongoing response and management of toxicity. However, patients with epithelial ovarian cancer and a prolonged treatment-free interval generally receive a platinum-based combination.

The decision to embark on antineoplastic drug therapy is obviously complex. Optimal patient care demands careful review of the multiple factors affecting therapy to maximize any opportunity for improving survival and quality of life.

Choice of Specific Chemotherapeutic Regimens

After the decision to use chemotherapy has been made, the appropriate regimen must be selected. The physician is aided in this task by the results of randomized trials and evolving standards of care, including published practice guidelines. However, not every patient can receive "standard" therapy because of idiosyncratic reactions, vital organ dysfunction, prior treatment, or other factors. Practical individualized decisions are facilitated by the logical grouping of chemotherapeutic agents in several classes with similar pharmacologic properties, mechanisms of action, and spectrum of toxicity. The most important classes are the platinum-based alkylating agents, non-platinum alkylating agents, antimetabolites, antitumor antibiotics, antimicrotubule agents, nucleoside analogs, hormones, and newer molecular targeted therapies.

A number of combinations have been evaluated in the management of gynecologic cancer, and some have been widely adopted as "standard of care" for primary management of advanced-stage or recurrent disease. Phase 3 trials have demonstrated the superiority of specific regimens, such as paclitaxel with either cisplatin (104) or carboplatin (105) in ovarian cancer; a triplet combination of paclitaxel, cisplatin, and doxorubicin with granulocyte colony-stimulating factor (G-CSF) in endometrial cancer (106); cisplatin with either paclitaxel (107) or topotecan in cervical cancer (108); and ifosfamide with paclitaxel in uterine mixed müllerian tumors (109).

However, none of the standard combinations for advanced ovarian, endometrial, or cervical cancer has been directly compared to sequential therapy with the best active single agents, and the superiority of combination therapy has not been fully established. In the setting of ovarian cancer, phase 3 trials have suggested that sequential therapy with platinum followed by paclitaxel may offer similar long-term outcomes to a combination of platinum and paclitaxel (110,111). Although the initial frequency of tumor response is often increased with combination therapy, long-term outcomes such as overall survival and symptom-adjusted quality of life can be similar for patients who receive optimal sequential therapy with single agents. This is primarily related to the advanced stage of disease at the time of initial treatment with systemic chemotherapy and the lack of curative therapy for the majority of patients. As such, if individual patient circumstances contraindicate the use of a standard combination regimen, it remains a reasonable option to begin therapy with one of the active single agents. In addition to their application as primary therapy for advanced disease, combinations can also be employed as adjuvant therapy for patients with early-stage disease at increased risk for recurrence and for patients with late recurrence after good response to initial therapy.

Adjuvant chemotherapy refers to the initial use of systemic chemotherapy after surgery and/or radiation therapy has been performed with curative intent and there is no evidence of residual disease. Adjuvant chemotherapy is considered if the subsequent risk for recurrence after initial definitive therapy is relatively high (generally greater than 20%), but it is not routinely recommended when the risk of recurrence is less than 10%. In the adjuvant therapy of epithelial ovarian cancer, long-term results from randomized trials have documented a reduction in the risk of recurrence after platinum-based chemotherapy (112,113). However, in carefully staged patients (to exclude occult advanced-stage disease), it has been difficult to establish an advantage in overall survival. Phase 3 studies in endometrial cancer (114) and uterine mixed müllerian tumors (115) have documented improved survival with the use of adjuvant combination chemotherapy compared to whole abdomen radiation in selected patients with high-risk disease, increasing the overall proportion of patients who receive adjuvant therapy.

Concurrent chemotherapy with radiation (chemoradiation) refers to the use of chemotherapy to sensitize tumor to the effects of radiation delivered with curative intent. This has been most extensively studied in the primary management of locally advanced cervical cancer, where platinum-based chemoradiation has been proven to be superior to radiation alone (116). In general, the duration of chemotherapy coincides with the duration of external beam radiation. Although the preferred weekly dose of cisplatin might appear to be low, these regimens generally exceed the overall dose intensity of cisplatin when used to treat advanced disease, and patients require monitoring to avoid cumulative toxicity and treatment interruptions.

Neoadjuvant chemotherapy generally refers to the use of chemotherapy in the management of locally advanced disease in situations where it would be difficult or impractical to perform immediate surgery or radiation. Following a response to initial chemotherapy, there is an expectation that morbidity associated with the overall treatment program can be minimized in conjunction with a reduction in radiation treatment volume or extent of surgery. This approach is most often considered in advanced cervical cancer, where high initial response rates to neoadjuvant therapy have been observed. However, the long-term benefit of this approach has not been established. Neoadjuvant therapy is also a consideration in advanced ovarian cancer, particularly in patients with large-volume ascites, pleural effusions, diffuse small-volume disease, or comorbidities that might increase surgical risk. In this setting, it has been difficult to conduct randomized neoadjuvant trials owing to impaired performance status, the desire to establish a definitive tissue diagnosis, and the bias toward initial cytoreductive surgery.

Monitoring of Tumor Response

Generally accepted criteria for evaluation of response are necessary to facilitate treatment decisions and comparisons among different regimens. Several standards have been used, including those developed by the World Health Organization (WHO). However, in 2000, an international working group including the European Organization for Research and Treatment of Cancer (EORTC), the National Cancer Institute of Canada (NCIC), and the National Cancer Institute (NCI) of the United States developed, validated, and published new Response Evaluation Criteria in Solid Tumors (RECIST), which have subsequently been widely adopted within clinical trials (117). RECIST is based on the prospective designation of at least one "target lesion" that measures at least 2 cm in one dimension, as well as "nontarget lesions" that are used to corroborate response. Radiographic imaging by helical computed tomography (CT) or magnetic resonance imaging (MRI) are the preferred techniques to monitor tumor response, and the same technique that is used for initial assessment should be used for subsequent measurements. The use of physical examination is restricted to cutaneous lesions or superficial adenopathy that can be directly measured. The omission of findings on bimanual pelvic examination posed a particular challenge for monitoring regional disease in patients with gynecologic tumors, and the criteria were subsequently modified by the Gynecologic Oncology Group (GOG) to include pelvic lesions measurable by physical examination, as summarized in Table 15.8.

TABLE 15.8

OVERALL DISEASE RESPONSE CATEGORIES (RECIST)

Category	Definition
Complete response (CR)[a]	Disappearance of all *target*[b] and *non-target* lesions, and normalization of tumor marker levels (if appropriate).
Partial response (PR)	Disappearance of all *target* lesions without progression of *non-target* lesions, without appearance of new lesions, and persistence of abnormal tumor marker levels. *Or* At least a 30% decrease in the sum LD of *target* lesions (taking as reference the baseline sum LD) without progression of *non-target* lesions or appearance of new lesions. *Note:* In the case where the only *target* lesion is a solitary pelvic mass measured by physical exam (not radiographically measurable), a 50% decrease in the LD is required.
Progressive disease (PD)	At least a 20% increase in the sum LD of *target* lesions, taking as reference the smallest sum LD recorded since the start of treatment, or the appearance of one or more new lesions, or progression of any *non-target* lesion. *Note:* In the case where the only *target* lesion is a solitary pelvic mass measured by physical exam (not radiographically measurable), a 50% increase in the LD is required.
Stable disease (SD)[c]	Neither sufficient shrinkage of *target* lesions to qualify for PR nor sufficient increase to qualify for PD, taking as reference the smallest sum LD since the start of treatment. No appearance of new lesions (*target* or *non-target*).

Note: Measurable lesions—lesions that can be accurately measured in at least one dimension with longest diameter (LD) ≥20 mm using conventional techniques or ≥10 mm with spiral CT scan. *Non-measurable lesions*—all other lesions, including small lesions (longest diameter <20 mm with conventional techniques or <10 mm with spiral CT scan), i.e., bone lesions, leptomeningeal disease, ascites, pleural/pericardial effusion, inflammatory breast disease, lymphangitis cutis/pulmonis, cystic lesions, and also abdominal masses that are not confirmed and followed by imaging techniques.

[a]To be assigned PR or CR, changes in tumor measurements must be confirmed by repeat assessments no less than 4 weeks after the criteria for response are first met. The duration of overall response is measured from the time that criteria are met for CR or PR (whichever status is recorded first) until the first date that recurrence or PD is objectively documented, taking as reference for PD the smallest measurements recorded since the treatment started.

[b]All measurable lesions up to a maximum of five lesions per organ and 10 lesions in total, representative of all involved organs, should be identified as *target* lesions and recorded and measured at baseline. *Target* lesions should be selected on the basis of their size (lesions with the longest diameter) and their suitability for accurate repeated measurements (either by imaging techniques or clinically). All other lesions (or sites of disease) should be identified as *non-target* lesions and should also be recorded at baseline. Measurements of these lesions are not required, but the presence or absence of each should be noted throughout follow-up.

[c]In the case of SD, follow-up measurements must have met the SD criteria at least once after study entry at a minimum interval (in general, not less than 6 to 8 weeks) that is defined in the study protocol. SD is measured from the start of the treatment until the criteria for disease progression are met, taking as reference the smallest measurements recorded since the treatment started.

The summary response designation within RECIST integrates the findings from target and nontarget lesions, as well as serum tumor markers (if applicable). Serum tumor markers are not sufficient to declare response, but if initially elevated, must normalize to designate a complete response. International criteria to declare disease progression on the basis of a serial elevation in CA125 have been widely adopted (118,119), but there is incomplete agreement on criteria to define a partial response during treatment (120). Overall, RECIST is more detailed and specific than previous response criteria, and is also more demanding of the clinical team and radiologist, particularly if there are a large number of target and nontarget lesions.

A *complete response* refers to the complete disappearance of all objective evidence of tumor and a resolution of all signs and symptoms referable to the tumor. Complete regressions of cancer are generally those associated with a prolongation of survival. A *partial response* refers to at least a 30% decrease in the sum of the longest diameter of all measurable lesions. Usually, this would be accompanied by some degree of subjective improvement and the absence of any new lesions during treatment. Partial remissions are generally accompanied by improved well-being for a period of time, but are not expected to improve overall survival. A variety of terms have been used to designate lesser responses (e.g., minor response, objective regression), but these are rarely associated with any significant clinical benefit. *Progressive disease* is defined as a 20% or greater increase in the sum of the longest diameter of all measurable lesions or the appearance of new lesions. *Stable disease* is the term applied to patients without measurable tumor response or progression fitting one of the prior criteria. Disease stabilization is an acceptable goal in the setting of palliative therapy for recurrent disease provided that symptoms have not progressed and the patient can tolerate continued therapy.

Changes in the volume of ascites or pleural fluid are not usually considered in the measurement of response, as a number of factors unrelated to cancer can influence third-space fluid accumulation, such as nutritional status, renal function, and treatment-related toxicity. However, appearance of a new fluid collection with cytologic verification would represent progressive disease. Similarly, the appearance of new symptoms, such as a partial small bowel obstruction, does not always indicate progression of disease, but could be related to prior surgery, irradiation, chemotherapy, or infection. In general, it is preferable to base decisions regarding treatment on objective measures of response as described rather than subjective findings or symptoms.

MANAGEMENT OF CHEMOTOXICITIES

Toxicity Assessment, Dose Modification, and Supportive Care

Chemotherapeutic regimens are universally toxic, with a narrow margin of safety, and it is often necessary to adjust doses individually in accordance with patient tolerance. Initial

TABLE 15.9

CTCAE GRADING OF MYELOSUPPRESSION

	Grade			
Element	1	2	3	4
Leukocytes (per mm^3)	LLN to 3,000	<3,000 to 2,000	<2,000 to 1,000	<1,000
Granulocytes (per mm^3)	LLN to 1,500	<1,500 to 1,000	<1,000 to 500	<500
Hemoglobin (g/dL)	LLN to 10.0	<10.0 to 8.0	<8.0 to 6.5	<6.5
Platelets (per mm^3)	LLN to 75,000	<75,000 to 50,000	<50,000 to 25,000	<25,000

Note: LLN, lower limit normal (institutional).
Source: CTCAE, Common Terminology Criteria for Adverse Events, version 3.0, Cancer Therapy Evaluation Program, National Cancer Institute. http://ctep.info.nih.gov/reporting/ctc.html. Published June 10, 2003.

chemotherapy dosing is based on body surface area, weight, renal function, and hepatic function, using guidelines from clinical trials. However, there are a number of other factors that could further influence host tolerance, including nutritional status, performance status, extent of disease, prior therapy, third-space fluid accumulations, metabolic polymorphisms, and uncharacterized drug interactions. Current dose algorithms generally fail to address these factors, although emerging pharmacodynamic and pharmacogenomic research has improved individualized dosing in selected cases. As such, it is necessary to monitor host toxicity with ongoing modifications to avoid serious acute and cumulative toxicity.

The Cancer Therapy Evaluation Program (CTEP) of the NCI has developed a detailed and comprehensive set of guidelines for the description and grading of acute and chronic organ-specific toxicity in collaboration with the FDA, international cooperative groups, and the pharmaceutical industry. Most clinical research protocols have incorporated these criteria, which are also applicable to the grading of toxicity for standard chemotherapy regimens outside of a clinical trial. The current version of the Common Terminology Criteria for Adverse Events (CTCAE) is available in electronic format from CTEP (http://ctep.info.nih.gov). Basic hematologic parameters have been summarized in Table 15.9.

An unintended consequence of our current regulatory environment is that most new medications receive single-agent FDA approval at a dose and schedule that is close to the maximally tolerated dose (MTD), essentially maximizing the risk of host toxicity. The association between dose and toxicity is usually dramatic at levels close to the MTD. As such, a modest reduction in dose, or an adjustment in schedule, can have a substantial impact on acute and cumulative toxicities. The impact of these minor modifications on efficacy is generally unknown, but unlikely to be as dramatic as the impact on toxicity, and many clinicians frequently make modifications in the starting dose and/or schedule of single agents or combinations, essentially deviating from FDA-approved indications. As these modifications become integrated with clinical practice, limited supporting data emerge, usually from nonrandomized trials, but the primary FDA-approved dose and schedule is rarely changed. Many agents in common use today, including polyethylene glycol (PEG)-liposomal doxorubicin, topotecan, paclitaxel, docetaxel, and gemcitabine, are frequently modified in accord with emerging clinical experience, but without changes in the FDA-approved regimen. It is thus important for the clinician to be aware of emerging data, as well as data from pivotal trials that were used to support original FDA registration.

In view of the narrow safety margin for chemotherapy, it is important that all orders be reviewed by a nurse and pharmacist with oncology experience. Height, weight, calculation of body surface area, pertinent laboratory values, and methods of dose calculation should be clearly indicated and verifiable. Pretemplated orders encourage systematic review and can reduce the risk of error. In addition, it is preferable to have predefined dose levels to account for expected treatment modifications rather than relying on percentage-based modifications. For example, it is not always obvious if a percentage refers to the degree of dose reduction or the amount of drug to be administered, which becomes compounded over multiple cycles, with the potential for more than one modification. One convenient method of structured dose modification is illustrated in Table 15.10. With this approach, modifications for the subsequent course of therapy are implemented according to the degree (grade), duration, and timing of toxicity experienced during the preceding course. Although treatment can be delayed on a week-by-week basis to allow for recovery, delays of greater than 2 weeks should be avoided through dose modification and utilization of hematopoietic growth factors. With expanded utilization of combination regimens, it is also helpful to know the patterns of toxicity associated with individual drugs, as it might be appropriate to modify one component rather than an entire regimen.

Bone Marrow Toxicity

Bone marrow toxicity is the most common dose-limiting side effect associated with cytotoxic drugs, and neutropenia is the most common manifestation of bone marrow toxicity, occurring 7 to 14 days after initial drug treatment and persisting for 3 to 10 days. CTCAE grading criteria are summarized in Table 15.9. For purposes of dose modification, the absolute neutrophil count (ANC) is preferred over total white blood count, as this more accurately reflects dose tolerance and risk of infection, which parallels the duration of grade 4 neutropenia (ANC $\leq$500/mm^3). Dose-limiting thrombocytopenia is less common than neutropenia, but has become more frequent with wider utilization of carboplatin and carboplatin-based combinations. A systematic approach to management of hematologic toxicity can help to reduce the risk of error and facilitate overall compliance with a treatment regimen (Table 15.10).

Radiation, alkylating agents (e.g., melphalan, carboplatin), and other DNA-damaging agents (e.g., nitrosoureas, mitomycin C), can have cumulative long-term effects on the bone marrow. Most other agents, including the taxanes and topotecan, show no evidence of cumulative toxicity and can be administered for multiple cycles without dose modification.

TABLE 15.10

REPRESENTATIVE DRUG DOSE MODIFICATIONS

Category (timing)	Parameters	CTCAE grade	Dose or schedule modifications
Granulocytes (day of therapy)	>1,500/mm^3	0, 1	Full doses of all drugs.
	<1,500/mm^3	2, 3, 4	Delay until recovered. If already delayed, reduce dose by one level or add G-CSF.
Platelets (day of therapy)	WNL	0	Full doses of all drugs.
	< LLN to 75,000/mm^3	1	Delay until recovered.
	<75,000/mm^3	2	Delay until recovered. If already delayed, reduce dose by one level.
Granulocytes (cycle nadir)	>1,000/mm^3	0, 1, 2	Full doses of all drugs.
	<500/mm^3 for ≥ 7 days	4	Reduce dose by one level. If already reduced, add G-CSF.
	<1,000/mm^3 with fever	3, 4	Reduce dose by one level. If already reduced, add G-CSF.
Platelets (cycle nadir)	≥50,000/mm^3	3	Full doses of all drugs.
	<50,000/mm^3 with bleed	3, 4	Reduce doses by one level.
	<25,000/mm^3	4	Reduce doses by one level.

Note: CTC, common toxicity criteria; G-CSF, granulocyte colony-stimulating factor; LLN, lower limit normal; WNL, within normal limits.

In view of the frequent occurrence of neutropenia and the risk of infectious complications, utilization of G-CSF, including filgrastim or the longer-acting PEG-filgrastim, has increased. Although these agents promote more rapid granulocyte recovery, thus avoiding potential complications and facilitating the maintenance of dose intensity, their use has not been shown to improve long-term survival for patients with gynecologic cancer compared to conservative management with dose reduction and cycle delay. In addition, G-CSF is not effective in the management of thrombocytopenia and may actually increase the degree of thrombocytopenia by diversion of immature marrow elements, a particular problem after multiple cycles of carboplatin. Recombinant megakaryocyte growth factor is an option to maintain platelet counts (121). However, current treatment programs are not associated with a high frequency of complicated grade 4 thrombocytopenia, and the value of aggressive support would appear to be limited.

Moderate degrees of anemia are quite common in cancer patients receiving chemotherapy, which may contribute to chronic fatigue. With increased recognition of blood-borne viral pathogens and limited supplies of banked blood, frequent transfusions are not practical or recommended, and many patients will adapt to chronic anemia with minimal symptoms. The availability of recombinant erythropoiesis-stimulating agents (ESA), including erythropoietin (epoietin alfa) and darbepoeitin, has provided a generally safe and effective alternative for the management of anemia associated with chemotherapy (122) and should be considered on a case-by-case basis, although financial costs at the recommended dose and schedule can be greater than the intermittent use of blood products (123). Emerging data with regard to the potential risks associated with ESA, including cardiovascular events, thrombosis, and reduced tumor-related survival in placebo-controlled, randomized trials (124), have prompted the FDA to reevaluate the role for ESAs in routine practice (125–127), including a Medicare decision memo (128) limiting reimbursement to patients with confirmed hemoglobin of less than 10 g/dL. Patients with anemia should undergo evaluation of iron stores, with appropriate use of iron replacement, prior to initiation of ESA. Based on available data, the initiation of ESA should be restricted to patients with hemoglobin of less than 10 g/dL, and should be avoided in patients with a hemoglobin of greater than 12 g/dL to avoid thrombotic complications.

Gastrointestinal Toxicity

Most anticancer agents are associated with some degree of nausea, vomiting, and anorexia. There are three major categories of nausea and vomiting: *anticipatory*, occurring prior to actual administration of chemotherapy; *acute onset*, beginning within 1 hour of chemotherapy administration and persisting for less than 24 hours; and *delayed*, beginning more than 1 day after chemotherapy administration and persisting for several days. Prophylactic management of these adverse effects improves patient acceptance and facilitates completion of therapy with full doses on schedule.

The antiemetic regimen is tailored to the emetogenic potential of the treatment, which reflects the incorporation of specific drugs, as well as the dose and schedule of drug administration. Mild nausea and vomiting can often be managed effectively with H_1 antihistamines (diphenhydramine), phenothiazines (prochlorperazine or thiethylperazine), butyrophenones (haloperidol), steroids (dexamethasone or methylprednisolone), benzamides (metoclopramide), or benzodiazepines (lorazepam). These are likely to be sufficient with drugs such as bleomycin, docetaxel, paclitaxel, Vinca alkaloids, 5-fluorouracil, methotrexate, mitomycin C, gemcitabine, PEG-liposomal doxorubicin, and topotecan.

For drugs with more severe emetogenic potential, including cisplatin, carboplatin, cyclophosphamide, or dactinomycin, a more aggressive prophylactic regimen is required. In general, these patients should receive a 5-hydroxytryptamine (5-HT3) receptor antagonist, such as ondansetron or granisetron, prior to chemotherapy and repeated at 8- to 12-hour intervals. Both compounds are also available in an oral formulation, which has been helpful in the management of delayed and/or chronic nausea after chemotherapy, or nausea associated with multi-day oral chemotherapy regimens. Longer acting 5-HT3 antagonists have also become available, including palonosetron and dolasetron, which require only a single intravenous or oral dose prior to chemotherapy. As a group, the 5-HT3 antagonists have been quite effective in controlling severe emesis with few side effects, but are more expensive than prochlorperazine (129). Chronic nausea and vomiting can be a particular problem after several cycles of cisplatin, and occasionally carboplatin (130). The mechanism is poorly understood, and symptoms can be difficult to control with currently available medications, prompting the use of extended steroid administration, cannabinoids, or repeated dosing with 5-HT3 receptor antagonists.

Anticipatory nausea and vomiting can become a significant problem during repeated cycles of chemotherapy, as patients associate environmental cues (such as odor, carpeting, or paint colors) with nausea. In addition to behavioral modification, it can sometimes be modulated by pretreatment with antiemetics and amnesic drugs, such as benzodiazepines, administered orally at home prior to arriving at the treatment center. Lorazepam (0.05 mg/kg) can also be given by slow intravenous push 1 hour before therapy, with doses being continued as needed every 4 hours for up to six doses (131). Unfortunately, this particular schedule produces significant sedation and can be used only in hospitalized patients or outpatients with independent transportation.

Diarrhea, oral stomatitis, esophagitis, and gastroenteritis are also potential problems. Patients with significant oral or esophagogastric symptoms may have symptoms managed with oral viscous lidocaine (2%), other topical anesthetics, or parenteral narcotics in severe cases. Randomized, controlled trials following 5-fluorouracil-based chemotherapy or radiation have failed to document any clinical improvement with sucralfate, which can bind to ulcerated mucosa (132,133). However, randomized, controlled trials have demonstrated that multiple intravenous doses of recombinant keratinocyte growth factor (palifermin) before and after treatment can reduce the incidence and severity of chemotherapy-induced oral stomatitis associated with bolus 5-fluorouracil (134) or high-dose chemotherapy. In general, dose-limiting mucosal injury is uncommon with platinum-based combinations, taxanes, and other single agents used in the treatment of gynecologic cancer. While many patients might develop some degree of diarrhea in the setting of concurrent chemoradiation, palifermin has not been specifically evaluated in that setting, although there are preclinical data to suggest benefit (135). In refractory cases, patients should be screened for secondary infectious complications, such as candidiasis and herpes simplex. Following treatment with irinotecan, noninfectious secretory diarrhea is a well-recognized dose-limiting toxicity associated with local exposure to the active metabolite SN-38, and is generally managed with prophylactic antimotility agents and intravenous hydration, with utilization of octreotide in severe cases. Diarrhea can also result from diffuse mucosal injury following administration of doxorubicin (including PEG-liposomal doxorubicin), 5-fluorouracil, methotrexate, and other agents. In the setting of recent surgery and chemotherapy, patients are also at increased risk for infectious diarrhea, and screening for *Clostridium difficile* is appropriate.

Alopecia

Scalp alopecia is one of the most emotionally taxing side effects of chemotherapy. Aside from long-lasting alopecia that follows cranial irradiation, it is almost always reversible, but it can be a major deterrent to successful chemotherapy. Total scalp alopecia is particularly common with drugs like doxorubicin and paclitaxel, and there is generally some degree of partial alopecia with cisplatin, carboplatin, cyclophosphamide, docetaxel, Vinca alkaloids, and 5-fluorouracil. In a minority of cases, patients treated with paclitaxel will also experience loss of eyelashes, eyebrows, and other body hair, which can be particularly distressing. A variety of physical techniques have been devised to minimize alopecia, including scalp tourniquets and ice caps designed to decrease scalp blood flow. Although partially effective, they are rarely successful with extended chemotherapy.

Skin Toxicity

Skin toxicities that occur during chemotherapy include allergic or hypersensitivity reactions, skin hyperpigmentation, photosensitivity, radiation recall reactions, nail abnormalities, folliculitis, palmar-plantar erythrodysesthesia (PPE, hand-foot syndrome), and local extravasation necrosis. Many of these are drug specific and self limited, but occasionally they may be dose limiting.

PPE is a reversible but painful erythema, scaling, swelling, or ulceration involving the hands and feet. This occurs more often with chronic oral or intravenous medications, weekly treatment regimens, and formulations that increase drug circulation time, such as prolonged oral etoposide, weekly and continuous-infusion 5-fluorouracil, capecitabine, and PEG-liposomal doxorubicin, where it has emerged as a major dose-limiting toxicity (136).

Extravasation necrosis is a serious complication seen after tissue infiltration of vesicant drugs such as doxorubicin, dactinomycin, mitomycin C, and vincristine (137,138). These drugs should always be administered through a freely flowing intravenous line with careful monitoring. Caution is also required during utilization of central venous ports, as malfunctions in the needle, hub, or tubing can be associated with gradual extravasation that will not be apparent for several hours (139). Any suspected infiltration should prompt immediate removal of the intravenous line and application of ice packs to the infiltrated area every 6 hours for 3 days. Small series have reported a limited experience with local infiltration or topical application of steroids, *n*-acetylcysteine, dimethyl sulfoxide (DMSO), and hyaluronidase with variable results, and recommendations are imprecise. However, single or multiple intravenous doses of dexrazoxane, a topoisomerase II catalytic inhibitor, appears to offer specific protection against injury from anthracyclines, including doxorubicin and daunorubicin (140,141). Skin necrosis from some extravasations may eventually require surgical debridement and skin grafting.

Neurotoxicity

Peripheral neuropathy is the most common neurotoxicity encountered in gynecologic oncology, and is a particular risk with administration of cisplatin, paclitaxel, docetaxel, nanoparticle albumin-bound (NAB) paclitaxel, epothilones, Vinca alkaloids, and hexamethylmelamine (142,143). Although less common with carboplatin than cisplatin, neuropathy can still occur, particularly in combination with paclitaxel. Peripheral neuropathy generally begins with symptoms of paresthesia accompanied by loss of vibratory and position sense in longer nerves associated with the feet and hands. It then progresses to functional impairment, with gait unsteadiness and loss of fine motor coordination, such as trouble buttoning clothes and writing. This is closely followed by loss of deep tendon reflexes and eventual development of motor weakness. With paclitaxel and other nonplatinum agents, this is almost always reversible, but may require several months posttherapy for substantial improvement. In more severe cases, accompanied by neuronal injury or demyelination, recovery may require active neuronal regeneration over an extended period of time, and symptoms may persist for the lifetime of the patient.

In current clinical practice, neurotoxicity from widely utilized microtubule-stabilizing agents is predominant (144,145). The frequency of moderate to severe toxicity is more common with paclitaxel, compared to docetaxel or epothilones. Risk appears related to peak levels associated with individual doses, as well as cumulative doses over multiple cycles, which is further complicated by alternative schedules and newer drug formulations. For example, although the risk associated with NAB-paclitaxel on the FDA-approved 3-week schedule is at least as high as paclitaxel (146), the risk is reduced with NAB-paclitaxel administered on a weekly schedule, even with higher cumulative doses. In addition, as the primary means of assessment is clinical, reported frequencies vary widely in clinical trials, reflecting variability in documenting history, subjective and objective findings.

If related to cisplatin, neuropathy can continue to progress after therapy has been discontinued owing to ongoing axonal demyelination and loss, with long-term persistence of symptoms. Cisplatin has also been associated with permanent ototoxicity, and at higher doses, with loss of color vision (147) and autonomic neuropathy. Oxaliplatin can produce a long-term peripheral neuropathy similar to cisplatin (148), but is also associated with transient acute reactions, including paresthesia and cold-sensitive laryngeal dysesthesia (149), which may reflect blockade of membrane ion channels (150). Of interest is that, although infusions of calcium and magnesium have been used to ameliorate the acute oxaliplatin reactions (151), an ongoing phase 3 randomized trial was terminated due to concerns about a reduction in clinical response rates at interim analysis, illustrating the potential interplay of toxicity and efficacy for some agents (152).

Although some patients report transient distal paresthesia after a single dose of paclitaxel (153), the onset of persistent neuropathy is generally more gradual. Neuropathy can become clinically apparent after two to three courses of therapy, with mild symptoms that resolve between cycles. Careful questioning and examination may reveal subtle findings at an earlier stage, and functional assessments have been developed that demonstrate good concordance with actual neuropathy (154). Patients with underlying neurologic problems, such as diabetes, alcoholism, or carpal tunnel syndrome, are particularly susceptible, and substitution of docetaxel for paclitaxel can be a useful strategy in some situations. All patients who receive potentially neurotoxic therapy, especially cisplatin and paclitaxel, should be routinely queried regarding proprioception and fine motor tasks and examined for loss of vibratory sense, high-frequency hearing, and deep tendon reflexes.

In view of the frequency of neurotoxicity and the impact on daily life, there has been interest in agents that might prevent nerve damage, encourage recovery, or ameliorate symptoms. Amifostine has been reported to reduce the frequency and severity of platinum-mediated neuropathy (155) and is being evaluated as a treatment to promote resolution of established neuropathy. However, a nonrandomized study in patients receiving cisplatin and paclitaxel in combination with amifostine failed to achieve a targeted reduction in the incidence of neuropathy (156). Widespread substitution of carboplatin for cisplatin has reduced but not eliminated the risk, and the value of amifostine in combination with carboplatin and paclitaxel, or paclitaxel as a single agent, has not been established. Thus far, small studies with glutamine, vitamin E, and other agents have been inconclusive, and there are no agents that can be recommended for prevention of neuropathy in routine practice. Clinical management of painful paresthesia has been reported with amitriptyline and gabapentin (157), prompting the empiric use of similar agents for relief of symptoms.

Other neurotoxicities include acute and chronic encephalopathies, usually associated with intrathecal chemotherapy, acute cerebellar syndromes, autonomic dysfunction, inappropriate secretion of antidiuretic hormone (SIADH), and cranial nerve paresis. Of particular relevance to the gynecologic cancer population, an acute reversible metabolic encephalopathy has been well described in association with ifosfamide and attributed to the toxic metabolite chloroacetaldehyde. Of note, this syndrome can potentially be prevented by infusion of methylene blue (158), which may act through inhibition of monoamine oxidase activity with reduced chloroacetaldehyde formation in the liver.

Genitourinary Toxicity

Renal toxicity is a well-recognized side effect of cisplatin (159), with implication of specific local metabolites, even though only a small fraction of cisplatin is cleared by renal excretion. In contrast, carboplatin undergoes extensive renal clearance with little risk of toxicity. Indeed, with increased substitution of carboplatin for cisplatin, and with a reduction in overall cisplatin dose intensity, there has been a decline in clinical familiarity with cisplatin-mediated nephrotoxicity. However, the expanded utilization of concurrent cisplatin and pelvic radiation for management of early-stage cervical cancer has renewed awareness of this potential problem, particularly as commonly utilized weekly dosing can exceed 100 mg/m^2 over a 3-week period. Careful attention to hydration status and saline-driven urinary output before, during, and immediately after therapy is required to reduce the risk associated with this serious complication (160).

Another troublesome side effect is hemorrhagic cystitis, which can be seen with cyclophosphamide or ifosfamide, attributed to the metabolite acrolein. With moderate-dose cyclophosphamide, this complication can be prevented by maintaining high urinary output, which reduces overall urothelial exposure to the toxic metabolites. However, patients receiving combination regimens often have reduced oral intake postchemotherapy, and selected patients receiving cyclophosphamide might benefit from supplemental intravenous hydration. The risk of cystitis is essentially 100% with ifosfamide, even with aggressive hydration, but this can be prevented with simultaneous administration of mesna, which binds and neutralizes acrolein in the urine (161).

Hypersensitivity Reactions

Increased utilization of paclitaxel, a natural product with poor solubility, has focused attention on the risk of hypersensitivity reactions (HSR). For intravenous administration, paclitaxel is formulated in Cremophor-EL, a mixture of polyoxyethylated castor oil and dehydrated alcohol, which has been associated with mast cell degranulation and clinical HSR. Over 80% of reactions occur within minutes during either the first or second cycle of drug administration and can usually be managed with prophylactic medication (corticosteroids, histamine H_1/H_2 blockade) followed by rechallenge beginning at a lower rate of infusion (162,163). Similar reactions have been reported with docetaxel and PEG-liposomal doxorubicin, but with lower frequency in the absence of Cremophor-EL. Ermerging data with NAB-paclitaxel indicate a marked reduction in the risk of HSR, further emphasizing the role of formulation, vehicle, and carriers.

With improved survival and an increased utilization of second-line therapy, patients can also experience more traditional allergic reactions to selected chemotherapy agents. Carboplatin, an organoplatinum compound, has emerged as a major source of late allergic reactions. These occur most often during the second cycle of a second course of therapy, suggesting a process of antigen recall and priming of the immune response (164). Patients receiving a second course of carboplatin-based therapy should be closely monitored for early signs of hypersensitivity to avoid more serious reactions. Unlike the situation with paclitaxel, carboplatin reactions are not readily prevented or circumvented with prophylactic medication, although inpatient (165) and outpatient strategies for desensitization have been reported (166) and successfully utilized for patients who are responding to retreatment. However, the desensitization routine must generally be repeated with each cycle of treatment.

Other Significant Toxicities

A comprehensive discussion of all potential toxicities for currently available chemotherapeutic agents is beyond the scope of this chapter, and additional information is available throughout the text. Nevertheless, a variety of other important toxicities are occasionally encountered in regimens commonly used in gynecologic oncology. These include cardiac toxicity from cumulative doxorubicin exposure, radiation recall vasculitis from doxorubicin, pulmonary fibrosis from bleomycin, gonadal dysfunction in premenopausal women from alkylating agents, and secondary acute leukemia from the chronic administration of alkylating agents, particularly melphalan in ovarian cancer.

DEVELOPMENTAL CHEMOTHERAPY

Background

The identification, evaluation, and regulatory approval of effective drugs for cancer treatment is a long, complicated, and expensive process. Of note, it has been argued that the expanded availability of only 17 existing generic chemotherapeutic agents would substantially improve worldwide mortality from cancer (167). However, most cases of advanced disease remain incurable with current treatments, and the search for new agents remains a high priority. Promising candidates are identified and prioritized through preclinical screening (168), utilizing derivatives of previously defined active agents or established drug classes or new compounds engineered to interact with a specific target. In addition, there continues to be broad screening of natural products isolated from terrestrial and marine sources (169). Some evidence of antitumor activity during screening must be demonstrated before clinical trials are undertaken. Thus far, all useful antitumor agents have demonstrated antitumor activity using *in vitro* or *in vivo* screening systems.

These traditional approaches are being increasingly challenged by the large number of new genes and potential targets identified through molecular biology, genomics, and proteomics. Principles of genomic libraries, solid-phase organic synthesis (170), and combinatorial chemical library generation (171) have been adopted by the pharmaceutical industry to promote high-throughput screening (172). As new targets are identified, a large number of related compounds can be created, beginning with lead natural products or known reagents (173), and then screened for improved target binding and/or inhibition of target function (174). Substantial bioinformatics resources are required to manage and analyze the large amount of data generated from these processes, but the accumulation of gene expression and proteomic data can facilitate "pre-discovery" modeling of potential targets and reagents prior to making decisions about actual development. To some extent, these processes have evolved in parallel, as it is clear that agents generated from a library or a database will still require some form of biologic validation prior to entering complex and expensive clinical studies.

After antitumor activity has been identified, the new agent must be formulated for human use and produced in sufficient quantities to support clinical trials. This is never a trivial achievement, as was evident from the natural supply limitations and formulation problems encountered in early trials with paclitaxel (175) and the camptothecins (176). Clinical-grade material is then subjected to detailed preclinical toxicology tests in animals. These toxicology trials are done in several animal species and may explore different schedules of drug administration to provide a basis for clinical development. As such, they are time consuming, complex, and expensive.

After all of the steps of preclinical testing are completed, new agents can enter clinical evaluation. As such, clinical trials are the primary means utilized to evaluate new agents in a systematic manner. All physicians and patients are urged to consider participation in clinical trials, which are available for almost all diagnoses and treatment circumstances. Sponsors of clinical trials include the NCI in collaboration with individual institutions and national groups, such as the GOG, as well as the pharmaceutical industry and individual institutions.

Clinical Trials

Detailed rationale and methodology for clinical trials design has been covered in other sections. This material is provided to highlight key concepts related to investigational drug development.

Phase 1 Trials

Phase 1 trials are typically first-in-human studies for new compounds and employ a dose- and/or schedule-escalating design to determine the dose-limiting toxicity (DLT), maximally tolerated dose (MTD), and pharmacokinetic parameters applicable to each regimen. In the most common model, accrual is suspended when more than one DLT event occurs within a dose level (two of six patients), as this would generally exceed predefined limits for the MTD. Modifications of the standard dose-escalation schema have been developed to enroll fewer patients at lower dose levels with greater dose increments between successive dose levels in the absence of toxicity. As the MTD is approached, the dose level increments are reduced and accrual can be expanded. These newer methods aim to minimize the number of patients treated at very low (nonefficacious and nontoxic) doses, while providing greater precision for estimating the MTD and DLT at higher doses (177).

With the shifting focus from conventional cytotoxic agents to non-cytotoxic molecular-targeted agents, the traditional phase 1 paradigm needs to be reexamined. Many newer agents, such as human monoclonal antibodies, may not demonstrate traditional dose-limiting and dose-related toxicities, and phase 1 studies can reach their highest dose level without achieving a conventional MTD. In addition, these agents are frequently destined for chronic administration in conjunction with chemotherapy, and/or following chemotherapy, and cumulative toxicity over multiple cycles appears more important than acute toxicity during the first cycle. Finally, with an identified biologic target, it is also important to consider the optimal biologic dose that achieves a desired level of receptor blockade or signal transduction inhibition. With these considerations, it is apparent that a modified phase 1 design utilizing expanded cohorts treated for multiple cycles would provide better data to guide large randomized trials.

Tumor response is not a primary endpoint within a phase 1 trial, which will typically include patients representing a variety of primary tumor types and multiple prior therapies.

Comprehensive analysis of aggregate phase 1 data, often from multiple trials, will generally determine a dose, schedule, and disease site profile for evaluation in phase 2 studies. In selected situations where the toxicity and appropriate tumor targets are well defined, some phase 1 studies have included an embedded phase 2 component to conserve patient resources, avoid delays associated with activation of a stand-alone phase 2 trial, and accelerate the overall development process. With the increased number of compounds that merit early phase testing, it is also important to prioritize these studies carefully within the limited clinical resources that are available.

Phase 1 studies can also serve to evaluate new combinations that build on standardized chemotherapy regimens to establish feasibility and tolerability of the proposed regimen before embarking on larger trials. In certain situations, such as epithelial ovarian cancer, disease-specific phase 1 trials may enroll newly diagnosed patients without prior therapy, as the experimental combinations generally incorporate other known active agents, such as platinum and a taxane.

Phase 2 Trials

After the recommended dose and schedule have been defined, the regimen can receive focused evaluation in patients with a specific cancer diagnosis, usually in the setting of measurable disease after one (or two) prior chemotherapy regimens. Phase 2 trials are designed and powered based on a surrogate endpoint that is thought to reflect clinical benefit, such as response rate, disease stabilization rate, biologic (tumor marker) response rate, or the proportion of patients alive and progression-free at a specific time interval. Although each of these endpoints may reflect antitumor activity, they are viewed as surrogate endpoints in comparison with overall survival or quality-adjusted survival, which provide a true measure of clinical benefit. In general, each phase 2 trial tests a single hypothesis, such as response rate, to determine if the new agent or regimen crosses a threshold based on historical data in the same patient population with an appropriate degree of power (type II or β error) and precision (type I or α error). Through this process, new agents are "selected" for further development based on historical controls. In order to conserve patient resources and minimize the number of patients who might receive ineffective therapy, most phase 2 studies utilize a multi-stage accrual design with early-stopping parameters, as proposed by Gehan (178) and modified by Simon (179).

Although most phase 2 trials are single-arm nonrandomized studies, there are circumstances where randomized phase 2 evaluations are appropriate (180–182). Randomized phase 2 trials allocate patients among two or more treatment arms to minimize potential differences in prognostic factors or other variables. Each arm is then independently tested against the same historical threshold value. Using this approach, one or both arms can be "selected" for further clinical development. Such randomized trials are generally underpowered for direct comparison of response rate and survival between each arm owing to the limited number of patients. Examples include looking at two different schedules of drug administration with comparative analysis of toxicity and noncomparative reporting of response data to facilitate the selection of experimental arms for future studies. This approach has been used to select between two different schedules of topotecan administration in recurrent ovarian cancer (183).

The traditional phase 2 paradigm has also been challenged by the availability of new molecular-targeted or biologic agents that are thought best to work in combination with conventional cytotoxic chemotherapy. Given the number of combinations that need to be evaluated, it has been appealing to consider randomized designs to select promising combinations. Indeed, in situations where the specific choice of chemotherapy might not be critical to evaluate clinical activity, pilot studies have allowed clinicians to select one of several chemotherapy regimens, and then randomly allocate patients to receive new agents in combination. In addition, where phase 2 data appear interesting but might not support a fully-powered phase 3 trial, there have been phase 3 designs that incorporate an embedded phase 2 study to confirm disease-specific activity and feasibility prior to enabling full accrual.

Phase 3 Trials

If a promising regimen is identified for further testing, it then moves toward a phase 3 randomized trial, in which it is directly compared with an existing standard regimen in a particular clinical setting, as defined by the type of cancer and stage at enrollment. Phase 3 trials generally require a minimum of 150 patients per arm to provide adequate *precision* for the comparison of primary study endpoints while avoiding false-positive conclusions (type I or α error) and adequate *power* to detect a difference while avoiding a false-negative result and potentially missing a true advantage of one arm over the other (type II or β error). In keeping with current drug registration guidelines of the FDA, the primary endpoint of most phase 3 trials is a true measure of clinical benefit, such as overall survival or quality-adjusted survival, with secondary endpoints of progression-free survival, response rate, and toxicity.

Owing to the large number of uniformly staged and treated patients required for a phase 3 trial, such studies are best conducted through a national clinical trials organization, such as GOG. To minimize potential sources of bias, phase 3 trials frequently stratify patients into groups according to key prognostic variables prior to randomization, such as stage or extent of residual disease, as well as other minor variables, such as location of the treating institution. Verification of patient diagnosis, stage of disease, eligibility, treatment delivered, and tumor response can further improve the reliability of results reported from clinical trials.

The traditional phase 3 endpoint of overall survival has been challenged by an increasing number of available treatment options for management of recurrent disease. This has prompted greater consideration of progression-free survival as the primary endpoint for phase 3 trials, as progression is not altered by secondary treatments. However, progression-free survival is subject to observer and detection bias, requiring better control over post-treatment monitoring. Regulatory authorities have also questioned if progression-free survival (as a surrogate endpoint) may not always translate into clinical benefit, and most registration trials include sufficient accrual to evaluate both progression-free and overall survival.

FDA Approval and Postmarketing Studies

Following a successful phase 3 trial or a group of trials, a sponsor can apply to the FDA for marketing approval for a specific disease indication. This triggers a detailed review of clinical trials and pharmaceutical data by the Oncology Drug Advisory Committee (ODAC), which then issues a recommendation to the FDA, followed by formal review and a decision by the FDA, which may grant approval or request additional data. In the United States, all marketing requires approval for at least one specific indication by the FDA. The average time from initial drug discovery to application for an FDA-approved indication is 10 to 12 years, involving considerable expense and effort, as noted above. Supplemental phase 4 or postmarketing studies can be required by the FDA as part of the approval process or be performed by the sponsor to evaluate alternative drug formulations or resolve questions regarding dose, schedule, or toxicity. In addition, phase 4 studies may involve substitution of the new agent in combination chemotherapeutic regimens already established for the disease. These studies are not commonly employed in the development of new chemotherapeutic regimens, but can provide confirmatory postmarketing evidence of safety and efficacy.

Development of Combination Regimens

With some notable exceptions, such as choriocarcinoma and childhood Burkitt's lymphoma, single agents are not sufficient to achieve prolonged survival or cure. Development of combination regimens has been accelerated by our knowledge of cell killing, pharmacokinetics, molecular targets, tumor heterogeneity, and drug resistance. Combinations can approach maximal cell kill by including drugs with minimal overlap of toxicities, such that antitumor effects can be summed but the toxicities dispersed. Combinations are also more likely to demonstrate activity against heterogeneous tumor populations, and effective combinations would prevent the emergence of drug resistance. However, in practice it may also encourage greater resistance among surviving cell fractions.

No direct evidence currently exists to indicate whether optimal combinations should utilize sequential single agents, doublets, or triplets. Utilization of single agents generally precludes any biologic interaction between the various components of a treatment regimen, but permits administration of each agent at the full active dose. The use of sequential doublets generally permits higher doses of individual drugs compared to a triplet regimen, but over a smaller number of cycles with each agent. Doublets have the potential advantage of sequentially introducing more than one regimen with a different mechanism of action and/or pattern of resistance, which has been postulated to prevent the emergence of drug resistance.

Development of combination chemotherapy has been guided by several principles (Table 15.11). However, much of the reported experience has been derived from empiric combinations evaluated in conventional phase 1 dose-escalating trials. Ideally, each of the drugs employed in a new combination should have independent activity as a single agent, as verified in phase 2 studies. Generally, drugs that can produce complete remissions are preferred to agents that produce only partial regressions, but complete remissions are uncommon in previously treated patients with recurrent disease. An attempt should be made to use drugs with minimal overlap of toxicities to avoid excessive dose reduction. Although this may broaden the range of toxicities encountered with each combination, it avoids cumulative and serious toxicity within individual organ systems. Bone marrow recovery usually proves to be the most dominant factor in cycle timing, and in practice, cycles of most combinations can be repeated every 3 to 4 weeks.

Several of these strategies are currently under evaluation in epithelial ovarian cancer based on preclinical models that have suggested an advantage for combinations with platinum, which has been attributed to inhibition of DNA repair (Table 15.12). Each of the selected agents (topotecan, gemcitabine, and PEG-liposomal doxorubicin) has also demonstrated independent single-agent activity against recurrent ovarian cancer, adding to the overall potential benefit of the combination. However, based on available phase 3 data in ovarian cancer, none of the newer combinations hase successfully translated into improved long-term clinical outcomes, providing additional support for a shift in developmental priorities toward molecular targeted agents and other novel approaches.

TABLE 15.11

PRINCIPLES OF COMBINATION CHEMOTHERAPY

Each component should have
- Activity against the target tumor as a single agent
- A different mechanism of action and cellular target
- A biochemical basis for additive or synergistic effects in combination with at least one of the other agents
- No evidence of antagonistic interactions
- Distinct patterns of resistance to discourage the emergence of drug-resistant phenotypes

Optimal dose, schedule, and sequence of drug administration should be determined from preclinical data and early clinical trials to maximize tumor response and minimize host toxicity.

Minimal overlap of nonhematologic toxicity is desirable to safely maintain full therapeutic doses of each component over multiple cycles.

TABLE 15.12

REPRESENTATIVE AGENTS FOR DEVELOPMENT OF COMBINATION REGIMENS

Agent	Cellular target	Mechanism of action	Schedule-dependent effects	Patterns of resistance	Interaction with platinum
Platinum	DNA	DNA adduct formation	Independent	↑GSH ↑DNA repair ↑Damage tolerance ↓Accumulation	NA
Paclitaxel	β tubulin	↑Tubulin aggregation	Dependent (toxicity)	↑*MDR 1* (P 170) β tubulin mutations	↓Heme toxicity, ↑Neuropathy
Topotecan	Topoisomerase-I	Stabilize DNA-topoisomerase complex	Dependent (efficacy)	↓Topoisomerase-I ↑*BCRP* (ABCG2)	↑Heme toxicity
Gemcitabine	Ribonucleotide reductase, DNA, nucleotide pool	↓DNA synthesis ↓Nucleotide pools Masked chain termination	Dependent (metabolism)	↑Ribonucleotide reductase	↑Heme toxicity
PEG-liposomal doxorubicin	Topoisomerase-II	↓DNA synthesis	Prolonged clearance	↑*MDR 1* (P 170)	↑Heme toxicity

Drug Interactions, Scheduling, and Sequence

Drugs should be used in their optimal dose and schedule. However, new combinations have the potential to alter the pharmacokinetics, bioavailability, toxicity, and efficacy of individual components based on substrate-dependent effects, such as a reduction in nucleotide pools or altered metabolism. Therefore, the optimal dose and schedule for individual agents within a combination might differ from their use as single agents, and regimen development would benefit from preclinical models and phase 1 trials with pharmacodynamic endpoints.

The impact of sequence variations using platinum with either paclitaxel or topotecan has been explored in phase 1 clinical trials with somewhat surprising results. For example, prior administration of cisplatin can delay subsequent clearance of paclitaxel when administered as a 24-hour infusion (184). The mechanism for this effect is unknown, but is not attributable to platinum-mediated renal dysfunction. Instead, it has been postulated to occur following cisplatin-mediated inhibition of cytochrome P450 mixed-function oxidases that participate in paclitaxel metabolism. This enzymatic effect is not shared by carboplatin, and prior carboplatin exposure has not been demonstrated to interfere with clearance of paclitaxel. However, most combinations with carboplatin have utilized a shorter (3-hour) paclitaxel infusion, which would tend to blunt the impact of sequencing. Earlier preclinical models had demonstrated enhanced cytotoxicity when paclitaxel was administered prior to cisplatin and antagonism by the reverse sequence (185,186). Thus, the schedule ultimately adopted in clinical practice (paclitaxel followed by cisplatin) is both less toxic and potentially more efficacious. Although this would appear to be firmly grounded in science, it is more likely due to practical considerations owing to the risk of acute paclitaxel HSR, which can require interruption of treatment in approximately 5% of cases, and it was more practical to administer the carboplatin after it was clear that the patient had already tolerated the paclitaxel.

A different pattern was observed with sequences of platinum and topotecan. Preclinical models have consistently favored the sequence of platinum followed by topotecan, which has been postulated to interfere with repair of platinum-mediated DNA damage. In a phase 1 clinical trial, treatment with cisplatin on day 1 was associated with increased bone marrow toxicity compared with the reverse sequence (187). In this instance, the sequence recommended for further clinical evaluation was clearly more toxic, but the question of antitumor efficacy remains to be resolved. When combined with carboplatin, the risk of hematologic toxicity was accentuated, and a similar sequence-dependent relationship was identified (188). Once again, higher doses of topotecan could be safely administered using the reverse sequence of drug administration (with carboplatin on day 3). Topotecan has also been evaluated in sequence with docetaxel (189), showing a reduction in docetaxel clearance associated with increased neutropenia when topotecan was administered prior to docetaxel, emphasizing that each new combination may require independent evaluation.

Even with a single drug, the schedule of administration can have a significant impact on host toxicity and potential efficacy (Table 15.13). Early studies with paclitaxel utilized an

TABLE 15.13A

IMPACT OF PACLITAXEL INFUSION DURATION AND SCHEDULE ON TOXICITY AND EFFICACY

Paclitaxel dose and schedule			Dose-limiting toxicities				
Infusion duration (hr)	Dose interval (wk)	Single-agent unit dose (mg/m²/d)	Neutropenia	Mucositis	Alopecia	Neuropathy	Antitumor efficacy
96	3–4	80–120	+++	++	+++	+	+++
24	3	135	++	0	+++	++	+++
3	3	175	+	0	+++	+++	+++
1	1	60–80	0	0	+	+	+++

TABLE 15.13B

IMPACT OF TOPOTECAN INFUSION DURATION AND SCHEDULE ON TOXICITY AND EFFICACY

Topotecan dose and schedule			Dose-limiting toxicities				
Infusion duration (days)	Dose interval (wk)	Single-agent unit dose (mg/m²/d)	Neutropenia	Mucositis	Alopecia	Neuropathy	Antitumor efficacy
21	4	0.40	+++	0	0	0	+++
5	3–4	1.25	+++	0	0	0	+++
3	3	2.00	+++	0	0	0	++
1	3	8.50	+++	0	0	0	+/−
1	1	1.75	++	0	0	0	+/−
1	1	4.00	+	0	0	0	(UA)[a]

[a]UA, under evaluation.

arbitrary 24-hour infusion, which was selected to reduce the risk of hypersensitivity reactions. Preclinical data suggested that prolonged exposure (96 hours) might have greater efficacy. Owing to increased bone marrow and mucosal toxicity, the MTD was lowered, and the frequency of serious neuropathy was reduced. However, the 96-hour regimen was not demonstrated to have significant activity in patients with recurrent ovarian cancer (190). In addition, the efficacy of a 3-hour infusion was comparable to a 24-hour infusion in a phase 3 trial (191), reinforcing a clinical shift toward the convenient 3-hour schedule, which achieved a higher MTD, primarily due to a marked decrease in bone marrow toxicity, but with an increased incidence of neuropathy. This was followed by phase 1 evaluation of a weekly low-dose 1-hour infusion, which was almost devoid of serious toxicity, including a decreased incidence of alopecia, with maintenance of clinical efficacy (192). Thus, the optimal preclinical regimen (96-hour exposure) was superseded in the clinical setting by an unexpected series of observations from empiric phase 1 trials, yielding decreased toxicity, improved convenience, and the potential for increased efficacy.

With topotecan, a different relationship was defined (Table 15.13B). Initial studies utilized an inconvenient daily infusion for 5 consecutive days, which was based on preclinical data suggesting that prolonged exposure would be more efficacious. This 5-day regimen achieved a 33% response rate in a GOG phase 2 trial in recurrent platinum-sensitive ovarian cancer with expected dose-limiting neutropenia and thrombocytopenia (193). This was followed by the evaluation of a single 24-hour infusion once every 3 weeks, achieving only a 7% response rate in a similar population (194). An attempt to define an intermediate 3-day regimen achieved only a 14% response rate (195). Topotecan was also evaluated as a prolonged intravenous infusion for 21 days to maximize the duration of exposure (196). Although conducted in a different patient population, the overall response rate (35%) was similar to the 5-day regimen, and once again there was equivalent hematologic toxicity without dose-limiting non-hematologic toxicity. Finally, a randomized phase 2 trial conducted by the NCIC and EORTC determined that the 5-day schedule was more appropriate for further clinical development owing to limited activity of an experimental weekly schedule (183). However, this has been challenged on the grounds of inadequate dosing for the weekly regimen, which clearly has reduced hematologic toxicity, and studies are ongoing to evaluate a revised weekly treatment program. In this situation, changes in drug schedule, over a wide range, were associated with substantial differences in efficacy, but without any change in the spectrum or severity of host toxicity, with the exception of reduced hematologic toxicity on the weekly schedule. Thus, each new agent needs to be independently evaluated in the appropriate clinical setting to select the optimal dose and schedule for cancer treatment.

References

1. Lissauer A. Zwei Falle von Leucaemie. *Berl Klin Wochenschr* 1865;2:403.
2. Cutler EG, Bradford EH. Action of iron, cod-liver oil, and arsenic on the globular richness of the blood. *Am J Med Sci* 1878;75:74–84.
3. Kandel EV, LeRoy GV. Chronic arsenical poisoning during the treatment of chronic myeloid leukemia. *Arch Intern Med* 1937;60:846–866.
4. Gilman A. The initial clinical trial of nitrogen mustard. *Am J Surg* 1963;105:574–578.
5. Farber S, Diamond LK, Mercer RD, et al. Temporary remissions in acute leukemia in children produced by folic acid antagonist, 4-aminopteroyl-glutamic acid (aminopterin). *N Engl J Med* 1948;238:787.
6. Hertz R, Ross GT, Lipsett MB. Primary chemotherapy of nonmetastatic trophoblastic disease in women. *Am J Obstet Gynecol* 1963;86:808–814.
7. Huggins C, Hodges CV. Studies on prostatic cancer. The effect of castration, of estrogen and of androgen injection on serum phosphatases in metastatic carcinoma of the prostate. *Cancer Res* 1941;1:293.
8. Adjei AA. Farnesyltransferase inhibitors. *Cancer Chemother Biol Response Modif* 2005;22:123–133.
9. Cell kinetics and the chemotherapy of cancer. *Cancer Chemother Rep* 1971;2:23.
10. Lotem J, Sachs L. Regulation by bc-l2, c-myc and p53 of susceptibility to induction of apoptosis by heat shock and chemotherapy compounds in differentiation-competent and -defective myeloid leukemic cells. *Cell Growth Differ* 1993;4:41–47.
11. Scheffner M, Munger K, Byrne JC, et al. The state of the p53 and retinoblastoma genes in human cervical carcinoma cell lines. *Proc Natl Acad Sci USA* 1991;88:5523–5527.
12. Collins VP, Loeffler RK, Tivey H. Observations on growth rates of human tumors. *AJR Am J Roentgenol* 1956;76:988–1000.
13. Charbit A, Malaise EP, Tubiana M. Relationship between the pathological nature and the growth rate of human tumors. *Eur J Cancer* 1971;7:307–315.
14. Baserga R. The relationship of the cell cycle to tumor growth and control of cell division: a review. *Cancer Res* 1965;25:581–595.
15. Jain RK. Normalization of tumor vasculature: an emerging concept in antiangiogenic therapy. *Science* 2005;307(5706):58–62.
16. Tannock I. Cell kinetics and chemotherapy: a critical review. *Cancer Treat Rep* 1978;62:1117–1133.
17. Steel GG. Cell loss as a factor in the growth rate of human tumors. *Eur J Cancer* 1967;3:381–387.
18. Reddy N, Cohen R, Whitehead B, et al. A phase I, open-label, three period, randomized crossover study to evaluate the effect of food on the pharmacokinetics of lapatinib in cancer patients. *Clin Pharmacol Ther* 2007;81:S16–S17.
19. Ratain MJ, Cohen EE. The value meal: how to save $1,700 per month or more on lapatinib. *J Clin Oncol* 2007;25:3397–3398.
20. Lown K, Bailey DG, Fontana RJ, et al. Grapefruit juice increases felodipine oral availability in humans by decreasing intestinal CYP3A protein expression. *J Clin Invest* 1997;99:2545–2253.
21. Murry DJ, Riva L, Poplack DG. Impact of nutrition on pharmacokinetics of anti-neoplastic agents. *Int J Cancer* 1998;11(Suppl):48–51.
22. Engels FK, Sparreboom A, Mathot RAA, et al. Potential for improvement of docetaxel-based chemotherapy: a pharmacological review. *Br J Cancer* 2005;93:173–177.
23. Markman M. Intraperitoneal antineoplastic drug delivery: rationale and results. *Lancet Oncol* 2003;4:277–283.
24. Myers C. The clinical setting and pharmacology of intraperitoneal chemotherapy: an overview. *Semin Oncol* 1985;12:12–16.
25. TenBokkel Huinink WW, Dubbelman R, Aartsen E, et al. Experimental and clinical results with intraperitoneal cisplatin. *Semin Oncol* 1985; 12:43–46.
26. Howell SB, Zimm S, Markman M, et al. Long-term survival of advanced refractory ovarian carcinoma patients with small-volume disease treated with intraperitoneal chemotherapy. *J Clin Oncol* 1987;5:1607–1612.
27. Markman M, Brady MF, Spirtos NM, et al. Phase II trial of intraperitoneal paclitaxel in carcinoma of the ovary, tube, and peritoneum: a Gynecologic Oncology Group study. *J Clin Oncol* 1998;16:2620–2624.
28. Knox RJ, Friedlos F, Lydall DA, et al. Mechanism of cytotoxicity of anticancer platinum drugs: evidence that cis-diamminedichloroplatinum(II) and cis-diammine-(1,1-cyclobutanedicarboxylato)platinum(II) differ only in the kinetics of their interaction with DNA. *Cancer Res* 1986;46: 1972–1979.
29. Natarajan G, Malathi R, Holler E. Increased DNA-binding activity of cis-1,1-cyclobutane-dicarboxylato-diammineplatinum(II) (carboplatin) in the presence of nucleophiles and human breast cancer MCF-7 cell cytoplasmic extracts: activation theory revisited. *Biochem Pharmacol* 1999;58:1625–1629.
30. Hurria A, Lichtman SM. Pharmacokinetics of chemotherapy in the older patient. *Cancer Control* 2007;14:32–43.
31. Muss HB, Biganzoli L, Sargent DJ, et al. Adjuvant therapy in the elderly: making the right decision. *J Clin Oncol* 2007;25:1870–1875.
32. Clase CM, Garg AX, Kiberd BA. Prevalence of low glomerular filtration rate in nondiabetic Americans: Third National Health and Nutrition Examination Survey (NHANES III). *J Am Soc Nephrol* 2002;13:1338–1349.
33. Gaspari F, Perico N, Matalone M, et al. Precision of plasma clearance of iohexol for estimation of GFR in patients with renal disease. *J Am Soc Nephrol* 1998;9:310–313.
34. Levey AS, Bosch JP, Lewis JB, et al. A more accurate method to estimate glomerular filtration rate from serum creatinine: a new prediction equation. Modification of Diet in Renal Disease Study Group. *Ann Intern Med* 1999;130:461–470.
35. Cockroft DW, Gault MH. Prediction of creatinine clearance from serum creatinine. *Nephron* 1976;16:31–41.
36. Jelliffe RW. Creatinine clearance: bedside estimate. *Ann Intern Med* 1973; 79:604–605.
37. National Kidney Foundation. K/DOQI clinical practice guidelines for chronic kidney disease: evaluation, classification and stratification. *Am J Kidney Dis* 2002;39(Suppl 1):S1–S266.
38. Li YF, Fu S, Hu W, et al. Systemic anticancer therapy in gynecologic cancer patients with renal dysfunction. *Int J Gynecol Cancer* 2007;17:739–763.
39. Gouyette A, Lemoine R, Adhemar JP, et al. Kinetics of cisplatin in an anuric patient undergoing hemofiltration dialysis. *Cancer Treat Rep* 1981; 65:665–668.

40. Motzer RJ, Niedzwiecki D, Isaacs M, et al. Carboplatin-based chemotherapy with pharmacokinetic analysis for patients with hemodialysis-dependent renal insufficiency. *Cancer Chemother Pharmacol* 1990;27:234–238.
41. Powis G. Effect of human renal and hepatic disease on the pharmacokinetics of anticancer drugs. *Cancer Treat Rev* 1982;9:85–124.
42. Lee Villano J, Mehta D, Radhakrishnan L. Abraxane induced life-threatening toxicities with metastatic breast cancer and hepatic insufficiency. *Invest New Drugs* 2006;24:455–456.
43. Hande KR, Wolff SN, Greco FA, et al. Etoposide kinetics in patients with obstructive jaundice. *J Clin Oncol* 1990;8:1101–1107.
44. Boisdron-Celle M, Remaud G, Traore S, et al. 5-fluorouracil-related severe toxicity: a comparison of different methods for the pretherapeutic detection of dihydropyrimidine dehydrogenase deficiency. *Cancer Lett* 2007;249:271–282.
45. Nagar S, Blanchard RL. Pharmacogenetics of uridine diphosphoglucuronosyltransferase (UGT) 1A family members and its role in patient response to irinotecan. *Drug Metab Rev* 2006;38:393–409.
46. Han JY, Lim HS, Shin ES, et al. Comprehensive analysis of UGT1A polymorphisms predictive for pharmacokinetics and treatment outcome in patients with non-small-cell lung cancer treated with irinotecan and cisplatin. *J Clin Oncol* 2006;24:2237–2244.
47. Rouits E, Boisdron-Celle M, Dumont A, et al. Relevance of different UGT1A1 polymorphisms in irinotecan-induced toxicity: a molecular and clinical study of 75 patients. *Clin Cancer Res* 2004;10:5151–5159.
48. Han JY, Lim HS, Yoo YK, et al. Associations of ABCB1, ABCC2, and ABCG2 polymorphisms with irinotecan-pharmacokinetics and clinical outcome in patients with advanced non-small cell lung cancer. *Cancer* 2007;110:138–147.
49. Tanaka E. Clinically important pharmacokinetic drug-drug interactions: role of cytochrome P450 enzymes. *J Clin Pharmacol Ther* 1998;23:403–416.
50. Kivisto KT, Kroemer HK, Eichelbaum M. The role of cytochrome P450 enzymes in the metabolism of anticancer agents: implications for drug interactions. *Br J Clin Pharmacol* 1995;40:523–530.
51. Fojo AT, Ueda K, Slamon DJ, et al. Expression of multidrug resistance gene in human tumors and tissues. *Proc Natl Acad Sci USA* 1987;84:265–269.
52. Nunberg JH, Kaufman RJ, Schimke RT, et al. Amplified dihydrofolate reductase genes are localized to a homogeneously staining region in a single chromosome in a methotrexate-resistant Chinese hamster ovary cell line. *Proc Natl Acad Sci USA* 1978;75:5553–5556.
53. Fojo AT, Whang-Peng J, Gottesman MM, et al. Amplification of DNA sequences in human multidrug-resistant KB carcinoma cells. *Proc Natl Acad Sci USA* 1985;82:7661–7665.
54. Ling V, Thompson LH. Reduced permeability in CHO cells as a mechanism of resistance to colchicine. *J Cell Physiol* 1974;83:103–116.
55. Kelland L. The resurgence of platinum-based cancer chemotherapy. *Nat Rev Cancer* 2007;7:573–584.
56. Schondorf T, Scharl A, Kurbacher CM, et al. Amplification of the mdr1-gene is uncommon in recurrent ovarian carcinomas. *Cancer Lett* 1999;146:195–199.
57. Rubin SC, Finstad CL, Hoskins WJ, et al. Expression of P-glycoprotein in epithelial ovarian cancer: evaluation as a marker of multidrug resistance. *Am J Obstet Gynecol* 1990;163:69–73.
58. Yusuf RZ, Duan Z, Lamendola DE, et al. Paclitaxel resistance: molecular mechanisms and pharmacologic manipulation. *Curr Cancer Drug Targets* 2003;3:1–19.
59. Lamendola DE, Duan Z, Penson RT, et al. Beta tubulin mutations are rare in human ovarian carcinoma. *Anticancer Res* 2003;23:681–686.
60. Bergman AM, Pinedo HM, Talianidis I, et al. Increased sensitivity to gemcitabine of P-glycoprotein and multidrug resistance-associated protein-overexpressing human cancer cell lines. *Br J Cancer* 2003;88:1963–1970.
61. Belinsky MG, Bain LJ, Balsara BB, et al. Characterization of MOAT-C and MOAT-D, new members of the MRP/cMOAT subfamily of transporter proteins. *J Natl Cancer Inst* 1998;90:1735–1741.
62. Maliepaard M, van Gastelen MA, de Jong LA, et al. Overexpression of the BCRP/MXR/ABCP gene in a topotecan-selected ovarian tumor cell line. *Cancer Res* 1999;59:4559–4563.
63. Ishida S, Lee J, Thiele DJ, et al. Uptake of the anticancer drug cisplatin mediated by the copper transporter Ctr1 in yeast and mammals. *Proc Natl Acad Sci USA* 2002;99:14298–14302.
64. Holzer AK, Howell SB. The internalization and degradation of human copper transporter 1 following cisplatin exposure. *Cancer Res* 2006;66:10944–10952.
65. McKeage MJ. Satraplatin in hormone-refractory prostate cancer and other tumour types: pharmacological properties and clinical evaluation. *Drugs* 2007;67:859–869.
66. Samimi G, Howell SB. Modulation of the cellular pharmacology of JM118, the major metabolite of satraplatin, by copper influx and efflux transporters. *Cancer Chemother Pharmacol* 2006;57:781–788.
67. Green JA, Vistica DT, Young RC, et al. Potentiation of melphalan cytotoxicity in human ovarian cancer cell lines by glutathione depletion. *Cancer Res* 1984;44:5427–5431.
68. Sadowitz PD, Hubbard BA, Dabrowiak JC, et al. Kinetics of cisplatin binding to cellular DNA and modulations by thiol-blocking agents and thiol drugs. *Drug Metab Dispos* 2002;30:183–190.
69. Daubeuf S, Balin D, Leroy P, et al. Different mechanisms for gamma-glutamyltransferase–dependent resistance to carboplatin and cisplatin. *Biochem Pharmacol* 2003;66:595–604.
70. Hanigan MH, Lykissa ED, Townsend DM, et al. Gamma-glutamyl transpeptidase-deficient mice are resistant to the nephrotoxic effects of cisplatin. *Am J Pathol* 2001;159:1889–1894.
71. O'Dwyer PJ, Hamilton TC, LaCreta FP, et al. Phase I trial of buthionine sulfoximine in combination with melphalan. *J Clin Oncol* 1996;14:249–256.
72. Bailey HH, Ripple G, Tutsch KD, et al. Phase I study of continuous-infusion L-S,R-buthionine sulfoximine with intravenous melphalan. *J Natl Cancer Inst* 1997;89:1789–1796.
73. Holford J, Beale PJ, Boxall FE, et al. Mechanisms of drug resistance to the platinum complex ZD0473 in ovarian cancer cell lines. *Eur J Cancer* 2000;36:1984–1990.
74. Gore ME, Atkinson RJ, Thomas H, et al. A phase II trial of ZD0473 in platinum-pretreated ovarian cancer. *Eur J Cancer* 2002;38:2416–2420.
75. Masuda H, Ozols RF, Lai GM, et al. Increased DNA repair as a mechanism of acquired resistance to cis-diamminedichloroplatinum (II) in human ovarian cancer cell lines. *Cancer Res* 1988;48:5713–5716.
76. Aebi S, Kurdihaidar B, Gordon R, et al. Loss of DNA mismatch repair in acquired resistance to cisplatin. *Cancer Res* 1996;56:3087–3090.
77. Gifford G, Paul J, Vasey PA, et al. The acquisition of hMLH1 methylation in plasma DNA after chemotherapy predicts poor survival for ovarian cancer patients. *Clin Cancer Res* 2004;10:4420–4426.
78. Plumb JA, Strathdee G, Sludden J, et al. Reversal of drug resistance in human tumor xenografts by 2′-deoxy-5-azacytidine-induced demethylation of the hMLH1 gene promoter. *Cancer Res* 2000;60:6039–6044.
79. Raymond E, Chaney SG, Taamma A, et al. Oxaliplatin: a review of preclinical and clinical studies. *Ann Oncol* 1998;9:1053–1071.
80. Vaisman A, Varchenko M, Umar A, et al. The role of hMLH1, hMSH3, and hMSH6 defects in cisplatin and oxaliplatin resistance: correlation with replicative bypass of platinum-DNA adducts. *Cancer Res* 1998;58:3579–3585.
81. Piccart MJ, Green JA, Lacave AJ, et al. Oxaliplatin or paclitaxel in patients with platinum-pretreated advanced ovarian cancer: a randomized phase II study of the European Organization for Research and Treatment of Cancer Gynecology Group. *J Clin Oncol* 2000;18:1193–1202.
82. Fracasso PM, Blessing JA, Morgan MA, et al. Phase II study of oxaliplatin in platinum-resistant and refractory ovarian cancer: a Gynecologic Oncology Group study. *J Clin Oncol* 2003;21:2856–2859.
83. Dabholkar M, Bostick-Bruton F, Weber C, et al. ERCC1 and ERCC2 expression in malignant tissues from ovarian cancer patients. *J Natl Cancer Inst* 1992;84:1512–1517.
84. Olaussen KA, Dunant A, Fouret P, et al. DNA repair by ERCC1 in non-small-cell lung cancer and cisplatin-based adjuvant chemotherapy. *N Engl J Med* 2006;355:983–991.
85. Zheng Z, Chen T, Li X, et al. DNA synthesis and repair genes RRM1 and ERCC1 in lung cancer. *N Engl J Med* 2007;356:800–808.
86. Cobo M, Isla D, Massuti B, et al. Customizing cisplatin based on quantitative excision repair cross-complementing 1 mRNA expression: A phase III trial in non–small-cell lung cancer. *J Clin Oncol* 2007;25:2747–2754.
87. Trent JM, Buick RN, Olson S, et al. Cytologic evidence for gene amplification in methotrexate-resistant cells obtained from a patient with ovarian adenocarcinoma. *J Clin Oncol* 1984;2:8–15.
88. Cowan KH, Jolivet J. A methotrexate-resistant human breast cancer cell line with multiple defects, including diminished formation of methotrexate polyglutamates. *J Biol Chem* 1984;259:10793–10800.
89. Obata T, Endo Y, Murata D, et al. The molecular targets of antitumor 2′-deoxycytidine analogues. *Curr Drug Targets* 2003;4:305–313.
90. Zhou B, Mo X, Liu X, et al. Human ribonucleotide reductase M2 subunit gene amplification and transcriptional regulation in a homogeneous staining chromosome region responsible for the mechanism of drug resistance. *Cytogenet Cell Genet* 2001;95:34–42.
91. Jung CP, Motwani MV, Schwartz GK. Flavopiridol increases sensitization to gemcitabine in human gastrointestinal cancer cell lines and correlates with down-regulation of ribonucleotide reductase M2 subunit. *Clin Cancer Res* 2001;7:2527–2536.
92. Johnston PG, Lenz HJ, Leichman CG, et al. Thymidylate synthase gene and protein expression correlate and are associated with response to 5-fluorouracil in human colorectal and gastric tumors. *Cancer Res* 1995;55:1407–1412.
93. Salonga D, Danenberg KD, Johnson M, et al. Colorectal tumors responding to 5-fluorouracil have low gene expression levels of dihydropyrimidine dehydrogenase, thymidylate synthase, and thymidine phosphorylase. *Clin Cancer Res* 2000;6:1322–1327.
94. Fidler IJ, Kripke ML. Metastasis results from preexisting variant cells within a malignant tumor. *Science* 1977;197:893–895.
95. Kern DH, Weisenthal LM. Highly specific prediction of antineoplastic drug resistance with an in vitro assay using suprapharmacologic drug exposures. *J Natl Cancer Inst* 1990;82:582–588.
96. Cortazar P, Johnson BE. Review of the efficacy of individualized chemotherapy selected by in vitro drug sensitivity testing for patients with cancer. *J Clin Oncol* 1999;17:1625–1631.
97. Nagourney RA, Brewer CA, Radecki S, et al. Phase II trial of gemcitabine plus cisplatin repeating doublet therapy in previously treated, relapsed ovarian cancer patients. *Gynecol Oncol* 2003;88:35–39.

98. Levin L, Hryniuk W. Dose intensity analysis of chemotherapy regimens in ovarian cancer. *J Clin Oncol* 1987;5:756–767.
99. McGuire WP, Hoskins WJ, Brady MF, et al. Assessment of dose-intensive therapy in suboptimally debulked ovarian cancer: a Gynecologic Oncology Group study. *J Clin Oncol* 1995;13:1589–1599.
100. Schilder RJ, Gallo JM, Millenson MM, et al. Phase I trial of multiple cycles of high-dose carboplatin, paclitaxel, and topotecan with peripheral-blood stem-cell support as front-line therapy. *J Clin Oncol* 2001;19:1183–1194.
101. Tiersten A, Selleck M, Smith DH, et al. Phase I/II study of tandem cycles of high-dose chemotherapy followed by autologous hematopoietic stem cell support in women with advanced ovarian cancer. *Int J Gynecol Cancer* 2006;16:57–64.
102. Mobus V, Wandt H, Frickhofen N, et al. High-dose sequential chemotherapy with peripheral blood stem cell support compared with standard dose chemotherapy for first-line treatment of advanced ovarian cancer: results of a phase III intergroup trial of the AGO-Ovar/AIO and EBMT. *J Clin Oncol* 2007;25(27):4187–4193.
103. Kummel S, Krocker J, Kohls A, et al. Randomised trial: survival benefit and safety of adjuvant dose-dense chemotherapy for node-positive breast cancer. *Br J Cancer* 2006;94:1237–1244.
104. McGuire WP, Hoskins WJ, Brady MF, et al. Cyclophosphamide and cisplatin compared with paclitaxel and cisplatin in patients with stage III and stage IV ovarian cancer. *N Engl J Med* 1996;334:1–6.
105. Ozols RF, Bundy BN, Greer BE, et al. Phase III trial of carboplatin and paclitaxel compared with cisplatin and paclitaxel in patients with optimally resected stage III ovarian cancer: a Gynecologic Oncology Group study. *J Clin Oncol* 2003;21:3194–3200.
106. Fleming GF, Brunetto VL, Cella D, et al. Phase III trial of doxorubicin plus cisplatin with or without paclitaxel plus filgrastim in advanced endometrial carcinoma: a Gynecologic Oncology Group study. *J Clin Oncol* 2004;22(11):2159–2166.
107. Moore DH, Blessing JA, McQuellon RP, et al. Phase III study of cisplatin with or without paclitaxel in stage IVB, recurrent or persistent squamous cell carcinoma of the cervix: a Gynecologic Oncology Group study. *J Clin Oncol* 2004;22(15):3113–3119.
108. Long HJ, Bundy BN, Grendys EC, et al. Randomized phase III trial of cisplatin (P) vs cisplatin plus topotecan (T) vs MVAC in stage IVB, recurrent or persistent carcinoma of the uterine cervix: a Gynecologic Oncology Group study. *J Clin Oncol* 2005;23(21):4626–4633.
109. Homesley HD, Filiaci V, Markman M, et al. Phase III trial of ifosfamide with or without paclitaxel in advanced uterine carcinosarcoma: a Gynecologic Oncology Group study. *J Clin Oncol* 2007;25:526–531.
110. Muggia FM, Braly PS, Brady MF, et al. Phase III randomized study of cisplatin versus paclitaxel versus cisplatin and paclitaxel in patients with suboptimal stage III or IV ovarian cancer: a Gynecologic Oncology Group study. *J Clin Oncol* 2000;18:106–115.
111. The International Collaborative Ovarian Neoplasm (ICON) Group. Paclitaxel plus carboplatin versus standard chemotherapy with either single-agent carboplatin or cyclophosphamide, doxorubicin, and cisplatin in women with ovarian cancer: the ICON3 randomised trial. *Lancet* 2002;360:505–515.
112. Young RC, Brady MF, Nieberg RK, et al. Adjuvant treatment for early ovarian cancer: a randomized phase III trial of intraperitoneal ^{32}P or cyclophosphamide-cisplatin. A Gynecologic Oncology Group study. *J Clin Oncol* 2003;21(23):4350–4355.
113. Trimbos JB, Vergote I, Bolis G, et al. EORTC-ACTION collaborators. European Organisation for Research and Treatment of Cancer—Adjuvant ChemoTherapy in Ovarian Neoplasm. Impact of adjuvant chemotherapy and surgical staging in early-stage ovarian carcinoma: European Organisation for Research and Treatment of Cancer—Adjuvant ChemoTherapy in Ovarian Neoplasm trial. *J Natl Cancer Inst* 2003;95:113–125.
114. Randall ME, Filiaci VL, Muss H, et al. Randomized phase III trial of whole-abdominal irradiation versus doxorubicin and cisplatin chemotherapy in advanced endometrial carcinoma: a Gynecologic Oncology Group study. *J Clin Oncol* 2006;24:36–44.
115. Wolfson AH, Brady MF, Rocereto T, et al. A Gynecologic Oncology Group randomized phase III trial of whole abdominal irradiation (WAI) vs. cisplatin-ifosfamide and mesna (CIM) as post-surgical therapy in stage I-IV carcinosarcoma (CS) of the uterus. *Gynecol Oncol* 2007; 107(2):177–185.
116. Rose PG, Ali S, Watkins E, et al. Long-term follow-up of a randomized trial comparing concurrent single agent cisplatin, cisplatin-based combination chemotherapy, or hydroxyurea during pelvic irradiation for locally advanced cervical cancer: a Gynecologic Oncology Group study. *J Clin Oncol* 2007;25:2804–2810.
117. Therasse P, Arbuck SG, Eisenhauer EA, et al. New guidelines to evaluate the response to treatment in solid tumors. European Organization for Research and Treatment of Cancer, National Cancer Institute of the United States, National Cancer Institute of Canada. *J Natl Cancer Inst* 2000;92:205–216.
118. Rustin GJ, Bast RC Jr, Kelloff GJ, et al. Use of CA-125 in clinical trial evaluation of new therapeutic drugs for ovarian cancer. *Clin Cancer Res* 2004;10:3919–3926.
119. Vergote I, Rustin GJ, Eisenhauer EA, et al. Re: new guidelines to evaluate the response to treatment in solid tumors (ovarian cancer). Gynecologic Cancer Intergroup. *J Natl Cancer Inst* 2000;92:1534–1535.
120. Rustin GJ. Use of CA-125 to assess response to new agents in ovarian cancer trials. *J Clin Oncol* 2003;21(10 Suppl):187–193.
121. Fanucchi M, Glaspy J, Crawford J, et al. Effects of polyethylene glycol-conjugated recombinant human megakaryocyte growth and development factor on platelet counts after chemotherapy for lung cancer. *N Engl J Med* 1997;336:404–409.
122. Del Mastro L, Venturini M, Lionetto R, et al. Randomized phase III trial evaluating the role of erythropoietin in the prevention of chemotherapy-induced anemia. *J Clin Oncol* 1997;15:2715–2721.
123. Barosi G, Marchetti M, Liberato NL. Cost-effectiveness of recombinant human erythropoietin in the prevention of chemotherapy-induced anaemia. *Br J Cancer* 1998;78:781–787.
124. Khuri FR. Weighing the hazards of erythropoiesis stimulation in patients with cancer. *N Engl J Med* 2007;356:2445–2448.
125. Food and Drug Administration. FDA alert. Information for healthcare professionals: erythropoiesis stimulating agents (ESA). http://www.fda.gov/cder/drug/InfoSheets/HCP/RHE2007HCP.htm. Published March 9, 2007.
126. Food and Drug Administration. Oncologic Drugs Advisory Committee. Continuing reassessment of the risks of erythropoiesis-stimulating agents (ESAs) administered for the treatment of anemia associated with cancer chemotherapy. http://www.fda.gov/ohrms/dockets/ac/07/briefing/2007-4301b2-00-index.htm. Published May 10, 2007.
127. Steinbrook R. Erythropoietin, the FDA, and oncology. *N Engl J Med* 2007;356:2448–2451.
128. Center for Medicare and Medicaid Services. Decision memo for erythropoiesis stimulating agents (ESAs) for non-renal disease indications (CAG-00383N). http://www.cms.hhs.gov/mcd/viewdecisionmemo.asp?id=203. Published July 30, 2007.
129. Bonneterre J, Chevallier B, Metz R, et al. A randomized double-blind comparison of ondansetron and metoclopramide in the prophylaxis of emesis induced by cyclophosphamide, fluorouracil, and doxorubicin or epirubicin chemotherapy. *J Clin Oncol* 1990;8:1063–1069.
130. du Bois A, Vach W, Kiechle M, et al. Pathophysiology, severity, pattern, and risk factors for carboplatin-induced emesis. *Oncology* 1996;53(Suppl 1):46–50.
131. Friedlander ML, Sims K, Kearsely JH. Impairment of recall improves tolerance of cytotoxic chemotherapy. *Lancet* 1983;2:686.
132. Dodd MJ, Miaskowski C, Greenspan D, et al. Radiation-induced mucositis: a randomized clinical trial of micronized sucralfate versus salt & soda mouthwashes. *Cancer Invest* 2003;21:21–33.
133. Nottage M, McLachlan SA, Brittain MA, et al. Sucralfate mouthwash for prevention and treatment of 5-fluorouracil-induced mucositis: a randomized, placebo-controlled trial. *Support Care Cancer* 2003;11:41–47.
134. Rosen LS, Abdi E, Davis ID, et al. Palifermin reduces the incidence of oral mucositis in patients with metastatic colorectal cancer treated with fluorouracil-based chemotherapy. *J Clin Oncol* 2006;24:5194–5200.
135. Booth D, Potten CS. Protection against mucosal injury by growth factors and cytokines. *J Natl Cancer Inst Monogr* 2001;29:16–20.
136. Muggia FM, Hainsworth JD, Jeffers S. Phase II study of liposomal doxorubicin in refractory ovarian cancer: antitumor activity and toxicity modification by liposomal encapsulation. *J Clin Oncol* 1997;15:987–993.
137. Dunagin WG. Dermatologic toxicity. *Semin Oncol* 1982;9:14–22.
138. Kassner E. Evaluation and treatment of chemotherapy extravasation injuries. *J Pediatr Oncol Nurs* 2000;17:135–148.
139. Schulmeister L, Camp-Sorrell D. Chemotherapy extravasation from implanted ports. *Oncol Nurs Forum* 2000;27:531–538.
140. Langer SW, Sehested M, Jensen PB. Treatment of anthracycline extravasation with dexrazoxane. *Clin Cancer Res* 2000;6:3680–3686.
141. Mouridsen HT, Langer SW, Buter J, et al. Treatment of anthracycline extravasation with Savene (dexrazoxane): results from two prospective clinical multicentre studies. *Ann Oncol* 2007;18:546–550.
142. Verstappen CC, Heimans JJ, Hoekman K, et al. Neurotoxic complications of chemotherapy in patients with cancer: clinical signs and optimal management. *Drugs* 2003;63:1549–1563.
143. Quasthoff S, Hartung HP. Chemotherapy-induced peripheral neuropathy. *J Neurol* 2002;249:9–17.
144. Lee JJ, Swain SM. Peripheral neuropathy induced by microtubule-stabilizing agents. *J Clin Oncol* 2006;24:1633–1642.
145. Hausheer FH, Schilsky RL, Bain S, et al. Diagnosis, management, and evaluation of chemotherapy-induced peripheral neuropathy. *Semin Oncol* 2006;33:15–49.
146. Gradishar WJ, Tjulandin S, Davidson N, et al. Phase III trial of nanoparticle albumin-bound paclitaxel compared with polyethylated castor oil-based paclitaxel in women with breast cancer. *J Clin Oncol* 2005;23: 7794–7803.
147. Wilding G, Caruso R, Lawrence TS, et al. Retinal toxicity after high-dose cisplatin therapy. *J Clin Oncol* 1985;3:1683–1689.
148. Land SR, Kopec JA, Cecchini RS, et al. Neurotoxicity from oxaliplatin combined with weekly bolus fluorouracil and leucovorin as surgical adjuvant chemotherapy for stage II and III colon cancer: NSABP C-07. *J Clin Oncol* 2007;25:2205–2211.
149. Pasetto LM, D'Andrea MR, Rossi E, et al. Oxaliplatin-related neurotoxicity: how and why? *Crit Rev Oncol Hematol* 2006;59:159–168.
150. Krishnan AV, Goldstein D, Friedlander M, et al. Oxaliplatin and axonal Na+ channel function in vivo. *Clin Cancer Res* 2006;12:4481–4484.

151. Gamelin L, Boisdron-Celle M, Delva R, et al. Prevention of oxaliplatin-related neurotoxicity by calcium and magnesium infusions: a retrospective study of 161 patients receiving oxaliplatin combined with 5-fluorouracil and leucovorin for advanced colorectal cancer. *Clin Cancer Res* 2004;10:4055–4061.
152. Hochster HS, Grothey A, Childs BH. Use of calcium and magnesium salts to reduce oxaliplatin-related neurotoxicity. *J Clin Oncol* 2007;25: 4028–4029.
153. Holmes FA, Walters RS, Theriault RL, et al. Phase II trial of Taxol, an active drug in the treatment of metastatic breast cancer. *J Natl Cancer Inst* 1991;83:1797–1805.
154. Calhoun EA, Welshman EE, Chang CH, et al. Psychometric evaluation of the functional assessment of cancer therapy/Gynecologic Oncology Group—neurotoxicity (Fact/GOG-Ntx) questionnaire for patients receiving systemic chemotherapy. *Int J Gynecol Cancer* 2003;13:741–748.
155. Mollman JE, Glover DJ, Hogan WM, et al. Cisplatin neuropathy. Risk factors, prognosis, and protection by WR-2721. *Cancer* 1988;61: 2192–2195.
156. Moore DH, Donnelly J, McGuire WP, et al. Limited access trial using amifostine for protection against cisplatin- and three-hour paclitaxel–induced neurotoxicity: a phase II study of the Gynecologic Oncology Group. *J Clin Oncol* 2003;21:4207–4213.
157. van Deventer H, Bernard S. Use of gabapentin to treat taxane-induced myalgias. *J Clin Oncol* 1999;17:434–435.
158. Pelgrims J, De Vos F, Van den Brande J, et al. Methylene blue in the treatment and prevention of ifosfamide-induced encephalopathy: report of 12 cases and a review of the literature. *Br J Cancer* 2000;82:291–294.
159. Arany I, Safirstein RL. Cisplatin nephrotoxicity. *Semin Nephrol* 2003;23: 460–464.
160. Santoso JT, Lucci JA 3rd, Coleman RL, et al. Saline, mannitol, and furosemide hydration in acute cisplatin nephrotoxicity: a randomized trial. *Cancer Chemother Pharmacol* 2003;52:13–18.
161. Andriole GL, Sandlund JT, Miser JS, et al. The efficacy of mesna as a uroprotectant in patients with hemorrhagic cystitis receiving further oxazaphosphorine chemotherapy. *J Clin Oncol* 1987;5:799–803.
162. Bookman MA, Kloth DD, Kover PE, et al. Short-course intravenous prophylaxis for paclitaxel-related hypersensitivity reactions. *Ann Oncol* 1997;8:611–614.
163. Weiss RB, Donehower RC, Weirnik PH, et al. Hypersensitivity reactions from Taxol. *J Clin Oncol* 1990;8:1263–1268.
164. Markman M, Kennedy A, Webster K, et al. Clinical features of hypersensitivity reactions to carboplatin. *J Clin Oncol* 1999;17:1141–1145.
165. Rose PG, Fusco N, Smrekar M, et al. Successful administration of carboplatin in patients with clinically documented carboplatin hypersensitivity. *Gynecol Oncol* 2003;89:429–433.
166. Lee CW, Matulonis UA, Castells MC. Rapid inpatient/outpatient desensitization for chemotherapy hypersensitivity: standard protocol effective in 57 patients for 255 courses. *Gynecol Oncol* 2005;99:393–399.
167. Sikora K, Advani S, Koroltchouk V, et al. Essential drugs for cancer therapy: a World Health Organization consultation. *Ann Oncol* 1999;10: 385–390.
168. Grever MR, Schepartz S, Chabner BA. The National Cancer Institute: cancer drug discovery and development program. *Semin Oncol* 1992;19: 622–638.
169. Cragg GM, Newman DJ, Weiss RB. Coral reefs, forests, and thermal vents: the worldwide exploration of nature for novel antitumor agents. *Semin Oncol* 1997;24:156–163.
170. Brocchini S. Combinatorial chemistry and biomedical polymer development. *Adv Drug Deliv Rev* 2001;53:123–130.
171. Geysen HM, Schoenen F, Wagner D, et al. Combinatorial compound libraries for drug discovery: an ongoing challenge. *Nat Rev Drug Discov* 2003;2:222–230.
172. Leonard KA, Deisseroth AB, Austin DJ. Combinatorial chemistry in cancer drug development. *Cancer J* 2001;7:79–83.
173. Breinbauer R, Manger M, Scheck M, et al. Natural product guided compound library development. *Curr Med Chem* 2002;9:2129–2145.
174. Batra S, Srinivasan T, Rastogi SK, et al. Identification of enzyme inhibitors using combinatorial libraries. *Curr Med Chem* 2002;9:307–319.
175. Wani MC, Taylor HL, Wall ME, et al. Plant antitumor agents. VI. The isolation and structure of Taxol, a novel antileukemic and antitumor agent from *Taxus brevifolia*. *J Am Chem Soc* 1971;93:2325–2327.
176. Wall ME, Wani MC, Cook CE, et al. Plant antitumor agents. I. The isolation and structure of camptothecin, a novel alkaloidal leukemia and tumor inhibitor from *Camptotheca accuminata*. *J Am Chem Soc* 1966;88: 3888–3890.
177. Babb J, Rogatko A, Zacks S. Cancer phase I clinical trials: efficient dose escalation with overdose control. *Stat Med* 1998;17:1103–1120.
178. Gehan EA. The determination of the number of patients required in a preliminary and follow-up trial of a new chemotherapeutic agent. *J Chronic Dis* 1961;13:346–353.
179. Simon R. Optimal two-stage designs for phase II clinical trials. *Controlled Clin Trials* 1989;10:1–10.
180. Estey EH, Thall PF. New designs for phase 2 clinical trials. *Blood* 2003;102:442–448.
181. Steinberg SM, Venzon DJ. Early selection in a randomized phase II clinical trial. *Stat Med* 2002;21:1711–1726.
182. Strauss N, Simon R. Investigating a sequence of randomized phase II trials to discover promising treatments. *Stat Med* 1995;14:1479–1489.
183. Hoskins P, Eisenhauer E, Beare S, et al. Randomized phase II study of two schedules of topotecan in previously treated patients with ovarian cancer: a National Cancer Institute of Canada Clinical Trials Group study. *J Clin Oncol* 1998;16:2233–2237.
184. Rowinsky EK, Gilbert M, McGuire WP, et al. Sequences of Taxol and cisplatin: a phase I and pharmacologic study. *J Clin Oncol* 1991;9:1692–1703.
185. Rowinsky EK, Citardi M, Noe DA, et al. Sequence-dependent cytotoxicity between cisplatin and the antimicrotubule agents Taxol and vincristine. *J Cancer Res Clin Oncol* 1993;119:737–743.
186. Jekunen AP, Christen RD, Shalinsky DR, et al. Synergistic interaction between cisplatin and Taxol in human ovarian carcinoma cells in vitro. *Br J Cancer* 1994;69:299–306.
187. Rowinsky EK, Kaufmann SH, Baker SD, et al. Sequences of topotecan and cisplatin: phase I, pharmacological and in vitro studies to examine sequence dependence. *J Clin Oncol* 1996;14:3074–3084.
188. Bookman MA, McMeekin DS, Fracasso P. Sequence-dependence of hematologic toxicity using carboplatin and topotecan for primary therapy of advanced epithelial ovarian cancer: a phase I study of the Gynecologic Oncology Group. *Gynecol Oncol* 2006;103:473–478.
189. Zamboni WC, Egorin MJ, Van Echo DA, et al. Pharmacokinetic and pharmacodynamic study of the combination of docetaxel and topotecan in patients with solid tumors. *J Clin Oncol* 2000;18:3288–3294.
190. Markman M, Rose PG, Jones E, et al. Ninety-six-hour infusional paclitaxel as salvage therapy of ovarian cancer patients previously failing treatment with 3-hour or 24-hour paclitaxel infusion regimens. *J Clin Oncol* 1998;16:1849–1851.
191. Eisenhauer EA, ten Bokkel Huinink WW, Swenerton KD, et al. European-Canadian randomized trial of paclitaxel in relapsed ovarian cancer: high-dose versus low-dose and long versus short infusion. *J Clin Oncol* 1994;12:2654–2666.
192. Fennelly D, Aghajanian C, Shapiro F, et al. Phase I and pharmacologic study of paclitaxel administered weekly in patients with relapsed ovarian cancer. *J Clin Oncol* 1997;15:187–192.
193. McGuire WP, Blessing JA, Bookman MA, et al. Topotecan has substantial antitumor activity as first-line salvage therapy in platinum-sensitive epithelial ovarian carcinoma: a Gynecologic Oncology Group study. *J Clin Oncol* 2000;18:1062–1067.
194. Markman M, Blessing JA, Alvarez RD, et al. Phase II evaluation of 24-h continuous infusion topotecan in recurrent, potentially platinum-sensitive ovarian cancer: a Gynecologic Oncology Group study. *Gynecol Oncol* 2000;77:112–115.
195. Miller DS, Blessing JA, Lentz SS, et al. Phase II evaluation of three-day topotecan in recurrent platinum-sensitive ovarian carcinoma: a Gynecologic Oncology Group study. *Cancer* 2003;98:1664–1669.
196. Hochster H, Wadler S, Runowicz C, et al. Activity and pharmacodynamics of 21-day topotecan infusion in patients with ovarian cancer previously treated with platinum-based chemotherapy: New York Gynecologic Oncology Group. *J Clin Oncol* 1999;17:2553–2561.

CHAPTER 16 ■ PHARMACOLOGY AND THERAPEUTICS IN GYNECOLOGIC CANCER

DAVID S. ALBERTS, LISA M. HESS, DANIEL D. VON HOFF, AND ROBERT T. DORR

The determinants of effective cancer drug therapies include drug disposition, tumor kinetics, and drug resistance. These factors profoundly influence the cytotoxicity of each anticancer drug and must be considered in designing therapeutic regimens. These principles are discussed in Chapter 15. In this chapter, we elaborate the basic and clinical pharmacology of cancer chemotherapeutic and biologic agents and provide a limited discussion of cytotoxic, molecularly targeted, antiangiogenesis, and modulating/supportive care drugs useful in the treatment of patients with gynecologic cancer.

DETERMINANTS OF EFFECTIVE DRUG THERAPIES

Drug Disposition Factors

The term *pharmacokinetics* describes the time course of drug disposition in body fluids and tissues through the use of mathematical models. These models use an equation or set of equations to describe the concentration versus time profile of a specific drug after administration into the body. The models are often illustrated by box diagrams, with each box or compartment corresponding to a region of the body, although the compartments may not represent real anatomic regions. A drug is considered to be uniformly distributed within a compartment if its concentration within tissues has reached homogeneity.

Pharmacokinetic models may be useful in predicting the plasma or tissue concentrations of drugs in the body after any one of several routes or methods of drug administration. The simplest model has one compartment into which the drug is assumed to be instantaneously introduced, and elimination occurs by one linear route. The disappearance of the drug from this compartment can be described by a straight line if plotted on semilogarithmic graph paper. As discussed by Tozer (1), no one-compartment pharmacokinetic model can be used to describe the disposition of commonly used anticancer drugs; nevertheless, the one-compartment pharmacokinetic model lends itself to an understanding of the concept of plasma half-life (i.e., $t_{1/2}$), which represents the time required for the concentration of a drug at any point on the plasma concentration · time elimination curve to achieve half its value. This constant may be applied repeatedly, so that, for instance, only 25% of the drug remains in two half-lives. The equation for plasma half-life that can be applied to any linear plasma concentration · time elimination curve is as follows: $t_{1/2}z = 0.693$/slope of the linear elimination curve (i.e., λ_z or rate constant for that part of the curve). Unfortunately, the determination of the terminal half-life of a drug is often poorly reproducible because it is highly dependent on measuring multiple plasma levels, often at the limit of drug assay sensitivity.

Pharmacokinetic Models

The pharmacokinetics of virtually all anticancer drugs require two- or three-compartment models for their mathematic description. These models are commonly referred to as biphasic or triphasic models (i.e., two or three phases observed on semilogarithmic plots). Conceptually, the one-compartment model relates to a drug that remains confined to the intravascular space after intravenous injection, and the two- or three-compartment model allows the pharmacokinetic description of anticancer drugs whose ultimate targets are beyond the intravascular space in tumor tissues.

Drug Clearance and AUC Concepts

Wisdom dictates using the simplest mathematical model that can provide the "best" fit of the actual plasma concentration · time data using nonlinear least squares regression. After the mathematic model is selected, it is possible to generate the important pharmacokinetic parameters that describe the disposition of a specific anticancer drug within the body. Besides the determination of the terminal-phase plasma half-life (i.e., half-life related to the second or third phase of biphasic or triphasic plasma concentration · time data), the area under the plasma disappearance curve ($AUC_0\infty$) and total body plasma clearance (Cl_T) are the most significant and clinically useful pharmacokinetic parameters. The relationship between AUC and clearance is simplified to dose = clearance × area.

Although the height of an anticancer drug's peak plasma level (C_{max}) generally correlates with peak dose and the degree of toxicity, the drug's plasma AUC tends to correlate better with its ultimate antitumor activity and normal tissue side effects. For example, when identical doses of melphalan are administered first orally and then intravenously at a 1-month interval, because of its poor oral availability, the melphalan plasma AUC after the oral dose would be only one third of that after the intravenous dose (Fig. 16.1). As would be anticipated, the equivalent intravenous dose of melphalan was associated with a twofold to threefold deeper nadir in granulocytes and a greater than twofold increase in objective response rates in various cancer types (e.g., myeloma).

The plasma AUC (in mg/mL · hour) can be estimated through the use of a pharmacokinetic model or measured directly by plotting the drug's plasma concentrations against time on semilogarithmic graph paper. Then, it is possible to calculate the

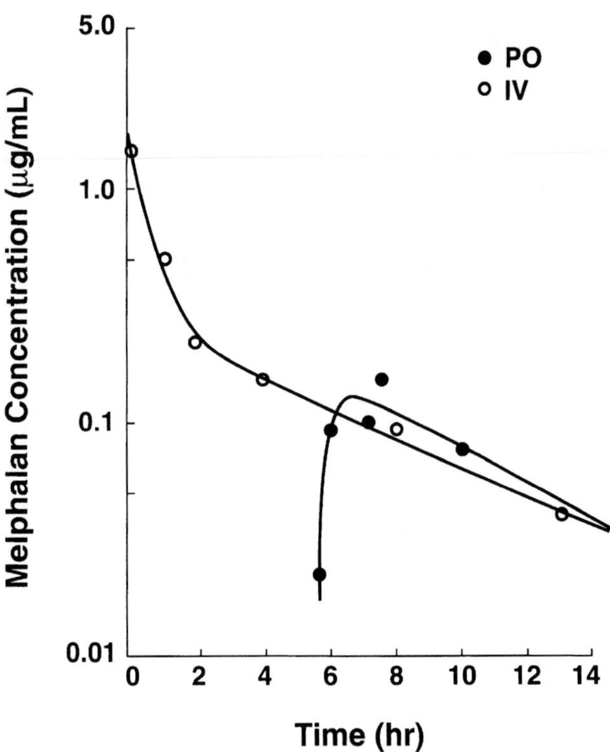

FIGURE 16.1. Plasma disappearance curves for intravenous and oral (tablets) melphalan (0.6 mg/kg) in a patient with ovarian cancer. The melphalan plasma AUC associated with the bolus oral dose was only one third of that associated with the intravenous dose. *Source:* Reprinted with permission from Alberts DS, Chang SY, Chen HS, et al. Oral melphalan kinetics. *Clin Pharmacol Ther* 1979;26:737–745.

areas of successive trapezoids under the concentration · time curve wherein the upper surface of the trapezoid is a line that connects two successive plasma concentration data points. By convention, when the plasma AUC is measured in this way, the terminal part of the AUC is calculated using a triangular area, rather than a trapezoid.

After the plasma AUC has been determined, it is possible to derive the anticancer drug's total body clearance rate based on the following formula: Cl_T = dose (mg)/AUC (mg/mL · hour). The resulting Cl_T is measured in units of milliliters or liters per minutes or hours, sometimes with normalization to the body surface area. The total body clearance of an anticancer drug depends on the drug's dose and plasma AUC and represents the rate at which the drug is eliminated from the entire body. The drug's total body clearance is made up of the combination of renal clearance (Cl_R) plus nonrenal clearance (Cl_{NR}). The renal clearance of a drug can be calculated by the following equation: $Cl_R = Ae_c/AUC$, where Ae_c is the total amount of the unchanged drug that is excreted in the urine. For many drugs that are glomerularly filtered but not reabsorbed, renal clearance is proportional to creatinine clearance. In a patient with severe renal impairment, if nonrenal clearance is unaltered, the total body clearance of the drug is diminished significantly. This phenomenon is observed in patients with relatively severe renal impairment who receive drugs like methotrexate and carboplatin, both of which are eliminated mainly through renal excretion.

Volume of Distribution

The volume of distribution (Vd) of an anticancer drug is another important pharmacokinetic parameter that relates the drug plasma concentration (measured at the time of administration through extrapolation of the terminal phase of the concentration · time curve to 0 time) to the total amount of drug in the body. Thus, Vd_{area} represents the volume of distribution of a drug in the terminal phase of its elimination from the body and in its simplest form, Vd = amount of drug in the body ÷ plasma concentration. Since drug levels are typically measured only in the plasma compartment and not in tissues, most reported Vd values represent the "apparent" Vd of the drug in the plasma. Thus, these Vd values represent a theoretic plasma volume that would account for the drug's plasma levels after administration. The volume of distribution in the terminal phase can be derived using the following equation: Vd_{area} = dose/AUC · slope (λ_z), where λ_z is the rate constant in the terminal phase of a biphasic or triphasic elimination curve.

Linear and Nonlinear Kinetics

Most drugs exhibit linear pharmacokinetics, which in its simplest configuration means that the C_{max} and AUC are proportionate to the dose, and the $T_{1/2}$ Vd and clearance are constant, that is, they do not change with the dose. Linearity helps make predictions about the effects of changes in doses since the AUC (and the biological effects) of the drug should change in proportion to the dose. Drugs with nonlinear pharmacokinetics such as aspirin, ethanol, and phenytoin have saturable elimination patterns. This means that small dose changes can disproportionately increase the AUC and the drug's biologic effects. Drugs with nonlinear pharmacokinetic patterns may therefore have longer $T_{1/2}$s and much lower clearance values when the dose is increased.

As discussed by Collins and Dedrick (2), there are at least two explanations for nonlinear kinetics. First, nonlinearity may be caused by changes in drug excretion at high doses. For example, at extremely high doses of methotrexate (i.e., 7 to 8 g/m^2), the drug load outstrips renal tubular secretion capacity. Second, nonlinearity may be observed for drugs that depend almost completely on elimination through a specific degradative enzyme system (e.g., antimetabolites). Drugs like cytarabine and 5-fluorouracil administered in high doses may overcome the capacity of their respective degradative enzymes with a resultant decrease in their total body clearance rates and an increase in plasma levels that are more than proportionate to their doses.

Intraperitoneal Drug Pharmacokinetics

Intraperitoneal drug administration has become an increasingly important therapeutic strategy in the management of patients with advanced ovarian cancer who have minimal residual intraperitoneal disease after primary or secondary exploratory laparotomies. Three large phase 3 trials in the Gynecologic Oncology Group (GOG) and the Southwest Oncology Group (GOG-104/SWOG-8501, GOG-114, and GOG-172) comparing various cisplatin-based combination chemotherapeutic regimens administered intravenously (IV) or intraperitoneally (IP) have documented significant survival advantages for the intraperitoneal cisplatin treatment arms (3–5). Most recently, in GOG-172, an intraperitoneal regimen (intravenous paclitaxel on day 1, intraperitoneal cisplatin on day 2, and intraperitoneal paclitaxel on day 8) was associated with a 25% reduction in the risk of death as compared to the intravenously administered regimen (intravenous paclitaxel plus cisplatin) ($p = 0.03$) (4). A meta-analysis of IP cisplatin-based randomized trials found that both overall and progression-free survival were significantly improved with IP regimens ($p = 0.0007$ and $p = 0.001$, respectively) (6).

Despite the superior activity of this intravenous paclitaxel/intraperitoneal cisplain-paclitaxel regimen evaluated in GOG-172, there was significantly more hematologic, gastrointestinal, metabolic, and neurologic toxicity in comparison to intravenous paclitaxel and cisplatin (7); however, the dose of cisplatin on the IP arm was 33% higher than on the IV arm. When combining the toxicity data across intraperitoneal randomized trials, only acute gastrointestinal toxicity ($p = 0.01$) and fever ($p = 0.04$) are significantly higher among patients treated IP, and ototoxicity is significantly higher among patients receiving IV treatment as compared to those receiving IP therapy ($p = 0.004$) (6). A study of patient quality of life within GOG-172 demonstrated that patient quality of life was significantly lower during IP treatment as compared to IV therapy, but 1 year after treatment, the overall quality of life of patients receiving IP or IV therapy was equivalent (8). However, long-term neurotoxicity remained higher among patients treated IP. These short- and long-term effects should be balanced against the documented 16-month improvement in survival as compared with intravenous cisplatin/paclitaxel ($p = 0.03$) (7). This increase in survival is similar to that which was achieved when intravenous cisplatin was initially added to primary combination chemotherapeutic regimens for the treatment of this disease (9).

The incremental increase in cisplatin efficacy associated with intraperitoneal administration likely results from the delivery of approximately 20-fold greater concentrations of cisplatin into the intraperitoneal space than are achievable with intravenous administration. Anticancer drugs with known activity against ovarian cancer that undergo slow clearance from the intraperitoneal space into the systemic circulation without causing significant chemical peritonitis are the favored intraperitoneal compounds. Clearly, paclitaxel falls into this category. Intraperitoneal administration of this large taxane molecule results in 1,000-fold greater concentration · time products in the intraperitoneal space than is achievable with intravenous administration (10). In contrast, cisplatin undergoes rapid clearance from the systemic circulation after administration by the intraperitoneal route. Caution must be taken when considering other agents for research-based intraperitoneal administration, as some cytotoxic agents have not demonstrated efficacy and have been associated with excessive toxicity when given IP (e.g., mitoxantrone, doxorubicin) (11–14).

As with intravenous administration of anticancer drugs, the drug clearance rate from the intraperitoneal space is the most useful pharmacokinetic parameter for comparing drugs that are administered by the intraperitoneal route in the treatment of ovarian cancer. The peritoneal clearance rate can be calculated by dividing the drug dose by its intraperitoneal concentration · time product, which must be measured with repeated intraperitoneal fluid content sampling. Intraperitoneal drugs with slow clearance rates are favored because they result in prolonged exposure of the intraperitoneal tumor bed to high concentrations of anticancer drug. It is also possible to assess the pharmacokinetic characteristics of drug doses by comparing their peak intraperitoneal concentration with peak plasma concentration after intraperitoneal dosing or comparing their intraperitoneal concentration · time product (AUC_{IP}), with their plasma concentration · time products (AUC_{IV}) after intraperitoneal dosing. Virtually all commonly used drugs administered intraperitoneally in patients with ovarian cancer have peak or concentration · time product ratios of more than 20. In some cases, the peritoneal exposures can be much greater. For example, paclitaxel intraperitoneal exposure with IP therapy is 300 to nearly 3,000 times greater than with IV treatment (15).

Except for drugs whose cytotoxicity depends on continuous exposure, such as cytarabine and methotrexate, drugs used by the intraperitoneal route should be administered relatively rapidly in at least 2 L of peritoneal dialysate and remain within the peritoneal space without removal. For schedule-independent drugs, it is important to maintain high concentrations as long as possible within the intraperitoneal space to improve efficacy. It is of considerable interest that as the intraperitoneal dialysate volume decreases, a drug's intraperitoneal clearance rate increases rapidly. Thus, large volumes of intraperitoneal fluid increase the chances for uniform drug distribution throughout the intraperitoneal space and optimize the intraperitoneal clearance rates. Generally, it is suggested to administer the IP drug dose in the first liter of peritoneal dialysate, followed by a second liter of dialysate to the point of mild abdominal discomfort.

Ultimately, the effectiveness of intraperitoneal therapy depends on the inherent cytotoxic potency of the individual agent and its ability to penetrate from the outer surface to the inner core of intraperitoneal tumors. The degree of tumor penetration depends on the molecular weight, charge, and chemical structure of the compound. There is an inverse relationship between molecular weight and tumor penetration. The higher the molecular weight of the anticancer drug, the lower the degree of the tumor penetration. Indeed, one advantage of cisplatin over carboplatin as an intraperitoneal agent is its lower molecular weight. Los et al. (14) have demonstrated in intraperitoneal ovarian cancer animal studies that it requires almost 10 times more intraperitoneal carboplatin than cisplatin to achieve similar intratumoral concentrations; however, there is renewed interest to develop intraperitoneal carboplatin plus intraperitoneal and intravenous paclitaxel regimens to reduce the potential for cisplatin-paclitaxel–induced peripheral neuropathy (see Special Applications, in the Carboplatin section below).

CLINICAL PHARMACOLOGY OF ACTIVE DRUGS AGAINST GYNECOLOGIC CANCERS

We discuss below in alphabetical order the clinical pharmacology of cytotoxic, biologic/molecularly targeted, and modulating/supportive care drugs with demonstrated activity against gynecologic cancers. We also include several Food and Drug Administration (FDA)-approved drugs for other indications that may prove active against gynecologic cancers.

Cytotoxic Agents

Albumin-Bound Paclitaxel

Chemistry. Albumin-bound paclitaxel (Abraxane, ABI-007) is a protein-bound form of paclitaxel that measures approximately 130 nanometers. Each vial of albumin-bound paclitaxel contains 100 mg of paclitaxel and 900 mg of human albumin. The chemical name of paclitaxel is 5β, 20-epoxy-1, 2α,4,7β,10β,13α-hexahydroxytax-11-en-9-one 4,10-diacetate 2-benzoate 13-ester with (2*R*,3*S*)-*N*-benzoyl-3-phenylisoserine and the empirical formula and molecular weight are $C_{47}H_{51}NO_{14}$ and 853.91, respectively. Albumin-bound paclitaxel is FDA approved for the treatment of breast cancer after failure of treatment for metastatic disease or recurrence within 6 months of adjuvant chemotherapy. Phase 3 trials have demonstrated superior efficacy to castor oil–based paclitaxel and a more favorable toxicity profile (16). Clinical trials in gynecologic cancer (e.g., ovarian and cervical cancer) are ongoing. Please refer to the Paclitaxel section for details on the mechanism of action of this agent.

Drug Disposition. According to the Abraxane package insert, comparison studies of the clearance of albumin-bound paclitaxel (260 mg/m^2 over 30 minutes) was larger (43%) than for the clearance of paclitaxel injection (175 mg/m^2 over 3 hours) and the volume of distribution of the albumin-bound form was 53% higher; however, there was no difference in the terminal half-life of the active agent.

Administration and Dosage. The recommended dosage of albumin-bound paclitaxel is 260 mg/m^2 IV over 30 minutes every 3 weeks. No premedication to prevent hypersensitivity reactions is needed. Albumin-bound paclitaxel should be carefully reconstituted following the manufacturer instructions. Each mL of the reconstituted formulation will contain 5 mg/mL paclitaxel. The exact total dosing volume of 5 mg/mL for the patient should be calculated using the following formula: total dose (mg) ÷ 5 (mg/mL). Reconstituted agent should be used immediately, but can be refrigerated for up to 8 hours. If precipitates are observed, the solution should be discarded.

Side Effects and Toxicities. Neutropenia and sensory neuropathy are dose dependent. In drug approval studies, grade 4 neutropenia occurred among approximately 9% of patients, as compared to 22% of patients receiving 175 mg/m^2 paclitaxel. Infection (generally oral candidiasis and respiratory system events) occurred in approximately 23% of patients receiving albumin-bound paclitaxel. Anemia occurred among 33% of patients (severe anemia in 1% of cases). Severe cardiotoxicity occurred in approximately 3% of patients. Dyspnea (12%) and cough (6%) were also reported among patients receiving albumin-bound paclitaxel. Patients with neutrophil counts of less than 1,500 cells/mm^3 should not receive albumin-bound paclitaxel, as it may lead to bone marrow suppression, which can result in infection.

Altretamine

Chemistry. Altretamine (hexamethylmelamine, Hexalen), a synthetic cytotoxic antineoplastic s-triazine derivative, has FDA approval for treatment of persistent or recurrent ovarian cancer after first-line chemotherapy with cisplatin or other alkylating agents. The drug also exhibits antitumor activity against breast cancer, lymphomas, small cell carcinoma of the lung, and endometrial and cervical cancer. The empiric formula of altretamine is $C_9H_{18}N_6$ (molecular weight = 210.28).

Mechanism of Action. The mechanism of action of altretamine is not completely elucidated. Although it bears structural similarity to and cross reactivity with triethylene-melamine, a classic alkylating agent, evidence demonstrating altretamine to be an alkylating agent is inconclusive. Altretamine does not consistently demonstrate cross resistance with classic alkylating agents used in rodent tumors or in human cancer treatment, but its clinical antitumor spectrum resembles that of an alkylating agent. Altretamine is inactive against most common murine and human tumor cell lines *in vitro*. Rutty and Connors (17,18) presented definitive evidence that metabolic activation of altretamine is necessary for its cytotoxic activity. It is extensively demethylated *in vivo* in the presence of liver enzymes and these N-methylolmelamine derivatives are more cytotoxic than the parent compound (18). Additional studies have shown that the reactive methyl intermediates, formed during altretamine N-demethylations, covalently bind to tissue macromolecules, including DNA, and that the cytotoxicity against certain human solid tumor cells *in vitro* is dependent on the metabolic formation of the reactive intermediates or their direct addition to cell culture incubate (17).

Drug Disposition. Altretamine is practically insoluble in water and, therefore, it has only been administered orally in clinical studies, precluding absolute bioavailability studies. After administration of altretamine to laboratory animals by any route, urinary recovery of parent drug was very low (<1%), and urinary recovery of total dose or total radioactivity after administration of ^{14}C-labeled drug was as high as 90%. Ames et al. (19) determined that the bioavailability of the parent compound in rabbits after oral administration was 25% of that obtained after intravenous administration. Moreover, after giving the rabbits labeled altretamine by stomach tube, 85% of labeled drug equivalents was recovered in the urine. The high rate of recovery suggests efficient gastrointestinal absorption.

The urinary recovery and bioavailability data demonstrate that altretamine is well absorbed after oral administration and that the drug is extensively metabolized regardless of route of administration. The low bioavailability of intact altretamine is due to first-pass metabolism rather than to poor absorption.

After oral administration in doses of 120 to 300 mg/m^2, peak plasma levels, measured by gas chromatographic assay, from 0.2 to 20.8 mg/L are reached between 0.5 and 3.0 hours. The terminal-phase plasma half-life ranges from 4.7 to 10.2 hours (20). The interpatient variability of AUCs, ranging from 1.2 to 60.1 mg/L · hour, is most likely due to the differences in the rate at which the drug is metabolized.

Administration and Dosage. The recommended dose for altretamine as a single agent for use in the palliative treatment of patients with ovarian cancer is 260 mg/m^2/day, orally, for 14 to 21 consecutive days in a 28-day cycle (21). The total daily doses should be given as four divided oral doses after meals and at bedtime. Compliance to this regimen in a small group of patients with relapsed ovarian cancer has been documented to be over 95% (22). There is no pharmacokinetic information on this dosing regimen and the effect of food on altretamine bioavailability in humans. In combination regimens, altretamine is typically used at a dose of 150 mg/m^2/day for 7 to 14 days of monthly cycles (23).

Altretamine should be temporarily discontinued for 14 days or longer and subsequently restarted with a 20% to 25% dose reduction for any of the following side effects: gastrointestinal intolerance unresponsive to symptomatic measures; leukocyte count less than 2,000/mm^3 or granulocyte count less than 1,000/mm^3; platelet count less than 75,000/mm^3; or progressive neurotoxicity. If neurologic symptoms fail to stabilize on the reduced-dose schedule, altretamine should be discontinued.

Side Effects and Toxicities. Altretamine is administered at a dose of 260 mg/m^2 (single agent) or 150 mg/m^2 (in combination) on an intermittent schedule and is relatively well tolerated. Single-agent data for this drug are available for 1,014 patients (24). With high, continuous daily dosing, nausea and vomiting were the dose-limiting toxic effects, and a form of reversible peripheral neurotoxicity occurred occasionally. Myelosuppression was mild to moderate. Leukocyte and platelet counts usually recovered within 1 week of therapy discontinuation.

In a study of 395 patients with advanced ovarian cancer treated with altretamine-containing combination regimens with or without cisplatin, no additional effect of altretamine on the incidence or severity of neurotoxicity could be demonstrated (25). Peripheral neuropathy and central nervous system symptoms are more likely to occur in patients receiving continuous, high-dose daily altretamine administered on an intermittent schedule than in those receiving moderate doses. Neurologic toxicity reverses after the drug is discontinued. Pyridoxine should not be used concomitantly with altretamine to reduce neurotoxicity because clinical trials data suggest it may inhibit cytotoxic activity. Concurrent administration of altretamine and antidepressants of the monoamine oxidase (MAO) inhibitor class may cause severe orthostatic hypotension. Cimetidine, an inhibitor of microsomal drug metabolism, increased altretamine's half-life and toxicity in a rat model.

In two phase 2 studies of single-agent altretamine, at a dose of 260 mg/m^2 for 14 to 21 days of each monthly cycle, the most common toxicity was grade 2 to 3 nausea (23%) (26,27). In a consolidation therapy phase 2 trial, only three patients (4%) experienced any grade 4 toxicity: granulocytopenia (two patients) and anxiety/depression (one patient). The most common grade 3 toxicities were malaise, fatigue, or lethargy in seven patients (7%) and nausea in six patients (6%). Aside from these, there were no other grade 3 or 4 toxicities that occurred in more than 5% of patients (27).

With continuous high-dose daily drug administration, nausea and vomiting of gradual onset occur frequently. Although in most instances these symptoms are controllable with antiemetics, the severity sometimes requires altretamine dose reduction or, rarely, discontinuation.

Data from three large clinical trials demonstrated that altretamine can be added to full therapeutic doses of cyclophosphamide, doxorubicin, and cisplatin (CHAP) without evidence of increased hematologic toxicity (28–30). Leukopenia below 3,000 cells/mm^3 occurred in fewer than 15% of the patients on a variety of intermittent- or continuous-dose altretamine regimens. Fewer than 1% had leukopenia below 1,000 cells/mm^3. When given in high doses over a 21-day course, nadirs of leukocyte and platelet counts were reached by 3 to 4 weeks, and normal counts were observed by 6 weeks. With continuous administration, nadirs are reached in 6 to 8 weeks.

Bleomycin

Chemistry. Bleomycin (Blenoxane), an antineoplastic, is a mixture of complex glycopeptides originally isolated from a strain of the fungus *Streptomyces verticillus*. The primary components are bleomycins A_2 and B_2. The family of bleomycin glycopeptides has a relatively high molecular weight and is quantitated in units of cytotoxic activity (i.e., roughly 1 U/1 mg of polypeptide protein). Bleomycin is used as palliative treatment in patients with advanced cervical (31) and vulvar cancers. Other clinical indications include squamous cell carcinomas of the head and neck, lymphomas, and testicular carcinoma. The molecular formula of bleomycin A_2 is $C_{55}H_{84}N_{17}O_{21}S_3$ (molecular weight = 1,414) and the molecular formula of bleomycin B_2 is $C_{55}H_{84}N_{20}O_{21}S_2$ (molecular weight = 1,425).

Mechanism of Action. Although the exact mechanism of action is unknown, a key to its activity is the isolation of native compounds from *S. verticillus* as coordinated Cu(II) complexes, which are inactive as antitumor agents. When complexed with ferrous iron, bleomycin becomes a potent oxidase, producing DNA strand breaks by oxygen free radicals. Its unique mechanism of action is schedule dependent and cell cycle dependent for the G_2 phase.

The oxygen radicals produced by the bleomycin-iron complex bound to DNA primarily cause single-strand breaks and a lesser degree of double-strand breaks. There is a subsequent release of base propenals of all four DNA bases: guanine, thymine, adenine, and cytosine. These modified free bases result from cleavage of the deoxyribose sugar at the 3′-4′ bond. There is an apparent specificity for the release of thymine and for DNA binding at guanine-rich sequences in actively transcribed genes (32). The linker regions of DNA between nucleosomes comprise an important site for specific strand cleavage by bleomycin (33). Several mechanisms have been theorized to explain the development of resistance to bleomycin. Less important mechanisms appear to include DNA repair, membrane alterations, and decreased drug accumulation. The primary mechanism probably involves metabolic inactivation of bleomycin by a cytosolic hydrolase, which is in the cysteine proteinase family. The enzyme inactivates bleomycin by replacing a terminal amine with a hydroxyl group. The distribution of bleomycin hydrolase appears to explain some of the relative resistance and sensitivity to bleomycin in normal tissues. Normal tissues with high intrinsic hydrolase activities, such as the liver, spleen, intestine, and bone marrow, are not targets for bleomycin's toxic effects. In contrast, lung tissues and skin have low levels of hydrolase activity and are particularly susceptible to bleomycin-induced toxicity. However, there appears to be no direct correlation between hydroxylase levels in tumor cells and bleomycin-induced cytotoxicity (33). The development of other methods of bleomycin metabolism by tumor cells may be responsible for the emergence of drug resistance (34).

Drug Disposition. Bleomycin is eliminated predominantly by urinary excretion. This accounts for 45% to 62% of a dose after 24 hours. In the blood, the drug is rapidly cleared, and two phases of elimination are apparent. As a practical point, this means that over 95% of a dose has been completely eliminated by 24 hours (about six half-lives) (35). If administered by an intracavitary route, a large percentage of a bleomycin dose is absorbed, and the fractional systemic bioavailability is about 45% for intrapleural or intraperitoneal injections. The drug appears to efflux more slowly from the peritoneal cavity. This suggests that there is significantly greater local drug retention in the intraperitoneal space. This may explain some of the drug's unique efficacy by intracavitary administration (36). An increased exposure to drug in these local compartments is also reflected by the tenfold higher drug levels achieved with intraperitoneal or intrapleural therapy than with equivalent intravenous dosing.

Renal insufficiency markedly alters bleomycin elimination (37). This effect becomes most pronounced in patients with creatinine clearance values less than 25 to 35 mL/min (37). In these patients, the volume of distribution is unaltered at about 20 L, but the half-life varies as the inverse exponent of creatinine clearance. Thus, significant bleomycin dose reductions are required in all patients with reduced renal function.

Dosage. Bleomycin (in combination with cisplatin and etoposide or vinblastine) is used most commonly by bolus intravenous administration at dosages of as high as 30 mg/week for up to 12 weeks in the treatment of patients with germ cell tumors of the ovary. These 30-mg doses often are associated with delayed febrile episodes that can be inhibited successfully with a morning dose of dexamethasone or prednisone.

Bleomycin continues to be used commonly by continuous intravenous infusion at dosages of 10 mg/m^2/day for 4 consecutive days, with courses repeated every 4 weeks. This schedule has been proven to be successful in the treatment of women with metastatic cervical cancer. Total bleomycin doses should usually not exceed 400 mg to avoid serious pulmonary toxicity.

Bleomycin can also be administered by the intramuscular route in doses of 15 to 30 mg. Absorption appears to be complete, and because of its lack of vesicant activity, the intramuscular route has been proven to be extremely safe (38).

Side Effects and Toxicities. Bleomycin's dose-limiting side effect is pulmonary toxicity, which occurs in approximately 10% of treated patients and in rare instances can result in death. The likelihood of lung damage increases with advanced age, chest irradiation (39), hyperoxia during surgical anesthesia (40), renal insufficiency, and cumulative doses greater than 400 U. However, pulmonary toxicity is variable and may occur in younger patients following low cumulative doses. Bleomycin-induced lung damage presents as pneumonitis with dry cough, dyspnea, and rales and may progress within weeks to pulmonary fibrosis. Bleomycin should be discontinued at the first clinical signs of lung toxicity. Acute pneumonitis is often responsive to corticosteroid therapy; however, there is no effective therapy for the chronic pulmonary fibrosis that may result from bleomycin therapy (41). Evidence from preclinical models of bleomycin-induced pulmonary thrombosis has documented that pretreatment with amifostine can abrogate this dose-limiting toxicity (42,43).

Bleomycin is nonmyelosuppressive (a factor that facilitates its use in combination chemotherapeutic regimens). Mucocutaneous toxicities, including mucositis, are the primary acute side effects of bleomycin. Manifestations of cutaneous reactions include hyperpigmentation, erythema, rash, striae, pruritus, thickening of the nail beds, and, in rare instances, scleroderma (44). Fever, chills, and alopecia are common. Mild nausea, vomiting, and anorexia may also occur, but are typically self-limiting. Infrequent side effects include headache, pain at tumor site, and anaphylactoid reactions. An idiosyncratic reaction consisting primarily of mucositis and skin rash has also been reported (45).

Special Precautions. Bleomycin should be used with extreme caution in patients with significant renal impairment or compromised pulmonary function; frequent radiographs are recommended. Because up to 70% of a bleomycin dose is eliminated by renal excretion, the bleomycin dose should be reduced for individuals with severe renal insufficiency. Unfortunately, there are no prospectively evaluated dosing nomograms for bleomycin dose adjustment. An empiric dose-adjustment formula has been described (37). The percentage dose reductions that are indicated by applying this formula to a "normal" creatinine clearance (CrCl) of 120 mL/min and a fractional urinary drug excretion of 0.45 are CrCl >35 mL/min, no dose reduction required; CrCl = 20 mL/min, 50% dose reduction; CrCl = 15 mL/min, 52% dose reduction; CrCl = 10 mL/min, 55% dose reduction; and CrCl = 5 mL/min, 60% dose reduction. This is only a general guide, and it has not been clinically validated in a prospective study or retrospective analysis. Patients over 65 years of age may be at increased risk of developing orthostatic hypotension, especially when the recommended rate of intravenous infusion is exceeded.

Drug Interactions. Nephrotoxic drugs may significantly reduce the rate of bleomycin clearance and thus increase toxicity. Yee et al. (46) observed markedly reduced bleomycin clearance in children who had received six courses of a regimen including cisplatin (cumulative dose 300 mg/m^2). In another case report, fatal bleomycin pulmonary toxicity occurred in a patient with cisplatin-induced acute renal failure (47). Similar toxic interactions should be anticipated for combinations of bleomycin with other nephrotoxic drugs, such as aminoglycosides, amphotericin, or cyclosporine.

Special Applications. Because of its nonvesicant nature, bleomycin has been administered by a number of nonvascular routes, including intramuscular (38), subcutaneous (48), and, most significantly, intrapleurally for the management of malignant effusions. When compared with tetracycline, intrapleurally administered bleomycin, 60 to 120 U, had greater therapeutic benefit for the management of malignant pleural effusions (36). When compared with tetracycline, intrapleurally administered bleomycin 60 to 120 U had greater therapeutic benefit as evidenced by a longer time to effusion recurrence (46 vs. 32 days, $p = 0.037$) and a lower 3-month effusion recurrence rate (30% vs. 53%, $p = 0.047$). Because toxicities were similar for both therapies, bleomycin was selected as the preferred intrapleurally administered therapy for malignant pleural effusions.

Capecitabine

Chemistry. Capecitabine (Xeloda) is an orally administered antineoplastic agent. In patients with metastatic breast cancer, capecitabine in combination with docetaxel is indicated after failure of prior anthracycline-containing chemotherapy, and monotherapy is indicated for those who are resistant to paclitaxel and are resistant to anthracycline-containing chemotherapy (or further anthracycline-containing chemotherapy is not indicated). Capecitabine is a fluoropyrimidine carbamate prodrug form of 5′-deoxy-5-fluorouridine (5′-DFUR) that is enzymatically converted to 5-fluorouracil (5-FU) *in vivo*. Its chemical name is 5′-deoxy-5-fluoro-N-[(pentyloxy) carbonyl]-cytidine and its molecular weight is 359.35.

Mechanism of Action. Capecitabine itself is inactive, but after absorption in the gastrointestinal tract is metabolized to 5-FU by three enzymes: carboxylesterase, which converts capecitabine to 5′-deoxy-5-fluorocytidine in the liver; cytidine deaminase in the liver and tumor tissue, which converts it to 5′-deoxy-5-fluorouridine; and thymidine phosphorylase, which in many cases is highly expressed in tumors, completes the final step of conversion to 5-FU. Theoretically, capecitabine therapy is likely to be most effective in patients with tumors that express high concentrations of thymidine phosphorylase (resulting in greater 5-FU being generated in the tumor) and low concentrations of dihydropyrimidine dehydrogenase (which rapidly breaks down 5-FU) (49). 5-FU acts as a false pyrimidine or antimetabolite ultimately to inhibit the formation of the DNA-specific nucleoside base thymidine. The metabolites of 5-FU, 5-fluoro-21-deoxyuridine-5′-monophosphate (FdUMP) and 5-fluorouridine triphosphate (FUTP), inhibit thymidylate synthase (FdUMP) and are incorporated into cellular RNA (FUTP). DNA synthesis and function are inhibited by the incorporation of FdUMP into cellular DNA (50).

Drug Disposition. After oral administration, capecitabine reaches peak blood levels in about 1.5 hours, and peak 5-FU levels are reached at about 2 hours. Food reduces the rate and extent of absorption for both capecitabine and 5-FU. Plasma protein binding is not dose dependent and is less than 60% for capecitabine and its metabolites. Capecitabine (95.5% of administered dose) and its metabolites are excreted in urine. Capecitabine has no effect on the pharmacokinetics of docetaxel or vice versa. The precise pharmacokinetics of capecitabine have been difficult to establish, which is thought to be due to the large interindividual and intraindividual variation in expression of the enzyme dihydropyrimidine dehydrogenase (44).

Administration and Dosage. Capecitabine is available as 150- and 500-mg tablets for oral use. The recommended dose is 2,500 mg/m^2 daily to be administered as two doses: 1,250 mg/m^2 in the morning and 1,250 mg/m^2 in the evening for 2 weeks followed by a 1-week rest (21-day cycle). Because of the high rate of grade 2 or greater capecitabine-induced palmar-plantar erythrodysesthesia (PPE), recommendations have been made to reduce the starting dose to 2,000 mg/m^2 daily. It should be taken with water within 30 minutes after a meal. The same dosage of capecitabine should be used when combined with docetaxel, which should be administered at 75 mg/m^2 as a 1-hour infusion on day 1 of the 21-day cycle. Premedication (per docetaxel labeling) should be started prior to docetaxel administration for patients receiving the combination therapy.

Side Effects and Toxicities. The only side effect that occurs more frequently with capecitabine than with intravenous 5-FU is PPE (15% to 20% of patients). The other more common side effects of capecitabine include diarrhea (40%) and nausea and vomiting (30% to 40%). Grade 3 hyperbilirubinemia occurred in 15.2% and grade 4 in 3.9% of patients in the clinical safety database of Xeloda. Of those patients experiencing grades 3 and 4 hyperbilirubinemia, many (64% and 71%, respectively) had liver metastases at baseline, and 57.5% and 35.5% had elevations in alkaline phosphatase or transaminases, respectively. Other less common side effects include myelosuppression (less frequent than with IV 5-FU), leukopenia, and cardiotoxicity. In general, capecitabine is relatively well tolerated.

Special Precautions. Because capecitabine is administered orally, patients should be informed how to monitor their toxicity symptoms and be instructed to maintain the prescribed dosing regimen. Capecitabine has been shown to alter coagulation parameters in patients undergoing treatment concomitantly with coumarin-derivative anticoagulants (e.g., warfarin) (49). Therefore, patients taking oral coumarin-derivative anticoagulant therapy should be monitored regularly with regard to coagulation parameters (international normalized ratio or prothrombin time). Patients over the age of 80 years and those with mild to moderate liver dysfunction should also be closely monitored.

Carboplatin

Chemistry. Carboplatin (Paraplatin) is an alkylating agent that is approved by the FDA for the treatment of patients with advanced ovarian cancer of epithelial origin. It is also active against metastatic endometrial and cervical cancer. Carboplatin has a molecular formula of $C_6H_{12}N_2O_7Pt$ and a molecular weight of 371.25. Its chemical name is platinum, diammine[1,1-cyclobutane-dicarboxylato(2-)0,0′]-,(SP-4-2). The water solubility of carboplatin (14 mg/mL) is approximately 10 times that of cisplatin.

Mechanism of Action. Carboplatin, like cisplatin, produces an equal number of predominantly interstrand DNA cross links rather than DNA-protein cross links, causing equivalent lesions and biologic effects. The differences in potencies appear to be related to the aquation rate, which is 14 mg/mL for carboplatin, as compared to 1 mg/mL for cisplatin. It covalently binds to DNA with preferential binding to the N-7 position of guanine and adenine (50). Like cisplatin, carboplatin must first undergo sequential losses of the nonamine carboxylato ligands. Although this process proceeds readily with the loss of the chlorides in cisplatin, the rate of leaving or "opening" of the carboxylato moieties in carboplatin is much slower (51). The molar potency of carboplatin in creating DNA lesions and cytotoxicity was observed to be roughly 2% of cisplatin *in vitro* and 25% to 33% of cisplatin *in vivo* (52,53). A more striking difference is the markedly delayed onset of peak cross linking for carboplatin compared with cisplatin. With carboplatin, maximal DNA cross linking occurs 18 hours after exposure compared with 6 to 12 hours for cisplatin (53). In addition, carboplatin-induced DNA cross links appear to have a slower rate of resolution than cisplatin-induced cross links. This slower onset and offset of carboplatin cross linking is believed to be a direct result of a slow rate of monofunctional adduct formation or a slower rate of conversion of monoadducts to cross links. Despite the pharmacokinetic differences between carboplatin and cisplatin, phase 3 studies and meta-analyses of clinical studies reveal equivalent activity between carboplatin and cisplatin in all prognostic subgroups of ovarian cancer patients (54,55).

Harrap (56) described nuclear protein phosphorylation after treatment with both cisplatin and carboplatin. These events appear to correlate with cell killing (57). Carboplatin reacts with two sites on DNA to produce cross links, as has been observed with cisplatin (58). The formation of DNA adducts results in the inhibition of DNA synthesis and function and inhibits transcription (50). These lesions involve a bifunctional platinum adduct to a single-strand DNA. This may produce transcriptional miscoding and an inhibition of DNA synthesis. It is possible that the cytotoxic effects of carboplatin are the result of binding to nuclear and cytoplasmic proteins. Carboplatin-induced cytotoxicity is not cell cycle phase specific, but it can be maximized by exposing cells in S phase to the drug.

Drug Disposition. The pharmacokinetics of carboplatin differ significantly from those of cisplatin. Table 16.1 shows that the plasma clearance of carboplatin is biphasic and slower than that of cisplatin, with a much higher percentage of drug being excreted in the urine. Unlike cisplatin, relatively little carboplatin is bound to plasma proteins. The major route of elimination of carboplatin is glomerular filtration and tubular secretion. There is little or no true metabolism of the drug. The carboxylato bonds in carboplatin are slowly hydrolyzed to yield transient aquated intermediates. These activated platinum species are believed to lead directly to irreversible adducts to DNA or protein. Overall, the rate of hydrolysis of carboplatin is significantly slower than that of cisplatin, leading to much slower reactivity with DNA (59). Because as much as 65% of a carboplatin dose is excreted in the urine, significant dose adjustments are recommended for patients with creatinine clearance values less than 60 mL/min.

TABLE 16.1

CARBOPLATIN PHARMACOKINETICS

Cumulative 24-hour urinary excretion	**65% (if creatinine clearance >60 mL/min)**
In vitro half-life (H_2O)	~24 hours
Plasma half-life	
β-phase (free drug)	180 minutes
Protein-bound drug	>5 days
Volume of distribution	1,620 L
Protein binding	30% (slow equilibration)

Carboplatin is widely distributed in body fluids and achieves good penetration into pleural effusions and ascites fluid (60). Pharmacokinetic studies in patients receiving continuous carboplatin infusions show that, although total platinum levels increase over the course of the infusion, free or active platinum levels can decrease from 78% on day 1 to 38% on day 4 of a 4-day infusion.

Administration and Dosage. Carboplatin is usually administered as a brief infusion over 15 minutes or longer in a solution of 0.9% sodium chloride or 5% dextrose in water. The drug is typically diluted in 500 mL of fluid and infused IV over 15 to 30 minutes to 1 hour without further hydration (61). Carboplatin has also been administered as a continuous 24-hour IV infusion for 1, 4, or 5 days, or as a continuous IV infusion for 21 days.

The Calvert equation is the most frequently used formula for carboplatin dosing, inasmuch as it requires minimal calculations, results in predictable levels of myelosuppression, and prevents underdosing or overdosing in patients with excellent or poor renal function, respectively (62). The Calvert formula appears below along with general guidelines for selecting the specific carboplatin AUC.

$$\text{Carboplatin total dose (mg)} = \text{AUC (mg/mL} \cdot \text{min)} \times [\text{GFR (mL/min)} + 25]$$

AUC = 7, when carboplatin is used as a single agent in patients with good bone marrow reserve; 6, when carboplatin is used in combination regimens in patients with good bone marrow reserve or when used as a single agent in patients who have had prior moderate chemotherapy; and 4, when carboplatin is used as a single agent in patients with prior heavy chemotherapy exposure.

Glomerular filtration rate (GFR) can be determined by measuring creatinine clearance (i.e., [^{51}Cr]-ethylenediaminetetraacetic acid) for all patients or estimated creatinine clearance for patients who have had no prior cisplatin exposure or have not had cisplatin for at least 2 months prior to carboplatin dose determination. As an example, if the desired carboplatin AUC is 6 for a patient with an estimated creatinine clearance (CrCl) of 75 mL/min, the total carboplatin dose would equal 6 × (75 + 25), or 600 mg.

As noted above, the Calvert formula uses the following estimate of carboplatin clearance: Cl = GFR + 25. Although the method may be optimal (63), isotopic determination of the GFR as measured by [^{51}Cr]-ethylenediamine-tetraacetic acid (^{51}Cr-EDTA) is a costly, invasive procedure and the estimated creatinine clearance is often substituted for the GFR. A commonly used method for estimating creatinine clearance is the Cockroft-Gault equation (64):

$$\text{CrCl} = [0.85 \times (140 - \text{age}) \times \text{Wt(kg)}] / [72 \times \text{Scr (mg/dL)}]$$

(CrCl as calculated by the above equation is reduced by 15% for women; Scr = serum creatinine.)

Both the Cockroft-Gault calculation of creatinine clearance and creatinine clearance based on a 24-hour urine collection result in a systematic underestimation of the carboplatin AUC by approximately 10% (65–67). This level of bias may be deemed to be acceptable in view of the clinical utility of substituting creatinine clearance for GFR.

The Calvert formula has been prospectively evaluated by Sorenson et al. (68) in 24 previously untreated ovarian cancer patients and was found to more accurately predict carboplatin exposure than calculation of dose based on body surface area. The AUC of carboplatin as calculated by the Calvert formula accurately predicted the level of myelosuppression as determined by the relative decrease in the platelet count (68).

The recommendation dosage for single-agent carboplatin in ovarian cancer patients with good bone marrow reserve, based on body surface area, is 360 mg/m^2 given intravenously every 4 weeks. Because renal excretion is the primary route of carboplatin elimination, the carboplatin dose must be reduced for patients with compromised kidney function. The drug manufacturer's package insert recommends carboplatin doses of 250 and 200 mg/m^2 for patients with creatinine clearances of 41 to 59 and 16 to 40 mL/min, respectively.

The most frequently used primary chemotherapeutic regimen for advanced ovarian cancer is a combination of paclitaxel (175 mg/m^2 by 3-hour IV infusion) followed by carboplatin (at a targeted AUC of 5 or 6 by 30- to 60-minute IV infusion) every 21 days (if blood counts are adequate) for six cycles (69).

Side Effects and Toxicities. Although the activity is comparable to cisplatin, carboplatin is better tolerated, as measured by toxicity (e.g., low incidence of alopecia [70]) and quality of life analysis (55). The usual dose-limiting toxicity of carboplatin is bone marrow suppression, particularly thrombocytopenia (71). Leukopenia and anemia also occur but are less severe.

The platelet nadir is achieved 3 weeks after an IV bolus injection, and recovery is generally complete 4 to 5 weeks after dosing. However, patients with poor bone marrow reserve from previous chemotherapy or radiation therapy can have more profound thrombocytopenia and leukopenia with carboplatin treatment. Cell depletion may persist for several weeks after dosing.

Nausea and vomiting induced by carboplatin is much less severe than with cisplatin and rarely lasts beyond 24 hours. In a study of 943 ovarian cancer patients randomized to carboplatin, only 9% experienced greater than grade 2 nausea and/or vomiting (70). Emesis can usually be blocked entirely with aggressive therapy using antiemetic drug combinations (72). Diarrhea has been reported in only 6% of patients and constipation in 3% of carboplatin-treated patients (73).

Nephrotoxicity has been reported with carboplatin, but it is much less common and less severe than with cisplatin. In a large review, transient elevations in serum creatinine and blood urea nitrogen were described in 7% and 16% of patients, respectively (73). Measured creatinine clearances dropped in 25% of patients, and a slight increase in uric acid was described in the same percentage of patients. However, there can be a significant loss of serum electrolytes, including potassium (16% of patients) and magnesium (37%). Serum calcium is only rarely decreased after carboplatin (73).

A few cases of carboplatin-induced hematuria have been described. Hepatic enzyme elevations occasionally occur with carboplatin (73). Alkaline phosphatase was transiently increased in 36% of patients and serum glutamic oxaloacetic transaminase (SGOT) or serum glutamic pyruvic transaminase (SGPT) in about 15% of patients. Serum bilirubin levels are rarely elevated (4%) (73).

Neurotoxicity is uncommon after carboplatin and was described in only 25 of 428 (6%) patients treated on a variety of schedules for different tumor types (73). Mild paresthesias have been reported in a few patients receiving cumulative carboplatin doses of more than 1.6 g/m^2 (71). Unlike cisplatin, these peripheral nerve toxicities rarely produce any disabling symptoms. In most cases, no neurotoxicity was attributed to the drug.

Ototoxicity does not appear to be problematic with carboplatin, and only 8 of 710 (1.1%) patients have described clinical hearing deficits, mainly tinnitus (73). However, if pretreatment and serial audiometric tests are performed, as many as 15% of patients may have some decrease in audio acuity. Fortunately, ototoxicity from carboplatin sometimes improves after therapy is halted. Like cisplatin, greater ototoxicity from carboplatin can be expected in patients with preexisting hearing loss or in those concurrently being given other ototoxic drugs, such as aminoglycosides.

Other rare carboplatin toxicities include alopecia (2% of patients), mucositis (2%), skin rash (1.7%), injection-site irritation without extravasation necrosis (0.4%), and a flu-like syndrome (1.3%) (73). The same study described alterations in taste sensation. Skin disorders from carboplatin treatment may appear as an erythematous rash in exposed areas and do not occur in all patients who had developed similar rashes on cisplatin (71).

Although carboplatin-associated hypersensitivity reactions rarely occur when the drug is administered as part of an initial chemotherapeutic regimen, subsequent administration of carboplatin in the setting of second-line or salvage therapy is associated with an increased risk of hypersensitivity. It has been estimated that over 25% of patients who receive more than six courses of platinum-based (i.e., cisplatin or carboplatin) chemotherapy develop sensitivity to carboplatin (74). The onset of symptoms may occur during the carboplatin infusion or up to 3 days after drug administration. Mild reactions consist of localized itching and erythema, primarily of the palms and soles, and/or facial flushing, whereas severe reactions can cause diffuse erythema, tachycardia, wheezing, facial edema, chills, rigors, throat and chest tightness, dyspnea, vomiting, alterations in blood pressure (both hypotension and hypertension), and, in extreme cases, respiratory arrest. Mild cases may respond to IV diphenhydramine (50 mg) or oral diphenhydramine (25 to 50 mg every 4 to 6 hours) and additional courses of carboplatin can be administered. Severe hypersensitivity reactions typically necessitate the discontinuance of carboplatin; however, some patients are able to receive additional courses of carboplatin with administration of corticosteroids for several days prior to carboplatin administration. Hypersensitivity reactions may also occur when carboplatin is administered by the intraperitoneal route (75).

Platinum-based chemotherapy (either cisplatin or carboplatin) has been shown to increase the risk of leukemia in ovarian cancer patients (76). Following carboplatin-based chemotherapy, the estimated relative risk of leukemia is 6.5 (95% confidence interval, 1.1 to 9.4). The relative risk increases as a function of both cumulative dose and duration of treatment. Patients who receive 4,000 mg or greater of carboplatin have a relative risk of 7.6 of developing leukemia, whereas patients who receive more than 12 months of carboplatin-based chemotherapy have a relative risk of 7.0. Although radiation therapy alone does not increase the risk of leukemia, radiation therapy administered in combination with platinum-based chemotherapy is associated with a significantly higher risk of leukemia than platinum-based chemotherapy without radiation ($p = 0.006$). The average time to onset of secondary leukemia is 4 years after the diagnosis of ovarian cancer. Although the potential benefits of platinum-based chemotherapy for ovarian cancer far outweigh the risk of secondary leukemia, the dose-dependent leukemogenic potential of platinum-based chemotherapy should be considered during its administration to patients with early-stage disease.

With the high doses of carboplatin used in autologous bone marrow transplantation programs, other severe toxicities may occur. These include hepatotoxicity (both hepatitis and cholestasis) and severe renal dysfunction (60,77). Nausea, vomiting, and electrolyte wasting are also more profound with high-dose carboplatin treatments. In addition, other unusual toxic effects may occur. These include hemorrhagic colitis, optic neuritis, and interstitial pneumonitis.

As noted below (see Drug Interactions), paclitaxel ameliorates carboplatin-induced thrombocytopenia.

Drug Interactions. Although the pharmacokinetics of carboplatin are not altered by coadministration of paclitaxel, patients who receive combination chemotherapy with carboplatin plus paclitaxel experience less thrombocytopenia than would be predicted if carboplatin was administered as a single agent (65,78). The relationship between free platinum exposure and thrombocytopenia following carboplatin/paclitaxel chemotherapy can be described by a sigmoid maximum effect model (65). In that the degree of neutropenia appears to be unaffected by coadministration of paclitaxel and carboplatin, this pharmacodynamic interaction is believed to occur at the megakaryocyte level (78).

The cytoprotective agent amifostine reduces carboplatin-induced thrombocytopenia (79) but also extends the plasma half-life of carboplatin (80). In a randomized trial of carboplatin with or without amifostine, the median platelet nadir of patients treated with carboplatin 500 mg/m^2 was 88,000/µL, whereas the nadir in patients who received amifostine 910 mg/m^2 was 127,000/µL ($p = 0.023$) (79). Pharmacokinetic studies have shown that amifostine administered just before the carboplatin infusion and 2 to 4 hours thereafter is associated with a significant increase in the terminal half-life of the ultrafiltrable platinum species (e.g., in patients with a creatinine clearance less than 80 mL/min the platinum half-life increased from 4.2 to 5.6 hours with the addition of amifostine). In patients with good renal function, the impact of the increase in terminal half-life was associated with a minimal effect on the AUC. However, patients with impaired renal function experienced significant increases in the AUC of the ultrafiltrable platinum species (80).

Special Applications. Patients with advanced ovarian cancer have been treated with intraperitoneal carboplatin in doses ranging from 200 to 650 mg/m^2 (81). Pharmacologic studies have demonstrated that serum concentrations are equivalent between intravenous and intraperitoneal carboplatin regimens, but IP administration results in more than ten times the concentration in the peritoneal cavity as compared to IV administration (82). However, cisplatin may be a better choice for intraperitoneal delivery in that it appears to have significantly better penetration into tumor masses than carboplatin (83). Several early phase trials show potentially promising results (15,84); however, there is a need for phase 3 research to determine the possible efficacy of IP carboplatin and trials to determine the optimal dosing schedule.

Because of its relative lack of nonhematologic side effects, carboplatin has become the platinum analog of choice for bone marrow transplantation regimens. A regimen developed at Loyola University that consists of high-dose carboplatin combined with cyclophosphamide, mitoxantrone, and autologous bone marrow support was selected for an intergroup phase 3 study of high-dose versus standard-dose chemotherapy for ovarian cancer patients with low-volume, persistent disease following primary chemotherapy (GOG-164). Although this study was closed in May 1999 because of inadequate patient accrual, the high-dose regimen was well tolerated among the 24 patients entered to the trial. With adequate hydration and mannitol diuresis to prevent nephrotoxicity, nonhematologic side effects were predominantly mucositis, ototoxicity, and diarrhea (77).

Cisplatin

Chemistry. Cisplatin (Platinol, *cis*-diamminedichloroplatinum) is a primary drug in the treatment of advanced cancer of the ovary, cervix, and endometrium. It has the molecular formula $PtCl_2H_6N_2$ (molecular weight = 300.1). It is a planar inorganic heavy metal complex containing a central atom of platinum surrounded by two chloride atoms and two ammonia molecules in the *cis* position. It is soluble in water at a concentration of 1 mg/mL. Only the *cis*-isomer is therapeutically active.

Mechanism of Action. Cisplatin's interaction with DNA is probably its primary mode of action. The antitumor effect of cisplatin has been correlated with binding to DNA and the production of intrastructural cross links and formation of DNA adducts, similar to carboplatin (58,85). Intrastrand cisplatin adducts can cause changes in DNA conformation that may affect DNA replication (86). Platinum DNA adduct levels have been measured in patients' leukocytes and correlated with clinical response (85).

Mechanisms of cisplatin drug resistance is an area of concentrated research. Methods by which tumor cells may develop resistance to platinum agents include decreased drug accumulation, increased glutathione levels, enhanced DNA repair, and increased capacity to tolerate DNA damage (86). Platinum resistance is related to expression of excision repair proteins, one of which (ERCC-1) has been identified as playing a critical role in the synergy of gemcitabine and cisplatin. Phase 2 data suggest that gemcitabine may reverse cisplatin resistance, as gemcitabine-cisplatin combination therapy was active in platinum-resistant ovarian cancer patients (87). Mechanisms of resistance also include the increased inactivation of thiol-containing proteins such as glutathione and glutathione-related enzymes, a deficiency in mismatch repair enzymes (e.g., hMHL1, hMSH2), and decreased drug accumulation due to alterations in cellular transport (50).

Drug Disposition. Cisplatin demonstrates a triphasic disappearance curve with a $t_{1/2\alpha}$ of 20 minutes, a $t_{1/2\beta}$ of 48 to 70 minutes, and a terminal-phase half-life of 24 hours (88). The first two phases of disappearance represent clearance of free drug from the plasma, and the third phase is probably removal of drug from the plasma proteins. The ratio of cisplatin to total free platinum in plasma has a great deal of interpatient variability, from 0.5 to 1.1 after a dose of 100 mg/m^2. Three hours after a bolus injection and 2 hours after a 3-hour infusion, 90% of the plasma protein is bound to the platinum in cisplatin, not the cisplatin itself. The complexes between albumin and platinum are slowly eliminated with a minimum half-life of 5 days or more (89). Ninety percent of the drug is removed by renal mechanisms (i.e., glomerular filtration and tubular secretion), and less than 10% is removed by biliary excretion. Fecal excretion appears to be insignificant. Platinum is present in tissues for as long as 180 days after the last administration. There is a potential for accumulation of ultrafilterable platinum plasma concentrations whenever cisplatin is administered on a daily basis, but not when dosed on an intermittent schedule.

Administration and Dosage. Cisplatin may be administered intravenously or intraperitoneally. Cisplatin should be mixed only in solutions containing 0.9% or more sodium chloride, because drug stability is directly related to the concentration of the salt. When admixed with dextrose-containing solutions, by chromatographic analysis, the drug appears to be relatively unstable, with decomposition evident by 2 hours (90). Platinum can also form significant, colored complexes if directly admixed with mannitol and stored for 2 to 3 days (91). Short-term (<24 hour) admixtures, however, have been successfully used. Needles or intravenous sets containing aluminum should not be used in the preparation or administration of cisplatin, because this drug rapidly reacts with aluminum, resulting in a loss of drug potency and the formation of a black precipitate (92).

To protect against nephrotoxicity, it is critical that a high urinary output be maintained during cisplatin therapy. Several methods of accomplishing this have been recommended; however, the most widely practiced method involves prehydration and mannitol diuresis (93). If cisplatin is administered in a hospital setting, patients should receive hydration with 1 to 2 L of fluid prior to cisplatin. Mannitol diuresis is accomplished by diluting the cisplatin in 2 L of normal saline containing 37.5 g of mannitol. The solution is then infused over 6 to 8 hours. Adequate hydration and urinary output should be maintained during the next 24 hours. A safe outpatient procedure using concurrent mannitol that appears to prevent serious nephrotoxicity has also been reported (94). The desired dose of cisplatin plus 50 g mannitol is diluted to 1 L with 5% dextrose plus 0.45% sodium chloride, USP. This solution may then be infused at a rate of no greater than 1 mg/min. For patients with known cardiac disease, the dose may be placed in 200 mL of a 10% mannitol solution and infused at a rate of no greater than 1 mg/min. This is followed by 200 mL of additional 10% mannitol. An alternative is to add the drug to 400 mL of 10% mannitol that is then brought up to a 1-L volume with normal saline containing 3 g of magnesium sulfate and administered intravenously over 1 hour (95).

IP cisplatin administration and nursing guidelines are described in detail elsewhere (96,97), using the GOG-172 regimen, adapted to a 3-hour paclitaxel infusion (IV paclitaxel 135 mg/m^2 over 3 hours day 1 + IP cisplatin 100 mg/m^2 day 2 + IV paclitaxel 60 mg/m^2 day 8). A totally implantable device (intravenous port, such as single-lumen venous-access catheter: 9.6F, Port-A-Cath or Bardport) is surgically placed in the intraperitoneal space at least 2 days before cisplatin administration. Placement can be done at the time of surgery or postoperatively (e.g., laparoscopically). It is important to note that peritoneal or fenestrated catheters can lead to fibrous sheath formation, small bowel obstruction, and perforation and should be avoided (98). Day 2 IP administration requires that cisplatin be mixed in 1 L of normal saline and then warmed to body temperature. The 1-L cisplatin solution is instilled as rapidly as possible into the intraperitoneal space via the catheter, and should be followed by up to 1 additional liter of saline to the point of mild abdominal discomfort. The cisplatin solution is allowed to remain in the intraperitoneal cavity (i.e., the fluid is not drained). Concurrently, at least 1 L normal saline must be administered IV along with 40 g mannitol to ensure a brisk diuresis to eliminate the cisplatin. Since cisplatin has the potential to be highly emetogenic, it is important to consider an aggressive antiemetic regimen (96,99).

Retrospective analysis by Levin and Hryniuk (100) strongly suggests that the cisplatin efficacy against ovarian cancer is directly correlated with cisplatin dose intensity (i.e., mg/m^2/week). Typical high-dose regimens include 20 mg/m^2 daily for 5 days repeated every 3 weeks, 100 to 120 mg/m^2 IV every 3 to 4 weeks, or 100 mg/m^2 on day 1 and day 8 repeated every 20 days (101,102). Holleran and DeGregorio (103) prepared an excellent review of high-dose (200 mg/m^2/course) cisplatin. Dose-limiting toxicities with the higher dose regimens include severe, relatively irreversible neurotoxicity and myelosuppression. Responses have been seen in conventional-dose cisplatin-refractory patients, but they generally are of relatively short duration.

Side Effects and Toxicities. Dose-related nephrotoxicity is the major dose-limiting toxicity of cisplatin. It is manifested by renal tubular damage resulting in an elevation of the BUN or serum creatinine. The peak detrimental effect on renal function usually occurs between the 10th and 20th days after treatment. The renal damage is usually reversible. Patients concomitantly receiving gentamicin and cephalothin have been shown to be at greater risk of developing acute renal failure (104).

Madias and Harrington (105) have characterized the renal damage of cisplatin as being similar to mercury nephrotoxicity. Pathologically, renal tubular necrosis, degeneration, and interstitial edema without glomerular changes are observed. Although clinically overt renal toxicity may be common, it is usually reversible. However, some degree of long-term damage is likely. The renal-protective effect of hydration and mannitol is well established in animals and humans, and renal impairment can be prevented (94).

Ototoxicity, manifested by high-frequency hearing loss (above the frequency of normal speech), may be seen in as many as 30% of patients treated with cisplatin (106). Hearing impairment may be dose related and can be unilateral or bilateral. Occasional tinnitus (but not vestibular dysfunction) has been reported. The ototoxicity may be partially reduced by adequate hydration and the use of mannitol diuresis. Patients with lower than average threshold before chemotherapy with cisplatin were more likely to experience greater threshold shifts (106).

Neurotoxicity can be a dose-limiting side effect of cisplatin, particularly with high-dose regimens (107). The range of cisplatin-induced neurologic deficits includes peripheral sensory neuropathy, ototoxicity, autonomic neuropathy manifested by orthostatic hypotension and gastric paresis, Lhermitte's syndrome, and rarely focal encephalopathy, often accompanied by cortical blindness. Peripheral neuropathy is by far the most common cisplatin-induced neurotoxicity. Neurotoxicity is dose dependent, with symptoms typically developing after cumulative doses of 300 mg/m^2 or greater. A review of published literature (108) found that neurotoxicity occurred in 85% of patients at cumulative doses of 300 mg/m^2 or greater, but occurred in only 15% of patients who had received a cumulative dose below this level. Initial symptoms are usually numbness and tingling in the distal fingers and toes. If cisplatin is continued, proximal extension of the peripheral neuropathy occurs, and the sense of joint position becomes impaired, resulting in more severe neurologic symptoms, including ataxia, gait disturbances, loss of manual dexterity, and wheelchair dependency. Symptoms may begin and progress up to 4 or more months after discontinuation of cisplatin. In 30% to 50% of patients, cisplatin neuropathy is irreversible.

Early clinical data suggest that a number of investigational agents may ameliorate cisplatin-induced neurotoxicity (107). Agents that have been associated with positive preclinical results include ORG2766 (109), an adrenocorticotropic hormone (ACTH) analog, and the sulfhydryl-based compounds amifostine and glutathione. Only amifostine has been associated with a significant reduction of grades 2 and 3 neurotoxicity in the setting of an adequately designed phase 3 trial

(110). Further development of a neuroprotective agent, such as amifostine, could significantly enhance the clinical effectiveness of cisplatin, enabling dose-intensive therapy and greater cumulative doses to be delivered to more patients with sensitive tumors. In 2003, the GOG initiated a phase 3 trial of low-dose, intravenous bolus amifostine three times weekly to reverse grade 2 or greater peripheral neuropathy (GOG-192).

Symptomatic hypomagnesemia frequently occurs with cisplatin. In a study to determine the effects of magnesium supplementation on cisplatin-induced hypomagnesemia, the administration of magnesium (oral and intravenous) with cisplatin to one group of patients produced less renal tubular damage and no compromise in efficacy than that seen in a group not supplemented with magnesium (111).

Without adequate antiemetic therapy, most patients who receive cisplatin experience nausea and vomiting. This reaction may be severe and usually starts within the first hour after treatment and may persist for 24 to 48 hours. Delayed nausea and vomiting, lasting from 3 to 5 days, also may occur. The combination of a 5-HT3 inhibitor (e.g., ondansetron or granisetron) with dexamethasone (10 to 40 mg IV) has reduced the incidence of severe nausea and vomiting by as much as 75% (112). Delayed nausea and vomiting can be eradicated by continuation of oral low-dose dexamethasone (with or without a 5-HT3 inhibitor) for the first 5 days after platinum treatment (113). Other less effective antiemetic regimens to prevent cisplatin-induced nausea and vomiting include prochlorperazine, dexamethasone, and lorazepam; metoclopramide and dexamethasone; metoclopramide and methylprednisolone; or metoclopramide and lorazepam (72,114).

Anaphylactic hypersensitivity reactions consisting of tachycardia, wheezing, hypotension, and facial edema occurring within a few minutes of IV administration have occurred occasionally after a dose of cisplatin given to previously treated patients (115). These hypersensitivity reactions have been controlled with corticosteroids, epinephrine, or antihistamines. Wiesenfeld et al. (116) reported successful retreatment with cisplatin after apparent allergic reactions in two patients. *In vivo* and *in vitro* tests in one patient could not demonstrate an immunologic basis for the initial reaction. Both patients were successfully rechallenged with cisplatin after only diphenhydramine pretreatment. This suggests a nonallergic cause of the acute hypersensitivity reactions occasionally seen with platinum.

Myelosuppression occurs in 25% to 30% of patients receiving the recommended dose, and is more pronounced at higher doses. Coombs-positive hemolytic anemia also occurs as a result of cisplatin treatment. Cisplatin-induced anemia has been shown to respond to recombinant erythropoietin (117).

Drug Interactions. When cisplatin is given in combination with other agents, the order of drug sequence can affect the severity of drug-induced myelosuppression. Rowinsky and Donehower (118) conducted a phase 1 study of sequential escalating doses of paclitaxel and cisplatin therapy and determined that myelosuppression was more severe when cisplatin administration preceded paclitaxel than when given after paclitaxel. Another phase 1 study was conducted to evaluate the effects of drug sequence of treatment with cisplatin in combination with topotecan (119). This study also found a significantly higher incidence of myelosuppression when cisplatin was administered first.

Cisplatin-induced nephrotoxicity should be considered whenever this agent is given prior to or in combination with other cytotoxic drugs that are cleared by renal elimination (e.g., bleomycin, ifosfamide, etoposide, methotrexate). Cisplatin reduces the renal clearance of these agents, resulting in an increased accumulation of these drugs. Yee et al. (46) observed markedly reduced bleomycin clearance in children who had received six courses of a regimen including cisplatin (cumulative dose 300 mg/m^2). In another case report, fatal bleomycin pulmonary toxicity occurred in a patient with cisplatin-induced acute renal failure (47).

Cisplatin is directly inactivated by mesna and amifostine (50). The FDA has approved amifostine to reduce the cumulative renal toxicity associated with repeated administration of cisplatin in patients with advanced ovarian cancer. In a phase 3 randomized study of ovarian cancer patients, amifostine treatment, prior to IV cisplatin plus cyclophosphamide, did not appear to reduce cisplatin's anticancer activity (120). However, there are only limited data in other chemotherapeutic settings, and the FDA recommends that amifostine should not be administered to patients in settings where chemotherapy could produce a significant survival advantage or cure except in a clinical trial (121).

Special Applications. The efficacy of cisplatin can be increased significantly in patients with stage III, optimal disease (i.e., <1 cm^2 residual tumor) epithelial ovarian cancer when it is administered by the IP route as part of a primary, combination chemotherapy regimen. A pivotal phase 3 trial (GOG-172) performed by members of the GOG determined that the IP administration of cisplatin 100 mg/m^2 (on day 2, preceded by IV paclitaxel 135 mg/m^2 over 24 hours on day 1 and followed by IP paclitaxel 60 mg/m^2 on day 8, every 3 weeks for six cycles) was associated with a highly significant 16-month increase in overall survival as compared with the standard treatment arm (IV cisplatin 75 mg/m^2 plus IV paclitaxel 135 mg/m^2 over 24 hours every 3 weeks for six cycles) in patients with advanced, optimal ovarian cancer (4). Despite the higher incidence of toxicity in the IP arm, these effects appear to be of short duration, as patients treated IP and IV reported equivalent quality of life 1 year post-treatment (8). As a result, the National Cancer Institute issued a Clinical Announcement on January 5, 2006, recommending IP therapy as the referred treatment for optimal, advanced ovarian cancer (122).

Intraperitoneal therapy is not recommended for patients who have suboptimal cytoreductive surgery (i.e., >1 cm in largest diameter of a tumor nodule), because IP cisplatin (as well as other cytotoxic agents) only penetrates a few millimeters into tumor plaques (16). Additional considerations regarding the appropriate patient selection for consideration of IP therapy are discussed in detail elsewhere (96,97,123).

Multiple phase 3 studies have shown that cisplatin-based chemotherapy as an adjunct to radiation therapy improves survival in cervical cancer patients (22,124,125).

Cyclophosphamide

Chemistry. Cyclophosphamide (Cytoxan, Neosar, CTX, CPM, and Endoxan) is an alkylating agent that before the advent of paclitaxel was used in the primary chemotherapy of advanced, epithelial-type ovarian and endometrial cancer. At this time, it is uncommonly used in the treatment of gynecologic cancers because of the more effective agents currently available (e.g., paclitaxel). It is occasionally used in the third-line treatment of ovarian cancer and as a second-line agent in the treatment of choriocarcinoma. It is a cyclic phosphamide ester of nitrogen mustard and is referred to chemically as 2-[bis-(2-chloroethyl)amino]tetrahydro-2H-1,3,2,-oxazaphosphorine 2-oxide monohydrate. Its molecular weight is 279.1. The monohydrate is unionized and lipid soluble; in normal saline or water, it is soluble to a maximum of 4% at room temperature.

Mechanism of Action. Cyclophosphamide, a bifunctional substituted nitrogen mustard, was synthesized in 1958 in an attempt to achieve greater selective toxicity for tumor tissue. The N-methyl moiety of nitrogen mustard is replaced with a cyclic phosphamide group, resulting in a stable, inactive compound. The bis-(2-chloroethyl) group cannot ionize until the cyclic phosphamide is opened at the phosphorus-nitrogen linkage.

Activation of cyclophosphamide is a multistep process. The liver microsomal P450 mixed-function oxidase system converts the parent drug to 4-hydroxycyclophosphamide. This metabolite exists in equilibrium with the acyclic tautomer, aldophosphamide. These compounds may be further oxidized by hepatic aldehyde oxidase to the inactive metabolites of carboxyphosphamide and 4-ketocyclophosphamide. Nonenzymatic conversion to the cytotoxic compounds of phosphoramide mustard and acrolein occurs in susceptible peripheral tissues.

Most of the alkylating agents, like cyclophosphamide, are bifunctional, which facilitates their reaction with two cellular molecules. Accordingly, they can cross link the two opposite strands of DNA to give an interstrand cross link, react with two sites on the same strand (intrastrand cross link), or cross link DNA to protein. The latter type of lesion is generally considered to be innocuous, but the relative significance of the other cross links is still in contention. DNA intrastrand cross links are more frequent than interstrand cross links and are more often considered to be the critical lesions.

These two classes can be differentiated by the structure of the cross links in DNA. Generally, the entire mustard is involved in the cross link, with the two mustard "arms" linked usually to the N7 position of guanine. Because these guanines can be separated by several bases in DNA, the linkages represent particularly bulky lesions.

Drug Disposition. After IV administration, approximately 15% of the drug is excreted unchanged in the urine and the remainder as metabolites. The plasma half-life of the parent compound after doses of 6 to 80 mg/kg appears to range from 4.0 to 6.5 hours (126). Approximately 50% of the alkylating metabolites (but not parent drug) is bound to plasma proteins.

Although cyclophosphamide is exclusively excreted by the kidneys, because of the unionized nature of the intact drug molecule, tubular reabsorption is avid. Hepatic inactivation appears to be the major mechanism of active drug elimination. The mean renal clearance of intact drug is approximately 11 mL/min, or 15% of creatinine clearance, but renal elimination remains the major route of disposition of the more polar, less lipid-soluble metabolites (127). There can be significantly prolonged retention of active (alkylating) metabolites in patients with severe renal failure, and doses should be adjusted accordingly.

Dosage. Cyclophosphamide is active in many different types of malignancies. The dosing schemes are numerous and depend on the particular disease. Two general categories of treatment schedules exist. In the method generally used to treat ovarian and endometrial cancers, an intermediate dose (600 to 1,000 mg/m^2) is given all at once over a short period. This treatment approach usually involves other drugs, such as cisplatin, carboplatin, or doxorubicin, whose additive toxic effects must be considered in selecting the dose and frequency of cyclophosphamide administration. Adequate hydration for 72 hours before and following high-dose treatment with cyclophosphamide is recommended to reduce cyclophosphamide-induced hemorrhagic cystitis (128).

Side Effects and Toxicities. Myelosuppression consisting primarily of leukopenia is the usual dose-limiting toxic effect of cyclophosphamide. Both the nadir and time of bone marrow recovery are rapid at 8 to 14 and 18 to 21 days, respectively. Although this drug has long been considered to be "platelet sparing," significant thrombocytopenia can also occur at very high doses (>1.5 g/m^2).

Acute, sterile hemorrhagic cystitis is an infrequent toxic manifestation but is occasionally dose limiting. It is understandably more common in poorly hydrated or renally compromised patients. The onset of this complication may be delayed from 24 hours to several weeks. It is detected by gross hematuria or a microscopic hematuria of greater than 20 erythrocytes per high-power field. The bleeding may persist but is usually transient. Prophylactic hydration with intake of at least 3 L/day appears to offer the best protection. With continued therapy, patients characteristically develop a fibrotic "small bladder," and urinary frequency may become a permanent problem. There is a definite increase in the risk of bladder cancer in these patients. The availability of the sulfhydryl mesna as a prophylactic treatment of patients at high risk for developing cyclophosphamide-induced cystitis has almost completely eliminated this side effect.

A syndrome of inappropriate antidiuretic hormone (SIADH), or "water intoxication," has been reported after cyclophosphamide treatment. This is more common with IV doses greater than 50 mg/kg and is both a limitation to and consequence of fluid loading (129). Alopecia occurs to some degree in all patients receiving cyclophosphamide and is significant in at least half of all patients treated. Regrowth of hair may occur even with continuing treatment. Gastrointestinal problems are more common with high doses given orally. Anorexia, nausea, and vomiting are all common reactions, but they are usually controlled with IV antiemetic regimens. A rare pulmonary toxic effect has been reported with a pneumonitis picture similar to "busulfan lung." The typical clinical presentation is that of an interstitial pneumonitis, usually occurring after long-term and continuous low-dose therapy (130). The onset of symptoms is insidious. Pathologically, there can be alveolitis with eventual fibrosis and atypical type II pneumocytes. Steroids may be beneficial. Other toxic effects include testicular atrophy, sometimes with reversible oligospermia and azoospermia. Amenorrhea also has been reported. As with all alkylating agents, drug-induced congenital abnormalities are possible. With high-dose therapy used for bone marrow transplant (120 to 180 mg/kg), cyclophosphamide-associated cardiac toxicity has been reported (131).

Special Precautions. It is important to keep the patient well hydrated during cyclophosphamide therapy to reduce the potential for hemorrhagic cystitis. It is advisable to administer at least 1 L of additional IV fluids (usually normal saline) to assure an adequate urine volume to excrete the cyclophosphamide metabolite acrolein, which can otherwise alkylate bladder mucosa and cause hemorrhagic cystitis. The patient should be instructed to drink at least eight glasses of fluid daily during the 2 days after cyclophosphamide administration. In patients prone to developing cystitis, consider administering prophylactic IV mesna, a sulfhydryl-containing compound that can neutralize acrolein.

Drug Interactions. Cyclophosphamide must be metabolized to be active. Although some cyclophosphamide may be activated by phosphatases and phosphamidases peripherally, most of the drug is metabolized by microsomal enzymes in the liver (132). These enzymes may be activated by drugs like phenobarbital or inhibited by drugs like proadifen (SKF 525A). Because active and toxic metabolites are generated by the reactions of these enzymes and cyclophosphamide, many potential drug interactions may exist.

Barbiturates and other inducers of hepatic microsomal enzymes, such as phenytoin and chloral hydrate, may increase the rate of hepatic conversion of cyclophosphamide to its toxic metabolites. Similarly, cyclophosphamide may block the metabolism of barbiturates, increasing sedative effects. Although the clinical significance of these reactions is not clear, cyclophosphamide toxicity may be increased by the H_2-histamine blocker cimetidine (133). Cimetidine, but not ranitidine, may increase cyclophosphamide's myelotoxicity through an increase in the concentration · time product of its active metabolites (e.g., 4-hydroxycyclophosphamide and phosphoramide mustard) (134). Thus, H_2-blockers like ranitidine may be safer to use than cimetidine when high doses of cyclophosphamide are administered.

Dactinomycin

Chemistry. Dactinomycin (actinomycin D, ACT-D, Cosmegen) has been shown to be active in the treatment of patients with germ cell tumors of the ovary and endometrium and of gestational trophoblastic disease (135,136). It has a molecular weight of 1,255 and an empiric formula of $C_{62}H_{86}N_{12}O_{16}$. The drug is an antitumor antibiotic isolated from *Streptomyces parvulus*. The molecular structure includes two peptide loops linked to a three-ring chromophoric phenoxazone ring system (actinomycin). The drug is highly soluble in water, forming an amber- to gold-colored solution.

Mechanism of Action. Dactinomycin becomes anchored into or around a purine-pyrimidine base pair in DNA by intercalation. DNA-dependent ribosomal RNA synthesis and new messenger RNA synthesis is inhibited. The peptide loops appear to allow tight drug binding to DNA because the actinomycin (phenoxazone) moiety alone is inactive. This can occur adjacent to any G-C pair in DNA.

Bound dactinomycin molecules dissociate very slowly from DNA owing to electrostatic interactions of the cyclic peptide rings with each strand of the DNA double helix. This process, which stabilizes the intercalative interaction, appears to be crucial for cytotoxicity.

Dactinomycin on a molar basis is one of the most potent antineoplastic agents available. The drug possesses some hypocalcemic activity, similar to mithramycin. Although maximal cell killing is observed in the G_1 phase, the cytotoxic action is thought to be primarily cell cycle nonspecific. Actively proliferating cells are more sensitive than quiescent cells to the lethal effects of the drug (137).

In that dactinomycin is a natural product, it is not surprising that the primary mode of tumor cell resistance to dactinomycin is mediated through overexpression of P-glycoprotein (138).

Drug Disposition. Tattersall et al. (139) studied the pharmacokinetics of radiolabeled [^{3}H]dactinomycin in patients, and the drug appeared to be only minimally metabolized and was concentrated in nucleated cells. There was a greater drug uptake into bone marrow than in plasma. Drug penetration into the central nervous system was not observed. Urinary and fecal recovery totaled only 30% each after 9 days, and there was significant drug retention in lymphocytes and granulocytes. This may explain the prolonged terminal plasma half-life of 36 hours observed after single dactinomycin doses. There appears to be little metabolism because approximately 90% of excreted drug is collected as the intact molecule. Some monolactone forms of dactinomycin are recovered in the urine.

Using a more specific radioimmunoassay, a much shorter dactinomycin half-life is described ($t_{1/2\alpha}$ = 0.78 minutes, $t_{1/2\beta}$ = 3.5 hours) (140). The discrepancies between these and Tattersall's findings reflect the differences in the assays used.

Administration and Dosage. Dactinomycin is administered intravenously by slow IV push or, preferably, into the tubing of a freely running IV solution. A 5- to 10-mL flush of 5% dextrose in water (D_5W) or normal saline is recommended before and after IV push administration to ensure vein patency and to flush any remaining drug from the tubing.

Dactinomycin is commonly given intravenously in short "pulse" doses of 500 μg/m^2 daily for as long as 5 days in adults. The dose for each 2-week cycle should not exceed 15 μg/kg/day or 400 to 600 μg/m^2/day for 5 days.

A wide variety of dosing regimens have been employed. Several clinical studies have documented equal efficacy and toxicity for single-dose dactinomycin regimens (141,142). In nonmetastatic gestational trophoblastic cancer, a single IV dose of 1.25 mg/m^2 every 14 days produced a 99% remission rate after four courses of therapy (142). Compared with five divided doses of 500 μg/m^2/day, the single-dose method produced slightly greater mild to moderate toxic effects.

Side Effects and Toxicities. Bone marrow depression is the usual dose-limiting toxic effect of dactinomycin. It is usually manifested 7 to 10 days after dosing. All blood elements are affected, but primarily the platelets and leukocytes are depressed. Combined with gastrointestinal reactions, myelosuppression appears to be dose limiting as well as dose dependent (143). Immunosuppression is another well-known effect of dactinomycin. Patients should not receive this drug during viral infection because of the risk of developing disseminated disease.

Severe gastrointestinal consequences, such as vomiting, can occasionally represent the acute dose-limiting toxic effects of dactinomycin. Vomiting can persist for 4 to 20 hours, but it can be controlled by combination antiemetic regimens (144). Mucositis can also be severe. It is characterized by severe oral ulcerations and diarrhea in 30% of patients. Reversible alopecia may occur with dactinomycin. A variety of other skin manifestations have been reported, including acneiform changes, erythema, and hyperpigmentation.

Dactinomycin is toxicologically similar to the anthracyclines and characteristically interacts with radiation therapy, producing delayed "radiation recall" skin damage. Previously irradiated or even irritated skin may become reddened and inflamed after drug administration. Frank necrosis is sometimes reported. Oral ulcers may also develop after radiation therapy. These reactions may occur months after radiation therapy. Experimentally, radiation therapy given after dactinomycin does not produce this effect.

Dactinomycin potentiates pulmonary radiation and decreases radiation tolerance by at least 20%. Reintroduction of dactinomycin following pulmonary radiation has resulted in fatal pulmonary fibrosis (145). As noted in the Special Precautions section below, dactinomycin is highly ulcerogenic if extravasated.

Special Precautions. Dactinomycin is extremely damaging to soft tissue and every effort should be made to ensure vein patency during administration. Extravasations characteristically result in immediate pain and swelling followed by indolent, poorly healing necrotic ulcers (144).

Dactinomycin is highly potent and is typically dosed in micrograms per kilogram. Doses must be calculated and prepared carefully to prevent inadvertent overdosage of this drug. No specific antidote to overdosage is known, although granulocyte colony-stimulating factors may be useful.

Dactinomycin is a potent immunosuppressant and can inhibit the effectiveness of vaccinations given after drug administration. The drug also produces radiation recall skin and soft-tissue damage if given after ionizing radiation.

Docetaxel

Chemistry. Docetaxel (Taxotere) is a semisynthetic analog of paclitaxel and has an FDA-approved indication for locally advanced or metastatic breast cancer after failure of prior chemotherapy. It is also FDA approved for locally advanced or metastatic non–small cell lung cancer after failure of prior platinum-based chemotherapy. It has also shown marked antitumor activity against a variety of solid tumors, including both platinum-sensitive and platinum-refractory epithelial ovarian cancer (146,147). The natural component of docetaxel is 10-deacetyl baccatin III, which is extracted from the needles of the European yew tree (*Taxus baccata* L.) (147). Docetaxel has a molecular weight of 861.9 and the empirical formula $C_{43}H_{53}NO_{14} \cdot 3H_2O$. Unlike paclitaxel, which uses a polyoxyl compound (Cremophor) as a diluent, docetaxel is formulated in Tween 80 and alcohol.

Mechanism of Action. In a manner similar to paclitaxel, docetaxel promotes microtubule assembly and inhibits the depolymerization of tubulin. However, compared with paclitaxel, the microtubules formed by docetaxel are more slowly reversible and there are differential effects on tau binding sites and on microtubule-associated proteins. Docetaxel-induced stabilization of microtubules halts cellular division in M phase, thereby preventing cell replication.

Drug Disposition. The pharmacokinetics of docetaxel when administered as an IV infusion lasting from 1 to 24 hours have been investigated in a number of studies (148). When administered as a typical 1-hour infusion at doses of 70 to 100 mg/m^2, pharmacokinetics reveal triphasic elimination with a plasma AUC of 3.13 to 4.83 mg/mL/hour, a peak plasma concentration of 2.57 to 3.67 μg/mL, and a terminal-phase plasma half-life of 13.6 hours. There is very limited renal excretion of docetaxel; the 24-hour urinary excretion was 1.4% of the dose administered. Plasma drug clearance was determined to be 21.3 L/h (149).

Administration and Dosage. All patients receiving docetaxel should be premedicated with oral corticosteroids such as dexamethasone 16 mg/day (e.g., 8 mg bid) for 3 days beginning 1 day prior to docetaxel administration in order to reduce fluid retention and the risk of hypersensitivity reactions.

Docetaxel is commercially available in single-dose 20- and 80-mg vials with accompanying diluent vials. Both the docetaxel vials and the diluent vials should stand at room temperature for approximately 5 minutes prior to mixing. The entire contents of the diluent vial should be aseptically transferred to the docetaxel vial and the resulting contents should be gently rotated for 15 seconds to promote complete mixture. The resulting concentration of docetaxel is 10 mg/mL. Foam may be present owing to the Tween 80; however, it should largely dissipate within a few minutes. The infusion solution is prepared by aseptically withdrawing the proper amount of docetaxel with a calibrated syringe and adding it to a 250-mL infusion bag or bottle containing either 0.9% sodium chloride or 5% dextrose solution to produce a final concentration of 0.3 to 0.9 mg/mL. The infusion solution should be mixed by manual rotation and inspected for particulate formation and/or discoloration. Solutions that are cloudy or that contain particulate matter should be discarded.

The recommended dose of docetaxel for salvage chemotherapy of breast cancer is 60 to 100 mg/m^2 IV as a continuous 1-hour infusion every 3 weeks. For non–small cell lung cancer, the recommended dose is 75 mg/m^2 IV as a continuous 1-hour infusion every 3 weeks. The optimal dosing schedule for docetaxel in gynecologic cancers is presently undefined. A 100-mg/m^2 dose administered as a 1-hour infusion every 3 weeks has been used in phase 2 trials. Other tolerable docetaxel dose schedules that have been identified in phase 1 studies are 50 mg/m^2/day on days 1 and 8 every 3 weeks; 70 to 90 mg/m^2 by 24-hour continuous IV infusion every 3 weeks; 80 to 100 mg/m^2 by 6-hour infusion every 3 weeks; 14 mg/m^2/day for 5 days by 1-hour infusion every 21 days (150); and 30 to 35 mg/m^2 weekly (151). Docetaxel has been administered in combination with cisplatin using the following schedule: docetaxel 85 to 100 mg/m^2 as a 1-hour IV infusion followed (3 hours after completion) by cisplatin 75 mg/m^2 as a 3-hour IV infusion, with cycles being repeated every 3 weeks (152).

The docetaxel dose should be reduced for patients with moderate liver impairment (see Special Precautions section below).

Side Effects and Toxicities. The major dose-limiting toxicity of docetaxel is neutropenia, which is noncumulative and generally resolves within 7 to 8 days. The combined results of early phase 2 studies of docetaxel (without steroid premedication) in ovarian cancer revealed that at a dose level of 100 mg/m^2 every 3 weeks, over 90% of patients developed grades 3 to 4 neutropenia, with febrile neutropenia occurring in 8% to 44% of patients (153). The incidence of other grade 3 to 4 toxicities were stomatitis 0% to 5%, diarrhea 6% to 20%, dermatitis 4% to 8%, acute hypersensitivity reactions 7% to 12%, and fluid retention 8% to 12%. Other docetaxel-induced side effects include alopecia, anemia, neurosensory effects (paresthesia, dysesthesia, pain), and asthenia (150).

In early phase 2 studies, slow-onset (i.e., after three to five courses) cumulative fluid retention leading to peripheral or generalized edema with possible development of pleural effusion and/or ascites was a common dose-limiting toxicity. However, a 5-day premedication regimen with corticosteroids, starting the day before docetaxel administration, significantly reduces this side effect. In a retrospective analysis, severe fluid retention occurred in 20% of patients who received no premedication compared with 5% of patients who received steroid prophylaxis. Additionally, the percentage of patients who discontinued treatment secondary to fluid retention was reduced from 32% to 2% ($p < 0.00001$) with the use of a 5-day corticosteroid regimen (150). Steroid prophylaxis also reduces the incidence and severity of dermatologic side effects and hypersensitivity reactions.

The spectrum of docetaxel-induced hypersensitivity reactions is less severe than that associated with paclitaxel. In the absence of prophylactic medication, mild hypersensitivity reaction as characterized by flushing, rash, and pruritus occurs in approximately 5% of docetaxel administrations. Moderate reactions with dyspnea and/or slight hypertension occur in 8% of treatments, and severe reactions (with bronchospasm, angioedema, and/or severe hypertension) occur in less than 2% of docetaxel administrations (154). Initial symptoms of hypersensitivity to docetaxel therapy generally occur within minutes of the start of the first or second course of docetaxel and resolve rapidly with interruption of the infusion. Patients can be successfully rechallenged with docetaxel therapy following medication with corticosteroids, antihistamines, and H_2-agonists.

Dermatologic toxicities typically appear as maculopapular eruptions and desquamation generally localized to the extremities. Nail changes, including onycholysis, may also occur. Skin changes are largely self-limiting and may be alleviated with glycerin/chlorhexidine ointment or oral pyridoxine. This side effect can often be prevented with prophylactic oral steroids and H_1- and H_2-agonists (155). Recurrent skin toxicity refractory to oral prophylactic medication and pyridoxine therapy may respond to local hypothermia during docetaxel administration (156).

Special Precautions. Patients with impaired liver function have a significant reduction in docetaxel clearance and an increased risk of life-threatening side effects. Analysis of the overall safety database revealed that patients with moderately impaired liver function (defined as transaminase levels more than 1.5 times the upper limit of normal and alkaline phosphatase more than 2.5 times the upper limit of normal) have a 27% reduction in docetaxel clearance and a 38% increase in the area under the concentration · time curve (150). When compared with patients with normal liver function, patients with at least moderately impaired liver function had a significantly greater incidence of febrile neutropenia (40% vs. 16%) and toxic death (20% vs. 1.4%). Grades 3 to 4 nausea/vomiting, stomatitis, and thrombocytopenia were also increased in patients with impaired liver function (150).

The recommended docetaxel dose level for a patient with moderate hepatic impairment (defined as transaminases between 1.5 and 3.5 times the upper limit of normal and an alkaline phosphatase between 2.5 and 6.0 times the upper limit of normal) is 75 mg/m^2 over 1 hour. No safe docetaxel dose can be recommended for patients with greater than moderate liver impairment (157).

Special Applications. Verschraegen et al. (158) have published preliminary evidence that patients with ovarian cancer may respond to docetaxel even though they have had progression of their disease on paclitaxel. They noted a partial response rate of 37.5% in eight eligible patients. A phase 2 study conducted by the GOG of 60 patients with paclitaxel-resistant ovarian and peritoneal carcinoma observed responses in 22.4% of patients, with 5.2% achieving complete response and 17.2% achieving partial response (at a dose of 100 mg/m^2 IV over 1 hour every 21 days) (159). However, the 75% incidence of grade 4 neutropenia in this study suggests that further study is needed to determine the appropriate dose and schedule.

Doxorubicin

Chemistry. Doxorubicin (Adriamycin), a primary agent in the treatment of metastatic endometrial cancer and advanced ovarian cancer, is an anthracycline antibiotic obtained from *Streptomyces peucetius* var. *caesius*. It has a molecular weight of 580. The doxorubicin structure includes a water-soluble basic reducing amino sugar, daunosamine, linked by a glycosidic bond to carbon atom number 7 on the D-ring of the water-insoluble chromophore aglycone, adrimycinone.

Structural changes in the side groups of doxorubicin alter antitumor potency and pharmacokinetic properties. The aglycone is inactive, and modifications in the amino sugar substituents can also alter antitumor or toxic potency (160).

In DNA, the amino sugar projects into the minor groove and can interact electrostatically with negatively charged phosphate groups in the DNA strand to stabilize the aglycone moiety. Doxorubicin can also form complexes with iron or copper by means of the hydroquinone moieties (161). Metal-iron doxorubicin complexes may contribute to cardiotoxicity by enhancing redox cycling of the quinone moiety to produce membrane-damaging oxygen free radicals (162). Doxorubicin hydrochloride is freely soluble in water, slightly soluble in normal saline, and very slightly soluble in alcohol.

Doxorubicin also is commercially available in a polyethylene glycol (PEG)-coated (pegylated, Stealth) liposomal form (see Liposomal Encapsulated Doxorubicin section below).

Mechanisms of Action

DNA Binding. The anthracyclines, including doxorubicin, probably have several modes of action. The anthracycline portion of the molecule appears to intercalate between stacked nucleotide pairs in the DNA helix by means of P-P–type bonds (163). The drug may also bind ionically around certain base pairs of DNA (adlineation). The overall effect of this is interference with nucleic acid synthesis, specifically an inhibition of DNA synthesis (164). However, preribosomal RNA synthesis is also affected by the drug binding to DNA, preventing DNA-directed RNA and DNA transcription (165).

Mechanisms other than intercalation may also contribute to the antitumor effect of the doxorubicin molecule. The contribution of alkylation to antitumor effects has not been established.

Free-Radical Formation. Oxygen free-radical intermediates containing an unpaired electron can be formed by doxorubicin. This can react rapidly with oxygen to form superperoxide, and with hydrogen peroxide, highly reactive hydroxyl radicals can form. These radicals damage membrane lipids by peroxidation, break DNA strands by attacking ribose-phosphate bonds, and directly oxidize purine or pyrimidine bases, thiols, and amines. Free-radical mechanisms have most often been associated with cardiotoxicity.

Doxorubicin appears to be active in all phases of the cell cycle, and although maximally cytotoxic in S phase, it is not phase specific (166). Cells exposed to lethal doxorubicin concentrations in G_1 can proceed through S phase but are then blocked and die in G_2. Higher concentrations can also produce an S-phase blockade (167).

Inhibition of DNA Topoisomerase II. Topoisomerases are enzymes capable of covalent binding to DNA, forming transient breaks in one strand (TOPO-I) or two strands (TOPO-II). This activity is highly phase dependent for G_2, and in the case of TOPO-II, normally mediates strand passage to facilitate DNA condensation or decondensation (168). Doxorubicin and other DNA intercalators inhibit the strand-passing activity of TOPO-II by increasing and stabilizing the initial enzyme-DNA (cleavable) complexes. This leads to protein-linked DNA double-strand breaks that are roughly proportional to the cytotoxic potency of the drug *in vitro* (169).

Drug Disposition. Doxorubicin pharmacokinetics are usually described using a two-compartment or three-compartment open model. The drug is rapidly distributed in body tissues, and about 75% of the drug is bound to plasma proteins, principally albumin (170). In the blood, the free doxorubicin fraction depends on the hematocrit, with more free drug being available in patients with a reduced hematocrit (171). The avid binding to DNA is believed to explain the prolonged terminal elimination half-life of 30 to 40 hours, the large apparent volume of distribution of up to 28 L/kg, and the incomplete (50%) total recovery of drug in urine, bile, and feces (172). Human tissues with high drug concentrations (in descending order) include liver, lymph nodes, muscle, bone marrow, fat, and skin (173). The drug does not distribute into the central nervous system.

There is a significant distribution of doxorubicin into human breast milk (174). Doxorubicin levels of 0.24 μM and 0.2 μM of doxorubicinol have been measured in human milk. They produce cumulative AUCs in breast milk of 9.9 and 16.5 μM · hour, respectively. Both of these values were greater than concurrent plasma AUC values. However, doxorubicin does not appear consistently to pass the placenta. Except for one study reporting low drug levels in placental blood of 0.78 to 1.19 nmol/g and no drug in cord blood plasma, several other trials detected no drug in amniotic fluid after doxorubicin administration to pregnant patients (175,176).

Doxorubicin is extensively metabolized and eliminated primarily as glucuronide conjugates of the parent aglycone or its hydroxylated congener doxorubicinol. The conjugated metabolites are exclusively excreted in the bile and feces. Overall, biliary excretion accounts for about 40% of an administered dose (177). Approximately 42% of the biliary drug is parent doxorubicin, 22% is doxorubicinol, and 36% is other metabolites (177). Only 5% to 10% of the administered drug is excreted in the urine as doxorubicin (40%), doxorubicinol (29%), and other metabolites (31%).

In liver disease, patients with cholestasis have delayed doxorubicin clearance and experience exaggerated toxic reactions from standard doses (178). However, hepatoma patients with cirrhosis or simple hepatocellular enzyme elevation appear to have normal doxorubicin clearance and toxic effects from standard doses (179). Although obesity reduces clearance of doxorubicin in adult cancer patients (180), there were no differences in doxorubicin toxicity between normal, mildly obese, and obese patients.

There is some evidence that repeated doxorubicin dosing alters pharmacokinetics (181). In these reports, doxorubicin levels were lower after repeated dosing, which suggests increased drug clearance. However, because neither toxicity nor response rates are altered, the clinical significance of these observations has not been established. Age may also be a factor. In one trial, the highest clearances of doxorubicin were observed in younger patients (182). These observations suggest that higher peak doxorubicin levels may be achieved in older patients.

TABLE 16.2

INTRAVENOUS DOSING GUIDELINES FOR DOXORUBICIN

Dose (mg/m²)[a]	Intravenous method	Schedule	Average cumulative tolerable dose (mg/m²)[b]
60 to 75[c]	Bolus	Every 3 weeks	550
30	Bolus	3 successive days, every 3 weeks	550
20	Bolus	Weekly	750
60	96-h infusion	Every 3 to 4 weeks	1,000

[a]Lower doses should be administered to patients with hepatobiliary dysfunction and for poor bone marrow reserve or performance status.
[b]Represents average total cumulative dose tolerated without clinical evidence of doxorubicin cardiotoxicity.
[c]Allows for greater dose intensity in breast cancer.

The hepatic extraction ratio for doxorubicin in humans is 0.45 to 0.50, and systemic drug levels are about 25% lower with intra-arterial administration compared with IV dosing (183). Several studies have shown that the pharmacokinetics of intra-arterial drug are similar to those after IV doses (173). The relatively low hepatic extraction rate and similar overall disposition patterns provide little pharmacokinetic rationale for intra-arterial administration as a means of localizing doxorubicin effects to the liver (184).

Administration and Dosage. Short IV push infusions and IV bolus injections have been used with doxorubicin. A slow IV push over several minutes with constant monitoring of the patient and blood return can help minimize the chance of serious tissue damage occurring because of extravasation. A 5- to 10-mL flush of normal saline or D_5W before and after administration is strongly recommended to test vein patency and flush any remaining drug from the tubing. Alternatively, injection into the side port of a running IV infusion has also been recommended. The patient should be asked to report immediately any change in sensation during the administration. Old venipuncture sites or infusion sites previously used for administering blood, antibiotics, or other medications should not be used to administer doxorubicin. Heparin locks (unless recently inserted) are not recommended because the drug is chemically incompatible with sodium heparin.

Prolonged infusions increase the incidence and severity of stomatitis and dermatologic reactions. Administration through tunneled central venous catheters or indwelling vascular access ports is mandatory for all prolonged infusions. Careful patient and site monitoring are required because doxorubicin extravasation from central vascular access devices can occur.

Numerous dosing schedules have been reported. The individual doxorubicin dose depends on clinical variables, including the cumulative dose administered to date and the potential for interaction with other drugs or radiation (Table 16.2). As a single agent, doses of 60 to 75 mg/m² as a single intravenous injection have been used and repeated no more often than every 3 weeks. An alternative scheme uses 20 to 30 mg/m² given daily for 3 consecutive days and repeated in 3 weeks (185). When used in combination therapy, the most commonly used dosage is 40 to 60 mg/m² given as a single intravenous injection every 21 to 28 days.

Both the dose and rate of dosing (dose intensity) can have therapeutic impacts for different agents and tumors (186). Clinical studies with doxorubicin show that greater dose intensity is associated with enhanced response rates in breast cancer (187). The doses compared in this trial were 70 mg/m² every 21 days for eight cycles versus 35 mg/m² every 21 days for 16 cycles.

Dose adjustments are required in a number of clinical settings (Table 16.3), specifically in the case of hyperbilirubinemia.

TABLE 16.3

MODIFICATIONS OF DOXORUBICIN DOSES[a]

Condition	Recommended dose modification
Prior doxorubicin	Limit total cumulative lifetime dose (by IV bolus) to 550 mg/m² (188)
Prior chest radiation therapy	Reduce total dose limit to 300 to 350 mg/m²
Obesity	Base dose on ideal body weight (180)
Hepatobiliary dysfunction	Reduce dose for elevated serum bilirubin (give 50% of dose for serum bilirubin of 1.2–1.9 μg/dL, and give 25% of dose for serum bilirubin ≥3.0 mg/dL) (178) Use indocyamine green disappearance rate as an indicator of doxorubicin clearance
Infusion method	Greater cumulative (total) dose may be afforded by weekly bolus doses or continuous (96-hr) infusions[b] (189)

[a]Average safe cumulative doxorubicin dose is 750 mg/m² using standard infusion schedules.
[b]Average safe cumulative doxorubicin dose is 1,000 mg/m² when administered with a 96-hr infusion schedule.

A 50% dose reduction is indicated if plasma bilirubin concentration is 1.2 to 3.0 mg/dL, and the dose must be reduced by 75% if plasma bilirubin concentration reaches 3.1 to 5.0 mg/dL.

Side Effects and Toxicities. The single acute dose-limiting toxicity for doxorubicin is bone marrow suppression. The most commonly seen dose-limiting toxicity is leukopenia, with a nadir at 10 to 14 days. Other hematologic toxicities, such as anemia and thrombocytopenia, have been reported, but they are rare and generally less severe. Recovery from myelosuppression is usually prompt, with resolution often within about 1 week after the nadir.

Doxorubicin is known to produce local skin and deep-tissue damage at the site of inadvertent extravasations (190). Ulcers may result after 33% of extravasations. The lesions undergo a slow, indolent expansion and occasionally involve tendons and other deep structures. They characteristically do not heal and are associated with prolonged local drug retention (191). Reilly et al. (190) recommend early surgical debridement, with skin grafting and tendon repair for serious infiltrations. Numerous pharmacologic antidotes have been evaluated, but few have demonstrated unequivocal clinical efficacy. The application of cold, topical dimethylsulfoxide is recommended (192).

Cardiac consequences from the drug have included acute effects, such as a rare pericarditis-myocarditis syndrome or electrophysiologic aberrations, and a total-dose–related cardiomyopathy (193). Nonspecific electrocardiographic changes during infusion or immediately afterward may be seen. These include T-wave flattening, ST depression, supraventricular tachyarrhythmias, and extra systolic contractions (194). These conduction abnormalities are generally transient, not associated with severe morbidity, and do not require dose modification.

Cardiomyopathy from doxorubicin is dose related. It presents initially as a clinical syndrome identical to classic congestive heart failure. It is usually irreversible, but symptoms can be managed with standard medical therapy involving digitalis, glycosides, and diuretics. Potential risk factors for doxorubicin cardiotoxicity include cumulative doses greater than 550 mg/m^2, prior mediastinal irradiation ($\geq$20 Gy), age greater than 70 years, and preexisting cardiovascular diseases, such as prior myocardial infarction or long-standing hypertension (189). Anthracycline-induced cardiomyopathy can also occur 4 to 20 years after the drug is stopped at standard dose limits (195). The administration of anthracyclines incorporated into liposomes is one method that may significantly reduce the risk of cardiac toxicity (see the Liposomal Encapsulated Doxorubicin section below) (196).

At total doses under 500 mg/m^2, the incidence of cardiomyopathy is less than 1%; between 501 and 600 mg/m^2, 11% are affected; and the incidence is 30% for doses above 600 mg/m^2. In a retrospective cardiotoxicity study of 4,018 patient records, Von Hoff et al. (188) described an overall incidence of 2.2% for doxorubicin-induced congestive heart failure. In this analysis, there was no influence of performance status, sex, race, and tumor type on the incidence of cardiomyopathy. However, elderly patients were at greater risk even after adjustment for the normally decreased cardiac function in this group. The major determinants were the dose, the schedule of administration, and the age of the patient. A weekly doxorubicin dosing schedule was associated with significantly less congestive heart failure than an every-3-weeks dosing schedule. Continuous IV infusions over 96 hours also can significantly lessen doxorubicin cardiotoxicity (197).

Dexrazoxane (Zinecard) is a chemoprotective agent with an FDA-approved indication for reducing doxorubicin-associated cardiomyopathy in women with metastatic breast cancer who have received a cumulative doxorubicin dose of $\geq$300 mg/m^2 and who, in their physician's opinion, would benefit from further doxorubicin therapy (see the Modulating Agents section below).

There is evidence that doxorubicin is a radiosensitizing or "radiomimetic" agent and can cause reactivation of tissue reactions in areas previously irradiated (198). Radiation recall reactions have also been reported in areas of previous drug infiltration. A particularly sensitive area for serious recall toxicity is the esophagus (199).

Other toxic effects are observed in rapidly proliferating normal tissues. These include marked alopecia in all hairy body areas. Stomatitis may occur at high doses and is more pronounced when the drug is given on consecutive days. It generally begins in the sublingual and lateral tongue regions as a burning sensation with noticeable erythema. The initial inflammation typically progresses to ulceration after a few days. Anal fissures or proctitis have been rarely reported. Nausea and vomiting are common but of moderate intensity. Diarrhea is rare with consecutive daily dosing, and the emetic effects are generally limited to the first day of treatment. Hyperpigmentation of the skin, especially the nail beds, may occur. Extravasations of doxorubicin are known to cause severe ulceration and soft tissue necrosis (190). Vein patency should be assured before injection and constantly monitored during administration.

As discussed later in this chapter, pegylated liposomal encapsulation dramatically alters the pharmacokinetic profile of doxorubicin and, hence, the drug's toxicity profile.

Drug Interactions. Doxorubicin is believed to interact with numerous other drugs. Most of these effects have been described only in experimental systems, and their clinical significance is, therefore, unknown. However, several potentially significant interactions have been described in cancer patients. Altered doxorubicin disposition is postulated with α-interferon, and substantial doxorubicin dose reductions are required (200). The combination of doxorubicin with H_2 antihistamines, such as ranitidine or cimetidine, may also increase toxicities significantly and necessitate drug dose reduction.

Special Applications. Doxorubicin has been investigationally administered intrapleurally to patients with malignant pleural effusions (201). Doses of 30 mg were diluted in 20 mL of saline and administered by paracentesis needle as a bolus. Eight of 11 patients responded to doxorubicin, including one complete response. This response rate was superior to nitrogen mustard or tetracycline. Toxicity included pain or fever in 20% of patients and nausea or vomiting in 45% of patients. No alopecia or hematologic toxicity was reported. Markman et al. (202) combined doxorubicin (3 mg) with cytarabine (61 mg) and cisplatin (100 mg/m^2) in the treatment of seven cancer patients with malignant pleural effusions. Two ovarian cancer patients responded, and no significant systemic toxicities were reported. All injections were given in 250 mL of saline, and aggressive hydration was given to counteract cisplatin nephrotoxicity.

Etoposide

Chemistry. Intravenous etoposide (VP-16) is used commonly in combination chemotherapy regimens for the treatment of patients with germ cell tumors of the ovary (136). Oral etoposide has activity as a salvage agent for refractory or recurrent ovarian cancer (203). It is a semisynthetic epipodophyllotoxin derived from the root of *Podophyllum* (the May apple plant, or mandrake). The chemical name is demethylepipodophyllotoxin 9-[4,6-O-(R)-ethylidene-β-D-glucopyranoside]. Etoposide has the molecular formula of $C_{29}H_{32}O_{13}$ and a molecular weight of 588.58. It is highly soluble in methanol and chloroform, slightly soluble in ethanol, and sparingly soluble in water. Because of poor water solubility, the commercial drug is dissolved in an ethanol-based cosolvent system.

Etoposide was originally synthesized from *Podophyllum embodi* (204). Structure-activity studies show that the hydroxyl group at the C-4′ position is required for activity and that alterations at this site can dramatically affect activity.

Mechanism of Action. There is marked schedule dependence for etoposide cell killing, and cytotoxic effects are maximal in G_2 phase (205). There is also some activity against cells in late S phase, and the drug can halt cell cycle traverse at the S-G_2 interphase (206).

Etoposide produces protein-linked DNA strand breaks by inhibiting DNA TOPO-II enzymes (207). This normal mammalian enzyme mediates double-strand–passing activities in G_2 phase to condense or decondense supercoiled DNA (208). Drug-induced inhibition of TOPO-II is an energy-dependent process that is influenced by dose and duration of exposure.

Etoposide does not bind directly to DNA, but rather stabilizes a transition form of the DNA–TOPO-II complex (207). The number of single and double DNA strand breaks reflects the cytotoxic dose-response curve (209). Etoposide and intercalative drugs such as doxorubicin "poison" TOPO-II enzymes by stabilizing an otherwise transient form of TOPO-II covalently linked with DNA (169). Normal TOPO-II strand-passing activity is thereby blocked, and cell progression out of G_2 phase is halted (168). The production of cytotoxicity by etoposide may ultimately involve chromosomal breaks characterized as sister chromatid exchanges (210).

Another postulated etoposide mechanism involves microsomal activation to reactive intermediates capable of generating oxygen free radicals (209). Nucleoside transport is also inhibited at high drug concentrations, but whether this makes a major contribution to the antitumor effect is unknown (211).

Drug Disposition. A two-compartment open pharmacokinetic model appears to adequately describe etoposide disposition in cancer patients (212). The terminal half-life of the drug appears to be about 7 hours and is independent of the dose, route, or method of administration (213). Renal excretion appears to account for about 30% of overall drug elimination. Forty-two to 66% of radiolabeled drug is recovered in the urine, of which less than half is parent etoposide.

With standard doses of etoposide, no drug is detectable in the cerebrospinal fluid (CSF), and even after doses of 400 to 800 mg/m^2, CSF levels were less than 2% of concurrent plasma levels (214). Despite the low distribution of drug into the CSF, mean levels of 1.4 μg/g (range undetectable to 5.9 μg/g) have been measured in brain tumor tissue (215). The drug also distributes into myometrial carcinoma and normal myometrium, achieving levels 50% of those in the blood (216).

Biliary secretion of parent drug accounts for 2% or less of the dose, although fecal recovery of drug and metabolites is variable, ranging from 1.5% to 16.3% (217). However, patients with obstructive jaundice excrete a larger fraction of the dose in urine (46%) than do unaffected patients (35%), which suggests that there is a slight decrease in hepatic drug metabolism with a commensurate increase in renal clearance (214).

The plasma protein binding of etoposide is normally high, averaging 95% in typical patients (218). The free (unbound) fraction of etoposide can vary from 6% to 37% among patients. Patients with increased bilirubin or decreased albumin may have an increase in the free fraction even though systemic clearance is unaltered (218). Myelosuppression may also be commensurately increased in these patients. Other conditions that may decrease etoposide clearance include prior cisplatin therapy, obesity, and elevated alkaline phosphatase levels (219).

The absolute oral bioavailability of etoposide gelatin capsules ranges from 25% to 74%, with a mean of 48% (220). Some patients experience a 30% change in overall bioavailability (both increased and decreased) with repeat dosing. Neither food nor other chemotherapeutic agents appear to alter etoposide absorption (221). Wide variations in peak levels and AUC values were also described in this trial.

Administration and Dosage. Etoposide must be diluted prior to use with either 0.5% dextrose or 0.9% sodium chloride to give a final concentration of 0.2 to 0.4 mg/mL. Etoposide should be given by IV infusion over a 30- to 60-minute period. Severe hypotension may occur if the drug is given too rapidly. Although not a vesicant, extravasation of the drug should be avoided (222). Examine all solutions for fine precipitates; mix before use. Precipitation may occur if the solution is prepared 0.4 mg/mL. Continuous infusions of etoposide have been used as a means of enhancing efficacy because of its phase-specific mode of antitumor action. Most infusions have used 5-day courses, although 72-hour infusions have also been employed (223).

Oral administration of etoposide capsules may be useful if patient compliance is high and low-emetogenic drug regimens are used. The capsules may be taken all at once to achieve the desired dose. Neither food nor other chemotherapeutic drugs appear to alter oral absorption of the drug (221). The GOG has investigated multiple trials of oral etoposide at various dosing regimens. Based on a cumulative review of these trials and schedules, it was found to be active in platinum-resistant ovarian cancer patients (overall response rate 26.8%; 7.3% clinical complete remission rate) and in platinum-sensitive patients (overall response rate 34.1%; 14.6% clinical complete remission rate) (223). One of these trials that demonstrated activity used an oral etoposide dosing schedule of 50 mg/m^2/day for 21 days every 28 days with dose escalation to 60 mg/m^2/day when feasible (224). Studies using similar oral etoposide dosing schedules in patients with cervical cancer and endometrial cancer failed to show significant activity in these tumor types (225,226).

The variety of doses and schedules that have been used with etoposide are presented in Table 16.4. General principles of dosing include more frequent administration to take advantage of cell cycle–dependent cytotoxicity, an approximate doubling of oral doses due to 50% bioavailability for the gelatin capsules, and significant dose reductions for combinations of etoposide with other myelosuppressive drugs or for patients with poor bone marrow reserve or poor performance status. In general, etoposide doses can be repeated every 3 to 4 weeks depending on the leukocyte count. A pharmacokinetic study in patients with obstructive jaundice showed that no significant dose reductions are needed if renal function is normal (229).

Side Effects and Toxicities. Side effects and toxicities for oral and intravenous administration of etoposide as a single agent are similar. The principal toxicity of etoposide is dose-related and dose-limiting bone marrow suppression. Leukopenia and thrombocytopenia occur, but leukopenia consistently predominates, with a nadir at approximately 16 days and with recovery usually beginning by days 20 to 22.

Gastrointestinal complaints of nausea, vomiting, or anorexia are usually minor and are more frequent with the oral preparations (230). Other adverse effects include alopecia in 20% to 90% of patients, headache, fever, and hypotension (231). Severe hypotension can occur if the drug is infused too rapidly (<30 minutes) (217). Stomatitis has been infrequently reported. Rare instances of generalized allergic reactions and anaphylaxis have occurred (232). A few episodes of cardiotoxicity, including myocardial infarction and congestive heart failure, have been described (233). Immune suppression appears to be minimal with this drug (231). Bronchospasm with severe wheezing has been rarely observed and has usually been responsive to antihistamines and glucocorticosteroids. Chemical phlebitis also has been associated with etoposide, although the reaction is most likely related to solubilizers in the diluent. Diluted solutions of etoposide are not vesicants.

TABLE 16.4

INTRAVENOUS AND ORAL DOSING SCHEDULES FOR ETOPOSIDE

	Dose			
Administration method	mg/m2/day	Days	Repeat dosing interval (wk)	Clinical application
Short single-dose IV infusion	200–250	1	7	Single agent, small cell lung cancer
Short multiple-dose IV infusion	100	1–5	3–4	Testicular cancer
	100	1,3,5	3–4	With other drugs
	45	1–7	3	Phase 1
Continuous IV infusion	125	1–5	4	Phase 1, single agent
	30	1–5	4	With cisplatin in advanced cancer
	80	1–5	4	Phase 1, good-risk patients
	50	1–5	4	Poor-risk patients
	125	1–3	4	Adult patients with advanced cancer (227)
	500	1 (24-hr)	3	Small cell lung cancer
Oral	160	1–5	3–4	Small cell lung cancer
	50	1–21	4	Ovarian cancer (228)

For inadvertent extravasations of highly concentrated etoposide solution, hyaluronidase may be effective (234).

Neurotoxicity has been rarely reported with etoposide. This has consisted of somnolence and fatigue in 3% of patients and peripheral neuropathy in less than 1% of patients. However, the drug may exacerbate preexisting neuropathy caused by vincristine (235). Predisposing factors included advanced age, impaired nutritional status, and poor performance status. Degradation of myelin lamellae has been observed in affected nerves.

Special Applications. Despite preclinical data showing peritonitis with intraperitoneal injections, combinations of etoposide and cisplatin have been administered safely by the intraperitoneal route. Barakat et al. (236) performed a phase 2 study of three courses of intraperitoneal cisplatin 100 mg/m^2 plus etoposide 200 mg/m^2 as consolidation therapy in patients with stages II to IV epithelial ovarian cancer with negative second-look surgeries. When compared with a similar group of contemporaneous patients who did not receive consolidation therapy, the disease-free survival distribution between the two groups (using the log-rank test) was found to be significant ($p = 0.03$) in favor of consolidation therapy (236). European researchers have used a combination of etoposide 350 mg/m^2 IP, followed by cisplatin 200 mg/m^2 IP with IV sodium thiosulfate (4 g/m^2 bolus, followed by 12 g/m^2 over 6 hours) protection every 4 weeks for four to six cycles in ovarian cancer patients with either no residual disease or minimal residual disease at second-look surgery. The regimen was fairly well tolerated, although there was one study-related patient death from a bowel perforation and resulting complications. Other major clinical complications were nausea, vomiting, and the formation of intraabdominal adhesions. Grade 3 to 4 leukopenia and thrombocytopenia occurred in 30% and 6% of cycles, respectively (237).

Etoposide in combination with other chemotherapeutic agents and autologous stem cell rescue is often used in salvage therapy for germ cell tumors or metastatic trophoblastic disease. Two commonly used regimens are bleomycin, etoposide, and cisplatin (BEP) and ifosfamide, carboplatin, and etoposide (ICE) (238).

5-Fluorouracil and Floxuridine

Chemistry. 5-Fluorouracil (5-FU) is a fluorinated pyrimidine differing from the normal DNA substrate, uracil, by a fluorinated number 5 carbon (chemically, 5-fluoro-2,4(1H, 3H)-pyrimidinedione). 5-FU has activity as a second-line agent in advanced ovarian and cervical cancers and, in combination with cisplatin, is used as an adjunct to radiation therapy in women with locally advanced cervical cancer. Floxuridine (FUDR) is highly similar to its prodrug, 5-FU. The discussion of FUDR in this chapter will be limited to its special application as an intraperitoneally administered agent for salvage therapy for ovarian cancer. 5-FU is light sensitive and precipitates at low temperatures or, occasionally, with prolonged standing at room temperature. It has the molecular formula of $C_4H_3FN_2O_2$ and a molecular weight of 130.08.

Mechanism of Action. 5-FU acts as a false pyrimidine or antimetabolite ultimately to inhibit the formation of the DNA-specific nucleoside base thymidine. There are at least three mechanisms of action: inhibition of thymidylate synthase by 5-fluoro21-deoxyuridine-5′-monophosphate (FdUMP), the active metabolite of 5-FU; incorporation of 5-fluorouridine triphosphate (FUTP) into cellular RNA; and incorporation of FUTP into cellular DNA (239). 5-FU is a cell cycle phase-specific agent with cytotoxic effects seen maximally in S phase.

Drug Disposition. There is disagreement over whether 5-FU is eliminated by a two-compartment or three-compartment model (2,240). Fraile et al. (241) demonstrated that plasma levels of 5-FU after oral administration are quite erratic. Schaaf et al. (227) documented that the pharmacokinetic characteristics of 5-FU are nonlinear. Doubling of the dose was accompanied by a decrease in nonrenal clearance. The half-life from the high dose was twice as long as that for the low dose of 5-FU. Their data were compatible with a product-inhibition model. Yoshida et al. (242) found positive correlations between the dose and serum steady-state levels (C_{SS}) and areas under the concentration · time curves (AUCs). Patients who developed toxic reactions had greater C_{SS}s and AUCs. However, there were no correlations between serum levels and patient response to therapy.

5-FU and FUDR are extensively metabolized in the liver (hepatic metabolism can detoxify up to 80% of the total dose). However, there is no absolute documentation that patients with impaired liver function require dose reductions of 5-FU (243); however, patients should be monitored as they may be at increased risk of toxicity. As much as 15% of a dose may be found intact in the urine by 6 hours, with 90% of this excreted in the first hour. Depressed renal function does not generally require dosage adjustment for 5-FU.

5-FU distributes to all areas of body water by simple diffusion. Significant quantities of the drug may enter the central nervous system, and after 15 mg/kg given IV, CSF levels of 6 to 8×10^{-6} M are obtained after 30 minutes. These levels persist for several hours and slowly subside. Although distribution to brain tissue is less rapid, abnormal areas, such as those with neoplasms, may more readily take up drug.

5-FU achieves high and persistent levels in effusions after IV administration. Hepatic administration through the portal vein or artery also achieves high concentrations in the liver parenchyma and produces relatively low systemic levels.

Santini et al. (228) showed that therapeutic monitoring of 5-FU levels in patients with head and neck cancer can be used to improve the therapeutic index of the drug (i.e., less toxicity with maximal efficacy).

Administration and Dosage. Doses of 5-FU to be given by the IV push route do not require further dilution from the commercial solution. Vein patency should be assured before giving a dose, with a 5- to 10-mL flush of normal saline or D_5W and another flush after the dose to rinse the remaining drug from the tubing. For short infusion (less than 24 hours), the rate of administration is not critical, and the dose should be given at a rate compatible with the particular vein selected. The patient should be continuously monitored to guard against extravasation. Most doses can be conveniently given over 1 to 2 minutes in this fashion.

Continuous infusions (over 4 to 5 days) may maximize efficacy of this cycle-specific drug and lessen hematologic toxicity (244). Infusions of the drug may be added to a convenient volume of D_5W or normal saline, and each reconstituted daily dose can be administered over 24 hours. Commonly, the daily dose of the drug is added to 1 L, although volume is not critical.

Regimens reported for the use of 5-FU include the use of a loading dose, weekly IV bolus, continuous infusions over 4 to 5 days or over 6 weeks, and oral dosing. 5-FU may be administered intravenously as a bolus, rapid injection on a monthly (425 to 450 mg/m^2 IV on days 1 to 5 every 28 days) or a weekly schedule (500 to 600 mg/m^2 every week for 6 weeks every 8 weeks), or continuous IV infusion (24-hour infusion 2,400 to 2,600 mg/m^2 every week; 96-hour infusion 800 to 1,000 mg/m^2/day; or 120-hour infusion 1,000 mg/m^2/day on days 1 to 5 every 21 to 28 days) (50). Oral doses of up to 15 to 20 mg/kg/day for 5 to 8 days have been used (245). However, the efficacy of oral 5-FU has not been confirmed at this time (see the Capecitabine section above for a discussion of the oral prodrug of 5-FU).

The loading dose scheme calls for one course of 400 to 500 mg/m^2 (12 mg/kg; maximum of 800 mg) daily for 5 days every 28 days given as a single daily bolus injection or as a 4-day continuous infusion. This is followed by a weekly maintenance regimen. Horton et al. (246) and Jacobs et al. (247), however, strongly associated the use of the loading dose with significant morbidity and occasional fatalities, and suggested that it offers no greater antitumor efficacy over a weekly bolus injection of 15 mg/kg given IV.

Maintenance 5-FU dosing regimens include the following: 200 to 250 mg/m^2 (6 mg/kg) every other day for 4 days, repeated in 4 weeks (if toxicity has resolved); or 500 to 600 mg/m^2 (15 mg/kg), given IV weekly as a continuous infusion or bolus injection (with and without the loading dose).

By continuous infusion, higher daily doses have been successfully used, and many investigators have reported lessened hematologic toxicity and enhanced efficacy. Most of a dose is eliminated by the liver and the remainder by the kidney. Therefore, marked dysfunction in either system probably requires a dose reduction.

There are two commonly used dosing regimens for 5-FU combined with leucovorin: 370 mg/m^2/day of 5-FU for 5 days plus leucovorin given as a continuous infusion of 500 mg/m^2/day, beginning 24 hours before the first dose of 5-FU and continuing for 12 hours after completion of therapy; or 5-FU given at doses of 500 to 1,000 mg/m^2 every 2 weeks, preceded by calcium leucovorin at a dose of 20 mg/m^2 given as a 10-minute infusion (248).

Phase 3 studies performed by the GOG, SWOG, and Radiation Therapy Oncology Group have documented the efficacy of cisplatin/5-FU chemotherapy as an adjunct to radiation therapy in women with high-risk cervical cancer (22,124,249). The regimen used in the SWOG study was cisplatin 70 mg/m^2 by 2-hour IV infusion on day 1 of radiation followed by 5-FU 1,000 mg/m^2/day by 96-hour continuous infusion on days 1 to 4 every 3 weeks for four cycles, with the first and second cycles given concurrently with radiation therapy (124). The addition of concurrent cisplatin-based therapy to radiation therapy significantly improved progression-free and overall survival in this study; however, no definitive study has compared cisplatin versus cisplatin/5-FU as an adjunct to radiation therapy for cervical cancer, and the relative importance of 5-FU remains to be addressed.

Side Effects and Toxicities. The most pronounced and dose-limiting toxic effects of 5-FU are on the normal, rapidly proliferating tissues of the bone marrow and the lining of the gastrointestinal tract. Some nausea and vomiting can be expected. These adverse effects may respond relatively well to antiemetic treatment. Stomatitis, however, is usually an early sign of impending severe toxicity that may become evident after 5 to 8 days of therapy. Symptoms include soreness, erythema, or ulceration of the oral cavity or dysphagia. Other reported gastrointestinal symptoms are diarrhea, proctitis, and esophagitis.

Leukopenia, primarily granulocytopenia, and thrombocytopenia occur with a nadir at 9 to 14 days for the granulocytes and 7 to 14 days for platelets. Patients who are poor candidates for 5-FU therapy are those with a total leukocyte count of 2,000/mm^3 or less or platelet count of 100,000/mm^3 or less or those with poor nutritional status at the outset of therapy.

Some degree of alopecia is expected, although hair regrowth has occurred even when successive doses are given. Partial loss of nails and hyperpigmentation of the nail beds and other body areas (e.g., face, hands) have been reported. These may resemble the hyperpigmentation seen in Addison's disease. A maculopapular rash may occur on the extremities and sometimes the trunk. The rash is usually reversible. Sunlight may heighten or initiate many dermatologic reactions to 5-FU.

Palmar-plantar erythrodysesthesia (PPE) or hand-foot syndrome PPEs have been reported with very long continuous infusion 5-FU (over several weeks). This has been reported in 42% to 82% of patients in various series. The syndrome is progressive and disrupts treatment (250). This has encouraged the development of prodrugs of 5-FU, such as 5′-deoxy-5-fluorouridine, capecitabine, BOF-A2, ftorafur, UFT, and S-1 (251,252). Although there is no indicated treatment for PPE, the incidence has been reduced to a few percentage points by limiting 5-FU continuous infusion durations to 21 days with at least 1 additional week off drug. Possible therapies that have yet to be evaluated in clinical trials include DMSO, systemic corticosteroids, and pyridoxine (vitamin B_6) (251,253).

Hyperpigmentation over the veins used for 5-FU administration has been observed (254). In one the veins remained patent, but there was marked darkening of the skin immediately over the vein.

5-FU may also cause an acute cerebellar syndrome that can persist beyond the period of actual treatment (255). Neurotoxicity may be evidenced by headache, minor visual disturbances, cerebellar ataxia, or all three. This is a rare complication. The neurotoxic metabolite is probably fluorocitrate.

Cardiotoxicity is a rare but potentially serious toxicity attributable to 5-FU. The incidence of cardiotoxicity may vary from 1.2% to 18.0% of patients (256), and includes cases of myocardial infarction, angina, dysrhythmias, cardiogenic shock, sudden death, and electrocardiographic changes. The mechanism producing 5-FU–induced cardiotoxicity is unknown.

Special Precautions. 5-FU should never be given to pregnant women. 5-FU may increase the cortisone requirement in patients who have had an adrenalectomy (e.g., for breast cancer), and consideration should be given to increased doses of cortisone for patients receiving 5-FU.

Because dihydropyrimidine dehydrogenase is the rate-limiting enzyme in the metabolism of 5-FU, patients with a familial deficiency of dihydropyrimidine dehydrogenase (familial pyrimidinemia) should not receive 5-FU. The administration of 5-FU to patients with this enzyme deficiency has led to severe toxicity and even death (257, 258).

Accidental splashing of 5-FU on the skin or eyes of personnel should be treated with immediate irrigation with saline solution or water. There have been no long-term sequelae of these accidents (259).

Because of the alkaline nature of the drug, admixture with any acidic agents (amino acids, penicillin, multivitamins, insulin, tetracycline) represents a theoretic incompatibility.

Special Applications. FUDR, a closely related analog of 5-FU, has efficacy as a salvage agent when administered as an intraperitoneal agent to stage III ovarian cancer patients with minimal residual disease (i.e., <1 cm) following second-look surgery. A SWOG study utilized intraperitoneal FUDR (3 g/day for 3 days every 3 weeks for six courses) as a salvage regimen in this patient population and documented a median overall survival of 38 months (260). Additionally, 69% of study patients had not progressed 12 months after receiving intraperitoneal FUDR. Because the majority of the intraperitoneal FUDR dose is extracted during "first pass," it is relatively well tolerated, although grade 4, uncomplicated neutropenia was observed in 14% of patients (260). Because of the favorable 1-year progression-free survival in this study, a subsequent phase 1-2 trial was conducted by the SWOG (261). The researchers recommend that the regimen of IP FUDR + IP cisplatin (or IP FUDR with both platinums) be tested in a phase 3 trial in comparison to IP cisplatin (261).

Speyer et al. (262) investigated intraperitoneal 5-FU in patients with ovarian and colon carcinomas. Using a Tenckhoff catheter, patients received repeated 36-hour courses of eight 2-L exchanges, each 4 hours long, or a 3- to 5-day course of single, daily 2-L instillations. 5-FU concentrations ranged from 10^{-6} M (130 μg/L) to 8 (10^{-3} M × 1 g/L).

The procedure was relatively well tolerated locally, although there were two instances of catheter-related bacterial peritonitis that were easily managed. Concentrations of 4×10^{-3} M for 36 hours caused mucositis, pancytopenia, and alopecia. The systemic toxicities were quite severe with the highest dose tested (8×10^{-3} M). Pharmacokinetic studies revealed first-order drug elimination, with an intraperitoneal half-life of 72 to 112 minutes. Intraperitoneal drug levels were 300-fold greater than simultaneous plasma levels. Intraperitoneal 5-FU administration appears to produce high drug concentrations with minimal systemic toxicity. Objective responses were documented in two of seven patients studied in this phase 1 investigation. The investigators recommended further intraperitoneal 5-FU investigation at initial drug concentrations of 4×10^{-3} M (500 mg/L) for 36 hours (262).

Suhrland and Weisberger (263) used intracavitary 5-FU to manage malignant pleural effusions from carcinoma of the breast and lung tumors and to control malignant ascites from ovarian carcinoma. Approximately 38% of the patients responded to a single intracavitary dose of 2 to 3 g. For pericardial effusions, doses of 500 to 1,000 mg were used. Repeat dosing was not necessary. Patients with pleural effusions also tended to respond better than those with ascites. Although side effects were minimal in this study, some systemic toxicity was consistently produced.

Gemcitabine

Chemistry. Gemcitabine (Gemzar) is a relatively new chemotherapeutic agent that was approved by the FDA in 1995 for treatment of patients with advanced pancreatic cancer based on an increase in survival and clinical benefit (improvement in pain and performance status). The combination of gemcitabine plus cisplatin also is FDA approved and is considered standard therapy for patients with advanced non–small cell lung cancer. Gemcitabine has demonstrated significant activity in advanced ovarian cancer patients and is active against refractory ovarian cancer and cervical cancer, as well as other solid tumors (264–266). Gemcitabine is a synthetic nucleoside analog with a structure that is highly similar to deoxycytidine and cytosine arabinoside (ara-C). Gemcitabine HCl is 2′-deoxy-2′,2′-difluorocytidine monohydrochloride (β isomer). The empiric formula for gemcitabine is $C_9H_{11}F_2N_3O_4 \cdot HCl$ and the agent has a molecular weight of 299.66.

Mechanism of Action. Gemcitabine is a prodrug and undergoes multiple phosphorylations by deoxycytidine kinase at the intracellular level to form the active diphosphate and triphosphate metabolites. The triphosphate is incorporated into DNA as a fraudulent base pair. Following the insertion of gemcitabine, one additional deoxynucleotide is added to the end of the DNA chain before replication is terminated. This process is known as "masked chain termination" and prevents exonucleases from excising off the fraudulent base pair (267,268). The diphosphate inhibits ribonucleotide reductase and thereby depletes the deoxynucleotide pools that are necessary for DNA synthesis and repair (269). Inactivation of gemcitabine occurs when the drug is metabolized by cytidine deaminase (both intracellulary and extracellulary) to form difluorodeoxyuridine (dFdU) (270).

Drug Disposition. Following administration of gemcitabine 1,000 mg/m^2 by 30-minute IV infusion, the parent compound undergoes rapid clearance in a diphasic manner. The plasma half-life and clearance are dose, age, and gender dependent. Gemcitabine pharmacokinetics were evaluted in 353 patients with varied solid tumors using short infusions (<70 minutes) and long infusions (70 to 285 minutes) at various total doses (500 to 3,600 mg/m^2) (271). There is a three- to fourfold interpatient variability in pharmacokinetics. As noted above, gemcitabine is metabolized intracellularly by deoxycytidine kinase to form the active diphosphate and triphosphate metabolites. The drug is inactivated both intracellularly and extracellularly by cytidine deaminase to form dFdU. Of the administered gemcitabine dose, 99% is excreted in the urine either as the parent compound (<10%) or as dFdU (272).

Dutch researchers have performed a pharmacokinetic schedule-finding study of gemcitabine plus cisplatin. Gemcitabine 800 mg/m^2 was administered as a 30-minute infusion either 4 hours before, 24 hours before, 4 hours after, or 24 hours after administration of cisplatin 50 mg/m^2 by 1-hour IV infusion. Neither of the dosing schedules that used a 4-hour interval between drug administrations resulted in significant pharmacokinetic or pharmacologic differences. However, when gemcitabine was administered 24 hours before cisplatin, there was a twofold decrease in the plasma AUC of platinum.

Furthermore, when the order of the drugs was reversed (i.e., cisplatin was administered 24 hours before gemcitabine), there was a 1.5-fold increase in the concentration · time product of the active triphosphate metabolite of gemcitabine within white blood cells. On the basis of these results, the investigators are conducting a phase 2 study of the cisplatin/gemcitabine combination wherein cisplatin is administered 24 hours prior to gemcitabine (273).

Administration and Dosage. Gemcitabine should be diluted in 0.9% sodium chloride to a concentration of no greater than 40 mg/mL (higher drug concentrations may result in incomplete dissolution). Gemcitabine is generally administered as a 30-minute IV infusion at a dose of 1,000 mg/m^2; infusion durations of greater than 60 minutes are associated with dose-limiting flu-like symptoms (274).

The standard dosing schedule used for treatment of pancreatic cancer is 1,000 mg/m^2 by 30-minute IV infusion once weekly for 7 weeks for cycle 1 followed by a 1-week rest and then 1,000 mg/m^2 once weekly for 3 weeks followed by a 1-week rest for subsequent cycles (275).

Multiple phase 2 studies of single-agent gemcitabine in refractory/recurrent ovarian cancer have used a dosing schedule of 800 to 1,250 mg/m^2 once weekly for 3 weeks followed by a week of rest; however, doses above 1,000 mg/m^2 may be associated with higher toxicity (266).

In vitro studies have shown synergism between gemcitabine and cisplatin in a variety of human cancer cell lines (276). It is believed that this synergism is primarily the result of increased platinum-DNA adduct formation (276). As noted (see the Drug Disposition section above), the interval between cisplatin and gemcitabine administration can affect both pharmacokinetic and pharmacologic parameters (273). This combination appears to be especially promising for patients with advanced ovarian cancer. Several phase 2 studies have been conducted in previously untreated ovarian cancer patients using a dosing schedule of cisplatin (75 to 100 mg/m^2) on day 1 followed by gemcitabine 1,250 mg/m^2 days 1 and 8 (264,277). Others have performed phase 2 studies of gemcitabine plus cisplatin for patients with relapsed ovarian cancer after prior platinum-based chemotherapy and have determined that cisplatin 30 mg/m^2 plus gemcitabine 600 to 750 mg/m^2 on days 1 and 8 every 21 days is an active and tolerable regimen that demonstrated activity in platinum-resistant patients (87,278).

Side Effects and Toxicities. Gemcitabine-induced toxicity is highly schedule dependent; small daily doses are associated with greater toxicity than large doses administered on a weekly basis (279). The dose, schedule, and duration of infusion of gemcitabine directly affects the toxicity profile (279). Infusion durations of greater than 60 minutes are associated with increased myelosuppression and hepatic toxicity, whereas the administration of small daily doses results in dose-limiting flu-like symptoms (270,274). When gemcitabine is administered using the standard weekly dosing schedule, therapy is generally well tolerated and bone marrow suppression is the major dose-limiting toxicity.

Analysis of safety data from 22 completed clinical trials in which gemcitabine was administered on a weekly basis to 979 patients revealed that neutropenia was the most significant hematologic side effect. Six percent of patients experienced grade 4 neutropenia and an additional 20% experienced grade 3 neutropenia. Grade 4 leukopenia was experienced by less than 1% of patients. Decreases in white blood cell counts were noncumulative, short-lived, and rarely resulted in complications. Only 6 of 979 patients (1.1%) developed severe infections, and no patient developed a life-threatening infection. Grades 3 and 4 anemia were experienced by 6.8% and 1.3% of patients, respectively, and only 2 of the 979 patients discontinued gemcitabine secondary to anemia. Grades 3 and 4 thrombocytopenia occurred in 4.1% and 1.1% of patients, respectively. Less than 1% of patients received platelet transfusions and only four patients (0.4%) discontinued therapy on account of thrombocytopenia (279).

Gemcitabine is associated with a low incidence of hepatic toxicity. Grade 3 elevations in alkaline phosphatase, alanine aminotransferase (ALT), or aspartate aminotransferase (AST) occurred in less than 8% of patients. Grade 4 elevations in these liver enzymes occurred in 2% or fewer of patients. Grade 3 or 4 increases in bilirubin occurred in 1.8% and 0.8% of patients, respectively. It is noteworthy that one third of patients in this study population had documented liver metastases (279).

Clinically significant renal toxicity rarely occurs with gemcitabine therapy. However, rare cases of hemolytic uremic syndrome have been reported with gemcitabine therapy. The incidence is believed to be approximately 0.6% (279).

Other nonhematologic toxicities that were reported in more than 5% of patients were nausea/vomiting (64.3% overall, 17.1% grade 3, 1.2% grade 4), fever (37.3% overall, 0.7% severe), edema (greater than 20% of patients), flu-like symptoms (18.9%, 0.9% severe), cutaneous reactions (24.8%, 0.2% severe), alopecia (14.1%, 0.4% severe), diarrhea (12.1%, 0.7% severe), somnolence (9.1%, 0.9% severe), infection (8.7%, 1.1% severe), mucositis (8.4%, 0.2% severe), constipation (7.8%, 0.7% severe), and dyspnea (7.7%, 1.2% severe). Nausea and vomiting rarely were dose limiting and only two (0.2%) patients discontinued gemcitabine therapy because of nausea. Fever was a fairly frequent toxicity and sometimes occurred in the absence of flu-like symptoms or infection. Subcutaneous edema, including peripheral edema and facial edema, occurred in a significant number of patients. Edema was generally mild to moderate in nature; few patients (0.6%) discontinued gemcitabine because of this side effect, and the edema resolved after drug discontinuation. Flu-like symptoms consisted of headache, back pain, chills, myalgia, asthenia, and anorexia and were generally short lived. Paracetamol was reported to provide relief to some patients. Cutaneous reactions consisted of erythema in mild cases (15.5%) and dry desquamation, vesiculation, and/or pruritus in moderate cases (9.1%). Only one patient developed severe cutaneous toxicity that was characterized as moist desquamation and ulceration. Dyspnea (with or without bronchospasm) occurs in less than 10% of patients following gemcitabine administration. This toxicity generally occurs within a few hours of treatment and resolves within 6 hours (279).

Fatal pulmonary toxicity (acute respiratory distress syndrome) has been reported as a rare side effect of gemcitabine therapy (280). Symptoms include progressive dyspnea, tachypnea, marked hypoxemia, and bilateral interstitial infiltrates consistent with pulmonary edema. Some patients have responded to the termination of gemcitabine therapy and treatment with corticosteroids and diuretics. Prior radiation therapy to the mediastinum may be a risk factor for gemcitabine-induced pulmonary edema (280,281).

Possible incompatibilities between gemcitabine solutions and other drug solutions have not been studied.

Ifosfamide

Chemistry. In combination with cisplatin, ifosfamide (IFEX, Holoxan) is a commonly used drug for the first-line treatment of patients with advanced cancer of the cervix, and in combination chemotherapy, it is a second-line treatment for patients with advanced cancer of the ovary (282,283). It also has activity in advanced or recurrent endometrial cancer (284). Chemically, ifosfamide is 3-(2-chloroethyl)-2-[(2-chloroethyl)amino]-tetrahydro-2H-1,3,2-oxazaphosphorine-2-oxide, and is chemically related to the nitrogen mustards and a structural analog of cyclophosphamide. It differs only in the position of one of the two chloroethyl groups, which is transposed to the endocyclic (ring) nitrogen in ifosfamide. The molecular formula is $C_7H_{15}Cl_2N_2O_2P$, and the compound has a molecular weight of 261.1.

Mechanism of Action. Ifosfamide is a metabolically activated alkylating agent. Like cyclophosphamide, it must first undergo hydroxylation by microsomal (mixed-function oxidase) enzyme systems (285). The activation of ifosfamide occurs more slowly than that of cyclophosphamide, and there is quantitatively greater oxidation of the chloroethyl side chains with ifosfamide. This leads to a greater production of chloracetaldehyde, a possible neurotoxin.

The activation process generates highly reactive metabolites, particularly 4-hydroxyifosfamide, which are capable of cellular uptake and, ultimately, covalent binding to protein and to DNA (286). Metabolites can spontaneously break down to yield the bladder irritant acrolein and the active alkylating moiety ifosforamide mustard. Cross linking of DNA strands proceeds from ifosforamide mustard, but acrolein binds nonspecifically and covalently to bladder epithelium. The DNA–cross-link distance is greater for ifosfamide (seven atoms) compared with cyclophosphamide (five atoms). Furthermore, the aziridine forms more slowly and is less reactive since it lacks a positive charge (287). Chain scission of DNA and inhibition of thymidine uptake also occur with ifosfamide. The primary mechanism of alkylation is not cell cycle specific.

Drug Disposition. The pharmacokinetics of ifosfamide appear to be qualitatively similar to those of cyclophosphamide. Creaven et al. (288) found a plasma half-life of radiolabeled ifosfamide (5,000 mg/m^2) of 13.8 hours, with 82% urinary (radioactivity) recovery.

The plasma decay pattern appears to be biexponential (two-compartment model) for large bolus doses and monoexponential (one-compartment model) with fractionated doses. In contrast to single-dose pharmacokinetics studies, Allen et al. (289) found that with sequential daily administration of 2,400 mg/m^2/day for 3 days, there is monoexponential plasma decay with a half-life of 6.9 hours and a metabolized urinary recovery fraction of 72.8%, in contrast to the biexponential decay (plasma half-life 15.2 hours) of a single-bolus dose of ifosfamide (5,000 mg/m^2). This finding suggests that the metabolic disposition of the drug may be dose dependent. These half-lives are approximately twice those reported for cyclophosphamide. Of note, a longer ifosfamide half-life may be seen in obese patients who are more than 20% over ideal body weight. The renal clearance rate of ifosfamide is about twice that for cyclophosphamide: 21.3 versus 10.7 mL/min in bolus dosing and 18.7 versus 10.7 mL/min with fractionated doses. Only about half of an ifosfamide dose is metabolized compared with about 90% for cyclophosphamide. This reflects a substantial difference in the metabolic clearance capacity for the two analogs. Although more intact (inactive) ifosfamide than cyclophosphamide is renally excreted, urinary alkylating activity persists longer with ifosfamide.

Creaven et al. (288) demonstrated that because unchanged ifosfamide, but not metabolites, penetrates the blood-brain barrier, alkylating activity in the CSF may occur but is probably negligible.

Administration and Dosage. Ifosfamide is reconstituted by the addition of sterile water to the vial, which should be shaken to dissolve. Ifosfamide may be further diluted to a concentration of 0.6 to 29.0 mg/mL in 5% dextrose or 0.9% sodium chloride. It is administered intravenously, usually by a short infusion. Ifosfamide may also be administered by slow IV push in a 75-mL minimal volume of sterile saline solution but not water and infused over at least 30 minutes or by continuous infusion over 5 days. Large single doses of ifosfamide produce much more toxicity than fractionated schedules, which are therefore preferred in solid-tumor treatment regimens. Adequate hydration of the patient before and for 72 hours after ifosfamide therapy is recommended to reduce the incidence of drug-induced hemorrhagic cystitis. The use of a concurrent prophylactic agent for hemorrhagic cystitis, such as mesna (Mesnex), is required to prevent severe hematuria from high-dose ifosfamide. At least 2 L of fluid each day is recommended to produce a copious urine output.

Continuous infusions of ifosfamide over 24 hours have also been given every 3 weeks (290). Mesna can be given concurrently in the same infusion container or as a 4-hour intermittent IV bolus (291). However, renal toxicities may be increased with the single, large infusions. Extravasation of the drug should not cause tissue necrosis, but one case report has been described (292).

The FDA-approved dose for testicular cancer is 1,200 mg/m^2/day for 5 consecutive days every 21 days. Other dosage schedules include 2,000 mg/m^2 IV continuous infusion on days 1 to 3 every 21 days as part of the MAID regimen (mesna, Adriamycin, ifosfamide, dacarbazine) for soft-tissue sarcoma; 1,000 mg/m^2 on days 1 and 2 every 28 days as part of the ICE regimen (ifosfamide, carboplatin, etoposide) for non-Hodgkin's lymphoma; and 1,000 mg/m^2 on days 1 to 3 every 21 to 28 days as part of the TIC regimen (paclitaxel, ifosfamide, carboplatin) for head and neck cancer (50).

A phase 2 study evaluated ifosfamide (1,500 mg/m^2 IV over 1 hour, days 1 to 3) with mesna in combination with paclitaxel (175 mg/m^2 IV over 3 hours on day 1) and cisplatin (75 mg/m^2 IV over 2 hours on day 2) as first-line therapy in advanced, suboptimally debulked epithelial ovarian cancer patients (293). This regimen was associated with an 85% objective response rate and a median overall survival of 52.8 months in 22 patients with stage III or IV disease. A regimen of paclitaxel (175 mg/m^2), ifosfamide (5,000 mg/m^2), and cisplatin (75 mg/m^2 or 50 mg/m^2 in irradiated patients) every 21 days in 45 recurrent or persistent cervical cancer patients was associated with a 67% objective response rate (294).

Morgan et al. (295) evaluated several IV push and infusion dose schedules in non–small cell lung cancer: 700 to 900 mg/m^2/day by IV push for 5 days repeated every 3 weeks; 700 to 1,000 mg/m^2/day for 5 days repeated every 3 weeks plus 1 g/day of oral ascorbic acid; 4 g/m^2 slow infusion repeated every 3 weeks; and 900 mg/m^2 by IV push weekly. There appeared to be less hematuria produced with the sequential 5-day schedule with concomitant ascorbic acid.

Rodriguez et al. (296) described a 47% response rate in leukemia patients with continuous infusions of ifosfamide at 1,200 mg/m^2/day given for 5 days. Significant genitourinary toxicity was not encountered, and myelosuppression predominated as the dose-limiting toxicity. In combination with other cytotoxic drugs, such as doxorubicin or lomustine (CCNU), a single IV push dose of 1,000 mg/m^2 (not to exceed 12,500 g total) has been recommended.

Side Effects and Toxicities. Creaven et al. (288) reviewed the clinical toxicity of ifosfamide given as a large bolus injection (200 to 10,000 mg/m^2) and in a fractionated 3-day (2,400 mg/m^2/day) schedule. Urinary tract toxicity is the dose-limiting factor with both schedules. The clinical hallmark is hemorrhagic cystitis, which is caused by excretion of active alkylating metabolites into the urinary bladder. Vigorous hydration with oral and intravenous fluids and concomitant mesna are needed to prevent serious ifosfamide-induced bladder damage. Hydration may also overcome the antidiuretic effects of this drug. Nelson et al. (291) used IV furosemide (20 to 40 mg) to maintain adequate urine flow in a phase 1 study of ifosfamide. Diuretic responses usually occurred within 1 hour.

Symptoms of dysuria and urinary frequency appear to parallel those of hematuria. The onset of symptoms is 1 to 2 days after injection, with an average duration of 9 days (range 1 to 41 days) (297). Dose-related ifosfamide-induced nephrotoxicity was detected by elevation of the BUN, producing a subsequent dose-related uremia in 66% of patients receiving 150 mg/kg. Other lesions seen at autopsy (four of seven patients) included evidence of acute tubular necrosis and pyelonephritis. At low daily doses, granular cylindruria was seen in all patients, denoting marked tubular damage. The cylindruria cleared within 10 days of drug discontinuance (298). DeFronzo et al. (298) also described glomerular dysfunction and a Fanconi-type picture in a patient treated with ifosfamide. Prior cisplatin therapy may also increase ifosfamide-induced nephrotoxicity (299,300).

Nausea and vomiting appear to be common and are more severe after a rapid injection of large ifosfamide doses. Emesis typically begins within a few hours of administration and persists an average of 3 days (range 1 to 28 days) (297).

Hematologic toxicity from ifosfamide usually involves only a mild to moderate degree of leukopenia in most patients. In a review by Creaven et al. (288), significant thrombocytopenia was not encountered for any of the dose schedules used.

Lethargy and confusion are seen with high doses of ifosfamide and may be caused by the chloracetaldehyde metabolite. Nelson et al. (291) observed that this lasted from 1 to 8 hours, was spontaneously reversible, and was related to the passage of intact drug into the central nervous system (CNS). Seizures, ataxia, stupor, and weakness have been reported after ifosfamide. These effects may be increased by concomitant neurotoxic drugs, such as certain antiemetics, tranquilizers, narcotics, and antihistamines. There is a single case report of nonconvulsive status epilepticus associated with ifosfamide therapy. The patient responded to discontinuation of the ifosfamide and phenytoin therapy (301). Although alkylating metabolites appear to penetrate the blood-brain barrier, the levels achieved are too low to be useful in the treatment of CNS tumors (288).

Alopecia is usually seen with ifosfamide, especially when large bolus doses are used. In a study by Van Dyk et al. (297), the average onset of maximal hair loss was 19 days (range 11 to 32 days) after the start of treatment.

Hepatic enzyme elevations have been described in some patients. The elevations in alkaline phosphatase and serum transaminase are transient and typically resolve rapidly without sequelae.

Special Precautions. The patient must be kept well hydrated during ifosfamide therapy to reduce the potential for hemorrhagic cystitis. The use of mesna given intravenously or orally is required to prevent hemorrhagic cystitis. Table 16.5 outlines the recommended mesna schedule for ifosfamide uroprotection.

TABLE 16.5

DOSING SCHEDULES FOR MESNA COMBINED WITH IFOSFAMIDE

Route of mesna administration	Dose (mg/kg) as a percentage of ifosfamide dose at times before and after ifosfamide: 15 minutes before	4 hours after	8 hours after
Intravenous	20%	20%	20%
Oral[a]	Not recommended, use IV route	40%[a]	40%[a]

[a]For highly reliable patients with total emetic control, mesna solution can be diluted 1:1 to 1:10 in carbonated cola drinks or in chilled fruit juices (e.g., apple, grape, tomato, and orange juice) and administered orally.

Patients who have received previous or concurrent therapy with radiation or cytotoxic drugs may require significant ifosfamide dosage reductions. Dose reductions should also be considered for patients with impaired renal function and/or serum albumin concentrations below 3.5 g/dL.

Drug Interactions. Several drug interactions are possible with ifosfamide. Because the compound undergoes hepatic activation by microsomal enzymes, induction is potentially possible by pretreatment with various enzyme-inducing drugs, such as phenobarbital, phenytoin, and chloral hydrate.

Nephrotoxic drugs like cisplatin may significantly increase ifosfamide renal damage (300). Other drug interactions reported for cyclophosphamide that may also occur with ifosfamide include reactions with metabolic alteration of H_2 antihistamines, such as cimetidine.

Irinotecan

Chemistry. Irinotecan (CPT-11, Camptosar), a TOPO-I inhibitor, is a water-soluble semisynthetic derivative of camptothecin, a natural product extracted from the stem wood of the *Camptotheca acuminata* tree that has significant antitumor activity. It was approved by the FDA in 1998 for treatment of patients with progressive metastatic colon or rectal cancer following 5-FU therapy. Early clinical development of camptothecin was halted because of severe, unpredictable hemorrhagic cystitis, vomiting, and myelosuppression. Subsequently, irinotecan was formulated as a prodrug to have greater water solubility, increased antitumor activity, and less toxicity than the parent compound. Its chemical name is (4S)-4,11-diethyl4-hydroxy-9-[(4-piperidino-piperidino)carbonyloxy]-1Hpyrano[3′,4′:6,7]indolizino[1,2-b] quinoline-3,14 (4H,12H) dione hydrochloride trihydrate. This drug has a molecular weight of 677.19 and the empirical formula is $C_{33}H_{38}N_4O_6 \cdot HCl \cdot 3H_2O$.

Mechanism of Action. Irinotecan's cytotoxicity is believed to be related to the inhibition of TOPO-I, an enzyme necessary for DNA replication (208). Irinotecan is activated to the active metabolite, SN-38, by the liver (302). Irinotecan and SN-38 bind to the transient TOPO-I–DNA complex, stabilize the complex, and thereby promote DNA single-strand breaks. These strand breaks prevent DNA replication and result in cell death (208,302). Current research suggests that the cytotoxicity of irinotecan is due to DNA damage produced during DNA synthesis. Mammalian cells cannot repair these double-strand breaks.

Drug Disposition. Pharmacokinetic studies performed by Rothenberg et al. (303) have determined that when irinotecan is administered as a 90-minute IV infusion at dose ranges of 50 to 180 mg/m^2, the plasma terminal-phase half-life for irinotecan (total) was 7.9 ± 2.8 hours, 6.3 ± 2.2 hours for irinotecan (lactone), and 11.5 ± 3.8 hours for SN-38 (the active metabolite). The time of peak plasma concentration for irinotecan was at infusion end, whereas the time of peak concentration for total SN-38 varied from 30 to 90 minutes after completion of the infusion. Plasma clearance was unrelated to dose, with a mean clearance of 15.3 ± 3.5 L/h/m^2 for the total and 45.6 ± 10.8 L/h/m^2 for the lactone. At the 150-mg/m^2 dose, the following pharmacokinetic parameters were observed: peak plasma concentration—1.97 μg/mL for total irinotecan, 0.83 μg/mL for the lactone form, and 36.7 ng/mL for total SN-38; and concentration · time product (AUC) 8.44 μg · h/mL for total irinotecan, 2.81 μg · h/mL for the lactone form, and 409.8 ng · h/mL for total SN-38. Renal excretion was not a major route of drug elimination.

Abigerges et al. (304) determined in their pharmacokinetic study of irinotecan (100 to 700 mg/m^2 by 30-minute IV infusion) that the plasma disposition of irinotecan was biphasic or triphasic. The mean plasma terminal-phase half-life, volume of distribution, and total body clearance of irinotecan were 14.2 ± 0.9 hours, 157 ± 8 L/m^2, and 15 ± 1 L/m^2/h, respectively. Both the irinotecan and SN-38 concentration · time product (AUC) increased linearly with dose. At the 350-mg/m^2 dose level, the irinotecan and SN-38 AUCs were 34.0 ± 4.1 μg · h/mL and 451 ± 100 ng · h/mL, respectively. The plasma terminal-phase half-life of SN-38 was 13.8 ± 1.4 hours.

Administration and Dosage. The appropriate dose of irinotecan should be diluted with 500 mL of dextrose (5%) to a final concentration of 0.12 to 1.1 mg/mL and administered IV over 90 minutes (303). Alternatively, French investigators have administered irinotecan by diluting the appropriate amount of drug in 250 mL of 0.9% sodium chloride solution and delivering the drug IV over 30 minutes (304).

In the United States, the recommended dose for irinotecan therapy in colon cancer patients is 125 mg/m^2 weekly by 90-minute infusion for 4 weeks followed by a 2-week rest. In Europe, the recommended dose is 300 to 350 mg/m^2 by 90-minute infusion every 21 days. The U.S. schedule has been used in three phase 2 clinical trials, wherein irinotecan displayed modest activity in cervical cancer patients (305–307). When administered as a single dose every 3 weeks, a 240-mg/m^2 dose is recommended (303,308). French investigators have determined that a 600-mg/m^2 30-minute IV infusion every 3 weeks can be administered if drug-induced diarrhea is aggressively managed by high-dose loperamide (e.g., up to 16 mg/day); however, these investigators recommended a dose level of 350 mg/m^2 every 3 weeks until further experience is gained with higher dose levels (304).

Side Effects and Toxicities. Diarrhea and neutropenia are the major dose-limiting toxicities associated with irinotecan (303,304,308). Other moderate to severe toxicities associated with irinotecan therapy include anemia, dehydration (secondary to diarrhea), nausea, vomiting, anorexia, abdominal cramping, cumulative asthenia, thrombocytopenia, renal insufficiency, elevations in liver transaminases, and alopecia.

The diarrhea associated with irinotecan appears to be due to two separate mechanisms. The diarrhea that may occur during irinotecan infusion is highly responsive to atropine therapy and, therefore, appears to be related to cholinergic activity. However, the subacute diarrhea that develops 2 to 3 weeks after irinotecan therapy is refractory to anticholinergic agents. The most effective treatment for the subacute diarrhea is institution of therapy with antimotility agents (i.e., loperamide or diphenoxylate hydrochloride with atropine sulfate) at the first signs of increased intestinal motility (e.g., loose bowels). If left untreated, subacute diarrhea can rapidly progress to grade 4 toxicity. This life-threatening diarrhea is refractory to antidiarrheal therapy and generally lasts for 5 to 7 days. Patients with grade 4 diarrhea should be hospitalized and receive supportive care with IV fluids and electrolyte replacement (303).

Special Precautions. As described above (see the Side Effects and Toxicities section), irinotecan can induce grade 4 diarrhea that is refractory to antidiarrheal medication. Patients who are receiving irinotecan must be monitored carefully for early symptoms of increased intestinal motility and should receive antimotility therapy (e.g., up to 16 mg/day loperamide) as soon as initial symptoms of diarrhea appear. A low level of glucuronidation in the biliary system has been associated with the development of severe diarrhea in some patients (309).

Special Applications. The TOPO-I inhibitor irinotecan also has been shown to have activity against advanced cervical cancer. Cottu et al. (310) reported response rates in patients with relapsed cervical cancer ranging from 20% to 22%. The GOG reported a response rate of 13.3% (6 of 45) in patients with advanced cervical cancer with no prior chemotherapy (306). No responses were reported in second-line (after resistance to cisplatin) treatment in a phase 2 study of 16 patients (305). However, Verschraegen et al. (307) reported a 21% response rate in the same patient population (n = 42). Reviews by Eisenhauer and Vermorken (311) and Verschraegen (312) have reported response rates ranging from 13% to 24%. The combination of irinotecan (60 mg/m^2 90-min IV on days 1, 8, and 15) followed by cisplatin (60 mg/m^2 on day 8) administered every 3 weeks has demonstrated activity in a phase 2 trial of first-line treatment of cervical cancer, with a 1-year disease-free and overall survival of 26.7 and 65.1%, respectively (313).

Liposomal Encapsulated Doxorubicin

Chemistry. Liposomal doxorubicin (Doxil, Caelyx) is FDA approved for the treatment of patients with metastatic, refractory ovarian cancer and AIDS-related Kaposi's sarcoma. Doxorubicin HCl, which is the established name for (8*S*,10*S*)-10-[(3-amino-2,3,6-trideoxy-α-L-*lyxo*-hexopyranosyl)oxy]-8-glycolyl-7,8,9,10-tetrahydro-6,8,11-trihydroxy-1-methoxy-5,12-naphthacenedione hydrochloride, has a molecular weight of 579.99 and the molecular formula $C_{27}H_{29}NO_{11}$ · HCl. The liposomal carriers are composed of N-(carbonyl-methoxypolyethylene glycol 2000)-1,2distearoyl-*sn*-glycero-3-phosphoethanolamine sodium salt (MPEG-DSPE), 3.19 mg/mL; fully hydrogenated soy phosphatidylcholine (HSPC), 9.58 mg/mL; and cholesterol, 3.19 mg/mL. Greater than 90% of the drug is encapsulated in the liposomes. The liposomal encapsulation of doxorubicin dramatically alters the pharmacokinetic and toxicity profiles of the drug.

Mechanism of Action. The mechanism of action of doxorubicin was discussed previously (see the Doxorubicin section). Liposomes are microscopic vesicles composed of a phospholipid bilayer that are capable of encapsulating active drugs. The liposomes of the encapsulated form of doxorubicin are formulated with surface-bound methoxypolyethylene glycol (MPEG), a process often referred to as pegylation, to protect liposomes from detection by the mononuclear phagocyte system (MPS) and to increase blood circulation time (314).

Drug Disposition. Liposomal doxorubicin is associated with a much longer plasma half-life, slower plasma clearance, and reduced volume of distribution than free doxorubicin. In a pharmacokinetics study performed in six patients with solid tumors, the area under the plasma disappearance curve was 1.0 mg/L · hour versus 609 mg/L · hour when 25 mg/m^2 of doxorubicin was administered as free drug or as a pegylated liposomal form, respectively. The initial half-life was 0.07 versus 3.2 hours, and the terminal half-life was 8.7 versus 45.2 hours for the free and liposomal forms of doxorubicin, respectively. Additionally, the steady-state volume of distribution was 254 L versus 4.1 L for the free and liposomal forms, respectively (315). Liposomal encapsulation of doxorubicin has also been shown to result in fourfold to 16-fold increases in tumor-tissue drug concentrations relative to that achieved following administration of the free form.

Administration and Dosage. Liposomal doxorubicin must be diluted in 250 mL of 5% dextrose prior to administration. Because liposomal doxorubicin contains no preservative or bacteriostatic agent, aseptic technique must be strictly observed. Liposomal doxorubicin may be administered as an IV infusion over 30 to 60 minutes. In that liposomal doxorubicin is not a vesicant, extravasation of the drug is not a critical concern. For ovarian cancer patients, liposomal doxorubicin should be administered at a dose of 50 mg/m^2 (every 4 weeks) at an initial rate of 1 mg/min to reduce the risk of infusion reactions. The rate may be increased to a 60-minute infusion if no adverse events are noted. The recommended dose in AIDS-related Kaposi's sarcoma patients is 20 mg/m^2 over 30 minutes, once every 3 weeks, for as long as patients respond and tolerate treatment.

Side Effects and Toxicities. Unlike the parent drug, liposomal doxorubicin is not a vesicant and is associated with minimal cardiotoxicity, alopecia, and nausea/vomiting. However, the liposomal encapsulation results in acute infusion reactions, and an increased rate of PPE and stomatitis (316). PPE is a dose-limiting toxicity that can occur in 26% of patients who receive 50 mg/m^2 every 4 weeks (317). Stomatitis is a second dose-limiting toxicity associated with liposomal doxorubicin. Current methods to prevent PPE and stomatitis include dose reduction and discontinuation. (Grade 1—redose; if patient has experienced previous grade 3 or 4 toxicity, delay the treatment by 2 weeks until resolution to grades 0 to 1 and reduce dose by 25% before returning to original dose level. Grades 2 to 4—delay up to 2 weeks until resolved; if no resolution to grades 0 to 1, discontinue. Grades 3 to 4—after delay and resolution to grades 0 to 1, decrease dose by 25%; if no resolution, discontinue.) To help relieve pain from PPE, topical wound care, elevation, and cold compresses may be used as supportive care (253). Topical DMSO has been used to treat skin extravasations (99% DMSO four times daily up to 14 days), but has yet to be evaluated in a randomized trial (251). Other possible therapies that have yet to be evaluated in clinical trials include systemic corticosteroids and pyridoxine (vitamin B_6) (253).

Infusion-related reactions occur in fewer than 10% of patients treated with liposomal doxorubicin and are most common during the first course of treatment. Symptoms may include flushing, shortness of breath, facial swelling, headache, chills, back pain, tightness in the chest and throat, and hypotension. Alopecia has been observed in only 15% of ovarian cancer patients treated with liposomal doxorubicin.

Melphalan

Chemistry. Melphalan (Alkeran, L-phenylalanine mustard, L-PAM) is a phenylalanine derivative of nitrogen mustard that acts as a bifunctional alkylating agent. Melphalan is FDA approved for the chemotherapy of patients with multiple myeloma. The agent's molecular formula is $C_{13}H_{18}Cl_2N_2O_2$ and its molecular weight is 305.2. It is known chemically as 4-[bis(2-chloroethyl)amino]-*L*-phenylalanine. Melphalan is water insoluble and previously was only commercially available in a 2-mg tablet form. However, a parenteral formulation was approved by the FDA in 1993. Melphalan for injection is supplied as a freeze-dried powder in single-use vials containing 50 mg melphalan and 20 mg povidone. A vial of sterile diluent (10 mL) is also supplied.

Mechanism of Action. Melphalan is an alkylating agent of the bischloroethylamine type. Its cytotoxicity appears to be related to the extent of its interstrand cross linking with tumor-cell DNA, probably by binding at the N^7 position of guanine (318). The cross-helical base pairing causes strain and possible rupture of the double-stranded DNA backbone.

Melphalan is relatively stable in media containing high concentrations of chloride ions and at acid pH (318). It has a relatively short *in vitro* half-life in plasma of approximately two hours owing to the rapid hydroxylation of the chloroethyl groups of the molecule. Melphalan may form a reactive immonium ion that can alkylate or hydroxylate the monohydroxy and dihydroxy metabolites. Monohydroxy melphalan possesses only 2% of the cytotoxicity of the parent compound, and the dihydroxy derivative is inactive (319).

Melphalan is usually transported into cells by two amino acid–transporting systems: the sodium-independent system that transfers leucine and a monovalent cation-dependent system similar to that which transfers alanine, serine, or cysteine (320). Melphalan efflux from cells appears to be sodium independent, to be stimulated by amino acids in the extracellular medium, and to occur by a simple diffusion mechanism.

Drug Disposition. Melphalan has extremely variable systemic availability after oral administration. In the average patient, approximately one third of an administered dose of melphalan can be recovered from plasma after a bolus oral dose. The range of systemic availability after oral dosing varies from none to over 90%. The terminal-phase plasma half-life of orally administered melphalan is approximately 90 minutes, and the 24-hour urinary excretion rate averages 11% (321). Melphalan penetration into cerebrospinal fluid is low. Plasma protein binding ranges from 60% to 90%, and approximately 30% is irreversibly bound to plasma proteins.

Studies of melphalan metabolism, using an isolated perfused rat liver model and *in vitro* rat microsomal enzyme preparations, have documented insignificant hepatic biotransformation (322).

Two groups of investigators have reported that the systemic availability of melphalan is increased if the drug is administered in the fasting state. The presence of a large meal appears to enhance melphalan degradation at the alkaline pH found in the upper small bowel before systemic absorption (323).

Patients with multiple myeloma receiving intravenously administered melphalan achieved longer durations of survival than those receiving the oral formulation. Furthermore, a significantly lower dose of intravenously administered drug was associated with life-threatening leukopenia and infectious complications compared with the oral formulation (323).

Administration and Dosage. The usual IV dose is 16 mg/m^2 (15- to 20-minute infusion) administered at 2-week intervals for four doses, then at 4-week intervals. The oral agent dose is 6 mg/day for 2 to 3 weeks, followed by up to 4 weeks without treatment. As a single agent, one-time IV doses of 1 mg/kg repeated at 4- to 6-week intervals are generally well tolerated. Although the manufacturer reports equal effects from intravenous or oral doses, bioavailability differences and the potential for lessened hepatic clearance of IV doses suggest IV dosing at reduced levels. In a surgical adjuvant setting for ovarian carcinoma, melphalan has been used in large cyclic doses of 1 mg/kg given IV over 8 hours and repeated in 4 weeks (324). The apparently equivalent therapeutic results with intravenous and oral dosing are surprising in light of the reported poor oral absorption of the compound.

Side Effects and Toxicities. Compared with other standard alkylating agents, melphalan is relatively well tolerated after oral administration. Except for dose-limiting bone marrow suppression (i.e., neutropenia, thrombocytopenia, anemia), other acute side effects are uncommon and include infrequent nausea and vomiting and, rarely, skin rash and pulmonary toxicity (325). Melphalan is characterized by its potential to cause cumulative bone marrow damage, as expressed by profound and prolonged depression of neutrophils and platelets. There is a slow reduction in peripheral leukocyte and platelet counts to their nadirs at 28 to 35 days after drug administration followed by a 14- to 21-day recovery period.

Acute nonlymphocytic leukemia has been reported in patients with multiple myeloma and ovarian cancer after prolonged melphalan therapy. In one Swedish study of 474 patients with ovarian carcinoma, there were four cases of acute nonlymphocytic leukemia among 12 patients who received 800 mg or more of melphalan (326). An evaluation of the relationship between alkylating agents and leukemic disorders in 3,363 one-year survivors of ovarian cancer revealed that the 10-year cumulative risk of acquiring leukemia was 11.2% after treatment with melphalan and 5.4% after cyclophosphamide treatment (327). The risk of developing leukemia after melphalan and cyclophosphamide treatment was significantly higher than in matched patient groups who received no chemotherapy. These data suggest that, to reduce the leukemia risk, the total dose of melphalan should not exceed 600 mg.

Special Applications. One major impediment to the success of cancer chemotherapy is the rapid development of drug resistance as manifested clinically by short objective responses and subsequent, progressive tumor growth despite aggressive chemotherapy. Several mechanisms have been postulated to explain this relatively universal phenomenon.

Melphalan therapy has been used in autologous bone marrow transplantation. A series of studies has been reported for high-dose (120 to 225 mg/m^2) IV administered melphalan against adult melanoma, breast, and colon cancers (328). Although the resulting high response rates appear to be promising, most have been partial, and survival advantages have not yet been established. In general, these high doses of melphalan have been tolerated relatively well, with diarrhea and stomatitis becoming severe and dose-limiting at doses greater than 200 mg/m^2.

Because ovarian cancer remains confined to the intraperitoneal space for most of its natural history, there has been increasing interest in the intraperitoneal administration of cytotoxic drugs to patients with minimal residual intraperitoneal disease (i.e., plaques <1 cm in diameter) after aggressive cytoreductive surgery or primary chemotherapy. Melphalan exhibits a high degree of *in vitro* cytotoxicity as compared with other standard chemotherapeutic agents when tested against fresh human ovarian cancer tumors at drug concentrations achievable by intraperitoneal administration (329). In addition to its high degree of cytotoxicity, melphalan's high molecular weight ensures a relatively low clearance from the peritoneal space.

In a phase 1 dose-finding study, Howell et al. (330) showed that an intraperitoneal melphalan dose of 70 mg/kg was tolerated, with only moderate leukopenia (median nadir 2,000 cells/µL) and thrombocytopenia (median nadir 69,000 platelets/µL) and no evidence of peritoneal irritation. The peak peritoneal concentration averaged 93-fold greater than the plasma concentration, and total drug exposure for the peritoneal cavity averaged 63-fold greater than that for the plasma.

Methotrexate

Chemistry. Methotrexate is an active drug in the first-line treatment of gestational choriocarcinoma, chorioadenoma destruens, and hydatidiform mole. It is used in the prophylaxis and treatment of meningeal leukemia, and is used in combination with other agents for the treatment of breast cancer, epidermoid cancers of the head and neck, advanced mycosis fungoides, advanced non-Hodgkin's lymphoma, lung cancer, and metastatic squamous cell cancer of the cervix. Methotrexate is a cell cycle–specific antifolate analog, which differs from folic acid in two substitutions: an amino group for a hydroxyl in the pteridine portion of the molecule and a methyl group on the amino nitrogen between the pteridine nucleus and the benzoyl group of 4-amino-10-methyl folic acid. Chemically, methotrexate is N-[4-[[(2,4-diamino-6-pteridinyl)methyl]benzoyl]-L-glutamic acid. It is a weak acid with a molecular weight of 454.45 and a molecular formula of $C_{20}H_{22}N_8O_5$. It is only slightly soluble in water and alcohol. Sodium methotrexate is water soluble and is used in injectable preparations.

Mechanism of Action. Free intracellular methotrexate tightly binds to dihydrofolate reductase, blocking the reduction of dihydrofolate to tetrahydrofolic acid, the active form of folic acid. As a result, thymidylate synthetase and various steps in *de novo* purine synthesis that require 1-carbon transfer reactions are halted. This in turn arrests DNA, RNA, and protein synthesis.

Amino acid syntheses blocked by methotrexate include those requiring 1-carbon transfer, such as the conversion of glycine to serine and homocysteine to methionine. Experimental studies have shown that thymidylate synthetase is inhibited at methotrexate concentrations of 10^{-8} M or less, but inhibition of purine synthesis requires concentrations of 10^{-7} M or greater (331).

Methotrexate undergoes a variable degree of polyglutamation intracellularly. The polyglutamated forms of the drug are positively charged and do not readily pass through cell membranes. Methotrexate polyglutamates form an intracellular pool of active drug that is retained for long periods, sometimes months, after a single dose (332). The ability of tumor cells to add t-glutamyl residues to methotrexate may be a key determinant of antitumor activity.

The effects of methotrexate are rapidly reversible as free methotrexate leaves the cells. The normal intracellular levels of dihydrofolate are very low (10^{-8} M) but increase greatly after methotrexate administration.

Resistance to methotrexate may develop as a result of elevated dihydrofolate reductase activity or defective transport of methotrexate into malignant cells. Increased dihydrofolate reductase enzyme levels may also result from amplification of the dihydrofolate reductase gene, a process associated with homogeneously staining regions of chromosomes and an unstable inheritance mediated by double minutes or extra chromosomal DNA fragments (333). Certain quinazolines have been shown to be effective inhibitors of thymidylate synthetase and may be useful clinically in overcoming this type of resistance (334). *In vitro* studies and clinical experimentation with high-dose therapy indicate that a major mechanism of resistance is probably secondary to decreased cellular uptake.

Methotrexate is classified as a cell cycle phase–specific antimetabolite with activity mostly in S phase. Experimentally, methotrexate synchronizes tumor cells in S phase about 36 to 72 hours after administration (335).

The enhanced toxic effect on tumors compared with normal tissue from high-dose methotrexate with leucovorin rescue may be a result of bypassing normal carrier-mediated cell membrane transport of methotrexate. Leucovorin and its metabolite, 5-methyltetrahydrofolate, share a common influx transport site with methotrexate. There appear to be at least two active transport carrier systems involved in the influx and efflux of methotrexate and folates (336). If normal cells are rescued with calcium leucovorin, methotrexate can then exert a relatively greater toxic effect on the tumor cells. Selective rescue of normal cells may be mediated by a slower rate of DNA synthesis relative to the tumor cell or to tissue-specific differences in transmembrane transport.

Drug Disposition. Orally administered methotrexate is rapidly but incompletely absorbed from the gastrointestinal tract. It reaches peak blood levels in approximately 1 hour. Approximately 50% to 60% of the drug in the blood is bound to plasma proteins. Methotrexate is widely distributed to body tissues. In conventional doses, methotrexate is excreted unchanged in the urine. In high doses, it is partially metabolized to 7-hydromethotrexate, which is only slightly soluble in acidic solutions. About 1% to 11% of a dose is excreted as the 7-hydroxy metabolite, and this may comprise as much as 35% of the drug level in the terminal elimination phase. Only about one third of an oral dose is absorbed, but intramuscular absorption is almost 100% (337).

The hepatic extraction coefficient for methotrexate appears to be very low and intra-arterial hepatic doses show metabolism and pharmacokinetics similar to IV doses (338). Methotrexate is both filtered at the glomerulus and actively secreted by the renal tubule. Drugs that interfere with renal excretion of weak acids, such as probenecid, sulfinpyrazone, and salicylates, may be expected to reduce the rate of methotrexate excretion. Probenecid has been used successfully in one study to produce a prolonged elevation of plasma methotrexate levels from otherwise low doses of methotrexate (339).

Plasma decay of methotrexate levels has been reported to be biphasic and possibly triphasic. Huffman et al. (340) reported half-lives after a 30 mg/m^2 dose to be triphasic: 0.750 ± 0.11, 3.49 ± 0.55, and 26.99 ± 4.44 hours, respectively. Stoller et al. (341) reported a biphasic plasma decay for high-dose therapy of 2.06 ± 0.16 and 10.4 ± 1.8 hours. Wang et al. (342) reported age-dependent biphasic elimination of high-dose methotrexate.

Patients with pleural effusions may accumulate methotrexate that slowly distributes from this compartment back into the plasma to increase systemic exposure and the risk of toxicity (343). Effusions should be drained before administration of methotrexate.

Administration and Dosage. Methotrexate may be given by the oral, intramuscular, intravenous (intravenous infusion or push), intra-arterial, or intrathecal routes. For treatment of neoplastic disease, oral administration of low-dose methotrexate is preferred owing to the rapid absorption of the tablet form of the agent. Methotrexate has been given by numerous dosing schedules. The usual starting doses are adjusted based on clinical response and hematologic monitoring. In general, methotrexate is administered orally or intramuscularly in doses of 15 to 30 mg daily for a 5-day course. Courses are usually repeated for three to five times as required, with rest periods of 1 or more weeks between courses until toxicities subside (344). Leucovorin is indicated following treatment with higher doses of methotrexate to diminish toxicity.

If the IV formulation is administered, the dose should be reduced by 50% for patients with renal insufficiency (BUN ≥30 mg/L). Similar dose reductions should be made for the oral form, although no specific guidelines are available. Methotrexate administration is contraindicated in patients with a creatinine clearance less than 40 mL/min and/or a serum creatinine greater than 2 mg/dL.

Side Effects and Toxicities. Hematologic effects of methotrexate include leukopenia, thrombocytopenia, and anemia. They occur rapidly and depend on the dose and schedule used. The nadir of hemoglobin depression occurs after 6 to 13 days and of reticulocyte at 2 to 7 days, with rebound between 9 and 19 days. Leukocyte nadir occurs within 4 to 7 days, followed by partial recovery and then, in rare instances, a second decrease in the leukocyte counts occurs during days 12 to 21. The platelet nadir is reached in 5 to 12 days. Hypogammaglobulinemia may also occur after methotrexate administration.

Nausea, vomiting, and anorexia are usually the earliest gastrointestinal symptoms. Gingivitis, glossitis, pharyngitis, stomatitis, and ulcerations with bleeding of the mucosal membranes of the mouth or other portions of the gastrointestinal tract may occur. If ulcerative stomatitis or diarrhea occurs, methotrexate therapy must be interrupted to prevent severe hemorrhagic enteritis or intestinal perforation.

Hepatotoxicity is more common in patients receiving high-dose therapy and in those receiving frequent small doses. Hepatocellular injury is indicated in liver function tests by a rise in serum glutamic oxaloacetic transaminase (SGOT) and serum glutamic pyruvic transaminase (SGPT), usually within the first 12 hours. Prothrombin times may rise with a decrease in plasma factor VII activity, and indirect hyperbilirubinemia may develop. All of these usually return to normal within 1 week. Hepatocytes appear to be protected by fractionated high-dose methotrexate treatments with leucovorin rescue if treatments are administered at intervals of less than 1 week. This may be due to leucovorin activity remaining from prior doses. Various pathologic hepatic changes can occur, including atrophy, necrosis, fatty changes, fibrosis, and cirrhosis. Liver biopsy is the only reliable means of assessing the degree of methotrexate hepatotoxicity.

Dermatologic side effects include erythematous rashes, pruritus, urticaria, folliculitis, vasculitis, photosensitivity, depigmentation, or hyperpigmentation. Alopecia may occur, with several months being required for regrowth. CNS effects include dizziness, malaise, and blurred vision. Encephalopathy also has been reported. Intrathecal administration has been followed by increased CSF pressure, convulsions, paresis, and a syndrome resembling the Guillain-Barré syndrome (342). Deaths have been reported after intrathecal therapy. Renal failure may occur in patients receiving methotrexate, especially in high doses. This risk may be decreased by alkalinization of the urine to increase methotrexate solubility and by giving large quantities of fluid. Other reactions rarely reported include chills and fever, osteoporosis, and pulmonary reactions, mainly fibrosis (345).

Drug Interactions. Potential drug interactions have been postulated to occur with other protein-bound drugs, such as salicylates, sulfonamides, phenytoin, and *p*-aminobenzoic acid. These drugs displace methotrexate from its protein-binding site in the blood, causing an increase in the levels of the free drug. However, the overall degree of binding is probably not high enough for major displacement interactions.

Antibiotics used in gut sterilization may also alter methotrexate pharmacokinetics in humans, eliminating the slow phase of excretion (346). Salicylates and probenecid may also compete with methotrexate for renal tubular secretion and increase its serum half-life.

Ethyl alcohol may increase the possibility of methotrexate-induced hepatotoxicity. Oral anticoagulants, such as warfarin, may be greatly potentiated by methotrexate. Methotrexate may alter the liver metabolism of these drugs.

There are several drug interactions described for methotrexate with other chemotherapeutic agents. For example, a clinically significant interaction between methotrexate and L-asparaginase involves the administration of methotrexate 3 to 24 hours before L-asparaginase. The methotrexate treatment is believed to block protein synthesis and reduce asparaginase toxicities, allowing larger doses to be given. Some sequential methotrexate combinations may produce enhanced therapeutic activity. For example, methotrexate given 4 to 9 hours before 5-FU may produce enhanced antitumor activity in breast cancer, but with a commensurate increase in toxic effects (132,347). The mechanism of this interaction involves a significant increase in 5-FU for at least 3 hours (347). The reverse sequence decreases therapeutic activity (348).

Methotrexate activity is enhanced, and thus toxicity increased, when it is used with aspirin, penicillins, nonsteroidal anti-inflammatory agents, cephalosporins, or phenytoin. These agents inhibit the renal excretion of methotrexate (50).

Special Applications. Very high doses of methotrexate have been administered for a variety of tumors. Although leucovorin rescue reduces toxicity, it is still not certain that high-dose therapy is superior to more conventional dosing without rescue. Specific dosing schemes vary, but a high dose of methotrexate is usually administered intravenously and followed by calcium leucovorin 24 to 36 hours after initiation of therapy to prevent toxicity. Table 16.6 presents specific dosing recommendations.

The dose range of methotrexate with leucovorin rescue is 100 mg/m^2 to 10 g/m^2 given every 1 to 3 weeks. The lower end of this dosing spectrum has been administered in four divided oral doses over a 24-hour period. Most frequently, the dose is given by IV infusion in 1 to 2 L of fluid as a rapid infusion or over 6 to 24 hours. Higher peak methotrexate levels occur with more rapid IV infusions, and this may be theoretically more efficacious. There does not appear to be a clinical difference in toxicity between rapid and prolonged infusions. Only the 500- and 1,000-mg vials with no preservative should be used for this purpose. Further dilution of methotrexate is necessary and can be accomplished with normal saline or D_5W.

High-dose methotrexate has been associated with reversible nephrotoxicity. At high concentrations, methotrexate may

TABLE 16.6

DETERMINATION OF LEUCOVORIN DOSE FOR HIGH-DOSE METHOTREXATE (50 TO 250 MG/KG OVER 6 HOURS) REGIMENS[a]

	Leucovorin administration	
Plasma methotrexate concentration at 48 hours (M)	mg/m² of leucovorin every 8 hours	No. of doses of leucovorin
$<5 \times 10^{-7}$	15	7
5×10^{-7}	15	8
1×10^{-6}	100	8
2×10^{-6}	200	8

[a]Plasma methotrexate concentration at 96 hours should be determined also. If the plasma concentration at 96 hours is $\geq 5 \times 10^{-6}$ M, the previously used leucovorin regimen should be continued until the plasma methotrexate concentration is $\leq 5 \times 10^{-7}$ M. All patients should also be prehydrated for 12 hours to establish an alkaline diuresis using 1.5 L/m² of fluid containing 10 mEq of bicarbonate and 20 mEq of KCl (pH of urine should be 7.0).

precipitate in the renal tubule, causing tubular dilatation and damage. The pK_a of methotrexate is 5.4. When the urine pH is near this value, methotrexate exists predominantly in its insoluble form and is likely to precipitate. Renal toxicity may be prevented by increasing urine alkalinity and flow. Sodium bicarbonate (3 g every 3 hours for 12 hours before therapy) is usually sufficient to induce an alkaline urine in adults. The sodium bicarbonate should be continued with frequent urine pH checks during the therapy and for 48 hours after the dose has been delivered. Methotrexate serum levels are useful in predicting toxic reactions and appropriately adjusting rescue doses of leucovorin (349). High-dose methotrexate with rescue is complicated and potentially extremely toxic. Only experienced teams using carefully designed protocols should attempt this treatment. Immediate methotrexate levels should be readily available. Fatal renal or hematologic reactions have occurred at major treatment centers despite the prophylactic precautions described (350).

Mitomycin

Chemistry. Mitomycin (Mutamycin, mitomycin C) is a purple antibiotic isolated from *Streptomyces caespitosus* that is indicated for disseminated adenocarcinoma of the stomach or pancreas in combination with other agents and as palliative treatment. It has also has been proven to be useful in combination chemotherapy as a third-line agent in the treatment of advanced cervical cancer. Its chemical name is [1*aR*]6-amino-8-[[(aminocarbonyl)oxy]methyl]-1,1*a*,2,8,8*a*,8*b*-hexahydro-8*a*-methoxy-5-methylazirino[2′,3′:3,4]-pyrrolo[1,2-*a*]indole-4,7-dione, and it has a molecular weight of 334. Mitomycin is heat stable, is soluble in water and other organic solvents, and has a unique absorption peak at 365 nM (351). In solution, it is slowly inactivated by visible but not ultraviolet light. It is very unstable in acidic and highly basic conditions. The aziridine and carbamate groups on mitomycin are necessary for alkylating activity but not for antibacterial activity. The compound is activated by reduction of the quinone moiety, which releases a methanol residue from the molecule. This allows the aziridine ring to open, exposing an electrophilic carbon at C_1 (alkylating site). The second (cross-linking) site for alkylation is exposed at C_{10} after an enzymatic or chemically mediated loss of the carbamate side chain.

Mechanism of Action. Mitomycin is activated *in vivo* to an alkylating agent that cross links complementary DNA strands, halting DNA synthesis. DNA is the major site of mitomycin activity, although at extremely high concentrations, RNA synthesis may also be affected. The active metabolites of mitomycin resulting from reduction of the quinone moiety yield an opened aziridine ring exposing the primary alkylating site at C_1. A second alkylating site at C_{10} is exposed with the enzymatic loss of the carbamate side chain (352). The molecular site of DNA binding has been identified at the N_2 and O_6 positions of adjacent guanines in the minor groove of DNA (353).

Activation of the drug can be mediated by chemical reducing agents, by microsomal enzymes, or even by brief exposure to an acidic pH. The extent of DNA binding appears to be related to the guanine and cytosine content of the particular DNA. Cytotoxicity probably results directly from DNA synthesis inhibition secondary to alkylation.

Oxygen free radicals may also contribute to the cytotoxicity of mitomycin by producing DNA strand breaks (354). Oxygen free radicals are produced by cyclic redox reactions of the quinone moiety. Mitomycin's cytotoxic action is not cell cycle phase–specific, but cytotoxic effects are maximized if cells are treated in late G_1 and early S phase. In addition to the direct cytotoxic effects of the drug, mitomycin also causes chromosomal aberrations (mutagenic activity), and in experimental systems, it is a potent carcinogen and teratogen.

Kennedy et al. (355) described selective activation of mitomycin by hypoxic cells, suggesting some drug selectivity for hypoxic tumors. Resistance to mitomycin involves an increase in specific cytosolic proteins (possibly a glutathione transferase) and collateral resistance with anthracyclines and dactinomycin (356). The latter type of multidrug resistance is mediated by P-glycoprotein expression, with resultant enhanced drug efflux, as observed in mitomycin C–resistant L-1210 cells (357).

Drug Disposition. Mitomycin is cleared rapidly from the vascular compartment. Peak serum concentrations of about 1 µg/mL are typically achieved after IV bolus doses of 10 mg/m². Less than 10% of the dose is excreted into the urine, and this is complete within a few hours after administration. Mitomycin also has been detected in the bile and feces, although animal studies demonstrate that the highest drug levels occur in the kidneys. Detectable levels were also found in muscle, lung, intestine, stomach, and eye, but not in the brain, spleen, or liver (351).

The primary means of mitomycin elimination is by liver metabolism, but the specific enzymes responsible are unknown. However, the enzymes responsible for metabolism do not appear to involve the P450 mixed-function oxide family. *In vitro* studies demonstrate drug inactivation on contact with tissue preparations from the spleen, liver, kidney, brain, and heart. This inactivation is further augmented by anaerobic conditions (357).

There is no detectable change in mitomycin pharmacokinetics in patients with altered hepatic function nor when other drugs, including furosemide, are given concurrently (358). Schilcher et al. (359) showed that the pharmacokinetics of mitomycin do not change after the administration of high doses.

Mitomycin distribution into bile and ascites fluids has been quantitated in patients receiving standard IV doses. The maximum biliary level of 0.5 µg/mL was achieved after 2 hours and was five- to eightfold higher than simultaneous plasma levels during the elimination phase (360). Mitomycin also rapidly penetrates into ascites fluid and reaches maximal concentrations of 0.05 µg/mL 1 hour after administration. This distribution represents about 40% of the total plasma exposure. The drug also appears to slightly concentrate in cervical tissues after IV administration (361).

With intra-arterial administration, the hepatic extraction of mitomycin averages only 23% (362). The calculated relative advantage for hepatic arterial infusions is only 2.5- to 3.6-fold greater than for other methods.

Administration and Dosage. Sterile water (10 mL) should be added to each 5-mg vial of mitomycin and shaken gently to dissolve. Mitomycin should be administered intravenously to avoid extravasation of the drug. If extravasation occurs, severe local tissue necrosis may occur (363). The drug is usually given by a slow IV push, with continuous patient monitoring to lessen the chance of extravasation. Short infusions in 100 to 150 mL of D_5W or normal saline have also been used. Vein patency should be checked before the administration of any dose, using 5 to 10 mL of fluid that does not contain the drug. The same procedure should follow the dose. This flushes any remaining drug from the tubing and the venipuncture site.

The recommended dose of mitomycin used as a single agent is 20 mg/m^2 given IV every 6 to 8 weeks. In combination with other myelosuppressive drugs, mitomycin doses are typically limited to 10 mg/m^2 every 6 to 8 weeks. Bolus doses greater than 20 mg/m^2 produce severe toxicity without greatly enhancing efficacy.

Repeat dosing of mitomycin should be based on adequate marrow recovery, including leukocytes, platelets, and erythrocytes. Leukocyte count should return to 4,000/mm^3 and platelet count to 100,000/mm^3.

An ambulatory continuous infusion of mitomycin has been administered at 0.75 mg/m^2/day for consecutive 50-day dosing (364). A dosing regimen of 3 mg/m^2/day for 5 days every 4 to 6 weeks has also been used (364). These regimens are believed to deliver greater dose intensity by reducing myelosuppression. Intra-arterial perfusion doses of 20 mg/m^2 have been given every 6 to 8 weeks (365).

Side Effects and Toxicities. Bone marrow suppression involving platelets, leukocytes, and erythrocytes is the most serious toxicity, and it can continue for 3 to 8 weeks after drug administration is halted (351). Myelosuppression, particularly anemia, can be cumulative. This has been minimized by keeping total lifetime doses under 50 to 60 mg/m^2.

Gastrointestinal disturbances in the form of nausea, vomiting, and anorexia occasionally develop. These reactions are usually not severe and have an onset within 1 to 2 hours after administration. They may persist for several hours. Stomatitis may also occur, but it is generally not severe.

Renal toxicity detected by increasing serum BUN and creatinine levels with glomerular dysfunction is occasionally seen. This does not appear to be dose- or treatment-duration related, and it is usually not severe. However, mitomycin can also induce a microangiopathic hemolytic anemia with progressive renal failure (hemolytic-uremic syndrome) and cardiopulmonary decompensation. This disease is fatal within 3 to 4 weeks of diagnosis, although the onset is typically delayed for months after mitomycin administration (366). The incidence of this toxic effect may approach 10% among patients given large cumulative doses (366). In one series, renal complications from mitomycin developed in 1.6% of 63 patients receiving a total dose of 50 mg/m^2 or less, 11% of 37 patients receiving 50 to 69 mg/m^2, and 28% of 18 patients receiving total doses greater than 70 mg/m^2 (367). This suggests that a threshold for inducing microangiopathic hemolytic anemia may be a cumulative dose of about 50 mg/m^2 of mitomycin. Signs of the disease include thrombocytopenia, circulating schistocytes, and acute renal failure. Histopathologic examinations of the kidneys reveal fibrin thrombi in arterioles, tubular atrophy, and widespread glomerular necrosis.

Veno-occlusive disease of the liver has been reported after high-dose mitomycin therapy and autologous bone marrow transplantation (368). Signs include progressive hepatic dysfunction, abdominal pain, and ascites. Although this rarely has been observed with low-dose therapy, it appears to be much more frequent after high-dose regimens.

Alopecia may occur after mitomycin therapy, but it is usually not severe. Rarely, purple bands in the nail beds correspond to sequential doses of the drug. Lethargy or weakness may occur and can last from several days to 3 weeks. Fatigue and some drowsiness or confusion have also been observed. Dose-related skin reactions and fever with drug administration are occasionally seen.

Severe soft-tissue ulcers may also be expected if the drug escapes the vein during administration. Mitomycin extravasation injuries can result in chronic ulcers that can expand over months (363). Particularly distressing aspects of some mitomycin extravasations include the delayed (3 to 4 months) and sometimes distal occurrence of soft-tissue ulceration after uneventful injections in a peripheral vein (369). In animals, the only effective antidote to mitomycin skin reactions was topical DMSO (99% DMSO). Mitomycin extravasations may be empirically treated with topical application of 1.5 mL of DMSO every 6 hours for 14 days (370).

Interstitial pneumonia thought to be secondary to mitomycin has been reported for a small number of patients. These patients showed rapid improvement after treatment with corticosteroids (371).

Special Precautions. Myelosuppression may be cumulative with successive doses of mitomycin and may necessitate dose reductions. Careful monitoring of blood counts is critical. Serious local ulceration may occur if the drug is delivered outside the vein. Extravasation of mitomycin must be avoided.

Clinically significant antitumor drug synergy in humans has yet to be described for mitomycin, although it is probably at least additive in several drug combinations, including the FAM regimen (5-FU, doxorubicin, mitomycin) used in gastrointestinal cancer, the MOB regimen (mitomycin, vincristine [Oncovin], bleomycin) used in carcinoma of the uterine cervix, and megestrol acetate in patients with advanced breast cancer.

Special Applications. Mitomycin and intraperitoneal hyperthermia were combined to prophylactically treat patients with gastric cancer (372). Mitomycin (8 to 100 μg/mL) was administered continuously in bags containing 2,000 mL of heated (40°C to 45°C) saline solution. The total perfusion was 8 to 12 L over 50 to 60 minutes, comprising a mitomycin C dose of 64 to 100 mg. Low peak plasma levels (0.1 μg/mL) were produced, and approximately 39% of the administered dose was retained intraperitoneally. The half-lives of mitomycin C in the perfusate are 10 to 17 minutes (α) and 70 to 120 minutes (β) (373). Serum protein levels decreased significantly during and after the procedure, indicating that serum protein reaccumulates in the peritoneal space.

Mitomycin (5 to 10 mg) has also been given every 28 days combined with cisplatin (100 mg/m^2) using the intraperitoneal route. Mitomycin was always given 1 week after cisplatin, and the dose was diluted in 2 L of normal saline. In 11 patients with malignant peritoneal mesothelioma, five of eight previously untreated patients had reduced fluid reaccumulation lasting from 2 to 32 months (median 5 months) (202). The major toxic reaction was pain, and catheter failure was related to the intraperitoneal mitomycin.

Oxaliplatin

Chemistry. Oxaliplatin (Eloxatin, diaminocyclohexane platinum, DACH platinum) is a third-generation platinum with the molecular formula $C_8H_{14}N_2O_4Pt$ and the chemical name of *cis*-[(1R,2R)-1,2-cyclohexanediamine-N,N′][oxalato (2-)O, O′]platinum, and it has a molecular weight of 397.3. Oxaliplatin is an organoplatinum complex in which the platinum atom is complexed with 1,2-diaminocyclohexane (DACH) and with an oxalate ligand as a leaving group. Oxaliplatin is slightly soluble in water (6 mg/mL), slightly soluble in methanol, and practically insoluble in ethanol and acetone. It is FDA approved for second-line treatment in metastatic colorectal cancer in combination with fluoropyrimidines.

Mechanism of Action. Oxaliplatin binds to DNA in a manner similar to cisplatin, in that it binds to repeating deoxyguanosines d(GpG) in a single DNA strand. It reacts with DNA to produce intrastrand cross links (>90%) at adenine-guanine d(ApC) sites and to produce intrastrand cross links (<5%) with guanosines of opposing DNA strands $(dG)_2$ (50,128). This results in inhibition of DNA synthesis, function, and transcription. Oxaliplatin reacts more rapidly with DNA to form these interlinks and intralinks (e.g., within 15 minutes) than the other platinum agents (12 hours for cisplatin and over 24 hours for carboplatin) (128). Furthermore, unlike the other platinum-DNA adducts, mismatch repair enzymes are unable to recognize the adducts formed by oxaliplatin because of their bulkier size (50).

Drug Disposition. In a summary of pharmacokinetic studies, plasma platinum C_{max} values have been shown to be in the range of 2.59 to 3.22 μg/mL, and mean $AUC_{0\text{-}48h}$ in the range of 50.4 to 71.5 μg/ mL · hour after an oxaliplatin dose of 130 mg/m^2 (2-hour infusion) (373). Intrapatient and interpatient variability was moderate to low (23% and 6%, respectively) (374). In 1-hour infusion studies, mean plasma platinum C_{max} and $AUC_{0\text{-}24h}$ increased in a dose-dependent fashion up to 180 mg/m^2. The pharmacokinetics of platinum in ultrafiltrate after administration of oxaliplatin are triphasic and characterized by short α (0.28 hour) and β (16.3 hours) distribution phases, which are followed by a long terminal γ phase (273 hours) (375). Oxaliplatin is primarily cleared from plasma by renal excretion (53.8%) and covalent tissue binding. Clearance is not affected by age, gender, or hepatic impairment (375).

Administration and Dosage. Reconstitute oxaliplatin by adding 10 mL sterile water for each 50-mg vial, or dextrose (5%). The solution must be further diluted in 250 to 500 mL of 5% dextrose prior to administration. The infusion line should be flushed with D_5W prior to administration of any concomitant medication (375). Premedication with antiemetics is recommended.

The recommended dose for metastatic colorectal cancer is as follows: on day 1 of every 2-week cycle, oxaliplatin (85 mg/m^2) is generally administered intravenously with leucovorin (200 mg/m^2) over 120 minutes at the same time in two separate bags using a Y-line, followed by 5-FU (400 mg/m^2 IV bolus), followed by 5-FU (600 mg/m^2) in 500 mL D_5W as a 22-hour continuous infusion. On day 2, the patient should receive leucovorin (200 mg/m^2) over 120 minutes at the same time in two separate bags using a Y-line, followed by 5-FU (400 mg/m^2 IV bolus), followed by 5-FU (600 mg/m^2) in 500 mL D_5W as a 22-hour continuous infusion.

In phase 2 trials for gynecologic cancers, the recommended dose of oxaliplatin is 130 mg/m^2 intravenously over 2 hours every 21 days (376,377).

Side Effects and Toxicities. Oxaliplatin produces dose-limiting peripheral neuropathy and gastrointestinal and hematologic adverse events. Neurotoxic symptoms usually resolve within a week of stopping therapy; however, symptom intensity is cumulative with repeated courses of oxaliplatin (28,374,378). Other common adverse events include mild leukopenia and mild to moderate thrombocytopenia. Nausea and vomiting are common, and antiemetic prophylaxis is required with oxaliplatin therapy.

Unlike other platinum-containing agents, oxaliplatin is not associated with nephrotoxicity. Alopecia has not been reported with oxaliplatin.

Special Applications. Oxaliplatin is an agent with substantial activity in platinum-sensitive ovarian cancer patients previously treated with cisplatin. Bougnoux et al. (379) noted two complete and eight partial responses in 24 patients who were platinum sensitive (41.7% response rate). Similar findings were seen in a phase 2 study, which also saw a 42% response rate in platinum-sensitive patients. Chollet et al. (380) studied similar populations of patients and noted six responses in 13 platinum-sensitive patients (46%) and a 17% response rate (3 of 18 patients) in platinum-resistant patients. Phase 2 studies have seen only minimal activity in platinum-resistant patients (less than 6% response rate) (377).

Paclitaxel

Chemistry. Paclitaxel (Taxol) is one of the most commonly used drugs in oncology, with FDA approval for primary or salvage therapy for epithelial ovarian cancer, as salvage therapy for metastatic breast cancer, in second-line treatment of AIDS-related Kaposi's sarcoma, and in the treatment of non–small cell lung cancer. It is also active against a variety of other solid tumors, including cervical and endometrial cancer (380,381). It is a diterpene plant product derived from the bark of the Pacific yew, *Taxus baccata*. It has a molecular weight of 853.9, is insoluble in water, and has an empiric formula of $C_{47}H_{51}NO_{14}$. Its chemical name is 5β,20-epoxy-1,2α,4,7β,10β,13α-hexahydroxytax-11-en-9-one4,10-diacetate 2-benzoate 13-ester with (2*R*,3*S*)-N-benzoyl-3-phenylisoserine.

Mechanism of Action. Paclitaxel acts as a mitotic spindle poison. In a manner contrary to known mitotic spindle inhibitors, such as colchicine and podophyllotoxin, paclitaxel promotes assembly of microtubules and stabilizes them, preventing depolymerization. This inability to depolymerize microtubules prevents cellular replication (118).

Drug Disposition. Early pharmacokinetic studies using standard doses and a 24-hour infusion suggested that paclitaxel pharmacokinetics were linear; however, with short infusions and/or high dose levels, paclitaxel's nonlinear pharmacokinetics become readily apparent (157). The nonlinearity is due to saturable distribution, metabolism, and elimination. Terminal elimination half-life is largely dependent on the dose and administration schedule. At a dose level of 175 mg/m^2 with a 3-hour infusion, mean pharmacokinetic parameters of paclitaxel include the following: plasma $t_{1/2\alpha}$, 16 minutes; plasma $t_{1/2\beta}$, 140 minutes; plasma $t_{1/2\gamma}$, 18.75 hours; plasma clearance, 12.69 L/h/m^2; plasma AUC, 16.81 μmol/L · hour; 48-hour urinary excretion, <10% of dose; and 48-hour fecal excretion, 70% of dose (157).

Clearance is rapid and not due to urinary excretion; the major route of paclitaxel elimination is believed to be via hepatic metabolism and subsequent biliary excretion (381). About 70% to 80% of the drug is eliminated by fecal excretion.

Administration and Dosage. All patients undergoing paclitaxel therapy should receive premedication to prevent severe hypersensitivity reactions. A recommended regimen is dexamethasone (either 20 mg orally the night before treatment and the morning of treatment or 20 mg IV 30 minutes before paclitaxel delivery) plus diphenhydramine (50 mg) and famotidine (20 mg) IV 30 minutes before chemotherapy (382). For the majority of patients, administration of dexamethasone 20 mg IV 30 to 60 minutes before paclitaxel is sufficient and has been proven to be effective in preventing hypersensitivity reactions.

Paclitaxel is commercially available as an injection concentrate in 30-mg (5 mL), 100-mg (16.7 mL), and 300-mg (50 mL) multidose vials. Before infusion, paclitaxel must be diluted with 0.9% sodium chloride, 5% dextrose, 5% dextrose and 0.9% sodium chloride injection, or 5% dextrose in Ringer's injection to a final concentration of 0.3 to 1.2 mg/mL. The solution is stable for up to 27 hours at room temperature. Paclitaxel should be administered through an in-line filter with a microporous membrane not greater than 0.22 μ to remove particulates that are present in paclitaxel solutions. Although particulate formation does not indicate loss of drug potency, solutions exhibiting excess particulate matter formation should be discarded. Because of the possibility of leaching of phthalate plasticizers with paclitaxel solutions, only non-polyvinylchloride (such as polyethylene or polyolefin) IV administration sets should be used.

As a result of an unacceptable level of severe hypersensitivity reactions in early phase 1 studies (most likely related to the Cremophor EL vehicle), a 24-hour infusion schedule and a premedication regimen with corticosteroids and histamine H_1- and H_2-antagonists were used in all phase 2 and 3 clinical trials conducted in the United States from 1987 to 1992. Later clinical studies established that a 3-hour paclitaxel infusion schedule can be administered safely without a significant increase in major hypersensitivity reactions and that the shortened infusion schedule is associated with significantly less grade 4 neutropenia than the 24-hour infusion (i.e., 71% vs. 18% for the 24- and 3-hour infusions, respectively) (383). Follow-up studies have determined that a 1-hour infusion schedule also is feasible; however, infusion durations less than 1 hour are associated with a prohibitively high rate of hypersensitivity reactions (384).

There were early concerns that the shorter infusion schedules might be associated with a decline in efficacy. However, results from GOG-158, a phase 3, randomized study in women with optimal disease, advanced ovarian cancer, revealed that paclitaxel 175 mg/m^2 by 3-hour infusion combined with carboplatin (targeted AUC of 7.5) (arm II) had similar activity with less toxicity than paclitaxel 135 mg/m^2 by 24-hour infusion plus cisplatin 75 mg/m^2 (arm I) (385). Median progression-free survival and overall survival were 19.4 and 48.7 months, respectively, for arm I (paclitaxel-cisplatin) compared with 20.7 and 57.4 months, respectively, for arm II (paclitaxel-carboplatin). Because of its ease of administration and lower toxicity profile (cisplatin plus short-infusion paclitaxel is associated with dose-limiting neurotoxicity), the recommended primary chemotherapy regimen for advanced ovarian cancer is paclitaxel 175 mg/m^2 by 3-hour infusion plus carboplatin (targeted AUC of 6.0 to 7.5) every 21 days for six cycles (385). Although this generally is a well-tolerated regimen, neurosensory toxicity and prolonged thrombocytopenia can prove to be dose limiting. The FDA-approved regimen for first-line treatment of ovarian cancer is paclitaxel 135 mg/m^2 over 24 hours plus cisplatin 75 mg/m^2 every 21 days for six cycles or paclitaxel 175 mg/m^2 over 3 hours plus cisplatin 75 mg/m^2.

The FDA-approved recommended regimen for salvage therapy for patients with platinum-refractory ovarian cancer is paclitaxel 135 or 175 mg/m^2 administered IV over 3 hours every 3 weeks, but the optimal regimen has not been clearly established. Paclitaxel has been administered by various other schedules during investigational studies in patients with solid tumors, including 135 to 250 mg/m^2 as a 24-hour continuous infusion every 3 weeks; 212 to 225 mg/m^2 as a 6-hour infusion every 3 weeks; 30 mg/m^2 as a 1-hour infusion daily for 5 days every 3 weeks; 30 mg/m^2 as a 6-hour infusion daily for 5 days every 3 weeks; 120 to 140 mg/m^2 as a 96-hour infusion every 3 weeks; and 150 mg/m^2 as a 120-hour infusion every 3 weeks (118). Most recently, IP therapy for optimally debulked advanced ovarian cancer has demonstrated a significant survival advantage with a regimen of intravenous paclitaxel on day 1, intraperitoneal cisplatin on day 2, and intraperitoneal paclitaxel on day 8 (see the Intraperitoneal Drug Pharmacokinetics and Cisplatin sections of this chapter for more details on this IP regimen) (4,96,97).

Special Precautions. Before the institution of standard prophylactic medications, the incidence of major hypersensitivity reactions associated with paclitaxel therapy approached 25% to 30%. With premedication, the incidence of severe hypersensitivity reactions has decreased to less than 2%. The majority of paclitaxel-induced hypersensitivity reactions can be categorized as grade 1, with symptoms of dyspnea with bronchospasm, urticaria, and hypotension. Major sensitivity reactions usually occur within the first 10 minutes after the first or second dose of paclitaxel (118). Minor symptoms of flushing and rashes are not predictive of the future development of severe manifestations (118,383). According to National Cancer Institute guidelines for paclitaxel administration, emergency equipment must be available and medical personnel should be in attendance during paclitaxel infusion, especially during the first 15 minutes of the first and second courses. Vital signs should be periodically monitored during the first several hours of drug infusion. The paclitaxel infusion should be discontinued immediately if symptoms of a major hypersensitivity reaction occur (including respiratory distress, hypotension, generalized urticaria, and angioedema). Severe hypersensitivity reactions may be treated with IV epinephrine, IV diphenhydramine, IV fluids, and nebulized beta-agonists. Steroid therapy may be helpful in the resolution of recurrent symptoms (386). There is strong evidence that patients who develop major hypersensitivity reactions may be successfully retreated with slow, low-dose infusions of paclitaxel after premedication with multiple high doses of corticosteroids and antihistamines (387).

Drug Interactions. Paclitaxel therapy appears to modify the hematologic toxicity associated with platinum agents. Rowinsky et al. (388) conducted a phase 1 study of sequential escalating doses of paclitaxel and cisplatin therapy and determined that myelosuppression was more severe when paclitaxel was administered immediately after cisplatin therapy than when given prior to cisplatin.

Concomitant medications that contain substrates or inhibitors of hepatic enzymes, principally cytochrome P450 isoenzymes CYP_2C_8 and CYP_3A_4, may increase paclitaxel clearance, and caution should be exercised when administering paclitaxel. In a study by Chang et al. (389), the pharmacokinetics of paclitaxel were significantly altered by the concomitant use of anticonvulsants (i.e., phenytoin, carbamazepine, and phenobarbital), and the maximum tolerated doses of paclitaxel in malignant glioma patients were 360 mg/m^2 for those on anticonvulsant therapy versus 240 mg/m^2 for those not receiving anticonvulsants. There was also a significant difference in paclitaxel metabolite and toxicity profiles between the two groups. Central neurotoxicity, rather than neutropenia, was the dose-limiting toxicity in patients on anticonvulsant therapy who received paclitaxel at a dose greater than 350 mg/m^2.

Special Applications. Paclitaxel is a particularly promising agent for intraperitoneal administration, in that this route of drug delivery results in a more than 3-log increased exposure of the peritoneal cavity relative to systemic circulation. Additionally, potentially cytotoxic levels of paclitaxel remain in the peritoneal cavity for 5 to 7 days following intraperitoneal (IP) administration, and thus weekly intraperitoneal treatment results in continuous drug exposure (390). A phase 2 study in women with ovarian, fallopian, or peritoneal cancer and small-volume residual disease following primary chemotherapy has shown that IP paclitaxel has significant activity as evidenced by a 61% surgically defined complete response rate (391). Three large phase 3 trials in the GOG and the Southwest Oncology Group (GOG-104/SWOG-8501, GOG-114, and GOG-172) comparing various combination chemotherapeutic regimens administered IV or IP have documented significant survival advantages for the intraperitoneal treatment arms (3–5). Most recently, in GOG-172, an intraperitoneal regimen (intravenous paclitaxel, 135 mg/m^2 over 24 hours on day 1, intraperitoneal cisplatin 100 mg/m^2 on day 2, and intraperitoneal paclitaxel 60 mg/m^2 on day 8, every 21 days) was associated with a 25% reduction in the risk of death as compared to the intravenously administered regimen (intravenous paclitaxel plus cisplatin) (p = 0.03) (4). The day 1 paclitaxel may alternatively be given over 3 hours to reduce the myelosuppressive activity of paclitaxel and to eliminate the need for a hospital stay (96).

Paclitaxel has demonstrated activity against both endometrial and cervical cancers (392). Woo et al. (393) reported a 43% response rate to paclitaxel (95% CI, 6% to 80%) in seven patients with advanced, progressive, or recurrent endometrial cancer following platinum analog treatment. A GOG study noted a 14.3% complete and 21.4% partial response rate in 28 evaluable patients with endometrial cancer not previously treated with chemotherapy (394). Leukopenia was the most prominent side effect noted. A response rate of 37% (95% CI, 16% to 62%) was reported in 19 patients pretreated with cisplatin, doxorubicin, and cyclophosphamide (395). A GOG phase 2 trial of paclitaxel (3-hour infusion of 200 mg/m^2 every 21 days or 175 mg/m^2 for patients with prior pelvic radiation therapy) found a 27.3% response rate (95% CI, 15% to 42.8%) in 44 persistent or recurrent endometrial cancer patients who failed prior chemotherapy (396).

A GOG phase 2 trial of single-agent paclitaxel in advanced cervix cancer has demonstrated a response rate of 31% (380). Trials of combination cisplatin-paclitaxel (IV paclitaxel 175 mg/m^2 by 3-hour infusion followed by cisplatin 75 mg/m^2) in metastatic and recurrent cervical cancer show moderate activity (47% response rate; 95% CI, 30% to 65%) (397). A similar response rate (45%) was seen in another phase 2 trial of first-line therapy of advanced cervical cancer (IV paclitaxel 135 mg/m^2 by 24-hour infusion followed by cisplatin 75 mg/m^2 every 28 days) (398).

Pemetrexed

Chemistry. Pemetrexed (Alimta) is an antifolate antineoplastic agent with the chemical name of L-glutamic acid, *N*-[4-[2-(2-amino-4,7-dihydro-4-oxo-1*H*-pyrrolo[2,3-*d*]pyrimidin-5-yl)ethyl]benzoyl]-, disodium salt, heptahydrate. It has a molecular weight of 597.49 and the molecular formula $C_{20}H_{19}N_5Na_2O_6 \cdot 7H_2O$. Pemetrexed is FDA approved for combination therapy with cisplatin for malignant pleural mesothelioma, and for single-agent therapy for non–small cell lung cancer.

Mechanism of Action. Pemetrexed inhibits the folate-dependent enzymes thymidylate synthase (TS), dihydrofolate reductase (DHFR), and glycinamide ribonucleotide formyltransferase (GARFT). The inhibition of GARFT, for example, is directly associated with a decrease in the rate of tumor cells (399). Although methotrexate was an early but potent inhibitor of DHFR, the antifolate activity of pemetrexed is quite different. The K_m for pemetrexed is one hundredth that of methotrexate for folylpolyglutamate synthetase (FPGS), making it possible to rapidly and completely block TS activity, whereas methotrexate acts in a more gradual and cumulative process, only impacting cellular proliferation at the point where more than 95% of the enzyme is inhibited (399). Additional details regarding the unique mechanism of action of pemetrexed, including features of membrane transport, its maintained activity in loss of transport activity, and its comparison with other antifolates (e.g., 5-FU, methotrexate, raltitrexed) are discussed in more detail elsewhere (399).

Drug Disposition. Pemetrexed is primarily excreted in the urine and is only minimally metabolized. The elimination half-life is approximately 3.5 hours among patients with normal renal function. Pemetrexed exposure increases with decreasing renal function. Pemetrexed is 81% bound to plasma proteins, and binding is not affected by renal function.

Administration and Dosage. Pemetrexed is administered IV at 500 mg/m^2 over 10 minutes on day 1 of every 21-day cycle. When used in combination therapy, cisplatin (75 mg/m^2 over 2 hours) should begin 30 minutes after the pemetrexed administration. The premedication regimen with pemetrexid includes corticosteroids (dexamethasone) to reduce skin rash reactions, and folate-containing vitamin supplementation (daily for at least 7 days prior to pemetrexed administration) to reduce some toxcities.

Side Effects and Toxicities. The most commonly occurring side effects associated with pemetrexed treatment include hematologic toxicity, fever and infection, stomatitis, pharyngitis, and rash. Although many toxicities appeared significantly lower among patients receiving folate supplementation (e.g., neutropenia, nausea, vomiting, fever, infection), hypertension (11% vs. 3%), chest pain (8%, vs. 6%), and thrombosis/embolism (6% vs. 3%) were higher among those receiving supplementation. Rare cases of colitis have been reported in post-marketing studies.

Topotecan

Chemistry. Topotecan (Hycamtin, topotecan hydrochloride) was approved by the FDA in 1996 for treatment of ovarian cancer patients after failure of primary chemotherapy. It is also indicated in the treatment of small cell lung cancer after failure of first-line chemotherapy. Topotecan is a semisynthetic analog of camptothecin. The parent compound is derived from the bark of an ornamental tree native to Asia, *Camptotheca acuminata*. Sodium camptothecin was studied in clinical trials in the late 1960s through the early 1970s. However, clinical development of this agent was halted despite evidence of a variety of tumor responses because of severe and unpredictable toxicities (e.g., myelosuppression and hemorrhagic cystitis) (400). Topotecan and other camptothecin analogs (e.g., irinotecan) have been formulated in an effort to overcome unacceptable toxicities and to increase cytotoxicity and water solubility. Topotecan incorporates a stable basic side chain at the 9-position of the A-ring of 10-hydroxycamptothecin, which increases aqueous solubility. The molecular weight is 457.9 (the HCl salt) and the formula is $C_{23}H_{23}N_3O_5 \cdot HCl$ (the free base has a molecular weight of 421.5). The chemical name of topotecan is (*S*)-10-[(dimethylamino)methyl]-4-ethyl-4, 9-dihydroxy-1*H*-pyrano[3′,4′:6,7] indolizino [1,2-*b*]quinoline-3,14-(4*H*,12*H*)-dione monohydrochloride.

Mechanism of Action. In a manner similar to camptothecin, topotecan's cytotoxicity results from the inhibition of TOPO-I, an enzyme that induces reversible single-strand breaks during DNA replication. Camptothecin analogs bind with and stabilize the transient TOPO-I–DNA complex, preventing religation of the single-strand breakage. The interaction of the ternary topotecan–TOPO-I–DNA complex with replication enzymes results in double-strand DNA breaks and cellular death. Topotecan exists in a pH-dependent equilibrium as both a closed lactone ring and a hydroxy acid; the hydroxy acid is formed by hydrolysis of the lactone ring. The active lactone form predominates at a pH below 7.0, and at a pH of 6.0, over 80% of topotecan exists in the lactone form. Slow reaction kinetics studies have shown that the hydroxy acid is inactive and only the closed lactone bonds with the TOPO-I–DNA complex (302).

Drug Disposition. After IV administration, plasma pharmacokinetics show that the lactone form, which is active as an inhibitor of TOPO-I, is rapidly converted to the hydroxy acid form. At the end of a brief infusion, approximately half of the dose administered exits as hydroxy acid (308). One hour after administration, less than 30% of the dose remains in the lactone form. Topotecan does not inhibit TOPO-II.

Both forms of topotecan are subject to rapid biphasic elimination. In a summary of pharmacokinetics studies, the mean half-life of topotecan lactone was only 3.0 hours (range 1.2 to 4.9 hours) (302). Binding to plasma proteins is approximately 35%. Renal excretion appears to account for 40% to 70% of drug clearance (50,128).

When topotecan was administered as a weekly 24-hour IV infusion of 1 to 2 mg/m^2, the plasma steady-state concentration and the AUC increased linearly with dose. The lactone to total-drug-concentration ratio was constant, which suggests that the total drug concentration may be used as a measure of active lactone exposure with weekly, long infusions (401). Additionally, comparison of day 1 pharmacokinetics values with blood counts showed that both the topotecan AUC and lactone AUC were predictive of the level of neutrophil reduction on days 15, 22, and 29 using the sigmoid E_{max} model (401). This led the investigators to suggest that topotecan-induced myelosuppression is noncumulative and that elimination probably remains unchanged with repeat dosing in individual patients. Other studies have also found a correlation between the topotecan AUC and level of neutropenia (308,402).

Limited sampling models for topotecan pharmacokinetics have been proposed that may facilitate tailoring of topotecan drug doses in individual patients and large pharmacodynamic studies of topotecan (403). Plasma concentrations of the lactone and hydroxy acid forms of topotecan at 2 hours, after a 30-minute infusion, reliably predicted the lactone form AUC, the hydroxy acid AUC, the total topotecan AUC, and the clearance rate.

Administration and Dosage. Each 4-mg vial of topotecan should be reconstituted with 4 mL of sterile water. The resulting solution can be further diluted with either 0.9% sodium chloride or 5% dextrose. Because the active lactone form of topotecan is subject to a pH-dependent hydrolysis to the inactive hydroxy acid, consideration should be given to maintenance of an acidic pH during drug infusion. When the topotecan lactone is dissolved in 5% dextrose, only approximately 10% is converted to the hydroxy acid (308). Because the product does not contain an antibacterial preservative, it should be used immediately once constituted.

Parenteral topotecan has been administered by IV infusions varying in length from 30 minutes to 21 days (302). As discussed below, the dosing schedule has a profound effect on the maximum tolerated dose (MTD).

An oral formulation has been evaluated in murine tumor models and in phase 1-2 trials. It has been associated with excellent bioavailability and similar efficacy as compared with parenteral topotecan in four of the five murine tumor models tested (404). In early-phase human trials, oral topotecan is well tolerated and active in second-line therapy of ovarian cancer and small cell lung cancer, and is associated with less neutropenia than the intravenous formulation (405,406).

The standard FDA-approved dosing regimen is 1.5 mg/m^2/day × 5 days by 30-minute IV infusion every 21 days, for a minimum of four courses owing to delayed tumor response, as tolerated (in the absence of tumor progression). However, this dosing schedule is associated with a more than 80% incidence of grade IV neutropenia. Many oncologists, therefore, use a dose of 1.25 mg/m^2/day for 5 days and/or administer prophylactic granulocyte colony-stimulating factor (G-CSF).

In phase 1 studies, the MTD of topotecan was highly dependent on the length of infusion schedules; longer infusions were generally associated with lower MTDs. The estimated MTD of topotecan when administered as a 30-minute, 72-hour, and 120-hour continuous infusion is 22.5 mg/m^2, 1.6 mg/m^2/day (4.8 mg/m^2 total), and 0.68 mg/m^2/day (3.4 mg/m^2 total), respectively. As a continuous 21-day infusion administered every 28 days, the MTD of topotecan appears to be 0.5 mg/m^2/day (10.5 mg/m^2/cycle) (302,407). A weekly dosing schedule has been developed that appears to maintain antitumor activity without causing severe myelosuppression (408,409).

Side Effects and Toxicities. Toxicity data are available from a phase 3, randomized study of topotecan 1.5 mg/m^2/day for 5 days every 21 days versus paclitaxel 175 mg/m^2 IV over 3 hours every 21 days in ovarian cancer patients with progressive or recurrent disease following primary platinum-based chemotherapy (410). Neutropenia was the predominant toxicity in this study: 79% of patients experienced grade 4 neutropenia, 25% of patients experienced febrile neutropenia, and 5% of patients developed sepsis (two patients [2%] died of sepsis). The onset of grade 4 neutropenia was on days 9 through 15 of a chemotherapy cycle and it did respond to G-CSF therapy. Thrombocytopenia also occurred frequently: 50% of patients experienced grades 3 to 4 thrombocytopenia (25% experienced grade 4). Grade 4 anemia occurred in 3.6% of patients.

The most common nonhematologic toxicities were cumulative, dose-related alopecia (76%) and nausea/vomiting (10%, grades 3 to 4), which was amenable to antiemetic therapy. Other frequent toxicities were fatigue (41%), constipation (43%), diarrhea (40%), abdominal pain (27%), fever in the absence of neutropenia (29%), stomatitis (24%), dyspnea (24%), and asthenia (22%) (410).

Although the results of the study described in the above paragraphs led to an FDA approval of topotecan as salvage therapy for patients with ovarian cancer with a recommended dose level of 1.5 mg/m^2/day for 5 days, it is important to note that the patients in this European study had only received one prior platinum-based chemotherapeutic regimen, and that most had received cisplatin (not carboplatin) and none had received prior paclitaxel. In general, topotecan-induced myelosuppression is more severe in patients who have previously received carboplatin and/or multiple prior chemotherapeutic regimens. For this reason, many clinicians use an initial topotecan dose of 1.25 mg/m^2/day and/or administer prophylactic G-CSF.

Special Precautions. Because topotecan has a high rate of renal excretion and a modest hepatic clearance, a clinical study was conducted to evaluate the impact of renal and hepatic dysfunction on toxicity in patients undergoing treatment with topotecan on a daily × 5 dosing schedule (411). Pharmacokinetic analyses showed clear correlations between creatinine clearance and plasma clearance of both topotecan and topotecan lactone ($r^2 = 0.65$, $p < 0.0001$). Although the standard dose for patients with good renal function is 1.5 mg/m^2/day × 5 days, this study determined that the recommended starting dose for patients with moderate hepatic dysfunction (creatinine clearance of 20 to 39 mL/min) was 0.75 mg/m^2. The investigators urged extreme caution with topotecan administration in patients with more profound renal insufficiency and recommend further dose reductions for heavily pretreated patients (411). Hepatic insufficiency did not appear to exacerbate hematologic toxicity (411). Nonhematologic toxicity appeared to be unaffected by either renal or hepatic insufficiency.

Drug Interactions. Drug sequence of the paclitaxel/topotecan combination had no apparent impact on hematologic toxicities or pharmacologic behavior (412). However, drug sequence of the cisplatin/topotecan combination did have a significant impact on toxicity and topotecan pharmacokinetics. Prior administration of cisplatin significantly reduced the clearance of topotecan (possibly as a result of subclinical nephrotoxicity) and increased hematologic toxicity (388). In GOG-182, carboplatin was administered on day 3 of a daily × 3 topotecan administration schedule, because administration of carboplatin on day 1 was associated with excessive neutropenia and thrombocytopenia (413).

There has been interest in sequential administration of topotecan (TOPO-I inhibitor) with TOPO-II inhibitors (e.g., doxorubicin, etoposide). The rationale is that administration of a TOPO-I inhibitor would induce up-regulation of TOPO-II in tumor cells and thus enhance cytotoxicity. One clinical/translational study of topotecan (0.17 to 1.05 mg/m^2/day as a 72-hour continuous infusion on days 1 to 3) followed by etoposide (75 or 100 mg/m^2/day as a 2-hour infusion daily on days 8 to 10) failed to show reliable down-regulation of TOPO-I and up-regulation of TOPO-II following administration of topotecan (414). Although significant clinical activity was observed in this phase 1 study in patients with various solid tumors, the investigators concluded that the toxicity and translational research results did not support a significant synergistic advantage of this combination. Another study of the TOPO-I and TOPO-II inhibitor combination therapy (IV topotecan 0.5 mg/m^2/day for 5 days and oral etoposide 50 mg twice daily for 7 days of every 21-day cycle, with dose escalation of topotecan 0.75 and 1.0 mg/m^2) found the combination to be safe and effective in small cell lung cancer patients; however, the incidence of grades 3 to 4 neutropenia was 25%, and two patients died from neutropenic sepsis (415).

TOPO-I is a biochemical mediator of radiosensitization in cultured mammalian cells by camptothecin derivatives (416). There are *in vitro* and *in vivo* data suggesting that topotecan may have activity as a radiation-sensitizing agent (417). However, this apparent synergistic relationship remains to be explored in clinical trials.

Special Applications. Phase 1 trials of IP topotecan have demonstrated the feasibility of IP administration and the favorable toxicity profile (418,419). Pharmacokinetic studies revealed that the pharmacologic advantage associated with IP administration of topotecan (expressed as the ratio of the peritoneal to plasma AUC) was 31.2 (419). In a Netherlands study, patients were treated with escalating doses (5 to 30 mg/m^2 every 21 days). The dose-limiting toxicity was acute hypotension, chills, and fever at the 30 mg/m^2 dose level (418). The University of California, San Diego, study treated patients with escalating doses from 2 to 4 mg/m^2 every 21 days. The MTD of IP topotecan was determined to be 4 mg/m^2 every 21 days and the recommended dose for further phase 2 study was 3 mg/m^2. The dose-limiting toxicity was neutropenia. Other toxicities included anemia, vomiting, fever, and abdominal pain (419).

Vinblastine Sulfate

Chemistry. Vinblastine (Velban) is used in the treatment of germ cell tumors of the ovary (420) and has demonstrated activity in early clinical trials of cervical, endometrial, and ovarian cancers (420). In combination with other agents, it has also demonstrated activity in early trials of ovarian cancer (421). Vinblastine is the sulfate salt of an alkaloid isolated from *Vinca rosea* (periwinkle). It is structurally related to vincristine, another alkaloid isolated from the same plant. Vinblastine sulfate is a white to off-white crystalline powder that is freely soluble in water, soluble in methane, and slightly soluble in ethanol. Its empiric formula is $C_{46}H_{58}N_4O_9 \cdot H_2SO_4$, and it has a molecular weight of 909.07.

Mechanism of Action. Vinblastine binds to tubulin and inhibits microtubule assembly. This inhibition prevents mitotic spindle formation and results in an accumulation of cells in metaphase (422).

Vinblastine is considered cell cycle phase specific for mitosis; however, the cytotoxic effect probably occurs in S phase and is expressed only in M phase. At high doses, direct effects may be expressed in S and G_1 phases. Vinblastine may be assumed to have stathmokinetic (cell cycle arrest) effects similar to vincristine.

Drug Disposition. After IV administration, vinblastine is rapidly cleared from the plasma and concentrated in various tissues. The apparent volume of distribution for the central compartment is quite large (three to four times the blood volume). Vincristine and vindesine approximate total body water in their distributions. There is a triphasic vinblastine elimination pattern, with average half-lives of 3.7 minutes, 1.6 hours, and 24.8 hours, respectively (423). The drug also localizes in platelet and leukocyte fractions of whole blood (424). A radiolabeled drug study has shown that urinary elimination accounts for approximately 33% of the total vinblastine radioactivity, with 21% appearing in the stool, both after 72 hours (424). A large portion of the radiolabel was retained in the body: 73% remained at 6 days after dosing. Apparently, insufficient amounts of the drug pass the blood-brain barrier to produce an effective concentration in the central nervous system. Vinblastine is partially metabolized in the liver. Most of the drug is, therefore, ultimately excreted intact in the bile or the urine. Toxicity may be increased if there is obstructive liver disease, and doses should be greatly reduced.

Administration and Dosage. The solution for administration is usually prepared by adding 10 mL of sodium chloride solution (which may be preserved with phenols or benzyl alcohol) to the 10-mg vial. The use of other solutions is not generally recommended. The resultant solution has a concentration of 1 mg/mL and a pH of 3.5 to 5.0. Solutions prepared with preserved sodium chloride injection may be stored in the refrigerator (protected from light) for 28 days without significant loss of potency.

Vinblastine is usually given by the IV push technique, with the total dose being delivered over approximately 1 minute. This is usually accomplished by slowly pushing the dose through the injection site of a running IV infusion. Alternatively, the drug may be given directly into the vein. If this method is followed, the double-needle technique should be used: Do not use the same needle to withdraw the dose from the vial that is used for the direct injection into the vein. Vinblastine is very irritating and should not be given intramuscularly or subcutaneously. Vein patency should be checked before drug administration by flushing with a small quantity of normal saline or D_5W. After the dose has been given, the site should be flushed again to ensure that all of the drug has been delivered into the vein.

Vinblastine has been given by several dosing schemes. The dose depends on the protocol being followed, condition of the patient, other drugs or irradiation being used, and individual patient response. Usually, the drug is given no more frequently than once every week. In general, the dosage range is 3.8 to 18.5 mg/m^2 when used in combination with other agents. Patients are customarily started at a low dose and worked up in 1.8- to 1.9-mg/m^2 increments, depending on the degree of resulting leukopenia (e.g., the dose should not be increased beyond the dose at which the white cell count reaches 3,000 cells/mm^3) (423). The dosage ranges for the indicated use of vinblastine are 6 mg/m^2 IV on days 1 and 15 as part of the doxorubicin-bleomycin-vinblastine-dacarbazine regimen (Hodgkin's disease) and 0.15 mg/kg IV on days 1 and 2 as part of the cisplatin-vinblastine-bleomycin regimen (testicular cancer) (50). In gynecologic malignancies, vinblastine is only rarely used for ovarian and trophoblastic disease.

Side Effects and Toxicities. The major toxic effect of vinblastine is a dose-related bone marrow depression. This is more frequent and severe than with the close structural analog, vincristine. Dose-related leukopenia occurs with a nadir of 4 to 10 days and with recovery occurring over another 7 to 14 days. Because of the relatively predictable nadir, it may be possible to administer vinblastine cautiously as often as every 7 to 10 days. Thrombocytopenia typically occurs; however, with standard dosing regimens, serious platelet depressions are infrequent. Erythrocytes are usually only slightly depressed.

Nausea and vomiting occur rarely with vinblastine therapy and are at least partially responsive to antiemetics. Severe stomatitis is occasionally observed. Gastrointestinal symptoms, which may be related to neurotoxicity, include constipation, adynamic ileus, and abdominal pain, especially if high doses (>20 mg) are used. These side effects are rarely seen with doses of less than 10 mg. Prophylactic stool softeners may prevent constipation. Generalized muscle and tumor pain are commonly experienced by patients receiving vinblastine, especially in high doses (425).

Neurotoxicity associated with vinblastine occurs less frequently than with vincristine and usually occurs in patients on prolonged therapy or in those receiving high individual doses. Symptoms include paresthesias, peripheral neuropathy, depression, headache, malaise, jaw pain, urinary retention, tachycardia, orthostatic hypotension, or convulsions. Extravasations of vinblastine may result in local soft-tissue necrosis. Treatment with subcutaneously administered hyaluronidase is recommended (192). Other side effects include a reversible and mild alopecia, rashes, and photosensitivity reactions. Transient hepatitis has also been reported on the continuous-infusion regimen.

There have been several reports of a Raynaud's phenomenon associated with vinblastine or bleomycin in treating testicular cancer. The reaction consists of a delayed presentation of a cold feeling in the hands with physical evidence of cyanosis (426). Ginsberg et al. (427) demonstrated a case of vinblastine-associated syndrome of inappropriate antidiuretic hormone (ADH) secretion, which was previously thought to occur only with vincristine.

The drug is well documented as a teratogen in humans, and as with most anticancer drugs, usage in pregnancy is strongly contraindicated (428).

Special Precautions. Avoid extravasation of vinblastine. If extravasation occurs, stop the administration of the remaining drug immediately. Dorr and Alberts (429) favor injection of a corticosteroid into the infiltration site with sodium chloride to dilute the drug. Only minor tissue damage has occurred when vinblastine extravasation was treated with 50 to 500 mg of hydrocortisone sodium succinate. This is followed by cold compresses to minimize spread of the reaction.

Liver disease may alter the elimination of vinblastine and necessitate a dosage reduction. Neurotoxicity may be more frequent in patients with underlying neurologic problems or those who are weak or cachectic at the start of treatment.

Vinblastine solution is topically irritating and has caused corneal irritation when inadvertently splashed in the eyes. Protective precautions should be used by all persons working with the drug.

Vinorelbine

Chemistry. Vinorelbine (Navelbine) is a third-generation semisynthetic Vinca alkaloid that has been commercially available in the United States since 1994 for treatment of non–small cell lung cancer. Vinorelbine also appears to have significant activity in breast cancer patients (430) and moderate activity in patients with cervical or ovarian cancer (431,432), as well as other tumor types (433). It has a molecular formula of $C_{45}H_{54}N_4O_8 \cdot 2C_4H_6O_6$ and a molecular weight of 1079.12. Vinorelbine's structure differs from that of the parent compounds, vincristine and vinblastine, in that it contains a nine-member (rather than eight-member) catharanthine ring (434). Its chemical name is 3′,4′-didehydro-4′-deoxy-C′-norvincaleukoblastine[*R*-(*R**,*R**)-2,3-dihydroxybut anedioate-(1:2)(salt)].

Mechanism of Action. Like other Vinca alkaloids, vinorelbine is classified as a "spindle poison" since it interacts with tubulin with resulting inhibition of microtubule assembly and cellular division during mitosis (435). Vinorelbine blocks cell cycle progression specifically in G_2 and M phases (128).

Drug Disposition. The pharmacokinetics of vinorelbine show large interpatient variability and are best described by a triphasic model. Following IV administration of a 30-mg/m^2 dose, a peak plasma level of 1,000 ng/mL is achieved, but the plasma level declines to 100 ng/mL within 2 hours. Vinorelbine rapidly binds to platelets (78% of total dose) and plasma proteins (13.5%), and only 1.7% is available as free drug (435). The drug readily diffuses into other tissues, and has a large volume of distribution (75.61 L/kg). The terminal half-life is approximately 45 hours (436).

The primary means of vinorelbine clearance appears to be hepatic metabolism. Approximately 18% and 46% is recovered in the urine and feces, respectively; however, recovery was incomplete in pharmacokinetic studies (437).

Administration and Dosage. Vinorelbine is a vesicant and requires careful administration. The drug should be diluted in a syringe or IV bag to a concentration of 1.5 to 3.0 mg/mL (syringe) or 0.5 to 2 mg/mL (IV bag). When using a syringe or IV bag, vinorelbine should be diluted with dextrose (5%) or sodium chloride (0.9%). When using an IV bag, it may also be diluted with sodium chloride (0.45%), Ringer's injection, or lactated Ringer's injection. Diluted vinorelbine should be administered over 6 to 10 minutes into a side port of a free-flowing IV line closest to the IV bag. Following vinorelbine administration, the vein should be flushed with at least 75 to 125 mL of IV solution. Longer IV infusions (e.g., 20 minutes) are associated with a higher incidence of phlebitis (438).

Vinorelbine solution is incompatible with fluorouracil, mitomycin, and thiotepa. It is also incompatible with several antibiotics (including a number of cephalosporins, amphotericin B, ampicillin, piperacillin, and trimethoprim-sulfamethoxazole), acyclovir, furosemide, ganciclovir, methylprednisolone, and sodium bicarbonate (439).

Vinorelbine is generally administered at a dose of 30 mg/m^2 every week. This dosing schedule has been used in combination chemotherapeutic regimens; however, the recommended dosing schedule in combination with cisplatin (100 mg/m^2 every 4 weeks) is weekly administration of vinorelbine at a dose of 25 mg/m^2. Attempts to increase vinorelbine dose intensity using a daily $\times$ 3 every 21 days dosing schedule with or without G-CSF have not been successful (440). However, Weiss et al. (441) have reported that continuous infusion of vinorelbine at doses of 8 to 10 mg/m^2/day with concurrent administration of G-CSF results in a twofold increase in vinorelbine dose intensity without increasing toxicity.

Side Effects and Toxicities. The primary dose-limiting toxicity of vinorelbine is myelosuppression, chiefly granulocytopenia (36% of patients, <500 cells/mm^3). A safety summary of data from North American clinical trials reported that when vinorelbine was administered at a dose of 30 mg/m^2/week to patients with breast cancer and non–small cell lung cancer, 64% of patients experienced grades 3 to 4 granulocytopenia, 50% experienced grades 3 to 4 leukopenia, and 9% developed grades 3 to 4 anemia. Despite the high incidence of granulocytopenia, most events were uncomplicated and only 7% of patients required hospitalization for fever and/or infection. The death rate due to sepsis was 1% to 2%. Myelosuppression was noncumulative, and the incidence of grades 3 and 4 granulocytopenia declined during later cycles of vinorelbine therapy. The granulocyte nadir typically occurred on day 14 of treatment, with recovery of the granulocyte count within 7 days (442).

Vinorelbine therapy is frequently associated with transient increases in liver enzymes, especially alkaline phosphatase. Virtually all patients experience a rise in alkaline phosphatase, with approximately 25% developing grade 3 toxicity and an additional 2% experiencing grade 4 elevations. Increases in AST and ALT also occur in more than half of all patients. However, most patients with liver enzyme increases remain asymptomatic and do not require dose modification of vinorelbine. Total bilirubin also can be elevated: 10% of patients experience some degree of increased bilirubin, with 2% experiencing grade 4 elevation. Because of the high incidence of liver and bone metastases in the study population (breast cancer and non–small cell lung cancer patients), the proportion of these toxicities that is directly attributable to vinorelbine therapy is unknown (442).

Other common toxicities associated with vinorelbine when administered as a single agent at a dose of 30 mg/m²/week by a 20-minute IV infusion include nausea (38% overall, 2% severe), vomiting (17% overall, 2% severe), constipation (31%, 3% severe), asthenia (29%, 5% severe), injection-site reactions (26%, 2% severe), anorexia (15%, 1% severe), diarrhea (15%, 1% severe), stomatitis (14%, 0% severe), pain (13%, 2% severe), paresthesia (13%, <1% severe), fever (11%, 1% severe), and alopecia (10%, <1% severe) (442). Vinorelbine-induced nausea and vomiting are generally mild and are readily controlled with standard antiemetic medication (442). Injection-site reactions include erythema, warmth, pain, and phlebitis. Repeated administration of vinorelbine can result in discoloration of the vein. As discussed above, shortening the injection duration to 6 to 10 minutes significantly reduces the incidence of injection-site reactions (438).

Injection-site pain and pain of unspecified etiology have been reported with administration of vinorelbine as a single agent (442). Additionally, acute tumor pain has been reported in several cancer patients who received treatment with vinorelbine plus a platinum-containing agent (either carboplatin or cisplatin) (443).

Pulmonary toxicity is an infrequent side effect of vinorelbine. Approximately 5% of patients experience dyspnea. Some cases of dyspnea are characterized by rapid onset during administration and resolve with bronchodilator therapy. Other cases occur usually within 1 hour of vinorelbine infusion and are characterized by life-threatening progressive dyspnea and the development of interstitial infiltrates (442,444). The coadministration of mitomycin may increase the pulmonary toxicity of vinorelbine (444).

Rare side effects of vinorelbine include pancreatitis, PPE (with prolonged infusions), paralytic ileus, and syndrome of inappropriate ADH secretion (445–448).

Special Precautions. Vinorelbine extravasation can result in severe local irritation, tissue necrosis, and phlebitis. If extravasation occurs, the injection should be halted immediately and any remaining portion of the dose should be injected into a different vein. Specific antidotes for vinorelbine extravasation have not been studied; however, vinblastine extravasation reactions may be ameliorated with the use of corticosteroid injections followed by cold compresses (429).

Drug Interactions. In that Vinca alkaloids are metabolized by the cytochrome P450 3A system, coadministration of strong P450 inhibitors, such as erythromycin and ketoconazole, could potentially reduce vinorelbine clearance and increase toxicity (449). Doxorubicin and etoposide also are metabolized by the P450 system, and coadministration of these drugs with vinorelbine could potentially affect vinorelbine metabolism (449).

Mitomycin is known to exacerbate Vinca alkaloid–induced pulmonary toxicity (450), and the combination of high-dose vinorelbine (50 mg/m² on days 1 and 21) plus mitomycin (15 mg/m² on day 1) has been associated with life-threatening acute pulmonary toxicity characterized by rapid onset of severe, progressive dyspnea and the development of bilateral interstitial infiltrates (444).

The combination of paclitaxel and vinorelbine has been associated with severe neurotoxicity including grade 4 motor neuropathy, irreversible ototoxicity, and vocal cord paresis (451). In one report of clinical experience in five patients with preexisting, mild to moderate, paclitaxel-induced sensory neuropathy, the combination of vinorelbine 25 to 30 mg/m² followed by paclitaxel 150 mg/m² by 3-hour infusion every 2 weeks resulted in severe, slowly reversing motor neuropathy in all five patients. Four of the five patients required the use of a wheelchair (451).

Special Applications. On a well-tolerated weekly dose schedule for vinorelbine, Bajetta et al. (452) noted four partial responses and one complete response in 31 patients (24 platinum resistant, 4 platinum sensitive, 5 with undetermined sensitivity) for an overall response rate of 15% (95% CI of 5.1, 37.9%). A phase 2 trial (vinorelbine 30 mg/m² weekly infusion) in persistent or recurrent ovarian cancer found a 29% objective response rate; granulocytopenia was a dose-limiting but manageable toxicity (431). This is consistent with previous findings of a 21% response rate in the population of heavily pretreated and platinum-resistant ovarian cancer patients (452).

Molecularly Targeted Agents

Erlotinib

Chemistry. Erlotinib (OSI-774, Tarceva) is an oral tyrosine kinase inhibitor (specifically, HER1/EGFR) that has the potential for inhibiting tumor-cell growth of a variety of tumors. Erlotinib has the molecular formula $C_{22}H_{23}N_3O_4 \cdot HCl$ and a molecular weight of 429.90. Erlotinib is FDA approved for the treatment of advanced or metastatic non–small cell lung cancer after failure or prior chemotherapy, and is approved for use in combination with gemcitabine for the first-line treatment of unresectable or metastatic pancreatic cancer. Phase 1 and 2 studies have demonstrated some activity in ovarian cancer and head and neck squamous cell cancer (453,454). There is also ongoing exploration of the use of erlotinib for maintenance of patients with ovarian cancer following front-line treatment (455).

Drug Disposition. Erlotinib is rapidly absorbed after administration, with peak plasma levels occurring at 4 hours. Plasma levels increase with dose, but daily administration does not cause unexpected drug accumulation (456). More than 90% of erlotinib is bound to plasma proteins. It is primarily metabolized by CYP3A4, which suggests that concomitant treatment with potent CYP3A4 inhibitors (e.g., ketoconazole, systemic antifungals, clarithromycin) may affect the metabolism of erlotinib (456).

Administration and Dosage. Erlotinib is administered orally. As a single agent, erlotinib is to be administered at 150 mg/day. Dosage should be reduced to 100 mg/day in combination therapy regimens. Food substantially increases the bioavailability of erlotinib; therefore, it should be taken at least 1 to 2 hours prior to the ingestion of food. When administered at 200 mg/day, diarrhea is dose limiting.

Side Effects and Toxicities. The dose-limiting toxicities associated with erlotinib include diarrhea and rash; however, at a dose of 150 mg/day, diarrhea can be effectively managed with loperamide. Other less common toxicities include headache, nausea and vomiting, and mucositis (453). It can be administered as a single agent, and has an additive effect on antitumor activity when combined with cisplatin, doxorubicin, gemcitabine, or low-dose paclitaxel without an associated increase in toxicity (457).

Sunitinib

Chemistry. Sunitinib (SU11248, Sutent), a multi-kinase inhibitor (e.g., VEGFR, PDGFR, FLT3, KIT, and RET inhibitor), was granted accelerated approval by the FDA in 2006 for the treatment of advanced renal cell carcinoma and for the treatment of gastrointestinal stromal tumor (GIST) after disease progression on or intolerance to imatinib (Gleevec) (458). Clinical trials are planned and ongoing to evaluate the efficacy of sunitinib in the treatment of uterine and ovarian cancers and sunitinib is also being evaluated for potential efficacy against hematologic malignancies (459). Chemically, it is a butanedioic acid, hydroxy-, (2S)-, compound with *N*-[2-(diethylamino)ethyl]-5-[(*Z*)-(5-fluoro-1, 2-dihydro-2-oxo-3*H*-indol-3-ylidine)methyl]-2,4-dimethyl-1*H*-pyrrole-3-carboxamide (1:1). The molecular formula of sunitinib is $C_{22}H_{27}FN_4O_2 \cdot C_4H_6O_5$ and the molecular weight is 532.6.

Drug Disposition. Maximum plasma concentration occurs within 6 to 12 hours following administration (458). The terminal half-life of sunitinib is approximately 40 to 60 hours, and the terminal half-life of its primary metabolite is 80 to 110 hours. Steady-state concentrations are achieved within 10 to 14 days. Concomitant treatment with CYP3A4 inducers (e.g., rifampin, St. John's Wort, dexamethasone) may decrease the concentration of sunitinib, whereas concomitant treatment with CYP3A4 inhibitors (e.g., ketoconazole, systemic antifungals) and grapefruit may increase the plasma concentration of sunitinib (458).

Administration and Dosage. Sunitinib is administered 50 mg/day for 4 weeks, followed by 2 weeks off medication. Sunitinib may be taken with or without food, as the pharmacokinetics are unaffected by food intake (460).

Side Effects and Toxicities. The most common side effects of sunitinib monotherapy include gastrointestinal (e.g., AST/ALT, lipase, amylase, bilirubin), rare cardiac (decreased left ventricular ejection fraction), renal/metabolic (e.g., creatinine, hypokalemia, hypernatremia, uric acid) and hematologic (e.g., neutrophils, platelets, hemoglobin) toxicities (458).

Lapatinib

Chemistry. The dual kinase inhibitor lapatinib (Tykerb) is FDA approved for combination therapy with capecitabine for the treatment of HER2-overexpressing breast cancers, as a post–first-line regimen. Lapatinib inhibits both HER2 and epidermal growth factor receptor (EGFR) kinases (461). It has the chemical name *N*-(3-chloro-4-{[(3-fluorophenyl)methyl] oxy}phenyl)-6-[5-({[2-(methylsulfonyl)ethyl]amino}methyl)-2-furanyl]-4-quinazolinamine bis(4-methylbenzenesulfonate) monohydrate, the molecular formula $C_{29}H_{26}ClFN_4O_4S$ $(C_7H_8O_3S)_2\ H_2O$, and a molecular weight of 943.5.

Drug Disposition. Peak plasma concentration occurs approximately 4 hours after administration. The half-life of lapatinib is estimated to be between 7 and 24 hours, and steady-state concentrations are achieved within 6 to 7 days (462). Divided dosing (versus the same dose given once per day) results in nearly double the exposure (steady-state serum AUC). Systemic exposure is also increased with food (three- to fourfold higher AUC). Similar to other kinase inhibitors, concomitant treatment with CYP3A4 inducers may decrease the concentration of lapatinib, whereas concomitant treatment with CYP3A4 inhibitors may increase the plasma concentration of lapatinib.

Administration and Dosage. The FDA-approved dosage of lapatinib is 1,250 mg given orally daily (days 1 to 21), 1 hour before or at least 1 hour after a meal, in combination with capecitabine 2,000 mg/m^2/day (administered orally in two doses approximately 12 hours apart) which is given on days 1 to 14 of the 21-day cycle.

Side Effects and Toxicities. Rash, nausea, and vomiting (grades 1 to 2) are the most common side effects associated with lapatinib (462). Lapatinib may decrease left ventricular ejection fraction. Serious adverse events have been rarely reported in clinical trials (462).

Estrogen Receptor/Progesterone Receptor–Targeted Agents

Anastrozole

Chemistry. Anastrozole (Arimidex) is FDA approved for the adjuvant treatment of postmenopausal patients with estrogen receptor positive (ER+) breast cancers following tamoxifen therapy, and is also indicated for postmenopausal women for the first-line treatment of ER+/ER-unknown breast cancer that is locally advanced or metastatic. Anastrozole is rarely associated with response in ER-negative disease. Anastrozole has been shown to have fewer side effects and a significant survival advantage as compared to megestrol acetate in the treatment of postmenopausal patients with breast cancer (463). Chemically, it is 1,3-benzenediacetonitrile, α,α,α′,α′-tetramethyl-5-(1H-1,2,4-triazol-1-ylmethyl). It has a molecular formula of $C_{17}H_{19}N_5$ and a molecular weight of 293.4.

Mechanism of Action. Anastrozole is a nonsteroidal aromatase inhibitor that prevents the peripheral conversion of androgens (androstenedione and testosterone) to estrogens (estrone, estrone sulfate, and estradiol) (50). Anastrozole has a significant effect on serum estradiol; as low as 1 mg/day has caused estradiol levels to be undetectable (464). In patients receiving 5 and 10 mg of anastrozole, there was no effect on adrenal corticosteroids or aldosterone.

Drug Disposition. Following oral administration, anastrozole is well absorbed into the systemic circulation and not affected by food ingestion. Pharmacokinetics are linear and not affected by repeated dosing. Steady-state concentration levels are achieved after approximately 7 days of treatment.

Administration and Dosage. Anastrozole is administered orally at a dose of 1 mg/day. For advanced disease, treatment should continue until disease progression.

Side Effects and Toxicities. When compared in a controlled clinical study to megestrol acetate, the principal side effect of anastrozole was diarrhea (occurred in 8.4% vs. 2.8% of patients treated with megestrol acetate). In general, it is very well tolerated, with the most frequent side effects (any grade) being asthenia (18%), nausea (18%), headache (14%), hot flushes (13.2%), and pain (10%).

Special Applications. It is hypothesized that anastrozole may play a role on a molecular level in the endometrium. Most endometrial carcinomas are associated with endometrial hyperplasia and are estrogen receptor (ER) and progesterone receptor (PR) positive. In addition to ER/PR status, there is a progressive increase in the expression of the protein pS2 from normal to hyperplastic to well-differentiated carcinoma (465). Aromatase inhibition may be able to alter the course of disease by preventing the endometrium from being exposed to estrogen. This may in turn alter the expression of the pS2 protein as there is a strong association between ER/PR expression and expression of pS2 protein (465). Aromatase activity has been demonstrated in both ER/PR–positive and ER/PR–negative endometrial carcinomas (466). Although much research has yet to be done, phase 1 and 2 trials have demonstrated safety and minimal activity in an unselected population of recurrent endometrial carcinoma patients (467). There is some evidence that it may have benefit in the treatment of endometrial hyperplasia (468).

Letrozole

Chemistry. Letrozole (Femara) is a nonsteroidal aromatase inhibitor that is FDA approved for the first-line treatment of postmenopausal women with locally advanced or metastatic breast cancer (hormone receptor positive or hormone receptor unknown). Letrozole is also used for the treatment of advanced breast cancer in postmenopausal women whose disease has progressed following antiestrogen therapy. Letrozole has also demonstrated some activity in palliative care for recurrent ovarian cancer (469,470). The chemical name of letrozole is 4,4′-(1H- 91,2,4-Triazol-1-ylmethylene) dibenzonitrile, and the empirical formula is $C_{17}H_{11}N_5$.

Mechanism of Action. Similar to other aromatase inhibitors, letrozole inhibits the conversion of androgens to estrogens via the aromatase enzyme. Letrozole treatment does not increase serum follicle stimulating hormone (FSH), and as a selective gonadal steroidogenesis inhibitor, does not impact adrenal mineralocorticoid or glucocorticoid synthesis.

Drug Disposition. Letrozole is not affected by food intake, and is rapidly and completely absorbed through the gastrointestinal tract. The terminal elimination half-life is 2 days. The major excretion route is via the kidneys. Steady-state plasma concentration is reached in 2 to 6 weeks of daily 2.5-mg dosing. These concentrations are up to two times higher than after a single dose. Steady-state levels can be maintained for long periods of time without continuous accumulation of letrozole.

Administration and Dosage. Letrozole is administered orally, at 2.5 mg per day. Letrozole can be taken at any time during the day regardless of food intake. Treatment is indicated until disease progression.

Side Effects and Toxicities. Letrozole has a more favorable toxicity profile as compared to tamoxifen, with greater or equivalent efficacy in breast cancer patients (471). The most common side effects include bone pain, hot flushes, back pain, nausea, arthralgia, and dyspnea, each occurring in no more than 20% of patients.

Medroxyprogesterone

Chemistry. The chemical name of the progestational agent medroxyprogesterone acetate (Provera) is pregn-4-ene-3,20-dione,17-(acetyloxy)-6-methyl-,(6α)-. Its empirical formula is $C_{24}H_{34}O_4$, with a molecular weight of 386.53. Medroxyprogesterone acetate (MPA) therapy is indicated with estrogen therapy for therapeutic use in women to reduce the incidence of atypical endometrial hyperplasia. There is some evidence that MPA may be used for endometrial hyperplasia or stage 1 endometrial cancer as an alternative to surgery to preserve fertility with some success (472,473). MPA has demonstrated activity when used with other agents in advanced or recurrent endometrial cancer (474).

Drug Disposition. MPA is absorbed through the gastrointestinal tract, and is primarily metabolized by the liver. Maximum concentrations are reached within 2 to 4 hours after oral administration. Food intake enhances the bioavailability of MPA (C_{max} by up to 70% and AUC up to 33% increase), but does not affect its half-life (12 to 16 hours).

Administration and Dosage. MPA is administered at 5 or 10 mg/day for endometrial hyperplasia for 12 to 14 consecutive days every month. For abnormal uterine bleeding or amenorrhea, MPA is generally administered for a shorter duration (e.g., 5 to 10 consecutive days). Patients experience withdrawal bleeding for 3 to 5 days following the treatment cycle. MPA is recommended to be used with 0.625 mg conjugated estrogens in women with a uterus to avoid the risk of endometrial cancer. Women without a uterus may receive estrogen without a progestin. In addition to the tablet form for oral intake, there is an intramuscular (IM) depot formulation that may permit alternative treatment regimens. The IM formulation of MPA was compared to oral megestrol acetate for the treatment of menopausal symptoms in breast cancer patients. In this short-term study, the IM formulation provided superior benefit to patients and may be an alternative to long-term oral progestin therapy (475).

Side Effects and Toxicities. MPA, similar to other progestins (e.g., megestrol acetate), may cause abnormal uterine bleeding, breast tenderness, or nausea. A Women's Health Initiative (WHI) study found that estrogen plus progesterone was associated with an increased risk of myocardial infarction, stroke, invasive breast cancer, pulmonary emboli, and deep vein thrombosis in postmenopausal women (476). A memory study embedded within the WHI study found that this combination may also be associated with an increased risk of developing dementia in women over the age of 65 (477). A black box warning now included on the MPA package insert recommends that estrogen/progesterone be used at the lowest possible dose for the shortest duration possible for the specific treatment goals of the patient.

Megestrol

Chemistry. The chemical name of megestrol acetate (Megace) is 17 ⟨-acetyloxy-6-methylpregna-4,6-diene-3,20-dione. Similar to MPA, it has the empirical formula $C_{24}H_{34}O_4$, and has a molecular weight of 384.51. Megestrol acetate is an FDA-approved progestin that is used for the palliative treatment of advanced carcinoma of the breast or endometrium (i.e., recurrent, inoperable, or metastatic disease). In general, progestational agents are currently used in the treatment of endometrial hyperplasia at a variety of doses and schedules. The GOG is currently investigating megestrol acetate in trial GOG-0224 (A Randomized, Controlled Phase II Evaluation Of Megestrol [Megace®] in Different Dose and Sequence in the Treatment of Endometrial Intraepithelial Neoplasia [EIN] from a Referred Cohort of Atypical Endometrial Hyperplasia [AEH] or EIN). GOG-0224 is designed to provide objective data toward a standard treatment regimen for the care of women with EIN or AEH in addition to understanding the actual mechanism of action of progestational agents in the endometrium.

Drug Disposition. Megestrol acetate is primarily excreted in the urine, and oral absorption rates are variable. Time to peak concentration ranges from 1.0 to 3.0 hours, and the plasma elimination half-life ranges from 13.0 to 104.9 hours. Steady-state plasma concentrations have not yet been established.

Administration and Dosage. Megestrol acetate is supplied in 20- and 40-mg tablets for oral intake. Although the recommended dosage for breast cancer is 160 mg/day (40 mg qid), and for endometrial carcinoma it is 40 to 320 mg/day in divided doses, there are a wide variety of dose and schedules implemented therapeutically for precancerous conditions (e.g., AEH).

Side Effects and Toxicities. The side effect profile of the progestational agents megestrol acetate and MPA is similar. However, weight gain is a common side effect with megestrol acetate. Thrombophlebitis and pulmonary embolism have been reported with megestrol acetate. Other toxicities include nausea and vomiting, edema, breakthrough menstrual bleeding, and dyspnea. In general, there are only rare severe toxicities reported with progestational agents.

Tamoxifen

Chemistry. Tamoxifen citrate (Nolvadex) is a nonsteroidal agent with antiestrogenic properties. It is indicated for the treatment of metastatic breast cancer and as adjuvant treatment in node-positive breast cancer in postmenopausal patients. Tamoxifen competes with estrogen for binding sites, which explains its increased effectiveness in ER+ tumors. Chemically, tamoxifen is (Z)2-[4-(1,2-diphenyl-1-butenyl) phenoxy]-N,N-dimethylethanamine 2-hydroxy-1,2,3-propanetricarboxylate (1:1), and has a molecular weight of 563.62.

Mechanism of Action. Tamoxifen is a nonsteroidal agent that has antiestrogenic properties in the breast and ovary, but acts like an estrogen agonist in the endometrium and bone (478). It may exert its antitumor effects by binding the estrogen receptors. Because of this mechanism, it is most beneficial in the treatment of ER+ tumors.

Drug Disposition. Peak plasma concentrations (average 40 ng/mL) take place approximately 5 hours after dosing. The decline in plasma concentrations is biphasic with a terminal elimination half-life of about 6 days. Steady-state concentrations for tamoxifen are achieved in about 4 weeks after initiation of therapy. Tamoxifen is extensively metabolized, with N-desmethyl tamoxifen being the major metabolite. Approximately 65% of the administered dose is eliminated in the feces within 2 weeks (479).

Administration and Dosage. Tamoxifen is available in 10- and 20-mg tablets for oral administration. The recommended dosage is 20 to 40 mg/day; when the higher daily dose is prescribed, it should be divided into two doses of 20 mg (morning and evening).

Side Effects and Toxicities. Tamoxifen causes estrogenic changes of the vaginal and cervical squamous epithelium and increases the incidence of cervical and endometrial polyps (480). It is associated with an increased risk of uterine malignancies (endometrial adenocarcinoma and uterine sarcoma). Other serious adverse events associated with tamoxifen treatment include stroke, deep vein thrombosis, and pulmonary embolism. A discussion weighing the benefits versus the risks should take place prior to treatment with tamoxifen; however, the benefits have been determined to outweigh the risks in women who take tamoxifen to reduce the risk of breast cancer recurrence. The National Adjuvant Breast and Bowel Project (NSABP P-1) found a higher incidence of the following side effects for tamoxifen versus placebo, respectively: vaginal discharge (54.7% vs. 34%); cold sweats (21.4% vs. 14.8%); hot flashes (77.7% vs. 65.1%); night sweats (66.8% vs. 54.9%); and genital itching (47.1% vs. 38.3%) (481). Serious adverse events reported more frequently among women taking tamoxifen as compared to placebo in the NSABP P-1 trial included uterine malignancy, uterine sarcoma, stroke, and pulmonary embolism.

Special Applications. Some ovarian cancers express hormonal receptors, a factor supporting the investigation of tamoxifen in the treatment of ovarian malignancies (482). It has demonstrated activity in patients with platinum-refractory ovarian cancer, with response rates ranging from 13% to 17% (with some complete responses), and with durations ranging from 4.4 months to more than 5 years (482–484). In the series by Hatch et al. (482), patients with ovarian cancer who had complete or partial responses on tamoxifen were more likely to have an ER+ tumor (89% ER+) than those who had stable disease or progression on tamoxifen (59% had elevated ER). The favorable toxicity profile of tamoxifen makes it an ideal agent to consider in patients with refractory ovarian cancer.

Antiangiogenesis Agents

Angiogenesis is the process by which new blood vessels are sprouted from preexisting ones. Endothelial cells must migrate, proliferate, and assemble into tubes during this process. In normal tissues, blood vessel growth is tightly controlled by numerous angiogenesis-stimulating factors and angiogenesis-inhibiting factors. Vascular endothelial growth factor (VEGF) and platelet-derived endothelial-cell growth factor (PD-ECGF) are two of the most extensively studied growth factors that appear to function primarily as angiogenesis-stimulating factors. Other growth factors and cytokines, such as basic fibroblast growth factor (bFGF), have multiple functions in addition to angiogenesis stimulation (485). Naturally occurring factors that suppress angiogenesis include angiostatin, endostatin, interferon-α, interferon-β, interferon-γ, interleukin-1, interleukin-12, platelet factor-4, thrombospondin-1, 1,2-methoxyestradiol, tissue inhibitor metalloproteinases (TIMPs), and, at high concentrations, tumor necrosis factor-α (486).

In the early 1970s, Folkman (487) pioneered the study of tumor angiogenesis with his observation that the growth of tumor nodules to a diameter of greater than 1 to 2 mm required neovascularization of the tumor. He hypothesized that pharmacologic suppression of tumor angiogenesis could induce tumor dormancy. Further research has shown that formation of new blood vessels within tumor nodules results in an exponential increase in tumor cell growth; the transition from hyperplasia to malignancy parallels the induction of neovascularization; and tumor angiogenesis is a prerequisite for metastatic spread (485,488). Additionally, blood vessel density of tumors has been shown to be a potentially important prognostic factor in multiple human neoplasms, including cancers of the ovary, cervix, and endometrium (489,490).

Obviously, this is a very brief discussion of tumor angiogenesis. The reader is referred to several reviews on angiogenesis inhibition and its potential for cancer treatment (486,491). Several angiogenetic agents that have FDA approval for various indications that may have potential for the treatment of gynecologic cancers are briefly discussed below.

Bevacizumab

Chemistry. Bevacizumab (Avastin) is recombinant humanized monoclonal IgG1 antibody that is designed to inhibit angiogenesis through targeting the human VEGF. Bevacizumab is FDA approved for treatment for first-line metastatic colorectal cancer in combination with 5-FU–based chemotherapy. Ovarian, endometrial, and cervical cancers have been shown to express VEGF-A (492). Early trials show promising results in refractory ovarian cancer and heavily pretreated cervical cancer patients (494–496); however, larger randomized trials are needed to demonstrate efficacy in gynecologic cancer populations.

Administration and Dosage. Bevacizumab is administered 5 mg/kg IV once every 14 days until disease progression.

Side Effects and Toxicities. The most common serious (grade 3 to 4) side effects of bevacizumab treatment include asthenia, pain, hypertension, diarrhea, and leukopenia. Bevacizumab has been associated with gastrointestinal perforation, wound healing complications, and hemorrhage. Hemorrhage was specifically pronounced among patients with recent hemoptysis; therefore, these patients should not receive bevacizumab. Patients receiving bevacizumab therapy have also demonstrated an increase in hypertension, proteinuria, and congestive heart failure. It is recommended that bevacizumab therapy be delayed at least 28 days following any major surgical procedure. The safety of bevacizumab in patients with cardiovascular disease is unknown.

Thalidomide

Chemistry. Thalidomide (Thalomid) is an antiangiogenic agent that is indicated for the treatment of cutaneous manifestations of erythema nodosum leprosum (ENL). However, thalidomide has been used in the treatment of various advanced malignancies and has demonstrated possible activity in ovarian and papillary-serous peritoneal carcinoma (497). Thalidomide has the chemical name α-(N-phthalimido)glutarimide. The molecular structure is $C_{13}H_{10}N_2O_4$, and it has a molecular weight of 258.2.

Mechanism of Action. Although the exact mechanism of action is not fully characterized, the immunologic effects of thalidomide may be related to suppression of excessive tumor necrosis factor-α (TNF-α) production and down-modulation of selected cell surface adhesion molecules involved in leukocyte migration (498).

Dosage and Administration. Thalidomide is an oral agent, which is supplied in 50-, 100-, and 200-mg gelatin capsules. When used in chemotherapeutic regimens, the dose of thalidomide is generally titrated up to 400 mg/day as an evening dose (50). When used in a pilot study of ovarian and peritoneal carcinoma, daily thalidomide was initiated at 200 mg, with doses increasing by 100 mg per day every 2 weeks until response or tolerance (493).

Side Effects and Toxicities. Thalidomide is teratogenic and should not be used at any time during pregnancy. Latex condoms should be used by sexually active males using the drug because thalidomide is present in semen. The most common side effects include somnolence, peripheral neuropathy, dizziness, neutropenia, rash, and HIV viral load increase.

MODULATING AGENTS/ SUPPORTIVE CARE DRUGS USED IN THE TREATMENT OF GYNECOLOGIC CANCERS

Defining approaches to improve the therapeutic index of cancer chemotherapy, such that tumor-cell kill is enhanced while toxicity to normal cells is minimized, remains a fundamental goal of cancer treatment. A major limiting factor in successful cancer therapy is the ability of the tumor to develop resistance to the drugs used for treatment. A second fundamental problem faced by the oncologist treating patients with chemotherapy is the acute and chronic toxic effects of the drugs to the normal tissues. One approach that holds promise for the improvement of the therapeutic index is the concept of modulation, or the use of drugs with little or no cytotoxic activity to modulate the efficacy of standard anticancer drugs. Modulating agents can be divided into three main classes based on their ability to (a) protect host tissue from the toxic effects of the cancer drugs; (b) potentiate anticancer drugs; and (c) reverse acquired drug resistance. In this section, we discuss agents with chemoprotective abilities used with chemotherapy in the treatment of gynecologic cancers. The drugs outlined are not meant to be fully inclusive and the reader is referred to Tew et al. (499) for a complete review on the subject of modulation of anticancer drug activities.

Chemoprotective Agents

Amifostine

Chemistry. Amifostine (Ethyol) is, to date, the most extensively developed broad-spectrum cytoprotective agent. Originally developed as a radioprotective compound, amifostine was selected from a series of over 4,400 synthetic thiol derivatives developed by the U.S. Army as having the most effective radioprotective effects and best safety profile (500). Subsequently, an extensive number of studies have demonstrated that amifostine selectively protects normal, but not tumor, tissue from the toxicities induced by radiation therapy and chemotherapy (499,501). Amifostine is FDA approved and indicated to reduce the cumulative renal toxicity associated with repeat cisplatin administration in patients with advanced ovarian cancer or non–small cell lung cancer. It is also approved for chronic, three times weekly dosing, 15 to 20 minutes prior to daily radiation therapy in patients with head and neck cancer. Chemically, it is 2-[(3-aminopropyl) amino]ethanethiol dihydrogen phosphate (ester), its empiric formula is $C_5H_{15}N_2O_3PS$, and it has a molecular weight of 214.22.

Mechanism of Action. Amifostine is an inactive prodrug that is dephosphorylated to the active, free thiol species, WR1065, at the tissue site by cell membrane–bound and capillary alkaline phosphatase. The higher specific activity of the membrane-bound enzyme in normal tissue versus tumor tissue promotes rapid transport of the active thiol metabolite into the normal cell, with negligible transport into the cancer cells. The higher pH and higher activity of capillary alkaline phosphatase in normal tissue also contribute to the preferential uptake of WR1065 by normal cells (502). A number of mechanisms of protection by WR1065 have been reported, including scavenging of oxygen free radicals, direct intracellular binding to and subsequent detoxification of the active species of alkylating and platinum compounds, prevention or reversal of cisplatin-DNA adduct formation, induction of hypoxia, and alterations in intracellular glutathione and polyamine levels.

In addition to protecting normal cells from the cytotoxic effects of chemotherapy, amifostine has been shown to stimulate bone marrow progenitor cells (503) and sensitize tumor cells both *in vitro* and *in vivo* to the cytotoxic effects of anticancer agents, including nitrogen mustard, paclitaxel, melphalan, and carboplatin (80,504,505). Thus, amifostine is unique in that it is the only known modulating agent that may improve the therapeutic index for antitumor agents by dual mechanisms, that is, decreasing toxicity to normal tissue and potentiating tumor-specific cytotoxicity.

Drug Disposition. Pharmacokinetic studies in humans have shown that following IV administration at a dose of 740 or 910 mg/m^2, amifostine is rapidly cleared from the plasma and taken up into normal tissues with an α half-life of less than 1 minute and a β half-life of less than 10 minutes (506). Within 5 to 10 minutes after completion of a 15-minute infusion, greater than 90% of the parent drug is cleared from the plasma. A terminal elimination phase with a half-life of 48 minutes has also been reported (507). However, the plasma levels were very low during the elimination phase, and repeat dosing with amifostine at 2-hour intervals did not lead to increasing peak values at the end of each infusion.

Analyses of the human pharmacokinetics of WR1065 and the symmetric disulfide WR33278 following a single dose or three doses of amifostine (740 or 910 mg/m^2) 15 minutes before and 2 and 4 hours after chemotherapy have also been reported (507). WR1065 is rapidly cleared from the plasma by fast uptake into the tissues and conversion to disulfides. The initial half-life of 0.18 hour is followed by a slower, second phase with a half-life of 7.3 hours, where only low plasma levels are present. The final half-life of the disulfides ranged from 8.4 to 13.4 hours, and these metabolites were detectable 24 hours after treatment. As such, the disulfides may serve as an exchangeable pool of WR1065. After repeat dosing with amifostine, peak levels of WR1065 were increased, but peak levels of the disulfides were slightly decreased. This may suggest a change in the uptake or elimination of WR1065 or a saturation of the disulfide formation.

Amifostine changes the pharmacokinetics of carboplatin in humans, resulting in a longer, final half-life of ultrafiltrable platinum species in patients with a normal creatinine clearance, and a small increase in the AUC value (80). One can speculate that amifostine's effect on carboplatin pharmacokinetics may increase the efficacy of carboplatin in patients, similar to what has been observed in tumor-bearing mice. The effect of amifostine on the pharmacokinetics of cisplatin is minor, resulting in an increase of the final half-life of ultrafiltrable platinum but not unchanged cisplatin (508).

Administration and Dosage. The originally recommended schedule of amifostine was as a 15-minute IV infusion administered 15 to 30 minutes before chemotherapy; however, a markedly lower incidence of both hypotension and emesis has been documented when amifostine is administered by rapid IV bolus (509). Although an optimal dose has not been defined, amifostine is generally given at the MTD ranging from 740 to 910 mg/m^2. The rapid IV bolus administration of these amifostine doses can be achieved in increments of 500 mg with 5 minutes separating each dose, up to three IV injections, markedly minimizing nausea and hypotension.

Special Applications. Amifostine has been shown in a number of clinical trials to protect against cisplatin-induced nephrotoxicity and neurotoxicity and cyclophosphamide-induced hematotoxicity (501). Results of a randomized, multicenter phase 3 trial of cyclophosphamide (1,000 mg/m^2) and cisplatin (100 mg/m^2) with or without amifostine (910 mg/m^2) every 3 weeks for six cycles in advanced epithelial ovarian cancer patients confirmed that pretreatment with amifostine reduces the cumulative renal, hematologic, and neurologic toxicities of the chemotherapy regimen (120). Final analysis of 242 patients (122 received amifostine) revealed that amifostine pretreatment yielded significant protection against the toxic effects of cisplatin. Twenty-six percent of patients (31 of 120) on the chemotherapy-alone arm compared with 10% of patients (12 of 122) pretreated with amifostine had treatment-limiting renal, neurologic, or ototoxicity requiring discontinuation of cisplatin treatment (p = 0.001). No patients on the amifostine arm discontinued therapy because of nephrotoxicity compared with seven patients on the chemotherapy-alone arm (p = 0.008). Significant hematoprotection also was observed, including a 53% reduction in the percentage of patients experiencing neutropenia-associated events (p = 0.019) and a 62% reduction in the total incidence of neutropenia-associated events (p = 0.005). The latter resulted in a 61% reduction in the number of days in the hospital (p = 0.019) and a 61% reduction in days on antibiotics (p = 0.031). No difference in survival was observed at a 41-month median follow-up period between patients on either arm of the study, suggesting that amifostine does not reduce the antitumor efficacy of chemotherapeutic treatment.

Results from a study in breast cancer patients receiving high-dose chemotherapy with autologous bone marrow support showed that amifostine treatment of bone marrow cells prior to *ex vivo* purging with 4-hydroxycyclophosphamide (4-HC) resulted in a significant decrease in time to leukocyte engraftment from 36 days (4-HC alone) to 26 days (p = 0.032) (510). Additionally, those patients treated with amifostine required significantly fewer platelet transfusions and days of antibiotic therapy. Results of a randomized phase 2 trial of carboplatin plus amifostine versus carboplatin alone in patients with advanced solid tumors indicated that amifostine can reduce the cumulative thrombocytopenia resulting from carboplatin treatment (79).

There have been several small, randomized studies of amifostine in combination with carboplatin plus paclitaxel in the management of advanced ovarian cancer (511–513). In each of these trials, amifostine demonstrated some activity against the development of grade 2 and/or grade 3 neurotoxicity. Within the randomized trial publication, De Vos et al. present a pooled analysis of three selected trials of amifostine with similar dosing schedules of carboplatin plus paclitaxel (511). There was statistically significant evidence in this analysis that IV amifostine pretreatment reduced the risk of grade 2/3 neurotoxicity.

Side Effects and Toxicities. The dose-limiting toxicities of amifostine include nausea, vomiting, and arterial hypotension. However, the emesis and hypotension can be reduced to relatively mild toxicities through rapid IV bolus administration together with the preadministration of IV fluids, dexamethasone (20 mg IV in adults), and ondansetron (0.15 mg/kg IV) within 1 hour prior to chemotherapy (514). Amifostine administered on a daily × 5 schedule at 825 mg/m^2, with cisplatin and radiation therapy, can result in hypocalcemic effects; however, these doses are no longer used in clinical trials. Wadler et al. (515) reported that amifostine in extremely high doses can lead to a cumulative effect on decreased serum ionized calcium levels, which is mediated by direct inhibition of parathyroid hormone (PTH) activity. Administration of oral calcium with vitamin D supplements and frequent monitoring of serum ionized calcium levels are recommended for patients treated with the higher doses of amifostine, cisplatin, and radiation therapy.

Special Applications. The complications associated with IV administration have led to the ongoing development of amifostine for subcutaneous (SC) administration at 200 mg/m^2 three times weekly. The SC administration of amifostine has been evaluated in a number of preclinical and clinical studies; safety and efficacy studies have been conducted and are ongoing (516). Amifostine by either the IV bolus or SC routes in low (i.e., 200 to 340 mg/m^2) daily to three times weekly dosing schedules reduces both the acute and chronic cystitis and enteritis associated with pelvic irradiation in gastrointestinal, gynecologic, and urologic cancers, as shown in Table 16.7.

Dexrazoxane

Dexrazoxane (Zinecard), a metal-chelating agent, belongs to the bis-dioxopiperazine family, and was originally designed as a potential antitumor agent. Although early clinical trials failed to provide significant evidence of cytotoxic activity (517), an observation was made that the drug caused a marked increase in the urine clearance of iron and zinc (518). These findings, coupled with preclinical studies that showed that dexrazoxane and other chelating agents could prevent the acute myocardial damage induced by anthracyclines (519) without reducing the antitumor effect of the drugs (520), led to the use of dexrazoxane as a cardioprotective agent. Animal studies have shown that dexrazoxane can offer significant protection against anthracycline-induced cardiotoxicity, and dexrazoxane was most effective when given from 30 minutes

TABLE 16.7

AMIFOSTINE EFFICACY IN COLORECTAL/PELVIC CANCERS: PHASE 2/3 TRIALS

Study	Phase; study population	Treatment outcomes
Anthanassiou, 2003 (537)	Phase 3; pelvic carcinomas with radiation therapy	Amifostine reduced radiation-induced bladder and lower gastrointestinal toxicity
Koukourakis, 2000 (516)	Phase 2 subcutaneous amifostine; pelvic carcinomas with radiation therapy	Subcutaneous amifostine reduced radiation-induced mucosal toxicity and treatment interruptions
Antonadau, 2004 (538)	Phase 3; advanced colorectal cancer radiation plus chemotherapy	Amifostine reduced grade 2 gastrointestinal toxicity

before to 15 minutes after doxorubicin (521). Subsequent studies demonstrated that the degree of cardioprotection elicited by dexrazoxane is dependent on the dose of the anthracycline and the severity of the cardiomyopathy (522). Results from the initial clinical study of dexrazoxane in patients with metastatic breast cancer were encouraging and confirmed those of the preclinical studies. Speyer et al. (523) conducted a randomized trial of FAC (fluorouracil 500 mg/m^2, doxorubicin 50 mg/m^2, cyclophosphamide 500 mg/m^2) versus FAC plus dexrazoxane 1,000 mg/m^2, administered as an IV bolus injection 30 minutes before FAC therapy. Pretreatment with dexrazoxane offered significant protection against doxorubicin-induced cardiotoxicity as assessed by clinical examination, radionuclide scan of left ventricular ejection fraction, and endomyocardial biopsy. Patients receiving dexrazoxane received higher cumulative doses of doxorubicin, and significantly fewer of these patients were removed from the study because of cardiotoxicity.

Chemistry. Dexrazoxane is an FDA-approved chemoprotective agent that reduces the severity and incidence of cardiomyopathy in women with metastatic breast cancer undergoing doxorubicin therapy. It is chemically known as (S)-4,4′-(1-methyl-1,2-ethanediyl)bis-2,6-piperazinedione, has the molecular formula $C_{11}H_{16}N_4O_4$, and has a molecular weight of 268.28.

Mechanism of Action. The proposed mechanism by which dexrazoxane reduces cardiotoxicity is through chelation of free or loosely bound iron by the hydrolyzed form of the drug (524). This prevents the binding of anthracyclines to intracellular iron and subsequent formation of toxic free radicals.

Administration and Dosage. Dexrazoxane is specifically indicated for women who have received a cumulative dose of 300 mg/m^2 or greater of doxorubicin and who, in the physician's opinion, would benefit from further doxorubicin therapy. Dexrazoxane must be reconstituted with 0.167 molar (M/6) sodium lactate to give a concentration of 10 mg dexrazoxane for each milliliter of sodium lactate. It may be further diluted with either 0.9% sodium chloride or 5.0% dextrose to a concentration range of 1.3 to 5.0 mg/mL in intravenous infusion bags. It should be given slow IV push or rapid drip IV infusion. Dexrazoxane should be administered no less than 30 minutes before doxorubicin, and the recommended dose ratio of dexrazoxane to doxorubicin is 10:1 (i.e., dexrazoxane 500 mg/m^2:doxorubicin 50 mg/m^2).

Side Effects and Toxicities. Although randomized studies have shown that myelosuppression was slightly greater in patients pretreated with dexrazoxane, this does not appear to be clinically significant. In addition to dose-limiting granulocytopenia, other toxicities associated with the drug include mild nausea/vomiting and alopecia.

A number of studies in patients with advanced breast cancer have confirmed the protective effects of dexrazoxane against anthracycline-induced cardiotoxicity (525). Additionally, dexrazoxane was shown to have a significant cardioprotective effect in pediatric patients treated up to a cumulative doxorubicin dose of 410 mg/m^2 (526).

Special Applications. In addition to the cardioprotection indication for dexrazoxane, there are a number of other potential applications for this agent (527). Of particular interest, relative to the treatment of gynecologic malignancies, is the finding that dexrazoxane can enhance the effects of cisplatin in both drug-sensitive and drug-resistant human ovarian cancer cell lines.

Leucovorin

Leucovorin, a chemically reduced derivative of folic acid, is also known as citrovorum factor or folinic acid and was the original chemoprotective agent employed to overcome high-dose methotrexate-induced bone marrow toxicity (528). Leucovorin can serve as a substitute for the endogenous reduced-folate cofactor (N^5,N^{10}-methylene tetrahydrofolate) that is diminished by methotrexate. Thus, leucovorin can "rescue" cells by replenishing intracellular reduced-folate pools and preventing methotrexate toxicity via blockade of thymidine synthesis. Leucovorin acts in a dose- and time-dependent fashion and must be given within 48 hours of methotrexate in order to elicit its rescue effects.

Leucovorin is also a successful modulatory agent used clinically to potentiate the antitumor activity of 5-FU (499). Leucovorin can enhance the DNA toxicity induced by 5-FU through the formation of a stable tertiary complex of 5, 10-methylene tetrahydrofolate, thymidylate synthase, and fluorodeoxyuridine monophosphate. Compared with 5-FU alone, this combination has been shown to produce higher response rates and, in some cases, longer survival for patients with metastatic gastrointestinal malignancies (529). The combination of 5-FU and leucovorin currently is being tested extensively in other malignancies, including metastatic breast cancer (530). A complete review of leucovorin as a modulating agent is beyond the scope of this chapter and the reader is referred to a number of excellent reviews on this topic (499,531).

Mesna

Mesna (Mesnex) is used clinically as a specific chemoprotective agent against bladder toxicity resulting from oxazophosphorine-based alkylating agents, such as cyclophosphamide and ifosfamide. It is sodium-2-mercaptoethane sulfonate, with the molecular formula $C_2H_5NaO_3S_2$ and a molecular weight of 164.18.

Mechanism of Action. Mesna inactivates the protein-reactive aldehyde, acrolein metabolite of ifosfamide and cyclophosphamide, which accumulates in the urinary bladder and results in dose-limiting urotoxicity (234). Plasma conversion of mesna to its inactive disulfide metabolite, dimesna, allows for the pretreatment and simultaneous administration of mesna as a urinary protector for ifosfamide and cyclophosphamide (high dose). Following renal filtration and secretion, dimesna is converted back to the active parent compound by glutathione reductase, which is subsequently delivered to the bladder. The mesna-free sulfhydryl groups in the urinary bladder can directly complex to and thus neutralize acrolein, in addition to potentially blocking acrolein formation in the urinary tract (532). The metabolic characteristic of mesna should preclude any potential protection to tumors. Indeed, there is no clinical evidence that mesna coadministration with ifosfamide results in decreased antitumor activity. However, mesna has been shown to prevent the cytotoxicity of platinum agents when given simultaneously with them in *in vitro* models. As such, careful scheduling of mesna is warranted for clinical trials using ifosfamide in combination with platinum compounds. Additionally, mesna should not be given simultaneously with cisplatin.

Drug Disposition. Proper scheduling of mesna has been based on pharmacokinetic analysis, which showed that mesna and dimesna have relatively short half-lives of approximately 1 hour and that peak urinary thiol accumulation following IV or oral mesna occurs at 1 and 3 hours, respectively (533). Because the half-life of mesna is much shorter than that of acrolein, it must be administered beyond the completion of ifosfamide.

Administration and Dosage. Mesna is available for IV bolus injection (100 mg/mL) or for oral use, available as 400-mg tablets. For IV administration, it should be diluted to obtain a final concentration of 20 mg/mL. The diluted solution is stable for 24 hours at room temperature. The approved schedule for IV administration of mesna is as a bolus dose (20% of the ifosfamide dose) prior to ifosfamide and two additional doses 4 and 8 hours after ifosfamide treatment (283). A combination of IV and oral mesna has been used to simplify outpatient ifosfamide therapy. The oral dose of mesna is given equal to 40% of the ifosfamide dosage in two doses at 2 and 6 hours after ifosfamide administration, based on a 50% urinary bioavailability of oral mesna. Oral doses of 3 g/m^2 have been well tolerated in patients; however, nausea was observed in healthy volunteers receiving oral doses greater than 2 g/m^2. Goren et al. (534) reviewed the dosing schedules and incidence of hematuria in 47 clinical studies in which oral mesna was administered to 1,986 patients who received greater than 6,475 courses of ifosfamide. Compilation of the data showed that a variety of doses and schedules of oral and IV mesna were effective at preventing hemorrhagic cystitis in patients treated with a number of different ifosfamide regimens. Although an optimal dose and schedule of mesna has not been established, adequate protection against ifosfamide-induced cystitis can be achieved using an initial IV dose of mesna that is equal to 20% of the ifosfamide dose, followed by two oral doses of mesna, each equal to 40% of the ifosfamide dose.

Side Effects and Toxicities. The most common side effects of mesna include headache, injection site reactions, flushing, dizziness, nausea, vomiting, flu-like symptoms, and coughing. Patients may develop hematuria (up to 6%) when administered ifosfamide plus mesna; a urine sample should be evaluated for hematuria each day prior to ifosfamide therapy.

Special Applications. The superiority of mesna as a chemoprotectant against ifosfamide- and cyclophosphamide-induced bladder toxicity has been demonstrated in a number of clinical trials (283). In a comparative study of patients treated with ifosfamide at a dose of 2 g/m^2/day for 5 days, only 20% of the patients treated with mesna (400 mg/m^2) exhibited hematuria compared with 60% of those treated with N-acetylcysteine (NAC, 1.5 g/m^2) (534). Similar results were reported by Munshi et al. (535), wherein 4.2% of patients treated with mesna developed hematuria compared with 27.9% of NAC patients. In a phase 2 trial of ifosfamide and mesna in patients with platinum/paclitaxel–refractory ovarian cancer, there were no documented episodes of hemorrhagic cystitis, but one patient experienced treatment-related microscopic hematuria (282).

Subcutaneous administration of mesna is also being explored as an alternative to IV and oral dosing (536). Patients with gynecologic cancers receiving ifosfamide were treated with an initial IV dose of mesna at 20% of the ifosfamide dose. A subcutaneous infusion of mesna was given approximately 30 minutes after the completion of the ifosfamide infusion. A total dose of mesna equal to 40% of the ifosfamide dose was infused at a rate of 4 mL/hr over 8 hours. The subcutaneous infusion of mesna was well tolerated, and no episodes of gross hematuria were observed.

Oprelvekin

Chemistry. Oprelvekin (Neumega) is FDA approved for the prevention of severe thrombocytopenia and to reduce the need for platelet transfusions in patients with nonmyeloid malignancies. The active ingredient is produced *Escherichia coli* by recombinant DNA technology. This protein has a molecular mass of 19,000 daltons and is similar to native interleukin 11 (IL-11) with the exception of its lack of the amino-terminal praline residue.

Mechanism of Action. IL-11 is a thrombopoietic growth factor that induces megakaryocyte maturation resulting in increased platelet production. Platelets that develop as a result of oprelvekin therapy are morphologically and functionally similar to those produced normally.

Dosage and Administration. Oprelvekin is administered subcutaneously (to the abdomen, thigh, hip, or upper arm) at a dose of 50 μg/kg daily. Patients with renal impairment (creatinine clearance less than 30 mL/min) should receive half the normal dose (e.g., 25 μg/kg daily). Oprelvekin should be initiated within 24 hours of the completion of chemotherapy until the patient's platelet count is at least 50,000/μL. Treatment generally lasts between 10 and 21 days, and is not recommended beyond 21 days.

Side Effects and Toxicities. Allergic reactions may occur with oprelvekin, and patients should be counseled to be aware of potential allergic symptoms. Treatment with oprelvekin may also cause severe fluid retention. Fluid balance should be monitored during treatment. Other serious adverse effects associated with oprelvekin treatment include cardiovascular events and anemia.

Palifermin

Chemistry. Palifermin (Kepivance) is a human keratinocyte growth factor (KGF) that is FDA approved to reduce the incidence and duration of severe oral mucositis in patients with hematologic malignancies who are receiving myelotoxic therapy requiring hematopoietic stem cell support. The active ingredient is produced in *E. coli* by recombinant DNA technology.

Mechanism of Action. The KGF receptor is present on many epithelial cells in the digestive system (e.g., tongue, buccal mucosa, stomach, esophagus, intestine, salivary glands), and other organs (e.g., lung, liver, pancreas, bladder, skin, and eye). Palifermin enhances the proliferation of KGF-expressing epithelial cells, and has demonstrated the ability to thicken the tongue, buccal mucosa, and gastrointestinal tract.

Administration and Dosage. Palifermin is administered as an IV bolus at a dose of 60 mcg/kg/day for 3 days prior (with dose three to be administered within 24 to 48 hours of therapy) to and 3 days following myelotoxic therapy (with the fourth dose to be administered following but on the same day as hematopoietic stem cell infusion), for a total of six doses. Additional palifermin therapy should not be initiated within 4 days since the most recent administration of palifermin. Palifermin should be reconstituted in 1.2 mL of sterile water for a final concentration of 5 mg/mL. Reconstitution should be performed aseptically and contents should be gently swirled during dissolution. Palifermin should be used immediately; the reconstituted solution should be discarded if left for over 1 hour. Reconstituted medication may be refrigerated for up to 24 hours and must be protected from light.

Side Effects and Toxicities. The most common toxicity reported with palifermin is skin rash. Severe toxicities reported with palifermin include fever, gastrointestinal events, and respiratory events, although these were reported at a similar rate as patients receiving placebo.

References

1. Tozer N. Pharmacokinetics concepts basic to cancer chemotherapy. In: Ames MM, Powis G, Covach JS, eds. *Pharmacokinetics of Anti-cancer Agents in Humans.* New York: Elsevier; 1983.
2. Collins JM, Dedrick RL. Pharmacokinetics of anticancer drugs. In: Chabner B, ed. *Pharmacologic Principles of Cancer Treatment.* Philadelphia: WB Saunders; 1982:73.
3. Alberts DS, Liu PY, Hannigan EV, et al. Intraperitoneal cisplatin plus intravenous cyclophosphamide versus intravenous cisplatin plus intravenous cyclophosphamide for stage III ovarian cancer [comment]. *N Engl J Med* 1996;335(26):1950–1955.
4. Armstrong DK, Bundy B, Wenzel L, et al. Intraperitoneal cisplatin and paclitaxel in ovarian cancer. *N Engl J Med* 2006;354(1):34–43.
5. Markman M, Bundy BN, Alberts DS, et al. Phase III trial of standard-dose intravenous cisplatin plus paclitaxel versus moderately high-dose carboplatin followed by intravenous paclitaxel and intraperitoneal cisplatin in small-volume stage III ovarian carcinoma: an intergroup study of the Gynecologic Oncology Group, Southwestern Oncology Group, and Eastern Cooperative Oncology Group. *J Clin Oncol* 2001;19(4):1001–1007.

6. Hess LM, Benham-Hutchins M, Herzog TJ, et al. A meta-analysis of the efficacy of intraperitoneal cisplatin for the front-line treatment of ovarian cancer. *Int J Gynecol Cancer* 2007;17(3):561–570.
7. Armstrong DK, Bundy BN, Baergen R, et al. Randomized phase III study of intravenous (IV) paclitaxel and cisplatin versus IV paclitaxel, intraperitoneal (IP) cisplatin and IP paclitaxel in optimal stage III epithelial ovarian cancer (OC): a Gynecologic Oncology Group trial (GOG 172). *Proc ASCO* 2002;21:201a(abstract 803).
8. Wenzel LB, Huang HQ, Armstrong DK, et al. Health-related quality of life during and after intraperitoneal versus intravenous chemotherapy for optimally debulked ovarian cancer: a Gynecologic Oncology Group study. *J Clin Oncol* 2007;25(4):437–443.
9. Omura G, Blessing JA, Ehrlich CE, et al. A randomized trial of cyclophosphamide and doxorubicin with or without cisplatin in advanced ovarian carcinoma. A Gynecologic Oncology Group study. *Cancer* 1986;57(9): 1725–1730.
10. Markman M. Intraperitoneal therapy of ovarian cancer. *Semin Oncol* 1998;25(3):356–360.
11. Markman M, Hakes T, Reichman B, et al. Phase II trial of weekly or biweekly intraperitoneal mitoxantrone in epithelial ovarian cancer. *J Clin Oncol* 1991;9(6):978–982.
12. Deppe G, Malviya VK, Boike G, et al. Intraperitoneal doxorubicin in combination with systemic cisplatinum and cyclophosphamide in the treatment of stage III ovarian cancer. *Eur J Gynaecol Oncol* 1991;12(2): 93–97.
13. Markman M, Rowinsky E, Hakes T, et al. Phase I trial of intraperitoneal taxol: a Gynecoloic Oncology Group study. *J Clin Oncol* 1992;10(9): 1485–1491.
14. Los G, Mutsaers PH, van der Vijgh WJ, et al. Direct diffusion of cis-diamminedichloroplatinum(II) in intraperitoneal rat tumors after intraperitoneal chemotherapy: a comparison with systemic chemotherapy. *Cancer Res* 1989;49(12):3380–3384.
15. Fujiwara K, Suzuki S, Ishikawa H, et al. Preliminary toxicity analysis of intraperitoneal carboplatin in combination with intravenous paclitaxel chemotherapy for patients with carcinoma of the ovary, peritoneum, or fallopian tube. *Int J Gynecol Cancer* 2005;15(3):426–431.
16. Gradishar WJ, Tjulandin S, Davidson N, et al. Phase III trial of nanoparticle albumin-bound paclitaxel compared with polyethylated castor oil-based paclitaxel in women with breast cancer. *J Clin Oncol* 2005; 23(31):7794–7803.
17. Rutty CJ, Connors TA. *In vitro* studies with hexamethylmelamine. *Biochem Pharmacol* 1977;26(24):2385–2391.
18. Rutty CJ, Connors TA, Nguyen Hoang N, et al. *In vivo* studies with hexamethylmelamine. *Eur J Cancer* 1978;14(6):713–720.
19. Ames MM, Powis G, Kovach JS, et al. Disposition and metabolism of pentamethylmelamine and hexamethylmelamine in rabbits and humans. *Cancer Res* 1979;39(12):5016–5021.
20. D'Incalci M, Bolis G, Mangioni C, et al. Variable oral absorption of hexamethylmelamine in man. *Cancer Treat Rep* 1978;62(12):2117–2119.
21. Markman M, Blessing JA, Moore D, et al. Altretamine (hexamethylmelamine) in platinum-resistant and platinum-refractory ovarian cancer: a Gynecologic Oncology Group phase II trial. *Gynecol Oncol* 1998;69(3): 226–229.
22. Morris M, Eifel PJ, Lu J, et al. Pelvic radiation with concurrent chemotherapy compared with pelvic and para-aortic radiation for high-risk cervical cancer. *N Engl J Med* 1999;340(15):1137–1143.
23. Kristensen GB, Baekelandt M, Vergote IB, et al. A phase II study of carboplatin and hexamethylmelamine as induction chemotherapy in advanced epithelial ovarian carcinoma. *Eur J Cancer* 1995;31A(11):1778–1780.
24. Division of Cancer Treatment N. Annual Report to the Food and Drug Administration. Hexamethylmelamine (NSC 13875;IND #954). Washington, DC: U.S. Government Printing Office; 1988.
25. van der Hoop RG, van der Burg ME, ten Bokkel Huinink WW, et al. Incidence of neuropathy in 395 patients with ovarian cancer treated with or without cisplatin. *Cancer* 1990;66(8):1697–1702.
26. Keldsen N, Havsteen H, Vergote I, et al. Altretamine (hexamethylmelamine) in the treatment of platinum-resistant ovarian cancer: a phase II study. *Gynecol Oncol* 2003;88(2):118–122.
27. Rothenberg ML, Liu PY, Wilczynski S, et al. Phase II trial of oral altretamine for consolidation of clinical complete remission in women with stage III epithelial ovarian cancer: a Southwest Oncology Group trial (SWOG-9326). *Gynecol Oncol* 2001;82(2):317–22.
28. Bruckner HW, Cohen CJ, Feuer E, et al. Modulation and intensification of a cyclophosphamide, hexamethylmelamine, doxorubicin, and cisplatin ovarian cancer regimen. *Obstet Gynecol* 1989;73(3 Pt 1):349–356.
29. Edmonson JH, Wieand HS, McCormack GW. Role of hexamethylmelamine in the treatment of ovarian cancer: where is the needle in the haystack? *J Natl Cancer Inst* 1988;80(14):1172–1173.
30. Hainsworth JD, Jones HW 3rd, Burnett LS, et al. The role of hexamethylmelamine in the combination chemotherapy of advanced ovarian cancer: a comparison of hexamethylmelamine, cyclophosphamide, doxorubicin, and cisplatin (H-CAP) versus cyclophosphamide, doxorubicin, and cisplatin (CAP). *Am J Clin Oncol* 1990;13(5):410–415.
31. Baker LH, Opipari MI, Wilson H, et al. Mitomycin C, vincristine, and bleomycin therapy for advanced cervical cancer. *Obstet Gynecol* 1978; 52(2):146–150.
32. Mirabelli CK, Huang CH, Crooke ST. Role of deoxyribonucleic acid topology in altering the site/sequence specificity of cleavage of deoxyribonucleic acid by bleomycin and talisomycin. *Biochemistry* 1983;22(2): 300–306.
33. Dorr RT. Bleomycin pharmacology: mechanism of action and resistance, and clinical pharmacokinetics. *Semin Oncol* 1992;19(2 Suppl 5):3–8.
34. Sebti SM, Jani JP, Mistry JS, et al. Metabolic inactivation: a mechanism of human tumor resistance to bleomycin. *Cancer Res* 1991;51(1):227–232.
35. Alberts DS, Chen HS, Liu R, et al. Bleomycin pharmacokinetics in man. I. Intravenous administration. *Cancer Chemother Pharmacol* 1978;1(3): 177–181.
36. Ruckdeschel JC, Moores D, Lee JY, et al. Intrapleural therapy for malignant pleural effusions. A randomized comparison of bleomycin and tetracycline. *Chest* 1991;100(6):1528–1535.
37. Crooke ST, Comis RL, Einhorn LH, et al. Effects of variations in renal function on the clinical pharmacology of bleomycin administered as an IV bolus. *Cancer Treat Rep* 1977;61(9):1631–1636.
38. Oken MM, Crooke ST, Elson MK, et al. Pharmacokinetics of bleomycin after IM administration in man. *Cancer Treat Rep* 1981;65(5–6):485–489.
39. Samuels ML, Johnson DE, Holoye PY, et al. Large-dose bleomycin therapy and pulmonary toxicity. A possible role of prior radiotherapy. *JAMA* 1976;235(11):1117–1120.
40. Ingrassia TS 3rd, Ryu JH, Trastek VF, et al. Oxygen-exacerbated bleomycin pulmonary toxicity. *Mayo Clin Proc* 1991;66(2):173–178.
41. Maher J, Daly PA. Severe bleomycin lung toxicity: reversal with high dose corticosteroids. *Thorax* 1993;48(1):92–94.
42. Nici L, Calabresi P. Amifostine modulation of bleomycin-induced lung injury in rodents. *Semin Oncol* 1999;26(2 Suppl 7):28–33.
43. Nici L, Santos-Moore A, Kuhn C, et al. Modulation of bleomycin-induced pulmonary toxicity in the hamster by the antioxidant amifostine. *Cancer* 1998;83(9):2008–2014.
44. Kerr LD, Spiera H. Scleroderma in association with the use of bleomycin: a report of 3 cases. *J Rheumatol* 1992;19(2):294–296.
45. Haerslev T, Avnstorp C, Joergensen M. Sudden onset of adverse effects due to low-dosage bleomycin indicates an idiosyncratic reaction. *Cutis* 1993; 52(1):45–46.
46. Yee GC, Crom WR, Champion JE, et al. Cisplatin-induced changes in bleomycin elimination. *Cancer Treat Rep* 1983;67(6):587–589.
47. Bennett WM, Pastore L, Houghton DC. Fatal pulmonary bleomycin toxicity in cisplatin-induced acute renal failure. *Cancer Treat Rep* 1980; 64(8–9):921–924.
48. Crooke ST, Bradner WT. Bleomycin, a review. *J Med* 1976;7(5):333–428.
49. Gerbrecht BM. Current Canadian experience with capecitabine: partnering with patients to optimize therapy. *Cancer Nurs* 2003;26(2):161–167.
50. Chu E, DeVita VT. *Physicians' Cancer Chemotherapy Drug Manual 2003.* Sudbury: Jones and Bartlett Publishers; 2003.
51. Horacek P, Drobnik J. Interaction of cis-dichlorodiammineplatinum (II) with DNA. *Biochim Biophys Acta* 1971;254(2):341–347.
52. DeNeve W, Valeriote F, Tapazoglou E, et al. Discrepancy between cytotoxicity and DNA interstrand crosslinking of carboplatin and cisplatin *in vivo*. *Invest New Drugs* 1990;8(1):17–24.
53. Micetich KC, Barnes D, Erickson LC. A comparative study of the cytotoxicity and DNA-damaging effects of cis-(diammino)(1,1-cyclobutanedicarboxylato)-platinum(II) and cis-diamminedichloroplatinum(II) on L1210 cells. *Cancer Res* 1985;45(9):4043–4047.
54. Aabo K, Adams M, Adnitt P, et al. Chemotherapy in advanced ovarian cancer: four systematic meta-analyses of individual patient data from 37 randomized trials. Advanced Ovarian Cancer Trialists' Group. *Br J Cancer* 1998;78(11):1479–1487.
55. du Bois A, Luck HJ, Meier W, et al. Carboplatin/paclitaxel versus cisplatin/paclitaxel as first-line chemotherapy in advanced ovarian cancer: an interim analysis of a randomized phase III trial of the Arbeitsgemeinschaft Gynakologische Onkologie Ovarian Cancer Study Group. *Semin Oncol* 1997;24(5 Suppl 15):S15-44–S15-52.
56. Harrap KR. Preclinical studies identifying carboplatin as a viable cisplatin alternative. *Cancer Treat Rev* 1985;12 Suppl A:21–33.
57. Wilkinson R, Cox PJ, Jones M, et al. Selection of potential second generation platinum compounds. *Biochem J* 1978;60:851–856.
58. Zwelling LA, Kohn KW. Mechanism of action of cis-dichlorodiammineplatinum(II). *Cancer Treat Rep* 1979;63(9–10):1439–1444.
59. Gaver RC, George AM, Deeb G. *In vitro* stability, plasma protein binding and blood cell partitioning of 14C-carboplatin. *Cancer Chemother Pharmacol* 1987;20(4):271–276.
60. Shea TC, Flaherty M, Elias A, et al. A phase I clinical and pharmacokinetic study of carboplatin and autologous bone marrow support. *J Clin Oncol* 1989;7(5):651–661.
61. Misset B, Escudier B, Leclercq B, et al. Acute myocardiotoxicity during 5-fluorouracil therapy. *Intensive Care Med* 1990;16(3):210–211.
62. Calvert AH, Newell DR, Gumbrell LA, et al. Carboplatin dosage: prospective evaluation of a simple formula based on renal function. *J Clin Oncol* 1989;7(11):1748–1756.
63. Martino G, Frusciante V, Varraso A, et al. Efficacy of 51Cr-EDTA clearance to tailor a carboplatin therapeutic regimen in ovarian cancer patients. *Anticancer Res* 1999;19(6C):5587–5591.
64. Cockroft DW, Gault MH. Prediction of creatinine clearance for serum creatinine. *Nephron* 1976;16:31–35.

65. Belani CP, Kearns CM, Zuhowski EG, et al. Phase I trial, including pharmacokinetic and pharmacodynamic correlations, of combination paclitaxel and carboplatin in patients with metastatic non-small-cell lung cancer. *J Clin Oncol* 1999;17(2):676–684.
66. Calvert AH, Boddy A, Bailey NP, et al. Carboplatin in combination with paclitaxel in advanced ovarian cancer: dose determination and pharmacokinetic and pharmacodynamic interactions. *Semin Oncol* 1995;22(5 Suppl 12):91–98; discussion 9–100.
67. Okamoto H, Nagatomo A, Kunitoh H, et al. Prediction of carboplatin clearance calculated by patient characteristics or 24-hour creatinine clearance: a comparison of the performance of three formulae. *Cancer Chemother Pharmacol* 1998;42(4):307–312.
68. Sorensen BT, Stromgren A, Jakobsen P, et al. Dose-toxicity relationship of carboplatin in combination with cyclophosphamide in ovarian cancer patients. *Cancer Chemother Pharmacol* 1991;28(5):397–401.
69. Neijt JP, du Bois A. Paclitaxel/carboplatin for the initial treatment of advanced ovarian cancer. *Semin Oncol* 1999;26(1 Suppl 2):78–83.
70. The International Collaborative Ovarian Neoplasm Group. Paclitaxel plus carboplatin versus standard chemotherapy with either single-agent carboplatin or cyclophosphamide, doxorubicin, and cisplatin in women with ovarian cancer: the ICON3 randomised trial. [Comment]. *Lancet* 2002;360(9332):505–515.
71. Calvert AH, Harland SJ, Newell DR, et al. Early clinical studies with cis-diammine-1,1-cyclobutane dicarboxylate platinum II. *Cancer Chemother Pharmacol* 1982;9(3):140–147.
72. Plezia PM, Alberts DS, Kessler J, et al. Immediate termination of intractable vomiting induced by cisplatin combination chemotherapy using an intensive five-drug antiemetic regimen. *Cancer Treat Rep* 1984;68(12):1493–1495.
73. Canetta R, Rozencweig M, Carter SK. Carboplatin: the clinical spectrum to date. *Cancer Treat Rev* 1985;12 Suppl A:125–136.
74. Markman M, Kennedy A, Webster K, et al. Clinical features of hypersensitivity reactions to carboplatin. *J Clin Oncol* 1999;17(4):1141.
75. Shukunami K, Kurokawa T, Kawakami Y, et al. Hypersensitivity reactions to intraperitoneal administration of carboplatin in ovarian cancer: the first report of a case. *Gynecol Oncol* 1999;72(3):431–432.
76. Travis LB, Holowaty EJ, Bergfeldt K, et al. Risk of leukemia after platinum-based chemotherapy for ovarian cancer. *N Engl J Med* 1999 4;340(5): 351–357.
77. Stiff PJ, McKenzie RS, Alberts DS, et al. Phase I clinical and pharmacokinetic study of high-dose mitoxantrone combined with carboplatin, cyclophosphamide, and autologous bone marrow rescue: high response rate for refractory ovarian carcinoma. *J Clin Oncol* 1994;12(1):176–183.
78. Calvert AH. A review of the pharmacokinetics and pharmacodynamics of combination carboplatin/paclitaxel. *Semin Oncol* 1997;24(1 Suppl 2):S2-85–S2-90.
79. Budd GT, Ganapathi R, Adelstein DJ, et al. Randomized trial of carboplatin plus amifostine versus carboplatin alone in patients with advanced solid tumors. *Cancer* 1997;80(6):1134–1140.
80. Korst AE, van der Sterre ML, Eeltink CM, et al. Pharmacokinetics of carboplatin with and without amifostine in patients with solid tumors. *Clin Cancer Res* 1997;3(5):697–703.
81. Markman M, Reichman B, Hakes T, et al. Evidence supporting the superiority of intraperitoneal cisplatin compared to intraperitoneal carboplatin for salvage therapy of small-volume residual ovarian cancer. *Gynecol Oncol* 1993;50(1):100–104.
82. Miyagi Y, Fujiwara K, Kigawa J, et al. Intraperitoneal carboplatin infusion may be a pharmacologically more reasonable route than intravenous administration as a systemic chemotherapy. A comparative pharmacokinetic analysis of platinum using a new mathematical model after intraperitoneal vs. intravenous infusion of carboplatin—a Sankai Gynecology Study Group (SGSG) study. *Gynecol Oncol* 2005;99(3):591–596.
83. Los G, Verdegaal EM, Mutsaers PH, et al. Penetration of carboplatin and cisplatin into rat peritoneal tumor nodules after intraperitoneal chemotherapy. *Cancer Chemother Pharmacol* 1991;28(3):159–165.
84. Muggia FM, Groshen S, Russell C, et al. Intraperitoneal carboplatin and etoposide for persistent epithelial ovarian cancer: analysis of results by prior sensitivity to platinum-based regimens. *Gynecol Oncol* 1993;50(2):232–238.
85. Reed E, Ozols RF, Tarone R, et al. Platinum-DNA adducts in leukocyte DNA correlate with disease response in ovarian cancer patients receiving platinum-based chemotherapy. *Proc Natl Acad Sci USA* 1987;84(14): 5024–5028.
86. Rice JA, Crothers DM, Pinto AL, et al. The major adduct of the antitumor drug cis-diamminedichloroplatinum(II) with DNA bends the duplex by approximately equal to 40 degrees toward the major groove. *Proc Natl Acad Sci USA* 1988;85(12):4158–4161.
87. Rose PG, Mossbruger K, Fusco N, et al. Gemcitabine reverses cisplatin resistance: demonstration of activity in platinum- and multidrug-resistant ovarian and peritoneal carcinoma. *Gynecol Oncol* 2003;88(1):17–21.
88. DeConti RC, Toftness BR, Lange RC, et al. Clinical and pharmacological studies with cis-diamminedichloroplatinum (II). *Cancer Res* 1973;33(6): 1310–1315.
89. Gensia Sicor Pharmaceuticals. Cisplatin Package Insert. 2000.
90. Earhart RH. Instability of cis-dichlorodiammineplatinum in dextrose solution. *Cancer Treat Rev* 1979;6(62):1105–1107.
91. Eshaque M, McKay MJ, Theophande T, et al. p-Mannitol platinum complexes. *Wadley Med Bull* 1976;7:338–341.
92. Prestayko AW, Cadiz M, Crooke ST. Incompatibility of aluminum-containing IV administration equipment with cis-dichlorodiammineplatinum(II) administration. *Cancer Treat Rep* 1979;63(11–12):2118–2119.
93. Hayes DM, Cvitkovic E, Golbey RB, et al. High dose cis-platinum diammine dichloride: amelioration of renal toxicity by mannitol diuresis. *Cancer* 1977; 39(4):1372–1381.
94. Rainey JM, Alberts DS. Safe, rapid administration schedule for cis-platinum-mannitol. *Med Pediatr Oncol* 1978;4(4):371–375.
95. Brock J, Alberts DS. Safe, rapid administration of cisplatin in the outpatient clinic. *Cancer Treat Rep* 1986;70(12):1409–1414.
96. Alberts DS, Delforge A. Maximizing the delivery of intraperitoneal therapy while minimizing drug toxicity and maintaining quality of life. *Semin Oncol* 2006;33(6 Suppl 12):S8–S17.
97. Alberts DS, Markman M, Muggia F, et al. Proceedings of a GOG workshop on intraperitoneal therapy for ovarian cancer. *Gynecol Oncol* 2006;103(3):783–792.
98. Walker JL, Armstrong DK, Huang HQ, et al. Intraperitoneal catheter outcomes in a phase III trial of intravenous versus intraperitoneal chemotherapy in optimal stage III ovarian and primary peritoneal cancer: a Gynecologic Oncology Group study. *Gynecol Oncol* 2006;100(1):27–32.
99. NCCN. NCCN Antiemesis Guidelines version 2. http://www.nccn.org/professionals/physican_gls/PDF/antiemesis.pdf. Accessed March 11, 2006.
100. Levin L, Hryniuk WM. Dose intensity analysis of chemotherapy regimens in ovarian carcinoma. *J Clin Oncol* 1987;5(5):756–767.
101. Bonomi P, Blessing JA, Stehman FB, et al. Randomized trial of three cisplatin dose schedules in squamous-cell carcinoma of the cervix: a Gynecologic Oncology Group study. *J Clin Oncol* 1985;3(8):1079–1085.
102. Gandara DR, Wold H, Perez EA, et al. Cisplatin dose intensity in non-small cell lung cancer: phase II results of a day 1 and day 8 high-dose regimen. *J Natl Cancer Inst* 1989;81(10):790–794.
103. Holleran WM, DeGregorio MW. Evolution of high-dose cisplatin. *Invest New Drugs* 1988;6(2):135–142.
104. Gonzalez-Vitale JC, Hayes DM, Cvitkovic E, et al. Acute renal failure after cis-dichlorodiammineplatinum(II) and gentamicin-cephalothin therapies. *Cancer Treat Rep* 1978;62(5):693–698.
105. Madias NE, Harrington JT. Platinum nephrotoxicity. *Am J Med* 1978; 65(2):307–314.
106. Fleming S, Peppard S, Ratanatharathorn V, et al. Ototoxicity from cis-platinum in patients with stages III and IV previously untreated squamous cell cancer of the head and neck. *Am J Clin Oncol* 1985;8(4):302–306.
107. Alberts DS, Noel JK. Cisplatin-associated neurotoxicity: can it be prevented? *Anticancer Drugs* 1995;6(3):369–383.
108. Cersosimo RJ. Cisplatin neurotoxicity. *Cancer Treat Rev* 1989;16(4): 195–211.
109. Stengs CH, Klis SF, Huizing EH, et al. Protective effects of a neurotrophic ACTH(4-9) analog on cisplatin ototoxicity in relation to the cisplatin dose: an electrocochleographic study in albino guinea pigs. *Hear Res* 1998;124(1–2):108–117.
110. Rose PG. Amifostine cytoprotection with chemotherapy for advanced ovarian carcinoma. *Semin Oncol* 1996;23(4 Suppl 8):83–89.
111. Willox JC, McAllister EJ, Sangster G, et al. Effects of magnesium supplementation in testicular cancer patients receiving cis-platin: a randomised trial. *Br J Cancer* 1986;54(1):19–23.
112. Morrow GR, Hickok JT, Rosenthal SN. Progress in reducing nausea and emesis. Comparisons of ondansetron (Zofran), granisetron (Kytril), and tropisetron (Navoban). *Cancer* 1995;76(3):343–357.
113. Latreille J, Pater J, Johnston D, et al. Use of dexamethasone and granisetron in the control of delayed emesis for patients who receive highly emetogenic chemotherapy. National Cancer Institute of Canada Clinical Trials Group. *J Clin Oncol* 1998;16(3):1174–1178.
114. Kris MG, Gralla RJ, Tyson LB, et al. Controlling delayed vomiting: double-blind, randomized trial comparing placebo, dexamethasone alone, and metoclopramide plus dexamethasone in patients receiving cisplatin. *J Clin Oncol* 1989;7(1):108–114.
115. Von Hoff DD, Slavik M, Muggia FM. Letter: Allergic reactions to cis platinum. *Lancet* 1976;1(7950):90.
116. Wiesenfeld M, Reinders E, Corder M, et al. Successful re-treatment with cis-dichlorodiammineplatinum(II) after apparent allergic reactions. *Cancer Treat Rep* 1979;63(2):219–221.
117. Abels RI. Use of recombinant human erythropoietin in the treatment of anemia in patients who have cancer. *Semin Oncol* 1992;19(3 Suppl 8): 29–35.
118. Rowinsky EK, Donehower RC. Paclitaxel (Taxol). *N Engl J Med* 1995; 332(15):1004–1014.
119. de Jonge MJ, Loos WJ, Gelderblom H, et al. Phase I pharmacologic study of oral topotecan and intravenous cisplatin: sequence-dependent hematologic side effects. *J Clin Oncol* 2000;18(10):2104–2115.
120. Kemp G, Rose P, Lurain J, et al. Amifostine pretreatment for protection against cyclophosphamide-induced and cisplatin-induced toxicities: results of a randomized control trial in patients with advanced ovarian cancer. *J Clin Oncol* 1996;14(7):2101–2112.
121. Schuchter LM, Hensley ML, Meropol NJ, et al. American Society of Clinical Oncology C, Radiotherapy Expert. 2002 update of recommendations for the use of chemotherapy and radiotherapy protectants: clinical practice guidelines of the American Society of Clinical Oncology. *J Clin Oncol* 2002;20(12):2895–2903.

122. NCI. NCI Clinical Announcement on Intraperitoneal Chemotherapy in Ovarian Cancer. 2006. http://ctep.cancer.gov/highlights/ovarian.html. Accessed May 1, 2007.
123. Hess LM, Alberts DS. What is the role of intraperitoneal therapy in advanced ovarian cancer? *Oncology* 2007;21(2):227–232.
124. Peters WA 3rd, Liu PY, Barrett RJ 2nd, et al. Concurrent chemotherapy and pelvic radiation therapy compared with pelvic radiation therapy alone as adjuvant therapy after radical surgery in high-risk early-stage cancer of the cervix. *J Clin Oncol* 2000;18(8):1606–1613.
125. Rose PG, Bundy BN, Watkins EB, et al. Concurrent cisplatin-based radiotherapy and chemotherapy for locally advanced cervical cancer. *N Engl J Med* 1999;340(15):1144–1153.
126. Struck RF, Alberts DS, Horne K, et al. Plasma pharmacokinetics of cyclophosphamide and its cytotoxic metabolites after intravenous versus oral administration in a randomized, crossover trial. *Cancer Res* 1987; 47(10):2723–2726.
127. Cohen JL, Jao JY, Jusko WJ. Pharmacokinetics of cyclophosphamide in man. *Br J Pharmacol* 1971;43(3):677–680.
128. Dorr RT. *Cancer Chemotherapy Handbook*. 2nd ed. Norwalk: Appleton & Lange; 1994.
129. DeFronzo RA, Braine H, Colvin M, et al. Water intoxication in man after cyclophosphamide therapy. Time course and relation to drug activation. *Ann Intern Med* 1973;78(6):861–869.
130. Topilow AA, Rothenberg SP, Cottrell TS. Interstitial pneumonia after prolonged treatment with cyclophosphamide. *Am Rev Respir Dis* 1973; 108(1):114–117.
131. Braverman AC, Antin JH, Plappert MT, et al. Cyclophosphamide cardiotoxicity in bone marrow transplantation: a prospective evaluation of new dosing regimens. *J Clin Oncol* 1991;9(7):1215–1223.
132. Wiemann MC, Cummings FJ, Kaplan HG, et al. Clinical and pharmacological studies of methotrexate-minimal leucovorin rescue plus fluorouracil. *Cancer Res* 1982;42(9):3896–3900.
133. Dorr RT, Soble MJ, Alberts DS. Interaction of cimetidine but not ranitidine with cyclophosphamide in mice. *Cancer Res* 1986;46(4 Pt 1):1795–1799.
134. Struck RF, Alberts DS, Plezia PM, et al. Effect of the antiulcer drug ranitidine on the pharmacokinetics and hematologic toxicity of cyclophosphamide and its cytotoxic metabolites in patients. [Abstract]. *Proc AACR* 1988;29:187.
135. Homesley HD. Single-agent therapy for nonmetastatic and low-risk gestational trophoblastic disease. *J Reprod Med* 1998;43(1):69–74.
136. Williams SD. Ovarian germ cell tumors: an update. *Semin Oncol* 1998;25(3):407–413.
137. Schwartz HS. Some determinants of the therapeutic efficacy of actinomycin D (NSC-3053), adriamycin (NSC-123127), and daunorubicin (NSC-83142). *Cancer Chemother Rep* 1974;58(1):55–62.
138. Knutsen T, Mickley LA, Ried T, et al. Cytogenetic and molecular characterization of random chromosomal rearrangements activating the drug resistance gene, MDR1/P-glycoprotein, in drug-selected cell lines and patients with drug refractory ALL. *Genes Chromosomes Cancer* 1998; 23(1):44–54.
139. Tattersall MH, Sodergren JE, Dengupta SK, et al. Pharmacokinetics of actinoymcin D in patients with malignant melanoma. *Clin Pharmacol Ther* 1975;17(6):701–708.
140. Brothman AR, Davis TP, Duffy JJ, et al. Development of an antibody to actinomycin D and its application for the detection of serum levels by radioimmunoassay. *Cancer Res* 1982;42(3):1184–1187.
141. Blatt J, Trigg ME, Pizzo PA, et al. Tolerance to single-dose dactinomycin in combination chemotherapy for solid tumors. *Cancer Treat Rep* 1981; 65(1–2):145–147.
142. Petrilli ES, Twiggs LB, Blessing JA, et al. Single-dose actinomycin-D treatment for nonmetastatic gestational trophoblastic disease. A prospective phase II trial of the Gynecologic Oncology Group. *Cancer* 1987;60(9): 2173–2176.
143. Philips RS, Schwartz HS, Sternberg SS, et al. The toxicity of actinomycin D. *Ann NY Acad Sci* 1970;89:348.
144. Frei E 3rd. The clinical use of actinomycin. *Cancer Chemother Rep* 1974; 58(1):49–54.
145. Cohen IJ, Loven D, Schoenfeld T, et al. Dactinomycin potentiation of radiation pneumonitis: a forgotten interaction. *Pediatr Hematol Oncol* 1991;8(2):187–192.
146. Francis P, Schneider J, Hann L, et al. Phase II trial of docetaxel in patients with platinum-refractory advanced ovarian cancer. *J Clin Oncol* 1994; 12(11):2301–2308.
147. Gelmon K. The taxoids: paclitaxel and docetaxel. *Lancet* 1994;344(8932): 1267–1272.
148. Bruno R, Sanderink GJ. Pharmacokinetics and metabolism of Taxotere (docetaxel). *Cancer Surv* 1993;17:305–313.
149. Aapro MS. Phase I and pharmacokinetic study of RP 56976 in a new ethanol-free formulation of Taxotere. *Ann Oncol* 1992;3:208–211.
150. Von Hoff DD. The taxoids: same roots, different drugs. *Semin Oncol* 1997;24(4 Suppl 13):S13-3–S13-10.
151. Stemmler HJ, Gutschow K, Sommer H, et al. Weekly docetaxel (Taxotere) in patients with metastatic breast cancer. *Ann Oncol* 2001;12(10):1393–1398.
152. Pronk LC, Schellens JH, Planting AS, et al. Phase I and pharmacologic study of docetaxel and cisplatin in patients with advanced solid tumors. *J Clin Oncol* 1997;15(3):1071–1079.
153. Kaye SB, Piccart M, Aapro M, et al. Phase II trials of docetaxel (Taxotere) in advanced ovarian cancer—an updated overview. *Eur J Cancer* 1997; 33(13):2167–2170.
154. Wanders J, Schrijvers D, Bruntsch U, et al. The EORTC-ECTG experience with acute hypersensitivity reactions (HSR) in Taxotere studies. [Abstract]. *Proc ASCO* 1993;12:73.
155. Galindo E, Kavanagh J, Fossella F, et al. Docetaxel (Taxotere) toxicities: analysis of a single institution experience with 168 patients (623 courses). [Abstract]. *Proc ASCO* 1994;13:164.
156. Zimmerman GC, Keeling JH, Lowry M, et al. Prevention of docetaxel-induced erythrodysesthesia with local hypothermia. *J Natl Cancer Inst* 1994;86(7):557–558.
157. Eisenhauer EA, Vermorken JB. The taxoids. Comparative clinical pharmacology and therapeutic potential. *Drugs* 1998;55(1):5–30.
158. Verschraegen CF, Kudelka AP, Steger M, et al. Randomized phase II study of two dose levels of docetaxel in patients with advanced epithelial ovarian cancer who have failed paclitaxel chemotherapy. [Abstract]. *Proc ASCO* 1997;16:381a.
159. Rose PG, Blessing JA, Ball HG, et al. A phase II study of docetaxel in paclitaxel-resistant ovarian and peritoneal carcinoma: a Gynecologic Oncology Group study. *Gynecol Oncol* 2003;88(2):130–135.
160. Henry DW. Structure-activity relationships among daunorubicin and adriamycin analogs. *Cancer Treat Rep* 1979;63(5):845–854.
161. Hasinoff BB, Davey JP. Adriamycin and its iron(III) and copper(II) complexes. Glutathione-induced dissociation; cytochrome c oxidase inactivation and protection; binding to cardiolipin. *Biochem Pharmacol* 1988; 37(19):3663–3669.
162. Myers CE, Gianni L, Simone CB, et al. Oxidative destruction of erythrocyte ghost membranes catalyzed by the doxorubicin-iron complex. *Biochemistry* 1982;21(8):1707–1712.
163. Di Marco A, Zunino F, Silverstrini R, et al. Interaction of some daunomycin derivatives with deoxyribonucleic acid and their biological activity. *Biochem Pharmacol* 1971;20(6):1323–1328.
164. Painter RB. Inhibition of DNA replicon initiation by 4-nitroquinoline 1-oxide, adriamycin, and ethyleneimine. *Cancer Res* 1978;38(12): 4445–4449.
165. Driscoll JS, Hazard GF Jr, Wood HB Jr, et al. Structure-antitumor activity relationships among quinone derivatives. *Cancer Chemother Rep 2* 1974; 4(2):1–362.
166. Kim SH, Kim JH. Lethal effect of adriamycin on the division cycle of HeLa cells. *Cancer Res* 1972;32(2):323–325.
167. Ritch PS, Occhipinti SJ, Cunningham RE, et al. Schedule-dependent synergism of combinations of hydroxyurea with adriamycin and 1-beta-D-arabinofuranosylcytosine with adriamycin. *Cancer Res* 1981;41(10): 3881–3884.
168. Glisson BS, Ross WE. DNA topoisomerase II: a primer on the enzyme and its unique role as a multidrug target in cancer chemotherapy. *Pharmacol Ther* 1987;32(2):89–106.
169. Tewey KM, Chen GL, Nelson EM, et al. Intercalative antitumor drugs interfere with the breakage-reunion reaction of mammalian DNA topoisomerase II. *J Biol Chem* 1984;259(14):9182–9187.
170. Eksborg S, Ehrsson H, Ekqvist B. Protein binding of anthraquinone glycosides, with special reference to adriamycin. *Cancer Chemother Pharmacol* 1982;10(1):7–10.
171. Piazza E, Broggini M, Trabattoni A, et al. Adriamycin distribution in plasma and blood cells of cancer patients with altered hematocrit. *Eur J Cancer Clin Oncol* 1981;17(10):1089–1096.
172. Benjamin RS, Riggs CE Jr, Bachur NR. Plasma pharmacokinetics of adriamycin and its metabolites in humans with normal hepatic and renal function. *Cancer Res* 1977;37(5):1416–1420.
173. Lee YT, Chan KK, Harris PA, et al. Distribution of adriamycin in cancer patients: tissue uptakes, plasma concentration after IV and hepatic IA administration. *Cancer* 1980;45(9):2231–2239.
174. Egan PC, Costanza ME, Dodion P, et al. Doxorubicin and cisplatin excretion into human milk. *Cancer Treat Rep* 1985;69(12):1387–1389.
175. D'Incalci M, Broggini M, Buscaglia M, et al. Transplacental passage of doxorubicin. *Lancet* 1983;1(8314–5):75.
176. Karp GI, von Oeyen P, Valone F, et al. Doxorubicin in pregnancy: possible transplacental passage. *Cancer Treat Rep* 1983;67(9):773–777.
177. Riggs CE Jr, Benjamin RS, Serpick AA, et al. Bilary disposition of adriamycin. *Clin Pharmacol Ther* 1977;22(2):234–241.
178. Benjamin RS. A practical approach to adriamycin (NSC-123127). *Cancer Chemother Rep* 1975;6:191–193.
179. Chan KK, Chlebowski RT, Tong M, et al. Clinical pharmacokinetics of adriamycin in hepatoma patients with cirrhosis. *Cancer Res* 1980;40(4): 1263–1268.
180. Rodvold KA, Rushing DA, Tewksbury DA. Doxorubicin clearance in the obese. *J Clin Oncol* 1988;6(8):1321–1327.
181. Morris RG, Reece PA, Dale BM, et al. Alteration in doxorubicin and doxorubicinol plasma concentrations with repeated courses to patients. *Ther Drug Monit* 1989;11(4):380–383.
182. Robert J, Hoerni B. Age dependence of the early-phase pharmacokinetics of doxorubicin. *Cancer Res* 1983;43(9):4467–4469.
183. Garnick MB, Ensminger WD, Israel M. A clinical-pharmacological evaluation of hepatic arterial infusion of adriamycin. *Cancer Res* 1979;39(10): 4105–4110.

184. Chen HS, Gross JF. Intra-arterial infusion of anticancer drugs: theoretic aspects of drug delivery and review of responses. *Cancer Treat Rep* 1980; 64(1):31–40.
185. Creasey WA, McIntosh LS, Brescia T, et al. Clinical effects and pharmacokinetics of different dosage schedules of adriamycin. *Cancer Res* 1976; 36(1):216–221.
186. Hryniuk W, Levine MN. Analysis of dose intensity for adjuvant chemotherapy trials in stage II breast cancer. *J Clin Oncol* 1986;4(8): 1162–1170.
187. Carmo-Pereira J, Costa FO, Henriques E, et al. A comparison of two doses of adriamycin in the primary chemotherapy of disseminated breast carcinoma. *Br J Cancer* 1987;56(4):471–473.
188. Von Hoff DD, Layard MW, Basa P, et al. Risk factors for doxorubicin-induced congestive heart failure. *Ann Intern Med* 1979;91(5):710–717.
189. Minow RA, Benjamin RS, Gottlieb JA. Adriamycin (NSC-123127) cardiomyopathy—an overview with determinants of risk factors. *Cancer Chemother Rep* 1975;195–201.
190. Reilly JJ, Neifeld JP, Rosenberg SA. Clinical course and management of accidental adriamycin extravasation. *Cancer* 1977;40(5):2053–2056.
191. Dorr RT, Dordal MS, Koenig LM, et al. High levels of doxorubicin in the tissues of a patient experiencing extravasation during a 4-day infusion. *Cancer* 1989;64(12):2462–2464.
192. Dorr RT. Antidotes to vesicant chemotherapy extravasations. *Blood Rev* 1990;4(1):41–60.
193. Lenaz L, Page JA. Cardiotoxicity of adriamycin and related anthracyclines. *Cancer Treat Rev* 1976;3(3):111–120.
194. Rinehart JJ, Lewis RP, Balcerzak SP. Adriamycin cardiotoxicity in man. *Ann Intern Med* 1974;81(4):475–478.
195. Steinherz LJ, Steinherz PG, Tan CT, et al. Cardiac toxicity 4 to 20 years after completing anthracycline therapy. *JAMA* 1991;266(12):1672–1677.
196. Speyer J, Wasserheit C. Strategies for reduction of anthracycline cardiac toxicity. *Semin Oncol* 1998;25(5):525–537.
197. Bielack SS, Erttmann R, Winkler K, et al. Doxorubicin: effect of different schedules on toxicity and anti-tumor efficacy. *Eur J Cancer Clin Oncol* 1989;25(5):873–882.
198. Greco FA, Brereton HD, Kent H, et al. Adriamycin and enhanced radiation reaction in normal esophagus and skin. *Ann Intern Med* 1976;85(3): 294–298.
199. Newburger PE, Cassady JR, Jaffe N. Esophagitis due to adriamycin and radiation therapy for childhood malignancy. *Cancer* 1978;42(2):417–423.
200. Sarosy GA, Brown TD, Von Hoff DD, et al. Phase I study of alpha 2-interferon plus doxorubicin in patients with solid tumors. *Cancer Res* 1986;46(10):5368–5371.
201. Kefford RF, Woods RL, Fox RM, et al. Intracavitary adriamycin nitrogen mustard and tetracycline in the control of malignant effusions: a randomized study. *Med J Aust* 1980;2(8):447–448.
202. Markman M, Howell SB, Green MR. Combination intracavitary chemotherapy for malignant pleural disease. *Cancer Drug Deliv* 1984; 1(4):333–336.
203. Rose PG, Blessing JA, Buller RE, et al. Prolonged oral etoposide in recurrent or advanced non-squamous cell carcinoma of the cervix: a Gynecologic Oncology Group study. *Gynecol Oncol* 2003;89(2):267–270.
204. Keller-Juslen C, Kuhn M, Stahelin H, et al. Synthesis and antimitotic activity of glycosidic lignan derivatives related to podophyllotoxin. *J Med Chem* 1971;14(10):936–940.
205. Misra NC, Roberts DW. Inhibition by 4′-demethyl-epipodophyllotoxin 9-(4,6-O-2-thenylidene-beta-D-glucopyranoside) of human lymphoblast cultures in G2 phase of the cell cycle. *Cancer Res* 1975;35(1):99–105.
206. Krishan A, Paika K, Frei E III. Cytofluorometric studies on the action of podophyllotoxin and epipodophyllotoxins (VM-26, VP-16-213) on the cell cycle traverse of human lymphoblasts. *J Cell Biol* 1975;66(3): 521–530.
207. Ross W, Rowe T, Glisson B, et al. Role of topoisomerase II in mediating epipodophyllotoxin-induced DNA cleavage. *Cancer Res* 1984;44(12 Pt 1): 5857–5860.
208. Chen AY, Liu LF. DNA topoisomerases: essential enzymes and lethal targets. *Annu Rev Pharmacol Toxicol* 1994;34:191–218.
209. Wozniak AJ, Ross WE. DNA damage as a basis for 4′-demethylepipodophyllotoxin-9-(4,6-O-ethylidene-beta-D-glucopyranoside) (etoposide) cytotoxicity. *Cancer Res* 1983;43(1):120–124.
210. Chatterjee S, Trivedi D, Petzold SJ, et al. Mechanism of epipodophyllotoxin-induced cell death in poly(adenosine diphosphate-ribose) synthesis-deficient V79 Chinese hamster cell lines. *Cancer Res* 1990;50(9): 2713–2718.
211. Wozniak AJ, Glisson BS, Hande KR, et al. Inhibition of etoposide-induced DNA damage and cytotoxicity in L1210 cells by dehydrogenase inhibitors and other agents. *Cancer Res* 1984;44(2):626–632.
212. Allen LM, Creaven PJ. Comparison of the human pharmacokinetics of VM-26 and VP-16, two antineoplastic epipodophyllotixin glucopyranoside derivatives. *Eur J Cancer* 1975;11(10):697–707.
213. D'Incalci M, Farina P, Sessa C, et al. Pharmacokinetics of VP16-213 given by different administration methods. *Cancer Chemother Pharmacol* 1982;7(2–3):141–145.
214. Hande KR, Wedlund PJ, Noone RM, et al. Pharmacokinetics of high-dose etoposide (VP-16-213) administered to cancer patients. *Cancer Res* 1984; 44(1):379–382.
215. Stewart DJ, Richard MT, Hugenholtz H, et al. Penetration of VP-16 (etoposide) into human intracerebral and extracerebral tumors. *J Neuro Oncol* 1984;2(2):133–139.
216. D'Incalci M, Sessa C, Rossi C, et al. Pharmacokinetics of etoposide in gestochoriocarcinoma. *Cancer Treat Rep* 1985;69(1):69–72.
217. Creaven PJ, Newman SJ, Selawry OS, et al. Phase I clinical trial of weekly administration of 4′-demethylepipodophyllotoxin 9-(4,6-O-ethylidene-beta-D-glucopyranoside) (NSC-141540; VP-16-213). *Cancer Chemother Rep* 1974;58(6):901–907.
218. Stewart CF, Arbuck SG, Fleming RA, et al. Changes in the clearance of total and unbound etoposide in patients with liver dysfunction. *J Clin Oncol* 1990;8(11):1874–1879.
219. Pfluger KH, Schmidt L, Merkel M, et al. Drug monitoring of etoposide (VP16-213). Correlation of pharmacokinetic parameters to clinical and biochemical data from patients receiving etoposide. *Cancer Chemother Pharmacol* 1987;20(1):59–66.
220. Smyth RD, Pfeffer M, Scalzo A, et al. Bioavailability and pharmacokinetics of etoposide (VP-16). *Semin Oncol* 1985;12(1 Suppl 2):48–51.
221. Harvey VJ, Slevin ML, Joel SP, et al. The effect of food and concurrent chemotherapy on the bioavailability of oral etoposide. *Br J Cancer* 1985; 52(3):363–367.
222. Dorr RT, Alberts DS. Skin ulceration potential without therapeutic anticancer activity for epipodophyllotoxin commercial diluents. *Invest New Drugs* 1983;1(2):151–159.
223. Ozols RF. Oral etoposide for the treatment of recurrent ovarian cancer. *Drugs* 1999;58(Suppl 3):43–49.
224. Rose PG, Blessing JA, Mayer AR, et al. Prolonged oral etoposide as second-line therapy for platinum-resistant and platinum-sensitive ovarian carcinoma: a Gynecologic Oncology Group study. *J Clin Oncol* 1998; 16(2):405–410.
225. Rose PG, Blessing JA, Lewandowski GS, et al. A phase II trial of prolonged oral etoposide (VP-16) as second-line therapy for advanced and recurrent endometrial carcinoma: a Gynecologic Oncology Group study. *Gynecol Oncol* 1996;63(1):101–104.
226. Rose PG, Blessing JA, Van Le L, et al. Prolonged oral etoposide in recurrent or advanced squamous cell carcinoma of the cervix: a Gynecologic Oncology Group study. *Gynecol Oncol* 1998;70(2):263–266.
227. Schaaf LJ, Dobbs BR, Edwards IR, et al. Nonlinear pharmacokinetic characteristics of 5-fluorouracil (5-FU) in colorectal cancer patients. *Eur J Clin Pharmacol* 1987;32(4):411–418.
228. Santini J, Milano G, Thyss A, et al. 5-FU therapeutic monitoring with dose adjustment leads to an improved therapeutic index in head and neck cancer. *Br J Cancer* 1989;59(2):287–290.
229. Hande KR, Wolff SN, Greco FA, et al. Etoposide kinetics in patients with obstructive jaundice. *J Clin Oncol* 1990;8(6):1101–1107.
230. Rozencweig M, Von Hoff DD, Henney JE, et al. VM 26 and VP 16-213: a comparative analysis. *Cancer* 1977;40(1):334–342.
231. Anonymous. Epipodophyllotoxin VP 16213 in treatment of acute leukaemias, haematosarcomas, and solid tumours. *Br Med J* 1973;3(5873): 199–202.
232. Dombernowsky P, Nissen NI, Larsen V. Clinical investigation of a new podophyllum derivative, epipodophyllotoxin, 4′-demethyl-9-(4,6-O-2-thenylidene- -D-glucopyranoside) (NSC-122819), in patients with malignant lymphomas and solid tumors. *Cancer Chemother Rep* 1972;56(1): 71–82.
233. Aisner J, Whitacre M, VanEcho DA, et al. Doxorubicin, cyclophosphamide and VP16-213 (ACE) in the treatment of small cell lung cancer. *Cancer Chemother Pharmacol* 1982;7(2–3):187–193.
234. Dorr RT. Chemoprotectants for cancer chemotherapy. *Semin Oncol* 1991;18(1 Suppl 2):48–58.
235. Thant M, Hawley RJ, Smith MT, et al. Possible enhancement of vincristine neuropathy by VP-16. *Cancer* 1982;49(5):859–864.
236. Barakat RR, Almadrones L, Venkatraman ES, et al. A phase II trial of intraperitoneal cisplatin and etoposide as consolidation therapy in patients with stage II-IV epithelial ovarian cancer following negative surgical assessment. *Gynecol Oncol* 1998;69(1):17–22.
237. van Rijswijk RE, Hoekman K, Burger CW, et al. Experience with intraperitoneal cisplatin and etoposide and i.v. sodium thiosulphate protection in ovarian cancer patients with either pathologically complete response or minimal residual disease. *Ann Oncol* 1997;8(12):1235–1241.
238. Fields KK, Elfenbein GJ, Lazarus HM, et al. Maximum-tolerated doses of ifosfamide, carboplatin, and etoposide given over 6 days followed by autologous stem-cell rescue: toxicity profile. *J Clin Oncol* 1995;13(2): 323–332.
239. Rustum YM. Biochemical rationale for the 5-fluorouracil leucovorin combination and update of clinical experience. *J Chemother* 1990;2 Suppl 1: 5–11.
240. McDermott BJ, van den Berg HW, Murphy RF. Nonlinear pharmacokinetics for the elimination of 5-fluorouracil after intravenous administration in cancer patients. *Cancer Chemother Pharmacol* 1982;9(3):173–178.
241. Fraile RJ, Baker LH, Buroker TR, et al. Pharmacokinetics of 5-fluorouracil administered orally, by rapid intravenous and by slow infusion. *Cancer Res* 1980;40(7):2223–2228.
242. Yoshida T, Araki E, Iigo M, et al. Clinical significance of monitoring serum levels of 5-fluorouracil by continuous infusion in patients with advanced colonic cancer. *Cancer Chemother Pharmacol* 1990;26(5):352–354.

243. Floyd RA, Hornbeck CL, Byfield JE, et al. Clearance of continuously infused 5-fluorouracil in adults having lung or gastrointestinal carcinoma with or without hepatic metastases. *Drug Intell Clin Pharm* 1982;16(9): 665–667.
244. Lokich JJ, Ahlgren JD, Gullo JJ, et al. A prospective randomized comparison of continuous infusion fluorouracil with a conventional bolus schedule in metastatic colorectal carcinoma: a Mid-Atlantic Oncology Program study. *J Clin Oncol* 1989;7(4):425–432.
245. Nadler SH. Oral administration of fluorouracil. A preliminary trial. *Arch Surg* 1968;97(4):654–656.
246. Horton J, Olson KB, Sullivan J, et al. 5-FU in cancer: an improved regimen. *Ann Intern Med* 1970;73:897–900.
247. Jacobs EM, Reeves WJ Jr, Wood DA, et al. Treatment of cancer with weekly intravenous 5-fluorouracil. Study by the Western Cooperative Cancer Chemotherapy Group (WCCCG). *Cancer* 1971;27(6):1302–1305.
248. Bruckner HW, Glass LL, Chesser MR. Dose-dependent leucovorin efficacy with an intermittent high-dose 5-fluorouracil schedule. *Cancer Invest* 1990;8(3–4):321–326.
249. Whitney CW, Sause W, Bundy BN, et al. Randomized comparison of fluorouracil plus cisplatin versus hydroxyurea as an adjunct to radiation therapy in stage IIB-IVA carcinoma of the cervix with negative para-aortic lymph nodes: a Gynecologic Oncology Group and Southwest Oncology Group study. *J Clin Oncol* 1999;17(5):1339–1348.
250. Curran CF, Luce JK. Fluorouracil and palmar-plantar erythrodysesthesia. *Ann Intern Med* 1989;111(10):858.
251. Lopez AM, Wallace L, Dorr RT, et al. Topical DMSO treatment for pegylated liposomal doxorubicin-induced palmar-plantar erythrodysesthesia. *Cancer Chemother Pharmacol* 1999;44(4):303–306.
252. Malet-Martino M, Martino R. Clinical studies of three oral prodrugs of 5-fluorouracil (capecitabine, UFT, S-1): a review. *Oncologist* 2002;7(4): 288–323.
253. Nagore E, Insa A, Sanmartin O. Antineoplastic therapy-induced palmar plantar erythrodysesthesia ("hand-foot") syndrome. Incidence, recognition and management. *Am J Clin Dermatol* 2000;1(4):225–234.
254. Hrushesky WJ. Serpentine supravenous 5-fluorouracil (NSC-19893) hyperpigmentation. *Cancer Treat Rep* 1976;60(5):639.
255. Gottlieb JA, Luce JK. Cerebellar ataxia with weekly 5-fluorouracil administration. *Lancet* 1971;1(7690):138–139.
256. Cianci G, Morelli MF, Cannita K, et al. Prophylactic options in patients with 5-fluorouracil-associated cardiotoxicity. *Br J Cancer* 2003;88(10): 1507–1509.
257. Diasio RB, Beavers TL, Carpenter JT. Familial deficiency of dihydropyrimidine dehydrogenase. Biochemical basis for familial pyrimidinemia and severe 5-fluorouracil-induced toxicity. *J Clin Invest* 1988;81(1):47–51.
258. Lu Z, Zhang R, Diasio RB. Population characteristics of hepatic dihydropyrimidine dehydrogenase activity, a key metabolic enzyme in 5-fluorouracil chemotherapy. *Clin Pharmacol Ther* 1995;58(5):512–522.
259. Curran CF, Luce JK. Accidental acute exposure to fluorouracil. *Oncol Nurs Forum* 1989;16(4):468.
260. Muggia FM, Liu PY, Alberts DS, et al. Intraperitoneal mitoxantrone or floxuridine: effects on time-to-failure and survival in patients with minimal residual ovarian cancer after second-look laparotomy—a randomized phase II study by the Southwest Oncology Group. *Gynecol Oncol* 1996; 61(3):395–402.
261. Muggia FM, Jeffers S, Muderspach L, et al. Phase I/II study of intraperitoneal floxuridine and platinums (cisplatin and/or carboplatin). *Gynecol Oncol* 1997;66(2):290–294.
262. Speyer JL, Sugarbaker PH, Collins JM, et al. Portal levels and hepatic clearance of 5-fluorouracil after intraperitoneal administration in humans. *Cancer Res* 1981;41(5):1916–1922.
263. Suhrland LG, Weisberger AA. Intracavitary 5-fluorouracil in malignant effusions. *Arch Intern Med* 1965;116:431–433.
264. Belpomme D, Krakowski I, Beauduin M, et al. Gemcitabine combined with cisplatin as first-line treatment in patients with epithelial ovarian cancer: a phase II study. *Gynecol Oncol* 2003;91(1):32–38.
265. Hansen SW, Tuxen MK, Sessa C. Gemcitabine in the treatment of ovarian cancer. *Ann Oncol* 1999;10 Suppl 1:51–53.
266. Markman M, Webster K, Zanotti K, et al. Phase 2 trial of single-agent gemcitabine in platinum-paclitaxel refractory ovarian cancer. *Gynecol Oncol* 2003;90(3):593–596.
267. Huang P, Chubb S, Hertel LW, et al. Action of 2′,2′-difluorodeoxycytidine on DNA synthesis. *Cancer Res* 1991;51(22):6110–6117.
268. Plunkett W, Huang P, Gandhi V. Preclinical characteristics of gemcitabine. *Anticancer Drugs* 1995;6 Suppl 6:7–13.
269. Heinemann V, Xu YZ, Chubb S, et al. Inhibition of ribonucleotide reduction in CCRF-CEM cells by 2',2'-difluorodeoxycytidine. *Mol Pharmacol* 1990;38(4):567–572.
270. Abbruzzese JL, Grunewald R, Weeks EA, et al. A phase I clinical, plasma, and cellular pharmacology study of gemcitabine. *J Clin Oncol* 1991; 9(3):491–498.
271. Eli Lilly and Company. Gemzar (gemcitabine HCI) for injection. Prescribing Information 2003. http://pi.lilly.com/us/gemzar.pdf. Accessed November 5, 2003.
272. Storniolo AM, Allerheiligen SR, Pearce HL. Preclinical, pharmacologic, and phase I studies of gemcitabine. *Semin Oncol* 1997;24(2 Suppl 7): S7-2–S7-7.
273. van Moorsel CJ, Kroep JR, Pinedo HM, et al. Pharmacokinetic schedule finding study of the combination of gemcitabine and cisplatin in patients with solid tumors. *Ann Oncol* 1999;10(4):441–448.
274. O'Rourke TJ, Brown TD, Havlin K, et al. Phase I clinical trial of gemcitabine given as an intravenous bolus on 5 consecutive days. *Eur J Cancer* 1994;30A(3):417–418.
275. Hui YF, Reitz J. Gemcitabine: a cytidine analogue active against solid tumors. *Am J Health Syst Pharm* 1997;54(2):162–170; quiz 97–98.
276. van Moorsel CJ, Pinedo HM, Veerman G, et al. Mechanisms of synergism between cisplatin and gemcitabine in ovarian and non-small cell lung cancer cell lines. *Br J Cancer* 1999;80:981–990.
277. Bauknecht T, Hefti A, Morack G, et al. Gemcitabine combined with cisplatin as first-line treatment in patients 60 years or older with epithelial ovarian cancer: a phase II study. *Int J Gynecol Cancer* 2003;13(2): 130–137.
278. Nagourney RA, Brewer CA, Radecki S, et al. Phase II trial of gemcitabine plus cisplatin repeating doublet therapy in previously treated, relapsed ovarian cancer patients. *Gynecol Oncol* 2003;88(1):35–39.
279. Aapro MS, Martin C, Hatty S. Gemcitabine—a safety review. *Anticancer Drugs* 1998;9(3):191–201.
280. Pavlakis N, Bell DR, Millward MJ, et al. Fatal pulmonary toxicity resulting from treatment with gemcitabine. *Cancer* 1997;80(2):286–291.
281. Sauer-Heilborn A, Kath R, Schneider CP, et al. Severe non-haematological toxicity after treatment with gemcitabine. *J Cancer Res Clin Oncol* 1999; 125(11):637–640.
282. Markman M, Kennedy A, Sutton G, et al. Phase 2 trial of single agent ifosfamide/mesna in patients with platinum/paclitaxel refractory ovarian cancer who have not previously been treated with an alkylating agent. *Gynecol Oncol* 1998;70(2):272–274.
283. Sutton G. Ifosfamide and mesna in epithelial ovarian carcinoma. *Gynecol Oncol* 1993;51(1):104–108.
284. Sutton GP, Blessing JA, DeMars LR, et al. A phase II Gynecologic Oncology Group trial of ifosfamide and mesna in advanced or recurrent adenocarcinoma of the endometrium. *Gynecol Oncol* 1996;63(1):25–27.
285. Allen LM, Creaven PJ. Activation of the antineoplastic drug isophosphamide by rat liver microsomes. *J Pharm Pharmacol* 1972;24(7):585–586.
286. Allen LM, Creaven PJ. Interaction of mechlorethamine and isophosphamide with bovine serum albumin and rat liver microsomes. *J Pharm Sci* 1973;62(5):854–856.
287. Boal JH, Williamson M, Boyd VL, et al. 31P NMR studies of the kinetics of bisalkylation by isophosphoramide mustard: comparisons with phosphoramide mustard. *J Med Chem* 1989;32(8):1768–1773.
288. Creaven PJ, Allen LM, Cohen MH, et al. Studies on the clinical pharmacology and toxicology of isophosphamide (NSC-109724). *Cancer Treat Rep* 1976;60(4):445–449.
289. Allen LM, Creaven PJ, Nelson RL. Studies on the human pharmacokinetics of isophosphamide (NSC-109724). *Cancer Treat Rep* 1976;60(4):451–458.
290. Stuart-Harris RC, Harper PG, Parsons CA, et al. High-dose alkylation therapy using ifosfamide infusion with mesna in the treatment of adult advanced soft-tissue sarcoma. *Cancer Chemother Pharmacol* 1983;11(2): 69–72.
291. Nelson RL, Creaven PJ, Cohen MH, et al. Phase I clinical trial of a 3-day divided dose schedule of ifosfamide (NSC 109724). *Eur J Cancer* 1976; 12(3):195–198.
292. Mateu J, Alzamora M, Franco M, et al. Ifosfamide extravasation. *Ann Pharmacother* 1994;28(11):1243–1244.
293. Papadimitriou CA, Kouroussis C, Moulopoulos LA, et al. Ifosfamide, paclitaxel and cisplatin first-line chemotherapy in advanced, suboptimally debulked epithelial ovarian cancer. *Cancer* 2001;92(7):1856–1863.
294. Zanetta G, Fei F, Parma G, et al. Paclitaxel, ifosfamide and cisplatin (TIP) chemotherapy for recurrent or persistent squamous-cell cervical cancer. *Ann Oncol* 1999;10(10):1171–1174.
295. Morgan LR, Harrison EF, Hawke JE, et al. Toxicity of single- vs. fractionated-dose ifosfamide in non-small cell lung cancer: a multi-center study. *Semin Oncol* 1982;9(4 Suppl 1):66–70.
296. Rodriguez V, McCredie KB, Keating MJ, et al. Isophosphamide therapy for hematologic malignancies in patients refractory to prior treatment. *Cancer Treat Rep* 1978;62(4):493–497.
297. Van Dyk JJ, Falkson HC, Van der Merwe AM, et al. Unexpected toxicity in patients treated with iphosphamide. *Cancer Res* 1972;32(5):921–924.
298. DeFronzo RA, Abeloff M, Braine H, et al. Renal dysfunction after treatment with isophosphamide (NSC-109724). *Cancer Chemother Rep* 1974; 58(3):375–382.
299. Goren MP, Wright RK, Pratt CB, et al. Potentiation of ifosfamide neurotoxicity, hematotoxicity, and tubular nephrotoxicity by prior cis-diamminedichloroplatinum(II) therapy. *Cancer Res* 1987;47(5):1457–1460.
300. Hartmann JT, Fels LM, Franzke A, et al. Comparative study of the acute nephrotoxicity from standard dose cisplatin +/− ifosfamide and high-dose chemotherapy with carboplatin and ifosfamide. *Anticancer Res* 2000;20:3767–3773.
301. Bhardwaj A, Badesha PS. Ifosfamide-induced nonconvulsive status epilepticus. *Ann Pharmacother* 1995;29(12):1237–1239.
302. Creemers GJ, Lund B, Verweij J. Topoisomerase I inhibitors: topotecan and irenotecan. *Cancer Treat Rev* 1994;20(1):73–96.
303. Rothenberg ML, Kuhn JG, Burris HA 3rd, et al. Phase I and pharmacokinetic trial of weekly CPT-11. *J Clin Oncol* 1993;11(11):2194–2204.

304. Abigerges D, Chabot GG, Armand JP, et al. Phase I and pharmacologic studies of the camptothecin analog irinotecan administered every 3 weeks in cancer patients. *J Clin Oncol* 1995;13(1):210–221.
305. Irvin WP, Price FV, Bailey H, et al. A phase II study of irinotecan (CPT-11) in patients with advanced squamous cell carcinoma of the cervix. *Cancer* 1998;82(2):328–333.
306. Look KY, Blessing JA, Levenback C, et al. A phase II trial of CPT-11 in recurrent squamous carcinoma of the cervix: a gynecologic oncology group study. *Gynecol Oncol* 1998;70(3):334–338.
307. Verschraegen CF, Levy T, Kudelka AP, et al. Phase II study of irinotecan in prior chemotherapy-treated squamous cell carcinoma of the cervix. *J Clin Oncol* 1997;15(2):625–631.
308. Rowinsky EK, Grochow LB, Ettinger DS, et al. Phase I and pharmacological study of the novel topoisomerase I inhibitor 7-ethyl-10- 4-(1-piperidino)-1-piperidino]carbonyloxycamptothecin (CPT-11) administered as a ninety-minute infusion every 3 weeks. *Cancer Res* 1994;54(2):427–436.
309. Gupta E, Lestingi TM, Mick R, et al. Metabolic fate of irinotecan in humans: correlation of glucuronidation with diarrhea. *Cancer Res* 1994; 54(14):3723–3725.
310. Cottu PH, Extra JM, Lerebours F, et al. Clinical activity spectrum of irinotecan. *Bull Cancer* 1998;Spec No:21–25.
311. Eisenhauer EA, Vermorken JB. New drugs in gynecologic oncology. *Curr Opin Oncol* 1996;8(5):408–414.
312. Verschraegen CF. Irinotecan for the treatment of cervical cancer. *Oncology (Huntingt)* 2002;16(5 Suppl 5):32–34.
313. Chitapanarux I, Tonusin A, Sukthomya V, et al. Phase II clinical study of irinotecan and cisplatin as first-line chemotherapy in metastatic or recurrent cervical cancer. *Gynecol Oncol* 2003;89(3):402–407.
314. Alza Corporation. DOXIL (doxorubicin HCl liposome injection) package insert; 2001.
315. Gabizon A, Catane R, Uziely B, et al. Prolonged circulation time and enhanced accumulation in malignant exudates of doxorubicin encapsulated in polyethylene-glycol coated liposomes. *Cancer Res* 1994;54(4): 987–992.
316. Alberts DS, Garcia DJ. Safety aspects of pegylated liposomal doxorubicin in patients with cancer. *Drugs* 1997;54 Suppl 4:30–35.
317. Gordon AN, Fleagle JT, Guthrie D, et al. Recurrent epithelial ovarian carcinoma: a randomized phase III study of pegylated liposomal doxorubicin versus topotecan. *J Clin Oncol* 2001;19(14):3312–3322.
318. Chang SY, Evans TL, Alberts DS. The stability of melphalan in the presence of chloride ion. *J Pharm Pharmacol* 1979;31(12):853–854.
319. Goodman GE, Chang SE, Alberts DS. The antitumor activity of melphalan and its hydrolysis products. [Abstract]. *Proc AACR* 1980;21:1207.
320. Goldenberg GJ, Lam HY, Begleiter A. Active carrier-mediated transport of melphalan by two separate amino acid transport systems in LPC-1 plasmacytoma cells *in vitro*. *J Biol Chem* 1979;254(4):1057–1064.
321. Alberts DS, Chang SY, Chen HS, et al. Oral melphalan kinetics. *Clin Pharmacol Ther* 1979;26(6):737–745.
322. Evans TL, Chang SY, Alberts DS, et al. *In vitro* degradation of L-phenylalanine mustard (L-PAM). *Cancer Chemother Pharmacol* 1982;8(2): 175–178.
323. Bosanquet AG, Gilby ED. Pharmacokinetics of oral and intravenous melphalan during routine treatment of multiple myeloma. *Eur J Cancer Clin Oncol* 1982;18(4):355–362.
324. Rutledge F. Chemotherapy of ovarian cancer with melphalan. *Clin Obstet Gynecol* 1968;11(2):354–366.
325. Taetle R, Dickman PS, Feldman PS. Pulmonary histopathologic changes associated with melphalan therapy. *Cancer* 1978;42(3):1239–1245.
326. Einhorn N. Acute leukemia after chemotherapy (melphalan). *Cancer* 1978;41(2):444–447.
327. Greene MH, Harris EL, Gershenson DM, et al. Melphalan may be a more potent leukemogen than cyclophosphamide. *Ann Intern Med* 1986; 105(3):360–367.
328. Lazarus HM, Gray R, Ciobanu N, et al. Phase I trial of high-dose melphalan, high-dose etoposide and autologous bone marrow re-infusion in solid tumors: an Eastern Cooperative Oncology Group (ECOG) study. *Bone Marrow Transplant* 1994;14(3):443–448.
329. Alberts DS, Young L, Mason N, et al. *In vitro* evaluation of anticancer drugs against ovarian cancer at concentrations achievable by intraperitoneal administration. *Semin Oncol* 1985;12(3 Suppl 4):38–42.
330. Howell SB, Pfeifle CE, Olshen RA. Intraperitoneal chemotherapy with melphalan. *Ann Intern Med* 1984;101(1):14–18.
331. Zaharko DS, Fung WP, Yang KH. Relative biochemical aspects of low and high doses of methotrexate in mice. *Cancer Res* 1977;37(6):1602–1607.
332. Jolivet J, Schilsky RL, Bailey BD, et al. Synthesis, retention, and biological activity of methotrexate polyglutamates in cultured human breast cancer cells. *J Clin Invest* 1982;70(2):351–360.
333. Alt FW, Kellems RE, Bertino JR, et al. Selective multiplication of dihydrofolate reductase genes in methotrexate-resistant variants of cultured murine cells. 1978. *Biotechnology* 1992;24:397–410.
334. Calvert AH, Jones TR, Jackman AL, et al. 2-Amino-4-hydroxyquinazolines with dual metabolic loci in methotrexate resistant cells. [Abstract]. *Proc AACR* 1979;20:24.
335. Weinstein G, Newburger A, Troner M. Cell kinetic synchronization of human malignant melanoma (MM) with low-dose methotrexate (MTX) *in vivo*. [Abstract]. *Proc AACR* 1979;20:403.
336. Chello PL, Sirotnak FM, Dorick DM. Alterations in the kinetics of methotrexate transport during growth of L1210 murine leukemia cells in culture. *Mol Pharmacol* 1980;18(2):274–280.
337. Campbell MA, Perrier DG, Dorr RT, et al. Methotrexate: bioavailability and pharmacokinetics. *Cancer Treat Rep* 1985;69(7-8):833–838.
338. Ignoffo RJ, Oie S, Friedman MA. Pharmacokinetics of methotrexate administered via the hepatic artery. *Cancer Chemother Pharmacol* 1981; 5(4):217–220.
339. Aherne GW, Piall E, Marks V, et al. Prolongation and enhancement of serum methotrexate concentrations by probenecid. *Br Med J* 1978; 1(6120):1097–1099.
340. Huffman DH, Wan SH, Azarnoff DL, et al. Pharmacokinetics of methotrexate. *Clin Pharmacol Ther* 1973;14(4):572–579.
341. Stoller RG, Jacobs SA, Drake JC, et al. Pharmacokinetics of high-dose methotrexate (NSC-740). *Cancer Chemother Rep* 1975;6:19–24.
342. Wang YM, Sutow WW, Romsdahl MM, et al. Age-related pharmacokinetics of high-dose methotrexate in patients with osteosarcoma. *Cancer Treat Rep* 1979;63(3):405–410.
343. Evans WE, Pratt CB. Effect of pleural effusion on high-dose methotrexate kinetics. *Clin Pharmacol Ther* 1978;23(1):68–72.
344. Ben Venue Laboratories. Methotrexate injection, USP. Package Insert; 2000.
345. Everts CS, Westcott JL, Bragg DG. Methotrexate therapy and pulmonary disease. *Radiology* 1973;107(3):539–543.
346. Creaven GB, Morgan RG. Alteration of methotrexate (MTX) pharamacokinetics by gut sterilization in man. [Abstract]. *Proc AACR* 1975;16:134.
347. Cadman E, Heimer R, Davis L. Enhanced 5-fluorouracil nucleotide formation after methotrexate administration: explanation for drug synergism. *Science* 1979;205(4411):1135–1137.
348. Bowen D, White JC, Goldman ID. A basis for fluoropyrimidine-induced antagonism to methotrexate in Ehrlich ascites tumor cells *in vitro*. *Cancer Res* 1978;38(1):219–222.
349. Stoller RG, Kaplan HG, Cummings FJ, et al. A clinical and pharmacological study of high-dose methotrexate with minimal leucovorin rescue. *Cancer Res* 1979;39(3):908–912.
350. Von Hoff DD, Penta JS, Helman LJ, et al. Incidence of drug-related deaths secondary to high-dose methotrexate and citrovorum factor administration. *Cancer Treat Rep* 1977;61(4):745–748.
351. Crooke ST, Bradner WT. Mitomycin C: a review. *Cancer Treat Ref* 1976; 3(3):121–139.
352. Lown JW, Weir G. Studies related to antitumor antibiotics. Part XIV. Reactions of mitomycin B with DNA. *Can J Biochem* 1978;56(5):269–304.
353. Tomasz M, Chowdary D, Lipman R, et al. Reaction of DNA with chemically or enzymatically activated mitomycin C: isolation and structure of the major covalent adduct. *PNAS* 1986;83(18):6702–6706.
354. Dusre L, Covey JM, Collins C, et al. DNA damage, cytotoxicity and free radical formation by mitomycin C in human cells. *Chem Biol Interact* 1989;71(1):63–78.
355. Kennedy KA, Rockwell S, Sartorelli AC. Preferential activation of mitomycin C to cytotoxic metabolites by hypoxic tumor cells. *Cancer Res* 1980;40(7):2356–2360.
356. Taylor CW, Brattain MG, Yeoman LC. Occurrence of cytosolic protein and phosphoprotein changes in human colon tumor cells with the development of resistance to mitomycin C. *Cancer Res* 1985;45(9): 4422–4427.
357. Dorr RT, Liddil JD, Trent JM, et al. Mitomycin C resistant L1210 leukemia cells: association with pleiotropic drug resistance. *Biochem Pharmacol* 1987;36(19):3115–3120.
358. Verweij J, den Hartigh J, Stuurman M, et al. Relationship between clinical parameters and pharmacokinetics of mitomycin C. *J Cancer Res Clin Oncol* 1987;113(1):91–94.
359. Schilcher RB, Young JD, Ratanatharathorn V, et al. Clinical pharmacokinetics of high-dose mitomycin C. *Cancer Chemother Pharmacol* 1984; 13(3):186–190.
360. den Hartigh J, McVie JG, van Oort WJ, et al. Pharmacokinetics of mitomycin C in humans. *Cancer Res* 1983;43(10):5017–5021.
361. Malviya VK, Young JD, Boike G, et al. Pharmacokinetics of mitomycin-C in plasma and tumor tissue of cervical cancer patients and in selected tissues of female rats. *Gynecol Oncol* 1986;25(2):160–170.
362. Hu E, Howell SB. Pharmacokinetics of intraarterial mitomycin C in humans. *Cancer Res* 1983;43(9):4474–4477.
363. Argenta LC, Manders EK. Mitomycin C extravasation injuries. *Cancer* 1983;51(6):1080–1082.
364. Lokich J, Perri J, Fine N, et al. Mitomycin C: phase I study of a constant infusion ambulatory treatment schedule. *Am J Clin Oncol* 1982;5(4): 443–447.
365. Tseng MH, Luch J, Mittelman A. Regional intra-arterial mitomycin C infusion in previously treated patients with metastatic colorectal cancer and concomitant measurement of serum drug level. *Cancer Treat Rep* 1984;68(11):1319–1324.
366. Hanna WT, Krauss S, Regester RF, et al. Renal disease after mitomycin C therapy. *Cancer* 1981;48(12):2583–2588.
367. Valavaara R, Nordman E. Renal complications of mitomycin C therapy with special reference to the total dose. *Cancer* 1985;55(1):47–50.
368. Lazarus HM, Gottfried MR, Herzig RH, et al. Veno-occlusive disease of the liver after high-dose mitomycin C therapy and autologous bone marrow transplantation. *Cancer* 1982;49(9):1789–1795.

369. Wood HA, Ellerhorst-Ryan JM. Delayed adverse skin reactions associated with mitomycin-C administration. *Oncol Nurs Forum* 1984;11(4):14–18.
370. Olver IN, Aisner J, Hament A, et al. A prospective study of topical dimethyl sulfoxide for treating anthracycline extravasation. *J Clin Oncol* 1988;6(11):1732–1735.
371. Chang AY, Kuebler JP, Pandya KJ, et al. Pulmonary toxicity induced by mitomycin C is highly responsive to glucocorticoids. *Cancer* 1986;57(12):2285–2290.
372. Koga S, Hamazoe R, Maeta M, et al. Prophylactic therapy for peritoneal recurrence of gastric cancer by continuous hyperthermic peritoneal perfusion with mitomycin C. *Cancer* 1988;61(2):232–237.
373. Fujimoto S, Shrestha RD, Kokubun M, et al. Pharmacokinetic analysis in intraperitoneal hyperthermic perfusion using mitomycin C in far-advanced gastric cancer. *Gan To Kagaku Ryoho* 1989;16(7):2411–2415.
374. Sanofi-Synthelabo. Eloxatin (oxaliplatin for injection) Package Insert. 2002.
375. Graham MA, Lockwood GF, Greenslade D, et al. Clinical pharmacokinetics of oxaliplatin: a critical review. *Clin Cancer Res* 2000;6(4):1205–1218.
376. Fracasso PM, Blessing JA, Morgan MA, et al. Phase II study of oxaliplatin in platinum-resistant and refractory ovarian cancer: a gynecologic group study. *J Clin Oncol* 2003;21(15):2856–2859.
377. Fracasso PM, Blessing JA, Wolf J, et al. Phase II evaluation of oxaliplatin in previously treated squamous cell carcinoma of the cervix: a Gynecologic Oncology Group study. *Gynecol Oncol* 2003;90(1):177–180.
378. Gamelin E, Gamelin L, Bossi L, et al. Clinical aspects and molecular basis of oxaliplatin neurotoxicity: current management and development of preventive measures. *Semin Oncol* 2002;29(5 Suppl 15):21–33.
379. Bougnoux P, Dieras V, Petit T, et al. A multicenter phase II study of oxaliplatin (OXA) as a single agent in platinum (PT) and/or taxanes (TX) pretreated advanced ovarian cancer (AOC): final results. [Abstract]. *Proc ASCO* 1999;18:368a.
380. Chollet P, Bensmaine MA, Brienza S, et al. Single agent activity of oxaliplatin in heavily pretreated advanced epithelial ovarian cancer. *Ann Oncol* 1996;7(10):1065–1070.
381. Dorr RT. Pharmacology of the taxanes. *Pharmacotherapy* 1997;17(5 Pt 2):96S–104S.
382. Markman M, Kennedy A, Webster K, et al. Paclitaxel-associated hypersensitivity reactions: experience of the gynecologic oncology program of the Cleveland Clinic Cancer Center. *J Clin Oncol* 2000;18(1):102–105.
383. Eisenhauer EA, ten Bokkel Huinink WW, Swenerton KD, et al. European-Canadian randomized trial of paclitaxel in relapsed ovarian cancer: high-dose versus low-dose and long versus short infusion. *J Clin Oncol* 1994;12(12):2654–2666.
384. Tsavaris NB, Kosmas C. Risk of severe acute hypersensitivity reactions after rapid paclitaxel infusion of less than 1-h duration. *Cancer Chemother Pharmacol* 1998;42(6):509–511.
385. Ozols RF, Bundy BN, Greer BE, et al. Phase III trial of carboplatin and paclitaxel compared with cisplatin and paclitaxel in patients with optimally resected stage III ovarian cancer: a Gynecologic Oncology Group study. *J Clin Oncol* 2003;21(17):3194–3200.
386. Rowinsky EK, Eisenhauer EA, Chaudhry V, et al. Clinical toxicities encountered with paclitaxel (Taxol). *Semin Oncol* 1993;20(4 Suppl 3):1–15.
387. Peereboom DM, Donehower RC, Eisenhauer EA, et al. Successful re-treatment with Taxol after major hypersensitivity reactions. *J Clin Oncol* 1993;11(5):885–890.
388. Rowinsky EK, Kaufmann SH, Baker SD, et al. Sequences of topotecan and cisplatin: phase I, pharmacologic, and *in vitro* studies to examine sequence dependence. *J Clin Oncol* 1996;14(12):3074–3084.
389. Chang SM, Kuhn JG, Rizzo J, et al. Phase I study of paclitaxel in patients with recurrent malignant glioma: a North American Brain Tumor Consortium report. *J Clin Oncol* 1998;16(6):2188–2194.
390. Francis P, Rowinsky E, Schneider J, et al. Phase I feasibility and pharmacologic study of weekly intraperitoneal paclitaxel: a Gynecologic Oncology Group pilot study. *J Clin Oncol* 1995;13(12):2961–2967.
391. Markman M, Brady MF, Spirtos NM, et al. Phase II trial of intraperitoneal paclitaxel in carcinoma of the ovary, tube, and peritoneum: a Gynecologic Oncology Group study. *J Clin Oncol* 1998;16(8):2620–2624.
392. Thigpen T, Vance RB, Khansur T. The platinum compounds and paclitaxel in the management of carcinomas of the endometrium and uterine cervix. *Semin Oncol* 1995;22(5 Suppl 12):67–75.
393. Woo HL, Swenerton KD, Hoskins PJ. Taxol is active in platinum-resistant endometrial adenocarcinoma. *Am J Clin Oncol* 1996;19(3):290–291.
394. Ball HG, Blessing JA, Lentz SS, et al. A phase II trial of paclitaxel in patients with advanced or recurrent adenocarcinoma of the endometrium: a Gynecologic Oncology Group study. *Gynecol Oncol* 1996;62(2):278–281.
395. Lissoni A, Zanetta G, Losa G, et al. Phase II study of paclitaxel as salvage treatment in advanced endometrial cancer. *Ann Oncol* 1996;7(8):861–863.
396. Lincoln S, Blessing JA, Lee RB, et al. Activity of paclitaxel as second-line chemotherapy in endometrial carcinoma: a Gynecologic Oncology Group study. *Gynecol Oncol* 2003;88(3):277–281.
397. Papadimitriou CA, Sarris K, Moulopoulos LA, et al. Phase II trial of paclitaxel and cisplatin in metastatic and recurrent carcinoma of the uterine cervix. *J Clin Oncol* 1999;17(3):761–766.
398. Piver MS, Ghamande SA, Eltabbakh GH, et al. First-line chemotherapy with paclitaxel and platinum for advanced and recurrent cancer of the cervix—a phase II study. *Gynecol Oncol* 1999;75(3):334–337.
399. Chattopadhyay S, Moran RG, Goldman ID. Pemetrexed: biochemical and cellular pharmacology, mechanisms, and clinical applications. *Mol cancer ther.* 2007;6(2):404–417.
400. Slichenmyer WJ, Rowinsky EK, Donehower RC, et al. The current status of camptothecin analogues as antitumor agents. *J Natl Cancer Inst* 1993;85(4):271–291.
401. O'Dwyer PJ, LaCreta FP, Haas NB, et al. Clinical, pharmacokinetic and biological studies of topotecan. *Cancer Chemother Pharmacol* 1994;34 Suppl:S46–S52.
402. Stewart CF, Baker SD, Heideman RL, et al. Clinical pharmacodynamics of continuous infusion topotecan in children: systemic exposure predicts hematologic toxicity. *J Clin Oncol* 1994;12(9):1946–1954.
403. van Warmerdam LJ, Verweij J, Rosing H, et al. Limited sampling models for topotecan pharmacokinetics. *Ann Oncol* 1994;5(3):259–264.
404. McCabe FL, Johnson RK. Comparative activity of oral and parenteral topotecan in murine tumor models: efficacy of oral topotecan. *Cancer Invest* 1994;12(3):308–313.
405. Clarke-Pearson DL, Van Le L, Iveson T, et al. Oral topotecan as single-agent second-line chemotherapy in patients with advanced ovarian cancer. *J Clin Oncol* 2001;19(19):3967–3975.
406. von Pawel J, Gatzemeier U, Pujol JL, et al. Phase II comparator study of oral versus intravenous topotecan in patients with chemosensitive small-cell lung cancer. *J Clin Oncol* 2001;19(6):1743–1749.
407. Von Hoff DD, Burris HA 3rd, Eckardt J, et al. Preclinical and phase I trials of topoisomerase I inhibitors. *Cancer Chemother Pharmacol* 1994;34 Suppl:S41–S45.
408. Morris RT. Weekly topotecan in the management of ovarian cancer. *Gynecol Oncol* 2003;90(3 Pt 2):S34–S38.
409. Rowinsky EK. Weekly topotecan: an alternative to topotecan's standard daily x 5 schedule? *Oncologist* 2002;7(4):324–330.
410. ten Bokkel Huinink W, Gore M, Carmichael J, et al. Topotecan versus paclitaxel for the treatment of recurrent epithelial ovarian cancer. *J Clin Oncol* 1997;15(6):2183–2193.
411. O'Reilly S, Rowinsky EK, Slichenmyer W, et al. Phase I and pharmacologic study of topotecan in patients with impaired renal function. *J Clin Oncol* 1996;14(12):3062–3073.
412. O'Reilly S, Fleming GF, Barker SD, et al. Phase I trial and pharmacologic trial of sequences of paclitaxel and topotecan in previously treated ovarian epithelial malignancies: a Gynecologic Oncology Group study. *J Clin Oncol* 1997;15(1):177–186.
413. Gordon AN, Hancock KC, Matthews CM, et al. Phase I study of alternating doublets of topotecan/carboplatin and paclitaxel/carboplatin in patients with newly diagnosed, advanced ovarian cancer. *Gynecol Oncol* 2002;85(1):129–135.
414. Hammond LA, Eckardt JR, Ganapathi R, et al. A phase I and translational study of sequential administration of the topoisomerase I and II inhibitors topotecan and etoposide. *Clin Cancer Res* 1998;4(6):1459–1467.
415. Mok TS, Wong H, Zee B, et al. A phase I-II study of sequential administration of topotecan and oral etoposide (toposiomerase I and II inhibitors) in the treatment of patients with small cell lung carcinoma. *Cancer* 2002;95(7):1511–1519.
416. Chen AY, Choy H, Rothenberg ML. DNA topoisomerase I-targeting drugs as radiation sensitizers. *Oncology (Huntingt)* 1999;13(10 Suppl 5):39–46.
417. Rave-Frank M, Glomme S, Hertig J, et al. Combined effect of topotecan and irradiation on the survival and the induction of chromosome aberrations *in vitro*. *Strahlenther Onkol* 2002;178(9):497–503.
418. Hofstra LS, Bos AM, de Vries EG, et al. A phase I and pharmacokinetic study of intraperitoneal topotecan. *Br J Cancer* 2001;85(11):1627–1633.
419. Plaxe SC, Christen RD, O'Quigley J, et al. Phase I and pharmacokinetic study of intraperitoneal topotecan. *Invest New Drugs* 1998;16(2):147–153.
420. Long HJ 3rd, Rayson S, Podratz KC, et al. Long-term survival of patients with advanced/recurrent carcinoma of cervix and vagina after neoadjuvant treatment with methotrexate, vinblastine, doxorubicin, and cisplatin with or without the addition of molgramostim, and review of the literature. *Am J Clin Oncol* 2002;25(6):547–551.
421. Aravantinos G, Bafaloukos D, Fountzilas G, et al. Phase II study of docetaxel-vinorelbine in platinum-resistant, paclitaxel-pretreated ovarian cancer. *Ann Oncol* 2003;14(7):1094–1099.
422. Noble RR, Beer CT. Experimental observations concerning the mode of action of vinca alkaloids. In: WIH S, ed. *The Vinca Alkaloids in the Chemotherapy of Malignant Disease.* Alburcham, England: John Sherrat & Sons; 1968:4–11.
423. Velban (vinblastine sulfate for injection, USP). *Physicians Desk Reference.* 55th ed. Montvale: Medical Economics Company; 2001.
424. Owellen RJ, Hartke CA. The pharmacokinetics of 4-acetyl tritium vinblastine in two patients. *Cancer Res* 1975;35(4):975–980.
425. Lucas VS, Huang AT. Vinblastine-related pain in tumors. *Cancer Treat Rep* 1977;61(9):1735–1736.
426. Teutsch C, Lipton A, Harvey HA. Raynaud's phenomenon as a side effect of chemotherapy with vinblastine and bleomycin for testicular carcinoma. *Cancer Treat Rep* 1977;61(5):925–926.
427. Ginsberg SJ, Comis RL, Fitzpatrick AV. Vinblastine and inappropriate ADH secretion. *N Engl J Med* 1977;296(16):941.

428. Cohlan SW, Kitay D. The teratogenic effect of vincaleukoblastine in the pregnant rat. *J Pediatr* 1965(66):541–544.
429. Dorr RT, Alberts DS. Vinca alkaloid skin toxicity: antidote and drug disposition studies in the mouse. *J Natl Cancer Inst* 1985;74(1):113–120.
430. Blajman C, Balbiani L, Block J, et al. A prospective, randomized phase III trial comparing combination chemotherapy with cyclophosphamide, doxorubicin, and 5-fluorouracil with vinorelbine plus doxorubicin in the treatment of advanced breast carcinoma. *Cancer* 1999;85(5):1091–1097.
431. Burger RA, DiSaia PJ, Roberts JA, et al. Phase II trial of vinorelbine in recurrent and progressive epithelial ovarian cancer. *Gynecol Oncol* 1999;72(2):148–153.
432. Morris M, Brader KR, Levenback C, et al. Phase II study of vinorelbine in advanced and recurrent squamous cell carcinoma of the cervix. *J Clin Oncol* 1998;16(3):1094–1098.
433. Peacock NW, Burris HA, Dieras V, et al. A phase I trial of vinorelbine in combination with mitoxantrone in patients with refractory solid tumors. *Invest New Drugs* 1998;16(1):37–43.
434. Mangeney P, Andriamialisoa RZ, Lallemand JY, et al. 5′Nor-anhydrovinblastine, prototype of a new class of vinblastine derivatives. *Tetrahedron* 1979;35:2175–2179.
435. Johnson SA, Harper P, Hortobagyi GN, et al. Vinorelbine: an overview. *Cancer Treat Rev* 1996;22(2):127–142.
436. Marquet P, Lachatre G, Debord J, et al. Pharmacokinetics of vinorelbine in man. *Eur J Clin Pharmacol* 1992;42(5):545–547.
437. Wargin WA, Lucas VS. The clinical pharmacokinetics of vinorelbine (Navelbine). *Semin Oncol* 1994;21(5 Suppl 10):21–27.
438. Lozano M, Muro H, Triguboff E, et al. A randomized trial for effective prevention of Navelbine (NVB) related phlebitis. [Abstract]. *Proc ASCO* 1995;14:535.
439. Trissel LA, Martinez JF. Visual, turbidimetric, and particle-content assessment of compatibility of vinorelbine tartrate with selected drugs during simulated Y-site injection. *Am J Hosp Pharm* 1994;51(4):495–499.
440. Gershenson DM, Burke TW, Morris M, et al. A phase I study of a daily x3 schedule of intravenous vinorelbine for refractory epithelial ovarian cancer. *Gynecol Oncol* 1998;70(3):404–409.
441. Weiss AJ, Sabol J, Lackman RD. Concurrent administration of vinorelbine with recombinant human granulocyte colony-stimulating factor: an effective method of increasing dose intensity. *Am J Clin Oncol* 1999;22(1):38–41.
442. Hohneker JA. A summary of vinorelbine (Navelbine) safety data from North American clinical trials. *Semin Oncol* 1994;21(5 Suppl 10):42–46; discussion 6–7.
443. Gebbia V, Testa A, Valenza R, et al. Acute pain syndrome at tumour site in neoplastic patients treated with vinorelbine: report of unusual toxicity. *Eur J Cancer* 1994;30A(6):889.
444. Raderer M, Kornek G, Hejna M, et al. Acute pulmonary toxicity associated with high-dose vinorelbine and mitomycin C. *Ann Oncol* 1996;7(9): 973–975.
445. Garrett CA, Simpson TA Jr. Syndrome of inappropriate antidiuretic hormone associated with vinorelbine therapy. *Ann Pharmacother* 1998;32(12): 1306–1309.
446. Hoff PM, Valero V, Ibrahim N, et al. Hand-foot syndrome following prolonged infusion of high doses of vinorelbine. *Cancer* 1998;82(5): 965–969.
447. Liebmann J, Friedman K. Adynamic ileus in a patient with non-small-cell lung cancer after treatment with vinorelbine. *Am J Med* 1996;101(6): 658–659.
448. Raderer M, Kornek G, Scheithauer W. Re: vinorelbine-induced pancreatitis: a case report. *J Natl Cancer Inst* 1998;90(4):329.
449. Budman DR. Vinorelbine (Navelbine): a third-generation Vinca alkaloid. *Cancer Invest* 1997;15(5):475–490.
450. Ozols RF, Hogan WM, Ostchega Y, et al. MVP (mitomycin, vinblastine, and progesterone): a second-line regimen in ovarian cancer with a high incidence of pulmonary toxicity. *Cancer Treat Rep* 1983;67(7–8):721–722.
451. Parimoo D, Jeffers S, Muggia FM. Severe neurotoxicity from vinorelbine-paclitaxel combinations. *J Natl Cancer Inst* 1996;88(15):1079–1080.
452. Bajetta E, Di Leo A, Biganzoli L, et al. Phase II study of vinorelbine in patients with pretreated advanced ovarian cancer: activity in platinum-resistant disease. *J Clin Oncol* 1996;14(9):2546–2551.
453. Herbst RS. Erlotinib (Tarceva): an update on the clinical trial program. *Semin Oncol* 2003;30(3 Suppl 7):34–46.
454. Gordon AN, Finkler N, Edwards RP, et al. Efficacy and safety of erlotinib HCl, an epidermal growth factor receptor (HER1/EGFR) tyrosine kinase inhibitor, in patients with advanced ovarian carcinoma: results from a phase II multicenter study. *Int J Gynecol Cancer* 2005;15(5):785–792.
455. Vasey PA, Paul J, Rustin G, et al. Maintenance erlotinib (E) following first-line treatment with docetaxel, carboplatin and erlotinib in patients with ovarian carcinoma. *J Clin Oncol* (Meeting Abstracts). 2007;25(18S):5560.
456. Hidalgo M, Bloedow D. Pharmacokinetics and pharmacodynamics: maximizing the clinical potential of erlotinib (Tarceva). *Semin Oncol* 2003; 30(3 Suppl 7):25–33.
457. Akita RW, Sliwkowski MX. Preclinical studies with erlotinib (Tarceva). *Semin Oncol* 2003;30(3 Suppl 7):15–24.
458. Goodman VL, Rock EP, Dagher R, et al. Approval summary: sunitinib for the treatment of imatinib refractory or intolerant gastrointestinal stromal tumors and advanced renal cell carcinoma. *Clin Cancer Res* 2007;13(5): 1367–1373.
459. Ikezoe T, Nishioka C, Tasaka T, et al. The antitumor effects of sunitinib (formerly SU11248) against a variety of human hematologic malignancies: enhancement of growth inhibition via inhibition of mammalian target of rapamycin signaling. *Mol Cancer Ther* 2006;5(10):2522–2530.
460. Bello CL, Sherman L, Zhou J, et al. Effect of food on the pharmacokinetics of sunitinib malate (SU11248), a multi-targeted receptor tyrosine kinase inhibitor: results from a phase I study in healthy subjects. *Anticancer Drugs* 2006;17(3):353–358.
461. Konecny GE, Pegram MD, Venkatesan N, et al. Activity of the dual kinase inhibitor lapatinib (GW572016) against HER-2-overexpressing and trastuzumab-treated breast cancer cells. *Cancer Res* 2006;66(3): 1630–1639.
462. Nelson MH, Dolder CR. Lapatinib: a novel dual tyrosine kinase inhibitor with activity in solid tumors. *Ann Pharmacother* 2006;40(2): 261–269.
463. Buzdar AU, Jonat W, Howell A, et al. Anastrozole versus megestrol acetate in the treatment of postmenopausal women with advanced breast carcinoma: results of a survival update based on a combined analysis of data from two mature phase III trials. Arimidex Study Group. *Cancer* 1998;83(6):1142–1152.
464. Plourde PV, Dyroff M, Dukes M. Arimidex: a potent and selective fourth-generation aromatase inhibitor. *Breast Cancer Res Treat* 1994;30(1): 103–111.
465. Koshiyama M, Yoshida M, Konishi M, et al. Expression of pS2 protein in endometrial carcinomas: correlation with clinicopathologic features and sex steroid receptor status. *Int J Cancer* 1997;74(3):237–244.
466. Watanabe K, Sasano H, Harada N, et al. Aromatase in human endometrial carcinoma and hyperplasia. Immunohistochemical, *in situ* hybridization, and biochemical studies. *Am J Pathol* 1995;146(2):491–500.
467. Rose PG, Brunetto VL, VanLe L, et al. A phase II trial of anastrozole in advanced recurrent or persistent endometrial carcinoma: a Gynecologic Oncology Group study. *Gynecol Oncol* 2000;78(2):212–216.
468. Agorastos T, Vaitsi V, Pantazis K, et al. Aromatase inhibitor anastrozole for treating endometrial hyperplasia in obese postmenopausal women. *Eur J Obstet Gynecol Reprod Biol* 2005;118(2):239–240.
469. Smyth JF, Gourley C, Walker G, et al. Antiestrogen therapy is active in selected ovarian cancer cases: the use of letrozole in estrogen receptor-positive patients. *Clin Cancer Res* 2007;13(12):3617–3622.
470. Rao GG, Miller DS. Hormonal therapy in epithelial ovarian cancer. *Expert Rev Anticancer Ther* 2006;6(1):43–47.
471. Li YF, Fu S, Hu W, et al. Systemic anticancer therapy in gynecologic cancer patients with renal dysfunction. *Int J Gynecol Cancer* 2007;17(4): 739–763.
472. Imai M, Jobo T, Sato R, et al. Medroxyprogesterone acetate therapy for patients with adenocarcinoma of the endometrium who wish to preserve the uterus—usefulness and limitations. *Eur J Gynaecol Oncol* 2001;22(3): 217–220.
473. Kobiashvili H, Charkviani L, Charkviani T. Organ preserving method in the management of atypical endometrial hyperplasia. *Eur J Gynaecol Oncol* 2001;22(4):297–299.
474. Thigpen JT, Brady MF, Alvarez RD, et al. Oral medroxyprogesterone acetate in the treatment of advanced or recurrent endometrial carcinoma: a dose-response study by the Gynecologic Oncology Group. *J Clin Oncol* 1999;17(6):1736–1744.
475. Bertelli G, Venturini M, Del Mastro L, et al. Intramuscular depot medroxyprogesterone versus oral megestrol for the control of postmenopausal hot flashes in breast cancer patients: a randomized study. *Ann Oncol* 2002;13(6):883–888.
476. Rossouw JE, Anderson GL, Prentice RL, et al. Risks and benefits of estrogen plus progestin in healthy postmenopausal women: principal results from the Women's Health Initiative randomized controlled trial. *JAMA* 2002;288(3):321–333.
477. Shumaker SA, Legault C, Rapp SR, et al. Estrogen plus progestin and the incidence of dementia and mild cognitive impairment in postmenopausal women: the Women's Health Initiative Memory Study: a randomized controlled trial. *JAMA* 2003;289(20):2651–2662.
478. Jordan VC, Assikis VJ. Endometrial carcinoma and tamoxifen: clearing up a controversy. *Clin Cancer Res* 1995;1(5):467–472.
479. PDR Electronic Library, Vol 6.0.0a. 2003 [cited; Available from:
480. Varras M, Polyzos D, Akrivis C. Effects of tamoxifen on the human female genital tract: review of the literature. *Eur J Gynaecol Oncol* 2003; 24(3–4):258–268.
481. Day R. Quality of life and tamoxifen in a breast cancer prevention trial: a summary of findings from the NSABP P-1 study. National Surgical Adjuvant Breast and Bowel Project. *Ann NY Acad Sci* 2001;949: 143–150.
482. Hatch KD, Beecham JB, Blessing JA, et al. Responsiveness of patients with advanced ovarian carcinoma to tamoxifen. A Gynecologic Oncology Group study of second-line therapy in 105 patients. *Cancer* 1991;68(2): 269–271.
483. Ahlgren JD, Ellison NM, Gottlieb RJ, et al. Hormonal palliation of chemoresistant ovarian cancer: three consecutive phase II trials of the Mid-Atlantic Oncology Program. *J Clin Oncol* 1993;11(10):1957–1968.
484. Markman M, Iseminger KA, Hatch KD, et al. Tamoxifen in platinum-refractory ovarian cancer: a Gynecologic Oncology Group Ancillary Report. *Gynecol Oncol* 1996;62(1):4–6.

485. Strohmeyer D. Pathophysiology of tumor angiogenesis and its relevance in renal cell cancer. *Anticancer Res* 1999;19(2C):1557–1561.
486. Malonne H, Langer I, Kiss R, et al. Mechanisms of tumor angiogenesis and therapeutic implications: angiogenesis inhibitors. *Clin Exp Metastasis* 1999;17(1):1–14.
487. Folkman J. Tumor angiogenesis: therapeutic implications. *N Engl J Med* 1971;285(21):1182–1186.
488. Folkman J, Watson K, Ingber D, et al. Induction of angiogenesis during the transition from hyperplasia to neoplasia. *Nature* 1989;339(6219):58–61.
489. Alvarez AA, Krigman HR, Whitaker RS, et al. The prognostic significance of angiogenesis in epithelial ovarian carcinoma. *Clin Cancer Res* 1999; 5(3):587–591.
490. Cooper RA, Wilks DP, Logue JP, et al. High tumor angiogenesis is associated with poorer survival in carcinoma of the cervix treated with radiotherapy. *Clin Cancer Res* 1998;4(11):2795–2800.
491. Sauer G, Deissler H. Angiogenesis: prognostic and therapeutic implications in gynecologic and breast malignancies. *Curr Opin Obstet Gynecol* 2003; 15(1):45–49.
492. Frumovitz M, Sood AK. Vascular endothelial growth factor (VEGF) pathway as a therapeutic target in gynecologic malignancies. *Gynecol Oncol* 2007; 104(3):768–778.
493. Folkman J. Seminars in Medicine of the Beth Israel Hospital, Boston. Clinical applications of research on angiogenesis. *N Engl J Med* 1995;333(26): 1757–1763.
494. Wright JD, Viviano D, Powell MA, et al. Bevacizumab combination therapy in heavily pretreated, recurrent cervical cancer. *Gynecol Oncol* 2006; 103(2):489–493.
495. Cohn DE, Valmadre S, Resnick KE, et al. Bevacizumab and weekly taxane chemotherapy demonstrates activity in refractory ovarian cancer. *Gynecol Oncol* 2006;102(2):134–139.
496. Monk BJ, Choi DC, Pugmire G, et al. Activity of bevacizumab (rhuMAB VEGF) in advanced refractory epithelial ovarian cancer. *Gynecol Oncol* 2005;96(3):902–905.
497. Abramson N, Stokes PK, Luke M, et al. Ovarian and papillary-serous peritoneal carcinoma: pilot study with thalidomide. *J Clin Oncol* 2002; 20(4):1147–1149.
498. Celgene Corporation. *Thalomid (Thalidomide): Balancing the Benefits and Risks*; 1998.
499. Tew KD, Houghton PJ, Houghton JA. *Preclincial and Clinical Modulation of Anticancer Drugs.* Boca Raton, FL: CRC Press; 1993.
500. Davidson DE, Grenan MM, Sweeney TR. Biological characteristics of some improved radioprotectors. In: Brady LW, ed. *Radiation Sensitizers.* New York: Masson Pub. USA; 1980:309–320.
501. Schucter LM, Glick JH. The current status of WR2721 (amifostine): a chemotherapy and radiation therapy protector. In: De Vita VT, Hellman S, Rosenberg SA, eds. *Biologic Therapy of Cancer Updates.* Philadelphia: J.B. Lippincott Co.; 1993:1–9.
502. Calabro-Jones PM, Aguilera JA, Ward JF, et al. Uptake of WR-2721 derivatives by cells in culture: identification of the transported form of the drug. *Cancer Res* 1988;48(13):3634–3640.
503. List AF, Heaton R, Glinsmann-Gibson B, et al. Amifostine stimulates formation of multipotent and erythroid bone marrow progenitors. *Leukemia* 1998;12(10):1596–1602.
504. Taylor CW, Wang LM, List AF, et al. Amifostine protects normal tissues from paclitaxel toxicity while cytotoxicity against tumour cells is maintained. *Eur J Cancer* 1997;33(10):1693–1698.
505. Valeriote F, Tolen S. Protection and potentiation of nitrogen mustard cytotoxicity by WR-2721. *Cancer Res* 1982;42(11):4330–4331.
506. Shaw LM, Glover D, Turrisi A, et al. Pharmacokinetics of WR-2721. *Pharmacol Ther* 1988;39(1–3):195–201.
507. Korst AE, Eeltink CM, Vermorken JB, et al. Pharmacokinetics of amifostine and its metabolites in patients. *Eur J Cancer* 1997;33(9):1425–1429.
508. Korst AE, van der Sterre ML, Gall HE, et al. Influence of amifostine on the pharmacokinetics of cisplatin in cancer patients. *Clin Cancer Res* 1998;4(2):331–336.
509. Wagner W, Radmard A, Schonekaes KG. A new administration schedule for amifostine as a radioprotector in cancer therapy. *Anticancer Res* 1999;19(3B):2281–2283.
510. Shpall EJ, Stemmer SM, Hami L, et al. Amifostine (WR-2721) shortens the engraftment period of 4-hydroperoxycyclophosphamide-purged bone marrow in breast cancer patients receiving high-dose chemotherapy with autologous bone marrow support. *Blood* 1994;83(11):3132–3137.
511. De Vos FY, Bos AM, Schaapveld M, et al. A randomized phase II study of paclitaxel with carboplatin +/− amifostine as first line treatment in advanced ovarian carcinoma. *Gynecol Oncol* 2005;97(1):60–67.
512. Hilpert F, Stahle A, Tome O, et al. Neuroprotection with amifostine in the first-line treatment of advanced ovarian cancer with carboplatin/paclitaxel-based chemotherapy—a double-blind, placebo-controlled, randomized phase II study from the Arbeitsgemeinschaft Gynakologische Onkologoie (AGO) Ovarian Cancer Study Group. *Support Care Cancer* 2005;13(10):797–805.
513. Lorusso D, Ferrandina G, Greggi S, et al. Phase III multicenter randomized trial of amifostine as cytoprotectant in first-line chemotherapy in ovarian cancer patients. *Ann Oncol* 2003;14(7):1086–1093.
514. Gall HE, Eeltink CM, Vermorken JB. Nursing protocol for effective administration of amifostine. *Eur J Cancer* 1995;31A:S286.
515. Wadler S, Haynes H, Beitler JJ, et al. Management of hypocalcemic effects of WR2721 administered on a daily times five schedule with cisplatin and radiation therapy. The New York Gynecologic Oncology Group. *J Clin Oncol* 1993;11(8):1517–1522.
516. Koukourakis MI, Kyrias G, Kakolyris S, et al. Subcutaneous administration of amifostine during fractionated radiotherapy: a randomized phase II study. *J Clin Oncol* 2000;18(11):2226–2233.
517. Creighton AM, Hellmann K, Whitecross S. Antitumour activity in a series of bisdiketopiperazines. *Nature* 1969;222(191):384–385.
518. Von Hoff DD, Howser D, Lewis BJ, et al. Phase I study of ICRF-187 using a daily for 3 days schedule. *Cancer Treat Rep* 1981;65(3–4):249–252.
519. Herman EH, Ferrans VJ. Reduction of chronic doxorubicin cardiotoxicity in dogs by pretreatment with (+/−)-1,2-bis(3,5-dioxopiperazinyl-1-yl) propane (ICRF-187). *Cancer Res* 1981;41(9 Pt 1):3436–3440.
520. Wadler S, Green MD, Muggia FM. Synergistic activity of doxorubicin and the bisdioxopiperazine (+)-1,2-bis(3,5-dioxopiperazinyl-1-yl)propane (ICRF 187) against the murine sarcoma S180 cell line. *Cancer Res* 1986;46(3):1176–1181.
521. Green MD, Alderton P, Gross J, et al. Evidence of the selective alteration of anthracycline activity due to modulation by ICRF-187 (ADR-529). *Pharmacol Ther* 1990;48(1):61–69.
522. Imondi AR, Della Torre P, Mazue G, et al. Dose-response relationship of dexrazoxane for prevention of doxorubicin-induced cardiotoxicity in mice, rats, and dogs. *Cancer Res* 1996;56(18):4200–4204.
523. Speyer JL, Green MD, Kramer E, et al. Protective effect of the bispiperazinedione ICRF-187 against doxorubicin-induced cardiac toxicity in women with advanced breast cancer. *N Engl J Med* 1988;319(12): 745–752.
524. Blum RH, Walsh C, Green MD, et al. Modulation of the effect of anthracycline efficacy and toxicity by ICRF-187. *Cancer Invest* 1990; 8(2):267–268.
525. Venturini M, Michelotti A, Del Mastro L, et al. Multicenter randomized controlled clinical trial to evaluate cardioprotection of dexrazoxane versus no cardioprotection in women receiving epirubicin chemotherapy for advanced breast cancer. *J Clin Oncol* 1996;14(12):3112–3120.
526. Wexler LH, Andrich MP, Venzon D, et al. Randomized trial of the cardioprotective agent ICRF-187 in pediatric sarcoma patients treated with doxorubicin. *J Clin Oncol* 1996;14(2):362–372.
527. Von Hoff DD. Phase I trials of dexrazoxane and other potential applications for the agent. *Semin Oncol* 1998;25(4 Suppl 10):31–36.
528. Bertino JR. "Rescue" techniques in cancer chemotherapy: use of leucovorin and other rescue agents after methotrexate treatment. *Semin Oncol* 1977;4(2):203–216.
529. Erlichman C. Fluorouracil and leucovorin for metastatic colorectal cancer. *J Chemother* 1990;2 Suppl 1:38–40.
530. Zaniboni A, Arcangeli G, Meriggi F, et al. Low-dose 6-S leucovorin and 5-fluorouracil as salvage treatment in metastatic breast cancer. [Abstract]. *Proc ASCO* 1994;13:91.
531. Kobayashi K, Schilsky RL. Update on biochemical modulation of chemotherapeutic agents. *Oncology (Huntingt)* 1993;7(5):99–106, 109; discussion 10–14, 17.
532. Brock N, Pohl J, Stekar J, et al. Studies on the urotoxicity of oxazaphosphorine cytostatics and its prevention—III. Profile of action of sodium 2-mercaptoethane sulfonate (mesna). *Eur J Cancer Clin Oncol* 1982; 18(12):1377–1387.
533. Burkert H. Clinical overview of mesna. *Cancer Treat Rev* 1983;10 Suppl A:175–181.
534. Goren MP, McKenna LM, Goodman TL. Combined intravenous and oral mesna in outpatients treated with ifosfamide. *Cancer Chemother Pharmacol* 1997;40(5):371–375.
535. Munshi NC, Loehrer PJ Sr, Williams SD, et al. Comparison of N-acetylcysteine and mesna as uroprotectors with ifosfamide combination chemotherapy in refractory germ tumors. *Invest New Drugs* 1992;10(3):159–163.
536. Markman M, Kennedy A, Webster K, et al. Continuous subcutaneous administration of mesna to prevent ifosfamide-induced hemorrhagic cystitis. *Semin Oncol* 1996;23(3 Suppl 6):97–98.
537. Athanassiou H, Antonadou D, Coliarakis N, et al. Protective effect of amifostine during fractionated radiotherapy in patients with pelvic carcinomas: results of a randomized trial. *Int J Radiat Oncol Biol Phys.* 2003;56(4):1154–1160.
538. Antonadou D, Athanassiou H, Sarris G, et al . Randomized phase III trial of chemoradiation treatment ± amifostine in patients with colorectal cancer. *ASCO Proc.* 2004:abstract 258.

CHAPTER 17 ■ HORMONES AND HUMAN MALIGNANCIES

G. LARRY MAXWELL, AMIR A. JAZAERI, AND LAUREL W. RICE

INTRODUCTION

Hormones have been linked to several of the most commonly occurring human malignancies, including breast, endometrium, ovary, and colon. The ability of hormones to stimulate cellular proliferation, leading to random genetic errors, is postulated as the basis by which these peptides promote the development of human neoplasia. The laboratory investigation of the pathways and mechanisms by which hormones affect their biologic responses is an exploding area of research, largely as a result of the tremendous potential for translational research and improved patient care. This chapter reviews the relationship between hormones and human malignancies, specifically as they relate to risk, prevention, and treatment.

HORMONE RECEPTOR PATHWAYS AND MECHANISMS

Overview

Steroid hormones are involved in a variety of growth and developmental processes and exert their physiologic effects by binding to their respective receptors. Steroid hormone receptors are part of the ligand-activated nuclear transcription factor superfamily whose members also include glucocorticoid, mineralocorticoid, androgen, thyroid, retinoid, progesterone (PR), and estrogen (ER) receptors (1). In the inactive state these receptors are bound to repressor/chaperone complexes within the cytoplasm. Upon binding to their respective ligands, the receptor-ligand complex undergoes dimerization followed by nuclear localization (leading to the name "nuclear receptor"). Inside the nucleus the steroid hormone-receptor complex binds to specific DNA sequences called response elements (2). Also participating in this interaction are nuclear receptor coactivators and corepressors, as well as the general transcription machinery (3). The net result of these interactions is the transcriptional activation or repression of hormone responsive genes. More recently, nongenomic actions of ER and other nuclear receptors have been documented. These effects result from protein-protein interactions and membrane-associated nuclear receptor action (4).

Steroid Hormone Biosynthesis

Although a detailed description of steroid biosynthesis is beyond the scope of this chapter, a brief overview is presented (Fig. 17.1) to highlight targets of therapeutic intervention. The rate-limiting and irreversible reaction in steroid synthesis is the conversion of cholesterol to pregnenolone by the P450-linked side chain-cleaving enzyme (P450 ssc) (5). In the ovary this reaction is regulated by follicle-stimulating hormone (FSH) and luteinizing hormone (LH) via cAMP and protein kinase A (PKA) signaling (6). This leads to increased production of androgen intermediates, androstenedione and testosterone, that are then converted by the P450-aromatase enzyme to estrone and estradiol (E2), respectively. The expression of P450-aromatase enzyme is not limited to the ovaries; its expression and action in a variety of tissues lead to local E2 production in these tissues (7). This local E2 biosynthesis may be especially significant in men and postmenopausal women, where ovarian hormone production is lacking. Furthermore, high levels of locally synthesized E2 have been implicated in breast carcinogenesis (8).

Examination of the transcription patterns of the gene encoding aromatase *CYP19* has revealed tissue-specific promoter usage. Promoter I.1 is used in the placenta; I.4 in adipose tissue, bone, and skin; and promoter II in breast cancer (CA), endometriosis, and ovary (9). The transcripts generated from these promoters are translated into the same protein. However, the presence of tissue-specific promoters has raised the possibility of developing tissue-selective aromatase inhibitors. Such agents would be able to block E2 in breast CA, for example, without affecting estrogenic pathways in bones (7,10).

Steroid Hormone Receptor Structure

Steroid receptors are comprised of six functional domains (Fig. 17.2) (11). The A/B domain is highly variable among the different members of this family and contains within it the hormone-independent activating 1, or AF-1, domain. The C region consists of the DNA-binding domain (DBD) and is relatively conserved. Within the central DBD two zinc fingers target the receptors to their corresponding hormone response elements. The DBD binds as a dimer with each monomer recognizing half of the palindromic DNA sequence of the response element. The D domain is a peptide linker that connects the DBD to the ligand-binding domain (LBD). The E region is a multifunctional domain and contains amino acids involved in ligand binding, receptor dimerization, nuclear localization, coactivator/corepressor interaction, and ligand-dependent activating function (AF-2). The F region is a variable extension of the E region.

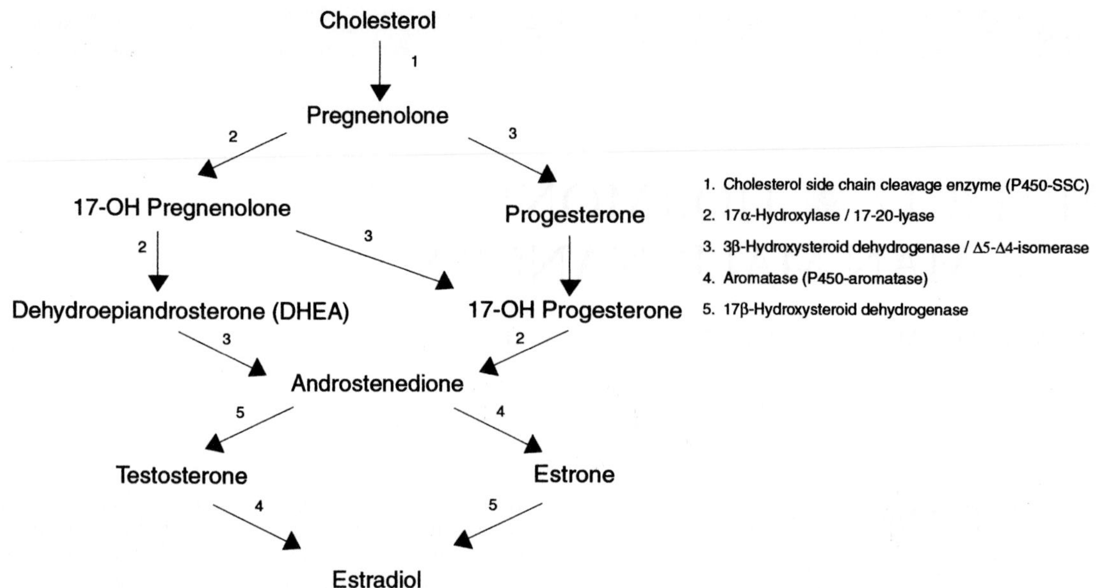

FIGURE 17.1. Steroid hormone biosynthesis. Notice the important role of aromatase in the conversion of androgens to E2s.

Estrogen Receptors

The two main isoforms of the human ER are ER-α and ER-β. ER-α is encoded by the *ESR1* gene, which maps to the 6q25.1 locus. This isoform was the only known ER until 1996 when a second isoform, now known as ER-β, was discovered. Estrogen receptor-β is encoded by the *ESR2* gene located on chromosome 14q23 (12). The human ERs exhibit 96% and 58% homology in their DBD and LBD, respectively, while the other domains show relatively little similarity. These structural differences result in distinct ligand affinities and physiological properties. For example, raloxifene has a significantly higher affinity for ER-α and genistein, a naturally occurring phyto-E2 that has a 30-fold higher affinity for ER-β compared to ER-α *in vitro*. Furthermore, tamoxifen and raloxifene exhibit partial agonist activities after binding to ER-α, while they act as pure antagonists when bound to ER-β (13). This is thought to result from distinct conformational changes induced by ligand binding in the two receptors (14).

ER-α is the predominant ER isoform in some tissues including breast, uterus, and pituitary gland, while ER-β has notably higher expression in ovarian granulosa cells, prostate gland, gastrointestinal tract, endothelial cells, and parts of the nervous system (15,16). However, in many tissues some expression of both receptors is observed. As noted above, ER-α and ER-β have been shown to have unique physiologic properties. In addition, they are capable of forming ER-α/ER-β heterodimers and thus influencing each other's function (17). In this context, ER-β has been shown to function as a dominant inhibitor of ER-α (18). Therefore, it is likely that normal physiologic function in E2 responsive tissues relies on the relative expression ratio of ER-α and ER-β in those tissues. There is evidence to suggest that perturbations of the normal ER-α-to-ER-β ratio correlate with neoplastic states. Cancers of the ovary, colon, and endometrium are all characterized by a relative loss of the normally predominant ER subtype when compared to normal tissue (19–22). Whether these changes predispose to or are a result of carcinogenesis remains to be elucidated. The development of ER-α, ER-β, and double knockout mice (ERKO, βERKO, and αβERKO, respectively) has helped with the identification of each receptor's physiologic role in their target organs (23). These findings are summarized in Table 17.1.

Both ER-α and ER-β have several isoforms resulting from exon deletions due to alternative splicing (24,25). Several of these ER-α and ER-β "splice variants" have been demonstrated to possess altered hormone binding and/or transcriptional properties. Some can act in a dominant negative fashion by dimerizing with the wild-type receptors and interfering with their function *in vitro* (26). The *in vivo* physiologic or pathophysiologic significance of these variants awaits further clarification.

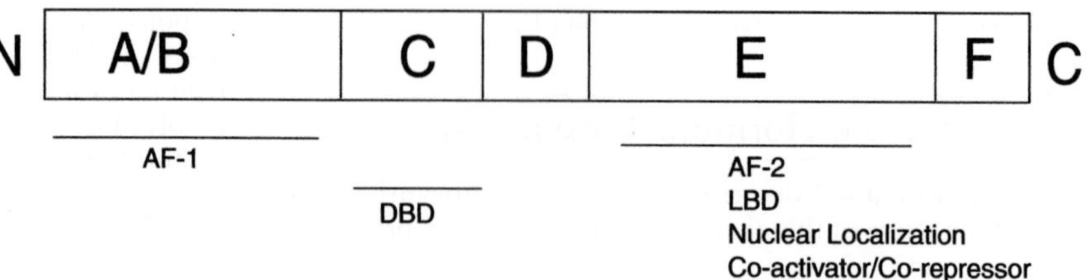

FIGURE 17.2. Functional domains common to steroid receptors. The A/B domain is highly variable among the different members of this family and contains the hormone-independent activating 1, or AF-1, domain. The C region consists of the DNA-binding domain (DBD). The D domain is a peptide linker that connects the DBD to the ligand-binding domain (LBD). The E region is a multifunctional domain and contains the LBD as well as amino acids involved in receptor dimerization, nuclear localization, coactivator/corepressor interaction, and ligand-dependent activating function (AF-2). The F region is a variable extension of the E region.

TABLE 17.1

SUMMARY OF FINDINGS FROM ESTROGEN-RECEPTOR KNOCKOUT MICE EXPERIMENTS

	Phenotype		
Organ	αERKO	βERKO	αβERKO
Pituitary gland	High LH	None	High LH
Ovary	Hemorrhagic cysts, high estrogen and testosterone due to high LH, anovulatory	Reduced ovulation	Anovulatory, "sex-reversed" follicles with Sertoli-like cells
Endometrium	Estrogen insensitive, no growth or induction of estrogen-responsive genes	Normal growth and response to estrogen	Estrogen insensitive, no growth or induction of estrogen-responsive genes
Breast	No pubertal development	Normal development and lactation	No pubertal development

LH, luteinizing hormone.

As mentioned above, ER-α and ER-β have been shown to regulate transcription by interacting with other transcription factors and signal mediators (27–29). This mechanism involves protein-protein interaction and does not require DNA binding. One example of this type of interaction is the influence of ERs on the transcriptional activity mediated by the components of the activating protein 1 (AP-1) pathway jun and fos (30). In the presence of ER-α, E2 stimulates, while tamoxifen and raloxifene inhibit AP-1–dependent transcription. In contrast ER-β produces the opposite effect, with estradiol inhibiting, and tamoxifen and raloxifene stimulating AP-1–mediated transcription. An additional mechanism of ER action involves "cross talk" with growth factors including insulin-like growth factor 1 (IGF-1), epidermal growth factor (EGF), and transforming growth factor β (TGF-β) (31,32). Epidermal growth factor can mimic the effects of E2 on the reproductive tract. This effect is dependent on ER-α since it can be blocked by ER antagonists and is absent in ERKO mice despite an intact EGF signaling cascade (32). Mechanisms for this cross talk involve signal transduction from growth factor receptors via the ras/raf/MAPK, as well as the AKT/PI3K cascade intermediaries culminating in the phosphorylation and activation of ER's AF-1 domain (33). AKT activation results in cell survival and inhibition of apoptosis. In normal tissue this pathway is kept in check by a phosphatase called PTEN. PTEN is a tumor suppressor that negatively regulates the PI3K/AKT pathway by dephosphorylating PIP3. The activation of the PI3K/AKT pathway is particularly relevant in endometrial adenocarcinoma where up to 80% of malignancies and 55% of premalignant lesions have been shown to harbor PTEN mutations (34,35). Most investigations of the growth factor–ER cross talk have involved ER-α. However, recently positive regulation of AKT over ER-β was reported via phosphorylation of glucocorticoid receptor-interacting protein 1 (GRIP1) transcriptional coactivator (36).

Finally, for decades it has been observed that exposure to estrogens can lead to immediate physiologic sequelae independent of transcriptional effects. These observations supported the presence of ERs outside the nucleus as the mediators of these nongenomic steroid hormone effects (37). While the details of this nongenomic effect of estrogens are still under investigation, there appear to be at least two major mechanisms involved. The first consists of interactions of ER-α and its splice variants with components of the growth factor signaling cascades including MAPK and PI3K pathways (38,39). The second mechanism involves a G protein coupled receptor, GPR30, an intracellular transmembrane receptor that localizes mainly to the endoplasmic reticulum. In this pathway estrogens diffuse through the plasma membrane and bind GPR30 at the endoplasmic reticulum. This results in intracellular calcium mobilization and synthesis of phosphatidylinositol 3,4,5-trisphosphate in the nucleus. Activation of this pathway has been demonstrated in cells that lack ER-α and ER-β expression (40).

Progesterone Receptors

The effects of progesterone are mediated by two PR proteins, PRA and PRB. The two PR proteins are products of the same gene, *PGR*, which has been mapped to chromosome 11q22-q23. These isoforms result from transcription from alternative promoters (41). The two PR forms are identical except that PRB has an additional 164 amino acids contained at its N-terminus compared to PRA. This unique region of PRB contains a transcription-activating functional domain, AF-3, in addition to AF-1 and AF-2, which are common to PRA (42). The two PRs exhibit differences in function that are cell context and promoter dependent. For example, PRB uniformly exhibits progestin-dependent transactivation in various cell types examined. However, PRA's transcriptional activity is cell and response element specific. When tested on simple progestin response elements (PRE), PRA and PRB display similar transactivational activity. However, PRA's activity is reduced or abolished on more complex response elements (43). In addition, PRA has been shown to act in a dominant negative fashion, antagonizing the transcriptional activity of not only PRB, but also other nuclear receptors such as the glucocorticoid, mineralocorticoid, androgen, and estrogen receptors (44).

In general, most tissues express equal levels of the two PR isoforms. However, differential expression can be observed as each promoter is regulated independently. For example, in the endometrium, stromal cells express predominantly PRA throughout the menstrual cycle, whereas the epithelial cells switch from PRA to PRB during the early secretory phase (45). It has been hypothesized that dysregulation of the normal PRA-to-PRB ratio may lead to disordered proliferation or neoplasia. In support of this hypothesis, PRA knockout mice (PRAKO) exhibit endometrial hyperplasia mediated by PRB following exposure to progestins (46). Similar studies using

PRB knockout mice (PRBKO) have shown that PRA is sufficient for eliciting progesterone's reproductive responses in the ovary and the uterus. In contrast, PRB is required to elicit normal proliferative responses of the mammary gland to progesterone (46). Finally, changes in PR isoform relative or overall expression have been described in endometrial, ovarian, and breast cancers (21,22,47). The significance of these alterations awaits further investigation.

Like estrogen receptors, progesterone receptors also possess nongenomic functions that are mediated through two general mechanisms. The first involves interaction with the Src/Ras/MAPK pathway (48), while the second pathway is mediated by plasma membrane–associated G protein–coupled receptors distinct from the classical PRs (49). Clinical significance and potential therapeutic implications of the two different pathways are active areas of steroid hormone research at this time.

HORMONES AS RISK FACTORS FOR HUMAN MALIGNANCIES

Endogenous Hormones and Modulation of CA Risk

Obesity

The prevalence of obesity, defined as a body mass index (BMI) >30, has become an epidemic health care issue, affecting 20% of Americans and approximately 35% of eastern Europeans. When overweight patients (BMI >25) are included, the prevalence of this problem in the United States approaches 56% (50). In women with endometrial CA, obesity is a comorbid condition in up to 40% of cases (50,51). Obesity has been associated with a two- to fivefold increase in endometrial CA risk in both pre- and postmenopausal women (50,52). A recent case-control study performed by the American Cancer Society reported that the cancer death rates were 62% higher for morbidly obese women compared to normal sized women. Specifically, the relative risk of CA-related mortality was significantly increased among obese women with breast CA (relative risk [RR] 1.63; 95% CI, 1.44 to 1.85) and colon CA (RR 1.33; 95% CI, 1.17 to 1.51). In patients with cervix and ovarian CA, a moderate (RR <2) yet significantly increased risk was observed. Uterine CA was most strongly associated with death: women with BMI >40 had an RR of CA-related mortality of 6.25 (95% CI, 3.75 to 10.42) (50,53). The results of recent epidemiologic studies have prompted the International Agency for Research on Cancer (IARC) to recommend avoidance of weight gain in order to minimize the risk of cancers of the colon, breast, and endometrium (50,54).

The relationship between obesity and endometrial carcinoma has been the most clearly elucidated. Progesterone deficiency, related to oligo- or anovulation, is one of the major risk factors for endometrial cancer in obese premenopausal women. The endometrium is chronically stimulated by unopposed E2, inducing neoplastic changes.

In both pre- and postmenopausal women, excess weight frequently results in increased androgen production, which decreases hepatic production of sex hormone binding protein (SHBG). Reducing SHBG increases bioavailable estrogens, including estrane. Obesity is also associated with greater bioavailability of estradiol (E2), but this effect is noted only among postmenopausal women. In premenopausal women, negative feedback of estradiol on FSH, a stimulator of ovarian estradiol synthesis and aromatase activity, helps maintain constant estradiol levels throughout the menstrual cycle. Peripheral conversion of androgens in premenopausal women is subsequently limited by decreased FSH and aromatase activity. Endometrial CA risk, therefore, does not appear to be directly related to plasma E2 levels prior to menopause.

Obesity may also induce insulin resistance, which can lead to elevated levels of IGF-1. Progestin deficiency, frequently accompanying obesity, can also lower levels of IGF binding protein (IGF-BP1), resulting in increased levels of IGF-1. The unregulated increase in serum IGF-1 provides a stimulus for continuous growth of the endometrium. Hyperinsulinemia can also lead to a reduction in SHBG. Hyperinsulinemia induces LH-mediated hypersecretion of ovarian androgens leading to oligoovulation and the polycystic ovary syndrome (PCOS), a disease process highly correlated with risk of endometrial cancer.

In postmenopausal obese women, peripheral conversion of androgens is an important source of serum estrogens. Elevated FSH levels typically present in postmenopausal women also contribute to the estrogenic state by the stimulation of aromatase activity. The increase in endogenous unopposed estrogens among obese postmenopausal women leads to the observed increased risk of developing endometrial carcinoma (50,55).

Perinatal E2 Levels

An association between perinatal exogenous estrogen exposure and an increased risk of CA in the offspring suggests that CA risk may be modulated *in utero*. The synthetic nonsteroidal estrogen diethylstilbestrol (DES) was administered during pregnancy to over two million women in the 1940s through the 1960s. Subsequently, DES was banned by the Food and Drug Administration (FDA) due to its teratogenic effects on limb bud development. Epidemiologic studies later revealed that there was a higher incidence of clear cell adenocarcinoma of the vagina and cervix in seemingly normal offspring of mothers who ingested DES prenatally (50,56,57). In a laboratory setting, DES has been found to induce gynecologic carcinomas in developmentally exposed rodents (50,58). Mice treated neonatally with DES on days 1 to 5 have a 90% to 95% incidence of endometrial carcinoma at 18 months of life (59). These data strongly implicate a direct role of estrogen exposure, even early in development, in gynecologic carcinogenesis.

The increased incidence of gynecologic CA associated with antenatal DES exposure would suggest that the developing fetus or neonate is particularly susceptible to the epigenetic effects of estrogen. Investigators recently evaluated the carcinogenic potential of neonatal exposure for another E2 compound, genistein, a naturally occurring phytoestrogen found in many soy products. In this study, treated mice received equivalent estrogenic doses of DES, genistein, or placebo on days 1 to 5. At 18 months, the incidence of uterine adenocarcinomas was 31% for DES and 35% for genistein, suggesting that estrogenic compounds other than DES may be carcinogenic if exposure occurs early during development (50,60).

A growing body of evidence suggests that elevated perinatal levels of endogenous estrogen also may lead to an increased risk of CA in the offspring (50,61). High birth weight, which is an indirect measurement of perinatal endogenous estrogen (50), is associated with an increased risk of breast CA in the newborn's adulthood (62). This increased breast CA risk is even more dramatic in twins, where the levels of perinatal estrogen are more pronounced compared to singleton pregnancies (50,63). Neonatal conditions, such as neonatal jaundice or prematurity, which are associated with increased estrogen, are also associated with a significantly increased risk of breast CA. In contrast, preeclampsia, a condition characterized by low E2 levels during pregnancy, is associated with a decreased risk of breast CA in the newborn's adulthood. Similar studies have been undertaken in evaluating possible associations between perinatal exposures and endometrial cancer later in adulthood. Using a Swedish population cohort of 11,000 singletons with obstetric and long-term medical follow-up, investigators found that women with higher birth weight had a 24% lower rate of endometrial cancer (64). Other investigators using similar Swedish cohorts and the data from the Nurses' Health Study have not found similar associations (65). Other studies have been undertaken in evaluating possible associations between perinatal exposures and endometrial cancer later in adulthood.

Exogenous Hormones and Modulation of CA Risk

Breast

Hormone Replacement Therapy

Women With No History of Breast CA. Multiple epidemiologic investigations have evaluated the relationship between hormone replacement therapy (HRT) and breast CA. In a meta-analysis of 51 studies of 52,705 women with breast CA and 108,411 women without breast CA, the Collaborative Group on Hormonal Factors in Breast Cancer (CGHFBC) determined that the risk of developing breast CA is increased in women using HRT, especially among women with >5 years of use (RR 1.3; 95% CI, 1.21 to 1.49). The cumulative incidence of breast CA was 45 per 1,000 women between the ages of 50 and 70, and use of HRT for >5 years was associated with an estimated cumulative excess of two breast CAs for every 1,000 users. The increased risk of breast CA risk associated with prolonged HRT was greater for women with low weight or BMI. Breast CAs diagnosed in women who had a history of HRT tended to be less advanced clinically compared to women with a negative history of use (66). The Breast Cancer Detection Demonstration Project, a cohort study with 46,355 postmenopausal women, 2,082 of whom were diagnosed with incident cases of breast CA, reported that women who had taken unopposed E2 had a 1.2-fold (95% CI, 1.0 to 1.4) increase in breast CA risk, while women taking combination E2 and progestin regimens had a 1.4-fold (95% CI, 1.1 to 1.8) increased risk. Breast CA risk was significantly elevated only in recent users with a BMI less than 24 (67). Finally, a recently reported case-control study involving 1,897 women with breast CA revealed that women using combination HRT had a statistically higher risk of breast CA (odds ratio [OR] 1.24; 95% CI, 1.07 to 1.45) than women taking unopposed E2 (OR 1.06; 95% CI, 0.97 to 1.15) (68).

The Women's Health Initiative (WHI), a randomized, double-blind, placebo-controlled trial, recently reported the interim analysis of 8,506 women who received continuous combination HRT (0.625 mg of conjugated equine estrogen plus 2.5 mg of medroxyprogesterone acetate) versus 8,102 women prescribed placebo. The Data and Safety Monitoring Board for the trial recommended early cessation of this trial arm secondary to the observed adverse effects. Interim results from the WHI study revealed that the risk of coronary heart disease (hazard ratio [HR] 1.29; 95% CI, 1.02 to 1.63), stroke (HR 1.41; 95% CI, 1.07 to 1.85), and pulmonary embolism (HR 2.13; 95% CI, 1.39 to 3.25) were all significantly elevated in patients receiving continuous combination HRT. The observed increased risk of breast CA (HR 1.26; 95% CI, 1.0 to 1.59) was similar to results from the aforementioned observational studies (69). A more detailed evaluation of the WHI data used a weighted Cox proportion hazards analysis in an effort to account for the lag in time required to achieve the full effects of the hormone on breast CA incidence. In this analysis, the rate of invasive breast CA was increased in patients receiving progestin plus estrogen (HR 1.24, weighted p <0.003). In addition, patients on HRT were diagnosed with larger tumors and at a more advanced stage when compared to patients who received placebo (70).

In the WHI trial, 10,739 postmenopausal women with prior hysterectomy were randomized to received 0.625 mg of conjugated equine estrogen (n = 5,310) versus placebo (n = 5,429). In the initial manuscript the WHI investigators reported that there was a possible reduction in breast CA incidence but the results did not reach statistical significance (HR 0.77; 95% CI, 0.59 to 1.01) (71). Further analysis of the data revealed that treatment with conjugated equine estrogen for 7 years does not appear to increase the incidence of breast CA (72).

Women With a History of Breast CA. There is apprehension among physicians to prescribe HRT to women with a positive personal history of breast CA. The *theoretical* concern has been that exogenous hormones may stimulate the growth of dormant microscopic disease and ultimately lead to a decreased disease-free interval and survival.

Several case-control studies have reported that the rates of breast CA recurrence among survivors taking HRT vary from 3% to 7% (73–75) and don't appear to significantly diverge from stage-specific population rates of recurrence. In a case-control study by DiSaia et al. (76), 41 sporadic breast CA patients taking HRT were matched to controls according to age, stage, and socioeconomic status. A majority of the patients had early-stage disease. Recurrences were detected in 12 patients with stage I disease, one with stage II, and two with stage III. No evidence of increased disease recurrence was noted among the patients receiving HRT. In a subsequent analysis by the same authors, 125 sporadic breast CA survivors receiving HRT were compared to 363 control subjects matched according to age at diagnosis, stage of breast CA, and year of diagnosis. The analysis revealed that the risk of death was lower among the breast CA patients receiving HRT (OR 0.28; 95% CI, 0.11 to 0.71) According to the American College of Obstetricians and Gynecologists, the projected absolute lifetime risk for non-HRT users is approximately 10 cases of breast CA per 100 women. This risk would increase to 12 cases per 100 women using unopposed E2 and 14 cases per 100 women using combined E2 and progestin (77). Data from a prospective, randomized trial is not available to answer this question.

Oral Contraceptives. Since their introduction in the 1960s, over 200 million women throughout the world have taken oral contraceptives (OCPs). The CGHFBC performed a meta-analysis of 54 epidemiologic studies on 53,297 women with breast CA and 100,239 women without breast CA. Women who were current users or had used OCPs in the previous 10 years were at an increased risk of breast CA (RR 1.24; 95% CI, 1.15 to 1.33). In women taking OCPs, the breast CAs that developed were less advanced than those diagnosed in women with no history of OCP use (78). Because the results from this meta-analysis reflected data from studies completed over the prior 25 years, the Women's Contraceptive and Reproductive Experiences (Women's CARE) study was initiated in an effort to provide a more contemporary analysis of the relationship between OCPs and breast CA risk (79). In this case-control study, a total of 4,574 women with breast CA and 4,682 controls were compared. The RR was 1.0 (95% CI, 0.8 to 1.3) for current OCP use and 0.9 (95% CI, 0.8 to 1.0) for previous use, suggesting that among women aged 35 to 64 years of age, current or former OCP use is not associated with a significantly increased risk of breast CA.

Women With BRCA Mutations. In the meta-analysis by the CGHFBC, the increased risk of breast CA associated with OCP use was *not* influenced by a family history of breast CA (78). However, a threefold increased risk of breast CA was observed among women taking OCPs who had a positive family history of breast CA. This increased risk was observed only in women using high estrogen potency formulations before 1975 (80). A subsequent matched case-control study by Narod et al. revealed that among *BRCA1* carriers, an increased risk of early-onset breast CA was evident in women who used OCPs prior to 1975 (OR 1.42; 95% CI, 1.17 to 1.75), used OCPs prior to age 30 (OR 1.29; 95% CI, 1.09 to 1.52), or who used OCPs for 5 or more years. Despite the increased risk associated with OCP usage among *BRCA1* carriers, an increased risk of breast CA was not observed among women with a *BRCA2* carrier status (81). In *BRCA1* carriers, the protective effects of OCPs against ovarian CA must be weighed against the possible increased risk of OCP use and breast CA.

Ovary

HRT

Women With No History of Ovarian CA. Recently, several well-designed case-control and cohort studies have evaluated the relationship between HRT and ovarian carcinoma. The American Cancer Society's Cancer Prevention Study II found that after accounting for OCP use and parity, postmenopausal women using HRT had higher rates of ovarian CA–related deaths compared to nonusers (RR 1.51; 95% CI, 1.16 to 1.96). The increased mortality risk was most notable for women using HRT for 10 or more years and persisted for up to 29 years after HRT cessation (82). This study is limited by the lack of information regarding estrogen and progestin potency. Another cohort study of 44,241 former participants in the Breast Cancer Detection Demonstration Project identified 329 women who developed ovarian CA during follow-up. Multivariant analysis revealed an increased association of estrogen-only HRT with ovarian CA (RR 1.6; 95% CI, 1.2 to 2.0) after accounting for age, menopause type, and OCP use (83). In contrast, an increased risk of ovarian CA was not noted among women who used estrogen and progestin. A Swedish case-controlled trial evaluated 655 case subjects with ovarian CA and 3,819 control subjects. An increased risk of ovarian CA was noted among women with a history of either estrogen (OR 1.43; 95% CI, 1.02 to 2.00) or estrogen with sequentially added progestins (OR 1.54; 95% CI, 1.15 to 2.05), particularly with hormone use exceeding 10 years. However, use of estrogen with continuously added progestin was *not* associated with an increased risk of ovarian CA when compared to nonusers (84). The latter two studies suggest that HRT regimens containing both E2 and progestin may not have the increased risk of ovarian CA observed with E2 therapy alone. However, the WHI recently identified, in women taking continuous combined HRT, an HR of 1.58 (95% CI, 0.77 to 3.24) for developing invasive ovarian carcinoma (85). The importance of the presence or absence of progesterone in HRT, as well as the type and potency, remains to be clearly elucidated.

Women With a History of Ovarian CA. Only one randomized, controlled clinical trial exists evaluating the risk of ovarian CA recurrence in patients receiving HRT. This study was designed to detect a 20% difference in survival between the two treatment groups. In this study, 130 patients less than 59 years of age with invasive ovarian CA were randomized to continuous E2 HRT or no supplementation. The median disease-free interval for women receiving HRT versus not was 34 months and 27 months, respectively, not reaching statistical significance (86).

OCPs. Multiple epidemiologic studies have revealed that OCPs are *not* a risk factor for ovarian CA, but rather a means of prevention. See below.

Endometrium

HRT

Women With No History of Endometrial CA. Multiple case-control and cohort studies also have suggested that the risk of endometrial CA is elevated among patients receiving unopposed estrogen. A meta-analysis of 30 studies indicated that the summary RR of endometrial CA was 2.7 for patients receiving unopposed estrogen (87). The use of unopposed estrogen has also been shown to be associated with the development of endometrial hyperplasia. In the Postmenopausal E2/Progestin Intervention (PEPI) trial, 875 patients were randomized to receive one of five regimens: (a) placebo; (b) conjugated equine E2 (CEE), 0.625 mg/day; (c) CEE, 0.625 mg/day plus continuous medroxyprogesterone (MPA), 2.5 mg/day; (d) CEE, 0.625 mg/day plus MPA, 10 mg for 12 days each month; or (e) CEE, 0.625 mg/day plus micronized progesterone (MP), 200 mg/day for 12 days per month. Patients receiving unopposed estrogen had a significantly increased risk of atypical adenomatous endometrial hyperplasia (34% vs 1%) (88).

The addition of progestin to HRT has been shown to eliminate the increased risk of hyperplasia associated with unopposed E2. Although progestins have been associated with the effective treatment of endometrial hyperplasia, the data supporting the protective effects of progestins in HRT are limited. Many of the initial HRT regimens combining progestin and estrogens utilized the progestin for 7 days a month (89). Subsequent studies have recommended prolongation of the progestin component to at least 10 days each month. A case-control study of 832 endometrial CA patients and 1,114 controls in Washington State revealed that patients using a combined regimen of estrogen combined with progestin (0.625 mg/day CEE, 2.5 mg/day MPA) had a significantly lower relative risk (RR 1.4; 95% CI, 1.0 to 1.9) of endometrial CA compared to patients who had taken unopposed estrogen (RR 4.0; 95% CI, 3.2 to 5.1). However, patients receiving less than 10 days of cyclic progestin had an RR that was much higher (RR 3.1; 95% CI, 1.7 to 5.7) than patients receiving 10 to 21 days of cyclic progestin (RR 1.3; 95% CI, 0.8 to 2.2). Patients using either regimen of cyclic combination HRT had an increased risk of endometrial CA when these regimens were taken for a duration exceeding 5 years (cyclic progestin <10 days per month; RR 3.7; 95% CI, 1.7 to 8.2; cyclic progestin 10 to 21 days each month, RR 2.5; 95% CI, 1.1 to 5.5) (90). Subsequent data from the same investigators suggested that use of a continuous progestin HRT regimen may actually be protective against endometrial CA (91). The largest case-control study of continuous HRT involved 79 case subjects and 88 control subjects and revealed that the relative risk of patients receiving continuous HRT was 1.07 (95% CI, 0.80 to 1.43) (92). Data from the WHI indicated that the HR for endometrioid endometrial cancer (EEC) was 0.81 (95% CI, 0.48 to 1.36) in patients receiving continuous HRT with average follow-up of 5.6 years (85).

There has recently been some suggestion that the degree of endometrial CA risk reduction may be dependent on the type of progestin used in the continuous HRT regimen. A Swedish case-control study found that patients with a continuous HRT involving testosterone-derived progestins (i.e., norhisterone, norhisterone acetate, levonorgestrel, lynestrenol) were associated with a lower RR of endometrial CA than those patients whose regimens involved progesterone-derived progestins (i.e., medroxyprogesterone) (93). Data from the Continuous Hormones as Replacement Therapy (CHART) study found no evidence of endometrial hyperplasia in participants who received norethindrone acetate (a testosterone derived progestin). In this clinical trial, 1,265 patients were randomized to placebo versus one of eight treatment groups involving either various doses of unopposed ethinyl estradiol or various combinations of ethinyl estradiol plus norethindrone. Approximately 1,134 endometrial biopsies were performed over a 2-year follow-up period among women who received the combination HRT regimen; 1,232 biopsies were performed in the women given unopposed E2. As the dose of unopposed ethinyl estradiol was increased, there were increased percentages of subjects with endometrial hyperplasia. There were no cases of hyperplasia noted among the subjects who received different doses of the testosterone-derived progestin norethindrone. The protective effect was noted even among patients randomized to receive doses of norethindrone as low as 0.2 mg (88). In contrast, the PEPI trial identified hyperplasia on a surveillance endometrial biopsy in 3 out of 339 patients who received E2 with a progesterone-derived progestin. Further studies are needed to determine the degree of endometrial CA risk influenced by the progestational activity of the progestin.

Women With a History of Endometrial CA. The use of E2 among patients with endometrial CA is controversial. *In vitro* treatment of Ishikawa endometrial CA cells with estrogen upregulates ER expression and augments growth in endometrial CA cells (94,95). However, *in vivo* growth of residual microscopic endometrial CA in patients has not been proven to date. Four retrospective cohort studies have evaluated patients with early-stage endometrial CA receiving E2 postoperatively. Creasman et al. evaluated 221 patients with stage I disease, of whom 47 received postoperative HRT and 174 did not (96). Patients receiving HRT were followed for a median of 26 months. Regression analysis revealed that there was no increased risk of recurrent disease associated with HRT use, even when adjusting for age, tumor grade, myometrial lymph node status, and peritoneal cytology. A subsequent study by Lee et al. (97) compared the outcomes of 44 low-risk endometrial CA patients (stage IA/IB G1/G2 disease) who received HRT following treatment to 62 patients who received no HRT. There were no recurrences observed among the endometrial CA patients receiving HRT for a median duration of 64 months. Investigators from the University of California, Irvine, have also failed to demonstrate an increased risk of recurrent disease associated with postoperative HRT (98). In the first study, investigators evaluated 123 women with surgical stage I and II endometrial CA. Sixty-one women received postoperative estrogen and the mean duration of follow-up was 40 months. The disease-free interval was not significantly shortened among the patients receiving E2 (98). The second study was a retrospective cohort study that involved 75 patients with stage I-III disease who received HRT (51% E2 only, 49% E2 with added progestin) postoperatively. This group of patients was then matched according to decade of age at diagnosis and stage of disease to a group of endometrial CA patients in the study cohort not receiving HRT. Both groups were comparable in terms of parity, tumor grade, depth of myometrial invasion, histology, lymph node status, surgical treatment, concurrent morbidities, and postoperative radiation. The patients receiving HRT were followed for a mean interval of 83 months and patients not receiving HRT were followed for a comparable interval of 69 months. Patients using HRT had a longer disease-free interval compared to non–hormone users. Among the 150 patients, only 8 patients had stage III disease (99).

In a Committee Opinion by the American College of Obstetricians and Gynecologists Committee of Gynecologic Practice, the members announced that "the decision to use HRT in these women [endometrial CA patients] should be individualized on the basis of potential benefit and risk to the patient" (100). The Gynecologic Oncology Group (GOG) initiated a multicenter randomized, controlled trial aimed at an enrollment of 2,100 patients with stage I and II endometrial CA. The study was closed after enrollment of 1,200 patients because the majority of the patients were low-risk with stage IA and G1 disease. In the absence of adequate enrollment of more intermediate-high risk early-stage endometrial CA patients, the number of recurrences used in the ad hoc sample size determination would be underestimated leading to suboptimal power for the clinical trial. With the closure of this GOG protocol, the safety of exogenous estrogen use in women who have undergone surgical management of endometrial CA may never be fully ascertained.

OCPs. Multiple epidemiologic studies have revealed that OCPs are *not* a risk factor for endometrial CA, but rather a means of prevention. See below.

Selective Estrogen Receptor Modulators. The anti-estrogen tamoxifen has been used in the adjuvant therapy of advanced breast CA for years and has recently been evaluated as a chemopreventive agent in patients at a high risk for developing this malignancy. Tamoxifen increases the risk of second primary malignancies at other sites. A randomized, controlled trial involving 2,729 women performed by the Stockholm Breast Cancer Study Group revealed that patients given tamoxifen (40 mg/d) had a nearly sixfold increased risk of endometrial CA and a threefold increased risk of gastrointestinal CA (50,101). These findings were confirmed in the National Surgical Adjuvant Breast and Bowel Project (NSABP). In this study, 2,843 patients with node negative invasive breast CA were randomized to receive tamoxifen (40 mg/d) or placebo. The RR of endometrial CA in patients receiving tamoxifen was 7.5 (CI, 1.7 to 32.7) (102) compared to placebo (50). When the population-based rates of endometrial CA from another NSABP trial (B-06), and data from the Surveillance, Epidemiology, and End Results (SEER) Program were used in the calculation of risk, the RR of endometrial CA associated with tamoxifen use was 2.3 and 2.2, respectively. In addition, the average annual HR during follow-up was only 1.6 out of 1,000 in the group receiving tamoxifen (50,102), suggesting that routine screening would not be cost-effective.

Other selective estrogen receptor modulators (SERMs) are being evaluated as adjuvant treatment for breast CA in an attempt to avoid the increased risk of secondary malignancies, while maintaining the same or greater effectiveness. Results from the Multiple Outcomes of Raloxifene Evaluation (MORE) study indicate that patients receiving raloxifene had a lower incidence of breast CA without any increase in endometrial CA risk (50,103). However, the primary endpoint in this investigation was risk reduction of fracture in postmenopausal women with osteoporosis. In the National Surgical Adjuvant Breast and Bowel Project Study of Tamoxifen and Raloxifene (STAR) P-2 trial, investigators found that raloxifene is as effective as tamoxifen in reducing the risk of invasive breast cancer. Although the overall risk of developing endometrial cancer was similar in patients on raloxifene versus tamoxifen (RR 0.62; 95% CI, 0.35 to 1.08), the incidence of hyperplasia was less often found in the raloxifene group (RR 0.16; 95% CI, 0.09 to 0.29) (104).

Several other SERMs are under investigation. The results of ongoing clinical trials will confirm these preliminary findings and establish the applicability of this contemporary generation of SERMs.

Colon

HRT. Multiple epidemiologic studies have revealed that HRT is *not* a risk factor for colon CA, but rather protects against this malignancy. See below.

OCPs. Multiple epidemiologic studies have revealed that OCPs are *not* a risk factor for colon CA, but rather protect against this malignancy. See below.

SERMs. *In vitro* evidence has revealed that both tamoxifen and raloxifene are effective in reducing cell proliferation and viability of colon CA cell lines, suggesting a possible application in the prevention of colon CA (105). Unfortunately, the available epidemiologic evidence is limited and controversial regarding the issue of tamoxifen's effects on colorectal CA risk. A meta-analysis by the Stockholm Breast Cancer Study Group analyzed 4,914 postmenopausal women participating in one of three Scandinavian clinical trials evaluating adjuvant tamoxifen: the

Stockholm Trial, the Danish Breast Cancer Group Trial, and the South-Swedish Trial (101). The joint analysis of these three trials revealed that adjuvant tamoxifen therapy in breast CA patients increased the risk of colorectal CAs (RR 1.9; 95% CI, 1.1 to 1.3) (101). In contrast, findings from the NSABP B-14 and the SEER Program (106) have failed to confirm an increased risk of colorectal CA among patients receiving adjuvant tamoxifen therapy. Additional epidemiologic trials are needed to resolve the issue of adjuvant tamoxifen therapy and the risk of secondary sporadic colorectal CAs.

Although some epidemiologic evidence suggests that tamoxifen may be associated with an increased risk of sporadic colorectal CA, SERMs have been used in the treatment of desmoid tumors associated with hereditary colorectal CA. Colorectal CA includes two main mechanisms of inheritance: familial adenomatous polyposis (FAP) and hereditary nonpolyposis colorectal CA (HNPCC). Desmoid tumors are fibroaponeurotic tumors that occur rarely in the general population but can be found in 12% to 17% of patients with FAP (107). Tamoxifen has been shown to have growth inhibition in desmoid tumor cell lines in an E2-independent mechanism (108). According to the practice guidelines of the Standard Task Force of Colon and Rectal Surgeons, high-dose tamoxifen (120 mg/day) and other SERMs may be used in the treatment of aggressive desmoid tumors. This recommendation is weak (level III) and based on limited descriptive European case series (109,110). The use of tamoxifen in the prevention or treatment of primary colorectal CA is not advocated.

Phytoestrogens. Increased rates of breast, colon, ovarian, and endometrial CA are found in Western societies. Phyto-E2s are possible dietary mediators of increased CA risk that are subdivided into two groups: isoflavonoids and lignans. Isoflavonoids are compounds with inherent E2-ic activity that can lead to low IGF expression and inhibition of aromatase and growth factors resulting in a possible chemoprotective effective in the breast. Lignans are compounds formed from plant lignan precursors by intestinal microflora. Both isoflavonoids and lignans are found in foods such as whole grain rye bread, soybeans, and red clover. Studies suggest that the development period during which the isoflavonoid is ingested is important in modulation of future CA risk. Ingestion of soy before or during adolescence may decrease the risk of future breast CA. However, there is no convincing evidence indicating that soy or other isoflavonoids are protective against breast CA or colon CA if ingested during adulthood (50,111). There is a paucity of data regarding the association between isoflavonoids and other CAs affecting women. A case-control study using a Hawaiian group revealed that the high consumption of soy products in adults significantly decreased the risk of endometrial CA even after accounting for confounding influences (50,112). Large, population-based studies are needed to determine the effects of isoflavonoids on specific CA risk, particularly since they are becoming a more common component of the American diet.

Consumption of whole grain products, berries, fruits, and vegetables can stimulate production of lignans, which can be indirectly measured via urinary enterolactone. Although women with breast CA have significantly lower levels of urinary enterolactone, it is unknown whether higher levels of enterolactone are protective against breast CA or whether they are a marker for an unknown chemoprotective compound associated with a healthier diet. High enterolactone production has been associated with inhibition of colon CA in animal models, but elevated levels have not been confirmed to be protective against colon CA in humans (50,111). In contrast, obesity as well as increased dietary fat intake is associated with decreased levels of urinary lignans, suggesting that the increased risk of CA associated with obesity may be in part related to lignan production.

HORMONES AND THE PREVENTION OF HUMAN CANCERS

Chemoprevention can be defined as the use of specific natural or synthetic chemical agents to reverse, suppress, or prevent the progression toward malignancies. Human carcinogenesis proceeds through multiple discernible stages of molecular and cellular alterations, thus providing the scientific rationale for clinical CA chemoprevention. The necessary requirements for evaluation of chemoprevention include (a) identification of high-risk individuals based on family history and/or genetic mutations; (b) identification of putative surrogate endpoints or biomarkers for CA; and (c) the possibility that relatively nontoxic agents may decrease the risk of a given malignancy. Prospective clinical trials are mandatory for evaluating potential strategies for preventing human malignancies.

Breast Cancer Chemoprevention

SERMs

Reducing the incidence of breast CA has the potential to provide a major impact on the morbidity of the disease and its treatment, cost to the individual and to society, and overall CA mortality. Epidemiologic studies indicate that E2-mediated events play a role in the development of breast CA. Tamoxifen, a SERM, has been utilized as a chemopreventive agent for breast CA in four randomized, prospective, placebo-controlled clinical trials. Raloxifene, a second-generation SERM, was investigated in the MORE trial, in which the primary endpoint was risk reduction of fracture in postmenopausal women with osteoporosis; the incidence of breast CA was a secondary endpoint. These five studies are reviewed and summarized below.

Breast Cancer Prevention Trial. In 1992, the National Cancer Institute in collaboration with the NSABP initiated the Breast Cancer Prevention Trial (BCPT, P-1) (113). The primary goal was to determine whether tamoxifen administered for 5 years prevented breast CA in women at high risk, including women 60 years or older, women 35 to 59 with a 5-year predicted risk of breast CA of at least 1.66%, or women who had a history of lobular carcinoma *in situ* (LCIS). Risk was estimated using the Gail model (114). Each of the 13,388 women enrolled was randomly assigned to receive tamoxifen 20 mg/day or placebo. The median follow-up time was 54.6 months, with 175 cases of invasive breast CA in the placebo group compared with 89 in the tamoxifen group (RR 0.51; 95% CI, 0.39 to 0.66; $P < 0.00001$). Tamoxifen reduced the incidence of ER+ tumors by 69%, but there was no difference in the incidence of ER− tumors.

Italian Tamoxifen Prevention Study. This double-blind, placebo-controlled, randomized trial began recruitment in October 1992 and ended in July 1997, and included healthy women aged 35 to 70 years of age (115). The trialist and data-monitoring committee ended recruitment because 26% of women dropped out of this study; 5,408 women were randomized to receive tamoxifen 20 mg/day or placebo for 5 years. Women were allowed to take HRT. The primary endpoints were reduction in the frequency and mortality of breast CA. At a median follow-up of 46 months, 19 CAs were diagnosed in the tamoxifen arm and 22 among women in the placebo arm ($P = 0.6$). An update was reported in 2002 (116). At 81.2 months of follow-up, 45 of 2,708 women receiving placebo and 34 of 2,700 women receiving tamoxifen developed breast CA (OR 0.76; 95% CI, 0.47 to 1.60). The difference was not statistically significant ($P = 0.215$). Among women who used HRT either at baseline or during the study, breast CA was diagnosed in 17 of 791 receiving placebo and six of 793 receiving tamoxifen ($P = 0.022$).

Royal Marsden Hospital Chemoprevention Trial. This trial was initiated in 1986 as a preliminary pilot study for the International Breast Cancer Intervention Study (IBIS-I) (117). The aim of this study was to assess whether tamoxifen would prevent breast CA in healthy women at increased risk for the disease based on family history only. Each participant had at least one first-degree relative under the age of 50 with breast CA, one first-degree relative with bilateral breast CA, or one affected first-degree relative of any age and another affected first-degree or second-degree relative. Women were allowed to take HRT during this study. Randomization of 2,494 women between the ages of 30 and 70 to tamoxifen 20 mg/day or placebo occurred. The median follow-up was 70 months and 2,471 of the women were analyzed. The frequency of breast CA was the same for women receiving tamoxifen and placebo (tamoxifen = 34, placebo = 36; RR 1.06; 95% CI, 0.7 to 1.7), and there appeared to be no interaction between the use of HRT and the effect of tamoxifen on breast CA occurrence. An update of this trial reported 75 cases of breast CA in the placebo group compared with 62 in the tamoxifen group (OR 0.83; 95% CI, 0.58 to 1.16) (118,119).

International Breast Cancer Intervention Study. Randomization occurred to tamoxifen 20 mg/day or placebo for 7,152 women, aged 35 to 70 years and at high risk for breast CA (120). Eligible women had risk factors for breast CA indicating at least a twofold relative risk among those aged 45 to 70 years, a fourfold relative risk among those aged 40 to 44 years, and a tenfold relative risk among those aged 35 to 39 years. The women enrolled in this study were at moderately increased risk of developing breast CA, with 60% of the study cohort having a 10-year risk ranging from 5% to 10%. The IBIS-I investigators used a model to predict the absolute 10-year risk of developing breast CA, but the details of their model have not been published. Use of HRT was permitted, and approximately 40% of women used such therapy at some point during the trial. The primary endpoint was the incidence of breast CA, including ductal carcinoma *in situ* (DCIS). At a median follow-up of 50 months (7,139 women analyzed), 69 women in the tamoxifen group compared to 101 women in the placebo group developed breast CA (overall 32% reduction in breast CA rate; 95% CI, 8 to 50; $P = 0.01$). The risk of developing ER+ invasive tumors was reduced by 31%, but there was no reduction in the risk of ER− tumors. There was no difference in the incidence of breast carcinoma among women taking HRT during the study. However, among women who received HRT before the trial, 21 cases of breast CA developed in the placebo group and nine in the tamoxifen group (OR 0.43; 95% CI, 0.80 to 6.06).

Multiple Outcome of Raloxifene Evaluation. The MORE study was a multicenter, randomized, double-blind trial, raloxifene 60 or 120 mg/day or placebo for 3 years, with the primary endpoint of rate of fracture in postmenopausal women with osteoporosis (121). Breast CA incidence was a secondary endpoint. A total of 7,705 women, at least 2 years postmenopausal and no older than 80 years of age, were enrolled. Women who were taking E2 during the previous 6 months were excluded, and 12.3% of women reported a family history of breast CA. There were 27 cases of invasive breast CA in the placebo group compared to 13 in the raloxifene group (RR 0.24; 95% CI, 0.13 to 0.44; $P < 0.001$). There was no difference in breast CA incidence between the two doses of raloxifene. Raloxifene reduced the risk of invasive ER+ breast CA by 90% (RR 0.10; 95% CI, 0.04 to 0.24), but did not reduce the risk of ER− breast CA. Four-year results from this study have now been reported (122). These results, with extension to 4 years after initiation of the trial, are consistent with the results based on the 3-year follow-up. The MORE trial was not designed to evaluate invasive breast CA as a primary endpoint. In addition, women in this trial were at lower risk of breast CA compared with women in the BCPT. Further study of raloxifene is indicated, and at this time this SERM cannot be recommended for chemoprevention outside of a clinical trial.

Summary of the Tamoxifen Chemoprevention Trials. The Royal Marsden and Italian studies failed to confirm the results of the BCPT, a reduction in the incidence of ER+ breast carcinoma in women taking tamoxifen. An updated report from the Italian Tamoxifen Prevention Study found a reduction in the incidence of ER+ breast CA among a subgroup of women. The results of the IBIS-I study confirmed that tamoxifen reduces the risk of breast CA. Numerous methodologic differences exist between the BCPT and European trials in trial design, trial implementation, and characteristics of the women studied. It is probable that both the Royal Marsden and Italian trials would fail to detect an overall effect for tamoxifen among the populations studied. Both of these trials were statistically less powerful and smaller than the BCPT, with fewer person-years of follow-up and fewer reported events. As well, the risk of breast CA among women in these trials was lower than the BCPT. The U.S. FDA approved the use of tamoxifen for breast CA risk reduction in women aged 35 years or older, with a 5-year risk of 1.66% or greater.

In January 2003, Cuzick et al. (119) published an overview of the above breast CA chemoprevention trials. The results are summarized in Figure 17.3. Tamoxifen reduced the incidence of ER+ breast CAs by 48% (95% CI, 36 to 58; $P < 0.0001$), with no reduction in the incidence of ER− breast CAs. Age had no effect on the degree of breast CA reduction. The rates of endometrial CA increased in all the tamoxifen prevention trials (consensus RR 2.4; 95% CI, 1.5 to 4; $P = 0.0005$); no increase in endometrial CA was observed with the use of raloxifene. Venous thromboembolic events were increased in all the tamoxifen prevention studies (RR 1.9; 95% CI, 1.4 to 2.6; $P < 0.0001$), with similar results seen in the MORE study. Overall, there was no effect on all-cause mortality in the tamoxifen prevention trials (HR 0.90; 95% CI, 0.70 to 1.17; $P = 0.44$). The authors concluded that the evidence clearly shows that tamoxifen can reduce the risk of ER+ breast CA.

The STAR trial (Study of Tamoxifen and Raloxifene), powered to demonstrate superior efficacy or equivalence of either tamoxifen (20 mg/day) or raloxifene (60 mg/day) in reducing the incidence of primary breast CA, was opened to accrual on July 1, 1999. The trial enrolled 19,747 women and data are available for 19,471 of them; 9,726 women in the tamoxifen arm and 9,745 women in the raloxifene arm. All women had a projected 5-year risk of developing breast CA of 1.66% or higher as determined by the Gail model. Eligible women included postmenopausal women 35 years or older with no prior history of invasive breast CA or DCIS. Postmenopausal women with a history of LCIS who are aged 35 years or older were also eligible. The number of invasive breast cancers was statistically equivalent (167 in the raloxifene group and 163 in the tamoxifen group). Both drugs reduced the risk of invasive breast cancer by around 50 percent.

Aromatase Inhibitors

Aromatase inhibitors (AIs) are being considered for use in breast CA chemoprevention. In contrast to SERMs, which are competitive inhibitors of E2 at its receptor, AIs suppress plasma E2 levels by inhibiting or inactivating aromatase, the enzyme responsible for the synthesis of E2s from androgenic substrates. This class of compounds has effectively challenged tamoxifen for use as adjuvant therapy in postmenopausal women with ER+ breast CAs, who constitute the majority of patients with breast CA. Evaluating women with early-stage

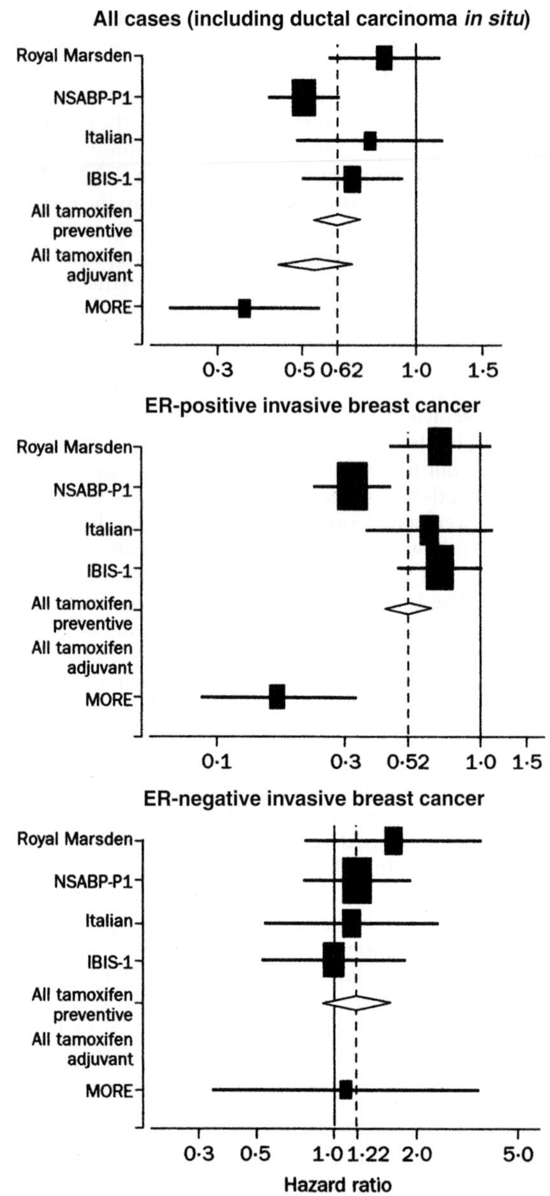

FIGURE 17.3. Incidence of breast CA. Note that the scale for the hazard ratio on the horizontal axis is different for each section of the figure. *Source:* Reprinted with permission from Cuzick J, Powles T, Veronesi U, et al. Overview of the main outcomes in breast-cancer prevention trials. *Lancet* 2003;361:296–300.

breast CA, the ATAC (Arimidex, Tamoxifen Alone or in Combination) Trialists' Group found that the incidence of contralateral invasive breast CA was lower in those receiving the third-generation AI (anastrozole [Arimidex]), when compared to tamoxifen, after a median of 33 months of follow-up (see below). By extrapolation, Arimidex might reduce the early incidence of breast CA to an even greater extent than tamoxifen and thus have potential in breast CA chemoprevention (116,123). The long-term effects of profound E2 suppression in postmenopausal women are unknown, and careful monitoring for bone demineralization and other potential problems is essential as the role of AIs evolves.

Prophylactic Oophorectomy

The potential role for oophorectomy as *chemoprevention* (decreased E2 levels) for breast CA in premenopausal women is an area of active investigation. In genetically uncharacterized premenopausal women, oophorectomy is associated with a 50% reduction in breast CA incidence, but also incurs the associated negative effects of a surgically induced early menopause (124,125). In this patient population, where the overall incidence of breast CA is one in eight, it is not standard practice to offer oophorectomy for breast CA prevention. However, in premenopausal women with germ-line *BRCA1* and *BRCA2* mutations, the cumulative lifetime risk (to 70 years of age) of invasive breast CA is 60% to 85%, allowing for more serious consideration for prophylactic oophorectomy as a *chemoprevention*. The prevalence of germ-line *BRCA1* or *BRCA2* in the general population is 0.1% to 0.2%, contributing to a small fraction of all cases of breast CA, but as many as 10% of cases diagnosed in women younger than 40 years of age and approximately 75% of familial cases. Two recent publications support the practice of recommending prophylactic oophorectomy after the completion of childbearing in premenopausal women (126,127). Kauff et al., in a prospective study, reported on 170 carriers of *BRCA* mutations with a mean follow-up of 24.2 months, 98 of whom underwent prophylactic salpingo-oophorectomy (126). A 70% risk reduction in breast CA incidence was identified. Rebbeck et al., in a multicenter retrospective analysis, reported on 551 carriers of *BRCA* mutations with 11 years of follow-up, 259 of whom underwent a prophylactic salpingo-oophorectomy. A 53% risk reduction in breast CA incidence was identified (127). The reduced risk of a subsequent diagnosis of breast CA in women with *BRCA* mutations, after salpingo-oophorectomy, confirms an earlier report of a 47% reduction in this patient population (128).

Phytochemicals

Phytochemicals with potential anti-CA properties span a wide range of chemical types and activities. Their presence, concentration, and bioavailability in any of thousands of plant species used by humans is variably and incompletely documented. Several studies have specifically examined the effects of vegetable and fruit intake on breast CA risk. These studies suggest a protective effect of vegetable intake, particularly those rich in carotenoids. Beta-carotene intake has been associated with lower breast CA risk in several studies (129–131). High dietary fiber intake has also been associated with a lower risk of breast CA (132). The multiplicity of phytochemical actions at different sites in the process of tumorigenesis complicates the investigative effort needed for the development of chemopreventive agents from this class of compounds.

Endometrial Cancer Chemoprevention

Chemoprevention strategies for endometroid endometrial cancer (EEC) have been based on the observation that exposure to E2 with insufficient progestational stimulation predisposes women to EEC and its precursor lesion, atypical endometrial hyperplasia. While marked obesity, use of exogenous E2, early menarche, and diabetes have been identified as risk factors for the development of EEC, only early menarche has been associated with serous carcinoma, as well as its precursor lesion, endometrial intraepithelial carcinoma (EIC) (133). This observation, as well as other investigational work, supports the existence of a dualistic model for endometrial carcinogenesis, where atypical endometrial hyperplasia and EEC are E2 related and EIC and serous carcinoma are E2 unrelated. Further delineation of E2-independent pathways of endometrial carcinogenesis will be necessary to develop chemoprevention strategies for serous carcinoma, which accounts for a minority of endometrial carcinomas, but a disproportionate number of endometrial CA deaths. Chemoprevention strategies for EEC, because of its clear association with E2, have been more easily identified, and are described below.

Continuous Combined HRT

Premature termination of one comparison (continuous combined HRT: daily conjugated equine E2 0.625 mg and medroxyprogesterone acetate 2.5 mg) in the WHI primary prevention trial occurred because cardiovascular disease and breast CA were increased, recognizing that colorectal CA, endometrial CA, and osteoporotic fractures were reduced (134). The reduction seen in the incidence of EEC with continuous HRT is in agreement with case-control studies that have documented a reduction in incidence of this malignancy in women taking continuous combined HRT (90,91,93).

OCPs

There is substantial evidence that ever-use of OCPs reduces the risk of EEC by approximately 50% (135). Numerous epidemiologic studies demonstrate that the reduced risk depends on the duration of OCP use. The risk is reduced by 20% with 1 year of use, 40% with 2 years of use, and 60% with 4 or more years of use (136).

A preliminary analysis of the Centers for Disease Control and Prevention (CDC) Cancer and Steroid Hormone (CASH) study attempted to characterize the protective effect of specific OCP formulations on EEC risk by comparing 187 endometrial CA cases with 1,320 controls (137). The CASH study determined that continuous OCP formulations provided protective effects (RR 0.4; 95% CI, 0.2 to 0.9) while sequential OCPs did not (RR 2.1; 95% CI, 0.8 to 5.8). Similarly, in the World Health Organization (WHO) Collaborative Study of Neoplasia and Steroid Contraceptives, 132 cases of EEC and 835 matched controls were evaluated to determine the protective effects of OCPs on endometrial CA. Investigators found that the risk of EEC was decreased among women who had a history of combination OCP use (OR 0.53; 95% CI, 0.29 to 0.97) (138). In both the CASH and the initial WHO study, combination OCP formulations were not categorized according to the potency of estrogen and progestin, thereby preventing an assessment of the effects on EEC risk according to the potency of the hormonal components.

In order to better understand the protective effects of combination OCPs, two case-control studies have attempted to evaluate progestin and estrogen potency of OCP formulations in relation to EEC risk. Following further enrollment of patients in the WHO Collaborative Study of Neoplasia and Steroid Contraceptives, investigators reported an analysis of 220 cases of EEC and 1,537 controls (139). In this study, a lower risk of EEC was observed with high progestin potency OCP formulations compared with low progestin potency. Although the number of patients using high potency progestin was very small in this study, the results suggested that high progestin potency OCP formulations could be more protective against EEC. A second case-control study evaluated 316 cases and 501 controls from women in the King or Pierce counties of Washington. Among these women, the relative risk for women who had used a high progestin potency OCP (RR 0.3; 95% CI, 0.1 to 0.9) was as low as the relative risk for women using a low potency progestin (RR 0.2; 95% CI, 0.1 to 0.8) (50). These results did not find a potency-dependent protective effect and suggested that the progestin potency was adequate to achieve a protective effect against endometrial CA in most combination OCP formulations. The methods of classifying progestin potency were the same in both the WHO study and the Washington State study, thereby eliminating differences in classification as a reason for the different findings from these two studies. Details regarding the specific OCPs taken by case and control subjects were not reported in the Washington State study. The OCP formulations used in the second WHO study contained progestins that are no longer used in OCPs marketed in the United States. A third case-control study using data from the CASH study included 434 endometrial CA cases and 2,557 control subjects. Overall, high potency OCPs did not confer more protection than low potency OCPs. However, among women with a BMI >22.1 kg/m^2, those who used high potency progestin potency OCPs had a lower risk of endometrial cancer than those who used low potency OCPs (OR 0.31; 95% CI, 0.11 to 0.92) while those with a BMI <22.1 kg/m^2 did not (OR, 1.36; 95% CI, 0.39 to 4.70) (140). The small number of cases that were overweight (BMI >25 kg/m^2) or obese (BMI >30 kg/m^2) prevented an analysis with sufficient power to detect a statistically significant modifying effect of overweight status or obesity on the relationship between progestin potency and endometrial CA risk. However, these findings suggest that high potency OCPs may be associated with a greater protective effect than low potency OCPs among women with a larger BMI who are at the greatest risk of endometrial CA.

Intrauterine Devices

Seven studies have reported the relationship between previous copper or nonmedicated intrauterine device (IUD) use and endometrial CA (141–147). In all but one study, previous IUD use was associated with a decreased risk of EEC. The one study where this relationship was not validated was based on research in China, where the steel ring IUD was utilized, suggesting that this type of IUD is not protective against this malignancy (146). The landmark CASH study of the CDC was one of the studies to report significant protection against EEC (141). The majority of the articles reported subgroup analyses regarding factors such as type of IUD and duration/timing of use. In general, no consistent pattern emerged from the articles to suggest that length or timing of use, or type of IUD was associated with an increase or decrease in the risk of EEC (148).

The levonorgestrel-releasing IUD was investigated by Gardner et al. in women taking tamoxifen as adjuvant therapy for breast CA (149). This preliminary investigation, which included 122 women, randomized 64 patients to the IUD group and 58 patients to the no-IUD group. The authors did an outpatient hysteroscopic assessment with endometrial sampling at entry and after 12 months. A uniform decidual response was seen in all women with the IUD in place. Similar histologic patterns were identified in both groups at baseline and after 12 months. A statement on the effect of this device on the incidence of EEC in women taking tamoxifen cannot be made, but warrants further prospective evaluation.

Phytochemicals

The effect of dietary phytochemical consumption on endometrial CA risk is not clearly delineated. Levi et al. found a strong negative association between beta-carotene and vitamin C intake and endometrial carcinoma among Swiss women, but no clear effect was seen in similar studies in China and the United States (150–152). Barbone et al. demonstrated a protective effect of carotene intake on endometrial CA (153). Zheng et al. found a weak negative correlation between endometrial CA and plant food intake in the Iowa Women's Health Study (154). In an analysis of phytoestrogen (i.e., isoflavones, coumestans, and lignans) consumption and endometrial CA risk, investigators found that a lower risk was associated with increased intake. Obese postmenopausal women consuming relatively low amounts of phytoestrogens had the highest risk of endometrial cancer (OR 6.9; 95% CI, 3.3 to 14.5) compared with nonobese postmenopausal women consuming high amounts of isoflavones (155). As is the case with breast CA, further investigative efforts are necessary to establish the role of phytochemicals in the prevention of endometrial CA.

Ovarian Cancer Chemoprevention

Although efforts to improve the survival of ovarian CA patients continue to focus on the development of more effective systemic therapies, the prevention of ovarian CA is an area of increasing interest. As is the case with breast CA, assessment of prevention efforts must be analyzed by genetic predisposition. In genetically uncharacterized U.S. women, the lifetime risk of developing ovarian CA is approximately 1.5%. *BRCA1* mutations increase the risk to 30% to 60%, while women who harbor a mutant *BRCA2* gene have an estimated risk of 10% to 30% (156). Precancerous lesions have not been well defined for ovarian CA, although phenotypic changes have recently been described (157). Future chemoprevention trials in ovarian CA have the potential to utilize biochemical markers of transformation, including cell cycle progression and apoptosis, as surrogate endpoint markers (158,159). Although hysterectomy alone, as well as tubal ligation, has been associated with a decreased risk of developing ovarian CA, this review will focus on *chemo*prevention.

OCPs

The ability of OCPs to reduce the risk of ovarian CA has been extensively studied and it is estimated that there is an overall reduction in risk approximating 40% (135). The adjusted odds ratio for *ever-use* of OCPs has consistently been shown to be between 0.6 and 0.7 (160–162). The degree of protection and the length of protection appear to be associated with the duration of OCP usage. Prolonged risk reduction has been reported when OCPs are used longer than 4 to 6 years, and minimal benefit has been observed if utilization is restricted to a period of 6 months to 2 years (163–166). One of the largest case-control studies to date is the CDC CASH study. In this study, 546 women with ovarian CA and 4,228 control subjects from eight population-based CA registries were compared. Women with a history of OCP use had a 40% reduced risk of epithelial ovarian CA (RR 0.6; 95% CI, 0.5 to 0.7) when compared to women with no history of OCP use. This protective effect was evident with as little as 3 months of OCP use and continued for up to 15 years following discontinuation of OCP use. OCP-mediated risk reduction was independent of the histologic type of ovarian CA (167).

It has been estimated that more than half of all ovarian CAs in the United States could be prevented by OCP usage for at least 4 to 5 years (161,162,168). The protective effect of OCPs appears to be consistent across races as John et al. demonstrated a reduction in risk of 0.6 in African American women with OCP use of 6 years or more (169). The estrogen/progestin content of any particular OCP and how it relates to protection against ovarian carcinoma needs further investigation. Ness et al. demonstrated identical risk reduction for OCPs with high-estrogen/high-progesterone content when compared with low-estrogen/low-progesterone content pills (170). Schildkraut et al., in an observational study, recently reported that low-progesterone OCP formulations were associated with a significantly higher risk of ovarian CA when compared with high-progesterone potency OCP formulations (171).

The lifetime risk of ovarian CA is approximately 45% in *BRCA1* carriers and 25% among *BRCA2* carriers (172). In women carrying *BRCA1* or -*2* mutations, Modan et al. concluded that OCPs did not protect against ovarian CA in Israeli Jewish women. However, Narod et al. showed that the use of OCPs in Jewish and non-Jewish women with *BRCA* mutations was strongly protective against this malignancy, with an odds ratio of 0.44 (95% CI, 0.28 to 0.68) (173,174). Important differences exist between the two studies, most notably that the controls in the Narod et al. study were all mutation carriers, while in the Modan et al. study only 1.7% of the controls carried the mutation. The use of OCP as a chemopreventive agent against ovarian CA should be considered in *BRCA* carriers.

Little is known about the mechanism of the protective effect of OCPs against ovarian CA, although it has been postulated that a major mechanism of OCP protection relates to a decrease in ovulatory cycles. There is data to suggest that an increased rate of apoptosis in aberrant epithelial cells secondary to the progestational component may also play an important role. Recently, Rodriguez et al. examined the effect on ovarian epithelium of levonorgesterol in 130 ovulatory macaque monkeys (175). These authors demonstrated significantly increased apoptotic cell counts in the ovarian epithelium of animals exposed to progesterone, leading to the hypothesis that progestin-induced apoptosis of the ovarian epithelium is responsible for the chemopreventive effect of OCPs.

Colon Cancer Chemoprevention

Colorectal CA is the fourth most common incident CA and the second most common cause of CA death in the United States. In 2000, there were an estimated 50,400 new cases of colon CA and 16,200 cases of rectal CA diagnosed in U.S. women; approximately 24,600 and 3,900 women died from these disorders, respectively (176).

HRT

Two recent meta-analyses have calculated an approximate one-third reduction in risk of *colon* CA among current or recent users of HRT, compared with about a 10% to 20% reduction among ever-users versus never-users of HRT (177,178). Although Nanda et al. determined that *rectal* CA was not related to HRT usage, Grodstein et al. determined a reduction in risk for ever-users versus never-users (RR 0.81; 95% CI, 0.72 to 0.92). Both meta-analyses are limited by lack of consistent and accurate reporting on type of HRT, as well as lack of control for potential confounders, such as diet, site of CA, family history, or screening. Adenomatous polyps precede colorectal CAs by a decade or more; thus any association between their presence and HRT is of obvious interest. Two case-control studies have found a protective effect of HRT on the development of adenomatous polyps (179,180). The prospective Nurses' Health Study reported a decreased risk of large adenomatous polyps for current users (RR 0.74; 95% CI, 0.55 to 0.99), whereas there was no association between small adenomatous polyps and HRT (181).

The WHI, a randomized, controlled primary prevention trial in which 16,608 postmenopausal women aged 50 to 79 years with an intact uterus at baseline were recruited by 40 U.S. clinical centers in 1993 to 1998, confirmed what other observational studies have suggested: a reduction in the incidence of colorectal CA in those women taking combined estrogen and progesterone therapy. In 8,506 women prescribed estrogen and progesterone, with a placebo control group of 8,102 women, a hazard ratio of 0.63 with a nominal 95% CI of 0.43 to 0.92 was observed. Colorectal CA rates were reduced by 37% (10 vs 16 per 10,000 person-years) (134,181).

There are several hypotheses regarding a protective effect of HRT on the risk of colorectal CA, including alteration of the predominant ER isoform, as well as E2's ability to decrease production of secondary bile acids.

OCPs

The relationship between OCPs and colorectal CA has not been clearly delineated. Recently, a large case-control study was conducted in northern Italy between the years 1985 and 1992, with 709 cases of colorectal CA and 992 control subjects (182). Ever-use of OCPs versus never-use through use of a multiple logistic regression was associated with a reduced risk of colorectal CA (RR 0.58; 95% CI, 0.36 to 0.92). Further, there was a suggestion that duration of use (i.e., more than 2 years) was associated with increased protection. More recently, the Nurses' Health Study cohort identified 502 cases of colorectal CA among participants between 1980 and 1992 (183). Among women using OCPs, use for 6 or greater years was associated with a 40% reduction in risk of colorectal CA (RR 0.60; 95% CI, 0.40 to 0.89). The trend for the duration effect was statistically significant ($P = 0.02$). Several smaller studies, all with serious limitations in study design and/or execution, have reported varying results regarding the relationship between OCPs and colorectal CA.

HORMONES AND THE TREATMENT OF HUMAN CANCERS

Whereas the role of hormones in the treatment of human malignancies has been most extensively examined in the management of breast carcinoma, the potential to exploit hormone-signaling pathways in the management of other malignancies, affecting both men and women, is rapidly becoming a reality. As our understanding both of the molecular biology of CA and of the human genome expands, targeted therapeutics, including hormonal manipulation, will undoubtedly assume a more critical role in the management of human malignancies.

Breast

Overview

When considering hormonal treatment (HT) of breast CA, it is important to distinguish between premenopausal women, in whom the primary source of estrogen is the ovaries, and postmenopausal women, in whom aromatization of androgens in the peripheral tissue is the major source of estrogen production. In premenopausal women, removal of the ovaries via surgical or radiologic ablation, or inhibition of ovarian estrogen production with a gonadotropin-releasing hormone (GnRH) analog, results in marked decrease in estrogen levels. SERMs, most notably tamoxifen, are a treatment option for both premenopausal and postmenopausal women with ER-positive disease; they reduce tumor cell proliferation by binding to and blocking the activation of ERs. In premenopausal women, treatment with tamoxifen plus ovarian ablation may provide added benefit by decreasing estrogen levels through two complementary mechanisms (184). Aromatase inhibitors (AIs) interfere with estrogen production by targeting the peripheral aromatization of androgens. In postmenopausal women, in whom peripheral tissue production of estrogen is responsible for the majority of circulating estrogen, AIs are a likely choice in the selection of HT. The role of AIs in premenopausal women is less clear owing to the high level of ovarian estrogen in this patient population.

Adjuvant Hormonal Therapy for Early-Stage Breast Cancer—Postmenopausal Women

Tamoxifen prescribed for approximately 5 years after surgery to patients with early, ER-positive breast CA is the current standard of adjuvant therapy worldwide. The Early Breast Cancer Trialists' Collaborative Group (EBCTCG) conducted a meta-analysis to assess recurrence and mortality rates among randomized trials of women with primary breast CA who received adjuvant tamoxifen therapy or placebo. Table 17.2 details the reduction in recurrence and mortality, stratified by ER and PR status, revealing that women with hormone receptor–positive tumors experience a more significant improvement in both endpoints. Conversely, women with hormone receptor–negative tumors received little, if any, benefit from HT (184). Furthermore, the EBCTCG established that hormone receptor–positive women receiving tamoxifen demonstrated a 21%, 28%, and 50% reduction in recurrence and a 14%, 18%, and 28% reduction in mortality in the treatment groups of 1 year, 2 years, and approximately 5 years, respectively, with consistent benefits across various tamoxifen dosing regimens (20 to 40 mg/day) (184). Although the efficacy of tamoxifen in the adjuvant setting has been established, the toxicity profile of this agent, including an increased risk of EEC and thromboembolic events, has prompted investigative efforts into alternative therapies.

In 2002, anastrozole alone was approved as adjuvant treatment for early breast CA. The ATAC trial included 9,366 postmenopausal women with operable, early, invasive breast CA who had completed primary treatment and were candidates for adjuvant HT. The data demonstrated superior efficacy of anastrozole when compared to tamoxifen in improving disease-free survival in postmenopausal women with hormone receptor–positive or unknown early-stage breast CA. Disease-free survival was significantly longer for patients on anastrozole alone than for those who received tamoxifen alone (HR 0.83; 95% CI, 0.71 to 0.96; $P = 0.013$) or the combination of both (HR 0.81; 95% CI, 0.70 to 0.94; $P = 0.006$). The combination was not significantly different

TABLE 17.2

HORMONE RECEPTOR STATUS: EFFECT ON RESPONSE RATE IN EARLY-STAGE DISEASE

Receptor status	N	Reduction in recurrence % (95% CI)	Reduction in mortality % (95% CI)
ER^+, PgR^+	7,000	37 (±6)	16 (±8)
ER^+, PgR^-	2,000	32 (±12)	18 (±14)
ER^-, PgR^+	602	23 (±24)	9 (±28)
ER^-, PgR^-	2,000	1 (±14)	1 (±14)

Note: All patients were treated with tamoxifen.
Source: Early Breast Cancer Trialists' Collaborative Group. *Lancet* 1998;351:1451–1467.

from tamoxifen alone (HR 1.02; 95% CI, 0.89 to 1.18; $P = 0.8$) (123). The disease-free survival estimates at 3 years were 89.4%, 87.4%, and 87.2% on anastrozole, tamoxifen, and the combination, respectively. Incidence of contralateral breast CA was significantly lower with anastrozole than with tamoxifen (OR 0.42 [0.22–0.79]; $P = 0.007$). After publication of the ATAC data, the American Society of Clinical Oncology (ASCO) Health Services Research Committee suggested that a 5-year course of tamoxifen remain the standard adjuvant HT pending updated data from the ATAC trial and other trials of third-generation AIs in the adjuvant setting (185). The panel further suggested that it would be reasonable for a patient to be treated with anastrozole if there was a history of cardiovascular disease or thromboembolic events, or if the patient developed complications or intolerable side effects attributable to tamoxifen. The ATAC data was recently updated, with 68 months of follow-up, and the benefit of anastrozole over tamoxifen was maintained (186).

Goss et al. conducted a double-blind, placebo-controlled trial evaluating the effectiveness of 5 years of letrozole in 5,187 postmenopausal women with early-stage breast CA who had completed 5 years of tamoxifen therapy (187). The estimated 4-year disease-free survival rates were 93% for the letrozole group and 87% for the control group ($P < 0.001$), suggesting that in this subset of breast CA patients, AI therapy after tamoxifen provides a survival advantage. An analysis of the post-unblinding data was recently presented. Among the 2,594 women initially randomized to placebo, 1,655 women chose to receive open-label letrozole. At 54 months, a statistically significant benefit in disease-free survival favored the crossover patients (HR 0.31; $P < 0.0001$) (188). The Breast International Group (BIG) 1-98 study, a randomized, phase 3, double-blind trial, compared 5 years of treatment with various adjuvant endocrine therapy regimens in postmenopausal women with hormone receptor–positive breast CA: letrozole, letrozole followed by tamoxifen, tamoxifen, and tamoxifen followed by letrozole. A total of 8,010 women with data that could be assessed were enrolled: 4,003 in the letrozole group and 4,007 in the tamoxifen group. After a median follow-up of 25.8 months, 351 events had occurred in the letrozole group and 428 events in the tamoxifen group, with 5-year disease-free survival estimates of 84.0% and 81.4%, respectively. As compared with tamoxifen, letrozole significantly reduced the risk of an event ending a period of disease-free survival (HR 0.81; 95% CI, 0.70 to 0.93; $p = 0.003$), especially the risk of distant recurrence (HR 0.73; 95% CI, 0.60 to 0.88; $P = 0.001$). In postmenopausal women with endocrine-responsive breast CA, adjuvant treatment with letrozole, as compared with tamoxifen, reduced the risk of recurrent disease, especially at distant sites (189). Multiple other studies investigating the role of AIs in the adjuvant treatment of ER-positive breast CA, including the investigation of exemestane, have shown survival benefit (190). Many issues regarding the adjuvant use of AIs remain unsettled, including the optimal duration of treatment, the optimal sequencing with tamoxifen, and the optimal AI. The ASCO concluded in 2004 that optimal adjuvant endocrine therapy for postmenopausal women with hormone receptor–positive breast CA should include an AI either as initial therapy or after a period of treatment with tamoxifen (185).

Adjuvant Hormonal Therapy for Early-Stage Breast Cancer—Premenopausal Women

The EBCTCG overview analysis has confirmed that adjuvant tamoxifen confers a survival benefit for ER-positive patients regardless of menopausal status. Accumulated clinical trial data as well as the EBCTCG overview analyses have confirmed that ablation of functioning ovaries significantly improves survival in breast CA patients younger than age 50, at least in the absence of chemotherapy (191). In premenopausal women with ER-positive, early-stage breast CA, significant investigation is ongoing regarding the role of AIs. Several investigations have suggested that young premenopausal women with hormone receptor–positive disease who fail to develop complete ovarian failure after chemotherapy may potentially benefit from ovarian suppression/ablation (OS/OA) (192). Several ongoing trials are expected to definitively address the various roles of combining chemotherapy, OS/OA, tamoxifen, and AIs in premenopausal patients with early-stage hormone receptor–positive breast CA. These trials include the Suppression of Ovarian Function Trial (SOFT), Tamoxifen and Exemestane Trial (TEXT), Premenopausal Endocrine Responsive Chemotherapy (PERCHE), and Austrian Breast and Colorectal Cancer Study Group (ABCSG).

Hormonal Therapy for Metastatic Breast Cancer

Regression of advanced breast CA as a result of prophylactic oophorectomy in premenopausal women was first described in 1896 (193). In unselected series of premenopausal women with metastatic breast CA, a 30% to 40% response with oophorectomy has been identified, whereas in ER-positive tumors, a 50% to 60% response has been noted.

Endocrine therapy for postmenopausal women with advanced hormonally responsive breast CA is based on the observation that greater than three fourths of these patients respond to HT, whereas only 11% of patients with hormone receptor–negative tumors show a response. Tamoxifen was the gold standard of first-line HT for metastatic breast CA until approximately 8 years ago. However, third-generation AIs have eclipsed tamoxifen in the treatment of postmenopausal women with metastatic estrogen-dependent breast cancer (194). Anastrozole and letrozole are both nonsteroidal AIs that compete with the substrate for binding to the enzyme active site. Mouridsen et al. compared tamoxifen to letrozole in 907 women with a median follow-up of 18 months. Letrozole was associated with a longer time to disease progression than tamoxifen (9.4 vs. 6.0 months; $P = 0.0001$) (195). Two trials compared tamoxifen to anastrozole, with conflicting results. Nabholtz et al. found that anastrozole provided longer time to disease progression compared to tamoxifen (11.1 vs 5.6 months; $P = 0.005$) (196). Bonneterre et al., in a similarly designed study, failed to confirm these findings; anastrozole was as effective as tamoxifen, but not superior (197). Exemestane, another third-generation AI, is a mechanism-based steroidal inhibitor that mimics the substrate, resulting in inactivation of aromatase and has been proven to be effective in the treatment of metastatic breast cancer, particularly when used sequentially with anastrozole or letrozole (198). In summary, the third-generation–specific AIs, which include anastrozole (Arimidex), letrozole (Femara), and exemestane (Aromasin), are now available in the United States and are approved as first-line therapy for the treatment of metastatic breast CA.

Endometrium

Hormonal Treatment of Endometrioid Endometrial Cancer

The median survival of women with advanced or recurrent endometrioid endometrial CA (EEC) is less than 1 year. Utilizing the best chemotherapeutic regimen available, the complete response rate in those patients with advanced-stage EEC is only 22%. Histologic grade is known to be a predictor of stage and survival, with grade 3, poorly differentiated CAs

TABLE 17.3

ENDOMETRIOID ENDOMETRIAL CARCINOMA CLINICAL ESTIMATES

	Grade 1	Grade 2	Grade 3	Total
Estimated new cases, 2003 (SEER)	12,030	17,243	10,827	40,100
Estimated deaths, 2003	2,040	2,924	1,836	6,800
% of cases with deep myometrial invasion	10%	20%	42%	22%
Extrauterine spread at diagnosis	10.40%	26.00%	59.60%	21.80%
5-year survival (all stages)	87%	75%	58%	68%

Note: SEER, Surveillance, Epidemiology, and End Results.

portending a higher risk of extrauterine disease and thus poorer survival. Estimates from the SEER data registry for 2003 for both incidence and mortality are provided in Table 17.3. Carcangiu et al. evaluated 183 patients with EEC, establishing a correlation between the International Federation of Gynecology and Obstetrics (FIGO) grade and hormone receptor expression (199). The recognized association of higher grade with lower ER/PR expression carries implications for the use of HT in advanced EEC. A majority of advanced cases of EEC are grade 3 lesions, limiting the use of HT in this patient population.

Advanced or Recurrent Endometrioid Endometrial Cancer

Progestational Agents. The use of progestational agents in women with advanced or recurrent EEC has been under investigation for several decades. Several different types of progestational agents have been investigated, including hydroxyprogesterone caproate (Delalutin), medroxyprogesterone acetate (MPA, Provera), and megestrol acetate (Megace). A majority of studies evaluating this treatment modality have included small numbers of patients with no stratification for well-recognized predictors of response. In the last decade, several studies with larger patient sample size, clearer eligibility criteria, and clearer definition of response and toxicity have evaluated the effectiveness of progestational agents in the treatment of advanced or recurrent EEC. The GOG, in GOG protocol 48, evaluated unselected patients with advanced or recurrent EEC. An overall response rate (MPA 50 mg three times daily) of 18% (32 complete and 26 partial responses among 331 patients with measurable disease) and median progression-free and overall survival times of 4.0 and 10.5 months, respectively, were identified (200). In another GOG protocol, 299 eligible women with advanced or recurrent EEC were randomized to receive either oral MPA 200 mg/day or oral MPA 1,000 mg/day until unacceptable toxicity or disease progression (201). Among the 145 patients receiving the low-dose regimen, there were 25 (17%) complete responses and 11 (8%) partial responses; 109 patients (75%) demonstrated no response. Among the 154 patients receiving the high-dose regimen, there were 14 (9%) complete responses and 10 (6%) partial responses; 130 patients (84%) had no response. The overall response rates (complete plus partial; 25% and 16% for low- and high-dose regimens, respectively) favored the low-dose regimen. The median progression-free survival time was 3.2 months for the low-dose regimen and 2.5 months for the high-dose regimen. There was an association, including patients receiving both dosing regimens of MPA, between response and histologic grade, with well-differentiated tumors responding more frequently than poorly differentiated lesions. The response rates were 37% (22 of 59 patients), 23% (26 of 113 patients), and 9% (12 of 127 patients) for those with grade 1, 2, or 3, respectively. As well, there was a noteworthy correlation between response and receptor content. The response rate was 8% (7 of 86 patients) for patients who were PR negative and 37% (17 of 46) for patients who were PR positive ($P < 0.001$). The response rate was 7% (4 of 55) for patients who were ER negative and 26% (20 of 77) for patients who were ER positive ($P = 0.005$). An association between receptor status and tumor grade was established as well. After tumor grade was adjusted for, PR concentration remained an important predictor of survival. In summary, the overall response rate for the progestational agents in women with advanced or recurrent EEC is relatively low. However, progestational agents remain a therapeutic alternative for this patient population, where significant comorbid conditions frequently exist, particularly in those women who can predictably expect a higher response based on grade and receptor content.

Combination Chemotherapy and Progestational Agents. Combining chemotherapy with hormonal therapy is an area of active research. Pinelli et al. prospectively treated 13 advanced EEC patients with carboplatinum 300 mg/mm^2 every 4 weeks for six cycles. Subsequently, Megace 80 mg/day for 3 weeks alternating with tamoxifen 40 mg/day for 3 weeks was prescribed. A complete response was obtained in 30% of patients, a partial response in 46%, stable disease in one patient, and disease progression in two patients (202). Work is ongoing investigating the role of combination cytotoxic chemotherapy and HT in the treatment of advanced or recurrent EEC.

Selective Estrogen Receptor Modulators. SERMs have been and continue to be investigated for HT of EEC. Tamoxifen was studied by the GOG in a phase 2 study of patients with advanced or recurrent EEC. At a dose of 20 mg twice daily, only 10% of 68 patients demonstrated objective response, but response occurred more commonly in grades 1 and 2 tumors (23% and 14%, respectively) compared to grade 3 tumors (3%) (203). From pooled reports of eight other studies including 257 patients, 22% of patients with advanced EEC responded to tamoxifen, but the range was wide in that it was from 0 to 53% (204). Tamoxifen can increase PgR content in endometrial CA tissues, which theoretically would enhance the activity of progestins, which frequently down-regulate PgR within the target tissue, prompting a relatively short duration of response. Clinical studies on alternating treatment with tamoxifen and progestin have provided conflicting results (Table 17.4) (201,203,205–208).

Other SERMs are also under investigation, including raloxifene and its metabolite, LY353381.HCl (arzoxifene). First-generation SERMs, such as tamoxifen, have mixed estrogenic agonist and antagonist activity, whereas second-generation SERMs, such as raloxifene, have more selective E2 antagonism. Arzoxifene (LY353381), a third-generation SERM, is a potent E2 antagonist in mammary and uterine tissues, with enhanced bioavailability and antiestrogenic activity compared

TABLE 17.4

HORMONAL THERAPY WITH PROGESTINS AND TAMOXIFEN IN ADVANCED OR RECURRENT ENDOMETRIAL CANCER

Reference	Hormonal agent	Patients	CR (%)	PR (%)	OR (%)
(201)	MPA (200 mg/day)	145	17	8	25
	MPA (1,000 mg/day)	154	9	6	15
(203)	TAM	68	4	6	10
(206)	MA	20	5	15	20
	TAM/MA	42	2	17	19
(207)	TAM/MPA	58	10	23	33
(205)	TAM/MA	56	21	5	26

Note: CR, complete response, MA, megestrole acetate; MPA, medroxyprogesterone acetate; OR, overall response; PR, partial response; TAM, tamoxifen.

with raloxifene. This SERM elicited a complete response in one and a partial response in eight of 29 patients with advanced EEC, with an overall response rate of 31%, a median duration of response of 13.9 months, and minimal toxicity. All responses occurred in progestin-sensitive patients. The relatively high response rate and the favorable toxicity profile make this agent worthy of further investigation (209,210).

Aromatase Inhibitors. Anastrozole and letrozole are active, highly selective nonsteroidal competitive inhibitors of the enzyme aromatase. It has been shown that significant amounts of aromatase are found in endometrial CA, with low amounts being present in the surrounding normal endometrial tissue. Rose et al. recently found in 23 patients that anastrozole at 1 mg a day for 28 days has minimal activity, with only a 9% partial response rate and a progression-free interval of 1 to 6 months in women with advanced EEC (211). The National Cancer Institute of Canada completed a multicenter phase 2 trial evaluating letrozole in postmenopausal women with recurrent or advanced endometrial carcinoma. Thirty-two eligible patients were treated with letrozole at 2.5 mg daily continuously. Of the 28 patients evaluated for response, one complete and two partial responses were noted; overall response was 9.4% (95% CI, 2 to 25). Eleven patients had stable disease for a median duration of 6.7 months (range 3.7 to 19.3 months). In conclusion, letrozole is well tolerated but has little overall activity in this cohort of women with endometrial cancer (212).

Antigonadotropins. Antigonadotropins, such as danazol, antagonize pituitary gonadotropin release and limit adrenal and estrogen production. Danazol has yet to be clinically tested in patients with endometrial CA. However, *in vitro* studies have shown it to inhibit endometrial tumor cell migration (similar to MPA) and inhibit invasive activity (not demonstrated by MPA) (213,214). The clinical effects of danazol on endometrial hyperplasia have been evaluated (215). Of 15 patients with pathologically proven hyperplasia, all were successfully converted to atrophic endometriums by day 90 of danazol 400 mg/day. Given the perceived low toxicity of danazol in comparison to conventional chemotherapy, the lack of effective agents in this disease, and a theoretical rationale for its activity in endometrial CA, a phase 2 trial has been initiated by the GOG (GOG-0180).

Adjuvant Therapy for Endometrioid Endometrial Cancer

The use of progestational agents as adjuvant therapy for stages I and II EEC has been investigated by von Minckwitz et al. (216). They conducted a randomized trial of 388 patients with early-stage EEC who received either MPA (n = 133) or tamoxifen (n = 121) orally for 2 years or were observed only (n = 134) after surgical therapy. After 56 months of follow-up, no benefit was observed from adjuvant progestin or tamoxifen therapy after surgical treatment in early-stage EEC. However, given the low frequency of recurrence in this patient population, larger randomized studies are needed to fully evaluate the role of progestational agents as adjuvant therapy in early EEC.

Progestational Agents as Primary Therapy for Endometrioid Endometrial Cancer

Several small series have retrospectively reported on the use of progestational agents alone, not preceded by hysterectomy, in the treatment of patients with EEC, either because of the desire to maintain fertility or because of comorbid conditions. No randomized, controlled studies exist evaluating progestational agents in either clinical scenario. Montz et al., in a prospective pilot study, reported on the use of the progesterone IUD in women with presumed stage IA, grade 1 EEC, who were at significant risk for perioperative morbidity (217). Follow-up endometrial biopsies were negative in 7 of 11 patients at 6 months and in 6 of 8 patients at 12 months. Recently, Ramirez et al. searched MEDLINE and other databases for English-language articles describing patients with grade 1 EEC who were treated with hormonal therapy. Ultimately, 81 patients in 27 articles were included in the study. Sixty-two patients (76%) responded to treatment. The median time to response was 12 weeks (range, 4 to 60 weeks). Fifteen patients (24%) who initially responded to treatment recurred. The median time to recurrence was 19 months (range, 6 to 44 months). Ten (67%) of the patients with recurrence ultimately underwent total abdominal hysterectomy. Residual endometrial carcinoma was found in six patients (60%). Nineteen patients never responded. Twenty patients were able to become pregnant at least once after completing treatment. The median follow-up was 36 weeks (range, 0 weeks to 30 years). No patients died of their disease. Further investigation is needed into this approach to the primary management of EEC (218).

Ovary

The ovary is an endocrine and end organ. Hormones and their receptors have been associated with ovarian CA and may be related to its causation. Some data suggest that hormonal therapies may have an effect on ovarian CA in palliative settings (219). Several investigators have established that hormone receptors are expressed in epithelial ovarian CA, and that significant alterations occur with malignant transformation (20).

Rao and Slotman reviewed 45 series, including 2,508 ovarian CA patients, and reported that 67% of tumors expressed ER and 47% expressed PR (220). Recently, one investigation found that the expression of the ERs and PRs correlated with long-term survival in invasive ovarian CA; the ER^-PR^+ phenotype predicted a more favorable tumor biology and long-term survival (221). Interestingly, many studies have demonstrated that ER-β is highly represented in normal epithelial cells or benign tumors (222), whereas ER-α is the main form expressed in malignant tumors. ER-β mRNA decreases in an inversely correlated way with tumor progression as compared with ER-α mRNA. The ER-α/ER-β mRNA ratio is markedly increased in ovarian CA (223). An increased ER-α/ER-β ratio has also been observed in different CAs, such as breast CA, prostatic CA, lung CA, and colorectal carcinoma. These data suggest that ER-β might play a protective role against ER-α mitogenic activity or that the loss of ER-β is a marker of cell dedifferentiation. However, multiple studies investigating the relationship between hormone receptor status in ovarian CA and prognostic factors, including disease-free interval and survival, have not produced consistent results. The ambiguous results in studies evaluating receptor status and survival in ovarian CA patients are due to several factors, including small numbers with heterogeneous groups of patients, different receptor assay methods, and heterogeneity in the receptor content within one tumor population.

A large number of hormonal agents have been evaluated in the treatment of ovarian CA, including SERMs, E2, progestogens, androgens, AIs, and GnRH agonists. Progestin therapy in patients with advanced ovarian CA has a global response rate of 8% to 15% (220,224). One of the most widely studied compounds in this clinical setting is tamoxifen. Preclinical studies have confirmed that tamoxifen inhibits ovarian cell growth *in vitro*, providing rationale for the use of this agent in the treatment of ovarian CA. Several studies have evaluated the activity of single-agent tamoxifen in the treatment of advanced ovarian CA (Table 17.5) (225–242). Perez-Garcia and Carrasco reviewed the literature evaluating single-agent tamoxifen in the treatment of patients with advanced ovarian CA, most of whom were heavily pretreated and refractory to chemotherapy (243). A total of 648 patients were included with an overall response rate (ORR) of 13% (95% CI, 10.4 to 15.6, range 0 to 56), including a 4% complete response rate and a 9% partial response rate. In 38% of patients, stable disease was noted. These results are not entirely dissimilar from those seen with progestins. The role of GnRH agonists in the management of refractory ovarian CA has been evaluated in multiple studies and has been summarized by Paskeviciute et al. (244). In this study, GnRH

TABLE 17.5

TAMOXIFEN THERAPY FOR ADVANCED OVARIAN CANCER

Study (reference)	No. of evaluable patients	Median no. of lines prior CT (%)	Dose (mg/n)	No. of patients responding (%)			
				OR	CR	SD	PR
Hatch et al. (228)	105	1 (100)	20/12	18 (17)	10 (10)	8 (8)	40 (38)
Marth et al. (231)	65[a]	1 (24) ≥2 (74)	30–40/24	4 (6)	2 (3)	2 (3)	50 (77)
Landoni et al. (230)	55	NS	40/24	0	0	0	19 (35)
Osborne et al. (232)	51	0 (2) 1 (41) 2 (57)	20/12[b]	1 (2)	0 (0)	1 (2)	5 (9)
Gennatas et al. (226)	50	0 (50) 1–2 (50)	20/12	28 (56)	2 (4)	26 (52)	NS
Rolski et al. (235)	47	1–4	40/24	3 (6)	1 (2)	2 (4)	22 (47)
Quinn (234)	40	1	20/12	9 (23)	5 (13)	4 (10)	12 (30)
Jager et al. (229)	33	NS (≥1)	30/24	0 (0)	0 (0)	0 (0)	2 (6)
Weiner et al. (242)	31	3	10/12[b]	3 (10)	1 (3)	2 (6)	6 (19)
Van der Velden et al. (240)	16	1	20/12	2 (13)	2 (13)	0 (0)	6 (38)
	14	2 or 3	20/12	0 (0)	0 (0)	0 (0)	4 (29)
Ahlgren et al. (225)	29	1 (50) ≥2 (50)	20/12[b]	5 (17)	2 (7)	3 (10)	18 (62)
Shirey et al. (238)	23	NS(≥1)	20–40/24	0 (0)	0 (0)	0 (0)	19 (83)
Slevin et al. (239)	22	2	20/12	0 (0)	0 (0)	0 (0)	1 (5)
Pagel et al. (233)	21	NS	NS	8 (38)	1 (5)	7 (3)	12 (57)
Hamerlynck et al. (227)	18	NS	20/12	1 (6)	0 (0)	1 (6)	2 (11)
Schwartz et al. (237)	13	≥2	10/12	1 (8)	0 (0)	1 (8)	4 (31)
Rowland et al. (236)	9	1–3	20/24	0 (0)	0 (0)	0 (0)	NS
Van der Vange et al. (241)	6	2	20/12	1 (17)	0 (0)	1 (17)	1 (17)
Total	648			84 (13.0)	26 (4.0)	58 (9.0)	223 (37.9)[c]

Note: CR, complete response; CT, chemotherapy; NS, not stated; OR, overall response; PR, partial response; SD, stable disease.
[a]Only evaluable patients are included (but prior CT lines refer to the whole population).
[b]With a loading dose of 100 mg/24 hours during 1 day (Osborne et al. [232]), 40 mg/24 hours during 7 days (Weiner et al. [242]), and 40 mg/24 hours during 30 days (Ahlgren et al. [225]).
[c]Calculated over the number of patients included in trials that report these data.

agonists induced an overall objective response in 8.5% of refractory ovarian CA patients with disease stabilization in 23% of these women.

Comparing chemotherapy alone to chemotherapy and hormonal therapy primarily in patients with advanced ovarian CA has been carried out by several investigators. However, these studies had small patient sample size and were not randomized, controlled studies. Schwartz et al. evaluated cisplatinum and doxorubicin, with or without tamoxifen after initial surgery, without finding significant overall survival (OS) or progression-free survival (PFS) differences between both groups (237). Emons et al. randomized 135 patients with advanced ovarian CA to receive the GnRH triptorelin, or placebo, following surgery and chemotherapy, until the patient's death or termination of the trial. There were no significant differences in OS or PFS between the groups, with documented gonadotropin suppression (245). At least four randomized studies comparing chemotherapy and MPA or a GnRH versus chemotherapy alone in ovarian CA patients have been reported. These studies contain many of the same flaws as noted throughout this discussion, namely, small sample size and no stratification for optimal versus suboptimal surgical status, menopausal status, and histologic status.

Combining cytotoxic chemotherapy and tamoxifen or other hormonal agents as salvage therapy for patients with advanced ovarian CA is an area of investigation that warrants further study (246).

As previously stated, in patients with ovarian CA, receptor status does not reproducibly correlate with prognostic factors, including survival or disease-free interval. However, receptor status may be useful in predicting response to hormonal agents. Although several investigators have approached this question, results are not conclusive. The ascertainment of receptor status as a predictor of hormonal activity in ovarian CA will require a randomized clinical trial comparing hormonal activity in patients expressing hormone receptors versus those with no receptor expression, controlling for the many variables recognized as important prognosticators in ovarian CA.

Colon

The clinical data available evaluating the relationship between hormones and colon CA relate primarily to hormones as risk factors for the development of this common human malignancy. There is a plethora of data in colon CA cell lines regarding the effect of hormonal agents on cell growth, as well as cell death. To date, there are no clinical studies evaluating the treatment of colon CA, either in the adjuvant setting or otherwise, with hormonal agents.

References

1. Evans RM. The steroid and thyroid hormone receptor superfamily. *Science* 1988;240:889–895.
2. O'Malley BW, Tsai SY, Bagchi M, et al. Molecular mechanism of action of a steroid hormone receptor. *Recent Prog Horm Res* 1991;47:1–24, discussion 24–26.
3. Molenda HA, Kilts CP, Allen RL, et al. Nuclear receptor coactivator function in reproductive physiology and behavior. *Biol Reprod* 2003;69(5): 1449–1457.
4. Bjornstrom L, Sjoberg M. Mechanisms of estrogen receptor signaling: convergence of genomic and nongenomic actions on target genes. *Mol Endocrinol* 2005;19:833–842.
5. Miller WL. Molecular biology of steroid hormone synthesis. *Endocr Rev* 1988;9:295–318.
6. Channing CP, Tsafriri A. Mechanism of action of luteinizing hormone and follicle-stimulating hormone on the ovary in vitro. *Metabolism* 1977;26:413–468.
7. Simpson ER. Aromatase: biologic relevance of tissue-specific expression. *Semin Reprod Med* 2004;22:11–23.
8. Pasqualini JR, Chetrite GS. Recent insight on the control of enzymes involved in estrogen formation and transformation in human breast cancer. *J Steroid Biochem Mol Biol* 2005;93:221–236.
9. Davis SR. Minireview: aromatase and the regulation of estrogen biosynthesis—some new perspectives. *Endocrinology* 2001;142:4589–4594.
10. Miller WR. Aromatase and the breast: regulation and clinical aspects. *Maturitas* 2006;54:335–341.
11. Kumar V, Green S, Stack G, et al. Functional domains of the human estrogen receptor. *Cell* 1987;51:941–951.
12. Mosselman S, Polman J, Dijkema R. ER beta: identification and characterization of a novem human estrogen receptor. *FEBS Lett* 1996;392:49–53.
13. Barkhem T, Carlsson B, Nilsson Y, et al. Differential response of estrogen receptor alpha and estrogen receptor beta to partial estrogen agonists/antagonists. *Mol Pharmacol* 1998; 54:105–112.
14. Christensen DJ, Gron H, Norris JD, et al. Estrogen receptor (ER) modulators each induce distinct conformational changes in ER alpha and ER beta. *Proc Natl Acad Sci USA* 1999;96:3999–4004.
15. Kuiper GG, Carlsson B, Grandien K, et al. Comparison of the ligand binding specificity and transcript tissue distribution of estrogen receptors alpha and beta. *Endocrinology* 1997;138:863–870.
16. Taylor AH, Al-Azzawi F. Immunolocalisation of oestrogen receptor beta in human tissues. *J Mol Endocrinol* 2000;24:145–155.
17. Matthews J, Gustafsson JA. Estrogen signaling: a subtle balance between ER alpha and ER beta. *Mol Interv* 2003;3:281–292.
18. Hall J, McDonell DP. The estrogen receptor beta-isoform (ERbeta) of the human estrogen receptor modulates ERalpha transcriptional activity and is a key regular of the cellular response to estrogens and antiestrogens. *Endocrinology* 1999;140:5566–5578.
19. Pujol P, Rey JM, Nirde P, et al. Differential expression of estrogen receptor-alpha and -beta messenger RNAs as a potential marker of ovarian carcinogenesis. *Cancer Res* 1998;58:5367–5373.
20. Li AJ, Baldwin RL, Karlan BY. Estrogen and progesterone receptor subtype expression in normal and malignant ovarian epithelial cell cultures. *Am J Obstet Gynecol* 2003;189:22–27.
21. Jazaeri AA, Nunes KJ, Dalton MS, et al. Well-differentiated endometrial adenocarcinomas and poorly differentiated mixed müllerian tumors have altered ER and PR isoform expression. *Oncogene* 2001;20:6965–6969.
22. Foley E, Jazaeri AA, Shupnik MA, et al. Selective loss of estrogen receptor beta in malignant human colon. *Cancer Res* 2000;60:245–248.
23. Hewitt S, Korach KS. Oestrogen receptor knockout mice: roles for oestrogen receptors alpha and beta in reproductive tissues. *Reproduction* 2003;125:143–149.
24. Poola I, Koduri S, Chatra S, et al. Identification of twenty alternatively spliced estrogen receptor alpha mRNAs in breast cancer cell lines and tumors using splice targeted primer approach. *J Steroid Biochem Mol Biol* 2000;72:249–258.
25. Zhao C, Toresson G, Xu L, et al. Mouse estrogen receptor beta isoforms exhibit differences in ligand selectivity and coactivator recruitment. *Biochemistry* 2005;44:7936–7944.
26. Palmieri C, Lam EW, Mansi J, et al. The expression of ER beta cx in human breast cancer and the relationship to endocrine therapy and survival. *Clin Cancer Res* 2004;10:2421–2428.
27. Paech K, Webb P, Kuiper GG, et al. Differential ligand activation of estrogen receptors ERalpha and ERbeta at AP1 sites. *Science* 1997;277:1508–1510.
28. Kumar P, Wu Q, Chambliss KL, et al. Direct interactions with G alpha i and G betagamma mediate nongenomic signaling by estrogen receptor alpha. *Mol Endocrinol* 2007;21:1370–1380.
29. Maruyama S, Fujimoto N, Asano K, et al. Suppression by estrogen recepta beta of AP-1 mediated transactivation through estrogen receptor alpha. *J Steroid Biochem Mol Biol* 2001;78:177–184.
30. Kushner PJ, Agard DA, Greene GL, et al. Estrogen receptor pathways to AP-1. *J Steroid Biochem Mol Biol* 2000;74:311–317.
31. Lee AV, Weng CN, Jackson JG, et al. Activation of estrogen receptor-mediated gene transcription by IGF-I in human breast cancer cells. *J Endocrinol* 1997;152:39–47.
32. Ignar-Trowbridge D, Nelson KG, Bidwell MC. Coupling of dual signaling pathways: epidermal growth factor action involves the estrogen receptor. *Proc Natl Acad Sci USA* 1992;89:4658–4662.
33. Manavathi B, Kumar R. Steering estrogen signals from the plasma membrane to the nucleus: two sides of the coin. *J Cell Physiol* 2006;207:594–604.
34. Hecht JL, Mutter GL. Molecular and pathologic aspects of endometrial carcinogenesis. *J Clin Oncol* 2006;24:4783–4791.
35. Maxwell GL, Risinger JI, Gumbs C. Mutation of the PTEN tumor supressor gene in endometrial hyperplasias. *Cancer Res* 1998;58:2500–2503.
36. Duong BN, Elliott S, Frigo DE, et al. AKT regulation of estrogen receptor [beta] transcriptional activity in breast cancer. *Cancer Res* 2006; 66: 8373–8381.
37. Losel RM, Falkenstein E, Feuring M, et al. Nongenomic steroid action: controversies, questions, and answers. *Physiol Rev* 2003;83:965–1016.
38. Song RX, Santen RJ. Membrane initiated estrogen signaling in breast cancer. *Biol Reprod* 2006;75:9–16.
39. Simoncini T, Hafezi-Moghadam A, Brazil DP, et al. Interaction of oestrogen receptor with the regulatory subunit of phosphatidylinositol-3-OH kinase. *Nature* 2000;407:538–541.

40. Revankar CM, Cimino DF, Sklar LA, et al. A transmembrane intracellular estrogen receptor mediates rapid cell signaling. *Science* 2005;307:1625–1630.
41. Kastner P, Krust A, Turcotte B, et al. Two distinct estrogen-regulated promoters generate transcripts encoding the two functionally different human progesterone receptor forms A and B. *Embo J* 1990;9:1603–1614.
42. Sartorius CA, Melville MY, Hovland AR, et al. A third transactivation function (AF3) of human progesterone receptors located in the unique N-terminal segment of the B-isoform. *Mol Endocrinol* 1994;8:1347–1360.
43. Graham JD, Clarke CL. Expression and transcriptional activity of progesterone receptor A and progesterone receptor B in mammalian cells. *Breast Cancer Res* 2002;4:187–190.
44. Huse B, Verca SB, Matthey P, et al. Definition of a negative modulation domain in the human progesterone receptor. *Mol Endocrinol* 1998;12: 1334–1342.
45. Mote PA, Balleine RL, McGowan EM, et al. Heterogeneity of progesterone receptors A and B expression in human endometrial glads and stroma. *Hum Reprod* 2002;3(15 Suppl):48–56.
46. Conneely OM, Mulac-Jericevic B, DeMayo F, et al. Reproductive functions of progesterone receptors. *Recent Prog Horm Res* 2002;57:339–355.
47. Arnett-Mansfield RL, deFazio A, Wain GV, et al. Relative expression of progesterone receptors A and B in endometroid cancers of the endometrium. *J Cancer Res* 2001;61:4576–4582.
48. Boonyaratanakornkit V, Scott MP, Ribon V, et al. Progesterone receptor contains a proline-rich motif that directly interacts with SH3 domains and activates c-Src family tyrosine kinases. *Mol Cell* 2001;8:269–280.
49. Zhu Y, Bond J, Thomas P. Identification, classification, and partial characterization of genes in humans and other vertebrates homologous to a fish membrane progestin receptor. *Proc Natl Acad Sci USA* 2003; 100:2237–2242.
50. Voigt LF, Deng Q, Weiss NS. Recency, duration, and progestin content of oral contraceptives in relation to the incidence of endometrial cancer (Washington, USA). *Cancer Causes Control* 1994;5:227–233.
51. Bianchini F, Kaaks R, Vainio H. Overweight, obesity, and cancer risk. *Lancet Oncol* 2002;3:565–574.
52. Bergstrom A. Overweight as an avoidable cause of cancer in Europe. *Int J Cancer* 2001;91:421–430.
53. Calle EE, Rodriguez C, Walker-Thurmond K, et al. Overweight, obesity, and mortality from cancer in a prospectively studied cohort of U.S. adults. *N Engl J Med* 2003;348:1625–1638.
54. *IARC Handbooks of Cancer Prevention, Volume 6: Weight Control and Physical Activity*; Oxford University Press. Oxford, England. 2002.
55. Kaaks R, Lukanova A, Kurzer MS. Obesity, endogenous hormones, and endometrial cancer risk: a synthetic review. *Cancer Epidemiol Biomarkers Prev* 2002;11:1531–1543.
56. Herbst AL. Adenocarcinoma of the vagina. Association of maternal stilbestrol therapy with tumor apearance in young women. *N Engl J Med* 1971;284:878–881.
57. Herbst AL, Cole P, Colton T, et al. Age-incidence and risk of diethylstilbestrol-related clear cell adenocarcinoma of the vagina and cervix. *Am J Obstet Gynecol* 1977;128:43–50.
58. McLachlan JA, Newbold RR, Bullock BC. Long-term effects on the female mouse genital tract associated with prenatal exposure to diethylstilbestrol. *Cancer Res* 1980;40:3988–3999.
59. Newbold RR, Bullock BC, McLachlan JA. Uterine adenocarcinoma in mice following developmental treatment with estrogens: a model for hormonal carcinogenesis. *Cancer Res* 1990;50:7677–7681.
60. Newbold RR, Banks EP, Bullock B, et al. Uterine adenocarcinoma in mice treated neonatally with genistein. *Cancer Res* 2001;61:4325–4328.
61. Ekbom A. Growing evidence that several human cancers may originate *in utero*. *Semin Cancer Biol* 1998;8:237–244.
62. Michels KB, Trichopoulos D, Robins JM, et al. Birthweight as a risk factor for breast cancer. *Lancet* 1996;348:1542–1546.
63. Kaijser M, Lichtenstein P, Granath F, et al. *In utero* exposures and breast cancer: a study of opposite-sexed twins. *J Natl Cancer Inst* 2001;93:60–62.
64. McCormack VA, Dos SS, Koupil I, et al. Birth characteristics and adult cancer incidence: Swedish cohort of over 11,000 men and women. *Int J Cancer* 2005;115:611–617.
65. Lof M, Sandin S, Hilakivi-Clarke L, et al. Birth weight in relation to endometrial and breast cancer risks in Swedish women. *Br J Cancer* 2007; 96:134–136.
66. Breast cancer and hormone replacement therapy: collaborative reanalysis of data from 51 epidemiological studies of 52,705 women with breast cancer and 108,411 women without breast cancer. Collaborative Group on Hormonal Factors in Breast Cancer. *Lancet* 1997;350:1047–1059.
67. Schairer C. Menopausal estrogen and estrogen-progestin replacement therapy and breast cancer risk. *JAMA* 2002;283:485–491.
68. Ross RK. Effect of hormone therapy on breast cancer risk: estrogen versus estrogen plus progestin. *J Natl Cancer Inst* 2000;92:328-332.
69. Writing Group for the Women's Health Initiative Investigators. Risks and benefits of estrogen plus progestin in healthy postmenopausal women. Principal results from the Women's Health Initiative Randomized Controlled Trial. *JAMA* 2002;288:321–333.
70. Chlebowski RT, Hendrix SL, Langer RD, et al. Influence of estrogen plus progestin on breast cancer and mammography in healthy postmenopausal women: the Women's Health Initiative Randomized Controlled Trial. *JAMA* 2003; 289:3243–3253.
71. Anderson GL, Limacher M, Assaf AR, et al. Effects of conjugated equine estrogen in postmenopausal women with hysterectomy: the Women's Health Initiative Randomized Controlled Trial. *JAMA* 2004;291:1701–1712.
72. Stefanick ML, Anderson GL, Margolis KL, et al. Effects of conjugated equine estrogens on breast cancer and mammography screening in postmenopausal women with hysterectomy. *JAMA* 2006;295:1647–1657.
73. Eden JA. A case-control study of combined continuous estrogen-progestin replacement therapy among women with a personal history of breast cancer. *Menopause* 1995;2:67–72.
74. Bluming AZ. Hormone replacement therapy in women with previously treated primary breast cancer: update III (abstract 131a). *Proc Am Soc Clin Oncol* 1997;(16A):463.
75. Vassilopoulou-Sellin R, Asmar L, Hortobagyi GN, et al. Estrogen replacement therapy after localized breast cancer: clinical outcome of 319 women followed prospectively. *J Clin Oncol* 1999;17:1482–1487.
76. DiSaia PJ, Brewster WR, Ziogas A, et al. Breast cancer survival and hormone replacement therapy: a cohort analysis. *Am J Clin Oncol* 2000;23:541–545.
77. *ACOG Committee Opinion: Estrogen Replacement Therapy in Women With Previously Treated Breast Cancer*. Washington DC: American College of Obstetricians and Gynecologists; 1994.
78. Breast cancer and hormonal contraceptives: collaborative reanalysis of individual data on 53,297 women with breast cancer and 100,239 women without breast cancer from 54 epidemiological studies. Collaborative Group on Hormonal Factors in Breast Cancer. *Lancet* 1996;347:1713–1727.
79. Marchbanks PA, McDonald JA, Wilson HG, et al. Oral contraceptives and the risk of breast cancer. *N Engl J Med* 2002;346:2025–2032.
80. Grabick DM. Risk of breast cancer with oral contraceptive use in women with a family history of breast cancer. *JAMA* 2000;284:1791–1798.
81. Narod SA, Dube MP, Klijn J, et al. Oral contraceptives and the risk of breast cancer in *BRCA1* and *BRCA2* mutation carriers. *J Natl Cancer Inst* 2002;94:1773–1779.
82. Rodriguez C, Patel AV, Calle EE, et al. Estrogen replacement therapy and ovarian cancer mortality in a large prospective study of US women. *JAMA* 2001;285:1460–1465.
83. Lacey JV Jr, Mink PJ, Lubin JH, et al. Menopausal hormone replacement therapy and risk of ovarian cancer. *JAMA* 2002;288:334–341.
84. Riman T. Hormone replacement therapy and the risk of invasive epithelial ovarian cancer in Swedish women. *JNCI* 2002;94:497–504.
85. Anderson G, Judd HL, Klaunitz AM, et al. Effect of estrogen plus progestin on gynecologic cancers and associated diagnostic procedures. *JAMA* 2003;290(13):1739–1748.
86. Guidozzi F, Daponte A. Estrogen replacement therapy for ovarian carcinoma survivors: a randomized controlled trial. *Cancer* 1999;86:1013–1018.
87. Grady D. Hormone replacement therapy and endometrial cancer risk: a meta-analysis. *Obstet Gynecol* 1995;85:302–313.
88. Speroff L, Rowan J, Symons J, et al. The comparative effect on bone density, endometrium, and lipids of continuous hormones as replacement therapy (CHART study). A randomized controlled trial. *JAMA* 1996; 276:1397–1403.
89. Flowers CE. Mechanisms of uterine bleeding in postmenopausal patients receiving estrogen alone or with a progestin. *Obstet Gynecol* 1983;61: 135–143.
90. Beresford SA, Weiss NS, Voigt LF, McKnight B. Risk of endometrial cancer in relation to use of oestrogen combined with cyclic progestagen therapy in postmenopausal women. *Lancet* 1997;349:458–461.
91. Hill DA, Weiss NS, Beresford SA, et al. Continuous combined hormone replacement therapy and risk of endometrial cancer. *Am J Obstet Gynecol* 2000;183:1456–1461.
92. Pike MC, Peters RK, Cozen W, et al. Estrogen-progestin replacement therapy and endometrial cancer. *J Natl Cancer Inst* 1997;89:1110–1116.
93. Weiderpass E, Adami HO, Baron JA, et al. Risk of endometrial cancer following estrogen replacement with and without progestins. *J Natl Cancer Inst* 1999;91:1131–1137.
94. Holinka CF, Hata H, Kuramoto H, et al. Responses to estradiol in a human endometrial adenocarcinoma cell line (ishikawa). *J Steroid Biochem* 1986;24:85–89.
95. Farnell YZ, Ing NH. The effects of estradiol and selective estrogen receptor modulators on gene expression and messenger RNA stability in immortalized sheep endometrial stromal cells and human endometrial adenocarcinoma cells. *J Steroid Biochem Mol Biol* 2003;84:453–461.
96. Creasman WT, Henderson D, Hinshaw W, et al. Estrogen replacement therapy in the patient treated for endometrial cancer. *Obstet Gynecol* 1986;67:326–330.
97. Lee RB. Estrogen replacement therapy following treatment for stage I endometrial carcinoma. *Gynecol Oncol* 1990;67:189–191.
98. Suriano KA, McHale M, McLaren CE, et al. Estrogen replacement therapy in endometrial cancer patients: a matched control study. *Obstet Gynecol* 2001;97:555–560.
99. Chapman JA. Estrogen replacement in surgical stage I and II endometrial cancer survivors. *Obstet Gynecol* 1996;175:1195–2000.
100. ACOG committee opinion. Hormone replacement therapy in women treated for endometrial cancer. Number 234, May 2000 (replaces number 126, August 1993). *Int J Gynaecol Obstet* 2001;73:283–284.
101. Rutqvist LE, Johansson H, Signomklao T, et al. Adjuvant tamoxifen therapy for early stage breast cancer and second primary malignancies. Stockholm Breast Cancer Study Group. *J Natl Cancer Inst* 1995;87:645–651.

102. Fisher B, Costantino JP, Redmond CK, et al. Endometrial cancer in tamoxifen-treated breast cancer patients: findings from the National Surgical Adjuvant Breast and Bowel Project (NSABP) B-14. *J Natl Cancer Inst* 1994;86:527–537.
103. Ettinger B, Black DM, Mitlak BH, et al. Reduction of vertebral fracture risk in postmenopausal women with osteoporosis treated with raloxifene: results from a 3-year randomized clinical trial. Multiple Outcomes of Raloxifene Evaluation (MORE) Investigators. *JAMA* 1999;282: 637–645.
104. Vogel VG, Costantino JP, Wickerham DL, et al. Effects of tamoxifen vs raloxifene on the risk of developing invasive breast cancer and other disease outcomes: the NSABP Study of Tamoxifen and Raloxifene (STAR) P-2 trial. *JAMA* 2006;295:2727–2741.
105. Picariello L, Fiorelli G, Martineti V. Growth response of colon cancer cell lines to selective estrogen receptor modulators. *Anticancer Res* 2003; 23:2419–2424.
106. Newcomb PA, Solomon C, White E. Tamoxifen and risk of large bowel cancer in women with breast cancer. *Breast Cancer* 1999;53:271–277.
107. Church J, Simmang C, Standards Task Force, American Society of Colon and Rectal Surgeons, Collaborative Group on Inherited Colorectal Cancer and the Standards Committee of the American Society of Colon and Rectal Surgeons. Practice parameters for the treatment of patients with dominantly inherited colorectal cancer (familial adenomatous polyposis and hereditary nonpolyposis colorectal cancer. *Dis Colon Rectum* 2003; 46:1001–1012.
108. Serpell JW, Paddle-Ledinek JE, Johnson WR. Modification of growth of desmoid tumors in tissue culture by anti-oestrogenic substances: a preliminary report. *Aust N Z J Surg* 1996;66:457–463.
109. Bus PJ, Verspaget HW, van Krieken JH. Treatment of mesenteric desmoid tumors with the antioestrogenic agent toremifene: case histories and an overview of the literature. *Eur J Gastroenterol Hepatol* 1999;11: 1179–1183.
110. Kadmon M, Moslein G, Buhr HJ, et al. Desmoid tumors in patients with familial adenomatous polyposis (FAP). Clinical and therapeutic observations from the Heidelberg polyposis register. *Chirurg* 1995;66:997–1005.
111. Adlercreutz H. Phyto-oestrogens and cancer. *Lancet Oncol* 2002;3: 364–373.
112. Goodman MT, Wilkens LR, Hankin JH, et al. Association of soy and fiber consumption with the risk of endometrial cancer. *Am J Epidemiol* 1997; 146(4):294–306.
113. Fisher B, Costantino JP, Wickerham DL, et al. Tamoxifen for prevention of breast cancer: report of the National Surgical Adjuvant Breast and Bowel Project P-1 Study. *J Natl Cancer Inst* 1998;90:1371–1388.
114. Gail MH, Brinton LA, Byar DP, et al. Projecting individualized probabilities of developing breast cancer for white females who are being examined annually. *J Natl Cancer Inst* 1989;81:1879–1886.
115. Veronesi U, Maisonneuve P, Costa A, et al. Prevention of breast cancer with tamoxifen: preliminary findings from the Italian randomized trial among hysterectomised women. *Lancet* 1998;352:93–97.
116. Veronesi U, Maisonneuve P, Sacchini V, et al. Tamoxifen for breast cancer among hysterectomised women. *Lancet* 2002;359:1122–1124.
117. Powles T, Eeles R, Ashley S, et al. Interim analysis of the incidence of breast cancer in the Royal Marsden Hospital tamoxifen randomised chemoprevention trial. *Lancet* 1998;352:98–101.
118. Chlebowski RT, Col N, Winer EP, et al. American Society of Clinical Oncology technology assessment of pharmacologic interventions for breast cancer risk reduction including tamoxifen, raloxifene, and aromatase inhibition. *J Clin Oncol* 2002;20:3328–3343.
119. Cuzick J, Powles T, Veronesi U, et al. Overview of the main outcomes in breast-cancer prevention trials. *Lancet* 2003;361:296–300.
120. Cuzick J, Forbes J, Edwards R, et al. First results from the International Breast Cancer Intervention Study (IBIS-I): a randomised prevention trial. *Lancet* 2002;360:817–824.
121. Cummings SR, Eckert S, Krueger KA, et al. The effect of raloxifene on risk of breast cancer in postmenopausal women. *JAMA* 1999;281(23): 2189–2197.
122. Cauley JA, Norton L, Lippman ME, et al. Continued breast cancer risk reduction in postmenopausal women treated with raloxifene: 4-year results from the MORE trial. Multiple outcomes of raloxifene evaluation. *Breast Cancer Res Treat* 2001;65:125–134.
123. Baum M, Budzar AV, Cuzi KJ, et al. Anastrozole alone or in combination with tamoxifen versus tamoxifen alone for adjuvant treatment of postmenopausal women with early breast cancer: first results of the ATAC randomised trial. *Lancet* 2002;359: 2131–2139.
124. Parazzini F, Braga C, La Vecchia C, et al. Hysterectomy, oophorectomy in premenopause, and risk of breast cancer. *Obstet Gynecol* 1997;90: 453–456.
125. Satagopan JM, Offit K, Foulkes WD, et al. The lifetime risks of breast cancer in Ashkenazi Jewish carriers of *BRCA1* and *BRCA2* mutations. *Cancer Epidemiol Biomarkers Prev* 2001;10:467–473.
126. Kauff ND, Satagopan JM, Robson ME, et al. Risk-reducing salpingo-oophorectomy in women with a *BRCA1* or *BRCA2* mutation. *N Engl J Med* 2002;346(21):1609–1615.
127. Rebbeck TR, Lynch HT, Neuhausen SL, et al. Prophylactic oophorectomy in carriers of *BRCA1* or *BRCA2* mutations. *N Engl J Med* 2002;346: 1616–1622.
128. Rebbeck TR, Levin AM, Eisen A, et al. Breast cancer risk after bilateral prophylactic oophorectomy in *BRCA1* mutation carriers. *J Natl Cancer Inst* 1999;91(17):1475–1479.
129. Buring JE, Hennekens CH. Beta-carotene and cancer chemoprevention. *J Cell Biochem* 1995;(Suppl 22):226–230.
130. Howe GR, Hirohata T, Hislop TG, et al. Dietary factors and risk of breast cancer: combined analysis of 12 case-control studies. *J Natl Cancer Inst* 1990;82(7):561–569.
131. Van't Veer P, Kolb CM, Verhoef P, et al. Dietary fiber, beta-carotene and breast cancer: results from a case-control study. *Int J Cancer* 1990;45(5): 825–828.
132. Shankar S, Lanza E. Dietary fiber and cancer prevention. *Hematol Oncol Clin North Am* 1991;5(1):25–41.
133. Sherman M, Sturgeon S, Brinton L, et al. Endometrial cancer risk factors differ by histopathologic type. (Abstract). *Mod Pathol* 1995;8:97A.
134. Rossouw JE, Anderson GL, Prentice RL, et al. Risks and benefits of estrogen plus progestin in healthy postmenopausal women. Writing Group of the Women's Health Initiative Investigators. *JAMA* 2002;288(3):321–333.
135. Prentice RL, Thomas DB. On the epidemiology of oral contraceptives and disease. *Adv Cancer Res* 1987;49:285–401.
136. Schlesselman JJ. Oral contraceptives and neoplasia of the uterine corpus. *Contraception* 1991;43:557–579.
137. Oral contraceptive use and the risk of endometrial cancer. The Centers for Disease Control Cancer and Steroid Hormone Study. *JAMA* 1983;249: 1600–1604.
138. The WHO Collaborative Study of Neoplasia and Steroid Contraceptives. *Int J Cancer* 1991;49:186–190.
139. Rosenblatt KA, Thomas DB. Hormonal content of combined oral contraceptives in relation to the reduced risk of endometrial carcinoma. The WHO Collaborative Study of Neoplasia and Steroid Contraceptives. *Int J Cancer* 1991;49:870–874.
140. Maxwell GL, Schildkraut JM, Calingaert B, et al. Progestin and estrogen potency of combination oral contraceptives and endometrial cancer risk. *Gynecol Oncol* 2006;103:535–540.
141. Castellsague X, Thompson WD, Dubrow R. Intra-uterine contraception and the risk of endometrial cancer. *Int J Cancer* 1993;54(6):911–916.
142. Hill DA, Weiss NS, Voigt LF, et al. Endometrial cancer in relation to intra-uterine device use. *Int J Cancer* 1997;70(3):278–381.
143. Parazzini F, La Vecchia C, Moroni S. Intrauterine device use and risk of endometrial cancer. *Br J Cancer* 1994;70(4):672–673.
144. Rosenblatt K, Thomas, DB. Intrauterine devices and endometrial cancer. *Contraception* 1996;54:329–332.
145. Salazar-Martinez E, Lazcano-Ponce EC, Lira-Lira GG, et al. Reproductive factors of ovarian and endometrial cancer risk in a high fertility population in Mexico. *Cancer Res* 1999;59:3658–3662.
146. Shu XO, Brinton LA, Zheng W, et al. A population-based case-control study of endometrial cancer in Shanghai, China. *Int J Cancer* 1991; 49(1):38–43.
147. Sturgeon S, Brinton LA, Berman ML, et al. Intrauterine device use and endometrial cancer risk. *Int J Epidemiol* 1997;26(3):496–500.
148. Hubacher D, Grimes DA. Noncontraceptive health benefits of intrauterine devices: a systematic review. *Obstet Gynecol Surv* 2002;57:120–128.
149. Gardner FJ, Konje JC, Abrams KR, et al. Endometrial protection from tamoxifen-stimulated changes by a levonorgestrel-releasing intrauterine system: a randomised controlled trial. *Lancet* 2000;356(9243):1711–1717.
150. Levi F, La Vecchia C, Gulie C, et al. Dietary factors and breast cancer risk in Vaud, Switzerland. *Nutr Cancer* 1993;19:327–335.
151. Potischman N, Swanson CA, Brinton LA, et al. Dietary associations in a case-control study of endometrial cancer. *Cancer Causes Control* 1993;4(3):239–250.
152. Shu XO, Zheng W, Potischman N, et al. A population-based case-control study of dietary factors and endometrial cancer in Shanghai, People's Republic of China. *Am J Epidemiol* 1993;137(2):155–165.
153. Barbone F, Austin H, Patridge EE. Diet and endometrial cancer: a case-control study. *Am J Epidemiol* 1993;137(4):393–403.
154. Zheng W, Kushi LH, Potter JD, et al. Dietary intake of energy and animal foods and endometrial cancer incidence. The Iowa Women's Health Study. *Am J Epidemiol* 1995;142:388–394.
155. Horn-Ross PL, John EM, Canchola AJ, et al. Phytoestrogen intake and endometrial cancer risk. *J Natl Cancer Inst* 2003;95:1158–1164.
156. Shaw PA, Deavers MT, Mills GB. Clinical characteristics of genetically determined ovarian cancer. In: Vogel IVG, ed. *Management of Patients at High Risk for Breast Cancer*. Blackwell Science; 2001:94–107.
157. Salazar H, Godwin AK, Daly MB, et al. Microscopic benign and invasive malignant neoplasms and a cancer-prone phenotype in prophylactic oophorectomies. *J Natl Cancer Inst* 1996;88(24):1810–1820.
158. van Hoeven KH, Ramondetta L, Kovatich AJ, et al. Quantitative image analysis of MIB-1 reactivity in inflammatory, hyperplastic, and neoplastic endocervical lesions. *Int J Gynecol Pathol* 1997;16(1):15–21.
159. Williams GT, Smith CA. Molecular regular of apoptosis: genetic controls of cell death. *Cell* 1993;74(5):777–779.
160. Ness RB, Grisso JA, Vergona R, et al. Oral contraceptives, other methods of contraception, and risk reduction for ovarian cancer. *Epidemiology* 2001;12:307–312.
161. Stanford JL. Oral contraceptives and neoplasia of the ovary. *Contraception* 1991;43(6):543–556.

162. Whittemore A. Characteristics relating to ovarian cancer risk: collaborative analysis of 12 US case-control studies. II. Invasive epithelial ovarian cancers in white women. Collaborative Ovarian Cancer Group. *Am J Epidemiol* 1992;136(10):1184–1203.
163. Gross TP, Schlesselman JJ, Stadel BV, et al. The risk of epithelial ovarian cancer in short-term users of oral contraceptives. *Am J Epidemiol* 1992;136(1):46–53.
164. Parazzini F, La Vecchia C, Negri E, et al. Oral contraceptive use and the risk of ovarian cancer: an Italian case-control study. *Eur J Cancer* 1993; 27(5):594–598.
165. Rosenberg L, Palmer JR, Zauber AG, et al. A case-control stud of oral contraceptive use and invasive epithelial ovarian cancer. *Am J Epidemiol* 1994;139(7):654–661.
166. Hartge P, Whittemore AS, Itnyre J, et al. Rates and risks of ovarian cancer in subgroups of white women in the United States. The Collaborative Ovarian Cancer Group. *Obstet Gynecol* 1994;84(5):760–764.
167. The Cancer and Steroid Hormone Study of the Centers for Disease Control and the National Institute of Child Health and Human Development: the reduction of risk of ovarian cancer associated with oral-contraceptive use. *N Engl J Med* 1987;316:650–655.
168. Hankinson SE, Colditz GA, Hunter DJ, et al. A quantitative assessment of oral contraceptive use and risk of ovarian cancer. *Obstet Gynecol* 1992;80(4):708–714.
169. John EM, Whittemore AS, Harris R, et al. Characteristics relating to ovarian cancer risk: collaborative analysis of seven U.S. case-control studies. Epithelial ovarian cancer in black women. Collaborative Ovarian Cancer Group. *J Natl Cancer Inst* 1993;85(2):142–147.
170. Ness RB, Grisso JA, Klapper J, et al. Risk of ovarian cancer in relation to estrogen and progestin dose and use characteristics of oral contraceptives. SHARE Study Group. Steroids, Hormones and Reproduction. *Am J Epidemiol* 2000;152(3);233–241.
171. Schildkraut JM, Calingaert B, Marchbanks PA, et al. Impact of progestin and estrogen potency in oral contraceptives on ovarian cancer risk. *J Natl Cancer Inst* 2002;94:32–38.
172. Ford D, Easton DF, Stratton M, et al. Genetic heterogeneity and penetrance analysis of the *BRCA1* and *BRCA2* genes in breast cancer families. *Am J Hum Genet* 1998;62:676–689.
173. Modan B, Hartge P, Hirsh-Yechezkel G, et al. Parity, oral contraceptives, and the risk of ovarian cancer among carriers and noncarriers of a *BRCA1* or *BRCA2* mutation. *N Engl J Med* 2001;345:235–240.
174. Narod SA, Risch H, Moslehi R, et al. Oral contraceptives and the risk of hereditary ovarian cancer. Hereditary Ovarian Cancer Clinical Study Group. *N Engl J Med* 1998;339:424–428.
175. Rodriguez GC, Walmer DK, Cline M, et al. Effect of progestin on the ovarian epithelium of macaques: cancer prevention through apoptosis? *J Soc Gynecol Invest* 1998;5:271–276.
176. Greenlee RT, Murray T, Bolden S, et al. Cancer statistics, 2000. *Cancer J Clin* 2000;50:7–33.
177. Grodstein F, Newcomb PA, Stampfer MJ. Postmenopausal hormone therapy and the risk of colorectal cancer: a review and meta-analysis. *Am J Med* 1999;106(5):574–582.
178. Nanda K, Bastian LA, Hasselblad V, et al. Hormone replacement therapy and the risk of colorectal cancer: a meta-analysis. *Obstet Gynecol* 1999;93(5 Pt 2):880–888.
179. Peipins LA, Newman B, Sandler RS. Reproductive history, use of exogenous hormones, and risk of colorectal adenomas. *Cancer Epidemiol Biomarkers Prev* 1997;6(9):671–675.
180. Potter JD, Bostick RM, Grandits GA, et al. Hormone replacement therapy is associated with lower risk of adenomatous polyps of the large bowel: the Minnesota Cancer Prevention Research Unit Case-Control Study. *Cancer Epidemiol Biomarkers Prev* 1996;(10):779–784.
181. Grodstein F, Martinez ME, Platz EA, et al. Postmenopausal hormone use and risk for colorectal cancer and adenoma. *Ann Intern Med* 1998; 128(9):705–712.
182. Fernandez E, La Vecchia C, D'Avanzo B, et al. Oral contraceptives, hormone replacement therapy and the risk of colorectal cancer. *Br J Cancer* 1996;73(11):1431–1435.
183. Martinez ME, Grodstein F, Giovannucci E, et al. A prospective study of reproductive factors, oral contraceptive use, and risk of colorectal cancer. *Cancer Epidemiol Biomarkers Prev* 1997;6(1):1–5.
184. Tamoxifen for early breast cancer: an overview of the randomised trials. Early Breast Cancer Trialists' Collaborative Group. *Lancet* 1998;351: 1451–1467.
185. Winer EP, Hudis C, Burstein HJ, et al. American Society of Clinical Oncology technology assessment on the use of aromatase inhibitors as adjuvant therapy for postmenopausal women with hormone receptor-positive breast cancer: status report 2004. *J Clin Oncol* 2005;23: 619–629.
186. Howell A, Cuzick J, Baum M, et al. Results of the ATAC (Arimidex, Tamoxifen, Alone or in Combination) trial after completion of 5 years' adjuvant treatment for breast cancer. *Lancet* 2005;365:60–62.
187. Goss PE, Ingle JN, Silvana, MD, et al. A ranomized trial of letrozole in postmenopausal women after five years of tamoxifen therapy for early-stage breast cancer. *N Engl J Med* 2003;349(19)1793–1802.
188. Robert N. Updated analysis of NCIC CTG MA.17. *J Clin Oncol* 2006;24:15S.
189. Thurlimann B, Keshaviah A, Coates AS, et al. A comparison of letrozole and tamoxifen in postmenopausal women with early breast cancer. *N Engl J Med* 2005;353:2747–2757.
190. Coombes R. First mature analysis of the Intergroup Exemestane Study (abstract LBA527). *J Clin Oncol* 2006;24:8S.
191. Breast Cancer Trialists' Collaborative Group: ovarian ablation in early breast cancer: overview of the randomized trials. *Lancet* 2002;348: 4628–4635.
192. Goldhirsch A, Gelber RD, Yothers G, et al. Adjuvant therapy for very young women with breast cancer: need for tailored treatments. *J Natl Cancer Inst Monogr* 2001;(30):44–51.
193. Beatson CT. Inoperable cases of carcinoma of the mamma. *Lancet* 1986;162–165.
194. Brueggemeier RW. Update on the use of aromatase inhibitors in breast cancer. *Expert Opin Pharmacother* 2006;7:1919–1930.
195. Mouridsen H, Gershanovich M, Sun Y, et al. Superior efficacy of letrozole versus tamoxifen as first-line therapy for postmenopausal women with advanced breast cancer: results of a phase III study of the International Letrozole Breast Cancer Group. *J Clin Oncol* 2001;19(10):2596–2606.
196. Nabholtz JM, Buzdar A, Pollak M, et al. Anastrozole is superior to tamoxofen as first-line therapy for advanced breast cancer in postmenopausal women: results of a North American multicenter randomized trial. Armidex Study Group. *J Clin Oncol* 2000;22(22):3758–3767.
197. Bonneterre J, Thurlimann B, Robertson JF, et al. Anastrozole versus tamoxifen as first-line therapy for advanced breast cancer in 668 postmenopausal women: results of the Tamoxifen or Arimidex Randomized Group Efficacy and Tolerability study. *J Clin Oncol* 2000;22(22): 3748–3757.
198. Chin YS, Beresford MJ, Ravichandran D, et al. Exemestane after non-steroidal aromatase inhibitors for post-menopausal women with advanced breast cancer. *Breast* 2007;16(4):436–439.
199. Carcangiu ML, Chambers JT, Voynick IM, et al. Immunohistochemical evaluation of estrogen and progesterone receptor content in 183 patients with endometrial carcinoma. Part I: Clinical and histologic correlations. *Am J Clin Pathol* 1990;94(3):247–254.
200. Thigpen JT, Blessing JA, DiSaia PJ, et al. A randomized comparison of doxorubicin alone versus doxorubicin plus cyclophosphamide in the management of advanced or recurrent endometrial carcinoma: A Gynecologic Oncology Group study. *J Clin Oncol* 1994;12:1408–1414.
201. Thigpen JT, Brady MF, Alvarez RD, et al. Oral medroxyprogesterone acetate in the treatment of advanced or recurrent endometrial carcinoma: a dose-response study by the Gynecologic Oncology Group. *J Clin Oncol* 1999;17:1736–1744.
202. Pinelli DM, Fiorica JV, Roberts WS, et al. Chemotherapy plus sequential hormonal therapy for advanced and recurrent endometrial carcinoma: a phase II study. *Gynecol Oncol* 1996;60:462–467.
203. Thigpen T, Brady MF, Homesley HD, et al. Tamoxifen in the treatment of advanced or recurrent endometrial carcinoma: a Gynecologic Oncology Group study. *J Clin Oncol* 2001;19:364–367.
204. Moore TD, Phillips PH, Nerenstone SR, et al. Systemic treatment of advanced and recurrent endometrial carcinoma: current status and future directions. *J Clin Oncol* 1991;9(6):1071–1088.
205. Fiorica JV, Brunetto VL, Hanjani P, et al. Phase II trial of alternating courses of megestrol acetate and tamoxifen in advanced endometrial carcinoma: a Gynecologic Oncology Group study. *Gynecol Oncol* 2004;92: 10–14.
206. Pandya KJ, Yeap BY, Weiner L, et al. Megestrol and tamoxifen in patients with advanced endometrial cancer: an Eastern Cooperative Oncology Group Study (E4882). *Am J Clin Oncol* 2001;24:43–46.
207. Whitney CW, Brunetto VL, Zaino RJ, et al. Phase II study of medroxyprogesterone acetate plus tamoxifen in advanced endometrial carcinoma: a Gynecologic Oncology Group study. *Gynecol Oncol* 2004;92:4–9.
208. Gadducci A, Cosio S, Genazzani AR. Old and new perspectives in the pharmacological treatment of advanced or recurrent endometrial cancer: hormonal therapy, chemotherapy and molecularly targeted therapies. *Crit Rev Oncol Hematol* 2006;58:242–256.
209. Burke TW, Walker CL. Arzoxifene as therapy for endometrial cancer. *Gynecol Oncol* 2003;90:S40–S46.
210. McMeekin D, Gordon A, Fowler J, et al. A phase II trial of arzoxifene, a selective estrogen response modulator, in patients with recurrent or advanced endometrial cancer. *Gynecol Oncol* 2003;1:64–69.
211. Rose PG, Brunetto VL, VanLe L, et al. A phase II trial of anastrozole in advanced recurrent or persistent endometrial carcinoma: a Gynecologic Oncology Group study. *Gynecol Oncol* 2000;78:212–216.
212. Ma BB, Oza A, Eisenhauer E, et al. The activity of letrozole in patients with advanced or recurrent endometrial cancer and correlation with biological markers—a study of the National Cancer Institute of Canada Clinical Trials Group. *Int J Gynecol Cancer* 2004;14:650–658.
213. Fujimoto J, Ichigo S, Hori M, et al. Progestins and danazol effect on cell-to-cell adhesion, and E-cadherin and alpha- and beta-catenin mRNA expressions. *J Steroid Biochem Mol Biol* 1996;57(5–6):275–282.
214. Ueda M, Fujii H, Yoshizawa K, et al. Effects of sex steroids and growth factors on migration and invasion of endometrial adenocarcinoma SNG-M cells in vitro. *Jpn J Cancer Res* 1996;87:524–533.
215. Soh E, Sato K. Clinical effects of danazol on endometrial hyperplasia in menopausal and postmenopausal women. *Cancer* 1990;66:983–988.

216. von Minckwitz G, Loibl S, Brunnert K, et al. Adjuvant endocrine treatment with medroxyprogesterone acetate or tamoxifen in stage I and II endometrial cancer: a multicentre, open, controlled, prospectively randomized trail. *Eur J Cancer* 2002;38:2265–2271.
217. Montz FJ, Bristow RE, Bovicelli A, et al. Intrauterine progesterone treatment of early endometrial cancer. *Am J Obstet Gynecol* 2002;186:651–657.
218. Ramirez PT, Frumovitz M, Bodurka DC, et al. Hormonal therapy for the management of grade 1 endometrial adenocarcinoma: a literature review. *Gynecol Oncol* 2004;95:133–138.
219. Rao GG, Miller DS. Hormonal therapy in epithelial ovarian cancer. *Expert Rev Anticancer Ther* 2006;6:43–47.
220. Rao BR, Slotman B. Endocrine role in ovarian cancer. *Cancer* 1996; 3:309–326.
221. Munstedt K, Steen J, Knauf AG, et al. Steroid hormone receptors and long term survival in invasive ovarian cancer. *Cancer* 2000;89:1783–1791.
222. Pujol P, Rey JM, Nirde P, et al. Differential expression of estrogen receptor-alpha and -beta messenger RNAs as a potential marker of ovarian carcinogenesis. *Cancer Res* 1998;58:5367–5373.
223. Brandenberger AW, Tee MK, Jaffe RB. Estrogen receptor alpha (ER-alpha) and beta (ER-beta) mRNAs in normal ovary, ovarian serous cystadenocarcinoma and ovarian cancer cell lines: down-regulation of ER-beta in neoplastic tissues. *J Clin Endocrinol Metab* 1998;83:1025–1028.
224. Schwartz PE, GDMWE. The role of hormonal therapy in the management of ovarian cancer. In: Gershenson DM, McGuire WP, eds. *Ovarian Cancer: Controversies in Management.* Churchill Livingstone; 1998:325–341.
225. Ahlgren JD, Ellison NM, Gottlieb RJ, et al. Hormonal palliation of chemoresistant ovarian cancer: three consecutive phase II trials of the Mid-Atlantic Oncology Program. *J Clin Oncol* 1993;11(10):1957–1968.
226. Gennatas C, Dardoufas C, Karvouni H, et al. Phase II trial of tamoxifen in patients with advanced epithelial ovarian cancer. *Proc Am Soc Clin Oncol* 1996;15:782.
227. Hamerlynck JV, Vermorken JB, Van der Burgh ME. Tamoxifen therapy in advanced ovarian cancer (abstract). *Proc Am Soc Clin Oncol* 1985;4:115.
228. Hatch KD, Beechan JB, Blessing JA, et al. Responsiveness of patients with advanced ovarian cancer to tamoxifen: a Gynecologic Oncology Group study. *Cancer* 1991;68:269–271.
229. Jager W, Sauerbrei W, Beck Maassen V, et al. A randomized comparison of triptorelin and tamoxifen as treatment of progressive ovarian cancer. *Anticancer Res* 1995;15:2639–2642.
230. Landoni F, Bonazzi C, Regallo M, et al. Antiestrogen as last-line treatment in epithelial ovarian cancer. *Chemioterapia* 1985;(4 Suppl 2):1059–1060.
231. Marth C, Sorheim N, Kaern J, et al. Tamoxifen in the treatment of recurrent ovarian carcinoma. *J Gynecol Cancer* 1997;7:256–261.
232. Osborne RJ, Malik ST, Slevin ML, et al. Tamoxifen in refractory ovarian cancer: the use of a loading dose schedule. *Br J Cancer* 1988;57: 115–116.
233. Pagel J, RCTSHI. Treatment of advanced ovarian carcinoma with tamoxifen: a phase II trial (abstract). *Proc 2nd Eur Conf Clin Oncol* 1983;42.
234. Quinn MA. Hormonal therapy of ovarian cancer. *London: Royal College of Obstetricians and Gynaecologists* 1987;383–393.
235. Rolski J, Pawlicki M. Evaluation of efficacy and toxicity of tamoxifen in patients with advanced chemotherapy resistant ovarian cancer. *Ginekol Pol* 1998;69:586–589.
236. Rowland K, Bonomi P, WGYEGJDC. Hormone receptors in ovarian cancer (abstract C-456). *Proc Am Soc Clin Oncol* 1985;4:117.
237. Schwartz PE, Chambers JT, Kohorn EI, et al. Tamoxifen in combination with cytotoxic chemotherapy in advanced epithelial ovarian cancer. A prospective randomized trial. *Cancer* 1989;63:1074–1078.
238. Shirey DR, Kavanagh JJ Jr, Gershenson DM, et al. Tamoxifen therapy of epithelial ovarian cancer. *Obstet Gynecol* 1985;66:575–578.
239. Slevin ML, Harvey VJ, Osborne RJ, et al. A phase II study of tamoxifen in ovarian cancer. *Eur J Cancer Clin Oncol* 1986;22:309–312.
240. Van Der Velden J, Gitsch G, Wain GV, et al. Tamoxifen in patients with advanced epithelial ovarian cancer. *Int J Gynecol Cancer* 1995;5:301–305.
241. van der Vange S, Greggi S, Burger CW, et al. Experience with hormonal therapy in advanced epithelial ovarian cancer. *Acta Oncol* 1995;34: 813–820.
242. Weiner SA, Alberts DS, Surwit EA, et al. Tamoxifen therapy in recurrent epithelial ovarian carcinoma. *Gynecol Oncol* 1987;27:208–213.
243. Perez-Gracia JL, Carrasco EM. Tamoxifen therapy for ovarian cancer in the adjuvant and advanced settings: systematic review of the literature and implications for future research. *Gynecol Oncol* 2002;84: 201–209.
244. Paskeviciute L, Roed H, Engelholm A. No rules without exception: a long-term complete remission observed in a study using a LH-RH agonist in platinum-refractory ovarian cancer. *Eur J Cancer* 2002; (38 Suppl 6):S73.
245. Emons G, Ortmann O, Teichert HM, et al. Luteinizing hormone-releasing hormone agonist triptorelin in combination with cytotoxic chemotherapy in patients with advanced ovarian carcinoma. A prospective double blind randomized trial. Decapeptyl Ovarian Cancer Study Group. *Cancer* 1996;78(7):1452–1460.
246. Benedetti Panici P, Greggi S, Amoroso M, et al. A combination of platinum and tamoxifen in advanced ovarian cancer failing platinum-based chemotherapy: results of phase II study. *Int J Gynecol Cancer* 2001; 11(6):438–444.

CHAPTER 18 ■ INNOVATIVE 21st CENTURY THERAPIES

ERIC K. ROWINSKY, ARNO J. MUNDT, AND NADEEM R. ABU-RUSTUM

The convergence of a plethora of recently acquired information about specific molecular abnormalities that "drive" the malignant phenotype with profound advances in biomedical technology has ushered in a wide range of novel therapeutic options to treat patients with gynecologic malignancies. It has also brought about many challenges for clinical investigators. As novel anticancer therapeutics are developed, prioritization of these therapies for efficient allotment of clinical trial resources, identification of patients whose malignancies most likely express the molecular constituents resembling the true target, and derivation of relevant endpoints for both screening and assessment will be critical to their successful incorporation into our therapeutic armamentarium (1). In this chapter, many promising novel systemic therapeutics, as well as advances in the delivery of radiotherapy, particularly intensity-modulated radiation therapy (IMRT), that are likely to make incremental improvements in outcome and therapeutic indices for patients with gynecologic malignancies are discussed. The section on novel systemic therapeutics does not include information on agents targeting malignant angiogenesis, which are reviewed in Chapter 16.

SYSTEMIC THERAPIES: ADVANCES IN THE 21st CENTURY

The number of rationally designed, target-based systemic therapeutics undergoing development is unprecedented. The cellular processes that are specifically being targeted for therapeutic development are those that principally confer autonomy, which is the hallmark of the malignant phenotype. Novel targets, many of which are listed in Table 18.1, include those that are involved in aberrant growth signal transduction, cell cycle dysregulation, evasion of apoptosis, sustained angiogenesis, tissue invasion, metastasis, and immune tolerance (2–4). Based on the results of preclinical studies and early clinical trials to date, more selective therapeutics are likely to result in less cytotoxicity to normal tissues, and hence more "breathing room" to maximize the therapeutic indices of multiagent regimens. Therefore, it is expected that the development of therapeutics that differentially affect malignant and normal tissues will more readily achieve high therapeutic indices. However, most new targets for antiproliferative therapies have not yet been validated in clinical practice, and prioritizing the long list of rationally designed, target-based therapeutics entering clinical evaluations, so that those with a high potential for improving clinical outcome are accurately identified for further study, is a formidable challenge.

Proliferative Signal Transduction Elements as Therapeutic Targets

The broad term "signal transduction" refers to the means by which regulatory molecules, which govern the fundamental processes of cell growth, differentiation, and survival (e.g., extracellular hormones, growth factors, cytokines, specialized proteins), communicate and induce responses within cells, resulting in the coordination of proliferative and other essential processes among various tissues. Cell signaling is complex, with a wide array of components interacting through cascades of chemical signals arranged in overlapping networks (5,6). These networks, consisting of parallel tracks and intricate interconnections, enhance the robustness and diversity of signaling, and permit fine tuning, and amplification and diminution of outputs, which may not be accomplished as efficiently by simpler linear cascades. However, the inherent redundancy and complexity of networks also confer protection against toxins, thereby decreasing the likelihood that any therapeutic manipulation against a single element will be highly successful, unless the element significantly contributes to the tumor's proliferative advantage.

Targeting aberrant and/or overactive proliferative cell signaling elements is perhaps the most important of ongoing developmental therapeutic endeavors against cancer, since aberrations in signal transduction processes enhance tumor cell proliferation, invasiveness, metastasis, and angiogenesis, and resist programmed cell death (apoptosis) despite insults caused by anticancer therapeutics (5–8). Furthermore, the development of therapeutics against such processes is projected to yield broadly generalizable results since most malignancies, including gynecologic cancers, possess at least one aberrant signaling element that confers a proliferative or survival advantage (5–7). The most common aberrations are those involving "loss of protein function," but others result in "gain of function" or unchecked, autonomous, or constitutive activity of elements that normally regulate cell signaling (2,5,6,8). In contrast to the situations represented by chronic myelogenous leukemia, gastrointestinal stromal cell tumors, and a small proportion of breast and lung carcinomas, in which a single aberration, such as a *bcr-abl* translocation, and a mutation in *c-kit*, *ErbB1*, or *ErbB2*, respectively, is the principal driver of tumor proliferation, and successful targeting results in profound antitumor effects, most malignancies possess many aberrations, several of which confer proliferative advantages (2,9–12). However, targeting any one specific "driver" in a tumor that has multiple relevant aberrations may result in therapeutic efficacy, the magnitude of which relates to the importance of the driver itself and its contribution

TABLE 18.1

NOVEL TARGETS AND THERAPEUTICS UNDER DEVELOPMENT AS ANTICANCER APPROACHES

General target	Specific target	Therapeutic
Growth signal transduction	Growth factor receptors ErbB family receptors Insulin growth factor–like receptor Platelet-derived growth factor receptor C-met family receptors	Anti-receptor antibodies Small-molecule inhibitors of receptor tyrosine kinases Anti-ligand antibodies
	Ras	Small molecule inhibitors of farnesyltransferase ASON (K-Ras, H-Ras, N-Ras)
	Raf	ASONs
	MAPK	Small molecule inhibitors
	Rapamycin-sensitive and PI3K/Akt/*PTEN* pathways	Small molecule inhibitors Rapamycin analogs Small molecule inhibitors against mTOR, PI3K, akt, p70s6k
Death-survival equilibrium	Bcl-2	ASONs Small-molecule inhibitors
	TRAIL and other death receptors	TRAIL agonist ligands TRAIL agonist antibodies
	Survival proteins	Therapeutics targeting survivin, clusterin, others
Epigenetic mechanisms	Histone deacetylation Histone methylation	HDAC inhibitors Methyltransferase inhibitors and ASONs
Cell cycle control	Cyclin-dependent kinases (cdk) Checkpoint kinases 1 and 2	Small molecule kinase inhibitors
Protein degradation	Heat shock protein (Hsp-90)	Geldanamycin derivatives and other small molecules
	Ubiquitin-proteasome degradation pathway	Proteasome inhibitors Ubiquitin ligase inhibitors
Immune tolerance	Targeting CTLA4	Monoclonal antibodies

Note: ASONs, antisense oligonucleotides; CTLA4, cytotoxic T-lymphocyte–associated antigen 4; HDAC, histone deacetylase; MAPK, mitogen-activated protein kinase; mTOR, molecular target of rapamycin; PI3K, phosphatidylinositol 3-kinase; TRAIL, tumor necrosis factor–related apoptosis-inducing ligand.

to the tumor's proliferative and/or survival advantage. Nevertheless, even if the overall efficacy achieved by targeting only one of many drivers may be somewhat limited, the importance of many types of signaling elements, several of which are shown in Figure 18.1, as well as the selectivity of their cognate therapeutic, may impart minimal toxicity and favorable therapeutic indices, rendering the agent an attractive addition to our therapeutic armamentarium. Furthermore, the development of genomic profiling to assess aberrant expression of genes that govern signaling pathways or critical cellular elements, as well as pathway mapping, may facilitate achieving the aforementioned goals (13,14).

Rationale for Targeting the ErbB Receptor Family

Most current development efforts directed against signal transduction processes involve either membrane receptors or elements that comprise downstream signaling cascades. With regard to signal transduction receptors, development efforts are predominantly being directed against receptor tyrosine kinases (RTKs) and G-protein receptors (GPCRs), which have secondary relay systems that permit signal amplification, diversification, and cross talk (1,5–9). The complexity of signal transduction networks and the challenges related to the development of therapeutics against these intricate systems are exemplified by the complex structural and functional aspects of the ErbB receptor family and related downstream processes, as well as the multifactoral determinants of each specific signal. The overexpression and/or constitutive activation of ErbB receptors favor cell proliferation, invasiveness, angiogenesis, and resistance to both chemotherapy and radiotherapy (3,5,6,8). Members of the ErbB receptor family include ErbB1 (also called EGFR or HER1), ErbB2 (HER2 or neu*)*, ErbB3 (HER3), and ErbB4 (HER4), which are commonly overexpressed, overactive, or constitutively active in ovarian and other epidermoid gynecologic malignancies (5,6,8,15–22). In addition to the extracellular domain of ErbB, which binds to growth factors and serves as a target for therapeutic antibodies, the ErbB receptor is comprised of a transmembrane domain and intracellular portions that consist of an RTK domain and a domain that regulates RTK activity (Fig. 18.2) (5,6,8,15,16). Ligand binding induces conformational changes in the receptor, which in turn activates the RTK, thereby facilitating dimerization with other ErbB receptors (5,6,8,15–21). Following dimerization, conformational changes result in phosphorylation or "activation" of specific tyrosine residues. Activated ErbB receptors, in turn, activate specific downstream signaling elements, thereby transducing mitogenic and other types of signals in the cell.

The specificity and potency and, in essence, the diversity of intracellular signals are determined, in part, by the effectors of ErbB, as well as by the identity of the ligand, dimer, and

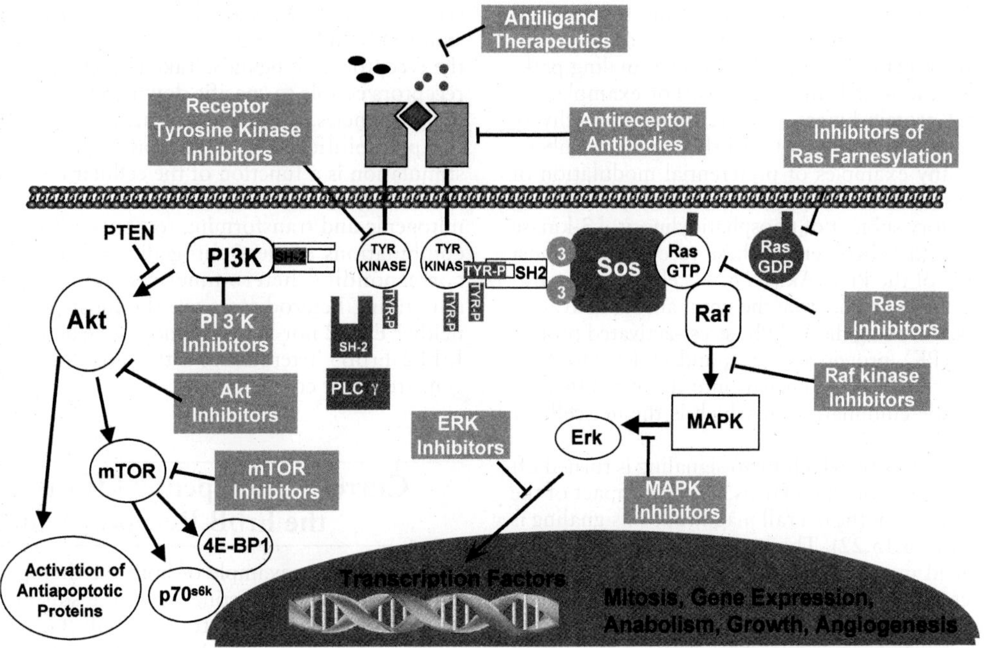

FIGURE 18.1. Schematic representation of critical signal transduction pathways and pathway elements that are being targeted with therapeutic strategies consisting of small molecules, antibodies, ASONs, and other novel approaches. The ErbB family of receptors, the insulin growth factor–like receptor (IGF-IR), the platelet-derived growth factor (PDGFR), and the c-met receptor family are examples of relevant upstream receptor targets for strategic therapeutic development.

specific structural determinants of the receptors. However, the principal determinant is the vast array of phosphotyrosine-binding (PTB) proteins that associate with the C-terminal "downstream docking" tail of each ErbB receptor after engagement into dimeric complexes (5,6,8,15–21). Whether a specific site is autophosphorylated, and hence which PTB signaling proteins are engaged, are determined by many factors, including the identity of the ligand and the specific heterodimer partner.

The diversity of signals generated through the ErbB receptor family is largely determined by the amino acid sequences of their C-terminal domains (8,16–21). These critical sequences, which contain tyrosine residues that undergo phosphorylation, represent docking sites for proteins that are involved in signal transduction. Docking sites are provided for proteins that recognize specific PTB residues in the context of their surrounding amino acids. Each ErbB receptor displays a distinct pattern of C-terminal autophosphorylation sites. At least for

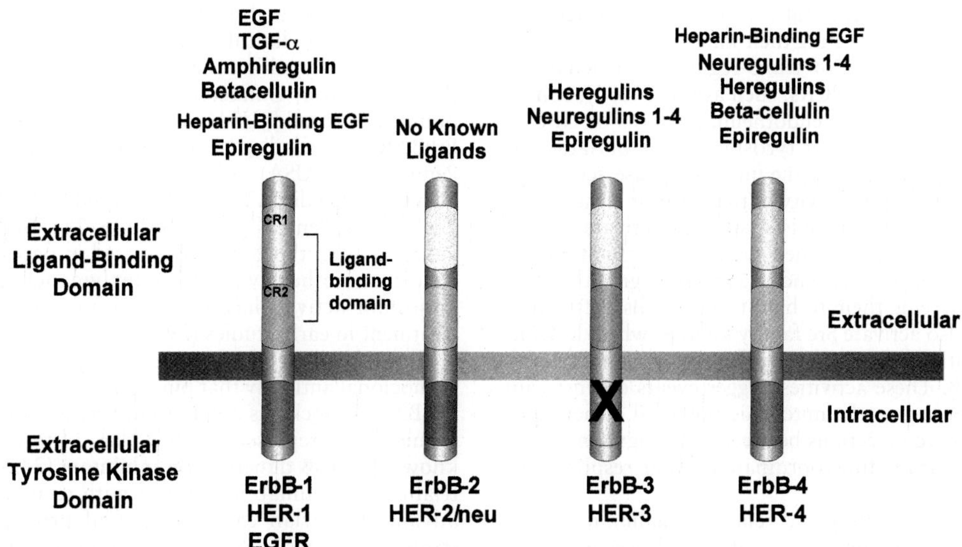

FIGURE 18.2. Structures of ErbB family receptor tyrosine kinase receptors and their cognate ligands. The receptor consists of three domains: a ligand-binding extracellular domain containing two cysteine-rich regions (CR1 and CR2), a transmembrane domain, and an intracellular domain containing a tyrosine kinase region.

ErbB2, which does not have a direct activating ligand, PTB sites are essential for the transforming properties of the receptor. There is also a great deal of overlap in the signaling pathways activated by the four ErbB receptors. For example, the mitogen-activated protein kinase (MAPK) signaling pathway is an invariable activation target of all ErbB family members. There are also many examples of preferential modulation of specific pathways such as the presence of multiple binding sites for the regulatory subunit of phosphatidylinositol 3-kinase (PI3K) on ErbB3 and ErbB4 render these receptors the most efficient activators of the PI3K/Akt/*PTEN* "cell survival pathway" (8,17–19). Signals arising from the simultaneous activation of linear cascades, including the MAPK, stress-activated protein kinase cascade (SAPK), protein kinase C, and PI3K/Akt/*PTEN* pathways, are integrated in the nucleus into distinct transcriptional programs, the culmination of which is the net cellular response.

The principal process by which ErbB signaling is turned off is ligand-mediated receptor endocytosis, and the impact of the kinetics of this process on the overall magnitude of signaling is often understated (5,6,15,22). The kinetics of signal degradation are determined in part by the composition of the receptors. ErbB1 receptors are more likely to be degraded via endosome formation and lysomsomal degradation, whereas the other ErbB receptors are relatively endocytosis impaired and are more often recycled (5,6,8,22). The rapid endocytosis and degradation of the activated ErbB receptor attenuate the signal generated at the cell surface in response to growth factor stimulation. The specific mode and site of degradation are also determined in part by the composition of the dimer. For example, ErbB1 homodimers are processed primarily by the lysosome; ErbB3 molecules are constitutively recycled; and heterodimerization with ErbB2 decreases the rate of endocytosis and increases recycling of its partners (5,6,8,22). ErbB2 homodimers, which are stable in the environment of the endosomal vacuole, are rapidly tagged with ubiquitin and processed for digestion, resulting in relatively weak signals, whereas ErbB2 heterodimers are unstable in the endosome, resulting in a lower rate of degradation and a higher rate of receptor recirculation. Networks also integrate heterologous signals from other networks and systems. In the case of ErbB, heterologous signals, including those induced by hormones, neurotransmitters, lymphokines, and stress inducers, are integrated into downstream messages (6,8). These interactions are mediated by protein kinases that directly phosphorylate the ErbB receptors, thereby affecting their kinase activity or endocytic transport. One type of *trans*-regulatory mechanism involves the activation of GPCRs, such as those for lysophosphatidic acid, thrombin, and endothelin. Agonists of GPCRs may result in a net increase of tyrosine phosphorylation of ErbB1 and ErbB2 by increasing the intrinsic kinase activity or inhibiting the phosphatase activity of the receptor. By a poorly defined mechanism, these agonists can also activate matrix metalloproteinases, which can then cleave membrane-tethered ErbB ligands (such as heparin-binding epidermal growth factor [EGF]), thereby freeing them to bind to the ErbBs. Activation of GPCRs may also activate Src family kinases, which leads to the phosphorylation of tyrosine residues on the intracellular domains of ErbB. These activities trigger events downstream of ErbB, contributing to the mitogenic potential of heterologous agonists. Interconnections between other signaling pathways help to integrate and coordinate cellular responses to extracellular stimuli.

The ErbB receptor family and related signaling networks provide enormous signaling diversity at many levels, including ligand specificity, receptor partnering, providing scaffolding sites for effector signaling proteins and substrate specificity for their kinase activities, receptor degradation, and integration of heterologous signals (5,6,8,16–24). Diversity between various types of cells and tissues also exists, depending on the expression levels and the preferred stoichiometry for interactions of the receptors and ligands. Taken together, it is clear that ErbB receptors couple to specific downstream pathways with differing efficiencies, thus affording an astonishing range of signaling possibilities. The particular cellular response to ErbB stimulation is a function of the cellular context, as well as the specific ligand and ErbB dimer. This has been shown best for mitogenic and transforming responses; homodimeric receptor combinations are less mitogenic and transforming than the corresponding heterodimeric combinations, and ErbB2-containing heterodimers are the most potent. For example, neither ErbB2 nor ErbB3 alone can be activated by ligand; the ErbB2-ErbB3 heterodimer is the most transforming and mitogenic receptor complex.

Current Therapeutic Efforts Targeting the ErbB Receptor Family

Perhaps the best example of both the therapeutic implications and limitations of targeting signal transduction elements is the situation represented by trastuzumab (Genentech, South San Francisco, California, USA) in targeting ErbB2 (HER2/neu) in patients with breast cancer (6,11,23–25). Targeting ErbB2 with trastuzumab results in impressive clinical activity, albeit limited to women with breast cancer whose tumors have amplified ErbB2, which drives proliferation (6,11,23–25). In contrast to the situation in breast cancer, trastuzumab treatment results in negligible antitumor activity in patients with advanced ovarian carcinoma, which commonly expresses ErbB2 (25–29). The lack of relevant activity despite receptor expression is due to the fact that *HER2/neu* gene amplification, which is a prominent driver of proliferation in breast cancer, is uncommon in gynecologic and most other malignancies. The same can be said about the profound responsiveness of only a small proportion of non–small cell lung cancers with mutations of ErbB1 following treatment with small molecule RTK inhibitors and other therapeutics target ErbB1 (12). Although these signal transduction inhibitors confer clinical benefit in patients with various cancers that do not have ErbB1 RTK mutations, much less impressive activity is generally noted.

In addition to therapeutic antibody approaches designed to target ErbB2, several small-molecule RTK inhibitors of ErbB2 are undergoing clinical development. They encompass agents that specifically inhibit the ErbB2 RTK, including CP724,714 (Pfizer, Groton, Connecticut, USA) and ARRY-380 (Array, Boulder, Colorado, USA); agents that inhibit both ErbB1 and ErbB2 RTKs, including lapatinib (Glaxo SmithKline, Philadelphia, Pennsylvania, USA), ARRY-543 (Array); and pan-ErbB RTK inhibitors, including CI-1033 (Pfizer) and EKB-569 (Wyeth Ayerst, Collegeville, Pennsylvania, USA) (26–28). To date, these agents have not been thoroughly evaluated in patients with ovarian cancer and other gynecologic malignancies, but impressive antitumor activity has not been observed with single-agent treatment in early studies (29–33).

Pertuzumab (2C4; Genentech), a recombinant humanized monoclonal antibody that binds to the extracellular domain of ErbB2 and blocks its ability to dimerize with other ErbB family members, represents a new class of targeted therapeutics known as ErbB dimerization inhibitors (34,35). In a phase 2 trial of pertuzumab in patients with recurrent or refractory advanced ovarian cancer, proof of principle was demonstrated, with 5 (4.3%) of 117 patients experiencing partial responses; 8 (6.8%) additional patients had stable disease lasting at least 6 months (35).

Still other approaches to targeting ErbB involve monoclonal antibodies and small-molecule inhibitors of ErbB1. Monoclonal antibodies, such as cetuximab (Imclone Systems, New York, New York, USA) and panitumumab (Amgen, Thousand Oaks, California, USA), bind to the extracellular domain of the ErbB1 subfamily and preferentially block binding of ErbB1 stimulatory ligands (36,37). However, monoclonal antibodies directed against ErbB1 have not yet demonstrated impressive antitumor activity following single-agent treatment in patients with refractory or recurrent ovarian cancer (38). Nevertheless, intriguing preliminary activity has been observed with cetuximab plus platinum-taxane–based chemotherapy in the first-line treatment of women with advanced ovarian cancer (39). Similar to the situation with ErbB2 targeting, approaches that target ErbB1 with small molecules include developing agents that competitively and reversibly inhibit the ErbB1 RTK activity. Small-molecule inhibitors targeting ErbB1 include those with specificity for ErbB1 RTK, including gefitinib (AstraZeneca London, UK) and erlotinib (OSI Pharmaceuticals, Mellville, New York, USA), and those targeting the RTKs of both ErbB1 and ErbB2 receptor subfamilies (e.g., lapatinib, ARRY-543) (23,36). Still others, as previously discussed, form irreversible covalent linkages with the cysteine residues in the RTK domains of several types of ErbB receptors. CI-1033 is an example of an irreversible inhibitor of all four ErbB family member RTKs, whereas EKB-569 irreversibly inhibits the RTK activity of both ErbB1 and ErbB2 (26–28,32,33). The relative therapeutic merits of antibodies versus small molecules, inhibitors of a single ErbB RTK versus multiple RTKs, and reversible versus irreversible receptor binding are not known, but antibodies, in contrast to small molecules, induce rapid receptor internalization and degradation (40). In clinical evaluations of small-molecule inhibitors of ErbB1 RTK in patients with advanced non–small cell lung, colorectal, renal, head and neck, and ovarian carcinomas, largely not prescreened for mutations and/or expression of ErbB1, low rates of tumor regression have been observed (36,41–44). Few studies have been performed to date in gynecologic malignancies; however, epidermoid carcinomas of gynecologic origin commonly express all ErbB receptor targets, but the ErbB family members do not appear to be major drivers of proliferation. Although ErbB1 mutations have been reported in some ovarian epithelial carcinomas, mutation rates are much lower compared to non–small cell lung cancer (43). In an early phase 2 study of erlotinib in previously treated patients with ErbB-expressing ovarian carcinoma, 3 (10%) of 30 heavily pretreated subjects had partial responses and 15 (50%) had stable disease as their best response (44). Thus far, negligible anticancer activity has also been observed with erlotinib and gefitinib administered as single agents in other studies, as well as with small-molecule inhibitors of ErbB1 (44). However, most clinical evaluations of signal transduction inhibitors in gynecologic malignancies to date have not been randomized and therefore have not been adequately designed to assess the degree to which these agents affect tumor growth rates, time to tumor progression, and overall survival. Another important challenge is to discern which patients have the highest likelihood of benefiting from treatment with ErbB-targeted therapies based on the biologic features of their tumors, as well as determining the optimal means to combine these novel therapies with other anticancer agents.

Targeting the MAPK Pathway (Ras/Raf/Mitogen-Activated ERK Kinase)

Following activation of membrane-bound members of the Ras family of small GPCRs, proliferative signals are relayed to downstream intracellular signaling elements along the MAPK pathway, most prominently to the Raf family kinases, which in turn trigger mitogen-activated ERK kinase (MEK)/extracellular signal–regulated kinase (ERK1/ERK2) (45–52). Likewise, Ras can directly relay survival signals by activating the PI3K/Akt/*PTEN* "cell survival" pathway (45–52). Ras activation through the MAPK pathway modulates the activity of nuclear transcription factors, including Fos, Jun, and AP-1, which regulate the transcription of genes required for proliferation (45,49–52).

MAPK represents the convergence of a broad array of signals from membrane receptors, and the network of phosphorylation-mediated signals emanating from MAPK is equally expansive. Functionally, MAPK circuits are three-tiered kinase modules (45–47,49–52). The Raf-1-MEK-ERK module is employed ubiquitously in the transduction of cell-type specific growth and differentiation signals from RTKs and GPCRs (45–47). Signaling through MAPK also mediates inflammatory and stress response to stimuli such as cytokines, FasL, and tumor necrosis factor (TNF). Additionally, the MAPK pathway does not function in isolation, but instead is integrated into other cellular signaling networks that impact upon MAPK signaling. Since cells are almost always receiving many types of stimuli, response outputs represent the integration of many signaling pathways, and slight modifications in the quality and quantity of stimuli can vastly alter transcriptional profiles, cell cycle commitment, and the equilibrium between cell survival and apoptosis. Corresponding to the prominence of MAPKs in numerous signaling events, perturbations in the MAPK signaling pathway can profoundly influence cellular integrity. Developmental therapeutic efforts are currently being directed at several components of the MAPK pathway, particularly the Raf-1-MEK-ERK module (45–47).

Targeting Raf

Since the Raf family of signaling elements is immediately downstream of Ras, which has not been successfully inhibited by targeting Ras maturation (i.e., Ras farnesylation), Ras expression (e.g., antisense oligonucleotides [ASONs]), and structural elements, and because Raf mutations result in autonomous growth and transformation, Raf has become an important target for therapeutic development (45–48,53). The Raf family is composed of three related serine-threonine protein kinases, Raf-1, A-Raf, and B-Raf, which act, in part, as downstream effectors of Ras signaling. Raf-1 is ubiquitous, whereas B-Raf is found mainly in neural tissue, and A-Raf is most abundant in urogenital organs, including the ovary, kidney, testes, and prostate. B-Raf and A-Raf, like Raf-1, are Ras effectors, but the specificity of their activities is not well understood. Raf mutations have also recently described and mutated B-Raf, which results in elevated kinase activity and transforming properties, which is found in 66% of malignant melanomas and at a lower frequency in many other cancers (45). Furthermore, Raf appears to play a role in tumorigenesis, as it can be activated independently of Ras by protein kinase C-α and promotes the expression of the multidrug resistance gene (53–55). Activated Ras interacts directly with the amino-terminal regulatory domain of the Raf kinase, resulting in a cascade of reactions that include direct activation of MEK (45–47,53–55). The serine-threonine kinase Raf-1, a well-characterized downstream effector of Ras, is activated in a stepwise sequence of events that include phosphorylation, recruitment to the plasma membrane, and binding to activated Ras (49–52). Following activation, Raf-1 in turn activates MEK through phosphorylation of two separate serines. Raf-1 is the protein product of the c-*raf* proto-oncogene.

Since Raf kinase is the first committed step in the MAPK pathway, it is an attractive target for therapeutic development since successful targeting may block growth signaling from a diverse array of stimuli (45–48,53). Furthermore, there is a large body of experimental evidence indicating that inhibition of Raf kinase can reverse the phenotype of Ras-transformed cells and block tumor growth (53).

Several approaches to targeting Raf, including ASONs and small molecules, are being evaluated. ISIS 5132 (CGP 69846A; ISIS, Carlsbad, California, USA) is a 20-base phosphorothioate ASON designed to hybridize to the 3′ untranslated sequences of the *c-raf-1* gene (56–58). Binding of ISIS 5132 to Raf-1 mRNA promotes RNAaseH-mediated mRNA degradation and reduced Raf-1 protein synthesis in a nucleotide sequence–specific and concentration-dependent fashion. ISIS 5132 inhibits expression of c-Raf mRNA, as well as the proliferation of ovarian, lung, colon, cervical, prostate, and colon carcinoma cell lines (53,56,57). Acute toxicities, including fever; fatigue; transient, asymptomatic prolongation of activated partial thromboplastin time; and activation of alternate complement activation, have been attributed to the phosphorothioate backbone (53,58). Another approach involves the development of small-molecule inhibitors of Raf kinase, such as sorafenib (Bayer Corporation Pharmaceutical Division, West Haven, Connecticut, USA), a bis-aryl urea designed to specifically inhibit the ATP-binding site of Raf kinase (53,59,60). The importance of therapeutics that effectively target cells driven by *ras* mutations cannot be overstated since *ras* mutations occur in 30% of human malignancies. Additionally, tumor cells with the predominant *ras* mutation *K-ras* are not effectively targeted by farnesyltransferase inhibitors due to alternative prenylation pathways that can take the place of farnesyltransferase, thereby conferring resistance. *Ras* mutations drive growth signals downstream through Raf and other MAPK signaling elements (45–47,53). Sorafenib is active in tumors that overexpress growth factor receptors, as well as in those with *K-ras* mutations, and the agent has shown robust activity against human colon, pancreatic, lung, and ovarian cancers in preclinical studies (53,59,60). However, sorafenib is promiscuous, inhibiting tyrosine kinase activity of vascular endothelial growth factor receptor (VEGFR) 1 and VEGFR2, and it is not known if Raf inhibition is responsible for the agent's anticancer activity *in vivo*. In fact, sorafenib has received regulatory approval in the United States and many other countries for treatment of advanced renal cancer, most likely due to its VEGFR2 inhibitory actions, and it has demonstrated clinical activity in liver, lung, breast, ovarian, and other solid malignancies in both early- and late-stage clinical trials (53). Toxicities include stomatitis, vomiting, diarrhea, fatigue, skin rash, hand-foot syndrome, lymphopenia, and anemia (53). Other small-molecule inhibitors of Raf kinase are also under development.

Targeting MEK

MEK (also called MAPK kinase [MAPKK]) is a dual-specificity kinase in that it activates ERK by phosphorylating both tyrosine and threonine residues. Two related genes code for MEK1 and MEK2 (45–47,49–52). Both MEK proteins play critical roles in Ras signaling. However, MEK1 and MEK2 differ in ERK binding affinities and, possibly, in their abilities to activate ERK. In the mitogen-activated Ras/Raf/MEK/ERK cascade, Raf generally activates the dual-specific serine-threonine and tyrosine kinases MEK1 and MEK2, which then activate ERK1 and ERK2. MEK has not been identified as an oncogene product in human malignancies; however, it is a critical point of integration of input from many other protein kinases. In addition, Ras is restricted in its substrate specificity, with the MAPKs being the only important substrates. Therefore, MEK is a target of great interest for cancer therapeutic development, and several small-molecule MEK inhibitors (ARRY-886, Array BioPharma; PD325901, Pfizer), which have been associated with impressive preclinical activity, are in clinical development (61–65).

Targeting ERK

In mammalian cells, there are two closely related genes that code for ERK1 and ERK2. Following activation, ERKs enter the nucleus of cells where they are phosphorylated and, in turn, activate transcription factors, which leads to the expression of genes involved in growth and differentiation (45–47, 49–52). Although no direct inhibitors of ERK are currently in clinical development, ERK is actively being pursued as a strategic target for therapeutic development.

Targeting the PI3K/Akt/*PTEN* Pathway

Cellular survival involves an active "decision" that is monitored continuously and determined by a balance of signals that promote either survival or apoptosis. These signals relay information about the availability of growth and survival factors, supply of nutrients and oxygen, cellular stress, and genomic integrity, and activate death receptors. Sufficient survival signaling enables cellular repair under conditions of limited cellular and genomic damage, whereas insufficient survival and/or heightened oppositional signaling can trigger cell death via the PI3K/Akt/*PTEN* pathway. On the other hand, irreparable DNA damage may lead to diminished survival signaling, resulting in apoptosis to prevent the propagation of deleterious mutations. Also, many types of amplified, overexpressed, and aberrant signaling elements in the PI3K/Akt/*PTEN* pathway increase survival signaling (66–72). For example, PI3K and the serine-threonine protein kinase Akt (also known as protein kinase B) are amplified or overexpressed in many ovarian, endometrial, and cervical cancers, and may even play a causal role in the development of several types of gynecologic cancer (66–76).

PI3K, a nonreceptor kinase, can be activated by numerous signals generated by growth factor receptors, including the ErbB family, platelet-derived growth factor receptor (PDGFR), insulin-like growth factor receptor (IGF-IR), VEGFRs, integrins, and GCPRs. The main effector of the PI3K/Akt/*PTEN* pathway, Akt, phosphorylates phosphoinositides, which in turn generate 3-phosphorylated phospholipids (PI3Ps) that act as membrane tethers for proteins with pleckstrin homology (PH) regions, including Akt and phosphoinositide-dependent kinase 1 (PDK1). Binding of Akt to membrane PI3Ps results in the translocation of Akt to the plasma membrane, bringing Akt in contact with PDK1, which is responsible for phosphorylation events required to activate Akt. Akt is the focal point for survival signals emanating from growth and survival receptors (66–72). In its activated state, Akt inhibits apoptosis by phosphorylating antiapoptotic substrates, including Bcl-2, Bcl_{XL}-antagonist causing cell death (BAD), forehead homolog 1, glycogen synthase-3, IκB kinase, and caspase-9. The PI3Ks, Akt, and PDK1 regulate many cellular processes, including proliferation, survival following antiapoptotic signaling, carbohydrate metabolism, and motility, and there is emerging evidence that these kinases are important components of the molecular mechanisms of disease such as cancer, diabetes, and chronic inflammation (66–68).

The dominant influence of Akt on cellular survival is suggested by the causal role of activating mutations of several elements of the Akt pathway in the development of many cancers (66,67). Growth factor RTKs, integrin-dependent cell adhesion elements, and GCPRs activate PI3K, both directly and indirectly, through adaptor molecules. The tumor suppressor oncogene *PTEN* is a negative regulator of Akt activation, and deletions or mutations of *PTEN,* in many types of cancer, particularly endometrial, ovarian (especially the endometrioid variant), and breast cancers, and high-grade astrocytomas, permit genomically compromised cells to survive and accumulate further DNA damage, which in turn leads to neoplastic transformation (66,77). Conversely, *PTEN* mutations are uncommon in cervical cancer, but loss of *PTEN* expression through epigenetic mechanisms is common in cervical cancer and appears to be associated with poor survival (78,79). In addition to the influence of PI3K/Akt hyperactivity on enhanced survival signaling in many types of cancer, including gynecologic malignancies, hyperactive signaling through the PI3K/Akt/*PTEN* pathway is associated with resistance to inhibitors of ErbB1 and ErbB2, as well as many other classes of molecular targeting and cytotoxic agents (66–76,80–82). Although efforts are being directed at developing specific small-molecule inhibitors of PI3K, PDK1, and Akt, they have largely resulted in nonspecific kinase inhibitors such as wortmannin and LY294002 (Eli Lilly, Indianapolis, Indiana, USA). Nevertheless, more specific inhibitor candidates, including PX-866 (ProlX, Tucson, Arizona, USA), SF1126 (Semafore, Indianapolis, Indiana, USA), a prodrug of LY294002, and p110alpha subunit inhibitors (Piramed; Slough, UK), are in preclinical or early clinical development. Therapeutics targeting signaling elements upstream of PI3K, such as inhibitors of the IGF-IR, and downstream of PI3K and Akt, such as molecular target of rapamycin (mTOR) and the antiapoptotic protein Bcl-2, are in more advanced stages of development.

Targeting mTOR-Dependent and Rapamycin-Sensitive Pathways

mTOR (also called FRAP, RAFT1, and RAPT1) is a member of the PI3K related kinase (PIKK) family of protein kinases, which link proliferative stimuli to cell cycle progression and nutrient utilization (7,83–88). mTOR, which plays a critical role in transducing proliferative signals mediated through the PI3K/Akt/*PTEN* signaling pathway, and vice versa, regulates protein translation by altering the phosphorylation state of the translational regulator eukaryotic initiation factor 4E-binding protein (4E-BP1) and a 70-kDa S6 kinase known as $p70^{s6k}$ (Fig. 18.3). In addition to its central role in modulating protein synthesis, mTOR plays a fundamental role in other critical cellular functions that affect cell growth and proliferation, such as angiogenesis and cytoskeletal organization (7,83–88). The regulation of mTOR is complex, involving several associated proteins and pathways. mTOR is repressed by tuberin, which is a product of the tuberous sclerosis complex-2 (TSC2) (7,83–88). Following Akt activation, TSC2 is inactivated by phosphorylation, which in turn results in mTOR activation. Effectors of mTOR include $p70^{s6k}$ and 4E-BP1. Phosphorylation of 4E-BP1 results in the dissociation of 4E-BP1 from eIF4E, thereby relieving the inhibition of 4E-BP1 on eIF4E-dependent translation initiation (7). eIF4E overexpression enhances cell growth and transforms cells by increasing the translation of key growth-promoting proteins, including cyclin D1, c-Myc, and the VEGF ligands. Deregulation of upstream growth-promoting pathways that converge on mTOR induce aberrant mTOR activity and relay unchecked growth signals that

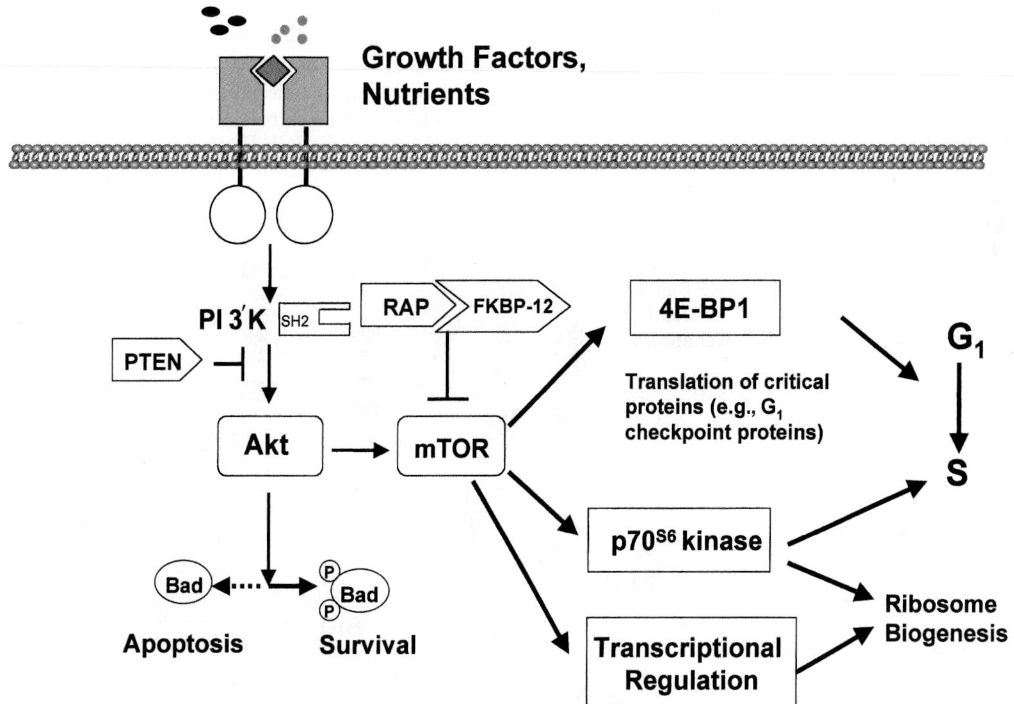

FIGURE 18.3. Rapamycin-sensitive signal transduction pathway. Growth factors and nutrients induce signaling along several pathways including the PI3K cell survival pathway, which relay proapoptotic signals downstream, as well as growth stimulatory signals downstream through mTOR. Rapamycin (RAP) and RAP analogs bind to the immunophilin FK506 binding protein-12 (FKBP-12). The RAP-FKBP-12 complex blocks the kinase activity of mTOR, which, in turn, inhibits 4E-BP1, $p70^{s6k}$, and other translational regulators. The inhibition of 4E-BP1 and $p70^{s6k}$ decreases ribosomal biosynthesis and the translational of mRNA of specific proteins essential for cell-cycle progression from G_1 to S phase.

result in cellular growth, proliferation, and carcinogenesis. Dysregulation of mTOR signaling occurs in many types of human cancer, and activation of the mTOR pathway occurs frequently in gynecologic malignancies, particularly ovarian and endometrial cancers (7,83–90). In fact, aberrant phosphorylation of mTOR has been detected in more than 70% of primary endometrial cancers, most likely through *PTEN* mutations and activation of other PI3K/Akt/*PTEN* pathway elements (7,83–90).

Targeting mTOR

In preclinical studies, inhibition of mTOR function abolishes the proliferative and nutrient utilization signals mediated through the PI3K/Akt/*PTEN* signaling pathway, resulting in cell cycle arrest and tumor growth inhibition (7,83–90). The prototypic mTOR inhibitor, rapamycin, a macrolide fungicide isolated from *Streptomyces hygroscopicus,* exerts potent antimicrobial, immunosuppressant, and antineoplastic actions (7,83–90). Because of its profound immunosuppressive actions, rapamycin was initially developed and received regulatory approval for prevention of allograft rejection following organ transplantation. However, rapamycin confers impressive antiproliferative activity in a diverse range of experimental cancers. Malignant tumors with aberrations of signaling elements that activate the PI3K pathway, particularly *PTEN* deletions and hyperactivation of PI3K and Akt, are especially sensitive to inhibition of mTOR following rapamycin treatment (7,84,85,87,89–94). Rapamycin strongly inhibits the growth of cervical, ovarian, and endometrial cancers *in vitro*, which is associated with reduced phosphorylation of downstream targets, as well as the reversal of resistance to chemotherapeutic agents (7,84,85,87,89–94).

The antiproliferative actions of rapamycin and rapamycin analogs appear to be principally due to their ability to bind to the intracellular immunophilin FKBP-12, thereby forming a complex that binds to and inhibits the activity of mTOR (7,83–88). The inhibition of mTOR blocks the activation of 4E-BP1, $p70^{s6k}$, and other translational modulators (Fig. 18.4), which in turn inhibits the synthesis of proteins required for G_1 to S phase traverse and ribosomal biosynthesis. However, the poor solubility and chemical instability of rapamycin preclude its administration on a variety of dose schedules, and several rapamycin analogs are more amenable to parenteral administration such as temsirolimus (CCI-779; Wyeth Ayerst), which has undergone regulatory approval for the treatment of renal cancer in the United States, and both everolimus (RAD001; Novartis, Basel, Switzerland) and AP23573 (Ariad, Cambridge, Massachusetts, USA), which are undergoing clinical development (7,84,85,93–96). The toxicities of these rapamycin analogs are similar to those of rapamycin (e.g., mild cytopenias, fatigue, elevations of serum triglycerides and liver functions), but infectious complications due to protracted immunosuppression have not been noted to date. In clinical studies, regression of several types of advanced cancer, including breast, renal, and lung carcinomas, lymphoma, and soft-tissue sarcoma, has been reported. In addition to conferring clinical benefit in renal cancer, robust activity in mantle cell lymphoma has also been noted with temsirolimus. Clinical evaluations in patients with endometrial and ovarian carcinomas are ongoing (7,84,85,93–96). Preliminary results of a phase 2 study of temsirolimus in patients with recurrent or metastatic endometrial cancer indicate modest activity, with confirmed partial responses in 5 (26%) of 19 evaluable patients, and stable disease as best response in 12 (63%) other patients. Responses have been observed irrespective of *PTEN* status (95).

Targeting Insulin-Like Growth Factor and Related Elements

The critical roles of IGF-IR and its related signaling elements in the growth and development of both normal and cancer cells are increasingly being recognized (96–100). These signaling elements are highly conserved and may have evolved to regulate cellular proliferation in response to nutrient availability. In addition to their roles in balancing cellular proliferation and apoptosis, the IGF-IR and its close counterpart, the insulin

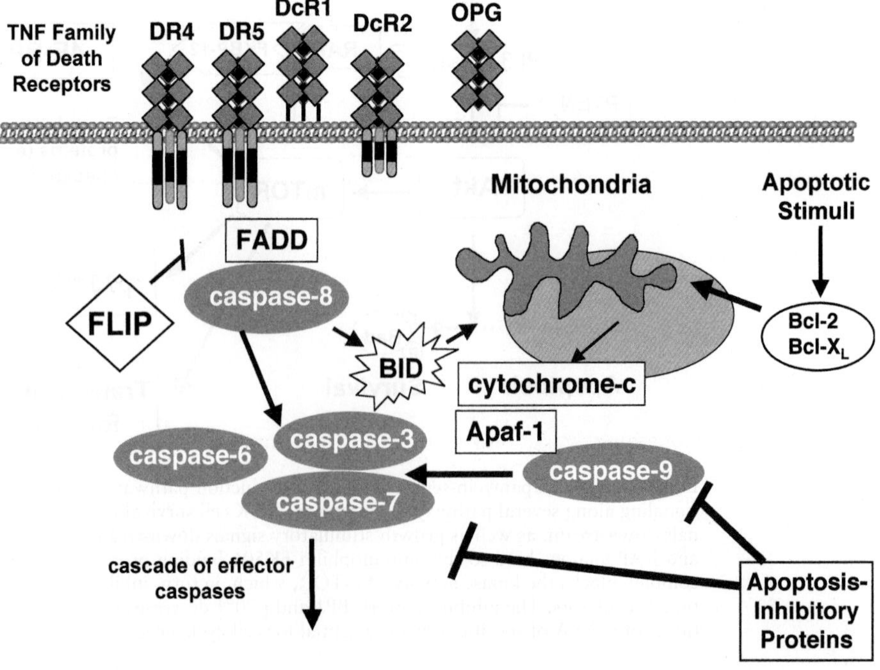

FIGURE 18.4. Schematic representation of the intrinsic and extrinsic pathways of apoptosis. The intrinsic pathway is mediated by Bcl-2 family members at the mitochondria that releases cytochrome-c and activates the proapoptotic protein apoptotic protease activating factor-1 (Apaf-1) and the cascade of caspases. The extrinsic pathway is mediated by the TNF family of receptors at the cellular membrane. *Note:* TNF, tumor necrosis family; FADD, Fas associated death domain.

receptor (IR), play key roles in regulating energy metabolism, body size, longevity, and various organ-specific functions (96–100). Experimental studies in animal model systems have provided evidence that the proliferative and metastatic potentials of cancer cells are enhanced by IGF-IR activation either due to higher levels of circulating IGF-1 or autocrine production of ligands by cancer cells (101). The critical role of IGF-IR signaling in controlling cellular renewal has led to interest in targeting the IGF-IR as a therapeutic strategy against cancer (96,98,101,102).

The IGF-IR and its ligands, IGF-1 and IGF-2, play key roles in the development, maintenance, and progression of cancer (98,101–108). IGF-IR activation stimulates cellular proliferation and differentiation and protects cells from undergoing apoptosis in the face of robust proapoptotic stimuli. Overexpression of the IGF-IR in cancer cells, often in concert with overexpression of IGF ligands, results in enhanced cancer cell proliferation and survival. In contrast, the IGF-2R does not transduce signals, but instead acts as a "sink" for IGF-2, which exerts its biologic effects through the IGF-IR (98,108).

IGF-1 and -2 are potent mitogens in a broad range of cancers, including those derived from human prostate, breast, colon, ovary, and lung cancers, melanoma, and multiple myeloma, and their growth stimulatory effects are mediated through the IGF-IR (98,101,109). Furthermore, high circulating levels of IGF-1 have been associated with an increased risk of developing many types of cancer (104). In experimental systems, the growth of cancers that express the IGF-IR is influenced by circulating IGF-1, which is produced by tissues remote from the cancer. However, some cancers appear to be controlled, at least to some extent, by locally synthesized IGF-1 and/or IGF-2, which act in an autocrine or paracrine manner. It has also been proposed that cancers may be highly dependent on the host for the ligand during early stages of cancer progression, but later acquire the capacity to produce ligands in an autocrine fashion, which relates to genotypic and phenotypic changes suggestive of a more aggressive behavior. IGF-IR signaling can also become exaggerated or aberrant due to molecular abnormalities involving downstream signaling elements. One example is the loss of function of the tumor-suppressor gene *PTEN*, which encodes a phosphatase that typically attenuates proliferative signals originating from the IGF-IR and other RTKs (98,110,111).

Signaling through the IGF-IR protects cancer cells from many types of insults, including those due to cytotoxic chemotherapeutic agents, ionizing radiation, and therapeutics targeting steroid and peptide-hormone receptors, and effective strategies against IGF-IR may thwart these protective effects (96,98,109,112). The hypothesis that targeting the IGF-1R will increase the efficacy of other anticancer therapeutics is largely based on evidence that survival signals originating at the receptor limit the efficacy of agents that may otherwise induce apoptosis. Furthermore, resistance to the anti-ErbB2 antibody trastuzumab is associated with activation of IGF-IR signaling, and IGF-1R blockade can restore sensitivity (112). These observations, together with other examples, such as synergistic induction of apoptosis when small cell lung cancer is targeted using inhibitors of c-KIT or IGF-IR, suggest that IGF-IR blockade sensitizes certain cancers to other kinase inhibitors (113). Consequently, inhibition of IGF-IR signaling has been shown to increase the susceptibility of tumor cells to chemotherapeutic agents and ionizing radiation, indicating that it is an attractive target for therapeutic development (114). Furthermore, IGF signaling can induce secretion of VEGF, which is central to the promotion of deregulated malignant angiogenesis, implying that there is an angiogenic component to the biologic activity of the IGF-IR signaling cascade (109). It would therefore follow that strategies designed to inhibit the IGF-IR would suppress VEGF secretion, potentially slowing vascular expansion in proliferating tumors. Indeed, therapeutics targeting IGF-IR may enhance the activity of anti-VEGF treatment by potentially suppressing secretion of tumor-associated VEGF.

Several therapeutic strategies, including small-molecule RTK inhibitors and monoclonal antibodies directed against the human IGF-IR, have been shown to inhibit the proliferation of a broad range of cancers both *in vitro* and *in vivo* (96,98,109). In response, there has been considerable interest to develop effective targeted agents to inhibit the IGF-IR signaling pathway. Antibody strategies targeting the extracellular domain of the IGF-IR may be more advantageous than small-molecule kinase inhibitors by being highly selective against the IGF-IR, given its close homology to the IR kinase domain.

Various fully human IgG1 monoclonal antibodies, including IMC-A12 (ImClone Systems), AMG-479 (Amgen), R-1507 (Roche, Nutley, New Jersey, USA), M-0646 (Merck, Whitehouse Station, New Jersey, USA), and AVE-1642 (Sanofi-Aventis, Paris, France) and an IgG2 fully human monoclonal antibody (CP-751,871, Pfizer), have been engineered to selectively bind to the IGF-IR, thereby antagonizing ligand binding and signaling through downstream MAPK and PI3K/Akt/*PTEN* pathways (115). Early clinical evaluations of these antibodies are ongoing (109,116–118). In addition, several small-molecule inhibitors of IGF-IR, including OSI-906 (OSI Pharmaceuticals) and BMS-536924 (Bristol-Myers Squibb, Princeton, New Jersey, USA), are also being evaluated. There is also extensive preclinical evidence that therapies directed against IGF-IR are effective against a wide range of cancers, but their antitumor activities appear to be enhanced when they are combined with cytotoxic chemotherapeutics and/or other types of targeted therapies. IgG1 monoclonal antibodies also have the capacity to engage host immune effectors, thereby inducing antibody-dependent cellular cytotoxicity and complement-mediated cellular cytotoxicity as supplemental anticancer mechanisms; however, the contributions of various immune effectors in conferring anticancer activity is not known.

Favorable cytotoxic interactions between inhibitors of IGF-IR and many types of chemotherapeutic agents, including alkylating agents, platinating agents, Vinca alkaloids, taxanes, antimetabolites, and inhibitors of topoisomerase I and II, *in vitro* and in xenograft and orthotopic models of human cancer have been noted (109,119,120). For example, impressive antitumor activity has been noted following treatment of well-established human tumor xenografts with the anti–IGF-IR antibody IMC-A12 combined with the anti-ErbB1 antibody cetuximab (109,121). Additionally, IGF-IR and related signaling elements have been demonstrated to be activated in trastuzumab-resistant *HER2/neu*-amplified breast cancer, and experimental results suggest that IGF-1R blockade can restore trastuzumab sensitivity (109,122,123). In addition, the anti-angiogenic effects noted when the IGF-IR pathway is blocked in preclinical studies suggest that combinations of therapeutics targeting both IGF-IR and malignant angiogenesis may produce favorable antitumor interactions (109). Lastly, favorable interactions between inhibitors of IGF-IR and therapeutics targeting Raf/MEK/ERK and PI3K/Akt/mTOR pathways have been reported (109). Perhaps the most impressive interactions to date have been demonstrated between inhibitors of mTOR (rapamycin analogs) and IGF-IR (110). There is experimental evidence that treatment of cancer cells with mTOR inhibitors induces expression and activation of IGF-IR and downstream signaling elements, especially Akt, which may ultimately impede the effectiveness of mTOR inhibitors (110). Interestingly, IGF-IR targeting sensitizes cancer cells to mTOR inhibitors, whereas treatment with IGF-1 reverses the antiproliferative effects of mTOR inhibitors. These observations suggest that feedback up-regulation of IGF-IR and downstream signaling in response to inhibiting mTOR may be thwarted by combined treatment with inhibitors of both mTOR and IGF-IR.

Targeting the Platelet-Derived Growth Factor Receptor

The platelet-derived growth factor (PDGF) family consists of four different polypeptide chains (PDGF-A, PDGF-B, PDGF-C, and PDGF-D) that exert cellular effects through two types of protein kinase receptors (PDGFRs), PDGF-α and PDGF-β (124–127). Ligand binding to the PDGFR induces receptor dimerization and phosphorylation of the RTK domain, which results in activation of several downstream signal transduction pathways, including MAPK, PI3K/Akt/*PTEN,* Src-family kinase, signal tranducers, and activators of transcription factors (Stat) and phospholipase C (124–126). Overexpression of PDGF and the PDGFR has been shown to play a role in the development of cancer through autocrine stimulation of cancer cells, development of angiogenesis, and modulation of tumor interstitial pressure (124–126). Overexpression of PDGFR seems to result principally from deregulated expression, but genetic abnormalities, including PDGFR-α amplification and a constitutive activating mutation characterized by a deletion in exons 8 and 9, have also been identified. *In situ* hybridization studies have shown that both PDGF-α and PDGF are expressed mainly in tumors, whereas endothelial cells appear to principally express PDGFR-β (127,128). These results suggest that the paracrine effects of PDGF and PDGFR may also be relevant. In many cancers, including ovarian carcinoma and malignant glioma, PDGFR-α overexpression is common and associated with a poor prognosis (129–131). Experimental studies of gliomagenesis have suggested that PDGFR pathways not only play a key role in cell proliferation, but modulate differentiation by de-differentiating mature cells, thereby preventing glial differentiation, and even promote expansion of cancer stem cells (132,133).

Targeting PDGFR

The utility of the PDGFR as a potential target for cancer treatment is suggested by the results of experimental studies evaluating both small molecules and antibodies designed to inhibit the PDGFR (124–127,134). Inhibition of PDGFR is associated with decreased phosphorylation of the downstream effectors ERK and Akt, principal signaling elements of the MAPK and PI3K/Akt/*PTEN* pathways, respectively. The PDGF ligand/PDGFR axis is also crucial for malignant angiogenesis. Several small-molecule inhibitors of RTK, including imatinib and sunitinib, block PDGFR signaling, but these and other known small-molecule RTK inhibitors are promiscuous, as they inhibit other kinases as well (128). However, phase 2 results with imatinib in PDGFR-expressing malignancies, including ovarian cancer and glioma, have demonstrated that these agents have limited activity in unselected patients (135). Nevertheless, the lack of clinical activity observed with these promiscuous small-molecule therapeutics may be explained by poor tumor penetration and/or preclusive toxicities due to off-target effects. Later generation small-molecule inhibitors of PDGFR, which are much more selective for the PDGFR, such as CP-868,596 (Pfizer), are in early clinical development (136). Furthermore, a neutralizing, fully human IgG1 monoclonal antibody to human PDGFR-α, IMC-3G3 (ImClone Systems), which does not cross-react with the PDGFR-β, is also under clinical evaluation (137). The Kd of IMC-3G3 is 40 pmol/L and it blocks both PDGF-AA and PDGF-BB ligands from binding to PDGFR-α. In addition to blocking ligand-induced cell mitogenesis and receptor autophosphorylation, IMC-3G3 inhibits phosphorylation of the downstream signaling in both the MAPK and PI3K/Akt/*PTEN* pathways in both transfected and tumor cell lines expressing PDGFR-α. Furthermore, IMC-3G3 significantly inhibits the growth of xenografts derived from PDGFR-α–expressing human glioma and sarcoma, indicating that the antibody may be useful in treating PDGFR-α expressing cancers.

Regulators of Apoptosis as Anticancer Targets

Enhancing or restoring apoptotic mechanisms to improve the effectiveness of chemotherapy, therapeutic radiation, and hormone therapy, particularly in malignancies with deficient apoptotic triggering mechanisms, is the principal goal of therapeutic strategies targeting apoptosis. Rationally derived therapeutics directed at the regulation of the Bcl-2 family members that are the main components of the *intrinsic pathway of apoptosis* are in late clinical trials, whereas therapeutics aimed at targeting the TNF receptor (TNFR) family, a main component of the *extrinsic pathway of apoptosis,* are in earlier clinical developmental stages.

There is a hierarchical organization to the pathways of cellular apoptosis, as shown in Figure 18.4. The intrinsic and extrinsic pathways of apoptosis converge on a final common biochemical pathway that executes apoptotic cell death and requires the activation of a family of tightly regulated intracellular cysteine proteases called caspases (138–141). These pathways utilize different downstream caspase family members to activate a series of common downstream caspases, including caspase-3, -6, -7, -8, and -9. These downstream caspases induce enzymatic activation of many other proteins involved in apoptosis, leading to a cascade of proteolysis of other caspases and cellular proteins. Caspase activation and downstream proteolysis either destroy or damage many cellular "housekeeping" elements such as protein kinases, signal transduction proteins, cytoskeletal proteins, chromatin-modifying proteins, repair proteins, and inhibitory subunits of endonucleases.

Targeting the Intrinsic Pathway of Apoptosis

The intrinsic pathway of apoptosis is a mitochondrial-membrane–dependent pathway mediated by the Bcl-2 family of proteins (138–143). The *bcl-2* gene was originally identified as the chromosomal breakpoint of the translocation of a protein of chromosome 18 to 14 in follicular B-cell non-Hodgkin's lymphoma, and its translated protein belongs to a superfamily of apoptosis regulatory gene products, including antagonists of apoptosis (Bcl-2, Bcl-X_L, Bcl-2, Bfl-1, and Mcl-1) and agonists (Bax, Bak, Bcl-X_s, Bad, Bid, Bik, Bim, and Hrk) (138–143). The interactions of death antagonist with agonist proteins, as well as their relative ratios, determine how cells respond to apoptotic signals. This death/life balance is mediated, at least in part, by the selective and competitive dimerization of both antagonists and agonists (138–143). Many of the pro- and anti-apoptotic members of this regulatory family, such as Bax, act at the level of the outer mitochondrial membrane (138–143). Following mitochondrial membrane disruption, cytochrome *c* and other protease activators, including caspases -2, -3, and -9, and apoptosis-inducing factors, particularly apoptosis protease activating factor-1 (Apaf-1), are released. Cytochrome *c*, along with deoxyadenosine triphosphate, binds to and modifies the conformation of the Apaf-1 complex, which results in the activation of caspase-9. Many novel therapeutic agents that perturb the dynamic equilibrium between pro- and antiapoptotic proteins enhance the effectiveness of chemotherapy, radiation, and hormonal therapy.

Targeting Bcl-2

Targeting the Bcl-2 antiapoptotic protein, which is overexpressed in gynecologic and many common human malignancies and impedes apoptosis following apoptotic stimuli, makes Bcl-2 an attractive target for therapeutic intervention (138,140,142–150). Oblimersen sodium (Genta, Berkeley Heights, New Jersey, USA) is an 18-mer phosphorothioate ASON directed at the first six codons of the human Bcl-2 open reading frame (138,140,143,147). ASONs hybridize to the complementary sequence present on the target mRNA, followed by RNaseH-mediated degradation of mRNA. Modifying the phosphate backbone of the ASON, such as with phosphorothioate substitutions, enables resistance to protein degradation and enhances stability in the plasma and intracellular environments. Experimental studies have suggested that oblimersen sodium treatment leads to sequence-specific and dose-dependent degradation of Bcl-2 mRNA with subsequent inhibition of Bcl-2 protein expression (138,140, 142,143,147). Furthermore, several lines of evidence suggest that oblimersen sodium treatment enhances the effectiveness of other anticancer therapeutics, particularly cytotoxics. Normal and aberrant Bcl-2 expression mediates cellular resistance to apoptosis produced following treatment with many types of chemotherapeutics, including alkylating agents, antimetabolites, mitomycin, irinotecan, Vinca alkaloids, and taxanes, and Bcl-2 ASON treatment has been shown to markedly enhance the antitumor activity of many of these agents, especially the taxanes and alkylating agents (138,140, 142,143,147,151,152). In fact, antimicrotubule agents like the taxanes and Vinca alkaloids induce Bcl-2, thereby reducing its ability to heterodimerize with Bax and ultimately inducing apoptosis. These actions are enhanced when oblimersen sodium is combined with antimicrotubule agents (138,140,151,152).

Many studies have examined the feasibility of administering oblimersen sodium alone or in combination with various chemotherapeutic agents (138,140,142,143,147). Its principal toxicities when administered as either a protracted intravenous infusion or subcutaneously include hyperglycemia, transient hepatic transaminase elevations, fever, fatigue, thrombocytopenia, leukopenia, and local inflammation at the injection site. The early observations of clinical activity against lymphomas and leukemias, particularly chronic lymphocytic leukemia, with oblimersen sodium administered as a single agent may be due to the pivotal role of Bcl-2 expression in the etiology of these disorders and provide "proof of principle" that Bcl-2 inhibition may restore normal apoptotic processes in tumors with Bcl-2 regulation (138,140,142,143,148). In many other malignancies, however, Bcl-2 expression may not be as critically important to cell survival, except in the presence of external apoptotic stimuli such as chemotherapy and irradiation. Other therapeutics under evaluation designed to decrease Bcl-2 expression include the RNA antagonist SPC2996 (Santaris, Copenhagen, Denmark), which is a 16-mer oligonucleotide that binds to Bcl-2 mRNA with high affinity and resists digestion by nucleases (153).

Small-molecule and peptide inhibitors of Bcl-2, which essentially inhibit Bcl-2-Bax heterodimer formation, are undergoing early clinical development (140,143,149,150,154–157). One small-molecule inhibitor, HA14-1, which was discovered using a computer screening strategy based on the predicted structure of the Bcl-2 protein surface, binds to a surface pocket of Bcl-2. Another small molecule, AT-101 (Ascenta Therapeutics, San Diego, California, USA), an orally bioavailable pan-Bcl-2 inhibitor that triggers apoptosis of cancer cells by directly inhibiting the activity of Bcl-2, Bcl-XL, and Mcl-1, is also undergoing evaluations in both solid and hematologic malignancies (156). Other small-molecule inhibitors of Bcl-2 structure and function in early clinical evaluations include ABT-263 and ABT-737 (Abbott Laboratories, Abbott Park, Illinois, USA), and GX15-070MS (Gemin X Biotechnologies, Montreal, Canada) (157).

Several agents targeting other components of the intrinsic pathway of apoptosis in preclinical or early clinical development include small molecules and ASONs that target Bcl-X_L and antiapoptotic regulatory proteins, including clusterin, survivin, and TRPM-2. Still other efforts are being directed at the antiapoptotic protein Bax by perturbing the proteosome and/or ubiquitin protein degradation pathways or Bax gene transfection (138,140,142,143,157–161; see section on Targeting Regulators of Protein Trafficking). Another class of promising targets for therapeutic development is the apoptosis interfering proteins, such as survivin and clusterin, which inhibit downstream apoptotic processes (140–143,158–161). Survivin is highly expressed in most cancers, including ovarian cancer, and has been associated with resistance to chemotherapeutic agents and poor clinical outcome. In experimental models, therapies targeting survivin often produce antitumor activity without overt toxicity; however, the consequences of prolonged survivin inhibition in normal cells have not been evaluated thoroughly. Promising therapeutic approaches include those that are aimed at suppressing survivin expression using ASON, ribozyme, siRNA, and shRNA technologies, as well as antagonizing survivin function by inhibiting specific cyclin-dependent kinases. Alternatively, small molecule suppressants of survivin, such as YM-155 (Astellas Pharma US, Inc., Deerfield, Illinois, USA), which has demonstrated preliminary clinical activity in both hematopoietic and solid malignancies, are in clinical development (161). Similar strategies that target clusterin, represented by the ASON OGX-011 (OncoGenex; Vancouver, Canada) (162), are also undergoing clinical evaluation.

Targeting the Extrinsic Pathway of Apoptosis

The extrinsic pathway of apoptosis refers to the activation of caspase-8 as a result of apoptosis-inducing ligands that bind to the TNFR family. The TNFR family consists of the receptors TNFR1, Fas (Apo1), DR3 (Apo2), DR4 (TNF-related apoptosis-inducing ligand [TRAIL] R1), DR5 (TRAILR2), and DR6 (71). Critical adaptor proteins, particularly TNF-α receptor associated death domain (TRADD) or Fas associated death domain (FADD) protein, mediate intracytoplasmic signals from the receptor using death domain proteins to interact with the receptor and death effector domains to interact with procaspase-8 (138,140,142,163–167). The proteins engage proteases and cleave the N-terminal of caspase-8, thereby activating the caspase cascade.

Targeting TRAIL Receptors

There are several homeostatic mechanisms that regulate cell death in the extrinsic pathway. Decoy receptors for Fas ligands and TRAIL (TRAIL R3/DcR1 and TRAIL R-4/DcR2) compete for ligand and modulate apoptotic signals. Moreover, several intracellular proteins interact with death domain proteins to inhibit the signal transduction of apoptosis. These proteins include the protein silencer of death domains and FAP1, which may represent a mechanism of resistance to Fas-inducing apoptosis (166). In addition, members of the death effect domain family (e.g., FLIP) compete with procaspase-8 for the binding with FADD and inhibit apoptosis (167). Deregulation of these mediators may lead to malignant transformation. Mutations or deletions in the FAS gene have been found in cells from patients with many types of malignancies. It is also likely that the intrinsic and extrinsic apoptotic pathways are linked at many critical juncture points. For example, abrogation of TRAIL-mediated apoptosis occurs in some cancer cell lines secondary to overexpression of Bcl-2 family proteins, whereas TNF-α mediated expression of nuclear factor (NF)-κB activates several Bcl-2 family genes that have antiapoptotic functions (168).

TNF, which has the potential to induce apoptosis in tumor cells and mediates inflammatory processes, is the prototypic ligand for the TNFR family (169). TNF-α and Fas ligands are not candidates for drug therapy due to their nonspecific activation of multiple TNFRs and their causality of septic shock and fulminant hepatic failure in animals (170). However, recombinant soluble human TRAIL has entered clinical development since it is capable of inducing apoptosis in a broad spectrum of human cancers *in vitro*, but not in normal cells (138,140,142,164–167). Moreover, antitumor activity without toxicity has been observed in xenograft models. The selectivity of TRAIL in mediating apoptosis in tumor cells and not normal cells has not been elucidated, but the overexpression of death receptors and/or a relative absence of decoy receptors in tumor cells have been proposed as explanations. However, preclinical studies demonstrating apoptosis in human hepatic cells *in vitro* have raised concerns about the clinical development of TRAIL, but recent evidence indicates that different versions of recombinant soluble human TRAIL may confer varying propensities for hepatocyte toxicity (171). In early clinical evaluations, recombinant soluble human TRAIL ligands against DR4 and DR5 (rhApo2L/TRAIL; Genentech and Amgen) have been well tolerated without relevant hepatotoxicity (172).

Monoclonal antibodies with agonist-like properties at the DR4 and DR5 sites may represent alternate strategies for the induction of apoptosis via the extrinsic pathway. Following antibody-antigen complex formation, caspase activation and apoptosis induction occur, resulting in tumor regression of human tumor xenograft (138,140,142,164–167,173,174). The affinity for DR4 binding appears to be less important for agonist activity than the specific binding site on the receptor (173). This implies that the specific agonist site exists within the receptor and suggests that widely divergent results may be achieved with different antibodies directed to the same target DR4 (174). Clinical investigations of humanized and fully human antibodies directed against DR4 (HGS-ETR1; Human Genome Sciences, Rockville, Maryland, USA) and DR5 (HGS-ETR2; lexatumumab; Human Genome Sciences; AMG-655; Amgen) have been ongoing (175–177).

Targeting Regulators of Protein Trafficking

Targeting the Heat-Shock Protein Complex

Since the structure and function of proteins are highly dependent on their precise three-dimensional structures, targeting chaperone proteins, which are responsible for protein folding, is a logical therapeutic strategy against cancer (178–180). Geldanamycin analogs target the adenosine triphosphate (ATP) binding site of Hsp-90, an abundant and highly conserved chaperone protein that plays an important role in generating, regulating, and degrading signaling elements and other critical proteins (181–183). Proteins that are folded by Hsp-90 include the cyclin-dependent kinases (cdks) 4 and 6, focal adhesion kinases that are involved in integrin signaling, components of the MAPK and PI3K/Akt/*PTEN* pathways, and the proangiogenic hypoxia-inducible factor-1α (178–180,184). During malignant transformation, the essential chaperoning functions of heat-shock proteins (HSPs) are subverted to facilitate rapid somatic evolution. Functioning as biochemical buffers for the numerous genetic lesions that are present within tumors, chaperones, especially Hsp-90, allow mutant proteins to retain or even gain function while permitting cancer cells to tolerate the imbalanced signaling that oncoproteins create. The first Hsp-90 inhibitor to enter clinical trials, 17-allylamino-17-demethoxygeldanamycin (17-AAG), is a less toxic derivative of geldanamycin, whose administration is precluded by hepatotoxicity and suboptimal pharmaceutical properties. However, more potent, water soluble geldanamycin analogs and unrelated agents, including 17-(demethyoxy), 17-dimethylaminoethylamino geldanamycin (17-DMAG), CNF1010 (Biogen IDEC, San Diego, California, USA), KOS-953 (Kosan Biosciences, Hayward, California, USA), IPI-504 (Infinity, Cambridge, Massachusetts, USA), and the totally synthetic, orally bioavailable Hsp-90 inhibitor CNF2024 (Biogen IDEC), are undergoing early clinical evaluations (181–188). Although objective antitumor activity has been reported with 17-AAG as a single agent, inhibitors of Hsp-90 are much more likely to confer relevant activity in combination with therapeutics that induce apoptosis since disruption of antiapoptotic signaling occurs following treatment with Hsp-90 inhibitors, which can enhance the proapoptotic effects of cytotoxic agents (181–184).

Targeting the Ubiquitin-Proteasome Protein Degradation Pathway

The principal mechanism that is responsible for intracellular protein degradation is the ubiquitin-proteasome pathway (183, 189–192). This pathway "tags" protein substrates with polyubiquitin chains, marking them for degradation into peptides and free ubiquitin. The process is modulated by the proteasome, which is a large multimeric protease that is found in all eukaryotic cells. Many important proteins, such as the cyclins, cyclin-dependent kinase inhibitors, and transcription factors (e.g., NF-κB) are tagged by the ubiquitin-proteasome pathway, and therefore the pathway plays a critical role in neoplastic growth and metastasis. Inhibiting the proteasome perturbs the cyclical degradation of these critical proteins, thereby resulting in the accumulation of cyclin-dependent kinase inhibitors and ultimately cell-cycle arrest and apoptosis. Several small-molecule inhibitors of the proteasome pathway have recently been identified, particularly the dipeptide boronate derivatives (189–192). Bortezomib (Millennium Pharmaceuticals, Cambridge, Massachusetts, USA), a peptidyl boronic acid and highly selective inhibitor of the chymotryptic site within the 20S proteasome, has recently received regulatory approval for treating patients with drug-refractory multiple myeloma (92,93). Bortezomib is capable of permeating the membrane of tumor cells, reversibly inhibiting the proteasome, and blocking cell division in the G_2/M phase of the cell cycle, which in turn leads to apoptosis. The agent also inhibits the degradation of wild-type p53 and stabilizes p21, which induces G_1 arrest by inhibiting cyclin D-, E-, and A-dependent kinases and activating NF-κB. In preclinical studies, bortezomib demonstrates broad anticancer activity, with mechanism-based toxicities related to the degree of proteasomal inhibition. These studies predicted that severe toxicity would occur when proteasome activity is inhibited by at least 70% to 80%, and therefore the achievement of this magnitude of proteasome inhibition was a pharmacologic goal in early clinical studies.

Based on impressive activity in preclinical studies when bortezomib is combined with a wide variety of cytotoxic agents, clinical evaluations of bortezomib and other proteasome pathway inhibitors, as well as relevant combination regimens, are being performed in patients with gynecologic and other malignancies.

Targeting Epigenetic DNA Modifications

Targeting processes that result in post-translational or *epigenetic* modifications in histone proteins associated with DNA is a rational approach to anticancer therapeutic development (193–195). To date, therapeutic targeting has focused on covalently modifying the amino-terminal tails of histones, which package eukaryotic DNA into units that are folded into chromatin fibers. Highly conserved histone proteins (H1, H2A, H2B, H3, and H4) and the nucleosomes they form with DNA are the basic blocks of eukaryotic chromatin, the organization of which determines gene expression (193–195).

Nucleosomes form the basic repeating unit of chromatin and consist of DNA wrapped around a histone octomer that is in turn formed by four histone partners including an H3-H4 tetramer and two H2A-H2B dimers. Extending out from the nucleosome are the charged amino-terminal tails of the histones. The tail of histone H4 appears to extend into the adjacent nucleosome to interact with the H2A-H2B complex, indicating that the histone tails might regulate higher order chromatin structure. As depicted in Figure 18.5, the amino acid histone tail domains are targets for various post-translational modifications, including acetylation, methylation, phosphorylation, ADP-ribosylation, and ubiquitination. How the code is established and maintained remains to be determined, but many modification sites are close enough to each other that modification of a histone tail by any one enzyme might influence the rate and efficiency at which subsequent enzymes use the newly modified tails as substrates. In essence, interfering with these modifications modulates histone-associated proteins and gene expression. Covalent modifications of core histone tails by histone acetyltransferases (HATs), histone methyltransferases (HMTs), kinases, and especially histone deacetylases (HDACs) regulate gene expression (193–195).

Targeting Histone Deacetylase

HATs catalyze the acetylation of the ε-NH2 group on lysine residues with histone tails leading to transcriptional activation, whereas HDACs function in opposition by deacetylating lysine residues and inducing transcriptional repression through chromatin condensation (196). Transcriptional aberrations may be among the leading contributors to conferring the neoplastic phenotype, which is the case in acute promyelocytic leukemia, in which aberrant transcriptional repression mediated by HDACs is a common mechanism utilized by oncoproteins. Alterations in chromatin structure can impact on normal cell differentiation and lead to malignant tumor formation. Furthermore, the fact that HDAC inhibitors are active against a wide variety of cancers *in vitro* and in human tumor xenograft models, and that defects in the acetylation machinery are found in most epithelial and hematologic malignancies, including ovarian cancer, suggest that the pharmacologic inhibition of HDAC may have broad therapeutic ramifications (197). In preclinical investigations, many structurally diverse compounds have been shown to bind to HDAC; promote histone acetylation; induce cell cycle arrest, differentiation, or apoptosis; and possess prominent antitumor activity. HDAC inhibitors that are currently approved for the treatment of underdevelopment as anticancer therapeutics include (a) short-chain fatty acids (e.g., butyrates); (b) hydroxamic acids (e.g., suberoylanilide hydroxamic acid [vorinostat; Merck], oxamflatin, LAH-824 [Novartis], LBH-589 [Novartis], PXD-101 [CuraGen, Branford, Connecticut, USA]), (c) benzamides (e.g., MS-275 [Mitsui, Chiba, Japan], MGCD0103 [MethylGene, Montreal, Canada]); and (d) cyclic peptides (e.g., depsipeptide [Gloucester, Cambridge, Massachusetts, USA], trapoxin A, apicidin) (195,196). The results of phase 1 studies, particularly of hydroxamic acid derivatives, demonstrated antitumor activity at doses below the maximum tolerated dose (MTD). The first evidence of robust antitumor activity with the HDAC inhibitors occurred in patients with persistent or recurrent cutaneous T-cell lymphoma, resulting in vorinostat receiving regulatory approval. Synergy has also been observed between the HDAC inhibitors and various classes of anticancer agents, and the spectrum of anticancer activity demonstrated in preclinical studies has been broad (195,196).

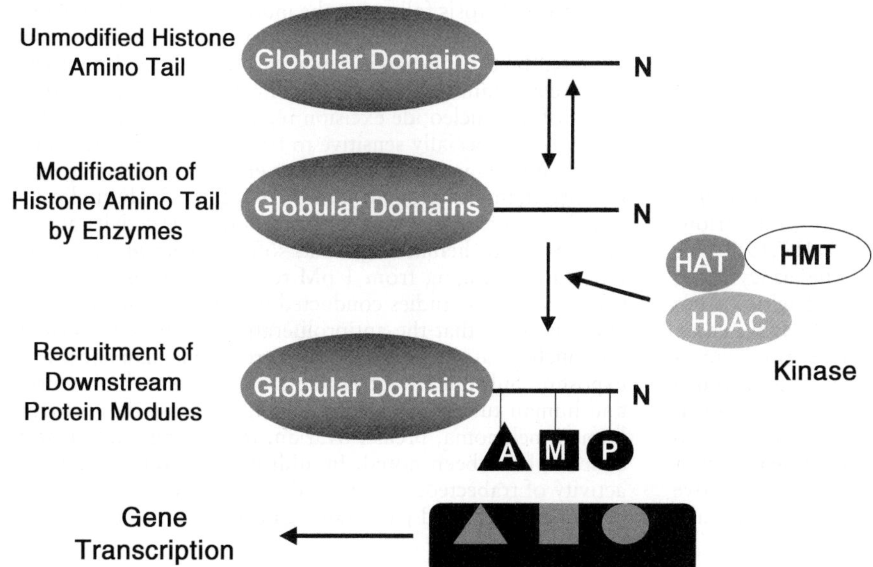

FIGURE 18.5. Covalent post-translational modifications on the histone amino tail domain. Pictured are the enzymes HAT, HDAC, HMT, and kinases that covalently modify histones. *Note:* HAT, histone acetyltransferase; HDAC, histone deaceyltransferase; HMT, histone methyltransferase; A, acetyl group; M, methyl group; and P, phosphate.

At a more fundamental level, it will be important to understand the nature of the molecular basis of the selectivity of HDAC inhibitors in altering gene transcription, and whether there are differences in the biologic function of different HDACs. Furthermore, it will be helpful to understand why normal cells are apparently more resistant to the apoptotic effects of HDAC inhibitors, as well as the role of non-histone substrates of HDACs, such as transcription factors, in the suppression of cell growth. Most importantly, the reasons for the differential sensitivity of the HDAC inhibitors must be understood. This knowledge will undoubtedly contribute to both the further understanding of the process of transformation and the development of effective agents to treat many types of cancer.

Targeting DNA Methylation

The most extensively characterized epigenetic alteration is DNA methylation (193–195,197). Cytosine methylation of the palindromic CpG dinucleotide sequence has been the most widely known and studied epigenetic modification; however, DNA methylation of non-CpG sequences has also been reported. CpG islands are defined as DNA regions with greater than 500 base pairs containing CG content of at least 55%. Hypermethylation of CpG islands near the promoter region of genes usually silences their expression. The biologic effects of the loss of gene function caused by promoter hypermethylation are analogous to those caused by genetic mutations. The gene silencing effects of hypermethylation of CpG islands have been explained by several mechanisms. Perhaps the most plausible one is that methylated CpG islands in the promoter region inhibit binding of transcription factors to their CpG-containing recognition sites. Another theory proposes the involvement of methylated CpG-binding proteins. The list of hypermethylated genes in all types of cancers, particularly hematologic malignancies, has increased tremendously over the last several decades, and more candidate tumor suppressor genes are expected to be identified (193–195,197). In ovarian cancer, for example, epigenetic silencing by hypermethylation of the connective tissue growth factor gene promoter results in a loss of gene function, which may be a factor in the carcinogenesis of ovarian cancer in a stage-dependent and/or histologic subtype–dependent manner (198). Aberrant DNA methylation that results in the transcriptional silencing of proapoptotic genes appears to be involved in conferring acquired resistance to many types of chemotherapy agents (199–201). In a study of plasma DNA from patients with ovarian cancer, methylation of the DNA mismatch repair gene *hMLH1* was demonstrated to be increased at relapse (201). For this reason, the methylating agent 2′-deoxy-5-azacytidine (decitabine; MGI Pharma, Minneapolis, Minnesota, USA) in combination with carboplatin is being evaluated in women with recurrent ovarian cancer in a phase 2 study (197,202).

The concept of modifying DNA methylation as a therapeutic strategy has been validated by the demonstration that demethylating agents induce clinical benefit in patients with various hematologic malignancies and premalignancies (197,198). The nucleoside analogs decitabine and 5-azacytidine (azacytidine; Pharmion, Boulder, Colorado, USA), both of which have received regulatory approval for treatment of myelodysplastic syndrome, do not directly inhibit DNA methyltransferases (DNMTs). Instead, they incorporate into DNA as cytidine analogs and form covalent intermediate complexes with DNMT, which ultimately undergoes degradation. 5-Azacytidine also incorporates into RNA, thereby interfering with protein translation, resulting in cell death. Development of more selective demethylating agents that may target cancer cells preferentially is under way (197,198).

Novel Cytotoxic Targets and Agents

A number of novel cytotoxic agents with unique mechanisms of action are being evaluated in patients with ovarian cancer in an effort to identify therapeutics that would not be cross-resistant with taxane and platinating compounds.

Targeting the DNA Minor Groove

Trabectedin

Trabectedin (ecteinascidin-743 [ET-743], Pharmamar, Madrid, Spain), a tetrahydroisoquinoline alkaloid isolated from the marine ascidian *Ecteinascidia turbinata,* is a DNA minor-groove interactive agent with specific affinity for guanine-cytosine–rich sequences (203,204). Trabectedin-guanine adducts are formed only in double-strand DNA and these adducts are reversible upon DNA denaturation. Nuclear magnetic resonance and x-ray crystallographic studies have demonstrated that two of three subunits (A and B) bind to nucleic acids in the minor groove of DNA, but subunit C, which lacks DNA binding capabilities, acts as a molecular hinge that facilitates binding of trabectedin to critical nuclear proteins (203–208). In essence, trabectedin's dual affinity for DNA and proteins produces DNA-trabectedin-protein cross links. Adducts induced by trabectedin are unique because no DNA repair machinery pathway examined to date is capable of removing them, whereas cells deficient in nucleotide excision repair show increased drug resistance (209). Because loss of repair proteins is common in human tumors, expression levels of selected repair factors may be useful in identifying patients who might benefit from trabectedin treatment. Recent studies have also indicated that trabectedin interacts with nuclear histones and transcription factors, including E2F1, c-fos, NF-y, and SP-1. Additionally, trabectedin perturbs cell cycle progression and induces G_1 arrest, delayed S-phase traverse, and G_2/M arrest (206,208). Cell cycle arrest induced by trabectedin has been observed in p53 mutated cell lines, suggesting that this effect is p53 independent. Trabectedin does not inhibit topoisomerase I and II, but does perturb microtubules and intermediate filament bundles.

Trabectedin is of particular interest for development in gynecologic malignancies because it has been demonstrated to enhance the cytotoxic effects of platinating agents (208). In contrast to apoptosis mediated by platinating agents, trabectedin-mediated apoptosis following the induction of DNA damage is enhanced by the nucleotide excision repair pathway and inhibited by the mismatch repair pathway (207). Tumor cells that are resistant to platinating agents because of the up-regulation of the nucleotide excision repair pathway are therefore likely to be especially sensitive to trabectedin, and the combination of both agents may be more effective at inducing cytotoxicity than either agent alone (207,209). Trabectedin has also demonstrated substantial antiproliferative activity against many types of hematologic and solid cancers *in vitro*, with IC_{50} values ranging from 1 pM to 10 nM. These investigations, as well as studies conducted in a human tumor-cloning assay, indicate that the antiproliferative effects of trabectedin are much greater with continuous treatment than short-term exposure. Substantial antiproliferative effects in both murine and human tumor xenografts, including those derived from human melanoma, breast, ovarian, renal, lung, and prostate cancers, have been noted. In addition, the antiproliferative activity of trabectedin has been demonstrated to be similar to that of cisplatin and paclitaxel against human ovarian tumor xenografts (208).

In early clinical evaluations, trabectedin's antitumor activity has been especially notable in patients with soft-tissue sarcoma, breast cancer refractory to the anthracyclines, and ovarian cancer resistant to platinating agents and taxanes (203,206,210,211). The principal toxicities include reversible transaminitis, emesis, and myelosuppression; however, these adverse effects appear less common on intermittent divided-dose schedules. A pooled analysis of 294 ovarian cancer patients who participated in three phase 2 trials of trabectedin as second- or third-line treatment, including 108 and 186 patients who were either resistant or sensitive to their last platinum treatment, respectively, demonstrated overall response rates and median time to progression of 8% and 2.1 months, respectively, in platinum-resistant patients, and respective values were 34% and 5.8 months in platinum-sensitive patients. The median duration of response was 5.8 months, and patients receiving the agent as a 3- or 24-hour infusion every 3 weeks demonstrated significantly higher response rates (33% vs. 16%, $p = <0.0001$) and median time to tumor progression (5.8 vs. 2.8 months, $p = 0.0001$) than those treated on a weekly divided-dose schedule. The most common drug-related adverse events were fatigue, noncumulative neutropenia, and transaminitis. Low incidences of febrile neutropenia, neurotoxicity, stomatitis, and alopecia were noted. The merits of trabectedin in patients with relapsed ovarian cancer were evaluated in a phase 3 trial in which 672 patients with advanced recurrent or refractory cancers were randomized to treatment with either liposomal doxorubicin plus trabectedin or liposomal doxorubicin alone. Progression-free survival was significantly increased in patients receiving the combination (7.3 versus 5.8 months; hazard ratio, 0.79; P value = 0.019).

Targeting the Folate Receptor Type α

There has been cumulative evidence that suggests that the folate receptor type α (FRA), which is a glycosylphosphatidylinositol-linked transmembrane protein with high affinity for folates and some antifolates, is overexpressed in mesothelioma and ovarian, uterine, some brain, and other cancers, and may confer the means by which selective tumor targeting can be achieved (212–216). Furthermore, expression of the FRA is very low in most adult normal tissues but is high in several types of cancer, providing the rationale for developing antifolates that are transported primarily by the FRA rather than by the reduced folate carrier. Among the approaches that are being used to target the FRA include the humanized monoclonal antibody MORAb-003 (Morphotek; Exton, Pennsylvania, USA) and the small-molecule thymidylate synthase inhibitor BGC945 (BTG, London, UK), which appears to be highly selective for the FRA (216–221). Binding of MORAb-003 to FRA can prevent phosphorylation of substrates specific for Lyn kinase, suppress proliferation of cells that overexpress the FRA, mediate tumoricidal effects via antibody-dependent cellular and complement-dependent mechanisms, and suppress growth *in vivo* of FRA-expressing tumor xenograft models. Toxicology studies in nonhuman primates found no evidence of toxicity with MORAb-003 at suprapharmacologic doses, which was confirmed in phase 1 studies in patients with advanced solid malignancies (218). A phase 2 study of MORAb-003 in patients with advanced ovarian cancer in first relapse has begun (219).

Along the same lines, a novel series of cyclopenta[*g*]quinazoline analogs of folic acid that are potent thymidylate synthase inhibitors (K_i ~0.2 to 1 nM) and at least 500-fold more selective for human cancer cell lines with high expression of the FRA compared to those with low expression, have been synthesized (220,221). Pharmacokinetic studies in KB tumor-bearing mice have demonstrated selective retention of BGC945, a lead compound in this series in tumors relative to normal tissues. Furthermore, pharmacodynamic measurements have demonstrated inhibition of thymidylate synthase only in tumor tissue. The agent is in late-stage preclinical development.

Targeting DNA Alkylation

Canfosfamide

Canfosfamide (TLK-286; Telik, Palo Alto, California, USA) is a small-molecule prodrug that is metabolically activated by glutathione S-transferase P1-1 (GST P1-1) to release a highly reactive alkylating nitrogen mustard moiety (222–224). The enzyme GST P1-1 is overexpressed in ovarian, breast, lung, and many other human cancers, and its enzyme activity in cancer appears to relate to resistance to commonly used chemotherapeutic drugs, especially alkylating agents (222–224). Following intratumoral uptake of canfosfamide, drug activation and DNA damage ensue, which is followed by apoptosis. Myelosuppression is the principal toxicity of the agent (224,225). In a phase 2 study of canfosfamide in recurrent ovarian cancer, 5 (15%) of 34 evaluable patients had objective responses, including one complete response lasting longer than 3 years, and 12 (35%) patients had stable disease as their best response (226). Sixty percent and 40% of patients were alive at 12 and 18 months, respectively. However, a phase 3 study known as ASSIST-1, which enrolled 461 patients with advanced ovarian cancer that had progressed following first-line platinum-based therapy plus second-line treatment with either liposomal doxorubicin or topotecan, did not meet its primary endpoint of improving overall survival nor its secondary endpoint of improving progression-free survival (227). Patients were randomized to treatment with canfosfamide or either topotecan or liposomal doxorubicin, provided that they had not received prior treatment with these agents (227). Median survival on the canfosfamide arm was 8.5 months compared with 13.6 months on the active control arm ($p < 0.01$). Median progression-free survival was 2.3 months on the canfosfamide arm compared with 4.3 months on the active control arm. Based on more recent phase 2 study results, in which the combination of carboplatin plus canfosfamide resulted in an impressive rate of objective responses in heavily pretreated ovarian cancer patients whose disease had either progressed during or shortly after platinum-based treatment, the efficacy of canfosfamide plus liposomal doxorubicin is being compared to liposomal doxorubicin alone in second-line platinum-refractory or -resistant ovarian cancer in a phase 3 trial known as ASSIST-5 (228). In a preliminary analysis of the platinum-resistant subset, response rates were 31.5% and 10.5% in patients treated with canfosfamide plus liposomal doxorubicin alone, respectively. Median progression-free survival had not been reached for the combination, whereas it was 3.5 months for liposomal doxorubicin alone.

Targeting Immune Tolerance

Cytotoxic T-Lymphocyte–Associated Antigen 4

Many cancer-associated gene products that induce immune recognition, and are potential targets for therapeutic development against cancer but host immune reactions, rarely impact upon the progression of most advanced human cancers. The weak immunogenicity of nascent tumors contributes to this failure.

Therapeutic vaccines that enhance dendritic cell presentation of cancer antigens increase specific cellular and humoral responses, resulting in tumor destruction in some cases. The attenuation of T-cell activation by cytotoxic T-lymphocyte–associated antigen 4 (CTLA4) further limits the therapeutic impact of tumor immunity (229,230). CTLA4, a CD28-family receptor expressed mainly on CD4+ T cells, binds the same ligands as CD28 (CD80 and CD86 on B cells and dendritic cells), but with higher affinity than CD28 (229–232). However, in contrast to CD28, which enhances cell function when bound at the same time as the T-cell receptor, CTLA4 inhibits T-cell function. CTLA4 is also found intracellularly in regulatory T cells, which may be of functional significance. In experimental systems, the administration of antibodies that block CTLA4 function inhibits the growth of moderately immunogenic tumors, and in combination with cancer vaccines, augments the rejection of poorly immunogenic tumors, albeit with a loss of tolerance to normal differentiation antigens (229–232).

Various antibodies to CTLA4 are currently being evaluated in late-stage clinical trials in patients with advanced melanoma, and in phase 2 trials in patients with ovarian and other cancer types (231). These fully human antibodies include the IgG_1 construct ipilimumab (MDX-010; Medarex, Princeton, New Jersey, USA, and Bristol-Myers Squibb) and the IgG_2 construct ticilimumab (CP675,206; Pfizer). Patients with advanced malignant melanoma who received treatment with either of these CTLA4 antibodies have experienced tumor regression with prolonged time to progression, and objective anticancer activity has also been observed in patients with advanced lymphoma and ovarian, prostate, and renal cancers (231–238). Interestingly, antitumor activity is often characterized by short-term tumor progression followed by delayed tumor regression, and an important, possibly unique clinical observation is the protracted nature of both objective responses and stable disease. Adverse effects, including rash, colitis, and hepatitis, appear to be immune mediated and may represent breaking of tolerance to self-antigens (239). Interestingly, these toxicities have been directly related to time to tumor progression in high-risk melanoma patients who have undergone resection of their primary tumor (239).

Targeting Mitosis

Targeting Microtubules

Several natural products, which are structurally different from the taxanes but share mechanisms of action and show comparable activities, have been identified. The furthest along from a clinical development standpoint are the epothilones, which are 16-member macrolides derived from myxobacterium (240–245). Similar to the taxanes, the epothilones induce formation of microtubules that are long, rigid, and resistant to destabilization by cold temperature and calcium. The epothilones are at least as potent as the taxanes and induce mitotic arrest and microtubule bundling. Furthermore, these agents exert prominent cytotoxic activity in tumors with multidrug resistance conferred by overexpression of P-glycoprotein and other resistance proteins. Experimental studies have also indicated that the epothilones and taxanes differ in terms of resistance conferred by point mutations in β-tubulin; however, the significance of tubulin mutations in conferring clinical resistance to antimicrotubule agents is not clear. Several members of the epothilone B family, including epothilone B itself (patupilone; EPO-0906, Novartis) and the epothilone B analog ixabepilone (BMS-247550; Bristol-Myers Squibb), that are furthest along in clinical development have demonstrated impressive activity against human xenografts derived from ovarian, breast, and colorectal cancers, many of which are clearly resistant to the taxanes (240–245). Objective antitumor activity has been noted in patients with many types of advanced cancer; however, notable activity has largely been restricted to tumor types that are known to be responsive to the taxanes. These include breast, ovarian, and non–small cell lung cancers, but activity has been noted in patients whose disease has failed to respond to treatment with taxane analogs (246–252). The most advanced studies of ixabepilone are in patients with metastatic breast cancer, and an impressive degree of clinical activity has been noted in breast cancer patients whose tumors are clearly refractory to taxanes (248). A phase 2 trial of patupilone in patients with ovarian cancer refractory to platinating agents has recently been completed and preliminary data indicate a modest degree of activity (247). Similarly, promising antitumor activity has been noted in ovarian cancer patients treated with other epothilone analogs, including major responses in 4 (31%) of 13 eligible ovarian cancer patients in first or second relapse and a platinum-free interval of less than 6 months following treatment with the fully synthetic epothilone B analog ZK-EPO (Scherring AG, Berlin, Germany) (240,252).

Other natural products and semisynthetic antimicrotubule agents that are in clinical development interact with tubulin in the Vinca-alkaloid or colchicine-binding domains (240,243). Among the best characterized are the dolastatins, which consist of a series of oligopeptides isolated from the sea hare *Dolabella auricularia* (253–255). Two of the most potent dolastatins, dolastatin-10 and -15, noncompetitively inhibit the binding of Vinca alkaloids to tubulin, inhibit tubulin polymerization and tubulin-dependent GTP hydrolysis, stabilize the colchicine-binding activity of tubulin, and have cytotoxic activity in the picomolar to low nanomolar range. Dolastatin-10 and the semisynthetic dolastatin analogs depsipeptide tasidotin (ILX651; Genzyme, Boston, Massachusetts, USA) and TZT-1027 (Daiichi, Tokyo, Japan), which bind in the Vinca domain, are undergoing clinical development (254–258).

Phomopsin A, halichondrin B, homohalichondrin B, and spongistatin 1, which competitively inhibit Vinca alkaloid binding to tubulin, are being evaluated in preclinical or early clinical evaluations (240,243,259–262). Halichondrin B (E7389; Eisai, Ridgefield Park, New Jersey, USA), a large polyether macrolide originally isolated from the marine sponge *Halichondria okadai*, and two less complex synthetic macrocyclic ketone analogs, ER-076349 and ER-086526, are in early clinical development (263,264). These compounds bind to tubulin, inhibit tubulin polymerization, disrupt mitotic spindle formation, induce mitotic arrest, and possess growth inhibitory properties in the subnanomolar range and show marked activity in preclinical studies. Experimental data also suggest that tumors expressing higher levels of the βIII tubulin isotype may be more responsive to treatment with both E7389 and the hemiasterlin analog E7974 (Eisai). If confirmed clinically, such preclinical insights may lay the foundation for preferentially treating patients whose tumors may be particularly sensitive to these agents. E7389 has also demonstrated clinical activity in patients with recurrent metastatic breast cancer following treatment with taxanes, and clinical evaluations are ongoing in ovarian cancer and other malignancies. E7389 and HTI-286 (Wyeth), which are synthetic forms of the natural product hemiasterlin derived from a marine sponge (261,262), are also in clinical development (265,266). Hemiasterlin and its analogs bind to the Vinca-peptide site in tubulin, disrupt normal microtubule dynamics, and depolymerize microtubules. HTI-286 also appears to be a much weaker substrate for the P-glycoproteins than the Vinca alkaloids and taxanes (240,243,261,262).

Targeting Established Tumor Vasculature

Most efforts targeting the tumor vasculature are aimed at inhibiting tumor angiogenesis, but several antimicrotubule agents disrupt existing tumor vasculature (267–270). Since the late 1990s, the combretastatins and *N*-acetylcolchicinol-*O*-phosphate, which bind to the colchicine-binding domain on tubulin, have undergone clinical development as antivascular agents. These agents include combretastatin-A-4 3-*O*-phosphate, combretastatin A-1-phosphate (Oxigene, Waltham, Massachusetts, USA), ZD6126 (AstraZeneca), and AVE8062A (Sanofi-Aventis). Although several of these agents have exhibited preliminary antitumor activity in early clinical evaluations, cardiovascular toxicity has been problematic. Another experimental agent, 5,6-dimethylxanthenone-4-acetic acid (DMXAA or ASA404; Antisoma, London, UK, and Novartis), a small molecule, has demonstrated robust antivascular and antitumor activity in preclinical studies (270). DMXAA induces a cascade of events leading to the release of vasoactive substances, including serotonin, TNF, and nitric oxide, from host cells, as well as hemorrhagic necrosis in experimental tumor models (270). Clinical evaluations of DMXAA plus chemotherapy in patients with ovarian cancer and other cancer types are in progress (271).

Targeting Mitotic Kinesins

Although tubulin is the most abundant protein component of the mitotic spindle apparatus, many other proteins, particularly mitotic kinesins, play critical roles in the mechanics of mitosis and in progression through the premitotic cell cycle checkpoint. Kinesins are motor proteins that translate chemical energy released by the hydrolysis of adenosine triphosphate into mechanical force for movement along microtubules, transport of many types of cargo, and the intracellular organization of the mitotic spindle and other microtubule-containing structures (272–274).

The mitotic kinesins are a subgroup of kinesin motor proteins that function exclusively in mitosis in proliferating cells (272). During mitosis, different, highly specialized mitotic kinesins play critical roles in various aspects of mitotic spindle assembly, including the establishment of spindle bipolarity, spindle pole organization, chromosome alignment and segregation, and regulation of microtubule dynamics. The establishment of mitotic spindle bipolarity is among the earliest events in spindle assembly and it requires the kinesin motor protein KSP (also known as Eg5), which has no known role other than that played in mitosis (272). The low expression of KSP mRNA in normal tissues is consistent with preferential expression of KSP in proliferating cells relative to normal adjacent tissues. As essential elements in mitotic spindle assembly and function, KSP and mitotic kinesins provide attractive targets for intervention to thwart the cell cycle. A therapeutic targeting KSP may prove at least as effective as the taxanes and Vinca alkaloids without the potential for neurotoxicity or other adverse effects associated with interfering with tubulin function in nondividing cells. Furthermore, combinations of therapeutics targeting KSP and tubulin dynamics may exhibit additive or synergistic cytotoxicity. Ispinesib (SB-715992; Glaxo SmithKline, and Cytokinetics, South San Francisco, California, USA), a polycyclic, nitrogen-containing heterocycle, was the first KSP-targeting therapeutic to enter clinical trials (273). The agent, which is 10,000-fold more selective for KSP relative to other members of the kinesin superfamily, blocks assembly of functional mitotic spindles, thereby causing cell cycle arrest in mitosis and cell death (273). Ispinesib has demonstrated objective antitumor activity in patients with breast and ovarian cancers; however, activity noted in ovarian cancer has been modest to date (275,276). Other KSP inhibitors, some of which have increased potency and/or specificity for KSP, including SB-743921 (Glaxo SmithKline and Cytokinetics), MK-0731 (Merck), ARRY-649 (Array Biopharma, Boulder, Colorado, USA), are in early clinical investigations (277–279).

Targeting Mitotic Kinases

Several mitotic kinases, particularly the aurora kinases, are being assessed as strategic targets for anticancer therapeutic development (274,280–284). The aurora kinases, which encompass three known family members known as aurora-A, -B, and -C, regulate chromosome segregation and cytokinesis during mitosis. Aberrant expression and activity of these kinases, which may lead to aneuploidy and tumorigenesis, occur in many types of human cancer. Additionally, aurora-A and -B kinases have distinct roles in mitosis. Aurora-A kinase, which is typically found in the pericentrosomal region, recruits several important components to the mitotic spindle, such as γ-tubulin, while the mitotic spindle is forming from the daughter centrosomes (285). In addition, aurora-A kinase is overexpressed in a large proportion of ovarian cancers and is associated with centrosome amplification and poor survival, rendering it a potential useful prognostic marker and therapeutic target (286). Alternatively, aurora-B kinase is localized to the interphase chromosomes proximal to the centromer, and as chromosome condensation occurs at the start of mitosis, both aurora-A and -B kinases share responsibility for phosphorylating histone H3 (274,280,281). In addition, both kinases have distinct roles in the function of the contractile ring that participates in the formation of two daughter cells. Aurora-C kinase appears to have a highly specialized, albeit as yet undetermined, role in mitosis. Recently, highly potent and selective small-molecule inhibitors of aurora-A and -B kinases, including VX-680 (also known as MK-0457, Cambridge, Massachusetts, USA), MLN-8054 (Millennium, Cambridge, Massachusetts, USA), AS703569 (R763) (Rigel Pharmaceuticals, South San Francisco, California, USA), and AZD1152 (AstraZeneca), which block cell cycle progression and induce apoptosis in experimental models of human cancer, have entered clinical development (287–290). Early results indicate that neutropenia is their principal toxicity.

Like the aurora family of kinases, the polo-like, Nek, and other kinase families participate in the centrosome cycle and modulate spindle function (274,280,282–284), while Bub1, BubR1, and Mps1 kinases regulate the spindle assembly checkpoint. Some members of these families, particularly the polo-like kinases, are being evaluated as potential targets for therapeutic intervention. Small-molecule inhibitors of polo-like kinase that are in early clinical development include BI2536 (Boehringer Ingelheim, Ingelheim, Germany) and ON01910.Na (Onconova, Lawrenceville, New Jersey, USA), and have demonstrated broad-spectrum antitumor activity against both solid and hematologic malignancy in preclinical studies, as well as synergistic activity when combined with some types of cytotoxic agents (291, 292).

RADIATION THERAPY: ADVANCES IN THE 21st CENTURY

Radiation therapy (RT) has been used in the treatment of gynecologic malignancies for more than a century (293). Over the years, numerous technologic advancements have been introduced, including high-energy (megavoltage) linear accelerators, high-dose-rate (HDR) brachytherapy, and computed tomography (CT)-based treatment planning. These and other important innovations have markedly improved the quality and delivery of radiation in women with gynecologic tumors.

Despite such advancements, the basic approach to the planning and delivery of radiation in these patients has remained relatively unchanged. This is particularly the case with external beam RT. After determining the site to be treated, a limited number of treatment fields (typically two to four) are selected. Select variables (e.g., beam energy, weighting) are then altered iteratively, producing a treatment plan that irradiates the target tissues while avoiding, as best as possible, the nearby normal tissues. Finally, fields are shaped with customized blocks to further reduce the dose to neighboring normal tissues.

Intensity-Modulated Radiation Therapy

In recent years, a novel approach to the planning and delivery of radiation has been introduced, known as intensity-modulated RT (IMRT) (294,295). Unlike conventional RT approaches, IMRT conforms the radiation dose to the shape of the target tissues in three dimensions (3D), thereby sparing the nearby normal tissues. While used predominantly in patients with head and neck tumors and prostate cancer, increasing interest has been focused recently on IMRT in gynecology patients. In fact, in a recent practice survey of IMRT use in the United States (296), gynecologic tumors were the fourth most common site treated with IMRT, with 35% of respondents reporting having treated a gynecology patient.

The majority of the IMRT literature to date has focused on head and neck tumors and prostate cancer (297–300). In these sites, IMRT has been associated with lower rates of adverse treatment sequelae due to reductions in the volume of normal tissues irradiated. Reducing the irradiation of normal tissues has also allowed the delivery of higher than conventional doses, improving tumor control. The rationale underlying IMRT in gynecology patients is similar. Standard approaches result in the irradiation of considerable volumes of normal tissues, exposing women to a wide range of untoward sequelae, particularly related to the gastrointestinal tract (301,302). Sparing of normal tissues also allows the use of higher doses, an appealing approach in patients at high risk for locoregional recurrence (303,304). IMRT may also provide a means of treating cervical cancer patients unable to undergo brachytherapy, improving their chance of cure (305).

IMRT and Inverse Planning

IMRT is an advanced form of 3D conformal RT (3DCRT) that utilizes computer-optimized intensity-modulated beams to generate highly conformal dose distributions (306). Although first used in the 1990s, the concepts underlying IMRT are not new. In fact, IMRT was first proposed in the 1960s (307). Its implementation in clinical practice, however, had to await the development of sophisticated computerized optimization programs (308).

Unlike conventional approaches, IMRT planning is an *inverse* process whereby the treatment planner delineates the target and normal tissues on a planning CT scan (309). Specific dose-volume constraints are then entered for the target and normal tissues and the optimization program generates a treatment plan that best satisfies these goals. This approach is distinguished from the trial-and-error forward conventional planning method. Inverse planning is a powerful tool. Whereas conventional approaches result in an acceptable plan, inverse planning generates the optimal one.

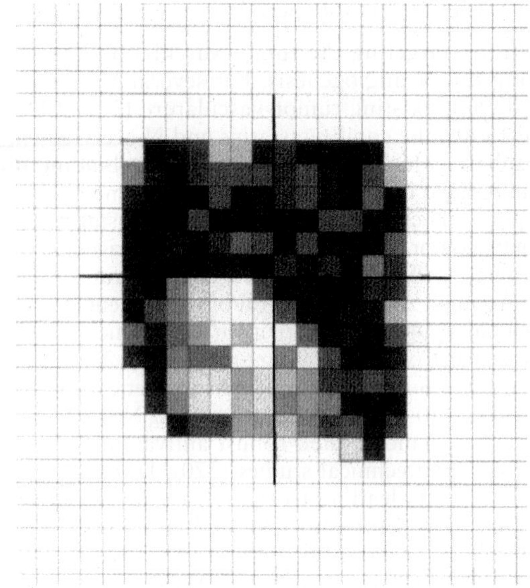

FIGURE 18.6. Intensity profile of an intensity-modulated radiation beam used in a patient with cervical cancer. Black regions represent areas of high intensity, and white regions represent areas of low intensity.

During the optimization process, each radiation beam is divided by the computer into small "beamlets" whose intensity is varied until the desired dose distribution is obtained. The resultant intensity profile of each beam is often quite complex and cannot be determined manually (Fig. 18.6). When cast into a patient, these intensity-modulated beams result in highly conformal dose distributions, which are nearly always superior to those achieved with conventional planning, particularly in patients with complex shaped targets (309). Such plans are distinguished by rapid dose gradients outside the target, resulting in considerable sparing of neighboring normal tissues (306). An example IMRT plan in a gynecologic patient is shown in Figure 18.7.

IMRT is typically delivered using a linear accelerator equipped with a multileaf collimator whose "leaves" (typically 0.5 to 1.0 cm in width) move in and out of the beam's path under computer control (306,309). The longer the leaves remain open at a particular position, the greater the intensity of radiation. Other available approaches include helical Tomotherapy and customized compensators.

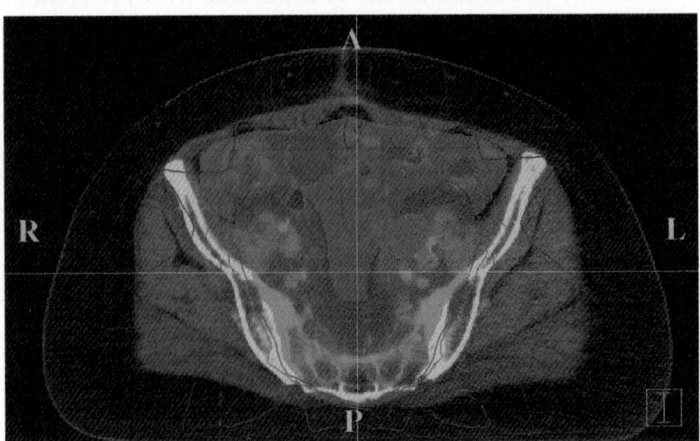

FIGURE 18.7. Example IMRT in a patient with cervical cancer undergoing posthysterectomy pelvic IMRT. Note that the high-dose isodose lines conform to the laterally situated internal and external iliac lymph nodes and the posteriorly situated presacral nodes.

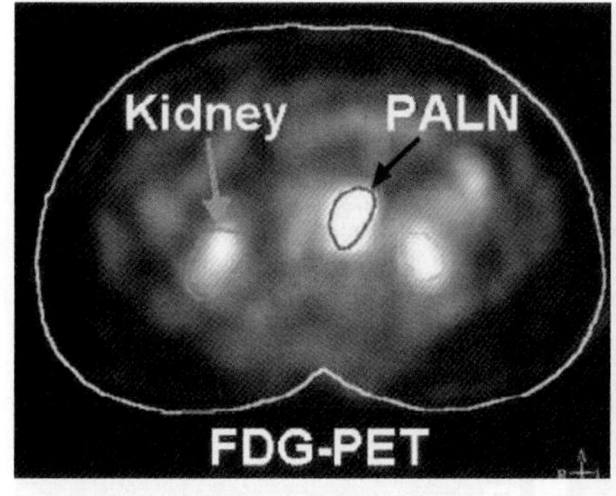

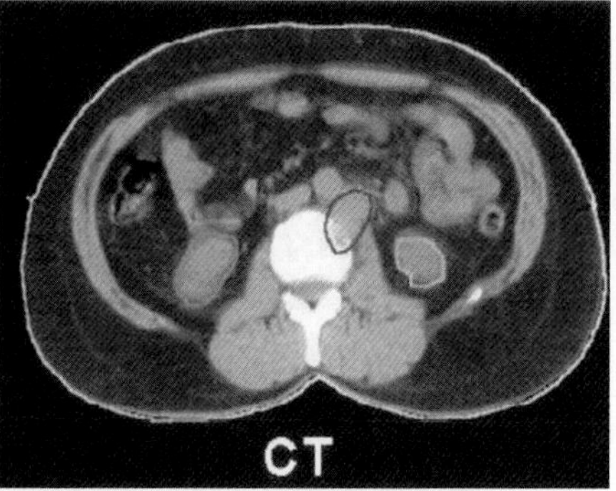

FIGURE 18.8. (*See color plate section.*) Axial PET and CT images showing a positive para-aortic lymph node and the kidneys in a patient with cervical cancer. *Source:* Printed with permission from Mutic S, Malyapa RS, Grigsby PW, et al. PET-guided IMRT for cervical carcinoma with positive para-aortic lymph nodes—a dose-escalation treatment planning study. *Int J Radiat Oncol Biol Phys* 2003;55:28–35.

IMRT Process

The IMRT process begins at simulation. Unlike in conventional approaches, a contrast-enhanced planning CT scan is performed, typically using a CT simulator. Attention is focused on optimal patient immobilization, given the rapid dose gradients in IMRT plans (306). At the University of Chicago, an upper and lower body alpha cradle is fabricated and indexed to the treatment table for gynecology patients undergoing IMRT (310,311). Such an approach has improved patient setup accuracy. Patients at most centers are simulated and treated in the supine position. Others, however, favor prone positioning (312).

At simulation, bladder, rectal, oral, and intravenous contrast may be used to add in the visualization of the target and normal tissues. Intravenous contrast is particularly useful since the pelvic vessels serve as surrogates for the lymph nodes. A vaginal marker is placed to identify the vaginal cuff. Two targets are delineated on the planning CT: a gross target (GTV) and a clinical target (CTV) volume (313). The GTV consists of all visualizable tumor (primary and other sites including enlarged lymph nodes). Unfortunately, the primary tumor is often poorly visualized even when contrast is used. Ongoing work is evaluating the incorporation of other imaging modalities, for example, magnetic resonance imaging (MRI) and positron emission tomography (PET) (314), into the planning process to improve target delineation (Fig. 18.8).

The CTV in an individual gynecology patient undergoing IMRT is a function of the tumor site treated. In women receiving adjuvant intensity-modulated pelvic RT, the CTV consists of the upper vagina, parametria, presacral region, and pelvic lymph nodes (common, internal, and external iliacs) (310,311). Contrast-enhanced vessels are included with a 0.5- to 1.0-cm margin to cover the pelvic lymph nodes. In patients with an intact uterus, the entire uterus is often included. If more comprehensive volumes are treated, the CTV may also include the para-aortic (315) and/or inguinal (316) lymph nodes. The CTV is uniformly expanded at most centers by 1 cm in three dimensions, creating a planning target volume (PTV) to account for setup uncertainty and organ motion.

Normal tissues contoured on the planning CT scan may include the bladder, rectum, and small bowel. The bone marrow within the iliac crests is often outlined, particularly when chemotherapy is planned (317–320). Controversy exists whether the iliac crests alone should be contoured or all the pelvic bone marrow sites (317). Recent data have suggested that delineation of the active (red) marrow sites is possible by incorporating a technetium 99m scan in the planning process (Fig. 18.9) (321). Depending on the site treated, other normal structures may include the kidneys (315) and femoral heads (316).

IMRT planning continues with dose specification. In most gynecology patients undergoing pelvic IMRT, 45 Gy is delivered in 1.8-Gy daily fractions. Given the inherent inhomogeneities of IMRT planning, larger fractions are not recommended. More complicated dose prescriptions are used in women undergoing a simultaneous integrated boost (SIB), where different parts of the target receive different daily (and total) doses (317,322). If the whole abdomen is treated, 30 Gy in 150-cGy daily fractions is recommended (311).

A more challenging task is the specification of dose-volume constraints for the PTV and normal tissues. Such constraints serve as input parameters used in the inverse planning optimization process and are entered in the form of dose-volume histograms (DVH), a graphical representation of the volume of an organ receiving a particular dose. Priority is given to PTV coverage. However, in all IMRT plans, a small percentage of the PTV may receive below the prescription dose. A common approach is to cover ≥98% of the PTV with the prescription dose. Input parameters for the normal tissues are less intuitive. The parameters used in intensity-modulated whole pelvic radiation therapy (IM-WPRT) patients treated at our center were derived empirically over a number of years (Table 18.2). The goal for most normal tissues is to minimize the volume receiving high doses (323). In other organs, however, the volume receiving low doses may be equally or more important (319).

Albeit many aspects of IMRT planning are automated, one still selects the number of beams, and their angles and energy. Typically, seven or nine equally spaced coplanar beams are used (51.4- and 40.0-degree increments, respectively) delivered with 6- or 15-MV photons. Fewer beams result in poorer conformity; more beams do not improve the overall quality of the plan. At other centers, other beam configurations are used. In the future, beam number and configuration may be incorporated in the optimization process (324).

Using inverse planning, the treatment-planning computer then generates a dose distribution that best satisfies the input constraints. At most centers, a number of potential plans are generated by varying the input parameters. Plan evaluation and selection is a time-consuming process. Each plan is evaluated qualitatively slice by slice for dose conformity and the presence and magnitude of hot and cold spots. Each plan is also evaluated quantitatively by assessing the PTV and normal tissue DVHs. A reasonable approach is to ensure that ≥98% of the PTV receives the prescription dose. Cold spots should only be considered acceptable along the periphery of the PTV; they are never acceptable within the CTV, particularly within the GTV. Similarly, hot spots should be minimized, particularly along the anterior rectal and posterior bladder walls in patients subsequently undergoing brachytherapy.

Both before and during IMRT, rigorous quality assurance (QA) is essential. A full discussion of QA procedures used in these patients is beyond the scope of this text and interested readers are referred elsewhere (311). Several QA procedures including independent monitor unit checks and verification of calculated IMRT dose distributions using both phantom and film dosimetry have been proposed.

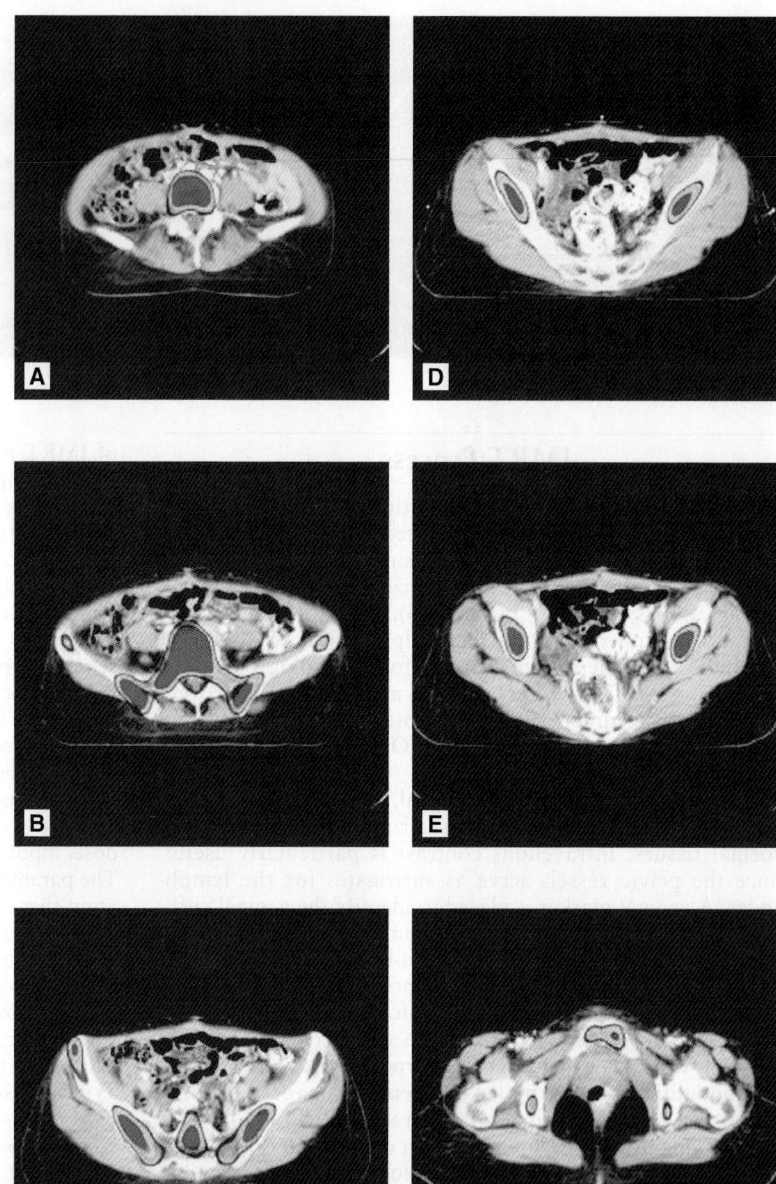

FIGURE 18.9. (*See color plate section.*) Overlay of SPECT bone marrow images on planning CT images. (**A**) Lumbar vertebrae; (**B**) lumbar vertebrae and iliac crests; (**C**) sacrum and iliac crest; (**D**) mid-pelvis; (**E**) hip; and (**F**) pubic symphysis. *Source:* Printed with permission from Roeske JC, Lujan AE, Mundt AJ. Incorporation of SPECT bone marrow imaging into IMRT planning in gynecology patients undergoing IM-WPRT. Presented at the 6th International Conference on Dose, Time and Fractionation. Madison, WI, September 23–26, 2001.

TABLE 18.2

INPUT PLANNING PARAMETERS FOR IM-WPRT PATIENTS, UNIVERSITY OF CHICAGO

	Goal (Gy)	Volume below goal (%)	Minimum (Gy)	Maximum (Gy)
PTV	45	3	42.8	47.3
Organ	**Limit (Gy)**	**Volume above limit (Gy)**	**Minimum (Gy)**	**Maximum (Gy)**
Bladder	35.1	40	27.9	42.8
Rectum	35.8	54	27.5	42.8
Small bowel	38.1	0	8.2	42.8

Note: IM-WPRT, intensity-modulated whole pelvic radiation therapy; PTV, planning target volume.

Preclinical Data

Numerous investigators have compared IMRT and conventional planning in gynecologic patients, demonstrating the benefits of IMRT planning. Of note, most have focused on women undergoing pelvic irradiation in an attempt to reduce the volume of small bowel irradiated. Representative studies are summarized in Table 18.3.

Roeske et al. (310) compared conventional and intensity-modulated pelvic RT plans in ten gynecologic patients. Although PTV coverage was similar, the volume of small bowel receiving the prescription dose in the IMRT plans was decreased by a factor of two (17.4% vs. 33.8%; $p = 0.0005$) compared with the conventional approach. The volumes of rectum and bladder irradiated were also reduced by 23%. Other investigators have reported reductions in small bowel irradiation using IMRT planning ranging from 40% to 70% (326–328). Marked reductions in the volume of bladder and rectum irradiated have also been reported (328).

While most attention has been focused on small bowel sparing, Lujan et al. (317) demonstrated that IMRT planning could also minimize the volume of pelvic bone marrow irradiated in gynecology patients undergoing pelvic RT (Fig. 18.10). Bone marrow (within the iliac crests) was contoured in ten women and added as a constraint in the planning process. Although the volume receiving 10 Gy was slightly increased, IMRT planning reduced the bone marrow volume treated at all dose levels above 15 Gy, an important finding given the exquisite radiosensitivity of bone marrow. Of note, the addition of bone marrow as a constraint did not compromise PTV coverage or the sparing of other normal tissues.

Several investigators have evaluated IMRT planning in gynecologic patients treated with more comprehensive fields. In ten locally advanced cervical cancer patients undergoing extended field (pelvic plus para-aortic) RT, Portelance et al. (315) noted significant reductions in the small bowel, bladder, and rectum using IMRT planning compared to conventional two- or four-field approaches. Hong et al. (329) evaluated IMRT planning in ten endometrial cancer patients undergoing whole abdomen radiation therapy (WART). PTV coverage was improved, particularly near the kidneys (under the conventional blocks). Moreover, the volume of pelvic bones (and thus bone marrow) receiving 21 Gy or higher was reduced by 60% (Fig. 18.11). Duthoy et al. similarly noted a benefit to IMRT planning in gynecology patients undergoing WART (328).

Several IMRT studies have focused on gynecologic patients undergoing pelvic-inguinal RT. In vulvar cancer patients, Beriwal et al. (330) noted improved sparing of the small bowel and rectum using IMRT. Garofalo et al. (316) reported that IMRT planning reduced the volume of all normal tissues irradiated, including the small bowel, bladder, rectum, and bone marrow. Of particular note, the dose to the femoral heads was also significantly reduced. In contrast, Gilroy et al. (331) noted that higher doses to the pelvic tissues and greater setup complexity were seen with IMRT. However, the sole goal of this study was to reduce the dose to the femoral heads. No attempt was made to spare the small bowel and other pelvic tissues.

IMRT has also been evaluated as a means to deliver higher than conventional doses in gynecology patients. Lujan et al. (320) found that dose escalation was feasible using an SIB technique in patients with involved pelvic nodes, without compromising normal tissue sparing. Mutic et al. (314) proposed a PET-guided SIB approach to irradiate involved para-aortic lymph nodes in advanced cervical cancer patients. In their exploratory study, 59.4 Gy could be delivered to PET-positive para-aortic nodes, while maintaining acceptable doses to the normal tissues. Kavanagh et al. (322,332) presented an SIB technique to treat the primary tumor and/or involved lymph nodes to higher dose in cervical cancer patients. Others have reported similar results using the SIB approach in patients with involved para-aortic lymph nodes (333).

IMRT as an alternative for brachytherapy has received considerable attention (305,334). In cervical cancer patients unable to receive brachytherapy, Roeske and Mundt (335) found that a total dose of 75 Gy or higher was feasible with IMRT. Select patients could receive doses as high as 81 Gy to the residual tumor. Low et al. (336) proposed a technique known as applicator-guided IMRT as a replacement for brachytherapy. As envisioned, an applicator would be placed in the cervix to localize the tumor and reproducibly position the bladder and rectum during treatment. MRI and/or PET imaging would be used to delineate the tumor with treatment delivered using conventional HDR dose schedules.

Clinical Studies

Mundt et al. (337,338) have provided a series of detailed analyses of acute gastrointestinal toxicity in gynecology patients undergoing intensity-modulated pelvic RT. In their most recent analysis (338), acute gastrointestinal sequelae were compared in 40 IMRT and 35 conventional RT patients, with the two groups well balanced in terms of tumor site, stage, surgery, radiation dose, and chemotherapy. IMRT was found to be associated with less grade 2 or higher acute gastrointestinal toxicity (60% vs. 91%; $p = 0.002$) than conventional RT. Moreover, the percentage of IMRT and conventional pelvic RT patients requiring no (or only infrequent) antidiarrheal

TABLE 18.3

DOSIMETRIC STUDIES COMPARING CONVENTIONAL AND INTENSITY-MODULATED PELVIC RADIOTHERAPY IN GYNECOLOGIC TUMOR PATIENTS

	Reduction in volume receiving prescription dose using IMRT		
Author	Bowel	Bladder	Rectum
Roeske et al. (310)	↓50%	↓23%	↓23%
Ahamad et al. (327)	↓40% to 63%[a]	NS	NS
Chen et al. (325)	↓70%	↓[b]	↓[b]
Heron et al. (326)	↓51%[c]	↓31%[c]	↓66%[c]

Note: IMRT, intensity-modulated radiation therapy, NS, not stated.
[a]Dependent on planning target volume expansion used.
[b]Data not shown.
[c]Reduction in percent volume receiving 30 Gy or higher.

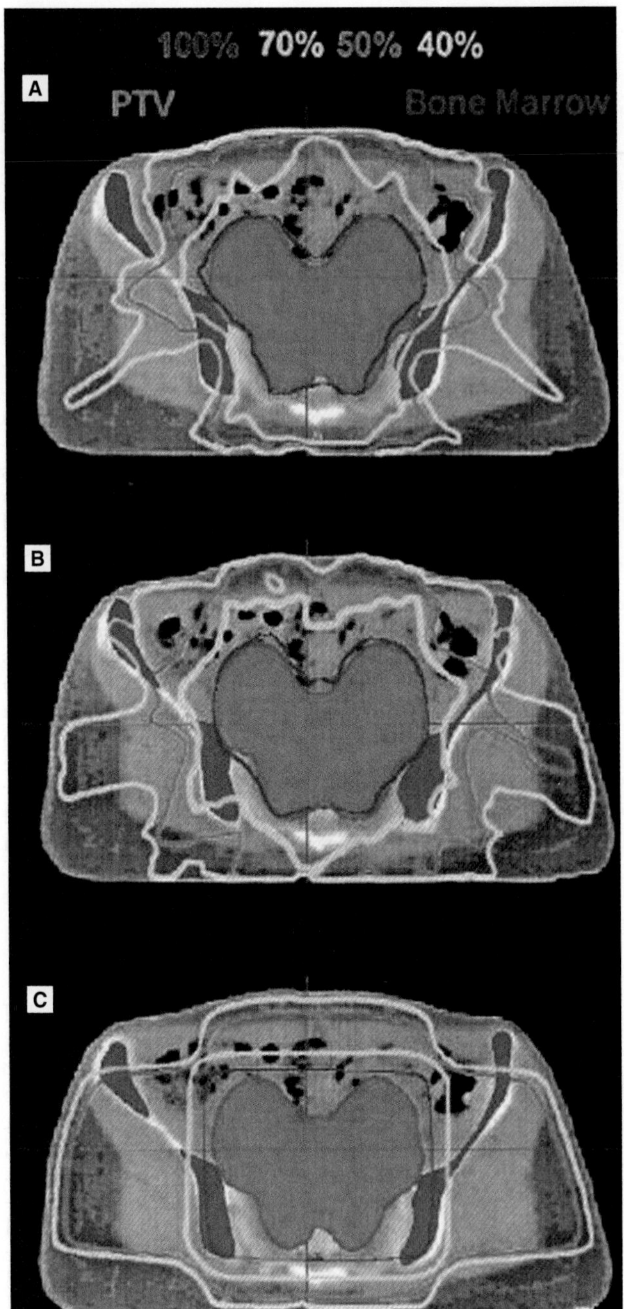

FIGURE 18.10. (*See color plate section.*) Axial CT slices of a cervical cancer patient undergoing postoperative IMRT: (A) bone marrow sparing IMRT plan with isodose lines bending medially away from the iliac crest bone marrow, (B) IMRT plan without bone marrow as a constraint, and (C) conventional four-field box pelvic RT plan showing bone marrow almost entirely enclosed by the 40% isodose line. *Source:* Printed with permission from Lujan AE, Mundt AJ, Yamada SD, et al. Intensity-modulated radiation therapy as a means of reducing dose to bone marrow in gynecologic patients receiving whole pelvic radiation therapy. *Int J Radiat Oncol Biol Phys* 2003;57:516–521.

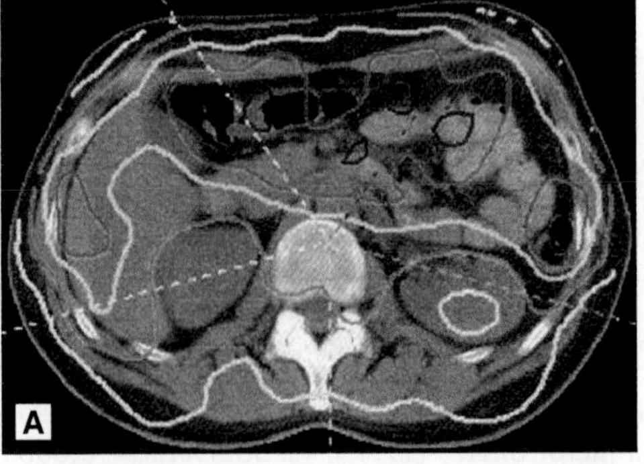

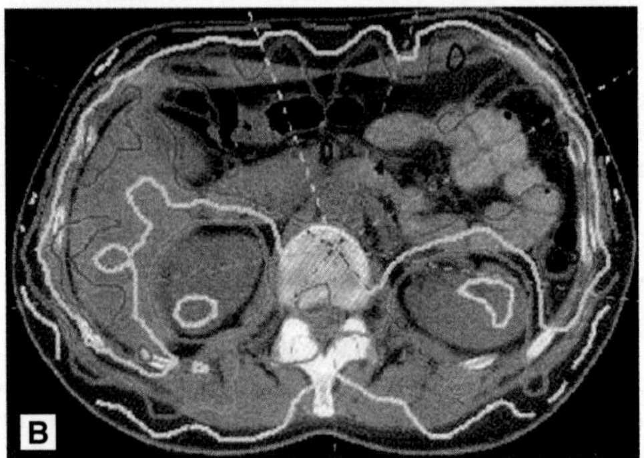

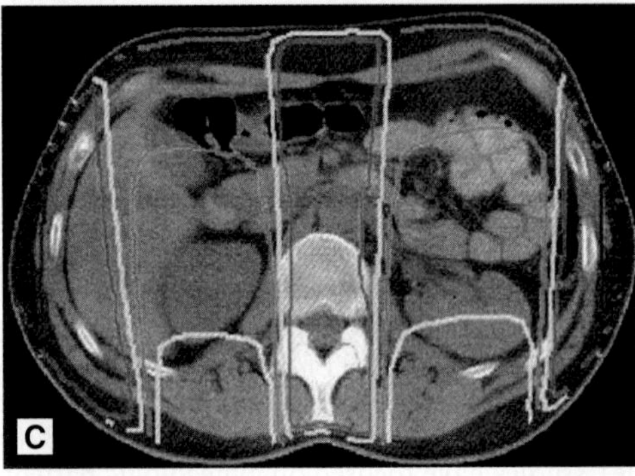

FIGURE 18.11. (*See color plate section.*) IMRT and conventional plan comparison in a gynecology patient treated with whole abdominal irradiation. **A:** IMRT plan with five gantry angles. **B:** IMRT plan with nine gantry angles. **C:** Conventional plan with kidney blocks. Source: Printed with permission from Hong L, Alektiar K, Chui C, et al. IMRT of large fields: whole abdomen irradiation. *Int J Radiat Oncol Biol Phys* 2002;54:278–289.

medications was 75% and 34%, respectively (p = 0.001). Although less urinary toxicity (10% vs. 20%) was observed, this difference failed to reach statistical significance (p = 0.22).

These investigators have recently evaluated chronic gastrointestinal toxicity in a cohort of 30 gynecology patients treated with intensity-modulated pelvic RT with a median follow-up of 19.6 months (339). Compared to conventional pelvic RT patients, IMRT patients experienced less chronic gastrointestinal sequelae (11.1% vs. 50.0%; p = 0.001). On multivariate analysis controlling for age, stage, chemotherapy, surgery, and length of follow-up, IMRT was correlated with less chronic toxicity (p = 0.01; odds ratio [OR] 0.16; 95% CI, 0.04 to 0.67).

Others have similarly reported favorable acute and chronic toxicity profiles in gynecology patients undergoing IMRT (340), even those treated to more comprehensive volumes (341,342). For example, Gerszten et al. treated 22 locally advanced cervical cancer patients with a SIB IMRT technique (341). PET-positive para-aortic lymph nodes received 55 Gy in 2.2-Gy fractions, while the remainder of the pelvis and para-aortic regions received 45 Gy in 1.8-Gy fractions. All patients received concomitant cisplatin. No patient developed grade 3 or higher acute sequelae. Grade 2 or higher acute gastrointestinal and genitourinary toxicity was noted in 10% and 10% of patients, respectively.

Brixey et al. (318) compared the acute hematologic toxicity in women undergoing intensity-modulated versus conventional pelvic RT. Whereas sequelae were infrequent in RT alone patients, conventional RT patients treated with concomitant chemotherapy developed more grade ≥2 leukopenia (60% vs. 31.2%; $p = 0.08$) and a lower white blood cell count nadir (2.8 vs. 3.6; $p = 0.05$) than IMRT plus chemotherapy patients. The conventional RT patients also developed a lower absolute neutrophil count nadir (1,874 vs. 2,669; $p = 0.04$). Of note, these benefits were realized even though bone marrow was not entered as a constraint in the planning process, but was simply spared owing to the highly conformal nature of the IMRT plans.

In a recent analysis, Mell et al. (319) reported the importance of sparing all pelvic bone marrow sites in gynecology patients undergoing concomitant chemotherapy and pelvic IMRT, not simply the bone marrow within the iliac crests. Patients in whom the total pelvic bone marrow receiving 10 Gy or higher (V_{10}) was >90% had a higher rate of grade ≥2 leukopenia (73.7% vs. 11.1%, $p < 0.01$) compared to those in whom the pelvic bone marrow V_{10} was <90%. The corresponding rates of having one or more chemotherapy cycles held were 47.4% and 16.7%, respectively ($p = 0.08$).

As gynecologic IMRT matures, an increasing number of studies focused on tumor control have been published. Knab et al. (343) treated 31 stage I-III endometrial cancer patients with adjuvant intensity-modulated pelvic RT following hysterectomy. At a median follow-up of 24 months, no pelvic recurrences were seen. Similarly, Beriwal et al. (340) noted no pelvic failures in 47 endometrial cancer patients undergoing adjuvant intensity-modulated pelvic RT at a median follow-up of 20 months.

Two series have reported the outcomes of intact cervical cancer patients undergoing IMRT (344,345). Kochanski et al. treated 44 stage IB-IIIB cervical cancer patients with intensity-modulated pelvic RT (nearly all received concomitant chemotherapy) followed by intracavitary brachytherapy (344). At a median follow-up of 23 months, the 3-year actuarial pelvic control in the stage I-IIA and stage IIB-IIIB patients was 93% and 53%, respectively. Beriwal et al. (345) reported an 80% pelvic control rate in 36 stage IB-IVA cervical cancer patients at a median follow-up of 18 months.

Excellent pelvic control rates have been reported in cervical cancer patients undergoing IMRT following radical hysterectomy. In a series of 18 clinical stage I-II patients (many with positive pelvic lymph nodes) treated with adjuvant pelvic IMRT, Kochanski et al. (344) reported a 3-year pelvic control of 94%. Chen et al. (346) noted a 93% pelvic control in a similar group of patients treated with intensity-modulated pelvic RT, all of whom received concomitant chemotherapy.

Based on these promising results, the Radiation Therapy Oncology Group (RTOG) has launched a multi-institution phase 2 trial (RTOG 0418) evaluating the tolerance and efficacy of IMRT in gynecology patients following hysterectomy. The results of this important trial will help establish the role of IMRT in these women.

Future Directions

Just as IMRT is becoming increasingly accepted in gynecologic cancer patients, the next revolution has begun, namely, *image-guided* RT (IGRT). IGRT involves the use of imaging to improve target delineation and treatment delivery.

In terms of its role in target delineation, as described earlier in this chapter, promising approaches have been developed incorporating PET (314,333) and SPECT (321) in the IMRT planning process. PET may be extended to the planning of brachytherapy in cervical cancer patients (347). MRI may also prove beneficial (348), in particular, nanoparticle-enhanced MRI techniques to improve the delineation of pelvic lymph node regions (Fig. 18.12) (348).

Numerous vendors have recently introduced in-room imaging solutions allowing patients to be imaged daily in the treatment room on the treatment table immediately prior to treatment. Several vendors have developed on-board imaging devices, consisting of x-ray imagers mounted to the linac gantry providing the means to generate high-quality planar and volumetric images (Fig. 18.13). Such techniques may substantially improve the ability to accurately align patients on the table, reducing the need for large safety margins around the target tissues. More importantly, daily imaging may address concerns about internal organ motion, particularly in patients with an intact uterus undergoing IMRT (349).

Perhaps the most exciting application of IGRT, however, is the potential to *adapt* treatment to changes in the tumor during treatment. It is well known that cervical cancers respond rapidly during pelvic RT. Consequently, the highly conformal IMRT plans generated *prior* to treatment may no longer be optimal *during* therapy. Van de Bunt et al. illustrated this problem by performing MRI scans on 14 cervical cancer patients undergoing definitive irradiation prior to treatment and after 30 Gy (349). On average, the cervical tumor decreased by 46% in size (Fig. 18.14). Replanning significantly improved the sparing of the rectum in these patients. Moreover, in patients with bulky cervical tumor (>30 cc), replanning also improved sparing of the small bowel.

The clinical application of adaptive IGRT approaches is not yet ready for prime time. Numerous hurdles need to be first overcome. For example, rapid and accurate automated segmentation programs are needed. Moreover, deformable image registration programs are required to allow doses to be accurately calculated as the anatomy changes. Finally, additional computational power is also needed to allow segmentation, deformable registration, and reoptimization to be performed in a timely fashion, preferably while the patient is on the treatment table. All of these topics are currently the subject of active research.

Conclusion

IMRT represents a true revolution in the treatment of gynecologic tumors. Preclinical and clinical data have been extremely promising to date, suggesting that IMRT can improve the planning and delivery of radiation in these patients. Nonetheless, carefully designed prospective clinical trials are needed to fully ascertain the potential benefits and risks of IMRT in gynecology patients. Attention is now turning to IGRT approaches, both to improve target delineation and treatment delivery, in patients undergoing IMRT. It is hoped one day that true adaptive image-guided IMRT will be a reality in these patients.

ADVANCES IN FERTILITY-SPARING SURGERY

Minimally invasive and laparoscopic surgery for gynecologic oncology are discussed in detail in other chapters. The utility of advanced operative laparoscopy in gynecologic oncology expanded following advancements in laparoscopic retroperitoneal surgery, particularly pelvic and aortic lymphadenectomy. The performance of a laparoscopic retroperitoneal dissection opened the door for more advanced laparoscopic gynecologic cancer applications and operations, including the

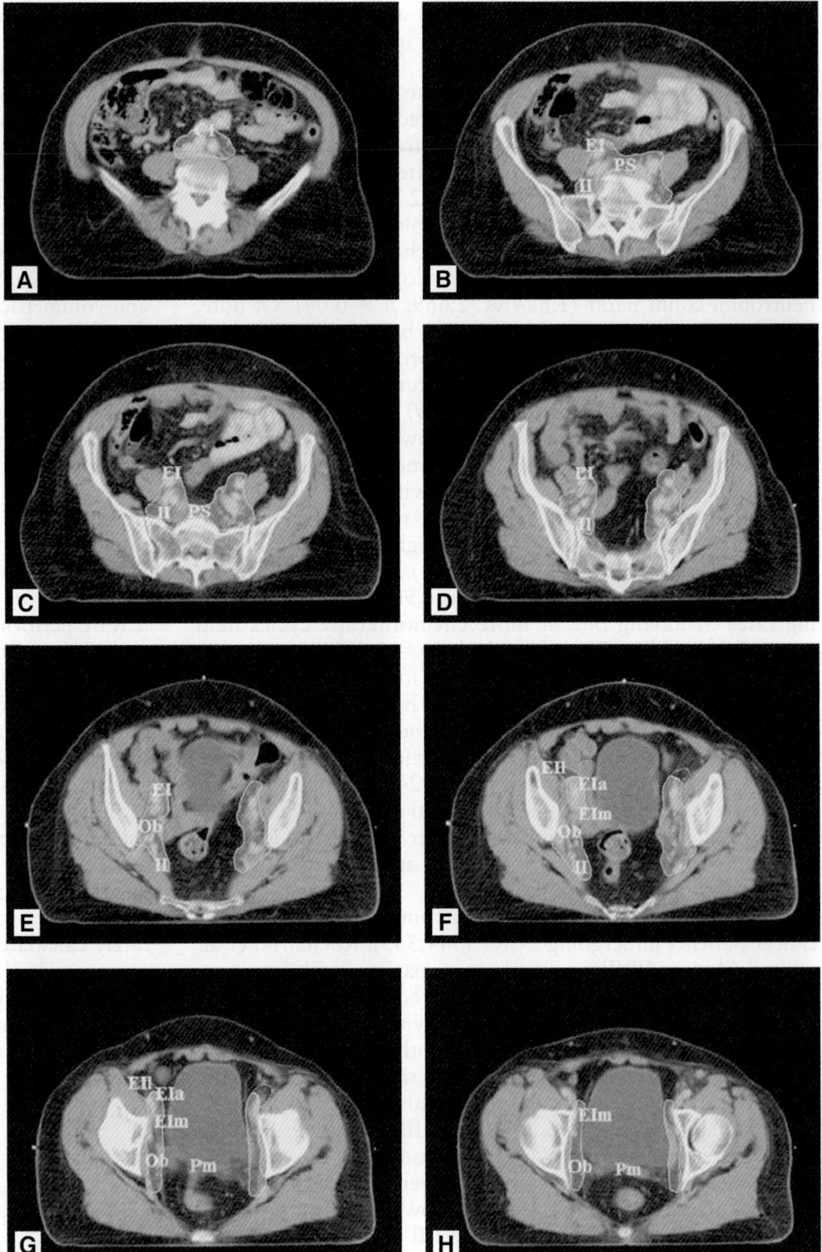

FIGURE 18.12. (*See color plate section.*) Guidelines for CTV delineation for gynecologic tumors to cover the common iliac (CI), subaortic presacral (PS), internal iliac (II), obturator (Ob), and medial (EIm) and anterior (EIa) external iliac lymph nodes based on nanoparticle-directed MR imaging. *Source:* Printed with permission from Taylor A, Rockall AG, Reznek RH, et al. Mapping pelvic lymph nodes: guidelines for delineation in intensity-modulated radiotherapy. *Int J Radiat Oncol Biol Phys* 2005;63:1604–1612.

revival of radical vaginal surgery (350) and the complete laparoscopic management and staging of selected patients with a variety of gynecologic malignancies. The potential oncologic effects of laparoscopy and pneumoperitoneum will continue to be debated (351); however, the results from emerging clinical trials and published retrospective series are reassuring.

Fertility-Sparing Radical Trachelectomy for Stage I Cervical Cancer

This operation is a major innovation in the surgical therapy of early cervical cancer, and the laparoscopic/vaginal approach is described well under the laparoscopy chapter in this book.

Although the concept of a radical abdominal trachelectomy was described and performed on women with cervical cancer by Aburel in Rumania in the last century (352,353), the abdominal procedure initially did not become popular, and fertility-sparing surgery in cervical cancer remained limited to conization for women with very early lesions and a strong desire to retain reproductive function. The radical vaginal approach to trachelectomy was developed by Professor Daniel Dargent in 1987 in France (354). It is a modification of the radical vaginal hysterectomy with two main purposes: treat early cervical cancer, and preserve uterine morphology and reproductive function. One of the main advantages in learning the radical vaginal hysterectomy is that the experience gained allows the surgeon to offer radical trachelectomy to selected young women with early invasive cervical cancer who wish to preserve their fertility (355). To date, several series are available in the English literature to document feasibility and safety, and many healthy births have been documented in women treated for early cervical cancer with this approach, including a case of pregnancy after radical trachelectomy and pelvic irradiation (356). The general eligibility criteria for

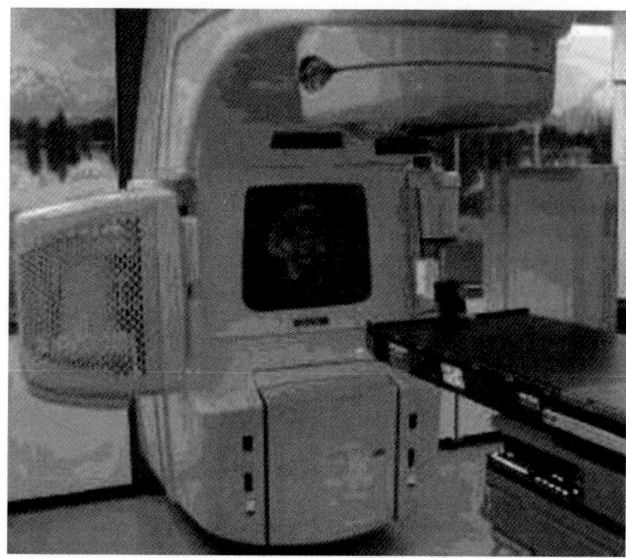

FIGURE 18.13. Varian Medical Systems on-board imaging (OBI) system with the electronic portal imaging device (EPID) mounted at right angles to the megavoltage beam.

radical vaginal trachelectomy vary but may include women age less than 44 with a very strong desire to preserve fertility, no clinical evidence of impaired fertility, lesion size less than 3 cm, FIGO stage IA-IB1 lesions, no involvement of the upper endocervical canal, and negative regional lymph nodes (357).

In a series of 96 radical trachelectomies performed between April 1987 and May 2002 at Hospital Edouard Herriot in Lyon, France, one second cancer (bilateral suprarenal glands cancer) and four recurrences were observed (358). The retrospective unifactorial analysis demonstrated that the maximal tumoral diameter (2 cm or more) and the depth of infiltration (1 cm or more) were the only two significant factors of risk. Age less than 30 years and the presence of lymphovascular space involvement were likely to be risk factors, but the level of statistical significance was not reached. Histology other than squamous, infiltration of the parametrium, and involvement of the vaginal cuff had no prognosis impact. The chances for recurrence were 19% for patients affected by a tumor 2 cm or more and 25% for the patients affected by a tumor 2 cm or more with a depth of infiltration 1 cm or more (358).

Technique of Radical Vaginal Trachelectomy

A laparoscopic pelvic with or without para-aortic node dissection is completed and multiple frozen sections are obtained from selected nodal packages and any suspicious nodes. Once all frozen sections are negative the vaginal component is started.

Cystoscopy and the insertion of bilateral temporary retrograde ureteral catheters are at the surgeon's discretion (359). The catheters may help identify the ureters in difficult cases and are removed at the end of the procedure. If there is concern of ureteral injury, the catheter can be changed over a guide wire to a double-J stent. The stent may be left in place for 4 to 6 weeks.

The radical vaginal trachelectomy is begun by delineating an adequate vaginal margin (usually 1 to 2 cm). Eight Kocher clamps are placed circumferentially around the cervix on the vaginal mucosa. A dilute solution of vasopressin is used to liberally inject the vaginal mucosa between the Kocher clamps (Fig. 18.15). This step helps separate the planes of dissection.

The assistants place two Brieski vaginal wall retractors at the 2 and 10 o'clock positions. A scalpel is now used to circumferentially incise the vaginal mucosa. The lateral incisions are shallow and the anterior and posterior incisions are deep. The

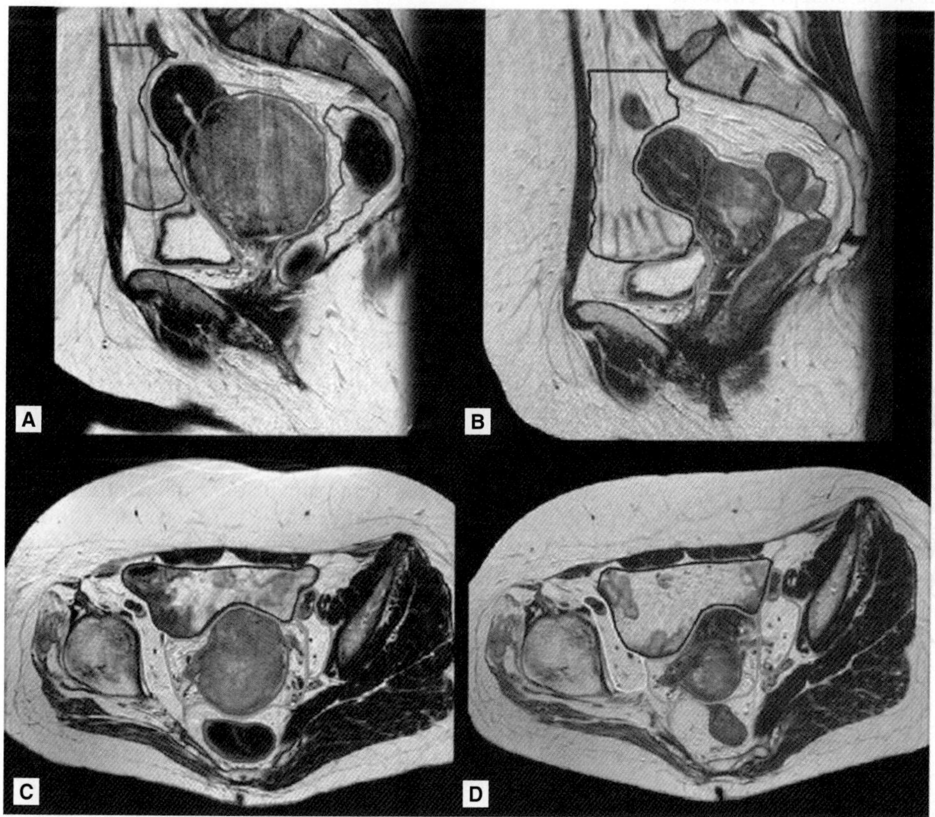

FIGURE 18.14. (*See color plate section.*) Delineation on magnetic resonance images of a patient with cervical cancer undergoing definitive RT: (**A**) pretreatment sagittal, (**B**) intratreatment sagittal, (**C**) pre-treatment axial, and (**D**) intratreatment axial. Note the significant decrease in size of the bulky central cervical tumor. Source: Reprinted with permission from van de Bunt L, van der Heide UA, Katelaars M, et al. Conventional, conformal and intensity-modulated radiation therapy treatment planning of external beam radiotherapy for cervical cancer: the impact of tumor regression. *Int J Radiat Oncol Biol Phys* 2006;64: 189–196.

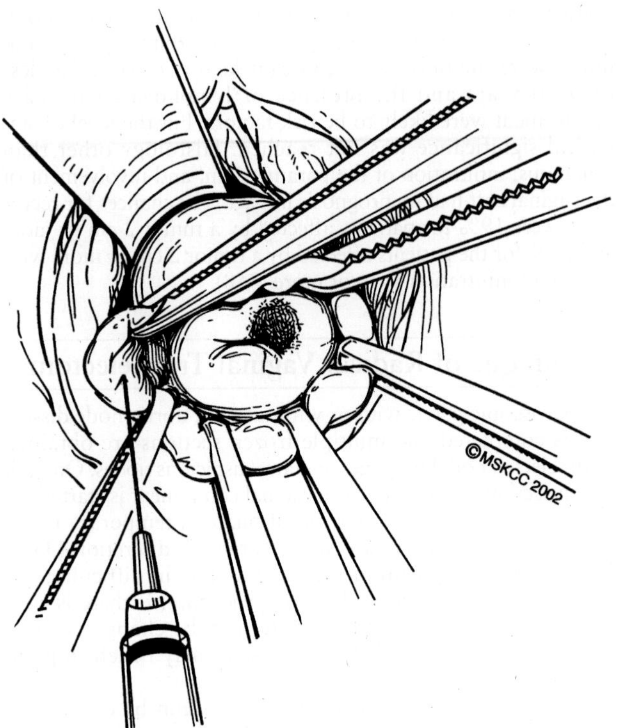

FIGURE 18.15. Preparing the vaginal margin.

shallow lateral incisions allow traction to be put on the parametria and pulled downward.

The Kocher clamps can now be removed, and the anterior and posterior vaginal mucosa can be folded over the ectocervix. The Krobach clamps are aligned horizontally to keep the ectocervix covered (Fig. 18.16).

The posterior cul de sac can now be sharply entered (Fig. 18.17). This allows the uterosacral ligaments to be isolated and the inferior portion of this ligament can be divided. By releasing the posterior attachments there is greater uterine descensus, which is helpful for the more difficult anterior dissection.

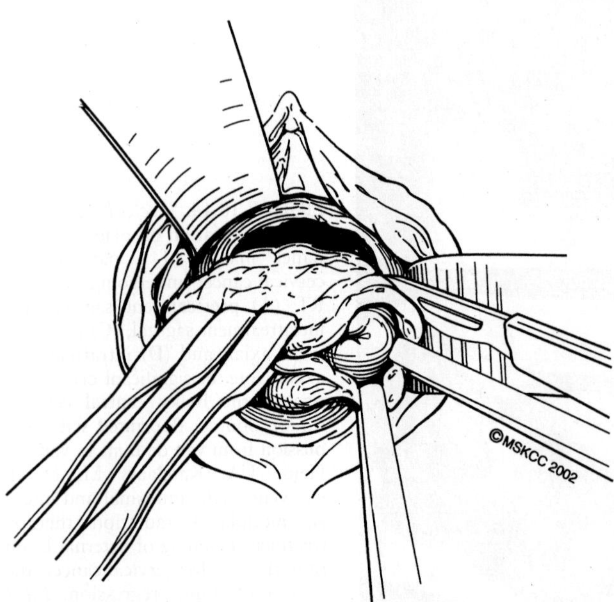

FIGURE 18.16. Incising the vaginal mucosa.

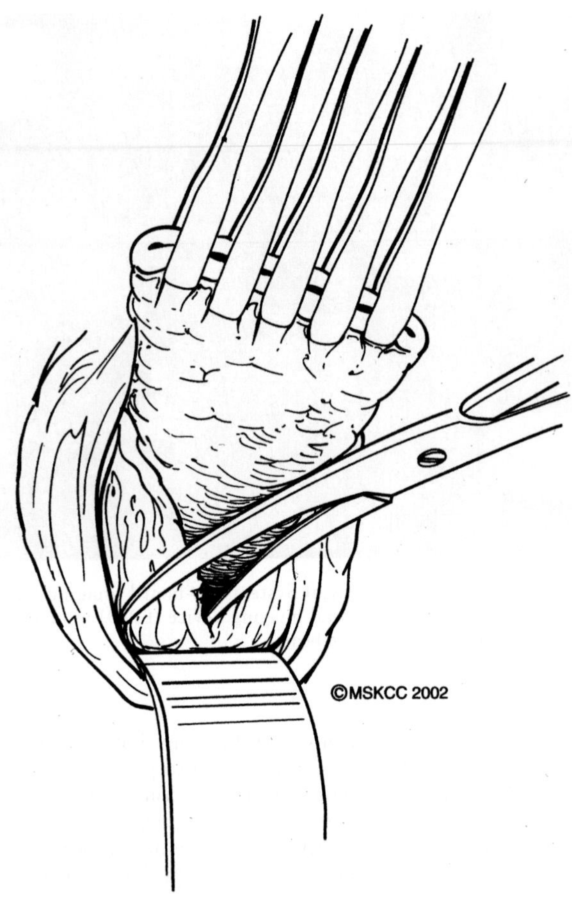

FIGURE 18.17. Posterior colpotomy.

The anterior portion of the dissection begins with sharply developing the vesicouterine space. The posterior vaginal retractor is removed, and the downward traction is placed on the specimen with the Krobach clamps. During this portion of the procedure, the surgeon should keep the axis of the scissors perpendicular to the axis of the vagina. This maneuver helps avoid tunneling into the bladder. Once the vesicouterine space is developed, the paravesical spaces must be opened. The left paravesical space is opened by placing two Kocher clamps on the vaginal mucosa at the 1 and 3 o'clock positions. By doing such, a small dimple is noted in between the two Kocher clamps. The Metzenbaum scissors are used to gently spread this dimple, tunnel under the vaginal mucosa, and enter the left paravesical space. The tissue between the paravesical and vesicouterine space is the left bladder pillar. The knee of the left ureter can now be palpated in the left bladder pillar (Fig. 18.18).

The inferior aspect of the left bladder pillar can now be transected. This frees the knee of the left ureter and allows it to be pushed superiorly. After doing such, two curved Heaney clamps can be placed across the parametrium to obtain an adequate margin. The parametrium is now divided between the two clamps, and the pedicle is secured with a suture ligature. The cervicovaginal branch of the left uterine artery is doubly clamped, divided, and secured with a suture ligature (Fig. 18.19).

The procedures of opening the paravesicle space, dividing the inferior aspect of the bladder pillar, and dividing the parametrium and cervicovaginal branch of the uterine artery are repeated on the right side. Once the branches of the uterine

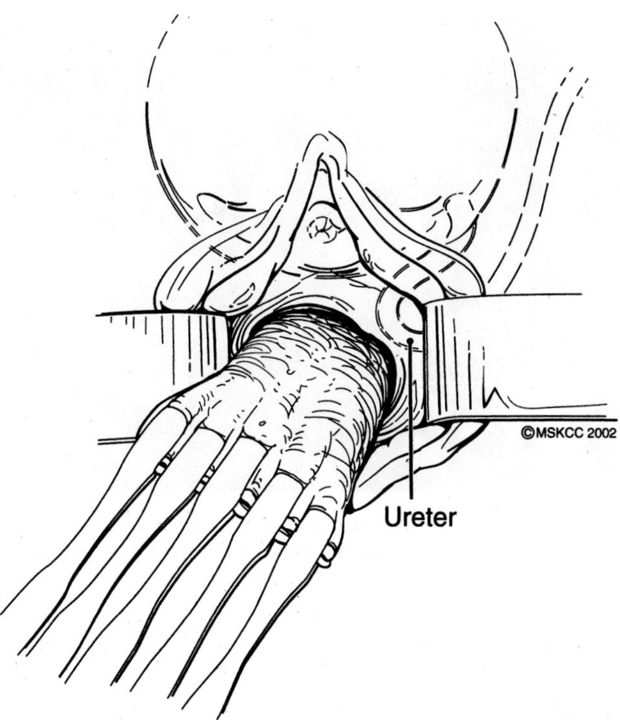

FIGURE 18.18. Identifying the ureter.

artery have been secured, the cervix can be amputated. An endocervical and endometrial curettage is performed, and frozen-section analysis is performed on the endocervical margin and endocervical/endometrial curettage. It is preferable to leave one centimeter of cervical stump to place a cerclage with permanent suture (Fig. 18.20).

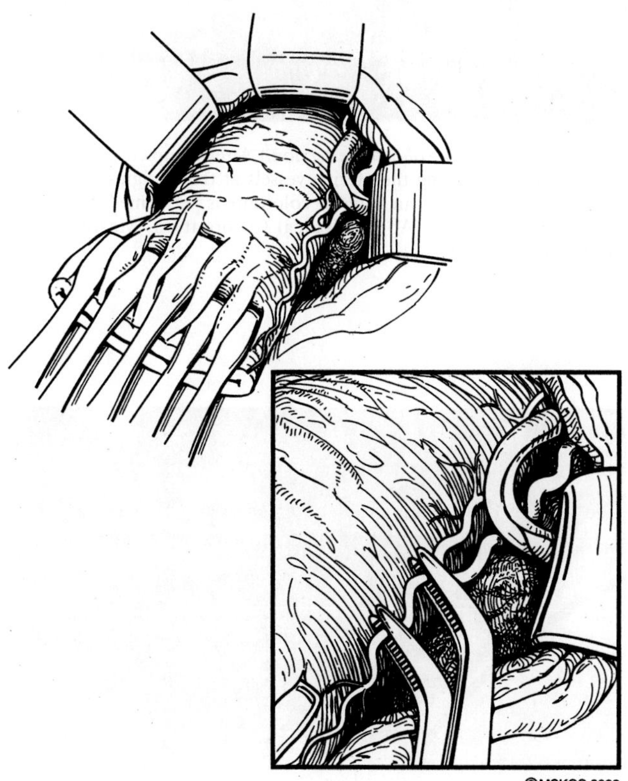

FIGURE 18.19. Ligating the paracervical vessels.

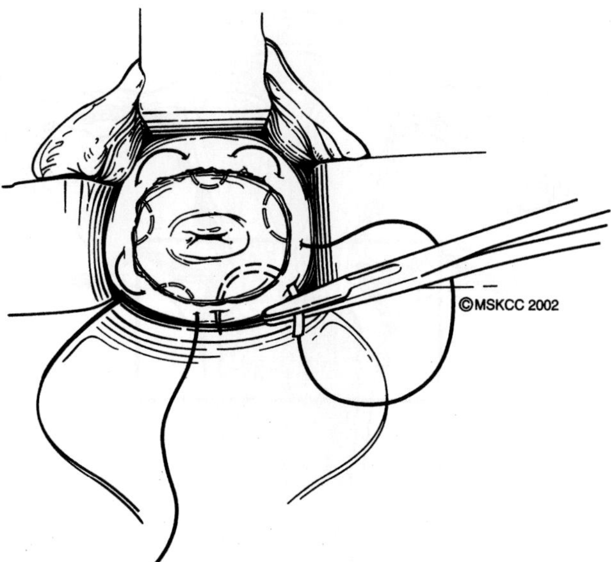

FIGURE 18.20. Inserting permanent cerclage.

The vaginal mucosa can now be reapproximated to the cervical stump to complete the vaginal portion of the procedure. Laparoscopy is the final step in the procedure to ensure pelvic hemostasis.

Fertility-Sparing Radical Abdominal Trachelectomy for Cervical Carcinoma

Technique of Fertility-Sparing Radical Abdominal Trachelectomy

A laparotomy and a bilateral complete pelvic lymphadenectomy are performed usually via a transverse lower abdominal incision in a similar manner to patients undergoing a radical abdominal hysterectomy. The limits of nodal dissection are the deep circumflex iliac vein caudally and the proximal common iliac artery cephalad. Any suspicious lymph nodes are sent for frozen-section analysis. A fertility-sparing approach should be abandoned if positive lymph nodes are identified. Sentinel lymph node identification is also a reasonable option and may allow for pathologic ultrastaging of these sentinel nodes. The removal of para-aortic nodes is also considered for lesions of stage IB1 or greater.

The intent of the radical abdominal trachelectomy is to resect the cervix, upper 1 to 2 cm of the vagina, parametrium, and paracolpos in a similar manner to a type III radical abdominal hysterectomy but sparing the uterine fundus or corpus (Figs. 18.21 and 18.22).

The procedure is begun by developing the paravesical and pararectal spaces and dissecting the bladder caudal to the mid vagina. The round ligaments are divided and large Kelly clamps are placed on the medial round ligaments to manipulate the uterus. Care is taken not to destroy the cornu or the utero-ovarian pedicles. The infundibulopelvic ligaments with ovarian blood supply are kept intact. Care is also taken not to injure the fallopian tubes or disrupt the utero-ovarian ligament. The uterus is manipulated with clamps at the round ligaments or using a Collin-Buxton–type clamp (Fig. 18.23).

The uterine vessels are then ligated and divided at their origin from the hypogastric vessels. The parametria and paracolpos with uterine vessels are mobilized medially with the specimen, and a complete ureterolysis is performed similar to

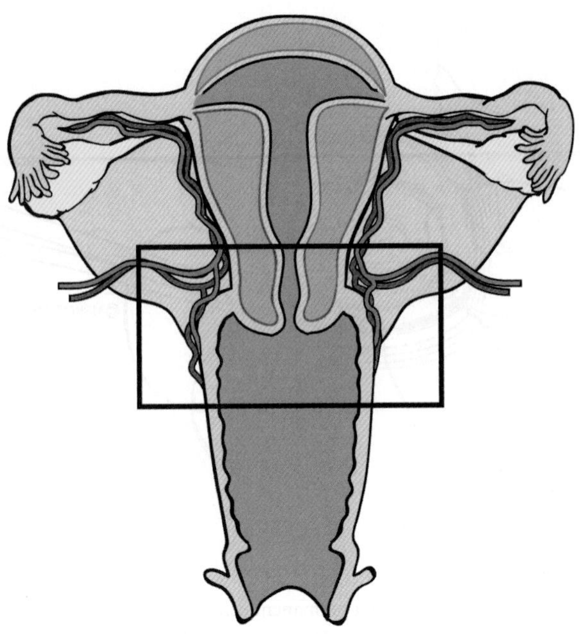

FIGURE 18.21. The intent of the radical abdominal trachelectomy is to resect the cervix and upper 1 to 2 cm of the vagina.

a type III radical abdominal hysterectomy. The posterior cul de sac peritoneum is incised and the uterosacral ligament divided; similarly, the parametria and paracolpos are divided. Using a vaginal cylinder (Apple Medical Corporation, Marlborough, Massachusetts, USA), the desired length of vaginectomy is performed, and the specimen is completely separated from the vagina (Fig. 18.24) and placed in the mid pelvis, keeping its attachment to the utero-ovarian ligaments. Alternatively, a Wertheim clamp can be placed at the desired length of the vagina and the specimen separated (Fig. 18.25).

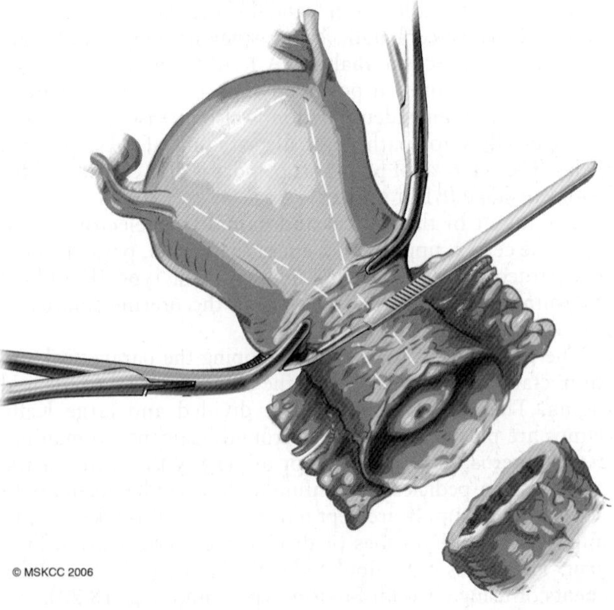

FIGURE 18.22. The intent of the radical abdominal trachelectomy is to resect the cervix and upper 1 to 2 cm of the vagina, parametrium, and paracolpos in a similar manner to a type III radical abdominal hysterectomy, but sparing the uterine corpus.

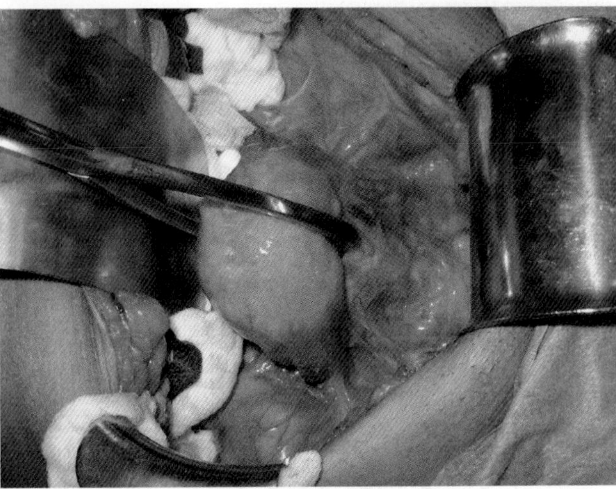

FIGURE 18.23. (*See color plate section.*) The uterus is manipulated by clamps on the round ligaments, avoiding the utero-ovarian pedicles or using a Collin-Buxton–type clamp.

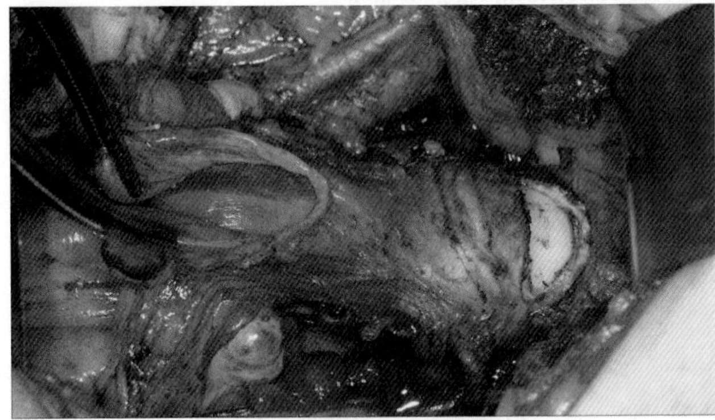

FIGURE 18.24. (*See color plate section.*) After completely separating the parametria, ligating the uterine vessels at their origins, and completing the ureterolysis, an anterior colotomy is performed, facilitated by a vaginal cylinder (Apple Medical Corporation, Marlborough, Massachusetts, USA).

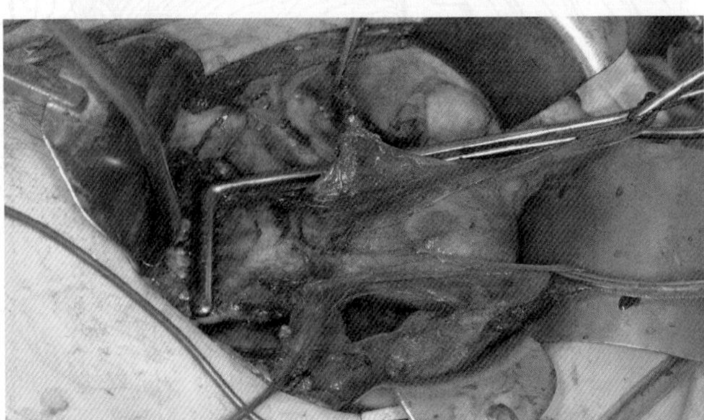

FIGURE 18.25. (*See color plate section.*) Alternatively, a Wertheim clamp can be used to determine the vaginal resection margin.

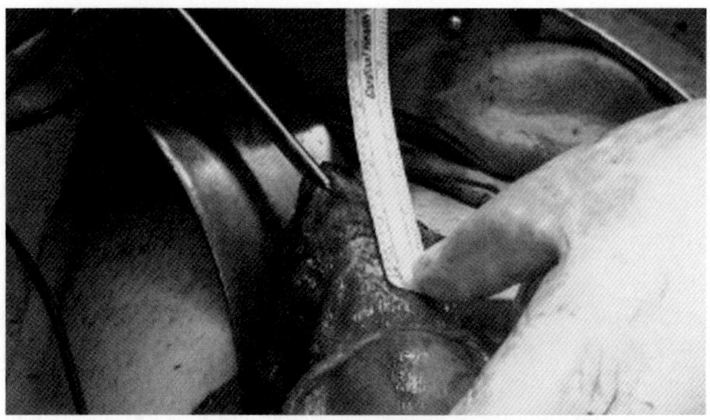

FIGURE 18.26. Estimating the resection margin of abdominal trachelectomy.

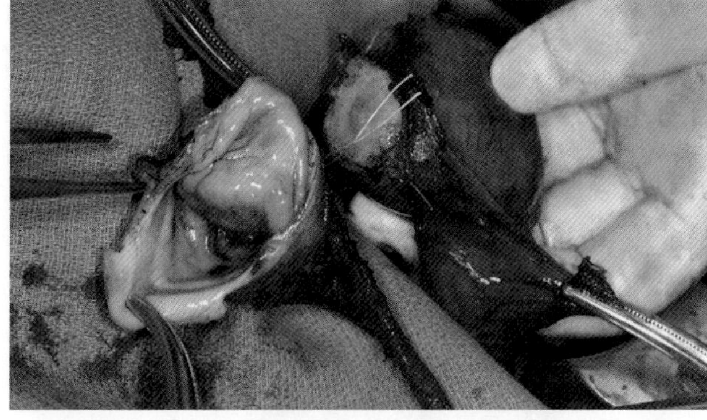

FIGURE 18.28. (*See color plate section.*) Using a knife, the radical trachelectomy is completed by separating the fundus from the isthmus or upper endocervix at approximately 5 mm below the level of the internal os, if possible.

The lower uterine segment is then estimated (Fig. 18.26), and clamps are placed at the level of the internal os. Using a knife, the radical trachelectomy is completed by separating the fundus from the isthmus or upper endocervix at approximately 5 mm below the level of the internal os, if possible (Figs. 18.27 and 18.28).

The uterine fundus with preserved attachments to the utero-ovarian ligaments, placed in the superior part of the pelvis, and the specimen, consisting of radical trachelectomy and parametria with suture marking the vaginal cuff at 12 o'clock, is sent for frozen-section evaluation of its endocervical margin. The uterine fundus is inspected and curettage of the endometrial cavity is performed as well as a shave disc margin on the remaining cervical tissue, which is sent for frozen-section analysis (Fig. 18.29A). This is performed to ensure that the reconstructed uterus to vagina is disease free. A frozen-section analysis is also obtained on the distal vaginal margin, if clinically indicated (Fig. 18.29B–C).

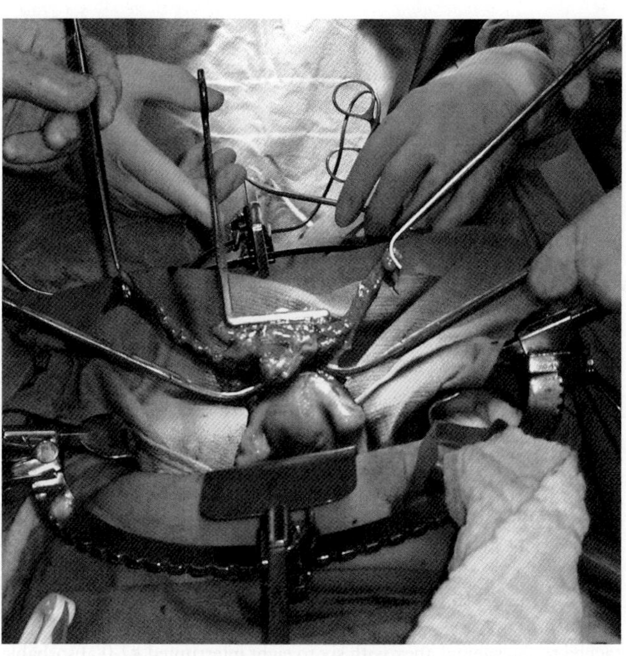

FIGURE 18.27. Clamps are placed at the level of the internal os.

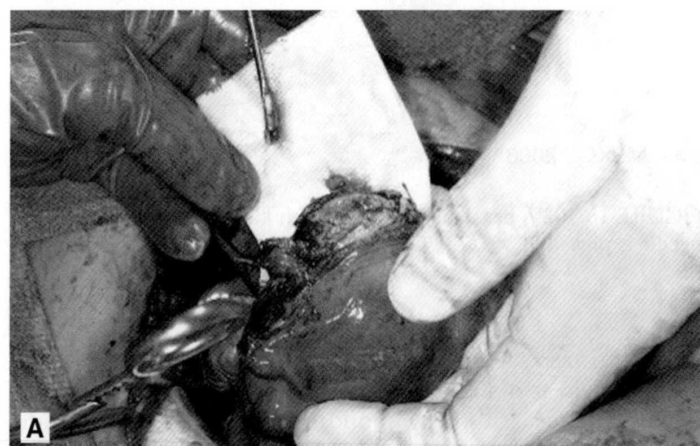

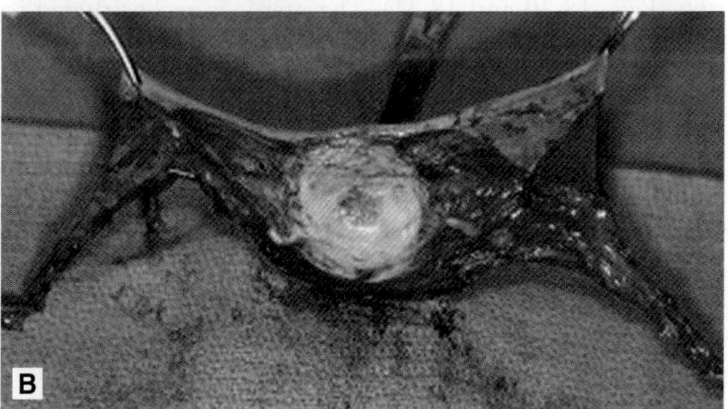

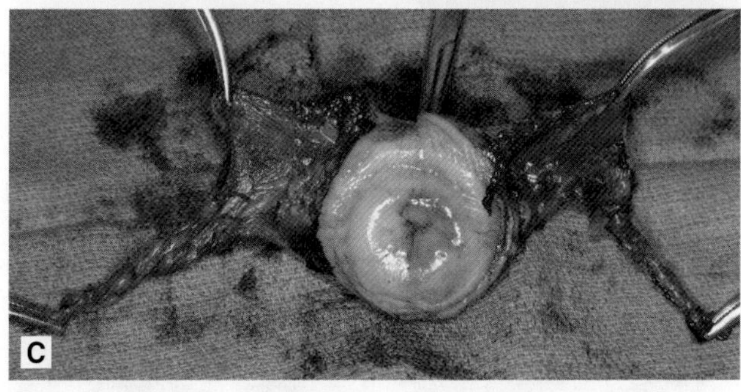

FIGURE 18.29. (*See color plate section.*) **A:** Endometrial and upper endocervical curettage as well as a shave margin on the remaining tissue, which is sent for frozen-section analysis prior to reconstruction. **B:** Frozen section is obtained on the endocervical margin. **C:** Frozen section is obtained circumferentially on the vaginal cuff, if needed.

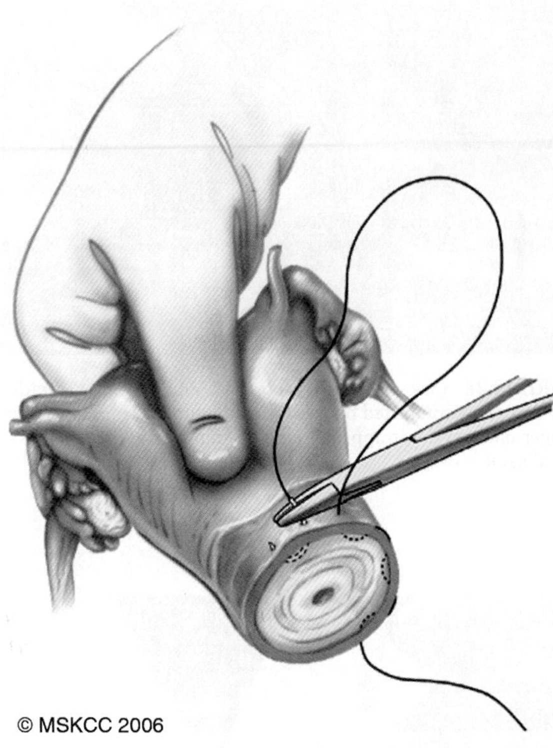

FIGURE 18.30. A permanent cerclage with #0 Ethibond on a Ferguson needle is placed.

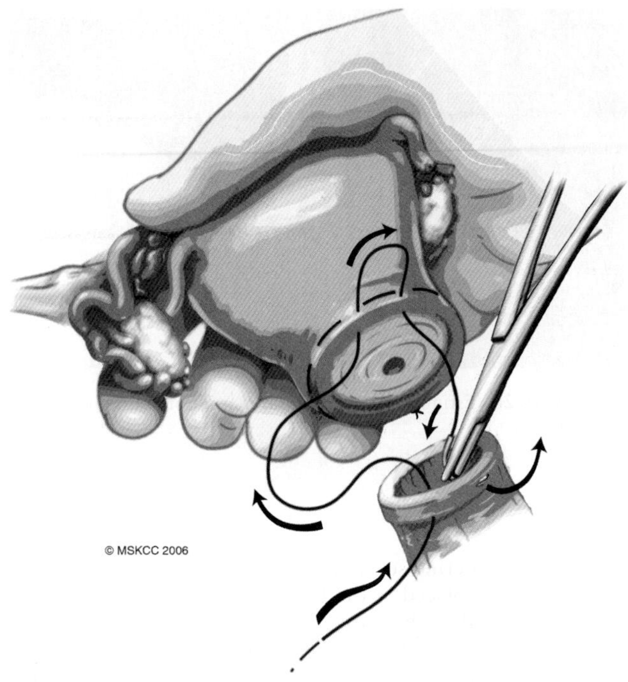

FIGURE 18.32. Reconstruction of the uterine corpus to upper vagina after the cerclage is placed.

If all frozen sections tested are benign and at least a 5 mm clear margin is obtained on the endocervical edge, a permanent cerclage with #0 Ethibond on a free Ferguson needle (knot tied posteriorly) may be placed prior to the reconstruction (Figs. 18.30 and 18.31). The uterus is reconstructed to the upper vagina with six to eight #2-0 absorbable sutures (Figs. 18.32–18.34). No drains are placed. Standard antibiotic prophylaxis and routine postoperative care are prescribed.

An alternative approach would be to separate the fundus from the cervix prior to the colpotomy, pack the fundus with the intact utero-ovarian blood supply in the upper pelvis, place retraction clamps on the cervix, and perform the radical trachelectomy. The role of cystourethroscopy with bilateral temporary ureteral catheterization is optional.

ROBOTICALLY ASSISTED LAPAROSCOPIC SURGERY

The etymology of the word robot is from Czech (robota) meaning compulsory labor. The word robot was first introduced in Karel Capel's play "Rossum's Universal Robots" in Prague in 1921 (360).

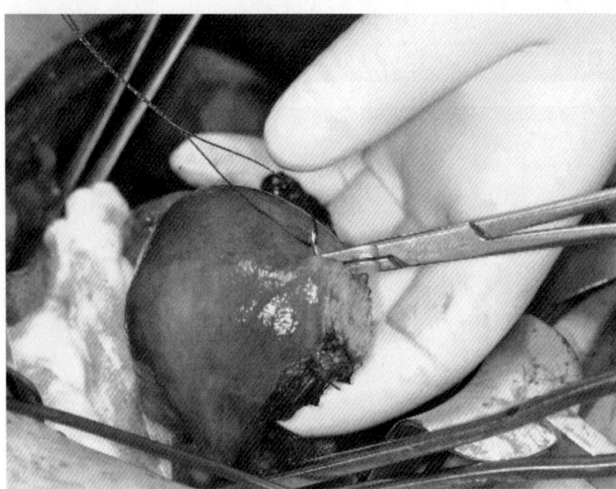

FIGURE 18.31. Once the permanent cerclage is placed, the knot is tied posteriorly.

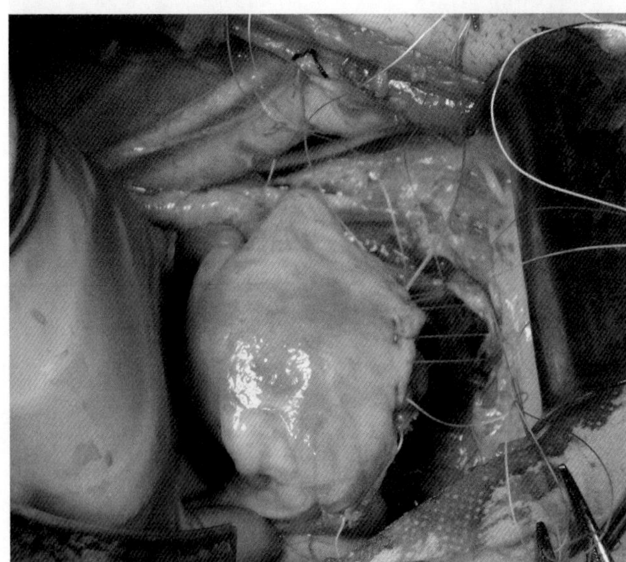

FIGURE 18.33. (*See color plate section.*) The uterine fundus is reattached to the vaginal apex with six to eight interrupted #2-0 absorbable sutures.

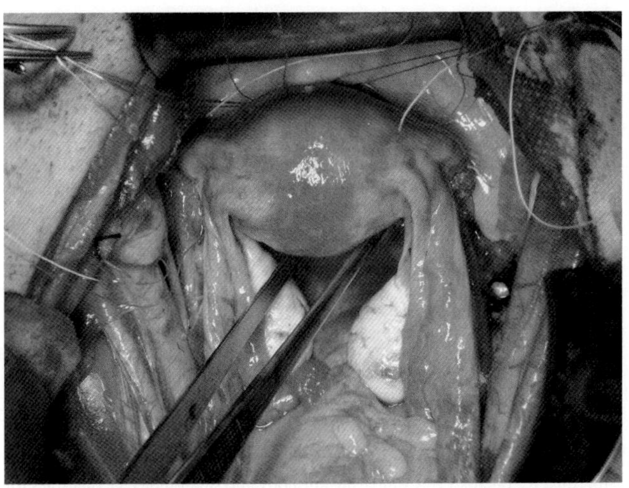

FIGURE 18.34. (*See color plate section.*) The reconstructed fundus with remaining blood supply from the intact utero-ovarian ligaments—uterine serosa without evidence of fundal ischemia.

Industry has used mechanical robots successfully for fine, delicate, repetitive tasks for decades. Recently, robots have been introduced into clinical medicine and surgery. The initial devices in the 1980s were used for stereotactic biopsies and neurosurgery; however, currently more advanced systems are routinely being used in cardiac, thoracic, orthopedic, urologic, general, and gynecologic surgery.

Voice activation of some types of equipment in the operating room, such as the laparoscope or the light source, has also become commonly available, and advances in computer software have allowed a computer controller to translate a surgeon's movements from the handles located in a console to the robotic arms that hold the surgical instruments. This remote console may be placed away from the surgical field.

Telerobotic surgery refers to the utilization of a surgical system where the robot is manipulated by input devices under the surgeon's control and the surgeon may be remote from the operating room. The approved telerobotic devices in the United States that are used in gynecologic surgery are the Intuitive Surgical daVinci System and the Computer Motion AESOP (automated endoscopic system for optimal positioning) system. The ease of accomplishing difficult tasks and the potential advantages over traditional laparoscopy are partly due to the increased number of degrees of freedom, the vividness of the three-dimensional imaging, band filtration with more precision, and less tremor. In addition, the sitting position provides improved ergonomics and comfort by recreating the eye-hand motor axis.

On the other hand, the potential disadvantages of the current models are size and weight, limitation in surgical field, cost, limited trocar and energy source options, and absence of haptics (no sense of force feedback from the instruments).

Animal trials in telerobotic surgery have demonstrated favorable results. Robotic technology has the potential to make laparoscopic microsuturing easier. Robotics have been used to perform uterine horn reanastomosis in a live porcine model, and this application appeared safe in creating laparoscopic microsurgical anastomoses with adequate lumen patency rates achieved during the acute phase and at 4-weeks follow-up (361). In another pilot animal study, the feasibility and safety of using a robotic device "Zeus" to perform complex gynecologic surgery such as adnexectomy and hysterectomy in ten female pigs was undertaken. After 1 week of observation the animals were sacrificed and the surgical site was explored. The procedures were uneventful and no complications were noted. The authors concluded that this technology has the potential to be used for more complex gynecologic procedures (362).

Clinical experience in gynecology is limited but increasing as more surgeons are accepting minimally invasive approaches. To date there are few published clinical trials. The initial trials have focused on laparoscopic microsuturing such as that performed during coronary bypass surgery or tubal anastomosis. Preliminary results have demonstrated that laparoscopic coronary bypass surgery with the internal mammary artery can be achieved.

In an initial study to compare robotic versus human laparoscopic camera control, the AESOP was utilized in 50 patients undergoing routine gynecologic endoscopic surgical procedures. The elimination of the camera holder allowed two surgeons to perform complex laparoscopic surgery faster than without the robotic arm (363).

Robotic surgery in gynecology appeared useful and applicable in performing laparoscopic microsurgical tubal reanastomosis after tubal sterilization. Eight patients with previous laparoscopic tubal sterilization who requested tubal reanastomosis underwent laparoscopic tubal reanastomosis using a remote-controlled robot. The robot, with three-dimensional vision, allows the surgeon to perform ultra-precise manipulations with intra-abdominal articulated instruments while providing the necessary degrees of freedom (364). Microsurgical applications in gynecologic general surgery (robotic tubal reanastomosis) appear to be acceptable indications for this technology (365).

Recently, a case series of 11 patients reporting the use of robotic surgery for performing hysterectomy and bilateral salpingo-oophorectomy demonstrated feasibility and safety. Four trocars were used: one for the camera, two for the robotic arms controlled by the operating surgeon from the surgeon's console, and an additional port for use by the surgical assistant. All patients tolerated the procedure and recovered satisfactorily (366). The daVinci surgical system (Intuitive Surgical, Mountainview, California, USA) has also been used to perform endoscopic ovarian transposition. The ovaries were mobilized on their respective infundibulopelvic ligaments and sutured to the ipsilateral pericolic gutters (367). Trials and pilot investigations of telerobotic surgery in gynecologic oncology are ongoing, and it appears that the utilization will continue to increase to applications where the current device can be used in part of the operation to perform a specific, highly precise objective such as fine suturing or dissection.

In experienced hands, robotic operative times for simple and radical hysterectomy appear shorter than those obtained by conventional laparoscopy, and robotic technology may be preferable to conventional laparoscopy for the surgical treatment of selected gynecologic malignancies and complex operations for benign disease such as hysterectomy, myomectomy, and extensive pelvic endometriosis (368).

In addition, robotic radical hysterectomy in early-stage cervical carcinoma patients was also recently reported (369). No conversions to laparotomy were observed in the robotic group. Median operation time was 241 minutes and the authors demonstrated technical feasibility of robotic-assisted laparoscopic radical hysterectomy in early-stage cervical carcinoma.

This technology will undoubtedly improve with full integration into new operating room systems, additional degrees of freedom, small size devices, easier use, and improved optics and surgical instrumentation.

From investigations in nongynecologic applications, it appears that the results of robotic-assisted surgery compare favorably with those of conventional laparoscopy with respect to mortality, complications, and length of stay. Robotic-assisted surgery, in the pilot phase, appears safe and effective and its role in surgery will likely expand as the technology evolves; however, there are currently limited data to justify the routine use of these systems over laparoscopy in terms of patient outcomes or reduced complications (370).

References

1. Rowinky EK. The challenges of developing therapeutics that target signal transduction in patients with gynecologic and other malignancies. *J Clin Oncol* 2003;21(10 suppl):175–186.
2. Hanahan D, Weinberg RA. The hallmarks of cancer. *Cell* 2000;100: 57–70.
3. Nam N-H, Parang K. Current targets for anti-cancer drug discovery. *Curr Drug Targets* 2003; 4:159–179.
4. Lane D. The promise of molecular oncology. *Lancet* 1998;351(suppl 2): 17–20.
5. Oved S, Yarden Y. Signal transduction: molecular ticket to enter cells. *Nature* 2002;416:133–136.
6. Yarden Y, Sliwkowski MX. Untangling the ErbB signalling network. *Nat Rev Mol Cell Biol* 2001;2:127–137.
7. Hidalgo M, Rowinsky EK. The rapamycin-sensitive signal transduction pathway as a target for cancer therapy. *Oncogene* 2000;19:6680–6686.
8. Citri A, Yarden Y. EGF-ErbB signaling: towards the systems level. *Nat Rev Mol Cell Biol* 2006;7:505–516.
9. Demetri GD, von Mehren M, Blanke CD, et al. Efficacy and safety of imatinib mesylate in advanced gastrointestinal stromal tumors. *N Engl J Med* 2002;347:472–480.
10. Kantarjian H, Sawyers C, Hochhaus A, et al. Hematologic and cytogenetic responses to imatinib mesylate in chronic myelogenous leukemia. *N Engl J Med* 2002;346:645–652.
11. Hudis CA. Trastuzumab—mechanism of action and use in clinical practice. *N Engl J Med* 2007;357:39–51.
12. Sharma SV, Bell DW, Settleman J, et al. Epidermal growth factor receptor mutations in lung cancer. *Nat Rev Cancer* 2007;7:169–181.
13. Ioannidis JP. Is molecular profiling ready for use in clinical decision making? *Oncologist* 2007;12;301–311.
14. Irish JM, Kotecha N, Nolan GP. Mapping normal and cancer cell signaling networks: towards single-cell proteomics. *Nat Rev Cancer* 2006;6: 146–155.
15. Schlessinger J. Cell signaling by receptor tyrosine kinases. *Cell* 2000;103: 211–225.
16. Walker RA. The erbB/HER type 1 tyrosine kinase receptor family. *J Pathol* 1998;185:234–235.
17. Simon MA. Receptor tyrosine kinases: specific outcomes from general signals. *Cell* 2000;103:13–15.
18. Daly RJ. Take your partners, please: signal diversification by the erbB family of receptor tyrosine kinases. *Growth Factors* 1999;16:255–263.
19. Riese DJ II, Stern DF. Specificity within the EGF family/ErbB receptor family signaling network. *Bioassays* 1998;20:41–48.
20. Olayioye MA, Neve RM, Lane HA, et al. The ErbB signaling network: receptor heterodimerization in development and cancer. *EMBO J* 2000;19: 3159–3167.
21. Riese DJ II, van Raaij TM, Plowman GD, et al. The cellular response to neuregulins is governed by complex interactions of the erbB receptor family. *Mol Cell Biol* 1995;15:5770–5776.
22. Shtiegman K, Yarden Y. The role of ubiquitylation in signaling by growth factors: implications to cancer. *Semin Cancer Biol* 2003;13:29–40.
23. Baselga J, Albanell J, Molina MA, et al. The ErbB receptor family: a therapeutic target for cancer. *Trends Mol Med* 2002;8(Suppl 4):S19–S26.
24. Ranson M, Sliwkowski MX. Perspectives on anti-HER monoclonal antibodies. *Oncology* 2002;63(Suppl 1):17–24.
25. Crijns AP, Duiker EW, de Jong S, et al. Molecular prognostic markers in ovarian cancer: toward patient-tailored therapy. *Int J Gynecol Cancer* 2006;16(Suppl 1):152–165.
26. Fry DW. Site-directed irreversible inhibitors of the erbB family of receptor tyrosine kinases as novel chemotherapeutic agents for cancer. *Anticancer Drug Des* 2000;15:3–16.
27. Greenberger LM, Discafani C, Wang Y-F, et al. EKB-569: a new irreversible inhibitor of EGFR tyrosine kinase for the treatment of cancer. *Clin Cancer Res* 2000;6(Suppl):4544s (abstract).
28. Reid A, Vidal L, Shaw H, et al. Dual inhibition of ErbB1 (EGFR/HER1) and ErbB2 (HER2/neu). *Eur J Cancer* 2007;43:481–489.
29. Ebert AD, Wechselberger C, Martinez-Lacaci I, et al. Expression and function of EGF-related peptides and their receptors in gynecologic cancer—from basic science to therapy. *J Recept Signal Transduct Res* 2000;20:1–46.
30. Meden H, Kuhn W. Overexpression of the oncogene c-erbB-2 (HER2/neu) in ovarian cancer: a new prognostic factor. *Eur J Obstet Gynecol Reprod Biol* 1997;71:173–179.
31. Flaherty KT, Brose MS. Her-2 targeted therapy: beyond breast cancer and trastuzumab. *Curr Oncol Rep* 2006;8:90–95.
32. Campos S, Hamid O, Seiden MV, et al. Multicenter, randomized phase II trial of oral CI-1033 for previously treated advanced ovarian cancer. *J Clin Oncol* 2005;23:5597–5604.
33. Baselga J. Is there a role for the irreversible epidermal growth factor receptor inhibitor EKB-569 in the treatment of cancer? A mutation-driven question. *J Clin Oncol* 2006;24:2225–2226.
34. Mullen P, Cameron DA, Hasmann M, et al. Sensitivity to pertuzumab (2C4) in ovarian cancer models: cross-talk with estrogen receptor signaling. *Mol Cancer Ther* 2007;6:93–100.
35. Gordon MS, Matei D, Aghajanian C, et al. Clinical activity of pertuzumab (rhuMAb 2C4), a HER dimerization inhibitor, in advanced ovarian cancer: potential predictive relationship with tumor HER2 activation status. *J Clin Oncol* 2006;24:4324–4332.
36. Mendelsohn J, Baselga J. Epidermal growth factor receptor targeting in cancer. *Semin Oncol* 2006;33:369–385.
37. Giusti RM, Shastri KA, Cohen MH, et al. FDA drug approval summary: panitumumab (Vectibix). *Oncologist* 2007;12:577–583.
38. Schilder RJ, Lokshin AE, Holloway RW, et al. Phase II trial of single-agent cetuximab in patients with persistent or recurrent epithelial ovarian or primary peritoneal carcinoma with the potential for dose escalation to rash. *Proc Am Soc Clin Oncol* 2007;25(Part 1):18S (abstract 5577).
39. Aghajanian C, Sabbatini P, Derosa F, et al. A phase II study of cetuximab/paclitaxel/carboplatin for the initial treatment of advanced stage ovarian, primary peritoneal, and fallopian tube cancer. *Proc Am Soc Clin Oncol* 2005;23(Part 1):16S (abstract 5047).
40. Imai K, Takaoka A. Comparing antibody and small-molecule therapies for cancer. *Nat Rev Cancer* 2006;6:714–727.
41. Arteaga, C. Targeting HER1/EGFR: a molecular approach to cancer therapy. *Semin Oncol* 2003;30(Suppl 7):3–14.
42. Arteaga C. Overview of epidermal growth factor receptor biology and its role as a therapeutic target in human neoplasia. *Semin Oncol* 2002; 5(Suppl 14):3–9.
43. Schilder RJ, Sill MW, Chen X, et al. Phase II study of gefitinib in patients with relapsed or persistent ovarian or primary peritoneal carcinoma and evaluation of epidermal growth factor receptor mutations and immunohistochemical expression: a Gynecologic Oncology Group study. *Clin Cancer Res* 2005;11:5539–5548.
44. Gordon AN, Finkler N, Edwards RP, et al. Efficacy and safety of erlotinib HCl, an epidermal growth factor receptor (HER1/EGFR) tyrosine kinase inhibitor, in patients with advanced ovarian carcinoma: results from a phase II multicenter study. *Int J Gynecol Cancer* 2005;15:785–792.
45. Roberts PJ, Der CJ. Targeting the Raf-MEK-ERK mitogen-activated protein kinase cascade for the treatment of cancer. *Oncogene* 2007;26: 3291–3310.
46. Dhillon AS, Hagan S, Rath O, et al. MAP kinase signalling pathways in cancer. *Oncogene* 2007;26:3279–3290.
47. Sebolt-Leopold JS. Development of anti-cancer drugs targeting the MAP kinase pathway. *Oncogene* 2000;19:6594–6599.
48. Lopez-Ilasaca M, Crespo P, Pellici PG, et al. Linkage of G protein-coupled receptors to the MAPK signaling pathway through PI3-kinase gamma. *Science* 1997;394–397.
49. Lewis TS, Shapiro PS, Ahn NG. Signal transduction through MAP kinase cascades. *Adv Cancer Res* 1998;74:49–139.
50. Ichijo H. From receptor to stress-activated MAP kinases. *Oncogene* 1999; 18:6087–6093.
51. Cobb MH. MAP kinase pathways. *Prog Biophys Mol Biol* 1999;71: 479–500.
52. Herrera R, Sebolt-Leopold JS. Unraveling the complexities of the Raf/MAP kinase pathway for pharmacological intervention. *Trends Mol Med* 2002;8(Suppl 4):S27–S31.
53. Beerham M, Patnaik A, Rowinsky EK. Regulation of c-Raf-1: therapeutic implications. *Clin Adv Hematol Oncol* 2003;1:476–481.
54. Kolch W, Heidecker G, Kochs G, et al. Protein kinase C α activates RAF-1 by direct phosphorylation. *Nature* 1993;364:249–252.
55. Cronwell MM, Smith DE. A signal transduction pathway for activation of the mdr1 promotor involves the proto-oncogene C-raf kinase. *J Biol Chem* 1993;268:15347–15350.
56. Phillips F, Mullen P, Monia BP, et al. Association of c-Raf expression with survival and its targeting with antisense oligonucleotides in ovarian cancer. *Br J Cancer* 2001;85:1753–1758.
57. Monia BP, Johnston JF, Geiger T, et al. Antitumor activity of a phosphorothioate antisense oligodeoxynucleotide targeted against C-raf kinase. *Nat Med* 1996:2:668–675.
58. Oza AM, Swenerton K, Faught W, et al. Phase II study of CGP 69846A (ISIS 5132) in recurrent epithelial ovarian cancer: an NCIC clinical trials group study (NCIC IND.116). *Gynecol Oncol* 2003;89:129–133.
59. Lyons JF, Wilhelm S, Hibner B, et al. Discovery of a novel raf kinase inhibitor. *Endocr Relat Cancer* 2001;8:219–225.
60. Wilhelm S, Chien DS. BAY 43-9006: preclinical data. *Curr Pharm Des* 2002;8:2255–2257.
61. Sebolt-Leopold JS. Development of anti-cancer drugs targeting the MAP kinase pathway. *Oncogene* 2000;19:6594–6599.
62. Sebolt-Leopold JS, English JM. Mechanisms of drug inhibition of signaling molecules. *Nature* 2006;441:457–462.
63. Sebolt-Leopold JS, Herrera R. Targeting the mitogen-activated protein kinase cascade to treat cancer. *Nat Rev Cancer* 2004;4:937–947.
64. Sebolt-Leopold JS. MEK inhibitors: a therapeutic approach to targeting the Ras-MAP kinase pathway in tumors. *Curr Pharm Des* 2004;10: 1907–1914.

65. Messersmith WA, Hidalgo M, Carducci M, et al. Novel targets in solid tumors: MEK inhibitors. *Clin Adv Hematol Oncol* 2006;4:831–836.
66. Vivanco I, Sawyers CL. The phosphatidylinositol 3-kinase Akt pathway in human cancer. *Nat Rev Cancer* 2002;2:489–501.
67. Cantley LC. The phosphoinositide 3-kinase pathway. *Science* 2002;296: 1655–1657.
68. Stein RC. Prospects for phosphoinositide 3-kinase inhibition as a cancer treatment. *Endocr Relat Cancer* 2001;8:237–248.
69. Manning BD, Cantley LC. AKT/PKB signaling: navigating downstream. *Cell* 2007;129:1261–1274.
70. Stein RC, Waterfield MD. PI3-kinase inhibition: a target for drug development? *Mol Med Today* 2000;6:347–357.
71. Cully M, You H, Levine AJ, et al. Beyond *PTEN* mutations: the PI3K pathway as an integrator of multiple inputs during tumorigenesis. *Nat Rev Cancer* 2006;6:184–192.
72. Bader AG, Kang S, Zhao L, et al. Oncogenic PI3K deregulates transcription and translation. *Nat Rev Cancer* 2005;5:921–929.
73. Wiener JR, Nakano K, Kruzelock RP, et al. Decreased Src tyrosine kinase activity inhibits malignant human ovarian cancer tumor growth in a nude mouse model. *Clin Cancer Res* 1999;5:2164–2170.
74. Nakayama K, Nakayama N, Kurman RJ, et al. Sequence mutations and amplification of PIK3CA and AKT2 genes in purified ovarian serous neoplasms. *Cancer Biol Ther* 2006;5:779–785.
75. Yuan ZQ, Sun M, Feldman RI, et al. Frequent activation of AKT2 and induction of apoptosis by inhibition of phosphoinositide-3-OH kinase/Akt pathway in human ovarian cancer. *Oncogene* 2000;19:2324–2330.
76. Ma YY, Wei SJ, Lin YC, et al. PIK3CA as an oncogene in cervical cancer. *Oncogene* 2000;19:2739–2744.
77. Konopka B, Paszko Z, Janiec-Jankowska A, et al. Assessment of the quality and frequency of mutations occurrence in *PTEN* gene in endometrial carcinomas and hyperplasias. *Cancer Lett* 2002;178:43–51.
78. Cheung TH, Lo KW, Yim SF, et al. Epigenetic and genetic alternation of *PTEN* in cervical neoplasm. *Gynecol Oncol* 2004;93:621–627.
79. Bertelsen BI, Steine SJ, Sandvei R, et al. Molecular analysis of the PI3K-Akt pathway in uterine cervical neoplasia: frequent PIK3CA amplification and Akt phosphorylation. *Int J Cancer* 2006;118:1877–1883.
80. Shayesteh L, Lu Y, Kuo WL, et al. PIK3CA is implicated as an oncogene in ovarian cancer. *Nat Genet* 1999;21:99–102.
81. Chakravarti A, Loeffler JS, Dyson NJ. Insulin-like growth factor receptor I mediates resistance to anti-epidermal growth factor receptor therapy in primary human glioblastoma cells through continued activation of phosphoinositide 3-kinase signaling. *Cancer Res* 2002;62:200–207.
82. Lu Y, Zi X, Zhao Y, et al. Insulin-like growth factor-I receptor signaling and resistance to trastuzumab (Herceptin). *J Natl Cancer Inst* 2001;19: 1852–1857.
83. Schmelzle T, Hall MN. TOR, a central controller of cell growth. *Cell* 2000;13(103):253–262.
84. Faivre S, Kroemer G, Raymond E. Current development of mTOR inhibitors as anti-cancer agents. *Nat Rev Drug Discov* 2006;5:671–688.
85. Easton JB, Houghton PJ. mTOR and cancer therapy. *Oncogene* 2006;25: 6436–6446.
86. Averous J, Proud CG. When translation meets transformation: the mTOR story. *Oncogene* 2006;25:6423–6435.
87. Mamane Y, Petroulakis E, LeBacquer O, et al. mTOR, translation initiation and cancer. *Oncogene* 2006;25:6416–6422.
88. Rohde J, Heitman J, Cardenas ME. The TOR kinases link nutrient sensing to cell growth. *J Biol Chem* 2001;276:9583–9586.
89. Altomare DA, Wang HQ, Skele KL, et al. Akt and mTOR phosphorylation is frequently detected in ovarian cancer and can be targeted to disrupt ovarian tumor cell growth. *Oncogene* 2004;23:5853–5857.
90. Wolf J, Slomovitz DM. Novel biologic therapies for the treatment of endometrial cancer. *Int J Gynecol Cancer* 2005;15:411–420.
91. Podsypanina K, Lee RT, Politis C, et al. An inhibitor of mTOR reduces neoplasia and normalizes p70/S6 kinase activity in Pten+/- mice. *Proc Natl Acad Sci USA* 2001;98:10320–10325.
92. Neshat MS, Mellinghoff IK, Tran C, et al. Enhanced sensitivity of *PTEN*-deficient tumors to inhibition of FRAP/mTOR. *Proc Natl Acad Sci USA* 2001;98:10314–10319.
93. Mita MM, Mita A, Rowinsky EK. Mammalian target of rapamycin: a new molecular target for breast cancer. *Clin Breast Cancer* 2003;4:126–137.
94. Pectasides D, Pectasides E, Economopoulos T. Systemic therapy in metastatic or recurrent endometrial cancer. *Cancer Treat Rev* 2007;33: 177–190.
95. Oza AM, Elit L, Biagi J, et al. Molecular correlates associated with a phase II study of temsirolimus (CCI-779) in patients with metastatic or recurrent endometrial cancer—NCIC IND 160. *Proc Am Soc Clin Oncol* 2006; 24(Part 1):18S (abstract 3003).
96. Colombo N, McMeekin S, Schwartz P, et al. A phase II trial of the mTOR inhibitor AP23573 as a single agent in advanced endometrial cancer. *Proc Am Soc Clin Oncol* 2007;25(Part 1):18S (abstract 5516).
97. Baserga R, Peruzzi F, Reiss K. The IGF-1 receptor in cancer biology. *Int J Cancer* 2003;107:873–877.
98. Nakae J, Kido Y, Accili D. Distinct and overlapping functions of insulin and IGF-I receptors. *Endocr Rev* 2001;22:818–835.
99. Pollak MN, Schernhammer ES, Hankinson SE. Insulin-like growth factors and neoplasia. *Nat Rev Cancer* 2004;4:505–518.
100. Khandwala HM, McCutcheon IE, Flyvbjerg A, et al. The effects of insulin-like growth factors on tumorigenesis and neoplastic growth. *Endocr Rev* 2000;21:215–244.
101. Zhang H, Yee D. Type I insulin-like growth factor receptor as a therapeutic target in cancer. *Cancer Res* 2005;12;10123–10127.
102. Burroughs KD, Dunn SE, Barrett JC, et al. Insulin-like growth factor-I: a key regulator of human cancer risk? *J Natl Cancer Inst* 1999;91: 579–581.
103. Pollak M. Insulin-like growth factors and prostate cancer. *Epidemiol Rev* 2001;23:59–66.
104. Pollak M. Insulin-like growth factor physiology and cancer risk. *Eur J Cancer* 2000;36,1224–1228.
105. Miyake H, Pollak M, Gleave ME. Castration-induced up-regulation of insulin-like growth factor binding protein-5 potentiates insulin-like growth factor-I activity and accelerates progression to androgen independence in prostate cancer models. *Cancer Res* 2000;60:3058–3064.
106. Elmlinger MW, Deininger MH, Schuett BS, et al. *In vivo* expression of insulin-like growth factor-binding protein in human gliomas increases with tumor grade. *Endocrinology* 2001;142;1652–1658.
107. Baron-Hay S, Boyle F, Ferrier A, et al. Elevated serum insulin-like growth factor binding protein-2 as a prognostic marker in patients with ovarian cancer. *Clin Cancer Res* 2004;10:1796–1806.
108. O'Gorman DB, Weiss J, Hettiaratchi A, et al. Insulin-like growth factor-II/mannose 6-phosphate receptor overexpression reduces growth of choriocarcinoma cells *in vitro* and *in vivo*. *Endocrinology* 2002;143:4287–4294.
109. Rowinsky EK, Tonra J, Solomon P, et al. IMCL-A12, a human IgG1 monoclonal antibody to the insulin-growth factor-like receptor. *Clin Cancer Res* 2007;13(18 Pt 2):5549s–5555s. Review.
110. O'Reilly KE, Rojo F, She QB, et al. mTOR inhibition induces upstream receptor tyrosine kinase signaling and activates Akt. *Cancer Res* 2006;66: 1500–1508.
111. McCampbell AS, Broaddus RR, Loose DS, et al. Overexpression of the insulin-like growth factor I receptor and activation of the Akt pathway in hyperplastic endometrium. *Clin Cancer Res* 2006;12:6373–6378.
112. Lu Y, Zi X, Zhao Y, et al. Insulin-like growth factor-I receptor signaling and resistance to trastuzumab (Herceptin). *J Natl Cancer Inst* 2001;93: 1852–1857.
113. Rubini M, Hongo A, D'Ambrosio C, et al. The IGF-I receptor in mitogenesis and transformation of mouse embryo cells: role of receptor number. *Exp Cell Res* 1997;1;230:284–292.
114. Benini S, Manara MC, Baldini N, et al. Inhibition of insulin-like growth factor I receptor increases the anti-tumor activity of doxorubicin and vincristine against Ewing's sarcoma cells. *Clin Cancer Res* 2001;7:1790–1797.
115. Burtrum D, Zhu Z, Lu D, et al. A fully human monoclonal antibody to the insulin-like growth factor I receptor blocks ligand-dependent signaling and inhibits human tumor growth *in vivo*. *Cancer Res* 2003;63: 8912–8921.
116. Higano CS, Yu EY, Whiting SH. A phase I, first in man study of weekly IMC-A12, a fully human insulin like growth factor-I receptor IgG1 monoclonal antibody, in patients with advanced solid tumors. *Proc Am Soc Clin Oncol* 2007; 25(Part 1):18S (abstract 3505).
117. Tolcher PU, Rothenberg M, Rodon J. A phase I pharmacokinetic and pharmacodynamic study of AMG 479, a fully human monoclonal antibody against insulin-like growth factor type 1 receptor (IGF-1R), in advanced solid tumors. *Proc Am Soc Clin Oncol* 2007;25(Part 1):18S (abstract 3002).
118. Karp DD, Paz-Ares LG, Blakely LJ, et al. Efficacy of the anti-insulin like growth factor I receptor (IGF-IR) antibody CP-751871 in combination with paclitaxel and carboplatin as first-line treatment for advanced non-small cell lung cancer (NSCLC). *Proc Am Soc Clin Oncol* 2007;25(Part 1): 18S (abstract 7506).
119. Tonra JR, Deevi DS, Corcoran E, et al. Combined antibody mediated inhibition of IGF-IR, EGFR, and VEGFR2 for more consistent and greater anti-tumor effects. *Eur J Cancer* 2006;4(Suppl):207.
120. Bertrand FE, Steelman LS, Chappell WH, et al. Synergy between an IGF-1R antibody and Raf/MEK/ERK and PI3K/Akt/mTOR pathway inhibitors in suppressing IGF-1R-mediated growth in hematopoietic cells. *Leukemia* 2006;20:1254–1260.
121. Tonra JR, Corcoran E, Makhoul G, et al. Synergistic anti-tumor effects of anti-EGFR monoclonal antibody Erbitux® combined with antibodies targeting IGF1R or VEGFR-2. *Proc Am Assoc Cancer Res* 2005;46:1193.
122. Best CJM, Ludwig DL, Steeg PS. Breast cancer cell lines resistant to either tamoxifen or Herceptin exhibit sensitivity to the anti-IGF receptor antibody A12 *in vitro*. *Proc Am Assoc Cancer Res* 2006;47:290.
123. Lu Y, Zi X, Zhao Y, et al. Insulin-like growth factor-I receptor signaling and resistance to trastuzumab (Herceptin). *J Natl Cancer Inst* 2001;93: 1852–1857.
124. Lewis NL. The platelet-derived growth factor receptor as a therapeutic target. *Curr Oncol Rep* 2007;9:89–95.
125. Alvarez RH, Kantarjian HM, Cortes JE. Biology of platelet-derived growth factor and its involvement in disease. *Mayo Clin Proc* 2006;81: 1241–1257.
126. Russell MR, Loizos N, Fatatis A, et al. Human bone marrow activates the Akt pathway in metastatic prostate cells through transactivation of the alpha-platelet-derived growth factor receptor. *Cancer Res* 2007;67: 555–562.

127. Board R, Jayson GC. Platelet-derived growth factor receptor (PDGFR): a target for anti-cancer therapeutics. *Drug Resist Update* 2005;8:75–83.
128. Shih AH, Holland EC. Platelet-derived growth factor (PDGF) and glial tumorigenesis. *Cancer Lett* 2006;232:139–147.
129. Apte SM, Bucana CD, Killion JJ, et al. Expression of platelet-derived growth factor and activated receptor in clinical specimens of epithelial ovarian cancer and ovarian carcinoma cell lines. *Gynecol Oncol* 2004;93: 78–86.
130. Lassus H, Sihto H, Leminen A, et al. Genetic alterations and protein expression of KIT and PDGFRA in serous ovarian carcinoma. *Br J Cancer* 2004;91:2048–2055.
131. Matei D, Emerson RE, Lai YC, et al. Autocrine activation of PDGFRalpha promotes the progression of ovarian cancer. *Oncogene* 2006;25: 2060–2069.
132. Dai C, Celestino JC, Okada Y, et al. PDGF autocrine stimulation dedifferentiates cultured astrocytes and induces oligodendrogliomas and oligoastrocytomas from neural progenitors and astrocytes *in vivo*. *Genes Dev* 2001;15:1913–1925.
133. Uhrbom L, Hesselager G, Nister M, et al. Induction of brain tumors in mice using a recombinant platelet-derived growth factor B-chain retrovirus. *Cancer Res* 1998;58:5275–5279.
134. Kilic T, Alberta JA, Zdunek PR, et al. Intracranial inhibition of platelet-derived growth factor-mediated glioblastoma cell growth by an orally active kinase inhibitor of the 2-phenylaminopyrimidine class. *Cancer Res* 2000;60:5143–5150.
135. Wen PY, Yung WKA, Lamborn KR, et al. Phase I/II study of imatinib mesylate for recurrent malignant gliomas: North American Brain Tumor Consortium Study 99-08. *Clin Cancer Res* 2006;12:4899–4907.
136. Lewis N, Eder JP, Guo F, et al. Phase 1 study of CP-868,596, an oral, highly specific PDGFR inhibitor. *Proc Am Soc Clin Oncol* 2007;25(Part 1): 18S (abstract 3524).
137. Dolloff NG, Russell MR, Loizos N, et al. Human bone marrow activates the Akt pathway in metastatic prostate cells through transactivation of the alpha-platelet-derived growth factor receptor. *Cancer Res* 2007;67: 555–562.
138. Rowinsky EK. Targeted induction of apoptosis in cancer management: the emerging role of tumor necrosis factor-related apoptosis-inducing ligand receptor activating agents. *J Clin Oncol* 2005;23:9394–9407.
139. Hockenbery D, Nunez G, Milliman C, et al. Bcl-2 Is an inner mitochondrial membrane protein that blocks programmed cell death. *Nature* 1990; 348:334.
140. Reed JC. Drug insight: cancer therapy strategies based on restoration of endogenous cell death mechanisms. *Nat Clin Pract Oncol* 2006;3(7): 388–398.
141. Korsmeyer SJ. Regulators of cell death. *Trends Genet* 1995;11:101–105.
142. Andersen MH, Becker JC, Straten P. Regulators of apoptosis: suitable targets for immune therapy of cancer. *Nat Rev Drug Discov* 2005;4: 399–409.
143. Fesik SW. Promoting apoptosis as a strategy for cancer drug discovery. *Nat Rev Cancer* 2005;5:876–885.
144. Tsujimoto Y, Finger LR, Yunis J, et al. Cloning of the chromosome breakpoint of neoplastic B cells with the t(14;18) chromosome translocation. *Science* 1984;226:1097–1099.
145. Krajewska M, Krajewski S, Epstein JI, et al. Immunohistochemical analysis of bcl-2, bax, bcl-X, and mcl-1 expression in prostate cancers. *Am J Pathol* 1996;148:1449–1457.
146. Silvestrini R, Veneroni S, Daidone MG, et al. The Bcl-2 protein: a prognostic indicator strongly related to p53 protein in lymph node-negative breast cancer patients. *J Natl Cancer Inst* 1994;86:499–504.
147. Gleave ME, Monia BP. Antisense therapy for cancer. *Nat Rev Cancer* 2005;5:468–479.
148. Stauffer SR. Small molecule inhibition of the Bcl-X(L)-BH3 protein-protein interaction: proof-of-concept of an *in vivo* chemopotentiator ABT-737. *Curr Top Med Chem* 2007;7(10):961–965.
149. Dai Y, Grant S. Targeting multiple arms of the apoptotic regulatory machinery. *Cancer Res* 2007;67:2908–2911.
150. Manion MK, Fry J, Schwartz PS, et al. Small-molecule inhibitors of Bcl-2. *Curr Opin Invest Drugs* 2006;7:1077–1084.
151. Jansen B, Schlagbauer-Wadl H, Brown BD, et al. Bcl-2 antisense therapy chemosensitizes human melanoma in SCID mice. *Nat Med* 1998;4: 232–234.
152. Haldar S, Chintapalli J, Croce CM. Taxol induces bcl-2 phosphorylation and death of prostate cancer cells. *Cancer Res* 1996;56:1253–1255.
153. Tilly H, Coiffier B, Michallet AS, et al. Phase I/II study of SPC2996, an RNA antagonist of Bcl-2, in patients with advanced chronic lymphocytic leukemia. *Proc Am Soc Clin Oncol* 2007;25(Part 1):18S (abstract 7036).
154. Wang JL, Zhang ZJ, Choksi S, et al. Cell permeable Bcl-2 binding peptides: a chemical approach to apoptosis induction in tumor cells. *Cancer Res* 2000;60:1498–1502.
155. Wang JL, Liu D, Zhang ZJ, et al. Structure-based discovery of an organic compound that binds Bcl-2 protein and induces apoptosis of tumor cells. *Proc Natl Acad Sci USA* 2000;97:7124–7129.
156. Pitot HC, Saleh M, Holmlund J, et al. Extended phase I trial of the oral pan-Bcl-2 inhibitor AT-101 by multiple dosing schedules in patients with advanced cancers. *Proc Am Soc Clin Oncol* 2007;25(Part 1):18S (abstract 3583).
157. Michels JE, Chi KN, Sinneman S, et al. Effect of GX15-070MS, a small molecule inhibitor of Bcl-2 proteins, on PSA expression in preclinical prostate cancer. *Proc Am Soc Clin Oncol* 2007;25(Part 1):18S (abstract 86).
158. Stauber RH, Mann W, Knauer SK. Nuclear and cytoplasmic survivin: molecular mechanism, prognostic, and therapeutic potential. *Cancer Res* 2007;67:5999–6002.
159. Fukuda S, Pelus LM. Survivin, a cancer target with an emerging role in normal adult tissues. *Mol Cancer Ther* 2006;5:1087–1098.
160. Gleave M, Jansen B. Clusterin and IGFBPs as antisense targets in prostate cancer. *Ann NY Acad Sci* 2003;1002:95–104.
161. Gonzalez R, Lewis K, Samlowski W, et al. A phase II study of YM155, a novel survivin suppressant, administered by 168 hour continuous infusion in patients with unresectable stage III or stage IV melanoma. *Proc Am Soc Clin Oncol* 2007;25(Part 1):18S (abstract 8538).
162. Schmitz G. Drug evaluation: OGX-011, a clusterin-inhibiting antisense oligonucleotide. *Curr Opin Mol Ther* 2006;8:547–554.
163. Li B, Dou QP. Bax degradation by the ubiquitin/proteasome-dependent pathway: involvement in tumor survival and progression. *Proc Natl Acad Sci USA* 2000;97:3850–3855.
164. Takeda K, Stagg J, Yagita H, et al. Targeting death-inducing receptors in cancer therapy. *Oncogene* 2007;26:3745–3757.
165. Pan G, O'Rourke K, Chinnaiyan AM, et al. The receptor for the cytotoxic ligand TRAIL. *Science* 1997;276:111–113.
166. Jiang Y, Woronicz JD, Liu W, et al. Prevention of constitutive TNF receptor 1 signaling by silencer of death domains. *Science* 1999;283:543–546.
167. Zapata JM, Pawlowski K, Haas E, et al. A diverse family of proteins containing tumor necrosis factor receptor-associated factor domains. *J Biol Chem* 2001;276:24242–24252.
168. Munshi A, Pappas G, Honda T, et al. TRAIL (APO-2L) induces apoptosis in human prostate cancer cells that is inhibitable by Bcl-2. *Oncogene* 2001;20:3757–3765.
169. Havell EA, Fiers W, North RJ. The antitumor function of tumor necrosis factor (TNF). I. Therapeutic action of TNF against an established murine sarcoma is indirect, immunologically dependent, and limited by severe toxicity. *J Exp Med* 1998;167:1067–1085.
170. Ashkenazi A, Pai RC, Fong S, et al. Safety and antitumor activity of recombinant soluble Apo2 ligand. *J Clin Invest* 1999;104:155–162.
171. Lawrence D, Shahrokh Z, Marsters S, et al. Differential hepatocyte toxicity of recombinant Apo2L/TRAIL versions. *Nat Med* 2001;7:383–385.
172. Pan Y, Xu R, Peach M, et al. Application of pharmacodynamic assays in a phase Ia trial of Apo2L/TRAIL in patients with advanced tumors. *Proc Am Soc Clin Oncol* 2007;25(Part 1):18S (abstract 3535).
173. Chuntharapai A, Dodge K, Grimmer K, et al. Isotype-dependent inhibition of tumor growth *in vivo* by monoclonal antibodies to death receptor 4. *J Immunol* 2001;166:4891–4898.
174. Ichikawa K, Liu W, Zhao L, et al. Tumoricidal activity of a novel anti-human DR5 monoclonal antibody without hepatocyte cytotoxicity. *Nat Med* 2001;7:954–960.
175. Chow LQ, Eckhardt SG, Gustafson DL, et al. HGS-ETR1, an antibody targeting TRAIL-R1, in combination with paclitaxel and carboplatin in patients with advanced solid malignancies: results of a phase 1 and PK study. *Proc Am Soc Clin Oncol* 2006;24(Part 1) (abstract 2515).
176. Sikic BI, Wakelee HA, von Mehren M, et al. A phase Ib study to assess the safety of lexatumumab, a human monoclonal antibody that activates TRAIL-R2, in combination with gemcitabine, pemetrexed, doxorubicin or FOLFIRI. *Proc Am Soc Clin Oncol* 2007;25(Part 1) (abstract 14006).
177. LoRusso P, Hong D, Heath E, et al. First-in-human study of AMG 655, a pro-apoptotic TRAIL receptor-2 agonist, in adult patients with advanced solid tumors. *Proc Am Soc Clin Oncol* 2007;25(Part 1):18S (abstract 3534).
178. Xu W, Neckers L. Targeting the molecular chaperone heat shock protein 90 provides a multifaceted effect on diverse cell signaling pathways of cancer cells. *Clin Cancer Res* 2007;13:1625–1629.
179. Sharp S, Workman P. Inhibitors of the HSP90 molecular chaperone: current status. *Adv Cancer Res* 2006;95:323–348.
180. Whitesell L, Lindquist SL. HSP90 and the chaperoning of cancer. *Nat Rev Cancer* 2005;5:761–772.
181. Chiosis G, Caldas Lopes E, Solit D. Heat shock protein-90 inhibitors: a chronicle from geldanamycin to today's agents. *Curr Opin Invest Drugs* 2006;7:534–541.
182. Xiao L, Rasouli P, Ruden DM. Possible effects of early treatments of hsp90 inhibitors on preventing the evolution of drug resistance to other anti-cancer drugs. *Curr Med Chem* 2007;14(2):223–232.
183. Dupont J, Aghajanian C, Sabbatini P, et al. New agents for the treatment of ovarian cancer: the next generation. *Int J Gynecol Cancer* 2005;15(Suppl 3): 252–257.
184. An WG, Schnur RC, Neckers L, et al. Depletion of p185erbB2, Raf-1 and mutant p53 proteins by geldanamycin derivatives correlates with antiproliferative activity. *Cancer Chemother Pharmacol* 1997;40:60–64.
185. Pacey SC, Wilson R, Walton M, et al. A phase I trial of the heat shock protein 90 (HSP90) inhibitor 17-dimethylaminoethylamino-17-demethoxygeldanamycin (17- DMAG, alvespimycin) administered weekly. *Proc Am Soc Clin Oncol* 2007;25(Part 1):18S (abstract 3568).
186. Kefford R, Millward M, Hersey P, et al. Phase II trial of tanespimycin (KOS-953), a heat shock protein-90 (Hsp90) inhibitor in patients with

metastatic melanoma. *Proc Am Soc Clin Oncol* 2007;25(Part 1);18S (abstract 8558).

187. Demetri GD, George S, Morgan JA, et al. Inhibition of the heat shock protein 90 (Hsp90) chaperone with the novel agent IPI-504 to overcome resistance to tyrosine kinase inhibitors (TKIs) in metastatic GIST: updated results of a phase I trial. *Proc Am Soc Clin Oncol* 2007;25(Part 1);18S (abstract 10024).
188. Steed PM, Fadden P, Hall S. A novel, selective, orally active, potent small molecule inhibitor of Hsp90. *Proc Am Soc Clin Oncol* 2006;24(Part 1): 18S (abstract 13067).
189. Ishii Y, Waxman S, Germain D. Targeting the ubiquitin-proteasome pathway in cancer therapy. *Anticancer Agents Med Chem* 2007;7:359–365.
190. Milano A, Iaffaioli RV, Caponigro F. The proteasome: a worthwhile target for the treatment of solid tumours? *Eur J Cancer* 2007;43:1125–1133.
191. Cusack JC. Rationale for the treatment of solid tumors with the proteasome inhibitor bortezomib. *Cancer Treat Rev* 2003;1(Suppl):21–31.
192. Adams J. Potential for proteasome inhibition in the treatment of cancer. *Drug Discov Today* 2003;8:307–315.
193. Brown R, Strathdee G. Epigenomics and epigenetic therapy of cancer. *Trends Mol Med* 2002;8(Suppl):S43–S48.
194. Yoo CB, Jones PA. Epigenetic therapy of cancer: past, present and future. *Nat Rev Drug Discov* 2006;5:37–50.
195. Kalebic T. Epigenetic changes: potential therapeutic targets. *Ann NY Acad Sci* 2003;983:278–285.
196. Bolden JE, Peart MJ, Johnstone RW. Anti-cancer activities of histone deacetylase inhibitors. *Nat Rev Drug Discov* 2006;5:769–784.
197. Bruceckner B, Kuck D, Lyko F. DNA methyltransferase inhibitors for cancer therapy. *Cancer J* 2007;13;17–22.
198. Kikuchi R, Tsuda H, Kanai Y, et al. Promoter hypermethylation contributes to frequent inactivation of a putative conditional tumor suppressor gene connective tissue growth factor in ovarian cancer. *Cancer Res* 2007;67:7095–7105.
199. Balch C, Huang TH, Brown R, et al. The epigenetics of ovarian cancer drug resistance and resensitization. *Am J Obstet Gynecol* 2004;191:1552–1572.
200. Wei SH, Brown R, Huang TH. Aberrant DNA methylation in ovarian cancer: is there an epigenetic predisposition to drug response? *Ann NY Acad Sci* 2003;983:243–250.
201. Strathdee G, MacKean MJ, Illand M, et al. A role for methylation of the hMLH1 promoter in loss of hMLH1 expression and drug resistance in ovarian cancer. *Oncogene* 1999;18:2335–2341.
202. Gifford G, Paul J, Vasey PA, et al. The acquisition of hMLH1 methylation in plasma DNA after chemotherapy predicts poor survival for ovarian cancer patients. *Clin Cancer Res* 2004;10:4420–4426.
203. van Kesteren CH, de Vooght MM, Lopez-Lazaro L, et al. Yondelis (trabectedin, ET-743): the development of an anti-cancer agent of marine origin. *Anticancer Drugs* 2003;14:487–502.
204. Garcia-Rocha M, Garcia-Gravalos MD, Avila JL. Characterisation of antimitotic products from marine organisms that disorganise the microtubule network: ecteinascidin 743, isohomohalichondrin and LL-15. *Br J Cancer* 1996;73:875–883.
205. Mantovani R, La Valle E, Bonfanti M, et al. Effect of ET-743 on the interaction between transcription factors and DNA. *Ann Oncol* 1998;9:534 (abstract).
206. Scotto KW. ET 743: more than just an innovative mechanism of action. *Anticancer Drugs* 2002;13:S3–S6.
207. D'Incalci M, Colombo T, Ubezio P, et al. The combination of yondelis and cisplatin is synergistic against human tumor xenografts. *Eur J Cancer* 2003;39:1920–1926.
208. Minuzzo M, Marchini S, Broggini M, et al. Interference of transcriptional activation by the antineoplastic drug ecteinascidin-743. *Proc Natl Acad Sci USA* 2000;97:6780–6784.
209. Soares DG, Escargueil AE, Poindessous V, et al. From the cover: replication and homologous recombination repair regulate DNA double-strand break formation by the antitumor alkylator ecteinascidin 743. *Proc Natl Acad Sci USA* 2007;104:13062–13067.
210. Colombo N, Capri G, Bauer J, et al. Phase II and pharmacokinetic study of 3-hr infusion of ET-743 in ovarian cancer patients failing platinum-taxanes. *Proc Am Soc Clin Oncol* 2002;21:221a (abstract 880).
211. McMeekin S, del Campo JM, Colombo N, et al. Trabectedin (T) in relapsed advanced ovarian cancer (ROC): a pooled analysis of three phase II studies. *Proc Am Soc Clin Oncol* 2007;25(Part 1) (abstract 5579)
212. Tomassetti A, Mangiarotti F, Mazzi M, et al. The variant hepatocyte nuclear factor 1 activates the P1 promoter of the human alpha-folate receptor gene in ovarian carcinoma. *Cancer Res* 2003;63:696–704.
213. Wu M, Gunning W, Ratnam M. Expression of folate receptor type alpha in relation to cell type, malignancy, and differentiation in ovary, uterus, and cervix. *Cancer Epidemiol Biomarkers Prev* 1999;8:775–782.
214. Parker N, Turk MJ, Westrick E, et al. Folate receptor expression in carcinomas and normal tissues determined by a quantitative radioligand binding assay. *Anal Biochem* 2005;338:284–293.
215. Weitman SD, Lark RH, Coney LR, et al. Distribution of the folate receptor GP38 in normal and malignant cell lines and tissues. *Cancer Res* 1992;52:3396–3401.
216. Kelley KM, Rowan BG, Ratnam M. Modulation of the folate receptor alpha gene by the estrogen receptor: mechanism and implications in tumor targeting. *Cancer Res* 2003;63:2820–2828.
217. Ebel W, Routhier EL, Foley B, et al. Preclinical evaluation of MORAb-003, a humanized monoclonal antibody antagonizing folate receptor-alpha. *Cancer Immun* 2007;7:6–10.
218. Phillips M, Armstrong D, Coleman R, et al. Novel phase II study design of MORAb-003, a monoclonal antibody against folate receptor alpha in platinum-sensitive ovarian cancer in first relapse. *Proc Am Soc Clin Oncol* 2007;25(Part 1):18S (abstract 5583).
219. Armstrong DK, Laheru D, Ma WW, et al. A phase 1 study of MORAb-009, a monoclonal antibody against mesothelin in pancreatic cancer, mesothelioma and ovarian adenocarcinoma. *Proc Am Soc Clin Oncol* 2007;25(Part 1):18S (abstract 14041).
220. Henderson EA, Bavetsias V, Theti DS, et al. Targeting the alpha-folate receptor with cyclopenta[g]quinazoline-based inhibitors of thymidylate synthase. *Bioorg Med Chem* 2006;14:5020–5042.
221. Gibbs DD, Theti DS, Wood N, et al. BGC 945, a novel tumor-selective thymidylate synthase inhibitor targeted to alpha-folate receptor-overexpressing tumors. *Cancer Res* 2005;65:11721–11728.
222. Townsend DM, Shen H, Staros AL, et al. Efficacy of a glutathione S-transferase pi-activated prodrug in platinum-resistant ovarian cancer cells. *Mol Cancer Ther* 2002;1:1089–1095.
223. Tew KD. TLK-286: a novel glutathione S-transferase-activated prodrug. *Expert Opin Invest Drugs* 2005;14:1047–1054.
224. Morgan AS, Sanderson PE, Borch RF, et al. Tumor efficacy and bone marrow-sparing properties of TER286, a cytotoxin activated by glutathione S-transferase. *Cancer Res* 1998;58:2568–2575.
225. Rosen LS, Brown J, Laxa B, et al. Phase I study of TLK286 (glutathione S-transferase P1-1 activated glutathione analogue) in advanced refractory solid malignancies. *Clin Cancer Res* 2003;9:1628–1638.
226. Kavanagh JJ, Gershenson DM, Choi H, et al. Multi-institutional phase 2 study of TLK286 (TELCYTA, a glutathione S-transferase P1-1 activated glutathione analog prodrug) in patients with platinum and paclitaxel refractory or resistant ovarian cancer. *Int J Gynecol Cancer* 2005;15: 593–600.
227. Vergote I, Finkler N, del Campo J, et al. Single agent, canfosfamide (C, TLK286) vs pegylated liposomal doxorubicin (D) or topotecan (T) in 3rd-line treatment of platinum (P) refractory or resistant ovarian cancer (OC): phase 3 study results. *Proc Am Soc Clin Oncol* 2007;25(Part 1):18S (abstract 5528).
228. Rose P, Edwards R, Finkler N, et al. Phase 3 study: canfosfamide (C, TLK286) plus carboplatin (P) vs liposomal doxorubicin (D) as 2nd line therapy of platinum (P) resistant ovarian cancer (OC). *Proc Am Soc Clin Oncol* 2007;25(Part 1):18S (abstract 5529).
229. Egen JG, Kuhns MS, Allison JP. CTLA-4: new insights into its biological function and use in tumor immunotherapy. *Nat Immunol* 2002;3: 611–618.
230. Chikuma S, Bluestone JA. CTLA-4 and tolerance: the biochemical point of view. *Immunol Res* 2003;28:241–253.
231. Phan GQ, Yang JC, Sherry RM, et al. Cancer regression and autoimmunity induced by cytotoxic T lymphocyte-associated antigen 4 blockade in patients with metastatic melanoma. *Proc Natl Acad Sci USA* 2003;100: 8372–8377.
232. Hodi FS, Mihm MC, Soiffer RJ, et al. Biologic activity of cytotoxic T lymphocyte-associated antigen 4 antibody blockade in previously vaccinated metastatic melanoma and ovarian carcinoma patients. *Proc Natl Acad Sci USA* 2003;100:4712–4717.
233. Ribas A, Camacho LH, Lopez-Berestein G, et al. Antitumor activity in melanoma and anti-self responses in a phase I trial with the anti-cytotoxic T lymphocyte-associated antigen 4 monoclonal antibody CP-675,206. *J Clin Oncol* 2005;23:8968–8977.
234. Ribas A, Antonia S, Sosman J. Results of a phase II clinical trial of 2 doses and schedules of CP-675,206, an anti-CTLA4 monoclonal antibody, in patients (pts) with advanced melanoma. *Proc Am Soc Clin Oncol* 2007;25:18S(Part 1) (abstract 3000).
235. Gomez-Navarro J, Sharma A, Bozon V, et al. Dose and schedule selection for the anti-CTLA4 monoclonal antibody ticilimumab in patients (pts) with metastatic melanoma. *Proc Am Soc Clin Oncol* 2006;24:18S(Part 1) (abstract 8032).
236. Attia P, Phan GQ, Maker AV, et al. Autoimmunity correlates with tumor regression in patients with metastatic melanoma treated with anti-cytotoxic T-lymphocyte antigen-4. *J Clin Oncol* 2005;23:6043–6053.
237. Fong L, Kavanaugh B, Rini BI, et al. A phase I trial of combination immunotherapy with CTLA-4 blockade and GM-CSF in hormone refractory prostate cancer. *Proc Am Soc Clin Oncol* 2006;24:18S(Part 1) (abstract 2508).
238. Yang JC, Beck KE, Blansfield JA, et al. Tumor regression in patients with metastatic renal cancer treated with a monoclonal antibody to CTLA4 (MDX-010). *Proc Am Soc Clin Oncol* 2006;23:18S(Part 1) (abstract 2501).
239. Weber J. Review: anti–CTLA-4 antibody ipilimumab: case studies of clinical response and immune-related adverse events. *Oncologist* 2007;12: 864–872.
240. Jordan MA. Mechanism of action of antitumor drugs that interact with microtubules and tubulin. *Curr Med Chem Anti-Cancer Agents* 2002;2: 1–17.
241. Wartmann M, Altmann KH. The biology and medicinal chemistry of epothilones. *Curr Med Chem Anti-Cancer Agents* 2002;2:123–148.

242. Cortes J, Baselga J. Targeting the microtubules in breast cancer beyond taxanes: the epothilones. *Oncologist* 2007;12:271–280.
243. Jordan MA, Wilson L. Microtubules as a target for anti-cancer drugs. *Nat Rev Cancer* 2004;4:253–265.
244. Lee FY, Borzilleri R, Fairchild CR, et al. BMS-247550: a novel epotholone analog with a mode of action similar to paclitaxel but possessing superior antitumor efficacy. *Clin Cancer Res* 2001;7:1429–1437.
245. Verrills NM, Flemming CL, Liu M, et al. Microtubule alterations and mutations induced by desoxyepothilone B: implications for drug-target interactions. *Chem Biol* 2003;10:597–607.
246. Abraham J, Agrawal M, Bakke S, et al. Phase I trial and pharmacokinetic study of BMS-247550, an epothilone B analog, administered intravenously on a daily schedule for five days. *J Clin Oncol* 2003;21: 1866–1873.
247. Kaye S. Preliminary results from a phase II trial of EPO906 in patients with advanced refractory ovarian cancer. *Eur J Cancer* 2002;38:127 (abstract).
248. Thomas E, Tabernero J, Fornier M, et al. Phase II clinical trial of ixabepilone (BMS-247550), an epothilone b analog, in patients with taxane-resistant metastatic breast cancer. *J Clin Oncol* 2007;25:3399–3406.
249. Vansteenkiste J, Lara PN Jr, Le Chevalier T, et al. Phase II clinical trial of the epothilone B analog, ixabepilone, in patients with non small-cell lung cancer whose tumors have failed first-line platinum-based chemotherapy. *J Clin Oncol* 2007;25:3448–3455.
250. Stopeck S, Moulder S, Jones, et al. Phase I trial of KOS-1584 (a novel epothilone) using two weekly dosing schedules. *Proc Am Soc Clin Oncol* 2007;25(Part 1):18S (abstract 2571).
251. Rustin GJ, Reed NS, Jayson G, et al. Phase II trial of the novel epothilone ZK-EPO in patients with platinum resistant ovarian cancer. *Proc Am Soc Clin Oncol* 2007;25(Part 1):18S (abstract 5527).
252. Chen T, Molina A, Moore S, et al. Epothilone B analog (BMS-247550) at the recommended phase II dose (RPTD) in patients (pts) with gynecologic (gyn) and breast. *Proc Am Soc Clin Oncol* 2004;22:14S(Part 1) (abstract 2115).
253. Poncet J. The dolastatins, a family of promising antineoplastic agents. *Curr Pharm Des* 1999;5:139–162.
254. Hashiguchi N, Kubota T, Koh J, et al. TZT-1027 elucidates antitumor activity through direct cytotoxicity and selective blockade of blood supply. *Anti-cancer Res* 2004;24:2201–2208.
255. Ray A, Okouneva T, Manna T, et al. Mechanism of action of the microtubule-targeted antimitotic depsipeptide tasidotin (formerly ILX651) and its major metabolite tasidotin C-carboxylate. *Cancer Res* 2007;67: 3767–3776.
256. Schoffski P, Thate B, Beutel G, et al. Phase I and pharmacokinetic study of TZT-1027, a novel synthetic dolastatin 10 derivative, administered as a 1-hour intravenous infusion every 3 weeks in patients with advanced refractory cancer. *Ann Oncol* 2004;15:671–679.
257. Tamura K, Nakagawa K, Kurata T, et al. Phase I study of TZT-1027, a novel synthetic dolastatin 10 derivative and inhibitor of tubulin polymerization, which was administered to patients with advanced solid tumors on days 1 and 8 in 3-week courses. *Cancer Chemother Pharmacol* 2007;60: 285–293.
258. Mita AC, Hammond LA, Bonate PL, et al. Phase I and pharmacokinetic study of tasidotin hydrochloride (ILX651), a third-generation dolastatin-15 analogue, administered weekly for 3 weeks every 28 days in patients with advanced solid tumors. *Clin Cancer Res* 2006;12:5207–5215.
259. Jordan MA, Kamath K, Manna T, et al. The primary antimitotic mechanism of action of the synthetic halichondrin E7389 is suppression of microtubule growth. *Mol Cancer Ther* 2005;4:1086–1095.
260. Kuznetsov G, Towle MJ, Cheng H, et al. Induction of morphological and biochemical apoptosis following prolonged mitotic blockage by halichondrin B macrocyclic ketone analog E7389. *Cancer Res* 2004;64: 5760–5766.
261. Ravi M, Zask A, Rush TS. Structure-based identification of the binding site for the hemiasterlin analogue HTI-286 on tubulin. *Biochemistry* 2005;44:15871–15879.
262. Loganzo F, Hari M, Annable T, et al. Cells resistant to HTI-286 do not overexpress P-glycoprotein but have reduced drug accumulation and a point mutation in alpha-tubulin. *Mol Cancer Ther* 2004;3:1319–1327.
263. Blum JL, Pruitt B, Fabian CJ. Phase II study of eribulin mesylate (E7389) halichondrin b analog in patients with refractory breast cancer. *Proc Am Soc Clin Oncol* 2007;25:18S(Part 1) (abstract 1034).
264. Wong H, Desjardins C, Silberman S, et al. Pharmacokinetics (PK) of E7389, a halichondrin B analog with novel anti-tubulin activity: results of two phase I studies with different schedules of administration. *Proc Am Soc Clin Oncol* 2005;23:16S (Part 1) (abstract 2013).
265. Madajewicz S, Zojwalla NJ, Lucarelli AG, et al. A phase I trial of E7974 administered on days 1 and 15 of a 28-day cycle in patients with solid malignancies. *Proc Am Soc Clin Oncol* 2007;25:18S(Part 1) (abstract 2550).
266. Ratain MJ, Undevia S, Janisch L, et al. Phase 1 and pharmacological study of HTI-286, a novel antimicrotubule agent: correlation of neutropenia with time above a threshold serum concentration. *Proc Am Soc Clin Oncol* 2003;22 (abstract 516).
267. Tozer GM, Kanthou C, Baguley BC. Disrupting tumour blood vessels. *Nat Rev Cancer* 2005;5:423–435.
268. Hinnen P, Eskens FA. Vascular disrupting agents in clinical development. *Br J Cancer* 2007;96:1159–1165.
269. Cooney MM, van Heeckeren W, Bhakta S, et al. Drug insight: vascular disrupting agents and angiogenesis—novel approaches for drug delivery. *Nat Clin Pract Oncol* 2006;3:682–692.
270. Baguley BC. Antivascular therapy of cancer: DMXAA. *Lancet Oncol* 2003;4:141–148.
271. Gabra H, AS1404-202 Study Group Investigators. Phase II study of DMXAA combined with carboplatin and paclitaxel in recurrent ovarian cancer. *Proc Am Soc Clin Oncol* 2006;24:18S (abstract 5032).
272. Wood KW, Cornwell WD, Jackson JR. Past and future of the mitotic spindle as an oncology target. *Curr Opin Pharmacol* 2001;4:370–377.
273. Sakowicz R, Finer JT, Beraud C, et al. Antitumor activity of a kinesin inhibitor. *Cancer Res* 2004;64:3276–3280.
274. Rowinsky EK, Calvo E. Novel agents that target tubulin and related elements. *Semin Oncol* 2006;33:421–435.
275. Chu Q, Holen KD, Rowinsky EK, et al. A phase I study to determine the safety and pharmacokinetics of IV administered SB-715992, a novel kinesin spindle protein (KSP) inhibitor, in patients (pts) with solid tumors. *Proc Am Soc Clin Oncol* 2003;22:131 (abstract).
276. Shahin MS, Braly P, Rose P, et al. A phase II, open-label study of ispinesib (SB-715992) in patients with platinum/taxane refractory or resistant relapsed ovarian cancer. *Proc Am Soc Clin Oncol* 2007;25:18S(Part 1) (abstract 5552).
277. Stein MN, Tan A, Taber K, et al. Phase I clinical and pharmacokinetic (PK) trial of the kinesin spindle protein (KSP) inhibitor MK-0731 in patients with solid tumors. *Proc Am Soc Clin Oncol* 2007;25:18S(Part 1) (abstract 2548).
278. Miglarese MR, Wallace E, Woessner R, et al. ARRY-649, a member of a novel class of Eg5 kinesin inhibitors. *Proc Am Soc Clin Oncol* 2006;24: 18S(Part 1) (abstract 13045).
279. Holen KD, Belani CP, Wilding G, et al. Phase I study to determine tolerability and pharmacokinetics (PK) of SB-743921, a novel kinesin spindle protein (KSP) inhibitor. *Proc Am Soc Clin Oncol* 2006;24:18S(Part 1) (abstract 2000).
280. Li JJ, Li SA. Mitotic kinases: the key to duplication, segregation, and cytokinesis errors, chromosomal instability, and oncogenesis. *Pharmacol Ther* 2006;111:974–984.
281. Fu S, Hu W, Kavanagh JJ, et al. Targeting Aurora kinases in ovarian cancer. *Expert Opin Ther Targets* 2006;10:77–85.
282. Martin BT, Strebhardt K. Polo-like kinase 1: target and regulator of transcriptional control. *Cell Cycle* 2006;5:2881–2885.
283. van de Weerdt BC, Medema RH. Polo-like kinases: a team in control of the division. *Cell Cycle* 2006;5:853–864.
284. Strebhardt K, Ullrich A. Targeting polo-like kinase 1 for cancer therapy. *Nat Rev Cancer* 2006;6:321–330.
285. LeRoy PJ, Hunter JJ, Hoar KM, et al. Localization of human TACC3 to mitotic spindles is mediated by phosphorylation on Ser558 by Aurora A: a novel pharmacodynamic method for measuring Aurora A activity. *Cancer Res* 2007;67:5362–5370.
286. Landen CN Jr, Lin YG, Immaneni A, et al. Overexpression of the centrosomal protein Aurora-A kinase is associated with poor prognosis in epithelial ovarian cancer patients. *Clin Cancer Res* 2007;13:4098–4104.
287. Renshaw JS, Patnaik A, Gordon M, et al. A phase I two arm trial of AS703569 (R763), an orally available aurora kinase inhibitor, in subjects with solid tumors: preliminary results. *Proc Am Soc Clin Oncol* 2007;25: 18S(Part 1) (abstract 4130).
288. Jones SF, Cohen RB, Dees EC, et al. Phase I clinical trial of MLN8054, a selective inhibitor of Aurora A kinase. *Proc Am Soc Clin Oncol* 2007;25: 18S(Part 1) (abstract 3577).
289. Schellens JH, Boss D, Witteveen PO, et al. Phase I and pharmacological study of the novel aurora kinase inhibitor AZD1152. *Proc Am Soc Clin Oncol* 2006;24:18S(Part 1) (abstract 3008).
290. Rubin EH, Shapiro GI, Stein MN, et al. A phase I clinical and pharmacokinetic (PK) trial of the aurora kinase (AK) inhibitor MK-0457 in cancer patients. *Proc Am Soc Clin Oncol* 2006;24:18S(Part 1) (abstract 3009).
291. Munzert G, Steinbild S, Frost A, et al. A phase I study of two administration schedules of the polo-like kinase 1 inhibitor BI 2536 in patients with advanced solid tumors. *Proc Am Soc Clin Oncol* 2006;24:18S(Part 1) (abstract 3069).
292. Jimeno A, Chan A, Zhang X, et al. Evaluation of ON 01910.Na, a novel modulator of polo-like kinase 1 (Plk1) pathway, and development of a cyclin-B1-based predictive assay in pancreatic cancer. *Proc Am Soc Clin Oncol* 2007;25:18S(Part 1) (abstract 3569).
293. Cleaves M. Radium: with a preliminary note on radium rays in the treatment of cancer. *Med Rec* 1903;64:1719–1723.
294. Leibel SA, Fuks Z, Zelefsky MJ. Intensity-modulated radiotherapy. *Cancer J* 2002;8:164–171.
295. Nutting C, Dearnaley DP, Webb S. Intensity modulated radiation therapy: a clinical review. *Br J Radiol* 2000;73:459–466.
296. Mell LK, Mehrotra AK, Mundt AJ. Intensity modulated radiotherapy use in the United States, 2004. *Cancer* 2005;104:1296–1303.
297. Teh BS, Mai WY, Augsburger ME, et al. Intensity modulated radiation therapy (IMRT) following prostatectomy: more favorable acute genitourinary toxicity profile compared to primary IMRT for prostate cancer. *Int J Radiat Oncol Biol Phys* 2001;49:465–471.

298. Zelefsky MJ, Fuks Z, Hunt M, et al. High-dose intensity modulated radiation therapy for prostate cancer: early toxicity and biochemical outcome in 772 patients. *Int J Radiat Oncol Biol Phys* 2002;53:1111–1119.
299. Chao KS, Ozyigit G, Tran BN, et al. Patterns of failure in patients receiving definitive and postoperative IMRT for head-and-neck cancer. *Int J Radiat Oncol Biol Phys* 2003;55:312–319.
300. Eisbruch A, Kim HM, Terrell JE, et al. Xerostomia and its predictors following parotid-sparing irradiation of head-and-neck cancer. *Int J Radiat Oncol Biol Phys* 2001;50:695–672.
301. Perez CA, Breaux S, Bedwinek JM, et al. Radiation therapy alone in the treatment of carcinoma of the uterine cervix. II. Analysis of complications. *Cancer* 1984;54:235–246.
302. Corn BW, Lanciano RM, Greven KM. Impact of improved irradiation technique, age, and lymph node sampling on the severe complication rate of surgically staged endometrial cancer patients: a multivariate analysis. *J Clin Oncol* 1994;12:510–517.
303. Stock RG, Chen AS, Flickinger JC, et al. Node-positive cervical cancer: impact of pelvic irradiation and patterns of failure. *Int J Radiat Oncol Biol Phys* 1995;31:31–36.
304. Mundt AJ, Murphy KT, Rotmensch J, et al. Surgery and postoperative radiation therapy in FIGO Stage IIIC endometrial carcinoma. *Int J Radiat Oncol Biol Phys* 2001;50:1154–1160.
305. Mundt AJ, Roeske JC. Could intensity modulated radiation therapy (IMRT) replace brachytherapy in the treatment of cervical cancer? *Brachytherapy J* 2002;1:195–196.
306. Intensity Modulated Radiation Therapy Collaborative Working Group. Intensity modulated radiotherapy: current status and issues of interest. *Int J Radiat Oncol Biol Phys* 2001;51:880–914.
307. Takahashi S. Conformation radiotherapy. Rotation techniques as applied to radiography and radiotherapy of cancer. *Acta Radiol Diagn (Stockh)* 1965;242:1–5.
308. Brahme A. Optimization of stationary and moving beam radiation therapy technique. *Radiother Oncol* 1998;12:129–133.
309. Purdy JA. 3D treatment planning and intensity-modulated radiation therapy. *Oncology* 1999;13:155–168.
310. Roeske JC, Lujan A, Rotmensch J, et al. Intensity-modulated whole pelvic radiation therapy in patients with gynecologic malignancies. *Int J Radiat Oncol Biol Phys* 2000;48:1613–1621.
311. Mundt AJ, Roeske JC, Lujan AE. Intensity modulated radiation therapy in gynecologic malignancies. *Med Dosim* 2002;27:131–134.
312. Adli M, Mayr NA, Kaiser HS, et al. Does prone positioning reduce small bowel dose in pelvic radiation with intensity-modulated radiotherapy for gynecologic cancer? *Int J Radiat Oncol Biol Phys* 2003;57:230–238.
313. International Commission on Radiation Units and Measurements (ICRU). *Report Number 50: Prescribing, Recording, and Reporting Photon Beam Therapy*. Washington, DC: ICRU; 1993.
314. Mutic S, Malyapa RS, Grigsby PW, et al. PET-guided IMRT for cervical carcinoma with positive para-aortic lymph nodes—a dose-escalation treatment planning study. *Int J Radiat Oncol Biol Phys* 2003;55: 28–35.
315. Portelance L, Chao KS, Grigsby PW, et al. Intensity-modulated radiation therapy (IMRT) reduces small bowel, rectum, and bladder doses in patients with cervical cancer receiving pelvic and para-aortic irradiation. *Int J Radiat Oncol Biol Phys* 2001;51:261–266.
316. Garofalo M, Lujan AE, Roeske JC, et al. Intensity modulated radiation therapy in the treatment of vulvar carcinoma. Presented at the 88th Annual Meeting of the Radiologic Society of North America, Chicago, December 1–6, 2002.
317. Lujan AE, Mundt AJ, Yamada SD, et al. Intensity-modulated radiation therapy as a means of reducing dose to bone marrow in gynecologic patients receiving whole pelvic radiation therapy. *Int J Radiat Oncol Biol Phys* 2003;57:516–521.
318. Brixey CJ, Roeske JC, Lujan AE, et al. Impact of intensity-modulated radiation therapy on acute hematologic toxicity in women with gynecologic malignancies. *Int J Radiat Oncol Biol Phys* 2002;54:1388–1396.
319. Mell LK, Kochanski JD, Roeske JC, et al. Dosimetric predictors of acute hematologic toxicity in cervical cancer patients treated with concurrent cisplatin and intensity-modulated pelvic radiotherapy. *Int J Radiat Oncol Biol Phys* 2006;66:1356–1365.
320. Lujan AE, Mundt AJ, Roeske JC. Sequential versus simultaneous boost in the female pelvis using intensity modulated radiation therapy. Presented at the 43rd Annual Meeting of the American Association of Physicists in Medicine, Salt Lake City, July 22–26, 2001.
321. Roeske JC, Lujan AE, Mundt AJ. Incorporation of SPECT bone marrow imaging into IMRT planning in gynecology patients undergoing IM-WPRT. Presented at the 6th International Conference on Dose, Time and Fractionation. Madison, WI, September 23–26, 2001.
322. Kavanagh B, Schefter TE, Wu Q, et al. Clinical application of intensity modulated radiotherapy for locally advanced cervical cancer. *Semin Radiat Oncol* 2002;12:260–271.
323. Roeske JC, Bonta D, Lujan AE, et al. Dose volume histogram analysis of acute gastrointestinal toxicity in gynecologic patients undergoing intensity modulated whole pelvic radiation therapy. *Radiother Oncol* 2003;69:201–207.
324. Pugachev A, Xing L. Computer-assisted selection of coplanar beam orientations in intensity-modulated radiation therapy. *Phys Med Biol* 2001;46:2467.
325. Chen Q, Izadifar S, King S. Comparison of IMRT with 3-D CRT for gynecologic malignancies. *Int J Radiat Oncol Biol Phys* 2001;51:332a (abstract).
326. Heron DE, Gerszten K, Selvaraj RN, et al. Conventional 3D versus intensity modulated radiotherapy for adjuvant treatment of gynecologic malignancies: a comparative study of dose-volume histograms and the potential impact on toxicities. *Gynecol Oncol* 2003;91:39–45.
327. Ahamad A, D'Souza W, Salehpour M. Intensity modulated radiation therapy for post-hysterectomy pelvic radiation: selection of patients and planning target volume. *Int J Radiat Oncol Biol Phys* 2002;54:42a (abstract).
328. Duthoy W, De Gersem W, Vergote K, et al. Whole abdominopelvic radiotherapy (WAPRT) using intensity-modulated arc therapy (IMAT): first clinical experience. *Int J Radiat Oncol Biol Phys* 2003;57:1019–1032.
329. Hong L, Alektiar K, Chui C, et al. IMRT of large fields: whole abdomen irradiation. *Int J Radiat Oncol Biol Phys* 2002;54:278–289.
330. Beriwal S, Heron DE, Kim H, et al. Intensity-modulated radiotherapy for the treatment of vulvar carcinoma: a comparative dosimetric study with early clinical outcome. *Int J Radiat Oncol Biol Phys* 2006;64:1395–1400.
331. Gilroy JS, Amdur RJ, Louis DA. Irradiating the inguinal nodes without breaking a leg. *Int J Radiat Oncol Biol Phys* 2002;54;68a (abstract).
332. Schefter TE, Kavanagh BD, Wu Q. Technical considerations in the application of intensity-modulated radiotherapy as a concomitant integrated boost for locally advanced cervix cancer. *Med Dosim* 2002;27:177–181.
333. Ahmed RS, Kim RY, Duan J, et al. IMRT dose escalation for positive para-aortic lymph nodes in patients with locally advanced cervical cancer while reducing dose to bone marrow and other organs at risk. *Int J Radiat Oncol Biol Phys* 2004;60:505–512.
334. Alektiar K. Could intensity modulated radiation therapy (IMRT) replace brachytherapy in the treatment of cervical cancer? *Brachytherapy J* 2002;1:194–195.
335. Roeske JC, Mundt AJ. A feasibility study of IMRT for the treatment of cervical cancer patients unable to receive intracavitary brachytherapy. *Med Phys* 2000;27:1382–1383.
336. Low DA, Grigsby PW, Dempsey JF, et al. Applicator-guided intensity modulated radiation therapy. *Int J Radiat Oncol Biol Phys* 2002;52: 1400–1406.
337. Mundt AJ, Roeske JC, Lujan AE, et al. Initial clinical experience with intensity-modulated whole pelvis radiation therapy in women with gynecologic malignancies. *Gynecol Oncol* 2001;456–463.
338. Mundt AJ, Lujan AE, Rotmensch J, et al. Intensity-modulated whole pelvic radiotherapy in women with gynecologic malignancies. *Int J Radiat Oncol Biol Phys* 2002;52:1330–1337.
339. Mundt AJ, Mell LK, Roeske JC. Preliminary analysis of chronic gastrointestinal toxicity in gynecology patients treated with intensity modulated whole pelvic radiation therapy. *Int J Radiat Oncol Biol Phys* 2003;56: 1354–1360.
340. Beriwal S, Jain SK, Heron DE, et al. Clinical outcome with adjuvant treatment of endometrial carcinoma using intensity-modulated radiation therapy. *Gynecol Oncol* 2006;102:195–199.
341. Gerszten K, Colonello K, Heron DE, et al. Feasibility of concurrent cisplatin and extended field radiation therapy (EFRT) using intensity-modulated radiotherapy (IMRT) for carcinoma of the cervix. *Gynecol Oncol* 2006;102:182–188.
342. Salama JK, Mundt AJ, Roeske J, et al. Preliminary outcome and toxicity report of extended-field, intensity-modulated radiation therapy for gynecologic malignancies. *Int J Radiat Oncol Biol Phys* 2006;65:1170–1176.
343. Knab BR, Roeske JC, Mehta N, et al. Outcome of endometrial cancer patients treated with adjuvant intensity modulated pelvic radiation therapy. *Int J Radiat Oncol Biol Phys* 2004;60(Suppl 1):S303–S304.
344. Kochanski JD, Mehta N, Mell LK, et al. Outcome of cervical cancer patients treated with intensity modulated radiation therapy. *Int J Radiat Oncol Biol Phys* 2005;63:S214–S215.
345. Beriwal S, Gan GN, Heron DE, et al. Early clinical outcome with concurrent chemotherapy and extended-field, intensity-modulated radiation therapy for cervical cancer. *Int J Radiat Oncol Biol Phys* 2007;68: 166–171.
346. Chen MF, Tseng CJ, Tseng CC, et al. Clinical outcome in post-hysterectomy cervical cancer patients treated with concurrent cisplatin and intensity-modulated pelvic radiotherapy: comparison with conventional radiotherapy. *Int J Radiat Oncol Biol Phys* 2007;67:1428–1444.
347. Lin LL, Mutic S, Low DA, et al. Adaptive brachytherapy treatment planning for cervical cancer using FDG-PET. *Int J Radiat Oncol Biol Phys* 2007;67:91–96.
348. Taylor A, Rockall AG, Reznek RH, et al. Mapping pelvic lymph nodes: guidelines for delineation in intensity-modulated radiotherapy. *Int J Radiat Oncol Biol Phys* 2005;63:1604–1612.
349. van de Bunt L, van der Heide UA, Katelaars M, et al. Conventional, conformal and intensity-modulated radiation therapy treatment planning of external beam radiotherapy for cervical cancer: the impact of tumor regression. *Int J Radiat Oncol Biol Phys* 2006;64:189–196.
350. Dargent D. A new future for Schauta's operation through presurgical retroperitoneal pelviscopy. *Eur J Gynaecol Oncol* 1987;8:292–296.
351. Abu-Rustum NR, Gemignani ML, Moore K, et al. Total laparoscopic radical hysterectomy with pelvic lymphadenectomy using the argon-beam coagulator: pilot data and comparison to laparotomy. *Gynecol Oncol* 2003;91(2):402–409.

352. Aburel E. Sub-corporeal extended colpohysterectomy in therapy of incipient cancer of cervix. *C R Soc Fr Gynecol* 1957;27(6):237–243.
353. Aburel E. Proceedings: extended abdominal exstirpation of cervix and isthmus in early stages of cervix carcinoma (carcinoma *in situ* and microcarcinoma). *Arch Gynakol* 1973;214(1):106–108.
354. Dargent D, Brun JL, Roy M, et al. Pregnancies following radical trachelectomy for invasive cervical cancer (Abstract). *Gynecol Oncol* 1994;52:105.
355. Roy M, Plante M, Renaud MC, et al. Vaginal radical hysterectomy versus abdominal radical hysterectomy in the treatment of early-stage cervical cancer. *Gynecol Oncol* 1996;62(3):336–339.
356. Martin XJ, Golfier F, Romestaing P, et al. First case of pregnancy after radical trachelectomy and pelvic irradiation. *Gynecol Oncol* 1999;74(2): 286–287.
357. Roy M, Plante M. Pregnancies after radical vaginal trachelectomy for early-stage cervical cancer. *Am J Obstet Gynecol* 1998;179(6 Pt 1):1491–1496.
358. Dargent D, Franzosi F, Ansquer Y, et al. Extended trachelectomy relapse: plea for patient involvement in the medical decision. *Bull Cancer* 2002;89(12):1027–1030.
359. Abu-Rustum NR, Sonoda Y, Black D, et al. Cystoscopic temporary ureteral catheterization during radical vaginal and abdominal trachelectomy. *Gynecol Oncol* 2006;103(2):729–731.
360. Margossian H, Garcia-Ruiz A, Falcone T, et al. Robotically assisted laparoscopic microsurgical uterine horn anastomosis. *Fertil Steril* 1998;70(3): 530–534.
361. Margossian H, Falcone T. Robotically assisted laparoscopic hysterectomy and adnexal surgery. *J Laparoendos Adv Surg Tech A* 2001;11(3): 161–165.
362. Mettler L, Ibrahim M, Jonat W. One year of experience working with the aid of a robotic assistant (the voice-controlled optic holder AESOP) in gynaecological endoscopic surgery. *Hum Reprod* 1998;13(10):2748–2750.
363. Degueldre M, Vandromme J, Huong PT, et al. Robotically assisted laparoscopic microsurgical tubal reanastomosis: a feasibility study. *Fertil Steril* 2000;75(5):1020–1023.
364. Falcone T, Steiner CP. Robotically assisted gynecologic surgery. *Human Fertil (Camb)* 2002;5(2):72–74.
365. Diaz-Arrastia C, Jurnalov C, Gomez G, et al. Laparoscopic hysterectomy using a computer-enhanced surgical robot. *Surg Endosc* 2002;16(9): 1271–1273.
366. Molpus KL, Wedergren JS, Carlson MA. Robotically assisted endoscopic ovarian transposition. *JSLS* 2003;7(1):59–62.
367. Molpus KL, Wedergren JS, Carlson MA. Robotically assisted endoscopic ovarian transposition. *JSLS* 2003;7(1):59–62.
368. Magrina JF. Robotic surgery in gynecology. *Eur J Gynaeol Oncol* 2007;28(2): 77–82.
369. Sert B, Abeler V. Robotic radical hysterectomy in early-stage cervical carcinoma patients, comparing results with total laparoscopic radical hysterectomy cases. The future is now? *Int J Med Robot* 2007;3(3):224–228.
370. Talamini MA. Robotic surgery: is it for you? *Adv Surg* 2002;36:1–13.

CHAPTER 19 ■ PATHOGENESIS AND DIAGNOSIS OF PREINVASIVE LESIONS OF THE LOWER GENITAL TRACT

THOMAS C. WRIGHT JR

INTRODUCTION

The high level of public and professional interest in various aspects of preinvasive lesions of the lower genital tract is due to many factors. Perhaps the most important is the marked increase over the last four decades in the number of patients in North America and Western Europe diagnosed with human papillomavirus (HPV)-associated disease. This increase is due partly to a heightened awareness of various clinical and pathologic manifestations of HPV infections, the recent introduction of prophylactic vaccines against specific high-risk types of HPV, and to the increased use of highly sensitive tests for the detection of HPV infections and cervical cancer precursors. In addition, a real increase in the prevalence of HPV infections appears to have taken place during this time. HPV-associated genital tract disease is the most commonly diagnosed sexually transmitted disease in the United States. Over half of men and women who are sexually active will be infected at some point in their lives. The Centers for Disease Control and Prevention (CDC) estimates that approximately 20 million Americans 15 to 49 years of age are infected with HPV (1). This represents approximately 15% of all individuals in this age group. About half of these are sexually active adolescents and young adults 15 to 24 years of age.

Cervical cancer precursors also appear to have increased in prevalence over the last 2 decades in the United States and Western Europe. According to the National Cancer Institute's Surveillance, Epidemiology, and End Results (SEER) program, an increase in the incidence of high-grade cervical cancer precursors began to be detected in the early 1980s in white women under the age of 50 in the United States (2). In 1980 the incidence of carcinoma *in situ* of the cervix in white women under the age of 50 years was 27 per 100,000; by 1995, it had increased to 41 per 100,000 women (3). Currently, the median reporting rate for abnormal cervical cytology in the United States is approximately 9%, with wide variations depending on the characteristics of the population screened and the particular cytology laboratory being used (4). Based on rates of cytologic abnormalities obtained by the College of American Pathologists, we can estimate that approximately 1,548,000 women receive a cytologic result of low-grade cervical cancer precursors each year in the United States, and another 2,790,000 have equivocal cytologic changes referred to as atypical squamous cells (4).

DEFINITIONS AND TERMINOLOGY OF PREINVASIVE LESIONS OF THE LOWER GENITAL TRACT

The terminology used to classify preinvasive lesions of the lower genital tract has changed many times over the last 50 years and is continuing to do so. Unfortunately, these changes, and the lack of a uniform terminology, have been an ongoing source of confusion for the clinician. Despite recent attempts to simplify the classification and make the terminology more uniform, as much controversy exists today as existed 30 years ago regarding the appropriate definitions of preinvasive lesions of the lower genital tract.

Cervix—Squamous Lesions

For more than a century, it has been recognized that invasive squamous cell carcinomas of the cervix are associated with lesions histologically and cytologically identical to invasive cervical carcinoma but that lack the capacity to invade the subepithelial stroma. Because of their unique spatial and temporal relationships with cervical cancer, these intraepithelial lesions were referred to as carcinoma *in situ*. As cytology-based cervical cancer screening programs were being introduced in the 1950s it became clear that there were also squamous epithelial abnormalities whose histologic and cytologic features were less severe than carcinoma *in situ*. These lesions were referred to as *dysplasia* and were often divided into three grades (e.g., *mild*, *moderate*, or *severe*) based on the degree of cytologic or histologic abnormality (5). Dysplastic lesions were believed to represent lesions that were biologically less ominous than carcinoma *in situ*. In the late 1960s a series of descriptive studies that used a variety of techniques, including electron microscopy, tissue culture, chromosome analysis, DNA ploidy analysis, and radioautography, suggested that dysplastic lesions, carcinoma *in situ*, and invasive carcinoma formed a continuum rather than a series of discrete steps. In 1973, based on follow-up studies of patients with cervical cancer precursor lesions and studies of the biology of these lesions, Richart proposed that the term *cervical intraepithelial neoplasia* (CIN) be used to encompass all forms of cervical cancer precursor lesions, including dysplasia and carcinoma *in situ* (6). The CIN terminology divided cervical cancer precursor lesions into three groups or grades. CIN 1 corresponded to mild dysplasia, and CIN 2 corresponded to moderate dysplasia. Since studies had shown that pathologists could not reproducibly distinguish between severe dysplasia and carcinoma *in situ*, CIN 3 encompassed both of these lesions. The CIN terminology stressed the concept that all cervical cancer precursors formed a continuum and that lesions of all grades of severity had the potential to progress to invasive cancer if left untreated. Since the risk for progression of any individual lesion is unknown (i.e., by light microscopy it is impossible to categorize the lesions as to which will persist or progress), the CIN terminology emphasized that all "precursor" lesions should be treated. Inherent in this reasoning was the acknowledgment that appropriate treatment and eradication of precursors (irrespective of their histologic grade) greatly reduces a patient's risk for subsequently developing invasive cervical cancer.

The CIN terminology provided information in a context that made approaches to clinical management straightforward and became the most widely used terminology for cervical cancer precursors. However, over the last 15 years, tremendous advances in our understanding of the pathogenesis of cervical cancer precursors have taken place. These advances have changed both our pathologic nomenclature and our approach to clinical management of cervical cancer precursor lesions. It is now clear that the CIN (continuum) concept of cervical cancer precursors has certain limitations. For example, the spectrum of histologic changes grouped together as CIN is now recognized to represent two distinct biologic entities. One entity is a productive HPV infection rather than a neoplasm or cancer precursor. The characteristic histologic feature of a productive HPV infection is the presence of HPV cytopathic effect (e.g., koilocytosis with multinucleation, perinuclear halos, nuclear enlargement, and nuclear atypia). These productive HPV infections can be associated with any HPV type including "low-risk" HPVs as well as "high-risk" or oncogenic HPV types. The other HPV-associated biologic entity should be considered to be an actual neoplasm or cancer precursor, rather than simply a productive viral infection. These neoplasms or "true precursors" are invariably monoclonal and are usually associated with "high-risk" or oncogenic HPV types such as 16, 18, 31, 33, 35, 39, 45, 51, 52, 56, 58, 59, 68, 73, or 82 (5,7). These lesions are frequently aneuploid and often demonstrate specific loss of heterozygosity (LOH) at chromosomal loci observed in invasive cervical cancers (8,9).

These advances in our understanding of the biology of preinvasive lesions of the cervix have led to suggestions that the terminology used to refer to cervical cancer precursors be modified (5). The proposed terminologies abolish the three-tiered CIN 1, 2, and 3 classification and replace it with a two-tiered classification. To allow histopathologic findings to be easily correlated with cytologic findings, one of the proposed classifications follows that of the Bethesda system for cytologic diagnosis, which uses the terms "high-grade squamous intraepithelial lesion" and "low-grade squamous intraepithelial lesion" to report cytologic diagnoses (10). In this proposed classification system, lesions previously classified as mild dysplasia, koilocytotic atypia, koilocytosis, flat condylomata, and CIN 1 are grouped together into a single entity termed *low-grade squamous intraepithelial lesion* (i.e., low-grade SIL or LSIL), and lesions previously classified as CIN 2 and 3 are grouped together into a single entity termed *high-grade squamous intraepithelial lesion* (i.e., high-grade SIL or HSIL). A similar modification of the CIN system of nomenclature was also suggested. In this modified scheme CIN 1 was termed low-grade CIN 1 and CIN 2 and 3 were combined under the high-grade CIN 2,3 rubric. Table 19.1 compares the different terminologies.

In this chapter we use a two-tiered terminology (e.g., CIN 1 and CIN 2,3) because it is the most widely used terminology in the United States and was adopted for clinical guidelines at the 2001 Consensus Conference, and a decision was made to continue with this terminology for the 2006 Consensus Guidelines (11,12). However, two points should be emphasized about the use of any terminology for cervical cancer precursors. First, it is important to remember that the histologic appearance of a lesion does not unequivocally predict whether it represents a simple productive viral infection or a neoplasm. Although the majority of histologically high-grade lesions contain "high-risk" or oncogenic HPV types, are monoclonal proliferations, and are aneuploid, the converse is not true. Lesions that are histologically low-grade are quite heterogeneous with respect to their associated HPV types, clonal status, and ploidy. Some histologically low-grade lesions can be classified as productive viral infections; others contain "high-risk" or oncogenic HPV types and have the biologic features of a precursor lesion. Therefore, histologic appearance does not necessarily predict the biologic behavior of an individual lesion. Second, it must be emphasized that different terminologies are currently in use by different pathology laboratories. Although most laboratories in the United States have switched

TABLE 19.1

COMPARISON OF DIFFERENT TERMINOLOGIES FOR CERVICAL SQUAMOUS NONINVASIVE LESIONS

Older terminology	CIN[a] terminology	The Bethesda system	Modified CIN terminology
Flat condyloma Koilocytosis Koilocytotic atypia Mild dysplasia	CIN 1	Low-grade squamous intraepithelial lesion (LSIL)	CIN 1 (low-grade CIN)
Moderate dysplasia	CIN 2	High-grade squamous intraepithelial lesion (HSIL)	CIN 2,3 (high-grade CIN)
Severe dysplasia Carcinoma *in situ*	CIN 3		

[a]CIN, cervical intraepithelial neoplasia.

to the two-tiered or modified CIN terminology, some continue to utilize the terms dysplasia and carcinoma *in situ*. This is expected to change over the next several years since the World Health Organization (WHO) recently switched to the CIN terminology (13).

Cervix—Glandular Lesions

Interest in glandular lesions of the cervix has been stimulated by an apparent increase in the number of women, especially those under the age of 35, who are being diagnosed with invasive adenocarcinoma of the cervix and glandular precursor lesions. Large series of women with invasive cervical cancers as well as cancer registries have demonstrated that the relative proportion of adenocarcinomas to squamous cell carcinomas of the cervix has been increasing over the last 3 decades. Most large series from the 1950s and 1960s reported that 95% of invasive cervical cancers were squamous cell carcinomas and only 5% were adenocarcinomas. However, beginning in the 1970s, case series began reporting that 75% to 80% of invasive cervical cancers were squamous cell carcinomas and that 20% to 25% of cases were either adenocarcinomas, adenosquamous cell carcinomas, or undifferentiated carcinomas. This relative increase is clearly demonstrated by the clinical series of Shingleton et al. (14). During the 1974 to 1978 period, adenocarcinomas accounted for 7% of all cervical cancers, whereas by 1979 to 1980 they accounted for 19%. Similarly, cancer registries from the United States and Europe have reported that the ratio of adenocarcinomas to squamous cell carcinomas has increased over the same period (15–17). During the 1996 to 2000 period adenocarcinomas accounted for 25% of all invasive cervical cancers in whites in the U.S. SEER database (3). In the Finnish Cancer Registry, 6% of cervical cancers were classified as adenocarcinomas in 1953 to 1957, whereas by 1978 to 1982, 17% were classified as adenocarcinomas (15).

In the U.S. SEER registry, the incidence of invasive adenocarcinoma of the cervix has increased from 1.23 per 100,000 in 1976 to 1980 to 1.76 per 100,000 in 1996 to 2000 (3). Much of this increase is due to young women 15 to 34 years of age. Among white women in this age group the incidence increased from 0.6 to 1.2 per 100,000. Cancer registries from Norway and the United Kingdom have also reported increases in the absolute incidence of invasive adenocarcinomas of the cervix in women 35 years or younger (16,18). It is important to note, however, that despite the increased incidence of invasive adenocarcinoma in young women and the clear increase in the relative proportions of adenocarcinomas to squamous cell carcinomas over the last 3 decades, the absolute number of invasive adenocarcinomas has not actually increased when women of all age groups are combined. Instead, the number of women with invasive squamous cell carcinomas has decreased, producing a relative increase.

The first indication that precursor lesions existed for invasive adenocarcinomas of the cervix was the description by Helper et al. in 1952 of highly atypical endocervical cells lining architecturally normal endocervical glands adjacent to frankly invasive adenocarcinomas of the cervix (19). Friedell and McKay subsequently described two additional patients with similar histologic findings and coined the term adenocarcinoma *in situ* (AIS) to refer to these glandular lesions that were histologically highly atypical, but noninvasive (20). Inherent in the use of the term adenocarcinoma *in situ* to refer to these lesions was the acknowledgment that these lesions were precursors to invasive adenocarcinoma of the cervix. In addition to the highly atypical glandular lesions referred to as adenocarcinoma *in situ*, glandular lesions with a lesser degree of histologic abnormality than adenocarcinoma *in situ* are also found in the cervix. These low-grade glandular lesions have been referred to by a variety of terms including *endocervical dysplasia*, *atypical hyperplasia*, and more recently, *endocervical glandular atypia* (5). By way of analogy to squamous lesions, some authors have suggested that the term *cervical intraepithelial glandular neoplasia* (CIGN) be used to refer to all of these noninvasive glandular lesions. Using the CIGN terminology, atypical hyperplasia is classified as either CIGN grade 1 or 2 depending on the degree of cytologic atypia and mitotic activity present and adenocarcinoma *in situ* is classified as CIGN grade 3. In the United States between 1976 and 2000 the incidence of adenocarcinoma *in situ* has increased steadily in women 15 to 74 years of age. In 1976 to 1980 the incidence in white women was 0.21 per 100,000; this increased to 1.25 per 100,000 by 1991 to 1995 (3). Increases were greatest among young women.

It is important to note that although there is considerable evidence indicating that adenocarcinoma *in situ* is a precursor for invasive adenocarcinoma of the cervix, there is little evidence to support such a role for the lower-grade glandular abnormalities. Because the terms endocervical dysplasia and CIGN imply a relationship between the low-grade lesions and invasive adenocarcinoma that is not documented, some prefer the more noncommittal term endocervical glandular atypia to refer to the low-grade lesions that lack the features of adenocarcinoma *in situ* (5).

Vulva and Vagina

The nomenclature used for preinvasive lesions of the vulva and vagina has tended to parallel that used for the cervix. The original description of preinvasive lesions of the vulva was made in 1912 by Bowen, who described a lesion of the thigh and buttock that he termed "precancerous dermatosis." These lesions were grossly red and scaly and were characterized microscopically by significant cellular atypia. Clinically, they either persisted or recurred. Bowen believed that these lesions, which subsequently came to be called *Bowen's disease*, were precursors to invasive squamous cell carcinomas of the vulva. Since this original description, a number of other terms have been used for lesions with significant cellular atypia that lack invasion. These include erythroplasia of Queyrat, atypical hyperplasia, dysplasia, atypia, carcinoma *in situ*, carcinoma *in situ* simplex, and intraepithelial carcinoma.

In the 1980s many clinicians and pathologists began to apply the intraepithelial neoplasia terminology widely used for describing cervical cancer precursors to the vulva. Thus the term *vulvar intraepithelial neoplasia* (VIN), together with a grade of 1 to 3, was adopted (21). Similarly, the term *vaginal intraepithelial neoplasia* (VAIN), together with a grade of 1 to 3, is widely used to describe preinvasive lesions of the vagina. It should be pointed out, however, that data that suggest a continuum between all grades of vulvar and vaginal preinvasive lesions and invasive squamous cell carcinoma at these sites are significantly less compelling than that for the cervix. In 2004 the International Society for the Study of Vulvar Disease (ISSVD) proposed a new terminology for vulvar lesions. In their new nomenclature, VIN 1 is eliminated and the term VIN is used to apply only to high-grade lesions, which are subdivided into *VIN, usual type* (which encompasses former VIN 2 or VIN 3 of the warty, basaloid, and mixed types) and *VIN, differentiated type* (22). This proposed nomenclature fails to take into account that a significant proportion of VIN 1 lesions are actually associated with "high-risk" types of HPV and this terminology has not been widely adopted for use in the United States (23).

NATURAL HISTORY OF PREINVASIVE LESIONS OF THE LOWER GENITAL TRACT

Cervix

A variety of epidemiologic and long-term follow-up studies support the concept that certain epithelial lesions are precursors of invasive squamous cell carcinoma of the cervix. Several different methods have been used to study the natural history of different types of cervical cancer precursors. When cytologic screening programs for cervical cancer were introduced to previously unscreened populations in the 1940s and 1950s, a large difference in the mean age of patients with invasive cervical cancer and patients with "dysplasia" became apparent (Table 19.2). In the study by Reagan et al., the mean age of patients with "dysplasia" was 34 years, the mean age of patients with carcinoma *in situ* was 42 years, and the mean age of patients with invasive cancer was 48 years (24). Similar age distributions were observed by Patten in his studies (25). These data were interpreted to imply that it takes over 10 years for a dysplastic lesion to progress to carcinoma *in situ* and invasive cancer.

The most direct way to study the natural history of cervical cancer precursors is to study cervical lesions prospectively without therapeutic intervention. Before widespread acceptance of the fact that a high percentage of carcinoma *in situ* lesions inevitably progress to invasive cancer, patients with carcinoma *in situ* were followed prospectively in several studies. These studies, with all their attendant methodologic problems (including lack of standardized histologic criteria, small patient numbers, inadequate and short patient follow-up, and wide differences in results) form the basis of our estimates of the premalignant potential of carcinoma *in situ*. Now that the premalignant potential of carcinoma *in situ* is universally accepted, it would obviously be unethical to repeat these prospective follow-up studies of carcinoma *in situ* lesions using more contemporary methods.

In 1961, Kottmeier reported on a group of 31 women with carcinoma *in situ* who were followed for at least 12 years (26). Twenty-two (72%) of these women subsequently developed invasive cancer. Similarly, Koss et al. in 1963 reported a long-term follow-up study of 67 women with biopsy-confirmed carcinoma *in situ* (27). In this study, a lower frequency of progression was detected than in the study by Kottmeier (Table 19.3). Sixty-one percent of carcinoma *in situ* lesions persisted, and only 6% progressed to invasive cancer. However, the follow-up time was only 3 years. A larger study of the natural history of carcinoma *in situ* was that of Green and Donovan from New Zealand (Table 19.3) (28). On the basis of a short-term follow-up study of patients with carcinoma *in situ*, it was initially proposed that carcinoma *in situ* either had a low malignant potential or took much longer than 20 years to develop into invasive cancer. However, on long-term follow-up of a group of 817 patients whose Pap smears reverted to normal, 12 patients (1.5%) subsequently developed invasive carcinoma (29). Of the group of 131 patients with persistently abnormal Pap smears (followed for 4 to 23 years), 29 (22%) developed invasive carcinoma of the cervix or vaginal vault, and 90 (69%) had persistent carcinoma *in situ*. This and other follow-up studies clearly demonstrate that, once established, carcinoma *in situ* has a significant potential for progression to invasive cancer, and progression is a slow process, usually requiring a decade or more.

Whether carcinoma *in situ*, once established, can spontaneously regress in the absence of therapy is controversial. Based on the studies of Kottmeier and Green it would appear that, once established, carcinoma *in situ* only rarely regresses spontaneously (26,29). However, other follow-up studies have found that about one third of carcinoma *in situ* lesions regress during follow-up (30). Evaluation of data obtained from the British Columbia population-based screening program suggests that the cumulative incidence of carcinoma *in situ* is significantly higher than the cumulative incidence of invasive cervical cancer (31). Similar data has been obtained from cytologic screening programs in Sweden. This cytologic data has been interpreted as indicating that many cases of carcinoma *in situ* regress spontaneously (31,32).

Many prospective studies have also followed the transitions between different grades of CIN. These studies have obtained quite different estimates of the frequency of mild dysplasia, the likelihood of progression from low-grade to high-grade precursors, and the time required for this progression. The major reasons for these differences include the use of cervical biopsy rather than cytology to document the presence

TABLE 19.2

AGE DISTRIBUTION OF CERVICAL CANCER PRECURSORS

	Mean age at diagnosis (yr)	
Cytology	Patten (25)	Reagan et al. (24)
Dysplasia	34.7	34
Slight	32	—
Moderate	35.7	—
Marked	38.4	—
Carcinoma *in situ*	42.3	41.5
Invasive cancer	51.7	48.2

TABLE 19.3

NATURAL HISTORY OF PATIENTS WITH CERVICAL CANCER PRECURSORS

		Diagnosis					
Reference	Patients (no.)	Method of diagnosis	Actual diagnosis	Regression (%)	Persistence (%)	Progression (%)	Follow-up period (yr)
Kottmeier (26)	31	Biopsy	CIS	—	—	72	>12
Koss et al. (27)	26	Biopsy	CIN 1,2	39	15	46	0.5–7
Koss et al. (27)	67	Biopsy	CIS	25	61	6	3
Green and Donovan (28)	576	Biopsy	CIS	—	—	0.17	1–12
McIndoe et al. (29)	131	Biopsy	CIS	8	69	22	1–28

TABLE 19.4

NATURAL HISTORY OF DYSPLASIA—TORONTO HISTORICAL COHORT STUDY

	% Occurring at		
	2 yr	5 yr	10 yr
PROGRESSION			
Mild to moderate or worse	11	20	29
Mild to severe or worse	2	6	9
Moderate to severe or worse	16	25	32
REGRESSION			
Mild to normal (×1)	44	74	88
Mild to normal (×2)	—	39	62
Moderate to normal (×1)	33	63	83
Moderate to normal (×2)	—	29	54

Source: Holowaty P, Miller AB, Rohan T, To T. Natural history of dysplasia of the uterine cervix. *J Natl Cancer Inst* 1999;91:252.

TABLE 19.5

NATURAL HISTORY OF CIN IS DEPENDENT ON LESIONAL GRADE

	% Regression	% Persist	Progress to CIS
CIN 1	57	32	11
CIN 2	43	35	22
CIN 3	32	56	12

Source: Mitchell MF, Tortolero-Luna G, Wright T, et al. Cervical human papillomavirus infection and intraepithelial neoplasia: a review. *J Natl Cancer Inst Monogr* 1996;21:17–25.

of an abnormality in some studies. Cervical biopsies can remove small precursor lesions in their entirety and therefore can alter natural history. In addition, prospective studies have differed in study design and pathologic criteria used to grade cervical lesions.

The two most widely quoted follow-up studies are the historical cohort study from Toronto published by Holowaty et al. and the prospective clinical trials of Nasiell et al. The Toronto study utilized a historical cohort of women whose cervical cytology was evaluated at a single large laboratory in an era (1962 to 1980) during which CIN lesions were managed conservatively in Canada (33). Rates of regression and progression were estimated using actuarial methods and through linkage to the Ontario cancer registry. Both mild and moderate dysplasias were found to be more likely to regress than progress. The risk of mild dysplasia progressing to severe dysplasia or worse was approximately 1% per year. In contrast, the risk of moderate dysplasia progressing was 16% at 2 years and 25% at 5 years (Table 19.4). The majority of both mild and moderate dysplasias showed spontaneous clearance and much of the clearance occurred within 2 years of diagnosis.

Nasiell et al. reported on 555 women with a single Pap smear showing mild dysplasia who were followed colposcopically and cytologically without major treatment (34). Biopsies were performed in only 14% of these patients. In this series, 62% of the patients with a mean follow-up time of 39 months developed normal Pap smears, with apparent regression of their mild dysplasia. Persistent dysplasia occurred in 22% of the patients, with a mean follow-up of 52 months. Progression to severe dysplasia, carcinoma *in situ*, and invasive carcinoma occurred in 16% of the patients, with a mean follow-up of 48 months. Two patients who were lost to follow-up in this study subsequently developed invasive carcinoma, which was detected 79 months and 125 months, respectively, after a diagnosis of mild dysplasia. A number of other studies have investigated cohorts of women with moderate dysplasia. In a study of identical design to that used to study the biologic behavior of mild dysplasia, Nasiell et al. followed patients originally diagnosed cytologically as having moderate dysplasia. By life table analysis, progression to severe dysplasia, carcinoma *in situ*, and invasive carcinoma occurred in 33% of the patients after 12 or more years of follow-up (35).

Melnikow et al. performed a comprehensive meta-analysis of studies in which women with a cytologic result of SIL were followed (36). The analysis included 13,226 women with a cytologic result of LSIL who were followed for at least 6 months and had a median weighted follow-up of 29 months. There were 10,026 women with HSIL who had a median weighted follow-up of 25 months. The pooled estimates for regression to normal were 47% for LSIL and 35% for HSIL (Fig. 19.1). Rates of progression of LSIL were 7% at 6 months and 21% at 24 months. For HSIL the 6- and 24-month pooled progression rates were 7% and 24%. The pooled progression rates for invasive cancer at 6 and 24 months for LSIL were 0.04% and 0.15%, respectively. For HSIL they were 0.15% at 6 months and 1.44% at 24 months.

Mitchell et al. performed a systematic review of the different studies investigating the natural history of untreated biopsy-confirmed CIN, most of which were conducted in the 1970s and 1980s (Table 19.5) (37). Many of these studies are older and used the carcinoma *in situ* terminology. The higher the grade of lesion, the more likely it is to persist and the less likely it is to regress. Overall, it appears that approximately 57% of CIN 1 spontaneously regresses in the absence of therapy, 32% persist as CIN, and 11% progress to carcinoma

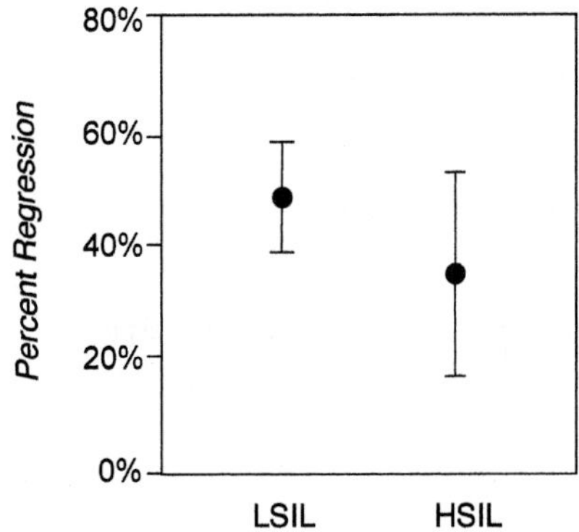

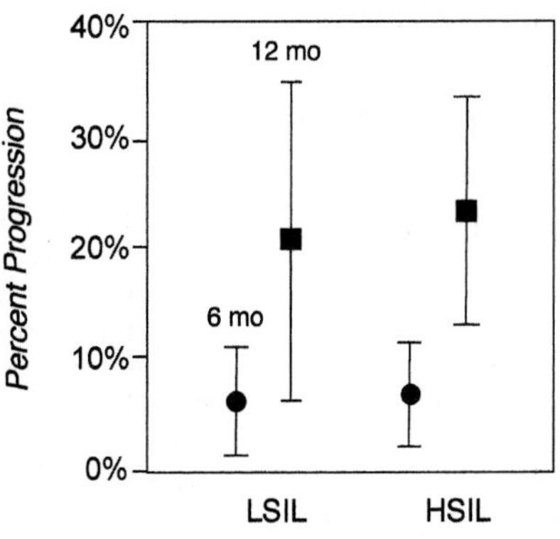

FIGURE 19.1. Pooled estimates of the rates of spontaneous regression (**left panel**) of a cytologic diagnosis of LSIL and HSIL obtained from the literature. Pooled estimates of the rates of spontaneous progression of LSIL and HSIL after 6 months (circles) and 12 months (squares) are shown (**right panel**). Progression for HSIL is from CIN 2 to CIN 3 or carcinoma *in situ*. Bars represent 95% confidence intervals. *Source:* Modified with permission from Melnikow J, Nuovo J, Willan AR, et al. Natural history of cervical squamous intraepithelial lesions: a meta-analysis. *Obstet Gynecol* 1998;92:727–735.

in situ. The rates of persistence and progression are greater for CIN 2,3. Forty-three percent of CIN 2 lesions regress, 35% persist, and 22% progress to carcinoma *in situ*. The equivalent rates for CIN 3 lesions were 32% regression, 56% persistence, and 12% progression to carcinoma *in situ*. Overall, the progression of all grades of CIN to invasive cancer in the published observational studies is 1.7%. The rate at which CIN progresses appears to be relatively slow.

Until recently it was generally believed that it took many years for a low-grade lesion to progress to a high-grade lesion. Mathematical modeling studies based on the prevalence of cytologic abnormalities in an unscreened population suggested that it takes on average almost 5 years for a mild dysplasia to progress to carcinoma *in situ* (5). More recent studies indicate, however, that high-grade lesions can develop quite rapidly after an incident HPV infection. A prospective study of college students found that the median length of time from first detection of an HPV infection to detection of CIN 2,3 was only 14.1 months (38). The finding that CIN 2,3 lesions can develop quite rapidly after initial HPV infections has been confirmed in the HPV vaccine trials (39).

Vulva

Studies on the natural history of VIN lesions are much fewer than for CIN. Partly because of the paucity of studies, the relationships between VIN and invasive squamous cell carcinoma of the vulva appear to be less straightforward than those documented between CIN and invasive squamous cell carcinoma of the cervix. Unlike the cervix, in which the majority of carcinomas are associated with a CIN lesion, only a third of invasive vulvar squamous carcinomas have a coexisting VIN 3 lesion (40). A review of six published follow-up studies found that only 16 of 330 patients (4.8%) with VIN progressed to invasive cancer (41). Solitary lesions in postmenopausal women had the highest risk of progression; multifocal lesions in women of reproductive age rarely progressed, although well-documented cases of young patients with VIN 3 who have developed cancer exist. In a series from Denmark, Hording et al. reported that only 4% of 73 women with VIN 3 developed invasive cancer during follow-up (median follow-up was 5 years) (42).

What is generally not emphasized when this data is discussed is that most of the patients in these follow-up studies were treated for their VIN or followed for relatively short periods of time. This fact explains, in part, the low incidence of progression. In one of the few long-term follow-up studies of women with VIN, Jones and Rowan found that only 3% of 105 women with treated VIN developed invasive vulvar cancer. In contrast, of eight women between the ages of 28 and 73 years with biopsy-documented VIN 3 who were followed without further treatment, seven developed invasive squamous cell carcinoma of the vulva within 8 years of diagnosis (43).

RISK FACTORS FOR THE DEVELOPMENT OF LOWER GENITAL TRACT CANCERS AND PREINVASIVE LESIONS OF THE LOWER GENITAL TRACT

Cervix

Risk Factors

A large number of epidemiologic studies have analyzed risk factors for the development of cervical cancer and its precursors. Although the risk factors are similar for both cervical cancer and its precursors, the association with the risk factors is generally much stronger for cervical cancer than for precursor lesions. The major risk factors found in most studies are markers of sexual behavior such as number of sexual partners, early age of first pregnancy and first intercourse, sexually transmitted diseases, and parity. In addition, lower socioeconomic class, cigarette smoking, oral contraceptive use, specific HLA-DR haplotypes, and immunosuppression from any cause are associated with both cervical cancer and its precursors (Table 19.6).

It has been known for almost a century that cervical cancer has many of the characteristics of a sexually transmitted disease. The observations that the disease is much more frequent in married women than in celibate women, that it was more common in prostitutes and incarcerated women than in the general population, and that it was highly associated with a woman's lifetime number of male sexual partners all argue for venereal transmission. The fact that a woman's risk is increased not only by the number of sexual partners that she has had, but also by the number of sexual partners that her male partner or partners has had, strengthens the epidemiologic evidence that cervical cancer behaves as a sexually transmitted disease (44). With so much evidence favoring the sexual transmission of cervical cancer, many investigators have searched for an etiologic agent among the known sexually transmitted diseases.

Virtually every known sexually transmitted infection has been suggested as the etiologic agent for cervical cancer and, in more recent times, for cervical cancer precursors. The list includes *Treponema pallidum, Trichomonas vaginalis, Candida albicans, Chlamydia trachomatis*, and the herpes simplex viruses (HSV). There is now considerable evidence for a role for both *C. trachomatis* and HSV as cofactors in the pathogenesis of HPV-associated cervical neoplasia. One recent case-control study found that among HPV-infected women there was a two-fold risk for cervical cancer associated with having antibodies to *C. trachomatis* (45). This risk is similar

TABLE 19.6

RISK FACTORS FOR CERVICAL CANCER AND ITS PRECURSOR LESIONS

DEMOGRAPHIC FACTORS
Older age
Race (e.g., black, Hispanic, American Indian)
Residence in selected parts of Africa, Asia, or Latin America
Low socioeconomic status
Low educational level
BEHAVIORAL AND SEXUAL FACTORS
Large number of sexual partners
Early age at first coitus
Cigarette smoking
Long-term contraceptive use
Diet low in folate, carotene
MEDICAL/GYNECOLOGIC FACTORS
Multiparity
Early age at first pregnancy
History of sexually transmitted diseases (especially herpes genitalis or HPV-associated lesions)
Lack of routine cytologic screening
Immunosuppression (any cause)
Specific HLA-DR haplotypes

to the 2.5-fold increased risk observed with seroconversion in a prospective seroepidemiologic study (46). The prevalence of antibodies to HSV is also increased among women with cervical cancer. Smith et al. performed a pooled analysis of clinical samples from seven case-control studies of cervical cancer. After adjusting for HPV status and sexual behavior, HSV seropositivity was associated with an approximately twofold increased risk of cervical cancer (45). It has been suggested that both *C. trachomatis* and HSV act as cofactors in HPV-associated neoplasia, possibly through the induction of cervical inflammation (47).

Human Papillomavirus

Over the last 15 years, considerable evidence has been accumulating rapidly to implicate HPV in the pathogenesis of cervical cancer and its preinvasive precursors. Epidemiologic and molecular studies have found that there is a consistent and strong relationship between HPV infection and cervical neoplasia, that the temporal sequence between infection and the development of cancer is correct, that the association between HPV and cervical cancer is relatively specific, and that the epidemiologic findings are consistent with the natural history and biologic behavior of HPV infections and cervical cancer (48).

Studies that use sensitive molecular methods to detect and type HPV in cervical lesions have found that almost all cervical cancers and their precursors contain "high-risk" HPV DNA. For example, in a large study that analyzed over 1,000 invasive cervical cancers from all over the world using polymerase chain reaction (PCR), high-risk types of HPV were identified in over 90% of the invasive cervical cancers (49). Morevover, the same types of HPV were identified in cancers from all different geographic locations. When cases that were initially classified as HPV DNA negative were re-tested with PCR methods, high-risk HPV types were identified in almost all (50). This indicates that essentially all cervical cancers are caused by specific high-risk types of HPV.

Large case-control studies have identified HPV infection as a risk factor in the development of CIN and cervical cancer. For example, a recent pooled analysis of data from 11 case-control studies shows that HPV was detected in 1,739 of 1,918 patients with cervical cancer (91%) compared to 259 of 1,928 control women (13%). The pooled odds ratio for cervical cancer associated with any HPV type was 158 (51). Prospective studies indicate that the temporal sequence between HPV infection and the development of cancer is what would be expected for a causal agent. HPV infection occurs first and high-grade cervical cancer precursors or cancer occur subsequently. For example, in a study of colposcopically negative women in New York City, the incidence of CIN was significantly higher in women who were HPV-16 or -18 DNA positive compared to those who lacked "high-risk" HPV DNA (52). Moreover, persistent infection with "high-risk" types of HPV was much more closely linked with the subsequent development of CIN 2,3 than was detection of high-risk HPV DNA at a single visit. In a recent study of college students it was found that over a 3-year period, 27% of those with incident HPV-16 or -18 infections developed CIN 2,3 lesions, whereas no CIN 2,3 lesions developed in HPV DNA negative women (38).

Taken together, these epidemiologic studies clearly demonstrate that there is a strong and consistent association between specific types of HPV DNA and invasive cervical cancer and its precursor lesions, and that exposure to HPV precedes the development of cervical disease. When combined with the enormous body of molecular evidence demonstrating a role for HPV in the development of cervical cancer and CIN, these findings clearly indicate that HPV infection, acquired through sexual contact, is a "necessary cause" of both CIN and invasive cervical cancer (53,54). Based on this data, the International Agency for Research on Cancer (IARC) of the WHO has classified HPV-16 and -18 and all of the other "high-risk" types of HPV as carcinogens in humans (55).

Smoking, Diet, and Oral Contraceptives

In addition to risk factors associated with sexual behavior, several other risk factors such as low socioeconomic class and cigarette smoking have also been associated with the development of cervical cancer (44). In a comprehensive review of the literature, Szarewski and Cuzick concluded that a positive association between cigarette smoking and the development of cervical cancer had been reported by the majority of studies designed to address this question (56). Several mechanisms could account for the association between cigarette smoking and cervical cancer. One is the secretion of cigarette smoke by-products, including nicotine and cotinine, in cervical mucous of tobacco users and women passively exposed to cigarette smoke (57). DNA adducts (e.g., structurally altered DNA sequences) are significantly more common in the cervical epithelium of smokers than in nonsmokers, and it has been suggested that the secretion of cigarette smoke by-products might have a direct mutagenic effect on the cervical epithelium (58). Another possible mechanism that could account for the association is the effect of smoke by-products on the number of Langerhan's cells in the cervix (59).

The use of combined oral contraceptives has also been found to be a risk factor for the development of cervical cancer and its precursors in some studies. In a meta-analysis of 28 studies evaluating the risk of cervical cancer in women on oral contraceptives, Smith et al. found that the relative risk of invasive cervical cancer increased with increasing duration of contraceptive use. After 10 years of use, the summary relative risks were 2.2 (95% CI, 1.9 to 2.2) for all women and 2.5 (95% CI, 1.6 to 3.9) for HPV-positive women (60). A recent reanalysis of epidemiologic studies involving over 50,000 women confirmed an increased risk of cervical cancer in oral contraceptive users (61). Associations between exogenous hormones and cervical disease could be explained by a number of mechanisms including direct promoting effects of estrogens and progestins on the HPV genome, as well as by indirect effects such as a reduction in blood folate levels, which is occasionally observed in women on oral contraceptives. Whether an association exists between endogenous hormone levels and invasive cervical cancer is even more controversial. There is no association between age at menarche or age at menopause and the risk of invasive cervical squamous cell carcinoma. It has been suggested that the strong association observed between early age of first parity and risk for cervical cancer reflects risk of exposure to a sexually transmitted agent at an early age, rather than an influence of endogenous hormones (62).

Only a few studies have focused on relationships between cervical cancer and diet, but some evidence suggests that a diet low in either vitamin A or C may be associated with an increased risk. Other studies have not detected an association between dietary intake of beta-carotene or retinol and CIN. A recent review of the role of antioxidant nutrients on cervical disease concluded that there are six studies that have properly controlled for HPV (47). In all six, an inverse relationship was observed between serum beta-carotene and cervical carcinogenesis. In studies that measured carotenoids other than beta-carotene, inverse associations between cervical neoplasia and serum lycopene and alpha-carotene have been observed (47). Folate deficiency has also been considered to be a risk factor. A recent case-control study reported that folate deficiency enhances the effects of other risk factors such as parity, HPV-16 infection, and cigarette smoking on the development of CIN (63).

Immunosuppression

Immunosuppression is another risk factor for the development of both CIN and cervical cancer. In studies of patients with renal transplants, transplant recipients have a relative risk of 13.6 for the development of cervical carcinoma *in situ* compared to women in the general population (64). Over the last decade it has become widely accepted that there is also an association between cervical disease and infection with the human immunodeficiency virus (HIV) (64). HPV infections are more prevalent and tend to be more persistent in HIV-infected women (65). Numerous studies have documented a higher prevalence of cervical neoplasia among HIV-infected women compared to various control groups of HIV-uninfected women (64). There also appears to be an increase in invasive cervical cancer. Among women in New York City, the standardized incidence ratio for cervical cancer is 9.2 times higher in HIV-infected compared to noninfected women (66). It is clear that the invasive cervical cancers that do develop in HIV-infected women act aggressively and respond poorly to standard forms of therapy (67). Invasive cervical cancer was designated in 1993 as an AIDS case-defining illness by the CDC (68).

HUMAN PAPILLOMAVIRUS

Classification

Papillomaviruses are a diverse group of viruses that are widely distributed in mammals and birds. Papillomavirus isolates are traditionally described as *types*. The characteristic features of papillomaviruses are a double-stranded, circular DNA genome of about 8,000 base pairs, a nonenveloped virion, and an icosahedral capsid composed of 72 capsomers. The papillomaviruses are now classified as a separate family of viruses termed Papillomavaviridae. To date 118 papillomavirus types have been completely described. Papillomaviruses are highly species specific and are classified based on their species of origin and the extent of DNA relatedness between viral isolates. Human papillomaviruses are epitheliotropic. They infect epithelial cells of the skin and mucous membranes, often producing local epithelial proliferation or warts at the sites of infection. There has been only limited success in propagating HPV in either tissue or culture.

Within a given species, many types and subtypes of papillomaviruses may exist. Since the capsid proteins of different papillomaviruses are antigenically similar, papillomaviruses are subdivided into genotypes and subtypes based on the extent of DNA relatedness as determined by DNA hybridization under stringent conditions, rather than into serotypes based on structural antigenic features. In order to be classified as a distinct type, the E6, E7, and L1 gene sequences (about one third of the genome) must differ by more than 10% from those of other, known HPV types. In addition to types, there also are subtypes or variants of specific types. In order to be considered a subtype or variant, the different viruses must differ by 2% to 5% from the original isolate. In humans, more than 100 types of papillomaviruses have been characterized. Although the different types are structurally similar, they have significant specificity with regard to the anatomic location of the epithelia that they infect and the type of lesions that they produce at the site of infection (69). For example, HPV types 1, 2, 4, 26, 27, 29, 41, and 57 are associated with common warts (verrucae vulgaris); types 1, 2, and 4 with deep plantar warts; and type 7 with common warts on the hands of meat handlers (butcher's warts). HPV types 5, 8, 9, 12, 14, and others are associated with flat warts and cancers in patients with epidermodysplasia verruciformis, which is a rare, heritable, lifelong skin disease characterized by the development of multiple flat warts throughout life. These warts may progress to skin cancer.

Over 30 types of HPV that infect the anogenital tract have been described (Table 19.7). These different types of HPV tend to be associated with different types of lesions. HPV-6 is the most common HPV type found in association with exophytic condylomata of the male and female anogenital tract in adults (70). Most exophytic condylomata that are not associated with HPV-6 are associated with HPV-11. Exophytic condylomata are occasionally associated with HPV types 16 or 31, but are almost never found in association with HPV-18. In adults, cutaneous HPV types such as HPV-1 or -2 are seldom associated with exophytic condylomata. However, a significant proportion of condylomata acuminata in children are associated with HPV-2, which is a common cutaneous HPV type (71). Small, raised, plaque-type warts on the penis are also commonly associated with "low-risk" HPV types (72).

More than 80% of CIN lesions are found to be associated with HPV when sensitive, molecular methods are used to detect HPV DNA. CIN 1 is quite heterogeneous with regard to associated HPV types (7,73). CIN 1 can be associated with any of the anogenital HPV types that have been identified in women in the general population. Although studies performed in the mid-1980s indicated that HPV-6 and -11 were the predominant types of HPV associated with CIN 1, subsequent studies have detected HPV-6 and -11 in less than 10% of CIN 1 lesions. HPV-16 and -18, combined, are detected in about one third of all CIN 1 lesions. Multiple types of HPV are often identified in women with CIN 1 (74).

In contrast to CIN 1, almost half of all CIN 2,3 lesions are associated with HPV-16 (7,75). The prevalence of HPV-16 in women with high-grade SIL (CIN 2,3) varies from 30% to 77% in different studies. A meta-analysis of the distribution of HPV types in CIN 2,3 lesions recently concluded that HPV-16 is identified in 45.3%, HPV-18 in 6.9%, and HPV-31 in 8.6% (Fig. 19.2) (75). Fifty-two percent of CIN 2,3 lesions are associated with either HPV-16 or -18. HPV types 31, 33, 58, and 52 are the next most common types found in CIN 2,3. Multiple types of HPV are uncommonly detected in women with CIN 2,3 (74). The associations between specific types of HPV and invasive cervical cancers are similar to those observed in women with CIN 2,3 (Fig. 19.2) (7,75). HPV-16 is

TABLE 19.7

CLASSIFICATION OF ANOGENITAL HPV TYPES

"Low-risk" types	6, 11, 40, 42, 43, 44, 53[a], 54, 61, 72, 81
"High-risk" types	16, 18, 31, 33, 35, 39, 45, 51, 52, 56, 58, 59, 68, 82
Possible high-risk types	26, 66, 73

[a]Classified as "low-risk" based on other data.
Source: From Munoz N, Bosch FX, de Sanjose S, et al. Epidemiologic classification of human papillomavirus types associated with cervical cancer. *N Engl J Med* 2003;348:518–527.

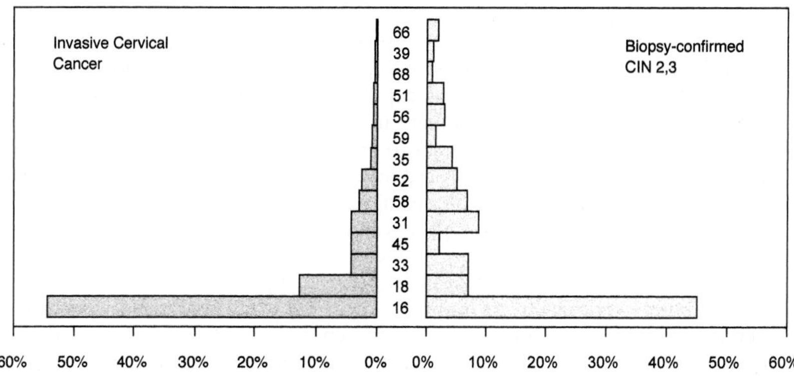

FIGURE 19.2. Distribution of HPV types determined by PCR in cases of invasive cervical cancer and biopsy-confirmed CIN 2,3. *Source:* Modified from Smith JS, Lindsay L, Hoots B, et al. Human papillomavirus type distribution in invasive cervical cancer and high-grade cervical lesions: a meta-analysis update. *Int J Cancer* 2007;121:621–632.

the most common HPV type found in association with invasive cervical squamous cell carcinomas, and HPV-18 is the second most common. All other types are much less commonly found.

Based on their associations with benign epithelial proliferations, high-grade cancer precursors, or invasive cancers of the vulva, vagina, anus, and cervix, human papillomaviruses have been categorized into three groups: "high-risk" viruses that are classified as "high risk" because infection with these HPV types is associated with a high relative risk of cancer; "low-risk" viruses that are associated with a relatively low risk of invasive cervical cancer; and "possible high-risk" types that are occasionally associated with cervical cancer (Table 19.7) (51). It is important to recognize that all of the 30 different types of anogenital HPV have been isolated from cervicovaginal secretions of women lacking any colposcopic or cytologic evidence of cervical disease. The most common HPV types detected in women with no cytologic evidence of cervical disease include high-risk types such as 16, 51, 52, 31, 58, and 56 (76–78).

Genomic Organization

The overall genomic organization of all sequenced HPV types is similar. The genome contains eight open reading frames (ORFs) that are transcribed from a single DNA strand as a polycistronic message (Fig. 19.3). ORFs are DNA segments that are transcriptional units and have the capacity to encode protein. The viral DNA can be divided into three regions. First, there is an upstream regulatory region (URR) of about 400 base pairs that contains binding sites for transcriptional activators and repressors. This region plays a role in regulating the production of viral proteins and infectious particles and possibly plays a central role in determining the host range of specific types of HPV (79,80). Transcriptional control appears to be quite complex, involving multiple promoters and repressors and binding sites for a number of transcriptional factors.

Downstream of the URR is the early region. The early region encodes for proteins that play a fundamental role in viral infection and replication. Within the early region are six ORFs designated E1, E2, E4, E5, E6, and E7. The E6 and E7 ORFs are important in the immortalizing and transforming functions of HPV (81). E1 encodes the only virally encoded enzyme, an adenosine 5′-triphosphate (ATP)-dependent helicase that is required for extrachromosomal DNA replication (79,80). The E2 protein has important transcriptional regulatory activities (82). Together with E1, E2 is also required for extrachromosomal DNA replication to occur—a fundamental role in viral infection and replication. E2 also acts as a key regulator of transcription of the E6 and E7 ORFs. The E4 protein has many characteristics of a structural viral protein and is similar to the protein products of the late region (83). Like the L1 and L2 capsid proteins, the E4 protein is expressed during the late stages of the viral life cycle at a time when complete virions are being produced. The E4 protein is thought to disrupt the normal intermediate filament matrix of infected epithelial cells and disrupt the cornified cell envelope. This is thought to facilitate the release of assembled virions from the infected epithelium and to produce the characteristic cytopathic infection (e.g., "koilocytosis") (79). E5 appears to play a role in the early course of infection. E5 is a short transmembrane protein that stimulates cell growth by forming complexes with epidermal growth factor receptor, platelet-derived growth factor receptor, and colony stimulating factor-1 receptor (80). Unlike E6 and E7, which are required for the development of cervical cancer, E5 is often lost during the development of cervical cancers.

The late region is downstream of the early region and includes two ORFs: L1, which encodes for the major capsid protein, and L2, which encodes for the minor capsid protein. The L1 major capsid protein is highly conserved among papillomaviruses of all species and serves as a convenient source of

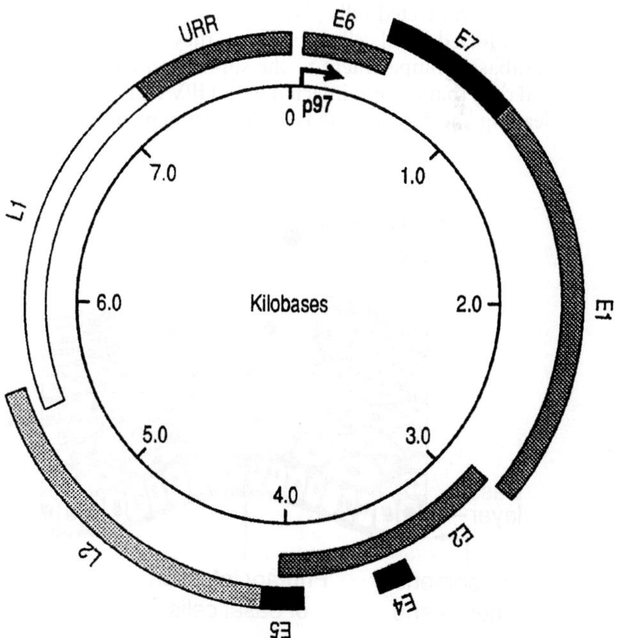

FIGURE 19.3. Schematic of genomic organization of HPV. *Source:* Reprinted with permission from Wright TC, Ferenczy AF, Kurman RJ. Precancerous lesions of the cervix. In: Kurman RJ, ed. *Balustein's Pathology of the Female Genital Tract.* 4th ed. New York: Spring-Verlag; 1994:229–241.

antigen for the production of antibodies to the papillomavirus. The minor capsid protein, L2, shows considerable sequence variation between different types of HPV and has been used as an antigen for the production of type-specific antibodies to HPV. Expression of L1 and L2 capsid proteins occurs late during the viral life cycle and coincides with the production of complete virions (84). Expression of L1 and L2 capsid proteins is post-transcriptionally regulated by cell-derived factors and occurs only in superficial and intermediate squamous epithelial cells. This helps explain why virion production and the resultant cytopathic effect of HPV infection are pronounced in CIN 1 and in condyloma acuminatum, but are less pronounced in CIN 2,3 and invasive cancer, which contain fewer differentiated cells. The current generation of prophylactic HPV vaccines is composed of L1 proteins that have been induced to fold into viral-like particles (VLPs) (85).

HPV Life Cycle

The life cycle of HPV infections is tightly coupled with the differentiation of the stratified epithelium that is the target of infection. Unlike any other known virus families, infection requires access to the actively proliferating basal cells of the epithelium (Fig. 19.4) (86). This occurs usually at sites of microtrauma to the epithelium. Binding of HPV to the basal cells appears to involve interactions with cell surface–associated alpha 6 integrin that may act as the receptor for binding and entry into the cells (87). After HPV has entered into the basal cell, the viral genome undergoes limited replication. Within the basal cells, replication of the HPV genome is tightly controlled by cellular mechanisms and appears to be linked to cellular replication so that the viral DNA co-replicates with the host's genome. Therefore, the HPV genome is maintained at a relatively low copy number in the basal cell's nucleus as a circular or episomal form, and virally encoded proteins are expressed at very low levels. As a result, HPV-infected basal cells show no specific cytologic or histologic changes and cannot be distinguished from uninfected cells (81).

As the infected basal cells proliferate, they migrate from the basal/parabasal compartment to the suprabasal compartment. Epithelial cells that are not infected with HPV exit the cell cycle when leaving the basal/parabasal compartment. However, in order to replicate in the differentiating epithelial cells, the virus needs to reactivate the cellular DNA replication machinery. Studies of cultured human keratinocytes have shown that the viral E7 protein is capable of reactivating the cellular DNA replication machinery in differentiated cells (88). The viral E6 protein also appears to play an important role by blocking the apoptosis that would normally occur in the differentiated cells (89). Together, these changes provide the S-phase environment necessary for vegetative viral DNA replication and complete virion formation. Coincident with the assembly of large numbers of infectious virions, the typical HPV-associated cytopathic effects occur. The cytopathic effects are most prominent in the upper layers of the epithelium and include multinucleation, nuclear enlargement, hyperchromasia, and regions of perinuclear clearing or halos (i.e., koilocytes).

Transforming Functions of HPV

HPV E7 Oncoprotein

Characterization of the regions of the HPV genome responsible for the immortalizing and transforming functions of "high-risk" HPV types indicates that both functions reside predominantly in the E6/E7 ORFs. Phylogenetic comparisons of the E5 genes of different HPVs show a correlation between DNA sequence and a type's capacity to form tumors, suggesting that E5 may play a role in carcinogenicity (90). The E6/E7 ORFs of HPV-16 and -18 encode for several distinct proteins. The E7 protein is the major transforming and immortalizing activity of HPV (81,83). E7 is a small zinc-binding protein composed of approximately 100 amino acids that is phosphorylated in the native state and lacks enzymatic activity. The HPV-16 E7 gene product can cooperate with activated *ras* oncogenes for transformation and contains a consensus sequence for casein kinase II–mediated serine phosphorylation and a binding site for the product of the retinoblastoma (*Rb*) gene, as well as the structurally related "Rb-like pocket proteins," p130 and p10 (88). These proteins (Rb, p130, and p107) all play an important role in regulating cell proliferation.

Although the exact mechanism of action of E7 within cells has not been fully worked out, it is clear that the binding of

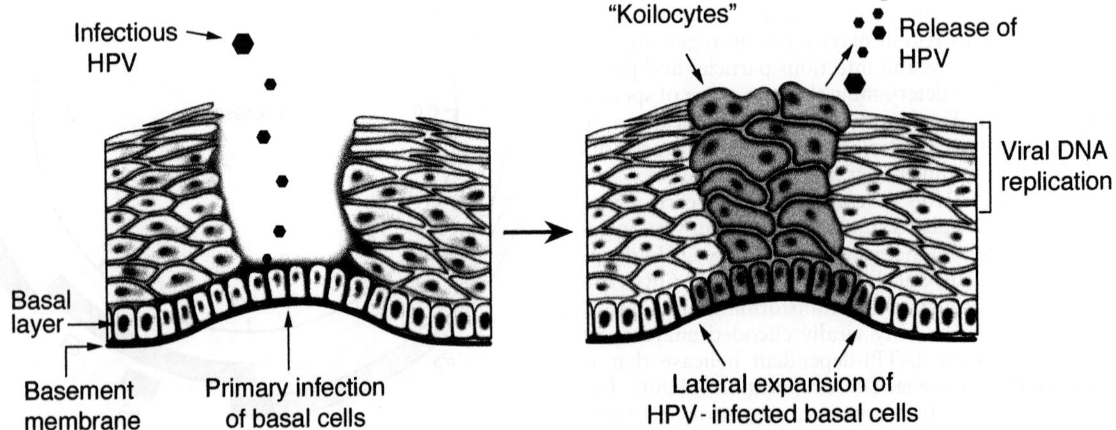

FIGURE 19.4. Life cycle of HPV infections. HPV infects cells of the basal layer where it exists in a low copy number in episomal form. It is thought that basal cells become exposed to HPV after microabrasions occur in the epithelium. Basal cells infected with HPV have a proliferative advantage and expand laterally. As HPV-infected cells progress through the more differentiated layers of the epithelium, viral replication is turned on and large numbers of copies of HPV DNA are produced. Late genes, including the viral capsid, are produced in the most superficial layers of the epithelium and infectious virions are assembled. This produces the characteristic cytopathic effects of HPV (e.g., koilocytosis).

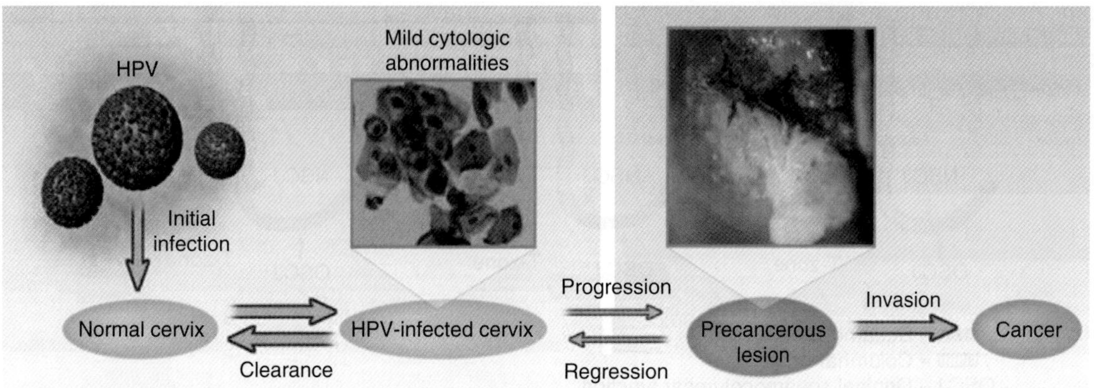

FIGURE 19.6. Natural history of HPV infections. *Source:* Adapted from Wright TC Jr, Schiffman M. Adding a test for human papillomavirus DNA to cervical-cancer screening. *N Engl J Med* 2003;348(6):489–490.

could also explain the increase in prevalence of HPV among cytologically negative older women (Fig. 19.5). The clinical significance of reactivation of latent infections in older women is probably minimal since the risk for CIN 2,3 or cancer among previously well-screened older women is quite low.

There is no accepted definition of what constitutes a clinically significant, persistent infection. Although spontaneous clearance can continue to occur even after 24 months, clinically significant, persistent infections should probably be defined as infections that last at least 2 years. Long-term, stable, persistent infections appear to occur in only about 10% of infected individuals (117). Since prevalence of infection in a population is determined by both the rate of new infections in the population and the rate of clearance of the infection, those HPV types that are most likely to become persistent will also tend to be the most commonly detected ones in the population. Persistent infections are the only clinically significant HPV infections since these are the only ones that can produce high-grade precursors that can progress to invasive cancers. Although newer studies suggest that CIN 2,3 lesions can develop within a relatively short period of time after initial infection, lesions that do not persist for at least 2 years are unlikely to have clinical significance.

PATHOLOGY OF PREINVASIVE LESIONS OF THE LOWER GENITAL TRACT

Cervix

Localization of CIN

The use of colposcopy to identify CIN and careful microscopic studies of the distribution of CIN in conization and hysterectomy specimens have greatly increased our knowledge of the clinical appearance and distribution of CIN. Colposcopic and histologic mapping studies of the position of CIN have shown that the vast majority of lesions develop in a region of the cervix called the *transformation zone*. At the time of menarche, most young women have some endocervical-type columnar epithelium present on the portio (vaginal portion) of the cervix. This endocervical-type epithelium appears salmon red to the naked eye and has been referred to as *cervical erosion, ectropion, cervical ectopy,* or *native columnar epithelium.* In response to a variety of stimuli including low

TABLE 19.8

PREVALENCE AND CUMULATIVE DETECTION RATES OF HPV IN YOUNG WOMEN

Author	No. of patients	Mean age	Type of infection	% Persistent at 6 mo	12 mo	24 mo
Sun et al.	231	34 yr	Incident and prevalent	50%	35%	18%
Ho et al.	608	20 yr	Incident	—	30%	8%
Moscicki et al.	618	20 yr	Prevalent	50%	30%	10%
Woodman et al.	1,075	20 yr	Incident	24%	4%	<1%
Richardson et al.	635	23 yr	Incident	—	62%	—

Sources: Adapted from Sun XW, Kuhn L, Ellerbrock TV, et al. Human papillomavirus infection in women infected with the human immunodeficiency virus. *N Engl J Med* 1997;337:1343; Ho GY, Bierman R, Beardsley L, et al. Natural history of cervicovaginal papillomavirus infection in young women. *N Engl J Med* 1998;338:423; Moscicki AB, Hills N, Shiboski S, et al. Risks for incident human papillomavirus infection and low-grade squamous intraepithelial lesion development in young females. *JAMA* 2001;285:2995; Woodman CB, Collins S, Winter H, et al. Natural history of cervical human papillomavirus infection in young women: a longitudinal cohort study. Lancet 2001;357:1831; Richardson H, Kelsall G, Tellier P, et al. The natural history of type-specific human papillomavirus infections in female university students. *Cancer Epidemiol Biomarkers Prev* 2003;12:485.

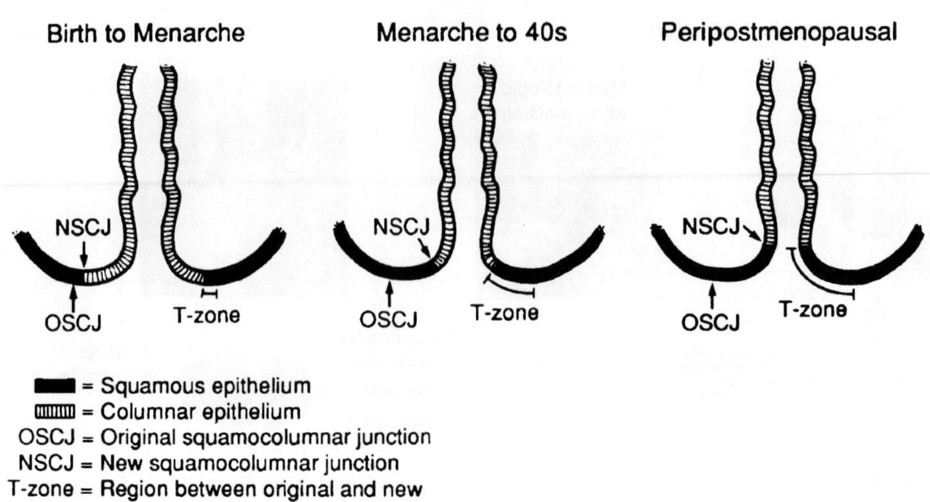

FIGURE 19.7. Impact of age on the location of the squamocolumnar junction. As females age, the location of the squamocolumnar junction on the cervix moves. The movement of the squamocolumnar junction defines the transformation zone.

pH, trauma, hormonal factors, and cervicovaginal infections, shortly after menarche the columnar epithelium gradually becomes replaced by a stratified squamous epithelium (Fig. 19.7). The replacement of columnar epithelium by a stratified squamous epithelium occurs by two different processes. One is called *squamous metaplasia* and the other is the direct ingrowth of squamous epithelium from the periphery of the portio, referred to as *epidermidization*. As these processes occur, the histologic junction between stratified squamous epithelium and endocervical-type columnar epithelium moves inward toward the external cervical os. By the age of 40 in most women the entire portio is covered by mature squamous epithelium.

The transformation zone is defined as the region of the cervix that lies between the original squamocolumnar junction and the current or anatomic squamocolumnar junction (Fig. 19.7). The transformation zone is of critical importance in cervical pathology and colposcopy because it is the site at which CIN usually develops as well as the major locus for cervical carcinomas. Although CIN often extends into the endocervical canal, it rarely extends out onto the native squamous epithelium of the portio. The mechanisms responsible for the restricted distribution of CIN on the cervix are unknown.

Origin of CIN

The majority of CIN arises in the transformation zone with one margin adjacent to the current squamocolumnar junction. Therefore, it would appear that the cell of origin of the majority of CIN is the basal cell of squamous metaplasia. The recent demonstration that alpha 6 integrin is a possible receptor for HPV supports this model since alpha 6 integrin is only expressed in basal cells and epidermal stem cells (87). Over the years, there has been some controversy as to whether CIN develops from a single focus or cell and then enlarges centrifugally over the cervix, or whether it can develop as a field effect from multiple foci. CIN 1 frequently develops from a latently-infected cervical epithelium, is often associated with multiple types of HPV, and has many of the features of a productive viral infection rather than a neoplasm. Therefore, it might be predicted that these lesions would be polyclonal in origin. Using more modern molecular techniques, Park et al. found that CIN 1 associated with "non-high-risk" HPV types are typically polyclonal, whereas CIN 1 associated with "high-risk" HPV types are typically monoclonal, as are almost all CIN 2,3 lesions (120). This indicates that CIN 1 associated with low-risk types of HPV are biologically different at their inception from lesions that are histologically low grade but associated with "high-risk" HPV types. There is now data to suggest that some CIN 2,3 lesions develop *de novo* without a preexisting CIN 1 (121,122). In a study of 54 cytologically negative women who were HPV-16 DNA positive, 17 (31%) developed CIN on follow-up and 41% of the incident cases were first identified as CIN 3 (122). In the recent HPV vaccine trials, some CIN 3 lesions developed very quickly after initial infection with HPV-16 and did not appear to go through a low-grade precursor phase (39).

Microscopic Appearance of CIN

The two histologic hallmarks of CIN, regardless of grade, are the presence of nuclear atypia and aberrant cytoplasmic differentiation. Nuclear atypia in CIN can take many forms. In most cases, the nuclei become enlarged and an increase in the nuclear-cytoplasmic ratio occurs. The extent of nuclear enlargement usually varies from cell to cell, leading to an irregular appearance of the epithelium. Multinucleation also often occurs. The nuclei of cells in CIN are usually hyperchromatic, and the chromatin is coarsely clumped. The nuclear outline is sometimes irregular and angulated rather than round.

Aberrant cytoplasmic differentiation is also invariably found in CIN, irrespective of grade. The normal, stratified, squamous epithelium of the cervix can be divided into three layers (Fig. 19.8). The basal layer is composed of a single layer of cells that is in contact with the basement membrane. The parabasal layer is the proliferative compartment and is one to two cell layers thick. This is the site at which mitoses are observed in the normal cervix. As cells leave the parabasal layer, they become progressively more mature and develop cytoplasmic flattening. Squamous intraepithelial lesions have aberrant differentiation and deviate from this normal pattern. The extent and type of aberrant differentiation varies greatly from lesion to lesion. In the original CIN terminology, lesions were graded 1 to 3 based on the extent to which the epithelium was replaced by undifferentiated basaloid cells. Lesions were classified as follows: CIN 1 if

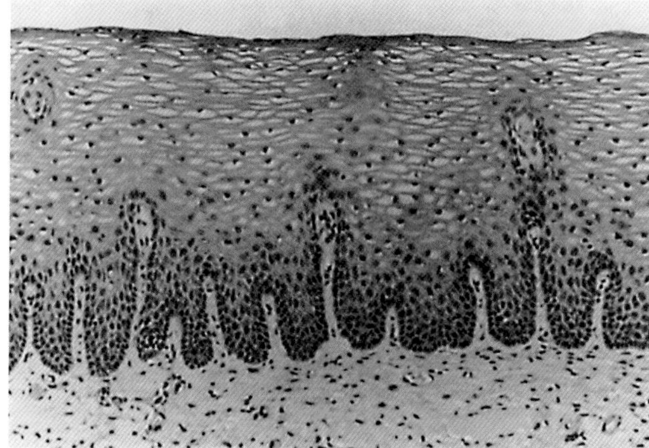

FIGURE 19.8. Normal statified squamous epithelium of the cervix.

the undifferentiated cells involved only the lower third of the epithelium (Fig. 19.9A); CIN 2 if undifferentiated cells and mitoses were present up to two thirds of the way through the epithelium (Fig. 19.9B); and CIN 3 if they extended through more than two thirds of the epithelium (Fig. 19.9C).

In CIN 1, HPV cytopathic effect is usually a prominent feature and immature basaloid cells and mitotic figures are restricted to the lower third of the epithelium. The cytopathic effect of HPV can best be described as the formation of a region of perinuclear clearing or vacuolization (Fig. 19.10). Cells with a combination of nuclear atypia and perinuclear clearing are called *koilocytes*, a term derived from the Greek word *koilos*, which means hollow or empty. Not all cells with perinuclear clearing are HPV infected. The presence of perinuclear clearing, or halos, in cells without significant nuclear atypia is seen in a variety of nonneoplastic disorders as well as HPV infections. These disorders include infections with *Trichomonas* organisms, *Gardnerella vaginalis*, and *Candida* organisms. In addition, perinuclear clearing can occasionally be a feature of the atrophic epithelial changes found in postmenopausal patients or in immature squamous metaplasia. Before the recognition that all CIN are associated with HPV infections, cervical condylomata and CIN 1 were generally classified as separate histopathologic entities. With the widespread application of HPV typing to cervical lesions, it has become evident that it is impossible to distinguish on histologic grounds alone between flat cervical condylomata and CIN 1 lesions associated with "low-risk" HPV types and those associated with "high-risk" HPV types (5). Since clinical and histologic criteria do not allow segregation of low-grade lesions on the basis of oncogenic potential, distinctions between flat cervical condylomata and low-grade CIN 1 lesions are no longer clinically meaningful and have been dropped from the Bethesda terminology.

Although HPV-induced cytopathic effects are often present, they are usually less prominent in CIN 2,3 than in CIN 1. CIN 2,3 is characterized by immature basaloid cells and mitotic figures that extend into the upper two thirds of the epithelium. The immature basaloid cells usually have nuclear crowding, pleomorphism, and loss of normal cell polarity. Cytoplasm is usually minimal, which results in a high nuclear-to-cytoplasmic ratio. Another feature found in most high-grade lesions is abnormal mitotic figures (Fig. 19.11). Most squamous cell carcinomas of the cervix have chromosomal abnormalities, and many are aneuploid. This suggests that aneuploid precursor lesions are highly significant and may

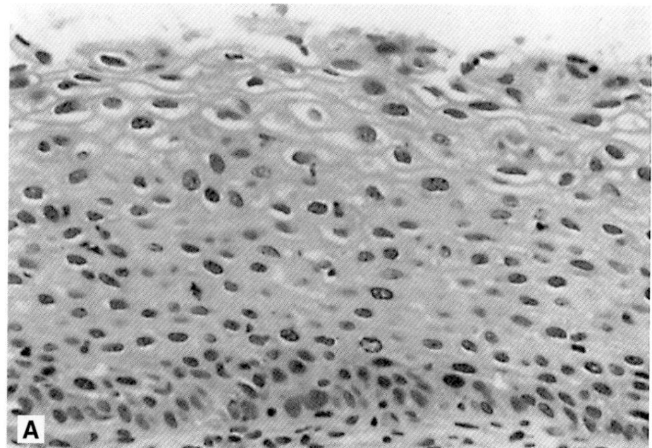

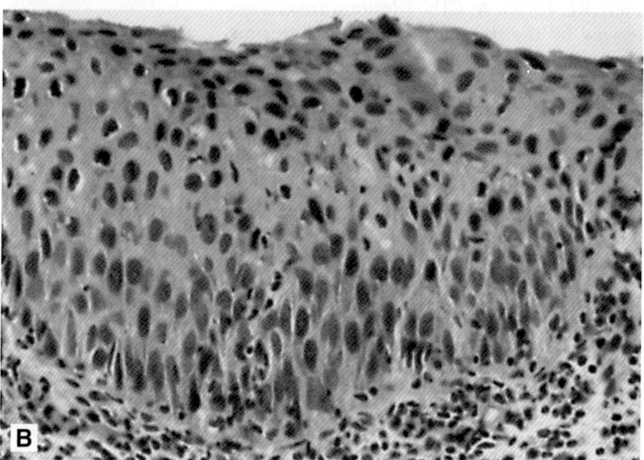

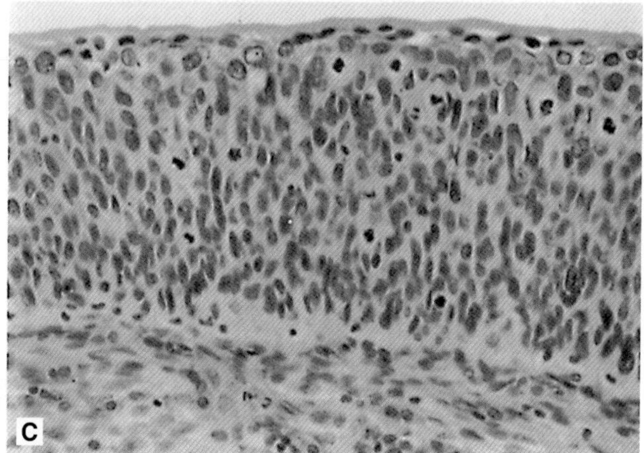

FIGURE 19.9. Histology of (A) CIN 1, (B) CIN 2, (C) CIN 3.

have the capacity to progress to an invasive carcinoma if left untreated. Support for such a hypothesis comes from studies that have documented that the percentage of aneuploid CIN lesions increases as the grade of the lesion increases (9). The best histologic predictor of an aneuploid lesion is the presence of abnormal mitotic figures.

Microscopic Appearance of Endocervical Glandular Atypia and Adenocarcinoma *In Situ*

Both endocervical glandular atypia and adenocarcinoma *in situ* of the endocervix are characterized by endocervical

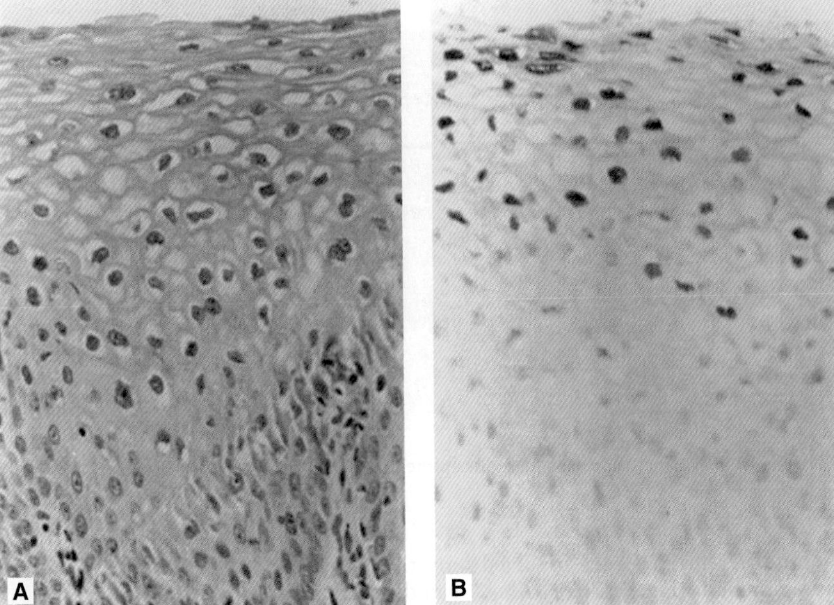

FIGURE 19.10. A: CIN 1 lesions are characterized by the presence of cells with perinuclear halos and nuclear atypia. B: *In situ* hybridization of a CIN 1 lesion using probes for HPV-16/18 defects HPV DNA appearing as dark staining of the nuclei of the superficial cells.

glands that are lined by atypical glandular cells and lack evidence of stromal invasion (Fig. 19.12A). In both lesions, individual endocervical cells have many of the histologic and cytologic features of invasive adenocarcinoma. The atypical endocervical cells are enlarged with hyperchromatic, elongated nuclei (Fig. 19.12B). Characteristically, the chromatin pattern is coarse and granular. There is a reduction in the amount of cytoplasm and only minimal intracellular mucin is present. A characteristic feature of both endocervical glandular atypia and adenocarcinoma *in situ* is crowding of the cells and pseudostratification. Abrupt transitions between involved and uninvolved epithelium are frequently observed.

Endocervical glandular atypia and adenocarcinoma *in situ* are differentiated from each other by their relative degrees of mitotic activity and pseudostratification. Mitotic figures are quite common and atypical mitotic figures are frequently observed in adenocarcinoma *in situ*. There is marked pseudostratification of the endocervical cells that form two or three cell layers. This results in cribriforming and complex papillary infoldings of the epithelium into the gland lumens. In contrast, mitotic figures are relatively uncommon in endocervical glandular atypia, and the atypical endocervical cells are not pseudostratified. Instead they form a single row of cells. Cribriforming and papillary infoldings are also infrequent in endocervical glandular atypia.

Architectural features are used to distinguish between adenocarcinoma *in situ* and invasive endocervical adenocarcinoma. Invasion is diagnosed when atypical glands extend beyond the depth of the normal, uninvolved endocervical glands. This is usually approximately 5 to 6 mm from the surface. Features suggestive of invasion include desmoplasia or stromal reaction around the involved glands, exuberant gland budding, back-to-back glands, and papillary projections from the endocervical surface.

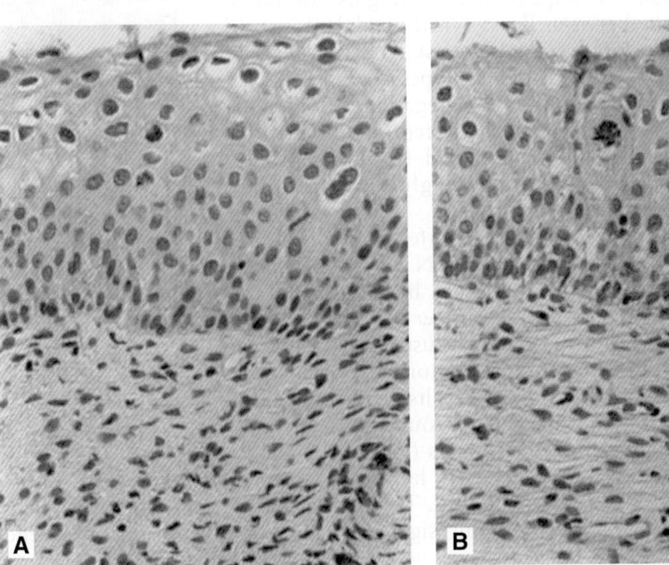

FIGURE 19.11. Histology of (A) CIN 1 that lacks abnormal mitotic figures and (B) CIN 2,3 that is classified as high-grade because it contains abnormal mitotic figures.

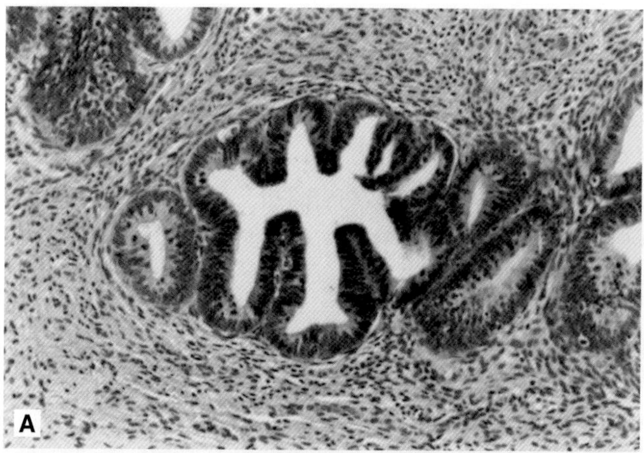

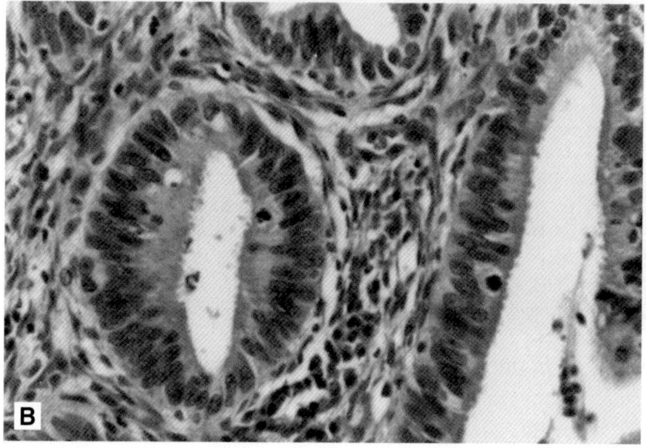

FIGURE 19.12. Adenocarcinoma *in situ* of the cervix. **A:** Adenocarcinoma *in situ* is characterized by glands lined by atypical endocervical cells that frequently form papillary projections into the glandular lumen. **B:** At higher magnification, the endocervical cells are pseudostratified and there are numerous mitotic figures.

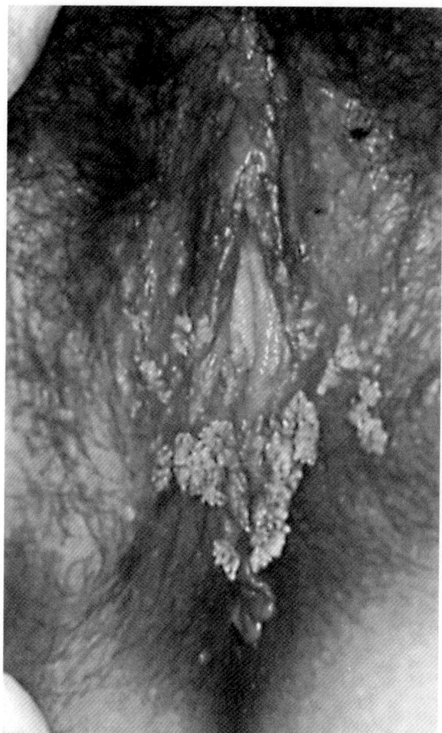

FIGURE 19.13. Gross features of vulvar condyloma acuminatum. *Source:* Used with permission courtesy of Dr. D. Townsend, University of California. From Wright TC, Richart RM. Pathology quiz: condyloma acuminatum. *Contemp OB/GYN* 1990;4:5.

Vulva

Gross Appearance of Vulvar HPV-Associated Lesions

Anogenital warts can be categorized into three separate types based on their gross appearances (123). One is a hyperplastic, cauliflower-like lesion called condyloma acuminatum. These raised exophytic lesions are pink to white and are found in moist areas such as the labia, perianal region, glans penis, inner aspect of the prepuce, and the urethral meatus. Another is a small sessile plaque type of wart. These are most common on the penile shaft. The final type is a keratotic, verruca vulgaris-like wart.

Vulvar condylomata occur in women of all age groups but have a peak incidence from ages 20 to 24. They vary in size from small, easily treated lesions to large, inflamed masses that tend to recur after treatment (Fig. 19.13). A key feature of HPV infection of the lower female genital tract is that it often involves multiple sites and is multifocal. For example, 22% to 32% of female patients with vulvar condylomata will have concurrent cervical lesions (124,125). Therefore, it is essential that the entire lower genital tract be examined carefully in all patients with vulvar condylomata. Vulvar lesions with a typical gross appearance of condylomata are readily recognized and are rarely confused with other lesions. However, when the appearance is atypical, the differential diagnosis can include almost any raised vulvar lesion, including condyloma latum, molluscum contagiosum, fibropapilloma, lymphoma, hidradenoma, and even verrucous carcinoma if the lesion is large. In atypical cases, a biopsy of the lesion is mandatory and usually diagnostic. The classic histologic features of condylomata acuminata are papillomatosis, acanthosis with hyperkeratosis, parakeratosis, and the presence of nuclear atypia with multinucleation and koilocytosis (Fig. 19.14). As mentioned previously, condylomata acuminata are usually associated with HPV types 6 and 11. Human papillomavirus DNA can be detected by *in situ* hybridization in more than 90% of cases of condylomata acuminata (Fig. 19.14) (126).

Many patients have small genital epithelial lesions that are clinically suggestive of plaque-type anogenital warts and are better visualized after the application of 4% acetic acid but histologically lack characteristic HPV-associated cytopathic effects. These lesions are particularly common in men and occur on the corona glandis and along each side of the frenulum of the penis. The term *pearly penile papules* has been used for these lesions (127). In females, a common mimic of condylomata acuminata is *micropapillomatosis labialis* (128). Micropapillomatosis labialis occurs at the introitus and appears as multiple, soft papillary projections that are characteristically bilateral and symmetric (Fig. 19.15). Although micropapillomatosis labialis can histologically be mistaken for an HPV-related lesion, multiple studies have failed to detect HPV DNA in a significant number of cases (128). Another common entity that is often confused with condyloma acuminatum, especially by pathologists, is benign fibropapilloma of the anogenital region.

Like CIN 2,3, vulvar intraepithelial neoplasia has been increasing in incidence over the last two decades (129,130). Vulvar intraepithelial neoplasia usually presents as a slightly raised, sharply demarcated lesion that can be black, white, gray, red, or brown, depending on the age, race, and complexion of the patient (Fig. 19.16). These lesions tend to be unifocal in older patients and multifocal in younger patients. The margins are often irregular, and the lesions vary in size from

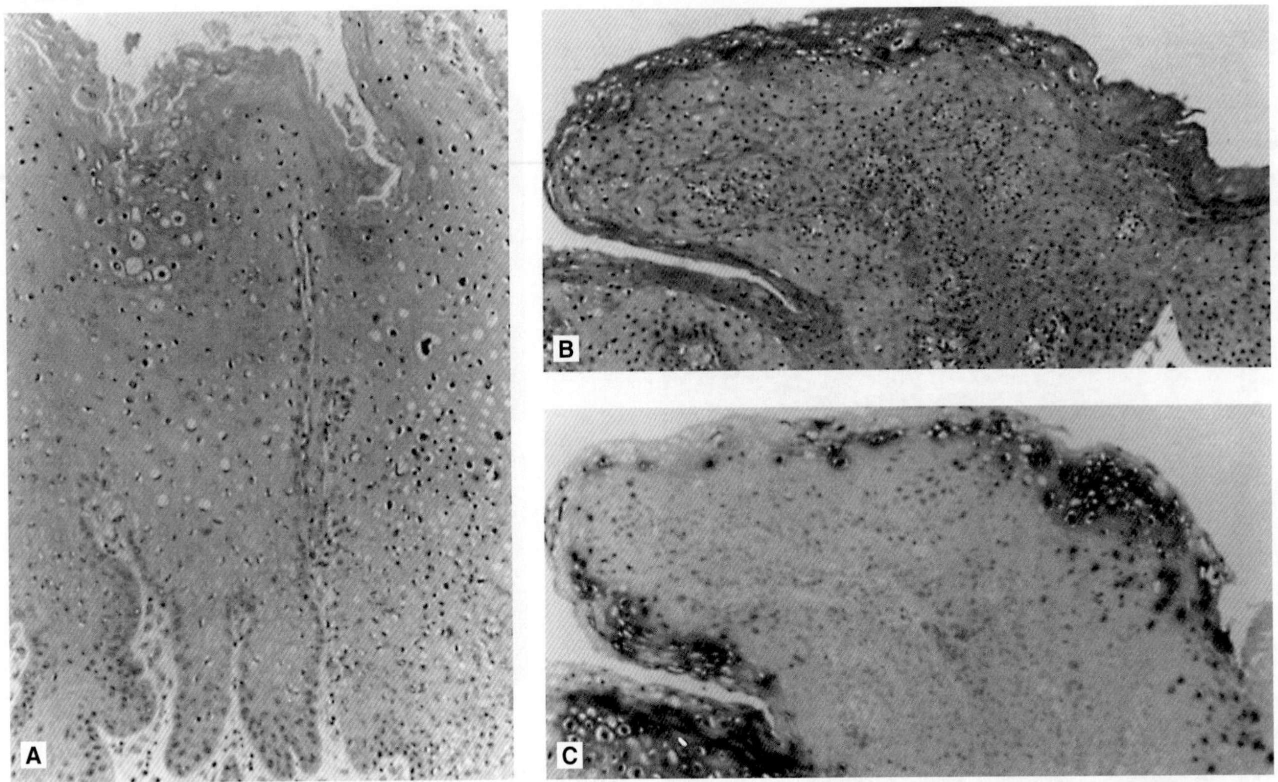

FIGURE 19.14. A, B: Histology of condyloma acuminatum. C: *In situ* hybridization of a vulvar condyloma using probes for HPV-6/11.

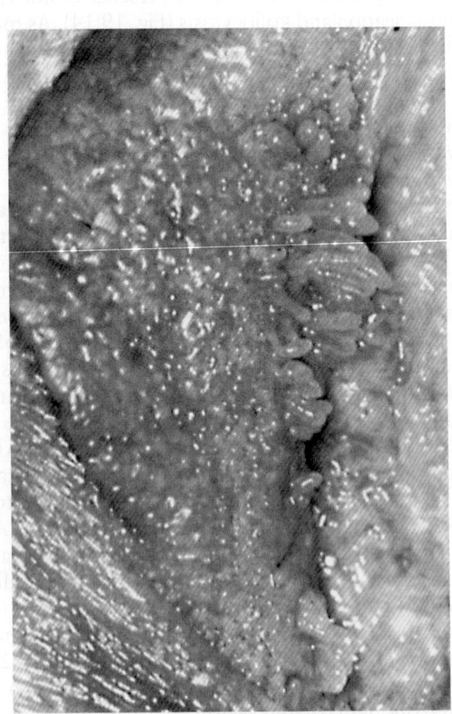

FIGURE 19.15. Characteristic gross features of micropapillomatosis labialis. *Source:* Courtesy of Dr. Alex Ferenczy, Jewish General Hospital, McGill University, Montreal, Quebec, Canada.

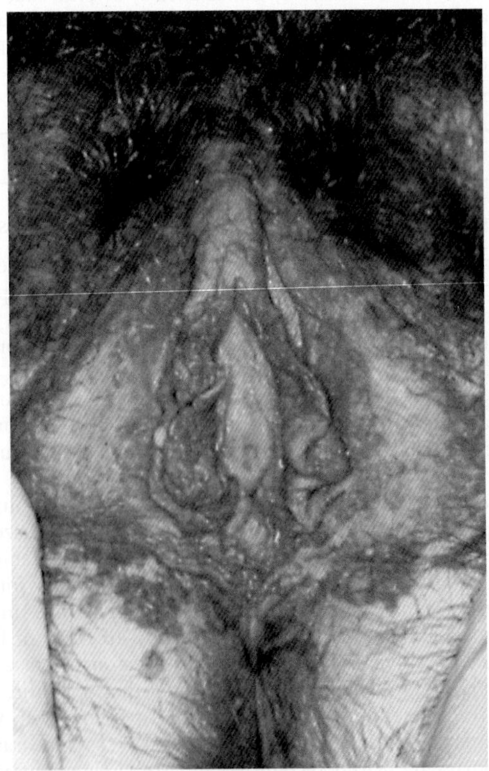

FIGURE 19.16. Gross features of vulvar intraepithelial neoplasia. *Source:* Used with permission courtesy of Dr. D. Townsend, University of California. From Wright TC, Richart RM. Pathology quiz: condyloma acuminatum. *Contemp OB/GYN* 1990;4:5.

several millimeters to large, confluent lesions that involve the entire vulva. The majority of lesions are 1 to 3 cm in diameter. Most commonly, VIN develops on the labia minora, around the anus, and at the introitus (131). The clitoris and urethra are less commonly involved.

Bowenoid papulosis is considered by many to be a separate entity. It is a disease characterized by multiple small papules that are often violaceous and occasionally coalesce to form large plaques. The lesions develop on the vulvar skin and occasionally on the abdomen. Bowenoid papulosis is a disease of young women, with a peak incidence in the third decade. However, despite the relatively innocuous gross appearance of bowenoid papulosis, this lesion is identical histologically to VIN 3. Invasive vulvar carcinoma may arise in untreated cases of bowenoid papulosis.

Microscopic Appearance of Vulvar Intraepithelial Neoplasia

Microscopically, VIN lesions are similar to CIN lesions. The four major histologic features are increased numbers of undifferentiated cells with nuclear atypia, alterations in epidermal maturation with disorganization, parakeratosis and hyperkeratosis, and the presence of abnormal mitotic figures (Fig. 19.17). Although the ISSVD has recommended that VIN lesions no longer be graded and that VIN 1 lesions not be diagnosed, in most centers VIN lesions continue to be histologically graded on a scale of 1 to 3, using criteria identical to those used for the original CIN terminology for cervical cancer precursors (22,132). Nuclear atypia in VIN typically involves the basal and parabasal cell layers as well as cells in the upper, more differentiated cell layers. Nuclear size in VIN varies from small and hyperchromatic to pleomorphic and large.

VIN lesions tend to have three histopathologic appearances termed *warty*, *basaloid*, and *differentiated* (133). Separation into these three subtypes is based predominately on nuclear size and the amount of cytoplasmic differentiation. In general, invasive vulvar cancers that are HPV DNA positive occur in younger women and are associated with the warty and basaloid variants of VIN (134). In the ISSVD terminology these histologic types of VIN are grouped together as *VIN, usual type* (22). In contrast to the warty and basaloid variants of VIN which are associated with HPV DNA positive vulvar cancers in younger women, differentiated VIN is found in older women and tends to be associated with HPV DNA negative invasive vulvar cancers (135). This type of VIN was originally referred to as *carcinoma in situ, simplex type*. Differentiated VIN often occurs adjacent to well-differentiated invasive vulvar cancers and is often associated with either squamous hyperplasia or lichen sclerosis of the vulva (133).

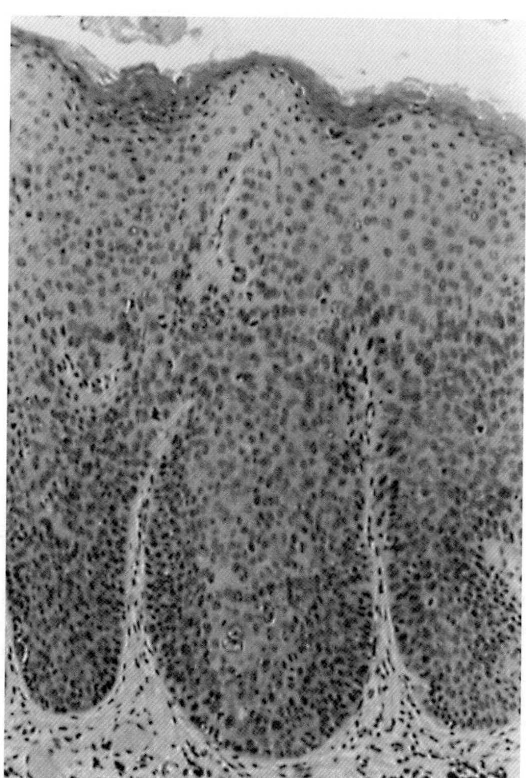

FIGURE 19.17. Microscopic features of VIN 3.

These histologic variants, especially the warty and basaloid forms, are frequently found together in the same patient. Moreover, there is no data to suggest that histopathologic type has a significant impact on either rates of progression to invasive vulvar cancer or response to standard therapies. One additional point needs further clarification. Although the histologic distinction between cervical condylomata and CIN 1 is no longer thought to be possible, vulvar condylomata and VIN are still distinguished from one another. The reason for retaining this distinction for the vulva is that the vast majority of vulvar condylomata are caused by HPV-6 or -11, which are low-oncogenic-risk HPV types (70). The development of invasive vulvar carcinoma from a preexisting condyloma acuminatum is an extremely rare event. Histologically, the distinction between vulvar condylomata and VIN is made on the basis of two features: the presence or absence of abnormal mitotic figures and the presence or absence of nuclear atypia that involve the basal and parabasal cell layers.

Vagina

Vaginal intraepithelial neoplasia lesions are generally white with sharp borders. They are best evaluated with colposcopy after the application of 4% acetic acid. In general, vascular changes are not striking in VAIN lesions, although punctation is occasionally seen. The histologic features of VAIN are identical to those of CIN and VIN.

CYTOLOGIC SCREENING FOR CERVICAL CANCER AND ITS PRECURSORS

Background

Cytology-based cervical cancer screening programs were first introduced in the mid-20th century and are now widely recognized as being able to reduce both the incidence of, and mortality from, invasive cervical cancer. Strong evidence for their effectiveness comes from comparison of incidence and mortality trends of invasive cervical cancer with screening activity in a given country or region. The Nordic countries provide some of the best evidence for a linkage between screening and reductions in both incidence and mortality from cervical cancer (54). In order to be effective, these programs require good coverage of the target population and appropriate management of screen-positive women (54). The importance of coverage is seen in the cervical cancer rates in the United Kingdom. Prior to 1988 there was a recommendation by the National Health Service (NHS) for routine cytologic screening, but coverage of the population was relatively low and cervical cancer rates

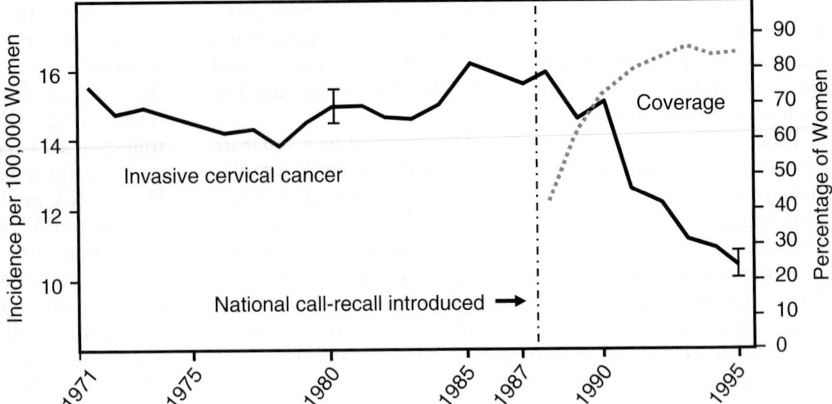

FIGURE 19.18. Impact of increasing screening coverage on the age-standardized incidence of invasive cervical cancer in the United Kingdom, 1971–1995. *Source:* Adapted from Quinn M, Babb P, Jones J, Allen E. Effect of screening on incidence of and mortality from cancer of cervix in England: evaluation based on routinely collected statistics. *BMJ* 1999;318;904.

remained relatively high (Fig. 19.18) (136). In 1988 the NHS introduced a national call-recall system, improved quality control in the laboratories, and provided financial incentives to general practitioners to encourage high rates of screening in their patients. As a result of this program, the incidence of invasive cervical cancer began to quickly drop.

Accuracy of Cervical Cytology

Despite the proven effectiveness of cervical cytology in reducing the incidence of cervical cancer, over the last several years the accuracy of cervical cytology has been questioned. Two factors need to be considered when assessing the accuracy of any diagnostic test including cervical cytology. One is whether the test is specific in detecting a given condition; the other is the sensitivity of the test for detecting a given condition. Several meta-analyses have been conducted and have concluded that both the sensitivity and specificity of cervical cytology is lower than previously thought (137,138). The first analysis by Fahey et al. estimated that the mean sensitivity of a conventional cervical cytology was 58% and the mean specificity was 69%, *when used in a screening setting* (Fig. 19.19) (137). The second meta-analysis by Nanda et al. considered different cytologic cut-offs and endpoints (138). When a cytologic cut-off of atypical squamous cells of undetermined significance (ASC-US) is used and the endpoint is biopsy-confirmed CIN 1 or worse, the average sensitivity of conventional cytology was 68% and the average specificity was 75% (Fig. 19.19). When the cytologic cut-off was LSIL and the endpoint was biopsy-confirmed CIN 2,3 or worse, the average sensitivity was 81% and the specificity was 77%.

A number of factors influence the false-negative rate of cervical cytology. Of key importance is the use of a proper technique for sampling the cervix. Since the majority of CIN and cancers involve the transformation zone, sampling devices have been specifically designed to sample this area. Sampling the endocervical canal also reduces the false-negative rate. This sample can be taken with an endocervical brush (e.g., Cytobrush) or one of the newer collection devices such as a cell broom. Saline-moistened cotton-tipped applicators should not be used since the number of endocervical cells that are obtained with a cotton-tipped applicator is less than the number obtained with a Cytobrush and several studies have reported a higher CIN detection rate when Cytobrushes are used (139). Other important factors for reducing the false-negative rate are the rapid fixation of cells to prevent artifactual changes secondary to air-drying and the use of a cytology laboratory with stringent quality control standards.

Although a false-negative rate of 20% to 40% for a cancer screening test appears to be unacceptably high, the test has been effective despite its limitations due to the natural history of the disease, and the use of cervical cytology has reduced the incidence of cervical cancer by almost 80% in the United States over the last 3 decades (140). The effectiveness of cervical cytology is attributable to the fact that invasive cervical cancer requires many years to develop from a CIN 2,3 lesion (5). If cervical cytology is performed on a routine basis, it is unlikely that a CIN 2,3 lesion will remain undetected, although such cases do rarely occur. The current screening recommendation from the American Cancer Society and the American College of Obstetricians and Gynecologists is that cervical cancer screening should be initiated approximately

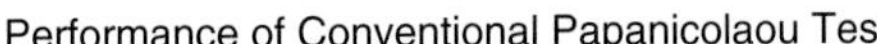

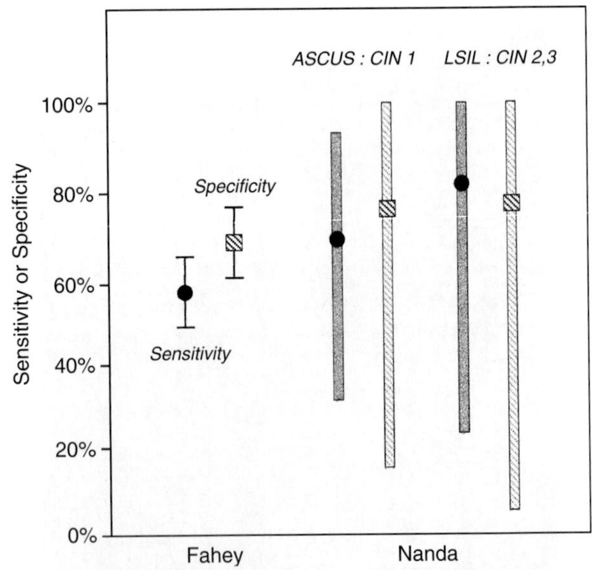

FIGURE 19.19. Estimates of the sensitivity (circles) and specificity (squares) of conventional cervical cytology obtained from two meta-analyses (those of Fahey et al. *left side with bars showing 95% confidence interals* and Nanda et al. *right side with bars representing range of values in different studies*). *Source:* Modified with permission from Fahey MT, Irwig L, Macaskill P. Meta-analysis of Pap test accuracy. *Am J Epidemiol* 1995;141:680, and Nanda K, McCrory DC, Myers ER, et al. Accuracy of the Papanicolaou test in screening for and follow-up of cervical cytologic abnormalities: a systematic review. *Ann Intern Med* 2000;132:810.

3 years after the initiation of sexual intercourse, but no later than age 21 years (141,142). After 30 years of age, the interval between cervical cytology examinations can be extended to 2 to 3 years in women who have had three consecutive negative cervical cytology screening test results, who have no history of CIN 2,3, and are neither immunocompromised nor exposed to diethylstilbestrol (DES) (141,142). There is currently no consensus as to when to stop screening. The American Cancer Society recommends that screening can be discontinued in women 70 years and older with three documented negative screening tests within the preceding 10 years and no history of cervical cancer, DES exposure, or immunosuppression (142). The U.S. Preventative Services Task Force recommends discontinuing screening at age 65 years in women who have had adequate recent screening and who are not otherwise at high risk for cervical cancer (143). Routine screening is not recommended for women who have undergone a hysterectomy for benign indications and who have no prior history of CIN 2,3.

Obtaining an Optimal Cervical Cytology

To obtain an optimal cervical cytology, it is necessary to observe several simple guidelines. The patient should be instructed not to douche, wash her vagina, or have intercourse for 24 hours before obtaining the specimen. Cervical cytology should not be obtained during menses or within 1 week after stopping intravaginal antibiotics or antifungal agents. Cervical cytology should be taken before a bimanual exam, using a minimal amount or no lubricant. It is preferable not to apply acetic acid to the cervix before the cervical cytology is taken. An Ayre-type spatula or cell broom type of device should be used and rotated around the cervix several times with firm pressure. A Cytobrush is immediately placed in the external os, rotated 180° only, and withdrawn. The sample is immediately fixed and labeled with the patient's name and date of birth.

Liquid-Based Cytology

Liquid-based cytology (LBC) is now widely used in the United States for cervical cytology. Three liquid-based cytology methods are currently available in the United States. These are the ThinPrep Pap Test marketed by Cytyc Corporation, SurePath marketed by BD Diagnostics, and MonoPrep Pap Test marketed by MonoGen, Inc. ThinPrep and MonoPrep use a filter method to collect a monolayer of epithelial cells and separate the epithelial cells from blood, mucus, and inflammatory debris. SurePath uses a density centrifugation method to enrich for epithelial cells and reduce blood and inflammatory cells.

A major reappraisal is underway in the screening community of the performance of LBC. When it was first introduced, LBC was believed to provide a significant advantage compared to conventional cervical cytology with respect to sensitivity for the identification of women with CIN 2,3 or cancer. However, most of the studies that compared LBC with conventional cytology had methodologic problems such as the use of historical controls, and others simply reported increases in the number of cases cytologically diagnosed as squamous intraepithelial lesions (SIL). Very few studies measured histologic endpoints and the few studies that actually utilized histologic endpoints did not blind the pathologists evaluating the histology to the cytologic findings. Only one small study was randomized.

Recently two systematic reviews of the published literature comparing the performance of LBC with conventional cytology were published (144,145). One included a total of 56 studies, 52 of which provided enough information to evaluate differences between LBC and conventional cytology (144). These 52 included more than a 1.25 million slides. Of the studies that were evaluated, none were of "ideal quality" and only five were of "high quality." When all of the studies were taken into account and combined it was concluded that they saw no evidence that LBC reduced the proportion of unsatisfactory slides nor that it has better performance than conventional cytology with respect to the identification of women with CIN 2,3. The reviews concluded that large randomized trials were needed.

TABLE 19.9

COMPARISON OF PERFORMANCE OF LIQUID-BASED AND CONVENTIONAL CYTOLOGY IN LARGE, WELL-CONTROLLED CLINICAL TRIALS

	Conventional cytology			Liquid-based cytology	
	No. of women	Sensitivity[a]	PPV	Sensitivity[a]	PPV
Taylor et al.	5,652	84%	11.4	71%	9.4
Ronco et al.	33,364	70%	11.4	74%	6.5

PPV, positive predictive value.
[a]For detection of CIN 2,3 or cancer.
Source: Adapted from Taylor S, Kuhn L, Dupree W, et al. Direct comparison of liquid-based and conventional cytology in a South African screening trial. *Int J Cancer* 2006;118:957; Ronco G, Segnan N, Giorgi-Rossi P, et al. Human papillomavirus testing and liquid-based cytology: results at recruitment from the new technologies for cervical cancer randomized controlled trial. *J Natl Cancer Inst* 2006;98:765.

Since the first systematic review was conducted, two large randomized trials comparing LBC with conventional cytology have been published. One was conducted in South Africa and no significant difference was observed in the sensitivity of LBC and conventional cytology in the detection of CIN 2,3 or cancer (Table 19.9) (146). An Italian randomized study also failed to find that LBC is more sensitive than conventional cytology but did find a 43% reduction in positive predictive value (PPV) with LBC due to an increase in the number of abnormals (Table 19.9) (147). After the publication of these two large trials, another systematic review and meta-analysis of LBC found that there were only six other published studies that were appropriately designed to allow a comparison of the performance of LBC and conventional cytology (148). This review concluded that there is no evidence that LBC is either more sensitive or more specific than conventional cytology.

Having said this, it is important for clinicians to recognize that there are other advantages of LBC. The greatest of these appears to be the availability of residual fluid for "reflex" HPV testing in women with ASC-US as well as testing for other pathogens such as *Chlamydia*. Moreover, almost all cytologists agree that it is easier to evaluate LBC specimens than conventional cytology specimens and it is unlikely that cytology laboratories will want to switch back to conventional cytology now that the conversion to LBC has taken place.

Terminology of Cytologic Reports

The Bethesda system terminology is used for reporting cervical cytology results in the United States. The Bethesda system underwent significant modifications in 2001 (Table 19.10) (10). The major features of the 2001 Bethesda system are that it requires (a) an estimate of the adequacy of the specimen for diagnostic evaluation; (b) a general categorization of the specimen as being either "negative for intraepithelial lesion or malignancy," as having an "epithelial cell abnormality," or as

TABLE 19.10

THE 2001 BETHESDA SYSTEM

SPECIMEN ADEQUACY
Satisfactory for evaluation (*note presence/absence of endocervical transformation zone component*)
Unsatisfactory for evaluation (*specify reason*)
Specimen rejected/not processed (*specify reason*)
Specimen processed and examined, but unsatisfactory for evaluation of epithelial abnormality because of (*specify reason*)

GENERAL CATEGORIZATION (*OPTIONAL*)
Negative for intraepithelial lesion or malignancy
Epithelial cell abnormality
Other

INTERPRETATION/RESULT
Negative for Intraepithelial Lesion or Malignancy
Organisms
- *Trichomonas vaginalis*
- Fungal organisms morphologically consistent with *Candida* species
- Shift in flora suggestive of bacterial vaginosis
- Bacteria morphologically consistent with *Actinomyces* species
- Cellular changes consistent with herpes simplex virus
- Other nonneoplastic findings (*optional to report; list not comprehensive*)
- Reactive cellular changes associated with inflammation (includes typical repair)
- Radiation
- Intrauterine contraceptive device
- Glandular cells status posthysterectomy
- Atrophy

Epithelial Cell Abnormalities
Squamous cell
- Atypical squamous cell (ASC)
  - of undetermined significance (ASC-US);
  - cannot exclude HSIL (ASC-H)
- Low-grade squamous intraepithelial lesion (LSIL)
- High-grade squamous intraepithelial lesion (HSIL)
- Squamous cell carcinoma

Glandular cell
- Atypical glandular cells (AGC) (*specify endocervical, endometrial, or not otherwise specified*)
- Atypical glandular cells, favor neoplastic (*specify endocervical or not otherwise specified*)
- Endocervical adenocarcinoma *in situ* (AIS)
- Adenocarcinoma

Other (*list not comprehensive*)
- Endometrial cells in a woman ≥40 years of age

Source: Solomon D, Davey D, Kurman R, et al. The 2001 Bethesda system: terminology for reporting results of cervical cytology. *JAMA* 2002;287:2114.

"other" (i.e., having endometrial cells in a woman 40 years of age and older); and (c) a descriptive diagnosis that includes a description of epithelial cell abnormalities. This system provides clear criteria for determining whether a specimen is adequate for evaluation. In addition, the terminology closely correlates with histopathologic terminology. The terms *low-grade squamous intraepithelial lesion* (LSIL) and *high-grade squamous intraepithelial lesion* (HSIL) are used to designate cytologic changes that correlate with CIN 1 and CIN 2,3, respectively. In addition, the Bethesda system attempts to separate epithelial changes secondary to inflammation or repair from those associated with cervical cancer precursors whenever possible. Nondiagnostic squamous cell abnormalities are included in a category of *atypical squamous cells* (ASC). ASC is used when a specimen has features suggestive, but not diagnostic, of an SIL. This category is further subdivided into two subcategories: atypical squamous cells of undetermined significance (ASC-US); and atypical squamous cells—cannot exclude HSIL (ASC-H). The risk of a woman with ASC-US having biopsy-confirmed CIN 2,3 is approximately 7% to 17% and the risk of a woman with ASC-H is approximately 40% (11). Nondiagnostic glandular cell abnormalities are included in a category of *atypical glandular cells* (AGC). This category is further subdivided into either *not further classified* or *atypical glandular cells, favor neoplasia.*

Cytologic Features of CIN

The features used to diagnose SIL cytologically are similar to those used to diagnose CIN in histopathologic specimens. These features include nuclear enlargement with an increase in the nuclear-cytoplasmic ratio, nuclear hyperchromaticity, irregular nuclear membranes, and multinucleation. Perinuclear clearing, or halos, is also commonly present. An example of normal superficial cells is shown in Figure 19.20A. In LSIL, cytologic changes are seen predominantly in superficial cells (i.e., more mature cell types, Fig. 19.20B). In HSIL, the cytologic changes are seen in intermediate and parabasal cells (i.e., less mature cell types, Fig. 19.20C).

USE OF COLPOSCOPY

Over the last 25 years, colposcopy combined with colposcopically directed cervical biopsies has become the primary modality by which women with abnormal Pap smears are evaluated. Colposcopic examination consists of viewing the cervix with a long-focal-length, dissecting-type microscope at a magnification of about 16× after a solution of dilute (4%) acetic acid has been applied to the cervix. The acetic acid solution acts to remove and dissolve the cervical mucus and causes CIN lesions to become whiter than the surrounding epithelium (acetowhite). This coloration allows the colposcopist to identify and biopsy epithelial lesions. In addition to allowing the detection of acetowhite areas, colposcopy also allows for the detection of blood vessel patterns that can indicate high-grade CIN lesions and the detection of invasive cancers. Colposcopy and appropriately directed biopsy have greatly facilitated the management of patients with preinvasive lesions of the cervix because they allow the clinician to rule out invasive cancer and determine the limits of preinvasive disease. Conservative ablative treatment modalities such as cryosurgery, laser ablation, and electrofulguration, as well as excisional methods such as loop electrosurgical excision procedure (LEEP) can then be used to treat preinvasive disease, with success rates similar to those obtained with cone biopsies.

MANAGEMENT OF CYTOLOGIC ABNORMALITIES AND CIN

Overview

In 2006 the American Society for Colposcopy and Cervical Pathology sponsored a consensus workshop to update the 2001 Consensus Guidelines for the Management of Women with Cytological Abnormalities and Cervical Cancer Precursors

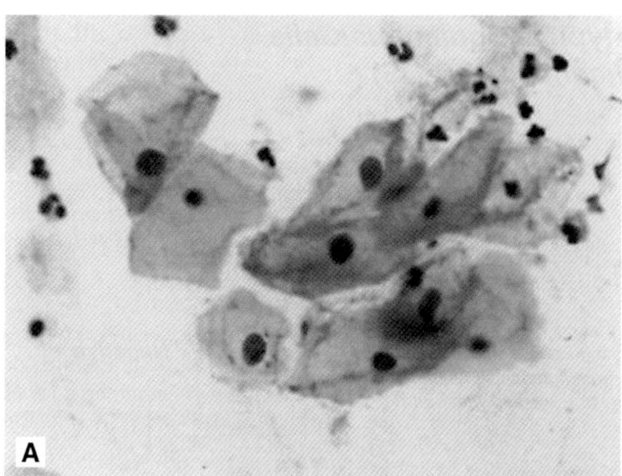

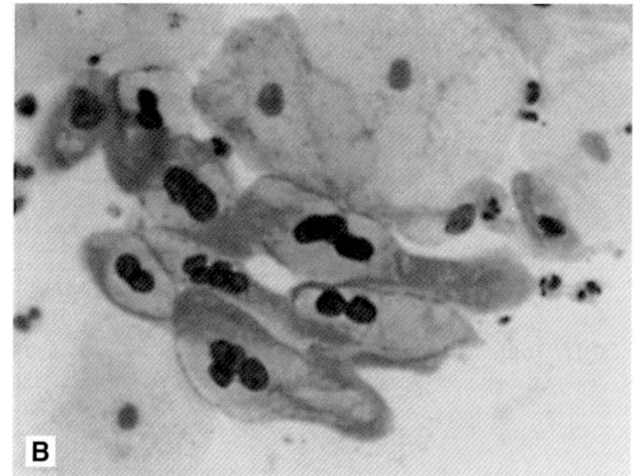

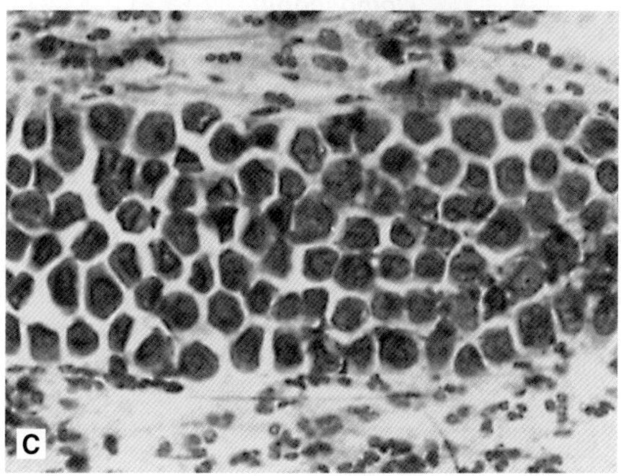

FIGURE 19.20. Cervical cytology. **A:** Normal superficial cells. **B:** Low-grade SIL (CIN 1) in which the cells are multinucleated with slightly enlarged hyperchromatic nuclei and perinuclear halos. **C:** High-grade SIL (CIN 2,3) with cells with high nucleocytoplasmic ratios.

(12,147). These guidelines are widely used in the United States and are evidence-based with each recommendation accompanied by a grading of both the strength of the recommendation and the strength of the data supporting the recommendation. The complete recommendations and management algorithms are available at www.asccp.org.

Atypical Squamous Cells

A vexing group of patients for both clinicians and cytologists are those whose cervical cytology is atypical (i.e., not normal) but lack the characteristic features of SIL or cancer. In the past, many cytology laboratories subdivided atypical smears into two categories: atypical, reparative-inflammatory changes (i.e., benign atypia); and atypical smears, suggestive but not diagnostic of CIN. The 2001 Bethesda system classifies specimens that have reparative-inflammatory changes as being "negative for intraepithelial lesion or malignancy." In the current terminology only those specimens that have features suggestive of SIL should be classified as ASC. Irrespective of the classification system used, clinicians need to be aware that a cytologic result of ASC is the least reproducible cytologic category (149). The number of cytology specimens that are diagnosed as ASC varies greatly among different cytology laboratories and patient populations. The reported incidence of atypical Pap smears that fall into this category varies greatly from 1% to over 10% (4). These differences reflect the difficulties encountered by cytologists in determining the significance of minor degrees of cytologic atypia and in reproducibly recognizing these changes. In the most recent report from the College of American Pathologists (CAP), the median ASC rate from reporting laboratories from the United States was 5% (4).

The clinical significance of an ASC result depends on a number of factors including the age of the patient, the patient's history, and the subclassification of the result (e.g., ASC-US or ASC-H). The prevalence of biopsy-confirmed CIN 2,3 found in women undergoing colposcopy for an ASC cytology is generally reported as being 5% to 17% (12). A study of 46,009 women undergoing routine cytologic screening in the Northern California Kaiser Permanente Medical Group found that 3.5% had a diagnosis of ASC-US (150). At colposcopy, 13% of these women were diagnosed with CIN 1, 7% with CIN 2,3, and one woman had invasive cervical cancer. In the large, multicenter ASC-US/LSIL Triage Study (ALTS), 15% of the women referred with ASC were found to have biopsy-confirmed CIN 2,3 at the initial colposcopic examination and 20% had biopsy-confirmed CIN 1 (151). Overall, it appears that between one third and one half of all women diagnosed as having CIN 2,3 have ASC as their initial abnormal cervical cytology result (152,153). Although the risk that a woman with ASC has invasive cervical cancer is quite low (about one per thousand) the very large number of women with this cytology interpretation (2.5 million annually) guarantees that each year approximately 2,500 women with invasive cervical cancer will have only equivocal results on their cervical cytology. Therefore, women with ASC-US need to receive some form of follow-up evaluation, but consideration should be given to preventing unnecessary inconvenience, anxiety, cost, and discomfort.

Atypical Squamous Cells of Undetermined Significance

Three methods are in widespread use for the management of women with ASC. These are immediate colposcopy, HPV DNA testing, and a program of repeat cervical cytology. A number of studies have directly compared the sensitivity and specificity of repeat cervical cytology and HPV DNA testing

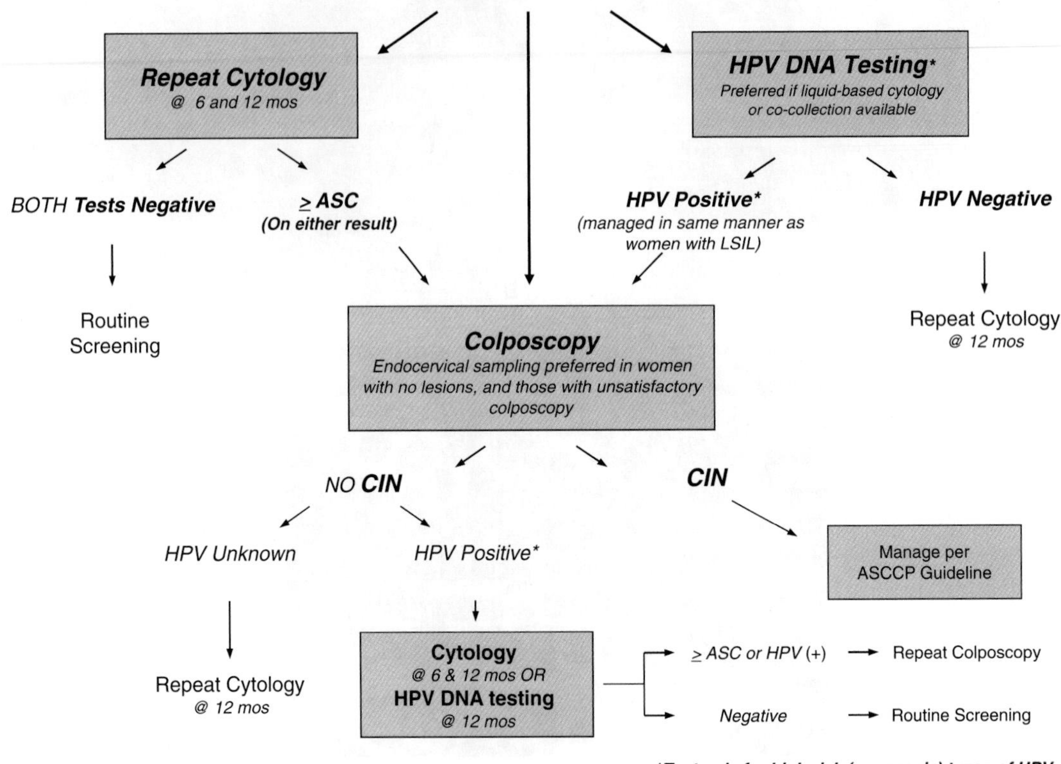

FIGURE 19.21. 2006 Consensus Guidelines for the management of women with ASC-US. *Source:* Used with permission from the American Society of Colposcopy and Cervical Pathology.

for identifying women with CIN 2,3 (154). In every single study, HPV DNA testing identified more cases of CIN 2,3 than did a single repeat cervical cytology, but referred approximately equivalent numbers of women for colposcopy. Moreover, cost-effectiveness modeling using mathematical models has demonstrated that HPV DNA testing for women with ASC-US is a highly attractive alternative to immediate colposcopy or a program of repeat cytology when the initial ASC-US cytology was obtained from a liquid-based sample or when a co-collected HPV test was taken at the time a conventional cytology was obtained (155,156). Based on this evidence, the 2006 American Society for Colposcopy and Cervical Pathology (ASCCP) Consensus Conference concluded that although all three of the methods traditionally used to manage women with ASC-US (i.e., colposcopy, repeat cytology, and HPV DNA testing) are safe and effective, high-risk HPV DNA testing is the preferred approach to managing women with ASC-US whenever liquid-based cytology is used for screening or co-collection of a sample for HPV DNA testing can be performed (12). Figure 19.21 provides the algorithm recommended for the management of women in the general population with ASC-US. This algorithm is appropriate for women of all ages with ASC-US.

The prevalence of HPV DNA positivity is much higher in young women with ASC-US than in older women. For example, in the ALTS study only 31% of women 29 years and older with ASC were HPV DNA positive compared to 65% of those under 29 years old (157). Rates are even higher in adolescents with ASC-US (158). Therefore, the 2006 Consensus Guidelines do not recommend the use of HPV DNA testing in adolescents, defined as females 13 to 20 years of age (12). Instead, adolescents should be managed using annual repeat cytologic examinations and only referred to colposcopy if the repeat Pap tests are diagnosed as HSIL or are persistently abnormal for a period of 2 years (12).

Management options for pregnant patients with ASC-US are identical to those for nonpregnant patients with the exception that it is acceptable to defer the colposcopic examination until the patient is 6 to 8 weeks post-partum (12).

Atypical Squamous Cells—Cannot Exclude HSIL

The prevalence of biopsy-confirmed CIN 2,3 is considerably higher among women referred for the evaluation of an ASC-H cervical cytology than it is for women referred for the evaluation of ASC-US. CIN 2,3 is identified in 24% to 94% of women with ASC-H (11). Therefore, for the purposes of management, ASC-H should be considered to be an equivocal HSIL result. Because of this high risk, the 2006 Consensus Guidelines recommend that all women with ASC-H be referred for a colposcopic evaluation (12). If CIN is not identified, follow-up utilizing either repeat cytology at 6 and 12 months or high-risk HPV DNA testing at 12 months is acceptable (Fig. 19.22).

Low-Grade Squamous Intraepithelial Lesions

As with ASC-US, there is considerable variation between populations and laboratories in the rate at which LSIL is reported. In 2003 the median rate of LSIL reported from the College of American Pathology survey was 2.6%, but rates as high as 7.0% were reported from 5% of the laboratories (4). In 1996

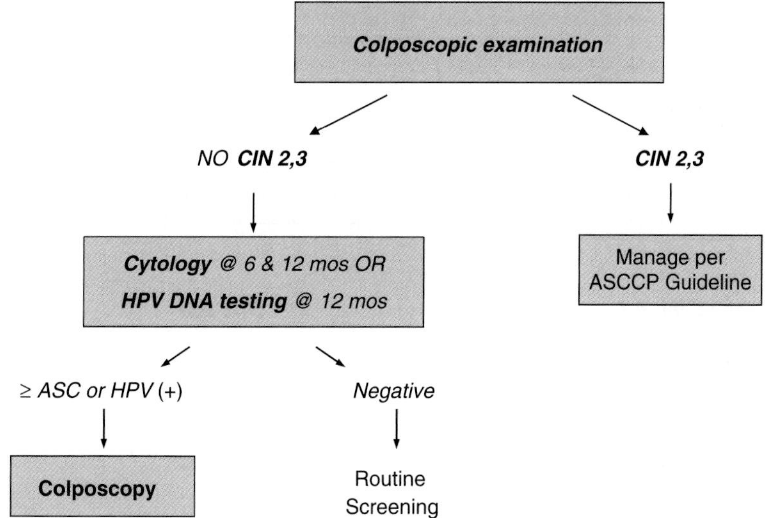

FIGURE 19.22. 2006 Consensus Guidelines for the management of women with ASC-H. *Source:* Used with permission from the American Society of Colposcopy and Cervical Pathology.

the median rate of LSIL in the United States was only 1.6% (159). The increase appears to be due to the introduction of liquid-based cytology (144). A cytologic result of LSIL is a very specific indicator of the presence of high-risk types of HPV. In ALTS, 83% of the women referred for the evaluation of LSIL were high-risk HPV DNA positive (160). However, a cytologic result of LSIL is a poor predictor of the grade of CIN that will be identified at colposcopy. CIN 2,3 is identified at colposcopy in 15% to 30% of women with LSIL on cervical cytology (152,159,161). Therefore, the 2006 Consensus Guidelines recommend that all women in the general population with a cytologic result of LSIL be referred for a colposcopic evaluation (Fig. 19.23) (12). This allows women with significant disease to be rapidly identified and reduces the risk of women being lost to follow-up. A diagnostic excisional procedure is not required when a woman with LSIL cytology is found to have an unsatisfactory colposcopic examination.

The risk of invasive cervical cancer is very low in adolescents and prospective studies have shown that over 90% of LSIL will spontaneously clear over a period of years in adolescents (162,163). Therefore, adolescents with LSIL (<21 years of age) are considered to be a "special population" and it is now recommended that they should not receive colposcopy, but instead should be followed using yearly Pap tests for a period of 2 years (12). Another special population is postmenopausal women with LSIL. In some studies, the prevalence of HPV DNA in postmenopausal women with LSIL is lower than in premenopausal women and the prevalence of CIN 2,3 also declines in postmenopausal women with LSIL (157,164). Therefore, the 2006 Consensus Guidelines indicate that postmenopausal women with LSIL can be managed in the same manner as women with ASC-US. This allows the use of reflex HPV DNA testing to determine which of these women require colposcopy.

High-Grade Squamous Intraepithelial Lesions

The cytologic result of HSIL is uncommon, accounting for only about 0.7% of all cervical cytology results, but the prevalence varies with age (4). In one U.S. study the prevalence of HSIL was 0.6% in women 20 to 29 years of age, but only 0.1% in women 50 to 59 years of age (165). A diagnosis of HSIL confers a significant risk for CIN 2,3 and invasive cervical cancer (4,166). CIN 2,3 or cancer has been identified at a single colposcopic examination in 53% to 66% of women with HSIL and in 84% to 97% of those evaluated using a loop electrosurgical excision procedure (LEEP) (12). Invasive cervical cancer is identified in approximately 2% of women with HSIL (167). Therefore, women with a cytologic result of HSIL should be referred for either a colposcopic evaluation or an immediate LEEP (Fig. 19.24) (12). Subsequent management depends on whether or not the patient is pregnant and whether the colposcopic examination is satisfactory. If CIN 2,3 is not identified after colposcopy, the colposcopic examination is satisfactory, and endocervical sampling is negative, either a diagnostic excisional procedure or follow-up using colposcopy and cytology at 6-month intervals is acceptable for 1 year. If a repeat HSIL cytologic result is found at either the 6- or 12-month visit, a diagnostic excisional procedure is recommended. Nonpregnant women with HSIL who have an unsatisfactory colposcopic examination also require a diagnostic excisional procedure.

Biopsy-Confirmed CIN 1

Women with a histologically confirmed CIN 1 lesion represent a heterogeneous group. A number of studies have clearly demonstrated a high level of variability in the histologic diagnosis of CIN 1. In the ALTS study, only 43% of biopsies that were originally diagnosed as CIN 1 at the clinical centers were subsequently classified as CIN 1 by the reference pathology committee. Forty-one percent were downgraded to normal, and 13% were upgraded to CIN 2,3 (149). It should also be noted that there is a very high rate of spontaneous regression of CIN 1 in the absence of treatment. One prospective Brazilian study found that 90% of women with a cytologic diagnosis of LSIL spontaneously regressed within 24 months (168). A Dutch study found that over 4 years, 70% of women with

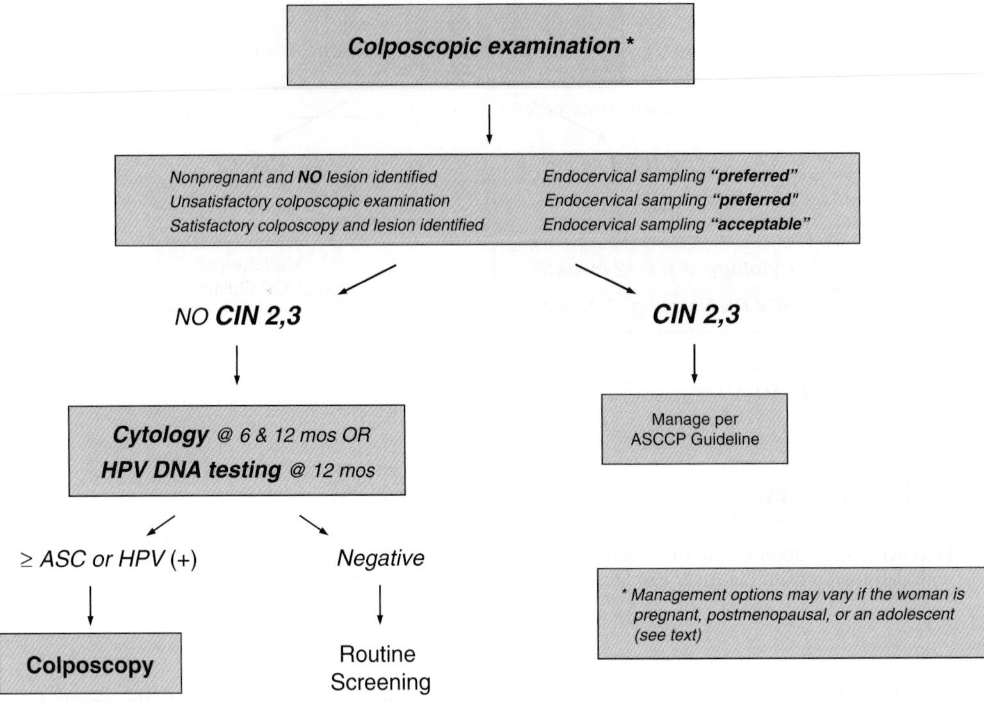

FIGURE 19.23. 2006 Consensus Guidelines for the management of women with LSIL. *Source:* Used with permission from the American Society of Colposcopy and Cervical Pathology.

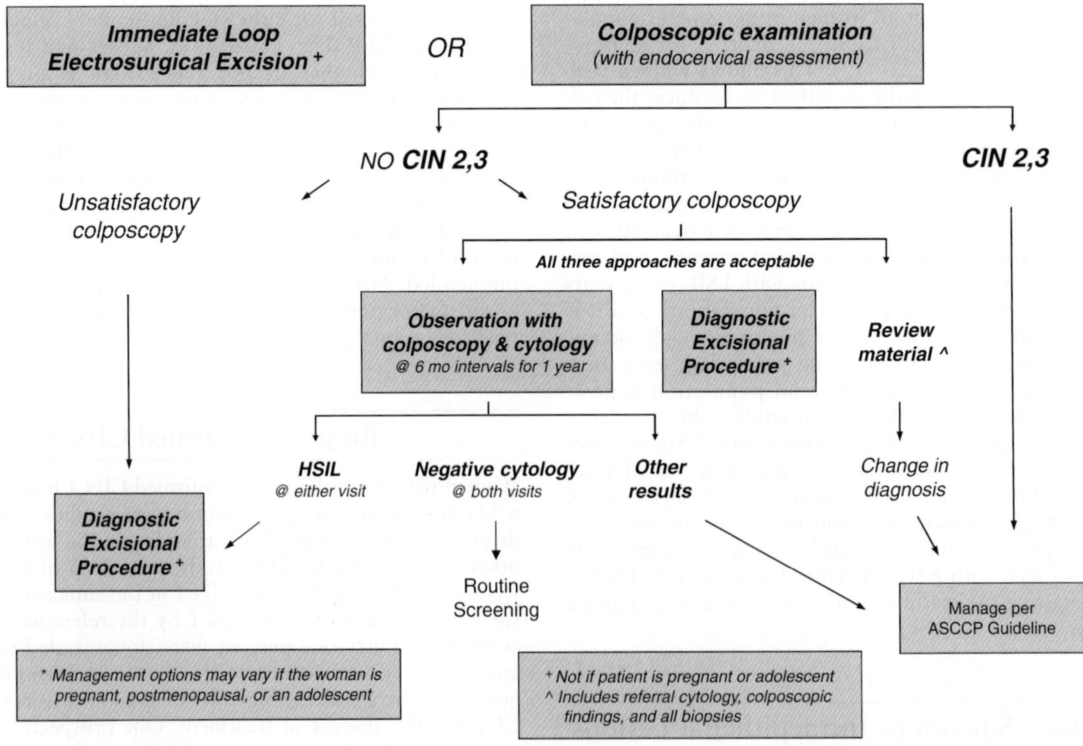

FIGURE 19.24. 2006 Consensus Guidelines for the management of women with HSIL. *Source:* Used with permission from the American Society of Colposcopy and Cervical Pathology.

LSIL infected with high-risk types of HPV spontaneously cleared their infections (169). Recent studies indicate that CIN 1 only rarely progresses to CIN 2,3. In the ALTS study most of the CIN 2,3 lesions that were subsequently diagnosed in women who had initially been diagnosed with CIN 1 appear to represent lesions that were missed at the time of the initial colposcopic examination (170). Since the risk of an undetected CIN 2,3 or glandular lesion is expected to be higher in women referred for the evaluation of an HSIL or AGC on cytology, women with CIN 1 preceded by HSIL or AGC cervical cytology can be managed more aggressively than women with CIN 1 preceded by ASC-US, ASC-H, or LSIL cytology.

Because of the above considerations, the 2006 Consensus Guidelines state that women with biopsy-confirmed CIN 1 preceded by ASC-US, ASC-H, or LSIL should have follow-up with either HPV DNA testing every 12 months or repeat cervical cytology every 6 to 12 months. If CIN 1 persists for at least 2 years, either continued follow-up or treatment is acceptable. For women with a satisfactory colposcopic examination, acceptable treatments include the use of ablative (e.g., cryotherapy, electrofulguration, or laser ablation) or excisional modalities such as loop electrosurgical excision (148). All treatment modalities are considered acceptable since randomized, controlled clinical trials comparing cryotherapy, laser ablation, and LEEP for treating biopsy-confirmed CIN have reported no significant differences in either complication rates or success rates and a comprehensive review of controlled and randomized trials of various treatment modalities found no significant differences in outcomes after treatment in women with CIN with satisfactory colposcopic examinations (171). Before treating any grade of CIN using an ablative modality such as cryotherapy, it is important to perform an endocervical sampling in order to ensure that an unsuspected lesion is not present in the endocervical canal. For women with biopsy-confirmed CIN 1 preceded by HSIL or AGC cytology, either a diagnostic excisional procedure or follow-up with colposcopy and cytology at 6-month intervals for 1 year is acceptable, provided the colposcopic examination is satisfactory and endocervical sampling is negative (148).

Biopsy-Confirmed CIN 2,3

Women with an untreated, histologically confirmed CIN 2,3 lesion are felt to have a significantly high risk of progressing to invasive cervical cancer to warrant routine treatment. Provided the colposcopic examination is satisfactory and there is no suggestion of invasive disease (e.g., by either colposcopy, cytology, or histology) both ablative and excisional treatment modalities are considered acceptable forms of treatment (148). In patients with recurrent CIN (either CIN 1 or CIN 2,3) it is preferred that an excisional treatment modality be used. A diagnostic excisional procedure is recommended for all women with biopsy-confirmed CIN 2,3 and an unsatisfactory colposcopic examination.

The risk of recurrent CIN 2,3 or invasive cancer after treatment remains elevated for many years after treatment. A large follow-up study from the United Kingdom reported that the cumulative risk of invasive cervical cancer was 5.8 per 1,000 after 8 years of follow-up, which is approximately 100 times higher than in women in the general population (172). The size of the original CIN 2,3 lesion appears to be an important determinant of the rate of recurrence. Large lesions have a higher failure rate than small lesions. The 2006 Consensus Guidelines recommend that after treatment for CIN 2,3 women be followed up using either (a) HPV DNA testing at 6 to 12 months, (b) cytology alone at 6-month intervals, or (c) a combination of cytology and colposcopy at 6-month intervals. After two negative cytology results are obtained, routine screening is recommended for at least 20 years (148). When CIN is identified at the margins of a diagnostic excisional procedure, it is preferred that the 4- to 6-month follow-up visit include endocervical sampling.

References

1. CDC. Human Papillomavirus: HPV Information for Clinicians. 2007. http://www.cdc.gov/std/HPV/common-clinicians/ClinicianBro-fp.pdf. Accessed January 2008.
2. Larsen NS. Invasive cervical cancer arising in young white females. *J Natl Cancer Inst* 1994;86:6.
3. Wang SS, Sherman ME, Hildesheim A, et al. Cervical adenocarcinoma and squamous cell carcinoma incidence trends among white women and black women in the United States for 1976-2000. *Cancer* 2004;100:1035.
4. Davey DD, Neal MH, Wilbur DC, et al. Bethesda 2001 implementation and reporting rates: 2003 practices of participants in the College of American Pathologists Interlaboratory Comparison Program in Cervicovaginal Cytology. *Arch Pathol Lab Med* 2004;128:1224.
5. Wright TC, Ferenczy AF, Kurman RJ. Precancerous lesions of the cervix. In: Kurman RJ, ed. *Blaustein's Pathology of the Female Genital Tract.* 5th ed. New York: Springer-Verlag; 2002:253.
6. Richart RM. Cervical intraepithelial neoplasia: a review. In: Sommers SC, ed. *Pathology Annual.* East Norwalk, CT: Appleton-Century-Crofts; 1973:301.
7. Clifford G, Franceschi S, Diaz M, et al. HPV type-distribution in women with and without cervical neoplastic diseases. *Vaccine* 2006;24(suppl 3): S26.
8. Chung TK, Cheung TH, Lo WK, et al. Loss of heterozygosity at the short arm of chromosome 3 in microdissected cervical intraepithelial neoplasia. *Cancer Lett* 2000;154:189.
9. Melsheimer P, Vinokurova S, Wentzensen N, et al. DNA aneuploidy and integration of human papillomavirus type 16 e6/e7 oncogenes in intraepithelial neoplasia and invasive squamous cell carcinoma of the cervix uteri. *Clin Cancer Res* 2004;10:3059.
10. Solomon D, Davey D, Kurman R, et al. The 2001 Bethesda system: terminology for reporting results of cervical cytology. *JAMA* 2002;287:2114.
11. Wright TC Jr, Cox JT, Massad LS, et al. 2001 consensus guidelines for the management of women with cervical cytological abnormalities. *JAMA* 2002;287:2120.
12. Wright TC Jr, Massad LS, Dunton CJ, et al. 2006 consensus guidelines for the management of women with abnormal cervical cancer screening tests. *Am J Obstet Gynecol* 2007;197:346.
13. Wells M, Ostor AG, Franceschi S, et al. Epithelial tumors of the uterine cervix. In: Tavassoli FA, Devilee P, eds. *Tumors of the Breast and Female Genital Organs.* Lyon: IARC; 2003:221.
14. Shingleton HM, Gore H, Bradley DH, et al. Adenocarcinoma of the cervix. I. Clinical evaluation and pathologic features. *Am J Obstet Gynecol* 1981;139:799.
15. Leminen A, Paavonen J, Forss M, et al. Adenocarcinoma of the uterine cervix. *Cancer* 1990;65:53.
16. Parazzini F, La Vecchia C. Epidemiology of adenocarcinoma of the cervix. *Gynecol Oncol* 1990;39:40.
17. Schwartz SM, Weiss NS. Increased incidence of adenocarcinoma of the cervix in young women in the United States. *Am J Epidemiol* 1986; 124:1045.
18. Eide TJ. Cancer of the uterine cervix in Norway by histologic type, 1970-1984. *J Natl Cancer Inst* 1987;79:199.
19. Helper TK, Dockerty MB, Randall LM. Primary adenocarcinoma of the cervix. *Am J Obstet Gynecol* 1952;63:800.
20. Friedell GH, McKay DG. Adenocarcinoma in situ of endocervix. *Cancer* 1953;6:887.
21. Ridley CM, Frankman O, Jones ISC, et al. New nomenclature for vulvar disease: International Society for the Study of Vulvar Disease (letter to the editor). *Lancet* 1989;20:495.
22. Sideri M, Jones RW, Wilkinson EJ, et al. Squamous vulvar intraepithelial neoplasia; 2004 modified terminology, ISSVD Vulvar Oncology Subcommittee. *J Reprod Med* 2005;50:807.
23. Srodon M, Stoler MH, Baber GB, et al. The distribution of low and high-risk HPV types in vulvar and vaginal intraepithelial neoplasia (VIN and VaIN). *Am J Surg Pathol* 2006;30:1513.
24. Reagan JW, Hicks DJ, Scott RB. Atypical hyperplasia of uterine cervix. *Cancer* 1955;8:42.
25. Patten SF. *Diagnostic Cytology of the Uterine Cervix.* 2nd ed. Baltimore: Williams and Wilkins; 1969.
26. Kottmeier H-L. *Annual Report on the Results of Treatment in Carcinoma of the Uterus, Vagina and Ovary.* International Federation of Gynecology and Obstetrics—Stockholm; 1976.
27. Koss LG, Stewart FW, Foote FW, et al. Some histological aspects of behavior of epidermoid carcinoma in situ and related lesions of the uterine cervix. *Cancer* 1963;16:1160.

28. Green GH, Donovan JW. The natural history of cervical carcinoma in situ. *J Obstet Gynaecol Br Commonw* 1970;77:1–9.
29. McIndoe WA, McLean MR, Jones RW, et al. The invasive potential of carcinoma in situ of the cervix. *Obstet Gynecol* 1984;64:451.
30. Koss LG. *Diagnostic Cytology and Its Histopathologic Basis, Vol. 1.* 3rd ed. New York: JB Lippincott Company; 1992.
31. Miller AB. *Cervical Cancer Screening Programmes: Managerial Guidelines.* Geneva: World Health Organization; 1992:50.
32. Ponten J, Adami H-O, Bergstrom R, et al. Strategies for global control of cervical cancer. *Int J Cancer* 1995;60:1.
33. Holowaty P, Miller AB, Rohan T, et al. Natural history of dysplasia of the uterine cervix. *J Natl Cancer Inst* 1999;91:252.
34. Nasiell K, Roger V, Nasiell M. Behavior of mild cervical dysplasia during long-term follow-up. *Obstet Gynecol* 1986;67:665.
35. Nasiell K, Nasiell M, Vaclavinkova V. Behavior of moderate cervical dysplasia during long-term follow-up. *Obstet Gynecol* 1983;61:609.
36. Melnikow J, Nuovo J, Willan AR, et al. Natural history of cervical squamous intraepithelial lesions: a meta-analysis. *Obstet Gynecol* 1998;92:727.
37. Mitchell MF, Tortolero-Luna G, Wright T, et al. Cervical human papillomavirus infection and intraepithelial neoplasia: a review. *J Natl Cancer Inst Monogr* 1996;21:17.
38. Winer RL, Kiviat NB, Hughes JP, et al. Development and duration of human papillomavirus lesions, after initial infection. *J Infect Dis* 2005;191:731.
39. Mao C, Koutsky LA, Ault KA, et al. Efficacy of human papillomavirus-16 vaccine to prevent cervical intraepithelial neoplasia: a randomized controlled trial. *Obstet Gynecol* 2006;107:18.
40. Buscema J, Stern J, Woodruff JD. The significance of the histological alterations adjacent to invasive vulvar carcinoma. *Am J Obstet Gynecol* 1987;156:212.
41. Roy M. VIN: latest management approaches. *Cont OB/Gyn* 1988;32:170.
42. Hording U, Junge J, Poulsen H, et al. Vulvar intraepithelial neoplasia III: a viral disease of undetermined progressive potential. *Gynecol Oncol* 1995;56:276.
43. Jones RW, Rowan DM. Vulvar intraepithelial neoplasia III: a clinical study of the outcome in 113 cases with relation to the later development of invasive vulvar carcinoma. *Obstet Gynecol* 1994;84:741.
44. Bosch FX, de Sanjose S. The epidemiology of human papillomavirus infection and cervical cancer. *Dis Markers* 2007;23:213.
45. Smith JS, Munoz N, Herrero R, et al. Evidence for *Chlamydia trachomatis* as a human papillomavirus cofactor in the etiology of invasive cervical cancer in Brazil and the Philippines. *J Infect Dis* 2002;185:324.
46. Anttila T, Saikku P, Koskela P, et al. Serotypes of *Chlamydia trachomatis* and risk for development of cervical squamous cell carcinoma. *JAMA* 2001;285:47.
47. Castle PE, Giuliano AR. Genital tract infections, cervical inflammation, and antioxidant nutrients—assessing their roles as human papillomavirus cofactors. *J Natl Cancer Inst Monogr* 2003;29.
48. Bosch FX, de Sanjose S. Human papillomavirus and cervical cancer—burden and assessment of causality. *J Natl Cancer Inst Monogr* 2003;3.
49. Bosch FX, Manos MM, Munoz N, et al. Prevalence of human papillomavirus in cervical cancer: a worldwide perspective. International Biological Study on Cervical Cancer (IBSCC) Study Group. *J Natl Cancer Inst* 1995;87:779.
50. Walboomers JM, Jacobs MV, Manos MM, et al. Human papillomavirus is a necessary cause of invasive cervical cancer worldwide. *J Pathol* 1999;189:12.
51. Munoz N, Bosch FX, de Sanjose S, et al. Epidemiologic classification of human papillomavirus types associated with cervical cancer. *N Engl J Med* 2003;348:518.
52. Ellerbrock TV, Chiasson MA, Bush TJ, et al. Incidence of cervical squamous intraepithelial lesions in HIV-infected women. *JAMA* 2000;283:1031.
53. Munoz N, Castellsague X, De Gonzalez AB, et al. HPV in the etiology of human cancer. *Vaccine* 2006;24(suppl 3):1–10.
54. *Cervix Cancer Screening*, Vol. 10. Lyons: IARC; 2005.
55. Cogliano V, Baan R, Straif K, et al. Carcinogenicity of human papillomaviruses. *Lancet Oncol* 2005;6:204.
56. Szarewski A, Cuzick J. Smoking and cervical neoplasia: a review of the evidence. *J Epidemiol Biostat* 1998;3:229.
57. McCann MF, Irwin DE, Walton LA, et al. Nicotine and cotinine in the cervical mucus of smokers, passive smokers, and nonsmokers. *Cancer Epidemiol Biomarkers Prev* 1992;1:125.
58. Simons AM, Phillips DH, Coleman DV. Damage to DNA in cervical epithelium related to smoking tobacco. *BMJ* 1993;306:1444.
59. Szarewski A, Maddox P, Royston P, et al. The effect of stopping smoking on cervical Langerhans' cells and lymphocytes. *BJOG* 2001;108:295.
60. Smith JS, Green J, Berrington de Gonzalez A, et al. Cervical cancer and use of hormonal contraceptives: a systematic review. *Lancet* 2003;361:1159.
61. Appleby P, Beral V, Berrington de Gonzalez A, et al. Cervical cancer and hormonal contraceptives: collaborative reanalysis of individual data for 16,573 women with cervical cancer and 35,509 women without cervical cancer from 24 epidemiological studies. *Lancet* 2007;370:1609.
62. Bornstein J, Rahat MA, Abramovici H. Etiology of cervical cancer: current concepts. *Obstet Gynecol Surv* 1995;50:146.
63. Butterworth CEJ, Hatch KD, Macaluso M, et al. Folate deficiency and cervical dysplasia. *JAMA* 1992;267:528.
64. Wright TC, Kuhn L. Immunosuppression and the cervix: human immunodeficiency virus (HIV). In: Jordan JA, Singer A, eds. *The Cervix*. Malden, MA: Blackwell; 2006:450.
65. Sun XW, Kuhn L, Ellerbrock TV, et al. Human papillomavirus infection in HIV-seropositive women: natural history and variability of detection. *N Engl J Med* 1997;337:1343.
66. Fordyce EJ, Wang Z, Kahn AR, et al. Risk of cancer among women with AIDS in New York City. *AIDS Public Policy J* 2000;15:95.
67. Maiman M. Management of cervical neoplasia in human immunodeficiency virus-infected women. *J Natl Cancer Inst* 1998;23:43.
68. CDC. 1993 revised classification system for HIV infection and expanded surveillance case definition for AIDS among adolescents and adults. *Morbidity Mortality Weekly Report* 1993;41:1.
69. de Villiers EM. Human pathogenic papillomavirus types: an update. *Curr Top Microbiol Immunol* 1994;186:1.
70. Lacey C, Lowndes CM, Shah KV. Burden and management of non-cancerous HPV-related conditions; HPV 6/11 disease. *Vaccine* 2006;24(suppl 3):35–41.
71. Aguilera-Barrantes I, Magro C, Nuovo GJ. Verruca vulgaris of the vulva in children and adults: a nonvenereal type of vulvar wart. *Am J Surg Pathol* 2007;31:529.
72. Bleeker MC, Hogewoning CJ, Voorhorst FJ, et al. HPV-associated flat penile lesions in men of a non-STD hospital population: less frequent and smaller in size than in male sexual partners of women with CIN. *Int J Cancer* 2005;113:36.
73. Clifford GM, Rana RK, Franceschi S, et al. Human papillomavirus genotype distribution in low-grade cervical lesions: comparison by geographic region and with cervical cancer. *Cancer Epidemiol Biomarkers Prev* 2005;14:1157.
74. Lungu O, Sun XW, Felix J, et al. Relationship of human papillomavirus type to grade of cervical intraepithelial neoplasia. *JAMA* 1992;267:2493.
75. Smith JS, Lindsay L, Hoots B, et al. Human papillomavirus type distribution in invasive cervical cancer and high-grade cervical lesions: a meta-analysis update. *Int J Cancer* 2007;121:621.
76. Jacobs MV, Walboomers JM, Snijders PJ, et al. Distribution of 37 mucosotropic HPV types in women with cytologically normal cervical smears: the age-related patterns for high-risk and low- risk types. *Int J Cancer* 2000;87:221.
77. Liaw KL, Glass AG, Manos MM, et al. Detection of human papillomavirus DNA in cytologically normal women and subsequent cervical squamous intraepithelial lesions. *J Natl Cancer Inst* 1999;91:954.
78. Peyton CL, Gravitt PE, Hunt WC, et al. Determinants of genital human papillomavirus detection in a US population. *J Infect Dis* 2001;183:1554.
79. Doorbar J. Papillomavirus life cycle organization and biomarker selection. *Dis Markers* 2007;23:297.
80. DiMaio D, Liao JB. Human papillomaviruses and cervical cancer. *Adv Virus Res* 2006;66:125.
81. Fehrmann F, Laimins LA. Human papillomaviruses: targeting differentiating epithelial cells for malignant transformation. *Oncogene* 2003;22:5201.
82. Ustav E, Ustav M. E2 protein as the master regulator of extrachromosomal replication of the papillomaviruses. *Papillomavirus Reports* 1998;9:145.
83. zur Hausen H. Papillomaviruses and cancer: from basic studies to clinical application. *Nat Rev Cancer* 2002;2:342.
84. Doobar J. Late stages of the papillomvirus life cycle. *Papillomavirus Reports* 1998;9:119.
85. Lowy DR, Schiller JT. Prophylactic human papillomavirus vaccines. *J Clin Invest* 2006;116:1167.
86. zur Hausen H. Papillomaviruses causing cancer: evasion from host-cell control in early events in carcinogenesis. *J Natl Cancer Inst* 2000;92:690.
87. Evander M, Frazer IH, Payne E, et al. Identification of the alpha6 integrin as a candidate receptor for papillomaviruses. *J Virol* 1997;71:2449.
88. Munger K, Howley PM. Human papillomavirus immortalization and transformation functions. *Virus Res* 2002;89:213.
89. Horner SM, DeFilippis RA, Manuelidis L, DiMaio D. Repression of the human papillomavirus E6 gene initiates p53-dependent, telomerase-independent senescence and apoptosis in HeLa cervical carcinoma cells. *J Virol* 2004;78:4063.
90. Schiffman M, Castle PE, Jeronimo J, et al. Human papillomavirus and cervical cancer. *Lancet* 2007;370:890.
91. McCluggage WG. Immunohistochemistry as a diagnostic aid in cervical pathology. *Pathology* 2007;39:97.
92. Durst M, Glitz D, Schneider A, et al. Human papillomavirus type 16 (HPV 16) gene expression and DNA replication in cervical neoplasia: analysis by in situ hybridization. *Virology* 1992;189:132.
93. Stoler MH, Rhodes CR, Whitbeck A, et al. Human papillomavirus type 16 and 18 gene expression in cervical neoplasias. *Hum Pathol* 1992;23:117.
94. Snijders PJ, Steenbergen RD, Heideman DA, et al. HPV-mediated cervical carcinogenesis: concepts and clinical implications. *J Pathol* 2006;208:152.
95. Mitra AB, Murty VV, Li RG, et al. Allelotype analysis of cervical carcinoma. *Cancer Res* 1994;54:4481.

96. Larson AA, Kern S, Curtiss S, et al. High resolution analysis of chromosome 3p alterations in cervical carcinoma. *Cancer Res* 1997;57:4082.
97. Iftner T, Villa LL. Human papillomavirus technologies. *J Natl Cancer Inst Monogr* 2003;80.
98. Cuzick J, Beverley E, Ho L, et al. HPV testing in primary screening of older women. *Br J Cancer* 1999;81:554.
99. Salmeron J, Lazcano-Ponce E, Lorincz A, et al. Comparison of HPV-based assays with Papanicolaou smears for cervical cancer screening in Morelos State, Mexico. *Cancer Causes Control* 2003;14:505.
100. Kuhn L, Denny L, Pollack A, et al. Human papillomavirus DNA testing for cervical cancer screening in low-resource settings. *J Natl Cancer Inst* 2000;92:818.
101. Belinson J, Qiao YL, Pretorius R, et al. Shanxi Province Cervical Cancer Screening Study: a cross-sectional comparative trial of multiple techniques to detect cervical neoplasia. *Gynecol Oncol* 2001;83:439.
102. Ratnam S, Franco EL, Ferenczy A. Human papillomavirus testing for primary screening of cervical cancer precursors. *Cancer Epidemiol Biomarkers Prev* 2000;9:945.
103. Kulasingam SL, Hughes JP, Kiviat NB, et al. Evaluation of human papillomavirus testing in primary screening for cervical abnormalities: comparison of sensitivity, specificity, and frequency of referral. *JAMA* 2002;288:1749.
104. Brown DR, Shew ML, Qadadri B, et al. A longitudinal study of genital human papillomavirus infection in a cohort of closely followed adolescent women. *J Infect Dis* 2005;191:182.
105. Winer RL, Koutsky LA. Human papillomavirus through the ages. *J Infect Dis* 2005;191:1787.
106. Bosch FX, Lorincz A, Munoz N, et al. The causal relation between human papillomavirus and cervical cancer. *J Clin Pathol* 2002;55:244.
107. de Sanjose S, Diaz M, Castellsague X, et al. Worldwide prevalence and genotype distribution of cervical human papillomavirus DNA in women with normal cytology: a meta-analysis. *Lancet Infect Dis* 2007;7:453.
108. Fife KH, Katz BP, Roush J et al. Cancer-associated human papillomavirus types are selectively increased in the cervix of women in the first trimester of pregnancy. *Am J Obstet Gynecol* 1996;174:1487.
109. Burk RD, Ho GY, Beardsley L, et al. Sexual behavior and partner characteristics are the predominant risk factors for genital human papillomavirus infection in young women. *J Infect Dis* 1996;174:679.
110. Kjaer SK, Chackerian B, van den Brule AJ, et al. High-risk human papillomavirus is sexually transmitted: evidence from a follow-up study of virgins starting sexual activity (intercourse). *Cancer Epidemiol Biomarkers Prev* 2001;10:101.
111. Winer RL, Hughes JP, Feng Q, et al. Condom use and the risk of genital human papillomavirus infection in young women. *N Engl J Med* 2006;354:2645.
112. Oriel JD. Natural history of genital warts. *Br J Ven Dis* 1971;47:1.
113. Roden RB, Lowy DR, Schiller JT. Papillomavirus is resistant to desiccation. *J Infect Dis* 1997;176:1076.
114. Ferris DG, Batish S, Wright TC, et al. A neglected lesbian health concern: cervical neoplasia. *J Fam Pract* 1996;43:581.
115. Armstrong LR, Preston EJ, Reichert M, et al. Incidence and prevalence of recurrent respiratory papillomatosis among children in Atlanta and Seattle. *Clin Infect Dis* 2000;31:107.
116. Smith EM, Swarnavel S, Ritchie JM, et al. Prevalence of human papillomavirus in the oral cavity/oropharynx in a large population of children and adolescents. *Pediatr Infect Dis J* 2007;26:836.
117. Wright TC, Schiffman M. Adding a test for human papillomavirus DNA to cervical-cancer screening. *N Engl J Med* 2003;348:489.
118. Strickler HD, Burk RD, Fazzari M, et al. Natural history and possible reactivation of human papillomavirus in human immunodeficiency virus-positive women. *J Natl Cancer Inst* 2005;97:577.
119. Sun XW, Kuhn L, Ellerbrock TV, et al. Human papillomavirus infection in women infected with the human immunodeficiency virus. *N Engl J Med* 1997;337:1343.
120. Park TW, Fujiwara H, Wright TC. Molecular biology of cervical cancer and its precursors. *Cancer* 1995;76:1902.
121. ter Haar-van Eck SA, Rischen-Vos J, Chadha-Ajwani S, et al. The incidence of cervical intraepithelial neoplasia among women with renal transplant in relation to cyclosporine. *Br J Obstet Gynecol* 1995;102:58.
122. Harmsel B, Smedts F, Kuijpers J, et al. Relationship between human papillomavirus type 16 in the cervix and intraepithelial neoplasia. *Obstet Gynecol* 1999;93:46.
123. Schneider A. Latent and subclinical genital HPV infections. *Papillomavirus Report* 1990;1:2.
124. Ward KA, Houston JR, Lowry BE, et al. The role of early colposcopy in the management of females with first episode anogenital warts. *Int J STD AIDS* 1994;5:343.
125. Coker R, Desmond N, Tomlinson D, et al. Screening for cervical abnormalities in women with anogenital warts in an STD clinic: an inappropriate use of colposcopy. *Int J STD AIDS* 1994;5:442.
126. Felix JC, Wright TC. Analysis of lower genital tract lesions clinically suspicious for condylomata using in situ hybridization and the polymerase chain reaction for the detection of human papillomavirus. *Arch Pathol Lab Med* 1994;118:39.
127. Ferenczy A, Richart RM, Wright TC. Pearly penile papules: absence of human papillomavirus DNA by the polymerase chain reaction. *Obstet Gynecol* 1991;78:118.
128. Bergeron C, Ferenczy A, Richart RM, et al. Micropapillomatosis labialis appears unrelated to human papillomavirus. *Obstet Gynecol* 1990;76:281.
129. Hemminki K, Li X, Vaittinen P. Time trends in the incidence of cervical and other genital squamous cell carcinomas and adenocarcinomas in Sweden, 1958-1996. *Eur J Obstet Gynecol Reprod Biol* 2002;101:64.
130. Iversen T, Tretli S. Intraepithelial and invasive squamous cell neoplasia of the vulva: trends in incidence, recurrence, and survival rate in Norway. *Obstet Gynecol* 1998;91:969.
131. McNally OM, Mulvany NJ, Pagano R, et al. VIN 3: a clinicopathologic review. *Int J Gynecol Cancer* 2002;12:490.
132. Skapa P, Zamecnik J, Hamsikova E, et al. Human papillomavirus (HPV) profiles of vulvar lesions: possible implications for the classification of vulvar squamous cell carcinoma precursors and for the efficacy of prophylactic HPV vaccination. *Am J Surg Pathol* 2007;31:1834.
133. Crum CP, Granter SR. Squamous neoplasia of the vulva. In: Crum CP, Lee KR, eds. *Diagnostic Gynecologic and Obstetric Pathology.* Elsevier; 2006:109.
134. Haefner HK, Tate JE, McLachlin CM, et al. Vulvar intraepithelial neoplasia: age, morphological phenotpe, papillomavirus DNA and coexisiting invasive carcinoma. *Hum Pathol* 1995;26:147.
135. Kaufman RH. Intraepithelial neoplasia of the vulva. *Gynecol Oncol* 1995;56:8.
136. Quinn M, Babb P, Jones J, et al. Effect of screening on incidence of and mortality from cancer of cervix in England: evaluation based on routinely collected statistics. *BMJ* 1999;318:904.
137. Fahey MT, Irwig L, Macaskill P. Meta-analysis of Pap test accuracy. *Am J Epidemiol* 1995;141:680.
138. Nanda K, McCrory DC, Myers ER, et al. Accuracy of the Papanicolaou test in screening for and follow-up of cervical cytologic abnormalities: a systematic review. *Ann Intern Med* 2000;132:810.
139. Koonings PP, Dickinson K, d'Ablaing G 3rd, et al. A randomized clinical trial comparing the Cytobrush and cotton swab for Papanicolaou smears. *Obstet Gynecol* 1992;80:241.
140. Miller AB. Failures of cervical cancer screening. *Am J Public Health* 1995;85:795.
141. ACOG Practice Bulletin: clinical management guidelines for obstetrician-gynecologists. Number 45, August 2003. Cervical cytology screening (replaces committee opinion 152, March 1995). *Obstet Gynecol* 2003;102:417.
142. Saslow D, Runowicz CD, Solomon D, et al. American Cancer Society guideline for the early detection of cervical neoplasia and cancer. *CA Cancer J Clin* 2002;52:342.
143. U.S. Preventive Services Task Force. *Guide to Clinical Preventive Services.* 3rd ed. Periodic updates ed. Washington, DC: U.S. Department of Health and Human Services; 2003.
144. Davey E, Barratt A, Irwig L, et al. Effect of study design and quality on unsatisfactory rates, cytology classifications, and accuracy in liquid-based versus conventional cervical cytology: a systematic review. *Lancet* 2006;367:122.
145. Arbyn M, Bergeron C, Klinkhamer P, et al. Liquid compared with conventional cervical cytology: a systematic review and meta-analysis. *Obstet Gynecol* 2008;111:167.
146. Taylor S, Kuhn L, Dupree W, et al. Direct comparison of liquid-based and conventional cytology in a South African screening trial. *Int J Cancer* 2006;118:957.
147. Ronco G, Segnan N, Giorgi-Rossi P, et al. Human papillomavirus testing and liquid-based cytology: results at recruitment from the new technologies for cervical cancer randomized controlled trial. *J Natl Cancer Inst* 2006;98:765.
148. Wright TC Jr, Massad LS, Dunton CJ, et al. 2006 consensus guidelines for the management of women with cervical intraepithelial neoplasia or adenocarcinoma *in situ*. *Am J Obstet Gynecol* 2007;197:340.
149. Stoler MH, Schiffman M. Interobserver reproducibility of cervical cytologic and histologic interpretations: realistic estimates from the ASCUS-LSIL Triage study. *JAMA* 2001;285:1500.
150. Manos MM, Kinney WK, Hurley LB, et al. Identifying women with cervical neoplasia: using human papillomavirus DNA testing for equivocal Papanicolaou results. *JAMA* 1999;281:1605.
151. Solomon D, Schiffman M, Tarrone R. Comparison of three management strategies for patients with atypical squamous cells of undetermined significance: baseline results from a randomized trial. *J Natl Cancer Inst* 2001;93:293.
152. Lonky NM, Sadeghi M, Tsadik GW, et al. The clinical significance of the poor correlation of cervical dysplasia and cervical malignancy with referral cytologic results. *Am J Obstet Gynecol* 1999;181:560.
153. Kinney WK, Manos MM, Hurley LB, et al. Where's the high-grade cervical neoplasia? The importance of minimally abnormal Papanicolaou diagnoses. *Obstet Gynecol* 1998;91:973.
154. Arbyn M, Sasieni P, Meijer CJ, et al. Clinical applications of HPV testing: a summary of meta-analyses. *Vaccine* 2006;24(Suppl 3):S78.
155. Kim JJ, Wright TC, Goldie SJ. Cost-effectiveness of alternative triage strategies for atypical squamous cells of undetermined significance. *JAMA* 2002;287:2382.
156. Kulasingam SL, Kim JJ, Lawrence WF, et al. Cost-effectiveness analysis based on the atypical squamous cells of undetermined significance/low-grade squamous intraepithelial lesion Triage Study (ALTS). *J Natl Cancer Inst* 2006;98:92.

157. Sherman ME, Schiffman M, Cox JT, et al. Effects of age and HPV load on colposcopic triage: data from the ASCUS LSIL Triage study (ALTS). *J Natl Cancer Inst* 2002;94:102.
158. Boardman LA, Stanko C, Weitzen S, et al. Atypical squamous cells of undetermined significance: human papillomavirus testing in adolescents. *Obstet Gynecol* 2005;105:741.
159. Jones BA, Novis DA. Follow-up of abnormal gynecologic cytology: a College of American Pathologists Q-Probes study of 16132 cases from 306 laboratories. *Arch Pathol Lab Med* 2000;124:665.
160. Human papillomavirus testing for triage of women with cytologic evidence of low-grade squamous intraepithelial lesions: baseline data from a randomized trial. The Atypical Squamous Cells of Undetermined Significance/Low-Grade Squamous Intraepithelial Lesions Triage Study (ALTS) Group. *J Natl Cancer Inst* 2000;92:397.
161. A randomized trial on the management of low-grade squamous intraepithelial lesion cytology interpretations. *Am J Obstet Gynecol* 2003;188:1393.
162. Moscicki AB, Schiffman M, Kjaer S, et al. Updating the natural history of HPV and anogenital cancer. *Vaccine* 2006;24(Suppl 3):S42.
163. Moscicki AB, Hills N, Shiboski S, et al. Risks for incident human papillomavirus infection and low-grade squamous intraepithelial lesion development in young females. *JAMA* 2001;285:2995.
164. Evans MF, Adamson CS, Papillo JL, et al. Distribution of human papillomavirus types in ThinPrep Papanicolaou tests classified according to the Bethesda 2001 terminology and correlations with patient age and biopsy outcomes. *Cancer* 2006;106:1054.
165. Insinga RP, Glass AG, Rush BB. Diagnoses and outcomes in cervical cancer screening: a population-based study. *Am J Obstet Gynecol* 2004;191:105.
166. Jones BA, Novis DA. Cervical biopsy-cytology correlation. A College of American Pathologists Q-Probes study of 22,439 correlations in 348 laboratories. *Arch Pathol Lab Med* 1996;120:523.
167. Jones BA, Davey DD. Quality management in gynecologic cytology using interlaboratory comparison. *Arch Pathol Lab Med* 2000;124:672.
168. Schlecht NF, Platt RW, Duarte-Franco E, et al. Human papillomavirus infection and time to progression and regression of cervical intraepithelial neoplasia. *J Natl Cancer Inst* 2003;95:1336.
169. Nobbenhuis MA, Helmerhorst TJ, van den Brule AJ, et al. Cytological regression and clearance of high-risk human papillomavirus in women with an abnormal cervical smear. *Lancet* 2001;358:1782.
170. Cox JT, Schiffman M, Solomon D. Prospective follow-up suggests similar risk of subsequent cervical intraepithelial neoplasia grade 2 or 3 among women with cervical intraepithelial neoplasia grade 1 or negative colposcopy and directed biopsy. *Am J Obstet Gynecol* 2003;188:1406.
171. Kyrgiou M, Tsoumpou I, Vrekoussis T, et al. The up-to-date evidence on colposcopy practice and treatment of cervical intraepithelial neoplasia: the Cochrane Colposcopy & Cervical Cytopathology Collaborative Group (C5 Group) approach. *Cancer Treat Rev* 2006;32:516.
172. Soutter WP, de Barros Lopes A, Fletcher A, et al. Invasive cervical cancer after conservative therapy for cervical intraepithelial neoplasia. *Lancet* 1997;349:978.

SECTION III:

DISEASE SITES

CHAPTER 20 ■ VULVA

DAVID H. MOORE, WUI-JIN KOH, WILLIAM P. MCGUIRE, AND EDWARD J. WILKINSON

Malignant tumors of the vulva are rare and account for less than 5% of all cancers of the female genital tract. In 2007 there were an estimated 3,490 new cases of, and 880 deaths from, invasive vulva carcinoma (1). Consequently, most physicians who provide primary health care for women may never encounter a patient with vulvar cancer. Although an occasional patient will present without symptoms, the vast majority of women with vulvar cancer initially present with complaints such as irritation, pruritis, pain, or a mass lesion that does not resolve. The time interval between the onset of symptoms and the diagnosis of cancer is usually protracted by the patient, who ignores her symptoms or attempts a number of self-remedies, and the physician, who may prescribe empiric topical therapies without proper physical examination or tissue biopsy confirmation. Jones and Joura evaluated the clinical events preceding the diagnosis of squamous cell carcinoma of the vulva and found that 88% of patients had experienced symptoms for more than 6 months, 31% of women had three or more medical consultations prior to the diagnosis of vulva carcinoma, and 27% had applied topical estrogen or corticosteroids to the vulva (2).

The vulva is covered by keratinized squamous epithelium, and expectedly the majority of malignant vulva tumors are squamous cell carcinomas. Consequently, our current understanding of the epidemiology, spread patterns, prognostic factors, and survival data for vulvar cancer is derived almost exclusively from retrospective observations and a few prospective studies of squamous cell carcinomas. Malignant melanoma is the second most common cancer of the vulva. Although there is some consensus regarding the behavior and treatment of vulva melanoma, its rarity precludes the conduct of prospective clinical trials. A number of other malignant tumors may also arise on the vulva including basal cell carcinoma, adenocarcinomas (derived from Bartholin's glands, eccrine sweat glands, Paget's disease, or ectopic breast tissue), and a host of very rare soft-tissue sarcomas, including leiomyosarcomas, malignant fibrous histiocytomas, liposarcomas, angiosarcomas, rhabdomyosarcomas, epithelioid sarcomas, and Kaposi's sarcomas. Finally, the vulva may be secondarily involved with malignant disease originating in the bladder, anorectum, or other genital organs.

The traditional therapeutic approach to vulvar cancer has been radical surgical excision of the primary tumor and inguinal femoral lymph nodes. As our clinical understanding of this disease evolved, it became evident that survival could be improved with the administration of postoperative radiation therapy to selected patients at high risk for local regional failure. More recent developments have included the administration of radiation therapy and concurrent chemotherapy in the postoperative setting, and as primary therapy for locally advanced tumors not amenable to radical surgery. An individualized approach to vulvar cancer management, often employing multiple modalities in an effort to achieve excellent disease control with better cosmetic results and sexual function, is now the norm. These and other topics pertinent to the principles of management of women with vulvar cancer are the subjects of this chapter.

ANATOMY

The vulva consists of the external genital organs including the mons pubis, labia minora and majora, clitoris, vaginal vestibule, perineal body, and their supporting subcutaneous tissues (3). The vulva is bordered superiorly by the anterior abdominal wall, laterally by the labiocrural fold at the medial thigh, and inferiorly by the anus. The vagina and urethra open onto the vulva. The mons pubis is a prominent mound of hair-bearing skin and subcutaneous adipose and connective tissue that is located anterior to the pubic symphysis. After puberty it is covered by coarse pubic hair. The labia majora are two elongated skin folds that course posterior from the mons pubis and blend into the perineal body. The skin of the labia majora is pigmented and contains hair follicles and sebaceous glands. The labia minora are a smaller pair of skin folds medial and parallel to the labia majora that extend inferiorly to form the margin of the vaginal vestibule. Superiorly, the labia minora separate into two components that course above and below the clitoris, fusing with those of the opposite side to form the prepuce and frenulum, respectively. The skin of the labia minora contains sebaceous glands, but is not hair-bearing and has little or no underlying adipose tissue. The clitoris is supported externally by the fusion of the labia minora (prepuce and frenulum) and is approximately 2 to 3 cm anterior to the urethral meatus. It is comprised of erectile tissue organized into the glans, body, and two crura. The glans has a concentration of nerve endings important for normal sexual response. Two loosely fused corpora cavernosa form the body of the clitoris and extend superiorly from the glans, ultimately dividing into the two crura. The crura course laterally beneath the ischiocavernosus muscles and attach to the ischial rami.

The vaginal vestibule is situated in the center of the vulva and is demarcated circumferentially by the labia minora and inferiorly by the perineal body. Both the vagina and urethra open onto the vestibule. Anteriorly, numerous small vestibular glands are located beneath the vestibular mucosa and open onto its surface adjacent to the urethral meatus. The vestibular bulbs, a loose collection of bilateral erectile tissue covered superficially by the bulbocavernosus muscle, are located laterally. The Bartholin's glands, two small, mucus-secreting glands situated within the subcutaneous tissue of the posterior labia majora, have ducts opening onto the posterolateral portion of the vestibule. The perineal body is a 3- to 4-cm band of skin and

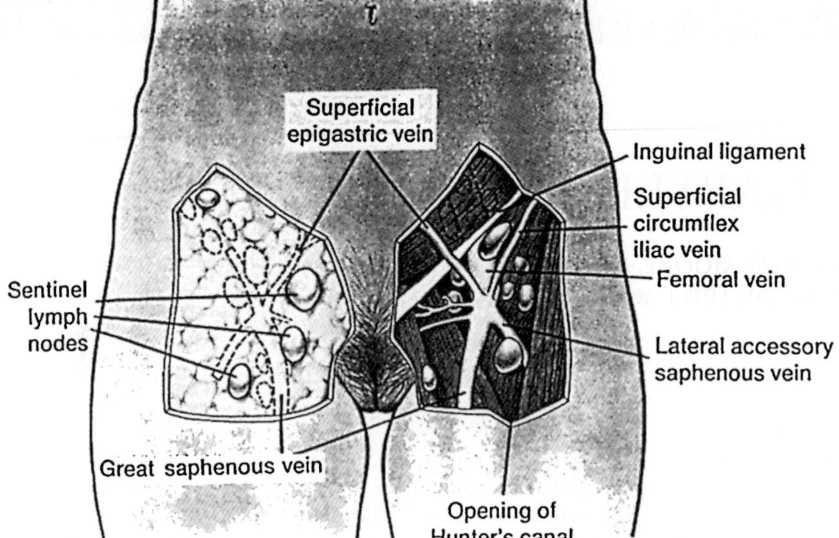

FIGURE 20.1. The superficial inguinal lymph nodes comprise eight to ten subcutaneous nodes located between Camper's fascia and the cribriform fascia. These nodes are immediately adjacent to the saphenous vein and its branches. *Source:* Reprinted from DiSaia PJ, Creasman WT, Rich WM. An alternative approach to early cancer of the vulva. *Am J Obstet Gynecol* 1979;133:825–832.

subcutaneous tissue located between the posterior extension of the labia majora, and separates the vaginal vestibule from the anus and forms the posterior margin of the vulva.

The vulva has a rich blood supply derived primarily from the internal pudendal artery, which arises from the anterior division of the internal iliac (hypogastric) artery, and the superficial and deep external pudendal arteries, which arise from the femoral artery. The internal pudendal artery exits the pelvis and passes behind the ischial spine to reach the posterolateral vulva, where it divides into several small branches to the ischiocavernosus and bulbocavernosus muscles, the perineal artery, artery of the bulb, urethral artery, and dorsal and deep arteries of the clitoris. Both external pudendal arteries travel medially to supply the labia majora and their deep structures. These vessels anastomose freely with branches from the internal pudendal artery. Innervation of the vulva is derived from multiple sources and spinal cord levels. The mons pubis and upper labia majora are innervated by the ilioinguinal nerve (L1) and the genital branch of the genitofemoral nerve (L1-2). Either of these nerves may be easily injured during pelvic lymph node dissection with resulting paresthesias. The pudendal nerve (S2-4) enters the vulva in parallel with the internal pudendal artery and gives rise to several branches that innervate the lower vagina, labia, clitoris, perineal body, and their supporting structures.

The vulva lymphatics run anteriorly through the labia majora, turn laterally at the mons pubis, and drain primarily into the superficial inguinal lymph nodes. Elegant lymphatic dye studies by Parry-Jones demonstrated that vulva lymphatic channels do not extend lateral to the labiocrural folds and generally do not cross the midline, unless the site of dye injection is at the clitoris or perineal body (4). Several small lymphatics may drain from the clitoris under the pubic symphysis directly into the pelvic nodes. Many of these observations have been substantiated by surgical-pathologic studies and sentinel lymph node mapping studies that are discussed later.

The vulva lymphatics drain to the superficial inguinal lymph nodes located within the femoral triangle formed by the inguinal ligament superiorly, the border of the sartorius muscle laterally, and the border of the adductor longus muscle medially. About ten superficial inguinal lymph nodes lie along the saphenous vein and its branches between Camper's fascia and the cribriform fascia overlying the femoral vessels (Fig. 20.1). The superficial nodes are located within the triangle formed by the inguinal ligament superiorly, the border of the sartorius muscle laterally, and the border of the adductor longus muscle medially (Fig. 20.2) (5). Lymphatic drainage proceeds from the superficial to the deep inguinal (or femoral) nodes, which are located beneath the cribriform fascia and medial to the femoral vein. There are usually three to five deep nodes, the most superior of which is Cloquet's node

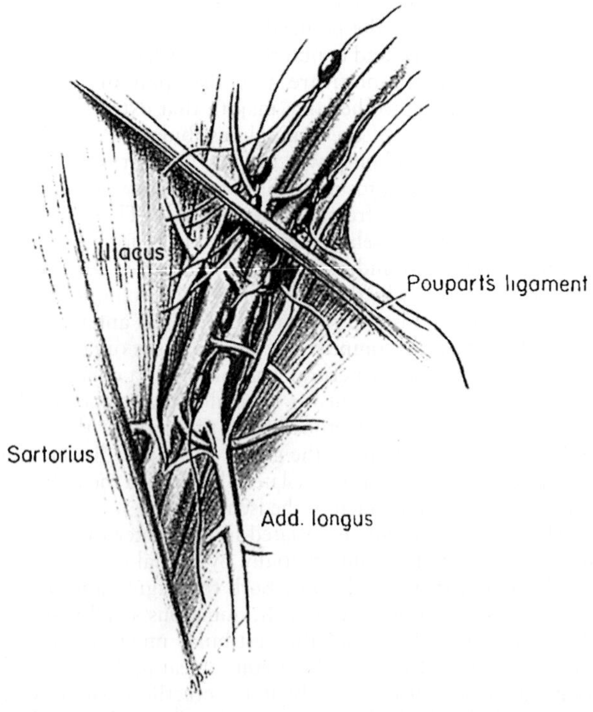

FIGURE 20.2. Anatomic diagram of the right groin with the superficial structures removed demonstrates the saphenous vein and the boundaries of inguinal dissection—the sartorius muscle, inguinal ligament, and adductor longus muscle. *Source:* Reprinted from Plentl AA, Friedman EA, eds. *Lymphatic System of the Female Genitalia.* Philadelphia: WB Saunders; 1971.

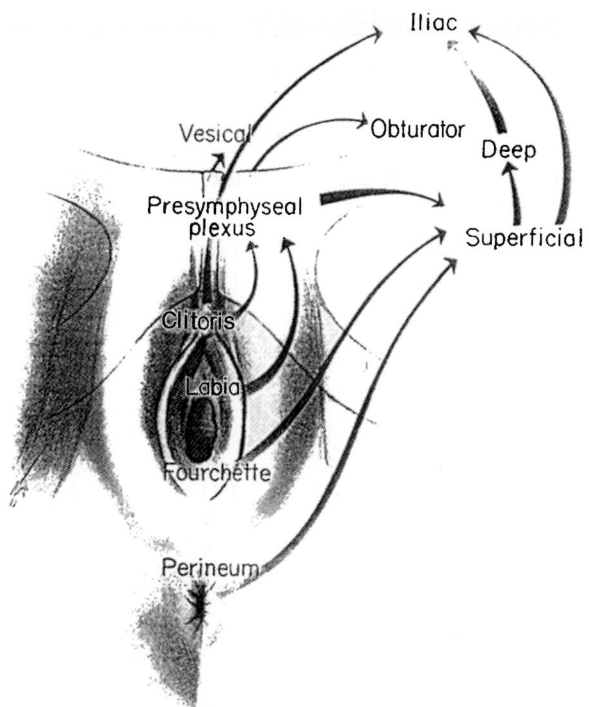

FIGURE 20.3. The lymphatic drainage of the vulva initially flows to the superficial inguinal nodes then to the deep femoral and iliac groups. Drainage from midline structures may flow directly beneath the symphysis to the pelvic nodes. *Source:* Reprinted from Plentl AA, Friedman EA, eds. *Lymphatic System of the Female Genitalia.* Philadelphia: WB Saunders; 1971.

located under the inguinal ligament. The deep inguinal nodes drain superiorly into the medial portion of the external iliac nodes and then upward through the pelvic and aortic lymph node chains (Fig. 20.3).

EPIDEMIOLOGY

Most vulvar cancers occur in postmenopausal women, although more recent reports suggest a trend toward younger age at diagnosis (6,7). Observational studies have suggested associations between hypertension, diabetes mellitus, and obesity with vulva carcinoma (8). However, it is not clear whether these represent independent risk factors or merely coexisting medical conditions common to the aging process. More recent analysis has not confirmed the prognostic significance of these diagnoses (9).

Several infectious agents have been proposed as possible etiologic agents in vulvar carcinoma, including granulomatous infections, herpes simplex virus, and human papillomavirus (HPV). Reports associating vulvar cancer with granuloma inguinale, lymphogranuloma venereum, or syphilis are largely historical and anecdotal (8). The observed coexistence of vulvar cancer with these granulomatous infections may only reflect such patients' risk for any sexually transmitted disease (9). Kaufman et al. identified serologic evidence of infection with herpes simplex virus type 2 and carcinoma *in situ* of the vulva in a small group of women (10). However, they were unable to isolate whole virus antigens, again suggesting an association with a sexually transmitted infection but failing to establish a direct causal link between the two.

Recent areas of investigation have focused on the neoplastic potential of HPVs. Strong associations between vulvar condylomata and the later development of vulvar cancer have been identified (9). In addition, HPV DNA has been isolated from both invasive and carcinoma *in situ* lesions (11,12). HPV type 16 appears to be most common, but types 6 and 33 have also been identified (13,14). HPV DNA can be identified in approximately 70% to 80% of intraepithelial lesions, but is seen in only 10% to 50% of invasive lesions. HPV-related cancers may exhibit distinguishing clinical and histologic features, leading some to suggest a stratification scheme for vulvar cancers based on the presence or absence of an HPV association (15). Although much of the information linking past or current vulvar HPV infection with neoplastic transformation is enticing, the evidence for a causative relationship is presently inconclusive.

Brinton et al. conducted a case-control analysis and identified women with a history of genital condylomata, those with a previous abnormal Papanicolaou smear, and those who smoked as having an increased risk for vulvar cancer (9). Those who both smoked and had a history of genital warts had a 35-fold increase in risk when compared with women without these factors (Table 20.1). Chronic immunosuppression has also been linked to invasive vulvar tumors (6). HPV infection and nonspecific immune suppression may act as cofactors in the development of some vulvar cancers.

Both chronic vulvar inflammatory lesions, such as vulvar dystrophy or lichen sclerosus, and squamous intraepithelial lesions, particularly carcinoma *in situ*, have been suggested as precursors of invasive squamous cancers (Fig. 20.4). Carli et al. suggested a possible role of lichen sclerosus as a precursor to vulvar cancer based on their observation that 32% of vulvar cancer cases not HPV related were associated with lichen sclerosis (16). However, Hart et al., in a large pathologic review, were unable to identify transitions from lichen sclerosus to vulvar cancer (17). In an observational study of women with carcinoma *in situ*, seven of eight untreated cases progressed to invasive carcinoma within 8 years, and four of 105 treated women presented with invasive tumors from 7 to 18 years later (18). In a subsequent study of 405 cases of vulvar intraepithelial neoplasia (VIN) 2 to 3, Jones et al. found that 3.8% of patients had developed invasive cancer despite therapy, and ten untreated patients had developed invasive cancer in 1.1 to 7.3 years (mean 3.9 years) (19). Although some intraepithelial lesions regress spontaneously, it appears that a significant number persist or progress to invasive cancer. Recent incidence analyses from the United States and Norway have identified a two- to threefold increase in carcinoma *in situ* lesions from the 1970s to the 1990s (20,21). However, a concomitant rise in the incidence of invasive vulvar cancers has not yet been seen. This discrepancy leads to several alternative hypotheses: (a) affected women have not reached the age at which invasive lesions are seen; (b) aggressive treatment of preinvasive disease has prevented the development of invasive tumors; or (c) the causes of *in situ* and invasive lesions are not strongly related (21).

Trimble et al. have postulated that squamous carcinoma of the vulva may represent a final common endpoint of heterogeneous etiologic pathways (22). According to their studies, two histologic subtypes—with basaloid or warty features—are associated with HPV, whereas keratinizing squamous carcinomas are not. Furthermore, basaloid or warty carcinomas are associated with classic risk factors for cervical carcinoma, including age at first intercourse, lifetime number of sexual partners, prior abnormal Papanicolaou smears, smoking, and lower socioeconomic status. Keratinizing squamous carcinomas are weakly linked to these factors, and in some cases not at all. Flowers et al. have reported that mutations in the p53 tumor suppressor gene are more frequently found in HPV negative vulvar carcinomas versus those associated with HPV (23). The p53 tumor suppressor gene has several key regulatory functions, including the control of cell growth and proliferation.

TABLE 20.1

RELATIVE RISKS OF *IN SITU* AND INVASIVE VULVAR CANCERS BY SELECTED RISK FACTORS

	In situ series			Invasive series		
	No. of cases	RR	95% CI	No. of cases	RR	95% CI
NO. OF SEXUAL PARTNERS						
0–1	17	1.00		48	1.00	
2	11	2.78	0.9–8.3	17	1.22	0.6–2.5
3–4	23	2.33	0.9–6.0	28	3.32	1.6–7.1
5–9	23	5.08	1.7–14.8	11	1.50	0.6–3.9
≥10	22	2.74	0.9–7.9	8	0.83	0.3–2.5
Trend test	$p = 0.03$			$p = 0.24$		
EVER HAD AN ABNORMAL PAP SMEAR						
No	64	1.00		90	1.00	
Yes	30	1.92	0.9–3.9	11	1.41	0.5–3.6
No previous Pap smear	2	0.37	0.1–1.9	10	2.46	0.9–6.7
EVER HAD GENITAL WARTS						
No	73	1.00		105	1.00	
Yes	23	18.50	5.5–62.5	8	14.55	1.71–25.6
CURRENT SMOKING STATUS						
Nonsmoker	22	1.00		46	1.00	
Current smoker	55	4.65	2.2–10.0	48	1.19	0.6–2.2
Ex-smoker	19	1.78	0.7–4.4	19	0.40	0.2–0.8

Note: CI, confidence interval; RR, relative risk.
Source: Reprinted from Brinton LA, Nasca PC, Mallin K, et al. Case-control study of cancer of the vulva. *Obstet Gynecol* 1990;75:864.

The common denominator in the development of vulvar carcinoma appears to be functional inactivation of the p53 tumor suppressor gene, either by genetic mutation in HPV negative tumors or by inactivation through the expression of HPV gene products (24).

Mitchell et al. evaluated 169 women with invasive vulvar cancers and noted that second genital squamous neoplasms occurred in 13% of cases (25). The risk of a second primary tumor was significantly increased in cancer cases with HPV DNA, intraepithelioid growth pattern, or adjacent dysplasia. These observations support the concept that some squamous lesions may be initiated by sexually transmitted viruses capable of producing neoplastic change within the entire field of the lower genital tract. The obvious clinical implication is that a patient with an established squamous lesion of the vulva, vagina, or cervix needs to be evaluated and monitored for new or coexistent lesions at other sites.

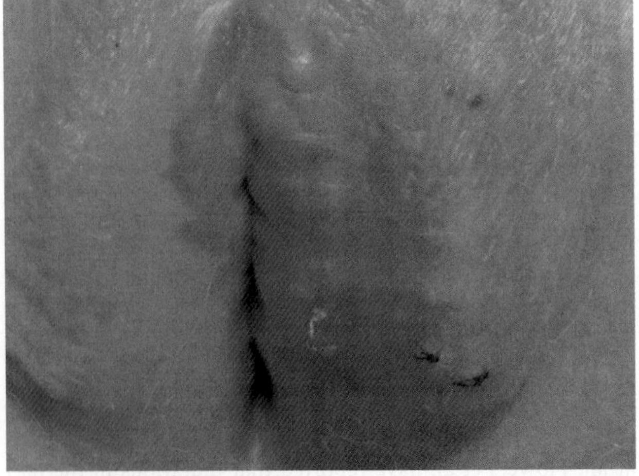

FIGURE 20.4. This T1 lesion arose from a background of lichen sclerosus and demonstrates the typical irregular surface features and superficial ulceration of a squamous-cell carcinoma. The biopsy site is marked with a suture.

CLINICAL PRESENTATION

Most women with vulvar cancer present with pruritus and a recognizable lesion. Selecting the most appropriate site for biopsy in women with condylomata, chronic vulvar dystrophy, multifocal dysplasia, or Paget's disease can be difficult, and multiple biopsies may be required. Optimal management for any patient presenting with a suspicious lesion is to proceed directly to biopsy under local analgesia. Tissue biopsies should include the cutaneous lesion in question and contiguous underlying stroma, so that the presence and depth of invasion can be accurately assessed.

Although other techniques to facilitate the assessment of vulvar lesions (e.g., toluidine blue stain or exfoliative cytology) have been described, they are less accurate than, and should not be considered a substitute for, tissue biopsy. As noted previously, one of the greatest clinical pitfalls in the management of women with vulvar cancer is delay in diagnosis. The goals of immediate evaluation with outpatient biopsy are to provide an accurate and definitive diagnosis and to avoid delay in the

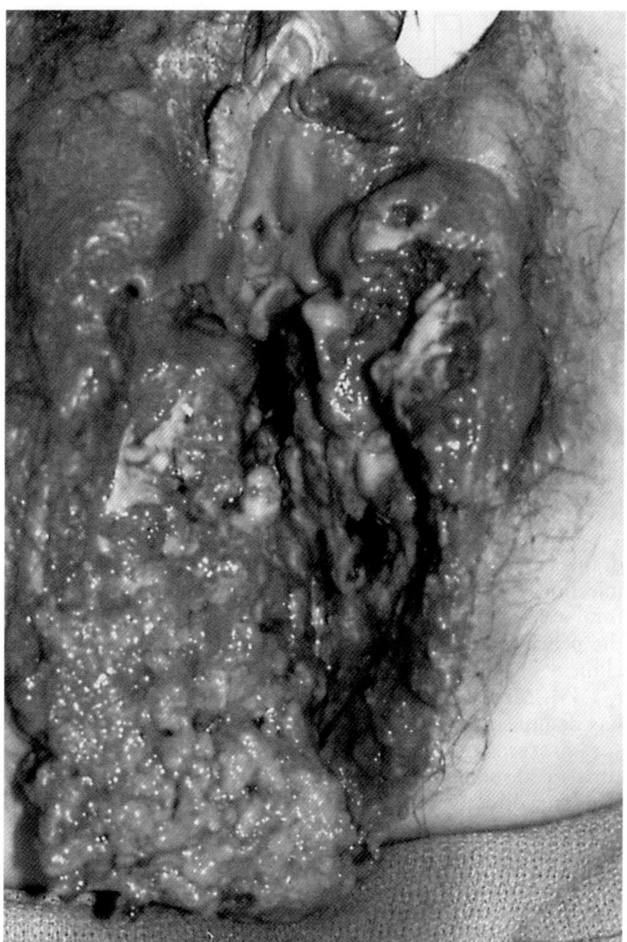

FIGURE 20.5. This patient ignored symptoms and an obvious tumor for more than a year. Although uncommon, such late presentations occur. Therapy options are limited.

planning of appropriate therapy. Unfortunately, some women ignore or deny obvious symptoms and lesions for long periods of time and present with advanced disease (Fig. 20.5). The presentation in such cases is generally dominated by local pain, bleeding, and surface drainage from the tumor. Metastatic disease in the groin lymph nodes or at distant sites may also be symptomatic.

DIAGNOSTIC EVALUATION

The evaluation of the patient with vulvar cancer must take into consideration the clinical extent of disease, the anticipated treatment plan, and the presence of coexisting medical illnesses. Initial evaluation should include a detailed physical examination with measurements of the primary tumor, assessment for extension to adjacent mucosal or bony structures, and possible involvement of the inguinal lymph nodes. Women with small cancers and clinically negative groin nodes require few diagnostic studies other than those for preoperative clearance. Additional radiographic and endoscopic studies should be considered for those with large primary tumors or suspected metastases. Potentially useful studies include barium enema, proctosigmoidoscopy, cystourethroscopy, computed tomography (CT) scan, and intravenous pyelography. Fine needle aspiration biopsy from sites of suspected metastases may eliminate the need for surgical exploration in some patients with advanced tumors. Because neoplasia of the female genital tract is often multifocal, evaluation of the vagina and cervix—including cervical cytologic screening—should always be performed in women with vulvar neoplasms.

STAGING SYSTEMS

The International Federation of Gynecology and Obstetrics (FIGO) adopted a modified surgical staging system for vulvar cancer in 1989, which remained relatively unchanged in their 1995 recommendations (Table 20.2) (26). The previous clinical system provided reliable information regarding the primary lesion but an inaccurate assessment of groin node involvement in 20% to 30% of cases. The frequent discrepancy between clinical staging and surgical-pathologic findings spurred the acceptance of the current surgical evaluation of the inguinal lymph nodes. The American Joint Committee on Cancer has published a tumor-node-metastasis (TNM) classification scheme that is correlated with the FIGO staging system (Table 20.3) (27). Tumor assessment is based on physical examination with endoscopy in cases of bulky disease. Nodal status is determined by the surgical evaluation of the groins. The presence or absence of distant metastases is based on an unspecified diagnostic workup tailored to the patient's clinical presentation.

A microinvasive substage (IA) is defined as tumors ≤2 cm in diameter and depth of invasion ≤1 mm. Prior attempts to define a microinvasive substage were hindered by the lack of uniformity in defining the techniques for measuring depth of invasion and the cut-off level for a depth of invasion that provided a reliably low risk of lymph node metastasis (28,29). The technique recommended by the International Society for the Study of Vulvar Disease and the International Society of Gynecologic Pathologists to assess depth of stromal invasion is to measure from the base of the epithelium at the nearest superficial dermal papillae to the deepest point of tumor penetration (30).

PATTERNS OF SPREAD

Vulvar cancers metastasize in three ways: (a) local growth and extension into adjacent organs; (b) lymphatic embolization to regional lymph nodes in the groin; and (c) hematogenous

TABLE 20.2

FIGO STAGING OF VULVAR CARCINOMA

Stage	Clinical findings
Stage 0	Carcinoma *in situ*; intraepithelial carcinoma
Stage I	Tumor confined to the vulva or perineum; 2 cm or less in greatest dimension; no nodal metastasis Stage IA: stromal invasion ≤1.0 mm Stage IB: stromal invasion >1.0 mm
Stage II	Tumor confined to the vulva or perineum; more than 2 cm in greatest dimension; no nodal metastasis
Stage III	Tumor of any size with adjacent spread to the urethra, vagina, or the anus or with unilateral regional lymph node metastasis
Stage IVA	Tumor invades upper urethra, bladder mucosa, rectal mucosa, pelvic bone, or bilateral regional node metastases
Stage IVB	Any distant metastasis, including pelvic lymph nodes

TABLE 20.3

AMERICAN JOINT COMMITTEE ON CANCER STAGING (1992)

PRIMARY TUMOR (T)

TX	Primary tumor cannot be assessed
T0	No evidence of primary tumor
Tis	Carcinoma *in situ* (preinvasive carcinoma)
T1	Tumor confined to the vulva or to the vulva and perineum, 2 cm or less in greatest dimension
T2	Tumor confined to the vulva or to the vulva and perineum, more than 2 cm in greatest dimension
T3	Tumor invades any of the following: lower urethra, vagina, or anus
T4	Tumor invades any of the following: bladder mucosa, upper urethral mucosa, or rectal mucosa, or is fixed to the bone

REGIONAL LYMPH NODES (N)

NX	Regional lymph nodes cannot be assessed
N0	No regional lymph node metastasis
N1	Unilateral regional lymph node metastasis
N2	Bilateral regional lymph node metastases

DISTANT METASTASIS (M)

MX	Presence of distant metastasis cannot be assessed
M0	No distant metastasis
M1	Distant metastasis (pelvic lymph node metastasis is M1)

STAGE GROUPINGS

Stage 0	Tis	N0	M0
Stage I	T1	N0	M0
Stage II	T2	N0	M0
Stage III	T1	N1	M0
	T2	N1	M0
	T3	N0	M0
	T3	N1	M0
Stage IVA	T1	N2	M0
	T2	N2	M0
	T3	N2	M0
	T4	Any N	M0
Stage IVB	Any T	Any N	M1

Source: Reprinted from Beahrs OH, Henson DE, Hutter RVP, et al., eds. *Manual for Staging Cancer.* 4th ed. Philadelphia: JB Lippincott; 1992.

dissemination to distant sites. Objective clinical descriptions of local growth have been categorized in the TNM staging system (Table 20.3). These descriptive definitions are clinically useful in that local surgical resection with a wide margin is almost universally feasible in women with T1 or T2 tumors, occasionally possible in those with T3 lesions, and impossible in those with T4 tumors without resorting to an exenterative operation.

A more precise understanding of the lymphatic drainage of the vulva has been key to developing an individualized surgical approach to vulvar cancer. The lymphatic dye studies described by Parry-Jones demonstrated that the dermal lymphatic network of the vulva courses superiorly to the area of the mons pubis and then turns laterally to drain into the superficial lymph nodes of the ipsilateral groin (4). Lymphatic channels from the superficial group then perforate the cribriform fascia to the deep inguinal (femoral) nodes. Observations following cutaneous dye injection showed that lymphatic drainage from lateral sites was to the ipsilateral groin. No lymphatic channels were located beyond the labiocrural fold, and crossover

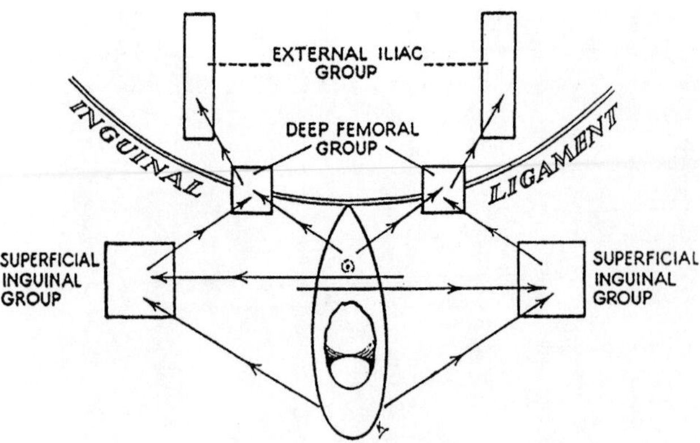

FIGURE 20.6. Stanley Way's schematic representation of the potential routes of lymphatic spread from vulvar cancer based on his clinical observations. *Source:* Reprinted from Way S. *Malignant Disease of the Female Genital Tract.* New York: Churchill Livingstone; 1951.

drainage to the opposite groin was rare. Drainage from midline injections could be bilateral (31). Some channels from the clitoral area appeared to drain beneath the symphysis directly to the pelvic nodes. These anatomic descriptions confirmed the clinical impressions originally outlined by Way (Fig. 20.6) (32,33). More recent experience with intraoperative mapping has demonstrated that lymphatic drainage from most vulvar sites proceeds initially to a "sentinel" node located within the superficial inguinal group (34). However, aberrant channels coursing directly to deep inguinal, contralateral superficial inguinal, and pelvic lymph nodes were observed in a few cases. These infrequent anatomic variations may ultimately provide the explanation for unanticipated lymph-node failure.

Inguinal node metastasis can be predicted by the presence of certain parameters, including lesion diameter >2 cm, poor differentiation, increasing depth of stromal invasion, and invasion of lymphovascular spaces (35). Clinically important observations regarding nodal metastases include the following: (a) the superficial inguinal nodes are the most frequent site of lymphatic metastasis; (b) in-transit metastases within the vulvar skin are exceedingly rare, suggesting that most initial lymphatic metastases represent embolic phenomena; (c) metastasis to the contralateral groin or deep pelvic nodes is unusual in the absence of ipsilateral groin metastases; and (d) nodal involvement generally proceeds in a stepwise fashion from the superficial inguinal to the deep inguinal and then to the pelvic nodes.

Spread beyond the inguinal lymph nodes is considered distant metastasis. This may occur as secondary or tertiary level lymphatic metastases to the pelvic/aortic nodes or as a result of hematogenous dissemination to more distant sites, such as bone, lung, or liver. Distant metastases are uncommon at initial presentation, and more often are seen in the context of recurrent vulvar cancer.

PATHOLOGY

Most vulvar malignancies arise within squamous epithelium. Although the vulva does not have an identifiable transformation zone, as in the cervix, squamous neoplasms arise most commonly on the labia minora, clitoris, fourchette, perineal body, or medial aspects of the labia majora areas in which keratinized stratified squamous epithelial junction with the nonkeratinized squamous mucosa of the vestibule (36).

Most vulvar squamous carcinomas arise within areas of epithelium involved by some recognized epithelial cell abnormality. Approximately 60% of cases have adjacent VIN. In cases of superficially invasive squamous carcinoma of the vulva, the frequency of adjacent VIN approaches 85%

(29,37). Lichen sclerosus, usually with associated squamous cell hyperplasia, and/or differentiated VIN, can be found adjacent to vulvar squamous cell carcinoma in 15% to 40% of the cases (38,39). Granulomatous disease is also associated with vulvar squamous cell carcinoma; however, this is not a commonly associated finding in the United States. Thus, vulvar squamous cell carcinoma precursors can be considered in two distinct groups: those associated with HPV, usually associated VIN, and those that are not (e.g., those associated with lichen sclerosus, chronic granulomatous disease).

Vulvar Carcinomas

Squamous Cell Carcinomas

The term microinvasive carcinoma is not recognized as meaningful in reference to the vulva because there are no commonly agreed on pathologic criteria established for this term. The International Society for the Study of Vulvar Disease (ISSVD) proposed a substage of FIGO stage I, stage IA, as a solitary squamous carcinoma of the vulva measuring 2 cm or less in diameter with clinically negative nodes, with depth of tumor invasion 1 mm or less (40). The depth of invasion is defined as the measurement from the epithelial dermal junction of the most superficial adjacent dermal papillae to the deepest point of invasion (41,42). Tumor thickness is measured from the overlying surface epithelium, or the bottom of the granular layer if the surface is keratinized, to the deepest point of invasion, as specified by the International Society of Gynecologic Pathologists (ISGYP), the World Health Organization, and FIGO (Fig. 20.7) (26,43).

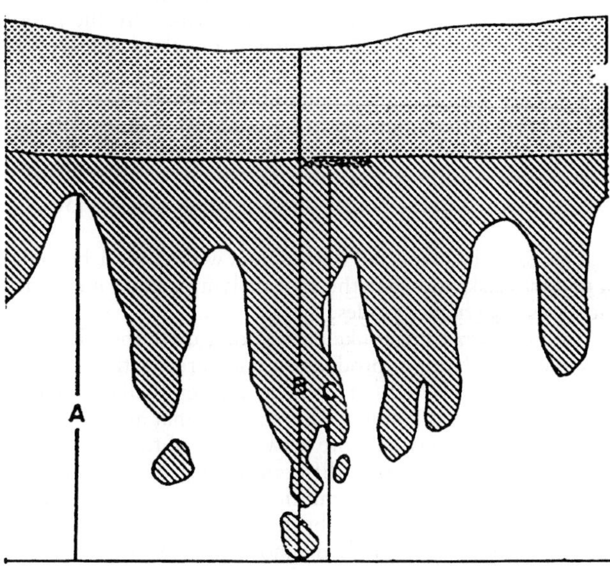

FIGURE 20.7. Methods for measurement for vulvar superficially invasive carcinomas: (A) Depth of invasion: the measurement from the epithelial stromal junction of the most superficial dermal papillae to the deepest point of invasion. This measurement is defined as the depth of invasion and is used to define stage IA vulvar carcinoma. The measurement (B) is the thickness of the tumor: from the surface of the lesion to the deepest point of invasion. Measurement (C) is from the bottom of the granular layer to the deepest point of invasion. This is also defined as thickness of the tumor in cases where there is a keratinized surface. The International Society of Gynecologic Pathologists and the World Health Organization recommend that both the depth of invasion and thickness of tumor, as well as method of measurement, be defined in the pathology reports. Source: Reprinted with permission by Edward J. Wilkinson, MD.

Stage I squamous carcinomas of the vulva, with a reported depth or thickness of 5 mm or more, have a lymph node metastasis rate of 15% or higher. Tumors with a depth or thickness of 3 mm have a lymph node metastasis rate averaging 12%. Therefore, a 3- or 5-mm tumor thickness is not acceptable as one considered superficial and of no or little risk of metastasis. Tumors with a depth or thickness of 1 mm or less carry little or no risk of lymph node metastasis (44,45).

The Gynecologic Oncology Group (GOG) correlated morphologic features of vulvar carcinoma with tumor invasion. Their findings were remarkably similar to those of the ISSVD (46). Because the GOG study did not measure tumor depth by the standards defined by the ISSVD, a reported case with 1-mm invasion with lymph node metastasis cannot be considered as an ISSVD stage IA tumor. The depth of invasion and thickness of tumor are seperately defined, because considerable variations can exist among measurements from various superficial points in tumors of approximately 1 mm (Fig. 20.8) (45). There are significant differences between tumor depth of invasion and thickness when superficially invasive tumors are measured; vulvar epithelium can be up to 0.77 mm thick, which can significantly influence the difference between the depth of invasion and the measurement of tumor thickness (47). Tumors with invasion deeper than 1 mm can be readily measured by determining thickness, but tumors with surface ulceration may have a thickness, as measured from the surface, significantly less than the depth of invasion. With large tumors, thickness may be the only reliable measurement because of the lack of identifiable adjacent dermal papillae.

In addition to tumor stage and depth or thickness, other pathologic features include vascular space invasion, growth pattern of the tumor, grade of the tumor, and tumor type. Vascular space involvement can be defined as tumor within an endothelial lined vascular space. Strict pathologic criteria require that the tumor be attached to the wall of the vessel, but this is not observed in all cases. Vascular space involvement by squamous cell carcinoma of the vulva is associated with a higher frequency of lymph node metastasis and a lower overall 5-year survival rate. No reliable methods unambiguously predict lymph node metastasis by quantitation of vascular space involvement by tumor.

Tumor growth pattern influences the rate of lymph node metastasis and survival in tumors exceeding 1 mm in depth of invasion. In stage IA vulvar carcinomas, tumor growth pattern does not influence the risk of node involvement (48). Three factors describe tumor growth patterns: confluent; compact (pushing pattern); and finger-like (or spray or diffuse), a pattern also described as poorly differentiated. Confluent growth

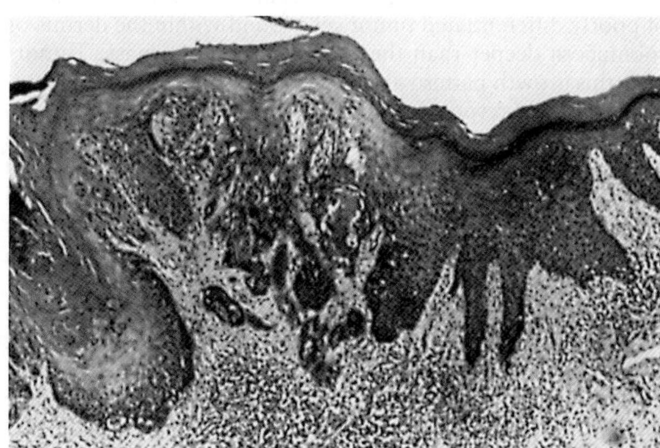

FIGURE 20.8. Microinvasive carcinoma of the vulva. The lesion is less than 2 cm across and the depth of invasion is less than 1 mm, measured from the overlying surface epithelium.

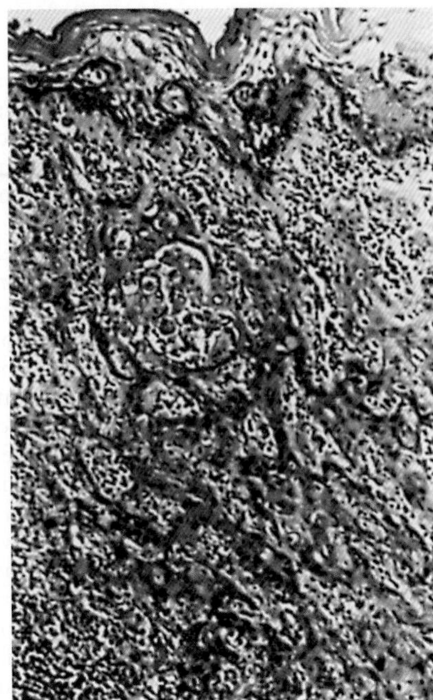

FIGURE 20.9. Confluent pattern of invasion. The tumor has a trabecular pattern of growth associated with a marked chronic inflammatory stromal infiltrate. The tumor diameter exceeds 1 cm.

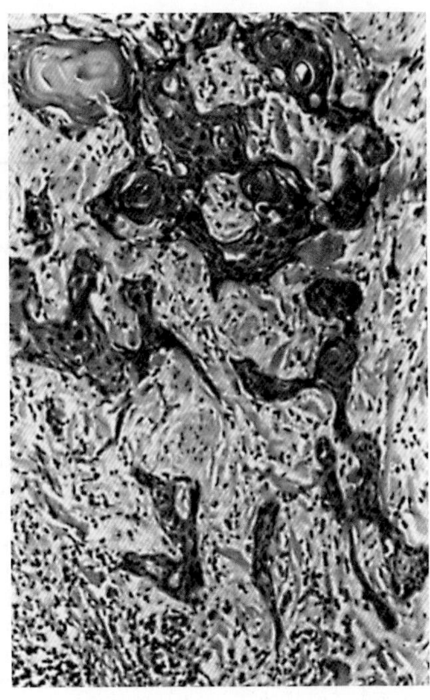

FIGURE 20.10. Finger-like growth. The tumor forms small nests surrounded by a desmoplastic stroma.

is defined as a tumor mass composed of interconnected tumor exceeding 1 mm in dimension (Fig. 20.9). Tumors with confluent growth, by definition, have a depth of invasion exceeding 1 mm. Confluent growth is characteristic of deeply invasive squamous cell carcinomas that are associated with stromal desmoplasia, resulting in fibrovascular stromal changes adjacent to the interconnected cords of tumor.

Compact (pushing; well differentiated) growth is squamous tumor growth that maintains continuity with the overlying epithelium and infiltrates as a well-defined and -circumscribed tumor mass, without islands of infiltrating tumor remote from the tumor mass. Tumors with compact growth typically have thickness of 5 mm or less and rarely invade vascular space. They are characteristically well differentiated, with the tumor cells resembling the squamous cells of the adjacent and overlying epithelium. There is usually minimal stromal desmoplasia, although there may be a lymphocytic inflammatory cell infiltrate.

Finger-like (spray or diffuse; poorly differentiated) growth is characterized by a trabecular appearance with small islands of poorly differentiated tumor cells found within the dermis or submucosa deeper than the bulk of the tumor mass. Tumors with this growth pattern are typically associated with a desmoplastic stromal response (Fig. 20.10) and a lymphocytic inflammatory cell infiltrate. Vascular space involvement is more commonly seen with this pattern of growth than with tumors with a compact pattern of growth (49). In tumors with a depth of invasion less than 5 mm, the finger-like pattern of growth is associated with a higher frequency of inguino femoral lymph node metastasis.

In some cases, a single tumor may have both compact and finger-like growth patterns. Mixed patterns, in our experience, are more commonly encountered in frankly invasive vulvar carcinomas and are rarely seen in superficially invasive tumors. The GOG has referred to tumors with a compact pattern of growth as well differentiated, and to tumors with the finger-like pattern of growth as poorly differentiated. Using this terminology, the GOG proposed the following grading system for vulvar squamous cell carcinoma:

- Grade 1 tumors are composed of well-differentiated tumor and contain no poorly differentiated element.
- Grade 2 tumors contain both patterns, with the poorly differentiated portions making up one third or less of the tumor.
- Grade 3 tumors also contain both components, with the poorly differentiated portion comprising more than one third but less than one half of the tumor.
- Grade 4 tumors have one half or more of the tumor composed of the poorly differentiated elements (50).

The GOG has reported that tumors with grade 1 histology have little risk and that the risk of lymph node metastasis increases with higher grades.

Tumors with a finger-like pattern of growth (poorly differentiated) lack laminin production compared with those that are well differentiated (51). Vulvar intraepithelial neoplasia also has associated laminin. This suggests that areas of tumor without laminin may be more active areas of tumor proliferation than areas with well-differentiated growth containing laminin. The absence of laminin in a questionable focus of invasion, as demonstrated by immunoperoxidase staining techniques, may support the diagnosis of invasion.

In a study of tumor cell proliferation using MIB-1 immunohistochemistry, a monoclonal antibody related to the proliferation-related protein KI-67, which is applicable in formation of fixed paraffin-embedded tissue, Hendricks et al. demonstrated that, in the well-differentiated tumors, the MIB-1 expression was detected in the tumor cells near the dermal tumor interface, but not in the tumor cells in the center of tumor foci or near the tumor epithelial surface (52). Poorly differentiated tumors demonstrated MIB-1 expression throughout the tumor cell population. This difference in pattern of expression in MIB-1 was statistically significant when related to survival and appeared somewhat more reliable than tumor growth pattern alone.

The ISGYP Committee of Terminology for Nonneoplastic Epithelial Disorders and Tumors recommended that the following information be included in the pathology report of all excised vulvar squamous cell carcinomas, information also supported by the College of American Pathologists, and often used by tumor registeries (53):

1. Depth of tumor invasion in millimeters
2. Thickness of the tumor in millimeters
3. Method of measurement of the depth of invasion and thickness
4. Presence or absence of vascular space (lymphatic) involvement by tumor
5. Diameter of the tumor, measured from the specimen in the fresh or fixed state
6. Clinical measurement of the tumor diameter, if available

In a multivariable retrospective analysis of 39 cases of vulvar squamous carcinoma, in addition to clinical stage and when corrected for treatment modality, pattern of tumor invasion, depth of tumor invasion, and lymph node status were all found to be significant prognostic factors. In addition, dermal desmoplasia associated with tumor invasion also had a suggestive association (54). Desmoplasia (a fibroblastic stromal tumor response) has been correlated with a higher risk of lymph node metastasis and poorer survival (55,56). Findings that did not correlate with survival were squamous cell carcinoma type, vascular space involvement by tumor, adjacent VIN, tumor nuclear grade, or associated degree of inflammatory response (54). DNA ploidy analysis (i.e., diploid versus aneuploid) of vulvar carcinoma does not appear to have significance in regard to survival (54).

Squamous cell carcinoma of the vulva, as well as VIN 3, overexpress p53 in approximately one half of the cases and have evidence of p16 methylation in approximately two thirds of the cases (57). However, p16 methylation appears to be an early event and a relatively frequent genetic change in vulvar neoplasia, whereas loss of pRb expression appears to be a late event being identified in invasive squamous carcinoma but not in VIN (57).

Several histopathologic types of vulvar squamous cell carcinoma are recognized. The usual types include squamous cell carcinoma, keratinizing type; squamous cell carcinoma, nonkeratinizing type; basaloid carcinoma; and warty (condylomatous) carcinoma (58). Less common types include acantholytic squamous cell carcinoma, squamous cell carcinoma with tumor giant cells and spindle cell squamous carcinoma, squamous cell carcinoma with sarcoma-like stroma, sebaceous carcinoma, verrucous carcinoma, and other rarer types (39,59).

Vulvar squamous cell carcinomas of the basaloid and warty types, as well as VIN of all but the differentiated type, are recognized to be associated with human papillomavirus, primarily HPV-16. The HPV can be detected within the tumor cells by a variety of techniques, including polymerase chain reaction (PCR), hybrid capture, and *in situ* hybridization. In addition, it is now recognized that approximately one quarter (27% ± 9%) of the women with vulvar squamous carcinoma have anti–HPV-16 antibodies expressed serologically as IgG antibodies to HPV-16 virus-like particles as measured by enzyme-linked immunosorbent assay (ELISA) (60).

The term acantholytic squamous cell carcinoma (*adenoid squamous cell carcinoma*; pseudoglandular squamous cell carcinoma) refers to squamous cell carcinomas with pseudoglandular features. These tumors are characterized by small gland-like spaces within a tumor that otherwise appears to be a poorly differentiated squamous cell carcinoma. This tumor should be differentiated from adenosquamous carcinomas that contain an obvious adenocarcinoma component (61). Adenoid squamous carcinoma does not contain sialomucin, but adenosquamous carcinoma typically contains mucin within the adenocarcinoma component. Although there are few reported cases of adenoid squamous carcinoma of the vulva, these tumors may have a more aggressive clinical behavior.

Squamous cell carcinoma with tumor giant cells has multinucleated tumor giant cells intermixed within the squamous carcinoma (62). This tumor may resemble amelanotic melanoma. Squamous cell carcinoma with tumor giant cells, unlike melanoma, does not express S100 antigen, HMB45, or Melan-A on immunoperoxidase studies. This tumor does express low-molecular-weight keratin, similar to other squamous carcinomas.

Sebaceous carcinoma of the vulva may be associated with VIN (63). These tumors have characteristics of squamous cell carcinoma but also have intermixed sebaceous elements.

Spindle cell squamous cell carcinomas consist of poorly differentiated neoplastic epithelial cells that have an elongated spindle shape and may mimic a spindle cell melanoma or a sarcoma (Fig. 20.11) (64). Squamous cell carcinoma with spindle cell stroma is a squamous cell carcinoma asociated with a sarcoma like stromal/dermal response that may mimic with a primary sarcoma (65). Spindle cell squamous cell carcinomas can be differentiated from sarcomas by immunoperoxidase techniques. Like other squamous cell carcinomas, the spindle cell variant contains keratin and lacks the antigens distinctive to sarcomas of various origin. S100 antigen, HMB 45, and Melan-A are usually immunoreactive in a spindle cell melanoma and lacking in a spindle cell squamous carcinoma.

Verrucous Carcinoma

Verrucous carcinoma of the vulva typically presents as an exophytic-appearing growth that can be locally destructive. Clinically, it may resemble condyloma acuminatum. The so-called Buschke-Lowenstein giant condyloma is classified as a variant of verrucous carcinoma by the World Health Organization.

Microscopically, verrucous carcinoma is characterized by well-differentiated epithelial cells. The tumor growth pattern is characterized by a "pushing" tumor-dermal interface with minimal stroma between the acanthotic epithelium (Fig. 20.12). The surface is often hyperkeratotic, and there may be parakeratosis. Observed mitoses are characteristically normal. Within the dermis, a mild lymphocytic inflammatory cell response is usually seen. Vascular space involvement by tumor is characteristically lacking. Because of its excellent prognosis, strict

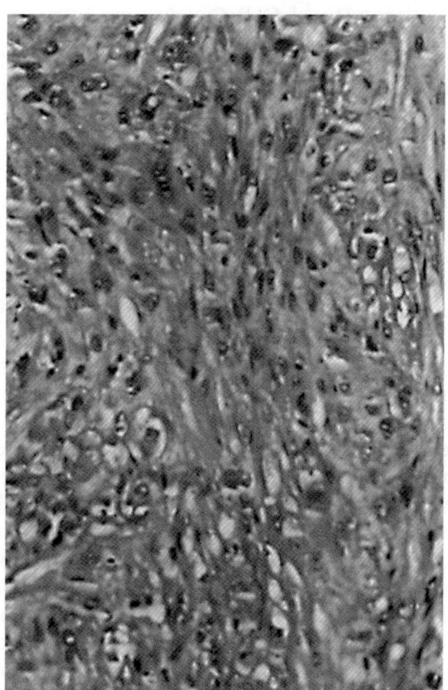

FIGURE 20.11. Spindle-cell squamous carcinoma. The tumor cells have a spindle shape and poorly defined cell junctions.

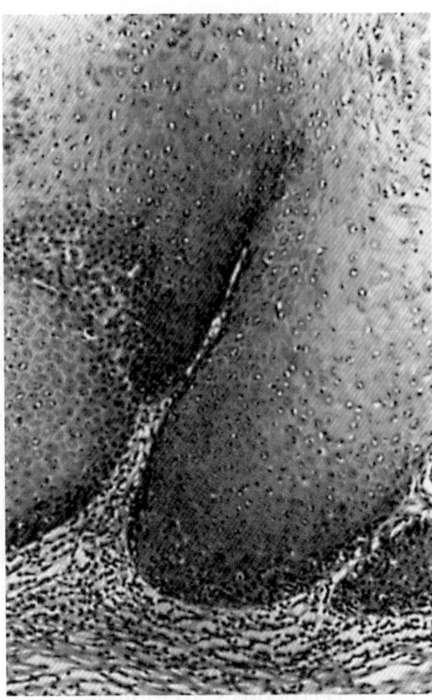

FIGURE 20.12. Verrucous carcinoma. The epithelial cells are well differentiated, and the tumor has a "pushing border" with a delicate vascular core between the epithelial elements.

histologic criteria should be used in the diagnosis of verrucous carcinoma. Squamous carcinomas with focal verrucous features should not be described or diagnosed as verrucous carcinoma.

Verrucous carcinomas are characteristically diploid, unlike typical squamous cell carcinomas of the vulva, which are usually aneuploid by DNA analysis. Verrucous tumors may be associated with HPV-6 or its variants (66).

The major differential diagnosis of squamous cell carcinoma includes keratoacanthomas, pseudocarcinomatous (pseudoepitheliomatous) hyperplasia, epithelioid sarcoma, and malignant rhabdoid tumor.

Basal Cell Carcinoma

Basal cell carcinoma is a relatively rare tumor in the vulva, comprising 2% to 4% of infiltrative neoplasms. These tumors are most commonly found in elderly women. The surface of the tumor appears granular and is well circumscribed; on palpation, the tumor is characteristically very firm. Vulvar basal cell carcinoma most commonly arises on the labia majora and is typically 2 cm or less in diameter; however, giant basal cell carcinomas have been described (67).

The epithelial cells comprising basal cell carcinoma are typically small and vary in form, with small hyperchromatic nuclei that may exhibit some nuclear pleomorphism. These tumors may have a variety of growth patterns (e.g., trabecular, insular), although peripheral nuclear palisading is a relatively consistent finding. Basal cell carcinomas often have an intraepthelial component that is contiguous with the infiltrative component, if present.

Metatypical basal cell carcinoma is a variant of basal cell carcinoma that usually occurs at mucocutaneous junctions. The term *basosquamous carcinoma* is applied to these tumors because of their microscopic features, which include basal cell carcinoma intermixed with a squamous cell carcinoma component. Nuclear pleomorphism is usually seen in metatypical basal cell carcinoma and in the basal cell and squamous cell components of the tumor. The deeper tumor cells, close to the underlying stroma, have the greatest degree of nuclear pleomorphism and the more prominent squamous features. These tumors have a more aggressive clinical behavior than typical basal cell carcinoma. A variant of vulvar basal cell carcinoma, *adenoid basal cell carcinoma,* has gland-like features (68).

The differential diagnosis of basal cell carcinoma includes basaloid squamous cell carcinoma, Merkel cell tumor of the skin, and metastatic small cell carcinoma. Basaloid squamous cell carcinoma can be distinguished by its lack of characteristic basal cell growth pattern, and the presence of intracellular bridges. Nuclear pleomorphism is typically much greater in basaloid squamous cell carcinoma than in basal cell carcinoma. Basal cell carcinomas express Ber EP4 on histochemical study, an antigen not expressed by basaloid squamous cell carcinomas. Basaloid squamous cell carcinomas are typically associated with HPV-16, which is not typically associated with basal cell carcinoma. Merkel cell tumors and other neuroendocrine tumors of the vulva are typically subcutaneous or dermal nodules, and not intraepithelial lesions (see the section on neuroendocrine tumors).

Neuroendocrine and Neuroectodermal Tumors: Merkel Cell Tumors and Peripheral Neuroectodermal Tumor/Extraosseous Ewing Sarcoma

Merkel Cell Tumor. Merkel cell tumors are neuroendocrine tumors of the skin occurring usually within the dermis. The tumor is composed of small, relatively uniform cells with little cytoplasm and hyperchromatic nuclei with a punctate chromatin pattern and has a high mitotic count. The tumor is infiltrative and often involves vascular spaces. Merkel cell tumors have been associated with squamous cell carcinoma and vulvar intraepithelial neoplasia (69). Merkel cell tumors are subclassified as carcinoid-like (trabecular), intermediate type, and small cell (oat cell) type. These tumors typically express neuron-specific enolase, synaptophysin, chromogranin, and low-molecular-weight keratin. Keratin study, such as with cytokeratin 20, demonstrates a distinct perinuclear cytoplasmic dot. Dense core neurosecretory granules are seen by electron microscopy. These features differentiate it from basal cell or squamous cell carcinoma. Merkle cell tumors frequently have both regional lymph node and distant metastases and are associated with a poor prognosis.

Peripheral Neuroectodermal Tumor/Extraosseous Ewing Sarcoma. Peripheral neuroectodermal tumor/extraosseous Ewing sarcoma (PNET) is a rare neuroendocrine vulvar neoplasm that has been reported in childhood and women of reproductive age. The tumor may present as a subcutaneous or polypoid mass and clinically may resemble a cyst, or be ulcerated (70,71). On microscopic examination the tumor is circumscribed and multilobulated, without capsule but nonencapsulated, and contains small cells with little cytoplasm and nuclei with hyperchromatic and finely granular nuclear chromatin. Some cells have small nucleoli, and mitotic figures are usually common, with mitotic counts from 3 to exceeding 10 per 10 high power fields. Numerous patterns of growth may be seen with highly cellular undifferentiated areas, areas with cyst formation containing eosinophilic proteinous material, rosettes with Homer-Wright rosettes, and follicle-like structures.

The cells of PNET have periodic-acid Schiff (PAS) staining cytoplasm that digests with diastase, and typically express CD99 and vimentin. Although, as in Merkle cell tumors, focal reactivity for synaptophysin and neuron specific enolase may be present; cytokeratin reactivity is not present but may be focally immunoreactive in some cases.

Dense core neurosecretory granules, as seen in Merkle cell tumor by electron microscopy, are not present. Cytogenetic study of these PNET tumors demonstrates translocation t(11;22)(q24;q12) in approximately 90% of cases. This translocation can also be demonstrated with fluorescence *in situ* hybridization, or reverse transcriptase polymerase chain reaction (RT-PCR) (70,71).

Urothelial/Transitional Cell Carcinoma

Urothelial carcinoma may be a primary tumor of the vulva, usually arising within the Bartholin's glands. More commonly, urothelial carcinoma is metastatic to the vulva, having arisen within the bladder or urethra (72). In rare instances the tumor presents as a Paget-like lesion of the vulva (see section on Paget's disease) (73).

Microscopically, urothelial carcinomas are composed of relatively uniform cells; nuclear pleomorphisms may be marked in high grade urothelial neoplasms. The cytoplasm is eosinophilic without apparent inclusions or keratin formations, although focal keratin formation may be seen. The tumors may exhibit papillary-like growth.

Adenocarcinoma and Carcinoma of Bartholin's Glands

Most primary adenocarcinomas of the vulva arise within Bartholin's glands. Adenocarcinoma may also arise from other glands or skin appendages of the vulva, including sweat glands and Skene's glands (74,75). Clear cell adenocarcinoma arising in endometriosis has been reported in the groin (76). Invasive vulvar Paget's disease has given rise to adenocarcinoma (Fig. 20.13). Primary malignant tumors arising within Bartholin's glands include adenocarcinoma and squamous cell carcinoma, which occur with approximately equal frequency and account for approximately 80% of all primary malignant tumors in this site. Adenoid cystic carcinomas comprise approximately 15% of all primary carcinomas, with adenosquamous carcinomas and transitional cell carcinomas each comprising approximately 5% of the primary Bartholin's gland tumors (77).

Carcinoma of the Bartholin's gland generally occurs in older women and is rare in women younger than 50. In clinical practice, it is generally advisable to excise an enlarged Bartholin's gland in a woman 50 years of age or older, especially if there is no known history of prior Bartholin's cyst. If a cyst is drained and a palpable mass persists, excision is also indicated. Fine needle aspiration of a Bartholin's mass for cytologic evaluation may help to establish a positive diagnosis.

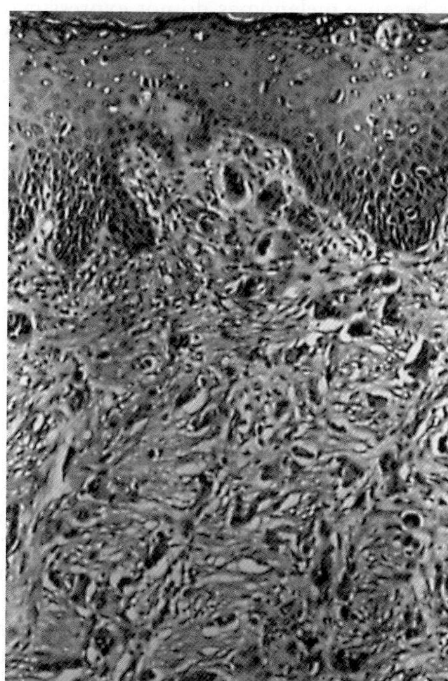

FIGURE 20.13. Adenocarcinoma underlying Paget's disease. The adenocarcinoma is composed of small tumor clusters within the underlying dermis.

Primary carcinomas within Bartholin's glands are usually solid tumors and are often deeply infiltrative. A variety of histologic types of adenocarcinoma have been described within Bartholin's glands. Mucinous, papillary, and mucoepidermoid carcinoma tumor types have been described in addition to adenosquamous, squamous, and transitional cell carcinoma. Adenocarcinoma of Bartholin's gland is typically immunoreactive for carcinoembryonic antigen (78). Histopathologic features that identify a carcinoma arising in Bartholin's glands include a recognizable transition from Bartholin's gland to tumor. The histopathologic tumor type must be consistent with an origin from a Bartholin's gland, and the tumor must not be metastatic to a Bartholin's gland.

These malignancies are characteristically deep and difficult to detect in their early growth. Approximately 20% of women with primary carcinoma of Bartholin's glands have metastatic tumor to the inguino femoral lymph nodes at the time of primary tumor diagnosis.

Adenocarcinoma Arising in Vulvar Skin Appendages

The vulvar labia majora were once thought to be within the milk line, but this has been significantly challenged by Van der Putte, who observed that the milk line did not involve the vulva in the human (79,80). The breast-like tumors found are believed to arise from specialized anogenital glands that reside in the intralabial sulci and may be the origin of papillary hidradenoma. Both benign and malignant breast-like tumors have been observed within the vulva (81). Fibroadenoma, intraductal papilloma, and lactating adenoma have been observed. Primary adenocarcinoma of the vulva may arise in specialized anogenital glands, which reside in the intralabial sulcus, and are believed to be the origin of papillary hidradenoma of the vulva as well as the breast-like tumors seen within the vulva, and these glands may resemble breast tissue (79,80,82).

Adenosquamous Carcinoma

Adenosquamous carcinomas are epithelial tumors composed of both malignant squamous and gland-forming elements. Adenosquamous carcinomas account for approximately 5% of all tumors of Bartholin's glands. These tumors may be composed of a poorly differentiated squamous component mixed with cells bearing small glandular lumens containing mucin (29).

Adenoid Cystic Carcinoma

Adenoid cystic carcinoma arising within the vulva most commonly arises within the Bartholin's glands and comprises approximately 15% of all carcinomas of Bartholin's glands. Microscopically, adenoid cystic carcinomas are composed of relatively uniform small cells with regular, round nuclei and minimal cytoplasm. The cord-like or "nested" arrangement contains gland-like lumens that include an acellular eosinophilic material (77). Electron microscopy has documented that this material is basement membrane–like material rather than a secretion. These tumors are therefore more properly considered a variant of squamous cell carcinoma than adenocarcinoma.

Carcinomas of Sweat Gland Origin

Primary carcinomas of sweat gland origin are relatively rare within the vulva, comprising approximately 10% of all vulvar malignant tumors. A variety of sweat gland carcinomas have been described in this site, including eccrine adenocarcinoma, eccrine porocarcinoma, and clear cell hidradenocarcinoma (75). Primary adenocarcinomas of apocrine gland origin have also been described arising within the vulva, and some of these have been associated with vulvar Paget's disease. These should be distinguished from the benign papillary hidradenoma, which typically arises in the intralabial papillary sulcus from specialized anogenital glands and contains a myoepithelial cell population, distinguishing it from adenocarcinoma (79,80,82).

Vulvar Paget's Disease and Paget-Like Lesions

Vulvar Paget's disease typically presents as an eczematoid, red, weeping area on the vulva, often localized to the labia majora, perineal body, clitoral area, or other sites. This disease typically occurs in older, postmenopausal Caucasian women, although it has been described in a premenopausal woman. Because of its eczematoid appearance, it is not unusual for vulvar Paget's disease to be misdiagnosed as eczema or contact dermatitis. Approximately 15% of women with vulvar Paget's disease have underlying primary adenocarcinoma, usually arising within apocrine glands or the underlying Bartholin's glands (Fig. 20.13). The Wilkinson and Brown etiologic classification of vulvar Paget's disease divides Paget's disease into two main groups: those of cutaneous origin and those of non-cutaneous origin (73). The two most common types of non-cutaneous Paget's disease are those associated with colorectal adenocarcinoma and those associated with bladder urothelial carcinoma. Women with Paget's disease of the colorectal type usually present with a lesion that involves the perianal skin, and this lesion is a manifestation of underlying colon or rectal adenocarcinoma. Women with Paget-like disease (Pagetoid urothelial intraepithelial neoplasia [PUIN]) typically present with a lesion involving the perurethral area and vulvar vestibule (73,82,83). In these cases there is associated bladder and/or urethral urothelial carcinoma with the extension of the neoplastic urothelial cells to the epithelium of the vulva (73,82). In cases of PUIN, total deep vulvectomy is not indicated because there is no associated underlying cutaneous adenocarcinoma. The tumor cells are from the bladder and/or urethra, representing an intraepithelial transitional cell neoplasm extending from the bladder and/or urethra (73). These cells have been reported from a vaginal cytology specimen from a woman with a PUIN lesion (84).

Cutaneous Paget's disease is most commonly a primary intraepithelial neoplasm. In such cases the intraepithelial Paget's disease may have an associated invasive Paget's disease. In rare cases, cutaneous Paget's disease may be a manifestation of an underlying cutaneous adenocarcinoma (73). Cutaneous Paget's disease is characterized by the presence of Paget's cells, which are found within the involved epithelium. A Paget's cell is relatively large, with a prominent nucleus that typically has coarse chromatin and a prominent nucleolus. On hematoxylin and eosin staining the cytoplasm is distinctly pale compared with the surrounding keratinocytes. The cytoplasm may be vacuolated or appear foamy and typically is somewhat basophilic. The Paget's cells are generally found in higher concentrations near the basement membrane, but are also seen throughout the epithelium. These cells may be clustered together and may have an acinar or gland-like arrangement (Fig. 20.14).

Paget's cells of cutaneous origin are rich in carcinoembryonic antigen (CEA), which can be identified with immunoperoxidase techniques (73). Paget's cells also express cytokeratin 7 (CK-7) and gross-cystic-disease fluid protein-15 (GCDFP-15) (73,85). More than one half of cases may also express c-erB2 (HER2/neu), but this was not found to influence metastasis risk (86,87). Paget's cells infrequently express CA-125, and estrogen receptor is generally negative (87,88). In some cases, Paget's disease may be associated with a distinctive squamous hyperplasia, or papillomatous hyperplasia, which must be distinguished from VIN. Immunohistochemical study for CK-7 is useful in many cases to identify the Paget's cells that are strongly CK-7 positive, whereas the adjacent epithelial cells are negative (89). Paget's cells may be aneuploid or diploid

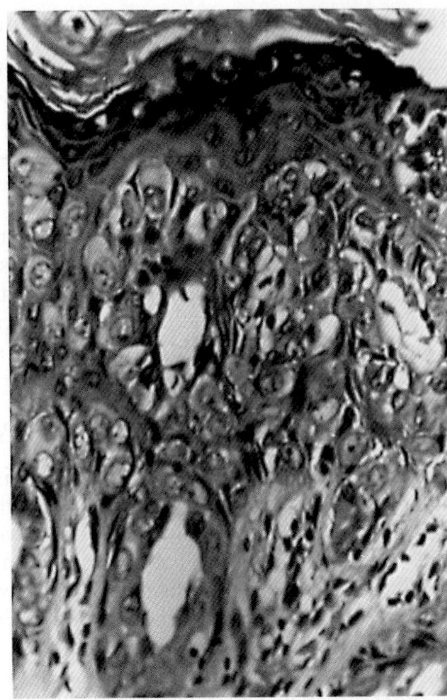

FIGURE 20.14. Paget's disease. The large cells with prominent cytoplasm and large nuclei represent the intraepithelial Paget's cells. A few small gland-like intraepithelial structures are formed by the Paget's cells.

by DNA ploidy analysis; however, prognosis does not appear to be influenced by DNA ploidy. Invasive Paget's disease 1 mm or less in depth of invasion has reportedly little risk for recurrence (87).

The differential diagnosis of Paget's disease of cutaneous origin includes PUIN/Paget's disease of urothelial origin, Paget's disease of colorectal origin/or other related adenocarcinoma, superficial spreading malignant melanoma, Pagetoid reticulosis, and the Pagetoid variant of vulvar intraepithelial neoplasia, which are keratinocytic cells resembling Paget's cells. These can all be differentiated by immunoperoxidase techniques because melanomas do not express cytokeratin, but usually express S100 protein, HMB-45, and Melan-A, which are absent in Paget's cells (90). The Paget-like cells in PUIN express uroplakin-3, but do not express GCDFP-15. CEA is expressed in approximately two thirds of urothelial neoplasms, but is expressed in both Paget's disease of cutaneous origin and Paget's disease of gastrointestinal origin. Adenocarcinoma cells of colonic, anal, or rectal origin express CEA, as well as caudal homeobox (CDX), whereas Paget's disease of cutaneous origin does not express CDX. Pagetoid reticulosis cells express leukocyte common antigen and some other lymphoproliferative markers, but lack CEA or cytokeratin. VIN of Pagetoid type may microscopically resemble Paget's disease or melanoma, but the cells of VIN do not express CEA, S100, or melanoma antigen (68,82).

Vulvar Malignant Melanoma

Malignant melanoma of the vulva accounts for approximately 9% of all primary malignant neoplasms on the vulva, and vulvar melanoma accounts for approximately 3% of all melanomas in women. This tumor occurs predominantly in Caucasian women, with approximately one third of the cases occurring in women younger than 50, and the mean age at diagnosis is 55 years of age (91). The peak frequency occurs between the sixth and seventh decades and the highest incidence is in women 75 years of age of older, where the age-specific incidence is reported to be 1.28 per 100,000 (92). The most common presenting symptom is bleeding; however, pruritus, pain, dysuria, and a palpable mass may all be symptoms (92). The tumor may arise from a preexisting pigmented lesion or from normal-appearing skin. The primary site on the vulva may be the clitoris, labia minora, and labia majora, where melanomas occur with approximately equal frequency (93). The tumor may be elevated, nodular, or ulcerated. Although usually pigmented, approximately one fourth are nonpigmented, amelanotic melanomas, a melanoma type that clinically and pathologically may resemble squamous carcinoma. In the clinical setting, the differential diagnosis includes pigmented condyloma acuminatum, pigmented VIN, atypical genital nevus, large vulvar nevi, melanosis of the vulva, or other malignant tumors including malignant soft-tissue tumors (82,94,95).

Vulvar malignant melanomas may be subclassified into three specific categories: superficial spreading malignant melanoma, nodular melanoma, and mucosal lentiginous melanoma, which is also referred to as mucosal/acral lentiginous melanoma (96,97). In the vulva some cases are mixed or cannot be specifically classified. Mucosal lentiginous melanomas are the type most commonly reported on the vulva, accounting for over one half the cases in larger series (92,96). Nodular melanomas are second in frequency, accounting for approximately one fifth of the cases, and have the overall worst prognosis of the melanoma types, usually related to the greater thickness and deeper invasion at the time of presentation. Superficial spreading melanomas are the least common type in the vulva. Some variation in the frequency of these types in the vulva is present in the literature, primarily related to some variations in pathologic classification (91–93,96,98–101).

Histopathologic differentiation of melanoma type is based on identification of a superficial spreading component. Mucosal lentiginous melanomas have the neoplastic melanocytes clustered in the dermal-epithelial junction and have both radial growth and vertical growth. Superficial spreading melanomas have radial growth involving four or more rete lateral to their vertical or infiltrative growth (82). Nodular melanomas show minimal or no radial growth. Superficial spreading malignant melanoma characteristically shows junctional melanocytes with radial growth, and a vertical growth pattern may be absent. The tumor cells are highly variable in appearance but commonly are relatively large, with nuclei showing minimal variation in size and containing prominent nucleoli (Fig. 20.15). These cells may or may not contain pigment. The form of the cells ranges from epithelioid to spindle shaped; in some cases, the spindle cell type may predominate. The spindle cells may be relatively small, with oval nuclei and elongated cytoplasm. They may infiltrate the adjacent dermis in cords and sheets.

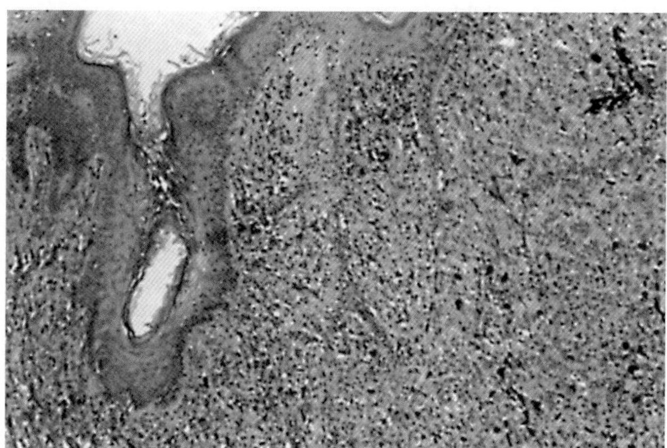

FIGURE 20.15. Malignant melanoma. The tumor is within the dermis and contains dark melanin pigment. Junctional growth is seen within the overlying epithelial dermal junction.

Malignant melanomas typically express S100 antigen, HMB-45, and Melan-A, and lack cytokeratin or CEA. The microscopic differential diagnosis for superficial spreading malignant melanoma is primarily vulvar Paget's disease. Immunohistochemical techniques are essential in discriminating superficial spreading melanoma from Paget's disease (see the section on vulvar Paget's disease) (90). Nonpigmented nodular melanomas may mimic squamous cell carcinoma or spindle cell neoplasms of various types. In these circumstances, immunoperoxidase procedures are of great value, because squamous cell carcinomas typically do not express S100 protein, HMB-45, or Melan-A, and melanomas do not express cytokeratin (82).

The level of invasion and tumor thickness are essential measurements in evaluating malignant melanoma (91,98,102). The Clark level definitions describe the extent of dermal and subcutanous involvement by the melanoma (102). Measurements for vulvar melanomas can be applied as for skin and mucous membranes, as described by Breslow (103). Malignant melanomas that have a thickness of less than 0.75 mm have little or no risk for metastasis and tumors up to 1 mm in thickness are generally considered of minimal risk of recurrence. Melanomas at Clark level 2 or thickness of 1.49 mm or less, or tumor volume of 100 mm^3 also correlate with good prognosis (104). A poor prognosis is correlated with Clark level 5, thickness >2 mm, or mitotic count exceeding $10/mm^2$. Other prognostic factors include a minimal or absent inflammatory reaction and surface ulceration (98).

Vulvar melanoma has been described associated with NRAS codon 12 mutation, as more commonly seen in sun exposure–related melanomas; however, most mucosal non-sun-exposure–related melanomas do not express Nras exon 2 mutations (105).

Melanomas arising in the vulva may metastasize to other sites within the lower female genital tract, including the cervix, vagina, urethra, and rectum. Distant metastasis is common with disseminated disease. Survival after recurrence is poor, approximately 5% (97).

Vulvar Sarcomas

Leiomyosarcoma. Leiomyosarcoma is the most frequent primary vulvar sarcoma. It most commonly arises in the labia majora or Bartholin's gland area, although these tumors may arise in the clitoris and labia minora. The tumors are generally larger than 5 cm in diameter when first diagnosed and may be deep within the subcutaneous tissue.

On microscopic examination, these tumors are composed of interlacing spindle shaped cells, sometimes with an epithelioid appearance. Features of leiomyosarcoma include an infiltrating border and metastasis. Microscopic criteria for diagnosis require determination of the mitotic figure count. In cases with minimal pleomorphism, it is generally accepted that the diagnosis of leiomyosarcoma can be made with a mitotic count of 10 or more per 10 high power fields. Tumors that have an infiltrating border or nuclear atypia with pleomorphism and mitotic count of 5 or more per 10 high power fields are classified as leiomyosarcoma. There are tumors that may show no significant atypia, have a diameter exceeding 5 cm, have an infiltrating margin, and have a low mitotic count, up to 5 per 10 high power fields. It is preferable to classify them as smooth muscle tumors of uncertain malignant potential, because the risk of recurrence is uncertain (39,106–108).

Malignant Fibrous Histiocytoma. Malignant fibrous histiocytoma arises from histiocytes with fibroblastic differentiation. It is considered the second most common sarcoma of the vulva and has its peak frequency in middle age. Malignant fibrous histiocytoma typically presents as a solitary mass that may appear somewhat brownish or pigmented, secondary to areas of focal hemorrhage within the tumor.

On microscopic examination, the tumor is characterized by a complex interlacing cellular growth pattern with marked nuclear pleomorphism, including multinucleated cells and large bizarre cells. Abnormal mitotic figures may be apparent. Microscopic variants of this tumor include inflammatory, giant cell, myxoid, and angiomatoid types (82,109). On immunoperoxidase study, these tumors contain α_1 antitrypsin and α_1 antichymotrypsin. Malignant fibrous histiocytoma is typically infiltrative, with infiltrative margins, and may involve the underlying fascia. Involvement of the fascia is associated with a higher risk of local spread and distant metastasis.

Epithelioid Sarcoma. Epithelioid sarcoma may arise within the labia majora, subclitoral area, and clitoris (110). Its microscopic features may resemble squamous carcinoma, malignant melanoma, malignant rhabdoid tumor, or lymphoma. Epithelioid sarcoma is usually relatively superficial, arising in and involving the reticular dermis, but it may occur in deeper structures.

On microscopic examination, the tumor is nodular and may have areas of necrosis. The tumor cells have an epithelioid appearance with eosinophilic cytoplasm, but there may be metaplastic components, including cartilage and bone. On immunohistochemical study, this tumor contains cytokeratin, which does not distinguish it from epithelial tumors, but is of value in differentiating it from malignant melanoma or other types of soft-tissue tumors. Epithelioid sarcoma rarely metastasizes, although local recurrence is a risk. Differential diagnosis for this tumor includes squamous cell carcinoma, malignant melanoma, lymphoma, and malignant rhabdoid tumor, all of which are capable of distant metastasis and aggressive behavior (110). Immunoperoxidase studies are of value in differentiation, but have not been of value in differentiating epithelioid sarcoma from malignant rhabdoid tumor. The distinction of these two tumors is based primarily on microscopic features.

Malignant Rhabdoid Tumor. Malignant rhabdoid tumor has been described in the vulva and, like epithelioid sarcoma, may be relatively superficial and contain tumor cells with an epithelioid appearance with eosinophilic cytoplasm. Unlike epithelioid sarcoma, malignant rhabdoid tumors have relatively pleomorphic nuclei. Metaplastic elements are usually not present. Malignant rhabdoid tumor also has eosinophilic cytoplasmic inclusions, which are not present in epithelioid sarcoma. These inclusions give some of the cells the appearance of signet ring cells. Electron microscopic evaluation of the rhabdoid tumor reveals that the eosinophilic inclusions are composed of intermediate filaments. Malignant rhabdoid tumor has a lobulated architecture but lacks necrosis or granulomatous features, which are often found in epithelioid sarcoma (107,108,110).

Malignant Schwannoma

Malignant schwannoma has been reported on the vulva, and approximately half of the cases are associated with neurofibromatosis. Most malignant schwannomas occur in women of reproductive age (111). This tumor is found primarily in the labia majora or minora, but may arise in other sites within the vulva.

On microscopic examination it is typically highly cellular and is composed of spindle cells with nuclear palisading. Metaplastic elements, such as cartilage, epithelial islands, and striated muscle, may be seen in approximately 50% of the cases. Malignant schwannoma is immunoreactive for S100 protein. In some cases, a nerve trunk can be identified adjacent to or within the tumor mass.

Yolk Sac Tumor

Yolk sac tumor (endodermal sinus tumor) is a rare germ cell tumor of the vulva, primarily arising in the labia or clitoral areas (39,112). The age range of patients is from just under 2 to 26 years. Distinctive microscopic features are similar to endodermal sinus tumor in the ovary, including the Schiller-Duval bodies, distinctive globules that are PAS positive, and the presence of α-fetoprotein within the tumor, as demonstrated by immunoperoxidase technique.

Other Sarcomas

A partial list of primary sarcomas of the vulva includes angiosarcoma, Kaposi's sarcoma, hemangiopericytoma, rhabdomyosarcoma, alveolar soft part sarcoma, and liposarcoma (39,107,108,113,114). Sarcoma botryoides is a variant of rhabdomyosarcoma that may involve the vulva, but most cases arise within the vagina or base of the bladder. Aggressive angiomyxoma, a locally aggressive but rarely metastatic sarcoma, has also been documented arising within the vulva (50,107). Kaposi's sarcoma and angiosarcoma should be differentiated from bacillary angiomatosis, which is a benign pseudoneoplastic infectious process (115). The reader is referred to additonal texts on these and other soft-tissue tumors of the vulva (39, 07,108).

Metastatic Tumors to the Vulva

Most metastatic tumors to the vulva involve the labia majora or Bartholin's glands. In the vulva they usually present as single or multiple intradermal or subcutaneous nodules, but may present as a Bartholin's gland mass (77,116–119). Metastatic tumors account for approximately 8% of all vulvar tumors, and in approximately one half of the cases the primary tumor was in the lower genital tract, including the cervix, vagina, endometrium, and ovary. Cervical carcinoma is the most common origin of contiguous metastasis. Local metastasis secondary to contiguous involvement of the vulva from urothelial carcinoma of the bladder or urethra, or ano-rectal carcinoma, may involve the vulva and present as a Paget-like lesion (see Paget's disease and Paget-like lesions in this section) or a vulvar or groin node mass (73,120). Contiguous involvement of tumors from the genital tract or ano-rectal areas are commonly associated with metastasis to regional lymph nodes and widespread metastases. Remote metastases have been observed from tumors arising in breast, kidney, stomach, lung, and other sites. Malignant melanoma and neuroblastoma can also metastasize to the vulva, as can gestational choriocarcinoma and malignant lymphomas. In approximately 10% of the cases the primary site of the metastatic tumor cannot be identified. Prognosis with metastatic tumor to the vulva is generally guarded, but is influenced by the type of tumor and the therapy available.

PROGNOSTIC FACTORS

Prognosis has been most extensively evaluated in women with squamous cell carcinomas. The major prognostic factors in vulvar cancer—tumor diameter, depth of tumor invasion, nodal spread, and distant metastasis—have been incorporated into the current FIGO staging system. These are clearly the most important predictors of tumor recurrence and death from disease (121–126). However, several additional features may be useful in refining prognosis in smaller subsets of patients.

Wharton et al. suggested the concept of "microinvasive" carcinoma of the vulva in their 1975 report and proposed eliminating groin dissection for patients with small tumors that invaded <5 mm (75). A number of later reports confirmed that 10% to 20% of patients meeting these criteria had occult groin metastases, making the elimination of inguinal lymph node evaluation undesirable for these patients (127–130). Several authors have further attempted to define a population of microinvasive tumors whereby the risk of inguinal metastasis is negligible (46,131–135). The consensus opinion is that only tumors with less than 1 mm invasion fulfill this requirement (18,46,65,136). This is reflected in the FIGO classification of tumors invading ≤1 mm into stage IA (26).

Risk of local recurrence, although clearly associated with tumor size and extent, is also related to the adequacy of the surgical resection margins. Heaps et al., in their analysis of formalin-fixed tissue specimens, were able to demonstrate a sharp rise in the incidence of local recurrence for tumors with microscopic margins less than 8 mm (59). They suggested that this would correspond to a minimum margin of 1 cm in fresh, unfixed tissue. These observations were confirmed in a retrospective multivariate analysis of clinical data by Chan et al., who showed that pathologic margin distance ≤8 mm is an important predictor of local recurrence (137). De Hullu et al. reported nine local recurrences among 40 patients with tumor-free margins ≤8 mm compared to no local recurrences among 39 patients with margins >8 mm (138). To aid the surgeon in planning surgical margins of resection, Hoffman et al. measured the radial occult microscopic spread of tumor in patients with invasive squamous cell carcinoma of the vulva. They found that the gross and microscopic periphery of most cancers were approximately the same; however, ulcerative tumors with an infiltrative pattern of invasion were more likely to extend beyond what is grossly apparent (139).

The single most important prognostic factor in women with vulvar cancer is metastasis to the inguinal lymph nodes, and most recurrences will occur within 2 years of primary treatment (140). The presence of inguinal node metastasis portends a 50% reduction in long-term survival (141,142). A number of noninvasive imaging modalities have been studied for the evaluation of inguinal femoral lymph node metastasis, including magnetic resonance imaging, computed tomography, positron emission tomography (PET), and ultrasound. There currently is no imaging modality with a sufficiently high negative predictive value to allow for exclusion of surgical groin lymph node evaluation (143,144). Because the clinical prediction of lymph node spread is inaccurate, node status is best determined via surgical biopsy. Prognostic issues that appear to be important in evaluating lymphatic involvement are (a) whether nodal spread is bilateral or unilateral, (b) the number of positive nodes, (c) the volume of tumor in the metastasis, and (d) the level of the metastatic disease. Multiple positive nodes, bilateral metastases, involvement beyond the groin, and bulky disease are associated with poor prognosis (44,145). Rutledge et al. provided the detailed analysis of prognostic factors outlined in Table 20.4 (146).

TABLE 20.4

SUMMARY OF COX PROPORTIONAL HAZARDS MODEL FOR VULVA DATA: PREDICTORS OF FAILURE TO SURVIVE

	Relative hazard	95% Confidence interval
TUMOR SIZE (cm) ($p = 0.005$)		
0–2	1.0000	
3–4	1.1312	(0.6364, 2.0108)
5–6	2.1833	(1.2116, 3.9342)
>6	2.3683	(1.2310, 4.5560)
TUMOR GRADE ($p = 0.182$)		
1	1.0000	
2	0.9556	(0.5716, 1.5974)
3	1.4748	(0.8653, 2.5136)
FIGO STAGE ($p = 0.000$)		
I	1.0000	
II	2.9842	(0.8694, 10.2431)
III	8.6452	(2.6973, 27.7087)
IV	40.9031	(12.2898, 136.1343)
THERAPY AIM ($p = 0.000$)		
Curative	1.0000	
Palliative	8.2821	(5.1064, 13.4328)
GROIN NODES ($p = 0.000$)		
Bilaterally negative	1.0000	
Unilaterally positive	6.8656	(3.5492, 13.2808)
Bilaterally positive	20.3212	(10.0935, 40.9127)
PELVIC NODES ($p = 0.000$)		
Bilaterally negative	1.0000	
Unilaterally positive	5.9230	(2.9335, 11.9590)
Bilaterally positive	10.9852	(2.4803, 48.6537)

(*continued*)

TABLE 20.4

SUMMARY OF COX PROPORTIONAL HAZARDS MODEL FOR VULVA DATA: PREDICTORS OF FAILURE TO SURVIVE (CONTINUED)

	Relative hazard	95% Confidence interval
CLOQUET'S NODE ($p = 0.631$)		
Negative	1.0000	
Positive	1.4548	(0.3424, 6.1807)
DEEP SURGICAL MARGINS ($p = 0.931$)[a]		
Negative	1.0000	
Invasive	1.0914	(0.1523, 7.8227)
VAGINAL SURGICAL MARGINS ($p = 0.906$)[b]		
Negative	1.0000	
Invasive	0.9063	(0.2233, 3.6779)
LATERAL SURGICAL MARGINS ($p = 0.010$)[c]		
Negative	1.0000	
Invasive	5.2267	(1.8889, 14.4626)
AGE ($p = 0.100$)		
<41	1.0000	
41–60	1.8266	(0.6416, 5.2002)
61–80	2.5600	(0.9264, 7.0745)
>80	3.0251	(0.9068, 10.0917)
SITE OF LESION ($p = 0.359$)		
Clitoris or mons	1.0000	
Labia	2.3082	(0.3045, 17.4957)
GROSS TUMOR APPEARANCE ($p = 0.668$)		
Nonulcerative	1.0000	
Ulcerative	1.0905	(0.7338, 1.6205)
CLINICAL STAGE (TUMOR) ($p = 0.000$)		
T1	1.0000	
T2	2.3574	(1.0462, 5.3119)
T3	4.2916	(1.9420, 9.4837)
T4	35.1826	(10.0462, 123.2127)
CLINICAL STAGE (NODES) ($p = 0.000$)		
N0	1.0000	
N1	1.3209	(0.7026, 2.4834)
N2	3.0702	(1.8513, 5.0916)
N3	11.2343	(6.3559, 19.8571)
CLINICAL STAGE (METASTASIS) ($p < 0.001$)		
M0	1.0000	
M1A or M1B	14.5149	(5.6785, 37.1022)
MEDICAL STATUS ($p = 0.289$)		
No illness	1.0000	
Obesity	0.7925	(0.3355, 1.8723)
Diabetes	0.2702	(0.0374, 1.9509)
Hypertension	1.1532	(0.6884, 1.9318)
Cardiovascular abnormalities	1.4235	(0.7582, 2.6725)

[a]Of the 133 patients with deep surgical margins, only 4 had invasive carcinoma.
[b]Of the 327 patients with vaginal surgical margins, only 8 had invasive carcinoma.
[c]Of the 331 patients with lateral surgical margins, only 6 had invasive carcinoma.
Source: Reprinted from Rutledge FN, Mitchell MF, Munsell MF, et al. Prognostic indicators for invasive carcinoma of the vulva. *Gynecol Oncol* 1991;42:239–244.

TREATMENT

Development of the radical vulvectomy with bilateral inguinofemoral lymphadenectomy during the 1940s and 1950s was a dramatic improvement over prior surgical options and greatly enhanced survival, particularly for women with smaller tumors and negative lymph nodes (147,148). The ability to successfully resect vulvar tumors eliminated prolonged survival marked by local and regional progression of disease and associated pain, drainage, and bleeding. Long-term survival of 85% to 90% can now be routinely obtained with radical surgery. However, radical surgery can be associated with postoperative complications such as wound breakdown and lymphedema.

More recently, surgical emphasis has evolved to an individualized approach for tumors at either end of the spectrum. Many gynecologists believe that smaller vulvar tumors can be acceptably managed by less radical surgical approaches and have proposed more limited resections for certain subsets considered to represent early or low-risk disease (65,149,150). The obvious advantages of such an approach are retention of a significant portion of the uninvolved vulva, less operative morbidity, and fewer late complications. In contrast, radical surgery is frequently ineffective in curing patients with bulky tumors or positive groin nodes. Multimodality programs that incorporate radiation, surgery, and chemotherapy are now being investigated in women with these high-risk tumors based upon success with similar approaches in women with squamous cancers of the cervix (151–154). It seems fair to state that "quality of life" issues predominate at the lower end of the disease scale, whereas "survival" concerns are most important at the upper end. At present, there are limited curative treatment options for women who present with disseminated disease.

Microinvasive Tumors

Tumors demonstrating early invasion of the vulvar stroma (≤1 mm) have minimal risk for lymphatic dissemination. Excisional procedures that incorporate a 1-cm normal tissue margin are likely to provide curative results (155). Patients in this category represent the only subset for whom the status of the groin lymph nodes can be ignored. These so-called microcarcinomas tend to arise in younger patients with multifocal preinvasive disease and are commonly associated with HPV infections. Occult invasion in lesions thought to be intraepithelial is common (156,157). Consequently, the entire lower genital tract and vulva should be carefully evaluated before surgical resection of these lesions is attempted. The risk of vulvar recurrence or development of a new lesion at another vulvar site is significant. After primary therapy these patients should undergo frequent follow-up examinations.

Stage I and II Cancers

Traditional management of stage I and II vulvar cancer has been radical vulvectomy with bilateral inguinofemoral lymphadenectomy. The operation removes the primary tumor with a wide margin of normal skin, along with the remaining vulva, dermal lymphatics, and regional nodes. This approach provides excellent long-term survival and local control in approximately 90% of patients (158,159). Disadvantages of radical surgery include loss of normal vulvar tissue with alterations in appearance and sexual function, a 50% incidence of wound breakdown, a 30% incidence of groin complications (breakdown, lymphocyst, lymphangitis), and a 10% to 15% incidence of lower extremity lymphedema (160,161). Additional postoperative therapy, primarily irradiation, should be considered in the 10% to 20% of patients with positive nodes with the understanding that this will further increase the incidence of lymphedema (162).

In an effort to reduce morbidity and enhance psychosexual recovery, several groups have espoused a more limited surgical approach for women with small vulvar cancers (163,164). Although some patients with T2 lesions have been treated in this manner, most have limited the conservative approach to women with T1 cancers. DiSaia et al. were the first to describe successful conservative resection of tumors measuring 1 cm or less with invasion of less than 5 mm (150). Additional reports have expanded this experience to include more patients with larger lesions and more significant invasion (Table 20.5) (65,165,166). The most frequent recommendation is to resect the primary lesion with a 1- to 2-cm margin of normal tissue and to carry the dissection to the deep perineal fascia. These operations should not be confused with the concept of excisional biopsy, which is used primarily as a diagnostic procedure.

Limited resection of the primary tumor is combined with a more conservative surgical approach to the groin, in which the ipsilateral superficial groin nodes are used as the sentinel group for lymphatic metastases (15,166,167). Bilateral superficial dissections are performed in patients whose tumors encroach on midline structures (clitoris or perineal body) (165). In patients with negative inguinal nodes, no further dissection or postoperative therapy is used. In their series of 61 patients with non-midline T1 and T2 squamous cell carcinomas of the vulva, DeSimone et al. found no patient with lymph node metastasis to the contralateral groin (168). Similarly, Gonzalez et al. reported that contralateral groin lymph node dissection was unnecessary for patients with non-midline lesions <2 cm in size and/or with negative ipsilateral groin lymph nodes (169). Patients with positive nodes can undergo additional nodal dissection of the deep nodes and the contralateral groin or be treated with postoperative irradiation, or both. The risk of chronic groin complications and lymphedema is related to the extent of groin dissection (149). Patients with superficial and deep lymphadenectomy followed by irradiation have the greatest likelihood of morbidity.

With limited resection, survival of 90% or better is attainable for patients with stage I vulva carcinoma with acceptable anatomic appearance and function. Critics of conservative surgical approaches cite several potential risks, including potential recurrence in retained vulvar skin, inadequate assessment of the groin nodes, inadequate surgical therapy in women with nodal spread, and the potential for leaving in-transit skin metastases. Examination of the published experience using a selective approach to inguinal lymphadenectomy would suggest that unanticipated ipsilateral groin failure occurs in ≤5% of cases (Table 20.6) (65,165,166,170), whereas contralateral groin failure is uncommon. Because randomized prospective evaluations of surgical therapy have not been performed, a critical comparison of radical vulvectomy and radical wide excision is not possible.

TABLE 20.5

PROPOSED CRITERIA FOR CONSERVATIVE SURGICAL RESECTION

Investigator	Tumor diameter	Depth of invasion	Groin dissection
Wharton et al. (75)	<2 cm	<5 mm	None
DiSaia et al. (150)	<1 cm	<5 mm	Superficial
Berman et al. (65)	<2 cm	<5 mm	Superficial
Burke et al. (149)	Resectable	Any	Superficial
Stehman et al. (166)	<2 cm	<5 mm	Superficial

TABLE 20.6

UNANTICIPATED GROIN FAILURE IN PATIENTS WITH NEGATIVE SUPERFICIAL LYMPHADENECTOMY

Investigators	No.	%
Burke et al. (165)	4/76	5.2
Berman et al. (65)	0/50	0
Stehman et al. (166)	6/121	5.0
Gordinier et al. (170)	9/104	8.6
Total	19/351	5.4

In an attempt to reduce treatment-related morbidity, yet retain the essential components of radical excision of the primary tumor plus groin lymph node assessment, some have introduced modifications of the classic radical operation. These include the use of "triple incision" techniques that separate the vulvectomy incision from the groin incisions, as well as techniques that use a more limited dissection of the deep inguinal nodes as compared to "complete" groin lymphadenectomy (171). Le et al. have suggested that a total of at least ten nodes from a bilateral groin dissection define an optimal surgical evaluation (172). Using anatomical groin dissections from cadavers, Hudson et al. showed that the incision or removal of deep fascia in the femoral triangle with "stripping" of the femoral vessels was unnecessary; however, some nodes of importance were present within fenestrations of the cribriform fascia covering the saphenous opening (173). Other surgical refinements that may reduce postoperative morbidity without compromising outcome include preservation of the saphenous vein (174–176). A prospective, randomized trial showed that sartorius transposition did not reduce the incidence of postoperative wound infection or lymphedema (177).

Another surgical concept that is undergoing evaluation is the potential for cutaneous lymphatic mapping to define and target the true sentinel groin nodes (178). Preliminary experience with both intraoperative lymphatic dye and radioisotope injections suggests that a sentinel node can often be identified in the groin (34,179,180). This early experience supports the concept that the assessment of lymphatic metastases may ultimately be reduced to the biopsy of one or two identifiable nodes (Fig. 20.16). Terada et al. performed sentinel lymph node mapping and biopsy for 21 patients with T1 vulvar cancer using preoperative lymphoscintigraphy and intraoperative isosulfan blue dye staining. Three patients proved to have positive sentinel lymph nodes. None of the patients with negative sentinel lymph nodes had developed a groin or distant recurrence with median follow-up of 4.6 years (181).

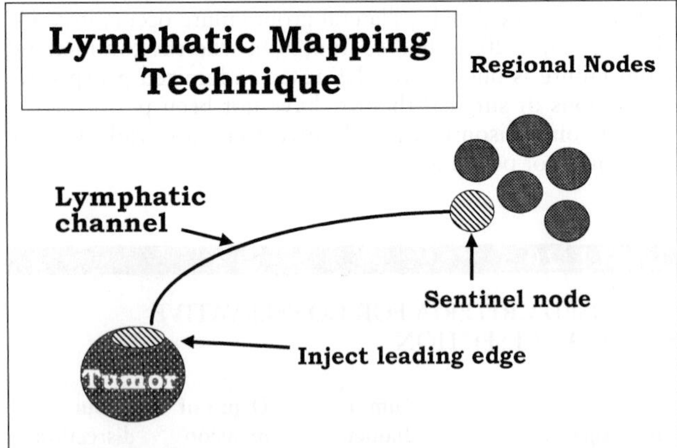

FIGURE 20.16. Intraoperative lymphatic mapping is accomplished by injecting the leading edge of the visible tumor with isosulfan blue dye. The dye is taken up by the specific node that drains the tumor site. This "sentinel" node can be visually identified and separated from other nodes within the regional group. In concept, all tumors with nodal metastases can be detected by biopsy of the sentinel node.

In summary, therapy for women with stage I and II cancers must be individualized to the patient and her tumor. Radical vulvectomy provides excellent local control and long-term survival, but has significant morbidity and sexual function limitations. More conservative approaches appear safe in most stage I settings and may be applicable in some stage II patients. The surgical approach to the groin nodes is evolving. The accuracy of the superficial inguinal nodes (or the "sentinel" node identified by intraoperative mapping) as predictors of nodal spread is currently being evaluated. If these concepts prove suitably sensitive and specific, more extensive inguinal lymphadenectomy might be abandoned.

Stage III and IV Cancers

By definition, stage III tumors extend to adjacent mucosal structures or the inguinal lymph nodes. Many are bulky, but some are of limited volume but considered high stage because of proximity to critical central structures. Some of these primary tumors can be curatively resected by radical operations, such as radical vulvectomy or some variation of pelvic exenteration and vulvectomy. Surgical resection of 1 to 1.5 cm of the distal urethra in order to achieve a negative surgical margin does not appear to compromise bladder continence (182). However, recent therapeutic efforts have focused on combined modality treatment programs involving sequenced radiation therapy or chemoradiation therapy and radical surgery. There are now ample data from retrospective series, and a few prospective trials, from which to conclude that vulvar cancers are radioresponsive and that function-sparing operations are feasible in selected patients with advanced disease who receive combined modality treatment (183,184). A similar experience has been reported for patients with stage IVA tumors. Ultraradical (exenteration) resection may also be considered for selected patients. Although occasional cures have been described with innovative combinations of surgery, irradiation, and chemotherapy, treatment of patients with stage IVB vulvar cancer should be considered palliative.

Node Positive Cancers

An optimal management strategy for node positive patients is yet to be defined. Two factors appear to be important in the management of regional disease: radiation therapy can have a significant impact on controlling or eradicating small volume nodal disease, and surgical resection of bulky nodal disease also improves regional control and probably enhances the curative potential of irradiation. In multivariate analysis, Hyde et al. found that, for patients with clinically positive groin nodes who underwent surgery followed by radiation therapy, the method of surgical groin node dissection (nodal "debulking" versus full groin dissection) had no prognostic signficance (185).

Patients who undergo bilateral inguinofemoral lymphadenectomy as initial therapy and are found to have positive nodes—particularly more than one positive node—are likely to benefit from postoperative irradiation to the groin and lower pelvis (162). Radiation therapy is superior to surgery in the management of patients with positive pelvic nodes. The morbidity of combining superficial and deep inguinal lymphadenectomy with irradiation is substantial. The highest incidences of chronic groin and extremity complications, primarily lymphedema, are seen in such cases.

Several management options are available for patients found to have positive nodes during the course of superficial lymphadenectomy when performed as a staging procedure: (a) no further surgical therapy may be performed; (b) the lymphadenectomy can be extended to include the ipsilateral deep nodes, the contralateral groin nodes, or both; or (c) postoperative irradiation can be added to any of these surgical options. Given the heterogeneity of vulvar cancer presentations, treatment individualization is necessary. If postoperative radiotherapy to the inguinal nodes is deemed necessary, it would be reasonable to limit resection to grossly positive nodes, thereby minimizing the likelihood of lymphedema following combined radical surgery and radiation. Postoperative radiation requires careful treatment planning, using CT imaging to evaluate for any measurable residual tumor and to determine appropriate groin node depth. Excellent local control and minimal morbidity have been achieved when selective inguinal lymphadenectomy and tailored postoperative adjuvant therapy were administered to carefully selected patients (165).

Recurrent Cancer

Regardless of initial treatment, vulvar cancer recurrences can be categorized into three clinical groups: local (vulva), groin, and distant. The reported experience with local recurrence on the vulva is surprisingly good. Recurrence-free survival can be obtained in up to 75% of cases when the recurrence is limited to the vulva and can be resected with a gross clinical margin (186,187). The observation that many of these vulva recurrences occur at sites remote from the initial primary tumor or that they occur years after apparently successful primary treatment suggests that some recurrences probably represent new primary tumors rather than the development of new disease. Recurrences in the groin are almost universally fatal. A few patients may be saved by resection of bulky disease and local irradiation. Patients who develop distant metastases are candidates for systemic cytotoxic therapy, which is largely palliative.

SURGICAL TECHNIQUES

Radical Vulvectomy and Bilateral Inguinofemoral Lymphadenectomy

Although a number of modifications have been described, the basic incisions for radical vulvectomy and bilateral lymphadenectomy can be described as based on either a "butterfly" or "longhorn" approach. The butterfly incisions use convex "wings" over the groin and around the anus to facilitate closure of the defect (Fig. 20.17). The longhorn incisions were developed to limit skin resection over the groin in an attempt to reduce wound breakdown (Fig. 20.18) (188). The arcing superior incision is placed from the lateral margins of the groin dissection across the mons pubis. The lateral vulvar incisions are placed at the labiocrural folds, because these topographical landmarks represent the most lateral location of the superficial vulvar lymphatics. The perianal incision is placed to allow resection of the perineal body. These incisions are taken to the level of the deep inguinal and perineal fascia and permit *en bloc* removal of both superficial and deep groin nodes, the entire vulva, and an intervening skin bridge.

After removal of the specimen, the skin and mucosal edges are undermined to permit mobilization and primary closure with delayed absorbable suture. Some degree of tension at the suture lines is unavoidable, particularly in the perineal body and periurethral areas. Closed suction drains are usually placed in the groin sites to remove excess lymphatic- and serous-fluid accumulations and are usually removed when drain output is minimal (5 to 14 days).

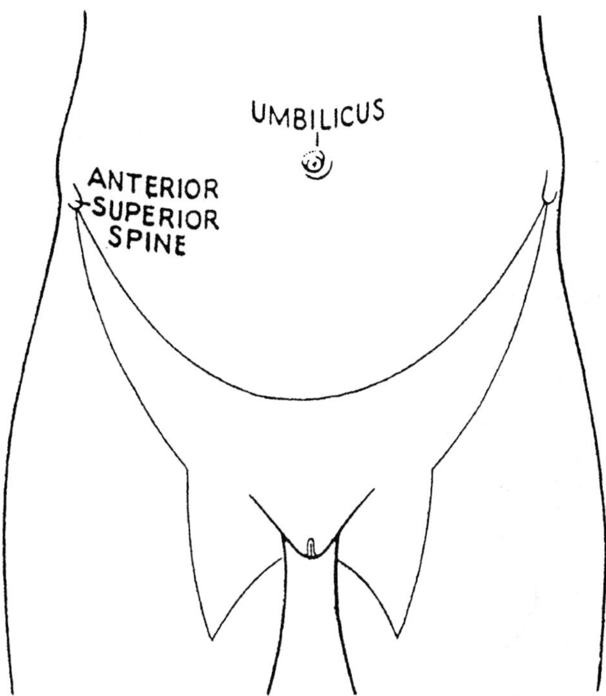

FIGURE 20.17. "Butterfly" incisions for the superior portion of a radical vulvectomy with bilateral inguinofemoral lymphadenectomy. *Source:* Reprinted from Way S. *Malignant Disease of the Female Genital Tract*. New York: Churchill Livingstone; 1951.

Some degree of wound breakdown is seen in approximately 50% of patients (161). Local wound care results in satisfactory secondary healing in most of these cases. Lymphocyst formation is relatively common and frequently presents as a tense but nontender groin mass. Percutaneous needle drainage is usually sufficient but occasionally replacement of a groin drain may be required. Inguinal cellulitis, lower extremity lymphangitis, and lymphedema are uncommon late sequelae. The incidence of these complications is related to the extent of groin therapy and is highest in patients treated with superficial and deep lymphadenectomy along with groin irradiation.

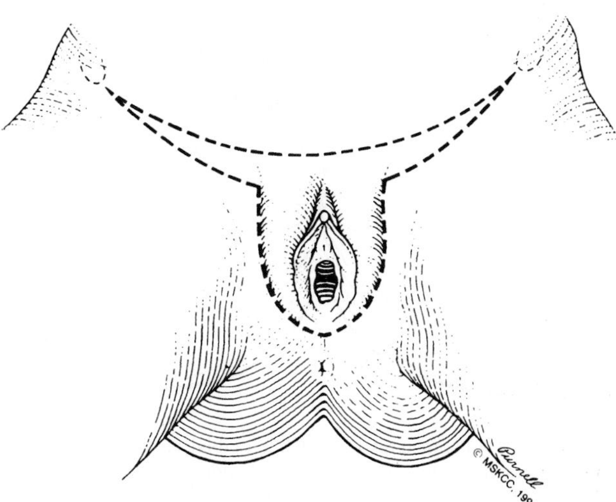

FIGURE 20.18. Modified skin-sparing "longhorn" incisions for *en bloc* radical resection.

Radical Wide Excision

Several names have been applied to the procedures used to resect small vulvar cancers: radical wide excision, radical local excision, wide local excision, modified radical vulvectomy, and hemivulvectomy. Regardless of preferred nomenclature, the surgical procedure should be adequately defined and described. Surgical incisions are devised to allow for at least a 2-cm resection margin encompassing the primary lesion (Fig. 20.19). Dissection is carried to the deep perineal fascia. Recent data suggest that a 1-cm margin may be adequate for some tumors (160). If this information is verified by other studies it will be most useful when planning the resection of tumors in close proximity to midline structures. Tumors that encroach on the anus or anal sphincters can be managed by radical wide excision with sphincter or flap repair, or they can be treated with combined modality therapy as outlined under the Radiation Therapy section. Most radical wide excision sites can be closed primarily. In some patients, rhomboid flaps can be used to facilitate coverage of the vulvar defect (189). Some form of inguinal lymphadenectomy, performed through a separate incision, is generally combined with radical wide excision. The necessary extent of the groin dissection is an area of current investigation.

Ambulation is begun on the day of surgery. Perineal irrigation and air drying are started 24 hours after operation. The average hospital stay for patients undergoing radical wide excision is usually 3 days or less. Wound breakdown, usually of minor degree, is reported in approximately 15% of cases (65,149). The incidence and severity of groin complications is proportional to the extent of the lymphadenectomy.

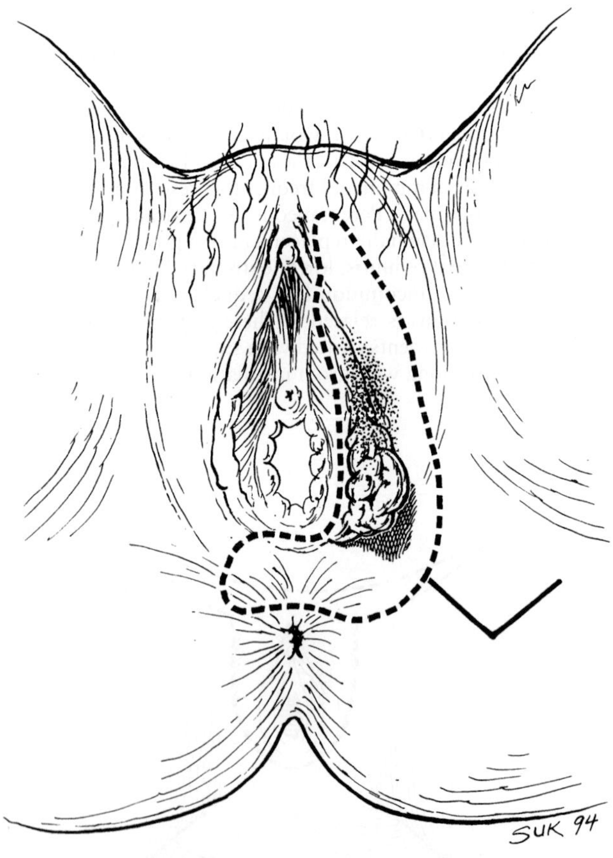

FIGURE 20.19. Planned resection of a left labial squamous carcinoma and adjacent carcinoma *in situ* by radical wide excision. A 2-cm margin is outlined. Rhomboid-flap repair using a V-incision is anticipated. *Source:* Reprinted from Burke TW, Morris M, Levenback C, et al. Closure of complex vulvar defects using local rhomboid flaps. *Obstet Gynecol* 1994;84:1043–1047.

Triple Incision Techniques

As a radical operation, the three incision technique represents an intermediate surgical procedure with radical vulvectomy and *en bloc* inguinofemoral lymphadenectomy on one end of the spectrum and radical wide excision on the other. For this approach, radical vulvectomy is accomplished using two elliptical incisions—an inner one circumscribing the vaginal introitus and vulvar vestibule and an outer one placed at the labiocrural folds and brought across the mons pubis and perineal body. When carried to the deep perineal fascia, this resection allows complete removal of the vulvar skin in a manner identical to that achieved with radical vulvectomy; however, bilateral inguinofemoral lymphadenectomy is accomplished via separate incisions parallel to the inguinal ligaments. The three incision concept preserves the radicality of the vulvar resection while retaining skin over the groin. Consequently, the incidence of major wound breakdown is significantly reduced to approximately 15% to 20% of cases (171,190,191). As with other techniques, the incidence and severity of groin complications such as infection, wound breakdown, or lymphocyst formation are still high (192).

Inguinal Lymphadenectomy

Appropriate surgical management of the inguinal nodes is controversial and evolving. Precise recommendations are not possible, because there is a wide range of treatment philosophies. Nevertheless, the surgical approaches to the groin lymph nodes can be readily defined and described.

Excisional Biopsy

Most preoperative diagnostic dilemmas related to enlarged groin nodes can be resolved simply and accurately using fine needle aspiration biopsy. However, surgical removal of one or two lymph nodes may occasionally be considered in the management of women with vulvar cancer. Selective excision of groin lymph nodes may be considered when fine needle aspiration biopsy results are negative or equivocal, or to remove bulky positive nodes before beginning a course of combined modality therapy. A small incision is made over the palpable node and dissection is carried to the level of the lymph node mass. The involved node is freed from the adjacent subcutaneous tissues and removed. The incision is closed with skin staples or absorbable sutures. The decision to electively place a closed suction drain depends upon the extent of the dissection, the amount of subcutaneous free space, and surgeon preference. Most lymph node biopsies can be performed as outpatient procedures, and some can be accomplished under local anesthesia.

Superficial Inguinal Lymphadenectomy

Superficial inguinal lymphadenectomy involves the removal of the eight to ten lymph nodes that lie superficial to the cribriform fascia and surround the branches of the saphenous vein. This is a more meticulous and complete lymphatic dissection than that described for excisional biopsy. The anatomic boundaries of the superficial lymphatic dissection are the inguinal ligament superiorly, the border of the sartorius muscle laterally, and the border of the adductor longus muscle medially. The anterior limit is the superficial subcutaneous fascia (Camper's fascia), and the posterior limit is the cribriform fascia overlying the femoral artery, vein, and deep nodes.

The skin incision used to provide access to the groin is made parallel to the inguinal ligament approximately from a point overlying the adductor longus tendon laterally to a point below the anterior superior iliac spine. The superficial subcutaneous fat is left attached to the skin to provide blood supply, but is separated from the underlying nodal tissue by dissecting inferiorly at the level of Camper's fascia. The lymphadenectomy specimen is developed by continuing the inferior dissection along the borders of the sartorius and adductor longus muscles. As the dissection proceeds, the specimen is mobilized off the cribriform fascia. Care should be taken to identify and individually ligate the vessels that perforate this fascia. The saphenous vein is encountered at the lower medial margin of the dissection, and whenever possible should be preserved to minimize the risk for postoperative lymphedema (Fig. 20.20). The dissected specimen is forwarded for pathologic assessment. The skin incision can be closed with either staples or absorbable sutures. A closed-suction drain is placed and removed when output is <25 mL per day.

Deep Inguinal (Femoral) Lymphadenectomy

The deep inguinal (femoral) lymph nodes lie medial to the femoral vein beneath the cribriform fascia. This space contains three to five nodes, the channels of which course beneath the inguinal ligament and continue in the pelvis as the external iliac nodal chain. The most superior deep inguinal node is known as Cloquet's node.

Surgical removal of the deep nodes is performed as an extension of a superficial lymphadenectomy rather than as an isolated procedure. The usual approach is to open the cribriform fascia along the sartorius muscle at the time of the superficial lymphadenectomy. The cribriform fascia is then mobilized medially as a part of the specimen. Once the superior aspect of the femoral vein is identified and exposed, the deep nodes are removed in continuity with the superficial nodes. Some surgeons then cover the exposed femoral vessels by removing the sartorius muscle from its insertion onto the anterior iliac spine and transposing the muscle over the femoral vessels by suturing the free edge of the muscle to the inguinal ligament.

Because all of the deep nodes are consistently located medial to the femoral vein, some surgeons have recommended eliminating the removal of the entire cribriform plate (193). They suggest opening the fascia medial to the vein and removing only the adjacent nodes. This modified approach to the deep nodes may help to reduce acute morbidity while providing a more definitive lymphatic resection. In a retrospective review of 194 patients undergoing various modifications of inguinofemoral lymphadenectomy, Rouzier et al. showed that techniques of groin node dissection that preserved the cribriform fascia and saphenous vein were associated with a decreased risk of postoperative morbidity without jeopardizing outcomes (194).

Sentinel Lymph Node Mapping and Biopsy

The concept of a "sentinel lymph node" was first introduced by Cabanas. Using lymphangiography for the clinical evaluation of penile carcinoma, he suggested that the sentinel lymph node was the first lymph node in the lymphatic pathway and the main site of metastasis (195). DiSaia et al. described the eight to ten superficial lymph nodes above the cribriform fascia as "sentinel nodes." When these lymph nodes proved negative, the risk for metastasis to the deep inguinal or pelvic lymph nodes was negligible (150). In 1992, Morton et al. introduced the use of vital blue dye (isosulfan blue) to identify lymphatic drainage from malignant melanoma (196). Levenback et al. utilized this intraoperative blue dye staining technique for sentinel lymph node identification in vulvar squamous cell carcinoma (Fig. 20.21) (178). Further work has demonstrated that blue dye staining alone has relatively low sensitivity in identifying the sentinel lymph node, particularly among patients with midline primary tumors. Lymphoscintigraphy using radioactive ^{99m}technetium administered shortly before surgery, combined with the intraoperative use of a handheld gamma probe, has significantly improved the sensitivity of sentinel lymph node identification (197).

Several earlier studies suggested that sentinel lymph node biopsy is a highly accurate procedure, with a negative predictive value approaching 100% (198–201). De Hullu et al. performed sentinel lymph node identification and biopsy in 59 women with primary vulvar carcinoma using the combination of intraoperative isosulfan blue dye staining plus preoperative lymphoscintigraphy (202). Only 60% of sentinel lymph nodes were visible with blue staining alone. With the addition of the handheld

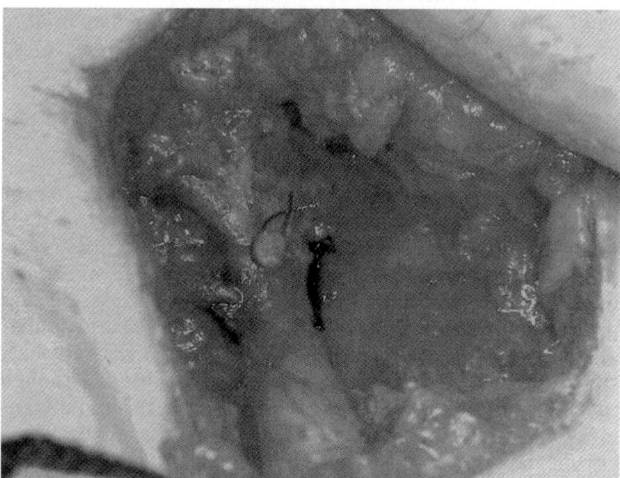

FIGURE 20.20. The patient is undergoing superficial and deep dissection of the right groin nodes. At this point in the procedure the saphenous vein, which is entering the surgical field from the right lower aspect, has been identified and preserved.

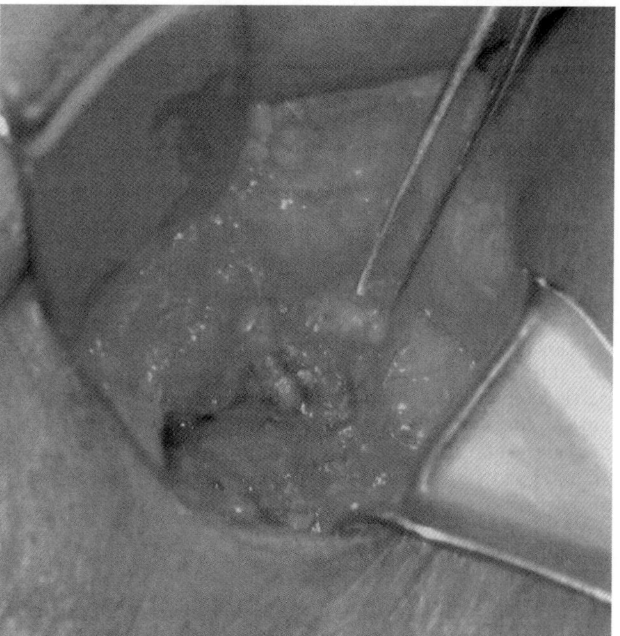

FIGURE 20.21. Following isosulfan blue dye injection, sentinel lymph node biopsy is performed. In this case the sentinel lymph node is easily identified by the visible presence of dye. *Source:* Photo courtesy of Charles Levenback, MD, Houston, Texas, USA.

gamma probe sentinel lymph nodes were identified in 89% of groins dissected. Lymph node metastases were present in 27 groins and all were detected using sentinel lymph node identification and biopsy. The negative predictive value of a negative sentinel lymph node was 100%. Others have also reported a negative predictive value of 100% with sentinel lymph node biopsy (203,204). Because sentinel lymph nodes are subjected to a more rigorous pathologic (ultra-staging) examination, Robison et al. showed that sentinel lymph node biopsy allowed for the detection of smaller tumor foci in patients undergoing the procedure compared to patients who underwent complete groin node dissection and traditional pathologic examination (205). Others have reported that the detection of a sentinel lymph node in one groin does not preclude the presence of lymph node involvement in the contralateral groin (false negative) (206,207). Factors that may contribute to failure of sentinel lymph node identification include midline location for the primary tumor (207), and stasis of lymph flow from a node completely replaced by tumor (206,208). The prognosis associated with groin relapse is poor, and sentinel lymph node identification and biopsy should be confirmed by a prospective, randomized, controlled trial before sentinel lymph node identification and biopsy may be considered part of the standard of surgical care for vulvar carcinoma.

Surgical Resection for Recurrent Disease

The site, extent, and volume of recurrent vulvar cancer have important implications on both resectability and potential for cure. Recurrences can be categorized as local (vulva), groin, or distant (lung, bone, liver, brain). Surgical therapy plays a curative or palliative role in selected subsets of patients with recurrent disease (209).

Radical Wide Excision

As many as 75% of patients with recurrent disease limited to the vulva can be salvaged by radical wide excision or re-excision of the tumor (126,186,187). Surgical principles of recurrent vulvar tumors are identical to those for primary tumors: wide excision with a measured normal tissue margin of at least 2 cm. Particular attention is also focused on obtaining a clear deep margin. Because most patients have had prior operative therapy, primary closure of the vulvar defect is frequently more difficult. More complex reconstructive efforts may be needed to restore tissue integrity.

Pelvic Exenteration

Curative resection may still be possible when vulvar recurrence extends to the vagina, proximal urethra, or anus. Selected patients have achieved long-term survival after pelvic exenteration for such recurrences (88,210–212). The surgical approach in these cases should be individualized to the size and location of the recurrent tumor, prior therapies, and the age and overall health of the patient. Patients considered for pelvic exenteration should have a thorough preoperative evaluation to exclude the presence of regional and/or distant metastases. Frequently, anterior or posterior exenteration with an extended vulvar phase will provide excellent resection margins while allowing preservation of one major excretory system. The techniques used to perform the exenteration are identical to those routinely used for the treatment of women with recurrent cervical carcinoma. Unilateral gracilis flap repair may be combined with tailored exenteration to provide coverage for the surgical defect (213).

Resection of Groin Recurrence

Patients who develop groin recurrence are rarely curable. Untreated groin recurrence follows a particularly morbid course characterized by pain, bleeding, skin breakdown, and infection. Palliative treatment should be considered for these patients. Surgical resection should be viewed with caution in the previously irradiated patient. Cure is unlikely with resection alone, and wound healing is impaired. The debility caused by a combination of unresolved recurrence and surgical wound breakdown is worse than that of progressive recurrence alone. Patients who develop groin recurrence without a history of prior irradiation should be considered for surgical resection in combination with preoperative or postoperative radiation therapy. The surgical approach is limited to the removal of gross tumor to the extent feasible. The operative goal is to resect or debulk the recurrence to a small volume in the hope that subsequent irradiation will achieve regional control. Tumor reduction is especially difficult when the recurrence arises within the deep compartment or encases the femoral vessels. Extended survival is possible for the few patients who achieve control of recurrent disease in the groin and do not later manifest distant metastasis. Isolated groin recurrence is a rare event, so the data to support the efficacy of this treatment are anecdotal.

Vulvar Reconstruction

With careful planning and adequate tissue mobilization, most vulvar defects can be closed primarily with absorbable sutures. When large portions of the vulva have been resected, when tissue mobility is poor, or when radiation therapy has been administered previously, primary closure may not be feasible. Alternate tissue sources must be considered for these difficult cases.

Rhomboid Flaps

The rhomboid flap is a local tissue advancement flap that draws its blood supply from the subcutaneous vascular network. These flaps can be developed at any level of the vulva. Single or combination flaps can be designed to cover a wide variety of defects. The maximal practical flap size is approximately 4 cm^2. Rhomboid flaps are particularly useful in providing closure of large midline defects following the radical wide excision of periclitoral or perineal body tumors (189,214,215).

The rhomboid flap is designed by marking a V-shaped incision adjacent to the tissue defect needing coverage (Fig. 20.22). Flap size should correspond to the measured size of the defect. The flap incision is carried approximately 1 to 1.5 cm into the subcutaneous tissue. The flap is then developed by dissection within the subcutaneous tissue. When the adjacent tissues have been undermined, the flap can be rotated over the defect and sutured in place. Rhomboid flap repairs provide full thickness padded coverage without tension.

Myocutaneous Flaps

Several types of myocutaneous flaps—gracilis, gluteus, tensor fascia lata, rectus abdominis—have been used to provide repair and reconstruction of large vulvar and groin defects (216–221). Myocutaneous flaps, unlike local advancement flaps, include a segment of muscle and receive their blood supply and innervation through a clearly defined neurovascular pedicle. These are large, thick tissue sources that are best suited for the reconstruction of substantial defects. Although each of the flaps listed has proponents and specific advantages, the widest degree of experience has been reported for gracilis flaps. A gracilis flap can be designed to cover virtually any vulvar defect (Fig. 20.23).

The gracilis muscle is a broad flat muscle that courses through the superficial portion of the medial thigh. It is a weak adductor whose absence produces little perceptible deficit. The flap design is initiated by drawing a line from the

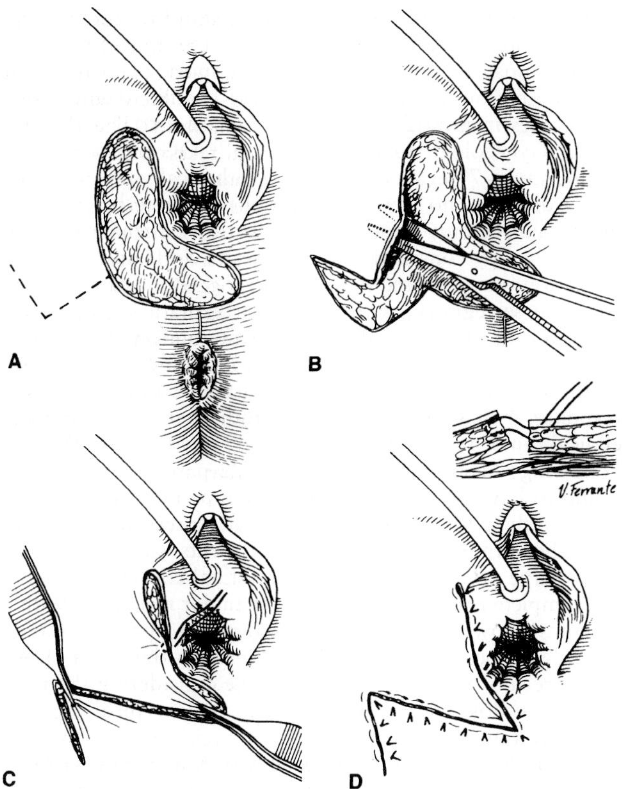

FIGURE 20.22. Technique for a unilateral rhomboid-flap repair. **A:** The flap is outlined. **B:** A 1-cm-thick flap of skin and subcutaneous tissue is raised. The area is undermined. **C:** The flap is rotated, and stay sutures are placed. **D:** Completed repair.

pubic tubercle to the medial femoral condyle. The gracilis muscle lies directly beneath this line. Flap size should be limited to a skin paddle of 6 to 8 cm × 10 to 12 cm. Smaller flaps have been associated with a lower incidence of necrosis and wound separation (213). The skin paddle incisions are carried to the gracilis fascia. The distal muscle is identified and transected 2 to 3 cm beyond the edge of the skin paddle. The myocutaneous unit is then developed by continuing the dissection more proximally. The main vascular bundle is usually encountered approximately 7 cm below the pubic tubercle. If possible, this pedicle should be preserved; however, if additional mobility is required, this vascular pedicle may be sacrificed. Flap viability is thought to be retained through blood supply derived from the more proximal obturator branches. Once developed, the flap is mobilized through a subcutaneous tunnel to reach the perineum or groin. The flap can be trimmed and sutured into position.

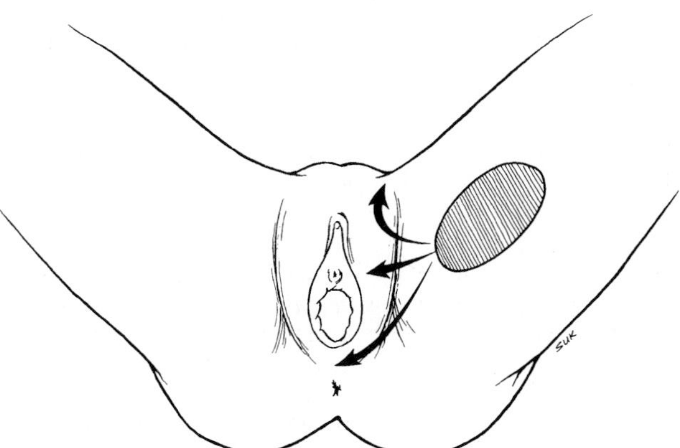

FIGURE 20.23. Diagrammatic representation of possible external placements for a gracilis myocutaneous flap. These flaps can be used to reconstruct large defects of the groin, labium majus, or perineal body. *Source:* Reprinted from Burke TW, Morris M, Roh MS, et al. Perineal reconstruction using single gracilis myocutaneous flaps. *Gynecol Oncol* 1995;57:221–225.

RADIATION THERAPY

Early reports of severe local reactions and poor survival rates with primary radiation therapy of vulvar carcinomas led some previous investigators to conclude that radiotherapy had a very limited role in the curative management of these patients (222–224). The use of high doses of radiation alone, delivered with low energy photons and electrons, in patients who were mostly poor surgical candidates, resulted in a suboptimal therapeutic window between tumor control probability and normal tissue complications (225). However, more contemporary experiences, emphasizing appropriate fractionation, attention to treatment planning detail, and recognition of vulvar and low pelvic radiation tolerance limits, have clearly demonstrated that relatively high doses of irradiation can be delivered safely. In selected patients, treatment of the vulva and/or regional lymph nodes improves locoregional control rates, survival rates, and may even reduce overall treatment morbidity. Radiation therapy is now accepted as an important element in the multidisciplinary management of patients with locoregionally advanced disease.

Treating Locally Advanced Disease in the Vulva

Following initial resection of a vulvar primary tumor, various surgicopathologic features have been identified that are associated with a higher risk of local recurrence. Podratz et al. reported a 24% incidence of vulvar recurrence in 71 patients with stage III carcinoma (126). Recurrence was correlated with tumor size and nodal status. Heaps et al. reported that a close surgical margin was the most powerful predictor of local recurrence in their patients (59). They observed 21 vulvar recurrences in 44 patients with tumor margins <8 mm (deep or at the skin surface) compared with no local recurrences in 91 patients with margins ≥8 mm (after fixation). The importance of a pathologic margin distance ≥8 mm in optimizing local vulvar control and 5-year disease specific survival has also been emphasized in a recent analysis by Chan et al. (137). Lymphovascular space invasion and deep tumor penetration are also associated with a greater and increased risk of recurrence (59,127,226). Although many local recurrences are controlled with additional surgery or irradiation, salvage surgery is often morbid, and local recurrences may provide additional opportunity for regional and distant tumor spread. While no prospective trials of postoperative vulvar site radiotherapy have been completed, adjuvant radiation of the primary tumor bed in selected patients with close margins or other high-risk features does improve vulvar tumor control (227).

Alternatively, in patients who present with more advanced primary tumors, radiation therapy may be delivered preoperatively. Advocates of this approach have listed several theoretical advantages for patients with locally advanced vulvar carcinomas:

1. Less radical resection of the vulva may be adequate to achieve local tumor control after preoperative treatment of the vulva with irradiation.
2. Tumor regression during radiation therapy may allow the surgeon to obtain adequate surgical margins without sacrificing important structures such as urethra, anus, and clitoris.

3. Radiation treatment alone may be sufficient to sterilize microscopic regional disease when the inguinal nodes are clinically normal and may mobilize fixed and matted nodes, facilitating subsequent surgical excision.

Although the published experiences with preoperative single-modality radiation therapy are small, several investigators have reported excellent responses and high local control rates after treatment of advanced tumors with relatively modest doses of radiation therapy followed by local resection (228–232). These reports provided emerging evidence that radiation could significantly debulk advanced local disease and allow for more conservative, viscera-sparing surgery, while preserving good local control.

More recently, a number of published series have suggested the therapeutic benefit of concurrent chemoradiation, typically followed by limited surgical resection, in addressing locally advanced disease (Table 20.7) (49,72,154,233–249). These trials were initially prompted by extrapolation from excellent results reported with chemoirradiation of carcinoma of the anus (250,251). Typical regimens have included combinations of irradiation with 5- fluorouracil (5-FU) and cisplatin or mitomycin C. Most studies included small numbers of patients with various disease presentations, including patients with very advanced or recurrent lesions, and none of these experiences can be compared meaningfully with results of treatment with preoperative irradiation alone. However, most investigators have observed impressive regressions of advanced lesions with chemoradiation, suggesting that responses may be better than would be expected with irradiation alone. Randomized trials of the role of chemoirradiation have not been done and are unlikely to be feasible given the small number of patients, and heterogeneity of clinical presentation, with this disease. However, recent trials that demonstrated improved local control and survival when concurrent cisplatin-containing chemotherapy was added to radiation treatment of cervical cancers (119,152,175) suggest that this approach may also be useful for women with other locally advanced lower genital tract neoplasms (151,152,252).

The most compelling data in support of concurrent chemoradiation in the management of locally advanced disease comes from a large prospective phase 2 trial performed by the Gynecologic Oncologic Group (GOG protocol 101). In this study, 71 evaluable patients with locally advanced T3 or T4 disease who were deemed not resectable by standard radical vulvectomy underwent preoperative chemoradiation. Chemotherapy consisted of two cycles of 5-FU and cisplatin. Radiation was delivered to a dose of 47.6 Gy, using a planned split-course regimen, with part of the radiation given twice daily during the 5-FU infusion. Patients underwent planned resection of the residual vulvar tumor, or incisional biopsy of the original tumor site in the case of complete clinical response, 4 to 8 weeks after chemoradiotherapy. A complete clinical tumor response was noted in 33 of 71 (47%) patients. Following vulvar excision or biopsy, 22 patients (31%) were found to have no residual tumor in the pathologic specimen. In all, only 2 of 71 patients (3%) had unresectable disease after chemoradiation, and in only 3 patients was it impossible to preserve urinary and/or gastrointestinal continuity following complete resection of the primary tumor residuum. With a median follow-up interval of 50 months, 11 patients (16%) have developed locally recurrent disease in the vulva (154). These results are all the more notable considering the relatively low dose of radiation used in these typically bulky, advanced tumors.

It is important to be cautious in designing aggressive treatment protocols for this group of patients, who are often elderly, with coexistent medical problems. Serious pulmonary toxicity has been observed in patients treated with bleomycin (237,243). In the largest published series of patients treated with mitomycin C and 5-FU, hematologic tolerance was acceptable, but the administered dose of mitomycin C was more conservative than is usually used in the treatment of anal cancers (244). Other investigators have confirmed the increased toxicity associated

TABLE 20.7

CONCURRENT CHEMOIRRADIATION IN THE MANAGEMENT OF LOCALLY ADVANCED OR RECURRENT CARCINOMA OF THE VULVA

Investigators	No. of patients	Chemotherapy	RT dose (Gy)	No. with recurrent or persistent local disease after RT □ surgery	Follow-up (months)
Moore et al. (154)	73	5-FU + CDDP	47.6	15 (21%)	22–72
Mulayim et al. (248)	11	Mito +/− 5-FU	45–62	6 (54%)	5–74
Gerszten et al. (249)	18	5-FU + CDDP	44.6	3 (17%)	1–55
Cunningham et al. (234)	14	5-FU + CDDP	45–50	4 (29%)	7–81
Landoni et al. (240)	58	5-FU + Mito	54	13 (22%)	4–48
Lupi et al. (241)	31	5-FU + Mito	54	7 (23%)	22–73
Whalen et al. (245)	19	5-FU + Mito	45–50	1 (5%)	3–70
Eifel et al. (235)	12	5-FU + CDDP	40–50	5 (42%)	17–30
Koh et al. (239)	20	5-FU ± CDDP or Mito	30–54	9 (45%)	1–75
Akl et al. (246)	12	5-FU + Mito	30–36	0	8–125
Russell et al. (49)	25	5-FU ± CDDP	47–72	6 (24%)	4–52
Han et al. (247)	14	5FU + CDDP or Mito	40–62	6 (43%)	4–273
Scheistroen and Trope (243)	42	Bleomycin	45	39 (93%)	7–60
Berek et al. (233)	12	5-FU + CDDP	44–54	0	7–60
Thomas et al. (244)	24	5-FU ± Mito	44–60	10 (42%)	5–43
Evans et al. (236)	4	5-FU + Mito	25.7	2 (50%)	2–29
Levin et al. (72)	6	5-FU + Mito	18.6	0	125
Iversen (237)	15	Bleomycin	15.4	11 (83%)[a]	4

Note: 5-FU, 5-fluorouracil; CDDP, cisplatin; Mito, mitomycin C; RT, radiation therapy.
[a]Most patients had unresectable, stage IV lesions.

with concurrent chemoradiation, especially with the use of mitomycin C–based regimens (248).

The use of concurrent weekly cisplatin with radiation has been widely tested in patients with locally advanced cervical cancer, and found to be therapeutically beneficial and well tolerated (151,153). In an attempt to further improve clinical and pathologic complete response, and ultimate local tumor control rates, the GOG is conducting another prospective phase 2 trial (GOG protocol 205), which combines weekly cisplatin with daily fractionated radiotherapy, followed by resection of residual primary tumor (or biopsy of the initial tumor bed if a clinical complete response is achieved). Radiation will be given to a total dose of 57.6 Gy (representing a 20% dose escalation over that used in GOG 101) to the gross tumor volume using careful treatment planning and boost techniques, and the previously used 2-week planned break has been eliminated. A stated objective of GOG 205 is to determine if the pathologic complete response can be increased to 45%, compared with the 31% pCR rate seen in the preceding GOG 101 study. Sufficient activity has been noted in the preliminary first accrual stage of 25 patients that the larger second stage of GOG 205 is now continuing active accrual.

Following chemoradiation for locally advanced disease, it remains undefined if surgery is necessary in those who achieve complete clinical response. In GOG 101, about 70% of patients who achieved complete clinical response were found to have no pathologic residual in the surgical specimen. At this point, we continue to recommend biopsies of the original tumor bed in patients who achieve complete clinical response. In those with residual vulvar disease after chemoradiation, surgical resection would be individualized and tailored to the extent and location of residuum.

Treatment of Regional Disease

Although radical inguinal lymphadenectomy has historically been considered the treatment of choice for regional management of invasive vulvar carcinoma, a number of retrospective studies have suggested that regional prophylactic radiation therapy is an effective method of preventing groin recurrences with minimal morbidity (253–257). In a review of 91 patients treated electively for cancers with primary drainage to the inguinal nodes, Henderson et al. observed only two failures after treatment with 45 to 50 Gy in 5 weeks, and both of these were outside the radiation treatment fields. Complications were rare, with only one case of mild leg edema, which may not have been treatment related (253). In another review of patients treated for vulvar carcinomas, Petereit et al. found no difference in the groin recurrence rate for clinically negative inguinal nodes treated with radical lymphadenectomy or radiation therapy, even though the irradiated patients had more advanced primary tumors (255). In a large single-institution retrospective analysis, Katz et al. reported no differences in the inguinal relapse rates for patients treated with prophylactic groin irradiation compared with those undergoing lymph node dissection (256). Leiserowitz et al. had no groin recurrences in 23 patients with locally advanced, clinically N0 vulvar cancers after prophylactic treatment of the groins with concurrent chemoirradiation (257).

The GOG tried to define the optimal approach to clinically negative inguinal nodes in a trial that randomized patients between inguinal node irradiation and radical lymphadenectomy (followed by inguinopelvic irradiation in patients with positive nodes) after resection of the primary tumor (258). This study was closed after entry of only 58 patients when there appeared to be a higher rate of groin recurrence in the radiation treatment arm. However, this study has been criticized because the treatment protocol was not CT-based, recommended combination photon and electron dosing to a depth of 3 to 4 cm, and likely delivered an inadequate dose to the inguinal nodes (259,260).

While the role of prophylactic radiotherapy in the undissected but high-risk groin remains controversial, there is strong evidence that adjunctive radiation therapy improves regional tumor control and survival in patients who have documented nodal metastases following inguinal node dissection. Retrospective studies suggested that patients with metastases to multiple nodes or extranodal tumor extension had an increased risk of groin recurrence after radical surgery and therefore may benefit from radiation therapy (261,262). However, the critical role of radiation therapy was not appreciated until 1986, when Homesley et al. published results of a prospective GOG trial in 114 patients with inguinal metastases (162). In that study, all patients underwent radical vulvectomy and inguinal lymphadenectomy. Patients who had positive inguinal nodes were randomized intraoperatively to receive either pelvic node dissection or postoperative irradiation to the pelvis and inguinal nodes. This trial was closed before the projected accrual goal because an interim analysis revealed a statistically significant overall survival advantage for the radiation treatment arm ($p = 0.03$). The differences between the 2-year survival rates of patients treated with radiation therapy or pelvic dissection were most marked for patients presenting with clinically positive nodes (59% and 31%, respectively) and for those with two or more positive groin nodes (63% and 37%, respectively). There was no significant difference in survival between the treatment groups for patients with only one microscopically positive node, although the authors commented that the number of patients in this subset was insufficient for reliable analysis. The most striking difference in the patterns of recurrence for the two treatment groups was the much larger number of inguinal failures among patients who were treated with surgery alone (Fig. 20.24). These groin recurrences were rarely if ever salvageable. The vulva, regardless of tumor pathologic risk factors, was not included in the radiation treatment fields in this study, and approximately 9% of patients in both treatment arms had recurrences at the primary site at the time of the analysis, raising the question of whether selective radiation to the vulva may have decreased local recurrences. It is important to recall that while subset analysis showed the most dramatic benefit to adjuvant radiotherapy for clinically positive adenopathy or ≥2 pathologically involved nodes in the the Homesley study (162), the trial was closed early because of an overall survival benefit before subset analysis. The role of adjuvant radiation for patients with a single positive groin node following inguinal node dissection remains unresolved. A recent retrospective review of patients with only a

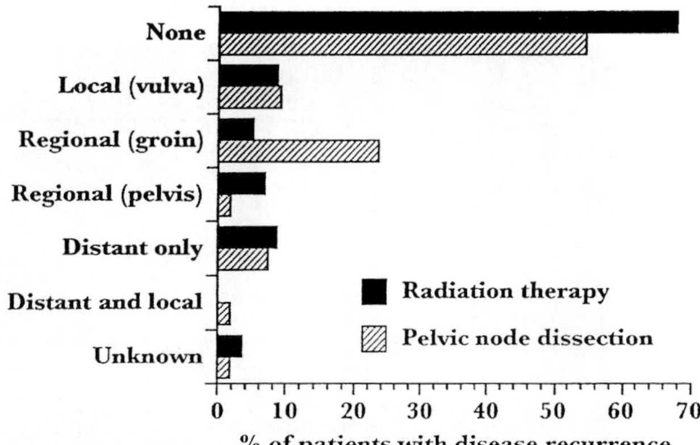

FIGURE 20.24. Sites of disease recurrence in patients treated with adjuvant radiation therapy to the pelvis and inguinal region or with pelvic node dissection following radical vulvectomy and bilateral inguinal lymphadenectomy. *Source:* Modified from Homesley HD, Bundy BN, Sedlis A, et al. Radiation therapy versus pelvic node resection for carcinoma of the vulva with positive groin nodes. *Obstet Gynecol* 1986;68:733–740.

single positive inguinal nodal metastasis from vulvar cancer suggests that adjuvant radiation may provide therapeutic benefit if the groin node dissection was less extensive in scope (263).

Successful use of concurrent chemotherapy and radiation therapy following radical hysterectomy in cervical cancer patients with positive lymph nodes suggests that concurrent chemoradiotherapy might be valuable for patients with node positive vulvar cancer (152). Although a randomized trial was initiated to address the role of adjuvant chemoradiation following resection of node positive tumors, the study was deemed infeasible and closed due to the relative rarity of these cancers and lack of patient accrual.

However, the role of preoperative chemoradiation has been assessed in patients who present with bulky, unresectable inguinal adenopathy. In the GOG 101 study of preoperative chemoradiation for local regionally advanced vulvar cancer, there was a cohort of 42 evaluable patients with N2 or N3 nodal disease that were deemed initially unresectable. Patients received 47.6 Gy of radiotherapy in split-course fashion, with two concurrent cycles of 5-FU and cisplatin as described above. Three to eight weeks later, planned inguino femoral lymph node dissection was performed. In only two patients (5%) did nodal disease remain unresectable. The surgical specimen showed histologic clearance of nodal disease in 15 patients (36%). At a median follow-up of 78 months only one of 37 (3%) patients who completed the full prescribed regimen of preoperative chemoradiation and bilateral inguino femoral node dissection relapsed in the groin (264). This study, while nonrandomized, provides further evidence of the efficacy of combined chemoradiotherapy in the management of locally regionally advanced vulvar cancer and in patients with significant regional adenopathy. Given the high risk of distant relapse with node positive vulvar cancer, especially in those with ≥2 involved nodes (265), it seems reasonable to consider adjuvant chemoradiation for such high-risk patients, provided that careful attention is paid to treatment planning and amelioration of toxicity.

Radiation Therapy Technique

Techniques commonly used for treatment of vulvar carcinoma reflect the need to encompass the lower pelvic and inguinal nodes as well as the vulva, while minimizing the dose to the femoral heads. One approach is to treat with an anterior field that encompasses the inguinal regions, lower pelvic nodes, and vulva, and a narrower posterior field that encompasses the lower pelvic nodes and vulva but excludes the majority of the femoral heads. If the fields are evenly weighted to the midplane of the pelvis using 6 MV photons, the contribution of the anterior field to the groin nodes (at 3 to 5 cm depth) will generally be 60% to 70% of the dose to the mid pelvis. The difference may be made up by supplementing the dose to the lateral groins with anterior electron fields of appropriate energy (Fig. 20.25). Kalnicki et al. described another technique, using a partial transmission block, that also reduces the dose to the femoral heads (266). CT scans are used to determine the appropriate electron energy and to detect enlarged nodes that may not be appreciated on clinical exam. Gross disease in the groin or vulva may be boosted with *en face* electron fields. In some cases, interstitial implants or *en face* electron fields may be used to boost the dose to the primary site (267,268). If radiation is directed to the regional nodes only, with intentional sparing of the vulva, care must be taken to avoid a large "midline" block, which may lead to higher medial groin and vulvar failures (269).

The complex anatomy of the vulva and its regional lymphatics, interwoven with adjacent critical normal tissues, has led some investigators to propose the use of intensity modulated radiation therapy (IMRT) in the management of vulvar cancer (Fig. 20.26) (270). IMRT theoretically and dosimetrically

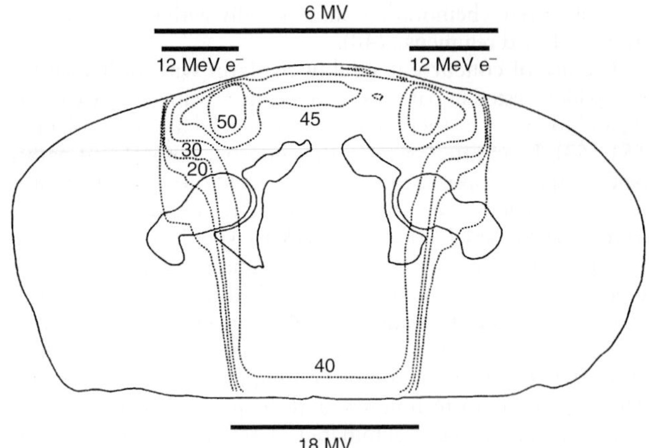

FIGURE 20.25. The radiation dose to the femoral heads can be reduced by delivering part of the dose to inguinal nodes with appropriate-energy electron fields. In this example, a wide anterior 6 MV field encompasses the primary site as well as the inguinal and pelvic nodes. Electron fields are placed anteriorly to overlap slightly with the exit of a narrower posterior 18 MV field that encompasses the primary and pelvic nodes.

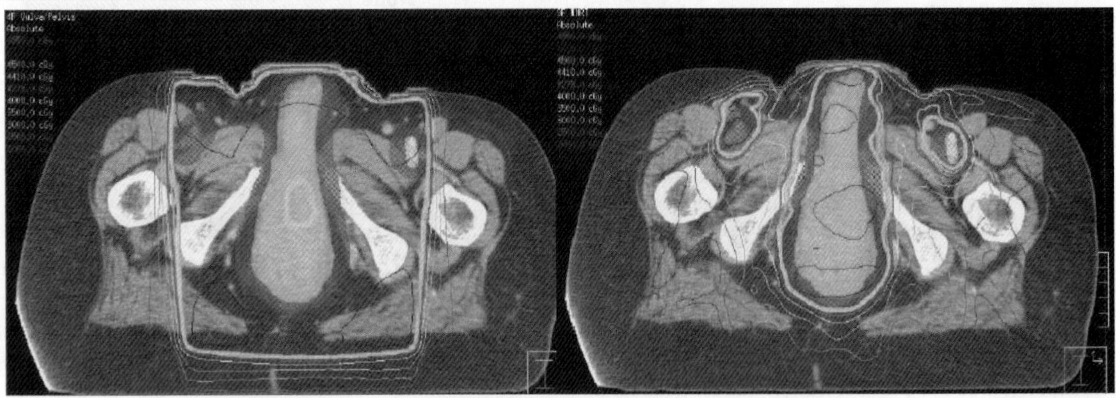

FIGURE 20.26. Intensity modulated radiation therapy (IMRT) in the management of vulvar cancer *Source:* From Beriwal S, Heron D, Kim H, et al. Intensity-modulated radiotherapy for the treatment of vulvar carcinoma: a comparative dosimetric study with early clinical outcome. *Int J Radiat Oncol Biol Phys* 2006;64:1395–1400.

allows for greater sparing of the bladder, rectum, and small bowel centrally, femoral necks laterally, and uninvolved buttock and perineal skin compared to traditional anteroposterior or four-field techniques. However, issues regarding the appropriate definition of target volumes at risk, including altered lymphatic pathways secondary to advanced tumor presentations, as well as patient and organ motion, will need to be carefully considered and assessed before IMRT can be deemed a standard radiotherapeutic approach in patients with vulvar cancer.

Acute Complications of Radiation Therapy

Acute radiation reactions are brisk, and doses of 35 to 45 Gy routinely induce confluent moist desquamation. However, with adequate local care, this acute reaction usually heals within 3 to 4 weeks. Sitz baths, steroid cream, and treatment of possible superimposed *Candida* infection all help to minimize the discomfort. If the patient is sufficiently flexible, she may be placed in a frog-leg position during treatment to minimize the dose and ensuing skin reaction on the medial thighs; care must then be taken, however, to deliver an adequate dose to the vulvar skin. Although most patients will develop confluent mucositis by the fourth week of treatment, this is usually tolerated if the patient is warned in advance and assured that the discomfort will resolve after treatment is completed. Although a treatment break is occasionally required, delays should be minimized, because they may allow time for repopulation of tumor cells.

Late Complications of Radiation Therapy

Many factors add to the late morbidity of radiation treatment in patients with vulvar carcinoma. Patients with advanced vulvar carcinomas often are treated with radiation therapy following radical surgery, which may include extensive dissection of the inguinal and possibly pelvic nodes. Large ulcerative cutaneous lesions frequently have superimposed infection. Patients are often elderly and may have complicating medical conditions, such as diabetes, multiple prior surgeries, and osteoporosis. The contribution of concurrent chemotherapy to local morbidity is not yet clearly defined, but may contribute to bowel and bone complications (271,272).

The incidence of lower extremity edema after inguinal irradiation alone is negligible (253,255,256,262). Although radiation therapy probably contributes to the incidence of peripheral edema following radical node dissection, no difference was evident in the GOG randomized study (162). However, the investigators admitted that evaluation of lymphedema was not a major consideration of the study and that the complication may have been underreported. Femoral head fractures have occasionally been reported in patients treated with irradiation to the inguinal nodes (231,244,253). Techniques that limit the dose to the femoral heads to less than 35 Gy should minimize the risk of this complication. It is not known whether severe osteoporosis contributes to femoral head complications. In general, with careful treatment planning techniques, the risk of major late complications following regional nodal radiation, either electively or adjuvant to lymph node dissection, is low (256). It has been suggested that concurrent chemotherapy may increase the risk, but this remains to be adequately substantiated (271).

The effect of radiation therapy on the long-term cosmesis and function of the vulva is poorly understood. Although treatment with irradiation or chemoradiation and wide excision is becoming a more accepted alternative to extensive surgery for selected patients, and major complication rates appear to be acceptable, very little has been reported regarding more subtle late effects of such treatment in the vulva. Late effects are dose related. Although Frischbier and Thomsen reported a 24% incidence of late ulceration in a large number of patients treated primarily with electron beam radiation therapy to the vulva, the relatively large dose per fraction (3 Gy/d) that was used probably contributed to this high incidence (273). Better information will become available only as treating physicians record and report the late cosmetic and functional results of treatment (274).

CHEMOTHERAPY

Data on the use of chemotherapeutic agents for the treatment of vulvar malignancies are limited; the incidence is low, the majority of patients are cured with surgery with or without postoperative radiation therapy, and thus chemotherapy has been used primarily as a salvage therapy. Patients with advanced vulvar cancers tend to be older, making them poor candidates for cytotoxic therapy because of concomitant diseases that increase the likelihood for significant adverse effects. Furthermore, recurrent vulvar cancer often occurs in the setting of extensive prior surgery and/or radiation therapy, making tolerance to cytotoxic therapy poor. No single institution has a large enough patient population to allow adequate phase 2 testing of cytotoxic agents.

Squamous Cell Carcinoma

Squamous carcinoma is the only cell type for which reproducible information exists on the value of cytotoxic therapy. Several drugs have undergone phase 2 testing in squamous vulvar cancer (Table 20.8) (111,275–278). Only doxorubicin and bleomycin appear to have activity as single agents. Although methotrexate has been claimed to have activity, data are inadequate for confirmation. Cisplatin, a drug that has demonstrated broad activity in most gynecologic tumors (e.g., epithelial ovary, endometrial adenocarcinoma, endometrial

TABLE 20.8

SINGLE-AGENT CYTOTOXICS IN SQUAMOUS VULVAR CANCER

		No. of patients		Partial	Investigators
Drug	Dose and schedule	Complete	response	response	
Doxorubicin	45 mg/m² IV q 3 weeks	4	0	3	Deppe et al. (275)
Bleomycin	15 mg IM twice weekly	11	2	3	Trope et al. (111)
Cisplatin	50 mg/m² q 3 weeks	22	0	0	Thigpen et al. (276)
Piperazinedione	9 mg/m² IV q 3 weeks	13	0	0	Thigpen et al. (276)
Mitoxantrone	12 mg/m² IV q 3 weeks	19	0	0	Muss et al. (277)
Etoposide	100 mg/m² IV days 1, 3, 5	18	0	0	Slayton et al. (278)

TABLE 20.9

COMBINATION CHEMOTHERAPY REGIMENS IN SQUAMOUS VULVAR CANCER

Regimen	Dose and schedule	No. of patients entered	Complete response	Partial response	Investigators
Bleomycin	15 mg/m^2 cont. IV days 1–3	22[a]	2	4	Belinson et al. (279)
Vincristine	1.4 mg/m^2 IV day 3				
Mitomycin C	10 mg/m^2 IV day 3				
Cisplatin	60 mg/m^2 IV day 3				
Bleomycin	5 mg IM days 1–5	28[b]	3	15	Durrant et al. (280)
Methotrexate	15 mg PO days 1 and 4				
CCNU	40 mg PO days 5–7				
Bleomycin	5 mg IV days 1–6	1	1	0	Shimizu et al. (47)
Vincristine	1 mg IV day 6				
Mitomycin C	10 mg IV day 6				
Cisplatin	100 mg IV day 6				

[a]Five of six responses with no prior therapy; one of 16 responses in refractory disease.
[b]No patient with prior radiation therapy or chemotherapy; responses were the same for primary therapy and recurrences; eight patients had resectable disease after chemotherapy.

mixed mesodermal tumors, and squamous carcinoma of the cervix), has notably little activity in vulvar and vaginal squamous tumors. This lack of activity, however, is based on treatment of refractory patients only. No trials of this agent as a presurgical cytoreductive regimen have been attempted. With the recent dramatic results obtained with concurrent cisplatin-based chemotherapy and radiation therapy in locally advanced squamous cancer of the cervix, one must consider a similar approach in the patient with locally advanced squamous cancer of the vulva.

Several drug combinations have also been used in squamous vulvar cancer. These combinations consisted principally of drugs without clear evidence of single-agent activity in phase 2 studies. Nevertheless, these combinations have been evaluated as initial therapy for patients with inoperable disease. Significant responses have allowed operative intervention in some patients. Combinations used in vulvar squamous cancer are inventoried in Table 20.9 (47,279,280). As noted above, the significant response rates observed with primary chemotherapy in inoperable disease presentations and the poor response rates in refractory disease should lead investigators to the earlier consideration of using cytotoxic therapy in stage III and IV vulvar cancers. Toxicity with these regimens has been reported as tolerable, although some patient selection for good performance status was probably operational. In the one well-reported trial, 64% of patients had mucositis (21% severe), and infections or fever occurred in 35% (280). Bleomycin lung disease was responsible for one death. Patients should be selected who are at lowest risk for chemotherapy associated toxicity (i.e., no concomitant disease, normal organ function, younger age).

There are some increasing reports of the concomitant use of cytotoxic therapy with irradiation, usually as primary therapy in advanced and inoperable disease (Table 20.7). This approach may have increased impetus based on recent reports from several large randomized trials demonstrating superior outcome for combined chemoirradiation over radiation therapy alone in locally advanced squamous cancer of the cervix (151–153,252). It is not possible from such study designs to specifically comment on the effects of chemotherapy on the disease. Nevertheless, these studies are cited because chemotherapy may have played a role in the end result. The largest experience was recently reported by the GOG, in which 73 patients with T3 or T4 cancers were treated with split-course radiation therapy with concomitant chemotherapy (cisplatin, 75 mg/m^2 on day 1, and 5-FU, 1,000 mg/m^2/d on days 1–5). Irradiation of the primary tumor in a split course was followed by resection of residual primary tumor and inguinofemoral nodes. Those patients with unresectable groin nodes received chemoirradiation to both the primary tumor and involved nodes. Seven patients never underwent surgery for various reasons. After chemoirradiation, 46% of patients were grossly tumor free. Of the 54% with gross residual disease, only five had positive margins at resection. Only 3% of the patients completing planned chemoirradiation and surgery had residual unresectable disease, and in only three patients was it not possible to preserve urinary and/or gastrointestinal continence. Survival data from this study remain immature, but demonstrated that this approach is feasible with acceptable toxicity (primarily decreased wound healing and enhanced cutaneous reactions) and with a possible decrease in the need for more radical surgery (154). Landoni et al. treated 58 advanced primary and 17 recurrent disease patients with 5-FU (750 mg/m^2/d on days 1–5) and mitomycin C (15 mg/m^2 on day 1) at the beginning of each of two courses of irradiation separated by 2 weeks (total dose of 54 Gy). Primary chemoradiation was followed by wide local excision and inguinal lymphadenectomy. A total of 89% of patients completed planned radiation therapy and chemotherapy, and 72% underwent surgery. Response was noted in 80%, and pathologic complete response was observed in both primary and nodes in 31%. Three treatment related deaths were also recorded (240). Lupi et al. treated 31 patients with mitomycin C and 5-FU using the same doses as in the previous study and split-course irradiation to only 36 Gy. Response was noted in 29 of 31 (94%), but postoperative morbidity was noted in 65% and mortality in 14%. Of patients with positive inguinal nodes, 55% (five of nine) were rendered pathologically disease free at surgery. Recurrence was noted in 32%, and survival was not reported (241). Whalen et al. treated 19 patients with clinical stage III/IV vulva carcinoma and clinically negative nodes with 45 to 50 Gy and 5-FU (1,000 mg/m^2/d continuous intravenous infusion over 96 hours at weeks 1 and 5) and mitomycin C (10 mg/m^2 on day 1 only). A response rate of 90% and a local control rate of 74% was observed. Survival was not reported (245). Cunningham et al. treated 14 patients who were not candidates for radical vulvectomy with cisplatin (50 mg/m^2) and 5-FU (1,000 mg/m^2/d over 96 hours) in combination with 50 to 65 Gy irradiation to vulva and bilateral

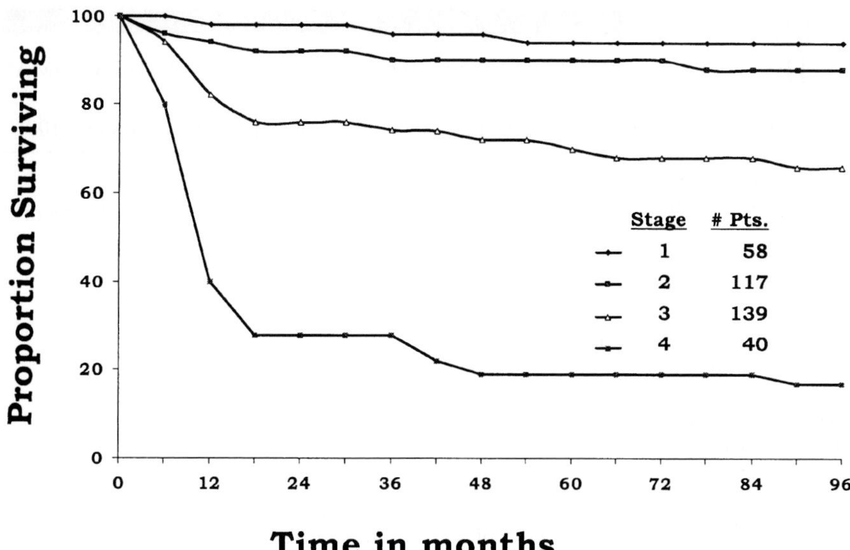

FIGURE 20.27. Invasive squamous vulvar carcinoma. Survival by FIGO stage. *Source:* Patients treated at M. D. Anderson Cancer Center 1944–1990; data courtesy of F. N. Rutledge.

groins and 45 to 50 Gy to the pelvis. Surgery was not performed in complete responders. There was a 64% complete response rate and only one recurrence in that group, with mean follow-up of 36 months. All partial responders died of disease. Toxicity was moderate, with five patients requiring treatment delay due to desquamative reactions and one late bowel complication (234). Thomas et al. treated 33 patients with stage II, III, or IV disease: 9 with definitive radiation therapy and chemotherapy as a preoperative adjuvant, 9 with definitive radiation therapy and chemotherapy, and 15 with radiation therapy and chemotherapy after local recurrence following surgery. Chemotherapy consisted of infusional 5-FU given at a dose of 1,000 mg/m^2/d over 4 to 5 days; six patients also received low-dose mitomycin C. Various doses and techniques of irradiation were used. Seven of nine patients treated with neoadjuvant therapy remained free of disease at 5 to 45 months, one after local excision of a vulvar recurrence. Of the nine patients receiving curative intent radiation therapy and chemotherapy, six were alive without evidence of disease at 5 to 43 months. Of the 15 patients treated after recurrence, 7 were alive without evidence of disease for 5 to 45 months. It is impossible to determine the role of chemotherapy in these patients, but it appears that combined modality therapy offers the potential for long-term disease control without radical surgery (244).

RESULTS OF THERAPY

The overall results of therapy for women with squamous cancers of the vulva are excellent. Approximately two thirds of patients present with early-stage tumors. Five-year survival rates of 80% to 90% are routinely reported for stage I and II disease (281). As anticipated, survival rates for patients with advanced disease are poor: 60% for stage III cases and 15% for stage IV (Fig. 20.27).

Several strategies to enhance survival for women with vulvar cancer are evident. High-risk patients can be educated and screened more consistently for the development of early cancer. Women with human papillomavirus infections, *in situ* vulvar disease, long smoking history, and other genital neoplasms are at risk for developing vulvar cancer. Careful screening targeted at women with these high-risk factors may lead to improvements in early diagnosis.

The survival rate for women with nodal spread is one half that of women without nodal disease who have similarly sized primary tumors (Fig. 20.28). A more precise understanding of lymphatic flow and tumor spread might enable us to better identify those patients with subclinical metastases who now present with unanticipated groin or distant failure. Better treatment options for node positive patients are needed, possibly multimodality therapy that incorporates irradiation, chemotherapy, or both with surgery.

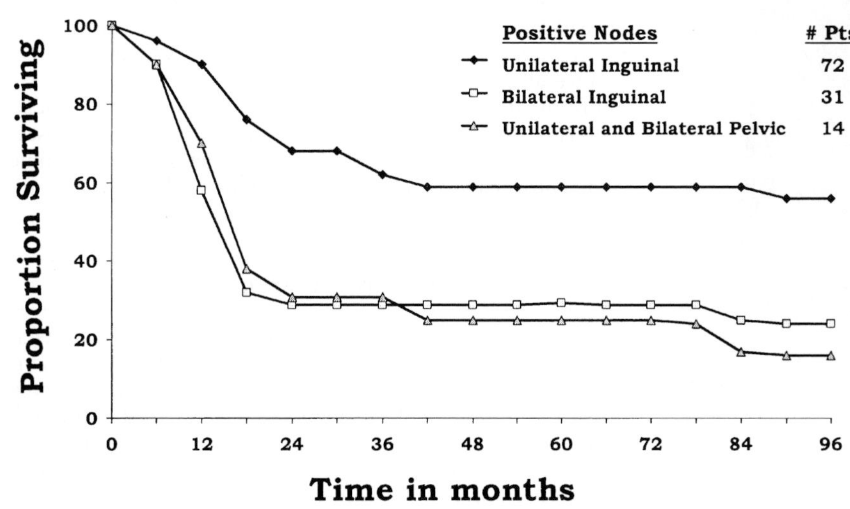

FIGURE 20.28. Invasive squamous vulvar carcinoma. Survival of patients with positive nodes. *Source:* Data courtesy of F. N. Rutledge.

MANAGEMENT OF OTHER VULVAR MALIGNANCIES

Because nonsquamous vulvar malignancies are exceedingly rare, relatively little definitive information is available regarding optimal treatment and long-term outcome. Most available information is derived from isolated case reports or small series spanning long periods of time.

Malignant Melanoma

Malignant melanoma is the second most common vulvar malignancy (97,282,283). Vulvar melanomas are most commonly seen in postmenopausal Caucasian women. Typical presentations include an asymptomatic pigmented lesion or an identified mass that may be painful or bleeding (Fig. 20.29). A definitive diagnosis is established by biopsy. Immunohistochemical staining for melanoma-specific antigen and S100 may be helpful in uncertain cases. Melanomas may arise from existing pigmented vulvar lesions or as new isolated primary tumors. Consequently, any pigmented vulvar lesion should be considered for biopsy. Melanomas are staged according to one of the three available microstaging systems, which base prognosis on either depth of local invasion or tumor thickness (Table 20.10) (103,284,285). Inguinal lymph node and distant metastases are frequent.

The primary treatment modality for vulvar melanoma is radical surgical excision. Radical vulvectomy with bilateral inguinofemoral lymphadenectomy has been the historical treatment of choice (282,283,286,287). Because most failures are distant, ultra-radical local resection does not appear to enhance survival. Furthermore, many patients with vulvar melanoma are elderly with coexisting medical problems, and less radical surgery may be a more realistic option without compromising survival (288). More recent reviews recommend some form of hemivulvectomy or radical wide excision, with or without inguinal lymphadenectomy (286,287). Depth of invasion and the presence of ulceration are significant prognostic factors, and should be considered in treatment planning. Look et al. reported that none of the patients with lesion depth of ≤1.75 mm experienced a recurrence, and suggested that these patients could be treated with wide local excision. In contrast, all patients with lesion depth of >1.75 mm recurred despite radical tumor excision (99). Based on information derived from large series of patients with cutaneous melanomas at nongenital sites, regional lymphadenectomy should probably be considered a prognostic rather than a therapeutic procedure (289). In a multivariate analysis of 644 patients with vulvar melanoma, Sugiyama et al. reported 5-year disease-specific survival rates of 68%, 29%, and 19% for patients with zero, one, and two or more positive lymph nodes, respectively (290). Lymphadenectomy can be avoided in patients with superficial melanomas (level III), for whom the risk of metastatic disease is negligible. Sentinel lymph node identification and biopsy have been increasingly applied to the surgical management of cutaneous malignant melanomas; however, data regarding sentinel lymph node biopsy for vulvar melanomas are insufficient.

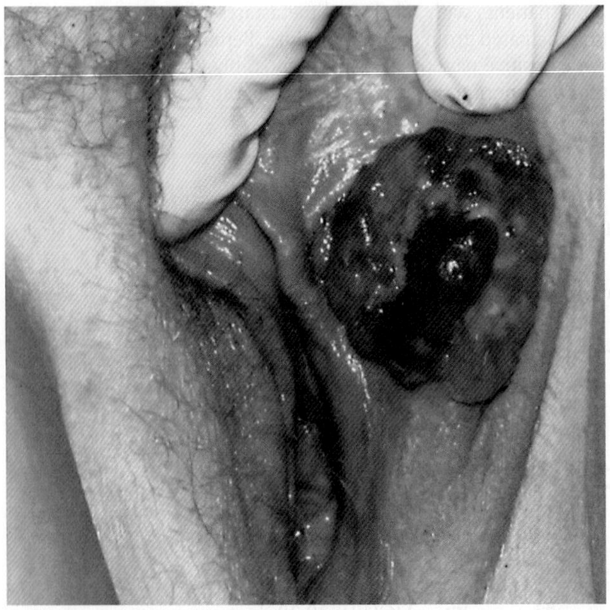

FIGURE 20.29. Nodular, darkly pigmented malignant melanoma of the left labium majus.

TABLE 20.10

MICROSTAGING SYSTEMS FOR VULVAR MELANOMAS

	Clark et al. (284)	Chung et al. (285)	Breslow (103)
I	Intraepithelial	Intraepithelial	<0.76 mm
II	Into papillary dermis	1 mm from granular layer	0.761.50 mm
III	Filling dermal papillae	12 mm from granular layer	1.512.25 mm
IV	Into reticular dermis	>2 mm from granular layer	2.263.0 mm
V	Into subcutaneous fat	Into subcutaneous fat	>3 mm

Radiation therapy may be useful in enhancing local and regional control for some high-risk patients. Despite reported complete clinical response rates and local tumor control rates of 50% to 70% for patients with localized recurrences treated with radiation therapy, alone or in combination with hyperthermia, these modalities have rarely been used in the primary treatment of vulvar melanoma (291,292). Doses in the range of 40 to 50 Gy, delivered in fractions of 4 to 8 Gy (one to three weekly fractions), have been described as more effective (293).

Systemic chemotherapy, in either an adjuvant or salvage setting, is considered palliative, but responses are truly rare and adverse effects may be significant. Biologic and immunologic approaches to the treatment of malignant melanoma are currently being evaluated. The Southwest Oncology Group reported their results of a randomized trial of an adjuvant allogeneic tumor vaccine in patients with intermediate thickness, node negative melanoma. There was no evidence of improved disease-free survival among patients randomized to receive vaccine (294).

Overall survival rates in women with vulvar melanoma are approximately 50% (97,282,287). Patients with superficial lesions have an excellent chance for cure after surgical resection, but patients with deeper lesions or metastases at the time of diagnosis have a more limited prognosis. These patients are good candidates for investigational trials.

Verrucous Carcinoma

Verrucous carcinomas are locally invasive and rarely metastasize (295). Consequently, treatment by radical wide excision is usually curative (296). Local recurrence can occur, especially when the tumor has been inadequately resected. Although radiation therapy has been reported to cause anaplastic transformation in some cases of verrucous carcinoma, this finding has not been observed by others (297,298).

Basal Cell Carcinoma

Basal cell carcinomas should be removed by excisional biopsy using a minimum surgical margin of 1 cm (299). Lymphatic or distant spread is exceedingly rare (300). Local recurrence may occur, particularly in tumors removed with suboptimal resection margins.

Adenocarcinoma

Patients presenting with apparent vulva adenocarcinoma should first undergo an extensive clinical evaluation to determine whether the lesion in question represents a primary versus metastatic tumor. Despite the paucity of data regarding the evaluation and treatment of vulva adenocarcinoma, resection of localized disease by radical wide excision, hemivulvectomy, or radical vulvectomy seems appropriate (301). The incidence of groin node metastases is approximately 30% (302). Some form of inguinal lymphadenectomy should be included with primary surgical resection. Radiation therapy may have a role in enhancing local control for women with large primary tumors or inguinal metastases. The effectiveness of chemotherapy is unknown, although a single case report documents a response with pegylated liposomal doxorubicin in adenocarcinoma of the vulva (303).

Paget's Disease

Paget's disease is associated with an underlying invasive adenocarcinoma component in approximately 15% of cases (304,305). As many as 20% to 30% of patients will have or will later develop an adenocarcinoma at another nonvulvar location (306,307), although more recent series suggest a lower incidence of secondary malignancies (308). Observed sites of non-vulvar malignancies developing in patients with extramammary Paget's disease include breast, lung, colorectum, gastric, pancreas, and upper female genital tract. Screening and surveillance for tumors at these sites should be considered in patients with Paget's disease.

Paget's disease should be resected with a wide margin. If underlying invasion is suspected, the deep margins should be extended to the perineal fascia. Some suggest careful assessment of the surgical margins using multiple frozen sections to ensure complete excision (309,310). This approach can be cumbersome and may not influence the long-term incidence of recurrence. Pierie et al. showed that patients with microscopic positive margins had a significantly higher rate of recurrence; however, with extended follow-up all patients eventually recurred (311). Others have shown that despite surgical efforts to the contrary, microscopically positive margins are frequent, and disease recurrence is common regardless of margin status (312). Repeat local excision of recurrent disease is usually effective in the absence of invasion (313).

Vulvar Sarcomas

The specific histologic types are described in the pathology section of this chapter. All types of vulvar sarcoma are rare, but leiomyosarcoma, malignant fibrous histiocytoma, and rhabdomyosarcoma predominate (106,314). Cures have occasionally been obtained with aggressive resection of either primary or locally recurrent disease. The results of regional and systemic therapy for leiomyosarcoma are disappointing. These patients are excellent candidates for clinical trials. Rhabdomyosarcoma seems to be more responsive to both

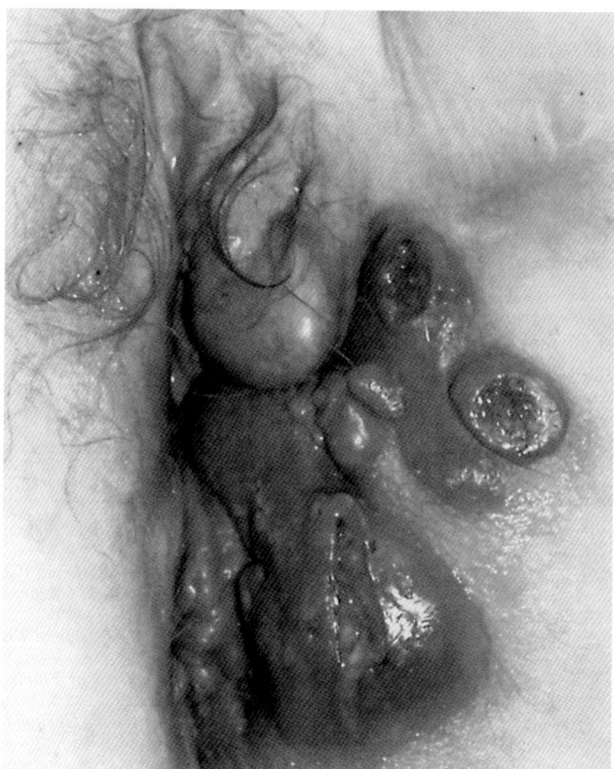

FIGURE 20.30. Multiple in-transit lymphatic metastases from a cloacogenic carcinoma of the rectum. A large constricting lesion was evident on rectal examination.

chemotherapy and radiation. The current treatment of choice is to combine chemoradiation with limited surgical resection of residual disease (314,315).

Metastatic Tumors to the Vulva

Treatment of secondary vulvar tumors should be directed against the primary tumor. As with bulky vulvar cancers, a multimodal approach seems to provide some opportunity for long-term survival along with enhanced local tumor control and organ preservation.

Cutaneous vulvar lymphatic metastases may occur as in transit tumor emboli from anorectal tumors or as retrograde flow metastases when bulky tumors of the cervix or uterus obstruct the normal lymphatic drainage patterns (Fig. 20.30). These metastases are multiple and are often bilateral. Their histology reflects that of the primary tumor. Because this metastatic pattern is associated with advanced tumors, the primary tumor should be readily detectable by examination.

FUTURE DIRECTIONS

Vulvar cancer is an uncommon neoplastic disease and its relative rarity is a major obstacle in designing prospective randomized trials. Current trends in its management are focusing on a more individualized approach that emphasizes conservative vulva surgical resection when feasible, the use of reconstructive procedures to preserve or restore vulva function, potential reduction in groin complications through sentinel lymph node biopsy, and multimodality therapy for advanced or disseminated disease. Most data supporting these concepts are preliminary. Further investigation is likely to result in ongoing refinement of the criteria used to select patients for specific surgical procedures. The greatest gaps in our present understanding of this disease and its treatment include (a) the uncertain role of infectious and epidemiologic factors in the development of the primary tumor; (b) the lack of consensus regarding the extent of groin dissection required to accurately assess lymphatic spread; (c) the lack of a well-defined management plan for patients with lymph node metastases; (d) the absence of proven systemic therapy for women with distant spread or recurrence; (e) scant information to evaluate the components and timing of combined modality treatment; and (f) poor understanding of different forms of treatment on the psychosexual adjustment of patients. These all represent areas of current investigation. Additional clinical experience should help to establish a rational approach to therapy that maximizes the potential for cure while minimizing morbidity.

References

1. American Cancer Society. *Cancer Facts and Figures 2007*. Atlanta: American Cancer Society; 2007.
2. Jones RW, Joura EA. Analyzing prior clinical events at presentation in 102 women with vulvar carcinoma: evidence of diagnostic delays. *J Reprod Med* 1999;44:766–768.
3. Warwick R, Williams PL, eds. *Gray's Anatomy*. 35th ed. Philadelphia: WB Saunders; 1973.
4. Parry-Jones E. Lymphatics of the vulva. *J Obstet Gynecol Br Empire* 1963;70:751–755.
5. Plentl AA, Friedman EA, eds. *Lymphatic System of the Female Genitalia*. Philadelphia: WB Saunders; 1971.
6. Carter J, Carlson J, Fowler J, et al. Invasive vulvar tumors in young women: a disease of the immunosuppressed? *Gynecol Oncol* 1993;51:307–310.
7. Messing MJ, Gallup DG. Carcinoma of the vulva in young women. *Obstet Gynecol* 1995;86:51–54.
8. Franklin EW, Rutledge FD. Epidemiology of epidermoid carcinoma of the vulva. *Obstet Gynecol* 1972;39:165–172.
9. Brinton LA, Nasca PC, Mallin K, et al. Case-control study of cancer of the vulva. *Obstet Gynecol* 1990;75:859–866.
10. Kaufman RH, Dreesman GR, Burke J, et al. Herpes-virus-induced antigens in squamous-cell carcinoma *in situ* of the vulva. *N Engl J Med* 1981;305:483–488.
11. Ansink AC, Krul MRL, DeWeger RA, et al. Human papillomavirus, lichen sclerosus, and squamous cell carcinoma of the vulva: detection and prognostic significance. *Gynecol Oncol* 1994;52:180–184.
12. Downey GO, Okagaki T, Ostrow RS, et al. Condylomatous carcinoma of the vulva with special reference to human papillomavirus DNA. *Obstet Gynecol* 1988;72:68–73.
13. Bloss JD, Liao S-Y, Wilczynski SP, et al. Clinical and histologic features of vulvar carcinomas analyzed for human papillomavirus status: evidence that squamous cell carcinoma of the vulva has more than one etiology. *Hum Pathol* 1991;22:711–716.
14. Kurman RJ, Trimble CL, Shah KV. Human papillomavirus and the pathogenesis of vulvar carcinoma. *Curr Opin Obstet Gynecol* 1992; 4:582–585.
15. Hording U, Junge J, Daugaard S, et al. Vulvar squamous cell carcinoma and papillomaviruses: indications for two different etiologies. *Gynecol Oncol* 1994;52:241–245.
16. Carli P, De Magnis A, Mannone F, et al. Vulvar carcinoma associated with lichen sclerosus: experience at the Florence, Italy vulvar clinic. *J Reprod Med* 2003;48:313–318.
17. Hart WR, Norris HJ, Helwig EB. Relation of lichen sclerosus et atrophicus of the vulva to development of carcinoma. *Obstet Gynecol* 1975;45:369–372.
18. Jones RW, Rowan DM. Vulvar intraepithelial neoplasia III: a clinical study of the outcome in 113 cases with relation to the later development of invasive vulvar carcinoma. *Obstet Gynecol* 1994;84:741–745.
19. Jones RW, Rowan DM, Stewart AW. Vulvar intraepithelial neoplasia: aspects of the natural history and outcome in 405 women. *Obstet Gynecol* 2005;106:1319–1326.
20. Iversen T, Tretli S. Intraepithelial and invasive squamous cell neoplasia of the vulva: trends in incidence, recurrence, and survival rate in Norway. *Obstet Gynecol* 1998;91:969–972.
21. Edwards CL, Tortolero-Luna G, Linares AC, et al. Vulvar intraepithelial neoplasia and vulvar cancer. *Obstet Gynecol Clin North Am* 1996;23:234–295.
22. Trimble CL, Hildesheim A, Brinton LA, et al. Heterogeneous etiology of squamous carcinoma of the vulva. *Obstet Gynecol* 1996;87:59–64.
23. Flowers LC, Wistuba II, Scurry J, et al. Genetic changes during multistage pathogenesis of human papillomavirus positive and negative vulvar carcinomas. *J Soc Gynecol Invest* 1999;6:213–217.
24. Hietanen SH, Kurvinen K, Syrjanen K, et al. Mutation of tumor suppressor gene p53 is frequently found in vulvar carcinoma cells. *Am J Obstet Gynecol* 1995;173:1477–1479.
25. Mitchell MF, Prasad CJ, Silva EG, et al. Second genital primary squamous neoplasms in vulvar carcinoma: viral and histopathologic correlates. *Obstet Gynecol* 1993;81:13–17.
26. Creasman WT. New gynecologic cancer staging. *Gynecol Oncol* 1995;58: 157–161.
27. Beahrs OH, Henson DE, Hutter RVP, et al., eds. *Manual for Staging of Cancer.* 4th ed. Philadelphia: JB Lippincott; 1992.
28. Wilkinson EJ. Superficial invasive carcinoma of the vulva. *Clin Obstet Gynecol* 1985;28:188–192.
29. Zaino RJ. Carcinoma of the vulva, urethra and Bartholin's gland. In: Wilkinson EJ, ed. *Pathology of the Vulva and Vagina: Contemporary Issues in Surgical Pathology*. Vol 9. New York: Churchill Livingstone; 1987:119–121.
30. Kneale BL. Microinvasive cancer of the vulva: Report of the International Society for Study of Vulvar Disease Task Force, 7th Congress. *J Reprod Med* 1984;29:457–458.
31. Iversen T, Aas M. Lymph drainage from the vulva. *Gynecol Oncol* 1983; 16:179–182.
32. Way S. The anatomy of the lymphatic drainage of the vulva and its influence on the radical operation of carcinoma. *Ann R Coll Surg Engl* 1948;187:3–8.
33. Way S. *Malignant Disease of the Female Genital Tract.* New York: Churchill Livingstone; 1951.
34. Levenback C, Burke TW, Morris M, et al. Potential applications of intraoperative lymphatic mapping in vulvar cancer. *Gynecol Oncol* 1995;59:216–220.
35. Homesley HD, Bundy BN, Sedlis A, et al. Prognostic factors for groin node metastasis in squamous cell carcinoma of the vulva (a Gynecologic Oncology Group study). *Gynecol Oncol* 1993;49:279–285.
36. Wilkinson EJ, Hardt NS. Vulva. In: Mills S, ed. *Histology for Pathologists.* 3rd ed. Philadelphia: Lippincott Williams & Wilkins; 2007:983–988.
37. Dvoretsky PM, Bonfiglio TA, Helmkamp F, et al. The pathology of superficially invasive thin vulvar squamous cell carcinoma. *Int J Gynecol Pathol* 1984;3:331–334.
38. Jones RW, Sadler L, Grant S, et al. Clinically identifying women with vulvar lichen sclerosus at increased risk of squamous cell carcinoma: a case-control study. *J Reprod Med* 2004;49:808–813.
39. Kurman RJ, Ronnett B, Wilkinson EJ, eds. *The Cervix, Vagina, and Vulva.* Fascicle, 3rd ed. American Registry of Pathology; 2009, in press.
40. Kneale BL. Microinvasive cancer of the vulva: Report of the International Society for Study of Vulvar Disease Task Force, 7th Congress. *J Reprod Med* 1984;29:457–458.
41. Wilkinson EJ, Kneale B, Lynch PJ. Report of the ISSVD Terminology Committee. *J Reprod Med* 1986;1:973–975.
42. Wilkinson EJ, Rico MJ, Pierson KK. Microinvasive carcinoma of the vulva. *Int J Gynecol Pathol* 1982;1:29–39.
43. Scully RE, Bonfiglio TA, Kurman RJ, et al. *Histological Typing of Female Genital Tract Tumors. World Health Organization International Histological Classification of Tumors.* 2nd ed. New York: Springer-Verlag; 1994.
44. Curry SL, Wharton JT, Rutledge F. Positive lymph nodes in vulvar squamous carcinoma. *Gynecol Oncol* 1980;9:63–67.
45. Wilkinson EJ. Superficial invasive carcinoma of the vulva. *Clin Obstet Gynecol* 1985;28:188–192.
46. Sedlis A, Homesley H, Bundy BN, et al. Positive groin lymph nodes in superficial squamous cell vulvar cancer. *Am J Obstet Gynecol* 1987;156:1159–1163.
47. Shimizu Y, Hasumi K, Masubuchi K. Effective chemotherapy consisting of bleomycin, vincristine, mitomycin C and cisplatin (BOMP) for a patient with inoperable vulvar cancer. *Gynecol Oncol* 1990;36:423–425.
48. Yoder B, Rufforny I, Massoll NA, et al. Stage IA vulvar squamous cell carcinoma: an analysis of tumor invasive characteristics and risk. *Am J Surg Pathol* 2008;32(5):765–772.
49. Russell AH, Mesic JB, Scudder SA, et al. Synchronous radiation and cytotoxic chemotherapy for locally advanced or recurrent squamous cancer of the vulva. *Gynecol Oncol* 1992;47:14–18.
50. Steeper TA, Rosai J. Aggressive angiomyxoma of the female pelvis and perineum. *Am J Surg Pathol* 1983;7:463–475.
51. Ehrmann RL, Dwyer IM, Yavner BA, et al. An immunoperoxidase study of laminin and type IV collagen distribution in carcinoma of the cervix and vulva. *Obstet Gynecol* 1988;72:257–265.
52. Hendricks JB, Wilkinson EJ, Drew P, et al. Ki-67 expression in vulvar carcinoma. *Int J Gynecol Pathol* 1994;13:205–210.
53. Wilkinson EJ. Protocol for the examination of specimens from patients with carcinomas and malignant melanomas of the vulva: a basis for checklists. Cancer Committee of the American College of Pathologists. *Arch Pathol Lab Med* 2000;124:51–56.
54. Drew PA, Al-Abbadi MA, Orlando C, et al. Prognostic factors in carcinoma of the vulva: a clinicopathologic and DNA flow cytometric study. *Int J Gynecol Pathol* 1996;15:235.
55. Ambros RA, Kallakury BVS, Malfetano JH, et al. Cytokine, cell adhesion receptor, and tumor suppressor gene expression in vulvar squamous carcinoma: correlation with prominent fibromyxoid stromal response. *Int J Gynecol Pathol* 1996;15:320–324.
56. Ambrose RM, Malfetano JL, Mihm MC. Clinicopathologic features of vulvar squamous cell carcinomas exhibiting prominent fibromyxoid stromal response. *Int J Gynecol Pathol* 1996;15:137–141.
57. Lerma E, Esteller M, Matis-Guiu X, et al. P16 methylation, pRb and P53 in squamous cell carcinoma of the vulva. *Mod Pathol* 1999;12: 119A.

58. Kurman RJ, Toki T, Schiffman MH. Basaloid and warty carcinomas of the vulva: distinctive types of squamous cell carcinoma frequently associated with human papillomaviruses. *Am J Surg Pathol* 1993;17:133–136.
59. Heaps JM, Fu YS, Montz FJ, et al. Surgical-pathologic variables predictive of local recurrence in squamous cell carcinoma of the vulva. *Gynecol Oncol* 1990;38:309–315.
60. Carter JJ, Koutsky LA, Wipf GC, et al. The natural history of human papillomavirus type 16 capsid antibodies among a cohort of university women. *J Infect Dis* 1996;174:927–934.
61. Underwood JW, Adcock LL, Okagaki T. Adenosquamous carcinoma of skin appendages (adenoid squamous cell carcinoma, pseudoglandular squamous cell carcinoma, adenoacanthoma of sweat gland of Lever) of the vulva: a clinical and ultrastructural study. *Cancer* 1978;42:1851–1863.
62. Wilkinson EJ, Croker BP, Friedrich EG Jr, et al. Two distinct pathologic types of giant cell tumor of the vulva: a report of two cases. *J Reprod Med* 1988;33:519–522.
63. Jacobs DM, Sandles LG, LeBoit PE. Sebaceous carcinoma arising from Bowen's disease of the vulva. *Arch Dermatol* 1986;122:1191–1192.
64. Copas P, Dyer M, Comas FV, et al. Spindle cell carcinoma of the vulva. *Diagn Gynecol Obstet* 1982;4:235–238.
65. Berman ML, Soper JT, Creasman WT, et al. Conservative surgical management of superficially invasive stage I vulvar carcinoma. *Gynecol Oncol* 1989;35:352–356.
66. Rando RF, Sedlacek TV, Hunt J, et al. Verrucous carcinoma of the vulva associated with an unusual type 6 human papillomavirus. *Obstet Gynecol* 1986;67:70S–75S.
67. Dudzinski MR, Askin FB, Fowler WC Jr. Giant basal cell carcinoma of the vulva. *Obstet Gynecol* 1984;63:57S–61S.
68. Merino MJ, LiVolsi VA, Schwartz PE, et al. Adenoid basal cell carcinoma of the vulva. *Int J Gynecol Pathol* 1982;1:299–304.
69. Bottles K, Lacey CG, Goldberg J, et al. Merkel cell carcinoma of the vulva. *Obstet Gynecol* 1984;63:61S–65S.
70. Takeshima N, Tabata T, Hishida H, et al. Peripheral primitive neuroectodermal tumor of the vulva: report of a case with imprint cytology. *Acta Cytol* 2001;45:1049–1052.
71. Vang R, Taubenberger JK, Mannion CM, et al. Primary vulvar and vaginal extraosseous Ewing's sarcoma/peripheral neuroectodermal tumor: diagnostic confirmation with CD99 immunostaining and reverse transcriptase-polymerase chain reaction. *Int J Gynecol Pathol* 2000;19:236–242.
72. Levin W, Goldberg G, Altaras M, et al. The use of concomitant chemotherapy and radiotherapy prior to surgery in advanced stage carcinoma of the vulva. *Gynecol Oncol* 1986;25:20–27.
73. Wilkinson EJ, Brown HM. Vulvar Paget disease of urothelial origin: a report of three cases and a proposed classification of vulvar Paget disease. *Hum Pathol* 2002;33:549–554.
74. Taylor RN, Lacey CG, Shuman MA. Adenocarcinoma of Skene's duct associated with a systemic coagulopathy. *Gynecol Oncol* 1985;22:250–253.
75. Wharton JT, Gallager S, Rutledge RN. Microinvasive carcinoma of the vulva. *Am J Obstet Gynecol* 1974;118:159–161.
76. Klein AE, Bauer TW, Marks KE, et al. Papillary clear cell adenocarcinoma of the groin arising from endometriosis. *Clin Orthop Relat Res* 1999; 361:192–195.
77. Woolcott RJ, Henry RJ, Houghton CR. Malignant melanoma of the vulva: Australian experience. *J Reprod Med* 1988;33:699–711.
78. Nadji M, Ganji P. The application of immunoperoxidase techniques in the evaluation of vulvar and vaginal disease in the evaluation of the vulva and vagina. In: Wilkinson EJ, ed. *Contemporary Issues in Surgical Pathology*. Vol 9. New York: Churchill Livingstone; 1987:239–278.
79. Van der Putte SCJ. Mammary-like glands of the vulva and their disorders. *Int J Gynecol Pathol* 1994;13:150–154.
80. Van der Putte SCJ, van-Gorp HM. Cysts of mammary-like glands in the vulva. *Int J Gynecol Pathol* 1995;14:184–188.
81. Cho D, Buscema J, Rosenshein NB, et al. Primary breast cancer of the vulva. *Obstet Gynecol* 1985;66:79S–87S.
82. Malik S, Wilkinson EJ. Pseudopaget's disease of the vulva: a case report. *J Lower Genital Dis* 1999;3:201–206.
83. Powell FC, Bjornsson J, Doyle JA, et al. Genital Paget's disease and urinary tract malignancy. *J Am Acad Dermatol* 1985;13:84–87.
84. Brown HM, Wilkinson EJ. Uroplakin-III to distinguish vulvar Paget disease secondary to urothelial carcinoma. *Hum Pathol* 2002;33:545–548.
85. Chan TY, Alt SZ, Mandavilli SR, et al. Immunohistochemical analysis of Paget's disease of the vulva: implications for histogenetics and diagnosis. *Mod Pathol* 1999;12:110A–111A.
86. Chen CH, Ji H, Suh KW, et al. Control of HPV-associated malignancies grown in liver with DNA vaccine. *Mod Pathol* 1999;112:53A–55A.
87. Crawford D, Nimmo M, Thomson T, et al. Vulvar Paget's disease: prognostic factors. *Mod Pathol* 1999;12:114A–115A.
88. Cavanagh D, Shepherd JH. The place of pelvic exenteration in the primary management of advanced carcinoma of the vulva. *Gynecol Oncol* 1982;13:318–324.
89. Brainard JA, Hart WR. Proliferative squamous cell lesions in anogenital Paget's disease. *Mod Pathol* 1999;12:113A–115A.
90. Shah KD, Tabibzadch SS, Gerber MA. Immunohistochemical distinction of Paget's disease from Bowen's disease and superficial spreading melanoma with the use of monoclonal cytokeratin antibodies. *Am J Clin Pathol* 1987;88:689–693.
91. Panizzon RG. Vulvar melanoma. *Semin Dermatol* 1996;15:67–70.
92. Ragnarsson-Olding BK, Nilsson BR, Kanter-Lewensohn LR, et al. Malignant melanoma of the vulva in a nationwide, 25-year study of 219 Swedish females: predictors of survival. *Cancer* 1999;86:1285–1293.
93. Piura B, Rabinovich A, Dgani R. Malignant melanoma of the vulva: report of six cases and review of the literature. *Eur J Gynaecol Oncol* 1999;20:182–186.
94. Chu J, Tamimi HK, Ek M, et al. Stage I vulvar cancer: criteria for microinvasion. *Obstet Gynecol* 1982;59:716–721.
95. Sison-Torre EQ, Ackerman AB. Melanosis of the vulva: a clinical simulator of malignant melanoma. *Am J Dermatopathol* 1985;7:51–55.
96. Benda JA, Platz CE, Anderson B. Malignant melanoma of the vulva: a clinical pathologic review of 16 cases. *Int J Gynecol Pathol* 1986;5: 202–216.
97. Podratz KC, Gaffey TA, Symmonds RE, et al. Melanoma of the vulva: an update. *Gynecol Oncol* 1983;16:153–157.
98. Johnson TL, Kumar N, White CD. Prognostic features of vulvar melanoma: a clinicopathologic analysis. *Int J Gynecol Pathol* 1986;5:110–119.
99. Look KY, Roth LM, Sutton GP. Vulvar melanoma reconsidered. *Cancer* 1993;72:143–146.
100. Morgan L, Joslyn P, Chafe W, et al. A report on 18 cases of primary malignant melanoma of the vulva. *Colposcopy Gynecol Laser Surg* 1988;4: 161–170.
101. Raspagliesi F, Ditto A, Paladini D, et al. Prognostic indicators in melanoma of the vulva. *Ann Surg Oncol* 2000;7:738–742.
102. Mihm MC Jr, Clark WH Jr, From L. The clinical diagnosis, classification and histogenetic concepts of the early stages of cutaneous malignant melanomas. *N Engl J Med* 1971;284:1078–1082.
103. Breslow A. Thickness, cross-sectional area and depth of invasion in the prognosis of cutaneous melanoma. *Ann Surg* 1970;172:902–907.
104. Beller U, Demopoulos RI, Bechnan EM. Vulvovaginal melanoma: a clinicopathologic study. *J Reprod Med* 1986;31:315–321.
105. Jiveskog S, Ragnarsson-Olding B, Platz A, et al. N-ras mutations are common in melanomas from sun-exposed skin of humans but rare in mucosal membranes or unexposed skin. *J Invest Dermatol* 1998;111:757–762.
106. Tavassoli FA, Norris HJ. Smooth muscle tumors of the vulva. *Obstet Gynecol* 1979;53:213–215.
107. Nielsen GP, Young RH. Mesenchymal tumors and tumor-like lesions of the female genital tract: a selective review with emphasis on recently described entities. *Int J Gynecol Pathol* 2001;20:105–127.
108. Nucci MR, Fletcher CDM. Vulvovaginal soft tissue tumors: update and review. *Histopathology* 2000;36:97–108.
109. Taylor RN, Bottles K, Miller TR, et al. Malignant fibrous histiocytoma of the vulva. *Obstet Gynecol* 1985;66:145–150.
110. Perrone T, Swanson PE, Twiggs L, et al. Malignant rhabdoid tumor of the vulva: is distinction from epithelioid sarcoma possible? *Am J Surg Pathol* 1989;13:848–851.
111. Trope C, Johnsson JE, Larsson G, et al. Bleomycin alone or combined with mitomycin C in treatment of advanced or recurrent squamous cell carcinoma of the vulva. *Cancer Treat Rep* 1980;64:639–643.
112. Ungerleider RS, Donaldson SS, Warnke RA, et al. Endodermal sinus tumor: the Stanford experience and the first reported case arising in the vulva. *Cancer* 1978;41:1627–1634.
113. Ehrmann RL, Dwyer IM, Yavner BA, et al. An immunoperoxidase study of laminin and type IV collagen distribution in carcinoma of the cervix and vulva. *Obstet Gynecol* 1988;72:257–260.
114. LiVolsi VA, Brooks JJ. Soft tissue tumors of the vulva. In: Wilkinson EJ, ed. *Pathology of the Vulva and Vagina: Contemporary Issues in Surgical Pathology*. Vol 9. New York: Churchill Livingstone; 1987:209.
115. Cockerell CJ, LeBoit PE. Bacillary angiomatosis: a newly characterized, pseudoneoplastic, infectious, cutaneous vascular disorder. *J Am Acad Dermatol* 1990;22:501–504.
116. Leiman G, Markowitz S, Veiga-Ferreira MM, et al. Renal adenocarcinoma presenting with bilateral metastases to Bartholin's glands: primary diagnosis by aspiration cytology. *Diagn Cytopathol* 1986;2:252–255.
117. Lerner LB, Andrews SJ, Gonzalez JL, et al. Vulvar metastases secondary to transitional cell carcinoma of the bladder: a case report. *J Reprod Med* 1999;8:729–732.
118. Neto AG, Deavers MT, Silva EG, et al. Metastatic tumors of the vulva: a clinicopathologic study of 66 cases. *Am J Surg Pathol* 2003;27: 799–812.
119. Vang R, Medeiros LJ, Malpica A, et al. Non-Hodgkin's lymphoma involving the vulva. *Int J Gynecol Pathol* 2000;19:236–242.
120. Levine RL. Urethral cancer. *Cancer* 1980;45:1965–1969.
121. Boutselis JG. Radical vulvectomy for invasive squamous cell carcinoma of the vulva. *Obstet Gynecol* 1972;39:827–831.
122. Collins CG, Lee FYL, Lopez JJ. Invasive carcinoma of the vulva with lymph node metastases. *Am J Obstet Gynecol* 1971;109:446–450.
123. Iversen T, Aalders JG, Christensen A, et al. Squamous cell carcinoma of the vulva: a review of 424 patients, 1956–1974. *Gynecol Oncol* 1980;9:271–279.
124. Kurzl R, Messerer D. Prognostic factors in squamous cell carcinoma of the vulva: a multivariate analysis. *Gynecol Oncol* 1989;32:143–147.
125. Malfetano JH, Piver S, Tsukada Y, et al. Univariate and multivariate analyses of 5-year survival, recurrence, and inguinal node metastases in stage I and II vulvar carcinoma. *J Surg Oncol* 1985;30:124–131.

126. Podratz KC, Symmonds RE, Taylor WF. Carcinoma of the vulva: analysis of treatment failures. *Am J Obstet Gynecol* 1982;143:340–346.
127. Binder SW, Huang I, Fu YS, et al. Risk factors for the development of lymph node metastasis in vulvar squamous carcinoma. *Gynecol Oncol* 1990;37:9–16.
128. Donaldson ES, Powell DE, Hanson MB, et al. Prognostic parameters in invasive vulvar cancer. *Gynecol Oncol* 1981;11:184–190.
129. Hacker NF, Berek JS, Lagasse LD, et al. Individualization of treatment for stage I squamous cell vulvar carcinoma. *Obstet Gynecol* 1984;63:155–160.
130. Parker RT, Duncan I, Rampone J, et al. Operative management of early invasive epidermoid carcinoma of the vulva. *Am J Obstet Gynecol* 1975;123:349–354.
131. Buscema J, Stern JL, Woodruff JD. Early invasive carcinoma of the vulva. *Am J Obstet Gynecol* 1981;140:563–570.
132. Chu J, Tamimi HK, Ek M, et al. Stage I vulvar cancer: criteria for microinvasion. *Obstet Gynecol* 1982;59:716–720.
133. Hoffman JS, Kumar NB, Morley GW. Microinvasive squamous carcinoma of the vulva: search for a definition. *Obstet Gynecol* 1983;61:615–619.
134. Magrina JF, Webb MJ, Gaffey TA, et al. Stage I squamous cell cancer of the vulva. *Am J Obstet Gynecol* 1979;134:453–459.
135. Ross MJ, Ehrmann RL. Histologic prognosticators in stage I squamous cell carcinoma of the vulva. *Obstet Gynecol* 1987;70:774–778.
136. Zucker PK, Berkowitz RS. The issue of microinvasive squamous cell carcinoma of the vulva: an evaluation of the criteria of diagnosis and methods of therapy. *Obstet Gynecol Surv* 1985;40:136–139.
137. Chan JK, Sugiyama V, Pham H, et al. Margin distance and other clinicopathologic prognostic factors in vulvar carcinoma: a multivariate analysis. *Gynecol Oncol* 2007;104:636–641.
138. De Hullu JA, Hollema H, Lolkema S, et al. Vulvar carcinoma. The price of less radical surgery. *Cancer* 2002;95:2331–2338.
139. Hoffman MS, Gunesakaran S, Arango H, et al. Lateral microscopic extension of squamous cell carcinoma of the vulva. *Gynecol Oncol* 1999;73:72–75.
140. Gonzalez Bosquet J, Magrina JF, Gaffey TA, et al. Long-term survival and disease recurrence in patients with primary squamous cell carcinoma of the vulva. *Gynecol Oncol* 2005;97:828–833.
141. Farias-Eisner R, Cirisano FD, Grouse D, et al. Conservative and individualized surgery for early squamous carcinoma of the vulva: the treatment of choice for stage I and II (T1-2 N0-1 M0) disease. *Gynecol Oncol* 1994;53: 55–58.
142. Figge DC, Tamimi HK, Greer BE. Lymphatic spread in carcinoma of the vulva. *Am J Obstet Gynecol* 1985;152:387–392.
143. Oonk MH, Hollema H, de Hullu JA, et al. Prediction of lymph node metastases in vulvar cancer: a review. *Int J Gynecol Cancer* 2006;16: 963–971.
144. Bipat S, Fransen GA, Spijkerboer AM, et al. Is there a role for magnetic resonance imaging in the evaluation of inguinal lymph node metastases in patients with vulva carcinoma? *Gynecol Oncol* 2006;103:1001–1006.
145. Hacker NF, Berek JS, Lagasse L, et al. Management of regional lymph nodes and their prognostic influence in vulvar cancer. *Obstet Gynecol* 1983;61:408–413.
146. Rutledge FN, Mitchell MF, Munsell MF, et al. Prognostic indicators for invasive carcinoma of the vulva. *Gynecol Oncol* 1991;42:239–245.
147. Taussig FJ. Cancer of the vulva: an analysis of 155 cases. *Am J Obstet Gynecol* 1940;40:764–770.
148. Way S. Carcinoma of the vulva. *Am J Obstet Gynecol* 1960;79:692–699.
149. Burke TW, Stringer CA, Gershenson DM, et al. Radical wide excision and selective inguinal node dissection for squamous cell carcinoma of the vulva. *Gynecol Oncol* 1990;38:328–334.
150. DiSaia PJ, Creasman WT, Rich WM. An alternative approach to early cancer of the vulva. *Am J Obstet Gynecol* 1979;133:825–829.
151. Keys HM, Bundy BN, Stehman FB, et al. Cisplatin, radiation, and adjuvant hysterectomy compared with radiation and adjuvant hysterectomy for bulky stage IB cervical carcinoma. *N Engl J Med* 1999;340: 1154–1162.
152. Peters WA, Liu PY, Barrett RJ, et al. Concurrent chemotherapy and pelvic radiation therapy compared with pelvic radiation therapy alone as adjuvant therapy after radical surgery in high-risk early-stage cancer of the cervix. *J Clin Oncol* 2000;18:1606–1610.
153. Rose PG, Bundy BN, Watkins EB, et al. Concurrent cisplatin-based radiotherapy and chemotherapy for locally advanced cervical cancer. *N Engl J Med* 1999;340:1144–1147.
154. Moore DH, Thomas GM, Montana GS, et al. Preoperative chemoradiation for advanced vulvar cancer: A phase II study of the Gynecologic Oncology Group. *Int J Radiat Oncol Biol Phys* 1998;42:1317–1321.
155. Kelley III JL, Burke TW, Tornos C, et al. Minimally invasive vulvar carcinoma: an indication for conservative surgical therapy. *Gynecol Oncol* 1991;144:240–245.
156. Chafe W, Richards A, Morgan L, et al. Unrecognized invasive carcinoma in vulvar intraepithelial neoplasia (VIN). *Gynecol Oncol* 1988;31:154–157.
157. Modesitt SC, Waters AB, Walton L, et al. Vulvar intraepithelial neoplasia III: occult cancer and the impact of margin status on recurrence. *Obstet Gynecol* 1998;92:962–970.
158. Morley GW. Infiltrative carcinoma of the vulva: results of surgical treatment. *Am J Obstet Gynecol* 1976;124:874–879.
159. Podratz KC, Symmonds RE, Taylor WF, et al. Carcinoma of the vulva: analysis of treatment and survival. *Obstet Gynecol* 1983;61:63–67.
160. Figge CD, Gaudenz R. Invasive carcinoma of the vulva. *Am J Obstet Gynecol* 1974;119:382–387.
161. Rutledge F, Smith JP, Franklin EW. Carcinoma of the vulva. *Am J Obstet Gynecol* 1970;106:1117–1121.
162. Homesley HD, Bundy BN, Sedlis A, et al. Radiation therapy versus pelvic node resection for carcinoma of the vulva with positive groin nodes. *Obstet Gynecol* 1986;68:733–739.
163. Hacker NF, Van der Velden J. Conservative management of early vulvar cancer. *Cancer* 1993;71:1673–1678.
164. Iversen T, Abeler V, Aalders J. Individualized treatment of stage I carcinoma of the vulva. *Obstet Gynecol* 1981;57:85–91.
165. Burke TW, Levenback C, Coleman RC, et al. Surgical therapy of T1 and T2 vulvar carcinoma: further experience with radical wide excision and selective inguinal lymphadenectomy. *Gynecol Oncol* 1995;57:215–219.
166. Stehman FB, Bundy BN, Dvoretsky PM, et al. Early stage I carcinoma of the vulva treated with ipsilateral superficial inguinal lymphadenectomy and modified radical hemivulvectomy: a prospective study of the Gynecologic Oncology Group. *Obstet Gynecol* 1992;79:490–494.
167. Morris JM. A formula for selective lymphadenectomy. *Obstet Gynecol* 1977;50:152–156.
168. DeSimone CP, Van Ness JS, Cooper AL, et al. The treatment of lateral T1 and T2 squamous cell carcinoma of the vulva confined to the labium majus or minus. *Gynecol Oncol* 2007;104:390–395.
169. Gonzalez BJ, Magrina JF, Magtibay PM, et al. Patterns of inguinal groin metastases in squamous cell carcinoma of the vulva. *Gynecol Oncol* 2007;105:742–746.
170. Gordinier ME, Malpica A, Burke TW, et al. Groin recurrence in patients with vulvar cancer with negative nodes on superficial inguinal lymphadenectomy. *Gynecol Oncol* 2003;90:625–628.
171. Hacker NF, Leuchter RS, Berek JS, et al. Radical vulvectomy and bilateral inguinal lymphadenectomy through separate groin incisions. *Obstet Gynecol* 1981;58:574–578.
172. Le T, Elsugi R, Hopkins L, et al. The definition of optimal inguinal femoral nodal dissection in the management of vulva squamous cell carcinoma. *Ann Surg Oncol* 2007;14:2128–2132.
173. Hudson CN, Shulver H, Lowe DC. The surgery of "inguino-femoral" lymph nodes: is it adequate or excessive? *Int J Gynecol Cancer* 2004;14:841–845.
174. Dardarian TS, Gray HJ, Morgan MA, et al. Saphenous vein sparing during inguinal lymphadenectomy to reduce morbidity in patients with vulvar carcinoma. *Gynecol Oncol* 2006;101:140–142.
175. Zhang X, Sheng X, Niu J, et al. Sparing of saphenous vein during inguinal lymphadenectomy for vulval malignancies. *Gynecol Oncol* 2007;105:722–726.
176. Rouzier R, Haddad B, Dubernard G, et al. Inguinofemoral dissection for carcinoma of the vulva: effect of modifications of extent and technique on morbidity and survival. *Am Coll Surg* 2003;196:442–450.
177. Judson PL, Jonson AL, Paley PJ, et al. A prospective, randomized study analyzing sartorius transposition following inguinal-femoral lymphadenectomy. *Gynecol Oncol* 2004;95:226–230.
178. Levenback C, Burke TW, Gershenson DM, et al. Intraoperative lymphatic mapping for vulvar cancer. *Obstet Gynecol* 1994;84:163–167.
179. Barton DPJ, Berman C, Cavanagh D, et al. Lymphoscintigraphy in vulvar cancer: a pilot study. *Gynecol Oncol* 1992;46:341–347.
180. DeCesare SL, Fiorica JV, Roberts WS, et al. A pilot study utilizing intraoperative lymphoscintigraphy for identification of the sentinel lymph nodes in vulvar cancer. *Gynecol Oncol* 1997;66:425–429.
181. Terada KY, Shimizu DM, Jiang CS, et al. Outcomes for patients with T1 squamous cell cancer of the vulva undergoing sentinel node biopsy. *Gynecol Oncol* 2006;102:200–203.
182. De Mooij Y, Burger MP, Schilthuis MS, et al. Partial urethral resection in the surgical treatment of vulvar cancer does not have a significant impact on urinary continence. A confirmation of an authority-based opinion. *Int J Gynecol Cancer* 2007;17:294–297.
183. Gerszten K, Selvaraj RN, Kelley J, et al. Preoperative chemoradiation for locally advanced carcinoma of the vulva. *Gynecol Oncol* 2005;99: 640–644.
184. Van Doorn HC, Ansink A, Verhaar-Langereis M, et al. Neoadjuvant chemoradiation for advanced primary vulvar cancer. *Cochrane Database Syst Rev* 2006;3:CD003752.
185. Hyde SE, Valmadre S, Hacker NF, et al. Squamous cell carcinoma of the vulva with bulky positive groin nodes—nodal debulking versus full groin dissection prior to radiation therapy. *Int J Gynecol Cancer* 2007;17: 154–158.
186. Hopkins MP, Reid GC, Morley GW. The surgical management of recurrent squamous cell carcinoma of the vulva. *Obstet Gynecol* 1990;75:1001–1007.
187. Piura B, Masotina A, Murdoch J, et al. Recurrent squamous cell carcinoma of the vulva: a study of 73 cases. *Gynecol Oncol* 1993;48:189–194.
188. Abitol MM. Carcinoma of the vulva: improvements in the surgical approach. *Am J Obstet Gynecol* 1973;117:483–489.
189. Burke TW, Morris M, Levenback C, et al. Closure of complex vulvar defects using local rhomboid flaps. *Obstet Gynecol* 1994;84:1043–1046.
190. Burrell MO, Franklin EW III, Campion MJ, et al. The modified radical vulvectomy with groin dissection: an eight-year experience. *Am J Obstet Gynecol* 1988;159:715–719.
191. Siller BS, Alvarez RD, Conner WD, et al. T2/3 vulva cancer: a case-control study of triple incision versus en bloc radical vulvectomy and inguinal lymphadenectomy. *Gynecol Oncol* 1995;57:335–340.

192. Gaarenstroom KN, Kenter GG, Trimbos JB, et al. Postoperative complications after vulvectomy and inguinofemoral lymphadenectomy using separate groin incisions. *Int J Gynecol Cancer* 2003;13:522–527.
193. Borgno G, Micheletti L, Barbero M, et al. Topographic distribution of groin lymph nodes: a study of 50 female cadavers. *J Reprod Med* 1990;35:1127–1132.
194. Rouzier R, Haddad B, Dubernard G, et al. Inguinofemoral dissection for carcinoma of the vulva: effect of modifications of extent and technique on morbidity and survival. *J Am Coll Surg* 2003;196:442–448.
195. Cabanas RM. An approach for the treatment of penile carcinoma. *Cancer* 1977;39:456–462.
196. Morton D, Wen D, Cochran A. Management of early-stage melanoma by intraoperative lymphatic mapping and selective lymphadenectomy: an alternative to routine elective lymphadenectomy or "watch and wait." *Surg Oncol Clin North Am* 1992;1:247–251.
197. Makar APH, Scheistroen M, van den Weyngaert D, et al. Surgical management of stage I and II vulvar cancer: the role of the sentinel node biopsy. *Int J Gynecol Cancer* 2001;11:255–261.
198. DeCicco C, Sideri M, Grana C, et al. Sentinel node biopsy in early vulvar cancer. *Br J Cancer* 2000;82:295–299.
199. Sliutz G, Reinthaller A, Lantzsch T, et al. Lymphatic mapping of sentinel nodes in early vulvar cancer. *Gynecol Oncol* 2002;84:449–454.
200. Levenback C, Coleman RL, Burke TW, et al. Intraoperative lymphatic mapping and sentinel node identification with blue dye in patients with vulvar cancer. *Gynecol Oncol* 2001;83:276–283.
201. Moore RG, Depasquale SE, Steinhoff MM, et al. Sentinel node identification and the ability to detect metastatic tumor to inguinal lymph nodes in squamous cell cancer of the vulva. *Gynecol Oncol* 2003;89:475–481.
202. De Hulla JA, Hollema H, Piers DA, et al. Sentinel lymph node procedure is highly accurate in squamous cell carcinoma of the vulva. *J Clin Oncol* 2000;18:2811–2820.
203. Nyberg RH, Iivonen M, Parkkinen J, et al. Sentinel node and vulvar cancer: a series of 47 patients. *Acta Obstet Gynecol Scand* 2007;86: 615–619.
204. Hauspy J, Beiner M, Harley I, et al. Sentinel lymph node in vulvar cancer. *Cancer* 2007;110:1015–1023.
205. Robison K, Steinhoff MM, Granai CO, et al. Inguinal sentinel node dissection versus standard inguinal node dissection in patients with vulvar cancer: a comparison of the size of metastasis detected in inguinal lymph nodes. *Gynecol Oncol* 2006;101:24–27.
206. Fons G, ter Rahe B, Sloof G, et al. Failure in the detection of the sentinel lymph node with a combined technique of radioactive tracer and blue dye in a patient with cancer of the vulva and a single positive lymph node. *Gynecol Oncol* 2004;92:981–984.
207. Louis-Sylvestre C, Evangelista E, Leonard F, et al. Sentinel node localization should be interpreted with caution in midline vulvar cancer. *Gynecol Oncol* 2005;97:151–154.
208. Louis-Sylvestre C, Evangelista E, Leonard F, et al. Interpretation of sentinel node identification in vulvar cancer. *Gynecol Obstet Fertil* 2006;34: 706–710.
209. Buechler DA, Kline JC, Tynes JC, et al. Treatment of recurrent carcinoma of the vulva. *Gynecol Oncol* 1979;8:180–185.
210. Miller B, Morris M, Levenback C, et al. Pelvic exenteration for primary and recurrent vulvar cancer. *Gynecol Oncol* 1995;58:189–193.
211. Phillips B, Buchsbaum JH, Lifshitz S. Pelvic exenteration for vulvovaginal carcinoma. *Am J Obstet Gynecol* 1981;141:1038–1043.
212. Thornton WN, Flanagan WL Jr. Pelvic exenteration in the treatment of advanced malignancy of the vulva. *Am J Obstet Gynecol* 1973;117: 774–780.
213. Burke TW, Morris M, Roh MS, et al. Perineal reconstruction using single gracilis myocutaneous flaps. *Gynecol Oncol* 1995;57:221–226.
214. Barnhill DR, Hoskins WJ, Metz P. Use of the rhomboid flap after partial vulvectomy. *Obstet Gynecol* 1983;62:444–448.
215. Helm CW, Hatch KD, Partridge EE, et al. The rhomboid flap for repair of the perineal defect after radical vulvar surgery. *Gynecol Oncol* 1993; 50:164–169.
216. Achauer BM, Braly P, Berman ML, et al. Immediate vaginal reconstruction following resection for malignancy using the gluteal thigh flap. *Gynecol Oncol* 1984;19:79–84.
217. Ballon SC, Donaldson RC, Roberts JA. Reconstruction of the vulva using a myocutaneous graft. *Gynecol Oncol* 1979;7:123–129.
218. Chafe W, Fowler WC, Walton LA, et al. Radical vulvectomy with use of tensor fascia lata myocutaneous flap. *Am J Obstet Gynecol* 1983;145:207–211.
219. Patsner B, Hetzler P. Postradical vulvectomy reconstruction using the inferiorly based transverse rectus abdominis (TRAM) flap: a preliminary experience. *Gynecol Oncol* 1994;55:78–82.
220. Potkul RK, Barnes WA, Barter JF, et al. Vulvar reconstruction using a mons pubis pedicle flap. *Gynecol Oncol* 1994;55:21–28.
221. Ragoowansi R, Yii N, Niranjan N. Immediate vulvar and vaginal reconstruction using the gluteal-fold flap: long-term results. *Br J Plast Surg* 2004;57:406–410.
222. Ellis F. Cancer of the vulva treated by radiation. *Br J Radiol* 1949;22:513.
223. Helgason NM, Hass AC, Latourette HB. Radiation therapy in carcinoma of the vulva. *Cancer* 1972;30:997–1004.
224. Tod MC. Radium implantation treatment of carcinoma vulva. *Br J Radiol* 1949;22:508–512.
225. Busch M, Wagener B, Duhmke E. Long term results of radiotherapy alone for carcinoma of the vulva. *Adv Ther* 1999;16:89–94.
226. Boyce J, Fruchter RG, Kasambilides E, et al. Prognostic factors in carcinoma of the vulva. *Gynecol Oncol* 1985;20:364–367.
227. Faul CM, Mirmow D, Huang Q, et al. Adjuvant radiation for vulvar carcinoma: improved local control. *Int J Radiat Oncol Biol Phys* 1997; 38:381–385.
228. Acosta AA, Given FT, Frazier AB, et al. Preoperative radiation therapy in the management of squamous cell carcinoma of the vulva: preliminary report. *Am J Obstet Gynecol* 1978;132:198–203.
229. Boronow RC, Hickman BT, Reagan MT, et al. Combined therapy as an alternative to exenteration for locally advanced vulvovaginal cancer: II. Results, complications and dosimetric and surgical considerations. *Am J Clin Oncol* 1987;10:171–176.
230. Fairey RN, MacKay PA, Benedet JL, et al. Radiation treatment of carcinoma of the vulva, 1950–1980. *Am J Obstet Gynecol* 1985;151:591–598.
231. Hacker NF, Berek JS, Julliard GJF, et al. Preoperative radiation therapy for locally advanced vulvar cancer. *Cancer* 1984;54:2056–2064.
232. Jafari K, Magalotti M. Radiation therapy in carcinoma of the vulva. *Cancer* 1981;47:686–691.
233. Berek JS, Heaps JM, Fu YS, et al. Concurrent cisplatin and 5-fluorouracil chemotherapy and radiation therapy for advanced-stage squamous carcinoma of the vulva. *Gynecol Oncol* 1991;42:197–204.
234. Cunningham MJ, Goyer RP, Gibbons SK, et al. Primary radiation, cisplatin, and 5-fluorouracil for advanced squamous carcinoma of the vulva. *Gynecol Oncol* 1997;66:258–264.
235. Eifel PJ, Morris M, Burke TW, et al. Preoperative continuous infusion cisplatinum and 5-fluorouracil with radiation for locally advanced or recurrent carcinoma of the vulva. *Gynecol Oncol* 1995;59:51–59.
236. Evans LS, Kersh CR, Constable WC, et al. Concomitant 5-fluorouracil, mitomycin C, and radiotherapy for advanced gynecologic malignancies. *Int J Radiat Oncol Biol Phys* 1988;15:901–907.
237. Iversen T. Irradiation and bleomycin in the treatment of inoperable vulval carcinoma. *Acta Obstet Gynecol Scand* 1982;61:195–200.
238. Kalra JK, Grossman AM, Krumholz BA, et al. Preoperative chemoradiotherapy for carcinoma of the vulva. *Gynecol Oncol* 1981;12:256–260.
239. Koh WJ, Wallace HJ, Greer BE, et al. Combined radiotherapy and chemotherapy in the management of local-regionally advanced vulvar cancer. *Int J Radiat Oncol Biol Phys* 1993;26:809–814.
240. Landoni F, Maneo A, Zanetta G, et al. Concurrent preoperative chemotherapy with 5-fluorouracil and mitomycin C and radiotherapy (FUMIR) followed by limited surgery in locally advanced and recurrent vulvar carcinoma. *Gynecol Oncol* 1996;61:321–326.
241. Lupi G, Raspagliesi F, Zucali R, et al. Combined preoperative chemoradiotherapy followed by radical surgery in locally advanced vulvar carcinoma: a pilot study. *Cancer* 1996;77:1472–1479.
242. Mäkinen J, Salmi T, Gronroos M. Individually modified treatment of invasive squamous cell vulvar cancer: 10-year experience. *Ann Chir Gynaecol* 1987;76(Suppl):68–72.
243. Scheistroen M, Trope C. Combined bleomycin and irradiation in preoperative treatment of advanced squamous cell carcinoma of the vulva. *Acta Oncol* 1992;32:657–663.
244. Thomas G, Dembo A, DePetrillo A, et al. Concurrent radiation and chemotherapy in vulvar carcinoma. *Gynecol Oncol* 1989;34:263–267.
245. Whalen SA, Slater JD, Wagner RJ, et al. Concurrent radiation therapy and chemotherapy in the treatment of primary squamous cell cancer of the vulva. *Cancer* 1995;75:2289–2294.
246. Akl A, Akl M, Boike G, et al. Preliminary results of chemoradiation as a primary treatment for vulvar carcinoma. *Int J Radiat Biol Phys* 2000;48:415–417.
247. Han SC, Kim DH, Higgins SA, et al. Chemoradiation as primary or adjuvant treatment for locally advanced carcinoma of the vulva. *Int J Radiat Oncol Biol Phys* 2000;47:1235–1239.
248. Mulayim N, Silver DF, Schwartz PE, et al. Chemoradiation with 5-fluorouracial and mitomycin C in the treatment of vulvar squamous cell carcinoma. *Gynecol Oncol* 2004;93:659–666.
249. Gerszten K, Selvaraj RN, Kelley J, et al. Preoperative chemoradiation for locally advanced carcinoma of the vulva. *Gynecol Oncol* 2005;99: 640–644.
250. Cummings B. Anal canal carcinomas. In: Meyer JL, Vaeth JM, eds. *Frontiers in Radiation Oncology*. Vol 26. Basel: Karger; 1992:131–135.
251. Rich TA, Ajani JA, Morrison WH, et al. Chemoradiation therapy for anal cancer: radiation plus continuous infusion of 5-fluorouracil with or without cisplatin. *Radiother Oncol* 1993;27:209–212.
252. Morris M, Eifel PJ, Lu J, et al. Pelvic radiation with concurrent chemotherapy compared with pelvic and paraaortic radiation for high-risk cervical cancer. *N Engl J Med* 1999;340:1137–1141.
253. Henderson RH, Parsons JT, Morgan L, et al. Elective ilioinguinal lymph node irradiation. *Int J Radiat Oncol Biol Phys* 1984;10:811–816.
254. Kucera H, Weghaupt K. The electrosurgical operation of vulva carcinoma with postoperative irradiation of inguinal lymph nodes. *Gynecol Oncol* 1988;29:158–164.
255. Petereit D, Mehta M, Buchler D, et al. A retrospective review of nodal treatment for vulvar cancer. *Am J Clin Oncol* 1993;16:38–42.
256. Katz A, Eifel PJ, Jhingran A, et al. The role of radiation therapy in preventing regional recurrences of invasive squamous cell carcinoma of the vulva. *Int J Radiat Oncol Biol Phys* 2003;57:409–413.

257. Leiserowitz GS, Russell AH, Kinney WK, et al. Prophylactic chemoradiation of inguinofemoral lymph nodes in patients with locally extensive vulvar cancer. *Gynecol Oncol* 1997;66:509–514.
258. Stehman F, Bundy B, Thomas G, et al. Groin dissection versus groin radiation in carcinoma of the vulva: a Gynecologic Oncology Group study. *Int J Radiat Oncol Biol Phys* 1992;24:39–42.
259. Eifel PJ. Vulvar carcinoma: radiotherapy or surgery for the lymphatics? *Front Radiat Ther Oncol* 1994;28:218–221.
260. Koh WJ, Chiu M, Stelzer KJ, et al. Femoral vessel depth and the implications for groin node radiation. *Int J Radiat Oncol Biol Phys* 1992;27:969–973.
261. Origoni M, Sideri M, Garsia S, et al. Prognostic value of pathological patterns of lymph node positivity in squamous cell carcinoma of the vulva stage III and IVA FIGO. *Gynecol Oncol* 1992;45:313–317.
262. Simonsen E, Nordberg UB, Johnsson JE, et al. Radiation therapy and surgery in the treatment of regional lymph nodes in squamous cell carcinoma of the vulva. *Acta Radiol Oncol* 1984;23:433–437.
263. Parthasarathy A, Cheung MK, Osann K, et al. The benefit of adjuvant radiation therapy in single-node-positive squamous cell vulvar carcinoma. *Gynecol Oncol* 2006;103:1095–1099.
264. Montana GS, Thomas GM, Moore DH, et al. Preoperative chemo-radiation for carcinoma of the vulva with N2/N3 nodes: a Gynecologic Oncology Group study. *Int J Radiat Oncol Biol Phys* 2000;48:1007–1010.
265. Lataifeh I, Nascimento MC, Nicklin JL, et al. Patterns of recurrence and disease-free survival in advanced squamous cell carcinoma of the vulva. *Gynecol Oncol* 2004;95:701–705.
266. Kalnicki S, Zide A, Malecki N, et al. Transmission block to simplify combined pelvic and inguinal radiation therapy. *Radiology* 1987;164:578–582.
267. Carlino G, Parisi S, Montemaggi P, Pastore G. Interstitial radiotherapy with ^{192}Ir in vulvar cancer. *Eur J Gynaecol Oncol* 1984;5:183–188.
268. Miyazawa K, Nori D, Hilaris BS, et al. Role of radiation therapy in the treatment of advanced vulvar carcinoma. *J Reprod Med* 1983;28:539–544.
269. Dusenbery KE, Carlson JW, LaPorte RM, et al. Radical vulvectomy with postoperative irradiation for vulvar cancer: therapeutic implications of a central block. *Int J Radiat Oncol Biol Phys* 1994;29:989–993.
270. Beriwal S, Heron D, Kim H, et al. Intensity-modulated radiotherapy for the treatment of vulvar carcinoma: a comparative dosimetric study with early clinical outcome. *Int J Radiat Oncol Biol Phys* 2006;64:1395–1400.
271. Jenkins PJ, Montefiore DJ, Arnott SJ. Hip complications following chemoradiotherapy. *Clin Oncol* 1995;7:123–128.
272. Thomas G, Dembo A, Fyles A, et al. Concurrent chemoradiation in advanced cervical cancer. *Gynecol Oncol* 1990;38:446–450.
273. Frischbier HJ, Thomsen K. Treatment of cancer of the vulva with high-energy electrons. *Am J Obstet Gynecol* 1971;111:431–440.
274. Barton DPJ. The prevention and management of treatment related morbidity in vulval cancer. *Best Practice Res Clin Obstet Gynecol* 2003;17: 683–701.
275. Deppe G, Bruckner HW, Cohen CJ. Adriamycin treatment of advanced vulvar carcinoma. *Obstet Gynecol* 1977;50:13–17.
276. Thigpen JT, Blessing JA, Homesley HD, et al. Phase II trials of cisplatin and piperzinedione in advanced or recurrent squamous cell carcinomas of the vulva: a Gynecologic Oncology Group study. *Gynecol Oncol* 1986; 23:358–362.
277. Muss HB, Bundy BN, Christopherson WA. Mitoxantrone in the treatment of advanced vulvar and vaginal carcinoma. *Am J Clin Oncol* 1989;12:142–147.
278. Slayton RE, Blessing JA, Beecham J, et al. Phase II trial of etoposide in the management of advanced or recurrent squamous cell carcinoma of the vulva and carcinoma of the vagina: a Gynecologic Oncology Group study. *Cancer Treat Rep* 1987;71:869–872.
279. Belinson JL, Stewart JA, Richards A, et al. Bleomycin, vincristine, mitomycin C, and cisplatin in the management of gynecologic squamous cell cancer. *Gynecol Oncol* 1985;20:387–392.
280. Durrant KR, Mangione C, Lacave AJ, et al. Bleomycin, methotrexate, and CCNU in advanced inoperable squamous cell carcinoma of the vulva: a phase II study of the EORTC Gynaecological Cancer Cooperative Group (GCCG). *Gynecol Oncol* 1990;37:359–363.
281. Kosary CL. FIGO stage, histology, histologic grade, age and race as prognostic factors in determining survival for cancers of the female gynecologic system: an analysis of 1973–87 SEER cases of cancers of the endometrium, cervix, ovary, vulva and vagina. *Semin Surg Oncol* 1994;10:31–36.
282. Morrow CP, Rutledge FN. Melanoma of the vulva. *Obstet Gynecol* 1972;39:745–750.
283. Jaramillo BA, Ganjei P, Averette HE, et al. Malignant melanoma of the vulva. *Obstet Gynecol* 1985;66:398–402.
284. Clark WH, From L, Bernardino EA, et al. The histogenesis and biologic behavior of primary human malignant melanomas of the skin. *Cancer Res* 1969;29:705–708.
285. Chung AF, Woodruff JM, Lewis JL Jr. Malignant melanoma of the vulva: a report of 44 cases. *Obstet Gynecol* 1975;45:638–642.
286. Phillips GL, Bundy BN, Okagaki T, et al. Malignant melanoma of the vulva treated by radical hemivulvectomy: a prospective study of the Gynecology Oncology Group. *Cancer* 1994;73:2626–2630.
287. Trimble EL, Lewis JL Jr, Williams LL, et al. Management of vulvar melanoma. *Gynecol Oncol* 1992;45:254–258.
288. Suwandinata FS, Bohle RM, Omwandho CA, et al. Management of vulvar melanoma and review of the literature. *Eur J Gynaecol Oncol* 2007;23: 220–224.
289. Balch CM. The role of elective lymph node dissection in melanoma: rationale, results, and controversies. *J Clin Oncol* 1988;6:163–167.
290. Sugiyama VE, Chan JK, Shin JY, et al. Vulvar melanoma: a multivariate analysis of 644 patients. *Obstet Gynecol* 2007;110:296–301.
291. Emami B, Perez CA. Combination of surgery, irradiation, and hyperthermia in treatment of recurrences of malignant tumors. *Int J Radiat Oncol Biol Phys* 1987;13:611–615.
292. Singhal RM, Narayana A. Malignant melanoma of the vulva: response to radiation. *Br J Radiol* 1991;64:846–850.
293. Habermalz HJ, Fischer JJ. Radiation therapy of malignant melanoma: experience with high individual treatment doses. *Cancer* 1976;38: 2258–2262.
294. Sondak VK, Liu PY, Tuthill RJ. Adjuvant immunotherapy of resected, intermediate-thickness, node-negative melanoma with an allogeneic tumor vaccine: overall results of a randomized trial of the Southwest Oncology Group. *J Clin Oncol* 2002;20:2058–2062.
295. Gallousis S. Verrucous carcinoma: report of three vulvar cases and a review of the literature. *Obstet Gynecol* 1972;40:502–506.
296. Japaze H, Dinh TV, Woodruff JD. Verrucous carcinoma of the vulva: study of 24 cases. *Obstet Gynecol* 1982;60:462–467.
297. Demian SDE, Bushkin FL, Echevarria RA. Perineural invasion and anaplastic transformation of verrucous carcinoma. *Cancer* 1973;32: 395–399.
298. Proffitt SD, Spooner TR, Kosek JC. Origin of undifferentiated neoplasm from verrucous carcinoma of the oral cavity following irradiation. *Cancer* 1970;26:389–394.
299. Breen JL, Neubecker RD, Greenwald E, et al. Basal cell carcinoma of the vulva. *Obstet Gynecol* 1975;46:122–125.
300. Hoffman MS, Roberts WS, Ruffolo EH. Basal cell carcinoma of the vulva with inguinal lymph node metastases. *Gynecol Oncol* 1988; 29:113–117.
301. Copeland LJ, Sneige N, Gershenson DM, et al. Bartholin gland carcinoma. *Obstet Gynecol* 1986;67:794–799.
302. Leuchter RS, Hacker NF, Voet RL, et al. Primary carcinoma of the Bartholin gland: a report of 14 cases and a review of the literature. *Obstet Gynecol* 1982;60:361–367.
303. Huang GS, Juretzka M, Ciaravino G, et al. Liposomal doxorubicin for treatment of metastatic chemorefractory vulvar adenocarcinoma. *Gynecol Oncol* 2002;87:313–317.
304. Creasman WT, Gallager HS, Rutledge F. Paget's disease of the vulva. *Gynecol Oncol* 1975;3:133–137.
305. Parmley TH, Woodruff JD, Julian CG. Invasive vulvar Paget's disease. *Obstet Gynecol* 1975;46:341–345.
306. Hart WR, Millman RB. Progression of intraepithelial Paget's disease of the vulva to invasive carcinoma. *Cancer* 1977;40:2333–2335.
307. Fanning J, Lambert L, Hale TM, et al. Paget's disease of the vulva: prevalence of associated vulvar adenocarcinoma, invasive Paget's disease, and recurrence after surgical excision. *Am J Obstet Gynecol* 1999; 180:24–30.
308. Niikura H, Yoshida H, Ito K, et al. Paget's disease of the vulva: clinicopathologic study of type 1 cases treated at a single institution. *Int J Gynecol Cancer* 2006;16:1212–1215.
309. Kodama S, Kaneko T, Saito M, et al. A clinicopathologic study of 30 patients with Paget's disease of the vulva. *Gynecol Oncol* 1995;56:63–67.
310. Stacy D, Burrell MO, Franklin EW III. Extramammary Paget's disease of the vulva and anus: use of intraoperative frozen-section margins. *Am J Obstet Gynecol* 1986;155:519–524.
311. Pierie JP, Choudry U, Muzikansky A, et al. Prognosis and management of extramammary Paget's disease and the association with secondary malignancies. *J Am Coll Surg* 2003;196:45–49.
312. Black D, Tornos C, Soslow RA, et al. The outcomes of patients with positive margins after excision for intraepithelial Paget's disease of the vulva. *Gynecol Oncol* 2007;104:547–550.
313. Bergen S, DiSaia PJ, Liao SY, et al. Conservative management of extramammary Paget's disease of the vulva. *Gynecol Oncol* 1989;33:151–155.
314. Hays DM, Shimada H, Raney RB, et al. Clinical staging and treatment results in rhabdomyosarcoma of the female genital tract among children and adolescents. *Cancer* 1988;61:1893–1899.
315. Bell J, Averette H, Davis J, et al. Genital rhabdomyosarcoma: current management and review of the literature. *Obstet Gynecol Surv* 1986; 41:257–262.

CHAPTER 21 ■ VAGINA

HIGINIA R. CÁRDENES, JEANNE M. SCHILDER, AND LAWRENCE M. ROTH

ANATOMY

The vagina is a muscular dilatable tubular structure averaging 7.5 cm in length that extends from the cervix to the vulva. It lies dorsal to the bladder and urethra, and ventral to the rectum. The upper portion of the posterior wall is separated from the rectum by a reflection of peritoneum, the pouch of Douglas. The vaginal wall is composed of three layers: the mucosa, muscularis, and adventitia. The inner mucosal layer is formed by a thick, nonkeratinizing, stratified squamous epithelium overlying a basement membrane containing many papillae. The epithelium normally contains no glands but is lubricated by mucous secretions originating in the cervix. Beneath the mucosa lies a submucosal layer of elastin and a double muscularis layer, highly vascularized with a rich innervation and lymphatic drainage. The muscularis layer is composed of smooth muscle fibers, arranged circularly on the inner portion and longitudinally in the outer portion. A vaginal sphincter is formed by skeletal muscle at the introitus. The adventitia is a thin, outer connective tissue layer that merges with that of adjacent organs.

The proximal vagina is supplied by the vaginal artery branch from the uterine or cervical branch of the uterine artery. It runs along the lateral wall of the vagina and anastamoses with the inferior vesical and middle rectal arteries from the surrounding viscera (1). The accompanying venous plexus, running parallel to the arteries, ultimately drains to the internal iliac vein. The lumbar plexus and pudendal nerve, with branches from sacral roots 2 to 4, provide innervation to the vaginal vault (Fig. 21.1). The lymphatic drainage of the vagina is complex, consisting of an extensive intercommunicating network. Fine lymphatic vessels coursing through the submucosa and muscularis coalesce into small trunks running laterally along the walls of the vagina. The lymphatics in the upper portion of the vagina drain primarily via the lymphatics of the cervix; the upper anterior vagina drains along cervical channels to the interiliac and parametrial nodes; the posterior vagina drains into the inferior gluteal, presacral, and anorectal nodes. The distal vaginal lymphatics follow drainage patterns of the vulva into the inguinal and femoral nodes and from there to the pelvic nodes. Lymphatic flow from lesions in the mid vagina may drain either way (2). However, because of the presence of intercommunicating lymphatics along the terminal branches of the vaginal artery and near the vaginal wall, the external iliac nodes are at high risk even in lesions of the lower third of the vagina. Such a complex lymphatic drainage pattern has significant implications for therapeutic planning. Therefore, bilateral pelvic nodes should be considered to be at risk in any invasive vaginal carcinoma, and bilateral groin nodes should be considered to be at risk in those lesions involving the distal third of the vagina.

EPIDEMIOLOGY AND ETIOLOGIC RISK FACTORS

Primary vaginal cancer, defined as a lesion arising in the vagina without involvement of the cervix or vulva, is a rare entity, representing only 1% to 2% of all female genital neoplasias (3). Most vaginal neoplasms, 80% to 90%, represent metastasis from other primary gynecologic (cervix or vulva) and nongynecologic sites, involving the vagina by direct extension or lymphatic or hematogenous routes. Creasman et al. (4) published the National Cancer Data Base (NCDB) report in 1998, based on 4,885 patients with primary diagnosis of vaginal cancer registered from 1985 to 1994. Approximately 92% of the patients were diagnosed with *in situ* or invasive squamous cell carcinoma (SCC) or adenocarcinomas, 4% with melanomas, 3% with sarcomas, and 1% with other or unspecified types of cancer. In the NCDB report, invasive carcinomas accounted for 72% of the carcinoma cases, or 66% of all vaginal cancers. *In situ* carcinomas accounted for 28%, SCC represented 79% of invasive vaginal carcinomas, and adenocarcinomas represented 14%. Adenocarcinomas represent nearly all the carcinomas in patients younger than 20 years of age and are seen less frequently with advanced age (4).

Carcinoma of the vagina is considered to be associated with advanced age, with the peak incidence occurring in the sixth and seventh decades of life. However, vaginal cancer is increasingly being seen in younger women, possibly due to human papillomavirus (HPV) infection or other sexually transmitted diseases. Only about 10% of patients are 40 years of age or younger (5). In the NCDB report, only 1% of the carcinoma patients were less than 20 years old at the time of diagnosis, and over 80% of those patients had *in situ* lesions. As patient age increased, the number of invasive tumors increased, reaching a peak in patients aged 70 to 79 years. The percentage of *in situ* carcinomas decreased to only 11% in patients over 80 years old (4). A decrease in the incidence of primary vaginal tumors has been noted in recent years, possibly because of early detection with cervical cytology or more rigid diagnostic criteria, which have eliminated from this category primary cancers arising from adjacent organs, such as the cervix, vulva, or endometrium.

Vaginal Intraepithelial Neoplasia and Squamous Cell Carcinoma

Potential risk factors for SCC include prior history of HPV infection, cervical intraepithelial neoplasia (CIN), vulvar intraepithelial neoplasia (VIN), immunosuppression, and possibly previous pelvic irradiation. HPV is the likely etiologic agent of

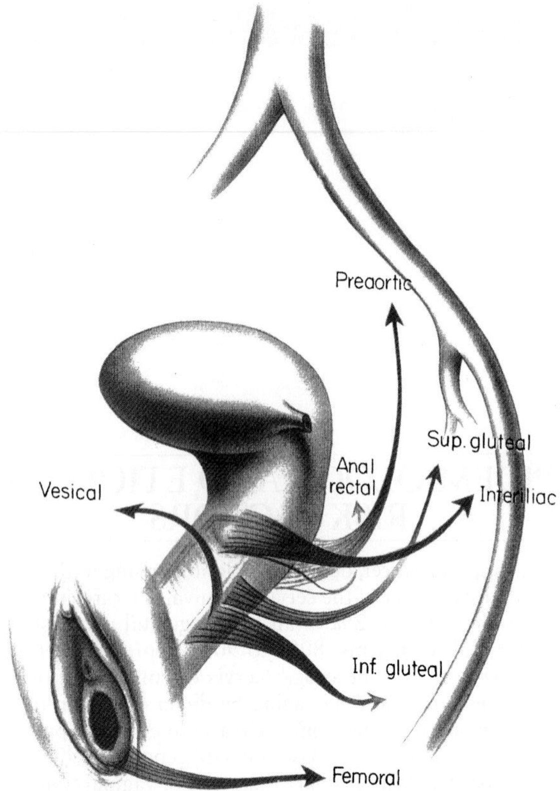

FIGURE 21.1. Lymphatic drainage of the vagina. *Source:* Reprinted from Plentl AA, Friedman EA. Lymphatic system of the female genitalia. In: Plentl AA, Friedman EA, eds. *The Morphologic Basis of Oncologic Diagnosis and Therapy*. Philadelphia: WB Saunders; 1971:55, Fig. 5-2. Used with permission.

SCC and its precursor lesion, vaginal intraepithelial neoplasia (VAIN). HPV has been recovered from 80% of VAIN lesions and 60% of invasive SCC of the vagina (6,7). In a case-control study of VAIN and early-stage cancer of the vagina, Brinton et al. (8) reported a 2.9-fold increase in therapy for genital warts and a 3.8-fold increase in prior abnormal Papanicolaou (Pap) smears in patients with VAIN compared to controls. This association likely represents the sequelae of infection with high-risk HPV strains (HPV-16, -18, -31, and -33) (9). The process most commonly occurs in the upper vagina, and it is frequently multifocal. Approximately one half of the lesions are associated with concomitant CIN or VIN (10).

In studies reporting on groups of women with VAIN and SCC of the vagina, the following risk factors have been identified: five or more sexual partners, sexual debut before age 17 years, smoking, low socioeconomic status, a history of genital warts, prior abnormal cytology, and prior hysterectomy (6–8). Weiderpass et al., in a population-based study of 36,856 women, found that alcoholic women had an excess risk for cancer of the vagina, probably related to higher incidence of HPV infection associated with lifestyle factors such as promiscuity, smoking, use of contraceptive hormones, and dietary deficiencies (11).

Patients with previous cervical carcinoma have a substantial risk of developing vaginal carcinoma, presumably because these sites share exposure and/or susceptibility to endogenous or exogenous carcinogenic stimuli. Ten percent to 50% of patients with VAIN–carcinoma *in situ* (CIS) or invasive carcinoma of the vagina have undergone prior hysterectomy or radiotherapy (RT) for CIS or invasive carcinoma of the cervix (12–23). The interval from therapy for cervical cancer or preinvasive disease to the development of carcinoma of the vagina averages nearly 14 years, but there have been cases with the vaginal primary manifesting 50 years after therapy for cervical cancer (15,24).

It is controversial as to whether or not prior pelvic RT is a risk factor. Boice et al. (25) reported a 14-fold increased risk of cancer of the vagina in previously irradiated women before the age of 45 years, and a dose-response relationship was found to be significant. However, Lee et al. (26) did not find prior RT to be associated with an increase in the incidence of pelvic second neoplasms. It is biologically plausible that there could be an apparent increase in risk given that prior pelvic RT would have likely been given for HPV-associated cervical carcinoma, and the antecedent HPV infection would increase the risk of SCC in the vagina. Such an association has led to the recommendation that patients treated for CIN or carcinoma of the cervix continue to undergo lifelong surveillance with vaginal cytologic evaluation even after hysterectomy (27). In addition, there is evidence that *in utero* exposure to diethylstilbestrol (DES) doubles the risk of development of VAIN. The putative mechanism is an enlargment of the transformation zone at risk, which is then at risk for infection with HPV (28).

Clear Cell Adenocarcinoma

An increased incidence of clear cell adenocarcinoma (CCA) of the vagina in young women related to *in utero* exposure to DES during the first 16 weeks of pregnancy was first reported in 1971 (29). Specific suggested mechanisms of carcinogenesis focus on the retention of nests of abnormal cells of müllerian duct origin, which, after stimulation by endogenous hormones during puberty, are promoted into adenocarcinomas. The median age at diagnosis in the DES-exposed patients is 19 years (29), whereas prior to this report, most patients with CCA of the vagina were elderly. The incidence of CCA in the exposed female population from birth to 34 years is estimated to be between 0.14 and 1.4 per 1,000. Approximately 90% of the patients had stage I-II disease at diagnosis (30,31). Hicks and Piver noted that 60% of CCA patients had been exposed to DES or similar agents *in utero*, that most cases involved the anterior upper third of the vaginal wall, and that DES-associated CCA cases had been reported from ages 7 to 34 (median, 19 years) (32). Fortunately, the incidence of this tumor has decreased in recent years, and may decrease even more since the practice of prescribing DES during pregnancy has been discontinued. Palmer et al. (33) assessed the influence of postnatal factors on the development of CCA in women exposed to DES in 244 cases compared with 244 age-matched non–DES-exposed women. Neither oral contraceptive use nor pregnancy was associated with risk of CCA (33).

Melanoma

Malignant melanoma is the second most common cancer of the vagina, accounting for 2.8% to 5% of all vaginal neoplasms (34–36). The most common location is the lower third and the anterior vaginal wall, although oftentimes it is multifocal (34–36). Trimble's examination of the Surveillance, Epidemiology, and End Results (SEER) data on 30,295 melanomas found 51 vaginal melanomas (0.3% of all melanomas), with an annual incidence of 0.026 per 100,000 and a median age at diagnosis of 66.3 years (37). In the NCDB report by Creasman et al. (4), vaginal melanomas represented 4% of primary vaginal cancers.

Sarcomas

Sarcomas represent 3% of primary vaginal cancers, and are most common in adults, with leiomyosarcoma representing 50% to 65% of vaginal sarcomas (4). Malignant mixed müllerian tumor (MMMT, carcinosarcoma), endometrial stromal sarcoma, and angiosarcoma are less common. Embryonal rhabdomyosarcoma (RMS)/sarcoma botryoides is a rare pediatric tumor. Prior pelvic RT is a risk factor, particularly for mixed mesodermal tumors and vaginal angiosarcomas (38). Unfortunately, most of the sarcomas are diagnosed at an advanced stage. Histopathologic grade appears to be the most important predictor of outcome (39).

NATURAL HISTORY

The majority (57% to 83%) of vaginal primaries occur in the upper third or at the apex of the vault, most commonly in the posterior wall; the lower third may be involved in as many as 31% of patients (15,21,40). Lesions confined to the middle third of the vagina are uncommon. The location of the vaginal carcinoma is an important consideration in planning therapy and determining prognosis. Vaginal tumors may spread along the vaginal walls to involve the cervix or the vulva. However, if biopsies of the cervix or the vulva are positive at the time of initial diagnosis, the tumor cannot be considered a primary vaginal lesion. A lesion on the anterior wall may infiltrate the vesicovaginal septum and/or the urethra; those on the posterior wall may eventually involve the rectovaginal septum and subsequently infiltrate the rectal mucosa. Lateral extension toward the parametrium and paracolpal tissues is not uncommon in more advanced stages of the disease.

The issue of regional nodal metastasis, both the incidence of occult nodal disease and the anatomic pathways of lymphatic spread, are somewhat controversial. Because the lymphatic system of the vagina is so complex, any of the nodal groups may be involved, regardless of the location of the lesion (2). Involvement of inguinal nodes is most common when the lesion is located in the lower third of the vagina. There does seem to be a significant risk of nodal metastasis for patients with disease beyond stage I. Although data on staging lymphadenectomy are sparse, two studies reported a significant incidence of nodal disease in early-stage vaginal carcinoma. In Al-Kurdi and Monaghan's series (41), the incidence of pelvic nodal metastasis was 14% and 32% for stages I and II, respectively, whereas in the Davis et al. series (24), the incidence was 6% and 26% for stages I and II, respectively. The incidence is expected to be higher for stage III, although no substantial data are available. Chyle et al. (14) noted a 10-year actuarial pelvic nodal failure rate of 28% and a 16% inguinal failure rate in patients who had local recurrence, in contrast to 4% and 2%, respectively, in the group without local recurrence ($P < 0.001$). The incidence of clinically positive inguinal nodes at diagnosis reported by several authors ranges from 5.3% to 20% (19,42).

Distant metastasis may occur, primarily in patients with advanced disease at presentation, or those who recurred after primary therapy. In the Perez et al. series (19), the incidence of distant metastasis was 16% in stage I, 31% in stage IIA, 46% in stage IIB, 62% in stage III, and 50% in stage IV. Robboy et al. reported that metastases to the lungs or supraclavicular lymph nodes represented 35% of recurrences in young women with CCA, a proportion much greater than found with squamous cell carcinoma of the cervix or vagina (43).

CLINICAL PRESENTATION

Vaginal Intraepithelial Neoplasia—Carcinoma *In Situ*

VAIN most often is asymptomatic (17). In modern practice, VAIN is usually detected by cytologic evaluation performed following hysterectomy as part of a surveillance strategy in patients with a history of CIN or invasive cervical carcinoma. In these cases, VAIN has a predilection for involvement of the upper vagina, likely secondary to a "field effect." A discharge may be present, but is likely secondary to superimposed vaginal infections. It should be noted that evidence-based guidelines do not support routine cytologic studies following hysterectomy for noncervical pathology. The American Cancer Society released guidelines in 2002 that said surveillance cytology in such patients is *not* necessary. Rather, surveillance cytology posthysterectomy should be limited to those patients with a prior history of CIN or invasive cervix cancer (44).

Invasive Squamous Cell Carcinoma

In patients with invasive disease, irregular vaginal bleeding, often postcoital, is the most common presenting symptom followed by vaginal discharge and dysuria. Pelvic pain is a relatively late symptom generally related to tumor extent beyond the vagina (15,40). In a series of 84 patients with invasive carcinoma, including 55 with SCC, Tjalma et al. noted that 62% of patients had vaginal discharge, 16% had positive cytology, 13% had a mass, 4% had pain, and 2% had dysuria. Forty-seven percent of the lesions were located on the posterior wall and 24% on the anterior wall; 29% had involvement of both walls (45). In 10% to 20%, no symptoms were reported, and the diagnosis was made by cytologic examination (45).

Other Histologies

The most common presenting symptom in patients with CCA is vaginal bleeding (50% to 75%) or abnormal discharge. More advanced cases may present with dysuria or pelvic pain (29). Cytology is abnormal in only 33% of cases. Therefore, in addition to four-quadrant cytology, Hanselaar et al. recommended palpation of the entire vaginal vault to assess for submucosal irregularity (46). The majority of CCA lesions are exophytic, superficially invasive in the upper third of the vault near the cervix. Ninety-seven percent will be associated with mucosal adenosis (47–49).

Embryonal RMS, the most common malignant vaginal tumor in children, presents as a protruding, edematous grape-like mass. Ninety percent of these sarcomas present before the age of 5 years. The average age at presentation was 23.5 months in the Maurer et al. series (50). In adults, symptoms most commonly noted were pain accompanied by a mass.

DIAGNOSTIC WORKUP

In general, in patients with suspected vaginal malignancy, thorough physical examination with detailed speculum inspection, digital palpation, colposcopic and cytologic evaluation, and biopsy constitute the most effective procedure for diagnosing primary, metastatic, or recurrent carcinoma of the vagina. In symptomatic patients, biopsy of any abnormal exophytic or endophytic lesion noted at the time of the examination is indicated. Examination under anesthesia is recommended for the thoroughness of evaluation of all of the vaginal walls and local extent of the disease, primarily if the patient is in great discomfort because of advanced disease, in order to obtain a biopsy. Biopsies of the cervix, if present, are recommended to rule out a primary cervical tumor. The speculum must be rotated as it is slowly withdrawn from the vaginal fornix, so that the total vaginal mucosa may be visualized, and, in particular, posterior wall lesions, which occur frequently, are not overlooked.

The patient with a history of preinvasive or invasive carcinoma of the cervix found to have abnormal cytology following prior hysterectomy or RT should be offered vaginoscopy with application of acetic acid to the entire vault, followed by biopsies as indicated by areas of white epithelium, mosaicism, punctation, or atypical vascularity. It can be very helpful for the menopausal patient or the patient previously irradiated to use a short course of topically applied estrogen into the vaginal vault once or twice a week for 1 month prior to the colposcopy in order to foster epithelial maturation. Another method of identifying the area(s) most in need of biopsy would be, after application of acetic acid, to apply half-strength Schiller's iodine to determine if the Schiller-positive (non-staining) areas correspond with the involved areas identified following acetic acid application.

STAGING

At present, primary malignancies of the vagina are all staged clinically. In addition to a complete history and physical examination, routine laboratory evaluations including complete blood cell count (CBC) with differential and platelets, and assessment of renal and hepatic function should be undertaken. In order to determine the extent of disease, the following tests are allowed by International Federation of Gynecology and Obstetrics (FIGO) criteria: chest radiograph, a thorough bimanual and rectovaginal examination, cystoscopy, proctoscopy, and intravenous pyelogram. Cystoscopy and/or proctosigmoidoscopy should be performed on patients with symptoms suggestive of bladder and/or rectal infiltration, respectively. If the patient is in significant discomfort the examination should be conducted under anesthesia, preferably by a radiation oncologist and gynecologic oncologist who will be involved in her ongoing care. However, it can be difficult even for the experienced examiner to differentiate between disease confined to the mucosa (stage I) and disease spread to the submucosa (stage II) (13,40).

Pelvic computed tomography (CT) scan is generally performed to evaluate inguinofemoral and/or pelvic lymph nodes, as well as extent of local disease. In patients with vaginal melanoma or sarcoma, chest, abdomen, and pelvic CT scans are often part of the workup. Magnetic resonance imaging (MRI) has emerged as a potentially important imaging modality in the evaluation of vaginal cancers, predominantly the T1-weighted with contrast and T2-weighted images (51). An additional role of MRI is differentiation of tumor from fibrotic tissue in patients with suspected recurrent vaginal carcinoma (51). Positron emission tomography (PET) is evolving as a modality of potential use in the evaluation of vaginal cancer that allows detection of the extent of the primary as well as abnormal lymph nodes more often than does CT scan (52). In modern practice, for the majority of patients with disease volume and/or location requiring definitive RT to achieve cure, therapeutic planning will be guided by disease volume assessment utilizing CT, MRI, and/or PET/CT, even though such radiologic modalities are not "allowed" for purposes of staging.

The two commonly used staging systems for carcinoma of the vagina are the FIGO (Table 21.1A) (53) and the American Joint Commission on Cancer (TNM) (Table 21.1B) (54) classifications. According to FIGO guidelines, patients with tumor involvement of the cervix or vulva should be classified as primary cervical or vulvar cancers, respectively. Patients with abnormal vaginal cytology are susceptible to a "field effect," that is, dysplasia of the urogenital epithelium, including the cervix and vulva. Therefore, cervical cytology should be obtained, and directed biopsies if indicated based on abnormal cytology. If a cervical abnormality is visualized or palpated, biopsy is recommended to rule out a primary cervical malignancy. Similarly, the vulva should be carefully inspected, including application of acetic acid, with directed biopsies of abnormally staining epithelium. Perez et al. (55) proposed in 1973 that FIGO stage II vaginal cancer should be subdivided

TABLE 21.1A

FIGO STAGING SYSTEM FOR CARCINOMA OF THE VAGINA

Stage	Description
Stage 0	Carcinoma *in situ*, intraepithelial neoplasia grade 3
Stage I	Limited to the vaginal wall
Stage II	Involvement of the subvaginal tissue but without extension to the pelvic side wall
Stage III	Extension to the pelvic side wall
Stage IV	Extension beyond the true pelvis or involvement of the bladder or rectal mucosa. Bullous edema as such does not permit a case to be allotted to stage IV
IVA	Spread to adjacent organs and/or direct extension beyond the true pelvis
IVB	Spread to distant organs

Source: From Pecorelli S, Beller U, Heintz AP, et al. FIGO annual report on the results of treatment in gynecologic cancer. *J Epidemiol Biostat* 2000;24:56–60.

TABLE 21.1B

AMERICAN JOINT COMMISSION ON CANCER (AJCC) STAGING OF VAGINAL CANCER

PRIMARY TUMOR (T)	
Tx	Primary tumor cannot be assessed
T0	No evidence of primary tumor
Tis/0	Carcinoma *in situ*
T1/I	Tumor confined to the vagina
T2/II	Tumor invades paravaginal tissues but not to the pelvic wall
T3/III	Tumor extends to the pelvic wall
T4/IVA	Tumor invades mucosa of the bladder or rectum and/or extends beyond the pelvis (bullous edema is not sufficient to classify a tumor as T4)
REGIONAL LYMPH NODES (N)	
Nx	Regional lymph nodes cannot be assessed
N0	No regional lymph nodes
N1/IVB	Pelvic or inguinal lymph node metastasis
DISTANT METASTASIS (M)	
Mx	Distant metastasis cannot be assessed
M0	No distant metastasis
M1/IVB	Distant metastasis
AJCC STAGE GROUPINGS	
Stage 0	Tis N0 M0
Stage I	T1 N0 M0
Stage II	T2 N0 M0
Stage III	T1-3 N1 M0, T3 N0 M0
Stage IVA	T4, any N, M0
Stage IVB	Any T, any N, M1

Source: American Joint Committee on Cancer (AJCC). Vagina. In: Greene FL, Page DL, Fleming ID, et al., eds. *AJCC Cancer Staging Manual*. 6th ed. New York: Springer-Verlag; 2002:251–257.

into stage IIA (tumor infiltrating the subvaginal tissues but not extending into the parametrium) and stage IIB (tumor infiltrating the parametrium but not extending to pelvic side walls). However, most investigators do not use this classification, and there are few published data to support it (19,56).

PATHOLOGIC CLASSIFICATION

The most common malignant tumor of the vagina is squamous cell carcinoma. Other epithelial neoplasms are uncommon since glands are not normally present in the vaginal mucosa. Melanoma is the second most frequent malignancy. A wide variety of tumors of other types have been described. The classification of neoplasms of the vagina is shown in Table 21.2.

Squamous Cell Carcinoma

SCC represents about 80% to 90% of primary vaginal cancers. These tumors occur in older women and are most often located in the upper, posterior wall of the vagina. According to the FIGO recommendations, a tumor of the vagina that involves the cervix or vulva should be classified as a primary cervical or vulvar cancer, respectively. Additionally, for a neoplasm to be considered a vaginal primary, there must not have been a cervical cancer for 5 years prior to the diagnosis (57). It may be difficult or impossible histologically to distinguish a primary vaginal SCC from recurrent cervical or vulvar disease. Histologically, keratinizing, nonkeratinizing, basaloid, warty, and verrucous variants have been described. Tumors may also be graded as being well, moderately, or poorly differentiated, based on a combination of cytologic and histologic features. However, there is little correlation between tumor grade and survival (3). Most cases are moderately differentiated and nonkeratinizing. Well-differentiated tumors show prominent keratin or squamous pearl formation and intercellular bridges (Fig. 21.2). Rarely, poorly differentiated tumors have a spindle-cell appearance. Warty SCC has a papillary appearance with hyperkeratosis and koilocytosis.

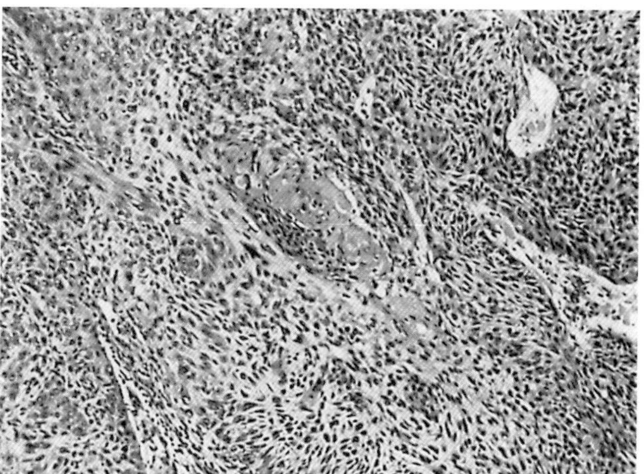

FIGURE 21.2. Well-differentiated vaginal squamous cell carcinoma with focal keratinization (center). *Source:* Courtesy of Dr. Deborah J. Gersell, St. Louis, Missouri, USA.

TABLE 21.2

HISTOLOGIC CLASSIFICATION OF MALIGNANCIES OF THE VAGINA

SQUAMOUS TUMORS AND PRECURSORS
Squamous cell carcinoma
Vaginal intraepithelial neoplasia 3/squamous cell carcinoma *in situ*

GLANDULAR TUMORS
Clear cell adenocarcinoma
Endometrioid adenocarcinoma
Mucinous adenocarcinoma
Serous adenocarcinoma

OTHER EPITHELIAL TUMORS
Adenosquamous carcinoma
Adenoid cystic carcinoma
Neuroendocrine carcinoma

MESENCHYMAL TUMORS
Sarcoma botyroides (embryonal rhabdomyosarcoma)
Leiomyosarcoma
Endometrioid stromal sarcoma (low grade)
Undifferentiated vaginal sarcoma

MIXED EPITHELIAL AND MESENCHYMAL TUMORS
Carcinosarcoma (malignant müllerian mixed tumor, metaplastic carcinoma)
Adenosarcoma
Malignant mixed tumor
Mesonephric carcinosarcoma

MISCELLANEOUS TUMORS
Melanoma
Yolk sac tumor (endodermal sinus tumor)
Peripheral primitive neuroectodermal tumor/Ewing tumor

LYMPHOID AND HEMATOPOETIC TUMORS
Malignant lymphoma (specify type)
Leukemia (specify type)

Verrucous carcinoma is a rare distinct variant of well-differentiated SCC, usually with the appearance of a large, well-circumscribed, soft, cauliflower-like mass. Microscopically, the tumor exhibits a papillary growth pattern, pushing borders, bulbous pegs of acanthotic epithelium with little or no atypia, and surface maturation in the form of parakeratosis and hyperkeratosis without koilocytosis. Because of its well-differentiated character, the histologic diagnosis of verrucous carcinoma may be difficult, especially if the biopsy is superficial (58). Verrucous carcinoma may recur locally after surgery, but rarely, if ever, metastasizes. This behavioral difference justifies separating verrucous carcinoma as a distinct tumor entity.

VAIN is a precursor of SCC and is graded from 1 to 3 depending upon the degree of nuclear atypia and crowding and the proportion of the epithelium involved. VAIN 1 typically involves the lower third to one half of the epithelium, VAIN 2 one half to two thirds the thickness of the epithelium, and VAIN 3 more than three fourths of the thickness. Alternatively, VAIN can be classified as low or high grade. High grade lesions indicate involvement of the outer third of the mucosa, and include CIS, which encompasses the entire thickness of the epithelium. The true incidence of VAIN and its rate of progression to invasive carcinoma are unknown, ranging in several series from 9% to 28% (8,10,59). High-risk HPV was found in 35% of VAIN 1 and 94% of VAIN 3 lesions (60). Comparison of the distribution of HPV types in the vagina, vulva, and cervix suggests that VAIN is more closely related to CIN than to VIN. A large epidemiologic study showed a two-fold relative risk for high-grade CIN and VAIN among women exposed prenatally to DES when compared to an unexposed control group (61).

Clear Cell Adenocarcinoma and Vaginal Adenosis

DES-associated CCA has a predilection for the upper third of the vagina and the exocervix. It is frequently located at or near the lower margin of the zone of glandular tissue in the vagina or cervix. Most CCAs are exophytic and superficially invasive (47). Ninety-seven percent will be associated with mucosal adenosis (47–49). CCA is arranged in tubulocystic, solid, papillary, or mixed cell patterns, and is mainly composed of clear and hobnail-shaped cells (Fig. 21.3A, B). The clear cells are cuboidal or columnar with abundant glycogen-rich cytoplasm and distinct cell membranes. The hobnail cells have large atypical protruding nuclei rimmed by a small amount of cytoplasm (47).

Vaginal adenosis is a condition in which müllerian-type glandular epithelium is present after vaginal development is complete. Although adenosis is the most common histologic abnormality in women exposed to DES *in utero*, it is not strictly confined to this population. Adenosis is associated with 97% of vaginal and 52% of cervical CCAs (62,63). The glandular epithelium may replace the surface epithelium and/or form glands in the superficial stroma. The glandular epithelium undergoes progressive squamous metaplasia (62–65) and ultimately only stromal nodules or pegs of immature squamous epithelium containing small mucin droplets may remain (65). A few CCAs have been detected among women under surveillance for adenosis (66). Atypical adenosis of tuboendometrial type appears to be a precursor lesion of CCA (49). Whether immature squamous metaplasia in adenosis is associated with an increased risk of vaginal intraepithelial neoplasia or SCC is controversial (66). Rarely, clear cell adenocarcinoma of the vagina occurs in older women unrelated to DES exposure *in utero*, but sometimes in association with vaginal endometriosis (67,68). The major determinant of outcome in CCA is stage, but some pathologic features are statistically associated with better outcome, including a tubulocystic growth pattern, size less than 3 cm^2, and less than 3 mm of stromal invasion (47).

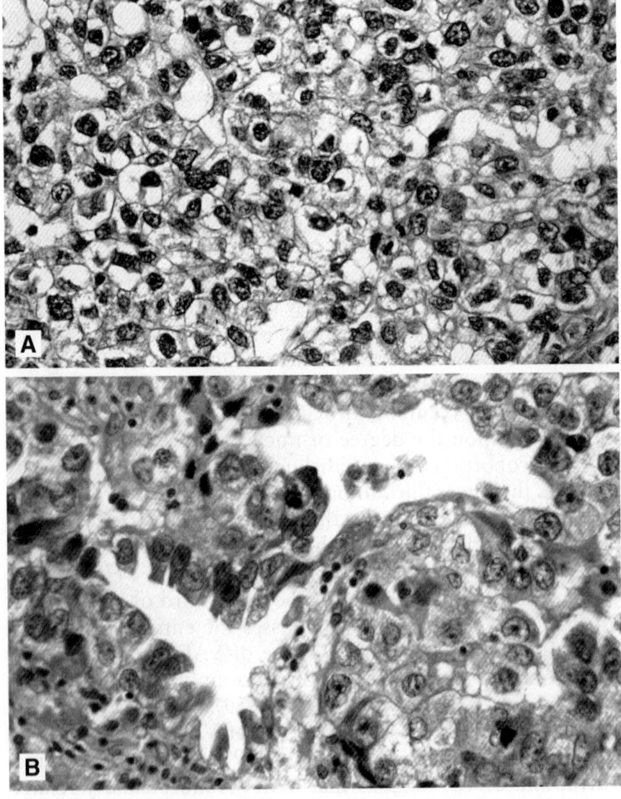

FIGURE 21.3. Clear cell adenocarcinoma. **A:** Neoplasm shows a solid growth pattern. Note the tumor cells with pleomorphic nuclei, clear cytoplasm, and distinct cell borders. **B:** Tumor has tubulocystic growth pattern with prominent hobnail cells lining the tubules.

Other Adenocarcinomas

Primary adenocarcinoma of the vagina is rare and occurs predominantly in postmenopausal women. Reported histologic subtypes have included endometrioid, mucinous, mesonephric, and papillary serous adenocarcinomas. Only a few cases of *mucinous adenocarcinoma* have been described (69). Histologically, the tumors can resemble typical endocervical adenocarcinoma and arise in endocervicosis (70,71). Cases of primary intestinal-type adenocarcinoma can be mistaken for metastatic colonic carcinoma and rarely arise from tubular adenoma (72,73). Some cases may be related to DES exposure (74). A relationship to vaginal adenosis has been described in a patient not exposed to DES (75). Rare cases of mucinous adenocarcinoma have been described in neovaginas (76).

Endometrioid adenocarcinoma of the vagina usually arises in endometriosis (77). *Mesonephric adenocarcinoma* is a rare variant that may arise from mesonephric duct remnants that are mostly situated deep in the lateral walls of the vagina (78). Primary *serous adenocarcinoma* of the vagina has rarely been reported (79). *Vaginal metastases* from adenocarcinoma of the breast, other gynecologic primaries, or renal cell carcinomas have been described (80).

Melanoma

Melanoma is the second most common cancer of the vagina, accounting for 2.8% to 5.0% of vaginal neoplasms. The most common locations are the lower third and the anterior vaginal wall (34–36,81). Grossly, these tumors are typically pigmented, and show considerable variation in size, color, and growth patterns, being polypoid or nodular in the majority of cases (35,36). Histologically, melanoma is composed of epithelioid cells, spindle cells, or nevus-like cells; melanin pigment is often observed. Junctional activity is usually present. Premelanosomes may be identified by electron microscopy. Immunohistochemical stains are frequently positive for S100 protein. HMB-45, and melan-A tyrosinase and MART-1 are useful markers when S100 is negative or only focally positive (81). Tumor thickness correlates with prognosis, and may be measured by the method of Breslow (82). Poorly differentiated melanomas may be difficult to distinguish from sarcoma or SCC. Primary melanoma must also be distinguished from metastatic melanoma, which also presents as a polypoid mass (83).

Mesenchymal Tumors

Embryonal rhabdomyosarcoma (RMS) is a rare pediatric tumor. The botryoid variant, or sarcoma botryoides, is the most common malignant vaginal tumor in infants and children (84). Ninety percent of cases occur in children younger than 5 years of age. Sarcoma botyroides has a characteristic macroscopic appearance consisting of multiple gray-red, translucent, edematous, grape-like masses that fill the vagina, and may protrude from it. Microscopically, there is a zone of condensed round or spindle cells (the cambium layer) immediately beneath the intact vaginal epithelium. Elsewhere, the

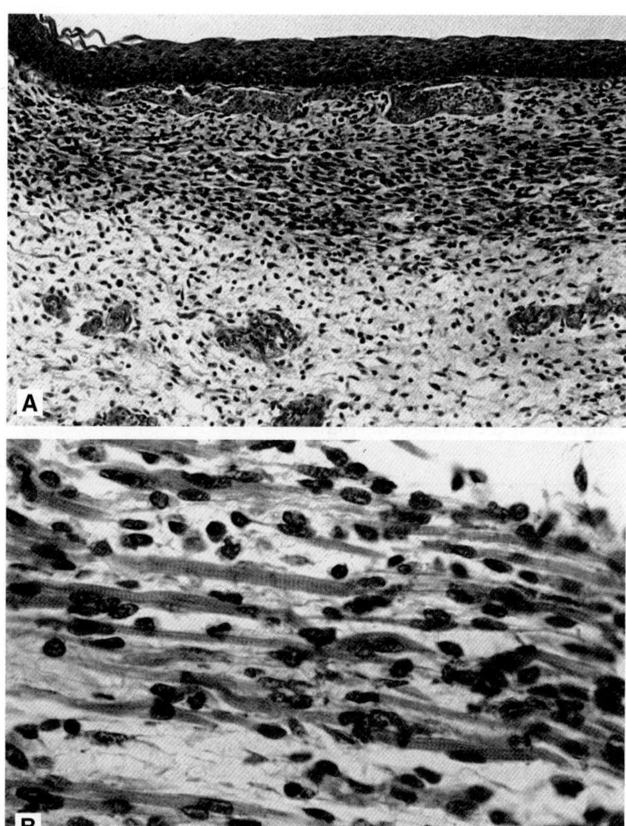

FIGURE 21.4. Embryonal rhabdomyosarcoma (sarcoma botyroides). A: Note the subepithelial cambium layer. B: The tumor is composed of strap cells with atypical, elongated, often tandem, nuclei and edematous stroma. The eosinophilic cytoplasm shows prominent cross striations.

tumor is composed of small, dark, spindle-shaped cells sparsely distributed in a myxoid stroma. Some cells may show skeletal muscle differentiation, evidenced by intensely eosinophilic cytoplasm with cross striations (Fig.21.4A, B). Immunohistochemical stains with antibodies directed against myogenic markers, including actin, desmin, myoD1, or myogenin, facilitate the recognition of muscle differentiation in these tumors.

Leiomyosarcoma is the most common vaginal sarcoma in adults (85). The frequency and behavior are uncertain because of the variable histologic criteria used to distinguish benign and malignant smooth muscle tumors. Smooth muscle tumors 3 cm or greater in diameter have an increased risk of recurrence. It is currently recommended that neoplasms with five or greater mitoses per ten high-power fields (HPFs), moderate or marked cytologic atypia, and/or infiltrating margins be classified as leiomyosarcoma (86). Although they may originate in any part of the vagina, most are submucosal. The macroscopic appearance varies greatly depending on cellularity, type, and extent of degenerative change and the amount of necrosis and hemorrhage (86). On histologic examination, leiomyosarcoma is typically composed of interlacing bundles of spindle-shaped cells with blunt-ended nuclei and fibrillar cytoplasm. An epithelioid pattern or extensive myxoid change occurs uncommonly (86,87). Because smooth muscle tumors vary from area to area, adequate sampling (one block, 1 to 2 cm of tumor diameter) is essential for accurate diagnosis. Rarely, cases of extragastrointestinal stromal tumors present as a vulvovaginal or rectovaginal septal mass (88). Histologically, they can be confused with benign or malignant smooth muscle tumors. Misdiagnosis can lead to inappropriate treatment, whereas specific therapy is available.

Other sarcomas that may occur in the vagina include *endometrioid stromal sarcoma*, which may arise in endometriosis (89–91); *alveolar soft part sarcoma* (92); *malignant fibrous histiocytoma* (93), a biphasic tumor interpreted as resembling synovial sarcoma (94) or *malignant mixed tumor* (95); angiosarcoma (38); *malignant peripheral nerve sheath tumor*; and *hemangiopericytoma* (96).

Malignant Lymphoma and Leukemia

Malignant lymphoma may be localized to the female genital tract or occur there as part of a widespread disease process (97,98). Approximately 6% of female genital tract lymphomas occur in the vagina and over 80% were primary in one study (99). The majority of primary lymphomas involving the vagina are of the diffuse large B-cell type, but lymphoplasmacytic, Burkitt lymphoma, and mucosa-associated lymphoid tissue (MALT) lymphoma also occur (100). The histologic diagnosis depends on the identification of monomorphous, cytologically atypical, mitotically active lymphoid cells deeply penetrating the stroma. Characteristically, the mucosa is intact. The tumors typically express CD20. Patients with vaginal lymphomas characteristically present with vaginal bleeding. Those with primary lymphomas also have a mass on clinical examination. Leukemic infiltrates, especially granulocytic sarcoma, can be histologically impossible to distinguish from lymphoma. Chloracetate esterase or myeloperoxidase stains may be helpful in some cases.

Uncommon Vaginal Tumors

Neuroendocrine small cell carcinoma may occur in the vagina either in pure form or associated with squamous or glandular elements (101,102). A high proportion of these tumors show immunohistochemical or ultrastructural evidence of neuroendocrine differentiation (103). Rarely, primary neuroendocrine carcinoma of the vagina has a Merkel cell carcinoma phenotype (104).

Adenosquamous carcinoma is an uncommon neoplasm of the vagina composed of an admixture of glandular and squamous elements (105). Tumors diagnosed as *carcinosarcoma* (malignant mixed müllerian tumor) of the female genital tract appear to be metaplastic carcinomas, and should be treated as epithelial neoplasms, although the prognosis is poor. This tumor is rare in the vagina, and typically occurs in postmenopausal women (106). Uncommonly, *yolk sac tumor* (endodermal sinus tumor) has been reported in the vagina of infants and young children (107,108). Rare cases of mesonephric adenocarcinoma or malignant mixed mesonephric tumor have been described (109). Rare cases of primary vaginal Ewing's sarcoma–primitive neuroectodermal tumor occur in younger women (110).

PROGNOSTIC FACTORS INFLUENCING CHOICE OF TREATMENT

Invasive Squamous Cell Carcinoma

As with most primaries, stage of disease is the dominant prognostic factor in terms of ultimate outcome (14,16,18,19,42, 111–118). In a report by Creasman et al., the 5-year survival rate was 96% for patients with stage 0, 73% for stage I, 58% for stage II, and 36% for those with stage III-IV disease, respectively (4). In the Perez et al. series including 165 patients with primary vaginal carcinomas treated with definitive RT, the 10-year actuarial disease-free survival (DFS) was 94% for stage 0, 75% for stage I, 55% for stage IIA, 43% for stage IIB, 32% for stage III, and 0% for those with stage IV disease (19).

The impact of lesion location has been controversial. Tarraza et al. (119) reported that upper-third lesions develop local recurrences more frequently, and lower-third lesions develop a disproportionate number of sidewall and distant recurrences. Chyle et al. (14) observed a 17% rate of pelvic relapse in patients with upper vaginal tumors, 36% in those with middle or lower vaginal tumors, and 42% with whole-vaginal involvement. However, a larger series failed to note any difference in site of recurrence based on primary lesion location (19). Several investigators (14,23,120,121) have shown better survival and decreased recurrence rates for patients with cancers involving the proximal half of the vagina when compared with those in the distal half or those involving the entire length of the vagina. In addition, lesions of the posterior wall have a worse prognosis than those involving other vaginal walls (10-year recurrence rates of 32% and 19%, respectively) (14), which probably reflects the greater difficulty of performing adequate brachytherapy procedures in this location.

The prognostic importance of lesion size has been controversial, with an adverse impact being noted by Tjalma et al. (45) and Chyle et al. (14) , which is contrary to the findings of Perez et al. (42). In the Chyle et al. series (14), lesions measuring less than 5 cm in maximum diameter had a 20% 10-year local recurrence rate compared to 40% for those lesions larger than 5 cm. Similarly, in the Princess Margaret Hospital experience, tumors larger than 4 cm in diameter fared significantly worse than smaller lesions (16). In the Perez et al. series (42), stage was an important predictor of pelvic tumor control and 5-year disease-free survival, but the size of the tumor in stage I patients was not a significant prognostic factor. However, in stage IIA disease, lower pelvic tumor control and survival were noted with tumors larger than 4 cm. In stages IIB and III, tumor size was not a significant prognostic factor, probably related to the difficulty in assessing size and the fact that higher doses of RT were delivered for larger tumors. Stock et al. (21) reported that disease volume, a likely surrogate for stage or lesion size, adversely impacted survival as well as local control.

Age was a significant prognostic factor in the Urbanski et al. series (23), with 5-year survival of 63.2% for patients below the age of 60 years compared with 25% for those over 60 years of age ($p < 0.001$). Similar findings were reported by Eddy et al. (115). However, most of these series do not correct for death secondary to intercurrent disease in the elderly population. No statistical significance of age to survival was found in the series of Dixit et al. (116) and Perez et al. (42).

With regard to the histologic type and grade, several series (16,23,121) have shown the histologic grade to be an independent, significant predictor of survival. Chyle et al. (14) noted a higher incidence of local recurrence in patients with adenocarcinoma compared with squamous cell carcinoma (52% and 20%, respectively, at 10 years), as well as a higher incidence of distant metastases (48% and 10%, respectively), and lower 10-year survival rate (20% vs 50%). Overexpression of *HER2/neu* oncogenes in squamous cancer of the lower genital tract is a rare event that may be associated with aggressive biologic behavior (122). Waggoner et al. (123), in a group of 21 women with CCA of the vagina and cervix, observed a more favorable prognosis in gynecologic tumors with an overexpression of wild-type p53 protein than in tumors containing mutated *TP53* genes.

Other Histologies

An increased propensity for distant metastases to the lung and supraclavicular nodes has been reported in patients with CCA (43). Stage, tubulocystic pattern, size less than 3 cm, and depth of invasion less than 3 mm were all noted to be associated with superior survival (47).

Vaginal melanoma has a higher propensity for development of distant metastases, and affected patients do more poorly than patients with SCC. A review by Reid et al. of 115 vaginal melanoma patients noted that depth of invasion and size of lesion (>3 cm) adversely impacted survival, but stage did not, perhaps because it was known for only 42 of the 115 patients in the series (36).

Patients with malignant mesenchymal tumors of the vagina do less well than those with invasive SCC. Specific, adverse prognostic factors for vaginal sarcoma identified by Tavassoli and Norris (86) included infiltrative versus pushing borders, high mitotic rate of five or more mitoses per ten HPFs, size >3 cm in diameter, and cytologic atypia.

GENERAL MANAGEMENT: TREATMENT OPTIONS AND OUTCOME BY FIGO STAGES

Owing to its rarity, data concerning the natural history, prognostic factors, and treatment of vaginal carcinoma derive from small, retrospective studies. Most of the currently available literature in terms of radiotherapeutic and surgical techniques refers to primary SCC of the vagina. It is important to recognize the complexity of the management of patients with carcinoma of the vagina and the need for an individualized approach after careful assessment by the gynecologic oncologist and radiation oncologist. In most patients, the primary treatment modality is RT, as reported by the Society of Gynecologist Oncologists in practice guidelines published in 1998 (4). RT provides excellent tumor control in early and superficial lesions and with satisfactory functional results.

Local excision and partial and complete vaginectomy have given way to a more individualized approach that takes into consideration the patient's age, the extent of the lesion, and whether it is localized or multicentric. There is evidence that patients with CIS-VAIN and early stage I, primarily with a lesion located in the upper or distal third of the vagina, and highly selected young women with stage II vaginal cancers can be successfully treated with surgery alone (13,21,24,45,124,125). In addition, surgery could be considered in younger patients with a desire to preserve ovarian function (126) and/or a functional vagina (21), patients with verrucous carcinoma (58), those with nonepithelial tumors, and patients with localized pelvic failures after radiation. For the most part, surgical resection often requires a radical approach resulting in urinary and fecal diversion in order to secure adequate margins. Given the potentially devastating functional results often associated with radical surgery, definitive RT has largely replaced surgery as primary therapeutic modality in patients with vaginal cancer, in order to maximize cure and improve quality of life. Furthermore, most patients are elderly, and a radical surgical approach is often not feasible.

Despite the acceptance of RT as the treatment of choice for this disease, the optimal therapy for each stage is not well defined in the literature. A combination of limited surgery and RT has been suggested to improve outcome, although the complication rates my increase (127). Intracavitary and interstitial irradiation is used in small superficial stage I disease. External beam RT (EBRT) in combination with intracavitary (ICB), and/or interstitial (ITB) brachytherapy is generally used for more extensive stage I-II disease. Data regarding the use of cytotoxic therapy in vaginal carcinomas are based on underpowered phase II trials of various monotherapies or extrapolated from SCC of the cervix, which has a similar biology.

FIGO Stage 0: Vaginal Intraepithelial Neoplasia–Carcinoma *In Situ*

VAIN has been approached both surgically and medically by multiple investigators. Treatment options range from partial or complete vaginectomy to more conservative approaches such as local excision, electro-coagulation, laser vaporization, topical 5% fluorouracil (5-FU) administration, or ICB. For patients in whom invasive disease cannot be ruled out, as well as for those who fail conservative therapy, surgical resection remains the treatment of choice. Overall, the reported control rates are very similar among the different approaches, ranging from 48% to 100% for laser, 52% to 100% for colpectomy, 75% to 100% for topical 5-FU, and 83% to 100% for RT (Table 21.3) (4,14,16,42,124,125,128–134). The degree of VAIN and the age and general health of the patient are important treatment considerations. A therapy appropriate for CIS in a woman with good performance status and many anticipated years of life expectancy may not be appropriate for a woman with multiple comorbid conditions who may succumb to one of her other illnesses before the CIS would be expected to progress to invasive carcinoma.

The anatomic constraints posed by the location of the vagina with the close proximity of the bladder and rectum led to the use of the CO_2 laser as a relatively noninvasive surgical approach (59,128). Data published by Hoffman et al. (124), who performed upper colpectomy in 32 patients, of whom 31 had undergone prior hysterectomy and 14 prior therapy for VAIN, and found a 28% risk of invasive disease, in addition to reports of invasive disease in the laser failures, and in patients who had undergone upper colpectomy for presumed VAIN, prompted some to begin to use the laser to effect colpectomy (128). Later series have used novel approaches with the Cavitron ultrasonic aspirator (CUSA) (133) to effect partial colpectomy with satisfactory results, at least in the reporting investigator's hands. In a series of 52 patients reported by Diakomanolis et al., in which 28 underwent laser and 24 had partial colpectomy, results were found to be operator dependent, but they favored partial colpectomy for unifocal disease and laser ablation for multifocal disease (135). Overall, the control rates following laser vaporization range from 58% to 100% (59,128). Patients most likely to fail after vaporization are those with anatomic distortion caused by scarring (124). In general, patient acceptance is high and scarring minimal (136).

Even though partial colpectomy has many advocates for focal VAIN without any prior history of pelvic RT, patients who had received prior pelvic RT for other gynecologic malignancies, wherein partial colpectomy would have high risk of fistula formation, may benefit from a medical approach with topical application of 5-FU. This acts by inciting a desquamation of the vaginal squamous epithelium, which later re-epithelializes with presumably normal cells. Multiple schedules have been suggested since the first use of 5-FU, including monthly, daily, twice a day, and weekly administrations, with control rates

TABLE 21.3

VAIN—CARCINOMA *IN SITU*: TREATMENT APPROACH AND RESULTS

Treatment modality, author(s)	No. of patients	Comments	Outcome—control
LASER THERAPY			
Julian et al. (128)	10	Used to effect colpectomy	80%
Hoffman et al. (59)	26	3 of 11 failures had invasive disease Recommended excision. Not ideal	58%
TOPICAL 5-FU			
Woodruff et al. (129)	9	1% to 2% 5-FU q month	88%
Piver et al. (130)	8	20% 5-FU bid × 5 days Could use 5% or 10%	75%
Petrilli et al. (131)	15	5% 5-FU bid × 5 days Repeat in 12 weeks	80%
Krebbs (132)	31	One-third applicator q week × 10 weeks	81%
SURGICAL EXCISION			
Creasman et al. (NCDB) (4)	23		96%
Fanning et al. (125)	15	Used LEEP, 1 patient had cancer	100%
Robinson et al. (133)	46	CUSA—29 primaries CUSA—17 recurrent	66% 52%
Hoffman et al. (124)	32	28% invasive cancer out of 23 with VAIN	83%
IRRADIATION			
Chyle et al. (14)	37		83%
Kirkbride et al. (16)	14		100%
Perez et al. (134)	20		94%

Note: 5-FU, 5-fluorouracil; bid, twice a day; CUSA, Cavitron ultrasonic aspirator; LEEP, loop electrosurgical excision procedure; NCDB, National Cancer Data Base.

ranging from 75% to 88% (129,130,132,137). However, we prefer the schedule suggested by Krebs et al. of one-third applicator weekly for 10 weeks (132). It is important that the perineal skin be protected with a topical ointment such as zinc oxide to prevent painful vulvar erosions regardless of which 5-FU application schedule is chosen. More recently, investigators have demonstrated the feasibility and likely efficacy of imiquimod in the treatment of VAIN, although large series remain to be performed (138). In the study by Haidopoulos et al., six out of seven patients with high-grade dysplasia (VIN 2-3) regressed to either no evidence of dysplasia or VIN 1 following imiquimod treatment (138). Application of 0.25 g of imiquimod 5% intravaginally once weekly for 3 weeks was effective and well tolerated. Larger studies are required, but this regimen appears to be promising, with a simpler dosing regimen, and lower toxicity when compared to 5-FU (138).

Partial or total vaginectomy has been considered by many to be an acceptable treatment for VAIN (139). However, one of its main drawbacks is shortening or stenosis of the vagina, frequently with poor functional results. Hoffman et al. (124) reported a 17% recurrence rate in a series of 32 patients with CIS of the vagina who underwent upper vaginectomy. In this series, 44% had received prior therapy, including laser vaporization, or topical 5-FU and local excision. Nine patients (28%) were found to have invasive cancer upon final pathologic examination. Four of nine patients with invasive carcinoma showing more than 3.5-mm infiltration were treated subsequently with RT, three of whom remained free of disease. Of the five patients with less than 2 mm invasion, one received RT for local recurrence, and the remaining four patients were without disease after surgery alone. Overall, five of nine patients with microinvasive carcinoma required RT in addition to surgery, and only 72% of all patients treated with surgery remained free of disease at last follow-up. Of 23 patients with VAIN 3, 19 (83%) remained without evidence of recurrence at a mean follow-up of 38 months. Hoffman et al. (124) advocated upper vaginectomy with 1 cm margins when there were concerns about possible invasion, and when the lesion was confined to the upper one third or one half of the vagina. To minimize postoperative stenosis, Hoffman et al. (124) recommended not closing the mucosa, using a dilator with estrogenic vaginal cream, and consideration of a skin graft. Prior RT is probably a contraindication to vaginectomy owing to significantly increased morbidity. Control rates of 66% to 100% following partial colpectomy effected either with a traditional surgical approach (124,139), with CUSA (133), or with the loop electrosurgical excision procedure (LEEP) (125) have been achieved.

RT has a long history of documented efficacy with control rates ranging between 80% and 100%, and a significantly better therapeutic ratio than other modalities (14,16,42,56). Using conventional low-dose-rate (LDR) ICB techniques, the entire vaginal mucosa should receive between 50 and 60 Gy, given the high incidence of multicentricity; the area of involvement should receive 70 to 80 Gy, in one or two implants, prescribed to the mucosal surface (134). Higher doses may cause significant vaginal fibrosis and stenosis. Perez et al. reported only one distal local failure in the 20 patients treated for CIS (134). Pelvic recurrences or distant failures have not been observed in the absence of invasive component, after ICB.

There have been some reports in the literature regarding the use of high-dose-rate (HDR) ICB for patients with VAIN 3. Ogino et al. (140) reported six patients treated with HDR to a mean dose of 23.3 Gy (range, 15 to 30 Gy), none of whom developed recurrent disease. Limited rectal bleeding and moderate to severe vaginal mucosa reactions were noted in patients treated to the entire length of the vagina. MacLeod et al. (141) reported on 14 patients with VAIN 3 treated with HDR-ICB to a dose of 34 to 45 Gy in 4.5- to 8.5-Gy fractions. With a median duration of follow-up of 46 months, one patient had persistent tumor and another showed progression of tumor with an overall local control of 78.5%; two patients developed grade 3 vaginal toxicity. Mock et al. (142) reported 100% recurrence-free survival in six patients with CIS treated with HDR-ICB. At the present time, no definite conclusions can be drawn from the limited data published in the literature regarding the use of HDR-ICB. Based on the excellent local control and functional results obtained with LDR-ICB, this remains, in our opinion, the treatment of choice when definitive RT is used.

Estrogen therapy should be considered in women who are postmenopausal or have undergone RT, provided the possibility of invasive disease has been eliminated. The effect of irradiation on ovarian function, as well as occasional fibrosis of the vaginal vault, makes this treatment currently unacceptable except in cases resistant to conservative therapy.

Invasive Squamous Cell Carcinoma

Surgical Approach and Outcomes

In general, SCC of the vagina has been treated with RT. However, several surgical series have reported acceptable to excellent outcomes in well-selected patients, with survival rates after radical surgery for stage I disease ranging from 75% to 100% (4,13,21,24,40,45). Cases in which surgery may be the preferred treatment include selected stage I-II patients, with lesions at the apex and upper third of the posterior or lateral vagina that could be approached with radical hysterectomy, upper vaginectomy, and pelvic lymphadenectomy providing adequate margins (13,15,21,24,40) and very superficial lesions that may be removed with wide local excision. Lesions in the lower third of the vagina would require vulvovaginectomy in addition to dissection of inguinofemoral node exenteration to achieve negative margins (13,15,21,40). If the margins are found to be close or positive after resection, adjuvant RT is recommended. However, for lesions at other sites, and those cases requiring more extensive resection, definitive RT is the treatment of choice since it offers excellent results (19), with isolated central failures post-radiation being offered exenteration (40).

Creasman et al. noted superior survival in those undergoing surgery (4). However, they and Tjalma et al. (45) recognized that there may be bias in surgical series, such that younger, healthier patients with better performance status are more likely to be offered radical surgery, whereas older patients with multiple comorbid medical conditions are offered RT.

Ball and Berman's series (13) included 58 patients: 27 stage I and 18 stage II disease. Twenty-seven patients were managed primarily with surgery, with an overall 78% 5-year survival rate, 84% in patients with stage I, and a 63% rate in those with stage II disease, which is comparable to the results reported by Perez et al. in their RT series (19). Rubin et al. (40) reported 75 cases of vaginal cancer: 14 patients with stage I and 35 patients with stage II. RT was the primary modality used in this series; however, eight patients (five with stage I and three with stage II) underwent primary surgery with curative intent. Six of these eight patients survived 5 years, and the local control rate for stage I patients was 80%. However, only one patient with stage II was a long-term survivor. This surgical outcome compares unfavorably with the remaining patients in whom RT was the primary modality. In general, patients with lesions that could be encompassed by radical vulvovaginectomy with or without hysterectomy did better than those requiring exenteration. Rubin et al. (40) advocated that exenteration should be reserved for those with central failure after RT, or as primary therapy in those with disease not fixed to the bone. Davis et al. (24) reported on 52 patients with cancer of the vagina treated with surgery alone in a series that included 89 cases. In this nonrandomized series, an 85% 5-year survival rate was achieved in stage I patients compared to 65% in those treated with RT (24). Of 45 patients with stage II disease, 49% survived after surgery, 50% after RT, and 69% after surgery and RT.

The Peters et al. series (112) included 86 vaginal carcinomas, with an overall survival rate of 56%. Most were treated with RT. However, 12 highly selected patients had surgery, with a 75% survival rate. The investigators suggested that vaginectomy with radical hysterectomy, if the uterus was still in place, should be limited to those with superficial disease because the closeness of the bladder and rectum limited the true radicality of surgical approaches. Gallup et al. (15) reported 28 cases, of which 57% were stage I-II lesions (only three patients had stage II), and of these, 83% survived. Most patients in this series received RT; however, all three patients with stage I disease who were treated with surgery survived. Extent of surgery and median follow-up were not stated.

In the largest single-institution series reported to date by Stock et al. (21), of 100 patients with carcinoma of the vagina (including 85 with SCC), a 47% 5-year survival rate was achieved. In this series, 40 patients were treated with surgery alone, 47 with radiation alone, and 13 with combination therapy. Overall, 5-year survival was 47%. Survival for stage I patients was 56% when treated with surgery versus 80% for those who recieved RT, whereas for stage II patients, a 68% survival was seen versus a 31% survival in those who underwent RT (21). The investigators acknowledged that the apparent surgical superiority for stage II patients may have been due to selection bias in that those treated with RT alone were more likely to have had stage IIB disease with extensive paracolpos involvement, and those with lesser involvement were preferentially offered surgery. Stock advocated RT for stage II patients with extensive paracolpos. Stock et al. concluded that for upper-third vault lesions, radical hysterectomy and pelvic lymphadenectomy with upper vaginectomy should be offered to those with stage I lesions, with a consideration for wide local excisions, and postoperative RT for patients with small lesions. If there was extension to the paracolpos, RT should be recommended; however, in very well-selected patients, there might be a role for surgery (21).

Tjalma et al. reported on 55 cases of SCC of the vagina, including 27 cases with stage I and 12 with stage II disease, with a median follow-up of 45 months (45). Of the 27 cases with stage I disease, 26 underwent surgery, and 4 of them received some form of postoperative RT. A 91% 5-year survival rate was achieved for stage I disease. Surgery was a part of the primary management for 6 of the 12 patients with stage II disease. In the multviariate analysis, age and lesion size were the only prognostic factors. Tjalma et al. concluded that surgery should be considered part of the therapeutic approach for stage I and minimal stage II disease (45). However, as Stock et al. suggested (21), and later Creasman et al. (4) and Tjalma et al. (45) concurred, such apparent improvement in small surgical series may be secondary to a selection bias such as patients with better performance status and smaller lesions are selected for surgery, whereas older patients with more comorbid medical conditions and larger stage I-II lesions undergo RT.

While several series have reported on primary surgical approaches, including exenterations for patients with advanced stage III-IV SCC, achieving control rates as high as 50% for highly selected patients (13,15,21,40), the number of patients treated in any single series is so small that in modern practice, primary exenteration for advanced disease would not be recommended as the preferred approach (127). Therefore, advanced-stage patients should receive definitive RT, probably in combination with concurrent chemotherapy, although the role of combined modality therapy is unknown.

With regard to the surgical technique, if a complete vaginectomy is to be undertaken, most experts have suggested a combined abdominoperineal approach, with the perineal incision in the pubocervicovesical fascia made beneath the urethra and above the rectum so as to avoid the hemorrhoidal plexus. Some have suggested that the perineal incision can be made before or after the abdominal incision to perform the radical abdominal resection. However, we would favor performing the abdominal incision, first mobilizing the bladder, urethra, and rectum down to the perineum, and dividing the paracolpos at the side wall, mobilizing the ureters, and harvesting the nodes such that if unresectable disease is found, the patient would be spared a perineal incision. Given the large defect that is left after surgical resection, placement of a gracilis myocutaneous flap allows not only coverage of the defect, but may serve as a neovagina in the sexually active woman (143,144). Alternatively, two new techniques have been described with excellent results. Vaginal reconstruction can be performed with the use of vicryl mesh combined with a pedicled omental graftor with a deep inferior epigastric perforator flap. Both techniques have been shown to be effective, and when performed at the time of pelvic exenteration, carry the additional benefit of avoiding an additional surgical incision, as required for creation of a gracilis flap. Long-term follow-up has been favorable for the former, while only preliminary data is available for the latter (145,146).

Radiation Therapy Techniques and Outcome

Stage I. In patients with stage I lesions, usually 0.5 to 1 cm thick, that may involve one or more vaginal walls, it is important to individualize radiation therapy techniques to obtain optimal functional results. Most investigators emphasize that brachytherapy alone is adequate for superficial stage I patients. Superficial lesions can be adequately treated with ICB alone using afterloading vaginal cylinders. The entire length of the vagina is generally treated to a mucosal dose of 60 Gy, and an additional mucosal dose of 20 to 30 Gy is delivered to the area of tumor involvement (134). For lesions thicker than 0.5 cm at the time of implantation, it is advisable to combine ICB and ITB with a single-plane implant to increase the depth dose and limit excessive irradiation to the vaginal mucosa. With LDR-ICB a dose of 60 to 65 Gy is delivered to the entire vaginal mucosa; the dose to 0.5 cm depth from the ICB should be calculated; an additional 15 to 20 Gy at a depth of 0.5 cm beyond the plane of the implant will be delivered with the ITB such that the base of the tumor receives between 65 and 70 Gy, with the involved vaginal mucosa receiving an estimated 80 to 100 Gy. The proximal and distal vaginal mucosal doses should be limited to 140 and 100 Gy, respectively (134).

There are no well-established criteria regarding the use of external beam RT (EBRT) in patients with stage I disease. Perez et al. (19,42) did not find a significant correlation between the technique of irradiation used and the probability of local or pelvic recurrence, probably since the treatment technique varied based on tumor-related factors. There is general consensus that EBRT is advisable for larger, more infiltrating or poorly differentiated tumors that may have a higher risk of lymph node metastasis. The whole pelvis is treated with 10 to 20 Gy; an additional parametrial dose should be delivered with a midline block (five half-value layer [HVL]) to give a total of 45 to 50 Gy to the parametria and pelvic side walls. Chyle et al. (14) recommended EBRT in addition to brachytherapy for stage I disease to cover at least the paravaginal nodes, and, in larger lesions, to cover the external and internal iliac nodes. Ninety-five percent to 100% local control has been achieved with intracavitary and interstitial techniques, with 5-year survival for patients with stage I disease treated with RT alone ranging from 70% to 95% (Table 21.4) (18,19,21,23,121,147).

TABLE 21.4

FIGO STAGE I-II VAGINAL CANCER: TREATMENT APPROACH AND RESULTS

Treatment modality, authors	No. of patients	Outcome—survival
IRRADIATION +/− SURGERY		
Chyle et al. (14)	59 St I	10 years, 76%
	104 St II	10 years, 69%
Creasman et al. (NCDB) (4)	169 St I	5-year survival: 73%; 79% S+RT (47), 63% RT (122)
	175 St II	5-year survival: 58%; 58% S+RT (39), 57% RT (136)
Davis et al. (24)	19 St I	5-year survival: 100% S+RT (5), 65% RT (14)
	18 St II	5-year survival: 69% S+RT (9), 50% RT (9)
Kirkbride et al. (16)	40 St I	5 years, 72%
	38 St II	5 years, 70%
Kucera and Vavra (121)	16 St I	5 years, 81%
	23 St II	5 years, 43.5%
Perez et al. (42)	59 St I	10 years, 80%
	63 St IIA	10 years, 55%
	34 St IIB	10 years, 35%
Stock et al. (21)	8 St I	5 years: 100% S+RT, 80% RT
	35 St II	5 years: 69% S+RT, 31% RT
Urbanski et al. (23)	33 St I	5 years, 73%
	37 St II	5 years, 54%
Frank et al. (147)	50 St I	5-year DSS, 85%
	97 St II	5-year DSS, 78%
		5-year survival
RADICAL SURGERY		
Ball and Berman (13)	19 St I	84%
	8 St II	63%
Creasman et al. (NCDB) (4)	76 St I	90%
	34 St II	70%
Davis et al. (24)	25 St I	85%
	27 St II	49%
Rubin et al. (40)	5 St I	80%
	3 St II	33%
Stock et al. (21)	17 St I	56%
	23 St II	68%
Tjalma et al. (45)	26[a]	91%

Note: DSS, disease-specific survival; NCDB, National Cancer Data Base; RT, radiotherapy; S, surgery; St, stage.
[a]Four patients received adjuvant irradiation.

Stage II. Patients with stage IIA tumors have more advanced paravaginal disease without extensive parametrial infiltration. These patients are uniformly treated with EBRT followed by ICB and/or ITB. Generally, the whole pelvis receives 20 Gy followed by an additional parametrial dose with a midline 2- to 4-cm-wide (five HVL) block, depending on the width of the implant, to deliver a total of 45 to 50 Gy to the pelvic side walls. A combination of LDR-ICB or LDR-ITB may be used to deliver a minimum of 50 to 60 Gy 0.5 cm beyond the deep margin of the tumor (in addition to the whole pelvis dose, to a total tumor dose of 70 to 80 Gy). Double-plane or volume implants may be necessary for more extensive disease. Perez et al. (42) showed that in stage IIA, the local tumor control was 70% (37 of 53) in patients receiving brachytherapy combined with EBRT, compared with 40% (4 of 10) in patients treated with either brachytherapy or EBRT alone. The superiority of the combination of EBRT and brachytherapy over EBRT or brachytherapy alone has been shown as well in other series (14,21,120).

Patients with stage IIB, with more extensive parametrial infiltration, will receive 40 to 50 Gy whole pelvis and 55 to 60 Gy total parametrial dose (with midline shielding). An additional boost of 30 to 35 Gy will be given with LDR interstitial and intracavitary brachytherapy, to deliver a total tumor dose of 75 to 80 Gy to the vaginal tumor (14,20,42,120) and 65 Gy to parametrial and paravaginal extensions. The pelvic side wall dose should be kept below 60 Gy (including the contributions of EBRT and brachytherapy). Patients with lesions limited to the upper third of the vagina can be treated with an intrauterine tandem and vaginal ovoids or cylinders. The local-regional control in patients with stage IIB in the Perez et al. series (42) was also superior with combined EBRT and brachytherapy (61% vs 50%, respectively).

The 5-year survival for patients with stage II disease treated with RT alone ranges between 35% and 70% for stage IIA, and 35% and 60% for stage IIB. The results of several series published in the literature using different treatment approaches for stage I and II vaginal cancer are shown in Table 21.4 (4,13,14,16,21,23,24,40,45,121,147).

Stage III-IVA. Generally, patients with stage III and IVA disease will receive 45 to 50 Gy EBRT to the pelvis, and in some cases, additional parametrial dose with midline shielding to deliver up to 60 Gy to the pelvic side walls. Ideally, ITB brachytherapy boost is performed, if technically feasible, to deliver a minimum tumor dose of 75 to 80 Gy. If brachytherapy is not feasible, a shrinking-field technique can be used, with fields defined using the three-dimensional treatment planning capabilities to deliver a tumor dose around 65 to 70 Gy. An alternative approach is intensity modulated RT (IMRT) using multiple beams of varying intensity that conform the high-dose region to the shape of the target tissues, with more adequate sparing of the surrounding normal tissues, primarily the bladder, rectum, and small bowel (148,149).

Boronow et al. (127) proposed an alternative to exenterative procedure for locally advanced vulvovaginal carcinoma, using RT to treat the pelvic disease and a radical vulvectomy with bilateral inguinal node dissection to treat the vulvar extension of the tumor. External irradiation to the pelvis and inguinal nodes consisted of 45 to 50 Gy, combined with LDR intracavitary insertions to deliver maximal doses of 80 to 85 Gy to the vaginal mucosa with both modalities.

The overall cure rate for patients with stage III disease is 30% to 50%. Stage IVA includes patients with rectal or bladder mucosa involvement, or in most series, positive inguinal nodes. Although some patients with stage IVA disease are curable, many patients are treated palliatively with EBRT only. Pelvic exenteration can also be curative in highly selected stage IV patients with small-volume central disease. Table 21.5 (4,13,14,16,21,23,40,42,121,147) shows the treatment results with different therapeutic modalities, including four series that reported the use of primary surgery in highly selected patients with advanced disease. However, each of these series reported a far greater number of patients with similar stage disease treated with RT, which represents the preferred approach in contemporary practice (19,56).

External Beam Radiotherapy

EBRT is advisable in patients with deeply infiltrating or poorly differentiated stage I lesions and in all patients with stages II to IVA disease. The treatment is generally delivered using opposed anterior and posterior fields (AP/PA). The pelvis receives between 20 and 45 Gy depending on the stage of the disease. This will be followed, in some cases, by bilateral pelvic sidewall boosts to 50 to 55 Gy. High-energy photons (≥10 MV) are usually preferred. CT simulation is highly encouraged since it allows a more accurate delineation of the regional lymph node areas, rather than relying on pelvic bony anatomy (150). Treatment portals cover at least the true pelvis with 1.5- to 2.0-cm margin beyond the pelvic rim. Superiorly, the field extends to either L4-5 or L5-S1 to cover the pelvic lymph nodes up to the common iliacs, and extends distally to the introitus to include the entire vagina. Lateral fields, if used, should extend anteriorly to adequately include the external iliac nodes, anterior to the pubic symphysis, and at least to the junction of S2-3 posteriorly.

In patients with tumors involving the middle and lower vagina with clinically negative groins, the bilateral inguinofemoral lymph node regions should be treated electively to 45 to 50 Gy (42). Planning CT is recommended to adequately determine the depth of the inguinofemoral nodes. A number of techniques have been used to treat the areas at risk without overtreating the femoral necks. Some of the most commonly used techniques include the use of unequal loading (2:1, AP/PA), a combination of low- and high-energy photons (4 to 6 MV, AP; and 15 to 18 MV, PA), or equally weighted beams with a transmission block in the central AP field, utilizing small AP photon or electron beams to deliver a daily boost to the inguinofemoral nodes (151). A technique has been developed and implemented at Indiana University that uses a narrow PA field to treat the pelvis and a wider AP field encompassing the pelvis and inguinofemoral nodes, with daily AP photon boost to the inguinal nodes being delivered using the asymmetric collimator jaws (152). Advantages of this technique include simplicity of setup and treatment (single isocenter, no need for transmission block), dose homogeneity, reduced dose to the femoral necks, low potential risk of nodal underdose, and elimination of dosimetric difficulties inherent in electron boosts (Fig. 21.5).

TABLE 21.5

FIGO STAGE III-IV VAGINAL CANCER OUTCOME WITH RADIATION THERAPY WITH/WITHOUT SURGERY

Treatment modality, authors	No. of patients	Outcome—survival
IRRADIATION +/− SURGERY		
Chyle et al. (14)	55 St III	10 years, 47%
	16 St IV	10 years, 27%
Creasman et al. (NCDB) (4)	180 St III-IV	5-year survival: 36%; 60% S+RT (36), 35% RT (144)
Kirkbride et al. (16)	42[a] St III-IV	5 years, 53%
Kucera and Vavra (121)	46 St III	5 years, 35%
	19 St IVA	5 years, 32%
Perez et al. (42)	20 St III	10 years, 38%
	15 St IV	0%
Stock et al. (21)	9 St III	5 years, 0%
	8 St IV	0%
Urbanski et al. (23)	40 St III	5 years, 22.5%
	15 St IVA	0%
Frank et al. (147)	46 St III-IVA	5-year DSS, 58%
RADICAL SURGERY		**5-YEAR SURVIVAL**
Ball and Berman (13)	2 St III	50%
Creasman et al. (NCDB) (4)	21 St III-IV	47%
Rubin et al. (40)	2 St III	50%

Note: DSS, disease-specific survival; NCDB, National Cancer Data Base; RT, radiotherapy; S, surgery; St, stage.
[a]Twenty patients with St III-IV were treated with chemotherapy (5-FU +/− mitomycin C) and radiotherapy.

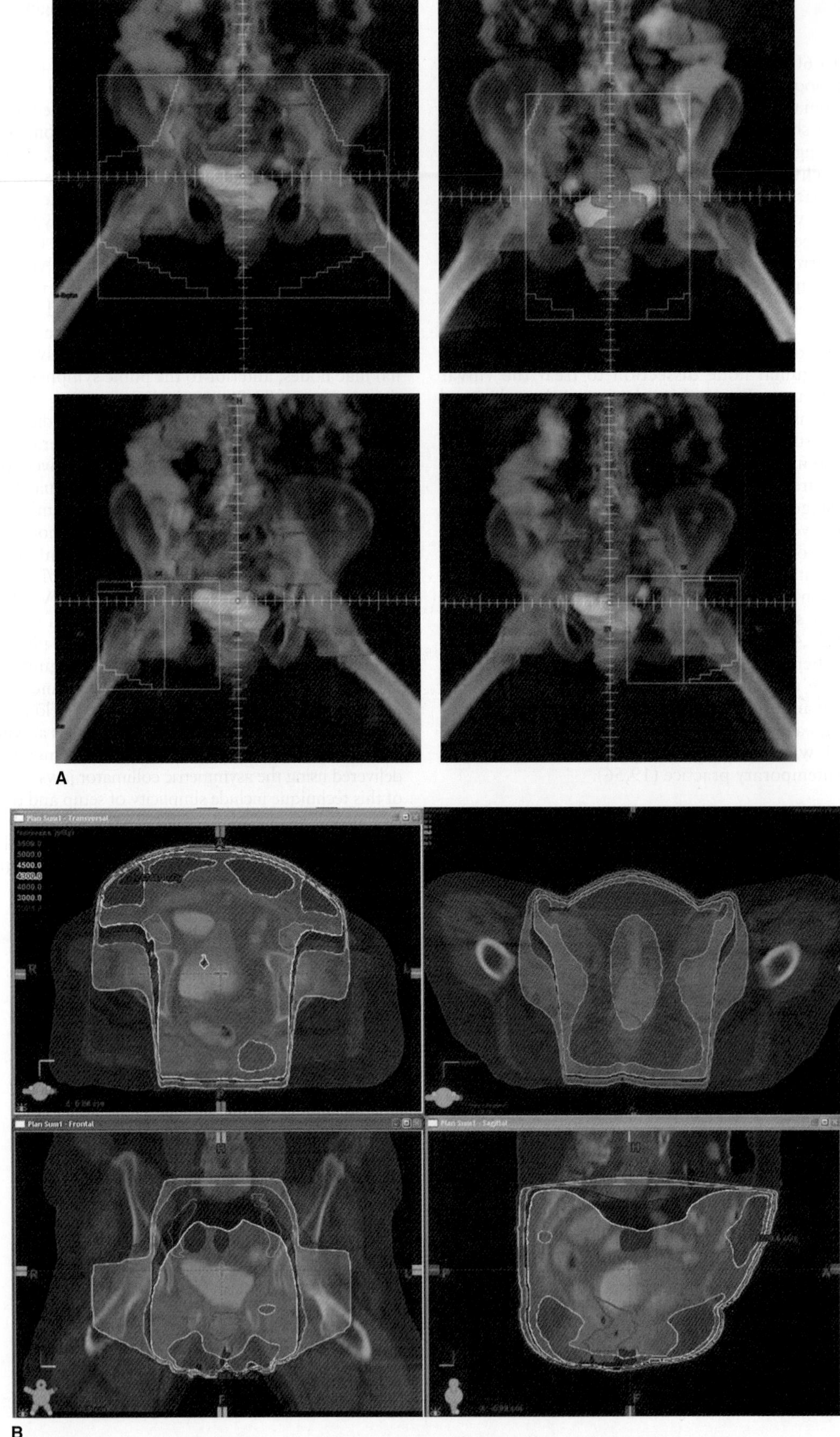

FIGURE 21.5. (*See color plate section.*) Vaginal cancer with distal-third vaginal involvement—squamous cell carcinoma. Technique for pelvic and inguinofemoral nodal irradiation. **A:** Digital reconstructed radiographs (DRRs) AP/PA and daily right and left inquinofemoral photon boost. **B:** Axial, sagittal, and coronal isodose distributions.

For patients with positive pelvic nodes or those patients with advanced disease not amenable to interstitial implant, additional boost to the areas of gross disease, as defined by CT scan, should be given using conformal therapy to deliver a total dose between 65 and 70 Gy, when feasible, with high-energy photons. Boost to the areas of gross nodal disease, as defined by CT scan, should be given using small fields (similar to the parametrial boost with midline shielding) to deliver a total dose between 60 and 65 Gy with high-energy photons. In patients with clinically palpable inguinal nodes, additional doses of 15 to 20 Gy (calculated at a depth determined by CT scan) are necessary with reduced portals. This is generally achieved by using low-energy photons or electron beam (12 to 18 MeV). IMRT techniques are now available to deliver higher doses to the gross disease while reducing the dose to the bladder and rectum (Fig. 21.6) (148,149).

Overall treatment time (7 to 9 weeks) has been found to be a significant treatment factor predicting tumor control (111,153), although this has not been universally recognized (42).

Low-Dose-Rate Intracavitary Brachytherapy

VAIN and small T1 lesions with less than a 0.5-cm depth can be adequately treated with intracavitary brachytherapy (ICB) alone. Low-dose-rate (LDR)-ICB is performed using vaginal cylinders such as Burnett, Bloedorn, Delclos (154), or MIRALVA (Nucletron Veenendaal, the Netherlands) (155,156) loaded with cesium 137 (^{137}Cs) radioactive sources. Choo et al. (157)

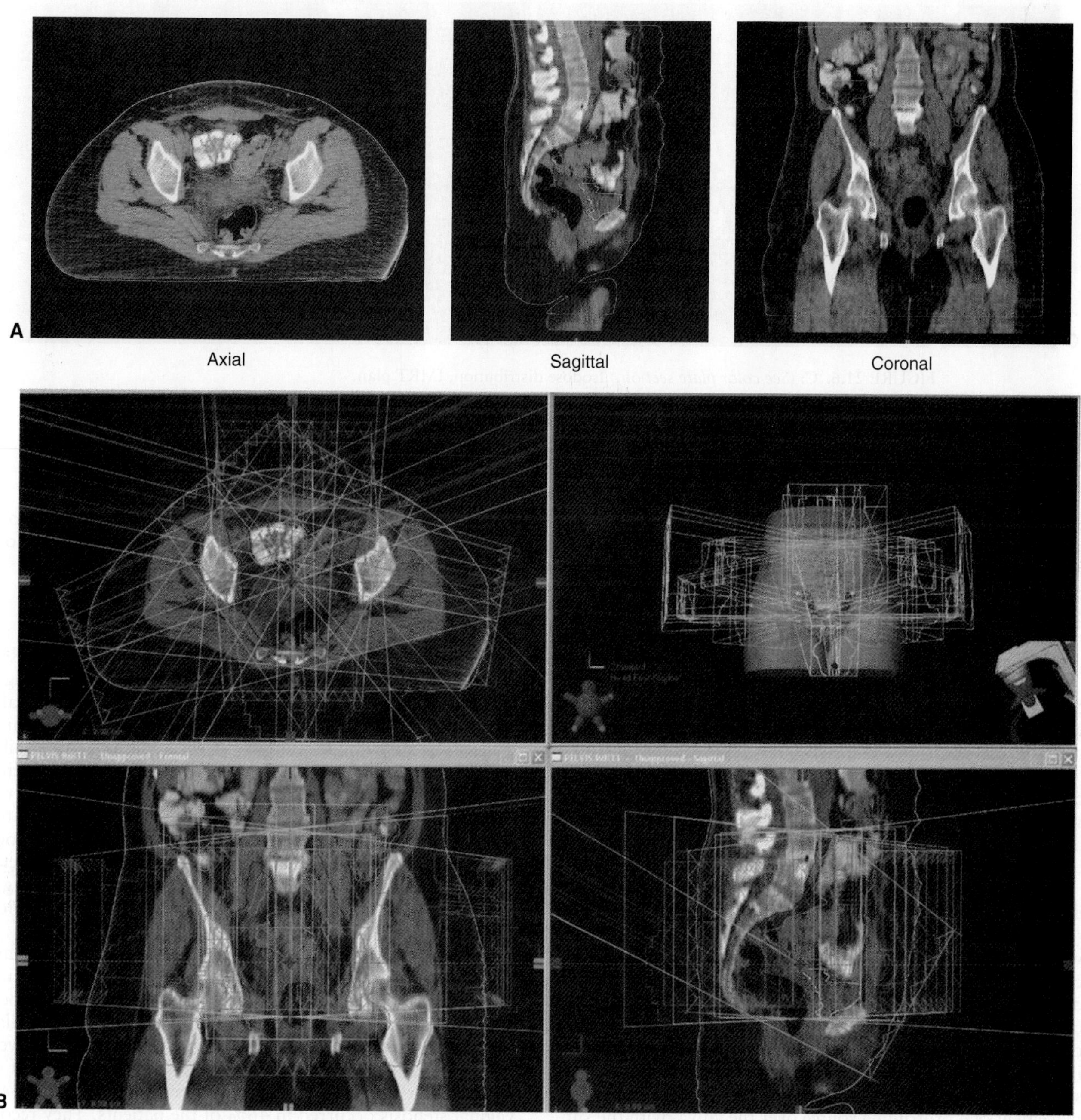

FIGURE 21.6. (*See color plate section.*) Intensity modulated radiotherapy (IMRT) in vaginal cancer. **A:** Axial, sagittal, and coronal reconstructions of the gross tumor volume (GTV). **B:** Beam arrangement, IMRT plan. (*Continued.*)

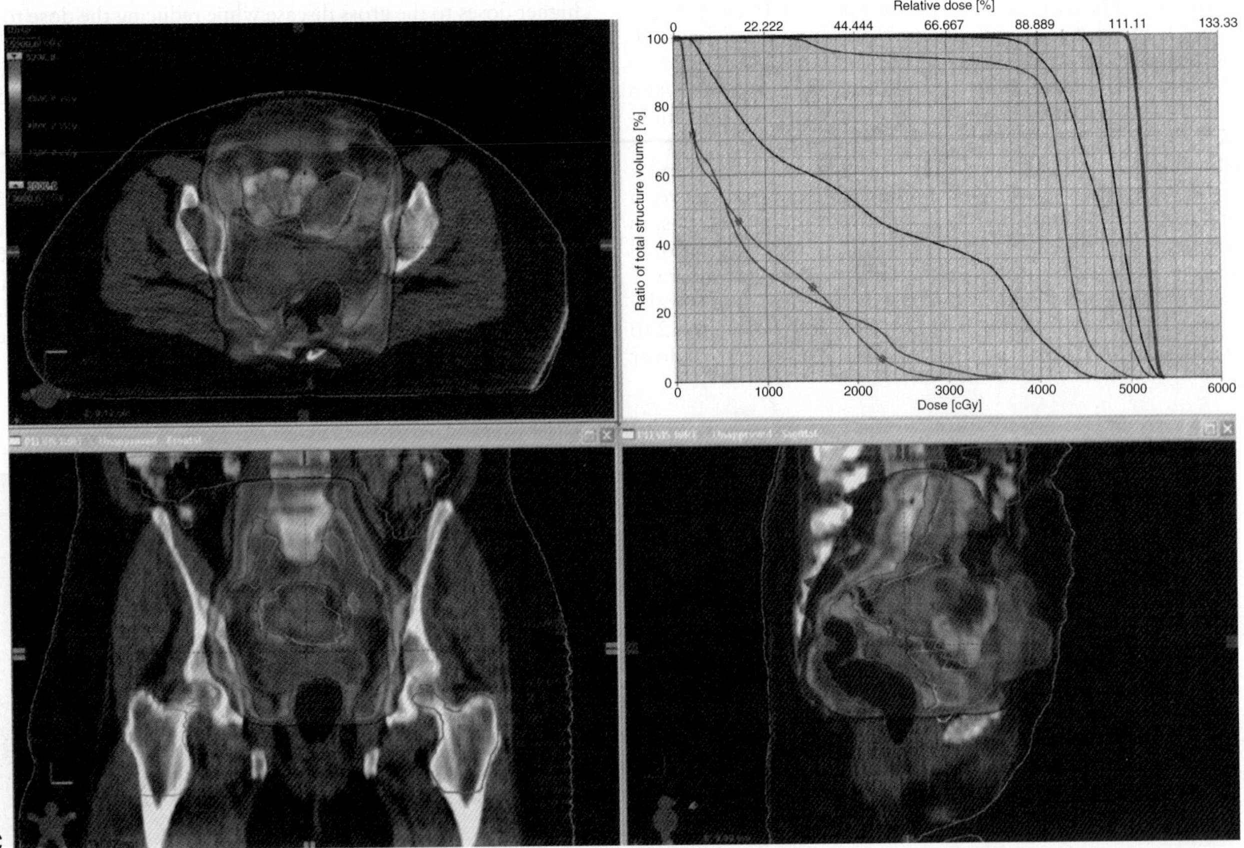

FIGURE 21.6. C: (*See color plate section.*) Isodose distribution, IMRT plan.

evaluated the depth distribution of lymphatics lying beneath the mucosal surface of the vagina in 31 patients who underwent full-thickness vaginal biopsy or resection for benign or malignant lesions. In their series, 95% of vaginal lymphatic channels were located within a 3 mm depth from the vaginal surface, confirming the adequacy of prescribing the dose to a depth of 5 mm for superficially invasive lesions (157).

It is recommended that the largest possible diameter that can be comfortably accommodated by the patient should be used to improve the ratio of mucosa to tumor dose, and eliminate vaginal rugations. In general, the vulva is sutured closed for the duration of the implant in order to secure the position of the applicators. Perez et al. (155,156) designed and constructed a vaginal applicator, MIRALVA, that incorporates two ovoid sources and a central tandem that can be used to treat the entire vagina (alone or in combination with the uterine cervix).

In patients with upper vagina lesions with less than a 0.5 cm depth of invasion, vaginal colpostats alone (after hysterectomy) or in combination with intrauterine tandem, loaded with ^{137}Cs sources similar to that used in treatment of cervical cancer, can be used to treat the proximal vagina to a minimum dose of 65 to 70 Gy, estimated to 0.5 cm depth, including the contribution of EBRT if given. When indicated, the remainder of the vagina can be treated by performing a subsequent implant using vaginal cylinders (generally 50 to 60 Gy prescribed to the vaginal surface). It is important to avoid the placement of a protruding source over the vulva, with the subsequent increased risk of complications. When appropriate dose specification points are chosen, a very uniform dose distribution over the entire length of the vagina can be obtained. The use of LDR remote control afterloading technology allows the reduction of radiation exposure to hospital personnel and optimization of the isodose distribution.

High-Dose-Rate Intracavitary Brachytherapy

The International Commission of Radiation Units (ICRU) defines HDR brachytherapy as exceeding 12 Gy/h (42). High-dose-rate intracavitary brachytherapy (HDR-ICB) is typically performed with a 10 Ci single iridium-192 (^{192}Ir) source (Micro-Selectron HDR, Nucletron). The applicators are similar to those described for LDR. Little information regarding HDR-ICB in the treatment of primary carcinoma of the vagina is available (22,158). Fewer patients have been treated compared with LDR-ICB, follow-up for most series is short, publication bias is likely, and there is no agreement on treatment regimen. Generally, the number of insertions ranges from one to six (median three), with the dose per fraction ranging from 300 to 800 cGy (median 700 cGy).

Nanavati et al. (158) reported 13 patients with primary vaginal cancer treated with external beam RT (45 Gy) and HDR-ICB. All 13 patients had a complete response, and local control was achieved in 92% of the patients with a median follow-up of only 2.6 years (range 0.7 to 5.2 years). The investigators did not observe any acute or chronic intestinal or bladder grade 3 or 4 toxicity. However, moderate to severe vaginal stenosis occurred in 46% of the patients. They recognize that "late-occurring toxicity could be missed at a medium follow-up of 2.6 years." Kucera et al. (159) reported on 190 patients with invasive carcinoma of the vagina. Eighty were treated with intracavitary HDR-ICB with or without EBRT. These patients are compared with a historical group of 110 patients treated with intracavitary LDR brachytherapy with or without EBRT. No significant differences were found for stages, tumor grade, or location between the two groups. The crude 5-year survival rates for all patients were 41% in the LDR group, 81% in stage I, and 43% in stage II. Overall actuarial 3-year survival and disease-specific survival rates for all patients in the HDR series were 51% and 66%, respectively. Disease-specific 3-year survival rates were 83% in stage I and 66% in stage II. There were no significant differences in local and distant recurrences between the treatment modalities. Complications analysis showed no significant differences between the HDR and LDR series. Similar results were published by Mock et al. (142) in 86 patients treated with HDR-ICB alone or in combination with EBRT with fairly good toxicity profile. However, Kushner et al. (160) reported on 19 patients with vaginal cancer treated with different combinations of EBRT and intracavitary and interstitial HDR brachytherapy, with a low 39.3% 2-year progression-free survival and 15.8% serious late complications including ureteral stenosis, painful vaginal necrosis, and small bowel obstruction.

Many aspects remain unknown or not well understood in the use of HDR-ICB in vaginal cancer treatment. These include the radiobiologic equivalency of HDR to LDR, fractionation schedule, total dose, specification of dose prescription, and how to combine HDR with EBRT and/or LDR brachytherapy. In addition, optimization approaches and methods of dose calculation, such as the inclusion of anisotropic corrections, are not well described in the sparse literature available to date (161,162). These factors could result in an increased incidence of severe complications, such as vaginal necrosis and rectovaginal or vesicovaginal fistulas (160,163,164). In our opinion, until further data are available with longer follow-up, as well as a better understanding of the physical and radiobiologic principles involved in HDR-ICB, its use should be cautiously considered in the radiotherapeutic management of primary vaginal carcinoma.

Interstitial Brachytherapy

Interstitial brachytherapy (ITB) is an important component in the treatment of more advanced primary vaginal carcinomas, typically in combination with EBRT and/or ICB. In the first place, a careful definition of the "target volume," which is the gross tumor volume (based on clinical, radiologic, and operative findings) and a margin of adjoining normal tissue, is required. Other considerations include whether a permanent (^{198}Au or ^{125}I) or temporary implant (^{192}Ir) is optimal, the geometry of the implant (e.g., single or double plane or volume implant), source distribution, dose rate, and total dose, based upon tumor size, location, local extent, and proximity of normal structures (165). The principal advantages of temporary implants are readily controlled distribution of the radioactive sources and easier modification of the dose distribution. The main advantages of a permanent seed implant include relative safety/simplicity, easy applicability, cost-effectiveness, and ability, in most cases, to be performed using local anesthesia. As a general rule, temporary implants are more commonly used in the curative treatment of larger gynecologic malignancies, whereas permanent implants are usually performed for smaller volume disease. When performing an interstitial procedure, freehand implants or template systems designed to assist in preplanning and to guide and secure the position of the needles in the target volume can be employed. Commercially available templates include the Syed-Neblett device (SNIT) (Alpha Omega Services, Bellflower, California, USA) (166), the modified Syed-Neblett (167), and the "MUPIT" (Martinez Universal Perineal Interstitial Template) (168). These templates generally consist of a perineal template, vaginal obturator, and 17-gauge hollow guides of various lengths that can be afterloaded with ^{192}Ir sources. The vaginal obturator is centrally drilled so that it can allow the placement of a tandem to be loaded with ^{137}Cs sources. This makes it possible to combine an interstitial and intracavitary application simultaneously (Fig. 21.7). The major advantage of these systems is greater control of the placement of the sources relative to tumor volume and critical structures owing to the fixed geometry provided by the template. In addition, improved dose-rate distributions are obtained by means of computer-assisted optimization of the source placement and strength during the planning and loading phase.

Owing to the inaccuracies of pelvic examination and close proximity of the rectum and bladder to the target volume, there exists a serious risk of either underdosing the target volume or causing bladder and rectal morbidity. In order to improve the accuracy of target localization and needle placement, several investigators have explored performing ITB under transrectal ultrasound (TRUS) (169), CT, MRI-planned implants with endorectal coil (170), laparotomy, and laparoscopic guidance (167–173). An open retropubic approach allows direct visualization of the bladder and urethra during interstitial implantation of anterior vaginal malignancies and facilitates negotiation of the pubic arch. Paley et al. (173) described a technique using an open retropubic approach for Syed template interstitial implants in anterior vaginal tumors under direct visualization.

Tewari et al. (174) described results in 71 patients who underwent ITB with (61 patients) or without (10 patients) EBRT. Patients included those with stage I (10 patients), Perez modification stage IIA (14 patients), Perez modification stage IIB (25 patients), stage III (15 patients), and stage IV (7 patients) disease. Each implant delivered a total tumor dose reaching 80 Gy integrated with EBRT. Local control was achieved in 53 patients (75%). With a median follow-up of 66 months the 5- and 10-year actuarial disease-free survival rates were both 58%. By stage, 5-year disease-free survival rates included stage I, 100%; stage IIA, 60%; stage IIB, 61%; stage III, 30%; and stage IV, 0%. Stage and primary lesion size independently influenced the survival rates. Significant complications occurred in nine patients (13%) including necrosis (n = 4), fistulas (n = 4), and small bowel obstruction (n = 1).

Stryker (175) treated 40 patients with vaginal carcinoma; 14 had a history of prior hysterectomy. There were four treatment groups: EBRT and intracavitary brachytherapy (group WPIC, n = 15), EBRT and interstitial brachytherapy (group WPIS, n = 10), EBRT alone (group WP, n = 7), and brachytherapy alone (group BA, n = 2).The 5-year disease-specific survival rates were 68% for 28 patients with squamous cell carcinoma and 50% for six patients with adenocarcinoma. The 5-year survival rates were 78% for stage I disease, 63% for stage II, 33% for stage III, and 50% for stage IV ($P = 0.2$). Local failure occurred in two patients (13%) in the WPIC group, two (20%) in WPIS, three (43%) in WP, and one (50%) in BA. Nine patients (26%) had late small/large intestine or bladder morbidity. Vaginal morbidity occurred in 15 patients (44%).

Role of Chemotherapy and Radiation

The control rate in the pelvis for stage III-IV patients is relatively low, and about 70% to 80% of the patients have persistent disease or recurrent disease in the pelvis in spite of high doses of EBRT and brachytherapy. Failure in distant sites does occur in about 25% to 30% of the patients with locally advanced tumors, which is much less than pelvic recurrences. Therefore, there is a need for better approaches to the management of advanced disease such as the use of concomitant chemoradiotherapy. Agents such as 5-FU, mitomycin-C, and cisplatin have shown promise when combined with RT, with complete response rates as high as 60% to 85% (176,177),

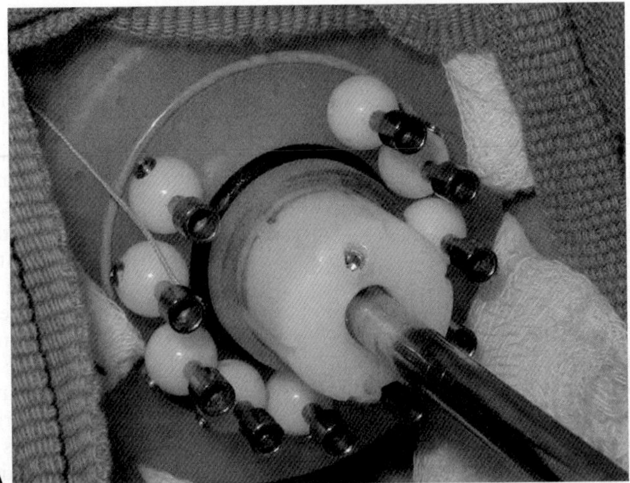

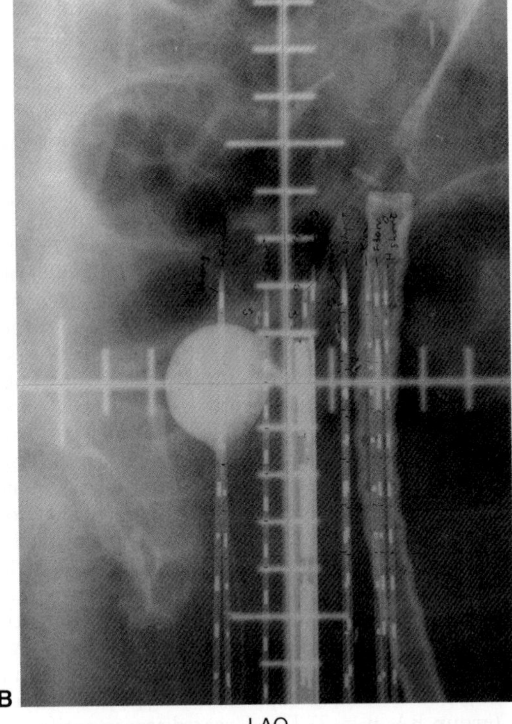

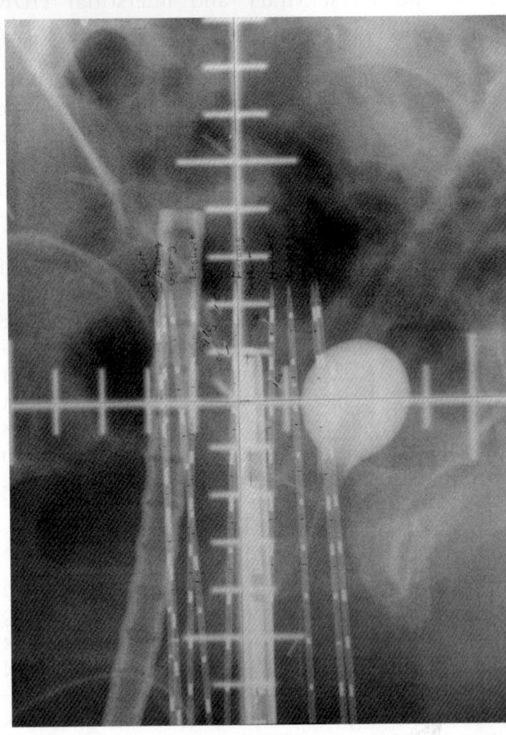

FIGURE 21.7. (*See color plate section.*) Interstitial plus endocavitary brachytherapy in a patient with vaginal cancer. **A.** Applicators in place. **B.** Oblique implant films.

but long-term results of such therapy have been variable. In these small studies, many of the patients had advanced (stage III) disease at the initiation of combined-modality therapy, perhaps explaining the lack of long-term disease control.

Evans et al. (176) found no local recurrences, however, among patients achieving a complete response with RT and 5-FU plus mitomycin C (12 of 25 patients), with a median follow-up period of 28 months, suggesting that local control may be improved with combined-modality therapy since local failure is common with radiation alone in large-volume pelvic disease. The survival for the entire population was 56% (66% for patients with primary vaginal cancer). Only two patients had severe complications, although the investigators recognize that longer follow-up is probably required to assess the true incidence of late effects. More sobering are the data from Roberts et al. (177), who reported 67 patients with advanced cancers of the vagina, cervix, and vulva treated with concurrent 5-FU, cisplatin, and RT. Although 85% experienced a complete response, 61% of the cancers recurred, with a median time to recurrence of only 6 months and an overall survival at 5 years of 22%. Further, 9 of 67 patients (13%) developed severe late complications, of which 8 required surgeries.

Kersh et al. (178) reported that five of eight vaginal cancer patients achieved local control with combined modality therapy. Dalrymple et al. (179) recently published a small study including 14 patients, primarily stages I and II SCC of the vagina, treated with reduced doses of RT (median 63 Gy)

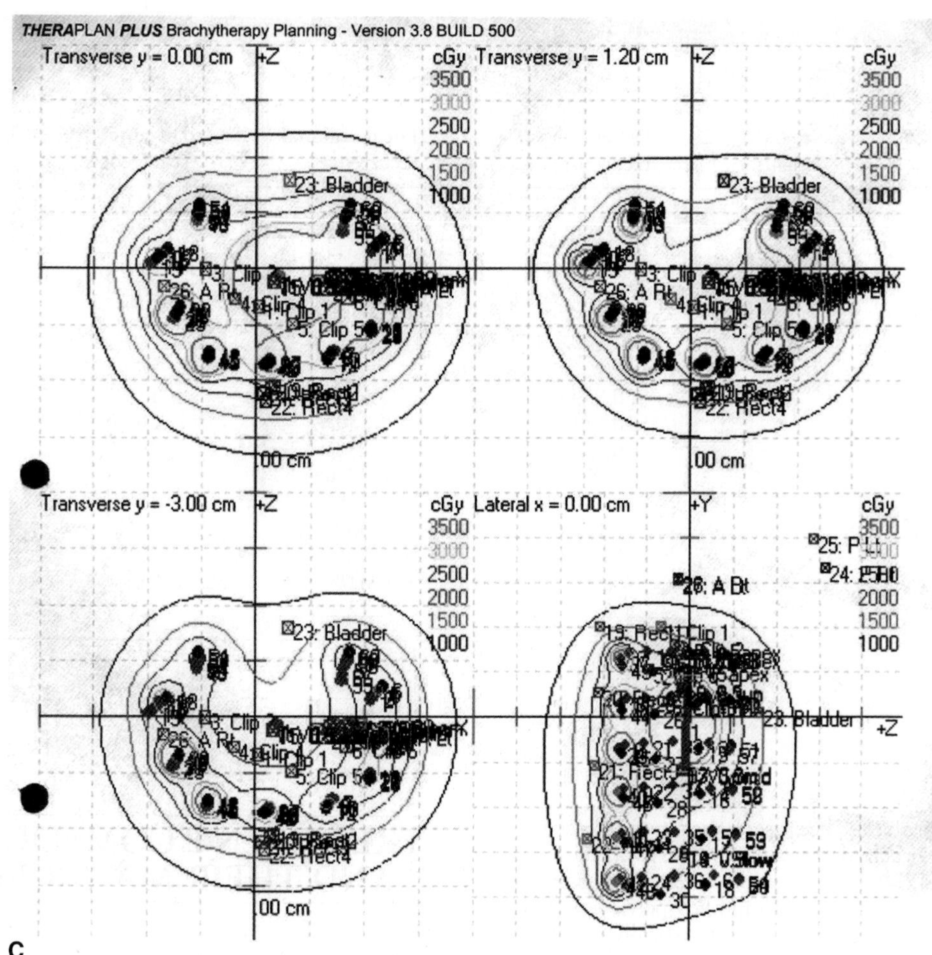

FIGURE 21.7. C: (*See color plate section.*) Dose Distribution.

concurrently with different 5-FU–based chemotherapeutic regimens. They reported a 93% control rate (four patients died of intercurrent disease with no evidence of tumor), probably reflecting a more favorable stage distribution. Interestingly, none of the patients required interstitial implants and no patients developed fistulas. The authors indicate that this approach, similar to the one used in the management of anal and vulvar cancer, would allow reducing the RT dose with the subsequent improvement in organ function and late toxicity.

Studies of primary chemoradiation in primary vaginal cancer are small or heterogeneous populations including cervical and vulvar cancers, making it difficult to truly assess the role of combined-modality therapy in the management of locally advanced disease. No randomized trials comparing radiation with or without chemotherapy have been reported. Further investigation is needed to determine the therapeutic efficacy of the concurrent chemoradiotherapeutic and the optimal chemotherapeutic regimen. Recently published data on locally advanced cervical cancer have demonstrated an advantage in locoregional control, overall survival, and disease-free survival for patients receiving cisplatin-based chemotherapy concurrently with RT (180–183). The only drug common to all the studies was cisplatin, suggesting it may be the only agent needed to improve radiation sensitivity. Based on these data, as well as data on locoregionally advanced vulvar cancer (184), consideration should be given to a similar approach in patients with advanced vaginal cancer. Randomized trials comparing radiation therapy alone to chemoradiation therapy, however, are unlikely because of small patient numbers.

PATTERNS OF FAILURE IN SQUAMOUS CELL CARCINOMA

At least 85% of patients who recur will have a component of locoregional failure, and the vast majority of these recurrences will be confined to the pelvis and vagina. The rate of locoregional recurrence in stage I is approximately 10% to 20% versus 30% to 40% in stage II. The pelvic control rate for patients with stage III and stage IV is relatively low and about 50% to 70% of the patients have recurrences or persistence in spite of well-designed RT. The median time to recurrence is 6 to 12 months. Tumor recurrence is associated with a dismal prognosis, with only a few long-term survivors after salvage therapy (185). Failure in distant sites alone or associated with locoregional failure does occur in about 25% to 40% of patients with locally advanced tumors (Table 21.6) (61,62,67, 68,91,101,147,185).

It is important to recognize that analysis of RT doses and techniques and their impact on local/pelvic tumor control are fraught with difficulty since the available data are retrospective and not the result of prospective randomized or dose escalation studies. Andersen (12) has shown that the combination of EBRT and brachytherapy and tumor dose over 70 Gy were associated with improved local control. In the Stanford experience (20), earlier stage and higher RT dose had a positive influence on survival. Nine of 16 patients receiving ≤75 Gy had recurrent disease versus 3 of 22 receiving >75 Gy. Larger series have not found a significant impact of the RT dose and

TABLE 21.6

PATTERNS OF FAILURE-SCC VAGINA

Authors	No. of patients	Percent of recurrence	Local-regional recurrence	Distant recurrence	Local + distant
Chyle et al. (14)	301	35%	21%	11%	3%
Davis et al. (24)	89	St I (23%)	18%	5%	Not shown
		St II (36%)	16%	20%	
Kirkbride et al. (16)	153	42%	32%	7%	3%
Kucera and Vavra (121)	110	24.5%	21%	4%	0.5%
Perez et al. (42)	212	St 0 (5%)	5%	0	0
		St I (22%)	8%	8%	5%
		St IIA (47%)	17%	13%	17%
		St IIB (71%)	15%	26%	29%
		St III (55%)	5%	20%	30%
		St IVA (73%)	27%	0	47%
		Total: 42%	13%	12%	17%
Tabata et al. (185)	51	St 0-II (36%)	36%	0%	Not shown
		St III-IV (92%)	50%	42%	
Urbanski et al. (23)	125	53%	41%	8%	4%
Frank et al. (147)	193	25%	12%	7%	13%

Note: St, stage.

recurrence rate, probably because larger tumors received higher EBRT and brachytherapy doses (14,42). The M. D. Anderson series (147) did not find dose lower than or greater than 75 Gy to be associated with improved pelvic control or disease-specific survival, the only two statistically significant factors being the stage of the disease and the size of the tumor over 4 cm.

Perez et al. (19,42) observed increased tumor control in patients with stages IIA to IVA with EBRT and brachytherapy compared to patients receiving brachytherapy alone. In patients with stage I disease, no correlation was found between the technique of RT used and the incidence of local or pelvic recurrences. In addition, they suggested that doses in the range of 70 to 75 Gy to the primary tumor volume and 55 and 65 Gy to the medial parametria for patients with more advanced disease are necessary to optimize tumor and pelvic control. Furthermore, of 100 patients with primary tumors involving the upper and middle third of the vagina who received no elective irradiation to the groins, none developed metastatic inguinofemoral lymph nodes, which is in contrast to 3 of 29 (10%) patients with lower-third primaries and 1 of 20 patients with tumors involving the entire length of the vagina. Of seven patients with initially palpable inguinal lymph nodes treated with doses to around 60 Gy, only one developed a nodal recurrence. The investigators recommended that elective RT of the inguinal lymph nodes should be carried out only in patients with primary tumors involving the lower third of the vagina. Similar results were published by Stock et al. (21) and Stryker (175). Lee et al. (111) identified overall treatment time as the most significant treatment factor predicting pelvic tumor control in 65 patients with carcinomas of the vagina treated with definitive RT. If the entire course of RT, including EBRT and brachytherapy, was completed within 9 weeks, pelvic tumor control was 97% in contrast to only 57% when treatment time extended beyond 9 weeks ($P < 0.01$). Conversely, Perez et al. (42) did not find a significant impact of prolongation of treatment time on pelvic tumor control. Nevertheless, these investigators advocate completion of treatment within 7 to 9 weeks.

TREATMENT COMPLICATIONS AND THEIR MANAGEMENT

The anatomic location of the vagina places the lower gastrointestinal and genitourinary tracts at greatest risk for complications after surgery or RT. Although in most of the retrospective series, the investigators comment on the nature of the complications encountered, little information is typically given regarding their prevention or manangement (13,15,21,40,112,124). In modern oncology, survival rate is the primary endpoint in treatment evaluation, but the analysis of treatment complications and quality of life is of crucial importance. The knowledge of common acute and late complications with standard RT and consideration of risk factors may improve the therapeutic ratio of RT for gynecologic malignancies in general, and for vaginal cancer in particular (186).

The acute and chronic pathophysiology of vaginal RT has been well described by Grigsby et al. (187). As an immediate response to high-dose RT, there is loss of most or all of the vaginal epithelium, especially in areas in proximity to brachytherapy sources. Clinically, the severity of the acute effects (edema, erythema, moist desquamation, and confluent mucositis with or without ulceration) varies in intensity and duration depending upon patient age, hormonal status, tumor size, stage, RT dose, and personal hygiene. These effects usually resolve within 2 to 3 months after completion of therapy. In some patients, there is progressive vascular damage with subsequent ulcer formation and mucosal necrosis, which may require up to 8 months for healing. Chemotherapy concurrently with RT enhances the acute mucosal response to both EBRT and brachytherapy. The effects of chemotherapy on the incidence of late complications, if any, are unclear. Over time, most patients will develop some degree of vaginal atrophy, fibrosis, and stenosis. Telangiectasis is commonly seen in the vagina. Vaginal narrowing or shortening, paravaginal fibrosis, loss of elasticity, and reduced lubrication often result in dyspareunia. More severe complications include necrosis with ulceration that can progress to fistula formation (rectovaginal, vesicovaginal, urethrovaginal).

The RT tolerance limits of the entire vagina are ill defined given the variety of techniques employed for the treatment of vaginal cancers. An irradiation tolerance level of the proximal vagina was suggested by Hintz et al. (188) based on a study of 16 patients whom received a maximum surface dose of 140 Gy, none of who developed severe complications or necrosis of the upper vagina. Based on their previous observation of a patient who developed a vesicovaginal fistula after receiving a 150-Gy mucosal dose to the anterior vaginal wall, they recommended a tolerance dose level of 150 Gy (direct summation of EBRT dose and ICB) to the anterior upper vaginal mucosa. They advocated dose rates of <0.8 Gy/h. These authors cautioned against placing radioactive needles on the surface of the vaginal cylinder because this may increase the frequency of vaginal necrosis. They also recommended keeping the total dose to the distal vagina less than 98 Gy. In addition, it was also observed that the posterior wall of the vagina is more prone to radiation injury than the anterior or lateral walls, and that the dose should be kept below 80 Gy in order to minimize the risk of rectovaginal fistula. Rubin and Casarett (189) suggested that the tolerance of the vaginal mucosa (Tolerance dose 5/5: 5% necrosis within 5 years) is approximately 90 Gy for ulceration and more than 100 Gy for fistula formation. This tolerance limit has been specified as a direct summation of dosage given by LDR-ICB and EBRT in the treatment of cervical cancer. Within the low-dose-rate range, whether a correction for the brachytherapy dose rate is necessary remains controversial. In a more recent series from Washington University, the traditional LDR tolerance dose of 150 Gy to the mucosa of the proximal vagina was shown to yield a nominal 11% and 4% grades 1, 2, and 3 sequelae, respectively (190).

The incidence of grade 2 or higher complications has been reported to be 15% to 25%, with the average of severe complications (those requiring surgery for correction or necessitating hospitalization) being approximately 8% to 10%. Table 21.7 (56,61,62,67,79,91,92,101,147) shows the incidence of complications greater than grade 2 in several large series of vaginal cancer patients. Host factors that may increase the risk of complications include prior pelvic surgery, pelvic inflammatory disease, immunosuppression status, collagen vascular disease, low body weight, patient age, significant smoking history, and comorbid illness (e.g., diabetes, hypertension, and cardiovascular disease) (19,42,147).

Perez et al. (19) reported grade 2-3 complications in approximately 5% of patients treated for stage 0 and I disease and in approximately 15% of patients with stage II lesions. No complications were reported in stage III and IV disease, probably because few patients lived long enough to manifest complications of treatment. The most common major complications were proctitis (two), rectovesicovaginal fistula (three), and vesicovaginal fistula (two). The most common minor complications were fibrosis of the vagina and small areas of mucosal necrosis, which were noted in approximately 10% of patients.

Lee et al. (111) showed that the total dose to the primary site was the most significant factor predicting the development of a severe complication (9% in patients receiving ≤80 Gy as compared with 25% in those receiving higher doses). Perez et al. (19) reported an increase in the rate of severe complications with higher clinical stage, probably reflecting the higher doses delivered with EBRT and brachytherapy.

Ball and Berman (13) reported on 58 patients with carcinoma of the vagina, including 30 who underwent surgery. There were four rectovaginal fistulae (one following RT and three after exenterative surgery) and two vesicovaginal fistulae (one following radical vaginectomy and the other following a recurrence, being managed with cystectomy and diversion). The single ureterovaginal fistula occurred after radical vaginectomy and partial cystectomy and was managed with ureteroneocystotomy.

In the Peters et al. report (112) of 86 vaginal primaries, there were two fistulae in the 57 patients who received primary RT. However, there was a 44% rate of fistula formation in the nine patients who underwent re-irradiation after having previously received RT for an earlier cancer. Rubin et al. (40) reported a 23% incidence of complications after RT, including a 13% rate of fistula formation and a 10% rate of cystitis/proctitis. Although two patients developed fistulae following combination therapy, the investigators did not think that the rate of complications following combination therapy was greater than that seen following RT alone.

In the Stock et al. series (21) of 100 patients with vaginal carcinoma, there was a 16% actuarial complication rate at 10 years. All patients undergoing vaginectomies or exenterations lost vaginal function. None of the patients was offered vaginal reconstruction in this series. The investigators emphasized that therapeutic options need to be individualized such that surgery is offered only to those most likely to benefit and least likely to suffer complications.

Chyle et al. (14) in 301 patients noted that 39 (13%) had 48 grade 2 or greater sequelae, including rectal ulceration or proctitis in 10 (3 requiring colostomy), small bowel obstruction in 7, rectovaginal fistula in 6, vesicovaginal fistula in 4,

TABLE 21.7

COMPLICATIONS OF THERAPY (≥GRADE 2)

Authors	No. of patients	Percent of complications (≥Grade 2)
Chyle et al. (14)	310	19% actuarial at 20 years
Kirkbrideet al. (16)	153	10%
Kucera and Vavra (121)	110	5.5%
Perez et al. (42)	212	13%
Peters et al. (112)	86	7 (8%)
Rubin et al. (40)	75	15 (23%)
Stock et al. (21)	100	16% actuarial at 10 years
Urbanski et al. (23)	125	13%
Frank et al. (147)	193	5 years, actuarial St I, 4% St II, 9% III-IVA, 21%

Note: St, stage.

vaginoperitoneal/cutaneous fistula in 2, and vaginal ulceration or necrosis in 8 patients. Fewer complications developed in patients with stage 0 or I tumors (8% to 9%) than with more advanced stages (14% to 40%). Vaginal ulceration occurred in 8 of 206 patients (4%) treated with brachytherapy, but in none of 95 patients who received no brachytherapy ($p = 0.06$).

Frank et al. (147) reported 10% and 17% 5- and 10-year cumulative rates of major (greater than grade 2) complications in a series of 193 patients treated with definitive RT with or without chemotherapy. They found FIGO stage and history of smoking to be the two factors significantly correlated with subsequent complications. Other clinical, dosimetric factors or the addition of chemotherapy did not correlate with the likelihood of complications. However, 73% of patients with major complications had tumors involving the posterior vaginal wall.

Treatment options for acute radiation vaginitis include daily vaginal douching with a diluted hydrogen peroxide/water mixture (187). This should continue for 2 to 3 months or until the mucosal reactions have subsided. Patients are then advised to continue douching once or twice per week for several months. Regular vaginal dilation is recommended as a way for patients to maintain vaginal health and good sexual function, although the compliance rate is low. The lack of resolution of vaginal ulceration or necrosis after several months of adequate therapy must be appropriately evaluated, considering the possibility of recurrent tumor. The use of topical estrogens following completion of RT appears to stimulate epithelial regeneration more than systemic estrogens. Some patients with severe radiation sequelae, such as fistula formation, will respond to conservative treatment with antibiotics and periodic limited debridement of necrotic tissue. More recently, Delanian et al. (191) published a randomized trial demonstrating the effectiveness of the combination of pentoxifyllin and vitamin E in the regression of radiation-induced fibrosis.

Patients with more severe gastrointestinal or urinary late effects will require urinary or fecal diversion with possible delayed re-anastomosis. Occasionally, repair of the fistula may be attempted by employing a myocutaneous graft in which the skin, subcutaneous fat, and muscle are mobilized using a vascular pedicle to maintain the blood supply to the pedicled graft (Martius flap), or by excision of the necrotic tissue with re-establishment of organ continuity (such as in the treatment of high rectovaginal fistula). A detailed review of the pathogenesis and management of potential late effects of treatment is not within the scope of this chapter, and may be found in the chapter on management of complications of gynecologic cancer treatment (see Chapter 31).

It is likely that improvements in modern practice such as advancements in surgical techniques (such as more generous use of myocutaneous flaps) (104,134), improved supportive care during the immediate postoperative stay, the use of more sophisticated RT field setting (three-dimensional conformal therapy and IMRT) and treatment delivery, more accurate brachytherapy techniques, and dose calculations have the potential to lessen complication rates posttherapy, regardless of which modality is used.

CLEAR CELL CARCINOMA OF THE VAGINA

Since Herbst and Scully's first report (192) of seven adenocarcinomas arising in the vagina of adolescent females after *in utero* exposure to DES, there have been several reports limited to DES-related vaginal CCA (28,29,47,193). In 1979, Herbst et al. (194) reported 142 cases of stage I CCA of the vagina. An 8% risk of recurrence was seen after radical surgery (N = 117), and an 87% survival was achieved. There was a 36% risk of recurrence after RT for stage I lesions; however, the investigators acknowledged that, in general, RT was reserved for large stage I lesions that involved more of the vault and were less amenable to surgical resection. Surgery for stage I CCA may have the advantage of ovarian preservation and, after skin graft, better vaginal function. As the majority of CCAs occur in the upper third of the vault, the largest series addressing the surgical approach to these lesions have advocated radical hysterectomy, pelvic and paraaortic lymphadenectomy, and sufficient colpectomy to achieve negative margins. Senekjian et al. have also reported a series of exenterations done for CCA (195). However, there have also been efforts to attempt fertility-sparing radical resections (196) or more limited wide local excisions followed by some form of RT (197). Wharton et al. (198) advocate intracavitary or transvaginal irradiation for the treatment of small tumors because this may yield excellent tumor control with a functional vagina and preservation of ovarian function.

Senekjian et al. (197) reported a series of 219 stage I CCA cases of which 176 had conventional therapy and 43 underwent local therapy. The two groups appear to be similar with respect to symptoms, stage, location of the lesion in the vagina, greatest tumor diameter, depth of invasion, predominant histologic pattern, grade, and number of mitoses. Actuarial survival rates at 5 and 10 years for the local therapy group (92% and 88%, respectively) were essentially equivalent to those for the conventional therapy group (92% and 90%, respectively). However, the recurrence experience after local therapy was less favorable; at 10 years, the actuarial recurrence rate for the local excision subgroup was 45%, in comparison with only 13% for patients treated with more radical surgery. Local therapy consisted of vaginectomy in 9 cases, local excision alone in 17 cases, and local irradiation (with or without local excision) in 17 cases. The subgroup of patients receiving local irradiation had a recurrence rate of 27%, similar to that of the conventional therapy group and more favorable than that of either the subgroup treated with vaginectomy or local excision alone. Recurrences were more frequently noted in patients with tumors >2 cm, with invasion of ≥ 3 mm, and with a predominant histologic pattern other than tubulocystic. Pelvic lymph node metastases were noted at death in 12% of patients. They advocated a combination of wide local excision and extraperitoneal node dissection followed by brachytherapy for patients desirous of fertility preservation (197).

In a subsequent report, Senekjian et al. (199) reviewed the experience with 76 cases with stage II CCA from the Registry for Research on Hormonal Transplacental Carcinogenesis. The overall 5- and 10-year survival rates were 83% and 65%, respectively. Of the 76 patients, 22 received surgery exclusively (either radical hysterectomy with vaginectomy, 13 patients, or exenterative type procedure, 9 patients), 38 received RT alone, 12 received combination therapy, and 4 underwent other approaches. Patients treated with primary RT achieved an 87% 5-year survival rate versus 80% for those treated with surgery and 85% for those receiving both treatments. The investigators concluded that most patients with stage II vaginal CCA should be treated with combination EBRT and brachytherapy; however, small, easily resectable lesions in the upper fornix might undergo resection, allowing better preservation of coital and ovarian function (199).

In 1989, Senekjian et al. (195) reported their experience of 20 pelvic exenterations for CCA of the vagina, including 13 for primary lesions and 7 for recurrent disease. The 9 patients with stage II disease treated with primary exenteration were compared with the 67 who had other modalities of therapy; no significant difference in the survival experience was noted between the two groups. They reported a 72% success rate if the exenterations were done as part of primary therapy. They advocated reserving exenterative approaches for those who have failed RT in order to maximize quality of life for the greatest number of patients (195).

There are few published reports regarding the use of systemic therapy for CCA. Fowler et al. (200) reported one complete and one partial response after treatment with melphalan (1 mg/kg qd × 5 days). Robboy et al. (43) reported responses in recurrent disease to both 5-FU and vinblastine.

NONEPITHELIAL TUMORS OF THE VAGINA

Melanoma of the Vagina

Vaginal melanoma is an exceedingly rare entity. It accounts for 2% to 3% of all primary tumors of the vagina and approximately 0.5% of all malignant melanomas in females. Therefore, the number of patients with vaginal melanoma is too small to permit prospective controlled trials. Melanoma of the vagina, with its propensity to develop distant metastases and its lack of a recognized precursor lesion, has presented therapeutic challenges for surgeons. Investigators have reported small series with generally disappointing results irrespective of treatment modality (34,201–206). Because of the reputation of melanoma as a radioresistant tumor, it is not surprising that radical surgery has been considered to be the treatment of choice in operable patients. However, limited data are available that validate its efficacy. Although 75% 2-year survival has been achieved after radical excision in small series (206), most series report 5-year survival rates of 5% to 30% regardless of radicality of surgery (34–36,201–206).

Morrow and DiSaia, in their review of all genital melanomas, noted no long-term survivors after isolated wide local excision for vaginal melanoma; however, 3 of 19 patients survived following exenteration (35). In the Chung et al. series of 19 patients, 7 were treated with radical surgery, including one exenteration and 6 radical vaginectomies, with or without hysterectomy, with an overall survival of 21%. All patients treated with wide local excision developed recurrences (34). On the other hand, Levitan et al. (205), in their review of the literature, argued that although the 2-year survival following radical surgery was better (20% to 40%) than with any other therapy, the 5-year survival rates were equally poor (average 8%) regardless of type of therapy. Furthermore, the incidence of distant recurrence was not influenced by the extent of surgical resection. Geisler et al. (203) published the Indiana University experience using pelvic exenteration for malignant melanomas of the vagina or urethra with more than 3 mm of invasion. None of the four patients included in this study had recurrences, and three patients remained alive with a minimum follow-up of 31 months. Conversely, Bonner et al. (201) reported nine cases of vaginal melanoma: Three received wide local excisions and six underwent radical surgery (including exenterations and radical vaginectomies with or without hysterectomies), with a 29% actuarial 5-year survival rate. All nine patients suffered locoregional recurrence. The investigators advocated that surgery alone was ineffective in obtaining local control, and that preoperative RT should be considered (201).

Reid et al. (36) reported an overall 17% 5-year survival rate in a report of 15 patients, including 13 who underwent surgery. In addition, they reviewed the literature, summarizing the results achieved in 115 patients with vaginal melanoma, and compared outcomes for the 55 patients who underwent some form of surgery, including the 24 treated conservatively with wide local excision or partial vaginectomy, to the 31 treated with more radical excisions. No difference in survival or disease-free survival was found among the different surgical procedures (36). In a meta-analysis of essentially the same patient population (n = 119 patients), Van Nostrand et al. (206), after adding eight of their own cases, reached different conclusions. They stated that radical surgery is recommended for patients with primary vaginal melanomas of less than 10 cm^2. In the Van Nostrand et al. series of their own eight patients with vaginal melanoma, including four treated conservatively and four undergoing radical surgery, the only long-term survivor was in the radical surgery group. In their review of the literature, comprising a total of 119 patients, there was 48% 2-year survival rate if treated with radical surgery (50 patients) versus only 20% if treated conservatively (69 patients) ($P < 0.005$). Therefore, Van Nostrand et al. advocated radical excision for those vaginal melanomas less than 10 cm^2 in area (206).

Not all authors support a radical resection approach. Buchanan et al. (202) performed a literature review of 66 cases reported since the publication of Reid et al. (36). Survival was influenced by tumor size, with a median survival time of 41 months of those with lesions <3 cm and 21 months in those with larger lesions. However, there was no statistically significant difference in median survival or 2- and 5-year survival among the various surgical strategies. Hence, many investigators have adopted the suggestion of Irvin et al. (204) that if distant failure and death are expected, quality of life should be optimized by wide excision followed by RT to affect local control, while obviating the need for disfiguring radical surgery (162). In the Irvin et al. series (204), all patients treated with wide local excision or brachytherapy alone developed recurrent disease locally, whereas those patients treated with radical surgical resection or with wide local excision followed by high-dose-per-fraction EBRT maintained locoregional control until death.

Recent retrospective data suggest that vaginal melanoma is reasonably radioresponsive and possibly radiocurable (204,207). Volumes and doses of irradiation are similar to those used for epithelial tumors, ranging from 50 Gy for subclinical disease to 75 Gy for gross tumors. Retrospective analysis suggested a dose-response curve of melanoma to external beam irradiation as the dose per fraction is increased and fractions of 3.5 Gy three times weekly to 5 Gy twice weekly have been used to treat melanoma because of a large D_q observed in *in vitro* studies (208,209). However, the Radiation Therapy Oncology Group conducted a prospective randomized study (RTOG 83-05) (210) evaluating the effectiveness of high-dose-per-fraction irradiation in the treatment of melanoma. Patients with measurable lesions were randomized to 4 × 8.0 Gy in 21 days once weekly to 20 × 2.5 Gy in 26 to 28 days, 5 days a week. One hundred thirty-seven patients were randomized and 126 patients were evaluable; stratification was performed on lesions <5 cm or ≥5 cm. There was no difference between the two arms in terms of response rate (complete responses 24.2% and 23.4% in the 4 × 8.0 Gy and in the 20 × 2.5 Gy arms, respectively) (210).

Chung et al. (34) reported on 19 cases of primary vaginal melanoma. Local tumor control was obtained by primary radical surgery in five of seven patients, three of whom later died of disseminated disease. Six of eight patients treated primarily with radiation therapy died with metastatic melanoma; another died after pelvic exenteration for persistent local disease. The overall 5-year survival rate for these 16 patients was 21%. Harwood and Cummings (211) described a complete response in four patients with vaginal melanoma treated with irradiation, although two subsequently relapsed; complete response to irradiation was seen in one patient who was alive and well 10 months after treatment. Harrison et al. (212)

reported that one of three patients with vaginal melanoma treated with irradiation survived 7.5 years; the other two died with distant metastases but had local tumor control. Rogo et al. (213) reported on 22 cases of vulvovaginal melanoma treated with conservation surgery or irradiation, or both. Eight patients (36%) were alive 5 years and four 10 years after treatment. Inguinal lymph node recurrences and distant metastases were the most common modes of failure. Results were comparable with those obtained with radical surgery.

In the Petru et al. series (207) of 14 patients, the three long-term survivors received either primary RT after biopsy only, or adjuvantly after local excision. Tumor size was found to be prognostically important, with 43% of patients with tumors ≤3 cm surviving longer than 5 years, compared with 0% of patients with tumors >3 cm. The median overall survival was 10 months, and the 5-year DFS and overall survival rates were 14% and 21%, respectively. The authors concluded that prolonged local control could be obtained with RT as an adjunct to more limited surgery, or even with RT alone, primarily in patients with lesions ≤3 cm in diameter.

In summary, given that the high incidence of distant metastasis remains a major factor in limiting curability, a more conservative treatment approach might be more reasonable in selected patients. Patients with vaginal melanoma should probably be managed in a manner similar to that recommended for cutaneous lesions (214). Wide local excision with 1- to 2-cm margins should be the surgical treatment of choice for most primary vaginal melanomas since radical surgery has failed to improve long-term survival. The role of adjuvant RT is unclear, but it appears to improve survival in some series. The use of systemic chemotherapy and/or immunotherapy has been very disappointing in the limited published data (215).

Sarcomas of the Vagina

Sarcomas represent 3% of vaginal primaries (4) with leiomyosarcoma representing 50% to 65% of vaginal sarcomas. Unfortunately, most of the sarcomas are diagnosed at an advanced stage. Histopathologic grade appears to be the most important predictor of outcome (39). Most vaginal leiomyosarcomas arise from the posterior wall of the vagina. Radical surgical resection, such as posterior pelvic exenteration, offers the best chance for cure for vaginal leiomyosarcomas (4,216). The largest series on vaginal sarcomas reported to date included 17 cases, of which 35% had received prior RT. This series, which included ten leiomyosarcomas, four malignant mixed müllerian tumors (MMMTs), and three other sarcoma types, noted that all were resistant to chemotherapy, and all of the failures were first noted as pelvic recurrences. There were only three survivors seen, and all had undergone exenterative surgery. The 5-year survival rate was 36% in patients with leiomyosarcoma and 17% in those with MMMT (85).

Vaginal MMMTs occur more commonly in postmenopausal women. In approximately half of the cases there is a history of prior pelvic RT (85,217). Despite surgery and adjuvant RT, patients usually do poorly, with a high incidence of local and distant recurrences. The treatment of choice is complete surgical resection, followed by EBRT and ICB in an attempt to decrease the local recurrence rate.

The roles of adjuvant chemotherapy and RT in vaginal sarcomas have not been clearly defined, primarily owing to limited patient numbers and even fewer data where chemotherapy was used as the primary treatment rather than as salvage therapy at recurrence. Adjuvant RT seems to be indicated in patients with high-grade tumors and locally recurrent low-grade sarcomas. According to Peters et al. (85) the most common site of failure is the pelvis. In 50% of patients with recurrence, it is the only site of failure. Extrapolating data from the Gynecologic Oncology Group (218) for uterine sarcomas and considering patterns of failure, patients with localized MMMTs would be appropriately treated with pelvic exenteration, or with more limited surgical resection followed by postoperative RT, unless the patient has received prior pelvic RT. Since patterns of failure suggest that local therapies only reduce the local recurrence rate and do not improve survival, consideration should be given to adjuvant treatments with agents that are active in similar tumors arising in the uterus. Agents found to be active in MMMT of the uterus include ifosfamide, cisplatin, and paclitaxel, although it remains unclear whether any combination of these agents is better than ifosfamide alone, which has produced the highest response rate among these agents (219,220). Doxorubicin remains the standard therapy for leiomyosarcoma (221).

Embryonal rhabdomyosarcoma (RMS) of the vagina, the most common pediatric vaginal tumor, is such a rare lesion that no single institution has sufficient experience to identify superior therapeutic strategies. Rather, cooperative efforts through the Intergroup Rhabdomyosarcoma Study Group (IRSG) through numerous clinical trials have demonstrated that the use of of multimodality therapy with wide local excision and cytotoxic chemotherapy with or without RT makes it possible to avoid exenterative surgery and optimize quality of life for these young patients (50,222–224). Prior to the modern era of multimodality therapy, Hilgers reported that only 20% to 30% 5-year survival rates were achieved with the use of exenterative-type surgery alone (225). Later, several small series noted that 70% survival could be achieved if RT and combination cytotoxic chemotherapy including vincristine, actinomycin D, and cyclophosphamide (VAC) were given in addition to radical surgery (84,225,226). After complete resection, irradiation of the entire pelvis is not required, thus avoiding its adverse effects.

In a series of reports from the IRSG, survival rates in excess of 85% have been achieved utilizing VAC chemotherapy and wide excision with or without adjuvant RT, sparing the great majority of patients from exenterative surgery (222–224, 227,228). In a subsequent report, Andrassy et al. (229) from the IRSG summarized the outcome of 72 patients with embryonal RMS of the vagina treated on four IRSG trials. Over the course of the four IRSG trials, the need for radical resection decreased from 100% to 13%, with continued improvement in disease-free survival (229). Andrassy et al. suggested that after biopsy to document RMS, multiagent induction chemotherapy with doxorubicin, cisplatin, vincristine, actinomycin D, and cyclophosphamide should be utilized, then local resection undertaken, with radical resection being reserved for those with persistent or recurrent disease (229). In addition, several non-IRSG series have shown that combination chemotherapy with or without RT leads to sufficient tumor shrinkage, and that less radical resections can become feasible (227,228), allowing preservation of anatomy and function.

Flamant et al. (227) reported 11 cases of vaginal RMS (8 stage I, 2 stage II, 1 stage III) in whom 100% survival was achieved with multimodality therapy. Eight patients received neoadjuvant chemotherapy, generally a VAC regimen, and all patients underwent brachytherapy (doses of 26 to 75 Gy), followed by maintenance chemotherapy and VAC alternating with VAD (vincristine, doxorubicin, dacarbazine). Seven patients underwent ovarian transposition in an attempt to preserve function. The investigators noted partial ovarian insufficiency in one patient without ovarian transposition. They recommended brachytherapy at a total dose of approximately 50 to 60 Gy (227).

Lymphomas and the Vagina

Lymphomatous involvement of the vagina most often represents metastatic spread from another primary site. Although surgery including radical hysterectomy, pelvic lymphadenectomy, vaginectomy, and exenteration has been performed in the past, more recent reports suggest that combination RT and chemotherapy can achieve excellent results. Radical surgery in such patients then should be avoided, as lymphoma represents a systemic disease. Following biopsy, patients with lymphoma should be managed with chemotherapy alone or combined chemoradiation. Extrapolation from patients with similar tumors arising in extranodal sites would suggest that RT has its primary role in preventing local recurrence in patients who present with bulky disease. In some patients who have a rapid and complete response to multiagent chemotherapy, RT may not be indicated since the combination of both modalities increases the risk of second malignancies. Harris and Scully noted in a clinicopathologic series of 25 lower genital tract lymphomas, including four vaginal lymphomas, that definitive local therapy prevented relapse (98). Prevot et al. (230) and Perren et al. (231) also advocated the use of less extensive surgery, with RT plus cytotoxic multiagent chemotherapy such as CHOP (cyclophosphamide, hydroxydaunomycin [doxorubicin], Oncovin [vincristine], prednisone) or BACOP (bleomycin, Adriamycin [doxorubicin], cyclophosphamide, Oncovin [vincristine], prednisone) for four to six cycles to affect local control with better preservation of fertility in patients with stage IE and nonbulky tumors of low and intermediate grade.

Yolk Sac (Endodermal Sinus) Tumors of the Vagina

Prior to the use of multiagent cytotoxic chemotherapy, less than 25% of patients with yolk sac tumor (YST), or endodermal sinus tumor (EST), of the vagina survived. However, Young and Scully noted 100% survival in a small series of six patients who had received chemotherapy (232). The VAC regimen in conjunction with surgery or RT was advocated by Copeland et al. (233). Collins et al. (234) reported on the use of combination bleomycin, vinblastine, and platinum (BVP) for patients with EST of the vagina. Aartsen et al. (235) reported a successful pregnancy following surgery and chemotherapy. Most recently, Hwang et al. have reported two cases, one of which did well with partial vaginectomy followed by 2 years of VAC; however, the second one developed a central persistence following wide local excision and VAC, but was salvaged with bleomycin, etoposide, and platinum (BEP) (236). Given the excellent results that three to four cycles of BEP have achieved in malignant germ-cell neoplasms of the ovary (237), it is likely that BEP will become the preferred regimen for EST of the vagina used in conjunction with parital vaginectomy, as it requires less prolonged administration and is less oophorotoxic than VAC. It appears that routine use of combination chemotherapy in the management of endodermal sinus tumor allows conservative surgery with preservation of sexual function in young patients, with excellent prospects for long-term survival.

The role of radiation in this disease is limited because of the younger age at presentation, and preservation of ovarian function is desired; in addition, RT would potentially increase the risk for secondary malignancies (238,239), which may be even more significant with the use of IMRT as the volume of irradiation receiving lower doses is generally larger (240). Brachytherapy may occasionally be used, and in one instance, preservation of hormonal function and subsequent pregnancy were reported (235).

OTHER UNCOMMON VAGINAL CANCERS

Squamous Cell Carcinoma of the Neovagina

In situ and invasive carcinomas arising in the neovagina are rare, and this type of malignancy seems to be related to the transplanted tissue. A few cases of squamous cell carcinoma have been described after split-thickness skin graft vaginoplasty in patients with vaginal agenesis (241–243), as well as after radical vulvo-vaginal resection for known malignancy (244). Mucinous adenocarcinoma has been described arising in the sigmoid colon used for the reconstruction of the neovagina (76). Neovaginal malignant melanoma following surgery and radiation therapy for vulvo-vaginal malignancies, although extremely rare, has been reported (245), suggesting the potential role of radiation-induced melanoma in non–sun-exposed areas such as the genital tract.

Malignant transformation occurs in the neovaginal epithelium, in relation with local carcinogenic environmental factors as well as possible viral infection, with the subsequent risk of malignancy. Therefore, it is important to emphasize the need for regular follow-up visits with Pap smears. The elapsed time between the construction of the neovagina and the development of malignancy ranges between 10 and 30 years. The optimal treatment is not well defined. Radical surgery resection when possible should be the treatment of choice, since definitive RT seems to be associated with higher failure rates (241). Adjuvant RT could be considered in patients with positive margins or positive nodes (76).

Carcinoma in Episiotomy Scar

Episiotomy scar tumor implantation from a cervical or vulvar carcinoma is a very rare event. Van Dam et al. (246) reported on three cases of primary or metastatic carcinoma in an episiotomy scar. One patient had a primary squamous cell carcinoma of the vulva in an episiotomy scar; a second patient was diagnosed with cervical carcinoma 6 months postpartum and was found to have a metastatic deposit in the episiotomy scar during the staging of her disease; the third patient developed adenocarcinoma metastatic from an endocervical primary in an episiotomy scar that presented as a small nodule at the introitus. These cases exemplify the need for careful inspection and biopsy of any nodular lesions in episiotomy scars as part of the initial assessment and follow-up of patients with premalignant or malignant lesions of the lower genital tract. Early initial stage, small size lesion, and early therapy appear to improve prognosis. Treatment needs to be individualized given the rarity of this entity. Patients with limited recurrent disease at the episiotomy site without any other evidence of locoregional recurrence could be treated with surgical resection followed by tailored radiation therapy. Patients with more advanced disease may be offered radiation with or without chemotherapy followed by surgical resection when feasible (247,248).

SALVAGE THERAPY

In general, the patient with recurrent cancer of the lower female genital tract presents a difficult clinical dilemma. Optimal therapy for patients with recurrent gynecologic cancer after potentially curative therapy has not been completely defined, partly owing to the difficulty of conducting prospective, randomized trials in this heterogeneous population. It must be determined if the disease is amenable to curative salvage therapy, implying some reasonable chance of cure, or whether palliation is the primary goal. Treatment selection factors include primary therapy, extent of the disease at presentation, site of recurrence, extent of the recurrence, disease-free interval, evidence of metastatic disease, patient age, performance status, and coexisting medical conditions. The presence of distant metastasis portends a poor prognosis, and although chemotherapy may result in objective responses and improvements in short-term survival, the current lack of curative systemic treatments focuses therapeutic attempts on symptom palliation and quality of life. In most cases, only patients with small volume local recurrences and no metastatic disease are curable. Therefore, careful workup to establish extent of disease is crucial. When salvage therapies are contemplated, local recurrences should be confirmed by biopsy, and, when possible, parametrial recurrences should be documented pathologically. Pelvic sidewall involvement can almost always be diagnosed in the presence of a symptom triad of sciatic pain, leg edema, and hydronephrosis. It is important to evaluate for regional and/or distant metastasis by physical examination and imaging studies such as CT or MRI scans. More recently, the positron emission tomography (PET) scan has been used to document the extent of recurrent disease (249), but both false-positive and false-negative results have been reported.

Generally, patients with isolated pelvic or regional recurrences after definitive surgery who have not received prior RT are managed with EBRT, often in conjunction with brachytherapy. Concurrent cisplatin-based chemotherapy may also be recommended. Salvage options for patients with central recurrence after definitive or adjuvant RT are limited to radical surgery, usually exenterative, or, in selected patients with small volume disease, reirradiation using interstitial radiation implants or highly conformal three-dimensional EBRT. Response rates with chemotherapy are low and the impact on survival is limited. Further, response to chemotherapy in central pelvic recurrences following RT tends to be less common than response at distant sites. Additionally, prior high-dose radiation therapy compromises bone marrow tolerance of many agents that are active in this tumor (e.g., ifosfamide and doxorubicin). However, chemotherapy-responsive patients can obtain meaningful palliation in many cases.

Surgical Considerations

Despite thorough clinical evaluation of patients considered to be excellent candidates for salvage surgery, this will be aborted in over 25% of the cases because of advanced disease found at the time of the exploratory laparotomy (250). Pelvic exenteration results in long-term functional and psychologic changes that have not been adequately studied (251). Surgical refinements have done much to improve body image changes associated with pelvic exenteration. The purposes of vaginal and perineal reconstruction following radical pelvic surgery for recurrent gynecologic cancer are primarily twofold: to restore or create vulvovaginal function, and thereby minimize the effects of surgical treatment on body image and normal sexual activity, and to minimize postoperative complications by transferring to the pelvic defect healthy tissue with a good blood supply (143,144). A detailed review of urinary diversion and pelvic reconstruction techniques is not within the scope of this chapter.

Radiation Therapy Considerations

Those patients who have not received prior RT should receive whole-pelvis EBRT followed, when feasible, by brachytherapy. Generally, the whole pelvis receives a dose of 40 to 50 Gy. Inguinofemoral lymph node regions should be included in patients with involvement of the distal third of the vagina or with vulvar recurrences. The gross tumor volume in the vagina, paravaginal tissues, and/or parametrium should receive an additional boost, preferably with an interstitial implant, to bring the total tumor dose to 75 to 80 Gy. The role of combined chemoradiotherapy in the management of patients with recurrent disease is unknown. Given the rarity of vaginal carcinoma and the heterogeneity within the population with recurrent disease, large randomized studies intended to answer this question will probably never be conducted. However, by extrapolation from the available data for locally advanced cervical and vulvar cancer (181–184), it seems that a combined modality approach may improve the locoregional control and survival in patients with isolated pelvic recurrences.

Reirradiation in previously irradiated patients must be undertaken with extreme caution. However, selected patients who are medically inoperable, technically unresectable, or refuse to undergo exenterative surgery are appropriately considered for reirradiation to limited volumes. A variety of techniques is available, and the choice is based on patient and tumor-related factors, as well as the experience of the radiation oncologist. When using EBRT, multiple-beam arrangements utilizing three-dimensional treatment planning are favored. Only limited doses are possible, and the physician might consider a hyperfractionated regimen in an attempt to decrease the incidence of late toxicity. In patients with small, well-defined vulvovaginal or pelvic recurrences, reirradiation using primarily interstitial techniques has been attempted with control rates between 50% and 75% and grade 3 or higher complication rates between 7% and 15% (252–256). The rationale, logistics, and selection of implant technique when performing an interstitial implant (ITI) were reviewed earlier in the chapter. Permanent radioactive seed implants (e.g., ^{198}Au) in patients with small vaginal recurrences often provide long-lasting tumor control in elderly or medically debilitated patients previously treated with definitive doses of RT (253).

Other potential treatment options include the use of surgery and intraoperative RT (IORT) with intraoperative electron beam (257,258), laparotomy, or laparoscopically guided placement of HDR catheters (172,257,259,260), which allows direct visualization of the target volume and displacement and/or shielding of the surrounding normal tissues. However, the published series are generally small, including a wide spectrum of patients with different gynecologic malignancies, varying amounts of residual disease, and disparate initial therapies. The locoregional recurrence and distant metastasis rates after IORT vary between 20% and 60% and 20% and 58%, respectively. The 3- to 5-year actuarial survival is poor, ranging from 8% to 25%. Grade 3 or higher toxicity has been reported in about 35% of patients (257,258). In the Memorial Sloan-Kettering Cancer Center experience using radical surgical resection and HDR-IORT, patients with complete gross resection had a 3-year local control rate of 83% compared to 25% in patients with gross residual disease. Interestingly, most of the failures in the microscopic group were distant, perhaps indicating a potential role for adjuvant chemotherapy (259).

Hockel et al. (260) described a combined operative and radiotherapeutic treatment (CORT) for the treatment of recurrent gynecologic malignancies infiltrating the pelvic side wall. The procedure involves gross complete resection of the tumor and a single plane interstitial implant. In order to improve the therapeutic index, well-vascularized tissue is transposed to the pelvis to protect the hollow organs and reduce the late effects of RT. Reconstruction of pelvic organs is performed as with exenteration. The tumor bed is irradiated postoperatively, days 10 to 14, using HDR brachytherapy. In a total of 48 patients treated with this technique, the overall severe complication rate was 33% at 5 years. The 5-year survival rate was 44%, and the absolute local control rate was 60% for the first 20 patients and 85% for the last 28 treated patients (260).

Stereotactic body radiotherapy (SBRT), also known as extracranial stereotactic radioablation (ESR), is a novel treatment paradigm that delivers a small number of high-dose fractions to extracranial targets using a linear accelerator with highly precise, accurate, and reproducible target localization based on the same principle as that of gamma-knife therapy. By means of better target localization and patient immobilization, smaller margins of normal tissue surrounding the gross tumor volume are required, which allows treatment complications to be minimized. Blomgren et al. (261) reported on 15 patients with 19 extrahepatic abdominal tumors who had a mean survival of 17.7 months. The toxicity was more often self-limited except for four patients with gastrointestinal bleeding. They concluded that this treatment, which is noninvasive, painless, rapid, and does not require hospitalization, does not impair the quality of life of the patients when used properly.

PALLIATIVE THERAPY

Radiation Therapy

At the present time, there is no curative option for patients who present with stage IVB disease. Many of these patients suffer from severe pelvic pain or bleeding. If vaginal bleeding is the main concern, ICB, if feasible, often offers good symptom control with relatively low morbidity. For patients who have received prior RT, intracavitary doses in the range of 35 to 40 Gy to point A should be prescribed. A short course of EBRT using high-dose fractionation schedules has been used, including single doses of 10 Gy per fraction, times three, with an interval of 4 to 6 weeks between courses, combined with misonidazole (RTOG clinical trial 79–05), resulting in significant palliation in selected patients with advanced gynecologic malignancies. The overall response rate was 41% for patients completing the three courses; however, the actuarial 45% incidence of grades 3 and 4 late gastrointestinal toxicity was unacceptable (262).

Spanos et al. (263) reported on a phase 2 study (RTOG 85–02) of daily multifraction split-course EBRT in patients with recurrent or metastatic disease. The regimen consisted of 3.7 Gy per fraction given twice daily for 2 consecutive days and repeated at 3- to 6-week intervals for a total of three courses (tumor dose 44.4 Gy). Occasionally, this regimen was combined with an intracavitary implant (ICI) (4,500 mgh), with a midline block in the last 14.4 Gy. Complete tumor response was noted in 15 patients (10.5%) and partial response in 32 (22.5%). In patients completing three courses of irradiation (59%), the rate of complete or partial response was 45%. Twenty-seven patients survived longer than 1 year. Late complications were significantly fewer, with a projected actuarial rate of 5% at 12 months. In a subsequent phase 3 study (210), 136 patients were randomized between rest intervals of 2 versus 4 weeks between the split courses of RT. Decreasing the interval between courses did not result in a significant improvement in tumor response (34% vs 26%). More patients in the 2-week rest group completed the three courses of therapy, and not surprisingly, patients completing all three courses had a higher overall response rate than patients completing less than three courses (42% vs 5%) and a higher complete response rate (17% vs 1%). This schedule offers significant logistic benefits, and has been shown to result in good tumor regression and excellent palliation of symptoms (264). Spanos et al. (265) reported a trend toward increased acute toxicity in patients with shorter rest periods, but late toxicity was not significantly different in the two groups.

Chemotherapy in Advanced and Recurrent Vaginal Cancer

Given its rarity, most chemotherapy reports for treatment of metastatic disease in vaginal cancer are anecdotal or combined with reports of treatment of advanced or recurrent cervical cancer. Concurrent chemoradiation is frequently employed in clinical practice in the treatment of unresectable, locoregionally advanced disease. Various chemotherapeutic agents have been used with limited success (176,177). Evans et al. (176) reported on seven patients with vaginal cancers who were treated with a combination of 5-FU 1,000 mg/m^2/d for 4 days, mitomycin C 10 mg/m^2 day 1, and primary irradiation, receiving 2,000 to 6,500 cGy. All of the vaginal cancer patients responded, and 66% were alive with a median follow-up of 28 months. Treatment of recurrent or metastatic disease is confined to a handful of phase 2 clinical trials and anecdotal reports. In general, regimens that are active in cervical cancer are usually active in vaginal cancer. Thigpen et al. (220) reported the results of a phase 2 trial of cisplatin 50 mg/m^2 every 3 weeks in 26 patients with advanced or recurrent vaginal cancer. There were 22 evaluable patients, 16 with SCC, two adenosquamous carcinoma, one clear cell carcinoma (CCC), one leiomyosarcoma, and two unspecified. Of the 16 SCC patients, there was one complete response (6.2%). It should be noted that these patients, for the most part, had received prior surgery and RT. Muss et al. (266) reported no responses in 19 evaluable patients who were treated with mitoxantrone 12 mg/m^2 every 3 weeks. Median survival of patients with vaginal cancer was 2.7 months. Other anecdotal reports of responses in trials that included advanced cervical cancer include a report by Long et al. (267) in which three patients with advanced vaginal SCC received treatment with methotrexate, vinblastine, doxorubicin, and cisplatin (MVAC). All three patients achieved a complete response of short duration. Patton et al. (268) reported the results of intra-arterial chemotherapy with mitomycin C, bleomycin, cisplatin, and vincristine, including six patients with primary vaginal cancer and 40 patients with cervical cancer. Seventy-six percent responded to intra-arterial chemotherapy and subsequently received primary RT. The report did not give details as to site of relapse, impact on disease-free survival, or overall survival.

At the present time, data on systemic treatment of advanced vaginal cancer outside of a clinical trial is purely anecdotal, although it might be reasonable to extrapolate from the experience reported with SCC of the cervix and vulva (180–184). Although published response rates are low, standard therapy should include cisplatin alone or in conjunction with RT in patients with locoregionally advanced vaginal cancer.

SUMMARY AND CONCLUSIONS

The malignant histologies of the vagina are so rare that randomized clinical trials have not been undertaken. It is difficult to establish strong, evidence-based recommendations in such a rare disease as cancer of the vagina. Therefore, future progress will likely come from reports from single institutions. Most of the available data refer to the treatment of primary invasive SCC of the vagina, since this represents the most common histology. The following management recommendations are made based on the available data.

Vaginal Intraepithelial Neoplasia

In patients with unifocal disease, partial colpectomy has come to be favored over laser vaporization, since there is an approximately 25% risk that there can be underlying invasive disease, and one quarter to one third of patients will require a second laser vaporization to effect long-term control. However, for patients who develop VAIN following radiation wherein colpectomy would be associated with a higher risk of fistulae development, there may be a role for laser vaporization and/or topical 5-FU application. Intracavitary brachytherapy alone has provided satisfactory functional and local control results as well.

Invasive Squamous Cell Carcinoma

Although RT can control many cases of vaginal cancer, local control remains a problem. The treatment of invasive SCC with RT should include the use of brachytherapy, with particular attention to technique that ensures that the treatment volume is adequately covered. In larger tumors, the dose that is needed to achieve local control may well exceed the tolerance of surrounding normal tissues. Although not specifically proven for patients with vaginal primaries, the addition of chemotherapy (i.e., weekly cisplatin) as a radiosensitizing agent may help to improve these results if the strong evidence in locally advanced cervical cancer can be extrapolated to vaginal cancer. Although there are multiple series that demonstrate excellent results with radical surgery for well-selected early-stage patients, RT will continue to be the primary modality even for early-stage disease and for those elderly patients with multiple comorbid conditions.

Clear Cell Adenocarcinoma

It has been suggested that patients with early-stage disease may be offered fertility-sparing combined modality local therapy with extraperitoneal node dissection and wide local excision followed by brachytherapy with acceptable local failure rates. However, advanced-stage disease would require primary RT. Patients who have completed childbearing would be best served by radical hysterectomy, colpectomy, and lymphadenectomy. Exenteration should be reserved for those patients who have isolated central failures following definitive RT.

Melanoma

The risk of distant metastases is high enough that most modern investigators have suggested that ultra-radical surgery, although it might improve 2-year survival rates, has not led to an increase in long-term survival. Wide excision followed by RT to effect local control may obviate the need of disfiguring surgery in those likely destined to develop distant metastases.

Sarcoma

The trials conducted by the IRSG and others have demonstrated that pediatric embryonal RMS of the vagina is best approached with induction multiagent-combination therapy, e.g., VAC, followed by local resection with or without brachytherapy, with radical surgery being reserved for those with persistent or recurrent disease. Patients with adult-onset vaginal sarcoma do not respond as well to chemotherapy, and the only long-term survivors are those who have been offered exenterative surgery.

References

1. Sedlis A, Robboy SJ. Diseases of the vagina. In: Kurman RJ, ed. *Blaustein's Pathology of the Female Genital Tract.* 3rd ed. New York: Springer-Verlag; 1987:98–140.
2. Plentl AA, Friedman EA. Lymphatic system of the female genitalia. In: Plentl AA, Friedman EA, eds. *The Morphologic Basis of Oncologic Diagnosis and Therapy.* Vol 2. Philadelphia: WB Saunders; 1971:51–74.
3. Herbst AL, Green TH Jr, Ulfelder H. Primary carcinoma of the vagina. *Am J Obstet Gynecol* 1970;106:210–218.
4. Creasman WT, Phillips JL, Menck HR. The National Cancer Data Base report on cancer of the vagina. *Cancer* 1998;83:1033–1040.
5. Di Domenico A. Primary vaginal squamous cell carcinoma in the young patient. *Gynecol Oncol* 1989;35:181–187.
6. Daling JR, Madeleine MM, Schwartz SM, et al. A population-based study of squamous cell vaginal cancer: HPV and cofactors. *Gynecol Oncol* 2002;84:263–270.
7. Okagaki T, Twiggs LB, Zachow KR, et al. Identification of human papillomavirus DNA in cervical and vaginal intraepithelial neoplasia with molecularly cloned virus-specific DNA probes. *Int J Gynaecol Pathol* 1983;2:153–159.
8. Brinton LA, Nasca PC, Mallin K, et al. Case-control study of *in situ* and invasive carcinoma of the vagina. *Gynecol Oncol* 1990;38:49–54.
9. Reeves WC, Brinton LA, Garcia M, et al. Human papilloma virus infection and cervical cancer in Latin America. *N Engl J Med* 1989;320: 1437–1441.
10. Aho MK, Vesterinen E, Meyer B, et al. Natural history of vaginal intraepithelial neoplasia. *Cancer* 1991;68:195–197.
11. Weiderpass E, Ye W, Tamimi R, et al. Alcoholism and risk for cancer for the cervix uteri, vagina, and vulva. *Cancer Epidemiol Biomarkers Prev* 2001;10:899–901.
12. Andersen ES. Primary carcinoma of the vagina: a study of 29 cases. *Gynecol Oncol* 1989;33:317–320.
13. Ball HG, Berman ML. Management of primary vaginal carcinoma. *Gynecol Oncol* 1982;14:154–163.
14. Chyle V, Zagars GK, Wheeler JA, et al. Definitive radiotherapy for carcinoma of the vagina. *Int J Radiat Oncol Biol Phys* 1996;35:891–905.
15. Gallup DG, Talledo OE, Shah KJ, et al. Invasive squamous cell carcinoma of the vagina. A 14-year study. *Obstet Gynecol* 1987;69:782–785.
16. Kirkbride P, Fyles A, Rawlings GA, et al. Carcinoma of the vagina—experience at the Princess Margaret Hospital (1974–1989). *Gynecol Oncol* 1995;56: 435–443.
17. Lenehan PM, Meffe F, Lickrish GM. Vaginal intraepithelial neoplasia: biologic aspects and management. *Obstet Gynecol* 1986;68:333–337.
18. Leung S, Sexton M. Radical radiation therapy for carcinoma of the vagina—impact of treatment modalities on outcome: Peter MacCallum Cancer Institute experience 1970–1990. *Int J Radiat Oncol Biol Phys* 1993;25:413–418.
19. Perez CA, Camel HM, Galakatos AE, et al. Definitive irradiation in carcinoma of the vagina: long-term evaluation and results. *Int J Radiat Oncol Biol Phys* 1988;15:1283–1290.
20. Spirtos NM, Doshi BP, Kapp DS, et al. Radiation therapy for primary squamous cell carcinoma of the vagina: Stanford University experience. *Gynecol Oncol* 1989;35:20–26.
21. Stock RG, Chen ASJ, Seski J. A 30-year experience in the management of primary carcinoma of the vagina: analysis of prognostic factors and treatment modalities. *Gynecol Oncol* 1995;56:45–52.
22. Stock RG, Mychalczak B, Armstrong JG, et al. The importance of the brachytherapy technique in the management of primary carcinoma of the vagina. *Int J Radiat Oncol Biol Phys* 1992;24:747–753.
23. Urbanski K, Kojs Z, Reinfuss M, et al. Primary invasive vaginal carcinoma treated with radiotherapy: analysis of prognostic factors. *Gynecol Oncol* 1996;60:16–21.
24. Davis KP, Stanhope CR, Garton GR, et al. Invasive vaginal carcinoma: analysis of early stage disease. *Gynecol Oncol* 1991;42:131–136.
25. Boice JD, Engholm G, Kleinerman RA, et al. Radiation dose and second cancer risk in patients treated for cancer of the cervix. *Radiat Res* 1988;116:3–55.
26. Lee JY, Perez CA, Ettinger N, et al. The risk of second primaries subsequent to irradiation for cervix cancer. *Int J Radiat Oncol Biol Phys* 1982;8:207–211.
27. Manetta A, Guttrecht EL, Berman ML, et al. Primary invasive carcinoma of the vagina. *Obstet Gynecol* 1990;76:639–642.
28. Bornstein J, Adam E, Adler-Storthz K, et al. Development of cervical and vaginal squamous neoplasia as a late consequence of *in utero* exposure to diethylstilbestrol. *Obstet Gynecol Surv* 1988;43:15–21.
29. Herbst AL, Ulfelder H, Poskanzer DC. Adenocarcinoma of the vagina: association of maternal stilbestrol therapy with tumor appearance in young women. *N Engl J Med* 1971;284:878–881.
30. Melnick S, Cole P, Anderson D, et al. Rates and risks of diethylstilbestrol-related clear-cell adenocarcinoma of the vagina and cervix. *N Engl J Med* 1987;316:514–516.
31. Hebrst AL, Anderson D. Clear cell adenocarcinoma of the vagina and cervix secondary to intrauterine exposure to diethylstilbestrol. *Semin Surg Oncol* 1990;6:343–346.

32. Hicks ML, Piver MS. Conservative surgery plus adjuvant therapy for vulvovaginal rhabdomyosarcoma, diethylstilbestrol clear cell adenocarcinoma of the vagina, and unilateral germ cell tumors of the ovary. *Obstet Gynecol Clin North Am* 1992;19:219–233.
33. Palmer JR, Anderson D, Helmrich SP, et al. Risk factors for diethylstilbestrol-associated clear cell adenocarcinoma. *Obstet Gynecol* 2000;95:814–820.
34. Chung AF, Casey MJ, Flannery JT, et al. Malignant melanoma of the vagina: report of 19 cases. *Obstet Gynecol* 1980;55:720–727.
35. Morrow CP, DiSaia PJ. Malignant melanoma of the female genitalia: a clinical analysis. *Obstet Gynecol Surv* 1976;31:233–271.
36. Reid GC, Schmidt RW, Roberts JA, et al. Primary melanoma of the vagina. A clinicopathologic analysis. *Obstet Gynecol* 1989;74:190–199.
37. Trimble EL. Melanomas of the vulva and vagina. *Oncology* 1996;10:1017–1023; discussion 1024.
38. Prempree T, Tang CK, Hatef A, et al. Angiosarcoma of the vagina: a clinicopathologic report: a reappraisal of radiation treatment of angiosarcomas of the female genital tract. *Cancer* 1983;51:618–622.
39. Curtin JP, Saigo P, Slucher B, et al. Soft-tissue sarcoma of the vagina and vulva: a clinicopathologic study. *Obstet Gynecol* 1995;86:269–272.
40. Rubin SC, Young J, Mikuta JJ. Squamous carcinoma of the vagina: treatment, complications and long-term follow-up. *Gynecol Oncol* 1985;20:346–353.
41. Al-Kurdi M, Monaghan JM. Thirty-two years experience in management of primary tumors of the vagina. *Br J Obstet Gynaecol* 1981;88:1145–1150.
42. Perez CA, Grigsby PW, Garipagaoglu M, et al. Factors affecting long-term outcome of irradiation in carcinoma of the vagina. *Int J Radiat Oncol Biol Phys* 1999;44:37–45.
43. Robboy SJ, Herbst AL, Scully RE. Clear cell adenocarcinoma of the vagina and cervix in young females: analysis of 37 tumors that persisted or recurred after primary therapy. *Cancer* 1974;34:606–614.
44. Saslow D, Runowicz CD, Solomon D, et al. American Cancer Society guideline for the early detection of cervical neoplasia and cancer. *CA Cancer J Clin* 2002;52:342–362.
45. Tjalma W, Monaghan JM, de Barros Lopes A, et al. The role of surgery in invasive carcinoma of the vagina. *Gynecol Oncol* 2001;81:360–365.
46. Hanselaar AG, Van Leusen ND, DeWilde PC, et al. Clear cell adenocarcinoma of the vagina and cervix. A report of the central Netherlands registry with emphasis on early detection and prognosis. *Cancer* 1991;67:1971–1978.
47. Herbst AL, Robboy SJ, Scully RE, et al. Clear-cell adenocarcinoma of the vagina and cervix in girls: analysis of 170 registry cases. *Am J Obstet Gynecol* 1974;119:713–724.
48. Robboy SJ, Welch WR, Young RH, et al. Topographic relation of cervical ectropion and vaginal adenosis to clear cell adenocarcinoma. *Obstet Gynecol* 1982;60:546–551.
49. Robboy SJ, Young RH, Welch WR, et al. Atypical vaginal adenosis and cervical ectropion associated with clear cell adenocarcinoma in diethylstilbestrol-exposed offspring. *Cancer* 1984;54:869–875.
50. Mauer HM, Beltangady M, Gehan EA. The Intergroup RMS Study I.A. Final Report. *Cancer* 1988;61:209–220.
51. Chang YCF, Hricak H, Thurnher S, et al. Vagina: evaluation with MR imaging. Part II. Neoplasms. *Radiology* 1988;169:175–179.
52. Lamoreaux WT, Grigsby PW, Dehdashti F, et al. FDG-PET evaluation of vaginal carcinoma. *Int J Radiat Oncol Biol Phys* 2005;62:733–737.
53. Pecorelli S, Beller U, Heintz A, et al. FIGO annual report on the results of treatment in gynecologic cancer. *J Epidemiol Biostat* 2000;24:56–60.
54. American Joint Committee on Cancer (AJCC). Vagina. In: Greene FL, Page DL, Fleming ID, et al., eds. *AJCC Cancer Staging Manual*. 6th ed. New York: Springer-Verlag; 2002:251–257.
55. Perez CA, Arneson AN, Galakatos A. Radiation therapy in carcinoma of the vagina. *Cancer* 1973;31:36–44.
56. Prempree T, Amommam R. Radiation therapy of primary carcinoma of the vagina. *Acta Radiol Oncol* 1985;24:51–56.
57. Zaino RJ, Robboy SJ, Kurman RJ. Diseases of the vagina. In: Kurman RJ, ed. *Blaustein's Pathology of the Female Genital Tract*. 5th ed. New York: Springer-Verlag; 2002:151–206.
58. Vayrynen M, Romppanen T, Koskela E, et al. Verrucous squamous cell carcinoma of the female genital tract: report of three cases and survey of the literature. *Int J Gynaecol Obstet* 1981;19:351–356.
59. Hoffman MS, Roberts WS, LaPolla JP, et al. Laser vaporization of grade 3 vaginal intraepithelial neoplasia. *Am J Obstet Gynecol* 1991;165:1342–1344.
60. Srodon M, Stoler MH, Baber GB, et al. The distribution of low and high-risk HPV types in vulvar and vaginal intraepithelial neoplasia (VIN and VAIN). *Am J Surg Pathol* 2006;30:1513–1518.
61. Hatch EE, Herbst AL, Hoover RN, et al. Incidence of squamous neoplasia of the cervix and vagina in women exposed prenatally to diethylstilbestrol (United States). *Cancer Causes Control* 2001;12:837–845.
62. Antonioli DA, Burke L. Vaginal adenosis: analysis of 325 biopsy specimens from 100 patients. *Am J Clin Pathol* 1975;64:625–638.
63. Robboy SJ, Scully RE, Welch WR, et al. Intrauterine diethylstilbestrol exposure and its consequences: pathologic characteristics of vaginal adenosis, clear cell adenocarcinoma and related lesions. *Arch Pathol Lab Med* 1977;101:1–5.
64. Hart WR, Townsend DE, Aldrich JO, et al. Histopathologic spectrum of vaginal adenosis and related changes in stilbestrol-exposed females. *Cancer* 1976;37:763–775.
65. Robboy SJ, Prat J, Welch WR, et al. Squamous cell neoplasia controversy in the female exposed to diethylstilbestrol. *Hum Pathol* 1977;8:843–485.
66. Kaufman RH, Korhonen MO, Strama T, et al. Development of clear cell adenocarcinoma in DES-exposed offspring under observation. *Obstet Gynecol* 1982;59:68S–72S.
67. Watanabe Y, Ueda H, Nozaki K, et al. Advanced primary clear cell carcinoma of the vagina not associated with diethylstilbestrol. *Acta Cytol* 2002;46:577–581.
68. Shah C, Pizer E, Veljovich DS, et al. Clear cell adenocarcinoma of the vagina in a patient with vaginal endometriosis. *Gynecol Oncol* 2006;103:1130–1132.
69. Ebrahim S, Daponte A, Smith TH, et al. Primary mucinous adenocarcinoma of the vagina. *Gynecol Oncol* 2001;80:89–92.
70. Clement PB, Benedet JL. Adenocarcinoma *in situ* of the vagina: a case report. *Cancer* 1979;43:2479–2485.
71. McCluggage WG, Price JH, Dobbs SP. Primary adenocarcinoma of the vagina arising in endocervicosis. *Int J Gynecol Pathol* 2001;20:399–402.
72. Fox H, Wells M, Harris M, et al. Enteric tumours of the lower female genital tract: a report of three cases. *Histopathology* 1988;12:167–176.
73. Mudhar HS, Smith JH, Tidy J. Primary vaginal adenocarcinoma of intestinal type arising from an adenoma: case report and review of the literature. *Int J Gynaecol Pathol* 2001; 20:204–209.
74. DeMars LR, Van Le L, Huang I, et al. Primary non-clear cell adenocarcinomas of the vagina in older DES-exposed women. *Gynecol Oncol* 1995;58:389–392.
75. Massen V, Lampe B, Untch M, et al. Adenocarcinoma and adenosis of the vagina. On the histogenesis, diagnosis and therapy of a rare genital neoplasm. *Geburtshilfe Frauneheilkd* 1993;53:308–315.
76. Hiroi H, Yasugi T, Matsumoto K, et al. Mucinous adenocarcinoma arising in a neovagina using the sigmoid colon thirty years after operation: a case report. *J Surg Oncol* 2001;77:61–64.
77. Haskel S, Chen SS, Spiegel G. Vaginal endometrioid adenocarcinoma arising in vaginal endometriosis: a case report and literature review. *Gynecol Oncol* 1989;34:232–236.
78. Hinchey WW, Silva EG, Guarda LA, et al. Paravaginal wolffian duct (mesonephros) adenocarcinoma: a light and electron microscopic study. *Am J Clin Pathol* 1983;80:539–544.
79. Riva C, Fabbri A, Facco C, et al. Primary serous papillary adenocarcinoma of the vagina: a case report. *Int J Gynaecol Pathol* 1997;16:286–290.
80. Tarraza MH Jr, Meltzer SE, DeCain M, et al. Vaginal metastases from renal cell carcinoma: report of four cases and review of the literature. *Eur J Gynecol Oncol* 1998;19:14–18.
81. Gupta D, Malpica A, Deavers MT, et al. Vaginal melanoma: a clinicopathologic and immunohistochemical study of 26 cases. *Am J Surg Pathol* 2002;26:1450–1457.
82. Breslow A. Tumor thickness, level of invasion and node dissection in stage I cutaneous melanoma. *Ann Surg* 1975;182:572–575.
83. Gupta D, Neto AG, Deavers MT, et al. Metastatic melanoma to the vagina: clinicopathologic and immunohistochemical study of three cases and literature review. *Int J Gynaecol Pathol* 2003;22:136–140.
84. Copeland LJ, Gersheson DM, Saul PB, et al. Sarcoma botryoides of the female genital tract. *Obstet Gynecol* 1985;66:262–266.
85. Peters WA, Kumar NB, Andersen WA, et al. Primary sarcoma of the adult vagina: a clinicopathologic study. *Obstet Gynecol* 1985;65:699–704.
86. Tavassoli FA, Norris HJ. Smooth muscle tumors of the vagina. *Obstet Gynecol* 1979;53:689–693.
87. Chen KT, Hafez GR, Gilbert EF. Myxoid variant of epithelioid smooth muscle tumor. *Am J Clin Pathol* 1980;74:350–353.
88. Lam MM, Corless Cl, Goldblum JR, et al. Extragastrointestinal stromal tumors presenting as vulvovaginal/rectovaginal septal masses: a diagnostic pitfall. *Int J Gynaecol Pathol* 2006;25:288–292.
89. Berkowitz RS, Ehrmann RL, Knapp RC. Endometrial stromal sarcoma arising from vaginal endometriosis. *Obstet Gynecol* 1978;51:34S–37S.
90. Granai CO, Walters MD, Safaii H, et al. Malignant transformation of vaginal endometriosis. *Obstet Gynecol* 1984;64:592–595.
91. Ulbright TM, Kraus FT. Endometrial stromal tumors of extrauterine tissue. *Am J Clin Pathol* 1981;76:371–377.
92. O'Toole RV, Tutle SE, Lucas JG, et al. Alveolar soft part sarcoma of the vagina: an immunohistochemical and electron microscopic study. *Int J Gynaecol Pathol* 1985;4:258–265.
93. Webb MJ, Symmonds RE, Weiland LH. Malignant fibrous hystiocytoma of the vagina. *Am J Obstet Gynecol* 1974;119:190–192.
94. Okagaki T, Ishida T, Hilgers RD. A malignant tumor of the vagina resembling synovial sarcoma: a light and electron microscopic study. *Cancer* 1976;37:2306–2320.
95. Shevchuk MM, Fenoglio CM, Lattes R, et al. Malignant mixed tumor of the vagina probably arising in mesonephric nests. *Cancer* 1978;24:214–223.
96. Buscema J, Rosenshein NB, Taqi F, et al. Vaginal hemangiopericytoma: a histopathological and ultrastructual evaluation. *Obstet Gynecol* 1985;66 82S–85S.
97. Chorlton I, Karnei RF, King FM, et al. Primary malignant reticuloendothelial disease involving the vagina, cervix and corpus uteri. *Obstet Gynecol* 1974;44:735–748.

98. Harris NL, Scully RE. Malignant lymphoma and granulocytic sarcoma of the uterus and vagina: a clinicopathologic analysis of 27 cases. *Cancer* 1984;53:2530–2545.
99. Kosari F, Daneshbod Y, Parwaresch R, et al. Lymphomas of the female genital tract: a study of 186 cases and review of the literature. *Am J Surg Pathol* 2005;29:1512–1520.
100. Yoshinaga K, Akahira J, Niikura H, et al. A case of primary mucosa-associated lymphoid tissue lymphoma of the vagina. *Hum Pathol* 2004;35: 1164–1166.
101. Kaminski JM, Anderson PR, Han AC, et al. Primary small cell carcinoma of the vagina. *Gynecol Oncol* 2003;88:451–455.
102. Ulich TR, Liao S-Y, Layfield K, et al. Endocrine and tumor differentiation markers in poorly differentiated small-cell carcinoids of the cervix and vagina. *Arch Pathol Lab Med* 1986;110:1054–1057.
103. Bing Z, Levine L, Lucci JA, et al. Primary small cell neuroendocrine carcinoma of the vagina: a clinicopathologic study. *Arch Pathol Lab Med.* 2004;128:857–862.
104. Coleman NM, Smith-Zagone MJ, Tanyl J, et al. Primary neuroendocrine carcinoma of the vagina with Merkel cell carcinoma phenotype. *Am J Surg Pathol* 2006;30:405–410.
105. Sulak P, Barnhill D, Heller P, et al. Nonsquamous carcinoma of the vagina. *Gynecol Oncol* 1988;29:309–320.
106. Shibata R, Umezawa A, Takehara K, et al. Primary carcinosarcoma of the vagina. *Pathol Int* 2003;53:106–110.
107. Clement PB, Young RH, Scully RE. Extraovarian pelvic yolk sac tumours. *Cancer* 1988;62:620–626.
108. Handel LN, Scott SM, Giller RH, et al. New perspectives on therapy for vaginal endodermal sinus tumors. *J Urol* 2002;168:687–690.
109. Bague S, Rodriguez IM, Prat J. Malignant mesonephric tumors of the female genital tract: a clinicopathologic study of 9 cases. *Am J Surg Pathol* 2004; 28:601–607.
110. Liao X, Xin X, Lu X. Primary Ewing's sarcoma-primitive neuroectodermal tumor of the vagina. *Gynecol Oncol* 2004;92:684–688.
111. Lee WR, Marcus RB Jr, Sombeck MD, et al. Radiotherapy alone for carcinoma of the vagina: the importance of overall treatment time. *Int J Radiat Oncol Biol Phys* 1994;29:983–988.
112. Peters WA, Kumar NB, Morely GW. Carcinoma of the vagina. Factors influencing treatment outcome. *Cancer* 1985;55:892–897.
113. Chu AM, Beechinor R. Survival and recurrence patterns in the radiation treatment of carcinoma of the vagina. *Gynecol Oncol* 1984;19:298–307.
114. MacNaught R, Symonds RP, Hole D, et al. Improved control of primary vaginal tumors by combined external beam and interstitial brachytherapy. *Clin Radiol* 1986;37:29–32.
115. Eddy GL, Marks RD, Miller MC, et al. Primary invasive vaginal carcinoma. *Am J Obstet Gynecol* 1991;165:292–296; discussion 296–298.
116. Dixit S, Singhal S, Baboo HA. Squamous cell carcinoma of the vagina. A review of 70 cases. *Gynecol Oncol* 1993;48:80–87.
117. Delclos L. In: Levitt SH, Tapley N, eds. *Technological Basis of Radiation Therapy—Practical Clinical Applications.* Philadelphia: Lea & Febiger; 1984.
118. Dancuart F, Delclos L, Wharton JT, et al. Primary squamous cell carcinoma of the vagina treated by radiotherapy: a failures analysis—the M. D. Anderson hospital experience 1955–1982. *Int J Radiat Oncol Biol Phys* 1988;14:745–749.
119. Tarraza MH Jr, Muntz H, DeCain M, et al. Patterns of recurrence of primary carcinoma of the vagina. *Eur J Gynecol Oncol* 1991;12:89–92.
120. Ali MM, Huang DT, Goplerud DR, et al. Radiation alone for carcinoma of the vagina. Variation in response related to the location of the primary tumor. *Cancer* 1996;77:1934–1939.
121. Kucera H, Vavra N. Radiation management of primary carcinoma of the vagina: clinical and histopathological variables associated with survival. *Gynecol Oncol* 1991;40:12–16.
122. Berchuck A, Rodriguez G, Kamel A, et al. Expression of epidermal growth factor receptor and HER-2/neu in normal and neoplastic cervix, vulva, and vagina. *Obstet Gynecol* 1990;76:381–387.
123. Waggoner SE, Anderson SM, Luce MC, et al. p53 protein expression and gene analysis in clear cell adenocarcinoma of the vagina and cervix. *Gynecol Oncol* 1996;60:339–344.
124. Hoffman MS, DeCesare SL, Roberts WS, et al. Upper vaginectomy for *in situ* and occult, superficially invasive carcinoma of the vagina. *Am J Obstet Gynecol* 1992;166:30–33.
125. Fanning J, Manahan KJ, McLean SA. Loop electrosurgical excision procedure for partial upper vaginectomy. *Am J Obstet Gynecol* 1999;181: 1382–1385.
126. Morice P, Thiam-Ba R, Castaigne D, et al. Fertility results after ovarian transposition for pelvic malignancies treated by external irradiation or brachytherapy. *Hum Reprod* 1998;13:660–663.
127. Boronow RC, Hickman BT, Reagan MT, et al. Combined therapy as an alternative to exenteration for locally advanced vulvovaginal cancer. II. Results, complications, and dosimetric and surgical considerations. *Am J Clin Oncol* 1987;10:171–181.
128. Julian TM, O'Connell BJ, Gosewehr JA. Indications, techniques, and advantages of partial laser vaginectomy. *Obstet Gynecol* 1992;80: 140–143.
129. Woodruff JD, Parmley THE, Julian CG. Topical 5-fluorouracil in the treatment of vaginal carcinoma *in situ*. *Gynecol Oncol* 1975;3:124–132.
130. Piver MS, Barlow JJ, Tsukada Y, et al. Postirradiation sqaumous cell carcinoma *in situ* of the vagina: treatment by topical 20% 5-fluorouracil cream. *Am J Obstet Gynecol* 1979;135:377–389.
131. Petrilli ES, Townsend DE, Morrow CP, et al. Vaginal intraepithelial neoplasia: biologic aspects and treatment with topical 5-fluorouracil and the carbon dioxide laser. *Am J Obstet Gynecol* 1980;138:321–328.
132. Krebs HB. Treatment of vaginal intraepithelial neoplasia with laser and topical 5-fluorouracil. *Obstet Gynecol* 1989;73:657–660.
133. Robinson JB, Sun CC, Bodurka-Bevers D, et al. Cavitational ultrasonic surgical aspiration for the treatment of vaginal intraepithelial neoplasia. *Gynecol Oncol* 2000;78:235–241.
134. Perez CA, Korba A, Sharma S. Dosimetric considerations in irradiation of carcinoma of the vagina. *Int J Radiat Oncol Biol Phys* 1977;2:639–649.
135. Diakomanolis E, Rodolakis A, Boulgaris Z, et al. Treatment of vaginal intraepithelial neoplasia with laser ablation and upper vaginectomy. *Gynecol Oncol Invest* 2002;54:17–20.
136. Wright VC, Riopelle MA. Laser surgery for vaginal disease. In: Wright VC, ed. *Gynecologic Laser Surgery: A Practical Handbook.* Houston: Biomedical Communications; 1986:155–160.
137. Daly JW, Ellis GE. Treatment of vaginal dysplasia and carcinoma *in-situ* with topical 5-fluorouracil. *Obstet Gynecol* 1980;55:350–352.
138. Haidopoulos D, Diakomanolis E, Rodolakis A, et al. Can local application of imiquimod cream be an alternative mode of therapy for patients with high-grade intraepithelial lesions of the vagina? *Int J Gynaecol Cancer* 2005;15(5):898–902.
139. Indermaur MD, Martino MA, Fiorica JV, et al. Upper vaginectomy for the treatment of vaginal intraepithelial neoplasia. *Am J Obstet Gynecol* 2005;193:577–580; discussion 580–591.
140. Ogino I, Kitarmura T, Okajima H, et al. High-dose-rate intracavitary brachytherapy in the management of cervical and vaginal intraepithelial neoplasia. *Int J Radiat Oncol Biol Phys* 1998;40:881–887.
141. MacLeod C, Fowler A, Dalrymple C, et al. High-dose-rate brachyherapy in the management of high-grade intraepithelial neoplasia of the vagina. *Gynecol Oncol* 1997;65:74–77.
142. Mock U, Kucera H, Fellner C, et al. High-dose-rate (HDR) brachytherapy with or without external beam radiotherapy in the treatment of primary vaginal carcinoma: long-term results and side effects. *Int J Radiat Oncol Biol Phys* 2003;56:950–957.
143. Magrina JF, Basterson BJ. Vaginal reconstruction in gynecologic oncology. A review in techniques. *Obstet Gynecol Surv* 1981;36:1–10.
144. Burke TW, Morris M, Roh MS, et al. Perineal reconstruction using single gracilis myocutaneous flaps. *Gynecol Oncol* 1995;57:221–225.
145. Elaffandi AH, Khalil HH, Aboul Kassem HA, et al. Vaginal reconstruction with a greater omentum-pedicled graft combined with a vicryl mesh after anterior pelvic exenteration. Surgical approach with long-term follow-up. *Int J Gynaecol Cancer* 2007;17(2):536–542.
146. Wang X, Qiao Q, Burd A, et al. A new technique of vaginal reconstruction with the deep inferior epigastric perforator flap: a preliminary report. *Plas Reconstruct Surg* 2007;119(6):1785–1790; discussion 1791.
147. Frank SJ, Jhingran A, Levenback C, et al. Definitive radiation therapy for squamous cell carcinoma of the vagina. *Int J Radiat Oncol Biol Phys* 2005;62:138–147.
148. Mundt AJ, Mell LK, Roeske JC. Preliminary analysis of chronic gastrointestinal toxicity in gynecology patients treated with intensity-modulated whole pelvic radiation therapy. *Int J Radiat Oncol Biol Phys* 2003;56: 1354–1369.
149. Mundt AJ, Lujan AE, Rotmensche J, et al. Intensity-modulated whole pelvic radiotherapy in women with gynecologic malignancies. *Int J Radiat Oncol Biol Phys* 2002;52:1330–1337.
150. Taylor A, Rockall AG, Rezneck RH, et al. Mapping pelvic lymph nodes: guidelines for delineation in intensity-modulated radiotherapy. *Int J Radiat Oncol Biol Phys* 2005;63:1604–1612.
151. Digel CA, Lastner GM, Zinreich ES. The use of transmission block in the radiation therapy portal treatment of the inguinal nodes in late stage pelvic malignancies. *Radiol Technol* 1987;58:227–231.
152. Dittmer PH, Randall ME. A technique for inguinal node boosts using photon fields defined by asymmetric collimator jaws. *Radiother Oncol* 2001;59:61–64.
153. Pingley S, Shrivastava SK, Sarin R, et al. Primary carcinoma of the vagina: Tata Memorial Hospital experience. *Int J Radiat Oncol Biol Phys* 2000;46:101–108.
154. Delclos L, Fletcher GH, Moore EB, et al. Minicolpostats, dome cylinders, other additions and improvements of the Fletsher-Suit afterloadable system: indications and limitations of their use. *Int J Radiat Oncol Biol Phys* 1980;6:1195–1206.
155. Perez CA, Slessinger ED, Grigsby PW. Design of an afterloading vaginal applicator (MIRALVA). *Int J Radiat Oncol Biol Phys* 1990;18: 1503–1508.
156. Slessinger ED, Perez CA, Grigsby PW, et al. Dosimetry and dose specification for a new gynecologic brachytherapy applicator. *Int J Radiat Oncol Biol Phys* 1992;22:1117–1124.
157. Choo JJ, Scudiere J, Bitterman P, et al. Vaginal lymphatic channel location and its implication for intracavitary brachytherapy radiation treatment. *Brachytherapy* 2005;4:236–240.
158. Nanavati PJ, Fanning J, Hilgers RD, et al. High-dose brachytherapy in primary stage I and II vaginal cancer. *Gynecol Oncol* 1993;51:67–71.

159. Kucera H, Mock U, Knocke TH, et al. Radiotherapy alone for invasive vaginal cancer: outcome with intracavitary high dose rate brachytherapy versus conventional low dose rate brachytherapy. *Acta Obstetricia et Gynecologica Scandinavica* 2001;80:355–360.
160. Kushner DM, Fleming PA, Kennedy AW, et al. High dose rate Ir afterloading brachytherapy for cancer of the vagina. *Br J Radiol* 2003;76: 719–725.
161. Gore E, Gillin MT, Albano KI, et al. Comparison of high dose-rate and low dose-rate dose distributions for vaginal cylinders. *Int J Radiat Oncol Biol Phys* 1995;31:165–170.
162. Li Z, Liu C, Palta JR. Optimized dose distribution of a high dose rate vaginal cylinder. *Int J Radiat Oncol Biol Phys* 1998;41:239–244.
163. Tyree WC, Cardenes H, Randall M, et al. High-dose rate brachytherapy for vaginal cancer: learning from treatment complications. *Int J Gynaecol Cancer* 2002;12:27–31.
164. Rutkowski T, Bialas B, Rembielak A, et al. Efficacy and toxicity of MDR versus HDR brachytherapy for primary vaginal cancer. *Neoplasma* 2002;49:197–200.
165. Hilaris BS, Nori D, Anderson LL. Brachytherapy treatment planning. *Front Radiat Ther Oncol* 1987;21:94–106.
166. Syed AMN, Puthawala AA, Neblett D, et al. Transperineal interstitial-intracavitary "Syed-Neblett" applicator in the treatment of carcinoma of the uterine cervix. *Endocuriether Hypertherm Oncol* 1986;2:1–13.
167. DiSaia PJ, Syed N, Puthwala AA. Malignant neoplasia of the upper vagina. *Endocuriether Hypertherm Oncol* 1990;6:251–256.
168. Martinez A, Cox RS, Edmundson GK. A multiple-site perineal applicator (MUPIT) for treatment of prostatic, anorectal and gynecologic malignancies. *Int J Radiat Oncol Biol Phys* 1984;10:297–305.
169. Stock RG, Chen K, Terk M, et al. A new technique for performing Syed-Neblett template interstitial implants for gynecologic malignancies using transrectal-ultrasound gudiance. *Int J Radiat Oncol Biol Phys* 1997;37: 819–825.
170. Corn BW, Lanciano RM, Rosenblum N, et al. Improved treatment planning for the Syed-Neblett template using endorectral-coil magnetic resonance and intraoperative (laparotomy/laparoscopy) guidance: a new intergrated technique for hysterectomized women with vaginal tumors. *Gynecol Oncol* 1995;56:255–261.
171. Childers JM, Surwit EA. Current status of operative laparoscopy in gynecologic oncology. *Oncology (Huntington)* 1993;7:47–51; discussion 53–54.
172. Orr JW Jr, Dosoretz DD, Mahoney D, et al. Surgically (laparotomy/ laparoscopy) guided placement of high dose rate interstitial irradition catheters (LG-HDRT): technique and outcome. *Gynecol Oncol* 2006;100: 145–148.
173. Paley PJ, Koh WJ, Stelzer KJ, et al. A new technique for performing Syed template interstitial implants for anterior vaginal tumors using an open retropubic approach. *Gynecol Oncol* 1999;73:121–125.
174. Tewari KS, Cappuccini F, Puthawala AA, et al. Primary invasive carcinoma of the vagina: treatment with interstitial brachytherapy. *Cancer* 2001;91:758–770.
175. Stryker JA. Radiotherapy for vaginal carcinoma: a 23-year review. *Br J Radiol* 2000;73:1200–1205.
176. Evans LS, Kersh CR, Constable WC, et al. Concomitant 5-fluorouracil, mitomycin-C and radiotherapy for advanced gynecologic malignancies. *Int J Radiat Oncol Biol Phys* 1988;15:901–906.
177. Roberts WS, Hoffman MS, Kavanagh JJ, et al. Further experience with radiation therapy and concomitant intravenous chemotherapy in advanced carcinoma of the lower female genital tract. *Gynecol Oncol* 1991;43:233–236.
178. Kersh CR, Constable W, Spaulding C, et al. A phase I-II trial of multimodality management of bulky gynecologic malignancy. Combined chemoradiosensitization and radiotherapy. *Cancer* 1990;66:30–34.
179. Dalrymple JL, Russell AH, Lee SW, et al. Chemoradiation for primary invasive squamous carcinoma of the vagina. *Int J Gynaecol Cancer* 2004;14:110–117.
180. Keys HM, Bundy BN, Stehman FB, et al. Cisplatin, radiation and adjuvant hysterectomy compared with radiation and adjvuvant hysterectomy for bulky stage IB cervical carcinoma. *N Engl J Med* 1999;340:1154–1161.
181. Morris M, Eifel PJ, Lu J, et al. Pelvic irradiation with concurrent chemotherapy compared with pelvic and para-aortic radiation for the high-risk cervical cancer. *N Engl J Med* 1999;340:1137–1143.
182. Rose PG, Bundy BN, Watkins EB, et al. Concurrent cisplatin-based radiotherapy and chemotherapy for locally advanced cervical cancer. *N Engl J Med* 1999;340:1144–1153.
183. Whitney CW, Sause W, Bundy BN, et al. Randomized comparison of fluorouracil plus cisplatin versus hydroxyurea as an adjunct to radiation therapy in stage IIB-IVA carcinoma of the cervix with negative para-aortic lymph nodes: a Gynecologic Oncology Group and Southwest Oncology Group study. *J Clin Oncol* 1999;17:1339–1348.
184. Moore DH, Thomas GM, Montana GS, et al. Preoperative chemoradiation for advanced vulvar cancer. A phase II study of the Gynecologic Oncology Group. *Int J Radiat Oncol Biol Phys* 1988;42:79–85.
185. Tabata T, Takeshima N, Nishida H, et al. Treatment failure in vaginal cancer. *Gynecol Oncol* 2002;84:309–314.
186. Cardenes H, Song G, Randall M. Late sequelae of radiation therapy in the management of gynecologic malignancies. Current medical literature. *Gynecol Oncol* 2001;2:1–10.
187. Grigsby PW, Russell A, Bruner D, et al. Late injury of cancer therapy on the female reproductive tract. *Int J Radiat Oncol Biol Phys* 1995;31: 1281–1299.
188. Hintz BL, Kagan AR, Gilbert HA, et al. Radiation tolerance of the vaginal mucosa. *Int J Radiat Oncol Biol Phys* 1980;6:711–716.
189. Rubin P, Casarett GW. The female genital tract. In: Rubin P, Casarett GW, eds. *Clinical Radiation Pathology*. Philadelphia: WB Saunders; 1968: 396–442.
190. Au SP, Grigsby PW. The irradiation tolerance dose of the proximal vagina. *Radiother Oncol* 2003;67:77–85.
191. Delanian S, Porcher R, Balla-Mekias, et al. Randomized, placebo-controlled trial of combined pentoxifylline and tocopherol for regression of superficial radiation-induced fibrosis. *J Clin Oncol* 2003;21:2545–2550.
192. Herbst AL, Scully RD. Adenocarcinoma of the vagina in adolescence: a report of seven cases including six clear-cell carcinomas (so-called mesonephromas). *Cancer* 1970;25:745–757.
193. Herbst AL, Anderson D. Clear cell adenocarcinoma of the vagina and cervix secondary to intrauterine exposure to diethylstilbestrol. *Semin Surg Oncol* 1990;6:343–346.
194. Herbst AL, Norusis MJ, Rosenow PJ, et al. An analysis of 346 cases of clear cell adenocarcinoma of the vagina and cervix with emphasis on recurrence and survival. *Gynecol Oncol* 1979;7(2):111–122.
195. Senekjian EK, Frey KW, Herbst AL. Pelvic exenteration in clear cell adencarcinoma of the vagina and cervix. *Gynecol Oncol* 1989;34:413–416.
196. Hudson CN, Findlay WS, Roberts H. Successful pregnancy after radical surgery for diethyl-stilbestrol (DES)-related vaginal adenocarcinoma. Case report. *Br J Obstet Gynaecol* 1988;95:818–819.
197. Senekjian EK, Frey KW, Anderson D, et al. Local therapy in stage I clear cell adenocarcinoma of the vagina. *Cancer* 1987;60:1319–1324.
198. Wharton JT, Rutledge FN, Gallager HS, et al. Treatment of clear cell adenocarcinoma in young females. *Obstet Gynecol* 1975;45:365–368.
199. Senekjian EK, Frey KW, Stone C, et al. An evaulation of stage II vaginal clear cell adenocarcinoma according to substages. *Gynecol Oncol* 1989;31:56–64.
200. Fowler WC, Brantley JC, Edelman DA. Clear cell adenocarcinoma of the genital tract. *South Med J* 1979;72:15–17.
201. Bonner JA, Perez-Tamayo C, Reid GC, et al. The management of vaginal melanoma. *Cancer* 1988;62:2066–2072.
202. Buchanan DJ, Schlaerth J, Kuroaki T. Primary vaginal melanoma: thirteen-year disease free survival after wide local excision and review of recent literature. *Am J Obstet Gynecol* 1998;178:1177–1184.
203. Geisler JP, Look KY, Moore DA, et al. Pelvic exenteration for malignant melanomas of the vagina or urethra with over 3 mm of invasion. *Gynecol Oncol* 1995;59:338–341.
204. Irvin WP, Bliss SA, Rice LW, et al. Malignant melanoma of the vagina and locoregional control: radical surgery revisited. *Gynecol Oncol* 1998;71: 476–480.
205. Levitan Z, Gordon AN, Kaplan AL, et al. Primary malignant melanoma of the vagina: report of four cases and review of the literature. *Gynecol Oncol* 1989;33:85–90.
206. Van Nostrand K, Lucci J, Schell M, et al. Primary vaginal melanoma: improved survival with radical pelvic surgery. *Gynecol Oncol* 1994;55: 234–237.
207. Petru E, Nagele F, Czerwenka K, et al. Primary malignant melanoma of the vagina: long-term remission following radiation therapy. *Gynecol Oncol* 1998;70:23–26.
208. Bentzen SM, Overgaard J, Thames HD, et al. Clinical radiobiology of malignant melanoma. *Radiother Oncol* 1989;16:169–182.
209. Overgaard J, Overgaard M, Hansen PV, et al. Some factors of importance in the radiation treatment of malignant melanoma. *Radiother Oncol* 1986;5:183–192.
210. Sause WT, Cooper JS, Rush S, et al. Fraction size in external beam radiation therapy in the treatment of melanoma. *Int J Radiat Oncol Biol Phys* 1991;20:429–432.
211. Harwood AR, Cummings BJ. Radiotherapy for mucosal melanomas. *Int J Radiat Oncol Biol Phys* 1982;8:1121–1126.
212. Harrison LB, Fogel T, Peschel R. Primary vaginal cancer and vaginal melanoma: a review of therapy with external beam radiation and a simple intracavitary brachytherapy system. *Endocuriether Hypertherm Oncol* 1987;3:67–72.
213. Rogo KO, Andersson R, Edbom G, et al. Conservative surgery for vulvovaginal melanoma. *Eur J Gynecol Oncol* 1991;12:113–119.
214. Das Gupta T, D'Urso J. Melanoma of the female genitalia. *Surg Obstet Gynecol* 1964;119:1074–1078.
215. Brand E, Fu YS, Lagasse LD, et al. Vulvovaginal melanoma: report of seven cases and literature review. *Gynecol Oncol* 1989;33:54–60.
216. Hachi H, Ottmany A, Bougtab A, et al. Leiomyosarcoma of the vagina: a rare case. *Bull Cancer* 1997;84:215–217.
217. Neesham D, Kerdemelidis P, Scurry J. Case report. Primary malignant mixed müllerian tumor of the vagina. *Gynecol Oncol* 1998;70:303–307.
218. Hornback NB, Omura G, Major FJ. Observations of the use of adjuvant radiation therapy in patients with stage I and II uterine sarcoma. *Int J Radiat Oncol Biol Phys* 1986;12:2127–2130.
219. Sutton GP, Blessing JA, Rosenshein N, et al. Phase II trial of ifosfamide and mensa in mixed mesodermal tumors of the uterus (a Gynecologic Oncology Group study). *Am J Obstet Gynecol* 1989;161:309–312.

220. Thigpen JT, Blessing JA, Homesley HD, et al. Phase II trial of cisplatin in advanced or recurrent cancer of the vagina: a Gynecologic Oncology Group study. *Gynecol Oncol* 1986;23:101–104.
221. Muss HB, Bundy B, DiSaia PJ, et al. Treatment of recurrent or advanced uterine sarcoma. A randomized trial of doxorubicin and cyclophosphamide (a phase III trial of the Gynecologic Oncology Group). *Cancer* 1985;55:1648–1653.
222. Hays DM, Shimada H, Raney RB Jr, et al. Sarcomas of the vagina and uterus: the Intergroup Rhabdomyosarcoma Study. *J Pediatr Surg* 1985;20:718–724.
223. Raney RB Jr, Gehan EA, Hays DM, et al. Primary chemotherapy with or without radiation and/or surgery for children with localized sarcoma of the bladder, prostate, vagina, uterus, and cervix: a comparison of the results in Intergroup Rhabdomyosarcoma Studies I and II. *Cancer* 1990;66:2072–2081.
224. Andrassy RJ, Hays DM, Raney RB, et al. Conservative surgical management of the vaginal and vulvar pediatric rhabdomyosarcoma: a report from the Intergroup Rhabdomyosarcoma Study III. *J Pediatr Surg* 1995;30:1034–1036; discussion 1036–1037.
225. Hilgers RD. Pelvic exenteration of vaginal embryonal rhabdomyosarcoma. A review. *Obstet Gynecol* 1975;45:175–180.
226. Grosfeld JL, Smith JP, Chatworthy HW. Pelvic rhabdomyosarcoma in infants and children. *J Urol* 1972;107:673–675.
227. Flamant F, Gerbaulet A, Nihol-Fekete C, et al. Long-term sequelae of conservative treatment by surgery, brachytherapy and chemotherapy for vulvar and vaginal rhabdomyosarcoma in children. *J Clin Oncol* 1990;8:1847–1853.
228. Friedman M, Peretz BA, Niseenbaum M, et al. Modern treatement of vaginal embryonal rhabdomyosarcoma. *Obstet Gynecol Surv* 1986;41:614–618.
229. Andrassy RJ, Wiener ES, Raney RB, et al. Progress in the surgical management of vagina rhabdomyosarcoma: a 25 year review from the Intergroup Rhabdomyosarcoma Study Group. *J Pediatr Surg* 1999;34:731–734; discussion 734–735.
230. Prevot S, Hugol D, Andouin J, et al. Primary non-Hodgkin's malignant lymphoma of the vagina: report of three cases and review of the literature. *Pathol Res Pract* 1992;188:78–85.
231. Perren T, Farrant M, McCarthy K, et al. Lymphomas of the cervix and upper vagina: a report of five cases and a review of the literature. *Gynecol Oncol* 1992;44:87–95.
232. Young RH, Scully RE. Endodermal sinus tumor of the vagina: a report of nine cases and review of the literature. *Gynecol Oncol* 1984;18:380–392.
233. Copeland LJ, Sneige N, Ordones N, et al. Endodermal sinus tumor of the vagina and cervix. *Cancer* 1985;55:2558–2565.
234. Collins HS, Burke TW, Heller PB, et al. Endodermal sinus tumor of the infant vagina treated exclusively by chemotherapy. *Obstet Gynecol* 1989;73:507–509.
235. Aartsen EJ, Delamarre JFM, Gerresten G. Endodermal sinus tumor of the vagina: radiation therapy and progeny. *Obstet Gynecol* 1993;81:893–895.
236. Hwang EH, Han SJ, Lee MK, et al. Clincial experience with conservative surgery for vaginal endodermal sinus tumor. *J Pediatr Surg* 1996;31:219–222.
237. Williams S, Blessing JA, Liao SY, et al. Adjuvant therapy of ovarian germ cell tumors with cisplatin, etoposide, and bleomycin: a trial of the Gynecologic Oncology Group. *J Clin Oncol* 1994;12:701–706.
238. Kleinerman RA, Boice JD Jr, Storm HH, et al. Second primary cancer after treatment for cervical cancer. An International Cancer Registries study. *Cancer* 1995;76:442–452.
239. Ohno T, Kakinuma S, Kato S, et al. Risk of second cancers after radiotherapy for cervical cancer. *Expert Rev Anticancer Ther* 2006;6:2306–2320.
240. Hall EJ, Wuu CS. Radiation-induced second cancers: the impact of 3D-CRT and IMRT. *Int J Radiat Oncol Biol Phys* 2003;56:83–88.
241. Hopkins MP, Morely GW. Squamous cell carcinoma of the neovagina. *Obstet Gynecol* 1987;69:525–527.
242. Schult M, Hecker A, Lelle RJ, et al. Recurrent rectoneovaginal fistula caused by an incidental squamous cell carcinoma of the neovagina in Mayer-Rokitansky-Kuster-Hauser syndrome. *Gynecol Oncol* 2000;77:210–212.
243. Bobin JY, Zinzindohoue C, Naba T, et al. Primary squamous cell carcinoma in a patient with vaginal agenesis. *Gynecol Oncol* 1999;74:293–297.
244. Guven S, Guvendag Guven ES, Ayhan A, et al. Recurrence of high-grade squamous intraepithelial neoplasia in neovagina: case report and review of the literature. *Int J Gynaecol Cancer* 2005;15:1179–1182.
245. Lara PN Jr, Hearn E, Leigh B. Neovaginal malignant melanoma following surgery and radiation for vulvar squamous cell carcinoma. *Gynecol Oncol* 1997;65:520–522.
246. Van Dam PA, Irvine L, Lowe DG, et al. Carcinoma in episiotomy scars. *Gynecol Oncol* 1992;44:96–100.
247. Heron DE, Axtel A, Gerszten K, et al. Villoglandular adenocarcinoma of the cervix recurrent in an episiotomy scar: a case report in a 32-year-old female. *Int J Gynaecol Cancer* 2005;15:366–371.
248. Khalil AM, Khatib RA, Mufarrij AA, et al. Squamous cell carcinoma of the cervix implanting in the episiotomy site. *Gynecol Oncol* 1993;51:408–410.
249. Sun SS, Chen TC, Yen RF, et al. Value of whole body 18F-fluoro-2-deoxyglucose positron emission tomography in the evaluation of recurrent cervical cancer. *Anticancer Res* 2001;21:2957–2961.
250. Miller B, Morris M, Rutledge E, et al. Aborted exenterative procedures in recurrent cervical cancer. *Gynecol Oncol* 1993;50:94–99.
251. Ratliff CR, Gershenson DM, Morris M, et al. Sexual adjustment of patients undergoing gracilis myocutaneous flap vagina reconstruction in conjunction with pelvic exenteration. *Cancer* 1996;78:2229–2235.
252. Russell AH, Koh WJ, Markette K, et al. Radical reirradiation for recurrent or second primary carcinoma of the female reproductive tract. *Gynecol Oncol* 1987;27:226–232.
253. Randall ME, Evans L, Greven KM, et al. Interstitial re-irradiation for recurrent gynecologic malignancies: results and analysis of prognostic factors. *Gynecol Oncol* 1993;48:23–31.
254. Wang X, Cai S, Ding Y, Wei K. Treatment of late recurrent vaginal malignancy after initial radiotherapy for carcinoma of the cervix: an analysis of 73 cases. *Gynecol Oncol* 1998;69:125–129.
255. Gupta AK, Vicini FA, Frazier AJ, et al. Iridium-192 transperineal interstitial brachytherapy for locally advanced for recurrent gynecologic malignancies. *Int J Radiat Oncol Biol Phys* 1999;43:1055–1060.
256. Charra C, Roy P, Coquard R, et al. Outcome of treatment of upper third vaginal recurrences of cervical and endometrial carcinomas with interstitial brachytherapy. *Int J Radiat Oncol Biol Phys* 1998;40:421–426.
257. Haddock MG, Martinez-Monge R, Petersen IA, et al. Locally advanced primary and recurrent gynecologic malignancies EBRT with or without IORT or HDR-IORT. In: Gunderson LL CF, Harrison LB, et al., eds. *Current Clinical Oncology: Intraoperative Irraditation: Techniques and Results.* New Totowa, NJ: Humana Press; 1999:397–419.
258. Garton GR, Gunderson LL, Webb MJ, et al. Intraoperative radiation therapy in gynecologic cancer: update of the experience at a single institution. *Int J Radiat Oncol Biol Phys* 1997;37:839–843.
259. Gemignani ML, Alektiar KM, Leitao M, et al. Radical surgical resection and high-dose intraoperative radiation therapy (HDR-IORT) in patients with gynecologic cancers. *Int J Radiat Oncol Biol Phys* 2001;50:687–694.
260. Hockel M, Schlenger K, Hamm H, et al. Five-year experience with combined operative and radiotherapeutic treatment of recurrent gynecologic tumors infiltrating the pelvic wall. *Cancer* 1996;77:1918–1933.
261. Blomgren J, Lax I, Goranson H, et al. Radiosurgery of tumors in the body: clinical experience using a new method. *J Radiosurg* 1998;1:63–74.
262. Spanos WJ, Wasserman T, Meoz R, et al. Palliation of advanced pelvic malignant disease with large fraction pelvic radiation and misonidazole: final report of RTOG phase I/II study. *Int J Radiat Oncol Biol Phys* 1987;13:1479–1482.
263. Spanos WJ, Guse C, Perez CA, et al. Phase II study of multiple daily fractionations in the palliation of advanced pelvic malignancies. Preliminary report of the RTOG 85-02. *Int J Radiat Oncol Biol Phys* 1989;17:659–662.
264. Spanos WJ, Perez CA, Marcus S, et al. Effect of rest interval on tumor and normal tissue response. A report of phase III study of accelerated split-course palliative radiation for advanced pelvic malignancies (RTOG 85-02). *Int J Radiat Oncol Biol Phys* 1993;25:399–403.
265. Spanos WJ, Clery M, Perez CA, et al. Late effect of multiple daily fraction palliation schedule for advanced pelvic malignancies (RTOG 85-02). *Int J Radiat Oncol Biol Phys* 1994;29:961–967.
266. Muss HB, Bundy BN, Christopherson WA. Mitoxantrone in the treatment of advanced vulvar and vaginal carcinoma: a Gynecologic Oncology Group study. *Am J Clin Oncol* 1989;12:142–144.
267. Long HJ 3rd, Cross WG, Wieand HS, et al. Phase II trial of methotrexate, vinblastine, doxorubicin, and cisplatin in advanced/recurrent carcinoma of the uterine cervix and vagina. *Gynecol Oncol* 1995;57:235–239.
268. Patton TJ Jr, Kavanagh JJ, Delclos L. Five-year survival in patients given intra-arterial chemotherapy prior to radiotherapy for advanced squamous carcinoma of the cervix and vagina. *Gynecol Oncol* 1991;42:54–59.

CHAPTER 22 ■ UTERINE CERVIX

MARCUS E. RANDALL, HELEN MICHAEL, HARRY LONG III, AND SEAN TEDJARATI

EPIDEMIOLOGY

Worldwide, cervical cancer is the third most common malignancy, and the second most common cancer (after breast cancer) in women. Nearly one-half million new cases occur each year (1). The majority of cases occur in developing countries without availability of routine Papanicolaou (Pap) smear screening. Cervical cancer is the leading cause of death of women from cancer in developing countries (1). The highest incidence of the disease is seen in Central and South America, southern and eastern Africa, and the Caribbean (2). There is a correlation between incidence and mortality in a given area, but Africa appears to have a disproportionately higher mortality (2). The incidence and mortality of this disease in North America have declined during the last half-century owing to both increased availability of Pap smear screening and a decrease in fertility rate. These declines in incidence have slowed in recent years, and there is a trend toward increasing incidence in some populations of white women in the United States (2). Cervical carcinoma is the 12th most common malignant tumor in women in the United States (3), but black and Hispanic women are disproportionately affected (4).

RISK FACTORS AND ETIOLOGY

Cervical cancer is a sexually transmitted disease associated with chronic infection by oncogenic types of human papillomavirus (HPV). Therefore, risk factors for cervical cancer are the same as those for sexually transmitted disease, including early age at onset of sexual activity, multiple pregnancies, long duration of oral contraceptive use, other sexually transmitted infections including chlamydia and herpes simplex virus, immunosuppressed states such as renal transplant, and multiple sexual partners. Tobacco smoking is also a risk factor for cervical cancer (5). Cigarette smoking may be a cofactor for development of high-grade cervical dysplasia in women who have chronic HPV infections (6). Patients infected with human immunodeficiency virus (HIV) are often also infected with HPV, and they have higher rates of cervical dysplasia and progression to invasive carcinoma than HIV-negative women (7).

Human Papillomavirus

Human papillomavirus is a double-stranded DNA virus of approximately 8 kd, and contains eight open reading frames and a non-coding region that contains transcriptional regulatory sequences (8). Over 30 recognized oncogenic strains of HPV and over 70 nononcogenic strains of HPV have been described to date (9,10). Oncogenic strains in order of decreasing prevalence include HPV-16, -18, -45, -31, -33, -58, -52, -35, -59, -56, -6, -51, -68, -39, -82, -73, -66, and -70. In the United States, HPV-16 and -18 account for approximately 70% of cervix cancers. The HPV genomes code for six early (E) and two late (L) open reading frame proteins (11). High-risk HPV genotypes code for three early proteins (E5, E6, and E7) with cellular growth–stimulating and transforming properties. The E5 protein is expressed during active HPV infection, and the open reading frame is often deleted in cervical carcinoma (11). It has weak transforming activity and can activate membrane-associated protein kinases. The E6 protein binds to p53, results in chromosomal instability, activates telomerase, inhibits apoptosis, and results in cellular immortalization (11). The E7 protein binds to retinoblastoma protein (Rb), inactivating the Rb protein-related pocket proteins, activates cyclins E and A, inhibits cyclin-dependent kinase inhibitors, and also results in cellular immortalization (11). In cells with p53 mutations, E7 exerts an antiapoptotic effect (11). HPV E6 and E7 have numerous other functions, and together with those outlined above, lead to dysplasia and malignant transformation of cervical epithelium. High-risk HPV types are identified in a high percentage of patients with adenocarcinoma of the cervix (12) and small cell carcinoma of the cervix (13) in addition to the more common squamous carcinoma of the cervix.

Cellular and humoral immune responses are likely to be involved in the resolution of HPV infection, and deficiencies may result in more rapid progression to dysplasia and carcinoma. CD4+ T-lymphocytes have been described with increased prevalence in the stroma and epithelium of regressing early cervical intraepithelial neoplasia (CIN) (14) compared to progressed CIN, CIN 3, and squamous cell carcinoma (SCC). Histologically determined CD4+/CD8+ ratios declined as HPV+ patients progressed from CIN 1 to SCC. (8).

Almost 50% of women will be infected with the HPV virus within 4 years after onset of sexual activity. Despite a high prevalence of HPV, only 5% to 15% will develop cervical dysplasia (15,16). HPV attaches to basal epithelial cells and remains elusive to the reticuloendothelial system. It can amplify to more than 1,000 genomes per cell without cell lysis, enhancing its ability to escape a host immune response.

The age-specific HPV prevalence peaks between 25 to 35 years of age when exposure is at its greatest. In a large cohort study, Ho et al. evaluated over 600 female college students and found a cumulative incidence of new HPV infection of 43%. The two-year clearance rate of HPV was over 90% and only 5% developed cytologic abnormality (15).

Concurrent Infection With HPV and HIV

HIV is a sexually transmitted virus that results in a decline in circulating CD4+ cells over time. It is not surprising, therefore, that concurrent HIV and HPV infections are commonly seen in sexually active patients, and that the HPV infection may more rapidly progress from chronic infection to dysplasia and cancer. Reports of abnormal cervical cytology as high as 78% have been reported in HIV+ patients compared to 38% of HIV– patients who are also HPV+ (17). HIV-infected women with low CD4+ lymphocyte counts (<200 cells/μL) were nearly twice as likely to have squamous intraepithelial lesion (SIL) than women with high CD4+ counts. This was confirmed in another report that noted no association with duration of HIV infection, antiretroviral therapy, or HIV viral load (18). HIV+ patients with concurrent HPV infection must be followed closely and should be aggressively treated for SIL. This combination is a particular problem in Equatorial Africa where the combination of HIV and HPV infections is prevalent. Antiretroviral therapy does not affect HPV-related disease in HIV-infected patients (7).

ANATOMY

The uterus, situated in the center of the pelvis, is composed of a muscular layer (myometrium) and mucosal layer (endometrium), which lines a hollow cavity extending from the top of the uterus (fundus) through the lower uterine segment connecting to the endocervical canal. The endometrial cavity is surrounded by the myometrium. The three segments of the uterus include the fundus, body, and isthmus (lower uterine segment). Anteriorly, the lower uterine segment is attached to the bladder peritoneum (vesicouterine pouch), which requires dissection and separation to expose the cervix. This compartment between the bladder and uterus is the anterior cul-de-sac. Posteriorly the peritoneum lines and separates the lower uterine segment and cervix from the rectum, creating the posterior cul-de-sac (pouch of Douglas). The cervix is an extension of the lower uterine segment and can be divided into vaginal and supra-vaginal components. The cervix varies in length, averaging 3 to 4 cm. Centrally in the vaginal portion is the external cervical os, which connects to the endocervical canal, the internal cervical os, and the endometrial canal.

The cervix is a fibrous organ lined by squamous and columnar cells. The transition from columnar cells to squamous cells occurs in the region of the cervical os in the transformation zone. Most cervical dysplasias and invasive cancers arise from this area. The endocervix contains mostly mucinous glandular epithelium.

The uterus has five ligamentous attachments. Specifically these include the round, broad, utero-ovarian, cardinal, and uterosacral ligaments. The round ligaments run from both sides of the fundus anterolaterally on top of the broad ligaments to the pelvic sidewall where they are closely related to the inferior epigastric vessels and continue on their path to leave the pelvis through the inguinal ring and canal. They contain a vessel known as Sampson's artery as well as other small vessels and nerves.

The broad ligaments attach to the lateral margin of the uterus on either side and extend underneath the round ligaments from above the cervicouterine junction and to the pelvic sidewall. These ligaments are covered by peritoneum anteriorly and posteriorly, and are relatively thinner above the cervicouterine junction. Within the leaves of the broad ligament are extraperitoneal connective tissues known as the parametrium.

The utero-ovarian ligaments originate just below the fallopian tubes and directly connect to the ovaries. The cardinal ligaments, also known as Mackenrodt's ligaments, are thickened extensions of the broad ligaments attaching laterally from the lower uterine segment (isthmus) and the cervix. They course to the lateral vaginal wall and rectal pillars and extend to the pelvic sidewalls.

Each cardinal ligament helps create and define two important anatomical spaces, the pararectal and paravesical spaces, which are important in the surgical treatment of early cervical cancer. The cardinal ligament covers a portion of the pelvic ureter, which lies underneath the uterine artery and above the uterine vein about 2 cm away from the isthmus. It contains uterine, vaginal, middle rectal, and inferior vesical arteries and veins as well as lymphatic tissue and channels.

The uterosacral ligaments connect laterally to the cervix and lower uterine segment medial to the ureters. They run from the posteriolateral segment of the cervix over the top of the anterolateral portion of the rectum and attach to the rectal wall and the sacrum. The cardinal and uterosacral ligaments provide the bulk of support for the uterus and cervix.

The blood supply of the uterus is mainly through the uterine artery, originating from the anterior division of the hypogastric artery. An important landmark during a radical hysterectomy, the uterine artery spawns cervical and vaginal branches that supply the cervix, and then extends superiorly to the fundus where its tributaries supply the fundus and the body of the uterus. The uterine artery also descends toward the vagina and gives off a vaginal branch. The ovarian vessels originating from the aorta also contribute to the blood supply of the uterus. There is a rich anastomosis between the uterine and ovarian arteries. Other potential collateral blood supply to the uterus may be from the branches of the posterior division of the hypogastric, the ilio-lumbar artery, or other vessels supplying the pelvis such as middle sacral artery, and pudendal and obturator arteries. The venous drainage follows the arterial supply.

The lymphatic drainage of the cervix is rich and complex. Laterally from the cervix, the lymphatics drain into the paracervical and parametrial lymph nodes and to the internal, external, and common iliac chains. The obturator lymph nodes are the most medial portion of the external iliac nodal region. Other lymphatic drainage routes include the inferior and superior gluteal lymph nodes and the superior rectal, presacral, and para-aortic lymph nodes. The innervations of the cervix are from the sacral roots (S2-4) crossing through the hypogastric plexuses.

Two important anatomical landmarks during radical hysterectomy for treatment of early cervical cancer are the paravesical and pararectal spaces. The paravesical space is lateral to the bladder and can be opened by dissection underneath the insertion of the round ligament into the pelvic wall. The anterior wall is bounded by the superior pubic ramus, the medial wall is the bladder and vagina, the lateral wall is composed of the external iliac vessels and parts of the obturator fossa, and the posterior wall is formed by the cardinal ligament, separating this space from the pararectal space. This space can be continuous with the space between the bladder and the pubic bone, known as the space of Retzius.

The pararectal space is found between the ureter laterally and the origin of the hypogastric artery medially and follows the curve of the sacrum. Anteriorly it is bounded by the cardinal ligament. The lateral wall is formed by the hypogastric vessels. Medially it is bounded by the ureter, and the floor is composed of the curve of the sacrum down to the levator muscles.

NATURAL HISTORY

Preinvasive Disease

Cervical cancer is preceded by an interval of epithelial dysplastic changes, typically in the transformation zone, known as cervical intraepithelial neoplasia (CIN), which may progress to invasive cancer. Low-grade dysplasia (CIN 1) is confined to the basal one third of the epithelium, whereas high-grade dysplasia (CIN 2-3) involves two thirds or greater of the epithelial thickness. Full thickness involvement is known as carcinoma *in situ* (CIS). Cytologic screening has helped in decreasing the incidence of cervical cancer in the United States and other developed nations by over 90%. Of approximately 50 million Pap smears performed in the United States annually, 5% to 7% are abnormal, and the majority of these are atypical squamous cells of undetermined significance (ASCUS) (19,20). The majority of the disease burden is in developing nations where screening and treatment programs are scarce (21).

Many studies have evaluated the natural history of cervical dysplasia. Holowaty et al. evaluated cervical dysplasia in about 17,000 women with mild, moderate, and severe dysplasia (22). The reported risk of progression from mild to severe dysplasia was 2% and 6% at years 2 and 5, respectively. However, progression from moderate to severe dysplasia was 16% and 25% at 2 and 5 years, respectively. The relative risks of progression from severe dysplasia to CIS and invasive cancer were 4.2 and 2.5, respectively, 2 years after diagnosis of dysplasia. The majority of mild dysplasias (CIN 1) regressed to normal within 2 years.

In a meta-analysis of 15 studies of 27,929 women, Melnikow et al. found 2-year progression rates to high-grade dysplasia to be 7% and 21% from ASCUS and low-grade dysplasia, respectively (23). The rate of progression to invasive cancer for ASCUS was 0.25%, as compared to low-grade dysplasia (0.15%) and high-grade dysplasia (1.4%). The regression rates to normal for ASCUS, low-grade, and high-grade dysplasias were 68%, 47%, and 35%, respectively.

The incidence of progression from CIS to invasive cancer in patients with persistent abnormal cytology after initial treatment was 24.8 times greater than in those who had normal cytology after initial treatment (24). Overall the reported rate of progression of CIS to invasive cancer ranges from 12% to 22% (24).

Most low-grade dysplasia will regress to normal in about 24 months. Therefore, only careful follow-up is warranted. However, women with high-grade disease or CIS should be more closely evaluated and treated aggressively as the risk of progression is higher (24).

Patterns of Spread

Cervical cancer can spread through direct extension to the endocervix, lower uterine segment, parametrium, vagina, and, less often, to the bladder and/or rectum. It can also spread lymphatically to the parametrial, obturator, and internal, external, and common iliac lymph nodes. Inferior and superior gluteal, superior rectal, presacral, and para-aortic lymph nodes can also become involved. The pattern of spread is usually predictable and orderly as the rate of para-aortic lymph node metastasis is very rare if the pelvic nodes were spared. The overall risk of pelvic lymph node metastasis in stage IB is about 17% (25,26). The risk of para-aortic nodal metastasis is higher with advanced stage with rates of 16% and 25% for stage II and III, respectively (27). Scalene nodal involvement is reported to be between 10% and 23% (28).

Girardi et al. reported data in 163 patients who had undergone radical hysterectomy, finding that when the parametrial nodes were not involved, the rate of pelvic nodal involvement was 26% (29). However, when the parametrial nodes were involved, the incidence of pelvic lymphatic spread was over 80%.

The most common sites of hematogenous spread include lung, mediastinum, bone, and liver. Other less common sites are spleen, brain, and adrenal. Most recurrences occur in the first 24 months with a median of 17 months (30).

CLINICAL PRESENTATION AND DIAGNOSTIC EVALUATION

Preclinical Invasive Disease

Screening and Cytology

In 2007, 11,150 women were expected to be diagnosed with invasive cervical cancer in the United States, and about 3,670 of them were expected to succumb to the disease (31). These statistics represent a dramatic reduction from statistics prior to introduction of cervical cytology screening programs in the 1950s. However, in developing nations it is one of the leading causes of cancer death (32). This disparity is essentially due to availability of cytologic screening programs in developed nations.

The effectiveness of screening cytology is related to the ease of obtaining specimens, the sensitivity of the test, and a long dysplastic phase that can be detected via cytology and effectively treated with high success rates. There are currently two primary means of obtaining and diagnosing cervical dysplasia. One is the conventional Pap smear and the other is liquid-based thin layer preparation.

Using classification as low-grade squamous intraepithelial lesion (LSIL) as the threshold, Nanda et al. reported a large variation in the sensitivity of conventional smears with published data ranging from 30% to 87%; specificity was much higher at 86% to almost 100% (33). Cytologic screening is a continuum in which sensitivity is increased through sequential testing. The most common reasons for false-negative smears are errors in sampling and preparation. In 1996, liquid-based cytology was introduced in the United States. Cells are obtained by a Cytobrush and transferred into a buffered alcohol medium. The suspended cells are then plated in a thin, evenly distributed layer, improving the clarity of the slide for evaluation. Another benefit is that the specimen can be tested for HPV, gonorrhea, and chlamydia. Although the data is conflicting, it appears that liquid-based cytology may be superior to conventional cytology in minimizing the number of unsatisfactory smears and increasing detection rates of low- and high-grade abnormalities (34). Sulik et al. reported no difference between the two methods in a large systematic review (35). The American Cancer Society (ACS) and U.S. Preventive Services Task Force (USPSTF) have concluded that, although liquid-based technology may be more sensitive than conventional cytology, there was insufficient evidence to recommend universal adoption. The American College of Obstetricians and Gynecologists (ACOG) does not support changing screening intervals based on the method of screening (36).

The current recommendation is to start cytologic screening within 3 years after onset of sexual activity or when a woman reaches the age of 21. The ACS recommends annual screening until age 30 with conventional Pap smear or every other year if liquid-based cytology is used. If a woman has two to three normal smears, the screening interval can be lengthened to every 2 to 3 years (37). The ACOG recommends annual testing and does not specify any testing methodology until age 30. Patients over 30 with no history of CIN 2 or 3, no immunocompromised state, and no diethylstilbestrol (DES) exposure who have three negative cytologies may be screened every 2 to 3 years. In women over 30 years of age with negative testing using both cytology and HPV screening, testing is recommended every 3 years (36,38). The USPSTF recommends that screening intervals be lengthened to every 3 years regardless of age in patients who have had two negative smears. Liquid-based cytologic screening and testing has not been adopted by the USPSTF due to insufficient data. High-risk women should be screened annually.

The upper age of screening is set at 65 by the USPSTF if there are previous normal smears and the woman is not at high risk. The ACS recommends stopping at age 70 if there have been three consecutive negative smears in the prior 10 years. The ACOG recommends individual assessment of risk factors and examination (36). Women who have undergone hysterectomy should be screened according to risk factors such as prior history of CIN 2 and 3 and others.

To provide a standard terminology when reporting cytologic findings, the Bethesda system set forth guidelines in 1988 with revisions in 2001 (39). This system describes the adequacy of the specimen, a general categorization of whether it falls within normal limits or not, and a description of the dysplastic cytologic abnormalities detected in three categories: ASCUS or atypical squamous cells—cannot rule out high-grade squamous intraepithelial lesion (ASC-H), LSIL (the same as CIN 1), and high-grade squamous intraepithelial lesion (HSIL), which is the same as CIN 2 or 3. It can also report squamous cell carcinoma directly. For glandular lesions, categories include atypical glandular cells (AGS), denoting origin if possible (endocervix, endometrial, or not otherwise specified), AGS favoring neoplastic, adenocarcinoma *in situ* (AIS), or frank adenocarcinoma.

It is estimated that approximately 10% to 20% of women with ASCUS or ASC-H have underlying CIN 2 or 3 and that 1 in 1,000 may have underlying invasive cancer. ASC-H is expected to be diagnosed in about 5% to 10% of all ASCUS readings. AGS is associated with a much higher percentage of high-grade disease when compared to ASCUS—as high as 39%.

The ASCUS/LSIL Triage Study (ALTS), a multicenter randomized trial of 3,488 women, compared immediate colposcopy versus triage to colposcopy based on HPV testing, and liquid-based cytology with a threshold of HSIL versus conservative management with triage based on repeat cytology with a threshold of HSIL (40,41). ASCUS was reproducible in repeat liquid-based cytology in only 32% of cases with an overall CIN 2 and 3 diagnosis of 15% when ASCUS cytology was further investigated. HPV testing was able to identify 92% of women who would ultimately have a diagnosis of CIN 3. Only 1.4% of women with negative HPV testing developed CIN 3 over 2 years. Repeat cytology for ASCUS would have referred almost 67% of women to colposcopy as compared to HPV testing, which referred about half the number of women for colposcopy. The American Society of Colposcopy and Cervical Pathology (ASCCP) endorsed HPV testing as the preferred method of triage for ASCUS smears detected by liquid-based cytology (42).

HPV Testing

HPV testing has been gaining more popularity in recent years. Methods of detecting HPV include hybrid capture II and polymerase chain reaction. Both tests have similar sensitivity and specificity, but the former is easier to perform technically, especially in a large screening program setting. Sherman et al. studied over 20,000 women, evaluating the role of conventional Pap smear and concurrent HPV testing to determine the risk of developing CIN 3 (43). In this study, 72% of women who developed CIN 3 had baseline abnormal cytology and positive HPV testing with a cumulative incidence of developing CIN 3 or invasive cancer of 4.5% in approximately 45 months of follow-up. This was compared with women with negative smears and HPV testing whose cumulative incidence of developing CIN 3 or invasive cancer was only 0.16%. The combination of negative cytology and HPV testing carries a high negative predictive value of over 95% regarding the development of CIN 3 or invasive cancer, providing great reassurance for low-risk women and lengthening the interval of screening in that population. The ACS and ACOG agreed that it would be reasonable to offer this combined modality screening to low-risk women aged 30 or greater and allow for screening intervals of 3 years (36).

Clavel et al. studied the role of HPV testing as a primary screening tool in almost 8,000 women (44). They reported 100% sensitivity of HPV testing in detecting histologically proven high-grade dysplasia compared to conventional smear (68%) and liquid-based cytology (87%). The specificity of HPV testing was 93% in women over 30, compared to conventional and liquid-based technologies with specificities of 86% and 95%, respectively. Overall it was found that HPV testing is much more sensitive in detecting high-grade disease compared to conventional smears but with a lower specificity rate. This approach requires further study; screening women younger than 30 may lead to unnecessary testing as many HPV infections are transient, and most women will not develop dysplasia with HPV infection. In LSIL, more than 85% of cases test positive for HPV. Therefore, HPV testing is not encouraged. CIN 2 and 3 require immediate referral for colposcopic evaluation. The overall 2-year cumulative risk of developing CIN 2 and 3 for LSIL and ASCUS with positive HPV testing was essentially the same (27.6% and 26.7%). The authors suggested that repeat HPV testing 12 months after diagnosis of LSIL and ASCUS with positive HPV yielded the highest sensitivity and lowest rate of referral for colposcopy. Repeat cytology with HPV testing did not significantly increase sensitivity and increased referral for colposcopy. HPV testing appears to be useful in triage of ASCUS smears, possibly reducing colposcopic referrals by almost 50% (40,41).

Colposcopy

Colposcopy examines the lower genital tract including the vulva, vagina, and epithelium of the cervix and opening of the endocervix. The use of acetic acid and Lugol's solution assists in highlighting abnormal and dysplastic changes. Changes such as aceto-white plaques and vascular abnormalities such as punctations, mosaicism, and abnormal branching may signify high-grade disease. Indications for colposcopy include an abnormal appearing cervix, persistent post-coital bleeding or discharge, persistent CIN 1, 2, or 3 on cytology, *in utero* exposure to DES, and ASCUS smears with positive high-risk HPV testing. In order to have an adequate colposcopic examination the entire transformation zone must be fully visualized. Endocervical curettage is recommended in all colposcopic evaluations.

Conization Biopsy

Cervical conization refers to the surgical removal of the squamo-columnar junction. This may be done in the operating suite through a classical cold knife conization technique or as an outpatient using thermal cautery with loop excision. Indications for conization include inadequate colposcopy, positive endocervical curettage, persistent CIN 1 (usually >1 year), CIN 2,3 or CIS, and discrepancy between cytologic, colposcopic, or pathologic findings.

Loop Electrosurgical Excision Procedure

Loop diathermy, an alternative to cold knife conization, is usually performed on an outpatient basis. Trials have demonstrated loop electrosurgical excision procedure (LEEP) to be as effective as cold knife conization with advantages in terms of cost, anesthesia, and ease of use (45). A disadvantage is that significant thermal artifact can hamper evaluation of margin status, which can be minimized with careful technique avoiding prolonged contact with the tissue.

Clinical Disease

Symptoms and Complaints

The most common presentations of invasive cervical cancer are abnormal vaginal bleeding, post-coital bleeding, and vaginal discharge. However, many women are asymptomatic and are found to have disease upon pelvic examination or cytologic evaluation. As the tumor enlarges it can cause local symptoms such as pelvic pain and difficulty with urination or defecation. As the disease metastasizes to regional lymph nodes, back pain, leg swelling (especially unilateral), and neuropathic pain may occur.

Physical Findings

The most common finding on physical examination is an abnormal lesion on the cervix, at times necrotic and friable. Possible extension onto the vaginal wall should be assessed. Determination of parametrial, sidewall, and uterosacral ligament involvement must be done through a rectovaginal examination. Other areas of concern are the superficial groin and femoral lymph nodes and the supraclavicular region.

Diagnostic Biopsy

Suspicious lesions on the cervix and surrounding areas should be biopsied with enough depth to assure adequate non-necrotic tissue to render diagnosis. Biopsy on the margin tends to yield better results.

Staging

Clinical Staging Procedures

The most critical component of staging is a through pelvic examination, including a rectovaginal exam. If necessary, an exam under anesthesia allows for a careful visual and digital examination as well as cystoscopy and proctoscopy.

Laboratory Studies

A complete peripheral blood count is indicated to evaluate for anemia, which might warrant correction. Thrombocytosis is found in up to 30% of patients with locally advanced disease and has been associated with larger tumor size, parametrial involvement, and poorer survival. Serum chemistries with attention to serum creatinine are essential to evaluate for renal failure or assess renal function in patients who will receive cisplatin-based chemoradiotherapy. Additional tests should include liver function and urinanalysis.

Serum Tumor Markers

The most commonly studied markers are squamous cell carcinoma antigen (SCCA), carcinoembryonic antigen (CEA), CA-125, and CYFRA 21-1. Molina et al. evaluated SCCA, CEA, and CYFRA 21-1 in 156 patients with invasive cervical cancer. They found a sensitivity at diagnosis of 43%, 25%, and 26%, respectively, and found that in squamous cell cancers the latter two did not add to SCCA alone (46). Reesink-Peters et al. studied preoperative SCCA levels in early-stage cervical cancer and found that patients with elevated SCCA had a higher chance of requiring postoperative radiation therapy (RT) (57% vs. 16%) and a higher relapse rate in those with elevated SCCA as compared to those with normal levels (15 % vs. 1.6%) (47). In any case, most clinicians will use parameters for postoperative RT such as margin status, lymph node and parametrial involvement, depth of invasion, size of tumor, and lymph vascular involvement, irrespective of SCCA levels, to assess the need for adjuvant RT. In one study CA-125 was a poor marker as only up to 21% of patients had elevated levels (48). In general, tumor markers currently have no role in management of advanced cervical cancer.

Radiographic Studies

Cervical cancer is clinically staged by physical examination and limited radiographic evaluation. Computed tomography (CT) and magnetic resonance imaging (MRI) are used extensively to delineate disease extent and improve treatment planning but do not change the assigned staging. Mitchell et al. compared CT versus MRI for measurement of tumor diameter in early-stage disease in 208 patients and found that MRI was superior to CT in preoperative evaluation of tumor size and uterine body involvement (49). Hirack et al. evaluated MRI in evaluating extent of disease in correlation with surgical findings. They reported an accuracy of 91% for detection of tumor location, 70% in determining tumor size, 93% for vaginal extension, and 88% for parametrial involvement (50). In a meta-analysis, Bipat et al. reported sensitivity of 74% for parametrial involvement with MRI as compared to 55% for CT; lymph node involvement was 60% versus 43%, respectively, and MRI was superior in detecting bladder and rectum invasion (51).

Narayan et al. studied International Federation of Gynecology and Obstetrics (FIGO) staging, tumor volume, and lymphatic metastasis using MRI and positron emission tomography (PET) scanning (52). They found that tumor invasion of the uterine body was a strong predictor of lymphatic invasion; uterine body invasion was present in 58%, 73%, 88%, and 100% of stages I, II, II, and IV, respectively. Node positivity was noted in 11% of patients with PET scanning without uterine body involvement on MRI versus 75% of those with uterine body involvement.

Choi et al. reported a preoperative accuracy of MRI in tumor staging of 77% and a sensitivity of 97% for pelvic node metastasis (53). Park et al. evaluated 36 patients with MRI and PET, reporting an accuracy of FIGO and MRI staging of 67% and 84%, respectively. PET was superior to MRI in detecting pelvic nodal metastasis (78% vs. 67%) (54).

Hricak et al. reported a multicenter trial of 172 patients. They found that surgico-pathologic findings correlated with FIGO staging in 76% of cases in stages IA to IIA and in 21% in stage IIB. Sensitivity for detecting advanced stage (>IIB) for FIGO staging, CT, and MRI were 29%, 42%, and 53%, respectively, with specificities of 99%, 82%, and 74%, respectively (55).

In comparing MRI to CT, Subak et al. reported that MRI was superior to CT in evaluating stage of disease, with an accuracy of 90% versus 65%, respectively (56). MRI was superior to CT in detecting parametrial invasion (94% vs. 76%). In evaluating pelvic adenopathy, both were equal. Contrast-enhanced T1-weighted images are superior to nonenhanced T2-weighted images.

Modern imaging techniques such as CT and MRI have low sensitivities for detecting disease in the para-aortic nodes less than 1 cm (57). PET has emerged as a superior method of imaging nodal disease in cervical cancer. The reported sensitivity is about 84% (58,59). Loft et al. completed a prospective study of PET/CT scanning in 120 patients with cervical cancer. There were several false negatives, resulting in a positive predictive value of only 63%. However, negative predictive value, sensitivity, and specificity were 100%, 100%, and 94%, respectively (60).

FIGO and American Joint Committee on Cancer Staging

The staging system used for cervical cancer is based on the 1995 FIGO staging system (61,62). Stage IA1 is defined as stromal invasion to <3 mm in depth and no wider than 7 mm, stage IA2 is defined as stromal invasion of 3 to 5 mm with width of no >7 mm. The Society of Gynecologic Oncologists (SGO) also considers negative lymphovascular space invasion (LVSI) and margin status as criteria for microinvasive disease (MID). The horizontal spread must be 7 mm or less to be considered MID according to FIGO, but SGO does not include lateral spread in defining MID. The diagnosis of MID must be made on a conization or hysterectomy specimen. Punch biopsies are not adequate. Stage IB is divided into IB1, which includes all lesions greater than IA2 and no more than 4 cm in greatest dimension, and stage IB2, a lesion limited to the cervix measuring greater than 4 cm.

Surgical findings and radiographically guided biopsies of suspected lesions cannot be used to change or modify clinical FIGO staging. Stage IVA requires biopsy confirmation of bladder or rectal mucosal involvement. For example, bullous edema of bladder mucosa is not sufficient to render staging as FIGO IVA. Stage IIIB indicates pelvic sidewall involvement or demonstration of a nonfunctioning kidney or hydronephrosis, irrespective of clinical detection of sidewall involvement, as long as there is no alternative explanation for the kidney abnormality.

A tumor-node-metastasis (TNM) staging system is proposed by the American Joint Committee on Cancer (AJCC) that corresponds well to the FIGO clinical staging. The current criteria for the various stages are defined in Table 22.1. TNM is mainly used in documenting findings on surgical and pathologic evaluations as the pathologic stage of the disease, and FIGO is used for clinical staging. All histologic types are included. If there is ambiguity regarding the correct stage, the lower stage is assigned.

Pretreatment Nodal Staging

The presence of para-aortic lymph node metastases is known to have a significant impact on progression-free and overall survival. Pretreatment knowledge of para-aortic spread could potentially direct treatment in a manner that could improve outcomes. Given the limitations of imaging in reliably detecting para-aortic micrometastases, surgical staging has been used. However, the role of surgical staging for locally advanced cervical cancer remains unclear. Leblanc et al. performed pretreatment laparoscopic nodal staging on 156 patients with stages IB2 to IVA with negative preoperative CT scans (63). The average number of

TABLE 22.1

DEFINITION OF TNM

TNM categories		FIGO stages
PRIMARY TUMOR (T)		
TX		Primary tumor cannot be assessed
T0		No evidence of primary tumor
Tis	0	Carcinoma *in situ*
T1	I	Cervical carcinoma confined to uterus (extension to corpus should be disregarded)
T1a[a]	IA	Invasive carcinoma diagnosed only by microscopy. Stromal invasion with a maximum depth of 5.0 mm measured from the base of the epithelium and a horizontal spread of 7.0 mm or less. Vascular space involvement, venous or lymphatic, does not affect classification
T1a1	IA1	Measured stromal invasion 3.0 mm or less in depth and 7.0 mm or less in horizontal spread
T1a2	IA2	Measured stromal invasion more than 3.0 mm and not more than 5.0 mm with a horizontal spread 7.0 mm or less
T1b	IB	Clinically visible lesion confined to the cervix or microscopic lesion greater than T1a/IA2
T1b1	IB1	Clinically visible lesion 4.0 cm or less in greatest dimension
T1b2	IB2	Clinically visible lesion more than 4.0 cm in greatest dimension
T2	II	Cervical carcinoma invades beyond uterus but not to pelvic wall or to lower third of vagina
T2a	IIA	Tumor without parametrial invasion
T2b	IIB	Tumor with parametrial invasion
T3	III	Tumor extends to pelvic wall and/or involves lower third of vagina, and/or causes hydronephrosis or nonfunctioning kidney
T3a	IIIA	Tumor involves lower third of vagina, no extension to pelvic wall
T3b	IIIB	Tumor extends to pelvic wall and/or causes hydronephrosis or nonfunctioning kidney
T4	IVA	Tumor invades mucosa of bladder or rectum, and/or extends beyond true pelvis (bullous edema is not sufficient to classify a tumor as T4)
REGIONAL LYMPH NODES (N)		
NX		Regional lymph nodes cannot be assessed
N0		No regional lymph node metastasis
N1		Regional lymph node metastasis
DISTANT METASTASIS (M)		
MX		Distant metastasis cannot be assessed
M0		No distant metastasis
M1	IVB	Distant metastasis

Note: The definitions of the T categories correspond to the stages accepted by the Fédération Internationale de Gynécologie et d'Obstetrique (FIGO). Both systems are included for comparison.

[a]All macroscopically visible lesions—even with superficial invasion—are T1b/IB.

Source: American Joint Committee on Cancer (AJCC). Cervix uteri. In: Greene FL, Page DL, Fleming ID, et al. eds. *AJCC Cancer Staging Manual.* 6th ed. New York: Springer; 2002:260.

nodes removed and length of stay were 21 and 1.4 days, respectively. The rate of para-aortic metastasis was 25.4%. Nearly a quarter of patients with stage IB2 required extended field RT due to surgical findings. Survival was not different between patients with microscopic versus resected macroscopic nodal disease.

Leblanc et al. evaluated 184 patients with stages IB2 through IVA with pretreatment extraperitoneal laparoscopic staging of para-aortic nodes (64). They found a 24% incidence of para-aortic nodal involvement and an operative complication rate of 2%. They had a 13% symptomatic lymphocyst rate that decreased to about 3% with modification of techniques. Findings of surgical staging changed the management of 20% of patients who would have only received pelvic RT to extended field RT. Data suggested a survival advantage in patients with resected positive nodes.

Lai et al. compared clinical staging versus surgical staging (laparoscopic or extraperitoneal approach) in 61 patients (65). Para-aortic nodal metastasis was detected in 25% of the surgical group. The study was terminated early as the surgical arm had a significantly worse progression-free and overall survival compared to the nonsurgical arm. The role of surgical staging remains unclear, particularly in the era of metabolic imaging. Gallup et al. described an extraperitoneal approach to dissect and evaluate para-aortic lymph nodes, and Querleu et al. have reported a laparoscopic staging technique (66,67). These approaches can minimize treatment delays and complications compared to the open approach.

Sentinel Lymphatic Mapping in Early Cervical Cancer

The standard surgical treatment for early cervical cancer (stages IA2 to IIA) is radical hysterectomy and pelvic lymphadenectomy (PL). The PL is complete and removes all nodal bearing tissues on the external iliac artery and vein (up to the circumflex iliac vein), internal iliac artery above the obturator nerve, and common iliac artery up to the iliac bifurcation. The procedure carries some risk of injury to vessels and nerves, can lead to lymphedema, and can predispose to a higher complication rate if postoperative RT is needed. Lymphatic mapping (LM) refers to the concept of delineating the path of malignant cells through the lymphatics, identifying the nodes primarily at risk for early spread, and determining if this knowledge will safely allow a limited rather than a complete regional lymphadenectomy.

Thompson and Uren described the sentinel node (SN) as "any lymph node that receives lymphatic drainage directly from primary tumor" (68). In cervical cancer, Medl et al. were the first to report LM with blue dye (69). Dargent et al. reported the laparoscopic identification of the SN (70). In a study of 20 patients, O'Boyle et al. noted a low SN detection rate of 60%, which is lower with larger tumors (71). Levenback et al. reported 39 patients with early cervix cancer who underwent radical hysterectomy (RH) and PL. Preoperative lymphoscintigraphy was performed, revealing at least one SN in 85%. Most SNs were iliac, obturator, and parametrial nodes; however, approximately 20% were in the common iliac and aortic chains. Eight (21%) had nodes involved with tumor, and five of these eight had SN as the only positive node. Sensitivity was 87.5% and negative predictive value (NPV) was 97% (72).

Using a laparoscopic approach to SN identification and dissection, Lambaudie et al. reported a sensitivity of 66%, specificity of 100%, positive predictive value of 100%, and NPV of 90% (73). Plante et al. followed with a larger series of 70 patients using laparoscopy. Bilateral SNs were found in 60% of cases. Using both a gamma probe and blue dye, the SN detection rate was 93%. Eighty-eight percent of SNs were in the external iliac, obturator, and the bifurcation area. Fifty-one percent had two SNs, and 24% had ≥ SNs. The NPV was 100% and sensitivity was 93%. The rate of allergy to blue dye was 3% (74). Darai et al. also investigated laparascopic SN identification and biopsy, finding an SN detection rate of 83%. Consistent with other work, the detection rate was considerably worse in patients with advanced tumors. The positive and negative predictive values were each 80%, and positive SNs tended to be associated with parametrial involvement (75). Use of both blue dye and technetium 99 enhances the detection rate of SN.

Using preoperative lymphoscintigraphy, Frumovitz et al. found that 71% of patients showing a solitary SN actually had multiple SNs during laparotomy, and 52% who had unilateral SNs had bilateral SNs noted during exploration. Given the poor concordance between lymphoscintigraphy and laparotomy findings, the authors questioned the utility of preoperative lymphoscintigraphy (76). Wydra et al. reported their findings on 100 patients and found that the detection rate of SN was 96% in patients with tumors <2 cm compared to 54% in those with tumors >2 cm. The false-negative rate was 3% (77).

PATHOLOGY

Squamous Cell Carcinoma

Squamous carcinoma of the cervix includes both microinvasive squamous carcinoma and more deeply invasive carcinoma. Variants of invasive squamous carcinoma, which may be associated with differences in biologic behavior, include verrucous carcinoma, papillary squamous and transitional carcinoma, warty carcinoma, and lymphoepithelioma-like carcinoma.

Preinvasive Disease

Squamous carcinoma *in situ* is a precursor lesion of invasive squamous carcinoma. Squamous carcinoma *in situ* is characterized by full-thickness atypia of the cervical epithelium. Endocervical glands may also be involved. The normal maturation of squamous epithelium is absent. The epithelium is replaced by atypical cells that often have enlarged, oval nuclei and increased nuclear-to-cytoplasmic ratios. Mitotic figures are present. There is no breach of the underlying basement membrane (Fig. 22.1). A recent study of cervical biopsies found excellent interpathologist and intrapathologist agreement in the diagnosis of cervical biopsy specimens (78).

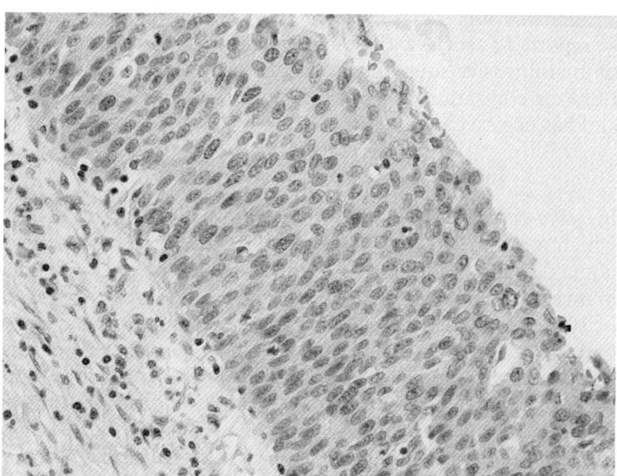

FIGURE 22.1. Squamous carcinoma *in situ*. The epithelium displays full thickness atypia. Cells have enlarged, hyperchromatic nuclei, and there is no evidence of maturation.

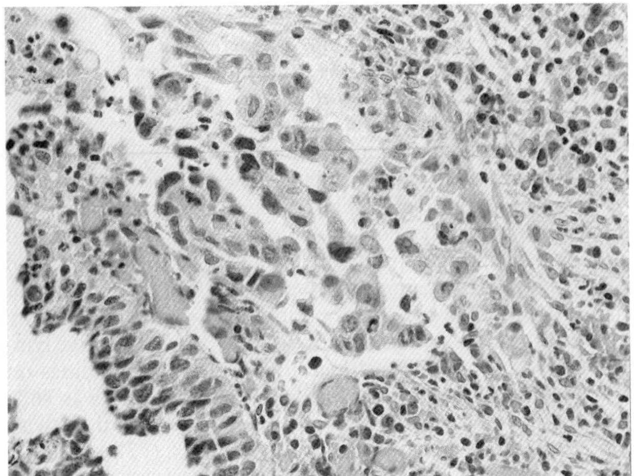

FIGURE 22.2. Microinvasive squamous carcinoma. There is an area of squamous carcinoma *in situ* (lower left). A nest of invasive carcinoma cells (center) has broken through the basement membrane. The invasive cells are larger, with more abundant cytoplasm and larger, more pleomorphic nuclei. A desmoplastic stroma response is present (right).

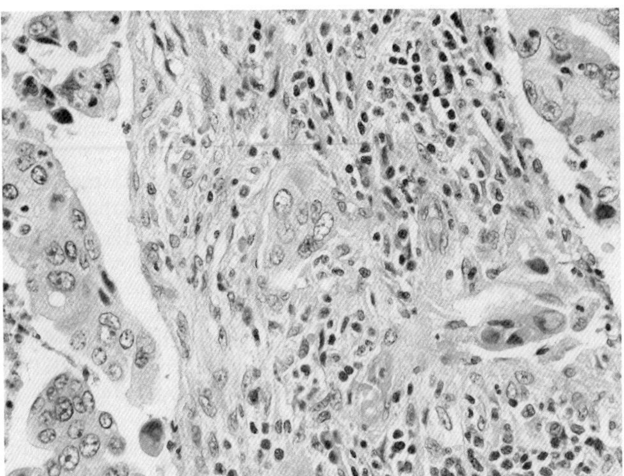

FIGURE 22.3. Invasive squamous carcinoma. Small, irregular nests of cells with markedly atypical nuclei are present. They are surrounded by desmoplastic stroma, containing inflammatory cells.

Microinvasive Carcinoma

Microinvasive squamous carcinoma is associated with squamous intraepithelial neoplasia, and may arise from either the surface epithelium or from endocervical glands involved by dysplasia. It is characterized by small nests of cells that have escaped the basement membrane of the surface or glandular epithelium. Microinvasive carcinoma often displays cells that are larger, with more abundant eosinophilic cytoplasm than cells in the adjacent dysplasia (Fig. 22.2). A desmoplastic stromal reaction is usually present. The nests of microinvasive tumor are irregular and haphazardly arranged. These features are useful in distinguishing microinvasion from rounded, well-circumscribed endocervical glands involved by squamous dysplasia.

Depth of invasion should be measured from the basement membrane of the site of origin. If the tumor arises from surface epithelium, depth is the distance from the basement membrane of the surface epithelium to the deepest nest of invasive neoplasm. If the tumor arises from an endocervical gland, depth is measured from the basement membrane of the gland. If the site of origin is not clear, depth is measured from the basement membrane of the surface epithelium.

Nests of superficial invasion seen in small biopsies should be reported as such, with dimensions of the tumor. A diagnosis of microinvasive squamous carcinoma of the cervix requires a LEEP or conization biopsy that encompasses the entire lesion and has negative margins.

Invasive Squamous Cell Carcinoma

Invasive cervical carcinoma arises from high-grade dysplasia, which may be detected up to 10 years before invasive carcinoma develops. Untreated squamous carcinoma *in situ* results in invasive carcinoma in about one third of cases over a period of 10 years. Invasive carcinoma occurs most often after the age of 40 years (15), although it may be seen in young women. It is associated with human papillomavirus infection in more than 99% of cases. These tumors may consist of firm, indurated masses, or they may be ulcerated or polypoid. Microscopic examination reveals irregular, haphazardly infiltrating nests of cells with eosinophilic cytoplasm and enlarged, atypical, hyperchromatic nuclei (Fig. 22.3).

Mitoses may be numerous, and atypical forms may be present. There is typically a desmoplastic stromal response around the nests of invasive neoplasm. Lymphatic and vascular space invasion may be present, especially in more deeply invasive tumors. Invasive squamous carcinomas are classified as keratinizing or nonkeratinizing, although this classification has no prognostic significance. Keratinizing squamous carcinomas display at least some keratin pearl formation. Nonkeratinizing squamous carcinomas are composed of irregular nests of cells that may display abundant eosinophilic cytoplasm and intercellular bridges but do not contain keratin pearls. Some squamous carcinomas are composed of smaller cells without evidence of neuroendocrine differentiation; these neoplasms should be classified as nonkeratinizing squamous carcinomas.

Invasive squamous carcinomas are also graded (79), although treatment protocols do not depend on grade, and the histologic grade may not correlate with prognosis. Grade 1 (well-differentiated) tumors are not very common in the cervix. They display keratin pearls and large numbers of keratinized cells. Nuclei display only mild to moderate atypia, and mitoses are typically not numerous. Grade 2 (moderately differentiated) tumors represent the majority of invasive squamous carcinomas of the uterine cervix, and are usually nonkeratinizing squamous carcinomas with nuclear pleomorphism, numerous mitoses, and an infiltrative pattern. Grade 3 (poorly differentiated) tumors either have smaller cells without neuroendocrine differentiation, or are pleomorphic with anaplastic nuclei and sometimes a tendency to form spindle cells that must be distinguished from sarcoma by positive cytokeratin stains.

Variants of Squamous Cell Carcinoma

Basaloid Squamous Cell Carcinoma. Basaloid squamous carcinoma is an invasive, highly aggressive tumor composed of basaloid cells resembling those seen in squamous carcinoma *in situ* (80).

Verrucous Carcinoma

Verrucous carcinoma occurs rarely in the uterine cervix (81). Examination of the cervix reveals a papillary excrescence that may resemble condyloma acuminatum. In fact, lesions termed "giant condyloma of Buschke and Lowenstein" in the past probably represent verrucous carcinomas. Microscopic examination displays papillary fronds of squamous epithelium not containing connective tissue cores. The fronds are often pointed and have a "church spire" appearance. Underlying connective

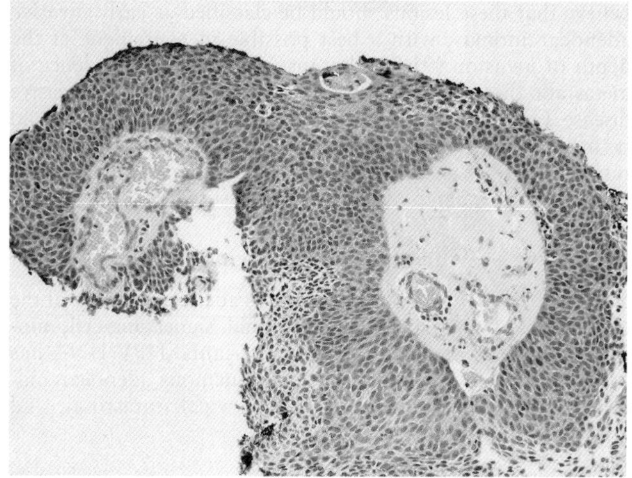

FIGURE 22.4. Papillary squamous carcinoma. Papillary fronds of tumor contain connective tissue cores, and are covered with multiple layers of atypical epithelial cells.

tissue displays bulbous nests of squamous epithelium that invade the stroma with a pushing margin but display little cytologic atypia. Any lesion displaying significantly atypical nuclei does not represent verrucous carcinoma. The distinction between verrucous carcinoma and regular squamous carcinoma is important because verrucous carcinoma invades locally but does not metastasize. In order to diagnose verrucous carcinoma, it is necessary to see the invasive portion of the neoplasm. Superficial biopsies are usually not diagnostic.

Papillary Squamous and Transitional Carcinoma

Some cervical neoplasms are characterized by papillary superficial architecture with substantial nuclear atypia not seen in verrucous carcinomas (82,83). The most common presenting symptoms are vaginal bleeding and abnormal Pap smears. Papillary, polypoid, or granular lesions are often evident upon examination of the cervix.

These tumors may have thin or thick papillae that contain a connective tissue core (Fig. 22.4). The papillary processes may be covered by highly atypical epithelium displaying keratinization, or the epithelium may consist of multiple layers of cells with oval, hyperchromatic nuclei that do not show keratinization, and resemble transitional cell epithelium. Nuclear grooves may be present. Some tumors display epithelium with mixed features. Immunohistochemical studies have shown that most of these tumors are cytokeratin 7 positive and cytokeratin 20 negative; these results are consistent with squamous differentiation (83). HPV-16 has been identified in these neoplasms (82). A recent study demonstrated that these tumors all have the same immunophenotype (uroplakin III negative, p63 positive, and p16^{INK4a} positive) regardless of light microscopic features (84). The authors concluded that these neoplasms lack true transitional cell differentiation and share features with squamous carcinoma.

Many papillary squamous and transitional carcinomas are associated with an underlying invasive carcinoma. The invasive neoplasm is often typical squamous carcinoma, but some cases of invasive transitional carcinoma have been described. Superficial biopsies display only the papillary portion of the neoplasm. LEEP or conization biopsy should be performed to evaluate the possibility of underlying invasive carcinoma.

The invasive form of this neoplasm may be associated with local recurrence and metastasis. These tumors must be distinguished from verrucous carcinomas, which display little atypia and have a much more indolent clinical course.

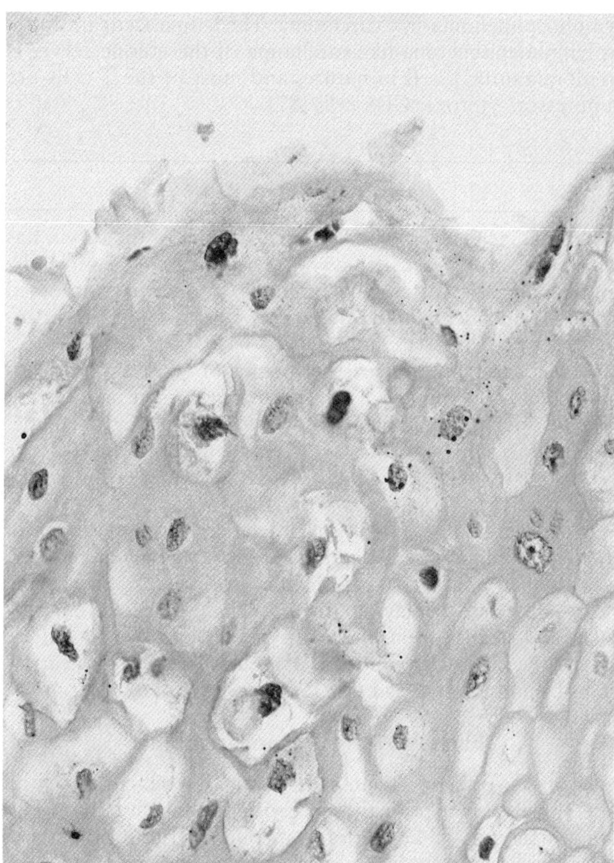

FIGURE 22.5. Human papillomavirus changes. This squamous epithelium displays cells with large halos surrounding atypical nuclei ("koilocytotic atypia").

Warty Carcinoma

Warty carcinoma of the cervix is a rare papillary neoplasm that displays marked condylomatous change but has features typical of routine invasive squamous carcinoma at its deep margin (85). These tumors are associated with HPV and may behave less aggressively than the usual type of invasive squamous carcinoma. Cellular change consistent with HPV infection ("koilocytotic atypia") is shown in Figure 22.5.

Lymphoepithelioma-Like Carcinoma

Lymphoepithelioma-like carcinoma, more commonly seen in the nasopharynx, also occurs in the uterine cervix. Some patients may present with abnormal bleeding and have cervical masses, whereas others may have abnormal Pap smears and no visible cervical lesions. Lymphoepithelioma-like carcinoma of the cervix is seen most often in Asian women, and it has been associated with Epstein-Barr virus infection in those patients (86). In contrast, studies from Europe have not demonstrated Epstein-Barr virus DNA (87,88), but some have suggested a role for HPV in the etiology of this neoplasm (88–90).

Microscopically, this tumor is characterized by nests of cells with lightly eosinophilic cytoplasm and large vesicular nuclei with prominent eosinophilic nucleoli. Cell borders are indistinct, giving the tumor cell nests a syncytial appearance. Aggregates of tumor cells are surrounded by a prominent inflammatory infiltrate that includes lymphocytes, plasma cells, and varying numbers of eosinophils. This neoplasm can be distinguished from glassy cell carcinoma (which is also accompanied by prominent inflammation) by the lack of prominent cell borders and granular eosinophilic cytoplasm in lymphoepithelioma-like carcinoma. The lymphocytic infiltrate in lymphoepithelioma-like carcinoma of the uterine cervix is predominantly T cell in nature, and most of the T cells are suppressor/cytotoxic CD8 cells (87).

Adenocarcinoma

While the incidence of squamous carcinoma of the cervix has decreased in past decades owing to cytologic screening, the number of cases of cervical adenocarcinoma has increased (91–93). Adenocarcinoma of various types accounts for 20% to 25% of cervical carcinomas (92).

Adenocarcinoma *in situ* is a precursor of invasive adenocarcinoma. It is found adjacent to many invasive adenocarcinomas, often accompanied by squamous dysplasia. Both adenocarcinoma *in situ* and invasive adenocarcinoma of the cervix are associated with HPV (usually type 18, but sometimes type 16).

Adenocarcinoma *in situ* is characterized by preservation of the overall endocervical gland architecture. However, endocervical glands and surface epithelium are replaced to varying degrees by cells displaying atypia, including nuclear enlargement and stratification, nuclear hyperchromasia, and mitotic figures (Fig. 22.6). Most adenocarcinomas *in situ* occur near the transformation zone, and skip lesions are unusual (93).

Early Invasive Adenocarcinoma

Early invasive adenocarcinoma of the uterine cervix displays an alteration from the normal endocervical gland architecture. This abnormality may take the form of solid or cribriform nests of cells, architecturally irregular or incomplete glands lined by malignant cells, or small buds of highly atypical cells arising from glands involved by adenocarcinoma *in situ*. A desmoplastic stroma may be present. Diagnosis of early invasive adenocarcinoma may be difficult because endocervical glands normally have a complex pattern. Wheeler and Kurman (94) have reported that close proximity of glands to thick-walled blood vessels is suggestive of an invasive neoplasm.

Technically, the definitions of microinvasive carcinoma, according to both SGO and FIGO, apply to all types of carcinoma. Application of this term to glandular lesions of the cervix has not been generally accepted. Some gynecologic pathologists believe that these lesions should be classified as early invasive adenocarcinomas, with a best possible measurement of the depth of invasion (91,93), because an increased incidence of metastatic disease correlates with increasing depth of invasive disease. One author has suggested that depth of invasion should be measured from the luminal surface to the deepest invasive tumor nest so that, as in malignant melanomas, tumor thickness rather than depth of invasion is measured (93).

Mucinous Adenocarcinoma

There are several variants of mucinous adenocarcinoma of the cervix, including endocervical, intestinal, signet ring cell, minimal deviation, and villoglandular variants. HPV DNA has been detected in more than 90% of mucinous adenocarcinomas of the cervix, including endocervical, intestinal, and endometrial subtypes (95).

Mucinous Adenocarcinoma, Endocervical Variant

The endocervical variant of mucinous adenocarcinoma is the most common type of cervical adenocarcinoma. It is composed of irregular, haphazardly arranged tubuloracemose glands lined by cells resembling those seen in normal endocervical glands, although they may sometimes have limited amounts of cytoplasmic mucin. Nuclei are basally located, stratified, and atypical (Fig. 22.7). Mitoses are present. Grade 1 (well-differentiated) tumors have uniform nuclei with minimal stratification and few mitotic figures. Grade 2 (moderately differentiated) adenocarcinomas have more marked cytologic atypia with frequent mitoses. They may also have solid areas accounting for less than half of the neoplasm. Grade 3 (poorly differentiated) adenocarcinomas contain more prominent solid areas, pleomorphic nuclei, and many mitoses. Desmoplastic stromal response is variable in this type of cervical adenocarcinoma.

Mucinous Adenocarcinoma, Intestinal Type, Signet Ring, and Colloid Variants

Rare endocervical adenocarcinomas have glands containing goblet cells; these tumors display intestinal differentiation. Signet ring cell carcinomas and colloid carcinomas are extremely rare and must be distinguished from metastatic tumors from the gastrointestinal tract.

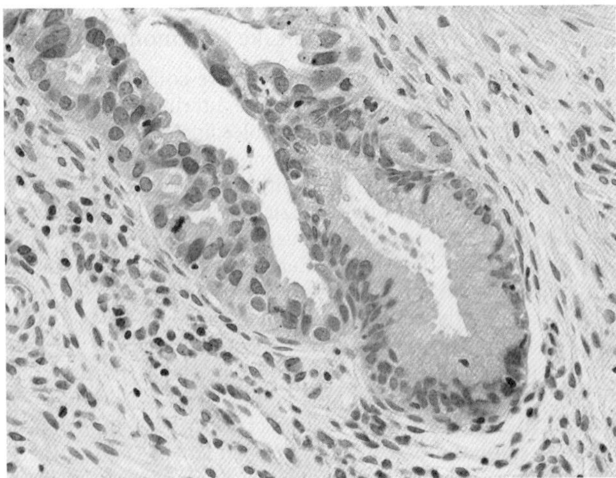

FIGURE 22.6. Adenocarcinoma *in situ*. Part of this endocervical gland is normal (upper left corner). The remainder of the gland has been replaced by stratified cells with atypical, large nuclei and mitotic figures.

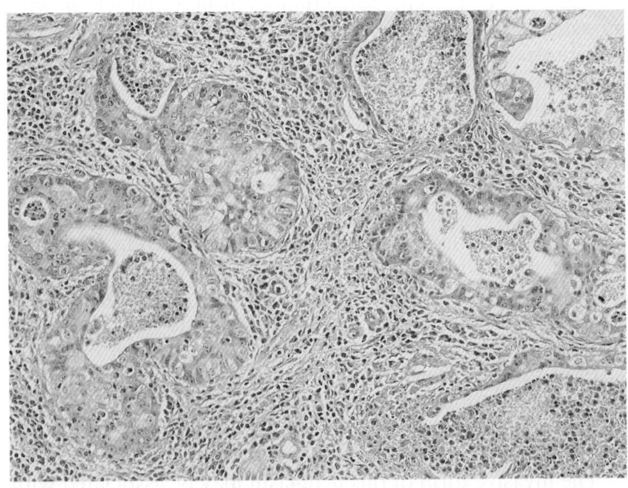

FIGURE 22.7. Invasive adenocarcinoma. There is a haphazard invasion of the cervix by irregular glands lined by multiple layers of atypical cells.

Mucinous Adenocarcinoma, Minimal Deviation Variant (Adenoma Malignum)

The term *adenoma malignum* was originally proposed by McKelvey and Goodlin (96) to describe a form of cervical adenocarcinoma that is so well differentiated that it may be difficult to recognize as a malignant lesion. The term *minimal deviation adenocarcinoma* is a more appropriate designation for this lesion. There is also a tendency for benign lesions of the uterine cervix to be overdiagnosed as minimal deviation adenocarcinoma (97), further emphasizing the difficulty of diagnosing this neoplasm.

This tumor is uncommon, and represents only about 1.3% of cervical adenocarcinomas (98). Patients range in age from 25 to 72 years. They may present with abnormal bleeding or a mucoid discharge. The cervix may appear normal, or it may display a firm area or a mass. The neoplasm is very difficult to diagnose on small biopsies because the infiltrative gland pattern cannot be appreciated. Conization specimens are more conducive to accurate diagnosis in this lesion, but some cases have been diagnosed only after hysterectomy. In contrast to most other types of cervical adenocarcinomas, minimal deviation adenocarcinomas are not associated with HPV infection (99).

Gross examination of hysterectomy specimens displays firm, tan-yellow neoplasms. Most cases contain mucinous glands, but some display endometrioid glands. Microscopically, glands infiltrate the cervical stroma in a haphazard manner; they do not conform to the normal endocervical gland pattern. They may display budding contours, and they typically have angular, sharply pointed outlines, in contrast to the rounded contours of benign endocervical glands. The glands of minimal deviation adenocarcinoma appear deceptively benign on low power. Lack of substantial cytologic atypia is a prerequisite for this diagnosis. However, high-power examination reveals at least some areas with mild to moderate atypia, in which some nuclear enlargement, stratification, and rare mitotic figures may be identified (Fig. 22.8). The infiltrating glands may be devoid of any surrounding desmoplastic reaction. Some authors (97) have described the utility of positive cytoplasmic staining for carcinoembryonic antigen (CEA) in these neoplasms after the possibility of squamous metaplasia has been excluded.

Minimal deviation adenocarcinoma may occur as a sporadic neoplasm, although patients with Peutz-Jeghers syndrome are at risk of developing this cervical tumor.

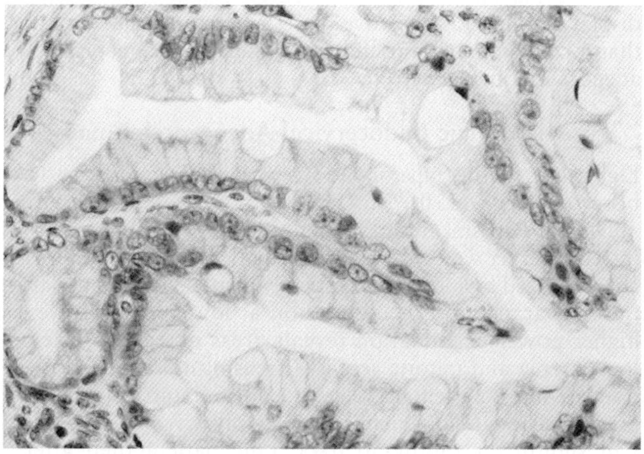

FIGURE 22.8. Minimal deviation adenocarcinoma. This gland has some very bland cytologic features (left side), but enlarged, atypical nuclei are evident in other areas.

Mucinous Adenocarcinoma, Well-Differentiated Villoglandular Variant

Well-differentiated villoglandular adenocarcinoma is a type of low-grade adenocarcinoma that displays similarities to villous adenomas of the intestine. Patients may present with polypoid or papillary endocervical masses upon pelvic examination, abnormal bleeding, or abnormal Pap smears. The age range has been 23 to 57 years, with most cases occurring in patients younger than 40 years of age (100,101).

Microscopic examination of these neoplasms reveals villous, papillary structures that may be either long and slender, or short and broad. These processes contain a connective tissue core that often displays inflammatory cells. The covering epithelium is a single layer of stratified cells with endocervical, endometrial, or intestinal differentiation. Nuclei display only mild to moderate atypia, and mitotic figures are infrequent (Fig. 22.9). Only tumors with low-grade cytologic atypia should receive this diagnosis, since other endocervical carcinomas may have papillary features. Invasive adenocarcinoma may be seen deep to the papillary areas, and is characterized by branching glands lined by atypical cells and surrounded by desmoplastic stroma. These neoplasms do not display the marked nuclear atypia and epithelial tufting seen in the much more aggressive papillary serous carcinoma of the cervix. They may be associated with typical adenocarcinoma *in situ* of the cervix.

Some authors have found an association between well-differentiated villoglandular adenocarcinoma of the cervix and oral contraceptive use (100). More recently, these tumors have been shown to contain high-risk types of HPV (types 16 and 18) (99,100). Neither oncogene amplification nor tumor suppressor gene loss was identified (101).

Well-differentiated villoglandular carcinoma has not metastasized unless it was associated with more aggressive types of carcinoma. A few cases have recurred (100). Some cases have been successfully treated by conization if the tumor is completely excised and the patient wishes to retain fertility. Generally, this diagnosis should not be suggested on the basis of small biopsy specimens; definitive diagnosis should be made only in tumors seen on conization or hysterectomy specimens. Diagnosis of this type of neoplasm on the basis of only a small biopsy specimen could result in undertreatment of a potentially more aggressive neoplasm (92). Villoglandular tumors associated with a high-grade cytologic component or

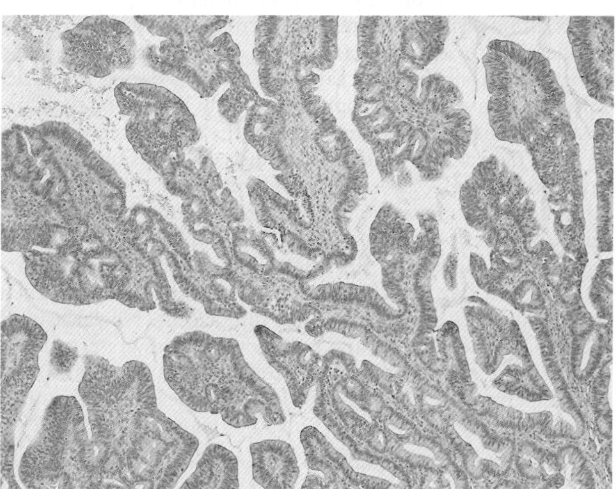

FIGURE 22.9. Well-differentiated villoglandular adenocarcinoma. Long, slender villous processes are covered with epithelium, displaying mild atypia. Nuclei are crowded, but they retain an oval shape, and are uniform in size.

an underlying obvious invasive adenocarcinoma may be associated with lymphovascular invasion, recurrences, and lymph node metastases (102,103).

Endometrioid Adenocarcinoma

Endometrioid carcinomas of the uterine cervix are rare, and have probably been overdiagnosed. These tumors make up about 7% of all cervical adenocarcinomas. These neoplasms display histologic features identical to endometrial carcinoma. Therefore, the possibility of a primary endometrial adenocarcinoma with endocervical extension or drop metastasis must be excluded before the diagnosis of a primary endocervical endometrioid adenocarcinoma is established. A rare case has arisen from endocervical endometriosis (104). In difficult cases, immunohistochemical stains may be helpful since a combination of CEA positivity, ER negativity, and vimentin negativity is most often seen in endocervical primary tumors, while the reverse is more often characteristic of endometrial primary tumors. Evidence of association with HPV also supports an endocervical primary neoplasm.

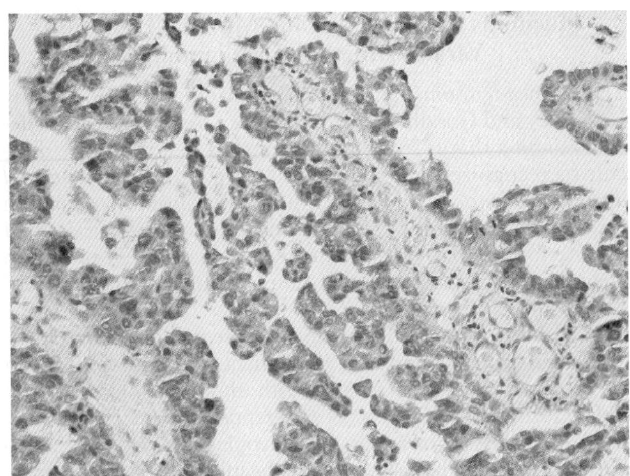

FIGURE 22.10. Papillary serous adenocarcinoma. The papillary structures have a connective tissue core. There is marked tufting and stratification, and the nuclei are markedly atypical.

Other Adenocarcinomas

Clear Cell Adenocarcinoma

Clear cell carcinoma of the cervix has been associated with intrauterine diethylstilbestrol (DES) exposure; however, it also occurs in the absence of DES exposure. Patients usually have a cervical mass. The solid pattern of tumor displays sheets of cells containing abundant glycogen-rich clear cytoplasm, atypical nuclei, and mitoses. The tubulocystic pattern contains tubules and cystic spaces lined by oxyphilic, hobnail, or clear cells. The papillary pattern is the least common variant and often coexists with solid or tubulocystic areas. Clear cell carcinomas of the cervix are not associated with HPV DNA (99).

Serous Adenocarcinoma

Papillary serous carcinoma of the uterine cervix (105,106) has a bimodal age distribution, occurring in patients younger than 40 years and patients older than 65 years. This age distribution has also been seen in well-differentiated villoglandular carcinoma but differs from the typical mid-life age of patients with cervical adenocarcinomas in general. Serous carcinomas of the cervix are not associated with HPV DNA (99).

Gross examination may reveal a nodular mass, an indurated cervix, or no visible abnormality. Microscopically, these tumors are identical to serous tumors of the ovary, endometrium, and primary peritoneal serous carcinomas. Considering the rarity with which this type of neoplasm is seen in the cervix, the diagnosis of primary serous carcinoma of the uterine cervix should be made only after excluding metastasis or extension of disease from another site, especially the endometrium.

Histologic examination of serous carcinoma of the uterine cervix reveals fibrous papillae lined by atypical epithelial cells; secondary papillae and tufts of neoplastic epithelial cells are often present (Fig. 22.10). Glandular structures have irregular luminal borders due to tufting of tumor cells. Nuclei usually show high-grade atypia, and numerous mitoses are present.

These are aggressive tumors (106) that may metastasize to pelvic, periaortic, and inguinal lymph nodes. Larger tumors (>2 cm diameter) and tumors invading more than 10 mm are associated with a worse prognosis.

Mesonephric Adenocarcinoma

Remnants of the mesonephric ducts persist and can be seen in the lateral aspects of the cervix. They are often not identified because uteri are traditionally bivalved along their lateral aspects, and most microscopic sections are taken from the anterior and posterior portions of the cervix. Mesonephric duct remnants are seen as lobules of small, round, glandular structures lined by flattened cuboidal epithelium and containing intraluminal periodic acid-Schiff stain (PAS)-positive material. The cells of mesonephric duct remnants do not contain intracytoplasmic mucin, unlike the cells lining endocervical glands. Mesonephric duct hyperplasia may occur in the cervix. Mesonephric adenocarcinomas are thought to arise from mesonephric duct remnants. Only about two dozen cases have been documented (107,108). Early reports of lesions termed mesonephric carcinoma are now known to represent clear cell carcinoma, with no relationship to the mesonephric duct remnants.

Patients have ranged in age from 52 to 55 years (98). Some patients have not had grossly apparent lesions, but most present with abnormal bleeding and have visible cervical masses. These neoplasms occur deep in the lateral cervical wall. Microscopically, most mesonephric carcinomas are adenocarcinomas (108), although some with a concomitant spindle cell component have been termed "malignant mesonephric mixed tumors" (107). Mesonephric carcinomas display a variety of histologic appearances, including ductal, tubular, retiform, solid, and sex cord–like patterns (107). Mesonephric hyperplasia may be associated with the carcinoma. Like mesonephric remnants, mesonephric carcinoma tumor cells contain no intracytoplasmic mucin; however, glandular structures may display luminal PAS-positive material. Recent studies suggest that CD10 staining is useful in diagnosing mesonephric-type adenocarcinomas (97,109).

Microcystic Endocervical Adenocarcinomas

Eight cases of this type of endocervical adenocarcinoma have been described (110). Most patients presented with either abnormal Pap smears or vaginal bleeding. Abnormalities of the endocervix were visible in three patients. These tumors are characterized by numerous cystically dilated glands simulating the appearance of a benign lesion at low power. However, higher power examination reveals areas of significant cytologic atypia and mitotic activity. Areas of more typical mucinous or intestinal endocervical adenocarcinoma may also be present. These lesions may be deeply invasive. Three patients had significant follow-up data. One patient died after a debulking procedure for a pelvic recurrence 2 years after her initial diagnosis, and two other patients are alive without evidence of tumor at 1 and 6.5 years after diagnosis.

Other Epithelial Tumors

Adenosquamous Carcinoma

Adenosquamous carcinoma is a tumor composed of admixed malignant glandular and squamous elements. This term should not be used for poorly differentiated squamous carcinomas, in which mucicarmine stains show only scattered mucin vacuoles. Likewise, it is different from collision tumors, which display adjacent adenocarcinoma and squamous carcinoma. A recent multi-institutional study found that adenosquamous carcinomas are more commonly associated with higher tumor grade ($p < 0.001$) and vascular invasion ($p = 0.002$) than are adenocarcinomas (111). Adenosquamous carcinomas appear to be either histologically more aggressive or diagnosed at a later stage than adenocarcinomas of the uterine cervix.

Glassy Cell Carcinoma

Glassy cell carcinoma is a rare form of poorly differentiated adenosquamous carcinoma that displays cells with eosinophilic cytoplasm, well-defined cell borders, prominent nucleoli, and a prominent infiltrate of eosinophils and plasma cells. Occasionally, this morphology may be seen in recurrences of adenocarcinomas or adenosquamous carcinomas that have been treated with radiation therapy (RT) (92).

Adenoid Cystic Carcinoma

Adenoid cystic carcinoma of the cervix is a rare but aggressive malignant neoplasm. These lesions are typically seen in elderly patients, many of whom present with postmenopausal bleeding. Examination of the cervix typically shows a lesion.

Microscopic examination of these tumors reveals a cribriform gland pattern. The glands may contain hyaline or mucinous material. Nuclei are larger and more pleomorphic than those seen in adenoid basal epithelioma, and numerous mitoses as well as areas of necrosis are present in adenoid cystic carcinoma. Electron microscopy has shown basement membrane–like material around the nests of tumor cells as well as in some gland lumina. The tumor cells stain with cytokeratin. In contrast to adenoid cystic carcinoma of the salivary glands, this neoplasm in the cervix has not displayed unequivocal evidence of myoepithelial cells, either by immunohistochemical staining for S100 protein or by electron microscopy.

Adenoid cystic carcinoma of the cervix often recurs, and may metastasize. In the largest series reported, the only patients who were free of tumor at last follow-up had stage IB tumor. No patient with higher stage disease was alive and well.

Adenoid Basal Epithelioma (Carcinoma)

Adenoid basal epithelioma is a rare cervical neoplasm. It was originally called adenoid basal carcinoma. The indolent behavior of most of these neoplasms led to the term "adenoid basal epithelioma." More recently, Parwani et al. reported ten tumors that had low-grade adenoid basal epitheliomas admixed or associated with invasive carcinomas of various types, including adenoid basal/squamous carcinoma, pure squamous carcinoma, adenoid cystic carcinoma, or small cell neuroendocrine carcinoma. Most adenoid basal epitheliomas and associated invasive carcinomas contain HPV-16 DNA. It now appears that adenoid basal epitheliomas may be precursor lesions that may give rise to carcinomas of various types. These tumors should now be subclassified as adenoid basal epitheliomas and carcinomas (112).

The age of patients with adenoid basal epithelioma ranges from 30 to 91 years (98,113). This neoplasm is often seen in postmenopausal women who are asymptomatic, with normal appearing cervices. These lesions are usually incidental findings in specimens obtained for the purpose of evaluating squamous intraepithelial neoplasia. A neoplastic squamous component is often an associated feature (98).

Microscopically, adenoid basal epithelioma is characterized by nests of cells that have a basaloid appearance, and may display peripheral palisading. Some gland lumina are present in the basaloid cell nests, although the number of glands is variable. Squamous metaplasia may also be seen. Mitotic figures are typically rare.

Adenoid basal epithelioma, in the absence of a coexisting invasive carcinoma, is a benign lesion with no reported cases of metastatic behavior (98). It must be distinguished from adenoid cystic carcinoma, which is an aggressive malignant neoplasm. Adenoid basal tumors with carcinomatous components should be reported as carcinomas.

Neuroendocrine Tumors

The College of American Pathologists and the National Cancer Institute (114) have proposed standard terminology for neuroendocrine tumors of the uterine cervix. The previous lack of uniform nomenclature and diagnostic criteria for these neoplasms made it difficult to study their incidence and biologic behavior. Immunohistochemical or electron microscopic evidence of neuroendocrine differentiation is necessary for diagnosis of all neuroendocrine tumors except small cell carcinoma. Chromogranin or synaptophysin stains are recommended for documentation of neuroendocrine differentiation. Chromogranin works best when cells contain numerous neuroendocrine granules; synaptophysin stains cells with fewer granules. Neuron-specific enolase is nonspecific by itself, but may be useful in conjunction with one of the other stains. Many cases of small cell carcinoma will also stain for these markers. CD56 (neural cell adhesion molecule) has recently been reported to be the most sensitive marker for the diagnosis of small cell carcinoma of the uterine cervix (115). Neuroendocrine granules can also be seen by electron microscopy if fresh tumor tissue is available.

Neuroendocrine Tumors

Typical Carcinoid Tumors

Typical carcinoids of the cervix are rare neoplasms. This diagnosis should be made with caution, because most cervical neuroendocrine tumors are aggressive neoplasms. They display organoid architecture without nuclear atypia, mitotic figures, or necrosis. Immunohistochemical stains for chromogranin and synaptophysin demonstrate neuroendocrine differentiation. There are not enough documented cases of this neoplasm to permit assessment of biologic behavior.

Atypical Carcinoid Tumors

Atypical carcinoid tumors also display organoid nests of cells, but the cells display nuclear atypia and a mitotic rate of 5 to 10 MF/10 HPF. Necrosis may be present. These tumors are also rare, precluding evaluation of biologic behavior. However, they may metastasize. Immunohistochemical evidence of neuroendocrine differentiation is required for diagnosis (116).

Large Cell Neuroendocrine Carcinoma

Large cell neuroendocrine carcinomas (Fig. 22.11) display organoid nests of cells with peripheral palisading of nuclei, prominent nucleoli, variable amounts of necrosis, eosinophilic cytoplasmic granules, and numerous mitotic figures (> 0 MF/10 HPF). Vascular/lymphatic space involvement is often seen, and many are associated with coexisting adenocarcinoma

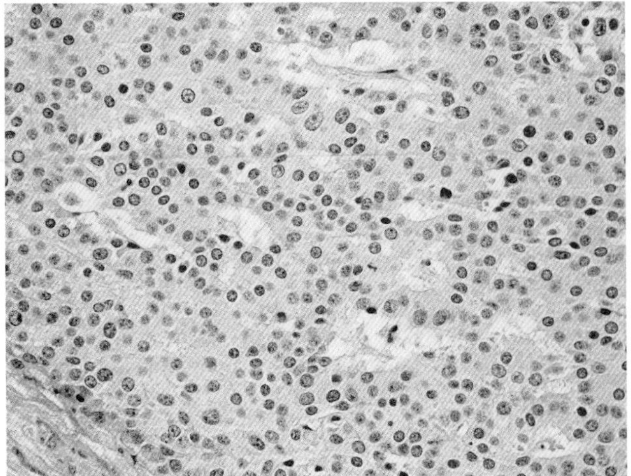

FIGURE 22.11. Large cell neuroendocrine carcinoma. This tumor displays organoid architecture. The tumor cells are much larger than those seen in small cell carcinoma. They have abundant eosinophilic cytoplasm, and there are numerous mitotic figures. Areas of necrosis were present elsewhere in the tumor.

in situ or adenocarcinoma of the cervix (117). These tumors are highly aggressive neoplasms (118). Evidence of neuroendocrine differentiation is necessary for diagnosis and is most easily obtained with immunohistochemical stains for chromogranin and synaptophysin.

Small Cell Carcinoma

Most neuroendocrine tumors seen in the uterine cervix represent small cell carcinomas. A recent study found that 1.3% of cervical cancers contain a small cell carcinoma component, and that even a small component of small cell carcinoma in a tumor of mixed type is associated with adverse outcome (118). Small cell carcinoma is characterized by cells with scant cytoplasm, inconspicuous nuclei with finely stippled chromatin, nuclear molding, extensive necrosis, crush artifact, and numerous mitotic figures (Fig. 22.12). Single cell infiltration of the stroma is common. Vascular/lymphatic space invasion is often seen. These tumors have morphology identical to that seen in small cell carcinoma of the lung. They are aneuploid tumors that show a strong association with type 18 HPV (116). Immunohistochemical stains for neuroendocrine markers such as chromogranin and synaptophysin may be helpful in the diagnosis (119). CD56 (neural cell adhesion molecule) is a sensitive marker for the diagnosis of small cell cancer in the cervix. A panel of antibodies should be used when this diagnosis is a possibility (120).

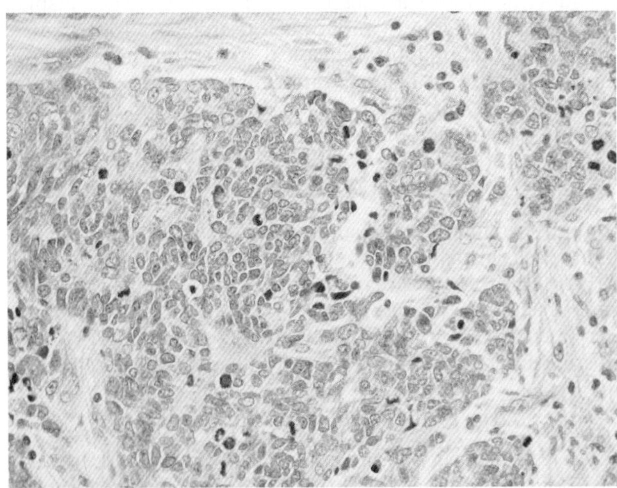

FIGURE 22.12. Small cell neuroendocrine carcinoma. This tumor displays cells that are smaller than those of squamous carcinoma. Nuclei are large and atypical with molding of adjacent nuclei. There is a very high mitotic rate.

Mixed Epithelial and Mesenchymal Tumors

Müllerian adenosarcomas occur in the cervix (121). Patients range in age from 13 to 67 years, with a mean age of 37 years. They may present with abnormal bleeding. These neoplasms consist of polypoid or papillary masses. Microscopically, they display benign glands and sarcomatous stroma with a periglandular cuff of condensed stroma. The sarcomatous component contains variable numbers of mitotic figures, and some cases display heterologous elements including cartilage and striated muscle. These tumors generally have a favorable prognosis, but deep invasion and sarcomatous overgrowth are adverse prognostic factors (121).

Malignant mixed müllerian tumors may involve the cervix, although only about 40 cases have been reported (122,123). Patients have ranged in age from 23 to 87 years; the mean age is 65 years. Patients have presented with abnormal bleeding or abnormal Pap smears, and all have had cervical masses. Various types of carcinoma can be seen in these tumors, including squamous carcinoma, basaloid carcinoma, adenocarcinoma, or adenoid cystic carcinoma (122). The sarcomatous component may be homologous or heterologous. Some have suggested that malignant mixed müllerian tumors arising in the cervix have a better prognosis than those arising in the uterine corpus (122). HPV DNA was detected by polymerase chain reaction in all cases of cervical malignant mixed müllerian tumors reported in one study (124).

Other Malignant Tumors

Various sarcomas have been reported in the uterine cervix, although they are uncommon. A recent review of 1,583 cervical malignant tumors revealed eight cervical sarcomas (125). Five were carcinosarcomas, and the remainder were unclassified sarcomas, leiomyosarcomas, or endometrial stromal sarcomas. Primary cervical malignant melanoma is rare (126). About a dozen cases of granulocytic sarcoma involving the uterine cervix have been reported in the past decade (127,128). Some represented the initial disease presentation, and others were identified during the course of acute myeloid leukemia (127). Primary extranodal lymphomas (129) of the uterine cervix are usually diffuse B-cell neoplasms. Primitive neuroectodermal tumors (130,131), desmoplastic small round cell tumors (132), and primary germ cell tumors of the cervix have also been described (133).

Secondary tumors of the cervix include those invading from contiguous organs and metastases from other sites. The former include tumors arising in the uterine corpus, urinary bladder, or rectum. Metastases can originate from many sites, including the ovary, uterus, and more distant primary tumors.

PROGNOSTIC FACTORS

Tumor Size, Volume, Margin Status

In a Gynecologic Oncology Group (GOG) study, Delgado et al. (134) described 3-year disease-free survival rates of 94.8%, 88.1%, and 67.6%, respectively, for occult, ≥3 cm, and >3 cm stage I squamous cell carcinomas of the cervix treated by radical operation. Survival strongly correlated with depth of tumor invasion of the stroma: 86% to 94% for less than 10 mm, 71% to 75% for 11 to 20 mm, and 60% for 21 mm or greater. In patients without parametrial involvement, the survival rate was 84.9%, but it was 69.6% for those with parametrial tumor extension. More recently, these findings were validated by Van de Putte et al. (135). Rutledge et al. compared patients with FIGO stage IB1 cancers with IB2 cancers treated with radical hysterectomy, finding that lymphovascular space invasion and depth of cervical stromal invasion were more significantly associated with poor prognosis in a multivariate analysis (136). In all these series, there was frequent use of postoperative RT with or without chemotherapy. The use of adjuvant treatment was preferentially given in higher risk patients, narrowing the differences in outcomes and affecting the analysis. In patients treated with curative intent RT, Perez et al. analyzed 1,499 patients treated curatively with RT, finding 10-year actuarial pelvic failure rates of 5%, 15%, and 35% for tumors <2 cm, 2 to 5 cm, and >5 cm, respectively, with the stage IB group. In stage IIB patients, medial parametrial involvement was significantly favorable compared to lateral paramentrial extension, and in stage IIIB disease unilateral sidewall extension was significantly favorable to bilateral extension (137). Similarly, Eifel et al. (138) noted a strong correlation between central and pelvic tumor control, disease-specific survival, and tumor size. Pelvic tumor control was 97% with tumors less than 5 cm, and 84% with tumors 5 to 7.9 cm.

In a multivariate analysis of prognostic factors related to nodal or distant metastases in 128 patients, Pitson et al. found that tumor size and tumor hypoxia were both independently predictive, whereas stage and hemoglobin concentration were not (139).

In patients with stage IB cervical cancer treated surgically, with or without RT, positive margin status conveyed a hazard ratio of 3.92 compared to negative margins. Also, margin status (distance in millimeters in patients with close margins) was significantly associated with an increased recurrence rate. In this series, postoperative RT eliminated local recurrences in patients with close margins and halved the recurrence rate in patients with positive margins (140).

Stage

The FIGO stage is universally accepted for its prognostic significance. For example, Fyles et al. (141), in 965 patients with invasive carcinoma of the cervix, identified FIGO stage as the most significant prognostic factor. Stehman et al., reporting for the GOG on 626 patients treated in phase 3 trials (142), confirmed the prognostic significance of tumor burden, whether measured by FIGO stage, centimeter size, or bilateral disease. Para-aortic node metastases conferred a much greater risk than any of the measures of volume of tumor, however. This emphasizes the fact that FIGO staging does not take into account important prognostic information such as nodal status. While some clinicians would place patients with known para-aortic nodal disease in the stage IV category, others would choose to stage according to approved clinical staging procedures, mainly pelvic examination. Furthermore, stage is only indirectly related to tumor volume, since there can be significant variability in this important prognostic factor within a given stage, resulting in substantial overlap within stage groupings.

Nodal Status

Lymph node involvement is, in most studies, the most significant negative prognostic factor. Reports emphasize higher 5-year survival rates (90% or higher) among surgically treated patients with no evidence of metastasis in the regional nodes, compared to patients with positive pelvic (50% to 60%) or para-aortic nodes (20% to 45%). Delgado et al. (134) reported a 3-year disease-free survival of 85.6% for 545 patients with negative pelvic lymph nodes, compared with 74.4% for patients with one or more positive nodes. In an extensive review of the literature, Creasman and Kohler found that lymph node involvement was reported as an independent risk factor for survival in 88% of series reporting multivariate analyses, versus tumor size/depth of invasion in 61% of series (143). Decreasing 5-year survival rates have been associated with increasing numbers of positive pelvic nodes.

Even micrometastases appear to negatively impact prognosis. Marchiole et al. reported that recurrence was tenfold more likely in an early-stage population of patients treated with radical surgery compared to those without micrometastases (144). Similarly, in a retrospective study from Stanford, a much higher rate of recurrence was seen in early-stage surgically treated patients in whom lymph node micrometastases were detected immunochemically (145).

Lymphovascular Space Invasion

Lymphovascular space invasion (LVSI) proved to be a significant prognostic factor in a surgical-pathologic study of 542 patients completed by the GOG (134). Disease-free survivals were 77% and 89%, respectively, in patients with and without LVSI. Furthermore, LVSI was shown to correlate strongly with pelvic adenopathy. In a case-control study, Marchiole et al. established a relative risk of recurrence of 2.64 in patients with LVSI compared to those without (144). Chernofsky et al. quantitated the amount of LVSI in 101 consecutive patients who underwent surgery for stages IA2-IIA cervical cancer, showing that amount of LVSI was an independent prognostic factor for time to recurrence (146). In a similar but smaller study, Sykes et al. evaluated the density of lymphovascular space invasion, finding that it offered no useful information in addition to presence versus absence (147). Milam et al. showed a very strong correlation between LVSI on preoperative biopsy specimen and nodal metastases in surgically treated early-stage cervical cancer (148).

Hypoxia and Anemia

Fyles et al. published an excellent review of the basic, translational, and clinical data regarding anemia and its potential impact on radiosensitivity and radiocurability (149). Clearly, the interactions are much more complex than previously believed. For example, in the presence of anemia, adaptive mechanisms come into play that shift the oxyhemoglobin dissociation curve to the right, providing a compensatory increase in oxygen released into the tissues. There is also an increase in tissue perfusion and oxygenation as hemoglobin decreases due to reduced blood viscosity. However, these effects are potentially less effective in patients with diabetes, smokers, or patients who are vasoconstricting in the presence of marginal cardiac output.

Furthermore, the work of Fyles et al. shows that the relationship between pretreatment hemoglobin levels and direct measurements of oxygen tension in cervical cancers is tenuous. Interestingly, there was a positive correlation between hemoglobin and tumor oxygenation in nonsmokers, but the correlation was negative in smokers. Fyles et al. suggested that the negative prognostic impact of tumor hypoxia might be present only in subgroups of patients. Specifically, they observed worse outcomes with tumor hypoxia only in node-negative patients, manifested by an increase in distant metastases rather than poorer pelvic tumor control (150).

Fuso et al. looked at the impact of pretreatment serum hemoglobin as a predictive factor of response to neoadjuvant chemotherapy in patients with locally advanced cervical cancer, finding hemoglobin level to be the most powerful predictor of response. A threshold of 12 mg/dL served to discriminate between optimal and nonoptimal response. However, the authors recognized that a lower hemoglobin level could also be simply a marker for more aggressive disease as opposed to a physiologic variable that could be manipulated for therapeutic benefit (151). The Southwest Oncology Group conducted a phase 2 study in 53 patients to determine whether erythropoietin along with oral iron therapy could safely correct anemia during chemoradiotherapy for cervical cancer. This study did show such an effect, at the cost of a higher than expected incidence of deep vein thrombosis (152).

A more important question therapeutically is whether correction of the anemia will improve oxygenation status and treatment outcomes. Human data from Sundfor et al. show that only 50% of transfused patients will show an increase in tumor oxygenation (153), similar to data from Fyles et al. (149). Furthermore, the significant association between tumor hypoxia and tumor size suggests that improving oxygen delivery is unlikely to improve outcomes owing to factors unrelated to oxygenation, such as number of clonogens, suboptimal brachytherapy dose distributions, and greater risk of metastatic disease.

In spite of the lack of a clear relationship between serum hemoglobin and tumor oxygenation status, various efforts have been directed to the correction of anemia as a therapeutic target. A common approach in cervical cancer and other malignancies has been the use of poietic proteins such as erythropoietin. However, two randomized studies (one in head and neck and one in breast cancer) showed a decrease in survival in the erythropoietic stimulation arm (154,155). A meta-analysis of randomized trials between 1985 and 2001, although not including the studies just mentioned, suggested the possibility of a small but difficult to measure improvement in survival (156).

Santin et al. investigated the effect of blood transfusion on immune function in patients receiving radiotherapy for cervical cancer. These investigators measured significant changes in percentages of lymphocyte populations that differed in transfused and nontransfused populations. Furthermore, interleukin-10, a potential dysregulator of lymphocyte function, was only observed in transfused patients. These findings provide a basis for implicating blood transfusion as a possible factor in diminished immune function (157). Additional basic and clinical research will be helpful in determining the reliability of these findings and the potential utility of altered hemoglobin and tumor oxygenation status on tumor sensitivity and treatment outcomes.

Another approach that has been used to potentially address tumor hypoxia is the application of hypoxic cytotoxins. Tirapazamine is one such agent that has shown promise in lung cancer and is currently under study (158).

A concern possibly related to the risk of decreased survival with poietic protein use is the associated risk of thromboembolic events. This topic is reviewed later in the chapter in the context of treatment complications. In addition, De Los Santos and Thomas have published an excellent review of the literature regarding the potential cellular and tissue responses to hypoxia (including angiogenesis), the potential advantages and disadvantages of anemia correction in the management of malignancies, and a review of the clinical data regarding the incremental increase in thromboembolism with the administration of hemopoietic factors (159).

Biomarkers and Bio-imaging

Multiple biomarkers with potential prognostic value have been evaluated in cervical cancer, often with conflicting results and conclusions (160). For example, measures of tumor proliferation parameters (e.g., potential doubling time, S phase fraction, labeling indices), apoptosis, and other cellular characteristics often correlate with clinical outcomes. What is less clear is how to use this information in a way that improves therapy in the individual patient. Gaffney et al. performed immunohistochemical staining for epidermal growth factor receptor (EGFR), vascular endothelial growth factor (VEGF), topoisomerase-II alpha (TOPO-II), and cyclooxygenase-2 (COX-2) on specimens from 55 patients, and evaluated potential correlations between expression and outcome (161). On multivariate analysis, increased staining for VEGF and COX-2 correlated with an increased risk of death.

More recently, metabolic bio-imaging has been explored as a possible prognostic marker. Using F-18 fluorodeoxyglucose (FDG) positron emission tomography (PET), Xue et al. found a significant correlation between the standardized uptake value and disease-free survival (162). As suggested by the authors, high FDG uptake could be useful in identifying patients requiring alternate or more aggressive initial treatment. Similarly, Grigsby et al. used PET scanning to show that patients who are node-negative by PET scan might not benefit from concurrent chemoradiation as compared to RT alone (163). In terms of prognostic information, the same group performed pre- and post-treatment PET scanning in 152 patients. Those whose PET scans became or remained negative had an 80% 5-year cause-specific survival estimate compared to only 32% for those patients who showed persistent abnormal uptake (164).

Histopathology

There have been several reports of similar survival rates for comparable stages of adenocarcinoma and squamous cell carcinoma. Look et al. found no additional risk associated with adenocarcinoma compared to squamous carcinoma among stage IB patients (165). Similar observations were reported by Eifel et al. (166) for 334 patients with adenocarcinoma of the cervix. The 5-year relapse-free survival and locoregional control rates were 88% and 94%, respectively, for 91 patients with normal-sized cervix, 64% and 82%, respectively, for 102 patients with lesions 3 to 5.9 cm in diameter, but only 45% and 81%, respectively, for 22 patients with tumors greater than 6 cm in diameter. In a surgical series, Ayhan et al. reviewed 67 patients with IB adenocarcinomas and compared them to a concurrent series of 454 squamous carcinomas. Although the percentage of patients with metastases to three or more nodes was significantly greater in the adenocarcinoma group, there were no differences in overall or disease-free survival (167).

However, Kleine et al. performed a matched-pair analysis of squamous carcinomas (268 patients) and adenocarcinomas (144 patients) of the cervix, finding significantly lower 5- and 10-year survival in stages I-II adenocarcinomas (168). Baalbergen et al. reported 5-year survival rates of 79% and 37% for stages I and II adenocarcinoma of the cervix and less than 9% for stages III and IV, results that would be generally considered inferior to those typically obtained in squamous lesions (169).

A study of 505 patients with non–squamous cell carcinoma of the cervix examined histologic features for prognostic significance (170). In comparison with tumor limited to the cervix, tumor extension to the uterine corpus was correlated with twice the risk of dying of tumor. The grade and specific type of adenocarcinoma were not of prognostic significance in this study, although well-differentiated villoglandular adenocarcinoma and minimal deviation adenocarcinoma were not evaluated. There is no prognostic significance in the distinction between mucinous and endometrioid adenocarcinoma of the cervix. There is evidence that adenosquamous carcinoma is either a histologically more aggressive tumor than cervical adenocarcinoma or it is diagnosed later in the disease course (111).

Higher tumor grade and vascular invasion are statistically more common in adenosquamous carcinoma than adenocarcinoma of the cervix. The presence of small cell neuroendocrine carcinoma in any amount, even when associated with other types of neoplasm, is an independent prognostic factor associated with aggressive tumor behavior.

GENERAL MANAGEMENT AND RESULTS OF TREATMENT

Prevention: HPV Vaccination

HPV is composed of a major capsid protein, L1, and a minor capsid protein, L2. L1's protein coat is transcribed at the superficial epithelial level and is capable of spontaneously assembling into an isometric capsid composed of 360 L1 molecules arranged in 72 pentameric capsomers. It is therefore capable of self-assembly into a virus-like particle (VLP) when expressed in recombinant systems. VLPs elicit strong adaptive immune responses, both B-cell and T-cell mediated, that are capable of protecting against subsequent type-specific infections (171).

L2 plays a critical role in incorporating the viral genome into the nucleus during the active phase of HPV infection and encapsulates the viral genome during the later stages of HPV replication. The underlying target and major site of the prophylactic vaccine against HPV is the L1-based VLPs. L1-based VLP vaccines are highly HPV type specific; evidence suggests that antibody responses to L2 may confer some protection against other oncogenic HPV types (172).

It is believed that most antibodies produced after exposure to HPV are type specific and do not necessarily cross react or protect against other types, although some data suggest some cross protection. HPV evades the reticuloendothelial system and does not undergo cytolysis; therefore, there is no release of immune modulators (173).

The efficacy of the HPV vaccine has been established in randomized clinical trials (172,174). A quadrivalent vaccine (QVV) targets HPV types 16, 18, 6, and 11, and bivalent vaccine (BVV) tartgets types16 and18.

Villa et al. (172) reported a double-blind, placebo-controlled, randomized trial evaluating the QVV in 277 young women (mean age of 20.2 years). Vaccine was given intramuscularly on day 1 and at 2 months and 6 months. The primary end point was combined incidence of infection with the types of HPV in the vaccine, cervical or external genital disease, HPV infection recorded, external warts, CIN, and invasive cancer. The combined incidence of persistent infection or disease with the HPV types in the vaccine was reduced by 90%.

Villa et al. (175) also reported highly sustained efficacy of the QVV in 552 women ages 16 to 23. The rate of persistent HPV-6, -11, -16, and -18 infection was reduced by 96% in the treated group. There were two cases of HPV infection in the vaccination arm versus 46 in the placebo arm. Protection against types 6, 16, and 18 was 100%, 86%, and 89%, respectively. No case of infection with HPV-11 was noted. The vaccine was 100% efficacious against CIN caused by all types 16 and 18. There was no case of genital warts in the vaccinated group. The seroconversion rate was high for all types (type 6, 94%; type 11, 96%; type 16, 100%; and type 18, 76%) at 3 years. Villa et al. (176) demonstrated a 12- to 26-fold higher antibody response following vaccination compared to that of a natural immune response after exposure to HPV.

Garland et al. reported a phase 3 study of the QVV in 5,455 women ages 16 to 24 years. The vaccine was 100% effective in preventing type-specific HPV-related genital warts, vulvar intraepithelial neoplasia (VIN), vaginal intraepithelial neoplasia (VAIN), CIN, AIS, and invasive cancers of the cervix, vulva, and vagina (177).

Olsson et al. evaluated the phenomenon of immune memory following the QVV in a randomized, placebo-controlled trial (178). This study confirmed the finding of high immunity from initial vaccination and a robust immune memory response following a subsequent challenge dose, suggesting long-lasting efficacy of the vaccine.

Harper et al. reported a randomized, double-blind, placebo-controlled trial of the BVV in 1,113 women ages 15 to 25 years (174). Vaccine efficacy was 91.6% against incident infection and 100% against persistent infection for HPV types 16 and 18. In an intent to treat analysis, the vaccine efficacy was 95.1% against persistent cervical infection and 92.9% against cytologic abnormalities. These authors subsequently reported sustained efficacy of the BVV (179).

In these trials the vaccine was generally very well tolerated with very few side effects. The most common adverse effect was pain at the injection site. The vaccine has not been fully tested in women with HIV, and the immune response is unknown in that population.

The Advisory Committee on Immunization Practices (ACIP), an arm of the Centers for Disease Control and Prevention (CDC), and the American College of Obstetrics and Gynecology have recommended the QVV for all women ages 9 to 26 years. As the vaccine does not contain live virus, it is classified as category B for pregnant women. Its use and implementation in that population are not recommended as not enough safety data are available. Lactating women can receive the vaccine safely (180).

All women who receive the vaccine are recommended to be followed according to guidelines already set for cytologic smears as discussed previously. This is a potential pitfall as women may have a false sense of security that the vaccine is effective against all strains. However, up to 30% of CIN and invasive cancers are caused by strains not in the vaccine.

The vaccine is given at 0, 2, and 6 months. The vaccine is not effective in women with active HPV infection and abnormal cytology. HPV testing is not recommended before initiating HPV vaccination (181).

Goldie et al. reviewed the cost effectiveness and projected clinical benefits of HPV vaccination. They reported that the most cost-effective strategy is combining vaccination at age 12 with triennial conventional cytologic screening beginning at age 25. This would reduce the absolute lifetime risk of cervical cancer by 94% compared with no intervention (182). Sanders et al. estimated that if all girls at 12 years of age were vaccinated in the United States, over 1,300 deaths from cervical cancer would be prevented (183).

Block et al. reported the use of the QVV in men ages 16 to 23 years. They reported a seroconversion rate of 99% and antibody titers that were similar to vaccinated females (184).

It is recognized that psychosocial factors could negatively impact efforts to implement HPV vaccination programs. Parents might not accept vaccinations of their young daughters or sons because this could imply early sexual activity. Furthermore, the male child is not at risk for cervical cancer. Because the general population is relatively naïve about HPV and cervical cancer, mass education is needed to inform the public and health professionals about the HPV vaccine and follow-up after inoculation.

The HPV vaccine has the potential of significantly reducing the burden of cervical cancer worldwide, and particularly in less developed countries where screening and treatment programs are scarce. The impact of HPV vaccine on rates of invasive cervical cancer has not been established.

Severe Dysplasia and Carcinoma *In Situ*

Patients with severe dysplasia/CIN and carcinoma *in situ* (CIS) have essentially no risk of lymphatic involvement and are often treated with local therapies such as conization, laser ablation, cryotherapy, or a simple hysterectomy. These various techniques have comparable efficacy. The more conservative approaches are preferentially used when a patient wishes to have more children. Patients with HIV infection, high HPV viral load, positive margins, older age, and residual high-risk infection following conservative management have a higher recurrence rate (185–187). Detection of residual high-risk HPV infection following conservative management predicts for a higher recurrence rate after conservative treatment (186,187). In 1976, Kolstad reported results of conization in treatment of CIS. Therapeutic conization was performed in 795 patients; 2.3% had recurrent CIS, and 0.9% developed invasive cancer (188). Two hundred thirty-eight patients were treated with hysterectomy and the corresponding rates were 1.2% and 2.1%, respectively. Luesley et al. reported a 91% success in over 600 patients treated with LEEP (189). Martin-Hirsch et al. in a review of the Cochrane Gynecologic Cancer Group registry, evaluated 23 trials in treatment of CIN. They concluded that there was no clearly superior surgical technique for treating CIN (190).

Instances in which conization might be preferred to ablative procedures such as laser or cryotherapy include presence of a positive endocervical curettage (ECC), treatment of adenocarcinoma *in situ* (AIS), and inadequate colposcopy due to the advantage of having a pathologic specimen. If the patient is not desirous of childbearing, a hysterectomy would also be a viable option. All uterus-sparing procedures have potential adverse effects including cervical stenosis, predisposition to preterm labor in subsequent pregnancies, persistent vaginal discharge, and possible infertility.

Temkin et al. reviewed 146 patients who had undergone cold knife conization after having been treated with LEEP for CIS (191). Of 146 patients, 133 had residual CIN on cone biopsy, and 15.8% had invasive carcinoma. Patients with residual CIN 3, ectocervical and endocervical margins with CIN, and positive endocervical curettings after conization were more likely to harbor or develop invasive disease. Lu et al. evaluated 449 patients with CIN 3 treated with conization (192). They found that a positive post-cone ECC was the most significant factor predicting persistent-disease-associated (65.5%) versus 7.6% with a negative post-conization ECC. Positive endocervical margins and multiquadrant disease had an odds ratio of 2.97 for persistent disease. The only preoperative indicator of persistent disease was age >50. Given these data, patients with positive ECC after conization or positive endocervical margins on a cone specimen for CIS should have repeat conization prior to hysterectomy to avoid inappropriate treatment for invasive disease.

Of interest is recent data reported by Case et al. evaluating CIN in adolescent women in which 192 patients with CIN 2,3 underwent conization. On follow-up, 55% had abnormal cytology but no invasive cancer was found (193). This may reflect a high infection rate and point prevalence with HPV in adolescents rather than true recurrence.

Since patients with CIS have virtually no risk of pelvic adenopathy, it is also appropriate to treat with only intracavitary RT. Tumor control rates of 100% have been reported. Grigsby and Perez successfully treated 21 such patients with a single intracavitary implant, delivering a mean point A dose of 46.12 Gy; no treatment sequelae were observed (194). Others might choose to use two separate low-dose-rate implants and slightly higher point A doses.

Stage IA

The concept of "microinvasion" (equating to FIGO stage IA) should define tumors that penetrate the basement membrane but have little or no risk of nodal involvement or dissemination. Elliott et al. reported a 0.8% rate of lymph node metastasis in stage IA1. All macroscopically visible lesions are considered stage IB tumors (195).

Controversies remain in regard to the clinically relevant definition of microinvasive squamous carcinoma of the cervix, particularly as conservative treatment options, including fertility sparing, have become more common. Takeshima et al. performed a clinico-pathologic analysis of 402 patients with invasive squamous carcinoma of the cervix whose tumors demonstrated no more than 5 mm of stromal invasion (196). Although the incidence of nodal metastasis was only 1% among 82 patients with invasion limited to 3 mm, it was nearly 7% in 73 patients with 3 to 5 mm of invasion. Nevertheless, recurrences were rare and were nearly exclusively limited to tumors with more than 7 mm of horizontal spread. In an accompanying editorial, Creasman noted that this work validated the FIGO definition of microinvasion and potentially opens up the IA2 patients for consideration of more conservative surgical approaches (197).

Stage IA1 carcinoma is usually treated with conization or hysterectomy. The control rate approaches 100% (188). Morris et al. demonstrated the efficacy and safety of cervical conization as definitive treatment for these patients (198). Absence of LVSI plays a key role in opting for conservative management of patients with MID as its presence may herald a higher incidence of lymphatic involvement. Buckley et al. found that tumor recurrence was greater in positive LVSI tumors as compared to those with no LVSI (9.7% vs. 3.2%) (199). Roman et al. found that LVSI was a significant factor in pelvic nodal metastasis (200). If fertility is not a consideration and prognostic factors for recurrence such as positive post-cone ECC or involved margins are present, a hysterectomy is the standard option for definitive treatment of stage IA1 (188).

Management of stage IA2 disease is more controversial. Patients with FIGO IA2 disease with LVSI are not candidates for conservative surgical approaches in most circumstances. The average pelvic lymphatic metastasis rate from reported data is 5% to 13% (199,201).

Presence and greater extent of LVSI are poor prognostic signs and predict a higher recurrence rate (199). The recommended treatment for stage IA2 squamous cell carcinoma is a modified (type II) radical hysterectomy and pelvic lymphadenectomy, although curative intent RT is an equivalent option. However, the role of radical hysterectomy and the need for parametrial resection have been challenged in this population. Covens et al. evaluated 842 patients (202). Six percent had positive pelvic nodes, and 4% had parametrial involvement. Parametrial invasion was associated with LVSI, tumor size >2 cm, higher tumor grade, greater depth of invasion (DOI), and pelvic node metastasis. The incidence of parametrial involvement in patients with tumors <2 cm, negative pelvic nodes, and DOI <10 mm was 0.6%. They concluded that because most patients with positive nodes and deep invasion will likely receive adjuvant pelvic RT, resection of the parametrium may not be necessary. Kodama et al. found that simple or modified radical hysterectomy alone may be sufficient in IA2 lesions with no LVSI (203). Gadducci et al. validated the role of conization in stage IA1 and found that simple hysterectomy with pelvic lymphadenectomy may be sufficient for stage IA2 (204). Some have advocated for conization and pelvic lymphadenectomy in stage IA2. Greer et al. evaluated 50 patients with stage IA2 treated with cone biopsy followed by radical hysterectomy, finding histologically positive margins in 66% of patients after conization. The rate of residual invasive disease discovered after radical hysterectomy was 24% in patients who had negative margins after conization (205). It is difficult to justify conization alone as definitive therapy for stage IA2 disease.

Nam et al. reported a comparative study of laparoscopico-vaginal radical hysterectomy and abdominal radical hysterectomy in patients with IA1 to IB cancers less than 2 cm in maximum dimension (206). These authors found excellent survival in both groups but higher recurrence rates among the larger lesions in the laparoscopic group.

In the absence of a clear consensus on the type of hysterectomy (simple vs. abdominal modified radical vs. laparoscopically assisted vaginal) in stage IA2 disease, a modified radical hysterectomy with pelvic lymphadenectomy is most easily supported until clearer data is presented.

In patients who are medically inoperable, intracavitary RT may be used successfully. Hamberger et al. studied 151 patients with stage I treated with intracavitary radium. None of the patients with stage IA recurred (207). Grigsby et al. treated 34 patients with stage IA with 13 receiving intracavitary RT only and the remaining 21 treated with pelvic RT. Only one patient with stage IA recurred. The overall complication rate was about 6% (194).

Adenocarcinoma—Early Disease

The incidence of cervical adenocarcinoma has increased in the past 40 years. Adenocarcinoma *in situ* (AIS) presents a potential diagnostic and therapeutic challenge. The term "microinvasion" is controversial in describing glandular lesions as accurate measurement of depth of invasion in glands may be difficult. Schorge et al. provided some parameters for defining stage IA1 adenocarcinoma in 1999 (208). Almost all AIS lesions are associated with HPV, with 18 being the predominant type. Management of AIS is controversial. Schorge et al. reported on five women who were treated with conization for stage IA1 adenocarcinoma (209). All had negative margins and no LVSI. No recurrence was seen in follow-up of 6 to 20 months. Schorge et al. also reported on ten patients with AIS treated with conization with negative margins and no LVSI; of seven evaluable patients, none had recurrence within 2 years (210). Shin et al. reported on 92 patients with AIS treated with conization with negative margins (211). During a 30-month follow-up, none had recurrent AIS. Sixty-two percent of those with positive margins after conization had residual disease on hysterectomy specimens. Wolf et al. reported their experience in which, out of 55 patients treated with conization, 80% had subsequent hysterectomy (212). Seven out of 21 (33%) patients with negative margins on conization had residual disease in the hysterectomy specimens, and three had invasive cancer. Of 19 with positive margins after conization, 10 (53%) had residual disease on hysterectomy specimen, and 5 had invasive cancer. The overall rate of residual disease in hysterectomy specimens after conization with negative margins is 25% and with positive margins around 50%. Lea et al. highlighted the importance of post-conization endocervical curettage, demonstrating a positive predictive value of 100% for detecting residual disease (213). Widrich et al. evaluated margin status of AIS lesions following cold knife conization and LEEP (214). The rates of positive margins were 33% and 50%, respectively. Given the critical role of margin status post-conization, a cold knife technique may be preferred in patients with AIS. The recommended surveillance after conization for AIS includes cytology and ECC every 4 months. The most successful conservative management protocols require negative margins and no LVSI. Therefore, careful counseling and follow-up are warranted.

Stage IB-IIA (Non-bulky)

Stage IB is divided into IB1 (lesions less than 4 cm) and IB2 (lesions confined to cervix >4 cm). IB1 lesions and selected IIA lesions without extensive vaginal involvement can be treated with either RH and pelvic lymph node dissection (PLD) (followed by tailored chemoradiation as indicated by surgical findings) or primary chemoradiation. The preference of one over the other depends on the institution, the oncologists involved, the general condition of the patient, and tumor characteristics. Surgery is the preferred option in younger women as ovarian function and vaginal length, and thus sexual function, can generally be maintained. Transposition of the ovaries to the abdominal wall or the gutters away from the field of RT may prevent radiation-induced ovarian failure. Chambers et al. reported that 71% of patients maintained ovarian function after ovarian transposition (OT) and pelvic RT (215). The preservation of function correlated with the estimated scatter dose to the ovaries. The rate of ovarian failure was 11% with doses ≤300 cGy, compared to 50% if the estimated dose was >300 cGy. Others have reported that up to a quarter of patients with OT had symptomatic ovarian cysts requiring operative interventions, and only 53% retained ovarian function (216).

Radical hysterectomy can be performed through an abdominal, vaginal, or minimally invasive approach (traditional laparoscopy and robotic assisted). As salpingooophorectomy is not part of RH, ovarian removal should be based on the patient's age or other factors. The rate of ovarian metastasis is very low, about 0.9% (217). The two most common types of RH used in treatment are classes II and III, described elsewhere in the chapter. Landoni et al. compared these two approaches in a prospective, randomized trial in 238 patients (218). Type II had a significantly decreased mean operative time (135 minutes vs. 180 minutes), and the rate of blood loss and transfusions was comparable. Immediate postoperative complications and length of hospital stay were also similar. The long-term complication rate was significantly less in type II versus type III (13% vs. 28%). The use of postoperative RT, recurrence rate, and death rate due to disease were similar in both arms. The overall survival was 81% and 77%, respectively.

Nam et al. performed a retrospective analysis of outcomes with laparoscopic radical hysterectomy with or without pelvic lymph node dissection with conventional radical hysterectomy (206). Operating time, complication rate, and number of lymph nodes obtained were similar with the two approaches. Hospital stay was shorter with the laparoscopic technique. Overall, recurrences were lower with the standard operative route, leading the authors to recommend limiting the laparoscopic approach to patients with tumor diameters less than 2 cm.

Radical operation will shorten the functional length of the vagina, but pliability and transudative lubrication are usually preserved. Jensen et al. documented a substantial negative impact on sexual function that is persistent following radical hysterectomy (219). Radiation therapy can reduce length, caliber, and lubrication of the vagina; however, these symptoms can be alleviated in some patients with hormonal replacement and vaginal dilatation. The evidence to differentiate between surgery and radiation based on sexual function is poor. A strong predictor of post-therapy sexual function is the level of activity prior to therapy. The postmenopausal patient who is not sexually active may have complete obliteration of the vagina, precluding follow-up examination. Combined modalities appear to have a more pronounced effect than either radiation or operation alone (220).

In terms of outcome, radical surgery and definitive chemoradiation have similar good outcomes. Typically, 5-year survival for stage IB patients is 85% to 90% and 65% to 75% for stage IIA. Landoni et al. reported a prospective study of RH versus RT (221). In the RH arm, patients with parametrial involvement, deep stromal invasion, and/or positive nodes received postoperative RT. Fifty-four percent (62 out of 114) and 84% (40 out of 55) of stages IB1 and IB2 received postoperative RT, respectively. Severe morbidity was seen (28%) in the surgical arm (mostly combined surgery and RT) compared to 12% in the RT arm. No difference was seen in disease-related outcomes.

Results of therapy comparing modalities should include all patients evaluated for each therapeutic modality. This applies particularly to surgical series. Findings revealed at operation may change the treatment plan, excluding some high-risk patients. This is exemplified by a report by Delgado et al. (222)

for the GOG. Member institutions entered 1,125 patients prior to operation. There were 80 ineligible patients after pathology review. An additional 129 patients were explored, but the hysterectomy was abandoned because of intraoperative complications in 49 patients, or because of extent of disease beyond the uterus in 80. Failure to account for these patients in other series overestimates the efficacy of the operative procedure.

It is best to select patients who can have a high chance of being adequately treated with only one modality, assuming equal oncologic outcomes.

Fertility-Sparing Surgery/Radical Vaginal and Abdominal Trachelectomy

Almost 30% of women diagnosed with cervical cancer will be less than 40 and 40% will have early stage I disease. Preservation of fertility can be a major consideration in treatment if an acceptable oncologic outcome can be obtained. Recently, there have been major advances in fertility-sparing surgery (FSS) in women with stage IA2 to IB1 cervical cancer. Dargent pioneered the procedure of transvaginal resection of cervical and paracervical tissue (vaginal radical trachelectomy, VRT) and proximal vaginal, placement of a permanent cerclage at the cervico-uterine junction, and a laparoscopic pelvic lymphadenectomy (LPL) (223).

Plante et al. reported on 72 patients treated with VRT and LPL (224). Median age was 32, with 74% being nulligravid. Fifty pregnancies occurred in 31 women. Miscarriage rates in the first and second trimester were 16% and 4%, respectively, and 72% of pregnancies reached the third trimester. The overall prematurity was rate was 16% to 19% versus 12% in the general population.

The overall recurrence rate in the literature is about 4%, comparing favorably with standard treatment (224). Bader et al. reported an isolated recurrence on residual uterine cervix in 6 months, and Bali et al. reported a central recurrence 7 years post VRT (225,226). In a review, Boss et al. reported that of patients electing FSS, 43% attempt conception, 70% conceive, 49% deliver at term, and 15% have cervical stenosis causing infertility (227).

Marchiole et al. compared VRT with LPL to radical vaginal hysterectomy (RVH) with LPL in patients with lesions <2 cm (228). They reported similar intraoperative complication rates (2.5 % vs. 5.8%, respectively) and postoperative complication rates of 21.2% and 19.4 %, respectively. The recurrence rates were also similar, 5.2% and 8.5%, respectively. Ungar et al., among others, have reported an abdominal approach to radical trachelectomy (ART) (229).

In terms of patient selection, appropriate lesions include FIGO stage IA1 without extensive LVSI and IA2 or IB1 lesions less than 2 cm with limited endocervical involvement. Although early data is encouraging, no level I evidence exists to adequately compare safety and efficacy between conservative and radical surgical approaches. Whether adenocarcinomas are appropriately managed in this fashion is subject to debate; however, in the literature, close to 40% of cases were of glandular histology.

Bulky IB Carcinoma of the Cervix

Bulky endocervical tumors and the so-called barrel-shaped cervical cancers have a higher incidence of central recurrence, pelvic and para-aortic lymph node metastasis, and distant dissemination. Historically, adjuvant extrafascial hysterectomy following preoperative RT was an accepted treatment approach.

The GOG performed a randomized trial in which 256 eligible patients with carcinomas of the cervix ≥4 cm were treated with external beam and intracavitary irradiation, or with a slightly lower dose of intracavitary irradiation and the same external beam pelvic irradiation followed by an extrafascial hysterectomy (230). The 3-year disease-free survival and overall survival rates were 79% and 83%, respectively, and were virtually identical in the irradiation alone and the combined irradiation and surgery groups. The incidence of progression was somewhat higher in the irradiation alone group (46%) compared to the combined therapy group (37%) ($p = 0.07$). However, it appears that surgery does not contribute to increased survival compared to RT alone in patients with "bulky" stage IB disease. A favorable impact on the local recurrence rate with adjuvant hysterectomy is likely, and an improvement in survival for patients with tumors 4 to 6 cm in diameter is suggested. Nevertheless, conventional management typically involves chemoradiation (231).

Boronow reported a survival rate of 71.3% in patients with tumors greater than 6 cm who were treated initially with radical hysterectomy and postoperative RT and chemotherapy in all cases (232). Complications were reported to be minimal. Havrilesky et al. reported an analysis of 72 patients who underwent radical hysterectomy and lymph node dissection for stage IB2 cervical cancer, followed by adjuvant RT for high-risk features (233). The 5-year survival was 72%, and the 5-year progression-free survival was 63%. Survival was particularly poor for high-risk patients. Yessian et al. also reported their experience with initial radical surgery and tailored postoperative RT in stage IB2 patients (234). As postoperative RT was used less frequently than suggested by currently reported randomized trials, the recurrence rate was 38%, and the estimated 5-year survival was only 62%. Interestingly, out of 21 recurrences, 11 were on the pelvic sidewall.

Kamelle et al. retrospectively analyzed 86 patients with IB2 tumors treated with radical hysterectomy (235). Over half the patients received postoperative RT. This study identified presence of LVSI as the only independent predictor of recurrence and argued for the utility of radical hysterectomy up front in the management of patients with intermediate-risk IB2 cervical cancers when there is no evidence of LVSI. Two accompanying editorials questioned several aspects of the analysis, including the diagnostic accuracy of a cervical biopsy in determining LVSI, the small numbers of patients and wide confidence intervals, the possible inferiority of radical hysterectomy compared to modern chemoradiation, and the wisdom of relying on a single variable to determine therapy when there are a number of other recognized considerations for prognosis and treatment selection (236,237).

Stages IIB, IIIB, and IVA

Most patients in the United States with stage IIB disease are treated with curative intent chemoradiation. With RT alone, the 5-year survival rate has historically been 60% to 65%, and the pelvic failure rate 18% to 39%. Similarly, most patients with stage III and IVA tumors are best treated with concurrent chemoradiation. Leung et al. reported long-term outcomes in 91 patients with stages IIIB (n = 84) and IVA (n = 7) tumors treated curatively with RT. With a median follow-up of 8.8 years, the 5- and 10-year local control rates were 53% and 53%, respectively, and 5- and 10-year survival rates were 29% and 21%, respectively (238). The severe complication rate was 13%.

Based on multiple randomized clinical trials, concurrent cisplatin is a standard agent to combine with RT. Other chemotherapy agents that have been used successfully include 5-fluorouracil (5-FU), mitomycin, carboplatin, paclitaxel, and epirubicin. This data is nicely summarized in an article by Eifel (Table 22.2) (231). As acute effects are increased when conventional chemotherapy is added to RT, the clinician must always

TABLE 22.2

PROSPECTIVE, RANDOMIZED TRIALS OF CONCURRENT RADIOTHERAPY AND CHEMOTHERAPY FOR PATIENTS WITH LOCOREGIONALLY ADVANCED CERVICAL CANCER

Author	Trial	Eligibility	Number of patients	CT in investigational arm	CT in control arm	Relative risk of recurrence (90% CI)	*p* value
Rose et al. (240)	GOG-120	FIGO IIB-IVA	526	Cisplatin 40 mg/m^2/wk (up to six cycles)	HU 3 g/m^2 (22 × week)	0.57 (0.42–0.78)	<0.001
				Cisplatin 50 mg/m^2 5-FU 4 g/m^2/96 h HU 2 g/m^2 (2 × week) (two cycles)	HU 3 g/m^2 (22 × week)	0.55 (0.40–0.75)	<0.001
Morris et al. (274) Eifel et al.	RTOG 90-01	FIGO IB-IIA (≥5 cm), IIB-IVA or pelvic nodes involved	403	Cisplatin 75 mg/m^2 5-FU 4 g/m^2/96 h (three cycles)	None[a]	0.48 (0.35–0.66)	<0.001
Keys et al. (230)	GOG-123	FIGO IB (≥4 cm)	369	Cisplatin 40 mg/m^2/wk (up to six cycles)	None[b]	0.51 (0.34–0.75)	0.001
Whitney et al.	GOG-85	FIGO IIB-IVA	368	Cisplatin 50 mg/m^2 5-FU 4 g/m^2/96 h (two cycles)	HU 3 g/m^2 (22 × week)	0.79 (0.62–0.99)	0.03
Peters et al. (246)	SWOG 87-97	FIGO I-IIA after radical hysterectomy with nodes, margins, or parametrium positive	268	Cisplatin 70 mg/m^2 5-FU 4 g/m^2/96 h (two concurrent + two adjuvant cycles)	None	0.50 (0.29–0.84)	0.01
Pearcey et al.	NCIC	FIGO IB-IIA (≥5 cm), IIB-IVA, or pelvic nodes involved	259	Cisplatin 40 mg/m^2/wk (up to six cycles)	None	0.91 (0.62–1.35)[c]	0.43
Lanciano et al.	GOG-165	FIGO IIB-IVA, clinically negative aortic nodes	268	PVI 5-FU 225 mg/m/day, 5 days/wk (six cycles)	Cisplatin 40 mg/m^2/wk (up to six cycles)		
Wong et al.		FIGO IB-IIA (>4 cm), IIB-III	220	Epirubicin 60 mg/m^2 then 90 mg/m^2 q 4 wks for five more cycles[d]	None	~0.65	0.02
Thomas et al.		FIGO IB-IIA (≥5 cm), IIB-IVA	234	5-FU 4 g/m^2/96 h × 2	None[e]		Not stated
Lorvidhaya et al.		FIGO IIB-IVA	926	Mitomycin 10 mg/m^2 and oral 5-FU 300 mg/m^2/d × 14 days (two cycles); ± adjuvant 5-FU	None or adjuvant 5-FU only	Not stated[f]	0.0001

Note: CI, confidence interval; CT, chemotherapy; FIGO, International Federation of Gynecology and Obstetrics; HU, hydroxyurea; PA, para-aortic; PVI, protracted venous infusion; RT, radiotherapy
[a]Patients in control arm had prophylactic para-aortic irradiation.
[b]All patients had extrafascial hysterectomy after radiotherapy.
[c]Survival.
[d]Chemotherapy was begun on day 1 and continued every 4 weeks through and after radiotherapy.
[e]Patients were also randomized to receive standard or hyperfractionated RT in a four-arm trial.
[f]Relative risks were not stated. Disease-free survival rates at 5 years for RT only and RT + concurrent chemotherapy only were 48.2% and 64.5%, respectively.
Source: Adapted from: Eifel PJ. Chemoradiotherapy in the treatment of cervical cancer. *Semin Rad Oncol* 2006;16:177–185.

weigh the risk of acute side effects and the threat posed by them with the potential benefit in patients with significant comorbid illnesses and poor performance status.

Chemoradiation should result in outcomes that compare favorably to these older series. Considering all eligible patients with stages IIB-IVA carcinomas enrolled in GOG #85, a 55% survival rate with platinum-based chemotherapy with RT was demonstrated after a median follow-up of 8.7 years (239). In this same group of patients, GOG #120 found a 66% to 67% survival rate with platinum-based chemoradiation (240).

External Irradiation Alone

Rarely, brachytherapy procedures cannot be performed because of medical reasons or unusual anatomic configuration of the pelvis or the tumor (e.g., extensive lesion and inability to identify the cervical canal, presence of a fistula). These patients may be treated with higher doses of external irradiation alone, although the results are inferior to those obtained with combined external beam and intracavitary irradiation.

Although speculative, results of external RT alone could be improved over historical results with the utilization of intensity-modulated RT (IMRT), which could allow higher doses to be delivered to the tumor volume while respecting normal tissue tolerances.

UNUSUAL CLINICAL SITUATIONS

Node-Positive Early-Stage (Operable) Cervical Carcinoma

Approximately 15% of patients with surgically amenable cervical carcinomas (FIGO stages I-IIA) will have positive pelvic nodes. Of these, a percentage less than 50% will have grossly positive nodes recognized intraoperatively. When this occurs, the dilemma becomes whether to proceed with the radical hysterectomy or to abandon the surgery and opt for curative intent chemoradiation. Whitney and Stehman reviewed the GOG #49 database and found that, in 98 of 1,127 patients with clinical stage IB tumors, the surgeon abandoned the operation. Sixty-eight of these were patients with squamous carcinomas whose surgery was abandoned due to tumor extension beyond the uterus rather than for medical reasons, forming the basis of their report (241). Of these, 17 (1.5% of the total group, 25% of the study group) patients had grossly positive pelvic lymph nodes, and 12 (1.1% of the total group, 17.6% of the study group) had this finding as the only manifestation of extrauterine disease. Most patients received curative intent RT when feasible. Patients with positive pelvic nodes did poorly, with 8 of 12 failing, including 3 with distant disease. The median recurrence-free interval was only 10 months, and the median survival was 17 months. The main conclusion from this study was that it is invalid to directly compare results of surgical treatment with results from RT, since surgical series typically exclude the patients with a poor prognosis in whom the operation is abandoned, while these patients would be included in the RT series.

Should the Hysterectomy Be Completed?

Leath et al. reviewed 23 patients with early-stage cervical cancer who had the radical hysterectomy aborted because of pelvic extension (11 patients) or positive nodes (12 patients) (242). All received RT as definitive treatment. The 5-year overall survival was 83%, suggesting that the aborted radical hysterectomy did not negatively impact outcome.

Bremer et al. reported considerably better outcomes in a series of 26 patients in whom the operation was aborted after the intraoperative finding of positive pelvic nodes. Five-year survival was 61% in this patient group (243). Morbidity was limited. Suprasert et al. compared 23 patients in whom the radical hysterectomy was aborted due to the intraoperative finding of grossly positive nodes with 35 patients whose positive nodes were detected after completion of the operation. Although the outcome was substantially better in the group completing surgical treatment, the authors recognized that the surgical group had much better prognostic factors (244).

Although older, probably the best data regarding whether to complete the hysterectomy come from Potter et al., who did a matched-pair analysis of 30 patients with positive pelvic nodes. Patients undergoing hysterectomy also received pelvic RT (245). There was no survival or local control advantage conferred by completing the radical hysterectomy; however, local control data suggested a trend favoring definitive RT.

In patients with positive nodes, the use of concurrent chemotherapy would be advised based on the possibility of distant spread and the need to optimize pelvic control. Randomized data support the addition of chemotherapy to postoperative RT in these patients (245).

Based on available data, it is difficult to conclude that completing the hysterectomy improves the outcome. Possible disadvantages of surgery include delaying the initiation of RT, adding surgical morbidity, and utilizing two treatment modalities when one (RT) would likely suffice. Furthermore, leaving the uterus in place provides an appropriate conduit for intracavitary RT and probably lessens the risk of complications. Clinicians who believe that completing the radical hysterectomy improves outcome, even with positive nodes, will point to data suggesting that patients who undergo radical hysterectomy, as a group, have a better outcome than the patients in whom the procedure is aborted (241,243). Others will point out that the groups are not prognostically similar and suggest that a reasonable approach is to have the surgeon resect or debulk grossly positive nodes and surgically stage the para-aortics but abort the radical hysterectomy. RT with chemotherapy would then become the primary therapy.

Should the Lymphadenopathy Be Debulked?

Data suggests an advantage for surgically resecting grossly positive lymph nodes prior to RT, although others have questioned the benefit in the vast majority of patients (247). Kupets et al. calculated that only 7 out of 300 patients undergoing surgical debulking of positive nodes could benefit in terms of survival. These calculations are based on assumptions suggested to be faulty by Tammela et al. (248), who calculated that 43 patients out of 300 would benefit.

Invasive Carcinoma Treated by Simple Hysterectomy

Given the frequency of simple hysterectomy or total abdominal hysterectomy (type I), it is not surprising that occasionally a patient is found to have an invasive cervical cancer unrecognized prior to surgery. Although this occurs uncommonly in an era of cytologic screening, it can occur in patients operated on for what is felt to be carcinoma *in situ,* "microinvasive" disease, or for "benign" indications.

If only microinvasive carcinoma is found, with no evidence of LVSI, no additional therapy is necessary. However, in patients with more advanced disease, simple extrafascial abdominal hysterectomy is not curative, because the paravaginal/paracervical soft tissue, vaginal cuff, and pelvic lymph nodes are not removed.

It may be technically difficult to perform an adequate radical operation after previous simple hysterectomy, but this alternative deserves consideration for selected patients. In 23 stage

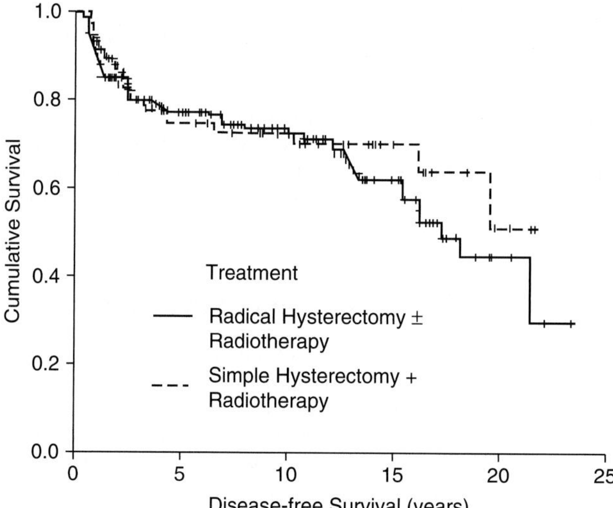

FIGURE 22.13. The influence of type of treatment on disease-free survival in patients undergoing radical hysterectomy with and without RT and those who had simple hysterectomy followed by adjuvant RT. (Kaplan-Meier analysis, p = not significant). *Source:* From Munstedt K, Johnson P, von Georgi R, et al. Consequences of inadvertent, suboptimal primary surgery in carcinoma of the uterine cervix. *Gynecol Oncol* 2004;94:515–520.

IA2 and IB1 patients, Leath et al. reported good results with a radical surgical approach, although three patients also received postoperative RT. The operative complication rate was 30% (249). Another approach favored by some is the use of adjuvant pelvic RT in patients with invasive disease of severity greater than microinvasive. A large series of 90 patients, including 18 stage II patients, treated with RT following inadvertent hysterectomy was reported by Hsu et al. (250). Overall 5- and 10-year survival rates were 85.5% and 74.1%, respectively. Long-term complications were rare. Munstedt et al. reviewed their experience with 80 patients who had inappropriate simple hysterectomies followed by postoperative RT and compared outcomes with those undergoing radical hysterectomy, with or without postoperative RT (251). These authors found that patients who had inadvertent hysterectomies followed by postoperative RT had outcomes at least equivalent to those who had radical hysterectomies up front (Fig. 22.13). In an exhaustive review of the literature comparing series of patients having reoperation with radical parametrectomy and lymph node dissection (LND) versus those having postoperative RT, the weighted average 5-year survival favored RT (68.7% vs. 49.2%) (Table 22.3)

If the postoperative RT approach is chosen, postoperative irradiation should be administered immediately after recovery from operation, as prognosis is much worse if therapy is delayed. When there is gross tumor present in the vaginal vault, external irradiation to the whole pelvis (40 to 45 Gy) is required. In some cases, a small external beam boost might be advisable for an additional 10 to 15 Gy. An intracavitary insertion, as outlined previously, should be performed (35 to 60 Gy mucosal dose). If there is residual tumor, an interstitial implant, when feasible, should be carried out to increase the dose to this volume. The brachytherapist should note the possibility that small bowel is adherent to the vaginal cuff in the hysterectomized patient, representing a risk factor for complications with interstitial implants. Laparotomy or laparoscopy can be helpful in guiding the implant in these circumstances.

The potential contribution of concurrent platinum-based chemotherapy must be considered, particularly in view of the randomized study of patients treated after radical hysterectomy with high-risk features (246). Although not directly comparable, it is reasonable to extrapolate these results favoring concurrent chemotherapy to patients treated after simple hysterectomy for invasive disease, particularly in patients with gross residual, positive margins, positive nodes, lymphovascular space invasion, and, possibly, adenocarcinoma.

TABLE 22.3

SERIES REPORTING OUTCOMES FOR OCCULT INVASIVE CERVICAL CARCINOMAS DISCOVERED AFTER SIMPLE HYSTERECTOMY COMPARING SUBSEQUENT TREATMENT WITH RT OR FURTHER SURGERY

Author	No. of patients	5-year survival (%)
RADIOTHERAPY		
Cosbie	86	54
Green and Morse	30	30
Andras et al.	118	89
Davy et al.	72	77
Papavasiliou et al.	36	89
Heller et al.	35	67
Roman et al.	122	65
Fang et al.	73	67
Choi et al.	64	76
Crane and Schneider	18	93
Huerta Bahena et al.	59	59
Current study	80	83
Overall average	**793**	**68.7**
FURTHER SURGERY		
Barber et al.	115	32
Green and Morse	21	67
Orr et al.	23	Not given
Kinney et al.	27	82
Chapman et al.	18	89
Ayhan et al.	15	Not given
Overall average	**219**	**49.2**

Source: Adapted from Munstedt K, Johnson P, von Georgi R, et al. Consequences of inadvertent, suboptimal primary surgery in carcinoma of the uterine cervix. *Gynecol Oncol* 2004;94:515–520.

Stage IIIA Carcinoma of the Cervix

Cervical carcinomas extending to the lower third of the vagina without pelvic sidewall extension or hydronephrosis are uncommon, representing less than 2% of patients with cervical cancer. As a result, these patients are often not reported separately, although management presents a significant challenge to the radiation oncologist. In general, these patients have a better prognosis than stage IIIB patients, especially when there is limited parametrial extension and the vaginal involvement is continuous with the cervix.

Kavadi and Eifel (252) found a local control rate of 72% in 44 patients, but 5- and 10-year actuarial survival rates were 37% and 34%, respectively, reflecting the impact of distant failure seen in 13 patients. In this series, patients with no parametrial extension and direct extension from the cervix (as opposed to "skip" lesions in the lower vagina) had a 5-year survival of 73%.

The inguinal lymph node areas must be assessed clinically and radiographically. When this assessment is negative, RT is

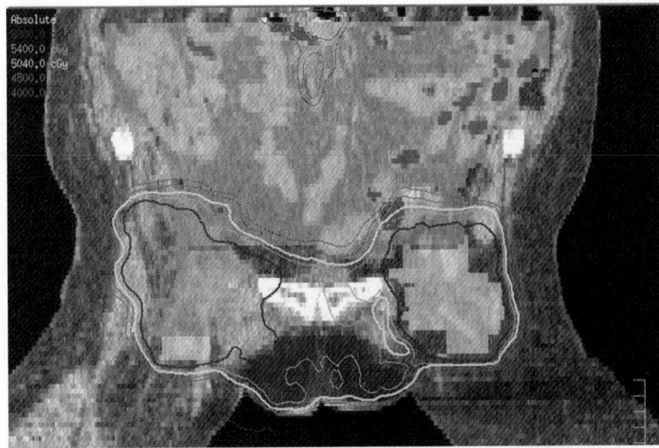

FIGURE 22.14. (*See color plate section.*) This coronal dose plot shows how IMRT can be used to deliver adequate radiation dose to inguinal areas while limiting dose to femoral heads, as might be necessary in a cervical cancer extending to the lower third of the vagina. *Source:* From Jhingran A. Potential advantages of intensity-modulated radiation therapy in gynecologic malignancies. *Semin Radiat Oncol* 2006;16:144–151.

given to the inguinofemoral nodes prophylactically. When the lymph node assessment suggests gross disease, it might be appropriate to confirm this with needle biopsy or consider the role of inguinal lymph node dissection following RT. Alternatively, RT doses can be escalated to reflect the presence of gross tumor.

Treating the inguinal nodes adequately while limiting the dose to the underlying femoral heads is a challenge. Understanding the location of the inguinal nodes is best accomplished by measuring the depth of the femoral vessels by a cross-sectional imaging technique. The depth of these nodes averages 6 cm and can vary substantially and be beyond the range of typical electron energies. Dittmer and Randall have reported a photon-only technique that provides good coverage of inguinal nodes at depth, minimizes "hot" and "cold" spots, and respects the tolerance of the femoral heads in most cases (Fig. 21.5A and B, previous chapter) (253). Intensity-modulated techniques are also possible (Fig. 22.14).

More difficult is the challenge of delivering tumoricidal doses of radiation to the entire vagina while respecting tolerances of the normal tissues, in particular the rectum. Given that virtually the entire length of rectum will be treated with an intracavitary approach encompassing the entire vagina, the tolerance will be lessened, and the risk of complications will increase. In addition, because of the typical "slope," or decrease, in patient thickness in the superior-inferior direction, there will be a dose gradient that can result in "hot" spots of 120% to 125%. This is potentially remediable with intensity-modulation techniques, although another approach is simply to measure the dose gradient and take it into account by raising the lower border accordingly, and/or taking the gradient into account during the brachytherapy portion of the treatment.

A general approach is to give external beam RT to the pelvis and entire vagina of approximately 40 to 44 Gy over 5 weeks (delivering 50 Gy to the inguinal areas at depth), and follow this with one or two intracavitary implants. An intrauterine tandem combined with Delclos rings permits delivery of a controlled, measurable dose to the vagina. One should aim for a total dose of approximately 65 Gy to the entire vagina, combining the external and intracavitary doses. One can consider a second implant that does not treat the entire vagina, typically with a Fletcher-Suit applicator, particularly when there is parametrial extension. Ideally, one will deliver 80 to 85 Gy to point A in this fashion, but if the maximum rectal dose is limited to 60 to 65 Gy some compromise in point A dose may be required. These doses are appropriate only for low-dose-rate techniques, which are to be preferred when treating the entire vagina.

It is appropriate to administer cisplatin-based chemotherapy with the external RT with the hope of improving survival. However, concurrent chemotherapy will likely increase acute toxicities, particularly given the increased volume encompassed by the RT port and the sensitivity of the vulva to RT. Considerable individualization of therapy is required.

Small Cell Carcinoma of the Cervix

The term "small cell" should be limited to those rare tumors with counterparts in the lung and other anatomic locations noted for a high proliferation rate, marked propensity to regional lymph node and distant metastases, and positive staining with neuroendocrine markers (116). These tumors account for less than 3% of cervical neoplasms.

Small cell carcinomas are not often confined to the cervix and surrounding tissues at diagnosis. Therefore, workup may include bone marrow aspiration and other tests to detect the metastatic spread characteristic of this histology. Lymph node involvement is present in over 50%, and vascular invasion is frequently present. Viswanathan et al. reviewed 21 patients meeting stringent criteria for neuroendocrine type small cell cervical carcinomas (254). Ten patients had IB1 disease (although 2 of these had radiographic evidence of nodal metastases), and 11 patients had IB2-IIIB disease. Six patients underwent radical hysterectomy (5 of these were IB1), and 15 patients had RT as curative intent treatment. Cisplatin-based chemotherapy was given to 62%, either neoadjuvantly and/or following surgery or RT. No patient with greater than stage IB1 survived, and even for stage IB1 patients, the survival was much worse than would be expected in more common histologies. In-field RT failures were uncommon, but metastatic failures were not. Given the propensity to distant metastasis, the use of combination chemotherapy has been widely accepted in these patients (255). Prophylactic cranial RT has also been given following this chemoradiation in the absence of progression. However, its role remains unclear.

Cervical Lymphoma

Lymphomas primarily arising and confined to the cervix are quite rare. Patients often present with signs and symptoms including vaginal bleeding, discharge, and pelvic pain. Cervical lymphomas typically develop and grow submucosally; therefore, Pap smears often do not detect these neoplasms. Generous punch biopsies or conizations are often required for diagnosis. Histologically, these lymphomas are typically of the diffuse, large B-cell variety (256,257).

Due to the rarity of this diagnosis, reports of management approaches are anecdotal and there is no clear consensus. However, general guidelines can be suggested. Clearly, treatment with systemic therapy using combination chemotherapy regimens is indicated in the majority of cases (256–259). The CHOP regimen (cyclophosphamide, doxorubicin, vincristine, prednisone) is commonly used. Surgery has been used as an adjunct to chemotherapy, either before or after chemotherapy, especially in patients with stage I or II disease. Radiation therapy following chemotherapy should be considered, particularly for larger tumors, tumors that do not completely respond to chemotherapy, and in patients with early-stage disease who are not candidates for or refuse hysterectomy (258,259).

Young patients who wish to preserve fertility can be counseled about the possibility of conization followed by fertility-preserving chemotherapy and close follow-up. Conception has been reported in patients treated in this fashion, although the outcome of these pregnancies is unclear due to their overall rarity (256,260).

Cervical Sarcomas

Primary sarcomas arising in the cervix are exceedingly rare. In a tumor registry of 1,583 patients with cervical malignancies conducted at Washington University, only eight sarcomas were identified. Five of these were carcinosarcomas. All six patients treated with curative intent remained alive with a mean follow-up of 2.5 years, although two patients had developed pulmonary metastases. Radical surgery and chemoradiation were both effective in curing patients with localized pelvic disease (125).

Granulocytic sarcoma can present as a cervical neoplasm. It is important to distinguish this lesion from primary cervical lymphoma, as this is a manifestation of acute myelocytic leukemia and the chemotherapy regimens are quite different. Outcomes for these patients are generally dismal (261).

Carcinoma of the Cervical Stump

Historically, in patients who have undergone subtotal or supracervical hysterectomy, carcinoma of the cervical stump made up nearly 4% of cases treated with RT. Although the incidence has greatly declined, these increasingly rare patients remain at risk of developing cervical carcinoma. The natural history and patterns of spread of these cancers are similar to those of the cervix in the intact uterus. The diagnostic workup, clinical staging, and basic principles of therapy are the same. However, there are potentially important differences in treatment.

Radical operation for stage I cervical stump carcinomas (trachelectomy) is made more difficult by the previous procedure. Barillot et al. prospectively accrued 213 cases of cervical stump carcinoma (262) and reported that stage for stage, local control and survival were equivalent among the surgically treated and the RT-treated patients. However, lethal complications were much more likely in the surgically treated patients. Patients receiving RT including brachytherapy had significantly better results than those having only external RT. Severe complications with RT were similar to those observed among patients with intact uteri.

The higher complication rate probably relates to the lack of adequate uterine cavity length to accommodate a tandem containing two or three sources. However, some patients with a history of supracervical hysterectomy retain enough lower uterine segment to insert two standard cesium-137 sources. As many sources as technically feasible should be inserted in the remaining cervical canal without protruding active source length through the cervical os. Comparably higher activity sources should be used in the tandem, allowing a greater contribution from these sources to the point A dose and a correspondingly lower vaginal mucosal dose.

In early-stage tumors, it is critical to maximize the brachytherapy portion of the treatment, because this allows higher doses to be delivered to the tumor while limiting dose to normal structures. Early midline shields (e.g., at 20 to 30 Gy) are desirable. Limiting the total external beam dose to 40 Gy, optimizing the intracavitary RT with proper packing and distribution of activity, and respecting the tolerances of the rectum and bladder will keep complication rates reasonably low. Limiting the maximum rectal dose to 65 or 66 Gy and the bladder dose to around 80 Gy is desirable, even if the point A dose is somewhat compromised (<80 Gy). More advanced stages should be treated with 40 Gy to the pelvis, combined with the maximum intracavitary doses permitted within tolerance. Platinum-based chemotherapy will be indicated in most cases. Limited sidewall boosts may be necessary, depending on the dose to the sidewalls from the brachytherapy and the radiographic evaluation of the nodes. When there is no opportunity to insert any sources in the cervical canal, the whole pelvis dose should be increased to 45 Gy, and the primary tumor boosted to around 60 to 65 Gy with shrinking fields. Stereotactic and intensity-modulated RT techniques can be used to escalate doses to the primary tumor.

The 5-year survival for carcinoma of the cervical stump treated with irradiation is similar to that reported for patients with carcinoma of the intact uterus.

MANAGEMENT OF CERVICAL CANCER DURING PREGNANCY

Of all patients with cervical cancer, about 1% are pregnant at diagnosis (263). Most will present with abnormal cytology or abnormal vaginal bleeding. Overall incidence of abnormal cytology in pregnancy is about 5% (264). The availability of cervical cytology in developed countries affords an opportunity to diagnose early dysplastic changes during pregnancy, which may contribute to a higher incidence (3:1) of stage I cervix cancer diagnosed during pregnancy compared to the nonpregnant state (263). Either conventional or liquid-based cytology is effective in pregnancy. The use of an endocervical brush is safe and can enhance the rate of optimal smears. Endocervical curettage is not recommended due to predisposition to premature rupture of membranes and bleeding.

Hopkins and Morley published their experience with cervical cancer during pregnancy and outcomes compared to those in nonpregnant state (265). They found similar survival rates when controlled for confounding factors such as age and stage.

Diagnosis

All abnormal cervical lesions during pregnancy require a biopsy. Colposcopy in pregnancy is used to rule out invasive disease. Colposcopic evaluation and directed biopsies are safe in pregnancy. In a series of 612 women with abnormal smears during pregnancy reported by Economos et al., 449 colposcopies were performed (239). All patients had satisfactory colposcopy by the 20th week of gestation, as the squamo-columnar junction (SCJ) everts during pregnancy. They reported a 95% concordance rate between colposcopic impression and directed biopsies within one degree of severity. No complications were noted. Failure to visualize the entire SCJ is not an indication to proceed to conization during pregnancy as most repeat colposcopies will be satisfactory due to eversion of the SCJ as the pregnancy progresses.

A diagnosis of cervical cancer during pregnancy requires a multidisciplinary approach involving gynecologic and radiation oncologists, perinatologist, neonatologist, and psychologic counselors.

Management of Dysplasia

Woodrow et al. reported only a 7% progression rate from dysplasia in pregnancy to higher-grade dysplasia in the postpartum period in 811 women (266). Given these data it is reasonable to manage abnormal cytology in pregnancy according to guidelines in nonpregnant states. Given the low rate of progression and high reliability and safety of colposcopy, a conservative approach is likely to be safe for the patient and the unborn child. Dysplasia diagnosed by colposcopy and biopsies in pregnancy should be followed conservatively with serial colposcopic examinations every 8 weeks and managed definitively in the postpartum period.

Conization During Pregnancy

In a series of 180 conizations during pregnancy, Averette et al. reported a first trimester fetal loss rate of 24% (267). Second trimester fetal loss was less than 10%. Hannigan et al. reported 13 conizations during the first trimester and no fetal loss. The rate of severe bleeding was 9%. Fetal loss rate in second trimester was less than 10% (268).

In a small series of 17 patients, Goldberg et al. reported a novel approach to conization in pregnancy. The cervix was injected with vasopressin, and lateral hemostatic sutures and a cerclage were placed following the conization. The mean gestational age was 18.8 weeks (10–32). There was no major bleeding or other complications and no second trimester loss (269). An argument against the use of a cerclage is that the majority of post-conization fetal deaths are delayed and presumably due to chorioamnionitis and not necessarily a function of cervical incompetence. The cerclage may also act as a nidus for infection.

Robinson et al. reported their experience with loop electrocautery excisional procedure (LEEP) excision during pregnancy in 20 patients with gestational ages ranging from 8 to 34 weeks (270). They found that 57% had involved margins and 47% had residual disease after LEEP. There were three preterm deliveries, two patients requiring blood transfusions, and one intrauterine fetal demise 4 weeks after LEEP excision (chorioamnionitis was found on autopsy). They concluded that LEEP excision during pregnancy does not yield consistent diagnostic specimens and is associated with a high complication rate. If conization is indicated during pregnancy, a cold knife technique may be the preferred method. The optimum timing would be sometime in the second trimester.

Treatment of Adenocarcinoma *In Situ* and Microinvasive Disease

Diagnosis of glandular abnormalities in pregnancy can be difficult as glandular hyperplasia and decidual and glandular cells may exhibit benign Arias-Stella reaction, which may appear ominous to someone who is not experienced with these conditions during pregnancy. An expert evaluation is mandated for accurate diagnosis of glandular disease in pregnancy.

There is a paucity of data on management of adenocarcinoma *in situ* (AIS) in pregnancy. Lacour et al. reported the safety of conization in the second trimester as treatment of AIS in pregnancy in five patients. All patients delivered at term and only one required radical hysterectomy for stage IB disease after delivery (271).

It is believed that there is no significant difference in outcome in squamous MID versus AIS. It is difficult to know how to best treat these lesions in pregnancy. It is recommended that similar guidelines be adopted as in nonpregnant patients.

Most patients with MID in pregnancy can be safely followed even if margins are involved with dysplasia (not invasive disease). Vaginal delivery should be safe in women with microscopic disease, and definitive management may be delayed safely until the postpartum period.

Management of Invasive Cancers During Pregnancy

Surgery

Over 70% of cervical cancers in pregnancy present with stage I disease and have an excellent survival rate. Key elements in therapeutic decision making include stage, tumor size, gestational age, and the patient's desire to maintain the pregnancy. Treatment options can be separated according to gestational age of <20 or >20 weeks.

Invasive disease diagnosed in a pregnant patient of less than 20 weeks gestation should generally be managed immediately, resulting in loss of the fetus. However, there are reports of delaying treatment until fetal maturity without harm to the mother or the fetus. Most of the reported cases of delay in treatment were stage I disease. The delay of treatment ranged from 3 to 32 weeks. The overall mortality is about 5% to 6% with a similar recurrence rate. These data are limited by small numbers of patients but are reassuring when considering a delay in treatment. This approach is only appropriate in selected well-counseled patients with early-stage, small volume disease.

Sood et al. published a case-control study of 30 pregnant women with cervical cancer with matched nonpregnant controls (272). Surgical treatment included either radical or simple hysterectomy. Eleven patients underwent surgical treatment in the third trimester after a mean delay in treatment of 16 weeks, and none developed recurrent disease. Radical hysterectomy in pregnancy was associated with increased blood loss but with no increased rate of blood transfusion. No difference was noted in postoperative complication rates.

Monk and Montz evaluated the safety and efficacy of radical hysterectomy with pelvic lymphadenectomy in 13 patients with fetus *in situ* and 8 with cesarean delivery followed by radical hysterectomy. No perioperative deaths were reported. The most common postoperative morbidity was febrile illness. The overall survival was 95% with over 40 months median follow-up (273).

For stage I disease, radical hysterectomy and pelvic lymphadenectomy can be safely performed prior to 20 weeks with fetus *in situ* or as a planned procedure after cesarean section in the third trimester after documentation of fetal lung maturity. Excellent oncologic outcomes are generally obtained.

Radiotherapy

Radiotherapy and platinum-based chemosensitization has become the standard of care for advanced cervical cancer (274), and it is an equivalent option to radical hysterectomy in stage I disease. Most reports of chemoradiation for cervical cancer during pregnancy are in patients with locally advanced disease.

Benhaim et al. reported the use of chemoradiation in two patients (275). The first patient was diagnosed with stage IVA squamous carcinoma at 12 weeks gestation. She was treated with RT and weekly cisplatin with the fetus *in situ*. Spontaneous miscarriage occurred at about 40 Gy, which is consistent with other reports in the literature. The patient died of metastatic disease 20 months after treatment. The second patient was diagnosed with stage IIB squamous cancer at 12 weeks gestation and received the same treatment regimen. Spontaneous miscarriage occurred 3 weeks after beginning RT. The patient remained disease-free at 29 months follow-up. Ostrom et al. reported two cases of stage IB2 disease diagnosed at 15 weeks gestational age. Fetal losses occurred 3 to 4 weeks after initiation of RT. Both patients were disease-free 12 months after completing treatment (276). Although experience is limited with chemoradiation in pregnancy, it seems to be feasible and safe. If RT is used in the postpartum setting, it should begin within 3 weeks after uterine involution.

Neoadjuvant Chemotherapy in Pregnancy

Use of neoadjuvant chemotherapy (NACT) has been reported in eight pregnant women with cervical cancer. Chemotherapeutic agents used included cisplatin, bleomycin, and vincristine. Gestational age ranged from 12 to 21 weeks at diagnosis and stages were IB1 to IIA. Seven of eight had clinical response including one complete response. Surgical treatment was delayed for a median of 16.5 weeks. Three of seven received adjuvant treatment after surgical resection. With a follow-up range of 5 to 80 months, four were alive disease-free and four were dead of disease. All children appeared to be normal (277,278). Although data are very limited, they do suggest that NACT could be cautiously considered and discussed with patients who have advanced-stage cervical cancer diagnosed during pregnancy when a delay in treatment is desired to allow fetal lung maturation.

Radical Trachelectomy During Pregnancy

Vaginal or abdominal trachelectomy and cerclage placement along with laparoscopic or pelvic lymphadenectomy is an option for treatment of stage I cervical cancers less than 2 cm in women interested in preserving pregnancy and fertility (224). Ungar et al. reported birth of two healthy term infants to two of five pregnant patients with stage IB disease who were so treated (229). Gestational age ranged from 13 to 18 weeks. Fetal losses were reported on postoperative days 1 and 16. All patients remained disease-free with follow-up ranging from 10 to 54 months.

Route of Delivery

Sood et al. studied outcomes of women diagnosed with cervical cancer during pregnancy or within 6 months after delivery. One of 7 women who had cesarean sections developed local and distant metastasis compared to 10 of 17 (59%) of those who delivered vaginally. In multivariate analysis, vaginal delivery was the strongest predictor of recurrence. They concluded that pregnant women with cervical cancer should deliver by cesarean section (279).

Except in stage IA1 where vaginal delivery is reasonable, a cesarean section should be performed in the presence of cervical cancer. This should be done through a classical uterine incision to avoid encroaching into the lower uterine segment or cervix. In addition, cesarean section can be followed by radical hysterectomy as definitive treatment or to allow surgical exploration to delineate extent of disease. Performing oophoropexy during the procedure may assist in preserving ovarian function after pelvic RT.

HUMAN IMMUNODEFICIENCY VIRUS/ACQUIRED IMMUNODEFICIENCY SYNDROME AND CERVICAL NEOPLASIA

About 2.1 million people live with HIV in North America of whom approximately 1.2 million are in the United States. Heterosexual transmission accounted for 34% of cases. The proportion of women among new HIV and AIDS diagnoses has increased greatly in the United States. Over 50% of HIV-positive women are infected with HPV. In 1993, the CDC designated high-grade dysplasia as a marker for early HIV infection and cervical cancer as an AIDS-defining illness (280).

Prevalence

Ahdieh et al. reported that the HPV point prevalence in HIV-positive women is as high as 60%, compared to about 30% in HIV-negative women (281). The relative risk (RR) of HPV-associated cancers in patients with HIV/AIDS is significantly increased with relative risks of 5.4 and 5.8 for cervical and vulvar/vaginal cancers, respectively (282,283). The clearance of HPV in an HIV-positive individual correlates directly with the CD4 count. HPV DNA prevalence is as high as 85% in those with CD4 counts of 0 to 500 and as high as 70% in those with CD4 counts over 500. This is compared to a range of 30% to 50% in HIV-negative women. Even with a normal CD4 count, HIV-positive women still have a twofold increase in incidence of HPV compared to HIV-negative women (281,282,284).

Pathophysiology

In HIV-infected women with no evidence of CIN on Pap smear and colposcopy and negative HPV testing, a prospective study found that the probability of developing CIN was much greater than women who were HIV negative (20% vs. 5%). The strongest predictor of development of CIN in HIV-positive women is the degree of immunosuppression delineated by CD4 counts (284). Ellerbrock et al., in a prospective study of HIV-positive and -negative women with normal cytology at onset, found a significantly higher rate of CIN development in HIV-positive patients over a 3-year interval (20% vs. 5%) (285). When matched for sexual behavior, HIV-positive women have a one- to twofold increase in HPV sero-prevalence compared to HIV-negative women. When controlled for exposure to HPV, the persistence and detection of HPV is much greater in HIV-positive women compared to HIV-negative women (286–288). In immunocompetent women, the rate of HPV clearance within 2 to 4 years is 80% to 90%. This is affected by multiple factors such as smoking, re-exposure, prolonged oral contraceptive use, and other sexually transmitted infections (e.g., *Chlamydia trachomatis*, herpes simplex virus). The clearance rate of HPV is twofold greater in HIV-negative women as compared to those infected with the virus, despite adequate CD4 counts and low HIV viremia (286,288,289). There are emerging data evaluating the effects of HIV and HPV coinfection and its effect on local immunity in the cervix and vagina. Infection of vaginal Langerhans cells (LC) by HIV is a primary mode of entry and propagation into systemic infection. LCs constitute an important local defense against HPV infection. The numbers of LCs are lowered significantly in patients with AIDS with a resultant decrease in their immunologic response to HPV (290).

HPV Genotype Distribution in HIV-Positive Women

Most HIV-positive women are infected with multiple types of high-risk HPV including 11, 16, 18, 33, 51, 52, 53, 58, and 61. Clifford et al. found HPV-16 to be the most common HPV subtype in HIV-positive women; however, when compared to HIV-negative women the rate of type 16 infection is lower (291). HIV-positive women showed a higher proportion of multiple and HPV types other than 16 as compared to HIV-negative women.

Screening

Despite conflicting reports in the literature regarding the reliability of cervical smears as a screening tool for CIN in HIV-infected patients, it remains an important tool in primary screening. In a study of 189 HIV-infected women versus 95 controls, Anderson et al. found that the incidence of biopsy-proven CIN, despite normal cytology, was greater for HIV-infected women (14.3% vs. 1.2%, $p < 0.01$) (292). However, in the small number of HIV-infected women with normal cytology and biopsy-proven CIN, 95% had an abnormal cytologic smear within the preceding 12 months, most commonly ASCUS. The authors concluded that these data did not support routine colposcopy in all HIV-infected women. These data also highlight the importance of vigilance in follow-up and colposcopic examination of even low-grade cytology including ASCUS in

HIV-infected women, especially those with low CD4 counts. A finding of ASCUS on cervical smears of HIV-infected women is more common than in uninfected women. The probability of development of CIN in those with ASCUS was greater in the infected group compared to controls (60% vs. 25%) (293). According to U.S. Preventive Services Task Force recommendations, women with HIV infection should undergo semiannual screening in the first 12 months after diagnosis and then annually if the results are normal. If any abnormality is detected, then closer follow-up and colposcopic examination are warranted.

In a low resource setting where cervical cytology and adequate follow-up is problematic, a new approach has been devised and tested called the "see and treat" or visual inspection with acetic acid (VIA) or visual inspection with Lugol's iodine (VILI). In this approach, health care extenders are trained to use immediate visual inspection to detect dysplastic changes on the cervix. If detected, immediate treatment of the area with cryotherapy is offered. Multiple studies addressing the accuracy of VIA demonstrated a sensitivity of 66% to 96% with median of 84% and a specificity of 64% to 98% with median of 82%. The positive predictive value was 10% to 20% with a negative predictive value of 92% to 97%. Overall VIA is found to be more sensitive but less specific than cytology. The overall sensitivity and specificity of VIA and VILI are 92% and 85%, respectively. Although these methods can be helpful in a low resource setting, debate continues on its use in HIV-positive women (294).

HPV Subtype Testing

Given the high prevalence of HPV in HIV-infected women, the value of HPV testing is unclear. Goldie et al. evaluated the cost effectiveness of HPV testing in this population, concluding that adding HPV testing to the initial two cervical cytologies in the first year after diagnosis of HIV may modify subsequent cytology screening intervals and may be cost effective (295). This would be true in patients with CD4 counts >500 with normal cytology whose risk would be equivalent to women without HIV infection. There is no consensus regarding its use, and the best recommendation is to individualize to the patient and specific risk factors.

Vaginal Cytology After Hysterectomy

There is a paucity of data regarding cytologic screening of the vaginal vault in women infected with HIV. Paramsothy et al. evaluated 102 HIV-infected women after hysterectomy for varying indications (296). Among those with a history of CIN prior to hysterectomy, 63% were found to have vaginal intraepithelial neoplasia (VAIN) in follow-up. CD4 count of <200 and HIV viral load of >10,000 copies/mL at time of hysterectomy were highly predictive of subsequent VAIN. Overall, out of 102 women, 16% developed VAIN in follow-up. The authors concluded that close follow-up with vaginal cytology is warranted in HIV-infected women after hysterectomy, particularly in those with severe immunodeficiency and a previous history of CIN.

Effects of Highly Active Antiretroviral Therapy on HPV

The introduction of highly active antiretroviral therapy (HAART) has made significant impact on the prognosis of patients with HIV but has not been shown to affect the rate of HPV detection, and data regarding its effect on cervical dysplasia are mixed. The close relationship of low CD4 count and cervical dysplasia makes HAART attractive in halting progression of HPV infection. Ahdieh-Grant et al. studied 2,059 HIV-infected women receiving HAART (297). In 312 women with CIN, 141 had regression of CIN to normal with a median time to regression of 2.7 years. After HAART, elevated CD4 counts were associated with greater regression of CIN. However, there are no clear data to support HAART's role in regression of high-grade dysplasias. Therefore, the recommendation remains active surveillance and aggressive treatment for HPV in HIV-positive women who have responded well to HAART with low viral loads and adequate CD4 levels.

HPV Vaccination and Its Effect on HIV-Positive Women

In phase 3 clinical trials, HPV vaccination has been shown to be effective in reducing the rate of HPV infection by over 90% by inducing a much higher antibody titer for almost 5 years compared to the natural immune response (172,174). None of these trials included women known to have HIV infection, and there are no data demonstrating the efficacy of HPV vaccines in HIV-positive women. A pilot study to evaluate the safety and immunogenicity of HPV vaccine is under way in HIV-positive women.

Treatment of Dysplasia

The indolent nature of low-grade CIN in HIV-positive women allows for a conservative treatment approach. These patients have a low rate of progression to high-grade CIN, especially if CD4 counts are above 500. Delmas et al., in a large study of the natural history of CIN in HIV-positive women, demonstrated that almost 30% of low-grade CIN lesions would regress (298). Close follow-up with cytology or colposcopy every 4 months will help in detecting progression. It is important to collaborate with other health care professionals caring for the patient, particularly to determine the CD4 count status. As mentioned, HAART therapy may also contribute to regression of low-grade CIN.

For high-grade CIN, cervical conization by cautery or cold knife technique, or ablative techniques such as cryotherapy or laser vaporization are adequate, provided that invasive disease has been ruled out and that a satisfactory colposcopy is documented.

Although these techniques are effective in treatment of CIN in patients with HIV, the rate of recurrence is higher than in HIV-negative women. Wright et al. reported outcomes from LEEP procedures, finding a recurrence rate of 56% in patients with HIV versus 10% in non-HIV patients (185). The quality and size of the LEEP was an issue as all HIV-positive patients had positive margins compared to only 32% of controls. However, even when controlling for margin status, the rate of recurrence was higher among HIV-positive women, highlighting other risk factors for disease recurrence, e.g., CD4 counts.

Role of Medical Therapy

Maiman et al. evaluated 5-fluorouracil (5-FU) as maintenance therapy in HIV-positive women after treatment for high-grade dysplasia (299). Women received either biweekly 5-FU (2 g) or no further therapy. The recurrence rate was 28% in the treatment arm compared to 47% in the observation arm. Those with CD4 counts <200 had a 46% recurrence rate versus 33% in patients with CD4 counts >200. There was no grade 3 or 4 toxicity.

Robinson et al. studied the effects of isotretinoin for low-grade dysplasia in women infected with HIV and found no significant effect on time to progression (300).

Treatment of Invasive Cancer

The age at which HIV-infected women present with cervical cancer is, on average, 15 years younger than HIV-negative cohorts. Lomalisa et al. found that CD4 <200 was an independent risk factor for advanced stage of presentation (301). The treatment of invasive cervical cancer in HIV-infected women differs little from that used in HIV-negative women. There is little data on the role and long-term follow-up of radical hysterectomy for early-stage disease. Gichangi et al. evaluated the impact of HIV status on morbidity and pelvic tumor control following pelvic RT and found that 53% had acute radiation-related grade 3 to 4 toxicity (302). HIV infection was associated with a sevenfold higher risk of multisystem toxicity, was found to be a major factor in treatment interruption, and was associated with a sixfold increased risk of residual tumor 4 to 7 months after treatment. Mugambe and Kavuma compared outcomes of HIV-infected women with cervical cancer treated with RT, finding that 4-year survival was significantly lower for sero-positive patients as compared with sero-negative (303).

SURGERY

A generally accepted classification of types of hysterectomy is given in Table 22.4 and described below.

Class I Extrafascial Hysterectomy

This is the most common hysterectomy performed for a variety of gynecologic disorders. It consists of removing the uterus by separating it from the adnexal structures and round ligaments, dissecting the bladder off of the vesicouterine fold past the level of the cervix, ligation of the uterine vessels at their insertion close to the cervicouterine junction, serial application of surgical clamps next to the uterine and cervical wall as the parametrial tissues are separated from these walls, and completed by removal of the cervix off the upper vaginal vault with very little removal of vaginal mucosa. The pubovesicocervical fascia is removed with the uterus. The opened vaginal cuff is usually closed with simple running or interrupted sutures. This hysterectomy is adequate for treatment of stage IA1 and advocated by some for stage IA2. This procedure can be accomplished abdominally, vaginally, or laparoscopically.

Class II or Modified Radical Hysterectomy

The modified radical hysterectomy (MRH) has gained popularity as the operation of choice for treatment of early-stage cervical cancer, depending on extent of the lesion. MRH involves opening the paravesical and pararectal spaces to determine resectability by palpating the parametrial tissues and surrounding structures. The pelvic nodal tissues are examined for gross involvement. Once resectability is established, the rest of the operation is carried forward.

Modified radical hysterectomy involves dissection of the uterine artery at its junction with the ureter. The ureters are partially dissected off the parametrial tissue and tunneled to their insertions into the bladder. The bladder is dissected off the lower uterine segment past the cervix. The parametrial tissue is resected medial to the ureter. The ureterosacral ligaments are isolated, and the proximal portions medial to the ureter are resected. A 1- to 2-cm vaginal margin is resected along with the cervix. A pelvic lymphadenectomy is typically performed along with MRH. Type II MRH is reserved for microscopic or smaller tumors depending on the surgeon's experience and preference.

Class III or Radical Abdominal Hysterectomy

The radical hysterectomy (RH) differs from the MRH in the amount of dissection and resection. The paravesical and pararectal spaces are opened. The uterine artery is ligated at its origin from the internal iliac artery. The ureters are dissected

TABLE 22.4

TYPES OF ABDOMINAL HYSTERECTOMY

Type of surgery	Intrafascial	Extrafascial type I	Modified radical type II	Radical type III
Cervical fascia	Partially removed	Completely removed	→	→
Vaginal cuff removal	None	Small rim removed	Proximal 1 to 2 cm removed	Upper one third to one half removed
Bladder	Partially mobilized	→	→	Mobilized
Rectum	Not mobilized	R-V septum partially mobilized	→	Mobilized
Ureters	Not mobilized	→	Unroofed in ureteral tunnel	Completely dissected to bladder entry
Cardinal ligaments	Resected medial to ureters	→	Resected at level of ureter	Resected at pelvic sidewall
Uterosacral ligaments	Resected at level of cervix	→	Partially resected	Resected at post-pelvic insertion
Uterus	Removed	→	→	→
Cervix	Partially removed	Completely removed	→	→

Note: Type IV, extended radical hysterectomy (partial removal of bladder or ureter), in addition to type III. (*Source:* Perez CA. Uterine cervix. In: Perez CA, Brady LW, eds. *Principles and Practice of Radiation Oncology.* 3rd ed. Philadelphia: Lippincott-Raven; 1998.)
Source: From Stehman FB, Perez CA, Kurman RJ, et al. Uterine cervix. In: Hoskins WJ, Perez CA, Young RC, eds. *Principles and Practice of Gynecologic Oncology*. 3rd ed. Philadelphia: Lippincott Williams & Wilkins; 2000:864.

with complete tunneling to their insertion into the bladder trigone. The ureterosacral ligaments are isolated after the rectovaginal space is developed. The bladder is dissected off the cervix anteriorly. The cardinal ligaments are resected to the pelvic sidewall. Complete resection of the ureterosacral ligaments to their attachment may not be necessary in all cases. An alternative is resection of the ureterosacral ligaments midway and resection of 2 to 3 cm of proximal vagina, but the operation can be tailored according to tumor size and patient anatomy.

The choice of abdominal incision for RH depends on body habitus. A Maylard incision keeps the fascia on the rectus muscles. The epigastric vessels are ligated and the muscle is transected in the middle to have greater access to the sidewall and to facilitate pelvic lymphadenectomy. The other option is a Cherney's incision, which involves detachment of the rectus muscle from its tendinous insertion, allowing for greater access to the pelvis and common iliac and lower para-aortic nodes. The muscle is reattached at the end of the procedure. The peritoneum is closed in both of these approaches. In properly selected patients, these incisions provide excellent exposure compared to a vertical incision with better cosmetic outcome and perhaps less discomfort to the patient.

Class IV or Extended Radical Hysterectomy

There is little indication for extended radical hysterectomy (ERH) with availability of modern RT and chemosensitization for locally advanced tumors. As distinct from type III RH, ERH involves complete dissection of the ureter off the vesicouterine ligament, sacrifice of the superior vesical artery, and resection of three fourths of the vagina. The risk of bladder dysfunction and fistula formation is greatly increased compared to types I-III hysterectomy.

Class V Hysterectomy

A rarely performed operation, a type V hysterectomy involves resection of the distal ureter or bladder with reimplantation of ureter if needed.

Nerve-Sparing Radical Hysterectomy

Radical hysterectomy can disrupt the hypogastric plexus, which contains sympathetic fibers that fuse with parasympathetic fibers located in the parametrium to control bladder contraction and compliance. Bladder dysfunction occurs in about 5% of patients, which may require continuous or intermittent drainage for several weeks. Some patients may also experience some rectal dysfunction depending on the extent of the dissection and resection. Nerve-sparing radical hysterectomy (NSRH) has been proposed as a possible technique to identify and spare nerves and preserve good oncologic outcomes (304,305).

Trimbos et al. described NSRH as identification of the hypogastric nerve beneath the ureteral sheath lateral to the ureterosacral ligament, identification of the inferior hypogastric plexus during resection of the cardinal ligament, and preservation of the distal inferior hypogastric plexus during dissection of the posterior aspect of the vesicouterine ligament (304).

Although intriguing, large studies to clearly define the benefit of NSRH are lacking. Charoenkwan et al. reported on post-void residual (PVR) of patients with NSRH versus standard RH (306). At 7 days, 36% and 27% of NSRH patients had PVRs <100 and <50 cc, respectively, increasing to 82% and 77% by day 14. Raspagliesi et al. reported that type III NSRH had a similar rate of bladder dysfunction as MRH, and both were lower than standard RH III (307). Papp et al. reported their experience with NSRH in 501 patients with stages IA2 to IIB and found no decrement in outcome (305).

Pelvic Exenteration

Total pelvic exenteration (TPE) is mainly used for patients with limited central recurrences and no metastatic disease following treatment with primary RT or combined surgery and RT. It involves *en bloc* removal of bladder, uterus, rectum, vagina, and at times vulva, depending on the exact site and extent of recurrence. The procedure can be tailored to remove only the anterior or posterior structures including the bladder (anterior exenteration) or rectum (posterior exenteration). In treatment of central recurrence of cervix cancer, TPE is the most common approach. Reported 5-year survival is approximately 40%, ranging from 18% to 70% in the literature (308,309). TPE has been employed in selected patients with stage IVA cervix cancer, although with modern chemoradiotherapy this is unusual.

As part of TPE, reconstruction can involve diversion of the urine through a conduit utilizing a segment of the bowel (ileum, transverse and sigmoid colon) and/or vaginal and pelvic reconstruction with placement of flaps using either transposed muscle (rectus or gracilis), segments of colon (rarely), or omentum. Depending on the location of tumor and the extent of resection, the colon may be reanastomosed with the rectal stump (supralevator) or a permanent colostomy placed (310).

TPE is a morbid operation that should only be undertaken in selected patients with limited recurrences. Sidewall extension, metastatic disease, and, usually, hydronephrosis are possible contraindications to the procedure. Even with appropriate workup and evaluation, 25% to 50% of candidates will have the procedure aborted due to intraoperative findings of metastatic or locally advanced disease. Equally important are evaluations of patients' overall health status and a careful psychological and social evaluation and counseling to ensure that the patient realizes the sequelae of TPE. Perioperative complications can include bleeding, infection, cardiac and pulmonary complications, gastrointestinal and urinary leaks, fistulas, bowel obstruction, and reconstruction flap failure. Sexual dysfunction and psychosocial effects are often longer-term sequelae that can be permanent. The mortality rate from TPE is about 5%, even with careful patient selection (308,309).

RADIATION THERAPY

External Irradiation

Standard Fields (Non-IMRT)

Treatment of invasive carcinoma of the uterine cervix requires delivery of adequate doses of irradiation to the pelvic lymph nodes. Greer et al. (311) reported on intraoperative retroperitoneal measurements carried out in 100 patients at the time of radical surgery. Both common iliac bifurcations were cephalad to the level of the lumbosacral prominence in 87% of patients. Therefore, the superior border of the pelvic portal should be at the L4-5 interspace to include the external iliac and hypogastric lymph nodes. This margin should generally be extended to the L3-4 or even the L2-3 interspace if common iliac nodal coverage is indicated. The width of the pelvis at the level of the obturator fossae averaged 12.3 cm, and the distance between the femoral arteries at the level of the inguinal rings averaged 14.6 cm. Posterior extension of the cardinal ligaments in their attachment to the pelvic wall was consistently posterior to the rectum

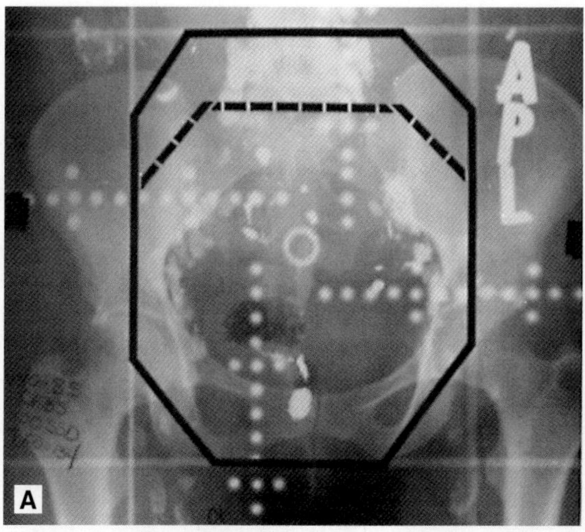

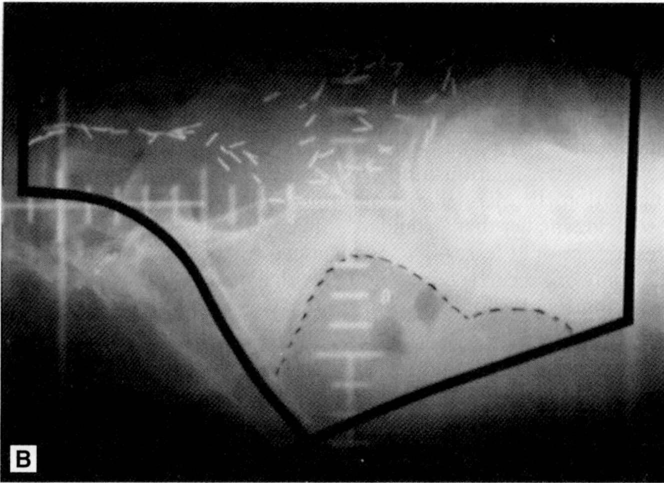

FIGURE 22.15. **A:** Anteroposterior simulation film of the pelvis illustrating portals used for external irradiation. The 15 × 15 cm portals at SSD (source-skin distance) are used for stage IB (broken line), and 18 × 15 cm portals are used for more advanced disease (solid line). This allows better coverage of the common iliac lymph nodes. The distal margin is usually placed at the bottom of the obturator foramina. **B:** Lateral simulation film of the pelvis illustrating portals used for external irradiation. *Source:* From Stehman FB, Perez CA, Kurman RJ, et al. Uterine cervix. In: Hoskins WJ, Perez CA, Young RC, et al., eds. *Principles and Practice of Radiation Oncology*. 3rd ed. Philadelphia: Lippincott-Raven; 2000:867.

and extended to the sacral hollow. The uterosacral ligaments also extended posteriorly to the sacrum. These anatomic landmarks must be kept in mind in the correct design of lateral pelvic portals. The upper margins of the portals in patients with small stage IB tumors can be placed at the L5-S1 interspace, and for more advanced stages at the L4-5, L3-4, or even L2-3 interspace (Fig. 22.15A and B). A 2-cm margin lateral to the bony pelvis is adequate. If there is no vaginal extension, the lower margin of the portal is at the midportion to inferior border of the obturator foramen. When there is vaginal involvement, the field should extend distally beyond the tumor a minimum of 4 cm, although some contend that the entire length of vagina should be treated down to the introitus. It is important to identify the distal extension of the tumor in some manner at the time of initial simulation, for example, by inserting a small rod with a radiopaque marker in the vagina. Often, vaginal extension will not be clearly defined by CT scan. For stage IB disease, 15 × 15 cm portals at the surface (about 16.5 cm at isocenter) usually will be sufficient. For patients with stage IIA, IIB, III, or IVA carcinoma, somewhat larger portals (18 × 15 cm at surface, 20.5 × 16.5 cm at isocenter) may be required to cover all of the common iliac nodes, in addition to the cephalad half of the vagina (312). Using placement of intraoperative clips to determine the extremes of nodal locations, McAlpine et al. essentially confirmed the findings of Greer et al. (313).

In patients with involvement of the distal third of the vagina, portals should cover the inguinal lymph nodes because of the increased probability of metastases. Dittmer and Randall have published a convenient method of treating inguinal-femoral nodes using anteroposterior-posteroanterior (AP-PA) photons only while limiting the dose to femoral heads and avoiding some of the problems with junctioning fields, e.g., electrons (Figure 21.5A and B, previous chapter) (253). Alternatively, IMRT approaches can be used (Fig. 22.14) (314).

The lateral portal anterior margin is placed anterior to the pubic symphysis to include the anterior extent of the external iliac nodes. A margin at the anterior edge of the symphysis pubis may not suffice for adequate coverage of primary tumor as well. The posterior margin usually covers at least 50% of the rectum in stage IB tumors, and will often extend to the sacral hollow in patients with more advanced tumors (Fig. 22.15B). Routinely placing the posterior border at the S2-3 interspace frequently results in inadequate coverage of the planning target volume. Ideally, three-dimensional imaging with CT, MRI, or both will be used to ensure adequate coverage (315).

The use of lateral fields allows significant protection of small bowel. With a four-field technique, some radiation oncologists choose to weight the AP-PA beams in relation to the lateral fields, e.g., 60:40. While this increases small bowel dose slightly, it can avoid giving very high doses laterally, particularly in larger patients.

Use of Midline Shield

Although common practice, the use of midline shields (MLSs) during external beam RT for cervical cancer has not been well described, and there is no consensus regarding their use. There is variability in opinions and practice patterns. The purpose of the MLS is to limit dose to the bladder and rectum in order to permit maximization of the intracavitary dose while still delivering sufficient doses to gross parametrial disease and microscopic or gross pelvic sidewall disease (nodal or tumor extension). In general terms, patients with earlier disease (stages I-IIA, or perhaps early IIB) benefit from earlier introduction of an MLS (20 to 30 Gy); patients with more advanced disease should not have an MLS placed before 40 Gy, and possibly not at all. By performing pelvic examinations on a weekly basis in patients receiving primary RT for cervical cancer, the physician might note an early favorable response that might permit earlier use of the MLS. Keeping in mind the purpose of the MLS, a frequent practice is to use a standard-width shield (4 cm), and place it in midline position. Generally, the pelvic dose delivered with the MLS is not added to the point A dose, but this dose is added to the nodal (sidewall, point B, point P) dose calculation. Unilateral sidewall boosts should be considered in patients who have only unilateral parametrial or sidewall involvement. Increasing parametrial doses correlate with risk of complications, particularly radiation proctitis (316).

Small Field RT

In patients treated postoperatively, a sensible approach to limiting complications in selected patients was piloted by Kridelka et al. (317). Pelvic failure is by far the most frequent site of failure in early-stage cervical cancer patients, regardless of the initial treatment. However, in node-negative patients, the risk factors that indicate adjuvant RT following radical surgery are overwhelmingly related to a risk of failure in the central pelvis, including the vaginal vault and paravaginal soft tissues. Given the well-known relationship between radiation volume and complication risk, Kridelka et al. limited the adjuvant pelvic RT to fields smaller than "standard." In 25 patients with a risk of recurrence of at least 40%, as suggested by the GOG study (222), only one recurrence was noted, with a median follow-up of 32 months. As predicted, morbidity was very limited in quantity and grade. The authors compared disease-free survival curves of their experience and that of the observation arm in the GOG trial by Sedlis et al. (318), finding small field pelvic RT to be significantly superior ($p = 0.005$).

A similar experience with small field pelvic RT was reported by Ohara et al. in 42 patients with stages I-II node-negative squamous carcinoma of the cervix at significant risk of local recurrence (319). All patients so treated had deep cervical stromal invasion, parametrial extension, and/or positive or close (<5 mm) surgical margins. Only three patients treated with small field RT suffered recurrences, all in the pelvis. Serious toxicity was rare. The analysis of Chen et al. supports the concept of treating only the lower pelvis with adjuvant RT in appropriately selected patients as a means of limiting non-rectal radiation-induced intestinal injury (320).

An alternative approach to limit small bowel dose in the postoperative RT situation is to utilize intensity-modulated RT (IMRT) approaches. D'Souza et al. compared IMRT plans to conventional four-field plans, finding that the mean volume of small bowel was 33% lower with the IMRT plans. However, the authors noted that these calculations did not account for interfraction organ motion and recognized the lack of data regarding safety and efficacy (312).

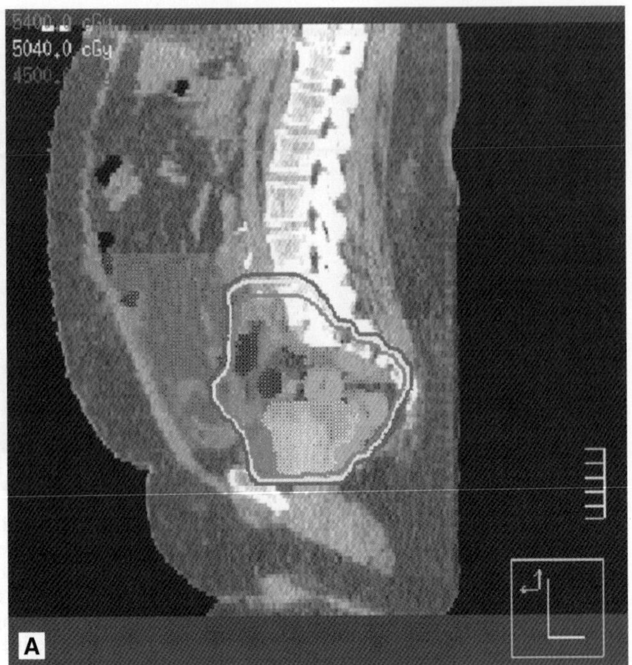

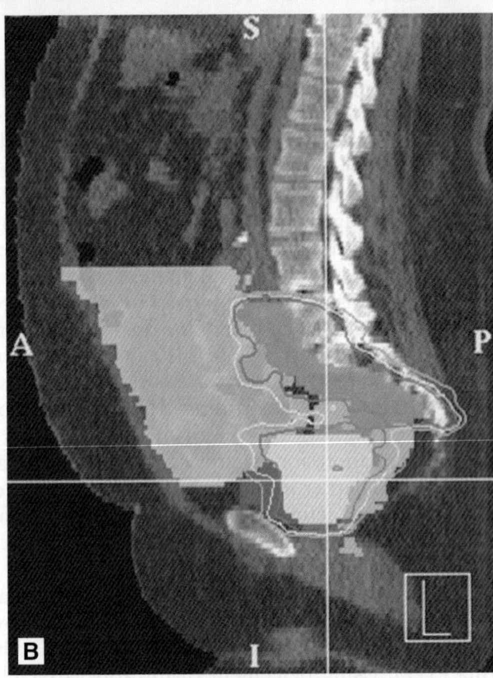

FIGURE 22.16. (*See color plate section.*) **A:** Dose distribution from a standard four-field box showing some volume of small bowel receiving full dose. **B:** IMRT approach in which the small bowel is almost excluded from the full dose region. *Source:* From Jhingran A. Potential advantages of intensity-modulated radiation therapy in gynecologic malignancies. *Semin Radiat Oncol* 2006;16:144-151.

Intensity-Modulated External Radiation Therapy

IMRT refers to the delivery of radiation beams that have varying intensity patterns that, when summed inside a patient, create a dose distribution in which the target receives near to the prescribed dose while tissues that are to be avoided receive much less radiation. Treatment planning is based on three-dimensional imaging utilizing CT, most commonly. MRI and PET images can also be incorporated into the determination of treatment volume.

Specially configured linear accelerators with multi-leaf collimators (MLCs) are used to create highly contoured dose distributions utilizing various techniques. "Step and shoot" IMRT uses multiple static fields, typically five to nine, with specific dose maps entering the patient from multiple beam angles. "Sliding window" IMRT utilizes an arcing motion of the radiation source along with movements of the MLC leafs. Helical TomoTherapy is a variation of the sliding window technique in which the radiation source is constantly moving around a patient and the patient is translated through the path of the beam while the MLCs rapidly open and close to create the desired dose distribution.

Potential benefits of IMRT include the ability to preferentially limit the dose of radiation to normal tissues, safely deliver higher tumor doses, and enable treatment and retreatment of tumors that are not otherwise treatable (Fig. 22.16A and B). Roeske et al. were the first to propose and test the hypothesis that IMRT could be used to lower small bowel dose in patients receiving pelvic RT (321). Subsequently, this approach has been popularized by Mundt et al. (322).

Dose-volume histograms (DVHs) plot the percent of a certain organ or volume of interest versus the dose received (Fig. 22.17). By looking at a DVH, the radiation oncologist can quickly and quantitatively assess whether the dose delivered to critical structures and tumor volumes is adequate for safety and efficacy of treatment. Furthermore, DVH analysis provides an objective method of comparing different treatment plans. The increasing use of IMRT requires a better understanding of radiation dose-volume relationships than has existed in the past. For the most part, consensus remains to be generated regarding proper dose-volume constraints for most normal tissues.

Jhingran has published an extensive review of IMRT use in gynecologic malignancies (314). Early data supports the ability

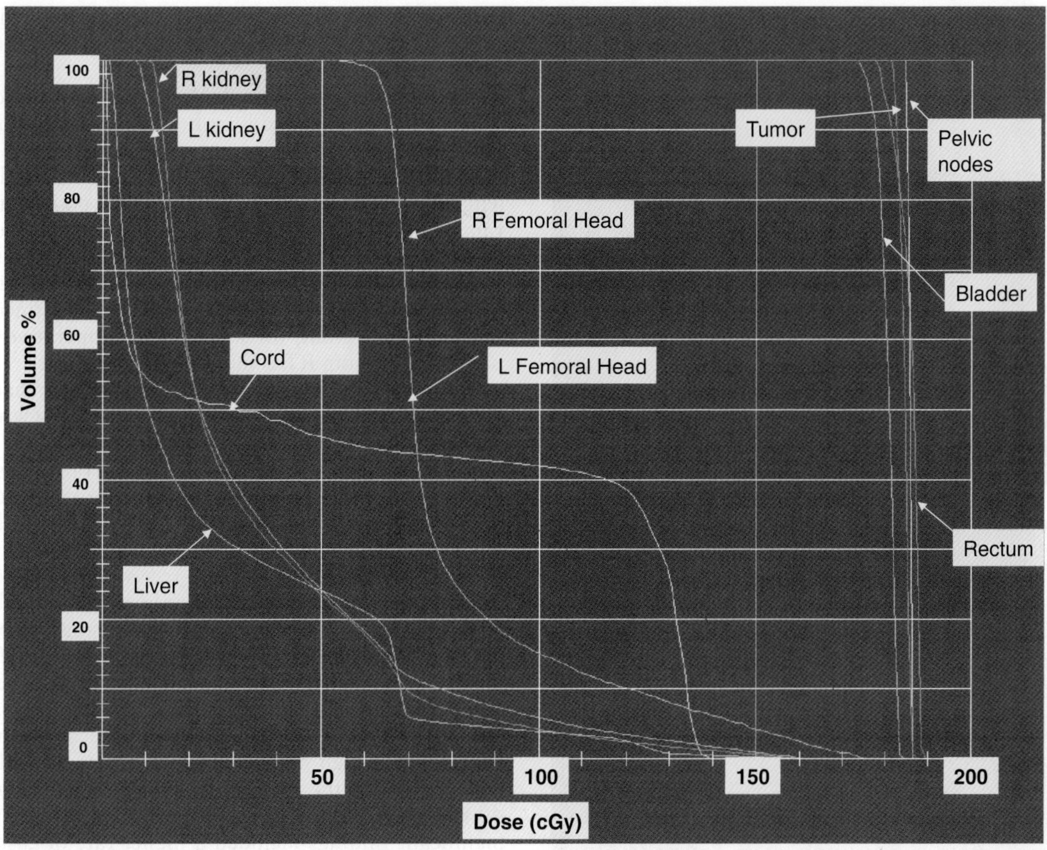

FIGURE 22.17. This dose-volume histogram from an extended field RT plan plots the volume of various organs or structures versus the dose received. It shows excellent coverage of tumor and nodal regions while the normal structures, e.g., kidneys, spinal cord, etc., receive limited dose. This provides quantitative measures of dose distribution for use in evaluating and comparing treatment plans.

of IMRT to reduce dose to normal tissues and thereby reduce acute and late toxicities. It can also facilitate treatment of recurrences in or near previous RT fields, dose escalation to grossly involved lymph nodes, and treatment of patients with vesico- or rectovaginal fistulae. There is active debate regarding the ability of IMRT techniques to replace intracavitary brachytherapy for treatment of cervical cancer (323–325). To date, the weight of opinion does not support this latter indication.

Randall and Ibbott have presented a discussion of possible pitfalls and hazards from implementation of IMRT for gynecologic cancers (326). Chief among these concerns is the problem of organ and tissue motion. In addition to respiratory motion, in the pelvis there is considerable motion with varying amounts of distension of the bladder and rectum (327). Ahamad et al. performed a systematic analysis of 10 patients with gynecologic cancers planned with both IMRT and four-field approaches. When IMRT margins were expanded to take into account internal motion and setup variation, the dosimetric advantage of IMRT largely disappeared (328). Han et al. completed a similar study, noting that significant differences in the small bowel dose-volume histogram can result, making strict protocols for bladder distention, margins, and image guidance necessary for IMRT implementation (329).

In addition, patient and tumor geometry often changes during treatment. Beadle et al. performed serial CTs during treatment of 16 patients with cervical cancer to assess tumor regression and organ motion. These authors found that the location of the tumor volume varied markedly during treatment from both these factors, and proper treatment would require large volumes initially, as is done with conventional treatment. As a result, it was felt that the potential value of IMRT was diminished and the risk of missing tumor was increased (330).

In general, there is lack of agreement regarding scanning parameters, necessity of intravenous contrast enhancement, appropriate volumes to contour, and dose-volume constraints. Taylor et al. have presented guidelines for contouring pelvic lymph nodes for patients undergoing RT, suggesting that a 7-mm margin around iliac vessels presents a reasonable trade-off in terms of maximizing nodal coverage while limiting small bowel dose (331). Other concerns include an increase in the incidence of secondary radiation-induced malignancies (332–335), limitations of imaging in accurately defining pelvic disease, increased dose heterogeneity, and problems with quality assurance (326). In addition there are concerns regarding deleterious effects of prolonged treatment times on the radiation-induced cell killing (336,337). Finally, many technical issues are of concern, including the fact that dose distributions are less reproducible and the fact that calculated dosimetry might not reflect what is actually delivered to the patient for many reasons (326).

Extended Field RT

The reluctance among some radiation oncologists to utilize extended field radiation therapy (EFRT) either prophylactically or therapeutically in some cases relates to concern over increased acute and late toxicities. This is largely because the para-aortic chain is surrounded by organs of limited radiation tolerance, i.e., spinal cord, kidneys, small intestine. The use of opposed anterior and posterior fields is the easiest technique but delivers to a significant portion of the small bowel a radiation dose that will generally exceed tolerance if an appropriate

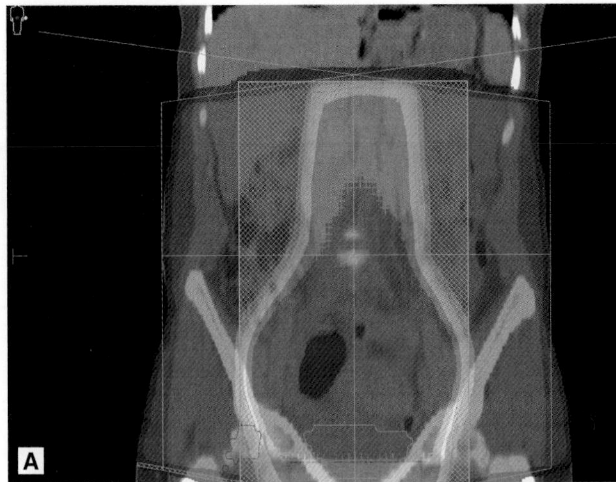

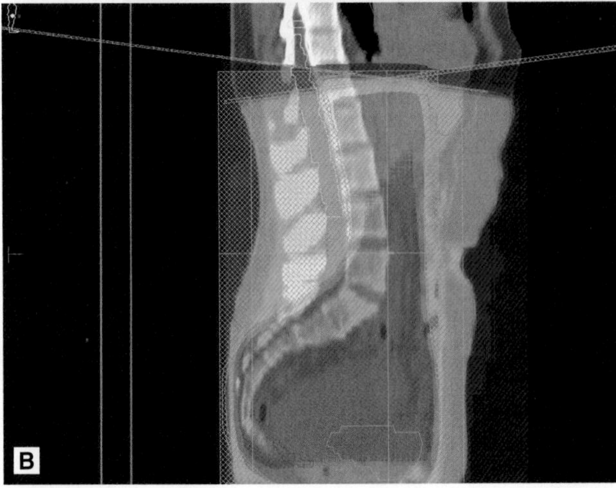

FIGURE 22.18. (*See color plate section.*) This shows dose distribution from extended field RT given with a four-field isocentric technique with all fields treated in continuity. The AP-PA fields (**A**) are weighted 70:30 in relation to the lateral fields (**B**), limiting the dose to kidneys, as shown in the DVH in Figure 22.17. This patient had a large pelvic mass, compromising the ability to spare rectum and bladder.

dose for microscopic disease is delivered. Various techniques have been utilized in an effort to deliver EFRT, all of which have both advantages and disadvantages. A four-field technique permits continuity with and use of a four-field approach in the pelvis, spares much of the small intestine, and shields the spinal cord and the vast majority of the kidneys from half of the beams (Fig. 22.18A and B). It is important to perform an intravenous pyelogram (IVP) or CT to accurately determine the kidneys' location. The dose to the kidneys can be kept within tolerance by preferentially weighting the anterior and posterior beams (e.g., 70:30 AP-PA to laterals). In most cases, this will be adequate to limit kidney doses within tolerance, even when delivering 40 to 45 Gy to the volume. Nevertheless, it is critical to know the kidney doses and the amount of the renal parenchyma receiving this dose when utilizing this technique. A DVH of such a treatment is shown in Figure 22.17.

Esthappan et al. used positron emission tomography (PET) data to assess for metastatic disease and to guide planning using IMRT techniques (338). In this fashion, it was feasible to escalate RT doses to 59.4 Gy while maintaining acceptable doses to surrounding tissues. Salama et al. reported the use of IMRT for extended field RT in 13 patients, finding the approach to be well tolerated (339). With limited follow-up, two patients reported grade 3 or higher toxicity, and the local control rate was high.

Elective Para-aortic Lymph Node Irradiation. Occult involvement of the para-aortic lymph nodes is a potential cause of treatment failure in carcinoma of the cervix. Given the orderly lymphatic spread of cervical carcinoma to pelvic and para-aortic lymph nodes, and its frequency in defined patient groups, adjuvant or EFRT is a logical treatment strategy that seeks to avoid the risks and treatment delays associated with surgical staging. Its use may be considered in patients with early-stage disease who have undergone appropriate surgical treatment and have risk factors arguing for adjuvant postoperative RT and in patients for whom RT is the primary treatment.

Retrospective and prospective data suggest that EFRT can be delivered safely and with reasonable efficacy in high-risk patients. In a large retrospective series from Japan, Horii et al. reported on patients who received adjuvant (in some cases, therapeutic) EFRT based on multiple positive pelvic lymph nodes, and/or radiographic evidence of para-aortic lymph node enlargement (340). The investigators found a significant survival advantage for patients receiving EFRT, compared to similar patients who received only pelvic RT. This survival advantage was particularly noticeable among stage II patients. No serious complications were reported. The European Organization for Research and Treatment of Cancer (EORTC) study reported by Haie et al. (341) included 441 patients with stages I-III disease who did not have surgical staging, but were considered at high risk of undetected para-aortic lymph node involvement. In the study group, the para-aortic area received 40 to 50 Gy with external beam radiation therapy (EBRT). Significant findings included a higher rate of gastrointestinal toxicity, a significantly lower rate of para-aortic failures in the EFRT group, and a significantly lower rate of distant metastases in patients receiving EFRT and achieving pelvic control. There was no statistically significant difference between the two treatment arms with regard to local control, distant metastases, disease-free survival at 4 years, or survival. The incidence of small bowel injury was 0.9% in the pelvic RT and 2.3% in the EFRT groups. A severe complication rate of 9% was observed in patients receiving EFRT, compared with 4.8% in those treated to the pelvis only. Rotman et al. published 10-year results from Radiation Therapy Oncology Group (RTOG) study 79–20 (342). In this study, 367 patients (stage IIB or stages IB-IIA ≥4 cm) were randomized to pelvic RT versus EFRT. Overall survival was 67% at 5 years and 55% at 10 years for the patients receiving elective EFRT, compared with 55% and 44%, respectively, for those treated to the pelvis only ($p = 0.02$). Locoregional failures were similar at 10 years for both arms (pelvic only, 35%; EFRT, 31%). When the first disease failure patterns were examined, more patients failed distally when treated only with pelvic RT compared to those receiving EFRT ($p = 0.053$). The EFRT arm was associated with more grade 4 and 5 complications, particularly in patients with prior abdominal surgery (11% vs. 2%).

Gerzten et al. reported the use of concurrent cisplatin with EFRT using IMRT techniques (343). In 22 consecutive patients, the median length of treatment was 39.5 days. Only two patients required short treatment breaks, and there was no acute or subacute grade 3 or 4 gastrointestinal (GI) or genitourinary (GU) toxicity.

Grigsby et al. looked at the ability to control nodal disease with RT in cervical cancer. In patients with subclinical para-aortic disease demonstrated by PET, there were no failures with a median dose of 43.3 Gy (344).

Results from RTOG 90–01 show that pelvic RT combined with platinum-based chemotherapy is superior to adjuvant EFRT in patients with locally advanced disease (274). However, given the apparent ability of EFRT to impact failure rates in the para-aortic chain and the improving therapeutic ratio, EFRT combined with chemotherapy could offer opportunities for improved outcomes in patients at high risk of metastatic para-aortic disease. Possible indications for its consideration include positive PET scans in the para-aortic region; high pelvic lymph nodes involved, e.g., common iliac; gross nodal metastases in the pelvis; bilateral positive pelvic lymph nodes; adenocarcinoma histology with any number of positive pelvic lymph nodes; and squamous cell histology with four or more positive pelvic lymph nodes. In all cases, the radiation oncologist must determine that the patient is in reasonably good general health, with no limited risk factors for RT injury. Furthermore, there should be an assessment that there is a good chance of pelvic control (in patients receiving primary RT), since the absence of pelvic control will render para-aortic control meaningless.

Therapeutic Para-aortic Lymph Node Irradiation. Data from the GOG suggests that patients with stages IB, II, III, and IVA cervical cancer will have spread to the para-aortic lymph nodes in 5%, 16% to 21%, 25% to 31%, and 13%, respectively (27). Tumor involvement in para-aortic lymph nodes is quite uncommon in the absence of pelvic lymph node metastasis (27). Grigsby et al. have demonstrated that para-aortic RT can control known metastatic nodal disease in a high percentage of patients (344). However, the degree to which RT demonstrates curative potential in this group of patients is quite variable, and is mostly related to selection factors in the patient population so treated.

Kim et al. reviewed 43 patients with known para-aortic lymph node spread who received curative intent RT following surgical staging and removal of gross para-aortic disease, in some cases (345). Pelvic tumor size (<6 cm vs. ≥6 cm) was a significant factor in survival. It was noted that patients with no residual para-aortic disease following surgery had significantly better outcomes than those patients with gross residual tumor, raising the question of whether surgical excision of bulky para-aortic lymph node disease is advisable in this situation. In contrast, Grigsby et al. did not find that tumor stage (reasonably correlated with pelvic tumor volume) was a significant factor in patients with para-aortic lymph node involvement (346). In a series of 43 patients, the overall survival rate was 32% and the median survival was 2.2 years, although only 20 patients manifested recurrence. The predominant failure pattern was distant spread, suggesting that effective systemic therapy is warranted. Severe toxicity occurred in only two patients.

Based on a retrospective review of 35 patients treated for documented para-aortic lymph node spread, Stryker and Mortel suggested that EFRT can contribute to cure in approximately 30% of these patients (347). Again, patients with only microscopic involvement had considerably better outcomes than those with gross disease (42% vs. 26% 5-year survival). Grade 4 morbidity was seen in 8.6%, although in all cases the morbidity was related to the pelvic portion of the treatment rather than the EFRT.

Varia et al. completed a phase 2 GOG study of EFRT plus chemotherapy (348). The protocol called for cisplatin to be given at 50 mg/m^2 on day 1, and 5-FU to be given at 1,000 mg/m^2 over 96 hours during weeks 1 and 5. Eighty-six evaluable patients were accrued, 85 of whom completed EFRT; 90% completed chemotherapy. Grade 3 to 4 gastrointestinal and hematologic toxicities were seen in 19% and 15%, respectively. The actuarial risk of late morbidity was 14% at 4 years, primarily from rectal injury. Three-year overall survival and progression-free survival rates were 39% and 34%, respectively. Overall survival was 50% among stage I patients. Approximately 40% of patients had a distant failure as the first site of relapse.

In terms of toxicity, the RTOG found much greater toxicity compared to the Varia-GOG study when giving extended field RT along with sensitizing chemotherapy. Small et al. observed very high acute and late toxicities. Differences in the treatment regimens included the use of weekly cisplatin at 40 mg/m^2 and more frequent boosting of para-aortic nodes in the RTOG study (349).

Therapeutic EFRT in patients with para-aortic metastases appears to be efficacious, resulting in long-term survivals of 25% to 50%. Definable subgroups may have an even higher rate of long-term survival. EFRT can reliably control microscopic disease in the para-aortic chain; however, the curability of the individual patient is more a function of the ability to gain control of the pelvic disease and the likelihood that the patient will develop other metastatic disease.

Chemotherapy can feasibly be added to EFRT in these patients, and it is reasonable to approach patients in this fashion unless comorbid illnesses contraindicate systemic therapy. The optimum chemotherapy agents and schedule remain to be determined, although weekly cisplatin is a reasonable suggestion, based on current knowledge. The potential impact of concurrent chemotherapy on complication rates is unclear.

Proton Beam Radiotherapy

There is increasing interest in and availability of proton beam RT, although the reported experience in cervical cancer is limited. Kagel et al. reported 25 patients, stages IIB-IVA, treated with curative intent by photon pelvic RT followed by a proton boost to the primary tumor. No intracavitary RT was given. Long-term survival and complication rates were considered similar to those of conventional photon RT plus intracavitary brachytherapy (350).

Brachytherapy

Brachytherapy refers to the placement of radioactive sources at a short distance from the intended target. Because the anatomy of cervical cancer typically facilitates brachytherapy, and because brachytherapy permits very high doses to be safely delivered, it has long been a major factor in the ability of RT to cure cervical cancer. Several isotopes are available for cervical cancer brachytherapy, although at the present time ^{137}Cs is the most popular for low-dose-rate (LDR) brachytherapy. ^{192}Ir is frequently used for high-dose-rate (HDR) brachytherapy because of its high specific activity. It is also frequently used in lower activity in removable LDR interstitial applications. Brachytherapy can be delivered with intracavitary techniques using applicators typically consisting of an intrauterine tandem and vaginal colpostats or, when necessary, vaginal cylinders. All state-of-the-art applicators are afterloading. Interstitial implants are typically done with permanent or removable isotopes, such as ^{198}Au and ^{192}Ir, respectively. Radiographs are obtained using dummy sources, and the active sources can be afterloaded following review of images, if the position of the applicators is judged to be satisfactory.

Intracavitary Implants

Intracavitary brachytherapy is generally used in combination with external beam RT, although it may be used alone in very early disease. LDR has been used since the early 1900s, but starting in the late 1950s, with the Cathetron Cobalt-60, HDR brachytherapy has become increasingly utilized.

Three brachytherapy systems were developed almost simultaneously: the Paris, Stockholm, and Manchester systems. The term "system" denotes a set of established rules, taking into account the source strength and the geometry, method, and duration of the application in order to obtain suitable dose distributions. In each of these systems, a brachytherapy insertion consisted of an intrauterine component (tandem) and a vaginal applicator. Treatment duration and loadings were developed empirically. Intracavitary treatment prescriptions were quantified in terms of milligram-hours, i.e., the product of the total mass of radium or radium equivalent (e.g., ^{137}Cs) contained in the sources, and the duration of the application in hours.

The classical Manchester system was the first system to use units of radiation exposure (roentgens) rather than milligram-hours to prescribe dose. The dose (in roentgens) was prescribed at specific points, termed A and B. Point A was originally defined as a point 2 cm lateral to the center of the uterine canal and 2 cm from the mucous membrane of the lateral fornix in the plane of the uterus. Point A was intended to represent the average dose to the "paracervical triangle." Point B was defined as 5 cm from the patient's midline at the same level as point A, and it was intended to quantify the dose received by the regional (obturator) lymph nodes. The various combinations of Manchester system ovoid dimensions and applicator loadings were designed to provide a reasonably constant point A dose rate of 50 to 55 cGy per hour. This approach heavily influenced intracavitary treatment practice patterns in the United States. The widely used Fletcher-Suit applicator system, Fletcher loadings, and the reference points A and B are all derived from this system.

Computer-generated isodose curves provide the best means of determining the doses to point A, point B, bladder, and rectum (Fig. 22.19A and B). International Commission on Radiation Units and Measurements (ICRU) Report No. 38 (351) defines the dose and volume specifications for reporting intracavitary therapy in gynecologic procedures. ICRU-38 recommended that reference points such as point A not be used, because "such points are located in a region where the dose gradient is high and any inaccuracy in the determination of the distance results in large uncertainties in the absorbed doses evaluated at those points." Instead, it introduced the concept of reference volume, i.e., the tissue volume encompassed by a reference isodose surface, recommending that the dimensions of the 60-Gy isodose surface be specified, including the contribution of EBRT. They proposed that this pear-shaped reference volume be described in terms of its three dimensions: height (maximum dimension along the intrauterine sources), width (maximum dimension perpendicular to the intrauterine sources), and thickness (maximum dimension perpendicular to the intrauterine sources in the oblique sagittal plane), measured in the oblique, coronal, and sagittal planes containing the intracavitary sources. A number of weaknesses of the ICRU-38 recommendations have been pointed out, including the absence of rationale for the choice of 60 Gy. Widespread adoption is, therefore, lacking (352). However, the ICRU definitions of rectal and bladder points are frequently used.

If the vaginal vault is narrow, making it impossible to insert regular colpostats, miniovoids can be used (usually loaded with 10 mCi RaEq sources). When miniovoids cannot be inserted, an option is to use a protruding source in the vaginal vault, which is inserted in the afterloading tandem (usually 20 to 30 mCi RaEq) with an overlying plastic sleeve (Delclos ring). Afterloaded vaginal cylinders are used in conjunction with an intrauterine tandem to irradiate the vagina when the disease extends from the uterine cervix along the vaginal walls. Cylinders are available in various diameters (1 to 5 cm) and lengths to fit any vaginal width and length.

For LDR implants, the first intracavitary insertion is generally scheduled after 20 to 45 Gy of EBRT if patient and tumor geometry permit an adequate implant (typically early-stage patients, e.g., IB to early IIB). Otherwise, 30 to 45 Gy are delivered before the first application to decrease the size of the lesion and improve the relationship of the applicators to the cervix and vagina. The second application is performed 1 or 2 weeks later. For HDR implants, there is more variability in number of implants used. However, generally, more implants are done, and a common practice is to do one implant each week during external beam RT.

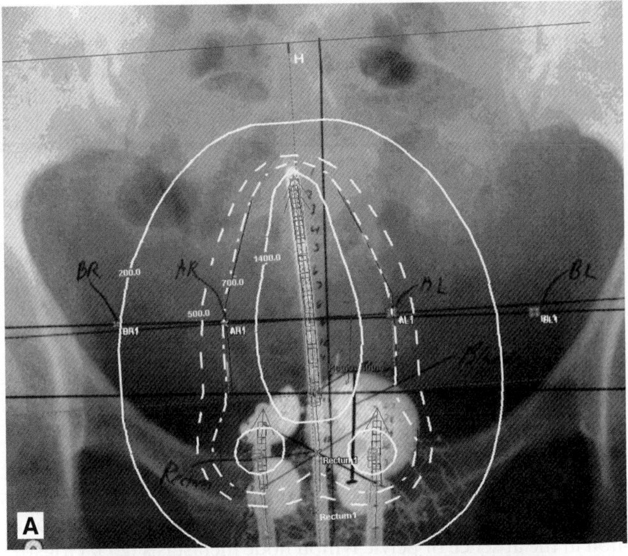

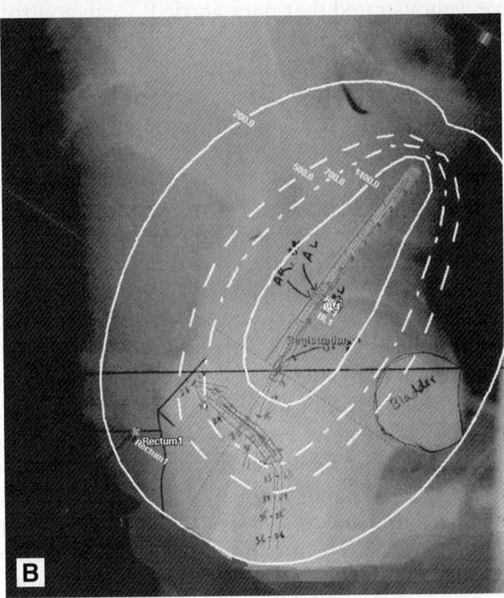

FIGURE 22.19. (A) Anteroposterior and (B) lateral radiographs of an HDR intracavitary insertion. Isodose lines reflect various dose levels, including the point A isodose of 700 cGy. A urinary catheter is in place with contrast material in the balloon, which is used to determine the maximum bladder dose. Radiopaque material in the vaginal packing helps determine the location of the anterior rectal wall to aid in determining the maximum rectal dose. Although not yet in common use, analysis of brachytherapy dose distributions based on cross-sectional imaging reconstructions, e.g., MRI, is an area of interest and research.

Intracavitary therapy, with its rapid dose fall-off with distance, yields a high dose to the uterus and paracervical tissues, but it is inadequate to treat the pelvic lymph nodes; external irradiation is necessary to supplement the dose. Therefore, the parametrial dose is primarily delivered with external irradiation. This combination technique affords a high central dose to the cervix, paracervical tissues, and parametria, as well as a moderate dose to the external iliac lymph nodes, without exceeding the bladder and rectal tolerance doses.

Image-Based Brachytherapy

Although the empiric point A has proven very useful in cervix cancer brachytherapy prescription, it has been suggested that better anatomic understanding of brachytherapy dose distribution using modern imaging techniques could allow better tumor coverage and lessen dose to normal tissues. The U.S.-based Image-Guided Brachytherapy Working Group and the Europe-based Gynecologic GEC-ESTRO Working Group have proposed similar guidelines for implementation of image-based brachytherapy (353,354). These investigators recommend T2-weighted MRI scans with contrast as the preferred method for imaging implant geometry. Limited availability of MRI-compatible applicators and expense have slowed adoption of this approach. Definitions of gross tumor volume (GTV), clinical tumor volume (CTV), and organs at risk (OAR) are suggested, enabling quantitative analysis of implant geometry through dose-volume histograms (DVHs), similar to external beam RT (355). Viswanathan et al. compared the results of contouring CTVs and OARs according to CT versus MRI images in ten patients following placement of a standard applicator (356). Both CT and MRI were adequate for contouring OARs. However, it was found that CT overestimated tumor width compared to MRI, and this could result in significant differences in dose prescription when compared to MRI contours. These investigators supported the use of MRI as the gold standard for CTV definition in image-based brachytherapy.

Dose Rate Considerations

The rate at which radiation is given is an important variable in the delivery of RT. Conventional EBRT typically uses dose rates of 100 to 300 cGy per minute but is fractionated. Brachytherapy dose rates can be much more variable, the exposure is often continuous, and dose gradients are infinitely greater than with external beam therapy.

The ICRU defines LDR as exposures between 40 and 200 cGy/hr, medium dose rate (MDR) as between 200 and 1,200 cGy/hr, and HDR as >1,200 cGy/hr (351). All agree that clinically significant differences exist between LDR, MDR, and HDR. In general, as the dose rate is lowered, the biologic effect of the radiation is decreased owing to the ability of tissues to repair sublethal radiation damage and to repopulate. While there is probably no inherent difference in these parameters between tumor and normal tissues, there is apparently a substantial difference when one considers acute-responding (rapidly proliferating) versus late-responding (slowly proliferating) tissues. Late-responding tissues have a greater capability for repair than tumor or early-responding tissues, but this repair does not take place as fully with high dose rates. Therein lies the radiobiologic dilemma: higher dose rate or large doses per fraction cause relatively more severe late damage than tumor cell kill during HDR brachytherapy or external beam therapy.

To a large degree, published data documenting the effectiveness of RT has been obtained with continuous LDR intracavitary techniques, which have been used for nearly a century. However, even within the dose-rate range considered LDR (0 to 200 cGy/hr), a strong dose-rate effect is likely (357,358). Using a slightly higher dose rate (in the low MDR range), Patel et al. suggested, based on analysis of their clinical experience, that a dose reduction factor of approximately 30%, in comparison to a typical LDR range of 50 to 55 cGy/hr, would be required when using a dose rate of 220 cGy/hr at point A (359).

Although the dose prescriptions for LDR brachytherapy are reasonably well established and practiced around the world, there remains some disagreement about whether the LDR intracavitary dose should be given in one or two implants (360). Rotman and Aziz have published a nice review of the literature regarding this controversy (361). Most radiation oncologists favor fractionating the intracavitary portion of the treatment (mostly two implants) because of theoretical and practical advantages that include (a) tumor shrinkage between implants, allowing better dose coverage in the relevant isodose (higher dose to the tumor periphery); (b) repair of normal tissues between fractions, leading to fewer late effects; and (c) limiting the duration of bed rest and potential complications that can result. The clinical data tend to support the superiority of two implants over one implant, but this is not uniformly the case.

Pulsed LDR brachytherapy has also been investigated as a possible means of preserving the radiobiologic advantages of LDR while taking advantage of dose optimization offered by HDR technology. Swift et al. reported their experience in 65 patients, 42 of who had cervical cancer (362). Median follow-up was only 15 months. In these patients with cervical cancer, 23 were alive without known disease at the time of the report. The 2-year actuarial survival rate was 65%, and the 2-year actuarial incidence of late complications was 14%. The authors concluded that pulsed LDR was feasible and produced good local control rates. Bachtiary et al. compared outcomes of patients treated with LDR (109 patients) and pulsed dose rate (PDR) (57 patients). Seventy patients also received concurrent cisplatin. No significant differences were noted in outcomes or toxicities (363).

The use of HDR in the curative management of cervical cancer is becoming more accepted, presumably because the outpatient treatment is more convenient. Other suggested advantages include better stability of the implant and source positions during the short duration of the implant and better ability to optimize dose distributions. The literature reflects considerable inconsistency in terms of whether complication rates are increased with HDR over LDR. Although many retrospective series and a few randomized trials have been reported, results are difficult to interpret. More recent studies include the results of Hareyama et al., who published a randomized trial of 132 patients with stage II or IIIB disease (364). External RT doses were identical, and a conversion factor of 0.588 was used to convert LDR to HDR. The 5-year disease-specific survival rates were 69% and 51% with HDR in stages II and III, respectively. This compared with 87% and 60% with LDR. Pelvic recurrence-free survival with HDR was 89% and 73% for stages II and III, versus 100% and 70%, respectively, in the LDR group. Actuarial complication rates (≥ grade 3) at 5 years were 10% with HDR and 13% with LDR. These differences did not reach statistical significance, although stage II patients had a better survival rate than those treated with HDR.

Ferrigno et al. published a retrospective series of 190 patients treated with LDR from 1989 to 1995 and 118 patients treated with HDR from 1994 to 2001. With median follow-ups of 70 and 33 months in the LDR and HDR groups, respectively, no significant differences were seen in overall survival (OS), disease-free survival (DFS), and local control among stage I-II patients. However, for stage III patients, OS and DFS were significantly better in the LDR group, and local control was also better, although not at a statistically significant level (365).

Falkenberg et al. reported a single institution study comparing outcomes of 103 patients treated with LDR versus 57 patients treated with HDR. No significant differences were seen in any stage in this series (366).

To facilitate multiple insertions, intrauterine stents can be used so that applicators can be placed quickly, without cervical dilatation, using little or no sedation. Treatment planning is performed on the initial insertion, and is duplicated for all fractions by verifying the applicator position with fluoroscopy or radiographs. In addition to fractionation, clinical experience has demonstrated that some method of increasing the distance from the HDR sources to the rectal wall is mandatory to keep rectal doses and subsequent sequelae at acceptable levels. Various techniques, including rectal retractors, vaginal speculums, gauze packing, and intravaginal Foley catheter balloons, are used to achieve this goal.

Interstitial Implants

Interstitial implants are an option when intracavitary implants are impossible (367). Implants are typically planned and facilitated using perineal templates such as the Syed-Neblett Interstitial Template or the Martinez Universal Perineal Template (MUPIT). The use of endorectal magnetic resonance coils and transrectal ultrasound can facilitate needle placement by improving visualization of tumor and normal tissues in relation to needle position. In some cases, this is done in conjunction with open laparotomy or laparoscopy.

Patients are typically selected for interstitial therapy on the basis of practical difficulties that preclude intracavitary therapy; thus, they may not be comparable to patients treated in a more conventional manner. However, until further improvements and better data supporting the efficiency and safety of this technique are available, its use in locally advanced cervical cancer should be only in exceptional circumstances, and by experienced brachytherapists. Furthermore, IMRT is likely to prove to be an effective alternative to interstitial therapy in patients who are not candidates for intracavitary therapy.

Doses of Irradiation

Invasive carcinoma of the cervix is treated with a combination of whole pelvis and intracavitary therapy. Some institutions use lower doses of pelvic RT (10 Gy for stage IB and 20 Gy for stages IIA, IIB, and III), in addition to parametrial doses to complete therapy with an MLS. This brings total doses to 50 Gy in stage IB and IIA, or 60 Gy to the involved parametrial tissues for more advanced stages.

Other institutions prefer higher doses of whole pelvis external irradiation (usually 40 to 45 Gy), delivered by four-field box or IMRT technique. This is usually combined with one or two LDR intracavitary insertions for approximately 40 to 55 Gy to point A, depending on tumor stage (volume). Usual doses to point A from both the external irradiation to the whole pelvis and the LDR intracavitary brachytherapy range from 70 Gy for small (≤1 cm) stage IB tumors to 90 to 95 Gy for stage IIB or IIIB tumors. An additional parametrial dose is administered in some patients with IIB, III, or IVA tumors (considering the dose delivered to the side wall by the brachytherapy). In patients with only unilateral parametrial involvement, consideration should be given to boosting only the involved side.

When using HDR brachytherapy, the greatest concern is the potential for increasing complication rates in a patient population in which the majority will be cured. To decrease the likelihood of increased late effects with HDR brachytherapy, it is necessary to use multiple HDR fractions and to decrease, as much as possible, the dose to late-responding tissues. Petereit and Pearcey (368) used 45 Gy/25 fractions of external beam irradiation to the pelvis, combined with five HDR fractions (5.5 to 6 Gy per fraction), or four fractions of HDR brachytherapy (6.5 to 7 Gy in each fraction). The equivalent LDR brachytherapy at point A is 80 Gy, with 67 Gy delivered to the bladder or the rectum, assuming that these tissues receive 70% of the prescribed point A dose. For advanced stages, such as IIB or IIIB, the intracavitary dose may be increased to 7.5 Gy per fraction, to have an LDR equivalent dose of 85 to 90 Gy to point A.

The recommended HDR brachytherapy prescription in GOG cervical cancer protocols is five fractions of 6 Gy (to point A) in addition to EBRT. Toita et al. from Japan have reported good results in their patients using significantly lower HDR doses (369). Whether this observation can be explained by anatomic variation, different tumor biology, or other reasons is not clear at this time. More clinical data with close observation and extended follow-up are needed to establish optimum brachytherapy treatment schedules using nonstandard dose rates.

Altered Fractionation

Conventional RT schedules typically employ fraction sizes of 180 to 200 cGy, given 5 days per week over a number of weeks. Altered fractionation refers to the use of nonstandard dose and fractionation schedules. Radiobiologic research and modeling suggest that these different fractionation schedules could favorably impact control rates, complication rates, or both. Examples include hypofractionation (larger doses per fraction, lower total dose), hyperfractionation (smaller doses per fraction given more frequently, e.g., two to three fractions per day, to a slightly higher total dose), accelerated fractionation (standard fraction sizes given more frequently, e.g., twice daily), and concomitant boost techniques (a larger volume is treated in standard fashion, while part of the volume, typically gross tumor, is treated with an additional smaller fraction on the same day, separated by 4 to 6 hours).

Hyperfractionation has been the most frequently investigated altered fractionation regimen (370). In general, the results have not been sufficiently positive to warrant its adoption.

Use of the concomitant boost technique in cervical cancer was reported by Kavanagh et al., who conducted a prospective trial in 22 patients (371). Pelvic RT of 45 Gy/25 fractions was given, and a concomitant boost of 14.4 Gy/9 fractions was given to gross tumor during weeks 3 to 5. Standard LDR brachytherapy was also given. Although the local control and survival rates were higher than a matched control group, the incidence of late bowel toxicity was sufficient to diminish enthusiasm for this approach until methods of lowering toxicity can be established.

Overall Treatment Time

Owing to the radiobiologic phenomena of tumor cell repopulation and accelerated repopulation, clinicians have long assumed that treatment prolongation, beyond some reasonable point, would likely have a deleterious effect on outcome in patients treated with RT. Several studies have supported this assumption by demonstrating lower pelvic tumor control and survival rates after definitive RT in invasive carcinoma of the uterine cervix when the overall treatment time is prolonged (372–374).

Combining the published results, one can suggest that pelvic control will suffer at an approximate rate of 1% per day that treatment extends beyond 52 to 55 days. This impact will be potentially seen in all stages of localized disease, and survival will be negatively affected. Erridge et al. have pointed out that there is probably a limit to the relationship between treatment time and outcome (375). In a cohort of patients, almost all of whom completed treatment within 7 weeks, no impact of overall treatment time was observed. However, grade 4 toxicities were more common among patients completing treatment on a compact schedule of 29 to 32 days.

Pallative or Emergent Irradiation

The radiation or gynecologic oncologist is often faced with treating a patient who requires palliation of pelvic pain, obstruction, or bleeding. If vaginal bleeding is the main concern, a single intracavitary implant with tandem and colpostats, about 50 to 55 Gy, to point A suffices. Alternatively, bleeding can be controlled by more conservative measures, such as vaginal packing, followed by the immediate institution of EBRT. In this circumstance, it can be appropriate to treat a slightly smaller pelvic volume and use doses per fraction slightly higher than standard, e.g., 250 to 300 cGy, allowing patients with localized disease to be approached with curative intent, without an excessive risk of complications.

Patients with stage IVB or incurable recurrent carcinoma often require palliation of pelvic pain or bleeding, and their general condition may not warrant a prolonged course of external irradiation. Spanos et al. (376) reported an RTOG phase 3 study of accelerated split-course palliative irradiation in 284 patients. Patients received three courses of 14.8 Gy in four fractions over 2 days, with a rest of 2 to 4 weeks between courses, up to 44.4 Gy total dose. There were 136 patients randomized to rest periods of 2 or 4 weeks. There was a trend toward increased acute toxicity in patients with shorter rest periods (5 of 68, versus 0 of 68; $p = 0.07$). Late toxicity was not significantly different in the two groups, although length of follow-up was not sufficient to accurately assess it. Pelvic tumor response was comparable in both groups (34% vs. 26%). More patients in the 2-week rest period group completed the three courses of therapy, but the most significant predictor for completion of therapy was Karnofsky performance status of 80 or higher. This schedule offers significant logistic benefits and has been shown to result in good tumor regression and excellent palliation of symptoms.

CHEMOTHERAPY

Chemotherapy is increasingly utilized in the management of cervical cancer, both in primary management and for recurrent and metastatic disease. Reviews have indicated that several chemotherapeutic agents from different classes are active in this disease (377). Conventional agents able to induce a response rate of at least 20% in measurable disease include cisplatin, paclitaxel, topotecan, ifosfamide, doxorubicin, epirubicin, and vinorelbine. Doublets that combine these agents with cisplatin result in a doubling of response rate and improved progression-free survival but little or no improvement in overall survival when compared to cisplatin as a single agent. Three and four drug chemotherapy regimens further increase the response rate without improvement in overall survival at the expense of increased toxicity.

COMBINED MODALITY TREATMENT

Adjuvant Hysterectomy after Radiation Therapy

Multiple retrospective series have been reported comparing preoperative RT plus adjuvant hysterectomy post–radiation therapy (AHPRT) with curative intent RT or chemo-RT without AHPRT. Most commonly, no improvement in tumor control or survival is noted (378). Other series report improved pelvic control rates and possibly improved survival (379). Given the retrospective nature of these series, the authors acknowledge likely biases in patient selection, limiting the ability to draw conclusions.

A randomized trial to address this question was performed by the GOG. Keys et al. reported 256 patients with cervix cancers >4 cm in size who were randomized to curative doses of pelvic RT with brachytherapy versus preoperative doses of RT and brachytherapy plus AHPRT. The relapse rate was significantly lower in the AHPRT arm versus RT alone (27% vs. 14%). The incidence of progression was somewhat higher in the RT alone group at 46% versus 37% ($p = 0.07$) in the AHPRT group. However, no overall survival advantage was seen, and the toxicities were similar in both groups. Pathologic evaluation of hysterectomy specimens revealed 48% with no residual disease, 40% with microscopic disease, and 12% with grossly positive tumor. Patients with grossly positive tumors had a death rate seven times higher than those with negative specimens (230).

The main impetus for AHPRT is to decrease the incidence of pelvic recurrence; however, its use remains controversial because overall survival appears to be unaffected. Patients who could potentially benefit include those with bulky endocervical lesions greater than 4 cm in size and patients with difficult anatomy that limits appropriate placement of brachytherapy applicators. Patients with persistent disease after RT may benefit from planned hysterectomy.

Adjuvant Postoperative Pelvic RT

The most common failure pattern following radical surgery for cervical carcinoma is pelvic relapse. Based on an extensive GOG clinico-pathologic study, Delgado et al. proposed separate intermediate- and high-risk groups (134). These definitions have become generally accepted and incorporated into the design of both prospective trials and retrospective reports. Intermediate-risk criteria relate to tumor size, depth of stromal invasion, and lymphovascular space invasion; these are presented in Table 22.5. High-risk criteria include positive pelvic nodes, close or positive margins, and parametrial extension. Retrospective and prospective data suggest that adjuvant pelvic RT significantly improves pelvic control rates and disease-free survival in patients with risk factors for recurrence who have completed radical surgery. The role of chemotherapy, particularly in high-risk patients, has also become established.

Intermediate Risk, Node Negative

The GOG conducted a phase 3 trial comparing radical hysterectomy alone with radical hysterectomy and postoperative pelvic RT in patients with node-negative stage IB cervical carcinomas, with prognostic features correlated with an intermediate risk of recurrence (GOG #92) (317). Eligibility criteria for this study are given in Table 22.5. There were 277 patients randomized after radical hysterectomy: 137 to pelvic RT, and 140 to no further therapy. RT consisted of 46 to 50.4 Gy to a whole pelvic field. No brachytherapy was used. After a median follow-up of 5 years for living patients, recurrence was observed in 28% of the patients in the control group and in 15% of the radiated patients. There was a statistically significant reduction in the risk of recurrence (relative risk = 0.53, $p = 0.008$) in the irradiated group. Cox model analysis adjusting for risk factor combinations indicated that the risk of recurrence was decreased by 44% in the RT arm. A trend toward lower mortality with RT was observed but had not reached statistical significance at the time of publication. Severe or life-threatening adverse effects were observed in 7% of the radiated patients, versus 2.1% of the controls.

TABLE 22.5

GOG 92 ELIGIBILITY CRITERIA

CLS (capillary lymphatic space involvement)	Stromal invasion	Tumor size
Positive	Deep 1/3	Any
Positive	Middle 1/3	≥2 cm
Positive	Superficial 1/3	≥5 cm
Negative	Deep or middle 1/3	≥4 cm

After additional follow-up and data maturation, Rotman et al. presented a final report from GOG #92 (380). It was shown that the RT arm had a 46% reduction in the risk of recurrence compared to the observation arm ($p = 0.007$) and a reduction in the risk of progression or death ($p = 0.009$). Particularly striking was the impact of postoperative RT in patients with adenocarcinoma or adenosquamous histologies: among this subset, only 8.8% recurred in the RT arm, versus 44% in the observation arm. There was a strong trend toward improved survival in the RT arm, but this did not reach statistical significance ($p = 0.074$).

Several reasons have been suggested for the inability of this study to conclusively demonstrate a survival benefit in the presence of such a strong impact on recurrence rate. For example, a number of patients randomized to the RT arm did not receive RT and additional patients had protracted treatment or inadequate doses. However, the strongest factor is probably that the study was powered for its primary end point, which was disease-free interval, and was not sufficiently powered to demonstrate a survival benefit.

A retrospective series from the Netherlands looked at 51 patients with intermediate-risk, node-negative tumors. Of these, 34 received RT and 17 did not. The 5-year disease-free survival was 86% in the group receiving RT, compared to 57% in the observation group (381).

Management of patients with stage IB2 tumors is somewhat controversial, in that some favor initial surgery followed by adjuvant RT, while others recommend curative intent chemoradiation, avoiding the use of two local modalities. This topic is discussed earlier in the chapter.

Node-Positive/High-Risk Patients

Metastatic disease in the pelvic lymph nodes is a poor prognostic sign. Pelvic nodal metastases may be associated with lesion size, deep stromal invasion, and involvement of capillary or lymphatic vascular spaces (134). Postoperative pelvic radiation therapy has been advocated in the presence of these prognostic factors.

An intergroup study was conducted by the Southwest Oncology Group (SWOG), GOG, and RTOG in women with FIGO stages IA2, IB, or IIA carcinoma of the cervix found to have metastatic disease in the pelvic lymph nodes, positive parametrial involvement, or positive surgical margins at time of primary radical hysterectomy, and total pelvic lymphadenectomy with confirmed negative para-aortic lymph nodes (245). One hundred twenty-seven patients were randomized between pelvic external beam radiation therapy with 5-FU infusion and cisplatin, and 116 were treated with pelvic external beam irradiation alone. The median follow-up for survivors was 43 months. The 3-year survival on the adjuvant cisplatin/5-FU and irradiation arm was 87%, compared with 77% on the pelvic irradiation arm. The difference is statistically significant. Chemotherapy appeared to reduce both pelvic and extrapelvic recurrences. Acute toxicities were more common in the chemotherapy arm. Monk et al. reviewed the data from this randomized intergroup trial to assess the benefit of adjuvant therapies in definable subgroups of patients and to better understand histologic and clinical risk factors for recurrence (382). With a median follow-up of 5.2 years, the survival rates were 80% and 66% for the chemo-RT and RT alone groups, respectively. In a univariate analysis, the benefit of chemotherapy was most significant in patients with tumors >2 cm and >1 nodal metastasis.

Although retrospective, a large and well-analyzed series of patients receiving postoperative RT was presented by Kim et al. (383). Death and recurrence rates increased with the number of positive lymph nodes. Five-year disease-free survival was 89% if no nodes were positive, decreasing to 85%, 74%, and 56% in patients with one, two to three, and four or more positive nodes, respectively. Similar data was reported by Uno et al. (384).

Close or Positive Margins/Parametrial Involvement

Eighty-five percent of patients accrued on the SWOG/GOG/RTOG Intergroup study were eligible based on pelvic node involvement. Only 5% of patients accrued to this intergroup study had positive margins, probably because of the reluctance of clinicians to put these patients on a trial that did not allow brachytherapy boosts. Nevertheless, patients with positive or close margins and/or parametrial involvement are considered to be at high risk and, based on this randomized trial, should be considered for adjuvant chemoradiation (245). Other data might suggest that some patients, particularly close or positive margin patients, might be adequately treated with only postoperative RT.

Estape et al. retrospectively analyzed 51 patients with close vaginal surgical margins following radical hysterectomy (defined as ≤5 mm) (385). Twenty-three patients with negative nodes and close vaginal margins were studied. Although the 16 patients receiving RT had a preponderance of other risk factors, recurrence rates (12.5% vs. 85.7%) and 5-year survival rates (81.3% vs. 28.6%) significantly favored the group receiving adjuvant pelvic RT.

Kim et al. (386) described results for 38 patients receiving postoperative RT after radical hysterectomy for close surgical margins and/or metastatic pelvic lymph nodes. Patients with close surgical margins were treated with intracavitary vaginal ovoid insertions. Patients with positive margins fell into two groups: those with positive parametrial margins and those with involved vaginal margins. All five patients with involved parametrial margins treated with only cuff brachytherapy suffered local failures, compared with no pelvic failure in similarly treated patients with only vaginal margins positive for tumor.

Uno et al. analyzed 117 patients with parametrial invasion who had undergone radical surgery and received adjuvant RT. Of 51 node-negative patients, only 6 developed extrapelvic recurrence, and the 5-year overall survival and recurrence-free survivals were 89% and 83%, respectively. Patients with positive nodes fared much worse (384). Similarly, Kodama et al. found excellent outcomes among parametrium-positive patients who were treated with RH and adjuvant RT if lymph node metastasis and vaginal invasion were not present (approximately 90% 5-year survival) (387).

Radiation Therapy Dose and Technique

Vaginal intracavitary RT alone can be appropriate for patients with carcinoma *in situ* with minimally invasive carcinoma at the vaginal margin of resection as the only risk factor. Outpatient HDR brachytherapy is commonly employed because it prevents the prolonged immobilization required for LDR brachytherapy. The usual dose per fraction prescribed at 0.5 cm depth is 7 Gy; three weekly fractions are typically given. The upper 3 to 5 cm of the vagina should be targeted.

When external RT is used, patients generally should not receive more than 45 Gy to the whole pelvis. Doses up to 50.4 Gy are acceptable when treating smaller fields that exclude more small bowel. Brachytherapy or small-field external beam boosts can be given, within tolerance, to increase dose to the central pelvis. The impact of concurrent chemotherapy on complication rates appears to be limited, but continued follow-up and research are needed.

The use of IMRT with chemotherapy has been reported to maintain excellent pelvic control rates, with better acute tolerance and fewer chronic toxicities compared to conventional four-field box RT (388).

TABLE 22.6

RANDOMIZED TRIALS OF NEOADJUVANT CHEMOTHERAPY FOLLOWED BY RADIOTHERAPY

First author	Stage of disease	No. of patients	Chemotherapy No. of cycles	Local CRR CT -> RT	% RT	Survival (FUP) CT -> RT	RT
Souhami, 1991	IIIB	107	VBMP × 3	47	32	23% (60)[a]	39% (60)[a]
Tattersall, 1992	IIB-IVA	71	PVB × 3	65	73	141 wk[b]	169 wk[b]
Chauvergne, 1993	IIB-III	151	VMCP × 2 to 4	77	75	42 mo[b]	45 mo[b]
Kumar, 1994, 1998	IIB-IVA	184	BIP × 2	63	69	38% (48)	36% (mo)
Tattersall, 1995	IIB-IVA	260	EP × 3	43[c]	65[c]	62% (18)	

Note: B, bleomycin; C, chlorambucil; E, epirubicin; FUP, follow-up in months; I, ifosfamide; Local CRR, local complete response rate; M, methotrexate; P, cisplatin; V, vincristine (in VBMP and VMCP), vinblastine (in PVB).
[a]$p = 0.02$
[b]Median
[c]Pelvic failures 29% versus 19% ($p < 0.003$)

Chemotherapy in Combinations for Localized Carcinoma of the Cervix

Neoadjuvant Chemotherapy Followed by Radiotherapy

Randomized trials of neoadjuvant chemotherapy (NACT) followed by radiation versus radiation alone in patients with locally advanced cervical cancer (mainly stages III and IV) have been disappointing, in terms of both complete response rates and increase in survival (389–394). In fact, none of the five reported studies showed any survival benefit (Table 22.6). Pelvic failure was more common on the NACT arm in some of these trials, and a negative influence on survival was reported in two trials (392,394). In addition, treatment morbidity was sometimes severe (392). Explanation for these negative results cannot be given with certainty, but it has been suggested that chemotherapy could lead to an accelerated regrowth of surviving clones of cells, thus lessening the effect of subsequent RT (395). Another possibility is the development of cross-resistance between certain chemotherapeutic agents and radiation (396). A meta-analysis of 18 randomized clinical trials of neoadjuvant chemotherapy including 2,074 patients compared NACT followed by RT to RT alone and demonstrated no advantage of neoadjuvant chemotherapy with regard to progression-free survival, locoregional disease-free survival, metastasis-free survival, or overall survival (397). Whatever the reason, NACT followed by RT for patients with locally advanced cervical cancer does not seem to be an option to follow any further.

Neoadjuvant Chemotherapy Followed by Surgery

Numerous nonrandomized studies reported in the 1990s suggested that NACT followed by surgery might be an attractive approach (398–403). Indeed, some but not all of the randomized trials show a trend in favor of this combined approach (Table 22.7) (404–408). A meta-analysis of five randomized clinical trials and 872 patients who received NACT followed by surgery ± RT were compared to RT alone (397). There was a significant improvement in progression-free survival, locoregional disease-free survival, metastasis-free survival, and overall

TABLE 22.7

RANDOMIZED TRIALS OF NEOADJUVANT CHEMOTHERAPY (NACT) FOLLOWED BY SURGERY

Author (ref.)	FIGO stage	No. of patients per study arm: NACT->S	NACT->RT	Control	Survival data
Sardi (404)	All IB	102		103+	81% vs. 66%, 8-year FUP ($p < 0.05$)
	IB1	41		47+	82% vs. 77%, 8-year FUP (NS)
	IB2	61		56+	80% vs. 61%, 9-year FUP ($p < 0.01$)
Sardi (405)	IIIB	53	54	54++	63% vs. 53% vs. 37%,[a] 4-year FUP ($p < 0.05$)
Benedetti-Pancini (406)	IB2-III	211		202++	OS: 68.5% vs. 60% ($p = 0.005$) PFS: 52% vs. 44% ($p = 0.02$) (median FUP 27 mo)
Sardi (407)	IIB	76		75+	OS: 65% vs. 41% ($p < 0.001$) (median FUP 84 mo)
Chang (408)	IB/IIA	68		52++	OS: 79% vs. 79% (NS) (median FUP 39 mo)

Note: +, surgery ± radiotherapy; ++, radiotherapy; FUP, follow-up; NS, not significant; OS, overall survival; PFS, progression-free survival; RT, radiotherapy; S, surgery.
[a]NACT -> S versus NACT -> RT, nonsignificant; NACT -> S versus control, $p = 0.005$; NACT -> RT versus control, $p = 0.025$.

survival for those who were resectable following NACT. Results of NACT were best for trials with cisplatin dose intensity greater than 25 mg/m^2/wk and dose density with treatment interval less than 14 days. Observations that have been made in the above-mentioned studies include the following: (a) cisplatin-based regimens are well tolerated, induce high response rates (particularly in earlier disease), and have little or no effect on surgical morbidity; (b) with NACT there is a reduced incidence of involved lymph nodes, capillary space involvement, deep invasion, or undiagnosed parametrial disease; and (c) recurrence rates are reduced. Nevertheless, based on the available data, NACT remains investigational.

Preoperative Chemoradiation in Advanced Disease

Houvenaeghel et al. have reported long-term results of neoadjuvant chemoradiation followed by radical surgery in 35 patients with locally advanced cervical cancer. Forty patients initially entered the study; however, five patients did not go on to have surgery following the preoperative regimen. Patients received cisplatin and 5-fluorouracil along with RT, typically 45 Gy. Twelve of 20 stage IB-IIB patients obtained a complete histologic response compared to 4 of 15 patients with stage III-IVA disease, and the pelvic control rate was 88.6%. The 10-year disease-free survival was 66.4%. Serious postoperative complications were seen in five patients (409).

Adjuvant Chemotherapy

Several nonrandomized studies suggest a beneficial effect of adjuvant chemotherapy given after radical surgery in patients at high risk for recurrence (410–412). Two randomized trials with a very limited number of patients have tried to evaluate the effect of adjuvant chemotherapy in patients with high-risk cervical cancer after radical hysterectomy. The first study, with only 71 patients (all with lymph node metastases) compared postoperative RT versus three cycles of postoperative chemotherapy (PVB; cisplatin, vinblastine, bleomycin) followed by RT. In the second study 76 patients (with pelvic lymph node metastases and/or vascular invasion) randomly received either adjuvant chemotherapy (carboplatin plus bleomycin) for six courses at 4-week intervals, standard RT, or no further treatment. The results of both studies are inconclusive, but there was no apparent difference in the recurrence rates and patterns of recurrences or survival between those treated and those not treated with adjuvant chemotherapy.

TREATMENT OF RECURRENT CARCINOMA OF THE CERVIX

General Considerations

The main cause of death among women with cervical cancer is uncontrolled disease in the pelvis. However, a subset of patients with recurrent disease confined to the pelvis following definitive therapy, whether that therapy is surgery or RT, are potentially curable. Treatment selection and the likelihood of success are functions of the primary therapy, extent of disease at presentation, site of recurrence, local extent of the recurrence, disease-free interval, performance status, and comorbidities.

When curative intent salvage treatment is contemplated, the local recurrence should be biopsy proven, and the patient should be evaluated for regional and distant metastasis by physical examination and imaging. A clinical diagnosis of pelvic sidewall involvement can almost always be made in the presence of a triad of sciatic pain, leg edema, and hydronephrosis. PET scanning may be the most accurate test in terms of assessing metastasis prior to embarking on local salvage therapy. Husain et al. enrolled 27 patients with recurrent cervical or vaginal cancer who were being considered for surgical resection on an imaging protocol consisting of PET with CT and/or MRI (413). Metabolic imaging was found to have a sensitivity of 100% and a specificity of 73% in detecting sites of extra-pelvic metastasis. However, biopsy confirmation of recurrence remains the gold standard for diagnosis.

Generally, patients with pelvic or regional recurrences after definitive surgery alone are managed with RT or chemoradiation, often with brachytherapy. Salvage options for patients with central recurrence after definitive or adjuvant RT are limited to radical, usually exenterative, surgery, and in selected patients, re-irradiation using interstitial radiation implants or highly conformal EBRT or IMRT. Chemotherapy-responsive patients can obtain meaningful palliation in many cases.

Salvage Treatment After Definitive Radiation Therapy: Re-irradiation

Recurrent cervical carcinoma following definitive RT within previously irradiated areas presents a difficult management problem. Although salvage surgery, usually exenterative, can be offered to patients with limited, centrally recurrent lesions if age and general condition permit, radical surgery following RT is accompanied by operative mortality in some, severe morbidity in many, and substantial loss of structure and function in all. Therefore, the applicability of salvage surgery is limited by physician and patient acceptance, as well as by clinical parameters. Even among patients meeting rigorous preoperative criteria, salvage surgery will be aborted in about one fourth of patients.

Previously irradiated tissues do not have the same tolerance as newly irradiated tissues. Therefore, severe late effects have been frequently observed, particularly in older series that predominantly used external beam techniques in poorly selected patients. More recently, evidence has been presented to suggest that re-irradiation can be curative in a significant percentage of patients with small-volume central recurrences, particularly when there has been a long disease-free interval since the earlier diagnosis and treatment.

Randall et al., in a series of 13 patients, observed a 69% complete response rate and a 46% NED (no evidence of disease) rate with a minimum 2-year follow-up, and median follow-up of 59 months (414). Interstitial re-irradiation (IRI) doses of 30 to 55 Gy were employed, with low-dose-rate permanent and temporary implants. Patients with squamous histology did significantly better than patients with adenocarcinoma histology. Other predictors for improved outcomes included smaller tumor volumes, higher implant doses, and vaginal wall/suburethra versus vaginal cuff location. Late morbidity was limited to one rectovaginal fistula in a patient who also had recurrent tumor.

In a series of 73 patients with late recurrences of squamous carcinoma of the cervix in the vaginal canal following radiation therapy, Wang et al. (415) reported a 5-year survival rate of 40%. Sixty-one patients received only RT, mainly with fractionated brachytherapy techniques such as vaginal molds. Doses of 20 to 40 Gy in three to five fractions over 3 to 5 weeks, using both LDR and HDR techniques, were typically employed, sometimes followed by more focused boosts. Favorable prognostic factors included proximal location in the vagina and tumor size <4 cm. Significant complications occurred in nearly 25%, including a 12% fistula rate. Complications were more common among patients with distally located tumors.

Jhingran has described the use of IMRT in the re-irradiation setting (314). In particular, IMRT can treat pelvic recurrences that cannot be treated with brachytherapy, because of size, location, or other factors (Fig. 22.20).

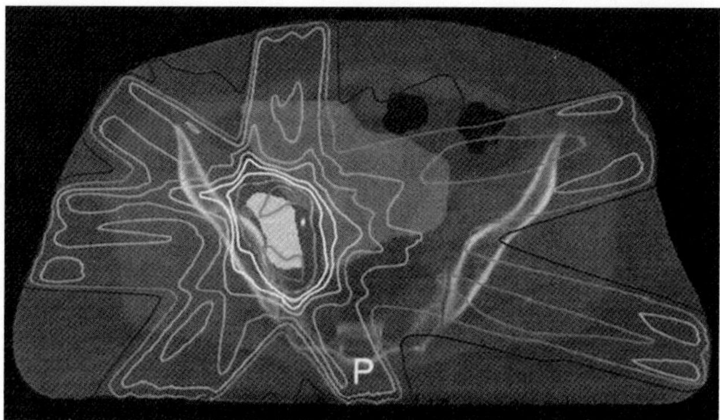

FIGURE 22.20. (*See color plate section.*) This demonstrates the use of multiple-field IMRT to retreat a painful pelvic sidewall recurrence after previous RT. After 35 Gy at 2.5 Gy per fraction, the patient became asymptomatic and remained stable for 2 years. *Source:* From Jhingran A. Potential advantages of intensity-modulated radiation therapy in gynecologic malignancies. *Semin Radiat Oncol* 2006;16:144–151.

Compared to exenterative surgery, re-irradiation is better tolerated acutely, has little operative mortality, and often preserves structure and function of pelvic organs. When contemplating re-irradiation, it is important to analyze the techniques used in the initial treatment (beam energy, volume, doses delivered with external or intracavitary irradiation). The period of time between the two treatments must be taken into consideration.

Re-irradiation is probably under-utilized in the management of locally recurrent cervical cancer. As chemotherapy does not have curative potential and many patients will not be candidates for exenterative surgery or will refuse such surgery, re-irradiation, in many cases, will be the only feasible curative intent therapy. Patient selection and careful brachytherapy technique are crucial to successful re-irradiation.

Recurrence in the Para-aortic Chain

Although unusual, recurrences limited to the para-aortic nodal region are reported following primary surgery or RT. Grigsby et al. reported 20 patients with recurrent cervical cancer confined to the para-aortic region following definitive RT (346). The median time between the initial diagnosis and the recurrence was 12 months. Although all patients died within 2 years after recurrence, median survivals were longer in patients receiving >45 Gy. A disease-free interval of >24 months was also a positive prognostic factor. However, a subsequent report from this group found a 100% salvage rate in patients with isolated para-aortic recurrences if the recurrences were asymptomatic and discovered by imaging follow-up and received full dose (>45 Gy) salvage RT combined with chemotherapy (416).

This observation was confirmed by the experience reported by Kim et al. (345). These investigators treated 12 patients with isolated para-aortic failures following RT with concurrent chemotherapy (mostly paclitaxel) and hyperfractionated RT. In patients who relapsed within 24 months of their initial treatment, the median survival following attempted salvage was 13 months. In contrast, patients having a disease-free interval >24 months had a median survival of 45 months with this therapy. A much larger series with encouraging results was presented by Hong et al., who reported 46 patients with isolated para-aortic failures, of whom 35 (76%) received salvage chemo-RT. The 3-year and 5-year survival rates were 34% and 27%, respectively. Patients who had supraclavicular relapse, with or without para-aortic relapse, had a 28% 3-year survival with salvage therapy (417).

An IMRT plan demonstrating treatment of gross recurrence and clinically high-risk areas in the para-aortic chain is shown in Figure 22.21.

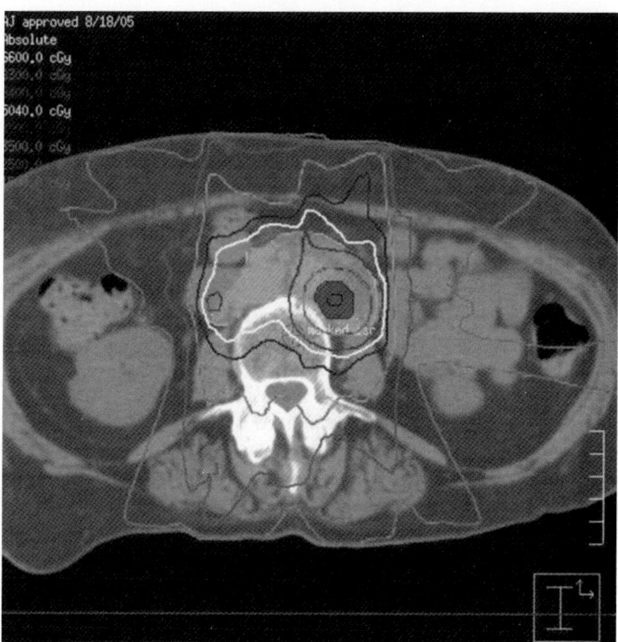

FIGURE 22.21. IMRT dose distribution in a patient treated for para-aortic lymph node recurrence. The gross nodal disease received 63 Gy at 2.5 Gy per fraction, and the nearby at-risk areas received 50 Gy. IMRT allows the creation of this sort of dose gradient to provide a "field within a field" boost. *Source:* From Jhingran A. Potential advantages of intensity-modulated radiation therapy in gynecologic malignancies. *Semin Radiat Oncol* 2006;16:144–151.

Salvage Treatment After Definitive Radiation Therapy: Radical Surgery

Pelvic Exenteration

Advances in perioperative and postoperative care and better techniques of pelvic, urinary, and GI reconstruction have lead to much improved outcomes and enhanced quality of life compared to early experiences with pelvic exenteration (PE). Survival rates have increased from 20% to about 60% with an average of 40% to 50% 5-year survival in reported series of patients completing the procedure (418,419).

Despite these advances, PE is still a very morbid operation with acute and late complications reported as high as 50% to 60% and a mortality rate of 5% to 7%. The procedure is most commonly used in patients with recurrent central pelvic disease after treatment with pelvic RT. In some cases patients with stage IVA disease may be offered primary PE, although modern chemoradiotherapy is probably preferred.

In patients undergoing PE, Marnitz et al. noted the importance of margin status: 5-year survival was 55% with negative margins compared to 10% if margins were positive (420). Given this fact and the potential morbidity and mortality from the procedure, proper patient selection requires that all efforts be made to assure that there is no site of metastatic disease and the isolated central recurrence can be resected with negative margins. Additional negative prognostic factors include disease-free interval <1 year, size of recurrence >3 cm, lymphatic spread, and parametrial and sidewall involvement. Patients with positive nodes have a survival rate of 20% or less. The presence of grossly positive lymph nodes during exploration is a poor indicator for survival and should be considered a contraindication to exenteration.

Historically, 40% to 50% of patients explored for PE will have the procedure abandoned. Husain et al. prospectively evaluated the role of PET scanning in identifying metastatic disease prior to PE. They found that PET scan had a sensitivity of 100% and specificity of 73% in detecting extra-pelvic metastatic sites and may be the most accurate imaging modality prior to PE (413). Other investigators have confirmed these findings (421). Kohler et al. found that laparoscopy was able to accurately identify cases that were eligible for PE, and their laparoscopic findings were not changed with laparotomy (422). Hopefully, better imaging and evaluation techniques will improve patient selection and minimize laparotomies in patients who are not candidates for PE.

Berek et al. reported 75 patients older than 45 years who underwent PE at a single institution. The operative time averaged 7.76 hours, the mean estimated blood loss was 2.5 liters, and the median length of stay was 23 days. Morbidities included intestinal fistulae in 15%, urinary fistulae in 8%, early bowel obstruction in 11%, and late bowel obstruction in 22%. When a J-pouch was used for colonic re-anastomosis, there was no reported fistula. Survival for patients with cervical and vaginal cancers was 73% at 1 year, 57% at year 3, and 54% at 5 years (419).

Goldberg et al. reported a 16-year experience in 103 patients. Complications included ureteral anastomotic leaks (14%, no difference between continent vs. incontinent), ureteral stricture (5%), pouch fistula (3%), pouch stones (2%), wound complications (17%), and GI fistula (11%). Other observations included that 46% of patients with primary low rectal re-anastomosis had pelvic recurrences, continent conduits were unsatisfactory in 54%, and use of mesh for pelvic floor reconstruction increased infection and fistula rates. The overall mortality was low at 1%. The 5-year survival in patients with recurrent cervical cancer was 48% (309).

Pelvic Reconstruction

In 1950, Bricker described a novel approach to diversion of urinary flow that involved isolating a segment of ileum, implanting the ureters into this segment, and bringing an open end to the abdominal wall as a separate urostomy (423). This technique was a major advancement and significantly reduced complications compared to the wet colostomy (reimplantation of ureters in the colostomy that diverts the fecal stream). This form of urinary conduit is incontinent, where the urine drains continuously to an external reservoir. The other option is to create an internal reservoir using bowel wall with a continent mechanism that allows for self-catheterization, which negates the need for an ostomy bag and affords more control to a motivated patient (423,424). The most common complications of continent reservoirs are acute and chronic pyelonephritis, ureteral stricture, urinary leak, fistula, stone formation, and, rarely, renal failure (424,425).

Segreti et al. reported their experience with transverse colon conduits and found no advantage for incontinent pouches (426). The choice depends most heavily on the surgeon's preference and the status of the distal ileum after RT. Penalver et al. reported complications in a series of patients undergoing construction of a Miami pouch. The early complication rate in 66 patients was 53% and included ten ureteral stricture/obstructions, four anastomotic leaks, and four fistulae. An additional five had difficulty with catheterization, and ten had pyelonephritis. Most complications were managed conservatively with antibiotics, percutaneous drainage, and nephrostomies. The operative mortality was 9%. The late complication rate was 37%. Out of 25 patients, 6 had strictures, 8 were incontinent, 7 had difficulty with catheterization, and 4 developed urinary stones. Again, most complications were managed conservatively (427). In a similar series from M. D. Anderson Cancer Center, 65% had postoperative complications related to the Miami pouch. Most complications were managed conservatively, and 90% retained normal continent conduit function (428).

Ungar and Palfalvi reported 29 patients who underwent orthotopic urinary reconstruction using ileocecal ascending colon reservoirs (the Budapest pouch). Although 77% of patients were able to void voluntarily without the need for self-catheterization, 23% to 47% had some incontinence (429). This is an attractive option as patients can potentially be free of any ostomies. However, only a select group of patients are candidates for these procedures.

The other component of pelvic reconstruction following PE is creation of a neovagina. Formation of a neovagina is an important component of reconstruction in several respects. For example, it fills the pelvis with well-perfused tissue and can significantly decrease the rate of pelvic infection and fistula formation (430). It also may restore some sense of normalcy in patients who are able to resume sexual activity after PE.

Many options are available for construction of a neovagina. These include the following flaps: gracilis myocutaneous, anterolateral thigh fasciocutaneous, bulbocavernosus myocutaneous, transverse rectus abdominis musculoperitoneal (TRAMP) or myocutaneous (TRAM), vertical rectus abdominis musculocutaneous (VRAM), femoris myocutaneous, tensor fasciae latae myocutaneous, inferior gluteal, and omental J flap. Portions of sigmoid colon have also been used. Myocutaneous flaps are favored due to better blood supply, ease of procedure, and functionality.

McCraw et al. first described the use of gracilis muscle for vaginal reconstruction (431). Burke et al. described perineal reconstruction using a single gracilis muscle, and 3 out of 17 had flap necrosis (432). Ratliff et al. evaluated sexual adjustment in these patients and found that 52.5% never resumed sexual activity even though 70% were thought to have adequate and functional neovagina length on examination. Self-consciousness about urostomy and colostomy was the most common reason cited for avoiding sexual activity (433). Soper et al. reported on a "short gracilis" flap based on the terminal branches of the obturator artery and found no difference between the traditional and "short gracilis" flaps (434).

O'Connell et al. reported a 100% success rate with no fistula formation, bowel obstruction, or pelvic infection using VRAM flaps. Almost 50% of women reported sexual activity after VRAM (435). Soper et al. reported that 62% of women reported sexual activity within 12 months after VRAM or TRAM flap reconstruction, concluding that both techniques give similar results and complication rates (436). Previous ligation of the inferior epigastric artery is an absolute contraindication of use of rectus flaps.

Sood et al. reported a modification to the VRAM using a smaller flap size anteriorly with a full thickness skin graft placed posteriorly. One of 18 had a partial flap loss that resolved with conservative management, and 8 of 18 remained sexually active (437). This technique allows for a smaller abdominal wall defect with minimal compromise of the neovagina. Goldberg et al. reported that gracilis flaps had a failure rate of 11% to 37%. As a group, VRAMs resulted in better outcomes with a vaginal stenosis rate of 11% and the majority of women remaining sexually active (309,310). Soper et al. compared gracilis muscle versus rectus abdominis flaps for vaginal reconstruction. Flap-specific complications and flap loss were significantly greater in gracilis muscle flaps. The authors have adopted rectus abdominis flaps as their preferred choice for vaginal reconstruction (438).

Re-anastomosis following rectosigmoid resection depends on many factors and is an option in patients undergoing supra-levator PE. Factors associated with anastomosic integrity include the length of remaining rectum/anus (<4 cm having a higher incidence of leaks versus >7 cm), blood supply to the region, and tension on the anastomosis. The use of low rectal anastomosis is controversial. Mirhashemi et al. found a 35% versus 7.5% rate of fistula formation or anastomosic breakdown in patients with previous RT compared to those who were radiation naïve. Protective colostomy was not associated with an improved outcome (439). Husain et al. reported a 54% anastomotic leak after low rectal anastomosis (440). This may be decreased by using a J pouch instead of an end-to-end re-anastomosis (419). However, some patients have difficulty emptying the pouch, particularly with shorter pouch lengths.

Wheeless described good results from neovaginal construction combining an omental J flap and a split thickness skin graft, an approach that may be considered in patients who are not candidates for rectus or gracilis flaps (441). No method of pelvic reconstruction is clearly superior to others or appropriate in all cases. The surgeon has many choices and should individualize according to each patient.

Radical Hysterectomy

Patients with very small central recurrences (less than 2 cm) after RT may be candidates for a less radical approach than PE, specifically RH. Maneo et al. evaluated the role of RH in patients with persistent or recurrent disease in 34 patients. They reported grade 3 to 4 toxicities in 44%, including five who developed fistulae. The overall 5-year survival was 49%, and 59% recurred with an average time to recurrence of 37 months. Patients with smaller tumors and lack of involvement of parametrium or vagina had better outcomes (442). Coleman et al. studied 50 patients treated with RH for persistent or recurrent central disease after RT. All patients with positive nodes died within 13 months. Severe toxicities occurred in 42%, and 28% developed either a GI or GU fistula. An additional 22% had ureteral injuries with 20% having severe long-term bladder dysfunction. The 5- and 10-year survival rates were 72% and 60%, respectively. Tumor size less than 2 cm was associated with a significantly greater survival compared to larger tumors. Overall recurrence rate was 48% (443).

RH may be a reasonable option for selected patients with persistent or recurrent central disease less than 2 cm with no extension to the parametrium or vagina. However, significant morbidity rates are relatively high (442–444).

Salvage Treatment After Previous Surgery—Definitive RT or Chemoradiation

Monk et al. (445) utilized EBRT followed by laparotomy and "open" interstitial implant for recurrent cancer in the upper vagina following hysterectomy. This approach provided the ability to accurately assess the extent of the disease and to separate bowel and bladder adhesions from the area of the implant, facilitated placement of the interstitial brachytherapy needles, and allowed the placement of an omental pedicle graft to separate the bladder and rectum from the implant volume. In 28 patients, local control was 71%, and the long-term complication rate was 11%. Long-term NED survival was 36%. Lesions <6 cm in patients with no previous RT had high control rates.

Ito et al. (446) reported on 90 patients with central recurrences from cervical cancer after surgery treated with HDR intracavitary brachytherapy (ICB), with or without EBRT. The 10-year survival for the entire series was 52%. They found survival to be greatly influenced by tumor size—72%, 48%, and 0% 10-year survival rates respectively, for small or no palpable tumor, medium (<3 cm), and large (≥3 cm). In addition, patients who achieved a complete response after RT had a 10-year survival of 63% versus 10% for those with residual disease.

Ijaz et al. (447) reported a 5-year survival of 39% in 43 patients with isolated locoregional recurrences treated with external RT and brachytherapy. In 16 patients with limited recurrences to the vagina and paravaginal tissues, the 5-year survival was 69% after radical RT.

Concurrent chemotherapy with RT has proven beneficial in locally advanced cervical cancer. Several studies also suggest a possible benefit in patients with recurrent disease (413,448). Grigsby reported a prospective trial of 22 patients with pelvic recurrences of cervical cancer following hysterectomy who received concurrent RT with 5-FU and cisplatin chemotherapy (449). None had received prior RT. The 10- and 15-year overall survival rates were 35%. Acute toxicity was limited; however, late toxicity was significant in some survivors, leading the author to recommend consideration of other chemotherapy regimens or RT alone.

In RT-naïve patients, pelvic RT of 40 to 50 Gy to the primary tumor and regional lymphatics is indicated. Inguinofemoral lymph node regions should be included in patients with involvement of the distal third of the vagina. The entire vagina should be treated in most patients with vaginal recurrences following hysterectomy. A vaginal dose of 60 to 65 Gy from external RT, with or without brachytherapy, is desirable. The gross tumor volume should receive additional radiation; doses of 15 to 30 Gy are administered with single, double-plane, or volume implants, or with intensity-modulated external RT. High-dose-rate brachytherapy techniques are also possible with appropriate dose modifications.

Salvage Treatment—Intraoperative Radiation Therapy

Patients with microscopically positive or close margins have a poor prognosis after salvage surgery. Intraoperative RT (IORT) has been used in this situation to potentially sterilize residual disease after tumor debulking. IORT allows direct visualization of the target volume, and displacement and/or shielding of the surrounding normal tissues. The IORT dose is generally limited because of prior RT, proximity of critical normal structures, and the single fraction nature of the treatment.

IORT has been used for treatment of locally advanced and recurrent carcinoma of the cervix. Most of this experience is based on the treatment of isolated central and nodal recurrences, generally amenable to surgical excision. Limitations in evaluating IORT include small patient numbers, short follow-up, and widely varying patient selection criteria. The available data seem to indicate that IORT, although feasible, does not dramatically improve prognosis and is associated with significant incidences of long-term complications. Patients with limited central recurrences who are candidates for pelvic exenteration but are found to have unfavorable prognostic factors for local recurrence, such as close positive margins, LVSI, or perineural invasion, may benefit from IORT or intraoperative interstitial brachytherapy (450).

Salvage Treatment—Role of Chemotherapy

Cisplatin, at present, is considered the single most active cytotoxic agent, and its preferred schedule of administration in metastatic or recurrent disease is 50 to 100 mg/m^2, given intravenously every 3 weeks. Overall, the duration of the objective responses to cisplatin in patients with metastatic or recurrent disease remains disappointing (4 to 6 months) and survival in such patients is only approximately 7 months. There is a suggestion of a dose-response relationship; in one trial comparing 50 mg/m^2 and 100 mg/m^2, the overall response rate increased

TABLE 22.8

RANDOMIZED STUDIES OF CISPLATIN-BASED COMBINATIONS VERSUS SINGLE-AGENT CISPLATIN IN PATIENTS WITH CERVICAL CANCER

Arms of studies and study drug	No. of patients	CR n (%)	PR n (%)	CR + PR n (%)	Median survival (mo)
MMC/VCR/BLM/CDDP	54	4 (7)	8 (15)	12 (22)	6.9
vs.					
MMC/CDDP	51	2 (4)	11 (21)	13 (25)	7
vs.					
CDDP	9	1 (11)	2 (22)	3 (33)	17
DVA/BLM/MMC/CDDP	143	11 (8)	33 (23)	44 (31)[a]	10
vs.					
CDDP	144	8 (6)	20 (14)	28 (19)[a]	9.4
DBD/CDDP	153 (147)[b]	14 (9)	17 (12)	31 (21)	7.3
vs.					
IFOSF/CDDP	155 (151)[b]	19 (12.5)	28 (18.5)	47 (31)[c]	8.3
vs.					
CDDP	146 (140)[b]	9 (6.5)	16 (11.5)	25 (18)[c]	8
BLM/IFOSF/CDDP	50 (46)[b]	12 (26)	12 (26)	24 (52)[d]	8
vs.					
CDDP	56 (51)[b]	5 (10)	10 (20)	15 (29)[d]	6

Note: BLM, bleomycin; CDDP, cisplatin (dose in all studies and in all arms 50 mg/m^2); DBD, dibromodulcitol; DVA, vindesine; IFOSF, ifosfamide; MMC, mitomycin C.
[a] $p = 0.03$
[b] Numbers evaluable for response
[c] $p = 0.004$
[d] $p < 0.01$

from 21% to 31% (451). However, there was only a minimal increase in the complete response rate (from 10% to 13%) and no improvement in response duration, progression-free interval, or survival. A small study performed at the Memorial Sloan-Kettering Cancer Center using 200 mg/m^2 of cisplatin (and sodium thiosulfate nephroprotection) suggested no further increase in response rate with these higher dosages, and toxicity was unacceptably high (452).

Response rates with combination chemotherapy have varied from 0% to nearly 100% in individual reports, reflecting sample size, differences in response assessment criteria, and patient characteristics. However, cumulative data indicate that a response rate of about 40% can be expected in well-selected patients. Randomized clinical trials that compared combination chemotherapy regimens to single-agent cisplatin have demonstrated improved objective response rates and progression-free survival without improvement in overall survival (Table 22.8) (453–455). A recent randomized clinical trial (456) was the first to demonstrate an overall survival advantage for combination chemotherapy over single-agent cisplatin. Topotecan (0.75 mg/m) days 1 to 3 with cisplatin (50 mg/m^2) day 1, repeated every 21 days demonstrated a significant improvement in objective response rate (27% vs. 13%; $p = 0.004$), progression-free survival (4.6 vs. 2.9 months; $p = 0.014$), and overall survival (9.4 vs. 6.5 months; $p = 0.017$). The figures for single-agent cisplatin were considerably lower than in previous trials with cisplatin, suggesting that the advantage for the combination could represent reduced efficacy of cisplatin in this patient population due to prior platin exposure during concurrent chemoradiation for primary treatment (57%). For those with no prior platin exposure the progression-free survival was 6.9 versus 3.2 months and overall survival 15.4 versus 8.8 months favoring the combination. Nevertheless, this was the first randomized clinical trial to demonstrate a survival advantage for combination chemotherapy over single-agent cisplatin in this patient population. Despite increased hematologic toxicity of this combination, a concurrent quality of life study failed to demonstrate any reduction in the quality of life of treated patients for the combination compared to the single agent (457). An individual approach to these patients is warranted. Identification of a subset of patients who might benefit from chemotherapy would be a major advance. Any decision for treatment of cervical cancer patients in the palliative setting should be assessed against the benefit of best supportive care, which may provide the best option for some of these patients.

COMPLICATIONS AND SEQUELAE OF TREATMENT

Surgery Related

The most common complications with conization include infection, bleeding, damage to surrounding structures (bladder, rectum, vagina), and cervical incompetence with predisposition to preterm labor in future pregnancies. Radical hysterectomy and lymphadenectomy may result in additional and somewhat unique complications. Urologic complications such as ureteral injuries and vesicovaginal or ureterovaginal fistulas are reported in 1% to 2% of cases, and this can be increased in patients requiring postoperative RT (318). Most vesicovaginal fistulas can be diagnosed with a voiding cystogram or clinically by infusion of a diluted methylene blue solution into the bladder and observation of leakage into the vaginal vault commonly known as the "tampon test." The majority will heal spontaneously with continuous bladder drainage for 6 to 8 weeks and treatment of any underlying infection. Ureterovaginal fistulas may be more difficult to diagnose. An intravenous pyelogram or CT scan may be indicated and demonstrate such a fistula in a patient with symptoms suggestive of a urinary fistula with a negative clinical exam or cystogram. Conservative management can include ureteral stenting and drainage of the urinary system via percutaneous nephrostomy, which may lead to healing of the fistula. Repeat imaging should be done prior to removal of the stent to assure ureteral healing. Repair of a persistent vesicovaginal fistula can be attempted vaginally, depending on the site of injury. The fistulous tract is excised and repaired in multiple layers, followed by continuous bladder drainage and repeat cystogram to ensure surgical success. Ureteral fistulas that do not resolve with conservative management may require reimplantation of the ureter into the bladder (ureteroneocystotomy). Fistulas that occur following pelvic RT are less likely to heal with conservative management and may require earlier surgical treatment. As surgical repair after RT has a lower success rate, urinary diversion may be required as definitive treatment.

Averette et al. published their experience with RH in 978 patients over 25 years. The surgical mortality was 1.4%, and the urinary fistula rate was 1.4% (458). Artman et al. published their experience with RH in 275 patients over 21 years. The average blood loss was 1,800 cc. The urinary fistula rate was 2.6%, and the surgical mortality rate was 0.7% (459). Lee et al. reported a fistula rate of 2.4% and an operative mortality of 0.4% in a series of 954 patients. Lymphocyst formation is about 1.6% and the lymphedema rate is about 3.6% following pelvic lymph node dissection (LND) (460).

Located over the sacral promontory, the hypogastric plexus contains sympathetic fibers that fuse with parasympathetic fibers located in the parametrium and allows for bladder contraction and compliance. Surgical disruption of this plexus results in bladder atony and dysfunction in about 5% of patients, possibly requiring continuous or intermittent drainage for a few weeks (461). Efforts have been made to incorporate nerve-sparing techniques into the radical hysterectomy procedure, and these efforts continue (462).

Farquharson et al. compared bladder function after RH versus RH plus RT. They found that bladder compliance was significantly reduced when RT was added to RH (463). Ralph et al. performed urologic evaluations in 40 patients at 2 weeks, 6 months, and 1 year after RH. At 2 weeks all had impaired bladder sensation and 68% had residual urine after voiding. At 1 year, 63% had impaired bladder sensation. Bladder capacity was lowest at 2 weeks (180 mL) and returned to baseline between 6 to 12 months. By 1 year, patients had residual urine after voiding. However, 62% had abnormal compliance and 85% used abdominal straining to void (464).

Rectal function can also be impacted by RH. Schreuder et al. used a questionnaire to evaluate rectal function after RH in 48 patients; 18% had constipation, 33% required chronic straining, and 60% required laxative or manual assistance with defecation. The incidence of chronic constipation was >20% (465). Barnes et al. used manometric studies to demonstrate that all patients had normal manometric studies preoperatively, and all had abnormal manometric studies postoperatively. Changes included altered relaxation of the internal sphincter, increased distention required to trigger relaxation, and decreased rectal sensation. Twelve of 15 patients reported rectal dysfunction (466).

It has been suggested that inflammatory change induced by conization increases the risk of complications from subsequent RH. A waiting period of 6 weeks between procedures has been advocated on this basis. Orr et al. reviewed 122 patients who had undergone conization followed by RH. The interval between conization and RH ranged from 48 hours to 6 weeks (467). Similarly, Samlal et al. evaluated 68 patients with conization followed by RH (468). Both reported no difference in complications related to differing intervals of time from conization to RH.

Levrant et al. evaluated the effects of obesity and age on RH outcomes. They reported no difference in survival or complications in obese versus nonobese patients. Similarly, age did not affect long-term complications and survival. However, patients older than 65 did have a higher incidence of postoperative ileus (469). Cohn et al. reported on 48 obese women (median body mass index [BMI] of 36 kg/m^2) who underwent RH. Median blood loss was 800 cc, and the median number of lymph nodes obtained was 26. Margins were uninvolved in 98%. This study also confirmed the safety and efficacy of RH in selected obese patients (470).

Methods to decrease postoperative complications following RH have been suggested. Franchi et al. evaluated the role of pelvic drains following RH with LND in a randomized trial of pelvic drainage versus none. No difference was noted in lymphocyst formation or postoperative complications, suggesting that drains can be safely omitted following RH (471). The omental J flap has been used in gynecologic oncology for pelvic reconstruction. Patsner and Hackett evaluated 140 patients who had an omental J flap placed following RH. No urinary complications or infections were noted, even in patients who received postoperative RT (472). These data suggest that an omental J flap may decrease postoperative complication rate, although there was no control arm for comparison.

Radiation Therapy Related

Acute effects during external pelvic RT most typically include diarrhea and bladder irritation. These are usually self-limited and can be managed effectively with conservative measures. Most late gastrointestinal and urologic complications occur within the first 3 years after RT, with an overall fistula rate of about 2%. Post-radiation fistulae can be difficult to manage as most will not heal spontaneously and local corrective procedures may prove unsuccessful. Patients with large fistulas may require diversion. Factors that may increase the rate of fistula are combined treatment (surgery and RT), smoking, thin habitus, inflammatory bowel diseases, and diabetes and other vasculopathies.

Late sequelae are often permanent or require some intervention to improve. Commonly reported late sequelae of pelvic RT involve the rectosigmoid, the small intestine, the genitourinary tract, the vagina, and other sites or organs, resulting, for example, in lymphedema, lumbosacral plexopathy, and pelvic insufficiency fractures. Rectosigmoid complications include chronic proctosigmoiditis, rectal stricture, and rectal ulcer. Complications involving the small intestine include obstruction and malabsorption syndrome. It is accepted that predisposing factors for injury, particularly to small bowel, include a history of abdominopelvic surgery and pelvic inflammatory disease. Furthermore, it appears that radiation enteritis is not a single disease entity, but rather a variety of diagnoses that manifest with similar symptoms. Accurate diagnosis is essential to proper management. It does not appear that specific symptoms have a reliable relationship to the underlying process (473). Genitourinary toxicity includes chronic cystitis, bladder contracture, urethral stricture, and incontinence. Late sequelae involving the vagina include vaginal stenosis/fibrosis, dyspareunia, vault necrosis, and rectovaginal or vesicovaginal fistulae.

There is approximately a 5% rate of major late sequelae in patients with stage I cervical carcinoma treated with RT, and approximately 10% in patients with stages II-IVA disease. Grade 2 complications are seen in 10% to 15% of patients with all stages treated with RT alone (474,475). However, the risk is related to a number of factors, mainly dose and volume treated.

Perez et al. reported a <2% risk of severe small bowel toxicity when the pelvic sidewall dose was <50 Gy, and a 5% incidence with doses >60 Gy (474). In a multivariate analysis, Perez et al. found only total doses to rectal and bladder points to significantly impact morbidity (475). Many investigators have found a significant relationship between radiation dose and complications. A greater incidence of pelvic complications has been consistently observed in patients treated with higher doses to the whole pelvis (above 40 to 50 Gy). Intracavitary dose from radium or cesium does not correlate closely with severe complications. Injury to the gastrointestinal tract is the most frequent late complication of RT for cervical cancer. The rate of chronic bowel injury is 5% to 15% in most series of patients treated with pelvic RT (476). Although these injuries may take years to manifest, Iraha et al. reported a median latency period of 10 months (476). A report by Eifel et al. (477) on 1,784 patients with stage IB carcinoma of the cervix indicates that the greatest risk is in the first 3 years after therapy. The risk of rectal complications declined after the first 2 years of follow-up to 0.06% per year. Major complications include intestinal obstruction, fistula formation, severe bleeding, and intractable diarrhea. Fortunately, these sequelae are relatively infrequent. These injuries generally result from fibrosis and ischemia secondary to the effect of RT on the small blood vessels and connective tissue. Conservative management might include a low residue diet, antidiarrheal medications, and steroid or sucralfate enemas. Some cases of partial small bowel obstruction can be managed by bowel rest, decompression, and diet modification. Obstruction refractory to conservative management may require surgery involving intestinal resection, and/or end-to-end anastomoses.

Chronic urinary symptoms (urgency, incontinence, and frequency) are frequently seen following RT. Parkin et al. (478) reported a 26% incidence of these symptoms in patients treated with RT alone for cervical carcinoma. The authors found that the mean volume of full bladder sensation was significantly lower in the post-RT group than in the pretreatment group, as was the mean maximum cystometric capacity.

Severe genitourinary toxicities secondary to RT include hemorrhagic cystitis and fistula in 2% to 3% (474,475). The latency period between RT and symptom onset is considerably longer than for gastrointestinal sequelae. In the longitudinal study by Eifel et al. (477), the risk of major urinary tract complications for survivors continued at 0.3% per year beyond 20 years. At 20 years, the actuarial risk of major complications was 14.4%. Lajer et al. prospectively gathered data regarding urologic morbidity in 177 consecutive patients treated curatively with RT (479). The 5-year actuarial incidences of grades 1 + 2 + 3, 2 + 3, and 3 were 62%, 32%, and 5%, respectively. In the long-term recurrence-free survivors, there was evidence of some reversibility of grade 1 and 2 morbidities.

Vaginal function can be affected by both radical surgery and RT. Surgery will shorten the functional length of the vagina, but pliability and transudative lubrication are often preserved. Radiation therapy can reduce length, caliber, and lubrication of the vagina; however, these symptoms can be alleviated in some patients with hormonal replacement and vaginal dilatation. Although some gynecologists feel that radical pelvic surgery may affect vaginal function to a lesser degree than RT, a large Swedish study found that the type of treatment had virtually no effect on the prevalence of vaginal changes and sexual distress (480).

Although extremely rare, lumbosacral plexopathy has been occasionally reported in patients treated for pelvic tumors with doses of 60 to 68 Gy. Characteristically, these patients have lower motor neuron weakness of the legs combined with loss of deep reflexes and muscular fasciculation. The differential diagnosis of lumbosacral plexopathy with recurrent tumors is sometimes difficult. Generally, weakness is more prominent in radiation-related plexopathy, and pain is more frequently seen in tumor-related cases. Muscular weakness, numbness, and paresthesias are common in both groups.

Insufficiency fracture occurs with normal stress in bone with diminished elastic flexibility, a condition that can exist in irradiated bones. The usual presenting symptom is moderate to severe pelvic pain. Huh et al. reported that 8 out of 463 patients (1.7%) developed this complication (481). All patients were postmenopausal, and seven of eight were treated with curative intent. Differential diagnosis can include metastatic disease, tumor recurrence, second malignancy, and benign causes. Because symptoms can resolve with conservative management, proper diagnosis is important.

High doses of RT can cause obliterative endarteritis, reactive fibrosis, and decreased vascularity and oxygenation. As a result, soft-tissue injury can occur, and this can be particularly problematic in the treatment of cervical cancer extending to the distal vagina. Careful attention to radiation planning and dosimetry, careful blocking, and avoidance of unnecessary dose to the perineum during brachytherapy will make these complications less common. Although these injuries can cause pain that can be difficult to distinguish clinically from recurrent disease, the possibility of radiation injury should be kept in mind, because it is advisable to try to avoid deep biopsies or other trauma to tissues in which perfusion is compromised. For refractory radiation-related ulceration and necrosis of the vagina, vulva, and soft tissues, hyperbaric oxygen therapy has been used with some success (482).

Low-dose-rate (and pulsed LDR) implants require hospitalization and bed rest. At typical dose rates of 50 to 60 cGy per hour, implants typically last 2 or 3 days. During this time, there is the potential for acute problems related to or during the hospital stay. However, Jhingran and Eifel reviewed 7,662 implants in 4,043 patients, finding fatal or life-threatening complications to be exceptionally rare (483).

Combined Modality Related

Irradiation Followed by Surgery

Eifel et al. reported a series of patients with stage IB cervical carcinoma treated with RT. At 3 and 5 years, 7.7% and 9.3% experienced major complications; the actuarial risk of major complications was 14.4% at 20 years. The rate of fistula formation was doubled in those who underwent adjuvant hysterectomy (5.3% vs. 2.6%) (477).

In a GOG study reported by Keys et al., 256 patients with stage IB carcinomas of the cervix ≥4 cm confined to the cervix were treated with either external RT and intracavitary irradiation, or with external RT and a lower dose of intracavitary irradiation followed by an extrafascial hysterectomy. The toxicities were similar in both groups with grade 3 and 4 toxicities of about 10% in each arm (230). Meticulous, sharp dissection is recommended in the performance of extrafascial hysterectomy following preoperative RT.

Coleman et al. studied 50 patients managed with RH for persistent or recurrent disease limited to the cervix after pelvic RT. Severe toxicities occurred in 42%, and 28% developed GI or GU fistulas (443).

Surgery Followed by Irradiation

Radical operation commonly results in intestinal adhesions to denuded surfaces in the pelvis. When postoperative RT is given, complications are more likely. The GOG demonstrated a significant increase in grade 2 to 4 late complications among patients undergoing pre-RT surgical staging, particularly with a transperitoneal approach compared with a retroperitoneal

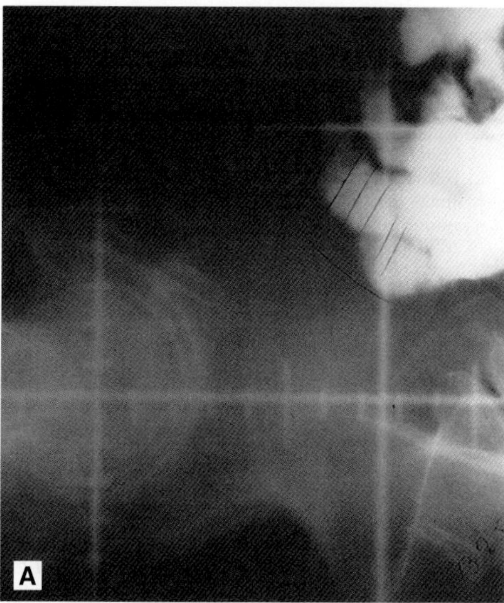
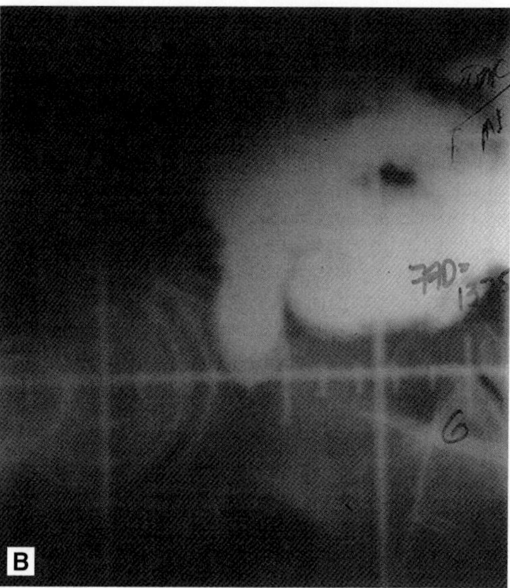

FIGURE 22.22. (A and B): Lateral radiographs with and without bladder distention in a patient with contrast in small intestine.

approach (484). Pretreatment laparotomy also increased the rate of fistula formation (5.2% vs. 2.9%) as well as small bowel obstruction (14.5% vs. 3.7%) (477). An extraperitoneal approach to lymph node staging purposes lessens these complications (67).

In a randomized study of postoperative RT versus no further treatment (NFT) after RH, Sedlis et al. found that grade 3 to 4 GU toxicities occurred in 3.1% in the RT versus 1.4% in the NFT arm. Grade 3 to 4 GI toxicities were 3.1% versus 0.8%, respectively. The overall grade 3 to 4 toxicity was 6% in the RT group versus 2.1% in the NFT arm (318).

Kim et al. presented an analysis of 800 patients with stages IB-IIB cervical cancer who received postoperative RT following RH and bilateral salpingo-oophorectomy (BSO). With a median follow-up of 100 months, the incidences of late injuries (grade 3 to 4) were 1.6%, 1.4%, and 1.0% for rectum, bladder, and small bowel, respectively (383).

Methods to decrease the volume of small bowel irradiated will further lessen enteric morbidity. Figures 22.22 and 22.23 show the effect of treating patients in the prone position with a full bladder as a means of limiting the volume of small bowel irradiated. Similarly, IMRT techniques can also be used to limit doses to normal tissues (Figs. 22.14 and 22.16A and B) (314).

Concurrent Chemoradiation

As concurrent chemoradiation has become standard management for most patients treated nonsurgically for cervical cancer, it is not surprising that additional hematologic toxicity has been seen. A major concern has been the possible need to delay treatment, thus potentially compromising outcomes. Typical RT fields radiate some pelvic bone marrow, and Mell et al. have shown that as the volume of marrow receiving ≥10 Gy (V_{10}) increases, the incidence of grade 2 or worse leucopenia and neutropenia increases (485). No association of V_{30} and V_{40} with hematologic toxicity was observed. A role for IMRT to limit hematologic toxicity in some patients was suggested but not proven in this study. On the contrary, Chen et al. reported 68 patients who received

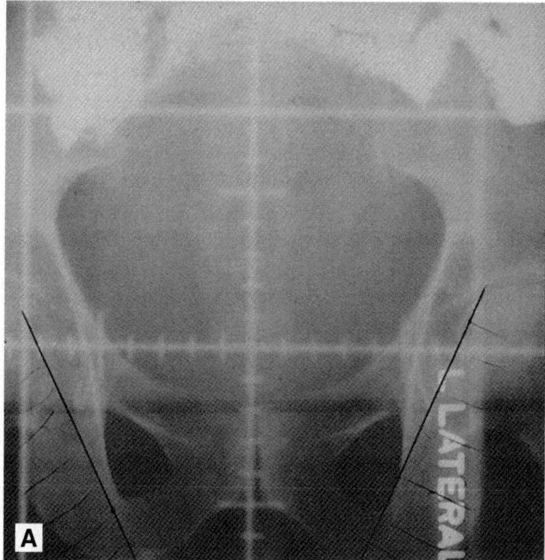

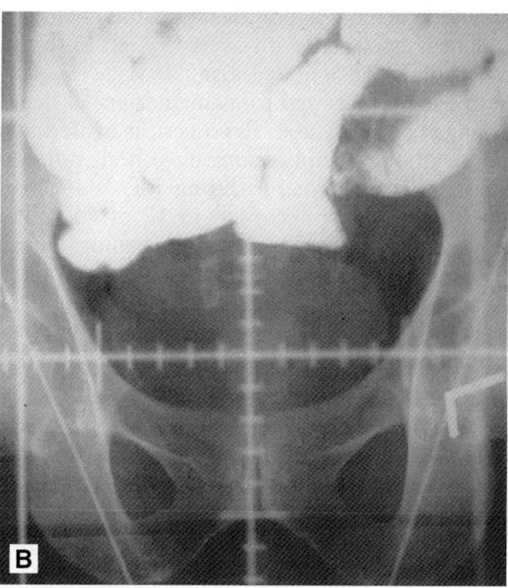

FIGURE 22.23. (A and B): Anterior-posterior radiographs with and without bladder distention in a patient with contrast in small intestine.

pelvic IMRT with concurrent chemotherapy. Compared to non-IMRT historic controls, patients receiving IMRT had significantly lower acute and late GI and GU effects (486). A possible role for single photon emission computed tomography (SPECT) in individualizing dose distribution to optimize functional marrow sparing has been suggested (484).

Although some early series suggested that concurrent chemotherapy increased late complications in patients receiving curative intent RT, most studies suggest no significant impact (487). However, some unusual complications have been reported that are rarely if ever seen with RT alone. Subacute neurologic toxicity including radiation myelitis can occur with extended field RT combined with chemotherapy. In a case reported by Bloss et al., this devastating complication was seen with only 45 Gy in 30 fractions given to the para-aortic chain along with cisplatin (50 mg/m^2) and 5-FU continuous infusion at 300 mg/m^2 per day during RT (488). A latent period of 4 months was observed in this case. Coulombe et al. reported an additional two patients who developed lower extremity weakness and paresthesia that began 1 and 4 months following extended field RT of 45 Gy in 25 fractions concurrent with weekly cisplatin at 40 mg/m^2 (489). Clinical and electromyography (EMG) findings were consistent with neuropathy, and potential causes other than chemoradiation were felt to be ruled out. One patient showed spontaneous improvement beginning at 10 months. A case of complete uterine necrosis following chemoradiation has also been reported (490).

Early studies suggest that amifostine, a cytoprotectant and radioprotectant, is reasonably well tolerated when combined with RT and cisplatin. Data is limited regarding its ability to decrease complications; however, clinical trials are ongoing (349).

Thromboembolic Complications

Clarke-Pearson et al. (491) reported the experience of thromboembolic complications in 281 consecutive patients who underwent radical surgery for cervical and uterine malignancies. Postoperative thromboembolic complications were experienced in 7.8% of patients despite regular use of low-dose heparin and antiembolism stockings during the postoperative hospitalization. Preoperative risk factors included weight in excess of 85.5 kg, clinical stage II malignancy, and preoperative RT within 6 weeks of the surgical procedure. Jacobson et al. (492) reported a 16.7% incidence of thromboembolic complications in 48 patients who received chemoradiation therapy without surgery. Brachytherapy alone is associated with a very low rate of thromboembolic complications, 0.3% in one series (483).

Erythropoietin has been utilized to maintain normal hemoglobin levels during chemoradiation. Reports of increased incidence of thromboembolic complications have been noted in patients who receive erythropoietin during RT. Wun et al. reported thromboembolic complications in 17 of 75 (23%) patients who received erythropoietin during chemoradiation compared to 2 of 72 (3%) who did not receive erythropoietin (493). A survey of the literature regarding this phenomenon has been presented (159). The routine use of erythropoietin to maintain normal hemoglobin levels during chemoradiation should be discouraged.

References

1. Ferlay J, Bray F, Pisani P, et al. *GLOBOCAN 2000: Cancer Incidence, Mortality, and Prevalence Worldwide*. Version 1.1, IARC Cancer Base No. 5. Lyon: IARC Press; 2001.
2. Franco EL, Duarte-Franco E, Ferenczy A. Cervical cancer: epidemiology, prevention and the role of human papillomavirus infection. *Can Med Assoc J* 2001;164:1017–1025.
3. Jemal A, Siegel R, Ward E, et al. Cancer statistics, 2007. *CA Cancer J Clin* 2007;57:43–66.
4. Saslow D, Castle PE, Cox JT, et al. American Cancer Society guideline for human papilloma virus (HPV) vaccine use to prevent cervical cancer and its precursors. *CA Cancer J Clin* 2007;57:7–28.
5. Winkelstein W. Smoking and cervical cancer: current status—a review. *Am J Epidemiol* 1990;131:945–957.
6. Tolstrup J, Munk C, Thomsen BL, et al. The role of smoking and alcohol intake in the development of high-grade squamous intraepithelial lesions among high-risk HPV-positive women. *Acta Obstet Gynecol Scand* 2006;85(9):1114–1119.
7. Jay N, Moscicki AB. Human papillomavirus infections in women with HIV disease: prevalence, risk and management. *AIDS Read* 2000;10: 659–668.
8. Smith JS, Lindsay L, Hoots B, et al. Human papillomavirus type distribution in invasive cervical cancer and high-grade cervical lesions: a meta-analysis update. *Int J Cancer* 2007;121:621–632.
9. Munoz N, Bosch FX, de Sanjose S, et al. Epidemiologic classification of human papillomavirus types associated with cervical cancer. *N Engl J Med* 2003;348(6):518–527.
10. Clifford GM, Smith JS, Plummer M, et al. Human papillomavirus types in invasive cervical cancer worldwide: a meta-analysis. *Br J Cancer* 2003;88(1): 63–73.
11. zur Hausen H. Papillomaviruses causing cancer: evasion from host-cell control in early events in carcinogenesis. *J Natl Cancer Inst* 2000;92: 690–698.
12. Castellsagué X, Diaz M, de Sanjosé S, et al. Worldwide human papillomavirus etiology of cervical adenocarcinoma and its cofactors: implications for screening and prevention. *J Natl Cancer Inst* 2006;98:303–315.
13. Horn L, Lindner K, Szepankiewicz G, et al. p16, p14, p53, and cyclin D1 expression and HPV analysis in small cell carcinomas of the uterine cervix. *Int J Gynecol Pathol* 2006;25:182–186.
14. Monnier-Benoit S, Mauny F, Riethmuller D, et al. Immunohistochemical analysis of CD4+ and CD8+ T-cell subsets in high risk human papillomavirus-associated pre-malignant and malignant lesions of the uterine cervix. *Gynecol Oncol* 2006;102:22–31.
15. Ho GY, Bierman R, Beardsley L, et al. Natural history of cervicovaginal papillomavirus infection in young women. *N Engl J Med* 1998;338: 423–428.
16. Franco EL, Villa LL, Sobrinho JP, et al. Epidemiology of acquisition and clearance of cervical human papillomavirus infection in women from a high-risk area for cervical cancer. *J Infect Dis* 1999;180:1415–1423.
17. Duerr A, Paramsothy P, Jamieson DJ, et al. Effect of HIV infection on atypical squamous cells of undetermined significance. *Clin Infect Dis* 2006;42:855–861.
18. Lehtovirta P, Finne P, Nieminen P, et al. Prevalence and risk factors of squamous intraepithelial lesions of the cervix among HIV-infected women: a long-term follow-up study in a low-prevalence population. *Int J Std AIDS* 2006;17:831–834.
19. Jones BA, Davey DD. Quality management in gynecologic cytology using interlaboratory comparison. *Arch Pathol Lab Med* 2000;124: 672–681.
20. ACOG Practice Bulletin. Clinical management guidelines for obstetricians-gynecologists. Human papillomavirus. *Obstet Gynecol* 2005;105(61):905.
21. Herrero R. Epidemiology of cervical cancer. *J Natl Cancer Inst Monogr* 1996;21:1–6.
22. Holowaty P, Miller AB, Rohan T, et al. Natural history of dysplasia of the uterine cervix. *J Natl Cancer Inst* 1999;91:252–258.
23. Melnikow J, Nuovo J, Willan AR, et al. Natural history of cervical squamous intraepithelial lesions: a meta-analysis. *Obstet Gynecol* 1998;92: 727–735.
24. McIndoe WA, McLean MR, Jones RW, et al. The invasive potential of carcinoma *in situ* of the cervix. *Obstet Gynecol* 1984;64:451–458.
25. Creasman WT, Soper JT, Clarke-Pearson D. Radical hysterectomy as therapy for early carcinoma of the cervix. *Am J Obstet Gynecol* 1986;155: 964–969.
26. Samlal RA, van der Velden J, Ten Kate FJ, et al. Surgical pathologic factors that predict recurrence in stage IB and IIA cervical carcinoma patients with negative pelvic lymph nodes. *Cancer* 1997;80:1234–1240.
27. Berman ML, Keys H, Creasman W, et al. Survival and patterns of recurrence in cervical cancer metastatic to periaortic lymph nodes (a Gynecologic Oncology Group study). *Gynecol Oncol* 1984;19:8–16.
28. Vasilev SA, Schlaerth JB. Scalene lymph node sampling in cervical carcinoma: a reappraisal. *Gynecol Oncol* 1990;37:120–124.
29. Girardi F, Lichtenegger W, Tamussino K, et al. The importance of parametrial lymph nodes in the treatment of cervical cancer. *Gynecol Oncol* 1989;34:206–211.
30. Takehara K, Shigemasa K, Sawasaki T, et al. Recurrence of invasive cervical carcinoma more than 5 years after initial therapy. *Obstet Gynecol* 2001;98:680–684.
31. Ries LAG, Melbert D, Krapcho M, et al., eds. *SEER Cancer Statistics Review, 1975-2004*. http://seer.cancer.gov/csr/1975_2004/. Bethesda, MD: National Cancer Institute. Based on November 2006 SEER data submission, posted to the SEER Web site, 2007.
32. Parkin DM, Pisani P, Ferlay J. Global cancer statistics. *CA Cancer J Clin* 1999;49:33–64.

33. Nanda K, McCrory DC, Myers ER, et al. Accuracy of the Papanicolaou test in screening for and follow-up of cervical cytologic abnormalities: a systematic review. *Ann Intern Med* 2000;132:810–819.
34. Hutchinson ML, Zahniser DJ, Sherman ME, et al. Utility of liquid-based cytology for cervical carcinoma screening: results of a population-based study conducted in a region of Costa Rica with a high incidence of cervical carcinoma. *Cancer* 1999;87:48–55.
35. Sulik SM, Kroeger K, Schultz JK, et al. Are fluid-based cytologies superior to the conventional Papanicolaou test? A systematic review. *J Fam Pract* 2001;50:1040–1046.
36. ACOG Practice Bulletin. Clinical management guidelines for obstetricians-gynecologists. Cervical cytology screening. *Obstet Gynecol* 2003;45.
37. Saslow D, Runowicz CD, Solomon D, et al. American Cancer Society guidelines for the early detection of cervical neoplasia and cancer. *CA Cancer J Clin* 2002;52:342–362.
38. ACOG Practice Bulletin. Clinical management guidelines for obstetricians-gynecologists. Human papillomavirus. *Obstet Gynecol* 2005;61.
39. Solomon D, Davey D, Kurman R, et al. The 2001 Bethesda system: terminology for reporting results of cervical cytology. *JAMA* 2002;287: 2114–2119.
40. Solomon D, Schiffman M, Tarone R, ALTS Study Group. Comparison of three management strategies for patients with atypical squamous cells of undetermined significance: baseline results from a randomized trial. *J Natl Cancer Inst* 2001;93:293–299.
41. Cox JT, Schiffman M, Solomon D, ASCUS-LSIL Triage Study (ALTS) Group. Prospective follow-up suggests similar risk of subsequent cervical intraepithelial neoplasia grade 2 or 3 among women with cervical intraepithelial neoplasia grade 1 or negative colposcopy and directed biopsy. *Am J Obstet Gynecol* 2003;188:1406–1412.
42. Ancheta E, Perry J, Bernard-Pearl L, et al. Participants at the ASCCP 2000 biennial meeting adhere to published guidelines in their management of atypical squamous cells and atypical glandular cells on Pap test. *J Low Genit Tract Dis* 2003;7:279–284.
43. Sherman ME, Lorincz AT, Scott DR, et al. Baseline cytology, human papillomavirus testing, and risk for cervical neoplasia: a 10-year cohort analysis. *J Natl Cancer Inst* 2003;95:46–52.
44. Clavel C. Value of cervical screening by HPV DNA testing. It is legitimate to type HPV for the primary screening of cervix neoplasms. *Gynecol Obstet Fertil* 2002;30:896–898.
45. Mathevet P, Chemali E, Roy M, et al. Long-term outcome of a randomized study comparing three techniques of conization: cold knife, laser, and LEEP. *Eur J Obstet Gynecol Reprod Biol* 2003;106:214–218.
46. Molina R, Filella X, Auge JM, et al. CYFRA 21.1 in patients with cervical cancer: comparison with SCC and CEA. *Anticancer Res* 2005;25: 1765–1771.
47. Reesink-Peters N, van der Velden J, Ten Hoor KA, et al. Preoperative serum squamous cell carcinoma antigen levels in clinical decision making for patients with early-stage cervical cancer. *J Clin Oncol* 2005;23: 1455–1462.
48. Takeda M, Sakuragi N, Okamoto K, et al. Preoperative serum SCC, CA125, and CA19-9 levels and lymph node status in squamous cell carcinoma of the uterine cervix. *Acta Obstet Gynecol Scand* 2002;81:451–457.
49. Mitchell DG, Snyder B, Coakley F, et al. Early invasive cervical cancer: tumor delineation by magnetic resonance imaging, computed tomography, and clinical examination, verified by pathologic results, in the ACRIN 6651/GOG 183 intergroup study. *J Clin Oncol* 2006;24:5687–5694.
50. Hricak H, Lacey CG, Sandles LG, et al. Invasive cervical carcinoma: comparison of MR imaging and surgical findings. *Radiology* 1988;166:623–631.
51. Bipat S, Glas AS, van der Velden J, et al. Computed tomography and magnetic resonance imaging in staging of uterine cervical carcinoma: a systematic review. *Gynecol Oncol* 2003;91:59–66.
52. Narayan K, McKenzie AF, Hicks RJ, et al. Relation between FIGO stage, primary tumor volume, and presence of lymph node metastases in cervical cancer patients referred for radiotherapy. *Int J Gynecol Cancer* 2003;13: 657–663.
53. Choi SH, Kim SH, Choi HJ, et al. Preoperative magnetic resonance imaging staging of uterine cervical carcinoma: results of prospective study. *J Comput Assist Tomogr* 2004;28:620–627.
54. Park W, Park YJ, Huh SJ, et al. The usefulness of MRI and PET imaging for the detection of parametrial involvement and lymph node metastasis in patients with cervical cancer. *Jpn J Clin Oncol* 2005;35:260–264.
55. Hricak H, Gatsonis C, Chi DS, et al. Role of imaging in pretreatment evaluation of early invasive cervical cancer: results of the intergroup study American College of Radiology Imaging Network 6651-Gynecologic Oncology Group 183. *J Clin Oncol* 2005;23:9329–9337.
56. Subak LL, Hricak H, Powell CB, et al. Cervical carcinoma: computed tomography and magnetic resonance imaging for preoperative staging. *Obstet Gynecol* 1995;86:43–50.
57. Scheidler J, Hricak H, Yu KK, et al. Radiological evaluation of lymph node metastases in patients with cervical cancer. A meta-analysis. *JAMA* 1997;278:1096–1101.
58. Havrilesky LJ, Kulasingam SL, Matchar DB, et al. FDG-PET for management of cervical and ovarian cancer. *Gynecol Oncol* 2005;97:183–191.
59. Grigsby PW, Siegel BA, Dehdashti F. Lymph node staging by positron emission tomography in patients with carcinoma of the cervix. *J Clin Oncol* 2001;19:3745–3749.
60. Loft A, Berthelsen AK, Roed H, et al. The diagnostic value of PET/CT scanning in patients with cervical cancer: a prospective study. *Gynecol Oncol* 2007; 06:29–34.
61. Creasman WT. New gynecologic cancer staging. *Gynecol Oncol* 1995;58: 157–158.
62. American Joint Committee on Cancer (AJCC). Cervix uteri. In: Greene FL, Page DL, Fleming ID, et al., eds. *AJCC Cancer Staging Manual.* 6th ed. New York: Springer; 2002:260.
63. Leblanc F, Narducci F, Chevalier A, et al. Pretherapeutic laparoscopic staging of locally advanced cervical carcinomas: technique and results. *Gynecol Oncol* 2005;99:S157–S158.
64. Leblanc E, Narducci F, Frumovitz M, et al. Therapeutic value of pretherapeutic extraperitoneal laparoscopic staging of locally advanced cervical carcinoma. *Gynecol Oncol* 2007;105:304–311.
65. Lai CH, Huang KG, Hong JH, et al. Randomized trial of surgical staging (extraperitoneal or laparoscopic) versus clinical staging in locally advanced cervical cancer. *Gynecol Oncol* 2003;89:160–167.
66. Gallup DG, King LA, Messing MJ, et al. Para-aortic lymph node sampling by means of an extraperitoneal approach with a supraumbilical transverse "sunrise" incision. *Am J Obstet Gynecol* 1993;169:307–311; discussion 311–312.
67. Querleu D, Dargent D, Ansquer Y, et al. Extraperitoneal endosurgical aortic and common iliac dissection in the staging of bulky or advanced cervical carcinomas. *Cancer* 2000;88:1883–1891.
68. Thompson JF, Uren RF. What is a "sentinel" lymph node? *Eur J Surg Oncol* 2000;26:103–104.
69. Medl M, Peters-Engl C, Schutz P, et al. First report of lymphatic mapping with isosulfan blue dye and sentinel node biopsy in cervical cancer. *Anticancer Res* 2000;20:1133–1134.
70. Dargent D, Martin X, Mathevet P. Laparoscopic assessment of the sentinel lymph node in early stage cervical cancer. *Gynecol Oncol* 2000;79:411–415.
71. O'Boyle JD, Coleman RL, Bernstein SG, et al. Intraoperative lymphatic mapping in cervix cancer patients undergoing radical hysterectomy: a pilot study. *Gynecol Oncol* 2000;79:238–243.
72. Levenback C, Coleman RL, Burke TW, et al. Lymphatic mapping and sentinel node identification in patients with cervix cancer undergoing radical hysterectomy and pelvic lymphadenectomy. *J Clin Oncol* 2002;20: 688–693.
73. Lambaudie E, Collinet P, Narducci F, et al. Laparoscopic identification of sentinel lymph nodes in early stage cervical cancer: prospective study using a combination of patent blue dye injection and technetium radiocolloid injection. *Gynecol Oncol* 2003;89:84–87.
74. Plante M, Renaud MC, Tetu B, et al. Laparoscopic sentinel node mapping in early-stage cervical cancer. *Gynecol Oncol* 2003;91:494–503.
75. Darai E, Lavoue' V, Rouzier R, et al. Contribution of the sentinel node procedure to tailoring the radicality of hysterectomy for cervical cancer. *Gynecol Oncol* 2007;106:251–256.
76. Frumovitz M, Coleman RL, Gayed IW, et al. Usefulness of preoperative lymphoscintigraphy in patients who undergo radical hysterectomy and pelvic lymphadenectomy for cervical cancer. *Am J Obstet Gynecol* 2006;194:1186–1193; discussion 1193–1195.
77. Wydra D, Sawicki S, Wojtylak S, et al. Sentinel node identification in cervical cancer patients undergoing transperitoneal radical hysterectomy: a study of 100 cases. *Int J Gynecol Cancer* 2006;16:649–654.
78. Malpica A, Matisic JP, Van Niekirk D, et al. Kappa statistics to measure interrater and intrarater agreement for 1790 cervical biopsy specimens among twelve pathologists: qualitative histopathologic analysis and methodologic issues. *Gynecol Oncol* 2005;99:S38–S52.
79. Kristensen GB, Abeler VM, Risberg B, et al. Tumor size, depth of invasion and grading of the invasive tumor front are the main prognostic factors in early squamous cell cervical carcinoma. *Gynecol Oncol* 1999;74:245–251.
80. Grayson W, Cooper K. A reappraisal of "basaloid carcinoma" of the cervix, and the differential diagnosis of basaloid cervical neoplasms. *Adv Anat Pathol* 2002;9:290–300.
81. Kashimura M, Tsukamoto N, Matsukuma K, et al. Verrucous carcinoma of the uterine cervix: report of a case with follow-up of 6 1/2 years. *Gynecol Oncol* 1984;19:204–215.
82. Randall ME, Andersen WA, Mills SE, et al. Papillary squamous cell carcinoma of the uterine cervix: a clinicopathologic study of nine cases. *Int J Gynecol Pathol* 1986;5:1–10.
83. Koenig C, Turnicky RP, Collins FK, et al. Papillary squamotransitional cell carcinoma of the cervix: a report of 32 cases. *Am J Surg Pathol* 1997;21: 915–921.
84. Drew PA, Hong B, Massoll NA, et al. Characterization of papillary squamotransitional cell carcinoma of the cervix. *J Lower Genital Tract Dis* 2005;9:149–153.
85. Kurman RJ, Norris HJ, Wilkinson E. Tumors of the cervix, vagina, and vulva. In: *Atlas of Tumor Pathology.* 3rd Series, Fascicle 4. Washington, DC: Armed Forces Institute of Pathology; 1992.
86. Tseng CJ, Pao CC, Tseng LH, et al. Lymphoepithelioma-like carcinoma of the uterine cervix: association with Epstein-Barr virus and human papillomavirus. *Cancer* 2000;80:91–97.
87. Martorell MA, Julian JM, Calabuig C, et al. Lymphoepithelioma-like carcinoma of the uterine cervix. A clinicopathologic study of 4 cases not associated with Epstein-Barr virus, human papillomavirus, or simian virus 40. *Arch Pathol Lab Med* 2002;126:1501–1505.

88. Noel J, Lespagnard L, Fayt I, et al. Evidence of human papilloma virus infection but lack of Epstein-Barr virus in lymphoepithelioma-like carcinoma of uterine cervix: report of two cases and review of the literature. *Hum Pathol* 2001;32:135–138.
89. Saylam K, Anaf V, Fayt I, et al. Lymphoepithelioma-like carcinoma of the cervix with prominent eosinophilic infiltrate: an HPV associated case. *Acta Obstet Gynecol Scand* 2002;81:564–566.
90. Bais AG, Kooi S, Teune TM, et al. Lymphoepithelioma-like carcinoma of the uterine cervix: absence of Epstein-Barr virus, but presence of a multiple human papillomavirus infection. *Gynecol Oncol* 2005;97:716–718.
91. Zaino RJ. Symposium part I: adenocarcinoma *in situ*, glandular dysplasia, and early invasive adenocarcinoma of the uterine cervix. *Int J Gynecol Pathol* 2002;21:314–326.
92. Young RH, Clement PB. Endocervical adenocarcinoma and its variants: their morphology and differential diagnosis. *Histopathology* 2002;41:185–207.
93. McCluggage WG. Endocervical glandular lesions: controversial aspects and ancillary techniques. *J Clin Pathol* 2003;56:164–173.
94. Wheeler D, Kurman RJ. The relationship of glands to thick-wall blood vessels as a marker of invasion in endocervical adenocarcinoma. *Int J Gynecol Pathol* 2005;24:125–130.
95. Pirog EC, Kleter B, Olgac S, et al. Prevalence of human papillomavirus DNA in different histological subtypes of cervical adenocarcinoma. *Am J Pathol* 2000;157:1055–1062.
96. McKelvey JL, Goodlin RR. Adenoma malignum of the cervix. *Cancer* 1963;16:549–557.
97. Michael H, Grawe L, Kraus FT. Minimal deviation endocervical adenocarcinoma: clinical and histologic features, immunohistochemical staining for carcinoembryonic antigen, and differentiation from confusing benign lesions. *Int J Gynecol Pathol* 1984;3:261–276.
98. Hart WR. Special types of adenocarcinoma of the uterine cervix. *Int J Gynecol Pathol* 2002;21:327–346.
99. An HJ, Kim KR, Kim IS, et al. Prevalence of human papillomavirus DNA in various histological subtypes of cervical adenocarcinoma: a population-based study. *Mod Pathol* 2005;18:528–534.
100. Jones MW, Silverberg SG, Kurman RJ. Well-differentiated villoglandular adenocarcinoma of the uterine cervix: a clinicopathological study of 24 cases. *Int J Gynecol Pathol* 1993;12:1–7.
101. Jones MW, Kounelis S, Papadaki H, et al. Well-differentiated villoglandular adenocarcinoma of the uterine cervix: oncogene/tumor suppressor gene alterations and human papillomavirus genotyping. *Int J Gynecol Pathol* 2000;19:110–117.
102. Fadare O, Zheng W. Well-differentiated papillary villoglandular adenocarcinoma of the uterine cervix with a focal high-grade component: is there a need for reassessment? *Virchows Arch* 2005;447:883–887.
103. Macdonald RD, Kirwan J, Hayat K, et al. Villoglandular adenocarcinoma of the cervix: clarity is needed on the histological definition for this difficult diagnosis. *Gynecol Oncol* 2006;100:192–194.
104. Chang SH, Maddox WA. Adenocarcinoma arising within cervical endometriosis and invading the adjacent vagina. *Am J Obstet Gynecol* 1971;110:1015–1017.
105. Gilks CB, Clement PB. Papillary serous adenocarcinoma of the uterine cervix: a report of three cases. *Mod Pathol* 1992;5:426–431.
106. Zhou C, Gilks CB, Hayes M, et al. Papillary serous carcinoma of the uterine cervix: a clinicopathologic study of 17 cases. *Am J Surg Pathol* 1998;22:113–120.
107. Clement PB, Young RH, Keh P, et al. Malignant mesonephric neoplasms of the uterine cervix: a report of eight cases, including four with a malignant spindle cell component. *Am J Surg Pathol* 1995;19;1158–1171.
108. Silver SA, Devouassoux-Shisheboran J, Mezzetti TP, et al. Mesonephric adenocarcinomas of the uterine cervix: a study of 11 cases with immunohistochemical findings. *Am J Surg Pathol* 2001;25:379–387.
109. Ordi J, Nogales FF, Palacin A, et al. Mesonephric adenocarcinoma of the uterine corpus: CD10 expression as evidence of mesonephric differentiation. *Am J Surg Pathol* 2001;25:1540–1545.
110. Tambouret R, Bell DA, Young RH. Microcystic endocervical adenocarcinomas: a report of eight cases. *Am J Surg Pathol* 2000;24:369–374.
111. Wang SS, Sherman ME, Silverberg SG, et al. Pathological characteristics of cervical adenocarcinoma in a multi-center U.S.-based study. *Gynecol Oncol* 2006;103:541–546.
112. Parwani AV, Sehdev AES, Kurman RJ, et al. Cervical adenoid basal tumors comprised of adenoid basal epithelioma associated with various types of invasive carcinoma: clinicopathologic features, human papillomavirus DNA detection, and P16 expression. *Hum Pathol* 2005;36:82–90.
113. Brainard JA, Hart WR. Adenoid basal epitheliomas of the uterine cervix: a re-evaluation of distinctive cervical basaloid lesions currently classified as adenoid basal carcinoma and adenoid basal hyperplasia. *Am J Surg Pathol* 1998;22:965–975.
114. Albores-Saavedra J, Gersell D, Gilks B, et al. Terminology of endocrine tumors of the uterine cervix. Results of a workshop sponsored by the College of American Pathologists and the National Cancer Institute. *Arch Pathol Lab Med* 1997;121:34–39.
115. Albores-Saavedra J, Shahnila L, Carrick KS, et al. CD56 reactivity in small cell carcinoma of the uterine cervix. *Int J Gynecol Pathol* 2005;24:113–117.
116. Ambros RA, Park JS, Shah KV, et al. Evaluation of histologic, morphometric, and immunohistochemical criteria in the differential diagnosis of small cell carcinomas of the cervix with particular reference to human papillomavirus types 16 and 18. *Mod Pathol* 1991;4:586–593.
117. Gilks CB, Young RH, Gersell DJ, et al. Large cell carcinoma of the uterine cervix: a clinicopathologic study of 12 cases. *Am J Surg Pathol* 1997;21:905–914.
118. Horn LC, Hentschel B, Bilek K, et al. Mixed small cell carcinomas of the uterine cervix: prognostic impact of focal neuroendocrine differentiation but not of Ki-67 labeling index. *Ann Diagn Pathol* 2006;10:140–143.
119. Conner MG, Richter H, Moran CA, et al. Small cell carcinoma of the cervix: a clinicopathologic and immunohistochemical study of 3 cases. *Ann Diagn Pathol* 2002;6:345–348.
120. Tsunoda S, Jobo T, Arai M, et al. Small-cell carcinoma of the uterine cervix: a clinicopathologic study of 11 cases. *Int J Gynecol Cancer* 2005;15:295–300.
121. Jones MW, Lefkowitz M. Adenosarcoma of the uterine cervix: a clinicopathological study of 12 cases. *Int J Gynecol Pathol* 1995;14:223–229.
122. Clement PB, Zubovits JT, Young RH, et al. Malignant müllerian mixed tumors of the uterine cervix: a report of nine cases of a neoplasm with morphology often different from its counterpart in the corpus. *Int J Gynecol Pathol* 1998;17:211–222.
123. Sharma NK, Sorosky JI, Bender D, et al. Malignant mixed müllerian tumor (MMMT) of the cervix. *Gynecol Oncol* 2005;97:442–445.
124. Grayson W, Taylor LF, Cooper K, et al. Carcinosarcoma of the uterine cervix: a report of eight cases with immunohistochemical analysis and evaluation of human papillomavirus status. *Am J Surg Pathol* 2001;25:338–347.
125. Wright JD, Rosenblum K, Huettner PC, et al. Cervical sarcomas: an analysis of incidence and outcome. *Gynecol Oncol* 2005;99:348–351.
126. Cantuaria G, Angioli R, Nahmias J, et al. Primary malignant melanoma of the uterine cervix: case report and review of the literature. *Gynecol Oncol* 1999;75:170–174.
127. Oliva E, Ferry JA, Young RH, et al. Granulocytic sarcoma of the female genital tract: a clinicopathologic study of 11 cases. *Am J Surg Pathol* 1997;21:1156–1165.
128. Tathak B, Bruchim I, Brisson ML, et al. Granulocytic sarcoma presenting as tumors of the cervix (Review). *Gynecol Oncol* 2005;98:493–497.
129. Chan JK, Loizzi V, Magistris A, et al. Clinicopathologic features of six cases of primary cervical lymphoma (Review). *Am J Obstet Gynecol* 2005;103:866–872.
130. Tsao AS, Roth LM, Sandler A, et al. Cervical primitive neuroectodermal tumor. *Gynecol Oncol* 2001;83:138–142.
131. Malpica A, Moran CA. Primitive neuroectodermal tumor of the cervix: a clinicopathologic and immunohistochemical study of two cases. *Ann Diagn Pathol* 2002;6:281–287.
132. Khalbuss WE, Bui M, Loya A. A 19-year-old woman with a cervicovaginal mass and elevated serum CA 125: desmoplastic small round cell tumor. *Arch Pathol Lab Med* 2006;130:e59–61.
133. Fox H, Wells M, Harris M, et al. Enteric tumours of the lower female genital tract: a report of three cases. *Histopathology* 1988;12:167–176.
134. Delgado G, Bundy B, Zaino R, et al. Prospective surgical-pathological study of disease-free interval in patients with stage IB squamous cell carcinoma of the cervix: a Gynecologic Oncology Group study. *Gynecol Oncol* 1990;38:352–357.
135. Van de Putte G, Lie AK, Vach W, et al. Risk grouping in stage IB squamous cell cervical cancer. *Gynecol Oncol* 2005;99:106–112.
136. Rutledge TL, Kamelle SA, Tillmanns TD, et al. A comparison of stages IB1 and IB2 cervical cancers treated with radical hysterectomy. Is size the real difference? *Gynecol Oncol* 2004;95:70–76.
137. Perez CA, Grigsby PW, Chao KSC, et al. Tumor size, irradiation dose, and long-term outcome of carcinoma of the uterine cervix. *Int J Radiat Oncol Biol Phys* 1998;41:307–317.
138. Eifel PJ, Morris M, Wharton JT, et al. The influence of tumor size and morphology on the outcome of patients with FIGO stage IB squamous cell carcinoma of the uterine cervix. *Int J Radiat Oncol Biol Phys* 1994;29:9–16.
139. Pitson G, Fyles A, Milosevic M, et al. Tumor size and oxygenation are independent predictors of nodal disease in patients with cervix cancer. *Int J Radiat Oncol Biol Phys* 2001;51:699–703.
140. Viswanathan AN, Lee H, Hanson E, et al. Influence of margin status and radiation on recurrence after radical hysterectomy in stage IB cervical cancer. *Int J Radiat Oncol Biol Phys* 2006;65:1501–1507.
141. Fyles AW, Pintilie M, Kirkbride P, et al. Prognostic factors in patients with cervix cancer treated by radiation therapy: results of a multiple regression analysis. *Radiother Oncol* 1995;35:107–117.
142. Stehman FB, Bundy BN, DiSaia PH, et al. Carcinoma of the cervix treated with irradiation therapy. I. A multi-variate analysis of prognostic variables in the Gynecologic Oncology Group. *Cancer* 1991;67:2776–2785.
143. Creasman WT, Kohler MF. Is lymph vascular space involvement an independent prognostic factor in early cervical cancer? *Gynecol Oncol* 2004;92:525–529.
144. Marchiole P, Buenerd A, Benchaib M, et al. Clinical significance of lymphovascular space involvement and lymph node micrometastases in early-stage cervical cancer: a retrospective case-control surgico-pathological study. *Gynecol Oncol* 2005;97:727–732.
145. Juretzka MM, Jensen KC, Longacre TA, et al. Detection of pelvic lymph node micrometastases in stage IA2-IB2 cervical cancer by immunohistochemical analysis. *Gynecol Oncol* 2004;93:107–111.

146. Chernofsky MR, Felix JC, Muderspach LI, et al. Influence of quantity of lymph node vascular space invasion on time to recurrence in women with early-stage squamous cancer of the cervix. *Gynecol Oncol* 2006;100: 288–293.
147. Sykes P, Allen D, Cohen C, et al. Does the density of lymphatic vascular space invasion affect the prognosis of stage IB and IIA node negative carcinoma of the cervix? *Int J Gynecol Cancer* 2003;13;313–316.
148. Milam MR, Frumovitz M, dos Reis R, et al. Preoperative lymphovascular space invasion is associated with nodal metastases in women with early-stage cervical cancer. *Gynecol Oncol* 2007;106:12–15.
149. Fyles AW, Milosevic M, Pintilie M, et al. Anemia, hypoxia and transfusion in patients with cervix cancer: a review. *Radiother Oncol* 2000;57:13–19.
150. Fyles M, Milosevic M, Hedley D, et al. Tumor hypoxia has independent predictor impact only in patients with node-negative cervix cancer. *J Clin Oncol* 2002;20:680–687.
151. Fuso L, Mazzola S, Marocco F, et al. Pretreatment serum hemoglobin as a predictive factor of response to neoadjuvant chemotherapy in patients with locally advanced squamous cervical carcinoma: a preliminary report. *Gynecol Oncol* 2005;99:S187–S191.
152. Lavey RS, Liu PY, Greer BE, et al. Recombinant human erythropoietin as an adjunct to radiation therapy and cisplatin for stage IIB-IVA carcinoma of the cervix: a Southwest Oncology Group study. *Gynecol Oncol* 2004;95:145–151.
153. Sundfor K, Lyng H, Kongsgard U, et al. Polarographic measurements of p02 in cervix carcinoma. *Gynecol Oncol* 1997;64:230–236.
154. Henke M, Laszig R, Rube C, et al. Erythropoietin to treat head and neck cancer patients with anaemia undergoing radiotherapy: randomized, double-blind, placebo-controlled trial. *Lancet* 2003;362:1255–1260.
155. Leyland-Jones B, Semiglazov V, Pawlicki M, et al. Maintaining normal hemoglobin levels with epoetin alfa in mainly nonanemic patients with metastatic breast cancer receiving first-line chemotherapy: a survival study. *J Clin Oncol* 2005;23:5960–5972.
156. Bohlius J, Langensiepen S, Schwarzer G, et al. Recombinant human erythropoietin and overall survival in cancer patients: results of a comprehensive meta-analysis. *J Natl Cancer Inst* 2005;97:489–498.
157. Santin AD, Bellone S, Palmieri M, et al. Effect of blood transfusion during radiotherapy on the immune function of patients with cancer of the uterine cervix: role of interleukin-10. *Int J Radiat Oncol Biol Phys* 2002; 54:1345–1355.
158. von Pawel J, von Roemeling R, Gatzemeier U, et al. Tirapazamine plus cisplatin versus cisplatin in advanced non-small-cell lung cancer: a report of the international CATAPULT I study group. *J Clin Oncol* 2000;18: 1351–1359.
159. De Los Santos JF, Thomas GM. Anemia correction in malignancy management: threat or opportunity? *Gynecol Oncol* 2007;105:517–529.
160. Lee IJ, Park KR, Lee KK, et al. Prognostic value of vascular endothelial growth factor in stage IB carcinoma of the uterine cervix. *Int J Radiat Oncol Biol Phys* 2002;54:768–779.
161. Gaffney DK, Haslam D, Tsodikov A, et al. Epidemal growth factor receptor (EDFR) and vascular endothelial growth factor (VEGF) negatively affect overall survival in carcinoma of the cervix treated with radiotherapy. *Int J Radiat Oncol Biol Phys* 2003;56:922–928.
162. Xue G, Lin LL, Dehdashti F, et al. F-18 fluorodeoxyglucose uptake in primary cervical cancer as an indicator of prognosis after radiation therapy. *Gynecol Oncol* 2006;101:147–151.
163. Grigsby PW, Mutch DG, Rader J, et al. Lack of benefit of concurrent chemotherapy in patients with cervical cancer and negative lymph nodes by FDG-PET. *Int J Radiat Oncol Biol Phys* 2005;61:444–449.
164. Grigsby PW, Siegel BA, Dehdashti F, et al. Posttherapy [^{18}F] fluorodeoxyglucose positron emission tomography in carcinoma of the cervix: response and outcome. *J Clin Oncol* 2004;22:2167–2171.
165. Look KY, Brunetto VL, Clarke-Pearson DL, et al. An analysis of cell type in patients with surgically staged stage IB carcinoma of the cervix: a Gynecologic Oncology Group study. *Gynecol Oncol* 1996;63:304–311.
166. Eifel PJ, Morris M, Oswald MJ, et al. Adenocarcinoma of the uterine cervix: prognosis and patterns of failure in 367 cases treated at the M. D. Anderson Cancer Center between 1965 and 1985. *Cancer* 1990;65:2507.
167. Ayhan A, Al RA, Baykal C, et al. A comparison of prognoses of FIGO stage IB adenocarcinoma and squamous cell carcinoma. *Int J Gynecol Cancer* 2004;14:279–285.
168. Kleine W, Rau K, Schwoeorer D, et al. Prognosis of the adenocarcinoma of the cervix uteri: a comparative study. *Gynecol Oncol* 1989;35:145–149.
169. Baalbergen A, Ewing-Graham PC, Hop WCJ, et al. Prognostic factors in adenocarcinoma of the uterine cervix. *Gynecol Oncol* 2004;92: 262–267.
170. Alfsen CG, Kristensen GB, Skovlund E, et al. Histologic subtype has minor importance for overall survival in patients with adenocarcinoma of the uterine cervix. A population-based study of prognostic factors in 505 patients with nonsquamous cell carcinomas of the cervix. *Cancer* 2001;92: 2471–2483.
171. Stubenrauch F, Laimins LA. Human papillomavirus life cycle: active and latent phases. *Semin Cancer Biol* 1999;9:379–386.
172. Villa LL, Costa RL, Petta CA, et al. Prophylactic quadrivalent human papillomavirus (types 6, 11, 16, and 18) L1 virus-like particle vaccine in young women: a randomised double-blind placebo-controlled multicentre phase II efficacy trial. *Lancet Oncol* 2005;6:271–278.
173. Lowy DR, Schiller JT. Papillomaviruses and cervical cancer: pathogenesis and vaccine development. *J Natl Cancer Inst Monogr* 1998;(23):27–30.
174. Harper DM, Franco EL, Wheeler C, et al. Efficacy of a bivalent L1 virus-like particle vaccine in prevention of infection with human papillomavirus types 16 and 18 in young women: a randomised controlled trial. *Lancet* 2004;364:1757–1765.
175. Villa LL, Costa RL, Petta CA, et al. High sustained efficacy of a prophylactic quadrivalent human papillomavirus types 6/11/16/18 L1 virus-like particle vaccine through 5 years of follow-up. *Br J Cancer* 2006;95: 1459–1466.
176. Villa LL, Ault KA, Giuliano AR, et al. Immunologic responses following administration of a vaccine targeting human papillomavirus types 6, 11, 16, and 18. *Vaccine* 2006;24:5571–5583.
177. Garland SM, Hernandez-Avila M, Wheeler CM, et al. Quadrivalent vaccine against human papillomavirus to prevent anogenital diseases. *N Engl J Med* 2007;356:1928–1943.
178. Olsson SE, Villa LL, Costa RL, et al. Induction of immune memory following administration of a prophylactic quadrivalent human papillomavirus (HPV) types 6/11/16/18 L1 virus-like particle (VLP) vaccine. *Vaccine* 2007;25:4931–4939.
179. Harper DM, Franco EL, Wheeler CM, et al. Sustained efficacy up to 4.5 years of a bivalent L1 virus-like particle vaccine against human papillomavirus types 16 and 18: follow-up from a randomised control trial. *Lancet* 2006;367:1247–1255.
180. Markowitz LE, Dunne EF, Saraiya M, et al. Quadrivalent human papillomavirus vaccine: recommendations of the Advisory Committee on Immunization Practices (ACIP). *MMWR Recomm Rep* 2007;56:1–24.
181. Committee on Adolescent Health Care, ACOG Working Group on Immunization. ACOG committee opinion no. 344: human papillomavirus vaccination. *Obstet Gynecol* 2006;108:699–705.
182. Goldie SJ, Kohli M, Grima D, et al. Projected clinical benefits and cost-effectiveness of a human papillomavirus 16/18 vaccine. *J Natl Cancer Inst* 2004;96:604–615.
183. Sanders GD, Taira AV. Cost-effectiveness of a potential vaccine for human papillomavirus. *Emerg Infect Dis* 2003;9:37–48.
184. Block SL, Nolan T, Sattler C, et al. Comparison of the immunogenicity and reactogenicity of a prophylactic quadrivalent human papillomavirus (types 6, 11, 16, and 18) L1 virus-like particle vaccine in male and female adolescents and young adult women. *Pediatrics* 2006;118:2135–2145.
185. Wright TC Jr, Koulos J, Schnoll F, et al. Cervical intraepithelial neoplasia in women infected with the human immunodeficiency virus: outcome after loop electrosurgical excision. *Gynecol Oncol* 1994;55:253–258.
186. Alonso I, Torne A, Puig-Tintore LM, et al. Pre- and post-conization high-risk HPV testing predicts residual/recurrent disease in patients treated for CIN 2-3. *Gynecol Oncol* 2006;103:631–636.
187. Verguts J, Bronselaer B, Donders G, et al. Prediction of recurrence after treatment for high-grade cervical intraepithelial neoplasia: the role of human papillomavirus testing and age at conization. *Br J Obstet Gynecol* 2006;113;1303–1307.
188. Kolstad P. Follow-up study of 232 patients with stage IA1 and 411 patients with stage IA2 squamous cell carcinoma of the cervix (microinvasive carcinoma). *Gynecol Oncol* 1989;33:265–272.
189. Luesley DM, Cullimore J, Redman CW, et al. Loop diathermy excision of the cervical transformation zone in patients with abnormal cervical smears. *Br Med J* 1990;300:1690–1693.
190. Martin-Hirsch PL, Paraskevaidis E, Kitchener H. Surgery for cervical intraepithelial neoplasia. *Cochrane Database Syst Rev* 2000;(2):CD001318.
191. Temkin SM, Hellmann M, Lee YC, et al. Dysplastic endocervical curettings: a predictor of cervical squamous cell carcinoma. *Am J Obstet Gynecol* 2007;196:469.e1–469.e4.
192. Lu CH, Liu FS, Kuo CJ, et al. Prediction of persistence or recurrence after conization for cervical intraepithelial neoplasia III. *Obstet Gynecol* 2006;107:830–835.
193. Case AS, Rocconi RP, Straughn JM Jr, et al. Cervical intraepithelial neoplasia in adolescent women: incidence and treatment outcomes. *Obstet Gynecol* 2006;108:1369–1374.
194. Grigsby PW, Perez CA. Radiotherapy alone for medically inoperable carcinoma of the cervix: stage IA and carcinoma *in situ*. *Int J Radiat Oncol Biol Phys* 1991;21:375–378.
195. Elliott P, Coppleson M, Russell P, et al. Early invasive (FIGO stage IA) carcinoma of the cervix: a clinico-pathologic study of 476 cases. *Int J Gynecol Cancer* 2000;10:42–52.
196. Takeshima N, Yanoh K, Tabata T, et al. Assessment of the revised International Federation of Gynecology and Obstetrics staging for early invasive squamous cervical cancer. *Gynecol Oncol* 1999;74:165–169.
197. Creasman WT. Stage IA cancer of the cervix: finally some resolution of definition and treatment? *Gynecol Oncol* 1999;74:163–164.
198. Morris M, Mitchell MF, Silva EG, et al. Cervical conization as definitive therapy for early invasive squamous carcinoma of the cervix. *Gynecol Oncol* 1993;51:193–196.
199. Buckley SL, Tritz DM, Van Le L, et al. Lymph node metastases and prognosis in patients with stage IA2 cervical cancer. *Gynecol Oncol* 1996;63:4–9.
200. Roman LD, Felix JC, Muderspach LI, et al. Influence of quantity of lymph-vascular space invasion on the risk of nodal metastases in women with early-stage squamous cancer of the cervix. *Gynecol Oncol* 1998;68:220–225.

201. Maiman MA, Fruchter RG, DiMaio TM, et al. Superficially invasive squamous cell carcinoma of the cervix. *Obstet Gynecol* 1988;72:399–403.
202. Covens A, Rosen B, Murphy J, et al. How important is removal of the parametrium at surgery for carcinoma of the cervix? *Gynecol Oncol* 2002;84:145–149.
203. Kodama J, Mizutani Y, Hongo A, et al. Optimal surgery and diagnostic approach of stage IA2 squamous cell carcinoma of the cervix. *Eur J Obstet Gynecol Reprod Biol* 2002;101:192–195.
204. Gadducci A, Sartori E, Maggino T, et al. The clinical outcome of patients with stage IA1 and IA2 squamous cell carcinoma of the uterine cervix: a cooperation task force (CTF) study. *Eur J Gynaecol Oncol* 2003;24: 513–516.
205. Greer BE, Figge DC, Tamimi HK, et al. Stage IA2 squamous carcinoma of the cervix: difficult diagnosis and therapeutic dilemma. *Am J Obstet Gynecol* 1990;162:1406–1409; discussion 1409–1411.
206. Nam JH, Kim JH, Kim DY, et al. Comparative study of laparoscopico-vaginal radical hysterectomy and abdominal radical hysterectomy in patients with early cervical cancer. *Gynecol Oncol* 2004;92:277–283.
207. Hamberger AD, Fletcher GH, Wharton JT. Results of treatment of early stage I carcinoma of the uterine cervix with intracavitary radium alone. *Cancer* 1978;41:980–985.
208. Schorge JO, Lee KR, Flynn CE, et al. Stage IA1 cervical adenocarcinoma: definition and treatment. *Obstet Gynecol* 1999;93:219–222.
209. Schorge JO, Lee KR, Sheets EE. Prospective management of stage IA(1) cervical adenocarcinoma by conization alone to preserve fertility: a preliminary report. *Gynecol Oncol* 2000;78:217–220.
210. Schorge JO, Lea JS, Ashfaq R. Postconization surveillance of cervical adenocarcinoma *in situ*: a prospective trial. *J Reprod Med* 2003;48:751–755.
211. Shin CH, Schorge JO, Lee KR, et al. Conservative management of adenocarcinoma *in situ* of the cervix. *Gynecol Oncol* 2000;79:6–10.
212. Wolf JK, Levenback C, Malpica A, et al. Adenocarcinoma *in situ* of the cervix: significance of cone biopsy margins. *Obstet Gynecol* 1996;88:82–86.
213. Lea JS, Shin CH, Sheets EE, et al. Endocervical curettage at conization to predict residual cervical adenocarcinoma *in situ*. *Gynecol Oncol* 2002;87: 129–132.
214. Widrich T, Kennedy AW, Myers TM, et al. Adenocarcinoma *in situ* of the uterine cervix: management and outcome. *Gynecol Oncol* 1996;61: 304–308.
215. Chambers SK, Chambers JT, Kier R, et al. Sequelae of lateral ovarian transposition in irradiated cervical cancer patients. *Int J Radiat Oncol Biol Phys* 1991;20:1305–1308.
216. Buckers TE, Anderson B, Sorosky JI, et al. Ovarian function after surgical treatment for cervical cancer. *Gynecol Oncol* 2001;80:85–88.
217. Landoni F, Zanagnolo V, Lovato-Diaz L, et al. Ovarian metastases in early-stage cervical cancer (IA2-IIA): a multicenter retrospective study of 1965 patients (a cooperative task force study). *Int J Gynecol Cancer* 2007;17:623–628.
218. Landoni F, Maneo A, Cormio G, et al. Class II versus class III radical hysterectomy in stage IB-IIA cervical cancer: a prospective randomized study. *Gynecol Oncol* 2001;80:3–12.
219. Jensen PT, Groenvold M, Klee MC, et al. Early-stage cervical carcinoma, radical hysterectomy, and sexual function. *Cancer* 2004;100:97–106.
220. Flay LD, Matthews JHL. The effects of radiotherapy and surgery on the sexual function of women treated for cervical cancer. *Int J Radiat Oncol Biol Phys* 1995;31:399–404.
221. Landoni F, Maneo A, Colombo A, et al. Randomised study of radical surgery versus radiotherapy for stage IB-IIA cervical cancer. *Lancet* 1997;350:535–540.
222. Delgado G, Bundy BN, Fowler WC, et al. A prospective surgical pathological study of stage I squamous carcinoma of the cervix: a Gynecologic Oncology Group study. *Gynecol Oncol* 1989;35:314–320.
223. Dargent D. Radical trachelectomy: an operation that preserves the fertility of young women with invasive cervical cancer. *Bull Acad Natl Med* 2001;185:1295–1304; discussion 1305–1306.
224. Plante M, Renaud MC, Hoskins IA, et al. Vaginal radical trachelectomy: a valuable fertility-preserving option in the management of early-stage cervical cancer. A series of 50 pregnancies and review of the literature. *Gynecol Oncol* 2005;98:3–10.
225. Bader AA, Tamussino KF, Moinfar F, et al. Isolated recurrence at the residual uterine cervix after abdominal radical trachelectomy for early cervical cancer. *Gynecol Oncol* 2005;99:785–787.
226. Bali A, Weekes A, Van Trappen P, et al. Central pelvic recurrence 7 years after radical vaginal trachelectomy. *Gynecol Oncol* 2005;96:854–856.
227. Boss EA, van Golde RJ, Beerendonk CC, et al. Pregnancy after radical trachelectomy: a real option? *Gynecol Oncol* 2005;99:S152–S156.
228. Marchiole P, Benchaib M, Buenerd A, et al. Oncological safety of laparoscopic-assisted vaginal radical trachelectomy (LARVT or Dargent's operation): a comparative study with laparoscopic-assisted vaginal radical hysterectomy (LARVH). *Gynecol Oncol* 2007;106:132–141.
229. Ungar L, Palfalvi L, Hogg R, et al. Abdominal radical trachelectomy: a fertility-preserving option for women with early cervical cancer. *Br J Obstet Gynecol* 2005;112:366–369.
230. Keys HM, Bundy BN, Stehman FB, et al. Radiation therapy with and without extrafascial hysterectomy for bulky stage IB cervical carcinoma: a randomized trial of the Gynecologic Oncology Group. *Gynecol Oncol* 2003;89:343–353.
231. Eifel PJ. Chemoradiotherapy in the treatment of cervical cancer. *Semin Radiat Oncol* 2006;16:177–185.
232. Boronow RC. The bulky 6-cm barrel-shaped lesion of the cervix: primary surgery and postoperative chemoradiation. *Gynecol Oncol* 2000;78: 313–317.
233. Havrilesky LJ, Leath CA, Huh W, et al. Radical hysterectomy and pelvic lymphadenectomy for stage IB2 cervical cancer. *Gynecol Oncol* 2004;93: 429–434.
234. Yessian A, Magistris A, Burger RA, et al. Radical hysterectomy followed by tailored postoperative therapy in the treatment of stage IB2 cervical cancer: feasibility and indications for adjuvant therapy. *Gynecol Oncol* 2004;94:61–66.
235. Kamelle SA, Rutledge TL, Tillmanns TD, et al. Surgical-pathologic predictors of disease-free survival and risk grouping for IB2 cervical cancer: do the traditional models still apply? *Gynecol Oncol* 2004;94:249–255.
236. Ackerman A. FIGO Stage IB2 cervix cancer and putting all your eggs in one basket. *Gynecol Oncol* 2004;94:245–246.
237. Stehman FB. A thousand several tongues. *Gynecol Oncol* 2004;94:247–248.
238. Leung AR, Amdur RJ, Morris CG, et al. Long-term outcome after radiotherapy for FIGO stage IIIB and IVA carcinoma of the cervix. *Int J Radiat Oncol Biol Phys* 2007;67:1445–1450.
239. Economos K, Perez Veridiano N, Delke I, et al. Abnormal cervical cytology in pregancy: a 17-year experience. *Obstet Gynecol* 1993;81:915–918.
240. Rose PG, Bundy BN, Watkins EB, et al. Concurrent cisplatin-based radiotherapy and chemotherapy for locally advanced cervical cancer. *N Engl J Med* 1999;340:1144–1153.
241. Whitney C, Stehman FB. The abandoned radical hysterectomy: a Gynecologic Oncology Group study. *Gynecol Oncol* 2000;79:350–356.
242. Leath CA, Straughn JM Jr, Estes JM, et al. The impact of aborted radical hysterectomy in patients with cervical carcinoma. *Gynecol Oncol* 2004:95:204–207.
243. Bremer GL, van der Putten HWHM, Dunselman GAJ, et al. Early stage cervical cancer: aborted versus completed radical hysterectomy. *Eur J Obstet Gynecol Reprod Biol* 1992;47:147–151.
244. Suprasert P, Srisomboon J, Charoenkwan K, et al. Outcomes of abandoned radical hysterectomy in patients with stages IB-IIA cervical cancer found to have positive nodes during the operation. *Int J Gynecol Cancer* 2005;15:498–502.
245. Potter ME, Alvarez RD, Shingleton HM, et al. Early invasive cervical cancer with pelvic lymph node involvement: to complete or not to complete radical hysterectomy? *Gynecol Oncol* 1990;37:78–81.
246. Peters WA III, Liu PY, Barrett RJ, et al. Concurrent chemotherapy and pelvic radiation therapy compared with pelvic radiation therapy alone as adjuvant therapy after radical surgery in high-risk early-stage cancer of the cervix. *J Clin Oncol* 2000;18:1606–1613.
247. Kupets R, Thomas GM, Covens A. Is there a role for pelvic lymph node debulking in advanced cervical cancer? *Gynecol Oncol* 2002;87:163–170.
248. Tammela J, Bundy B, Odunsi K. Reassessment of pelvic lymph node debulking in advanced cervical cancer. *Gynecol Oncol* 2004;92:1014–1015.
249. Leath CA, Straughn JM, Bhoola SM, et al. The role of radical parametrectomy in the treatment of occult cervical carcinoma after extrafascial hysterectomy. *Gynecol Oncol* 2004;92:215–219.
250. Hsu W-L, Shueng P-W, Jen Y-M, et al. Long-term treatment results of invasive cervical cancer patients undergoing inadvertent hysterectomy followed by salvage radiotherapy. *Int J Radiat Oncol Biol Phys* 2004;59:521–527.
251. Munstedt K, Johnson P, von Georgi R, et al. Consequences of inadvertent, suboptimal primary surgery in carcinoma of the uterine cervix. *Gynecol Oncol* 2004;94:515–520.
252. Kavadi VS, Eifel PJ. FIGO stage IIIA carcinoma of the uterine cervix. *Int J Radiat Oncol Biol Phys* 1992;24:211–215.
253. Dittmer PH, Randall ME. A technique for inguinal node boost using photon fields defined by asymmetric collimator jaws. *Radiother Oncol* 2001;59:61–64.
254. Viswanathan AN, Deavers MT, Jhingran A, et al. Small cell neuroendocrine carcinoma of the cervix: outcome and patterns of recurrence. *Gynecol Oncol* 2004;93:27–33.
255. Hoskins PJ, Swenerton KD, Pike JA, et al. Small-cell carcinoma of the cervix: fourteen years of experience at a single institution using a combined-modality regimen of involved-field irradiation and platinum-based combination chemotherapy. *J Clin Oncol* 2003;21:3495–3501.
256. Garavaglia E, Taccagni G, Montoli S, et al. Primary stage I-IIE non-Hodgkin's lymphoma of the uterine cervix and upper vagina: evidence for a conservative approach in a study on three patients. *Gynecol Oncol* 2005;97:214–218.
257. Dursun P, Gultekin M, Bozdag G, et al. Primary cervical lymphoma: report of two cases and review of the literature. *Gynecol Oncol* 2005;98:484–489.
258. Kendrick JE IV, Straughn JM Jr. Two cases of non-Hodgkin's lyhmphoma presenting as primary gynecologic malignancies. *Gynecol Oncol* 2005;98: 490–492.
259. Heredia F, Bravo M, Pierotic M, et al. Neoadjuvant combined chemotherapy followed by external whole pelvic irradiation in two cases of primary extranodal non-Hodgkin's lymphoma of the uterine cervix. *Gynecol Oncol* 2005;97:285–287.
260. Sandvei R, Lote K, Svendsen E, et al. Successful pregnancy following treatment of primary malignant lymphoma of the uterine cervix. *Gynecol Oncol* 1990;38:128–131.

261. Pathak B, Bruchim I, Brisson M-L, et al. Granulocytic sarcoma presenting as tumors of the cervix. *Gynecol Oncol* 2005;98:493–497.
262. Barillot I, Horiot JC, Cuisenier J, et al. Carcinoma of the cervical stump: a review of 213 cases. *Eur J Cancer* 1993;29A:1231–1236.
263. Duggan B, Muderspach LI, Roman LD, et al. Cervical cancer in pregnancy: reporting on planned delay in therapy. *Obstet Gynecol* 1993;82:598–602.
264. Campion MJ, Sedlacek TV. Colposcopy in pregnancy. *Obstet Gynecol Clin North Am* 1993;20:153–163.
265. Hopkins MP, Morley GW. The prognosis and management of cervical cancer associated with pregnancy. *Obstet Gynecol* 1992;80:9–13.
266. Woodrow N, Permezel M, Butterfield L, et al. Abnormal cervical cytology in pregnancy: experience of 811 cases. *Aust Nz J Obstet Gynaecol* 1998; 38:161–165.
267. Averette HE, Nasser N, Yankow SL, et al. Cervical conization in pregnancy: analysis of 180 operations. *Am J Obstet Gynecol* 1970;106:543–549.
268. Hannigan EV, Whitehouse HH III, et al. Cone biopsy during pregnancy. *Obstet Gynecol* 1982;60:450–455.
269. Goldberg GL, Altaras MM, Block B. Cone cerclage in pregnancy. *Obstet Gynecol* 1991;77:315–317.
270. Robinson WR, Webb S, Tirpack J, et al. Management of cervical intraepithelial neoplasia during pregnancy with LOOP excision. *Gynecol Oncol* 1997;64:153–155.
271. Lacour RA, Garner EI, Molpus KL, et al. Management of cervical adenocarcinoma *in situ* during pregnancy. *Am J Obstet Gynecol* 2005;192: 1449–1451.
272. Sood AK, Sorosky JI, Krogman S, et al. Surgical management of cervical cancer complicating pregnancy: a case-control study. *Gynecol Oncol* 1996;63:294–298.
273. Monk BJ, Montz FJ. Invasive cervical cancer complicating intrauterine pregnancy: treatment with radical hysterectomy. *Obstet Gynecol* 1992;80:199–203.
274. Morris M, Eifel PJ, Lu J, et al. Pelvic radiation with concurrent chemotherapy compared with pelvic and para-aortic radiation for high-risk cervical cancer. *N Engl J Med* 1999;340:1137–1143.
275. Benhaim Y, Haie-Meder C, Lhomme C, et al. Chemoradiation therapy in pregnant patients treated for advanced-stage cervical carcinoma during the first trimester of pregnancy: report of two cases. *Int J Gynecol Cancer* 2007;17:270–274.
276. Ostrom K, Ben-Arie A, Edwards C, et al. Uterine evacuation with misoprostol during radiotherapy for cervical cancer in pregnancy. *Int J Gynecol Cancer* 2003;13:340–343.
277. Bader AA, Petru E, Winter R. Long-term follow-up after neoadjuvant chemotherapy for high-risk cervical cancer during pregnancy. *Gynecol Oncol* 2007;105:269–272.
278. Caluwaerts S, Van Calsteren K, Mertens L, et al. Neoadjuvant chemotherapy followed by radical hysterectomy for invasive cervical cancer diagnosed during pregnancy: report of a case and review of the literature. *Int J Gynecol Cancer* 2006;16:905–908.
279. Sood AK, Sorosky JI, Mayr N, et al. Cervical cancer diagnosed shortly after pregnancy: prognostic variables and delivery routes. *Obstet Gynecol* 2000;95:832–838.
280. Maiman M, Fruchter RG, Clark M, et al. Cervical cancer as an AIDS-defining illness. *Obstet Gynecol* 1997;89:76–80.
281. Ahdieh L, Klein RS, Burk R, et al. Prevalence, incidence, and type-specific persistence of human papillomavirus in human immunodeficiency virus (HIV)-positive and HIV-negative women. *J Infect Dis* 2001;184: 682–690.
282. Frisch M, Biggar RJ, Goedert JJ. Human papillomavirus-associated cancers in patients with human immunodeficiency virus infection and acquired immunodeficiency syndrome. *J Natl Cancer Inst* 2000;92:1500–1510.
283. Frisch M, Biggar RJ, Engels EA, et al. AIDS-Cancer Match Registry Study Group. Association of cancer with AIDS-related immunosuppression in adults. *JAMA* 2001;285:1736–1745.
284. Harris TG, Burk RD, Palefsky JM, et al. Incidence of cervical squamous intraepithelial lesions associated with HIV serostatus, CD4 cell counts, and human papillomavirus test results. *JAMA* 2005;293:1471–1476.
285. Ellerbrock TV, Chiasson MA, Bush TJ, et al. Incidence of cervical squamous intraepithelial lesions in HIV-infected women. *JAMA* 2000;283: 1031–1037.
286. Koshiol JE, Schroeder JC, Jamieson DJ, et al. Time to clearance of human papillomavirus infection by type and human immunodeficiency virus serostatus. *Int J Cancer* 2006;119:1623–1629.
287. Viscidi RP, Schiffman M, Hildesheim A, et al. Seroreactivity to human papillomavirus (HPV) types 16, 18, or 31 and risk of subsequent HPV infection: results from a population-based study in Costa Rica. *Cancer Epidemiol Biomarkers Prev* 2004;13:324–327.
288. Viscidi RP, Snyder B, Cu-Uvin S, et al. Human papillomavirus capsid antibody response to natural infection and risk of subsequent HPV infection in HIV-positive and HIV-negative women. *Cancer Epidemiol Biomarkers Prev* 2005;14:283–288.
289. Strickler HD, Burk RD, Fazzari M, et al. Natural history and possible reactivation of human papillomavirus in human immunodeficiency virus-positive women. *J Natl Cancer Inst* 2005;97:577–586.
290. Spinillo A, Tenti P, Zappatore R, et al. Langerhans' cell counts and cervical intraepithelial neoplasia in women with human immunodeficiency virus infection. *Gynecol Oncol* 1993;48:210–213.
291. Clifford GM, Goncalves MA, Franceschi S, HPV and HIV Study Group. Human papillomavirus types among women infected with HIV: a meta-analysis. *AIDS* 2006;20:2337–2344.
292. Anderson JR, Paramsothy P, Heilig C, et al. Accuracy of Papanicolaou test among HIV-infected women. *Clin Infect Dis* 2006;42:562–568.
293. Duerr A, Paramsothy P, Jamieson DJ, et al. Effect of HIV infection on atypical squamous cells of undetermined significance. *Clin Infect Dis* 2006;42:855–861.
294. Parashari A, Singh V, Sehgal A, et al. Low-cost technology for screening uterine cervical cancer. *Bull World Health Org* 2000;78:964–967.
295. Goldie SJ, Freedberg KA, Weinstein MC, et al. Cost effectiveness of human papillomavirus testing to augment cervical cancer screening in women infected with the human immunodeficiency virus. *Am J Med* 2001;111:140–149.
296. Paramsothy P, Duerr A, Heilig CM, et al. Abnormal vaginal cytology in HIV-infected and at-risk women after hysterectomy. *J Acquir Immune Defic Syndr* 2004;35:484–491.
297. Ahdieh-Grant L, Li R, Levine AM, et al. Highly active antiretroviral therapy and cervical squamous intraepithelial lesions in human immunodeficiency virus-positive women. *J Natl Cancer Inst* 2004;96:1070–1076.
298. Delmas MC, Larsen C, van Benthem B, et al. Cervical squamous intraepithelial lesions in HIV-infected women: prevalence, incidence and regression. *AIDS* 2000;14:1775–1784.
299. Maiman M, Watts DH, Andersen J, et al. Vaginal 5-fluorouracil for high-grade cervical dysplasia in human immunodeficiency virus infection: a randomized trial. *Obstet Gynecol* 1999;94:954–961.
300. Robinson WR, Andersen J, Darragh TM, et al. Isotretinoin for low-grade cervical dysplasia in human immunodeficiency virus-infected women. *Obstet Gynecol* 2002;99:777–784.
301. Lomalisa P, Smith T, Guidozzi F. Human immunodeficiency virus infection and invasive cervical cancer in South Africa. *Gynecol Oncol* 2000;77: 460–463.
302. Gichangi P, Bwayo J, Estambale B, et al. HIV impact on acute morbidity and pelvic tumor control following radiotherapy for cervical cancer. *Gynecol Oncol* 2006;100:405–411.
303. Mugambe JB, Kavuma A. Effect of HIV serological status on outcome in patients with cancer of cervix treated with radiotherapy. *East Afr Med J* 2006;83:416–423.
304. Trimbos JB, Maas CP, Deruiter MC, et al. A nerve-sparing radical hysterectomy: guidelines and feasibility in western patients. *Int J Gynecol Cancer* 2001;11:180–186.
305. Papp Z, Csapo Z, Hupuczi P, et al. Nerve-sparing radical hysterectomy for stage IA2-IIB cervical cancer: 5-year survival of 501 consecutive cases. *Eur J Gynaecol Oncol* 2006;27:553–560.
306. Charoenkwan K, Srisomboon J, Suprasert P, et al. Nerve-sparing class III radical hysterectomy: a modified technique to spare the pelvic autonomic nerves without compromising radicality. *Int J Gynecol Cancer* 2006;16: 1705–1712.
307. Raspagliesi F, Ditto A, Fontanelli R, et al. Type II versus type III nerve-sparing radical hysterectomy: comparison of lower urinary tract dysfunctions. *Gynecol Oncol* 2006;102:256–262.
308. Berek JS, Howe C, Lagasse LD, et al. Pelvic exenteration for recurrent gynecologic malignancy: survival and morbidity analysis of the 45-year experience at UCLA. *Gynecol Oncol* 2005;99:153–159.
309. Goldberg GL, Sukumvanich P, Einstein MH, et al. Total pelvic exenteration: the Albert Einstein College of Medicine/Montefiore Medical Center experience (1987 to 2003). *Gynecol Oncol* 2006;101:261–268.
310. Goldberg GL. Total pelvic exenteration: the reconstructive phase. *Gynecol Oncol* 2005;99:S149.
311. Greer BE, Koh WJ, Figge DC, et al. Gynecologic radiotherapy fields defined by intraoperative measurements. *Gynecol Oncol* 1990;38:421–424.
312. D'Souza WD, Ahamad AA, Iyer RB, et al. Feasibility of dose escalation using intensity-modulated radiotherapy in posthysterectomy cervical carcinoma. *Int J Radiat Oncol Biol Phys* 2005;61:1062–1070.
313. McAlpine J, Schlaerth JB, Lim P, et al. Radiation fields in gynecologic oncology: correlation of soft tissue (surgical) to radiologic landmarks. *Gynecol Oncol* 2004;92:25–30.
314. Jhingran A. Potential advantages of intensity-modulated radiation therapy in gynecologic malignancies. *Semin Radiat Oncol* 2006;16:144–151.
315. Nagar YS, Singh S, Kumar S, et al. Conventional 4-field box radiotherapy technique for cancer cervix: potential for geographic miss without CECT scan-based planning. *Int J Gynecol Cancer* 2004;14:865–870.
316. Huang EY, Lin H, Hsu HC, et al. High external parametrial dose can increase the probability of radiation proctitis in patients with uterine cervix cancer. *Gynecol Oncol* 2000;79:406–410.
317. Kridelka FJ, Berg DO, Neuman M, et al. Adjuvant small field pelvic radiation for patients with high risk, stage IB lymph node negative cervix carcinoma after radical hysterectomy and pelvic lymph node dissection. *Cancer* 1999;86:2059–2065.
318. Sedlis A, Bundy BN, Rotman MZ, et al. A randomized trial of pelvic radiation therapy versus no further therapy in selected patients with stage IB carcinoma of the cervix after radical hysterectomy and pelvic lymphadenectomy: a Gynecologic Oncology Group study. *Gynecol Oncol* 1999;73:177–183.
319. Ohara K, Tsudoda H, Nishida M, et al. Use of small pelvic field instead of whole pelvic field in postoperative radiotherapy for node-negative, high-risk

stages I and II cervical squamous cell carcinoma. *Int J Gynecol Cancer* 2003;13:170–176.
320. Chen S-W, Liang J-A, Yang S-N, et al. Radiation injury to intestine following hysterectomy and adjuvant radiotherapy for cervical cancer. *Gynecol Oncol* 2004;95:208–214.
321. Roeske JC, Lujan A, Rotmensch J, et al. Intensity-modulated whole pelvic radiation therapy in patients with gynecologic malignancies. *Int J Radiat Oncol Biol Phys* 2000;48:1613–1621.
322. Mundt AJ, Lujan AE, Rotmensch J, et al. Intensity-modulated whole pelvic radiotherapy in women with gynecologic malignancies. *Int J Radiat Oncol Biol Phys* 2002;52:1330–1337.
323. Alektiar KM. Can intensity-modulated radiation therapy replace brachytherapy in the management of cervical cancer—point. *Brachytherapy* 2002;1:191–192.
324. Guerrero M, Li XA, Ma L, et al. Simultaneous integrated intensity-modulated radiotherapy boost for locally advanced gynecologic cancer: radiobiological and dosimetric considerations. *Int J Radiat Oncol Biol Phys* 2005;62:933–939.
325. Mundt AJ, Roeske JC. Can intensity-modulated radiation therapy replace brachytherapy in the management of cervical cancer—counterpoint. *Brachytherapy* 2002;1:192–194.
326. Randall ME, Ibbott GS. Intensity-modulated radiation therapy for gynecologic cancers: pitfalls, hazards, and cautions to be considered. *Semin Radiat Oncol* 2006;16:138–143.
327. Buchali A, Koswig S, Dinges S, et al. Impact of the filling status of the bladder and retum on their integral dose distribution and the movement of the uterus in the treatment planning of gynecologic cancer. *Radiother Oncol* 1999;52:29–34.
328. Ahamad A, D'Souza W, Salehpour M, et al. Intensity-modulated radiation therapy after hysterectomy: comparison with conventional treatment and sensitivity of the normal-tissue-sparing effect to margin size. *Int J Radiat Oncol Biol Phys* 2005;62:1117–1124.
329. Han Y, Shin E, Huh SJ, et al. Interfractional dose variation during intensity-modulated radiation therapy for cervical cancer assesses by weekly CT evaluation. *Int J Radiat Oncol Biol Phys* 2006;65:617–623.
330. Beadle BM, Jhingran A, Salehppour M, et al. Tumor regression and organ motion during the course of chemoradiation for cervical cancer: implications for treatment planning and use of IMRT. *Int J Radiat Oncol Biol Phys* 2006;66:S44.
331. Taylor A, Rockall AG, Reznek RH, et al. Mapping pelvic lymph nodes: guidelines for delineation in intensity-modulated radiotherapy. *Int J Radiat Oncol Biol Phys* 2005;63:1604–1612.
332. Dorr W, Herrmann T. Second primary tumors after radiotherapy for malignancies. Treatment-related parameters. *Strahlenth und Onk* 2002;178:357–362.
333. Hall EJ. Intensity-modulated radiation therapy, protons, and the risk of second cancers. *Int J Radiat Oncol Biol Phys* 2006;65:1–7.
334. Kry SF, Salehpour M, Followill DS, et al. The calculated risk of fatal secondary malignancies from intensity-modulated radiation therapy. 2005;62: 1195–1203.
335. Guerrero Urbano MT, Nutting MC. Clinical use of intensity-modulated radiotherapy: part II. *Br J Radiol* 2004;77:177–192.
336. Fowler JF, Welsh JS, Howard SP. Loss of biological effect in prolonged fraction delivery. *Int J Radiat Oncol Biol Phys* 2004;59:242–249.
337. Shibamoto Y, Ito M, Sugie C, et al. Recovery from sublethal damage during intermittent exposures in cultured tumor cells: implications for dose modification in radiosurgery and IMRT. *Int J Radiat Oncol Biol Phys* 2004;59:1484–1490.
338. Esthappan J, Mutic S, Malyapa RS, et al. Treatment planning guidelines regarding the use of CT/PET-guided IMRT for cervical carcinoma with positive para-aortic lymph nodes. *Int J Radiat Oncol Biol Phys* 2004; 58:1289–1297.
339. Salama JK, Mundt AJ, Roeske J, et al. Preliminary outcome and toxicity report of extended-field intensity-modulated radiation therapy for gynecologic malignancies. *Int J Radiat Oncol Biol Phys* 2006;65:1170–1176.
340. Horii T, Mitsumoto T, Noda K. Significance of para-aortic node irradiation in the treatment of cervical cancer. *Gynecol Oncol* 1988;31:371–383.
341. Haie C, Pejovic MH, Gerbaulet A, et al. Is prophylactic para-aortic irradiation worthwhile in the treatment of advanced cervical carcinoma? Results of a controlled clinical trial of the EORTC radiotherapy group. *Radiother Oncol* 1988;11:101–112.
342. Rotman M, Pajak TF, Choi K, et al. Prophylactic extended-field irradiation of para-aortic lymph nodes in stages IIB and bulky IB and IIA cervical carcinoma. *JAMA* 1995;274:387–390.
343. Gerzten K, Colonello K, Heron DE, et al. Feasibility of concurrent cisplatin and extended field radiation therapy (EFRT) using intensity-modulated radiotherapy (IMRT) for carcinoma of the cervix. *Gynecol Oncol* 2006; 102:182–188.
344. Grigsby PW, Singh AK, Siegel BA, et al. Lymph node control in cervical cancer. *Int J Radiat Oncol Biol Phys* 2004;59:706–712.
345. Kim JS, Kim SY, Kim KH, et al. Hyperfractionated radiotherapy with concurrent chemotherapy for para-aortic lymph node recurrence in carcinoma of the cervix. *Int J Radiat Oncol Biol Phys* 2003;55:1247–1253.
346. Grigsby PW, Vest ML, and Perez CA. Recurrent carcinoma of the cervix exclusively in the para-aortic nodes following radiation therapy. *Int J Radiat Oncol Biol Phys* 1994;28:451–455.
347. Stryker JA, Mortel R. Survival following extended field irradiation in carcinoma of cervix metastatic to para-aortic lymph nodes. *Gynecol Oncol* 2000;79:99–405.
348. Varia MA, Bundy BN, Deppe G, et al. Cervical carcinoma metastatic to para-aortic nodes: extended field radiation therapy with concomitant 5-fluorouracil and cisplatin chemotherapy: a Gynecologic Oncology Group study. *Int J Radiat Oncol Biol Phys* 1998;42:1015–1023.
349. Small W Jr, Winter K, Levenback C, et al. Extended-field irradiation and intracavitary brachytherapy with cisplatin chemotherapy for cervical cancer with positive para-aortic or high common iliac lymph nodes: results of arm 1 of RTOG 0116. *Int J Radiat Oncol Biol Phys* 2007;68:1081–1087.
350. Kagel K, Tokuuye K, Okumura T, et al. Long-term results of proton beam therapy for carcinoma of the uterine cervix. *Int J Radiat Oncol Biol Phys* 2003;55:1265–1271.
351. International Commission of Radiation Units and Measurements. *Dose and Volume Specification for Reporting Intracavitary Therapy in Gynecology*. ICRU Report 38. Bethesda, MD: ICRU; 1985.
352. Potter R, Limbergen EV, Gerstner N, et al. Survey of the use of the ICRU 38 in recording and reporting cervical cancer brachytherapy. *Radiother Oncol* 2001;58:11–18.
353. Haie-Meder C, Potter R, Van Limbergen E, et al. Recommendation from Gynecologic (GYN) GEC ESTRO Working Group: concepts and terms in 3D image-based treatment planning in cervix cancer brachytherapy with emphasis on MRI assessment of GTV and CTV. *Radiother Oncol* 2005;74:235–245.
354. Nag S, Cardenes H, Chang S, et al. Proposed guidelines for image-based intracavitary brachytherapy for cervical carcinoma: report from Image-Guided Brachytherapy Working Group. *Int J Radiat Oncol Biol Phys* 2004;60:1160–1172.
355. Nag S. Controversies and new developments in gynecologic brachytherapy: image-based intracavitary brachytherapy for cervical carcinoma. *Semin Radiat Oncol* 2006;16:164–167.
356. Viswanathan AN, Dimopoulos J, Kirisits C, et al. Computed tomography versus magnetic resonance imaging-based contouring in cervical cancer brachytherapy: results of a prospective trial and preliminary guidelines for standardized contours. *Int J Radiat Oncol Biol Phys* 2007;68:491–498.
357. Rodrigus P, Winter KD, Venselaar JLM, et al. Evaluation of late morbidity in patients with carcinomas of the uterine cervix following a dose rate change. *Radiother Oncol* 1997;42:137–141.
358. Newman G. Increased morbidity following the introduction of remote afterloading, with increased dose rate, for cancer of the cervix. *Radiother Oncol* 1996;39:97–103.
359. Patel FD, Negi PS, Sharma SC, et al. Dose rate correction in medium dose rate brachytherapy for carcinoma of the cervix. *Radiother Oncol* 1998;49:317–323.
360. Rotmensch J, Connell PP, Yamada D, et al. One versus two intracavitary brachytherapy applications in early-stage cervical cancer patients undergoing definitive radiation therapy. *Gynecol Oncol* 2000;78:32–38.
361. Rotman M, Aziz H. Techniques in the radiation treatment of carcinoma of the uterine cervix. *Int J Radiat Oncol Biol Phys* 1991;20:173–175.
362. Swift PS, Purser P, Roberts LW, et al. Pulsed low dose rate brachytherapy for pelvic malignancies. *Int J Radiat Oncol Biol Phys* 1997;37:811–817.
363. Bachtiary B, Dewitt A, Pintilie M, et al. Comparison of late toxicity between continuous low-dose-rate and pulsed-dose-rate brachytherapy in cervical cancer patients. *Int J Radiat Oncol Biol Phys* 2005;63:1077–1082.
364. Hareyama M, Sakata KI, Oouchi A, et al. High-dose-rate versus low-dose-rate intracavitary therapy for carcinoma of the uterine cervix: a randomized trial. *Cancer* 2002;94:117–124.
365. Ferrigno R, Nishimoto IN, Novaes PE, et al. Comparison of low and high dose rate brachytherapy in the treatment of uterine cervix cancer: retrospective analysis of two sequential series. *Int J Radiat Oncol Biol Phys* 2005;62:1108–1116.
366. Falkenberg E, Kim RY, Meleth S, et al. Low-dose-rate vs. high-dose-rate intracavitary brachytherapy for carcinoma of the cervix: the University of Alabama at Birmingham (UAB) experience. *Brachytherapy* 2006;5:49–55.
367. Agrawal PP, Singhal SS, Neema JP, et al. The role of interstitial brachytherapy using template in locally advanced gynecologic malignancies. *Gynecol Oncol* 2005;99:169–175.
368. Petereit DG, Pearcey R. Literature analysis of high dose rate brachytherapy fractionation schedules in the treatment of cervical cancer: is there an optimal fractionation schedule? *Int J Radiat Oncol Biol Phys* 1999; 43:359–366.
369. Toita T, Kakinohana Y, Ogawa K, et al. Combination external beam radiotherapy and high-dose-rate intracavitary brachytherapy for uterine cervical cancer: analysis of dose and fractionation schedule. *Int J Radiat Oncol Biol Phys* 2003;56:1344–1353.
370. Calkins AR, Harrison CR, Fowler WC Jr, et al. Hyperfractionated radiation therapy plus chemotherapy in locally advanced cervical cancer: results of two phase I dose-escalation Gynecologic Oncology Group trials. *Gynecol Oncol* 1999;75:349–355.
371. Kavanagh BD, Segreti EM, Koo D, et al. Long-term local control and survival after concomitant boost accelerated radiotherapy for locally advanced cervix cancer. *Am J Clin Oncol* 2001;24:113–119.
372. Girinsky T, Rey A, Roche B, et al. Overall treatment time in advanced cervical carcinomas: a critical parameter in treatment outcome. *Int J Radiat Oncol Biol Phys* 1994;27:1051–1056.

373. Petereit DG, Sarkaria JN, Chappel R, et al. The adverse effect of treatment prolongation in cervical carcinoma. *Int J Radiat Oncol Biol Phys* 1995;32: 1301–1307.
374. Perez CA, Grigsby PW, Castro-Vita H, et al. Carcinoma of the uterine cervix I. Impact of prolongation of treatment time and timing of brachytherapy on outcome of radiation therapy. *Int J Radiat Oncol Biol Phys* 1995;32:1275–1288.
375. Erridge SC, Kerr GR, Downing D, et al. The effect of overall treatment time on the survival and toxicity of radical radiotherapy for cervical carcinoma. *Radiother Oncol* 2002;63:59–66.
376. Spanos WJ, Clery M, Perez CA, et al. Late effect of multiple daily fraction schedule for advanced pelvic malignancies (RTOG 8502). *Int J Radiat Oncol Biol Phys* 1994;29:961–967.
377. Long HJ III. Management of metastatic cervical cancer: review of the literature. *J Clin Oncol* 2007;25:2966–2974.
378. Mendenhall WM, McCarty PJ, Morgan LS, et al. Stage IB or IIA-B carcinoma of the intact uterine cervix greater than or equal to 6 cm in diameter: is adjuvant extrafascial hysterectomy beneficial? *Int J Radiat Oncol Biol Phys* 1991;21:899–904.
379. Thoms WW Jr, Eifel PJ, Smith TL, et al. Bulky endocervical carcinoma: a 23-year experience. *Int J Radiat Oncol Biol Phys* 1992;23:491–499.
380. Rotman M, Sedlis A, Piedmonte MR, et al. A phase III randomized trial of postoperative pelvic irradiation in stage IB cervical carcinoma with poor prognostic features: follow-up of a Gynecologic Oncology Group study. *Int J Radiat Oncol Biol Phys* 2006;65:169–176.
381. Pieterse QD, Trimbos JBMZ, Kijkman A, et al. Postoperative radiation therapy improves prognosis in patients with adverse risk factors in localized, early-stage cervical cancer: a retrospective comparative study. *Int J Gynecol Cancer* 2006;16:1112–1118.
382. Monk BJ, Wang J, Im S, et al. Rethinking the use of radiation and chemotherapy after radical hysterectomy: a clinical-pathologic analysis of a Gynecologic Oncology Group/Southwest Oncology Group/Radiation Therapy Oncology Group trial. *Gynecol Oncol* 2005;96:721–728.
383. Kim JH, Kim HJ, Hon S, et al. Post-hysterectomy radiotherapy in FIGO stage IB-IIB uterine cervical carcinoma. *Gynecol Oncol* 2005;96:407–414.
384. Uno T, Ito H, Isobe K, et al. Postoperative pelvic radiotherapy for cervical cancer patients with positive parametrial invasion. *Gynecol Oncol* 2005;96:335–340.
385. Estape RE, Angioli R, Madrigal M, et al. Close vaginal margins as a prognostic factor after radical hysterectomy. *Gynecol Oncol* 1998;68:229–232.
386. Kim RY, Salter MM, Shingleton HM. Adjuvant postoperative radiation therapy following radical hysterectomy in stage IB carcinoma of the cervix: analysis of treatment failure. *Int J Radiat Oncol Biol Phys* 1988;14:445–449.
387. Kodama J, Seki N, Nakamura K, et al. Prognostic factors in pathologic parametrium-positive patients with stage IB-IIB cervical cancer treated by radical surgery and adjuvant therapy. *Gynecol Oncol* 2007;105:757–761.
388. Chen M-F, Tseng C-J, Tseng C-C, et al. Clinical outcome in posthysterectomy cervical cancer patients treated with concurrent cisplatin and intensity-modulated pelvic radiotherapy: comparison with conventional radiotherapy. *Int J Radiat Oncol Biol Phys* 2007;67:1438–1444.
389. Chauvergne J, Lhommé C, Rohart J, et al. Chimiothérapie néoadjuvante des cancers du col utérin aux stades Iib et III. Résultats éloignés d'un essai randomize pluricentrique portant sur 151 patients. *Bull Cancer (Paris)* 1993;80:1069–1079.
390. Kumar L, Kaushal R, Nandy M, et al. Chemotherapy followed by radiotherapy versus radiotherapy alone in locally advanced cervical cancer. A randomized study. *Gynecol Oncol* 1994;54:307–315.
391. Kumar L, Grover R, Pokharel YH, et al. Neoadjuvant chemotherapy in locally advanced cervical cancer: Two randomized studies. *Aust Nz J Med* 1998;28:387–390.
392. Souhami L, Gil RA, Allan SE, et al. A randomized trial of chemotherapy followed by pelvic radiation therapy in stage IIIB carcinoma of the cervix. *J Clin Oncol* 1991;9:970–977.
393. Tattersall MHN, Ramirez C, Coppleson MA. A randomized trial comparing platinum-based chemotherapy followed by radiotherapy vs. radiotherapy alone in patients with locally advanced cervical cancer. *Int J Gynecol Cancer* 1992;2:244–251.
394. Tattersall MHN, Lorvidhaya V, Vootiprux V, et al. Randomized trial of epirubicin and cisplatin chemotherapy followed by pelvic radiation in locally advanced cervical cancer. *J Clin Oncol* 1995;13:444–451.
395. Withers HR, Taylor JM, Maciejewski B. The hazard of accelerated tumor clonogen repopulation during radiotherapy. *Acta Oncol* 1988;27:131–146.
396. Ozols RF, Masuda H, Hamilton TC. Mechanisms of cross-resistance between radiation and antineoplastic drugs. *NCI Monogr* 1988;6:159–165.
397. Tierney J, Neodajuvant Chemotherapy for Cervical Cancer Meta-analysis Collaboration. Neoadjuvant chemotherapy for locally advanced cervical cancer: a systematic review and meta-analysis of individual patient data from 21 randomized trials. *Eur J Cancer* 2003;39:2470–2486.
398. Eddy GL, Manetta A, Alvarez RD, et al. Neoadjuvant chemotherapy with vincristine and cisplatin followed by radical hysterectomy and pelvic lymphadenectomy for FIGO stage IB bulky cervical cancer: a Gynecologic Oncology Group pilot study. *Gynecol Oncol* 1995;57:412–416.
399. Zanetta G, Lissoni A, Pellegrino A, et al. Neoadjuvant chemotherapy with cisplatin, ifosfamide and paclitaxel for locally advanced squamous cell cervical cancer. *Ann Oncol* 1998;9:977–980.
400. Sugiyama T, Nishida T, Muraoka Y, et al. Radical surgery after neoadjuvant intra-arterial chemotherapy in stage IIIb squamous cell carcinoma of the cervix. *Int Surg* 1999;84:67–73.
401. Marth C, Sundfor K, Kaern J, et al. Long-term follow-up of neoadjuvant cisplatin and 5-fluorouracil chemotherapy in bulky squamous cell carcinoma of the cervix. *Acta Oncol* 1999;38:517–520.
402. Minagawa Y, Kigawa J, Irie T, et al. Radical surgery following neoadjuvant chemotherapy for patients with stage IIIB cervical cancer. *Ann Surg Oncol* 1998;5:539–543.
403. Meden H, Fattahi-Meibodi A, Osmers R, et al. Wertheim's hysterectomy after neoadjuvant carboplatin-based chemotherapy in patients with cervical cancer stage IIB and IIIB. *Anticancer Res* 1998;18:4575–4579.
404. Sardi J, Giaroli A, Sananes C, et al. Long term follow-up of the first randomized trial using neoadjuvant chemotherapy in stage IB squamous carcinoma of the cervix: the final results. *Gynecol Oncol* 1997;67: 61–69.
405. Sardi J, Giaroli A, Sananes C, et al. Randomized trial with neoadjuvant chemotherapy in stage IIIB squamous carcinoma cervix uteri: an unexpected therapeutic management. *Int J Gynecol Cancer* 1996;6:85–93.
406. Benedetti-Panici P, Landoni F, Greggi S, et al. Randomized trial of neoadjuvant chemotherapy (NACT) followed by radical surgery (RS) vs. exclusive radiotherapy (RT) in locally advanced squamous cell cervical cancer (LASCCC). An Italian multicenter study. *Int J Gynecol Cancer* 1997;7(Suppl 2):18 (abstract).
407. Sardi JE, Sananes CE, Giaroli AA, et al. Neoadjuvant chemotherapy in cervical carcinoma stage IIB: a randomized controlled trial. *Int J Gynecol Cancer* 1998;8:441–450.
408. Chang TC, Lai CH, Hong JH, et al. Randomized trial of neoadjuvant cisplatin, vincristine, bleomycin, and radical hysterectomy versus radiation therapy for bulky stage IB and IIA cervical cancer. *J Clin Oncol* 2000; 18:1740–1747.
409. Houvenaeghel G, Lelievre L, Gonzague-Casabianca L, et al. Long-term survival after concomitant chemoradiotherapy prior to surgery in advanced cervical carcinoma. *Gynecol Oncol* 2006;100:338–343.
410. Killackey MA, Boardman L, Carroll DS. Adjuvant chemotherapy and radiation in patients with poor prognostic stage IB/IIA cervical cancer. *Gynecol Oncol* 1993;49:377–379.
411. Lai CH, Lin TS, Soong YK, et al. Adjuvant chemotherapy after radical hysterectomy for cervical carcinoma. *Gynecol Oncol* 1989;35: 193–198.
412. Sivanesaratnam V. Adjuvant chemotherapy in high-risk patients after Wertheim hysterectomy—10 year survivals. *Ann Acad Med Singapore* 1998;27:622–626.
413. Husain A, Akhurst T, Larson S, et al. A prospective study of the accuracy of ^{18}fluorodeoxyglucose positron emission tomography (^{18}FDG PET) in identifying sites of metastasis prior to pelvic exenteration. *Gynecol Oncol* 2007;106:177–180.
414. Randall ME, Evans L, Greven KM, et al. Interstitial re-irradiation for recurrent gynecologic malignancies: results and analysis of prognostic factors. *Gynecol Oncol* 1993;48:23–31.
415. Wang CJ, Lai CH, Huang HJ, et al. Recurrent cervical carcinoma after primary radical surgery. *Am J Obstet Gynecol* 1999;181:518–524.
416. Singh AK, Grigsby PW, Rader JS, et al. Cervix carcinoma, concurrent chemoradiotherapy, and salvage of isolated para-aortic lymph node recurrence. *Int J Radiat Oncol Biol Phys* 2005;61:450–455.
417. Hong J-H, Tsai C-S, Lai C-H, et al. Recurrent squamous cell carcinoma of cervix after definitive radiotherapy. *Int J Radiat Oncol Biol Phys* 2004; 60:249–257.
418. Shingleton HM, Soong SJ, Gelder MS, et al. Clinical and histopathologic factors predicting recurrence and survival after pelvic exenteration for cancer of the cervix. *Obstet Gynecol* 1989;73:1027–1034.
419. Berek JS, Howe C, Lagasse LD, et al. Pelvic exenteration for recurrent gynecologic malignancy: survival and morbidity analysis of the 45-year experience at UCLA. *Gynecol Oncol* 2005;99:153–159.
420. Marnitz S, Kohler C, Muller M, et al. Indications for primary and secondary exenterations in patients with cervical cancer. *Gynecol Oncol* 2006;103:1023–1030.
421. Lai CH, Huang KG, See LC, et al. Restaging of recurrent cervical carcinoma with dual-phase [18F]fluoro-2-deoxy-D-glucose positron emission tomography. *Cancer* 2004;100:544–552.
422. Kohler C, Tozzi R, Possover M, et al. Explorative laparoscopy prior to exenterative surgery. *Gynecol Oncol* 2002;86:311–315.
423. Bricker EM. Bladder substitution after pelvic evisceration. *Surg Clin North Am* 1950;30:1511–1521.
424. Kock NG, Nilson AE, Nilsson LO, et al. Urinary diversion via a continent ileal reservoir: clinical results in 12 patients. *J Urol* 1982;128:469–475.
425. Rowland RG, Mitchell ME, Bihrle R, et al. Indiana continent urinary reservoir. *J Urol* 1987;137:1136–1139.
426. Segreti EM, Morris M, Levenback C, et al. Transverse colon urinary diversion in gynecologic oncology. *Gynecol Oncol* 1996;63:66–70.
427. Penalver MA, Angioli R, Mirhashemi R, et al. Management of early and late complications of ileocolonic continent urinary reservoir (Miami pouch). *Gynecol Oncol* 1998;69:185–191.
428. Ramirez PT, Modesitt SC, Morris M, et al. Functional outcomes and complications of continent urinary diversions in patients with gynecologic malignancies. *Gynecol Oncol* 2002;85:285–291.

429. Ungar L, Palfalvi L. Pelvic exenteration without external urinary or fecal diversion in gynecologic cancer patients. *Int J Gynecol Cancer* 2006;16: 364–368.
430. Miller B, Morris M, Gershenson DM, et al. Intestinal fistulae formation following pelvic exenteration: a review of the University of Texas M D Anderson Cancer Center experience, 1957–1990. *Gynecol Oncol* 1995;56: 207–210.
431. McCraw JB, Massey FM, Shanklin KD, et al. Vaginal reconstruction with gracilis myocutaneous flaps. *Plast Reconstr Surg* 1976;58: 176–183.
432. Burke TW, Morris M, Roh MS, et al. Perineal reconstruction using single gracilis myocutaneous flaps. *Gynecol Oncol* 1995;57:221–225.
433. Ratliff CR, Gershenson DM, Morris M, et al. Sexual adjustment of patients undergoing gracilis myocutaneous flap vaginal reconstruction in conjunction with pelvic exenteration. *Cancer* 1996;78:2229–2235.
434. Soper JT, Larson D, Hunter VJ, et al. Short gracilis myocutaneous flaps for vulvovaginal reconstruction after radical pelvic surgery. *Obstet Gynecol* 1989;74:823–827.
435. O'Connell C, Mirhashemi R, Kassira N, et al. Formation of functional neovagina with vertical rectus abdominis musculocutaneous (VRAM) flap after total pelvic exenteration. *Ann Plast Surg* 2005;55:470–473.
436. Soper JT, Havrilesky LJ, Secord AA, et al. Rectus abdominis myocutaneous flaps for neovaginal reconstruction after radical pelvic surgery. *Int J Gynecol Cancer* 2005;15:542–548.
437. Sood AK, Cooper BC, Sorosky JI, et al. Novel modification of the vertical rectus abdominis myocutaneous flap for neovagina creation. *Obstet Gynecol* 2005;105:514–518.
438. Soper JT, Secord AA, Havrilesky LJ, et al. Comparison of gracilis and rectus abdominis myocutaneous flap neovaginal reconstruction performed during radical pelvic surgery: flap-specific morbidity. *Int J Gynecol Cancer* 2007;17:298–303.
439. Mirhashemi R, Averette HE, Estape R, et al. Low colorectal anastomosis after radical pelvic surgery: a risk factor analysis. *Am J Obstet Gynecol* 2000;183:1375–1379; discussion 1379–1380.
440. Husain A, Curtin J, Brown C, et al. Continent urinary diversion and low-rectal anastomosis in patients undergoing exenterative procedures for recurrent gynecologic malignancies. *Gynecol Oncol* 2000;78: 208–211.
441. Wheeless CR Jr. Neovagina constructed from an omental J flap and a split thickness skin graft. *Gynecol Oncol* 1989;35:224–226.
442. Maneo A, Landoni F, Cormio G, et al. Radical hysterectomy for recurrent or persistent cervical cancer following radiation therapy. *Int J Gynecol Cancer* 1999;9:295–301.
443. Coleman RL, Keeney ED, Freedman RS, et al. Radical hysterectomy for recurrent carcinoma of the uterine cervix after radiotherapy. *Gynecol Oncol* 1994;55:29–35.
444. Rutledge S, Carey MS, Prichard H, et al. Conservative surgery for recurrent or persistent carcinoma of the cervix following irradiation: is exenteration always necessary? *Gynecol Oncol* 1994;52:353–359.
445. Monk BJ, Walker JL, Tewari KS, et al. Open interstitial brachytherapy for the treatment of local-regional recurrences of uterine corpus and cervix cancer after primary surgery. *Gynecol Oncol* 1994;52:222–228.
446. Ito H, Shigematsu N, Kawada T, et al. Radiotherapy for centrally recurrent cervical cancer of the vaginal stump following hysterectomy. *Gynecol Oncol* 1997;67:154–161.
447. Ijaz T, Eifel PJ, Burke T, et al. Radiation therapy of pelvic recurrence after radical hysterectomy for cervical carcinoma. *Gynecol Oncol* 1998;70: 241–246.
448. Cerrotta A, Gardan G, Cavina R, et al. Concurrent radiotherapy and weekly paclitaxel for locally advanced or recurrent squamous cell carcinoma of the uterine cervix. A pilot study with intensification of the dose. *Eur J Gynaecol Oncol* 2002;23:115–119.
449. Grigsby PW. Prospective phase I/II study of irradiation and concurrent chemotherapy for recurrent cervical cancer after radical hysterectomy. *Int J Gynecol Oncology* 2004;14:860–864.
450. Beitler JJ, Anderson PS, Wadler S, et al. Pelvic exenteration for cervix cancer: would additional intraoperative interstitial brachytherapy improve survival? *Int J Radiat Oncol Biol Phys* 1997;38:143–148.
451. Bonomi P, Blessing JA, Stehman FB, et al. Randomized trial of three cisplatin dose schedules in squamous cell carcinoma of the cervix: a Gynecologic Oncology Group study. *J Clin Oncol* 1985;3:1079–1085.
452. Reichman B, Markman M, Hakes T, et al. Phase II trial of high-dose cisplatin with sodium thiosulfate nephroprotection in patients with advanced carcinoma of the uterine cervix previously untreated with chemotherapy. *Gynecol Oncol* 1991;43:159–163.
453. Omura GA, Blessing JA, Vaccarello L, et al. Randomized trial of cisplatin versus cisplatin plus mitolactol (Dibromodulcitol) versus cisplatin plus ifosfamide in advanced squamous carcinoma of the cervix: a Gynecologic Oncology Group study. *J Clin Oncol* 1997;15:165–171.
454. Kumar L, Pokharel YH, Kumar S, et al. Single agent versus combination chemotherapy in recurrent cervical cancer. *J Obstet Gynaecol Res* 1998;24:401–409.
455. Moore DH, Blessing JA, McQuellon RP, et al. Phase III study of cisplatin with or without paclitaxel in stage IVB, recurrent or persistent squamous cell carcinoma of the cervix: a Gynecologic Oncology Group study. *J Clin Oncol* 2004;22:3113–3119.
456. Long HJ III, Bundy BN, Grendys EC Jr, et al. Randomized phase III trial of cisplatin with or without topotecan in carcinoma of the uterine cervix: a Gynecologic Oncology Group study. *J Clin Oncol* 2005;23:4625–4633.
457. Monk BJ, Huang HQ, Cella D, et al. Quality of life outcomes from a randomized phase III trial of cisplatin with or without topotecan in advanced carcinoma of the uterine cervix: a Gynecologic Oncology Group study. *J Clin Oncol* 2005;23:4617–4625.
458. Averette HE, Nguyen HN, Donato DM, et al. Radical hysterectomy for invasive cervical cancer: a 25-year prospective experience with the Miami technique. *Cancer* 1993;71:1422–1437.
459. Artman LE, Hoskins WJ, Bibro MC, et al. Radical hysterectomy and pelvic lymphadenectomy for stage IB carcinoma of the cervix: 21 years experience. *Gynecol Oncol* 1987;28:8–13.
460. Lee YN, Wang KL, Lin MH, et al. Radical hysterectomy with pelvic lymph node dissection for treatment of cervical cancer: a clinical review of 954 cases. *Gynecol Oncol* 1989;32:135–142.
461. Raspagliesi F, Ditto A, Fontanelli R, et al. Type II versus type III nerve-sparing radical hysterectomy: comparison of lower urinary tract dysfunctions. *Gynecol Oncol* 2006;102:256–262.
462. Ercoli A, Delmas V, Gadonneix P, et al. Classical and nerve-sparing radical hysterectomy: an evaluation of the risk of injury to the autonomous pelvic nerves. *Surg Radiol Anat* 2003;25:200–206.
463. Farquharson DI, Shingleton HM, Orr JW Jr, et al. The short-term effect of radical hysterectomy on urethral and bladder function. *Br J Obstet Gynaecol* 1987;94:351–357.
464. Ralph G, Tamussino K, Lichtenegger W. Urological complications after radical abdominal hysterectomy for cervical cancer. *Baillieres Clin Obstet Gynaecol* 1988;2:943–952.
465. Schreuder HW, Vierhout ME, Veen HF. Disabling constipation following Wertheim's radical hysterectomy. *Ned Tijdschr Geneeskd* 1993;137: 1059–1062.
466. Barnes W, Waggoner S, Delgado G, et al. Manometric characterization of rectal dysfunction following radical hysterectomy. *Gynecol Oncol* 1991;42:116–119.
467. Orr JW Jr, Shingleton HM, Hatch KD, et al. Correlation of perioperative morbidity and conization to radical hysterectomy interval. *Obstet Gynecol* 1982;59:726–731.
468. Samlal RA, van der Velden J, Schilthuis MS, et al. Influence of diagnostic conization on surgical morbidity and survival in patients undergoing radical hysterectomy for stage IB and IIA cervical carcinoma. *Eur J Gynaecol Oncol* 1997;18:478–481.
469. Levrant SG, Fruchter RG, Maiman M. Radical hysterectomy for cervical cancer: morbidity and survival in relation to weight and age. *Gynecol Oncol* 1992;45:317–322.
470. Cohn DE, Swisher EM, Herzog TJ, et al. Radical hysterectomy for cervical cancer in obese women. *Obstet Gynecol* 2000;96:727–731.
471. Franchi M, Trimbos JB, Zanaboni F, et al. Randomised trial of drains versus no drains following radical hysterectomy and pelvic lymph node dissection: a European Organisation for Research and Treatment of Cancer-Gynaecological Cancer Group (EORTC-GCG) study in 234 patients. *Eur J Cancer* 2007;43:1265–1268.
472. Patsner B, Hackett TE. Use of the omental J-flap for prevention of postoperative complications following radical abdominal hysterectomy: report of 140 cases and literature review. *Gynecol Oncol* 1997;65:405–407.
473. Andreyev HJ, Vlavianos P, Blake P, et al. Gastrointestinal symptoms after pelvic radiotherapy: role for the gastroenterologist. *Int J Radiat Oncol Biol Phys* 2005;62:1461–1471.
474. Perez CA, Grigsby PW, Castro-Vita H, et al. Carcinoma of the uterine cervix. II. Lack of impact of prolongation of overall treatment time on morbidity of radiation therapy. *Int J Radiat Oncol Biol Phys* 1996;34:3–11.
475. Perez CA, Grigsby PW, Lockett MA, et al. Radiation therapy morbidity in carcinoma of the uterine cervix: dosimetric and clinical correlation. *Int J Radiation Oncol Biol Phys* 1999;44:855–866.
476. Iraha S, Ogawa K, Moromizato H, et al. Radiation enterocolitis requiring surgery in patients with gynecologic malignancies. *Int J Radiat Oncol Biol Phys* 2007;68:1088–1093.
477. Eifel PJ, Levenback C, Wharton JT, et al. Time course and incidence of late complications in patients treated with radiation therapy for FIGO stage IB carcinoma of the uterine cervix. *Int J Radiat Oncol Biol Phys* 1995;32:1289–1300.
478. Parkin DE, Davis JA, Symonds RP. Urodynamic findings following radiotherapy for cervical carcinoma. *Br J Urol* 1988;61:213–217.
479. Lajer H, Thranov KR, Skovgaard LT, et al. Late urologic morbidity in 177 consecutive patients after radiotherapy for cervical carcinoma: a longitudinal study. *Int J Radiat Oncol Biol Phys* 2002;54:1356–1361.
480. Bergmark K, Avall-Lundqvist E, Dickman PW, et al. Vaginal changes and sexuality in women with a history of cervical cancer. *N Engl J Med* 1999;340:1383–1389.
481. Huh SJ, Kim B, Kang MK, et al. Pelvic insufficiency fracture after pelvic irradiation in uterine cervix cancer. *Gynecol Oncol* 2002;86:264–268.
482. Fink D, Chetty N, Lehm JP, et al. Hyperbaric oxygen therapy for delayed radiation injuries in gynecologic cancers. *Int J Gynecol Cancer* 2006;16:638–642.
483. Jhingran A, Eifel PJ. Perioperative and postoperative complications of intracavitary radiation for FIGO stage I-III carcinoma of the cervix. *Int J Radiat Oncol Biol Phys* 2000;46:1177–1183.

484. Roeske JC, Lujan A, Reba RC, et al. Incorporation of SPECT bone marrow imaging into intensity modulated whole-pelvic radiation therapy treatment planning for gynecologic malignancies. *Radiother Oncol* 2005;77:11–17.
485. Mell LK, Kochanski JD, Roeske JC, et al. Dosimetric predictors of acute hematologic toxicity in cervical cancer patients treated with concurrent cisplatin and intensity-modulated radiotherapy. *Int J Radiat Oncol Biol Phys* 2006;66:1356–1365.
486. Chen M-F, Tseng C-J, Tseng C-C, et al. Clinical outcome in posthysterectomy cervical cancer patients treated with concurrent cisplatin and intensity-modulated pelvic radiotherapy: comparison with conventional radiotherapy. *Int J Radiat Oncol Biol Phys* 2007;67:1438–1444.
487. Novetsky AP, Einstein MH, Goldbergy GL, et al. Efficacy and toxicity of concomitant cisplatin with external beam pelvic radiotherapy and two high-dose-rate brachytherapy insertions for the treatment of locally advanced cervical cancer. *Gynecol Oncol* 2007;105:635–640.
488. Bloss JD, DiSaia PJ, Mannel RS, et al. Radiation myelitis: a complication of concurrent cisplatin and 5-fluorouracil chemotherapy with extended field radiotherapy for carcinoma of the uterine cervix. *Gynecol Oncol* 1991;43:305–308.
489. Coulombe G, Thiessen B, Balkwil S, et al. Polyradiculopathy post-concomitant chemoradiation for carcinoma of the uterine cervix treated with pelvic and para-aortic fields. *Gynecol Oncol* 2005;99:774–777.
490. Matthews KS, Rocconi RP, Straughn JM Jr. Complete uterine necrosis following chemoradiation for advanced cervical cancer: a case report. *Gynecol Oncol* 2007;106:265–267.
491. Clarke-Pearson DL, Jelovsek FR, Creasman WT. Thromboembolism complicating surgery for cervical and uterine malignancy: incidence, risk factors, and prophylaxis. *Obstet Gynecol* 1983;61:87–94.
492. Jacobson GM, Kamath RS, Smith BJ, et al. Thromboembolic events in patients treated with definitive chemotherapy and radiation therapy for invasive cervical cancer. *Gynecol Oncol* 2005;96:470–474.
493. Wun T, Law L, Harvey D, et al. Increased incidence of symptomatic venous thrombosis in patients with cervical carcinoma treated with concurrent chemotherapy, radiation, and erythropoietin. *Cancer* 2003;98: 1514–1520.

CHAPTER 23 ■ CORPUS: EPITHELIAL TUMORS

D. SCOTT McMEEKIN, KALED M. ALEKTIAR, PAUL J. SABBATINI, AND RICHARD J. ZAINO

Endometrial cancer accounts for nearly 50% of all new gynecologic cancers diagnosed in the United States. It is the fourth most common malignancy in women, and the eighth most common cause of cancer death. The American Cancer Society (ACS) estimated that there were 39,000 new cases of endometrial carcinoma and 7,400 deaths from advanced or recurrent disease in 2007 (1). The death rate per 100,000 women from all malignancies in the United States was 160.49, with uterine cancers contributing at a rate of 4.13 (1). Worldwide, endometrial cancer is only second to cervical cancer in frequency. Endometrial carcinoma occurs most often in the sixth and seventh decades of life, with an average age at onset of 60 years. It is estimated that 75% to 85% of the cases occur in patients 50 years old and older, and 95% occur in patients over 40 years of age (2,3). The disease, although reported in patients as young as age 16 years, is rare in patients younger than 30 years of age.

Endometrial cancer is commonly confined to the uterus at diagnosis. Data from the National Cancer Institute's Surveillance, Epidemiology, and End Results (SEER) program demonstrated that stage I disease was found in 73% of patients, and 10% had stage II disease (4). The 26th Annual Report of the International Federation of Gynecology and Obstetrics (FIGO) on 9,386 endometrial cancer patients demonstrated that 83% of patients were stage I-II (5). With the favorable disease distribution at presentation, it is not surprising that most patients have a favorable prognosis. Results from FIGO show that 85% to 91% of stage I patients are alive at 5 years, and patients in the SEER database with localized disease have 96% 5-year survival (4,5). As a result, endometrial cancer has been considered a "good cancer"; that is, most patients present with early-stage, highly curable disease. Despite the favorable characteristics for most patients, those with high-risk factors including increased age, higher tumor grade, aggressive histology, and advanced stage face real challenges.

The understanding and management of endometrial cancer has undergone continued evolution. In the past, most patients would receive some form of pre- or postoperative radiation in combination with a simple hysterectomy; postoperative treatment decisions were guided by pathologic factors identified following selective use of surgical staging. We are now in an era where, increasingly, surgical therapy has expanded to routine use of pelvic and para-aortic lymphadenectomy and acceptance of laparoscopic management. Understanding tumor biology as it relates to predicting recurrence and survival, and how molecular and genetic changes can be exploited to direct postoperative therapies, represent our next challenge. In 2001, the National Cancer Institute convened an expert panel to develop a national 5-year plan for research priorities in gynecologic cancers. The resulting report, Priorities of the Gynecologic Cancer Progress Review Group (PRG), specified that understanding tumor biology was the central key toward controlling gynecologic cancers (6). For endometrial cancer, one of the top research priorities defined by the PRG was to identify prognostic and predictive markers for treatment efficacy and toxicity.

Current clinical controversies center on the extent of nodal surgery and the changing roles of radiation therapy and chemotherapy. Increased use of surgical staging has translated to less frequent use of radiation therapy and to changes away from pelvic radiation (7). There have been important developments in chemotherapy in endometrial cancer. Combination chemotherapy is increasingly used in the primary management of advanced and recurrent disease, and may hold promise in an adjuvant setting (8). Hormonal therapy remains an important option and our understanding of steroid receptors at a molecular level may help to determine which patients may benefit most (9). Enhanced understanding of biologically relevant targets has fostered the development of new classes of agents that attempt to exploit susceptible pathways in tumor cells (10,11).

ANATOMY

The uterus is a fibromuscular pelvic organ situated between the bladder and the rectum and enveloped by peritoneal reflections. It is divided into the fundus, isthmus, and cervix. The uterine wall is composed of the outer smooth muscle myometrium and inner cavity lined by glandular endometrial epithelium with supporting stroma (endometrium). Five paired ligaments cover or support the uterus: broad, round, utero sacral, cardinal, and vesico uterine. The utero-sacral and cardinal ligaments provide the greatest support within the pelvis and, contrary to cervical cancer, are infrequently involved with tumor spread. Blood is supplied to the uterus by the uterine artery, a branch of the hypogastric artery, which enters the wall of the uterus at the isthmus after it crosses over the ureter. It anastomoses with the ovarian artery in the ovarian ligament.

Malignant transformation of the endometrium is manifest in many fashions based on the anatomical relationships. Tumor growth may be confined to the endometrium, invade the underlying myometrium, penetrate to the uterine serosal surface or adjacent bladder or rectum, or extend into the cervical canal and invade cervical glands or stroma. Peritoneal disease spread may occur via transmigration from the fallopian tubes or through serosal penetration. Hematogenous spread is not uncommon in endometrial cancer.

The lymphatics of the myometrium drain into the subserosal network of lymphatics, which coalesce into larger channels before leaving the uterus. Lymph flows from the fundus toward the adnexa and infundibulopelvic ligaments. The lymph flow from the lower and middle thirds of the uterus tends to spread in the base of the broad ligaments toward the lateral pelvic sidewall (12). There are four drainage channels from the uterus: from the fundus; in the folds of the broad ligament, along the mesosalpinx and fallopian tubes; and along the round ligaments. The drainage sites are principally reflected in metastatic potential to pelvic and para-aortic lymph nodes, and occasionally involve inguinal nodes.

EPIDEMIOLOGY AND RISK FACTORS

The most important risk factor for the development of endometrial cancer is age. Endometrial cancer is primarily a disease of postmenopausal woman, with median age at cancer diagnosis of 60 years (5). Approximately 85% of cases occur after the age of 50, the peak age-specific incidence is from 75 to 79 years (109 per 100,000), and only 5% of cases are from patients younger than 40 years of age (2,3,13). The ACS showed probability of developing a uterine cancer to be one in 142 from age 40 to 59, one in 124 from age 60 to 69, and one in 78 from age 70 and older (1). Not unexpectedly, with an aging U.S. population, the total number of cases of endometrial cancer has shown yearly increases, whereas the annual age-adjusted incidence rate peaked in the mid 1970s (33.8 per 100,000) and has remained stable at 23 to 25 cases per 100,000 women over the last 10 years (1).

Race also appears to play a role in the development of endometrial cancer. The rates of endometrial cancer are highest in North America and northern Europe, lower in eastern Europe and Latin America, and lowest in Asia and Africa (14). Factors accounting for these findings include differences in rates of obesity, use of hormone replacement therapy, and reproductive factors. In the United States, non-Hispanic white women have the highest age-adjusted incidence of endometrial cancer at 25.4 (per 100,000 women), compared to women of African American (19.5), Asian (15.8), or Hispanic (17) heritage (15). African American women, however, have a much higher mortality rate (7.1 vs. 3.9 per 100,000) and lower 5-year survival (61% vs. 84%) compared to non-Hispanic white women. Multiple explanations have been suggested to explain the differences in outcomes between racial groups including differences in frequency of high-risk tumor types, differences in access to care (reduced use of surgery and radiation), and differences in medical comorbidities among races. Data from SEER demonstrated that African American women were more frequently diagnosed with higher stage, grade, and high-risk histologies than non-Hispanic white women, but there was no difference in the frequency of recommended therapy types between races (4). In two analyses of nearly 1,200 patients with advanced or recurrent endometrial cancer participating in phase 3 chemotherapy trials conducted by the Gynecologic Oncology Group (GOG), African American race was independently associated with a lower likelihood of response to chemotherapy (relative odds of response 0.62) and decreased overall survival (hazard ratio, 1.26) compared to white women (16,17). These results suggest that racial disparity in outcomes exist even though patients were treated in similar fashion. Interestingly, one small study comparing microarray-based expression profiling between stage-, grade-, and histology-matched African American and Caucasian patients found no clear differences in global gene expression profiles, suggesting that environmental or social issues played a greater role in explaining disparity (18).

Most cases of endometrial carcinoma are thought to be sporadic; however, some cases clearly have a hereditary basis. The Lynch syndrome (hereditary nonpolyposis colorectal cancer [HNPCC]) is an autosomal-dominant cancer susceptibility syndrome associated with early-onset colon, rectal, ovary, small bowel, ureter/renal pelvis cancers, and endometrial cancer. Lynch syndrome–related endometrial cancers account for 2% to 5% of all endometrial cancers, and occur in nearly 10% of women diagnosed with endometrial cancer less than 50 years of age (19). The lifetime risk of endometrial cancer in Lynch syndrome women is 40% to 60%, a risk similar to that of developing colon cancer. The risk of ovarian cancer is 10% to 12%. In about 50% of cases where patients have both colonic and gynecologic cancers (endometrial or ovarian), the gynecologic cancer precedes the diagnosis of colon cancer (20). The syndrome is most commonly due to germ-line mutations of one of the DNA mismatch repair genes *MSH2, MLH1, or MSH6.* In one study, 23% of endometrial cancer patients diagnosed at <50 years of age with one relative having a Lynch type cancer had a mismatch repair gene mutation (21). Prophylactic hysterectomy and bilateral salpingo-oophorectomy has been shown to be an effective strategy for preventing ovarian and endometrial cancers in these high-risk patients (22).

Controversy exists regarding the relationship between *BRCA1 and BRCA2* mutations and the risk of endometrial cancer. Germ-line mutations of *BRCA1 and BRCA2* account for a large proportion of hereditary breast and ovarian/primary peritoneal cancers. In 1999, Hornreich et al. presented a case report of sisters with the same *BRCA1* mutation who were diagnosed with serous carcinomas of the uterus and suggested a possible association (23). Several larger studies have attempted to address this hypothesis. In one study of 199 Ashkenazi Jewish patients with endometrial cancer from a single institution, Levine et al. genotyped all patients for founder *BRCA1 and BRCA2* mutations that existed in that patient population. The frequency of germ-line mutations (3 per 199, 1.5%) in endometrial cancer patients was comparable to the baseline rate of 2% in the Ashkenazi population, suggesting no increased risk (24). In a large prospective study by Beiner et al., 857 known *BRCA1 and BRCA2* carriers aged 45 to 70 were followed over time for the development of endometrial cancer (25). With an average length of follow-up of 3.3 years, six women developed endometrial cancer. Four of the six patients had used tamoxifen. Compared to the expected rate of endometrial cancer in a general population, *BRCA* carriers who did not receive tamoxifen did not have a significant increase in risk of developing endometrial cancer, whereas those patients who had received tamoxifen had a 11.6 incidence ratio ($p = 0.0004$).

The clinical picture in endometrial carcinoma is as varied as are the associated risk factors for its development. One of the paradigms for bridging the gaps between epidemiologic, clinical-pathologic, and molecular factors seen in endometrial cancer types is the relatively simple, yet attractive classification system of endometrial cancers suggested by Bokhman (26). Endometrial cancers are thought to broadly arise from one of two different pathways: estrogen dependent or estrogen independent (Table 23.1). Based on the clinical and histologic features, endometrial cancers have been divided into type I and type II tumors. Type I tumors are more common (85%), tend to be found in younger women, and develop via a precursor lesion of atypical hyperplasia. These tumors are associated with a predisposing history of hyperestrogenism. They tend to be well differentiated and have minimal myometrial invasion, and as a result typically have a favorable outcome. Type II tumors account for a small percentage of endometrial carcinomas, occur in an older population, and frequently develop in the face of an atrophic endometrium. About half of all relapses occur in this group. Serous, clear cell, and perhaps grade 3 tumors fit into the type II category. Despite the broad generalizations of the two categories, translational science data lends support for a separation into these groups at a molecular level.

TABLE 23.1

COMPARISON BETWEEN TYPE I AND TYPE II ENDOMETRIAL CANCERS

	Type I	Type II
CLINICAL FEATURES		
Risk factors	Unopposed estrogen	Age
Race	White > black	White = black
Differentiation	Well differentiated	Poorly differentiated
Histology	Endometrioid	Non-endometrioid
Stage	I/II	III/IV
Prognosis	Favorable	Not favorable
MOLECULAR FEATURES		
Ploidy	Diploid	Aneuploid
K-ras overexpression	Yes	Yes
HER2/neu overexpression	No	Yes
P53 overexpression	No	Yes
PTEN mutations	Yes	No
Microsatellite instability	Yes	No

For example, mutations of *TP53* are common in uterine papillary serous carcinoma (UPSC), and rare in type I tumors (27). In type I tumors, *PTEN* mutations are common, but are rare with UPSC tumors. Global gene expression profiles have also been shown to be different between type I and II tumors (28).

Endogenous or exogenous exposure to estrogen is believed to be an important risk factor for the development of endometrial hyperplasia and type I cancers (29). Estrogens not opposed by progestins lead to increased mitotic activity of endometrial cells, resulting in more frequent errors in DNA replication and somatic mutations (30,31). These genetic changes are manifest clinically in endometrial hyperplasia and cancer. Estrogen excess as an etiology for cancers is supported by epidemiologic features of the disease. Patients with chronic anovulation, nulliparity, early age of menarche, and late menopause have classically been identified with endometrial cancer. Occasionally, endometrial hyperplasia or cancer develops in the setting of an estrogen-producing ovarian tumor (granulosa cell tumor) (32). The use of unopposed estrogens as part of hormone replacement strategies was first defined as an important risk factor in 1975 when the age-adjusted rate for endometrial cancer peaked at nearly 33.8 per 100,000 (33,34). A meta-analysis of 30 studies showed that the relative risk of ever users of estrogen therapy was 2.3 compared to non-users, and it increased to 9.5 in users of 10 or more years (35).

Obesity is an increasingly common problem in the United States, and is estimated to account for 17% to 46% of endometrial cancer incidence in postmenopausal women (36). Studies have shown that plasma concentrations of androstenedione and estrogens are correlated with body weight in postmenopausal women (37,38). Aromatization of androstenedione to estrone in adipose cells is believed to be the principle mechanism of excess estrogen production (39). While much of the data suggests that the relationship is strongest between estrogen exposure and type I cancers, Weiss et al. demonstrated in a case-control study that the risk of more aggressive tumors (higher grade or higher stage) was also seen with unopposed estrogen therapy, obesity, low parity, and history of diabetes. The authors suggested that the risk of endometrial cancer was influenced by similar risk factors regardless of tumor aggressiveness (40). Diabetes has also been associated classically with type I endometrial cancers (41,42). Only non–insulin dependent diabetes (type 2 diabetes mellitus [DM]), characterized by insulin resistance and elevated insulin levels, appears to be associated with endometrial cancer (43). Hyperinsulinemia and higher levels of insulin-like growth factor 1 are thought to have neoplastic potential and, coupled with increased estrogen, are responsible for cancer development (44–46).

Tamoxifen and Endometrial Cancer

Tamoxifen is a selective estrogen receptor modulator (SERM) with antiestrogenic properties in the breast and estrogenic effects in tissues such as bone, the cardiovascular system, and the uterus. It has been used in prevention and treatment for all stages of breast cancer. An association with tamoxifen and endometrial cancer was first reported by Killackey et al. in 1985 (47). The strongest data initially implicating tamoxifen use and the subsequent development of endometrial cancer were published in 1989 by Fornander et al. (48). The investigators reviewed the frequency of new primary cancers as recorded in the Swedish Cancer Registry for a group of 1,846 postmenopausal women with early breast cancer who were included in a randomized trial of adjuvant tamoxifen. They noted a 6.4-fold increase in the relative risk of endometrial cancer in 931 tamoxifen-treated patients compared to 915 patients in the control group. The dose of tamoxifen in this study was 40 mg/d, and the greatest cumulative risk of developing endometrial cancer was after 5 years of tamoxifen use.

Fisher et al. published data regarding the association between tamoxifen use and the development of endometrial cancer when they reported the findings of the National Surgical Adjuvant Breast and Bowel Project (NSABP) B-14 trial (49). Data regarding the rates of endometrial and other cancers were analyzed on 2,843 patients with node-negative, estrogen receptor (ER)-positive, invasive breast cancer randomly assigned to placebo or tamoxifen (20 mg/d) and on 1,220 tamoxifen-treated patients registered in NSABP B-14 subsequent to randomization. The average annual hazard rate for endometrial cancer in the placebo group was 0.2 out of 1,000 and 1.6 out of 1,000 for the randomized tamoxifen-treated group. The relative risk of an endometrial cancer occurring in the randomized, tamoxifen-treated group was 7.5. Similar results were seen in the 1,220 registered patients who received tamoxifen. The mean duration of tamoxifen therapy was 35 months, with 36% of the endometrial cancers developing within 2 years of therapy and six occurring less

TABLE 23.2

CLINICOPATHOLOGIC DATA FROM SERIES REPORTING ON TAMOXIFEN-ASSOCIATED UTERINE CANCER

	Magriples (39)	Barakat (34)	Fisher (35)	van Leeuwen (44)	van Leeuwen (43)	Total (%)
No. patients	15	23	25	17	23	103
FIGO stage						
I	7	15	21	14	17	74 (71.8)
II	0	2	1	2	3	8 (7.8)
III	2	5	1	0	0	8 (7.8)
IV	0	1	1	1	0	3 (2.9)
Unstaged	6	0	1	0	3	10 (9.7)
Histology						
Endometrioid	9	17	18	16	17	77 (74.8)
High-risk[a]	6	6	7	1	6	26 (25.2)
Grade (adenocarcinoma)						
Low (grade 1,2)	5	13	18	15	Not given	51 (72.9)[b]
High (grade 3)	10	4	5	0	Not given	19 (27.1)[b]
Deaths from uterine cancer	5 (33%)	5 (22%)	4 (16%)	3 (10%)	0 (0%)	17 (16.5)

[a]Includes papillary serous, clear cell, sarcoma.
[b]Grade only known for 70 patients.
Source: Reprinted with permission from Barakat RR. The effect of tamoxifen on the endometrium. *Oncology* 1995;9:129–134.

than 9 months after treatment was initiated, suggesting that some of the cancers may have been present prior to starting tamoxifen therapy.

Any conclusions drawn regarding the risks of tamoxifen treatment in inducing endometrial cancer must weigh the benefits of tamoxifen in reducing breast cancer recurrence and new contralateral breast cancers. In the B-14 trial, the cumulative rate per 1,000 women with breast cancer relapse was reduced from 227.8 in the placebo group to 123.5 in the randomized tamoxifen-treated group. In addition, the cumulative rate of contralateral breast cancer was reduced from 40.5 to 23.5, respectively, in the two groups. Taking into account the increased cumulative rate of endometrial cancer, there was a 38% reduction in the 5-year cumulative hazard rate in the tamoxifen-treated group. Thus, the benefit of tamoxifen therapy for breast cancer outweighs the potential increase in endometrial cancer being reported.

The suspected mechanism for endometrial cancer development following tamoxifen exposure is thought to be related to its estrogenic effects on the endometrium. As such, type I, low-grade/early-stage cancers would be expected. A report from the Yale Tumor Registry by Magriples et al. suggested that uterine cancers occurring in breast cancer patients on tamoxifen may behave more aggressively and carry a worse prognosis (50). Other studies, however, have not been able to confirm these findings (Table 23.2) (49,51–53). It would appear from the available literature that there is no difference in the stage, grade, or prognosis of endometrial cancers associated with tamoxifen use.

More commonly, breast cancer patients are being managed with a different strategy compared to SERMs by preventing estrogen synthesis by inhibiting the conversion of androgens to estrogens. Third-generation aromatase inhibitors (anastrozole, letrozole, exemestane) are replacing tamoxifen for many breast cancer patients with ~50% of postmenopausal estrogen receptor–positive patients receiving aromatase inhibitors (54). In clinical trials, compared to tamoxifen, aromatase inhibitors have lower incidences of vaginal bleeding or endometrial cancer (55,56). In premenopausal patients, aromatase inhibitors have little activity, and tamoxifen will continue to have a role.

Protective Factors

Factors that reduce circulating estrogen levels (weight loss/exercise, cigarette smoking) appear to be protective against endometrial cancer. Similarly, progestins antagonize the effects of estrogen on the endometrium and prevent the development of hyperplasia and cancer when added to estrogens (endogenous or exogenous) (57). Combined estrogen-progestin hormone replacement therapy has been associated with reductions in the risk of endometrial cancer in most, but not all, studies. Prior use of oral contraceptives also appears to be protective against the development of endometrial cancer (58,59).

NATURAL HISTORY OF DISEASE

A better understanding of the natural history of endometrial cancer has developed through evaluation of the patterns of spread. In a landmark study, the GOG performed a surgical pathologic study (GOG 33) in 621 patients with clinical stage I–occult stage II endometrial cancer who underwent a standardized surgical procedure including exploration of the abdomen with biopsy of suspicious findings, collection of peritoneal fluid for cytologic evaluation, abdominal hysterectomy and bilateral salpingo-oophorectomy, and pelvic and para-aortic nodal dissection (60). The results of this study demonstrated important relationships regarding uterine tumor characteristics and spread of disease, and should be ingrained into the memory of those caring for patients with endometrial cancers.

Overall, 22% of patients with seemingly uterine confined disease were found to have extrauterine spread. Pelvic and/or para-aortic metastases were found in 11% of patients, 12% had positive peritoneal cytology, 5% had adnexal involvement, and 6% had gross intraperitoneal spread. Nodal metastases were related to tumor grade and depth of myometrial invasion, and patients with positive cytology, or adnexal or intraperitoneal spread also had increased frequency of nodal disease.

Patterns of failure in patients with recurrent endometrial cancer demonstrate, alone or in combination, hematogenous, lymphatic, intraperitoneal, or local/contiguous spread. As attention has increasingly focused on therapies (surgical, radiation, chemotherapy) to reduce particular sites of recurrences, several have argued for defining relationships between initial disease spread and subsequent risk of recurrence (61). In GOG 33, treatment was not specified by protocol, but results showed that outcomes could be predicted by extent of disease found at surgery, thus demonstrating the important relationship between what is learned at surgical staging and recurrence risk (62).

DIAGNOSTIC EVALUATION

Screening

Many endometrial cancers develop by way of a precursor lesion. Estrogen-related cancers frequently develop secondary to atypical endometrial hyperplasia (AEH) or demonstrate AEH in the uterus at the time of hysterectomy. Serous tumors also may develop through a precursor lesion, endometrial intraepithelial carcinoma (EIC) (63,64). Prompt recognition of precursor lesions with institution of proper treatment will prevent cancers and their sequelae. The relatively low prevalence of endometrial cancer in the population (5 per 1,000 women >45 years) makes standardized screening inefficient. There are a few uncontrolled studies lending some support to the efficacy of screening programs (65,66). No randomized trials have been published. No health economic data have been presented in relation to the published reports. The American College of Obstetrics and Gynecology (ACOG) and the Society of Gynecologic Oncology do not recommend routine screening of patients for uterine cancer (67,68). The American Cancer Society does recommend annual endometrial biopsies starting at age 35 for women known to have or be at risk for HNPCC.

In lieu of routine screening, prompt assessment of symptomatic patients and those at high risk should be considered. Because 95% of endometrial carcinomas occur in women 40 years old and older, and because endometrial hyperplasia tends to occur in premenopausal and perimenopausal women, it is appropriate to evaluate individuals past their fourth decade of life if there is abnormal bleeding. Similarly, a higher degree of suspicion should be held for younger patients with high-risk characteristics including significant obesity, polycystic ovarian syndrome/chronic anovulation, or tamoxifen exposure.

Prevention

Due to the increased risk of endometrial cancer associated with unopposed estrogens, women with an intact uterus should rarely, if ever, be prescribed estrogen-only replacement therapy. The addition of progestins to the regimens of patients treated with exogenous estrogen may prevent endometrial hyperplasia and protect against the development of carcinoma (57,58). Continuous or sequential progestin regimens may be used, but the most important factor is administration of a progestin for at least 10 to 14 days each month. In patients with chronic endogenous estrogen exposure such as obese women with polycystic ovarian syndrome or chronic anovulation, and perimenopausal women with menometrorrhagia, periodic treatment with a progestin to create scheduled withdrawal bleeding and prevent hyperplasia may be considered (69,70).

In most cases, patients with hyperplasia with atypia should be treated by vaginal or abdominal hysterectomy to prevent the development of endometrial cancer (71). Surgery is the definitive therapy as it stops bleeding, prevents cancer, and alleviates the potential of medical failure. Patients with AEH remain at high risk for recurrence of AEH or cancer during their lifetime, even after successful medical therapy (72). Most importantly, despite a preoperative diagnosis of AEH many patients will be found to have a cancer at the time of hysterectomy (72,73). Older data suggested that if the endometrial sample is obtained by a biopsy or curettage, 15% to 25% of patients with the diagnosis of atypical hyperplasia may have a uterine carcinoma (74,75). Prospective data from a large surgical-pathologic trial conducted by the GOG demonstrated that, of 289 patients with a community diagnosis of AEH, 40% had an endometrial cancer (73). Neither the type of preoperative endometrial biopsy (office endometrial biopsy [EMB] or dilatation and curettage [D&C]) nor the use of an expert pathology panel was associated with a better prediction of who had cancer or not. Patients with significant medical comorbidities, advanced age, or those desiring future fertility may be managed with progestational therapy (76). It has been suggested that a D&C should be performed in those patients who will be medically managed with progestins for therapeutic effect (surgical curettage of tissue) and to better define the risk of an unrecognized cancer, while the data to support these practices are limited. When progestins are used to manage AEH, the specific agents, doses, and schedules may mirror those used to manage dysfunctional uterine bleeding or advanced or recurrent cancer. To assess the success of medical therapy, endometrial biopsies should be performed at 3- to 4-month intervals provided cancer is not identified (77,78).

Screening and prevention strategies for women on tamoxifen are more challenging. Women with intact uteri who are taking tamoxifen for either treatment or prevention of breast cancer should be informed of the increased relative risk of developing endometrial cancer with the use of tamoxifen. This risk is balanced by the reductions in recurrence or development of a contralateral breast cancer. Women on tamoxifen should be encouraged to report abnormal bleeding or vaginal discharge. Screening of asymptomatic women on tamoxifen therapy with ultrasound or endometrial biopsies is not recommended (79,80).

CLINICAL PRESENTATION

The classic symptom of endometrial carcinoma is abnormal uterine bleeding. A variety of conditions give rise to abnormal bleeding, but particular suspicion should be held for postmenopausal women, and women age 40 and over with high-risk factors. Approximately 10% of symptomatic postmenopausal patients will be found to have a cancer on biopsy (81). In one series, using age >70 years, diabetes, or nulliparity as risk factors, patients with all three factors had an 87% chance of having an AEH/carcinoma diagnosis, whereas only 3% had significant pathology in the absence of all risk factors (82). Additionally, patients with endometrial cancer may present with vaginal discharge or have a thickened endometrium incidentally noted on ultrasound performed for another reason. Pap smear screening is not designed to identify endometrial cancer, but occasionally patients will have abnormal cervical cytology (atypical glandular cells of undetermined significance [AGUS], adenocarcinoma *in situ* [AIS]). Patients with intraperitoneal disease may present with similar complaints to patients with ovarian cancer such as abdominal distension, pelvic pressure, and pain.

Historically, when endometrial cancer was a clinically staged disease (FIGO 1971) fractional D&C was the procedure of choice to evaluate abnormal bleeding. Fractional D&C permitted assessment of the uterine size and allowed for endocervical curettage, important steps in the staging process. The standard procedure starts with curettage of the endocervix prior to cervical dilatation. Careful sounding of the uterus is performed followed by dilatation of the cervix, followed by systematic curetting of the entire endometrial cavity. Cervical and endometrial specimens should be kept separate and forwarded for pathologic interpretation.

Pathologic evaluation of the endometrium provides histologic diagnosis and can identify other etiologies of bleeding such as chronic endometritis, atrophy, polyps, cervical cancer, or unusual histologic variants (carcinosarcoma, serous carcinoma, placental nodule), which may alter management. Tissue evaluation by office EMB or D&C offer similar information when adequately performed. Today EMB has largely replaced D&C as the diagnostic procedure of choice. In the GOG hyperplasia study, 63% of the specimens were from EMB (Vabra, Novak, Pipelle) and 37% were from D&C (73). Results of endometrial biopsies correlate well with endometrial curettings, and the accuracy to detect cancer is 91% to 99% (83,84). The accuracy of identifying cancers with EMB is higher in postmenopausal patients than in premenopausal, and a positive study showing cancer is more accurate for identifying disease than it is in excluding it. Cases where office biopsy cannot be obtained (cervical stenosis, patient intolerance of procedure) or results are nondiagnostic should be followed by D&C. In cases of abnormal bleeding that persists despite negative biopsy, additional investigation is warranted.

Hysteroscopy has been advocated as an adjuvant to D&C to improve detection of pathology in the evaluation of postmenopausal bleeding. Whether it improves the sensitivity to detect hyperplasia and cancers is controversial (85–87). Hysteroscopy is more accurate in postmenopausal patients, and is more accurate in detecting cancer versus other pathology than it is in identifying cancer or hyperplasia versus other pathology. One concern is that hysteroscopy may promote transtubal migration of tumor cells, which can be detected as malignant pelvic washings on cytology. In one retrospective study, an odds ratio of 3.88 for positive cytology was seen in hysteroscopic D&Cs compared to D&C alone, and the authors cautioned against hysteroscopy to evaluate endometrial cancer (88). Similarly, a review of literature suggested that water-based hysteroscopy was associated with increased frequency of positive cytology at time of hysterectomy (89). Positive peritoneal cytology has the potential to upstage a patient (stage IIIA) resulting in additional/different adjuvant therapy being recommended. No prospective studies have been performed to date, and it remains uncertain what effect positive washing produced by hysteroscopy has, if any, on prognosis.

Ultrasound is commonly used as a less invasive tool to evaluate abnormal bleeding. The measurement of endometrial thickness (ET) has been shown to best predict the absence of carcinoma, with a false-negative rate of 4%, using a threshold value of <5 mm (90,91). The specific endometrial thickness used for a cutoff value depends on the menopausal status of the patient population evaluated and on the use of hormone replacement (HRT). For example, postmenopausal patients on HRT have a median ET 2 to 3 mm more than those not on HRT (92,93). In a meta-analysis of 85 studies, Smith-Bindman et al. reported that a cutoff level of >5 mm would detect 96% of cancers, and would have a 39% false-positive rate (91). Transvaginal ultrasound measuring the lining thickness of the endometrium has excellent negative predictive value for ruling out endometrial cancers or hyperplasia when the thickness is <5 mm, but provides less information when >5 mm. Given a pretest probability of having endometrial cancer in a postmenopausal patient with vaginal bleeding of 10%, a normal endometrial stripe is associated with a 1% chance of a cancer. A consensus panel, composed of radiologists, pathologists, and gynecologic oncologists, suggested that when ET is <5 mm, the test can be considered negative for endometrial cancer (94). For patients with ET >5 mm, endometrial biopsy, D&C with hysteroscopy, or saline infusion sonohysteroscopy should be performed. Saline infusion sonohysteroscopy has been suggested to better define findings in the endometrial cavity noted on ultrasound and provide clearer distinction of polyps, fibroids, and cancers (95). It is more likely to be successful in pre- than postmenopausal patients. The role of vaginal ultrasound in the evaluation of bleeding remains somewhat controversial due to the belief of the importance of histology is defining treatment (for benign and malignant conditions) and of the concern for missed cancers. Good clinical judgment would suggest that patients with ET <5 mm who have persistent bleeding undergo tissue biopsy.

DIAGNOSTIC WORKUP

Preoperative Assessment

Following the diagnosis of endometrial cancer, the surgeon must assess the surgical risks of the patient, evaluate the patient for possible metastatic spread, and determine the most appropriate surgical procedure. Endometrial cancer patients are frequently elderly and suffer from obesity, hypertension, diabetes, or cardiac disease. In a series of 595 consecutive patients, Marziale et al. found an operability rate of 87% (96). Preoperative assessment must be performed, occasionally requiring consultation with additional specialists. At a minimum, patients require a thorough examination to evaluate for evidence of cardiac or pulmonary disease, and to determine the surgical approach. A chest x-ray and electrocardiogram (EKG), complete blood count, and assessment of electrolytes and renal function are standard in this population. Preoperative counseling includes obtaining permission to remove the uterus, tubes, and ovaries and permission for thorough intra-abdominal exploration with biopsy and tumor removal as necessary including removal of the pelvic and para-aortic lymph nodes.

Evaluation of Metastatic Spread

A thorough physical examination may discover suspicious supraclavicular, inguinal, and/or occasional pelvic lymph nodes as well as suggest the presence of pleural effusions, ascites, or omental caking. The pelvic examination can suggest cervical, vaginal, or adnexal spread. An assessment of uterine size and mobility is important, particularly in patients being considered for vaginal approaches (laparoscopic-assisted vaginal hysterectomy [LAVH], total vaginal hysterectomy [TVH]). A chest radiograph is done to search for metastatic tumor as well as to evaluate the cardiopulmonary status of the patient. For patients without obvious extrauterine disease, surgery is the next step. In cases where intra-abdominal, gross cervical, or distant disease spread is suspected, additional studies such as CT scans, magnetic resonance imaging (MRI), or cystoscopy and proctoscopy may be needed to assist with surgical planning.

In general there is very limited need for imaging studies prior to surgery since findings typically do not result in management changes as most patients present with stage I-II disease, and the surgery is essentially the same for stage I-III patients. Imaging studies have significant limitations in detecting nodal disease, which tends to be microscopic in 90% of cases (97,98). Patient review of systems and clinical examination frequently lead to suspicion of gross extrauterine disease. Imaging studies may be of better use in certain situations. Serous and clear cell tumors have a greater frequency of extrauterine disease spread, and imaging studies may offer additional information in some cases. In some settings, imaging studies may help some to determine whether to refer to a gynecologic oncologist or perform surgical staging when it would not otherwise be considered. In addition, imaging studies may have their greatest utility in helping to counsel young patients who are considering fertility preservation options. Magnetic resonance imaging has been suggested to have more value than computed tomography (CT) scans in assessing myometrial invasion, cervical invasion, and nodal disease with several reports indicating a 75% to 90% accuracy rate for determining muscle involvement (99–102). However, limitations do exist, making routine use more difficult to recommend (103,104). At the present time, the only way to accurately diagnose the extent and depth of intrauterine invasion is by histologic examination of the hysterectomy specimen.

Attempts have been made to correlate the tumor marker CA-125 with extent of extrauterine disease as serum levels are frequently elevated in patients with advanced or metastatic endometrial cancer (105). This observation was first reported by Niloff et al. in 1984 (106). Values exceeding 35 U/mL were found in 14 (78%) of 18 patients with stage IV or recurrent disease, although none of 11 patients with stage I disease had elevations. Patsner et al., in 1988, reported 81 patients with endometrial cancer that appeared to be confined to the uterus (107). At laparotomy, 20 (87%) of 23 of their patients with elevated CA-125 were found to have occult extrauterine disease. Conversely, only 1 of 58 patients with a normal value had occult extrauterine disease. In a large study, Hsieh et al. (108) reviewed preoperative serum CA-125 levels, operative records, and pathologic reports in 141 patients diagnosed with endometrial carcinoma to find out if the preoperative level of CA-125 can provide additional information to determine the extent of lymphadenectomy required in the surgical staging and which cutoff is optimal in this respect. Of 141 patients, 124 were staged surgically and 24 (19%) were found to have lymph node metastasis. In the node-positive group, median preoperative serum levels were 94 U/mL (range 17 to 363 U/mL). Multivariate analysis showed lymph node metastasis had the most significant effect on the elevation of CA-125 levels (>40 U/mL). The sensitivity and specificity for screening lymph node metastasis were 78% and 84%, respectively. The data of Hsieh et al. give evidence that preoperative CA-125 levels greater than 40 U/mL can be considered an indication for full pelvic and para-aortic lymphadenectomy in the surgical staging of endometrial carcinoma. These results are in accordance with others (109–113). Rose et al. (114) found serial CA-125 measurements to be most useful in patients with high-risk disease whose initial stage was II, III, or IV, or whose tumor was grade 3 or of clear cell or serous histology. Fifteen (94%) of 16 patients with recurrent disease had an elevated CA-125 level. Serial measurements of CA-125 are also used to monitor for recurrence and to assess response to tumor therapy in patients whose levels were initially elevated at diagnosis.

Determining the Surgical Procedure

Of all the female pelvic malignancies, endometrial cancer seems to have more advocates for different treatment plans than any other. The standard treatment for this disease has been and remains a hysterectomy. However, through the years, preoperative and postoperative irradiation has had an important role in the management of this disease. The first significant report of employing irradiation in the management of patients with endometrial cancer was the publication of the "Stockholm technique" by Heyman in 1935 (115). The use of intracavitary implants using Heyman's method became increasingly popular in the ensuing years. Subsequently, reports comparing results in patients treated with a single intrauterine tandem with those treated with multiple intrauterine capsules revealed a lower incidence of residual disease and an improved 5-year survival rate, favoring the patients treated with capsules (116–118). Lewis et al. (119), in cooperative studies in the late 1960s, showed that 25% of patients had deep myometrial invasion if treated initially by surgery, and only 8% had deep invasion if treated by preoperative irradiation. Patients frequently were managed with preoperative radiation (whole pelvic radiation [WPR], low-dose-rate [LDR] implant with or without WPR) followed within 4 to 6 weeks by a complete hysterectomy. While surgical evaluation of lymph nodes in endometrial cancer was reported in the 1960s, it was not widely embraced (120–123). The GOG undertook the large surgical-pathologic study, GOG 33, of clinical stage I endometrial cancer to better define patterns of spread with the hope that defining pathologic relationships would lead to a tailored (rather than a universal) approach to radiation (60,122). The results of this study subsequently led to the incorporation of a surgical staging system (FIGO 1988).

Contemporary management for most patients with endometrial cancer remains surgical and includes, at the minimum, an initial surgical exploration with collection of peritoneal fluid for cytologic evaluation (intraperitoneal cell washings), through inspection of the abdominal and pelvic cavities with biopsy or excision of any extrauterine lesions suspicious for tumor, and total extrafascial hysterectomy with bilateral salpingo-oophorectomy. Where the tradition has been to perform this surgery abdominally (typically through a vertical midline incision), laparoscopic management has increasingly been integrated into the forefront. The uterus should be particularly observed for tumor breakthrough of the serosal surface. The distal ends of the fallopian tubes are clipped or ligated to prevent possible tumor spill during uterine manipulation. To complete the surgical staging of endometrial cancer, the removal of bilateral pelvic and para-aortic lymph nodes is also required.

When surgical staging is performed, a bilateral pelvic and para-aortic nodal lymphadenectomy is increasingly performed (9,123). The margins of the pelvic nodal dissection are comparable to what is used for a pelvic nodal dissection with cervical cancer and is outlined by the margins of the circumflex iliac vein distally, the bifurcation of the iliac vessels proximally, the lateral margin is the genitofemoral nerve, and the medial margin is the superior vesical artery. The floor of the dissection is the obturator nerve. Nodal/fatty tissue is skeletonized from these structures. In cases of bulky nodal disease, complete resection/debulking rather than biopsy to solely demonstrate metastatic disease is favored where possible. The common iliac nodes can be removed as a separate specimen, or divided at a midpoint along the vessels, submitting the inferior half with the pelvic nodes, and the superior half with the para-aortic nodes. Particularly on the left side, the common iliac nodes will be quite lateral in location and will require sufficient mobilization to visualize the nodes. Removal of para-aortic nodes can be performed through a midline peritoneal incision over the common iliac arteries and aorta or by mobilizing the right and left colon medially (124,125). In each case, lymph nodes are resected along the upper common iliac vessels on either side and from the lower portion of the aorta and vena cava.

At the present time, the inferior mesenteric artery is used to demark the superior extent of the para-aortic nodal dissection. Suspicious nodes extending to the renal vessels are removed.

In cases with gross omental or intraperitoneal disease spread, cytoreductive surgery with total omentectomy, radical peritoneal stripping, and occasionally bowel resection are required. The goal of reducing the residual disease to no or small volumes akin to what is performed for ovarian cancer is increasingly considered. In cases complicated by medical comorbidity, advanced age, or obesity, or when nodal dissection cannot or will not be performed, total vaginal hysterectomy with or without laparoscopic assistance may also be utilized. Following surgical assessment, patients may be classified based on pathologic features as to their risk of recurrence, and those deemed to be at sufficient risk may be offered adjuvant therapies.

Nonsurgical Management

The management of most patients with endometrial cancer is surgical. The decision to use surgery is a function of patient and disease status. Patients with significant medical comorbidities who are not acceptable candidates for surgery (markedly advanced age, diminished performance status, severe cardiac/pulmonary disease, massive obesity) may be managed by alternative means. Primary radiation therapy without surgery has been used, and is discussed later in this chapter. Progestational therapy may be used for those who are inoperable or in younger patients who elect for fertility preservation (76,126,127). If the pretreatment studies are complete, the patient may be clinically staged if she is not a surgical staging candidate. The clinical staging system proposed by the FIGO in 1971 (Table 23.3) is still applicable for cases that do not go to primary operative staging while those that do undergo initial hysterectomy are staged by the 1988 FIGO system (Table 23.4) (128). Patients who are obese, but otherwise surgical candidates may undergo an abdominal panniculectomy to enhance surgical expose to facilitate hysterectomy and nodal dissection (129,130). For patients presenting with disseminated or nonresectable disease, nonsurgical options including radiation, chemotherapy, or hormonal therapy have also been used. Surgery may be required to control vaginal bleeding in some of these cases.

Approximately 5% of women with endometrial cancer are diagnosed under the age of 40 (4). For some younger women, the standard treatment of hysterectomy is unacceptable due to desires to maintain fertility. Endometrial cancer in younger women is usually associated with early-stage, low-grade disease and carries a favorable prognosis, making medical management an attractive option to some (77,78,127,131,132). Patients without myometrial invasion are thought to be the best candidates, and may undergo pelvic MRI to assess for myometrial involvement. Progestational therapy, most commonly with medroxyprogesterone acetate or megestrol acetate, has been successful in reversing malignant changes in up to 76% of cases (76,127,131). Because response may be temporary or incomplete, periodic sampling of the endometrium is advised.

Vaginal Hysterectomy

Vaginal hysterectomy with or without postoperative radiation may be another option for managing complicated patients. Vaginal hysterectomy has often been cited as the simplest and least morbid approach to hysterectomy, and has produced similar treatment outcomes in patients with clinical stage I endometrial cancer (133–135). It is often used as an alternative to an abdominal approach in obese and poor-surgical-risk patients (136,137). Limitations include the lack of exploration of the intraperitoneal cavity, inability to procure cytologic washings, greater difficulty in performing an oophorectomy, and inability to perform lymph node sampling. As lymph node metastasis is related to such high-risk features as poor differentiation, unfavorable histologic subtypes, and deep myometrial invasion, the risk of extrauterine disease following TVH must be estimated based on uterine pathology (60). Accurate assessment requires surgical staging, and understaging in clinical stage I disease has been reported to occur in 19% to 22% of cases (138).

Nodal Dissection

The value of staging any malignancy relates to the ability to describe the extent of disease at diagnosis, and to define comparable patient populations for whom prognosis and therapy are similar. Given the inability to accurately detect disease spread for many gynecologic malignancies, solely based on clinical examination and imaging studies, surgical staging systems that require pathologic evaluation of sampled sites have been largely incorporated into practice. The value of surgical staging as it relates to endometrial cancers has been the subject

TABLE 23.3

CORPUS CANCER CLINICAL STAGING, FIGO 1971

Stage	Characteristics
I	Carcinoma is confined to the corpus
IA	Length of the uterine cavity is 8 cm or less
IB	Length of the uterine cavity is more than 8 cm
Histologic subtypes of adenocarcinoma	
G1	Highly differentiated adenomatous carcinoma
G2	Differentiated adenomatous carcinoma with partly solid areas
G3	Predominantly solid or entirely undifferentiated carcinoma
II	Carcinoma involves the corpus and cervix
III	Carcinoma extends outside the uterus but not outside the true pelvis
IV	Carcinoma extends outside the true pelvis or involves the bladder or rectum

Note: FIGO, International Federation of Gynecology and Obstetrics.

TABLE 23.4

CORPUS CANCER SURGICAL STAGING, FIGO 1988

Stages/grades	Characteristics
IA G123	Tumor limited to endometrium
IB G123	Invasion to less than half of the myometrium
IC G123	Invasion to less than half of the myometrium
IIA G123	Endocervical glandular involvement only
IIB G123	Cervical stromal invasion
IIIA G123	Tumor invades serosa or adnexae or positive peritoneal cytology
IIIB G123	Vaginal metastases
IIIC G123	Metastases to pelvic or para-aortic lymph nodes
IVA G123	Tumor invades bladder and/or bowel mucosa
IVB	Distant metastases including intra-abdominal and/or inguinal lymph node

HISTOPATHOLOGY, DEGREE OF DIFFERENTIATION

Cases should be grouped by the degree of differentiation of the adenocarcinoma:

G1	5% or less of a nonsquamous or nonmorular solid growth pattern
G2	6% to 50% of a nonsquamous or nonmorular solid growth pattern
G3	More than 50% of a nonsquamous or nonmorular solid growth pattern

NOTES ON PATHOLOGIC GRADING

Notable nuclear atypia, inappropriate for the architectural grade, raises the grade of a grade 1 or grade 2 tumor by 1.

In serous adenocarcinomas, clear cell adenocarcinomas, and squamous cell carcinomas, nuclear grading takes precedence.

Adenocarcinomas with squamous differentiation are graded according to the nuclear grade of the glandular component.

RULES RELATED TO STAGING

Because corpus cancer is now surgically staged, procedures previously used for determination of stages are no longer applicable, such as the finding of fractional D&C to differentiate between stages I and II.

It is appreciated that there may be a small number of patients with corpus cancer who will be treated primarily with radiation therapy. If that is the case, the clinical staging adopted by FIGO in 1971 would still apply, but designation of that staging system would be noted.

Ideally, width of the myometrium should be measured, along with the width of tumor invasion.

Note: D&C, dilatation and curettage; FIGO, International Federation of Gynecology and Obstetrics.

of increased scrutiny and debate over the last several years. For endometrial cancers, the ability of surgical staging to accurately identify spread to draining lymph node basins and how this information (or lack of it) changes prognosis and alters the use of postoperative therapies are a source of controversy. Proponents of routine surgical staging suggest that the ability to identify otherwise unrecognized disease spread to the nodes changes the postoperative therapies that are given, and is the most accurate way to assess risk. Most controversial is the assertion that surgical staging has a therapeutic benefit independent of the node status (positive or negative for metastatic disease).

Fundamentally, surgeons must determine for themselves whether or not they believe that surgical staging has sufficient value to offer it for all patients or only selectively based on risk factors identified pre- and intra-operatively. If a patient will not be offered surgical staging/nodal dissection, then minimizing surgical morbidity with a vaginal or laparoscopic-assisted approach seems warranted. In this case, lower risk/quicker recovery comes at the cost of less information. In cases where nodal dissection will or potentially will be performed, patients must be adequately counseled regarding the risks and benefits. The principle risks attributable to nodal dissections include increased operative time, potential for blood loss associated with vascular injury, genitofemoral nerve injury with resulting numbness and paresthesias over medial thighs, lymphocyst formation, and lymphedema (Table 23.5) (62,139–141). In general, the risks associated with nodal dissections are low and acceptable. Patients who have nodal dissections and receive pelvic radiation therapy may be at a greater risk of bowel morbidity than those without dissections (142,143). Nodal dissections also require the involvement of someone trained and skilled to perform the procedure. The principle advantage of comprehensive staging is that the physician and patient are provided with the greatest amount of information. In the contemporary management of endometrial cancer, this information results in less use of radiation, and substitution of vaginal cuff brachytherapy for pelvic radiation (9,123,144).

The importance, extent, and technique of nodal dissection are hotly debated. Questions relate to which patients should be offered and could benefit from surgical staging (all, some, none), and what is the optimal surgical procedure to be performed (biopsy of enlarged/visible nodes, lymphadenectomy). Controversy also exists between those surgeons who perform only pelvic dissections and those who advocate pelvic and para-aortic nodal dissection. If para-aortic nodes are removed, are bilateral nodes required, and to what superior extent (inferior mesenteric artery, renal vessels) should the dissection proceed?

TABLE 23.5

RISKS ASSOCIATED WITH NODAL DISSECTION: SURGICAL COMPLICATION RATES ASSOCIATED WITH ABDOMINAL HYSTERECTOMY + PELVIC AND PARA-AORTIC LYMPH NODE DISSECTION

Study	N	Hemorrhage (%)	GU injury (%)	DVT/PE (%)	Lymphocyst (%)	Other
Morrow 1991(62)	895	2.2	0.4	2	1.2	—
Homesley 1992(140)	196	6% transfused	—	4	—	"Serious" 6%
Orr 1997(139)	396	4.2% transfused	0.6	1.5	1.2	—
Mariani 2006(182)	96 node (+) patients	—	1	1	3.1	—

Note: DVT/PE, deep vein thrombosis/pulmonary embolism; GU, genitourinary.

Nodal Dissection—None

In the United States, comprehensive surgical staging of endometrial cancer is infrequently performed. Only 30% to 40% of patients undergo nodal assessment, indicating that the majority of U.S. patients are not staged (6,145). Many gynecologists are neither trained in the techniques of lymphadenectomy nor familiar with the concept of full surgical staging. Full staging is more commonly performed by specialized surgeons, such as gynecologic oncologists (146,147). Philosophically, those opposed to nodal dissections suggest that most patients are at low risk for nodal disease, treatment decisions can be based on final pathologic information, and despite node dissection the majority of patients who are node negative do not get benefit (148). Most patients with endometrial cancer do present with low-risk features. In the entire GOG 33 study population of 621 patients, 75% had grade 1-2 tumors, 59% had inner one third or less myometrial invasion, and only 9% of patients had positive lymph nodes (60). The Post Operative Radiation Therapy in Endometrial Cancer (PORTEC) trial evaluated patients with stage IC, grade 1; stage IB-C, grade 2; or stage IB, grade 3 who underwent hysterectomy without lymph node dissection and compared observation to postoperative pelvic radiation (149). Of note, based on grade and depth of invasion, approximately 60% of patients enrolled in GOG 33 would have had disease characteristics required for eligibility in the PORTEC trial. This patient population managed without nodal dissection had favorable outcomes with or without radiation therapy (5-year survival rates of 85% observation, 81% with pelvic radiation) in the PORTEC study (149). Trimble et al. reported on data from stage I endometrial cancer patients collected by SEER from 1988 to 1993 and showed that 5-year relative survival for patients without nodal dissection was 98% compared to 96% in those undergoing nodal dissection and suggested that nodal dissection did not convey a benefit for the overall population (150). Unfortunately, data on adjuvant therapy use was not available. It is suspected that increased use of radiation in unstaged patients may produce similar outcomes to patients who are staged and who avoid radiation therapy.

In a nonrandomized trial comparing hysterectomy with or without pelvic lymphadenectomy, followed by radiation therapy, 14% of patients (N = 207) with negative nodes treated with vaginal cuff brachytherapy (VCB) recurred compared to 16% who did not have a lymphadenectomy (N = 660) (151). While the authors noted similar cancer-free survival between the groups, all patients who did not have nodal dissections received both pelvic radiation and VCB to attain these results. The only randomized trial comparing lymphadenectomy to no nodal assessment has recently concluded enrollment. A Study in the Treatment of Endometrial Cancer (ASTEC) randomized patients with endometrial cancer treated with hysterectomy to pelvic lymphadenectomy or not. Following surgery, patients with stage I-IIA disease were then randomized again to observation or pelvic radiation therapy if they had grade 3, serous, or clear cell histology; >50% myometrial invasion; or endocervical glandular invasion (stage IIA). Treatment centers were also permitted to use VCB regardless of pelvic radiation assignment based on institutional preference. As a result, a patient with unknown nodal status and >50% invasion could receive VCB and not be considered to have received radiation therapy. This may produce a potential bias as groups treated with lymphadenectomy and no radiation may be compared to those which had no nodal dissection and received VCB. Preliminary results suggest that there was no advantage of routine lymphadenectomy (152). The final results of this study are eagerly awaited.

Without nodal information, physicians must rely on uterine factors to estimate the probability for nodal disease and pelvic failure to determine the need for postoperative radiation. Risk assessments may be based on nodal positivity estimates from GOG 33 or on patient risk groups treated with or without radiation therapy (PORTEC, for example). This estimation can result in a substantial increase in the use of radiation, particularly if the primary benefit of postoperative radiation is in node-positive patients. As a result, the lack of nodal information can lead to overtreatment of patients. The absence of nodal dissection may also lead to poorer outcomes. For example, a subset of 99 patients with stage IC, grade 3 endometrial cancer, who did not have lymph node dissection, were not eligible, but were treated with pelvic radiation and followed prospectively within the PORTEC trial (153). Five-year survival for this group of patients was 58%, and 12% had vaginal or pelvic failures despite whole pelvic radiation. It is interesting to note that the outcome of this group is poorer than what has been reported in patients with stage IIIC endometrial cancer managed by lymphadenectomy followed by radiation (154–156). If patients are not to have nodal dissection, then it would seem reasonable to consider vaginal approaches (TVH, LAVH) to reduce morbidity.

Nodal Dissection—Selective

Increasingly some form of nodal assessment has been integrated into the up-front management of endometrial cancer, and nodal assessment has been incorporated into the staging of endometrial cancer since 1988. Surgical staging is the most accurate way to determine the extent of disease spread. Palpation of pelvic lymph nodes is not sufficiently accurate, with a sensitivity of 72% in a recent prospective study (157,158).

TABLE 23.6

HISTOLOGIC GRADE AND DEPTH OF INVASION

	Grade, no. of patients			
Depth	Grade 1 (%)	Grade 2 (%)	Grade 3 (%)	Total (% of total)
Endometrium only	44 (24)	31 (11)	11 (7)	86 (14)
Superficial	96 (53)	131 (45)	54 (35)	281 (45)
Middle	22 (12)	69 (24)	24 (16)	115 (19)
Deep	18 (10)	57 (20)	64 (42)	139 (22)
Total	180 (100)	288 (100)	153 (100)	621 (100)

Source: Reprinted from Creasman WT, Morrow CP, Bundy BN, et al. Surgical pathologic spread patterns of endometrial cancer: a Gynecologic Oncology Group study. *Cancer* 1987;60:2035–2041.

Many believe that nodal dissections should be reserved for those with sufficient risk of nodal disease (60,62,159,160). What risk of nodal disease (3%, 5%, 10%, etc.) warrants the procedure is debated. Data from GOG 33 demonstrated important relationships between tumor grade and depth of invasion and frequency of nodal disease that can be used to decide whether to perform nodal assessments (Tables 23.6 and 23.7) (60). For example, the risk of pelvic nodal disease was 3% for all patients with grade 1 tumors, but was 11% with deeply invasive (outer one-third myometrial invasion) tumors. Patients with grade 3 tumors had a risk of pelvic nodal metastases of 18%, and 34% with deep invasion. With cervical invasion, the rate of pelvic nodal disease was 16%. Patients with serous or clear cell histology also warrant nodal dissection as ~30% to 50% will have nodal disease, and even in the absence of myometrial invasion, nodal metastases have been reported in up to 36% of patients (161). Some advocate that lymph nodes need not be sampled for tumor limited to the endometrium, regardless of grade, because less than 1% of these patients have disease spread to pelvic or para-aortic lymph nodes (60,162). A gray zone in deciding about lymph node sampling is represented by patients whose only risk factor is inner one-half myometrial invasion, particularly if the grade is 2 or 3. This group has 5% or less chance of node positivity (62). The overall surgical complication rate after this type of staging is approximately 20%. The serious complication rate

TABLE 23.7

FREQUENCY OF NODAL METASTASIS AMONG RISK FACTORS

Risk factor	No. of patients	Pelvic no. (%)	Aortic no. (%)
Histology			
Endometrioid adenocarcinoma	599	56 (9)	30 (5)
Others	22	2 (9)	4 (18)
Grade			
1 Well	180	5 (3)	3 (2)
2 Moderate	288	25 (9)	14 (5)
3 Poor	153	28 (18)	17 (11)
Myometrial invasion			
Endometrial	87	1 (1)	1 (1)
Superficial	279	15 (5)	8 (3)
Middle	116	7 (6)	1 (1)
Deep	139	35 (25)	24 (17)
Site of tumor location			
Fundus	524	42 (8)	20 (4)
Isthmus-cervix	97	16 (16)	14 (14)
Capillary-like space involvement			
Negative	528	37 (7)	19 (9)
Positive	93	21 (27)	15 (19)
Other extrauterine metastasis			
Negative	586	40 (7)	26 (4)
Positive	35	18 (51)	8 (23)
Peritoneal cytology[a]			
Negative	537	38 (7)	20 (4)
Positive	75	19 (25)	14 (19)

[a]Nine patients did not have cytology reported.
Source: Modified with permission from Creasman WT, Morrow CP, Bundy BN, et al. Surgical pathologic spread patterns of endometrial cancer: a Gynecologic Oncology Group study. *Cancer* 1987;60:2035.

is ≤6%, and the rate of complications should be balanced by the probability of finding nodal disease (62,139–141).

An assessment of pelvic and para-aortic lymph nodes is required to assign stage according to FIGO 1988. Two principal nodal basins drain the uterus; the lower and middle portion of the uterus drains laterally to the pelvic lymph nodes, the upper corpus and fundus drain to the para-aortic nodes. In GOG 33, the rate of para-aortic nodal involvement was roughly 50% of the pelvic node rate. As an isolated finding, para-aortic nodes were involved in only 2% of cases. Para-aortic nodal dissection is more difficult to perform than pelvic dissection, by laparotomy or by laparoscopy, and is associated with greater risk. As such, some advocate for pelvic nodal dissections with only performing para-aortic nodal dissections selectively. In GOG 33, 46% of the positive para-aortic lymph nodes were enlarged, and 98% of the cases with aortic node metastases came from patients with positive pelvic nodes, adnexal or intra-abdominal metastases, or outer one-third myometrial invasion (62). These risk factors affected only 25% of the patients, yet they yielded most of the positive para-aortic node patients.

Intraoperative assessment of the uterus has been used to guide the surgeon as to when to perform a nodal dissection. Gross inspection of the uterus immediately following its removal can be used to estimate the degree of myometrial invasion. If the uterus is opened by the operating surgeon, care should be employed to avoid distortion of the anatomy. Optimally, the unfixed uterus should be opened by the surgical pathologist, who can grossly estimate the depth of invasion, assess involvement of the cervix, and later sample the tumor for histologic assessment. There is no typical gross appearance of an endometrial carcinoma. Most are polypoid or ulcerative. Carcinoma usually differs in texture and color from the surrounding normal endometrium. The normal endometrium is irregular and tan, but a carcinoma is usually shaggy, white to gray-white, and focally hemorrhagic. Areas of myometrial invasion may be visible as gray-white to white, with yellow areas disclosing necrosis (Figs. 23.1 and 23.2). The texture may be soft, friable, or firm depending on the degree of necrosis.

Doering et al. reported a 91% accuracy rate for 148 patients for determining the depth of myometrial invasion by gross visual examination of the cut uterine surface (163). A prospective study indicated that visual inspection of < or >50% correlated with microscopic assessment in 85% cases (158). However, the sensitivity of determining >50% was lower at 72%. Invasion of the myometrium may be more extensive microscopically than is evident visibly because of the characteristic infiltrative growth pattern of the tumor. In a retrospective study by Goff and Riche, the gross estimation by pathologists of myometrial invasion in grades 2 and 3 tumors was poor (164). With invasion, the uterine cavity usually enlarges and the myometrium thickens, but a small uterus may have myometrial penetration to the serosa.

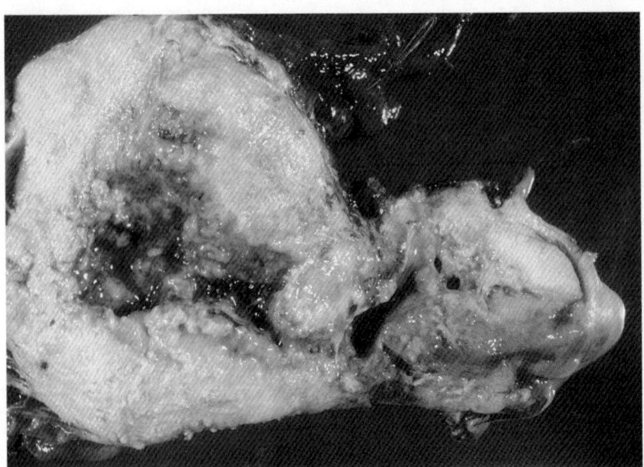

FIGURE 23.1. An ulcerating and deeply invasive adenocarcinoma that extends into the uterine cervix.

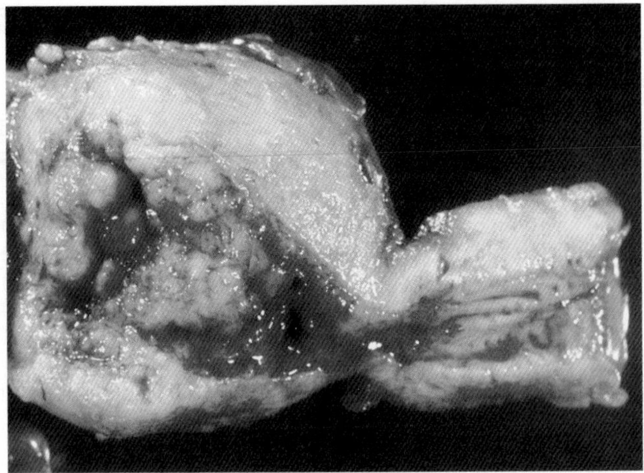

FIGURE 23.2. A polypoid adenocarcinoma of the endometrium that fills much of the lumen and superficially invades the myometrium.

Nodal Dissection—Routine

Many gynecologic oncologists have moved toward performing uniform comprehensive surgical staging for nearly all patients with endometrial cancer (9). The rationale for uniform staging includes the lack of a patient population for whom nodal disease is so low that nodes should be omitted, the inaccuracy of preoperative or intraoperative assessments predicting the risk for nodal disease, the potential for therapeutic benefit in node-positive and -negative patients, and the lack of significant morbidity associated with the procedure. Postoperative adjuvant decisions are best made with the most complete information. If nodal assessment is the predominant factor by which to categorize patients into risk groups, routine nodal dissection is the best method by which to determine which few patients will require adjuvant therapy.

What constitutes an acceptable rate of nodal disease in endometrial cancer to warrant the procedure is surgeon dependent. In cervical cancer, routine pelvic lymphadenectomy is advocated for all stage IA2 tumors where nodal positivity rates are 3% to 5% (165). For clinical stage I ovarian cancer, para-aortic dissection is recommended for all given the 6% risk of para-aortic disease (166). In endometrial cancer, major complication rates associated with nodal dissection are 2% to 6%, suggesting that this might be an appropriate level of risk to balance against the risk of nodal metastases. Data from GOG 33 show that only patients with tumor limited to the endometrium had a risk of pelvic nodal disease ≤3%, and this group accounted for only 14% of the entire study population.

Frozen section assessment has been the traditional tool to facilitate decisions on selective nodal dissections. Several studies have demonstrated inaccuracies with frozen sections in the interpretation of grade and depth of myometrial invasion compared to final pathology (167–169). In one prospective evaluation, frozen section determination of depth of invasion correlated with final pathology in 67% of cases but resulted in up-staging in 28% of cases (167). Patients with grade 1 endometrial cancer or AEH were up-staged in 61% of cases.

The clinical significance of these errors has been debated (148), but many believe that such unexpected up-staging justifies routine staging even in seemingly low-risk patients (167,168). Data also suggests that the strategy of routine nodal dissection is more cost effective than either no staging or selective staging based on frozen section results (170,171).

The technique of nodal dissection has undergone evolution. In an era where everyone was to receive radiation therapy, there was little value for a complete evaluation of lymph nodes. Removal of palpably enlarged nodes, "plucking" of visibly noted nodes, and "sampling" have given way to a more thorough assessment. Only 10% of patients with metastases to lymph nodes will have grossly enlarged nodes and frequently, even in these cases, direct palpation through the overlying peritoneum will fail to identify them (60). Today, adjuvant therapies are based on the extent of disease, and often only reserved for node-positive patients. Nodal assessments should sufficiently examine sites at risk including external iliac, hypogastric, and obturator nodes in the pelvis, common iliac nodes, and para-aortic nodes. Moving from a sampling technique to a more thorough lymphadenectomy is not associated with increased complication rates (172). Nodal dissection should be bilateral given the frequency of both left and right para-aortic involvement (173,174). It is interesting to note that GOG 33 only specified right-sided para-aortic removal in the surgical protocol. Likewise, the nodal dissection is more apt to be representative when a larger number of nodes are removed.

The importance of para-aortic nodal spread in node-positive endometrial cancer cannot be ignored (Table 23.8). Data from GOG 33 showing that of all patients, isolated para-aortic nodal metastases occurred in 2% is often taken out of context (60). If the goal of nodal dissection is to identify the node-positive patient population, para-aortic disease is seen in 40% to 66% of patients with node-positive/stage IIIC endometrial cancer, including isolated positive para-aortic nodes in 7% to 21% of cases. If only pelvic nodes are removed, when they are positive, para-aortic nodes will be positive in addition in nearly 30% to 40% of cases. It makes little sense to remove only pelvic or only para-aortic nodes given this data. Data would also suggest that when positive, outcomes are improved in patients who have complete surgical resection of para-aortic nodes. Chuang et al. reported on their experience with selective pelvic and or para-aortic dissections and found that failure to systematically remove pelvic and para-aortic nodes resulted in an increased frequency of recurrence in undissected retroperitoneal sites (175). Similarly, Mariani et al. showed that patients at high risk for para-aortic nodal disease (based on invasion >50%, palpable positive pelvic nodes, positive adnexa) who did not have para-aortic dissection or who had biopsy only and who were managed as though para-aortic nodes were positive had 5-year survival of 71% compared to 85% for those patients with positive para-aortic nodes who did undergo complete resection (172). Lymph node recurrences were detected in 37% of those not having para-aortic dissection compared to none in patients with positive but resected para-aortic nodes, suggesting a possible therapeutic effect of removing involved para-aortic nodes.

At the present time, the superior extent of para-aortic dissection should be at least to the level of the inferior mesenteric artery. Some suggest that dissections should proceed to the level of the renal vessels given the venous and lymphatic drainage following the infundibulopelvic ligament. In one series, 7 out of 11 patients had positive para-aortic nodes identified above the inferior mesenteric artery (176). This extended para-aortic dissection is feasible laparoscopically as well (177). Prospective data describing the frequency of high para-aortic/para-renal nodes are awaited.

No prospective data exist to adequately evaluate the claim that lymphadenectomy in endometrial cancer is therapeutic. The only prospective trial evaluating the role of lymphadenectomy (ASTEC trial) required only a pelvic lymphadenectomy and utilized a second randomization for pelvic radiation (152). Unfortunately, the study specified pelvic radiation for disease characteristics, which, following a negative nodal dissection, is typically avoided. Likewise, vaginal cuff radiation was permitted as per institutional practice irrespective of the assignment to pelvic radiation or not, making interpretations of any results likely difficult.

The retrospective data suggesting a therapeutic benefit supports but does not prove the hypothesis that lymphadenectomy is therapeutic. These studies are largely from single institutions, have short follow-up, suffer from selection biases, and do not clearly account for stage migration. Despite these limitations, the therapeutic value of lymphadenectomy is supported by several

TABLE 23.8

RELATIONSHIP BETWEEN PELVIC AND PARA-AORTIC NODAL INVOLVEMENT IN PATIENTS WITH NODE-POSITIVE ENDOMETRIAL CANCER

Study	N	Surgical technique	Pelvic (+) only (%)	Pelvic and para-aortic (+) (%)	Para-aortic only (%)	Any involvement of para-aortic nodes (%)
Creasman 1987(60)	70	Routine: sampling	51	31	17	48
Schorge 1996(108)	35	Selective: lymphadenectomy	74	17	9	26
Hirahatake 1997(176)	42	Routine: systematic lymphadenectomy	57	38	5	42
Onda 1997(154)	30	Routine: systematic lymphadenectomy	33	60	6.6	66
McMeekin 2001(155)	47	Routine: lymphadenectomy	38	41	21	62
Otsuka 2002(609)	23	Selective: systematic lymphadenectomy	66	33	10	43
Havrilesky 2005(183)	96	Selective: lymphadenectomy	52	30	18	48

reports. Kilgore et al. were among the first to report a therapeutic effect of nodal dissections in a series of 649 clinical stage I–occult II patients who were classified based on the extent of nodal dissection (178). Patients who underwent multiple site pelvic nodal dissection (defined by nodal dissection of at least four pelvic nodal sites) and had a mean of 11 nodes removed had improved survival over those patients who did not have nodes sampled. The survival advantage for multiple site dissection persisted even when patients were stratified into low-risk (uterine-confined disease) and high-risk (extrauterine disease) groups who received radiation. An explanation for this may be the removal of unrecognized micrometastasis, which goes undetected by standard pathologic processing techniques. Girardi et al. performed complete pelvic lymphadenectomies in 76 patients with endometrial cancer (mean 37 nodes removed) and reported a 36% nodal positivity rate (179). Nodal tissue was processed as step serial sections and 37% of positive nodes were <2 mm in diameter, suggesting that nodal metastases may be missed in a proportion of node-positive patients processed in a less extensive manner. Others have shown improvement in outcomes following a more complete nodal dissection in node-negative populations. Cragan et al. evaluated 509 stage I-IIA patients who underwent selective pelvic+/– para-aortic lymphadenectomy and found a survival advantage for patients with grade 3 tumors who had >11 pelvic nodes removed, compared to those with ≤11 nodes removed (hazard ratio 0.25) (180). For patients with high-risk features (grade 3, >50% myometrial invasion, serous/clear cell tumors) 5-year survival was 82% when >11 nodes were removed versus 64% when ≤11 nodes were removed. Chan et al. reported on the effect of a more complete nodal dissection in over 12,000 women with endometrial cancer tracked in the SEER data system. In patients with high-risk disease (IB/grade 3, IC, II-IV), 5-year survival was proportional to the number of nodes removed, increasing from 75% to 87% when 1 versus >20 nodes were removed (181). In a multivariate analysis, a more extensive nodal assessment was an independent predictor of survival.

In patients with positive pelvic and/or para-aortic nodes, complete resection followed by adjuvant therapy results in superior outcomes. Mariani et al. showed that pelvic sidewall failure at 5 years was 57% for patients who had inadequate nodal dissection and/or no adjuvant radiation compared to 10% when patients had adequate (removal >10 nodes) lymphadenectomy and received radiation (182). Patients with bulky residual nodes have poorer survival compared to those who have the nodes successfully resected (183). The best outcomes reported for node-positive patients follow complete nodal dissection. For example, in one series, of 30 stage IIIC patients managed with systematic pelvic and para-aortic lymphadenectomy (average number nodes removed, 66) followed by radiation therapy and chemotherapy, 5-year survival was 100% for patients with positive pelvic nodes and 75% for positive para-aortic nodes (154).

The most cogent argument for routine staging is that following thorough nodal assessment, most patients with node-negative disease can accurately be classified as low risk, and may avoid pelvic radiation or receive vaginal cuff brachytherapy in lieu of pelvic radiation therapy. Three randomized trials comparing radiation to observation have failed to demonstrate a survival advantage for adjuvant pelvic radiation therapy in patients with stage I-II disease, suggesting that in the absence of nodal disease no therapy is a reasonable option (143,149,184). Retrospective studies have shown how the incorporation of a strategy using lymphadenectomy changes the use of postoperative radiation (9,123,139,144,185,186). In the absence of nodal disease, recurrence risk is low and overall survival is high, with no radiation or with the substitution of vaginal cuff brachytherapy.

Laparoscopic Management

Laparoscopic management of endometrial cancer has increasingly been integrated into standard practice. Laparoscopic techniques are utilized in the initial treatment of endometrial cancer (LAVH, total laparoscopic hysterectomy [TLH]) to stage patients with laparoscopic pelvic and para-aortic nodal dissection, and to re-stage patients following incomplete surgical staging. The decade of the 1990s advanced the use of minimally invasive surgery and introduced the laparoscopic techniques and tools required for comprehensive surgical staging of endometrial cancer. As the initial debate on laparoscopic vaginal hysterectomy focused on whether laparoscopic techniques could be substituted for abdominal ones, in endometrial cancer, debate has focused on whether laparoscopic surgical staging could be substituted for open procedures. Initial case reports and small single institutional series describing technique and demonstrating feasibility were replaced by large series, small randomized trials, and subsequently a multi-institutional randomized controlled trial (187–197).

Improvements in laparoscopic equipment facilitated the development of LAVH. Building on that experience, and coupled with the introduction of better optics for visualization, laparoscopic resection of lymph nodes became possible. Querleu et al. were the first to report pelvic lymphadenectomy for cervical cancer in 1991 (198), followed by Nezhat et al. who reported in 1992 on the use of laparoscopic pelvic and para-aortic lymphadenectomy with radical hysterectomy in cervical cancer (199). When first utilized in endometrial cancer, laparoscopic para-aortic node dissection only evaluated right-sided nodes (187). Techniques have subsequently been developed allowing for dissection to include the left para-aortic nodes (177,200–202).

Arguments have been advanced for and against each of the surgical approaches to endometrial cancer. Vaginal hysterectomy was once a favored operation, but it did not allow for routine removal of the ovaries in some patients, permit inspection of the peritoneal cavity or the retroperitoneum for metastatic disease, or allow collection of peritoneal fluid for cytology (203). Laparoscopic-assisted or total laparoscopic approaches overcome these limitations, however. Compared to open procedures, LAVH/TLH are thought to lead to reduced incisional complications, wound infections, ileus, hospital stay, cost, and improved rate of recovery and quality of life (194,195). In patients requiring postoperative radiation, laparoscopic surgical staging followed by radiation therapy is suggested to result in fewer bowel adhesions and radiation-induced bowel injuries (204). Criticisms of LAVH/TLH with laparoscopic nodal dissection relate to the learning curve required to learn new or unfamiliar procedures, the increased length of operative times, and concerns about the adequacy of the nodal dissection. Studies do suggest that with increased experience, operative times decrease and nodal counts increase (200,205). Laparoscopy also introduced different procedural-related complications (206–208). For example, the technique has the potential to produce port-site recurrences (209) or intraperitoneal dissemination (210) of disease by laparoscopic gas and/or uterine manipulation, although the frequency of these events is low. Results of long-term survival in laparoscopically treated endometrial cancer patients are still limited (190,193).

Childers et al. (187,188) described the initial experience of LAVH in 59 patients with clinical stage I endometrial carcinoma. Laparoscopic pelvic and right-sided aortic lymph node samplings were performed in patients with grade 2 or 3 lesions, or with grade 1 lesions and greater than 50% myometrial invasion on frozen section. For the group, the mean weight was 153 pounds, and in two patients, laparoscopic lymphadenectomy was precluded by obesity. Six patients had the procedure converted to open due to intraperitoneal disease, and two patients required laparotomy to manage complications, including a transected ureter and a cystotomy. The mean hospital stay was 2.9 days. Since that time many retrospective series have appeared in the literature (242,303–307). Gemignani et al. compared the clinical outcomes and hospital charges for 69 women with early-stage endometrial cancer who underwent laparoscopically assisted vaginal hysterectomy compared to 251 who underwent an abdominal approach (194). Although the mean operating time was longer for the laparoscopic group, the overall complication rates, length of stay, and hospital charges were lower. With short follow-up, there was no significant difference in disease recurrence between the two groups.

A small prospective, randomized trial comparing laparoscopic-assisted vaginal versus abdominal surgery in patients with endometrial cancer was reported by Malur et al. (192). They randomized 70 patients with endometrial cancer FIGO stage I-III to laparoscopy-assisted simple or radical vaginal hysterectomy or simple or radical abdominal hysterectomy with or without lymph node resection. Thirty-seven patients were treated in the laparoscopic versus 33 patients in the laparotomy group. Lymph node resection was performed in 25 patients by laparoscopy and in 24 patients by laparotomy. Blood loss and transfusion rates were significantly lower in the laparoscopic group. The number of pelvic and para-aortic lymph nodes, duration of surgery, and incidence of postoperative complications were similar for both groups. No significant differences in disease recurrence rate and long-term survival were found between the laparoscopic and laparotomy groups (97.3% vs. 93.3% and 83.9% vs. 90.9%, respectively). There was no difference in duration of surgery between the two groups. Malur et al. explain this by an extensive exposure by laparoscopic surgery and laparoscopic lymphadenectomy in their team over the past 5 years, which helped to save time (192). They also found a significantly shorter duration of hospital stay in the laparoscopic group, which also has been reported by others (189,190,211). The conclusion of Malur et al. was that laparoscopic staging combined with laparoscopically assisted vaginal hysterectomy can be recommended for the treatment of women with endometrial cancer, offering a less invasive approach that is associated with less intraoperative and postoperative morbidity (192).

The largest and most comprehensive data set to date comes from the large prospective, randomized trial conducted by the GOG (Lap II trial) (196,197). The study was designed to compare laparoscopic hysterectomy with comprehensive surgical staging to the traditional laparotomy technique (using a 2:1 randomization favoring the laparoscopic arm) to determine the complete staging rates, safety, short-term surgical outcomes, and long-term cancer recurrence and survival. The study enrolled 920 patients to the open arm, and 1,696 to laparoscopy. The rate of conversion from laparoscopy to open procedure was 26%, and was most frequently related to poor visibility (15%), extrauterine cancer spread (4%), and bleeding (3%). The conversion rate increased with increasing patient obesity, with the laparoscopic success rate being 90% with a body mass index (BMI) <20, 65% with BMI = 35, and 34% with BMI = 50. Median number of removed nodes was similar between each technique as were the frequencies of patients found to have positive lymph nodes. Complication rates (combined rates of vascular, urinary, bowel, nerve, or other complications) for those who had an open procedure were 7.6%, compared to 9.5% of patients randomized to laparoscopy. Of the 1,242 patients randomized to laparoscopy who had the procedure successfully completed laparoscopically, the complication rate was 4.9%. Comparing patients who underwent open surgery versus successful completion of laparoscopy, operative time was longer (median 70 minutes), but hospital time was shorter (2 vs. 4 days) with laparoscopy. Postoperative arrhythmia, pneumonia, ileus, antibiotic use, and any complication > grade 2 were lower in the laparoscopic group. Long-term recurrence and survival data are maturing. The authors concluded that laparoscopic surgical staging is an acceptable and possibly a better option, particularly when the surgery can be successfully completed laparoscopically.

Age and obesity have been suggested as relative contraindications to laparoscopic surgery. In the GOG Lap II trial, the median age was 63 years. Scribner et al. evaluated the surgical experience of uterine cancer patients age ≥65 years who underwent LAVH with pelvic and para-aortic lymphadenectomy (N = 67) or abdominal hysterectomy with pelvic and para-aortic lymphadenectomy (N = 45) (212). Laparoscopic staging could be completed in 78% of patients. In the laparoscopic group, the BMI was 29.5 kg/m^2 (range 15.9 to 54.7), and 33% had a history of prior laparotomy. For the 22% of patients who required a conversion to laparotomy, obesity (10%), bleeding (6%), and intraperitoneal disease (5%) were the most frequent reasons. Similar nodal counts (29 laparoscopy, 29 open) were noted, the operative time was longer (236 minutes vs. 148 minutes), and hospital stay was shorter (median 3 vs. 5.6 days) with laparoscopy. The authors concluded that with the anticipated growth of an aging patient population, laparoscopic management is a viable option.

Obese patients have also been suggested to be poor laparoscopic candidates due to difficulties in establishing pneumoperitoneum, poorer visualization, inability to tolerate steep Trendelenburg positioning needed to facilitate the surgery, and difficulties with ventilation. In the report by Childers et al. mean patient weight was only 153 pounds (187,188). It is important to recognize that regardless of surgical approach, complete surgical staging is more difficult in an obese patient. Scriber et al. compared 55 obese patients (median weight 96.6 kg, median BMI 40) who underwent LAVH with pelvic and para-aortic lymphadenectomy to 45 patients (median weight 101 kg, median BMI 39) who had abdominal hysterectomy with pelvic and para-aortic lymphadenectomy (213). Successful completion of laparoscopy was possible in 64%, with patients with a BMI <35 kg/m^2 having an 82% success rate compared to 44% when the BMI was >35 kg/m^2. Eltabbakh et al. evaluated 40 women with BMI between 28 and 60 who were treated with LAVH and compared them to 40 similar women treated by abdominal approach (214). Laparoscopic conversion was only required in 8% of patients. Laparoscopic surgery was associated with a longer operative time (195 minutes vs. 138 minutes), but more pelvic nodes (mean 11 vs. 5), less pain medicine requirement, and shorter hospital stay (2.5 vs. 5.6 days) were recorded. Total laparoscopic hysterectomy has also been shown to be feasible in heavier patients (215). In the prospective GOG series, there was ≥80% success rate with patients with a BMI of 27 or less, but even at a BMI of 35, 65% could have successful laparoscopic surgery (196).

Whether an LAVH/TLH procedure is comparable to an open approach must be judged by the ability to accurately dissect appropriate nodal basins, to remove an adequate/representative number of lymph nodes, to identify metastatic disease, and by the rates of recurrence. The technique used to remove the uterus/ovaries is not the source of controversy. Comprehensive surgical staging allows for appropriate risk stratification to make appropriate treatment recommendations. Multiple reports demonstrated similar node counts for open and laparoscopic technique in the surgical staging of endometrial cancer (189,194). Possover et al., reporting on 150 patients undergoing pelvic and para-aortic lymphadenectomy, demonstrated the adequacy of lymph node counts utilizing the laparoscopic procedure (216). The average pelvic lymph node count was 26 per patient and ranged between 10 and 56. Spirtos et al. documented 40 women who his group attempted to stage surgically, limiting the size to a BMI of 30 (200). Thirty-five completed the procedure and two of those failed to have left para-aortic nodes sampled, resulting in an 82.5% success rate. The node count was 12 to 42 with 27.7 being the average nodes per patient, and 20.8 pelvic nodes (11 right, 9.8 left). There was an average of 7.9 aortic nodes (3.8 right, and 4.1 left). In the GOG Lap II trial, median numbers of nodes from pelvic and para-aortic basins, and frequencies of positive nodes were comparable in the surgical arms (196,197). Despite the potential benefits of laparoscopic surgery, if laparoscopic nodal dissection cannot be performed, conversion to laparotomy is advised when incomplete staging results would yield inadequate information for treatment planning.

The laparoscopic surgery must be performed with an acceptable complication rate to be considered a viable option. In one series reporting on complication rates with an institution's first 100 pelvic and para-aortic nodal dissections, conversion to manage complications was required in five to control bleeding, and one to repair a ureteral injury (217). In another group's experience with 150 patients, seven major vascular injuries were reported, but only four patients required laparotomy (216). Querleu et al. reported on intraoperative and postoperative complications of laparoscopic node dissection from 1,192 pelvic and para-aortic nodal dissections (218). Only 13 open procedures were required to complete the nodal dissections, and a laparotomy was required in seven cases to manage complications. Eleven intraoperative vascular injuries were noted, but none required laparotomy to manage. In the GOG Lap II study, intraoperative complications were comparable (7.6% open, 9.5% randomized to laparoscopy, 4.9% successful completion of laparoscopy). Postoperative complications and short-term quality of life improvements favored laparoscopy.

Restaging

One of the more useful roles of laparoscopic surgery is in restaging patients who underwent hysterectomy only. Patients who undergo hysterectomy without nodal dissection and who have pathologic risk factors for potential nodal spread face a difficult dilemma. Patients may elect to receive radiation or chemotherapy (presume nodes are positive), elect observation (presume nodes are negative), or undergo a second operation. A second laparotomy can be difficult to accept. Laparoscopic staging offers the patient a less invasive option to collect information. Childers et al. reported the initial experience with restaging in 13 patients, finding disease in 3 patients (219).

Laparoscopic Recommendations

Laparoscopic surgery has demonstrated an important role in the management of endometrial cancer. Just as with an abdominal procedure, hysterectomy with pelvic and para-aortic nodal assessment is standard. Additional training and experience are required for successful completion of the procedure, just as they are with open procedures. The demonstration of comparable surgical endpoints (similar numbers of nodes removed, similar frequency of positive nodes) along with shortened hospital stay and quicker recovery compared to open procedures suggest that appropriate patients should be counseled regarding this option. Challenges remain on how to increase the laparoscopic training of gynecologic oncologists in practice and fellows in training programs. Long-term follow-up demonstrating recurrence rates and survival are also required.

Surgical Management of Intraperitoneal Disease

The management of patients with stage IV disease depends on the ability to resect disease. In patients with distant metastasis, there may be a limited role for surgery such as to provide control of vaginal bleeding. In patients with intraperitoneal disease, options include resecting easily removable disease (uterus, adnexa, omentum) versus a more extensive cytoreductive effort. The value of extensive cytoreductive surgery in endometrial cancer has not been as well studied as it has in ovarian cancer. Historically, limitations in postoperative therapies (lack of enthusiasm for whole abdominal radiation, marginally effective chemotherapy regimens, reliance on hormonal therapy) perhaps reduced interest. Several retrospective reports suggest that survival correlates with volume of residual disease (220–222). Chi et al. showed that median survival was 31 months following cytoreduction to ≤2 cm residual disease compared to 12 months when debulked, but residuals were >2 cm. Bristow et al. demonstrated that optimal cytoreduction (<1 cm) could be obtained in 55% of stage IV patients, and required omentectomy (93%), peritoneal stripping (65%), and bowel resection (29%) to do it (221,222). In patients with serous histology, similar survival improvements were seen with optimal debulking of intraperitoneal disease (223).

Surgical Recommendations

The contemporary management of endometrial cancer has significantly changed. We believe the benefits of routine nodal dissections should be extended to all patients who are appropriate candidates for surgery. Patients who *a priori* are deemed not to be candidates for staging should be considered for vaginal or laparoscopic-assisted vaginal hysterectomies. We seldom perform simple abdominal hysterectomy without nodal dissection for this disease. Surgical therapy for endometrial cancer removes the disease and defines populations at risk for recurrence and death. Surgical staging, or the lack of it, defines patient groups into surgically staged node positive or negative, or unstaged. Comprehensive staging most accurately assigns stage and associated prognosis. Staging also allows for a more tailored approach to the use of adjuvant therapies. Laparoscopic techniques have been shown to result in comparable surgery to open procedures. Whether nodal dissections are therapeutic remains controversial, but retrospective data suggest that this potential may exist and should be explored in well-designed studies. For patients with resectable intraperitoneal disease, cytoreductive surgery can result in optimal volumes of residual disease, and perhaps improved outcomes.

PATHOLOGY

Hyperplasia

The current classification of endometrial hyperplasia accepted by both the International Society of Gynecologic Pathologists (ISGP) and the World Health Organization (WHO) is based on the schema of Kurman and Norris (224), which divides

TABLE 23.9

CLASSIFICATION OF ENDOMETRIAL HYPERPLASIA

Types of hyperplasia	Progressing to cancer (%)
Simple (cystic without atypia)	1
Complex (adenomatous without atypia)	3
Atypical	
Simple (cystic with atypia)	8
Complex (adenomatous with atypia)	29

hyperplasia on the basis of architectural features into simple or complex and on the basis of cytologic features into typical or atypical (Table 23.9). The resulting classification has four categories as follows: *simple hyperplasia* (SH), *complex hyperplasia* (CH), *simple atypical hyperplasia* (SAH), and *complex atypical hyperplasia* (CAH). Simple hyperplasia is defined as an increase in the number of endometrial glands, which may be dilated with little crowding or have an irregular outline and exhibit crowding. Complex hyperplasia is characterized by glands with irregular outlines, marked structural complexity, and back-to-back crowding. The designation atypical hyperplasia is used to denote a proliferation of glands exhibiting cytologic atypia, recognized as nuclear enlargement, the presence of nucleoli, or a change from an elongated to a more ovoid or round nucleus. The chromatin may be either evenly or irregularly dispersed. The justification for this classification system rests on three retrospective studies that demonstrate a higher rate of progression of CAH to adenocarcinoma (224–226). It is sometimes difficult to apply this system, which requires one to make a distinction between cytologically atypical nuclei and those without atypical nuclei since a spectrum of nuclear variability actually exists. As noted by Kendall et al. (227), the definitions of architectural complexity and nuclear atypia potentially rest on a multitude of criteria, and some but not all criteria may be fully developed in any given case.

Several reports have addressed the reproducibility of diagnoses of hyperplasia (227–229). Intraobserver reproducibility was generally found to be moderate to good, whereas interobserver reproducibility was poor to moderate for various diagnostic categories. These studies probably overestimate the interobserver reproducibility since they used expert gynecologic pathologists and specified the classification to be used. In a prospective study by the GOG, neither community-based nor expert panel diagnosis of atypical hyperplasia was highly accurate (73). The current classification of hyperplasia relies on a combination of multiple architectural and cytologic criteria. It is hardly surprising that interobserver reproducibility is relatively low when multiple criteria are used to classify a lesion since each pathologist must assign a relative value or weight to each potentially conflicting criterion. Other factors contributing to low reproducibility include (a) the fragmentary nature of curettings, (b) the presence of borderline lesions, (c) uncertainty about the significance of focal hyperplasia, (d) the inadequacy of published descriptions and understanding of terms used to define architectural or cytologic atypia, and (e) the difficulty associated with the translation of verbal descriptions into light microscopic interobserver reproducibility for images.

The gross manifestations of endometrial hyperplasia are highly varied. The endometrium is often of diffusely increased thickness (5 to 10 mm or greater), vaguely nodular, tan, and soft without hemorrhage or necrosis. However, hyperplasia may be focal or multifocal in a background of polyps or cycling endometrium, or even occasionally may be associated with a diffusely thin endometrial lining. Part of the variability may reflect a reduction in the endometrial thickness due to prior endometrial sampling. Coexistent adenocarcinoma is present in 1% to 40% of hysterectomies performed to treat hyperplasia, with the latter number reflecting the frequent co-occurrence of carcinoma with atypical complex hyperplasia.

Endometrial Intraepithelial Neoplasia

Based on a combination of morphologic, molecular, and morphometric information, Mutter et al. have proposed an alternative classification scheme to replace the current WHO hyperplasia terminology (230–233). They have presented data that endometrial intraepithelial neoplasia (EIN) is the histopathologic presentation of a monoclonal endometrial preinvasive glandular proliferation that is the immediate pathologic precursor of endometrioid endometrial adenocarcinoma. Monoclonality and forward carryover of EIN mutations into subsequent carcinoma were the original molecular standards used for EIN diagnosis. Computer-assisted morphometric analysis of more than 20 features was carried out initially and the three features seen in molecularly defined precancers enabled an objective delineation of histologic diagnostic criteria (the D-score). The principal components assessed included a reduction in the volume of stroma, an increased variability in nuclear shape gland contour. Several of these features have been translated to characteristics that can be assessed subjectively by the surgical pathologist (Fig. 23.3). These features include the following: (a) the area of the glands

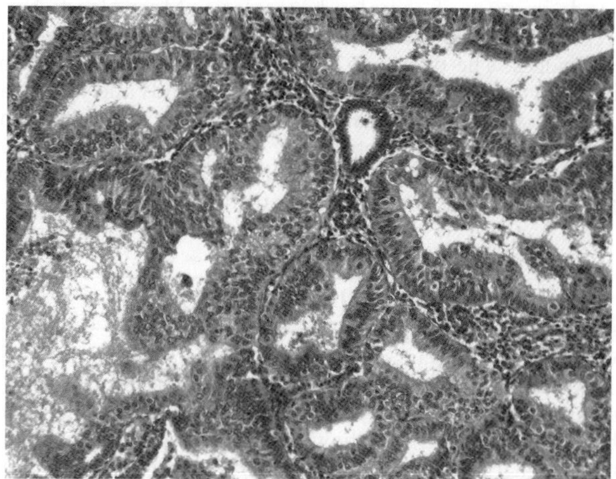

FIGURE 23.3. A lesion that could be classified in two different systems as either endometrial intraepithelial carcinoma (EIN) or complex atypical hyperplasia based on gland crowding and cytologic atypia. Note the presence of a residual inactive endometrial gland that may be used as a reference for estimating cytologic atypia.

exceeds that of stroma; (b) nuclear and cytoplasmic features of the affected glandular cells differ from those of the background glands, and may include loss of nuclear polarity or increased nuclear pleomorphism; in the absence of any background glands, a highly abnormal cytology is sufficient; (c) the maximum diameter exceeds 1 mm; (d) benign conditions including disordered proliferation, polyps, and repair are excluded; and (e) the cribriform or maze-like pattern of carcinoma is excluded. There is a high degree of concordance between EIN diagnoses rendered by computer and those made subjectively by pathologists, and either has superior cancer predictive value when compared to the 14-fold increased cancer risk conferred by the presence of atypia compared to lack thereof in the WHO hyperplasia schema. Clinical outcome studies have shown that almost 40% of women with an EIN diagnosis will be diagnosed with endometrial carcinoma within 1 year and, and for those who do not develop cancer within 12 months, a 45-fold increased risk of future endometrial cancer exists. Correspondingly, absence of an EIN lesion in an initial representative biopsy, including those with only benign hyperplasia, confers very high (99%) negative predictive value for concomitant or future adenocarcinoma.

While EIN shares many features with atypical complex hyperplasia, the two entities are not entirely overlapping. The concept of EIN is appealing since there appears to be a strong biologic basis, with EIN representing a clonal process, while disordered proliferation and hyperplasia remain as diffuse endometrial physiologic responses to an abnormal stimulus (unopposed estrogen stimulation).

Simple Hyperplasia

In simple hyperplasia, the endometrium is thicker than usual, with dilated glands that have outpouchings and invaginations, producing an irregular outline to the enlarged glands. The glands are crowded, the stroma is more densely cellular than usual, and some foam cells may exist within the stroma. Follow-up of patients with this condition reveals little or no progression to carcinoma.

Complex Hyperplasia

The endometrium is increased in thickness by back-to-back glands in cases of complex hyperplasia. Most glands have irregular outlines. There are papillary processes and intraluminal bridges. The two main features differentiating this from simple hyperplasia are the back-to-back glands and the intraluminal papillae. Epithelial pseudostratification is a frequent finding, producing an appearance of two to four cell layers. Mitotic activity is highly variable, but may range to up to ten mitotic figures per ten high-power fields.

Atypical Hyperplasia

Atypical hyperplasia is characterized by cytologic atypia of the glands. The gland outlines may reflect simple or complex hyperplasia, although it is usually complex. The cells lining the glands are enlarged, show nuclear hyperchromatism and nuclear enlargement, and have an increased nucleus-cytoplasm ratio. Nuclei are irregular in size and shape and have a thickened nuclear membrane, prominent nucleoli, and a coarse chromatin texture. The nuclei may appear clear with scattered, coarse chromatin clumps.

Progression From Hyperplasia to Cancer

The natural history of endometrial hyperplasia is difficult to define for a variety of reasons, four of which follow: (a) pathologic criteria—criteria and terminology for the various forms of hyperplasia have changed repeatedly; (b) initial sampling—the method of initial diagnosis is often curettage, which removes part or all of the lesion to be studied; (c) coexisting lesions—other lesions such as adenocarcinoma may coexist at the time of diagnosis without our knowledge, since the curettage or biopsy samples only a minority of the endometrium; and (d) subsequent intervention—hormonal or surgical intervention usually interrupts observations of the natural history of the hyperplasia. Nevertheless, there are reasonably good data to support the following assertions: (a) endometrial hyperplasia is commonly a consequence of unopposed prolonged estrogen stimulation; (b) some hyperplasias may regress if the estrogenic stimulus is removed or in response to progestational or antiestrogenic treatment; (c) some hyperplasias coexist with, or progress to, invasive adenocarcinoma; and (d) the probability of progression to adenocarcinoma is related to the degree of architectural or cytologic atypia. Progression from hyperplasia to carcinoma occurs in only 1% of patients with simple hyperplasia and in 3% of patients with complex hyperplasia (72). Progression from atypical hyperplasia is much higher; 8% of patients with simple atypical hyperplasia and 29% of those with complex atypical hyperplasia develop carcinoma (Table 23.9) (72,224). Glandular complexity superimposed on atypia probably places the patient at greater risk than does cytologic atypia alone, but the point is unsettled.

Pathologic Diagnosis

The ISGP and the WHO last revised the classification of uterine tumors in 1992 (234), and the portion pertaining to carcinomas of the endometrium is presented in Table 23.10. This relatively simple classification scheme accommodates the vast majority of endometrial carcinomas and distinguishes among neoplasms of significantly different prognosis. Mixed carcinomas with two distinctive cell types are relatively common, and are defined as those carcinomas in which the secondary component constitutes at least 10% of the neoplasm.

In most endometrial samples, the distinction of adenocarcinoma from hyperplasia is straightforward. However, a small fraction of problematic cases with complex proliferations

TABLE 23.10

CLASSIFICATION OF ENDOMETRIAL CARCINOMA

Endometrioid adenocarcinoma
- Papillary villoglandular
- Secretory
- Ciliated cell
- Adenocarcinoma with squamous differentiation

Mucinous carcinoma
Serous carcinoma
Clear cell carcinoma
Squamous carcinoma
Undifferentiated carcinoma
Mixed types
Miscellaneous carcinomas
Metastatic carcinoma

truly tax the abilities of experts as well as novices to classify them correctly. The diagnosis of a well-differentiated adenocarcinoma is made in the presence of any of the following criteria: (a) irregular infiltration of glands in an altered fibroblastic stroma, (b) a confluent glandular pattern that results in either a cribriform arrangement or confluent interconnected glands, or (c) extensive papillary growth of epithelium and stroma into glandular lumina (224).

Histologic Grade

The differentiation of a carcinoma is expressed as its grade. Grade 1 lesions are well differentiated and are generally associated with a good prognosis. Grade 2 tumors (Fig. 23.4) are moderately well differentiated and have an intermediate prognosis, and grade 3 reflects poorly differentiated lesions, which frequently have a poor prognosis. Both architectural criteria and nuclear grade are used in the FIGO and ISGP-WHO committee (235) classification of tumors and are easily applied to most cell types (Table 23.10). The architectural grade is determined as follows: grade 1—an adenocarcinoma in which less than 5% of the tumor growth is in solid sheets; grade 2—an adenocarcinoma in which 6% to 50% of the neoplasm is arranged in solid sheets of neoplastic cells; grade 3—an adenocarcinoma in which greater than 50% of the neoplastic cells are in solid masses. Regions of squamous differentiation are excluded from this assessment. The FIGO rules for grading state that notable nuclear atypia, inappropriate for architectural grade, raises the grade of a grade 1 or grade 2 tumor by one. However, FIGO did not define notable nuclear atypia. Justification and clarification for this modification based on extreme nuclear pleomorphism were provided in a recent GOG study. For 715 women with nonserous endometrial carcinomas, three nuclear grades were defined as follows: grade 1—round to oval nuclei with even distribution of chromatin and inconspicuous nucleoli; grade 2—irregular, oval nuclei with chromatin clumping and moderate-size nucleoli; and grade 3—large, pleomorphic nuclei with coarse chromatin and large, irregular nucleoli. Patients with tumors of architectural grade 1 or 2, but with a majority of cells having nuclei of grade 3, had a significantly worse behavior, justifying an upgrading by one grade (236).

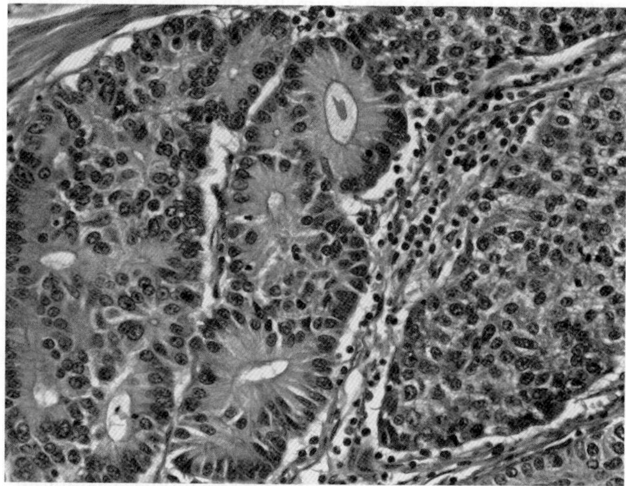

FIGURE 23.4. Endometrioid adenocarcinoma, grade 2. The glandular component is a caricature of proliferative phase glands, with stratification and a shared luminal border to the neoplastic cells. In grade 2 carcinomas, regions of solid neoplastic growth occupy between 5% and 50% of the surface area of the carcinoma.

Taylor et al. (237) proposed a two-tiered system for grading endometrial carcinoma based on a study of 85 patients with stage I and II endometrial cancer. They divided tumors at 10% intervals based on the percentage of solid tumor growth, and found that tumor recurrences were confined to the subset with greater than 20% solid tumor. They also found that this binary division yielded a higher degree of interobserver agreement than three architectural grades. Lax et al. (238) have presented preliminary data on a binary architectural grading system based on the presence of greater than 50% solid growth, a diffusely infiltrative growth pattern, and tumor cell necrosis. These methods will need to be replicated in a larger patient population before an assessment of their prognostic utility can be made. Some cell types (i.e., serous, clear cell, ciliated, and undifferentiated) are not easily architecturally graded because their growth patterns are architecturally limited. In these, the nuclear grading is more universally applicable (239).

Cell Types

Endometrioid Adenocarcinoma. Endometrioid adenocarcinoma is the most common form of carcinoma of the endometrium, comprising 75% to 80% of the cases (60,240). It varies from well differentiated to undifferentiated. Characteristically, the glands of endometrioid adenocarcinoma are formed of tall columnar cells that share a common apical border, resulting in a smoothly delineated, round or oval luminal contour. With decreasing differentiation, there is a preponderance of solid growth rather than gland formation, and the cells lining glandular lumina become more numerous but not necessarily clearly stratified. Stromal invasion manifested by a desmoplastic host response or vascular invasion is often not evident in the biopsy or curettage specimen.

Villoglandular Carcinoma. There has been considerable confusion about the definition and significance of papillary carcinoma of the endometrium. A variety of cell types of endometrial adenocarcinoma with differing biologic behavior, including serous, clear cell, mucinous, and villoglandular carcinoma, may grow in a papillary fashion. Thus, the adjective *papillary* does not represent a cell type but rather an architectural pattern (240,241).

Villoglandular carcinoma is a relatively common subtype of endometrioid adenocarcinoma characterized by neoplastic columnar cells covering delicate fibrovascular cores. The apical cytoplasmic borders are straight, the nuclei are usually low grade, and the tumor cells architecturally resemble those of other endometrioid adenocarcinomas, with which they are often admixed. In the largest study to date, villoglandular carcinomas were better differentiated than endometrioid carcinomas, but the age at diagnosis, depth of myometrial invasion, nodal spread, and survival were similar to those of endometrioid carcinomas, justifying their classification as a subtype of endometrioid adenocarcinoma (242).

Secretory Carcinoma. Secretory carcinoma is a variant of endometrial carcinoma, but it is unusual and represents no more than 2% of the cases (243,244). It is identified by its well-differentiated glandular pattern, consisting of columnar epithelial cells containing intracytoplasmic vacuoles similar to secretory endometrium. It is usually grade 1 architecturally and by nuclear features. There is minimal cellular atypia, stratification, and pleomorphism. The intracellular secretions are not mucin but glycogen. The cellular features of secretory carcinoma differentiate it from clear cell carcinoma, which is more papillary with more pleomorphic nuclei. By its lack of mucin, secretory carcinoma may be differentiated from mucinous carcinoma. Recognition of secretory carcinoma is important because it has a less virulent clinical course (244,245), although the clinical profile of patients is similar to that of patients with adenocarcinoma. Confused identification may occur in patients who have been given progestogens before tissue sampling in what would have otherwise been an atypical hyperplasia or a well-differentiated endometrioid carcinoma. Atypical hyperplasia and endometrioid carcinoma may retain responsiveness to progestins and develop a secretory appearance. A good clinical history should be provided for the pathologist to avoid this confusion.

Ciliated Carcinoma. Ciliated carcinoma is rare. Grossly, it does not differ from ordinary endometrial carcinoma. Ciliated cells are more commonly identified in endometrial hyperplasia and in benign metaplasia (tubal metaplasia), but they may occur in endometrial carcinomas. Associated with prior exogenous estrogen use, this cell type is reported to have a good prognosis (246).

Adenocarcinoma With Squamous Differentiation. Foci of squamous differentiation are found in about 25% of endometrial adenocarcinomas (Fig. 23.5). Historically, the tumors were sometimes separated into adenoacanthoma or adenosquamous carcinoma based on whether the squamous component appeared histologically benign or malignant (247–251). However, in about 30% of cases, the squamous component is not clearly benign or malignant. In a GOG study of early-stage disease, it was noted that these tumors with squamous regions behave in a fashion similar to endometrioid carcinomas without squamous differentiation (252). The squamous areas usually mirror the degree of differentiation, which, coupled with assessment of histologic grade and other conventional prognostic factors, is thus more useful for prognostication and determination of adjuvant therapy than the historic terms *adenoacanthoma* and *adenosquamous carcinoma*, which are confusing and should be abandoned.

Mucinous Carcinoma. Mucinous adenocarcinoma is rare in the endometrium in contrast to its high frequency in the endocervix. It has been reported to represent between 1% and 9% of endometrial adenocarcinomas (253–255), but the former figure is probably more accurate. If present as the major cellular component of an endometrial carcinoma, this tumor resembles mucinous carcinoma seen in the ovary and endocervix. Two patterns occur: In one, the cells are columnar with basally oriented nuclei; in the other, the cells are more pseudostratified, as in an adenocarcinoma of the colon or mucinous carcinoma of the ovary (Fig. 23.6). The characteristic cellular pattern should represent over 50% of the entire tumor. Typically, there are papillary processes and cystically dilated glands lined by columnar or pseudostratified columnar epithelium. The cytoplasm is positive for carcinoembryonic antigen (CEA), mucicarmine, and periodic acid-Schiff stain (PAS), but it is diastase resistant (255). This tumor differs from clear cell carcinoma and secretory endometrium by having more mucin and less glycogen. Ordinarily, atypia and mitotic figures are not prominent features. The glandular architecture is usually well maintained, and most are well differentiated (253). To establish the origin in the endometrium, exclusion of a primary endocervical tumor is required. If the endocervical sample demonstrates the same neoplasm, the site of origin must be carefully established because this cell type is common in the endocervix (256). Neither the pattern nor the type of mucin staining nor the presence of CEA can reliably distinguish mucinous adenocarcinoma of the endometrium from its more common counterpart in the endocervix (257,258). Mucinous carcinoma of the endometrium has the same prognosis as common endometrial carcinoma (254).

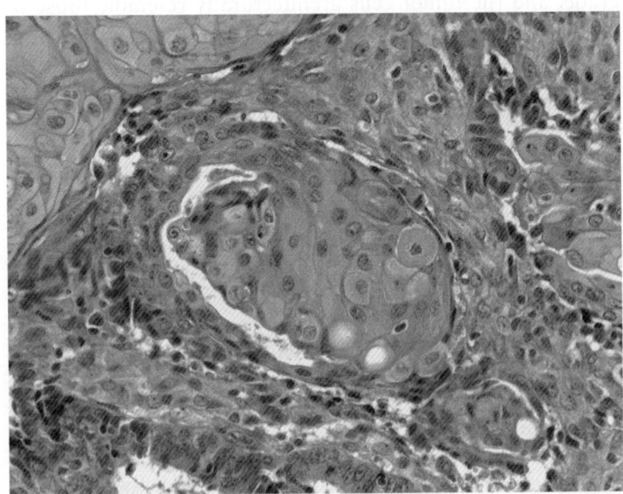

FIGURE 23.5. Endometrioid adenocarcinoma with squamous differentiation. The squamous component may form keratin pearls, but more often simply is characterized by acquisition of more abundant, deeply eosinophilic cytoplasm and distinct cell borders. The squamous component may appear histologically benign or malignant.

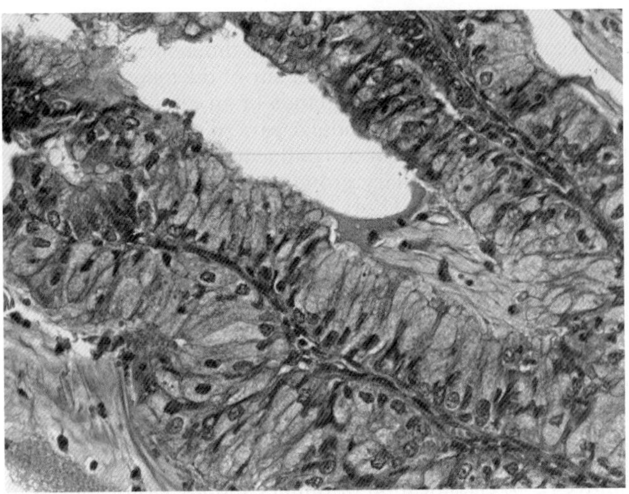

FIGURE 23.6. Mucinous adenocarcinoma. The apical cytoplasm cells as well as the lumens of glands are filled with a pale basophilic mucoid product.

Serous Carcinoma. Serous carcinoma of the endometrium closely resembles serous carcinoma of the ovary and fallopian tube because its papillary growth and cellular features are similar (Figs. 23.7 and 23.8). It is usually found in an advanced stage in older women (259). Fibrous papillary fronds are lined by epithelial cells, which are almost devoid of cytoplasm, but which manifest stratification, atypism, pleomorphism, mitotic figures, and bizarre forms. These fronds often detach or demonstrate a terminal growth of tiny papillary excrescences and individual cells, which detach easily. A second pattern of irregular gaping glands lined by cuboidal cells with scalloped, apical borders may be present, particularly in the deeper aspect of the tumor. Lymphatic invasion is commonplace in the myometrium. Distinction from clear cell carcinoma may be difficult but can usually be accomplished on the basis of a greater degree of papillary processes, greater nuclear atypia, and less cytoplasm in papillary serous carcinoma. Psammoma bodies are frequently observed in serous carcinoma, but solid growth is more common in clear cell carcinoma.

Serous carcinoma represents approximately 10% of endometrial carcinomas, which is fortunate because it is an aggressive tumor. The tumors often deeply invade the myometrium, and unlike typical endometrioid adenocarcinoma, there is a propensity

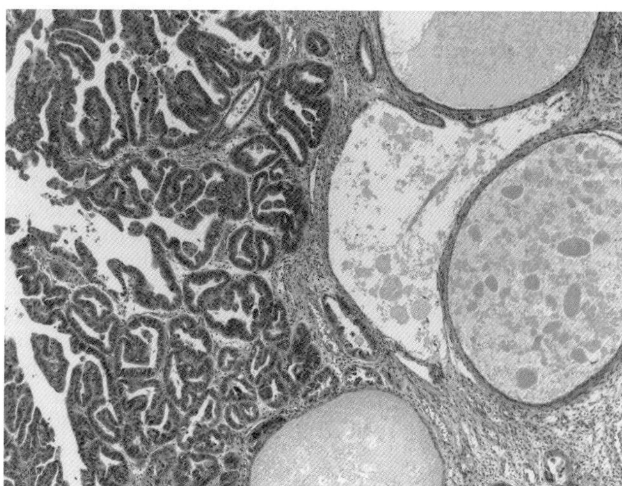

FIGURE 23.7. Serous carcinoma often arises in an otherwise atrophic polyp of older women.

for peritoneal spread. Unfortunately, advanced-stage disease or recurrence is common even when serous carcinomas are apparently only minimally invasive or even confined to the endometrium in polyps (161,260,261). Since the metastatic disease is often identified only microscopically, about 60% of patients are up-staged following complete surgical staging (161,259,262). A report by Wheeler et al. (263) stressed the prognostic importance of meticulous surgicopathologic staging. They and others found that serous carcinoma truly confined to the uterus had an overall excellent prognosis, whereas patients with extrauterine disease, even if only microscopic in size, almost always suffered recurrence and death from tumor (264,265).

Endometrial intraepithelial carcinoma (EIC) has recently been recognized as a histologically distinctive lesion that is specifically associated with serous carcinoma of the endometrium (Fig. 23.9) (266–270). Serous carcinomas most often arise from a background of atrophy or polyps rather than hyperplasia (266,267,269), and they are not epidemiologically related to unopposed estrogen stimulation. EIC has been proposed to represent a form of intraepithelial tumor characteristic of serous carcinoma, and it is the likely precursor to invasive serous carcinoma. EIC is usually found in the endometrium harboring a serous carcinoma (267), but occasionally occurs in the absence of any invasive carcinoma. In such cases, it may be associated with synchronous serous carcinoma in the peritoneum (268).

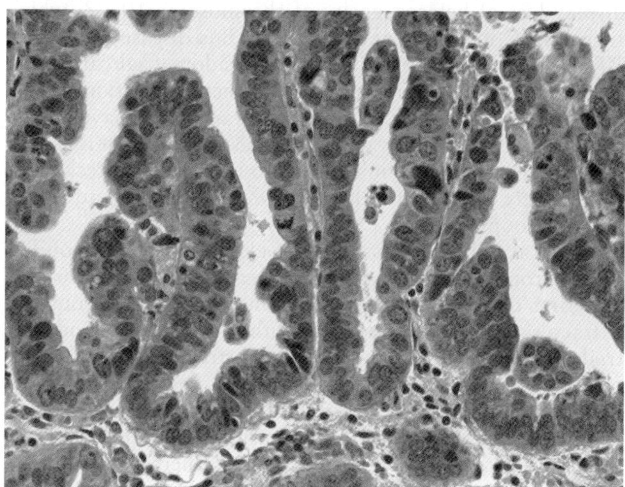

FIGURE 23.8. Serous carcinoma is characterized by high-grade cytologic atypia in cells that do not share a common apical border. A papillary architecture is common, but sometimes relatively subtle.

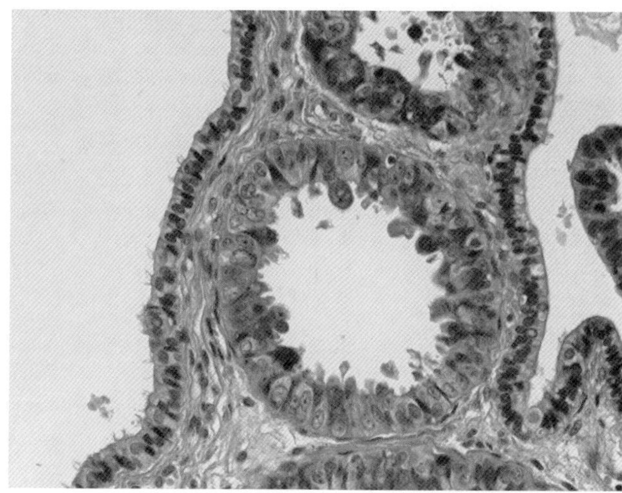

FIGURE 23.9. Endometrial intraepithelial carcinoma (EIC) is considered the precursor of serous carcinoma. Highly atypical cells resembling those of serous carcinoma are present in glands immediately adjacent to atrophic endometrium.

Clear Cell Carcinoma. Clear cell adenocarcinoma of the endometrium is generally recognized and defined on the basis of the distinctive clearing of the cytoplasm of neoplastic cells growing in any combination of solid, glandular, tubulocystic, or papillary configurations. About 4% of endometrial adenocarcinomas are of clear cell type (271–278). In contrast with the diethylstilbestrol (DES)-related clear cell carcinomas of the vagina and cervix, clear cell carcinoma of the endometrium is almost exclusively a disease of menopausal women. The mean age at diagnosis is about 68 years, which is similar to that of serous adenocarcinoma and about 6 years older than that of typical endometrial adenocarcinoma (271,274,278). It is a biologically aggressive neoplasm, with a 5-year survival rate varying from only about 20% to 65% (5,271,274,276,278).

The hallmark of clear cell carcinoma is the presence of neoplastic cells with optically clear cytoplasm, reflecting an abundance of glycogen. Four basic architectural patterns of clear cell adenocarcinoma exist, including solid, glandular, tubulocystic, and papillary, but most cases display an admixture of patterns. The solid pattern consists of masses of large neoplastic cells of polygonal shape with clear to faintly eosinophilic cytoplasm and distinct cell membranes. The glandular pattern is reminiscent of the tubular glands of endometrioid adenocarcinoma, whereas the tubulocystic pattern is formed of dilated spherical-appearing glands. The papillary pattern is architecturally identical to that of serous carcinoma, with generally short, branching fibrovascular cores, often hyalinized, covered by neoplastic cells. The latter three patterns often have lining cells with a hobnail appearance, resulting from the scalloped apex of individual neoplastic cells that project along the surface (Fig. 23.10).

Squamous Carcinoma. Although focal squamous differentiation is common in endometrial adenocarcinoma, pure squamous carcinoma of the endometrium is extremely rare, representing less than 1% of endometrial carcinoma, and with only about 60 reported cases (279–283). Most patients are postmenopausal, and the average age at diagnosis is about 65 years (279,281). Squamous carcinoma of the endometrium is established as primary in the endometrium after a cervical origin is ruled out. There must be no connection with or spread from benign or malignant cervical squamous epithelium. It is

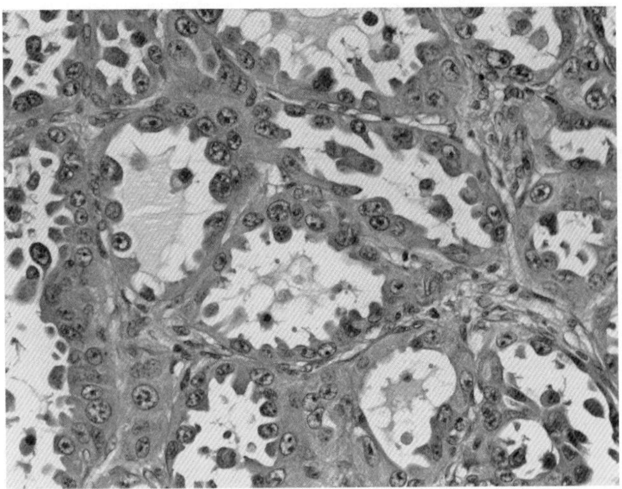

FIGURE 23.10. Clear cell carcinoma. A tubulocystic pattern with a lining of hobnail cells is present in this case, but other tumors may be solid or papillary, lined by clear or hobnail cells.

often associated with cervical stenosis, pyometra, and chronic inflammation. About 60% of the cases have been confined to the uterus, and the prognosis for these patients has been relatively good (279). In contrast, less than 15% of women with advanced-stage disease have survived 2 years after diagnosis. Histologic grade does not appear to correlate with the probability of survival.

Undifferentiated Carcinoma. Undifferentiated carcinoma of the endometrium has no glandular, squamous, or sarcomatous differentiation in routinely stained sections. Most contain epithelial antigens detected by immunologic stains. Selected cases may contain argyrophilic cells or neurosecretory granules demonstrated by immunohistochemical stains or electron microscopy. Neurosecretory products are apparently not released into the patient's circulation or are not in an active form because no affected women have manifested symptoms. Neuroendocrine granules, therefore, have no clinical or prognostic significance (284,285).

A *glassy cell carcinoma* has also been described, which comprises less than 1% of endometrial carcinomas. It is characterized by cytoplasm that has a ground-glass appearance, as in the cervix. Although few cases have been reported, like serous and clear cell carcinomas, glassy cell carcinoma appears to be aggressive (286,287).

Mixed Cell Type. If an endometrial carcinoma manifests two or more different cell types, each representing at least 10% or more of the tumor, the term *mixed cell type* is appropriate.

Metastatic Carcinoma to the Endometrium. Malignancies in other organs may metastasize to the endometrium. The most common extragenital sites are breast, stomach, colon, pancreas, and kidney, although any disseminated tumor could involve the endometrium. The ovaries are the most likely genital sources of metastasis. Metastatic carcinoma presents as abnormal vaginal bleeding, and the initial specimen for evaluation is usually a biopsy or curetting. Although the metastatic disease may appear as a large focus, individual and small groups of malignant cells may subtly intermingle with normal endometrium or myometrium. Lymphatics are usually involved. Special stains for mucin, CEA, or melanin may suggest that the cells are not of endometrial origin. In some instances, unusual cell types, such as signet-ring cells, may be present, suggesting a metastasis from the gastrointestinal (GI) tract. It is uncommon but not exceptional for the endometrial sample to be the first indication of an occult primary lesion (288,289).

Simultaneous Tumors. Cancers of an identical cell type may be discovered in the ovary and endometrium simultaneously (290). Usually, the primary site is assigned to the area having the largest tumor mass and most advanced stage. In certain situations, primary malignancies in the endometrium and ovary may coexist. This "field effect" of the "extended müllerian system" may occur in 15% to 20% of endometrioid carcinomas of the ovary (291,292). In a review of a GOG study of 74 patients with simultaneously detected endometrial and ovarian carcinoma with disease grossly limited to the pelvis, only 16% of women suffered a recurrence of disease, with a median follow-up of 80 months. This group of patients was atypical, with 86% having endometrioid histology in both sites. Recurrence was statistically related to the presence of microscopic metastases or high histologic grade (293).

Carcinomas of more advanced histologic grade and cell type are more difficult to assign to the field effect because of a higher probability of invasion and metastasis at the time of surgery (245). If the endometrial tumor is less than 5 cm in diameter, the ovarian lesion is unilateral, invasion is less than the middle third, vessels are not involved, and the endometrial carcinoma is well differentiated, metastasis to the ovary is unlikely (294).

MOLECULAR ALTERATIONS IN THE PATHOGENESIS AND PROGRESSION OF ENDOMETRIAL ADENOCARCINOMA

Deletions or mutations of the *PTEN* gene, and microsatellite instability (MSI) due to hypermethylation of the promoter for the mismatch repair gene, *hMLH1*, are both relatively common and early events in the development of a significant proportion of endometrioid adenocarcinomas. In contrast, these molecular alterations do not appear to be critical in the pathogenesis of serous or clear cell carcinoma. However, mutations in the p53 gene are found with high frequency not only in invasive serous carcinoma but also in endometrial intraepithelial carcinoma (270,295), the noninvasive precursor of serous carcinoma, suggesting that a different pathway is followed in the development of the second type of endometrial adenocarcinoma.

The function of the tumor-suppressor gene *PTEN* (MMAC1) includes inhibition of cell migration, spreading, and adhesion (296–300). The *PTEN* gene is located on chromosome 10q23 and about 40% of endometrial carcinomas display loss of heterozygosity of chromosome 10q23, which suggests the involvement of *PTEN* in this disease (296,301). *PTEN* mutations in 30% to 50% of endometrial carcinoma tumors make this the most frequent genetic alteration known in this disease (302–304). Risinger et al. (305) have in one study shown that inactivation of *PTEN* by mutation is associated with early disease in contrast to the study of Steck et al. (306) where *PTEN* gene alteration was linked to an advanced disease group.

MSI caused by shifts in allelic electrophenetric mobility results from replication error of repeated sequences (307). It was first described in HNPCC. One of the most common extracolonic tumors associated with this disease is endometrial cancer, and MSI has been demonstrated in both hereditary and sporadic tumors (308). MSI in endometrial cancer has been reported to be between 9% and 43% (309–313). In 71% to 92% of sporadic endometrial carcinoma, MSI has been found to be associated with hypermethylation of the *hMLH1* promoter region, whereas it seems to be less common in the promoter region of *hMSH2* (314,315). It is likely that methylation of the promoter region is an important mechanism of *hMLH1* gene inactivation in endometrial carcinoma

(316–320) and a precursor to MSI. Too few studies have been done to reach any conclusion regarding the importance of MSI as a prognostic factor in endometrial cancer.

TP53 is a tumor-suppressor gene, the product of which is a protein involved in the regulation of the cell cycle at the G_1 checkpoint, permitting replication of cells that have acquired various mutations (321). Mutations of the p53 gene often result in a protein with a longer half-life, which accumulates in the cell. Up-regulation of wild-type (i.e., nonmutated) p53 may occur after DNA damage and also results in overexpression that is detectable by immunohistochemistry. This appears to be an early event in the development of serous carcinoma, but it is a late event in endometrioid carcinomas for which it serves as an indicator of poor prognosis. In addition to the very frequent overexpression of p53 protein in serous carcinoma (322), it has also been related to a higher FIGO stage, clear cell histology, higher histologic grade, and increased depth of myometrial invasion (276,323–335). Lundgren et al. (336) studied p53 in relation to clinicopathologic variables in 376 consecutive patients with endometrial cancer stages I-IV. p53 overexpression was found to be a strong significant factor with regard to relapse-free survival in univariate analysis, but it failed to retain its significance when submitted to multivariate analysis.

In contrast, p53 mutations are not often found in low-grade endometrioid tumors (337). This suggests that different subgroups of endometrial cancers have different genetic pathways. Much more work is needed to understand the genetic mechanics at play and to translate this into use within the clinical and therapeutic field (338).

HER2/neu is a proto-oncogene, the product of which is a transmembrane growth factor receptor, p185erb-2, which shares some homology with the epidermal growth factor receptor. It is normally expressed at low levels in the cycling endometrium. Gene amplification and/or overexpression occurs in about 20% to 40% of endometrial carcinomas, and has been associated with advanced stage (339), decreased differentiation, aggressive cell types particularly including the clear cell type (340–343), and deep myometrial invasion (327). The significance of HER2/neu amplification or overexpression as a predictor of survival is somewhat unclear, with no apparent association of overexpression to outcome being identified in several studies (322,330,340,344,345), but a statistically significant relationship in most others (326,330,341,346–349) even after adjusting for other known risk factors (326,341,347). In addition to its potential utility as an indicator of poor prognosis, systemic therapy using antibodies directed against the HER2/neu protein is currently being investigated for patients with tumors that express the protein at high levels.

Abnormal expression of the oncogenes *beta*- and *gamma-catenin* and *E*- and *P-cadherin* may play a critical role in the initiation and progression of endometrioid neoplasia (350,351). Moreno-Bueno et al. (351) have evaluated the immunoreactivity of *beta*- and *gamma-catenin* and *E*- and *P-cadherin* in 149 patients with premalignant and malignant endometrioid lesions to correlate their membranous expression with clinical pathologic data. Their data indicate that abnormal expression of catenin and cadherin was common in premalignant and malignant endometrial lesions. Nonendometrioid endometrial cancer showed a greater reduction in *E-cadherin* expression, up-regulation of *P-cadherin*, and loss of heterozygosity at 16q21 than endometrial cancers. In contrast, nuclear accumulation of *beta-catenin* was frequently associated with a gene mutation characteristic of endometrioid lesions and may be an early event that is present in atypical endometrial hyperplasia. Reduced *E-cadherin* expression in endometrioid carcinomas is related to advanced stages, indicating a role for this molecule in tumor progression. Nuclear *beta-catenin* expression was found in 31.2% of endometrioid cancers and 3% of nonendometrioid cancers ($p = 0.002$) and was significantly associated with *beta-catenin* gene exon 3 mutations. *Beta-catenin* gene exon 3 mutations were associated with the endometrioid phenotype and were detected in 14 (15%) endometrioid cancers, but none of the nonendometrioid cancers ($p = 0.02$). *Gamma-catenin* nuclear expression was found in ten endometrial cancers. It was not associated with the histologic type but was associated with more advanced stages ($p = 0.04$) (350).

The activation of *RAS* proto-oncogenes through either point mutations or gene amplification has been identified in various malignant tumors. Mutations in the K-*ras* oncogene have been reported in endometrioid cancer and also in endometrial hyperplasia, suggesting that K-*ras* activation may be an early event in the development of endometrioid malignancy. Mutations in codon 12 of K-*ras* occur in only about 10% to 15% of endometrial carcinomas, and their significance is unknown. In most studies, the presence of K-*ras* mutations has not been related to stage, grade, depth of invasion, or survival (352–355).

Further studies have identified mutations in several tumor-related genes such as p16, *hMLH1*, *hMSH2*, and *hMSH6* in endometrial cancer (356–358). Salvesen et al. (359) have shown that loss of nuclear p16 protein expression is not associated with promoter methylation but defines a subgroup of aggressive endometrial carcinoma with a poor prognosis and found to be a strong independent prognostic factor.

PATHOLOGIC FACTORS OF PROGNOSTIC SIGNIFICANCE

Pathologic information has been used to estimate risk of nodal metastasis and to define prognosis (recurrence, survival) in endometrial cancer. Prognostic factors have been identified within each stage of endometrial cancer, and the discussion of prognostic factors is probably best served by discussing factors within comparably staged groups, more so than as isolated factors. For example, in GOG 99, which compared observation to pelvic radiation therapy in patients with stage I-II endometrial cancer and pathologically negative lymph nodes, a model based on combinations of patient age and tumor grade, depth of invasion, and lymphovascular space invasion (LVSI) could predict patients at highest risk for recurrence (143).

Predicting Nodal Disease

Based on pathologic information available at the time of surgery, the risk for nodal metastasis may be estimated. Physicians who selectively perform nodal dissections frequently do so based on the presence of uterine risk factors that suggest the potential for nodal disease. In patients who did not undergo a nodal dissection at the time of hysterectomy, decisions to offer radiation therapy are commonly based on the estimation of risk for nodal disease based on uterine risk factors. In the surgical pathologic study GOG 33, pelvic and para-aortic nodal disease was more frequent with increasing grade (percentage of pelvic nodal metastases: 3% grade I, 9% grade II, 18% grade 3), depth of invasion (1% endometrium only, 5% inner one third, 6% middle one third, 25% outer one third myometrial invasion), and LVSI (27% with LVSI, 7% without LVSI) (60). Pelvic and para-aortic nodal metastases were also more common with cervical involvement, when peritoneal cytology was positive, and when extranodal (adnexal, intraperitonal sites) disease was found. In a multivariate model, grade, depth of invasion, and intraperitoneal disease were independent predictors of pelvic nodal disease. In a further analysis of patients participating in GOG 33, 47 of 48 patients with para-aortic nodal disease had one or more factors of palpably enlarged para-aortic nodes, grossly positive pelvic nodes, gross adnexal disease, or outer one-third invasion (62). Despite the use of pathology to help predict nodal disease, many believe that routine lymph node assessment is superior as it provides actual information on nodal status, as opposed to an estimate, which can then be used to tailor therapy.

Prognostic Factors

FIGO Stage

Prognostic factors may be used to categorize patients into high- and low-risk groups and to guide the use of adjuvant therapies. Understanding these factors also allows for the development of novel strategies to reduce risk of recurrence or alter patterns of disease failure. Overall, the patients at highest risk for recurrence and death have spread of disease outside of the uterus, which is reflected by FIGO stage (62). The prognostic utility of surgicopathologic stage has been confirmed in multiple studies of large numbers of patients, using both univariate and multivariate analysis (60,232,271,360–365). FIGO surgical stage is often the single strongest predictor of outcome for women with endometrial adenocarcinoma in studies using multivariate analyses (271). Although the FIGO clinical staging system of 1971 was generally useful, retrospective comparison of the two methods demonstrated the clear superiority of surgicopathologic staging over clinical staging in predicting outcome.

Patients with intraperitoneal or distant metastases (stage IV) have the poorest prognosis with 5-year survival ranging from 20% to 25% (5). In GOG 122 comparing whole abdominal radiation therapy to doxorubicin/cisplatin chemotherapy as primary therapy for endometrial cancer patients with <2 cm residual disease stage III-IV, stage IV (compared to stage III) disease was an independent predictor of shorter progression-free survival (PFS) (hazard ratio [HR] 2.2.9) and survival (HR 1.9) (8). Gross intraperitoneal spread frequently indicates the presence of larger tumor burden as many patients with intraperitoneal disease also have adnexal and nodal disease. In GOG 33, 51% of patients with gross intraperitoneal spread had positive pelvic nodes, whereas only 7% without spread had positive pelvic nodes (60). Prognosis may be modified by the volume of residual disease after cytoreductive surgery (220–222).

Patients with nodal metastases (stage IIIC disease) also have poorer prognosis compared to node-negative populations. FIGO data shows 5-year survival to be 57% in stage IIIC patients compared to 74% to 91% when nodes are negative (stage I-II) (5). Patients with positive pelvic but negative para-aortic nodes have a better prognosis compared to those with para-aortic disease (62,366). Two retrospective series have also suggested that patients with nodal disease in addition to positive cytology, adnexa, or serosa have poorer PFS or survival compared to those patients with positive nodes alone (155,366). Lymphadenectomy (154,175,182), complete surgical resection of bulky nodes (367), and use of chemotherapy (8,152,368) have been suggested to improve outcomes in patients and modify the prognostic effect of nodal disease.

Patients with stage IIIA disease represent a heterogeneous population having adnexal, peritoneal cytology, and/or serosal involvement, but with negative lymph nodes. Positive peritoneal cytology or adnexal involvement may be prognostic factors, but must be interpreted in the setting of whether a patient was completely staged or not. In the GOG 33 study, 12% of all patients had positive cytology, and of these, 25% had positive pelvic nodes and 19% had metastases to para-aortic lymph nodes (60). Six percent of clinical stage I-II patients have spread of tumor to the adnexa, and of these, 32% have pelvic node metastases compared with 8% pelvic node positivity if adnexal involvement is not present (60). Twenty percent have positive para-aortic node metastases, which is four times greater than if adnexal metastases were not present.

For patients who are completely staged and found to have no extrauterine disease, 4% to 6% of patients have positive cytology as an isolated finding (60,191,369). Published opinions are mixed about the significance of this finding (370–378). Kadar et al. (379) found that positive peritoneal cytology had an adverse outcome on survival only if the endometrial cancer had spread to the adnexa, peritoneum, or lymph nodes, but not if disease was confined to the uterus, suggesting that not all cells that are found in the peritoneal cavity are capable of independent growth. Positive peritoneal cytology associated with extrauterine disease is a marker for aggressive disease and carries a worse prognosis. Cytology appears to carry the same significance as adnexal involvement (380).

Histologic Cell Types

The histologic classification of endometrial adenocarcinoma is important not only because it facilitates the recognition of lesions as carcinoma, but also because the cell type has consistently been recognized as being important in predicting the biologic behavior and probability of survival. Endometrioid adenocarcinoma accounts for the majority of tumors in the uterine corpus and carries a relatively favorable prognosis. Consequently, the virulence of other cell types is usually related to endometrioid adenocarcinoma.

Adenocarcinoma with squamous differentiation is similar to typical endometrioid adenocarcinoma with respect to the distribution by age and frequency of nodal metastasis, and is associated with a slightly increased probability of survival. *Villoglandular carcinoma* has a biologic behavior similar to that of endometrioid adenocarcinoma (242,381). *Serous carcinoma* has been considered an aggressive histologic type, with overall survival rates varying from 40% to 60% at 5 years (5,260,262,274,382–385). *Clear cell carcinoma* also has a highly aggressive behavior, with 5-year survival rates of 30% to 75% (272,273,278,386–389). One of the problems with using histology as a marker for prognosis is that serous cancers are more likely to have spread at presentation than endometrioid tumors. Patients with serous or clear cell tumors present with stage III-IV disease in 41% and 33%, respectively, compared to 14% with endometrioid type (5). Studies suggest that 40% to 70% of serous tumors will have extrauterine spread at presentation; therefore, complete surgical staging is warranted in this tumor type (161). Given this level of disease spread, it is not surprising that unstaged/clinical stage I serous patients appear to have similar prognosis to stage III-IV endometrioid types. Once patients with serous or clear cell tumors are appropriately allocated into the correct stage, the importance of histology appears to be less (390–393). For example, Creasman et al. evaluated FIGO data and showed that patients with stage I serous tumors had comparable outcomes to those with stage I, grade 3 endometrioid tumors. Five-year survival for stage IB and IC serous tumors was 81% and 55% compared to 84% and 66% for grade 3 tumors (393). In advanced and recurrent endometrial cancer patients participating in phase 3 GOG chemotherapy trials, response rate to chemotherapy was not associated with histologic type, and serous tumor type was not independently associated with PFS (17).

Grade

The degree of histologic differentiation has been considered to be an indicator of tumor spread. The GOG and other studies have confirmed that as grade becomes less differentiated, there is a greater tendency for deep myometrial invasion and, subsequently, higher rates of pelvic and para-aortic lymph node involvement (60,394–396). Survival has also been consistently related to histologic grade, and in a GOG study of more than 600 women with clinical stage I or occult stage II endometrioid adenocarcinoma, the 5-year relative survival was as follows: grade 1% to 94%; grade 2% to 84%; grade 3% to 72% (62). In patients with early-stage endometrial cancer participating in the Post Operative Radiation Therapy in Endometrial Carcinoma (PORTEC) trial, the risk of cancer-related death for patients with grade 3 tumors was 4.9 compared to grade 1–2 tumors (149).

Myometrial Invasion

Deep myometrial invasion is one of the more important factors correlated with a higher probability of extrauterine tumor spread, treatment failure, and recurrence, and with diminished probability of survival (Fig. 23.11) (143,360,397,398). In a GOG study of over 400 women with clinical stage I and occult stage II endometrioid adenocarcinoma, the 5-year relative survival was 94% when tumor was confined to the endometrium, 91% when tumor involved the inner third of the myometrium, 84% when the tumor extended into the middle third, and 59% when the tumor invaded into the outer third of the myometrium (62). Even in node-negative patients, deep myometrial invasion retains prognostic information. For example, Mariani et al. reported that for stage I (node-negative) patients, deep invasion (>66% myometrial invasion) was an independent predictor for recurrence and distant site of failure (399).

Lymphovascular Space Invasion

Several studies have suggested that lymphatic space invasion (LVSI) is a strong predictor of recurrence and death, and is independent of depth of myometrial invasion or histologic differentiation (Fig. 23.12) (271,400–403). In one investigation of FIGO stage I endometrial adenocarcinoma, 9 of 15 patients with LVSI died of tumor, whereas none of the 78 without identified vascular invasion died of cancer (400). Zaino et al. (365) found that LVSI was a statistically significant indicator of death from tumor in early clinical stage but not early surgical stage endometrial adenocarcinoma. This suggests that lymphatic invasion helps to identify patients likely to have spread to lymph nodes or distant sites, but that its importance is diminished for those in whom thorough sampling of nodes has failed to identify metastasis. Vascular space invasion or capillary-like space (CLS) involvement with tumor exists in approximately 15% of uteri containing adenocarcinoma (60,401,403). Pelvic lymph nodes are positive in 27% of cases, which is four times more often if malignant cells are found in the CLS than if absent. The risk of para-aortic node metastases when LVSI was present was 19%, which is a sixfold increase over negative CLS involvement (60). Lymphovascular invasion is identified in 35% to 95% of serous carcinomas of the endometrium, where it has generally been associated with an elevated risk of tumor recurrence or death from disease (262,382,384).

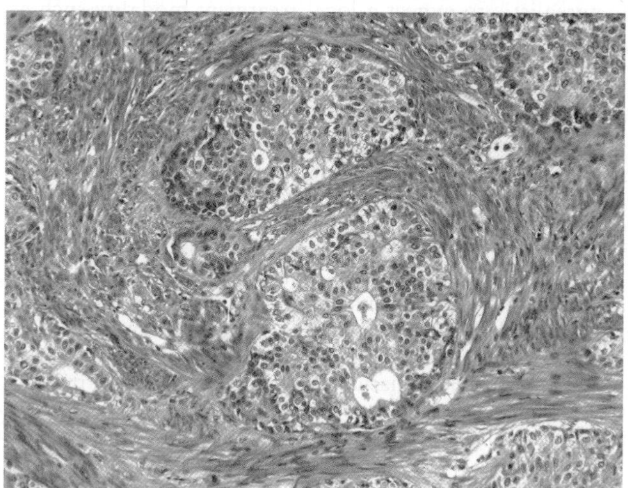

FIGURE 23.11. Myometrial invasion by endometrial adenocarcinoma may be accompanied by a desmoplastic reaction, but often no such reaction is present, as in this case.

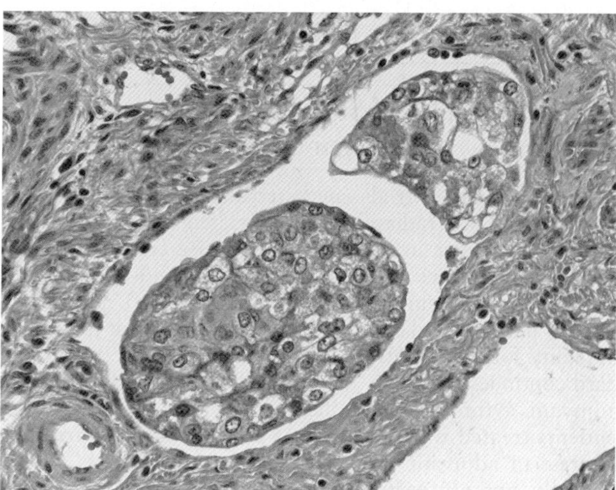

FIGURE 23.12. Lymphatic or capillary invasion by endometrial adenocarcinoma. Nests of neoplastic cells occupy the lumen of an endothelial-lined space.

Patterns of Failure

Another way to approach pathologic information is to understand the pathologic relationships that predict particular patterns of failure. For example, in patients with pathologic negative-node, stage I endometrial cancer, pelvic sidewall recurrences are rare, and failures occur most frequently at the vaginal cuff or at distant sites (143,404,405). High-risk stage I patients who do not undergo nodal dissections have both pelvic sidewall and distant sites of failure, even with routine use of radiation therapy (153). Patients with node-positive disease frequently have recurrences at distant sites, with rare intra-abdominal failures (155,156). Patients with stage IV/intraperitoneal disease most commonly fail in the peritoneal cavity. The implications of patterns of failure data are that we may choose our postoperative therapies better by defining patterns of failure for a particular stage distribution or based on the presence of risk factors. The Mayo Clinic group has advocated this approach following a review of patterns of failure data from their group (399,406–409). For example, these investigators suggested that hematogenous, lymphatic, and peritoneal failures could be predicted based on pathologic factors, and that therapy should be directed to reduce failures at these sites depending on pathologic information (61). Whether their finding can be validated in a prospective manner, or if existing therapies effectively control disease at particular sites needs to be evaluated.

GENERAL MANAGEMENT

Results of Standard Therapy and Their Sequelae

Early uncontrolled trials suggested that progestin therapy after surgery or irradiation was associated with a decreased risk of recurrence in patients with disease confined to the uterus (410). However, large prospective, randomized trials failed to show a survival advantage (411–413). Radiation therapy has been and remains the standard adjuvant treatment modality for most patients at risk for recurrence. This standard continues to evolve, however. An older, poorly designed adjuvant cytotoxic chemotherapy showed no benefit for patients treated with single-agent doxorubicin and arrested interest in adjuvant chemotherapy for many years (414). Recently, two prospective trials comparing radiation therapy to chemotherapy have since shown similar outcomes for patients treated with chemotherapy or radiation therapy (415,416). Adjuvant chemotherapy improved PFS and survival in patients with advanced-stage disease compared to whole abdominal radiotherapy, suggesting an important role for first-line therapy that includes chemotherapy (7). Current research focuses on whether outcomes may be improved by adding chemotherapy either sequentially or concomitantly with radiation.

ADJUVANT RADIATION THERAPY

Radiation therapy plays a significant role in the management of endometrial cancer. It is often used as an adjuvant treatment after surgery or as definitive treatment for patients who are medically inoperable or with local recurrence. In the past, most patients were treated with preoperative intracavitary brachytherapy with or without external beam radiotherapy followed by hysterectomy. This approach is not without its merit, especially in patients with gross cervical involvement. However, most patients nowadays undergo surgery first; then, depending on the prognostic features obtained from the pathology review, the need for radiotherapy is determined.

Early-Stage Disease

Most of the data on adjuvant radiation in endometrial cancer pertain to patients with early-stage (I-II) disease. The role of radiation in this group of patients, however, has been undergoing significant scrutiny in the last 10 years. Most of the debate focuses on the benefit of adjuvant radiation and to a lesser extent on the type of radiation that needs to be used.

Benefit of Adjuvant Radiation

Two prospective, randomized trials compared surgery alone to surgery and postoperative external beam radiation. The first trial was conducted by the GOG (study 99) where 392 patients with stage IB-IIB endometrial cancer who underwent total abdominal hysterectomy/bilateral salpingo-oophorectomy (TAH/ BSO) and pelvic/para-aortic lymph node sampling were randomized to observation (n = 202) or postoperative pelvic radiation (n = 190) to a total dose of 50.4 Gy in 28 fractions (143). With a median follow-up of 69 months, the 4-year survival rate was 92% in the radiation arm compared with 86% in the observation arm (Relative hazard: 0.86; $p = 0.557$). The estimated 2-year cumulative incidence of recurrence was 3% versus 12% in favor of the irradiation arm (RH: 0.42; $p = 0.007$). Specifically, the rate of vaginal recurrence was 6.4% (13 out of 202) in the surgery alone arm compared to 1.05% (2 out of 190) in the radiation arm. Of interest, these two patients were randomized to radiation but refused it. The second trial was the PORTEC study where 714 patients with stage IB grade 2,3 and IC grade 1,2 were randomized after TAH/BSO and no lymph node sampling to observation (n = 360) or pelvic radiation (n = 354) to a total dose of 46 Gy in 23 fractions (149). With a median follow-up of 52 months, the 5-year vaginal/pelvic recurrence rate was 4% in the radiation arm compared to 14% in the observation arm ($p < 0.001$). The corresponding 5-year survival rates were 81% and 85%, respectively ($p = 0.37$).

Despite the fact that adjuvant radiation significantly improved locoregional control, most of the debate focuses on the lack of improvement in overall survival. Obviously, the endpoint of overall survival is the gold standard for any randomized trial in cancer, but when dealing with early-stage endometrial cancer, the data should be interpreted with caution. First, in GOG 99, the primary endpoint was not overall survival but rather progression-free survival, which was significantly better in the radiation arm. Second, because of the relatively high incidence of other comorbidities such as hypertension, diabetes mellitus, and obesity as well as other cancers, the chance of dying from an intercurrent illness is as high if not higher than dying from endometrial cancer. In the radiotherapy (RT) arm of the PORTEC trial (149), the 8-year mortality rate from endometrial cancer was 9.6% compared to 14.4% from other causes and 5.3% from other cancers. In the no-RT arm, the corresponding rates were 7.5%, 10.6%, and 5.3%. Similar data that emerged from GOG 99 were that approximately half of the deaths were due to causes other than endometrial cancer or treatment. This led the authors of GOG 99 to state the following: "With this number of intercurrent deaths in both arms, even if RT reduces the risk of endometrial cancer–related deaths, the size of this trial is not adequate to reliably detect an overall survival difference." Thus, it is clear that the competing causes of death in this group of patients who have a low mortality rate to start with make overall survival a very elusive endpoint to attain. Third, even in patients who die from endometrial cancer, the most common cause is distant rather than local relapse. In the PORTEC trial, the 8-year mortality rate from local versus distant relapse was 1.1% and 7.9%, respectively, in the RT group and 2% and 5.2% in the surgery alone group (149). It is unrealistic to expect a local treatment modality such as radiation to alter this pattern of relapse. Fourth, in both GOG 99 and PORTEC trials most of the patients did not have poor prognostic features, thus making it difficult to demonstrate any survival advantage to adjuvant radiation. When the impact of adjuvant radiation in GOG 99 was assessed in the subset of patients with high-risk features (based on age, grade, depth of myometrial invasion, and presence of lymphovascular invasion) the death rate was somewhat lower in the radiation arm (RH: 0.73; 90% CI, 0.43 to 1.26). Lee et al. in their analysis of the SEER data also showed an overall survival advantage to pelvic radiation for patients with IC grade 1 and grade 3/4 ($p < 0.001$) endometrial cancer over those treated with surgery alone. This survival advantage of adjuvant pelvic radiation was significant even in patients who had surgical lymph node staging (417). All these issues need to be considered when assessing the benefit of adjuvant radiation. Such debate is not new in the field of oncology, but it is important to note that other oncologists treating cancers of the breast or rectum, to name a few, when faced with similar results from prospective, randomized trials, have recognized the importance of a multimodality approach.

Type of Radiation

There are two types of radiation (intravaginal brachytherapy or pelvic external beam radiation) that could be used either alone or in combination for early-stage endometrial cancer. Over the last three decades, the debate about the type of radiation to use has undergone a full circle. In the 1970s and mid-1980s, there was a shift from intravaginal brachytherapy alone to pelvic radiation plus intravaginal brachytherapy. Then, in the late 1980s and early 1990s, there was a shift toward pelvic radiation alone. More recently, and with the increase in surgical lymph node staging, there has been resurgence in the use of intravaginal brachytherapy alone.

Intravaginal Brachytherapy Alone or Combined With Pelvic Radiation. Aalders et al. (418) reported on 540 patients with stage IB-IC endometrial cancer who underwent TAH/BSO without lymph node sampling, and postoperative intravaginal brachytherapy to 60 Gy to the vaginal mucosa. The patients then were randomized to observation (n = 277) or to supplemental pelvic radiation to 40 Gy (n = 263). A significant reduction in local recurrence rates was seen with the addition of pelvic radiation (1.9% vs. 6.9%; $p < 0.01$). With regard to overall survival, there was no significant difference between the two arms of the study, but in the subset of patients with grade 3 disease and deep myometrial penetration, there was a survival advantage (cause-specific survival) of 18% versus 7% in favor of the pelvic radiation arm (418). The data from this trial somewhat contributed to the shift in treatment policies from intravaginal brachytherapy alone to external beam pelvic radiation.

Pelvic Radiation Alone or Combined With Intravaginal Brachytherapy. Greven et al. (419) reviewed the experience of two institutions in order to compare the outcome of the two approaches. In that study, there were 270 patients with stage I-II endometrial cancer: 173 were treated with postoperative pelvic radiation alone and 97 with a combination of intravaginal and pelvic radiation (419). The corresponding 5-year pelvic control and disease-free survival rates were 96% versus 93% ($p = 0.32$) and 88% versus 83% ($p = 0.41$). This study as well as others called into question whether the addition of vaginal radiation is needed (420,421). A number of other reports (422,423), however, suggest that vaginal vault radiation can be added to pelvic radiation with minimal morbidity and a very low rate of recurrences. Of interest, the two randomized trials (143,149) comparing surgery to adjuvant radiation both employed pelvic radiation alone with a local recurrence of only 2% to 4%. At Memorial Sloan-Kettering Cancer Center (MSKCC), when postoperative pelvic radiation is indicated it is often used alone to a dose of 50.4 Gy.

Intravaginal Brachytherapy Alone. With the increase in surgical lymph node staging, the use of postoperative intravaginal brachytherapy alone regained its appeal, the rationale being that full surgical lymph node staging could potentially eliminate the need for pelvic radiation, whereas vaginal brachytherapy could still address the risk of vaginal cuff recurrence. Several reports in the past 10 years indeed showed a very low rate of recurrence either in the vagina or in the pelvis with such an approach (139,186,424–427).

From the above discussion, it is clear that the options available for patients with early-stage endometrioid endometrial cancer are numerous. Perhaps it is better to consider different options based on the following factors: first, according to stage and grade; second, whether surgical lymph node staging was done; and third, based on the risk of nodal versus vaginal recurrence.

Stage IA Grade 1,2. The risk of pelvic lymph node positivity (60) is ≤3% and the 5-year progression-free survival rate in this group is of the order of 95% to 98%. It is unlikely that postoperative pelvic external beam radiation would add anything to the final outcome (422,428). The role of intravaginal radiation in these patients is also of questionable benefit because of an almost negligible risk of vaginal recurrence with surgery alone. Straughn et al. reported no vaginal recurrence in 103 patients with stage IA grade 1,2 treated with surgery alone (404).

Stage IA Grade 3. In GOG 33, there were only eight patients with stage IA grade 3 disease, making it difficult to draw any meaningful conclusion (60). There were no relapses in the three patients receiving postoperative radiation as compared with one failure in the five patients who received no postoperative therapy. The risk of lymph node metastasis in this group of patients is negligible. Straughn et al. reported on eight patients with stage IA grade 3 disease treated with surgery alone, with two of the patients developing isolated vaginal recurrence (404). At MSKCC, these patients are offered either intravaginal brachytherapy alone or observation (Table 23.11).

Stage IB Grade 1,2. This group of patients constitutes the most common stage subgroup of all endometrial cancers. The outcome of patients who have lymph node dissection and no adjuvant radiation seems to be very good. Straughn et al. reported on 296 patients with IB grade 1,2 and found only nine (3%) vaginal recurrences and one (0.3%) pelvic recurrence (404). Horowitz et al. reported on 62 patients who had surgical lymph node staging and received adjuvant intravaginal brachytherapy. There was one (1.6%) vaginal recurrence and no pelvic recurrence (424). In comparison, data from the MSKCC on 233 patients with IB grade 1,2 showed a vaginal recurrence rate of only 1% and pelvic recurrence of 2% using

TABLE 23.11

TREATMENT RECOMMENDATIONS AT MSKCC FOR SURGICALLY STAGED I-II PATIENTS

Stage/grade	1	2	3
IA	Observation	Observation	IVRT or observation[a]
IB	IVRT or observation[a]	IVRT or observation[a]	IVRT
IC	IVRT	IVRT	IVRT or IMRT[b]
IIA	IVRT	IVRT	IVRT
IIB < 50% CSI	IVRT	IVRT	IVRT
IIB > 50% CSI	IMRT	IMRT	IMRT

Note: CSI, cervical stromal invasion; IMRT, intensity-modulated radiation therapy; IVRT, intravaginal radiotherapy;.

[a]Observation is offered to patients <60 years old and without LVI (lymphovascular invasion).

[b]IMRT if outer third invasion and/or positive LVI.

TABLE 23.12

OUTCOME FOR IB GRADE 3 ENDOMETRIAL CANCER AFTER SURGICAL LYMPH NODE STAGING AND INTRAVAGINAL RADIATION THERAPY (IVRT) ALONE

Author	Year	No. of patients	Median F/U	Vaginal rec	Pelvic rec
Fanning (185)	2001	21	52 mo	0%	0%
Horowitz (424)	2002	31	65 mo	0%	0%
Alektiar (429)	2007	21	46 mo	4.8% (1/21)	4.8% (1/21)
Total	—	73	—	1.3% (1/73)	1.3% (1/73)

Note: F/U, follow-up.

postoperative intravaginal brachytherapy alone without routine surgical lymph node staging (429). In addition, Sorbe et al. reported on 110 patients with IB grade 1,2 who were part of a prospective, randomized trial evaluating two different intravaginal brachytherapy doses; the rate of vaginal recurrence was 0.9% and pelvic recurrence 1.8% where pelvic lymph node sampling was not routinely done either (430). Thus, it seems reasonable to suggest that either observation or intravaginal brachytherapy (irrespective of surgical staging) is a reasonable option. But when deciding on whether adjuvant radiation is needed, it is important to address three issues. First, older patients tend to have higher rates of relapse. In the study by Straughn et al., eight of the ten vaginal/pelvic recurrences were in patients ≥60 years old (404). Second, patients with lymphovascular invasion (LVI) have a higher chance of vaginal recurrence as demonstrated by Mariani et al. (406) who reported on 508 patients with stage I endometrial cancer treated with surgery alone (152 out of 508 were stage IA). The presence of LVI increased the vaginal relapse rate from 3% to 7% ($p = 0.02$). Third, often the indications for adjuvant radiation are rather arbitrarily based on the amount of myometrial invasion defined in thirds and on whether the tumor is grade 1 versus 2. Yet the amount of myometrial invasion in this group of patients and whether an endometrial cancer is assigned as grade 1 as opposed to 2 in general do not appear to be significant predictors of outcome (431,432). At MSKCC, patients with IB grade 1,2 without LVI and <60 years old are offered observation or intravaginal radiation while those with LVI or ≥60 years old are offered intravaginal radiation.

Stage IB Grade 3 to IC Grades 1,2,3. Up until the last 10 years, most data in the literature on this group of patients were based on pelvic radiation either alone or in combination with intravaginal brachytherapy (421,422,433,434). But with the increase in surgical lymph node staging, a shift has occurred with regard to the role of radiation for stage IB grade 3 and even in stage IC disease. Therefore, the treatment decision is primarily based on whether the patient had surgical lymph node staging. The adequacy of the lymph node sampling/dissection should, at a minimum, meet the GOG guidelines of sampling the obturator, external iliacs, internal iliacs, common iliacs, and para-aortic lymph node stations and the minimum number of nodes sampled should be ≥10.

Surgically Staged Patients. For patients with IB grade 3 disease the data on intravaginal brachytherapy alone after surgical staging is encouraging (Table 23.12). The average rate of vaginal recurrence and pelvic recurrence is 1.3% for both. This compares favorably with the data from the PORTEC trial where the 5-year rates for vaginal and pelvic recurrence, in the subset of patients with IB grade 3 disease treated with pelvic radiation (n = 35), were 0% and 3%, respectively. A multi-institutional review of 220 patients with stage IC endometrial cancer by Straughn et al. compared adjuvant radiation to no radiation in patients with negative nodes on surgical staging (405). The investigators concluded that adjuvant radiation is not needed even though the 5-year disease-free survival was 74.5% for those treated with surgery alone compared to 92.5% for those treated with adjuvant radiation ($p = 0.0134$). It is unlikely that observation alone, even in those patients with full surgical staging, will be accepted by the radiation oncology community or even the patients when they see an 18% statistically significant difference in disease-free survival from a retrospective study in which most likely those patients with the worst prognostic features were the ones who received radiation.

A better alternative to observation in those patients who had surgical lymph node staging is intravaginal brachytherapy alone (Table 23.13). Several investigators have shown the feasibility of such an approach with an average vaginal recurrence rate of 1.6% and pelvic control rate of 2.1%. Thus, intravaginal brachytherapy alone after surgical staging in patients with IB grade 3 and IC endometrial cancer, the preferred approach at MSKCC, seems to provide better local/regional control than surgery alone and an equivalent control to adjuvant pelvic radiation (424,435–438). The exception to this would be patients with stage IC with a combination of other poor prognostic factors such as age ≥60 years, grade 3, outer third myometrial invasion, and LVI where pelvic radiation ought to be considered. In the study from MSKCC of 40 patients with surgical stage IC treated with intravaginal brachytherapy alone, the 2 patients with vaginal/pelvic relapse both had the above-mentioned poor risk factors (436).

No Surgical Lymph Node Staging. In those patients with stage IB grade 3 IC and any grade without surgical lymph node staging, intravaginal brachytherapy alone does not seem to be adequate. In the Aalders et al. randomized trial, the rate of local recurrence in the subset of patients with IB grade 3 to IC was 9.3% (13 of 137) for those treated with brachytherapy alone compared to 1.3% (2 of 146) for those treated with brachytherapy and external radiation (418). This is not surprising since no lymph node sampling was done in that trial. Whether intravaginal brachytherapy needs to be added to external beam therapy in this group of patients is debatable. Weiss et al. reported on 61 patients with stage IC endometrial cancer who were treated with postoperative pelvic radiation alone. With a median follow-up of 69.5 months, there was only one recurrence in the pelvis (1.6%). Their review of the published data from the literature on patients with stage IC showed a pelvic recurrence of 1.04% in 240 patients treated with pelvic radiation alone compared to 0.97% in 301 patients treated with pelvic and intravaginal radiation. Their conclusion was that

TABLE 23.13

OUTCOME FOR IC ENDOMETRIAL CANCER GRADE 1-3 AFTER SURGICAL LYMPH NODE STAGING AND INTRAVAGINAL RADIATION THERAPY (IVRT) ALONE

Author	Year	No. of patients	Median F/U	Vaginal rec	Pelvic rec
Horowitz (424)	2002	50	65 mo	2% (1/50)	4% (2/50)
Rittenberg (438)	2003	53	32 mo	0%	1.8% (1/53)
Solheim (437)	2005	40	23 mo	0%	0%
Alektiar (436)	2007	40	46 mo	5% (2/40)	2.5% (1/40)
Total	—	183	—	1.6% (3/183)	2.1% (4/183)

Note: F/U, follow-up; rec=recurrence.

pelvic radiation alone is sufficient, and efforts should focus instead on trying to reduce the risk of distant relapse in this group of patients (439).

Stage II. It is important to recognize the distinction between gross and occult cervical involvement in endometrial cancer. Gross cervical involvement increases the risk of parametrial extension as well as spread to pelvic lymph nodes in a fashion similar to primary cervical cancer. Patients with gross cervical involvement from endometrial cancer could undergo radical hysterectomy and pelvic lymph node dissection or preoperative radiation including pelvic radiation and intracavitary brachytherapy followed by simple hysterectomy. For occult cervical involvement, the treatment often consists of simple hysterectomy with or without lymph node surgical staging and adjuvant radiation. The type of radiation most often utilized is pelvic radiation and intravaginal brachytherapy. Pitson et al. reported on 120 patients treated with such a combination (440). The 5-year disease-free survival rate was 68% and the rate of pelvic relapse was 5.8% (7 of 120).

There are also emerging data on the role of intravaginal brachytherapy alone in patients with occult cervical involvement who also had surgical lymph node staging. The rate of pelvic recurrence in four such series ranged from 0% to 6%, but the data need confirmation on a larger number of patients and longer follow-up (424,426,441,442). Another important distinction to make in stage II endometrial cancer is the difference between glandular versus stromal invasion. Intravaginal brachytherapy alone could be used for surgically staged IIA patients (424,443), whereas those with IIB disease should be treated with pelvic radiation with or without intravaginal brachytherapy boost, especially if there is more than half cervical stromal invasion.

Advanced-Stage Disease

Radiation

The outcome of patients with isolated adnexal involvement (stage IIIA) treated with pelvic radiation is reasonably good. Connell et al. reported on 12 patients treated with postoperative pelvic radiation with a 5-year disease-free survival of 70.9%. The weighted average of 5-year disease-free and overall survival rates from literature review in that study were 78.6% and 67.1%, respectively (444). Patients with isolated serosal involvement (stage IIIA) do worse than those with isolated adnexal involvement. Ashman et al. reported on 15 patients with isolated serosal involvement who were treated with pelvic radiation (445). The 5-year disease-free survival was only 41.5%. If pelvic node involvement (IIIC) is the only major risk factor, treatment with postoperative pelvic radiotherapy can yield a 60% to 72% long-term survival rate in these patients (156,446,447). Patients with stage IIIC disease, by virtue of para-aortic node involvement, represent a particularly high-risk group. Following surgery, these patients are generally treated with extended field radiation to encompass the pelvis and the para-aortic regions. With this aggressive approach, several investigators have reported 30% to 40% survival rates in small patient populations (448–450). The question of whether it is safe to omit radiation even after adequate surgical lymph node staging in patients with IIIC endometrial cancer was addressed in a study from the Mayo Clinic. Mariani et al. reported on 122 patients with node-positive disease; at 5 years the risk of pelvic recurrence was 57% after inadequate lymph node dissection and/or no RT compared to 10% with adequate lymph node dissection (>10 pelvic nodes and ≥5 para-aortic nodes) and radiation. This difference was statistically significant on univariate ($p <$ 0.001) and multivariate analysis ($p = 0.03$), indicating the need for postoperative radiation even after adequate surgical staging (182).

The recognition that a significant number of patients with stage III disease fail in the abdomen (407,446) has prompted a number of investigators to evaluate whole abdominal radiotherapy in these patients (451,452). The GOG also did a pilot study (GOG study 94) on patients with maximally debulked stage III and IV disease using whole abdominal radiotherapy to a total dose of 30 Gy at 1.5 Gy per fraction followed by a pelvic boost for an additional 19.8 Gy at 1.8 Gy per fraction. The 3-year disease-free and overall survival rates for the 58 patients with stage III typical adenocarcinoma were 34.5% for both, and for stage IV the corresponding rates were 10.4% and 21.1%, respectively (453). Using a different technique capable of delivering higher doses of radiation to the areas at risk for relapse in the abdomen, Stewart et al. reported 5-year disease-free and overall survival rates of 62% and 67%, respectively, in 62 patients with stage III endometrioid adenocarcinoma (454).

Chemoradiation

In the GOG 122 trial, there were 396 patients with stage III and optimally debulked stage IV disease who were randomized to whole abdomen radiation (n = 202) or to doxorubicin-cisplatin chemotherapy (n = 194). With a median follow-up of 74 months, there was significant improvement in both progression-free (50% vs. 38%; $p = 0.007$) as well as overall survival (55% vs. 42%; $p = 0.004$), respectively, in favor of chemotherapy (8).

At first glance the results of this trial seem to seal the fate of adjuvant radiation in advanced endometrial cancer; however, before concluding that chemotherapy alone is the answer a closer examination of the data is warranted. First, the overall absolute rate of relapse was 54% in the radiation arm compared to 50% in the chemotherapy arm, a small difference if any, yet the corresponding 5-year progression-free survival rates were 38% and 50% ($p = 0.007$), respectively. Why the discrepancy? The answer is that the 5-year progression-free survival rate for the radiation arm was 38% while the chemotherapy arm has two separate 5-year rates. The first one, called unadjusted, was 42%, which is not that significantly different from the 38% rate with radiation, and the second, called "adjusted for stage," was 50%, which was significantly different from the radiation arm. This led us to the second issue: Was the adjustment for stage warranted? The answer is no. Numerically, there were more patients with lymph node involvement in the chemotherapy than the radiation arm, but having positive lymph nodes was not an independent predictor of poor outcome in this study. Therefore, the adjustment was not warranted, and if any adjustment was needed it should have gone to the radiation arm since there were more patients with positive cytology in this arm, a factor with a hazard ratio of 1.8 (95% CI, 0.89 to 1.55) in predicting poor outcome. Third, what should be made of the significant difference in overall survival? There were 15 deaths unrelated to endometrial cancer or protocol treatment in the radiation arm compared to only to 6 in the chemotherapy arm, raising a question about whether the two arms of the study were truly balanced. Another randomized trial comparing adjuvant radiation to chemotherapy (doxorubicin-cisplatin-cyclophosphamide) in patients with stage I-III was recently reported and showed no difference in outcome between the two arms (415). With a median follow-up of 95.5 months, the 5-year disease-free survival was 63% in both arms ($p = 0.44$) and the 5-year overall survival rates were 69% in the radiation arm compared to 66% in the chemotherapy arm ($p = 0.77$). What those two trials show is that chemotherapy at a minimum is equivalent to radiation in this group of patients and ought to be used, not alone, but rather in combination with radiation. Greven et al. reported the results of Radiation Therapy Oncology Group (RTOG) 9708 on 44 patients with stage I-III endometrial cancer who were treated with pelvic radiation and intravaginal brachytherapy given concurrently with cisplatin 50 mg/m^2 on days 1 and 28 of radiation followed by four cycles of cisplatin (50 mg/m^2) and paclitaxel (Taxol) (175 mg/m^2). The 4-year disease-free and overall survival for those with stage III disease (66% of patients) were 72% and 77% respectively (455).

SPECIAL SITUATIONS

Stage IIIA Disease (Positive Cytology Without Adnexal or Serosal Involvement)

In this subset of patients, the presence of other adverse features such as aggressive histologies or deep myometrial invasion should be determined first. If they are present, then the patients should be considered to be in a true advanced stage and be treated as such. On the other hand, if they are absent, then the true prognostic value of positive peritoneal cytology is still unclear (456). The literature regarding the benefits of treatment in this setting is mixed; even if treatment is beneficial, the appropriate modality still has to be defined. Based on the concept that the entire peritoneal cavity is at risk, intraperitoneal radioactive colloidal ^{32}P has been used by some with results that were better than in historic controls (457). Eltabbakh et al. reported on 27 patients with FIGO grade 1,2 and <50% myometrial invasion who were treated with intravaginal brachytherapy and megestrol acetate (Megace). None of the patients relapsed or died from their disease. Megace was given for 1 year, and at the end of therapy, 24 patients underwent second-look laparoscopy and peritoneal cytology. In 23 patients, the cytology was negative and the remaining patient with persistent positive cytology received an additional year of Megace after which cytology was confirmed to be negative (458).

Definitive Radiation for Inoperable Disease

Patients with medically inoperable stage I-II uterine cancer are usually treated in a fashion similar to those with cervical cancer by using intracavitary applicators with or without pelvic radiation. For patients with clinical stage I grade 1 or 2 and no evidence of myometrial invasion or lymph node metastasis on MRI, intracavitary brachytherapy alone is sufficient. Usually a Fletcher-Suit or Henschke applicator with one or two tandems (depending on uterus size) and ovoids is used to deliver 70 to 75 Gy to point A. The loading of the tandems is usually different than that in cervical cancer. This is done in order to provide wider coverage of the uterus laterally and superiorly. When pelvic radiation is added, the dose is usually 45 to 50 Gy supplemented with 30 to 35 Gy from intracavitary brachytherapy to bring the total dose to point A to 80 to 85 Gy. Rouanet et al. (462) treated 250 patients with endometrial cancer according to this approach, which yielded a 5-year disease-specific survival of 76.5%. An alternative brachytherapy approach would be to use the Hymen or Simon afterloading system, which consists of multiple Teflon tubes that are inserted into the uterine cavity. With such a treatment approach, Grigsby et al. (463) reported that the 5-year progression-free survival rate of patients with clinical stage I disease treated with a combination of external and intracavitary radiotherapy was 94% for grade 1 disease, 92% for grade 2 disease, and 78% for grade 3 disease. More recently, high-dose-rate brachytherapy is also being employed (464,465). For patients with stage IIIB disease (vaginal involvement), an uncommon presentation, these patients are usually not surgical candidates and are also treated with definitive radiation including a combination of external beam and intracavitary/interstitial radiotherapy tailored to the extent of their disease (466).

RADIATION THERAPY TECHNIQUES

Intravaginal Brachytherapy

The purpose of this treatment modality is to deliver the highest dose of radiation to the vaginal mucosa while limiting the dose to the surrounding normal structures such as the bladder, rectum, and small intestines. Intravaginal brachytherapy could be delivered with low-dose-rate ^{137}Cs sources, which requires admission to the hospital for a few days. The dose is usually 60 Gy prescribed to the vaginal mucosa or 30 to 35 Gy prescribed to 0.5 cm depth from the vaginal mucosa. The type of applicator used is generally the two ovoids from a Fletcher-Suit applicator, where only the vaginal cuff is irradiated. Alternatively, a cylinder could be used to treat one half to two thirds of the length of the vagina. Occasionally, the whole length of the vagina needs to be treated, especially in patients with grade 3 tumors, which have the tendency for relapse in the distal periurethral region. High-dose-rate brachytherapy using ^{192}Ir sources has been shown to be an attractive alternative to low-dose-rate brachytherapy. The treatment is given on an outpatient basis without the need for anesthesia and without the radiation exposure to medical personnel. At MSKCC, patients start their treatment 4 to 6 weeks postoperatively depending on the vaginal cuff healing. The treatment is given in three fractions of 7 Gy to a total dose of 21 Gy. The interval between each fraction is 1 to 2 weeks. The dose is prescribed to 0.5 cm depth from the mucosal surface. The treatment is usually delivered using a 3-cm diameter cylinder to treat one half to two thirds of the length of the vagina, or the whole vagina in grade 3 tumors. Occasionally, the dose per fraction is lowered to 6 Gy instead of 7 Gy if the diameter of the cylinder is less than 3 cm. This is usually done to avoid a very high dose of radiation to the vaginal mucosa. The dose per fraction is also lowered to 4 to 5 Gy when pelvic radiation is added.

External Beam Radiation

Pelvic Radiation

Most patients are treated in the postoperative setting. At the time of simulation, the small bowel is opacified using oral contrast, a vaginal marker is used to define the vaginal cuff, and the rectum is opacified with barium or CT-compatible contrasts. Patients are usually placed in the prone position to displace the small intestines from the radiation field. The target volume consists of the pelvic lymph nodes, including obturator, external, internal, and lower common iliac groups, and the proximal two thirds of the vagina. High-energy linear accelerators (15 MV) are preferred because of their sparing of the skin and subcutaneous tissue. The ideal beam arrangement with conventional radiation is the four-field pelvic-box technique to reduce the dose to the small intestines and to some extent the bladder and rectum. For the anteroposterior/posteroanterior (AP/PA) fields, the superior border is L5-S1, the inferior border is the bottom of the obturator foramina, and the lateral border is 2 cm beyond the widest point of the inlet of the true bony pelvis. For the lateral fields, the anterior border is in front of the pubis symphysis and the posterior border at least at S2-3. The superior and inferior borders are the same for the AP/PA fields. All fields are treated daily to a dose of 1.8 Gy. A total dose of 50.4 Gy is generally used when pelvic radiation is used alone or 45 Gy when combined with intravaginal brachytherapy.

Extended Field

This technique is mainly used for patients with documented positive para-aortic nodes. The preferred approach is the four-field box technique in order to lower the dose to the small intestines. However, attention should be paid to the dose that the kidneys might receive with the four-field arrangement. The lower border is the same as in pelvic radiation but the upper border is extended usually to the T12-L1 interspace. The typical dose is 45.0 Gy at 1.8 Gy perfraction or 1.5 Gy perfraction if patients develop acute gastrointestinal toxicity.

Whole Abdomen Radiation

The standard approach is AP/PA open fields with five half-value layer (HVL) kidney blocks placed over the PA field only (if patient is lying supine) from the start of the treatment. The dose is usually 30.0 Gy at 1.5 Gy per fraction followed by a 19.8 Gy boost to the pelvis at 1.8 Gy per fraction. The upper border is usually placed 1 cm above the diaphragm, and the lateral borders should extend beyond the peritoneal reflections. The lower border is usually at the bottom of the obturator foramen.

Complications of Radiation

Pelvic Radiation

In the PORTEC randomized trial (149), the overall (grades 1 to 4) rate of late complications was 26% in the RT group compared to 4% in the observation group ($p < 0.0001$). Most of the late complications in the RT group, however, were grades 1,2 (22%) and only 3% were grades 3,4. It is also important to note that many patients in this trial were treated with AP/PA fields in which the overall rate of complications was 30% compared to 21% for those treated with the four-field box ($p = 0.06$). The morbidity rate of pelvic radiation could be reduced even further by using intensity-modulated radiation therapy (IMRT). Mundt et al. demonstrated a significant reduction in acute and chronic gastrointestinal toxicity when IMRT was compared to conventional radiation (467,468). At MSKCC, postoperative IMRT is used for most patients with endometrial cancer who need pelvic radiation (Fig. 23.13).

Whole Abdomen Radiation

The toxicity of whole abdomen radiation is more pronounced than that of pelvic radiation but not as high as expected. In the radiation arm of GOG study 122, the GI toxicity did not exceed 2% for grade 4 and 11% for grade 3, whereas in the chemotherapy arm the corresponding figures were 7% and 13%. Grade 4 liver toxicity was seen in 1% of patients in the radiation arm while the grade 4 cardiac grade toxicity was 4% in the chemotherapy arm (8).

Intravaginal Brachytherapy

The main advantage of intravaginal brachytherapy is its ability to deliver a relatively high dose of radiation to the vagina while limiting the dose to the surrounding normal structures such as the bowels and bladder. This advantage is manifested with the low rate of severe late toxicity seen with this treatment technique, ranging from 0% to 1% (469–471). But such a very low rate of severe complications cannot be taken for granted because special attention needs to be paid to the depth of prescription, the dose per fraction, the length of vagina treated, and the diameter of the cylinder used (472).

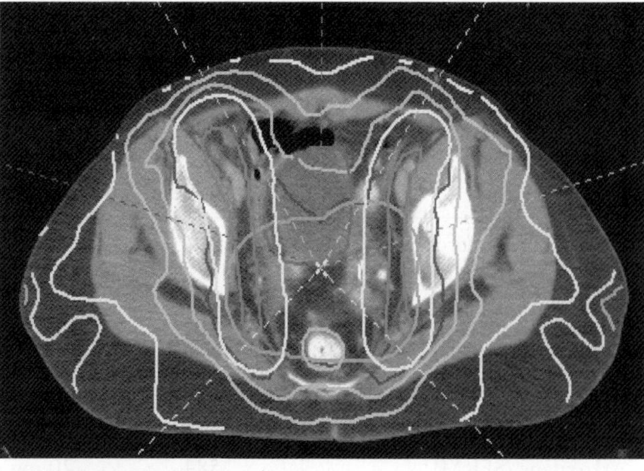

FIGURE 23.13. (*See color plate section.*) Pelvic IMRT demonstrating the sparing of bladder and bowel.

Radiation Therapy for Local Recurrence

Radiation therapy can be curative in a select group of patients with small vaginal recurrences who have not received prior radiation. The 5-year local control rate ranges from 42% to 65% and the 5-year overall survival rate from 31% to 53% (473–475). Creutzberg et al. reported on survival after relapse from the PORTEC randomized trial (476). In patients who were initially randomized to surgery alone (n = 46 out of 360), the 5-year survival after vaginal relapse was 65%. But before adopting salvage radiation as a treatment policy for all early-stage endometrial cancer, a few aspects of this trial need to be addressed. First, the 5-year survival rate from the PORTEC trial is much higher than what is reported in the literature. Most likely, the vaginal recurrences in this trial were detected very early, unlike patients in the community. The extent and size of local recurrence in endometrial cancer are very significant predictors of outcome (473). Second, this high rate of salvage pertains only to isolated vaginal recurrence. The rate of survival at 3 years for pelvic recurrence in the PORTEC trial was 0%. Third, although the trial does not mention any data on complications, it is not unrealistic to expect a higher complication rate than what is normally seen with adjuvant radiation. With salvage radiation, external beam RT and brachytherapy are often combined and the doses of radiation required are much higher than those used with adjuvant radiation. A recent study from the M. D. Anderson Cancer Center by Jhingran et al. clearly highlights these issues (477). They reported on 91 patients who were treated with definitive radiation for isolated vaginal recurrence. The 5-year local control and overall survival rates were 75% and 43%, respectively. The median dose of radiation was 75 Gy, which often included external radiation and brachytherapy. The rate of grade 4 complications (requiring surgery) was 9%. Thus, when talking with a patient about adjuvant radiation versus radiation reserved for salvage, these issues need to be addressed and compared to the excellent local control and low morbidity obtained with adjuvant intravaginal brachytherapy.

SYSTEMIC THERAPIES

Endocrine Therapy

Hormonal agents have been found to be valuable, particularly in the patient with recurrent disease, and reviews of their use have been extensively published. Response rates to a variety of endocrine agents including progestins, antiestrogens, and aromatase inhibitors are presented in Table 23.14 (478–485).

The overall response to progestins is approximately 25%. However, some trials demonstrate lower response rates, usually in the range of 15% to 20%. These studies generally used more rigorous response criteria and had multi-institutional participation. A higher dose of progestin does not appear to increase the response rate. In one randomized trial of 200 mg/d versus 1,000 mg/d of medroxyprogesterone acetate (MPA), the overall response rate was actually 25% versus 15% favoring the low-dose arm (486). The time to treatment failure and median overall survival of the low- versus high-dose regimen, respectively, were 3.2 versus 2.5 months and 11.1 versus 7.0 months, all showing no advantage for an increased dose. Prognostic factors related to response were performance status, grade, and progesterone receptor level. The response rate was only 8% in poorly differentiated tumors. A phase 2 trial of high-dose megestrol (800 mg orally daily) in 63 patients was associated with a response rate of 24% overall, which is similar to lower-dose regimens with doses of 40 mg po qid (487). As in the majority of studies with hormonal agents, response rates were statistically higher in patients with grade 1 or 2 lesions (37%) versus grade 3 lesions (8%); $p = 0.02$ (400). In addition to grade, a long disease-free interval (exceeding 2 or 3 years) and positive estrogen or progesterone receptor status have all been associated with an increased frequency of response (Table 23.15) (478,481,486,487). Age, location of metastatic disease, number of metastatic sites, prior therapy, and weight have also been analyzed by several investigators, but they have not been convincingly linked with response.

Tamoxifen has been investigated in patients with recurrent disease in several studies (484,488). Results have varied, but in general, response rates have been modest in untreated patients. A GOG study evaluated 68 patients with advanced or recurrent disease receiving tamoxifen at 20 mg po bid and showed an overall response rate of 10% (90% CI, 5.7 to 17.9) (484). The median progression-free interval was short at 1.9 months (90% CI, 1.7 to 3.2 months) and the overall survival was 8.8 months (90% CI, 7.0 to 10.1 months). One small randomized phase 2 study comparing megestrol acetate to megestrol acetate with tamoxifen showed no advantage in response rate for the combination, with response rates of 20% versus 19%, respectively (489). The lack of synergistic response is supported by observations of endometrial carcinoma treated in a nude mouse model. Tumors treated with medroxyprogesterone or tamoxifen plus medroxyprogesterone were devoid of progesterone receptor during the growth inhibitory and regrowth phase of the tumor resulting from receptor down-regulation (490). The possibility

TABLE 23.14

RESPONSE TO ENDOCRINE THERAPY

Hormonal agent	References	Average dose	Response rate (%)	Range (%)
Hydroxyprogesterone caproate (Delalutin)	478,479	1–3 g IM q wk	29	9–34
Medroxyprogesterone acetate (Provera)	476	200–1,000 mg IM q wk or po qd	22	14–53
Megestrol acetate (Megace)	479	40–800 mg po qd	20	11–56
Tamoxifen (Nolvadex)	481,482	20–40 mg po qd	10	0–53
Goserelin acetate	477	3.6 mg SC q mo	11	NA
Anastrozole (SERM)	480	1 mg po q d	9	NA
Arzoxifene (SERM)	584	20 mg po q d	31	NA

Note: IM, intramuscularly; NA, not applicable; SC, subcutaneously; SERM, selective estrogen receptor modulator.

TABLE 23.15

RESPONSE TO PROGESTATIONAL THERAPY AS A FUNCTION OF TUMOR GRADE

Study	Treatment	Grade	N	RR
Podratz 1985	Various progestins	1	10	40%
		2	71	15%
		3	73	2%
Lentz 1996	MA 800 mg/d	1	14	37% (grade 1-2)
		2	17	
		3	27	8%
Thigpen 1999	MPA 200 mg/d vs. 1,000 mg/d	1	59	37%
		2	113	23%
		3	127	9%
Whitney 2003	Tam 40 mg/d + alternating weekly MPA 200 mg/d	1	15	Overall RR 33%
		2	17	
		3	27	
Fiorica 2003	MA 160 mg/d × 3 wk, alternating with Tam 40 mg/d × 3 wk	1	16	38%
		2	17	24%
		3	22	22%

Note: MA, megestrol acetate; MPA, medroxyprogesterone acetate; RR, response rate; Tam, tamoxifen.

of alternating tamoxifen with megestrol acetate in order to exploit the recruitment of progesterone receptors by tamoxifen is an interesting strategy. The GOG performed a phase 2 study with 56 patients with advanced or recurrent endometrial cancer who had not previously received chemotherapy or hormonal manipulation (491). Patients were treated with megestrol acetate at 160 mg/d for 3 weeks alternating with tamoxifen 40 mg po q d for 3 weeks. An overall response rate of 27% (90% CI, 17.3 to 38.4) with a 21.4% complete response rate was seen, with the duration of response exceeding 20 months in 8 of 15 responders. The response rate was 38% for patients with grade 1 disease and 22% for those with grade 3 disease. In another phase 2 GOG study, a similar patient population was treated with tamoxifen 40 mg po daily plus alternating weekly cycles of medroxyprogesterone acetate 200 mg po daily (492). Of the 58 evaluable patients, the response rate was 33% (6 complete, 13 partial). Although these phase 2 results are intriguing, a randomized study would be required to determine if alternating hormones is superior to single-hormone approaches. Positive receptor status has been associated with improved disease-free and overall survival rates (126,493,494). These data indicate that the receptor status provides important biologic information and that receptor-positive tumors tend to be better differentiated and slower growing than are their receptor-negative counterparts. Chemotherapy had no effect on hormone receptor capacity in a nude mouse model of xenografted endometrial cancer (495). Other factors, such as changes in vaginal cytology during treatment (496), and results in the subrenal capsule chemosensitivity assay (497) and in the nude mouse model (498) may help predict response to progestins.

Several studies have evaluated gonadotropin-releasing hormone analogs in patients with metastatic endometrial cancer. Gallagher et al. (499) noted one complete and five partial responses to leuprolide or goserelin in 17 patients (35% response; 95% CI, 13% to 58%) with metastatic disease. Of note, the duration of remission ranged from 7 to 30 months, and 14 of the 17 patients had been previously treated with progestins. Another report described four responses in seven postmenopausal patients with endometrial cancer treated with goserelin (500). *In vitro* studies in human endometrial cancer cell lines have suggested that such growth inhibition may have been due to apoptosis (501). The GOG recently studied goserelin at 3.6 mg subcutaneously monthly in 40 patients with advanced or recurrent disease. Seventy-one percent of patients had received prior radiotherapy. There were two complete (5%) and three partial (7%) responses with an overall response rate of 11% (95% CI, 4% to 27%). Goserelin is felt to have limited activity in this patient population, and no additional single-agent studies are planned (479).

Investigation is under way in patients with uterine cancer to evaluate the activity of selective estrogen receptor modulators (SERMs). These agents have estrogen receptor (ER)-antagonist activity in breast and uterine tissues and ER-agonist activity in bone. The first reported study to date is from the GOG and evaluated anastrozole at 1 mg po daily orally in 23 unselected patients (i.e., 9 patients had grade 2 tumors and 14 patients had grade 3 tumors). A partial response rate of 9% was seen (90% CI, 3% to 23%). It is noted that the partial response rate of 9% in this study is similar to the 8% reported in grade 3 patients treated with standard progestins (487,493). A more recent study evaluated the investigational SERM arzoxifene in 37 patients. Twenty-six patients were ER positive and 22 were progesterone receptor (PR) positive. A response rate of 31% (95% CI, 25% to 51%) was seen in this selected patient population with a median duration of response of 13.9 months (480). Additional study of these agents in patients with well-differentiated tumors is warranted (502).

Cytotoxic Chemotherapy

Both single-agent and combination regimens are capable of inducing objective responses, yet the median time to treatment failure is on average 3 to 6 months and the overall survival of patients with metastatic endometrial cancer is generally less than 12 months. The role of chemotherapy in the recurrent disease setting remains palliative, and minimizing side effects is of equal importance when selecting a regimen. Responses to treatment are usually partial and have lasted an average of only 3 to 6 months. Also, the time to progression in most trials tends to be short, ranging from 4 to 6 months, with median survival averaging 7 to 10 months. Patients with complete response may have long progression-free intervals lasting 1 to 2 years, but such patients comprise only a minority of those treated. Particularly for patients with grade 1 histology, or small-volume asymptomatic metastatic disease, hormonal therapy may provide better initial palliation, reserving chemotherapy for rapidly progressive or symptomatic disease (503,504).

Single-Agent Trials

The wide variety of single agents that have been tested are presented in Table 23.16 (505–508). Despite the number of drugs evaluated, the most commonly used single agents today based on response rates of at least 20% include cisplatin, carboplatin, doxorubicin, epirubicin, ifosfamide, docetaxel, and paclitaxel, and more recently topotecan has been added to this list.

The response rate to cisplatin dosages of 50 to 60 mg/m^2 given every 3 weeks was similar in patients with prior (25%) (509,510) and no prior chemotherapy (21%) (511–513). Carboplatin given in dosages of 300 to 400 mg/m^2 every 4 weeks has been associated with response rates of 29% (514–516), which is similar to cisplatin. Doxorubicin in dosages of 55 to 60 mg/m^2 has been associated with an overall response rate of 26% (517–519) and epirubicin with a response rate of 26% (520). Liposomal doxorubicin was recently reported in a GOG study of 46 patients receiving 50 mg/m^2 every 4 weeks with an overall response rate of 9.5%

TABLE 23.16

SINGLE-AGENT TRIALS

Agent (reference)	n	Prior treatment	No. of CR + PR	(%)	95% CI
ALKYLATING AGENTS					
Cyclophosphamide (585)	37	Some	4	11	3–25
Chlorambucil (585)	11	NS	0	0	0–28
Ifosfamide (586,587)	56	Some	4 + 4	14	6–26
Hexamethylmelamine (588,589)	54	Few	2 + 7	17	8–29
CISPLATIN					
No prior Rx (509,513)	63	No	3 + 10	21	11–33
Prior chemo (510,511,512)	64	Yes	3 + 13	25	15–37
Carboplatin (514,515,516)	82	No	5 + 18	28	19–39
ANTHRACYCLINES/ANTHRAQUINONES					
Doxorubicin (517,518,519)	161	No	18 + 24	26	19–34
Epirubicin (520)	27	No	2 + 5	26	11–46
Liposomal doxorubicin (521)	42	Yes	0 + 4	9.5	2.7–22.6
Pirarubicin (590)	28	7	2 + 0	7	1–30
Mitoxantrone (591,592,593)	46	32	0 + 2	4	1–15
ANTIMETABOLITES					
Fluorouracil (585)	34	NS	7	21	9–38
Methotrexate (523)	33	No	1 + 1	6	2–20
6-Mercaptopurine (524)	10	NS	0	0	0–31
VINCAS/EPIPODOPHYLLOTOXINS					
Vincristine (525,592)	38	5	1 + 5	16	6–31
Vinblastine (593,594)	48	Most	1 + 3	8	2–20
Etoposide (VP-16) (595)	29	Yes	0 + 1	3	1–29
Teniposide (VM-26) (596)	22	17	0 + 2	9	1–26
TOPOISOMERASE I INHIBITOR					
Topotecan (528)	42	No	3 + 5	20	nr
TAXANES					
Paclitaxel (526)	44	Yes	3 + 9	27.3	15–42.8
Docetaxel (508)	35	No	3 + 4	21	nr
REPORTED INVESTIGATIONAL STUDIES					
Aminothiodiazole (505)	21	12	0	0	0–16
Amonafide (597)	38	4	2 + 0	6	1–20
Amsacrine (AMSA) (591,598)	23	1	1 + 1	9	1–28
Cytembina (524)	30	Yes	10	33	17–53
Diaziquone (AZQ) (595)	26	20	1 + 1	8	1–25
Echinomycin (599)	21	Yes	1 + 0	5	1–23
Fludarabine (507)	19	Yes	0	0	0–18
Methyl-G (600)	21	11	3	14	3–36
Piperazinedione (601)	20	Most	0 + 1	5	1–25
Razoxane (ICRF-159) (602)	24	Yes	0	0	0–14
Semustine (MeCCNU) (603)	5	NS	0 + 2	40	5–85

Note: 95% CI, the 95% confidence interval for complete and partial response; CR, complete response; NS, not stated; PR, partial response.

(95% CI, 2.7% to 26%) (521). It is important to note that 32 patients had received prior doxorubicin therapy. A second study evaluated its efficacy in 19 patients without prior chemotherapy treatment and resulted in a 21% response rate (522). Of the antimetabolites, 5-fluorouracil given in dosages of 15 mg/kg for 5 consecutive days and then every other day until dose-limiting toxicity occurred. It has displayed a 21% response rate in 34 patients, whereas methotrexate (523) and mercaptopurine (524) have been inactive. Vincristine given on a weekly schedule was associated with a response rate of 18% in 33 untreated patients (525), but dose-limiting neurotoxicity was substantial. In a phase 2 trial of paclitaxel conducted by the GOG (506), 28 patients with recurrent or advanced endometrial cancer received a dose of 250 mg/m^2 every 21 days. Patients who had received prior pelvic irradiation were treated at an initial dose of 200 mg/m^2. Complete responses were noted in four patients (14%) and partial responses in six (21%) for an overall response rate of 36%. A more contemporary GOG study evaluated paclitaxel at 200 mg/m^2 (175 mg/m^2 with prior radiotherapy) every 3 weeks in pretreated patients showing an overall response rate of 27.3% (95% CI, 15% to 42.8%). The median duration of response was 4.2 months with an overall survival of 10.3 months (526). A similar study showed a response rate of 43% (95% CI, 6% to 80%) in patients who had all previously been treated with platinum-based therapy (527). A multicenter trial recently reported showed a response rate of 21% with PFS of 12 weeks and overall survival (OS) of 43 weeks in 35 patients receiving weekly docetaxel at 35 mg/m^2 (508).

Topotecan was evaluated in a phase 2 trial of untreated advanced or recurrent endometrial cancer administered initially at 1.5 mg/m^2 every day for 5 days every 3 weeks. The trial was suspended for toxicity, but reopened and completed at 1 mg/m^2 q day for 5 days (or 0.8 mg/m^2/d for patients with prior radiotherapy). An overall response rate of 20% was seen with median duration of response of 8.0 months and overall survival of 6.5 months (528). A subsequent smaller study by Traina et al. using weekly topotecan dosing of 2.5 to 4.0 mg/m^2 on a 2 of 3 weeks schedule followed by 1 week off showed one partial response for 54 weeks with two patients having stable disease for 15 weeks each. Only two patients required dose reduction for toxicity using the weekly schedule (552).

The frequent variability in response rate noted for the same agent is probably related to several factors, including prior treatment, performance status, extent of disease, and the response criteria used for evaluation. No current data suggest that dose-response relationships exist for single-agent therapy, and doses and schedules are generally adjusted to minimize toxicity for an individual patient.

Combination Therapy

The results of treatment with combination regimens are presented in Table 23.17 (509,518,529–544). The first combination to be explored was cyclophosphamide with doxorubicin in four trials in chemotherapy-naïve patients (518,533, 538,542) using doxorubicin dosages of 40 to 50 mg/m^2 repeated every 3 to 4 weeks. The objective response rates for these trials were similar to single-agent doxorubicin and showed no advantage for the addition of cyclophosphamide. The GOG also compared doxorubicin alone with the same dose and schedule of doxorubicin plus cyclophosphamide (518). All patients had failed progestin therapy, had measurable lesions, and had no prior chemotherapy. The complete and partial response rates for patients receiving the doxorubicin (132 patients) and combination regimens (144 patients) were 22% and 30%, with a median progression-free interval of 3.2 and 3.9 months and a median survival of 6.9 and 7.3 months, respectively.

The addition of cyclophosphamide and doxorubicin to cisplatin (CAP) (509,532,535,536) and doxorubicin to cisplatin (AP) (530,539,541,543,544) has been associated with response rates ranging from 38% to 76%. The overlap of the 95% confidence intervals for CAP and AP regimens suggests no significant difference in response rates, thus allowing the AP regimen to become the "standard" to which more contemporary approaches are compared. Barrett et al. (530) studied a chronobiologically defined schedule of doxorubicin (60 mg/m^2 at 6:00 AM) and cisplatin (60 mg/m^2 at 6:00 PM) in an attempt to maximize the therapeutic index of the combination. The regimen in a phase 2 trial produced a 60% response rate, similar to other AP trials (539,541,544), but the median survival of 14 months was somewhat longer than in other AP trials. Toxicity was substantial, with 43% of patients developing white blood cell (WBC) counts of >1,000/mm^3. GOG 139 represented a randomized trial of standard versus circadian-timed cisplatin and doxorubicin, and found no difference in response rate (46% vs. 49%) or progression-free (6.5 vs. 5.9 months) or overall survival (11.2 vs. 13.2 months) (545). The results of GOG 107 comparing doxorubicin (60 mg/m^2 every 3 weeks) with the same doxorubicin dose and cisplatin (50 mg/m^2 every 3 weeks) in 223 patients with advanced or recurrent endometrial cancer have shown a significantly higher response rate for the combination (42% vs. 25%; p = 0.004), but a progression-free and overall survival of 5.7 versus 3.8 months and 9.2 versus 9.0 months, respectively (543). Moderate to severe nausea and vomiting (16% vs. 2%), platelet counts of 50,000 mm^3 (14% vs. 2%), and WBCs of 2,000 mm^3 (61% vs. 39%) were more common for the combination regimen. This study confirms a higher response rate with combination therapy, but the difference in progression-free survival is modest and likely not clinically meaningful; the overall survival is identical in the two groups.

Given the increased response rate of the doxorubicin combination, and the phase 2 activity of single-agent paclitaxel, the GOG conducted a randomized trial (GOG 163) for patients with primary stage III and IV or recurrent endometrial cancer comparing doxorubicin and cisplatin to doxorubicin with 24-hour paclitaxel and granulocyte colony-stimulating factor (G-CSF). There were no significant differences in response rate (40% vs. 43%), PFS (median 7.2 vs. 6 months), or OS (median 12.6 vs. 13.6 months) for arm 1 and 2, respectively (546).

The disadvantage of GOG 163 was the lack of platinum in the taxane-containing arm, however. The addition of a taxane was subsequently studied in GOG 177. Doxorubicin (60 mg/m^2 or 45 mg/m^2 in patients with prior radiotherapy) with cisplatin (50 mg/m^2) as the standard arm versus paclitaxel (160 mg/m^2) with doxorubicin (45 mg/m^2) and cisplatin (50 mg/m^2) and G-CSF as the investigational regimen (547). The primary objective was to determine if the addition of paclitaxel improved response rate and progression-free and overall survival, and a secondary objective explored the relationship between HER2/*neu* overexpression and outcome with doxorubicin-based therapy. Two hundred and seventy-three patients were enrolled, and the study was balanced for history of prior RT (50% vs. 46%), serous carcinoma (15% vs. 19%), stage, grade, and body surface area (BSA). Grade 3 and 4 platelet toxicity was higher in the three-drug arm (21% vs. 2%), but other hematologic toxicity was ameliorated with G-CSF: absolute neutrophil count (ANC) 36% versus 50% and neutropenic fever 3% versus 2%. Nonhematologic grade 3,4 toxicity was higher in the three-drug arm: gastrointestinal 59% versus 39% and metabolic 25% versus 13%. Response rates were better with the triplet: complete response 22% versus 7%, partial response 36% versus 27%, and overall response rate (RR) 57% versus 34%. Median PFS was 8.3 months versus 5.3 months ($p < 0.0005$) and median overall survival was 15.3 months versus 12.1 months (p = 0024).

TABLE 23.17

COMBINATION CHEMOTHERAPY

Reference	Drug	Dose (mg/m²)	Schedule	Chemotherapy	n	CR + PR (%)
CYCLOPHOSPHAMIDE-DOXORUBICIN-CISPLATIN (CAP)						
536	CYC	500	q 4 wk	No	18	55 (56)
	DOX	50				
	CIS	50				
509	CYC	400	q 3 wk	No	16	05 (31)
	DOX	40				
	CIS	40				
532	CYC	500	q 4 wk	No	87	1227 (45)
	DOX	50				
	CIS	50				
535	CYC	500	q 3 wk	5	17	35 (47)
	DOX	50				
	CIS	50				
DOXORUBICIN-CISPLATIN						
541	DOX	50	q 3 wk	No	9	12 (33)
	CIS	50				
544	DOX	50	q 4 wk	No	20	210 (60)
	CIS	50				
539	DOX	60	q 4 wk	4/16	16	67 (81)
	CIS	60				
530	DOX	60[a]	q 4 wk	No	30	612 (60)
	CIS	60				
CYCLOPHOSPHAMIDE-DOXORUBICIN						
538	CYC	500	q 3 wk	No	11	32 (45)
	DOX	37.5				
542	CYC	400–500	q 4 wk	No	26	08 (31)
	DOX	40–50				
518	CYC	500	q 3 wk	No	105	1519 (32)
	DOX	50				
533	CYC	600	q 3 wk	No	13	15 (46)
	DOX	50				
OTHER						
529	DOX	30	q 34 wk	No	42	310 (31)
	CIS	50				
	VLB	5				
	VCR	1.5	q 3 wk	No	44	914 (52)
	VM-26	100				
	CIS	60				
	CYC	500	q 3 wk	No	20	55 (50)
	DOX	40				
	VCR	1.5				
	FU	500 (d2,3)				
537	MTX	30 (d1,15,22)	q 4 wk	No	25	15 (60)
	VLB	3 (d2,15,22)				
	DOX	30 (d2)				
	CIS	70 (d2)				
RANDOMIZED TRIALS—CHEMOTHERAPY						
518	DOX	—	q 3 wk	No	90	(24)
	vs.					
	CYC			No	105	(32)
	DOX					
543	DOX	60	q 3 wk	No	122	(27)
	vs.					
	DOX	60		No	101	(45)
	CIS	50				

(*continued*)

TABLE 23.17

(CONTINUED)

Reference	Drug	Dose (mg/m²)	Schedule	Chemotherapy	n	CR + PR (%)
546	DOX	60	q 3 wk	No	157	40 (15 + n/a 35)
	CIS	50				
	vs.					
	DOX	50			157	43 (17 + 26)
	PAC	150				
547	DOX	60			133	33 (7 + n/a 26)
	CIS	50				
	vs.					
	DOX	45			133	57 (22 + 35)
	CIS	50				
	PAC	160				

Note: CIS, cisplatin; CR, complete response; CYC, cyclophosphamide; DOX, doxorubicin; FU, fluorouracil; MTX, methotrexate; PAC, paclitaxel; PR, partial response; VCR, vincristine; VLB, vinblastine; VM-26, teniposide.
[a]Circadian timed regimen doxorubicin at 0600 (6 AM) and cisplatin at 1800 (6 PM) hours.

Responses were similar in serous (48%) versus nonserous histology (45%). Overall, paclitaxel doxorubicin cisplatin (TAP) chemotherapy increased 12-month survival to 59% compared to 50% with AP with an HR of 0.75 (0.56 to 0.998). As the secondary objective using available specimens (HER2/neu testing was not done in approximately 12% of patients) approximately 20% stained 3+, which was neither prognostic nor predictive of outcome in this patient population (547).

Although the TAP regimen produced an improvement in response rate and PFS, survival was minimally increased, and it is associated with greater toxicity. The combination of paclitaxel and carboplatin as a doublet has also been evaluated in a variety of phase 2 trials and retrospective studies with response rates in the 43% to 80% range (548,549). No direct phase 3 comparisons between doxorubicin and platinum versus paclitaxel with platinum are currently available. A randomized phase 2 study was presented in abstract form evaluating doxorubicin with cisplatin versus paclitaxel with carboplatin in 70 patients with advanced or recurrent endometrial cancer showing a response rate of 27.9% versus 35.3%, respectively, but a phase 3 study would be required to comment on a progression-free or overall survival advantage (550). GOG 209 is currently accruing patients and comparing doxorubicin, cisplatin, and paclitaxel with cisplatin and paclitaxel and will provide an important comparison of efficacy and toxicity between these two regimens.

The results of combining chemotherapy with progestin therapy are presented in Table 23.18 (551–557). Complete and partial remission rates have ranged from 17% to 86%, although none is convincingly different than for chemotherapy alone. There are no data to suggest that endocrine therapy in conjunction with chemotherapy is superior to chemotherapy or endocrine therapy alone. Many of these trials have included small numbers of patients, and median survival rates have generally been less than 1 year. In most combined progestin-chemotherapy regimens, most patients had no prior progestin treatment, although in almost all of the chemotherapy trials most patients had prior progestins before entry.

Two other randomized trials compared different chemotherapy regimens with all patients receiving megestrol acetate (Megace) (534,555). Response rates for both these regimens were similar, with median survival times of approximately 7 and 10 months, respectively. In the trial of Horton et al. (555), many patients had prior progestins, but this did not appear to affect the response to chemotherapy, and the response to prior progestin therapy was not related to treatment results. In the study by Cohen et al. (534), response rate was also not related to prior progestin therapy, age, disease-free interval, metastatic site, or tumor grade.

Investigational Agents

A variety of investigational agents have been proposed as appropriate for evaluation in patients with endometrial cancer. These agents have generally failed to demonstrate sufficient activity for further development. More recently, as in other tumor types, agents targeting specific molecular pathways are in various early stages of evaluation.

mTOR Inhibitors. The *PTEN* tumor suppressor gene has been shown to be inactivated in a variety of tumors including 36% to 83% of endometrial carcinomas (558,559). Loss of *PTEN* leads to constitutive activation of AKT, which in turn leads to up-regulation of the mammalian target of rapamycin (mTOR) (296,560). Preclinical data has shown the activity of rapamycin in various cell endometrial cancer cell lines by inhibiting cell proliferation (561). Proposed mechanisms of mTOR blockade include inhibition of S6K1 and 4E-BP1 phosphorylation and the prevention of cyclin-dependent kinase activation, which leads to an arrest of the cell cycle in the G_1 to S transition. Preclinical studies have suggested that the degree of S6K1 inhibition in peripheral blood mononuclear cells (PBMCs) is identical to sampled tissue levels in mice, and PBMC levels may be able to be used as a surrogate for tissue levels in humans as phase 1 trials are performed (552). Rapamycin as a parent compound has poor solubility and stability in solution and several analogues (CCI-799 or tensirolimus, RAD-001 or everolimus, and AP-23573 or ARIAD) have been produced and are being evaluated in a variety of tumor types including endometrial carcinoma (562).

c-Kit, Abl, and Platelet-Derived Growth Factor Inhibitors. An immunohistochemical study of 63 patients showed positive staining for Abl, c-Kit, and platelet-derived growth factor receptor (PDGFR) in 85%, 0%, and 91% of the 33 primary endometrioid cancers; 92%, 25%, and 100% of the recurrent endometrioid cancers; and 73%, 0%, and 73% of the primary uterine papillary serous carcinomas (563). As data

TABLE 23.18

COMBINATION CHEMOTHERAPY AND PROGESTIN THERAPY

Reference	Drug	Dose (mg/m²)	Schedule[a]	Chemotherapy	n	CR + PR (%)
556	CYC	300	q 4 wk	No	15	54 (60)
	DOX	30				
	CIS	50				
	MEG	120	Daily			
554	CYC	250–500	q 3 wk	No	15	41 (33)
	DOX	30				
	CIS	50				
	MEG	80–160	Daily			
370	CYC	500	q 4 wk	No	15	8 (53)
	DOX	50				
	CIS	50				
	MPA	300	Daily			
553	CYC	400	q 3 wk	No	29	85 (45)
	FU	400				
	MEG	160	Daily			
531	CYC	400	d1,8 q 4 wk	No	7	06 (86)
	DOX	30				
	FU	400				
	MPA	400 (IM)	TIW			
RANDOMIZED TRIALS—CHEMOTHERAPY PLUS ENDOCRINE THERAPY						
555	CYC	400	q 4 wk	No	56	411 (27)
	DOX	40				
	MEG	80	tid			
	vs.					
	CYC	250	q 4 wk		58	36 (16)
	DOX	30				
	FU	300	(d1-3)			
	MEG	80	tid			
534	L-PAM	7	4d q 4 wk	No	77	1217 (38)
	FU	525[b]				
	MEG	180	q day 8 wk			
	vs.					
	CYC	400	q 3 wk		78	1615 (36)
	DOX	40				
	FU	400				
	MEG	180	q day 8 wk			

Note: alt q 3 wk, MPA and TAM alternate q 3 wk; CR, complete response; CIS, cisplatin; CYC, cyclophosphamide; DOX, doxorubicin; FU, fluorouracil; IM, intramuscular; L-PAM, melphalan; MEG, megestrol acetate; MPA, medroxyprogesterone acetate; PR, partial response; TIW, three times weekly.

[a]For chemotherapy and progestin therapy, the progestin schedule is listed separately at the bottom of the column.

[b]Total dose.

regarding imatinib has emerged, it is clear that the presence of targets as demonstrated by immunohistochemistry is not a surrogate for activity. Trials with uterine papillary serous carcinoma have been proposed, but enthusiasm has diminished for this agent given the negative data in serous ovarian carcinoma (564).

Epidermal Growth Factor–Targeted Agents. Epidermal growth factor (EGF) is expressed in normal epithelium and is overexpressed in 60% to 80% of endometrial carcinomas. It has been associated with advanced stage and poor outcome (565). Multiple downstream targets of the EGF pathway have been identified. Furthermore, the relationship between loss of function mutations for key tumor suppressors and resistance to EGF inhibitors is being explored (566). Preclinical models have shown differences in responses to EGF inhibitors between type I (Ishiwaka H) and II (Hec50co) endometrial cancer models. While gefitinib blocked the autophosphorylation of epidermal growth factor receptor (EGFR) in both models with demonstrable downstream effector consequences, continued growth of type II tumors suggested constitutive activation of other signaling pathways. This supports the hypothesis that for optimal clinical effectiveness, multiple pathway interruptions may be required (565,566). Single-agent studies have shown limited clinical activity, and trials evaluating combination treatment with EGF inhibitors and chemotherapy are ongoing.

HER2/neu-Targeted Agents. HER2/neu gene overexpression and amplification have been shown in the subset of uterine cancers with serous histology (342,567,568). An oligonucleotide microarray study with the objective of detecting differences in genes between uterine papillary serous carcinomas and ovarian serous carcinomas showed that HER2/neu is the most strikingly overexpressed gene in tumors of uterine origin when the two are compared (569). *In vitro* uterine papillary serous carcinoma cell lines resistant to natural killer cells were found to be sensitive to trastuzumab-mediated antibody-dependent cytotoxicity (570). Clinical trials evaluating trastuzumab in uterine papillary serous cancers are ongoing. It is noted that in the GOG study of trastuzumab in ovarian serous cancers, the frequency of HER2/neu overexpression was low, and the objective response rate was only 7.3% with a median PFS of 2 months, showing limited clinical value in serous tumors of ovarian origin (571).

Vascular Endothelial Growth Factor–Targeted Agents. The importance of vascular endothelial growth factor (VEGF) and angiogenesis in tumorigenesis is underscored by its overexpression in the majority of solid tumors as well as in lymphomas and hematologic malignancies (572). The prognostic and therapeutic implications of VEGF expression have been clearly shown in patients with ovarian cancer and particularly in those with malignant ascites, but the data in endometrial cancer have been less straightforward (573–575). Increased tumor VEGF levels in patients with endometrial cancer have been associated with higher-grade tumors, deep myometrial invasion, nodal metastasis, and more advanced-stage disease in some series (576,577). However, another study reported a lack of association between VEGF and its receptor expression and overall survival in 115 patients with endometrioid histology (578). A recent phase 2 trial of thalidomide in 27 patients with chemotherapy refractory endometrial cancer showed partial and stable disease responses of 12.5% and 8.3%, respectively, with a progression-free and overall survival of 1.7 months and 6.3 months (579). Thalidomide did not decrease VEGF or basic fibroblast growth factor (bFGF) levels in these patients, and elevated levels were associated with increased risk of progression or death in this study. Clinical trials with more potent inhibitors of angiogenesis such as bevacizumab are currently ongoing.

MANAGEMENT OF PATIENTS WITH SEROUS AND CLEAR CELL HISTOLOGIES

Serous cancer and, to a lesser extent, clear cell cancer tend to spread in a fashion similar to ovarian cancer with a high propensity for upper abdominal relapse. Therefore, whole abdomen radiation has been extensively studied in this group of patients (459). Lim et al. (460) reported on 78 patients with stage I-IIIA papillary serous carcinoma: 58 were treated with whole abdomen radiation and 20 were not. The corresponding 5-year disease-specific survival rates were 74.9% and 41.3%, respectively ($p = 0.04$). In GOG study 94, the 3-year disease-free and overall survival for the 60 patients with stage III papillary serous or clear cell carcinomas were 40.9% and 45.0%, respectively (453). The data on whole abdomen are somewhat encouraging, but the rate of relapse is still substantial, indicating the need for effective systemic therapy.

Based on the response rates of paclitaxel and carboplatin in other tumors of serous histology, trials investigating paclitaxel and carboplatin in uterine papillary serous carcinomas have reported response rates of 60% to 70% (580,581). No randomized, prospective trials evaluating multi-modality therapy for either early- or late-stage uterine papillary serous carcinomas have been reported. The GOG protocol 184 closed in 2004. This study randomized women with optimally stage III or IV endometrial carcinoma (including uterine papillary serous carcinoma [UPSC]) to doxorubicin and cisplatin chemotherapy versus doxorubicin, cisplatin, and paclitaxel chemotherapy following volume-directed radiation therapy. The data is not yet mature, and at recent follow-up only approximately 13% of patients in either arm had serous histology, so definitive conclusions regarding the best treatment for UPSC will not likely be possible from this study. A single-institution phase 2 trial for advanced-stage uterine papillary serous histology administered paclitaxel and platinum-based chemotherapy for three cycles followed by volume-directed radiation therapy. Patients then received an additional three cycles of chemotherapy. The most common toxicity was hematologic and occurred during chemotherapy following radiation therapy. The PFS for the nine women treated is 46.4 months (582). A similar study administered four cycles of platinum with paclitaxel or epirubicin followed by whole pelvic and vaginal brachytherapy. The 5-year overall survival for this group was 58.9% (583).

With regard to stage I disease, the available data for designing a treatment plan is retrospective. A study of 74 stage I patients with UPSC between 1987 and 2004 who underwent complete staging at Yale University was reported (461). Patients were divided into those who had no residual cancer in the hysterectomy specimen versus those who did. Stage IA patients who had residual in the hysterectomy specimen and who were treated with platinum-based chemotherapy had no recurrences ($n = 7$) versus 6 of 14 (43%) who did not receive treatment. Of 15 patients with stage IB disease, there were no recurrences in the treated group but 10 of 13 nontreated patients (77%) recurred. Platinum-based chemotherapy was associated with improved progression-free ($p < 0.01$) and overall survival ($p < 0.05$). Furthermore, no patient who received radiation to the vaginal cuff recurred at the cuff versus 6 of 31 (19%) of those who did not receive vaginal cuff irradiation (461). Recognizing the limits of retrospective studies, these data support the potential benefit of a regimen of platinum-based chemotherapy with cuff irradiation in patients with UPSC. Randomized, prospective data is needed to accurately define the best approach in these patients.

FUTURE DIRECTIONS

In 2001, the National Cancer Institute convened an expert panel to develop a national 5-year plan for research priorities in gynecologic cancers. The resulting report, Priorities of the Gynecologic Cancer Progress Review Group (PRG), specified that understanding tumor biology was the central key toward controlling gynecologic cancers (6). For endometrial cancer, one of the top research priorities defined by the PRG was to identify prognostic and predictive markers for treatment efficacy and toxicity. One of the key research issues in endometrial cancer relates to developing a more comprehensive and detailed understanding of cancers at a genetic and molecular level. By understanding these factors, a more rational development of targeted agents is hoped. One such large research effort involves a 3,500 patient trial conducted by the GOG, including patients with endometrial cancer who are to undergo hysterectomy with pelvic and para-aortic lymphadenectomy. Blood, urine, and cancer tissue at the time of initial surgery and at the time of recurrence are being collected to create a large tumor bank for translational research. The primary goals are to determine what biologic, molecular, and genetic changes are responsible for metastasis, and to develop biomarkers that predict response and prognosis. Epidemiologic information is also being collected and will be linked to molecular/genetic information and clinical outcome. Through this unprecedented study, researchers hope to foster new understanding of this cancer that will lead to promising avenues for treatment and prevention.

SUMMARY

Endometrial cancer is the most common gynecologic malignancy, and an understanding of presentation, surgical management, and treatment options is required for gynecologic oncologists. Surgical therapy is a mainstay of endometrial cancer with lymphadenectomy and laparoscopy increasingly integrated. A thorough knowledge of the relationships between uterine factors and extrauterine disease spread is essential (60). Surgical staging defines extent of disease and largely defines risk of recurrence. Pelvic radiation is associated with better local control, but no improvement in survival for patients with stage I-II endometrial cancer in randomized trials (143,149,184).

Chemotherapy is increasingly integrated into up-front management of advanced-stage endometrial cancer, and may have a role in early-stage disease (8,416). Combination therapy with radiation and chemotherapy is under evaluation. Targeted agents hold promise; however, a better understanding of molecular and genetic changes is required to improve efficacy.

References

1. Jemal A, Siegel R, Ward E, et al. Cancer statistics, 2007. *CA Cancer J* 2007;57:43–66.
2. Gallup DG, Stock RJ. Adenocarcinoma of the endometrium in women 40 years of age or younger. *Obstet Gynecol* 1984;64:417–420.
3. Norris HJ, Tavassoli FA, Kurman RJ. Endometrial hyperplasia and carcinoma, diagnostic consideration. *Am J Surg Pathol* 1988;7:839–847.
4. Trimble EL, Harlan LC, Clegg L, et al. Pre-operative imaging, surgery, and adjuvant therapy for women diagnosed with cancer of the corpus uteri in community practice in the US. *Gynecol Oncol* 2005;96:741–748.
5. Creasman W, Odicino F, Maisonneuve P, et al. Carcinoma of the corpus uteri. *Int J Gynecol Obstet* 2006;95(Suppl 1):S105–S143.
6. National Cancer Institute. Priorities of the Gynecologic Cancer Progress Review Group. http://planning.cancer.gov.pdfprgreports/gynreport.pdf. November 2001.
7. Naumann RW, Coleman R. The use of adjuvant radiation therapy in early endometrial cancer by members of the Society of Gynecologic Oncologists in 2005. *Gynecol Oncol* 2007;105:7–12.
8. Randall M, Filiaci V, Muss H, et al. Randomized phase III trial of whole abdominal radiation therapy versus doxorubicin and cisplatin chemotherapy in advanced endometrial carcinoma: a Gynecologic Oncology Group study. *J Clin Oncol* 2006;24:36–44.
9. Singh M, Zaino R, Filiaci V, et al. Relationship of estrogen and progesterone receptors to clinical outcome in metastatic endometrial carcinoma: a Gynecologic Oncology Group study. *Gynecol Oncol* 2007;106(2):325–333.
10. Salverson HB, Akslen LA. Molecular pathogenesis and prognostic factors in endometrial cancer. *APMIS* 2002;110:673–689.
11. Shiozawa T, Konishi I. Early endometrial carcinoma: clinicopathology, hormonal aspects, molecular genetics, diagnosis, and treatment. *Int J Clin Oncol* 2006;11:13–21.
12. Plentl AA, Friedman EA. *Lymphatic System of the Female Genitalia: The Morphologic Basis of Oncologic Diagnosis and Therapy.* Philadelphia: WB Saunders; 1971:116.
13. Ries LAG, Eisner CL, Kosary, et al., eds. *SEER Cancer Statistics Review, 1973–1997.* National Cancer Institute. NIH Pub #00-27 89. Bethesda, MD: NIH; 2000:171–181.
14. Parkin DM, Whelan SL, Ferlay J, et al., eds. *Cancer Incidence in Five Continents.* Vol. VII. IARC Sci. Pub. No. 143. Lyon: IARC; 1997.
15. Yap S, Matthews R. Racial and ethnic disparities in cancer of the uterine corpus. *J Nat Med Assoc* 2006;98:1930–1933.
16. Maxwell GL, Tian C, Risinger J, et al. Racial disparity in survival among patients with advanced/recurrent endometrial adenocarcinoma: a Gynecologic Oncology Group study. *Cancer* 2006;107:2197–2205.
17. McMeekin DS, Filiaci V, Thigpen JT, et al. Importance of histology in advanced and recurrent endometrial cancer patients participating in first-line chemotherapy trials: a Gynecologic Oncology Group study. *Gynecol Oncol* 2007;106:16–22.
18. Ferguson S, Olshen A, Levine D, et al. Molecular profiling of endometrial cancers from African American and Caucasian women. *Gynecol Oncol* 2006;101:209–213.
19. Watson P, Lynch H. Extracolonic cancer in hereditary nonpolyposis colorectal cancer. *Cancer* 1993;71:677–685.
20. Lu K, Dinh M, Kohlman W, et al. Gynecologic cancer as a "sentinel cancer" for women with hereditary nonpolyposis colorectal cancer syndrome. *Obstet Gynecol* 2005;105:569–574.
21. Berends M, Wu Y, Sijmons R, et al. Toward new strategies to select young endometrial cancer patients for mismatch repair gene mutation analysis. *J Clin Oncol* 2003;23:4364–4370.
22. Schmeler K, Lynch H, Chen L, et al. Prophylactic surgery to reduce the risk of gynecologic cancers in the Lynch syndrome. *N Engl J Med* 2006; 354:261–269.
23. Hornreich G, Beller U, Lavie O, et al. Is uterine serous papillary carcinoma a *BRCA1*-related disease? Case report and review of the literature. *Gynecol Oncol* 1999;75:300–304.
24. Levine D, Lin O, Barakat R, et al. Risk of endometrial cancer associated with BRCA mutation. *Gynecol Oncol* 2001;80:395–398.
25. Beiner M, Fich A, Rosen B, et al. The risk of endometrial cancer in women with *BRCA1* and *BRCA2* mutations. A prospective study. *Gynecol Oncol* 2007;104:7–10.
26. Bokhman JV. Two pathologenic types of endometrial carcinoma. *Gynecol Oncol* 1983;10:237–246.
27. Kovalev S, Marchenko ND, Gugliotta BG, et al. Loss of p53 function in uterine papillary serous carcinoma. *Hum Pathol* 1998;29:613–619.
28. Cao QJ, Belbin T, Socci N, et al. Distinctive gene expression profiles by cDNA microarrays in endometrioid and serous carcinomas of the endometrium. *Int J Gynecol Pathol* 2004;23:321–329.
29. Akhmedkhanov A, Zeleniuch-Jaquotte A, Toniolo P. Role of exogenous and endogenous hormones in endometrial cancer. *Ann NY Acad Sci* 2001; 943:296–315.
30. Key TJA, Pike MC. The dose effect relationship between unopposed estrogens and endometrial mitotic rate: its central role in explaining and predicting endometrial cancer risk. *Br J Cancer* 1998;57:205–212.
31. Henderson BE, Feigelson HS. Hormonal carcinogenesis. *Carcinogenesis* 2000;21:427–433.
32. McDonald TW, Malkasian GD, Gaffey TA. Endometrial cancer associated with feminizing ovarian tumor and polycystic ovarian disease. *Obstet Gynecol* 1977;49:654–658.
33. Smith DC, Prentice R, Thompson DJ, et al. Association of exogenous estrogen and endometrial carcinoma. *N Engl J Med* 1975;293:1164–1167.
34. Ziel HK, Finkle WD. Increased risk of endometrial carcinoma among users of conjugated estrogens. *N Engl J Med* 1975;293:1167–1170.
35. Grady D, Gebretsadik DT, Kerlikowske K, et al. Hormone replacement therapy and endometrial cancer risk: a meta-analysis. *Obstet Gynecol* 1995;85:304–313.
36. Schottenfeld D. Epidemology of endometrial neoplasia. *J Cell Biochem Suppl* 1995;23:151–159.
37. MacDonald PC, Edman CD, Hemsell DL, et al. Effect of obesity on conversion of plasma androstenedione to estrone in postmenopausal women with and without endometrial cancer. *Am J Obstet Gynecol* 1978;130: 448–455.
38. Judd HL, Lucas WE, Yen SS. Serum 17 beta-estradiol and estrone levels in postmenopausal women with and without endometrial cancer. *J Clin Endocrinol Metab* 1976;43:272–278.
39. Grodin, JM, Siiteri PK, MacDonald PC. Source of estrogen production in postmenopausal women. *J Clin Endocrinol Metab* 1973;36:207–214.
40. Weiss J, Saltzman B, Doherty J, et al. Risk factors for the incidence of endometrial cancer according to the aggressiveness of disease. *Am J Epidemiol* 2006;164:56–62.
41. Elwood JM, Cole P, Rothman KJ, et al. Epidemiology of endometrial cancer. *J Natl Cancer Inst* 1977;59:1055–1060.
42. O'Mara BA, Byers T, Schoenfeld E. Diabetes mellitus and cancer risk: a multisite case-control study. *J Chronic Dis* 1985;38:435–441.
43. Parazzini F, La Vecchia C, Negri E, et al. Diabetes and endometrial cancer: an Italian case-control study. *Int J Cancer* 1999;81:539–542.
44. Kazer RR. Insulin resistance, insulin-like growth factor I and breast cancer: a hypothesis. *Int J Cancer* 1995;62:403–406.
45. Rutanen EM. Insulin-like growth factors in endometrial function. *Gynecol Endocrinol* 1998;12:399–406.
46. Nagamani M, Stuart CA. Specific binding and growth-promoting activity of insulin in endometrial cancer cells in culture. *Am J Obstet Gynecol* 1998;179:6–12.
47. Killackey MA, Hakes TB, Pierce VK. Endometrial adenocarcinoma in breast cancer patients receiving antiestrogens. *Cancer Treat Rep* 1985;69:237–238.
48. Fornander T, Cedermark B, Mattsson A, et al. Adjuvant tamoxifen in early breast cancer: occurrence of new primary cancers. *Lancet* 1989;21: 117–120.
49. Fisher B, Costantino JP, Redmond CK, et al. Endometrial cancer in tamoxifen-treated breast cancer patients: findings from the National Surgical Adjuvant Breast and Bowel Project (NSABP) B-14. *J Natl Cancer Inst* 1994;86:527–537.
50. Magriples U, Naftolin F, Schwartz PE, et al. High-grade endometrial carcinoma in tamoxifen-treated breast cancer patients. *J Clin Oncol* 1993; 11:485–490.
51. Barakat RR, Wong G, Curtin JP, et al. Tamoxifen use in breast cancer patients who subsequently develop corpus cancer is not associated with a higher incidence of adverse histologic features. *Gynecol Oncol* 1994; 55:164–168.
52. van Leeuwen FE, Benraadt J, Coebergh JW, et al. Risk of endometrial cancer after tamoxifen treatment of breast cancer. *Lancet* 1994;343:448–452.
53. Fornander T, Hellstrom A-C, Moberger B. Descriptive clinicopathologic study of 17 patients with endometrial cancer during or after adjuvant tamoxifen in early breast cancer. *J Natl Cancer Inst* 1993;85:1850–1855.
54. Perez E. Appraising adjuvant aromatase inhibitor therapy. *Oncologist* 2006;11:1058–1069.

55. Breast International Group 1-98 Collaborative Group. A comparison of letrozole and tamoxifen in postmenopausal women with early breast cancer. *N Engl J Med* 2005;353:2747–2757.
56. Kaufmann M, Jonat W, Hilfrich J, et al. Improved overall survival in postmenopausal women with early breast cancer after anastrozole initiated after 2 years of treatment with tamoxifen compared with continued tamoxifen: the ARNO 95 study. *J Clin Oncol* 2007;25:2664–2670.
57. The Writing Group for the PEPI Trial. Effects of hormone replacement therapy on endometrial histology in postmenopausal women: the postmenopausal estrogen/progestin interventions trial. *JAMA* 1996;275: 370–375.
58. Maxwell GL, Schildkraut J, Calingaert B, et al. Progestin and estrogen potency of combination oral contraceptives and endometrial cancer risk. *Gynecol Oncol* 2006;103:535–540.
59. Stanford JL, Brinton LA, Berman ML, et al. Oral contraceptives and endometrial cancer: do other risk factors modify the association. *Int J Cancer* 1993;54:243–248.
60. Creasman WT, Morrow CP, Bundy BN, et al. Surgical pathologic spread patterns of endometrial cancer: a Gynecologic Oncology Group study. *Cancer* 1987;60:2035–2041.
61. Mariani A, Dowdy S, Keeney G, et al. High-risk endometrial cancer subgroups: candidates for target based adjuvant therapy. *Gynecol Oncol* 2004;95:120–126.
62. Morrow CP, Bundy BN, Kumar RJ, et al. Relationship between surgical-pathological risk factors and outcome in clinical stages I and II carcinoma of the endometrium. A Gynecologic Oncology Group study. *Gynecol Oncol* 1991;40:55.
63. Rabban JT, Zaloudek CJ. Minimal uterine serous carcinoma: current concepts in diagnosis and prognosis. *Pathology* 2007;39:125–133.
64. Wheeler DT, Bell KA, Kurman RJ, et al. Minimal uterine serous carcinoma: diagnosis and clinicopathologic correlation. *Am J Surg Pathol* 2000;24:797–806.
65. Nakagawa-Okamura C, Sato S, Tsuji I, et al. Effectiveness of mass screening for endometrial cancer. *Acta Cytol* 2002;46:277–283.
66. Vuento MH, Maatela JI, Tyrkko JE, et al. A longitudinal study of screening for endometrial cancer by endometrial biopsy in diabetic females. *Int J Gynecol Cancer* 1995;5:390–395.
67. ACOG Committee Opinion. Routine cancer screening. *Obstet Gynecol* 2006;108:1611–1613.
68. Society of Gynecologic Oncologists. Practice guidelines: uterine corpus-endometrial cancer. *Oncology* 1998;12:122–126.
69. Gambrell RD Jr, Massey FM, Castenada TA, et al. Use of the progesterone challenge test to reduce the risk of endometrial cancer. *Obstet Gynecol* 1980;55:732–738.
70. Gorodeski IG, Geier A, Lunenfeld B, et al. Progesterone challenge test in postmenopausal women with pathological endometrium. *Cancer Invest* 1988;6:481–485.
71. Hunter JE, Tritz DE, Howell MG, et al. The prognostic and therapeutic implications of cytologic atypia in patients with endometrial hyperplasia. *Gynecol Oncol* 1994;55:66–71.
72. Kurman R, Kaminski P, Norris H. The behavior of endometrial hyperplasia. A long-term study of "untreated" hyperplasia in 170 patients. *Cancer* 1985;56:403–411.
73. Trimble CL, Kauderer J, Zaino R, et al. Concurrent endometrial carcinoma in women with a biopsy diagnosis of atypical endometrial hyperplasia: a Gynecologic Oncology Group study. *Cancer* 2006;106:812–819.
74. King A, Seraj IM, Wagner RJ. Stromal invasion in endometrial adenocarcinoma. *Am J Obstet Gynecol* 1984;149:10–14.
75. Tavassoli F, Kraus FT. Endometrial lesions in uteri resected for atypical endometrial hyperplasia. *Am J Clin Pathol* 1978;70:770.
76. Randal TC, Kurman RJ. Progestin treatment of atypical hyperplasia and well-differentiated carcinoma of the endometrium under age 40. *Obstet Gynecol* 1997;90:434–440.
77. Ushijima K, Yahata H, Yoshikawa H, et al. Multicenter phase II study of fertility-sparing treatment with medroxyprogesterone acetate for endometrial carcinoma and atypical hyperplasia in young women. *J Clin Oncol* 2007;25:2798–2803.
78. Leitao M, Chi D. Fertility sparing options for patients with gynecologic malignancies. *Oncologist* 2005;10:613–622.
79. Runowicz CD. Gynecologic surveillance of women on tamoxifen: first do no harm. *J Clin Oncol* 2000;18:3457–3458.
80. ACOG Committee Opinion. Tamoxifen and uterine cancer. *Obstet Gynecol* 2006;107:1475–1478.
81. Gredmark T, Kvint S, Harvel G, et al. Histopathologic findings in women with post-menopausal bleeding. *Br J Obstet Gynaecol* 1995;102: 133–136.
82. Feldman S, Cook F, Harlow B, et al. Predicting endometrial cancer among women who present with abnormal vaginal bleeding. *Gynecol Oncol* 1995;56:376–381.
83. Clark TJ, Mann CH, Shah N, et al. Accuracy of outpatient endometrial biopsy in the diagnosis of endometrial cancer: a systematic quantitative review. *Br J Obstet Gynaecol* 2002;109:313–321.
84. Dijkhuizen FP, Mol B, Brolmann H, et al. The accuracy of endometrial sampling in the diagnosis of patients with endometrial carcinoma and hyperplasia: a meta-analysis. *Cancer* 2000;89:1765–1772.
85. Iossa A, Cianferoni L, Ciatto S, et al. Hysteroscopy and endometrial cancer diagnosis: a review of 2007 consecutive examinations in self-referred patients. *Tumori* 1991;77:479–483.
86. Ben-Yehuda O, Kim Y, Leuchter R. Does hysteroscopy improve upon the sensitivity of dilatation and curettage in the diagnosis of endometrial hyperplasia or carcinoma? *Gynecol Oncol* 1998;68:4–7.
87. Clark TJ, Voit D, Gupta J, et al. Accuracy of hysteroscopy in the diagnosis of endometrial cancer and hyperplasia. A systematic quantitative review. *JAMA* 2002;288:1610–1621.
88. Bradley WH, Boente MP, Brooker D, et al. Hysteroscopy and cytology in endometrial cancer. *Obstet Gynecol* 2004;104:1030–1033.
89. Revel A, Tsafrir A, Anteby SO, et al. Does hysteroscopy produce intraperitoneal spread of endometrial cancer cells? *Obstet Gynecol Surv* 2004;59: 280–284.
90. Tabor A, Watt H, Wald N. Endometrial thickness as a test for endometrial cancer in women with post-menopausal vaginal bleeding. *Obstet Gynecol* 2002;99:663–670.
91. Smith-Bindman R, Kerlikowske K, Feldstein K, et al. Endovaginal ultrasound to exclude endometrial cancer and other endometrial abnormalities. *JAMA* 1998;280:1510–1517.
92. Conoscenti G, Mier YJ, Fischer-Tamaro L, et al. Endometrial assessment by transvaginal sonography and histological findings after D&C in women with post-menopausal bleeding. *Ultrasound Obstet Gynecol* 1995;6:108–115.
93. Tongsong T, Pongnarisorn C, Mahanuphap P. Use of vaginosongraphic measurements of endometrial thickness in the identification of abnormal endometrium in pari- and post-menopausal bleeding. *J Clin Ultrasound* 1994;22:479–482.
94. Goldstein R, Bree R, Benson C, et al. Evaluation of the woman with postmenopausal bleeding. Society of Radiologists in Ultrasound—consensus conference statement. *J Ultrasound Med* 2001;20:1025–1036.
95. deKroon CD, deBrock GH, Dieben SW, et al. Saline contrast hysterosonography in abnormal uterine bleeding: a systematic review and meta-analysis. *Br J Obstet Gynaecol* 2003;110:938–947.
96. Marziale P, Atlante G, Pozzi M, et al. 426 cases of stage I endometrial carcinoma: a clinicopathological analysis. *Gynecol Oncol* 1989;32:278.
97. Ozalp S, Yalcin OT, Polay S, et al. Diagnostic efficacy of the preoperative lymphoscintigraphy, Ga-67 scintigraphy, and computed tomography for the detection of lymph node metastasis in cases of ovarian or endometrial cancer. *Acta Obstet Gynaecol Scand* 1999;78:155–159.
98. Zerbe M, Bristow R, Grumbine F, et al. Inability of preoperative computed tomography scans to accurately predict the extent of myometrial invasion and extracorporal spread in endometrial cancer. *Gynecol Oncol* 2000;78:67–70.
99. Gordon AN, Fleischer AC, Dudley BS, et al. Preoperative assessment of myometrial invasion of endometrial adenocarcinoma by sonography (US) and magnetic resonance imaging (MRI). *Gynecol Oncol* 1989;34: 175–179.
100. Yazigi R, Cohen J, Munoz AK, et al. Magnetic resonance imaging determination of myometrial invasion in endometrial carcinoma. *Gynecol Oncol* 1989;34:94–97.
101. Messiou C, Spencer JA, Swift SE. MR staging of endometrial cancer. *Clin Radiol* 2006;61:822–832.
102. Hardesty LA, Sumkin JH, Hakim C, et al. The ability of helical CT to preoperatively stage endometrial carcinoma. *Am J Roentgenol* 2001;176: 603–606.
103. Chung HH, Kang SB, Cho JY, et al. Accuracy of MR imaging for the prediction of myometrial invasion of endometrial cancer. *Gynecol Oncol* 2007;104:654–659.
104. Rockall AG, Meroni R, Sohaib SA, et al. Evaluation of endometrial carcinoma on magnetic resonance imagining. *Int J Gynecol Cancer*, 2007:17: 188–196.
105. Olt G, Berchuck A, Bast RC Jr. The role of tumor markers in gynecologic oncology. *Obstet Gynecol Surv* 1990;45:570–577.
106. Niloff JM, Klug TL, Schaetzl E, et al. Elevation of serum CA 125 in carcinomas of the fallopian tube, endometrium, and endocervix. *Am J Obstet Gynecol* 1984;148:1057.
107. Patsner B, Mann WJ, Cohen H, et al. Predictive value of preoperative serum CA 125 levels in clinically localized and advanced endometrial carcinoma. *Am J Obstet Gynecol* 1988;158:399–402.
108. Hsieh CH, Chang Chien CC, Lin H, et al. Can a preoperative CA 125 level be a criterion for full pelvic lymphadenectomy in surgical staging of endometrial cancer? *Gynecol Oncol* 2002;86:28–33.
109. Dotters DJ. Preoperative CA125 in endometrial cancer: is it useful? *Am J Obstet Gynecol* 2000;182:1328–1334.
110. Duk JM, Aalders JG, Fleuren GJ, et al. CA125: a useful marker in endometrial carcinoma. *Am J Obstet Gynecol* 1986;155:1097–1102.
111. Koper NP, Massuger LF, Thomas CM, et al. Serum CA 125 measurements to identify patients with endometrial cancer who require lymphadenectomy. *Anticancer Res* 1998;18:1897–1902.
112. Sood AK, Buller RE, Burger RA, et al. Value of preoperative CA125 level in the management of uterine cancer and prediction of clinical outcome. *Obstet Gynecol* 1997;90:441–447.
113. Soper JT, Berchuk A, Olt GJ, et al. Preoperative evaluation of serum CA125, TAG 72 and CA 15–3 in patients with endometrial carcinoma. *Am J Obstet Gynecol* 1990;163:1204–1209.
114. Rose PG, Sommers RM, Reale FR, et al. Serial serum CA-125 measurements for evaluation of recurrence in patients with endometrial carcinoma. *Obstet Gynecol* 1994;84:12–16.
115. Heyman J. The so-called Stockholm Method and the results of treatment of uterine cancer at the Radiumhemmet. *Acta Radiol* 1935;16:129.

116. Arneson AN, Stanbro WW, Nolan JF. The use of multiple sources of radium within the uterus in the treatment of endometrial cancer. *Am J Obstet Gynecol* 1948;55:64–78.
117. Asbury RF, Blessing JA, McGuire WP, et al. Aminothiadiazole (NSC 4728) in patients with advanced carcinoma of the endometrium. A phase II study of the Gynecologic Oncology Group. *Am J Clin Oncol* 1990;13:39–41.
118. Nolan J, Arneson A. An instrument for inserting multiple capsules of radium within the uterus in the treatment of corpus cancers. *Am J Roentgenol* 1943;49:504.
119. Lewis GC Jr, Slack NH, Mortel R, et al. Adjuvant progestogen therapy in the primary definitive treatment of endometrial cancer. *Gynecol Oncol* 1974;2:368–376.
120. Dobbie BMW, Taylor C, Waterhouse J. Study of carcinoma of the endometrium. *J Obstet Gynaecol Br Commonw* 1973;114:106–109.
121. Gray LA. Lymph node excision in treatment of gynecologic malignancies. *Am J Surg* 1964;108660–108663.
122. Lewis GC, Bundy B. Surgery for endometrial cancer. *Cancer* 1981;48: 568–574.
123. Barakat RR, Lev G, Hummer A, et al. Twelve-year experience in the management of endometrial cancer: a change in surgical and postoperative radiation approaches. *Gynecol Oncol* 2007;105:150–156.
124. Morrow CP. Curtin JP. *Surgery for Ovarian Neoplasia in Gynecologic Cancer Surgery.* New York: Churchill Livingstone Inc.; 1996:627–716.
125. Morrow CP. Curtin JP. *Surgery for Cervical Neoplasia in Gynecologic Cancer Surgery*. New York: Churchill Livingstone Inc.; 1996:451–568.
126. Ehrlich CE, Toung P, Stehman F, et al. Steroid receptors and clinical outcome in patients with adenocarcinoma of the endometrium. *Am J Obstet Gynecol* 1988;158:796–807.
127. Jadoul P, Donnez J. Conservative treatment may be beneficial for young women with atypical endometrial hyperplasia or endometrial adenocarcinoma. *Fert Steril* 2003;80:1315–1324.
128. International Federation of Gynecology and Obstetrics: classification and staging of malignant tumors in the female pelvis. *Int J Gynaecol Obstet* 1971;9:172.
129. Tillmanns T, Kamelle S, Abudayyeh I, et al. Panniculectomy with simultaneous gynecologic oncology surgery. *Gynecol Oncol* 2001;83:518–522.
130. Wright J, Powell M, Herzog T, et al. Panniculectomy: improving lymph node yield in morbidly obese patients with endometrial neoplasms. *Gynecol Oncol* 2004;94:436–441.
131. Ramirez P, Frumovitz M, Bodurka D, et al. Hormonal therapy for the management of grade 1 endometrial adenocarcinoma: a literature review. *Gynecol Oncol* 2004;95:133–138.
132. Soliman PT, Oh J, Schmeler K, et al. Risk factors for young premenopausal women with endometrial cancer. *Obstet Gynecol* 2005;105:575–580.
133. Candiani GB, Belloni C, Maggi R, et al. Evaluation of different surgical approach in the treatment of endometrial cancer at FIGO stage I. *Gynecol Oncol* 1990;37:6–8.
134. Massi G, Savino L, Susini T. Vaginal hysterectomy versus abdominal hysterectomy for treatment of stage I endometrial adenocarcinoma. *Am J Obstet Gynecol* 1996;174:1320–1326.
135. Scarselli G, Savino L, Ceccherini R, et al. Role of vaginal surgery in the 1st stage endometrial cancer. Experience of the Florence School. *Eur J Gynaecol Oncol* 1992;13:15–19.
136. Bloss JD, Berman ML, Bloss LP, et al. Use of vaginal hysterectomy for the management of stage I endometrial cancer in the medically compromised patient. *Gynecol Oncol* 1991;40:74–77.
137. Pitkin RM. Vaginal hysterectomy in obese women. *Obstet Gynecol* 1977; 49:567–569.
138. Vardi JR, Tadros GH, Anselmo MT, et al. The value of exploratory laparotomy in patients with endometrial carcinoma according to the new International Federation of Gynecology and Obstetrics Staging. *Obstet Gynecol* 1992;80:204–208.
139. Orr JW, Holimon J, Orr P. Stage I corpus cancer: is teletherapy necessary. *Am J Obstet Gynecol* 1997;176:777–789.
140. Homesley HD, Kadar N, Barrett RJ, et al. Selective pelvic and periaortic lymphadenectomy does not increase morbidity in surgical staging of endometrial carcinoma. *Am J Obstet Gynecol* 1992;167:1225–1230.
141. Abu-Rustum N, Alektiar K, Iasonos A, et al. The incidence of symptomatic lower-extremity lymphedema following treatment of uterine corpus malignancies: a 12-year experience at Memorial Sloan-Kettering Cancer Center. *Gynecol Oncol* 2006;103:714–718.
142. Lewandowski G, Torrisi J, Potkul R, et al. Hysterectomy with extended surgical staging and radiotherapy versus hysterectomy alone and radiotherapy in stage I endometrial cancer: a comparison of complication rates. *Gynecol Oncol* 1990;36:401–404.
143. Keys HM, Roberts JA, Brunetto VL, et al. A phase III trial of surgery with or without adjunctive external pelvic radiation therapy in intermediate risk endometrial adenocarcinoma: a Gynecologic Oncology Group study. *Gynecol Oncol* 2004;92:744–751.
144. Goudge C, Bernhard S, Cloven N, et al. The impact of complete surgical staging on adjuvant treatment decisions in endometrial cancer. *Gynecol Oncol* 2004;93:536–539.
145. Partridge EE, Shingleton H, Menck H. The National Cancer Data Base report on endometrial cancer. *J Surg Oncol* 1996;61:111–123.
146. MacDonald OK, Sause W, Lee J, et al. Does oncologic specialization influence outcomes following surgery in early stage adenocarcinoma of the endometrium. *Gynecol Oncol* 2005;99:730–735.
147. Roland PY, Kelly FJ, Kulwicki C, et al. The benefits of a gynecologic oncologist: a pattern of care study for endometrial cancer treatment. *Gynecol Oncol* 2004;93:125–130.
148. Aalders JG, Thomas G. Endometrial cancer—revisiting the importance of pelvic and para-aortic lymph nodes. *Gynecol Oncol* 2007;104:222–231.
149. Creutzberg CL, van Putten WL, Koper PC, et al. Surgery and postoperative radiotherapy versus surgery alone for patients with stage-1 endometrial carcinoma: multicentre randomised trial. PORTEC Study Group. Post Operative Radiation Therapy in Endometrial Carcinoma. *Lancet* 2000;355:1404–1411.
150. Trimble E, Kosary C, Park R. Lymph node sampling and survival in endometrial cancer. *Gynecol Oncol* 1998;71:340–343.
151. COSA-NZ-UK Endometrial Cancer Study Groups. Pelvic lymphadenectomy in high-risk endometrial cancer. *Int J Gynecol Cancer* 1996;6:102–107.
152. Kitchener H, Redman CW, Swart AM, et al. ASTEC—a study in the treatment of endometrial cancer: a randomized trial of lymphadenectomy in the treatment of endometrial cancer. *Gynecol Oncol* 2006;101(S1): abstr. 45.
153. Creutzberg C, van Putten W, Warlam-Rodenhuis C, et al. Outcome of high-risk stage IC, grade 3 compared with stage I endometrial carcinoma patients: the postoperative radiation therapy in endometrial carcinoma trial. *J Clin Oncol* 2004;22:1234–1241.
154. Onda T, Yoshikawa H, Mizutani K, et al. Treatment of node positive endometrial cancer with complete node dissection, chemotherapy and radiation therapy. *Br J Cancer* 1997;75:1836–1841.
155. McMeekin DS, Lashbrook D, Gold M, et al. Analysis of FIGO stage IIIc endometrial cancer patients. *Gynecol Oncol* 2001;81:273–278.
156. Nelson G, Randall M, Sutton G, et al. FIGO stage IIIC endometrial carcinoma with metastases confined to pelvic lymph nodes: analysis of treatment outcomes, prognostic variables, and failure patterns following adjuvant radiation therapy. *Gynecol Oncol* 1999;75:211–214.
157. Arango HA, Hoffman Marit Scheistrøen, Roberts WS, et al. Accuracy of lymph node palpation to determine need for lymphadenectomy in gynecologic malignancies. *Obstet Gynecol* 2000;95:553–556.
158. Franchi M, Ghezzi F, Melpigano M, et al. Clinical value of intraoperative gross examination in endometrial cancer. *Gynecol Oncol* 2000;76:357–361.
159. Kim Y, Niloff J. Endometrial carcinoma: analysis of recurrence in patients treated with a strategy minimizing lymph node sampling and radiation therapy. *Obstet Gynecol* 1993;82:175–180.
160. Faught W, Krepart G, Loctocki R, et al. Should selective para-aortic lymphadenectomy be part of surgical staging for endometrial cancer. *Gynecol Oncol* 1994;55:51–55.
161. Goff B, Kato D, Schmidt R, et al. Uterine papillary serous carcinoma: patterns of metastatic spread. *Gynecol Oncol* 1994;54:264–268.
162. Podratz KC, Mariani A, Webb M. Staging and therapeutic value of lymphadenectomy in endometrial cancer. *Gynecol Oncol* 1998;70:163–164.
163. Doering DL, Barnhill DR, Weiser EB, et al. Intraoperative evaluation of depth of myometrial invasion in stage I endometrial adenocarcinoma. *Obstet Gynecol* 1989;74:930–933.
164. Goff BA, Riche LW. Assessment of depth of myometrial invasion in endometrial adenocarcinoma. *Gynecol Oncol* 1990;38:46–48.
165. Creasman WT, Zaino R, Major FL, et al. Early invasive carcinoma of the cervix (3–5 mm invasion): risk factors and prognosis: a Gynecologic Oncology Group study. *Am J Obstet Gynecol* 1998;178:62–65.
166. Leblanc E, Querleu D, Narducci F, et al. Surgical staging of early invasive epithelial ovarian tumors. *Semin Surg Oncol* 2000;19:36–41.
167. Case AS, Rocconi RP, Straughn JM, et al. A prospective blinded evaluation of the accuracy of frozen section for the surgical management of endometrial cancer. *Obstet Gynecol* 2006;108:1375–1379.
168. Frumovitz M, Slomovitz BM, Singh DK, et al. Frozen section analyses as predictors of lymphatic spread in patients with early-stage uterine cancer. *J Am Coll Surg* 2004;199:388–393.
169. Frumovitz M, Singh DK, Meyer L, et al. Predictors of final histology in patients with endometrial cancer. *Gynecol Oncol* 2004;95:463–468.
170. Cohn D, Huh D, Fowler J, et al. Cost-effectiveness analysis of strategies for the surgical management of grade 1 endometrial cancer. *Obstet Gynecol* 2007;109:1388–1395.
171. Barnes MN, Roland P, Straughn M, et al. Comparison of treatment strategies for endometrial adenocarcinoma: analysis of financial impact. *Gynecol Oncol* 1999;74:443–447.
172. Mariani A, Webb M, Galli L, et al. Potential therapeutic role of para-aortic lymphadenectomy in node positive endometrial cancer. *Gynecol Oncol* 2000;76:348–356.
173. McMeekin DS, Lashbrook D, Gold M, et al. Nodal distribution and its significance in FIGO stage III endometrial cancer. *Gynecol Oncol* 2001;82:375–379.
174. Flanigan C, Mannel R, Walker J, et al. Incidence and location of para-aortic lymph node metastases in gynecologic malignancies. *J Am Coll Surg* 1995; 181:72–74.
175. Chuang L, Burke T, Tornos C, et al. Staging laparotomy for endometrial carcinoma: assessment of retroperitoneal lymph nodes. *Gynecol Oncol* 1995;58:189–193.
176. Hirahatake K, Hareyama H, Sakuragi N, et al. A clinical and pathologic study on para-aortic lymph node metastasis in endometrial carcinoma. *J Surg Oncol* 1997;65:82–87.
177. Kohler C, Tozzi R, Klemm P, et al. Laparoscopic para-aortic left-sided transperitoneal infrarenal lymphadenectomy in patients with gynecologic malignancies: techniques and results. *Gynecol Oncol* 2003;91:139–148.

178. Kilgore L, Partidge E, Alvarez R, et al. Adenocarcinoma of the endometrium: survival comparisons of patients with and without pelvic node sampling. *Gynecol Oncol* 1995;56:29–33.
179. Girardi F, Petru E, Heydarfadai M, et al. Pelvic lymphadenectomy in the surgical treatment of endometrial cancer. *Gynecol Oncol* 1993;49: 177–180.
180. Cragan J, Havrilesky L, Calingaert B, et al. Retrospective analysis of selective lymphadenectomy in apparent early-stage endometrial cancer. *J Clin Oncol* 2005;23:3668–3675.
181. Chan J, Cheung M, Huh W, et al. Therapeutic role of lymph node resection in endometrioid corpus cancer: a study of 12,333 patients. *Cancer* 2006;107:1823–1830.
182. Mariani A, Dowdy S, Cliby W, et al. Efficacy of systematic lymphadenectomy and adjuvant radiotherapy in node-positive endometrial cancer patients. *Gynecol Oncol* 2006;101:200–208.
183. Havrilseky LJ, Cragun J, Calingaert B, et al. Resection of lymph node metastases influences survival in stage IIIC endometrial cancer. *Gynecol Oncol* 2005;99(3):689–695.
184. Orton J, Blake P. Adjuvant external beam radiotherapy (EBRT) in the treatment of endometrial cancer: results of the randomized MRC ASTEC and NCIC CTG EN.5 trial. *J Clin Oncol* 2007;25(182), abstr 5504.
185. Fanning J, Nanavati P, Hilgers R. Surgical staging and high dose rate brachytherapy for endometrial cancer: limiting external radiotherapy to node positive tumors. *Obstet Gynecol* 1996;87:1041–1044.
186. Mohan D, Samuels M, Selim M, et al. Long term outcomes of therapeutic pelvic lymphadenectomy for stage I endometrial adenocarcinoma. *Gynecol Oncol* 1998;70:165–171.
187. Childers JM, Brzechffa P, Hatch K, et al. Laparoscopically assisted surgical staging of endometrial cancer. *Gynecol Oncol* 1993;51:33–38.
188. Childers JM, Surwit EA. Combined laparoscopic and vaginal surgery for the management of two cases of stage I endometrial cancer. *Gynecol Oncol* 1992;45:46–51.
189. Boike G, Lurain J, Bruke J. A comparison of laparoscopic management of endometrial cancer with a traditional laparotomy. *Obstet Gynecol* 1994; 52:105.
190. Magrina JF, Mutone NF, Weaver AL, et al. Laparoscopic lymphadenectomy and vaginal or laparoscopic hysterectomy with bilateral salpingo-oophorectomy for endometrial cancer: morbidity and survival. *Am J Obstet Gynecol* 1999;181:376–381.
191. Homesley HD, Boike G, Spiegel G. Feasibility of laparoscopic management of presumed stage I endometrial carcinoma and assessment of accuracy of myoinvasion estimates by frozen section: a Gynecologic Oncology Group study. *Int J Gynecol Cancer* 2004;14:341–347.
192. Malur S, Possover M, Michels W, et al. Laparoscopic assisted vaginal hysterectomy versus abdominal surgery in patients with endometrial cancer—a prospective randomized trial. *Gynecol Oncol* 2001;80:239–244.
193. Eltabbakh G. Analysis of survival after laparoscopy in women with endometrial cancer. *Cancer* 2002;95:1894–1901.
194. Gemignani ML, Curtin J, Zelmanovich J, et al. Laparoscopic assisted vaginal hysterectomy for endometrial cancer: clinical outcomes and hospital charges. *Gynecol Oncol* 1999;73:5–11.
195. Spirtos NM, Schlaerth J, Gross G, et al. Cost and quality of life analyses of surgery for early endometrial cancer: laparotomy versus laparoscopy. *Am J Obstet Gynecol* 1996;174(6):1795–1799.
196. Walker J, Mannel R, Piedmonte M, et al. Phase III trial of laparoscopy versus laparotomy for surgical resection and comprehensive surgical staging of uterine cancer: a Gynecologic Oncology Group study. *Gynecol Oncol* 2006;101(S1):11–12; abstr 22.
197. Walker J, Piedmonte M, Spirtos N, et al. Surgical staging of uterine cancer: randomized phase III trial of laparoscopy versus laparotomy: a Gynecologic Oncology Group study. *J Clin Oncol* 2006;24:5010; abstr 5010.
198. Querleu D, Leblanc E, Castelain B. Laparoscopic pelvic lymphadenectomy in the staging of early carcinoma of the cervix. *Am J Obstet Gynecol* 1991;164:579–581.
199. Nezhat CR, Burrell MO, Nezhat FR, et al. Laparoscopic radical hysterectomy with para-aortic and pelvic node dissection. *Am J Obstet Gynecol* 1992;166:864–865.
200. Spirtos N, Schlaerth J, Spirtos T, et al. Laparoscopic bilateral pelvic and para-aortic lymph node sampling: an evolving technique. *Am J Obstet Gynecol* 1995;172:105–111.
201. Childers JM, Hatch KD, Tran A, et al. Laparoscopic para-aortic lymphadenectomy in gynecologic malignancies. *Obstet Gynecol* 1993;82: 741–747.
202. Scribner D, Walker J, Johnson G, et al. Laparoscopic pelvic and para-aortic lymph node dissection: analysis of first 100 cases. *Gynecol Oncol* 2001;82:498–503.
203. Massi G, Savino L, Susini T. Vaginal hysterectomy versus abdominal hysterectomy for the treatment of stage I endometrial adenocarcinoma. *Am J Obstet Gynecol* 1996;174:1320–1326.
204. Fowler JM, Carter JR, Carlson JW, et al. Lymph node yield from laparoscopic lymphadenectomy in cervical cancer: a comparative study. *Gynecol Oncol* 1993;51:187–192.
205. Eltabbakh G. Effect of surgeon's experience on the surgical outcome of laparoscopic surgery for women with endometrial cancer. *Gynecol Oncol* 2000;78:58–61.
206. Harkki-Siren P, Kurki T. A nationwide analysis of laparoscopic complications. *Obstet Gynecol* 1997;89:108–112.
207. Harkki-Siren P, Sjoberg J. Evaluation and the learning curve of the first one hundred laparoscopic hysterectomies. *Acta Obstet Gynecol Scand* 1995;74:638–641.
208. Chapron C, Dubuisson JB, Querleu D, et al. Complications of laparoscopy: a prospective multicentre observational study. *Br J Obstet Gynaecol* 1997;104:1419–1420.
209. Wang PH, Yuan CC, Lin G, et al. Risk factors contributing to early occurrence of port site metastases of laparoscopic surgery for malignancy. *Gynecol Oncol* 1999;72:38–44, 310–312.
210. Sonoda Y, Zerbe M, Smith A, et al. High incidence of positive peritoneal cytology in low-risk endometrial cancer treated by laparoscopically assisted hysterectomy. *Gynecol Oncol* 2001;80:378–382.
211. Schribner DR, Mannel RS, Walker JL, et al. Cost analysis of laparoscopy versus laparotomy for early endometrial cancer. *Gynecol Oncol* 1999;75: 460–463.
212. Scribner D, Walker J, Johnson G, et al. Surgical manangement of early stage endometrial cancer in the elderly: is laparoscopy feasible? *Gynecol Oncol* 2001;83:563–568.
213. Scribner D, Walker J, Johnson G, et al. Laparoscopic pelvic and para-aortic lymph node dissection in the obese. *Gynecol Oncol* 2002;84:426–430.
214. Eltabbakh G, Shamonki M, Moody J, et al. Hysterectomy for obese women with endometrial cancer: laparoscopy or laparotomy. *Gynecol Oncol* 2000;78:329–335.
215. O'Hanlan K, Dibble S, Fisher D. Total laparoscopic hysterectomy for uterine pathology: impact of body mass index on outcomes. *Gynecol Oncol* 2006;103:938–941.
216. Possover M, Krause N, Plaul K, et al. Laparoscopic para-aortic and pelvic lymphadenectomy: experience with 150 patients and review of literature. *Gynecol Oncol* 1998;71:19–28.
217. Scribner D, Walker J, Johnson G, et al. Laparoscopic pelvic and para-aortic lymph node dissection: analysis of the first 100 cases. *Gynecol Oncol* 2001;82:498–503.
218. Querleu D, Lebanc E, Cartron G, et al. Audit of preoperative and early complications of laparoscopic lymph node dissection in 1000 cancer patients. *Am J Obstet Gynecol* 2006;195:1287–1292.
219. Childers JM, Spirtos N, Brainard P, et al. Laparoscopic staging of the patient with incompletely staged early adenocarcinoma of the endometrium. *Obstet Gynecol* 1994;83:597–600.
220. Goff BA, Goodman A, Muntz HG, et al. Surgical stage IV endometrial carcinoma: a study of 47 cases. *Gynecol Oncol* 1994;52:237–240.
221. Chi DS, Welshinger M, Venkatraman ES, et al. The role of surgical cytoreductive surgery in stage IV endometrial carcinoma. *Gynecol Oncol* 1997; 6756–6760.
222. Bristow RE, Zerbe MJ, Rosenshein N, et al. Stage IVb endometrial carcinoma: the role of cytoreductive surgery and determinants of survival. *Gynecol Oncol* 2000;78:85–91.
223. Bristow R, Duska L, Montz F. The role of cytoreductive surgery in the management of stage IV uterine papillary serous carcinoma. *Gynecol Oncol* 2001;81:92–99.
224. Kurman R, Norris H. Evaluation of criteria for distinguishing atypical endometrial hyperplasia from well-differentiated carcinoma. *Cancer* 1982;49:2547–2559.
225. Huang S, Amparo E, Fu Y. Endometrial hyperplasia: histologic classification and behavior. *Surg Pathol* 1988;1:215–225.
226. Hunter JE, Tritz DE, Howell MG, et al. The prognostic and therapeutic implications of cytologic atypia in patients with endometrial hyperplasia. *Gynecol Oncol* 1994;55:66–71.
227. Kendall BS, Ronnett BM, Isacson C, et al. Reproducibility of the diagnosis of endometrial hyperplasia, atypical hyperplasia, and well-differentiated carcinoma. *Am J Surg Pathol* 1998;22:1012–1019.
228. Bergeron C, Nogales F, Masseroli M, et al. A multicentric European study testing the reproducibility of the WHO classification of endometrial hyperplasia with a proposal of a simplified working classification for biopsy and curettage specimens. *Am J Surg Pathol* 1999;23: 1102–1108.
229. Skov BG, Broholm H, Engel U, et al. Comparison of the reproducibility of the WHO classifications of 1975 and 1994 of endometrial hyperplasia. *Int J Gynecol Pathol* 1997;16:33–37.
230. Mutter GL, The Endometrial Collaborative Group. Endometrial intraepithelial neoplasia (EIN): will it bring order to chaos? *Gynecol Oncol* 2000;76:287–290.
231. Baak JP, Mutter GL. EIN and WHO94. *J Clin Pathol* 2005;58:1–6.
232. Baak JP, Mutter G, Robboy S, et al. The molecular genetics and morphometry-based endometrial intraepithelial neoplasia classification system predicts disease progression in endometrial hyperplasia more accurately than the 1994 World Health Organization classification system. *Cancer* 2005;103:2304–2312.
233. Mutter GL, Zaino R, Baak J, et al. Benign endometrial hyperplasia sequence and endometrial intraepithelial neoplasia. *Int J Gynecol Pathol* 2007;26:103–114.
234. Silverberg S, Kurman R. *Tumors of the Uterine Corpus and Gestational Trophoblastic Disease*. Vol 3. Washington, DC: Armed Forces Institute of Pathology; 1992.
235. Zaino RJ, Silverberg SG, Norris HJ, et al. The prognostic value of nuclear versus architectural grading in endometrial adenocarcinoma: a Gynecologic Oncology Group study. *Int J Gynecol Pathol* 1994;13: 29–36.

236. Zaino RJ, Kurman RJ, Diana KL, et al. The utility of the revised International Federation of Gynecology and Obstetrics histologic grading of endometrial adenocarcinoma using a defined nuclear grading system. *Cancer* 1995;75:81–86.
237. Taylor R, Zeller J, Lieberman R, et al. An analysis of two versus three grades for endometrial carcinoma. *Gynecol Oncol* 1999;74:3–6.
238. Lax S, Ronntet B, Pizer E, et al. A binary grading system for uterine endometrioid carcinoma is comparable to FIGO grading for predicting prognosis and has superior interobserver reproducibility. *Mod Pathol* 1999;12:118A.
239. Connelly PJ, Albershasky RC, Christopherson WW. Carcinoma of the endometrium. III. Analysis of 865 cases of adenocarcinoma and adenoacanthoma. *Obstet Gynecol* 1982;59:569.
240. Fanning J, Evans MC, Peters AJ, et al. Endometrial adenocarcinoma histologic subtypes: clinical and pathologic profile. *Gynecol Oncol* 1989;32:288–291.
241. Sutton GP, Brill L, Michael H, et al. Malignant papillary lesions of the endometrium. *Gynecol Oncol* 1987;27:294–304.
242. Zaino FJ, Kurman RJ, Brunetto VL, et al. Villoglandular adenocarcinoma of the endometrium: a clinicopathologic study of 61 cases. *Am J Surg Pathol* 1998;22:1379.
243. Kusuyama J, Yoshida M, Imai H, et al. Secretory carcinoma of the endometrium. *Acta Cytol* 1989;33:127.
244. Toban H, Watkins GJ. Secretory adenocarcinoma of the endometrium. *Int J Gynecol Pathol* 1985;4:328.
245. Christopherson WM, Alberhasky RC, Connelly PF. Carcinoma of the endometrium. I. A clinicopathologic study of clear-cell carcinoma and secretory carcinoma. *Cancer* 1982;49:1511.
246. Hendrickson MR, Kempson RL. Ciliated carcinoma—a variant of endometrial adenocarcinoma. A report of 10 cases. *Int J Gynecol Pathol* 1983;2:1–12.
247. Alberhasky RC, Connelly PJ, Christopherson WM. Carcinoma of the endometrium. IV. Mixed adenosquamous carcinoma. A clinical-pathological study of 68 cases with long-term follow-up. *Am J Clin Pathol* 1982; 77:655–664.
248. Julian CG, Daikoku NH, Gillespie A. Adenoepidermoid and adenosquamous carcinoma of the uterus. A clinicopathologic study of 118 cases. *Am J Obstet Gynecol* 1977;128:106–116.
249. Ng AB, Reagan JW, Storaasli JP, et al. Mixed adenosquamous carcinoma of the endometrium. *Am J Clin Pathol* 1973;59:765–781.
250. Salazar OM, DePapp EW, Bonfiglio T, et al. Adenosquamous carcinoma of the endometrium. An entity with an inherently poor prognosis? *Cancer* 1977;40:119–130.
251. Silverberg SG, Bolin MG, DeGiorgi LS. Adenoacanthoma and mixed adenosquamous carcinoma of the endometrium. A clinicopathologic study. *Cancer* 1972;30:1307–1314.
252. Zaino R, Kurman R, Herbold D, et al. The significance of squamous differentiation in endometrial carcinoma. *Cancer* 1991;68:2293–2302.
253. Melhem MF, Tobon H. Mucinous adenocarcinoma of the endometrium: a clinicopathological review of 18 cases. *Int J Gynecol Pathol* 1987;6:347.
254. Ross J, Eifel P, Cox R, et al. Primary mucinous adenocarcinoma of the endometrium. *Am J Surg Pathol* 1983;7:715–729.
255. Tiltman A. Mucinous carcinoma of the endometrium. *Obstet Gynecol* 1980;55:244–247.
256. Maier RC, Norris HJ. Coexistence of cervical intraepithelial neoplasia with primary adenocarcinoma of the endocervix. *Obstet Gynecol* 1980;56:361.
257. Maes G, Fleuren GJ, Bara J, Nap M. The distribution of mucins, carcinoembryonic antigen, and mucus-associated antigens in endocervical and endometrial adenocarcinomas. *Int J Gynecol Pathol* 1988;7:112–122.
258. McCluggage WG, Roberts N, Bharucha H. Enteric differentiation in endometrial adenocarcinomas: a mucin histochemical study. *Int J Gynecol Pathol* 1995;14:250–254.
259. Wilson TO, Podratz KC, Gaffey TA, et al. Evaluation of unfavorable histologic subtypes in endometrial adenocarcinoma. *Am J Obstet Gynecol* 1990;162:418–423.
260. Carcangiu ML, Chambers JT. Uterine papillary serous carcinoma: a study on 108 cases with emphasis on the prognostic significance of associated endometrioid carcinoma, absence of invasion, and concomitant ovarian carcinoma. *Gynecol Oncol* 1992;47:298–305.
261. Chan JK, Loizzi V, Youssef M, et al. Significance of comprehensive surgical staging in noninvasive papillary serous carcinoma of the endometrium. *Gynecol Oncol* 2003;90:181–185.
262. Chambers JT, Merino M, Kohorn EI, et al. Uterine papillary serous carcinoma. *Obstet Gynecol* 1987;69:109–113.
263. Wheeler D, Bell K, Kurman R, et al. Minimal uterine serous carcinoma: diagnostic and clinicopathologic correlation. *Am J Surg Pathol* 2000;24: 797–806.
264. Huh W, Powell M, Leath C, et al. Uterine papillary serous carcinoma: comparisons of outcomes in surgical stage I patients with and without adjuvant therapy. *Gynecol Oncol* 2003;91:470–475.
265. Havrilesky L, Alvarez Secord A, Bae-Jump V, et al. Outcomes in surgical stage I uterine papillary serous carcinoma. *Gynecol Oncol* 2007;105:677–682.
266. Ambros RA, Sherman ME, Zahn CM, et al. Endometrial intraepithelial carcinoma: a distinctive lesion specifically associated with tumors displaying serous differentiation. *Hum Pathol* 1995;26:1260–1267.
267. Sherman ME, Bitterman P, Rosenshein NB, et al. Uterine serous carcinoma. A morphologically diverse neoplasm with unifying clinicopathologic features. *Am J Surg Pathol* 1992;16:600–610.
268. Soslow R, Pirong E, Isacson C. Endometrial intraepithelial carcinoma with associated peritoneal carcinomatosis. *Am J Surg Pathol* 2000;24: 726–732.
269. Spiegel G. Endometrial carcinoma *in situ* in postmenopausal women. *Am J Surg Pathol* 1995;19:417–431.
270. Zheng W, Khurana R, Farahmand S, et al. p53 immunostaining as a significant adjunct diagnostic method for uterine serous carcinoma. *Am J Surg Pathol* 1998;22:1463–1473.
271. Abeler V, Kjørdstad K, Berle E. Carcinoma of the endometrium in Norway: a histopathological and prognostic survey of a total population. *Int J Gynecol Cancer* 1992;2:9–22.
272. Abeler VM, Kjorstad KE. Clear cell carcinoma of the endometrium: a histopathological and clinical study of 97 cases. *Gynecol Oncol* 1991;40: 207–217.
273. Abeler VM, Vergote IB, Kjorstad KE, Trope CG. Clear cell carcinoma of the endometrium. Prognosis and metastatic pattern. *Cancer* 1996;78:1740–1747.
274. Christopherson W, Alberhasky R, Connelly P. Carcinoma of the endometrium. II. Papillary adenocarcinoma: a clinicopathological study of 46 cases. *Am J Clin Pathol* 1982;77:534–540.
275. Kurman RJ, Scully RE. Clear cell carcinoma of the endometrium. An analysis of 21 cases. *Cancer* 1976;37:872–882.
276. Lax SF, Pizer ES, Ronnett BM, et al. Clear cell carcinoma of the endometrium is characterized by a distinctive profile of p53, Ki-67, estrogen, and progesterone receptor expression. *Hum Pathol* 1998;29:551–558.
277. Miller B, Umpierre S, Tornos C, et al. Histologic characterization of uterine papillary serous adenocarcinoma. *Gynecol Oncol* 1995;56:425–429.
278. Webb GA, Lagios MD. Clear cell carcinoma of the endometrium. *Am J Obstet Gynecol* 1987;156:1486–1491.
279. Goodman A, Zukerberg LR, Rice LW, et al. Squamous cell carcinoma of the endometrium: a report of eight cases and a review of the literature. *Gynecol Oncol* 1996;61:54–60.
280. Melin JR, Wanner L, Schulz, DM, et al. Primary squamous cell carcinoma of the endometrium. *Obstet Gynecol* 1979;53:115.
281. Simon A, Kopolovic J, Beyth Y. Primary squamous cell carcinoma of the endometrium. *Gynecol Oncol* 1988;31:454–461.
282. Tagsjo EB, Rosenberg P, Simonsen E. Primary squamous cell carcinoma of the endometrium. Case report. *Eur J Gynaecol Oncol* 1993;14:308–310.
283. Yamashina M, Kobara TY. Primary squamous cell carcinoma with its spindle cell variant in the endometrium. A case report and review of literature. *Cancer* 1986;57:340–345.
284. Scully RE, Aguirre P, DeLellis RA. Argyrophilia, serotonin, and peptide hormones in the female genital tract and its tumor. *Int J Gynecol Pathol* 1984;3:51–70.
285. Ueda G, Yamasaki M, Inoue M, et al. A clinicopathologic study of endometrial carcinomas with argyrophil cells. *Gynecol Oncol* 1979;7:223.
286. Christopherson WM, Alberhasky PC, Connelly PJ. Glassy cell carcinoma of the endometrium. *Hum Pathol* 1982;13:418–421.
287. Hachisuga T, Sugimori H, Kaku T, et al. Glassy cell carcinoma of the endometrium. *Gynecol Oncol* 1990;36:134–138.
288. Kumar NB, Hart WR. Metastases to the uterine corpus from extravaginal cancers. A clinicopathologic study of 63 cases. *Cancer* 1982;50:2163.
289. Kumar NB, Schneider V. Metastases to the uterus from extrapelvic primary tumors. *Int J Gynecol Pathol* 1983;2:134.
290. Piura B, Glezerman M. Synchronous carcinomas of endometrium and ovary. *Gynecol Oncol* 1989;33:261–264.
291. Eifel P, Hendrickson M, Ross J, et al. Simultaneous presentation of carcinoma involving the ovary and uterine corpus. *Cancer* 1982;50:163–170.
292. Scully RE. *Tumors of the Ovary and Maldeveloped Gonad.* AFIP Pamphlet No. 16. Washington, DC: Armed Forces Institute of Pathology; 1982:92.
293. Zaino RJ, Whitney C, Brady MF. Simultaneously detected endometrial and ovarian carcinomas: a clinicopathologic study of 74 cases. *Mod Pathol* 1998;11:118.
294. Ulbright T, Roth L. Metastatic and independent cancers of the endometrium and ovary. A clinicopathologic study of 34 cases. *Hum Pathol* 1985;16: 28–34.
295. Moll UM, Chalas E, Auguste M, et al. Uterine papillary serous carcinoma evolves via a p53 driven pathway. *Hum Pathol* 1996;27:1295–1300.
296. Sansal I, Sellers W. The biology and clinical relevance of the *PTEN* tumor suppressor pathway. *J Clin Oncol* 2004;22:2954–2963.
297. Lee JO, Yang H, Georgescu MM, et al. Crystal structure of the *PTEN* tumor suppressor: implications for its phosphoinositide phosphatase activity and membrane association. *Cell* 1999;99:323–334.
298. Li J, Yen C, Liaw D, et al. *PTEN*, a putative protein tyrosine phosphatase gene mutated in human brain, breast, and prostate cancer. *Science* 1997; 275:1943–1947.
299. Maxwell GL, Risinger JI, Gumbs C, et al. Mutation of the *PTEN* tumor suppressor gene in endometrial hyperplasias. *Cancer Res* 1998;58: 2500–2503.
300. Tamura M, Gu J, Matsumoto K, et al. Inhibition of cell migration, spreading, and focal adhesions by tumour suppressor *PTEN*. *Science* 1998;280:1614–1617.
301. Peiffer SL, Herzog TJ, Tribune DJ, et al. Allelic loss of sequences from the long arm of chromosome 10 and replication errors in endometrial cancers. *Cancer Res* 1995;55:1922–1926.

302. Kong D, Suzuki A, Zou TT, et al. *PTEN1* is frequently mutated in primary endometrial carcinomas. *Nat Genet* 1997;17:143–144.
303. Risinger JI, Hayes AK, Berchech A, et al. *PTEN*/MMAC1 mutations in endometrial cancers. *Cancer Res* 1997;57:4736–4738.
304. Tashiro H, Blazes MS, Wu R, et al. Mutations in *PTEN* are frequent in endometrial carcinoma but rare in other gynecological malignancies. *Cancer Res* 1997;57:3935–3940.
305. Risinger JI, Hayes K, Maxwell GL, et al. PTEN mutation in endometrial cancers is associated with favorable clinical and pathologic characteristics. *Clin Cancer Res* 1998;4:3005–3010.
306. Steck PA, Pershouse MA, Jasser SA, et al. Identification of a candidate tumor suppressor gene, MMAC1, at chromosome 10q23.3 that is mutated in multiple advanced cancers. *Nat Genet* 1997;15:356–362.
307. Peltomäki P. Role of DNA mismatch repair defects in the pathogenesis of human cancer. *J Clin Oncol* 2003;21:1174–1179.
308. Dunlop MG, Farrington SM, Carothers AD, et al. Cancer risk associated with germline DNA mismatch repair gene mutations. *Hum Mol Genet* 1977;6:105–110.
309. Black D, Soslow R, Levine D, et al. Clinicopathologic significance of defective DNA mismatch repair in endometrial carcinoma. *J Clin Oncol* 2006;24:1745–1753.
310. Caduff RF, Johnston CM, Svoboda-Newman SM, et al. Clinical and pathological significance of microsatellite instability in sporadic endometrial carcinoma. *Am J Pathol* 1996;148:1671–1678.
311. Duggan BD, Felix JC, Muderspach LI, et al. Microsatellite instability in sporadic endometrial carcinoma. *J Natl Cancer Inst* 1994;86:1216–1221.
312. Helland A, Børresen-Dale AL, Peltomäki P, et al. Microsatellite instability in cervical endometrial carcinomas. *Int J Cancer* 1997;70:499–501.
313. Risinger JI, Berchuck A, Kohler MF, et al. Genetic instability of microsatellite in endometrial carcinoma. *Cancer Res* 1993;53:5100–5103.
314. Esteller M, Levine R, Baylin SB, et al. *MLH1* promoter hypermethylation is associated with the microsatellite instability phenotype in sporadic carcinomas. *Oncogene* 1998;17:2413–2417.
315. Gurin CC, Federici MG, Kang L, et al. Causes and consequences of microsatellite instability in endometrial carcinoma. *Cancer Res* 1999;59: 462–466.
316. Baylin SB, Herman JG, Graff JR, et al. Alterations in DNA methylation: a fundamental aspect of neoplasia. *Adv Cancer Res* 1998;72:141–196.
317. Herman JG, Latif F, Weng Y, et al. Silencing of the VHL tumor-suppressor gene by DNA methylation in real carcinoma. *Proc Natl Acad Sci USA* 1994;91:9700–9704.
318. Jones PA, Laird PW. Cancer epigenetics comes of age. *Nat Genet* 1999;21:163–167.
319. Kowalski LD, Mutch DG, Herzog TJ, et al. Mutational analysis of *MLH1* and *MSH2* in 25 prospectively acquired RER+ endometrial cancers. *Genes Chromosomes Cancer* 1997;18:219–227.
320. Merlo A, Herman JG, Mao L, et al. 51 CpG island methylation is associated with transcriptional silencing of the tumour suppressor p16/CDKN2/MTS1 in human cancers. *Nat Med* 1995;1:686–692.
321. Levine AJ. p53, the cellular gatekeeper for growth and division. *Cell* 1997; 88:323–331.
322. Tahiro H, Isacson C, Levine R, et al. p53 mutations are common in uterine serous carcinoma and occur as an early event in their pathogenesis. *Am J Pathol* 1997;150:177–185.
323. Lukes AS, Kohler MF, Pieper CF, et al. Multivariable analysis of DNA ploidy, p53, and HER-2/neu as prognostic factors in endometrial cancer. *Cancer* 1994;73:2380–2385.
324. Ambros RA, Sheehan CE, Kallakury BV, et al. MDM2 and p53 protein expression in the histologic subtypes of endometrial carcinoma. *Mod Pathol* 1996;9:1165–1169.
325. Geisler JP, Wiemann MC, Zhou Z, et al. p53 as a prognostic indicator in endometrial cancer. *Gynecol Oncol* 1996;61:245–248.
326. Hamel NW, Sebo TJ, Wilson TO, et al. Prognostic value of p53 and proliferating cell nuclear antigen expression in endometrial carcinoma. *Gynecol Oncol* 1996;62:192–198.
327. Jones MW, Kounelis S, Hsu C, et al. Prognostic value of p53 and K-ras-2 topographic genotyping in endometrial carcinoma: a clinicopathologic and molecular comparison. *Int J Gynecol Pathol* 1997;16:354–360.
328. Khalifa MA, Mannel RS, Haraway SD, et al. Expression of EGFR, HER-2/neu, p53, and PCNA in endometrioid, serous papillary, and clear cell endometrial adenocarcinomas. *Gynecol Oncol* 1994;53:84–92.
329. Kihana T, Hamada K, Inoue Y, et al. Mutation and allelic loss of the p53 gene in endometrial carcinoma. Incidence and outcome in 92 surgical patients. *Cancer* 1995;76:72–78.
330. Kohler MF, Carney P, Dodge R, et al. p53 overexpression in advanced-stage endometrial adenocarcinoma. *Am J Obstet Gynecol* 1996;175: 1246–1252.
331. Nielsen AL, Nyholm HC. p53 protein and c-erbB-2 protein (p185) expression in endometrial adenocarcinoma of endometrioid type. An immunohistochemical examination on paraffin sections. *Am J Clin Pathol* 1994;102:76–79.
332. Nordstrom B, Strang P, Lindgren A, et al. Endometrial carcinoma: the prognostic impact of papillary serous carcinoma (UPSC) in relation to nuclear grade, DNA ploidy and p53 expression. *Anticancer Res* 1996;16:899–904.
333. Risinger JI, Dent GA, Ignar-Trowbridge D, et al. p53 gene mutations in human endometrial carcinoma. *Mol Carcinog* 1992;5:250–253.
334. Tashiro H, Isacson C, Levine R, et al. p53 gene mutations are common in uterine serous carcinoma and occur early in their pathogenesis. *Am J Pathol* 1997;150:177–185.
335. Yamauchi N, Sakamoto A, Uozaki H, et al. Immunohistochemical analysis of endometrial adenocarcinoma for bcl-2 and p53 in relation to expression of sex steroid receptor and proliferative activity [published erratum appears in *Int J Gynecol Pathol* 1996;15:369]. *Int J Gynecol Pathol* 1996;15:202–208.
336. Lundgren C, Auer G, Frankendal B, et al. Nuclear DNA content, proliferative activity, and p53 expression related to clinical and histopathologic features in endometrial carcinoma. *Int J Gynecol Cancer* 2002;12:110–118.
337. Lax SF, Kendall B, Tashiro H, et al. The frequency of p53, K-ras mutation and microsatellite instability differs in uterine endometrioid and serous carcinoma. *Cancer* 2000;88:814–824.
338. Lalloo F, Evans G. Molecular genetics and endometrial cancer. *Best Pract Res Clin Gynaecol* 2001;15:355–363.
339. Berchuck A, Rodriguez G, Kinney R, et al. Overexpression of HER-2/neu in endometrial cancer is associated with advanced stage disease. *Am J Obstet Gynecol* 1991;164:15–21.
340. Reinartz JJ, George E, Lindgren BR, et al. Expression of p53, transforming growth factor alpha, epidermal growth factor receptor, and c-erbB-2 in endometrial carcinoma and correlation with survival and known predictors of survival. *Hum Pathol* 1994;25:1075–1083.
341. Rolitsky C, Theil K, McGaughy V, et al. HER-2/neu amplification and overexpression in endometrial carcinoma. *Int J Gynecol Pathol* 1999;18:138–143.
342. Santin A, Bellone S, Van Stedum S, et al. Determination of HER2/neu status in uterine serous papillary carcinoma: Comparative analysis of immunohistochemistry and fluorescence *in situ* hybridization. *Gynecol Oncol* 2005;98:24–30.
343. Slomovitz B, Broaddus RR, Burke TW, et al. Her-2/neu overexpression and amplification in uterine papillary serous carcinoma. *J Clin Oncol* 2004;22:3126–3132.
344. Backe J, Gassel AM, Krebs S, et al. Immunohistochemically detected HER-2/neu—expression and prognosis in endometrial carcinoma. *Arch Gynecol Obstet* 1997;259:189–195.
345. Pisani AL, Barbuto DA, Chen D, et al. HER-2/neu, p53, and DNA analyses as prognosticators for survival in endometrial carcinoma. *Obstet Gynecol* 1995;85:729–734.
346. Hetzel DJ, Wilson TO, Keeney GL, et al. HER-2/neu expression: a major prognostic factor in endometrial cancer. *Gynecol Oncol* 1992;47:179–185.
347. Nazeer T, Ballouk F, Malfetano JH, et al. Multivariate survival analysis of clinicopathologic features in surgical stage I endometrioid carcinoma including analysis of HER-2/neu expression. *Am J Obstet Gynecol* 1995;173:1829–1834.
348. Saffari B, Jones L, el-Naggar A, et al. Amplification and overexpression of HER-2/neu (c-erbB-2) in endometrial cancers: correlation with overall survival. *Cancer Res* 1995;55:5693–5698.
349. Morrison C, Zanagnolo V, Ramirez N, et al. HER-2 is an independent prognostic factor in endometrial cancer: association with outcome in a large cohort of surgically staged patients. *J Clin Oncol* 2006;24: 2376–2385.
350. Moreno-Bueno G, Hardisson D, Sánchez C, et al. Abnormalities of the APC/β-catenin pathway in endometrial cancer. *Oncogene* 2002;21:7981–7990.
351. Moreno-Bueno G, Hardisson D, Sarrió D, et al. Abnormalities of E- and P-cadherin and catenin (beta-, gamma-catenin, and p120ctn) expression in endometrial cancer and endometrial atypical hyperplasia. *J Pathol* 2003;199:471–478.
352. Caduff RF, Johnston CM, Frank TS. Mutations of the K-ras oncogene in carcinoma of the endometrium. *Am J Pathol* 1995;146:182–188.
353. Esteller M, Garcia A, Martinez-Palones JM, et al. The clinicopathological significance of K-RAS point mutation and gene amplification in endometrial cancer. *Eur J Cancer* 1997;33:1572–1577.
354. Ito K, Watanabe K, Nasim S, et al. K-ras point mutations in endometrial carcinoma: effect on outcome is dependent on age of patient. *Gynecol Oncol* 1996;63:238–246.
355. Semczuk A, Berbec H, Kostuch M, et al. K-ras gene point mutations in human endometrial carcinomas: correlation with clinicopathological features and patients' outcome. *J Cancer Res Clin Oncol* 1998;124:695–700.
356. Katabuchi H, van Rees B, Lambers AR, et al. Mutations in DNA mismatch repair genes are not responsible for microsatellite instability in most sporadic endometrial carcinomas. *Cancer Res* 1995;55:5556–5560.
357. Nakashima R, Fujita M, Enomoto T, et al. Alteration of p16 and p15 genes in human tumours. *Br J Cancer* 1999;80:458–467.
358. Winjen J, Leeuwen W, Vasen H, et al. Familial endometrial cancer in female carriers of *MSH6* germline mutations. *Nat Genet* 1999;23:142–144.
359. Salvesen HB, Das S, Akslen LA. Loss of nuclear p16 protein expression is not associated with promoter methylation but defines a subgroup of aggressive endometrial carcinomas with poor prognosis. *Clin Cancer Res* 2000;6:153–159.
360. Boronow R, Morrow C, Creasman W, et al. Surgical staging in endometrial cancer: clinical-pathologic findings of a prospective study. *Obstet Gynecol* 1984;63:825–832.
361. Gal D, Recio FO, Zamurovic D. The new International Federation of Gynecology and Obstetrics surgical staging and survival rates in early endometrial carcinoma. *Cancer* 1992;69:200–202.

362. Homesly H, Zaino R. Endometrial cancer: prognostic factors. *Semin Oncol* 1994;21:71–8.
363. Kosary CL. FIGO stage, histology, histologic grade, age and race as prognostic factors in determining survival for cancers of the female gynecological system: an analysis of 1973–87 SEER cases of cancers of the endometrium, cervix, ovary, vulva, and vagina. *Semin Surg Oncol* 1994;10:31–46.
364. Wolfson A, Sightler S, Markoe A, et al. The prognostic significance of surgical staging for carcinoma of the endometrium. *Gynecol Oncol* 1992;45:142–146.
365. Zaino RJ, Kurman RJ, Diana KL, et al. Pathologic models to predict outcome for women with endometrial adenocarcinoma. *Cancer* 1996;77:1115–1121.
366. Mariani A, Webb M, Keeney G, et al. Stage IIIC endometrioid corpus cancer includes distinct subgroups. *Gynecol Oncol* 2002;87:112–117.
367. Havrilesky LJ, Cragun J, Calingaert B, et al. Resection of lymph node metastases influences survival in stage IIIc endometrial cancer. *Gynecol Oncol* 2005;99:689–695.
368. Takeshima N, Umayahara K, Fujiwara K, et al. Effectiveness of postoperative chemotherapy for para-aortic lymph node metastasis of endometrial cancer. *Gynecol Oncol* 2006;102:214–217.
369. Kennedy A, Peterson G, Becker S, et al. Experience with pelvic washings in stage I and II endometrial carcinoma. *Gynecol Oncol* 1987;28:50–60.
370. Yazigi R, Piver M, Blumenson I. Malignant peritoneal cytology as an indicator in stage I endometrial cancer. *Obstet Gynecol* 1983;62:359–362.
371. Creasman W, DiSaia P, Blessing J, et al. Prognostic significance of peritoneal cytology in patients with endometrial cancer and preliminary data concerning therapy with intraperitoneal radiopharmaceuticals. *Am J Obstet Gynecol* 1981;141:921–929.
372. Grimshaw R, Tupper W, Fraser R, et al. Prognostic value of peritoneal cytology in endometrial carcinoma. *Gynecol Oncol* 1990;36:97–100.
373. McLellan R, Dillon MB, Currie JL, et al. Peritoneal cytology in endometrial cancer: a review. *Obstet Gynecol Surv* 1989;44:711–719.
374. Sutton GP. The significance of positive peritoneal cytology in endometrial cancer. *Oncology* 1990;4:21–26.
375. Szpak C, Creasman W, Vollmer R, et al. Prognostic value of cytologic examination of peritoneal washings in patients with endometrial carcinoma. *Acta Cytol* 1981;25:640–646.
376. Harouny V, Sutton G, Clark S, et al. The importance of peritoneal cytology in endometrial carcinoma. *Obstet Gynecol* 1988;72:394–398.
377. Konski A, Poulter C, Keys H, et al. Absence of prognostic significance, peritoneal dissemination and treatment advantage in endometrial cancer patients with positive peritoneal cytology. *Int J Radiat Oncol Biol Phys* 1988;14:49–55.
378. Turner D, Gershenson D, Atkinson N, et al. The prognostic significance of peritoneal cytology for stage I endometrial cancer. *Obstet Gynecol* 1989;74:775–780.
379. Kadar N, Homesley H, Malfetano J. Positive peritoneal cytology is an adverse risk factor in endometrial carcinoma only if there is other evidence of extrauterine disease. *Gynecol Oncol* 1992;46:145–149.
380. Havrilesky L, Cragun J, Calingaert B, et al. The prognostic significance of positive peritoneal cytology and adnexal/serosal metastasis in stage IIIa endometrial cancer. *Gynecol Oncol* 2007;104:401–405.
381. Esteller M, Garcia A, Martinez-Palones JM, et al. Clinicopathologic features and genetic alterations in endometrioid carcinoma of the uterus with villoglandular differentiation. *Am J Clin Pathol* 1999;111:336–342.
382. Abeler VM, Kjorstad KE. Serous papillary carcinoma of the endometrium: a histopathological study of 22 cases. *Gynecol Oncol* 1990;39:266–271.
383. Chen J, Trost D, Wilkinson E. Endometrial papillary adenocarcinomas: two clinicopathologic types. *Int J Gynecol Pathol* 1985;4:279–288.
384. Hendrickson M, Martinez A, Ross J, et al. Uterine papillary serous carcinoma: a highly malignant form of endometrial adenocarcinoma. *Am J Surg Pathol* 1982;6:93–108.
385. Ward BG, Wright RG, Free K. Papillary carcinomas of the endometrium. *Gynecol Oncol* 1990;39:347–351.
386. Aquino-Parsons C, Lim P, Wong F, et al. Papillary serous and clear cell carcinoma limited to endometrial curettings in FIGO stage 1a and 1b endometrial adenocarcinoma: treatment implications. *Gynecol Oncol* 1998;71:83–86.
387. Carcangiu ML, Chambers JT. Early pathologic stage clear cell carcinoma and uterine papillary serous carcinoma of the endometrium: comparison of clinicopathologic features and survival. *Int J Gynecol Pathol* 1995;14:30–38.
388. Kanbour-Shakir A, Tobon H. Primary clear cell carcinoma of the endometrium: a clinicopathologic study of 20 cases. *Int J Gynecol Pathol* 1991;10:67–78.
389. Malpica A, Tornos C, Burke TW, et al. Low-stage clear-cell carcinoma of the endometrium. *Am J Surg Pathol* 1995;19:769–774.
390. Havrilesky L, Alvarez Secord A, Bae-Jump V, et al. Outcomes in surgical stage I uterine papillary serous carcinoma. *Gynecol Oncol* 2007;105:677–682.
391. Alektiar A, McKee A, Lin O, et al. Is there a difference in outcome between stage I-II endometrial cancer of papillary serous/clear cell and endometrioid FIGO grade 3 cancer? *Int J Radiat Oncol Biol Phys* 2002;54:79–85.
392. Huh W, Powell M, Leath C, et al. Uterine papillary serous carcinoma: comparisons of outcomes in surgical stage I patients with and without adjuvant therapy. *Gynecol Oncol* 2003;91:470–475.
393. Creasman WT, Kohler M, Odicino F, et al. Prognosis of papillary serous, clear cell, and grade 3 stage I carcinoma of the uterus. *Gynecol Oncol* 2004;95:593–596.
394. Chambers SK, Kapp DS, Peschel RE, et al. Prognostic factors and sites of failure in FIGO stage I, grade 3 endometrial carcinoma. *Gynecol Oncol* 1987;27:180–188.
395. Sutton GP, Geiser HE, Stehman FB, et al. Features associated with survival and disease-free survival in early endometrial cancer. *Am J Obstet Gynecol* 1989;160:1385–1393.
396. Wharton JT, Mikuta JJ, Mettlin C, et al. Risk factors and current management in carcinoma of the endometrium. *Surg Gynecol Obstet* 1986;162:515–520.
397. Bucy GS, Mendenhall WM, Morgan LS, et al. Clinical stage I and II endometrial carcinoma treated with surgery and/or radiation therapy: analysis of prognostic and treatment-related factors. *Gynecol Oncol* 1989;33:290.
398. Jones HW III. Treatment of adenocarcinoma of the endometrium. *Obstet Gynecol Surv* 1975;30:147.
399. Mariani A, Webb M, Keeney G, et al. Surgical stage I endometrial cancer: predictors of distant failure and death. *Gynecol Oncol* 2002;87:274–280.
400. Gal D, Recio FO, Zamurovic D, et al. Lymphovascular space involvement—a prognostic indicator in endometrial adenocarcinoma. *Gynecol Oncol* 1991;42:142–145.
401. Hanson M, van Nagell J, Powell D. The prognostic significance of lymph-vascular space invasion in stage I endometrial cancer. *Cancer* 1985;55:1753–1757.
402. Inoue Y, Obata K, Abe K, et al. The prognostic significance of vascular invasion by endometrial carcinoma. *Cancer* 1996;78:1447–1451.
403. Sivridis E, Buckley CH, Fox H. The prognostic significance of lymphatic vascular space invasion in endometrial adenocarcinoma. *Br J Obstet Gynaecol* 1987;94:991–994.
404. Straughn JM, Huh W, Kelly J, et al. Conservative management of stage I endometrial carcinoma after surgical staging. *Gynecol Oncol* 2002;84:194–200.
405. Straughn JM, Huh W, Orr J, et al. Stage IC adenocarcinoma of the endometrium: survival comparisons of surgically staged patients with and without adjuvant therapy. *Gynecol Oncol* 2003;89:295–300.
406. Mariani A, Dowdy S, Keeney G, et al. Predictors of vaginal relapse in stage I endometrial cancer. *Gynecol Oncol* 2005;97:820–827.
407. Mariani A, Webb M, Kenney G, et al. Endometrial cancer: predictors of peritoneal failure. *Gynecol Oncol* 2003;89:236–242.
408. Mariani A, Webb M, Keeney G, et al. Predictors of lymphatic failure in endometrial cancer. *Gynecol Oncol* 2002;84:437–442.
409. Mariani A, Webb M, Rao S, et al. Significance of pathologic patterns of pelvic lymph node metastases in endometrial cancer. *Gynecol Oncol* 2001;80:113–120.
410. Kauppila A, Kujansuu E, Vihko R. Cytosol estrogen and progestin receptors in endometrial carcinoma of patients treated with surgery, radiotherapy, and progestin. Clinical correlates. *Cancer* 1982;50:2157–2162.
411. Macdonald RR, Thorogood J, Mason MK. A randomized trial of progestogens in the primary treatment of endometrial carcinoma. *Br J Obstet Gynaecol* 1988;95:166–174.
412. Vergote I, Kjorstad K, Abeler V, et al. A randomized trial of adjuvant progestogen in early endometrial cancer. *Cancer* 1989;64:1011.
413. von Minckwitz G, Loibl S, Brunnert K, et al. Adjuvant endocrine treatment with medroxyprogesterone acetate or tamoxifen in stage I and II endometrial cancer—a multicentre, open, controlled, prospectively randomised trial. *Eur J Cancer* 2002;38:2265–2271.
414. Morrow C, Bundy B, Homesley H, et al. Doxorubicin as an adjuvant following surgery and radiation therapy in patients with high-risk endometrial carcinoma, stage I and occult stage II: a Gynecologic Oncology Group study. *Gynecol Oncol* 1990;36:166–171.
415. Maggi R, Lissoni A, Spina F, et al. Adjuvant chemotherapy vs. radiotherapy in high-risk endometrial carcinoma: results of a randomised trial. *Br J Cancer* 2006;95(3):266–271.
416. Sagae S, Udagawa Y, Susumu N, et al. Randomized phase III trial of whole pelvic radiotherapy vs. cisplatin-based chemotherapy in patients with intermediate risk endometrial cancer. *J Clin Oncol* 2005;23(16S); abstr 5002.
417. Lee CM, Szabo A, Shrieve DC, et al. Frequency and effect of adjuvant radiation therapy among women with stage I endometrial adenocarcinoma. *JAMA* 2006;295(4):389–397.
418. Aalders J, Abeler V, Kolstad P, et al. Postoperative external irradiation and prognostic parameters in stage I endometrial carcinoma: clinical and histopathologic study of 540 patients. *Obstet Gynecol* 1980;56:419–427.
419. Greven KM, D'Agostino RB Jr, Lanciano RM, et al. Is there a role for a brachytherapy vaginal cuff boost in the adjuvant management of patients with uterine-confined endometrial cancer? *Int J Radiat Oncol Biol Phys* 1998;42:101–104.
420. Randall ME, Wilder J, Greven K, et al. Role of intracavitary cuff boost after adjuvant external irradiation in early endometrial carcinoma. *Int J Radiat Oncol Biol Phys* 1990;19:49–54.

421. Rush S, Gal D, Potters L, et al. Pelvic control following external beam radiation for surgical stage I endometrial adenocarcinoma. *Int J Radiat Oncol Biol Phys* 1995;33:851–854.
422. Kucera H, Vaura N, Weghoupt K. Benefit of external irradiation in pathologic stage I endometrial carcinoma: a prospective clinical trial of 605 patients who received postoperative vaginal irradiation and additional pelvic irradiation in the presence of unfavorable prognostic factors. *Gynecol Oncol* 1990;38:99–104.
423. Nori D, Merimsky O, Batata M, et al. Postoperative high dose-rate intravaginal brachytherapy combined with external irradiation for early stage endometrial cancer: a long-term follow-up. *Int J Radiat Oncol Biol Phys* 1994;30:831–837.
424. Horowitz NS, Peters WA 3rd, Smith MR, et al. Adjuvant high dose rate vaginal brachytherapy as treatment of stage I and II endometrial carcinoma. *Obstet Gynecol* 2002;99:235–240.
425. Anderson JM, Stea B, Hallum AV, et al. High-dose-rate postoperative vaginal cuff irradiation alone for stage IB and IC endometrial cancer. *Int J Radiat Oncol Biol Phys* 2000;46:417–425.
426. MacLeod C, Fowler A, Duval P, et al. High-dose-rate brachytherapy alone post-hysterectomy for endometrial cancer. *Int J Radiat Oncol Biol Phys* 1998;42:1033–1039.
427. Petereit DG, Tannehill SP, Grosen EA, et al. Outpatient vaginal cuff brachytherapy for endometrial cancer. *Int J Gynecol Cancer* 1999;9: 456–462.
428. Elliot P, Green D. The efficacy of postoperative vaginal irradiation in preventing vaginal recurrence in endometrial cancer. *Int J Gynecol Cancer* 1994;4:84.
429. Alektiar KM, McKee A, Venkatraman E, et al. Intravaginal high-dose-rate brachytherapy for stage IB (FIGO grade 1, 2) endometrial cancer. *Int J Radiat Oncol Biol Phys* 2002;53:707–713.
430. Sorbe B, Staumits A, Karlsson L. Intravaginal high-dose-rate brachytherapy for stage I endometrial cancer: a randomized study of two dose-perfraction levels. *Int J Radiat Oncol Biol Phys* 2005;62(5):1385–1389.
431. Alektiar KM, McKee A, Lin O, et al. The significance of the amount of myometrial invasion in patients with stage IB endometrial carcinoma. *Cancer* 2002;95:316–321.
432. Scholten AN, Creutzberg CL, Noordijk EM, et al. Long-term outcome in endometrial carcinoma favors a two—instead of a three—tiered grading system. *Int J Radiat Oncol Biol Phys* 2002;52:1067–1074.
433. Irwin C, Levin W, Fyles A, et al. The role of adjuvant radiotherapy in carcinoma of the endometrium—results in 550 patients with pathologic stage I disease. *Gynecol Oncol* 1998;70:247–254.
434. Piver M, Hempling R. A prospective trial of post-operative vaginal radium/cesium for grade 1–2 less than 50% myometrial invasion and pelvic radiation therapy for grade 3 or deep myometrial invasion in surgical stage I endometrial adenocarcinoma. *Cancer* 1990;66:133.
435. Chadha M, Nanavati PJ, Liu P, et al. Patterns of failure in endometrial carcinoma stage IB grade 3 and IC patients treated with postoperative vaginal vault brachytherapy. *Gynecol Oncol* 1999;75:103–107.
436. Alektiar KM, Chi D, Barakat RR. Risk stratification of death from endometrial cancer in patients with early stage disease. *IJROBP* 2007; abstract.
437. Solhjem MC, Petersen IA, Haddock MG. Vaginal brachytherapy alone is sufficient adjuvant treatment of surgical stage I endometrial cancer. *Int J Radiat Oncol Biol Phys* 2005;62(5):1379–1384.
438. Rittenberg PVC, Lotocki RJ, Heywood MS, et al. High-risk surgical stage 1 endometrial cancer: outcomes with vault brachytherapy alone. *Gynecol Oncol* 2003;89(2):288–294.
439. Weiss MF, Connell PP, Waggoner S, et al. External pelvic radiation therapy in stage IC endometrial carcinoma. *Obstet Gynecol* 1999;93:599–602.
440. Pitson G, Colgan T, Levin W, et al. Stage II endometrial carcinoma: prognostic factors and risk classification in 170 patients. *Int J Radiat Oncol Biol Phys* 2002;53:862–867.
441. Fanning J. Long-term survival of intermediate risk endometrial cancer (stage IG3, IC, II) treated with full lymphadenectomy and brachytherapy without teletherapy. *Gynecol Oncol* 2001;82:371–374.
442. Ng TY, Nicklin JL, Perrin LC, et al. Postoperative vaginal vault brachytherapy for node-negative stage II (occult) endometrial carcinoma. *Gynecol Oncol* 2001;81:193–195.
443. Rittenberg PVC, Lotocki RJ, Heywood MS, et al. Stage II endometrial carcinoma: limiting post-operative radiotherapy to the vaginal vault in node-negative tumors. *Gynecol Oncol* 2005;98(3):434–438.
444. Connell PP, Rotmensch J, Waggoner S, et al. The significance of adnexal involvement in endometrial carcinoma. *Gynecol Oncol* 1999;74:74–79.
445. Ashman JB, Connell PP, Yamada D, et al. Outcome of endometrial carcinoma patients with involvement of the uterine serosa. *Gynecol Oncol* 2001;82:338–343.
446. Greven K, Corn B, Lanciano RM. Pathologic stage III endometrial carcinoma. *Cancer* 1993;71:3697.
447. Mariani A, Webb MJ, Keeney GL, et al. Stage IIIC endometrioid corpus cancer includes distinct subgroups. *Gynecol Oncol* 2002;87:12–17.
448. Corn BW, Lanciano RM, Greven KM, et al. Endometrial carcinoma with para-aortic lymphadenopathy: patterns of failure and opportunity for cure. *Int J Radiat Oncol Biol Phys* 1992;24:223.
449. Hicks ML, Piver S, Jeffrey LP, et al. Survival in patients with para-aortic lymph node metastases from endometrial adenocarcinoma clinically limited to the uterus. *Int J Radiat Oncol Biol Phys* 1993;26:607.
450. Rose PG, Cha SD, Tak WK, et al. Radiation therapy for surgically proven para-aortic node metastasis in endometrial carcinoma. *Int J Radiat Oncol Biol Phys* 1992;24:229–233.
451. Gibbons S, Martinez A, Schary M, et al. Adjuvant whole abdominopelvic irradiation for high-risk endometrial carcinoma. *Int J Radiat Oncol Biol Phys* 1991;21:1019–1025.
452. Martinez A, Podratz K. Results of whole abdomino-pelvic radiation with nodal boost for patients with endometrial cancer at high risk of failure in the peritoneal cavity. *Hematol Oncol Clin North Am* 1988;2:431.
453. Sutton G, Axelrod J, Bundy B, et al. Whole abdominal radiotherapy in the adjuvant treatment of patients with stage III and IV endometrial cancer: a Gynecologic Oncology Group study. *Gynecol Oncol* 2005;97(3): 755–763.
454. Stewart KD, Martinez AA, Weiner S, et al. Ten-year outcome including patterns of failure and toxicity for adjuvant whole abdominopelvic irradiation in high-risk and poor histologic feature patients with endometrial carcinoma. *Int J Radiat Oncol Biol Phys* 2002;54:527–535.
455. Greven K, Winter K, Underhill K, et al. Final analysis of RTOG 9708: adjuvant postoperative irradiation combined with cisplatin/paclitaxel chemotherapy following surgery for patients with high-risk endometrial cancer. *Gynecol Oncol* 2006;103(1):155–159.
456. Milosevic MF, Dembo AJ, Thomas GM. The clinical significance of malignant peritoneal cytology in stage I endometrial carcinoma. *Int J Gynecol Cancer* 1992;2:225–235.
457. Soper JT, Creasman WT, Clarke-Pearson DL, et al. Intraperitoneal chromic phosphate ^{32}P suspension therapy of malignant peritoneal cytology in endometrial carcinoma. *Am J Obstet Gynecol* 1985;153:191–196.
458. Eltabbakh GH, Piver MS, Hempling RE, et al. Excellent long-term survival and absence of vaginal recurrences in 332 patients with low-risk stage I endometrial adenocarcinoma treated with hysterectomy and vaginal brachytherapy without formal staging lymph node sampling: report of a prospective trial. *Int J Radiat Oncol Biol Phys* 1997;38:373–380.
459. Smith RS, Kapp DS, Chen Q, et al. Treatment of high-risk uterine cancer with whole abdominopelvic radiation therapy. *Int J Radiat Oncol Biol Phys* 2000;48:767–778.
460. Lim P, Al Kushi A, Gilks B, et al. Early stage uterine papillary serous carcinoma of the endometrium: effect of adjuvant whole abdominal radiotherapy and pathologic parameters on outcome. *Cancer* 2001;91:752–757.
461. Kelly MG, O'Malley DM, Hui P, et al. Improved survival in surgical stage I patients with uterine papillary serous carcinoma (UPSC) treated with adjuvant platinum-based chemotherapy. *Gynecol Oncol* 2005;98(3): 353–359.
462. Rouanet P, Dubois JB, Gely S, et al. Exclusive radiation therapy in endometrial carcinoma. *Int J Radiat Oncol Biol Phys* 1993;26:223–228.
463. Grigsby P, Kuske R, Perez CA, et al. Medically inoperable stage I adenocarcinoma of the endometrium treated with radiotherapy alone. *Int J Radiat Oncol Biol Phys* 1986;13:483.
464. Knocke TH, Kucera H, Weidinger B, et al. Primary treatment of endometrial carcinoma with high-dose-rate brachytherapy: results of 12 years of experience with 280 patients. *Int J Radiat Oncol Biol Phys* 15; 37:359–365.
465. Nguyen TV, Petereit DG. High-dose-rate brachytherapy for medically inoperable stage I endometrial cancer. *Gynecol Oncol* 1998;71:196–203.
466. Nicklin JL, Petersen RW. Stage 3B adenocarcinoma of the endometrium: a clinicopathologic study. *Gynecol Oncol* 2000;78:203–207.
467. Mundt AJ, Lujan AE, Rotmensch J, et al. Intensity-modulated whole pelvic radiotherapy in women with gynecologic malignancies. *Int J Radiat Oncol Biol Phys* 2002;52(5):1330–1337.
468. Mundt AJ, Mell LK, Roeske JC. Preliminary analysis of chronic gastrointestinal toxicity in gynecology patients treated with intensity-modulated whole pelvic radiation therapy. *Int J Radiat Oncol Biol Phys* 2003;56(5): 1354–1360.
469. Horowitz NS, Peters WA 3rd, Smith MR, et al. Adjuvant high dose rate vaginal brachytherapy as treatment of stage I and II endometrial carcinoma. *Obstet Gynecol* 2002;99:235–240.
470. Alektiar KM, McKee A, Venkatraman E, et al. Intravaginal high-dose-rate brachytherapy for stage IB (FIGO grade 1, 2) endometrial cancer. *Int J Radiat Oncol Biol Phys* 2002;53:707–713.
471. Petereit DG, Tannehill SP, Grosen EA, et al. Outpatient vaginal cuff brachytherapy for endometrial cancer. *Int J Gynecol Cancer* 1999;9:456–462.
472. Sorbe BG, Smeds AC. Postoperative vaginal irradiation with high dose-rate afterloading technique in endometrial carcinoma stage I. *Int J Radiat Oncol Biol Phys* 1990;18:305–314.
473. Curran WJ, Whittington R, Peters AJ, et al. Vaginal recurrences of endometrial carcinoma: the prognostic value of staging by a primary vaginal carcinoma system. *Int J Radiat Oncol Biol Phys* 1988;15:803–808.
474. Sears J, Greven K. Prognostic factors and treatment outcome for patients with locally recurrent endometrial cancer. *Cancer* 1994;74:1303–1308.
475. Wylie J, Irwin C, Pintilie M, et al. Results of radical radiotherapy for recurrent endometrial cancer. *Gynecol Oncol* 2000;77:66–72.
476. Creutzberg CL, van Putten WL, Koper PC, et al. PORTEC Study Group. Survival after relapse in patients with endometrial cancer: results from a randomized trial. *Gynecol Oncol* 2003;89:201–209.
477. Jhingran A, Burke TW, Eifel PJ, et al. Definitive radiotherapy for patients with isolated vaginal recurrence of endometrial carcinoma after hysterectomy. *Int J Radiat Oncol Biol Phys* 2003;56:1366–1372.

478. Podratz KC, O'Brien PC, Malkasian GD Jr, et al. Effects of progestational agents in treatment of endometrial carcinoma. *Obstet Gynecol* 1985;66: 106–110.
479. Asbury RF, Brunetto VL, Lee RB, et al. Goserelin acetate as treatment for recurrent endometrial carcinoma: a Gynecologic Oncology Group study. *Am J Clin Oncol* 2002;25:557–560.
480. McMeekin DS, Gordon A, Fowler J, et al. A phase II trial of arzoxifene, a selective estrogen response modulator, in patients with recurrent or advanced endometrial cancer. *Gynecol Oncol* 2003;90:64–69.
481. Piver MS, Barlow JJ, Lurain JR, et al. Medroxyprogesterone acetate (Depo-Provera) vs. hydroxyprogesterone caproate (Delalutin) in women with metastatic endometrial adenocarcinoma. *Cancer* 1980;45:268–272.
482. Quinn MA, Cauchi M, Fortune D. Endometrial carcinoma: steroid receptors and response to medroxyprogesterone acetate. *Gynecol Oncol* 1985;21: 314–319.
483. Rose PG, Brunetto VL, et al. A phase II trial of anastrozole in advanced recurrent or persistent endometrial carcinoma: a Gynecologic Oncology Group study. *Gynecol Oncol* 2000;78(2):212–216.
484. Slavik M, Petty WM, Blessing JA, et al. Phase II clinical study of tamoxifen in advanced endometrial adenocarcinoma: a Gynecologic Oncology Group study. *Cancer Treat Rep* 1984;68:809–811.
485. Thigpen T, Brady MF, Homesley HD, et al. Tamoxifen in the treatment of advanced or recurrent endometrial carcinoma: a Gynecologic Oncology Group study. *J Clin Oncol* 2001;19:364–367.
486. Thigpen JT, Brady MF, Alvarez RD, et al. Oral medroxyprogesterone acetate in the treatment of advanced or recurrent endometrial carcinoma: a dose-response study by the Gynecologic Oncology Group. *J Clin Oncol* 1999;17:1736–1744.
487. Lentz SS, Brady MF, Major FJ, et al. High-dose megestrol acetate in advanced or recurrent endometrial carcinoma: a Gynecologic Oncology Group Study. *J Clin Oncol* 1996;14:357–361.
488. Quinn MA, Campbell JJ, Murray R, et al. Tamoxifen and aminoglutethimide in the management of patients with advanced endometrial carcinoma not responsive to medroxyprogesterone. *Aust N Z J Obstet Gynaecol* 1981;21:226–229.
489. Pandya KJ, Yeap BY, Weiner LM, et al. Megestrol and tamoxifen in patients with advanced endometrial cancer: an Eastern Cooperative Oncology Group study (E4882). *Am J Clin Oncol* 2001;24:43–46.
490. Satyaswaroop PG, Clarke CL, Zaino RJ, et al. Apparent resistance in human endometrial carcinoma during combination treatment with tamoxifen and progestin may result from desensitization following downregulation of tumor progesterone receptor. *Cancer Lett* 1992;62:107–114.
491. Fiorica JV, Brunetto VL, Hanjani P, et al. Phase II trial of alternating courses of megestrol acetate and tamoxifen in advanced endometrial carcinoma: a Gynecologic Oncology Group study. *Gynecol Oncol* 2004;92: 10–14.
492. Whitney C, Brunetto V, Zaino R, et al. Phase II study of medroxyprogesterone acetate plus tamoxifen in advanced endometrial carcinoma: a Gynecologic Oncology Group study. *Gynecol Oncol* 2004;92:4–9.
493. Geisinger K, Homesely H, Morgan T, et al. Endometrial adenocarcinoma. A multiparameter clinicopathologic analysis including the DNA profile and the sex steroid hormone receptors. *Cancer* 1986;58:1518–1525.
494. Kauppila A. Oestrogen and progestin receptors as prognostic indicators in endometrial cancer. A review of the literature. *Acta Oncol* 1989; 28:561–566.
495. Vering A, Michel RT, Mitze M, et al. Influence of chemotherapy on hormone receptor concentration in a xenotransplanted endometrial cancer. *Eur J Obstet Gynecol Reprod Biol* 1992;45:131–138.
496. Bonte J, Decoster JM, Ide P. Vaginal cytologic evaluation as a practical link between hormone blood levels and tumor hormone dependency in exclusive medroxyprogesterone treatment of recurrent or metastatic endometrial adenocarcinoma. *Acta Cytol* 1977;21:218–224.
497. Stratton JA, Mannel RS, Rettenmaier MA, et al. Treatment of advanced and recurrent endometrial carcinoma: correlation of patient response to hormonal and cytotoxic chemotherapy and the response predicted by the subrenal capsule chemosensitivity assay. *Gynecol Oncol* 1989;32:55–59.
498. Zaino RJ, Satyaswaroop PG, Mortel R. Hormonal therapy of human endometrial adenocarcinoma in a nude mouse model. *Cancer Res* 1985;45:539–541.
499. Gallagher CJ, Oliver RT, Oram DH, et al. A new treatment for endometrial cancer with gonadotrophin releasing-hormone analogue. *Br J Obstet Gynaecol* 1991;98:1037.
500. De Vriese G, Bonte J. Possible role of goserelin, an LH-RH agonist, in the treatment of gynaecological cancers. *Eur J Gynaecol Oncol* 1993; 14:187–191.
501. Kleinman D, Douvdevani A, Schally AV, et al. Direct growth inhibition of human endometrial cancer cells by the gonadotropin-releasing hormone antagonist SB-75: role of apoptosis. *Am J Obstet Gynecol* 1994; 170:96–102.
502. Chan S. A review of selective estrogen receptor modulators in the treatment of breast and endometrial cancer. *Semin Oncol* 2002;29(3 Suppl 11):129–133.
503. Levine DA, Hoskins WJ. Update in the management of endometrial cancer. *Cancer J* 2002;8(Suppl 1):S31–S40.
504. Sonoda Y. Optimal therapy and management of endometrial cancer. *Expert Rev Anticancer Ther* 2003;3:37–47.
505. Asbury RF, Blessing JA, McGuire WP, et al. Aminothiadiazole (NSC 4728) in patients with advanced carcinoma of the endometrium. A phase II study of the Gynecologic Oncology Group. *Am J Clin Oncol* 1990; 13:39–41.
506. Ball H, Blessing JA, Lentz S, et al. A phase II trial of Taxol in advanced and recurrent adenocarcinoma of the endometrium: a Gynecologic Oncology Group study. *Gynecol Oncol* 1996;62:278.
507. Von Hoff DD, Green S, Alberts DS, et al. Phase II study of fludarabine phosphate (NSC-312887) in patients with advanced endometrial cancer. A Southwest Oncology Group study. *Am J Clin Oncol* 1991;14:193–194.
508. Gunthert AR, Ackermann S, Beckmann MW, et al. Phase II study of weekly docetaxel in patients with recurrent or metastatic endometrial cancer: AGO Uterus-4. *Gynecol Oncol* 2007;104:86–90.
509. Edmonston JH, Krook JE, Holton JF, et al. Randomized phase II studies of cisplatin and a combination of cyclophosphamide-doxorubicin-cisplatin (CAP) in patients with progestin-refractory advanced endometrial carcinoma. *Gynecol Oncol* 1987;28:20–24.
510. Thigpen JT, Blessing JA, Lagasse LD, et al. Phase II trial of cisplatin as second-line chemotherapy in patients with advanced or recurrent endometrial carcinoma. A Gynecologic Oncology Group study. *Am J Clin Oncol* 1984;7:253–256.
511. Deppe G, Cohen CJ, Bruckner HW. Treatment of advanced endometrial adenocarcinoma with cis-dichlorodiamine platinum (II) after intensive prior therapy. *Gynecol Oncol* 1980;10:51–54.
512. Seski JC, Edwards CL, Herson J, et al. Cisplatin chemotherapy for disseminated endometrial cancer. *Obstet Gynecol* 1982;59:225–228.
513. Thigpen JT, Blessing JA, Homesley H, et al. Phase II trial of cisplatin as first-line chemotherapy in patients with advanced or recurrent endometrial carcinoma: a Gynecologic Oncology Group study. *Gynecol Oncol* 1989;33:68–70.
514. Burke TW, Munkarah A, Kavanagh JJ, et al. Treatment of advanced or recurrent endometrial carcinoma with single-agent carboplatin. *Gynecol Oncol* 1993;51:397–400.
515. Green JB, Green S, Alberts DS, et al. Carboplatin therapy in advanced endometrial cancer. *Obstet Gynecol* 1990;75:696–700.
516. Long HJ, Pfeifle DM, Wieand HS, et al. Phase II evaluation of carboplatin in advanced endometrial carcinoma. *J Natl Cancer Inst* 1988;80: 276–278.
517. Horton J, Begg CB, Arseneault J, et al. Comparison of Adriamycin with cyclophosphamide in patients with advanced endometrial cancer. *Cancer Treat Rep* 1978;62:159–161.
518. Thigpen JT, Blessing JA, Ball H, et al. Hexamethylmelamine as first-line therapy in the treatment of advanced or recurrent carcinoma of the endometrium: a phase II trial of the Gynecologic Oncology Group. *Gynecol Oncol* 1988;31:435–438.
519. Thigpen JT, Buchsbaum HJ, Mangan C, et al. Phase II trial of Adriamycin in the treatment of advanced or recurrent endometrial carcinoma: a Gynecologic Oncology Group study. *Cancer Treat Rep* 1979;63:21–27.
520. Calero F, Asins-Codoner E, Jimeno J, et al. Epirubicin in advanced endometrial adenocarcinoma: a phase II study of the Grupo Ginecologico Espanol para el Tratamiento Oncologico (GGETO). *Eur J Cancer* 1991; 27:864–866.
521. Muggia FM, Blessing JA, Sorosky J, et al. A phase II trial of the pegylated liposomal doxorubicin in previously treated metastatic endometrial cancer: a Gynecologic Oncology Group study. *J Clin Oncol* 2002;20:2360–2364.
522. Escobar PF, Markman M, Zanotti K, et al. Phase 2 trial of pegylated liposomal doxorubicin in advanced endometrial cancer. *J Cancer Res Clin Oncol* 2003;129:651–654.
523. Muss HB, Blessing JA, Hatch KD, et al. Methotrexate in advanced endometrial carcinoma. A phase II trial of the Gynecologic Oncology Group. *Am Clin Oncol* 1990;13:61–63.
524. Dvorak O. Cytembena treatment of advanced gynecological carcinomas. *Neoplasm* 1971;18:461.
525. Broun GO, Blessing JA, Eddy GL, et al. A phase II trial of vincristine in advanced or recurrent endometrial carcinoma. A Gynecologic Oncology Group study. *Am J Clin Oncol* 1993;16:18.
526. Lincoln S, Blessing JA, Lee RB, et al. Activity of paclitaxel as second-line chemotherapy in endometrial carcinoma: a Gynecologic Oncology Group study. *Gynecol Oncol* 2003;88:277–281.
527. Woo HL, Swenerton KD, Hoskins PJ. Taxol is active in platinum-resistant endometrial adenocarcinoma. *Am J Clin Oncol* 1996;19:290–291.
528. Wadler S, Levy DE, Lincoln ST, et al. Topotecan is an active agent in the first-line treatment of metastatic or recurrent endometrial carcinoma: Eastern Cooperative Oncology Group Study E3E93. *J Clin Oncol* 2003; 21(11):2110–2114.
529. Alberts DS, Mason NL, O'Toole RV, et al. Doxorubicin-cisplatin-vinblastine combination chemotherapy of advanced endometrial carcinoma: a Southwest Oncology Group study. *Gynecol Oncol* 1987;26:193.
530. Barrett RJ, Blessing JA, Homesley HD, et al. Circadian-timed combination doxorubicin-cisplatin chemotherapy for advanced endometrial carcinoma. A phase II study of the Gynecologic Oncology Group. *Am J Clin Oncol* 1993;16:494–496.
531. Bruckner HW, Deppe G, et al. Combination chemotherapy of advanced endometrial adenocarcinoma with Adriamycin, cyclophosphamide, 5-fluorouracil, and medroxyprogesterone acetate. *Obstet Gynecol* 1977; 50:10s–12s.

532. Burke TW, Stringer CA, Morris M, et al. Prospective treatment of advanced or recurrent endometrial carcinoma with cisplatin, doxorubicin, and cyclophosphamide. *Gynecol Oncol* 1991;40:264.
533. Campora E, Vidali A, Mammoliti S, et al. Treatment of advanced or recurrent adenocarcinoma of the endometrium with doxorubicin and cyclophosphamide. *Eur J Gynaecol Oncol* 1990;11:181.
534. Cohen CJ, Bruckner HW, Deppe G, et al. Multidrug treatment of advanced and recurrent endometrial carcinoma: a Gynecologic Oncology Group study. *Obstet Gynecol* 1984;63:719–726.
535. Dunton CJ, Pfeifer SM, Braitman LE, et al. Treatment of advanced and recurrent endometrial cancer with cisplatin, doxorubicin, and cyclophosphamide. *Gynecol Oncol* 1991;41:113–116.
536. Hancock KC, Freedman RS, Edwards CL, et al. Use of cisplatin, doxorubicin, and cyclophosphamide to treat advanced and recurrent adenocarcinoma of the endometrium. *Cancer Treat Rep* 1986;70:789–791.
537. Long, H. J, Langdon RM. Phase II trial of methotrexate, vinblastine, doxorubicin, and cisplatin in advanced/recurrent endometrial carcinoma. *Gynecol Oncol* 1995;58:240–243.
538. Muggia FM, Chia G, Reed LJ, et al. Doxorubicin-cyclophosphamide: effective chemotherapy for advanced endometrial adenocarcinoma. *Am J Obstet Gynecol* 1977;128:314–319.
539. Pasmantier MW, Coleman M, Silver RT, et al. Treatment of advanced endometrial carcinoma with doxorubicin and cisplatin: effects on both untreated and previously treated patients. *Cancer Treat Rep* 1985;69: 539–542.
540. Piver MS, Fanning J, Baker TR. Phase II trial of cisplatin, Adriamycin, and etoposide for metastatic endometrial adenocarcinoma. *Am J Clin Oncol* 1991;14:200–202.
541. Seltzer V, Vogl SE, Kaplan BH. Adriamycin and cis-diamminedichloroplatinum in the treatment of metastatic endometrial adenocarcinoma. *Gynecol Oncol* 1984;19:308–313.
542. Seski JC, Edwards CL, Gershenson DM, et al. Doxorubicin and cyclophosphamide chemotherapy for disseminated endometrial cancer. *Obstet Gynecol* 1981;58:88–91.
543. Thigpen JT, Brady MF, Homesley HD, et al. Phase III trial of doxorubicin with or without cisplatin in advanced endometrial carcinoma: a Gynecologic Oncology Group study. *J Clin Oncol* 2004;22:3902–3908.
544. Tropë C, Johnsson JE, Simonsen E, et al. Treatment of recurrent endometrial adenocarcinoma with a combination of doxorubicin and cisplatin. *Am J Obstet Gynecol* 1984;149:379–381.
545. Gallion HH, Brunetto VL, Cibull M, et al. Randomized phase III trial of standard timed doxorubicin plus cisplatin versus circadian timed doxorubicin plus cisplatin in stage III and IV or recurrent endometrial carcinoma: A Gynecologic Oncology Group study. *J Clin Oncol* 2003;21: 3808–3813.
546. Fleming GF, Filiaci VL, Bentley RC, et al. Phase III randomized trial of doxorubicin + cisplatin versus doxorubicin + 24-h paclitaxel + filgrastim in endometrial carcinoma: a Gynecologic Oncology Group study. *Ann Oncol* 2004;15:1173–1178.
547. Fleming GF, Brunetto VL, Cella D, et al. Phase III trial of doxorubicin plus cisplatin with or without paclitaxel plus filgrastim in advanced endometrial carcinoma: a Gynecologic Oncology Group study. *J Clin Oncol* 2004;22:2159–2166.
548. Hoskins PJ, Swenerton KD, Pike JA, et al. Paclitaxel and carboplatin, alone or with irradiation, in advanced or recurrent endometrial cancer: a phase II study. *J Clin Oncol* 2001;19(20):4048–4053.
549. Sovak MA, Dupont J, Hensley ML, et al. Paclitaxel and carboplatin in the treatment of advanced or recurrent endometrial cancer: a large retrospective study. *Int J Gynecol Cancer* 2007;17:197–203.
550. Weber B, Mayer F, et al. What is the best chemotherapy regimen in recurrent or advanced endometrial carcinoma? Preliminary results. *Proc ASCO* 2003;22:1819; abst.
551. Bruckner HW, Deppe G. Combination chemotherapy of advanced endometrial adenocarcinoma with Adriamycin, cyclophosphamide, 5-fluorouracil, and medroxyprogesterone acetate. *Obstet Gynecol* 1977; 50:10s–12s.
552. Peralba JM, DeGraffenried L, Friedrichs W, et al. Pharmacodynamic evaluation of CCI-779, an inhibitor of mTOR, in cancer patients. *Clin Cancer Res* 2003;9:2887–2892.
553. Deppe G, Jacobs AJ, Bruckner H, et al. Chemotherapy of advanced and recurrent endometrial carcinoma with cyclophosphamide, doxorubicin, 5-fluorouracil, and megestrol acetate. *Am J Obstet Gynecol* 1981; 140:313–316.
554. Hoffman MS, Roberts WS, Cavanagh D, et al. Treatment of recurrent and metastatic endometrial cancer with cisplatin, doxorubicin, cyclophosphamide, and megestrol acetate. *Gynecol Oncol* 1989;35:75.
555. Horton J, Elson P, Gordon P, et al. Combination chemotherapy for advanced endometrial cancer. An evaluation of three regimens. *Cancer* 1982;49:2441–2445.
556. Lovecchio JL, Averette HE, Lichtinger M, et al. Treatment of advanced or recurrent endometrial adenocarcinoma with cyclophosphamide, doxorubicin, cis-platinum, and megestrol acetate. *Obstet Gynecol* 1984; 63:557–560.
557. Piver MS, Lele SB, Patsner B, et al. Melphalan, 5-fluorouracil, and medroxyprogesterone acetate in metastatic endometrial carcinoma. *Obstet Gynecol* 1986;67:261–264.
558. Mutter GL, Lin MC, Fitzgerald JT, et al. Altered *PTEN* expression as a diagnostic marker for the earliest endometrial precancers. *J Natl Cancer Inst* 2000;92:924–930.
559. An HJ, Lee YH, Cho NH, et al. Alteration of *PTEN* expression in endometrial carcinoma is associated with down-regulation of cyclin-dependent kinase inhibitor, p27. *Histopathology* 2002;41:437–445.
560. Vogelstein B, Kinzler KW. Cancer genes and the pathways they control. *Nat Med* 2004;10:789–799.
561. Zhou C, Gehrig PA, Whang YE, et al. Rapamycin inhibits telomerase activity by decreasing the hTERT mRNA level in endometrial cancer cells. *Mol Cancer Ther* 2003;2:789–795.
562. Dutcher JP. Mammalian target of rapamycin inhibition. *Clin Cancer Res* 2004;10(18 Pt 2):6382S–6387S.
563. Slomovitz BM, Broaddus RR, Schmandt R, et al. Expression of imatinib mesylate-targeted kinases in endometrial carcinoma. *Gynecol Oncol* 2004;95:32–36.
564. Coleman RL, Broaddus RR, Bodurka DC, et al. Phase II trial of imatinib mesylate in patients with recurrent platinum- and taxane-resistant epithelial ovarian and primary peritoneal cancers. *Gynecol Oncol* 2006;101: 126–131.
565. Albitar L, Laidler LL, Abdallah R, et al. Regulation of signaling phosphoproteins by epidermal growth factor and Iressa (ZD1839) in human endometrial cancer cells that model type I and II tumors. *Mol Cancer Ther* 2005;4:1891–1899.
566. Albitar L, Carter MB, Davies S, et al. Consequences of the loss of p53, RB1, and *PTEN*: relationship to gefitinib resistance in endometrial cancer. *Gynecol Oncol* 2007;106(1):94–104.
567. Santin AD, Zhan F, Bellone S, et al. Gene expression profiles in primary ovarian serous papillary tumors and normal ovarian epithelium: identification of candidate molecular markers for ovarian cancer diagnosis and therapy. *Int J Cancer* 2004;112:14–25.
568. Villella JA, Cohen S, Smith DH, et al. HER-2/neu overexpression in uterine papillary serous cancers and its possible therapeutic implications. *Int J Gynecol Cancer* 2006;16:1897–1902.
569. Santin AD, Zhan F, Cane S, et al. Gene expression fingerprint of uterine serous papillary carcinoma: identification of novel molecular markers for uterine serous cancer diagnosis and therapy. *Br J Cancer* 2005;92: 1561–1573.
570. Santin AD, Bellone S, Gokden M, et al. Overexpression of HER-2/neu in uterine serous papillary cancer. *Clin Cancer Res* 2002;8:1271–1279.
571. Bookman MA, Darcy KM, Clarke-Pearson D, et al. Evaluation of monoclonal humanized anti-HER2 antibody, trastuzumab, in patients with recurrent or refractory ovarian or primary peritoneal carcinoma with overexpression of HER2: a phase II trial of the Gynecologic Oncology Group. *J Clin Oncol* 2003;21:283–290.
572. Dvorak HF. Angiogenesis: update 2005. *J Thromb Haemost* 2005;3: 1835–1842.
573. Monk BJ, Han E, Josephs-Cowan CA, et al. Salvage bevacizumab (rhuMAB VEGF)-based therapy after multiple prior cytotoxic regimens in advanced refractory epithelial ovarian cancer. *Gynecol Oncol* 2006;102:140–144.
574. Numnum TM, Rocconi RP, Whitworth J, et al. The use of bevacizumab to palliate symptomatic ascites in patients with refractory ovarian carcinoma. *Gynecol Oncol* 2006;102:425–428.
575. Ma WW, Jimeno A. Strategies for suppressing angiogenesis in gynecological cancers. *Drugs Today (Barc)* 2007;43:259–273.
576. Salvesen HB, Iversen OE, Akslen LA. Independent prognostic importance of microvessel density in endometrial carcinoma. *Br J Cancer* 1998;77: 1140–1144.
577. Lee CN, Cheng WF, Chen CA, et al. Angiogenesis of endometrial carcinomas assessed by measurement of intratumoral blood flow, microvessel density, and vascular endothelial growth factor levels. *Obstet Gynecol* 2000;96:615–621.
578. Talvensaari-Mattila A, Soini Y, Santala M. VEGF and its receptors (flt-1 and KDR/flk-1) as prognostic indicators in endometrial carcinoma. *Tumour Biol* 2005;26:81–87.
579. McMeekin DS, Sill MW, Darcy KM, et al. A phase II trial of thalidomide in patients with refractory endometrial cancer and correlation with angiogenesis biomarkers: a Gynecologic Oncology Group study. *Gynecol Oncol* 2007;105:508–516.
580. Zanotti KM, Belinson JL, Kennedy AW, et al. The use of paclitaxel and platinum-based chemotherapy in uterine papillary serous carcinoma. *Gynecol Oncol* 1999;74:272–277.
581. Ramondetta L, Burke TW, Levenback C, et al. Treatment of uterine papillary serous carcinoma with paclitaxel. *Gynecol Oncol* 2001;82:156–161.
582. Gehrig PA. Uterine papillary serous carcinoma: a review. *Expert Opin Pharmacother* 2007;8:809–816.
583. Low JS, Wong EH, Tan HS, et al. Adjuvant sequential chemotherapy and radiotherapy in uterine papillary serous carcinoma. *Gynecol Oncol* 2005;97:171–177.
584. Gadducci A, Cosio S, Genazzani AR. Old and new perspectives in the pharmacological treatment of advanced or recurrent endometrial cancer: hormonal therapy, chemotherapy and molecularly targeted therapies. *Crit Rev Oncol Hematol* 2006;58:242–256.
585. Carbone PP, Carter SK. Endometrial cancer: approach to development of effective chemotherapy. *Gynecol Oncol* 1974;2:348–353.

586. Barton C, Buxton EJ, Blachledge G, et al. A phase II study of ifosfamide in endometrial cancer. *Cancer Chemother Pharmacol* 1990;26(Suppl):S4.
587. Sutton GP, Blessing JA, Homesley HD, et al. Phase II study of ifosfamide and mesna in refractory adenocarcinoma of the endometrium. A Gynecologic Oncology Group study. *Cancer* 1994;73:1453–1455.
588. Seski JC, Edwards CL, Copeland LJ, et al. Hexamethylmelamine chemotherapy for disseminated endometrial cancer. *Obstet Gynecol* 1981;58:361–363.
589. Thigpen JT, Blessing JA, Ball H, et al. Hexamethylmelamine as first-line therapy in the treatment of advanced or recurrent carcinoma of the endometrium: a phase II trial of the Gynecologic Oncology Group. *Gynecol Oncol* 1988;31:435–438.
590. Chauvergne J, Fumoleau P, Cappelaere P, et al. Phase II study of pirarubicin (THP) in patients with cervical, endometrial and ovarian cancer: study of the Clinical Screening Group of the European Organization for Research and Treatment of Cancer (EORTC). *Eur J Cancer* 1993;29A:350–354.
591. Boadle DJ, Tattersall MH. Phase II study of mitoxantrone in advanced or metastatic endometrial carcinoma. *Aust N Z J Obstet Gynaecol* 1987;27:341–342.
592. Hilgers RD, Von Hoff DD, Stephens RL, et al. Mitoxantrone in adenocarcinoma of the endometrium: a Southwest Oncology Group study. *Cancer Treat Rep* 1985;69:1329–1330.
593. Muss HB, Bundy BN, DiSaia PJ, et al. Mitoxantrone for carcinoma of the endometrium: a phase II trial of the Gynecologic Oncology Group. *Cancer Treat Rep* 1987;71:217–218.
594. Thigpen JT, Kronmal R, Vogel S, et al. A phase II trial of vinblastine in patients with advanced or recurrent endometrial carcinoma. A Southwest Oncology Group study. *Am J Clin Oncol* 1987;10:429–431.
595. Slayton RE, Blessing JA, Delgado G. Phase II trial of etoposide in the management of advanced or recurrent endometrial carcinoma: a Gynecologic Oncology Group study. *Cancer Treat Rep* 1982;66:1669–1671.
596. Muss HB, Bundy BN, Adcock L. Teniposide (VM-26) in patients with advanced endometrial carcinoma. A phase II trial of the Gynecologic Oncology Group. *Am J Clin Oncol* 1991;14:36–37.
597. Malviya VK, Liu PY, O'Toole R, et al. Phase II trial of amonafide in patients with advanced metastatic or recurrent endometrial adenocarcinoma. A Southwest Oncology Group study. *Am J Clin Oncol* 1994;17:37–40.
598. Hilgers RD, Legha SS, Johnson GA Jr, et al. m-AMSA and adenocarcinoma of the endometrium. A Southwest Oncology Group study. *Invest New Drugs* 1984;2:335–338.
599. Muss HB, Blessing JA, DuBeshter B. Echinomycin in recurrent and metastatic endometrial carcinoma. A phase II trial of the Gynecologic Oncology Group. *Am J Clin Oncol* 1993;16:492–493.
600. Slayton R, Faraggi D. A phase II clinical trial of methly-glyoxal-bisguanylhydrazone (MGBG) in advanced endometrial cancer. *Proc Am Soc Clin Oncol* 1986;5:119.
601. Thigpen JT, Blessing JA, Homesley HD, et al. Phase II trial of peperazinedione in the treatment of advanced or recurrent endometrial carcinoma. A Gynecologic Oncology Group study. *Am J Clin Oncol* 1986;9:21.
602. Homesley HD, Blessing JA, Conroy J, et al. ICRF-159 (razoxane) in patients with advanced adenocarcinoma of the endometrium. A Gynecologic Oncology Group study. *Am J Clin Oncol* 1986;9:325–326.
603. Omura GA, Shingleton HM, Creasman WT, et al. Chemotherapy of gynecologic cancer with nitrosoureas: a randomized trial of CCNU and methyl-CCNU in cancers of the cervix, corpus, vagina, and vulva. *Cancer Treat Rep* 1978;62:833–835.

CHAPTER 24 ■ CORPUS: MESENCHYMAL TUMORS

GREGORY SUTTON, JOHN KAVANAGH, AARON WOLFSON, AND CARMEN TORNOS

Uterine sarcomas are rare malignancies accounting for as few as 6% of the estimated over 40,000 cases of cancer of the uterine corpus in the United States in 2009 (1). In contrast to the generally favorable prognosis in endometrial adenocarcinomas, uterine sarcomas are generally aggressive; overall mortality rates approached 90% in early reports (2). In a 1997 Norwegian survey, uterine sarcomas accounted for 26% of all deaths from uterine malignancies (3). Uterine sarcomas encompass a broad spectrum of neoplasms from pure mesenchymal tumors and endometrial stromal tumors (leiomyosarcomas and endometrial stromal sarcomas) to mixed epithelial/stromal tumors such as adenosarcoma and carcinosarcoma. Several classification systems exist (4), most of which are based upon the original work of Ober (5); the World Health Organization histologic classification system of uterine sarcomas is summarized in Table 24.1.

EPIDEMIOLOGY AND RISK FACTORS

Leiomyosarcoma and Carcinosarcoma

The two major sarcomas, leiomyosarcoma and carcinosarcoma, are distinguishable in several ways including clinical presentation, spread patterns, mean age at diagnosis, racial distribution, apparent relative incidence, method of diagnosis, and history of prior radiotherapy.

Median Age at Diagnosis

Figure 24.1 demonstrates mean ages at diagnosis for common uterine sarcomas and endometrial adenocarcinomas. Patients with carcinosarcomas are on the average older (mean 65 [2], 67 [6] years) than those with endometrial adenocarcinomas (mean 59.1 years [7]), müllerian adenosarcomas (mean 57.4 [8], 58 [9] years), leiomyosarcomas (mean 53.5 [1], 55 [10, 11, 56.2 [12] years), and endometrial stromal tumors (mean 41 [13], 46 [14], 48 [15] years). Olah et al. (6) observed a bimodal age distribution among 423 cases of uterine sarcoma; they attributed this to a premenopausal peak for patients with leiomyosarcomas and a postmenopausal maximum for those with carcinosarcomas. Thus, many patients with carcinosarcomas are postmenopausal, whereas those with leiomyosarcomas may be premenopausal or perimenopausal at the time of diagnosis. In a review of 208 patients with leiomyosarcomas from the Mayo Clinic (11), only 41% were postmenopausal.

Racial Distribution

Zelmanowicz et al. (16) are the most recent investigators to note that women with carcinosarcomas are more likely to be of African American descent (among 453 patients and controls, 28% versus 4%, $p = 0.001$) than those with endometrial adenocarcinomas. In the reviews of Mortel et al. and Norris et al. (17,18), 33% and 24% of patients with carcinosarcomas were nonwhite, respectively. Brooks et al. (12) reported that the age-adjusted incidence of uterine sarcomas in African American women was twice that of controls. The age-adjusted incidences of leiomyosarcomas for black and white women, respectively, were 1.5 and 0.9 per 100,000. Those for carcinosarcomas in black and white women, respectively, were 4.3 and 1.7 per 100,000.

Relative Incidence

Carcinosarcomas and leiomyosarcomas constitute about 4% and 1.5% of all uterine malignancies in clinical series, respectively (6). Echt et al. (19) reported on 66 patients diagnosed with uterine sarcomas over a 21-year period at the University of Southern California and found carcinosarcomas in 48%, leiomyosarcomas in 36%, and endometrial stromal sarcomas in 15%. Because the risk profile of carcinosarcomas so closely parallels that of endometrial adenocarcinomas with regard to obesity, diabetes, anovulation, and low parity, Silverberg et al. (20) have suggested that they be regarded as "metaplastic" endometrial carcinomas instead of true sarcomas. Many other pathologists agree with this notion (21).

In series of uterine sarcomas referred for histopathologic diagnosis, leiomyosarcomas are seen more commonly than carcinosarcomas. The differentiation between benign, malignant, and "of uncertain malignant potential" smooth muscle tumors is more subtle than the diagnosis of carcinosarcoma.

Prior Radiotherapy

Although as many as a third of patients with carcinosarcomas in some series have a history of antecedent pelvic radiotherapy, this is rarely, if ever, an etiologic factor in patients with leiomyosarcoma of the uterus. Christopherson et al. (22) described two cases among 33 patients with uterine leiomyosarcoma who had a history of radiotherapy. In the series of carcinosarcomas reported by Norris et al. (18), 9 of 31 patients (29%) had received pelvic radiotherapy from 7 to 26 years prior to diagnosis. Among 1,208 uterine malignancies in the report by Meredith et al. (23), 30, or 2.4%, occurred in patients exposed to pelvic radiotherapy. Only 8 of these 30 patients had been irradiated for a gynecologic malignancy, with the others

TABLE 24.1

WORLD HEALTH ORGANIZATION CLASSIFICATION SYSTEM OF UTERINE SARCOMAS

MESENCHYMAL TUMORS
Endometrial stromal and related tumors
Endometrial stromal sarcoma, low grade
Endometrial stromal nodule
Undifferentiated endometrial sarcoma
Smooth muscle tumors
Leiomyosarcoma
Epithelioid variant
Myxoid variant
Smooth muscle tumor of uncertain malignant potential
Leiomyoma, not otherwise specified
Histologic variants
Mitotically active variant
Cellular variant
Hemorrhagic cellular variant
Epithelioid variant
Myxoid
Atypical variant
Lipoleiomyoma variant
Growth pattern variants
Diffuse leiomyomatosis
Dissecting leiomyoma
Intravenous leiomyomatosis
Metastasizing leiomyoma
Miscellaneous mesenchymal tumors
Mixed endometrial stromal and smooth muscle tumor
Perivascular epithelioid cell tumor
Adenomatoid tumor
Other malignant mesenchymal tumors
Other benign mesenchymal tumors
MIXED EPITHELIAL AND MESENCHYMAL TUMORS
Carcinosarcoma (malignant müllerian mixed tumor, metaplastic carcinoma)
Adenosarcoma
Carcinofibroma
Adenofibroma
Adenomyoma
Atypical polypoid variant

being treated for uterine bleeding, polyps, or fibroids. Of irradiated patients, five (17%) developed carcinosarcomas, for a crude association of 11%. The risk of endometrial adenocarcinoma arising after radiation was 2%. It has been suggested that postirradiation carcinosarcomas occur at a younger average age than those arising *de novo* (24). Latency to diagnosis of malignancy is generally shorter in older patients, however (23). Carcinosarcomas in previously irradiated patients also tend to present in advanced stage, perhaps because radiotherapy is often associated with cervical stenosis and, thus, no telltale uterine bleeding.

Müllerian Adenosarcoma

Clinically, these neoplasms occur in women aged 14 to 89 years (median 58 years) (25), with no racial predilection or noteworthy reproductive characteristics. The most common symptoms were bleeding, pelvic pain, prolapse, and vaginal discharge. On clinical examination, about 40% of patients had tissue protruding from the cervical os (25). In the series of Clement and Scully, five patients had a history of radiation therapy 8 to 30 years before diagnosis. In 1996 Clement et al. (9) reported six patients who developed müllerian adenosarcomas of the uterine corpus after taking tamoxifen for periods of 6 months to 4 years. An additional such case was reported by Bocklage et al (26).

CLINICAL PRESENTATION

Vaginal bleeding is the most common presenting symptom in women with uterine sarcomas in general (27,28) and is nearly universal in those with carcinosarcomas (29). Vaginal bleeding occurs in as few as 40% of women with leiomyosarcomas, however. A typical presentation of carcinosarcoma is vaginal bleeding associated with a protuberant, fleshy mass from the cervix. Uterine enlargement is common with carcinosarcomas. These neoplasms arise in the endometrial lining but often grow in an exophytic pattern within the endometrial cavity (Fig. 24.2). Bleeding and uterine cramping are common.

Uterine enlargement and a presumptive diagnosis of uterine *leiomyomata* are nearly universal findings in patients with leiomyosarcoma (Figs. 24.3 and 24.4). The incidence of leiomyosarcoma in all patients with a clinical picture of myomas is less than 1% but increases with age to slightly over 1% in the sixth decade of life (30).

DIAGNOSIS AND EVALUATION

Whereas the diagnosis of carcinosarcoma is confirmed, or at least suggested, at the time of endometrial biopsy or curettage, leiomyosarcomas are rarely diagnosed before hysterectomy (11). Although positron emission tomography and magnetic resonance imaging offer the potential of differentiating between benign and malignant smooth muscle tumors of the uterus, these techniques are not sufficiently sensitive and specific at the present time.

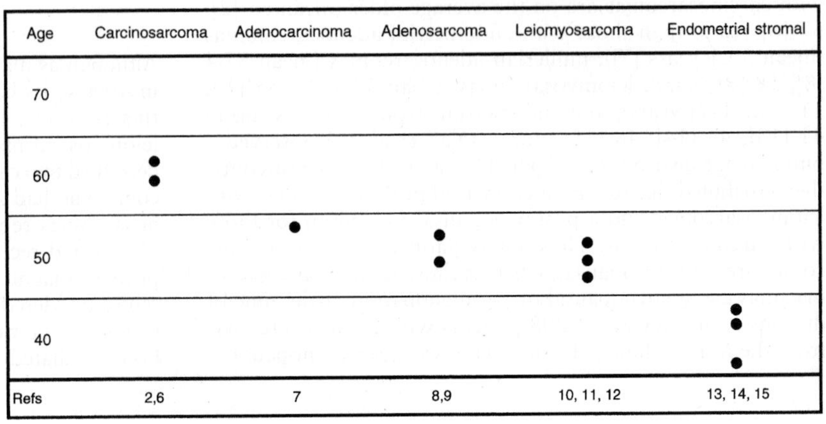

Age	Carcinosarcoma	Adenocarcinoma	Adenosarcoma	Leiomyosarcoma	Endometrial stromal
70					
60	• •				
50		•	• •	• • •	
40					• • •
Refs	2,6	7	8,9	10, 11, 12	13, 14, 15

FIGURE 24.1. Mean age at diagnosis of common uterine sarcomas and endometrial adenocarcinomas.

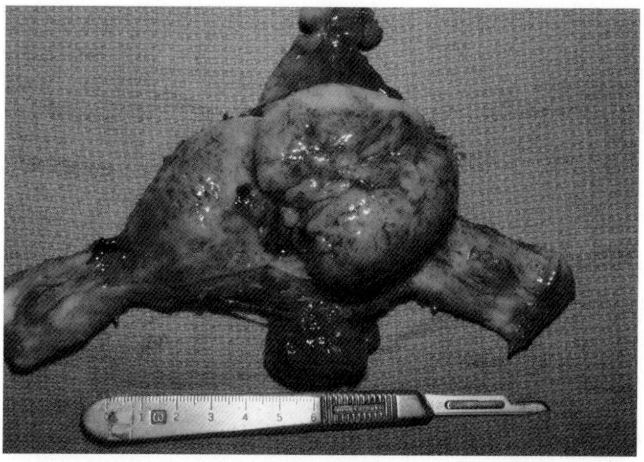

FIGURE 24.2. Exophytic pattern of growth in carcinosarcoma.

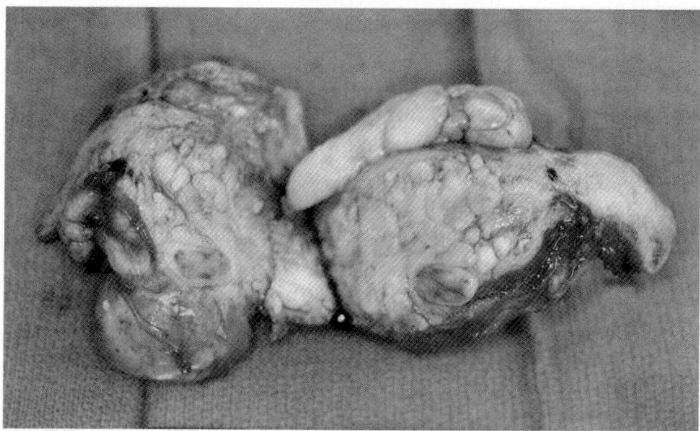

FIGURE 24.4. Leiomyosarcoma, gross, showing heterogenous appearance.

Berchuck et al. reported that in 14 patients with leiomyosarcomas undergoing dilatation and curettage, a prehysterectomy diagnosis was made in only 8 (31). Although the diagnosis of carcinosarcoma may be missed because endometrial biopsy or curettage does not adequately sample both the epithelial and stromal components of the tumor, appropriate preoperative referral is made because of the presence of a malignancy, and staging is accomplished at the time of hysterectomy. Conversely, most leiomyosarcomas are diagnosed after hysterectomy at the time of histologic review of the surgical specimen. Referral and disposition decisions are therefore made *a posteriori*. More often than not, staging is omitted from the initial procedure. This dichotomy in the presentation of the two main uterine sarcomas was highlighted in a staging study published by the Gynecologic Oncology Group (GOG) (32). Far fewer patients with leiomyosarcomas were referred for enrollment in the study than those with the diagnosis of carcinosarcoma (301 carcinosarcomas, 59 leiomyosarcomas, and 93 endometrial stromal tumors and adenosarcomas). Restaging after primary surgery may have been an obstacle to entry of patients with leiomyosarcoma. In fact, the investigators who performed this study, Major et al. (32), deigned that "[i]n light of the small number of leiomyosarcoma cases with positive lymph nodes, re-exploration [*solely for staging*] is not recommended in patients with leiomyosarcomas."

Patients with uterine carcinosarcomas, much like high-grade endometrial lesions, unless presenting with clinical metastases, should be managed in referral centers where appropriate surgical staging can be performed. Although vaginal sonography and magnetic resonance imaging may reveal myometrial involvement, the frequency of occult nodal, omental, and peritoneal metastases makes appropriate surgical evaluation paramount. Yamada et al. (33) underscored this fact in their staging study of 62 patients, 38 (61%) of whom had surgically detected extrauterine metastases.

Since the most common sites of metastases for uterine sarcomas other than leiomyosarcoma are pelvic and para-aortic lymph nodes, studies such as computed tomography (CT) of the abdomen and pelvis are probably not justified in patients with clinical stages I and II disease; on the other hand, if an extensive uterine mass is present, these evaluations may identify findings that suggest a palliative rather than curative approach to the patient. Radionuclide bone scans and imaging of the brain are of little value in the absence of pulmonary metastases. Preoperative radiographs are helpful in excluding pulmonary metastases and are often medically indicated in patients of advanced age or with compromised health. The utility of chest tomography in uterine sarcomas has not been formally addressed but should be considered in patients with high-grade lesions, especially if there is evidence that palliation rather than curative therapy would be appropriate.

Porter et al. (34) reviewed 600 patients with nonthoracic T2 soft-tissue sarcomas and concluded that routine chest CT identified metastases in 19.2% of patients but at a cost of $27,594 per patient with metastases. If scanning were limited to patients with high-grade histologies only, the cost per patient with metastases was reduced to $418 per patient with metastases. Since no specific data are in place for uterine sarcomas, CT scanning may be indicated in patients with high-grade sarcomas to determine extent of surgery.

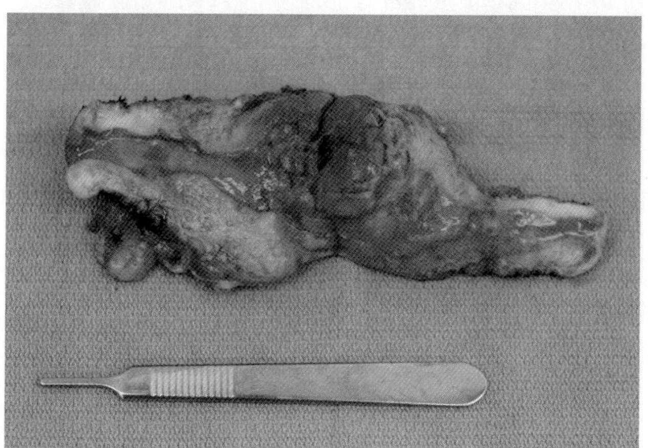

FIGURE 24.3. Leiomyosarcoma, gross.

STAGING AND NODAL INVOLVEMENT

By convention, the 1988 International Federation of Obstetrics and Gynecology (FIGO) staging criteria for endometrial cancer (see Table 23.4) are used to assign stages in uterine sarcomas.

Whereas carcinosarcomas, like endometrial adenocarcinomas, commonly metastasize to pelvic or para-aortic lymph nodes, leiomyosarcomas rarely spread to nodal sites. In the review of 203 stage I and II carcinosarcomas surgically staged as part of a GOG study reported by Silverberg et al. (20), nodal metastases were detected in 34 cases (16.7%). Nearly all subjects had lymphatic or vascular involvement in the myometrium; lymphatic channel involvement was a much better predictor of nodal metastases than tumor grade or mitotic index. Doss et al. (2) confirmed that pelvic lymph nodes were the most common site of metastasis in carcinosarcomas, and others have confirmed a rate of nodal spread in clinically localized disease between 13.2% and 31.0% (33,35).

Multiple nodal metastases were noted in 66% of patients with any nodal spread in Chen's report (36), and Norris et al. (18) described lymph node disease in 90% of fatal cases.

Lymph node metastases were identified in only 3.5% of patients with clinically localized leiomyosarcomas at the time of surgical staging in the GOG study reported by Major et al. (32). In the recent Mayo Clinic series (11), 4 of 36 (11%) patients had nodal spread, but only 1 of these (2.6%) had isolated nodal metastases. Data from three series (28,30,37) indicate that lymph nodes were histologically positive only if clinically enlarged or associated with obvious intra-abdominal spread. Thus, the need for lymph node dissection in patients with leiomyosarcomas remains unsubstantiated.

Among patients with müllerian adenosarcomas who underwent surgical staging including lymph node sampling (38), 20% were found to have spread outside the uterus to involve lymph nodes, vagina, parametrium, ovary, and malignant peritoneal washings. Similar yields are reported for endometrial stromal sarcomas.

PATHOLOGY

Malignant mesenchymal tumors can be classified into pure mesenchymal tumors and tumors with a mixed epithelial and mesenchymal components. In the first group the most common is leiomyosarcoma, followed by endometrial stromal sarcoma, and rarely others including rhabdomyosarcoma, liposarcoma, angiosarcoma, chondrosarcoma, osteosarcoma, and alveolar soft part sarcoma. Mixed epithelial and mesenchymal tumors include carcinosarcoma and adenosarcoma. In addition, there are two rare mesenchymal tumors occurring in the uterus: uterine tumors resembling ovarian sex-cord tumors (UTROSCTs) and perivascular epithelioid cell tumors (PEComas).

Leiomyosarcoma and Other Smooth Muscle Tumors

Leiomyosarcomas are malignant smooth muscle tumors that usually arise *de novo*. Recent studies have shown that some tumors show areas with benign morphology, suggesting some progression from leiomyoma to leiomyosarcoma (39) but clonality studies only support this progression in a small percentage of cases (40). Unlike leiomyoma, leiomyosarcoma is rarely a solitary poorly circumscribed mass with a soft and fleshy consistency. The cut surface is variegated with gray areas intermixed with yellow areas of necrosis and sometimes hemorrhagic areas. The epicenter of the tumor is the myometrium and most leiomyosarcomas are intramural. Occasionally, they can extend into the cervix or beyond the uterus (Fig. 24.5).

Microscopically, most leiomyosarcomas are overtly malignant and have hypercellularity, coagulative tumor cell necrosis, abundant mitoses (more than 10/10 high power fields [hpf]), atypical mitoses, marked cytologic atypia, and infiltrative borders (Fig 24.6). Some cases lack some of these features, and occasionally the differential diagnosis between a benign and a malignant lesion can be controversial. The three most important criteria are coagulative tumor cell necrosis, high mitotic rate, and significant cytologic atypia (41). Coagulative tumor cell necrosis (FCN) has an abrupt transition from viable to necrotic tissue (Fig. 24.7). In contrast, the hyaline necrosis seen in some leiomyomas has an area of hyalinized

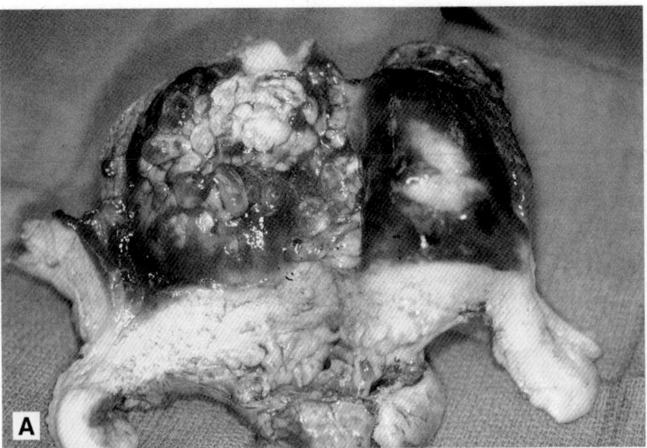

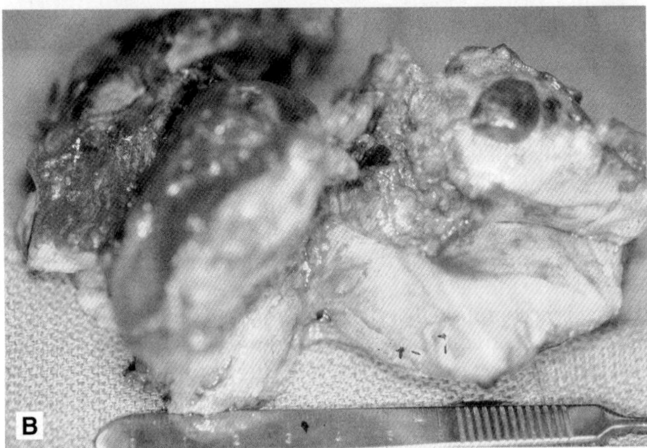

FIGURE 24.5. Leiomyosarcoma, gross, with extension beyond uterus.

tissue between the necrotic and viable tumor. Some smooth muscle tumors have histologic features that are not worrisome enough to render an unequivocal diagnosis of sarcoma. These tumors can be classified as atypical leiomyomas, smooth muscle tumors with low malignant potential (low probability of an unfavorable outcome), or smooth muscle tumors of uncertain malignant potential (STUMP) (insufficient numbers have been studied to predict their behavior). Figure 24.8 summarizes the classification of uterine smooth muscle tumors based on their histologic characteristics. This classification is based in large part upon a large retrospective study from Stanford

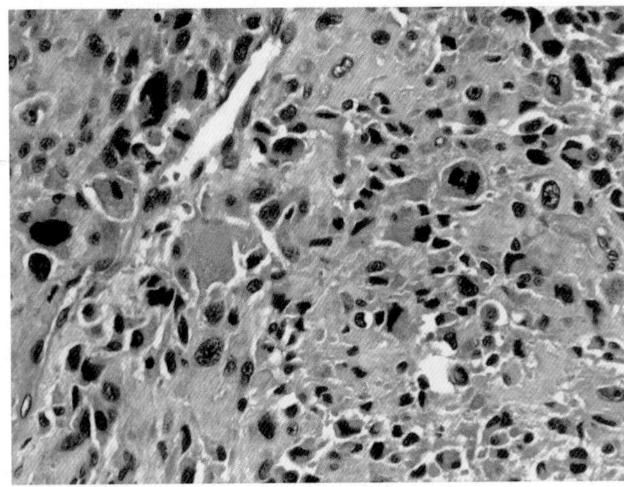

FIGURE 24.6. Leiomyosarcoma, microscopic.

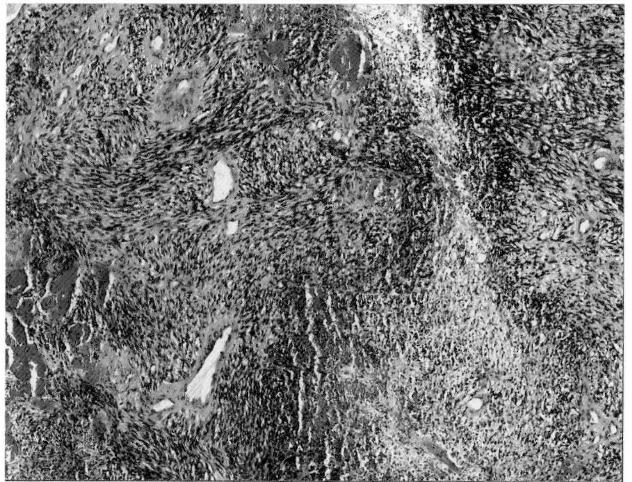

FIGURE 24.7. Leiomyosarcoma, microscopic, with abrupt transition from viable to necrotic tissue.

University published in 1994 (39), the largest to date. A multi-institutional study of 77 leiomyosarcomas presented at the United States Clinical and Anatomic Pathology meeting in 2006 (42) reported three leiomyosarcomas with minimal atypia and no tumor cell necrosis. This same study found the presence of tumor cell necrosis coexisting with areas of hyaline necrosis typical of leiomyosarcomas. Tumors that clinically and pathologically appear to be leiomyomas but have up to 15 mitoses per 10 hpf behave in a benign fashion and are classified as mitotically active leiomyomas (43,44). Leiomyomas are more likely to have a high mitotic count if they are excised during the secretory phase of the menstrual cycle, during pregnancy, or while patients are receiving exogenous progesterone therapy.

There are some tumors that are not represented in Figure 24.8, for example, tumors without tumor necrosis, with focal or multifocal atypia, and with more than 20 mitoses per 10 hpf. These tumors are rare but some behave as sarcomas (42). Since there are few of these cases reported they should be considered at least STUMPs. There are tumors that lack one of the three major diagnostic criteria (mitoses, atypia, necrosis) but have other worrisome features such as infiltrative borders, lymphovascular invasion, or atypical mitoses. Classification of such cases is always problematic. It is recommended that these unusual cases be reviewed by a gynecologic pathologist.

Infarcted necrosis of benign leiomyomas can be seen sometimes during pregnancy, after uterine artery embolization, thermal balloon endometrial ablation, therapy with tranexamic acid, or therapy with high-dose progestins. In addition, pedunculated submucosal leiomyomas can undergo spontaneous torsion, and infarction, even with protrusion through the cervix. Infarcted leiomyomas should not be confused with leiomyosarcoma. The infarcted necrosis is not tumor cell necrosis, as mentioned before. In addition, infarcted leiomyomas are not associated with significant cytologic atypia, high mitotic rate, atypical mitoses, or invasive borders. An accurate clinical history can be very useful in many of these cases.

Classification critieria of smooth muscle tumors with either myxoid or epithelioid features differ from those used for spindle cell tumors. Epithelioid tumors have cells that are round rather than spindle shaped and have round nuclei mimicking epithelial cells (hence the term "epithelioid") (Fig. 24.9). Epithelioid leiomyosarcomas have significant cytologic atypia, at least three mitoses per 10 hpf and tumor cell necrosis in 50% of cases (45). At least one previous study suggests that epithelioid tumors may behave more aggressively than spindle cell tumors and have a higher tendency to metastasize (46).

Myxoid leiomyosarcomas are rare and may be deceiving because of minimal atypia and a low mitotic rate. However, they are always infiltrative and this feature can be used to render the diagnosis of sarcoma (Fig. 24.10). Lymphovascular invasion is also indicative of malignancy. Myxoid leiomyosarcoma has a clinical behavior similar to other leiomyosarcomas (47,48).

Histologic parameters of leiomyosarcomas that have been shown to be prognostic indicators include grade, mitotic rate, extensive tumor cell necrosis, and lymphovascular invasion. However, multivariate analyses from large studies vary in their

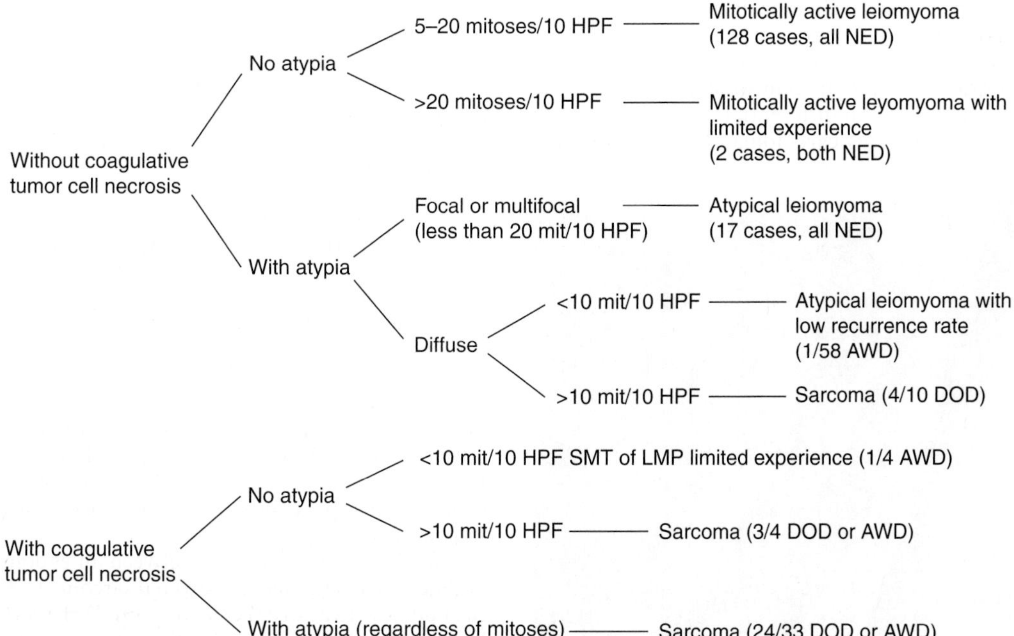

FIGURE 24.8. Uterine smooth muscle tumors (excluding epithelioid and myxoid types and cervical tumors). *Note:* AWD, alive with disease; DOD, dead of disease; HPF, high power fields; LMP, low malignant potential; NED, no evidence of disease; SMT, smooth muscle tumor.

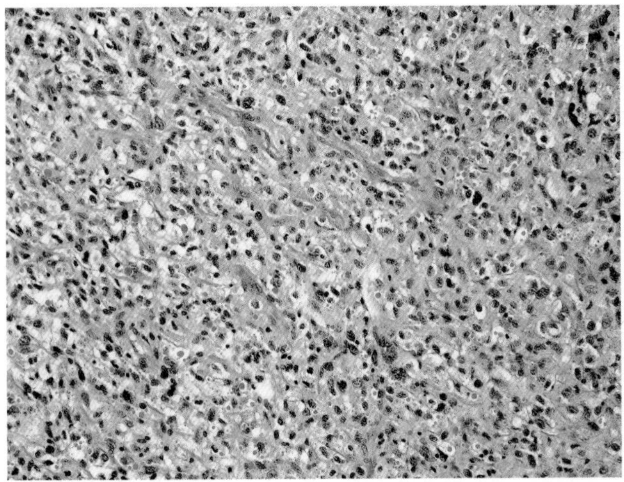

FIGURE 24.9. Epithelioid leiomyosarcoma, microscopic appearance.

results (11,49). Estrogen and progesterone receptors are expressed in a large percentage of leiomyosarcomas (38% to 60%), but this does not seem to correlate with overall survival (50,51), nor does it suggest that hormonal therapy is beneficial.

Carcinosarcoma

Uterine carcinosarcomas, also called malignant mixed müllerian tumors, are lesions containing carcinomatous and sarcomatous elements (Fig. 24.11). Numerous studies have shown that these tumors are clonal malignancies derived from a single stem cell (52–54) and should be considered "metaplastic carcinomas."

Most carcinosarcomas are polypoid tumors that fill the endometrial cavity and may protrude through the cervical os (Fig. 24.12). The tumors are soft and fleshy with areas of necrosis and hemorrhage. Occasionally, they show gross myometrial invasion, and may extend into or through the cervix. The size of the tumor is quite variable and may range from less than 2 cm to over 20 cm in diameter.

Microscopically, the tumors have a typical biphasic pattern with carcinomatous and sarcomatous elements. The carcinoma is usually high grade and reminiscent of serous carcinoma, although some cases have undifferentiated, endometrioid, clear cell, or even squamous carcinoma. The sarcomatous

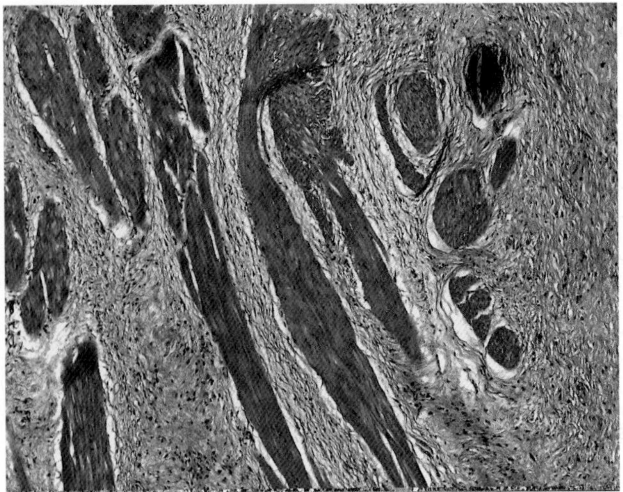

FIGURE 24.10. Myxoid leiomyosarcoma, microscopic appearance.

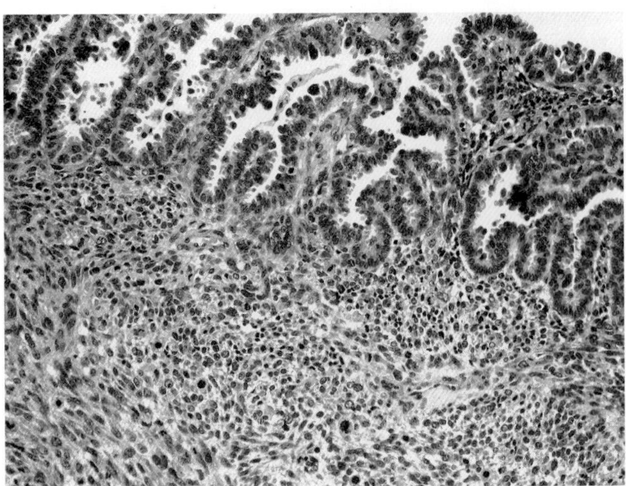

FIGURE 24.11. Carcinosarcoma, microscopic appearance.

component is always high grade and may be homologous or heterologous. In homologous tumors, the sarcomatous component is usually high-grade fibrosarcoma, although varieties such as leiomyosarcoma, malignant fibrous histiocytoma, or undifferentiated sarcoma may be found as well. Heterologous elements are seen in half of the cases. The most common heterologous sarcoma is rhabdomyosarcoma, followed by chondrosarcoma, and less often osteosarcoma and liposarcoma (55). Most carcinosarcomas have myometrial invasion (85% in a recent study), most commonly into less than half of the wall (55). Lymphovascular invasion is present in 60% (55) and the carcinomatous element is usually the component invading myometrium and lymphovascular spaces.

Most studies suggest that the behavior of carcinosarcomas is predicted by the carcinomatous component. Tumors typically metastasize through lymphatic channels similar to endometrial carcinomas. Most metastases and recurrences are composed of pure carcinoma (20,56,57). In two recent studies, adverse prognostic factors included heterologous elements (in stage I tumors) and a high percentage of sarcomatous components in the main tumor and in the recurrences (55,58); these factors did not affect prognosis according to other studies (20,59–61).

Müllerian carcinosarcomas may arise in extrauterine sites. Most cases have been reported in the peritoneum (62–65) or retroperitoneum (66,67). Some cases occur at the site of previous radiotherapy, and some cases arise in areas of endometriosis (67).

Endometrial Stromal Neoplasms

In the current World Health Organization classification, endometrial stromal tumors are classified into endometrial stromal nodules, endometrial stromal sarcomas (by definition low grade), and undifferentiated endometrial sarcoma. Both endometrial stromal nodules and endometrial stromal sarcomas are composed of cells identical to those found in the stroma of proliferative endometrium. Undifferentiated endometrial sarcomas, on the other hand, are high-grade sarcomas that do not resemble endometrial stroma and diagnosis is by excluding other uterine sarcomas.

The differential diagnosis between an endometrial stromal nodule and an endometrial stromal sarcoma is important since the nodules are always benign lesions. Differential diagnosis is based upon the presence of infiltrating margins with or without angioinvasion in endometrial stromal sarcoma. These two features are not seen in stromal nodules, which are always well circumscribed and have pushing margins (68). It is impossible

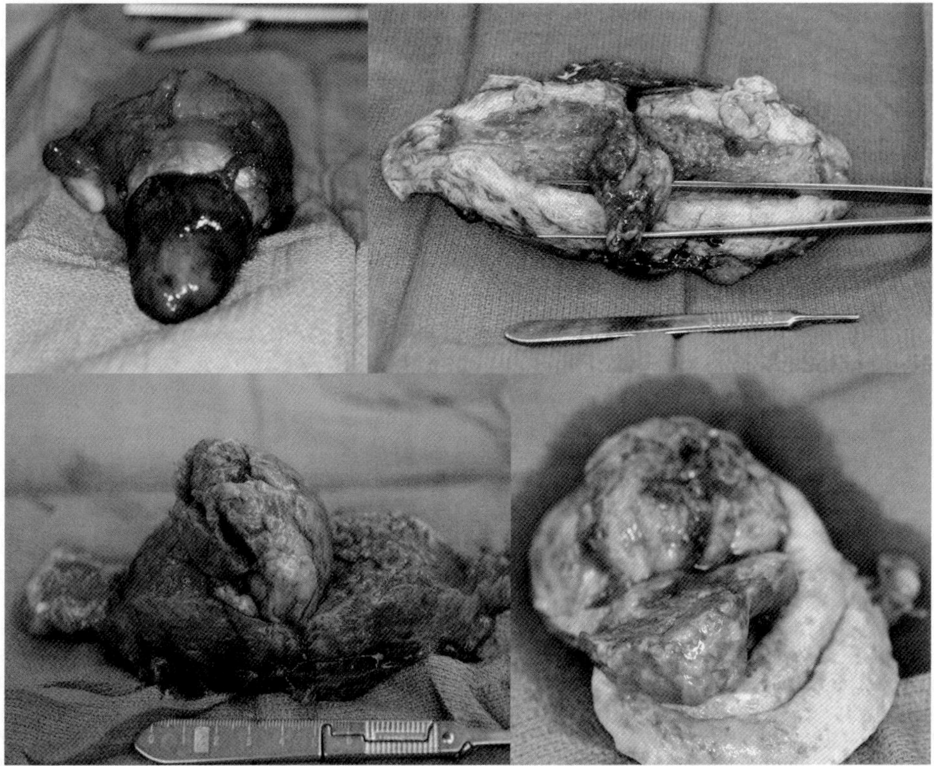

FIGURE 24.12. Carcinosarcomas, gross photographs of four cases demonstrating polypoid nature of lesions.

to render a definitive diagnosis based upon curettage material alone; final diagnosis requires a hysterectomy specimen. If the patient is young and wants to preserve fertility, a combination of diagnostic imaging and hysteroscopy must be used to monitor tumor growth and direct excision (69).

Stromal Nodule

Stromal nodules are by far the least common of the pure endometrial stromal neoplasms. They are usually solitary masses with diameter varying from 1.2 to 22 cm with an average of 7.1 cm (70).

On cut section, endometrial stromal nodules are fleshy and often tan-yellow. Microscopically, they are composed of uniform bland, small cells resembling normal endometrial stromal cells with fusiform nuclei and scant cytoplasm. Abundant arterioles reminiscent of the spiral arterioles of the normal endometrium are also present. The mitotic rate is low, with most tumors having fewer than five mitoses per 10 hpf. Most endometrial stromal nodules are cellular, and some have variable amounts of intercellular collagen, which occasionally forms dense collagen bands or nodules (Fig. 24.13). Another common finding is the presence of clusters of foamy histiocytes within the tumor. The borders between the tumor and the adjacent myometrium are microscopically well defined (pushing). Occasionally, they may have more irregular borders with minimal areas of tumor extending into adjacent myometrium, usually within 3 mm of the main tumor mass (70,71). Endometrial stromal nodules lack associated lymphovascular invasion. Other changes that can be seen in endometrial stromal nodules include smooth muscle metaplasia, cystic degeneration, sex-cord–like areas, and necrosis.

Endometrial stromal nodules may be confused with cellular leiomyomas. Since both tumors are benign, the misdiagnosis of one for the other is probably of no clinical consequence as long as the tumor is found in a hysterectomy specimen. If the tumor is found in a curettage specimen, it is impossible for the pathologist to distinguish a stromal nodule from a stromal sarcoma. If the tumor is misdiagnosed as a cellular leiomyoma in a curettage, the consequences may be dramatic. There are some histologic features that favor a leiomyoma: blood vessels with thick muscular walls, cleft-like spaces, and merging with the adjacent myometrium. In addition, a battery of immunohistochemical stains may be of use. CD10 is usually present in endometrial stromal cells, and smooth muscle tumors stain positively for desmin and h-caldesmon (72,73).

Endometrial Stromal Sarcoma

Endometrial stromal sarcomas (ESSs) are, by definition, always of low grade and have uniformly bland cells reminiscent of endometrial stromal cells. On gross examination, some are comprised of a single visible mass, and others have multiple

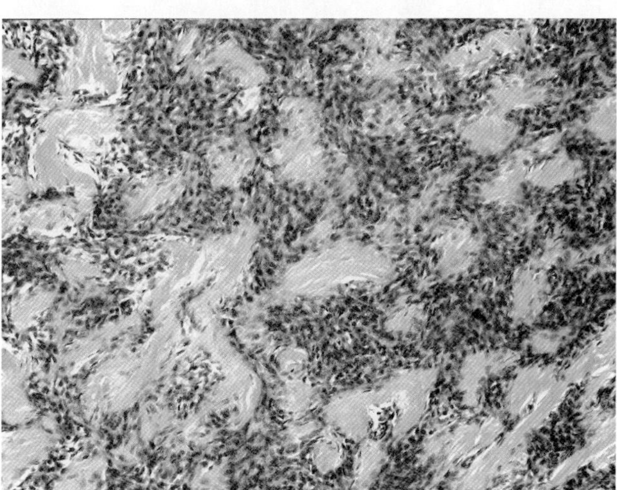

FIGURE 24.13. Endometrial stromal nodule, microscopic appearance.

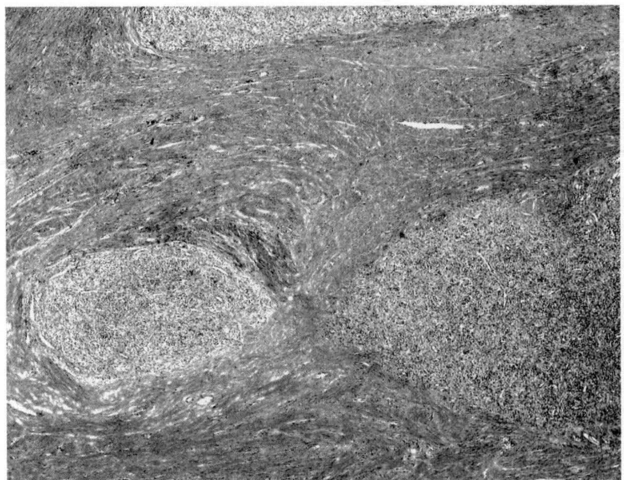

FIGURE 24.14. Endometrial stromal sarcoma, low grade, microscopic appearance.

masses or diffuse myometrial infiltration by worm-like masses (Fig. 24.14). Typically, these tumors show permeation of the myometrial wall, in some cases up to the serosa (Fig. 24.15). Most tumors have fewer than ten mitoses per 10 hpf, but even mitotically active variants behave in a similar indolent manner. Some ESSs have unusual histologic features that may confound the diagnosis. These features include myxoid changes, fibroblastic and/or smooth muscle differentiation, epithelioid changes,

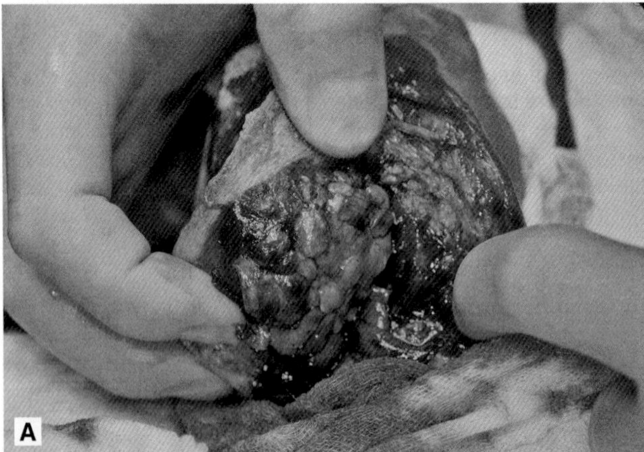

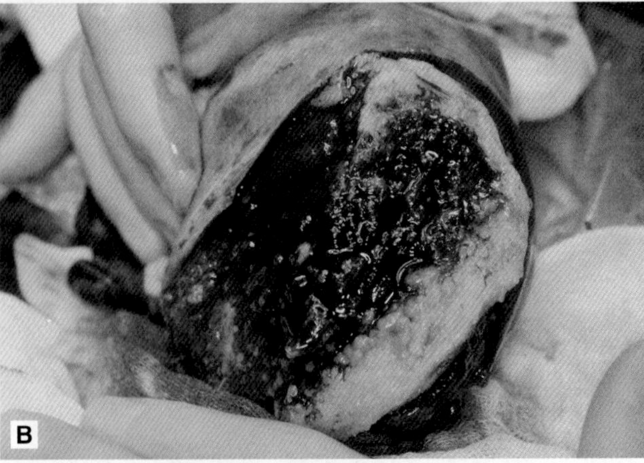

FIGURE 24.15. Endometrial stromal sarcoma, low grade, gross appearance.

and extensive endometrioid glandular differentiation (73–75). No single histologic parameter can be used to predict behavior of low-grade ESSs, including mitotic rate and lymphovascular invasion. However, in a recent study, all low-grade ESSs with high androgen or low estrogen receptor expression behaved aggressively (76).

Low-grade ESSs may occur in extrauterine sites including ovary, fallopian tube, cervix, vagina, vulva, pelvis, abdomen, retroperitoneum, placenta, sciatic nerve, or round ligament (77–84). Some of these cases have been associated with endometriosis. Histologically, they are similar to uterine ESSs, and a uterine tumor needs to be excluded before accepting the lesion as a primary extrauterine ESS. The relapse rate for extrauterine ESS is 62%, which is similar to advanced low-grade uterine ESS. Mitosis and atypia do not correlate with prognosis.

Sixty percent of low-grade endometrial stromal tumors (including ESS and stromal nodule) have cytogenetic abnormalities involving rearrangements of chromosomes 6, 7, and 17. The most characteristic translocation of these tumors, t(T7;17) (Tp15;q21), generates a fusion of the *JAZF1* and *JJAZ1* genes. The presence of this chromosomal abnormality may be of use in the diagnosis of difficult cases or recurrent tumors (85).

Undifferentiated endometrial sarcomas have cytologic atypia to the extent that they cannot be recognized as arising from endometrial stroma. Morphologically, these high-grade lesions resemble undifferentiated mesenchymal tumors and behave as high-grade sarcomas (86). It is advisable to use a term such as "high-grade sarcoma," "undifferentiated sarcoma," or "poorly differentiated uterine sarcoma" (86) rather than "endometrial stromal sarcoma." This last term may inaccurately suggest an indolent tumor. Undifferentiated uterine sarcomas are usually seen in patients older than 50 years, have a recurrence rate of over 85%, and are usually fatal. There have been reports of synchronous or metachronous low-grade ESS with undifferentiated endometrial sarcoma. These cases behave like high-grade tumors and should be diagnosed as such (87).

Müllerian Adenosarcoma

Clement and Scully (8) described müllerian adenosarcomas in 1974 and updated their experience with 100 cases in 1990 (25). These are mixed müllerian tumors composed of malignant stromal and benign epithelial components.

Most adenosarcomas arise in the endometrium and rarely in the endocervix, lower uterine segment, and myometrium (88). Grossly, the majority are solitary polypoid masses with a spongy appearance secondary to the presence of small cysts. Occasional cases appear as multiple polyps or masses and can be multicentric. Their size is variable, being from 1 to 17 cm (mean 5 cm).

Microscopically, the tumors have a benign epithelial component usually covering the surface of the polyps and in the form of benign glands uniformly distributed throughout the tumor. The mesenchymal component is usually a low-grade sarcoma that resembles endometrial stroma. The presence of hypercellular stroma around the glands is common, and some tumors have a leaf-like papillary growth pattern (Fig. 24.16). Sometimes the diagnosis of adenosarcoma may be difficult because of the very low-grade nature of the sarcoma. Minimal criteria were described by Clement and Scully in a review of 100 cases of adenosarcoma published in 1990 (25). They include at least one of the following: two or more stromal mitoses per 10 hpf, marked stromal hypercellularity, and significant stromal cell atypia. Even with these criteria, some cases are deceivingly bland, and several cases have been seen

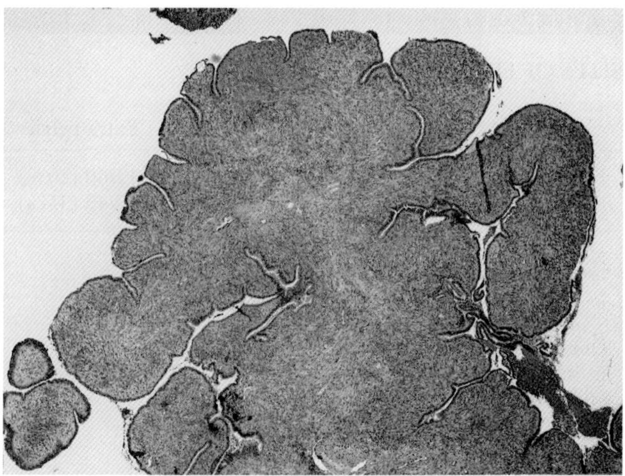

FIGURE 24.16. Müllerian adenosarcoma, microscopic appearance.

in which the diagnosis was only possible after multiple "recurrences" of uterine polyps were reviewed. A minority of cases have "sarcomatous overgrowth," when more than 25% of the tumor is composed of pure sarcoma. In these cases, the sarcoma is typically high grade and the lesions are aggressive (Fig. 24.17) (88).

Most adenosarcomas without stromal overgrowth express estrogen receptors in the sarcomatous component and this may be used for therapeutic purposes (89,90).

Müllerian adenosarcomas have been described in extrauterine sites including the ovary and areas of endometriosis in the vagina, rectovaginal-septum, gastrointestinal tract, urinary bladder, pouch of Douglas, peritoneum, and liver (91–98).

Uterine Tumor Resembling Ovarian Sex-Cord Tumor

In 1976, Clement and Scully (99) coined the term uterine tumors resembling ovarian sex-cord tumors (UTROSCTs) to describe a series of uterine neoplasms with sex-cord–like patterns. Since then, sex-cord–like patterns have been demonstrated in endometrial stromal neoplasms, smooth muscle

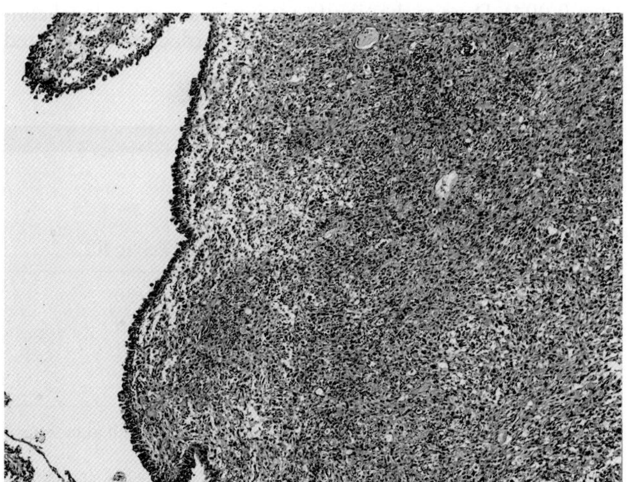

FIGURE 24.17. Müllerian adenosarcoma with sarcomatous overgrowth, microscopic appearance.

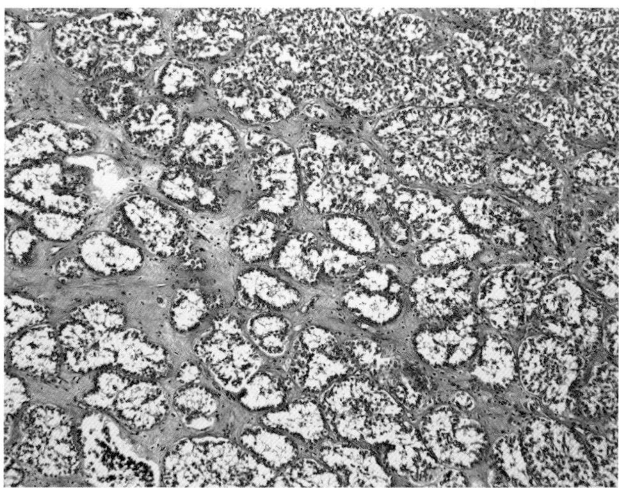

FIGURE 24.18. Uterine tumor resembling ovarian sex-cord tumor (UTROSCT), microscopic appearance.

neoplasms, and in cases lacking clear endometrial stroma and smooth muscle differentiation. The term UTROSCT should be reserved for this last category (100). True UTROSCTs are rare tumors, usually submucosal and well circumscribed, with a yellow cut surface. Histologically, they are composed of sertoliform tubules with low mitotic activity and little nuclear atypia (Fig. 24.18) (100). These tumors behave in a benign fashion.

Perivascular Epithelioid Cell Tumors

Perivascular epithelioid cell tumors (PEComas) are rare neoplasms presumably derived from perivascular epithelioid cells that co-express melanocytic and smooth muscle markers. Other tumors that belong to the same family include angiomyolipoma (AML), clear cell/sugar tumor of the lung, lymphangioleiomyomatosis (LLM), and myelomelanocytic tumor of ligamentum teres/falciform ligament. PEComas have been described in a variety of locations including visceral organs, soft tissues, skin, oral mucosa, orbit, and base of skull (101). Uterus and gastrointestinal tract are the most common locations for visceral PEComas. About 8% of PEComas occur in patients with the tuberous sclerosis complex. Most uterine PEComas are histologically and clinically benign. They can be either grossly well-circumscribed or focally infiltrative masses. Histologically, they are composed of epithelioid cells with clear or eosinophilic cytoplasm, sometimes associated with spindle cells, and a prominent vasculature (102,103).

Approximately 25% of reported cases developed metastases and/or recurrences. Most malignant tumors have more than one of these three histologic features: necrosis, mitoses >2 per 50 hpf, and lymphovascular invasion, but there is not a single reliable prognostic indicator other than the presence of lymphovascular invasion.

The concept of PEComa as a true entity is debatable and some authors believe that the tumor represents a variant of smooth muscle neoplasm (104–106).

RADIATION THERAPY

Since the utilization of radiation therapy for patients with uterine sarcomas has been almost exclusively in the postoperative setting (107), the role of primary or palliative radiotherapy will not be presented. As they are more fully explored in the chapter on epithelial tumors of the corpus, a detailed discussion of the techniques and complications of adjuvant radiation therapy will not be presented in this section.

Uterine Sarcomas

Most of the published papers on sarcomas of the uterus have been retrospective in nature, often requiring many years, if not decades, to accumulate enough patients to perform meaningful statistical analyses. Furthermore, these studies have often had to combine many types of sarcomas to attain numbers sufficient for evaluation (12,108–118). Thus, most of these retrospective studies have not achieved statistical power to reach definite conclusions. However, the data from the nonrandomized review of the Surveillance, Epidemiology, and End Results (SEER) analyses of 2,677 cases of uterine sarcoma did demonstrate a statistically significant improvement in survival favoring adjuvant radiotherapy for stage II, III, and IV (but not stage I) uterine sarcomas (12).

The GOG previously conducted two prospective clinical trials involving selected patients with uterine sarcomas. The earliest study reported on 156 evaluable patients with surgically staged I or II sarcomas of the uterus (119). Patients were enrolled from 1973 to 1982 and randomized (GOG protocol 20) to receive either at least one cycle of adjuvant doxorubicin or no adjuvant chemotherapy. Prior to study randomization, patients could receive optional adjuvant radiotherapy either preoperatively (external pelvic treatment of 40 Gy in 4 to 5 weeks with intracavitary vaginal brachytherapy of 20 Gy to point A) or postoperative pelvic external beam irradiation alone to 50 Gy in 5 to 6 weeks (120).

It should be noted that 11 of 48 (23%) patients with leiomyosarcomas in GOG 20 underwent adjunctive radiotherapy. Furthermore, 49 of 109 patients (45%) with "nonleiomyosarcomas" (85.3% were carcinosarcomas) had adjuvant external beam therapy of the pelvis. Radiotherapy did not seem to affect recurrence in general. However, Table 24.2 shows that there was a notable decrease (119) in vaginal recurrences in patients with carcinosarcomas. Moreover, Table 24.2 also demonstrates an increase in extravaginal failures in the group receiving radiotherapy. Furthermore, Table 24.3 demonstrates a significant reduction in pelvic relapses (10%) in treated patients compared with those untreated (23%) (120).

The second main GOG trial for patients with uterine sarcomas involved a clinicopathologic evaluation of patients with clinical stage I and II disease (GOG protocol 40). This study opened in February 1979 and subsequently closed in October 1988 (32). Of the 453 eligible patients, 430 (95%) had the mandated extrafascial hysterectomy, bilateral salpingo-oophorectomy, and selective retroperitoneal lymphadenectomy. Of this latter group, there were 301 (70%) patients with carcinosarcomas, of which 240 (80%) had surgical stage I/II disease. From this subset, Table 24.4 depicts the locations of first relapse(s). Although adjuvant pelvic external beam therapy was not mandated in this surgical trial, there appeared to be a possibility that adjuvant radiation plays a role in reducing pelvic relapses.

Currently, there is one completed prospective phase III clinical trial that focused on the role of adjuvant radiation therapy for patients with all three main cell types of uterine sarcomas (protocol 55874 of the European Organization for Research and Treatment of Cancer [EORTC]). When initially published in abstract form (121), this trial reported on 224 patients, of which 91 had carcinosarcomas, 103 leiomyosarcomas, and 28 endometrial stromal sarcomas. This study opened in July 1987 and closed to patient accrual in July 2001. Eligible patients underwent an initial surgical resection that involved mandatory total abdominal hysterectomy and bilateral salpingo-oophorectomy. Retroperitoneal lymph node dissection was optional. Due to the time period of the inception of this trial, there were no recommendations regarding either collection of peritoneal washings or omentectomy.

Those subjects in EORTC 55874 with surgical stage I or II disease were then randomized to either no further treatment or external beam irradiation of the whole pelvis. At the time of the abstract, there was a significant reduction in local recurrences (14 of 112 or 12.5%) in the adjuvantly treated arm versus 21.4% (24 out of 112) local relapses in the observation group ($p = 0.004$). Despite the significant improvement in local control, there was no survival benefit afforded the irradiated

TABLE 24.2

SITES OF FIRST RECURRENCE[a]

	None	Vaginal	Extravaginal
No RT	28	11	10
RT	23	2	19

Note: RT, radiation therapy.
[a]Patients with stage I/II uterine carcinosarcomas.
Source: Modified from Omura GA, Blessing JA, Major F, et al. A randomized clinical trial of adjuvant Adriamycin in uterine sarcomas: a Gynecologic Oncology Group study. *J Clin Oncol* 1985;3:1240–1245.

TABLE 24.3

SITES OF FIRST RECURRENCE[a]

	Pelvic	Extra-pelvic
No RT	14/60 (23%)	12/60 (20%)
Pelvic RT	5/49 (10%)	17/49 (35%)

Note: RT, radiation therapy.
[a]85% of this group (93 patients) with non-leiomyosarcomas of the uterus were stage I/II uterine carcinosarcomas.
Source: Modified from Hornback NB, Omura G, Major FJ. Observations on the uterine sarcomas of adjuvant radiation therapy in patients with stage I and II uterine sarcoma. *Int J Radiat Oncol Biol Phys* 1986;12:2127–2130.

TABLE 24.4

SITES OF FIRST RECURRENCE(S)[a]

	No RT	Pelvic RT
Pelvis	43	20
Abdomen	43	19
Distant	38	31
None	83	59

[a]For patients with uterine carcinosarcomas who may have had more than one relapse.
Source: Modified from Major FJ, Blessing JA, Silverberg SG, et al. Prognostic factors in early-stage uterine sarcoma: a Gynecology Oncology Group study. *Cancer* 1993;71:1702–1709.

cohort. Of further note was the fact that this impact on pelvic control was only present in patients with carcinosarcomas. Moreover, due to the lack of rigorous sarcomas surgical staging, it is impossible to know the proportion of patients with occult higher-stage disease in each study arm, which may have affected the results.

EORTC 55874 has been recently updated (122). Compared to the initial report, there are now 221 evaluable patients—92 with carcinosarcomas, 99 with leiomyosarcomas, and 30 with endometrial stromal sarcomas. The dose fractionation for EORTC 55874 centered upon delivering approximately 50.4 Gy in 28 fractions for 5 to 6 weeks to the whole pelvis with all fields being treated daily. The number of "any local recurrence" for carcinosarcomas was 11 out of 46 (23.9 %) and 21 out of 45 (46.7%) for irradiated and nonirradiated patients, respectively. In addition, for leiomyosarcomas there were 10 of 50 (20%) and 12 of 49 (24.5%) with "some aspect" of local failure for the corresponding adjuvant and nonadjuvant arms. For carcinosarcomas, there were 2 of 46 (4.4%) in the adjuvantly irradiated arm and 11 of 45 (24.4%) in the observation subset with isolated local relapses. For leiomyosarcomas, 1 of 50 (2%) in the radiotherapy group and 7 of 49 (14.3%) in the untreated cohort developed isolated local failures.

Thus, it is apparent that patients with isolated local failures evaluated in EORTC 55874 are in the minority for both carcinosarcomas (13 out 32 [40.6%]) and leiomyosarcomas (8 out of 22 [36.4%]), respectively. In fact, distant metastases as any component of relapse occurred in 29 out of 91 (31.9%) and in 45 out of 99 (45.5%) for carcinosarcomas and leiomyosarcomas, respectively. Finally, the 3-year progression-free survival was not statistically significant between the two study arms (57.7% and 51.9% for the irradiated and nonirradiated subsets, respectively). By the same token, the patients treated postoperatively had a nonsignificant median survival advantage of 8.5 years versus 6.7 years for the observational cohort with a hazard ratio of 1.02 (95% confidence interval [CI], 0.68 to 1.53; $p = 0.92$).

However, in a novel pilot study from France (123), 18 patients (13 of 18 with leiomyosarcomas) with optimally debulked surgical stage I, II, and III sarcomas received adjuvant doxorubicin, cisplatin, and ifosfamide (three cycles) followed by sequential external beam radiotherapy to a total dose of approximately 45 Gy in 5 weeks with or without vaginal brachytherapy. These investigators then performed a matched case-control study utilizing 18 patients of whom 16 underwent pelvic radiotherapy alone and 2 received no adjuvant treatment. With a median follow-up of 43 months (range, 23 to 56 months), this study found that only five patients (27.8%) had suffered recurrences. All failed solely in extrapelvic sites. Moreover, neither median survival nor disease-free survival had been reached for study patients at last follow-up.

Uterine Carcinosarcomas

Other reports have been limited to one histologic type of sarcoma. The most common of these pertained to what is currently being termed as "mixed epithelial and stromal tumors of the uterus" (124) or historically known as uterine carcinosarcomas (110,125–134). Results are inconsistent with some studies demonstrating no benefit for radiotherapy (110,128,130,131,133), while others have shown a significant impact of adjuvant pelvic radiotherapy on survival for patients with carcinosarcomas (125,127,132,134). One of these studies (134) involved a review of the nonrandomized SEER database of 2,461 women with carcinosarcomas from 1973 to 2003. In this data set, 890 patients received adjuvant radiotherapy. The overall 5-year survivals of those receiving radiotherapy versus no irradiation were 41.5% and 33.2%, respectively ($p < 0.001$). Furthermore, a significant improvement in survival in this study was observed for all stages of disease, including stage IV. Finally, there have been several published retrospective reports suggesting that combined adjuvant radiotherapy and chemotherapy may impart even longer survival, especially in stage I and II disease (35,129,135).

There has been one randomized phase III prospective trial of adjuvant radiotherapy in carcinosarcomas, (GOG 150). This study compared whole abdominal irradiation to three cycles of cisplatin-ifosfamide chemotherapy with respect to recurrence rates, and disease-free and overall survival. Also evaluated were therapeutic toxicities. Eligible were patients with carcinosarcomas confined to the abdomen who underwent optimal surgical debulking with no postsurgical residual disease greater than 1 cm. Patients randomized to receive radiotherapy were prescribed a total dose of 30 Gy to the whole abdomen using external beam therapy followed by a pelvic boost to an approximate cumulative pelvic dose of 50 Gy. The first published report (136) of the two treatment cohorts was based upon an analysis done in December 2005. There were 224 patients enrolled, of whom 206 were evaluable. In this latter group, 105 patients underwent adjuvant radiotherapy, while 101 were given chemotherapy. The estimated death rate for patients receiving chemotherapy was 32.8% lower than for those receiving radiotherapy ($p = 0.042$). A subsequently published update (137) of this study based upon a May 2006 analysis demonstrated that this reduction in estimated death rate by chemotherapy had dropped to 31% relative to radiotherapy ($p = 0.046$).

The most recent evaluation of the data of patients on GOG 150 occurred in November 2006 (138). At the time of this analysis, the median duration of follow-up for patients alive at last contact was 63 months. The breakdown of surgical stages for patients in the radiotherapy versus chemotherapy arms is as follows: stage I—35 out of 105 (33.3%) versus 29 out of 101 (28.7%); stage II—11 out of 105 (10.5%) versus 15 out of 101 (14.9%); stage III—45 out of 105 (42.9%) versus 47 out of 101 (46.5%); and stage IV—14 out of 105 (13.3%) versus 10 out of 101 (9.9%). The estimated crude probability of relapse within 5 years was a nonsignifcant 58% versus 52% for the radio- and chemotherapy groups, respectively. The sites of first failure are presented in Table 24.5. Although not statistically significant, there were fewer vaginal but more abdominal relapses in the adjuvant radiotherapy group as

TABLE 24.5

PATTERNS OF FAILURE

Sites of recurrence[a]	WAI (n = 105), number of cases	Chemotherapy (n = 101), number of cases
Vagina	4	10
Pelvis	14	14
Abdomen	29	19
Distant	27	24

Note: n, total number of cases in each arm; WAI, whole abdominal irradiation.
[a]Some patients had multiple sites of relapse.
Source: Modified from Wolfson AH, Brady MF, Rocereto T, et al. A Gynecologic Oncology Group randomized phase III trial of whole abdominal irradiation (WAI) vs. cisplatin-ifosfamide and mesna (CIM) as postsurgical therapy in stage I-IV carcinosarcoma (CS) of the uterus. *Gynecol Oncol* 2007;107:177–185.

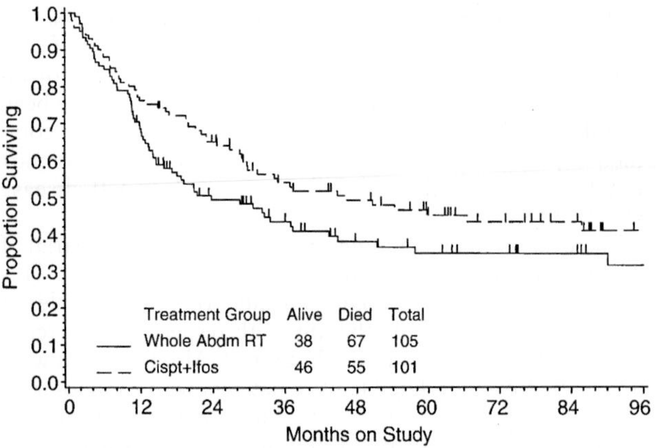

FIGURE 24.19. Overall survival in Gynecologic Oncology Group protocol 150, whole abdomen radiotherapy versus cisplatin plus ifosfamide chemotherapy.

compared to the chemotherapy arm. Figure 24.19 demonstrates that the estimated 5-year survival was approximately 35% for those randomized to adjuvant radiotherapy versus 45% for those receiving chemotherapy. After adjusting for stage and age at diagnosis, there was a further death rate reduction to 23% for those receiving chemotherapy compared with radiotherapy (HR = 0.712; 95% CI, 0.484 to 1.048; $p = 0.085$; two-tail test). Of interest is the fact that those patients who received adjuvant radiotherapy had more late complications, mainly gastrointestinal, than those having cytotoxic therapy ($p < 0.001$). In addition, two patients undergoing radiotherapy died as a direct result of radiation-induced hepatitis.

Based upon the results of GOG protocol 150, the role of adjuvant radiotherapy for the management of patients with carcinosarcomas continues to remain uncertain. Since there were more vaginal failures in the chemotherapy arm of GOG protocol 150 and other sites of relapse were similar or less common in frequency (abdominal recurrences) than those in the radiotherapy arm, then perhaps postoperative vaginal brachytherapy (either high or low dose rate) with chemotherapy should be considered for any patient having optimally debulked carcinosarcomas in future trials. It is anticipated that the next GOG-led adjuvant trial will compare two chemotherapy regimens, with radiation chosen by the treating physician.

Uterine Leiomyosarcomas

The second most frequent type of uterine sarcomas is leiomyosarcomas. Table 24.6 presents the overall pelvic/extrapelvic relapse rates of 16.6% and 42.0% for patients with uterine leiomyosarcoma. There still remains a paucity of information that specifies between upper abdominal and extra-abdominal distant sites of tumor involvement. The respective pelvic/extrapelvic percentages were 18.5% (22 out of 119)/41.2% (49 out of 119) for nonirradiated and 12.9% (8 out of 62)/43.5% (27 out of 62) for patients treated with postoperative radiotherapy (32,139,140). From this overview, it does not appear that postoperative radiotherapy has any real effect on reducing recurrences for patients with uterine leiomyosarcoma. However, two of the listed series (32,139) combined to yield an 11.1% (4 out of 36) pelvic relapse rate with radiation versus 61.1% (22 out of 36) without the implementation of adjuvant radiation therapy. Yet the major problem is that the majority of these patients have distant extra-abdominal metastases, such as the lung, despite having local control (32,139). In addition, a more recent retrospective study from a single institution (11) performed a case-control study of patients with uterine leiomyosarcomas that "showed a trend toward improved survival in the 31 cases with adjuvant pelvic irradiation compared with the controls who did not receive adjuvant radiation therapy." This would suggest that adjuvant systemic therapy must be added in order to have an impact on the outcome of these patients.

Endometrial Stromal Sarcomas

Table 24.7 focuses on patients with endometrial stromal sarcomas (ESSs), the third most common type of uterine sarcomas. This class of endometrial sarcoma can be subdivided (141) by mitotic index into either a low-grade category (endometrial stromal sarcoma) or a high-grade sarcoma now termed undifferentiated uterine sarcoma. The total pelvic and extrapelvic rates of relapse depicted in Table 24.7 are 42.2% and 33.3%, respectively. Only one (142) of the listed studies clearly attempts to subdivide the sites of disease relapse by sarcoma type.

It can be ascertained from this latter report (142) that there were no reported abdominal or distant recurrences independent of the administration of adjuvant irradiation for all stages of

TABLE 24.6

PATTERNS OF FAILURE FOR PATIENTS WITH SURGICALLY STAGED UTERINE LEIOMYOSARCOMAS MANAGED BY SURGERY WITH OR WITHOUT EXTERNAL BEAM PELVIC IRRADIATION (+/− VAGINAL BRACHYTHERAPY +/− CHEMOTHERAPY)

Reference	Stage	Vagina	Pelvis	Extrapelvic	Abdomen	Distant	Adjuvant treatment
32	I, II, III, IV	Not stated	0/13	Not stated	1/13	7/13	Yes[a]
32	I, II, III, IV	Not stated	8/50	Not stated	9/50	17/50	No[a]
140	I, II	Not stated	4/26	10/26	Not stated	Not stated	Mainly yes[a]
11	I, II, III	Not stated	4/23	9/23	Not stated	Not stated	Yes[a]
11	I, II	Not stated	14/69	23/69	Not stated	Not stated	No[a]
Subtotals	—	—	30/181 (16.6%)	42/118 (35.6%)	10/63 (15.9%)	24/63 (38.1%)	—
Totals	—	—	30/181 (16.6%)	76/181 (42.0%)	—	—	—

[a]Nonrandomized.

TABLE 24.7

PATTERNS OF FAILURE FOR PATIENTS WITH SURGICALLY STAGED ENDOMETRIAL STROMAL SARCOMAS MANAGED BY SURGERY WITH OR WITHOUT EXTERNAL BEAM PELVIC IRRADIATION (+/− VAGINAL BRACHYTHERAPY +/− CHEMOTHERAPY)

Reference	Stage	Vagina	Pelvis	Extrapelvic	Abdomen	Distant	Adjuvant treatment
143	I, II, III, IV	2/31	7/31	Not stated	0/31	6/31	Yes[a]
141	I, II, III, IV	4/29	10/29	Not stated	6/29	4/29	Yes[a]
144	I, II—low grade	Not stated	0/5	Not stated	0/3	0/3	Yes[a,b]
142	I, II—low grade	Not stated	5/15	Not stated	0/15	0/15	No[a]
142	III, IV—low grade	Not stated	1/3	Not stated	0/3	0/3	Yes[a,c]
142	III, IV—low grade	Not stated	0/1	Not stated	0/1	0/1	No[a]
142	I, II—high grade	Not stated	7/20	Not stated	8/20	5/20	Yes and no[a]
142	III—high grade	Not stated	6/12	Not stated	3/12	6/12	Yes and no[a]
Subtotals	—	6/60 (10%)	43/116 (37.1%)	—	17/114 (14.9%)	21/114 (18.4%)	—
Totals	—	—	49/116 (42.2%)	38/114 (33.3%)	—	—	—

[a]Nonrandomized.
[b]No RT for three patients.
[c]No RT for one patient.

low-grade ESS. Yet, there was a 33.3% (6 out of 18) pelvic recurrence rate, of which the majority did not undergo any radiation therapy. This latter finding suggests that postoperative external pelvis radiotherapy should at least be considered for the subset of patients with low-grade ESS.

A more recent report (143) retrospectively reviewed 28 patients with endometrial stromal sarcomas of which 19 were low grade and 9 were high grade. Fifty percent of the patients in this series underwent adjuvant pelvic radiotherapy with no difference in the survival of the patients. In addition, almost 30% of those receiving adjuvant radiotherapy relapsed within the treatment field. Regarding undifferentiated endometrial sarcomas, one study documented multiple sites of recurrence, including abdominal (34.8% [11 out of 32]), distant (34.8% [11 out of 32]), and pelvic (40.6% [13 out of 32]) sites of relapse (144). Thus, unless vaginal brachytherapy finds a niche, there appears to be no definite indication for postoperative radiotherapy for patients with these high-grade lesions.

CHEMOTHERAPY

Uterine sarcomas, although far less common than endometrial carcinomas, exhibit two features that increase the need for systemic therapy: a recurrence rate of at least 50%, even in early-stage disease, and a high propensity for distant failure. The comparatively low incidence of uterine sarcomas has made randomized, controlled trials difficult. Despite this, cooperative group studies have provided data from phase II and III trials for the rational selection of systemic chemotherapy.

Crucial to the understanding of the use of chemotherapy in uterine sarcomas is the observation that these neoplasms are heterogeneous. The first two subtypes, malignant mixed müllerian tumors (carcinosarcomas) and leiomyosarcomas, constitute 90% of cases entered into clinical trials. These two histologic subtypes are usually the only uterine sarcomas with sufficient numbers to permit meaningful phase III studies; however, as these two histologic subtypes appear to respond differently to chemotherapy, they should be studied separately.

Limited Disease

Uterine sarcoma has a high rate of distant metastases even in the absence of intraperitoneal or lymph node metastases. It has been concluded that this is due to the high rate of hematogenous and lymphatic dissemination (145). Even for surgical stage I disease, the recurrence is as high as 53% (32). To date, the largest randomized trial of adjuvant chemotherapy in patients with uterine sarcoma did not segregate different histologic subtypes. Although the recurrence rate and median survival of patients treated with doxorubicin compared to no therapy were 39% versus 51% and 73 months versus 55 months, respectively, this GOG trial concluded that there was no significant difference (119). As with advanced disease, more recent trials began to segregate the histologic subtypes. A nonrandomized study using adjuvant combination chemotherapy of etoposide, cisplatin, and doxorubicin demonstrated a 2-year survival of 92% of 23 patients with surgical stage I and stage II uterine malignant mixed müllerian tumors. The fact that seven patients also received radiation therapy makes the result controversial (146). A pilot study concluded that multimodality treatment consisting of chemotherapy with epirubicin and cisplatin as well as radiation resulted in a 74% overall survival at a median follow-up of 55 months in 38 patients with surgical stages I and II malignant mixed müllerian tumors (35). However, the high dropout made the conclusion of multimodality treatment controversial. A more recent GOG study by Sutton et al. reported that 65 patients with completely resected stage I and II malignant mixed müllerian tumors of the uterus were treated with adjuvant ifosfamide and cisplatin Fig. 24.20 (147). The 2- and 5-year survivals were 82% and 62%, respectively. Since more than half of the recurrences involved the pelvis, the study suggested that a combined sequential approach with chemotherapy and radiotherapy might be beneficial for this group of patients, which should be verified in a randomized phase III study.

Previous studies reported that an effective adjuvant chemotherapy regimen was a combination of cyclophosphamide, vincristine, doxorubicin, and dacarbazine (DTIC) with 68% to 89% 5-year survival in stage I uterine sarcomas (148–151).

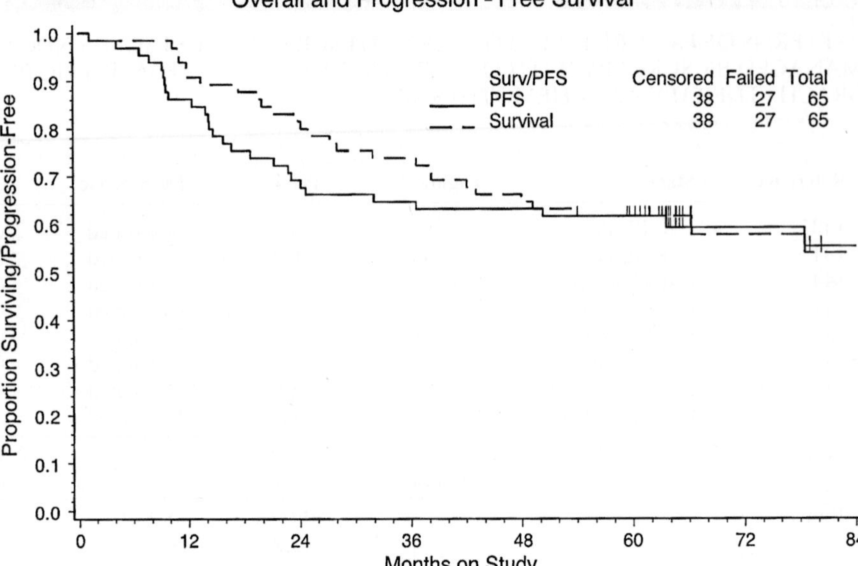

FIGURE 24.20. Survival in patients with stage I and II carcinosarcomas treated with adjuvant cisplatin and ifosfamide.

To date, there have been no separate prospective studies on patients with uterine leiomyosarcomas. Two factors continue to limit the study of adjuvant therapy in patients with uterine leiomyosarcomas: the relatively low frequency of the disease, which makes it difficult to complete randomized trials in a reasonable period of time, and the lack of highly active agents.

Advanced and Recurrent Disease

Leiomyosarcomas

Numerous single agents have been and continue to be tested in patients with leiomyosarcomas (Table 24.8) (152–174). Doxorubicin and ifosfamide are the most active agents investigated as primary single-agent chemotherapy in recurrent and advanced uterine leiomyosarcomas. As shown in other types of soft-tissue sarcoma, gemcitabine has demonstrated its activity in one (2.3%) complete response and eight (18.2%) partial responses in persistent or recurrent uterine leiomyosarcomas (162). Unfortunately, the results have been unimpressive. In 1983, the GOG demonstrated seven responses among 28 patients (25%) treated with doxorubicin every 3 weeks as a single agent (158). To date, this has been considered to be the most active single agent. Later the GOG reported that treatment with liposomal doxorubicin yielded one complete (3.2%) and four partial (12.9%) responses and no advantage over historical results with doxorubicin (152). The GOG demonstrated that ifosfamide had moderate activity, with six partial responses among 35 patients (17%) (155), whereas limited activity was seen with single-agent paclitaxel, which was associated with a 9% overall response in 33 patients (154). Intravenous single-agent etoposide was shown to have an overall response of 10.7% in 28 patients (171), whereas prolonged oral etoposide had an overall response of 6.9% among 29 patients (170). However, no complete or partial responses were observed in another GOG phase II study with single-agent intravenous etoposide 100 mg/m^2 daily for 3 days every 3 weeks (156). Topotecan was tested in 36 patients with complete response in 1 (3%), partial response in 3 (8%), stable disease in 12 (33%), and increasing tumor in 20 (56%) (153). Single-agent cisplatin also had a poor overall response of 3% to 5% in phase II trials (157,174). The antifolate compound trimetrexate was used in a small study reported in 2002, which was associated with an overall response of 4.3% in 28 patients who had received prior treatment (169). Mitoxantrone (173), diaziquone (161), amonafide (172), aminothiadiazole (160), and piperazinedione (159) were inactive as single agents.

Combination chemotherapy yields greater response rates (Table 24.8) (158,175–181). In 1983, the GOG demonstrated that the combination of doxorubicin and dacarbazine resulted in an overall response rate of 30%. Two years later, the same group demonstrated a 19% response rate using the combination of doxorubicin and cyclophosphamide (181). Both of the phase III trials were too small to make any definite conclusions. However, as mentioned, the trials did serve the purpose of allowing researchers to observe that leiomyosarcomas had a different chemotherapeutic response profile compared to malignant mixed müllerian tumors, resulting in the separation of the two different histologic entities in subsequent trials.

In 1996, the same group demonstrated an 18% overall response with a combination of dacarbazine, etoposide, and hydroxyurea (178). In the same year, using a combination of ifosfamide and doxorubicin, the GOG demonstrated an overall response of 30.3% in patients with advanced leiomyosarcoma with no history of prior treatment (179). The most recent study from the GOG showed that the use of mitomycin, doxorubicin, and cisplatin produced an overall response rate of 23% in 35 patients. Pulmonary toxicity was appreciable, however (177). Based on this study, the GOG conducted a phase II study with dacarbazine, doxorubicin, mitomycin, and cisplatin (DAMP), which produced a 27.8% response rate, but the complexity and toxicity of the regimen precluded further investigation, and the study was closed after the first stage of accrual (175). Gemcitabine plus docetaxel was proven highly active and tolerable (53% overall response rate) in treated and untreated patients with leiomyosarcomas (180). The effort in leiomyosarcomas continues to focus on the identification of active drugs and combinations in phase II trials. Given the paucity of survival data available from the randomized trials to compare various chemotherapy regimens, a pooled analysis of phase II studies was undertaken to compare the difference of response rate between single-agent and combination therapy. It showed that patients who received first- or second-line chemotherapy for the treatment of metastatic leiomyosarcoma had a higher response rate with combination chemotherapy than with single-agent chemotherapy (182). However, current phase III randomized clinical trials are only suggestive of the role of combination chemotherapy in advanced or recurrent uterine leiomyosarcomas.

TABLE 24.8

CHEMOTHERAPY IN LEIOMYOSARCOMA OF THE UTERUS

Drug	N	Prior therapy	Schedule	Overall response (%)	Reference
SINGLE-AGENT CHEMOTHERAPY					
Primary chemotherapy					
Liposomal doxorubicin	32	11 RT	50 mg/m² q 4 weeks	16.1	152
Topotecan	36	8 RT	1.5 mg/m² × 5 days q 3 weeks	11	153
Paclitaxel	33	8 RT	175 mg/m² q 3 weeks	9	154
Ifosfamide	35	15 RT	1.5 g/m² × 5 days q 4 weeks	17	155
Etoposide	28	7 RT	100 mg/m² × 3 days q 3 weeks	0	156
Cisplatin	33	8 RT	50 mg/m² q 3 weeks	3	157
Doxorubicin	28	N/A	60 mg/m² q 3 weeks	25	158
Piperazinedione	19	N/A	9 mg/m² q 3 weeks	5[a]	159
Aminothiadiazole	20	N/A	125 mg/m² q 1 week	0	160
Diaziquone	24	N/A	22.5 mg/m² q 3 weeks	0	161
Non-primary chemotherapy					
Gemcitabine	44	11 RT, 35 CT	1,000 mg/m² weekly × 3 q 4 weeks	20.5	163
	31	31 CT	1,250 mg/m² weekly × 2 q 3 weeks	3.2[b]	163
	29	15 RT, 19 CT	1,250 mg/m² weekly × 3 q 4 weeks	3[b]	164
	56	N/A	1,000 mg/m² weekly × 3 q 4 weeks	18[b]	165
Paclitaxel	48	15 RT, 33 CT	175 mg/m² q 3 weeks	8.4[b]	166
Ecteinascidin-743	54	54 CT	1.5 mg/m² q 3 weeks	4[b]	167
	49	49 CT	1–1.8 mg/m² q 3 weeks	4.1[b]	168
Trimetrexate	23	7 RT, 10 CT	5 mg/m² orally × 5 days q 2 weeks	4.3	169
Etoposide	29	6 RT, 27 CT	50 mg/m² orally × 21 days q 4 weeks	6.9	170
	28	7 RT, 27 CT	100 mg/m² days 1, 3, 5 q 4 weeks	10.7	171
Amonafide	26	8 RT, 25 CT	300 mg/m² × 5 days q 3 weeks	4	172
Mitoxantrone	12	12 CT	12 mg/m² q 3 weeks	0	173
Cisplatin	19	19 CT	50 mg/m² q 3 weeks	5	174
COMBINATION CHEMOTHERAPY					
Doxorubicin *plus* Dacarbazine	20	N/A	60 mg/m² q 3 weeks 250 mg/m² × 5 days q 3 weeks	30	158
Dacarbazine *plus* Mitomycin Doxorubicin Cisplatin	18	7 RT	750 mg/m² q 4 weeks 6 mg/m² q 4 weeks 40 mg/m² q 4 weeks 60 mg/m² q 4 weeks	27.8	175
Dacarbazine *plus* Mitomycin Doxorubicin Cisplatin	10	10 No CT	750 mg/m² q 4 weeks 6 mg/m² q 4 weeks 40 mg/m² q 4 weeks 60 mg/m² q 4 weeks	80	176
Mitomycin *plus* Doxorubicin Cisplatin	35	8 RT	8 mg/m² q 3 weeks 40 mg/m² q 3 weeks 60 mg/m² q 3 weeks	23	177
Hydroxyurea *plus* Dacarbazine Etoposide	38	11 RT	2 g orally × 1 day q 4 weeks 700 mg/m² q 4 weeks 300 mg/m² × 2 days q 4 weeks	18	178
Ifosfamide *plus* Doxorubicin	33	9 RT	5 mg/m² q 3 weeks 50 mg/m² q 3 weeks	30	179
Gemcitabine *plus* Docetaxel	34	14 RT, 16 CT	900 mg/m² days 1, 8 q 3 weeks 100 mg/m² day 8 q 3 weeks	53	180
Doxorubicin *plus* Cyclophosphamide	38	38 No CT	60 mg/m² q 3 weeks 500 mg/m² q 3 weeks	19[a]	181

Note: All chemotherapy agents were given intravenously unless specified. CT, chemotherapy; N/A, not available; RT, radiation therapy.
[a]Uterine sarcoma.
[b]Adult soft-tissue sarcoma.

TABLE 24.9

CHEMOTHERAPY IN CARCINOSARCOMAS OF THE UTERUS

Drug	N	Prior therapy	Schedule	Overall response (%)	Reference
SINGLE-AGENT CHEMOTHERAPY					
Primary chemotherapy					
Cisplatin	63	28 RT	50 mg/m² q 3 weeks	19	157
Ifosfamide	91	34 RT	2 g/m² × 3 days q 3 weeks	29	184
	102	27 RT	1.5 g/m² × 5 days q 3 weeks	36	185
	28	8 RT	1.5 g/m² × 5 days q 4 weeks	32	186
Doxorubicin	21	21 No CT	60 mg/m² q 3 weeks	19[a]	181
	9	6 No CT	50–90 mg/m² q 3 weeks	0	187
Piperazinedione	19	19 No CT	9 mg/m² q 3 weeks	5.3	159
Non-primary chemotherapy					
Doxorubicin	41	N/A	60 mg/m² q 3 weeks	10	158
Topotecan	48	16 RT, 44 CT	1.5 mg/m² × 5 days q 3 weeks	10	188
Trimetrexate	21	N/A	5 mg/m² orally × 5 days q 2 weeks	4.8	189
Paclitaxel	44	15 RT, 33 CT	170 mg/m² q 3 weeks	18.2	190
Amonafide	16	5 RT, 14 CT	300 mg/m² × 5 days q 3 weeks	6	191
Aminothiadiazole	22	10 RT, 18 CT	125 mg/m² q 1 week	5	192
Diaziquone	23	11 RT, 18 CT	22.5 mg/m² q 3 weeks	4	193
Mitoxantrone	17	17 CT	12 mg/m² q 3 weeks	0	173
Etoposide	31	14 RT, 29 CT	100 mg/m² days 1, 3, 5 q 4 weeks	6.5	194
Cisplatin	28	28 CT	50 mg/m² q 3 weeks	18	195
	12	7 CT	75–100 mg/m² q 3 weeks	42	195
COMBINATION CHEMOTHERAPY					
Doxorubicin *plus* Dacarbazine	31	N/A	60 mg/m² q 3 weeks 250 mg/m² × 5 days q 3 weeks	23	158
Doxorubicin *plus* Cyclophosphamide	30	30 No CT	60 mg/m² q 3 weeks 500 mg/m² q 3 weeks	19[a]	181
Ifosfamide *plus* Cisplatin	92	25 RT	1.5 g/m² × 5 days q 3 weeks 20 mg/m² × 5 days q 3 weeks	54	185
Ifosfamide *plus* Paclitaxel	88	26 RT	1.6 g/m² × 3 days q 3 weeks 135 mg/m² q 3 weeks	45	184
Ifosfamide *plus* Cisplatin	65	65 No CT	1.5 g/m² × 5 days q 3 weeks 20 mg/m² × 5 days q 3 weeks	N/A	197
Hydroxyurea *plus* Dacarbazine Etoposide	32	11 RT	2 g orally q 4 weeks 700 mg/m² q 4 weeks 100 mg/m² × 3 days q 4 weeks	15	198
Etoposide *plus* Cisplatin Doxorubicin	4	N/A	100 mg/m² × 2 days q 4 weeks 50 mg/m² q 4 weeks 50 mg/m² q 4 weeks	100	199
Cyclophosphamide *plus* Vincristine Doxorubicin Dacarbazine	26	14 CT	400 mg/m² day 2 q 4 weeks 1 mg/m² days 1, 5 q 4 weeks 40 mg/m² day 2 q 4 weeks 200 mg/m² × 5 days q 4 weeks	23	200
Cisplatin *plus* Doxorubicin Ifosfamide	32	32 No CT	50 mg/m² q 3 weeks 45 mg/m² q 3 weeks 5 g/m² q 3 weeks	56[b]	201

Note: All chemotherapy agents were given intravenously unless specified. CT, chemotherapy; N/A, not available; RT, radiation therapy.
[a]Uterine sarcoma.
[b]Female genital tract.

Uterine Carcinosarcomas

Several drugs have been studied in this group of tumors as single agents (Table 24.9) (158,173,175,183–196). However, only three drugs have demonstrated clear-cut activity: ifosfamide, cisplatin, and paclitaxel (183–186,190,195,196). Of the three drugs ifosfamide is the most active single agent studied to date. In a 5-day schedule, ifosfamide produced 25 complete and 12 partial responses (overall response of 36%) among 102 patients with no prior chemotherapy (185).

In patients with prior chemotherapy, cisplatin produced an 18% response in 28 patients (195). A repeat trial in patients with no prior chemotherapy documented essentially the same response rate of 19% among a larger group of patients (183).

Both trials used cisplatin at 50 mg/m^2 every 3 weeks. Investigators at the M. D. Anderson Cancer Center employed a higher dose ranging from 75 mg/m^2 to 100 mg/m^2 every 3 weeks. Only 12 patients with measurable disease were entered into the trial, but one complete and four partial responses were observed (overall responses 42%) (196). The lack of randomization and the small number of cases in this trial preclude conclusions about the merits of the higher dose. Paclitaxel as a single agent was associated with a response rate of 21.2% in a group of 33 patients with uterine sarcoma who had prior chemotherapy, with an 8.2% response rate in patients who failed appropriate local therapy (190).

Doxorubicin, generally regarded as the most active agent in soft-tissue sarcomas, unfortunately demonstrated inconsistent activity in three trials of patients with malignant mixed müllerian tumors. The first two studies constituted one arm of each of two randomized trials. In the first, four responses among 41 patients (10%) with mixed mesodermal tumors (158) were observed. The other demonstrated a 19% response rate utilizing a dose of 60 mg/m^2 every 3 weeks in recurrent or advanced uterine sarcomas (181). The third, which employed a range of doses from 50 mg/m^2 to 90 mg/m^2 every 3 weeks, resulted in no response among the nine patients with measurable disease (187). Topotecan 1.5 mg/m^2 daily for 5 days had unimpressive activity (10% response rate) in patients with advanced or recurrent uterine malignant mixed müllerian tumors previously treated with chemotherapy (188). Demonstrating negligible activity in phase II studies were etoposide (200), mitoxantrone (173), piperazinedione (164), diaziquone (193), amonafide (191), trimetrexate (93), and aminothiadiazole (192).

In the history of chemotherapy development, combination therapy usually results in a higher response rate than single-agent treatment. However, not all combination regimens have had an impact upon survival. This is clearly seen in the treatment of uterine carcinosarcomas.

There have been numerous reports of combination chemotherapy for uterine carcinosarcomas (Table 24.9) (158, 181, 185, 189, 197–201). A combination of cyclophosphamide, vincristine, doxorubicin, and DTIC had a reported 23% (61) overall response rate. A combination of etoposide, hydroxyurea, and DTIC resulted in a response of 15% in 32 patients (198). Later EORTC reported a trial based upon 48 patients with unresectable or recurrent malignant mixed müllerian tumor who were treated with a combination of cisplatin, doxorubicin, and ifosfamide. The overall response rate was an impressive 56%. Unfortunately, this regimen was also associated with a high incidence of nephrologic and hematologic toxicities. The group concluded that alternative platinum-based regimens with more favorable toxicity profiles should be explored (201). Indeed, evaluation of the true value of combination chemotherapy requires randomized phase III trials.

The first randomized study in 1983 by the GOG, which combined malignant mixed müllerian tumors with other sarcomas, resulted in patient numbers being too small for subset analysis (158). Nonetheless, combining doxorubicin and DTIC resulted in an overall response of 23% and a trend toward greater response as compared to single-agent doxorubicin (10%). A significant improvement in progression-free and overall survival could not be demonstrated, but two conclusions could be drawn from this trial. The first was the fact that a greater response to chemotherapy was significantly associated with an increase in overall survival and the disease-free survival. The second observation was that malignant mixed müllerian tumors had a different response profile compared to leiomyosarcomas. Two years later, the GOG compared cyclophosphamide plus doxorubicin to single-agent doxorubicin. A response of 25% was observed in malignant mixed müllerian tumors; again, however, numbers were inadequate to show any significant benefit compared with single-agent doxorubicin. The trial was also closed early because of failure to reach statistical significance (181).

With the recognition of the difference in response to therapy between malignant mixed müllerian tumors and leiomyosarcomas, randomized trials began to regard each of the two major histologic subtypes as separate patient populations. Unfortunately, this increased the time necessary to complete clinical trials. Nonetheless, a large randomized trial was performed and reported in 2000. The GOG evaluated the addition of cisplatin to ifosfamide in 194 eligible patients and found that this improved the overall response rate from 36% to 54% and prolonged the median progression-free interval by an absolute 2 months. However, this advantage was not associated with a significant overall survival gain (185).

More recently and based upon the finding of moderate activity (18% response rate) of paclitaxel for this disease, the GOG carried out a phase III trial of ifosfamide with or without paclitaxel in advanced uterine malignant mixed müllerian tumors. The group found that the addition of paclitaxel produced a 45% response rate compared with 29% in the ifosfamide single-agent arm with overall survival significantly improved. There was a significant decrease in the hazard of death and progression but more sensory neuropathy, as expected (189).

In conclusion, there is moderate evidence to support the use of combination chemotherapy in advanced or recurrent uterine carcinosarcomas (Table 24.10). Combination regimens that result in significant improvements in survival are needed.

Endometrial Stromal Sarcoma

Randomized phase III trials with stromal sarcomas are limited due to the rarity of this disease. Only two randomized trials compared single-agent and combination chemotherapy in advanced uterine sarcoma, without response rate of stromal sarcomas reported separately. The GOG reported a phase II study of ifosfamide treatment in 21 cases with recurrent or metastatic endometrial stromal sarcomas. Three patients experienced complete response and four had partial responses, for an overall response of 33.3% (202). Another noncontrolled study observed a 50% response rate to doxorubicin therapy in ten patients with recurrent endometrial stromal sarcomas (203). Many other literatures are case reports and retrospective studies with a small number of cases. Published chemotherapy regimens include carboplatin and paclitaxel (204); doxorubicin, cisplatin, and ifosfamide (205); doxorubicin and ifosfamide (206); doxorubicin, vincristine, and cyclophosphamide (207); and prolonged oral etoposide (208).

Interest in endometrial stromal sarcomas continues owing to the difference in the prognosis of patients with low-grade disease versus those with high-grade disease. In recurrent stromal sarcoma, reports support hormone therapy for patients with low-grade subgroup and chemotherapy for high-grade tumors (209). Current definitions do not include high-grade lesions as a component of endometrial stromal sarcoma.

Toxicity

The most common toxicities of chemotherapy are hematologic and gastrointestinal toxicity. The grade 3-4 adverse effects of chemotherapy with overall response rate higher than 5% in leiomyosarcomas and mixed mesodermal tumors are listed in Tables 24.11 and 24.12. Combination chemotherapy has a much higher incidence of grade 3-4 side effects compared with the single-agent regimen. The overall response rate of combination with ifosfamide plus cisplatin is 54%; however, the grade 3-4 of leukopenia is 97%, and six deaths occurred before the first dose reduction of ifosfamide (185). The current phase III trial with ifosfamide plus paclitaxel reported a 45%

TABLE 24.10

PHASE III CLINICAL TRIAL IN UTERINE SARCOMAS

Drug	N	Prior therapy	Schedule	Overall response (%)	Median PFS (months)	Median overall survival (months)	Leuko-penia (%)	Neutro-penia (%)	Thrombo-cytopenia (%)	Anemia (%)	GI (%)	Neuro-pathy (%)	Reference
Doxorubicin	41 MMT/28 LMS	N/A	60 mg/m² q 3 weeks	10/25	3.5[a]	7.7[a]	16	N/A	4	N/A	2	N/A	158
Doxorubicin *plus* Dacarbazine	31 MMT/20LMS	N/A	60 mg/m² q 3 weeks 250 mg/m² × 5 days q 3 weeks	23/30	5.5[a]	7.3[a]	35	N/A	13	N/A	9	N/A	
Doxorubicin	21 MMT/21LMS	8 RT	60 mg/m² q 3 weeks	19[a]	5.1[a]	11.6[a]	10	N/A	0	N/A	N/A	N/A	181
Doxorubicin *plus* Cyclophos-phamide	30 MMT/17LMS	9 RT	60 mg/m² q 3 weeks 500 mg/m² q 3 weeks	19[a]	4.9[a]	10.9[a]	35	N/A	0	N/A	N/A	N/A	
Ifosfamide	102 MMT		1.5 g/m² × 5 days q 3 weeks	36	4	7.6	59	36	5	8	5	20	185
Ifosfamide *plus* Cisplatin	92 MMT	25 RT	1.5 g/m² × 5 days q 3 weeks 20 mg/m² × 5 days q 3 weeks	54	6	9.4	97	67	64	19	18	29	
Ifosfamide	91 MMT		2 g/m² × 3 days q 3 weeks	29	3.6	8.4	42	53	3	9	7	0	184
Ifosfamide *plus* Paclitaxel	88 MMT	26 RT	1.6 g/m² × 3 days q 3 weeks 135 mg/m² q 3 weeks	45	5.8	13.5	36	44	3	15	8	3	

Note: All chemotherapy agents were given intravenously. GI, gastrointestinal; MMT, malignant mixed müllerian tumor; N/A, not available; LMS, leiomyosarcoma system; PFS, progression-free survival; RT, radiation therapy.
[a]Uterine sarcoma.

TABLE 24.11

GRADE 3-4 ADVERSE EFFECTS OF CHEMOTHERAPY IN LEIOMYOSARCOMA (RESPONSE RATE > 5%)

Drug	N	Prior therapy	Schedule	Overall response (%)	Leuko-penia (%)	Neutro-penia (%)	Thrombo-cytopenia (%)	Anemia (%)	GI (%)	Others	Reference
Liposomal *plus* doxorubicin	32	11 RT	50 mg/m^2 q 4 weeks	16.1	12.9	16.1	N/A	22.6	19.4	Dermatotoxicity 6.5%	152
Topotecan	36	8 RT	1.5 mg/m^2 × 5 days q 3 weeks	11	33	90	13	16	16.7		153
Paclitaxel	33	8 RT	175 mg/m^2 q 3 weeks	9	9.1	33.3	3	3	0	No neurotoxicity	154
	48	15 RT, 33 CT	175 mg/m^2 q 3 weeks	8.4	6.3	16.7	0	16.7	41.7		166
Ifosfamide	35	15 RT	1.5 g/m^2 × 5 days q 4 weeks	17	34	N/A	0	0	3	Neurotoxicity 3%, granulocytopenia 11%, dermatotoxicity 14%	155
Doxorubicin	28	N/A	60 mg/m^2 q 3 weeks	25	16	N/A	4	N/A	2		158
	29	6 RT, 27 CT	50 mg/m^2 orally × 21 days q 4 weeks	6.9	24	35	18	12	6	Neurotoxicity 6%	160
Gemcitabine	44	11 RT, 35 CT	1,000 mg/m^2 weekly × 3 q 4 weeks	20.5	27.3	34.1	11.4	6.8	13.6		162
Doxorubicin *plus* Dacarbazine	20	N/A	60 mg/m^2 q 3 weeks 250 mg/m^2 × 5 days q 3 weeks	30	35	N/A	13	N/A	9		158
Dacarbazine *plus* Mitomycin *plus* Doxorubicin *plus* Cisplatin	18	7 RT	750 mg/m^2 q 4 weeks 6 mg/m^2 q 4 weeks 40 mg/m^2 q 4 weeks 60 mg/m^2 q 4 weeks	27.8	67	78	94	61.1	44.4		175

(*continued*)

TABLE 24.11

GRADE 3-4 ADVERSE EFFECTS OF CHEMOTHERAPY IN LEIOMYOSARCOMA (RESPONSE RATE > 5%) (CONTINUED)

Drug	N	Prior therapy	Schedule	Overall response (%)	Leuko-penia (%)	Neutro-penia (%)	Thrombo-cytopenia (%)	Anemia (%)	GI (%)	Others	Reference
Mitomycin *plus* Doxorubicin *plus* Cisplatin	35	8 RT	8 mg/m² q 3 weeks 40 mg/m² q 3 weeks 60 mg/m² q 3 weeks	23	N/A	N/A	N/A	N/A	N/A	Pulmonary toxicity 8%	177
Hydroxyurea *plus* Dacarbazine *plus* Etoposide	38	11 RT	2 g orally × 1 day q 4 weeks 700 mg/m² q 4 weeks 300 mg/m² × 2 days q 4 weeks	18	29	N/A	3	N/A	N/A		178
Ifosfamide *plus* Doxorubicin	33	9 RT	5 mg/m² q 3 weeks 50 mg/m² q 3 weeks	30	0	49	0	0	0	Cardiac toxicity 3%	179
Gemcitabine *plus* Docetaxel	34	14 RT, 16 CT	900 mg/m² days 1, 8 q 3 weeks 100 mg/m² day 8 q 3 weeks	53	N/A	21	29	15	12	Dyspnea 21%, fatigue 21%	180

Note: All chemotherapy agents were given intravenously unless specified. CT, chemotherapy; GI, gastrointestinal system; N/A, not available; RT, radiation therapy.

TABLE 24.12

GRADE 3-4 ADVERSE EFFECTS OF CHEMOTHERAPY IN MIXED MÜLLERIAN TUMOR (RESPONSE RATE > 5%)

Drug	N	Prior therapy	Schedule	Overall response (%)	Leukopenia (%)	Neutropenia (%)	Thrombocytopenia (%)	Anemia (%)	GI (%)	Others	Reference
Doxorubicin	41	N/A	60 mg/m^2 q 3 weeks	10	16	N/A	4	N/A	2		158
	21	21 No CT	60 mg/m^2 q 3 weeks	19[a]	10	N/A	0	N/A	0		181
Cisplatin	63	28 RT	50 mg/m^2 q 3 weeks	19	2	N/A	0	N/A	N/A		157
	28	28 CT	50 mg/m^2 q 3 weeks	18	0	N/A	0	N/A	4.2	Nephrotoxicity 22.2%	195
Ifosfamide	91	34 RT	2 g/m^2 × 3 days q 3 weeks	29	42	53	3	9	7		184
	102	27 RT	1.5 g/m^2 × 5 days q 3 weeks	36	59	36	5	8	5	Neuropathy 20%	185
	28	8 RT	1.5 g/m^2 × 5 days q 4 weeks	32	45	24	7	0	0	Dermatotoxicity 35%	186
Topotecan	48	16 RT, 44 CT	1.5 mg/m^2 × 5 days q 3 weeks	10	83.3	85.4	39.6	25	8.3		188
Paclitaxel	44	15 RT, 33 CT	170 mg/m^2 q 3 weeks	18.2	30	43	7	9	2	Neurotoxicity 7%	190
Doxorubicin *plus* Dacarbazine	31	N/A	60 mg/m^2 q 3 weeks 250 mg/m^2 × 5 days q 3 weeks	23	35	N/A	13	N/A	9		158
Doxorubicin *plus* Cyclophosphamide	30	30 No CT	60 mg/m^2 q 3 weeks 500 mg/m^2 q 3 weeks	19[a]	35	N/A	0	N/A	N/A		181
Ifosfamide *plus* Cisplatin	92	25 RT	1.5 g/m^2 × 5 days q 3 weeks 20 mg/m^2 × 5 days q 3 weeks	54	97	67	64	19	18	Neuropathy 29%	185
Ifosfamide *plus* Cisplatin	65	65 No CT	1.5 g/m^2 × 5 days q 3 weeks 20 mg/m^2 × 5 days q 3 weeks	N/A	70.8	26.2	63.1	7.7	10.8	Cardiotoxicity 4.6%, neurotoxicity 4.6%, nephrotoxicity 3.1%	197
Ifosfamide *plus* Paclitaxel	88	26 RT	1.6 g/m^2 × 3 days q 3 weeks 135 mg/m^2 q 3 weeks	45	36	44	3	15	8	Neuropathy 3%	184

(*continued*)

TABLE 24.12

GRADE 3-4 ADVERSE EFFECTS OF CHEMOTHERAPY IN MIXED MÜLLERIAN TUMOR (RESPONSE RATE > 5%) (CONTINUED)

Drug	N	Prior therapy	Schedule	Overall response (%)	Leuko-penia (%)	Neutro-penia (%)	Thrombo-cytopenia (%)	Anemia (%)	GI (%)	Others	Reference
Hydroxyurea *plus* Dacarbazine *plus* Etoposide	32	11 RT	2 g orally q 4 weeks 700 mg/m^2 q 4 weeks 100 mg/m^2 × 3 days q 4 weeks	15	24	N/A	6	3	3	Dermatotoxicity 33%, fever 3%	198
Etoposide *plus* Cisplatin *plus* Doxorubicin	4	N/A	100 mg/m^2 × 2 days q 4 weeks 50 mg/m^2 q 4 weeks 50 mg/m^2 q 4 weeks	100	9.5	N/A	N/A	N/A	21.4	Aloplacia 100%	199
Cyclophos-phamide *plus* Vincristine *plus* Doxorubicin *plus* Dacarbazine	26	14 CT	400 mg/m^2 day 2 q 4 weeks 1 mg/m^2 days 1, 5 q 4 weeks 40 mg/m^2 day 2 q 4 weeks 200 mg/m^2 × 5 days q 4 weeks	23	34.6	N/A	15.4	N/A	N/A	Septicemia 15.4%, neurotoxicity 7.7%	200
Cisplatin *plus* Doxorubicin *plus* Ifosfamide	32	32 No CT	50 mg/m^2 q 3 weeks 45 mg/m^2 q 3 weeks 5 g/m^2 q 3 weeks	56[b]	94.6	84.8	64.8	43.2	53.8	Neurotoxicity 15.4%, aloplacia 64.1%	201

Note: All chemotherapy agents were given intravenously unless specified. CT, chemotherapy; N/A, not available; RT, radiation therapy.
[a]Uterine sarcoma.
[b]Female genital tract.

overall response rate with tolerable toxicities (189), which seems a relatively effective and safe regimen. Among other phase II trials of different chemotherapeutic regimens, liposomal doxorubin, paclitaxel, doxorubicin, cisplatin, and etoposide plus cisplatin plus doxorubicin were reported to have less toxicity with moderate effect.

Hormonal Therapy

Although the role of hormonal therapy is clear in breast and endometrial cancers, few uterine sarcomas contain sufficient estrogen- or progesterone-receptor protein to influence therapy, the only exception being low-grade endometrial stromal sarcomas or stromal nodules. It has been found that estrogen and progesterone receptors were found in 55.5% and 55.8%, respectively, of samples from patients with various types of uterine sarcomas, but the median concentrations were substantially lower than those observed in breast or endometrial cancers. Endometrial stromal sarcomas had higher receptor levels (210). Uniquely, low-grade endometrial stromal sarcomas are hormonally responsive in roughly two thirds of cases and long-term maintenance therapy should be beneficial.

Progestins, gonadotropin-releasing hormone (GnRH) analogues (211), or aromatase inhibitors (209,212) have been used in the treatment of patients with advanced or recurrent stromal sarcomas and successfully gain long-term stability in case reports. Several papers reported that long-term use of tamoxifen for the treatment of breast cancer was related to the development of uterine sarcoma (213,214).

Lantta et al. (215) published two cases of extensive intraperitoneal low-grade endometrial stromal sarcoma associated with high levels of progesterone receptors in complete remission with hormonal therapy. Three patients reported by Baker et al. (216) had partial responses or stabilization of disease on oral megestrol acetate; all had concentrations of progesterone receptors exceeding 674 fmol/mg. Piver et al. (217), in a collaborative survey of endolymphatic stromal myosis, recorded complete or partial responses to hormonal therapy in 6 of 13 patients (46%) treated with progestational agents. Scribner and Walker (218) reported a patient with an extensive endometrial stromal sarcoma of the uterus whose tumor was reduced to resectable size by the administration of leuprolide acetate and megestrol acetate. Endometrial stromal sarcomas of a lower grade have also been reported to express srp27, an estrogen-induced 24-DK protein suggesting hormone responsiveness (219). Medroxyprogesterone acetate has induced major responses in pulmonary metastatic lesions from endometrial stromal sarcoma (130,220,221). GnRH analogues were reported to control the progression of a recurrent low-grade endometrial stromal sarcoma with moderate estrogen and progesterone receptor positivity (211). Medroxyprogesterone acetate and aromatase inhibitors, such as letrozole, were observed to be highly effective and have sustained progression control in six of ten cases with low-grade stromal sarcoma (222). Spano et al. presented two cases of endometrial stromal sarcoma with lung metastases treated with aminoglutethimide who achieved complete response and remained disease-free for 14 and 7 years, respectively (209). However, there presently is no prospective study on hormonal treatment for stromal sarcoma published.

Hormonal therapy has not been extensively evaluated in mesenchymal uterine tumors. There are anecdotal reports of responses to hormonal therapy in adenosarcomas and low-grade leiomyosarcomas (223). One case of letrozole therapy in high-grade malignant mixed müllerian tumor with marked tumor control was reported, but the area has not been well studied (224).

Biologic Therapy

Since the high recurrence and poor response to radiotherapy and chemotherapy, biologic therapy may have more promise in the area of uterine sarcoma, as well as other types of soft-tissue sarcoma. The recent advances in the biology of uterine sarcoma related to probable treatment target have concentrated on tyrosine kinase receptors and vascular endothelial growth factor (VEGF).

Since the discovery that high proto-oncogene *c-kit* expression in gastrointestinal stromal tumors (GISTs) may be amenable to control with tyrosine kinase inhibitors, such as imatinib mesylate and sunitinib, some interest has been focused upon uterine sarcomas (225). However, the expression of *c-kit* in the uterine sarcoma varies greatly in different studies. Some studies demonstrated the presence of *c-kit* in 41.3% to 83% of uterine leiomyosarcoma (226–228), but other studies documented little presence (229–232). Given the great progress made in the GISTs with imatinib mesylate, a GOG phase II evaluation of sunitinib maleate in the treatment of recurrent or persistent leiomyosarcoma of the uterus was completed with negative results.

Emoto et al. demonstrated inhibition of a VEGF-expressing malignant mixed tumor cell line by TNP-470, an angiogenesis inhibitor (232). Another angiogenesis inhibitor, thalidomide, was studied in recurrent or persistent malignant mixed müllerian tumor of the uterus by the GOG. No activity was seen.

Advances in the understanding of the biology of uterine sarcomas may provide more treatment targets and make long-term control of the disease possible.

Systemic Therapy Summary

The current role of chemotherapy in the management of uterine sarcomas involves the treatment of patients with advanced or recurrent disease, and an emphasis on palliative intent. In leiomyosarcomas, the active drugs are doxorubicin, ifosfamide, gemcitabine, and docetaxel. For malignant mixed müllerian tumors, the drugs of choice are ifosfamide, cisplatin, and paclitaxel. Hormonal therapy, including progestational agents, GnRH analogues, and aromatase inhibitors, may have a role in the treatment of advanced or recurrent endometrial stromal sarcomas. The use of hormonal agents in the treatment of other histologic subtypes has not been well studied. Efforts to identify additional active agents continue.

LONG-TERM RESULTS OF THERAPY

Leiomyosarcoma

The prognosis of patients with uterine leiomyosarcoma is uniformly poor. The reported 5-year survival of uterine leiomyosarcoma varies between 30% and 48% (6, 233–236). However, leiomyosarcoma may tender a worse prognosis than malignant mixed müllerian tumor when adjusting for stage and mitotic count (6,233).

Major et al. reported a progression-free survival at 3 years of 31% and the recurrence rate was 71% in 59 patients with leiomyosarcomas. The mitotic index was the only factor significantly related to progression-free interval (32). In the study of 423 uterine sarcomas of Olah et al. (6), overall 5-year survival was 31%; 42% of patients with endometrial stromal sarcomas, 34% of those with leiomyosarcomas, and 33% with malignant mixed müllerian tumors were alive at the end of the study period with median survival times of 30, 17, and 13 months, respectively. These researchers also found that stage, degree of differentiation, age, and histologic type were the four common factors influencing survival in a multiple regression analysis (6,11).

Carcinosarcomas and Müllerian Adenosarcomas

Major et al. (32) reported a recurrence rate of 53% for 301 patients with clinical stage I and II malignant mixed müllerian tumors. This included 61 patients (20%) who were "upstaged" based upon surgical findings. The prognostic factors based on multivariate analysis were adnexal spread, lymph node metastases, histologic cell type, and grade of sarcoma. Median survival in patients with clinically recurrent or advanced-stage malignant mixed müllerian tumors ranged from 4 to 13 months (2,8,237,238) despite therapy.

Kaku et al. (239), in a review of GOG materials, indicated that müllerian adenosarcomas were usually locally invasive; 30% of the 31 cases in their review suffered recurrences. Among the 100 patients reported by Clement and Scully (25), 26.1% developed recurrent disease. Generally, müllerian adenosarcomas are regarded as locally invasive and are managed in some cases with local excision. However, sarcomatous overgrowth has been described in as many as 57% of cases (90,239) and is associated with a fulminant clinical course and death.

Endometrial Stromal Sarcoma

Virtually no endometrial stromal nodule will recur after hysterectomy. In the series of Dionigi et al. (240), there were no reported relapses in patients followed for a median of 43.5 months and a maximum of 214 months.

In comparison with leiomyosarcoma and malignant mixed müllerian tumor, patients with endometrial stromal sarcoma tend to present with low-grade and early-stage disease with favorable prognosis (236,241). Denschlag et al. (236) reported a 5-year survival of 82% among women with endometrial stromal sarcoma, which was significantly better than other subgroups. It may be difficult to determine the prognosis of endometrial stromal sarcoma in a given patient, however. Although mitotic count may be important, Chang et al. (242) suggested that stage (stage I versus stages II-IV) was more important in determining survival. Their series was largely referral material, and few patients had undergone complete surgical staging. Perhaps as a result, 36% of patients with stage I in their paper experienced relapse and 23% of these died of the disease. Remarkably, median time to relapse in patients with stage I tumors was 69 months. Patients with stage I endometrial stromal sarcomas most commonly experienced recurrences in the pelvis or abdomen, strongly suggesting a role for complete surgical staging and, perhaps, adjuvant radiotherapy. Eight of 73 patients (11%) with stage I disease either presented with or developed pulmonary metastases. However, the median time to pulmonary relapse was 116 months.

In the large series of Chang et al. (242), mitotic count successfully predicted outcome in patients with stage II-IV endometrial stromal sarcomas. Utilizing the ten mitoses per 10 hpf criteria, 8 of 13 (62%) patients with undifferentiated endometrial sarcomas experienced disease recurrence compared with 35 of 77 (45%) of those with low-grade tumors.

Young et al. (243) and Berchuck et al. (203) have suggested that patients with ovarian preservation at the time of hysterectomy for endometrial stromal sarcoma were more likely to develop recurrences. Although this was not the case in the report of Chang et al. (242) (seven cases with no recurrences after hysterectomy), bilateral salpingo-oophorectomy would seem to be prudent given the potential for low-grade endometrial stromal sarcomas to express estrogen receptors and respond to hormonal therapy.

Patterns of Failure

Although Echt et al. (19) reported no difference in recurrent patterns between patients with malignant mixed müllerian tumors and leiomyosarcomas, others have reported a propensity for malignant mixed müllerian tumor to relapse in the abdomen or pelvis and leiomyosarcomas to metastasize to the lung (120). In the follow-up of the GOG staging study reported by Major et al. (32), 28 of 301 patients with malignant mixed müllerian tumors developed lung metastases (9.3%) versus 24 of 59 (40.7%) of those with leiomyosarcomas. Recurrences with a pelvic component were 63 (20.9%) and 8 (13.6%), respectively, for the two tumor types. The decision to use postoperative irradiation in this study was made by treating physicians.

In patients whose tumors were initially confined to the uterus, there were purely distant recurrences in only 4 of 51 (7.8%) patients with malignant mixed müllerian tumors reported by Nielsen et al. (244) and Shaw et al. (245), but 22 of 35 (62.9%) in the patients with leiomyosarcoma reported by Punnonen et al. (246) and Yu et al. (247). In a 10-year review of uterine leiomyosarcomas at Massachusetts General Hospital, Dinh et al. (248) reported that 20 of 27 patients either presented with or developed pulmonary metastases.

CLINICAL TRIALS

The GOG has played a leading role in developing new drugs for advanced and metastatic leiomyosarcomas and uterine malignant mixed müllerian tumors through a series of phase II studies in both previously treated and chemotherapy-naïve patients. It will be important to include available biologic and immunologic agents in this series of studies. The GOG has also completed one phase III study of ifosfamide with or without paclitaxel in patients with persistent or recurrent mixed müllerian tumors (185). Several existing GOG phase II studies are ongoing, such as trabectedin in advanced, persistent, or recurrent leiomyosarcoma of the uterus.

MOLECULAR BIOLOGY, GENETICS, FUTURE DIRECTIONS, AND CONCLUSIONS

There has been a slow evolution in the understanding of the basic science of uterine sarcomas. The majority are felt to be sporadic with no specific etiology and most have complex karyotypes (249). However, in an increasing number of nonuterine sarcomas, specific chromosomal translocations resulting in fusion genes that are constitutive and involve activation of transcription factors have been identified. Clear cell sarcomas, myxoid liposarcomas, alveolar rhabdomyosarcomas, and alveolar soft-part sarcomas all have been associated with translocation-induced fusion genes that result in activated transcription factors and uncontrolled growth (249). Perhaps the most striking advance was the identification of c-*kit* tyrosine kinase activation in GISTs, which are histologically indistinguishable from leiomyosarcomas of the small bowel. The specific inhibitor of c-*kit*, imatinib mesylate (KSTI-571), may produce long-term responses in patients with metastatic GISTs.

The reported c-*kit* immunoreactivity was present in 0% to 83% of uterine leiomyosarcomas (226–231). Whether this finding will translate into a role for sunitinib maleate in these malignancies remains to be seen in future clinical trials.

In leiomyosarcomas, other avenues may be explored. Human immunodeficiency virus–immunocompromised pediatric patients are unusually susceptible to leiomyosarcomas. The causative agent in these tumors appears to be the Epstein-Barr virus (250). Similar smooth muscle tumors associated with the Epstein-Barr virus have been described in a few adult organ transplant recipients (251). Only one report about this virus is expressed in an immunocompetent adult with leiomyosarcomas (252). A common intermediary factor may exist, which is as yet unrecognized.

Trials of adjuvant chemotherapy are appropriate in early-stage, resected leiomyosarcomas. Recurrence rates after surgery alone are unacceptably high; the risk of mortality associated with recurrent leiomyosarcoma easily offsets any morbidity derived from adjuvant chemotherapy in this population of relatively young patients. One ongoing study utilizes sequential docetaxel plus gemcitabine followed by doxorubicin in women with high-grade, stage I and II leiomyosarcomas.

A variety of potential markers are overexpressed in uterine malignant mixed müllerian tumors and include p53, *mdm*-2 (253), platelet-derived growth factor receptor-β, c-*abl* (254), HER2/*neu* (255,256), vascular endothelial growth factor (257), and insulin-like growth factor (IGF)-II (258). None is associated with prognostic implications (259,260); the evolving concept of malignant mixed müllerian tumors as metaplastic endometrial carcinomas may result in elucidation of new means of prevention and therapy. Combination or sequential radiation and chemotherapy have a great deal of appeal (31).

Endometrial stromal sarcomas have been associated with the translocation t(7;17) (p15–21;q12–21) in over a third of cases (261); this information, in addition to the established hormone responsiveness of low-grade stromal sarcomas, may provide a basis for therapeutic strategies in the future.

A basic understanding of uterine sarcomas and their differences is paramount to the understanding of surgical and adjuvant therapy as well as palliative treatment in patients with these rare neoplasms; this knowledge is essential to the practice of gynecologic oncology.

References

1. Jemal A, Siegel R, Ward E, et al. Cancer statistics, 2007. *CA Cancer J Clin* 2007;57:43–66.
2. Doss LL, Llorens AS, Henriquez EM. Carcinosarcoma of the uterus: a 40-year experience from the state of Missouri. *Gynecol Oncol* 1984;18:43–53.
3. Nordal RR, Thoresen SO. Uterine sarcomas in Norway 1956–1992: incidence, survival, and mortality. *Eur J Cancer* 1997;33:907–911.
4. Scully RE, Bonfiglio TA, Kurman RJ, et al. *World Health Organization International Classification of Tumour: Histological Typing of Female Genital Tract Tumors.* 2nd ed. Berlin: Springer; 1994.
5. Ober WB. Uterine sarcomas: histogenesis and taxonomy. *Ann NY Acad Sci* 1959;75:689–703.
6. Olah KS, Dunn JA, Gee H. Leiomyosarcomas have a poorer prognosis than mixed mesodermal tumours when adjusting for known prognostic factors: the result of a retrospective study of 423 cases of uterine sarcoma. *Br J Obstet Gynaecol* 1992;99:590–594.
7. Ronnett BM, Zaino RJ, Ellenson LH, et al. Endometrial cancer. In: Kurman RJ, ed. *Blaustein's Pathology of the Female Genital Tract.* 5th ed. New York: Springer; 2002:501–560.
8. Clement PB, Scully RE. Müllerian adenosarcoma of the uterus: a clinicopathologic analysis of ten cases of distinctive type of müllerian mixed tumor. *Cancer* 1974;34:1138–1149.
9. Clement PB, Oliva E, Young RH. Müllerian adenosarcoma of the uterine corpus associated with tamoxifen therapy: a report of six cases and review of tamoxifen-associated endometrial lesions. *Int J Gynecol Pathol* 1996;15:222–229.
10. Bartsich EG, Bowe ET, Moore JG. Leiomyosarcoma of the uterus. *Obstet Gynecol* 1968;32:101–106.
11. Giuntoli RL, Metzinger DS, DiMarco CS, et al. Retrospective review of 208 patients with leiomyosarcoma of the uterus: prognostic indicators, surgical management, and adjuvant therapy. *Gynecol Oncol* 2003;89:460–469.
12. Brooks SE, Zhan M, Cote T, et al. Survival epidemiology and end results analysis of 267 cases of uterine sarcomas, 1989–1999. *Gynecol Oncol* 2004;93:204–208.
13. Chang KL, Crabtree GS, Kim Lim-Tan S, et al. Primary uterine endometrial stromal neoplasms. A clinicopathologic study of 117 cases. *Am J Surg Pathol* 1990;14:415–438.
14. Evans HL. Endometrial stromal sarcoma and poorly differentiated endometrial sarcoma. *Cancer* 1982;50:2170–2182.
15. Dionigi A, Oliva E, Clement PB, et al. Endometrial stromal nodules and endometrial stromal tumors with limited infiltration: a clinicopathologic study of 50 cases. *Am J Surg Pathol* 2002;26:567–581.
16. Zelmanowicz A, Hildesheim A, Sherman MA, et al. Evidence for a common etiology for endometrial carcinomas and malignant mixed müllerian tumors. *Gynecol Oncol* 1998;69:253–257.
17. Mortel R, Nedwich A, Lewis GC, et al. Malignant mixed müllerian tumors of the uterine corpus. *Obstet Gynecol* 1970;35:469–480.
18. Norris HJ, Roth E, Taylor HB. Mesenchymal tumors of the uterus. *Obstet Gynecol* 1966;28:57–63.
19. Echt G, Jepson J, Steel J, et al. Treatment of uterine sarcomas. *Cancer* 1990;66:35–39.
20. Silverberg SG, Major FJ, Blessing JA, et al. Carcinosarcoma (malignant mixed mesodermal tumor) of the uterus. A Gynecologic Oncology Group pathologic study of 203 cases. *Int J Gynecol Pathol* 1990;9:1–19.
21. Kurman RJ, ed. *Blaustein's Pathology of the Female Genital Tract.* 5th ed. New York: Springer; 2001.
22. Christopherson WM, Williamson EO, Gray LA. Leiomyosarcoma of the uterus. *Cancer* 1972;29:1512–1517.
23. Meredith RJ, Eisert DR, Kaka Z, et al. An excess of uterine sarcomas after pelvic irradiation. *Cancer* 1986;58:2003–2007.
24. Varala-Duran J, Nochomovitz LE, Prem KA, et al. Post irradiation mixed müllerian tumors of the uterus. *Cancer* 1980;45:1625–1631.
25. Clement PB, Scully RE. Müllerian adenosarcoma of the uterus: a clinicopathologic analysis of 100 cases with a review of the literature. *Hum Pathol* 1990;21:363–381.
26. Bocklage T, Lee KR, Belinson JL. Uterine müllerian adenosarcoma following adenomyoma in a woman on tamoxifen therapy. *Gynecol Oncol* 1993;44:104–109.
27. Larson B, Silfversward C, Nilsson B, et al. Mixed müllerian tumors of the uterus—prognostic factors: a clinical and histopathologic study of 147 cases. *Radiother Oncol* 1990;17(2):123–132.
28. Goff BA, Rice LW, Fleischhacker D, et al. Uterine leiomyosarcoma and endometrial stromal sarcoma: lymph node metastases and sites of recurrence. *Gynecol Oncol* 1993;50:105–109.
29. Iwasa Y, Haga H, Konishi I, et al. Prognostic factors in uterine carcinosarcoma: a clinicopathologic study of 25 patients. *Cancer* 1998;82:512–519.
30. Leibsohn S, d'Ablain G, Mischell DR, et al. Leiomyosarcoma in a series of hysterectomies performed for presumed uterine leiomyomas. *Am J Obstet Gynecol* 1990;162:968–974.
31. Berchuck A, Rubin SC, Hoskins WJ, et al. Treatment of uterine leiomyosarcoma. *Obstet Gynecol* 1988;71:845–854.
32. Major FJ, Blessing JA, Silverberg SG, et al. Prognostic factors in early-stage uterine sarcoma. *Cancer* 1993;71:1702–1709.
33. Yamada DS, Burger RA, Brewster WR, et al. Pathologic variables and survival for patients with surgically evaluated carcinosarcoma of the uterus. *Cancer* 2000;88:2782–2786.
34. Porter GA, Cantor SB, Ahmad SA, et al. Cost-effectiveness of staging computed tomography of the chest in patients with T2 soft tissue sarcomas. *Cancer* 2002;94:197–204.
35. Manolitsas T, Wain GV, Williams KE, et al. Multimodality therapy for patients with clinical stage I and II malignant mixed müllerian tumors of the uterus. *Cancer* 2001;91:1437–1443.
36. Chen SS. Propensity of retroperitoneal lymph node metastases in stage I sarcoma of the uterus. *Gynecol Oncol* 1989;32:215–219.
37. Gard GB, Mulvany NJ, Quinn MA. Management of uterine leiomyosarcoma in Australia. *Aust N Z J Obstet Gyneaecol* 1999;39:93–98.
38. Kaku T, Silverberg SG, Major FJ, et al. Adenosarcoma of the uterus: a Gynecologic Oncology Group clinicopathologic study of 31 cases. *Int J Gynecol Pathol* 1992;11:75–88.
39. Mittal K, Joutovsky A. Areas with benign morphologic and immunohistochemical features are associated with some uterine leiomyosarcomas. *Gynecol Oncol* 2007;104:362–365.
40. Zhang P, Zhang C, Hao J, et al. Use of X-chromosome inactivation pattern to determine clonal origins of uterine leiomyoma and leiomyosarcoma. *Hum Pathol* 2006;37:1350–1356.
41. Bell SW, Kempson RL, Hendrickson MR. Problematic uterine smooth muscle neoplasms. A clinicopathologic study of 213 cases. *Am J Surg Pathol* 1994;18:535–558.
42. Wang WL, Soslow RA, Zannoni GF, et al. The utility of tumor cell necrosis in the diagnosis of primary leiomyosarcoma of the uterus: an analysis of 77 cases. *Mod Pathol* 2006;19(Suppl 1):201A.
43. Perrone T, Dehner LP. Prognostically favorable "mitotically active" smooth muscle tumors of the uterus. A clinicopathologic study of ten cases. *Am J Surg Pathol* 1988;12:1–8.

44. O'Connor DM, Norris HJ. Mitotically active leiomyoma of the uterus. *Hum Pathol* 1990;21:223–227.
45. Prayson RA, Goldblum JR, Hart WR. Epithelioid smooth muscle tumors of the uterus. A clinicopathologic study of 18 patients. *Am J Surg Pathol* 1997;21:383–391.
46. Jones MW, Norris HJ. Clinicopathologic study of 28 uterine leiomyosarcomas with metastases. *Int J Gynecol Pathol* 1995;14:243–249.
47. Kugami S, Kashimura M, Toki N, et al. Myxoid leiomyosarcoma of the uterus with subsequent pregnancy and delivery. *Gynecol Oncol* 2002;85:538–542.
48. Kindelberger D, Hollowell M, Otis C, et al. Myxoid leiomyosarcomas: a clinicopathologic study of 10 cases. *Mod Pathol* 2007;20(Suppl 2): 203A.
49. Wang WL, Soslow RA, Hensley M, et al. Histopathologic prognostic factors in stage I uterine leiomyosarcomas: a clinicopathologic study of 28 cases. *Mod Pathol* 2007;20(Suppl 2):217A.
50. Leitao MM, Soslow RA, Nonaka D, et al. Tissue microarray immunohistochemical expression of estrogen, progesterone, and androgen receptors in uterine leiomyomata and leiomyosarcoma. *Cancer* 2004;101: 1455–1462.
51. Bodner K, BodnerpAdler B, Kimberger O, et al. Estrogen and progesterone receptor expression in patients with uterine leiomyosarcoma and correlation with different clinicopathological parameters. *Anticancer Res* 2003;23:729–732.
52. McCluggage WG. Malignant biphasic uterine tumors: carcinosarcomas or metaplastic carcinomas? *J Clin Pathol* 2002;55:321–325.
53. Torenbeek R, Hermsen MA, Meijer GA, et al. Analysis by comparative genomic hybridization of epithelial and spindle cell components in sarcomatoid carcinoma and carcinosarcoma: histogenetic aspects. *J Pathol* 1999;189:338–343.
54. Taylor NP, Zighelboim I, Huettner PC, et al. DNA mismatch repair and TP53 defects are early events in uterine carcinosarcoma tumorigenesis. *Mod Pathol* 2006;19:1333–1338.
55. Ferguson SE, Tornos C, Hummer A, et al. Prognostic features of surgical stage I uterine carcinosarcoma. *Am J Surg Pathol* 2007;31(11):1653–1661.
56. McCluggage WG. Malignant biphasic uterine tumors: carcinosarcomas or metaplastic carcinomas? *J Clin Pathol* 2002;55:321–325.
57. Torenbeek R, Hermsen MA, Meijer GA, et al. Analysis by comparative genomic hybridization of epithelial and spindle cell components in sarcomatoid carcinoma and carcinosarcoma: histogenetic aspects. *J Pathol* 1999;189:338–343.
58. Euscher ED, Deavers MT, Ramondetta L, et al. Clinicopathologic features of malignant mixed müllerian tumors in patients with and without prolonged survival. *Mod Pathol* 2006;19(Suppl 1):177A.
59. Pautier P, Genestie C, Rey A, et al. Analysis of clinicopathologic prognostic factors for 157 uterine sarcomas and evaluation of a grading score validated for soft tissue sarcoma. *Cancer* 2000;88:1425–1431.
60. Inthasorn P, Carter J, Valmadre S, et al. Analysis of clinicopathologic factors in malignant mixed müllerian tumors of the uterine corpus. *Int J Gynecol Cancer* 2002;12;348–353.
61. Temkin SM, Hellmann M, Lee YC, et al. Early stage carcinosarcoma of the uterus: the significance of lymph node count. *Int J Gynecol Cancer* 2007;17:215–219.
62. Garamvoelgyi E, Guillou L, Gebhard S, et al. Primary malignant mixed müllerian tumor of the female peritoneum. A clinical, pathologic and immunohistochemical study of three cases and review of the literature. *Cancer* 1994;74:854–863.
63. Rose PG, Rodriguez M, Abdul-Karim FW. Malignant mixed müllerian tumor of the female peritoneum: treatment and outcome of three cases. *Gyneol Oncol* 1997;65:523–525.
64. Sumathi VP, Murnaghan M, Dobbs SP, et al. Extragenital müllerian carcinosarcoma arising from the peritoneum: report of two cases. *Int J Gynecol Cancer* 2002;12:764–767.
65. Ko ML, Huang SH, Shen J, et al. Primary peritoneal carcinosarcoma: report of a case with five year disease free survival after surgery and chemoradiation and review of the literature. *Acta Oncol* 2005;44:756–760.
66. Shintaku M, Matsumoto T. Primary müllerian carcinosarcoma of the retroperitoneum: report of a case. *Int J Gynecol Pathol* 2001;20:191–195.
67. Booth C, Zahn CM, McBroom J, et al. Retroperitoneal müllerian carcinosarcoma associated with endometriosis: a case report. *Gynecol Oncol* 2004;93:546–549.
68. Norris HJ, Taylor HB. Mesenchymal tumors of the uterus. I. A clinical and pathological study of 53 endometrial stromal tumors. *Cancer* 1966;19:755–766.
69. Schilder JM, Hurd WW, Roth LM, et al. Hormonal treatment of an endometrial stromal nodule followed by local excision. *Obstet Gynecol* 1999;93:805–807.
70. Dionigi A, Oliva E, Clement PB, et al. Endometrial stromal nodules and endometrial stromal tumors with limited infiltration: a clinicopathologic study of 50 cases. *Am J Surg Pathol* 2002;26:567–581.
71. Chang KL, Crabtree GS, Kim Lim-Tan S, et al. Primary uterine endometrial stromal neoplasms: a clinicopathologic study of 117 cases. *Am J Surg Pathol* 1990;14:415–438.
72. Oliva E, Young RH, Clement PB, et al. Myxoid and fibrous endometrial stromal tumors of the uterus: a report of 10 cases. *Int J Gynecol Pathol* 1999;18:310–319.
73. Yilmaz A, Rush DS, Soslow RA. Endometrial stromal sarcomas with unusual histologic features: a report of 24 primary and metastatic tumors emphasizing fibroblastic and smooth muscle differentiation. *Am J Surg Pathol* 2002;26:1142–1150.
74. Oliva E, Clement PB, Young RH. Epithelioid endometrial and endometrioid stromal tumors: a report of four cases emphasizing their distinction from epithelioid smooth muscle tumors and other oxyphilic uterine and extrauterine tumors. *Int J Gynecol Pathol* 2002;21:48–55.
75. Clement PB, Scully RE. Endometrial stromal sarcomas of the uterus with extensive endometrioid glandular differentiation: a report of three cases that caused problems in differential diagnosis. *Int J Gynecol Pathol* 1992;11:163–173.
76. Dahiya S, Felix A, Branton P, et al. Low grade endometrial stromal sarcoma: is there an immunophenotype predictive of clinical behavior? *Mod Pathol* 2007;20(Suppl 2):194A.
77. Chang KL, Crabtree GS, Soo Kim LT, et al. Primary extrauterine endometrial stromal neoplasms: a clinicopathologic study of 20 cases and a review of the literature. *Int J Gynecol Oncol* 1993;12:282–296.
78. Irvin W, Pelkey T, Rice L, et al. Endometrial stromal sarcoma of the vulva arising in extraovarian endometriosis: a case report and literature review. *Gynecol Oncol* 1998;71:313–316.
79. Katsanis WA, O'Connor DM, Gibb RK, et al. Endometrial stromal sarcoma involymphovascular invasion the placenta. *Ann Diagn Pathol* 1998;2:301–305.
80. Kondi-Paphitis A, Smyrniotis B, Liapis A, et al. Stromal sarcoma arising in endometriosis. A clinicopathologic and immunohistochemical study of 4 cases. *Eur J Gynaecol Oncol* 1998;19:588–590.
81. Boardman CH, Jefferies JA. Low grade endometrial stromal sarcoma of the ectocervix after therapy for breast cancer. *Gynecol Oncol* 2000;79: 120–123.
82. Lacroix-Triki M, Beyris L, Martel P, et al. Low-grade endometrial stromal sarcoma arising from sciatic nerve endometriosis. *Obstet Gynecol* 2004;104:1147–1149.
83. Androulaki A, Papathomas TG, Alexandrou P, et al. Metastatic low-grade endometrial stromal sarcoma of clitoris: report of a case. *Int J Gynecol Cancer* 2007;17:290–293.
84. Sato K, Ueda Y, Sugaya J, et al. Extrauterine endometrial stromal sarcoma with JAZF1/JJAZ1 fusion confirmed by RT-CPR and interphase FISH presenting as an inguinal tumor. *Virchows Arch* 2007;450:349–353.
85. Nucci MR, Harburger D, Koontz J, et al. Molecular analysis of the JAZF1-JjAZ1 gene fusion by RT-CPR and fluorescence in situ hybridization in endometrial stromal neoplasms. *Am J Surg Pathol* 2007;31:65–70.
86. Evans HL. Endometrial stromal sarcoma and poorly differentiated endometrial sarcoma. *Cancer* 1982;50:2170–2182.
87. Malpica A, Deavers MT, Silva EG. High-grade sarcoma in endometrial stromal sarcoma: dedifferentiated endometrial stromal sarcoma. *Mod Pathol* 2006;19(Suppl 1):188A.
88. Clement PB. Müllerian adenosarcoma of the uterus with sarcomatous overgrowth. A clinicopathologic analysis of 10 cases. *Am J Surg Pathol* 1989;13:28–38.
89. Soslow RA, Ali A, Negron E, et al. Müllerian adenosarcomas: an immunophenotypic analysis of 35 cases. *Mod Pathol* 2006;19(Suppl 1): 197A.
90. Amant F, Shurmans K, Steenkiste E, et al. Immunohistochemical determination of estrogen and progesterone receptor positivity in uterine adenosarcoma. *Gynecol Oncol* 2004;93:680–685.
91. Anderson J, Behbakht K, De Geest K, et al. Adenosarcoma in a patient with vaginal endometriosis. *Obstet Gynecol* 2001;98:964–966.
92. Liu L, Davidosmon S, Singh M. Müllerian adenosarcoma of vagina arising in persistent endometriosis: report of a case and review of the literature. *Gynecol Oncol* 2003;90:486–490.
93. Raffaelli R, Piazzola E, Zanconato G, et al. A rare case of extrauterine adenosarcoma arising in endometriosis of the rectovaginal septum. *Fertil Steril* 2004;81:1142–1144.
94. Yantiss RK, Clement PB, Young RH. Neoplastic and pre-neoplastic changes in gastrointestinal endometriosis: a study of 17 cases. *Am J Surg Pathol* 2000;24:513–524.
95. Vara AR, Ruzis EP, Moussabeck O, et al. Endometrioid adenosarcoma of the bladder arising from endometriosis. *J Urol* 1990;143:813–815.
96. Murugasu A, Miller J, Proietto A, et al. Extragenital müllerian adenosarcoma with sarcomatous overgrowth arising in an endometriotic cyst in the pouch of Douglas. *Int J Gynecol Pathol* 2003;13:371–375.
97. Dincer AD, Timmins P, Pietrocola D, et al. Primary peritoneal adenosarcoma with sarcomatous overgrowth associated with endometriosis. *Int J Gynecol Pathol* 2002;21:65–68.
98. N'Senda P, Wendum D, Balladur P, et al. Adenosarcoma arising in hepatic endometriosis. *Eur Radiol* 2000;10:1287–1289.
99. Clement PB, Scully RE. Uterine tumors resembling ovarian sex-cord tumors. A clinicopathologic analysis of fourteen cases. *Am J Clin Pathol* 1976;66:512–525.
100. Rollins SE, Clement PB, Young RH. Uterine tumors resembling ovarian sex cord tumors frequently have incorporated mature smooth muscle imparting a pseudoinfiltrative appearance. *Mod Pathol* 2007;20(Suppl 2): 212A.
101. Hornick JL, Fletcher CDM. Pecoma: what do we know so far? *Histopathology* 2006;48:75–82.

102. Folpe AL, Mentzel T, Lehr H, et al. Perivascular epithelioid neoplasms of soft tissue and gynecologic origin. *Am J Surg Pathol* 2005;29:1558–1575.
103. Vang R, Kempson RL. Perivascular epithelioid cell tumor (PEComa) of the uterus. A subset of HMB-45 epithelioid mesenchymal neoplasms with an uncertain relationship to pure smooth muscle tumors. *Am J Surg Pathol* 2002;26:1–13.
104. Silva EG, Deavers MT, Bodurka DC, et al. Uterine epithelioid leiomyosarcoma with clear cells. Reactivity with HMB45 and the concept of Pecoma. *Am J Surg Pathol* 2004;28:244–249.
105. Oliva E, Wang WL, Branton S, et al. Expression of melanocytic (PEComa) markers in smooth muscle tumors of the uterus: an immunohistochemical analysis of 86 cases. *Mod Pathol* 2006;19(Suppl 1):191A.
106. Simpson KW, Albores-Saavedra J. HMB-45 reactivity in conventional uterine leiomyosarcoma. *Am J Surg Pathol* 2007;31:95–98.
107. Sutton G, Kavanagh J, Wolfson AH, et al., Corpus: mesenchymal tumors. In: Hoskins WJ, Perez CA, Young RC, et al., eds. *Principles and Practice of Gynecologic Oncology.* 4th ed. Philadelphia: Lippincott, Williams & Wilkins; 2004:884.
108. Vongtama V, Karlen JR, Piver SM, et al. Treatment, results and prognostic factors in stage I and II sarcomas of the corpus uteri. *Am J Obstet Gynecol* 1976;126:139–147.
109. Salazar OM, Bonfiglio TA, Patten SF, et al. Uterine sarcomas: natural history, treatment and prognosis. *Cancer* 1978;42:1152–1160.
110. Perez CA, Askin F, Baglan RJ, et al. Effects of irradiation on mixed müllerian tumors of the uterine sarcomas. *Cancer* 1979;43:1274–1284.
111. Hoffmann W, Schmandt S, Koradiotherapymann RD, et al. Radiotherapy in the treatment of uterine sarcomas: a retrospective analysis of 54 cases. *Gynecol Obstet Invest* 1996;42:49–57.
112. Knocke TH, Kucera H, Dorfler D, et al. Results of postoperative radiotherapy in the treatment of sarcomas of the corpus uteri. *Cancer* 1998;83:1972–1979.
113. Ferrer F, Sabater S, Farruterine B, et al. Impact of radiotherapy on local control and survival in uterine sarcomas: a retrospective study from the GRUP Oncologic Catala-Occita. *Int J Radiat Oncol Biol Phys* 1999;44:47–52.
114. Chauveinc L, Deniaud E, Plancher C, et al. Uterine sarcomas: the Curie Institut experience. Prognostic factors and adjuvant treatments. *Gynecol Oncol* 1999;72:232–237.
115. Soumarova R, Horova H, Seneklova Z, et al. Treatment of uterine sarcoma: a survey of 49 patients. *Arch Gynecol Obstet* 2002;266:92–95.
116. Livi L, Paiar F, Shah N, et al. Uterine sarcoma: twenty-seven years of experience. *Int J Radiat Oncol Biol Phys* 2003;57:1366–1373.
117. Dusenbery KE, Potish RA, Agenta PA, et al. On the apparent failure of adjuvant pelvic radiotherapy to improve survival for women with uterine sarcomas confined to the uterus. *Am J Clin Oncol* 2005;28:295–300
118. Dusenberry KE, Potish RA, Judson P. Limitations of adjuvant radiotherapy for uterine sarcomas spread beyond the uterus. *Gynecol Oncol* 2004;94:191–196
119. Omura GA, Blessing JA, Major F, et al. A randomized clinical trial of adjuvant Adriamycin in uterine sarcomas: a Gynecologic Oncology Group study. *J Clin Oncol* 1985;3:1240–1245.
120. Hornback NB, Omura G, Major FJ. Observations on the uterine sarcomas of adjuvant radiation therapy in patients with stage I and II uterine sarcoma. *Int J Radiat Oncol Biol Phys* 1986;12:2127–2130.
121. Reed NS, Mangioni C, Malmstrom H, et al. First results of a randomized trial comparing radiotherapy versus uterine sarcomas observation postoperatively in patients with uterine sarcomas: an EORTC-GCG study. *Int J Gynecol Cancer* 2003;13:4.
122. Reed NS, Mangioni C, Malmstrom H, et al. Phase III randomized study to evaluate the role of adjuvant pelvic radiotherapy in the treatment of uterine sarcoma stages I and II: an EORTC Gynecologic Cancer Group study (protocol 55874). *Eur J Cancer* 2008;44(6):808–818.
123. Pautier P, Rey A, Haie-Meder C, et al. Adjuvant chemotherapy with cisplatin, ifosfamide, and doxorubicin followed by radiotherapy in localized uterine sarcomas: results of a case-controlled study with radiotherapy alone. *Int J Gynecol Cancer* 2004;14:1112–1117.
124. *WHO: Pathology and Genetics of Tumors of the Breast and Female Genital Organs.* Lyon: IARC Press; 2003.
125. Gerszten K, Faul C, Kounelis S, et al. The impact of adjuvant radiotherapy on carcinosarcoma of the uterus. *Gynecol Oncol* 1998;68:8–13.
126. Wong L, See HT, Khoo-Tan HS, et al. Combined adjuvant cisplatin and ifosfamide chemotherapy and radiotherapy for malignant mixed müllerian tumors of the uterine sarcomas. *Int J Gynecol Cancer* 2006;16:1364–1369.
127. Molpus KL, Redline-Frazzier S, Reed G, et al. Postoperative pelvic irradiation in early stage uterine mixed müllerian tumors. *Eur J Gynaec Oncol* 1998;19:541–546.
128. Le T. Adjuvant pelvic radiotherapy for uterine carcinosarcoma in a high risk population. *Eur J Surg Oncol* 2001;27:282–285.
129. Menczer J, Levy T, Piura B, et al. A comparison between different postoperative treatment modalities of uterine carcinosarcoma. *Gynecol Oncol* 2005;97:166–170.
130. Chi DS, Mychalczak B, Saigo PE, et al. The role of whole-pelvic irradiation in the treatment of early-stage uterine carcinosarcoma. *Gynecol Oncol* 1997;65:493–498.
131. Callister M, Ramondetta LM, Jhingran A, et al. Malignant mixed müllerian tumors of the uterus: analysis of patterns of failure, prognostic factors, and treatment outcome. *Int J Radiat Oncol Biol Phys* 2004; 58:786–796.
132. Knocke TH, Weitmann HD, Kucera H, et al. Results of primary and adjuvant radiotherapy in the treatment of mixed müllerian tumors of the corpus uteri. *Gynecol Oncol* 1999;73:389–395.
133. Sartori E, Bazzurini L, Gadducci A, et al. Carcinosarcoma of the uterine sarcomas: a clinicopathological multicenter CTF study. *Gynecol Oncol* 1997;67:70–75.
134. Smith DC, MacDonald OK, Gaffney DK. The impact of adjuvant radiation therapy on survival in women with uterine carcinosarcoma. *Int J Gynecol Cancer* 2008;18(2):255–261.
135. Wong L, See HT, Khoo-Tan HS, et al. Combined adjuvant cisplatin and ifosfamide chemotherapy and radiotherapy for malignant mixed müllerian tumors of the uterine corpus. *Int J Gynecol Cancer* 2006;16:1364–1369.
136. Wolfson AH, Brady MF, Rocereto TF, et al. A Gynecologic Oncology Group radomized trial of whole abdominal irradiation (WWAI) vs. cisplatin-ifosfamide+mesna (WCIM) in optimally debulked stage I-IV carcinosarcoma (WCS) of the uterine sarcomas. *J Clin Oncol* 2006;24:256.
137. Wolfson AH, Brady MF, Rocereto TF, et al. A Gynecologic Oncology Group randomized trial of whole abdominal irradiation versus chemotherapy in optimally debulked carcinosarcomas of the uterus. *Int J Gynecol Cancer* 2006;16:45.
138. Wolfson AH, Brady MF, Rocereto T, et al. A Gynecologic Oncology Group randomized phase III trial of whole abdominal irradiation (WWAI) vs. cisplatin-ifosfamide and mesna (CIM) as postsurgical therapy in stage I-IV carcinosarcoma (CS) of the uterus. *Gynecol Oncol* 2007;107:177–185.
139. Gadducci A, Landoni F, Saradiotherapyori E, et al. Uterine leiomyosarcoma: analysis of treatment failures and survival. *Gynecol Oncol* 1996;62:25–32.
140. Gadducci A, Fabrini MG, Bonuccelli A, et al. Analysis of treatment failures in patients with early-stage uterine leiomyosarcoma. *Anticancer Res* 1995;15:485–488.
141. Berchuck A, Rubin SC, Hoskins WJ, et al. Treatment of endometrial stromal tumors. *Gynecol Oncol* 1990;36:60–65.
142. Gadducci A, Saradiotherapyori E, Landoni F, et al. Endometrial stromal sarcoma: analysis of treatment failure and survival. *Gynecol Oncol* 1996;63:247–253.
143. Bodner K, Bodner-Adler B, Obermair A, et al. Prognostic parameters in endometrial stromal sarcoma: a clinicopathologic study in 31 patients. *Gynecol Oncol* 2001;81(2):160–165.
144. Geller MA, Argenta P, Bradley W, et al. Treatment and recurrence patterns in endometrial stromal sarcomas and the relation to c-kit. *Gynecol Oncol* 2004;95:632–636.
145. Rose PG, Piver MS, Tsukada Y, et al. Patterns of metastasis in uterine sarcoma: an autopsy study. *Cancer* 1989;63:935–938.
146. Resnik E, Chambers SK, Carcangiu ML, et al. A phase II study of etoposide, cisplatin, and doxorubicin chemotherapy in mixed müllerian tumors (MMT) of the uterus. *Gynecol Oncol* 1995;56:370–375.
147. Sutton G, Kauderer J, Carson LF, et al. Adjuvant ifosfamide and cisplatin in patients with completely resected stage I or II carcinosarcomas (mixed mesodermal tumors) of the uterus: a Gynecologic Oncology Group study. *Gynecol Oncol* 2005;96:630–634.
148. Odunsi K, Moneke V, Tammela J, et al. Efficacy of adjuvant CYVADIC chemotherapy in early-stage uterine sarcomas: results of long-term follow-up. *Int J Gynecol Cancer* 2004;14:659–664.
149. Piver MS, Lele SB, Marchetti DL, et al. Effect of adjuvant chemotherapy on time to recurrence and survival of stage I uterine sarcomas. *J Surg Oncol* 1988;38:233–239.
150. Hempling RE, Piver MS, Baker TR. Impact on progression-free survival of adjuvant cyclophosphamide, vincristine, doxorubicin (Adriamycin), and dacarbazine (CYVADIC) chemotherapy for stage I uterine sarcoma. A prospective trial. *Am J Clin Oncol* 1995;18:282–286.
151. Wong C, Lele SB, Natarajan N. Effect of adjuvant chemotherapy on long-term survival of stage I uterine sarcoma. *Proc Am Soc Clin Oncol* 1999;18:386 (abstract 1492).
152. Sutton G, Blessing J, Hanjani P, et al. Phase II evaluation of liposomal doxorubicin (Doxil) in recurrent or advanced leiomyosarcoma of the uterus: a Gynecologic Oncology Group study. *Gynecol Oncol* 2005;96:749–752.
153. Miller DS, Blessing JA, Ball H, et al. Phase II trial of topotecan in patients with advanced, persistent, or recurrent uterine leiomyosarcomas: a Gynecologic Oncology Group study. *Am J Clin Oncol* 2000;23:355–357.
154. Sutton G, Blessing JA, Ball H. Phase II trial of paclitaxel in leiomyosarcoma of the uterus: a Gynecologic Oncology Group study. *Gynecol Oncol* 1999;74:346–349.
155. Sutton G, Blessing JA, Barrett RJ, et al. Phase II trial of ifosfamide and mesna in leiomyosarcoma of the uterus: a Gynecologic Oncology Group study. *Am J Obstet Gynecol* 1992;166:556–559.
156. Thigpen T, Blessing JA, Yordan E, et al. Phase II trial of etoposide in leiomyosarcoma of the uterus: a Gynecologic Oncology group study. *Gynecol Oncol* 1996;63:120–122.
157. Thigpen T, Blessing JA, Beecham J, et al. Phase II trial of cisplatin as first-line chemotherapy in patients with advanced or recurrent uterine

sarcomas: a Gynecologic Oncology Group study. *J Clin Oncol* 1991;9: 1962–1966.
158. Omura GA, Major FJ, Blessing JA, et al. A randomized study of Adriamycin with and without dimethyl triazenoimidazole carboxamide in advanced uterine sarcomas. *Cancer* 1983;52:626–632.
159. Thigpen JT, Blessing JA, Homesley HD, et al. Phase II trial of piperazinedione in patients with advanced or recurrent uterine sarcoma. A Gynecologic Oncology Group study. *Am J Clin Oncol* 1985;8:350–352.
160. Asbury R, Blessing JA, Smith DM, et al. Aminothiadiazole in the treatment of advanced leiomyosarcoma of the uterine corpus. A Gynecologic Oncology Group study. *Am J Clin Oncol* 1995;18:397–399.
161. Slayton RE, Blessing JA, Look K, et al. A phase II clinical trial of diaziquone (AZQ) in the treatment of patients with recurrent leiomyosarcoma of the uterus, a Gynecologic Oncology Group study. *Invest New Drugs* 1991;9:207–208.
162. Look K, Sandler A, Blessing JA, et al. Phase II trial of gemcitabine as second-line chemotherapy of uterine leiomyosarcoma: a Gynecologic Oncology Group study. *Gynecol Oncol* 2004;92:644–647.
163. Svancarova L, Blay JY, Judson IR, et al. Gemcitabine in advanced adult soft-tissue sarcomas. A phase II study of the EORTC Soft Tissue and Bone Sarcoma Group. *Eur J Cancer* 2002;38:556–559.
164. Okuno S, Edmonson J, Mahoney M, et al. Phase II trial of gemcitabine in advanced sarcomas. *Cancer* 2002;94:3225–3229.
165. Patel SR, Gandhi V, Jenkins J, et al. Phase II clinical investigation of gemcitabine in advanced soft tissue sarcomas and window evaluation of dose rate on gemcitabine triphosphate accumulation. *J Clin Oncol* 2001;19: 3483–3489.
166. Gallup DG, Blessing JA, Andersen W, et al. Evaluation of paclitaxel in previously treated leiomyosarcoma of the uterus: a Gynecologic Oncology Group study. *Gynecol Oncol* 2003;89:48–51.
167. Yovine A, Riofrio M, Blay JY, et al. Phase II study of ecteinascidin-743 in advanced pretreated soft tissue sarcoma patients. *J Clin Oncol* 2004;22: 890–899.
168. Twelves C, Hoekman K, Bowman A, et al. Phase I and pharmacokinetic study of YondelisTM (Ecteinascidin-743; ET-743) administered as an infusion over 1 h or 3 h every 21 days in patients with solid tumours. *Eur J Cancer* 2003;339:1842–1851.
169. Smith HO, Blessing JA, Vaccarello L. Trimetrexate in the treatment of recurrent or advanced leiomyosarcoma of the uterus: a phase II study of the Gynecologic Oncology Group. *Gynecol Oncol* 2002;84:140–144.
170. Rose PG, Blessing JA, Soper JT, et al. Prolonged oral etoposide in recurrent or advanced leiomyosarcoma of the uterus: a Gynecologic Oncology Group study. *Gynecol Oncol* 1998;70:267–271.
171. Slayton RE, Blessing JA, Angel C, et al. Phase II trial of etoposide in the management of advanced and recurrent leiomyosarcoma of the uterus: a Gynecologic Oncology Group study. *Cancer Treat Rep* 1987;71: 1303–1304.
172. Asbury R, Blessing JA, Buller R, et al. Amonafide in patients with leiomyosarcoma of the uterus: a phase II gynecologic oncology group study. *Am J Clin Oncol* 1998;21:145–146.
173. Muss HB, Bundy BN, Adcock L, et al. Mitoxantrone in the treatment of advanced uterine sarcoma. A phase II trial of the Gynecologic Oncology Group. *Am J Clin Oncol* 1990;13:32–34.
174. Thigpen JT, Blessing JA, Wilbanks GD. Cisplatin as second-line chemotherapy in the treatment of advanced or recurrent leiomyosarcoma of the uterus. A phase II trial of the Gynecologic Oncology Group. *Am J Clin Oncol* 1986;9:18–20.
175. Long H III, Blessing JA, Sorosky J. Phase II trial of dacarbazine, mitomycin, doxorubicin, and cisplatin with sargramostim in uterine leiomyosarcoma: a Gynecologic Oncology Group study. *Gynecol Oncol* 2005;99:339–342.
176. Edmonson JH, Marks RS, Buckner JC, et al. Contrast of response to dacarbazine, mitomycin, doxorubicin, and cisplatin (DMAP) plus GM-CSF between patients with advanced malignant gastrointestinal stromal tumors and patients with other advanced leiomyosarcomas. *Cancer Invest* 2002;20:605–612.
177. Edmonson JH, Blessing JA, Cosin JA, et al. Phase II study of mitomycin, doxorubicin and cisplatin in the treatment of advanced uterine leiomyosarcoma: a Gynecologic Oncology Group study. *Gynecol Oncol* 2002;85: 507–510.
178. Currie J, Blessing JA, Muss HB, et al. Combination chemotherapy with hydroxyurea, dacarbazine (DTIC), and etoposide in the treatment of uterine leiomyosarcoma: a Gynecologic Oncology Group study. *Gynecol Oncol* 1996;61:27–30.
179. Sutton G, Blessing JA, Malfetano JH. Ifosfamide and doxorubicin in the treatment of advanced leiomyosarcoma of the uterus: a Gynecologic Oncology Group study. *Gynecol Oncol* 1996;62:226–229.
180. Hensley ML, Maki R, Venkatraman E, et al. Gemcitabine and docetaxel in patients with unresectable leiomyosarcoma: results of a phase II trial. *J Clin Oncol* 2002;20:2824–2831.
181. Muss HB, Bundy B, DiSaia PJ, et al. Treatment of recurrent or advanced uterine sarcoma. A randomized trial of doxorubicin versus doxorubicin and cyclophosphamide (a phase III trial of the Gynecologic Oncology Group). *Cancer* 1985;15:1648–1653.
182. Kanjeekal S, Chambers A, Fung MF, et al. Systemic therapy for advanced uterine sarcoma: a systemic review of the literature. *Gynecol Oncol* 2005;97:624–637.
183. Thigpen JT, Blessing JA, Beecham J, et al. Phase II trial of cisplatin as first-line chemotherapy in patients with advanced or recurrent uterine sarcomas: a Gynecologic Oncology Group study. *J Clin Oncol* 1991;9: 1962–1966.
184. Homesley HD, Filiaci V, Markman M, et al. Phase III trial of ifosfamide with or without paclitaxel in advanced uterine carcinosarcomas: a Gynecologic Oncology Group study. *J Clin Oncol* 2007;25:526–531.
185. Sutton G, Brunetto VL, Kilgore L, et al. A phase III trial of ifosfamide with or without cisplatin in carcinosarcomas of the uterus: a Gynecologic Oncology Group study. *Gynecol Oncol* 2000;79:147–153.
186. Sutton G, Blessing JA, Rosenshein N, et al. Phase II trial of ifosfamide and mesna in mixed mesodermal tumors of the uterus: a Gynecologic Oncology Group study. *Am J Obstet Gynecol* 1989;161:309–312.
187. Gershenson DM, Kavanagh JJ, Copeland LJ, et al. High-dose doxorubicin infusion therapy for disseminated mixed mesodermal sarcoma of the uterus. *Cancer* 1987;59:1264–1267.
188. Miller DS, Blessing JA, Schilder J, et al. Phase II evaluation of topotecan in carcinosarcomas of the uterus: a Gynecologic Oncology Group study. *Gynecol Oncol* 2005;98:217–221.
189. Fowler JM, Blessing JA, Burger RA, et al. Phase II evaluation of oral trimetrexate in mixed mesodermal tumors of the uterus: a Gynecologic Oncology Group study. *Gynecol Oncol* 2002;85:311–314.
190. Curtin JP, Blessing JA, Soper JT, et al. Paclitaxel in the treatment of carcinosarcoma of the uterus: a Gynecologic Oncology Group study. *Gynecol Oncol* 2001;83:268–270.
191. Asbury R, Blessing JA, Podczaski E, et al. A phase II trial of amonafide in patients with mixed mesodermal tumors of the uterus: a Gynecologic Oncology Group study. *Am J Clin Oncol* 1998;21:306–307.
192. Asbury R, Blessing JA, Moore D. A phase II trial of aminothiadiazole in patients with mixed mesodermal tumors of the uterine corpus: a Gynecologic Oncology Group study. *Am J Clin Oncol* 1996;19:400–402.
193. Slayton RE, Blessing JA, Clarke-Pearson D. A phase II trial of diaziquone (AZQ) in mixed mesodermal sarcomas of the uterus. *Invest New Drugs* 1991;9:93–94.
194. Slayton RE, Blessing JA, DiSaia PJ, et al. Phase II trial of etoposide in the management of advanced or recurrent mixed mesodermal sarcomas of the uterus: a Gynecologic Oncology Group study. *Cancer Treat Rep* 1987;71: 661–662.
195. Thigpen JT, Blessing JA, Orr JW Jr, et al. Phase II trial of cisplatin in the treatment of patients with advanced or recurrent mixed mesodermal sarcomas of the uterus: a Gynecologic Oncology Group study. *Cancer Treat Rep* 1986;70:271–274.
196. Gershenson DM, Kavanagh JJ, Copeland LJ, et al. Cisplatin therapy for disseminated mixed mesodermal sarcoma of the uterus. *J Clin Oncol* 1987;5:618–621.
197. Sutton G, Kauderer J, Carson LF, et al. Adjuvant ifosfamide and cisplatin in patients with completely resected stage I or II carcinosarcomas (mixed mesodermal tumors) of the uterus: a Gynecologic Oncology Group study. *Gynecol Oncol* 2005;96:630–634.
198. Currie J, Blessing JA, McGehee R, et al. Phase II trial of hydroxyurea, dacarbazine (DTIC), and etoposide (VP-16) in mixed mesodermal tumors of the uterus: a Gynecologic Oncology Group study. *Gynecol Oncol* 1996;61:94–96.
199. Resnik E, Chambers SK, Carcangiu, ML, et al. A phase II study of etoposide, cisplatin, and doxorubicin chemotherapy in mixed müllerian tumors (MMT) of the uterus. *Gynecol Oncol* 1995;56:370–375.
200. Piver MS, DeEulis TG, Lele SB, et al. Cyclophosphamide, vincristine, Adriamycin, and dimethyl-triazeno imidazole carboxamide (CYVADIC) for sarcomas of the female genital tract. *Gynecol Oncol* 1982;14: 319–323.
201. van Rijswijk RE, Vermorken JB, Reed N, et al. Cisplatin, doxorubicin and ifosfamide in carcinosarcomas of the female genital tract. A phase II study of the European Organization for Research and Treatment of Cancer Gynaecological Cancer Group (EORTC 55923). *Eur J Cancer* 2003;39: 481–487.
202. Sutton G, Blessing JA, Park R, et al. Ifosfamide treatment of recurrent or metastatic endometrial stromal sarcomas previously unexposed to chemotherapy: a study of the Gynecologic Oncology Group. *Obstet Gynecol* 1996;87:747–750.
203. Berchuck A, Rubin SC, Hoskins WJ, et al. Treatment of endometrial stromal tumors. *Gynecol Oncol* 1990;36:60–65.
204. Szlosarek PW, Lofts FJ, Pettengell R, et al. Effective treatment of a patient with a high-grade endometrial stromal sarcoma with an accelerated regimen of carboplatin and paclitaxel. *Anticancer Drugs* 2000;11:275–278.
205. Yamawaki T, Shimizu Y, Hasumi K. Treatment of stage IV "high-grade" endometrial stromal sarcoma with ifosfamide, Adriamycin, and cisplatin. *Gynecol Oncol* 1997;64:265–269.
206. Ihnen M, Mahner S, Janicke F, Schwartz J. Current treatment options in uterine endometrial stromal sarcoma: report of a case and review of the literature. *Int J Gynecol Cancer* 2007;17(5):957–963.
207. Lehner LM, Miles PA, Enck RE. Complete remission of widely metastatic endometrial stromal sarcoma following combination chemotherapy. *Cancer* 1979;433:1189–1194.
208. Lin YC, Kudelka AP, Tresukosol D, et al. Prolonged stabilization of progressive endometrial stromal sarcoma with prolonged oral etoposide therapy. *Gynecol Oncol* 1995;58:262–265.

209. Spano JP, Soria JC, Kambouchner M, et al. Long-term survival of patients given hormonal therapy for metastatic endometrial stromal sarcoma. *Med Oncol* 2003;20:87–93.
210. Sutton GP, Stehman FB, Michael H, et al. Estrogen and progesterone receptors in uterine sarcomas. *Obstet Gynecol* 1986;68:709–714.
211. Burke C, Hickey K. Treatment of endometrial stromal sarcoma with a gonadotropin-releasing hormone analogue. *Obstet Gynecol* 2004;104: 1182–1184.
212. Maluf FC, Sabbatini P, Schwartz L, et al. Endometrial stromal sarcoma: objective response to letrozole. *Gynecol Oncol* 2001;82:384–388.
213. McCluggage WG, Abdulkader M, Price JH, et al. Uterine carcinosarcomas in patients receiving tamoxifen. A report of 19 cases. *Int J Gynecol Cancer* 2000;10:280–284.
214. Kloos I, Delaloge S, Pautier P, et al. Tamoxifen-related carcinosarcomas occur under/after prolonged treatment: report of five cases and review of the literature. *Int J Gynecol Cancer* 2002;12:496–500.
215. Lantta M, Kahanpaa K, Karkkainen J, et al. Estradiol and progesterone receptors in two cases of endometrial stromal sarcoma. *Gynecol Oncol* 1984;18:233–239.
216. Baker TR, Piver MS, Lele SB, et al. Stage I uterine adenosarcoma: a report of six cases. *J Surg Oncol* 1988;37:128–132.
217. Piver MS, Rutledge FN, Copeland L, et al. Uterine endolymphatic stromal myosis. *Obstet Gynecol* 1984;63:725–745.
218. Scribner DR Jr, Walker JL. Low-grade endometrial stromal sarcoma: preoperative treatment with depo-lupron and megace. *Gynecol Oncol* 1998;71:458–460.
219. Navarro D, Cabrera JJ, Leon L, et al. Endometrial stromal sarcoma expression of estrogen receptors, progesterone receptors and estrogen-induced srp27 (24K) suggests hormone responsiveness. *J Steroid Biochem Mol Biol* 1992;41:589–596.
220. Mansi JL, Ramachandra S, Wiltshaw E, et al. Endometrial stromal sarcomas. *Gynecol Oncol* 1990;36:113–118.
221. O'Brien AA, O'Briain DS, Daly PA. Aggressive endometrial stromal sarcoma responding to medroxyprogesterone following failure of tamoxifen and combination chemotherapy. Case report. *Br J Obstet Gynaecol* 1985;92:862–866.
222. Pink D, Lindner T, Mrozek A, et al. Harm or benefit of hormonal treatment in metastatic low-grade endometrial stromal sarcoma: single center experience with 10 cases and review of the literature. *Gynecol Oncol* 2006;101:464–469.
223. Krumholz BA, Lobovsky FY, Halitsky V. Endolymphatic stromal myosis with pulmonary metastases. Remission with progestin therapy: report of a case. *J Reprod Med* 1973;10:85–89.
224. Wang X, Tangjitgamol S, Liu J, et al. Response of recurrent uterine high-grade malignant mixed müllerian tumor to letrozole. *Int J Gynecol Cancer* 2005;15:1243–1248.
225. Maki RG. Recent advances in therapy for gastrointestinal stromal tumors. *Curr Oncol Rep* 2007;9:165–169.
226. Wang L, Felix JC, Lee JL, et al. The proto-oncogene c-kit is expressed in leiomyosarcomas of the uterus. *Gynecol Oncol* 2003;90:402–406.
227. Raspollini MR, Villanucci A, Amunni G, et al. c-KIT expression in leiomyosarcomas of the uterus: an immunocytochemical study on 29 cases of malignant smooth muscle tumors of the uterus. *J Chemother* 2003;15(1):81–84.
228. Rushing RS, Shajahan S, Chendil D, et al. Uterine sarcomas express KIT protein but lack mutation(s) in exon 11 or 17 of c-KIT. *Gynecol Oncol* 2003;91:9–14.
229. Oliva E, Young RH, Amin MB, et al. An immunohistochemical analysis of endometrial stromal and smooth muscle tumors of the uterus: a study of 54 cases emphasizing the importance of using a panel because of overlap in immunoreactivity for individual antibodies. *Am J Surg Pathol* 2002;26:403–412.
230. Klein WM, Kurman RJ. Lack of expression of c-kit protein (KCD117) in mesenchymal tumors of the uterus and ovary. *Int J Gynecol Pathol* 2003;22:181–184.
231. Winter WE III, Seidman JD, Krivak TC, et al. Clinicopathological analysis of c-kit expression in carcinosarcomas and leiomyosarcomas of the uterine corpus. *Gynecol Oncol* 2003;91:3–8.
232. Emoto M, Ishiguro M, Iwasaki H, et al. Effect of angiogenesis inhibitor TNP-470 on the growth, blood flow, and microvessel density in xenografts of human uterine carcinosarcoma in nude mice. *Gynecol Oncol* 2003;89:88–94.
233. Gadducci A, Sartori E, Landoni F, et al. The prognostic relevance of histological type in uterine sarcomas: a Cooperation Task Force (CTF) multivariate analysis of 249 cases. *Eur J Gynaecol Oncol* 2002;23:295–299.
234. Livi L, Andreopoulou E, Shah N, et al. Treatment of uterine sarcoma at the Royal Marsden Hospital from 1974 to 1998. *Clin Oncol (Coll Radiol)* 2004;16:261–268.
235. Kelly KL, Craighead PS. Characteristics and management of uterine sarcoma patients treated at the Tom Baker Cancer Centre. *Int J Gynecol Cancer* 2005;15:132–139.
236. Denschlag D, Masoud I, Stanimir G, et al. Prognostic factors and outcome in women with uterine sarcoma. *EJSO* 2007;33:91–95.
237. Gerszten K, Faul C, Kounelis S, et al. The impact of adjuvant radiotherapy on carcinosarcoma of the uterus. *Gynecol Oncol* 1998;68:8–13.
238. Hannigan EV, Gomez IG. Uterine leiomyosarcomas: a review of prognostic clinical and pathologic factors. *Am J Obstet Gynecol* 1979;134: 557–562.
239. Kaku T, Silverberg SG, Major FJ, et al. Adenosarcoma of the uterus: a Gynecologic Oncology Group clinicopathologic study of 31 cases. *Int J Gynecol Pathol* 1992;11:75–88.
240. Dionigi A, Oliva E, Clement PB, et al. Endometrial stromal nodules and endometrial stromal tumors with limited infiltration: a clinicopathologic study of 50 cases. *Am J Surg Pathol* 2002;26:567–581.
241. Sagae S, Yamashita K, Ishioka S, et al. Preoperative diagnosis and treatment results in 106 patients with uterine sarcoma in Hokkaido, Japan. *Oncology* 2004;67:33.
242. Chang KL, Crabtree GS, Kim Lim-Tan S, et al. Primary uterine endometrial stromal neoplasms. A clinicopathologic study of 117 cases. *Am J Surg Pathol* 1990;14:415–438.
243. Young RH, Prat J, Scully RE. Endometrioid stromal sarcomas of the ovary: a clinicopathologic analysis of 23 cases. *Cancer* 1984;53(5): 1143–1155.
244. Nielsen SN, Podratz KC, Scheithauer BW, et al. Clinical-pathologic analysis of uterine malignant mixed müllerian tumors. *Gynecol Oncol* 1988;34: 372–378.
245. Shaw RW, Lynch PF, Wade-Evans T. Müllerian mixed tumour of the uterine corpus: a clinical histopathological review of 28 patients. *Br J Obstet Gyneaecol* 1983;90:562–570.
246. Punnonen R, Lauslahti K, Pystynen P, et al. Uterine sarcomas. *Ann Chir Gynaecol* 1985;74(Supp):11–15.
247. Yu KJ, Ho DM, Ng HT, et al. Leiomyosarcoma of the uterus: a review of 14 cases. *Zhonghua Yi Xue Za Zhi (KTaipei)* 1989;44:109–115.
248. Dinh TA, Oliva EA, Fuller AF, et al. The treatment of gynecologic leiomyosarcoma. Results from a 10-year experience (1990–1999) at the Massachusetts General Hospital. *Gynecol Oncol* 2004;92:684–692.
249. Helman LJ, Meltzer P. Mechanisms of sarcoma development. *Nat Rev Cancer* 2003;3:685–694.
250. Rogatsch H, Bonatti H, Menet A, et al. Epstein-Barr virus–associated multicentric leiomyosarcoma in an adult patient after heart transplantation: case report and review of the literature. *Am J Surg Pathol* 2000;24: 614–621.
251. Boman F, Gultekin H, Dickman PS. Latent Epstein-Barr virus infection demonstrated in low-grade leiomyosarcomas of adults with acquired immunodeficiency syndrome, but not in adjacent Kaposi's lesion or smooth muscle tumors in immunocompetent patients. *Arch Pathol Lab Med* 1997;121:834–838.
252. Yokoi S, Iizasa T, Hiroshima K, et al. Pulmonary artery leiomyosarcoma expressing Epstein-Barr virus in an immunocompetent individual. *Ann Thorac Surg* 2006;81:1897–1899.
253. Seki A, Kodama J, Miyagi Y, et al. Amplification of the mdm-2 gene and p53 abnormalities in uterine sarcomas. *Int J Cancer* 1997;26:33–37.
254. Ramondetta LM, Burke TW, Jhingran A, et al. A phase II trial of cisplatin, ifosfamide and mesna in patients with advanced or recurrent malignant mixed müllerian tumors with evaluation of potential molecular targets. *Gynecol Oncol* 2003;90:529–536.
255. Nasu K, Kawano Y, Hirota Y. Immunohistochemical study of c-*erb*B-2 expression in MMMT of the female genital tract. *Int J Obstet Gynecol* 1996;22:347–351.
256. Costa MJ, Walls J. Epidermal growth factor receptor and c-*erb*B-2 oncoprotein expression in female genital tract carcinosarcomas (malignant mixed müllerian tumors): a clinicopathologic study of 82 cases. *Cancer* 1996;77:533–542.
257. Emoto M, Iwasaki H, Ishiguro M, et al. Angiogenesis in carcinosarcomas of the uterus: differences in the microvessel density and expression of vascular endothelial growth factor between the epithelial and mesenchymal elements. *Hum Pathol* 1999;30:1232–1241.
258. Roy RN, Gerulath AH, Cecutti A, et al. Loss of IGF-II imprinting in endometrial tumors: overexpression in carcinosarcomas. *Cancer Lett* 2000;153:67–73.
259. Anderson SE, Nonaka D, Chuai S, et al. p53, epidermal growth factor, and platelet-derived growth factor in uterine leiomyosarcoma and leiomyomas. *Int J Gynecol Cancer* 2006;16:849–853.
260. Iwasa Y, Haga H, Konishi I, et al. Prognostic factors in uterine carcinosarcoma: a clinicopathologic study of 82 cases. *Cancer* 1998;82:512–519.
261. Hibshoosh H, Lattes R. Immunohistochemical and molecular genetic approaches to soft tissue tumor diagnosis: a primer. *Semin Oncol* 1997; 24:515–525.

CHAPTER 25 ■ EPITHELIAL OVARIAN CANCER

GINI F. FLEMING, BRIGITTE M. RONNETT, JEFFREY SEIDMAN, RICHARD J. ZAINO, AND STEPHEN C. RUBIN

Epithelial ovarian cancer is the leading cause of death from gynecologic cancer in the United States. Data from the Surveillance, Epidemiology, and End Results (SEER) program of the U.S. National Cancer Institute (NCI) suggest that 21,650 new cases of ovarian cancer and 15,520 deaths from ovarian cancer are expected in the United States for 2008 (1). This makes ovarian cancer the eighth most common major cancer and the fifth most common cause of cancer death in U.S. women. It has been estimated that, in the United States, one woman in 70 will develop ovarian cancer, and one woman in 100 will die of the disease.

Worldwide, ovarian cancer is the sixth most common form of cancer in women. In general, the highest incidence rates are found in European and North American population groups with the lowest rates in Asian population groups (Fig. 25.1). In Japan, the incidence has increased since the 1970s, although it remains lower than in many Western countries (2). In the United States, rates for black American women are about two thirds of those for white women, and rates for women of Asian/Pacific Islander descent are similar to those of black women (3). Rates of hysterectomy and oophorectomy in a population will affect the rate of ovarian cancer; 40% to 50% of women in the United States have a hysterectomy by age 60 to 70, and about half of them have their ovaries removed at the same time (4).

Despite some apparent advances in therapy, survival in the United States from ovarian cancer has increased only slightly over the past decades. Small but significant improvements in survival have been noted for white women but not for black women. Overall 5-year relative survival rates increased from 37% during 1975 to 1977 (36% for whites and 43% for blacks) to 45% during 1996 to 2002 (45% for whites and 39% for blacks). These numbers are affected by the exclusion of borderline tumors from the 1996 to 2002 survival rates (1). Outcomes in black women are worse even when controlling for age, stage, and histology. The reasons for this are not clear. However, in a retrospective analysis of six Gynecologic Oncology Group (GOG) studies for women with advanced-stage disease, race was not associated with progression-free survival or overall survival in the clinical trial setting after controlling for other prognostic factors (5).

RISK FACTORS AND PATHOGENESIS

Established risk factors (reviewed in more detail in Chapter 1) for ovarian cancer include increasing age, family history, nulliparity, early menarche, and late menopause. Breast-feeding is protective. Aside from having a first-degree relative with the disease, age is the most important risk factor for ovarian cancer (Fig. 25.2). Fifty percent of all U.S. cases occur in women over the age of 65 (6). Older women have a much worse prognosis overall (Fig. 25.3), which is in part because they have an increased incidence of high-stage and high-grade disease at the time of diagnosis (Table 25.1) (7). However, in an analysis of the SEER database, age remained a poor prognostic factor even when results were adjusted for stage, grade, histologic cell type, race, and surgical treatment. The relative risks (RR) associated with endocrinologic factors are much smaller, though important, because they are potentially subject to modulation.

Risk Factors for Mucinous Tumors

The epidemiologic risks associated with mucinous tumors may be different from those associated with serous or other histologic subtypes (8), although the infrequency of this histologic subtype and the potential for contamination of the sample with metastatic tumors from other organ sites make it difficult to draw firm conclusions. The Danish MALOVA case-control study reported that the overall risk (OR) of ovarian cancer decreased with ever being pregnant (OR 0.40), with increasing number of pregnancies, and with use of oral contraceptives (OR 0.67) and risk increased with ever use of hormone replacement therapy (HRT) (OR 1.3). These effects were all present for serous tumors, endometrioid tumors, and tumors of other histologies, but not for mucinous tumors. In contrast, current smoking was an increased risk factor only for mucinous tumors (OR 1.78) (9). Smoking has also been associated with a threefold increased risk of benign mucinous ovarian tumors (10). Both invasive mucinous tumors and borderline mucinous tumors are more common in women of Asian descent.

Dietary and Environmental Factors

There have been no consistent relationships reported of specific dietary components to ovarian cancer risk. Although some studies have associated a diet high in meat and animal fat or a diet high in lactose with development of ovarian cancer (8,10), most large recent studies, including the European prospective investigation into cancer and nutrition (EPIC) study, which recruited 366,521 European women (11), and the California Teachers Study, which included 97,275 women with 280 ovarian cancer cases (12), failed to demonstrate any relationship between consumption of animal foods and the development of ovarian cancer. The investigators for the California Teachers Study concluded that while dietary consumption of isoflavones may be marginally associated with decreased

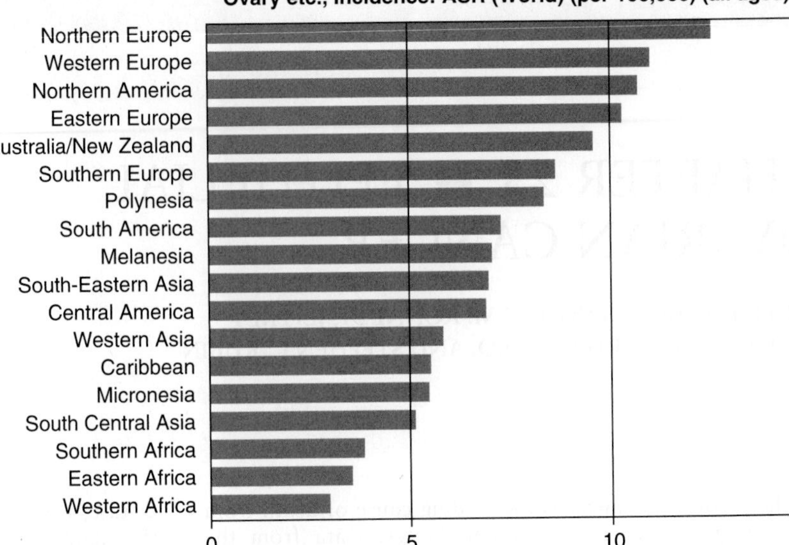

FIGURE 25.1. Age-standardized incidence rates of ovarian cancer in the world. *Source:* Ferlay J, Bray F, Pisani P, et al. GLOBOCAN 2000: cancer incidence, mortality and prevalence worldwide, version 1.0. IARC Cancer Base No. 5. Lyon: IARC, 2001.

ovarian cancer risk, most dietary factors are unlikely to play a major role in ovarian cancer development. Coffee has not been consistently associated with ovarian cancer. A few studies have suggested a relationship between alcohol intake and ovarian cancer (13), but this has not been consistent (12). Smoking is a risk factor for mucinous tumors (14). There does appear to be a modest inverse correlation between moderate physical activity and ovarian cancer risk (15,16,17), and obesity has shown a positive association with ovarian cancer risk in 24 of 28 studies reviewed in a recent meta-analysis (15). One interesting cohort control study showed that both recent obesity (OR 1.93; 95% CI, 1.3 to 2.88) and obesity at age 20 (OR 4.38; 95% CI, 1.88 to 10.2) were associated with an increased risk of benign serous tumors (16).

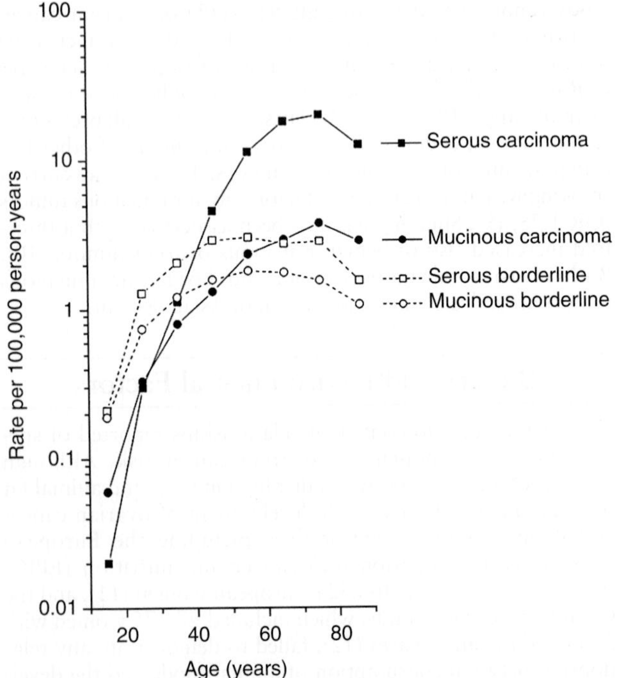

FIGURE 25.2. Incidence of invasive and borderline ovarian tumors in the United States by age. *Source:* Sherman ME, Berman J, Birrer MJ, et al. Current Challenges and Opportunities for Research on Borderline Ovarian Tumors. *Human Pathology* 2004;35:961–970.

Reproductive and Hormonal Factors

The protective effects of parity and oral contraceptive use support both the "incessant ovulation" hypothesis and the "gonadotropin" hypothesis of ovarian cancer etiology. According to the "incessant ovulation" hypothesis, ovarian cancer develops from an aberrant repair process of the surface epithelium, which is ruptured and repaired during each ovulatory cycle (17). The probability that ovarian cancer will develop is therefore a function of the total number of ovulatory cycles together with a genetic predisposition and undefined environmental factors. In support of this theory, it is well known that domestic egg-laying hens, which are forced to ovulate incessantly, have a high incidence of what are believed to be ovarian-derived tumors with peritoneal carcinomatosis (18). However, it fails to account for the increased risk of ovarian cancer with obesity and polycystic ovary syndrome (19). Alternatively, excessive gonadotropin secretion has been theorized to play a role in ovarian oncogenesis (20). Under excessive gonadotropin stimulation and resulting estrogenic stimulation, the surface epithelium is entrapped in inclusion cysts where it proliferates and undergoes malignant transformation. However, not all epidemiologic evidence supports this hypothesis. In particular, HRT, which suppresses postmenopausal gonadotropin levels, has been shown to increase, not decrease, the risk of ovarian cancer.

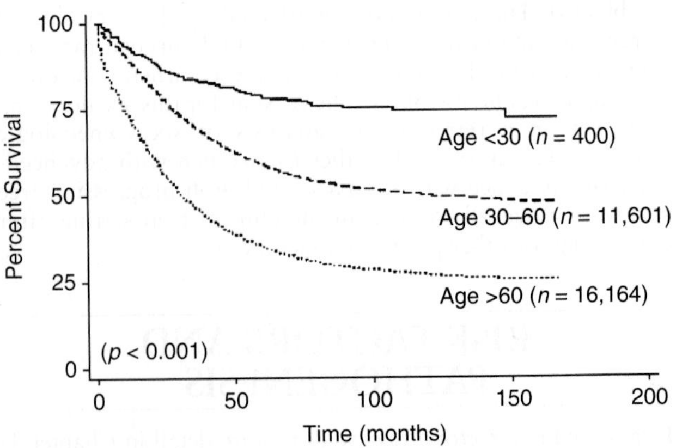

FIGURE 25.3. Disease-specific survival of patients based on age at diagnosis. *Source:* Chan JK, Urban R, Cheung MK, et al. Ovarian cancer in younger vs older women: a population-based analysis. *Br J Cancer* 2006;95:1314–1320.

TABLE 25.1

INCIDENCE OF STAGE AND GRADE BY AGE GROUPING IN SEER DATA 1988–2001

	Total (n = 28,165) (%)	Age <30 (n = 400) (%)	Age 30–60 (n = 11,601) (%)	Age >60 (n = 16,164) (%)
STAGE				
I	22	58	31	15
II	8	8	9	8
III	36	19	34	38
IV	34	16	26	40
GRADE				
1	9	34	12	5
2	18	24	21	16
3	44	13	44	45
Unknown	29	29	23	34

Source: Adapted from Chan JK, Urban R, Cheung MK, et al. Ovarian cancer in younger vs. older women: a population-based analysis. *Br J Cancer* 2006;95(10):1314–1320.

Another hypothesis has suggested a role for androgens and progestins in ovarian cancer development (21). Ovaries contain androgen receptors, and elevated androgen levels have been associated with an increased risk of ovarian cancer. Cottreau et al. reported that women who took danazol (a synthetic androgen) for endometriosis had a 3.2-fold higher risk of developing ovarian cancer than those who took a gonadotropin-releasing hormone (GnRH) agonist (22). Progestins, on the other hand, may be protective. Ovaries also contain progesterone receptors. Progestin levels are increased during pregnancy, and progestin-only oral contraceptives that do not suppress ovulation have a protective effect similar to that observed with contraceptive preparations with a greater suppressive effect on ovulation (23). These effects, however, are not simple; another case-control study suggested that users of the progestin norethindrone at low doses (0.5 mg or less) had a significantly reduced risk of ovarian cancer compared to women using 10 mg norethindrone (24). Cramer et al. have hypothesized that ovarian cancer risk is associated with "stromal hyperactivity" (25). He theorizes that granulosa and theca cells remain in the ovarian stroma after ovulation and control steroid production. By reducing ovulatory cycles, the number of residual follicles in the stroma with functioning granulosa-theca cells would also be decreased.

Another hypothesis for ovarian cancer development is based on the association of endometriosis and pelvic inflammatory disease with increased risk of ovarian cancer. Endometriosis is particularly associated with clear cell and endometrioid histotypes (26). The "inflammation" hypothesis states that any inflammatory agent or condition increases the risk of ovarian cancer. Some (27,28), but not all (29), epidemiologic data suggest that the use of anti-inflammatory agents, including aspirin and nonsteroidal anti-inflammatory drugs, protects against ovarian cancer development. Smith and Xu have provided an alternative hypothesis based on their observation that loss of basement membrane is an early event leading to morphologic transformation of ovarian surface epithelium (30,31). In preovulatory stimulation of the ovarian surface epithelium by gonadotropins, the basement membrane of the ovarian surface is similarly degraded. As loss of basement membrane is mediated through prostaglandins produced by gonadotropin-induced cyclo-oxygenase-2 (COX-2), this observation provides another mechanism for the possible preventive effect of nonsteroidal anti-inflammatory agents against ovarian cancer.

Oral Contraceptive Use

Case-control studies have consistently documented that users of oral contraceptives have a 30% to 60% smaller chance of developing ovarian cancer than do women who have never used oral contraceptives (OCPs) (31). The largest study reported, the Cancer and Steroid Hormone study (CASH) reported that OCP use for even a few months reduced the risk by 40% for women between the ages of 20 and 54 years (32). The World Health Organization (WHO) reported on 368 women with ovarian cancer and 2,397 matched controls (33). The relative risk for women who had ever used OCP was 0.75. The risk further decreased with increasing time since cessation of use and, in contrast to some other studies (34), the risk decreased with longer duration of use. In addition, the decreased risk was substantially greater in nulliparous compared to parous women (0.16 vs. 0.85, respectively).

Ovulation-Inducing Drugs

Some, but not all, studies have shown a link between fertility-inducing drugs such as clomiphene, and an increased risk of ovarian cancer. An older pooled analysis of 12 case-control studies found an odds ratio of 2.8 (95% CI, 1.3 to 6.1) for women who had ever used fertility drugs compared to those who had no history of infertility (35). The odds ratio for low malignant potential (LMP, borderline) tumors was 4.0. The risk was highest among nulliparous women, with an odds ratio of 27 (95% CI, 2.3 to 315.6). More recent studies have found either a weak association or no association between infertility treatment and ovarian cancer risk; the literature is well summarized in some comprehensive reviews (36,37).

Tubal Ligation

The Nurses' Health Study of 121,700 nurses was used to determine the effect of tubal ligation and hysterectomy on the subsequent risk of ovarian cancer (38). There was a strong inverse association between tubal ligation and ovarian cancer (RR 0.33). There was a weaker protective effect of hysterectomy (RR 0.67). The mechanism for the protective effects is unclear. Tubal ligation may affect circulating hormone levels by interfering with ovarian circulation. Statistically significant reductions in the risk of ovarian cancer after tubal ligation were also observed in a collaborative analysis of 12 U.S. case-control studies (OR 0.59; 95% CI, 0.38 to 0.53) (39). There was no association between age at surgery or time since surgery.

Hormone Replacement Therapy

Numerous studies have reported a modest association between HRT and risk of ovarian cancer, and a meta-analysis of nine published studies (only one of which did not show a relationship between HRT and ovarian cancer) confirms this (40). Included among these is a prospective, randomized study, the Women's Health Initiative (WHI) (41). Almost 17,000 postmenopausal women who had not had a hysterectomy were randomized to placebo or one tablet per day of 0.625 mg unconjugated estrogen plus 2.5 mg of medroxyprogesterone acetate. The hazard ratio for invasive ovarian cancer in the women receiving HRT was 1.58, but the overall number of ovarian cancer cases was small (n = 32), and the confidence interval was wide (95% CI, 0.77 to 3.24). In the largest analysis, a publication from the Million Women Study, 1.3 million women who had been invited for screening for breast cancer completed questionnaires that included information about HRT (40). Current users of HRT were significantly more likely to develop and die from ovarian cancer than never users (relative risk 1.2 for incident disease and 1.23 for death). The risk appeared to be primarily for serous tumors. Past users were not at increased risk, and there did not appear to be any significant risk with less than 5 years of use. Because of the lack of association with past risk, it has been suggested that HRT stimulates the growth of pre-existing, undiagnosed cancers, rather than increasing the risk of malignant transformation.

Progestins, as noted above, have been proposed to be protective against ovarian cancer, and the risk of ovarian cancer may be greater for estrogen-only HRT than for estrogen-progestin combinations. A Swedish case-control study reported an increased risk associated with the use of unopposed estrogens and sequential estrogen-progestin preparations, but not with the use of continuous progestin regimens (42). The risk of ovarian cancer in the Million Women Study did not differ significantly between those using estrogen-only and those using estrogen-progestin combinations, but the trend was for lower risk with the estrogen-progestin combination (RR 1.53 for more than 5 years of use for estrogen-only preparations versus RR 1.17 for more than 5 years of use of estrogen-progestin combinations).

Hereditary Ovarian Cancer

The clinical genetics of ovarian cancer are reviewed in more detail in Chapter 2. Approximately 10% of cases of invasive epithelial ovarian cancer are estimated to be the result of autosomal dominant high-penetrant genetic factors, predominantly germ-line mutations in the *BRCA1* or *BRCA2* genes. The *BRCA* genes function as classic tumor suppressors, with loss of function of both alleles required for cancer formation. The gene products appear to function in the cellular response to certain types of DNA damage. The lifetime risk of ovarian cancer for women with *BRCA1* mutations and *BRCA2* mutations has been estimated to be 40% and 20%, respectively (43,44).

Hereditary Nonpolyposis Colorectal Cancer Syndrome

Epithelial ovarian cancer is also a component of the hereditary nonpolyposis colorectal cancer syndrome (HNPCC; Lynch syndrome II). This syndrome is a result of germ-line mutations in genes involved in the DNA mismatch repair pathway, and mutation carriers have a predisposition not only to colorectal cancer, but to endometrial and ovarian carcinoma as well as other cancers, including those of the small bowel and biliary tract. HNPCC-related tumors frequently exhibit microsatellite instability (MSI). Not all tumors exhibiting MSI, however, are associated with hereditary syndromes; hypermethylation of the *MLH1* promoter region has been found in MSI-positive cancers of the ovary that do not contain germ-line *MLH1* mutations (45). Five genes are known to be involved in HNPCC: *MLH1, MSH2, MSH6,* PMS1, and *PMS2*. Mutations in *MLH1* and *MSH2* account for about 90% of the mutations detected in families with HNPCC, with *MSH2* being particularly associated with an excess of endometrial and ovarian carcinomas. Ovarian cancer occurs in approximately 10% of women with HNPCC (46), and tends to occur at an earlier age than sporadic ovarian cancer. Domanska et al. reviewed the Swedish Cancer Registry for epithelial ovarian cancer developing in women under the age of 40 years, and evaluated mismatch-repair status using immunohistochemical evaluation for *MLH1, PMS2, MSH2,* and *MSH6*. Among 98 cases there was loss of expression of *MLH1/PMS2* in 2, loss of *MSH2/MSH6* in 1, and loss of *MSH6* in 3 tumors. Five of the six demonstrated a microsatellite instability–high phenotype (47).

Clinical Features of *BRCA*-Associated Ovarian Cancer

In 1996 Rubin et al. reported results of a retrospective analysis suggesting that there are distinct clinical and pathologic features of *BRCA1*-associated ovarian cancer (48). Among 53 patients with germ-line *BRCA1* mutations, the average age at diagnosis was only 48 years, and the vast majority of cancers were serous adenocarcinomas. Cancers associated with *BRCA1* mutations had a relatively favorable prognosis, with an actuarial median survival of 77 months compared to 29 months for matched controls (Fig. 25.4).

Most subsequent reports have confirmed that *BRCA1* carriers with ovarian cancer have a younger age at diagnosis, are more likely to have cancers of serous histology and less likely to have borderline or mucinous tumors, and have a somewhat better prognosis than matched controls (49). The number of *BRCA2*-associated ovarian cancers is smaller, and it is not clear if there are differences in the clinical features of *BRCA2*- versus *BRCA1*-associated ovarian cancers. Boyd et al. performed a retrospective cohort study of invasive ovarian cancers in patients of Jewish origin (67 *BRCA1* and 21 *BRCA2*) (50). The average age at diagnosis was 54 years for *BRCA1* mutation carriers, 62 years for *BRCA2* mutation carriers, and 63 years for Jewish women with sporadic ovarian cancers. The histology, grade, stage, and success of cytoreductive surgery were similar for hereditary and sporadic cases, although there were no mucinous tumors and only two clear cell tumors observed among 88 *BRCA*-associated cases, versus five mucinous and seven clear cell tumors among 101 sporadic cases. The median disease-free interval after initial chemotherapy was 14 months for the *BRCA*-associated group and 7 months for the sporadic group ($p < 0.001$). Advanced-stage (III and IV) *BRCA*-linked cases also survived significantly longer than sporadic cases. These observations do not hold only for Ashkenazi-related mutations. A recent report notes that odds of a complete response to initial chemotherapy were 3.2-fold greater in non-Ashkenazi mutation

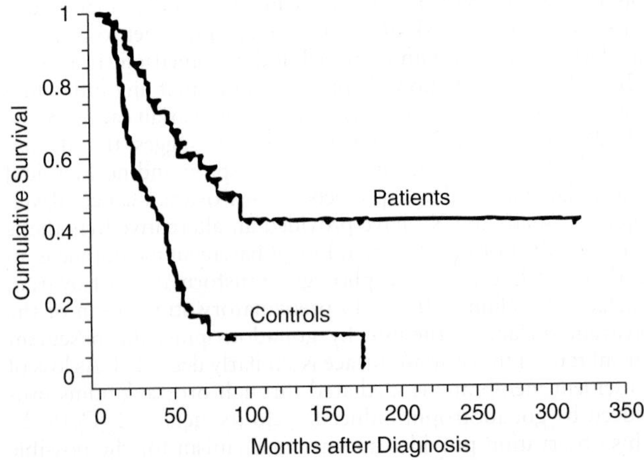

FIGURE 25.4. Actuarial survival among 43 patients with advanced ovarian cancer and *BRCA1* mutations compared to matched controls without known mutations. *Source:* Rubin SC, Benjamin I, Behbakht K, Takahashi H, et al. Clinical and pathological features of ovarian cancer in women with germ-line mutations of *BRCA1*. *N Engl J Med* 1996;335:1413–1416.

carriers compared to women with sporadic tumors, with a median overall survival of 101 months versus 51 months (51).

It has been hypothesized that the longer survival of women with *BRCA*-associated ovarian cancers is related to the fact that loss of function of *BRCA* proteins, which are believed to participate in DNA damage recognition and repair, results in a more favorable response to DNA-damaging chemotherapy. Decrease in *BRCA1* mRNA levels (PCR-based measurement) was associated with a significantly longer survival in 57 unselected ovarian cancers (52). Decrease in *BRCA1* protein expression, as measured by immunohistochemistry, was also associated with prolonged survival in a separate series of 230 sporadic ovarian cancers (53). On the other hand, women with ovarian cancers exhibiting methylation of the *BRCA1* gene promoter region, which might be expected to have decreased *BRCA1* gene expression, have been reported to have a worse survival than women with sporadic ovarian cancers (54). Further exploration of these observations will be important as specific targeted agents are developed that may be more active in subsets of cancers. For example, reports of preclinical studies suggest that deficiency in either *BRCA1* or *BRCA2* induces profound cellular sensitivity to the inhibition of poly(ADP-ribose) polymerase (PARP) activity (55). An early report of a phase 1 trial using the PARP inhibitor KU-0059436 suggested preferential single-agent activity in ovarian cancer patients who are known carriers of a *BRCA* mutation (56).

Effect of Reproductive Risk Factors on *BRCA* Mutation Carriers

In general, most studies have shown that the reproductive and hormonal factors that affect ovarian cancer risk in the general population also affect the ovarian cancer risk for women who carry *BRCA1* and *BRCA2* mutations. Narod et al. from Toronto initially reported a 60% reduction in risk of ovarian cancer for carriers of the *BRCA1* or *BRCA2* mutation with use of OCPs for 6 or more years (57). Three smaller studies confirmed this observation (58–60), but in a large population-based study from Israel no protective effect was seen (61), and the use of OCPs as a means to prevent ovarian cancer in *BRCA* mutation carriers prior to oophorectomy has therefore remained controversial. More recently, the Toronto group has reported their results from a greatly expanded database including 670 women with a history of *BRCA1*-associated ovarian cancer, 124 with a history of *BRCA2*-associated ovarian cancer, and 2,424 mutation carriers with no history of ovarian cancer (43). Use of OCPs reduced the risk of ovarian cancer both in women with *BRCA1* mutations (OR 0.56) and in those with *BRCA2* mutations (OR 0.39). Breast-feeding was protective for carriers of a *BRCA1* mutation (OR 0.74). An effect of similar magnitude was seen for breast-feeding in *BRCA2* mutation carriers, although it was not statistically significant (OR 0.72). Although the Toronto group had previously reported that tubal ligation was protective against ovarian cancer in mutation carriers as well as noncarriers, the association in this expanded cohort was not significant for carriers of either a *BRCA1* mutation (OR 0.8) or a *BRCA2* mutation (OR 0.63). Pregnancy, which had previously been reported to be protective for women carrying a *BRCA* mutation (61), was found to be protective for carriers of *BRCA1* mutations (OR 0.67), but was associated with increased risk for carriers of *BRCA2* mutations (OR 2.74). The reasons for this are not clear.

Prophylactic Oophorectomy for Prevention of Hereditary Ovarian Cancer

No current screening techniques, including serum CA-125 levels, pelvic ultrasound, and frequent pelvic examinations, have been shown to decrease the risk of death from ovarian cancer in women who carry *BRCA1* or *BRCA2* mutations. The U.S. National Institutes of Health (NIH) Consensus Development Panel recommended that prophylactic oophorectomy be considered in women with ovarian cancer syndromes at age 35 years or after childbearing is completed (62). This appears to substantially decrease ovarian cancer risk, although some risk of primary peritoneal cancer remains. In one large study 1,828 known carriers of a *BRCA1* or *BRCA2* mutation were identified from an international registry and asked to complete questionnaires at baseline and follow-up. The overall reduction in risk of cancer of ovaries, fallopian tubes, or peritoneum as a result of oophorectomy was 80%; the estimated cumulative incidence of peritoneal cancer was 4.3% at 20 years after oophorectomy (63). It is important to remove (and completely pathologically examine) the fallopian tubes at the time of oophorectomy, as an excess of invasive and noninvasive fallopian tube carcinomas, particularly involving the tubal fimbria, has been reported in prophylactic adnexectomy specimens from women with *BRCA* mutations undergoing prophylactic surgery (64). Removal of the ovaries may also reduce the risk of breast cancer in *BRCA* mutation carriers (65).

The Pathologic Examination of Risk-Reducing Salpingo-oophorectomy Specimens

In the largest series of *BRCA*-associated ovarian cancers with centralized pathology review (66), cancers in *BRCA* carriers were compared to those in noncarriers. Among 220 women, mutation-associated tumors were of significantly higher grade and stage and less often mucinous as compared to non–mutation-associated tumors. No mucinous and no borderline tumors were found in the mutation-associated group. Primary peritoneal carcinoma occurred rarely in both groups. Nonserous histology also appears to be less common in mutation carriers.

Microscopic occult carcinomas have been identified in risk-reducing salpingo-oophorectomy (RRSO) specimens in about 2% of *BRCA* mutation carriers. In one prospective series, seven ovarian and three tubal carcinomas (and one case in which washings showed malignant cells but no primary cancer was identified) were found among 490 women who underwent RRSO (63). The appropriate examination of RRSO specimens begins with efforts by the surgeon to avoid contact with the surface of the ovary intraoperatively, in order that the delicate surface epithelium not be abraded. The pathologist should submit for microscopic examination the entirety of the fallopian tubes and ovaries. This is best accomplished by serial cross sections across the short diameter of the ovaries and fallopian tubes. Levels of some sections should be obtained if foci of atypia are identified histologically, since foci of *in situ* or invasive occult carcinoma may be very subtle and less than 1 mm in maximum diameter.

Peritoneal lavage is becoming a standard portion of the procedure with RRSO. Occult carcinoma is occasionally identified in these cytology specimens. Colgan et al. found malignant cells in 3 of 35 specimens. One microscopic ovarian surface carcinoma and one *in situ* tubal carcinoma were found; no carcinoma could be identified in the third patient. Twenty-two percent of specimens showed endosalpingiosis (67). In rare cases, others have also reported malignant cells in washings at RRSO without an identifiable carcinoma by histology (63), and in two studies, positive cytology specimens led to the discovery of early-stage tubal carcinomas (64,68).

Ovaries derived from RRSO have been examined by several groups for potential precursor lesions of high-grade serous carcinoma. Surface epithelial inclusions, invaginations (clefts), papillomatosis, calcifications, and other features have been studied. The inclusion epithelium has been examined for atypia, and the inclusions and clefts have been counted and measured. Published studies of these high-risk ovaries have generated conflicting results. Some studies suggest that these ovaries have more cortical inclusions, surface epithelial invaginations, surface papillomatosis and/or deeper cortical invaginations than control ovaries (69–72), but these findings have not been confirmed by others (70,73–75). Some investigators have found a higher degree of cytologic atypia in the epithelium lining these inclusions (74,76) or the surface epithelium (70), but again these findings have not been confirmed (73). Some studies have significant methodologic limitations involving the methods of counting and measuring inclusions, control group issues, and in many studies it is not clear whether the data were collected by an experienced pathologist who can reliably separate inclusions and clefts from their mimics, which include rete ovarii, peritoneal folds, and adherent tubal plicae (77). At present, none of these features are conclusively identified as features predictive of significant risk of cancer development.

Genetic Counseling

The level of potential risk reduction with salpingo-oophorectomy makes awareness of the potential that a patient carries a *BRCA1* or *BRCA2* mutation very important. While treatment for *BRCA* mutation–associated ovarian cancers is not currently different from treatment of sporadic ovarian cancers, genetic counseling for relatives of index patients may save lives. Factors that should trigger consideration of genetic counseling/testing in women with invasive ovarian cancer include Ashkenazi Jewish ancestry, very young age, personal history of breast cancer, or a family history of ovarian cancer or breast cancer (particularly multiple first-degree relatives, or relatives with breast cancer at a young age, including paternal relatives). In Ontario, Canada, 20% of women diagnosed with ovarian cancer between the ages of 30 and 40 years were found to carry a mutation in the *BRCA1* or *BRCA2* genes (78). Among Ashkenazi Jewish women with ovarian cancer there is about a 40% to 50% chance that the disease is related to a *BRCA1* or *BRCA2* mutation (79). Even in Ashkenazi Jewish ovarian cancer patients with no family history of breast or ovarian cancer, the risk of a mutation is 13% to 23% and warrants genetic counseling (80).

PATHOLOGY

This section addresses the general pathologic classification and features of ovarian borderline tumors and carcinomas, but it also specifically emphasizes several areas of high clinical impact in which our understanding of ovarian cancer has recently advanced, as follows: the pathogenesis of ovarian carcinoma, the distinction between low-grade and high-grade serous carcinoma; the definition and significance of types of implants and micropapillary architecture in serous borderline tumors; the significance of stromal microinvasion; primary peritoneal carcinoma; and the criteria and the distinction of primary from metastatic mucinous carcinoma involving the ovary.

Pathologic Classification

Ovarian cancer, although inappropriately often considered as a single entity, consists of many types, each with subtypes. The classification in Table 25.2, presented in detail for the common

TABLE 25.2

HISTOLOGIC CLASSIFICATION OF COMMON EPITHELIAL TUMORS OF THE OVARY

SEROUS TUMORS
- Benign
  - Cystadenoma and papillary cystadenoma
  - Surface papilloma
  - Adenofibroma and cystadenofibroma
  - Borderline tumor (atypical proliferative tumor)
  - Cystadenoma and papillary cystadenoma
  - Surface papilloma
- Malignant
  - Adenocarcinoma
  - Surface papillary adenocarcinoma

MUCINOUS TUMORS
- Benign
  - Cystadenoma
  - Adenofibroma and cystadenofibroma
  - Borderline tumor (atypical proliferative tumor)
  - Intestinal type
  - Endocervical-like
- Malignant
  - Adenocarcinoma
  - Malignant adenofibroma
  - Mural nodule arising in mucinous cystic tumor

ENDOMETRIOID TUMORS
- Benign
  - Adenoma and cystadenoma
  - Adenofibroma and cystadenofibroma
  - Borderline tumor (atypical proliferative tumor)
- Malignant
  - Adenocarcinoma
  - Adenoacanthoma
  - Adenosquamous carcinoma
  - Malignant adenofibroma with a malignant stromal component
  - Adenosarcoma
  - Endometrial stromal sarcoma
  - Carcinosarcoma, homologous and heterologous
  - Undifferentiated sarcoma

CLEAR CELL TUMORS
- Benign
  - Borderline tumor (atypical proliferative tumor)
- Malignant
  - Adenocarcinoma

TRANSITIONAL CELL TUMORS
- Brenner's tumor
- Proliferating Brenner's tumor
- Malignant Brenner's tumor
- Transitional cell carcinoma (non-Brenner type)

SQUAMOUS CELL CARCINOMA

MIXED EPITHELIAL TUMORS (SPECIFY TYPES)
- Benign
  - Borderline tumor (atypical proliferative tumor)
- Malignant
  - Undifferentiated carcinoma

Source: Modified with permission from Tavassoli FA, Devilee P. *Tumours of the Breast and Female Genital Organs*. World Health Organization Classification of Tumors. Lyon, France: IARC Press; 2003, page 114.

TABLE 25.3

CONSECUTIVE PRIMARY OVARIAN EPITHELIAL TUMORS: WHC, 1999–2007

	Benign	Atypical proliferative	Malignant	Totals
Serous	431	12	113	556
Ser-peritoneal[a]	—	—	28	28
Carcinosarcoma	—	—	21	21
Endometrioid	7	4	17	28
Mucinous	71	12	6	89
Clear cell	0	2	20	22
Transitional	80	1	3	84
Squamous	10	—	1	11
Undifferentiated	—	—	0	0
Mixed	16	0	9	25
Totals	615	31	218	864

Notes: WHC, Washington Hospital Center, Washington, D.C. Atypical proliferative includes those with microinvasion and/or intraepithelial carcinoma. Epidermoid cysts (nonteratomatous) are classified as benign squamous tumors. Seromucinous are included in mucinous.
[a]Two "serous peritoneal" tumors were carcinosarcomas. The total number of cases differs from that in the text due to slightly differing time periods.

epithelial tumors, has been developed and updated under the auspices of WHO, the International Federation of Gynecology and Obstetrics (FIGO), the International Society of Gynecologic Pathologists, and the Society of Gynecologic Oncologists (SGO) (81).

The surface epithelial tumors are the most frequently encountered form of ovarian tumors, and they account for more than 90% of all ovarian cancer in adults (Tables 25.3 and 25.4). However, accurate determination of the relative frequencies of ovarian epithelial neoplasms is relatively limited, with very few published series of ovarian tumors that are population based and include all cell types that have been reviewed in a uniform manner according to standardized criteria (82). A recent review of unselected cases seen at a large community hospital included 1,287 consecutive ovarian tumors from 2000 through 2007, of which 802 were surface epithelial tumors (Table 25.3) and 485 were nonepithelial tumors (237 germ cell, 85 stromal, 163 metastatic). Notable differences from historical reports include the low frequency of primary ovarian mucinous carcinoma (<1% of primary epithelial tumors), the high frequency of ovarian carcinosarcoma, and the high proportion of primary peritoneal serous carcinoma (83). Serous carcinoma represented 52% of the total, and this is significant since it appears that both the pathogenesis and response to therapy differ according to the cell type.

Pathogenesis of Ovarian Carcinoma

During embryonic life, the coelomic cavity forms and is lined by a mesothelial lining of mesodermal origin, part of which becomes specialized to form the serosal epithelium covering the gonadal ridge. By a process of invagination, this same mesothelial lining gives rise to the müllerian ducts, from which

TABLE 25.4

CONSECUTIVE PRIMARY INVASIVE OVARIAN CARCINOMAS BY FIGO STAGE AND CELL TYPE 1991–2007

	I	II	III	IV	Totals
Serous	5	5	132	41	186
Peritoneal[a]	—	0	41	12	53
Carcinosarcoma	1	3	17	4	25
Endometrioid	12	5	6	2	26
Mucinous	6	0	2	0	8
Clear cell	11	8	8	5	32
Transitional	2	1	1	0	4
Squamous	0	0	0	1	1
Undifferentiated	0	0	1	0	1
Mixed	7	0	9	3	19
Totals	44	22	217	68	355

Notes: FIGO, International Federation of Gynecology and Obstetrics. Excludes microinvasive tumors, noninvasive micropapillary serous carcinoma, and carcinomas arising in nonsurface epithelial tumors (i.e., squamous cell carcinoma in teratoma).
Three serous tumors and one endometrioid were of unknown stage.
[a]Two were carcinosarcoma, one was transitional cell carcinoma.

arise the fallopian tubes, uterus, and wall of the vagina. As repair follows multiple ovulations, the surface epithelium of the ovary often extends into the ovarian stroma to form inclusion glands and cysts. Other mechanisms may also contribute to the formation of intraparenchymal epithelial inclusions. The epithelium, in the process of neoplastic transformation, may exhibit differentiation toward a variety of müllerian-type cells, which are, in order of decreasing frequency, (a) serous (resembling the fallopian tube); (b) mucinous (resembling the endocervix); (c) endometrioid (resembling endometrium); (d) clear cell (glycogen-rich cells sometimes resembling either embryonic müllerian epithelium and at other times secretory phase endometrial glands); and (e) urothelial or transitional (resembling Walthard's rests and bladder).

For the purpose of understanding pathogenesis, it is important to recognize that ovarian carcinoma may be separated into two broad divisions: those that arise *de novo*, i.e., without an identifiable precursor lesion, and those that arise via a stepwise progression in an adenoma-carcinoma sequence as occurs in the colon.

The vast majority of fatal ovarian cancers are high-grade serous carcinomas. These tumors are believed to arise *de novo* from the surface epithelium of the ovary, or perhaps sometimes from the mucosa of the fallopian tube, and progress rapidly. Accordingly, diagnosis of high-grade serous carcinoma in stage I is a rare and fortuitous event. Regrettably, this hinders our understanding of the early phase of this process and also makes screening and early detection difficult.

Most of the remaining cell types of ovarian carcinomas appear to follow an adenoma-carcinoma sequence. Nearly all clear cell carcinomas and a large proportion of endometrioid carcinomas arise in endometriosis, and appear to progress through an adenoma (or hyperplasia)–borderline tumor–carcinoma sequence. Similarly, mucinous carcinomas most probably transit through a mucinous cystadenoma–borderline tumor–intraepithelial carcinoma sequence before invasion occurs. Since a mass is often detected while still in the early phases of the sequence, such tumors are much more likely to be diagnosed while still confined to the ovary, and they therefore comprise most curable ovarian carcinomas. Low-grade serous carcinoma is a recently described and relatively small subset of ovarian serous carcinoma that also often appears to follow a stepwise progression from borderline tumor to invasive carcinoma. Its morphology and behavior are described later in this chapter.

Molecular biologic evidence (84) provides support for this dualistic model of ovarian carcinogenesis. High-grade serous carcinomas typically have p53 mutations in contrast to low-grade serous carcinomas, which usually have mutations in K-ras and *BRAF* genes. The identification of Pten mutations in endometrioid tumors and K-ras in mucinous tumors also supports the stepwise progression model.

Very recently, Lee et al. have proposed that many high-grade serous carcinomas thought to be of ovarian or peritoneal origin actually arise in the mucosa of the fimbriated end of the fallopian tube (85). This concept results from a convergence of data obtained from meticulous studies in which the fallopian tubes were sequentially sectioned and blocked for microscopic and molecular analysis. Much of the work has only been presented in abstract form, and it has not been corroborated by other investigators to date, but it is highly provocative and reasonably compelling. In brief, they found that in eight cases of ovarian carcinoma with coexisting *in situ* carcinoma of the fallopian tube mucosa, the same p53 mutations were identified in both sites (86). In cases diagnosed according to WHO criteria for primary peritoneal carcinoma, more than half of the fallopian tubes displayed tubal mucosal involvement, often with *in situ* carcinoma (87). In a series of RRSO specimens from women with *BRCA* mutations, clusters of p53-positive cells and intraepithelial carcinomas were identified in the mucosa of the fallopian tubes of about 30% of the women, while they were not present on the ovarian surface (64). Although all of these data are open to other interpretation, it is likely that the mucosa of the fimbriated end of the fallopian tube serves as the source of some of the carcinomas that previously have been considered to be of ovarian or primary peritoneal origin.

Specimen Examination

Although thorough sampling of an ovarian tumor for microscopic analysis is an often-stated requirement for optimal pathologic examination, thoroughness cannot be equated with a formula for a specified number of slides taken randomly, which often provides little additional information (88). Instead, careful gross examination and directed sampling of any unusual-appearing areas in addition to representative areas are essential (89). For example, adhesions on the surface of an ovary, although usually inflammatory in origin, are sometimes an indication that a tumor has penetrated the capsule. While four or five sections may be sufficient to provide the grade and histologic type of a grossly obvious malignant ovarian neoplasm, it is recommended that at least one section of neoplasm be taken for each centimeter of the maximum diameter (for tumors up to 10 cm in diameter and two per centimeter for those greater than 10 cm in diameter) of the lesion for suspected borderline tumors in order to establish the diagnosis and reduce the possibility of occult invasion. At the NCI-sponsored consensus conference on borderline tumors in 2003, it was suggested that grossly normal omentum removed from women with borderline tumors be submitted for histologic examination at a proportion of one block per 2 cm maximum diameter of omentum (89a).

The ovarian tumor specimen should be serially sectioned at close intervals and each piece carefully examined for differences in texture. Serous tumors tend to show greater uniformity than mucinous tumors, which are notorious for great variation, with only a small percentage of slides disclosing features diagnostic of cancer. Mucinous adenocarcinomas are commonly composed almost exclusively of cysts typical of adenoma or borderline tumors, whereas only a few areas are solid and show the diagnostic features of carcinoma. Solid areas preferentially should be submitted for microscopic examination. Benign serous tumors tend to be unilocular. Serous borderline tumors tend to have clusters of numerous papillae that are larger and more edematous than those of adenocarcinomas, which are solid or relatively fine. Blocks taken from the base of papillary processes are particularly helpful to avoid overlooking occult areas of poorly differentiated carcinoma. As transition forms between benign and malignant epithelia are well documented (90), careful gross examination of the specimen is mandatory to help identify both the regions of borderline tumor and the invasive carcinoma.

Borderline Tumors

Despite disagreement about the optimal terminology for borderline tumors (which are also known as atypical proliferative tumors or tumors of low malignant potential), there is widespread agreement on the histologic appearances and behavior of these tumors. Their reproducible identification among pathologists is not considered a major problem, but it must be recognized that extensive sampling (one or two sections of tissue per maximum diameter in centimeters of the neoplasm) is required to firmly establish the diagnosis. Consequently, underestimation in the severity of the process is frequent at the time of intraoperative diagnosis, and this needs to be recognized by both the pathologist and the operating surgeon. Effective communication of pathologists with gynecologic oncologists is essential to minimize inappropriate initial surgical therapy.

An appreciation of heterogeneity is critical to understanding the biologic behavior of borderline tumors. Accordingly, the natural history, recurrence and survival rates, and treatment of patients with borderline tumors should be considered according to five features, as follows: (a) cell type, (b) stage, (c) implant type (for serous borderline tumors), (d) the presence of a micropapillary architecture (for serous borderline tumors), and (e) microinvasion. Three decades ago, serous and mucinous borderline tumors were described, with 5-year survival rates of about 75% to 90%. More subtypes and special features have been recognized in the past 10 years, and the borderline category is now much better understood. No tumor deaths from the three rare subtypes of endometrioid, clear cell, and transitional borderline tumors have been well documented, and they are very uncommon (representing from less than 1% to 10% of borderline tumors). Consequently, no definitive conclusions can be drawn regarding their natural history, but no cancer deaths have been reported for women with borderline tumors of these three cell types.

Serous Tumors

About 20% of serous tumors are malignant, 2% are borderline tumors, and about 78% are benign. The mean age for patients with cancer is 56 years. Patients with benign and borderline tumors are generally younger, with mean ages at diagnosis of 45 and 48 years, respectively. Approximately one of six serous adenomas is bilateral. Serous borderline tumors are bilateral in one third of cases. Serous adenocarcinomas that are stage I are bilateral in one third of cases. Those of higher stage are bilateral in two thirds of cases.

Serous Borderline Tumors

Well-staged borderline tumors that are confined to the ovary are associated with a survival that approaches 100% at 10 years. However, the prognosis for women with tumors that have associated peritoneal lesions is diminished, and it varies according to the type of implant that is identified histologically. A fundamental source of potential confusion results from the presence of peritoneal lesions associated with a primary ovarian tumor in which invasion cannot be demonstrated. The designation of these lesions as "implants" is entrenched and implies the unproved assumption that the peritoneal lesions are derived from the ovarian neoplasm. (In fact, limited molecular biologic evidence suggests that in some cases, the peritoneal lesions arise independently.) The division of implants into invasive and noninvasive (epithelial and desmoplastic) types represented a tremendous advance in providing prognostic information.

Gross Appearance. Serous borderline tumors are similar in most respects to their benign counterparts, usually formed of a unilocular or paucilocular cyst with clear fluid and lining that varies from smooth to papillary. The papillations are usually more numerous, larger, and softer in texture in borderline tumors. Polypoid structures, 1 to 10 mm in greatest dimension, are frequently seen (Fig. 25.5). Their surfaces frequently are covered by relatively fine papillae. Necrosis is absent. Serous borderline tumors may secrete a fluid that has a higher mucin content than serous cystadenomas, and this can cause confusion with a mucinous neoplasm at the time of gross examination.

Microscopic Appearance. Serous borderline tumors are characterized microscopically by dichotomously branching, fine to coarse papillary fronds in which atypical, stratified neoplastic cells cover a thick core of fibrovascular stroma (Fig. 25.6). The general histologic features used to diagnose borderline tumors include (a) architectural complexity of glandular structures; (b) epithelial papillae (especially in serous tumors), with detached atypical cell clusters as single or small groups of cells; (c) cellular stratification (especially in mucinous tumors); (d) increased mitotic activity; and (e) nuclear atypia (increased nuclear:cytoplasmic ratios, hyperchromatism, and prominent

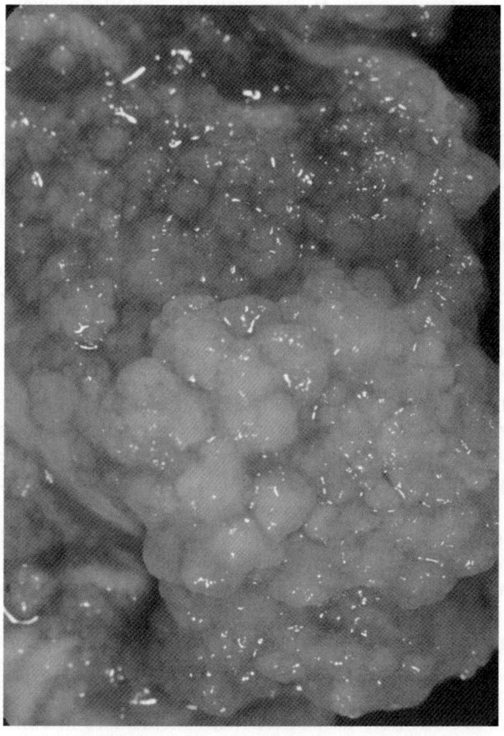

FIGURE 25.5. Serous borderline tumor. This 10-cm-diameter unilocular cystic neoplasm has a lining that varies from finely granular to rough and polypoid. In contrast, most serous cystadenomas have a smooth lining and most serous carcinomas have solid areas with foci of necrosis.

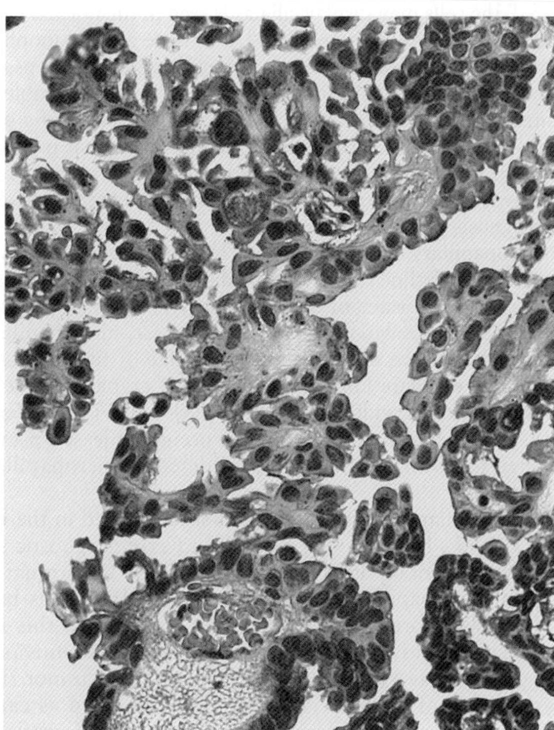

FIGURE 25.6. Serous borderline tumor. The fibrovascular papillae correspond to the rough or granular lining that is visible grossly. The papillae branch dichotomously into progressively smaller fibrovascular cores that are covered by a multilayered atypical epithelium.

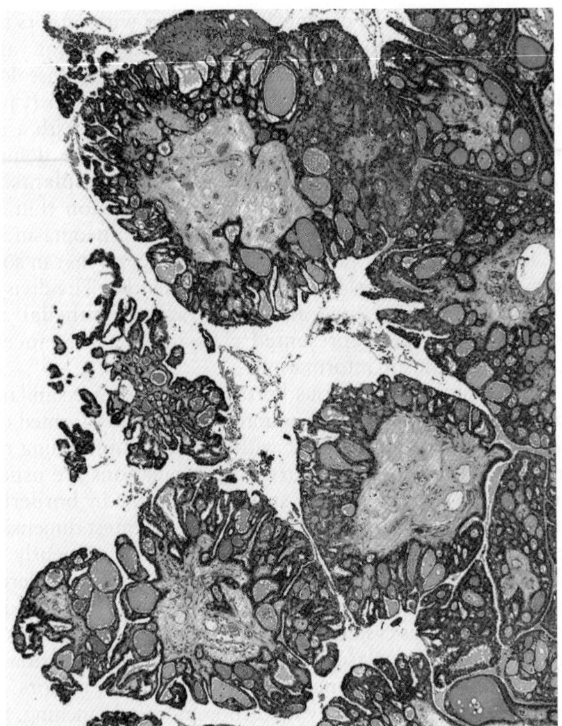

FIGURE 25.7. Micropapillary serous tumor. In contrast to the dichotomously branching fibrovascular cores of the usual serous borderline tumor, micropapillary tumors have relatively large papillae of fibrous tissue from which long, thin columns of atypical epithelium emanate directly.

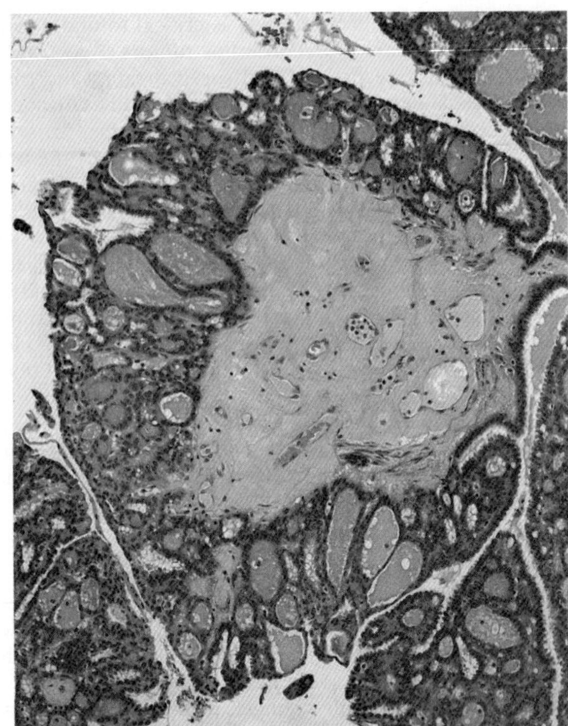

FIGURE 25.8. Micropapillary serous tumor. At higher magnification, it is evident that the height:width ratio of the atypical epithelium exceeds 5:1. In this case, bridging of atypical epithelium results in a cribriform or sieve-like pattern.

nucleoli). The epithelium that characterizes serous tumors resembles the lining of the normal fallopian tube. If well differentiated, the cells may display cilia as is seen in the normal tubal epithelium. If less well differentiated, they have only eosinophilic cytoplasm. Laminated, calcific concretions, known as psammoma bodies, are often numerous. Mucin, if demonstrable, is confined to the apical border of the cell. The diagnosis of a borderline tumor requires that no area contain stromal invasion that exceeds 5 mm in diameter. The presence of smaller foci of microinvasive tumor does not alter the patient's otherwise excellent prognosis (91).

Micropapillary Serous Tumors. The fibrovascular fronds of the typical borderline serous tumors display a mantle of epithelial cells on the surface of dichotomously branching, progressively smaller fibrovascular cores. In contrast, micropapillary serous tumors have relatively large papillae of fibrous tissue from which emanate long, thin columns of atypical epithelial cells, with a height:width ratio that exceeds 5:1 (Figs. 25.7 and 25.8). This architectural pattern must occupy at least a 5-mm-diameter focus in order to be considered a micropapillary serous tumor.

Micropapillary architecture was first recognized in the late 1970s (92,93), but data suggesting its adverse prognostic significance were not reported until 1996 (94,103). Unfortunately, the term micropapillary serous carcinoma (MPSC) has been used for two morphologically distinct entities and this has caused some confusion among clinicians. The noninvasive form of MPSC is a variant of serous borderline tumor. The invasive form of MPSC has always been classified as carcinoma and is the typical form of invasive well-differentiated serous carcinoma (see above). Thus, invasive MPSC is essentially synonymous with low-grade serous carcinoma (95).

Ten percent to 15% of serous borderline tumors display the micropapillary pattern (defined as a 5 mm area uninterrupted by typical serous borderline tumor [SBT]). The behavior of serous borderline tumors with a micropapillary pattern is clear. Stage I patients have 100% survival, based on over 2,000 reported SBTs among which 10% to 15% can be assumed to be micropapillary tumors (97). For advanced-stage patients, the survival depends upon the type of implants present and is similar to that of typical SBT with similar types of implants. More importantly, the micropapillary architecture is strongly associated with invasive implants. In eight studies of advanced-stage tumors with a total of over 300 patients, 49% of micropapillary tumors were associated with invasive peritoneal implants as compared to 6% of typical SBTs (98–105).

Advanced-stage patients with MPSC have a 10-year survival of 50% to 60%. These data have been confirmed by multiple investigators. Proponents of continuing to classify MPSC as borderline tumors contend that noninvasive MPSC has the same behavior as all other serous borderline tumors with similar implants. This is correct; the survival rates are virtually identical. The weakness of this argument becomes apparent as follows. It is now agreed that invasive implants are invasive carcinomas. So the argument is essentially this: MPSC has the same behavior as usual borderline serous tumor once the presence or absence of carcinoma is accounted for. That is like saying that the behavior of benign and malignant tumors is basically the same once the presence or absence of metastases (including occult micrometastases) is accounted for. The critical point is that MPSC is strongly associated with invasive implants, i.e., invasive carcinoma, in contrast to usual borderline serous tumors, which only rarely are associated with invasive carcinoma, just as malignant tumors are strongly associated with metastases in contrast to benign tumors, which very rarely produce metastases.

Microinvasion. Microinvasion (defined variously as a maximal invasive focus size of 2, 3 or 5 mm, or an area of 10 square mm) can be found in up to 10% of borderline

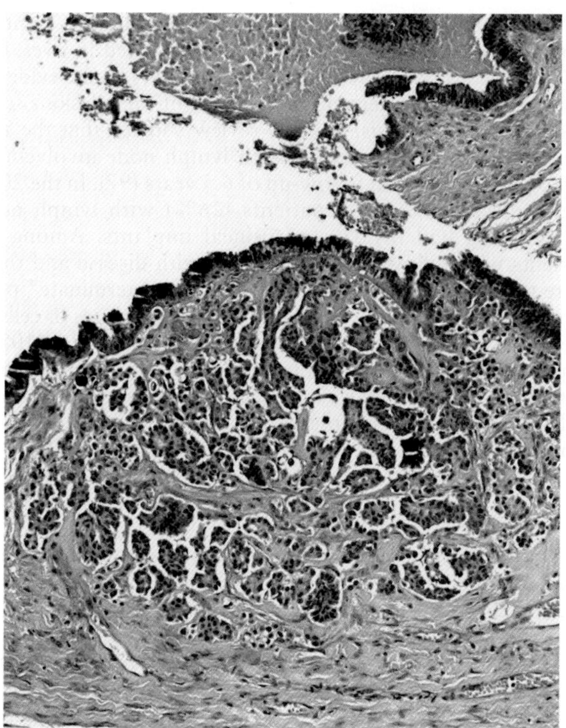

FIGURE 25.9. Microinvasion—microinvasion in a serous borderline tumor. A small focus of destructive stromal invasion is present in an otherwise typical serous borderline tumor. The stromal margins appear retracted around the purely epithelial papillae. This focus is less than 3 mm in maximum diameter. Its presence is not associated with any significant decrease in the survival rate.

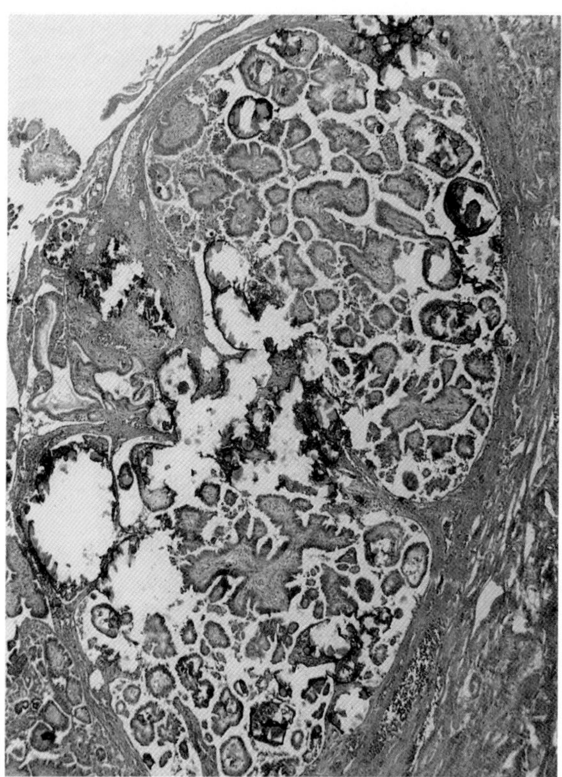

FIGURE 25.10. Noninvasive epithelial implant. This form of implant is characterized by a well-circumscribed proliferation of atypical epithelium on the surface of the peritoneum or between fat lobules of the omentum.

tumors (Fig. 25.9). Review of 94 reported cases as of 2000 showed a survival of 100% (97). More recently, a few tumors with microinvasion have been reported to have demonstrated malignant behavior. In that report, however, most of the patients had either invasive or indeterminate implants, and therefore the independent prognostic significance of microinvasion in these cases is not clear (101). The overall prognosis for the patient with microinvasion in a borderline tumor is currently considered to be no different from that of a borderline tumor without microinvasion. Larger foci of destructive invasion in a borderline tumor are considered to represent the presence of a serous carcinoma. When papillae invade into the stroma, the stromal margins may appear to be retracted and display relatively pointed contours in relief. Solid clusters of cells may exhibit a cribriform pattern (intraglandular bridging) indicative of autonomous growth and, hence, adenocarcinoma. Usually, invasion is accompanied by a fibrous stromal reaction.

Implants. *Noninvasive epithelial implants* are characterized by papillary proliferation of epithelium present on the surface of the peritoneum or in smoothly contoured submesothelial invaginations or between fat lobules, in the absence of a significant stromal response (Fig. 25.10). The papillae are composed of stratified cuboidal or columnar cells with varying degrees of cytologic atypia. *Noninvasive desmoplastic implants* are characterized by a marked stromal reaction to tumor cells in a similar distribution (Fig. 25.11). *Invasive implants* are recognized by an irregular, aggressive-appearing infiltration into the underlying submesothelial tissue or within lobules of fat from the omentum by small glands or solid nests of cells or papillae (Fig. 25.12) (106). There is now a consensus that invasive implants are associated with a poor outcome and behave as low-grade carcinoma. According to the NCI-sponsored Borderline Tumor Conference (89a), the terms "invasive serous carcinoma" and "invasive

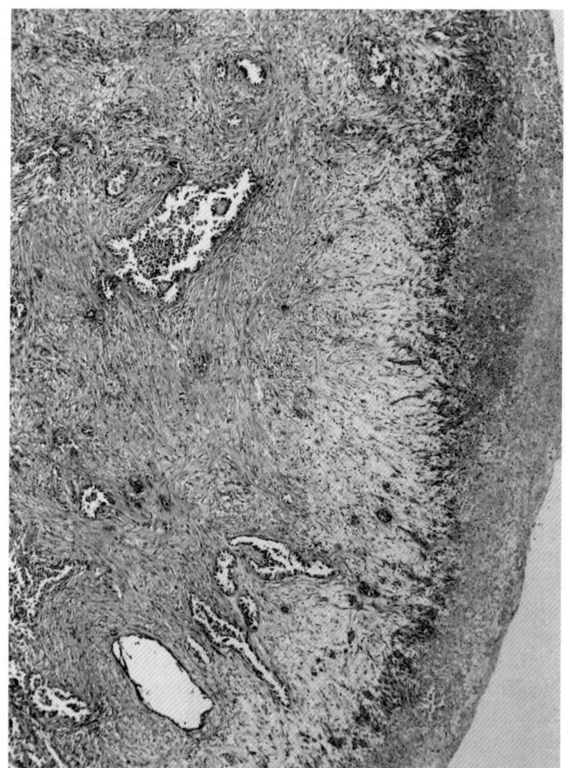

FIGURE 25.11. Noninvasive desmoplastic implant. These implants are characterized by a marked stromal granulation tissue-like reaction to tumor cells, in the absence of any irregular infiltration of underlying tissue.

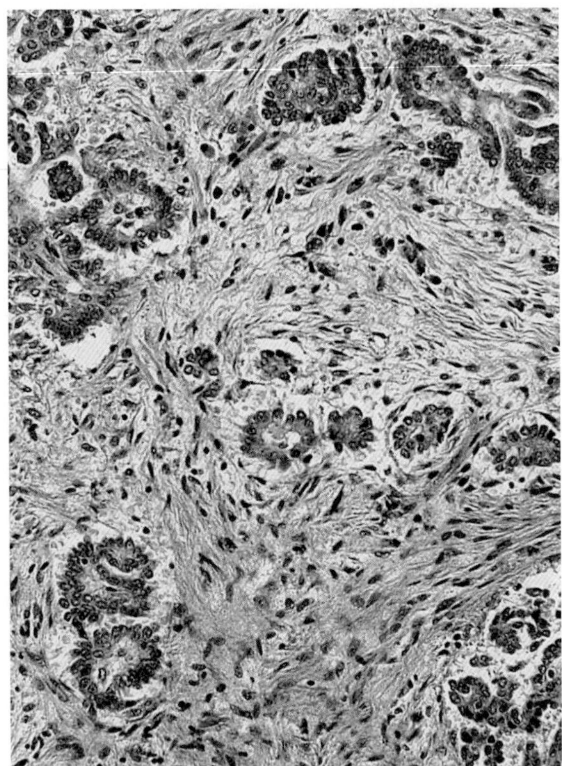

FIGURE 25.12. Invasive implants. This type of implant can be recognized by an irregular, aggressive-appearing infiltration of the omental fat or underlying submesothelial tissues by small glands or solid nests of atypical epithelial cells or papillae.

implant" can be used synonymously. The survival at 5 years for women with noninvasive implants exceeds 95%, while for those with invasive implants it is 67% (97). The clear separation of these groups might not have been possible without the recognition of the desmoplastic noninvasive implant, which is histologically pseudoinvasive and highly deceptive to pathologists unfamiliar with it.

The accuracy of implant subclassification has been a frequently raised issue. The highly significant difference in survival rates ($p < 0.001$) in published reports of about 500 women with invasive versus noninvasive implants suggests that they are being separated reliably (97). In some cases, a small biopsy of an implant makes it difficult to assess for invasion, and it has been suggested that one can classify a small implant without underlying tissue as noninvasive based on the assumption that it had been easily removed (107,108). However, surgeons with sharp knives tend to disagree with this statement. At the 2006 annual meeting of the U.S. and Canadian Academy of Pathology, five experts independently classified implants from photomicrographs. Despite concerns about reproducibility, the results were extremely encouraging and indicated very good reproducibility among experts.

In evaluating peritoneal biopsies, implants of borderline tumors must be distinguished from reactive peritoneal hyperplasia and benign epithelial inclusions, and endosalpingiosis. Müllerian inclusion cysts are another finding to be considered when dealing with serous borderline tumors. These occur in the form of individual round to oval glands with an obvious lumen and are found in both the omentum and lymph nodes. A peripheral basement membrane is present and cilia may be prominent. The epithelium is usually only one cell layer thick, and stratification, if present, is minimal. The nuclei are basally situated, mitotic activity is absent, and there is no nuclear atypia.

Lymph Node Involvement in Serous Borderline Tumors. Lymph node "involvement" has been reported in over 100 cases of serous borderline tumors (97,98,109). Some evidence suggests an independent origin of some of these lesions from nodal endosalpingiosis. A 2000 review showed that the survival of 43 reported patients with lymph node involvement was 98% after a mean follow-up of 6.5 years (97). In the 2006 Stanford series, 8 of 31 patients (26%) with lymph node involvement had invasive peritoneal implants. Among 22 patients with follow-up, 4 were alive with disease and there were two deaths, one in a patient with "indeterminate" peritoneal implants. The presence of nodular aggregates of cells in the nodes was found to be an adverse prognostic factor (109a). If patients with invasive implants in other sites or indeterminate implants (histologically indeterminate or slides unavailable) are excluded, then the overall survival for patients with lymph node involvement is 97%.

Serous Carcinoma

Histologically malignant epithelial tumors are uncommon in women under the age of 35 years. By the time a carcinoma reaches clinical detection, it has often already spread beyond the ovary and seeded the peritoneum.

Destructive growth, an important feature of malignancy, helps to distinguish frank malignancies from borderline tumors. Infiltrative destructive growth is best demonstrated by individual or small clusters of cells growing in a disorganized pattern with angulated, sharp borders that dissect into stromal planes and are usually associated with desmoplasia.

Gross Appearance. Serous adenocarcinomas have the most variegated appearance. They range in size from small (2 to 3 cm) to quite large. Serous carcinomas often present as solid masses bounded by a capsule, often containing areas of necrosis and hemorrhage. The ovary from which the neoplasm has arisen is frequently not apparent grossly or microscopically. Cysts and foci of papillarity are commonly present. If one postulates an origin from the surface epithelium that covers the ovary, it is surprising that so few serous carcinomas display substantial surface papillary growth covering an otherwise normal ovary. It is hypothesized that the neoplastic transformation actually occurs either in inclusion cysts or the tubal mucosa. The gross appearance of a typical high-grade serous carcinoma is not distinctive, and it may be mimicked by other high-grade epithelial ovarian neoplasms, granulosa cell tumors, and carcinomas metastatic to the ovary.

Microscopic Appearance. Serous adenocarcinomas are distinguished from borderline serous tumors by the presence of stromal invasion. The tumor may appear as large sheets of polygonal cells growing autonomously without stromal support or as broad to fine clusters of cells related to papillae that irregularly dissect through the stroma, accompanied by a host desmoplastic response. The nuceli are typically large and pleomorphic, with variably sized nucleoli, and numerous mitotic figures.

Two grading systems for serous carcinomas have been proposed and tested in the past decade: a three-grade system by Shimizu et al. (110), and more recently, a binary system of high-grade and low-grade serous carcinoma by Malpica et al. from the M. D. Anderson Cancer Center (MDACC) (111). The MDACC system appears to be both easy for the pathologist to use in routine practice and corresponds more closely to the dichotomous morphologic appearance, molecular features, and clinical behavior of serous carcinoma (Figs. 25.13 and 25.14) (96). In contrast to high-grade serous carcinoma, low-grade neoplasms are characterized by cells with only mild to moderate nuclear atypia, evenly distributed chromatin, variable nucleoli, and fewer than ten mitoses per ten high-power fields (HPF). A micropapillary architecture is very frequently

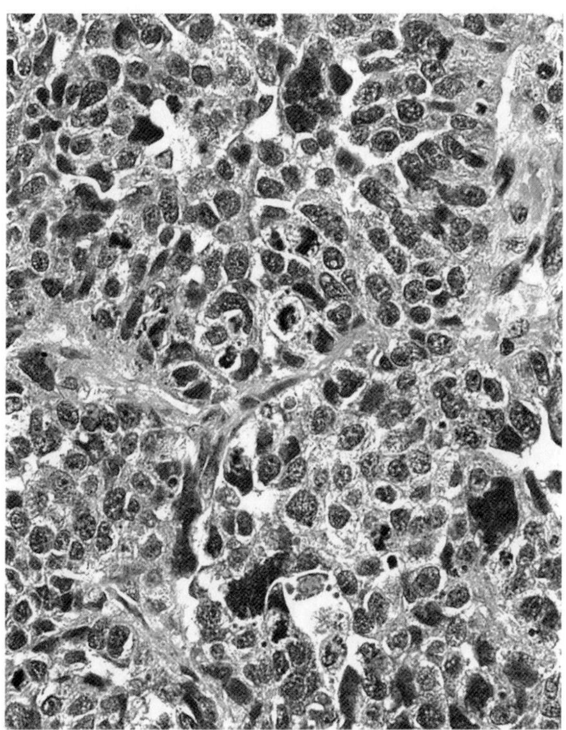

FIGURE 25.13. Serous carcinoma. The vast majority of serous carcinomas are of high grade, with marked cytologic atypia, large nucleoli, and more than ten mitoses per ten high power fields.

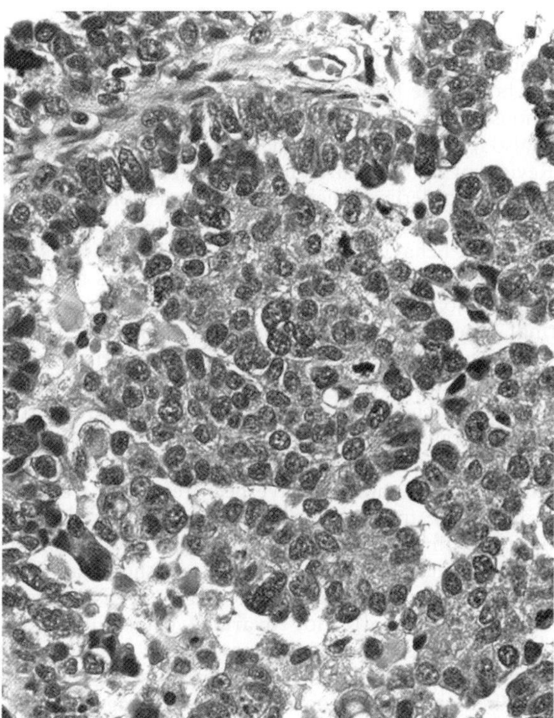

FIGURE 25.14. Serous carcinoma. Less than 10% of serous carcinomas of the ovary are of low grade, and many of them are of micropapillary type. They are characterized by mild to moderate cytologic atypia, variable nucleoli, and fewer than ten mitoses per ten high power fields.

observed (see above). The binary system separates over 90% of advanced-stage serous carcinomas into the high-grade group. This distribution is reflected in the overall behavior of advanced-stage serous carcinoma, which is associated with a 5-year survival of about 25%. In contrast, the 5- and 10-year survivals for women with advanced-stage low-grade serous carcinoma are about 85% and 50% to 60%, respectively.

Serous carcinomas nearly always stain positively with immunohistochemistry for WT1, cytokeratin (CK) 7, and negative or only focally positive for CK20 and calretinin. A panel that includes these antibodies is frequently employed to evaluate a carcinoma whose primary site is uncertain. Pancreatic and breast carcinomas have the same CK7/20 profile and thus other markers are needed for these sites. GCDFP-15 (gross cystic disease fluid protein) is often positive in breast carcinoma and only rarely positive in ovarian. Immunohistochemistry is rarely needed for serous carcinoma and is much more useful for the problematic mucinous tumors (see Mucinous Tumors).

Serous Psammocarcinoma. This is considered to be a rare variant of serous adenocarcinoma that is characterized by massive psammoma body formation. It is categorized as a carcinoma since it often displays destructive invasion or vascular invasion on microscopic examination; in half the cases, the extraovarian tumor also invades peritoneal sites. Despite these features, the cytologic attributes are more in keeping with a low-grade neoplasm, and the behavior is generally similar to that of serous borderline tumors.

Mucinous Tumors

Primary ovarian mucinous tumors represent about 10% of all common epithelial tumors and include three types: cystadenomas, borderline tumors, and carcinomas. The cystadenomas (81%), followed by the borderline tumors (13%), are the most commonly encountered, whereas primary ovarian mucinous carcinomas are much less common (5%). The mean age for patients with mucinous adenocarcinoma is 52 years, which, as with serous adenocarcinoma, is greater than the mean age of patients with benign and borderline tumors (44 and 49 years, respectively).

The cystadenomas and borderline tumors are noninvasive and are distinguished from one another primarily by their degree of complexity and epithelial proliferation. The carcinomas are distinguished from these two types of tumors by the presence of stromal invasion, which is required for a diagnosis of carcinoma. Intermediate forms exist, such as cystadenomas with focal epithelial proliferation and borderline tumors with intraepithelial carcinoma and/or microinvasion, providing evidence that these tumors form a morphologic spectrum with individual types representing steps in the sequence of mucinous carcinogenesis in the ovary.

The other types of mucinous tumors encountered in the ovary include metastatic mucinous carcinomas derived from various sites, most commonly the gastrointestinal tract, and low-grade mucinous tumors of appendiceal origin secondarily involving the ovary in association with the clinical syndrome of pseudomyxoma peritonei. Both metastatic mucinous carcinomas and low-grade mucinous tumors of appendiceal origin in the ovary can simulate primary ovarian mucinous tumors, including both the borderline (atypical proliferative) mucinous tumors and the primary ovarian mucinous carcinomas. Refined diagnosis of ovarian mucinous tumors in recent years, with distinction of these nonovarian tumors from true primary ovarian mucinous tumors, has been instrumental in clarifying the behavior of ovarian mucinous tumors. Accurate diagnosis and understanding of tumor behavior are essential for determining proper therapy, including both surgical management and chemotherapeutic regimens.

Mucinous Borderline Tumors

Mucinous borderline tumors differ in some respects from serous borderline tumors. There are two types of borderline mucinous tumors: the gastrointestinal type and the endocervical type (also referred to as the müllerian or seromucinous type).

Review of the literature on tumors meeting the diagnostic criteria for borderline mucinous tumor, gastrointestinal type, reveals that these tumors have demonstrated an overwhelmingly benign behavior (93,112–130). Specific aspects of the behavior of these tumors can be summarized as follows: (a) The vast majority of borderline mucinous tumors of gastrointestinal type are stage I; (b) of over 600 stage I tumors reported, less than 1% of these patients have been reported to have died of disease (most of these fatal tumors had inadequate or an unknown degree of sampling and are reported in the older literature; most recent studies report 100% survival); (c) a smaller number (~100) of so-called "advanced-stage borderline mucinous tumors" have been reported, with nearly 50% mortality; more than 85% of these tumors have been associated with the clinical syndrome of pseudomyxoma peritonei. However, recent studies have established that virtually all cases of pseudomyxoma peritonei are of gastrointestinal (usually appendiceal), not ovarian, origin (see below) (128–136). Therefore, the existence of true primary ovarian borderline mucinous tumors of advanced stage is questionable. When these questionable advanced-stage tumors are removed from the primary ovarian borderline mucinous tumor category, the remainder consists overwhelmingly of stage I tumors with benign behavior.

The endocervical (or seromucinous) type mucinous borderline tumors are much less common than the gastrointestinal type of mucinous borderline tumors. Based on a small number of studies, these tumors, including those with implants and intraepithelial and microinvasive carcinomas, have also demonstrated a benign behavior (137–141).

Gross Appearance. Mucinous tumors can grow to extremely large sizes, being among the largest of any recorded tumor in the body. Sizes exceeding 40 kg and 30 cm in greatest diameter are not uncommon.

The *gastrointestinal type of mucinous borderline tumor* is typically a large, multicystic tumor with a smooth capsule. This type of mucinous tumor is unilateral in >95% of cases, with mean and median sizes of 20 to 22 cm (126,142). The locules of the tumor are usually filled with mucinous material and the lining appears smooth, without grossly evident papillations.

The *endocervical (or seromucinous) type of mucinous borderline tumors* are grossly, microscopically, and immunophenotypically distinct from the gastrointestinal type tumors (143). The former are more frequently bilateral, can be intracystic or exophytic, and architecturally are identical to serous borderline tumors.

Microscopic Appearance. Microscopically, the *gastrointestinal type of mucinous borderline tumor* is composed of cysts that are lined by stratified, proliferative, gastrointestinal type mucinous epithelium exhibiting tufted and villoglandular or papillary intraglandular growth and displaying variable (usually mild to moderate) nuclear atypia; by definition, these tumors lack stromal invasion (Figs. 25.15 and 25.16).

The *endocervical (seromucinous) type of mucinous borderline tumors* have hierarchical branching of papillae, similar to serous tumors, but are lined by endocervical type mucinous as well as serous (ciliated cell) type epithelium. The epithelium exhibits tufting and stratification, with generally mild nuclear atypia and low mitotic activity.

Tumors composed predominantly of cystadenoma with a minor component of borderline tumor (<10%) are probably best diagnosed as a mucinous cystadenoma. The presence of focal borderline tumor should not generate overly aggressive treatment, given the literature indicating that *bona fide* mucinous borderline tumors are virtually always stage I, have an overwhelmingly benign behavior, and can be managed conservatively.

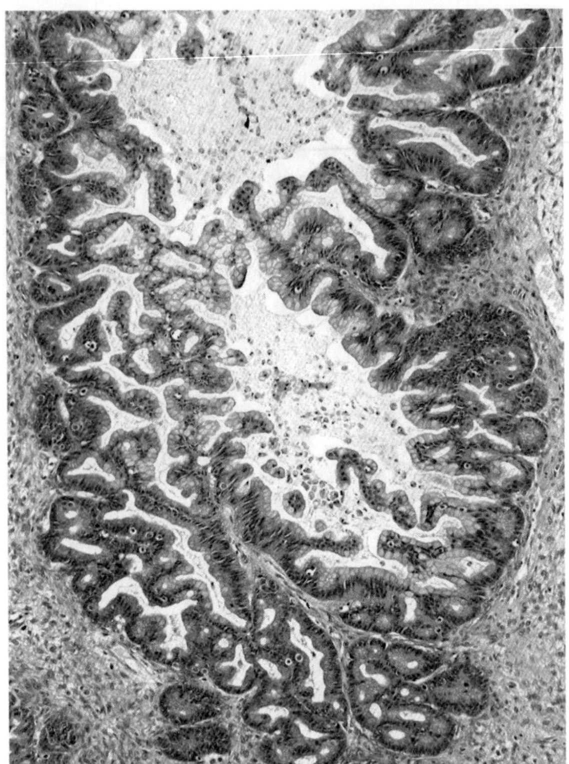

FIGURE 25.15. Borderline (atypical proliferative) mucinous tumor, gastrointestinal type. The tumor is composed of cysts lined by stratified and tufted mucinous epithelium with gastrointestinal-type differentiation; the periphery of the cyst is composed of crypts, but stromal invasion is lacking.

Mucinous Borderline Tumors With Intraepithelial Carcinoma. Based on the FIGO and WHO classification schemes of the early 1970s, the sole criterion for distinguishing a mucinous borderline tumor from mucinous carcinoma was the absence of stromal invasion. Shortly thereafter, the criteria for mucinous carcinoma were expanded to include tumors displaying marked overgrowth of atypical epithelial cells manifested as epithelial cell stratification in excess of three layers, cribriform intraglandular proliferations, or finger-like projections of solid cellular masses without connective tissue support; these patterns were often accompanied by marked nuclear atypia. In addition, the presence of marked nuclear atypia alone was added as a diagnostic feature of mucinous carcinoma (144,145). Since then, mucinous tumors lacking stromal invasion but displaying epithelial overgrowth and atypia have been referred to as intraglandular or intraepithelial carcinomas. Proposed diagnostic criteria for intraepithelial carcinoma vary slightly (Fig. 25.17) among different studies, but all studies (115,120,126,127,146) consider tumors with marked nuclear atypia as intraepithelial carcinomas. Stage I intraepithelial carcinomas have demonstrated an excellent prognosis (~95% survival overall in the literature, with most recent studies reporting 100% survival) (112–115,117,118,120,126,127, 141,146,147).

Mucinous Borderline Tumors With Microinvasion. Microinvasion in borderline mucinous tumors has been defined as either small foci of stromal invasion characterized

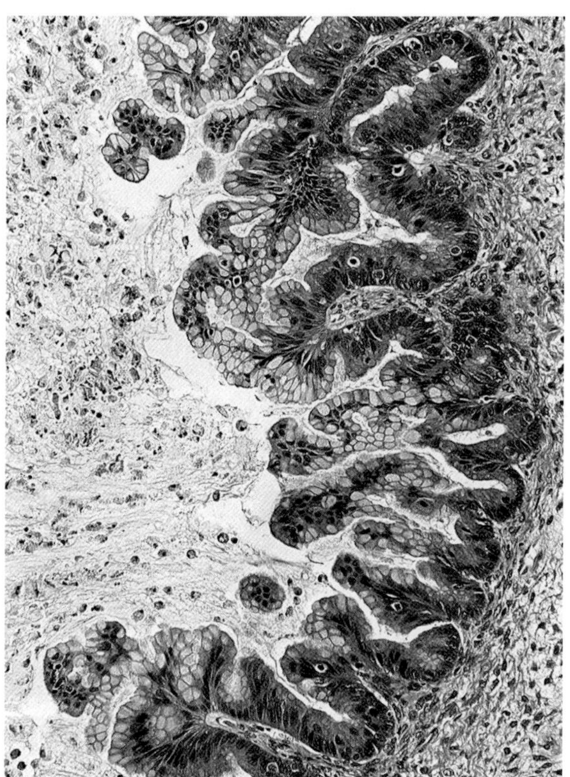

FIGURE 25.16. Borderline (atypical proliferative) mucinous tumor, gastrointestinal type. Mucinous epithelium displays stratification and papillary tufts, with mild to moderate nuclear atypia, differentiation toward the papillary tips, and proliferative activity primarily confined to the crypts.

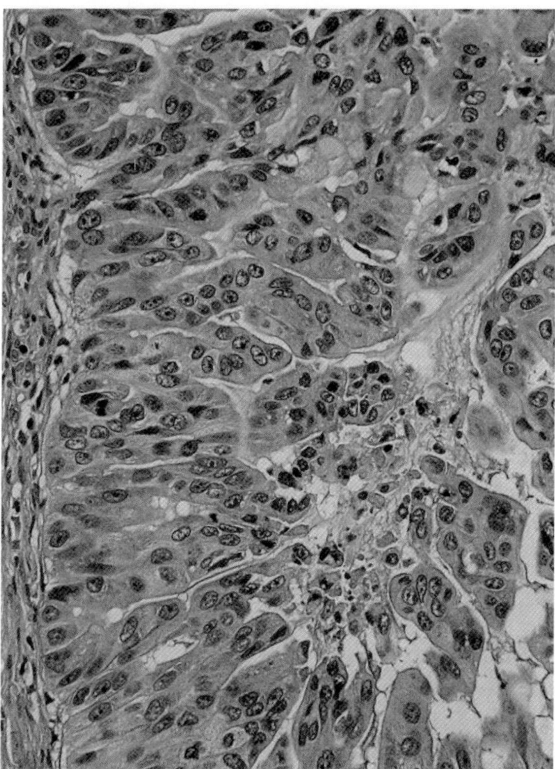

FIGURE 25.17. Borderline (atypical proliferative) mucinous tumor, gastrointestinal type, with intraepithelial carcinoma. The epithelium lining the cyst exhibits excessive stratification and marked nuclear atypia.

by single cells, glands, or small clusters/nests of mucinous epithelial cells within the stroma or as small foci of confluent glandular or cribriform growth within the stroma (Fig. 25.18). Some investigators have variably used 1, 2, 3, and 5 mm in greatest linear extent or 10 square mm as the size limit for each individual focus with no requirement regarding the number of such foci allowed (114,115,120,126,127,146,148,149). Irrespective of the size criterion chosen, based on the relatively small number of microinvasive tumors with follow-up that have been reported, no recurrences or deaths due to disease have been observed, with the exception of one inadequately sampled tumor (114,115,118,120,126,127,146,148,149).

Mucinous Adenocarcinoma

Studies focused on refined diagnosis of ovarian mucinous tumors have established that primary ovarian mucinous carcinomas are much less common than previously believed. It is important to recognize that when evaluating the literature on behavior and therapeutic responses of primary ovarian mucinous carcinomas, some reports likely include a subset of misclassified metastatic mucinous carcinomas from the gastrointestinal tract to the ovary (see below).

Gross Appearance. Primary ovarian mucinous carcinomas are often grossly similar to borderline mucinous tumors in that they are typically large, unilateral, multicystic mucinous tumors with smooth capsules and have mean and median sizes of 18 to 22 cm (126,142). They may contain solid areas, and regions of necrosis and rupture with surface involvement can occur. A thick, tenacious mucinous material may fill the cysts. Bilaterality is very uncommon, occurring in less than 5% of cases.

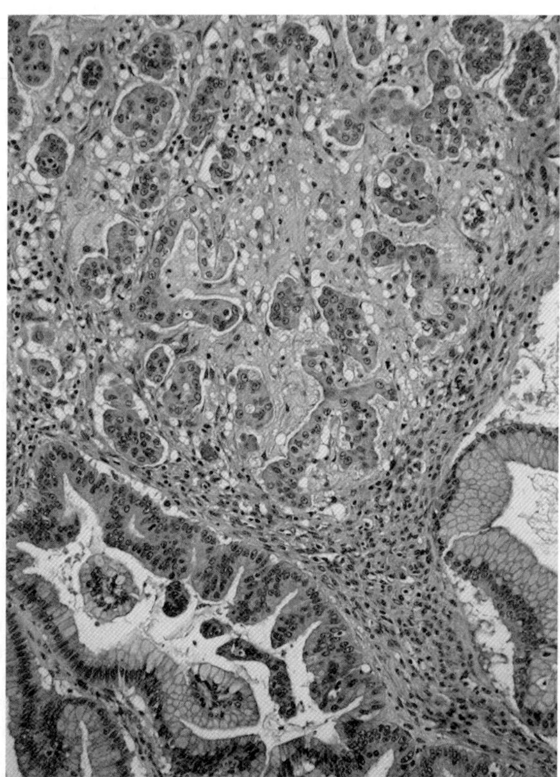

FIGURE 25.18. Borderline (atypical proliferative) mucinous tumor, gastrointestinal type, with microinvasion. A small area containing clusters of mucinous epithelial cells haphazardly arranged within edematous/reactive stroma is present adjacent to areas of typical borderline tumor.

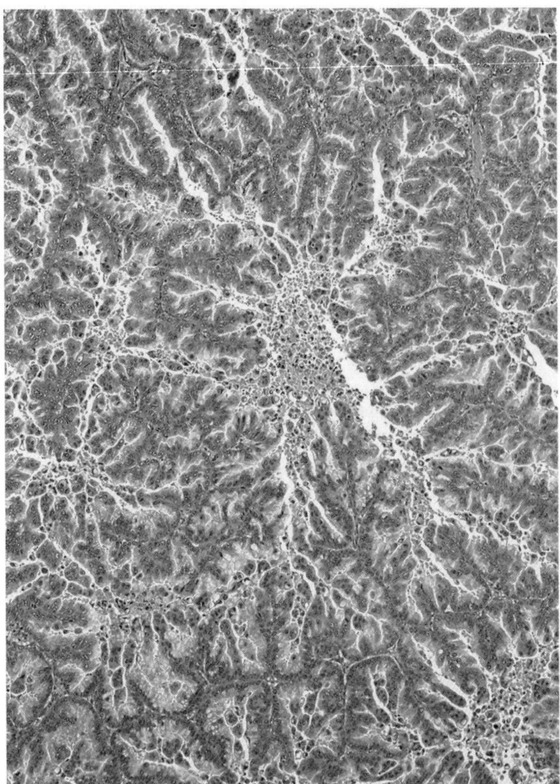

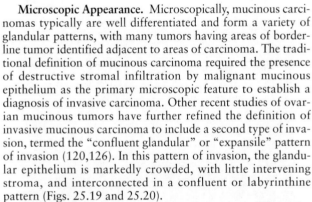

FIGURE 25.19. Primary ovarian mucinous carcinoma. Mucinous tumor is characterized by a confluent glandular proliferation exhibiting a labyrinthine pattern that is sufficiently complex to indicate a form of invasive carcinoma.

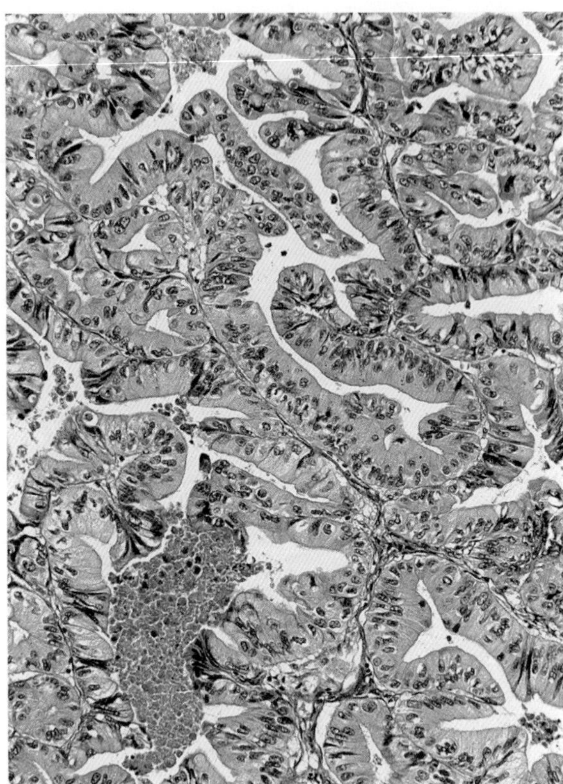

FIGURE 25.20. Primary ovarian mucinous carcinoma. Mucinous glands are well differentiated, moderately atypical, and sufficiently back to back to qualify as invasive mucinous carcinoma.

Microscopic Appearance. Microscopically, mucinous carcinomas typically are well differentiated and form a variety of glandular patterns, with many tumors having areas of borderline tumor identified adjacent to areas of carcinoma. The traditional definition of mucinous carcinoma required the presence of destructive stromal infiltration by malignant mucinous epithelium as the primary microscopic feature to establish a diagnosis of invasive carcinoma. Other recent studies of ovarian mucinous tumors have further refined the definition of invasive mucinous carcinoma to include a second type of invasion, termed the "confluent glandular" or "expansile" pattern of invasion (120,126). In this pattern of invasion, the glandular epithelium is markedly crowded, with little intervening stroma, and interconnected in a confluent or labyrinthine pattern (Figs. 25.19 and 25.20).

Primary ovarian mucinous carcinomas commonly exhibit this pattern of invasion and the presence of an infiltrative pattern of stromal invasion should raise concern for metastatic mucinous carcinoma (see below). Based on recent studies recognizing this pattern of invasion, it appears that patients with stage I mucinous carcinomas of this type have a survival rate of ~90%; despite a few exceptions, adverse prognosis is much more commonly associated with the infiltrative rather than the confluent glandular pattern of invasion (120,126,127,150,151). Most pathologists agree that the confluent glandular pattern reflects a type of invasive well-differentiated mucinous carcinoma which should be diagnosed as such, although some pathologists might classify tumors with this pattern as borderline tumor with intraepithelial carcinoma rather than as invasive carcinoma. For tumors comprised predominantly of borderline tumor the focus of confluent growth should measure more than the upper size limit allowed for a diagnosis of microinvasion to qualify for the diagnosis of invasive carcinoma.

Ovarian Mucinous Tumors Associated With Pseudomyxoma Peritonei. Recent studies have redefined pseudomyxoma peritonei as a specific clinicopathologic syndrome in which mucinous ascites is accompanied by low-grade neoplastic mucinous epithelium (not carcinoma), intimately associated with pools of extracellular mucin and fibrosis (131,133,153). Morphologic, immunohistochemical, and molecular genetic studies have provided compelling evidence that virtually all cases of pseudomyxoma peritonei are derived from appendiceal low-grade (adenomatous) mucinous tumors and the ovarian involvement is secondary (128–136). This concept is further supported by other studies showing that ruptured primary ovarian mucinous tumors have not been associated with the subsequent development of pseudomyxoma peritonei. Because the ovarian mucinous tumors associated with pseudomyxoma peritonei are almost invariably derived from the gastrointestinal tract, usually the appendix, they are reported as secondary involvement of the ovary by low-grade (adenomatous) mucinous tumor; such tumors should not be labeled with the same diagnostic terms used for primary ovarian tumors (cystadenoma or borderline tumor) so that clinicians are not confused about the established or suspected primary site. When intraoperative consultation with frozen section leads to diagnosis of a mucinous ovarian tumor in the setting of pseudomyxoma peritonei, the need for appendectomy should be conveyed to the surgeon and the pathologist should examine the entire appendix microscopically. The rare exception to this theory of the appendiceal origin of pseudomyxoma peritonei is the occurrence of mucinous tumors arising in ovarian mature cystic teratomas associated with pseudomyxoma peritonei (152).

The terms "disseminated peritoneal adenomucinosis" (131,133) and "involvement by low-grade appendiceal mucinous neoplasm" (153) are recommended as specific pathologic diagnostic terms for these low-grade peritoneal mucinous tumors. This recommendation is based on studies demonstrating that peritoneal mucinous tumors with the histologic features of the low-grade tumors are pathologically and prognostically distinct from mucinous carcinomas, with the latter having significantly worse survival (133,134,154).

Metastatic Mucinous Carcinomas

Despite improved recognition of metastases, the problem of distinguishing primary from metastatic mucinous carcinomas in the ovary persists. The difficulty in recognizing metastases that morphologically simulate primary ovarian mucinous tumors not only at the time of intraoperative frozen section analysis but also on permanent sections is compounded by the fact that some metastases present first in the ovary, without a clinically evident extraovarian primary mucinous tumor. In addition, ancillary techniques such as immunohistochemical analysis with currently available markers, while useful in certain situations (e.g., colorectal carcinomas vs. primary ovarian carcinomas), are limited in their ability to distinguish some metastases from primary ovarian mucinous tumors (e.g., pancreaticobiliary tract carcinomas vs. primary ovarian mucinous tumors). Metastatic mucinous carcinomas are usually readily recognized as such when the ovarian tumors exhibit any or all of the following features: bilaterality, smaller size (typically less than 10 cm), ovarian surface involvement, a nodular pattern of involvement, and an infiltrative pattern of stromal invasion (126,142,155,156). It is important to recognize that some metastatic mucinous carcinomas, especially those derived from the colorectum, pancreaticobiliary tract, appendix, and endocervix, can exhibit deceptive patterns of invasion simulating primary ovarian mucinous borderline tumors with intraepithelial carcinoma or well-differentiated mucinous carcinomas of confluent glandular type (Fig. 25.21) (157–160). Not infrequently, some of these metastases display highly differentiated areas adjacent to carcinoma, simulating benign and "borderline" precursor lesions and suggesting origin in the ovary. Recognizing such tumors as metastatic is especially problematic when the ovarian tumor represents the presenting finding of disease, is unilateral and large, and a primary mucinous carcinoma of another organ is not identified. Recent studies have found that when mucinous tumors in the ovary are rigorously classified based on refined criteria and awareness of the deceptive patterns mentioned above, metastatic mucinous carcinomas are much more commonly encountered than primary ovarian mucinous carcinomas (142,156). The presence of any of the above-mentioned features characteristic of metastatic mucinous carcinoma in the ovary, or the presence of extraovarian disease at the time of intraoperative evaluation of a mucinous tumor in the ovary, should prompt the pathologist to consider the possibility of metastatic mucinous carcinoma and suggest that the surgeon examine the gastrointestinal tract, including pancreaticobiliary tract and appendix, for a primary tumor. Immunohistochemical analysis with antibodies such as CK7, CK20, CDX-2, and p16 can be useful for identifying some metastatic mucinous carcinomas; however, the utility of currently available markers is limited due to overlapping immunoprofiles of primary ovarian mucinous tumors (particularly with those of upper gastrointestinal tract origin) (157,161–164). Thus, further clinical evaluation is often required to exclude metastatic mucinous carcinoma in the ovary derived from a clinically occult nonovarian source.

Endometrioid Tumors

Endometrioid tumors account for a relatively small proportion of the common epithelial tumors, but most endometrioid tumors are malignant. About 15% of the endometrioid tumors are of borderline type. The mean age of patients with cancer is 57 years, which is substantially higher than that associated with benign and borderline tumors (40 and 48 years, respectively). Approximately 10% of cases, with reports of up to 40% (165), are associated with endometriosis, implying that, in at least some cases, this tumor arises as neoplastic transformation of the endometriosis (166). Over 10% of endometrioid tumors of the ovary are also associated with endometrial tumors of an identical histologic variant, each appearing as if it were primary in its respective organ (167). Features that favor metastasis to the ovary include bilateral involvement; small, solid, multinodular ovaries; surface and hilar spread of tumor; and high-grade or deeply invasive tumor in the endometrium associated with lymphatic invasion. A large, cystic, unilateral ovarian tumor of low histologic grade arising in a background of endometriosis of the ovary with a low-grade, superficially invasive carcinoma of the endometrium is likely to represent a separate primary tumor. However, no single feature can clearly distinguish a metastasis from a second primary tumor. The similar histology and subtype and high survival rate of these patients (80% at 10 years) suggest that the majority are synchronous primaries rather than metastases (168). Many of these patients also have coexisting endometriosis (168,169).

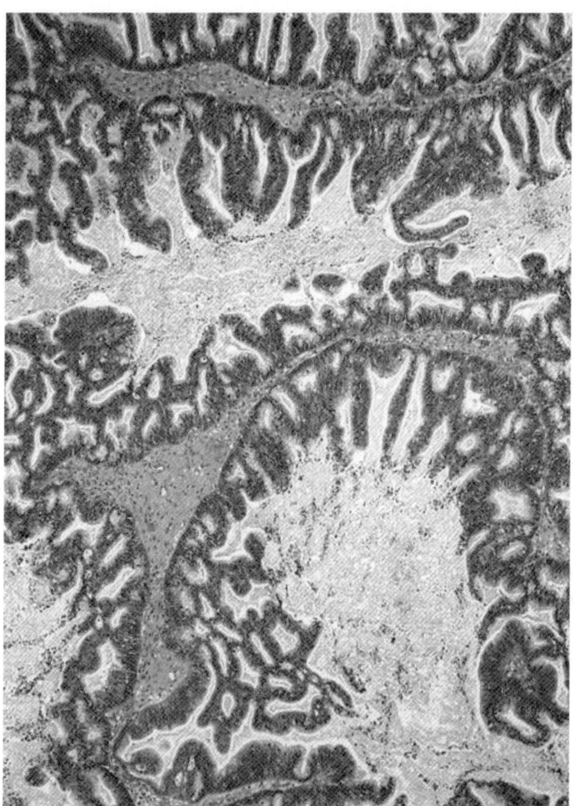

FIGURE 25.21. Metastatic endocervical adenocarcinoma in the ovary. The tumor exhibits a growth pattern that appears noninvasive, simulating a primary ovarian borderline (atypical proliferative) tumor and making recognition as a metastasis exceedingly difficult.

Gross Appearance

Borderline tumors range in size from small to large. They average 10 cm in diameter and are predominantly solid (170). Necrosis is rare. The cysts vary from small to about 9 cm in size and are filled with fluid that may be serous, mucinous, or hemorrhagic.

Endometrioid adenocarcinomas, like serous carcinomas, vary in size with an average of 10 cm. Wide zones of necrosis are common, especially if the tumor is large or poorly differentiated. Endometrioid tumors are more cystic than serous tumors and surface papillations are relatively infrequent.

Microscopic Appearance

Two variants of borderline tumors are recognized: the more common, which arises in adenofibromas, and the less common, which arises as a papilla. About 15% of the patients have associated endometriosis. An occasional borderline tumor may show only microscopic foci of invasion. The few recorded cases have behaved in a clinically benign fashion, suggesting that, as with serous tumors, tiny microscopic foci of invasive endometrioid tumor have little influence on later clinical behavior.

Endometrioid adenocarcinomas resemble adenocarcinomas of the endometrium. Like endometrial tumors, they can vary from well differentiated (grade 1) to poorly differentiated (grade 3) and may contain squamous cells of varying degrees of differentiation (endometrioid adenocarcinoma with squamous differentiation). Endometrioid carcinomas are more commonly well differentiated and of lower stage than serous carcinomas, which may also account for the overall better prognosis of endometrioid compared to serous tumors. When controlled for stage, the survival rate for endometrioid tumors is similar to that of serous adenocarcinoma in some studies (171) but better in others (172).

Endometrioid Neoplasms With Stromal Component

The classification of endometrioid neoplasms includes a subset of tumors that contain an endometrial-type stromal component. Endometrioid stromal sarcomas are tumors in which the neoplasm is composed exclusively of malignant endometrial-type stroma. The müllerian adenosarcoma displays a malignant stromal component and an epithelial component that appears proliferative or hyperplastic. As expected, spontaneous tumor rupture, high grade, or the presence of a high-grade sarcomatous component is associated with a poor prognosis (173). The ovarian carcinosarcoma is composed of malignant cells that display both mesenchymal and epithelial differentiation. The gross and microscopic features of these tumors are identical to carcinosarcomas arising in the endometrium (174). The clinical behavior also mirrors that of uterine carcinosarcoma, with a very poor prognosis when spread occurs beyond the ovary.

Clear Cell Tumors

Clear cell tumors are uncommon. The mean age for patients with clear cell adenocarcinoma is 53 years (175), which is similar to the other categories of cancers of common epithelial origin. About half of the cases are associated with endometriosis.

Gross Appearance

Clear cell tumors resemble endometrioid tumors on gross examination and cannot be distinguished with any reliability from serous tumors. Sometimes clear cell tumors, when arising within an endometriotic cyst, may appear as a pedunculated polyp. Clear cell adenocarcinoma is bilateral in under one sixth of cases (13%).

Microscopic Appearance

The ability to distinguish the rare clear cell borderline tumor from the frankly malignant tumor is difficult or impossible, since the latter, especially when small, may appear to be deceptively benign. A tumor is considered to be malignant when (a) the glands and islands of epithelial cells manifest high-grade cytologic characteristics of malignancy; and (b) invasion is present as evidenced by a desmoplastic or myxoid response of the stroma to the cells or a haphazard extension of cells into the stroma.

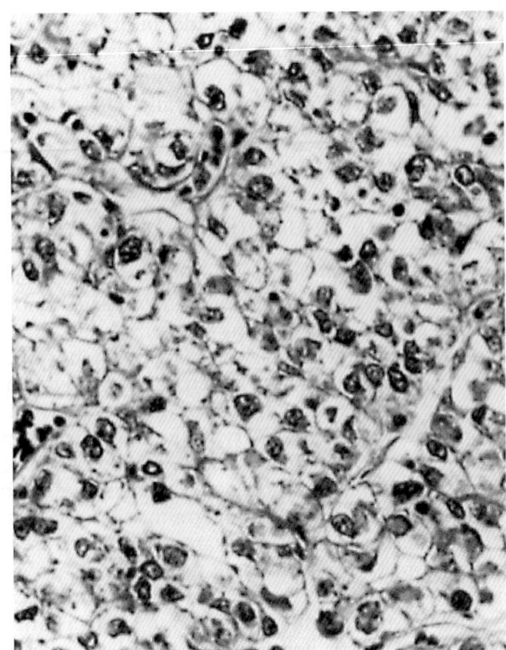

FIGURE 25.22. Clear cell adenocarcinoma. The sheets of tumor cells have clear cytoplasm.

Clear cell adenocarcinoma of the ovary is morphologically similar to the clear cell adenocarcinoma that occurs sporadically in the endometrium of older women and in the vagina and cervix of young women who were exposed prenatally to diethylstilbestrol (DES) (Fig. 25.22). Clear and "hobnail" cells are its hallmark, but it is important to recognize that the diagnosis rests upon architecture as well as optically clear cytoplasm. When present, the clear appearance of the cytoplasm results from glycogen that has leached as the tissue specimen is prepared for microscopic examination. The hobnail cells contain bulbous nuclei that protrude into the lumen at the apparent cytoplasmic limits of the cell. The clear cells usually appear as sheets of cells that have the appearance of a solid growth, but may also line tubules. The hobnail cells, and sometimes flat cells, are encountered more commonly in the pattern of growth showing tubules and cysts.

The clear cell carcinoma may also resemble the endodermal sinus (yolk sac) tumor. Historically, the two tumors were considered as being the same until it was recognized that clear cell tumors are müllerian in origin and endodermal sinus tumors are of germ cell origin. Immunohistochemistry has been of limited value in this distinction, since some keratins and alpha-fetoprotein can be expressed in both neoplasms. Recently, the presence of staining for the onco-fetal protein glypican-3 has been suggested as a means to distinguish yolk sac tumor from clear cell carcinoma (176).

Uncertainty exists whether ovarian clear cell adenocarcinoma is more aggressive than the other common epithelial malignancies. In some studies specifically addressing correlates of survival, advancing stage, and increased mitotic rate (>six mitoses per ten HPF or high MIB1 activity) were adverse prognostic indicators (177). Other investigators (178) emphasize young age, stage, or vascular invasion as being poor prognostic factors and the presence of a predominantly (>75%) papillary or tubulocystic morphology as a favorable prognostic factor. Many of the differences found in analyses appear to reflect the relative compositions of stage and grade and whether the more poorly differentiated tumors are correctly categorized by their true cell type.

Transitional Cell Tumors

Brenner Tumor

Brenner tumor, a tumor of urothelial differentiation, is the rarest of the common epithelial tumors. It is believed to arise from the pelvic mesothelium through transitional cell metaplasia, much in the same manner as Walthard's rests arise. Most of these tumors are small, benign, and discovered incidentally. Rarely are these borderline tumors or frankly malignant. Malignant tumors are of two types. Malignant Brenner tumor, which is exceedingly rare, consists of a poorly differentiated transitional cell–type epithelium in which definitive foci of benign Brenner tumor are present. The transitional cell carcinoma, which in some cases may be a malignant Brenner tumor in which foci of benign Brenner tumor cannot be found, is an entity that has been separated from the categories of malignant Brenner tumor and undifferentiated carcinoma.

Gross Appearance. Borderline Brenner tumors usually occur as large cysts, with a coarse papillary lining. Malignant Brenner tumors tend to be substantially more solid, but sometimes contain cysts.

Microscopic Appearance. Brenner tumors, unlike other common epithelial tumors, have two components. One is epithelial cords, which are composed of ovoid to polyhedral cells with large, longitudinally grooved nuclei (coffee-bean shaped). The cellular arrangement often resembles urothelium (179), with the most superficial layer of cells often displaying copious, mucin-rich cytoplasm. The second component is a dense, fibrous stroma in which are found the nests of transitional cells. The stroma is typically prominent and at times so massive as to nearly obscure the epithelial component. Minute foci of stromal calcification are found in over half the tumors.

The distinction between borderline and malignant Brenner tumor may be difficult. Borderline Brenner tumors exhibit papillae lined by a proliferating transitional epithelium typical of that found in low-grade bladder tumors. Malignant Brenner tumors have transitional epithelium that may be high grade or focally resemble squamous cell carcinoma. By definition, both borderline and malignant Brenner tumors have foci of a clearly identifiable benign Brenner's component.

Transitional Cell Carcinoma

Transitional cell carcinoma is a second form of ovarian cancer with urothelial differentiation. Unlike malignant Brenner tumor, which by definition arises from demonstrable pre-existing benign or proliferative Brenner tumor, the transitional cell carcinoma lacks such a component.

The transitional cell carcinoma is considered to be a separate variant of ovarian cancer based on both clinical and histologic grounds, although some consider it a variant of serous carcinoma.

Transitional cell tumors of the ovary, although appearing as urothelial-like, show immunoreactivity differences from true urothelium. The tumor of ovarian origin is immunoreactive with cytokeratin 7, whereas the bladder tumors show no such reactivity (180).

Squamous Cell Carcinoma

Squamous cell carcinoma is the newest category of surface epithelial-stromal tumors recognized by the WHO classification scheme for ovarian tumors. As for most epithelial tumors, the diagnosis is usually made in postmenopausal women, with an average age of about 56 years, and most of the tumors are stage II or III. The stage and grade of the tumor correlate best with overall survival (181). Pure squamous carcinomas are exceedingly rare, and some arise in endometriosis. Other squamous carcinomas reflect a teratomatous origin and arise consequent to malignant degeneration in a mature cystic teratoma.

Undifferentiated Carcinoma

Undifferentiated carcinoma refers to epithelial tumors that are so poorly differentiated based on examination of hematoxylin and eosin stained slides as to preclude further classification into any of the types described above. However, several subtypes of undifferentiated carcinoma display immunohistochemical and biochemical evidence of differentiation.

Small Cell Carcinoma

Small cell carcinoma is a subgroup of undifferentiated tumor. This tumor, which is of at least two types, the hypercalcemic and pulmonary types, is enigmatic in both its histogenesis and classification (182). The *hypercalcemic tumor* typically occurs in young women (mean age 24 years) (183). Two thirds have systemic hypercalcemia, which is commonly reversed after the tumor has been excised (184). This variety of small cell carcinoma is virtually always unilateral, but has spread beyond the ovary in half of patients by the time of diagnosis. Diffuse sheets of small, closely packed cells punctuated by variable numbers of follicle-like spaces characterize its histology. The individual cells have scant cytoplasm and a single nucleus. Mitotic activity is typically brisk. Although the DNA content is nearly always diploid, over 60% of patients with stage IA tumors die of the disease or have recurrences. Features in stage IA tumors associated with a more favorable outcome are age <30 years, normal preoperative serum calcium, and small tumor size. A large cell variant of the small cell type has also been described (185).

The second form of small cell carcinoma resembles small cell carcinoma of the lung (186). The tumor occurs in older women (mean, 59 years), and half of the tumors are bilateral. Neuron-specific enolase and reactivity are common, whereas chromogranin reactivity are only occasionally found. The majority of tumors are aneuploid. The mean survival is 8 months following diagnosis.

A third and rare form of undifferentiated carcinoma is *the neuroendocrine tumor of the non–small cell type* (187). Microscopically, the neuroendocrine component immunoreactive for chromogranin is in sheets, usually as closely packed islands, cords, or trabeculae of epithelial cells with little intervening stroma. The prognosis is poor (188). Metastasis from a respiratory origin must be excluded when the diagnosis of small cell or large cell undifferentiated carcinoma of the ovary is entertained.

Mixed Carcinoma

Perhaps as many as 10% of all ovarian tumors of common epithelial origin are mixed, when defined as a carcinoma in which more than 10% of the neoplasm exhibits a second histologic cell type. It has been commonly underreported since there is a tendency to place all high-grade carcinomas in the category of serous carcinoma. One common specific malignant combination is mixed clear cell and endometrioid carcinoma, both being related to endometriosis. Serous and endometrioid carcinomas are also commonly encountered. The behavior of mixed carcinomas of the ovary has not been elucidated.

Primary Peritoneal Serous Carcinomatosis

About 80% to 90% of women with peritoneal serous carcinomatosis (excluding advanced-stage endometrial serous carcinomas) have normal-sized ovaries with only surface implants of tumor. These are classified as primary peritoneal serous carcinomas, although a small proportion may represent primary tubal carcinomas (see below). Primary peritoneal carcinoma was defined by the GOG as follows: (a) ovaries are of normal size or enlarged by a benign process; (b) ovarian involvement is absent or limited to the surface and/or superficial cortex with no tumor nodule within the ovarian cortex exceeding 5 × 5 mm; (c) serous histology; and (d) volume of extraovarian disease significantly exceeds that of ovarian disease.

Primary peritoneal serous carcinomas may be more common than previously appreciated. A recent large series from a community hospital found that 22% of cases of peritoneal serous carcinomatosis were classified as peritoneal (83). In addition, there is reason to believe that the GOG criteria are too restrictive. A 5 or 6 mm nodule of serous carcinoma can be seen with tumors that fulfill all of the other criteria for peritoneal origin, and may even display the characteristic multi-nodular pattern of metastatic tumor to the ovary. The pathology and response to treatment of peritoneal serous carcinomas are essentially identical to that of ovarian serous carcinomas. However, the true relative incidence of ovarian versus peritoneal carcinoma is of pivotal importance because it directly impacts on the type of surgery recommended for prophylaxis in high-risk women as well as on the precise risk of developing serous carcinoma after prophylactic surgery.

The contribution of the fallopian tube to peritoneal serous carcinomatosis is unknown. It has recently become apparent that the tubal fimbriae may be an important source of carcinomatosis in the absence of the typical features of primary tubal carcinomas (i.e., a dilated fallopian tube with a large mucosal lesion). Furthermore, the intramural portion of the tube is not removed if there is no hysterectomy, and therefore this segment is theoretically a potential source of serous carcinoma even after prophylactic bilateral salpingo-oophorectomy.

In conclusion, lesions designated as primary peritoneal carcinoma are likely a heterogeneous collection of carcinomas that have arisen from the ovary, fimbria of the fallopian tube, or the pelvic peritoneum.

Fallopian Tube Carcinoma

Gross Appearance

The gross appearance of the fallopian tube affected by papillary carcinoma is typically described as enlarged, deformed, or fusiform, with agglutination of the fimbriae and, frequently, distal obstruction (Fig. 25.23) (188–191). When the tumor is confined to the mucosa, the tube is generally soft to palpation, and the initial impression of the surgeon is often hematosalpinx, pyosalpinx, or hydrosalpinxeale. Turbid fluid frequently fills the lumen, with a friable, exophytic, papillary, or nodular mass affixed to the mucosal surface. The most frequent site of origin is the ampulla, followed by the infundibulum (192,193). In about 10% of cases in a recent large study, the tumor arose in the fimbriated end of the fallopian tube. All of these tumors were less than 3 cm in diameter (194,195). Sometimes, multiple minute tumors stud the mucosal surface, or the entire lumen may be replaced by a necrotic mass. With more advanced disease, neoplastic cells penetrate the muscular wall and serosa of the tube, and extension to the ovary may result in a tubo-ovarian complex. In the latter situation, it is usually obvious that a malignant neoplasm has infiltrated the

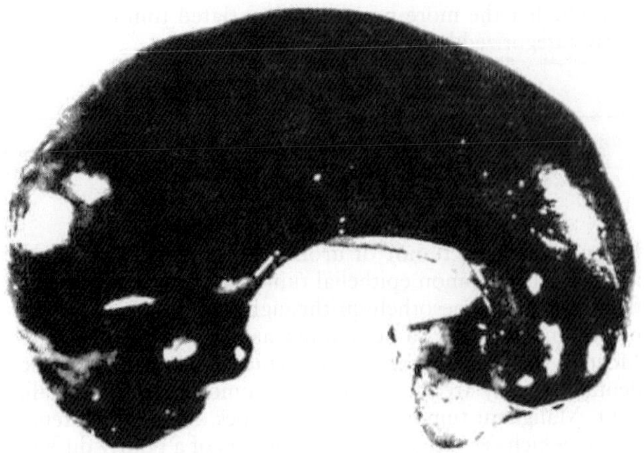

FIGURE 25.23. Carcinoma of the fallopian tube.

organs, but the distinction of tubal carcinoma from that of the ovary may not be possible, and reliance on arbitrary criteria usually results in the classification of the tumor as being ovarian in origin (see below). The carcinoma affects the left and right tube with about equal frequency and displays bilateral involvement in about 5% to 30% of cases (196–201).

Recently, a radically different presentation of fallopian tube carcinoma has been reported. Occult invasive or *in situ* carcinoma has been found to involve the fallopian tube in risk-reducing salpino-oophorectomy (RRSO) specimens obtained from women with a strong family history of ovarian cancer or known *BRCA1* or *BRCA2* germ-line mutations (67,202,203). Such tumors may not be visible macroscopically, and it is suggested that the entire fallopian tube as well as the ovary be serially sectioned and examined microscopically in this clinical setting.

Microscopic Appearance

The current WHO histologic classification of epithelial tumors of the fallopian tube is similar to that of other sites in the upper female genital tract and is divided into serous, mucinous, endometrioid, clear cell, transitional, squamous, glassy cell, and mixed carcinomas (195). This change in terminology reflects an increased recognition of both endometrioid and transitional cell differentiation in carcinomas of the fallopian tube during the past 10 years.

Papillary serous adenocarcinoma is the most frequent primary malignant neoplasm of the fallopian tube, and was previously reported to represent about 90% of the 300 new cases annually occurring in the United States (188). In more recent studies, its frequency has been lower, reflecting the increasing recognition by pathologists that tumors of other cell types may legitimately arise in the fallopian tube (189,190). In superficial lesions, the plicae, which are ordinarily covered by a simple columnar epithelium of ciliated and secretory cells, are replaced by multiple layers of columnar or cuboidal cells with pleomorphic and hyperchromatic nuclei (Figs. 25.24 and 25.25). The papillary configuration of the epithelium is usually preserved, but secretory activity and cilia are usually not preserved at the light microscopic level. Mitotic figures are frequent. Invasion of the muscular wall occurs early in the course of disease, and, as the tumor enlarges, necrosis becomes a common feature. It is critical for the pathologist to examine and liberally section the site of tumor carefully since the probability of survival is markedly different for women whose tumors are confined to the mucosa compared with those whose tumors either invade the muscular wall or extend to the serosa of the tube (201). Capillary or lymphatic vascular invasion is common even in

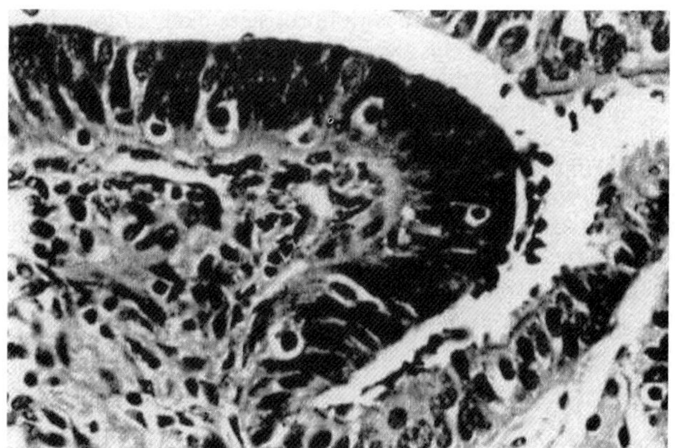

FIGURE 25.24. Hyperplasia of the fallopian tube. Pseudostratification of cells and crowding of nuclei discovered as an incidental finding in a fallopian tube removed from a 49-year-old female with stress incontinence.

early-stage disease, and has also been associated with a diminished probability of survival (200).

Endometroid carcinomas involving the fallopian tube are more common than previously reported, and over 50 cases have been documented in the literature (204). They are formed of tubular glands, sometimes with foci of either benign or malignant-appearing squamous differentiation (189,191,205). In at least one case, the tumor arose in tubal endometriosis. The tumor usually resembles typical adenocarcinoma of the endometrium, but it may simulate female adnexal tumors of probable wolffian origin (195,206,207). It may be distinguished from the latter by the greater degree of cytologic atypia, mitotic activity, and at least focal endometrial-type gland formation (206,208). Many of the endometrioid carcinomas are either noninvasive or only superficially invasive, and appear to have a more favorable prognosis than serous carcinomas.

Transitional cell carcinomas resemble tumors of urothelial type, with papillae formed of broad masses of cells covering a fibrovascular core (189,204–210). These papillae are distinguished from those of serous carcinomas by having a smooth surface rather than the scalloped surface of serous carcinoma, and by the presence of longitudinal grooves in the nuclei of some cells. This was the predominant histologic pattern in 12 of 21 primary tubal carcinomas from Japan (210), but represented only about 10% of cases in a large series from the United States (189). The survival has been reported to be either better than or similar to that of serous carcinoma (201,210).

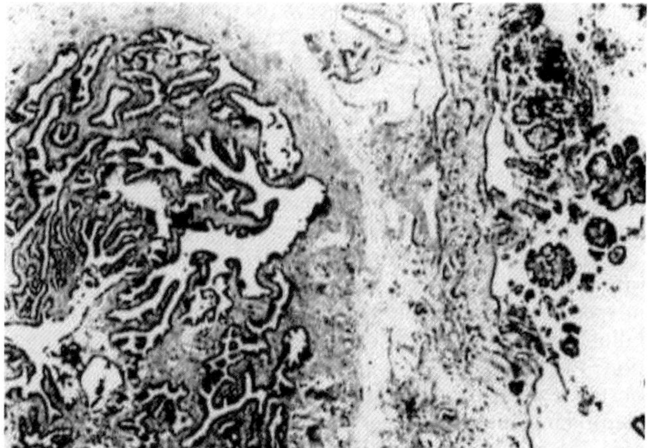

FIGURE 25.25. Multifocal neoplasia involving the fallopian tube. Papillary carcinoma of low malignant potential is depicted on the serosa of the fallopian tube, whereas psammoma bodies are noted in the lumen.

Too few cases of clear cell, undifferentiated, or mixed types of carcinoma have been reported to characterize their behavior.

The histologic grade of fallopian tube carcinoma is usually simply designated as well, moderately, or poorly differentiated. In contrast to the depth of invasion, the degree of histologic differentiation has generally not been related to prognosis (192,193,196,198,200,211), although a few series have demonstrated a better probability of survival when the tumor was well differentiated (177). It is unclear whether this inability to prognosticate reflects the lack of biologic importance of histologic grade or simply the absence of reproducible criteria for grading.

No distinctive immunohistochemical markers of fallopian tube differentiation exist. Carcinoembryonic antigen is widely distributed in the lower intestinal tract during embryonic development and is present in mucinous neoplasms of the cervix and ovary, but it is absent from the postnatal normal or neoplastic fallopian tube. CA-125 can be detected immunohistochemically in both the benign and malignant fallopian tube (211,212); however, it is also found in endometrial and ovarian serous carcinomas, and thus cannot help the pathologist to discriminate whether a carcinoma has arisen in the fallopian tube or ovary.

The data are insufficient to offer conclusions about the frequency or significance of oncogene overexpression in fallopian tube carcinoma. In one study of HER2/neu using a quantitative polymerase chain reaction assay, no tumors displayed amplification of the oncogene (213). The frequency of HER2/neu overexpression has varied from 26% to 89%, whereas that of p53 has ranged from 60% to 83% (202,214). In contrast to ovarian carcinoma, their overexpression in fallopian tube carcinoma has not been associated with a worsened prognosis. Immunohistochemical overexpression of *c-myc* has also been reported in 61% of cases in one study (214). K-*RAS* point mutations in codon 12 have been reported to be present in seven of eight carcinomas of the fallopian tube (215).

Estrogen receptors have been identified in the nuclei of fallopian tube epithelium and in a minority of fallopian tube carcinomas (216,217); however, no data on the relationship between the presence of estrogen receptors and response to hormonal therapy for fallopian tube cancer exist.

Rare Malignant Neoplasms of the Fallopian Tube

Most types of tumors found in the uterine corpus have also been reported to occur in the fallopian tube. About 50 cases of malignant mixed mesodermal tumors have been described (215,218–221). The average age at diagnosis is 58 years. The lesions grossly resemble those of fallopian tube carcinoma, with a dilated tube that contains an intraluminal papillary mass. However, in addition to a carcinoma arranged as glands or papillae, there is also a malignant stromal component. The tumors are further divided into homologous or heterologous types according to the absence or presence of differentiation of the stromal elements into cell types not normally found within the müllerian duct system, such as skeletal muscle or cartilage. The overall 5-year survival is about 15%, with a mean survival of about 17 months. The presence or absence of heterologous elements has not been related to outcome. A single positive observation is the markedly better probability of survival for women with tumors confined to the muscularis (220).

Three examples of primary squamous cell carcinoma (222), immature teratoma (223), glassy cell carcinoma (224), Wilms' tumor, and rare pure sarcomas, including leiomyosarcoma, angiosarcoma, malignant fibrous histiocytoma, stromal sarcoma, and fibrosarcoma, have been reported to occur in the fallopian tube (225–229). Other pure squamous carcinomas in the fallopian tube have been generally described as part of an extended *in situ* transformation that involves uterine cervix and corpus, frequently associated with cervical stenosis (see section Multifocal Carcinoma of the Müllerian System, Including the Fallopian Tubes below).

Serous, mucinous, and endometrioid tumors of low malignant potential occasionally occur in the fallopian tube (194,230–232). Their biologic behavior appears to mimic that of low malignant tumors of the ovary.

About 100 cases of gestational choriocarcinoma arising in an ectopic tubal pregnancy have been reported (233). It displays pathologic and biologic characteristics identical to those of uterine choriocarcinoma (233,234). Nongestational choriocarcinoma of the fallopian tube has been reported in a prepubertal girl.

Papillary carcinoma of the tube typically occurs in menopausal women; however, in a handful of cases, it occurred in adolescent females or was discovered during pregnancy or at postpartum tubal ligation (224,235–237).

The precise, but awkward, appellation "female adnexal tumors of probable wolffian origin" has been given by Young and Scully to a rare neoplasm identified along the serosal surface of the distal portion of the fallopian tube or within the broad ligament or ovary (238). About 20 such tumors have been reported in women between 28 and 79 years of age. These tumors are typically unilateral, lobulated, grossly encapsulated, solid, or partially cystic masses that measure from 1 to 20 cm in diameter. A variety of microscopic patterns have been described, including cystic, closely packed tubules, sieve-like spaces, or diffuse proliferation. Usually, the cells have bland, oval nuclei and little mitotic activity. It is these cytologic features that help distinguish them from mesotheliomas or common epithelial malignancies. Intracytoplasmic mucin is absent. Although the majority of the tumors behave in a benign fashion, the presence of nuclear pleomorphism and, especially, increased mitotic activity (>10 mitoses per ten HPF) has been associated with more aggressive behavior.

Distinction of Fallopian Tube Carcinoma From Ovarian Carcinoma

Because the gross and microscopic characteristics, as well as spread, of carcinoma of the fallopian tube is identical to those of the ovary, the determination of the site of origin of a tumor that forms a solid or cystic tubo-ovarian mass is arbitrary. In the past, some investigators have quite reasonably designated such tumors as tubo-ovarian carcinoma (205). Hu et al., in 1950, proposed criteria for differentiating primary from metastatic carcinoma that involves the fallopian tube. These criteria, slightly modified, are outlined in Table 25.5 (239). Many tumors of probable tubal origin fail to meet these stringent criteria, and the fault with this approach is the possibility that the incidence of fallopian tube carcinoma is greatly underestimated. This may simply reflect the rigidity of our definitions. Carcinomas that occur in a scarred tube or those that provoke an inflammatory response with fibrosis are likely to form localized masses that we classify as primary to the fallopian tube. In contrast, early dissemination of cells from carcinomas arising in the mucosa of the fimbriated end of a fallopian tube that is not sealed may result in a mass that is larger in the ovary or the peritoneum than in the fallopian tube. By convention, these carcinomas would be classified as primary ovarian or primary peritoneal carcinomas, although the neoplasm may have had an origin in the tube. The recent studies of Crum et al. suggest that this may be a very frequent occurrence, and the fallopian tube may actually be the source of many high-grade serous carcinomas that are considered as primary to the ovary (239a).

TABLE 25.5

CRITERIA FOR PATHOLOGIC DIAGNOSIS OF PRIMARY FALLOPIAN TUBE CARCINOMA

1. The main tumor is in the tube and arises from the endosalpinx.
2. The pattern histologically reproduces the epithelium of the mucosa and usually shows a papillary pattern.
3. If the wall is involved, the transition between benign and malignanat tubal epithelium should be demonstrable.
4. The ovaries and endometrium are either normal or contain less tumor than the tubes.

Hyperplasia and Preinvasive Carcinoma of the Fallopian Tube

The sequence of histologic changes that precedes the development of invasive adenocarcinoma of the fallopian tube has not been well described. Proliferation of the pseudostratified columnar cells in the absence of marked cytologic atypia or mitotic activity is referred to as epithelial hyperplasia (Fig. 25.24). The degree of proliferation varies and may result in a multilayered epithelium with focal tufting and, rarely, a cribriform pattern of cells. Tubal hyperplasia is more commonly observed as an incidental finding in patients with salpingitis (particularly tuberculous salpingitis), endogenous or exogenous estrogen stimulation, or serous ovarian tumors of low malignant potential (239–240). Moore and Enterline (241) prospectively sectioned entire oviducts from 124 nonselected hysterectomies and found hyperplasia in 19% of women, frequently as a focal lesion. The significance of hyperplasia is thus unknown, but the pathologist should be cautious not to overinterpret proliferative lesions as intraepithelial carcinoma.

In a very recent series of studies using serial sectioning of fallopian tubes from a variety of conditions, Crum et al. have suggested that mutations in the p53 tumor suppressor gene, either as an isolated finding or in association with cytologic atypia and increased proliferation, may serve to identify a molecular signature of various precursors of tubal carcinoma.

Preinvasive carcinoma (dysplasia, carcinoma *in situ*) of the fallopian tube was rarely reported prior to the practice of RRSO for women with *BRCA* mutations (241,242). In contrast to hyperplasia, the diagnosis of carcinoma *in situ* requires the presence of marked cytologic atypia. The proliferation usually results in the formation of multilayered epithelium composed of cells with large, pleomorphic nuclei, often prominent nucleoli, and interspersed mitotic activity. The evidence that supports the designation of lesions as carcinoma *in situ* is their frequent occurrence in the transition between normal tubal epithelium and invasive carcinoma and their presence as part of multifocal *in situ* and early invasive neoplasia that involves the fallopian tube and ovary (242). *In situ* carcinoma of the fallopian tube is one of the most common findings in grossly normal ovaries and fallopian tubes removed for cancer risk reduction in women with *BRCA* mutations (67,203,243–245) (see The Pathologic Examination of Risk-Reducing Salpingo-oophorectomy Specimens).

Chronic inflammation commonly coexists in fallopian tubes that contain carcinoma (201,246); this fact has resulted in speculation that acute and chronic salpingitis is a cause of fallopian tube cancer. However, it is more likely that inflammation is a response to the presence of the neoplasm coupled with obstruction of the fallopian tube rather than a carcinogenic factor. First, although acute salpingitis is usually a bilateral disease, the tube contralateral to the one that contains the carcinoma is frequently free of salpingitis. Second, fallopian tube carcinoma is a disease of postmenopausal women, a group with a low incidence of tubal infection. Nevertheless, in a pathologically based case-control study of the nonneoplastic contralateral tube from 14 women with fallopian tube carcinoma, changes significantly more common included luminal dilatation, plical atrophy, and chronic inflammation, which are all changes consistent with chronic, healed salpingitis (247).

In contrast to chronic salpingitis, the relationship between tuberculous salpingitis and carcinoma is more complex. More than two dozen cases of carcinoma arising in the tube affected by tuberculosis have been reported (248). Although some of the examples are well documented, with evidence of metastatic spread occasionally, there is some concern that not all of the cases truly represent coexisting invasive neoplasia. The diagnosis of invasive carcinoma should be made cautiously in the fallopian tube afflicted with tuberculosis and should be reserved for cases in which infiltration of the muscularis with a desmoplastic host response is obvious.

Cytology in Diagnosis of Fallopian Tube Carcinoma

Although exfoliative cervicovaginal cytology has been reported to be positive in as many as 40% to 60% of women with tubal carcinoma (200,239,249), in most series, abnormal Papanicolaou (Pap) smears were distinctly uncommon (0% to 18%) (193,250,251). When present, the neoplastic cells are indistinguishable from those shed from endometrial adenocarcinoma, although several features may suggest that the tumor has arisen in the tube rather than the uterus. The malignant cells are scant in number and degenerate; malignant cells often present a spherical or papillary configuration; and the background is free of cellular debris (tumor diathesis) (252).

Because occult spread of tubal carcinoma outside the pelvis with serosal seeding occurs frequently, cytologic examination of peritoneal washings has been recommended (253). The presence of ascites or positive peritoneal cytology correlates well with an advanced stage of disease (252,254). A significantly worse prognosis has been reported for patients with exfoliated malignant cells in the peritoneum. In one study, the 5-year survival was 67% when the cytologic findings were negative but only 20% when malignant cells were present (241). Peritoneal fluid or washings should routinely be obtained at surgery for cytologic examination.

Multifocal Carcinoma of the Müllerian System, Including the Fallopian Tube

Multifocal carcinomas that involve the fallopian tube can be divided into three patterns: synchronously detected multifocal neoplasia within the fallopian tubes; multifocal neoplasia that involves various genital organs, including the fallopian tube; and direct spread of carcinoma (frequently intraepithelial) along the mucosa of the cervix and endometrium to involve the fallopian tube.

About 20% of patients with fallopian tube carcinoma have bilateral involvement. Although many specimens display a distinct site of mucosal tumor in each tube, it is unclear what percentage of patients reported to have bilateral disease actually have two, synchronously detected primary tubal neoplasms rather than metastasis from the contralateral tube (255). Unfortunately, most series do not include sufficient information to resolve this issue.

Multifocal carcinoma of the upper genital tract, including the fallopian tube, is relatively common (256,257). Sometimes, multiple papillary serous carcinomas are found in the ovary and on the serosa or in the lumen of the fallopian tube. These findings may reflect neoplastic transformation of the common embryologic field, which includes the coelomic epithelium that covers the ovary, fallopian tube, and other pelvic peritoneum (Fig. 25.25). At other times, endometrioid carcinomas are present in the endometrium, in the ovary, and in the mucosa of the tube. The frequent presence of endometriosis in these patients has led to the suggestion that it is the site of multifocal neoplastic transformation (257). Multifocal neoplasia may be even more common than generally noted. In one series of 133 women with serous ovarian carcinoma, carcinoma *in situ* or early invasive carcinoma of the serially embedded fallopian tube was found in 4. The lesions were often focal, and none was grossly detected (155).

However, it is sometimes difficult to distinguish multiple primary neoplasms that arise in the fallopian tube and ovary or endometrium from endometrial or ovarian carcinoma metastatic to the tubal mucosa. For example, retrograde reflux of aggregates of neoplastic cells into the lumen of the fallopian tube may be observed in the hysterectomy specimen resected for endometrial adenocarcinoma (258). Occasionally, these refluxed tumor cells may implant and grow in the tubal mucosa since tumor types rarely observed primarily in the tube (such as clear cell carcinoma or endometrioid carcinoma) coexist with endometrial carcinomas of these types. Direct spread of carcinoma *in situ* or invasive squamous carcinoma of the cervix along the mucosa of the endometrium and into the fallopian tubes has been occasionally reported (221). This extensive surface growth of malignant cells may reflect either horizontal spread with displacement of glandular epithelium by neoplasm or concurrent squamous metaplasia and neoplastic transformation in the cervix, endometrium, and fallopian tube. In view of the rarity of primary squamous carcinoma of the fallopian tube, the first hypothesis seems much more plausible.

Carcinoma Metastatic to the Fallopian Tube

The most common carcinoma that involves the fallopian tube is metastatic, generally from another site in the female genital tract. Carcinoma of the ovary is particularly likely to spread to the fallopian tube and may be found in up to half of patients with ovarian cancer (199,259). Metastasis to the fallopian tube is reported to occur in 12% of patients with uterine corpus carcinoma and 4% of patients with cervical carcinomas (260). Although the tubal mucosa or muscular wall may be affected, primary involvement of the serosa is typical of ovarian carcinoma. Lymphatic or vascular space involvement is frequently identified in tumors metastatic from the uterus, and the entire wall of the fallopian tube may be permeated by tumor (260). Isolated examples of breast and bladder carcinoma metastatic to the fallopian tube have also been reported (261,262).

Endometrial stromal sarcomas, leiomyosarcomas, and malignant mixed mesodermal tumors that arise in the uterine corpus may invade directly into the adnexa and secondarily involve the fallopian tube. Lymphoma and leukemia also may spread to the fallopian tubes but usually do so as part of widespread organ involvement.

Lesions That Mimic Primary Carcinoma of the Fallopian Tube

The difficulty in distinguishing primary carcinoma of the fallopian tube from metastatic tumor has been addressed. In addition, several conditions, both neoplastic and nonneoplastic, may be confused with fallopian tube carcinoma (263–265).

Salpingitis isthmica nodosa is the term given to a localized diverticulosis of the isthmic portion of the fallopian tube. The gross appearance, when visible, is of a firm, nodular expansion of the isthmus, with a diameter of less than 2 cm. Microscopically, a complex proliferation of branching glandular arrays is seen extending from the lumen to deep within the muscular wall (Fig. 25.26), often associated with hypertrophy of the muscularis. In spite of this architectural abnormality with pseudoinvasion, no cytologic atypia occurs, and the normal epithelial cell types of the fallopian tube mucosa may be readily identified.

Adenomatoid tumors represent benign mesotheliomas, which may occur along the serosa or deep muscularis of the

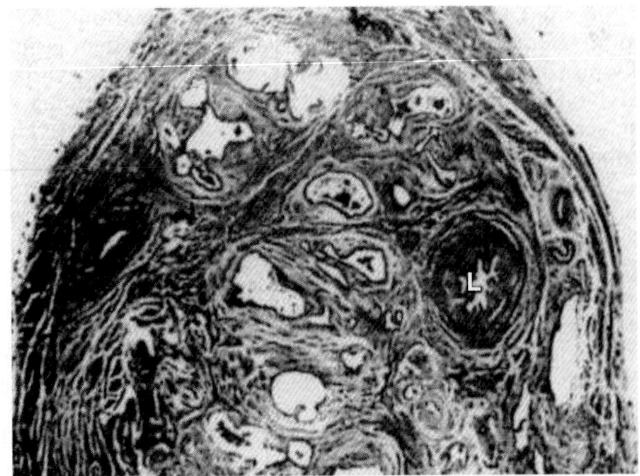

FIGURE 25.26. Salpingitis isthmica nodosa. In this cross section of the fallopian tube, the luminal mucosa (L) appears unremarkable.

TABLE 25.6

SUBCLINICAL METASTASES IN APPARENT EARLY OVARIAN CANCER

Site	No. of patients with involvement	Total patients	% involved
Diaphragm	17	223	7.6
Omentum	21	294	7.1
Cytology	13	69	18.8
Peritoneal	6	61	9.8
Pelvic nodes	18	202	8.9
Aortic nodes	35	285	12.3

Source: Modified with permission from Moore DH. Primary surgical management of early epithelial ovarian carcinoma. In: Rubin SC, Sutton GP, eds. *Ovarian Cancer*. New York: McGraw-Hill; 1993.

fallopian tube (Fig. 25.27). They are usually small (1 to 2 cm in diameter) nodular masses, formed of multiple, spherical, or slit-like channels lined by an attenuated layer of cells. The absence of cytologic atypia or significant mitotic activity permits the distinction from carcinoma. Immunohistochemical and ultrastructural studies provide convincing evidence of mesothelial cell differentiation for these lesions.

Metaplastic papillary tumor of the fallopian tube is a rare, incidental finding in pregnant or postpartum women. Focal, noncircumferential replacement of normal mucosa is accomplished by small papillae covered with large epithelial cells with abundant eosinophilic cytoplasm. Mitotic activity, severe cytologic atypia, and invasion are not seen. The behavior of these lesions is benign (266).

Natural History and Patterns of Spread

Ovarian carcinomas are distinctive by virtue of their propensity to exfoliate malignant cells into the peritoneal cavity. There the cells follow the normal circulation of peritoneal fluid up the right paracolic gutter and to the undersurface of the right hemidiaphragm, where they may implant and grow as surface nodules. The omentum is also a frequent site of involvement, and, indeed, all intraperitoneal surfaces are at risk. Such exfoliation and implantation are one of two primary modes of spread of ovarian cancer. The other is via the retroperitoneal lymphatics that drain the ovary. These follow the ovarian blood supply in the infundibulopelvic ligament to terminate in lymph nodes lying along the aorta and vena cava up to the level of the renal vessels. Lymph channels also pass laterally through the broad ligament and parametrial channels to terminate in the pelvic sidewall lymphatics, including the external iliac, obturator, and hypogastric chains (267). Spread may also occur along the course of the round ligament, resulting in involvement of the inguinal lymphatics. Lymph node metastases are correlated with the stage of disease, and retroperitoneal node involvement has been found in the majority of advanced ovarian cancer cases (268).

The initial spread of ovarian cancer, by both the intraperitoneal and lymphatic routes, is clinically occult. As many as 30% of women with ovarian cancer that grossly appears to be confined to one or both ovaries have widespread disease. The extent of their disease can be detected only by histologic examination of visually normal tissues sampled during careful surgical staging (269). It has been estimated that approximately 10% of patients with apparently localized ovarian cancer that appears to be confined to the ovaries will have metastases to the aortic nodes (269). Many patients with apparently localized disease will also have occult disease in peritoneal washings or in biopsies of the diaphragm and omentum (Table 25.6).

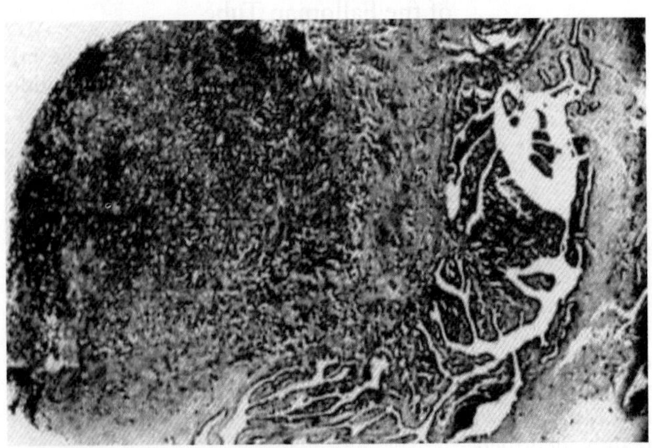

FIGURE 25.27. Adenomatoid tumor. An eccentrically located subserosal mass is present in the fallopian tube.

Fallopian Tube: Patterns of Spread and Prognostic Factors

The spread of fallopian tube carcinoma is identical to that of the ovary, with frequent involvement of the peritoneum, omentum, bowel, and ovaries (192,239,270–272). In some series, half or more of all recurrences presented outside the peritoneal cavity, most often in the liver, lungs, and pleura, as well as in the vagina, kidney, brain, cervix, and skin. Although some investigators have reported that lymphatic spread is uncommon, this finding in part may have reflected a tendency not to perform lymph node dissections (201,239). The principal lymphatic drainage of the fallopian tube appears to be via the para-aortic lymph nodes. Pelvic or para-aortic lymph node involvement has been identified in 10% to 30% of patients at initial operation (253), in about one third of women with recurrent disease (273), and in 75% (9 of 12) of patients at autopsy (253). As previously stated, the presence of capillary or lymphatic space involvement in early tubal carcinoma has been associated with diminished probability of survival at 5 years compared with patients in whom vascular invasion is not identified (29% vs. 83%) (241).

Transcoelomic spread of tumor is an important mode of spread of fallopian tube carcinoma (196). Initially, exfoliation of neoplastic cells from the distal fimbriated end of the tube has been suggested as the mechanism by which this occurred (239). It is difficult to reconcile this theory with the typical gross appearance of a dilated tube with a sealed distal tubal ostium (201). Schiller and Silverberg (201), in a retrospective review of 76 published cases of fallopian tube carcinoma, documented the important relationship between the depth of invasion by tumor and survival. A crude 5-year survival of 91% was found for intramucosal lesions, 53% for tumors with mucosal wall invasion, and 25% or less for cases in which the tumors penetrated the tubal serosa. Using these data, they proposed a staging system for fallopian tube carcinoma based in part on the depth of invasion. Very similar 5-year survival rates by stage were recently reported in a study of 151 patients treated at the Norwegian Radium Hospital (190). In a univariate analysis of survival, the stage, presence of residual disease, ascites, depth of tubal invasion, a hydrosalpinx-like appearance, age, and vascular invasion were all of statistical significance. However, several of these factors, such as depth of invasion and vascular space invasion, are interrelated. When subjected to a multivariate analysis, residual disease, stage, and a hydrosalpinx-like appearance retained strong statistical significance (190). In a subgroup analysis of 41 patients with stage I disease, depth of invasion and intraoperative tumor rupture were independent prognosticators. A study by Peters et al. (274) confirmed the importance of depth of invasion in predicting survival. Thus, the pathologist who examines a fallopian tube that contains carcinoma is recommended to provide information on the depth of invasion, the presence of lymphatic or capillary space involvement, and the degree of histologic differentiation.

DIAGNOSIS AND CLINICAL EVALUATION

Approximately 75% to 85% of patients with epithelial ovarian cancer are diagnosed at the time when their disease has spread throughout the peritoneal cavity. Several organizations, including the Gynecologic Cancer Foundation, the Society of Gynecologic Oncologists, and the American Cancer Society, released a consensus statement on the symptoms of ovarian cancer in June 2007. It urges women to seek medical attention if they have new and persistent symptoms of bloating, pelvic or abdominal pain, difficulty eating, or early satiety, or urinary urgency or frequency. These symptoms were found to be much more likely to occur in women with ovarian cancer than in the general population. Such symptoms are, however, vague and associated with many other conditions. However, they have been reported to be more recent and of greater severity and frequency in women with the disease than in women without (275). Fatigue, indigestion, back pain, pain with intercourse, constipation, and menstrual irregularities were also noted by ovarian cancer patients, but were equally common in the general population. There is, however, no evidence that detection based on these factors will shift diagnosis early enough to affect mortality.

The diagnosis of early-stage ovarian cancer (when the tumor is still confined to the pelvis) usually occurs by palpation of an asymptomatic adnexal mass during a routine pelvic examination. However, the vast majority of palpable adnexal masses are not malignant and, in premenopausal women, ovarian cancer represents less than 5% of adnexal neoplasms. In these women, the ovarian enlargement is usually due to either follicular or corpus luteum cysts. The vast majority of these functional cysts will regress in one to three menstrual cycles and, consequently, the initial approach to management for a palpable adnexal mass less than 8 cm in size in a premenopausal woman is to repeat the pelvic examination and imaging studies in 1 to 2 months.

In contrast, an adnexal mass in a premenarchal or postmenopausal woman, particularly when complex, has a higher likelihood of being a malignant tumor, and surgical exploration is usually indicated.

Ultrasonography is frequently used to aid in the evaluation of adnexal pelvic masses. Features that are more frequently associated with malignancy include irregular borders, multiple echogenic patterns due to the presence of solid elements with prominent papillary projections, dense multiple irregular septa, and bilateral tumors. Other radiographic techniques, including computed tomography (CT) scans and magnetic resonance imaging (MRI), are not routinely necessary for preoperative evaluation of ovarian cancer but may provide useful information. The CT scan may provide additional evidence of the exact size of liver and pulmonary nodules, as well as abdominal and pelvic masses, which can be used to monitor the response of therapy. CT scans are also currently used to evaluate para-aortic and pelvic adenopathy.

Positron emission tomography (PET) utilizes a differential in metabolic activity between benign and malignant cells using the radiopharmaceutical 2-[^{18}F]fluoro-2-deoxy-D-glucose (^{18}FDG). Some studies have suggested that PET/CT imaging is useful in the differential diagnosis of ovarian cancer (276), and it may have a role in detecting residual or recurrent disease (277).

The use of other radiographic studies is dependent upon the results of the initial physical examination and the presence of patient symptoms. Brain scans and bone scans are unnecessary unless suggested by the patient's symptoms; metastases to these sites are extremely uncommon, particularly at the time of diagnosis. Barium studies of the gastrointestinal tract are not routinely indicated in premenopausal women unless there is occult blood in the rectum or symptoms to suggest intestinal obstruction. In postmenopausal women, in whom there is a higher likelihood that colorectal carcinoma is producing symptoms similar to those which can be observed with ovarian cancer, barium enema and proctoscopy may be useful in the differential diagnosis. Because of the association of ovarian cancer with breast cancer and because metastatic breast cancer can produce intra-abdominal carcinomatosis as well, mammography is often performed to exclude the presence of primary breast cancer. A Pap smear should be obtained, although ovarian cancer cells are unlikely to exfoliate through the uterus to the cervix, and their presence is associated with advanced stage.

The preoperative evaluation of patients with suspected ovarian carcinoma should include a determination of the serum CA-125 level. CA-125 has proven to be the most useful, currently available marker for epithelial ovarian cancer, primarily because of its utility in monitoring the results of therapy. CA-125 determinants are glycoproteins, with molecular weights from 220 to >1,000 kD. OC-125 is a murine monoclonal antibody that recognizes the antigenic determinants of CA-125. A double-determinant immunoradiometric assay has been developed against these CA-125 determinants. It has been demonstrated that <1% of normal nonpregnant women have serum CA-125 levels >35 U/mL. In contrast, 80% to 85% of patients with epithelial ovarian cancer have elevated serum levels (278). The serous histologic subset of epithelial ovarian cancer has the highest incidence of elevated CA-125 levels (>85%), whereas mucinous tumors are associated with a low incidence of abnormally elevated serum CA-125 levels.

In postmenopausal women with asymptomatic pelvic masses, an elevated serum CA-125 (>65 U/mL) had a sensitivity of 97% and a specificity of 78% for ovarian cancer (279). In contrast, in premenopausal women, there is a higher prevalence of nonmalignant conditions that can produce elevated serum CA-125 levels (e.g., pregnancy, endometriosis, uterine fibroids, and pelvic inflammatory disease). In postmenopausal women with an adnexal mass, an elevated CA-125 level indicates the need for prompt surgical exploration, whereas in premenopausal women, additional noninvasive studies as described above are indicated.

SCREENING

No reliable procedures are currently available for the early detection of ovarian cancer. Available potential screening techniques have included pelvic examination (ovarian palpation), ultrasound examinations, CA-125 and other tumor markers, and combined modality approaches. Criteria have been established for useful screening tests (280). Besides being accurate, a screening test should be inexpensive, safe, simple, and tolerable. Successful screening should result in a decrease in site-specific morbidity and mortality from a disease. The usefulness of a test can be assessed by measures of sensitivity, specificity, and positive predictive value. The sensitivity refers to the probability of a positive test when the disease is present, whereas the specificity represents the probability that the test will be negative in the absence of the disease and is a measure of the false-positive rate. The positive predictive value represents the number of diagnostic procedures (i.e., laparotomies) performed in women who do not have the disease for each woman who has ovarian cancer. Mathematically: sensitivity = true positives/(true positives false negatives); specificity = true negatives/(true negatives false positives); positive predictive value = true positives/(true positives false positives).

What constitutes an acceptable positive predictive value for ovarian cancer has not been agreed upon, although some investigators feel that 10% is the minimum level (281). The positive predictive value varies with the incidence of the disease and, consequently, will be markedly affected by the population screened (Fig. 25.28). Assuming 100% sensitivity, a test will have to have a specificity of 99.6% and 90.0% for screening all women over 45 years of age and *BRCA1* mutant gene carriers, respectively, to achieve a 10% positive predictive value.

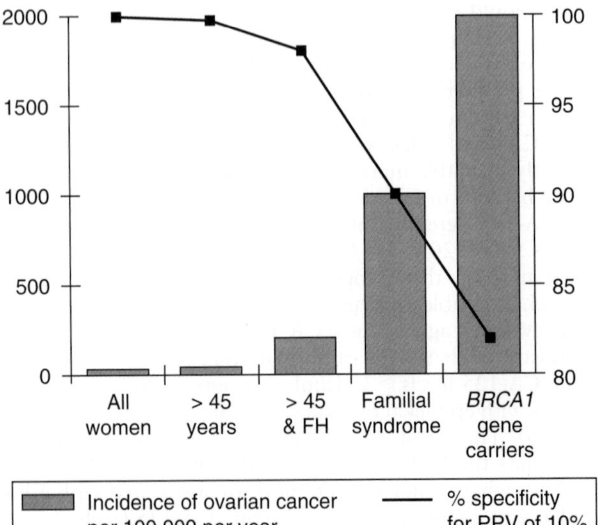

FIGURE 25.28. The incidence of ovarian cancer in various population groups with different risks for ovarian cancer and the specificity required of screening tests to achieve a positive predictive value (PPV) of 10%. *Source:* Jacobs I. Genetic, biochemical, and multimodal approaches to screening for ovarian cancer. *Gynecol Oncol* 1994;S22–S27.

Pelvic Examinations

The detection of an asymptomatic pelvic mass on routine physical examination may identify an ovarian carcinoma before abdominal dissemination, but there are no data on the frequency with which ovarian cancer is detected in asymptomatic women on the basis of an annual pelvic examination. Furthermore, there is no evidence that ovarian cancer detected in asymptomatic women on the basis of an abnormal pelvic examination alters morbidity or mortality. Thus, although frequent pelvic examination continues to be a common recommendation for women past the age of 40 years, its benefit as a screening procedure for ovarian cancer has not been established.

Ultrasonography

Transabdominal ultrasonography is a screening procedure that is easy to perform, has a good patient acceptability, and is essentially free of complications. However, ultrasonography is not sufficiently specific for use as a routine screening procedure. In a prospective study of 5,479 self-referred asymptomatic women undergoing annual transabdominal ultrasonography at King's College Hospital in London (282), five patients with primary ovarian cancer (three with LMP tumors) were identified from a total of 15,977 scans, of which 338 (2.3%) were initially abnormal. Of note, 326 laparotomies were performed to diagnose these five cases. An additional four patients were found to have metastatic ovarian cancer. Although the apparent detection rate was 100%, the false-positive rate was 2.3%, and the specificity was 97.7%. The odds that an abnormal transabdominal ultrasound indicated the presence of primary ovarian cancer were 1 in 67.

Transvaginal sonography has been proposed as a more specific alternative to abdominal sonography as a screening test (283,284) because of increased resolution capable of detecting minimal morphologic changes in the ovary. Transvaginal ultrasonography also does not require any patient preparation. At the University of Kentucky, 3,220 asymptomatic postmenopausal women were so screened (283,284). Surgery was performed in 44 women with ovarian abnormalities, with the following findings: two stage I ovarian cancers (one granulosa cell and one epithelial carcinoma); one stage IIIB ovarian cancer; and 41 benign pathologies, including 21 serous cystadenomas. Thus, the sensitivity was 100%, specificity 98.7%, and positive predictive value 6.7% (i.e., 15 laparotomies were needed to find one ovarian cancer). These investigators have proposed that removal of cystadenomas may also decrease the risk of ovarian cancer since, based upon their histologic review, they feel that such tumors may be precursors of invasive epithelial cancers.

Transvaginal ultrasonography has been combined with Doppler flow studies (285,286) in an effort further to improve the accuracy of sonography and reduce the unacceptably high rate of false-positive results that currently have been reported with ultrasonography alone. Such a procedure detects intraovarian vascular changes, which principally are neovascularization and changes in impedance of blood flow that may help discriminate benign from malignant tumors. Initial results have demonstrated that morphologically normal ovaries show no neovascularization. Similarly, benign masses lacked neovascularization and had a pulsatility index markedly different from invasive ovarian cancers (even early-stage disease), which had clear evidence of neovascularization and marked differences in pulsatility index. Unfortunately, Doppler technology did not improve diagnostic accuracy when the transvaginal sonogram assessed both tumor volume and wall structure (morphology index [MI]) (286). Four hundred forty-two ovarian tumors were assigned a score of 0 to 10 based on increasing volume and morphologic complexity. Doppler flow studies were performed on 371 of these tumors. Only one malignancy was found in 315 tumors with an MI less than 5, whereas there were 52 malignancies in 127 tumors with an MI ≥ 5. The positive predictive value was 0.409. The addition of Doppler flow indices to MI did not improve the accuracy of predicting malignancy.

CA-125 Screening

Approximately one half of women with stage I and stage II ovarian cancer have serum CA-125 levels >65 U/mL (287). In a group of 915 Roman Catholic nuns, when the upper limit of normal for CA-125 was raised to 65 U/mL, only 0.5% of women past the age of 50 years had elevated tests (288). As previously noted, false-positive test results have been reported in a number of nonmalignant gynecologic conditions, such as peritonitis, pancreatitis, renal failure, and alcoholic hepatitis. Owing to the high false-positive rate relative to the low incidence of epithelial ovarian cancer, a single CA-125 assay is not useful in detecting early-stage disease. In a large study from Sweden, serum CA-125 levels were measured annually in 5,550 women over the age of 40 years (289). In women who had CA-125 levels >30 U/mL, surveillance was undertaken with sequential CA-125 levels every 3 months, and pelvic examinations and transabdominal ultrasounds were performed every 6 months. If the CA-125 doubled or was >95 U/mL at the time of screening, or if an adnexal mass was detected by either ultrasound or pelvic examination, the patients underwent a laparotomy. One hundred seventy-five women were found to have elevated CA-125 levels, and six ovarian cancers were detected clinically or sonographically (two stage IA, two stage IIB, and two stage III). Three women with normal CA-125 levels developed ovarian cancer. For women less than 50 years old, a CA-125 value >35 U/mL had a specificity of 97% compared to 99% for women more than 50 years of age. Specificity was increased to 99.8% for both groups if the serum CA-125 level was set at 95 U/mL.

It is hoped that sequential measurements of CA-125 levels over a period of time can lead to substantial improvement of screening programs. The risk of ovarian cancer algorithm (ROCA) calculates the risk of ovarian cancer for an individual comparing each individual serial CA-125 level to the pattern in known cases of ovarian cancer and controls. The result is presented as the individual's estimated risk of having ovarian cancer during the year following the test. Currently, ROCA is being evaluated in a large United Kingdom screening trial as well as in a small pilot study of 2,400 high-risk women in the United States. Preliminary results of the U.S. pilot trial, in which CA-125 was measured every 3 months, suggested that among 2,343 women enrolled between 2001 and 2006, nine cancers were detected. Three were prevalent (found at first screen, one early and two late stage), three had not yet been found by screening and were incidentally found at the time of prophylactic salpingo-oophorectomy, and three were found as a result of screening, two early and one late stage (290). Full publication is awaited, but the early results do not suggest that even intensive CA-125 screening in high-risk women will catch all ovarian cancers at an early stage.

Multimodal Screening

The NCI-sponsored Prostate, Lung, Colorectal, and Ovarian (PLCO) Cancer Screening Trial enrolled over 74,000 women aged 55 to 74 from 1993 through 2000 at ten screening sites throughout the United States. Women were randomly assigned to either the intervention arm, which included baseline measurements of CA-125 levels and transvaginal ultrasonography followed by annual CA-125 readings for 5 years and transvaginal ultrasounds (TVUs) for 3 years, or an observation arm. Baseline screening in the 28,816 women randomized to screening who received at least one test detected 29 neoplasms (26 ovarian, 2 fallopian, and 1 primary peritoneal) (291). Nine were of low malignant potential. Only two of the invasive cancers were stage I; one of these was a granulosa cell tumor. Five hundred seventy surgical procedures, including 325 laparotomies, were performed. The authors calculated the positive predictive value for invasive cancer of an abnormal CA-125 as 3.7%, of an abnormal transvaginal ultrasound as 1.0%, and of having both tests abnormal as 23.5%. However, if only subjects in whom both tests were abnormal had been evaluated, 12 of the 20 invasive cancers would have been missed. Participants will be followed for a minimum of 13 years. A large English study examined a single screening with the sequential continuation of serum CA-125 and ultrasonography in 22,000 volunteers without a family history of ovarian cancer (292). If the serum CA-125 level was ≥ 30 U/mL in the initial determination, women underwent abdominal ultrasonography. If that was abnormal they underwent laparotomy. Forty-one women underwent surgery, and 11 had ovarian cancer: two stage IA, one stage IB, one stage IIA, and seven stage III or IV. Eight of the 21,959 women who had a negative screen developed ovarian cancer. In this study, the positive predictive value was 26.8% for ovarian cancer of all stages (these numbers do not include two women with fallopian tube carcinoma and one with abdominal carcinomatosis of uncertain origin). Seven women who did not have an elevated CA-125 (and one with a CA-125 of 80 who declined abdominal ultrasound) presented with ovarian cancer within the next 22 months. Of these, five had a stage I tumor and three had a stage III tumor.

Based on these results, the same group of investigators performed a pilot randomized trial of screening in 22,000 postmenopausal women aged 45 years or older (293). Women randomized to screening underwent three annual screens that involved measurement of serum CA-125 levels, pelvic ultrasonography if the CA-125 was elevated, and referral to a gynecologist if there was an increased ovarian volume on sonography. In the screened group, there were 468 women with elevated CA-125 levels; 29 were referred for a gynecologic opinion, and cancer was detected in 6 of these women with 23 false-positive screening results. The positive predictive value was 21%. During the 7-year follow-up of this study, an additional 10 women were identified with ovarian cancer in the screened group and 20 in the control group. The median survival for women with cancer in the screened group was 73 months and in the control group was 42 months (p = 0.0112). However, the number of deaths from cancer did not significantly differ between the two groups. These results demonstrate that a multimodality approach to screening is feasible. Based on these results, a large-scale screening trial has begun, termed the United Kingdom Collaborative Trial of Ovarian Cancer Screening (UKCTOCS). This is a randomized trial with a control group undergoing no screening, a multimodal group undergoing annual screening with serum CA-125 as the primary test and ultrasound as a secondary test, and an ultrasound-only group undergoing annual screening with an ultrasound as the primary test and repeat ultrasound in 6 to 8 weeks as a secondary test. An estimated 200,000 women are expected to enroll up until 2010, and ovarian cancer mortality will be assessed 7 years later.

These preliminary studies using serum CA-125 levels, pelvic examinations, and ultrasonography have demonstrated that ovarian cancer can be detected in asymptomatic women. However, these procedures are associated with a significant false-positive rate such that an unacceptably large number of negative laparotomies would result if each "positive" screening test resulted in surgical exploration aimed at diagnosing early ovarian cancer. Since a surgical procedure is required to diagnose ovarian cancer, there is a defined morbidity and mortality associated with screening. When the positive predictive value is below 10%, more harm (complications of unnecessary laparotomy) than good (diagnosing early-stage ovarian cancer) may come to a screened population. Furthermore, in a review of uncontrolled trials of ovarian cancer screening (294) in 36,208 women, 29 cases of ovarian cancer were identified, but only 12 (41%) were stage I. Survival is unlikely to be significantly affected by an earlier diagnosis of advanced-stage disease. Until the completion of the large randomized trials described above, the recommendations of the NIH Consensus Conference against routine screening of the general population remain in effect (62).

Even in women with a positive family history of ovarian cancer, there is no evidence that screening can affect mortality from this disease. In 1,502 asymptomatic women who were screened by transvaginal ultrasonography and who had at least one close relative with ovarian cancer, seven ovarian cancers (three of LMP) were found (295). Screening is also not established to be of value in high-risk women such as those who have two first-degree relatives with ovarian cancer or who are carriers of the *BRCA1* or *BRCA2* gene. The U.K. Familial Ovarian Cancer Screening Study (UKFOCSS) is currently accruing. Despite the lack of evidence for benefit of screening high-risk women, it seems prudent to follow them with pelvic and ultrasound examinations with serum CA-125 determinations on a regular basis until/unless they elect a prophylactic oophorectomy.

SURGICAL STAGING

Our understanding of the early natural history and patterns of spread of epithelial ovarian cancer forms the basis for a rational system for staging the disease and for the surgical management of apparent early ovarian cancer. The widely used FIGO staging system, revised in 1985, is presented in Table 25.7 (296).

The stage, defined as the extent of disease at the time of diagnosis, can be determined only following exploratory laparotomy and thorough evaluation of all areas at risk. Operations on women with a pelvic or adnexal mass that may represent ovarian cancer should generally be carried out through a vertical abdominal incision to allow access to the upper abdomen, which is difficult to visualize through a low transverse incision. On entering the abdomen, aspiration of ascites or peritoneal lavage should be performed to obtain specimens for cytologic examination. Separate specimens should be obtained from the pelvis, right and left paracolic gutters, and the undersurfaces of the right and left hemidiaphragms. An encapsulated adnexal mass should be removed intact, if possible, since rupture and spillage of malignant cells within the peritoneal cavity will increase the patient's stage and may adversely affect her prognosis. Adhesions should be noted and biopsied since they may represent occult areas of microscopic disease. If frozen section indicates the presence of ovarian cancer, a complete abdominal exploration should be carried out, including evaluation of all intestinal surfaces. Any suspicious areas should be biopsied. Omentectomy and random peritoneal biopsies should be performed. Aortic lymph node sampling (Fig. 25.29) should also be performed. Several reports (268,297) have demonstrated that the pelvic lymph nodes are involved by ovarian cancer at the same frequency as are para-aortic nodes and suggest the need for routine pelvic node sampling as well. The technique for surgical staging of apparent early ovarian cancer is summarized in Table 25.8.

Standardized protocols are used to record the specific details of operative and pathologic findings that have prognostic and therapeutic bearing on treatment and natural history. When a rigorous staging laparotomy is performed, a substantial number of patients initially felt to have localized disease will be upstaged. Young et al. (298) reported on ovarian cancer patients believed to have stage I or II disease following initial surgery who underwent repeat staging procedures. Almost a third

TABLE 25.7

CARCINOMA OF THE OVARY: FIGO NOMENCLATURE (RIO DE JANEIRO, 1988)

Stage I	Growth limited to the ovaries
IA	Growth limited to one ovary; no ascites present containing malignant cells. No tumor on the external surface; capsule intact
IB	Growth limited to both ovaries; no ascites present containing malignant cells. No tumor on the external surfaces; capsules intact
IC[a]	Tumor either stage IA or IB, but with tumor on surface of one or both ovaries, or with capsule rupture, or with ascites present containing malignant cells, or with positive peritoneal washings
Stage II	Growth involving one or both ovaries with pelvic extension
IA	Extension and/or metastases to the uterus and/or tubes
IIB	Extension to other pelvic tissues
IIC[a]	Tumor either stage IIA or IIB, but with tumor on surface of one or both ovaries; or with capsule(s) rupture; or with ascites present containing malignant cells or with positive peritoneal washings
Stage III	Tumor involving one or both ovaries with histologically confirmed peritoneal implants outside the pelvis and/or positive retroperitoneal or inguinal nodes. Superficial liver metastases equals stage III. Tumor is limited to the true pelvis, but with histologically proven malignant extension to small bowel or omentum
IIIA	Tumor grossly limited to the true pelvis, with negative nodes, but with histologically confirmed microscopic seeding of abdominal peritoneal surfaces, or histologically proven extension to small bowel or mesentery
IIIB	Tumor of one or both ovaries with histologically confirmed implants, peritoneal metastasis of abdominal peritoneal surfaces, not exceeding 2 cm in diameter; nodes are negative
IIIC	Peritoneal metastasis beyond the pelvis >2 cm in diameter and/or positive retroperitoneal or inguinal nodes
Stage IV	Growth involving one or both ovaries with distant metastases. If pleural effusion is present, there must be positive cytology to allot a case to stage IV. Parenchymal liver metastasis equals stage IV

[a]In order to evaluate the impact on prognosis of the different criteria for allotting cases to stage IC or IIC, it would be of value to know if rupture of the capsule was spontaneous or caused by the surgeon, and if the source of malignant cells detected was peritoneal washings or ascites.

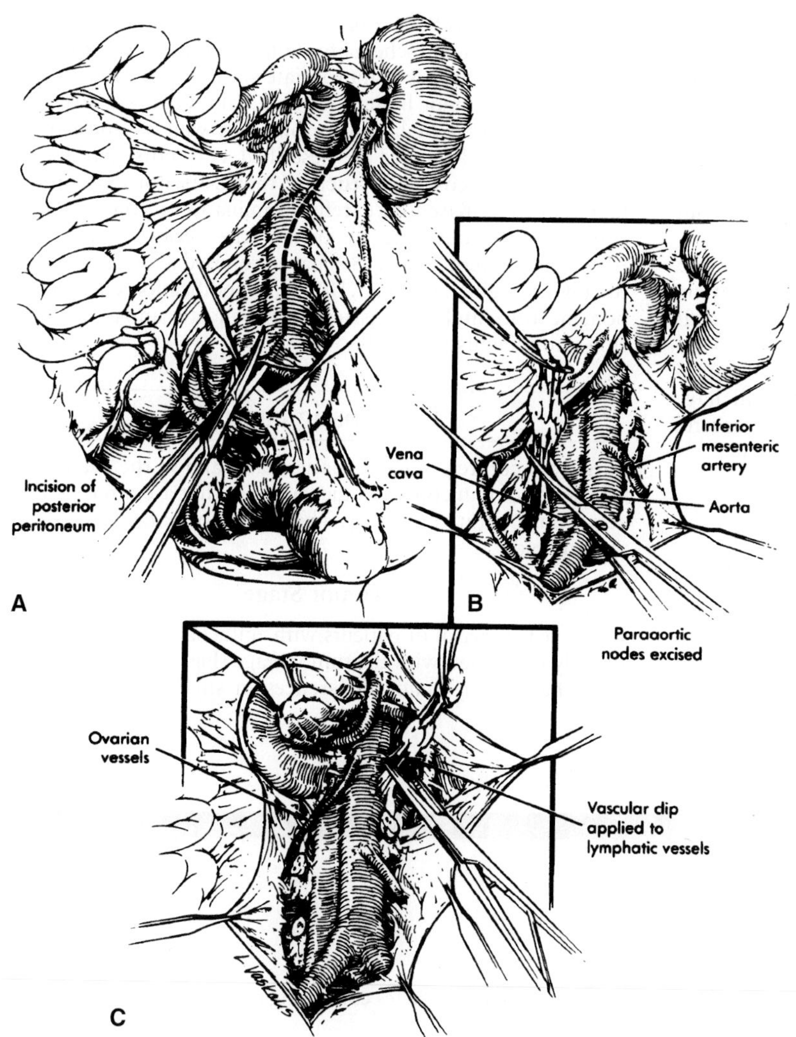

FIGURE 25.29. Para-aortic node dissection for staging of apparent early ovarian cancer.

(31%) of these women were upstaged following the second procedure (Table 25.9), and 77% of the upstaged patients actually had stage III disease. Before referral, only 25% of patients had an initial surgical incision that was adequate for proper staging. Similarly, McGowan et al. (299) examined the completeness of surgical staging in 291 women with ovarian cancer and concluded that 46% had been inadequately evaluated. When staging was performed by gynecologic oncologists, 97% of patients were properly staged as compared to 52% and 35% of cases operated on by obstetricians/gynecologists and general surgeons, respectively. These observations underscore the critical importance of having an experienced physician involved in the surgical staging of all patients with ovarian cancer.

The importance of meticulous staging cannot be overemphasized, since postoperative therapy is based upon anatomic stage,

TABLE 25.8

SURGICAL STAGING OF APPARENT EARLY OVARIAN CANCER

Vertical incision
Multiple cytologic washings
Intact tumor removal
Complete abdominal exploration
Removal of remaining ovaries, uterus, tubes[a]
Omentectomy
Lymph node sampling
Random peritoneal biopsies, including diaphragm

[a]May be preserved in selected patients.

TABLE 25.9

RESULTS OF REPEAT STAGING IN APPARENT STAGE I AND II OVARIAN CANCER

Initial stage	No. of patients	% upstaged
IA	37	16
IB	10	30
IC	2	0
IIA	4	100
IIB	38	39
IIC	9	33
Total	100	31

Source: Reprinted with permission from Young RC, Decker DG, Wharton JT, et al. Staging laparotomy in early ovarian cancer. *JAMA* 1983;250:3072–3076.

as well as other factors, discussed in the section on therapy below. In the past, inadequate surgery often led to understaging and subsequent inadequate postoperative therapy in a significant proportion of ovarian cancer patients. For example, patients were frequently treated with pelvic irradiation at a time when they already had distant, undetected metastases outside the radiation ports. A 1997 report from the NCI's SEER database indicated that only about 10% of American women with apparent early-stage ovarian cancer had received appropriate surgical staging and recommended postoperative therapy (273).

Although ovarian cancer is surgically staged primarily on the basis of the anatomic sites of disease documented at laparotomy, stage IV disease may be documented by cytologically positive pleural fluid or fine-needle aspiration of supraclavicular adenopathy. The majority of patients will have advanced-stage disease (FIGO stages III to IV) after careful staging. The stage distribution is depicted in Table 25.1.

Staging of Fallopian Tube Carcinoma

Because fallopian tube carcinoma has the propensity to spread intra-abdominally, the most widely accepted staging system used in this malignancy is a modification of the FIGO surgical staging of ovarian carcinoma. In 1992, FIGO formally established a staging classification for fallopian tube cancer.

Scully et al. (189,195) have pointed out deficiencies in the current FIGO staging schema for fallopian tube carcinoma. The definition of stage 0 is inappropriate since *in situ* carcinoma is described as a tumor limited to the tubal mucosa—a structure that is composed of lamina propria as well as epithelium. Similarly, stage I tumors are described as tumors that extend into the submucosa—a structure that does not exist in the fallopian tube. Based on careful examination of the histology coupled with outcome in their large series of patients, Alvarado-Cabrero et al. (189) have proposed a modification to the FIGO staging (Table 25.10). This modification corrects the nomenclature and emphasizes the prognostic impact of invasion into the muscular wall.

Prognostic Factors

Surgery accurately stages a patient and allows the evaluation of a series of clinicopathologic variables that are often used to select postoperative therapy. These prognostic factors are discussed below.

Tumor Stage

The 5-year survival of patients with epithelial ovarian cancer is directly correlated with the tumor stage (Fig. 25.30). However, there have been major differences in survival reported for

TABLE 25.10

MODIFIED FIGO STAGING FOR FALLOPIAN TUBE CARCINOMA[a]

Stage	Description
Stage 0:	Carcinoma *in situ* (limited to tubal epithelium[b])
Stage I:	Growth limited to tube
Stage IA:	Growth limited to one tube without extension through or onto serosa, ascites containing malignant cells, or positive peritoneal washings
Stage IA-0[c]:	Growth limited to one tube with no extension into lamina propria[b]
Stage IA-1[c]:	Growth limited to one tube with extension into lamina propria[a] but no extension into muscularis
Stage IA-2[c]:	Growth limited to one tube with extension into muscularis
Stage IB:	Growth limited to both tubes without extension through or onto serosa, ascites containing malignant cells, or positive peritoneal washings
Stage IB-0[c]:	Growth limited to both tubes with no extension into lamina propria[b]
Stage IB-1[c]:	Growth limited to both tubes with extension into lamina propria,[b] but no extension into muscularis
Stage IB-2[c]:	Growth limited to both tubes with extension into muscularis
Stage IC:	Tumor either stage IA or IB but with extension through or onto tubal serosa or with ascites containing malignant cells or with positive peritoneal washings
Stage I(F):	Tumor limited to fimbriated end of tube(s) without invasion of tubal wall
Stage II:	Tumor involving one or both fallopian tubes with pelvic extension
Stage IIA:	Extension and/or metastasis to uterus and/or ovaries
Stage IIB:	Extension to other pelvic tissues
Stage IIC:	Tumor either stage IIA or IIB with ascites containing malignant cells or with positive peritoneal washings
Stage III:	Tumor involving one or both fallopian tubes with peritoneal implants outside pelvis, including superficial liver metastasis, and/or positive retroperitoneal or inguinal nodes. Tumor limited to pelvis except for histologically proven extension to small bowel or omentum
Stage IIIA:	Tumor grossly limited to pelvis with negative nodes but with histologically confirmed microscopic seeding of abdominal peritoneal surfaces
Stage IIIB:	Tumor involving one or both fallopian tubes with grossly visible, histologically confirmed implants of abdominal peritoneal surfaces, none >2 cm in diameter. Lymph nodes are negative
Stage IIIC:	Abdominal implants >2 cm in diameter and/or positive retroperitoneal or inguinal nodes
Stage IV:	Growth involving one or both fallopian tubes with distant metastases including parenchymal liver metastases. If pleural effusion is present, fluid must be positive cytologically for malignant cells

[a]As suggested by Alvarado-Cabrero et al (189).
[b]Modification in terminology.
[c]Modifications to accommodate subsets of tumors that otherwise cannot be assigned a stage or to distinguish among subsets that may differ in their associated prognosis.

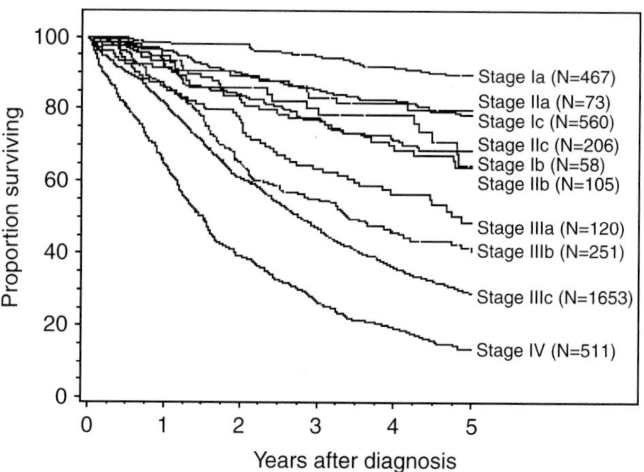

FIGURE 25.30. Carcinoma of the ovary; patients treated in 1996 to 1998. Survival of FIGO stage. *Source:* Heintz AP, Odicino F, Maisonneve P, et al. Carcinoma of the ovary. *Int J Gynecol Obstet* 2003;83:135–166.

patients with the same FIGO stage, reflecting the inadequacy of early staging procedures that led to the frequent understaging of patients. Whereas early studies reported 5-year survivals for patients with stage I disease of approximately 60% to 80%, current studies utilizing a comprehensive staging laparotomy demonstrate that some subsets of patients with stage I disease have a 90% 5-year survival (273). Similarly, initial studies of patients with stage II disease reported the range of 5-year survival from 0% to 40%. However, stage II disease frequently is upstaged to stage III disease, particularly when patients present with large-volume disease in the pelvis. The small number of patients who are found to have stage II disease following completion of a comprehensive laparotomy have a 5-year survival rate of approximately 80%. Patients with stage III disease have 5-year survival of approximately 15% to 20%, whereas patients with stage IV disease have less than a 5% 5-year survival (300).

Volume of Residual Disease

The volume of residual disease following cytoreductive surgery is directly correlated with survival (301–308). Patients who have been optimally cytoreduced have a 22-month improvement in median survival compared to those patients undergoing less than optimum resection. In these retrospective analyses of the importance of residual volume upon survival, the size of the largest residual mass, and not the total number of lesions, has been believed to be the primary factor correlating with prognosis. Yet, the number of residual masses may be an important prognostic factor as well (309,310). Patients who have only a single residual mass following cytoreductive surgery have a significantly greater chance of achieving a surgically confirmed complete remission compared with those patients with multiple small nodules even though each nodule is less than 2 cm in size. Randomized trial data confirming the importance of debulking surgery in the survival of patients with advanced disease, however, is lacking, and such trials are not likely ever to be performed. It is possible that there are underlying biologic features that distinguish those tumors for which optimal cytoreduction is feasible from those for which it is not.

Histologic Subtype and Grade

In general, the histologic type has less prognostic significance than the other clinical factors, such as stage, volume of disease, and histologic grade. But this is confounded by a high correlation between histologic type, stage, and grade. In some series, patients with mucinous adenocarcinomas have an overall better survival in comparison to endometrioid or serous adenocarcinomas. These findings reflect the rarity with which high-grade mucinous adenocarcinoma of the ovary is diagnosed. Few poorly differentiated tumors of advanced stage can clearly be identified as mucinous adenocarcinomas; patients with those tumors so identified have a 5-year survival rate near 0%. Similarly, endometrioid carcinoma also has been suggested to have a better prognosis than serous adenocarcinoma, as well as presenting with a lower histologic grade and clinical stage. Again, poorly differentiated endometrioid carcinomas cannot be differentiated with ease from poorly differentiated serous tumors and are generally classified as serous. Well-differentiated endometrioid carcinomas are, therefore, proportionally more common, which may account for the overall better prognosis for endometrioid than for serous tumors. Some analyses have suggested that ovarian clear cell adenocarcinoma may be more aggressive than the other common epithelial malignancies on a stage-for-stage basis (311). However, as discussed below, not all data support this, and it is possible that clear cell and mucinous tumors are less sensitive to chemotherapy but not faster growing.

The histologic grade of the tumor is a particularly important prognostic factor in patients with early-stage disease. As will be discussed, stage I patients with well- or moderately well-differentiated tumors have a greater than 90% 5-year survival when treated with surgery alone (312). In contrast, patients with stage I disease with poorly differentiated tumors have a significantly worse survival, and postoperative therapy is indicated. In advanced-stage patients treated with cisplatin-based chemotherapy, most studies have failed to demonstrate a significant correlation between histologic grade and survival (301). This may reflect variable degrees of intraobservational and interobservational variation in grading of ovarian tumors (313,314). In addition, different grading systems have been used at different institutions. It should also be recognized that grade 1 advanced-stage tumors are relatively uncommon. Gershenson et al. reported on a group of low-grade stage II-IV serous ovarian carcinomas, noting that they occurred at a younger age (median 43 years) and were associated with prolonged survival, consistent with the hypothesis that they are in a continuum with borderline serous tumors (95).

Surgical Prognostic Factors

Controversy remains about the prognostic importance of other surgical observations (315–317). Tumor size, bilaterality, and ascites without cytologically positive cells are not considered to be of prognostic significance in patients with early-stage disease. However, tumor spillage, capsular penetration, and cytologically malignant ascites (FIGO stage IC) are generally believed to be associated with a worse prognosis.

Prognostic Value of CA-125 Levels

The prognostic significance of preoperative and postoperative CA-125 levels has been established (318). Serum levels of CA-125 generally reflect volume of disease. Whereas prechemotherapy CA-125 levels have been shown on univariate analysis to be of prognostic significance, on multivariate analysis, they are usually not an independent prognostic factor owing to their association with volume of disease (318). In addition, high CA-125 levels may predict for unresectability and an inferior survival. Postoperative CA-125 levels appear to have greater prognostic significance. In a multivariate analysis, postoperative CA-125 levels were of independent prognostic significance in patients with or without residual disease (319).

Controversy also remains regarding the prognostic accuracy of the rate of decline of serum CA-125 levels and the absolute levels after one to three cycles of chemotherapy.

In one study, a level greater than 100 U/mL after the third cycle of treatment was associated with a median survival of 7 months compared to a 50% 5-year survival for patients with a CA-125 level of 10 U/mL or less (320). In another study, there was a marked difference in prognosis for patients who had a greater than sevenfold decrease in CA-125 levels 1 month after chemotherapy compared to those with a lesser reduction (318). In a multicenter study from England, the predictive value of CA-125 levels after the third cycle of chemotherapy was confirmed (320). However, the false-positive rate for accurately predicting progression was 19%. The investigators in this study concluded that, although CA-125 levels are useful for predicting group outcomes, they do not have the predictive power to guide treatment decisions in individual patients. Consequently, although CA-125 levels are frequently drawn before each course of therapy, if the patient shows clinical improvement, treatment should be continued despite the level of CA-125. If there is no change clinically, and if the CA-125 level markedly increases, changing treatment is a consideration. However, if there is no clinical change but the CA-125 is dropping or is not changing, treatment with the same regimen should continue.

An elevated CA-125 has also been increasingly used as an indicator of progression following completion of chemotherapy. Clinical trial groups have established criteria for progression of disease based on elevations of CA-125 levels or the observance of physical or radiographic evidence of disease. The use of serum CA-125 levels to initiate second-line therapy will be discussed subsequently.

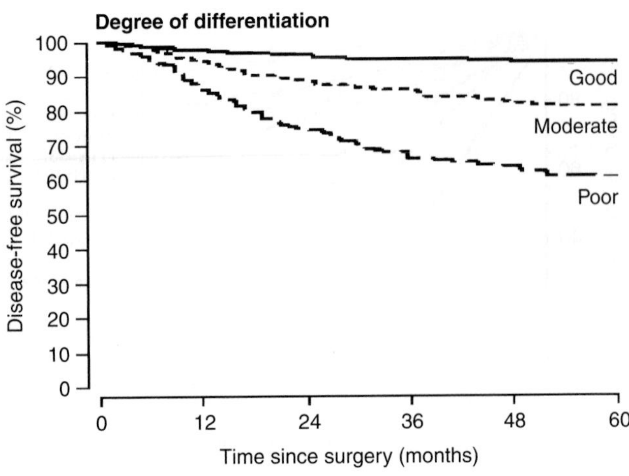

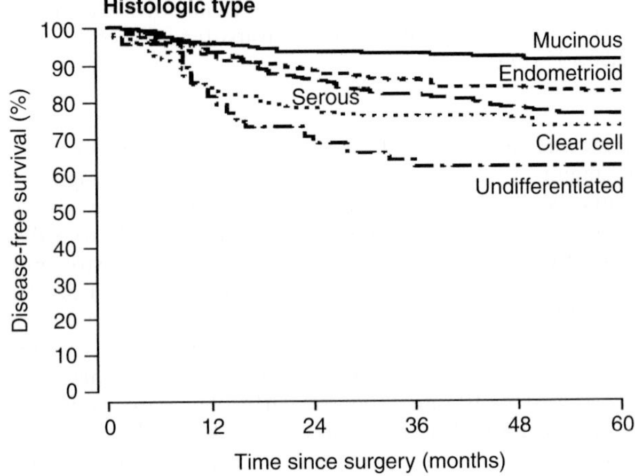

FIGURE 25.31. Actuarial disease-free survival according to prognostic variable. *Source:* Vergote I, De Brabanter J, Fyles A, et al. Prognostic importance of degree of differentiation and cyst rupture in stage I invasive epithelial ovarian carcinoma. *Lancet* 2001;357:176–182.

TREATMENT CONSIDERATIONS

The selection of therapy for patients with epithelial ovarian tumors is based upon anatomic stage and the previously described clinicopathologic features. Therapeutic options may include cytoreductive surgery, chemotherapy, radiation therapy, or a combination of these modalities. However, most patients with advanced ovarian cancer are not cured with these treatments. Clinical trials are evaluating new treatment approaches in virtually all stages of ovarian cancer in an effort to define more effective treatments, and patients should be encouraged to participate in these studies.

Early-Stage Ovarian Cancer

Prognosis in Early-Stage Disease

Survival by FIGO stage in surgically staged patients is shown in Figure 25.30. About one third of patients present with stage I or II epithelial ovarian cancer (Table 25.1). As noted above, both the incidence of and survival rates for early-stage disease vary, particularly in older publications, depending on (a) whether or not patients have been completely staged, and (b) whether borderline tumors (tumors of low malignant potential), which were not recognized as a separate entity by FIGO until 1971 and by the World Health Organization until 1973) are reliably excluded. From 4% to 25% of patients with apparent stage I ovarian cancer will have nodal involvement when lymph nodes are pathologically examined; the risk for lymph node involvement correlates with histology (higher risk with serous and clear cell types) and grade (higher risk with higher grade). The issue regarding borderline tumors is illustrated by a well-known early GOG trial that randomized women with early-stage disease to observation versus melphalan from 1976 to 1986. Although the design of the trial was to exclude borderline tumors, one third of the patients were declared to have tumors of borderline malignancy after central pathologic review (312).

Vergote et al. performed a large retrospective study using an international database of over 1,500 women with stage I invasive epithelial ovarian cancer to identify the most important prognostic variables in patients with stage I disease. Routine para-aortic and pelvic lymphadenectomy were not performed, but palpable nodes were sampled. The overall actuarial 5-year survival was 83% (disease-free survival 80%). As seen in Figure 25.31, women with mucinous tumors did best with a 5-year disease-free survival of 91% versus 82% for endometrioid, 76% for serous, 73% for clear cell, and 62% for undifferentiated histologies (321). However, histologic type was not independently prognostic. Multivariate analysis identified degree of differentiation as the most powerful prognostic indicator of disease-free survival: moderately versus well differentiated (hazard ratio [HR] 3.13), poorly versus well differentiated (HR 8.89). This translates into a 5-year disease-free survival of 94% for grade 1 tumors, 81% for grade 2 tumors, and 61% for grade 3 tumors. The other significant factors were rupture before surgery (HR 2.65); rupture during surgery (HR 1.65); FIGO stage IB versus IA (HR 1.70); and age (HR 1.02 per year). None of the following was of prognostic value when the effects of these additional factors were accounted for: histologic type, dense adhesions, extracapsular growth, ascites, FIGO stage (1988), and site of the tumor. It should be pointed out that ascites was defined as in the FIGO 1973 classification (i.e., ascites in the opinion of the surgeon was pathologic or clearly exceeded normal amounts, or malignant cells were detected on peritoneal cytology).

Although the literature has emphasized the importance of thorough intraoperative exploration (staging) in patients with disease apparently localized to the ovaries, scant recognition has been made of the semantic difficulty presented by the concept of "extension to other pelvic (equals stage II disease) or abdominal (equals stage III disease) organs." No problem exists when the surgeon encounters discrete implants separate from the primary tumor or when solid tumor is found growing into adjacent structures. However, more often, apparently benign adherence of a cyst to adjacent structures, in the absence of metastatic implants or obvious direct tumor extension, is found. There is a considerable body of evidence suggesting that such "benign" adherence, when it is dense, is associated with a relapse risk equivalent to stage II, and that these patients should be considered not as having stage I but rather stage II disease (322). Adherence is considered to be dense when so described by the surgeon, when sharp dissection was required to mobilize the tumor, when a raw area was left in the place of adherence, or when cyst rupture resulted from dissecting the adhesions free. Some clinical trials have advanced the stage of nonmetastatic but densely adherent tumors to stage II (171). However, as noted, the recent large retrospective international study failed to identify dense adhesions as an independent prognostic factor and adhesions are not used by the GOG to "upgrade" apparent stage I patients without histologic confirmation of disease.

The importance of grade is not merely that it predicts occult disease (more patients with presumed stage I grade 3 disease have lymph node involvement than do patients with presumed stage I grade 2 disease). Grade remains an important prognostic factor in surgically staged patients. In surgically staged patients from the FIGO database the overall 5-year survivals are similar to those described above, being 87%, 82%, and 69% for stage I grade 1, 2, and 3 tumors, respectively. For patients with stage II disease, the corresponding survivals were 84%, 67%, and 63% (323). As noted above, histologic grade and type have both been associated with a variable degree of interobserver consistency. One publication from 1984 reported that interobserver agreement was 66% in assigning grade and 66% in assigning histologic type (324).

A recent report analyzing data from 600 surgically staged (including lymphadenectomy) FIGO stage I epithelial ovarian cancer patients proposed that preoperative serum CA-125 was prognostic. The series included patients who did and did not receive chemotherapy. Overall 5-year survival was 88%. The only independent predictors for overall survival were preoperative serum CA-125 ≥30 U/mL (HR 2.7) and age at diagnosis >70 years (HR 2.6). Clear cell and mucinous tumors had somewhat lower preoperative CA-125 levels (325).

Future studies will focus on molecular prognostic markers in early-stage disease, to better determine which tumors have such a good prognosis that no adjuvant therapy is needed, and which will be sensitive to chemotherapy.

Surgical Therapy for Early-Stage Ovarian Carcinoma

The optimal surgical procedure for all epithelial ovarian carcinomas is removal of the uterus along with both fallopian tubes and ovaries. Complete surgical staging, as described above, is also indicated in most circumstances. In the younger patient who wishes to retain her childbearing potential and who appears to have a curable cancer (i.e., a localized tumor with favorable histology), it may be appropriate to preserve the uterus and other ovary if a wedge biopsy of this ovary confirms the absence of disease. However, there is a risk that women undergoing such a procedure may have a higher recurrence rate, and completion of the more standard operation is indicated following childbearing.

Postoperative Observation for Stage I Ovarian Carcinoma

The data sets discussed above include patients treated with a variety of adjuvant therapies. Three prospective observational studies have been published in which patients did not receive further therapy after surgery and borderline tumors were excluded.

Investigators at the Royal Marsden Hospital (326) prospectively observed all patients with stage I disease (not necessarily adequately surgically staged) referred to their institution from 1980 to 1994 following surgery only. Thirty percent of the deaths in the 10 years following diagnosis were from causes other than ovarian cancer. Sixty-one (31%) of 194 patients relapsed at a median of 17 months (range, 6 months to 15.7 years). At a median observation time of 54 months, the 5-year disease-free survival rates were 87%, 65%, and 62% for stage IA, IB, and IC disease and 90%, 85%, and 45% for grade 1, grade 2, and grade 3 tumors. Clear cell histology was not predictive of relapse.

The National Cancer Institute of Canada (NCIC) recruited 82 patients (68 evaluable) with FIGO stage I ovarian carcinoma. Patients were surgically staged; lymph node biopsies were recommended but not required. With a median follow-up time of 4 years, only 3 patients with disease progression were identified (2 had clear cell tumors of a total of 16 with clear cell tumors on study) and 1 patient died of disease. Very few of the patients in this series had grade 3 (n = 3) disease (327).

Finally, a multicenter Dutch trial followed 67 evaluable patients with early-stage well-differentiated ovarian cancer for a median of 50 months. Only 24 patients had complete surgical staging. Five-year disease-free survival for patients with complete surgical staging was 100%; for the remaining patients it was 88% (four recurrences total) (328).

Adjuvant Therapy of Early-Stage Disease

Although the benefits of chemotherapy in advanced-stage ovarian cancer have been well demonstrated, they have been much harder to show in early-stage disease. The number of patients available is smaller and the prognosis better than with more advanced-stage disease, making adequately powered randomized trials difficult to complete. Much of the published literature is old. The thoroughness of staging in the trials has been variable and has raised questions about whether the benefit of chemotherapy is seen only in less well-staged patients, presumably because their risk of recurrence is higher due to a percentage of occult stage IIIC disease. In addition, early-stage epithelial ovarian cancer is composed of a rather different mix of grades and histologies than advanced-stage disease, in particular a much larger percentage of low-grade, mucinous, and clear cell carcinomas and a smaller percentage of serous carcinomas. Nearly 90% of tumors that extend to the pelvic peritoneum, omentum, or beyond are grades 2 and 3. In contrast, 72% of tumors stages I to IIA are grade 1 (329). The FIGO data from 1996 (Table 25.11) report that serous histology accounts for 67% of stage IIIC carcinomas versus only 23% of stage IA carcinomas; mucinous histology accounts for 38% of stage IA carcinomas versus 7% of stage IIIC carcinomas (309). This is of concern because advanced-stage mucinous (330) and clear cell (331) carcinomas of the ovary appear to have a poorer response rate to front-line chemotherapy than serous carcinomas. However, histology has not yet been demonstrated to be of importance in predicting benefit from chemotherapy in early-stage disease.

External Beam Radiotherapy. Early randomized trials of pelvic radiotherapy were small and included patients without surgical staging. However, they suggested that pelvic radiotherapy compared to observation, while reducing the rate of

TABLE 25.11

HISTOLOGY AND STAGE IN OVARIAN CANCER

	IA (n = 550) (%)	IIIC (n = 1,793) (%)
Serous	23	67
Mucinous	38	7
Endometrioid	19	14
Clear cell	10	4
Undifferentiated	3	7
Mixed	6	2

Source: Adapted from Heintz AP, Odicino F, Maisonneuve P, et al. Carcinoma of the ovary. *Int J Gynaecol Obstet* 2003;83(Suppl 1): 135–166.

relapse in the pelvis, had no impact on overall recurrence rate or survival because relapses occurred throughout the peritoneal cavity (332). Interest turned to abdominopelvic radiotherapy (whole abdominal radiotherapy [WAR]) after Dembo from the Princess Margaret Hospital in Canada published results of a study randomizing 147 patients with incompletely staged IB, II, or III optimally debulked ovarian cancer to pelvic radiotherapy plus WAR to pelvic radiotherapy followed by chlorambucil. Among those with less than 2 cm or no residual disease, there was a statistically significant benefit in 10-year overall survivors favoring the WAR group (78% vs. 51% 5-year survival) (333). However, two subsequent small, randomized cooperative group trials of the NCIC and the Danish Ovarian Cancer Group (DACOVA) failed to show superiority of combining pelvic radiotherapy with WAR versus combining pelvic radiotherapy with cyclophosphamide or melphalan (334–336). In addition, investigators at the M. D. Anderson Cancer Center randomized 156 patients with FIGO stage I, II, or III disease to melphalan alone versus abdominopelvic radiotherapy, and found similar relapse-free survival for either treatment in women with stage I or stage II disease (337).

The late effects of WAR include asymptomatic basal pneumonitis or fibrosis detectable in 15% to 20% of patients on radiographic films. This results from the necessity of including 1 to 2 cm of lung field in the radiation portal in order to adequately encompass the leaves of the diaphragms. With upper abdominal doses of 2250 to 2500 cGY in 20 to 22 fractions, about 50% of patients will develop transient elevations of alkaline phosphatase from hepatic irradiation a few months after radiation therapy. Fewer than 1% of patients develop jaundice or ascites (338).

Late gastrointestinal toxicity, particularly obstruction requiring surgical correction, is the complication concerning most investigators. The frequency and severity are dependent on the total dose of radiation, the dose per fraction, and the extent and number of previous operations. There appears to be an increased risk of late complications if lymph node sampling was performed as part of the initial operation. Generally, about 10% to 15% of patients may report some diarrhea or persistent bloating related to particular dietary intolerance, but frank malabsorption is extremely rare. In four studies with almost 1,100 patients in total, 5.6% (range, 1.4% to 14%) of the patients required bowel surgery for late treatment-associated complications of radiation. In these collected series, less than 0.5% (four patients) died as a result of radiation-induced bowel damage.

No large trial has directly compared WAR to platinum-based chemotherapy in women with early-stage ovarian carcinoma; one very small trial showed a trend for superiority of chemotherapy (339). However, given the technical expertise required for and potential long-term bowel toxicity of this type of therapy, the difficulty in combining WAR with chemotherapy, and the fact that a trial in endometrial cancer suggested superiority of chemotherapy over WAR (340), it is not likely that this modality will be studied further in this situation. Given that pelvic radiotherapy can decrease local relapse, it is possible that the addition of pelvic radiotherapy to chemotherapy would improve disease control in some patients, such as those with bulky stage II disease. However, no studies have addressed this issue.

Intraperitoneal Radiocolloid Therapy. Since transcoelomic spread is the main route of dissemination of ovarian cancer, the intraperitoneal (IP) instillation of radiocolloids, which deliver high doses of radiation to the peritoneal surfaces, would seem intuitively attractive. Most trials have used colloids labeled with a radioactive isotope of phosphorus, ^{32}P, which is a pure beta emitter (short penetration electrons). Difficulties include the fact that experimental data show that the radiation dose distribution of the peritoneal surface is quite variable and unpredictable. Penetration of useful doses of radiation does not occur beyond 2 to 3 mm depth, and dose to lymph nodes, retroperitoneum, or nodules larger than 2 mm thick is negligible. When intraperitoneal ^{32}P is given together with pelvic radiotherapy, the risk of bowel toxicity has been reported to be unacceptable.

There have been no randomized trials of ^{32}P against a no-treatment control arm in early-stage ovarian cancer, although a randomized comparison of ^{32}P versus observation did not show any decrease in the risk of relapse or improve survival in patients with more advanced-stage disease who had a surgically confirmed complete remission (341). Nonetheless, a number of early trials randomized women between chemotherapy and intraperitoneal ^{32}P.

Chemotherapy. An early GOG trial (312) randomized 141 women with high-risk early-stage disease (stage IA or IB grade 3, stage IC any grade, or stage II optimally debulked) to ^{32}P versus oral melphalan. With a median follow-up of over 6 years, the 5-year disease-free survival in both groups was 80%; 5-year overall survival was 81% with melphalan and 78% with ^{32}P. Four patients receiving ^{32}P underwent surgery for bowel obstruction; no tumor was identified. Six of the patients assigned to receive ^{32}P did not receive it, in five of the cases because of difficulties with intraperitoneal catheter placement. Technical issues with IP catheter problems were consistent issues in trials of IP ^{32}P, and remain an issue for administration of intraperitoneal therapy today. One of the patients on the melphalan arm developed myelodysplastic syndrome, and one developed acute myelogenous leukemia. Patients with clear cell tumors had worse outcomes in this trial, and it is for this reason that all patients with clear cell tumors, regardless of grade, were included in subsequent GOG trials for high-risk, early-stage disease.

Randomized trials of cisplatin-based chemotherapy in early-stage ovarian cancer are summarized in Table 25.12. While individual trial results vary somewhat, as a group they have shown fairly consistent improvement in disease-free survival for chemotherapy, with the ICON1 trial also demonstrating a benefit in overall survival.

The Norwegian Radium Hospital performed a trial randomizing 347 women with completely resected stages I, II, or III ovarian cancer to either intraperitoneal ^{32}P or six cycles of single-agent cisplatin (50 mg/m^2). There was no significant difference in 5-year actuarial survival rates. However, late bowel complications occurred more often in patients treated with ^{32}P (9% vs. 2%) (342).

A multicenter group in Italy (Gruppo Interregionale Collaborativo in Ginecologia Oncologica; GICOG) randomized 152 women with stage IC ovarian cancer to intraperitoneal ^{32}P

TABLE 25.12

RANDOMIZED TRIALS OF PLATINUM-BASED CHEMOTHERAPY IN EARLY-STAGE OVARIAN CARCINOMA

Author (year)	N	Eligibility	Arms	Outcome
Vergote (1991) (Ref 342)	347	Stage I, II, III without residual disease	^{32}P vs. Cisplatin	No difference in OS or DFS
Chiara (1994) (Ref 339)	70	Stage IA/B Gr 3, Any IC, II	WAR vs. cisplatin/ cyclophosphamide	5-yr OS 53% vs. 71% RFS 50% vs. 74% p = NS Only 67% of patients completed WAR
Bolis (1995) (Ref 343)	83	Stage IA/B Gr 2/3	Observation vs. cisplatin	5-yr DFS 65% vs. 83% 5-yr OS 82% vs. 88%
Bolis (1995) (Ref 343)	152	Stage IC	^{32}P vs. cisplatin	5-yr DFS 65% vs. 85% 5-yr OS 79% vs. 81%
Trope (2000) (Ref 345)	162	Stage I Gr 2/3 or Gr 1 aneuploid/clear cell	Observation vs. carboplatin	5-yr DFS 80% vs. 85% 5-yr OS 70% vs. 71% p = NS
Young (2003) (Ref 344)	251	Stage IA/B Gr 3 or clear cell IC, II	^{32}P vs. cisplatin/ cyclophosphamide	10-yr RFS 65% vs. 72% 10-yr OS: HR chemo 0.83 p = NS
ICON1 (2003) (Ref 346)	477	Physician uncertain about need for chemotherapy	Observation vs. platinum-based chemotherapy	5-yr RFS 62% vs. 73% p = 0.01 5-yr OS 70% vs. 79% p = 0.03
ACTION (2003) (Ref 346)	448	Stage IA/B Gr 2-3 All IC, IIA, and clear cell	Observation vs. platinum-based chemotherapy	5-yr RFS 68% vs. 76% p = 0.02 5-yr OS 78% vs. 85% p = NS
Bell (2006) (Ref 350)	427	Stage IA/B Gr 3 or clear cell All IC, II	Carboplatin/paclitaxel three cycles vs. six cycles	HR RFS 0.761 p = NS 5-yr OS no difference
GOG		Stage IA/B Gr 3 or clear cell, IC, II	Carboplatin/paclitaxel three cycles followed by observation vs. followed by weekly paclitaxel × 26	Pending

Note: DFS, disease free survival; Gr, grade; HR, Hazard Ratio; NS, ; OS, overall survival; RFS, relapse free survival; WAR, whole abdominal radiotherapy.

versus six cycles (50 mg/m^2) of single-agent cisplatin (343). While 5-year disease-free survival was significantly improved with chemotherapy (85% vs. 65%), 5-year overall survival was not significantly different (81% vs. 79%). The risk of dying after relapse appeared to be greater for patients receiving cisplatin: 11 of 12 patients who relapsed after cisplatin had died of their disease at the time of data analysis versus 18 of 26 after ^{32}P.

The GOG performed a trial of intraperitoneal ^{32}P versus three cycles of cisplatin (100 mg/m^2) plus cyclophosphamide (1,000 mg/m^2) in 251 evaluable patients with unfavorable early-stage disease (stage IA or IB grade 3 or clear cell tumors, or stage IC or stage II disease of any grade or histology) (344). The 10-year recurrence rate was 29% lower (72% vs. 65%) and the death rate was 17% lower for patients receiving chemotherapy, but these differences were not statistically significant. However, based on the better progression-free interval with chemotherapy and the technical problems associated with IP therapy (three patients experienced bowel perforation during insertion of the IP catheter) it was felt that chemotherapy should be the future standard for women with high-risk, early-stage disease. Women with clear cell tumors did not fare worse on this trial; even after adjusting for stage (most of the clear cell tumors were stage I), the recurrence rate of clear cell tumors was similar to that of patients with grade 1 tumors.

Several trials have also randomized early-stage patients to chemotherapy versus observation.

A Nordic Cooperative Ovarian Cancer Group (NOCOVA) study randomizing women to no adjuvant therapy versus six cycles of adjuvant carboplatin was closed prematurely because of poor accrual (345). Although the confidence intervals were wide, no difference in disease-free or overall survival between the treatment groups was observed. In another small study, the GICOG, randomized 83 women with stage IA or IB grade 2 or grade 3 disease to observation versus six cycles of cisplatin and observed a significant benefit in disease-free survival but no difference in overall survival (343).

The only clear demonstration of a survival benefit in the treatment of early-stage ovarian cancer comes from two large European trials (the combined ACTION and ICON-1 trials), which together randomized 923 patients with early-stage disease to receive either platinum-based chemotherapy or no initial adjuvant treatment. Results of a preplanned combined analysis

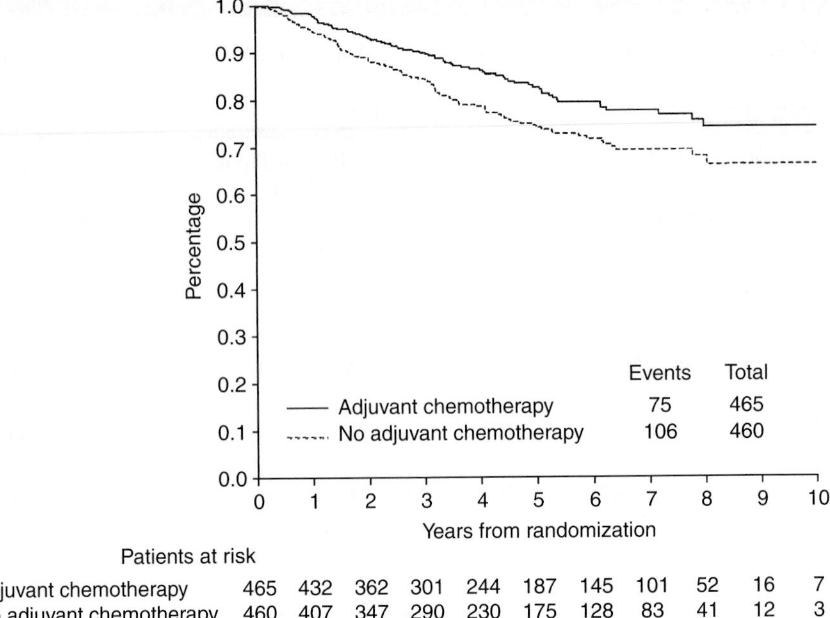

FIGURE 25.32. Kaplan-Meier curves for overall survival in early-stage ovarian cancer patients treated with adjuvant chemotherapy (*solid line*) and no adjuvant chemotherapy (*dotted line*). *Source:* Trimbos JB, Parmar M, Vergote I, et al. International Collaborative Ovarian Neoplasm Trial 1 and Adjuvant Chemotherapy in Ovarian Neoplasm Trial: two parallel randomized phase III trials of adjuvant chemotherapy in patients with early-stage ovarian carcinoma. *J Natl Cancer Inst* 2003;95:105–112.

indicated a statistically significant improvement in both disease-free survival and overall survival with adjuvant platinum-based therapy (Fig. 25.32). Neither tumor grade nor histologic cell type predicted for relative benefit from treatment. However, even these trials have left uncertainty about the benefit of chemotherapy in a woman with comprehensively staged early-stage disease. In the one third of patients on the ACTION trial with optimal surgical staging there was no benefit to treatment. However, this was a retrospective subset analysis, and this subset of patients was not large enough for the result to reach statistical significance (346–348).

The discrepancy between the benefits in disease-free survival and benefits in overall survival seen in several of the randomized chemotherapy trials has been suggested to result from increased salvage rates for chemotherapy in patients who recur after observation or intraperitoneal ^{32}P. In a GICOG trial randomizing women to chemotherapy versus no adjuvant therapy, 1 of 7 women who relapsed after adjuvant chemotherapy was alive at the time of reporting, whereas 6 of 14 who relapsed after observation were still alive (343). Investigators at the Royal Marsden Hospital examined the salvage rate after relapse in their series of prospective observation for patients with stage I disease (326). Sixty-one (31%) of 194 patients relapsed at a median of 17 months (range, 6 months to 15.7 years), and 55 of these received platinum-based chemotherapy at the time of relapse. Progression-free survival at 5 years after relapse was 24%. Interestingly, although clear cell histology was not predictive of relapse, it was a poor prognostic factor for survival after relapse (349).

Duration of Chemotherapy for Early-Stage Disease. The GOG randomized 427 eligible patients with unfavorable early-stage disease to receive either three or six cycles of carboplatin (Area under the curve [AUC] 7.5)/paclitaxel (175 mg/m^2) chemotherapy. Overall 5-year survival was 84% for stage I disease and 73% for stage II disease, and did not differ by treatment regimen (HR 1.02; 95% CI, 0.662 to 1.57; p = 0.94). Adjusting for initial FIGO stage and tumor grade, the recurrence rate was 25% lower for patients getting six cycles (relative hazard 0.761, 95% CI, 0.512 to 1.13; p = 0.18). The statistics of the study were designed to capture only very large differences in recurrence; there was an 85% chance of identifying a treatment regimen as active if it reduced the recurrence rate by 50%. Although surgical staging was required, 126 patients did not have a documented complete staging procedure. The estimated recurrence benefit of six cycles of chemotherapy among patients having a complete staging procedure was slightly less (HR 0.796 vs. 0.660 for those not completely staged), but there was no significant evidence of heterogeneity in the treatment effect. Toxicity was increased with six cycles of chemotherapy; in particular grade 3 or 4 neurotoxicity was seen in 11% of patients versus only 2% on the three-cycle arm (350). Based on the lack of survival benefit and the increased toxicity with six cycles of chemotherapy, the GOG conducted a subsequent trial in the same patient population randomizing women to either three cycles of carboplatin (AUC 6)/paclitaxel (175 mg/m^2) or three cycles of the same regimen followed by weekly paclitaxel 40 mg/m^2 for 24 weeks. Results of this study are pending.

At this time it is recommended that patients with comprehensively staged stage IA or IB grade 1 epithelial ovarian cancer receive no postoperative chemotherapy. Patients with grade 3 or stage IC disease have a relapse risk of at least 20%, and this can be reduced with platinum-based chemotherapy. Paclitaxel/carboplatin for three to six cycles is the usual treatment in the United States. It is hoped that future data will better address which women with early-stage ovarian cancers actually derive benefit from therapy.

Early-Stage Fallopian Tube Carcinomas

Unlike ovarian carcinoma, in which two thirds of patients present with advanced-stage disease, about half of patients with fallopian tube carcinoma are diagnosed in stage I or II (351). A review of eight series published over the past decade confirms the preponderance of early-stage disease in fallopian tube carcinoma (192,196,198,200,254). Of 558 patients, 33% were stage I, 33% were stage II, and 34% were stage III or IV. Prognosis of early-stage disease has been reported to be dependent on depth of invasion of the tumor into the fallopian tube (201). Some older series described high recurrence rates in early-stage disease, in particular one series in the radiation oncology literature which reported local recurrence rates of 35% and 70% in untreated stage I and stage II disease (196). However, most recent data have suggested that the survival for women with fallopian tube cancer is similar or superior to that of women with ovarian cancer when standardized for stage (351–353). No meaningfully sized series to inform about benefits of treatment exist. Radiotherapy including whole abdominal irradiation, intraperitoneal ^{32}P, and pelvic/para-arotic nodal radiotherapy has been used. As advanced-stage fallopian tube carcinomas appear to respond to platinum-based therapies in a manner similar to that of ovarian carcinomas, adjuvant chemotherapy is currently used for early-stage fallopian tumor in most situations.

Management of Borderline Tumors

Borderline (low malignant potential; LMP) tumors comprise 10% to 20% of ovarian malignancies, and most are of serous or mucinous histology. Their histology is discussed in detail above in the section on pathology. Serous borderline tumors are more common than mucinous borderline tumors in the United States, but mucinous borderline tumors are more common in Japan (354). Numerous large series attest to their good prognosis (97,355,356). Unlike invasive epithelial ovarian cancer, approximately 75% to 80% of borderline tumors are diagnosed in early stages. Even when they present with more advanced-stage disease, they progress very slowly. A review of borderline tumors entered into the NCI SEER database between 1988 and 1997 (when SEER stopped collecting data on ovarian borderline tumors) showed 10-year relative survivals of 99% for stage I, 98% for stage II, 96% for stage III, and 77% for stage IV disease (357). Given the good prognosis, no postoperative treatment is indicated for early-stage borderline tumors. Borderline tumors are particularly likely to affect young women (Fig. 25.2), in whom therapeutic decisions regarding fertility-sparing, premature hormonal deprivation, and adjuvant chemotherapeutic treatments are particularly pertinent.

Surgery is the cornerstone of treatment for early-stage borderline ovarian tumors of LMP. It is important to note that the same principles of surgical staging detailed earlier in this chapter with regard to invasive cancers apply equally to borderline tumors. Since many women with borderline tumors are in the childbearing years, the efficacy and safety of conservative surgery have been important. There is no evidence that a conservative surgical approach has an adverse effect on survival in patients with stage I borderline tumors of borderline (358). Even though patients treated with a unilateral oophorectomy have a higher recurrence rate than patients treated with a total hysterectomy and bilateral oophorectomy, effective surgery for recurrent disease leads to equivalent survival. Whether even more conservative surgery (e.g., cystectomy) has an adverse impact on survival remains a subject of debate. Although cystectomy may increase the recurrence rate, it may not have an adverse effect on survival. However, in order to avoid recurrences and still maintain fertility, there appears to be little, if any, disadvantage to performing a unilateral oophorectomy. In patients who present with stage II borderline tumors, a total abdominal hysterectomy and bilateral salpingo-oophorectomy with appropriate staging of the peritoneal cavity is recommended.

Chemotherapy is not indicated for stage I or II borderline tumors.

Serous Borderline Tumors

Approximately 5% to 10% of early-stage serous borderline tumors will ultimately recur. Recurrences can present 10 to 15 years after the initial diagnosis, making long-term follow-up necessary (and raising the question as to whether the relapses represent new primary disease). In one report of 160 stage I serous borderline tumors, 11 patients developed recurrent tumor at a median of 16 years after initial surgery (range, 7 to 39 years), and 8 died of the disease (359). It has been proposed that the majority of recurrences among serous borderline tumors are attributable to the subset with micropapillary histology, and that these have a higher frequency of invasive implants (103). This emphasizes the need for careful surgery in this subset of tumors. This is to be distinguished from the rare group of borderline tumors that exhibit stromal microinvasion; focal microinvasion (less than 3 to 5 mm) does not appear to have prognostic importance (360), and this subset can be managed in the same way as typical borderline tumors.

The optimal adjuvant treatment of more advanced-stage recurrent disease is unknown. The very long natural history of borderline tumors makes prospective clinical trials difficult. Tumors with invasive implants (the minority) have a worse prognosis than those with noninvasive implants, but longer follow-up will reveal more recurrences in patients with more indolent disease. Seidman and Kurman reported on a review of 97 reports including 4,129 patients and noted that after 7.4 years of follow-up, the survival of patients with noninvasive peritoneal implants was 95.3% as compared with 66% for those with invasive implants. Lymph node involvement did not appear to portend a particularly dire prognosis, and was associated with a 98% survival rate at 6.5 years (97).

The M. D. Anderson group retrospectively identified 39 patients with ovarian serous borderline tumors with invasive implants. At a median follow-up of 111 months, 12 (31%) had progressed or recurred with median time from diagnosis to recurrence of only 24 months (361). They also reviewed 80 cases of stage II-IV ovarian serous borderline tumors with noninvasive implants (362). Fifty received postoperative chemotherapy. Thirty-five (44%) developed recurrences, 10% within 5 years, 19% between 5 and 10 years, 10% between 10 and 15 years, and 5% more than 15 years after primary resection. The only statistically significant feature associated with recurrence was the presence of a micropapillary/cribriform pattern, although this pattern was present in only 26% of the cases that recurred.

Although their very slow growth would seem to predispose them to resistance to traditional cytotoxic agents, serous borderline tumors are not completely chemotherapy resistant. Gershenson et al. reported on a series of patients with metastatic serous borderline ovarian tumors who had macroscopic residual disease after initial surgery, received chemotherapy, and subsequently underwent second-look laparotomy. Three of 20 (15%) patients with noninvasive implants (363) and 4 of 7 (57%) patients with invasive peritoneal implants had a response to chemotherapy (361). Barakat et al. summarized several series in which second-look surgery was peformed to document response to initial platinum-based therapy and found that 6 of 23 patients (26%) with macroscopic residual disease had complete responses (364). However, the effect of treatment on survival is very uncertain. Surgery is often used as sole primary treatment for women with serous borderline tumor of the ovary with noninvasive implants, for whom 5-year survivals are 94% to 95% (365), and chemotherapy is often used in women with invasive implants. Aneuploidy has also been reported to predict for poor survival but appears to be related to the presence of invasive implants (366). However, there is no clear evidence that chemotherapy can decrease relapse rates or improve survival in any subset of patients.

Recurrences of serous borderline tumors may be histologically similar to the original tumor or can be invasive tumors, usually of low grade. In the M. D. Anderson series of borderline tumors with noninvasive implants described above, 2 of the 35 recurrences were not histologically examined. Six were recurrent borderline tumors, and the patients with these recurrences were all alive without evidence of disease 7 to 14 years after surgery. Twenty-seven patients had low-grade serous carcinomas at the time of recurrence, and 20 of these died of disease between 3 and 25 years after surgery (362). Crispens et al. reported that of 49 patients with recurrent borderline serous tumors, 73% of the recurrences were low-grade carcinomas, and that optimal cytoreduction in this group was associated with improved survival. Thirty-six percent of women with progressive or recurrent serous borderline tumors died of their disease. Six complete responses and four partial responses in 45 evaluable patients (22% response rate) were reported with use of a platinum/taxane-based regimen. One patient had a partial response to leuprolide, and one had a partial response to pelvic irradiation. Given the fact that women may live a very long time with advanced-stage borderline tumors, even those recurring as low-grade invasive serous carcinomas, use of chemotherapy should be judicious, and use of agents such as oral etoposide with a propensity to cause leukemia should be avoided. Over 90% of serous borderline ovarian tumors are estrogen-receptor positive (367), and there are case reports of major responses to tamoxifen (367), leuprolide (368), and anastrozole (369). The effect of antiangiogenic or other newer targeted agents on these tumors is not known. There is a high frequency of *BRAF* mutations in borderline serous tumors (370), and agents directed against this or other genetic alterations may be of interest.

Mucinous Borderline Tumors

The pathology and classification of mucinous borderline tumors are covered earlier in this chapter. Most mucinous borderline ovarian tumors are stage I and present as large unilateral ovarian masses; bilaterality suggests the possibility of metastatic tumor from another site. Appendectomy and evaluation of the GI tract should be performed to rule out a primary gastrointestinal tumor. Mucinous tumors need to be sampled thoroughly to avoid missing an area of invasion. However, as with serous borderline tumors, microinvasion is not thought to have prognostic significance. Risk of recurrence for stage I mucinous borderline tumors of either the more typical intestinal type or the less common endocervical type is very low, with metastatic rates of 0% to 7%. For many years pseudomyxoma peritonei was thought to result from ovarian borderline tumors, but pathologists now believe that most ovarian tumors associated with pseudomyxoma peritonei are metastatic from primary neoplasms of the appendix (153). High-stage pure borderline mucinous tumors are exceedingly uncommon.

Advanced Epithelial Ovarian Cancer

Cytoreductive Surgery

Despite decades of effort aimed at improving methods of early detection and diagnosis, the majority of cases of cancer of the ovary are not diagnosed until the disease has spread beyond the ovary. Often, patients with advanced disease will present with an abdomen distended with ascites and obviously bulky tumor masses in the pelvis and upper abdomen. For most human solid tumors, aggressive surgical resection is justified only if all known tumor can be removed, rendering the operation potentially curative. For epithelial cancer of the ovary, however, there is substantial theoretical and clinical support for the concept that debulking, or cytoreduction, of large tumor masses can be beneficial to the patient even in the absence of complete tumor removal. Griffiths (371) has reviewed the theoretical basis for cytoreductive surgery. Removal of bulky tumor masses in a patient with advanced ovarian cancer may improve the patient's comfort, reduce the adverse metabolic consequences of the tumor, and enhance the patient's ability to maintain her nutritional status. Such effects are likely to increase her ability to tolerate the intensive chemotherapy that is required. Perhaps, more importantly, removal of large tumor masses may enhance the response of the remaining tumor to chemotherapy. Large tumor masses with a relatively poor blood supply may provide a pharmacologic sanctuary where viable tumor cells can escape exposure to adequate concentrations of cytotoxic drugs. Additionally, such poorly vascularized masses may have a low growth fraction (i.e., a larger proportion of cells in the nonproliferating [G_0] phase of the cell cycle) when they are relatively insensitive to the effects of cytotoxic drugs.

In 1968, Munnell (372), who introduced a concept of the "maximum surgical effort" for ovarian cancer, reported an improved survival in patients who had a "definitive operation" compared to "partial removal" or "biopsy only." In 1969, Delclos and Quinlan (373) reported 25% versus 9% survival in stage III ovarian cancer patients when disease was cytoreduced surgically to "nonpalpable" versus "palpable." Griffiths (371) was the first to accurately quantify residual disease following primary surgery and to correlate this with survival in a group of 102 patients receiving chemotherapy (single-agent melphalan) for stage II or III ovarian cancer. Using a multiple linear regression model, he found that survival duration was significantly related to residual tumor size, and he reported a median survival of 39 months for patients with no residual tumor compared to 12.7 months for patients with residual tumor >1.45 cm in maximum diameter. He also noted an important limitation of cytoreductive surgery: Extensive resection of tumor bulk with failure to remove all masses >1.5 cm in diameter did not influence survival.

In 1978, Young et al. (374) reported the first randomized trial of multiagent nonplatinum chemotherapy versus single-agent alkylating therapy of advanced ovarian cancer, showing that patients reduced to "optimal disease" were more likely to achieve a complete clinical response, as well as a pathologic complete response. Other investigators utilizing platinum-based regimens have also supported the role of primary cytoreductive surgery. Omura et al. (375), reporting a GOG study comparing two cisplatin-based regimens, found a statistically significant difference in progression-free interval, survival, and proportion of patients achieving negative second-look laparotomy in those with no gross residual disease compared to those with gross residual ≤1 cm. In clinical trials in which the percentage of patients who were optimally cytoreduced was reported, the median survival for optimally cytoreduced patients was 39 months as compared to 17 months for those not optimally cytoreduced. In addition, Fuks et al. (375a) and Dembo (332) have reported beneficial effects of primary cytoreduction when radiation is used following surgery.

More recently, several investigators have published results supporting the role of primary cytoreduction. Hoskins et al. (376), analyzing GOG data, reported on the effect of residual disease size on survival after primary cytoreductive surgery. The patient population studied was relatively homogeneous because it included only patients with suboptimal residual disease according to the GOG definition (>1 cm). This removes an important source of bias present in most prior studies since patients found to have only small-volume disease (or debulked to very small-volume disease) are excluded. Among their study group of 294 patients, they noted a statistically significant improvement in survival in patients who had 1- to 2-cm residual disease as compared to those with >2-cm residual disease ($p < 0.01$). These data, when combined with data from GOG protocol 52, in which patients with stage III or IV disease had optimal (<1 cm) residual disease, provide a striking example of the prognostic importance of the extent of residual disease (Fig. 25.33) (376). Eisenkop et al. (377), in a small study, found a survival benefit to the complete elimination of all visual peritoneal implants using such modalities as CO_2 laser, argon-beam coagulator, and the cavitron ultrasonic surgical aspirator. Retrospective reports confirm that aggressive primary

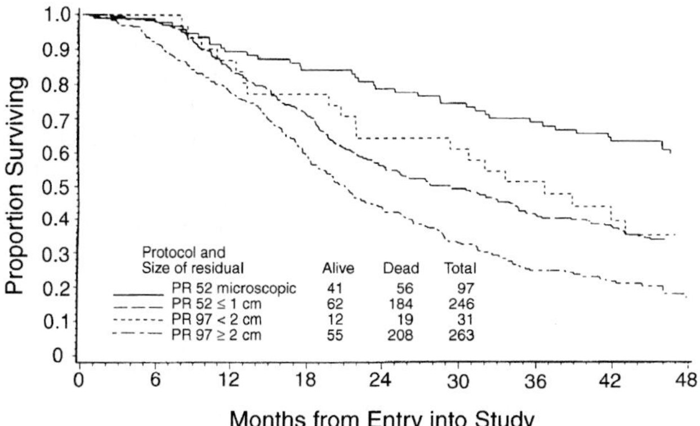

FIGURE 25.33. Survival time by initial abdominal tumor description (except omentum). *Source:* Hoskins WJ, McGuire WP, Brady MF, et al. The effect of diameter of largest residual disease on survival after primary cytoreductive surgery in patients with suboptimal residual epithelial ovarian carcinoma. *Am J Obstet Gynecol* 1994;170:974–980.

(and secondary) cytoreductive operations are associated with minimal morbidity and mortality when performed by experienced surgeons (378). The National Institutes of Health Consensus Development Conference on Ovarian Cancer held in April 1994 concluded that "aggressive attempts at cytoreductive surgery as the primary management of ovarian cancer will improve the patient's opportunity for long-term survival" (Final Statement, NIH Consensus Development Conference on Ovarian Cancer, Bethesda, 1994) (62).

None of the above reports represents randomized clinical trial data, and it is not likely ever to be feasible to conduct a randomized trial testing the value of aggressive debulking surgery. It has been suggested that patients who present with small-volume disease that is optimally cytoreduced following hysterectomy with bilateral salpingo-oophorectomy and omentectomy have disease that is biologically less aggressive than do patients who are anatomically cytoreduced to the same amount of residual disease but require a maximal tumor reduction with removal of bulky disease throughout the peritoneal cavity. For example, in a study from Roswell Park Cancer Institute, it was demonstrated that cytoreductive surgery was successful in debulking 87% of patients with stages III and IV disease to less than 2-cm residual tumor masses (379). The percentage of patients in this study who were optimally cytoreduced was markedly higher than the 17% to 40% successful debulking rate reported in many other series. However, only 30% of patients in this study achieved a complete remission with chemotherapy even though only 13% of the patients had any residual mass greater than 2 cm after debulking surgery. Furthermore, progression-free survival was only 29% at 3 years. These results suggest that, in addition to the volume of disease, other unknown biologic factors influence survival in patients with advanced disease.

The current FIGO staging system subdivides stage III disease into three groups, based upon the volume of disease before any attempt at surgical debulking (Table 25.7).

Stage IV ovarian cancer patients present special considerations with regard to cytoreduction. Most of the studies supporting cytoreductive surgery have included both stage III and stage IV patients but have not analyzed them separately. Four retrospective studies that have examined the prognostic significance of optimal debulking in stage IV ovarian cancer have all shown a statistically significant improvement in survival in patients with small-volume residual tumor (Table 25.13) (380–383). Based on these data, it seems reasonable to attempt cytoreduction in medically fit patients with stage IV disease if optimal residual disease is achievable.

The actual percentage of patients with advanced ovarian cancer who can successfully be cytoreduced remains to be established. The percentage of patients optimally cytoreduced has ranged from 87% to 17% in different studies in the literature, with a mean of 35%. This wide range is due to several factors in addition to the skill and experience of the surgeon. There has not been universal agreement as to the size of residual masses that place the patient in the "optimal" category. Furthermore, the patient populations may not be comparable with regard to volume of disease at surgery or are not controlled for surgery prior to referral to the investigator.

Preoperative Chemotherapy/Interval Cytoreduction

Since many patients cannot be successfully cytoreduced at initial surgery, the benefit of a brief induction course of chemotherapy prior to debulking surgery has been explored. Two to three cycles of chemotherapy substantially increase the percentage of patients who will be successfully cytoreduced. Several studies (384,385) have provided retrospective comparisons of advanced-stage patients treated with neoadjuvant chemotherapy compared to patients treated with surgery followed by chemotherapy. All have demonstrated the feasibility of neoadjuvant chemotherapy. Everett et al. (386) reported on a retrospective series of 98 patients with initial chemotherapy and 102 with initial surgery. Patients who received initial chemotherapy were more likely to have stage IV and grade 3 disease. Interestingly, there was no difference in surgical morbidity between the groups (as a neoadjuvant approach would generally seem attractive for patients who are ill enough that aggressive primary surgery is risky). Optimal cytoreduction was achieved in 86% of patients who received initial chemotherapy versus 54% of patients who received initial surgery. Optimal cytoreduction but not treatment choice was statistically associated with median survival. However, initial surgery was associated with a

TABLE 25.13

EFFECT OF DEBULKING ON SURVIVAL IN STAGE IV OVARIAN CANCER

Study (ref.)	Year	Surgical result	No. of patients	Optimal (%)	Median survival (months)	p
Curtin et al. (381)	1997	Optimal (<2 cm)	41	45	40	0.01
		Suboptimal	51		18	
Liu et al. (382)	1997	Optimal (<2 cm)	14	30	37	0.02
		Suboptimal	33		17	
Munkarah et al. (383)	1997	Optimal (<2 cm)	31	34	25	0.02
		Suboptimal	61		15	
Bristow et al. (380)	1998	Optimal (1 cm)	25	30	38	0.0004
		Suboptimal	59		10	

longer progression-free interval. There are currently two randomized trials under way of neoadjuvant chemotherapy versus surgical debulking followed by chemotherapy (EORTC-55971, UK CHORUS). Results will be very interesting.

There is conflicting evidence from two large prospective, randomized trials whether interval debulking can improve survival in certain patients with advanced ovarian cancer (387,388). In a multicenter trial conducted by the EORTC (388), patients with suboptimal (>1 cm) disease remaining after primary cytoreduction were treated with three cycles of cyclophosphamide and cisplatin. Those without progression were randomized to interval debulking surgery and additional chemotherapy versus additional chemotherapy alone. With approximately 150 patients randomized to each arm, patients undergoing the interval debulking showed a statistically significant improvement in both progression-free interval and median survival (Fig. 25.34A). The interval surgery was generally well tolerated.

More recently, the GOG has reported the results of protocol 152, a prospective, randomized trial of interval secondary cytoreduction in patients with advanced ovarian cancer with suboptimal residual disease (387). Five hundred fifty patients were enrolled in this study within 6 weeks of initial surgery. After three cycles of paclitaxel and cisplatin, patients without evidence of tumor progression were randomized to receive either secondary cytoreduction and three additional cycles of chemotherapy or chemotherapy alone. At the time of the report, median progression-free survival and overall survival for the interval cytoreduction group were 10.5 months and 33.9 months, respectively, compared to 10.7 months and 33.7 months for the chemotherapy-alone group. The overall survival for the two groups is shown in Figure 25.34B.

Several possibilities have been advanced to explain the difference in outcome between the GOG and European studies, both large prospective, randomized trials. Probably most important of these is the difference in the training and experience of the surgeons involved. In the GOG trials, both the initial and interval cytoreductive operations were performed almost exclusively by trained gynecologic oncologists, whereas in the EORTC trial the initial surgery was most often done by general gynecologists. As a result, residual disease following primary surgery measured <5 cm in about two thirds of the GOG patients as compared to one third of the patients in the EORTC trial. Following chemotherapy, residual disease >1 cm was found in 56% of the GOG patients versus 65% of the European patients. This resulted in a higher likelihood of successful cytoreduction in the EORTC trial, with conversion from suboptimal to optimal residual tumor in 45% of patients as compared to 36% in the GOG trial.

Additionally, the chemotherapeutic regimen used in the GOG trial, paclitaxel and platinum, may have reduced the benefit of interval cytoreduction relative to the EORTC trial, which used a platinum and cyclophosphamide combination. Differences in outcome may also be related to differing post-treatment surveillance and to the availability of more effective second-line therapies since the EORTC trial completed accrual in May 1993. It is of interest to note that the similar median and overall survivals in both arms of the GOG trial were substantially longer than those reported in the best (interval cytoreduction) arm of the EORTC trial.

The available evidence from the prospective trials of interval cytoreduction suggests that, although this technique should not be a routine management strategy, certain selected patients may benefit depending on the aggressiveness of the initial cytoreductive surgery, the geographic distribution and size of the remaining disease, and the response to the initial several cycles of chemotherapy.

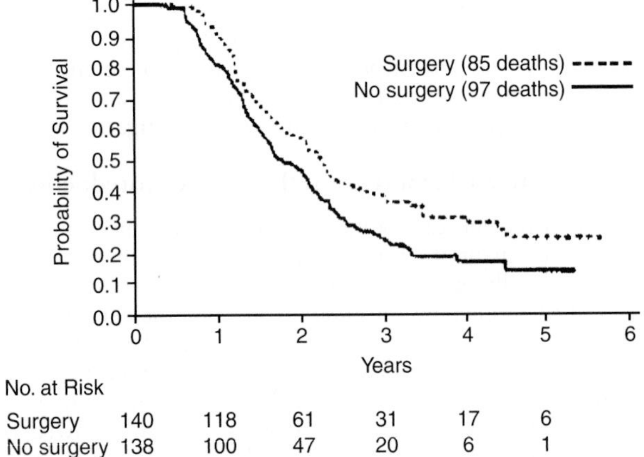

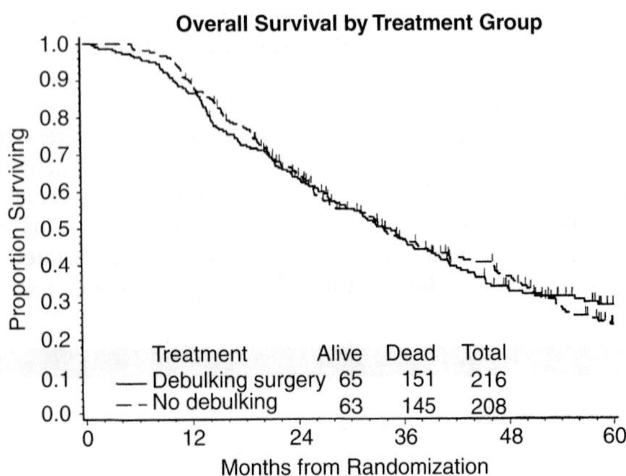

FIGURE 25.34. **A:** Survival of patients with advanced ovarian cancer who underwent internal debulking surgery compared to treatment with chemotherapy only. *Source:* van der Burg ME, van Lent M, Buyse M, et al. The effect of debulking surgery after induction chemotherapy on the prognosis in advanced epithelial ovarian cancer. Gynecologic Cancer Cooperative Group of the European Organization for Research and Treatment of Cancer. *N Engl J Med* 1995;332:629–634. **B:** Survival of patients with advanced ovarian cancer who underwent internal debulking surgery compared to treatment with chemotherapy only. *Source:* Rose PG, Nerenstone S, Brady M, et al. A phase III randomized study of interval secondary cytoreduction in patients with advanced stage ovarian carcinoma with suboptimal residual disease: a Gynecologic Oncology Group study. *Proc Am Soc Clin Oncol* 2002;21:201a.

Postoperative Chemotherapy

Surgery is rarely curative for women with advanced-stage ovarian carcinoma, even when there is no residual disease. Many chemotherapy agents have some activity against ovarian cancer, and a great deal of effort has been spent on trying to optimize adjuvant chemotherapy regimens to improve survival. A recent meta-analysis of 198 trials involving 38,440 women suggested that the regimen that best prolonged survival is a platinum and taxane combination with intraperitoneal administration; this resulted in a 55% relative risk reduction for mortality as compared with nonintraperitoneal monotherapy containing neither platinum nor taxane (389). The most standard regimen in the United States currently is six cycles of postoperative intravenous (IV) paclitaxel/carboplatin; areas of uncertainty exist not only regarding use of neoadjuvant therapy, but regarding the role of single-agent carboplatin, use of intraperitoneal chemotherapy, and use of maintenance taxane therapy.

Platinum Use. Platinum agents represent the most active group of chemotherapy agents in the treatment of ovarian cancer. The GOG performed the largest comparative trial of a platinum-containing regimen versus a non–platinum-containing regimen in the pretaxane era (390). Two hundred twenty-seven patients with advanced ovarian cancer were randomized to receive doxorubicin/cyclophosphamide treatment with or without the addition of cisplatin. Complete response rate (51% vs. 26%) and median overall survival (15.7 vs. 9.7 months) both were superior for the cisplatin-containing regimen. The meta-analysis of Kyrgiou et al. confirmed that platinum-based combination or monotherapy produces a survival benefit compared to non–platinum-based therapy. A relatively small increased risk of secondary leukemia has been identified in ovarian cancer patients treated with platinum-based chemotherapy (389). However, the clinical benefits of platinum treatment outweigh the risks.

Choice of Platinum Agent. As discussed in Chapter 15 (Principles of Chemotherapy in Gynecologic Cancer), the early trials of platinum in ovarian cancer all used the first available platinum agent, cisplatin, which is associated with troublesome nausea/vomiting, neurotoxicity, and nephrotoxicity. Carboplatin, while more myelotoxic, is otherwise substantially better tolerated than cisplatin. Multiple randomized trials comparing carboplatin to cisplatin in ovarian carcinoma have been performed, and meta-analyses have confirmed that there is no difference in efficacy between the two agents (391). Three trials have specifically compared the combination of intravenous cisplatin plus paclitaxel to intravenous carboplatin plus paclitaxel, and noninferiority for carboplatin/paclitaxel versus cisplatin/paclitaxel has been convincingly demonstrated (392–394). In general, carboplatin is the first-line platinum agent in the treatment of ovarian cancer in the United States. However, as discussed below, there are no randomized data showing that intraperitoneal carboplatin produces benefits similar to those seen with intraperitoneal cisplatin, and cisplatin remains the standard platinum drug for intraperitoneal administration.

Oxaliplatin, a third-generation platinum agent that produces an unusual cold-triggered neurotoxicity, is FDA approved in the United States for use in colon cancer. It has a theoretical benefit in activity against tumors that exhibit mismatch repair deficiency and preclinical data suggested that cell lines resistant to cisplatin might be sensitive to oxaliplatin (395). However, there is no clinical evidence of non–cross resistance with other platinum agents; a GOG trial of oxaliplatin in women with platinum-resistant tumors revealed negligible activity (396). A small ($n = 177$) randomized trial comparing oxaliplatin/ cyclophosphamide to cisplatin/cyclophosphamide as first-line therapy in women with ovarian cancer showed no difference in progression-free or overall survival between the two treatment groups (397).

Platinum Dose and Dose Intensity. To date no evidence supports the use of doses of cisplatin above 50 to 100 mg/m^2 every 3 weeks or carboplatin AUC 5 to 7.5 every 3 weeks. An influential early meta-analysis of over 60 published trials showed a correlation between dose intensity of cisplatin and observed response rate, but the correlation held only over a range of doses lower than those used in clinical practice today (398).

Numerous prospective clinical trials have compared different platinum doses and dose intensities over a clinically relevant range, and the majority of these have shown no benefit for higher dose or greater dose intensity (399–401). The largest was the GOG trial that tested dose intensity while keeping the total dose fixed. Four hundred fifty-eight patients with bulky stage III or stage IV disease were randomized to receive either eight cycles of cisplatin (50 mg/m^2) plus cyclophosphamide (500 mg/m^2) every 3 weeks or four cycles of cisplatin (100 mg/m^2) plus cyclophosphamide (1,000 mg/m^2) every 3 weeks. There was no difference between the regimens in response rate or survival (401). The outlier among the studies was a randomized Scottish trial that compared cyclophosphamide 750 mg/m^2 plus cisplatin either 50 mg/m^2 or 100 mg/m^2 every 3 weeks for six cycles, and found a better response rate, progression-free survival, and overall survival on the high-dose arm (402). Nonetheless, because neurotoxicity was still evident in patients treated with the higher dose of cisplatin 4 years after chemotherapy, investigators recommended that the dose of cisplatin not be increased beyond 75 mg/m^2 (400). No other reasonably sized trial has supported importance of cisplatin dose intensity or total dose beyond six cycles (see Prolongation of Primary Therapy/Consolidation/Maintenance below). Randomized trials have also failed to show benefit for escalated doses of carboplatin, although they produce less neurotoxicity than high doses of cisplatin. Danish investigators randomized patients with advanced-stage ovarian cancer to receive cyclophosphamide 500 mg/m^2 with carboplatin at an AUC of either 4 or 8. There was no difference in either surgically confirmed complete remission rate or overall survival (403). Very high doses of carboplatin requiring hematopoietic stem cell support have also been tested in ovarian cancer without any evidence of benefit (404).

Despite all of the above, as discussed below under Addition of a Taxane to Platinum Chemotherapy, doubt about the optimal dose of platinum for front-line use persists. Perhaps a subset of patients or ovarian cancers exists for which different doses would be appropriate. The Scottish clinical trials group has launched a large trial (SCOTROC4) of single-agent carboplatin in women who do not desire platinum/taxane combination therapy or in whom such therapy is contraindicated. Patients are randomized to a flat carboplatin dose or a dose that is individually escalated in each patient.

Addition of a Taxane to Platinum Chemotherapy. In the 1980s a great deal of excitement was generated by the demonstration that single-agent paclitaxel had substantial activity against platinum-resistant ovarian cancer. Initial trials of paclitaxel used prolonged infusion durations to reduce the incidence of acute hypersensitivity reactions. A GOG trial tested single-agent paclitaxel at 200 mg/m^2 given intravenously over 24 hours with growth factor support in 43 patients with recurrent, persistent, or progressive ovarian cancer during or after a platinum-based chemotherapy. The overall response rate was 37% with 18% complete responses (405). Twenty-seven of the patients were platinum resistant, and the response rate to paclitaxel in this group was 33%. When premedication with corticosteroids and histamine blockers was found to prevent most hypersensitivity reactions, shorter infusion durations were also tested. In an influential trial performed by a group of European and Canadian collaborators 391 eligible patients were randomized in a 2×2 factorial design to receive paclitaxel as either a 3-hour or a 24-hour infusion at a dose of either 135 mg/m^2 or 175 mg/m^2 every 3 weeks. Shorter infusions were found to be safe and to result in less myelosuppression but more neurotoxicity (406). There was a slight increase in time to progression (TTP) for patients who received the higher dose (19 weeks vs. 14 weeks; response rate 20% vs. 15%) and 175 mg/m^2 over 3 hours became the accepted dose in patients with recurrent disease.

A number of randomized trials were rapidly launched comparing platinum-based regimens with and without taxane in the first-line treatment of ovarian cancer. The four largest studies are summarized in Table 25.14. The results of the first two of these trials completed (GOG 111 and OV-10) clearly demonstrated that combination chemotherapy with paclitaxel and cisplatin prolongs both progression-free and overall survival as compared with cyclophosphamide/cisplatin (407,408). In GOG 111, which treated women with suboptimally debulked or stage IV cancer using a paclitaxel dose of 135 mg/m^2 over 24 hours, the median overall survival was 37 months for those treated with paclitaxel and cisplatin as compared with 25 months for those receiving cyclophosphamide and cisplatin (407). Similar results were found in the more inclusive (stage IIB-IV) European trial, although it produced 18% grade 3 neurotoxicity in the paclitaxel-containing arm (vs. 4% neurotoxicity in the GOG trial), as paclitaxel was used at a dose of 175 mg/m^2 (with the possibility of escalating to 200 mg/m^2) over 3 hours (408).

TABLE 25.14

RANDOMIZED TRIALS ± TAXANE IN FIRST-LINE CHEMOTHERAPY FOR OVARIAN CANCER

Author (year)	N	Eligibility	Regimens	Median PFS	Median OS
McGuire (1996) (Ref 407) GOG 111	386	Suboptimal III Any IV	Cisplatin 75 mg/m^2 + paclitaxel 135 mg/m^2/24 hr vs. Cisplatin 75 mg/m^2 + cyclophosphamide 750 mg/m^2	18 mo vs. 13 mo $p < 0.001$	38 mo vs. 24 mo $p < 0.001$
Piccart (2000) (Ref 408) OV-10	680	IIB-IV	Cisplatin 75 mg/m^2 + paclitaxel 175 mg/m^2/3 hr vs. Cisplatin 75 mg/m^2 + cyclophosphamide 750 mg/m^2	15.5 mo vs. 11.5 mo $p = 0.0005$	36 mo vs. 26 mo $p = 0.0016$
Muggia (2000) (Ref 409) GOG 132	614	Suboptimal III Any IV	Cisplatin 75 mg/m^2 + paclitaxel 135 mg/m^2/24 hr	14 mo	26 mo
			vs. Paclitaxel 200 mg/m^2/24 hr	11 mo	26 mo
			vs. Cisplatin 100 mg/m^2	16 mo Paclitaxel worse $p < 0.001$	30 mo $p = N$
ICON3 (2002) (Ref 411)	2,075	I-IV	Carboplatin AUC 6 + paclitaxel 175 mg/m^2	> 17 mo	39 mo
			vs. Carboplatin AUC 6 or Cyclophosphamide 500 mg/m^2 + cisplatin 50 mg/m^2 + doxorubicin 50 mg/m^2	16 mo p = NS	36 mo p = NS

Note: AUC, area under the curve; NS, not significant; OS, overall survival; PFS, progression-free survival; RR, response rate; mo, months.

The other two trials did not clearly support the addition of paclitaxel to front-line therapy. The GOG trial compared single-agent paclitaxel to single-agent cisplatin to the combination in the same subgroup of patients treated in GOG 111 (409). The response rate to single-agent paclitaxel in patients with measurable disease was significantly lower than to either of the platinum-containing regimens (42% vs. 67%, $p < 0.01$). However, the difference in median durations of overall survival (30.2, 25.9, and 26.3 months for patients randomized to cisplatin, paclitaxel, and the combination) was not statistically significant. Single-agent therapies were discontinued more frequently (cisplatin because of toxicity or patient refusal [17%] and paclitaxel because of progression [20%]) compared to combination chemotherapy in which 7% of patients discontinued because of toxicity and 6% because of disease progression. The relative hazard of first progression or death was significantly greater among those randomized to paclitaxel when compared with either of the cisplatin-containing regimens, but did not differ significantly between the two cisplatin regimens. Since overall survival was similar in the three arms, and the combination regimen had a better toxicity profile than single-agent cisplatin at 100 mg/m^2, the investigators concluded that the combination of cisplatin and paclitaxel should remain the preferred therapy. They speculated that the lack of benefit for the combination arm related to the fact that almost 50% of patients began subsequent treatment prior to overt clinical progression, presumably on the basis of a rising CA-125. The first nonprotocol treatment for those randomized to cisplatin included paclitaxel 52% of the time, and for women randomized to paclitaxel it included cisplatin or carboplatin 69% of the time. By way of contrast, paclitaxel was seldom used as salvage therapy in GOG 111 because of its limited availability at the time, and while 48% of patients in the cisplatin/cyclophosphamide arm of OV-10 crossed over to paclitaxel as first salvage treatment, it appears that they did so after overt clinical progression. The results of GOG 132 have raised the question of whether appropriately designed sequential therapy would be as effective as combination therapy. An Eastern Cooperative Oncology Group (ECOG) study of single-agent doxorubicin versus single-agent paclitaxel versus the combination for women with metastatic breast cancer had built in crossover at the time of progression, and showed that the combination produced more toxicity and a higher response rate, but no improvement in overall survival (410). However, no trial has formally tested the question of sequential versus concomitant agents in the treatment of ovarian cancer. Moreover, it is noteworthy that the response rate to single-agent cisplatin 100 mg/m^2 in GOG 132 was the same as that to the combination therapy (which used a cisplatin dose of 75 mg/m^2), again raising uncertainties about the role of platinum dose in the treatment of ovarian cancer.

ICON3, a large multinational trial which randomized women with stage I-IV disease to carboplatin/paclitaxel chemotherapy versus single-agent carboplatin or CAP (cisplatin/doxorubicin/cyclophosphamide) chemotherapy found no superiority for the taxane-containing combination in either progression-free or overall survival (hazard ratio for overall survival 0.98; 95% CI, 0.87 to 1.10) (411). About a third of patients on carboplatin in the control group went on to receive a taxane at some stage, mostly after the disease had progressed. The results of this trial also appear to contradict those of OV-10 and GOG 111, and the explanation remains unclear. It has been suggested that cisplatin/cyclophosphamide is an inferior control arm to optimal dose single-agent platinum. However, a trial comparing cisplatin 50 mg/m^2 to cisplatin 50 mg/m^2 plus cyclophosphamide 650 mg/m^2 repeated every 4 weeks for six cycles did not show any difference between treatment groups (412). ICON3 included stage I/II patients, a group in which, as discussed above, it has been very difficult to demonstrate the benefit of any chemotherapy, and in which the differences between different chemotherapy regimens might be blunted. However, they made up only about 20% of the study population and statistical analysis of ICON3 did not reveal any heterogeneity of treatment effect when analyzed by stage, cell type, grade, or country of origin.

Alternate Taxanes/Taxane Schedules. The Scottish Gynaecological Cancer Trials Group compared a docetaxel-containing primary regimen to a paclitaxel-containing primary regimen (412a). One thousand seventy-seven women with stage IC-IV ovarian or primary peritoneal carcinoma were randomized to six cycles of carboplatin AUC 5 and either docetaxel 75 mg/m^2 or paclitaxel 175 mg/m^2. At a median follow-up of 23 months, there was no difference in progression-free (15 months for docetaxel, 14.8 months for paclitaxel) or overall survival (2-year overall survival 64% for docetaxel and 69% for paclitaxel). This was confirmed in a subsequent report with longer follow-up. Docetaxel was associated with less neurotoxicity (11% vs. 30% grade $\geq$ 2 neurosensory toxicity) and more myelotoxicity (11 patients vs. 3 patients with neutropenic fever). This represents an attractive option for patients with or at risk for neurotoxicity.

A formulation of paclitaxel as protein-bound nanoparticles (ABI-007, Abraxane) has been approved for use in breast cancer in the United States. It has shown activity in ovarian cancer, but randomized trials of its use in front-line therapy have not been performed.

Given the slightly superior response rates observed for more prolonged infusion of a given dose of paclitaxel in the European-Canadian trial, interest in very prolonged infusion schedules was stimulated. The GOG completed a trial (GOG 162) randomizing women with ovarian cancer to cisplatin 75 mg/m^2 plus paclitaxel 135 mg/m^2 administered as either a 24- or a 96-hour infusion. There was no difference in overall or progression-free survival (413).

GOG investigators performed a randomized trial of a 24-hour infusion of paclitaxel at different doses in previously treated patients with advanced disease (414). For 271 patients with measurable disease, high-dose paclitaxel (250 mg/m^2 plus granulocyte colony-stimulating factor [G-CSF]) gave a higher response rate than the lower dose of 175 mg/m^2 (36% vs. 27%). However, progression-free survival and overall survival were similar. The median duration of overall survival was 13.1 months and 12.3 months for paclitaxel 175 and 250 mg/m^2, respectively. Despite cytokine support, high-dose paclitaxel is associated with increased platelet toxicity, anemia, neurotoxicity, and gastrointestinal toxicity, and there appears to be, at best, a modest dose-response effect for paclitaxel in previously treated patients. A subsequent prospective, randomized trial in previously untreated advanced ovarian cancer patients compared two different doses of paclitaxel (175 vs. 225 mg/m^2), with all patients receiving carboplatin at an AUC of 5. No improvement in survival was reported for the higher-dose paclitaxel regimen (415).

Fennelly et al. (416) performed a phase 1 pharmacologic study of paclitaxel administered weekly in patients with relapsed ovarian cancer. Maximum tolerated dose was 80 mg/m^2 in this heavily pretreated group of patients. Partial responses were observed in 30% of assessable patients including patients with progressive disease on a standard 3-week paclitaxel schedule. Weekly paclitaxel was associated with less toxicity, particularly alopecia. Subsequent phase 2 trials have reported response rates of 32% to 47% for weekly paclitaxel in platinum-refractory patients (417,418). Current and future trials will address the role of weekly paclitaxel in front-line therapy.

Addition of a Third Agent to Front-Line Chemotherapy. There are no data that addition of any third cytotoxic agent to front-line chemotherapy of ovarian cancer improves outcomes, despite an immense amount of investigation of this strategy.

Doxorubicin produces single-agent response rates of 20% to 30% in women with chemotherapy-naïve ovarian cancer. In the pretaxane era, two meta-analyses suggested that there was benefit to the addition of doxorubicin to cisplatin/cyclophosphamide therapy. The large ICON2 trial therefore randomized 1,526 patients with stage I-IV ovarian cancer to either single-agent carboplatin AUC 5 or CAP (cyclophosphamide 500 mg/m^2 plus doxorubicin 50 mg/m^2 plus cisplatin 50 mg/m^2). There was no evidence of a difference in survival between the two therapies (HR for survival 1.00) (419). Subsequently two large randomized studies tested the addition of epirubicin to paclitaxel/carboplatin therapy, and neither found any benefit for the addition of anthracycline (420).

Topotecan also seemed a reasonable candidate to improve results with first-line therapy of ovarian cancer. Topotecan has efficacy very similar to that of paclitaxel against ovarian cancer in women naïve to both agents; a large randomized trial reported a response rate of 20.5% for topotecan 1.5 mg/m^2/day $\times$ 5 and 13.2% for paclitaxel 175 mg/m^2 every 3 weeks (421). Moreover, there is some non–cross resistance between paclitaxel and topotecan. One hundred ten patients crossed over to the alternative drug as third-line therapy; 13.1% of topotecan-treated patients responded to paclitaxel and 10.2% of paclitaxel-treated patients responded to topotecan. Three hundred twenty-six patients with stage III/IV ovarian cancer were randomized to six cycles of either carboplatin/paclitaxel every 21 days or the same combination plus IV topotecan 1 mg/m^2 days 1 to 3 every 21 days. There was no difference in response rate (RR of 84% on carboplatin/paclitaxel vs. 94% for the triplet) or median TTP (70.4 and 71.8 weeks, respectively). There was more anemia with topotecan (23.3% vs. 9.4% of courses required transfusions) (422).

After a substantial number of preliminary studies to establish safe regimens for administering three drugs without unduly compromising the dose of any one agent, particularly platinum, an international multiarm randomized study was led by the GOG (GOG 182-ICON5) to definitively answer whether triplet cytotoxic chemotherapy improves survival (423). A total of 4,312 advanced-staged ovarian cancer patients were randomized to carboplatin/paclitaxel or carboplatin/paclitaxel combined with gemcitabine, liposomal doxorubicin, or topotecan. Progression-free survival ranged from 15.4 to 17.5 months across the four treatment arms, with an HR of 0.94 to 1.07, which was not statistically different among any of the combination regimens studied.

Recent interest has focused on the role of combining some of the newer molecular targeted agents with chemotherapy. The most promising agent to date has been bevacizumab, a monoclonal antibody targeting vascular endothelial growth factor (VEGF). It has produced single-agent response rates in the range of 15% to 20% in the setting of recurrent ovarian cancer, and has improved survival when combined with chemotherapy in the treatment of colon cancer and lung cancer. Two trials have been launched, a placebo-controlled three-arm trial in the GOG (GOG 218; Fig. 25.35), which separately tests the value of bevacizumab in combination with carboplatin/paclitaxel chemotherapy and the value of bevacizumab as consolidation/maintenance after primary therapy, and a two-arm trial (ICON7; carboplatin/paclitaxel vs. carboplatin/paclitaxel with concomitant and consolidation bevacizumab) with no placebo in the European cooperative groups.

Intraperitoneal Chemotherapy. Intraperitoneal (IP) chemotherapy provides a means by which high concentrations of drugs and long durations of tissue exposure can be attained at the peritoneal surface. As intraperitoneal progression of disease remains the major source of morbidity and mortality in ovarian cancer, it is a theoretically attractive approach in the treatment of this disease. Many chemotherapeutic agents, including those used for the treatment of ovarian cancer such as cisplatin, carboplatin, topotecan, and paclitaxel have been tested for feasibility with

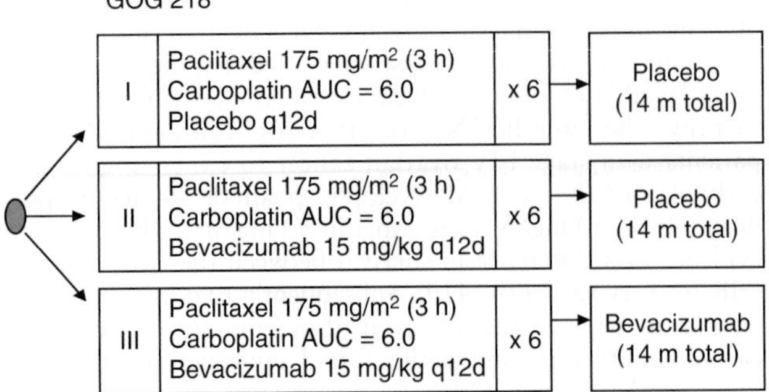

FIGURE 25.35. Design of GOG 218 with incorporation of bevacizumab, concurrently with primary chemotherapy and as maintenance until there is evidence of disease. *Source:* Personal communication, Robert Burger.

intraperitoneal administration. Larger or less water-soluble molecules will stay longer in the peritoneal cavity, and have a higher peritoneal cavity–to–plasma concentration ratio (sometimes referred to as "pharmacologic advantage"), but may not get into the bloodstream. The direct penetration of chemotherapy agents into tumor masses is limited to 1 to 2 mm from the tumor surface. Early work by Los et al., using a rat intraperitoneal tumor model, found that the concentration of cisplatin at the periphery of tumor nodules was higher after IP administration of cisplatin, but the concentration at the center of the nodules was identical after IP and IV administration (424). Hence (a) the theoretical benefit is only for very small tumor volumes, and (b) agents that do not reach therapeutic systemic levels when given by the intraperitoneal route need to be administered intravenously as well. Cisplatin has a 10- to 20-fold pharmacologic advantage when given intraperitoneally. For a given dose of cisplatin, peak concentrations are higher with IV cisplatin, and this has resulted in somewhat decreased toxicity in a randomized comparison of the same doses of cisplatin given intraperitoneally versus intravenously, including less hearing loss and neuromuscular toxicity (425). However, the amount of cisplatin recovered in the urine, reflecting total systemic exposure, is similar regardless of whether the administration is intravenous or intraperitoneal. Similarly, carboplatin given IP at an AUC of 6 has been shown to give an AUC in the peritoneal cavity about 17 times higher than that of carboplatin given intravenously while producing a very similar serum AUC (426). Paclitaxel, on the other hand, has a pharmacologic advantage of about 1,000, and significant levels persist in the peritoneal cavity 1 week after drug administration. However, the dose that can be given is limited by abdominal pain, and serum paclitaxel concentrations detected in patients treated with intraperitoneal paclitaxel at feasible doses are low (427).

Surgical Considerations for Intraperitoneal Chemotherapy. The three methods of obtaining access to the peritoneal cavity that have been examined are single-use percutaneous catheters, semipermanent percutaneous catheters, and implanted subcutaneous port and catheter systems. Reported complications for all catheters include intestinal injury, catheter blockage, and infections involving the peritoneal cavity or the abdominal wall. The implanted subcutaneous port and catheter systems have the advantages of a lower risk of infection and better patient acceptance. In one large single institutional series, Davidson et al. (428) analyzed data on 249 catheters placed in 227 patients. No injuries occurred at the time of catheter placement. Significant complications occurred in 17.6% of patients, including catheter blockage (8.8%) and infection (8.8%). In eight patients, late erosion of the catheter into the intestinal lumen was noted. Recommendations from this study concluded that catheters should not be placed at the time of colon surgery because of a possible increase in the risk of infection, and that intraperitoneal chemotherapy should not be administered until 7 to 14 days following catheter placement to allow time for wound healing. Strict aseptic technique should be used when catheters are accessed.

In a publication from GOG 172, which randomized patients with optimal stage III ovarian cancer to IV versus IP chemotherapy, Walker et al. reported on the IP catheter outcomes in 205 patients allocated to the IP arm (429). One third of patients on that trial discontinued IP therapy primarily related to catheter-related problems including infection in 21 women, catheter blockage in 9, catheter leak in 3, access problems in 5, and drainage per vagina in 1.

The evidence suggests that implanted subcutaneous port and catheter systems have an acceptable level of morbidity for delivery of intraperitoneal therapy. The major technical impediment to successful intraperitoneal therapy is the formation of adhesions within the peritoneal cavity, which leads to catheter blockage and poor distribution of drugs instilled into the cavity. Recent experience suggests that catheters designed for intravenous use may be used for intraperitoneal chemotherapy. The smaller diameter of the IV catheter, together with the absence of side holes, may produce fewer intraperitoneal adhesions as compared to the catheters designed for IP use. Guidance on the selection and placement of catheters is available on the GOG Web site, www.GOG.org.

Clinical Use of IP Therapy for Ovarian Cancer. In January 2006, the NCI issued a clinical alert suggesting the use of intraperitoneal cisplatin chemotherapy in women with optimally debulked ovarian cancer (430). A meta-analysis of eight trials comparing intraperitoneal to intravenous platinum-based chemotherapy (all but one used cisplatin) showed an average 21.6% decrease in the risk of death (hazard ratio 0.79; 95% CI, 0.70 to 0.89). As the expected median duration of survival for women with optimally debulked ovarian cancer receiving standard treatment is approximately 4 years, this size reduction in death rate was estimated to translate into about a 12-month increase in overall median survival. The power of this analysis was based primarily on the survival benefits for intraperitoneal chemotherapy observed in each of the three relatively large randomized trials summarized in Table 25.15 (425,431,432).

Despite these results, intraperitoneal therapy has not yet been consistently adopted for the treatment of women with optimally debulked ovarian cancer in the United States, and has not been widely adopted internationally. There are several reasons for this.

First, intraperitoneal therapy, as used in the reported trials, is technically demanding. Administration of paclitaxel over 24 hours, which is necessary to reduce the neurotoxicity when paclitaxel is combined with cisplatin, is inconvenient and, if it requires hospitalization, expensive. Use of IP catheters is not routine in many oncology practices, and is associated with a number of complications, as discussed above. In the report by Armstrong et al. (431), only 42% of patients on the IP arm received the six planned cycles of intraperitoneal therapy due either to cisplatin related toxicities or catheter problems. It has been suggested that icodextrin, which has a clinical record of use as an exchangeable peritoneal dialysis solution in humans, can reduce adhesion formation in a rat model of intraperitoneal chemotherapy (433). A trial using intraperitoneal 5-FU in 4% icodextrin in patients with colon cancer showed the regimen to be safe, but problems with peritoneal access still occurred in 20% of patients (434).

Second, all of the large randomized studies used cisplatin in both the intraperitoneal and intravenous arms, whereas carboplatin, which is less toxic and easier to administer, has become the standard intravenous platinum agent in the treatment of ovarian cancer. It has even been suggested, based on nonsignificant trends in two of the randomized trials comparing cisplatin/paclitaxel to carboplatin/paclitaxel, that the cisplatin/paclitaxel regimen is inferior to carboplatin/paclitaxel in optimally debulked patients, and that IP therapy must be compared to intravenous carboplatin/paclitaxel before it

TABLE 25.15

SELECTED RANDOMIZED TRIALS OF INTRAPERITONEAL VERSUS INTRAVENOUS CHEMOTHERAPY IN OPTIMALLY DEBULKED OVARIAN CANCER

Author (year)	N	Regimens	Median PFS	Median OS	Comments
Alberts (1996) (Ref 425)	546	IV cyclophosphamide 600 mg/m^2 plus IP cisplatin 100 mg/m^2 × 6 vs. IV cyclophosphamide 600 mg/m^2 plus IV cisplatin 100 mg/m^2 × 6	N/A	49 mo vs. 41 mo $p = 0.02$	<2 cm residual disease permitted; 58% of patients in both groups completed 6 cycles of cisplatin
Markman (2001) (Ref 432)	462	IV carboplatin AUC 9 × 2 followed by IV paclitaxel 135 mg/m^2/24 hr plus IP cisplatin 100 mg/m^2 × 6 vs. IV paclitaxel 135 mg/m^2/24hr plus IV cisplatin 75 mg/m^2 × 6	28 mo vs. 22 mo $p = 0.01$	63 mo vs. 52 mo $p = 0.05$	18% of patients on IP arm got ≤2 cycles of IP therapy
Armstrong (2006) (Ref 431)	416	D1 IV paclitaxel 135 mg/m^2/24 hr D2 IP cisplatin 100 mg/m^2 D8 IP paclitaxel 60 mg/m^2 vs. D1 IV paclitaxel 135 mg/m^2/24 hr D2 IV cisplatin 75 mg/m^2	24 mo vs. 19 mo $p = 0.027$	67 mo vs. 50 mo $p = 0.0076$	49% of patients received ≤3 cycles of IP therapy

Note: IP, intraperitoneal; OS, overall survival; PFS, progression-free survival; mo, months.

can be adopted (435). Although intraperitoneal carboplatin can be safely used and appears to have favorable pharmacokinetics (pharmacologic advantage combined with good systemic drug exposure), there is no clinical trial evidence that it will provide the same survival benefits as intraperitoneal cisplatin.

Finally, the heterogeneity and toxicity of the intraperitoneal regimens used have left some confusion as to what the most important elements of the ideal IP therapy regimen are, and which could be modified to improve safety and tolerability while maintaining efficacy. For example, the Markman et al. trial used two cycles of carboplatin AUC 9 (as "chemical debulking" prior to starting intraperitoneal therapy), which resulted in significant hematologic toxicity and difficulty delivering the IP regimen (432). The Armstrong et al. trial incorporated both IP cisplatin and IP paclitaxel. Despite these uncertainties, a potential 1-year survival advantage is certainly meaningful, and the option of intraperitoneal therapy should be discussed with healthy patients who have optimally debulked ovarian cancer.

It is possible that intraperitoneal therapy might benefit women other than those with initially optimally debulked disease. It is of note that the Alberts trial (perhaps the cleanest test of intraperitoneal therapy in that all variables were the same in both arms except the route of cisplatin administration) permitted accrual of women with up to 2 cm of residual disease. Benefit of therapy was not influenced by extent of residual disease ($p = 0.93$ for interaction of treatment and residual disease, microscopic vs. ≤0.5 cm vs. >0.5 to 2 cm) (425). Other groups that might stand to benefit are those with an excellent response to intravenous treatment after three cycles or those who have only minimal disease remaining after interim debulking surgery. However, no randomized trials have addressed these scenarios. One small trial did test IP cisplatin as consolidation therapy. The EORTC randomized women with a pathologic complete remission to front-line platinum-based therapy to no further therapy versus four cycles of intraperitoneal cisplatin at 100 mg/m^2. The trial closed due to poor accrual with less than half of its planned accrual. After a median follow-up of 8 years, the hazard rates for progression-free survival (PFS) and overall survival (OS) were 0.89 (95% CI, 0.59 to 1.33) and 0.82 (0.52 to 1.29). These results were felt to be suggestive of a treatment benefit but insufficient to change practice (436).

Use of Neuroprotectants. As discussions of cisplatin and paclitaxel above make obvious, neurotoxicity is one of the most bothersome long-term side effects of current therapy for ovarian cancer. Reporting of neurotoxicity is notoriously variable, depending both on the scale used and the awareness of the investigator. The intraperitoneal regimen (IV paclitaxel plus IP paclitaxel plus IP cisplatin) used by Armstrong et al. reported 19% grade 3/4 neurotoxicity. In GOG 132 the rate of grade 3/4 neurotoxicity for six cycles of carboplatin/paclitaxel chemotherapy was 5% (10% grade 2). A group of Italian investigators reported on long-term neurologic evaluations on 120 ovarian cancer patients treated with a front-line carboplatin AUC 5/paclitaxel 175 mg/m^2–based regimen. There was a 15% chance of residual neurotoxicity 6 months after the completion of chemotherapy (437). One potential neuroprotectant commercially available is amifostine (WR-2721). Two hundred forty-two patients with advanced ovarian cancer were randomized to receive six cycles of cyclophosphamide (1,000 mg/m^2) plus cisplatin (100 mg/m^2) with or without amifostine (910 mg/m^2 15 minutes prior to chemotherapy). There was a clear reduction in neutropenia requiring hospitalization ($p = 0.005$) and in nephrotoxicity (defined as a ≥40% reduction in creatinine clearance, $p = 0.004$). However, the reduction in neurotoxicity, while statistically significant, was less impressive; 29 versus 35 patients experienced grade 2 neurotoxicity and 9 versus 15 experienced grade 3 neurotoxicity. The trial was not powered to detect any potential loss of antitumor activity; however, median survival time was the same (31 months) in both arms. Infusion-related hypotension was the major toxicity observed (438).

No adequately sized studies have studied amifostine with paclitaxel-based therapy or with the lower amifostine doses currently used (which produce less hypotension). However, a placebo-controlled, randomized phase 2 study in which patients were treated with either carboplatin/paclitaxel or carboplatin/paclitaxel/epirubicin found worse nausea and vomiting with amifostine (740 mg/m^2); Common toxicitycriteria (CTC) graded sensory neuropathy was improved with amifostine, but there were almost no differences in patient-reported motor or sensory symptoms (439). Other potential neuroprotectants, such as vitamin E or glutamine, have not been tested in the setting of ovarian cancer. Early identification of neurotoxicity and dose reduction or switching to a less neurotoxic agent remain the best-established ways to manage this side effect.

Prolongation of Primary Therapy/Consolidation/ Maintenance. Many women with ovarian cancer have an excellent response to first-line chemotherapy, but most will nonetheless relapse and die of their disease. Approximately two thirds of patients with advanced ovarian cancer will achieve a clinical complete remission following chemotherapy, that is, have no evidence of disease on physical examination or in radiographic studies together with a serum CA-125 in the normal range. One third of all patients with advanced ovarian cancer will be free of disease at a second-look laparotomy following primary cisplatin-based therapy. The most important prognostic factor that influences the likelihood of achieving a surgically confirmed complete remission is the volume of disease at the time chemotherapy was initiated. Patients who have suboptimally debulked disease have a four- to fivefold decreased likelihood of achieving a complete remission as compared to those patients who were optimally cytoreduced. In addition, patients with large-volume disease who do achieve a complete remission have a higher likelihood of a subsequent relapse than do patients with small-volume disease (440). Among all patients who have a surgically documented complete remission, at least 50% will recur and die of their disease.

Further therapy after a clinical complete remission would clearly be warranted for many women if an effective treatment could be found. However, no trials of consolidation or maintenance therapy have produced any survival benefit to date.

Whole Abdominal Radiotherapy After Chemotherapy. Nonrandomized data have suggested that consolidative radiotherapy may be curative in a small percentage of patients with small-volume residual disease after primary chemotherapy. For example, Petit et al. recently reported on long-term (median 14 years) follow-up of consolidative whole abdominal radiotherapy (WAR) in a series of 106 stage III patients who had no (33%) or less than 1 cm (46%) residual disease after primary therapy, or who were debulked to less than 1 cm at the time of second-look surgery (21%) (441). Radiation was stopped for acute toxicity in 11 patients. Long-term toxicities included radiation enteritis in 21 patients with 9 patients requiring surgery for bowel obstruction. Four deaths were related to enteritis complications. Overall survival at 5 and 10 years was, respectively, 53% and 36%.

Several very small, randomized trials have examined the role of consolidative WAR after primary chemotherapy. Bruzzone et al. (442) randomly assigned patients who had minimal or no residual disease after chemotherapy to WAR or three more cycles of chemotherapy. The study was stopped after only 41 patients had accrued, because disease progression had been observed in 55% of patients treated with radiation versus 29% of those treated with additional chemotherapy (p = 0.08) Lambert et al. (443) randomized 117 patients with residual disease of 2 cm or less after secondary cytoreduction to WAR or five additional courses of carboplatin. There was no statistical difference in disease-free or overall survival between the two arms. Kapp et al. randomized 64 women with a complete clinical response after primary surgery and chemotherapy to WAR versus no further therapy (444). No second-look laparotomy was performed. Patients who had WAR had a significantly better 5-year survival than patients who had chemotherapy alone (59% vs. 33%, p = 0.03). Most recently the Swedish-Norwegian Ovarian Cancer Study Group (445) randomly assigned 98 patients who received four courses of cisplatin/anthracycline chemotherapy and had a pathologic complete response (CR) at second-look surgery to no further therapy, continued chemotherapy with cisplatin/anthracycline to ten courses total, or whole abdominal radiotherapy. Progression-free survival was significantly better (5-year PFS, WAR = 56%, chemotherapy = 36%, control = 35%, p = 0.032) and overall survival trended toward better in the group receiving WAR. No benefit for WAR was observed in a separate group of patients with microscopic residual disease, who were randomized to chemotherapy versus WAR. Late grade 3 bowel complications occurred in 10% of patients receiving WAR. In general, the studies of abdominopelvic radiotherapy after chemotherapy have reported higher complication rates than studies of abdominopelvic radiotherapy alone, which has dampened enthusiasm for further investigation of consolidative WAR (446). It has been suggested that there is cross-resistance between platinum chemotherapy and irradiation, as human ovarian cancer cell lines with acquired resistance to cisplatin develop relative radiation resistance *in vitro* (447). As discussed above, a randomized trial conducted by the GOG of ^{32}P versus observation after pathologic complete response to primary therapy was negative (341).

Consolidative/Maintenance Chemotherapy. Three small, randomized trials of prolonged duration of primary therapy have been conducted. Investigators at Memorial Sloan-Kettering Cancer Center in New York randomized 78 women to five versus ten cycles of CAP (cyclophosphamide, doxorubicin, cisplatin) chemotherapy (448). Danish investigators randomized women to 6 versus 12 cycles of CAP chemotherapy (449). North Thames investigators randomized women to five versus eight cycles of single-agent platinum therapy (450). None of these studies showed a survival benefit, and all showed more toxicity with prolonged therapy.

Like use of a third cytotoxic agent in front-line combination therapy, use of a third cytotoxic agent for consolidation therapy has not proven effective to date. Two large trials of four cycles of consolidative topotecan after primary chemotherapy have both been negative. A randomized phase 3 trial performed by the AGO-OVAR and the GINECO together randomized 1,308 patients with previously untreated FIGO stage IIB-IV ovarian cancer to six cycles of carboplatin/paclitaxel followed by surveillance or four cycles of topotecan (1.25 mg/m^2 IV days 1 to 5 on a 3-week schedule) (451). Complete response was not required to proceed to topotecan therapy. There was no difference in median PFS (18.2 months for topotecan vs. 18.5 months for control) or OS (43.1 months for topotecan vs. 44.5 months for control). A similar phase 3, multicenter Italian trial (452) randomized 273 patients to observation versus topotecan 1.5 mg/m^2 days 1 to 5 every 21 days for four cycles after primary carboplatin/paclitaxel chemotherapy. PFS did not differ between the treatment arms (18.2 months for topotecan vs. 28.4 months for controls). Consolidation therapy with epirubicin also failed to improve survival in patients who achieved a clinical complete remission following platinum-based induction therapy (453). As discussed above, the EORTC tested intraperitoneal cisplatin in women with a pathologic complete remission and found hazard rates for PFS and OS relative to observation of 0.89 and 0.82 (436).

Two small prospective trials of high-dose consolidation therapy with hematopoietic stem cell support have both been negative. In the larger trial a collaboration of French and Italian investigators randomized women in remission after front-line chemotherapy to either three further cycles of conventionally dosed carboplatin or a single high-dose cycle (carboplatin 1,600 mg/m^2 plus cyclophosphamide 6,000 mg/m^2) with peripheral stem cell support. No survival benefit was observed for the women receiving high-dose therapy (453a, 453b).

The most promising trial of maintenance therapy to date was a Southwest Oncology Group (SWOG)/GOG trial randomizing women in clinical complete remission to either 3 or 12 cycles of

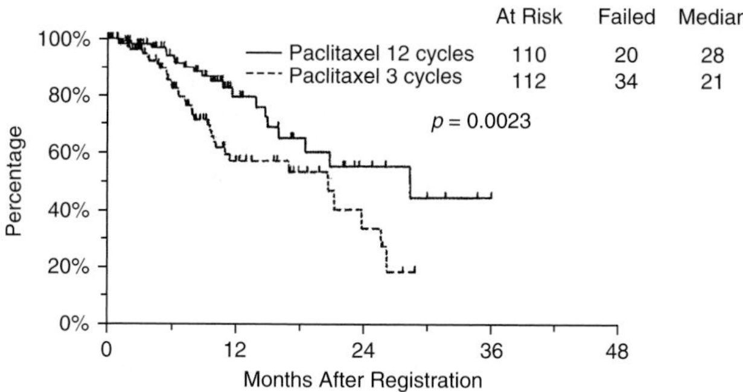

FIGURE 25.36. Progression-free survival of patients treated with either 3 monthly cycles or 12 monthly cycles of paclitaxel as maintenance therapy of advanced-stage ovarian cancer who were in a clinical complete remission after platinum/paclitaxel-based chemotherapy.

intravenous paclitaxel 175 mg/m^2 every 4 weeks (454). The trial was halted by its data and safety monitoring board after a planned interim efficacy analysis at a point when there was a statistically significant improvement in time to progression but no difference in overall survival between the treatment arms (PFS 28 vs. 21 months, one sided $p = 0.0035$) (Fig. 25.36). Because insufficient patients to detect a survival difference had been randomized at the time the study was stopped (n = 262), and because patients receiving 3 cycles of therapy were allowed the option of crossing over to 12 cycles, a survival comparison will not be possible. In addition, the neurotoxicity observed was so substantial, even though patients with >grade 1 neurotoxicity were excluded from the trial, that the dose of paclitaxel on the study had been modified to 135 mg/m^2 every 4 weeks. However, not very many patients had accrued to this dose at the time of study closure, and they were not included in the analysis, so the effect of this dose reduction on therapy efficacy is uncertain. An unplanned retrospective subgroup analysis suggested a trend toward survival benefit in the group of patients who started maintenance therapy with a CA-125 level of less than ten (455). A preliminary report on results of an Italian trial randomizing women in complete remission after front-line therapy to observation or six cycles of paclitaxel 175 mg/m^2 every 3 weeks showed no benefit in either progression-free or overall survival (456). The GOG is attempting to confirm the beneficial results it observed with a larger study randomizing women after clinical complete remission to one of three arms: no further therapy, paclitaxel 135 mg/m^2 every 4 weeks for 12 cycles, or Xyotax (a microparticle-bound paclitaxel) 135 mg/m^2 every 4 weeks for 12 cycles. This trial currently has overall survival as the endpoint.

Maintenance With Noncytotoxic Agents. Noncytotoxic agents such as interferon, a monoclonal antibody targeting CA-125 (oregovomab) (457), radioimmunoconjugates, and matrix metalloproteinase inhibitors have also all been tested in randomized trials with no survival benefit. The SWOG randomized 70 evaluable patients to six doses of 50 million IU of intraperitoneal interferon alpha versus observation after pathologic complete remission to primary therapy. There was no difference in progression-free survival between the two groups (435). A trial of subcutaneous interferon was also negative (458). No improvement in progression-free or overall survival was observed following a single intraperitoneal administration of 90Y-conjugated antimucin antibody in a large phase 3 trial, although intraperitoneal recurrences were decreased (459,460). Other current maintenance trials include a trial being conducted by the EORTC of the epithelial growth factor receptor (EGFR) tyrosine kinase inhibitor, erlotinib, and the ongoing trials of maintenance anti-VEGF monoclonal antibody described above.

Implications of Clear Cell and Mucinous Histology

It has long been realized that ovarian cancers of serous histology appear to be more chemotherapy sensitive than other histologic subtypes. For example, in an analysis of multiple different agents used in published phase 2 trials, serous histology (vs. all other histologies) was reported to be one of the most important factors predicting a response to second-line therapy (461). A review of all patients entered into advanced-stage GOG ovarian cancer trials from 1976 to 1982, when response was commonly surgically assessed, revealed no negative second-look laparotomies among women with clear cell or mucinous histology (462).

Clear Cell Carcinomas

Advanced clear cell carcinomas are unusual in the United States. Clear cell carcinoma is more common in Japan, where it accounts for about 20% of epithelial ovarian carcinomas (463). Women of Japanese descent living in the United States continue to have a higher incidence of clear cell carcinoma than is found in Western countries or other Asian countries (464). Even in Japan, early-stage clear cell carcinoma is more common than advanced-stage clear cell carcinoma; in one review, stage I made up 39% of clear cell disease, stage II 13%, stage III 30%, and stage IV 6% (465). As discussed above (Adjuvant Therapy of Early-Stage Disease), the implications of clear cell histology in early disease are not clear; in some reports it seems to portend a high risk of recurrence, and in others it appears to have little prognostic significance. However, it has become increasingly clear that advanced-stage clear cell tumors, which make up only a small percentage of advanced-stage ovarian cancers in the United States, may not respond well to platinum chemotherapy. As early as 1996, Goff et al. reported that 52% of stage III clear cell tumors of the ovary versus 29% of serous tumors progressed clinically while on primary platinum chemotherapy (466). Sugiyama et al. reported a response rate for clear cell carcinomas to primary platinum-based therapy of only 11% (467). The Hellenic Cooperative Oncology Group (331) reviewed patients with advanced clear cell carcinoma of the ovary treated on protocols from 1987 and 2003 (n = 35), and compared them to serous tumors treated on the same trials. Response rates were 45% versus 81% ($p = 0.008$) and median survival was 25.1 months versus 49.1 months ($p = 0.141$). The difference in response was significant; the difference in survival was not, and not all series have reported inferior survival even in advanced stages of disease (468). Ho et al. reported that patients with pure advanced clear cell carcinoma had a much worse prognosis (median survival, 11 months) than patients with mixed clear cell and other histologic types (median survival, over 48 months) (469). Similar results have been reported in the setting of recurrent disease. Investigators from M. D. Anderson published a retrospective review of 51 patients treated at their institution for recurrent clear cell carcinoma. Among those with platinum-sensitive disease, only 2 (9%) of 22 patients had a partial response to retreatment with carboplatin and paclitaxel; none of 29 patients given second-line therapy for platinum-resistant disease responded (470).

Unfortunately, the realization that these tumors may be resistant to platinum does not automatically indicate a superior option. Some authors have proposed that clear cell carcinomas have a low proliferation rate, and therefore general resistance to chemotherapy (471). However, Cloven et al. reported that human clear cell tumors (at variable times during therapy) sent for commercial testing for drug resistance had lower rates of extreme drug resistance to paclitaxel, doxorubicin, and cyclophosphamide than papillary serous tumors (472). An *in vitro* study (473) suggested that paclitaxel and irinotecan were effective against three of five clear cell cancer cell lines, whereas cisplatin was effective against only one. Shimizu et al. reported that irinotecan/mitomycin C chemotherapy produced a response rate of 52% against platinum-resistant clear cell and mucinous carcinomas (473a). Some (463,469) but not all (465) authors have suggested that the response rate might be higher with taxane-containing regimens; all the series are exceedingly small. A multinational phase 3 study for stage I-IV clear cell carcinoma of the ovary has been launched by the Japanese Gynecologic Oncology Group (JGOG). Women are randomized to therapy with either carboplatin/paclitaxel or cisplatin/irinotecan.

Interestingly, multiple reports suggest that women with clear cell carcinomas are more likely to have a thromboembolic event. Goff et al. noted that 42% of patients with stage III clear cell tumor had deep venous thrombosis (DVT) or pulmonary embolus (PE) versus 18% of patients with serous tumors (466); another more recent retrospective study reported that 27.3% of patients with clear cell carcinoma had a DVT or PE versus only 6.8% of patients with other histologies (474).

Molecular studies suggest a different profile for clear cell carcinomas. For example, they have been reported to have high levels of hepatocyte nuclear factor-1 beta (HNF-1 beta) (475) and high levels of ABCF2, which belongs to the ATP-binding cassette gene superfamily, and is highly expressed in nonresponders to chemotherapy (476). In addition, gene expression profiling suggests that clear cell tumors have a very different profile than other epithelial ovarian cancers, one which could not be statistically distinguished from clear cell carcinomas originating in other tissues, including endometrium and kidney (477).

Mucinous Tumors

Early-stage mucinous tumors tend to be low grade and have a good prognosis. Advanced-stage mucinous tumors are uncommon in the United States. They respond poorly to chemotherapy and are associated with a short survival. Investigators from the Royal Marsden Hospital reviewed all patients with stage III or IV mucinous epithelial ovarian cancer (n = 27, 19 with measurable disease) treated with first-line platinum-based therapy at their unit between 1992 and 2001 and compared them to controls with nonmucinous epithelial ovarian cancer (478). The response rate for patients with measurable mucinous cancer was 26% with one complete response; 63% of patients experienced disease progression while on platinum-based chemotherapy. The response rate for the controls with measurable disease was 65% ($p = 0.009$ for response). Median overall survival was 12 months versus 37 months ($p < 0.001$). Specific trials for patients with advanced-stage mucinous tumors, possibly using chemotherapeutic agents directed against gastrointestinal tumors, are being considered by the GOG.

Primary Peritoneal Carcinoma

As described in the section above on pathology of serous carcinomas, serous carcinomas may present as diffuse carcinomatosis of the peritoneal cavity with minimal or no involvement of the ovaries or fallopian tubes ("small ovary syndrome") and may be seen in women who have had prior surgical removal of their ovaries and fallopian tubes. This presentation is referred to as primary peritoneal serous carcinoma (PPSC). Up to 18% of laparotomies performed for presumed ovarian carcinoma are felt to be PPSC on final pathology review (479). CA-125 levels will be elevated in most patients with PPSC. In the older literature these were often misclassified as peritoneal mesotheliomas. Typically, mesotheliomas will express mesothelial markers such as calretinin or cytokeratin 5/6, which are rarely expressed in PPSC; CA-125 and S100 are common in PPSC and are rarely expressed on mesothelioma (480). The epithelium of the ovary and the peritoneal lining are histologically the same, and factors that induce ovarian epithelium to undergo malignant degeneration may have the same effect on the peritoneal lining. As discussed above, women who carry the *BRCA1* mutation are at increased risk for the development of primary peritoneal cancer (481). The risk of primary peritoneal carcinoma for *BRCA1* carriers after prophylactic oophorectomy is unknown but is estimated to be from 1% to 10% (482).

The GOG performed a retrospective case-control study of patients with PPSC and suboptimal cytoreduction, comparing them to patients with ovarian carcinoma with suboptimal cytoreduction. Both groups were treated with cisplatin and cyclophosphamide. Median overall survival and disease-free interval of the two groups appeared very similar (483). Current treatment recommendations for women with PPSC are the same as for women with stage III ovarian carcinoma, and women with PPSC are eligible for most ovarian cancer clinical trials. Peritoneal cancers with nonserous histologies similar to other subtypes of ovarian cancer (mucinous, endometrioid) may also be encountered. They are less common and optimal therapy is not known.

Fallopian Tube Carcinoma

Series of results of chemotherapy for advanced-stage fallopian tube carcinoma are small. It has recently been suggested that many serous tumors thought to be of ovarian or primary peritoneal origin may, in fact, be of fallopian tube origin. In general, advanced-stage fallopian tube carcinomas are treated in the same manner as advanced-stage ovarian cancers and have similar survival. A recent retrospective case-control study reported by Moore et al. identified 96 women with stage IA to IV fallopian tube carcinoma and two ovarian carcinoma controls for each patient with fallopian tube cancer matched by age, stage, and residual disease (n = 190). All patients underwent primary surgery with lymph node dissection followed by platinum/taxane combination chemotherapy. Forty-six of the women with fallopian tube cancer had early-stage (I/II) disease. Five-year overall survival for patients with early-stage fallopian tube carcinoma was 95% and for patients with early stage ovarian cancer it was 81%. Among women with advanced-stage (III/IV) disease, median time to recurrence and overall survival were 8.7 months and 32 months for patients with fallopian tube cancer and 7.2 months and 30 months for women with ovarian cancer (484).

Second-Look Laparotomy and Laparoscopy

In the past, patients with advanced ovarian cancer frequently underwent abdominal explorations after induction chemotherapy to assess whether or not residual disease remained. However, although surgery is the most accurate way to assess the response to therapy, there is no evidence that any type of routine surgical procedure after initial chemotherapy prolongs overall survival. The term *second-look laparotomy* has been incorrectly used to refer to several distinctly different types of surgery. These include secondary operations to resect known residual or recurrent disease and secondary operations performed for relief of cancer-related symptoms, such as intestinal obstruction. In current usage, the term should be reserved for a systematic surgical exploration in asymptomatic patients who have completed a planned course of chemotherapy for ovarian cancer.

In 1966, during an era when single-agent alkylating therapy for advanced ovarian cancer was standard, Rutledge and Burns (485) reported on 288 patients treated with melphalan and asked the question: Should laparotomy be used more often when a patient has an unusually good response to determine whether the drug should be discontinued? In their report, 28 patients underwent surgery for this reason; 12 had no tumor detected. The investigators felt that "good response to the drugs is the reason for laparotomy," but pointed out that patients with a negative re-exploration may relapse, as did two in their series (486). Interest in second-look laparotomy as a means of determining when chemotherapy could be discontinued was stimulated during the 1970s, when reports began to appear linking the long-term use of alkylating agents to the development of acute leukemia (486,487).

With the introduction of platinum-based chemotherapy in the mid to late 1970s and the use of aggressive primary debulking, up to 50% of patients treated with chemotherapy for advanced cancer had no clinically detectable tumor at the completion of their chemotherapy. Since it was known that many of these women harbored occult residual cancer, a number of investigators tested noninvasive methods of detecting such disease. Imaging techniques such as CT, sonography, MRI, and PET are generally unable to detect intraperitoneal tumor masses smaller than 1 cm and, in fact, may miss larger masses (488). Some investigators (489) have suggested that the cytologic analysis of peritoneal fluid obtained by culdocentesis may be a means of assessing response in women under treatment for ovarian cancer. The accuracy of this technique in detecting residual disease is quite low, however. In a study of 96 women re-explored for ovarian cancer who had multiple cytologic washings taken at the time of laparotomy, only 34% of patients with biopsy-proven gross intraperitoneal disease had positive washings (490). In patients with only microscopic disease, 28% had positive washings.

Several groups have used laparoscopy as an alternative to second-look laparotomy. In 1981, Berek et al. (491) reported 119 consecutive laparoscopic examinations performed in 57 patients. Fourteen percent of their patients had major complications requiring laparotomy, most of which involved bowel perforation. At the NCI, laparoscopy was routinely used to assess response to chemotherapy (492). In their series, no patient required a surgical exploration because of a laparoscopy complication. In 66 restaging laparoscopies, residual tumor was found in 33 (50%) and provided the only evidence for disease in 24 cases (36%). These latter patients were spared an unnecessary second-look laparotomy. However, if the laparoscopy was negative, residual disease was documented in 55% of patients at laparotomy.

More recently, the group from the Memorial Sloan-Kettering Cancer Center has reported their experience with the use of laparoscopy for second-look evaluation in 150 patients with advanced ovarian cancer following chemotherapy (493). The majority of patients (87%) had stage III or IV disease at initial surgery; the remainder had stage II disease or were unstaged. Eighty-two patients (54%) had optimal cytoreduction at the time of their initial surgery. All patients had completed primary chemotherapy and were clinically disease-free based on imaging studies and CA-125 levels at the time of second look. Sixty-nine patients (46%) were found to have pathologically negative second looks; thus, the rate of positive second-look evaluations was 54%. The rate of conversion to laparotomy was 18 of 150 (12%). In three cases, this was secondary to bowel injury; one patient sustained a bladder injury; the remainder of conversions to laparotomy was for secondary cytoreduction. There was only one case in which the patient was found to have extensive adhesions and laparoscopy was abandoned. The overall rate of major complications was 2.7%. Although long-term follow-up is not available, the rate of negative evaluations and the rate of recurrences in patients with negative second looks appear to be equivalent to those described in studies of second-look assessment by laparotomy.

Even with a normal serum CA-125 level, a significant number of patients in clinical complete remission will have residual disease at laparotomy. Rubin et al. (494) measured CA-125 levels at the time of secondary surgery in 96 ovarian cancer patients, all of whom had had documentation of an elevated CA-125 level at the time when the tumor was first diagnosed and were therefore "marker positive." Persistent disease was found in 62% of patients who had a normal CA-125 level at the time of surgery. These findings have been confirmed in other studies (495). Consequently, if the primary purpose of the second-look laparotomy is to determine whether the patient has residual ovarian cancer, an elevated CA-125 level makes such a procedure unnecessary.

A second-look laparotomy itself is intended as a thorough re-exploration of the peritoneal cavity and selected retroperitoneal structures. Immediately prior to surgery, a pelvic examination under anesthesia is performed. Cystoscopy and proctoscopy may be useful in symptomatic patients or in those with prior tumor involvement of the bladder or lower gastrointestinal tract.

The abdomen should be entered through a generous vertical excision, extending from the pubic symphysis to well above the umbilicus. If obvious tumor is found, frozen-section confirmation should be obtained. The goal of the operation becomes removal of as much tumor as possible. If no obvious tumor is found, the surgeon must undertake a meticulous, systematic search for areas of occult tumor. Saline washings are obtained from multiple sites within the peritoneal cavity, usually including the pelvis, both paracolic gutters, and the undersurfaces of both hemidiaphragms. All adhesions should be lysed and portions submitted for histologic analysis since adhesions often form at the site of tumor nodules. The upper abdomen should be explored carefully, with any suspicious areas biopsied. The residual omentum should be palpated, as should the aortic lymph nodes. The intestines must be carefully examined. A thorough exploration of the pelvic cavity is performed. Throughout this evaluation, particular attention should be paid to areas where residual disease was left at the initial operation. If suspicious areas are identified, frozen-section confirmation should be obtained and areas of tumor resected as completely as possible.

If no tumor is identified, a series of biopsies is performed from areas that may harbor occult disease. The stumps of the infundibulopelvic ligaments, which carry the ovarian blood and lymphatic supplies, should be identified in the retroperitoneum and biopsied. Other surgical pedicles in the pelvis should be examined and biopsied if suspicious. If the uterus was not removed at the initial operation, hysterectomy should be performed. Peritoneal biopsies should be taken from multiple sites within the abdominal cavity, including the pelvis, paracolic gutters, and both hemidiaphragms. Some have suggested the use of a laparoscope or sterile proctoscope to facilitate inspection of the diaphragms. Any remaining areas of omentum should be removed. Many surgeons remove the appendix if present. Para-aortic and pelvic lymph nodes should be thoroughly sampled. A second-look operation at which no tumor is identified will take several hours and will produce 20 to 30 individual biopsy specimens.

In previous years, there have been many published series on second-look laparotomy. Table 25.16 summarizes several reports in which about 55% of the patients with no clinical evidence of disease were found to have cancer present at re-exploration (496). These findings are a clear indication of our current inability to identify persistent cancer by noninvasive means.

Several clinical and histologic factors have been shown to relate to the likelihood of tumor being found at the time of second-look laparotomy. The most important factors are stage and the volume of tumor remaining following initial cytoreductive

TABLE 25.16

FINDINGS AT SECOND-LOOK LAPAROTOMY FROM 71 COMBINED SERIES

Finding	Number	%
No tumor found	2,417	47
Tumor found	2,773	53
Total	5,190	100

Source: Modified with permission from Barter JF, Barnes WA. Second-look laparotomy. In: Rubin SC, Sutton GP, eds. *Ovarian Cancer.* New York: McGraw-Hill; 1993:269–300.

TABLE 25.18

FINDINGS AT SECOND-LOOK LAPAROTOMY BY EXTENT OF RESIDUAL DISEASE FOLLOWING PRIMARY CYTOREDUCTION

Residual	No. negative	Total patients	% negative
None	331	460	72
Optimal[a]	330	655	50
Suboptimal[a]	158	682	23

[a]Original investigator's definition.
Source: Modified with permission from Barter JF, Barnes WA. Second-look laparotomy. In: Rubin SC, Sutton GP, eds. *Ovarian Cancer.* New York: McGraw-Hill; 1993:269–300.

surgery. As shown in Table 25.17, patients with stage III and IV disease had a substantially lower proportion of negative second-look operations than did those with stage I and II, 33% versus 70% to 80%, respectively.

The amount of residual disease remaining following the initial operation for ovarian cancer is also a major determinant of the likelihood of disease being found at the time of second-look laparotomy. Table 25.18 summarizes pooled data on 1,797 patients, providing information on the relationship of the extent of residual disease following primary surgery to findings at second look. Patients with suboptimal residual disease after primary surgery had only a 23% likelihood of a negative second look as compared to 50% for those with optimum residual and 72% in those with no known residual tumor. Many series have included stage I patients in their analysis of the effect of residual disease on findings at second-look laparotomy. As all stage I patients would be included in the no-residual-disease group, this would account, in part, for the improved prognosis of this group. Even considering this bias, there seems to be a strong correlation between extent of residual disease and the likelihood of finding disease at re-exploration.

The histologic grade of the tumor, as distinct from the cell type, has been shown to be a significant prognostic factor, although it has been suggested that, in advanced-stage patients treated with platinum-containing chemotherapy, grade may be of less importance. Numerous series have correlated the surgical findings at a re-exploration with tumor grade (Table 25.19). Earlier series demonstrated a stronger relationship between grade and second-look findings, perhaps because more of the patients in these series were treated with chemotherapeutic regimens that did not contain platinum. Overall, women with poorly differentiated tumors seem to have a somewhat lower chance of having a negative second-look laparotomy, although it should be remembered that these data are not controlled for other important prognostic variables, including stage and the amount of residual tumor.

Second-look laparotomy is a highly invasive diagnostic procedure that results in significant expense, discomfort, and time in the hospital for the patient; however, it is associated with little serious medical morbidity. Although many reports on second-look surgery have not discussed complications, among seven major series published since 1980 that specifically report complications, no deaths were seen in 682 operations (376). The most common complications were infections of the surgical wound (6.3%), the urinary tract (5.6%), and the lungs (2.8%).

The finding of large-volume residual tumor carries a grave prognosis. In some series, when survival is reported separately for patients with gross tumor, approximately 80% died within 3 years of second-look laparotomy. Patients who have only microscopic disease detected at second look fare considerably better. Copeland et al. (497) reported on 50 patients with microscopic disease followed for a median of 40 months from second look. Survival rates were 96% and 71% at 2 and 5 years, respectively.

Because even the most carefully performed second-look operation may miss microscopic areas of tumor, and because ovarian cancer may occasionally spread beyond the areas assessed at surgery, a negative second-look operation is not synonymous with cure of cancer. Papers reporting the incidence of recurrence following negative second-look laparotomy have often included patients treated with different chemotherapeutic regimens for variable durations and followed for relatively short periods of time. This has made the true incidence of and the risk factors for recurrence following negative second-look laparotomy difficult to determine. In an

TABLE 25.17

FINDINGS AT SECOND-LOOK LAPAROTOMY RELATED TO STAGE OF DISEASE FROM 31 COMBINED SERIES

Stage	No. negative	Total patients	% negative
I	268	331	81
II	190	276	69
III	441	1,120	39
IV	59	177	33

Source: Modified with permission from Barter JF, Barnes WA. Second-look laparotomy. In: Rubin SC, Sutton GP, eds. *Ovarian Cancer.* New York: McGraw-Hill; 1993:269–300.

TABLE 25.19

FINDINGS AT SECOND-LOOK LAPAROTOMY RELATED TO HISTOLOGIC GRADE

Grade	No. negative	Total patients	% negative
1	163	283	58
2	167	389	43
3	259	619	42

Source: Modified with permission from Barter JF, Barnes WA. Second-look laparotomy. In: Rubin SC, Sutton GP, eds. *Ovarian Cancer.* New York: McGraw-Hill; 1993:269–300.

old review that included 12 reports published from 1980 to 1986, it was calculated that the overall recurrence rate was 18%, including 10.9% in stages I and II and 26% for patients with stage III or IV disease (316). In 1988, Rubin et al. (498) reported a 50% risk of recurrence following a negative second-look laparotomy in patients treated with platinum-based chemotherapy. A multivariate analysis demonstrated that stage, histologic grade, and extent of residual disease remaining after primary cytoreduction were significant predictors of recurrence following a negative second look.

These results have been substantiated in the multicenter setting. In the GOG trial of intraperitoneal ^{32}P versus observation after negative second-look laparotomy, 64% of patients relapsed at a median follow-up of 63 months (341); in the EORTC trial of intraperitoneal cisplatin versus observation after negative second-look laparotomy, 52% of patients had relapsed with a median follow-up of 8 years (436).

There is presently no evidence that any type of additional therapy can improve survival in patients who do achieve a surgically confirmed complete remission, or that introducing further treatment earlier for patients who have residual disease without clinical signs or symptoms is of benefit. There is also no evidence that second-look laparotomy *per se* is a therapeutic procedure (499). Although there are no prospective trials in which patients in a clinical complete remission have been randomized either to a second-look operation or to medical follow-up, retrospective studies comparing the survival of patients who underwent a second-look laparotomy versus patients in whom a second-look was not performed have failed to show any difference in survival. Consequently, most gynecologic oncologists no longer consider second-look laparotomy a routine procedure in patients who achieve a complete remission.

An alternative to second-look laparotomy is second-look laparoscopy. A second-look laparoscopy is usually performed as a same-day procedure with patients being discharged home the day of surgery or 1 day postoperatively. With modern laparoscopic techniques, a second-look laparoscopy provides excellent visualization and access to the peritoneal and extraperitoneal spaces where ovarian cancer may be detected. The laparoscopic approach is associated with less operating time, fewer complications, less blood loss, fewer or less costly hospital charges, and shorter hospitalization than laparotomy. The majority of cases can be completed by the laparoscopic approach, with approximately 10% to 15% of cases requiring conversion to laparotomy to complete the procedure satisfactorily. If a second-look operation is planned, the laparoscopic approach should be considered as the initial step as it may provide all the necessary information and avoid the potential morbidity and hospitalization associated with the open approach.

Data from GOG protocol 158, comparing carboplatin and paclitaxel versus cisplatin and paclitaxel in optimal residual stage III ovarian cancer patients, have a bearing on the issue of second-look laparotomy (394). Although not randomly allocated to a second look, almost 400 patients (50%) in this study elected the procedure. Approximately half of them had no evidence of disease at second-look laparotomy. Patients with residual disease at the second look underwent a variety of treatments with the majority of patients receiving more systemic chemotherapy with paclitaxel and carboplatin. There was no difference in progression-free or overall survival between the patients electing second-look laparotomy and those declining the procedure and treated only at the time of clinical progression. The group with the pathologically documented complete remission had better overall survival than the group with residual disease at the second look. Consequently, the potential value of a second-look surgery to identify patients who could benefit from immediate treatment of residual disease was not substantiated in this study. Given the fact that many of these patients who had optimal residual disease following their initial surgery had no disease or only small-volume disease found at the second look, relatively few, if any, would be expected to benefit from secondary cytoreduction during the operation. The usefulness of a second-look laparotomy to assess the results of therapy accurately in the setting of a clinical trial is unequivocal. However, in a nonclinical trial situation, there appears to be little justification for a second-look laparotomy merely to obtain prognostic information. If, on the other hand, therapeutic decisions will be based upon findings at second look, such a procedure may be justified. However, the patient must be aware that there is no evidence that any form of subsequent therapy has been shown to significantly prolong survival. These observations are consistent with the recommendations from the 1994 NIH Consensus Conference.

As second-look procedures are not commonly performed, recent reports have explored the prognostic use of stratifying CA-125 levels within the normal range at completion of chemotherapy. Juretzka et al. found that patients with a CA-125 of less than or equal to 12 U/mL at the completion of primary chemotherapy had median overall and progression-free survivals of 5.8 years and 2.8 years versus 3.7 years and 1.7 years for those with a CA-125 of greater than 12 U/mL (500).

Follow-Up of Patients in Remission

Most patients with ovarian cancer who enter a clinical complete remission have been followed with a combination of pelvic examinations, computerized abdominal tomograms, and monitoring of serum CA-125 levels. However, none of these has been shown to decrease symptoms or improve survival. Unlike the situation in general screening, rise in CA-125 after primary treatment for ovarian cancer is fairly specific, particularly if a confirmatory test is obtained. One older study reported the median lead time to clinical progression from a doubling of CA-125 above the upper limits of normal was 63 days (501). However, a significant proportion of patients (approximately 30%) may have lead times of greater than 6 months. How early salvage therapy should be started in this situation remains controversial. On the one hand, general belief is that treatment is likely to be more effective when disease burden is smaller. On the other hand, second-line chemotherapy is not curative, and many women, once started on salvage chemotherapy, will be on chemotherapy for the rest of their lives. In Europe, the Medical Research Council (OV-05) and the European Organization for the Research and Treatment of Cancer (EORTC 55955) have completed accrual to a phase 3 trial in which women with clinical response to first-line platinum therapy are followed with serial CA-125 levels and are randomized to initiate treatment at the time of biochemical recurrence versus waiting until the time of clinical evidence of recurrence. Results should help determine if there is any benefit to starting treatment earlier. In addition, the GOG has conducted a randomized trial comparing tamoxifen to thalidomide for the therapy of women who have CA-125 marker elevation but no measurable recurrence of disease; results should be available soon.

In premenopausal women with ovarian cancer, the initial staging and cytoreductive laparotomy results in a surgical castration. Consequently, these women frequently experience hot flashes, and those who do achieve long-term survival are at increased risk for osteoporosis. There is epidemiologic evidence (described above) that estrogen replacement therapy slightly increases the risk of developing ovarian cancer *de novo*, and antiestrogens, such as tamoxifen, may produce tumor shrinkage in a small subset of women with advanced ovarian cancer. However, one small randomized, controlled trial (502) has reported that estrogen replacement therapy has no detrimental effect on disease-free or overall survival in women with ovarian cancer. The risks of deep venous thrombosis must be weighed against the symptomatic benefits. Short-term use of estrogen replacement therapy, particularly in symptomatic women who were premenopausal prior to their surgery for ovarian cancer, is reasonable.

Uses of CA-125 in Ovarian Cancer Treatment

As discussed above, the current usefulness of CA-125 for screening is limited, in part because many stage I ovarian cancers are not associated with an elevated serum level of CA-125, and a variety of nonmalignant conditions can elevate CA-125, particularly in premenopausal women. It is clear that CA-125 nadir after completion of primary therapy has prognostic value, but as there are no clinical interventions known to improve outcomes for those women who do not have a low nadir. CA-125 is widely used to monitor for cancer recurrence, as described above.

CA-125 may also be useful to monitor the effectiveness of second-line chemotherapy, decreasing the need for supplementing imaging. A number of studies have created CA-125 response definitions, such as 50% or 75% decline to qualify as a response (503). These have been compared to radiographic outcomes, suggesting that they may be similar to standard response criteria (504), may overestimate response compared to WHO criteria (505), or may be better at predicting prognostic outcomes compared to response evaluation criteria in solid tumors (RECIST) (506). In general these criteria have been developed to assist in providing clinical trial outcomes data, not as guidance for treatment of individual patients. False-positive rates (i.e., CA-125 is decreasing, but disease is clearly progressing) are 2% to 3% and false-negative rates (i.e., disease is responding but CA-125 is not decreasing) are about 20% with platinum/paclitaxel therapy (504). The false-positive rate would be higher if more minor decreases in CA-125 were used to indicate clinical benefit. Particular caution should be used in discontinuing a therapy prematurely based solely on rise in CA-125. Sabbatini et al. reported that only half of patients who eventually had a CA-125 decline with liposomal doxorubicin therapy had a decline prior to the second cycle of therapy (507). Removal of ascites will affect CA-125 levels; renal dysfunction does not (508).

TREATMENT OF PERSISTENT/ RECURRENT DISEASE

Secondary Cytoreductive Surgery

The benefit of secondary cytoreductive operations in ovarian cancer, at the time of second-look laparotomy or otherwise, has not been clearly demonstrated. Since about one half of patients who do undergo second-look laparotomy will have disease found, and in about 80% of these patients macroscopic disease will be present, approximately 40% of all patients having second-look laparotomy are candidates for secondary cytoreduction. Technically, secondary cytoreduction can be accomplished, with reported success rates ranging from 24% to 84% (509–512). There is less information available, however, on the effect of secondary cytoreduction on survival. Chambers et al. (513) concluded that residual tumor size following secondary cytoreduction did not influence survival after comparing 23 patients with microscopic residual disease and 6 with macroscopic disease. Luesley et al. (511) found no survival benefit in patients cytoreduced to microscopic disease compared to patients with residual macroscopic disease or small-volume gross residual disease. On the other hand, Podratz et al. (514) reported an actuarial 4-year survival rate of 55% in patients with microscopic residual disease compared to 19% for those with macroscopic disease. In a series reported by Hoskins et al. (510), patients cytoreduced to microscopic residual disease at the time of the second look had a 5-year survival of 51%. This was similar to the survival of patients found to have only microscopic disease at the second look, and was significantly better than the survival in patients left with gross disease. Lippman et al. (515) examined the effect of extensive tumor resection at second-look laparotomy on survival for patients with >2 cm gross residual disease. Patients undergoing optimum resection (<2 cm residual tumor) had a significantly better survival than those undergoing suboptimal resection, suggesting that there is a survival benefit associated with optimal cytoreduction at second-look laparotomy.

Segna et al. (512) reported on 100 patients with advanced ovarian cancer initially treated with cisplatin-based therapy who were explored at the time of recurrence. Sixty-one percent of patients were left with optimal (<2 cm) disease after secondary cytoreduction. These patients had a significant improvement in their median survival compared with patients with suboptimal residual disease (27 vs. 9 months, $p = 0.0001$).

More recently, Salani et al. (516) reported on 55 patients who underwent secondary cytoreduction for recurrent epithelial ovarian cancer after a complete response to initial chemotherapy, at least a 12-month interval from initial diagnosis to recurrence, and in whom preoperative imaging studies showed five or fewer sites of recurrence. Complete macroscopic cytoreduction was achieved in 41 patients (74.5%). Independent predictors of overall survival were a diagnosis-to-recurrence interval of 18 months or greater, only one to two sites of recurrence on preoperative imaging, and no macroscopic residual disease after the secondary surgery.

In a recent review article on secondary cytoreductive surgery for recurrent ovarian cancer, Hauspy and Covens (517) examined 17 publications on the subject, and concluded that patients with favorable characteristics such as a long disease-free interval, good performance status, and a single or few small intra-abdominal sites of recurrence may benefit from secondary cytoreduction. It appears that, in patients whose tumors remain sensitive to chemotherapy, cytoreduction to small-volume disease prior to secondary chemotherapy can be of benefit. The GOG is currently conducting a trial assessing the value of secondary cytoreductive surgery in the setting of platinum-sensitive disease.

Second-Line Chemotherapy

Ovarian cancer that is resistant to primary chemotherapy or recurs at some point after primary chemotherapy is generally not curable. Nonetheless, a group of women with recurrent disease will have tumors that remain very sensitive to chemotherapy, and will clearly benefit from further treatment. Eisenhauer et al. analyzed results for 704 patients who had recurrence or persistent disease after primary platinum-based therapy and were treated on a variety of second-line chemotherapy trials (461). Independent predictors of response to second-line therapy were bulk of disease less than 5 cm, fewer sites of disease, and serous histology. Time to recurrence since primary therapy, when analyzed as a continuous variable, was not independently prognostic, and was closely correlated with tumor size. However, time to recurrence from completion of primary platinum-based chemotherapy is clinically readily available and quantifiable, and has come into common use as the primary means of predicting which patients are most likely to benefit from further treatment, in particular from further platinum-based treatment. In 1991 Markman et al. published results of an influential retrospective review of 72 patients who had responded to an initial platinum-based therapy and were subsequently retreated with a platinum-based regimen (518). Response rate for women with a "platinum-free interval" of 5 to 12 months was 27%, for 13 to 24 months was 33%, and for over 24 months was 59%. Women who had a greater than 24-month interval with no therapy (as opposed to just no platinum-based therapy) had a 77% response rate with a 32% rate of surgical complete remission. The terms "platinum resistant" and "platinum refractory" are used somewhat variably in the literature, and are sometimes subdivided into "primary" and "secondary" platinum resistance, which may have different implications for survival or benefit to future therapies. Perhaps the most common usage is to define "platinum-resistant" tumors as those with a treatment-free interval of less than 6 months since previous platinum therapy. The GOG defines ovarian cancers with progression on platinum-based therapy as "platinum refractory," those that recur less than 6 months after completion of platinum-based therapy as "platinum resistant," and those that recur more than 6 months after completing treatment with a platinum-based regimen as "platinum sensitive" (short for "potentially platinum sensitive"). In general, tumors resistant to platinum are more resistant to any cytotoxic agent. Women with primary platinum-refractory therapy have a very poor prognosis, and response to any subsequent treatment is unlikely. Patients with a complete response to second-line platinum therapy will usually have a shorter time to recurrence after the second treatment regimen than after the first (519), and recurrent ovarian cancers eventually become resistant to platinum and all other therapies.

While the categories of "platinum sensitivity" are useful shorthand predictors of likelihood of response to further treatment, and are practical for designing and reporting clinical trials to estimate whether similar groups of patients are being studied across studies, they must be combined with clinical judgment in selecting therapy in individual cases. For example, a woman with stage I clear cell carcinoma that recurs with diffuse disease 7 months after completion of adjuvant chemotherapy probably had no response to treatment at all, and her cancer will likely be refractory to further therapy. On the other hand, a woman with suboptimally debulked stage IV serous carcinoma that responds completely to primary chemotherapy and has a rise in CA-125 five months later probably has chemotherapy-sensitive disease and is very likely to have some tumor shrinkage with a second line of treatment. The effects of prolonged consolidation therapy on future disease sensitivity have not been well studied, and are likely to vary with the agent used. Women who have tumors that repeatedly respond to a variety of therapies can sometimes be retreated with an agent to which their tumor had previously developed resistance after sufficient time has elapsed. For example, Kavanagh et al. published results describing 3 women with less than a complete response to primary platinum therapy who had a subsequent response to taxane therapy and over a year since their previous platinum therapy who then obtained a partial response to single-agent carboplatin (520). Finally, survival and sensitivity to treatment may sometimes be separable issues, and this should be taken into account in therapy planning. A few ovarian cancers (borderline tumors being one end of the spectrum) will be unresponsive to treatment but slow growing and associated with relatively longer survival.

General principles of treating recurrent disease include:

1. Although platinum-sensitive tumors are more sensitive than platinum-resistant tumors to any cytotoxic agent tested to date, most data suggest platinum compounds are the most active single agents in women with platinum-sensitive recurrent disease.
2. Platinum-based combinations produce superior response rates and progression-free survival compared with single-agent platinum therapy in women with platinum-sensitive disease; the effect on overall survival is less certain. In women with platinum-resistant disease, combination therapy has never been shown to provide any benefit.
3. No agents except possibly taxanes have consistently produced response rates over 20% in women with platinum-resistant disease.
4. Treatment must be recognized as primarily palliative, and decisions about treatment regimens should include patient convenience and toxicity as well as efficacy.

Single Agents in Platinum-Sensitive Disease

Response rates in multicenter trials testing single-agent cisplatin or carboplatin in women with platinum-sensitive disease are 30% to 50% (521,522), and, as discussed above, tend to be higher in women with a longer platinum-free interval. Response rates in multicenter trials to single-agent paclitaxel, topotecan, or liposomal doxorubicin in platinum-sensitive disease have generally been in the range of 20% to 30% (521,523), although one randomized phase 2 study comparing single-agent paclitaxel to a cyclophosphamide, doxorubicin, cisplatin combination therapy in women with platinum-sensitive disease reported a response rate of 45% for single-agent paclitaxel (vs. 55% for the platinum-based combination) (524). It is always difficult to compare activity of agents across trials because of bias as to which patients are entered on the various studies and variation in the rigidity of determination of response and progression-free interval. There are few randomized data comparing single-agent platinum compounds to other single agents in women with platinum-sensitive disease. The EORTC randomized 86 women to either single-agent paclitaxel or single-agent oxaliplatin. Responses among the 63 platinum-resistant patients were 5 out of 31 (16%) for paclitaxel and 2 out of 32 (6%) for oxaliplatin. Responses among the platinum-sensitive patients were 2 out of 10 (20%) for paclitaxel and 5 out of 13 (38%) for oxaliplatin (525).

Repeated courses of carboplatin therapy place patients at risk for hypersensitivity reactions. The incidence in patients treated with seven or more cycles of platinum-based therapy (typically the second dose of the second regimen) has been reported to be 27% (526). These reactions occur during drug infusion and are associated with flushing, nausea, and hypertension. Atypical hypersensitivity reactions, occurring after drug infusion, have also been described (527). A number of desensitization protocols have been published and appear to be generally effective (528); moreover, not all patients allergic to carboplatin will be allergic to cisplatin. However, the reactions are frightening and may be fatal, and desensitization protocols are time consuming for the patient and decrease the convenience of carboplatin therapy. Routine use of diphenhydramine premedication has been reported to produce a non-significant decrease in reaction rate (529).

Platinum-Based Combination Therapy in Platinum-Sensitive Disease

Results of several retrospective analyses of carboplatin/paclitaxel combination therapy in women with platinum-sensitive disease showed strikingly high response rates of 70% to 90% (530,531), and raised the question of whether combination therapy was superior to single-agent therapy in this setting. There have now been several randomized trials comparing platinum-based combination therapy to single-agent platinum therapy (Table 25.20) (521,522,524,532,533,534). As a group they show a superior response rate and superior progression-free survival with combination therapy. Results regarding overall survival are conflicting. Only the ICON4/AGO-OVAR-2.2, a combined analysis of two parallel trials comparing paclitaxel

TABLE 25.20

SINGLE-AGENT THERAPY VERSUS COMBINATION THERAPY IN PLATINUM-SENSITIVE RECURRENT OVARIAN CANCER

Author (year)	n	Regimen	RR	Median PFS	Median OS
Bolis 2001 (Ref 532)	190	Carboplatin	56%	3 yr 12%	3 yr 29%
		Carboplatin + epidoxorubicin	62% p = NS	3 yr 25%	3 yr 42% p = NS
Cantu 2002 (Ref 524)	97	Paclitaxel CAP	45% 55% p = NS	9 mo 16 mo	26 mo 35 mo
Parmar (ICON4/AGO-OVAR 2.2) (2003) (Ref 534)	802	Platinum[a] Platinum + paclitaxel	54% 66% p = 0.06	10 mo 13 mo	24 mo 29 mo
Pfisterer (2006) (Ref 522)	356	Carboplatin Carboplatin + gemcitabine	31% 47% p = 0.0016	5.8 mo 8.6 mo p = 0.0031	17.3 mo 18 mo
Gonzalez-Martin (2005) (Ref 521)	81	Carboplatin Carboplatin + paclitaxel	50% 75%	— —	73 wk Not yet reached
Alberts (2008) Ref 533	61	Carboplatin Carboplatin + liposomal/doxorubicin	32% 67% p = 0.02	8 mo 12 mo p = 0.06	18 mo 26 mo p = 0.02

Note: CAP, cisplatin/doxorubicin/cyclophosphamide; NS, not significant; OS, overall survival; PFS, progression-free survival; RR, response rate.
[a]control arm in CAP or single agent carboplatin

plus platinum to "conventional platinum-based chemotherapy" (71% received single-agent carboplatin, 17% cisplatin/ doxorubicin/ cyclophosphamide, and 12% other nontaxane platinum-based regimens), showed convincing survival benefit; the absolute improvement in overall survival was 5 months (from 24 months to 29 months) (534). Seventy-five percent of patients entered had a treatment-free interval of more than 12 months. The rate of grade 2 or greater neuropathy on the combination arm was 20%. Only about 40% of the patients had received prior taxane therapy, and this has raised concerns about the generalizability of the results (although there was no significant statistical interaction between survival benefit and prior taxane therapy). This trial also does not in any way address the question of whether sequential therapy might produce the same overall survival results as combination therapy. It was noted that only 31% of patients in the nontaxane arm received taxane therapy at the time of progression.

It is interesting that the ICON4 trial showed superior survival with a platinum/taxol combination compared to single-agent platinum in women with relapsed disease, whereas the ICON3 trial conducted by the same investigators showed no advantage with the addition of paclitaxel to front-line therapy. It is possible that the recurrent group of tumors, albeit noncurable, are overall more chemotherapy sensitive than the group of tumors initially presenting, as the majority of completely resistatant to therapy will not have survived to recur. Hence the differences between combination and single-agent therapy will be more obvious. However, there may be other unexplained factors as well.

The GCIC trial randomizing women to carboplatin and to carboplatin plus gemcitabine was not powered to show an overall survival difference; however, despite a superior response rate and progression-free interval with combination treatment, there is no evidence of a trend to survival benefit (530). There were no differences in quality of life scores between the two arms of that trial; the primary difference in toxicities was increased hematologic toxicity of the combination regimen, with 27% versus 8% grade 3/4 anemia, 70% versus 12% grade 3/4 neutropenia, and 35% versus 11% grade 3/4 thrombocytopenia.

As with front-line therapy, it could be hypothesized that combination therapy in the second-line setting will not produce any overall survival when compared to an appropriately designed sequential regimen, and may well produce more toxicity. The argument could be made that combination therapy is appropriate even if there is no survival benefit since (a) there would be more likely resolution of symptoms (if there are any symptoms to resolve); (b) improved quality of life due to decreased anxiety during the time of nonprogressing disease might overcome any decreased quality of life due to increased toxicity (not proven); (c) most convincingly, if a complete response is obtained, there would be higher likelihood of a meaningful period of time off chemotherapy (as the majority of patients in the United States are not given prolonged chemotherapy holidays in the presence of visible disease). It should be kept in mind that only a minority of patients achieve a complete response even with combination therapy; CR rate was 14.6% to the gemcitabine/carboplatin combination in the GCIG trial, and 27% to carboplatin/

paclitaxel in the GEICO trial. Nonetheless, platinum-based combinations have become the usual treatment in the United States for women who relapse more than 12 months after the completion of primary therapy, with single-agent therapy usual in women who have an initial treatment-free interval of less than 6 months, and individualized decisions in those with a 6- to 12-month treatment-free interval.

Treatment of Platinum-Resistant Disease—Randomized Trials of Nonplatinum Chemotherapy

Several phase 3 randomized trials have been informative in guiding our treatment of platinum-resistant disease, although several of them also included women with platinum-sensitive tumors (Table 25.21). Together they show that response rates to conventional single-agent therapy in this group of women are about 10%, median progression-free survival is about 3 to 4 months, and median overall survival is 9 to 12 months.

In 1997 ten Bokkel Huinink et al. published a trial performed before paclitaxel was a part of standard front-line therapy. Patients who progressed during or after platinum-based therapy received either topotecan 1.5 mg/m^2 daily for 5 days or paclitaxel 175 mg/m^2. Overall response rates were 20.5% and 13.2% in the topotecan and paclitaxel group, respectively (p = 0.138). Response rates in the platinum-resistant subgroup were 13% for topotecan and 7% for paclitaxel. Twenty-five percent of patients treated with topotecan experienced neutropenic fever, and 25% had grade 4 thrombocytopenia. A large number of patients (110) crossed over to the alternative drug as third-line therapy. Thirteen percent of topotecan-treated patients responded to paclitaxel and 10% of paclitaxel-treated patients responded to topotecan (535).

Another phase 3 trial in women who were platinum pretreated but paclitaxel naïve has been reported in abstract form only (536). O'Byrne et al. randomized women to paclitaxel versus liposomal doxorubicin; the trial is underpowered as it stopped early when paclitaxel became commercially available. No significant differences between the agents were seen in either platinum-sensitive or platinum-resistant patients.

Topotecan and pegylated liposomal doxorubicin were compared in a phase 3 trial of 474 women who did not respond to or progressed after first-line platinum-based therapy. The majority had received prior paclitaxel. Patients were randomized to topotecan 1.5 mg/m^2 days 1 to 5 every 3 weeks versus liposomal doxorubicin 50 mg/m^2 every 4 weeks (523). Overall response rates to liposomal doxorubicin and topotecan were 20% and 17%; in the platinum-resistant group they were 12% and 7%. Progression-free survival for platinum-resistant patients was 9 weeks for liposomal doxorubicin and 14 weeks for topotecan; overall survivals were 36 weeks and 41 weeks. At final analysis, there was an 18% reduction in the risk of death for patients treated with liposomal doxorubicin (537). However, this was observed primarily in women with platinum-sensitive disease; survival with the two agents was similar in platinum-refractory disease. This trial confirmed that there are a small number of patients with platinum-refractory disease who have relatively prolonged survival. The 3-year survival for women with platinum-refractory disease treated with liposomal doxorubicin was 13.8% (9.5% for topotecan). Twenty-two percent of patients treated with liposomal doxorubicin experienced grade 3 palmar-plantar erythrodysesthesia. Seventy-seven percent of patients on topotecan experienced grade 3/4 neutropenia and 28% had grade 3/4 thrombocytopenia.

A small trial randomized 234 women who had recurred within 12 months of initial platinum-based therapy (median 3 months) to single-agent paclitaxel versus epidoxorubicin plus paclitaxel (537). The response rate was 37% for the combination and 47% for single-agent paclitaxel; median survival was 12 months and 14 months, respectively.

Mutch et al. (538) compared pegylated liposomal doxorubicin 50 mg/m^2 every 4 weeks to gemcitabine 1,000 mg/m^2 on days 1 and 8 every 21 days in 195 women with platinum-resistant or refractory ovarian cancer. One or two prior chemotherapy regimens were permitted, and platinum resistance was defined according to exposure to the most recent platinum-based regimen. Response rates were 6.1% for gemcitabine and 8.3% for liposomal doxorubicin; progression-free and overall survivals were similar for the two regimens. One hundred thirty patients crossed over to the alternate therapy; the response rate in those who crossed over to gem-citabine was 7.6%; in those who crossed over to liposomal doxorubicin it was 4.7%. Liposomal doxorubicin was associatd with more grade 2/3 mucositis (16%) and palmar-plantar erythrodysesthesia (20%); gemcitabine was associated with more grade 3/4 neutropenia (38%), fatigue (11%), and nausea and vomiting (12%). Four patients in each arm experienced febrile neutropenia.

TABLE 25.21

PHASE 3 TRIALS OF SINGLE-AGENT THERAPY

Author (year)	n	Regimen	Overall RR	Platinum sensitive RR	Platinum-resistant RR	Median PFS	Median OS
ten Bokkel Humink (1997) (Ref 535)	226 (119 res)	Paclitaxel Topotecan	13% 21%	20% 29%	7% 13%	14 wk 23 wk	43 wk 61 wk
Gordon (2001) (Ref 523)	474 (154 res)	Liposomal doxorubicin Topotecan	20% 17%	28% 29%	12% 7%	18 wk 17 wk	60 wk 57 wk
O'Byrne (2002) (Ref 536)	214 (n/a)	Liposomal doxorubicin Paclitaxel	18% 22%	n/a n/a	n/a n/a	22 wk 22 wk	46 wk 56 wk
Gore (2002) (Ref 549)	266 (152 res)	Oral topotecan IV topotecan	13% 20%	19% 36%	8% 8%	13 wk 17 wk	51 wk 58 wk
Mutch (2007) (Ref 538)	195 (all res)	Liposomal doxorubicin Gemcitabine	— —	— —	8.3% 6.1%	3.1 mo 3.6 mo	13.5 mo 12.7 mo

Note: IV, intravenous; n/a, not available; OS, overall survival; PFS, progression-free survival; res, platinum-resistant; RR, response rate; wk, weeks; mo, months.

TABLE 25.22

AGENTS IN TREATMENT OF PLATINUM-REFRACTORY OVARIAN CANCER

Hexamethamelamine
Bevacizumab
Docetaxel
Epirubicin
po Etoposide
Gemcitabine
Ifosfamide
Tamoxifen
Weekly paclitaxel
Topotecan
Vinorelbine
Pegylated liposomal doxorubicin
Irinotecan

Agents Useful in Treatment of Platinum-Resistant Disease

A list of agents with some activity in the treatment of platinum-resistant recurrent ovarian cancer is shown in Table 25.22. Taxanes, liposomal doxorubicin, topotecan, and gemcitabine have been studied in randomized trials, as discussed above. They are discussed in slightly more detail below. Hexamethamelamine (altretamine) is an older alkylating agent with the advantages (patient convenience) and disadvantages (inappropriate for patients with episodic or partial small bowel obstruction, limited availability for patients without good insurance coverage for outpatient medication) of an oral therapy. It is rarely used, as it produces significant amounts of neuropathy, nausea, and vomiting. A GOG phase 2 trial of single-agent hexamethamelamine in women with platinum-resistant ovarian cancer demonstrated a 10% response rate and a 21% rate of grade 3 emesis (539). Oral etoposide, a topoisomerase II inhibitor, is better tolerated and may be slightly more active; however, it is leukemogenic, which has limited enthusiasm for attempts to incorporate it into front-line therapy. Interestingly, IV etoposide appears to have minimal activity in women with pretreated ovarian cancer. Ifosfamide has produced response rates of 10% to 20%, but the toxicities, hematologic and neurologic, are excessive compared to those of other available agents, and it is also rarely used (540). Response rates were not noticeably better in women who had not received a prior alkylating agent (i.e., cyclophosphamide). Irinotecan is associated with substantial diarrhea and nausea (541), which can be particularly troublesome in ovarian cancer patients with some preexisting level of bowel dysfunction; it will hopefully be better tolerated as part of the ongoing front-line international trial for clear cell carcinoma. Epothilones are a group of investigational antitubulin agents with activity against platinum-refractory ovarian cancer. However, they cause neuropathy, and their eventual place in the armamentarium against ovarian cancer remains to be established.

Hormonal therapies such as tamoxifen and antiangiogenics such as bevacizumab are discussed below. Response rates to hormonal treatment by modern standards are hard to gauge, as most of the trials are quite old; however, it does appear that selected patients may respond and toxicities are minimal. Antiangiogenics appear very promising in the treatment of ovarian cancer. None, including bevacizumab, are currently FDA approved for the treatment of ovarian cancer, all are exceedingly expensive, and bevacizumab has been associated with a number of toxicities, including an increased number of bowel perforations.

Taxanes. Although in most parts of the world, taxane therapy is part of front-line treatment for ovarian cancer, taxanes remain very useful in treating recurrent disease. Both weekly paclitaxel (542,543) and docetaxel (544) have shown response rates of 20% to 30% in women who recurred within 6 months of primary platinum-taxane–based combination therapy. Weekly paclitaxel is particularly useful, as it tends to be less myelotoxic than many other regimens.

Interest in the use of weekly paclitaxel had been stimulated by results in women with metastatic breast cancer in whom weekly paclitaxel at a dose of 80 mg/m^2 per week produced less myelosuppression and a superior response rate and overall survival when compared to a schedule of 175 mg/m^2 per week (545). However, the same superiority has not yet been documented in ovarian cancer. Rosenberg et al. randomized 208 patients with pretreated ovarian cancer to every-3-week paclitaxel at 200 mg/m^2 per week or weekly paclitaxel at a dose of 67 mg/m^2 per week (with the goal to have similar total doses of paclitaxel in the trial arm). There was no difference in efficacy between the two arms, but less toxicity (other than fingernail toxicity) in the weekly arm (546). This paclitaxel dose, however, is lower than the 80 mg/m^2 most commonly used in current therapy. Weekly administration of paclitaxel has resulted in about a 20% objective response rate in ovarian cancer patients with clinically defined resistance to platinum and standard every-3-week paclitaxel (543).

ABI-007 is a newer taxane with the advantage that it does not require steroid premedication to avoid hypersensitivity reactions. However, its activity in patients resistant to platinum/paclitaxel therapy remains to be defined.

Topotecan. Topotecan, a topoisomerase I inhibitor, is FDA approved for the treatment of recurrent ovarian cancer, and as discussed above, is as effective as or more effective than paclitaxel or liposomal doxorubicin in women with platinum-resistant disease. However, the FDA-approved schedule of 1.5 mg/m^2 daily $\times$ 5 every 3 weeks is not a convenient regimen and has proved more myelosuppressive than most treating physicians deem reasonable in the palliative setting. Lower starting doses of 1.0 to 1.25 mg/m^2 are more commonly employed, although their efficacy is not as well documented. Individuals at increased risk for myelotoxicity include those with impaired renal function, older age, extensive prior therapy, or prior pelvic irradiation.

Weekly bolus topotecan has been shown to have some activity in a number of small trials, and has come into common use (547). The maximum tolerated dose (MTD) in phase 1 studies was 4 mg/m^2 with dose-limiting toxicities of anemia, chronic fatigue, and gastrointestinal distress. However, there are no data showing that the weekly schedule is as effective as the daily $\times$ 5 schedule. A preliminary report presented on a randomized phase 2 trial of topotecan 4 mg/m^2 3 weeks out of 4 versus topotecan 1.25 mg/m^2 daily $\times$ 5 in women with platinum-resistant ovarian cancer showed a numerically lower response rate for the weekly schedule (2 of 28 vs. 5 of 21 for the daily $\times$ 5 regimen) (548).

As shown in Table 25.21, Gore et al. randomized women who had failed one prior platinum-based regimen to oral topotecan (which is not currently available) or IV topotecan 1.5 mg/m^2 per day every 21 days. The authors separated out response rates for platinum-refractory (progressive or stable disease during primary chemotherapy) and platinum-resistant disease (initial response but relapse within 6 months of completing chemotherapy; these two categories are combined in the table). For women with platinum-refractory disease, the response to IV topotecan was 5%; for those with platinum-resistant disease it was 11% (549).

Liposomal Doxorubicin. Liposomal doxorubicin is also FDA approved for the treatment of recurrent ovarian cancer. The every-4-week schedule of administration is convenient, and the lack of alopecia is attractive to patients. However, the high incidence of palmar-plantar erythrodysesthesia is unappealing for a palliative regimen. Markman et al. published a nonrandomized phase 2 trial suggesting that the there was only a 12% incidence of grade 2 and no grade 3 palmar-plantar erythrodysesthesia when the starting dose was lowered from 50 mg/m^2 to 40 mg/m^2. The response rate was 9%; all patients were platinum/paclitaxel resistant with a median of two prior regimens (550).

Gemcitabine. As discussed above, gemcitabine has modest activity in the treatment of recurrent ovarian cancer. Based on experimental models, it was hypothesized that combining gemcitabine with cisplatin might reverse platinum resistance. Cisplatin-resistant cells upregulate nucleotide excision repair complexes, which are thought to be inhibited by gemcitabine. Preclinical models suggested synergy between cisplatin and gemcitabine in platinum-resistant cell lines. However, while some early clinical reports appeared promising, a multicenter GOG trial of the combination as second-line therapy in women with platinum-resistant ovarian cancer reported a response rate of only 16% (551).

Hormonal Therapy

The ovary is an endocrine organ. There is evidence (discussed above) for the role of endocrine factors in the etiology of ovarian cancer, and ovarian cancers frequently express estrogen and progesterone receptors. Multiple attempts have therefore been made to treat ovarian carcinoma with hormonal therapy, including progestins, antiestrogens, and gonadotropin-releasing hormone (GnRH) analogs. The response rates generally are quite low, in the range of 10% (552). It seems clear that some patients respond, but there are no good means of selecting them. Many of the trials were performed decades ago, before steroid receptor analysis was available, and the role of steroid receptors in predicating response of ovarian carcinomas to hormonal therapy remains unclear. Of note, over 90% of serous borderline ovarian tumors are estrogen-receptor positive (367), and there are case reports of major responses to tamoxifen (553,554), leuprolide (368), and anastrozole (369).

Progestins/Antiprogestins

As discussed above, progesterone appears to play a protective role in the etiology of ovarian cancer. The protective role of pregnancy may be due to the tenfold increase in maternal circulating progesterone levels as well as suppression of ovulation. Combination oral contraceptive formulations with high progestin potency appear to be associated with a greater reduction in ovarian cancer risk than those with low progestin potency. In addition, overexpression of progesterone receptor (PR) has been found to be a favorable prognostic factor in women with invasive ovarian cancer. The most commonly reported progestins in the treatment of gynecologic malignancies are medroxyprogesterone acetate and megestrol acetate. A review of 13 trials of 10 patients or more (432 patients total) revealed a major response rate of 7.2%, with stable disease in 10.9%. Progestins have well-documented activity in the treatment of recurrent endometrial carcinoma, and it has therefore been hypothesized that they will have activity in the endometrioid subset of ovarian cancers, which tend to express high levels of progesterone receptors. One series of 43 patients with ovarian endometrioid carcinoma using medroxyprogesterone acetate as first-line therapy postsurgery or postradiotherapy was reported in 1982. Eighty-four percent of the patients had well-differentiated disease. Forty-one of them underwent second-look laparotomy after 6 to 8 months of therapy. Twenty-three had evidence of tumor regression and eight had no evidence of disease. Tumor regression was observed in 68% of the 31 cancers that were positive for both estrogen receptor (ER) and PR and in none of the cancers that did not express either receptor (553). In one phase 2 study of megestrol acetate in 36 platinum-refractory ovarian cancer patients, three complete responders were observed; all had tumors of endometrioid histology (554).

RU486 (mifepristone) is a synthetic antiprogestin that competitively binds the progesterone receptor (as well as the glucocorticoid receptor) and inhibits ovarian cancer cell growth *in vitro*. One phase 2 trial using RU486 in the treatment of platinum-resistant ovarian cancer patients has been reported with a 26.5% response rate, including one complete response of over 3 years' duration (555). Seven of the nine responders had grade 3 tumors. Rash was the primary treatment-limiting toxicity.

Estrogen Therapy/Estrogen Progestin Combinations

Diethylstilbestrol (DES), which was formerly used to treat endocrine-response breast cancer, has also been tested in the management of ovarian cancer, based on the hypothesis that it would inhibit gonadotropin production. One series published in 1963 reported on 14 ovarian carcinoma patients treated with 15 to 30 mg DES daily. There were two objective responses lasting more than a year and two patients with disappearance of ascites and an increased sense of well-being (556).

Estrogens and tamoxifen have the ability to upregulate progesterone receptor expression, and have therefore been used to try to improve the benefit observed with progestin therapy. Two trials treated women with sequential ethinyl estradiol 50 µg per day and medroyprogesterone acetate 200 mg per day with response rates of 14% and 17% (557,558). Some patients required dose reduction of the ethinyl estradiol because of severe nausea. Two trials have also treated women with sequential tamoxifen and progestins; no responses were observed (559,560).

Tamoxifen

Tamoxifen is a selective estrogen receptor modulator (SERM) with estrogen agonist activity on some tissues (such as bone) and antagonist activity on breast cancers. One review of 18 trials including 648 patients testing tamoxifen in the treatment of advanced ovarian cancer found an overall 13% response rate (561). There was marked heterogeneity in the response rates, suggesting that selection bias (for unknown factors) may be very important. A randomized controlled trial comparing tamoxifen to triptorelin showed no responses in either arm (562). The relationship between hormone receptor status and response to tamoxifen (or other hormonal therapy) is not clear. In the 1980s the GOG conducted a trial of tamoxifen 20 mg po bid (twice the dose commonly used in the treatment of breast cancer) in 105 women with previously treated ovarian cancer. There was an overall 17% response rate, including 13% complete responses. Eight of the nine patients achieving a complete response had elevated levels of estrogen receptor (563). However, the difference in response by estrogen receptor status was not statistically significant. It has been suggested that tamoxifen might be an appropriate therapy for women with small-volume asymptomatic recurrences. The GOG has completed a randomized trial comparing tamoxifen to thalidomide for the therapy of women who have CA-125 marker elevation but no measurable recurrence of disease, and results should be available soon.

GnRH Agonists

GnRH receptors are expressed on about 80% of ovarian cancers. A summary of 12 published trials using GnRH agonists in women with recurrent ovarian cancer noted an overall 5.7% response rate and a disease stabilization rate of 21% with only one complete responder (552). In the largest trial, which was conducted by the EORTC, there were no responders among 68 evaluable patients. One report suggested that responses may be more frequent in low-grade tumors. As low-grade ovarian cancers may respond less well to chemotherapy, and as GnRH agonists have very low toxicity in postmenopausal women, they are a reasonable option for this group of tumors. Like other hormonal therapies, they may also be active against stromal tumors. Of 12 patients treated in four reports of the use of GnRH agonists for ovarian granulosa cell tumors, there were 4 patients with a partial response and 4 with stable disease (552).

GnRH antagonists cause rapid suppression of gonadotropin secretion without the initial gonadotropin release caused by GnRH agonists. There has been one trial of the GnRH antagonist cetrorelix in 17 patients with ovarian or müllerian carcinoma refractory to platinum chemotherapy. Three patients (18%) experienced a partial remission (564).

Aromatase Inhibitors

The major source of estrogen (principally estrone) in postmenopausal women is aromatization of androstenedione in the skin and adipose tissues. Commercially available third-generation aromatase inhibitors include anastrazole, letrozole, and exemestane. Five phase 2 trials of aromatase inhibitors have reported 7 major responses among 179 patients with measurable disease by RECIST (Response Evaluation Criteria in Solid Tumors) critera (4%) and 16 CA-125 responses among 124 patients with CA-125 evaluable disease (13%) (552). One report suggested that higher ER, lower HER2, and higher EGFR were associated with CA-125 stable or responsive disease (565).

Androgen/Antiandrogen Therapy

About half of ovarian cancers have been reported to express the androgen receptor (552). As discussed above (under Pathogenesis) there is also some epidemiologic evidence supporting a role of androgens in the genesis of ovarian cancer. Two studies of androgen therapy did not report any objective responses (566). Two small studies of the nonsteroidal antiandrogen flutamide noted response rates of 4.3% and 8.7% and disease stabilization rates of 8.7% and 28%.

Front-Line Chemohormonal Therapy

Most of the trials of single-agent hormonal therapy have been in pretreated patients. There have been several small negative randomized studies comparing chemohormonal therapy to chemotherapy in patients with previously untreated advanced disease. Schwartz et al. treated 100 patients with the combination of doxorubin plus cisplatin. Half were randomized to concomitant tamoxifen. There was no difference in overall or progression-free survival between the groups (567). Similarly, Emons et al. enrolled 135 patients to a prospective double-blinded, randomized trial comparing chemotherapy with chemotherapy plus triptorelin (568). There was no difference between the groups in response, survival, or time to disease progression. Finally, a small randomized trial of 71 patients showed no differences between chemotherapy and chemotherapy plus medroxyprogesterone acetate (569).

SELECTED ISSUES IN PALLIATIVE CARE

Palliative Radiotherapy

Radiation therapy as a palliative modality in ovarian cancer is often neglected, but may be very useful if the sole or dominant symptomatic problem for the patient is localized to a site and volume that may be safely encompassed in a radiation field. For example, a fixed pelvic mass eroding the vaginal mucosa causing bleeding, pain, or bowel or bladder dysfunction may occur without obvious disseminated symptomatic peritoneal disease. Tumor regression or symptomatic relief can often be obtained in these situations from local irradiation. Similarly, radiation may be employed to treat localized masses elsewhere in the abdomen, such as the retroperitoneal nodes. Palliative irradiation may also be useful for extra-abdominal disease, particularly supraclavicular or inguinal node masses and bony or brain metastases.

Limited data are available from the literature concerning the palliative efficacy of radiation therapy in these settings (570–572). Using large single-fraction irradiation, one to three fractions of 10 Gy, investigators at the M.D. Anderson Cancer Center reported overall response rates of 55% and 71% among ovarian cancer patients palliated for pain and bleeding, respectively. However, 6 of 42 patients so treated did develop severe bowel radiation injury that may be attributable to the large fractions employed. Another report of palliative radiation therapy used after initial management with cisplatin-containing regimens documented that radiation therapy produced a mean symptom-free interval of 8.5 months in a group of patients with a median survival of 19.5 months (572). A study from Fox Chase Cancer Center (570) reported the use of fractionated palliative irradiation in 33 patients with symptomatic ovarian cancer in 47 irradiated sites. For the entire group, complete palliative response was seen in 51% of patients, and overall palliative responses occurred in 79%. The median duration of palliation was 4 months, which reflected palliation until death in 90% of cases. Vaginal or rectal bleeding was controlled in 90% and 85%, respectively, and pain relief occurred in 83%. A range of radiation doses was employed, but it is unclear whether patients with better performance status received the higher doses. Palliation was improved in those with higher Karnofsky performance status and in those who received biologically effective doses (BED) of at least 44 Gy (e.g., 35 Gy in 14 fractions). In a recently reported study from the Memorial Sloan-Kettering Cancer Center, variable doses of palliative irradiation were given to a group of 33 patients with platinum-refractory disease who had not previously received paclitaxel. Complete subjective or objective responses were observed in 70% (571). Firm recommendations on the optimal dose for palliation cannot be made; none of the papers provides sufficient detail to do a multivariate analysis of factors predictive of the observed palliative response. Also, the palliative dose fractionation schemes employed do not allow the construction of a dose-response curve. However, it is clear that durable palliation may be achieved with local radiation therapy for ovarian cancer recurring after cisplatin-based chemotherapy, particularly in patients with good performance status.

Palliative Surgery for Obstruction

For the majority of women with ovarian cancer, the disease eventually progresses within the abdominal cavity. Such tumor growth often produces compromise of the intestinal lumen, leading to intestinal obstruction that requires hospitalization for intravenous hydration and decompression of the intestinal tract. Since these patients generally have no impairment of other vital organ systems, they are often completely alert and in little or no pain. If conservative measures fail to result in relief of the obstruction, the patient and her physician must then confront a difficult decision: prolonged in-hospital (or at-home) intravenous hydration and gastric decompression, or an attempt at surgical relief of the obstruction. In making this decision, one must consider a number of factors, including the patient's overall physical condition, the current status of her cancer and future therapeutic options, the site of the intestinal obstruction, and the extent of her prior therapy, including prior surgical procedures, intraperitoneal chemotherapy, and radiation therapy. A number of investigators have attempted to identify clinical factors that would allow selection of patients unlikely to benefit from surgery for intestinal obstruction so that these women might be saved exploration. Krebs and Goplerud (574) identified a series of variables, including advanced age, poor nutritional status, the presence of palpable tumor masses, the presence of ascites, and a history of previous radiation therapy to the pelvis or whole abdomen, that were associated with a poor outcome. Other studies (515) have reported that the serum albumin level, nutritional status, and the amount of residual ovarian cancer at the completion of bowel obstruction surgery were significantly associated with postoperative survival. On the other hand, in one study (575), no clinical features could be identified that would predict operability or survival following surgery. These differences may be accounted for, in part, by variation in patient selection and preoperative and postoperative care.

The site of intestinal obstruction in ovarian cancer patients is most commonly the small intestine. If the patient is felt to be an operative candidate, consideration should be given to the use of preoperative total parenteral nutrition to improve the patient's nutritional status and decrease the risk of perioperative complications related to malnutrition. Total parenteral nutrition is generally not indicated in patients in whom no surgery is planned. In a series of 54 operations performed for intestinal obstruction in ovarian cancer patients, Rubin et al. (576) reported that the site of obstruction was in the small intestine in 44%, the large intestine in 33%, and involved both small and large intestines in the remaining 22% of cases. A definitive surgical procedure for relief of obstruction was performed in 79% of the patients in this series; the remaining patients were explored and judged to be inoperable. Among the patients undergoing a definitive procedure, about 80% were discharged from the hospital with restoration of intestinal function sufficient to allow a regular or low-residue diet. The mean postsurgical survival among these patients was 6.8 months. In a more recent report from the Memorial Sloan-Kettering Cancer Center (577), the investigators retrospectively reviewed all patients undergoing surgery for intestinal obstruction due to recurrent ovarian cancer from 1994 to 1999. During the study period, 68 operations were performed on 64 patients. The mean time from original diagnosis of ovarian cancer to obstruction was 2.8 years. Surgical correction (intestinal surgery performed for relief of obstruction) was attained in 57 of 68 (84%) cases. Successful palliation (the ability to tolerate a regular or low-residue diet at least 60 days postoperatively) was achieved in 71% of cases in which surgical correction was possible. The rate of major surgical morbidity was 22%. There was one death from pulmonary embolus and one from peritonitis. Two other deaths occurred because of progression of disease, for an overall perioperative mortality rate of 6%. Postoperative chemotherapy was administered in 45 of 57 (79%) cases in which surgical correction was possible. The median survival of the entire cohort was 8 months. If surgery resulted in successful palliation, median survival was 11.6 versus 3.9 months for all other patients. Although survival is relatively brief, by restoring intestinal function, at least temporarily, these patients can leave the hospital and enjoy an improved quality of life for their remaining months. In the absence of criteria that clearly predict operability, survival, and quality of life following surgery for intestinal obstruction in ovarian cancer patients, an active surgical approach should remain a management option. For patients who are deemed to be unsuitable for surgical exploration or found to be inoperable at exploration, gastrostomy, which can usually be accomplished percutaneously, offers a more comfortable alternative to prolonged nasogastric drainage (577).

Management of Ascites

Ascites is a common finding at the time of initial presentation in patients with advanced ovarian cancer. Generally, ascites does not produce any significant discomfort or respiratory embarrassment. Although the fluid may reaccumulate in the days following initial surgery, once chemotherapy is begun, it usually resolves quickly. In the occasional patient in whom massive ascites causes respiratory compromise, either before or after surgery, paracentesis may be performed safely for temporary relief prior to the initiation of chemotherapy. Cruikshank and Buchsbaum (578), using hemodynamic monitoring, showed that large quantities of ascites can be rapidly removed from ovarian cancer patients without untoward effects. This also appears to have little significant effect on serum proteins. The failure of ascites to resolve after the initiation of chemotherapy or its reappearance later in the course of treatment is an indication of lack of response to treatment and a grave prognostic sign.

Although the majority of patients with advanced ovarian cancer will eventually experience progression of disease, most do not develop clinically significant ascites. For those who do, therapeutic options are limited. Instillation of bleomycin into the peritoneal cavity as a nonspecific sclerotic agent has been reported but has been minimally effective in ovarian cancer (579,580). Experience with implanted peritoneovenous shunts has been poor, with a significant rate of blockage and the risk of embolization and implantation of tumor cells (581). In the absence of effective therapy for the patient's underlying cancer, it is usually not currently possible to control ascites other than on a temporary basis. The potential antiascites effects of the antiangiogenic agents are intriguing. An ongoing double-blind randomized trial is testing the effectiveness of single-agent intravenous VEGF trap for the control of ascites in women who have failed all other therapy for ovarian cancer. A preliminary abstract reported on nine patients (three with colon cancer, three with breast cancer, two with uterine cancer, and one with ovarian cancer) who had ascites that had reaccumulated within 2 weeks of paracentesis and were treated with a single dose of intraperitoneal bevacizumab monthly. No patient had a major antitumor response, but no patient had reaccumulation of ascites within 2 months (582).

NEW DIRECTIONS

Molecular Targeted Therapies

The group of newer targeted therapies with the most promise in the treatment of epithelial ovarian cancer to date is the antiangiogenic agents. None of the other available agents has shown appreciable activity, even though ovarian cancers express a number of the putative targets.

Agents Targeting Angiogenesis

Angiogenesis is crucial in the development of many cancers, including ovarian cancer. The most clinically advanced antiangiogenic therapeutics target vascular endothelial growth factor and its receptors, and a few of these are discussed below. Many other antiangiogenic agents are in various stages of development, and are of interest for the treatment of ovarian cancer. Most currently available anti-VEGF and anti-VEGF receptor (VEGFR) agents share (to a varying degree) a tendency to cause hypertension, and appropriate monitoring and treatment of blood pressure is critical to the safe use of these drugs.

Anti-VEGF Agents. Elevated vascular endothelial growth factor (VEGF or VEGF-A) expression occurs in all stages of ovarian cancer and is associated with poor prognosis, including shorter survival. In addition, VEGF (which is also known as vascular permeability factor) overexpression is directly associated with the production of ascitic fluid.

Bevacizumab is a humanized anti-VEGF monoclonal antibody that is currently FDA approved in the United States for the treatment of advanced colon cancer in combination with chemotherapy. Prospective trials have reported activity of single-agent bevacizumab against pretreated ovarian cancer to be in the range of 15% to 20%. The GOG evaluated single-agent bevacizumab in 63 patients who had one to two prior regimens of cytotoxic chemotherapy. The overall response rate was 21% with a median response duration of 10 months (583). Twenty-five of 62 patients had a progression-free survival (PFS) of ≥6 months. Cannistra et al. evaluated 44 patients with platinum-resistant disease that progressed after second-line topotecan or liposomal doxorubicin. The overall response rate was 16% (7 out of 44) (584). Another trial evaluated the combination of bevacizumab and metronomic (daily low-dose) oral cyclophosphamide. Fifty-six percent of patients were progression-free at 6 months and the overall response rate was 24% (585).

There has been caution in rapidly introducing bevacizumab into clinical use because (a) like many other newer anticancer agents, it is exceedingly expensive, and (b) it appears to cause an increased rate of bowel perforation. The study of Cannistra et al. described above closed early due to the higher than expected number of gastrointestinal perforations (5 out of 44), 1 of which was fatal. This led the NCI to alert investigators via an investigational new drug (IND) action letter dated October 4, 2005, of the risk of gastrointestinal perforation in ovarian cancer patients treated with bevacizumab (586). Despite this risk, the responses seen in heavily pretreated women and the durability of some of the responses observed have raised considerable interest in the treatment of ovarian cancer with bevacizumab. As discussed above, two randomized trials are currently testing the addition of bevacizumab to first-line therapy, one in the GOG (GOG 218) (Fig. 25.35) and one in the European Cooperative Group (ICON7). In the GOG trial bevacizumab/placebo is not given until the second cycle of chemotherapy to allow for adequate postoperative healing, and patients with any evidence of bowel obstruction are excluded. An early safety analysis was part of the study design, and the data and safety monitoring board did not recommend early stopping of the trial.

Another anti-VEGF agent of interest, which is not currently commercially available, is VEGF-Trap. VEGF-Trap is a high affinity soluble decoy receptor that comprises portions of the extracellular domains of both VEGFR-1 and VEGFR-2. Preliminary clinical trial reports suggest it has some activity against ovarian cancers that are platinum resistant (587). Preclinical data suggest that VEGF-Trap inhibits ascites in animal models, and it is currently being tested for the control of ascites in ovarian cancer patients who have failed other available treatments.

VEGF Receptor Tyrosine Kinase Inhibitors. VEGF actions are mediated through binding to receptor tyrosine kinases, including VEGFR-1(Flt-1) and VEGFR-2(KDR; whose murine form is known as Flk-1). Both are found predominantly on the surfaces of vascular endothelial cells. Numerous small molecule inhibitors of VEGF receptor tyrosine kinase are in clinical development. Many of these also inhibit other kinases of relevance, such as platelet-derived growth factor (PDGF) receptors. Single-agent phase 2 trials of sorafenib, sunitinib, and AZD2171 are under way or completed, and results are awaited with interest.

Thalidomide. Thalidomide is an interesting agent with documented activity in the treatment of erythema nodosum leprosum and multiple myeloma. Its mechanism of action is not well understood; it possesses both antiangiogenic and immunomodulatory properties. Complications are generally dose related and include somnolence, constipation, neuropathy, and thrombosis. An initial phase 2 trial including 19 patients with ovarian cancer showed no responses (588), but subsequent studies have documented CA-125 decreases and up to 18% partial responses in heavily pretreated ovarian cancer patients, with some of the responses lasting over a year (589,590). A phase 2 trial of the thalidomide derivative lenalidomide in 20 patients produced no major responses and only 4 patients with stable disease for 6 months or more. However, this was a particularly heavily pretreated group of patients with a median of five prior chemotherapy regimens (591). The GOG is currently conducting a randomized trial comparing tamoxifen to thalidomide for the therapy of women who have CA-125 marker elevation but no measurable recurrence of disease.

Agents Targeting Human Epidermal Growth Factor Receptor Family

The human epidermal growth factor receptor (HER) family comprises four transmembrane receptors, HER-1 (also called EGFR), HER-2 (HER2/neu, the target of trastuzumab), HER-3, and HER-4. The HER-1, -2, and -4 proteins are transmembrane tyrosine kinases that are autophosphorylated after homo- or heterodimerization, triggering a series of downstream events that ultimately affect cellular proliferation and survival. HER-3 does not possess tyrosine kinase activity, but can dimerize with other HER proteins. HER-1, -3, and -4 require ligand binding to dimerize; HER-2 has no known ligand, and can adopt a fixed conformation resembling a ligand-activated state, making it constitutively available for dimerization in the absence of a ligand (592). HER receptors are overexpressed or dysregulated in a variety of solid tumors, and a number of monoclonal antibodies and small molecule tyrosine kinase inhibitors of this pathway have been approved for use in different solid tumors. However, with the exception of HER2 gene amplification in breast cancer, molecular predictors of tumor response to these agents have been elusive. EGFR overexpression is no longer believed to accurately predict for response to the anti-EGFR monoclonal antibodies in colon cancer. While mutations in the tyrosine kinase domain of EGFR may predict response of lung cancers to the EGFR tyrosine kinase inhibitors (593), there also appears to be benefit in patients whose lung cancers do not have such a mutation. Results of immunohistochemical staining for EGFR in epithelial ovarian cancer tumor samples have varied widely, with detectable expression reported in 19% to 92% (594). Most studies suggest that dysregulation of EGFR in ovarian cancer is associated with worse survival. However, therapy targeting EGFR or HER2 has had minimal activity against ovarian cancers to date.

EGFR Tyrosine Kinase Inhibitors. As a group, the EGFR tyrosine kinase inhibitors tend to cause acneiform rash and diarrhea. It has been suggested that development of a rash predicts for longer survival with EGFR tyrosine kinase inhibitor treatment across tumor types. Several phase 2 trials using single-agent anti-EGFR small molecule tyrosine kinase inhibitors in women with pretreated ovarian cancer have been reported. Gordon et al. used single-agent erlotinib to treat 34 patients with refractory (up to three prior regimens with disease progression within 6 months of most recent therapy) EGFR-positive disease

(594). Two of 34 patients achieved a partial response (PR) (6%). Neither responder had strong EGFR expression; both had grade 2 rash. Patients with any grade rash had a significantly longer survival than those without (9.9 vs. 3.6 months, $p = 0.009$). The GOG reported on a phase 2 trial of gefitinib in women with up to two prior regimens and a platinum-free interval of less than 12 months (595). One of 27 evaluable patients (4%) had an objective partial response with a progression-free survival time of about 27 months. Forty-two percent of patients had EGFR expression (1+ or higher); exploratory analysis suggested an association between EGFR expression and progression-free survival. Grade 3 skin toxicity was also associated with improved progression-free survival. Only one of the 25 tumors examined had a mutation in exons 18-21 of the *EGFR*; this was in the patient with a partial response. The investigators also sequenced exons 18-21 of the *EGFR* in 32 additional cases of invasive epithelial ovarian cancer; one mutation was found. Two other phase 2 trials of gefitinib, one of which combined it with tamoxifen, reported no clinical responses (596,597).

The EORTC/GCIG is currently conducting a phase 3 trial of erlotinib for 2 years versus observation in women with responding or stable disease after first-line platinum-based therapy.

Anti-EGFR Monoclonal Antibodies. Cetuximab is an anti-EGFR monoclonal antibody FDA approved in the United States for the treatment of colon cancer. A phase 2 trial of cetuximab in women with pretreated ovarian cancer and was stopped after first stage as it produced only one response among the first 25 women treated (598). A phase 2 trial of matuzumab (EMD72000), a humanized anti-EGFR monoclonal antibody, produced no responses in 37 women with platinum-resistant EGFR-positive ovarian cancer (599).

Anti-HER2 Monoclonal Antibodies. Trastuzumab is an anti-HER2 monoclonal antibody approved for the treatment of breast cancer. The best predictor for response to trastuzumab in breast cancer patients appears to be tumor amplification of the HER2 gene. This is clinically tested by fluorescent *in situ* hybridization (FISH). Immunohistochemical staining for HER2 overexpression appears to be less predictive. HER2 overexpression has been reported in 11% to 30% of primary ovarian carcinomas, but in a higher percentage of women with metastatic or recurrent disease, including some in whom the primary tumor did not overexpress HER2 (600). In a phase 2 trial of trastuzumab conducted by the GOG only 11.2% of women with progressive or recurrent ovarian cancer had tumors that stained 2+ or 3+ for HER2 (601). Among women whose cancers were HER2 2+ or 3+, only 7.3% had a major response to trastuzumab (one CR, two PR). Gene amplification was not assessed in this study.

Pertuzumab is a monoclonal antibody that binds to an epitope on HER2 distinct from the trastuzumab-binding site, and prevents dimerization of HER2 with other receptors. HER2 amplification or overexpression does not appear to be necessary for antitumor activity. A randomized phase 2 trial testing two different doses of pertuzumab enrolled heavily pretreated ovarian cancer patients (median of five prior chemotherapy regimens). Five of 123 patients treated had a partial response. Where possible, fresh tumor biopsies were obtained for development of predictive testing, and there was a trend to improved progression-free survival for women with phospho-HER2+ tumors (602). Preliminary results of a subsequent trial that randomized women with platinum-resistant disease to gemcitabine or gemcitabine plus pertuzumab showed a 5% response rate for gemcitabine versus 14% for the combination (603).

Other Targeted Agents

Imatinib is a receptor tyrosine kinase inhibitor with potent activity against abl (including the bcr-abl fusion protein found in chronic myelogenous leukemia [CML]), platelet-derived growth factor receptor, and c-kit. It is FDA approved in the United States for use in the treatment of CML and gastrointestinal stromal tumors (GIST, many of which have gain-of-function c-kit mutations). While numerous reports have suggested that many ovarian carcinomas express c-kit and its ligand, stem cell factor (SCF), and they may also express platelet-derived growth factor receptor (PDGFR) (604,605), trials of imatinib in ovarian cancer have not reported any activity to date (604,606,607).

Src tyrosine kinase has been found to be overexpressed in both mouse and human ovarian cancer cells as well as in human primary ovarian cancers, and trials of *src inhibitors*, such as dasatinib, are planned or under way in ovarian cancer. Likewise, abnormalities of the PI3K/Akt pathway are common, and agents affecting this pathway, such as the mTOR inhibitor temsirolimus, are being tested in ovarian cancer.

Immunologic Therapies

It has long been known that immune therapies, such as IL2, have some activity in the treatment of ovarian cancer. Immune therapy has been of particular interest in ovarian cancer since the provocative observation by Zhang et al. that among patients in clinical complete remission the presence of intratumoral T cells was a strongly favorably prognostic factor (Fig. 25.37) (608). $CD3^{+}$ tumor-infiltrating T cells were detected within tumor cell islets in 102 of 186 tumors (54.8%). The 5-year survival rate was 38% for patients whose tumors contained T cells compared to 4.5% for patients without tumor-infiltrating T cells. While clinical results of immune therapy have been disappointing to date, vigorous investigation of a large number of immune strategies has continued, and these have recently been reviewed (609). Several phase 3 trials are planned or ongoing.

Oregovomab is a murine monoclonal antibody that binds with high affinity to circulating CA-125. The oregovomab–CA-125 complex is processed by antigen-processing cells, such as macrophages and dendritic cells. CA-125–specific antibodies, T-helper cells, and cytotoxic T cells (CTLs) are subsequently produced, demonstrating both a humoral and cellular response. This is referred to as an "anti-idiotype vaccine" approach. In a randomized, placebo-controlled trial, 145 patients with stage III

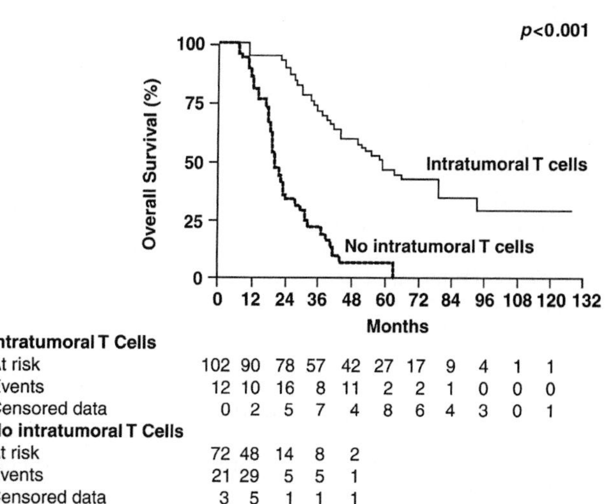

FIGURE 25.37. Kaplan-Meier curve for duration of survival according to presence or absence of intratumoral T cells in 173 patients with stage III or IV epithelial ovarian cancer. *Source:* Zhang L, Conejo-Garcia JR, Katsaros D, et al. Intratumoral T cells, recurrence and survival in epithelial ovarian cancer. *N Engl J Med* 2003;348:203–213.

or IV epithelial ovarian cancer received intravenous oregovomab at first clinical remission (457). There was no overall difference in time to progression between the two groups. However, in a retrospective analysis, it was found that for a subgroup of patients (≤2 cm of residual tumor at debulking, CA-125 ≤65 U/mL before third cycle, and CA-125 ≤35 U/mL at entry), time to progression for those receiving oregovomab was significantly better (24 vs. 10.8 months). Using the eligibility criteria of the subgroup, the investigators have completed enrollment to the phase 3 Immunotherapy Pivotal Ovarian Cancer Trials I and II with 354 patients. These results should be available soon.

Another anti-idiotypic monoclonal antibody is abagovomab (formerly ACA-125). An international, multicenter, randomized phase 3 trial of abagovomab versus placebo in stage III or IV epithelial ovarian cancer patients, with an accrual goal of 870 patients, began accruing patients in 2007 under the direction of the Arbeitsgemeinschaft Gynäkologische Onkologie group and the Cooperative Ovarian Cancer Group for Immunotherapy. Eligible patients have completed standard debulking and platinum with taxane-based chemotherapy (intravenous or intraperitoneal) and are in complete remission. The end points of this study are progression-free and overall survival.

Another vaccine trial planned is a phase 3 randomized study of a multivalent antigen-KLH construct by investigators at Memorial Sloan-Kettering Cancer Center for patients with epithelial ovarian cancer in second complete remission with progression-free survival as the study end point.

Other New Directions

Aberrant DNA methylation is a frequent epigenetic event in ovarian cancer and represents an additional source of potential molecular markers. Wei et al. (610) investigated CpG island hypermethylation across stages III and IV ovarian tumors. Hierarchical clustering revealed two tumor groups with distinctly different methylation profiles. The duration of progression-free survival after chemotherapy was significantly shorter for patients whose tumors contained high levels of concurrent methylation compared to patients whose tumors had lower tumor methylation levels. These data suggest that CpG island methylation is associated with early disease recurrence after chemotherapy. The differential methylation hybridization assay they developed also identified a group of CpG island loci that are potentially useful as epigenetic markers for predicting treatment outcome in ovarian cancer patients. Demethylating agents and histone deacetylase inhibitors are currently being studied in ovarian cancer.

Additional large-scale studies are in progress to correlate the gene expression profiles in patients with advanced ovarian cancer and survival. Such analyses may identify patients with advanced-stage disease in whom standard therapy is likely to be ineffective and who may be candidates for experimental treatments. Differential gene expression profiles will also be essential in the identification of novel molecular targets.

References

1. Jemal A, Siegel R, Ward E, et al. Cancer statistics, 2008. *CA Cancer J Clin* 2008;58:71–96.
2. Niwa Y, Yatsuya H, Tamakoshi K, et al. Relationship between body mass index and the risk of ovarian cancer in the Japanese population: findings from the Japanese Collaborate Cohort (JACC) study. *J Obstet Gynaecol Res* 2005;31:452–458.
3. Goodman MT, Howe HL, Tung KH, et al. Incidence of ovarian cancer by race and ethnicity in the United States, 1992–1997. *Cancer* 2003;97:2676–2685.
4. Merrill RM. Impact of hysterectomy and bilateral oophorectomy on race-specific rates of corpus, cervical, and ovarian cancers in the United States. *Ann Epidemiol* 2006;16:880–887.
5. Farley J, Risinger JI, Rose GS, et al. Racial disparities in blacks with gynecologic cancers. *Cancer* 2007;110:234–243.
6. Stat bite. Age-specific incidence and mortality rates for ovarian cancer, 1998–2002. *J Natl Cancer Inst* 2002;98:511.
7. Chan JK, Urban R, Cheung MK, et al. Ovarian cancer in younger vs older women: a population-based analysis. *Br J Cancer* 2006;95:1314–1320.
8. Chiaffarino F, Parazzini F, Bosetti C, et al. Risk factors for ovarian cancer histotypes. *Eur J Cancer* 2007;43:1208–1213.
9. Soegaard M, Jensen A, Hogdall E, et al. Different risk factor profiles for mucinous and nonmucinous ovarian cancer: results from the Danish MALOVA study. *Cancer Epidemiol Biomarkers Prev* 2007;16:1160–1166.
10. Genkinger JM, Hunter DJ, Spiegelman D, et al. Dairy products and ovarian cancer: a pooled analysis of 12 cohort studies. *Cancer Epidemiol Biomarkers Prev* 2006;15:364–372.
11. Schulz M, Nothlings U, Allen N, et al. No association of consumption of animal foods with risk of ovarian cancer. *Cancer Epidemiol Biomarkers Prev* 2007;16:852–855.
12. Chang ET, Lee VS, Canchola AJ, et al. Diet and risk of ovarian cancer in the California Teachers Study cohort. *Am J Epidemiol* 2007;165:802–813.
13. Modugno F, Ness RB, Allen GO. Alcohol consumption and the risk of mucinous and nonmucinous epithelial ovarian cancer. *Obstet Gynecol* 2003;102:1336–1343.
14. Jordan SJ, Whiteman DC, Purdie DM, et al. Does smoking increase risk of ovarian cancer? A systematic review. *Gynecol Oncol* 2006;103:1122–1129.
15. Biesma RG, Schouten LJ, Dirx MJ, et al. Physical activity and risk of ovarian cancer: results from the Netherlands Cohort Study (the Netherlands). *Cancer Causes Control* 2006;17:109–115.
16. Patel AV, Rodriguez C, Pavluck AL, et al. Recreational physical activity and sedentary behavior in relation to ovarian cancer risk in a large cohort of US women. *Am J Epidemiol* 2006;163:709–716.
17. Casagrande JT, Louie EW, Pike MC, et al. "Incessant ovulation" and ovarian cancer. *Lancet* 1979;2:170–173.
18. Fredrickson TN. Ovarian tumors of the hen. *Environ Health Perspect* 1987;73:35–51.
19. Schildkraut JM, Schwingl PJ, Bastos E, et al. Epithelial ovarian cancer risk among women with polycystic ovary syndrome. *Obstet Gynecol* 1996;88:554–559.
20. Choi JH, Wong AS, Huang HF, et al. Gonadotropins and ovarian cancer. *Endocr Rev* 2007;28:440–461.
21. Risch HA. Hormonal etiology of epithelial ovarian cancer, with a hypothesis concerning the role of androgens and progesterone. *J Natl Cancer Inst* 1998;90:1774–1786.
22. Cottreau CM, Ness RB, Modugno F, et al. Endometriosis and its treatment with danazol or lupron in relation to ovarian cancer. *Clin Cancer Res* 2003;9:5142–5144.
23. Schildkraut JM, Calingaert B, Marchbanks PA, et al. Impact of progestin and estrogen potency in oral contraceptives on ovarian cancer risk. *J Natl Cancer Inst* 2002;94:32–38.
24. Lurie G, Thompson P, McDuffie KE, et al. Association of estrogen and progestin potency of oral contraceptives with ovarian carcinoma risk. *Obstet Gynecol* 2007;109:597–607.
25. Cramer DW, Barbieri RL, Fraer AR, et al. Determinants of early follicular phase gonadotrophin and estradiol concentrations in women of late reproductive age. *Hum Reprod* 2002;17:221–227.
26. Kontoravdis A, Augoulea A, Lambrinoudaki I, et al. Ovarian endometriosis associated with ovarian cancer and endometrial-endocervical polyps. *J Obstet Gynaecol Res* 2007;33:294–298.
27. Schildkraut JM, Moorman PG, Halabi S, et al. Analgesic drug use and risk of ovarian cancer. *Epidemiology* 2006;17:104–107.
28. Sorensen HT, Friis S, Norgard B, et al. Risk of cancer in a large cohort of nonaspirin NSAID users: a population-based study. *Br J Cancer* 2003;88:1687–1692.
29. Bonovas S, Filioussi K, Sitaras NM. Do nonsteroidal anti-inflammatory drugs affect the risk of developing ovarian cancer? A meta-analysis. *Br J Clin Pharmacol* 2005;60:194–203.
30. Smith ER, Xu XX. Etiology of epithelial ovarian cancer: a cellular mechanism for the role of gonadotropins. *Gynecol Oncol* 2003;91:1–2.
31. Rufford B, Jacobs IJ. Screening and diagnosis of ovarian cancer in the general population. In: Gershenson DM, McGuire WP, Gore M, et al., eds. *Gynecologic Cancer: Controversies in Management.* London: Churchill Livingstone; 2004:355–368.
32. The reduction in risk of ovarian cancer associated with oral-contraceptive use. The Cancer and Steroid Hormone Study of the Centers for Disease Control and the National Institute of Child Health and Human Development. *N Engl J Med* 1987;316:650–655.
33. Epithelial ovarian cancer and combined oral contraceptives. The WHO Collaborative Study of Neoplasia and Steroid Contraceptives. *Int J Epidemiol* 1989;18:538–545.
34. Cramer DW, Hutchison GB, Welch WR, et al. Factors affecting the association of oral contraceptives and ovarian cancer. *N Engl J Med* 1982;307:1047–1051.
35. Whittemore AS, Wu ML, Paffenbarger RS Jr, et al. Epithelial ovarian cancer and the ability to conceive. *Cancer Res* 1989;49:4047–4052.

36. Kashyap S, Moher D, Fung MF, et al. Assisted reproductive technology and the incidence of ovarian cancer: a meta-analysis. *Obstet Gynecol* 2004;103:785–794.
37. Lukanova A, Kaaks R. Endogenous hormones and ovarian cancer: epidemiology and current hypotheses. *Cancer Epidemiol Biomarkers Prev* 2005;14:98–107.
38. Hankinson SE, Hunter DJ, Colditz GA, et al. Tubal ligation, hysterectomy, and risk of ovarian cancer. A prospective study. *JAMA* 1993;270: 2813–2818.
39. Whittemore AS, Harris R, Itnyre J. Characteristics relating to ovarian cancer risk: collaborative analysis of 12 US case-control studies. II. Invasive epithelial ovarian cancers in white women. Collaborative Ovarian Cancer Group. *Am J Epidemiol* 1992;136:1184–1203.
40. Beral V, Bull D, Green J, et al. Ovarian cancer and hormone replacement therapy in the Million Women Study. *Lancet* 2007;369:1703–1710.
41. Anderson GL, Judd HL, Kaunitz AM, et al. Effects of estrogen plus progestin on gynecologic cancers and associated diagnostic procedures: the Women's Health Initiative randomized trial. *JAMA* 2003;290:1739–1748.
42. Riman T, Dickman PW, Nilsson S, et al. Hormone replacement therapy and the risk of invasive epithelial ovarian cancer in Swedish women. *J Natl Cancer Inst* 2002;94:497–504.
43. McLaughlin JR, Risch HA, Lubinski J, et al. Reproductive risk factors for ovarian cancer in carriers of *BRCA1* or *BRCA2* mutations: a case-control study. *Lancet Oncol* 2007;8:26–34.
44. Chen S, Iversen ES, Friebel T, et al. Characterization of *BRCA1* and *BRCA2* mutations in a large United States sample. *J Clin Oncol* 2006;24: 863–871.
45. Gras E, Catasus L, Arguelles R, et al. Microsatellite instability, MLH-1 promoter hypermethylation, and frameshift mutations at coding mononucleotide repeat microsatellites in ovarian tumors. *Cancer* 2001;92:2829–2836.
46. Lynch HT, de la Chapelle A. Hereditary colorectal cancer. *N Engl J Med* 2003;348:919–932.
47. Domanska K, Malander S, Masback A, et al. Ovarian cancer at young age: the contribution of mismatch-repair defects in a population-based series of epithelial ovarian cancer before age 40. *Int J Gynecol Cancer* 2007;17(4):789–793.
48. Rubin SC, Benjamin I, Behbakht K, et al. Clinical and pathological features of ovarian cancer in women with germ-line mutations of *BRCA1*. *N Engl J Med* 1996;335:1413–1416.
49. Lakhani SR, Manek S, Penault-Llorca F, et al. Pathology of ovarian cancers in *BRCA1* and *BRCA2* carriers. *Clin Cancer Res* 2004;10:2473–2481.
50. Boyd J, Sonoda Y, Federici MG, et al. Clinicopathologic features of *BRCA*-linked and sporadic ovarian cancer. *JAMA* 2000;283:2260–2265.
51. Lacour RA, Westin SN, Daniels MS, et al. Survival in advanced-stage ovarian cancer patients with non-Ashkenazi Jewish *BRCA* mutations. *J Clin Oncol* 2007;25:277s.
52. Quinn JE, James CR, Stewart GE, et al. *BRCA1* mRNA expression levels predict for overall survival in ovarian cancer after chemotherapy. *Clin Canc Res* 2007;13:7413–7420.
53. Thrall M, Gallion HH, Kryscio R, et al. *BRCA1* expression in a large series of sporadic ovarian carcinomas: a Gynecologic Oncology Group study. *Int J Gynecol Cancer* 2006;16(Suppl 1):166–171.
54. Chiang JW, Karlan BY, Cass L, et al. *BRCA1* promoter methylation predicts adverse ovarian cancer prognosis. *Gynecol Oncol* 2006;101:403–410.
55. McCabe N, Turner NC, Lord CJ, et al. Deficiency in the repair of DNA damage by homologous recombination and sensitivity to poly(ADP-ribose) polymerase inhibition. *Cancer Res* 2006;66:8109–8115.
56. Yap TA, Boss DS, Fong PC, et al. First in human phase I pharmacokinetic (PK) and pharmacodynamic (PD) study of KU-0059436 (Ku), a small molecule inhibitor of poly ADP-ribose polymerase (PARP) in cancer patients (p), including *BRCA* 1/2 mutation carriers. *J Clin Oncol* 2007;25:145s, Abtr #3529.
57. Narod SA, Risch H, Moslehi R, et al. Oral contraceptives and the risk of hereditary ovarian cancer. Hereditary Ovarian Cancer Clinical Study Group. *N Engl J Med* 1998;339:424–428.
58. Whittemore AS, Balise RR, Pharoah PD, et al. Oral contraceptive use and ovarian cancer risk among carriers of *BRCA1* or *BRCA2* mutations. *Br J Cancer* 2004;91:1911–1915.
59. McGuire V, Felberg A, Mills M, et al. Relation of contraceptive and reproductive history to ovarian cancer risk in carriers and noncarriers of *BRCA1* gene mutations. *Am J Epidemiol* 2004;160:613–618.
60. Gronwald J, Byrski T, Huzarski T, et al. Influence of selected lifestyle factors on breast and ovarian cancer risk in *BRCA1* mutation carriers from Poland. Breast *Cancer Res Treat* 2006;95:105–109.
61. Modan B, Hartge P, Hirsh-Yechezkel G, et al. Parity, oral contraceptives, and the risk of ovarian cancer among carriers and noncarriers of a *BRCA1* or *BRCA2* mutation. *N Engl J Med* 2001;345:235–240.
62. National Institutes of Health Consensus Development Conference Statement. Ovarian cancer: screening, treatment, and follow-up. *Gynecol Oncol* 1994;55:S4–S14.
63. Finch A, Beiner M, Lubinski J, et al. Salpingo-oophorectomy and the risk of ovarian, fallopian tube, and peritoneal cancers in women with a *BRCA1* or *BRCA2* mutation. *JAMA* 2006;296:185–192.
64. Medeiros F, Muto MG, Lee Y, et al. The tubal fimbria is a preferred site for early adenocarcinoma in women with familial ovarian cancer syndrome. *Am J Surg Pathol* 2006;30:230–236.
65. Kramer JL, Velazquez IA, Chen BE, et al. Prophylactic oophorectomy reduces breast cancer penetrance during prospective, long-term follow-up of *BRCA1* mutation carriers. *J Clin Oncol* 2005;23:8629–8635.
66. Werness BA, Ramus SJ, DiCioccio RA, et al. Histopathology, FIGO stage, and *BRCA* mutation status of ovarian cancers from the Gilda Radner Familial Ovarian Cancer Registry. *Int J Gynecol Pathol* 2004;23: 29–34.
67. Colgan TJ, Murphy J, Cole DE, et al. Occult carcinoma in prophylactic oophorectomy specimens: prevalence and association with *BRCA* germline mutation status. *Am J Surg Pathol* 2001;25:1283–1289.
68. Agoff SN, Mendelin JE, Grieco VS, et al. Unexpected gynecologic neoplasms in patients with proven or suspected *BRCA*-1 or -2 mutations: implications for gross examination, cytology, and clinical follow-up. *Am J Surg Pathol* 2002;26:171–178.
69. Kaur TB, Shen T, Gaughan J, et al. Premalignant lesions in the contralateral ovary of women with unilateral ovarian carcinoma. *Gynecol Oncol* 2004; 93:69–77.
70. Kerner R, Sabo E, Gershoni-Baruch R, et al. Expression of cell cycle regulatory proteins in ovaries prophylactically removed from Jewish Ashkenazi *BRCA1* and *BRCA2* mutation carriers: correlation with histopathology. *Gynecol Oncol* 2005;99:367–375.
71. Resta L, Russo S, Colucci GA, et al. Morphologic precursors of ovarian epithelial tumors. *Obstet Gynecol* 1993;82:181–186.
72. Salazar H, Godwin AK, Daly MB, et al. Microscopic benign and invasive malignant neoplasms and a cancer-prone phenotype in prophylactic oophorectomies. *J Natl Cancer Inst* 1996;88:1810–1820.
73. Sherman ME, Lee JS, Burks RT, et al. Histopathologic features of ovaries at increased risk for carcinoma. A case-control analysis. *Int J Gynecol Pathol* 1999;18:151–157.
74. Werness BA, Afify AM, Bielat KL, et al. Altered surface and cyst epithelium of ovaries removed prophylactically from women with a family history of ovarian cancer. *Hum Pathol* 1999;30:151–157.
75. Westhoff C, Murphy P, Heller D, et al. Is ovarian cancer associated with an increased frequency of germinal inclusion cysts? *Am J Epidemiol* 1993;138:90.
76. Deligdish L, Gil J, Kerner H, et al. Ovarian dysplasia in prophylactic oophorectomy specimens: cytogenetic and morphometric correlations. *Cancer* 1999;86:1544–1550.
77. Seidman JD, Wang BG. Evaluation of normal-sized ovaries associated with primary peritoneal serous carcinoma for possible precursors of ovarian serous carcinoma. *Gynecol Oncol* 2007;106(1):201–206.
78. Risch HA, McLaughlin JR, Cole DE, et al. Population *BRCA1* and *BRCA2* mutation frequencies and cancer penetrances: a kin-cohort study in Ontario, Canada. *J Natl Cancer Inst* 2006;98:1694–1706.
79. Struewing JP, Hartge P, Wacholder S, et al. The risk of cancer associated with specific mutations of *BRCA1* and *BRCA2* among Ashkenazi Jews. *N Engl J Med* 1997;336:1401–1408.
80. Tobias DH, Eng C, McCurdy LD, et al. Founder *BRCA* 1 and 2 mutations among a consecutive series of Ashkenazi Jewish ovarian cancer patients. *Gynecol Oncol* 2000;78:148–151.
81. Robboy SJ, Anderson MC, Russell P. *Pathology of the Female Reproductive Tract*. London: Churchill Livingstone; 2002.
82. Platz CE, Benda JA. Female genital tract cancer. *Cancer* 1995;75:270–294.
83. Seidman JD, Horkayne-Szakaly I, Haiba M, et al. The histologic type and stage distribution of ovarian carcinomas of surface epithelial origin. *Int J Gynecol Pathol* 2004;23:41–44.
84. Shih Ie M, Kurman RJ. Ovarian tumorigenesis: a proposed model based on morphological and molecular genetic analysis. *Am J Pathol* 2004;164:1511–1518.
85. Lee Y, Medeiros F, Kindelberger D, et al. Advances in the recognition of tubal intraepithelial carcinoma: applications to cancer screening and the pathogenesis of ovarian cancer. *Adv Anat Pathol* 2006;13:1–7.
86. Lee Y, Miron A, Drapkin R, et al. A candidate precursor to serous carcinoma that originates in the distal fallopian tube. *J Pathol* 2007;211: 26–35.
87. Kindelberger DW, Lee Y, Miron A, et al. Intraepithelial carcinoma of the fimbria and pelvic serous carcinoma: evidence for a causal relationship. *Am J Surg Pathol* 2007;31:161–169.
88. Raab SS, Robinson RA, Jensen CS, et al. Mucinous tumors of the ovary: interobserver diagnostic variability and utility of sectioning protocols. *Arch Pathol Lab Med* 1997;121:1192–1198.
89. Robboy SJ, Anderson MC, Russell P. Cutup. In: Robboy SJ, Anderson MC, Russell P, eds. *Pathology of the Female Reproductive Tract*. London: Churchill Livingstone; 2002:861–875.

89a. Seidman JD, Soslow RA, Vang R, et al. Borderline ovarian tumors: diverse contemporary viewpoints on terminology and diagnostic criteria with illustrative images. *Hum Pathol* 2004;35:918–33.

90. Puls LE, Powell DE, DePriest PD, et al. Transition from benign to malignant epithelium in mucinous and serous ovarian cystadenocarcinoma. *Gynecol Oncol* 1992;47:53–57.
91. Bell KA, Kurman RJ. A clinicopathologic analysis of atypical proliferative (borderline) tumors and well-differentiated endometrioid adenocarcinomas of the ovary. *Am J Surg Pathol* 2000;24:1465–1479.
92. Katzenstein AL, Mazur MT, Morgan TE, et al. Proliferative serous tumors of the ovary. Histologic features and prognosis. *Am J Surg Pathol* 1978;2:339–355.

93. Russell P. The pathological assessment of ovarian neoplasms. II: The proliferating "epithelial" tumours. *Pathology* 1979;11:251–282.
94. Burks RT, Sherman ME, Kurman RJ. Micropapillary serous carcinoma of the ovary. A distinctive low-grade carcinoma related to serous borderline tumors. *Am J Surg Pathol* 1996;20:1319–1330.
95. Gershenson DM, Sun CC, Lu KH, et al. Clinical behavior of stage II-IV low-grade serous carcinoma of the ovary. *Obstet Gynecol* 2006;108: 361–368.
96. Seidman JD, Horkayne-Szakaly I, Cosin JA, et al. Testing of two binary grading systems for FIGO stage III serous carcinoma of the ovary and peritoneum. *Gynecol Oncol* 2006;103:703–708.
97. Seidman JD, Kurman RJ. Ovarian serous borderline tumors: a critical review of the literature with emphasis on prognostic indicators. *Hum Pathol* 2000;31:539–557.
98. Deavers MT, Gershenson DM, Tortolero-Luna G, et al. Micropapillary and cribriform patterns in ovarian serous tumors of low malignant potential: a study of 99 advanced stage cases. *Am J Surg Pathol* 2002;26:1129–1141.
99. Eichhorn JH, Bell DA, Young RH, et al. Ovarian serous borderline tumors with micropapillary and cribriform patterns: a study of 40 cases and comparison with 44 cases without these patterns. *Am J Surg Pathol* 1999;23: 397–409.
100. Goldstein NS, Ceniza N. Ovarian micropapillary serous borderline tumors. Clinicopathologic features and outcome of seven surgically staged patients. *Am J Clin Pathol* 2000;114:380–386.
101. Longacre TA, McKenney JK, Tazelaar HD, et al. Ovarian serous tumors of low malignant potential (borderline tumors): outcome-based study of 276 patients with long-term (> or =5-year) follow-up. *Am J Surg Pathol* 2005;29:707–723.
102. Prat J, De Nictolis M. Serous borderline tumors of the ovary: a long-term follow-up study of 137 cases, including 18 with a micropapillary pattern and 20 with microinvasion. *Am J Surg Pathol* 2002;26:1111–1128.
103. Seidman JD, Kurman RJ. Subclassification of serous borderline tumors of the ovary into benign and malignant types. A clinicopathologic study of 65 advanced stage cases. *Am J Surg Pathol* 1996;20:1331–1345.
104. Slomovitz BM, Caputo TA, Gretz HF 3rd, et al. A comparative analysis of 57 serous borderline tumors with and without a noninvasive micropapillary component. *Am J Surg Pathol* 2002;26:592–600.
105. Smith Sehdev AE, Sehdev PS, Kurman RJ. Noninvasive and invasive micropapillary (low-grade) serous carcinoma of the ovary: a clinicopathologic analysis of 135 cases. *Am J Surg Pathol* 2003;27:725–736.
106. Bell DA, Weinstock MA, Scully RE. Peritoneal implants of ovarian serous borderline tumors. Histologic features and prognosis. *Cancer* 1988;62: 2212–2222.
107. Bell DA, Longacre TA, Prat J, et al. Serous borderline (low malignant potential, atypical proliferative) ovarian tumors: workshop perspectives. *Hum Pathol* 2004;35:934–948.
108. Gilks CB, Alkushi A, Yue JJ, et al. Advanced-stage serous borderline tumors of the ovary: a clinicopathological study of 49 cases. *Int J Gynecol Pathol* 2003;22:29–36.
109a. McKenney J, Balzer BL, Longacre TA. Lymph node involvement in ovarian serous tumors of low malignant potential (borderline tumors): pathology, prognosis, and proposed classificiation. *Am J Surg Pathol* 2006;30: 614–624.
109. Morice P, Joulie F, Camatte S, et al. Lymph node involvement in epithelial ovarian cancer: analysis of 276 pelvic and paraaortic lymphadenectomies and surgical implications. *J Am Coll Surg* 2003;197:198–205.
110. Shimizu Y, Kamoi S, Amada S, et al. Toward the development of a universal grading system for ovarian epithelial carcinoma: testing of a proposed system in a series of 461 patients with uniform treatment and follow-up. *Cancer* 1998;82:893–901.
111. Malpica A, Deavers MT, Lu K, et al. Grading ovarian serous carcinoma using a two-tier system. *Am J Surg Pathol* 2004;28:496–504.
112. Chaitin BA, Gershenson DM, Evans HL. Mucinous tumors of the ovary. A clinicopathologic study of 70 cases. *Cancer* 1985;55:1958–1962.
113. de Nictolis M, Montironi R, Tommasoni S, et al. Benign, borderline, and well-differentiated malignant intestinal mucinous tumors of the ovary: a clinicopathologic, histochemical, immunohistochemical, and nuclear quantitative study of 57 cases. *Int J Gynecol Pathol* 1994;13:10–21.
114. Guerrieri C, Hogberg T, Wingren S, et al. Mucinous borderline and malignant tumors of the ovary. A clinicopathologic and DNA ploidy study of 92 cases. *Cancer* 1994;74:2329–2340.
115. Hoerl HD, Hart WR. Primary ovarian mucinous cystadenocarcinomas: a clinicopathologic study of 49 cases with long-term follow-up. *Am J Surg Pathol* 1998;22:1449–1462.
116. Kaern J, Trope CG, Abeler VM. A retrospective study of 370 borderline tumors of the ovary treated at the Norwegian Radium Hospital from 1970 to 1982. A review of clinicopathologic features and treatment modalities. *Cancer* 1993;71:1810–1820.
117. Kikkawa F, Kawai M, Tamakoshi K, et al. Mucinous carcinoma of the ovary. Clinicopathologic analysis. *Oncology* 1996;53:303–307.
118. Kim KR, Lee HI, Lee SK, et al. Is stromal microinvasion in primary mucinous ovarian tumors with "mucin granuloma" true invasion? *Am J Surg Pathol* 2007;31:546–554.
119. Kuoppala T, Heinola M, Aine R, et al. Serous and mucinous borderline tumors of the ovary: a clinicopathologic and DNA-ploidy study of 102 cases. *Int J Gynecol Cancer* 1996;6:302–308.
120. Lee KR, Scully RE. Mucinous tumors of the ovary: a clinicopathologic study of 196 borderline tumors (of intestinal type) and carcinomas, including an evaluation of 11 cases with "pseudomyxoma peritonei." *Am J Surg Pathol* 2000;24:1447–1464.
121. Michael H, Sutton G, Roth LM. Ovarian carcinoma with extracellular mucin production: reassessment of "pseudomyxoma ovarii et peritonei." *Int J Gynecol Cancer* 1987;6:298–312.
122. Nikrui N. Survey of clinical behavior of patients with borderline epithelial tumors of the ovary. *Gynecol Oncol* 1981;12:107–119.
123. Nomura K, Aizawa S, Hano H. Ovarian mucinous borderline tumors of intestinal type without intraepithelial carcinoma: are they still tumors of low malignant potential? *Pathol Int* 2004;54:420–424.
124. Piura B, Dgani R, Blickstein I, et al. Epithelial ovarian tumors of borderline malignancy: a study of 50 cases. *Int J Gynecol Cancer* 1992;2:189–197.
125. Rice LW, Berkowitz RS, Mark SD, et al. Epithelial ovarian tumors of borderline malignancy. *Gynecol Oncol* 1990;39:195–198.
126. Riopel MA, Ronnett BM, Kurman RJ. Evaluation of diagnostic criteria and behavior of ovarian intestinal-type mucinous tumors: atypical proliferative (borderline) tumors and intraepithelial, microinvasive, invasive, and metastatic carcinomas. *Am J Surg Pathol* 1999;23:617–635.
127. Rodriguez IM, Prat J. Mucinous tumors of the ovary: a clinicopathologic analysis of 75 borderline tumors (of intestinal type) and carcinomas. *Am J Surg Pathol* 2002;26:139–152.
128. Cuatrecasas M, Matias-Guiu X, Prat J. Synchronous mucinous tumors of the appendix and the ovary associated with pseudomyxoma peritonei. A clinicopathologic study of six cases with comparative analysis of c-Ki-ras mutations. *Am J Surg Pathol* 1996;20:739–746.
129. Guerrieri C, Franlund B, Fristedt S, et al. Mucinous tumors of the vermiform appendix and ovary, and pseudomyxoma peritonei: histogenetic implications of cytokeratin 7 expression. *Hum Pathol* 1997;28: 1039–1045.
130. Prayson RA, Hart WR, Petras RE. Pseudomyxoma peritonei. A clinicopathologic study of 19 cases with emphasis on site of origin and nature of associated ovarian tumors. *Am J Surg Pathol* 1994;18:591–603.
131. Ronnett BM, Kurman RJ, Zahn CM, et al. Pseudomyxoma peritonei in women: a clinicopathologic analysis of 30 cases with emphasis on site of origin, prognosis, and relationship to ovarian mucinous tumors of low malignant potential. *Hum Pathol* 1995;26:509–524.
132. Ronnett BM, Shmookler BM, Diener-West M, et al. Immunohistochemical evidence supporting the appendiceal origin of pseudomyxoma peritonei in women. *Int J Gynecol Pathol* 1997;16:1–9.
133. Ronnett BM, Yan H, Kurman RJ, et al. Patients with pseudomyxoma peritonei associated with disseminated peritoneal adenomucinosis have a significantly more favorable prognosis than patients with peritoneal mucinous carcinomatosis. *Cancer* 2001;92:85–91.
134. Ronnett BM, Zahn CM, Kurman RJ, et al. Disseminated peritoneal adenomucinosis and peritoneal mucinous carcinomatosis. A clinicopathologic analysis of 109 cases with emphasis on distinguishing pathologic features, site of origin, prognosis, and relationship to "pseudomyxoma peritonei." *Am J Surg Pathol* 1995;19:1390–1408.
135. Szych C, Staebler A, Connolly DC, et al. Molecular genetic evidence supporting the clonality and appendiceal origin of pseudomyxoma peritonei in women. *Am J Pathol* 1999;154:1849–1855.
136. Young RH, Gilks CB, Scully RE. Mucinous tumors of the appendix associated with mucinous tumors of the ovary and pseudomyxoma peritonei. A clinicopathological analysis of 22 cases supporting an origin in the appendix. *Am J Surg Pathol* 1991;15:415–429.
137. Dube V, Roy M, Plante M, et al. Mucinous ovarian tumors of müllerian-type: an analysis of 17 cases including borderline tumors and intraepithelial, microinvasive, and invasive carcinomas. *Int J Gynecol Pathol* 2005;24:138–146.
138. Rodriguez IM, Irving JA, Prat J. Endocervical-like mucinous borderline tumors of the ovary: a clinicopathologic analysis of 31 cases. *Am J Surg Pathol* 2004;28:1311–1318.
139. Rutgers JL, Scully RE. Ovarian müllerian mucinous papillary cystadenomas of borderline malignancy. A clinicopathologic analysis. *Cancer* 1988;61:340–348.
140. Shappell HW, Riopel MA, Smith Sehdev AE, et al. Diagnostic criteria and behavior of ovarian seromucinous (endocervical-type mucinous and mixed cell-type) tumors: atypical proliferative (borderline) tumors, intraepithelial, microinvasive, and invasive carcinomas. *Am J Surg Pathol* 2002;26:1529–1541.
141. Siriaunkgul S, Robbins KM, McGowan L, et al. Ovarian mucinous tumors of low malignant potential: a clinicopathologic study of 54 tumors of intestinal and müllerian type. *Int J Gynecol Pathol* 1995;14: 198–208.
142. Yemelyanova A, Vang R, Judson K, et al. Distinction of primary and metastatic mucinous tumors involving the ovary: analysis of size and laterality data by primary site with re-evaluation of an algorithm for tumor classification. *Am J Surg Pathol* 2008;32(1):128–138.
143. Vang R, Gown AM, Barry TS, et al. Ovarian atypical proliferative (borderline) mucinous tumors: gastrointestinal and seromucinous (endocervical-like) types are immunophenotypically distinctive. *Int J Gynecol Pathol* 2006;25:83–89.
144. Hart WR. Ovarian epithelial tumors of borderline malignancy (carcinomas of low malignant potential). *Hum Pathol* 1977;8:541–549.

145. Hart WR, Norris HJ. Borderline and malignant mucinous tumors of the ovary. Histologic criteria and clinical behavior. *Cancer* 1973;31:1031–1045.
146. Nomura K, Aizawa S. Noninvasive, microinvasive, and invasive mucinous carcinomas of the ovary: a clinicopathologic analysis of 40 cases. *Cancer* 2000;89:1541–1546.
147. Watkin W, Silva EG, Gershenson DM. Mucinous carcinoma of the ovary. Pathologic prognostic factors. *Cancer* 1992;69:208–212.
148. Khunamornpong S, Russell P, Dalrymple JC. Proliferating (LMP) mucinous tumors of the ovaries with microinvasion: morphologic assessment of 13 cases. *Int J Gynecol Pathol* 1999;18:238–246.
149. Nayar R, Siriaunkgul S, Robbins KM, et al. Microinvasion in low malignant potential tumors of the ovary. *Hum Pathol* 1996;27:521–527.
150. Chen S, Leitao MM, Tornos C, et al. Invasion patterns in stage I endometrioid and mucinous ovarian carcinomas: a clinicopathologic analysis emphasizing favorable outcomes in carcinomas without destructive stromal invasion and the occasional malignant course of carcinomas with limited destructive stromal invasion. *Mod Pathol* 2005;18:903–911.
151. Ludwick C, Gilks CB, Miller D, et al. Aggressive behavior of stage I ovarian mucinous tumors lacking extensive infiltrative invasion: a report of four cases and review of the literature. *Int J Gynecol Pathol* 2005;24:205–217.
152. Ronnett BM, Seidman JD. Mucinous tumors arising in ovarian mature cystic teratomas: relationship to the clinical syndrome of pseudomyxoma peritonei. *Am J Surg Pathol* 2003;27:650–657.
153. Misdraji J, Yantiss RK, Graeme-Cook FM, et al. Appendiceal mucinous neoplasms: a clinicopathologic analysis of 107 cases. *Am J Surg Pathol* 2003;27:1089–1103.
154. Yan TD, Black D, Savady R, et al. A systematic review on the efficacy of cytoreductive surgery and perioperative intraperitoneal chemotherapy for pseudomyxoma peritonei. *Ann Surg Oncol* 2007;14:484–492.
155. Lee KR, Young RH. The distinction between primary and metastatic mucinous carcinomas of the ovary: gross and histologic findings in 50 cases. *Am J Surg Pathol* 2003;27:281–292.
156. Seidman JD, Kurman RJ, Ronnett BM. Primary and metastatic mucinous adenocarcinomas in the ovaries: incidence in routine practice with a new approach to improve intraoperative diagnosis. *Am J Surg Pathol* 2003;27:985–993.
157. Ji H, Isacson C, Seidman JD, et al. Cytokeratins 7 and 20, Dpc4, and MUC5AC in the distinction of metastatic mucinous carcinomas in the ovary from primary ovarian mucinous tumors: Dpc4 assists in identifying metastatic pancreatic carcinomas. *Int J Gynecol Pathol* 2002;21:391–400.
157a.Judson K, McCormick C, Vang R, et al. Women with undiagnosed colorectal adenocarcinomas presenting with ovarian metastases: clinicopathologic features and comparison with women having known colorectal adenocarcinomas and ovarian involvement. *Int J Gynecol Pathol* 2008;27:182–190.
157b.Ronnett BM, Yemelyanova AV, Vang R, et al. Endocervical adenocarcinomas with ovarian metastases: analysis of 29 cases, with emphasis on minimally invasive cervical tumors and the ability of the metastases to simulate primary ovarian neoplasms. *Am J Surg Pathol* 2008;32:1835–1853.
158c.Ronnett BM, Kurman RJ, Shmookler BM, et al. The mophologic spectrum of ovarian metastases of appendiceal adenocarcinomas: a clinicopathologic and immunohistochemical analysis of tumors often misinterpreted as primary ovarian tumors or metastatic carcinoma from other gastrointestinal sites. *Am J Surg Pathol* 1997;21:1144–1155.
158. Lash RH, Hart WR. Intestinal adenocarcinomas metastatic to the ovaries. A clinicopathologic evaluation of 22 cases. *Am J Surg Pathol* 1987;11:114–121.
159. Young RH, Scully RE. Mucinous ovarian tumors associated with mucinous adenocarcinomas of the cervix. A clinicopathological analysis of 16 cases. *Int J Gynecol Pathol* 1988;7:99–111.
160. Young RH, Scully RE. Ovarian metastases from carcinoma of the gallbladder and extrahepatic bile ducts simulating primary tumors of the ovary. A report of six cases. *Int J Gynecol Pathol* 1990;9:60–72.
161. Vang R, Gown AM, Barry TS, et al. Immunohistochemistry for estrogen and progesterone receptors in the distinction of primary and metastatic mucinous tumors in the ovary: an analysis of 124 cases. *Mod Pathol* 2006;19:97–105.
162. Vang R, Gown AM, Barry TS, et al. Cytokeratins 7 and 20 in primary and secondary mucinous tumors of the ovary: analysis of coordinate immunohistochemical expression profiles and staining distribution in 179 cases. *Am J Surg Pathol* 2006;30:1130–1139.
163. Vang R, Gown AM, Farinola M, et al. p16 expression in primary ovarian mucinous and endometrioid tumors and metastatic adenocarcinomas in the ovary: utility for identification of metastatic HPV-related endocervical adenocarcinomas. *Am J Surg Pathol* 2007;31:653–663.
164. Vang R, Gown AM, Wu LS, et al. Immunohistochemical expression of CDX2 in primary ovarian mucinous tumors and metastatic mucinous carcinomas involving the ovary: comparison with CK20 and correlation with coordinate expression of CK7. *Mod Pathol* 2006;19:1421–1428.
165. Takahashi K, Kurioka H, Irikoma M, et al. Benign or malignant ovarian neoplasms and ovarian endometriomas. *J Am Assoc Gynecol Laparosc* 2001;8:278–284.
166. Stern RC, Dash R, Bentley RC, et al. Malignancy in endometriosis: frequency and comparison of ovarian and extraovarian types. *Int J Gynecol Pathol* 2001;20:133–139.
167. Grosso G, Raspagliesi F, Baiocchi G, et al. Endometrioid carcinoma of the ovary: a retrospective analysis of 106 cases. *Tumori* 1998;84:552–557.
168. Zaino R, Whitney C, Brady MF, et al. Simultaneously detected endometrial and ovarian carcinomas—a prospective clinicopathologic study of 74 cases: a Gynecologic Oncology Group study. *Gynecol Oncol* 2001;83:355–362.
169. McMeekin DS, Burger RA, Manetta A, et al. Endometrioid adenocarcinoma of the ovary and its relationship to endometriosis. *Gynecol Oncol* 1995;59:81–86.
170. Norris HJ. Proliferative endometrioid tumors and endometrioid tumors of low malignant potential of the ovary. *Int J Gynecol Pathol* 1993;12:134–140.
171. Zwart J, Geisler JP, Geisler HE. Five-year survival in patients with endometrioid carcinoma of the ovary versus those with serous carcinoma. *Eur J Gynaecol Oncol* 1998;19:225–228.
172. Tornos C, Silva EG, Khorana SM, et al. High-stage endometrioid carcinoma of the ovary. Prognostic significance of pure versus mixed histologic types. *Am J Surg Pathol* 1994;18:687–693.
173. Eichhorn JH, Young RH, Clement PB, et al. Mesodermal (müllerian) adenosarcoma of the ovary: a clinicopathologic analysis of 40 cases and a review of the literature. *Am J Surg Pathol* 2002;26:1243–1258.
174. Le T, Krepart GV, Lotocki RJ, et al. Malignant mixed mesodermal ovarian tumor treatment and prognosis: a 20-year experience. *Gynecol Oncol* 1997;65:237–240.
175. Behbakht K, Randall TC, Benjamin I, et al. Clinical characteristics of clear cell carcinoma of the ovary. *Gynecol Oncol* 1998;70:255–258.
176. Esheba GE, Pate LL, Longacre TA. Oncofetal protein glypican-3 distinguishes yolk sac tumor from clear cell carcinoma of the ovary. *Am J Surg Path* 2008;32:600–607.
177. Morimura Y, Hoshi K, Hang XL, et al. Evaluation with MIB1 antibody of proliferative activity in ovarian clear cell adenocarcinoma. *Int J Gynecol Pathol* 1996;15:315–319.
178. Kennedy AW, Biscotti CV, Hart WR, et al. Histologic correlates of progression-free interval and survival in ovarian clear cell adenocarcinoma. *Gynecol Oncol* 1993;50:334–338.
179. Riedel I, Czernobilsky B, Lifschitz-Mercer B, et al. Brenner tumors but not transitional cell carcinomas of the ovary show urothelial differentiation: immunohistochemical staining of urothelial markers, including cytokeratins and uroplakins. *Virchows Arch* 2001;438:181–191.
180. Soslow RA, Rouse RV, Hendrickson MR, et al. Transitional cell neoplasms of the ovary and urinary bladder: a comparative immunohistochemical analysis. *Int J Gynecol Pathol* 1996;15:257–265.
181. Pins MR, Young RH, Daly WJ, et al. Primary squamous cell carcinoma of the ovary. Report of 37 cases. *Am J Surg Pathol* 1996;20:823–833.
182. Dickersin GR, Scully RE. Ovarian small cell tumors: an electron microscopic review. *Ultrastruct Pathol* 1998;22:199–226.
183. Young RH, Oliva E, Scully RE. Small cell carcinoma of the ovary, hypercalcemic type. A clinicopathological analysis of 150 cases. *Am J Surg Pathol* 1994;18:1102–1116.
184. Matias-Guiu X, Prat J, Young RH, et al. Human parathyroid hormone-related protein in ovarian small cell carcinoma. An immunohistochemical study. *Cancer* 1994;73:1878–1881.
185. Ferlicot S, Bessoud B, Martin V, et al. Large cell variant of small cell carcinoma of the ovary with hypercalcemia. *Ann Pathol* 1998;18:197–200.
186. Eichhorn JH, Young RH, Scully RE. Primary ovarian small cell carcinoma of pulmonary type. A clinicopathologic, immunohistologic, and flow cytometric analysis of 11 cases. *Am J Surg Pathol* 1992;16:926–938.
187. Eichhorn JH, Lawrence WD, Young RH, et al. Ovarian neuroendocrine carcinomas of non-small-cell type associated with surface epithelial adenocarcinomas. A study of five cases and review of the literature. *Int J Gynecol Pathol* 1996;15:303–314.
188. Strobel SL, Graham R. Primary non-small cell neuroendocrine carcinoma of the ovary. *J Histotechnol* 2003;26:73–76.
189. Alvarado-Cabrero I, Young RH, Vamvakas EC, et al. Carcinoma of the fallopian tube: a clinicopathological study of 105 cases with observations on staging and prognostic factors. *Gynecol Oncol* 1999;72:367–379.
190. Baekelandt M, Jorunn N, Kristensen GB, et al. Carcinoma of the fallopian tube. *Cancer* 2000;89:2076–2084.
191. Moore DH, Woosley JT, Reddick RL, et al. Adenosquamous carcinoma of the fallopian tube. A clinicopathologic case report with verification of the diagnosis by immunohistochemical and ultrastructural studies studies. *Am J Obstet Gynecol* 1987;157:903–905.
192. Podratz KC, Podczaski ES, Gaffey TA, et al. Primary carcinoma of the fallopian tube. *Am J Obstet Gynecol* 1986;154:1319–1326.
193. Semrad N, Watring W, Fu YS, et al. Fallopian tube adenocarcinoma: common cancer of the fallopian tube to *BRCA* 1 germline mutations. *Gynecol Oncol* 2000;76:45–50.
194. Alvarado-Cabrero I, Navani SS, Young RH, et al. Tumors of the fimbriated end of the fallopian tube: a clinicopathologic analysis of 20 cases, including 9 carcinomas. *Int J Gynecol Pathol* 1998;16:189.
195. Scully R, Young R, Clement P. *Tumors of the Ovary, Maldeveloped Gonads, Fallopian Tube, and Blood Ligament*. Washington DC: Armed Forces Institute of Pathology; 1998:23;466.
196. Denham JW, Maclennan KA. The management of primary carcinoma of the fallopian tube. Experience of 40 cases. *Cancer* 1984;53:166–172.
197. Kinzel GE. Primary carcinoma of the fallopian tube. *Am J Obstet Gynecol* 1976;125:816–820.

198. McMurray EH, Jacobs AJ, Perez CA, et al. Carcinoma of the fallopian tube. Management and sites of failure. *Cancer* 1986;58:2070–2075.
199. Nordin AJ. Primary carcinoma of the fallopian tube: a 20-year literature review. *Obstet Gynecol Surv* 1994;49:349–361.
200. Pfeiffer P, Mogensen H, Amtrup F, et al. Primary carcinoma of the fallopian tube. A retrospective study of patients reported to the Danish Cancer Registry in a five-year period. *Acta Oncol* 1989;28:7–11.
201. Schiller HM, Silverberg SG. Staging and prognosis in primary carcinoma of the fallopian tube. *Cancer* 1971;28:389–395.
202. Heselmeyer K, Hellstrom AC, Blegen H, et al. Primary carcinoma of the fallopian tube: comparative genomic hybridization reveals high genetic instability and a specific, recurring pattern of chromosomal aberrations. *Int J Gynecol Pathol* 1998;17:245–254.
203. Zweemer RP, van Diest PJ, Verheijen RH, et al. Molecular evidence linking primary cancer of the fallopian tube to *BRCA1* germline mutations. *Gynecol Oncol* 2000;76:45–50.
204. Chin H, Matsui H, Mitsuhashi A, et al. Primary transitional cell carcinoma of the fallopian tube: a case report and review of the literature. *Gynecol Oncol* 1998;71:469–475.
205. Seraj IM, King A, Chase D. Malignant mixed müllerian tumor of the oviduct. *Gynecol Oncol* 1990;37:296–301.
206. Daya D, Young RH, Scully RE. Endometrioid carcinoma of the fallopian tube resembling an adnexal tumor of probable wolffian origin: a report of six cases. *Int J Gynecol Pathol* 1992;11:122–130.
207. Navani SS, Alvarado-Cabrero I, Young RH, et al. Endometrioid carcinoma of the fallopian tube: a clinicopathologic analysis of 26 cases. *Gynecol Oncol* 1996;63:371–378.
208. Williamson JM, Armour A. Microcystic endometrioid carcinoma of the fallopian tube simulating an adnexal tumour of probable wolffian origin. *Histopathology* 1993;23:578–580.
209. Koshiyama M, Konishi I, Yoshida M, et al. Transitional cell carcinoma of the fallopian tube: a light and electron microscopic study. *Int J Gynecol Pathol* 1994;13:175–180.
210. Uehira K, Hashimoto H, Tsuneyoshi M, et al. Transitional cell carcinoma pattern in primary carcinoma of the fallopian tube. *Cancer* 1993;72: 2447–2456.
211. Neunteufel W, Breitenecker G. Tissue expression of CA 125 in benign and malignant lesions of ovary and fallopian tube: a comparison with CA 19-9 and CEA. *Gynecol Oncol* 1989;32:297–302.
212. Puls LE, Davey DD, DePriest PD, et al. Immunohistochemical staining for CA-125 in fallopian tube carcinomas. *Gynecol Oncol* 1993;48: 360–363.
213. Stuhlinger M, Rosen AC, Dobianer K, et al. HER-2 oncogene is not amplified in primary carcinoma of the fallopian tube. Austrian Cooperative Study Group for Fallopian Tube Carcinoma. *Oncology* 1995;52:397–399.
214. Chung TK, Cheung TH, To KF, et al. Overexpression of p53 and HER2/neu and c-myc in primary fallopian tube carcinoma. *Gynecol Obstet Invest* 2000;49:47–51.
215. Mizuuchi H, Mori Y, Sato K, et al. High incidence of point mutation in K-ras codon 12 in carcinoma of the fallopian tube. *Cancer* 1995;76:86–90.
216. Press MF, Holt JA, Herbst AL, et al. Immunocytochemical identification of estrogen receptor in ovarian carcinomas. Localization with monoclonal estrophilin antibodies compared with biochemical assays. *Lab Invest* 1985;53:349–361.
217. Press MF, Nousek-Goebl NA, Greene GL. Immunoelectron microscopic localization of estrogen receptor with monoclonal estrophilin antibodies. *J Histochem Cytochem* 1985;33:915–924.
218. Carlson JA Jr, Ackerman BL, Wheeler JE. Malignant mixed müllerian tumor of the fallopian tube. *Cancer* 1993;71:187–192.
219. Imachi M, Tsukamoto N, Shigematsu T, et al. Malignant mixed müllerian tumor of the fallopian tube: report of two cases and review of literature. *Gynecol Oncol* 1992;47:114–124.
220. Muntz HG, Rutgers JL, Tarraza HM, et al. Carcinosarcomas and mixed müllerian tumors of the fallopian tube. *Gynecol Oncol* 1989;34:109–115.
221. Weber AM, Hewett WF, Gajewski WH, et al. Malignant mixed müllerian tumors of the fallopian tube. *Gynecol Oncol* 1993;50:239–243.
222. Cheung AN, So KF, Ngan HY, et al. Primary squamous cell carcinoma of fallopian tube. *Int J Gynecol Pathol* 1994;13:92–95.
223. Aziz S, Kuperstein G, Rosen B, et al. A genetic epidemiological study of carcinoma of the fallopian tube. *Gynecol Oncol* 2001;80:341–345.
224. Herbold DR, Axelrod JH, Bobowski SJ, et al. Glassy cell carcinoma of the fallopian tube. A case report. *Int J Gynecol Pathol* 1988;7:384–390.
225. Abrams J, Kazal HL, Hobbs RE. Primary sarcoma of the fallopian tube; review of the literature and report of one case. *Am J Obstet Gynecol* 1958;75:180–182.
226. Barakat RR, Rubin SC, Saigo PE, et al. Second-look laparotomy in carcinoma of the fallopian tube. *Obstet Gynecol* 1993;82:748–751.
227. Chang KL, Crabtree GS, Lim-Tan SK, et al. Primary extrauterine endometrial stromal neoplasms: a clinicopathologic study of 20 cases and a review of the literature. *Int J Gynecol Pathol* 1993;12:282–296.
228. Halligan AW, McGuinness EP. Malignant fibrous histiocytoma of the fallopian tube. *Br J Obstet Gynaecol* 1990;97:275–276.
229. Jacoby AF, Fuller AF Jr, Thor AD, et al. Primary leiomyosarcoma of the fallopian tube. *Gynecol Oncol* 1993;51:404–407.
230. Kayaalp E, Heller DS, Majmudar B. Serous tumor of low malignant potential of the fallopian tube. *Int J Gynecol Pathol* 2000;19:398–400.
231. Seidman JD. Mucinous lesions of the fallopian tube. A report of seven cases. *Am J Surg Pathol* 1994;18:1205–1212.
232. Zheng W, Wolf S, Kramer EE, et al. Borderline papillary serous tumour of the fallopian tube. *Am J Surg Pathol* 1996;20:30–35.
233. Ober WB, Maier RC. Gestational choriocarcinoma of the fallopian tube. *Diagn Gynecol Obstet* 1981;3:213–231.
234. Patton GW Jr, Goldstein DP. Gestational choriocarcinoma of the tube and ovary. *Surg Gynecol Obstet* 1973;137:608–612.
235. Gatto V, Selim MA, Lankerani M. Primary carcinoma of the fallopian tube in an adolescent. *J Surg Oncol* 1986;33:212–214.
236. Schinfeld JS, Winston HG. Primary tubal carcinoma in pregnancy. *Am J Obstet Gynecol* 1980;137:512–514.
237. Starr AJ, Ruffolo EH, Shenoy BV, et al. Primary carcinoma of the fallopian tube: a surprise finding in a postpartum tubal ligation. *Am J Obstet Gynecol* 1978;132:344–345.
238. Young RH, Scully RE. Ovarian tumors of probable wolffian origin. A report of 11 cases. *Am J Surg Pathol* 1983;7:125–135.
239. Sedlis A. Primary carcinoma of the fallopian tube. *Obstet Gynecol Surv* 1961;16:209–226.
239a. Crum CP, Drapkin R, Kindelberger D, et al. Lessons from *BRCA:* the tubal fimbria emerges as origin for pelvic serous cancer. *Clin Med Res* 2007;5:35–44.
240. Robey SS, Silva EG. Epithelial hyperplasia of the fallopian tube. Its association with serous borderline tumors of the ovary. *Int J Gynecol Pathol* 1989;8:214–220.
241. Moore SW, Enterline HT. Significance of proliferative epithelial lesions of the uterine tube. *Obstet Gynecol* 1975;45:385–390.
242. Bannatyne P, Russell P. Early adenocarcinoma of the fallopian tubes. A case for multifocal tumorigenesis. *Diagn Gynecol Obstet* 1981;3: 49–60.
243. Hartley A, Rollason T, Spooner D. Clear cell carcinoma of the fimbria of the fallopian tube in a *BRCA1* carrier undergoing prophylactic surgery. *Clin Oncol (R Coll Radiol)* 2000;12:58–59.
244. Paley PJ, Swisher EM, Garcia RL, et al. Occult cancer of the fallopian tube in *BRCA*-1 germline mutation carriers at prophylactic oophorectomy: a case for recommending hysterectomy as surgical prophylaxis. *Gynecol Oncol* 2001;80:176–180.
245. Rose PG, Shrigley R, Wiesner GL. Germline *BRCA2* mutation in a patient with fallopian tube carcinoma: a case report. *Gynecol Oncol* 2000;77: 319–320.
246. Yeung HH, Bannatyne P, Russell P. Adenocarcinoma of the fallopian tubes: a clinicopathological study of eight cases. *Pathology* 1983;15:279–286.
247. Demopoulos RI, Aronov R, Mesia A. Clues to the pathogenesis of fallopian tube carcinoma: a morphological and immunohistochemical case control study. *Int J Gynecol Pathol* 2001;20:128–132.
248. Wiskind AK, Dudley AG, Majmudar B, et al. Primary fallopian tube carcinoma with coexistent tuberculous salpingitis: a case report. *J Med Assoc Ga* 1992;81:77–81.
249. Muntz HG, Tarraza HM, Granai CO, et al. Primary adenocarcinoma of the fallopian tube. *Eur J Gynaecol Oncol* 1989;4:239–249.
250. Harrison CR, Averette HE, Jarrell MA, et al. Carcinoma of the fallopian tube: clinical management. *Gynecol Oncol* 1989;32:357–359.
251. Pinto MM, Bernstein LH, Brogan DA, et al. Immunoradiometric assay of CA 125 in effusions. Comparison with carcinoembryonic antigen. *Cancer* 1987;59:218–222.
252. Hirai Y, Chen JT, Hamada T, et al. Clinical and cytologic aspects of primary fallopian tube carcinoma. A report of ten cases. *Acta Cytol* 1987;31:834–840.
253. Maxson WZ, Stehman FB, Ulbright TM, et al. Primary carcinoma of the fallopian tube: evidence for activity of cisplatin combination therapy. *Gynecol Oncol* 1987;26:305–313.
254. Eddy GL, Copeland LJ, Gershenson DM, et al. Fallopian tube carcinoma. *Obstet Gynecol* 1984;64:546–552.
255. Lootsma-Miklosova E, Aalders JG, Willemse PH, et al. Levels of CA 125 in patients with recurrent carcinoma of the fallopian tube: two case histories. *Eur J Obstet Gynecol Reprod Biol* 1987;24:231–235.
256. Jackson-York GL, Ramzy I. Synchronous papillary mucinous adenocarcinoma of the endocervix and fallopian tubes. *Int J Gynecol Pathol* 1992;11:63–67.
257. Woodruff JD, Solomon D, Sullivant H. Multifocal disease in the upper genital canal. *Obstet Gynecol* 1985;65:695–698.
258. Creasman WT, Lukeman J. Role of the fallopian tube in dissemination of malignant cells in corpus cancer. *Cancer* 1972;29:456–457.
259. Rauthe G, Vahrson HW, Burkhardt E. Primary cancer of the fallopian tube. Treatment and results of 37 cases. *Eur J Gynaecol Oncol* 1998;19: 356–362.
260. Anbrokh GB, Anbrokh Ya M. Morphology of metastatic cancer of the fallopian tube in uterine cervix carcinoma. *Neoplasma* 1975;22:73–79.
261. Andriole GL, Garnick MB, Richie JP. Unusual behavior of low-grade, low-stage transitional cell carcinoma of bladder. *Urology* 25:524–526.
262. Case TC. Cancer of the breast with metastasis to the fallopian tube. *J Am Geriatr Soc* 1968;16:832–834.
263. Krebs HB, Walsh J. An unusual case of ruptured tubo-ovarian abscess simulating ovarian carcinoma. *Diagn Gynecol Obstet* 1982;4:63–68.
264. Puflett D. Tuberculous salpingitis resembling adenocarcinoma. *Med J Aust* 1972;2:149–151.

265. Silverberg SG, Frable WJ. Prolapse of fallopian tube into vaginal vault after hysterectomy. Histopathology, cytopathology, and differential diagnosis. *Arch Pathol* 1974;97:100–103.
266. Scharl A, Crombach G, Vierbuchen M, et al. Antigen CA 19-9: presence in mucosa of nondiseased müllerian duct derivatives and marker for differentiation in their carcinomas. *Obstet Gynecol* 1991;77:580–585.
267. Mangan CE, Rubin SC, Rabin DS, et al. Lymph node nomenclature in gynecologic oncology. *Gynecol Oncol* 1986;23:222–226.
268. Burghardt E, Pickel H, Lahousen M, et al. Pelvic lymphadenectomy in operative treatment of ovarian cancer. *Am J Obstet Gynecol* 1986;155:315–319.
269. Piver MS, Barlow JJ, Lele SB. Incidence of subclinical metastasis in stage I and II ovarian carcinoma. *Obstet Gynecol* 1978;52:100–104.
270. Gadducci A, Landoni F, Sartori E, et al. Analysis of treatment failures and survival of patients with fallopian tube carcinoma: a Cooperation Task Force (CTF) study. *Gynecol Oncol* 2001;81:150–159.
271. Hebert-Blouin MN, Koufogianis V, Gillett P, et al. Fallopian tube cancer in a *BRCA1* mutation carrier: rapid development and failure of screening. *Am J Obstet Gynecol* 2002;186:53–54.
272. Hirai Y, Kaku S, Teshima H, et al. Clinical study of primary carcinoma of the fallopian tube: experience with 15 cases. *Gynecol Oncol* 1989;34:20–26.
273. Munoz KA, Harlan LC, Trimble EL. Patterns of care for women with ovarian cancer in the United States. *J Clin Oncol* 1997;15:408–415.
274. Peters WA 3rd, Andersen WA, Hopkins MP, et al. Prognostic features of carcinoma of the fallopian tube. *Obstet Gynecol* 1988;71:757–762.
275. Black SS, Butler SL, Goldman PA, et al. Ovarian cancer symptom index: possibilities for earlier detection. *Cancer* 2007;109:167–169.
276. Risum S, Hogdall C, Loft A, et al. The diagnostic value of PET/CT for primary ovarian cancer—a prospective study. *Gynecol Oncol* 2007;105: 145–149.
277. Bristow RE, del Carmen MG, Pannu HK, et al. Clinically occult recurrent ovarian cancer: patient selection for secondary cytoreductive surgery using combined PET/CT. *Gynecol Oncol* 2003;90:519–528.
278. Davis HM, Surawski VR Jr, Bast RC, et al. Characterization of the CA 125 antigen associated with human epithelial ovarian carcinomas. *Cancer Res* 1986;46:6143–6148.
279. Niloff JM, Bast RC Jr, Schaetzl EM, et al. Predictive value of CA 125 antigen levels in second-look procedures for ovarian cancer. *Am J Obstet Gynecol* 1985;151:981–986.
280. Hulka BS. Cancer screening. Degrees of proof and practical application. *Cancer* 1988;62:1776–1780.
281. Jacobs I. Genetic, biochemical, and multimodal approaches to screening for ovarian cancer. *Gynecol Oncol* 1994;55:S22–S27.
282. Campbell S, Bhan V, Royston P, et al. Transabdominal ultrasound screening for early ovarian cancer. *BMJ* 1989;299:1363–1367.
283. van Nagell JR Jr, DePriest PD, Puls LE, et al. Ovarian cancer screening in asymptomatic postmenopausal women by transvaginal sonography. *Cancer* 1991;68:458–462.
284. van Nagell JR Jr, Higgins RV, Donaldson ES, et al. Transvaginal sonography as a screening method for ovarian cancer. A report of the first 1000 cases screened. *Cancer* 1990;65:573–577.
285. Karlan BY, Platt LD. The current status of ultrasound and color Doppler imaging in screening for ovarian cancer. *Gynecol Oncol* 1994;55:S28–S33.
286. Ueland FR, DePriest PD, Pavlik EJ, et al. Preoperative differentiation of malignant from benign ovarian tumors: the efficacy of morphology indexing and Doppler flow sonography. *Gynecol Oncol* 2003;91:46–50.
287. Olt GJ, Berchuck A, Bast RC Jr. Gynecologic tumor markers. *Semin Surg Oncol* 1990;6:305–313.
288. Zurawski VR Jr, Broderick SF, Pickens P, et al. Serum CA 125 levels in a group of nonhospitalized women: relevance for the early detection of ovarian cancer. *Obstet Gynecol* 1987;69:606–611.
289. Einhorn N, Sjovall K, Knapp RC, et al. Prospective evaluation of serum CA 125 levels for early detection of ovarian cancer. *Obstet Gynecol* 1992;80:14–18.
290. Skates SJ, Drescher CW, Isaacs C, et al. A prospective multi-center ovarian cancer screening study in women at increased risk. *J Clin Oncol* 2007; 25:276s.
291. Buys SS, Partridge E, Greene MH, et al. Ovarian cancer screening in the Prostate, Lung, Colorectal and Ovarian (PLCO) cancer screening trial: findings from the initial screen of a randomized trial. *Am J Obstet Gynecol* 2005;193:1630–1639.
292. Jacobs I, Davies AP, Bridges J, et al. Prevalence screening for ovarian cancer in postmenopausal women by CA 125 measurement and ultrasonography. *BMJ* 1993;306:1030–1034.
293. Jacobs IJ, Skates SJ, MacDonald N, et al. Screening for ovarian cancer: a pilot randomised controlled trial. *Lancet* 1999;353:1207–1210.
294. Westhoff C. Current status of screening for ovarian cancer. *Gynecol Oncol* 1994;55:S34–S37.
295. Bourne TH, Campbell S, Reynolds K, et al. The potential role of serum CA 125 in an ultrasound-based screening program for familial ovarian cancer. *Gynecol Oncol* 1994;52:379–385.
296. Odicino F, Pecorelli S, Zigliani L, et al. History of the FIGO cancer staging system. *Int J Gynaecol Obstet* 2008;101:205–210.
297. Burghardt E, Pickel H, Holzer E, et al. The significance of lymphadenectomy in therapy of ovarian carcinoma. *Am J Obstet Gynecol* 1983;146:111–112.
298. Young RC, Decker DG, Wharton JT, et al. Staging laparotomy in early ovarian cancer. *JAMA* 1983;250:3072–3076.
299. McGowan L, Lesher LP, Norris HJ, et al. Misstaging of ovarian cancer. *Obstet Gynecol* 1985;65:568–572.
300. Heintz AP, Odicino F, Maisonneuve P, et al. Carcinoma of the ovary. *Int J Gynecol Oncol* 2003;83:S135–S166.
301. Delgado G, Oram DH, Petrilli ES. Stage III epithelial ovarian cancer: the role of maximal surgical reduction. *Gynecol Oncol* 1984;18:293–298.
302. Hacker NF, Berek JS, Lagasse LD, et al. Primary cytoreductive surgery for epithelial ovarian cancer. *Obstet Gynecol* 1983;61:413–420.
303. Louie KG, Ozols RF, Myers CE, et al. Long-term results of a cisplatin-containing combination chemotherapy regimen for the treatment of advanced ovarian carcinoma. *J Clin Oncol* 1986;4:1579–1585.
304. Neijt JP, ten Bokkel Huinink WW, van der Burg ME, et al. Long-term survival in ovarian cancer. Mature data from the Netherlands Joint Study Group for Ovarian Cancer. *Eur J Cancer* 1991;27:1367–1372.
305. Pohl R, Dallenbach-Hellweg G, Plugge T, et al. Prognostic parameters in patients with advanced ovarian malignant tumors. *Eur J Gynaecol Oncol* 1984;5:160–169.
306. Redman JR, Petroni GR, Saigo PE, et al. Prognostic factors in advanced ovarian carcinoma. *J Clin Oncol* 1986;4:515–523.
307. Sutton GP, Stehman FB, Einhorn LH, et al. Ten-year follow-up of patients receiving cisplatin, doxorubicin, and cyclophosphamide chemotherapy for advanced epithelial ovarian carcinoma. *J Clin Oncol* 1989;7:223–229.
308. Vogl SE, Pagano M, Kaplan BH, et al. Cis-platin based combination chemotherapy for advanced ovarian cancer. High overall response rate with curative potential only in women with small tumor burdens. *Cancer* 1983; 51:2024–2030.
309. Heintz AP, Van Oosterom AT, Trimbos JB, et al. The treatment of advanced ovarian carcinoma (I): clinical variables associated with prognosis. *Gynecol Oncol* 1988;30:347–358.
310. Piver MS, Lele SB, Marchetti DL, et al. Surgically documented response to intraperitoneal cisplatin, cytarabine, and bleomycin after intravenous cisplatin-based chemotherapy in advanced ovarian adenocarcinoma. *J Clin Oncol* 1988;6:1679–1684.
311. Vergote IB, Kaern J, Abeler VM, et al. Analysis of prognostic factors in stage I epithelial ovarian carcinoma: importance of degree of differentiation and deoxyribonucleic acid ploidy in predicting relapse. *Am J Obstet Gynecol* 1993;169:40–52.
312. Young RC, Walton LA, Ellenberg SS, et al. Adjuvant therapy in stage I and stage II epithelial ovarian cancer. Results of two prospective randomized trials. *N Engl J Med* 1990;322:1021–1027.
313. Baak JP, Langley FA, Talerman A, et al. The prognostic variability of ovarian tumor grading by different pathologists. *Gynecol Oncol* 1987;27: 166–172.
314. Cramer SF, Roth LM, Ulbright TM, et al. Evaluation of the reproducibility of the World Health Organization classification of common ovarian cancers. With emphasis on methodology. *Arch Pathol Lab Med* 1987;111: 819–829.
315. Friedlander ML. Prognostic factors in ovarian cancer. *Semin Oncol* 1998;25:305–314.
316. Rubin SC, Lewis JL Jr. Second-look surgery in ovarian carcinoma. *Crit Rev Oncol Hematol* 1988;8:75–91.
317. Sevelda P, Vavra N, Schemper M, et al. Prognostic factors for survival in stage I epithelial ovarian carcinoma. *Cancer* 1990;65:2349–2352.
318. Makar AP, Kristensen GB, Kaern J, et al. Prognostic value of pre- and postoperative serum CA 125 levels in ovarian cancer: new aspects and multivariate analysis. *Obstet Gynecol* 1992;79:1002–1010.
319. Mogensen O. Prognostic value of CA 125 in advanced ovarian cancer. *Gynecol Oncol* 1992;44:207–212.
320. Rustin GJ, Gennings JN, Nelstrop AE, et al. Use of CA-125 to predict survival of patients with ovarian carcinoma. North Thames Cooperative Group. *J Clin Oncol* 1989;7:1667–1671.
321. Vergote I, De Brabanter J, Fyles A, et al. Prognostic importance of degree of differentiation and cyst rupture in stage I invasive epithelial ovarian carcinoma. *Lancet* 2001;357:176–182.
322. Dembo AJ, Davy M, Stenwig AE, et al. Prognostic factors in patients with stage I epithelial ovarian cancer. *Obstet Gynecol* 1990;75:263–273.
323. Heintz AP, Odicino F, Maisonneuve P, et al. Carcinoma of the ovary. *Int J Gynecol Obstet* 2003;83(Suppl 1):135–166.
324. Hernandez E, Bhagavan BS, Parmley TH, et al. Interobserver variability in the interpretation of epithelial ovarian cancer. *Gynecol Oncol* 1984;17: 117–123.
325. Obermair A, Fuller A, Lopez-Varela E, et al. A new prognostic model for FIGO stage 1 epithelial ovarian cancer. *Gynecol Oncol* 2007;104: 607–611.
326. Ahmed FY, Wiltshaw E, A'Hern RP, et al. Natural history and prognosis of untreated stage I epithelial ovarian carcinoma. *J Clin Oncol* 1996;14: 2968–2975.
327. Monga M, Carmichael JA, Shelley WE, et al. Surgery without adjuvant chemotherapy for early epithelial ovarian carcinoma after comprehensive surgical staging. *Gynecol Oncol* 1991;43:195–197.
328. Trimbos JB, Schueler JA, van der Burg M, et al. Watch and wait after careful surgical treatment and staging in well-differentiated early ovarian cancer. *Cancer* 1991;67:597–602.
329. Scully RE, Young RH, Clement RB. Tumors of the ovary, maldeveloped gonads, fallopian tube, and broad ligament. In: *Atlas of Tumor Pathology*. Washington DC: Armed Forces Institute of Pathology; 1998:23.

330. Pectasides D, Fountzilas G, Aravantinos G, et al. Advanced stage mucinous epithelial ovarian cancer: the Hellenic Cooperative Oncology Group experience. *Gynecol Oncol* 2005;97:436–441.
331. Pectasides D, Fountzilas G, Aravantinos G, et al. Advanced stage clear-cell epithelial ovarian cancer: the Hellenic Cooperative Oncology Group experience. *Gynecol Oncol* 2006;102:285–291.
332. Dembo AJ. Radiotherapeutic management of ovarian cancer. *Semin Oncol* 1984;11:238–250.
333. Dembo AJ. The role of radiotherapy in ovarian cancer. *Bull Cancer* 1982;69:275–283.
334. Dent SF, Klaassen D, Pater JL, et al. Second primary malignancies following the treatment of early stage ovarian cancer: update of a study by the National Cancer Institute of Canada—Clinical Trials Group (NCIC-CTG). *Ann Oncol* 2000;11:65–68.
335. Klaassen D, Shelley W, Starreveld A, et al. Early stage ovarian cancer: a randomized clinical trial comparing whole abdominal radiotherapy, melphalan, and intraperitoneal chromic phosphate: a National Cancer Institute of Canada Clinical Trials Group report. *J Clin Oncol* 1988;6:1254–1263.
336. Sell A, Bertelsen K, Andersen JE, et al. Randomized study of whole-abdomen irradiation versus pelvic irradiation plus cyclophosphamide in treatment of early ovarian cancer. *Gynecol Oncol* 1990;37:367–373.
337. Smith JP. Chemotherapy in gynecologic cancer. *Clin Obstet Gynecol* 1975;18:109–124.
338. Dembo AJ. Abdominopelvic radiotherapy in ovarian cancer. A 10-year experience. *Cancer* 1985;55:2285–2290.
339. Chiara S, Conte P, Franzone P, et al. High-risk early-stage ovarian cancer. Randomized clinical trial comparing cisplatin plus cyclophosphamide versus whole abdominal radiotherapy. *Am J Clin Oncol* 1994;17:72–76.
340. Randall ME, Filiaci VL, Muss H, et al. Randomized phase III trial of whole-abdominal irradiation versus doxorubicin and cisplatin chemotherapy in advanced endometrial carcinoma: a Gynecologic Oncology Group study. *J Clin Oncol* 2006;24:36–44.
341. Varia MA, Stehman FB, Bundy BN, et al. Intraperitoneal radioactive phosphorus (^{32}P) versus observation after negative second-look laparotomy for stage III ovarian carcinoma: a randomized trial of the Gynecologic Oncology Group. *J Clin Oncol* 2003;21:2849–2855.
342. Vergote IB, Vergote-De Vos LN, Abeler VM, et al. Randomized trial comparing cisplatin with radioactive phosphorus or whole-abdomen irradiation as adjuvant treatment of ovarian cancer. *Cancer* 1992;69:741–749.
343. Bolis G, Colombo N, Pecorelli S, et al. Adjuvant treatment for early epithelial ovarian cancer: results of two randomised clinical trials comparing cisplatin to no further treatment or chromic phosphate (^{32}P). GICOG: Gruppo Interregionale Collaborativo in Ginecologia Oncologica. *Ann Oncol* 1995;6:887–893.
344. Young RC, Brady MF, Nieberg RK, et al. Adjuvant treatment for early ovarian cancer: a randomized phase III trial of intraperitoneal ^{32}P or intravenous cyclophosphamide and cisplatin—a Gynecologic Oncology Group study. *J Clin Oncol* 2003;21:4350–4355.
345. Trope C, Kaern J, Hogberg T, et al. Randomized study on adjuvant chemotherapy in stage I high-risk ovarian cancer with evaluation of DNA-ploidy as prognostic instrument. *Ann Oncol* 2000;11:281–288.
346. Colombo N, Guthrie D, Chiari S, et al. International Collaborative Ovarian Neoplasm trial 1: a randomized trial of adjuvant chemotherapy in women with early-stage ovarian cancer. *J Natl Cancer Inst* 2003;95:125–132.
347. Trimbos JB, Parmar M, Vergote I, et al. International Collaborative Ovarian Neoplasm trial 1 and Adjuvant Chemotherapy In Ovarian Neoplasm trial: two parallel randomized phase III trials of adjuvant chemotherapy in patients with early-stage ovarian carcinoma. *J Natl Cancer Inst* 2003;95:105–112.
348. Trimbos JB, Vergote I, Bolis G, et al. Impact of adjuvant chemotherapy and surgical staging in early-stage ovarian carcinoma: European Organisation for Research and Treatment of Cancer—Adjuvant Chemotherapy in Ovarian Neoplasm trial. *J Natl Cancer Inst* 2003;95:113–125.
349. Kolomainen DF, A'Hern R, Coxon FY, et al. Can patients with relapsed, previously untreated, stage I epithelial ovarian cancer be successfully treated with salvage therapy? *J Clin Oncol* 2003;21:3113–3118.
350. Bell J, Brady MF, Young RC, et al. Randomized phase III trial of three versus six cycles of adjuvant carboplatin and paclitaxel in early stage epithelial ovarian carcinoma: a Gynecologic Oncology Group study. *Gynecol Oncol* 2006;102:432–439.
351. Heintz AP, Odicino F, Maisonneuve P, et al. Carcinoma of the fallopian tube. FIGO 6th Annual Report on the Results of Treatment in Gynecologic Cancer. *Int J Gynecol Obstet* 2006;95(Suppl 1):S145–S160.
352. Gemignani ML, Hensley ML, Cohen R, et al. Paclitaxel-based chemotherapy in carcinoma of the fallopian tube. *Gynecol Oncol* 2001;80:16–20.
353. Kosary C, Trimble EL. Treatment and survival for women with fallopian tube carcinoma: a population-based study. *Gynecol Oncol* 2002;86:190–191.
354. Yokoyama Y, Moriya T, Takano T, et al. Clinical outcome and risk factors for recurrence in borderline ovarian tumours. *Br J Cancer* 2006;94:1586–1591.
355. Bjorge T, Engeland A, Hansen S, et al. Prognosis of patients with ovarian cancer and borderline tumours diagnosed in Norway between 1954 and 1993. *Int J Cancer* 1998;75:663–670.
356. Zanetta G, Rota S, Chiari S, et al. Behavior of borderline tumors with particular interest to persistence, recurrence, and progression to invasive carcinoma: a prospective study. *J Clin Oncol* 2001;19:2658–2664.
357. Trimble CL, Kosary C, Trimble EL. Long-term survival and patterns of care in women with ovarian tumors of low malignant potential. *Gynecol Oncol* 2002;86:34–37.
358. Barnhill DR, Kurman RJ, Brady MF, et al. Preliminary analysis of the behavior of stage I ovarian serous tumors of low malignant potential: a Gynecologic Oncology Group study. *J Clin Oncol* 1995;13:2752–2756.
359. Silva EG, Tornos C, Zhuang Z, et al. Tumor recurrence in stage I ovarian serous neoplasms of low malignant potential. *Int J Gynecol Pathol* 1998;17:1–6.
360. McKenney JK, Balzer BL, Longacre TA. Patterns of stromal invasion in ovarian serous tumors of low malignant potential (borderline tumors): a re-evaluation of the concept of stromal microinvasion. *Am J Surg Pathol* 2006;30:1209–1221.
361. Gershenson DM, Silva EG, Levy L, et al. Ovarian serous borderline tumors with invasive peritoneal implants. *Cancer* 1998;82:1096–1103.
362. Silva EG, Gershenson DM, Malpica A, et al. The recurrence and the overall survival rates of ovarian serous borderline neoplasms with noninvasive implants is time dependent. *Am J Surg Pathol* 2006;30:1367–1371.
363. Gershenson DM, Silva EG, Tortolero-Luna G, et al. Serous borderline tumors of the ovary with noninvasive peritoneal implants. *Cancer* 1998;83:2157–2163.
364. Barakat RR, Benjamin I, Lewis JL Jr, et al. Platinum-based chemotherapy for advanced-stage serous ovarian carcinoma of low malignant potential. *Gynecol Oncol* 1995;59:390–393.
365. Lackman F, Carey MS, Kirk ME, et al. Surgery as sole treatment for serous borderline tumors of the ovary with noninvasive implants. *Gynecol Oncol* 2003;90:407–412.
366. Seidman JD, Sherman ME, Kurman RJ. Recurrent serous borderline tumors of the ovary. *Int J Gynecol Pathol* 1998;17:387–389.
367. Abu-Jawdeh GM, Jacobs TW, Niloff J, et al. Estrogen receptor expression is a common feature of ovarian borderline tumors. *Gynecol Oncol* 1996;60:301–307.
368. Tresukosol D, Kudelka AP, Edwards CL, et al. Leuprolide acetate in advanced ovarian serous tumor of low malignant potential. A case report. *J Reprod Med* 1996;41:363–366.
369. Lee EJ, Deavers MT, Hughes JI, et al. Metastasis to sigmoid colon mucosa and submucosa from serous borderline ovarian tumor: response to hormone therapy. *Int J Gynecol Cancer* 2006;16(Suppl 1):295–299.
370. Mayr D, Hirschmann A, Lohrs U, et al. KRAS and *BRAF* mutations in ovarian tumors: a comprehensive study of invasive carcinomas, borderline tumors and extraovarian implants. *Gynecol Oncol* 2006;103:883–887.
371. Griffiths CT. Surgical resection of tumor bulk in the primary treatment of ovarian carcinoma. *Natl Cancer Inst Monogr* 1975;42:101–104.
372. Munnell EW. The changing prognosis and treatment in cancer of the ovary. A report of 235 patients with primary ovarian carcinoma 1952–1961. *Am J Obstet Gynecol* 1968;100:790–805.
373. Delclos L, Quinlan EJ. Malignant tumors of the ovary managed with postoperative megavoltage irradiation. *Radiology* 1969;93:659–663.
374. Young RC, Chabner BA, Hubbard SP, et al. Advanced ovarian adenocarcinoma. A prospective clinical trial of melphalan (L-PAM) versus combination chemotherapy. *N Engl J Med* 1978;299:1261–1266.
375. Omura GA, Bundy BN, Berek JS, et al. Randomized trial of cyclophosphamide plus cisplatin with or without doxorubicin in ovarian carcinoma: a Gynecologic Oncology Group study. *J Clin Oncol* 1989;7:457–465.
375a. Fuks Z, Rizel S, Anteby SO, et al. Current concepts in cancer: ovary-treatment for stages III and IV. The multimodal approach to the treatment of stage III ovarian carcinoma. *Int J Rad Oncol Biol Phys* 1982;8:903–908.
376. Hoskins WJ, McGuire WP, Brady MF, et al. The effect of diameter of largest residual disease on survival after primary cytoreductive surgery in patients with suboptimal residual epithelial ovarian carcinoma. *Am J Obstet Gynecol* 1994;170:974–979; discussion 979–980.
377. Eisenkop SM, Nalick RH, Wang HJ, et al. Peritoneal implant elimination during cytoreductive surgery for ovarian cancer: impact on survival. *Gynecol Oncol* 1993;51:224–229.
378. Venesmaa P, Ylikorkala O. Morbidity and mortality associated with primary and repeat operations for ovarian cancer. *Obstet Gynecol* 1992;79:168–172.
379. Piver MS, Lele SB, Marchetti DL, et al. The impact of aggressive debulking surgery and cisplatin-based chemotherapy on progression-free survival in stage III and IV ovarian carcinoma. *J Clin Oncol* 1988;6:983–989.
380. Bristow RE, Montz FJ, Lagasse LD, et al. Survival impact of surgical cytoreduction in stage IV epithelial ovarian cancer. *Gynecol Oncol* 1999;72:278–287.
381. Curtin JP, Malik R, Venkatraman ES, et al. Stage IV ovarian cancer: impact of surgical debulking. *Gynecol Oncol* 1997;64:9–12.
382. Liu PC, Benjamin I, Morgan MA, et al. Effect of surgical debulking on survival in stage IV ovarian cancer. *Gynecol Oncol* 1997;64:4–8.
383. Munkarah AR, Hallum AV 3rd, Morris M, et al. Prognostic significance of residual disease in patients with stage IV epithelial ovarian cancer. *Gynecol Oncol* 1997;64:13–17.

384. Schwartz PE, Rutherford TJ, Chambers JT, et al. Neoadjuvant chemotherapy for advanced ovarian cancer: long-term survival. *Gynecol Oncol* 1999;72:93–99.
385. Vergote I, De Wever I, Tjalma W, et al. Neoadjuvant chemotherapy or primary debulking surgery in advanced ovarian carcinoma: a retrospective analysis of 285 patients. *Gynecol Oncol* 1998;71:431–436.
386. Everett EN, French AE, Stone RL, et al. Initial chemotherapy followed by surgical cytoreduction for the treatment of stage III/IV epithelial ovarian cancer. *Am J Obstet Gynecol* 2006;195:568–574; discussion 574–576.
387. Rose PG, Nerenstone S, Brady M, et al. Secondary surgical cytoreduction for advanced ovarian carcinoma. *N Engl J Med* 2004;351:2489–2497.
388. van der Burg ME, van Lent M, Buyse M, et al. The effect of debulking surgery after induction chemotherapy on the prognosis in advanced epithelial ovarian cancer. Gynecologic Cancer Cooperative Group of the European Organization for Research and Treatment of Cancer. *N Engl J Med* 1995;332:629–634.
389. Kyrgiou M, Salanti G, Pavlidis N, et al. Survival benefits with diverse chemotherapy regimens for ovarian cancer: meta-analysis of multiple treatments. *J Natl Cancer Inst* 2006;98:1655–1663.
390. Omura G, Blessing JA, Ehrlich CE, et al. A randomized trial of cyclophosphamide and doxorubicin with or without cisplatin in advanced ovarian carcinoma. A Gynecologic Oncology Group study. *Cancer* 1986;57:1725–1730.
391. Aabo K, Adams M, Adnitt P, et al. Chemotherapy in advanced ovarian cancer: four systematic meta-analyses of individual patient data from 37 randomized trials. Advanced Ovarian Cancer Trialists' Group. *Br J Cancer* 1998;78:1479–1487.
392. du Bois A, Luck HJ, Meier W, et al. A randomized clinical trial of cisplatin/paclitaxel versus carboplatin/paclitaxel as first-line treatment of ovarian cancer. *J Natl Cancer Inst* 2003;95:1320–1329.
393. Neijt JP, Engelholm SA, Tuxen MK, et al. Exploratory phase III study of paclitaxel and cisplatin versus paclitaxel and carboplatin in advanced ovarian cancer. *J Clin Oncol* 2000;18:3084–3092.
394. Ozols RF, Bundy BN, Greer BE, et al. Phase III trial of carboplatin and paclitaxel compared with cisplatin and paclitaxel in patients with optimally resected stage III ovarian cancer: a Gynecologic Oncology Group study. *J Clin Oncol* 2003;21:3194–3200.
395. Mani S, Graham MA, Bregman DB, et al. Oxaliplatin: a review of evolving concepts. *Cancer Invest* 2002;20:246–263.
396. Fracasso PM, Blessing JA, Morgan MA, et al. Phase II study of oxaliplatin in platinum-resistant and refractory ovarian cancer: a Gynecologic Oncology Group study. *J Clin Oncol* 2003;21:2856–2859.
397. Misset JL, Vennin P, Chollet PH, et al. Multicenter phase II-III study of oxaliplatin plus cyclophosphamide vs. cisplatin plus cyclophosphamide in chemonaive advanced ovarian cancer patients. *Ann Oncol* 2001;12: 1411–1415.
398. Levin L, Hryniuk WM. Dose intensity analysis of chemotherapy regimens in ovarian carcinoma. *J Clin Oncol* 1987;5:756–767.
399. Conte PF, Bruzzone M, Carnino F, et al. High-dose versus low-dose cisplatin in combination with cyclophosphamide and epidoxorubicin in suboptimal ovarian cancer: a randomized study of the Gruppo Oncologico Nord-Ovest. *J Clin Oncol* 1996;14:351–356.
400. Kaye SB, Paul J, Cassidy J, et al. Mature results of a randomized trial of two doses of cisplatin for the treatment of ovarian cancer. Scottish Gynecology Cancer Trials Group. *J Clin Oncol* 1996;14:2113–2119.
401. McGuire WP, Hoskins WJ, Brady MF, et al. Assessment of dose-intensive therapy in suboptimally debulked ovarian cancer: a Gynecologic Oncology Group study. *J Clin Oncol* 1995;13:1589–1599.
402. Kaye SB, Lewis CR, Paul J, et al. Randomised study of two doses of cisplatin with cyclophosphamide in epithelial ovarian cancer. *Lancet* 1992;340:329–333.
403. Jakobsen A, Bertelsen K, Andersen JE, et al. Dose-effect study of carboplatin in ovarian cancer: a Danish Ovarian Cancer Group study. *J Clin Oncol* 1997;15:193–198.
404. Cure H, Battista C, Guastalla JP, et al. Phase III randomized trial of high-dose chemotherapy (HD) and peripheral blood stem cell (PBSC) support as consolidation in patients (pts) with advanced ovarian cancer (AOC): 5-year follow-up of a GINECO/FNCLCC/SFGM-TC study. *Proc Am Soc Clin Oncol* 2004;23:449, abstr 5006.
405. Thigpen JT, Blessing JA, Ball H, et al. Phase II trial of paclitaxel in patients with progressive ovarian carcinoma after platinum-based chemotherapy: a Gynecologic Oncology Group study. *J Clin Oncol* 1994;12:1748–1753.
406. Eisenhauer EA, ten Bokkel Huinink WW, Swenerton KD, et al. European-Canadian randomized trial of paclitaxel in relapsed ovarian cancer: high-dose versus low-dose and long versus short infusion. *J Clin Oncol* 1994;12:2654–2666.
407. McGuire WP, Hoskins WJ, Brady MF, et al. Cyclophosphamide and cisplatin compared with paclitaxel and cisplatin in patients with stage III and stage IV ovarian cancer. *N Engl J Med* 1996;334:1–6.
408. Piccart MJ, Bertelsen K, James K, et al. Randomized intergroup trial of cisplatin-paclitaxel versus cisplatin-cyclophosphamide in women with advanced epithelial ovarian cancer: three-year results. *J Natl Cancer Inst* 2000;92:699–708.
409. Muggia FM, Braly PS, Brady MF, et al. Phase III randomized study of cisplatin versus paclitaxel versus cisplatin and paclitaxel in patients with suboptimal stage III or IV ovarian cancer: a Gynecologic Oncology Group study. *J Clin Oncol* 2000;18:106–115.
410. Sledge GW, Neuberg D, Bernardo P, et al. Phase III trial of doxorubicin, paclitaxel, and the combination of doxorubicin and paclitaxel as front-line chemotherapy for metastatic breast cancer: an intergroup trial (E1193). *J Clin Oncol* 2003;21:588–592.
411. The International Collaborative Ovarian Neoplasm (ICON) Group. Paclitaxel plus carboplatin versus standard chemotherapy with either single-agent carboplatin or cyclophosphamide, doxorubicin, and cisplatin in women with ovarian cancer: the ICON3 randomised trial. *Lancet* 2002;360:505–515.
412. Randomised comparison of cisplatin with cyclophosphamide/cisplatin and with cyclophosphamide/doxorubicin/cisplatin in advanced ovarian cancer. Gruppo Interegionale Cooperativo Oncologico Ginecologia. *Lancet* 1987;2:353–359.
412a. Vasey PA, Jaysen GC, Gordon A, et al. Phase III ransomized trial of docetaxel-carboplatin versus paclitaxel-carboplatin as first-line chemotherapy for ovarian carcinoma. *J Natl Cancer Inst* 2004;96:1682–1691.
413. Spriggs DR, Brady MF, Vaccarello L, et al. A phase III randomized trial of intravenous cisplatin plus a 24- or 96-hour infusion of paclitaxel in epithelial ovarian cancer: a Gynecologic Oncology Group study. *J Clin Oncol* 2007;25:4466–4471.
414. Omura GA, Brady MF, Look KY, et al. Phase III trial of paclitaxel at two dose levels, the higher dose accompanied by filgrastim at two dose levels in platinum-pretreated epithelial ovarian cancer: an intergroup study. *J Clin Oncol* 2003;21:2843–2848.
415. Bolis G, Scarfone G, Polverino G, et al. Paclitaxol 175 or 223 mg per meters squared with carboplatin in advanced ovarian cancer: a randomized trial. *J Clin Oncol* 2004;22:686–690.
416. Fennelly D, Aghajanian C, Shapiro F, et al. Phase I and pharmacologic study of paclitaxel administered weekly in patients with relapsed ovarian cancer. *J Clin Oncol* 1997;15:187–192.
417. Kaern J, Baekelandt M, Trepe CG. A phase II study of weekly paclitaxel in platinum and paclitaxel-resistant ovarian cancer patients. *Eur J Gynaecol Oncol* 2002;23:383–389.
418. Markman M, Blessing J, Rubin SC, et al. Phase II trial of weekly paclitaxel (80 mg/m^2) in platinum and paclitaxel-resistant ovarian and peritoneal cancers: a Gynecologic Oncology Group Study. *Gynecol Oncol* 2006;101: 436–440.
419. The International Collaborative Ovarian Neoplasm (ICON) Group. ICON2: randomised trial of single-agent carboplatin against three-drug combination of CAP (cyclophosphamide, doxorubicin, and cisplatin) in women with ovarian cancer. ICON Collaborators. International Collaborative Ovarian Neoplasm Study. *Lancet* 1998;352:1571–1576.
420. du Bois A, Weber B, Rochon J, et al. Addition of epirubicin as a third drug to carboplatin-paclitaxel in first-line treatment of advanced ovarian cancer: a prospectively randomized gynecologic cancer intergroup trial by the Arbeitsgemeinschaft Gynaekologische Onkologie Ovarian Cancer Study Group and the Groupe d'Investigateurs Nationaux pour l'Etude des Cancers Ovariens. *J Clin Oncol* 2006;24:1127–1135.
421. ten Bokkel Huinink W, Gore M, Carmichael J, et al. Topotecan versus paclitaxel for the treatment of recurrent epithelial ovarian cancer. *J Clin Oncol* 1997;15:2183–2193.
422. Scarfone G, Scambia G, Raspagliesi F, et al. A multicenter, randomized, phase III study comparing paclitaxel/carboplatin (PC) versus topotecan/ paclitaxel/carboplatin (TPC) in patients with stage III (residual tumor > 1 cm after primary surgery) and IV ovarian cancer (OC). *J Clin Oncol* 2006; 24:256S, Abst #5003.
423. Bookman MA. GOG0182-ICON5: 5-arm phase III randomized trial of paclitaxel (P) and carboplatin (C) vs combinations with gemcitabine (G), PEG-liposomal doxorubicin (D), or topotecan (T) in patients with advanced stage epithelial ovarian (EOC) or primary peritoneal (PPC) carcinoma. *J Clin Oncol* 2006;24:256, abstr #5002.
424 Los G, Mutsaers PH, van der Vijgh WJ, et al. Direct diffusion of cis-diamminedichloroplatinum(II) in intraperitoneal rat tumors after intraperitoneal chemotherapy: a comparison with systemic chemotherapy. *Cancer Res* 1989;49:3380–3384.
425. Alberts DS, Liu PY, Hannigan EV, et al. Intraperitoneal cisplatin plus intravenous cyclophosphamide versus intravenous cisplatin plus intravenous cyclophosphamide for stage III ovarian cancer. *N Engl J Med* 1996;335:1950–1955.
426. Miyagi Y, Fujiwara K, Kigawa J, et al. Intraperitoneal carboplatin infusion may be a pharmacologically more reasonable route than intravenous administration as a systemic chemotherapy. A comparative pharmacokinetic analysis of platinum using a new mathematical model after intraperitoneal vs. intravenous infusion of carboplatin—a Sankai Gynecology Study Group (SGSG) study. *Gynecol Oncol* 2005;99:591–596.
427. Fujiwara K, Armstrong D, Morgan M, et al. Principles and practice of intraperitoneal chemotherapy for ovarian cancer. *Int J Gynecol Cancer* 2007;17:1–20.
428. Davidson SA, Rubin SC, Markman M, et al. Intraperitoneal chemotherapy: analysis of complications with an implanted subcutaneous port and catheter system. *Gynecol Oncol* 1991;41:101–106.
429. Walker JL, Armstrong DK, Huang HQ, et al. Intraperitoneal catheter outcomes in a phase III trial of intravenous versus intraperitoneal chemotherapy in optimal stage III ovarian and primary peritoneal cancer: a Gynecologic Oncology Group study. *Gynecol Oncol* 2006;100: 27–32.

430. Trimble EL. NCI Clinical Announcement on Intraperitoneal Chemotherapy in Ovarian Cancer. http://ctep.cancer.gov/highlights/ovarian.html. Accessed January 5, 2006.
431. Armstrong DK, Bundy B, Wenzel L, et al. Intraperitoneal cisplatin and paclitaxel in ovarian cancer. *N Engl J Med* 2006;354:34–43.
432. Markman M, Bundy BN, Alberts DS, et al. Phase III trial of standard-dose intravenous cisplatin plus paclitaxel versus moderately high-dose carboplatin followed by intravenous paclitaxel and intraperitoneal cisplatin in small-volume stage III ovarian carcinoma: an intergroup study of the Gynecologic Oncology Group, Southwestern Oncology Group, and Eastern Cooperative Oncology Group. *J Clin Oncol* 2001;19:1001–1007.
433. Conroy SE, Baines L, Rodgers K, et al. Prevention of chemotherapy-induced intraperitoneal adhesion formation in rats by icodextrin at a range of concentrations. *Gynecol Oncol* 2003;88:304–308.
434. Seymour MT, Trigonis I, Finan PJ, et al. A feasibility, pharmacokinetic and frequency-escalation trial of intraperitoneal chemotherapy in high risk gastrointestinal tract cancer. *Eur J Surg Oncol* 2008;34(4):403–409.
435. Alberts DS, Hannigan EV, Liu PY, et al. Randomized trial of adjuvant intraperitoneal alpha-interferon in stage III ovarian cancer patients who have no evidence of disease after primary surgery and chemotherapy: an intergroup study. *Gynecol Oncol* 2006;100:133–138.
436. Piccart MJ, Floquet A, Scarfone G, et al. Intraperitoneal cisplatin versus no further treatment: 8-year results of EORTC 55875, a randomized phase III study in ovarian cancer patients with a pathologically complete remission after platinum-based intravenous chemotherapy. *Int J Gynecol Cancer* 2003;13(Suppl 2):196–203.
437. Pignata S, De Placido S, Biamonte R, et al. Residual neurotoxicity in ovarian cancer patients in clinical remission after first-line chemotherapy with carboplatin and paclitaxel: the Multicenter Italian Trial in Ovarian Cancer (MITO-4) retrospective study. *BMC Cancer* 2006;6:5.
438. Kemp G, Rose P, Lurain J, et al. Amifostine pretreatment for protection against cyclophosphamide-induced and cisplatin-induced toxicities: results of a randomized control trial in patients with advanced ovarian cancer. *J Clin Oncol* 1996;14:2101–2112.
439. Hilpert F, Stahle A, Tome O, et al. Neuroprotection with amifostine in the first-line treatment of advanced ovarian cancer with carboplatin/paclitaxel-based chemotherapy—a double-blind, placebo-controlled, randomized phase II study from the Arbeitsgemeinschaft Gynakologische Onkologoie (AGO) Ovarian Cancer Study Group. *Support Care Cancer* 2005;13:797–805.
440. Rubin SC, Hoskins WJ, Saigo PE, et al. Prognostic factors for recurrence following negative second-look laparotomy in ovarian cancer patients treated with platinum-based chemotherapy. *Gynecol Oncol* 1991;42:137–141.
441. Petit T, Velten M, d'Hombres A, et al. Long-term survival of 106 stage III ovarian cancer patients with minimal residual disease after second-look laparotomy and consolidation radiotherapy. *Gynecol Oncol* 2007;104: 104–108.
442. Bruzzone M, Repetto L, Chiara S, et al. Chemotherapy versus radiotherapy in the management of ovarian cancer patients with pathological complete response or minimal residual disease at second look. *Gynecol Oncol* 1990;38:392–395.
443. Lambert HE, Rustin GJ, Gregory WM, et al. A randomized trial comparing single-agent carboplatin with carboplatin followed by radiotherapy for advanced ovarian cancer: a North Thames Ovary Group study. *J Clin Oncol* 1993;11:440–448.
444. Kapp KS, Kapp DS, Poschauko J, et al. The prognostic significance of peritoneal seeding and size of postsurgical residual in patients with stage III epithelial ovarian cancer treated with surgery, chemotherapy, and high-dose radiotherapy. *Gynecol Oncol* 1999;74:400–407.
445. Sorbe B. Consolidation treatment of advanced (FIGO stage III) ovarian carcinoma in complete surgical remission after induction chemotherapy: a randomized, controlled, clinical trial comparing whole abdominal radiotherapy, chemotherapy, and no further treatment. *Int J Gynecol Cancer* 2003;13:278–286.
446. Thomas GM. Is there a role for consolidation or salvage radiotherapy after chemotherapy in advanced epithelial ovarian cancer? *Gynecol Oncol* 1993;51:97–103.
447. Louie KG, Behrens BC, Kinsella TJ, et al. Radiation survival parameters of antineoplastic drug-sensitive and -resistant human ovarian cancer cell lines and their modification by buthionine sulfoximine. *Cancer Res* 1985;45:2110–2115.
448. Hakes TB, Chalas E, Hoskins WJ, et al. Randomized prospective trial of 5 versus 10 cycles of cyclophosphamide, doxorubicin, and cisplatin in advanced ovarian carcinoma. *Gynecol Oncol* 1992;45:284–289.
449. Bertelsen K, Jakobsen A, Stroyer J, et al. A prospective randomized comparison of 6 and 12 cycles of cyclophosphamide, adriamycin, and cisplatin in advanced epithelial ovarian cancer: a Danish Ovarian Study Group trial (DACOVA). *Gynecol Oncol* 1993;49:30–36.
450. Lambert HE, Rustin GJ, Gregory WM, et al. A randomized trial of five versus eight courses of cisplatin or carboplatin in advanced epithelial ovarian carcinoma. A North Thames Ovary Group Study. *Ann Oncol* 1997;8:327–333.
451. Pfister J, Weber B, Reuss A, et al. Randomized phase III trial of topotecan following carboplatin and paclitaxel in first-line treatment of advanced ovarian cancer: a gynecologic cancer intergroup trial of the AGO-OVAR and GINECO. *J Natl Cancer Inst* 2006;98:1036–1045.
452. De Placido S, Scambia G, Di Vagno G, et al. Topotecan compared with no therapy after response to surgery and carboplatin/paclitaxel in patients with ovarian cancer: Multicenter Italian Trials in Ovarian Cancer (MITO-1) randomized study. *J Clin Oncol* 2004;22:2635–2642.
453. Bolis G, Danese S, Tateo S, et al. Epidoxorubicin versus no treatment as consolidation therapy in advanced ovarian cancer: results from a phase II study. *Int J Gynecol Cancer* 2006;16(Suppl 1):74–78.
453a. Papadimitriou C, Dafni U, Anagnostopoulos A, et al. High-dose melphalan and autologous stem cell transplantation as consolidation treatment in patients with chemosensitive ovarian cancer: results of a single institution randomized trial. *Bone Marrow Transp* 2008;41:547–554.
453b. Cure H, Battista J, Guastalla J, et al. Phase III trial of high-dose chemotherapy (HDC) and peripheral blood stem cell (PBSC) support as consolidation in patients with responsive low-burden advanced ovarian cancer (AOC): 5-year follow-up of a GINECO/FNCLCC/SFGM-TC study. *Proc Am Soc Clin Oncol* 2004;23:449.
454. Markman M, Liu PY, Wilczynski S, et al. Phase III randomized trial of 12 versus 3 months of maintenance paclitaxel in patients with advanced ovarian cancer after complete response to platinum and paclitaxel-based chemotherapy: a Southwest Oncology Group and Gynecologic Oncology Group trial. *J Clin Oncol* 2003;21:2460–2465.
455. Markman M, Liu P, Wilczynski S, et al. Survival (S) of ovarian cancer (OC) patients (pts) treated on SWOG9701/GOG178: 12 versus (v) 3 cycles (C) of monthly single-agent paclitaxel (PAC) following attainment of a clinically-defined complete response (CR) to platinum (PLAT)/PAC. *J Clin Oncol* 24:257s.
456. Conte PF, Favilli G, Gadducci A, et al. Final results of after-6 protocol 1: a phase III trial of observation versus 6 courses of paclitaxel (Pac) in advanced ovarian cancer patients in complete response (CR) after platinum-paclitaxel chemotherapy (CT). *J Clin Oncol* 2007;25:275s.
457. Berek JS, Taylor PT, Gordon A, et al. Randomized, placebo-controlled study of oregovomab for consolidation of clinical remission in patients with advanced ovarian cancer. *J Clin Oncol* 2004;22:3507–3516.
458. Hall GD, Brown JM, Coleman RE, et al. Maintenance treatment with interferon for advanced ovarian cancer: results of the Northern and Yorkshire Gynaecology Group randomised phase III study. *Br J Cancer* 2004;91:621–626.
459. Oei AL, Verheijen RH, Seiden MV, et al. Decreased intraperitoneal disease recurrence in epithelial ovarian cancer patients receiving intraperitoneal consolidation treatment with yttrium-90-labeled murine HMFG1 without improvement in overall survival. *Int J Cancer* 2007;120:2710–2714.
460. Verheijen RH, Massuger LF, Benigno BB, et al. Phase III trial of intraperitoneal therapy with yttrium-90-labeled HMFG1 murine monoclonal antibody in patients with epithelial ovarian cancer after a surgically defined complete remission. *J Clin Oncol* 2006;24:571–578.
461. Eisenhauer EA, Vermorken JB, van Glabbeke M. Predictors of response to subsequent chemotherapy in platinum pretreated ovarian cancer: a multivariate analysis of 704 patients [see comments]. *Ann Oncol* 1997;8:963–968.
462. Omura GA, Brady MF, Homesley HD, et al. Long-term follow-up and prognostic factor analysis in advanced ovarian carcinoma: the Gynecologic Oncology Group experience. *J Clin Oncol* 1991;9:1138–1150.
463. Utsunomiya H, Akahira J, Tanno S, et al. Paclitaxel-platinum combination chemotherapy for advanced or recurrent ovarian clear cell adenocarcinoma: a multicenter trial. *Int J Gynecol Cancer* 2006;16:52–56.
464. McGuire V, Jesser CA, Whittemore AS. Survival among U.S. women with invasive epithelial ovarian cancer. *Gynecol Oncol* 2002;84:399–403.
465. Takano M, Kikuchi Y, Yaegashi N, et al. Clear cell carcinoma of the ovary: a retrospective multicentre experience of 254 patients with complete surgical staging. *Br J Cancer* 2006;94:1369–1374.
466. Goff BA, Sainz de la Cuesta R, Muntz HG, et al. Clear cell carcinoma of the ovary: a distinct histologic type with poor prognosis and resistance to platinum-based chemotherapy in stage III disease. *Gynecol Oncol* 1996;60: 412–417.
467. Sugiyama T, Kamura T, Kigawa J, et al. Clinical characteristics of clear cell carcinoma of the ovary: a distinct histologic type with poor prognosis and resistance to platinum-based chemotherapy. *Cancer* 2000;88:2584–2589.
468. Kennedy AW, Markman M, Biscotti CV, et al. Survival probability in ovarian clear cell adenocarcinoma. *Gynecol Oncol* 1999;74:108–114.
469. Ho CM, Huang YJ, Chen TC, et al. Pure-type clear cell carcinoma of the ovary as a distinct histological type and improved survival in patients treated with paclitaxel-platinum-based chemotherapy in pure-type advanced disease. *Gynecol Oncol* 2004;94:197–203.
470. Crotzer DR, Sun CC, Coleman RL, et al. Lack of effective systemic therapy for recurrent clear cell carcinoma of the ovary. *Gynecol Oncol* 2007; 105:404–408.
471. Itamochi H, Kigawa J, Sugiyama T, et al. Low proliferation activity may be associated with chemoresistance in clear cell carcinoma of the ovary. *Obstet Gynecol* 2002;100:281–287.
472. Cloven NG, Kyshtoobayeva A, Burger RA, et al. *In vitro* chemoresistance and biomarker profiles are unique for histologic subtypes of epithelial ovarian cancer. *Gynecol Oncol* 2004;92:160–166.
473. Itamochi H, Kigawa J, Sultana H, et al. Sensitivity to anticancer agents and resistance mechanisms in clear cell carcinoma of the ovary. *Jpn J Cancer Res* 2002;93:723–728.
473a. Shimizu Y, Umezawa S, Hasumi K. A phase II study of combined CPT-11 and mitomycin-C in platinum-refractory clear cell and mucinous ovarian carcinoma. *Ann Acad Med Singapore* 1998;27:650–656.

474. Matsuura Y, Robertson G, Marsden DE, et al. Thromboembolic complications in patients with clear cell carcinoma of the ovary. *Gynecol Oncol* 2007;104:406–410.
475. Tsuchiya A, Sakamoto M, Yasuda J, et al. Expression profiling in ovarian clear cell carcinoma: identification of hepatocyte nuclear factor-1 beta as a molecular marker and a possible molecular target for therapy of ovarian clear cell carcinoma. *Am J Pathol* 2003;163:2503–2512.
476. Tsuda H, Ito YM, Ohashi Y, et al. Identification of overexpression and amplification of ABCF2 in clear cell ovarian adenocarcinomas by cDNA microarray analyses. *Clin Cancer Res* 2005;11:6880–6888.
477. Zorn KK, Bonome T, Gangi L, et al. Gene expression profiles of serous, endometrioid, and clear cell subtypes of ovarian and endometrial cancer. *Clin Cancer Res* 2005;11:6422–6430.
478. Hess V, A'Hern R, Nasiri N, et al. Mucinous epithelial ovarian cancer: a separate entity requiring specific treatment. *J Clin Oncol* 2004;22:1040–1044.
479. Halperin R, Zehavi S, Langer R, et al. Primary peritoneal serous papillary carcinoma: a new epidemiologic trend? A matched-case comparison with ovarian serous papillary cancer. *Int J Gynecol Cancer* 2001;11:403–408.
480. Attanoos RL, Webb R, Dojcinov SD, et al. Value of mesothelial and epithelial antibodies in distinguishing diffuse peritoneal mesothelioma in females from serous papillary carcinoma of the ovary and peritoneum. *Histopathology* 2002;40:237–244.
481. Bandera CA, Muto MG, Schorge JO, et al. *BRCA1* gene mutations in women with papillary serous carcinoma of the peritoneum. *Obstet Gynecol* 1998;92:596–600.
482. Piver MS, Jishi MF, Tsukada Y, et al. Primary peritoneal carcinoma after prophylactic oophorectomy in women with a family history of ovarian cancer. A report of the Gilda Radner Familial Ovarian Cancer Registry. *Cancer* 1993;71:2751–2755.
483. Bloss JD, Liao SY, Buller RE, et al. Extraovarian peritoneal serous papillary carcinoma: a case-control retrospective comparison to papillary adenocarcinoma of the ovary. *Gynecol Oncol* 1993;50:347–351.
484. Moore KN, Gold MA, Moxley KM, et al. Serous fallopian tube carcinoma: a retrospective, multi-institutional case-control comparison to serous adenocarcinoma of the ovary. *Gynecol Oncol* 2007;107:398–403.
485. Rutledge F, Burns BC. Chemotherapy for advanced ovarian cancer. *Am J Obstet Gynecol* 1966;96:761–772.
486. Reimer RR, Hoover R, Fraumeni JF Jr, et al. Acute leukemia after alkylating-agent therapy of ovarian cancer. *N Engl J Med* 1977;297:177–181.
487. Kaldor JM, Day NE, Pettersson F, et al. Leukemia following chemotherapy for ovarian cancer. *N Engl J Med* 1990;322:1–6.
488. Lund B, Jacobsen K, Rasch L, et al. Correlation of abdominal ultrasound and computed tomography scans with second- or third-look laparotomy in patients with ovarian carcinoma. *Gynecol Oncol* 1990;37:279–283.
489. McGowan L, Bunnag B. The evaluation of therapy for ovarian cancer. *Gynecol Oncol* 1976;4:375–383.
490. Rubin SC, Dulaney ED, Markman M, et al. Peritoneal cytology as an indicator of disease in patients with residual ovarian carcinoma. *Obstet Gynecol* 1988;71:851–853.
491. Berek JS, Griffiths CT, Leventhal JM. Laparoscopy for second-look evaluation in ovarian cancer. *Obstet Gynecol* 1981;58:192–198.
492. Ozols RF, Fisher RI, Anderson T, et al. Peritoneoscopy in the management of ovarian cancer. *Am J Obstet Gynecol* 1981;140:611–619.
493. Husain A, Chi DS, Prasad M, et al. The role of laparoscopy in second-look evaluations for ovarian cancer. *Gynecol Oncol* 2001;80:44–47.
494. Rubin SC, Hoskins WJ, Hakes TB, et al. Serum CA 125 levels and surgical findings in patients undergoing secondary operations for epithelial ovarian cancer. *Am J Obstet Gynecol* 1989;160:667–671.
495. Berek JS, Knapp RC, Malkasian GD, et al. CA 125 serum levels correlated with second-look operations among ovarian cancer patients. *Obstet Gynecol* 1986;67:685–689.
496. Barter JF, Barnes WA. Second-look laparotomy. In: Rubin SC, Sutton GP, eds. *Ovarian Cancer*. New York: McGraw-Hill; 1993.
497. Copeland LJ, Gershenson DM, Wharton JT, et al. Microscopic disease at second-look laparotomy in advanced ovarian cancer. *Cancer* 1985;55:472–478.
498. Rubin SC, Hoskins WJ, Hakes TB, et al. Recurrence after negative second-look laparotomy for ovarian cancer: analysis of risk factors. *Am J Obstet Gynecol* 1988;159:1094–1098.
499. Ho AG, Beller U, Speyer JL, et al. A reassessment of the role of second-look laparotomy in advanced ovarian cancer. *J Clin Oncol* 1987;5: 1316–1321.
500. Juretzka MM, Barakat RR, Chi DS, et al. CA125 level as a predictor of progression-free survival and overall survival in ovarian cancer patients with surgically defined disease status prior to the initiation of intraperitoneal consolidation therapy. *Gynecol Oncol* 2007;104:176–180.
501. Rustin GJ, Nelstrop AE, Tuxen MK, et al. Defining progression of ovarian carcinoma during follow-up according to CA 125: a North Thames Ovary Group study. *Ann Oncol* 1996;7:361–364.
502. Guidozzi F, Daponte A. Estrogen replacement therapy for ovarian carcinoma survivors: A randomized controlled trial. *Cancer* 1999;86:1013–1018.
503. Duffy MJ, Bonfrer JM, Kulpa J, et al. CA125 in ovarian cancer: European Group on Tumor Markers guidelines for clinical use. *Int J Gynecol Cancer* 2005;15:679–691.
504. Bridgewater JA, Nelstrop AE, Rustin GJ, et al. Comparison of standard and CA-125 response criteria in patients with epithelial ovarian cancer treated with platinum or paclitaxel. *J Clin Oncol* 1999;17:501–508.
505. Gronlund B, Hansen HH, Hogdall C, et al. Do CA125 response criteria overestimate tumour response in second-line treatment of epithelial ovarian carcinoma? *Br J Cancer* 2004;90:377–382.
506. Gronlund B, Hogdall C, Hilden J, et al. Should CA-125 response criteria be preferred to response evaluation criteria in solid tumors (RECIST) for prognostication during second-line chemotherapy of ovarian carcinoma? *J Clin Oncol* 2004;22:4051–4058.
507. Sabbatini P, Mooney D, Iasonos A, et al. Early CA-125 fluctuations in patients with recurrent ovarian cancer receiving chemotherapy. *Int J Gynecol Cancer* 2007;17:589–594.
508. Menzin AW, Kobrin S, Pollak E, et al. The effect of renal function on serum levels of CA 125. *Gynecol Oncol* 1995;58:375–377.
509. Berek JS, Hacker NF, Lagasse LD, et al. Survival of patients following secondary cytoreductive surgery in ovarian cancer. *Obstet Gynecol* 1983; 61:189–193.
510. Hoskins WJ, Rubin SC, Dulaney E, et al. Influence of secondary cytoreduction at the time of second-look laparotomy on the survival of patients with epithelial ovarian carcinoma. *Gynecol Oncol* 1989;34:365–371.
511. Luesley DM, Chan KK, Fielding JW, et al. Second-look laparotomy in the management of epithelial ovarian carcinoma: an evaluation of fifty cases. *Obstet Gynecol* 1984;64:421–426.
512. Segna RA, Dottino PR, Mandeli JP, et al. Secondary cytoreduction for ovarian cancer following cisplatin therapy. *J Clin Oncol* 1993;11:434–439.
513. Chambers SK, Chambers JT, Kohorn EI, et al. Evaluation of the role of second-look surgery in ovarian cancer. *Obstet Gynecol* 1988;72: 404–408.
514. Podratz KC, Schray MF, Wieand HS, et al. Evaluation of treatment and survival after positive second-look laparotomy. *Gynecol Oncol* 1988;31:9–24.
515. Lippman SM, Alberts DS, Slymen DJ, et al. Second-look laparotomy in epithelial ovarian carcinoma. Prognostic factors associated with survival duration. *Cancer* 1988;61:2571–2577.
516. Salani R, Santillan A, Zahurak ML, et al. Secondary cytoreductive surgery for localized, recurrent epithelial ovarian cancer: analysis of prognostic factors and survival outcome. *Cancer* 2007;109:685–691.
517. Hauspy J, Covens A. Cytoreductive surgery for recurrent ovarian cancer. *Curr Opin Obstet Gynecol* 2007;19:15–21.
518. Markman M, Rothman R, Hakes T, et al. Second-line platinum therapy in patients with ovarian cancer previously treated with cisplatin. *J Clin Oncol* 1991;9:389–393.
519. Markman M, Markman J, Webster K, et al. Duration of response to second-line, platinum-based chemotherapy for ovarian cancer: implications for patient management and clinical trial design. *J Clin Oncol* 2004;22: 3120–3125.
520. Kavanagh J, Tresukosol D, Edwards C, et al. Carboplatin reinduction after taxane in patients with platinum-refractory epithelial ovarian cancer. *J Clin Oncol* 1995;13:1584–1588.
521. Gonzalez-Martin AJ, Calvo E, Bover I, et al. Randomized phase II trial of carboplatin versus paclitaxel and carboplatin in platinum-sensitive recurrent advanced ovarian carcinoma: a GEICO (Grupo Espanol de Investigacion en Cancer de Ovario) study. *Ann Oncol* 2005;16:749–755.
522. Pfisterer J, Plante M, Vergote I, et al. Gemcitabine plus carboplatin compared with carboplatin in patients with platinum-sensitive recurrent ovarian cancer: an intergroup trial of the AGO-OVAR, the NCIC CTG, and the EORTC GCG. *J Clin Oncol* 2006;24:4699–4707.
523. Gordon AN, Fleagle JT, Guthrie D, et al. Recurrent epithelial ovarian carcinoma: a randomized phase III study of pegylated liposomal doxorubicin versus topotecan. *J Clin Oncol* 2001;19:3312–3322.
524. Cantu MG, Buda A, Parma G, et al. Randomized controlled trial of single-agent paclitaxel versus cyclophosphamide, doxorubicin, and cisplatin in patients with recurrent ovarian cancer who responded to first-line platinum-based regimens. *J Clin Oncol* 2002;20:1232–1237.
525. Piccart MJ, Green JA, Lacave AJ, et al. Oxaliplatin or paclitaxel in patients with platinum-pretreated advanced ovarian cancer: a randomized phase II study of the European Organization for Research and Treatment of Cancer Gynecology Group. *J Clin Oncol* 2000;18(6):1193–1202.
526. Lee CW, Matulonis UA, Castells MC. Carboplatin hypersensitivity: a 6-h 12-step protocol effective in 35 desensitizations in patients with gynecologic malignancies and mast cell/IgE-mediated reactions. *Gynecol Oncol* 2004;95:370–376.
527. McAlpine JN, Kelly MG, O'Malley DM, et al. Atypical presentations of carboplatin hypersensitivity reactions: characterization and management in patients with gynecologic malignancies. *Gynecol Oncol* 2006;103: 288–292.
528. Lee CW, Matulonis UA, Castells MC. Rapid inpatient/outpatient desensitization for chemotherapy hypersensitivity: standard protocol effective in 57 patients for 255 courses. *Gynecol Oncol* 2005;99:393–399.
529. Kushner DM, Connor JP, Sanchez F, et al. Weekly docetaxel and carboplatin for recurrent ovarian and peritoneal cancer: a phase II trial. *Gynecol Oncol* 2007;105:358–364.
530. Dizon DS, Dupont J, Anderson S, et al. Treatment of recurrent ovarian cancer: a retrospective analysis of women treated with single-agent carboplatin originally treated with carboplatin and paclitaxel. The Memorial Sloan-Kettering Cancer Center experience. *Gynecol Oncol* 2003;91:584–590.
531. Gronlund B, Hogdall C, Hansen HH, et al. Results of reinduction therapy with paclitaxel and carboplatin in recurrent epithelial ovarian cancer. *Gynecol Oncol* 2001;83:128–134.

532. Bolis G, Scarfone G, Giardina G, et al. Carboplatin alone vs carboplatin plus epidoxorubicin as second-line therapy for cisplatin- or carboplatin-sensitive ovarian cancer. *Gynecol Oncol* 2001;81:3–9.
533. Alberts DS, Liu PY, Wilczynski S, et al. Randomized trial of pegylated liposomal doxorubicin (PLD) plus carboplatin versus carboplatin in platinum-sensitive (PS) patients with recurrent epithelial ovarian or peritoneal carcinoma after failure of initial platinum-based chemotherapy: Southwest Oncology Group Protocol SO200. *Gynecol Onc* 2008;108: 90–94.
534. Parmar MK, Ledermann JA, Colombo N, et al. Paclitaxel plus platinum-based chemotherapy versus conventional platinum-based chemotherapy in women with relapsed ovarian cancer: the ICON4/AGO-OVAR-2.2 trial. *Lancet* 2003;361:2099–2106.
535. ten Bokkel Huinink WW, Gere M, Carmichael J, et al. Topotecan versus paclitaxel for the treatment of recurrent epithelial ovarian cancer. *J Clin Oncol* 1997;15:2183–2193.
536. O'Byrne KJ, Bliss P, Graham JD, et al. A phase III study of Doxil/Caelyx versus paclitaxel in platinum-treated, taxane-naive relapsed ovarian cancer. *Proceedings of ASCO* 2002;21:203a.
537. Buda A, Flioriani I, Rossi R, et al. Randomized controlled trial comparing single agent paclitaxel vs epidoxorubicin plus paclitaxel in patients with advanced ovarian cancer in early progression after platinum-based chemotheraphy: an Italian Collaborative Study fromt he Mario Negri Institute, Milan, G.O.N.O. group and I.O.R. group. *Br J Cancer* 2004;90: 2112–2117.
538. Mutch DG, Orlando M, Goss T, et al. Randomized phase III trial of gemcitabine compared with pegylated liposomal doxorubicin in patients with platinum-resistant ovarian cancer. *J Clin Oncol* 2007;25:2811–2818.
539. Markman M, Blessing JA, Moore D, et al. Altretamine (hexamethylmelamine) in platinum-resistant and platinum-refractory ovarian cancer: a Gynecologic Oncology Group phase II trial. *Gynecol Oncol* 1998;69: 226–229.
540. Markman M, Hakes T, Reichman B, et al. Ifosfamide and mesna in previously treated advanced epithelial ovarian cancer: activity in platinum-resistant disease. *J Clin Oncol* 1992;10:243–248.
541. Bodurka DC, Levenback C, Wolf JK, et al. Phase II trial of irinotecan in patients with metastatic epithelial ovarian cancer or peritoneal cancer. *J Clin Oncol* 2003;21:291–297.
542. Kaern J, Baekelandt M, Trope CG. A phase II study of weekly paclitaxel in platinum and paclitaxel-resistant ovarian cancer patients. *Eur J Gynaecol Oncol* 2002;23:383–389.
543. Markman M, Hall J, Spitz D, et al. Phase II trial of weekly single-agent paclitaxel in platinum/paclitaxel-refractory ovarian cancer. *J Clin Oncol* 2002;20:2365–2369.
544. Markman M, Zanotti K, Webster K, et al. Phase 2 trial of single agent docetaxel in platinum and paclitaxel-refractory ovarian cancer, fallopian tube cancer, and primary carcinoma of the peritoneum. *Gynecol Oncol* 2003;91:573–576.
545. Seidman AD, Berry D, Cirrincione C, et al. Randomized phase III trial of weekly compared with every-3-weeks palitaxel for metastatic breast cancer, with trastuzumab for all HER-2 overexpressors and random assignment to trastuzumab or not in HER-2 nonoverexpressors: final results of cancer and Leukeumia Group B protocol 9840. *J Clin Oncol* 2008;26: 1642–1649.
546. Rosenberg P, Andersson H, Boman K, et al. Randomized trial of single agent paclitaxel given weekly versus every three weeks and with peroral versus intravenous steroid premedication to patients with ovarian cancer previously treated with platinum. *Acta Oncol* 2002;41:418–424.
547. Homesley HD, Hall DJ, Martin DA, et al. A dose-escalating study of weekly bolus topotecan in previously treated ovarian cancer patients. *Gynecol Oncol* 2001;83:394–399.
548. Sehouli J, Oskay-Oezcelik G, Stengel D, et al. Topotecan weekly versus routine 5-day schedule in patients with platinum-resistant ovarian cancer (TOWER): a randomized, two-stage phase-II study of the North-Eastern German Society of Gynaecological Oncology (NOGGO). *J Clin Oncol* 2007;25:280s.
549. Gore M, Oza A, Rustin G, et al. A randomised trial of oral versus intravenous topotecan in patients with relapsed epithelial ovarian cancer. *Eur J Cancer* 2002;38:57–63.
550. Markman M, Kennedy A, Webster K, et al. Phase 2 trial of liposomal doxorubicin (40 mg/m(2)) in platinum/paclitaxel-refractory ovarian and fallopian tube cancers and primary carcinoma of the peritoneum. *Gynecol Oncol* 2000;78:369–372.
551. Brewer CA, Blessing JA, Nagourney RA, et al. Cisplatin plus gemcitabine in platinum-refractory ovarian or primary peritoneal cancer: a phase II study of the Gynecologic Oncology Group. *Gynecol Oncol* 2006;103:446–450.
552. Zheng H, Kavanagh JJ, Hu W, et al. Hormonal therapy in ovarian cancer. *Int J Gynecol Cancer* 2007;17:325–338.
553. Rendina GM, Donadio C, Giovannini M. Steroid receptors and progestinic therapy in ovarian endometrioid carcinoma. *Eur J Gynaecol Oncol* 1982;3:241–246.
554. Wilailak S, Linasmita V, Srisupundit S. Phase II study of high-dose megestrol acetate in platinum-refractory epithelial ovarian cancer. *Anticancer Drugs* 2001;12:719–724.
555. Rocereto TF, Saul HM, Aikins JA Jr, et al. Phase II study of mifepristone (RU486) in refractory ovarian cancer. *Gynecol Oncol* 2000;77:429–432.
556. Long RT, Evans AM. Diethylstilbestrol as a chemotherapeutic agent for ovarian carcinoma. *Mo Med* 1963;60:1125–1127.
557. Freedman RS, Saul PB, Edwards CL, et al. Ethinyl estradiol and medroxyprogesterone acetate in patients with epithelial ovarian carcinoma: a phase II study. *Cancer Treat Rep* 1986;70:369–373.
558. Fromm GL, Freedman RS, Fritsche HA, et al. Sequentially administered ethinyl estradiol and medroxyprogesterone acetate in the treatment of refractory epithelial ovarian carcinoma in patients with positive estrogen receptors. *Cancer* 1991;68:1885–1889.
559. Belinson JL, McClure M, Badger G. Randomized trial of megestrol acetate vs. megestrol acetate/tamoxifen for the management of progressive or recurrent epithelial ovarian carcinoma. *Gynecol Oncol* 1987;28: 151–155.
560. Jakobsen A, Bertelsen K, Sell A. Cyclic hormonal treatment in ovarian cancer. A phase-II trial. *Eur J Cancer Clin Oncol* 1987;23:915–916.
561. Perez-Gracia JL, Carrasco EM. Tamoxifen therapy for ovarian cancer in the adjuvant and advanced settings: systematic review of the literature and implications for future research. *Gynecol Oncol* 2002;84:201–209.
562. Jager W, Sauerbrei W, Beck E, et al. A randomized comparison of triptorelin and tamoxifen as treatment of progressive ovarian cancer. *Anticancer Res* 1995;15:2639–2642.
563. Markman M, Iseminger KA, Hatch KD, et al. Tamoxifen in platinum-refractory ovarian cancer: a Gynecologic Oncology Group Ancillary Report. *Gynecol Oncol* 1996;62:4–6.
564. Verschraegen CF, Westphalen S, Hu W, et al. Phase II study of cetrorelix, a luteinizing hormone-releasing hormone antagonist in patients with platinum-resistant ovarian cancer. *Gynecol Oncol* 2003;90:552–559.
565. Bowman A, Gabra H, Langdon SP, et al. CA125 response is associated with estrogen receptor expression in a phase II trial of letrozole in ovarian cancer: identification of an endocrine-sensitive subgroup. *Clin Cancer Res* 2002;8:2233–2239.
566. Kavanagh JJ, Wharton JT, Roberts WS. Androgen therapy in the treatment of refractory epithelial ovarian cancer. *Cancer Treat Rep* 1987;71:537–538.
567. Schwartz PE, Chambers JT, Kohorn EI, et al. Tamoxifen in combination with cytotoxic chemotherapy in advanced epithelial ovarian cancer. A prospective randomized trial. *Cancer* 1989;63:1074–1078.
568. Emons G, Ortmann O, Teichert HM, et al. Luteinizing hormone-releasing hormone agonist triptorelin in combination with cytotoxic chemotherapy in patients with advanced ovarian carcinoma. A prospective double blind randomized trial. Decapeptyl Ovarian Cancer Study Group. *Cancer* 1996;78:1452–1460.
569. Senn HJ, Lei D, Castano-Almendral A, et al. Chemo-(hormonal)-therapy of advanced ovarian neoplasms in FIGO stages III and IV. Prospective SAKK-study 20/71. *Schweiz Med Wochenschr* 1980;110:1202–1208.
570. Corn BW, Lanciano RM, Boente M, et al. Recurrent ovarian cancer. Effective radiotherapeutic palliation after chemotherapy failure. *Cancer* 1994;74:2979–2983.
571. Gelblum D, Mychalczak B, Almadrones L, et al. Palliative benefit of external-beam radiation in the management of platinum refractory epithelial ovarian carcinoma. *Gynecol Oncol* 1998;69:36–41.
572. May LF, Belinson JL, Roland TA. Palliative benefit of radiation therapy in advanced ovarian cancer. *Gynecol Oncol* 1990;37:408–411.
573. Menczer J, Modan M, Brenner J, et al. Abdominopelvic irradiation for stage II-IV ovarian carcinoma patients with limited or no residual disease at second-look laparotomy after completion of cisplatinum-based combination chemotherapy. *Gynecol Oncol* 1986;24:149–154.
574. Krebs HB, Goplerud DR. Surgical management of bowel obstruction in advanced ovarian carcinoma. *Obstet Gynecol* 1983;61:327–330.
575. Clarke-Pearson DL, DeLong ER, Chin N, et al. Intestinal obstruction in patients with ovarian cancer. Variables associated with surgical complications and survival. *Arch Surg* 1988;123:42–45.
576. Rubin SC, Hoskins WJ, Benjamin I, et al. Palliative surgery for intestinal obstruction in advanced ovarian cancer. *Gynecol Oncol* 1989;34:16–19.
577. Pothuri B, Vaidaya A, Aghajanian C, et al. Palliative surgery for bowel obstruction in recurrent ovarian cancer: an updated series. *Gynecol Oncol* 2003;89:306.
578. Cruikshank DP, Buchsbaum HJ. Effects of rapid paracentesis. Cardiovascular dynamics and body fluid composition. *JAMA* 1973;225: 1361–1362.
579. Ostrowski MJ, Halsall GM. Intracavitary bleomycin in the management of malignant effusions: a multicenter study. *Cancer Treat Rep* 1982;66: 1903–1907.
580. Paladine W, Cunningham TJ, Sponzo R, et al. Intracavitary bleomycin in the management of malignant effusions. *Cancer* 1976;38:1903–1908.
581. Souter RG, Wells C, Tarin D, et al. Surgical and pathologic complications associated with peritoneovenous shunts in management of malignant ascites. *Cancer* 1985;55:1973–1978.
582. El-Shami K, Elsaid A, El-Kerm Y. Open-label safety and efficacy pilot trial of intraperitoneal bevacizumab as palliative treatment in refractory malignant ascites. *J Clin Oncol* 2007;25:503s, abstr #9043.
583. Burger RA, Sill M, Monk B, et al. Phase II trial of bevacizumab in persistent or recurrent epithelial ovarian cancer or primary peritoneal cancer: a Gynecologic Oncology Group Study. *J Clin Oncol* 2007;25:5165–5171.
584. Cannistra SA, Matulonis U, Penson R, et al. Phase II study of bevacizumab in patients with platinum-resistant ovarian cancer or peritoneal serous cancer. *J Clin Oncol* 2007;25:5180–5186.

585. Garcia AA, Hirte H, Fleming G, et al. Phase II clinical trial of bevacizumab and low-dose metronomic oral cyclosphosphamide in recurrent ovarian cancer: a trial of the California, Chicago, and Princess Margaret Hospital phase II consortia. *J Clin Oncol* 2008;26:76–82.
586. Aghajanian C. The role of bevacizumab in ovarian cancer—an evolving story. *Gynecol Oncol* 2006;102:131–133.
587. Tew WP, Colombo N, Ray-Coquard I, et al. VEGF-Trap for patients (pts) with recurrent platinum-resistant epithelial ovarian cancer (EOC): preliminary results of a randomized, multicenter phase II study. *J Clin Oncol* 2007;25:276s, abstr #5508.
588. Eisen T, Boshoff C, Mak I, et al. Continuous low dose thalidomide: a phase II study in advanced melanoma, renal cell, ovarian and breast cancer. *Br J Cancer* 2000;82:812–817.
589. Chan JK, Manuel MR, Ciaravino G, et al. Safety and efficacy of thalidomide in recurrent epithelial ovarian and peritoneal carcinoma. *Gynecol Oncol* 2006;103:919–923.
590. Gordinier ME, Dizon DS, Weitzen S, et al. Oral thalidomide as palliative chemotherapy in women with advanced ovarian cancer. *J Palliat Med* 2007;10:61–66.
591. Zhang MM, Chan JK, Husain A, et al. Safety and efficacy of lenalidomide (Revlimid) in recurrent ovarian and primary peritoneal carcinoma. *Gynecol Oncol* 2007;105:194–198.
592. Hudis CA. Trastuzumab—mechanism of action and use in clinical practice. *N Engl J Med* 2007;357:39–51.
593. Lynch TJ, Bell DW, Sordella R, et al. Activating mutations in the epidermal growth factor receptor underlying responsiveness of non-small-cell lung cancer to gefitinib. *N Engl J Med* 2004;350:2129–2139.
594. Gordon AN, Finkler N, Edwards RP, et al. Efficacy and safety of erlotinib HCl, an epidermal growth factor receptor (HER1/EGFR) tyrosine kinase inhibitor, in patients with advanced ovarian carcinoma: results from a phase II multicenter study. *Int J Gynecol Cancer* 2005;15:785–792.
595. Schilder RJ, Sill MW, Chen X, et al. Phase II study of gefitinib in patients with relapsed or persistent ovarian or primary peritoneal carcinoma and evaluation of epidermal growth factor receptor mutations and immunohistochemical expression: a Gynecologic Oncology Group study. *Clin Cancer Res* 2005;11:5539–5548.
596. Posadas EM, Liel MS, Kwitkowski V, et al. A phase II and pharmacodynamic study of gefitinib in patients with refractory or recurrent epithelial ovarian cancer. *Cancer* 2007;109:1323–1330.
597. Wagner U, du Bois A, Pfisterer J, et al. Gefitinib in combination with tamoxifen in patients with ovarian cancer refractory or resistant to platinum-taxane based therapy—a phase II trial of the AGO Ovarian Cancer Study Group (AGO-OVAR 2.6). *Gynecol Oncol* 2007;105: 132–137.
598. Schilder RJ, Pathak HB, Lokshin AE, et al. Phase II trial of single agent cetuximab in patients with persistent or recurrent epithelial ovarian or primary peritoneal carcinoma with the potential of dose escalation to rash. *Gynecol Oncol* 2009; epub ahead of print.
599. Seiden MV, Burris HA, Matulonis U, et al. A phase II trial of EMD72000 (matuzumab), a humanized anti-EGFR monoclonal antibody, in patients with platinum-resistant ovarian and primary peritoneal malignancies. *Gynecol Oncol* 2007;104:727–731.
600. Hellstrom I, Goodman G, Pullman J, et al. Overexpression of HER-2 in ovarian carcinomas. *Cancer Res* 2001;61:2420–2423.
601. Bookman MA, Darcy KM, Clarke-Pearson D, et al. Evaluation of monoclonal humanized anti-HER2 antibody, trastuzumab, in patients with recurrent or refractory ovarian or primary peritoneal carcinoma with overexpression of HER2: a phase II trial of the Gynecologic Oncology Group. *J Clin Oncol* 2003;21:283–290.
602. Gordon MS, Matei D, Aghajanian C, et al. Clinical activity of pertuzumab (rhuMAb 2C4), a HER dimerization inhibitor, in advanced ovarian cancer: potential predictive relationship with tumor HER2 activation status. *J Clin Oncol* 2006;24:4324–4332.
603. Gordon MS, Matei D, Aghajanian C, et al. Clinical activity of pertuzumab (rhuMAb 2C4), a HER dimerization inhibitor, in advanced ovarian cancer: a potential predictive relationship with tumor HER2 activation status. *J Clin Oncol* 2006;24:4324–4332.
604. Posadas EM, Kwitkowski V, Kotz HL, et al. A prospective analysis of imatinib-induced c-kit modulation in ovarian cancer: a phase II clinical study with proteomic profiling. *Cancer* 2007;110:309–317.
605. Schmandt RE, Broaddus R, Lu KH, et al. Expression of c-ABL, c-KIT, and platelet-derived growth factor receptor-beta in ovarian serous carcinoma and normal ovarian surface epithelium. *Cancer* 2003;98:758–764.
606. Alberts DS, Liu PY, Wilczynski SP, et al. Phase II trial of imatinib mesylate in recurrent, biomarker positive, ovarian cancer (Southwest Oncology Group Protocol S0211). *Int J Gynecol Cancer* 2007;17(4):784–788.
607. Coleman RL, Broaddus RR, Bodurka DC, et al. Phase II trial of imatinib mesylate in patients with recurrent platinum- and taxane-resistant epithelial ovarian and primary peritoneal cancers. *Gynecol Oncol* 2006;101:126–131.
608. Zhang L, Conejo-Garcia JR, Katsaros D, et al. Intratumoral T cells, recurrence, and survival in epithelial ovarian cancer. *N Engl J Med* 2003; 348:203–213.
609. Sabbatini P, Odunsi K. Immunologic approaches to ovarian cancer treatment. *J Clin Oncol* 2007;25:2884–2893.
610. Wei SH, Chen CM, Strathdee G, et al. Methylation microarray analysis of late-stage ovarian carcinomas distinguishes progression-free survival in patients and identifies candidate epigenetic markers. *Clin Cancer Res* 2002;8:2246–2252.

CHAPTER 26 ■ OVARIAN GERM CELL TUMORS

DANIELA E. MATEI, HELEN MICHAEL, ANTHONY H. RUSSELL, AND DAVID M. GERSHENSON

INTRODUCTION

Significant improvements in the management of ovarian germ cell tumors have been achieved during the past two decades. The development of more effective chemotherapy regimens is clearly the leading cause for improved outcome for these patients. In addition, advancements in other disciplines led to the development of a more precise surgical staging system, improved radiographic imaging, more sophisticated pathology techniques, as well as improved supportive care and symptom control. A substantial majority of patients with ovarian germ cell tumors are long-term survivors and suffer minimal morbidity from treatment. Fertility-sparing surgical procedures enable a large proportion of young women with ovarian germ cell tumors to preserve their reproductive potential. These results illustrate the value of collaboration between different specialties (surgery, medical oncology, pathology, imaging).

PATHOLOGY

The current World Health Organization (WHO) classification of ovarian germ cell tumors includes dysgerminoma, yolk sac tumor, embryonal carcinoma, polyembryoma, nongestational choriocarcinoma, mixed germ cell tumors, and teratomas (immature, mature, and monodermal types) (1). Primitive germ cell tumors account for 2% to 3% of all ovarian cancers and occur usually in young women. The peak age incidence for development of these tumors is the early 20s. The pathology of these neoplasms is discussed in the same order as the listing in the current WHO classification.

Dysgerminoma

Dysgerminoma represents the most common ovarian malignant germ cell tumor (2). Most dysgerminomas are seen in patients with a normal karyotype, but dysgerminoma is the most frequent ovarian neoplasm in patients with gonadal dysgenesis. Five percent to 10% are associated with gonadoblastomas in sexually maldeveloped patients. Most dysgerminomas occur in normal females who usually present with abdominal enlargement, a mass, or pain due to torsion. About 10% of dysgerminomas are bilateral on gross examination and another 10% have microscopic involvement of the contralateral ovary. Association with gonadoblastoma increases the risk of bilateral involvement by dysgerminoma.

On gross examination, dysgerminomas are usually large, white to gray, fleshy, lobulated masses that usually have no more than very focal areas of hemorrhage or necrosis on cut section. Abundant hemorrhage, necrosis, or cystic areas in a well-fixed tumor should raise the question of a mixed germ cell tumor. Microscopically, dysgerminomas display nests and cords of primitive-appearing germ cells with clear to eosinophilic cytoplasm and prominent cytoplasmic borders (Fig. 26.1). Nuclei are enlarged but they are not pleomorphic. Mitoses may be numerous, and the number of mitotic figures does not have any therapeutic or prognostic significance. Nests of tumor cells are separated by fibrous trabeculae that contain lymphocytes and, sometimes, granulomas. Syncytiotrophoblast cells are present in about 3% of dysgerminomas.

Dysgerminomas contain cytoplasmic glycogen that can be demonstrated with a periodic acid-Schiff (PAS) stain. These tumors display diffuse staining for placenta-like alkaline phosphatase (PLAP), usually with accentuation of the cytoplasmic membrane. Positive staining of dysgerminomas for c-kit (3) and the nuclear transcription factor OCT 3/4 (4) is helpful in confirming this diagnosis. Dysgerminoma is the only ovarian germ cell tumor that displays c-kit staining (5). Both dysgerminoma and embryonal carcinoma stain for OCT 3/4. In contrast to embryonal carcinoma, dysgerminoma does not stain for CD30. Syncytiotrophoblast cells present in dysgerminomas display human chorionic gonadotropin (hCG) staining. In contrast to choriocarcinoma, the syncytiotrophoblast cells in dysgerminomas are not admixed with cytotrophoblast cells. Dysgerminomas do not produce alpha fetoprotein (AFP), a finding that may be helpful in distinguishing them from the solid variant of yolk sac tumor. Optimal and prompt fixation of the surgical specimen facilitates the correct diagnosis. Poor fixation can result in artifacts that mimic embryonal carcinoma and yolk sac tumor histology.

Yolk Sac Tumor

Yolk sac tumor (endodermal sinus tumor) is the second most common ovarian germ cell tumor, accounting for 22% of ovarian germ cell tumors studied at the Armed Forces Institute of Pathology (AFIP) (2,6). These tumors grow very rapidly, often becoming clinically evident in less than one month.

Ovarian yolk sac tumors are typically large and unilateral, although metastasis to the opposite ovary may occur. These tumors have a smooth external surface unless rupture or invasion into surrounding structures has occurred. On cut section, these neoplasms are tan to gray, with abundant hemorrhage and necrosis. They may be partially solid, but they usually contain cysts that vary in size from a few millimeters to several centimeters in diameter. The cut surface appears mucoid, slimy, or gelatinous. Yolk sac tumor (6) displays many different histologic patterns (7). The most common microscopic

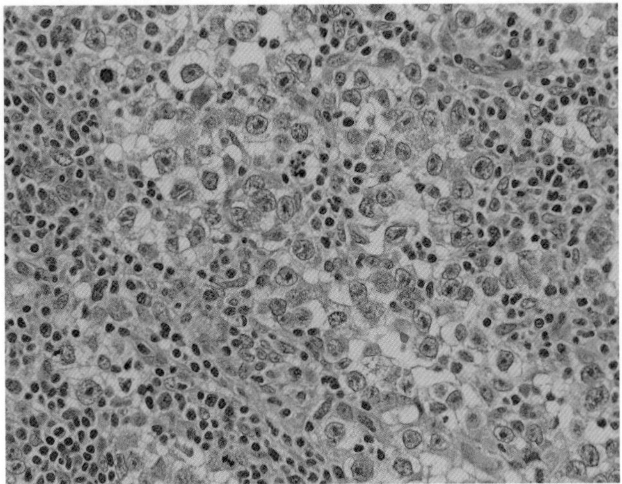

FIGURE 26.1. Dysgerminoma. This neoplasm has nests of cells with clear cytoplasm and enlarged hyperchromatic nuclei. Fibrous septae containing lymphocytes separate nests of tumor.

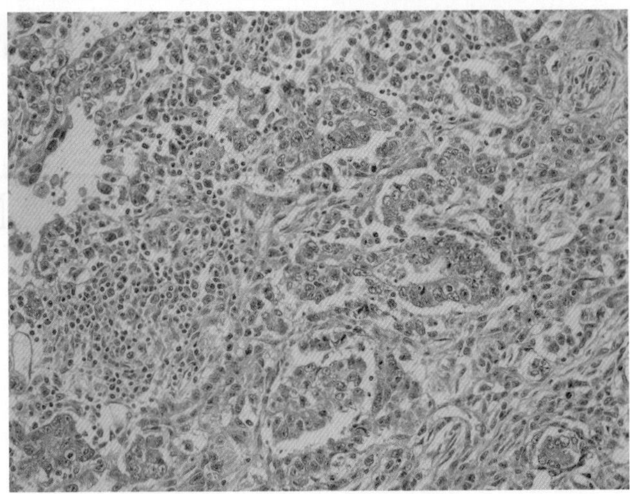

FIGURE 26.3. Schiller-Duvall bodies, papillary structures with central blood vessels, are seen in the endodermal sinus pattern of yolk sac tumor.

pattern in primary ovarian tumors is the reticular or microcystic pattern (Fig. 26.2). The tumor has a mesh-like pattern and it displays a network of flattened or cuboidal epithelial cells with varying degrees of atypia. The endodermal sinus (festoon) pattern contains Schiller-Duvall bodies (Fig. 26.3) that have a central capillary surrounded by connective tissue and a peripheral layer of columnar cells. These structures are situated in cavities lined by yolk sac tumor cells. When present, Schiller-Duvall bodies are diagnostic of yolk sac tumor. Other less common variants of yolk sac tumor include hepatoid, polyvesicular vitteline, enteric, endometrioid, solid, parietal, and mesenchymal patterns. Most patterns of yolk sac tumor may contain eosinophilic hyaline globules that are PAS positive and diastase resistant. These globules may be seen in non–germ cell tumors and they are not specific for yolk sac tumor. They do not contain AFP. Yolk sac tumors generally display cytoplasmic staining for cytokeratin and AFP, although the parietal pattern of yolk sac tumor typically does not contain AFP. Therefore, serum AFP is a useful marker for yolk sac tumor, although a negative serum AFP does not exclude the disease. Chemotherapy has resulted in the appearance of AFP-negative parietal yolk sac tumor after eradication

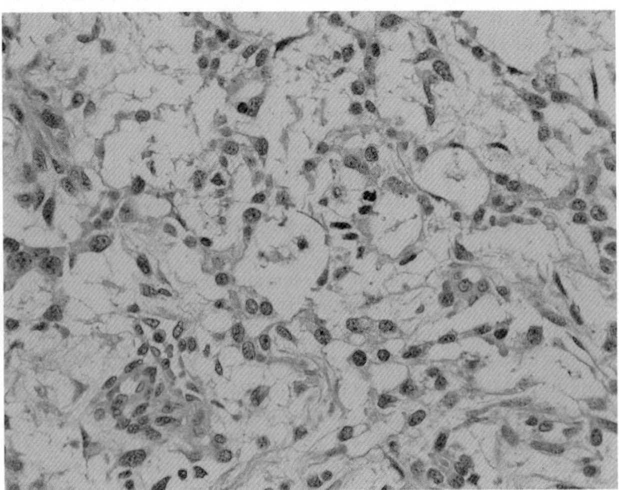

FIGURE 26.2. Reticular pattern of yolk sac tumor. There is a mesh-like arrangement of cuboidal tumor cells.

of AFP positive patterns of the tumor (8). Enteric glands in yolk sac tumor may be carcinoembryonic antigen (CEA) positive. Some types of yolk sac tumor need to be differentiated from endometrioid and clear cell tumors of the ovary. Germ cell tumors usually occur in younger patients than epithelial ovarian tumors, but the lack of staining for cytokeratin 7 and epithelial membrane antigen supports a diagnosis of yolk sac tumor (9) in controversial neoplasms.

Embryonal Carcinoma

Embryonal carcinoma is rarely seen in the ovary, in contrast to its frequent occurrence in the testis. Only 14 cases were identified during a period of 30 years at the AFIP (10), and there have been no recent large series of these tumors. Embryonal carcinoma of the ovary is usually associated with yolk sac tumor in mixed germ cell tumors. On gross examination, embryonal carcinoma characteristically displays areas of hemorrhage and necrosis. Microscopically, this tumor is composed of very crowded cells that display overlapping nuclei in paraffin sections. The nuclei are very pleomorphic and they contain large, prominent nucleoli. The mitotic rate is high in these tumors. Glandular, solid, and papillary patterns may be seen. Vascular invasion is common. Embryonal carcinoma stains positively for PLAP, pancytokeratin (AE1/AE3 and CAM 5.2), CD30, and OCT 3/4. In contrast to seminoma, embryonal carcinoma does not display c-kit staining. Some embryonal carcinomas display focal AFP positivity that may represent partial transformation to yolk sac tumor. Syncytiotrophoblast cells may be present. They produce hCG, but they are not accompanied by admixed cytotrophoblast cells unless choriocarcinoma is also present.

Polyembryoma

Polyembryoma is a very rare malignant ovarian tumor (2). In the few cases reported, the embryoid bodies characteristic of this germ cell tumor have coexisted with other germ cell tumor types. The microscopic appearance of embryoid bodies (11) with an embryonic disc separating a yolk sac and an amniotic cavity may actually be due to an admixture of yolk sac tumor and embryonal carcinoma.

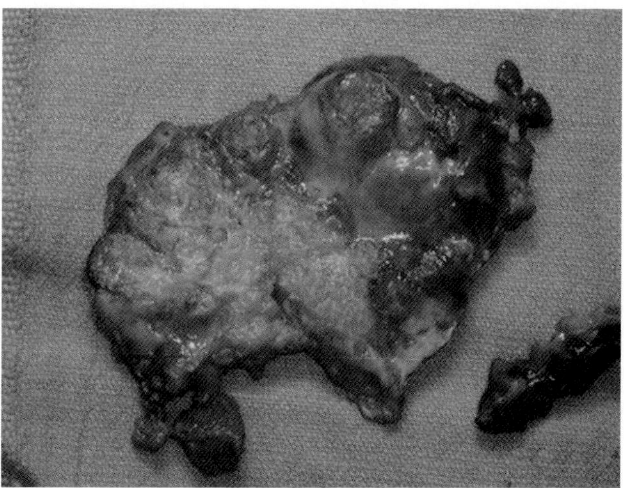

FIGURE 26.4. Choriocarcinoma. This ovarian neoplasm is extremely hemorrhagic.

Choriocarcinoma

Primary nongestational ovarian choriocarcinoma is rare (12). It is most often seen as a component of mixed germ cell tumors of the ovary (13,14). Choriocarcinomas display abundant hemorrhage and necrosis on gross examination (Fig. 26.4). Microscopically, these neoplasms show a plexiform pattern composed of an admixture of syncytiotrophoblast and cytotrophoblast cells (Fig. 26.5). Syncytiotrophoblastic giant cells have abundant eosinophilic to amphophilic cytoplasm that contains multiple atypical, hyperchromatic nuclei. Cytotrophoblast cells are round and often have well-defined cell borders, clear to lightly eosinophilic cytoplasm, and single, atypical nuclei. Numerous mitoses are present. Choriocarcinoma spreads by blood vessel invasion that is easy to identify in these tumors. Cytotrophoblast cells do not produce hCG. Syncytiotrophoblast cells are formed from cytotrophoblast cells, and syncytiotrophoblast does produce hCG. Choriocarcinoma may also stain for cytokeratins, epithelial membrane antigen, and carcinoembryonic antigen. Nongestational choriocarcinoma must be distinguished from gestational choriocarcinoma because the former has a worse prognosis and requires more aggressive therapy. Identification of paternal genetic material indicates that the tumor is of gestational origin (15).

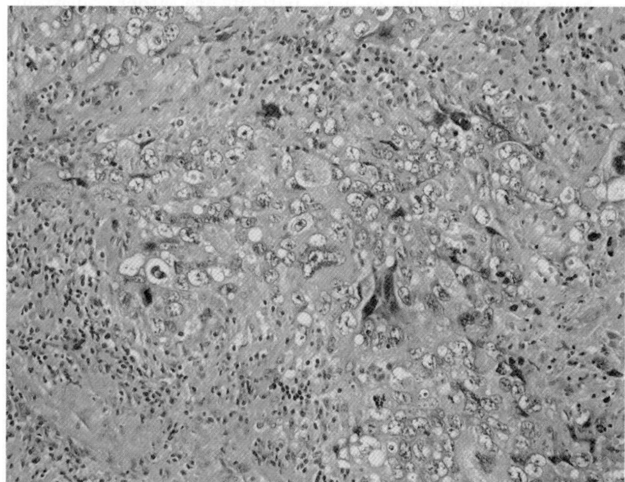

FIGURE 26.5. Choriocarcinoma. Syncytiotrophoblast cells have dark cytoplasm and multiple atypical nuclei. Cytotrophoblast cells have lighter cytoplasm and single atypical nuclei. Both cell types are admixed in choriocarcinoma. Areas of hemorrhage and necrosis are common.

Mixed Germ Cell Tumors

Mixed germ cell tumors of the ovary contain two or more different types of germ cell neoplasm, either intimately admixed or as separate foci within the tumor (13,14). They are much less common in the ovary than in the testis. They accounted for only 8% of malignant ovarian germ cell tumors accessioned at the AFIP over a period of 30 years (13).

Malignant mixed germ cell tumors are large, unilateral neoplasms, but the gross appearance on the cut surface depends on the particular type of germ cell tumor present. The most common germ cell tumor element in the AFIP series was dysgerminoma (80%), followed by yolk sac tumor (70%), teratoma (53%), choriocarcinoma (20%), and embryonal carcinoma (13%) (13). The most frequent combination has been dysgerminoma and yolk sac tumor. Syncytiotrophoblast may occur either as a component of choriocarcinoma or as isolated cells in other germ cell tumor elements. The diagnosis and prognosis of malignant mixed germ cell tumors depend on adequate tumor sampling in order to detect small areas of different types of germ cell tumor. Thorough sampling is essential because the types of tumor identified may affect therapy and prognosis.

Teratomas

Teratomas are germ cell tumors that contain tissue derived from two or three embryonic layers. Teratomas are subclassified according to whether the tumor elements represent mature or immature tissue types. In addition, monodermal and highly specialized teratomas are composed of a predominance of one tissue type such as thyroid tissue (struma ovarii). This discussion of the pathology of ovarian tumors will address predominantly mature and immature teratomas in adult women. In contrast to other ovarian germ cell tumor types, ovarian teratomas do not contain 12p amplification (16,17). Ovarian teratomas apparently arise by parthenogenesis.

Most teratomas are mature cystic teratomas that contain differentiated tissue components such as skin, cartilage, glia, glandular elements, and bone. Any tissue type present in adults may be represented in teratomas. The widest variety of tissue types is characteristically identified in a nodule in the wall of the cystic neoplasms. Mature cystic teratomas represent benign neoplasms unless they contain a somatic malignancy such as squamous carcinoma, papillary thyroid carcinoma, or other non–germ cell tumors arising in differentiated elements of the teratoma.

Immature teratomas in adult women, in contrast to mature cystic teratomas, are uncommon tumors. They represent about 3% of all ovarian teratomas, but immature teratomas are the third most common form of malignant ovarian germ cell tumors. Very limited amounts of immature tissue occurring in mature cystic teratomas does not seem to alter the prognosis of those tumors (18), but immature tissue in solid teratomas represents a malignant tumor that can disseminate and metastasize.

Most immature ovarian teratomas are unilateral neoplasms, although they can metastasize to the opposite ovary and they can also be associated with mature teratoma in the opposite ovary. Immature teratomas are predominantly solid tumors, but they may contain some cystic areas. The cut surface of immature teratomas is soft and fleshy or encephaloid in appearance (Fig. 26.6). Areas of hemorrhage and necrosis are common. Microscopically, these tumors contain a variety

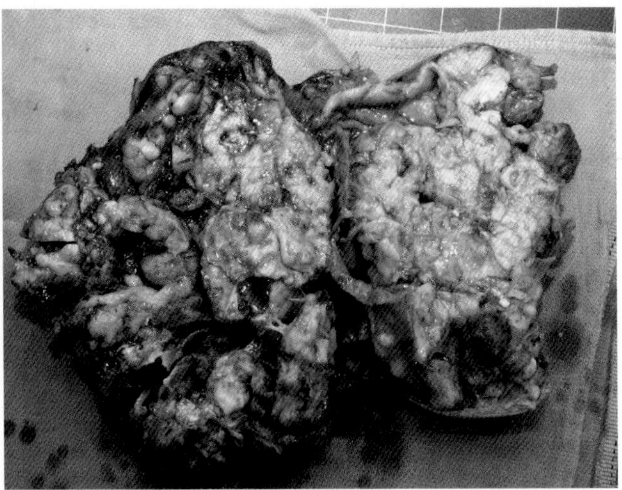

FIGURE 26.6. Ovarian immature teratoma. The neoplasm is predominantly solid and has a soft, encephaloid appearance.

of mature and immature tissue components. The immature elements almost always consist of immature neural tissue in the form of small, round blue cells focally organized into rosettes and tubules (Fig. 26.7). There is a correlation between disease prognosis and the degree of immaturity in the teratoma. The three-tiered grading system is still the one most often used (19). Grade 1 neoplasms display some immaturity, but the immature neural tissue does not exceed in aggregate the area of one low-power field (40×) in any slide. Grade 2 teratomas contain more immaturity, but immature neural tissue occupies no more than an area equal to three low-power fields in any slide. Grade 3 neoplasms contain immature neural tissue that occupies an area greater than three low-power fields in at least one slide (20). Mature tissue is easily identified in grade 1 tumors. It is present to a lesser extent in grade 2 neoplasms and may be absent altogether in grade 3 immature teratomas. The amount of mitotic activity and immature neural tissue with rosettes and tubules also increases with increasing tumor grade. Some authors prefer classifying immature teratomas as either low (grade 1) or high (grades 2 and 3) grade teratomas. In patients whose neoplasm has disseminated beyond the ovary, the grade of the tumor metastasis is important in predicting survival and determining treatment.

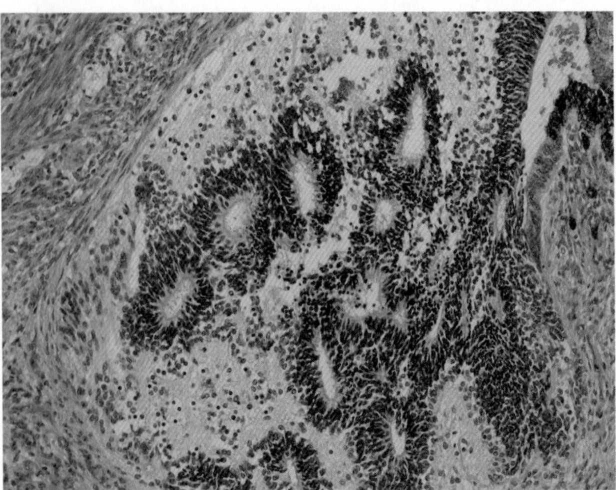

FIGURE 26.7. Ovarian immature teratoma. Immature neural tissue forms tubules.

Occasionally, patients may have peritoneal implants that contain only mature tissue, but these mature glial implants may represent host tissue and not actual tumor implants (21). It is extremely important to sample peritoneal disease thoroughly in order that foci of immature teratoma (that may coexist with mature glia) are identified.

A rare, but distinct entity deserves mention. The poorly differentiated small cell carcinoma of the ovary, classically associated with hypercalcemia (22), may have germ cell origin, as suggested by immunostaining for alpha-1-antitrypsin, presence of PAS-positive intracellular globules, presence of foci of intercellular basement membrane material, and focal laminin immunoreactivity (23). These tumors usually occur in young women and are invariably associated with a dismal prognosis (24,25). Treatment with germ cell type chemotherapy regimen is probably justified, although data are scant and inconclusive, given the rarity of such tumors.

Biologically, ovarian germ cell tumors, like testis cancer, are derived from primordial germ cells, which undergo defective meiosis. Karyotypic abnormalities are common and include aneuploidy or chromosomal rearrangements. In contrast, benign teratomas have a normal karyotype. One report notes chromosomal abnormalities in 7% of mature teratomas (26,27). Analysis of centromeric heteromorphisms suggests that 65% to 70% of benign teratomas result from a post-meiosis I type error (homozygotes), while the remaining 30% to 35% are caused by defective meiosis I, as demonstrated by heterozygosity of centromeric markers (26). Among malignant ovarian germ cell tumors, aneuploidy and chromosomal translocations or truncations similar to those encountered in testicular carcinoma have been widely reported (28,29). The presence of an isochromosome 12p (i12p) has been noted in ovarian tumors (30), albeit less commonly than in testis cancer. Other chromosomal aberrations such as loss or gain in chromosomes 1, 11, 12, 16, and X can be identified (31). The association between dysgerminoma and dysgenetic gonads (32) is well recognized and should be managed accordingly, as will be discussed.

CLINICAL FEATURES

Malignant germ cell tumors of the ovary occur mainly in girls and young women. In the University of Texas M. D. Anderson Cancer Center (UTMDACC) series, the age of the patients ranged from 6 to 40 years, with a median age of 16 to 20 years, depending upon histologic type (33).

Signs and symptoms in these patients are rather consistent. Abdominal pain associated with a palpable pelvic-abdominal mass is present in approximately 85% of patients (14,34,35). Approximately 10% of patients present with acute abdominal pain, usually caused by rupture, hemorrhage, or ovarian torsion. This finding is somewhat more common in patients with endodermal sinus tumor or mixed germ cell tumors and is frequently misdiagnosed as acute appendicitis. Less common signs and symptoms include abdominal distention (35%), fever (10%), and vaginal bleeding (10%). A few patients exhibit isosexual precocity, presumably due to hCG production by tumor cells.

In a small percentage of cases, ovarian germ cell tumors occur during pregnancy or in the immediate postpartum period (34). In the series reported by Gordon et al., 20 of 158 patients with dysgerminoma were diagnosed during pregnancy or after delivery (36). Nondysgerminomatous ovarian tumors occur less frequently during pregnancy, but rare cases have been reported (37–40). Marked increase in AFP heralds the presence of a germ cell tumor with yolk sac component. By and large, patients with ovarian tumors diagnosed during pregnancy can be treated successfully, without compromising the health of the fetus. Surgical resection of tumors and

TABLE 26.1

SERUM TUMOR MARKERS IN MALIGNANT GERM CELL TUMORS OF THE OVARY

Histology	AFP	hCG
Dysgerminoma	−	±
Endodermal sinus tumor	+	−
Immature teratoma	±	−
Mixed germ cell tumor	±	±
Choriocarcinoma	−	+
Embryonal carcinoma	±	+
Polyembryoma	±	+

chemotherapy have been performed safely in mid and third trimesters. However, rapid disease progression or pregnancy termination/miscarriage have been recorded, especially for nondysgerminomatous tumors (41).

Many germ cell tumors possess the unique property of producing biologic markers that are detectable in serum. The development of specific and sensitive radioimmunoassay techniques to measure hCG and AFP led to dramatic improvement in patient monitoring. Serial measurements of serum markers aid the diagnosis and, more importantly, are useful for monitoring response to treatment and detection of subclinical recurrences. Table 26.1 illustrates typical findings in the sera of patients with various tumor histologic types. Endodermal sinus tumor and choriocarcinoma are prototypes for AFP and hCG production, respectively. Embryonal carcinoma can secrete both hCG and AFP, but most commonly produces hCG. Mixed tumors may produce either, both, or none of the markers, depending on the type and quantity of elements present. Dysgerminoma is commonly devoid of hormonal production, although a small percentage of tumors produce low levels of hCG, if multinucleated syncytiotrophoblastic giant cells are present. The presence of an elevated level of AFP or high level of hCG (>100 U/mL) denotes the presence of tumor elements other than dysgerminoma. Therapy should be adjusted accordingly (see below). Although immature teratomas are associated with negative markers, a few tumors can produce AFP. A third tumor marker is lactic dehydrogenase (LDH), which is frequently elevated in patients with dysgerminoma or other germ cell tumors. Unfortunately, it is less specific than hCG or AFP, which limits its usefulness. CA-125 can also be nonspecifically elevated in patients with ovarian germ cell tumors (42).

SURGERY

Operative Findings

Malignant germ cell tumors of the ovary tend to be quite large. In the UTMDACC series, these tumors ranged in size from 7 to 40 cm, with a median size of 16 cm (14). Predominance of right-sided over left-sided involvement was noted. Bilaterality of tumor involvement (especially true stage IB disease) is exceedingly rare except for dysgerminoma. Bilateral involvement occurs in 10% to 15% of dysgerminoma patients (36,43–46). For nondysgerminomatous tumors, bilateral involvement signifies either advanced disease with metastatic spread to the contralateral ovary or the presence of a mixed germ cell tumor with prominent dysgerminoma component.

Ascites may be noted in approximately 20% of cases. Rupture of tumors, either preoperatively or intraoperatively, can occur in approximately 20% of cases. Torsion of the ovarian pedicle was documented in 5% of patients in the UTMDACC series.

Benign cystic teratoma is associated with malignant germ cell tumors in 5% to 10% of cases. These coexistent teratomas may occur in the ipsilateral ovary, in the contralateral ovary, or bilaterally. Likewise, a pre-existing gonadoblastoma may be noted in association with dysgerminoma and dysgenetic gonads related to a 46,XY karyotype (32,47–49).

Malignant germ cell tumors generally spread in one of two ways: along the peritoneal surface or through lymphatic dissemination. Although the relative frequency of these two principal mechanisms is difficult to discern, it is generally accepted that these neoplasms more commonly metastasize to lymph nodes than epithelial tumors. The high prevalence of inadequate staging procedures makes the true incidence of lymph node involvement uncertain. It is our impression that although still uncommon, malignant germ cell tumors have a somewhat greater predilection than epithelial tumors to metastasize hematogenously to parenchyma of liver or lung. The stage distribution is also very different from that of epithelial tumors. In most large series, approximately 60% to 70% of tumors will be stage I (36). The next most common stage is III, accounting for 25% to 30% of tumors. Stages II and IV are relatively uncommon.

Extent of Primary Surgery

The initial treatment approach for a patient suspected of having a malignant ovarian germ cell tumor is surgery, both for diagnosis and for therapy. After an adequate vertical midline incision, a thorough determination of disease extent by inspection and palpation should be made. If the disease is confined to one or both ovaries, it is imperative that proper staging biopsies be performed (see below).

The type of primary operative procedure depends upon the surgical findings. Because many of these patients are young women, for whom preservation of fertility is a priority, minimizing the surgical resection while ensuring removal of tumor bulk must be thoughtfully balanced. As noted previously, bilateral ovarian involvement is rare, except for the case of pure dysgerminoma. Bilateral involvement may be found in cases of advanced disease (stages II-IV), in which there is metastasis from one ovary to the opposite gonad, or in cases of mixed germ cell tumors with dysgerminoma component. Therefore, fertility-sparing unilateral salpingo-oophorectomy with preservation of the contralateral ovary and of the uterus can be performed in most patients (50–52). If the contralateral ovary appears grossly normal on careful inspection, it should be left undisturbed. However, in the case of pure dysgerminoma, biopsy may be considered, because occult or microscopic tumor involvement occurs in a small percentage of patients. Unnecessary biopsy, however, may result in future infertility due to peritoneal adhesions or ovarian failure. If the contralateral ovary appears abnormally enlarged, a biopsy or ovarian cystectomy should be performed. If frozen examination reveals a dysgenetic gonad, or if there are clinical indications suggesting a hermaphrodite phenotype, then bilateral salpingo-oophorectomy is indicated. However, it is difficult to establish this diagnosis on frozen section. This determination should preferably be made by determining a normal female karyotype preoperatively. If benign cystic teratoma is found in the contralateral ovary, an event that can occur in 5% to 10% of patients, then ovarian cystectomy with preservation of remaining normal ovarian tissue is recommended.

An important problem, albeit rare, is bilateral gonadal involvement in a patient who desires to preserve fertility and who is a candidate for postoperative chemotherapy. There are no data regarding the ability of chemotherapy to eradicate a primary ovarian tumor. In testis cancer, there are presumptive data suggesting that tumor may persist after chemotherapy in the gonad and that the testis may be a drug sanctuary. In exceptional situations, it may be reasonable to preserve an involved ovary in a patient who will be receiving chemotherapy. However, it is conceivable that ovarian preservation could increase the risk for recurrence in these selected cases. The decision to preserve an involved ovary is difficult and must be made carefully considering the patient's wishes.

The advent of *in vitro* fertilization technology also has an impact on operative management (53). Convention has dictated that if a bilateral salpingo-oophorectomy is necessary, a hysterectomy should also be performed. However, with current assisted reproduction technologies (ART) involving donor oocyte and hormonal support, a woman without ovaries could potentially sustain a normal intrauterine pregnancy. Similarly, if the uterus and one ovary are resected because of tumor involvement, current techniques provide the opportunity for oocyte retrieval from the remaining ovary, *in vitro* fertilization with sperm from her male partner, and embryo implantation into a surrogate's uterus. As the field of ART is evolving, traditional guidelines concerning surgical treatment in young patients with gynecologic tumors have to be thoughtfully adapted to individual circumstances.

Surgical Staging

Surgical staging information is essential for determining extent of disease, providing prognostic information, and guiding postoperative management. A meticulous approach is important for every patient, but is of critical importance for those patients with early clinical disease in order to detect the presence of occult or microscopic metastases. Staging of ovarian germ cell tumors follows the same principles applicable to epithelial ovarian tumors, as described by the International Federation of Gynecologists and Obstetricians (FIGO, Table 26.2). Proper staging procedures consist of the following:

1. Although a transverse incision is cosmetically superior, a vertical midline incision is usually necessary for adequate exposure, appropriate staging biopsies, and resection of large pelvic tumors or metastatic disease in the upper abdomen.
2. Ascites, if present, should be evacuated and submitted for cytologic analysis. If no peritoneal fluid is noted, cytologic washings of the pelvis and bilateral paracolic gutters should be performed prior to manipulation of the intraperitoneal contents.
3. The entire peritoneal cavity and its structures should be carefully inspected and palpated in a methodical manner. We generally prefer to start with the subphrenic spaces and move caudad toward the pelvis. The subdiaphragmatic areas, omentum, colon, all peritoneal surfaces, the entire retroperitoneum, and small intestinal serosa and mesentery should be checked. If any suspicious areas are noted, they should be submitted for biopsy or excised.
4. Next, the primary ovarian tumor and pelvis should be examined. Both ovaries should be carefully assessed for size, presence of obvious tumor involvement, capsular rupture, external excrescences, or adherence to surrounding structures.
5. If disease seems to be limited, i.e., confined to the ovary or localized to the pelvis, then random staging biopsies of structures at risk should be performed. These sites should include the omentum (with generous biopsies from multiple areas) and the peritoneal surfaces of the following sites: bilateral paracolic gutters, cul-de-sac, lateral pelvic walls, vesicouterine reflection, and subdiaphragmatic areas. Any adhesions should also be generously sampled.
6. The para-aortic and bilateral pelvic lymph node–bearing areas should be carefully palpated. Any suspicious nodes should be excised or sampled. If no suspicious areas are detected, these areas should be sampled. There is no evidence that a complete para-aortic and/or pelvic lymphadenectomy is advantageous.
7. If obvious gross metastatic disease is present, it should be excised if feasible, or at least sampled to document disease extent. The concept of cytoreductive surgery is discussed below.

TABLE 26.2

FIGO STAGING OF OVARIAN GERM CELL TUMORS

Stage	Description
I	Tumor limited to ovaries.
IA	Tumor limited to one ovary, no ascites, intact capsule.
IB	Tumor limited to both ovaries, no ascites, intact capsule.
IC	Tumor either stage IA or IB, but with ascites present containing malignant cells or with ovarian capsule involvement or rupture or with positive peritoneal washings.
II	Tumor involving one or both ovaries with extension to the pelvis.
IIA	Extension to uterus or tubes.
IIB	Involvement of both ovaries with pelvic extension.
IIC	Tumor either stage IIA or IIB, but with ascites present containing malignant cells or with ovarian capsule involvement or rupture or with positive peritoneal washings.
III	Tumor involving one or both ovaries with tumor implants outside the pelvis or with positive retroperitoneal or inguinal lymph nodes. Superficial liver metastases qualify as stage III.
IIIA	Tumor limited to the pelvis with negative nodes but with microscopic seeding of the abdominal peritoneal surface.
IIIB	Negative nodes, tumor implants in the abdominal cavity <2 cm.
IIIC	Positive nodes or tumor implants in the abdominal cavity >2 cm.
IV	Distant metastases present.

Note: FIGO, International Federation of Gynecologists and Obstetricians.

The gynecologic literature is replete with examples of inadequate surgical staging. Most patients still undergo initial surgery in community hospitals and are inadequately staged. Upon referral of such a patient to a university or tertiary care center, the oncologist is faced with the dilemma of inadequate staging information. In such cases, postoperative studies including computed tomography (CT) of the abdomen are recommended. If histopathologic and limited anatomic information from the first surgery clearly indicates the use of systemic chemotherapy, it is generally inadvisable to consider re-exploration solely for the purpose of precise staging information. Reoperation to complete comprehensive staging may be appropriate under clinical circumstances where careful surveillance observation after complete staging may be a sensible alternative to chemotherapy.

Cytoreductive Surgery

If widely spread tumor is encountered at initial surgery, it is recommended that the same principles concerning cytoreductive surgery applied in the surgical management of advanced epithelial ovarian cancer be followed. Specifically, as much tumor should be resected as is technically feasible and safe. However, because of their rarity, there is scant information in the literature on the impact of cytoreductive surgery of malignant germ cell tumors.

In a study of the Gynecologic Oncology Group (GOG), Slayton et al. found that 15 of 54 (28%) patients with completely resected disease at primary surgery failed chemotherapy with a combination of vincristine, dactinomycin, and cyclophosphamide (VAC), as opposed to 15 of 22 (68%) patients with incompletely resected disease treated with the same regimen (54). Furthermore, a higher percentage of patients with bulky postoperative residual disease (82%) failed chemotherapy compared to those with minimal residual disease (55%). In a subsequent GOG study reported by Williams et al., patients received the combination regimen of cisplatin, vinblastine, and bleomycin (PVB). In this study patients with nondysgerminomatous tumors and clinically nonmeasurable disease after surgery had a greater likelihood of remaining progression-free than those with measurable disease (65% vs. 34%) (55). In addition, patients who had been surgically debulked to optimal disease had an outcome intermediate between patients with suboptimal disease and those with optimal disease without debulking.

Even with epithelial tumors, the relative influence of tumor biology, surgical skill, and tumor aggressiveness remains uncertain. Germ cell tumors, especially dysgerminomas, are generally much more chemosensitive than epithelial ovarian tumors. Therefore, aggressive resection of metastatic disease in these cases, especially resection of bulky retroperitoneal nodes, is questionable. The surgeon must exercise thoughtful and mature intraoperative judgment when encountering such situations, carefully weighing the risks of cytoreductive maneuvers in the setting of chemosensitive tumors. There is no substitute for surgical experience and a clear understanding of the biologic behavior of these neoplasms. Even in the face of extensive metastatic disease, it is possible to perform a fertility-sparing procedure with preservation of a normal contralateral ovary.

The value of secondary cytoreductive surgery in the management of malignant ovarian germ cell tumors is even less clear than that of primary cytoreductive surgery. Although secondary cytoreduction is of questionable benefit for patients with refractory epithelial ovarian cancer (56,57), germ cell tumors are relatively more chemosensitive than epithelial tumors and more likely to respond to second-line therapy. Therefore, if a patient has an isolated focus of persistent tumor after first-line chemotherapy in an area such as the lung, liver, retroperitoneum, or brain, then surgical extirpation should be considered before changing chemotherapy regimens. Although this clinical situation is extremely rare, it has been observed in other situations involving chemosensitive tumors, such as gestational trophoblastic disease and testicular cancer.

Unlike testis cancer, the finding of a residual mass after completion of chemotherapy is less common in patients with ovarian germ cell tumors because these women are likely to have considerable tumor debulking at the time of the diagnostic surgical procedure and thus enter chemotherapy with significantly less tumor burden. At completion of chemotherapy, men with nonseminomatous tumors or seminoma may have persistent mature teratoma or desmoplastic fibrosis. In patients with bulky dysgerminoma, residual masses after chemotherapy are very likely to represent desmoplastic fibrosis. Although a number of patients with pure ovarian immature teratomas or mixed germ cell tumors have persistent mature teratoma at the completion of chemotherapy, as documented by second-look laparotomy (58), the majority are left with multiple small peritoneal implants rather than with a dominant mass. However, it is now recognized that occasional patients who have received chemotherapy for immature teratoma or mixed germ cell tumor containing teratoma will have bulky residual teratoma after chemotherapy. The natural history or biologic implications of this finding are not clear. In testis cancer, patients with bulky residual teratoma may experience slow progression of tumor (59) or may develop overtly malignant tumors over time (60–63). There are similar anecdotal reports of progressive mature teratoma in ovarian germ cell tumor patients after chemotherapy (64–66). Considering this information, it seems appropriate to resect persistent masses in patients with negative markers after chemotherapy for germ cell tumors containing immature teratoma. If viable neoplasm is found, additional chemotherapy should be considered. However, if only mature teratoma is resected, observation is generally recommended.

Second-Look Laparotomy

Since 1960, second-look laparotomy was included in the routine management of patients with epithelial ovarian cancer to assess disease status after a fixed interval of chemotherapy. It was only natural that such an approach would be extrapolated to the management of patients with malignant ovarian germ cell tumors. In a review of the experience with second-look laparotomy at UTMDACC, findings were negative in 52 of 53 patients (67). The one patient with positive findings at second-look laparotomy had an elevated AFP level prior to surgery, which accurately predicted residual disease. This patient received subsequent chemotherapy with PVB, entering prolonged remission. Of the patients with negative findings, one woman relapsed 9 months after the negative second-look surgery and subsequently died. Thirteen patients in this series had biopsy-proven evidence of residual mature teratoma (so-called "chemotherapeutic retroconversion") at second-look laparotomy; treatment was discontinued in all patients and none developed recurrence. Thus, in this series, second-look surgery did not add prognostic information or alter the therapeutic management of patients. The role of second-look surgery is further obscured in the setting of advancement in imaging techniques (CT scanning, positron emission tomography [PET], magnetic resonance imaging [MRI]) and in an era where tumor marker measurements are part of routine care of patients with germ cell tumors.

The GOG experience with second-look laparotomy in ovarian germ cell tumors has been reviewed (58). One hundred and seventeen patients enrolled prospectively on one of three GOG protocols using cisplatin-based chemotherapy after initial surgical staging and cytoreduction (GOG protocols 45, 78, and 90) underwent second-look surgical procedures. Of these, 45 surgical procedures were performed in patients who received three courses of bleomycin, etoposide, and cisplatin (BEP) after complete tumor resection. In this subgroup, 38 patients had negative findings, 2 patients had immature teratoma, and 5 patients had mature teratoma. One of the patients with residual immature teratoma received further chemotherapy and one did not. Both of them and the rest of the patients are disease-free. One patient with negative second-look surgery findings subsequently relapsed and succumbed to disease. Hence, in the subgroup of patients with completely resected primary ovarian germ cell tumors, the benefit of second-look surgery is nil. In contrast, 72 patients in this series treated with similar chemotherapy had advanced, incompletely resected tumor before beginning adjuvant treatment. In this subgroup, 48 patients did not have teratoma elements in their primary tumor. At second-look surgery, 45 patients had no residual tumor and 3 patients displayed persistent endodermal sinus tumor or embryonal carcinoma. All three of the latter patients are dead despite further treatment. Five patients with negative second-look laparotomies recurred, of which only one was salvaged with chemotherapy. Thus, the value of second-look surgery in patients with incompletely resected germ cell tumors not containing teratoma is arguably minimal. However, in the subgroup of patients with incompletely resected tumors containing teratoma elements (total of 24 patients), second-look surgery had an impact on subsequent management. Of these patients, 16 were found to have mature teratoma at second look, which was bulky or progressive in 7 cases. Four additional patients were found to have residual immature teratoma. Fourteen of the total 16 patients with teratoma and 6 of the 7 women with bulky residual tumor remain disease-free after surgical resection. Therefore, while second-look laparotomy is not necessary in patients with tumor completely resected primarily or in those patients with initially incompletely resected tumor not containing teratoma, clinical benefit can be derived in those patients with incompletely resected primary tumor that contains elements of teratoma (Table 26.3).

Advances in imaging technology, including the advent of PET scanning, may further obviate the need for surgical re-exploration. While PET scan is sensitive for detecting active (malignant) tumor, its usefulness in evaluating residual mature teratoma is more limited (68–71). A positive PET scan in the setting of a residual mass after treatment is highly indicative of viable tumor, and when used in conjunction with traditional radiographic techniques (CT scan, MRI) and tumor marker determinations, it can predict relapses with accuracy (72). A recent series demonstrates that in patients with residual masses after treatment for seminoma, a positive PET scan is strong evidence that the residual mass contains persistent tumor. In contrast, if the PET scan is negative, the residual mass is very unlikely to contain tumor. The specificity of the PET scan in this situation was 100%, the sensitivity was 80%, and the positive and negative predictive values were 100% and 95%, respectively (73). Although studies using PET scanning in ovarian germ cell tumors are scant, the concepts are very similar and can be extrapolated from the testis cancer literature.

CHEMOTHERAPY FOR OVARIAN GERM CELL TUMORS

Chemotherapy: From VAC to PEB

One of the great triumphs of cancer treatment in the 1970s and 1980s was the development of effective chemotherapy for testicular germ cell tumors (74,75). The lessons learned from prospective, randomized trials in testis cancer have been applied to ovarian germ cell tumors. Presently, the overwhelming majority of patients with ovarian germ cell tumors survive their disease with the judicious use of surgery and cisplatin-based combination chemotherapy. There are many similarities, but also a few important differences between testis cancer and ovarian germ cell tumors.

Historically, the first regimens used successfully for women with ovarian germ cell tumors were VAC (vincristine, dactinomycin, and cyclophosphamide) or VAC-type regimens. Such treatment had curative potential, especially in early-stage disease. However, among patients with advanced disease, the number of long-term survivors after VAC therapy remained under 50%. In the series reported from UTMDACC, although 86% of patients with stage I tumors were cured with VAC, the efficacy of the regimen was significantly less for patients with advanced disease (33). Only 57% of stage II patients and 50% of patients with stage III achieved long-term control. The two patients with stage IV tumors succumbed to disease. Similarly, in a study of the GOG, only 7 out of 22 patients with incompletely resected ovarian tumors achieved long-term disease control after treatment with VAC, as compared to 39 of 54 patients with completely resected tumors (76). In this report, 11 of 15 patients with stage III and both patients with stage IV

TABLE 26.3

RESULTS OF SECOND-LOOK SURGERY IN PATIENTS ENROLLED ON GOG PROTOCOLS

Primary surgery	Total number	Positive second look: progression-free/ total number	Negative second look: progression-free/ total number
Completely resected tumor	45	7/7[a]	37/38
Incompletely resected tumor			
Teratoma present	24	16/20[b]	4/4
Teratoma absent	48	0/3[c]	41/45

Note: GOG, Gynecologic Oncology Group.
[a]Five mature teratomas and two immature teratomas.
[b]Sixteen mature teratomas and four immature teratomas.
[c]Three embryonal carcinoma and yolk sac tumors.
Source: Reprinted with permission from Williams SD, Blessing JA, DiSaia PJ, et al. Second-look laparotomy in ovarian germ cell tumors: the Gynecologic Oncology Group experience. *Gynecol Oncol* 1994;52:287–291.

disease failed within 12 months of follow-up. These data suggest that VAC chemotherapy was insufficient for the treatment of advanced-stage and/or incompletely resected ovarian germ cell tumors.

Because of the experience gained from the treatment of testicular germ cell tumors demonstrating the superiority of cisplatin-based regimens, new platinum-based regimens were tested in patients with ovarian germ cell tumors. Gershenson et al. reported the efficacy of cisplatin, vinblastine, and bleomycin (PVB) in a small series of patients treated at UTMDACC (77). Among 15 patients, 7 received PVB in the adjuvant setting and 9 received the combination at the time of recurrence. Six of seven patients treated with PVB up front are long-term survivors. Among them, three patients had optimally debulked stage III disease.

Subsequently, the PVB combination was evaluated prospectively in a GOG protocol (GOG 45) (55). In this series, 47 of 89 patients with nondysgerminomatous ovarian tumors (53%) were disease-free with a median follow-up of 52 months. The latest treatment failure occurred at 28 months. Eight other patients had durable remissions with second-line therapy and a few other patients had nonprogressive or slowly progressive immature teratoma. Thus, the 4-year overall survival was approximately 70%. Of note, 29% of patients enrolled in this trial had received prior radiation or chemotherapy, which might have negatively affected the overall outcome. As discussed previously, patients who were debulked to optimal disease fared better than those who were not. Histologic type and marker elevation before treatment were not associated with adverse outcome. However, even among patients with nonmeasurable, and presumably small-volume disease, and without prior treatment, 8 of 30 patients treated with PVB ultimately failed.

In testis cancer, subsequent experience documented that etoposide is at least equivalent to vinblastine and produces improved survival in patients with high tumor volume (75). Furthermore, the use of etoposide in place of vinblastine led to reduced neurologic toxicity, abdominal pain, and constipation. The latter two adverse effects are particularly important for patients with ovarian tumors, as many will have had recent abdominal surgery. These observations led to the evaluation of the combination of bleomycin, etoposide, and cisplatin (BEP; Table 26.4) in patients with ovarian germ cell tumors. In a series from UTMDACC, long-term remissions were recorded in 25 of 26 patients treated with BEP (78). The only patient who succumbed to disease had been incompliant with treatment, monitoring, and follow-up. In this report, four patients with measurable disease after surgery had complete remissions after BEP treatment. This led to a prospective GOG study evaluating BEP in patients with ovarian germ cell tumors (79). The regimen was highly effective, with 91 of 93 enrolled patients being free of disease at follow-up. Based on these data, although BEP and VAC have not been prospectively compared, BEP emerged as the preferred regimen for patients with ovarian germ cell tumors.

The inclusion of cisplatin in the treatment of ovarian tumors resulted indisputably in an improvement in survival and disease control, as shown by the results of GOG studies, as well as by other clinical series (80–82). The results of therapy are summarized in Table 26.5.

TABLE 26.4

THE BEP REGIMEN[a]

Cisplatin	20 mg/m^2 days 1–5
Etoposide (VP-16)	100 mg/m^2 days 1–5
Bleomycin	30 units IV weekly

Note: BEP, bleomycin, etoposide, and cisplatin; IV, intravenously.
[a]Three to four courses given at 21-day intervals.

TABLE 26.5

ADJUVANT CHEMOTHERAPY

Institution	Regimen	Progression-free/total (%)
GOG (66)	BEP	89/93 (96)
Australia (51)	Multiple	9/10 (90)
Hospital 12 de Octubre (32)	PVB or BEP	9/9 (100)
M. D. Anderson (18)	PVB	4/4 (100)
Instituto Nazionale Tumori (3)	PVB	9/10 (90)
M. D. Anderson (19)	BEP	20/20 (100)

Note: BEP, bleomycin, etoposide, and cisplatin; GOG, Gynecologic Oncology Group; PVB, cisplatin, vinblastine, bleomycin.

Differences in Outcome for Patients With Completely Resected Tumors Versus Advanced-Stage Disease

It is clear that several prognostic factors impact the outcome of patients with ovarian germ cell tumors and that there are important differences between testicular and ovarian germ cell neoplasms. Debulking surgery plays a central role in the management of ovarian tumors, but has a less important role in testis cancer. In the hands of an experienced surgeon, the majority of women with ovarian tumors are debulked to minimal and often clinically undetectable disease before starting chemotherapy. Therefore, unlike patients with testis cancer, most women who are candidates for chemotherapy have minimal or no residual disease. However, even in this circumstance, there seems to be little doubt that adjuvant therapy is appropriate in the majority of cases. The anticipated risk of relapse with surgery alone in patients with advanced disease is as high as 75% to 80%. Particularly, patients with embryonal carcinoma, endodermal sinus tumors, and mixed tumors containing these elements are considered to be at very high risk of recurrence without postoperative therapy. This risk can be minimized by the use of adjuvant chemotherapy. In GOG protocol 78, 50 of 51 patients with completely resected ovarian germ cell tumors remained without evidence of disease when three cycles of BEP were given adjuvantly. Other studies using cisplatin-based therapy have given similar results (Table 26.6). The recommended

TABLE 26.6

CHEMOTHERAPY OF ADVANCED DISEASE

Institution	Regimen	Progression-free/total (%)
GOG (67)	PVB	47/89 (53)
Australia (51)	Multiple	42/46 (91)
Hospital 12 de Octubre (32)	PVB or BEP	15/19 (79)
M. D. Anderson (18)	PVB	7/11 (64)
Instituto Nazionale Tumor (13)	PVB	7/14 (50)
M. D. Anderson (19)	BEP	5/6 (83)

Note: BEP, bleomycin, etoposide, and cisplatin; GOG, Gynecologic Oncology Group; PVB, cisplatin, vinblastine, bleomycin.

TABLE 26.7

A TYPICAL ANTIEMETIC REGIMEN

Granisetron 1 mg IV 30 min prior to cisplatin daily for 5 days
or
Ondanesietron 0.15 mg/kg IV 30 min prior and 4 hours after cisplatin daily for 5 days
plus
Dexamethasone 20 mg IV 30 min prior to cisplatin on days 1 and 2
Plus
Aprepitant 125 mg po on day 1 and 80 mg po on days 2 and 3, prior to cisplatin infusion

treatment for most patients (with the exception of patients with grade 1, stage IA immature teratoma or stage IA dysgerminoma) is adjuvant chemotherapy with three courses of BEP. Virtually all patients with early-stage or completely resected disease will survive after careful surgical staging and cisplatin-based adjuvant chemotherapy. More recently, clinical series and observations are beginning to suggest that surveillance with careful follow-up after surgery may be an acceptable alternative for carefully selected patients, as discussed below. Given the fact that surgery followed by chemotherapy is curative for most patients, this course of action should be taken only after very careful consideration. Further studies are needed in this area.

In contrast, most clinical series have shown worse clinical outcome for patients with metastatic disease or with incompletely resected tumors (Table 26.7). Current clinical trials in testicular cancer separate patients with small tumor volume and a resultant excellent prognosis from those with bulky tumor or liver and brain involvement (83). Patients in the former group are usually complete responders to chemotherapy and long-term survivors, whereas only about 50% to 60% of the latter patients are cured. Hence, clinical trials for patients with good prognostic factors investigate shorter or less toxic chemotherapy aiming at minimizing toxicity (84), while preserving efficacy. In contrast, clinical trials for patients with high-risk disease evaluate more intensive chemotherapy regimens with the goal of improving the likelihood of cure (85,86). For instance, high-dose chemotherapy (HDCT) with stem-cell rescue was investigated for patients with high-risk testicular cancer in a multi-institutional clinical protocol (Eastern Cooperative Oncology Group [ECOG] protocol 3894). Patients considered to have high risk for relapse were randomized to receive four cycles of BEP (control arm) versus two cycles of BEP followed by HDCT with autologous stem-cell rescue in the form of two (tandem) courses using carboplatin, etoposide, and cyclophosphamide as a conditioning regimen (experimental arm). The 1-year durable complete response rate was 52% after BEP + HDCT and 48% after BEP alone ($p = 0.53$) (87). The trial disproved the concept that more aggressive chemotherapy in the first-line setting improves outcome of high-risk testicular cancer patients.

This is not the case for patients with incompletely resected or advanced ovarian germ cell tumors. Except for the subgroup of patients with dysgerminoma, there are no identifiable patients who have a sufficiently high cure rate to warrant less intensive therapy. Clinical prognosticators for outcome of malignant ovarian germ cell tumors are stage at diagnosis and increase in tumor markers (88). However, a dependable risk stratification, such as the one used for testis tumors, is not currently in use. Whether this reflects an inherent biologic difference between ovarian germ cell tumors and testis cancer or merely an underestimation of tumor volume because of intraperitoneal spread is not clear.

Management of Residual or Recurrent Disease

The large majority of patients with ovarian germ cell tumors are cured with surgery and platinum-based chemotherapy. However, a small percentage of patients have persistent or progressive disease during treatment or recur after completion of treatment. Like in testis cancer, these treatment failures are categorized as platinum-resistant (progression during or within 4 to 6 weeks of completing treatment) or platinum-sensitive (recurrence beyond 6 weeks from platinum-based therapy).

Most recurrences occur within 24 months from primary treatment. In a series from the UTMDACC, 42 treatment failures were identified among 160 patients with ovarian germ cell tumors treated between 1970 and 1990 (89). Treatment failure in these patients was attributed to inadequate surgery in 14 patients, inadequate radiation in 5 patients, inadequate chemotherapy in 16 patients (underdosing and noncompliance), treatment-related toxicity in 1 patient, and unidentifiable causes in 6 patients. A significant number of patients included in this series had received VAC-based chemotherapy, which might have accounted for the higher than expected rate of recurrence.

Given the high curability rate of ovarian germ cell tumors with primary treatment, the management of recurrent disease represents a complex and often difficult issue, and should preferably be performed in a specialized center. Data to guide the management of patients with recurrent ovarian germ cell tumors are scant and largely extrapolated from the clinical experience with testicular cancer. The single most important prognostic factor in patients with testis cancer is whether or not they are refractory to cisplatin. The likelihood of cure with high-dose salvage therapy in patients who relapse from a complete remission after initial therapy is as high as 60% or more. On the other hand, in patients who are truly cisplatin refractory, the likelihood of long-term survival and cure is significantly less, but fully 30% to 40% of these patients will be long-term survivors. Approximately 30% of patients with recurrent platinum-sensitive testis cancer can be salvaged with second-line chemotherapy (vinblastine, ifosfamide, platinum [VeIP]) (85). However, there is now strong evidence that high-dose therapy with carboplatin, etoposide with or without cyclophosphamide or ifosfamide, and stem-cell rescue is superior to standard dose salvage therapy for these patients (90,91). Generally, in patients who are not cisplatin refractory, one course of standard dose therapy, usually cisplatin, vinblastine, and ifosfamide, is given. If an initial response is seen, then two subsequent courses of high-dose chemotherapy (carboplatin and etoposide) with stem-cell rescue are given (92). A recent report from Indiana University describes this approach among 184 patients with recurrent testicular cancer. At a median follow-up of 48 months, 116 patients were in complete remission. Remarkably, of 40 patients who were platinum refractory, 18 are disease-free after high-dose chemotherapy (93). While this approach has not been prospectively tested in women with recurrent platinum-sensitive ovarian germ cell tumors, because of the small numbers of patients, the concepts are very similar and support the use of high-dose therapy in this setting. Referral to a specialized center for management of recurrent disease is desirable.

Active agents in the setting of recurrence after high-dose chemotherapy include ifosfamide, taxane, and gemcitabine (94–97). In a phase 2 trial from Indiana University, the combination of gemcitabine and paclitaxel induced objective responses in 10 of 31 patients who had recurred after high-dose chemotherapy. Of those, five patients were free of disease at 2 years after treatment (97). Referral for treatment with investigational agents for recurrent, refractory disease is appropriate.

Immediate Toxicity of Chemotherapy

Acute adverse effects of chemotherapy can be substantial and these patients should be treated by physicians experienced in their management. About 25% of patients develop febrile neutropenic episodes during chemotherapy and require hospitalization and broad-spectrum antibiotics (98). Cisplatin can be associated with nephrotoxicity. This adverse event can be avoided by ensuring adequate hydration during and immediately after chemotherapy and by avoidance of aminoglycoside antibiotics. Bleomycin can cause pulmonary fibrosis (98). Pulmonary function testing is frequently used to follow these patients. However, the value of carbon monoxide diffusion capacity to predict early lung disease has been challenged (99). The most effective method for monitoring germ cell tumor patients is careful physical examination of the chest. Findings of early bleomycin lung disease are a lag or diminished expansion of one hemithorax or fine basilar rales that do not clear with cough. These findings can be very subtle but if present mandate immediate discontinuation of bleomycin. It is important to note that randomized trials in good-prognosis testis cancer have suggested that bleomycin is an important component of the treatment regimen, particularly if only three courses of therapy are given (100,101). Other randomized trials have shown that carboplatin is inferior to cisplatin and cannot be substituted for cisplatin without worsening therapeutic outcome (102,103).

Patients with advanced ovarian germ cell tumors should receive three to four courses of treatment given in full dose and on schedule. There is presumptive evidence in testis cancer that the timeliness of chemotherapy may be associated with outcome. Thus, treatment is given regardless of hematologic parameters on the scheduled day of treatment. The impact of the hematopoietic growth factors (granulocyte colony-stimulating factor [G-CSF], granulocyte-macrophage colony-stimulating factor [GM-CSF]) on the management of the myelosuppressive complications of this chemotherapy has not been precisely defined. As most patients will not develop neutropenic fever or infection, hematopoietic growth factors are not routinely necessary (104). It is reasonable to use hematopoietic growth factors to avoid dose reductions for patients with previous episodes of neutropenic fever or in unusually ill patients who are at a higher risk of myelosuppressive complications, or those who received prior radiotherapy. Modern antiemetic therapy, an example of which is shown in Table 26.7, has greatly lessened chemotherapy-induced emesis. By following these guidelines and providing supportive care as indicated, virtually all patients can be treated on schedule, in full or nearly full dose. Chemotherapy-related mortality should be less than 1%. Late effects of chemotherapy are discussed below.

Immature Teratoma

The situation of patients with immature teratoma (IT) is more complex. Immature teratomas are categorized as grade 1, 2, or 3 depending on the amount of immature neuroepithelium in the tumor, based on Kurman and Norris's system (2), which was later modified by Norris (19). Our current appreciation of recurrence risk in these patients is based on an early study by Norris (19). This report demonstrated that prognosis of patients with IT directly relates to tumor grade. Specifically, only 1 of 14 patients with grade 1 IT recurred, while 13 of 26 patients with grade 2 and 3 tumors recurred. This study set the current standard of care for women with stage I teratoma, which is surveillance for grade 1 immature teratoma and adjuvant chemotherapy with three courses of BEP for patients with grade 2 and 3 tumors (4). However, a significant limitation of the Norris report is the probable underestimation of tumor stage. Hence, in the modern era of complete surgical staging of ovarian neoplasms, it might be appropriate to reconsider the role of routine adjuvant therapy in these patients. Obviously, such an approach must be done with great caution, as surgery followed by adjuvant therapy cures virtually all patients with localized high-grade teratoma. However, it is possible that the risk of relapse is sufficiently low in a defined population of well-staged patients as to warrant clinical observation. This could be accomplished with careful follow-up, such that relapsing patients would be diagnosed with small-volume tumor and cured with subsequent salvage chemotherapy. While some issues are different in testis cancer, a deferral of chemotherapy has been shown to be an appropriate therapeutic alternative for resected stage II tumors and clinical stage I disease. Surveillance for stage I ovarian IT is supported by experience from several groups.

First, an Intergroup study of the Pediatric Oncology Group and the Children's Cancer Group reported that surveillance after complete surgical resection in 41 girls with ovarian immature teratoma was sufficient (105,106). Only one recurrence (which was salvaged with BEP) was noted during 24 months of follow-up. Of note is that in this series, 13 patients had grade 2 and 3 IT, and 10 patients had mixed tumors containing IT plus yolk sac tumor (5).

Second, investigators at Mount Vernon and Charing Cross Hospitals in England have observed 15 patients with stage IA tumors after initial surgical treatment (107). Of these, nine patients had grade 2 or 3 immature teratoma and six had elements of endodermal sinus tumor. There were three recurrences in this series, one of nine in the pure immature teratoma group and two of six in the mixed histology group. Two of these patients were salvaged with chemotherapy and one patient died of pulmonary embolus. Of note is that the patient who died became pregnant 4 months after diagnosis and could not be followed adequately due to her pregnancy.

Third, investigators at the University of Milan reported the clinical outcome in a group of 32 patients with pure ovarian IT followed prospectively (108). In this group, nine patients had grade 2 and 3 stage IA immature teratomas and were treated with surgery and intensive surveillance. Only two recurrences were noted in this group. They consisted of one case of mature teratoma and one case of gliosis. The mature teratoma was resected and the patient with gliosis was followed without treatment. Both patients are alive and well and never received chemotherapy. Furthermore, among four patients with stage IC tumors treated with surgical resection and surveillance, there was one case of gliosis and one recurrence with mature tissue, which was resected (no chemotherapy). All patients are currently free of disease.

When considering these issues, it is important to not overstate the toxicities of adjuvant therapy. In earlier times, chemotherapy-induced emesis was a very significant problem. However, with modern antiemetics such as the 5HT3 antagonists, emesis is greatly reduced and, while unpleasant, rarely is a major complication of chemotherapy. Acute treatment-related mortality, particularly from bleomycin-related lung disease, is also rare. In GOG protocol 78, there were no toxic deaths among 93 patients. Nonetheless, chemotherapy is certainly unpleasant, produces universal alopecia and occasionally severe emesis, and has a remote risk of serious acute toxicity and drug-induced mortality. Considering this information, it may be appropriate to consider surveillance with careful follow-up in well-staged adult patients with ovarian stage IA immature teratoma. While this concept is supported by evidence derived from the pediatric literature and two small clinical series as discussed, this hypothesis has not been tested prospectively and should be approached with caution.

DYSGERMINOMA

Dysgerminoma is the female equivalent of seminoma. This disease differs from its nondysgerminomatous counterparts in several respects. First, it is more likely to be localized to the ovary at the time of diagnosis (stage I). Bilateral involvement is more common, as is its spread to retroperitoneal lymph nodes. While less relevant now than before the era of modern chemotherapy, dysgerminoma is very sensitive to radiation (36,45,109).

Observation for Stage I Tumors

As many as 75% to 80% of dysgerminoma patients used to be considered stage I at diagnosis (44,110). However, with more precise surgical staging, as done currently, the true figure is probably somewhat less. Traditionally, most of these women received postoperative radiotherapy. Given the fact that pelvic radiotherapy is associated with a high incidence of gonadal dysfunction and sterility, an alternative option for low-risk patients who desire to maintain fertility is postsurgical clinical surveillance (111). In a previous era, clinical observation was deemed appropriate for women with tumors less than 10 cm and without contralateral ovarian involvement, while adjuvant radiotherapy was recommended for larger tumors (112). The size-based distinction was subsequently called into question (110,113). In a series reported by LaPolla et al., seven of nine patients with stage IA dysgerminoma followed without postoperative radiotherapy remained disease-free (110). All but one had tumors greater than 10 cm. In another report, among 14 patients with stage IA dysgerminoma treated with surveillance, 5 recurred. Of those, four patients were salvaged with radiation and one was salvaged with radiation followed by chemotherapy. All stage IA patients are alive, free of disease (109). Similarly, Gordon et al. reported that the 5-year survival among 72 patients with stage IA pure dysgerminoma treated conservatively was 95% (36). The recurrence rate in this case series was 17%, with four deaths attributable to disease. However, in this series salvage chemotherapy was offered to only one patient, which may explain the unfavorable outcomes. A report from Mount Vernon and Charing Cross Hospitals quoted two relapses among nine patients with stage IA dysgerminoma treated with observation. Both were cured with salvage chemotherapy (114). A summary of reports using observation after surgery in stage I dysgerminoma is presented in Table 26.8.

Currently, patients with well-staged IA dysgerminoma can be observed after unilateral salpingo-oophorectomy, regardless of the size of the primary tumor, if preservation of fertility is an issue. Careful follow-up is required, because as many as 15% to 25% of patients will experience a recurrence. However, because of the tumor's chemosensitivity, virtually all dysgerminoma patients can be salvaged successfully at the time of recurrence, if adequate follow-up and early detection have been accomplished.

Radiation Therapy

In the past, many stage I patients and all patients with higher stage tumors received radiotherapy. DePalo et al. recommended radiation therapy for all stage I-III patients (44). Radiation therapy was delivered to the ipsilateral hemipelvis (with shielding of the contralateral ovary and the head of the femur) and to the para-aortic nodes. A single field incorporating these areas was used. In either case, the upper limit of the field was set at T10-11. The lower limit of the spinal field was at the L4-5 level. They recommended that all stage IB patients receive postoperative radiation therapy to the whole pelvis and para-aortic nodes. For stage III retroperitoneal disease they offered curative radiation therapy set up in the same fashion as for stage I with the addition of a prophylactic field including the mediastinum and supraclavicular nodes. In the presence of peritoneal involvement, the whole abdomen and pelvis, mediastinum, and supraclavicular nodes were irradiated. They gave 30 Gy (7.5 to 9 Gy per week) as prophylactic irradiation. For curative irradiation, 35 to 40 Gy total dose was given and a boost (10 Gy) was delivered to involved nodes. When irradiating above the diaphragm, DePalo et al. gave 30 Gy 3 to 6 weeks after completion of irradiation below the diaphragm. When irradiating the entire abdominal cavity the fields were similar to those used for epithelial tumors. They gave a total dose of 25 Gy (6 to 7.5 Gy per week). The kidneys were shielded. Similarly, Lawson and Adler reported giving 30 Gy (10 Gy per week) to pelvic and para-aortic fields (115). In their series, only two patients were treated to the whole abdomen, one with moving strip technique and one with open fields. The patient treated with moving strip technique received 22.5 Gy to the whole abdomen and 45 Gy to the pelvis.

Others reported similar treatment plans. Freed et al. gave external pelvic irradiation for disease limited to the pelvis (20 to 30 Gy in 2 to 3 weeks) (116). If the para-aortic nodes were positive histologically or by lymphangiogram, the fields were extended to cover this area. In this case, prophylactic radiation therapy to the mediastinum and supraclavicular nodes was also given. If extranodal spread or intra-abdominal disease was found, total abdominal therapy (25 to 30 Gy in 3 to 5 weeks) with a pelvic boost (15 to 20 Gy in 1.5 to 3 weeks) and para-aortic boost (15 Gy in 2 weeks) were recommended (112,116,117).

Historically, patients with testicular seminoma received prophylactic treatment to the mediastinum. However, over

TABLE 26.8

RESULTS OF CLINICAL SURVEILLANCE AFTER SURGERY IN PATIENTS WITH STAGE IA DYSGERMINOMA

Institution	Period	Progression-free/ total number (%)	Overall survival/ total number (%)
AFIP (34)	−1969	46/57 (80%)	52/57 (91%)
Hopkins (36)	1930–1981	58/72 (80%)	67/72 (94%)
Mayo Clinic (109)	1950–1984	9/14 (64%)	14/14 (100%)
Iowa Hospitals (110)	1935–1985	7/7 (100%)	7/7 (100%)
M. D. Anderson (112)	−1976	5/5 (100%)	5/5 (100%)
Mount Vernon Hospital (107)	1973–1995	6/9 (66%)	9/9 (100%)

Note: AFIP, Armed Forces Institute of Pathology.

time this line of reasoning has been challenged (118). Currently, most investigators consider that this form of treatment is obsolete because of the small number of patients who would derive a potential benefit and because of the subsequent reduced tolerance for chemotherapy in this population. Furthermore, considering the recent developments in the field of chemotherapy, it is accepted that primary chemotherapy is equally or more effective than irradiation of extensive normal tissue volumes, and is substantially less likely to compromise salvage therapy when patients relapse after primary therapy. Given that most patients will be cured of their ovarian tumors, and that most patients are young at the time of diagnosis, some consideration should also be given to the delayed carcinogenic effects of intermediate-dose radiation. Although this issue has not been specifically addressed in women with ovarian germ cell tumors, it is logical to extrapolate from the experience of younger women who are frequently successfully treated with radiation for cancer of the uterine cervix, and in whom the risk of second malignancies (both within and remote from the primary radiation fields) is increased 2 or 3 decades following successful initial treatment (119).

Results of radiation therapy are reasonably good. DePalo et al. reported that all 13 stage I patients (12 stage IA and 1 with stage IB) treated with radiotherapy were alive and free of disease with a median follow-up of 77 months (44). The 5-year relapse-free survival for 12 stage III patients was 61.4% and the overall survival was 89.5%. Median follow-up was 67 months. Only one death was reported in this group. Earlier, DePalo et al. reported 100% overall 5-year survival and 90% recurrence-free 5-year survival in 31 stage IA, IB, and IC patients (44). At 4 years, the overall survival was 80% and the recurrence-free survival was 57% in stage III patients. Lawson and Adler reported that 10 of 14 stage I-III patients were alive with a median follow-up of 54 months (115). In this small series there was no correlation between survival and the stage of disease or the size of the primary tumor. Others reported similar results with overall progression-free rates varying between 70% and 90% (Table 26.9) (45,46). However, despite the remarkable radiosensitivity of dysgerminoma, radiotherapy is rarely performed nowadays, since chemotherapy is equally or more effective, less toxic, and less likely to compromise gonadal function.

Chemotherapy

There is an increasing amount of information available about chemotherapy for patients with advanced ovarian dysgerminoma. Dysgerminoma is very responsive to cisplatin-based chemotherapy, even more so than tumors other than dysgerminoma (78,121). Since 1984, patients with advanced dysgerminoma were eligible for GOG protocols. Patients enrolled in these studies received three to four courses of PVB or BEP. In a combined analysis, 20 patients were evaluated (122). All had stage III or IV disease and most of them had suboptimal (greater than 2 cm) residual tumor. Overall, with a median follow-up of 26 months, 19 of the 20 women were disease-free. Among 11 patients with clinically measurable tumor, 10 had complete responses to chemotherapy. Fourteen patients who underwent second-look laparotomy had completely negative results. Thus, it appears that nearly all patients with advanced dysgerminoma treated with chemotherapy will be durable complete responders.

Considering that patients with stage III dysgerminoma would require extensive radiation and still carry a risk of failure and that such patients probably fare worse with subsequent chemotherapy, it is clear that these patients should be treated primarily with chemotherapy. For most, the preferred adjuvant therapy is BEP. This regimen almost invariably prevents recurrence in nondysgerminomatous tumors and certainly will do so in dysgerminoma. Most patients treated with BEP will retain fertility. An alternative regimen tested by the GOG consists of a 3-day regimen with carboplatin and etoposide. On this protocol, all 39 patients with pure dysgerminoma remained free of disease at a median follow-up of 7.8 years (123). Although highly active, this regimen is not recommended for routine use, because significantly less experience has been accumulated with its use and because of the concern that this regimen is not as effective in tumors containing nondysgerminomatous elements.

The implications of elevated hCG or AFP levels in patients with dysgerminoma should be emphasized. These tumor markers are usually increased in patients with nondygerminomatous tumors. Therefore, AFP elevation denotes the presence of elements other than dysgerminoma and treatment should be tailored accordingly. An elevated hCG level can occasionally be seen in pure dysgerminoma. This finding should not alter therapy, but prompt reexamination of the tumor specimen to determine whether syncytiotrophoblastic cells are present, or if the tumor contains nondysgerminomatous elements.

In summary, the majority of dysgerminoma patients have stage I disease at diagnosis. These patients can be treated with unilateral salpingo-oophorectomy, and if fertility is an issue, they can be observed carefully with regular pelvic exams, abdominal computerized tomography, and tumor markers including LDH. Fifteen percent to 25% of patients treated with surveillance recur and will require chemotherapy. In patients with more advanced disease, the risk of recurrence is significant

TABLE 26.9

EFFECTS OF RADIOTHERAPY IN WOMEN WITH PURE DYSGERMINOMA

Institution	Period	Stage	Progression-free/total number of patients (%)
AFIP (34)	1969	I-III	12/14 (85%)
Mayo Clinic (109)	1950–1984	I-IV	16/20 (80%)
M. D. Anderson (112)	1947–1974	I-III	26/31 (84%)
Florence (46)	1960–1983	IC-III	21/26 (80%)
NCI Milan (44)	1970–1982	I-III	21/25 (84%)
Iowa Hospitals (110)	1935–1985	I-III	12/13 (92%)
Sweden (45)	1927–1984	I-IV	49/60 (83%)
Egypt (120)	1978–1989	II-III	10/15 (66%)
Prince of Whales Hospital (115)	1969–1983	II-III	10/14 (72%)

Note: AFIP, Armed Forces Institute of Pathology; NCI, National Cancer Institute.

enough to warrant adjuvant treatment. Alternatives are chemotherapy or radiation. For the majority of patients, chemotherapy is the clear choice because of ease of administration, predictable and minimal toxicity, and fertility-sparing properties. Chemotherapy is recommended also for patients with metastatic or incompletely resected tumor and for patients who recur after previous radiotherapy. Radiation might be considered as initial treatment in unusual circumstances, such as older patients or in those with serious concomitant illness that would preclude the use of systemic chemotherapy.

LATE EFFECTS OF TREATMENT

As the prognosis of patients with malignant ovarian germ cell tumors has dramatically improved with the evolution of modern combination chemotherapy, attention is focused on late effects of therapy. There is a considerable body of literature on the late effects of treatment in testicular cancer patients, yet the information available for women with ovarian germ cell tumors remains scant. However, many analogies can be drawn.

Sequelae of Surgery

Young patients with malignant ovarian germ cell tumors undergo at least one, if not multiple, surgical procedures. Although there is no available information on the long-term effects of surgery on these patients, future infertility related to pelvic surgery with subsequent peritoneal and tubal adhesions is well described. Therefore, meticulous surgical technique and avoidance of unnecessary operative maneuvers (e.g., biopsy of a normal contralateral ovary) are required for preventing future complications (50,124,125). Another cause of infertility in this population is unnecessary bilateral salpingo-oophorectomy and hysterectomy. The UTMDACC series includes several patients who underwent surgical sterilization without good indication before referral to their center. It is expected that this phenomenon will be less frequent, as information concerning the outcome of treated patients with ovarian germ cell tumors will be more widely disseminated. In a series from Milan, among 55 patients treated with fertility-sparing surgery, without further chemotherapy, 12 out of 12 patients who attempted conception became pregnant and 12 normal deliveries were recorded (126). Two additional pregnancies occurred in this group and resulted in termination, one of which was due to in-uterus detection of fetal malformation. Recently, Gershenson et al. reported the findings of GOG protocol 9901 (127). Among 132 survivors of ovarian germ cell tumors treated with surgery and platinum-based chemotherapy, 71 patients had fertility-sparing procedures. Of those fertile survivors, 62 (87.3%) maintained menstrual periods and 24 survivors reported 37 successful pregnancies. Although the survivors reported increased incidence of gynecologic problems and diminished sexual pleasure, they also tended to have stronger, more positive relationships with their significant others (127).

As with any group of patients with history of pelvic surgery, patients with malignant ovarian germ cell tumors may develop functional cysts in the residual ovary. Muram et al. reported his experience with 27 patients with ovarian germ cell tumors who underwent unilateral salpingo-oophorectomy and were followed for 12 to 215 months after completion of therapy (128). Of the 18 patients who maintained ovarian function, 13 (72%) developed functional cysts during follow-up. A trial of oral contraceptives and serial ovarian surveillance with sonography is helpful in distinguishing functional cysts from tumor recurrence.

Sequelae of Radiation Therapy

There is limited information about the late effects of radiotherapy in dysgerminoma patients. In a review of the late effects of radiotherapy in patients receiving abdominal therapy for ovarian dysgerminoma at UTMDACC, there was a small increase in reported dyspareunia and the number of bowel movements (111). Somewhat surprisingly, at a median follow-up of 12 years, none of 43 patients treated with radiotherapy developed small-bowel obstruction. No other significant intestinal or bladder problems were recorded. As expected, none of the patients treated with radiation conceived.

Although the late effects of radiotherapy in this population seem to be few with the notable exception of gonadal failure (129), these observations may soon be of only historical interest. As discussed earlier, there has been a strong trend away from radiotherapy and toward chemotherapy as the preferred postoperative therapy of dysgerminoma patients. Concern over preservation of gonadal function has been the driving force behind this transition (43,130).

Sequelae of Chemotherapy

The evolutionary development and refinement of combination chemotherapy have resulted in the cure of a high percentage of patients with chemosensitive tumors, such as lymphomas, testicular cancer, gestational trophoblastic disease, and malignant ovarian germ cell tumors. Within the last few years, several reports have described the long-term effects of chemotherapy in cancer survivors. As expected, most reports refer to the more common lymphomas and testicular cancers.

A recently recognized effect of chemotherapy used for the treatment of germ cell tumors is the risk of secondary malignancies. The epipodophyllotoxins teniposide and etoposide are associated with the development of acute myelogenous leukemia (AML) with certain morphologic and cytogenetic features (131–135). This treatment complication appears to be dose (131,132) and schedule dependent (134). Of 348 male germ cell tumor patients receiving three to four courses of BEP as first-line therapy at Indiana University, 2 developed etoposide-related leukemia. None of 67 patients who received only three courses developed AML (131). Similarly, in the study reported by Pedersen-Bjergaard et al., 5 of 212 patients developed acute leukemia or myelodysplastic syndrome after etoposide therapy (132). However, all patients who developed AML received more than 2,000 mg/m^2 of etoposide. None of the 130 patients who received less than this dose developed AML. Morphologically, these leukemias are monocytic or myelomonocytic (M4 or M5). Characteristic chromosomal translocations (mostly involving the 11q23 region) are frequently, but not always, present. Leukemia after etoposide treatment occurs within 2 to 3 years compared to alkylating agent–induced AML, which has a longer latency period. Late occurrence of chronic myelogenous leukemia after treatment of testis cancer was reported (136). In the GOG protocol testing the efficacy of BEP in women with ovarian germ cell tumors, one case of AML was recorded among 91 patients treated (79). An additional case of lymphoma was diagnosed during follow-up in this series, yet a correlation between chemotherapy and lymphoproliferative disorders has not been reported to date.

Taking these issues into account, most clinicians consider BEP as the chemotherapy regimen of choice. The incidence of second neoplasms is quite low, particularly in patients receiving low cumulative etoposide doses. The continued use of etoposide over vinblastine is based on its superior efficacy demonstrated in testis cancer (75). Furthermore, vinblastine-induced abdominal pain and ileus are troublesome for some patients, particularly for those who underwent abdominal surgery, such as women with ovarian germ cell tumors. The risk/benefit ratio continues to favor etoposide over vinblastine.

There also continues to be considerable focus on the long-term effects of chemotherapy on gonadal function. Studies of patients with a variety of cancers suggest that, although ovarian dysfunction or failure is a risk of chemotherapy, the majority of survivors can anticipate normal menstrual and reproductive function (137–139). Factors such as older age at initiation of therapy, greater cumulative drug dose (140), and longer duration of therapy (139) have an adverse effect on future gonadal function. Successful pregnancies after treatment with combination chemotherapy have been well documented in other types of malignancies, including Hodgkin's disease, non-Hodgkin's lymphomas, and leukemia. There are similar reports in patients with malignant ovarian germ cell tumors (126,141–144).

In a review of the UTMDACC series (141), 27 (68%) of 40 patients who had retained a normal contralateral ovary and uterus maintained regular menses consistently after completion of chemotherapy, and 33 (83%) were having regular menses at the time of follow-up. Of 16 patients who had attempted to become pregnant, 12 were successful. One patient had an elective first-trimester abortion and the other 11 patients bore 22 healthy infants over time, none of which had a major birth defect. In a series from Milan, among 169 patients with ovarian germ cell tumors, 138 underwent fertility-sparing surgery, and of these 81 underwent adjuvant chemotherapy (126). After treatment, all but one woman recovered menstrual function and 55 conceptions were recorded. Forty normal full-term babies were delivered. There were four babies with congenital malformations, one in a patient who did not receive chemotherapy and three in women who had received chemotherapy (the difference was not statistically significant).

Although limited reports are available concerning other late effects of chemotherapy in patients with ovarian germ cell tumors (145,146), there are several articles on this topic involving patients with testicular cancer (147–152). In male patients who received cisplatin-based combination regimens, principally PVB, late toxicities included high-tone hearing loss (147), neurotoxicity (147,150,152), Raynaud's phenomenon (148,152), ischemic heart disease (152,153), hypertension (152), renal dysfunction (152), and pulmonary toxicity (149,151). Fortunately, despite these observations, most patients have excellent overall health and functional status (151). Indeed, in a prospective study of immediate chemotherapy versus observation and chemotherapy at the time of relapse in patients with early-stage testis cancer, the patients treated with chemotherapy had only an increased incidence of paresthesias compared to the patients who were monitored without chemotherapy (154). Hypertension, cardiac disease, and stroke were rare and of similar incidence in chemotherapy-treated and untreated patients at a median follow-up of 5.1 years. Interestingly, the late effects of treatment are more pronounced among children receiving treatment for germ cell tumors (145). Specifically, neurotoxicity, growth abnormalities, pulmonary toxicity, and gastrointestinal toxicity have been reported in a higher proportion than in adult patients. The GOG recently completed an analysis evaluating the quality of life and psychosocial characteristics of survivors of ovarian germ cell tumors compared to matched controls. In this analysis, the survivors appeared to be well adjusted, were able to develop strong relationships, and were free of significant depression (155). The impact on fertility was modest or none in patients undergoing fertility-sparing surgeries (127). Overall, these women appeared to be free of any major physical illnesses at a median follow-up of 10 years (Williams SD, personal communication).

SUMMARY

Virtually all patients with early-stage, completely resected ovarian germ cell tumors survive after careful surgical staging and three courses of adjuvant BEP. Furthermore, 50% to 80% of patients with incompletely resected or advanced tumors are expected to be long-term survivors. Current and future clinical trials should address the latter group of patients in an effort to improve therapeutic results. Acute toxicity of treatment is relatively modest. An important, but fortunately unusual late complication of treatment is etoposide-induced leukemia. However, patients receiving the usually administered cumulative dose of etoposide are at low risk for developing AML. Otherwise, late consequences of chemotherapy are limited. Efforts should concentrate on fertility preservation for patients who desire subsequent pregnancies.

The majority of dysgerminoma patients have stage I disease at diagnosis. These patients usually can be treated with unilateral salpingo-oophorectomy and careful postoperative observation without adjuvant treatment. Chemotherapy is offered at the time of recurrence. In patients with more advanced but resected disease, risk of recurrence is significant enough to warrant up-front adjuvant treatment, which for most patients is chemotherapy because of its near universal effectiveness and limited impact on fertility. In patients with incompletely resected tumor or for patients who recur after previous radiation, chemotherapy similar to that given for tumors other than dysgerminoma is appropriate.

Surgery continues to have a pivotal role in the management of all patients with ovarian germ cell tumors. Initial careful surgical staging is important for selection of appropriate subsequent therapy. The role of cytoreductive surgery is under study but the evidence supports its judicious use. However, an operation done strictly for debulking when the diagnosis is established does not seem warranted. Second-look laparotomy is not necessary in patients who have no residual tumor after their initial surgical procedure and who receive adjuvant chemotherapy. This procedure also does not seem warranted in patients with advanced tumors without elements of teratoma. However, patients with incompletely resected tumors containing teratoma elements are likely to benefit from such surgery.

The judicious use of surgery followed by chemotherapy will cure the majority of patients with ovarian germ cell tumors, at the expense of minimal and predictable immediate and late toxicities. In most circumstances fertility can be preserved.

References

1. Tavassoli FA, Devilee P, eds. *World Health Organization Classification of Tumors: Pathology and Genetics of Tumours of the Breast and Female Genital Organs*. Lyon, France: IARC Press; 2003.
2. Kurman RJ, Norris HJ. Malignant germ cell tumors of the ovary. *Hum Pathol* 1977;8:551–564.
3. Sever M, Jones TD, Roth LM, et al. Expression of CD117 (c-kit) receptor in dysgerminoma of the ovary: diagnostic and therapeutic implications. *Mod Pathol* 2005;18:1411–1416.
4. Cheng L, Thomas A, Roth LM, et al. OCT4: a novel biomarker for dysgerminoma of the ovary. *Am J Surg Pathol* 2004;28:1341–1346.
5. Hoei-Hansen CE, Kraggerud SM, Abeler VM, et al. Ovarian dysgerminomas are characterised by frequent KIT mutations and abundant expression of pluripotency markers. *Mol Cancer* 2007;2:6–12.
6. Kurman RJ, Norris HJ. Endodermal sinus tumor of the ovary: a clinical and pathologic analysis of 71 cases. *Cancer* 1976;38:2404–2419.
7. LM R. Variants of yolk sac tumor. *Pathol Case Rev* 2004;10:186–192.
8. Damjanov I, Amenta PS, Zarghami F. Transformation of an AFP-positive yolk sac carcinoma into an AFP-negative neoplasm. Evidence for in vivo cloning of the human parietal yolk sac carcinoma. *Cancer* 1984;53: 1902–1907.
9. Ramalingam P, Malpica A, Silva EG, et al. The use of cytokeratin 7 and EMA in differentiating ovarian yolk sac tumors from endometrioid and clear cell carcinomas. *Am J Surg Pathol* 2004;28:1499–1505.

10. Kurman RJ, Norris HJ. Embryonal carcinoma of the ovary: a clinicopathologic entity distinct from endodermal sinus tumor resembling embryonal carcinoma of the adult testis. *Cancer* 1976;38:2420–2433.
11. Beck JS, Fulmer HF, Lee ST. Solid malignant ovarian teratoma with "embryoid bodies" and trophoblastic differentiation. *J Pathol* 1969;99:67–73.
12. Vance RP, Geisinger KR. Pure nongestational choriocarcinoma of the ovary. Report of a case. *Cancer* 1985;56:2321–2325.
13. Kurman RJ, Norris HJ. Malignant mixed germ cell tumors of the ovary. A clinical and pathologic analysis of 30 cases. *Obstet Gynecol* 1976;48:579–589.
14. Gershenson DM, Del Junco G, Copeland LJ, et al. Mixed germ cell tumors of the ovary. *Obstet Gynecol* 1984;64:200–206.
15. Lorigan PC, Grierson AJ, Goepel JR, et al. Gestational choriocarcinoma of the ovary diagnosed by analysis of tumour DNA. *Cancer Lett* 1996;104: 27–30.
16. Riopel MA, Spellerberg A, Griffin CA, et al. Genetic analysis of ovarian germ cell tumors by comparative genomic hybridization. *Cancer Res* 1998;58:3105–3110.
17. Kraggerud SM, Szymanska J, Abeler VM, et al. DNA copy number changes in malignant ovarian germ cell tumors. *Cancer Res* 2000;60:3025–3030.
18. Yanai-Inbar I, Scully RE. Relation of ovarian dermoid cysts and immature teratomas: an analysis of 350 cases of immature teratoma and 10 cases of dermoid cyst with microscopic foci of immature tissue. *Int J Gynecol Pathol* 1987;6:203–212.
19. Norris HJ, Zirkin HJ, Benson WL. Immature (malignant) teratoma of the ovary: a clinical and pathologic study of 58 cases. *Cancer* 1976;37: 2359–2372.
20. O'Connor DM, Norris HJ. The influence of grade on the outcome of stage I ovarian immature (malignant) teratomas and the reproducibility of grading. *Int J Gynecol Pathol* 1994;13:283–289.
21. Ferguson AW, Katabuchi H, Ronnett BM, et al. Glial implants in gliomatosis peritonei arise from normal tissue, not from the associated teratoma. *Am J Pathol* 2001;159:51–55.
22. Dickersin GR, Kline IW, Scully RE. Small cell carcinoma of the ovary with hypercalcemia: a report of eleven cases. *Cancer* 1982;49:188–197.
23. Ulbright TM, Roth LM, Stehman FB, et al. Poorly differentiated (small cell) carcinoma of the ovary in young women: evidence supporting a germ cell origin. *Hum Pathol* 1987;18:175–184.
24. Seidman JD. Small cell carcinoma of the ovary of the hypercalcemic type: p53 protein accumulation and clinicopathologic features. *Gynecol Oncol* 1995;59:283–287.
25. Scully RE. Small cell carcinoma of hypercalcemic type. *Int J Gynecol Pathol* 1993;12:148–152.
26. Surti U, Hoffner L, Chakravarti A, et al. Genetics and biology of human ovarian teratomas. I. Cytogenetic analysis and mechanism of origin. *Am J Hum Genet* 1990;47:635–643.
27. Deka R, Chakravarti A, Surti U, et al. Genetics and biology of human ovarian teratomas. II. Molecular analysis of origin of nondisjunction and gene-centromere mapping of chromosome I markers. *Am J Hum Genet* 1990;47: 644–655.
28. Baker BA, Frickey L, Yu IT, et al. DNA content of ovarian immature teratomas and malignant germ cell tumors. *Gynecol Oncol* 1998;71:14–18.
29. Murty VV, Dmitrovsky E, Bosl GJ, et al. Nonrandom chromosome abnormalities in testicular and ovarian germ cell tumor cell lines. *Cancer Genet Cytogenet* 1990;50:67–73.
30. Speleman F, De Potter C, Dal Cin P, et al. i(12p) in a malignant ovarian tumor. *Cancer Genet Cytogenet* 1990;45:49–53.
31. Shen DH, KU Zhang Y, Cheung ANY. Cytogenetic study of malignant ovarian germ cell tumors by chromosome in situ hybridization. *Int J Gynecol Cancer* 1998;8:222–232.
32. Hart WR, Burkons DM. Germ cell neoplasms arising in gonadoblastomas. *Cancer* 1979;43:669–678.
33. Gershenson DM, Copeland LJ, Kavanagh JJ, et al. Treatment of malignant nondysgerminomatous germ cell tumors of the ovary with vincristine, dactinomycin, and cyclophosphamide. *Cancer* 1985;56:2756–2761.
34. Asadourian LA, Taylor HB. Dysgerminoma. An analysis of 105 cases. *Obstet Gynecol* 1969;33:370–379.
35. De Backer A, Madern GC, Oosterhuis JW, et al. Ovarian germ cell tumors in children: a clinical study of 66 patients. *Pediatr Blood Cancer* 2006;46: 459–464.
36. Gordon A, Lipton D, Woodruff JD. Dysgerminoma: a review of 158 cases from the Emil Novak Ovarian Tumor Registry. *Obstet Gynecol* 1981;58: 497–504.
37. Christman JE, Teng NN, Lebovic GS, et al. Delivery of a normal infant following cisplatin, vinblastine, and bleomycin (PVB) chemotherapy for malignant teratoma of the ovary during pregnancy. *Gynecol Oncol* 1990; 37:292–295.
38. Farahmand SM, Marchetti DL, Asirwatham JE, et al. Ovarian endodermal sinus tumor associated with pregnancy: review of the literature. *Gynecol Oncol* 1991;41:156–160.
39. Horbelt D, Delmore J, Meisel R, et al. Mixed germ cell malignancy of the ovary concurrent with pregnancy. *Obstet Gynecol* 1994;84:662–664.
40. Rajendran S, Hollingworth J, Scudamore I. Endodermal sinus tumour of the ovary in pregnancy. *Eur J Gynaecol Oncol* 1999;20:272–274.
41. Bakri YN, Ezzat A, Akhtar, et al. Malignant germ cell tumors of the ovary. Pregnancy considerations. *Eur J Obstet Gynecol Reprod Biol* 2000;90: 87–91.
42. Sekiya S, Seki K, Nagai Y. Rise of serum CA 125 in patients with pure ovarian yolk sac tumors. *Int J Gynaecol Obstet* 1997;58:323–324.
43. Ayhan A, Bildirici I, Gunalp S, et al. Pure dysgerminoma of the ovary: a review of 45 well staged cases. *Eur J Gynaecol Oncol* 2000;21:98–101.
44. De Palo G, Lattuada A, Kenda R, et al. Germ cell tumors of the ovary: the experience of the National Cancer Institute of Milan. I. Dysgerminoma. *Int J Radiat Oncol Biol Phys* 1987;13:853–860.
45. Bjorkholm E, Lundell M, Gyftodimos A, et al. Dysgerminoma. The Radiumhemmet series 1927-1984. *Cancer* 1990;65:38–44.
46. Santoni R, Cionini L, D'Elia F, et al. Dysgerminoma of the ovary: a report on 29 patients. *Clin Radiol* 1987;38:203–206.
47. Berg FD, Kurzl R, Hinrichsen MJ, et al. Familial 46,XY pure gonadal dysgenesis and gonadoblastoma/dysgerminoma: case report. *Gynecol Oncol* 1989;32:261–267.
48. Fisher RA, Salm R, Spencer RW. Bilateral gonadoblastoma/dysgerminoma in a 46 XY individual: case report with hormonal studies. *J Clin Pathol* 1982;35:420–424.
49. Kingsbury AC, Frost F, Cookson WO. Dysgerminoma, gonadoblastoma, and testicular germ cell neoplasia in phenotypically female and male siblings with 46 XY genotype. *Cancer* 1987;59:288–291.
50. Schwartz PE. Surgery of germ cell tumours of the ovary. *Forum (Genova)* 2000;10:355–365.
51. Peccatori F, Bonazzi C, Chiari S, et al. Surgical management of malignant ovarian germ-cell tumors: 10 years' experience of 129 patients. *Obstet Gynecol* 1995;86:367–372.
52. Gershenson DM. Fertility-sparing surgery for malignancies in women. *J Natl Cancer Inst Monogr* 2005;43–47.
53. Saunders DM, FA a. RJ. Fertility preservation in female oncology patients. *Int J Gynecol Cancer* 1996;6:161–167.
54. Slayton RE, Hreshchyshyn MM, Silverberg SC, et al. Treatment of malignant ovarian germ cell tumors: response to vincristine, dactinomycin, and cyclophosphamide (preliminary report). *Cancer* 1978;42:390–398.
55. Williams SD, Blessing JA, Moore DH, et al. Cisplatin, vinblastine, and bleomycin in advanced and recurrent ovarian germ-cell tumors. A trial of the Gynecologic Oncology Group. *Ann Intern Med* 1989;111:22–27.
56. Scarabelli C, Gallo A, Carbone A. Secondary cytoreductive surgery for patients with recurrent epithelial ovarian carcinoma. *Gynecol Oncol* 2001;83:504–512.
57. Parazzini F, Raspagliesi F, Guarnerio P, et al. Role of secondary surgery in relapsed ovarian cancer. *Crit Rev Oncol Hematol* 2001;37:121–125.
58. Williams SD, Blessing JA, DiSaia PJ, et al. Second-look laparotomy in ovarian germ cell tumors: the gynecologic oncology group experience. *Gynecol Oncol* 1994;52:287–291.
59. Andre F, Fizazi K, Culine S, et al. The growing teratoma syndrome: results of therapy and long-term follow-up of 33 patients. *Eur J Cancer* 2000;36:1389–1394.
60. Chen RJ, Huang PT, Lin MC, et al. Advanced stage squamous cell carcinoma arising from mature cystic teratoma of the ovary. *Acta Obstet Gynecol Scand* 2001;80:84–86.
61. Ronnett BM, Seidman JD. Mucinous tumors arising in ovarian mature cystic teratomas: relationship to the clinical syndrome of pseudomyxoma peritonei. *Am J Surg Pathol* 2003;27:650–657.
62. Vartanian RK, McRae B, Hessler RB. Sebaceous carcinoma arising in a mature cystic teratoma of the ovary. *Int J Gynecol Pathol* 2002;21:418–421.
63. Shen DH, Khoo US, Xue WC, et al. Ovarian mature cystic teratoma with malignant transformation. An interphase cytogenetic study. *Int J Gynecol Pathol* 1998;17:351–357.
64. Geisler JP, Goulet R, Foster RS, et al. Growing teratoma syndrome after chemotherapy for germ cell tumors of the ovary. *Obstet Gynecol* 1994;84:719–721.
65. Itani Y, Kawa M, Toyoda S, et al. Growing teratoma syndrome after chemotherapy for a mixed germ cell tumor of the ovary. *J Obstet Gynaecol Res* 2002;28:166–171.
66. Kattan J, Droz JP, Culine S, et al. The growing teratoma syndrome: a woman with nonseminomatous germ cell tumor of the ovary. *Gynecol Oncol* 1993;49:395–399.
67. Gershenson DM, Copeland LJ, del Junco G, et al. Second-look laparotomy in the management of malignant germ cell tumors of the ovary. *Obstet Gynecol* 1986;67:789–793.
68. Albers P, Bender H, Yilmaz H, et al. Positron emission tomography in the clinical staging of patients with stage I and II testicular germ cell tumors. *Urology* 1999;53:808–811.
69. Hain SF, O'Doherty MJ, Timothy AR, et al. Fluorodeoxyglucose positron emission tomography in the evaluation of germ cell tumours at relapse. *Br J Cancer* 2000;83:863–869.
70. Kollmannsberger C, Oechsle K, Dohmen BM, et al. Prospective comparison of [18F]fluorodeoxyglucose positron emission tomography with conventional assessment by computed tomography scans and serum tumor markers for the evaluation of residual masses in patients with nonseminomatous germ cell carcinoma. *Cancer* 2002;94:2353–2362.
71. Sanchez D, Zudaire JJ, Fernandez JM, et al. 18F-fluoro-2-deoxyglucose-positron emission tomography in the evaluation of nonseminomatous germ cell tumours at relapse. *BJU Int* 2002;89:912–916.
72. Sugawara Y, Zasadny KR, Grossman HB, et al. Germ cell tumor: differentiation of viable tumor, mature teratoma, and necrotic tissue with FDG PET and kinetic modeling. *Radiology* 1999;211:249–256.

73. De Santis M, Becherer A, Bokemeyer C, et al. FDG-PET as prognostic indicator for seminoma residuals: an update from the SEMPET study. *Proceedings of ASCO*; 2003.
74. Einhorn LH, Donohue J. Cis-diamminedichloroplatinum, vinblastine, and bleomycin combination chemotherapy in disseminated testicular cancer. *Ann Intern Med* 1977;87:293–298.
75. Williams SD, Birch R, Einhorn LH, et al. Treatment of disseminated germ-cell tumors with cisplatin, bleomycin, and either vinblastine or etoposide. *N Engl J Med* 1987;316:1435–1440.
76. Slayton RE, Park RC, Silverberg SG, et al. Vincristine, dactinomycin, and cyclophosphamide in the treatment of malignant germ cell tumors of the ovary. A Gynecologic Oncology Group study (a final report). *Cancer* 1985;56:243–248.
77. Gershenson DM, Kavanagh JJ, Copeland LJ, et al. Treatment of malignant nondysgerminomatous germ cell tumors of the ovary with vinblastine, bleomycin, and cisplatin. *Cancer* 1986;57:1731–1737.
78. Gershenson DM, Morris M, Cangir A, et al. Treatment of malignant germ cell tumors of the ovary with bleomycin, etoposide, and cisplatin. *J Clin Oncol* 1990;8:715–720.
79. Williams S, Blessing JA, Liao SY, et al. Adjuvant therapy of ovarian germ cell tumors with cisplatin, etoposide, and bleomycin: a trial of the Gynecologic Oncology Group. *J Clin Oncol* 1994;12:701–706.
80. Culine S, Lhomme C, Kattan J, et al. Cisplatin-based chemotherapy in the management of germ cell tumors of the ovary: the Institut Gustave Roussy Experience. *Gynecol Oncol* 1997;64:160–165.
81. Segelov E, Campbell J, Ng M, et al. Cisplatin-based chemotherapy for ovarian germ cell malignancies: the Australian experience. *J Clin Oncol* 1994;12:378–384.
82. Dimopoulos MA, Papadopoulou M, Andreopoulou E, et al. Favorable outcome of ovarian germ cell malignancies treated with cisplatin or carboplatin-based chemotherapy: a Hellenic Cooperative Oncology Group study. *Gynecol Oncol* 1998;70:70–74.
83. Einhorn LH. Curing metastatic testicular cancer. *Proc Natl Acad Sci USA* 2002;99:4592–4595.
84. Einhorn LH, Williams SD, Loehrer PJ, et al. Evaluation of optimal duration of chemotherapy in favorable-prognosis disseminated germ cell tumors: a Southeastern Cancer Study Group protocol. *J Clin Oncol* 1989;7:387–391.
85. Einhorn LH. Salvage therapy for germ cell tumors. *Semin Oncol* 1994;21: 47–51.
86. Bokemeyer C, Kollmannsberger C, Meisner C, et al. First-line high-dose chemotherapy compared with standard-dose PEB/VIP chemotherapy in patients with advanced germ cell tumors: a multivariate and matched-pair analysis. *J Clin Oncol* 1999;17:3450–3456.
87. Motzer RJ, Nichols CJ, Margolin KA, et al. Phase III randomized trial of conventional-dose chemotherapy with or without high-dose chemotherapy and autologous hematopoietic stem-cell rescue as first-line treatment for patients with poor-prognosis metastatic germ cell tumors. *J Clin Oncol* 2007;25:247–256.
88. Murugaesu N, Schmid P, Dancey G, et al. Malignant ovarian germ cell tumors: identification of novel prognostic markers and long-term outcome after multimodality treatment. *J Clin Oncol* 2006;24:4862–4866.
89. Messing MJ, Gershenson DM, Morris M, et al. Primary treatment failure in patients with malignant ovarian germ cell neoplasms. *Int J Gynecol Cancer* 1992;2:295–300.
90. Broun ER, Nichols CR, Turns M, et al. Early salvage therapy for germ cell cancer using high dose chemotherapy with autologous bone marrow support. *Cancer* 1994;73:1716–1720.
91. Broun ER, Nichols CR, Gize G, et al. Tandem high dose chemotherapy with autologous bone marrow transplantation for initial relapse of testicular germ cell cancer. *Cancer* 1997;79:1605–1610.
92. Lotz JP, Andre T, Donsimoni R, et al. High dose chemotherapy with ifosfamide, carboplatin, and etoposide combined with autologous bone marrow transplantation for the treatment of poor-prognosis germ cell tumors and metastatic trophoblastic disease in adults. *Cancer* 1995;75:874–885.
93. Einhorn LH, Williams SD, Chamness A, et al. High dose chemotherapy and stem cell rescue for metastatic germ cell rumors. *N Engl J Med* 2007;357(4):340–348.
94. Loehrer PJ Sr, Gonin R, Nichols CR, et al. Vinblastine plus ifosfamide plus cisplatin as initial salvage therapy in recurrent germ cell tumor. *J Clin Oncol* 1998;16:2500–2504.
95. Hinton S, Catalano P, Einhorn LH, et al. Phase II study of paclitaxel plus gemcitabine in refractory germ cell tumors (E9897): a trial of the Eastern Cooperative Oncology Group. *J Clin Oncol* 2002;20:1859–1863.
96. Nichols CR, Roth BJ, Loehrer PJ, et al. Salvage chemotherapy for recurrent germ cell cancer. *Semin Oncol* 1994;21:102–108.
97. Einhorn LH, Brames MJ, Juliar B, et al. Phase II study of paclitaxel plus gemcitabine salvage chemotherapy for germ cell tumors after progression following high-dose chemotherapy with tandem transplant. *J Clin Oncol* 2007;25:513–516.
98. Mann JR, Raafat F, Robinson K, et al. The United Kingdom Children's Cancer Study Group's second germ cell tumor study: carboplatin, etoposide, and bleomycin are effective treatment for children with malignant extracranial germ cell tumors, with acceptable toxicity. *J Clin Oncol* 2000;18:3809–3818.
99. McKeage MJ, Evans BD, Atkinson C, et al. Carbon monoxide diffusing capacity is a poor predictor of clinically significant bleomycin lung. New Zealand Clinical Oncology Group. *J Clin Oncol* 1990;8:779–783.
100. Loehrer PJ Sr, Johnson D, Elson P, et al. Importance of bleomycin in favorable-prognosis disseminated germ cell tumors: an Eastern Cooperative Oncology Group trial. *J Clin Oncol* 1995;13:470–476.
101. de Wit R, Stoter G, Kaye SB, et al. Importance of bleomycin in combination chemotherapy for good-prognosis testicular nonseminoma: a randomized study of the European Organization for Research and Treatment of Genitourinary Tract Cancer Cooperative Group. *J Clin Oncol* 1997;15: 1837–1843.
102. Bajorin DF, Sarosdy MF, Pfister DG, et al. Randomized trial of etoposide and cisplatin versus etoposide and carboplatin in patients with good-risk germ cell tumors: a multi-institutional study. *J Clin Oncol* 1993;11:598–606.
103. Horwich A, Sleijfer DT, Fossa SD, et al. Randomized trial of bleomycin, etoposide, and cisplatin compared with bleomycin, etoposide, and carboplatin in good-prognosis metastatic nonseminomatous germ cell cancer: a Multi-institutional Medical Research Council/European Organization for Research and Treatment of Cancer Trial. *J Clin Oncol* 1997;15:1844–1852.
104. American Society of Clinical Oncology. Recommendations for the use of hematopoietic colony-stimulating factors: evidence-based, clinical practice guidelines. *J Clin Oncol* 1994;12:2471–2508.
105. Cushing B, Giller R, Ablin A, et al. Surgical resection alone is effective treatment for ovarian immature teratoma in children and adolescents: a report of the Pediatric Oncology Group and the Children's Cancer Group. *Am J Obstet Gynecol* 1999;181:353–358.
106. Marina NM, Cushing B, Giller R, et al. Complete surgical excision is effective treatment for children with immature teratomas with or without malignant elements: a Pediatric Oncology Group/Children's Cancer Group Intergroup Study. *J Clin Oncol* 1999;17:2137–2143.
107. Dark GG, Bower M, Newlands ES, et al. Surveillance policy for stage I ovarian germ cell tumors. *J Clin Oncol* 1997;15:620–624.
108. Bonazzi C, Peccatori F, Colombo N, et al. Pure ovarian immature teratoma, a unique and curable disease: 10 years' experience of 32 prospectively treated patients. *Obstet Gynecol* 1994;84:598–604.
109. Buskirk SJ, Schray MF, Podratz KC, et al. Ovarian dysgerminoma: a retrospective analysis of treatment, sites of treatment failure, and radiosensitivity. *Mayo Clin Proc* 1987;62:1149–1157.
110. LaPolla JP, Benda J, Vigliotti AP, et al. Dysgerminoma of the ovary. *Obstet Gynecol* 1987;69:859–864.
111. Mitchell MF, Gershenson DM, Soeters RP, et al. The long-term effects of radiation therapy on patients with ovarian dysgerminoma. *Cancer* 1991;67:1084–1090.
112. Krepart G, Smith JP, Rutledge F, et al. The treatment for dysgerminoma of the ovary. *Cancer* 1978;41:986–990.
113. Thomas GM, Dembo AJ, Hacker NF, et al. Current therapy for dysgerminoma of the ovary. *Obstet Gynecol* 1987;70:268–275.
114. Patterson DM, Murugaesu N, Holden L, et al. A review of the close surveillance policy for stage I female germ cell tumors of the ovary and other sites. *Int J Gynecol Cancer* 2008;18(1):43–50.
115. Lawson AP, Adler GF. Radiotherapy in the treatment of ovarian dysgerminomas. *Int J Radiat Oncol Biol Phys* 1988;14:431–434.
116. Freel JH, Cassir JF, Pierce VK, et al. Dysgerminoma of the ovary. *Cancer* 1979;43:798–805.
117. Marks RD, Underwood PB, Othersen HB, et al. Dysgerminoma—100% control with combined therapy in six consecutive patients with advanced disease. *Int J Radiat Oncol Biol Phys* 1978;4:453–456.
118. Thomas GM, Rider WD, Dembo AJ, et al. Seminoma of the testis: results of treatment and patterns of failure after radiation therapy. *Int J Radiat Oncol Biol Phys* 1982;8:165–174.
119. Boice JD Jr, Engholm G, Kleinerman RA, et al. Radiation dose and second cancer risk in patients treated for cancer of the cervix. *Radiat Res* 1988; 116:3–55.
120. Zaghloul MS, Khattab TY. Dysgerminoma of the ovary: good prognosis even in advanced stages. *Int J Radiat Oncol Biol Phys* 1992;24:161–165.
121. Culine S, Lhomme C, Kattan J, et al. Cisplatin-based chemotherapy in dysgerminoma of the ovary: thirteen-year experience at the Institut Gustave Roussy. *Gynecol Oncol* 1995;58:344–348.
122. Williams SD, Blessing JA, Hatch KD, et al. Chemotherapy of advanced dysgerminoma: trials of the Gynecologic Oncology Group. *J Clin Oncol* 1991;9:1950–1955.
123. Williams SD, Kauderer J, Burnett AF, et al. Adjuvant therapy of completely resected dysgerminoma with carboplatin and etoposide: a trial of the Gynecologic Oncology Group. *Gynecol Oncol* 2004;95:496–499.
124. Perrin LC, Low J, Nicklin JL, et al. Fertility and ovarian function after conservative surgery for germ cell tumours of the ovary. *Aust NZ J Obstet Gynaecol* 1999;39:243–245.
125. Kanazawa K, Suzuki T, Sakumoto K. Treatment of malignant ovarian germ cell tumors with preservation of fertility: reproductive performance after persistent remission. *Am J Clin Oncol* 2000;23:244–248.
126. Zanetta G, Bonazzi C, Cantu M, et al. Survival and reproductive function after treatment of malignant germ cell ovarian tumors. *J Clin Oncol* 2001;19:1015–1020.
127. Gershenson DM, Miller AM, Champion VL, et al. Reproductive and sexual function after platinum-based chemotherapy in long-term ovarian germ cell tumor survivors: a Gynecologic Oncology Group study. *J Clin Oncol* 2007;25(19):2792–2797.
128. Muram D, Gale CL, Thompson E. Functional ovarian cysts in patients cured of ovarian neoplasms. *Obstet Gynecol* 1990;75:680–683.

129. Howell S, Shalet S. Gonadal damage from chemotherapy and radiotherapy. *Endocrinol Metab Clin North Am* 1998;27:927–943.
130. Casey AC, Bhodauria S, Shapter A, et al. Dysgerminoma: the role of conservative surgery. *Gynecol Oncol* 1996;63:352–357.
131. Nichols CR, Breeden ES, Loehrer PJ, et al. Secondary leukemia associated with a conventional dose of etoposide: review of serial germ cell tumor protocols. *J Natl Cancer Inst* 1993;85:36–40.
132. Pedersen-Bjergaard J, Daugaard G, Hansen SW, et al. Increased risk of myelodysplasia and leukaemia after etoposide, cisplatin, and bleomycin for germ-cell tumours. *Lancet* 1991;338:359–363.
133. Pui CH. Epipodophyllotoxin-related acute myeloid leukaemia. *Lancet* 1991;338:1269–1270.
134. Pui CH, Ribeiro RC, Hancock ML, et al. Acute myeloid leukemia in children treated with epipodophyllotoxins for acute lymphoblastic leukemia. *N Engl J Med* 1991;325:1682–1687.
135. Ratain MJ, Kaminer LS, Bitran JD, et al. Acute nonlymphocytic leukemia following etoposide and cisplatin combination chemotherapy for advanced non-small-cell carcinoma of the lung. *Blood* 1987;70:1412–1417.
136. Pedersen-Bjergaard J, Brondum-Nielsen K, Karle H, et al. Chemotherapy-related - late occurring - Philadelphia chromosome in AML, ALL and CML. Similar events related to treatment with DNA topoisomerase II inhibitors? *Leukemia* 1997;11:1571–1574.
137. Horning SJ, Hoppe RT, Kaplan HS, et al. Female reproductive potential after treatment for Hodgkin's disease. *N Engl J Med* 1981;304:1377–1382.
138. Byrne J, Mulvihill JJ, Myers MH, et al. Effects of treatment on fertility in long-term survivors of childhood or adolescent cancer. *N Engl J Med* 1987;317:1315–1321.
139. Siris ES, Leventhal BG, Vaitukaitis JL. Effects of childhood leukemia and chemotherapy on puberty and reproductive function in girls. *N Engl J Med* 1976;294:1143–1146.
140. Nicosia SV, Matus-Ridley M, Meadows AT. Gonadal effects of cancer therapy in girls. *Cancer* 1985;55:2364–2372.
141. Gershenson DM. Menstrual and reproductive function after treatment with combination chemotherapy for malignant ovarian germ cell tumors. *J Clin Oncol* 1988;6:270–275.
142. Brewer M, Gershenson DM, Herzog CE, et al. Outcome and reproductive function after chemotherapy for ovarian dysgerminoma. *J Clin Oncol* 1999;17:2670–2675.
143. Pektasides D, Rustin GJ, Newlands ES, et al. Fertility after chemotherapy for ovarian germ cell tumours. *Br J Obstet Gynaecol* 1987;94:477–479.
144. Rustin GJ, Pektasides D, Bagshawe KD, et al. Fertility after chemotherapy for male and female germ cell tumours. *Int J Androl* 1987;10:389–392.
145. Hale GA, Marina NM, Jones-Wallace D, et al. Late effects of treatment for germ cell tumors during childhood and adolescence. *J Pediatr Hematol Oncol* 1999;21:115–122.
146. Swenson MM, MacLeod JS, Williams SD, et al. Quality of life after among ovarian germ cell cancer survivors: a narrative analysis. *Oncol Nurs Forum* 2003;30:380.
147. Hansen SW, Helweg-Larsen S, Trojaborg W. Long-term neurotoxicity in patients treated with cisplatin, vinblastine, and bleomycin for metastatic germ cell cancer. *J Clin Oncol* 1989;7:1457–1461.
148. Hansen SW, Olsen N. Raynaud's phenomenon in patients treated with cisplatin, vinblastine, and bleomycin for germ cell cancer: measurement of vasoconstrictor response to cold. *J Clin Oncol* 1989;7:940–942.
149. Hansen SW, Groth S, Sorensen PG, et al. Enhanced pulmonary toxicity in smokers with germ-cell cancer treated with cis-platinum, vinblastine and bleomycin: a long-term follow-up. *Eur J Cancer Clin Oncol* 1989;25:733–736.
150. Roth BJ, Greist A, Kubilis PS, et al. Cisplatin-based combination chemotherapy for disseminated germ cell tumors: long-term follow-up. *J Clin Oncol* 1988;6:1239–1247.
151. Boyer M, Raghavan D, Harris PJ, et al. Lack of late toxicity in patients treated with cisplatin-containing combination chemotherapy for metastatic testicular cancer. *J Clin Oncol* 1990;8:21–26.
152. Stoter G, Koopman A, Vendrik CP, et al. Ten-year survival and late sequelae in testicular cancer patients treated with cisplatin, vinblastine, and bleomycin. *J Clin Oncol* 1989;7:1099–1104.
153. Nichols CR, Roth BJ, Williams SD, et al. No evidence of acute cardiovascular complications of chemotherapy for testicular cancer: an analysis of the Testicular Cancer Intergroup Study. *J Clin Oncol* 1992;10:760–765.
154. Williams SD, Stablein DM, Einhorn LH, et al. Immediate adjuvant chemotherapy versus observation with treatment at relapse in pathological stage II testicular cancer. *N Engl J Med* 1987;317:1433–1438.
155. Champion V, Williams SD, Miller A, et al. Quality of life in long-term survivors of ovarian germ cell tumors: a Gynecologic Oncology Group study. *Gynecol Oncol* 2007;105(3):687–694.

CHAPTER 27 ■ OVARIAN SEX CORD–STROMAL TUMORS

DAVID M. GERSHENSON, LYNN C. HARTMANN, AND ROBERT H. YOUNG

The intraovarian matrix that supports the germ cells and is covered by the surface epithelium consists of cells originating from the sex cords and mesenchyme of the embryonic gonad. Granulosa cells and Sertoli cells, generally considered to be homologous, are derived from the sex cord cells, whereas the pluripotential mesenchymal cells are the precursors of the theca cells, Leydig cells, and fibroblasts. Neoplastic transformation of these cellular constituents, either singly or in various combinations collectively, results in neoplasms that are termed sex cord–stromal tumors (SCSTs). The classification of the sex cord–stromal tumors provides the template from which this chapter endeavors to stratify and define these tumor entities according to their morphologic characteristics (Table 27.1).

The SCSTs are estimated to account for approximately 7% of all malignant ovarian neoplasms (1). Although SCSTs account for a decreasing proportion of all ovarian malignancies with advancing age, the annual age-related incidence continues to increase through the seventh decade of life (2). Overall, the majority of these tumors are benign or of low malignant potential and are associated with a favorable long-term prognosis. In addition, a significant proportion of SCSTs are diagnosed in patients prior to age 40 years and have the potential to produce a variety of steroid hormones. Hence, adequate knowledge of the natural history of each of these tumors is imperative to diagnose and individualize appropriately definitive surgical and adjuvant therapy.

Sex cord–stromal tumors account for nearly 90% of all functioning ovarian neoplasms (3). With the exception of fibromas, the clinical presentation of patients with SCSTs is frequently governed by the clinical manifestations resulting from the endocrinologic abnormalities. Excessive estrogen production, whether from increased tumor synthesis or peripheral conversion of androgens, influences end-organ responses, which are usually age-dependent and can range from isosexual precocious puberty to menometrorrhagia to postmenopausal bleeding. In addition, the associated risks for endometrial cancer and possibly breast cancer must be recognized (4–6). Conversely, the rapid onset of signs ranging from early defeminization to frank virilization heralds a hyperandrogenic state. Elevated circulating levels of testosterone and/or androstenedione provide strong evidence for the presence of an SCST. Although granulosa cell, theca cell, and Sertoli cell tumors are generally considered to be estrogenic, and Sertoli–Leydig cell and steroid cell tumors are predominantly androgenic, the functional endocrinologic capacities of these tumors are impossible to predict based on their morphologic features. It should also be noted that miscellaneous ovarian tumors, both primary and metastatic, that are not in the SCST family may be androgenic or estrogenic if their stroma is stimulated to undergo luteinization.

GRANULOSA CELL TUMORS

Although granulosa cell tumors (GCTs) of the ovary were initially described by Rokitansky in 1859 (7), the etiopathogenesis of these neoplasms remains ill defined. At least in part, this is a reflection of the low incidence of GCTs, and hence the limited number of cases witnessed at any single institution. To our knowledge, there are no recognized risk factors for the development of GCTs (4,8). Reproductive factors, including the use of fertility-promoting agents and oral contraceptives, do not correlate consistently with the development of disease. Unkila-Kallio et al. (9) studied a possible link between fertility-promoting agents and GCTs using the nationwide Finnish Cancer Registry. They analyzed the occurrence of GCTs in Finland during the time period 1965 to 1994 against sales statistics for ovulation inducers. In fact, the incidence of GCTs declined by nearly 40% from 1965–1969 to 1985–1994, whereas the use of clomiphene citrate increased 13-fold and that of human menopausal gonadotropin increased 200-fold. Of interest, oral contraceptive use increased fivefold. No hereditary predisposition for any of the sex cord–stromal tumors has been identified (10). Of note, a recent case report described the occurrence of adult GCTs in two first-degree relatives (11). Granulosa cell tumors comprise only 5% of all ovarian malignancies and account for approximately 70% of malignant sex cord–stromal tumors (4–6,12–19). The annual incidence of GCTs in the United States and other developed countries varies from 0.4 to 1.7 cases per 100,000 women (5,6,8,18,20,21). Quirk and Natarajan reported histology-specific age-adjusted ovarian cancer incidence rates that were standardized to the recently adopted year 2000 U.S. standard population (22). They utilized data gathered from the Surveillance, Epidemiology, and End Results (SEER) Program for the years 1992–1999. Out of a total of 23,484 microscopically confirmed cases of primary ovarian cancer, 293 (1.2%) were of sex cord–stromal origin. Although GCTs have been diagnosed from infancy through the tenth decade of life, the peak incidence for these tumors occurs during the perimenopausal decade. The average age at the time of diagnosis in over 750 cases was 52 years (4–6,13,15–18). Considering that GCTs occurring after the third decade of life appear to be histologically distinct in most instances from those occurring in children and younger adults, the clinical and pathologic characteristics for the juvenile and adult GCTs will be addressed separately.

TABLE 27.1

CLASSIFICATION OF SEX CORD–STROMAL TUMORS

GRANULOSA-STROMAL CELL TUMORS
Granulosa cell tumor
Adult type
Juvenile type
Tumors in the thecoma-fibroma group
Thecoma
Fibroma-fibrosarcoma
Sclerosing stromal tumor
SERTOLI-STROMAL CELL TUMORS
Sertoli cell tumor
Leydig cell tumor
Sertoli–Leydig cell tumor
Well differentiated
Of intermediate differentiation
Poorly differentiated
With heterologous elements
Retiform
Mixed
SEX CORD TUMOR WITH ANNULAR TUBULES
Unclassified
Gynandroblastoma
Steroid cell tumors
Stromal luteoma
Leydig cell tumor
Hilus cell tumor
Leydig cell tumor, nonhilar type
Steroid cell tumor not otherwise specified

Granulosa Cell Tumors: Adult Type

Adult-type granulosa cell tumors (AGCTs), as histologically described below, account for 95% of all GCTs. The majority of patients will present with one or a combination of the following clinical symptoms: abnormal vaginal bleeding, abdominal distention, and abdominal pain (5,6,15–18,23). The latter symptoms are most frequently attributable to the gross size of the tumor at the time of diagnosis, with the majority exceeding 10 cm in diameter and many exceeding 15 cm (5,16,18). In one series, 12% had ascites at diagnosis (23). In many series, menometrorrhagia, oligomenorrhea, or amenorrhea in premenopausal women or bleeding in postmenopausal women is the most common reason for seeking medical assistance. These and other clinical manifestations such as breast tenderness, uterine myohypertrophy, and endometrial hyperplasia are consistent with the presence of an estrogen-secreting tumor.

The endocrine function of AGCTs, specifically the production of estrogens, has been repeatedly demonstrated by assessment of the end organ, the endometrium, and measurements of peripheral levels of estrogen before and after surgery. In a detailed retrospective analysis of endometrial specimens from patients (n = 69) with GCTs, Gusberg and Kardon (24) observed histologic features consistent with unopposed estrogen, including atypical adenomatous hyperplasia in 42% of the evaluated cohort, adenocarcinoma *in situ* (4) in 5%, and invasive adenocarcinoma in 22%. Similarly, Evans et al. (4) noted endometrial hyperplasia in 55% and adenocarcinoma in 13% of their GCT study population. Other investigators have corroborated the high prevalence of glandular hyperplasia and have reported adenocarcinoma frequencies ranging from 3% to 27% (5,6,13,15–18,25,26). Selective ovarian venous catheterizations during surgery have documented hormonal production, including the secretion of large quantities of estrogen from the ovary harboring the GCT. The return of serum estrogen to physiologic levels after definitive treatment has been witnessed repeatedly. Occasionally, patients with GCTs present with endometrial changes (decidual reaction of the stroma or secretory characteristics of the glands) consistent with tumor production of progesterone (27). Rarely, virilizing changes such as oligomenorrhea, hirsutism, and other masculinizing signs may accompany GCTs (28–30).

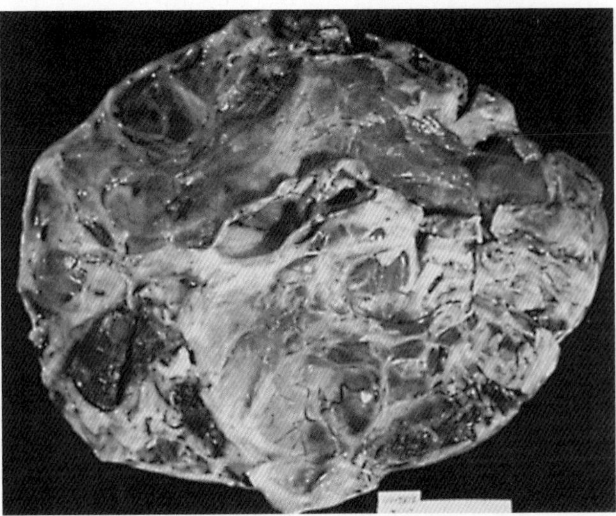

FIGURE 27.1. Granulosa cell tumor. The sectioned surface is composed predominantly of multiple cysts filled with blood. *Source:* Reprinted with permission from Case Records of the Massachusetts General Hospital, Case 89–1961. *N Engl J Med* 1961;265:1210–1214.

Pathology

AGCTs have an average diameter of approximately 12 cm, but a subset, 10% to 15% of the cases, are small and not appreciated on pelvic examination (31). Most characteristically, they are predominantly cystic with numerous locules filled with fluid or clotted blood and separated by solid tissue (Fig. 27.1), or they are solid with large areas of hemorrhage. The solid tissue may be gray-white or yellow and soft or firm. A rare tumor is cystic, usually thin walled, but occasionally thick walled, and multilocular or unilocular (29).

Microscopic examination reveals an almost exclusive population of granulosa cells or, more often, an additional component of theca cells, fibroblasts, or both. The granulosa cells grow in a wide variety of patterns. The better-differentiated tumors usually have microfollicular, macrofollicular, insular, or trabecular patterns. The microfollicular pattern is characterized by numerous small cavities (Call-Exner bodies) (Fig. 27.2) that may contain eosinophilic fluid, one or a few degenerating nuclei, hyalinized basement-membrane material, or rarely, basophilic fluid. The microfollicles are typically separated by well-differentiated granulosa cells that contain scanty cytoplasm and pale, angular or oval, often grooved nuclei arranged haphazardly in relation to one another and to the follicles. The uncommon macrofollicular pattern is characterized by cysts lined by well-differentiated granulosa cells beneath which theca cells are present. The trabecular and insular forms of granulosa cell tumors are characterized by bands and islands of granulosa cells separated by fibromatous or thecomatous stroma. The less well-differentiated forms of the adult granulosa cell tumor typically have a water silk (moire silk), gyriform, or diffuse (sarcomatoid) pattern alone or in combination. The first two patterns are manifested by parallel undulating or zigzag rows of granulosa cells,

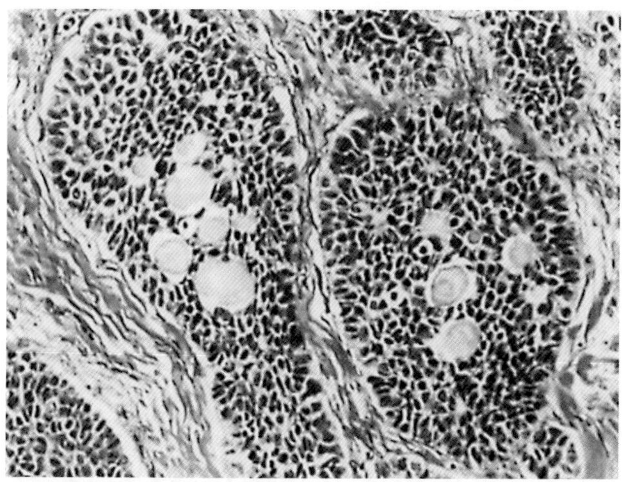

FIGURE 27.2. Granulosa cell tumor, adult type, microfollicular pattern. Several nests of granulose cells with small oval and angular nuclei enclose multiple Call-Exner bodies.

generally in single file, whereas the diffuse form is characterized by a monotonous, patternless cellular growth. In some adult granulosa cell tumors, the neoplastic cells have moderate to abundant quantities of dense or vacuolated cytoplasms; the term *luteinized granulosa cell tumor* is appropriate when such cells predominate (27). The cells in GCTs usually have round to oval, pale, and often grooved nuclei (Fig. 27.2), but rarely the cells are spindle shaped, resembling a cellular fibroma or low-grade fibrosarcoma; mitotic figures may be numerous, but are rarely atypical. There is usually only mild nuclear atypia, but approximately 2% of tumors contain mononucleate and multinucleate cells with large, bizarre, hyperchromatic nuclei, the presence of which does not appear to worsen the prognosis (32).

Natural History

Adult granulosa cell tumors are low-grade malignancies with a propensity to remain localized and demonstrate indolent growth. Ninety percent are stage I at diagnosis (26). The 10-year survival rate for stage I disease ranges from 86% to 96%; for more advanced disease at diagnosis, 26% to 49% (26). Bilaterality is infrequent (less than 10%) (23). For patients who recur, the median time to recurrence is 6 years. The median survival after recurrence is 5.6 years, consistent with indolent growth features (4,13). Tumor rupture occurred in 22% of a series of 97 cases (23). A unique feature of GCTs is the occurrence of recurrences at extended time intervals from primary therapy, suggesting the presence of persistent occult disease with a very indolent growth rate. Numerous investigators have witnessed recurrences more than a decade after primary treatment (33,34).

Prognostic Factors

The staging system for GCTs is the same as that used for epithelial ovarian cancer (International Federation of Gynecology and Obstetrics, FIGO). Whereas surgical stage has been recognized as the most important prognostic factor for GCTs, tumor size, rupture, histologic subtype, nuclear atypia, and mitotic activity have been correlated with survival with varying degrees of success (8,35,36). As noted above, GCTs are large and therefore prone to rupture. Rupture appears to adversely impact survival in stage I patients, justifying stratification as stage IC (13). However, the prognostic importance of positive cytology and surface involvement is less defined in stage I GCTs (8). Larger, well-characterized series are necessary to clarify these apparent discrepancies. Traditionally, tumor size was considered to be prognostically significant but appears to lose independent predictability when assessed according to stage (5,14,18,20). Both the increasing degree of nuclear atypia and the increasing mitotic frequency per 10 high-power fields (HPFs) have been correlated inversely with prognosis. Specimens from patients with more advanced disease were associated with a higher grade of atypia and/or more mitotic figures (5,13,14,18). Of note is the observation that nuclear grade, despite its somewhat subjective assessment, has been reported to be a reliable prognostic indicator in stage I cases (13,18). The significance of histologic subtypes and ploidy status has been debated and they appear to be of minimal value. Several investigative groups (4,5,12–14,18) have failed to confirm Kottmeier's (37) report of the prognostic importance of histologic patterns alone in GCTs. Similarly, the reported studies utilizing flow cytometric analysis of DNA content have been inconsistent. Klemi et al. (38) reported a significant survival advantage for patients with tumors demonstrating normal ploidy and/or an S-phase fraction of less than 6%. In contrast, other investigators have suggested that nondiploid GCTs are infrequently encountered (39,40). Chadha et al. (39) observed three of five aneuploid tumors from a sample population of 43 pathologically diagnosed GCTs to be vimentin negative but positive for cytokeratin and epithelial membrane antigen, and therefore cautioned that such highly aneuploid tumors may represent undifferentiated carcinomas. Indeed, it is clear that some series of GCTs in the literature are "contaminated" by the inclusion of undifferentiated carcinomas not otherwise specified or recently recognized entities, such as the large cell carcinoma of hypercalcemic type. Series with unusually large numbers of late-stage or poor-prognosis cases should accordingly be evaluated cautiously.

Investigators have analyzed several potential molecular markers, including p53 status, telomerase, Ki-67, c-myc, and HER2/neu in GCTs (41–45). To date, no molecular marker provides prognostic information for GCTs beyond what is known from stage and histopathologic parameters.

Ala-Fossi et al. stained 30 GCTs for the inhibin subunit. All 24 stage I and II tumors were positive, whereas 4 of 6 stage II to IV tumors were negative. Those that were negative were poorly differentiated and exhibited rapid disease progression. Whether other observers would have accepted these tumors as valid granulosa cell tumors is a concern. Stage was the sole independent prognostic factor (46).

Serum Markers

Recognizing that the majority of patients presenting with advanced GCTs will recur, the identification of a specific serum tumor marker(s) would facilitate early detection of recurrent disease and monitoring of treatment effectiveness (4,5,16,18). As noted above, serum estrogens are generally produced by GCTs and have been utilized as an indicator of disease status (47). Unfortunately, serum estradiol levels are occasionally not elevated, and more frequently are only marginally increased. Hence, they are not ideal for monitoring in a significant number of cases. Several proteins derived from granulosa cells, including inhibin, follicle-regulating protein, and müllerian-inhibiting substance, are readily assayable in serum and forwarded as useful diagnostic monitoring markers (48–56). In a prospective evaluation of 27 patients with GCTs, Jobling et al. (50) demonstrated that serum inhibin levels are typically elevated sevenfold above normal follicular phase levels prior to primary surgical management and can become elevated again several months prior to clinical detection of recurrent disease. In recent years, inhibin and calretinin have become available as markers that can be evaluated immunohistochemically to assist in the diagnosis of GCTs and, for that matter, other SCSTs (57).

Granulosa Cell Tumors: Juvenile Type

Ovarian neoplasms are relatively rare in childhood and adolescence, and when encountered, the majority are of germ cell origin, with only 5% to 7% being SCSTs. The latter, which consists predominantly of the granulosa cell type in this age group, demonstrates a tumor biology that appears to be different from the typical granulosa cell tumor (AGCT) considered above (58). Approximately 90% of the granulosa cell tumors diagnosed in prepubertal girls and in most women less than 30 years of age will be of the juvenile type (JGCT). In a clinicopathologic analysis of 125 cases of JGCT, 44% of the tumors occurred prior to age 10 years and only 3% after the third decade of life (59). The majority of prepubertal patients present with clinical evidence of isosexual precocious pseudopuberty, which may include breast enlargement, development of pubic hair, increased vaginal secretions, advanced somatic development, and other secondary sex characteristics (59–63). Serum estradiol levels were reported as being elevated in 17 of 17 cases of JGCTs and pseudopuberty (61). In addition, elevated levels of serum progesterone (six of ten) and testosterone (six of eight) were likewise observed, as well as suppressed levels of luteinizing hormone and follicle-stimulating hormone. The occasional patient will harbor an androgen-secreting JGCT accompanied by virilization (59,61,62). Although the signs of either precocious pseudopuberty or virilization are dramatic, the most consistent clinical sign at presentation in patients with JGCTs is increasing abdominal girth. Young et al. (59) indicated that in only 2 of 113 nonpregnant patients with JGCTs was the treating physician unable to palpate a mass on abdominal, pelvic, and/or rectal examination. Abdominal pain, dysuria, and constipation may occur. Infrequently, a surgical emergency is encountered following spontaneous rupture or torsion of the enlarged ovary. Juvenile granulosa cell tumors can occur in infants, in whom the prognosis appears to be more favorable than in older individuals (64). Hasiakos et al. describe a recent case of JGCT associated with pregnancy and review the literature (65).

The frequency of bilaterality for JGCTs is estimated to be 5%, similar to AGCTs (66). When stage was assigned based on surgical and histologic parameters, 88% were stage IA, 2% stage IB, 8% stage IC, and 3% stage II. As noted, extraovarian spread is infrequently encountered at exploration, whereas rupture of the tumor is noted in approximately 10% of cases. Ascites contributes to the abdominal distention in 10% to 36% of cases (59,61).

JGCTs have been reported in association with enchondromatosis alone (Ollier's disease) or concomitantly with hemangiomas (Maffucci's syndrome) (61,67–69). Individuals with these relatively uncommon mesodermal dysplasias generally present prior to puberty and frequently develop secondary neoplasms, most commonly sarcomas, after the second decade of life. Juvenile granulosa cell tumors are the next most frequent tumor associated with these disorders and become evident during the first and second decades of life. These observations appear to imply more than coincidental occurrences and suggest a generalized mesodermal dysplasia, perhaps contributing to the pathogenesis of these neoplastic processes. In addition, congenital bilateral JGCTs of the ovary have been reported in leprechaunism, a disease characterized by insulin resistance resulting from an insulin-receptor defect (70).

Pathology

The appearances of JGCTs are similar to the adult form; a solid and cystic neoplasm, in which the cysts contain hemorrhagic fluid, is common (59,60,63). Uniformly solid and uniformly cystic neoplasms are also encountered; the latter may be multilocular or, in rare instances, unilocular. The solid component is typically yellow-tan or gray and occasionally exhibits extensive necrosis, hemorrhage, or both.

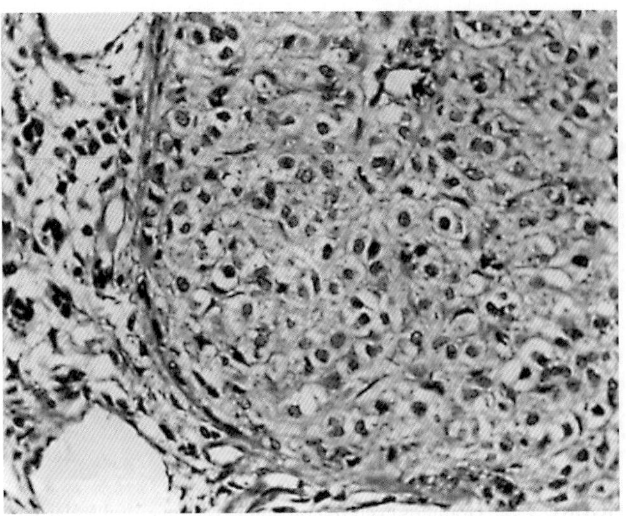

FIGURE 27.3. Granulosa cell tumor, juvenile type. A nodule of tumor is composed of large cells with abundant cytoplasm and slightly pleomorphic, hyperchromatic nuclei.

Microscopic examination typically reveals a predominantly solid cellular tumor with focal follicle formation, but occasionally, a uniformly solid or a uniformly follicular pattern is seen. In the solid areas, the neoplastic cells may be arranged diffusely or as multiple nodules of various sizes. The follicles typically vary in size and shape; Call-Exner bodies are rarely encountered, and the follicles rarely reach the large size of those in the macrofollicular AGCT. The follicular lumens in the juvenile tumor contain eosinophilic or basophilic fluid, which stains with mucicarmine in approximately two of three cases.

The two characteristic cytologic features of the neoplastic juvenile granulosa cells that distinguish them from those of AGCT are their generally rounded, hyperchromatic nuclei, which almost always lack grooves, and their almost invariable moderate to abundant eosinophilic or vacuolated (luteinized) cytoplasm (Fig. 27.3). Nuclear atypia in JGCTs varies from minimal to marked; in approximately 13% of the cases, severe degrees are present. The mitotic rate also varies greatly but is generally higher than that seen in AGCTs, often being five or more per HPF (59,63).

Natural History

In the initial series by Young et al., 98% of 125 patients with JGCTs were less than 35 years of age, and 78% were 20 years or less (59). Notwithstanding the customary presenting complaint of increased abdominal girth and the clinical documentation of a large mass (64% >10 cm), 90% of the JGCTs analyzed by Young et al. (59) were stage IA or IB. The corresponding survival rate for these patients with an average follow-up of 3.5 years was 97%. Included were nine stage IA2 patients with rupture of the tumor, all of whom were alive and free of disease. Patients presenting with associated isosexual pseudoprecocious puberty may have a more favorable prognosis. Assessing 80 such cases accrued from 212 reported JGCTs, only two cancer-related deaths (2.5%) were observed. Presumably, the clinical manifestations lead to early medical intervention and reflect the excellent outcomes (59,61–63).

Although the early symptoms and presentation with localized disease are similar to AGCTs, several behavioral characteristics are notably different when comparing these histologic variants. Although the natural history of the adult form frequently includes a latency period with recurrences remote from initial diagnosis, the juvenile counterpart is characteristically aggressive in advanced stages and the time to relapse and death of limited duration. Thirteen cases of stage II, III, or IV disease were abstracted from three analyses with a combined sample size of 180 patients (59,61,62). Of these 13 cases, only three patients (23%) were alive when reported, and notably, the recurrences and deaths occurred within a relatively brief interval. In contrast to the AGCTs, recurrences of JCGTs occur early, usually within 3 years of the diagnosis (59,61,63).

Prognostic Factors

Young et al. (59) noted surgical stage to represent the most reliable prognostic indicator. Tumor size, mitotic activity, and nuclear atypia appeared to be significant when tumors were analyzed without regard to stage. However, these parameters lost discriminating value when applied to only stages IA1 and IB1 tumors. In that series, rupture did not correlate with outcome. Schneider et al. reported on a group of 54 sex cord–stromal tumors in children and adolescents from Germany (45 JGCTs and 9 others) (71). They addressed the outcome of patients with "accidental" stage IC disease, defined as violation of the tumor capsule during surgery, versus "natural" stage IC tumors, with preoperative rupture or malignant ascites. Among 12 patients with accidental stage IC disease, there were no recurrences. In contrast, five of the nine patients with natural stage IC disease recurred ($p = 0.001$). Assessment of DNA content via flow cytometry in JGCTs demonstrated that nearly half of such tumors harbored nondiploid patterns (72,73). Jacoby et al. (72) were unable to correlate DNA ploidy or S-phase fraction (SPF) with either stage of disease or prognosis in patients with localized disease. In the series by Schneider et al., mitotic activity correlated with prognosis (71). There were no relapses in 35 patients whose tumors exhibited low or moderate mitotic activity. Among those with high mitotic activity (>19 mitoses per 10 HPFs), approximately half recurred.

Although the information in the literature is limited, the various tumor markers as discussed above for AGCTs would appear to be applicable to JGCTs for the monitoring of advanced disease.

TUMORS IN THE THECOMA-FIBROMA GROUP

Considering that the ovarian stromal cell is the precursor of both fibroblasts and theca cells, pure thecomas and pure fibromas appear to represent extremes in a continuum, with a significant percentage of the tumors having admixtures of lipid-laden, steroid-secreting cells and collagen-producing spindle cells. Nonetheless, the vast majority of tumors in the thecoma-fibroma group are readily subcategorized based on relatively distinct clinical and histologic characteristics. The major subcategories include thecoma, fibroma-fibrosarcoma, and the sclerosing stromal cell tumor.

Thecoma

Theca cell tumors (TCTs), or thecomas (Fig. 27.4), are composed of lipid-laden stromal cells, occasionally demonstrating luteinization, and are almost invariably clinically benign (4,74,75). Thecomas account for approximately 1% of ovarian neoplasms and occur at a more advanced age than other sex cord–stromal tumors. The majority of patients are in their sixth and seventh decades at the time of diagnosis (4,74). Combining two large series totaling over 140 patients, less than 10% presented prior to age 30 years. Notably, the luteinized tumors are an exception to this generalization, with

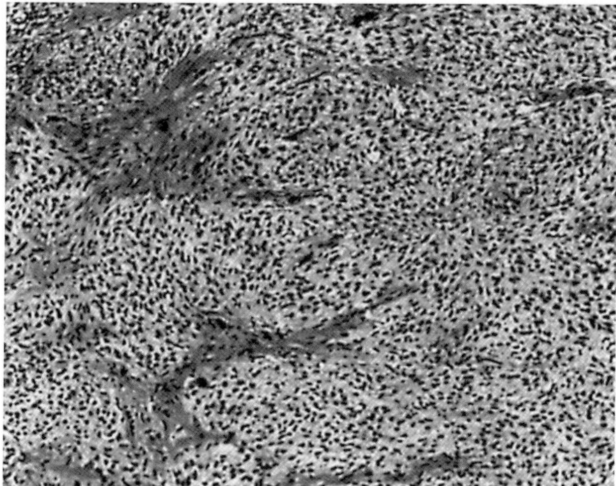

FIGURE 27.4. Thecoma. The tumor is composed of a mass of clear, vacuolated cells with round to oval nuclei intersected by bands of fibromatous tissue. *Source:* Reprinted with permission from Morris JM, Scully RE. *Endocrine Pathology of the Ovary*. St. Louis: Mosby; 1958.

30% occurring in women before their fourth decade of life (76). Assessing a compendium of nearly 300 cases, bilaterality occurs with a frequency of approximately 2% and extraovarian spread occurs rarely if at all (4,74,75,77).

The primary presenting signs and symptoms in patients with TCTs are abnormal genital bleeding and/or an abdominal/pelvic mass (74,75,77). The former urges initiation of medical intervention in the majority of postmenopausal patients, whereas an increasing abdominal girth or a palpable mass is more frequently the main presenting complaint of premenopausal patients. Lesion size has been reported to vary from <1 to 40 cm in diameter (74,75,77). Ascites is occasionally encountered.

Thecomas are considered to be among the most hormonally active of the sex cord–stromal tumors. The abnormal bleeding encountered in 60% of patients is presumably attributable to excess estrogen production (74,75). In the series reported by Evans et al. (4), endometrial hyperplasia was observed in 37% of the evaluable patients, and adenocarcinoma consistent with an unopposed estrogen effect was documented in an additional 27%. All the uterine cancers were well differentiated and minimally invasive, but two patients subsequently died of endometrial carcinoma. Other coexisting uterine pathologic findings potentially influenced by elevated circulating estrogen levels included leiomyomata, myohypertrophy, and endometrial polyps. Conversely, Zhang et al. (76) noted that nearly one half of the evaluated luteinized thecomas were either nonfunctional or androgenic, resulting in a relatively significant frequency of masculinization.

An enigmatic tumor that has been considered to be a variant of luteinized thecoma has been associated with sclerosing peritonitis (78). These tumors are often bilateral and frequently have a brisk mitotic rate, but have not been shown to have a metastatic potential. Sclerosing peritonitis has, however, been fatal owing to complications pursuant to it.

Fibroma-Fibrosarcoma

Fibromas represent the most commonly encountered sex cord–stromal tumor, accounting for approximately 4% of all ovarian neoplasms. These endocrine-inert tumors are seldom bilateral and vary in size from microscopic to extremely large masses. Although infrequently diagnosed prior to age 30 years, fibromas can occur at any age; the average age of diagnosis is the latter half of the fifth decade of life (79). These tumors become more edematous as their size increases, which is frequently accompanied by the escape of increasing quantities of fluid from the tumor surfaces. Ascites is detected in association with 10% to 15% of ovarian fibromas exceeding a diameter of 10 cm (80). Furthermore, 1% of patients develop a hydrothorax in addition to the hydroperitoneum, both resulting from excessive fluid loss from the ovarian fibroma (Meigs' syndrome) (81). Gorlin's syndrome represents an inherited predisposition to the development of ovarian fibromas along with several other abnormalities, the most frequent of which is the appearance of basal-cell nevi at an early age (82).

Although ovarian fibromas are generally considered to be benign lesions, approximately 10% will demonstrate increased cellularity and varying degrees of pleomorphorism and mitotic activity. Fibromatous tumors characterized histologically by an increased cellular density and brisk mitotic activity are designated cellular fibromas and are considered to be tumors of low malignant potential, particularly if ruptured or associated with adhesions (83). In contrast, fibrosarcomas are highly malignant neoplasms. These tumors are distinguished by their greater cellular density and, most notably, moderate to marked pleomorphorism (84).

Sclerosing Stromal Cell Tumors

Sclerosing stromal cell tumors (SSTs) were initially described by Chalvardjian and Scully (85) in 1973 as a distinct subgroup within the thecoma-fibroma family of ovarian tumors. Accounting for less than 5% of sex cord–stromal tumors, this relatively rare tumor characteristically differentiates itself histologically and clinically from both thecomas and fibromas (86,87). Histologically, the presence of pseudolobulation of cellular areas separated by edematous connective tissue, increased vascularity, and prominent areas of sclerosis are distinguishing features. Clinically, SSTs commonly become manifest during the second and third decades of life, with 80% being diagnosed prior to age 30 years, which is unique among ovarian stromal tumors (88). The signs and symptoms that most commonly necessitate medical evaluation include menstrual irregularities and/or pelvic pain (89). Despite the relatively large tumor size, which ranges from clinically undetectable to 20 cm or more in greatest diameter, ascites is seldom encountered; this further contrasts SSTs from fibromas (89). In contrast to thecomas, SSTs were originally considered to be inactive endocrinologically (85). However, a limited number of cases have been subsequently reported in which steroidogenic activity has been clinically demonstrable (89–92). To date, all SSTs have been clinically benign, and with one exception (93), all have been unilateral. Although a recent report noted an elevated CA-125 level, which the investigators speculated was perhaps nonspecific (94), no specific tumor marker has been identified for SSTs to date.

Natural History

Thecomas, fibromas, and sclerosing stromal tumors are considered to be benign ovarian neoplasms, and any associated morbidity or mortality that would be encountered would be attributed to the treatment modalities or the sequelae of concurrent disease (4,74,77,79,95). Examples of the latter are deaths from endometrial carcinoma resulting from the unopposed estrogen produced by the thecomas (4). Although several cases of "malignant thecomas" have been reported, critical reappraisal of such tumors invariably results in histologic reassignment as sarcomas or diffuse granulosa cell tumors (96). Furthermore, DNA ploidy assessment in both thecomas and fibromas not infrequently demonstrates aneuploid patterns that do not correlate with prognosis, rendering the significance of these observations questionable (97).

Prognostic Factors

The prognosis for patients diagnosed with cellular fibromas is generally considered to be quite favorable. Recurrences of these tumors of low malignant potential are generally correlated with adherent disease, rupture, or incomplete removal at the time of primary cytoreduction (83). Fibrosarcomas are associated with an extremely poor prognosis, but are fortunately rare.

SERTOLI STROMAL CELL TUMORS

Neoplasms arising in the ovary exhibiting morphologic characteristics similar to those of the testes during various stages of gonadogenesis were recognized and elegantly described by Meyer (98,99). He reasoned that the origin of these tumors was the male blastema and coined the term *arrhenoblastoma*. Considering the functional nature of these male homologs and the varying degrees of associated defeminization and/or masculinization, the term *androblastoma* was also adopted. However, Morris and Scully (100), in 1958, contended that both designations implied masculinization, which is frequently absent, and furthermore facilitated the inclusion of a variety of unrelated androgen-producing ovarian tumors. Therefore, they recommended the adoption of the morphologic designation Sertoli–Leydig cell tumor (SLCT), which also allowed a consistent nomenclature for the general classification of sex cord–stromal tumors of the ovary. The SLCTs include tumors composed of Sertoli cells only, Leydig cells only, and a combination of Sertoli and Leydig cells.

Sertoli Cell Tumors

Sertoli cell tumors are rare, accounting for less than 5% of all SLCTs (88). The average age at presentation is about 30 years, but this lesion can occur at any age. Evidence of estrogen production has been observed in approximately two thirds of the reported cases. Consistent with excess estrogen production, isosexual precocious puberty has been witnessed during the first decade of life, menstrual disorders during the reproductive decades, and postmenopausal bleeding in the decades after the climacteric. Reflecting tumor size (average 9 cm), capsular distention and/or adnexal torsion, and abdominal distention and/or pain are frequent complaints. Pelvic examination generally confirms the presence of the tumor under these circumstances. The frequency with which excessive renin production has been associated with Sertoli cells appears to exceed mere chance (101–103). Evaluation of refractory hypertension and hypokalemia has rarely eventuated in the discovery of a Sertoli cell tumor as the origin of the excess renin. An occasional Sertoli cell tumor has arisen in a patient with the Peutz-Jeghers syndrome (PJS) (104).

Pathology

On gross examination, these rare tumors are typically solid, lobulated, and yellow (88,105). Microscopic examination typically shows hollow or solid tubules lined by cells that usually have relatively bland cytologic features, but rare tumors exhibit moderate to severe nuclear atypia. In most tumors, a tubular pattern predominates, but occasionally a diffuse pattern is conspicuous.

Prognosis

The great majority of these rare tumors have been unilateral stage I lesions. The greater majority of Sertoli cell tumors are well differentiated, and only rare tumors are malignant (88). Excision of the tumor results in prompt resolution of the hyperestrogenic state. (Leydig cell tumors are discussed in the section on steroid cell tumors below.)

Sertoli–Leydig Cell Tumors

SLCTs are extremely uncommon, accounting for less than 0.2% of all ovarian tumors. As implied by their designation, the tumors contain both Sertoli and Leydig cell elements. Many of the clinical characteristics are related to the degree of histologic differentiation and the presence of a retiform pattern and/or heterologous elements (described below). The average patient age at diagnosis is approximately 25 years, with the majority (70% to 75%) of the tumors becoming clinically manifest during the second and third decades of life. Less than 10% occur either prior to menarche or after the climacterium. Patients harboring well-differentiated tumors present at an average age of 35 years, or 10 years later than patients with intermediate or poorly differentiated lesions. Conversely, tumors with retiform patterns are generally detected 10 years earlier than the intermediate and poorly differentiated tumors (106–108). Based on the compiled data from three reported series totaling over 300 patients, the frequency of extraovarian spread of disease at the time of diagnosis is approximately 2% to 3%. In addition, the likelihood of encountering bilateral tumors is even less frequent (106–108).

The most frequent complaints at the time of presentation of these generally healthy adolescents and young adults are menstrual disorders, virilization, and nonspecific symptoms resulting from an abdominal mass. Nearly one half of the patients experience sufficient abdominal pain or discomfort or note abdominal distention or palpate a mass on self-examination to prompt professional assessment. Whereas capsular distention and/or intralesional hemorrhage or necrosis of the tumor and/or adjacent visceral compression by the tumor account for the associated chronic or intermittent pain, acute abdominal pain necessitating emergency intervention invariably reflects vascular compromise from torsion. While lesion size varies according to histologic differentiation (approximately 5 cm for well-differentiated tumors to >15 cm for poorly differentiated tumors), abdominal, vaginal, and/or rectal examination readily identifies an adnexal mass in approximately 95% of symptomatic patients. The most common premonitory symptoms, namely, menstrual disorders and subtle androgenic manifestations, predate by several months, and less often, by years, the recognition of the overt clinical signs or symptoms. Irregular bleeding, oligomenorrhea, and postmenopausal bleeding, retrospectively, have been attributed to either excess androgens or estrogens. The etiology of the latter is presumably the peripheral conversion of androgens to estrogens or, rarely, from an estrogen-secreting SLCT. Frank virilization occurs in 35% of the patients with SLCTs, and another 10% to 15% have some clinical manifestations consistent with androgen excess. The most frequent androgenic symptom complex encountered includes amenorrhea, voice deepening, and hirsutism. In addition, breast atrophy, clitorimegaly, loss of female contour, and temporal hair recession, for example, are signs of masculinization witnessed in patients with SLCTs (106–108). The prevalence of androgenic manifestations appears to be independent of the degree of histologic differentiation but is observed less frequently in heterologous SLCTs and only occasionally in patients harboring retiform lesions (107,109–112). Although the preoperative diagnosis of SLCT in the absence of androgenic excess may be impossible, this neoplastic entity should constitute the primary preoperative diagnosis in patients with androgenic manifestations presenting during the second through the fourth decades of life with a unilaterally palpable adnexal mass.

Uncommonly, estrogen manifestations are witnessed in the context of presumed end-organ estrogenic responses, including postmenopausal bleeding and endometrial polyp formation, hyperplasia, and adenocarcinoma. Cautious interpretation of such observations is required, realizing that peripheral conversion of androgens to estrogens may be as plausible as a primary estrogen-secreting SLCT. As expected from the clinical findings, most patients demonstrating signs of defeminization or virilization have elevated plasma testosterone levels (106–108). Whereas plasma androstenedione may occasionally be elevated, the urinary 17-ketosteroids, including dehydroepiandrosterone, are usually normal, with the occasional patient presenting with a slightly elevated level. An elevated testosterone/androstenedione ratio generally suggests the presence of an androgen-secreting ovarian tumor, most likely an SLCT. Recognizing that certain gonadotropin-releasing hormone (GnRH) agonists modulate androgen production by down-regulating gonadotropin levels and through a direct effect on the ovary, Pascale et al. (113) demonstrated successful suppression of testosterone and androstenedione in five virilized women with the administration of GnRH agonists. Their data suggest that androgen-secreting tumors of the ovary appear to be less autonomous than such tumors originating in the adrenal gland. Surgical excision of the SLCTs results in a precipitous drop in androgen levels and, over time, partial to complete resolution of the clinical manifestations associated with androgen excess is observed.

The coexistence of other diseases with SLCTs has been chronicled. The frequency with which thyroid disease is observed in these patients appears to exceed mere chance. Furthermore, several cases of other mesenchymal tumors have occurred in patients with SLCTs, including sarcoma botryoides of the cervix as well as Ollier's disease (107,114). The latter is a rare disease, but it is associated with other sex cord–stromal tumors, specifically JGCTs, as noted above. Finally, a tendency toward familial occurrence appears to exist (107).

Pathology

Gross Features. Sertoli–Leydig cell tumors vary in size from small to huge masses, but most are between 5 and 15 cm in diameter. The majority are solid, often yellow, and lobulated (Fig. 27.5), but many are solid and cystic. Pure cystic tumors are exceptionally rare, in contrast to the situation with granulosa cell tumors. Poorly differentiated tumors tend to be larger than those more differentiated, and contain areas of hemorrhage and necrosis more frequently (107). Tumors with heterologous or retiform components are more often cystic than other tumors in this category (109,110,112,115). The heterologous tumors occasionally simulate mucinous cystic tumors on gross examination, and retiform tumors may contain large edematous intracystic papillae, resembling serous papillary tumors, or may be soft and spongy with varying degrees of cystification (112).

Microscopic Features. Well-differentiated SLCTs are characterized by a predominantly tubular pattern (116). On low-power examination, a nodular architecture is often conspicuous, with fibrous bands intersecting lobules composed of small, round, hollow, or, less often, solid tubules lined by well-differentiated cells and separated by variable numbers of Leydig cells. Rarely the tubules appear pseudoendometrioid (117).

Sertoli–Leydig cell tumors of intermediate and poor differentiation form a continuum characterized by a variety of patterns and combinations of cell types (106–108). Some tumors exhibit intermediate differentiation in some areas and poor differentiation in others, and less commonly, tumors of intermediate

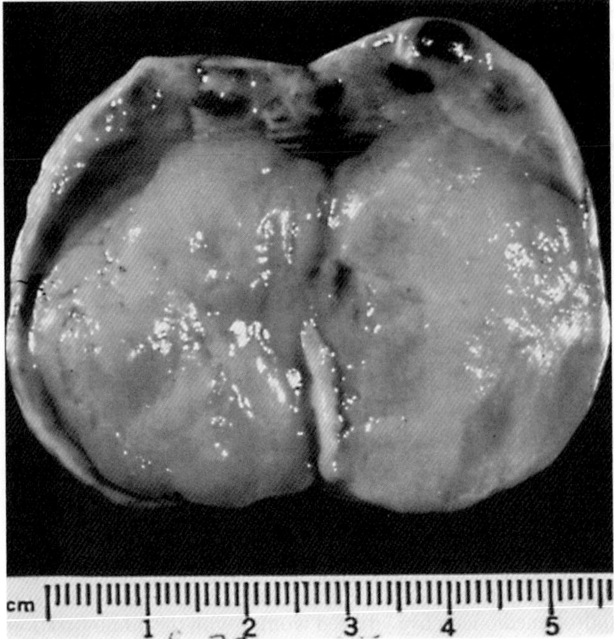

FIGURE 27.5. Sertoli–Leydig cell tumor. The sectioned surface of the tumor is focally lobulated and was yellow in the fresh state.

differentiation contain well-differentiated foci. Both the Sertoli cells and the Leydig cells may exhibit varying degrees of immaturity. In tumors of intermediate differentiation, immature Sertoli cells have small, round, oval, or angular nuclei and generally scanty cytoplasm and are arranged typically in ill-defined masses, often creating a lobulated appearance on low power; solid and hollow tubules, nests, broad columns of Sertoli cells, and, most characteristically, thin cords resembling the sex cords of the embryonic testis are often present (Fig. 27.6). These structures are separated by stroma, which ranges from fibromatous to densely cellular to edematous, and typically contains clusters of well-differentiated Leydig cells (Fig. 27.6). Cysts containing eosinophilic secretion may be present and create a thyroid-like appearance, and follicle-like spaces are encountered rarely. The Sertoli cell and Leydig cell elements, singly or in combination, may contain varying and sometimes large amounts of lipid in the form of small or large droplets. When a significant amount of the stromal component is made up of immature cellular mesenchymal tissue with high mitotic activity resembling a nonspecific sarcoma, the tumor is poorly differentiated.

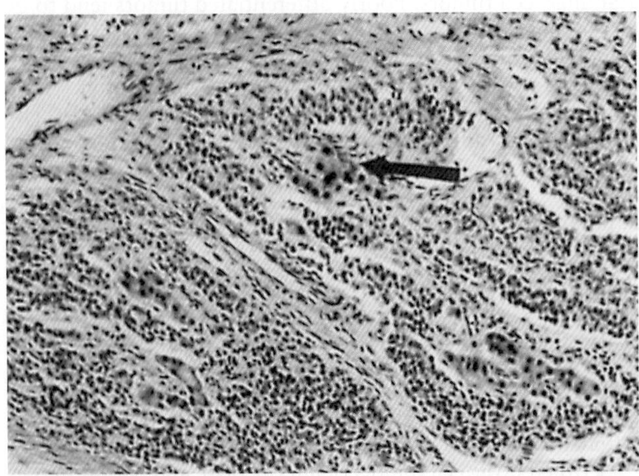

FIGURE 27.6. Sertoli–Leydig cell tumor, intermediate differentiation. Nests of large Leydig cells (*arrow*) lie among bands of immature Sertoli cells. *Source:* Reprinted with permission from Morris JM, Scully RE. *Endocrine Pathology of the Ovary*. St. Louis: Mosby; 1958.

Fifteen percent of SLCTs have a substantial retiform component, and are so designated because they are composed of a network of elongated tubules and cysts, both of which may contain papillae, resembling the rete testis (32). This pattern is usually accompanied by other patterns of SLCTs, but sometimes an entire tumor has a retiform pattern.

Heterologous elements occur in approximately 20% of Sertoli cell tumors (113,118). In a series of these tumors, 18% contain glands and cysts lined by moderately to well-differentiated intestinal-type epithelium (113). Mesenchymal heterologous elements, encountered in 5% of Sertoli cell tumors, include islands of cartilage arising on a sarcomatous background, areas of embryonal rhabdomyosarcoma, or both (118).

Natural History

SLCTs display characteristics that differ markedly from their epithelial counterparts, notably in regard to their malignant potential. Despite an average size of approximately 16 cm, only 2% to 3% of SLCTs have demonstrable extraovarian spread at the time of detection. Furthermore, Young et al. (59) identified only 29 clinically malignant cases in their series of 220 SLCTs having variable observation intervals, and they noted an 18% malignancy rate among 164 patients with adequate follow-up. At least in part, the more favorable prognosis reflects the abrupt onset of androgenic manifestations and the early detection of nonspecific symptoms, which promote prompt medical assessment. Nevertheless, the natural history of the malignant variant includes early recurrences, with approximately two thirds becoming evident within 1 year of treatment and only 6% to 7% recurring after 5 years. The abdominal cavity (including the pelvis) and the retroperitoneal nodes are the most frequent sites for recurrences. In addition, the contralateral ovary, lungs, liver, and bone are other reported sites of recurrent metastatic disease. The collective salvage rates in patients with clinically malignant disease are low, with extrapolated estimates being less than 20%.

Prognostic Factors

Stage is the most important predictor of outcome in SLCTs. Fortunately, 97% of SLCTs are reportedly stage I at diagnosis, and less than 20% of these localized tumors become clinically malignant. The most cogent phenotypic prognostic determinant for stage I SLCTs is the degree of histologic differentiation (106–108). Approximately one half of the reported SLCTs are of intermediate differentiation, 10% are well differentiated, 20% are heterologous, and the remainder are poorly differentiated. No extraovarian spread or subsequent recurrences were encountered by Young and Scully (116) among 23 well-differentiated SLCTs. However, approximately 10% of intermediate and 60% of poorly differentiated tumors as well as 20% of heterologous tumors demonstrated clinically malignant behavior (107). The heterologous tumors contain either endodermal elements such as gastrointestinal epithelium and carcinoids or mesenchymal elements including skeletal muscles and/or cartilage. The endodermal elements are typically associated with intermediately differentiated homologous elements and represent 75% of the heterologous SLCTs. Their corresponding prognosis parallels that of the intermediately differentiated homologous tumors. In contrast, heterologous tumors containing mesenchymal elements account for 5% of all SLCTs and invariably coexist with a poorly differentiated homologous component. The clinically aggressive malignant behavior of poorly differentiated heterologous tumors is witnessed in the extremely low survival (107).

Retiform patterns, tumor size, mitotic activity, and tumor rupture appear to increase in frequency as the degree of tumor differentiation decreases (106–108). Approximately 10% of neoplasms express histologic patterns resembling the rete testis. They are more commonly observed in younger patients (average age 15 years) and are generally larger, possibly secondary to the less frequent association of androgenic manifestations and hence a later clinical presentation (109–112). Sertoli–Leydig cell tumors harboring a retiform pattern are associated with a 20% malignancy rate, significantly higher than the 12% nonretiform SLCT rate. Young and Scully (112) noted that 14 of 25 retiform cases were of intermediate differentiation, with 1 demonstrating poorly differentiated homologous histology and 10 exhibiting heterologous elements (3 intermediate and 7 poorly differentiated). Arguably, the less favorable prognosis reflects the frequency of associated heterologous and/or poorly differentiated homologous lesions. This concept is supported by the findings that the majority of the metastatic lesions do not contain retiform patterns (112). However, the adverse characteristics of the retiform component are witnessed when examining tumors of intermediate differentiation. Although only 4 of over 100 reported intermediately differentiated SLCTs were clinically malignant, 3 of the 4 contained retiform patterns (107).

Tumor size, mitotic activity, and tumor rupture have been reported to influence prognosis (106,107). The size, mitotic index, and rupture frequency appear to increase as histologic dedifferentiation increases. Notwithstanding these associations, substratification of intermediate and poorly differentiated lesions according to these parameters identifies significant prognostic differences.

The frequency of androgen excess has been addressed above, with 50% or more of patients diagnosed with SLCTs either directly or indirectly displaying clinical manifestations of hyperandrogenism. Serum testosterone levels are invariably elevated when virilization is present, and selective venous catheterization has documented the ovary as the site of origin (119,120). In addition, immunostaining was positive for testosterone in eight SLCTs analyzed, including a limited number of tumors from patients without clinical signs or symptoms of androgen excess (2,121). The Leydig cells, as anticipated, were shown to be the cell of origin for the synthesis of testosterone. Following cytoreductive surgery, the serum testosterone levels are rapidly cleared from the circulation and have been reported on occasion to increase again as a function of the burden of recurrent metastatic disease.

Other unique secretory products, namely, inhibin and alpha fetoprotein (AFP), have been reported in a limited number of SLCTs and are proteins generally equated with GCTs and germ cell tumors, respectively (110,112,120–122). In addition to GCTs, the Sertoli and Leydig cells have been shown to produce inhibin in testicular tissues, and presumably these same cell types are the site of origin in the SLCTs. Motoyama et al. (122) summarized the literature and reported the 14th case of an elevated serum AFP accompanying SLCTs. A clinically malignant course was appreciated in 43% of the described population, which had a mean age of 16 years. In addition, the majority (57%) was described as having a retiform component, a frequency substantially higher than the 10% usually seen in larger SLCT samples. Perhaps preferential AFP sampling accounts for a portion of this seemingly unusually high frequency in that, histologically, the retiform pattern may be confused with an endodermal sinus tumor, particularly in the absence of clinical androgenic manifestations. The Sertoli and Leydig cells appear to be the cells of origin for AFP within the tumor. Employing immunostaining, Gagnon et al. (121) confirmed that Leydig cells appear to be the predominant site for AFP synthesis, but Sertoli cells are also capable of producing this oncoprotein. Testing four retiform and four nonretiform SLCTs, they demonstrated a 50% positivity rate in both histologic subtypes. The precise frequency of both inhibin and AFP positivity and their correlation with disease activity await larger confirmatory assessments.

OVARIAN SEX CORD TUMOR WITH ANNULAR TUBULES

In 1970, Scully (66) described a limited series of unique ovarian tumors characterized by either simple or complex ring-shaped tubules and proposed the morphologic designation ovarian sex cord tumor with annular tubules (SCTATs). The distinctive cellular elements of these neoplasms were judged to be histologically representative of an intermediate between Sertoli cell and granulosa cell tumors. Shen et al. (123) reported that SCTATs accounted for 6% of the sex cord tumors treated at their institution. An association with PJS was likewise recognized, and in a subsequent report of 74 cases of SCTAT, Young et al. (124) noted that approximately one in three SCTATs occurred in patients with PJS. Ovarian sex cord tumors with annular tubules occurring in association with PJS are typically small (many microscopic), multifocal, calcified, and bilateral. The average age of presentation is the early to mid portion of the fourth decade of life (124,125). The non-PJS tumors are considerably larger, seldom multifocal or calcified, and invariably unilateral. The average age of these patients is the mid to latter portion of the third decade of life.

Abnormal vaginal bleeding is the most common presenting complaint, including menstrual irregularities during the reproductive era and postmenopausal bleeding during the mature years. Menometrorrhagia followed by prolonged episodes of amenorrhea is commonly experienced in the non-PJS patients. Abdominal pain or discomfort is less frequently encountered but generally accompanies grossly involved adnexa or other incidental pelvic pathology. In addition, the signs and symptoms accompanying intussusception secondary to colonic polyp formation may be manifested in PJS-associated patients. The majority of PJS-associated SCTATs are not detectable via clinical examination and are appreciated unexpectedly during surgical or pathologic assessment. In contrast, the majority of non-PJS SCTATs are palpable on abdominal and/or vaginal examination. Although these tumors are seldom encountered during the first decade of life, isosexual precocity is invariably witnessed when SCTATs are diagnosed in affected children (124–127).

Considering the rarity of both PJS, an autosomal dominant disorder, and SCTAT, the frequency of concurrency of these two processes suggests a potential linkage in their pathogenesis. Approximately 36% of SCTATs are observed in patients with PJS. In addition, 15% of PJS-associated SCTATs also develop adenoma malignum of the cervix, a neoplasm that defies early diagnosis and is associated with a relatively high mortality rate (124,128–130). A recent report of 34 patients with PJS demonstrated a significantly elevated risk (relative risk = 20.3) of breast and gynecologic malignancies in women (131); 1 patient had a Sertoli–Leydig tumor and 3 had sex cord tumors with annular tubules. The PJS gene was mapped to chromosome 19p13.3 (132) and was later identified as a novel serine threonine kinase, STK11 (133). Because of the wide variety of malignancies occurring in individuals with PJS, STK11 is believed to function as a general tumor-suppressor gene.

Contingent on the patient's age, precocious puberty, menstrual irregularities, or postmenopausal bleeding are clinical manifestations of SCTATs, indirectly attesting to their endocrine activity (124–128,130,134,135). These signs of hyperestrogenism and the corresponding effects on the endometrium were readily recognized in the initial description of these unique tumors (58). Numerous reports have confirmed the presence of endometrial hyperplasia and/or polyp formation, particularly in PJS-associated SCTATs. Although similar signs in endometrial histology can be observed in non-PJS SCTATs, clinical histories of menorrhagia followed by episodes of amenorrhea are more frequently obtained (123–126,134,135). Endometrial sampling in a limited population of such patients has demonstrated a spectrum from atrophic glandular to secretory or decidualized endometrium suggestive of significant levels of progesterone production (123,125,135). Assessment of circulating steroid levels has confirmed the presence of excessive estrogen in essentially all SCTAT cases (123,134–136). However, normal progesterone levels have been observed in PJS-associated tumors, but elevated quantities of progesterone have been documented in non-PJS patients (123,134–136). Shen et al. (123) demonstrated elevated estrogen and progesterone levels (and normal testosterone levels) in two SCTAT patients without PJS having documented glandular atrophy and decidual stromal changes. Utilizing selective ovarian venous sampling, Crain (135) demonstrated a significant progesterone gradient between peripheral and ovarian venous serum in a non-PJS patient with pseudodecidual changes of the endometrium. Complete resolution of the manifestations attributed to these hormonal imbalances has been routinely witnessed with surgical extirpation of the ovarian neoplasm.

Pathology

Grossly, the PJS-associated tumors are solid and yellow. The non–PJS-associated neoplasms may be similar, but in some cases, they are solid and cystic or mostly cystic. This tumor is characterized microscopically by the presence of simple and complex annular tubules (Fig. 27.7). The simple tubules have the shape of a ring, with the nuclei oriented around the periphery and around a central hyalinized body composed of basement membrane material; an intervening anuclear cytoplasmic zone forms the major component of the ring. The more numerous complex tubules are rounded structures made up of intercommunicating rings revolving around multiple hyaline bodies. In patients with PJS, the tumors are typically multifocal and exhibit calcification.

Prognostic Factors

Notwithstanding their histologic similarities, the differences in the natural history and hence long-term prognosis for SCTATs associated with PJS and SCTATs independent of PJS are readily apparent. Those detected in women with PJS are benign. Important in the management of this entity, however, is the recognition that approximately 15% of these patients will harbor an adenoma malignum of the cervix (AMC). As a result of delayed declaration of symptoms, the diagnosis of AMC is frequently made following examination of the hysterectomy specimen. As evident in the recent review by Srivatsa et al. (130), the prognosis for PJS patients with SCTAT and AMC is ominous, reflecting high AMC recurrence rates and refractoriness to treatment.

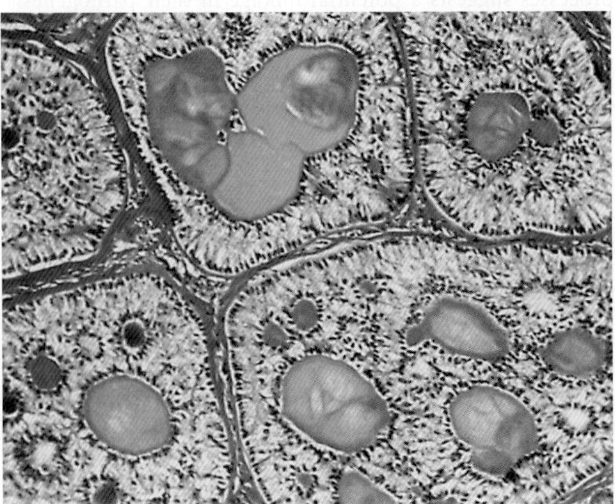

FIGURE 27.7. Sex cord tumor with annular tubules. Numerous rounded tubules encircle multiple hyaline bodies.

Based on the compiled data from four reported series totaling 63 patients with SCTATs without clinically apparent PJS, the clinical malignancy rate approximated 20% (123–126). Primary extraovarian extension and/or the recurrence frequency has been correlated with the original tumor size and mitotic activity. The tumor characteristically has a relatively long doubling time, a propensity for lymphatic dissemination, and an aptness to remain lateralized. As the primary ovarian lesion is invariably unilateral, the lymphatic metastases are invariably ipsilateral, extending within the confines from the paraaortic region to the supraclavicular area. The nature of the retroperitoneal metastases generally facilitates surgical resection and repeat cytoreduction. The tumor's indolent growth pattern, coupled with the relative ease of resection, affords patients extended palliation.

Because SCTATs possess characteristics of both granulosa cells and Sertoli cells, tumor markers elicited by either or both cell types might find utility in the diagnosis and surveillance of these tumors as well. The observed increased serum estrogen levels and the corresponding clinical manifestations recognized with SCTATs suggest utility in monitoring hormone levels. Unfortunately, serum estradiol lacks adequate sensitivity, particularly when the residual tumor volume is limited. However, recent reports demonstrate the potential value and sensitivity of two unique secretory proteins as tumor markers for SCTATs. Gustafson et al. (136) illustrated the applicability of monitoring serum inhibin and müllerian-inhibiting substance (MIS) in the management of a patient with advanced, recurrent SCTAT. More recently, Puls et al. (137) likewise reported an excellent correlation between serum inhibin and MIS levels and the clinical status of a patient with SCTAT during chemotherapy administration. The ultimate utility of these tumor markers awaits accrual of sufficient numbers of patients with SCTATs to address adequately sensitivity and specificity issues.

SEX CORD–STROMAL TUMORS, UNCLASSIFIED

This ill-defined group of tumors, which accounts for less than 10% of those in the sex cord–stromal category, comprises those in which a predominant pattern of testicular or ovarian differentiation is not clearly recognizable. Talerman et al. (138) have recently segregated from within this category a group of tumors for which they have proposed the designation "diffuse nonlobular androblastoma." The six ovarian tumors they reported were mostly estrogenic and had a predominant diffuse proliferation of cells resembling theca cells, granulosa cells, or both, but five of the six cases also contained steroid-type cells and tubules typical of Sertoli cell neoplasia.

Sex cord–stromal tumors may be particularly difficult to subclassify when they occur in pregnant patients because of alterations in their usual clinical and pathologic features (139). Their nature is rarely suggested clinically because during pregnancy estrogenic manifestations are not recognizable, and androgenic manifestations are rare. In one study, 17% of 36 SCSTs that were removed during pregnancy were placed in the unclassified group, and many of those that were classified in the granulosa cell or Sertoli–Leydig cell category had large areas with an indifferent appearance (139).

Gynandroblastoma

Gynandroblastoma is an extremely rare SCST if strict morphologic criteria are followed to establish the diagnosis. Microscopically, these tumors must demonstrate readily identifiable (at least 10%) granulosa cells and tubules of Sertoli cells. Not surprisingly, the corresponding stromal cells, namely, theca and/or Leydig cells, may also be present in varying degrees. Martin-Jimenez et al. (140) recently reviewed the world literature and were able to identify only 17 authenticated cases of gynandroblastoma. Patients presented at an average age of 29.5 years (range 16 to 65 years) with primary symptoms of menstrual disturbances consistent with the predominant functional status of the tumor. Commonly, a hyperandrogenic clinical profile is elicited, but signs and symptoms of excessive estrogens or no endocrine manifestations can be encountered. Amenorrhea, hirsutism, and clitorimegaly are frequently noted in association with elevated testosterone levels. Conversely, the common end-organ responses to hyperestrogenism include menometrorrhagia, postmenopausal bleeding, and endometrial hyperplasia. Although the unilateral masses are typically small, 75% are palpable prior to surgical exploration and are characterized by well-differentiated ovarian and testicular constituent elements. Regardless of the associated hormonal activity, gynandroblastomas are considered to be tumors of low malignant potential. To date, only a single case was reported to have been clinically malignant and resulted in death of the patient (141). Recently, a gynandroblastoma in pregnancy was reported (142).

Steroid Cell Tumors

Steroid cell tumors (SCTs) constitute only 0.1% of all ovarian neoplasms. The predominant components of these tumors are steroid hormone–secreting cells including lutein cells, Leydig cells, and adrenocortical cells. Until recently, the term *lipid cell tumors* was applied to these neoplasms, but Hayes and Scully (143) noted that 25% of such designated tumors did not contain appreciable intracellular fat. Hence, the functional designation steroid cell tumors was suggested and stratified into three subclasses: stromal luteoma, Leydig cell tumor, and steroid cell tumors not otherwise specified. The first two categories are essentially invariably benign, but some in the third group are malignant.

Stromal Luteoma

In 1964, Scully et al. (144) described the stromal luteoma as a distinctive type of steroid cell tumor. These relatively small (<3 cm) tumors are localized within the parenchyma of the ovary and account for approximately 25% of SCTs. They are thought to arise from luteinized stromal cells or their precursors. Histologically, the adjacent ovarian matrix as well as the contralateral ovary demonstrate stromal hyperthecosis in the vast majority of cases. The distinction between nodular hyperthecosis and stromal luteomas has been arbitrarily based on size, with lesions <5 mm being referred to as nodular hyperthecosis. In contrast to stromal hyperthecosis, stromal luteomas are rarely bilateral.

The average age at which stromal luteomas are diagnosed is the latter half of the sixth decade of life, with 80% occurring after the climacterium (143). Considering that the predominant functional profile is estrogenic, the result of either direct tumor secretion or peripheral conversion of androgens, it is not surprising that abnormal vaginal bleeding is the primary complaint. In a series of 25 cases reported by Hayes and Scully (143), information regarding the histologic architecture of the endometrium was known for 17 cases, which included 14 cases of hyperplasia and a single case of a well-differentiated adenocarcinoma of the endometrium. Conversely, 12% of the patients presented with clinical manifestations of hyperandrogenism. In their analysis, 20% of the tumors were functionally quiescent and were detected incidentally during histologic assessment of surgical specimens processed for a variety of other indications.

Prognostic Factors. Considering the small size and lack of atypical histology, the posttreatment course is benign. To date, we are unaware of a single adverse outcome. Any untoward sequelae related to the stromal luteoma would presumably reflect secondary events from prolonged excessive hormone secretions such as an endometrial carcinoma.

Leydig Cell Tumors

Leydig cell tumors account for only 15% to 20% of SCTs. Histologically, the cellular elements are indistinguishable from lutein cells or adrenocortical cells except for the presence of crystals of Reinke, a requirement based on either light or electron microscopy for definitive diagnosis. Roth and Sternberg (145) subdivided these tumors according to location and possibly the cell of origin, namely, Leydig cell tumors of hilar type versus nonhilar type. Whereas the latter presumably arise from ovarian stromal cells and are extremely rare, the former tumors are located in the hilus of the ovary and encroach on or extend into the ovarian stroma in varying degrees. Other tumors containing features of Leydig cell tumors (such as location in the ovarian hilus or adjacent to nonmedullated nerve fibers, location within a continuum of hilar cell hyperplasia, fibrinoid vascular changes in the tumor, clustering of cells around vessels) but lacking crystals of Reinke are preferably categorized as steroid cell tumors not otherwise specified (146). By combining two reviews (146,147) that summarize the English-language literature prior to and after 1966, 38 Reinke-positive cases affording adequate abstraction were identified. These invariably unilateral tumors are typically small, ranging in size from 0.7 to 15 cm, with a mean of 2.7 cm, and are therefore frequently not detectable via clinical examination or pelvic imaging. Similar to stromal luteomas, the age of diagnosis is 58 years (range, 37 to 86 years), with only a small percentage occurring prior to the climacterium. The initial clinical manifestations are usually consistent with a hyperandrogenic state. Overt signs of virilization are observed in greater than 80% of the patients. These include one or more of the following: hirsutism, acne, deepening of the voice, breast atrophy, clitorimegaly, and male-pattern baldness. In contrast to the frequently dramatic onset and progression of virilization witnessed with SLCTs, ovarian Leydig cell tumors are generally characterized by a more indolent course. Paraskevas and Scully (146) reported an interval of 7 years between recognized onset of signs and symptoms of androgen excess and diagnosis. Analysis of serum androgens demonstrated testosterone to be consistently elevated while urinary 17-ketosteroids were normal or marginally increased. These observations suggest minimal production of androstenedione or dehydroepiandrosterone by these tumors.

Conversely, estrogenic manifestations are occasionally witnessed, such as irregular menses or postmenopausal bleeding (146,147). Pathologic assessment of the uterus may reveal endometrial hyperplasia, polyp formation, and/or carcinoma in the presence or absence of leiomyomata and/or myohypertrophy. Whether the hyperestrogenic features are a result of tumor secretion of estrogens or peripheral conversion of androgens to estrogens remains to be ascertained.

Prognostic Factors. In a review of the English literature through 1988, 38 Reinke-positive cases were accrued and only a single case of a clinically malignant lesion was identified (146,147). Based on tumor size (15 cm) alone, this sole example might be considered to be an outlier. Hence, similar to stromal luteomas, ovarian Leydig cell tumors are essentially benign neoplasms with the primary postsurgical concerns consisting of regression of the androgen-induced alterations.

Generally speaking, significant regression is witnessed, but significant residual sequelae are appreciated in approximately one half of the patients.

Steroid Cell Tumors Not Otherwise Specified

Neoplasms identified as steroid cell tumors but lacking the specific characteristics of stromal luteomas or Leydig cell tumors are collectively classified as steroid cell tumors not otherwise specified (SCTNOS). These tumors constitute the majority of steroid cell tumors and undoubtedly include both Leydig cell tumors and stromal luteomas that fail to meet specific identification criteria already noted. Although serving as a catchment for an undefined percentage of steroid hormone–secreting tumors, as a group, the SCTNOS have nonetheless unique characteristics. The natural history and biology of these tumors are significantly different when compared to Leydig cell tumors or stromal luteomas.

Although the average age at presentation of patients harboring SCTNOS is 43 years (10 to 15 years earlier than stromal luteomas and/or Leydig cell tumors), these tumors have been diagnosed from early childhood to the ninth decade of life (148). In addition, these generally solid yellow tumors are larger than the other SCTs. The average size at diagnosis approximates 8.5 cm (range, 1.2 to 45.0 cm). Furthermore, a higher frequency of bilaterality (5%) in advanced disease is encountered with these neoplasms. In their review of 63 collated cases, Hayes and Scully (148) reported that 81% of cases had localized disease (stage I), 6% had stage II disease, and 13% had stage III or IV disease. Curiously, they noted the average age (54 years) of patients with advanced disease was 10 years older than the group as a whole. At least in part, these findings reflect the absence of documented advanced malignancies during the first two decades of life.

Clinical signs and/or symptoms of androgen excess ranging from heterosexual precocity in prepubertal girls to amenorrhea, hirsutism, and/or virilization during the reproductive and/or postmenopausal ages prompt the majority of patients to seek medical advice (148,149). Not infrequently, the duration of these androgenic changes may have extended over many years (150). Additional concerns at presentation include increasing abdominal girth reflecting tumor size and, rarely, ascites, abdominal pain, cushingoid symptoms, and irregular uterine bleeding. The latter may represent clinical manifestations of estrogen excess (148,151), which has been suggested to occur at a frequency of 6% to 23%. Whether the source of estrogen is *de novo* synthesis by the tumor or from peripheral conversion of androgens remains to be determined. Isosexual precocious pseudopuberty has been detected in young girls harboring SCTNOS (148,152,153). An additional 10% to 15% of patients are asymptomatic, with tumors being detected incidentally during routine pelvic examination or at the time of hysterectomy or other surgical interventions.

The steroid hormone–secreting capacities of SCTNOS are more diverse than those of most sex cord–stromal tumors. Whereas approximately one in four patients does not demonstrate clinical manifestations of hormonal imbalances, the majority of patients with SCTNOS have evidence of androgen excess (10% to 15% estrogen excess) and a lesser percentage of cortisol excess. These excesses are demonstrable via assessment of end-organ responses and serum/plasma steroid levels. Whereas elevated plasma levels of corticosteroids are typically observed in conjunction with SCTNOS, the number of overt presentations with Cushing's syndrome is limited (152,154–156). However, 17% of the clinically malignant tumors reported by Hayes and Scully (148) were associated with Cushing's syndrome. The serum testosterone and androstenedione levels are invariably elevated, as are urinary 17-ketosteroids; presumably, the latter reflect the level of excess androstenedione production.

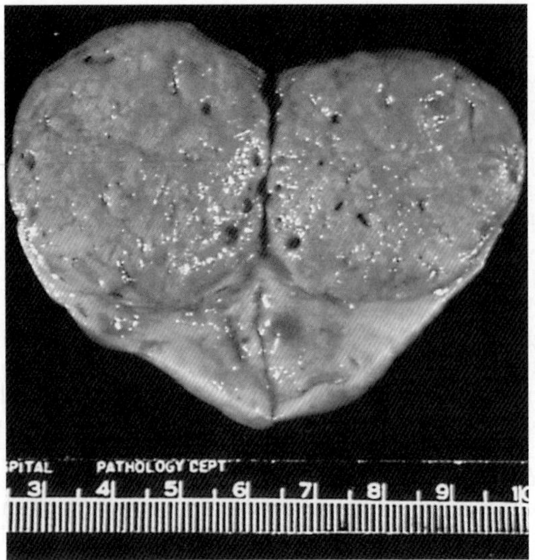

FIGURE 27.8. Steroid cell tumor, unclassified. The sectioned surface of the tumor is lobulated and was yellow-orange in the fresh state. This tumor was from a 9-year-old virilized girl.

Pathology.

Gross Features. The tumors are typically solid, well circumscribed, occasionally lobulated (Fig. 27.8), and average 8.4 cm in diameter (148). Approximately 5% are bilateral. They are typically yellow or orange but are occasionally red, dark brown, or black. Necrosis, hemorrhage, and cystic degeneration are occasionally observed.

Microscopic Features. On microscopic examination, the tumor cells are typically arranged diffusely but occasionally grow in nests, irregular clusters, thin cords, and columns. The polygonal to rounded tumor cells have distinct cell borders, central nuclei, and moderate to abundant amounts of cytoplasm that varies from eosinophilic and granular to vacuolated and spongy (Fig. 27.9). In approximately 60% of the cases, nuclear atypia is absent or minimal and mitotic activity is low (less than two mitotic figures [MFs] per 10 HPFs). In the remaining cases, grades 1 to 3 nuclear atypia (Fig. 27.3) is present, usually associated with an increase in mitotic activity (up to 15 MFs per 10 HPFs).

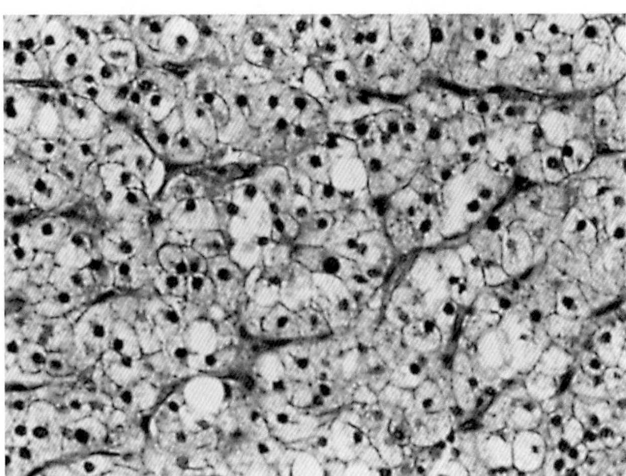

FIGURE 27.9. Steroid cell tumor. The tumor cells are large and rounded and laden with lipid vacuoles. *Source:* Reprinted with permission from Hayes MC, Scully RE. Ovarian steroid cell tumors not otherwise specified [lipid cell tumors]: a clinicopathologic analysis of 63 cases. *Am J Surg Pathol* 1987;11:835–845.

Prognosis. In contrast to the benign natural history of both ovarian Leydig cell tumors and stromal luteomas, SCTNOS are associated with a relatively high rate of clinical malignancy. In the largest series in the literature, 43% of patients with follow-up of 3 or more years demonstrated extraovarian disease either at primary surgery or during subsequent follow-up (157). Unfortunately, to date, salvage therapy has been abysmal. Multiple factors appear to correlate with the frequency of disseminated disease including age, stage, tumor size, mitotic activity, tumor necrosis, hemorrhage, and symptoms of Cushing's syndrome. The average age of patients with clinical malignancies was 16 years older than patients without metastatic disease and having had 3 or more years of observation. No clinically malignant cases have been reported to date in patients less than 20 years of age. All malignant SCTNOS were reported to measure 7 cm or more in greatest diameter (148). In fact, 78% of all tumors 7 cm or larger were malignant, whereas only 21% of all benign tumors exceeded this dimension. The most cogent determinant correlating with malignant potential was mitotic activity, with 92% of malignant tumors displaying two or more MFs per 10 HPFs. Similarly, in the presence of necrosis, 86% were malignant; if hemorrhage was present, 77% were malignant. In addition, three of four patients (17% of all malignant cases) with recognizable Cushing's syndrome harbored clinically malignant disease (148).

Although the majority of recurrences become clinically manifest within 3 years of diagnosis, Hayes and Scully (148) reported that 22% of recurrences occurred after 3 years and that, in fact, all of these cases occurred after 5 years; the longest interval witnessed was 19 years. Therefore, the duration of posttreatment surveillance should be adjusted accordingly. The only currently available utilizable markers for SCTNOS include the steroid hormones that were elevated prior to definitive treatment.

TREATMENT

The definitive management of sex cord–stromal tumors is dependent on one or more of the following therapeutic determinants: surgical stage, histologic subtype, patient's age and desire for fertility preservation, and various prognostic factors. Surgery alone is sufficient for several SCSTs lacking malignant potential, whereas postoperative adjunctive therapy generally should be considered for patients with advanced disease and Sertoli–Leydig cell tumors with poor differentiation or heterologous elements (158).

Operative Management

Surgery remains the cornerstone of treatment for patients with SCSTs. Definitive therapy for SCSTs commences with an abdominal exploration through an adequate vertical midline incision. Following securing of peritoneal washings for cytologic assessment, inspection and palpation of the viscera are conducted to detect macroscopic disease. Fertility-sparing surgery with unilateral salpingo-oophorectomy seems to be appropriate management for patients with stage IA disease who are desirous of retaining their reproductive potential. In a review of the 1988 to 2001 SEER database, Zhang et al. identified 376 patients with ovarian SCST (159). The survival for the group of 110 patients with stage I-II disease who underwent conservative surgery without hysterectomy was similar to that of patients who underwent standard surgery. For older patients or those with advanced-stage disease or bilateral ovarian involvement, abdominal hysterectomy and bilateral salpingo-oophorectomy are usually indicated. Frozen section examination of the ovarian tumor should be performed to confirm the diagnosis of a sex cord–stromal tumor. Resection of the ovarian tumor will constitute sufficient therapy for the essentially benign neoplasms, including thecomas; fibromas; gynandroblastomas; stromal luteomas; and Leydig cell, sclerosing stromal, Sertoli cell, and well-differentiated SLCTs. Furthermore, sex cord tumors with annular tubules associated with PJS are also considered to be benign and can be similarly managed, but it is imperative that the endocervix be evaluated and subsequently monitored for the potential development of an adenoma malignum of the cervix. Conversely, histologic confirmation of granulosa cell tumors, intermediate or poorly differentiated Sertoli–Leydig cell tumors, sex cord–stromal tumors with annular tubules (independent of PJS), and steroid cell tumors not otherwise specified will require definitive surgical staging. This includes multiple biopsies from high-yield sites, omentectomy, and pelvic and para-aortic lymph node sampling/dissection, although the benefit of comprehensive staging in those tumors has not been established. However, recent evidence from a retrospective review of the Memorial Sloan-Kettering Cancer Center experience calls into question the necessity of performing a retroperitoneal lymphadenectomy in the absence of any grossly suspicious lymph nodes (160). Of 68 patients with granulosa cell tumors, 16 (24%) underwent a pelvic lymph node sampling, and 13 (19%) also had a para-aortic lymph node sampling at primary surgery or re-staging surgery. All lymph nodes in these cases were negative for metastatic tumor. In addition, of 34 patients with recurrent granulosa cell tumors, 2 recurred in the retroperitoneum only; 2 in the pelvis and retroperitoneum; and 1 in the pelvis, abdomen, and retroperitoneum. Overall, approximately 15% of first recurrences appeared to involve the retroperitoneum.

Following careful surgical staging and in the absence of extraovarian disease, conservation of the uterus and contralateral ovary is reasonable in patients wishing preservation of fertility. However, when electing conservative, fertility-sparing treatment, a thorough curettage must be performed in all patients with estrogen-producing tumors whether they are considered to be benign or potentially malignant (4). If fertility is not an issue or if extraovarian spread of disease is documented, a hysterectomy and residual salpingo-oophorectomy should be performed. Although no scientific evidence exists pertaining to the efficacy of cytoreduction in SCSTs, based on the benefits observed with their epithelial counterparts, we endorse an aggressive maximum effort at primary surgery if metastatic disease is encountered. The value of secondary tumor reduction continues to be controversial but appears to be meritorious in the more indolent tumor types such as GCTs and SCTATs (those not associated with PJS). Repeat cytoreduction frequently affords these patients extended palliation. It is therefore mandatory that the surgeon have adequate familiarity with the natural history of the various SCSTs and the technical expertise to facilitate optimal surgical management.

Postoperative Management and Management of Recurrent Disease

Granulosa Cell Tumors (Adult)

The vast majority of women with stage I disease have an excellent prognosis after surgery alone and do not require adjuvant therapy. For those with stage IC disease, consideration can be given to adjuvant therapy on an individualized basis. Most women presenting with stages II to IV disease would be advised to have postoperative therapy depending on their individual characteristics.

Whereas some investigators have reported improved outcomes in patients treated with adjuvant radiation therapy, other investigators have found no clear value to the use of adjuvant radiation therapy (4,6,16,161). Because of the rarity of granulosa cell tumor, it is difficult to conduct prospective trials in these patients. Two retrospective reports provide some data on the use of radiotherapy. Savage et al. reviewed the courses of 62 women treated for adult GCTs at the Royal Marsden Hospital from 1969 to 1995 (162). Thirty-eight (61%) had stage I disease. Eleven of the stage I patients had adjuvant pelvic radiation. The 10-year disease-free survival of these patients was 77% versus 78% for stage I patients treated with surgery alone. Unfortunately, neither complete surgical staging information nor the features that led to the selection of patients for adjuvant radiation was provided. For eight patients with inoperable disease (or residual disease postoperatively), radiation resulted in complete responses in four (50%) that lasted 16 months to 5 years.

Wolf et al. reported on 34 patients with GCTs treated with radiation at the M. D. Anderson Cancer Center, 14 of whom had measurable disease (161). Six of the 14 (43%) had a clinical complete response. Three of the responders were alive without evidence of disease 10 to 21 years after radiation.

The Gynecologic Oncology Group (GOG) has reported the largest series of women with ovarian SCSTs treated with chemotherapy. They used four cycles of cisplatin, bleomycin, and etoposide (BEP) (163). Eligible patients had incompletely resected stage II to IV or recurrent disease. Seventy-five patients entered but 18 were ineligible because of incorrect histology or disease status. Of the 57 eligible patients, 41 had recurrent disease and 16 had primary disease. Thirty-nine had gross residual disease following surgery. Forty-eight had GCTs, seven had SLCTs, one had a malignant thecoma, and one had an unclassified SCST. This chemotherapy combination was considered to be active, with 11 of 16 primary-disease patients and 21 of 41 recurrent-disease patients remaining progression free at a median follow-up of 3 years. Recognizing the prolonged natural history of these tumors, longer follow-up of this cohort will be important. The regimen was fairly toxic, with two bleomycin-related fatalities among the first six patients treated with the initial bleomycin dose of 20 U/m^2 (maximum 30 U) weekly for 9 weeks. The bleomycin dose was then reduced (20 U/m^2 every 3 weeks × four cycles) with no mention of further toxicity. Grade 4 myelotoxicity occurred in 61% of the patients. The value of bleomycin in the treatment of this tumor type remains in question (164).

Gershenson et al. (165) also reported on the use of BEP in a group of nine women with poor-prognosis SCSTs of the ovary (seven had metastatic disease). The median progression-free survival was 14 months, with a median survival time of 28 months. These investigators, in the same publication, describe activity with paclitaxel in patients with granulose cell tumors who have failed platinum-based therapies. In an earlier series, Gershenson et al. (157) found that cisplatin, doxorubicin, and cyclophosphamide were shown to have activity in the treatment of metastatic ovarian stromal tumors, including two Sertoli–Leydig cell tumors. The overall response rate was 63% in this series.

The management of patients with recurrent disease must be individualized. Given the characteristic indolent growth pattern of GCTs, with long disease-free intervals, surgical resection of disease recurrence is often the initial step in the management of appropriate patients. Pecorelli et al. treated 38 patients with advanced (n = 7) or recurrent (n = 31) GCTs with cisplatin, vinblastine, and bleomycin (PVB) on a prospective trial through the European Organization for Research and Treatment of Cancer (EORTC) (166). Of the seven women who presented with advanced disease (stages II to IV), one was alive and disease-free at 81 months. Five died between 4 and 12 months after the start of PVB, and another was alive with disease at 2 months. Among the 31 women with recurrent disease, 7 were alive without further evidence of disease from 24 to 81 months from the start of PVB. Consistent with the indolent course observed with GCTs in some women, another 11 women were alive with disease at a mean of 45 months from the start of PVB (median 39 months).

The wisdom of using a germ cell–like regimen for stromal tumors is questionable. Uygun et al. reported on a small series of 11 women with recurrent GCTs (167). Most had cyclophoshamide, Adriamycin (doxorubicin), and cisplatin (CAP) in the adjuvant setting. Four were treated with cyclophosphamide and cisplatin for recurrence and survived 35 to 73 months after recurrence.

Recently, there has been increasing interest in the use of taxanes in SCSTs. A case report documented a dramatic response to paclitaxel in a patient with a GCT 2 years following cessation of platinum-based therapy (168). Subsequently, Brown et al. reported a retrospective review of the M. D. Anderson Cancer Center experience with taxane therapy in 44 patients with newly diagnosed or recurrent SCSTs (169). Eleven patients received paclitaxel and a platinum drug for newly diagnosed SCST; all were alive at the time of the study, with a median follow-up of 52 months. Of 37 patients treated with a taxane for recurrent SCST, 7 had no measurable disease after secondary cytoreductive surgery, and 30 had measurable disease. The response rate in the latter cohort was 42%. In a follow-up study, Brown et al. retrospectively compared the efficacy and side effects of taxanes, with or without platinum, to the combination of BEP (170). The outcomes of the two groups were similar, but the side effects associated with the BEP regimen appeared to be greater. The authors concluded that taxane and platinum chemotherapy warrants further investigation in SCSTs. The GOG is currently conducting a phase 2 trial of paclitaxel in women with stromal tumors with measurable disease (GOG protocol 187)—either previously untreated or recurrent. In addition, a GOG randomized phase 2 study of paclitaxel and carboplatin versus BEP in patients with SCSTs is planned in the near future.

Considerable rationale exists for the utilization of hormone-based approaches in GCTs. A proportion of these tumors express steroid hormone receptors (171). Responses of GCTs, occasionally long term, to medroxyprogesterone acetate and to GnRH antagonists have been reported (172–176). Fishman et al. (177) treated six patients with recurrent or persistent GCTs with monthly intramuscular injections of leuprolide acetate. Four patients had received prior cisplatinum-based chemotherapy. Five patients had evaluable disease: two had partial responses and three had stable disease. The leuprolide was well tolerated.

Granulosa Cell Tumors (Juvenile)

Calaminus et al. (178) reported the outcome of 33 patients with JGCTs—24 treated with surgery alone and 9 with surgery and cisplatinum-based chemotherapy. There have been six relapses, with 60 months median follow-up: 2 of 20 stage IA, 2 of 8 stage IC, and 2 of 5 stage IIC to IIIC. Three patients with stage IIC to IIIC disease treated with adjuvant cisplatinum-based therapy remain disease free at 46 to 66 months after diagnosis. Furthermore, Powell and Otis (179) reported short-term disease control in two teenagers with stage III JGCTs following surgery and cisplatinum-based chemotherapy.

German investigators published their 15-year experience (1985 to 2000) with 54 sex cord–stromal tumors in children and adolescents (71). Forty-five were JGCTs. Twelve received adjuvant chemotherapy for stages IC to IIIC disease. BEP and cisplatin, etoposide, and ifosfamide (PEI) were the most commonly used regimens. Six patients remained in remission after adjuvant chemotherapy from 15 to 106 months later. A seventh developed a contralateral JGCT 10 years after her initial primary tumor. Five of the 12 have recurred, 3 of whom died 16 to 28 months from diagnosis.

Powell et al. have reported a patient with long-term disease-free survival following salvage chemotherapy for recurrent JGCT (180). The patient had presented with stage IIIC disease initially treated by resection of all gross disease followed by carboplatin and etoposide for six cycles. She recurred 13 months later with limited disease in the liver and a mass at the inferior aspect of the spleen. She underwent gross total resection followed by six cycles of bleomycin and paclitaxel. She was disease-free 44 months later, delivering a normal baby at cesarean section.

Sertoli–Leydig Cell Tumors

Therapy for those few individuals presenting with high-stage SLCTs, as well as for individuals with recurrent disease, must be individualized. The effectiveness of radiation therapy is unknown (108). Reports exist of responses to vincristine, actinomycin D, and cyclophosphamide (VAC) and cisplatinum, doxorubicin, and cyclophosphamide (157,181). Schneider et al. reported three patients with SLCTs who were treated with platinum-based chemotherapy (71). One patient with stage IC disease with intermediate differentiation received two cycles of the combination of cisplatin and etoposide and was disease free at 47 months. Two other patients, both of whom had stage IC poorly differentiated SLCTs, were dead of tumor at 7 and 19 months after receiving either BEP or PEI. Given the functional hormonal nature of many of these neoplasms, consideration could also be given to some form of hormonal manipulation, such as luteinizing hormone–releasing agonists or antagonists (182).

Sex Cord Tumor With Annular Tubules

Given the rarity of this tumor, the collective experience with systemic therapy for SCTATs is scant. Their endocrine activities suggest that the tumors may retain responsiveness to perturbation of gonadotropin levels. A recent case report documents a complete response to etoposide, bleomycin, and cisplatinum in a patient with recurrent SCTAT (137).

MOLECULAR PATHOGENESIS

Our current knowledge regarding various autocrine and endocrine regulatory mechanisms influencing ovarian function, the overexpression of inhibin in several SCSTs, the alterations in ovarian steroidogenesis, and the changes in circulating gonadotropin levels in SCSTs provide several probable clues regarding the pathogenesis of these tumors. Investigations to date exploring the interactive regulatory mechanisms of inhibin, activin, follistatin, and follicle-stimulating hormone (FSH) have predominantly utilized GCTs. Follicle-stimulating hormone provides a fundamental regulatory role in the differentiation processes of granulosa cells during the early stages of follicle development. Specifically, FSH stimulates cell proliferation (mitosis), increases the availability of cell-surface prolactin and luteinizing hormone receptors, and induces aromatase activity, resulting in increased estradiol production. Other growth-regulatory factors such as insulin-like growth factor and epidermal growth factor modulate these actions, including the enhancement of the mitogenic effects of FSH. In addition, FSH secretion from the anterior pituitary is modulated in part by the serum levels of inhibin, activin, and estrogens and/or androgens.

Inhibin, a heterodimeric glycoprotein hormone composed of an alpha-subunit and one of two beta-subunits, is secreted by the granulosa cells of the ovary (183). Inhibin A consists of alpha and beta A; inhibin B, alpha and beta B. Petraglia et al. (184) studied the molecular form of inhibin in adult GCTs and epithelial ovarian cancers. Serum inhibin B was dramatically increased in eight of nine patients with GCTs. Inhibin A was slightly increased in all patients. Its major physiologic function is to inhibit the secretion of FSH by the anterior pituitary gland (185). Inhibin is expressed in excessive quantities by GCTs. Although it maintains its regulatory function pertaining to FSH suppression, it appears to be ineffective in controlling estrogen production and cell proliferation within the gonad. Robertson et al. have recently reviewed the various serum-based assays for inhibin (186).

Activin, also a peptide hormone of ovarian granulosa cell origin, is composed of two beta subunits that are identical to those of inhibin. In contrast to inhibin, activin stimulates the secretion of FSH, induces the production of estradiol while having a negative impact on progesterone production, and serves as a promoter of differentiation of granulosa cells (185).

Several investigative teams are pursuing studies to elucidate the underlying genetic and biologic changes that give rise to sex cord–stromal tumors, especially granulosa cell tumors. Lin et al. performed comparative genomic hybridization of a set of 37 adult-type granulosa cell tumors (36 primaries, 1 recurrence) obtained from five hospitals in Taiwan (187). All patients had stage I disease except for one stage III patient with limited disease at initial diagnosis. Twenty-two (61%) of the 36 primary tumors had chromosomal imbalances. The nonrandom changes included loss of 22q in 31% of tumors, gain of chromosome 14 in 25% of tumors, and gain of chromosome 12 in 14% of tumors. Monosomy 22 frequently coexisted with trisomy 14. High-level amplification, as can be seen in many aggressive carcinomas, was not detected in any of these granulosa cell tumors. Findings were similar to those reported by Mayr et al. (188). As a sole abnormality, trisomy 12 has also been found in fibromas and fibroepitheliomas, in addition to granulosa cell tumors (189,190). Menczer et al. looked for HER2/neu expression in 12 granulosa cell tumors and saw no immunohistochemical staining (191). An Austrian group looked at the immunohistochemical expression of the HER family of receptors—HER1 (EGFR), HER2, HER3, and HER4—in 38 adult granulosa cell tumors and two of the juvenile type (192). Thirty-one cases (77.5%) were positive for at least one of the receptors (EGFR, HER3, or HER4). None of the 40 cases showed a positive reaction for HER2. Twenty-six of 40 (65%) showed reactivity for EGFR. HER3 and HER4 expression were observed in 18 (45%) and 23 (57.5%) tumors, respectively. Kusamura et al. also looked for HER2 expression in 18 granulosa cell tumors: all cases were negative (193). They also showed a markedly low likelihood of immunohistochemical staining for p53 and low proliferative indices in these tumors.

Chu et al. examined the estrogen receptor isoform gene expression in a small series of granulosa cell tumors and serous cystoadenocarcinomas of the ovary (four of each) (194). They saw widespread expression of estrogen receptor (ER)-alpha in both tumor types but at relatively low levels, similar to or less than what is seen in the endometrium. ER-beta expression in the granulosa cell tumors, however, was several-fold higher than that of ER-alpha. Fuller and Chu have provided an informative review of various signaling pathways that are important in the regulation of growth, differentiation, and apoptosis of normal granulosa cells, which may contribute to the molecular pathogenesis of GCTs (195). Because of the important role of the insulin-like growth factor (IGF) system in development of the dominant follicle, and its contribution to epithelial ovarian cancer, Alexiadis et al. characterized the expression of several components of the IGF system in a series of nine granulosa cell tumors (196). Interestingly, pregnancy-associated plasma protein-A expression was highest in the granulosa cell tumors. PAPP-A is a metalloproteinase synthesized by granulosa cells, the activity of which leads to increased IGF bioavailability. Antonen et al. studied samples from a cohort of 80 GCT patients from the University of Helsinki and examined several growth regulatory factors known to be important in normal granulosa cell function, including anti-müllerian hormone, inhibin alpha, and GATA transcription factors (197). They found a correlation between high GATA-4 expression and higher likelihood of recurrence.

The natural history of sex cord–stromal tumors is uniquely different from that of their epithelial counterparts and provides an intriguing tumor model. The vast majority of these neoplasms are characteristically of low malignant potential. They are typically unilateral and remain localized, retain hormone-secreting functions, and infrequently develop recurrences, many of which are delayed. In contrast, a small percentage of otherwise phenotypically similar tumors demonstrate a more virulent course and are generally refractory to therapy. The SCST subtypes display a bimodal age distribution, notably with JGCTs, SSCTs, SLCTs, and SCTATs occurring predominantly during the first three decades of life. Furthermore, the association of these tumors with several uncommon congenital disease entities, such as enchondromatosis, leprechaunism, and PJS, occurs at frequencies that exceed mere chance. Uniquely, several of these functioning neoplasms, including AGCTs, JGCTs, SLCTs, and SCTATs, overexpress growth-regulatory substances including inhibin, müllerian-inhibiting substance, and follicle-regulating protein. Given the limited number of ovarian SCSTs available for study, our current understanding of the mechanism of oncogenesis in these tumors is understandably limited.

SUMMARY

The principal problem related to the study of SCSTs and the development of effective therapy is their rarity. Although this interesting group of tumors has been studied extensively from a histologic standpoint, there are surprisingly few features that distinguish tumors that are more likely to recur or have aggressive behavior, and much of the information is conflicting.

Surgery remains the cornerstone of treatment for patients with SCSTs. Furthermore, for young patients desirous of fertility preservation, fertility-sparing surgery is possible in a large proportion related to the propensity of these tumors to be unilateral and nonmetastatic. Patients who appear to have a worse prognosis and for whom postoperative therapy would appear to be indicated include those with metastatic SCSTs of any histotype and those with stage I poorly differentiated Sertoli–Leydig cell tumors. For patients with SCSTs confined to the ovary, postoperative therapy is not recommended. For those with stage IC disease, the issue of postoperative therapy is unresolved.

Standard postoperative treatment consists of platinum-based chemotherapy. The BEP regimen is currently the most popular combination. However, this is a relatively toxic regimen; hence, the interest in alternative combinations, such as taxane/platinum chemotherapy. However, more study of this latter combination is warranted. An upcoming GOG study should help resolve this issue.

Beyond platinum-based chemotherapy, there is no consensus concerning recommended second-line or salvage therapy. Hormonal medications clearly have some degree of activity in granulosa cell tumors. In addition, there is probably a limited role for radiation. This gap in our armamentarium underscores the need for novel target-based therapeutics developed through the study of the genes and pathways involved in the pathogenesis of these neoplasms.

References

1. Koonings PP, Campbell K, Mishell DR Jr, et al. Relative frequency of primary ovarian neoplasms: a 10-year review. *Obstet Gynecol* 1989;74:921–926.
2. Cramer DW, Devesa SS, Welch WR. Trends in the incidence of endometrioid and clear cell cancers of the ovary in the United States. *Am J Epidemiol* 1981;114:201–208.
3. Tavassoli FA. Ovarian tumors with functioning manifestations. *Endocrinol Pathol* 1994;5:137–148.
4. Evans AT, Gaffey TA, Malkasian GD Jr, et al. Clinicopathologic review of 118 granulosa and 82 theca cell tumors. *Obstet Gynecol* 1980;55:231–238.
5. Malmstrom H, Hogberg T, Risberg B, et al. Granulosa cell tumors of the ovary: prognostic factors and outcome. *Gynecol Oncol* 1994;52:50–55.
6. Ohel G, Kaneti H, Schenker JG. Granulosa cell tumors in Israel: a study of 172 cases. *Gynecol Oncol* 1983;15:278–286.
7. Rokitansky CV. Über abnormalities des corpus luteum. *Allg Wien Med Z* 1859;4:253–254.
8. Schumer ST, Cannistra SA. Granulosa cell tumor of the ovary. *J Clin Oncol* 2003;21:1180–1189.
9. Unkila-Kallio L, Leminen A, Tiitinen A, et al. Nationwide data on falling incidence of ovarian granulosa cell tumours concomitant with increasing use of ovulation inducers. *Hum Reprod* 1998;13:2828–2830.
10. Werness BA, Ramus SJ, Whittemore AS, et al. Histopathology of familial ovarian tumors in women from families with and without germline *BRCA1* mutations. *Hum Pathol* 2000;31:1420–1424.
11. Stevens TA, Brown J, Zander DS, et al. Adult granulosa cell tumors of the ovary in two first-degree relatives. *Gynecol Oncol* 2005;98:502–505.
12. Bjorkholm E. Granulosa cell tumors: a comparison of survival in patients and matched controls. *Am J Obstet Gynecol* 1980;138:329–331.
13. Bjorkholm E, Silfversward C. Prognostic factors in granulosa-cell tumors. *Gynecol Oncol* 1981;11:261–274.
14. Fox H, Agrawal K, Langley FA. A clinicopathologic study of 92 cases of granulosa cell tumor of the ovary with special reference to the factors influencing prognosis. *Cancer* 1975;35:231–241.
15. Pankratz E, Boyes DA, White GW, et al. Granulosa cell tumors. A clinical review of 61 cases. *Obstet Gynecol* 1978;52:718–723.
16. Piura B, Nemet D, Yanai-Inbar I, et al. Granulosa cell tumor of the ovary: a study of 18 cases. *J Surg Oncol* 1994;55:71–77.
17. Schweppe KW, Beller FK. Clinical data of granulosa cell tumors. *J Cancer Res Clin Oncol* 1982;104:161–169.
18. Stenwig JT, Hazekamp JT, Beecham JB. Granulosa cell tumors of the ovary. A clinicopathological study of 118 cases with long-term follow-up. *Gynecol Oncol* 1979;7:136–152.
19. Young RH, Scully RE. Ovarian sex cord–stromal tumours: recent advances and current status. *Clin Obstet Gynaecol* 1984;11:93–134.
20. Bjorkholm E, Silfversward C. Granulosa- and theca-cell tumors. Incidence and occurrence of second primary tumors. *Acta Radiol Oncol* 1980;19:161–167.
21. Muir CS, Waterhouse JAH, Mack TM, et al. *Cancer Incidence in Five Continents*. IARC Scientific Publication No. 88, Vol V. Lyon, France: International Agency for Research on Cancer; 1987.
22. Quirk JT, Natarajan N. Ovarian cancer incidence in the United States, 1992–1999. *Gynecol Oncol* 2005;97:519–523.
23. Cronje HS, Niemand I, Bam RH, et al. Review of the granulosa-theca cell tumors from the Emil Novak Ovarian Tumor Registry. *Am J Obstet Gynecol* 1999;180:323–327.
24. Gusberg SB, Kardon P. Proliferative endometrial response to theca-granulosa cell tumors. *Am J Obstet Gynecol* 1971;111:633–643.
25. Stuart GC, Dawson LM. Update on granulosa cell tumours of the ovary. *Curr Opin Obstet Gynecol* 2003;15:33–37.
26. Chen VW, Ruiz B, Killeen J, et al. Pathology and classification of ovarian tumors. *Cancer* 2003;97(10 Suppl):2631–2642.
27. Young RH, Oliva E, Scully RE. Luteinized adult granulosa cell tumors of the ovary: a report of four cases. *Int J Gynecol Pathol* 1994;13:302–310.
28. Zanagnolo V, Pasinetti B, Sartori E. Clinical review of 63 cases of sex cord stromal tumors. *Eur J Gynaecol Oncol* 2004; 25(4):431–438.
29. Nakashima N, Young RH, Scully RE. Androgenic granulosa cell tumors of the ovary. A clinicopathologic analysis of 17 cases and review of the literature. *Arch Pathol Lab Med* 1984;108:786–791.
30. Norris HJ, Taylor HB. Virilization associated with cystic granulosa tumors. *Obstet Gynecol* 1969;34:629–635.
31. Fathalla MF. The occurrence of granulosa and theca tumours in clinically normal ovaries. *J Obstet Gynaecol Br Commonw* 1967;74:279–282.
32. Young RH, Scully RE. Ovarian sex cord–stromal tumors with bizarre nuclei: a clinicopathologic analysis of 17 cases. *Int J Gynecol Pathol* 1983;1:325–335.
33. Spencer HW, Mullings AM, Char G, et al. Granulosa-theca cell tumor of the ovaries. A late metastasizing tumour. *West Indian Med J* 1999:48:33–35.
34. Dubuc-Lissoir J. Case report: bone metastasis from a granulosa cell tumor of the ovary. *Gynecol Oncol* 2001;83:400–404.
35. Miller BE, Barron BA, Wan JY, et al. Prognostic factors in adult granulosa cell tumor of the ovary. *Cancer* 1997;79:1951–1955.

36. Fujimoto T, Sakuragi N, Okuyama K, et al. Histopathological prognostic factors of adult granulosa cell tumors of the ovary. *Acta Obstet Gynecol Scand* 2001;80:1069–1074.
37. Kottmeier HL. *Carcinoma of the Female Genitalia*. Baltimore: Williams & Wilkins; 1953.
38. Klemi PJ, Joensuu H, Salmi T. Prognostic value of flow cytometric DNA content analysis in granulosa cell tumor of the ovary. *Cancer* 1990;65: 1189–1193.
39. Chadha S, Cornelisse CJ, Schaberg A. Flow cytometric DNA ploidy analysis of ovarian granulosa cell tumors. *Gynecol Oncol* 1990;36:240–245.
40. Evans MP, Webb MJ, Gaffey TA, et al. DNA ploidy of ovarian granulosa cell tumors. Lack of correlation between DNA index or proliferative index and outcome in 40 patients. *Cancer* 1995;75:2295–2298.
41. Ala-Fossi SL, Maenpaa J, Aine R, et al. Prognostic significance of p53 expression in ovarian granulosa cell tumors. *Gynecol Oncol* 1997;66: 475–479.
42. Kappes S, Milde-Langosch K, Kressin P, et al. p53 mutations in ovarian tumors, detected by temperature-gradient gel electrophoresis, direct sequencing and immunohistochemistry. *Int J Cancer* 1995;64:52–59.
43. King LA, Okagaki T, Gallup DG, et al. Mitotic count, nuclear atypia, and immunohistochemical determination of Ki-67, c-myc, p21-ras, c-erbB2, and p53 expression in granulosa cell tumors of the ovary: mitotic count and Ki-67 are indicators of poor prognosis. *Gynecol Oncol* 1996;61:227–232.
44. Liu FS, Ho ES, Lai CR, et al. Overexpression of p53 is not a feature of ovarian granulosa cell tumors. *Gynecol Oncol* 1996;61:50–53.
45. Dowdy SC, O'Kane DJ, Keeney GL, et al. Telomerase activity in sex cord–stromal tumors of the ovary. *Gynecol Oncol* 2001;82:257–260.
46. Ala-Fossi SL, Aine R, Punnonen R, et al. Is potential to produce inhibins related to prognosis in ovarian granulosa cell tumors? *Eur J Gynaecol Oncol* 2000;21:187–189.
47. Kaye SB, Davies E. Cyclophosphamide, Adriamycin, and cis-platinum for the treatment of advanced granulosa cell tumor, using serum estradiol as a tumor marker. *Gynecol Oncol* 1986;24:261–264.
48. Boggess JF, Soules MR, Goff BA, et al. Serum inhibin and disease status in women with ovarian granulosa cell tumors. *Gynecol Oncol* 1997;64:64–69.
49. Gustafson ML, Lee MM, Asmundson L, et al. Müllerian inhibiting substance in the diagnosis and management of intersex and gonadal abnormalities. *J Pediatr Surg* 1993;28:439–444.
50. Jobling T, Mamers P, Healy DL, et al. A prospective study of inhibin in granulosa cell tumors of the ovary. *Gynecol Oncol* 1994;55:285–289.
51. Lane AH, Lee MM, Fuller AF Jr, et al. Diagnostic utility of müllerian inhibiting substance determination in patients with primary and recurrent granulosa cell tumors. *Gynecol Oncol* 1999;73:51–55.
52. Lappohn RE, Burger HG, Bouma J, et al. Inhibin as a marker for granulosa cell tumor. *Acta Obstet Gynecol Scand Suppl* 1992;155:61–65.
53. Lappohn RE, Burger HG, Bouma J, et al. Inhibin as a marker for granulosa cell tumors. *N Engl J Med* 1989;321:790–793.
54. Rey RA, L'homme C, Marcillac I, et al. Antimüllerian hormone as a serum marker of granulosa cell tumors of the ovary: comparative study with serum alpha-inhibin and estradiol. *Am J Obstet Gynecol* 1996;174:958–965.
55. Rodgers KE, Marks JF, Ellefson DD, et al. Follicle regulatory protein: a novel marker for granulosa cell cancer patients. *Gynecol Oncol* 1990;37:381–387.
56. Sluijmer AV, Heineman MJ, Evers JL, et al. Peripheral vein, ovarian vein and ovarian tissue levels of inhibin in a postmenopausal patient with a granulosa cell tumour. *Acta Endocrinol (Copenh)* 1993;129:311–324.
57. McCluggage WG, Young R. Immunohistochemistry as a diagnostic aid in the evaluation of ovarian tumors. *Semin Diagn Pathol* 2005;22(1):3–32.
58. Scully RE. Stromal luteoma of the ovary: a distinctive type of lipoid-cell tumor. *Cancer* 1964;17:769–778.
59. Young RH, Dickersin GR, Scully RE. Juvenile granulosa cell tumor of the ovary. A clinicopathological analysis of 125 cases. *Am J Surg Pathol* 1984;8:575–596.
60. Lack EE, Perez-Atayde AR, Murthy AS, et al. Granulosa theca cell tumors in premenarchal girls: a clinical and pathologic study of ten cases. *Cancer* 1981;48:1846–1854.
61. Plantaz D, Flamant F, Vassal G, et al. Granulosa cell tumors of the ovary in children and adolescents. Multicenter retrospective study in 40 patients aged 7 months to 22 years. *Arch Fr Pediatr* 1992;49:793–798.
62. Vassal G, Flamant F, Caillaud JM, et al. Juvenile granulosa cell tumor of the ovary in children: a clinical study of 15 cases. *J Clin Oncol* 1988;6:990–995.
63. Zaloudek C, Norris HJ. Granulosa tumors of the ovary in children: a clinical and pathologic study of 32 cases. *Am J Surg Pathol* 1982;6:513–522.
64. Bouffet E, Basset T, Chetail N, et al. Juvenile granulosa cell tumor of the ovary in infants: a clinicopathologic study of three cases and review of the literature. *J Pediatr Surg* 1997;32:762–765.
65. Hasiakos D, Papakonstantinou K, Goula K, et al. Juvenile granulosa cell tumor associated with pregnancy: report of a case and review of the literature. *Gynecol Oncol* 2006;100:426–429.
66. Scully RE. Sex cord tumor with annular tubules: a distinctive ovarian tumor of the Peutz-Jeghers syndrome. *Cancer* 1970;25:1107–1121.
67. Asirvatham R, Rooney RJ, Watts HG. Ollier's disease with secondary chondrosarcoma associated with ovarian tumour. A case report. *Int Orthop* 1991;15:393–395.
68. Tamimi HK, Bolen JW. Enchondromatosis (Ollier's disease) and ovarian juvenile granulosa cell tumor. *Cancer* 1984;53:1605–1608.
69. Tanaka Y, Sasaki Y, Nishihira H, et al. Ovarian juvenile granulosa cell tumor associated with Maffucci's syndrome. *Am J Clin Pathol* 1992;97:523–527.
70. Brisigotti M, Fabbretti G, Pesce F, et al. Congenital bilateral juvenile granulosa cell tumor of the ovary in leprechaunism: a case report. *Pediatr Pathol* 1993;13:549–558.
71. Schneider DT, Calaminus G, Wessalowski R, et al. Ovarian sex cord–stromal tumors in children and adolescents. *J Clin Oncol* 2003;21:2357–2363.
72. Jacoby AF, Young RH, Colvin RB, et al. DNA content in juvenile granulosa cell tumors of the ovary: a study of early- and advanced-stage disease. *Gynecol Oncol* 1992;46:97–103.
73. Swanson SA, Norris HJ, Kelsten ML, et al. DNA content of juvenile granulosa tumors determined by flow cytometry. *Int J Gynecol Pathol* 1990;9: 101–109.
74. Bjorkholm E, Silfversward C. Theca-cell tumors. Clinical features and prognosis. *Acta Radiol Oncol* 1980;19:241–244.
75. Norris HJ, Taylor HB. Prognosis of granulosa theca tumors of the ovary. *Cancer* 1968;21:255–260.
76. Zhang J, Young RH, Arseneau J, et al. Ovarian stromal tumors containing lutein or Leydig cells (luteinized thecomas and stromal Leydig cell tumors)—a clinicopathological analysis of fifty cases. *Int J Gynecol Pathol* 1982;1:270–285.
77. Barrenetxea G, Schneider J, Centeno MM, et al. Pure theca cell tumors. A clinicopathologic study of 29 cases. *Eur J Gynaecol Oncol* 1990;11:429–432.
78. Clement PB, Young RH, Hanna W, et al. Sclerosing peritonitis associated with luteinized thecomas of the ovary. *Am J Surg Pathol* 1994;18:1–13.
79. Dockerty MB, Mason JC. Ovarian fibromas: clinical and pathologic study of 283 cases. *Am J Obstet Gynecol* 1944;47:741–752.
80. Samanth KK, Black WC. Benign ovarian stromal tumors associated with free peritoneal fluid. *Am J Obstet Gynecol* 1970;107:538–545.
81. Meigs JV. Fibroma of the ovary with ascites and hydrothorax: Meigs' syndrome. *Am J Obstet Gynecol* 1954;67:962–987.
82. Raggio M, Kaplan AL, Harberg JF. Recurrent ovarian fibromas with basal cell nevus syndrome (Gorlin syndrome). *Obstet Gynecol* 1983; 61(Suppl 3):95S–96S.
83. Prat J, Scully RE. Cellular fibromas of the ovary: a comparative clinicopathologic analysis of seventeen cases. *Cancer* 1981;47:2663–2670.
84. Irving JA, Alkushi A, Young RH, et al. Cellular fibromas of the ovary: a study of 75 cases including 40 mitotically active tumors emphasizing their distinction from fibrosarcoma. *Am J Surg Pathol* 2006;30:929–938.
85. Chalvardjian A, Scully RE. Sclerosing stromal tumors of the ovary. *Cancer* 1973;31:664–670.
86. Gee DC, Russell P. Sclerosing stromal tumours of the ovary. *Histopathology* 1979;3:367–376.
87. Lam RM, Geittmann P. Sclerosing stromal tumor of the ovary. A light, electron microscopic and enzyme histochemical study. *Int J Gynecol Pathol* 1988;7:280–290.
88. Young RH, Scully RE. Ovarian Sertoli cell tumors: a report of 10 cases. *Int J Gynecol Pathol* 1984;2:349–363.
89. Suit PF, Hart WR. Sclerosing stromal tumor of the ovary. An ultrastructural study and review of the literature to evaluate hormonal function. *Cleve Clin J Med* 1988;55:189–194.
90. Cashell AW, Cohen ML. Masculinizing sclerosing stromal tumor of the ovary during pregnancy. *Gynecol Oncol* 1991;43:281–285.
91. Ismail SM, Walker SM. Bilateral virilizing sclerosing stromal tumours of the ovary in a pregnant woman with Gorlin's syndrome: implications for pathogenesis of ovarian stromal neoplasms. *Histopathology* 1990;17: 159–163.
92. Katsube Y, Iwaoki Y, Silverberg SG, et al. Sclerosing stromal tumor of the ovary associated with endometrial adenocarcinoma: a case report. *Gynecol Oncol* 1988;29:392–398.
93. Healy DL, Burger HG, Mamers P, et al. Elevated serum inhibin concentrations in postmenopausal women with ovarian tumors. *N Engl J Med* 1993;329:1539–1542.
94. Van Winter JT, Podratz KC, Gaffey TA. Sclerosing stromal tumor of the ovary in a 13-year-old girl. *Adolesc Pediatr Gynecol* 1993;6:164–165.
95. Mancuso A, Grosso M, D'Anna R, et al. Anatomo-clinical considerations on the ovarian fibroma. *Clin Exp Obstet Gynecol* 1995;22:115–119.
96. Waxman M, Vuletin JC, Urcuyo R, et al. Ovarian low-grade stromal sarcoma with thecomatous features: a critical reappraisal of the so-called "malignant thecoma." *Cancer* 1979;44:2206–2217.
97. Lage JM, Weinberg DS, Huettner PC, et al. Flow cytometric analysis of nuclear DNA content in ovarian tumors. Association of ploidy with tumor type, histologic grade, and clinical stage. *Cancer* 1992;69:2668–2675.
98. Meyer R. Pathology of some special ovarian tumors and their relation to sex characteristics. *Am J Obstet Gynecol* 1931;22:697–713.
99. Novak E. Life and works of Robert Meyer. *Am J Obstet Gynecol* 1947;53:50–64.
100. Morris M, Scully RE. *Endocrine Pathology of the Ovary*. St. Louis: Mosby; 1958;82–96.
101. Aiba M, Hirayama A, Sukurada M, et al. Spironolactone body-like structure in rennin-producing Sertoli-cell tumors of the ovary. *Surg Pathol* 1990;3:143–149.
102. Ehrlich EN, Dominguez OV, Samuels LT, et al. Aldosteronism and precocious puberty due to an ovarian androblastoma (Sertoli cell tumor). *J Clin Endocrinol Metab* 1963;23:358–367.

103. Korzets A, Nouriel H, Steiner Z, et al. Resistant hypertension associated with a rennin-producing ovarian Sertoli cell tumor. *Am J Clin Pathol* 1986;85:242–247.
104. Ferry JA, Young RH, Engel G, et al. Oxyphilic Sertoli cell tumor of the ovary: a report of three cases, two in patients with the Peutz-Jeghers syndrome. *Int J Gynecol Pathol* 1994;13:259–266.
105. Tavassoli FA, Norris HJ. Sertoli tumors of the ovary. A clinicopathologic study of 28 cases with ultrastructural observations. *Cancer* 1980;46: 2281–2297.
106. Roth LM, Anderson MC, Govan AD, et al. Sertoli-Leydig cell tumors: a clinicopathologic study of 34 cases. *Cancer* 1981;48:187–197.
107. Young RH, Scully RE. Ovarian Sertoli-Leydig cell tumors with a retiform pattern: a problem in histopathologic diagnosis. A report of 25 cases. *Am J Surg Pathol* 1983;7:755–771.
108. Zaloudek C, Norris HJ. Sertoli-Leydig tumors of the ovary. A clinicopathologic study of 64 intermediate and poorly differentiated neoplasms. *Am J Surg Pathol* 1984;8:405–418.
109. Roth LM, Slayton RE, Brady LW, et al. Retiform differentiation in ovarian Sertoli-Leydig cell tumors. A clinicopathologic study of six cases from a Gynecologic Oncology Group study. *Cancer* 1985;55:1093–1098.
110. Talerman A. Ovarian Sertoli-Leydig cell tumor (androblastoma) with retiform pattern. A clinicopathologic study. *Cancer* 1987;60:3056–3964.
111. Young RH. Sertoli-Leydig cell tumors of the ovary: review with emphasis on historical aspects and unusual variants. *Int J Gynecol Pathol* 1993;12: 141–147.
112. Young RH, Scully RE. Ovarian Sertoli-Leydig cell tumors. A clinicopathological analysis of 207 cases. *Am J Surg Pathol* 1985;9:543–569.
113. Pascale MM, Pugeat M, Roberts M, et al. Androgen suppressive effect of GnRH agonist in ovarian hyperthecosis and virilizing tumours. *Clin Endocrinol (Oxf)* 1994;41:571–576.
114. Weyl-Ben Arush M, Oslander L. Ollier's disease associated with ovarian Sertoli-Leydig cell tumor and breast adenoma. *Am J Pediatr Hematol Oncol* 1991;13:49–51.
115. Young RH, Prat J, Scully RE. Ovarian Sertoli-Leydig cell tumors with heterologous elements. I. Gastrointestinal epithelium and carcinoid: a clinicopathologic analysis of thirty-six cases. *Cancer* 1982;50:2448–2456.
116. Young RH, Scully RE. Well-differentiated ovarian Sertoli-Leydig cell tumors: a clinicopathological analysis of 23 cases. *Int J Gynecol Pathol* 1984;3:277–290.
117. McCluggage WG, Young RH. Ovarian Sertoli-Leydig cell tumors with pseudoendometrioid tubules (pseudoendometrioid Sertoli-Leydig cell tumors). *Am J Surg Pathol* 2007;31:592–597.
118. Prat J, Young RH, Scully RE. Ovarian Sertoli-Leydig cell tumors with heterologous elements. II. Cartilage and skeletal muscle: a clinicopathologic analysis of twelve cases. *Cancer* 1982;50:2465–2475.
119. Cohen I, Shapira M, Cuperman S, et al. Direct *in-vivo* detection of atypical hormonal expression of a Sertoli-Leydig cell tumour following stimulation with human chorionic gonadotrophin. *Clin Endocrinol (Oxf)* 1993;39:491–495.
120. Ohashi M, Hasegawa Y, Haji M, et al. Production of immunoreactive inhibin by a virilizing ovarian tumour (Sertoli-Leydig tumour). *Clin Endocrinol (Oxf)* 1990;33:613–618.
121. Gagnon S, Tetu B, Silva EG, et al. Frequency of alpha-fetoprotein production by Sertoli-Leydig cell tumors of the ovary: an immunohistochemical study of eight cases. *Mod Pathol* 1989;2:63–67.
122. Motoyama I, Watanabe H, Gotoh A, et al. Ovarian Sertoli-Leydig cell tumor with elevated serum alpha-fetoprotein. *Cancer* 1989;63:2047–2053.
123. Shen K, Wu PC, Lang JH, et al. Ovarian sex cord tumor with annular tubules: a report of six cases. *Gynecol Oncol* 1993;48:180–184.
124. Young RH, Welch WR, Dickersin GR, et al. Ovarian sex cord tumor with annular tubules: review of 74 cases including 27 with Peutz-Jeghers syndrome and four with adenoma malignum of the cervix. *Cancer* 1982;50:1384–1402.
125. Hart WR, Kumar N, Crissman JD. Ovarian neoplasms resembling sex cord tumors with annular tubules. *Cancer* 1980;45:2352–2363.
126. Ahn GH, Chi JG, Lee SK. Ovarian sex cord tumor with annular tubules. *Cancer* 1986;57:1066–1073.
127. Solh HM, Azoury RS, Najjar SS. Peutz-Jeghers syndrome associated with precocious puberty. *J Pediatr* 1983;103:593–595.
128. Nomura K, Furusato M, Nikaido T, et al. Ovarian sex cord tumor with annular tubules. Report of a case. *Acta Pathol Jpn* 1991;41:701–706.
129. Podczaski E, Kaminski PF, Pees RC, et al. Peutz-Jeghers syndrome with ovarian sex cord tumor with annular tubules and cervical adenoma malignum. *Gynecol Oncol* 1991;42:74–78.
130. Srivatsa PJ, Keeney GL, Podratz KC. Disseminated cervical adenoma malignum and bilateral ovarian sex cord tumors with annular tubules associated with Peutz-Jeghers syndrome. *Gynecol Oncol* 1994;53:256–264.
131. Boardman LA, Thibodeau SN, Schaid DJ, et al. Increased risk for cancer in patients with the Peutz-Jeghers syndrome. *Ann Intern Med* 1998;128: 896–899.
132. Hemminki A, Tomlinson I, Markie D, et al. Localization of a susceptibility locus for Peutz-Jeghers syndrome to 19p using comparative genomic hybridization and targeted linkage analysis. *Nat Genet* 1997;15:87–90.
133. Jenne DE, Reimann H, Nezu J, et al. Peutz-Jeghers syndrome is caused by mutations in a novel serine threonine kinase. *Nat Genet* 1998;18: 38–43.
134. Benagiano G, Bigotti G, Buzzi M, et al. Endocrine and morphological study of a case of ovarian sex-cord tumor with annular tubules in a woman with Peutz-Jeghers syndrome. *Int J Gynaecol Obstet* 1988;26: 441–452.
135. Crain JL. Ovarian sex cord tumor with annular tubules: steroid profile. *Obstet Gynecol* 1986;68(Suppl 3):75S–79S.
136. Gustafson ML, Lee MM, Scully RE, et al. Müllerian inhibiting substance as a marker for ovarian sex-cord tumor. *N Engl J Med* 1992;326:466–471.
137. Puls LE, Hamous J, Morrow MS, et al. Recurrent ovarian sex cord tumor with annular tubules: tumor marker and chemotherapy experience. *Gynecol Oncol* 1994;54:396–401.
138. Talerman A, Hughesdon PE, Anderson MC. Diffuse nonlobular ovarian androblastoma usually associated with feminization. *Int J Gynecol Pathol* 1982;1:155–171.
139. Young RH, Dudley AG, Scully RE. Granulosa cell, Sertoli-Leydig cell, and unclassified sex cord–stromal tumors associated with pregnancy: a clinicopathological analysis of thirty-six cases. *Gynecol Oncol* 1984;18: 181–205.
140. Martin-Jimenez A, Condor-Munro E, Valls-Porcel M, et al. Gynandroblastoma of the ovary. Review of the literature. *J Gynecol Obstet Biol Reprod* 1994;23:391–394.
141. Novak ER. Gynandroblastoma of the ovary: review of 8 cases from the Ovarian Tumor Registry. *Obstet Gynecol* 1967;30:709–715.
142. Kalir T, Friedman F Jr. Gynandroblastoma in pregnancy: case report and review of literature. *Mt Sinai J Med* 1998;65:292–295.
143. Hayes MC, Scully RE. Stromal luteoma of the ovary: a clinicopathological analysis of 25 cases. *Int J Gynecol Pathol* 1987;6:313–321.
144. Scully RE, Young RH, Clement PB. *Tumors of the Ovary, Maldeveloped Gonads, Fallopian Tube, and Broad Ligament.* Washington, DC: Armed Forces Institute of Pathology; 1998.
145. Roth LM, Sternberg WH. Ovarian stromal tumors containing Leydig cells. II. Pure Leydig cell tumor, non-hilar type. *Cancer* 1973;32:952–960.
146. Paraskevas M, Scully RE. Hilus cell tumor of the ovary. A clinicopathological analysis of 12 Reinke crystal-positive and nine crystal-negative cases. *Int J Gynecol Pathol* 1989;8:299–310.
147. Dunnihoo DR, Grieme DL, Woolf RB. Hilar-cell tumors of the ovary. Report of 2 new cases and a review of the world literature. *Obstet Gynecol* 1966;27:703–713.
148. Hayes MC, Scully RE. Ovarian steroid cell tumors (not otherwise specified). A clinicopathological analysis of 63 cases. *Am J Surg Pathol* 1987;11:835–845.
149. Harris AC, Wakely PE Jr, Kaplowitz PB, et al. Steroid cell tumor of the ovary in a child. *Arch Pathol Lab Med* 1991;115:150–154.
150. Davidson BJ, Waisman J, Judd HL. Long-standing virilism in a woman with hyperplasia and neoplasia of ovarian lipidic cells. *Obstet Gynecol* 1981;58:753–759.
151. Taylor HB, Norris HJ. Lipid cell tumors of the ovary. *Cancer* 1967;20: 1953–1962.
152. Adeyemi SD, Grange AO, Giwa-Osagie OF, et al. Adrenal rest tumour of the ovary associated with isosexual precocious pseudopuberty and cushingoid features. *Eur J Pediatr* 1986;145:236–238.
153. Dengg K, Fink FM, Heitger A, et al. Precocious puberty due to a lipid-cell tumour of the ovary. *Eur J Pediatr* 1993;152:12–14.
154. Clement PB, Young RH, Scully RE. Clinical syndromes associated with tumors of the female genital tract. *Semin Diagn Pathol* 1991;8: 204–233.
155. Donovan JT, Otis CN, Powell JL, et al. Cushing's syndrome secondary to malignant lipoid cell tumor of the ovary. *Gynecol Oncol* 1993;50: 249–253.
156. Young RH, Scully RE. Ovarian steroid cell tumors associated with Cushing's syndrome: a report of three cases. *Int J Gynecol Pathol* 1987;6:40–48.
157. Gershenson DM, Copeland LJ, Kavanagh JJ, et al. Treatment of metastatic stromal tumors of the ovary with cisplatin, doxorubicin, and cyclophosphamide. *Obstet Gynecol* 1987;70:765–769.
158. Gershenson DM. Chemotherapy of ovarian germ cell tumors and sex cord stromal tumors. *Semin Surg Oncol* 1994;10:290–298.
159. Zhang M, Cheung MK, Shin JY, et al. Prognostic factors responsible for survival in sex cord stromal tumors of the ovary—an analysis of 376 women. *Gynecol Oncol* 2007;104:296–400.
160. Abu-Rustum N, Restivo A, Ivy J, et al. Retroperitoneal nodal metastasis in primary and recurrent granulosa cell tumors of the ovary. *Gynecol Oncol* 2006;103:31–34
161. Wolf JK, Mullen J, Eifel PJ, et al. Radiation treatment of advanced or recurrent granulosa cell tumor of the ovary. *Gynecol Oncol* 1999;73: 35–41.
162. Savage P, Constenla D, Fisher C, et al. Granulosa cell tumours of the ovary: demographics, survival and the management of advanced disease. *Clin Oncol* 1998;10:242–245.
163. Homesley HD, Bundy BN, Hurteau JA, et al. Bleomycin, etoposide, and cisplatin combination therapy of ovarian granulosa cell tumors and other stromal malignancies: a Gynecologic Oncology Group study. *Gynecol Oncol* 1999;72:131–137.
164. Colombo N, Parma G, Franchi D. An active chemotherapy regimen for advanced ovarian sex cord–stromal tumors. *Gynecol Oncol* 1999;72: 129–130.

165. Gershenson DM, Morris M, Burke TW, et al. Treatment of poor-prognosis sex cord–stromal tumors of the ovary with the combination of bleomycin, etoposide, and cisplatin. *Obstet Gynecol* 1996;87:527–531.
166. Pecorelli S, Wagenaar HC, Vergote IB, et al. Cisplatin (P), vinblastine (V) and bleomycin (B) combination chemotherapy in recurrent or advanced granulosa (-theca) cell tumours of the ovary. An EORTC Gynaecological Cancer Cooperative Group Study. *Eur J Cancer* 1999;35:1331–1337.
167. Uygun K, Aydiner A, Saip P, et al. Clinical parameters and treatment results in recurrent granulosa cell tumor of the ovary. *Gynecol Oncol* 2003;88:400–403.
168. Tresukosol D, Kudelka AP, Edwards CL, et al. Recurrent ovarian granulosa cell tumor: a case report of a dramatic response to Taxol. *Int J Gynecol Cancer* 1995;5:156–159.
169. Brown J, Shvartsman HS, Deavers MT, et al. The activity of taxanes in the treatment of sex cord-stromal ovarian tumors. *J Clin Oncol* 2004;22: 3517–3523.
170. Brown J, Shvarftsman HS, Deavers MT, et al. The activity of taxanes compared with bleomycin, etoposide, and cisplatin in the treatment of sex cord-stromal ovarian tumors. *Gynecol Oncol* 2005;97:489–496.
171. Chadha S, Rao BR, Slotman BJ, et al. An immunohistochemical evaluation of androgen and progesterone receptors in ovarian tumors. *Hum Pathol* 1993;24:90–95.
172. Fishman A, Kudelka A, Edwards C, et al. GnRH agonist (Depot-Lupron) in the treatment of refractory or persistent ovarian granulosa cell tumor (GCT). *Proc Am Soc Clin Oncol* 1994;13:236(abst).
173. Isaacs R, Forgeson G, Allan S. Progestogens for granulosa cell tumours of the ovary [Letter]. *Br J Cancer* 1992;65:140.
174. Malik ST, Slevin ML. Medroxyprogesterone acetate (MPA) in advanced granulosa cell tumours of the ovary—a new therapeutic approach? *Br J Cancer* 1991;63:410–411.
175. Martikainen H, Penttinen J, Huhtaniemi I, et al. Gonadotropin-releasing hormone agonist analog therapy effective in ovarian granulosa cell malignancy. *Gynecol Oncol* 1989;35:406–408.
176. Hardy RD, Bell JG, Nicely CJ, et al. Hormonal treatment of a recurrent granulosa cell tumor of the ovary: case report and review of the literature. *Gynecol Oncol* 2005;96:865–869.
177. Fishman A, Kudelka AP, Tresukosol D, et al. Leuprolide acetate for treating refractory or persistent ovarian granulosa cell tumor. *J Reprod Med* 1996;41:393–396.
178. Calaminus G, Wessalowski R, Harms D, et al. Juvenile granulosa cell tumors of the ovary in children and adolescents: results from 33 patients registered in a prospective cooperative study. *Gynecol Oncol* 1997;65:447–452.
179. Powell JL, Otis CN. Management of advanced juvenile granulosa cell tumor of the ovary. *Gynecol Oncol* 1997;64:282–284.
180. Powell JL, Connor GP, Henderson GS. Management of recurrent juvenile granulosa cell tumor of the ovary. *Gynecol Oncol* 2001;81:113–116.
181. Schwartz PE, Smith JP. Treatment of ovarian stromal tumors. *Am J Obstet Gynecol* 1976;125:402–411.
182. Emons G, Schally AV. The use of luteinizing hormone releasing hormone agonists and antagonists in gynaecological cancers. *Hum Reprod* 1994;9:1364–1379.
183. Burger HG. Inhibin. *Reprod Med Rev* 1992;1:1–20.
184. Petraglia F, Luisi S, Pautier P, et al. Inhibin B is the major form of inhibin/activin family secreted by granulosa cell tumors. *J Clin Endocrinol Metab* 1998;83:1029–1032.
185. Ying SY. Inhibins, activins, and follistatins: gonadal proteins modulating the secretion of follicle-stimulating hormone. *Endocr Rev* 1988;9:267–293.
186. Robertson DM, Stephenson T, Pruysers E, et al. Characterization of inhibin forms and their measurement by an inhibin alpha-subunit ELISA in serum from postmenopausal women with ovarian cancer. *J Clin Endocrinol Metab* 2002;87:816–824.
187. Lin YS, Eng HL, Jan YJ, et al. Molecular cytogenetics of ovarian granulosa cell tumors by comparative genomic hybridization. *Gynecol Oncol* 2005;97:68–73.
188. Mayr D, Kaltz-Wittmer C, Arbogast S, et al. Characteristic pattern of genetic aberrations in ovarian granulosa cell tumors. *Mod Pathol* 2002;15:951–957.
189. Fletcher JA, Gibas Z, Donovan K, et al. Ovarian granulosa stromal cell tumors are characterized by trisomy 12. *Am J Pathol* 1991;138: 515–520.
190. Halperin D, Visscher DW, Wallis T, et al. Evaluation of chromosome 12 copy number in ovarian granulosa cell tumors using interphase cytogenetics. *Int J Gynecol Pathol* 1995;14:319–323.
191. Menczer J, Schreiber L, Czernobilsky B, et al. Is Her-2/neu expressed in nonepithelial ovarian malignancies? *Am J Obstet Gynecol* 2007; 196:79e1–79e4.
192. Leibl S, Bodo K, Gogg-Kammerer M, et al. Ovarian granulosa cell tumors frequently express EGFR (Her-1), Her-3, and Her-4: an immunohistochemical study. *Gynecol Oncol* 2006;101:18–23.
193. Kusamura S, Derchain S, Alvarenga M, et al. Expression of p53, c-erbB-2, Ki-67, and CD34 in granulosa cell tumor of the ovary. *Int J Gynecol Cancer* 2003;13:450–457.
194. Chu S, Mamers P, Burger HG, et al. Estrogen receptor isoform gene expression in ovarian stromal and epithelial tumors. *J Clin Endocrinol Metab* 2000;85(3):1200–1205.
195. Fuller PJ, Chu S. Signalling pathways in the molecular pathogenesis of ovarian granulosa cell tumours. *Trends Endocrinol Metab* 2004;15(3): 122–128.
196. Alexiadis M, Mamers P, Chu S, et al. Insulin-like growth factor, insulin-like growth factor-binding protein-4, and pregnancy-associated plasma protein-A gene expression in human granulosa cell tumors. *Int J Gynecol Cancer* 2006;16:1973–1979.
197. Anttonen M, Unkila-Kallio L, Leminen A, et al. High GATA-4 expression associates with aggressive behavior, whereas low anti-müllerian hormone expression associates with growth potential of ovarian granulosa cell tumors. *J Clin Endocrinol Metab* 2005;90(12):6529–6535.

CHAPTER 28 ■ MOLAR PREGNANCY AND GESTATIONAL TROPHOBLASTIC NEOPLASMS

ROSS S. BERKOWITZ AND DONALD P. GOLDSTEIN

Molar pregnancy and gestational trophoblastic neoplasms (GTN) comprise a group of interrelated diseases including complete and partial molar pregnancy, invasive mole, placental-site trophoblastic tumor (PSTT), and choriocarcinoma (CCA) that have varying propensities for local invasion and metastasis. GTN are one of the rare human malignancies that are highly curable with chemotherapy even with widespread metastases (1–4). Although GTN most commonly follow a molar pregnancy, they may develop after any gestation. Important advances have been made in the diagnosis, treatment, and follow-up of patients with molar pregnancy and GTN over the past 5 years. This chapter reviews these advances and discusses basic principles in the management of patients with molar pregnancy and persistent GTN.

EPIDEMIOLOGY

The reported incidence of GTN varies dramatically in different regions of the world (5). The frequency of molar pregnancy in Asian countries is seven to ten times greater than the reported incidence in North America or Europe (6). Whereas hydatidiform mole occurs in Taiwan in 1 per 125 pregnancies, the incidence of molar gestation in the United States is about 1 per 1,500 live births. Variations in the incidence rates of molar pregnancy partly result from differences between reporting hospital-based versus population-based data. Jeffers et al. (7), reporting a study from Ireland where all products of conception from first- and second-trimester abortions were referred for pathologic examination, found the incidence of complete and partial mole was 1:1,945 and 1:695 pregnancies, respectively.

The high incidence of molar pregnancy in some populations has been attributed to socioeconomic and nutritional factors. We have observed in a case-control study that the risk for complete molar pregnancy progressively increases with decreasing levels of consumption of dietary carotene (vitamin A precursor) and animal fat (8). Parazzini et al. (9) also reported from Italy that low carotene consumption was associated with an increased risk of molar gestations and their sequelae. Global regions with a high incidence of vitamin A deficiency correspond to areas with a high frequency of molar pregnancy. Vitamin A deficiency in the rhesus monkey produces degeneration of the seminiferous epithelium with production of primitive spermatogonia and spermatocytes (10). Dietary factors such as carotene may therefore partly explain the regional variations in the incidence of complete molar pregnancy.

The risk of having a complete hydatidiform mole (CHM) also increases with advanced maternal age (6). Women older than age 40 years have a five- to tenfold greater risk of having a complete molar gestation. In fact, one out of three pregnancies in women over 50 years of age are molar and the risk of developing GTN is significantly increased as well. Ova from older women may be more susceptible to abnormal fertilizations.

The risk for both complete and partial molar pregnancy (partial hydatidiform mole [PHM]) is increased in women with a history of prior spontaneous abortion and infertility (11). Compared with women with no previous miscarriage, the risk for complete and partial mole was 3.1 and 1.9, respectively, among women with two or more prior miscarriages. Difficulty in conception or infertility problems were associated with an odds risk of 2.4 and 3.2, respectively, for complete and partial mole.

Certain epidemiologic features of complete and partial molar pregnancy differ markedly. Parazzini et al. (12) reported that the risk for partial mole was not associated with maternal age. Additionally, the risk for partial mole has been reported to be associated with the use of oral contraceptives and a history of irregular menstruation, but not with dietary factors (13). Therefore, in contrast to CHM, the risk for partial mole appears to be associated with reproductive history rather than dietary factors.

The risk for CCA and GTN has been observed in a case-control study to be related to hormonal factors (14). Women with light menstrual flow and menarche after the age of 12 years were noted to be at increased risk for CCA. Additionally, Palmer et al. (15) reported that the prior use of oral contraceptives was associated with an increased risk for CCA.

Immunobiology

The remarkable curability of GTN may be partly attributable to a host immunologic response to paternal antigens expressed on trophoblastic cells (16). The prognosis of patients with gestational CCA has been related to the intensity of lymphocytic and monocytic infiltration at the tumor-host interface (17). Because the lymphocytes and macrophages that infiltrate gestational CCA are probably exposed to paternal antigens and oncoproteins, the immune cells may become activated. Immunologically active cells may promote the regression of GTN through their release of cytokines. Cytokines have been reported to inhibit the proliferation of CCA cells *in vitro* and to increase the human leukocyte antigen (HLA) expression of CCA cells *in vitro*, thereby increasing immunogenicity (18–20).

It has been theorized that the development and progression of persistent GTN may be favored by histocompatibility between the patient and her partner. If the patient and her partner are histocompatible, the trophoblastic tumor that bears paternal antigens may not be immunogenic in the maternal host. The intensity of the host's immunologic response may depend upon the immunogenicity of the trophoblastic tumor. However, histocompatibility between the patient and her partner does not appear to be a prerequisite for the development or persistence of GTN (21,22). The HLA system may, however, influence the clinical course of rapidly progressive and fatal GTN. Tomoda et al. (23) reported that drug-resistant CCA was associated with increased histocompatibility between the patient and her partner. Similarly, Morgensen et al. (24) observed that histocompatibility between patients and partners was associated with a greater risk of metastatic disease.

Because all chromosomes in a CHM are paternal in origin, a CHM is a complete allograft and may stimulate a vigorous immunologic response by the maternal host. There is evidence for both a cellular and humoral immune response to CHM. As compared with normal placentas, molar implantation sites have a fivefold increased infiltration by helper T cells (25). Circulating immune complexes have also been measured in patients with CHM and have been noted to increase as the patient entered gonadotropin remission (26).

Circulating immune complexes in patients with complete moles have been demonstrated to contain paternal HLA antigen (27). The maternal host with a complete mole is therefore sensitized to paternal HLA. The distribution of HLA antigen in molar chorionic villi has been determined by immunofluorescence assays (28). HLA A, B, and C antigens were detected on the stromal cells of molar chorionic villi but not on the villous trophoblast. However, the molar villous fluid that bathes the stromal cells does not contain soluble HLA antigen (29). The maternal host may therefore be sensitized to paternal HLA antigen when the villous trophoblast layer is disrupted and HLA-positive villous stromal cells are released into the maternal circulation.

Molecular Pathogenesis

Several growth factors and oncogenes have been studied in molar tissues and CCA (11). Increased expression of p53 and c-*fms* has been observed in CHM and increased *ras* and c-*myc* RNA has been measured in CCA (30–32).

We have investigated the expression of various growth factors and oncogenes in normal placenta, complete and partial mole, and CCA (33,34). Complete mole and CCA were characterized by overexpression of c-*myc*, c-*erbB2*, and *bcl-2* and these oncoproteins may be important in the pathogenesis of GTN. Expression of c-fms protein did not differ between normal placenta and GTN. CHM and CCA were also characterized by increased expression of p53, *p21*, *Rb*, and *MdM2*. The p53 gene was studied to detect any mutation in 22 complete moles and 11 CCAs that had increased expression of p53. Because only one nonsense mutation in p53 was detected by polymerase chain reaction analysis, it is likely that the overexpressed p53 protein was wild type. Although studies have identified increased expression of several growth factors in GTN, the precise molecular pathogenesis has not been determined (35).

It was observed that the level of expression of epidermal growth factor receptor (EGFR) in CCA and the syncytiotrophoblast and cytotrophoblast of CHM was significantly greater than the expression of EGFR in syncytiotrophoblast and cytotrophoblast of placenta and PHM (36). This observation was consistent in both immunohistochemical and *in situ* hybridization studies. In CHM, strong expression of EGFR and c-*erbB3* in the extravillous trophoblasts was significantly associated with the development of postmolar tumor. The EGFR-related family of oncogenes may be important in the pathogenesis of GTN.

Extracellular proteinases such as matrix metalloproteinases (MMPs) are thought to be important in modulating both cell-matrix interactions and the degradation of the basement membrane necessary for invasion and metastasis. CCA exhibits significantly stronger expression of MMP-1 and MMP-2 and decreased expression of tissue inhibitor of MMP-1 (TIMP-1) than the syncytiotrophoblast of complete and partial mole and normal placenta (37). The increased expression of MMP-1 and MMP-2 and decreased expression of TIMP-1 in CCA may contribute to the invasiveness of choriocarcinoma cells.

Certain genes are normally expressed on either the maternal or paternal allele, and this occurrence is described as parental imprinting. Modification of parental imprinting has been associated with tumor formation, and CHMs and CCAs have relaxation of parental imprinting (38). Relaxation in parental imprinting may be important in the pathogenesis of GTN.

cDNA microarray analysis has been utilized to study differential gene expression in GTN. Kim et al. investigated differential gene expression in CHMs as compared to normal placenta and identified 91 upregulated genes and 122 downregulated genes (39). The differentially expressed genes need to be further studied to determine which may play an important role in the biology of GTN. Vegh et al. studied differential gene expression in CCA as compared to normal placenta using cDNA expression assay. CCA cells have marked downregulation of heat shock protein-27, which may contribute to the marked sensitivity of this tumor to chemotherapy (40).

Studies of loss of heterozygosity have been performed to identify potential tumor suppressor genes that may be important in the pathogenesis of GTN. Matsuda et al. demonstrated homozygous deletions of one or more markers in the 7p12-q11.23 region of seven of eight CCA cell lines indicating that deletion in this region may be important in the pathogenesis of this malignancy (41). In contrast, Ahmed et al. (42) did not identify significant loss of heterozygosity in chromosome 7 in a series of 12 choriocarcinomas. Furthermore, Burke et al. (43) reported no detectable deletions on 7q11.2 and 8p12-p21 in 14 cases of GTN after CHM. Molecular biologic studies continue to try to identify the key genetic events that are critical in the pathogenesis of GTN.

MOLAR PREGNANCY

Pathologic and Chromosomal Features

Hydatidiform moles may be categorized as either complete or partial based upon gross morphology, histopathology, and karyotype (Table 28.1). CHMs have no identifiable embryonic or fetal tissues. The chorionic villi have generalized swelling and diffuse trophoblastic hyperplasia and the implantation-site trophoblast has diffuse, marked atypia (Fig. 28.1) (44,45). Complete moles usually have a 46,XX karyotype, and the molar chromosomes are derived entirely from paternal origin (46). Most complete moles appear to arise from an anuclear empty ovum that has been fertilized by a haploid (23X) sperm, which then duplicates its own chromosomes (47). Whereas most complete moles have a 46,XX chromosomal pattern, approximately 10% of complete moles have a 46,XY karyotype (48). The 46,XY complete mole arises from fertilization of an anuclear empty ovum by two sperm. Whereas chromosomes in the complete mole are entirely of paternal origin, the mitochondrial DNA is of maternal origin (49).

Recent reports have shed light on the rare occurrence of familial recurrent hydatidiform mole (FRHM), which is characterized

TABLE 28.1

COMPLETE VERSUS PARTIAL MOLAR PREGNANCY: HISTOPATHOLOGIC AND CHROMOSOMAL FEATURES

	Complete mole	Partial mole
Fetal or embryonic tissue	Absent	Present
Hydropic swelling of villi	Diffuse	Focal
Trophoblastic hyperplasia	Diffuse	Focal
Scalloping of chorionic villi	Absent	Present
Trophoblastic stromal inclusions	Absent	Present
Implantation-site trophoblast	Marked atypia	Mild atypia
Karyotype	46, XX (mainly); 46, XY	Triploid, 69, XXY, 69, XYY

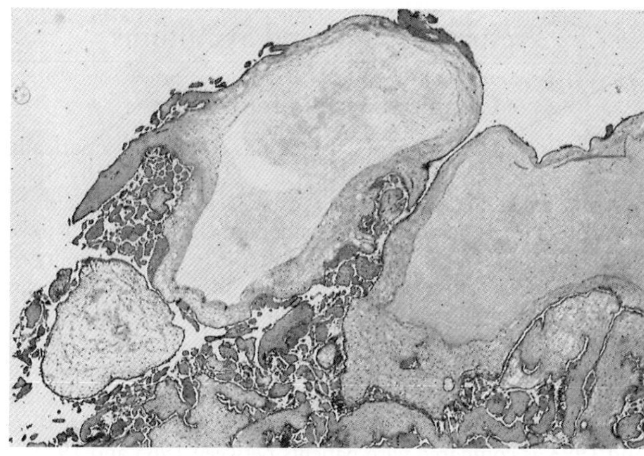

FIGURE 28.2. Photomicrograph of a partial hydatidiform mole demonstrating varying-sized chorionic villi with focal swelling and focal trophoblastic hyperplasia. (Magnification × 50)

by recurrent complete hydatidiform moles of biparental, rather than the more usual androgenetic, origin. Although the specific gene defect in these families has not been identified, genetic mapping has shown that in most families the gene responsible is located in a 1.1 Mb region on chromosome 19q13.4 (50). Mutations in this gene result in dysregulation of imprinting in the female germ line with abnormal development of both embryonic and extraembryonic tissue. Subsequent pregnancies in women diagnosed with this condition are likely to be CHM. Molar pregnancies in women with FRHM are associated with consanguinity and have a risk of progressing to GTN similar to that of androgenetic CHM.

During the 1960s and 1970s, CHMs were primarily diagnosed in the second trimester. However, currently, most patients with complete moles are diagnosed in the first trimester both in the United States and abroad (51–53). The pathologic characteristics of a first-trimester complete mole are different from the classic features in the second trimester. Mosher et al. (54) compared pathologic findings of 23 current complete moles (1994 through 1997; mean gestational age, 8.5 weeks) with 20 historic complete moles (1969 through 1975; mean gestational age, 17 weeks). Histologically, current complete moles had a smaller mean maximal villous diameter (5.7 vs. 8.2 mm), less circumferential trophoblastic hyperplasia (39% vs. 75%), more primitive villous stroma (70% vs. 10%), and less global necrosis (22% vs. 54%). Currently, complete moles are often characterized by subtle morphologic alterations that may result in their misclassification as partial moles or nonmolar spontaneous abortions. Similarly, Keep et al. (55) described that early complete moles were characterized by focal trophoblastic hyperplasia, minimal villous cavitation, and a hypercellular primitive stroma.

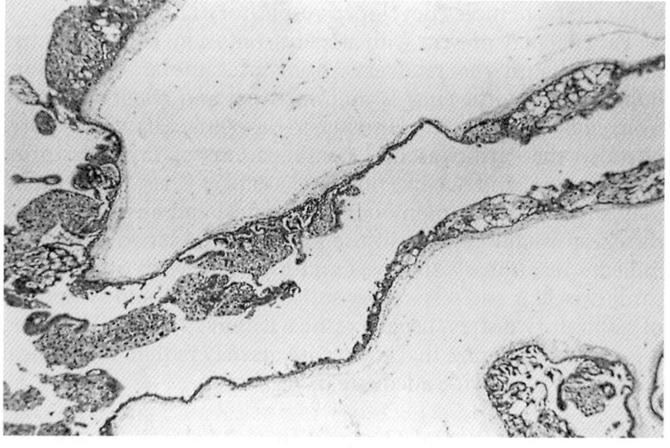

FIGURE 28.1. Photomicrograph of a complete hydatidiform mole showing chorionic villi with generalized swelling and diffuse trophoblastic hyperplasia. (Magnification × 20)

PHMs are characterized by the following pathologic features: (a) varying-sized chorionic villi with focal swelling and focal trophoblastic hyperplasia; (b) focal, mild atypia of implantation-site trophoblast; (c) marked villous scalloping and prominent stromal trophoblastic inclusions; and (d) identifiable fetal or embryonic tissues (Fig. 28.2) (56). Partial moles generally have a triploid karyotype, which results from the fertilization of an apparently normal ovum by two sperm (57). Lawler et al. (58) and Lage et al. (59) reported that 93% and 90%, respectively, of partial moles were triploid. When fetuses are identified with partial moles, they generally have stigmata of triploidy including growth retardation and multiple congenital anomalies. Genest et al. (60) reviewed 19 putative nontriploid PHMs using standardized histologic diagnostic criteria and repeat flow cytometry, and none of these cases on re-evaluation was convincingly a nontriploid partial mole. Nontriploid partial moles may not exist.

Early diagnosis and intervention has made the pathologic diagnosis of CHM challenging because the characteristic histologic features have become more subtle. Recently biomarkers have emerged that take advantage of imprinted genes to distinguish CHM from other entities. Because CHM results from diandry, paternally imprinted gene products, which are normally expressed only from maternally derived chromosomes, should be absent. Studies have recently shown that immunohistochemistry for p57 (paternally imprinted, maternally expressed gene products) is useful for confirming the diagnosis of CHM (61). Nuclei of decidua (maternally derived tissue) and extra villous trophoblast of all types of gestations stain positively for p57. Almost all complete moles have absent (or near absent) villous stromal and cytotrophoblastic nuclear activity for p57, while all other types of gestations (including partial moles) show nuclear reactivity in more than 25% of villous stromal and cytotrophoblastic nuclei. Fisher et al. (62) have shown that maternal chromosome 11 is retained in the rare cases of CHM exhibiting p57 staining.

Presenting Signs and Symptoms

Complete Hydatidiform Mole

The clinical presentation of a CHM has changed dramatically over the past two decades. Whereas CHM was usually diagnosed in the second trimester in the 1960s and 1970s, the diagnosis of CHM is now generally made in the first trimester (63). Earlier diagnosis is most likely attributable to the availability of accurate and sensitive tests for human chorionic gonadotropin (hCG) and the widespread use of ultrasound. The diagnosis of CHM is now often made before the classic clinical signs and symptoms develop. Soto-Wright et al. (53) investigated the clinical presentation and outcome of patients with CHM at the New England Trophoblastic Disease Center (NETDC) between 1988 and 1993 as compared with patients between 1965 and 1975.

Vaginal Bleeding. Vaginal bleeding is the most common presenting symptom in patients with CHM, occurring in 89% to 97% of cases (63–65). Retained blood may undergo oxidation and prune juice–like fluid may leak from the endometrial cavity. Molar chorionic villi may separate from the decidua and disrupt vessels, leading to the distension of the endometrial cavity by large volumes of retained blood. Because bleeding used to be prolonged, occult, and considerable, 54% of our patients used to present with anemia (hemoglobin <10 g/100 mL). Vaginal bleeding continues to be the most common presenting symptom, occurring in 84% of our current patients. However, anemia was present in only 5% of our current patients with complete mole.

Theca Lutein Ovarian Cysts. The reported frequency of theca lutein ovarian cysts depends upon the method of diagnosis. Ultrasonography detected theca lutein ovarian cysts (>5 cm in diameter) in 23 (46%) of 50 patients with molar pregnancy (66). However, clinical examination detected theca lutein ovarian cysts in 26% of patients with molar pregnancy (67). Although theca lutein cysts are generally 6 to 12 cm in diameter, they may enlarge to more than 20 cm in size. They are usually multicystic and bilateral and contain serosanguineous or amber-colored fluid. Although theca lutein cysts are usually detected at the time of presentation, they may develop rapidly after molar evacuation.

Theca lutein cysts are detected exclusively in patients with very high serum hCG levels and result from hyperstimulation of the ovaries by high circulating levels of hCG (68). Other signs of ovarian hyperstimulation may infrequently develop, including ascites and pleural effusion. Theca lutein cysts generally resolve over an interval of 8 weeks (67).

Torsion or rupture of theca lutein ovarian cysts occurs infrequently. Kohorn (69) reported that 3 (2.3%) of 127 patients with molar pregnancy developed torsion of ovarian theca lutein cysts. Similarly, Montz et al. (67) noted that only 2 of 102 patients with theca lutein cysts developed torsion or rupture. If patients develop severe symptoms of pelvic or abdominal pressure or pain, theca lutein cysts may be decompressed by ultrasound-directed or laparoscopic aspiration (70). Ovarian rupture or torsion may also be managed by laparoscopy.

Excessive Uterine Size. Uterine size was excessively enlarged as compared with gestational age in about 38% to 51% of patients with complete moles (44,64,65). Both retained blood and chorionic tissues may expand the uterine cavity. Excessive uterine enlargement is commonly associated with markedly elevated hCG values from trophoblastic proliferation and overgrowth. Among current patients at the NETDC, excessive uterine size was diagnosed at presentation in only 28% of patients.

Hyperemesis Gravidarum. Hyperemesis requiring antiemetic therapy used to develop in 20% to 26% of patients with complete moles (44,69). Hyperemesis was associated with excessive uterine enlargement and high hCG values. High circulating levels of estrogen have been proposed as a cause of hyperemesis (71). Although hyperemesis used to be a common problem, only 8% of our current patients present with hyperemesis.

Preeclampsia. Preeclampsia used to be observed in 12% to 27% of patients with complete moles (64,72). Preeclampsia primarily developed in patients with excessive uterine size and high hCG levels. Eclamptic convulsions developed rarely. In contrast, between 1988 and 1993, only 1 of 74 patients with CHM presented with preeclampsia at the NETDC.

Hyperthyroidism. Laboratory evidence of hyperthyroidism commonly used to be present in patients with complete moles. Galton et al. (73) reported that all 11 patients with CHM had elevated thyroid function tests before molar evacuation. Hyperthyroidism occurred almost exclusively in patients with very high hCG values. There are conflicting data whether hCG is a thyroid stimulator in patients with molar pregnancy. Amir et al. (74) found no significant correlation between serum hCG levels and free T_4 and T_3 index values in 47 patients with complete mole. Similarly, Nagataki et al. (75) found no correlation between free T_4 and hCG in ten patients. However, highly purified hCG may have intrinsic thyroid-stimulating activity, and some studies do report correlations between serum levels of hCG and total T_4 and T_3 (76).

Patients with poorly controlled or untreated hyperthyroidism may develop thyroid storm at the time of anesthesia induction and evacuation. Thyroid storm may be characterized by hyperthermia, delirium, coma, atrial fibrillation, and cardiovascular collapse. The diagnosis of thyroid storm must be made clinically so that treatment can be promptly instituted and not await the return of laboratory confirmation. Many of the cardiovascular and metabolic complications of thyroid storm may be prevented or reversed by the administration of beta-adrenergic blocking agents. A pulmonary artery catheter may be helpful to guide fluid replacement and to monitor cardiovascular status.

Between 1988 and 1993, none of our 74 patients with complete moles had clinical evidence of hyperthyroidism. However, during the past decade, one patient with a complete mole and a pre-evacuation hCG level of 1.4 million mIU/mL developed clinical and laboratory evidence of hyperthyroidism and required beta-adrenergic blockers to treat tachyarrhythmia.

Respiratory Insufficiency. Twiggs et al. (77) observed that 12 (27%) of 44 patients with a CHM of at least 16-weeks size developed pulmonary complications. Respiratory insufficiency used to develop in 2% of our patients with complete moles (72). Pulmonary compromise was generally observed in patients with excessive uterine size and high hCG levels—the same group of patients who are at risk for preeclampsia and hyperthyroidism. During the past decade, none of our patients with complete moles developed respiratory failure.

Patients may present with anxiety, confusion, tachypnea, and tachycardia in the recovery room after molar evacuation. Pulmonary insufficiency is multifactorial and results not only from embolization of molar tissue to the pulmonary vasculature, but also the cardiovascular complications of thyroid storm, preeclampsia, and massive fluid replacement. Chest radiography may show bilateral pulmonary infiltrates, and auscultation of the chest usually reveals diffuse rales. Arterial blood gases may indicate respiratory alkalosis and hypoxia. With appropriate cardiovascular and respiratory support, the signs and symptoms of respiratory distress usually resolve within 72 hours. However, it is vital to recognize that some patients may require mechanical ventilation to provide adequate oxygenation.

Partial Hydatidiform Mole

Patients with PHM usually do not present with the classic clinical features that are characteristic of a CHM. These patients generally present with the signs and symptoms of missed or incomplete abortion. Eighty-one patients were followed with partial moles at the NETDC between January 1979 and August 1984 (78). Excessive uterine size and preeclampsia were detected in only three and two patients, respectively. Szulman and Surti (56) and Czernobilsky et al. (79) reported that only 9 (11%) of 81 and 2 (8%) of 25 patients with partial moles had excessive uterine enlargement. Preeclampsia was reported in both studies in only 4% of patients. None of our patients had prominent theca lutein ovarian cysts, hyperthyroidism, or hyperemesis. The diagnosis of partial mole is usually made after histologic review of curettage specimens. In contrast to CHM, the gestational age at diagnosis and presenting symptoms of PHM have not appreciably changed in recent years (80).

Ultrasonography and Diagnosis of Hydatidiform Mole

Ultrasonography is a sensitive and reliable technique for detecting CHM. Because of marked swelling of the chorionic villi, a complete mole produces a characteristic vesicular sonographic pattern. However, it may be difficult to distinguish an early complete mole from degenerating chorionic tissues, since small molar chorionic villi in the first trimester may be difficult to visualize on ultrasound. However, despite smaller chorionic villi, ultrasound is still able to detect most first-trimester complete moles (81). An elevated hCG measurement at the time of sonography may help to differentiate an early complete mole from a missed abortion (82).

Ultrasonography may also contribute to the diagnosis of PHM. Two sonographic findings are significantly associated with the diagnosis of partial mole: focal cystic changes in the placenta and a ratio of the transverse to anteroposterior dimension of the gestational sac >1.5 (83). Changes in the shape of the gestational sac may be part of the embryopathy of triploidy. When both findings were present, the positive predictive value for partial mole was 87%. On rare occasions, the sonogram will show the presence of a fetus with multiple congenital anomalies associated with a focally hydropic placenta. Naumoff et al. (84) also reported that partial moles may exhibit cystic spaces within the placenta with a growth-retarded fetus.

hCG Measurement and Diagnosis of Hydatidiform Mole

Patients with CHM commonly have markedly elevated pre-evacuation hCG levels. Menczer et al. (85) reported that 30 (41%) of 74 patients with complete moles had pre-evacuation hCG values greater than 100,000 mIU/mL. Similarly, Genest et al. (86) noted that 46% of 153 patients with complete moles who were managed at the NETDC between 1980 and 1990 had pre-evacuation hCG levels above 100,000 mIU/mL. The measurement of markedly elevated hCG values is therefore suggestive of the diagnosis of complete mole.

Patients with PHM less commonly present with markedly elevated hCG values. Czernobilsky et al. (79) reported that only 1 of 17 patients with partial moles presented with a urinary hCG value >300,000 mIU/mL. Likewise, we noted that only 2 of 30 patients with partial moles at the NETDC presented with hCG levels >100,000 mIU/mL (78).

Complete and partial moles also differ in their levels of free β- and α-subunits of hCG. Whereas complete moles have higher levels of percentage free β-hCG, partial moles have higher levels of percentage free α-hCG (87,88). The mean ratios of percentage free β-hCG to free α-hCG in complete and partial moles are 20.9 and 2.4, respectively.

Natural History of Molar Pregnancy and Prognostic Factors

CHMs are well recognized to have the potential for developing uterine invasion or distant spread. Following molar evacuation, uterine invasion and metastasis occur in 15% and 4% of the patients, respectively (89). Although complete moles are now being diagnosed earlier in pregnancy, the incidence of postmolar tumors has not been affected (52,53).

Whereas the incidence of postmolar tumor is reported from 18% to 29% in the United States, the incidence of postmolar GTN in Western Europe is reported from 8% to 10% of patients (2,64,69,90–94). Most centers in the United States define postmolar persistent GTN by the presence of a re-elevation or persistent plateau in hCG for at least 3 consecutive weeks. However, the definition of persistent disease does vary among American centers (95). The criteria for persistent GTN in Western Europe have been more stringent than American definitions. At the Charing Cross Hospital in London, the criteria for postmolar persistent tumors were (a) hCG >20,000 IU/L more than 4 weeks after evacuation; (b) progressively rising hCG levels, with a minimum of three rising values over 2 to 3 weeks; (c) metastasis to the liver, kidney, brain, or gastrointestinal tract; (d) metastasis to lung larger than 2 cm in diameter or three or more in number; or (e) persistent hCG level 4 to 6 months after evacuation. The use of less stringent diagnostic criteria for postmolar tumors in the United States is partly motivated by the concern that some patients may be lost to follow-up. Among 333 recent patients with molar pregnancy at our center, 122 (37%) patients did not complete the entire hormonal follow-up and 13 (4%) patients were lost to follow-up without attaining even one undetectable hCG value (96). Furthermore, Massad et al. (97) observed that among 40 indigent women with molar pregnancy, 33 (82%) did not fully comply with hCG follow-up and 5 (13%) were lost to follow-up before remission.

We reviewed 858 patients with CHM to identify factors that predispose to postmolar tumors (63). At the time of presentation, 41% of the patients had the following signs of marked trophoblastic proliferation: (a) hCG level >100,000 mIU/mL; (b) uterine size greater than gestational age; and (c) theca lutein cysts >6 cm in diameter. After evacuation, 31.0% of these patients developed uterine invasion and 8.8% developed metastases. The risk for persistent tumors is considerably less for patients who do not present with signs of marked trophoblastic growth. Following molar evacuation, only 3.4% of these patients developed invasion and 0.6% developed metastases. Similarly, Curry et al. (64) and Morrow (98) reported postmolar tumors in 57% and 55% of patients, respectively, with excessive uterine size and theca lutein ovarian cysts. Therefore, patients with CHM who exhibit markedly elevated hCG levels and excessive uterine size are at increased risk of developing postmolar tumors, and are categorized as "high risk."

An increased risk of postmolar GTN has also been observed in women older than age 40 years. Tow (99) and Xia et al. (100) reported that 37% and 33%, respectively, of women more than 40 years old with complete molar pregnancy developed persistent tumors. In women over age 50 years, postmolar tumors were reported to have developed in 56% of patients (101). Complete moles in older women are more frequently aneuploid, and this may be related to their increased potential for local invasion and metastasis (102).

Patients with repetitive molar pregnancy are also at increased risk of developing persistent tumors in their later episodes of molar gestation. Between June 1965 and December 2001, we treated 34 patients with repeat molar gestations at the NETDC (103). Postmolar tumors developed following their first mole in 4 (20%) of 20 complete moles and in none of 14 partial moles. However, postmolar tumors developed following the second mole in 8 (44.4%) of 18 complete moles and 2 (12.5%) of 16 partial moles. Parazzini et al. (104) also reported a threefold increased risk of postmolar tumors in patients with repetitive molar disease.

The risk for persistent GTN has been reported to be increased in CHM with marked trophoblastic hyperplasia and atypia, high free β-hCG levels, and heterozygous genotype. However, data concerning these three potential prognostic variables are inconsistent and conflicting (58,86,87,104–109).

The risk of developing GTN following PHM has been reported from 0% to 11%. Hancock et al. (110), summarizing the data from ten centers, reported that 73 of 7,155 patients (1.0%) required chemotherapy after evacuation of a partial mole. In a series of 240 patients who were followed for PHM at the NETDC, 16 (6.6%) developed nonmetastatic GTN (111). Only one of these patients presented with the classic signs and symptoms of molar disease including excessive uterine enlargement, theca lutein ovarian cysts, and high hCG levels. Fifteen (94%) patients were thought to have a missed abortion before evacuation. Our patients with partial moles who developed persistent disease did not have clinical features that distinguished them from other patients with partial moles. Flow cytometric studies of partial moles that developed persistent tumors showed a triploid pattern in 11 (85%) of 13 cases with interpretable histograms (112). A recent update of our experience with partial moles found that 22 of 390 patients (5.6%) developed GTN, and that pre-evacuation clinical symptoms did not distinguish those patients at risk for persistence (113).

Multiple Conceptions With Molar Pregnancy and Coexisting Fetuses

Twin pregnancy consisting of a CHM and a coexisting fetus has been estimated to occur in 1 per 22,000 to 100,000 pregnancies (114). We have reported our experience with 8 cases of twin pregnancy with complete mole and a coexisting fetus and reviewed 14 additional published cases by other researchers (115). Furthermore, we described one case of a partial mole coexisting with a normal fetus and placenta. As compared with singleton complete moles, twin pregnancies consisting of complete moles and coexisting fetuses have higher pre-evacuation hCG levels, have larger uteri, and are diagnosed later in pregnancy (116–118). GTN developed in 12 (55%) of 22 cases and 5 (22.7%) had metastatic tumor. Limited information is available to guide antenatal management of multiple gestations with complete moles and coexisting fetuses. These pregnancies are at risk for hemorrhage and preeclampsia. However, no patient died from obstetric or neoplastic complications, and five fetuses survived and no anomalies were detected. The increased availability of ovulation-induction drugs may result in more multiple gestations involving a molar pregnancy. While patients should be advised of the potential risks of neoplastic and obstetrical complications, it is appropriate in many cases to carefully monitor the course of the pregnancy in the hope that delivery at viability can be accomplished.

Surgical Evacuation

After diagnosing a molar pregnancy, the patient should be carefully evaluated to identify the potential presence of medical complications including preeclampsia, electrolyte imbalance, hyperthyroidism, and anemia that might complicate surgical evacuation. The patient is first stabilized and then a decision must be made concerning the most appropriate method of evacuation.

If the patient no longer desires to preserve fertility, hysterectomy may be performed. Prominent theca lutein ovarian cysts may be aspirated at the time of surgery. Patients should be counseled that although hysterectomy eliminates the risks of local invasion, it does not prevent metastasis.

Suction curettage is the preferred method of evacuation regardless of uterine size in patients who desire to preserve fertility (119,120). As the cervix is being dilated, the surgeon may encounter brisk uterine bleeding due to the passage of retained blood. Shortly after commencing suction evacuation, uterine bleeding is generally well controlled and the uterus rapidly regresses in size. If the uterus is larger than 14-weeks size, one hand should be placed on top of the fundus and the uterus should be massaged to stimulate uterine contraction. When suction evacuation is thought to be complete, a sharp curettage should be performed to remove any residual chorionic tissue. Patients who are Rh negative should receive Rh immune globulin at the time of evacuation because Rh D factor is expressed on trophoblast.

Role of Prophylactic Chemotherapy

The use of prophylactic chemotherapy at the time of molar evacuation remains controversial (121). However, several investigators have reported that chemoprophylaxis reduces the risk of postmolar tumor (91,122).

Kim et al. (123) performed a randomized, prospective trial of chemoprophylaxis in patients with complete mole. Chemoprophylaxis significantly reduced the incidence of postmolar tumor from 47% to 14% in patients with high-risk complete moles. However, chemoprophylaxis did not significantly influence the occurrence of persistent tumors in patients with low-risk complete moles. Similarly, Limpongsanurak (124) demonstrated in a double-blind randomized, controlled trial that actinomycin D (ACT D) reduced postmolar tumor in patients with high-risk complete moles from 50.0% to 13.8%.

We have also reported that prophylactic ACT D reduces the risk of persistent GTN in patients with high-risk complete moles (89). Only 10 (11%) of 93 patients with high-risk complete moles developed postmolar tumor after prophylactic ACT D. Chemoprophylaxis failure more commonly occurred in patients with markedly elevated hCG values. Prophylactic chemotherapy may be of benefit in patients with high-risk complete moles, particularly when hormonal follow-up is unavailable or unreliable.

Hormonal Follow-Up

After molar evacuation, all patients must be followed with hCG measurements to ensure remission. Patients should be followed with weekly hCG values until they are normal for 3 weeks and then monthly values until they are normal for 6 months. After achieving nondetectable hCG levels, the risk of relapse appears to be very low (113,125). In fact, several recent studies have confirmed that after obtaining a nondetectable serum hCG level, the risk of developing GTN following molar evacuation approaches zero (113,126). As more data is published it is possible that hCG follow-up can be safely abbreviated.

It is also possible to utilize hCG regression curves to develop criteria that determine a patient's risk of developing GTN or achieving remission after molar evacuation. Growdon et al. (127) observed that an hCG level of >199 mIU/mL in the 3rd through 8th week following partial molar evacuation was associated with at least a 35% risk of GTN. Similarly, Wolfberg et al.

(128) reported that postevacuation hCG levels could be used to predict both GTN and remission within a few weeks of molar evacuation in a study of 1,029 women diagnosed with CHM between 1973 and 2001. These data demonstrated that within 3 weeks of molar evacuation, more than half the women in the cohort had their risk of GTN modified to either >50% or <9%.

Patients are encouraged to use effective contraception during the entire interval of follow-up. Intrauterine devices should not be inserted until the patient achieves normal hCG levels because of the risk of uterine perforation, bleeding, and infection if residual tumor is present. If the patient does not desire surgical sterilization, she is then confronted with the choice of using either hormonal contraceptives or barrier methods.

The incidence of postmolar tumor has been reported to be increased in patients who used oral contraceptives (129). However, data from the NETDC (130), the Gynecologic Oncology Group (131), and the Brewer Center (130) indicate that oral contraceptives do not increase the risk of postmolar trophoblastic disease. Ho Yuen and Burch (132) also reported that the use of oral contraceptives containing 50 μg or less of estrogen was not associated with an increased risk of postmolar tumor. They speculated that the conflicting data concerning the use of oral contraceptives and the risk of postmolar tumor may be explained by differences in the dosage of estrogen. We therefore believe that oral contraceptives may be safely prescribed after molar evacuation.

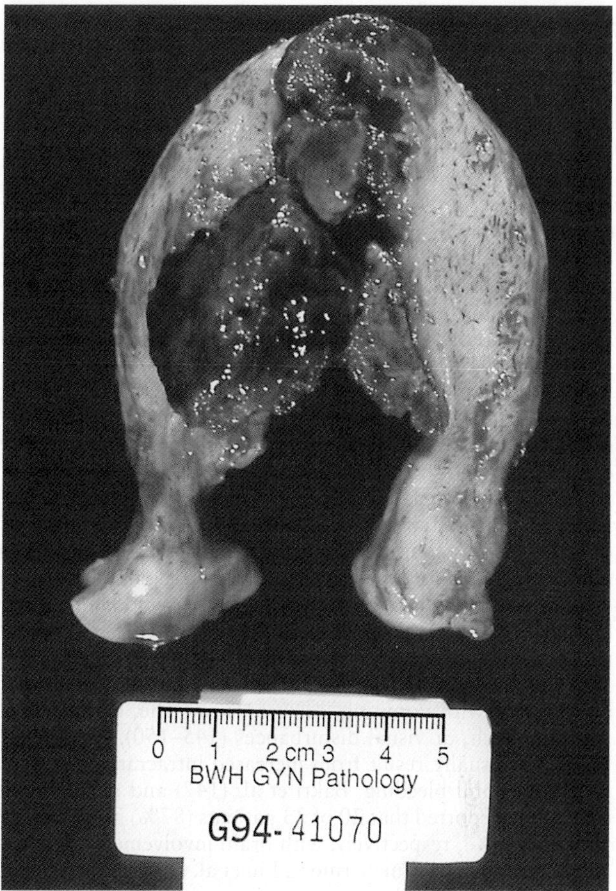

FIGURE 28.3. Uterine choriocarcinoma invading and replacing fundal myometrium.

GESTATIONAL TROPHOBLASTIC NEOPLASMS

Pathologic Considerations

After a molar pregnancy, persistent GTN may have the histologic pattern of either molar tissue or CCA. However, following a miscarriage or term pregnancy, GTN characteristically has only the histologic features of CCA (133). Gestational CCA does not contain chorionic villi, but is composed of sheets of both anaplastic cyto- and syncytiotrophoblasts. Since tubal moles can metastasize, the histologic pattern of GTN following an ectopic pregnancy can be either molar or CCA.

Placental-site trophoblastic tumor (PSTT) is an uncommon variant of CCA (134). This tumor is composed almost entirely of mononuclear intermediate trophoblast and does not contain chorionic villi. Because PSTTs secrete very small amounts of hCG, a large tumor burden may be present before hCG levels are detectable (135). PSTTs are associated with a higher percentage of free β-hCG, which can contribute to diagnosis (136,137).

Natural History

Nonmetastatic Disease

Locally invasive GTN develops in 15% of patients following evacuation of a complete mole and infrequently after other gestations (89). An invasive trophoblastic tumor may perforate through the myometrium, producing intraperitoneal bleeding, or erode into uterine vessels, causing vaginal hemorrhage (Fig. 28.3). A bulky necrotic tumor may also serve as a nidus for infection.

Metastatic Disease

Metastatic GTN occurs in 4% of patients after evacuation of CHM and infrequently after other pregnancies (89). GTN usually metastasizes as CCA because of its propensity for early vascular invasion with widespread dissemination. The most common metastatic sites are the lung (80%), vagina (30%), brain (10%), and liver (10%). Because trophoblastic tumors are perfused by fragile vessels, metastases are often hemorrhagic. Patients may present with signs and symptoms of bleeding from metastases such as hemoptysis, intraperitoneal bleeding, or acute neurologic deficits. Cerebral and hepatic metastases are uncommon unless there is concurrent involvement of the lungs and/or vagina.

Trophoblastic tumors produce four principal radiologic patterns in the lung: (a) pleural effusion, (b) alveolar or snowstorm pattern, (c) discrete rounded densities, or (d) embolic pattern caused by pulmonary arterial occlusion (138–141). Patients may develop pulmonary hypertension in the absence of substantial parenchymal involvement. The extent of pulmonary involvement may differ greatly among centers owing to differences in the frequency of early detection. In Saudi Arabia, Bakri et al. (141) reported that >50% opacification of the lungs, pleural effusion, and more than ten metastases were present in 33%, 48%, and 43% of patients, respectively, with pulmonary involvement. In contrast, in the United States, patients with pulmonary metastases generally have small nodules on chest radiography and infrequently present with prominent respiratory symptoms.

Patients with pulmonary metastases commonly have asymptomatic lesions on chest radiography or may present with dyspnea, chest pain, cough, or hemoptysis. Trophoblastic emboli may cause pulmonary arterial occlusion and lead to right-heart strain and pulmonary hypertension (142). Gynecologic symptoms may be minimal or absent and the antecedent pregnancy may be remote in time. The patient may be thought to have a primary pulmonary disease because respiratory symptoms may be dramatic. Unfortunately, the diagnosis of GTN may only be considered and established after the performance of a thoracotomy. *The diagnosis of GTN should be considered in any woman in the reproductive age group with unexplained systemic or pulmonary symptoms.*

Early respiratory failure requiring mechanical ventilation may develop in patients with extensive pulmonary involvement. Kelly et al. (143) and Bakri et al. (141) reported 100% mortality in 11 and 8 patients, respectively, with early respiratory failure. However, Vaccarello et al. (144) reported one patient who was cured following mechanical ventilation for respiratory failure. Risk factors for early respiratory failure within 1 month of presentation include >50% lung opacification, dyspnea, anemia, cyanosis, and pulmonary hypertension. With chemotherapy, patients may develop bleeding into metastatic sites and potentially worse pulmonary symptoms and radiologic findings. Importantly, Kelly et al. (143) also noted that reducing the initial dose of chemotherapy did not protect against early respiratory failure and recommended administering intensive chemotherapy at the outset.

Vaginal lesions may present with irregular bleeding or purulent discharge and are most commonly located in the fornices or suburethrally. Vaginal metastases are highly vascular and may bleed vigorously if biopsied. Biopsy of vaginal metastases should be absolutely avoided; the desire to avoid hemorrhage should supersede the interest of obtaining an unequivocal pathologic diagnosis.

Most patients with cerebral metastases are symptomatic and present with vomiting, seizures, headache, hemiparesis, slurred speech, or visual disturbances (145–150). Neurologic symptoms usually result from increased intracranial pressure or intracerebral bleeding. Bakri et al. (147) and Athanassiou et al. (149) reported that 20 of 23 patients (87%) and 66 of 69 patients (96%), respectively, with brain involvement had neurologic complaints. Furthermore, Liu et al. (150) reported that all 34 patients with brain metastases presented with neurologic symptoms.

Patients with liver metastases less commonly present with symptoms that are related to hepatic involvement. Bakri et al. (151) noted that only 5 (26%) of 19 patients with liver metastases presented with jaundice, intra-abdominal bleeding, or epigastric pain. Patients with liver metastases generally presented with symptoms related to pulmonary, vaginal, or cerebral involvement.

TABLE 28.2

FIGO ANATOMIC STAGING FOR GESTATIONAL TROPHOBLASTIC NEOPLASIA

Stage I	Disease confined to the uterus
Stage II	GTN extends outside of the uterus, but is limited to the genital structures (adnexa, vagina, broad ligament)
Stage III	GTN extends to the lungs, with or without known genital tract involvement
Stage IV	All other metastatic sites

Note: FIGO, International Federation of Gynecology and Obstetrics; GTN, gestational trophoblastic neoplasia.

Staging System

The International Federation of Gynecology and Obstetrics (FIGO) reports data on GTN using an anatomic staging system (Table 28.2). Staging enables a comparable reporting of data, which is critical to allow objective comparison of treatment results (152). Stage I includes all patients with persistently elevated hCG levels and tumor confined to the uterus. Stage II comprises all patients with tumor outside of the uterus but localized to the vagina and/or pelvis. Stage III includes all patients with pulmonary metastases with or without uterine, vaginal, or pelvic involvement. Stage IV patients have far-advanced disease with involvement of the brain, liver, kidneys, or gastrointestinal tract. Patients with stage IV disease are most likely to be resistant to chemotherapy. Stage IV tumors generally have the histologic pattern of CCA and commonly follow a nonmolar pregnancy, with protracted delays in diagnosis and large tumor burdens.

It is also helpful to use prognostic variables to predict the likelihood of drug resistance and to assist in selecting appropriate chemotherapy. The World Health Organization (WHO) has published a prognostic scoring system based on one published by Bagshawe in 1976 (1) that reliably predicts the potential for chemotherapy resistance (Table 28.3). The current

TABLE 28.3

MODIFIED WHO PROGNOSTIC SCORING SYSTEM AS ADAPTED BY FIGO

Scores	0	1	2	4
Age	<40	>40	—	—
Antecedent pregnancy	Mole	Abortion	Term	—
Interval months from index pregnancy	<4	4–7	7–13	>13
Pretreatment serum hCG (IU/L)	<1000	<10,000	<100,000	>100,000
Largest tumor size (including uterus)	—	3 to <5 cm	>5 cm	—
Site of metastases	Lung	Spleen/kidney	GI	Liver/brain
Number of metastases	—	1–4	5–8	>8
Previous failed chemotherapy	—	—	Single drug	Two or more drugs

Note: Format for reporting to FIGO Annual Report: In order to stage and allot a risk factor score, a patient's diagnosis is allocated to a stage as represented by a Roman numeral: I, II, III, and IV. This is then separated by a colon from the sum of all the actual risk factor scores expressed in arabic numerals, e.g., stage II:4, stage IV:9. This stage and score will be alloted for each patient. FIGO, International Federation of Gynecology and Obstetrics; WHO, World Health Organization.

FIGO staging system combines both anatomic staging and the prognostic scoring system. When the prognostic score is 7 or greater, the patient is considered to be "high-risk" and requires intensive combination chemotherapy for optimal results. In general, patients with stage I disease have a low-risk score and patients with stage IV disease have a high-risk score. Therefore, the distinction between low and high risk primarily applies to stages II and III. The variables that are included in the prognostic score include (a) tumor volume (hCG level, size of metastases, and number of metastases); (b) site of involvement; (c) prior chemotherapy exposure; and (d) duration of disease. In 1965, Ross et al. (153) reported that patients with high hCG levels, prolonged delays in diagnosis, and brain or liver metastases were relatively resistant to single-agent chemotherapy. Hammond et al. (154) further observed in 1973 that patients with prior chemotherapy or an antecedent term pregnancy were also relatively unresponsive to single-agent chemotherapy. Several investigators have since strongly confirmed the importance and reliability of these prognostic factors (155–162).

Choriocarcinoma following term pregnancy has been noted to be a poor-prognosis factor and to have some distinctive clinical features (163–167). We reviewed our experience with post-term CCA at the NETDC from 1964 to 1996 (164). Seven (16%) of 44 patients presented with clinical evidence of maternal-fetal bleeding, resulting in severe anemia and nonimmune hydrops or third-trimester bleeding. Although none of the infants had evidence of metastatic CCA, rare cases of fetal involvement have been reported and generally have resulted in fetal death. The time interval from delivery to diagnosis, sites of metastases, and pretreatment hCG level were all significant risk factors in predicting outcome. All 31 patients with a WHO score ≤8 survived, whereas 6 of 13 (46%) patients with a WHO score >8 died. A recent retrospective multicenter cohort study in the Netherlands of 68 patients with CCA by Lok et al. (167) concluded that although antecedent term pregnancy is considered an adverse prognostic factor in GTN, current survival is comparable to the general survival in high-risk patients with optimal therapy.

Diagnostic Evaluation

The optimal management of a GTN requires a thorough evaluation of the extent of the disease prior to treatment. All patients should undergo a thorough assessment including a complete history and physical examination; a baseline hCG level; hepatic, thyroid, and renal function tests; and chest radiograph. If the chest x-ray is negative a computed tomographic (CT) scan should be obtained. Asymptomatic patients with a normal pelvic examination and negative chest CT are very unlikely to have liver or brain metastases identified by further radiographic studies. However, patients with vaginal or lung metastases and/or a pathologic diagnosis of choriocarcinoma should undergo either a CT scan or magnetic resonance imaging (MRI) scan of the head and abdomen to exclude brain and liver involvement.

Cerebral involvement may also be assessed by measuring hCG levels in the cerebrospinal fluid (CSF). Bagshawe and Harland (168) reported that the plasma/CSF hCG ratio tends to be <60 in the presence of brain metastases. However, a single plasma/CSF hCG ratio may be misleading because very rapid changes in plasma hCG values may not be promptly reflected in the CSF (169). For example, Bakri et al. (170) observed that the serum/CSF hCG ratio was >60 in five of ten patients with cerebral involvement.

Pelvic ultrasonography may be useful to detect extensive uterine involvement by trophoblastic tumor and to identify sites of resistant uterine disease (171). However, ultrasound should not be performed merely to document nonmetastatic disease (172). The sensitivity of ultrasonography may be further enhanced by the use of color flow Doppler as well as the vaginal probe (173–175). Ultrasonography may be helpful to select patients who will benefit from hysterectomy because it can accurately detect an extensive uterine trophoblastic tumor (176).

Management

Stage I

Tables 28.4 and 28.5 review the NETDC protocol for the management of stage I disease and the results of therapy. The selection of treatment is based mainly on the patient's desire to preserve fertility. If the patient no longer wishes to retain fertility, hysterectomy with adjuvant single-agent chemotherapy may be performed as primary treatment. Adjuvant chemotherapy is administered for three reasons: (a) to reduce the likelihood of disseminating viable tumor cells at surgery, (b) to maintain a cytotoxic level of chemotherapy in the bloodstream and tissues in case viable tumor cells are disseminated at surgery, and (c) to treat any occult metastases that may already be present at the time of surgery. Occult pulmonary metastases may be detected by CT scan in about 40% of patients with presumed nonmetastatic disease (177,178). Chemotherapy may be safely administered at the time of hysterectomy without increasing operative complications. Thirty-two patients were treated by primary hysterectomy and adjuvant chemotherapy at the NETDC and all achieved complete remission with no additional therapy.

Single-agent chemotherapy is the preferred treatment in patients with stage I disease who desire to retain fertility. Primary single-agent chemotherapy induced complete remission in 419 (84%) of 502 patients with stage I GTN. The remaining 83 resistant patients subsequently attained remission with either combination chemotherapy or surgical intervention. If the patient is resistant to chemotherapy and wants to preserve fertility, local uterine resection may be considered. When local resection is planned, ultrasound, MRI, arteriography, and/or positron emission tomography (PET) scan may

TABLE 28.4

TREATMENT PROTOCOLS FOR STAGE I GTN (NEW ENGLAND TROPHOBLASTIC DISEASE CENTER)

INITIAL
Sequential MTX/ACT D
Hysterectomy (with adjunctive single-agent chemotherapy)
RESISTANT TO BOTH SINGLE AGENTS
MAC
EMACO, if MAC fails
Hysterectomy (with adjunctive multiagent chemotherapy)
Local uterine resection (for localized lesion, to preserve fertility)
FOLLOW-UP
Twelve consecutive months of normal hCG levels
Contraception mandatory

Note: ACT D, actinomycin D; EMACO, etoposide, methotrexate, actinomycin D, cyclophosphamide (Cytoxan), vincristine (Oncovin); GTN, gestational trophoblastic neoplasia; hCG, human chorionic gonadotropin; MAC, methotrexate, actinomycin D, cyclophosphamide (Cytoxan); MTX, methotrexate.

TABLE 28.5

STAGE I. CONFINED TO THE UTERINE CORPUS (NEW ENGLAND TROPHOBLASTIC DISEASE CENTER, JULY 1965 TO JUNE 2006)

Remission therapy	No. of patients (%)	No. of remissions (%)
INITIAL THERAPY	460 (85)	
Sequential MTX/ACT D		419 (77)
Hysterectomy, local resection		32 (6)
Other		9 (2)
RESISTANT THERAPY	83 (5)	
MAC		17 (3)
EMA, EMACO, other		51 (9)
Hysterectomy, local resection, etc.		15 (3)
TOTAL	543 (100)	543 (100)

Note: ACT D, actinomycin D; EMA, etoposide, methotrexate, actinomycin D; EMACO, etoposide, methotrexate, actinomycin D, cyclophosphamide (Cytoxan), vincristine (Oncovin); MAC, methotrexate, actinomycin D, cyclophosphamide (Cytoxan); MTX, methotrexate.

identify the site of resistant tumor (179,180). Two of our patients who underwent local uterine resection achieved remission, and one of these patients had a later term delivery by cesarean section.

Nonmetastatic PSTT should be treated with primary hysterectomy because this tumor responds poorly to chemotherapy. However, despite its relative resistance to chemotherapy, long-term survivors with metastatic disease have been reported with the use of combination chemotherapy (134,181–184). Papadopoulos et al. (181), in reviewing the clinical experience with 34 patients with PSTT at the Charing Cross Hospital, found that a long interval from the antecedent pregnancy to clinical presentation was the most important prognostic factor. Whereas all 27 patients survived when the interval from the antecedent pregnancy was less than 4 years, all 7 patients died when the time interval exceeded 4 years. Similarly, Lathrop et al. (135) reported in a review of 43 patients that all ten fatal cases of PSTT had a more than 2-year interval from antecedent pregnancy to diagnosis. However, whereas Lathrop et al. reported that the mitotic rate was prognostically important, Papadopoulos et al. also observed that the mitotic rate of PSTT was not related to outcome.

Stages II and III

The NETDC protocol for the management of stage II and III disease and the results of treatment are outlined in Tables 28.6, 28.7, and 28.8. Low-risk patients (prognostic score <7) can be optimally treated with primary single-agent chemotherapy. High-risk patients (prognostic score 7 or above) should receive combination chemotherapy as the primary modality (185).

Between July 1965 and June 2006, 28 patients with stage II disease were treated at the NETDC and all achieved remission. Single-agent chemotherapy induced complete remission in 16 of 20 (80%) low-risk patients. In contrast, only two of eight high-risk patients achieved remission with single-agent treatment.

Single-agent chemotherapy is well recognized to be effective as primary treatment in low-risk metastatic GTN (185,186). Summarizing the experience from four centers, single-agent chemotherapy induced complete remission in 128 (87.1%) of 147 patients with low-risk metastatic GTN (186–190). All patients who were resistant to single-agent chemotherapy later achieved remission with combination chemotherapy except two patients reported by Ayhan et al. (188).

Vaginal metastases may bleed profusely because they are highly vascular and friable. Bleeding may be controlled by packing the hemorrhagic lesion or performing wide local excision. Infrequently, angiographic embolization of the hypogastric arteries may be required to control hemorrhage from vaginal metastases. Yingna et al. (191) reported that 18 (35.3%) of 51 patients with vaginal metastases presented with vaginal hemorrhage. Bleeding was controlled by vaginal packing in 16 patients and angiographic embolization in 2 patients. Tse et al. (192) in a 20-year retrospective study confirmed that angiographic embolization appeared to be an attractive and promising alternative to hysterectomy and arterial ligation.

TABLE 28.6

TREATMENT PROTOCOL FOR STAGES II AND III GTN (NEW ENGLAND TROPHOBLASTIC DISEASE CENTER)

LOW RISK	
Initial therapy	Sequential MTX/ACT D
Resistant therapy	MAC or EMACO
	Surgery, as indicated
HIGH RISK	
Initial therapy	EMACO
Resistant therapy	EMAEP; VBP
FOLLOW-UP	
Twelve consecutive months of nondetectable hCG levels	
Contraception for 12 months	

Note: ACT D, actinomycin D; EMACO, etoposide, methotrexate, actinomycin D, cyclophosphamide (Cytoxan), vincristine (Oncovin); EMAEP, etoposide, methotrexate, actinomycin D, carboplatin; GTN, gestational trophoblastic neoplasia; hCG, human chorionic gonadotropin; MAC, methotrexate, actinomycin D, cyclophosphamide (Cytoxan); MTX, methotrexate; VBP, vinblastine (Velban), bleomycin, carboplatin.

TABLE 28.7

STAGE II. METASTASES TO PELVIS AND VAGINA (NEW ENGLAND TROPHOBLASTIC DISEASE CENTER, JULY 1965 TO JUNE 2006)

Remission therapy	No. of patients (%)	No. of remissions (%)
LOW RISK	20 (72)	
Initial therapy		
Sequential MTX/ACT D		16 (80)
Resistant therapy		
MAC, EMACO		4 (20)
HIGH RISK	8 (28)	
Initial therapy		
Sequential MTX/ACT D		2 (25)
MAC		4 (50)
Resistant therapy		
MAC, other		2 (25)
TOTAL	28 (100)	28 (100)

Note: ACT D, actinomycin D; EMACO, etoposide, methotrexate, actinomycin D, cyclophosphamide (Cytoxan), vincristine (Oncovin); MAC, methotrexate, actinomycin D, cyclophosphamide (Cytoxan); MTX, methotrexate.

Between July 1965 and June 2006, 161 patients with stage III tumors were managed at the NETDC and 160 (99.3%) attained complete remission. Single-agent chemotherapy induced complete remission in 82% of patients with low-risk disease and in 27% with high-risk disease. All but one patient who was resistant to single-agent treatment later achieved remission with combination chemotherapy.

Thoracotomy has a limited role in the management of stage III GTN. Thoracotomy should be performed if the diagnosis is seriously in doubt. Furthermore, if a patient has a persistent viable pulmonary nodule despite intensive chemotherapy, pulmonary resection may be performed (193). However, an extensive metastatic survey should be obtained to exclude other sites of persistent tumor. It is important to emphasize that fibrotic nodules may persist indefinitely on the chest radiograph after complete hCG remission is achieved (194). If a metastasis is persistent on radiography, but is of questionable viability, either a scan with a radioisotope-labeled antibody to hCG or a PET scan may be useful (180). A radioisotope hCG or PET scan may also be helpful in identifying occult sites of viable tumor (195). Tomoda et al. (196) reviewed their experience with pulmonary resection in 19 patients with chemotherapy-resistant GTN. They proposed the following guidelines for successful resection: (a) good surgical candidate, (b) primary malignancy is controlled, (c) no evidence of other metastatic sites, (d) pulmonary metastasis is limited to one lung, and (e) hCG level is <1,000 mIU/mL. Complete remission was achieved in 14 of 15 patients who met all five criteria, but in none of the 4 patients who had one or more unfavorable clinical features. Similarly, Jones

TABLE 28.8

STAGE III. METASTASES TO LUNG (NEW ENGLAND TROPHOBLASTIC DISEASE CENTER, JULY 1965 TO JUNE 2006)

Remission therapy	No. of patients (%)	No. of remissions (%)
LOW RISK	110 (68)	
Initial therapy		
Sequential MTX, ACT		90 (82)
Resistant therapy		
MAC, EMACO, EMAEP		20 (18)
HIGH RISK	51 (32)	
Initial therapy		
Sequential MTX/ACT D		14 (27)
MAC, EMACO		27 (53)
Resistant therapy		
EMAEP, VBP		9 (18)
TOTAL	161 (100)	160/161 (99)

Note: ACT D, actinomycin D; EMACO, etoposide, methotrexate, actinomycin D, cyclophosphamide (Cytoxan), vincristine (Oncovin); EMAEP, etoposide, methotrexate, actinomycin D, carboplatin; MAC, methotrexate, actinomycin D, cyclophosphamide (Cytoxan); MTX, methotrexate; VBP, vinblastine (Velban), bleomycin, carboplatin.

TABLE 28.9

TREATMENT PROTOCOL FOR STAGE IV GTN (NEW ENGLAND TROPHOBLASTIC DISEASE CENTER, JULY 1965 TO JUNE 2006)

INITIAL
EMACO
With brain metastases—radiation; craniotomy for peripheral lesions
With liver metastases—embolization; resection to manage complications

RESISTANT
Salvage chemotherapy—EMAEP; VBP; experimental protocols
Surgery, as indicated

FOLLOW-UP
Weekly hCG levels until undetectable for 3 weeks, then monthly for 24 months
Contraception for 24 months

Note: EMACO, etoposide, methotrexate, actinomycin D, cyclophosphamide (Cytoxan), vincristine (Oncovin); EMAEP, etoposide, methotrexate, actinomycin D, carboplatin; GTN, gestational trophoblastic neoplasia; hCG, human chorionic gonadotropin; VBP, vinblastine (Velban), bleomycin, carboplatin.

et al. (197) reported that six (66.7%) of nine carefully selected patients with drug-resistant pulmonary GTN attained complete remission following lung resection. Several investigators have reported that undetectable hCG levels within 1 to 2 weeks of resection of a solitary pulmonary nodule are highly predictive of a favorable outcome (198–202). Survival following salvage surgery is influenced by the number of preoperative chemotherapy regimens, number of disease sites, and the WHO score.

Hysterectomy may be required in patients with metastatic GTN to control uterine hemorrhage or sepsis. Furthermore, in patients with bulky uterine tumor, hysterectomy may reduce the tumor burden and thereby limit the need for chemotherapy. Hammond et al. (203) reported that patients who underwent hysterectomy had a shorter duration of hospitalization and chemotherapy. Angiographic embolization can also be effective in the management of profuse uterine bleeding in lieu of hysterectomy, especially in those patients who are hemodynamically stable and wish to retain their fertility potential (192).

Stage IV

Tables 28.9 and 28.10 outline the NETDC protocol for the management of stage IV disease and the results of treatment. These patients are at high risk for developing rapidly progressive disease despite intensive therapy.

All patients with stage IV disease should be treated with intensive combination chemotherapy and the selective use of radiation therapy and surgery (2,37). Before 1975, only 6 (30%) of 20 patients with stage IV disease attained complete remission. However, after 1975, 16 (80%) of 20 patients with stage IV tumors achieved remission. This dramatic improvement in survival resulted from the introduction of intensive multimodal therapy early in the course of treatment.

The management of hepatic metastases is particularly difficult and challenging. Hepatic resection may be required to control bleeding or to excise resistant tumor. Grumbine et al. (204) reported the use of selective occlusion of the hepatic arteries and concurrent combination chemotherapy in a patient with bleeding liver metastases who ultimately attained remission. Importantly, Wong et al. (205) noted that nine of ten patients with hepatic involvement achieved complete remission with primary intensive combination chemotherapy without any hepatic irradiation. Bakri et al. (151) similarly reported that five of eight (62.5%) patients with liver metastases who were treated with combination chemotherapy alone attained complete remission.

If cerebral metastases are detected, irradiation is promptly instituted at the NETDC. The presence of multiple lesions requires treatment to the whole head, while a solitary lesion can be treated locally. Solitary lesions can also be resected (206). The risk of spontaneous cerebral hemorrhage is reduced by the concurrent use of chemotherapy and brain

TABLE 28.10

STAGE IV. DISTANT METASTASES (NEW ENGLAND TROPHOBLASTIC DISEASE CENTER, JULY 1965 TO JUNE 2006)

Remission therapy	No. of patients (%)	No. of remissions (%)
Before 1975	20	
Sequential MTX/ACT D		5 (25)
MAC		1 (5)
After and including 1975	20	
Sequential MTX/ACT D		2 (10)
MAC, EMA, EMACO, etc.		14 (70)

Note: ACT D, actinomycin D; EMACO, etoposide, methotrexate, actinomycin D, cyclophosphamide (Cytoxan), vincristine (Oncovin); EMA, etoposide, methotrexate, actinomycin D; MAC, methotrexate, actinomycin D, cyclophosphamide (Cytoxan); MTX, methotrexate.

irradiation (207). Brain irradiation may also be tumoricidal. Yordan et al. (208) reported that deaths due to central nervous system involvement occurred in 11 (44%) of 25 patients treated with chemotherapy alone, but in none of 18 patients treated with brain irradiation and chemotherapy.

However, Newlands et al. (145) have reported excellent remission rates in patients with cerebral metastases who were treated with chemotherapy alone. Thirty of 35 (86%) patients with cerebral lesions achieved sustained remission with intensive combination chemotherapy including high-dose intravenous and intrathecal methotrexate (MTX). None of their patients received external beam brain irradiation.

In addition to its efficacy in removing solitary peripheral metastases, craniotomy is most useful for the management of life-threatening complications, which then allows the opportunity for chemotherapy to induce a complete remission. Infrequently, cerebral metastases that prove resistant to chemotherapy may be amenable to resection. Evans et al. (206) reported complete remission in three of four patients who underwent craniotomy to relieve intracranial pressure, and in two of three patients undergoing craniotomy for resection of chemotherapy-resistant tumor. Athanassiou et al. (149) similarly reported that four of five patients undergoing craniotomy for acute intracranial complications were ultimately cured. They also observed that most patients with cerebral metastases who achieve remission generally have no residual neurologic deficits.

Follow-Up

All patients with stage I, II, and III GTN should be followed with weekly hCG tests until normal for 3 consecutive weeks, and then monthly for 12 months. Patients are encouraged to use contraception during the entire interval of follow-up. Patients with stage IV disease are followed with weekly hCG values until normal for 3 weeks and then monthly for 24 months. These patients require prolonged follow-up because they have an increased risk of late recurrence.

False-Positive hCG Tests

It is important for clinicians to recognize that hCG molecules in GTN are more degraded or heterogeneous in serum than they are in normal pregnancy (209). Trophoblastic disease samples contain high proportions of free β-hCG, nicked hCG, and β-core fragment (210). When monitoring patients with GTN, it is therefore desirable to use an assay that detects not only intact hCG, but also all of its metabolites and fragments (211–214).

Many hCG assays have a degree of cross reactivity with luteinizing hormone. Following multiple courses of combination chemotherapy, ovarian steroidal function may be damaged, particularly in patients in their late 30s and 40s. When ovarian function is damaged, luteinizing hormone levels may rise, and owing to cross reactivity, the patient may be falsely thought to have persistent low levels of hCG. Patients who receive combination chemotherapy should therefore be placed on oral contraceptives to suppress luteinizing hormone levels and prevent problems with cross reactivity.

It is important to emphasize that some patients may have a false-positive elevation in serum hCG measurement owing to the presence of circulating heterophilic antibody called "phantom hCG" (211). These patients with phantom hCG or phantom CCA often have no clear antecedent pregnancy and no progressive rise in their hCG levels. The possibility of false-positive hCG measurement should be assessed by sending both serum and urine samples to a reference hCG laboratory. Patients with phantom hCG generally have no measurable hCG in a parallel urine sample.

Quiescent GTN

Low-level "real" hCG has recently been recognized as a new clinical entity called quiescent GTN that presents a clinical challenge to physicians who treat patients with GTN. These patients have had a molar pregnancy or other type of GTN and the hCG level initially regresses, but persists at very low levels (mostly in the nonhyperglycosylated form) for many weeks or months. In these women, extensive workup reveals no lesion in the uterus or elsewhere, and administering chemotherapy is not effective. In these patients careful follow-up is recommended, since approximately 6% to 10% will ultimately relapse with rising hCG levels. At that point in time, chemotherapy will prove effective. In all such patients who develop active disease, hyperglycosylated hCG is the major component of the hCG present (214–217).

Recurrent GTN

Mutch et al. (218) reported recurrences after initial remission in 2% of patients with nonmetastatic GTN, 4% of patients with good-prognosis metastatic GTN, and 13% of patients with poor-prognosis disease. Relapses developed within 3 and 18 months in 50% and 85% of patients, respectively. Similarly, we observed relapse after initial remission in 2.9% of stage I, 8.3% of stage II, 4.2% of stage III, and 9.1% of stage IV patients (219). The mean time to recurrence from the last nondetectable hCG level was 6 months, and this did not differ among the four FIGO stages. All patients with stage I, II, and III GTN who developed recurrence were subsequently cured, whereas both stage IV patients with recurrences died. Recently, Ngan et al. (220), reporting on a 20-year experience treating GTN in Hong Kong, observed that the median interval from remission to relapse was 6.5 months. They concluded that the most important risk factors for recurrence were attributable to patients who defaulted treatment or follow-up, and those who presented with massive disease. Yang et al. (221) in studying 901 patients with GTN who received treatment in Beijing reported a mean interval from remission to relapse of 15.3 months. The four recurrence-associated risk factors in this study identified by multivariate analysis were (a) clinical stage, (b) an interval of >12 months between the antecedent pregnancy and the start of chemotherapy, (c) a negative blood β-hCG titer after seven courses of chemotherapy, and (d) less than two courses of consolidation chemotherapy .

Chemotherapy

Single-Agent Chemotherapy

In 1956, Li et al. (222) reported the dramatic cure of metastatic CCA in three women by using MTX. In 1961, Hertz et al. (223) reviewed the initial 5-year experience with chemotherapy in treating metastatic GTN. Importantly, MTX alone induced complete remission in 28 (44%) of 63 patients with metastatic disease. After achieving impressive results in patients with metastatic disease, Hertz et al. (224) used MTX as the primary treatment of nonmetastatic GTN. Complete remission was attained in all 16 women with nonmetastatic disease by administering MTX alone. Chemotherapy, therefore, obviated the need for hysterectomy and enabled patients to attain cure while retaining their fertility. Although MTX induced cure in many patients, it was still necessary to identify other active chemotherapeutic agents. Ross et al. (225) first used actinomycin D (ACT D) in 13 patients with MTX-resistant GTN and 6 (46%) patients attained complete remission.

Since the early 1960s, MTX and ACT D have remained the two central drugs in the treatment of patients with GTN.

Single-agent chemotherapy with either ACT D or MTX has induced comparable and excellent remission rates in both nonmetastatic and metastatic GTN (226). An optimal regimen should maximize the cure rate while minimizing toxicity. Many protocols have been evaluated for administering ACT D and MTX as single agents in nonmetastatic and low-risk metastatic GTN (190,226–236). Several regimens of ACT D and MTX have induced complete remission in 70% to 100% of patients with nonmetastatic GTN and in 50% to 70% of patients with low-risk metastatic disease. Fortunately, if a patient develops resistance to the initial single-agent chemotherapeutic treatment, it is still likely that the patient may achieve remission with an alternative single agent.

In 1964, Bagshawe and Wilde (237) first reported administering MTX with folinic acid (MTX/FA) to reduce chemotherapeutic toxicity. MTX/FA has remained the primary treatment of nonmetastatic and low-risk metastatic GTN at the Charing Cross Hospital. Although MTX/FA is highly effective, resistance develops in 20%, and ACT D is then used sequentially.

MTX/FA has been the preferred single-agent regimen in the treatment of GTN at the NETDC since 1974 (238–240). Between September 1974 and September 1984, 185 patients with GTN were treated with primary MTX/FA at the NETDC. Complete remission was induced with MTX/FA in 162 (87.6%) patients, and 132 (81.5%) of these patients required only one course of MTX/FA to achieve remission. MTX/FA induced remission in 147 (90.2%) of 163 patients with stage I and in 15 (68.2%) of 22 patients with low-risk stages II and III. Among the 23 patients who were resistant to MTX/FA, 14 (61%) achieved remission with ACT D and remission was accomplished with combination chemotherapy in the remaining 9. Toxicity to MTX/FA including thrombocytopenia, granulocytopenia, and hepatotoxicity occurred in only 11 (5.9%), 3 (1.6%), and 26 (14.1%) patients, respectively. No patient required platelet transfusions or developed sepsis due to myelosuppression, and no patient developed alopecia. MTX/FA not only induces an excellent remission rate with minimal toxicity, but also effectively limits chemotherapy exposure (241). The MTX/FA regimen is administered over 8 days (MTX 1 mg/kg intramuscularly on days 1, 3, 5, and 7 and folinic acid 0.1 mg/kg intramuscularly or orally on days 2, 4, 6, and 8), and its effectiveness may be partly attributable to the prolonged exposure to MTX. When we infused MTX at a higher dosage (300 mg/m^2) over 12 hours and 30 minutes, the remission rate declined to 69% in patients with nonmetastatic disease (242).

Whereas MTX and ACT D are the two most commonly used single agents in the treatment of GTN in the United States and in most of the world, 5-fluorouracil (5FU) has been the preferred single-agent chemotherapy in China. Sung et al. (243) reported that 5FU induced complete remission in 93% of patients with stage I and in 86% of patients with stage II GTN. Etoposide has also been utilized as a single agent in the management of both nonmetastatic and metastatic disease with considerable success (244).

Combination Chemotherapy

Modified triple therapy with MTX/FA, ACT D, and cyclophosphamide had been the preferred combination drug regimen at the NETDC (245). However, triple therapy is inadequate as an initial treatment in patients with high-risk metastatic disease (prognostic score 7 or >7). Summarizing the experience from six centers, triple therapy induced complete remission in 47 (51%) of 92 patients with metastatic GTN and a high-risk WHO score (154–158,160, 188,189,245–247).

Etoposide (VP16) has been demonstrated to be a highly active antitumor agent in GTN. Primary oral etoposide induced complete sustained remission in 56 (93.3%) of 60 patients with nonmetastatic or low-risk metastatic disease (244). Bagshawe (248) reported an 83% remission rate in patients with metastatic disease and a high-risk score using a combination regimen that included etoposide. This regimen (EMACO) includes etoposide, MTX, ACT D, cyclophosphamide, and vincristine (Oncovin) and is currently the preferred treatment for patients with high-risk metastatic GTN. Bolis et al. (249), Lurain et al. (250), and Soper et al. (251) have similarly reported that EMACO induced complete remission in 13 (76%) of 17, in 20 (67%) of 30, and in 4 (67%) of 6 patients, respectively, with metastatic GTN and a high-risk score. Furthermore, Bower et al. (252) and Kim et al. (253) reported that primary EMACO induced remission in 130 (86.1%) of 151 patients and in 87 (90.6%) of 96 patients, respectively, with high-risk metastatic GTN. Therefore, EMACO is highly effective as primary therapy, inducing complete remission in 70% to 90% of patients with high-risk metastatic GTN.

If patients experience resistance to EMACO, they may then successfully be treated with a modification of this regimen by substituting etoposide and cisplatin on day 8 (EMAEP) (250–255). Bower et al. (252) reported that EMAEP induced remission, alone or in conjunction with surgery, in 16 (76%) of 21 patients who were resistant to EMACO. Lurain et al. (250) also noted the efficacy of using platinum. He observed that eight of ten patients (80%) resistant to EMACO were placed in remission with platinum-based chemotherapy. When patients develop resistance to EMACO, surgical intervention may also be necessary to remove sites of resistant tumor (255,256).

Unfortunately, the use of etoposide has been reported to increase the risk of later secondary tumors including myeloid leukemia, melanoma, colon cancer, and breast cancer (257). The relative risk for leukemia, melanoma, colon cancer, and breast cancer was increased by 16.6%, 3.4%, 4.6%, and 5.8%, respectively, in patients who received >2 gms/M^2. The increased risk for breast cancer did not become apparent until after 25 years. Among all patients who were treated with etoposide, 1.5% subsequently developed leukemia. Etoposide should therefore be used only with high-risk metastatic disease. When patients with nonmetastatic and low-risk metastatic GTN experience resistance to MTX and ACT D, it is reasonable to consider administering triple therapy before treatment with regimens containing etoposide (258).

Second-line therapy with cisplatin, vinblastine, and bleomycin (PUB) may also be effective in patients with drug-resistant GTN. Gordon et al. (259), DuBeshter et al. (260), and Azab et al. (261) reported that PUB induced complete remission in 2 of 11 patients, 4 of 7 patients, and 5 of 8 patients, respectively, with drug-resistant GTN.

The potential role of autologous bone marrow transplantation or stem-cell rescue in GTN has yet to be defined. However, individual cases have been reported where high-dose chemotherapy with autologous bone marrow or stem-cell support has induced complete remission in patients with refractory GTN (262,263).

Despite the efficacy of the well-recognized regimens used in treating GTN, efforts continue to identify new agents that are effective in treating patients with resistance. Although ifosfamide and paclitaxel (Taxol) are both active in treating GTN, further studies must be performed to determine their potential role in either primary treatment or second-line therapy (264,265). Osborne et al. (266) have reported that a novel three-drug doublet regimen, consisting of paclitaxel, etoposide, and cisplatin (TE/TO), induced complete remission in two patients with relapsed high-risk GTN. Wan et al. (267) analyzed the efficacy of floxuridine (FUDR)-containing regimens in the treatment of patients with invasive mole and CCA, some of whom had shown resistance to other regimens. Twenty-one

TABLE 28.11

SUBSEQUENT PREGNANCIES IN PATIENTS WITH COMPLETE MOLE (NEW ENGLAND TROPHOBLASTIC DISEASE CENTER, JUNE 1, 1965, TO NOVEMBER 20, 2001)

Outcome	No. of patients	%
Term delivery	877	68.6
Stillbirth	7	0.5
Premature delivery	95	7.4
Spontaneous abortion		
First trimester	221	17.3
Second trimester	8	0.6
Therapeutic abortion	41	3.2
Ectopic pregnancy	11	0.9
Repeat molar pregnancy	18	1.4
Total pregnancies	1,278	
Congenital malformations (major and minor)		40/979 (4.1)
Primary cesarean section		70/373 (18.8)[a]

[a]January 1979 to November 2001.

patients with drug-resistant GTN received FUDR-containing regimens and all patients achieved remission. Matsui et al. (268) found that 5FU in combination with ACT D could also be used as salvage therapy and induced complete remission in 9 of 11 (82%) patients with drug-resistant GTN.

Patients who require combination chemotherapy should be treated intensively to attain remission. Treatment delay or dose reduction due to chemotherapy-induced neutropenia may contribute to tumor resistance and treatment failure. Since the goal of therapy is cure of the disease, unnecessary treatment delays and dose reduction must be avoided, particularly in high-risk patients. Recombinant hematopoietic growth factors and platelet transfusion should be used. We administer combination chemotherapy as frequently as toxicity permits until the patient attains three consecutive normal hCG values. After the patient achieves normal hCG levels, three additional courses of chemotherapy are administered to reduce the risk of relapse.

Subsequent Pregnancies

Pregnancies After Hydatidiform Mole

Patients with CHM can anticipate normal reproduction in the future (103). Patients with complete moles who were treated at the NETDC had 1,278 later pregnancies between June 1965 and November 2001. These pregnancies resulted in 877 (68.6%) full-term live births, 95 (7.4%) premature deliveries, 11 (0.9%) ectopic pregnancies, and seven (0.5%) stillbirths (Table 28.11). First-trimester spontaneous abortion occurred in 221 (17.3%) pregnancies, and major and minor congenital malformations were detected in only 40 (4.1%) infants. Primary cesarean section was performed in only 70 (18.8%) of 373 subsequent full-term and premature births between January 1979 and November 2001.

Limited information is available regarding the later pregnancy experience in patients with partial moles (Table 28.12).

TABLE 28.12

SUBSEQUENT PREGNANCIES IN PATIENTS WITH PARTIAL MOLE (NEW ENGLAND TROPHOBLASTIC DISEASE CENTER, JUNE 1, 1965, TO NOVEMBER 20, 2001)

Outcome	No. of patients	%
Term delivery	189	75.3
Stillbirth	1	0.4
Premature delivery	4	1.6
Spontaneous abortion		
First trimester	38	15.1
Second trimester	1	0.4
Therapeutic abortion	11	4.4
Ectopic pregnancy	1	0.4
Repeat molar pregnancy	6	2.4
Total pregnancies	251	
Congenital malformations (major and minor)		3/194 (1.5)
Primary cesarean section		29/194 (14.9)[a]

[a]January 1979 to November 2001.

Between June 1965 and November 2001, patients with partial moles at the NETDC had 251 subsequent gestations that resulted in 189 (75.3%) full-term live births, one (0.4%) stillbirth, one (0.4%) ectopic pregnancy, and four (1.6%) premature deliveries. First-trimester spontaneous abortion occurred in 38 (15.1%) pregnancies, and major or minor congenital anomalies were detected in only three (1.5%) infants. The preliminary data concerning subsequent conceptions after partial moles are therefore reassuring.

When a patient has had a molar pregnancy, she is at increased risk of developing molar disease in later conceptions (269,270). Thirty-four (1:150) of our patients have had at least two molar gestations between June 1965 and November 2001 (101). Patients may have an initial complete or partial mole and then in a later pregnancy develop the other type of molar disease. Following two episodes of molar pregnancy, our 34 patients had 35 later conceptions, resulting in 20 (57.1%) full-term deliveries, seven (20%) molar pregnancies (six complete, one partial), three (8.6%) spontaneous abortions, one (2.9%) ectopic pregnancy, one intrauterine fetal death, and three (8.6%) therapeutic abortions. Bagshawe et al. (271) also reported that the risk of molar disease following two episodes of molar pregnancy was 15%. In six of our cases, the medical records clearly indicated that the patient had a different partner at the time of conception of different molar pregnancies (272). Patients with molar gestation appear to be at increased risk for later molar disease even with a different partner.

It therefore seems prudent to obtain an ultrasound in the first trimester of any subsequent pregnancy to confirm normal gestational development. An hCG measurement should also be obtained 6 weeks after the completion of any future pregnancy to exclude occult trophoblastic disease.

Pregnancies After GTN

Patients with successfully treated GTN can also generally expect normal reproduction in the future (103). Patients with GTN who were treated with chemotherapy at the NETDC had 581 pregnancies between June 1965 and November 2001. These later pregnancies resulted in 393 (67.6%) full-term live births, 35 (6.0%) premature deliveries, seven (1.2%) ectopic pregnancies, and nine (1.5%) stillbirths (Table 28.13). First-trimester spontaneous abortion occurred in 92 (15.8%) pregnancies and major and minor congenital anomalies were detected in only ten (2.3%) infants. It is particularly reassuring that the frequency of congenital malformations is not increased because chemotherapy may be teratogenic and mutagenic. Primary cesarean section was performed in only 68 (20.3%) of 335 subsequent full-term and premature deliveries between January 1979 and November 2001. Later pregnancies have no increased risk for obstetric complications either prenatally or intrapartum.

Summarizing the experience from the NETDC with eight other centers, following chemotherapy for GTN, data have been reported concerning the outcome of 2,657 later pregnancies (273–280). These subsequent pregnancies resulted in 2,038 (76.7%) live births, 71 (5.3%) premature deliveries, 34 (1.3%) stillbirths, and 378 (14.2%) spontaneous abortions. Although the frequency of stillbirth appears to be somewhat increased, congenital malformations were noted in only 37 infants (1.8%), which is consistent with the general population. Woolas et al. (280) noted that there was no difference in either the conception rate or pregnancy outcome between women treated with single-agent MTX and those receiving combination chemotherapy. Furthermore, only 7% of women who wished to become pregnant following chemotherapy for GTN failed to conceive.

In general, patients who achieve primary remission with various kinds of chemotherapy may anticipate a normal future reproductive outcome. Patients occasionally become pregnant before the recommended 12-month follow-up period has elapsed. When a patient's hCG level re-elevates after completing chemotherapy, the use of ultrasound enables the clinician to distinguish between an intercurrent pregnancy and disease recurrence. Matsui et al. (281) have reported that pregnancies that occur within 6 months following remission are at increased risk of abnormalities, including spontaneous miscarriage, stillbirths, and repeat moles.

Psychosocial Consequences of GTN

Women who develop GTN may experience significant mood disturbance, marital and sexual problems, and concerns over future fertility (282–285). Because GTN is a consequence of pregnancy, patients and their partners must confront the loss of a pregnancy at the same time they face concerns regarding

TABLE 28.13

SUBSEQUENT PREGNANCIES IN PATIENTS WITH GESTATIONAL TROPHOBLASTIC TUMORS (NEW ENGLAND TROPHOBLASTIC DISEASE CENTER, JUNE 1, 1965, TO NOVEMBER 30, 2001)

Outcome	No. of patients	%
Term delivery	393	67.6
Stillbirth	9	1.5
Premature delivery	35	6.0
Spontaneous abortion		
First trimester	92	15.8
Second trimester	7	1.2
Therapeutic abortion	28	4.8
Ectopic pregnancy	7	1.2
Repeat molar pregnancy	8	1.4
Total pregnancies	581	
Congenital malformations (major and minor)		10/437 (2.3)
Primary cesarean section		68/335 (20.3)[a]

[a]January 1979 to November 2001.

malignancy. Patients may experience clinically significant levels of anxiety, fatigue, anger, confusion, sexual problems, and concern for future pregnancy that may last for protracted periods of time. Particularly, patients with metastatic disease and active disease are at risk for severe psychologic reactions. Psychosocial assessments and interventions should be provided to patients with GTN and their partners, and should be targeted particularly to patients in the metastatic and active disease groups. The psychologic and social stresses related to persistent GTN may last for many years beyond achieving complete remission. Even 5 to 10 years after attaining complete remission, 51% of patients indicate that they would be somewhat likely to very likely to participate in a counseling program today to discuss psychosocial issues raised by having had GTN.

References

1. Bagshawe KD. Risks and prognostic factors in trophoblastic neoplasia. *Cancer* 1976;38:1373–1385.
2. Goldstein DP, Berkowitz RS. *Gestational Trophoblastic Neoplasms—Clinical Principles of Diagnosis and Management.* Philadelphia: WB Saunders; 1982:1–3.
3. Lurain JR. Advances in the management of high-risk gestational trophoblastic tumors. *J Reprod Med* 2002;47:451–459.
4. Martin BH, Kim JM. Changes in gestational trophoblastic tumors over four decades: a Korean experience. *J Reprod Med* 1998;43:60–68.
5. Palmer JR. Advances in the epidemiology of gestational trophoblastic disease. *J Reprod Med* 1994;39:155–162.
6. Bracken MB. Incidence and aetiology of hydatidiform mole: an epidemiologic review. *Br J Obstet Gynaecol* 1987;94:1123–1135.
7. Jeffers MD, O'Dwyer P, Curran B, et al. Partial hydatidiform mole: a common but underdiagnosed condition. *Int J Gynecol Pathol* 1993;12: 315–323.
8. Berkowitz RS, Cramer DW, Bernstein MR, et al. Risk factors for complete molar pregnancy from a case-control study. *Am J Obstet Gynecol* 1985; 152:1016–1020.
9. Parazzini F, LaVecchia C, Mangili G, et al. Dietary factors and risk of trophoblastic disease. *Am J Obstet Gynecol* 1988;158:93–99.
10. O'Toole BA, Fradkin R, Warkany J. Vitamin A deficiency and reproduction in rhesus monkeys. *J Nutr* 1974;104:1513–1524.
11. Fulop V, Mok SC, Berkowitz RS. Molecular biology of gestational trophoblastic neoplasia: A review. *J Reprod Med* 2004;49:415–422.
12. Parazzini F, Mangili G, LaVecchia C, et al. Risk factors for gestational trophoblastic disease: a separate analysis of complete and partial hydatidiform moles. *Obstet Gynecol* 1991;78:1039–1045.
13. Berkowitz RS, Bernstein MR, Harlow BL. Case-control study of risk factors for partial molar pregnancy. *Am J Obstet Gynecol* 1995;173:788–794.
14. Buckley JD, Henderson BE, Morrow CP, et al. Case-control study of gestational choriocarcinoma. *Cancer Res* 1988;48:1004–1010.
15. Palmer JR, Driscoll SG, Rosenberg L, et al. Oral contraceptive use and risk of gestational trophoblastic tumors. *J Natl Cancer Inst* 1999;91:635–640.
16. Berkowitz RS, Goldstein DP, Anderson DJ. Recent advances in understanding the immunobiology of gestational trophoblastic disease—a review. *Trophoblast Res* 1987;2:123–137.
17. Ito H, Sekine T, Komuro N, et al. Histologic stromal reaction of the host with gestational choriocarcinoma and its relation to clinical stage, classification and prognosis. *Am J Obstet Gynecol* 1981;140:781–786.
18. Anderson DJ, Berkowitz RS. Gamma-interferon enhances expression of class I MHC antigens in the weakly HLA-positive human choriocarcinoma cell line BeWo but does not induce MHC expression in the HLA-negative choriocarcinoma cell line Jar. *J Immunol* 1985;135:2498–2501.
19. Berkowitz RS, Hill JA, Kurtz CB, et al. Effects of products of activated leukocytes (lymphokines and monokines) on the growth of malignant trophoblast cells *in vitro*. *Am J Obstet Gynecol* 1988;158:199–203.
20. Steller MA, Mok S, Yeh J, et al. Effects of cytokines on epidermal growth receptor expression by malignant trophoblast cells *in vitro*. *J Reprod Med* 1994;39:209–216.
21. Berkowitz RS, Hornig-Rohan J, Martin-Alosco S, et al. HLA antigen frequency distribution in patients with gestational choriocarcinoma and their husbands. *Placenta Suppl* 1981;3:263–267.
22. Lawler SD, Klouda PT, Bagshawe KD. The HL-A system in trophoblastic neoplasia. *Lancet* 1971;2:834–837.
23. Tomoda Y, Fuma M, Saiki N, et al. Immunologic studies in patients with trophoblastic neoplasia. *Am J Obstet Gynecol* 1976;126:661–667.
24. Morgensen B, Kissmeyer-Nielsen F, Hauge M. Histocompatibility antigens on the HL-A locus in gestational choriocarcinoma. *Transplant Proc* 1969;1:76–82.
25. Berkowitz RS, Mostoufizadeh M, Kabawat SE, et al. Immunopathologic study of the implantation site in molar pregnancy. *Am J Obstet Gynecol* 1982;144:925–930.
26. Berkowitz RS, Lahey SJ, Rodrick ML, et al. Circulating immune complex levels in patients with molar pregnancy. *Obstet Gynecol* 1983;61:165–168.
27. Lahey SJ, Steele G Jr, Berkowitz RS, et al. Identification of material with paternal HLA antigen immunoreactivity from purported circulating immune complexes in patients with gestational trophoblastic neoplasia. *J Natl Cancer Inst* 1984;72:983–990.
28. Berkowitz RS, Anderson DJ, Hunter NJ, et al. Distribution of major histocompatibility (HLA) antigens in chorionic villi of molar pregnancy. *Am J Obstet Gynecol* 1983;146:221–222.
29. Berkowitz RS, Hoch EJ, Goldstein DP, et al. Histocompatibility antigens (HLA-A, B, C) are not detectable in molar villous fluid. *Gynecol Oncol* 1984;19:74–98.
30. Cheung ANY, Srivastava G, Chung LP, et al. Expression of the p53 gene in trophoblastic cells in hydatidiform moles and normal human placentas. *J Reprod Med* 1994;39:223–227.
31. Cheung ANY, Srivastava G, Pittaluga S, et al. Expression of c-myc and c-fms oncogenes in hydatidiform mole and normal human placenta. *J Clin Pathol* 1993;46:204–207.
32. Sarkar S, Kacinski BM, Kohorn EI, et al. Demonstration of myc and ras oncogene expression by hybridization *in situ* in hydatidiform mole and in the BeWo choriocarcinoma cell line. *Am J Obstet Gynecol* 1986; 154:390–393.
33. Fulop V, Mok SC, Genest DR, et al. p53, p21, Rb, and MdM2 oncoproteins: expression in normal placenta, partial and complete mole and choriocarcinoma. *J Reprod Med* 1998;43:119–127.
34. Fulop V, Mok SC, Genest DR, et al. c-myc, c-erb B-2, c-fms, and bcl-2 oncoproteins—expression in normal placenta, partial and complete mole and choriocarcinoma. *J Reprod Med* 1998;43:101–110.
35. Batorfi J, Ye B, Mok SC, et al. Protein profiling of complete mole and normal placenta using protein chain analysis on laser capture microdissected cells. *Gynecol Oncol* 2003;424–428.
36. Tuncer ZS, Vegh GL, Fulop V, et al. Expression of epidermal growth factor receptor related family products in gestational trophoblastic diseases and normal placenta and its relationship with development of postmolar tumor. *Gynecol Oncol* 2000;77:389–393.
37. Vegh GL, Tuncer ZS, Fulop V, et al. Matrix metalloproteinases and their inhibitors in gestational trophoblastic diseases and normal placenta. *Gynecol Oncol* 1999;75:248–253.
38. Mutter GL, Stewart CL, Chaponot ML, et al. Oppositely imprinted genes H19 and insulin-like growth factor 2 are co-expressed in human androgenetic trophoblast. *Am J Hum Genet* 1993;53:1096–1107.
39. Kim SJ, Lee SY, Lee C, et al. Differential expression profiling of genes in a complete hydatidiform mole using cDNA microarray analysis. *Gynecol Oncol* 2006;103:654–660.
40. Vegh GL, Fulop V, Lin Y, et al. Differential gene expression pattern between normal human trophoblast and choriocarcinoma cell lines: downregulation of heat shock protein-27 in choriocarcinoma *in vitro* and *in vivo*. *Gynecol Oncol* 1999;75:391–396.
41. Matsuda T, Sasaki M, Kato H, et al. Human chromosome 7 carries a putative tumor suppressor gene (s) involved in choriocarcinoma. *Oncogene* 1997;15:2773–2781.
42. Ahmed MN, Kim K, Haddad B, et al. Comparative genome hybridization studies in hydatidiform moles and choriocarcinoma: amplification of 7q21-q31 and loss of 8p12-p21 in choriocarcinoma. *Cancer Genet Cytogenet* 2000;116:10–15.
43. Burke B, Sebire NJ, Moss J, et al. Evaluation of deletions in 7q11.2 and 8p12-p21 as prognostic indicators of tumor development following molar pregnancy. *Gynecol Oncol* 2006;103:642–648.
44. Berkowitz RS, Goldstein DP, Bernstein MR. Evolving concepts of molar pregnancy. *J Reprod Med* 1991;36:40–44.
45. Montes M, Roberts D, Berkowitz RS, et al. Prevalence and significance of implantation site trophoblast atypia in hydatidiform moles and in spontaneous abortions. *Am J Clin Pathol* 1996;105:411–416.
46. Kajii T, Ohama K. Androgenetic origin of hydatidiform mole. *Nature* 1977;268:633–645.
47. Yamashita K, Wake N, Araki T, et al. Human lymphocyte antigen expression in hydatidiform mole: androgenesis following fertilization by a haploid sperm. *Am J Obstet Gynecol* 1979;135:597–600.
48. Pattillo RA, Sasaki S, Katayama KP, et al. Genesis of 46, XY hydatidiform mole. *Am J Obstet Gynecol* 1981;141:104–105.
49. Azuma C, Saji F, Tokugawa Y. Application of gene amplification by polymerase chain reaction to genetic analysis of molar mitochondrial DNA: the detection of anuclear empty ovum as the cause of complete mole. *Gynecol Oncol* 1991;40:29–33.
50. Fisher RA, Hodges MD, Newlands ES. Familial recurrent hydatidiform mole: a review. *J Reprod Med* 2004;49:595–601.
51. Felemban AA, Bakri YN, Alkharif HA, et al. Complete molar pregnancy—clinical trends at King Fahad Hospital, Riyadh, Kingdom of Saudi Arabia. *J Reprod Med* 1998;43:11–13.
52. Paradinas FJ, Browne P, Fisher RA, et al. A clinical, histopathologic and flow cytometric study of 149 complete moles, 146 partial moles, 107 nonmolar hydropic abortions. *Histopathology* 1996;28:101–109.
53. Soto-Wright V, Bernstein MR, Goldstein DP, et al. The changing clinical presentation of complete molar pregnancy. *Obstet Gynecol* 1995;86:775–779.
54. Mosher R, Goldstein DP, Berkowitz RS, et al. Complete hydatidiform mole—comparison of clinicopathologic features, current and past. *J Reprod Med* 1998;43:21–27.

55. Keep D, Zaragoza MV, Hasold T, et al. Very early complete hydatidiform mole. *Hum Pathol* 1996;27:708–713.
56. Szulman AE, Surti U. The syndromes of hydatidiform mole: II. Morphologic evolution of the complete and partial mole. *Am J Obstet Gynecol* 1978;132:20–27.
57. Szulman AE, Surti U. The syndromes of hydatidiform mole: I. Cytogenetic and morphologic correlations. *Am J Obstet Gynecol* 1978;131:665–671.
58. Lawler SD, Fisher RA, Dent J. A prospective genetic study of complete and partial hydatidiform moles. *Am J Obstet Gynecol* 1991;164:1270–1277.
59. Lage JM, Mark SD, Roberts D, et al. A flow cytometric study of 137 fresh hydropic placentas: correlation between types of hydatidiform moles and nuclear DNA ploidy. *Obstet Gynecol* 1992;79:403–410.
60. Genest DR, Ruiz RE, Weremowicz S, et al. Do nontriploid partial hydatidiform moles exist? A histologic and flow cytometric reevaluation of nontriploid specimens. *J Reprod Med* 2002;47:363–368.
61. Thaker HM, Berlin A, Tycko B, et al. Immunohistochemistry for the imprinted gene product IPL/PHLDA2 for facilitating the differential diagnosis of complete hydatidiform mole. *J Reprod Med* 2004;49:630–636.
62. Fisher RA, Nucci MR, Thaker HM, et al. Complete hydatidiform mole retaining a chromosome 11 of maternal origin: analysis of a case. *Mod Pathol* 2004;17:1155–1160.
63. Berkowitz RS, Goldstein DP. Presentation and management of molar pregnancy. In: Hancock BW, Newlands ES, Berkowitz RS, eds. *Gestational Trophoblastic Disease*. London: Chapman and Hall; 1997:127–142.
64. Curry SL, Hammond CB, Tyrey L, et al. Hydatidiform mole: diagnosis, management and long-term follow up of 347 patients. *Obstet Gynecol* 1975;45:1–8.
65. Kohorn EI. Molar pregnancy: presentation and diagnosis. *Clin Obstet Gynecol* 1984;27:181–191.
66. Santos-Ramos R, Forney JP, Schwartz BE. Sonographic findings and clinical correlations in molar pregnancy. *Obstet Gynecol* 1980;56:186–192.
67. Montz FJ, Schlaerth JB, Morrow CP. The natural history of theca lutein cysts. *Obstet Gynecol* 1988;72:247–251.
68. Osathanondh R, Berkowitz RS, de Cholnoky C, et al. Hormonal measurements in patients with theca lutein cysts and gestational trophoblastic disease. *J Reprod Med* 1986;31:179–182.
69. Kohorn EI. Hydatidiform mole and gestational trophoblastic disease in southern Connecticut. *Obstet Gynecol* 1982;59:78–84.
70. Berkowitz RS, Goldstein DP, Bernstein MR. Laparoscopy in the management of gestational trophoblastic neoplasia. *J Reprod Med* 1980;24:261–264.
71. Depue RH, Bernstein L, Ross RK, et al. Hyperemesis gravidarum in relation to estradiol levels, pregnancy outcome and other maternal factors: a seroepidemiologic study. *Am J Obstet Gynecol* 1987;156:1137–1141.
72. Berkowitz RS, Goldstein DP. Pathogenesis of gestational trophoblastic neoplasms. *Pathobiol Ann* 1981;11:391–411.
73. Galton VA, Ingbar SH, Jimenez-Fonseca J, et al. Alterations in thyroid hormone economy in patients with hydatidiform mole. *J Clin Invest* 1971;50:1345–1354.
74. Amir SM, Osathanondh R, Berkowitz RS, et al. Human chorionic gonadotropin and thyroid function in patients with hydatidiform mole. *Am J Obstet Gynecol* 1984;150:723–728.
75. Nagataki S, Mizuno M, Sakamoto S, et al. Thyroid function in molar pregnancy. *J Clin Endocrinol Metab* 1977;44:254–263.
76. Nisula BC, Taliadouros GS. Thyroid function in gestational trophoblastic neoplasia: evidence that the thyrotropic activity of chorionic gonadotropin mediates the thyrotoxicosis of choriocarcinoma. *Am J Obstet Gynecol* 1980;138:77–85.
77. Twiggs LB, Morrow CP, Schlaerth JB. Acute pulmonary complications of molar pregnancy. *Am J Obstet Gynecol* 1979;135:189–194.
78. Berkowitz RS, Goldstein DP, Bernstein MR. Natural history of partial molar pregnancy. *Obstet Gynecol* 1986;66:677–681.
79. Czernobilsky B, Barash A, Lancet M. Partial mole: a clinicopathologic study of 25 cases. *Obstet Gynecol* 1982;59:75–77.
80. Feltmate CM, Growdon WB, Wolfberg AJ, et al. Clinical characteristics of persistent gestational trophoblastic neoplasia after partial hydatidiform molar pregnancy. *J Reprod Med* 2006;51:902–906.
81. Benson CB, Genest DR, Bernstein MR, et al. Sonographic appearance of first trimester complete hydatidiform moles. *J Ultrasound Obstet Gynecol* 2000;16:188–191.
82. Romero R, Horgan JG, Kohorn EI, et al. New criteria for the diagnosis of gestational trophoblastic disease. *Obstet Gynecol* 1985;66:553.
83. Fine C, Bundy AL, Berkowitz RS, et al. Sonographic diagnosis of partial hydatidiform mole. *Obstet Gynecol* 1989;73:414–418.
84. Naumoff P, Szulman AE, Weinstein B, et al. Ultrasonography of partial hydatidiform mole. *Radiology* 1981;140:467–470.
85. Menczer J, Modan M, Serr DM. Prospective follow-up of patients with hydatidiform mole. *Obstet Gynecol* 1980;55:346–349.
86. Genest DR, Laborde O, Berkowitz RS, et al. A clinicopathologic study of 153 cases of complete hydatidiform mole (1980–1990): histologic grade lacks prognostic significance. *Obstet Gynecol* 1991;78:402–409.
87. Berkowitz RS, Ozturk M, Goldstein DP, et al. Human chorionic gonadotropin and free subunits' serum levels in patients with partial and complete hydatidiform moles. *Obstet Gynecol* 1989;74:212–216.
88. Ozturk M, Berkowitz RS, Goldstein DP, et al. Differential production of human chorionic gonadotropin and free subunits of gestational trophoblastic disease. *Am J Obstet Gynecol* 1988;158:193–198.
89. Berkowitz RS, Goldstein DP. Management of molar pregnancy and gestational trophoblastic tumors. In: Knapp RC, Berkowitz RS, eds. *Gynecologic Oncology*. New York: McGraw-Hill; 1993:328–350.
90. Bagshawe KD. Trophoblastic neoplasia. In: Holland JF, Frei E III, Bast R Jr, et al., eds. *Cancer Medicine*. 3rd ed. Baltimore: Williams & Wilkins; 1993:1691–1703.
91. Fasoli M, Ratti E, Francheschi S, et al. Management of gestational trophoblastic disease: results of a cooperative study. *Obstet Gynecol* 1982;60:205–209.
92. Franke HR, Risse EKJ, Kenemans P, et al. Epidemiologic features of hydatidiform mole in the Netherlands. *Obstet Gynecol* 1983;62:613–616.
93. Lurain JR, Brewer JI, Torok EE, et al. Natural history of hydatidiform mole after primary evacuation. *Am J Obstet Gynecol* 1983;145:591–595.
94. Morrow CP, Kletzky OA, DiSaia PJ, et al. Clinical and laboratory correlates of molar pregnancy and trophoblastic disease. *Am J Obstet Gynecol* 1977;128:424–430.
95. Kohorn EI. Evaluation of the criteria used to make the diagnosis of nonmetastatic gestational trophoblastic neoplasia. *Gynecol Oncol* 1993;48:139.
96. Feltmate CM, Batorfi J, Fulop V, et al. Human chorionic gonadotropin follow-up in patients with molar pregnancy: a time for reevaluation. *Obstet Gynecol* 2003;101:732–736.
97. Massad LS, Abu-Rustum NR, Lee SS, et al. Poor compliance with postmolar surveillance and treatment protocols by indigent women. *Obstet Gynecol* 2000;96:940–944.
98. Morrow CP. Postmolar trophoblastic disease: diagnosis, management and prognosis. *Clin Obstet Gynecol* 1984;27:211–220.
99. Tow WSH. The influence of the primary treatment of hydatidiform mole on its subsequent course. *J Obstet Gynaecol Br Commonw* 1966;73:545–552.
100. Xia Z, Song H, Tang M. Risk of malignancy and prognosis using a provisional scoring system in hydatidiform mole. *Chin Med J* 1980;93:605–612.
101. Tsukamoto N, Iwasaka T, Kashimura Y, et al. Gestational trophoblastic disease in women aged 50 or more. *Gynecol Oncol* 1985;20:53–61.
102. Tsuji K, Yagi S, Nakano RI. Increased risk of malignant transformation of hydatidiform moles in older gravidas: a cytogenetic study. *Obstet Gynecol* 1981;58:351–355.
103. Garner EIO, Lipson E, Bernstein MR, et al. Subsequent pregnancy experience in patients with molar pregnancy and gestational trophoblastic tumors. *J Reprod Med* 2002;47:380–386.
104. Parazzini F, Mangili G, Belloni C, et al. The problem of identification of prognostic factors for persistent trophoblastic disease. *Gynecol Oncol* 1988;30:57–62.
105. Ayhan A, Tuncer ZS, Halilzade H, et al. Predictors of persistent disease in women with complete hydatidiform mole. *J Reprod Med* 1996;41:591–594.
106. Khazeli MB, Hedayat MM, Hatch KD, et al. Radioimmunoassay of free-beta subunit of human chorionic gonadotropin as a prognostic test for persistent trophoblastic disease in molar pregnancy. *Am J Obstet Gynecol* 1986;155:320–324.
107. Murad TM, Longley JV, Lurain JR, et al. Hydatidiform mole: clinicopathologic associations with the development of postevacuation trophoblastic disease. *Int J Gynecol Obstet* 1990;32:359–367.
108. Mutter G, Pomponio RJ, Berkowitz RS, et al. Sex chromosome composition of complete hydatidiform moles: relationship to metastasis. *Am J Obstet Gynecol* 1993;168:1547–1551.
109. Wake N, Fujino T, Hoshi S, et al. The propensity to malignancy of dispermic heterozygous moles. *Placenta* 1987;8:319–326.
110. Hancock BW, Nazir K, Everard JE. Persistent gestational trophoblastic neoplasia after partial hydatidiform mole: incidence and outcome. *J Reprod Med* 2006;51:764–766.
111. Rice LW, Berkowitz RS, Lage JM, et al. Persistent gestational trophoblastic tumor after partial hydatidiform mole. *Gynecol Oncol* 1990;36:358–362.
112. Lage JM, Berkowitz RS, Rice LW, et al. Flow cytometric analysis of DNA content in partial hydatidiform moles with persistent gestational trophoblastic tumors. *Obstet Gynecol* 1991;77:111–115.
113. Wolfberg AJ, Growdon WB, Feltmate CM, et al. Low risk of relapse after achieving undetectable hCG levels in women with partial molar pregnancy. *Obstet Gynecol* 2006;108:393–396.
114. Vejerslev LO. Clinical management and diagnostic possibilities in hydatidiform mole with coexistent fetus. *Obstet Gynecol Surv* 1991;46:577–588.
115 Steller M, Genest DR, Bernstein MR, et al. Clinical features of multiple conception with partial or complete molar pregnancy and coexisting fetuses. *J Reprod Med* 1994;39:147–154.
116. Fishman DA, Padilla LA, Keh P, et al. Management of twin pregnancies consisting of a complete hydatidiform mole and normal fetus. *Obstet Gynecol* 1998;91:546–550.
117. Miller D, Jackson R, Ehlen T, et al. Complete hydatidiform mole coexistent with a twin live fetus: clinical course of four cases with complete cytogenetic analysis. *Gynecol Oncol* 1993;50:119–122.
118. Steller M, Genest DR, Bernstein MR, et al. Natural history of twin pregnancy with complete hydatidiform mole and coexisting fetus. *Obstet Gynecol* 1994;83:35–42.
119. Berkowitz RS, Goldstein DP. Chorionic tumors. *N Engl J Med ing* 1996;335:1740–1749.
120. Hancock BW, Tidy JA. Current management of molar pregnancy. *J Reprod Med* 2002:47:347–354.
121. Goldstein DP, Berkowitz RS. Prophylactic chemotherapy of complete molar pregnancy. *Semin Oncol* 1995;22:157–160.

122. Kashimura Y, Kashimura M, Sugimori H, et al. Prophylactic chemotherapy for hydatidiform mole: five to 15 years follow-up. *Cancer* 1986;58:624–629.
123. Kim DS, Moon H, Kim KT, et al. Effects of prophylactic chemotherapy for persistent trophoblastic disease in patients with complete hydatidiform mole. *Obstet Gynecol* 1986;67:690–694.
124. Limpongsanurak S. Prophylactic actinomycin D for high-risk complete hydatidiform mole. *J Reprod Med* 2001;46:110–116.
125. Wolfberg AJ, Feltmate CM , Goldstein DP, et al. Low risk of relapse after achieving undetectable hCG levels in women with complete molar pregnancy. *Obstet Gynecol* 2004;104:551–554.
126. Lavie I, Rao G, Castrillon DH, et al. Duration of human chorionic gonadotropin surveillance for partial hydatidiform moles. *Am J Obstet Gynecol* 2005;192:1362–1364.
127. Growdon WB, Wolfberg AJ, Feltmate CM, et al. Postevacuation hCG levels and risk of gestational trophoblastic neoplasia among women with partial molar pregnancies. *J Reprod Med* 2006;51:871–874.
128. Wolfberg AJ, Berkowitz RS, Goldstein DP, et al. Postevacuation hCG levels and risk of gestational trophoblastic neoplasia in women with complete molar pregnancy. *Obstet Gynecol* 2005;106:548–552.
129. Stone M, Dent J, Kardana A, et al. Relationship of oral contraception to development of trophoblastic tumour after evacuation of a hydatidiform mole. *Br J Obstet Gynaecol* 1976;83:913–916.
130. Berkowitz RS, Goldstein DP, Marean AR, et al. Oral contraceptives and postmolar trophoblastic disease. *Obstet Gynecol* 1981;58:474–478.
131. Curry SL, Schlaerth JB, Kohorn EI, et al. Hormonal contraception and trophoblastic sequelae after hydatidiform mole (a Gynecologic Oncology Group study). *Am J Obstet Gynecol* 1989;160:805–811.
132. Ho Yuen B, Burch P. Relationship of oral contraceptives and the intrauterine contraceptive devices to the regression of concentrations of the beta subunit of human chorionic gonadotropin and invasive complications after molar pregnancy. *Am J Obstet Gynecol* 1983;145:214–217.
133. Paradinas FJ, Fisher RA. Pathology and molecular genetics and trophoblastic disease. *Current Obstet Gynecol* 1995;5:6–12.
134. Feltmate CM, Genest DR, Wise L, et al. Placental site trophoblastic tumor. A 17-year experience at the New England Trophoblastic Disease Center. *Gynecol Oncol* 2001;82:415–419.
135. Lathrop JC, Lauchlan S, Nayak R, et al. Clinical characteristics of placental site trophoblastic tumor (PSTT). *Gynecol Oncol* 1988;31:32–42.
136. Cole LA, Khanlian SA, Muller CY, et al. Gestational trophoblastic diseases: 3. Human chorionic gonadotropin-free *B*-subunit, a reliable marker of placental site trophoblastic tumors. *Gynecol Oncol* 2006;102:160–164.
137. Cole LA, Khanlian SA, Riley JM, et al. Hyperglycosylated hCG in gestational implantation and in choriocarcinoma and testicular germ cell malignancy tumorigenesis. *J Reprod Med* 2006;51:919–929.
138. Bagshawe KD, Garnett ES. Radiologic changes in the lungs of patients with trophoblastic tumours. *Br J Radiol* 1963;36:673–679.
139. Libshitz HI, Baber CE, Hammond CB. The pulmonary metastases of choriocarcinoma. *Obstet Gynecol* 1977;49:412–416.
140. Sung HC, Wu PC, Hu MH, et al. Roentgenologic manifestations of pulmonary metastases in choriocarcinoma and invasive mole. *Am J Obstet Gynecol* 1982;142:89–97.
141. Bakri YN, Berkowitz RS, Khan J, et al. Pulmonary metastases of gestational trophoblastic tumor: risk factors for early respiratory failure. *J Reprod Med* 1994;39:175–178.
142. Bagshawe KD, Noble MIM. Cardio-respiratory aspects of trophoblastic tumors. *Q J Med* 1966;137:39–54.
143. Kelly MP, Rustin GJS, Ivory C, et al. Respiratory failure due to choriocarcinoma: a study of 103 dyspneic patients. *Gynecol Oncol* 1990;38:149–154.
144. Vaccarello L, Apte SM, Diaz PT, et al. Respiratory failure from metastatic choriocarcinoma: a survivor of mechanical ventilation. *Gynecol Oncol* 1997;67:111–114.
145. Newlands ES, Holden L, Seckl MJ, et al. Management of brain metastases in patients with high-risk gestational trophoblastic tumors. *J Reprod Med* 2002;47:465–471.
146. Hongzhao S, Baozhen W. Brain metastasis in choriocarcinoma and malignant mole. *Chin Med J* 1979;92:164–174.
147. Bakri YN, Berkowitz RS, Goldstein DP, et al. Brain metastases of gestational trophoblastic tumor. *J Reprod Med* 1994;39:179–184.
148. Cagayan SF, Lu-Lasala LR. Management of gestational trophoblastic neoplasia with metastasis to the central nervous system. *J Reprod Med* 2006;51:785–792.
149. Athanassiou A, Begent RHJ, Newlands ES, et al. Central nervous system metastases of choriocarcinoma: 23 years' experience at Charing Cross Hospital. *Cancer* 1983;52:1728–1735.
150. Liu TL, Deppe G, Chang QT, et al. Cerebral metastatic choriocarcinoma in the People's Republic of China. *Gynecol Oncol* 1983;15:166–170.
151. Bakri YN, Subhi J, Amer M, et al. Liver metastases of gestational trophoblastic tumor. *Gynecol Oncol* 1993;48:110–113.
152. Kohorn EI. Negotiating a staging and risk factor scoring system for gestational trophoblastic neoplasia: a progress report. *J Reprod Med* 2002;47:445–450.
153. Ross GT, Goldstein DP, Hertz R, et al. Sequential use of methotrexate and actinomycin D in the treatment of metastatic choriocarcinoma and related trophoblastic diseases in women. *Am J Obstet Gynecol* 1965;93:223–229.
154. Hammond CB, Borchert LG, Tyrey L, et al. Treatment of metastatic trophoblastic disease: good and poor prognosis. *Am J Obstet Gynecol* 1973;115:451–457.
155. Azab MB, Prejovic M-H, Theodore C, et al. Prognostic factors in gestational trophoblastic tumors. *Cancer* 1988;62:585–592.
156. Dijkema HE, Aalders JG, DeBruiju HWA, et al. Risk factors in gestational trophoblastic disease and consequences for primary treatment. *Eur J Obstet Gynecol Reprod Biol* 1986;22:145–152.
157. DuBeshter B. High-risk factors in metastatic gestational trophoblastic neoplasia. *J Reprod Med* 1991;36:9–.
158. Dubuc-Lissoir L, Sweizig S, Schlaerth JB, et al. Metastatic gestational trophoblastic disease: a comparison of prognostic classification. *Gynecol Oncol* 1992;45:40–45.
159. Lurain JR, Casanova LA, Miller DS, et al. Prognostic factors in gestational trophoblastic tumors: a proposed new scoring system based on multivariate analysis. *Am J Obstet Gynecol* 1991;164:611–616.
160. Mortakis AE, Braga CA. Poor prognosis metastatic gestational trophoblastic disease: the prognostic significance of the scoring system in predicting chemotherapy failures. *Obstet Gynecol* 1990;76:272–277.
161. Ngan HYS, Lopes ADB, Lauder IJ, et al. An evaluation of the prognostic factors in metastatic gestational trophoblastic disease. *Int J Gynecol Cancer* 1994;4:36–42.
162. Soper JT, Clarke-Pearson DL, Hammond CB. Metastatic gestational trophoblastic disease: prognostic factors in previously untreated patients. *Obstet Gynecol* 1988;71:338–343.
163. Berkowitz RS, Goldstein DP, Bernstein MR. Choriocarcinoma following term gestation. *Gynecol Oncol* 1984;17:52–57.
164. Miller JM, Surwit EA, Hammond CB. Choriocarcinoma following term pregnancy. *Obstet Gynecol* 1979;53:207–212.
165. Olive DL, Lurain JR, Brewer JI. Choriocarcinoma associated with term gestation. *Am J Obstet Gynecol* 1984;148:711–716.
166. Rodabaugh KJ, Bernstein MR, Goldstein DP, et al. Natural history of postterm choriocarcinoma. *J Reprod Med* 1998;43:780.
167. Lok CA, Ansink AC, Grootfaam D, et al. Treatment and prognosis of post term choriocarcinoma in the Netherlands. *Gynecol Oncol* 2006;103:698–702.
168. Bagshawe KD, Harland S. Immunodiagnosis and monitoring of gonadotropin-producing metastases in the central nervous system. *Cancer* 1976;38:112–116.
169. Berkowitz RS, Osathanondh R, Goldstein DP, et al. Cerebrospinal fluid human chorionic gonadotropin levels in normal pregnancy and choriocarcinoma. *Surg Gynecol Obstet* 1981;153:687–689.
170. Bakri YN, Al-Hawashim N, Berkowitz RS. Cerebrospinal fluid/serum beta-subunit human chorionic gonadotropin ratio in patients with brain metastases of gestational trophoblastic tumor. *J Reprod Med* 2000;45:94–96.
171. Berkowitz RS, Birnholz J, Goldstein DP, et al. Pelvic ultrasonography and the management of gestational trophoblastic disease. *Gynecol Oncol* 1983;15:403–412.
172. Kohorn EI, McCarthy SM, Taylor KJW. Nonmetastatic gestational trophoblastic neoplasia: role of ultrasonography and magnetic resonance imaging. *J Reprod Med* 1998;43:14–20.
173. Dobkin GR, Berkowitz RS, Goldstein DP, et al. Duplex ultrasonography for persistent gestational trophoblastic tumor. *J Reprod Med* 1991;36:14–16.
174. Hsieh FJ, Wu CC, Chen CA, et al. Correlation of uterine hemodynamics with chemotherapy response in gestational trophoblastic tumors. *Obstet Gynecol* 1994;83:1021–1025.
175. Long MG, Boultbee JE, Langley R, et al. Preliminary Doppler studies on the uterine artery and myometrium in trophoblastic tumors requiring chemotherapy. *Br J Obstet Gynaecol* 1990;97:686–689.
176. Mangili G, Spagnolo D, Valsecchi L, et al. Transvaginal ultrasound in persistent trophoblastic tumor. *Am J Obstet Gynecol* 1993;169:1218–1223.
177. Mutch DG, Soper JT, Baker ME, et al. Role of computed axial tomography of the chest in staging patients with nonmetastatic gestational trophoblastic disease. *Obstet Gynecol* 1986;68:348–352.
178. Garner EIO, Garrett A, Goldstein DP , et al. Significance of chest computed tomography findings in the evaluation and treatment of persistent gestational trophoblastic neoplasia. *J Reprod Med* 2004;49:411–414.
179. Roja-Espaillat L, Houck KL, Hernandez E, et al. Fertility-sparing surgery for persistent gestational trophoblastic neoplasia in the myometrium. *J Repro Med* 2007;52:431–434.
180. Dhillon T, Palmieri C, Sebire NJ, et al. Value of whole body 18 FDG-PET to identify the active site of gestational trophoblastic neoplasia. *J Reprod Med* 2006;51:879–887.
181. Papadopoulos AJ, Foskett M, Seckl MJ, et al. Twenty-five years clinical experience with placental site trophoblastic tumors. *J Reprod Med* 2002;47:460–464.
182. Hoekstra AV, Keh P, Lurain JR. Placental site trophoblastic tumor: a review of 7 cases and their implications for prognosis and treatment. *J Reprod Med* 2004;49:447–452.
183. Zhao J, Xiang Y, Wan XR, et al. Clinical and pathologic characteristics and prognosis of placental site trophoblastic tumor. *J Reprod Med* 2006;51:939–944.
184. Bonazzi C, Urso M, Dell'Anna T, et al. Placental site trophoblastic tumor: an overview. *J Reprod Med* 2004;49:585–588.
185. Berkowitz RS, Goldstein DP. Gestational trophoblastic disease. *Cancer* 1995;76:2079–2085.

186. Sekharan PK, Sreedevi NS, Radhadevi VP, et al. Management of postmolar gestational trophoblastic disease with methotrexate and folinic acid: 15 years experience. *J Reprod Med* 2006;51:835–840.
187. Feldman S, Goldstein DP, Berkowitz RS. Low-risk metastatic gestational trophoblastic tumors. *Semin Oncol* 1995;22:166–171.
188. Ayhan A, Yapar EG, Deren O, et al. Remission rates and significance of prognostic factors in gestational trophoblastic tumors. *J Reprod Med* 1992;37:461–465.
189. DuBeshter B, Berkowitz RS, Goldstein DP, et al. Metastatic gestational trophoblastic disease: experience at the New England Trophoblastic Disease Center, 1965–1985. *Obstet Gynecol* 1987;9:390–395.
190. Soper JT, Clarke-Pearson DL, Berchuck A, et al. Five day methotrexate for women with metastatic gestational trophoblastic disease. *Gynecol Oncol* 1994;54:76–79.
191. Yingna S, Yang X, Xiuyu Y, et al. Clinical characteristics and treatment of gestational trophoblastic tumor with vaginal metastasis. *Gynecol Oncol* 2002;84:416–419.
192. Tse KY, Chan KKL, Tam KF, et al. 20-year experience of managing profuse bleeding in gestational trophoblastic disease. *J Reprod Med* 2007;52;397–401.
193. Soper JT. Surgical therapy for gestational trophoblastic disease. *J Reprod Med* 1994;39:168–174.
194. Yang J, Xiang Y, Wan X, et al. The prognosis of gestational trophoblastic neoplasia in a patient with residual lung tumor after completing treatment. *Gynecol Oncol* 2006:103:479–482.
195. Begent RH, Bagshawe KD, Green AJ. The clinical value of imaging with antibody to human chorionic gonadotropin in the detection of residual choriocarcinoma. *Br J Cancer* 1987;55:657–660.
196. Tomoda Y, Arii Y, Kaseki S, et al. Surgical indications for resection in pulmonary metastasis of choriocarcinoma. *Cancer* 1980;46:2723–2730.
197. Jones WB, Romain K, Erlandson RA, et al. Thoracotomy in the management of gestational choriocarcinoma: a clinicopathologic study. *Cancer* 1993;72:2175–2181.
198. Edwards JL, Makey AR, Bagshawe KD. The role of thoracotomy in the management of pulmonary metastases of gestational choriocarcinoma. *Clin Oncol* 1975;1:329–339.
199. Shirley RL, Goldstein DP, Collins JJ Jr. The role of thoracotomy in management of patients with chest metastases from gestational trophoblastic disease. *J Thorac Cardiovasc Surg* 1972;63:545–550.
200. Sink JD, Hammond CB, Young WG. Pulmonary resection in the management of metastases from choriocarcinoma. *J Thorac Cardiovasc Surg* 1981;81:830–834.
201. Wang Y, Song H, Xia Z. Drug resistant pulmonary choriocarcinoma metastasis treated by lobectomy. *Chin Med J* 1980;93:758–766.
202. Lehman E, Gershenson DM, Burke TW, et al. Salvage surgery for chemorefractory gestational trophoblastic disease. *J Clin Oncol* 1994;12:2737–2742.
203. Hammond CB, Weed JC, Currie JL. The role of operation in the current therapy of gestational trophoblastic disease. *Am J Obstet Gynecol* 1980;136:844–856.
204. Grumbine FC, Rosenshein NB, Brereton HD, et al. Management of liver metastases from gestational trophoblastic neoplasia. *Am J Obstet Gynecol* 1980;137:959–961.
205. Wong LC, Choo YC, Ma HK. Hepatic metastases in gestational trophoblastic disease. *Obstet Gynecol* 1986;67:107.
206. Evans AC Jr, Soper JT, Clarke-Pearson DL, et al. Gestational trophoblastic disease metastatic to the central nervous system. *Gynecol Oncol* 1995;59:226.
207. Brace KC. The role of irradiation in the treatment of metastatic trophoblastic disease. *Radiology* 1968;91:540.
208. Yordan EL Jr, Schlaerth J, Gaddis O, et al. Radiation therapy in the management of gestational choriocarcinoma metastatic to the central nervous system. *Obstet Gynecol* 1987;69:627.
209. Cole LA. hCG, its free subunits and its metabolites—roles in pregnancy and trophoblastic disease. *J Reprod Med* 1998;43:3.
210. Cole LA. New perspectives in measuring human chorionic gonadotropin levels for measuring and monitoring trophoblastic disease. *J Reprod Med* 1994;39:193.
211. Cole LA, Butler S. Detection of hCG in trophoblastic disease—the USA hCG Reference Service Experience. *J Reprod Med* 2002;47:433–444.
212. Hancock BW. hCG measurement in gestational trophoblastic neoplasia: a critical appraisal. *J Reprod Med* 2006;51:859.
213. Mitchell H, Bagshawe KD, Newlands ES, et al. Importance of accurate human chorionic gonadotropin measurement in the treatment of gestational trophoblastic disease and testicular cancer. *J Reprod Med* 2006;51:868.
214. Cole LA, Kohorn EI. The need for an hCG assay that appropriately detects trophoblastic disease and other hCG-producing tumors. *J Reprod Med* 2006;51:793.
215. Kohorn EI. What we know about low-level hCG: definition, classification and management. *J Reprod Med* 2004;49:433.
216. Hwang D, Hancock BW. Management of persistent, unexplained, low-level human chorionic gonadotropin elevation: a report of 5 cases. *J Reprod Med* 2004;49:559.
217. Khanlian SA and Cole LA. Management of gestational trophoblastic disease and other cases with low serum levels of human chorionic gonadotropin. *J Reprod Med* 2006;51:812.
218. Mutch DG, Soper JT, Babcock CJ, et al. Recurrent gestational trophoblastic disease. Experience of the Southeastern Regional Trophoblastic Disease Center. *Cancer* 1990;66:978.
219. Goldstein DP, Zanten-Przybysz I, Bernstein MR, et al. Revised FIGO staging system for gestational trophoblastic tumors; recommendations regarding therapy. *J Reprod Med* 1998;43:37.
220. Ngan HYS, Tam K-F, Lam K-W, et al. Relapsed gestational trophoblastic neoplasia: a 20-year experience. *J Reprod Med* 2006;51;829–834.
221. Yang J, Xiang Y, Wan X, et al. Recurrent gestational trophoblastic tumor: management and risk factors for recurrence. *Gynecol Oncol* 2006; 103:587–590.
222. Li MC, Hertz R, Spencer DB. Effect of methotrexate therapy on choriocarcinoma and chorioadenoma. *Proc Soc Exp Biol Med* 1956;93:361–366.
223. Hertz R, Lewis JL Jr, Lipsett MB. Five year's experience with chemotherapy of metastatic choriocarcinoma and related trophoblastic tumors in women. *Am J Obstet Gynecol* 1961;82:631–637.
224. Hertz R, Ross GT, Lipsett MB. Primary chemotherapy of nonmetastatic trophoblastic disease in women. *Am J Obstet Gynecol* 1963;86:808–814.
225. Ross GT, Stolbach LL, Hertz R. Actinomycin D in the treatment of methotrexate-resistant trophoblastic disease in women. *Cancer Res* 1962;22:1015–1017.
226. Homesley HD. Single-agent therapy for nonmetastatic and low-risk gestational trophoblastic disease. *J Reprod Med* 1998;43:69–74.
227. Bagshawe KD, Dent J, Newlands ES, et al. The role of low-dose methotrexate and folinic acid in gestational trophoblastic tumours (GTT). *Br J Obstet Gynaecol* 1989;96:795–802.
228. DuBeshter B, Berkowitz RS, Goldstein DP, et al. Management of low-risk metastatic gestational trophoblastic tumor. *J Reprod Med* 1991;36:36–39.
229. Homesley HD, Blessing JA, Schlaerth J, et al. Rapid escalation of weekly intramuscular methotrexate for nonmetastatic gestational trophoblastic disease: a Gynecologic Oncology Group study. *Gynecol Oncol* 1990; 39:305–308.
230. Kohorn EI. Single-agent chemotherapy for nonmetastatic gestational trophoblastic neoplasia. *J Reprod Med* 1991;36:49–55.
231. Osathanondh R, Goldstein DP, Pastorfide GB. Actinomycin D as the primary agent for gestational trophoblastic disease. *Cancer* 1975;36:863–866.
232. Szigetvari J, Szepesi J, Vegh G, et al. 25 years' experience in the treatment of gestational trophoblastic neoplasia (GTN) in Hungary. *J Reprod Med* 2006;51:841–848.
233. Petrilli ES, Twiggs LB, Blessing JA, et al. Single-dose actinomycin-D treatment for nonmetastatic gestational trophoblastic disease: a prospective phase II trial of the Gynecologic Oncology Group. *Cancer* 1987;60:2173–2176.
234. Roberts JP, Lurain JR. Treatment of low risk metastatic gestational trophoblastic tumors with single agent chemotherapy. *Am J Obstet Gynecol* 1996;174:1917–1922.
235. Rose PG, Piver MS. Alternating methotrexate and dactinomycin in nonmetastatic gestational trophoblastic disease. *J Surg Oncol* 1989;41:149–153.
236. Wong LC, Choo YC, Ma HK. Methotrexate with citrovorum factor rescue in gestational trophoblastic disease. *Am J Obstet Gynecol* 1985; 152:59–62.
237. Bagshawe KD, Wilde CE. Infusion therapy for pelvic trophoblastic tumors. *J Obstet Gynaecol Br Commonw* 1964;71:565–570.
238. Berkowitz RS, Goldstein DP. Methotrexate with citrovorum factor rescue and non-metastatic gestational trophoblastic neoplasms. *Obstet Gynecol* 1979;54:725–728.
239. Berkowitz RS, Goldstein DP, Bernstein MR. Methotrexate with citrovorum factor rescue as a primary therapy for gestational trophoblastic disease. *Cancer* 1982;50:2024–2027.
240. Berkowitz RS, Goldstein DP, Bernstein MR. Ten years experience with methotrexate and folinic acid as primary therapy for gestational trophoblastic disease. *Gynecol Oncol* 1986;23:111–118.
241. Berkowitz RS, Goldstein DP, Jones MA, et al. Methotrexate with citrovorum factor rescue: reduced chemotherapy toxicity in the management of gestational trophoblastic neoplasms. *Cancer* 1980;45:423–425.
242. Garrett AP, Garner EIO, Goldstein DP, et al. Methotrexate infusion and folinic acid as primary therapy for nonmetastatic and low-risk metastatic gestational trophoblastic tumors—15 years of experience. *J Reprod Med* 2002;47:355–362.
243. Sung HC, Wu PC, Yang HY. Reevaluation of 5-fluorouracil as a single therapeutic agent for gestational trophoblastic neoplasms. *Am J Obstet Gynecol* 1984;150:69–75.
244. Wong LC, Choo YC, Ma HK. Primary oral etoposide therapy in gestational trophoblastic disease: an update. *Cancer* 1986;58:14–17.
245. Berkowitz RS, Goldstein DP, Bernstein MR. Modified triple chemotherapy in the management of high-risk metastatic gestational trophoblastic tumors. *Gynecol Oncol* 1984;19:173–181.
246. Curry SL, Blessing JA, DiSaia PJ, et al. A prospective randomized comparison of methotrexate, dactinomycin and chlorambucil versus methotrexate, dactinomycin, cyclophosphamide, doxorubicin, melphalan, hydroxyurea, and vincristine in poor prognosis metastatic gestational trophoblastic disease: a Gynecologic Oncology Group study. *Obstet Gynecol* 1989;73:357–362.
247. Gordon AN, Gershenson DM, Copeland LJ, et al. High-risk metastatic gestational trophoblastic disease: further stratification into two clinical entities. *Gynecol Oncol* 1989;34:54–56.

248. Bagshawe KD. Treatment of high-risk choriocarcinoma. *J Reprod Med* 1984;29:813–820.
249. Bolis G, Bonazzi C, Landoni F, et al. EMA/CO regimen in high-risk gestational trophoblastic tumor (GTT). *Gynecol Oncol* 1988;31:439–444.
250. Lurain JR, Singh DK, Schink JC. Primary treatment of metastatic high-risk gestational trophoblastic neoplasia with EMA-CO chemotherapy. *J Reprod Med* 2006;51:767–772.
251. Soper JT, Evans AC, Clarke-Pearson DL, et al. Alternating weekly chemotherapy with etoposide-methotrexate-dactinomycin/cyclophosphamide-vincristine for high-risk gestational trophoblastic disease. *Obstet Gynecol* 1994;83:113–117.
252. Bower M, Newlands ES, Holden L, et al. EMA/CO for high-risk gestational trophoblastic tumors: results from a cohort of 272 patients. *J Clin Oncol* 1997;15:2636–2643.
253. Kim SJ, Bae SN, Kim JH, et al. Risk factors for the prediction of treatment failure in gestational trophoblastic tumors treated with EMA/CO regimen. *Gynecol Oncol* 1998;71:247–251.
254. Newlands ES, Bower M, Holden L, et al. Management of resistant gestational trophoblastic tumors. *J Reprod Med* 1998;43:111–118.
255. Xiang Y, Sun Z, Wan X, et al. EMA/EP chemotherapy for chemorefractory gestational trophoblastic tumor. *J Reprod Med* 2004;49:443–446.
256. Lurain JR, Singh DK, Schink JC. Role of surgery in the management of high-risk gestational trophoblastic neoplasia. *J Reprod Med* 2006;51:773–776.
257. Rustin GJS, Newlands ES, Lutz JM, et al. Combination but not single-agent methotrexate chemotherapy for gestational trophoblastic tumors increases the incidence of second tumors. *J Clin Oncol* 1996;14:2769–2773.
258. Soto-Wright V, Goldstein DP, Bernstein MR, et al. The management of gestational trophoblastic tumors with etoposide, methotrexate and actinomycin D. *Gynecol Oncol* 1997;64:156–159.
259. Gordon AN, Kavanaugh JJ, Gershenson DM, et al. Cisplatin, vinblastine, and bleomycin combination therapy in resistant gestational trophoblastic disease. *Cancer* 1986;58:1407–1410.
260. DuBeshter B, Berkowitz RS, Goldstein DP, et al. Vinblastine, cisplatin and bleomycin as salvage therapy for refractory high-risk metastatic gestational trophoblastic disease. *J Reprod Med* 1989;34:189–192.
261. Azab M, Droz JP, Theodore C, et al. Cisplatin, vinblastine and bleomycin combination in the treatment of resistant high-risk gestational trophoblastic tumors. *Cancer* 1989;64:1829–1832.
262. Giacalone PL, Benos P, Donnadio D, et al. High-dose chemotherapy with autologous bone marrow transplantation for refractory metastatic gestational trophoblastic disease. *Gynecol Oncol* 1995;58:383–385.
263. VanBesien K, Verschraegen C, Mehra R, et al. Complete remission of refractory gestational trophoblastic disease with brain metastases treated with multicycle ifosfamide, carboplatin, and etoposide (ICE) and stem cell rescue. *Gynecol Oncol* 1997;65:366–369.
264. Jones WB, Schneider J, Shapiro F, et al. Treatment of resistant gestational choriocarcinoma with Taxol: a report of two cases. *Gynecol Oncol* 1996;61:126–130.
265. Sutton GP, Soper JT, Blessing JA, et al. Ifosfamide alone and in combination in the treatment of refractory malignant gestational trophoblastic disease. *Am J Obstet Gynecol* 1992;167:489–495.
266. Osborne R, Covens A, Merchandani DE, et al. Successful salvage of relapsed high-risk gestational trophoblastic neoplasia patients using a novel paclitaxel-containing doublet. *J Reprod Med* 2004;49:655–661.
267. Wan X, Yang Y, Wu Y, et al. Floxuridine-containing regimens in the treatment of gestational trophoblastic tumor. *J Reprod Med* 2004;49:453–456.
268. Matsui H, Iitsuka Y, Suzuka K, et al. Salvage chemotherapy for high-risk gestational trophoblastic tumor. *J Reprod Med* 2004;49:438–442.
269. Lurain JR, Sand PK, Carson SA, et al. Pregnancy outcome subsequent to consecutive hydatidiform moles. *Am Obstet Gynecol* 1982;142:1060–1061.
270. Rice LW, Lage JM, Berkowitz RS, et al. Repetitive complete and partial hydatidiform mole. *Obstet Gynecol* 1989;74:217–219.
271. Bagshawe KD, Dent J, Webb J. Hydatidiform mole in England and Wales 1973–1983. *Lancet* 1986;2:673–677.
272. Tuncer ZS, Bernstein MR, Wang J, et al. Repetitive hydatidiform mole with different male partners. *Gynecol Oncol* 1999;75:224–226.
273. Ayhan A, Ergeneli MH, Yuce K, et al. Pregnancy after chemotherapy for gestational trophoblastic disease. *J Reprod Med* 1990;35:522–524.
274. Kim JH, Park DC, Bae SN, et al. Subsequent reproductive experience after treatment for gestational trophoblastic disease. *Gynecol Oncol* 1998;71:108–112.
275. Kjer JJ, Iversen T. Malignant trophoblastic tumors in Norway: fertility rate after chemotherapy. *Br J Obstet Gynaecol* 1990;97:623–625.
276. Kobayashi O, Matsui H, Takamizawa H. Analysis of pregnancy outcome after chemotherapy of trophoblastic disease. *Nippon Sanka Fujinka Gakkai Zasshi* 1986;38:181–186.
277. Ngan HYS, Wong LC, Ma HK. Reproductive performance of patients with gestational trophoblastic disease in Hong Kong. *Acta Obstet Gynecol Scand* 1988;67:11–14.
278. Song HZ, Wu PC, Wang Y, et al. Pregnancy outcome after successful chemotherapy for choriocarcinoma and invasive mole: long-term follow-up. *Am J Obstet Gynecol* 1988;158:538–545.
279. VanThiel DH, Ross GT, Lipsett MB. Pregnancies after chemotherapy of trophoblastic neoplasms. *Science* 1970;169:1326–1327.
280. Woolas RP, Bower M, Newlands ES, et al. Influence of chemotherapy for gestational trophoblastic disease on subsequent pregnancy outcome. *Br J Obstet Gynaecol* 1998;105:1032–1035.
281. Matsui H, Iitsuka Y, Suzuka K, et al. Early pregnancy outcome after chemotherapy for gestational trophoblastic tumor. *J Reprod Med* 2004;49:531–534.
282. Wenzel LB, Berkowitz RS, Robinson S, et al. The psychological, social, and sexual consequences of gestational trophoblastic disease. *Gynecol Oncol* 1992;46:74–81.
283. Wenzel LB, Berkowitz RS, Robinson S, et al. Psychological, social, and sexual effects of gestational trophoblastic disease on patients and partners. *J Reprod Med* 1994;39:163–167.
284. Wenzel L, Berkowitz RS, Newlands E, et al. Quality of life after gestational trophoblastic disease. *J Reprod Med* 2002;47:387–390.
285. Wenzel L, Berkowitz RS, Habbal R, et al. Predictors of quality of life among long-term survivors of gestational trophoblastic disease. *J Reprod Med* 2004;49:589–594.

CHAPTER 29 ■ BREAST CANCER

DON S. DIZON, TREVOR TEJADA-BERGES, MARGARET M. STEINHOFF, C. JAMES SUNG, SUSAN L. KOELLIKER, HANAN I. KHALIL, BRIGID O'CONNOR, STEPHANIE MacAUSLAND, CHARU TANEJA, ROBERT D. LEGARE, AND JENNIFER S. GASS

INTRODUCTION

Breast cancer is a worldwide problem and affects more than 1.2 million women every year, making it the most common cancer diagnosis in women. Treatment paradigms require an understanding of the natural history of the disease including the various patterns of metastases and recurrence, and both the prognostic and predictive factors that may influence both response to treatment and overall survival. In addition, the complexities that govern medical and surgical decisions make the management of breast cancer far more complicated than that of other disease sites. This chapter provides the essential information regarding breast cancer with an emphasis on recent developments. It stresses an interdisciplinary view of disease management by providing the foundational aspects of breast disease and treatment.

EPIDEMIOLOGY

Each year about 180,510 women and 2,030 men are diagnosed with breast cancer in the United States (1). It is estimated that one in eight women will be diagnosed with breast cancer in their lifetime. Beginning in the late 1990s a shift in the incidence of breast cancer in the United States was noted. The steady increase in breast cancer diagnosis seen in the 1950s started to decline in 1999 and continued into 2003. The decline in the annual incidence between 2002 and 2003 was limited to women over the age of 50. Whether the declining use of hormone replacement therapy following publication of the Women's Health Initiative (WHI) results, utilization of mammographic screening and earlier diagnosis of disease, or a combination of these factors explains this trend continues to be an area of investigation. Mortality from breast cancer has been steadily declining since 1990, at a rate of 3.3% in women under 50 and 2.0% per year in older women (1). Still, over 40,000 women will succumb to breast cancer, making it second only to lung cancer.

RISK FACTORS

Risk factors for breast cancer have been well characterized. Breast cancer is 100 times more frequent in *women* than in men. Factors associated with an increased exposure to *estrogen* have also been elucidated including early menarche, late menopause, later age at first pregnancy, or nulliparity. The use of hormone replacement therapy has been confirmed as a risk factor, although mostly limited to the combined use of estrogen and progesterone, as demonstrated in the WHI (2). Analysis showed that the risk of breast cancer among women using estrogen and progesterone was increased by 24% compared to placebo. A separate arm of the WHI randomized women with a prior hysterectomy to conjugated equine estrogen (CEE) versus placebo, and in that study, the use of CEE was not associated with an increased risk of breast cancer (3). Unlike hormone replacement therapy, there is no evidence that oral contraceptive (OCP) use increases risk. A large population-based case-control study examining the risk of breast cancer among women who previously used or were currently using OCPs included over 9,000 women aged 35 to 64 (half of whom had breast cancer) (4). The reported relative risk was 1.0 (95% CI, 0.8 to 1.3) among women currently using OCPs and 0.9 (95% CI, 0.8 to 1.0) among prior users. In addition, neither race nor family history was associated with a greater risk of breast cancer among OCP users.

Apart from endocrine risk factors, sociodemographic risks have also been established. Breast cancer is an *age*-related phenomenon, with peak incidence after 40. Family history is also a strong epidemiologic risk factor, although it accounts for less than 10% of cases of breast cancer. Clinical models can now be employed to predict the risk of breast cancer. Among those in common use are the Gail and Claus models (Table 29.1) (5,6). Although they have been widely used in the African American and other minority populations, they have not been validated sufficiently.

Beyond classification of risk based on family history, the identification of genetic mutations that are passed in an autosomal-dominant fashion has been an important scientific breakthrough. Among the most significant was the identification of mutations at *BRCA1*, localized to chromosome 17q21, and *BRCA2* on chromosome 13q12-13, both of which confer a risk for breast cancer as high as 80% among carriers (7,8). A specific *BRCA1* mutation, 185delAG, has been identified in over 20% of Jewish women younger than 40 years of age. Other mutations known to carry an increased risk are those involving p53 in the Li-Fraumeni syndrome (associated with other cancers including sarcoma, leukemia, melanoma, gastrointestinal carcinomas, and brain tumors), CHEK-2, and *PTEN* mutations associated with Cowden syndrome (mental retardation associated with increased incidence of hamartomas, endometrial cancer, and noncancerous brain tumors).

Work evaluating the long-term effects of environmental factors has established prior radiation exposure as an additional risk factor. The therapeutic use of mantle-field radiation in women with Hodgkin's disease and the sequelae of the atomic bombing of Japan in World War II identified the heightened risks of breast cancer, particularly in young women (9,10).

TABLE 29.1

MODELS FOR ESTIMATING RISK FOR BREAST CANCER

	Gail[a]	Claus[b]
Source	Breast Cancer Detection Demonstration Project (n = 284,780)	Cancer and Steroid Hormone Study (n = 9,418)
Personal risk factors	Age Age at menarche Prior breast biopsies Age at first live birth	Age
Family history	Number of *maternal* first-degree relatives with breast cancer	Number of relatives with breast cancer (beyond first-degree relatives) and ages of onset
Calculations	Absolute risk[c] at 5 years Lifetime risk up to 90 years old	Lifetime risk up to 80 years old
Limitations	Excludes paternal history Excludes ovarian cancer history Does not use pathologic findings from breast biopsy Does not account for age of onset of breast cancer among family Not validated in other ethnic groups	Excludes other risk factors May underestimate risk in families with three or more family members with breast cancer

[a]Gail MH, Brinton LA, Byar DP, et al. Projecting individualized probabilities of developing breast cancer for white females who are being examined annually. *J Natl Cancer Inst* 1989;81(24):1879–1886.
[b]Claus EB, Risch N, Thompson WD. Autosomal dominant inheritance of early-onset breast cancer. Implications for risk prediction. *Cancer* 1994;73(3):643–651.
[c]Risk defined for invasive breast cancer only.

Among modifiable risk factors, obesity, weight gain in later life, and the consumption of alcohol have been identified in prospective observational studies (11). The association of environmentally found trace elements and breast cancer risk has also been evaluated with unconvincing results in general.

An association has been made between breast cancer risk and breast findings. Among the best described risk factors is the association between breast cancer and a history of biopsies for benign breast disease. In a study by Hartmann et al. the relative risk for breast cancer ranged from 1.27 for nonproliferative lesions to 1.88 for proliferative lesions without atypia to 4.24 in lesions with atypia, and this risk persisted for as long as 25 years after biopsy (12). A recent report from Worsham et al. evaluated the same risks in an inner-city clinic and reported that African American women with benign breast lesions faced similar risks in developing breast cancer (13). More recently, Boyd et al. reported on the association between risk and breast density (measured in percentage of the total breast) (14). Using 1,112 matched case-control pairs they determined the association between risk and reported that women with density of 75% or greater had a significantly increased risk of breast cancer (odds ratio, 4.7; 95% CI, 3.0 to 7.4), with younger women notably at greatest risk.

ANATOMY

The breast is a modified sweat gland composed of two components: the large ducts and the terminal duct–lobular unit (TDLU), surrounded by adipose and fibrous tissue, lymphatics, nerves, and blood vessels. The surface of the breast is attached to the underlying fibrous tissue by way of Cooper's ligaments, and the mammary gland lies over the pectoralis major muscle, extending vertically along the second to sixth ribs and horizontally from the sternum to the anterior midaxillary line. The axillary tail comprises mammary tissue as well and extends laterally from the chest wall into the axilla. The large duct system of subsegmental, segmental, and lactiferous ducts converge and empty onto the nipple. The TDLU is the most distal part of this branching ductal system, and is felt to be the site of origin of most pathologic entities of the breast, including fibrocystic changes, ductal hyperplasias, and the majority of carcinomas (15,16). It is connected to the subsegmental ducts and represents the secretory unit of the gland (Fig. 29.1).

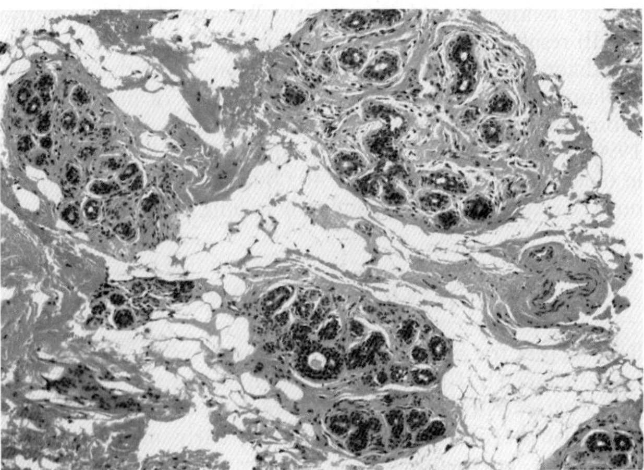

FIGURE 29.1. Normal breast lobules. Three terminal duct–lobular units are surrounded by adipose and fibrous tissue.

Mobility of the breast tissue over the chest wall is through the retromammary bursa, which lies between the superficial and deep fascia. The lymphatic system of the breast is vast, comprising a network over the entire surface of the chest, neck, and abdomen, with increased density under the axilla. There are three main lymphatic pathways of the breast: (a) the axillary pathway, which drains the upper and lower halves of the breast into the lateral axillary nodal chain; (b) the transpectoral pathway, which drains into the supraclavicular nodes; and (c) the internal mammary pathway, draining the inner halves of the breast, into the nodes of the internal mammary chain.

NATURAL HISTORY OF BREAST CANCER

Breast cancers can occur with predictable features. For example, it is more likely to be diagnosed in the central or outer quadrants of the breast than in the inner regions (17). It has also been reported to be more commonly involving the left breast; a study of 2,139 cases of breast cancer in Iceland showed that 13% more breast cancers occurred in the left breast versus the right (18).

Within the breast, cancer travels along ducts (intraductal carcinoma), and the process of invasion begins when the tumor erodes through the basement membrane. Continued growth results as the tumor spreads along adjacent lobules, breast lymphatics, perineural tumors, and vascular spaces. When it involves the dermal lymphatics, the overlying dermis becomes edematous and red with the classic appearance of *peau d'orange*. Continued growth of the primary tumor can result in the involvement of the pectoralis and intercostal muscles, ribs, and the clavicle.

While less frequently encountered, locally advanced or metastatic disease at diagnosis still occurs in clinical practice. Tumor spread can occur locally by direct extension, lymphatically, or via intravascular means. Lymphatic spread of tumor from the breast travels to the locoregional nodes of the chest—the axillary, intramammary, and supraclavicular nodal basins—and increasing tumor size is a well-known predictor of nodal involvement. A medial or central lesion of the breast is more likely to metastasize to the internal mammary nodes than outer quadrant lesions, and this has been theorized to explain their worse prognosis compared to upper outer breast tumors (17). Vascular invasion can be observed, even with small tumors.

Metastatic disease from breast cancer can occur in any organ site. Lee reported on presentations of metastatic breast cancer among over 2,000 women who had died of disease (Fig. 29.2) (19). The most commonly involved organs were the lungs, bones, nodes, and liver. The pleural space, adrenal glands, and brain represented the next most commonly involved sites. Regarding survival, bloom compared a group of women with untreated breast cancer to a cohort of patients treated with radical or modified radical mastectomy, with or without irradiation, and reported an overall 10-year survival of 3.6% in the untreated cohort, versus 34% in the treated group (20).

Theories on the spread of breast cancer have been used as a foundation for subsequent treatment, and have evolved over time. Under Halsted, the notion that cancer arose from one location and travelled contiguously by lymphatics to reach local and distant locations was borne. Hence, treatment with the *en bloc* resection of the breast and lymphatics was felt to present the best opportunity for cure. Still, it was clear that even with agressive surgery and removal of the lymphatics from the breast, women still died of breast cancer. In a seminal paper by Valagussa et al. the overall survival among women with node-negative disease was reported to be 60%, those with up to three nodes positive at 54%, and at 26% in those with more than three positive nodes. This showed that contiguous lymphatic spread alone could not explain survival outcomes (21).

The theory of breast cancer as a systemic disease was brought forward in 1980 by Dr. Bernard Fisher (22). Breast tumors were seen as a marker of this systemic syndrome, just as neuropathy would be a marker of advanced diabetes mellitus. Hence, nodal disease was not simply an extension of a primary breast cancer process, but rather a marker of disease already spread. This theory holds that achieving local control will not have an impact on overall survival and argues for the use of systemic treatment in order to effect the best outcome. Recently, however, a meta-analysis on the use of adjuvant radiation by the Early Breast Cancer Trialists' Collaborative has called this theory into question. In that analysis the use of adjuvant radiation not only improved local control but also reduced annual mortality by 13% after the 2nd year of follow-up (23).

It is likely that breast tumors express variable degrees of malignancy. Hellman argued that "synthesis" between Halsted and Fisher's theories was required (24). Recognizing that the size of tumor is proportional to the risk of metastases, he suggested that small and large tumors behave differently, and carried different prognoses. Whereas small tumors were a manifestation of a locoregional process and therefore were curable with treatment, larger tumors included a heterogenous population of cell types, including those more likely to proliferate and be more malignant—features that made them more likely to metastasize. As such, the larger tumors were likely to be associated with systemic disease. Defining cure as "that proportion of the treated group that has the same survival as an age-adjusted peer population," he estimated that over 80% of women with tumors less than 1 cm in size were curable and that this was manifest at 10 years of follow-up (24). In summary, he again stressed the importance of local control for small tumors, while emphasizing the importance of systemic control in larger breast cancers.

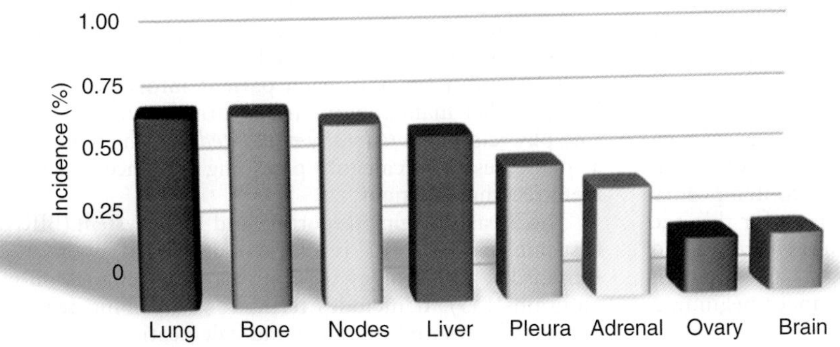

FIGURE 29.2. Pattern of metastatic disease from breast cancer based on an autopsy series of over 2,000 women.

CLINICAL PRESENTATION OF BREAST CANCER

Today the most common presentation is with an abnormal mammogram, although patients continue to present with a painless or slightly tender breast mass. In younger women, a delay in diagnosis may be attributed to benign causes such as recent trauma, changes with pregnancy, or due to breast-feeding. For those women presenting with a mass, the patient may ultimately present with breast tenderness, skin changes, bloody nipple discharge, or changes in the shape and size of the breast, with or without axillary adenopathy. Rarely will women present with axillary nodal disease but no evidence of a breast primary, otherwise known as occult breast carcinoma. Lastly, inflammatory breast cancer (IBC) presents as a tender, red, and swollen breast, often mistaken for mastitis. A crusting rash emanating from the nipple is *sine qua non* for Paget's disease of the breast, which is almost uniformly associated with an underlying malignancy. Fortunately, with the increase in screening following publication of the National Institutes of Health (NIH) Consensus Statement in 1978, patients rarely present with metastatic disease (25).

IMAGING STUDIES OF THE BREAST

Introduction

Breast imaging is performed as a screening tool in asymptomatic women to detect early cancer or as a diagnostic examination in women suspected of having breast cancer or previously treated for breast cancer. Mammography remains the most widely used technique for screening, and is the only modality proven to decrease mortality. Computer-aided detection (CAD), a tool designed to help the radiologist improve the detection of breast cancer, is now available and more frequently used by interpreting radiologists. In addition to mammography, ultrasound (US) and magnetic resonance imaging (MRI) now serve as adjunct tools in the diagnostic setting or for high-risk screening. Finally, breast tomosynthesis may prove to be an important tool in detection of early breast cancer.

Mammography

The purpose of screening mammography is the early detection of clinically unsuspected breast cancer in asymptomatic women. The efficacy has been widely established by multiple randomized, controlled trials, which have analyzed large-scale populations with and without screening over long time intervals. These studies show that screening mammography is associated with an 18% to 45% reduction in breast cancer mortality compared with unscreened groups (26–28). In 2003, the American Cancer Society (ACS) updated its guidelines for early detection of breast cancer based on results of an expert panel that reviewed evidence of early detection trials since the last guidelines were published in 1997 (29). A prior controversy regarding screening mammography in women 40 to 49 years of age was addressed as part of this review with the finding that contemporary studies did demonstrate the benefit of screening for this age group (28–30). Therefore, current guidelines recommend annual screening mammography beginning at age 40, with women at high risk of developing breast cancer beginning earlier than age 40.

There is no recommendation for age at which screening should stop; if an older individual is in reasonably good health, would be a candidate for treatment, and has a life expectancy of more than 3 to 5 years, continuing with screening mammography is recommended. There is consensus with the ACS, American College of Radiology (ACR), and the National Cancer Institute (NCI) for routine screening beginning at age 40. However, the NCI recommends mammography only every 1 to 2 years after age 40. The cost-effectiveness of age-related screening mammography has been assessed using the Markov model (30). The marginal cost per year–life saved varies from \$18,800 to \$16,100 for age groups including women ages 40 to 79, which is within the range of other generally acceptable diagnostic and therapeutic medical procedures.

Despite the success of screening mammography, the sensitivity of mammography ranges from 80% to 90%, largely because of insufficient contrast between normal and abnormal breast tissue (31–33). In a screening population, approximately 10% of patients will be "recalled" for additional imaging (i.e., additional mammographic views, spot compression views, or ultrasound evaluation). Of all positive screening examinations, approximately 5% to 10% will have a diagnosis of cancer, and of all recommended biopsies, 25% to 40% will be positive for cancer.

The screening mammogram is an x-ray of the breast, with two views of each breast obtained, a top-to-bottom (craniocaudad, or CC) view and an angled side-to-side (mediolateral oblique, MLO) view. The images can be recorded on film or stored digitally on a computer. Two views of each breast are needed to optimize the amount of breast tissue included on each mammogram, minimize overcalling disease because of superimposed tissue on a single view, and decreasing the likelihood of obscuring a cancer by overlapping tissue on a single view. In some patients, particularly those with larger breasts, more than four views are obtained by the technologist to ensure that all the breast tissue is included on the images.

Patients who present with concerning signs or symptoms such as mastalgia, a palpable mass, skin thickening, nipple retraction, or nipple discharge require a mammogram as a diagnostic study. Diagnostic mammograms are also indicated in patients recalled for further mammographic evaluation, and those with a personal history of breast cancer, and may be considered in patients with breast augmentation. In the latter, this may be considered diagnostic because of the increased effort and time involved with obtaining necessary views. However, given that this is a procedural reason (as opposed to the workup of a suspicious finding), patients with breast augmentation should be audited within the group undergoing mammography as a screening test.

Mammography practice in the United States is rigidly regulated by the Food and Drug Administration (FDA) under the Mammography Quality Standards Act (MQSA) of 1992 (34). The MQSA mandates extensive follow-up and outcome monitoring of all facilities and interpreting radiologists. Recall rates, biopsy recommendations and results, and cancer detection rates must be analyzed for each interpreting radiologist. Cancer staging must be recorded to include histologic type, size, nodal status, and grade. It also requires analysis of any known false-negative mammograms and mandates that the facility send a letter to each patient informing her of the results of her mammogram and a formal report to the referring physician. It is *federally mandated* that the report include a final assessment category providing guidance and management recommendations.

The Breast Imaging Reporting and Data System (BIRADS), first published in 1993, is a lexicon developed by the ACR to standardize terminology used in reporting findings on mammograms (35). It includes terms for describing features of masses (shapes and margins) and calcifications (morphology

TABLE 29.2

BIRADS (BREAST IMAGING AND REPORTING DATA SYSTEM) ASSESSMENT CATEGORIES

Category	Interpretation
0	**Mammographic assessment is incomplete** Additional imaging evaluation and/or prior mammograms required for comparison Used in screening situations
1	**Negative** No mammographic evidence of malignancy
2	**Normal, but describes a benign finding** No mammographic evidence of malignancy
3	**Probably benign finding—initial short interval follow-up suggested** Finding with less than 2% risk of malignancy, not expected to change over interval
4	**Suspicious abnormality—biopsy should be considered** Findings do not have classic appearance of malignancy, but greater probability than category 3
5	**Highly suggestive of malignancy—appropriate action should be taken** Finding had greater than 95% probability of being malignant
6	**Known biopsy-proven malignancy-appropriate action should be taken** Used for lesions identified on imaging studies with biopsy proof of malignancy prior to definitive therapy

Note: It is federally mandated that all mammography reports give a final assessment category.
Source: American College of Radiology BIRADS—Mammography. 4th ed. Reston, VA: American College of Radiology; 2003.

and distribution). It defines final assessment categories to describe the radiologist's level of suspicion about a mammographic abnormality, to comply with the federally mandated MQSA regulations. All mammograms must be assessed with a final BIRADS category of 0 to 6 (Table 29.2). The report must include the date of comparison films, the indication for the examination (screening, recall, clinical finding, or follow-up), an assessment of overall breast composition to indicate the relative possibility that a lesion may be hidden by normal tissue, limiting the sensitivity of the examination (Table 29.3), a description of any significant findings, and an overall summary impression.

A mammographic mass is defined as a space-occupying lesion seen in two projections, whereas an "asymmetry" is a potential mass seen only in a single projection (Fig. 29.3). Describing a mass must encompass its shape, margins, and density. Masses that are irregular in shape, with indistinct or spiculated margins, and of high density are the most worrisome for malignancy, whereas round or oval masses with circumscribed (well-defined) margins are more likely benign. Calcifications are described by type and distribution. Those that are larger, coarser, smoothly marginated, and more easily seen are likely benign, while those that are very fine, pleomorphic, or linear are more likely to be malignant (Fig. 29.4). The distribution may be telling as well;

TABLE 29.3

MAMMOGRAPHIC ASSESSMENT OF OVERALL BREAST COMPOSITION—THE OVERALL ASSESSMENT OF VOLUME OF ATTENUATING TISSUES IN BREAST, WHICH INDICATES THE RELATIVE POSSIBILITY THAT A LESION IS HIDDEN BY NORMAL TISSUE AND INDICATES THE SENSITIVITY OF THE EXAMINATION

Mammographic description	Glandular proportion of total breast tissue (%)
The breast is almost entirely fat	<25
Scattered fibroglandular densities present	25–50
The breast tissue is heterogeneously dense; this may obscure detection of small masses	51–75
The breast tissue is extremely dense; this may lower the sensitivity of mammography	>75

Source: American College of Radiology BIRADS—Mammography. 4th ed. Reston, VA: American College of Radiology; 2003.

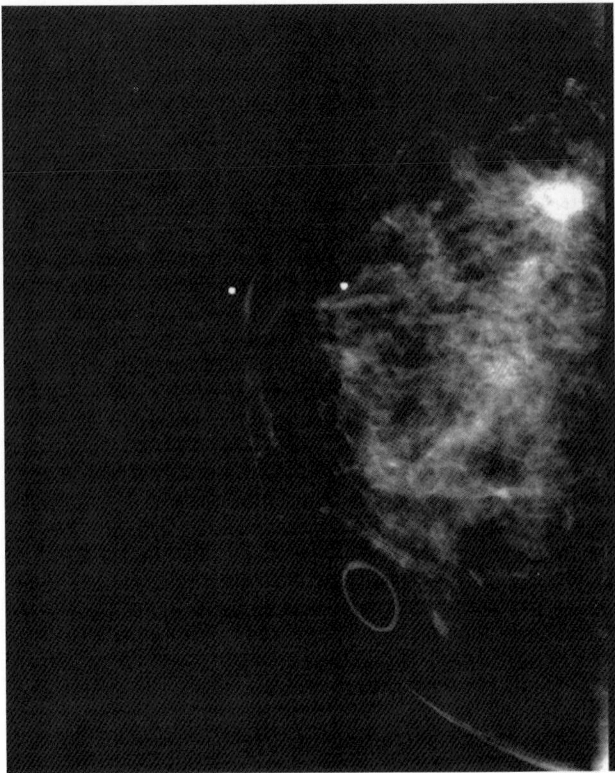

FIGURE 29.3. Right craniocaudad mammographic view shows a spiculated mass in the outer breast. Biopsy showed poorly differentiated invasive mixed ductal and lobular carcinoma.

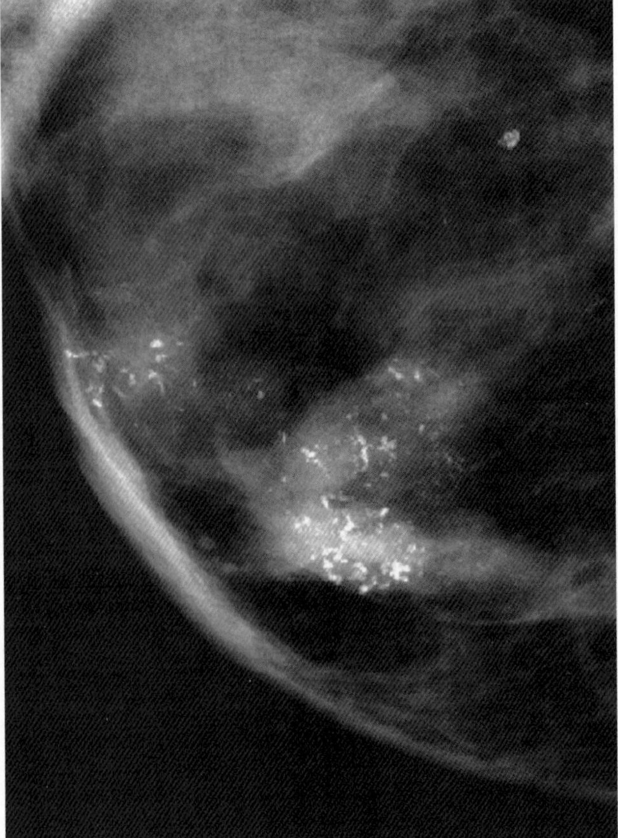

FIGURE 29.4. Magnification view of right breast calcifications shows linear and branching calcifications, which at biopsy were duct carcinoma *in situ*.

diffuse and scattered calcifications are more likely benign, while grouped or clustered, linear, or segmental calcifications are more worrisome. The side of any abnormality, location by quadrant or clock face, and depth should be included in the description.

Film Versus Digital Mammography

Film mammography is extremely effective and has been widely accepted as a screening modality for the past 20 to 30 years. With this technique, the mammography images are recorded as hard copy on film and developed by the technologist, then presented to the radiologist for review. Digital mammography, however, uses a digital detector to replace the screen film of conventional mammography. Radiation transmitted through the breast is absorbed by an electronic detector, with a response faithful over a wide range of intensities. The recorded information can be displayed using computer image–processing techniques to allow selective settings of image brightness and contrast without need for further exposure to patients. The lower system noise would be expected to enhance the visibility of subtle contrast differences between tumors and normal background tissue. With digital imaging, the processes of image acquisition, storage, and display are separated, allowing optimization of each (36,37). In addition, the average patient dose of radiation is slightly lower than that of film mammography, and examination time for each patient is shorter. The disadvantages of digital mammography are the cost of equipment, which is 1.5 to four times as much as film systems, and the slightly longer interpretation time by the radiologist (38).

Early clinical trials showed equivalent diagnostic accuracy between digital and screen-film mammography (39–43). The Senographe 2000D screening trial demonstrated a significant decrease in recall rate for digital (11.8%) versus screen film (14.9%), as well as a decrease in biopsy rate (43). In the Digital Mammographic Imaging Screening Trial (DMIST), 49,528 asymptomatic women presenting for screening mammography at 33 sites in the United States and Canada underwent both digital and film mammography, with the examinations interpreted independently by two radiologists (38). While the diagnostic accuracy of digital and film mammography was similar overall, the accuracy of digital mammography was significantly higher than that of film mammography in the following groups: women under the age of 50 years, women with heterogeneously dense or extremely dense breasts on mammography, and premenopausal or perimenopausal women. This finding is significant because it is widely recognized that increased density on mammography decreases the sensitivity of the technique (44–48). In addition, the major limitation of mammography is that cancer can be hidden by adjacent breast tissue. Digital mammography addresses this issue by allowing for contrast adjustment, which can bring out the visibility of a mass in this setting.

Computer-Aided Detection

CAD was first approved by the FDA in 1998. It aims to identify suspicious findings on mammogram which can assist radiologic interpretation. Initial studies demonstrated increased sensitivity of cancer detection when CAD was added to screening programs, with increased rates of cancer detection reported between 7.62% to 19.5% (49–52). Cupples et al. showed a particular improvement of small cancer detection by CAD, with a 164% increased cancer detection rate of invasive cancers less than 1 cm (49). Because of the reported improvement of breast cancer detection, Medicare and many insurers reimburse for use of CAD.

However, the increased detection rate with CAD has come at the cost of increased recalls and increased rate of biopsy (53–55). Recently a large-scale study conducted by Fenton et al. determined the association between use of CAD at mammographic facilities and performance of screening mammography during 1998 to 2002 (56). In that study, 223,135 women were screened at 43 facilities in three states, with and without the assistance of CAD. The specificity of screening decreased from 90.2% without CAD to 87.2% with CAD, and the biopsy rate increased by 19.7% with CAD. There was no statistically significant change in sensitivity with or without CAD, although there was a trend toward an increase in sensitivity. Overall, the increased rate of biopsy resulting from use of CAD was not clearly associated with improved detection of invasive cancer. Of the cancer detected by CAD, there was a trend toward more ductal carcinoma *in situ* detection than invasive cancer, which may be clinically important. Although there were a large number of women included in the study, the number of cancers was still relatively small, making it difficult to judge whether the benefits of routine use of CAD outweigh its harms (i.e., increased biopsy rate).

Ultrasound

Ultrasonography is used as a targeted examination, most often to determine the cystic versus solid nature of a mass. It has been shown to be effective in determining the likelihood of benign versus malignant breast masses (Fig. 29.5) (57). Prevalence studies in women with radiographically dense breasts have shown that three to four cancers per 1,000 women are detected by ultrasound only (57–62). However, the limitations of breast ultrasound as a screening tool are well known: it requires a skilled operator, is labor intensive, and there is currently no standardized examination technique or interpretation criteria. Moreover, it does not detect microcalcifications, which may be the hallmark of *in situ* breast cancer. Finally, it has a high false-positive rate and is less sensitive than breast MRI (59,60,62). Therefore, it is unlikely that screening breast US will become widely used in the United States.

Tomosynthesis

Tomosynthesis is a three-dimensional mammographic technique that allows improved visualization over mammography by minimizing effects of overlapping tissue. The acquisition of images mimics conventional mammography with breast positioning and compression. The x-ray tube takes multiple low-dose exposures from many angles, resulting in a digital data set that can be reconstructed into tomographic sections through the breast. The images can be obtained in a CC, MLO, or 90-degree lateral projection. It is currently undergoing testing, but shows great promise. Tomosynthesis may reduce the rate of false-positive mammograms, and thus decrease the recall rate, by minimizing the effects of overlapping tissue. In this way it may have more impact in women with dense breasts.

Poplack et al. compared the image quality of tomosynthesis with conventional mammography (63). Ninety-eight women with 99 screening recalls were evaluated with tomosynthesis of the affected breast. Image quality by tomosynthesis was found to be equivalent in 52% and superior in 37% of patients compared to mammogram. In addition, many findings on mammogram would not be recalled with tomosynthesis, suggesting that it could reduce recall rates by 40%.

Of breast findings, masses are better seen on tomosynthesis, but calcifications are better seen on diagnostic mammography. This may be attributed to motion-related blur due to the somewhat long (19 seconds) exposure time of the tomosynthesis. In addition, images are reconstructed at 1 mm thickness slices, which may be too thin to ably demonstrate the clustered distribution of calcifications.

It remains to be seen whether tomosynthesis can be performed in one projection, which would minimize radiation dose and the length of examination, or whether two views will be needed. Rafferty et al. presented data on 34 patients scheduled for biopsy by performing tomosynthesis in both the CC and MLO projections, finding that most lesions (65%) were equally visible on both, but 9% were only seen on the CC view; all of these potentially missed lesions were malignant (64). Today, we believe that tomosynthesis will require imaging in both projections for optimal lesion visualization.

The cost of tomosynthesis has yet to be determined. It is expected that the technique will be substantially less expensive than breast MRI and will not require an injection, which may make this advantageous in screening high-risk women. Larger-scale trials will need to be performed to evaluate who will best benefit from the examination as opposed to conventional mammography.

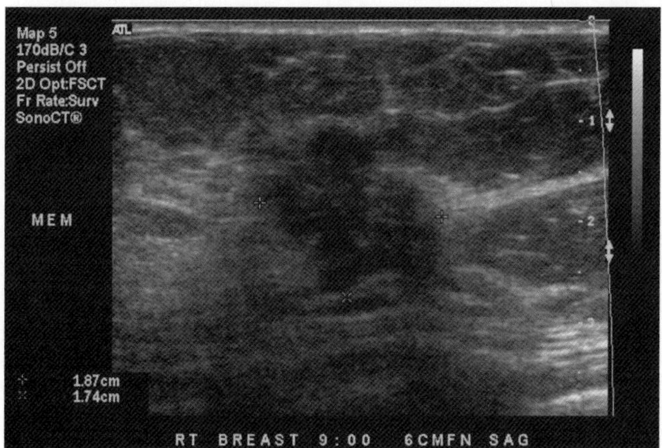

FIGURE 29.5. Targeted breast ultrasound demonstrating a heterogeneous solid mass with irregular margins measuring 1.9 cm. Ultrasound guidance was used to place a wire for subsequent localization and wide local excision of the patient's known infiltrating ductal carcinoma.

Breast MRI

MRI of the breast has evolved over the past 2 decades from a research tool to the most sensitive imaging modality in the detection of invasive breast cancer. Contrast-enhanced breast MRI is increasingly being incorporated in the clinical evaluation of breast cancer (65). For breast lesion detection, intravenous injection of gadolinium-based contrast is needed as contrast enhancement to allow visualization of breast cancer against the background of glandular tissue. This distinction relies on the determination that tumor angiogenesis and surrounding tissue permeability allow contrast uptake within cancer (66). That is, a significant number of invasive tumors demonstrate rapid wash in of contrast and wash out with time (67). Significant overlap between enhancement pattern of benign and malignant processes exists, which must be recognized, and which lowers the specificity of breast MRI. As such, analysis of breast MR-enhancing lesions involves analyzing both lesion morphology and kinetics of enhancement to provide the most specificity in lesion characterization (68). For example, spiculated morphology and rim enhancement are features highly predictive of malignancy, while circumscribed margins with persistent kinetics (increasing enhancement with time) suggest a benign etiology (Fig. 29.6) (69,70).

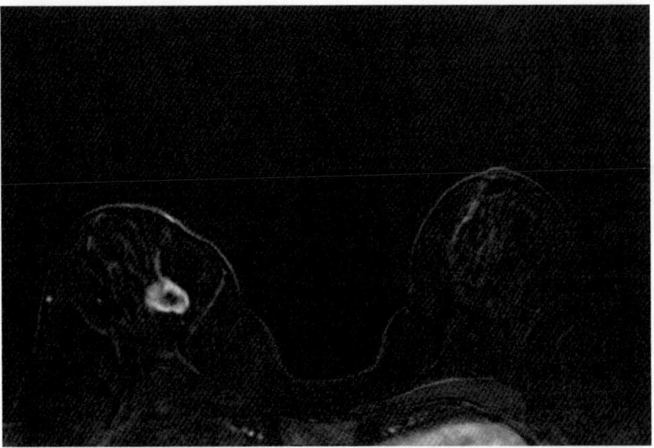

FIGURE 29.6. Breast MRI in a 55-year-old woman with biopsy-proven infiltrating ductal carcinoma. It shows spiculated morphology and rim enhancement, features that are highly specific for carcinoma.

Variable protocols for MRI imaging of the breast exist. However, technical prerequisites for standard imaging have been set by the ACR for proper imaging and diagnosis. In general, MRI breast imaging should be performed with a dedicated breast coil, using at least a 1.5-tesla magnet and imaging extents to optimize high spatial and temporal resolution.

Technical advances in breast MRI have led to improved sensitivity for the detection of invasive breast cancer currently reported to be between 89% and 100% (71,72). Although previous studies in ductal carcinoma *in situ* (DCIS) (Fig. 29.7A,B) showed low and variable sensitivities, with improved techniques contemporary studies report higher sensitivity of up to 89% (73,74). In one multicenter prospective study, MRI had higher sensitivity than mammography in detecting DCIS, including both DCIS with associated invasive component and multicentric disease (75). Recent advances introduced the use of a CAD system in interpretation of breast MRI and data suggest that CAD significantly improves discrimination between benign and malignant masses (76). As the first step in regulating analysis and reporting of this new technique, the ACR developed a new BIRADS MRI lexicon incorporating new terminology and specific descriptors of breast MRI findings. Continued effort for standardization is a work in progress.

Screening Breast MRI

Breast MRI may be used as a screening modality and mammography. In a study by Morris et al., mammographically occult breast cancer was detected by screening breast MRI in 4% of high-risk women, with a positive predictive value (PPV) of 24% (77). A subsequent meta-analysis by Liberman including 1,305 women at high risk found that MRI detected cancer in 34% (range 24% to 89%) of women who had a biopsy based on MRI findings and in 4% (range 2% to 7%) of all high-risk women (78). For women with *BRCA1* gene mutations, MRI is a very sensitive screening tool when used in conjunction with mammography. In a multicenter multimodality prospective trial by Sardanelli et al. that looked at screening in women with genetic-familial risk for breast cancer, MRI had a sensitivity of 94% and a PPV of 63% (79).

Recently, the American Cancer Society published new guidelines for high-risk screening with MRI, based on scientific evidence and expert opinion (Table 29.4) (80). According to the new guidelines, high risk is defined as a lifetime risk of 20% to 25% or more, BRCA gene mutation carrier or first-degree relative of BRCA carrier, women treated at an early age with chest radiation, and hereditary syndromes that put women at high risk for breast cancer. Currently there are no data to support or refute annual breast MRI in women with a personal history of breast cancer or with high-risk lesions, and these patients are to be assessed on a case-by-case basis and may be referred by the breast specialist to a screening breast MRI if deemed necessary.

Breast MRI also serves to screen the contralateral breast in women with recently diagnosed breast cancer. A recent multicenter, prospective trial evaluating contralateral breast cancer in women with recently proven breast cancer found clinically and mammographically occult breast cancer in 3.1% of 969 women, with a sensitivity of 91% and a negative predictive value of 99% (81).

Diagnostic Breast MRI

There are several clinical scenarios in which breast MRI may serve as an adjunct to mammography. One of the most common is preoperative staging of a newly diagnosed invasive cancer or DCIS. Breast MRI can delineate clinically and mammographically occult additional disease including *in situ*

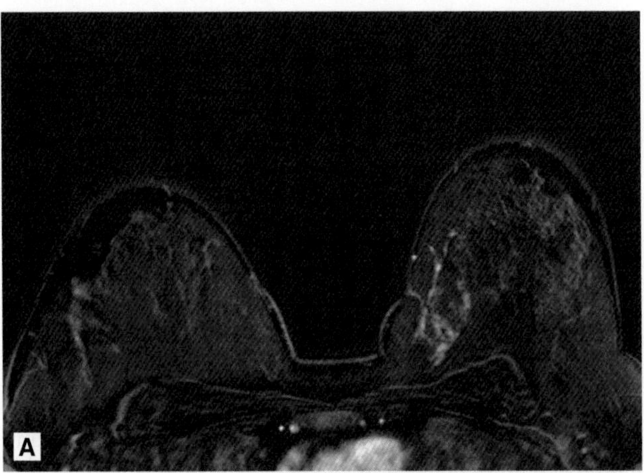

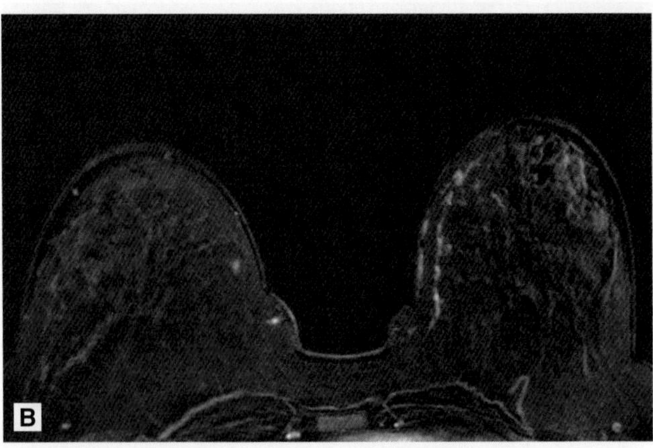

FIGURE 29.7. Breast MRI demonstrating DCIS in a 45-year-old woman with a positive biopsy for high-grade DCIS. **A:** Preoperative breast MR with post contrast subtraction image shows clumped linear non-mass enhancement in the medial breast corresponding to known DCIS. **B:** Post contrast subtraction image more inferiorly shows more extensive involvement than the mammogram with linear enhancement extending in a ductal distribution from posterior depth to the nipple.

TABLE 29.4

INDICATIONS FOR ANNUAL BREAST MRI SCREENING IN ASSOCIATION WITH MAMMOGRAPHY

EVIDENCE-BASED RECOMMENDATIONS
Confirmed BRCA mutation carrier status
Untested but with first-degree relative with positive BRCA mutation status
Estimated lifetime risk of developing disease >20% (based on risk models)
EXPERT OPINION
Recommended
Prior radiotherapy to the chest wall (between ages 10 and 30)
Patients (and first-degree relatives) with predisposing cancer syndromes:
Li-Fraumeni syndrome
Cowden sydrome
Bannayan-Riley-Ruvacalba sydrome
No recommendation (for or against)
Estimated lifetime risk 15% to <20% (based on risk models)
Lobular proliferative disease (LCIS or ALH)
Atypical ductal hyperplasia (ADH)
Mammographic heterogeneity or density
Women with personal history of breast cancer (including DCIS)
Not recommended
Estimated lifetime risk <15%

Note: ALH, atypical lobular hyperplasia; DCIS, ductal carcinoma *in situ;* LCIS, lobular carcinoma *in situ.*
Source: Saslow D, Boetes C, Burke W, et al. American Cancer Society guidelines for breast screening with MRI as an adjunct to mammography. *CA Cancer J Clin* 2007;57(2):75–89.

disease associated with invasive cancer and its extent, and it can detect noncalcified DCIS. Liberman et al. found that 48% of women who underwent preoperative MRI of the breast had additional foci of disease unsuspected by mammography (82). As such, the addition of breast MRI can aid in surgical planning, including decisions regarding the role of mastectomy or the consideration for neoadjuvant chemotherapy. In one study by Fischer et al., surgical management of patients was changed by 14.3% (83). It is advisable to biopsy additional suspicious foci detected by MRI to avoid overestimation of disease and unnecessary mastectomy.

Breast MRI can be added to the workup of an inconclusive mammographic finding. In this setting, however, the negative predictive value of MRI is imperfect and a negative MRI should be interpreted cautiously. If a mammographic or sonographic finding is suspicious, a stereotactic or sonographic biopsy should be performed, regardless of the MRI results.

MRI is not the best test for the exclusion of malignancy in the workup of mammographic calcifications, and suspicious microcalcifications should undergo core biopsy. A helpful role of MRI in such clinical scenarios would be to delineate the extent of disease and to rule out an underlying occult invasive component. For women presenting with suspicious clinical findings for breast cancer and negative conventional imaging tests, MRI of the breast has an added value. These instances include a woman with a palpable suspicious mass, women with metastatic axillary lymph nodes but no mammographically defined breast primary, and those with pathologic unilateral nipple discharge or Paget's disease and a negative mammogram and ultrasound.

MRI: Other Indications

In patients presenting with an increasing mammographic density at the lumpectomy site following breast conservation therapy, MRI is the most sensitive test for evaluating for recurrent disease with high specificity and negative predictive value. In addition, MRI has a role in determining the response to neoadjuvant chemotherapy and it is more reliable than mammography or US in that respect. However, while MRI may not show residual enhancement following chemotherapy, it is not 100% accurate in the detection of residual disease, and a 23% risk of underestimation has been reported (84).

THE WORKUP FOR SUSPECTED BREAST CANCER

The diagnostic workup begins with the mammogram, with a marker placed at the site of the lesion (if not already done). Focal compression, magnification, and tangential images may be required to allow for better visualization of the mass, evaluate any associated calcifications, and to displace it from the surrounding breast. Ultrasound of the lesion is typically performed to further characterize the lesion as solid or cystic, and to give its dimensions. This may be particularly indicated in nonspiculated lesions, and those in which the differential includes benign lesions, such as fibroadenoma.

Patients presenting with a suspicious breast mass or other concerning imaging should undergo image-guided core needle biopsy using a large-gauge needle to establish diagnosis. This has been championed as the preferred technique over fine-needle aspiration or diagnostic excision for many reasons. First, it avoids unnecessary surgery in approximately 80% of BIRADS category 4 patients who require biopsy to establish if a lesion is benign. It also allows the surgeon to plan an oncologic procedure at the time of the index operation. Further, in cases of invasive carcinoma, it allows characterization of histology, grade, hormone-receptor status, and HER2/neu status, all of which are necessary to develop medical and surgical planning, including the role of nodal mapping. Although fine-needle aspiration provides a quick and inexpensive means of evaluation, it is rarely sufficient to distinguish *in situ* from invasive disease and provides insufficient material for characterization of hormone and HER2/neu receptor status.

Core biopsy may be performed with stereotactic, sonographic, or MRI guidance, and all are acceptable methods. If the mammographic abnormality consists of suspicious calcifications without a mass, then stereotactic biopsy is performed. A specimen radiograph is required to document that calcifications are present in the specimen. With the increased refinement of ultrasonography and the increased portability of ultrasound units, there has been a shift to ultrasound core biopsy performed in radiology or in the surgeon's office. MRI-guided core biopsy is performed for MRI-detected lesions that have no mammographic or sonographic correlate. In all cases, a clip should be deployed at the end of the procedure followed by a mammogram to confirm its placement. Evaluation for concordance between pathology and imaging is then required. If a lack of concordance is discovered, excisional biopsy is required. For patients presenting with a palpable mass, biopsy under image guidance is still preferred.

TABLE 29.5

AJCC CLASSIFICATION OF BREAST CANCER

TUMOR (T)	
Tx	Cannot be assessed
T0	No primary tumor
Tis	*In situ* disease
T1	Tumor ≤2 cm
T1mic	Microinvasive, ≤0.1 cm
T1a	0.1 cm < T ≤0.5 cm
T1b	0.5 cm < T ≤1.0 cm
T1c	1.0 cm < T ≤2.0 cm
T2	Tumor >2 cm, but ≤5 cm
T3	Tumor >5 cm
T4	Tumor of any size with:
T4a	Chest wall extension
T4b	Edema or ulceration of skin, or satellite nodules
T4c	Both (a) and (b)
T4d	Inflammatory carcinoma

REGIONAL NODES (N)[a]	Clinical (c)	Pathologic (p)
Nx	Cannot be assessed	No nodes assessed
N0	No nodes involved	Designations in N0 (+ or –): N0(I): detected by IHC N0(mol): detected by RT-PCR
N1	Movable axillary node(s)	N1mic: micrometastases, up to 2 mm N1a: 1–3 nodes N1b: microscopically involved internal mammary node, not clinically apparent N1c: both a and b
N2		
N2a	Fixed or matted node(s)	Four to nine nodes positive
N2b	Clinically apparent mammary nodes; axillary node negative	Clinically apparent internal mammary node involvement, no axillary nodes (+)
N3		
N3a	Positive infraclavicular node(s)	Ten or more positive nodes
N3b	Positive mammary + axillary node(s)	Internal mammary nodes and axillary nodes involved
N3c	Positive supraclavicular node(s)	Supraclavicular nodes involved

METASTASES (M)	
Mx	Not assessed
M0	No distant metastases
M1	Distant metastases

Note: AJCC, American Joint Commission on Cancer; IHC, immunohistochemistry; RT-PCR, reverse transcription polymerase chain reaction.
[a]Regional nodal involvement refers to ipsilateral disease only.

The major complications of biopsy are predominantly hemorrhage and infection, although these are rare and occur in less than 0.5% of biopsies performed (85).

An ultrasound of the axilla with fine-needle aspiration (US-FNA) may also be considered as part of the workup of a woman with a confirmed breast cancer on biopsy. Sonographic characteristics of the suspicious node includes size greater than 1 cm, loss of fatty hilum, cortical hypertrophy, and hypoechogenic parenchyma. In a study from the M. D. Anderson Cancer Center, the overall sensitivity of US-FNA was 86%, specificity was 100%, positive predictive value was 100%, and the negative predictive value was 67% (86). Identification of a positive node by fine-needle aspiration negates the need for a sentinel node biopsy and commits the patient to axillary dissection, and the identification of node-positive disease by US-FNA has been shown to reduce the number of sentinel node biopsy procedures by up to 15%. For those with a negative fine-needle aspiration, sentinel node biopsy is still required (87,88).

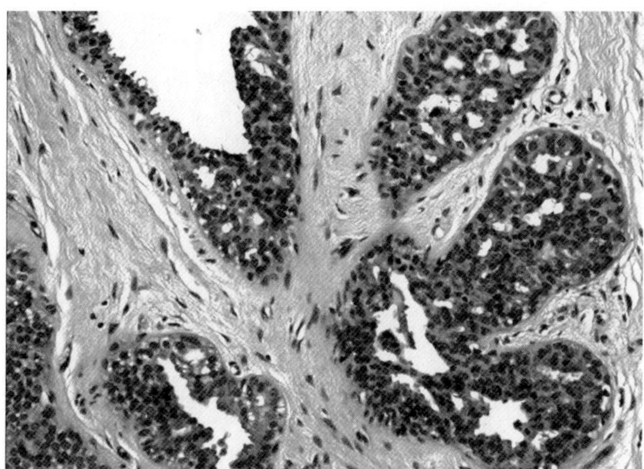

FIGURE 29.8. Ductal hyperplasia. Slightly expanded ducts are filled with hyperplastic ductal epithelial cells and myoepithelial cells in an irregular fenestrated growth pattern.

STAGING

The staging of breast cancer requires a full characterization of the primary tumor, including size, grade, biologic characterization of estrogen and progesterone receptor expression, and whether overamplification of overexpression of the HER2/neu oncogene is present. Lymphatic or vascular invasion of the primary tumor should be characterized as well as the nodal status of the tumor. In the asymptomatic patient, metastatic involvement can be ruled out clinically by physical exam, routine hematologic and chemistry profiles, and chest x-ray. For patients presenting with concerning symptoms, further evaluation with positron emission tomography (PET), bone scan, and/or computed tomography (CT) scan of the chest and abdomen may be required.

The staging of breast cancer follows the American Joint Commission on Cancer (AJCC) system which uses the tumor (T), node (N), and metastasis (M) classification (TNM, Tables 29.5 and 29.6) (89). The new classification moves supraclavicular nodal involvement from M1 to N3 disease. In addition, the revised 2003 version of the staging system includes new technologies for nodal evaluation using immunohistochemistry (IHC) and reverse transcription polymerase chain reaction (RT-PCR) (mol) in the node-negative category. For example, a patient can be node negative but positive by these techniques, allowing for a designation of N0(I+) if positive by IHC or N0(mol+) if positive by RT-PCR. Within node-positive patients, classification also allows the designation of microscopic tumor deposits up to 0.1 cm in diameter as node positive with isolated tumor cells [N0(ITC)]. If a patient undergoes sentinel node evaluation only without formal axillary node dissection, the prefix "sn" is used [pN(sn)], and if staging occurs after primary chemotherapy the designation of "y" is used (yTNM).

TABLE 29.6

STAGING OF BREAST CANCER

AJCC	T	N	M
Stage 0	Tis	N0	M0
Stage I	T1	N0	M0
Stage IIA	T0-1	N1	M0
	T2	N0	M0
Stage IIB	T2	N1	M0
	T3	N0	M0
Stage IIIA	T0-T3	N2	M0
	T3	N1	M0
Stage IIIB	T4	N0-N2	M0
Stage IV	Any T	Any N	M1

Note: AJCC, American Joint Commission on Cancer; M, metastases; N, node; T, tumor.

BREAST PATHOLOGY

Fibrocystic Changes

The breast ducts and lobules can show a wide range of benign nonproliferative and proliferative epithelial lesions. Nonproliferative lesions include cysts (macroscopic and microscopic), duct ectasia, fibrosis, and apocrine metaplasia. Proliferative lesions were first separated into different risk categories based on the work of Dupont and Page (90). Patterns associated with a mildly increased risk (~twofold) of subsequent breast carcinoma are considered proliferative changes, and include usual ductal epithelial hyperplasia (Fig. 29.8), lobular hyperplasia, sclerosing adenosis, radial scars, and intraductal papillomas (12,90). Both sclerosing adenosis (Fig. 29.9) and radial

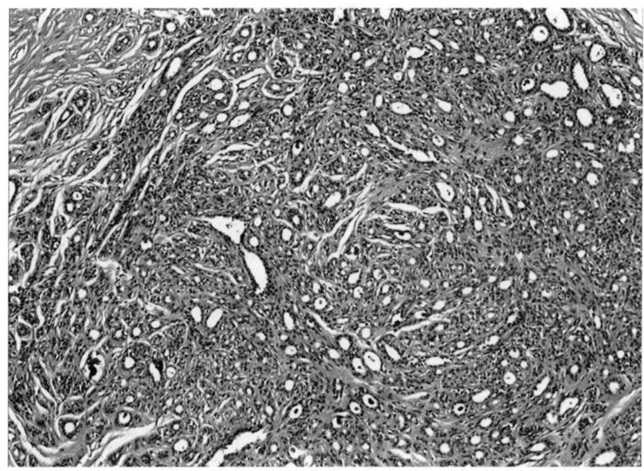

FIGURE 29.9. Sclerosing adenosis. A well-developed lobulocentric distribution of dilated ducts and overgrowth of spindly myoepithelial cells may be mistaken as malignancy in core biopsy or frozen section.

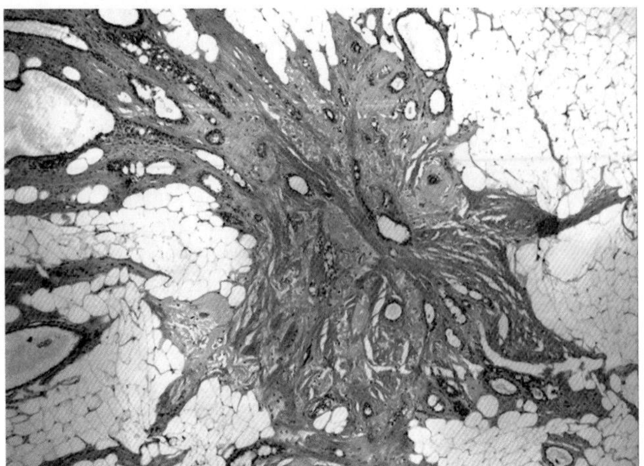

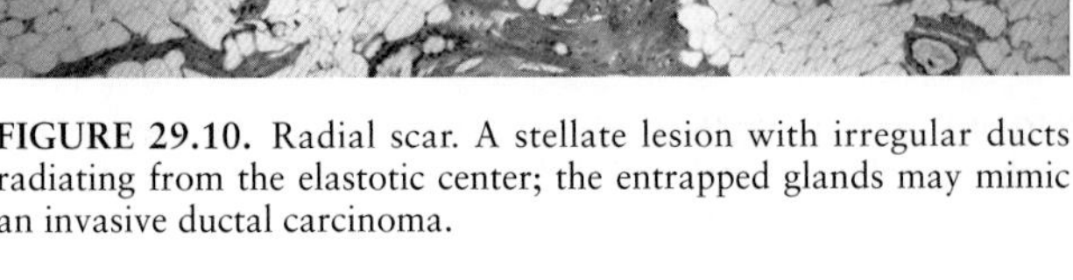

FIGURE 29.10. Radial scar. A stellate lesion with irregular ducts radiating from the elastotic center; the entrapped glands may mimic an invasive ductal carcinoma.

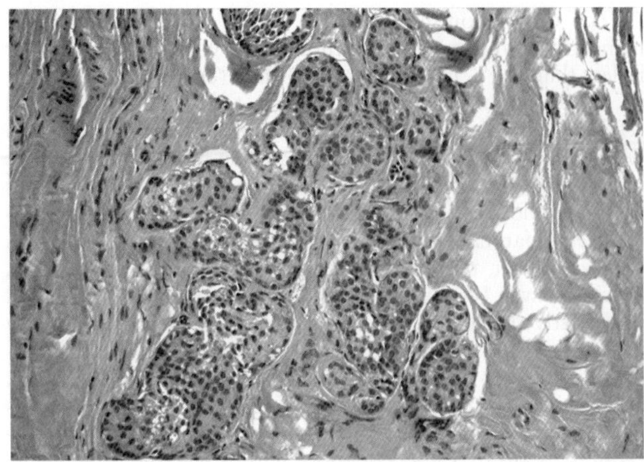

FIGURE 29.12. Atypical lobular hyperplasia. The lobular glands are somewhat expanded with a loose monomorphic cell population.

scar (Fig. 29.10) show distortion of normal breast architecture, and this irregular gland pattern may mimic an invasive carcinoma. These benign proliferations maintain a normal myoepithelial cell layer, which can be highlighted by special stains. Intraductal papillomas have fibrovascular cores lined by myoepithelial cells and one or more layers of epithelial cells. Papillomas involving large ducts near the nipple are the most frequent cause of bloody nipple discharge.

Atypical ductal hyperplasia (ADH) and atypical lobular hyperplasia (ALH) are associated with a higher increased risk of subsequent breast cancer, and in most studies it is increased fivefold (12,90,91). ADH is characterized by architectural patterns approaching those of *in situ* carcinoma (Fig. 29.11), while ALH shows expansion of the lobule by a loose, monomorphic cell population (Fig. 29.12). Reproducibility of the diagnosis of atypical ductal hyperplasia has been aided by more uniform criteria now used by most pathologists (92). However, there is still controversy as to whether size criteria should be used to separate ADH from low-grade ductal carcinoma *in situ* (two completely involved ducts or 2 mm). Excision is recommended for ADH found on core biopsy, as up to 30% of cases will have carcinoma (*in situ* or invasive) found on evaluation of the surrounding tissue (93). ADH can also involve a radial scar or intraductal papilloma (Fig. 29.13).

A newly appreciated group of lesions are columnar cell change, columnar cell hyperplasia, and flat epithelial atypia (FEA, Fig. 29.14). These lesions were originally described by Azzopardi and their significance has been reappraised due to their frequent association with mammographically detected microcalcifications (94–96). More recently, it has been noted that flat epithelial atypia has a high association with low-grade ductal carcinoma *in situ* and invasive tubular carcinoma (97–99). Molecular studies may be able to further characterize these lesions and their role in breast carcinogenesis. Currently, excision is recommended for atypical lesions (ADH, lobular carcinoma *in situ* [LCIS], FEA, and radial scar) identified on needle core biopsy.

In Situ Carcinoma

Ductal Carcinoma *In Situ*

Ductal carcinoma *in situ* (DCIS) or intraductal carcinoma is a heterogenous group of lesions with the proliferation of malignant cells confined within the ductal system. It is the most common type of noninvasive breast cancer currently. Historically, DCIS presented as a palpable mass and accounted for 1% to 2%

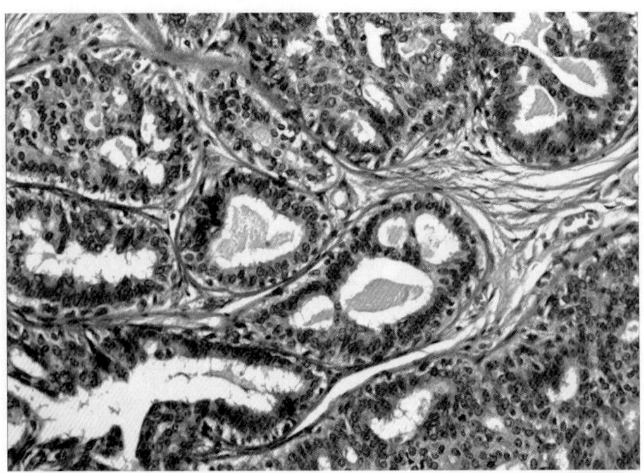

FIGURE 29.11. Atypical ductal hyperplasia. The proliferation has a cribriform growth pattern approaching that of a ductal carcinoma *in situ* but the microlumens are more irregular in sizes and shapes.

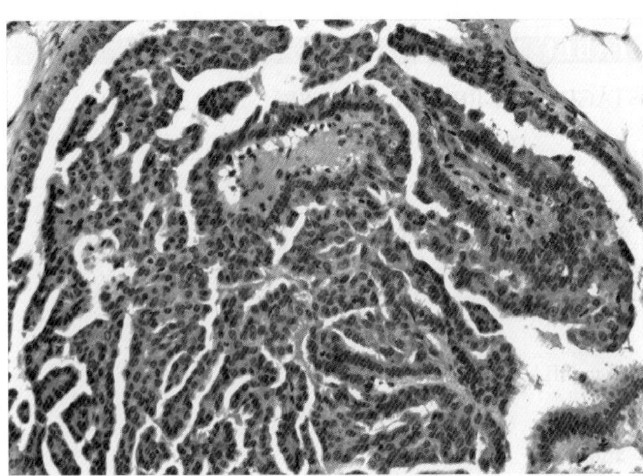

FIGURE 29.13. Intraductal papilloma. A well-circumscribed papillary proliferation fills a dilated duct. The presence of fibrovascular core of the papillae indicates a benign lesion.

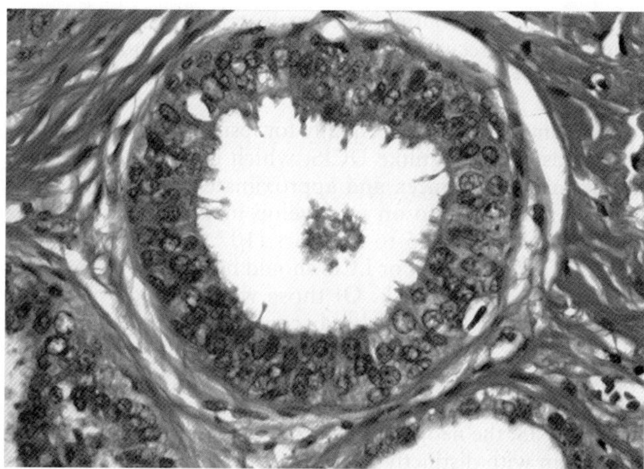

FIGURE 29.14. Flat epithelial hyperplasia. This is a columnar lesion characterized by mildly atypical epithelial cells which may represent a precursor of or the earliest morphologically recognizable form of low-grade ductal carcinoma *in situ*.

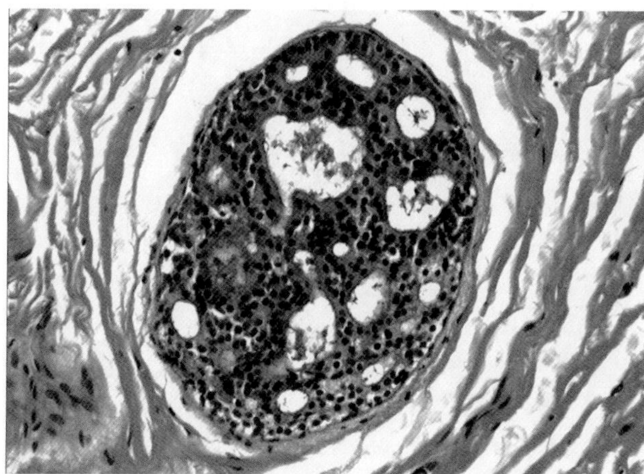

FIGURE 29.16. Cribriform ductal carcinoma *in situ*. Expanded duct is filled with low- to intermediate-grade neoplastic cells forming secondary rigid cribriform microlumens.

of positive biopsies. With screening it is now most commonly identified as clustered microcalcifications on a mammogram and accounts for approximately 20% of all mammographic abnormalities. DCIS is considered a precancerous lesion and it is estimated that approximately 30% of untreated DCIS cases become invasive within 10 years with almost all invasive lesions occurring in the same quadrant as the index lesion (100).

Traditionally, DCIS was classified on its architectural pattern, often dichotomized as comedo and noncomedo types, and solid, cribriform, micropapillary, clinging, and papillary types of noncomedo patterns were described (101). However, it is recognized that combinations of these patterns are not uncommon in a biopsy. Several grading schemes incorporating both architectural and nuclear features have been proposed, but the Holland version, where nuclear features predominate, was most reproducible in one study (102,103). The presence of intraluminal necrosis and calcifications is usually noted, along with the nuclear grade and pattern(s).

Comedo-type DCIS (comedocarcinoma) shows a solid proliferation of large, pleomorphic nuclear grade 3 epithelial cells with numerous mitoses and central necrosis containing cellular debris, so-called "comedo-necrosis" (Fig. 29.15). The necrotic material often becomes calcified and these coarse calcifications have a distinctive mammographic appearance outlining the ductal system ("casting calcifications"). Periductal fibrosis and inflammation is common in comedo-type DCIS and can be a diagnostic problem, as microinvasion is a feature more likely associated with comedo-type DCIS than other patterns (104,105). Extension of the large pleomorphic cells into the distal lobular unit is a pattern known as "cancerization of lobules."

The solid, cribriform, papillary, and micropapillary patterns of noncomedo DCIS are usually composed of uniform low-grade or intermediate-grade nuclei. Cribriform patterns show smooth, rounded, "punched-out" spaces (Fig. 29.16). The micropapillary subtype (Fig. 29.17) does not contain fibrovascular cores, whereas papillary DCIS does. The "clinging" or "flat" type of DCIS may have either low- or high-grade nuclei. Microcalcifications may be associated with these noncomedo patterns and may be detected by mammography. Their pattern of distribution is less specific than that of comedo DCIS and may be similar to that seen in benign conditions.

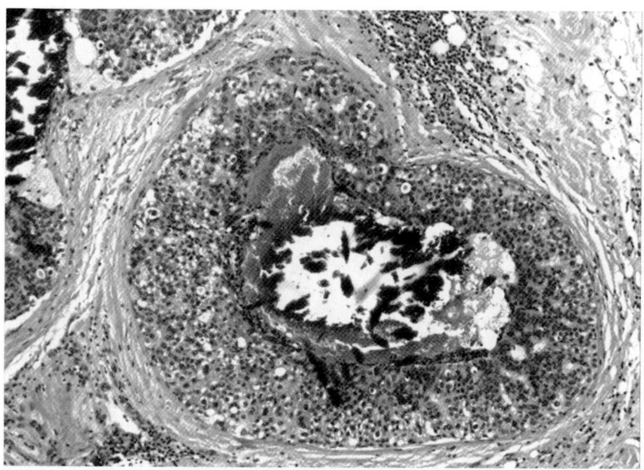

FIGURE 29.15. Comedo-type ductal carcinoma *in situ*. Markedly expanded ducts are filled with high-grade neoplastic ductal cells with central necrosis and calcifications.

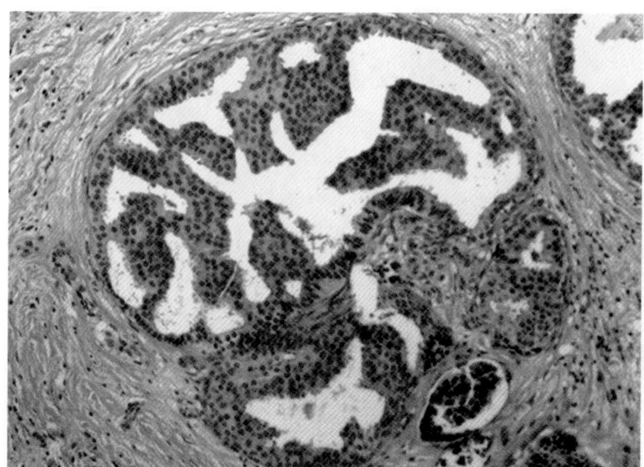

FIGURE 29.17. Micropapillary ductal carcinoma *in situ*. Low-grade neoplastic ductal cells form papillary fronds in an expanded duct. The papillary fronds lack fibrovascular core.

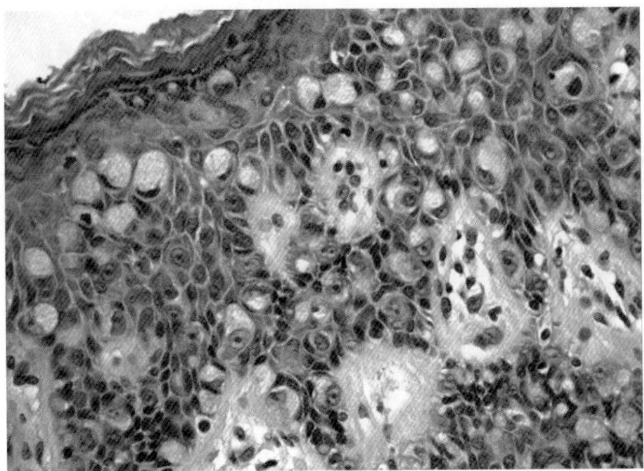

FIGURE 29.18. Paget's disease. Large, round, pale neoplastic cells occur singly within the epidermis, mimicking malignant melanoma, which could be easily distinguished using positive immunohistochemical staining for carcinoembryonic antigen and negative for Melan-A and HMB-45.

Paget's Disease of the Nipple

Paget's disease of the nipple reflects direct extension of ductal carcinoma *in situ,* usually high grade, into the lactiferous ducts and adjacent skin (Fig. 29.18). The DCIS may or may not be accompanied by invasive carcinoma. Histologically, the Paget cells are large, round cells with prominent nucleoli and pale cytoplasm. They occur singly within the layers of the epidermis, or may form groups at the dermal-epidermal junction. Treatment is dictated by whether the underlying tumor is *in situ* or invasive.

Lobular Carcinoma *In Situ*

LCIS was first described by Foote and Stewart in 1941 and has been an enigma ever since (106). It is a multicentric lesion, with no identifying features on gross or radiographic evaluation, and is often found as an incidental finding in biopsies performed for another reason. In classic LCIS, the lobule is distended by a monomorphic population of small uniform cells with round nuclei and scant cytoplasm (Fig. 29.19). The cells may extend into the adjacent duct, growing beneath the normal ductal epithelium, a pattern known as "pagetoid spread." There is continuing controversy as to whether LCIS is an obligate precursor of invasive lobular carcinoma, or just a marker of overall increased cancer risk in either breast (107,108).

LCIS increases the risk equally for ipsilateral and contralateral breast cancer, unlike DCIS, which increases the risk of ipsilateral breast cancer, and approximately 20% to 30% of LCIS patients will go on to develop invasive breast cancer within a median of 15 to 20 years (107,109). Patients with biopsy-diagnosed ALH or LCIS should be referred for surgical treatment given this risk. Of those who undergo definitive excision, carcinoma will be discovered at final pathologic analysis in 14% to 38% of patients (93,110,111). Plemorphic LCIS is a recently described subtype of LCIS that may confer a more agressive phenotype. While similar in architecture to typical LCIS, the neoplastic cells show a larger degree of pleomorphism with distinctly larger nuclei (112).

Invasive Carcinoma

Invasive carcinoma of the breast is defined by the presence of stromal invasion, usually manifest by a fibrotic, desmoplastic stromal reaction around the invading cells. Tumor may be microinvasive (<1 mm) within an area of DCIS, or may form an obvious tumor mass, clinically or radiographically. Tumors are classified by the pattern of growth into ductal and lobular forms. Breast carcinoma is surgically staged using the AJCC staging system based on the size of the invasive component, and synoptic checklist reporting using templates devised by the College of American Pathologists aids in ensuring that all important pathologic features are documented. DCIS may be focally present next to the invasive component or intermixed with invasive tumor. The term "EIC" denotes a tumor with an extensive *in situ* component, defined as at least 25% of the tumor mass.

Invasive Ductal Carcinoma

The majority of invasive tumors of the breast are ductal and have varying morphologic patterns that have led to several subclassifications. Most of the special types listed below are distinguished because they have an extremely good prognosis. The majority of tumors (~75%) have no specific features and are designated carcinoma, not otherwise specified (NOS) or carcinoma of no special type (NST). These tumors may be composed of small glands, tubules, solid cords, or

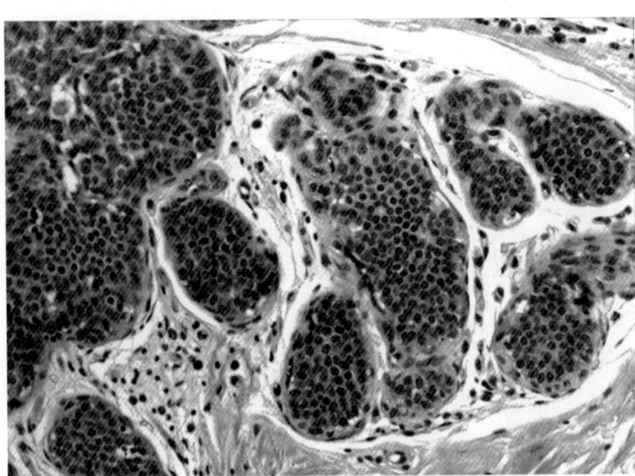

FIGURE 29.19. Lobular carcinoma *in situ.* An expanded lobule is markedly distended by a monomorphic population of small uniform cells. The underlying lobular architecture is still recognizable.

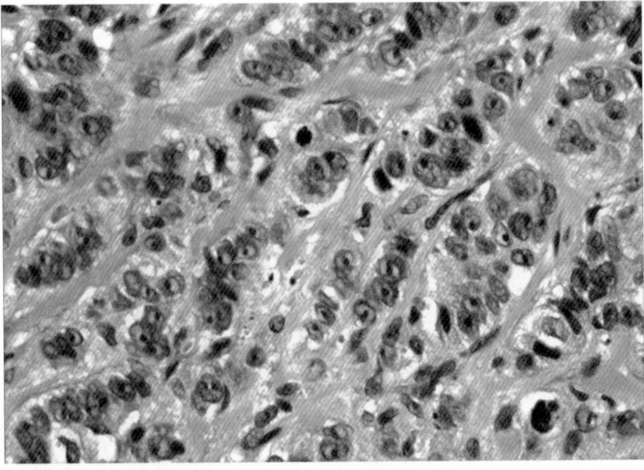

FIGURE 29.20. Invasive ductal carcinoma. Small solid cords of neoplastic cells with moderate to severe cytologic atypia are surrounded by a fibrous stroma.

TABLE 29.7

MODIFIED BLOOM-RICHARDSON GRADING SCHEME

	Score
TUBULE AND GLAND FORMATION	
Majority of tumor (>75%)	1
Moderate degree (10% to 75%)	2
Little or none (<10%)	3
NUCLEAR PLEOMORPHISM	
Small, regular, uniform cells	1
Moderate increase in size and variablity	2
Marked variation	3
MITOTIC COUNT (0.152 mm FIELD AREA)[a]	
0–5	1
6–10	2
>11	3

[a]Adjust for different field areas.

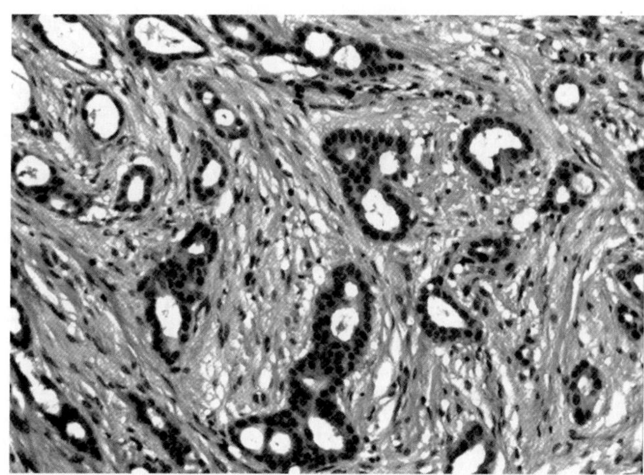

FIGURE 29.22. Tubular carcinoma. Well-formed angular, oval, and tubular glands with a single layer of neoplastic ductal cells diffusely infiltrate a desmoplastic fibrous stroma.

nests of cells with varying degrees of cytologic atypia surrounded by a reactive (desmoplastic) fibrous stroma (Fig. 29.20). The recommended grading system is the Nottingham modification of the Bloom-Richardson system, which is based on adding scores for architectural pattern, nuclear pleomorphism, and mitotic count (Table 29.7) (113). Grade 1 tumors (well differentiated) have 3 to 5 points, grade 2 tumors (moderately differentiated) have 6 to 7 points, and grade 3 tumors (poorly differentiated) have 8 to 9 points. Although initially applied only to invasive ductal carcinoma, this system can also be applied to invasive lobular carcinomas and has been validated in numerous studies (114).

Mucinous Carcinoma. Mucinous (or colloid) carcinoma usually occurs in postmenopausal women. The tumor is well circumscribed and may have a gelatinous gross appearance. Microscopically, nests of uniform small cells are surrounded by pools of mucin (Fig. 29.21). The *in situ* component is minimal, but may also show intraductal mucin production. Pure mucinous tumors are low grade and have an excellent prognosis with a low rate of lymph node metastasis (115). This is not true, however, of mixed carcinomas with a prominent nonmucinous, usual invasive ductal carcinoma component.

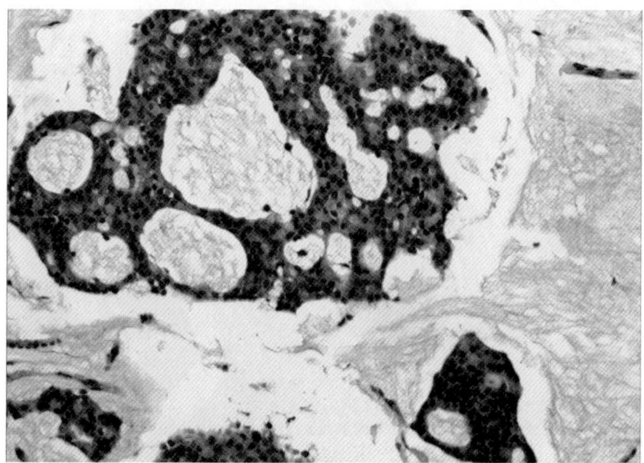

FIGURE 29.21. Mucinous carcinoma. Nests of low-grade neoplastic cells in a cribriform pattern are surrounded by a large pool of mucin.

Tubular Carcinoma. Tubular carcinoma is a well-differentiated invasive carcinoma composed of small glands or tubules that can be difficult to distinguish from some benign lesions, especially radial scars. The tubules are arranged haphazardly, often with a surrounding cellular stroma (Fig. 29.22). They are somewhat angular with open lumens and are lined by a single layer of monomorphic epithelial cells. Myoepithelial cells are absent, and immunohistochemistry for myoepithelial markers is helpful in confirming the diagnosis on needle biopsy. If the tumor is composed of at least 75% tubules and has grade 1 nuclei, the prognosis is considered to be excellent (116). Invasive tubular carcinoma is often associated with a low-grade micropapillary or cribriform ductal carcinoma *in situ* or adjacent atypical columnar cell lesions (98). Tubular carcinomas are small, usually less than 1 cm, and are frequently detected by screening mammography. Tumors with a component of usual invasive ductal carcinoma should not be included in this category. Invasive cribriform carcinoma, which also has a good prognosis, may be mixed with tubular carcinoma.

Medullary Carcinoma. Medullary carcinomas occur more commonly in women under 50 and have a higher frequency in *BRCA1* mutation carriers. Clinically, the tumor is well circumscribed and may mimic a fibroadenoma. Microscopically, the tumor is composed of solid syncytial sheets of large anaplastic cells with pleomorphic nuclei, prominent nucleoli, and abundant mitotic figures (Fig. 29.23). Gland formation is absent. The tumor has a pushing border and is surrounded by a dense lymphoplasmacytic infiltrate. Despite being anaplastic, however, tumors with this strict morphology and no component of typical invasive ductal carcinoma have a good prognosis.

Micropapillary Carcinoma. Micropapillary carcinoma is a recently described entity with a characteristic morphology, high incidence of positive nodes at presentation despite small tumor size, and poor overall survival (117,118). The tumor is composed of small clusters of malignant cells floating within small clear spaces resembling lymphatic channels (Fig. 29.24). Most tumors have high nuclear grade and true lymphatic space invasion. A component of usual invasive ductal carcinoma may be present.

Papillary Carcinoma. Papillary carcinoma is a rare subtype, and the majority of cases are felt to represent an *in situ* tumor, frequently termed "intracystic papillary carcinoma."

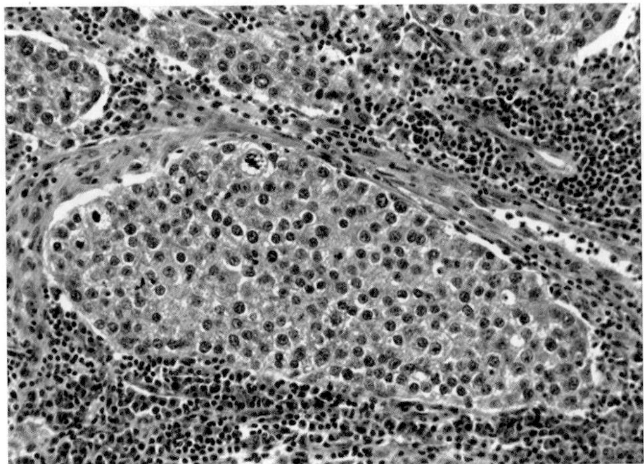

FIGURE 29.23. Medullary carcinoma. Highly pleomorphic neoplastic cells in a syncytial pattern are surrounded by a diffuse lymphocytic infiltrate.

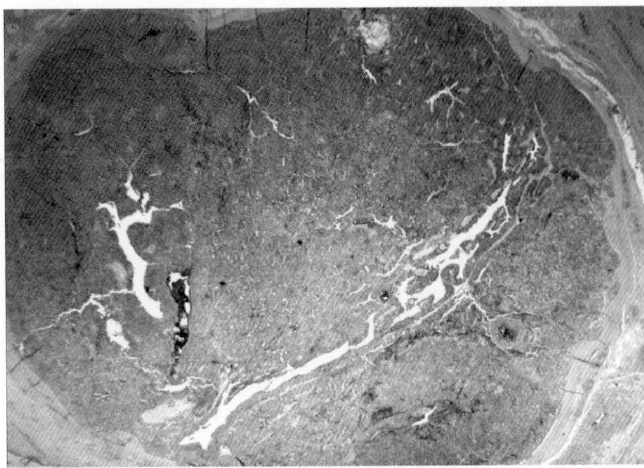

FIGURE 29.25. Solid or intracystic papillary carcinoma. Whole-mount section shows a well-circumscribed tumor with branching network of fibrovascular stroma. A cystic formation is not necessary for the diagnosis.

The lesion forms a well-circumscribed mass, and may have ductal carcinoma *in situ* present in adjacent ducts or foci of typical invasive carcinoma around the periphery of the main mass (Fig. 29.25). A recent study suggests that these are indeed invasive carcinomas without the myoepithelial layer that defines an *in situ* lesion (119). They have traditionally been treated as *in situ* lesions and have an overall excellent prognosis (120).

Inflammatory Carcinoma. The term "inflammatory carcinoma" originated as a clinical term to describe a patient presenting with a reddened edematous breast suggesting mastitis. Skin biopsies from such patients often show tumor thrombi in dermal lymphatic channels (Fig. 29.26), but this is not true in every case.

Invasive Lobular Carcinoma

Invasive lobular carcinoma comprises about 10% of all breast cancers. The classic form of invasive lobular carcinoma is composed of small monotonous tumor cells with scant cytoplasm growing in linear columns ("Indian file") or in concentric ("targetoid") patterns around normal ducts and lobules (Fig. 29.27). A mild stromal desmoplastic reaction may be present around the tumor cells, but many invasive lobular carcinomas do not form a discrete tumor mass. This diffuse growth pattern can be a problem when attempting conservative surgical excision, and tumors are frequently upstaged after surgery (121).

Variant forms of lobular carcinoma include alveolar, solid, and trabecular patterns composed of the same monomorphic small cells. Signet ring–cell carcinoma, in which the cells contain prominent intracytoplasmic vacuoles, is considered a variant of invasive lobular carcinoma due to its similar growth patterns. Another variant is pleomorphic lobular carcinoma, where the columns of cells show marked nuclear atypia.

Tubulolobular Carcinoma. This tumor shows a mixture of invasive lobular and tubular carcinoma growth patterns with low-grade nuclei. The mixed architectural pattern parallels the expression of markers of ductal and lobular differentiation, and these tumors appear to have a good prognosis (122).

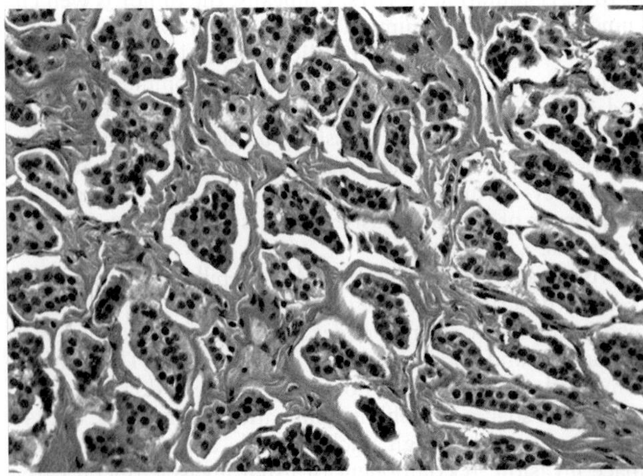

FIGURE 29.24. Invasive micropapillary carcinoma. Small clusters of intermediate-grade neoplastic cells lie within small, clear spaces of a fibrocollagenous stroma mimicking tumor cells in lymphatic spaces.

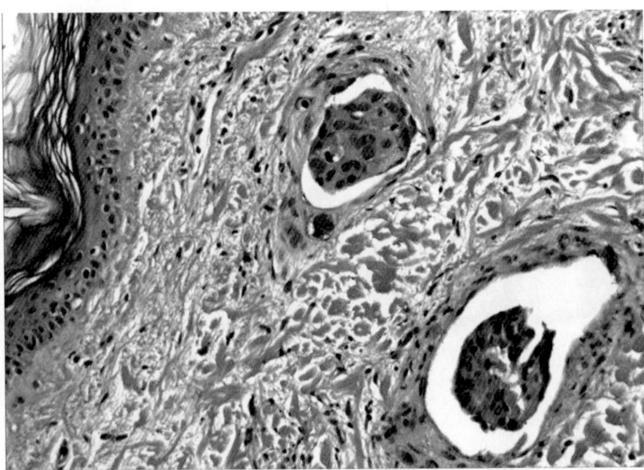

FIGURE 29.26. Inflammatory carcinoma. Carcinomatous emboli are present in dilated dermal lymphatics.

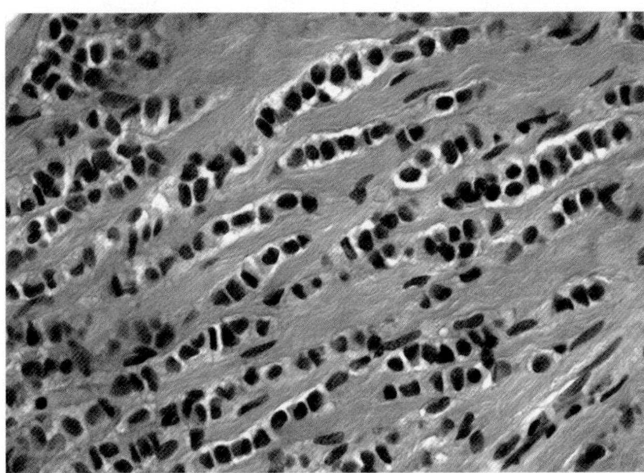

FIGURE 29.27. Invasive lobular carcinoma. Small monotonous tumor cells invade in linear "Indian file" pattern.

Other Tumors

Metaplastic Carcinoma

The term "metaplastic carcinoma" is used to describe tumors with prominent morphologic patterns different from usual ductal and lobular patterns (Fig. 29.28). The term encompasses epithelial tumors (carcinomas) showing squamous cell differentiation, monophasic spindle cell carcinoma, and biphasic tumors with both epithelial and mesenchymal elements. Spindle cell (sarcomatoid) carcinomas express epithelial markers (cytokeratins) despite their spindle cell morphology, and are aggressive tumors with a high rate of extranodal metastases (123). Biphasic tumors (biphasic sarcomatoid carcinoma or carcinosarcoma) may contain heterologous elements, such as malignant cartilage or bone. These rare but aggressive tumors tend to be estrogen receptor (ER), progesterone receptor (PR), and HER2/neu negative, but in a case series from the Swedish Cancer Institute, survival outcomes did not appear different from matched typical breast cancer cases (124).

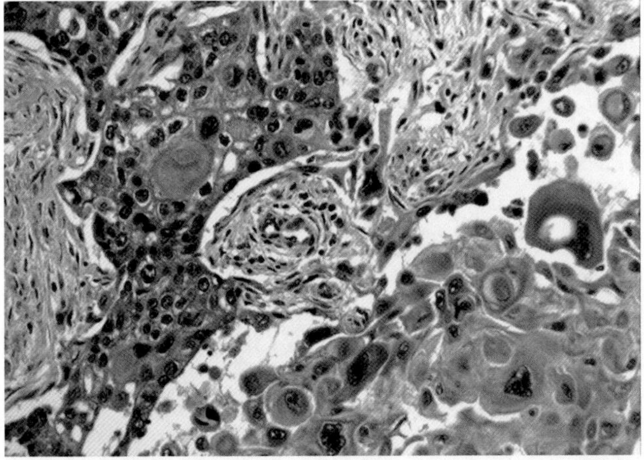

FIGURE 29.28. Metaplastic carcinoma. This is a poorly differentiated invasive carcinoma. To the right is an area of squamous differentiation.

Phyllodes Tumors

Phyllodes tumors, formerly known as "cystosarcoma phyllodes," are biphasic tumors similar to fibroadenomas with a spectrum of morphology and biologic behavior. The median age is 45, which is several decades higher than fibroadenoma. These tumors are grossly well circumscribed, but are infiltrative on microscopic examination. They are composed of benign glandular elements with a prominent stromal component showing varying degrees of hypercellularity, nuclear atypia, and mitotic activity. The older term "cystosarcoma phyllodes" refers to the leaf-like architectural pattern with intervening cystic spaces. Although features such as size, mitotic activity, and cellular atypia correlate with clinical behavior, attempts to reliably divide these tumors into benign and malignant forms are not always successful. The lower- grade tumors tend to recur, especially if incompletely excised, due to the subtle infiltrative margin. Obvious malignant tumors may have stromal overgrowth, which portends a worse prognosis (125,126). Overall, lymph node metastases are uncommon and surgery is the primary treatment.

Angiosarcoma

Angiosarcoma is the most common primary sarcoma of the breast, and may be associated with previous radiation therapy. The tumors are composed of anastomosing vascular channels lined by endothelial cells that range from mildly atypical to frankly malignant. The distinction between a benign angioma and a low-grade angiosarcoma can be difficult on a small biopsy. Overall 5-year survival is around 60% with multimodality therapy (127,128). Other histologic patterns of primary breast sarcoma also occur.

GENOMIC CLASSIFICATION OF BREAST CANCER

Our understanding of breast cancer has begun to evolve with the use of modern technology, and gene expression studies have heightened our understanding of breast cancers as being composed of heterogenous tumor subtypes with distinct biologic features. In a seminal paper, Perou et al. characterized 65 breast specimens from 42 patients with breast cancer, including 20 sampled pre- and postchemotherapy and 2 with node-positive disease (129). They demonstrated that breast tumors could be subdivided based on their genomic signature into distinct molecular types: luminal/ER positive, normal breast-like, basal/epithelial cell enriched, erb/B2 amplified, and an unknown cohort. Sorlie et al. later expanded this study into a classification of 78 tumors, and were able to separate the luminal group into three subtypes: luminal A tumors had the highest expression of ER genes; luminal B had low to moderate expression of luminal-specific genes; and luminal C was characterized by low expression of the luminal-specific genes and expression of genes of unknown function, but were also seen in the erb/B2 and basal classes of breast tumors (130). Inclusion of a *BRCA1* cohort into a later study also demonstrated the propensity of these tumors to fall into the basal subgroup (131).

Bertucci et al. sought to correlate molecular subtypes with pathologic characteristics routinely evaluated in breast cancer (132). Statistically significant differences in tumor grade, ER status, PR status, HER2/neu status, and p53 staining were noted in luminal A tumors, erb/B2 amplified, and basal-like tumors. The vast majority of luminal A tumors in this study were non–high grade (73%), ER positive (100%), PR positive

(96%), HER2/neu negative (96%), and p53 negative (85%). In contrast, the basal tumors were predominantly the opposite: grade 3 (88%), ER negative (94%), PR negative (94%), HER2/neu positive (100%), and p53 positive (53%). The erb/B2 amplified cohort had the biggest mix of features: grade 2 or 3 (100%), ER negative (93%), PR negative (80%), HER2/neu positive (100%), and p53 negative (53%). Even more important than the determination of these molecular subtypes, Sorlie et al. demonstrated that the classification also separated tumors prognostically, with luminal A tumors being associated with the highest probability of remaining alive and disease-free while basal tumors were associated with poor survival outcomes (130). These data have been replicated in other reports (132,133).

PROGNOSTIC AND PREDICTIVE FACTORS

In breast cancer, there are clinical and biologic factors that can inform the anticipated responses to a given therapy (*predictive* factors) and those that are independently associated with survival outcomes, whether it be recurrence or death from breast cancer (*prognostic* factors). Understanding such factors holds the key to making decisions regarding therapy for the patient with breast cancer. For patients whose prognosis is good, chemotherapy may hold little benefit and may not be recommended. Alternatively, endocrine therapy and the use of biologic agents, such as trastuzumab, may depend on the presence of factors that will predict tumor responsiveness, which may ultimately translate into a survival advantage.

Of the known prognostic factors in breast cancer, the most widely accepted are defined surgically. Axillary node involvement is a strong predictor of both relapse risk and mortality, and risks increase with the number of nodes involved by metastatic breast cancer. Tumor size is also a well-established prognostic factor, with increasing size associated with a greater number of involved nodes and a shorter time to recurrence. The presence of lymphovascular invasion and high tumor grade also portends a worse prognosis.

Histologically, tumors associated with mutations in either *BRCA1* or *BRCA2* are high-grade invasive ductal carcinomas. *BRCA1* mutation–associated breast cancers are usually triple negative and express basal markers (134). This is in contrast to *BRCA2* mutation–associated tumors, which are usually ER positive and express a luminal A phenotype (135).

The most commonly cited biologic factor associated with prognosis is the estrogen and progesterone receptor status. Estrogen interacting with nuclear ERs regulates cell growth, proliferation, and differentiation of normal breast epithelium, and those carcinomas that express ER. PR is an ER-regulated gene product with similar implications. Hormone receptors can be measured biochemically by ligand binding assays or by IHC techniques using monoclonal antibodies directed against the receptor protein, and correlation between the two techniques is high (136). With today's smaller tumors usually diagnosed by needle core biopsy, IHC is the preferred method of analysis. This method also allows distinction between invasive tumor, *in situ* tumor, and nontumor elements. Heterogeneity exists within tumors, and most laboratories now report positivity by the percentage of cells stained or use a semiquantitative scale (137). However, hormonal status is a relatively weak prognostic indicator, and measurement of ER in breast cancers is performed to predict the response of an invasive tumor to endocrine therapy, or the benefit of hormonal therapy for risk reduction in cases of *in situ* carcinoma. Patients with ER- and/or PR-positive disease are expected to benefit from hormonal agents. Alternatively, patients with hormone-positive disease may not derive a significant benefit from chemotherapy (138).

Recently, survivin, a member of the inhibitor of apoptosis (IAP) family, has been proposed as a prognostic factor. In one study, 293 cases of invasive breast cancer were assayed for survivin, showing that 60% were positive (139). In a multivariate analysis, survivin was shown to be significantly associated with relapse-free ($p < 0.001$) and overall survival ($p = 0.01$). This was independent of age, tumor size, tumor grade, nodal status, and estrogen receptor.

Other biologic factors have been proposed as prognostic, including Ki-67, a nuclear antigen that is not expressed at G_0 but is detected in the G_1 through M phases, the fraction of cells in S phase, and DNA ploidy analysis. However, these factors have yet to be validated in statistically robust studies, and are not recommended for use in daily practice (140).

HER2/neu or c-erbB2 is an oncogene whose protein product is a membrane receptor tyrosine kinase. Amplification of HER2/neu is seen in most cases of comedo-type ductal carcinoma *in situ* and in about 20% to 30% of invasive ductal carcinoma, usually of high grade. It can be detected by immunohistochemistry for the protein product or by gene amplification techniques, such as fluorescence *in situ* hybridization (FISH) or chromogenic *in situ* hybridization (CISH). Increased copy number is closely associated with elevated protein expression. Amplification of HER2/neu, and this used to confer a poor prognosis in breast cancer (141). However, with the advent of trastuzumab, a monoclonal antibody directed against the HER2/neu receptor, women with HER2/neu amplified breast cancers have gained significantly in their survival outcomes; as such it is no longer correct to consider it a prognostic factor, but rather to use it as a predictive factor for the selection of treatment (142–144).

The American Society of Clinical Oncology and College of American Pathologists recently published a joint guideline containing an algorithm for testing, interpretation, and reporting, as well as requirements for standardization and validation of testing techniques (145). A positive HER2/neu result is 3+ IHC staining, defined as uniform intense membrane staining of >30% of invasive tumor cells (Fig. 29.29) *or* a FISH result of more than six HER2 gene copies per nucleus *or* a FISH ratio (HER2 signals to chromosome 17 signals) of more than 2.2. Implementation of these guidelines will result in more reproducible results between laboratories.

A subset of breast carcinomas is negative for the usual markers ER, PR, and HER2/neu, and are referred to as triple negative. These tumors express cytokeratins 5/6, which

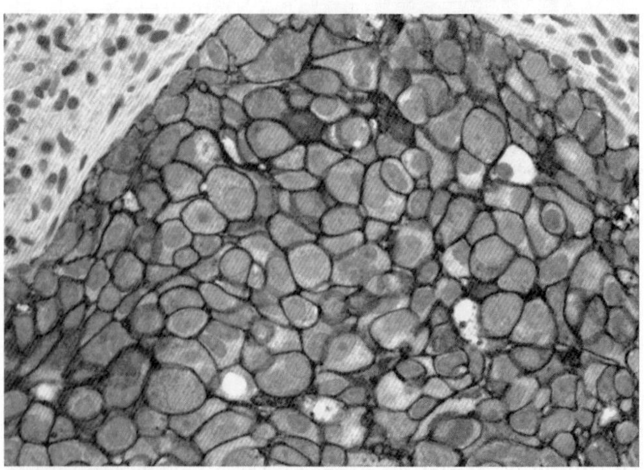

FIGURE 29.29. Positive HER2/neu. Strong (3+) HER2/neu membrane immunoreactivity is seen in this invasive ductal carcinoma.

denotes a basal phenotype, in contrast to the luminal cell phenotype of most breast carcinomas (146,147). These tumors are characteristically high grade, have a central hyalinized scar or necrosis, occur in younger women, and are associated with poor survival (148,149). Many metaplastic carcinomas fall into this group of tumors. Most triple-negative tumors are positive for epidermal growth factor receptor (EGFR), which may provide a target for future therapy (146).

GENERAL MANAGEMENT OF BREAST CANCER

SURGICAL CONSIDERATIONS

Historical Perspective

Early descriptions of breast disease date back to ancient Chinese and Egyptian civilizations, and those of breast malignancy date back to Hippocrates and Celsus. The predominating theories of Hippocrates and Galen's four bodily humours were taken as dogma until the 1700s, when LeDran proposed the revolutionary concept of lymphatic spread. Evolutions in surgical treatment of breast cancer, however, awaited the introduction of anesthesia and Listerian antisepsis.

Faced with a high incidence of local recurrence and the understanding that cancer growth and spread occurred in an "orderly sequential process," the radical mastectomy was championed as an attempt to get at "the roots" of the tumor. At the same time, surgeons suggested that the axillary nodes be removed as part of the operation on breast cancer, given the propensity of nodal involvement.

The earliest description of the mastectomy was by Jean Petit, but Charles Moore and Sir Joseph Lister are credited with advocating the more radical approach by incorporating the division of the pectoral muscles when performing a mastectomy, which allowed for improved exposure of the axillary contents. The subsequent groundwork by Pancoast, Gross, and Moore of London led to the reports of Willie Meyer and William Halsted, who simultaneously published papers advocating the systematic removal of nodes in continuity with the primary cancer in 1894 (150,151). These papers presented a systemically applied approach to the radical mastectomy and offered a standardized technique of lymphadenectomy in breast cancer in an anatomically logical and exact manner. Technically, the procedure involved an *en bloc* resection of the breast, the pectoralis major and minor, and a full axillary dissection, levels I-III. In so doing, the local recurrence rate dropped from nearly 50%–80% to 6%, and the reported 3-year cure rate was 38.3% (152). So successful was this operation that it became the yardstick against which all other interventions would be measured. Even with this breakthrough, Halsted recognized that node negativity did not ensure survival.

The extension of the operation was explored by surgeons in Europe and the United States, including operations that involved resection of the supraclavicular nodes (Halsted) or the internal mammary nodes (Handey), and extension of surgery into the neck and/or mediastinum (Urban and Wangensteen) (153,154). However, these increasingly extensive surgeries did not improve overall survival, but did increase operative mortality, and thus were largely abandoned. Simultaneously, Sir Geoffrey Keynes first described the role of radiation therapy (RT) in local control of cancer in 1930, and Robert McWhirter first demonstrated that axillary radiation was effective in locoregional control in breast cancer (155). This presaged the controversy regarding surgical resection versus radiotherapy for locoregional control and its relationship to survival.

Advances in medicine and public health between 1880 and the mid-1900s led to improvements in breast cancer detection and smaller tumors, which led surgeons to explore options beyond the radical mastectomy. It was not until the 1970s, however, that the surgical trend for breast cancer management was deliberately directed toward less aggressive approaches (156).

Modern History

Over a decade after the first randomized clinical trial evaluating the outcomes of breast conservation combined with postoperative radiation versus mastectomy revealed no difference in either overall survival or in breast recurrence between treatment groups, the National Surgical Breast and Bowel Project (NSABP) launched a series of trials where the underlying construct was that breast cancer was systemic at origin, and therefore the technique of surgery was less important than systemic therapy. Because the dogma was that it is the systemic disease that controls survival, the group accepted negative margins delineated as "no tumor at ink" and this qualification would distinguish NSABP trials from other investigations. In total, six major prospective, randomized trials were initiated between 1972 and 1983 and are summarized in Table 29.8.

The NSABP B-06 trial compared modified radical mastectomy to lumpectomy with or without breast irradiation in 1,851 patients with stage I-II breast cancer (157). At 20 years

TABLE 29.8

RANDOMIZED TRIALS COMPARING BREAST CONSERVATION THERAPY (BCT) AND MASTECTOMY (MAS)

	Local recurrence (%)		Overall survival (%)		Follow-up (years)
Trial	BCT	Mas	BCT	Mas	
Milan (158)	7	4	65	65	18
Institut Gustave-Roussy (160)	9	14	73	65	15
NSABP B-06 (157)	10	8	63	59	20
NCI (161)	19	6	77	75	10
EORTC (162)	20	12	65	66	10
Danish Breast Cancer Group (159)	3	4	79	82	6

Note: EORTC, European Organization for Research and Treatment of Cancer; NCI, National Cancer Institute; NSABP, National Surgical Breast and Bowel Project.

of follow-up, there was no significant difference in either disease-free or overall survival. Additionally, whole breast irradiation was found to reduce local recurrence in patients who received breast conservation. With these results, breast conservation therapy (BCT) was rightfully established as the standard of care. A similar trial was reported by Veronesi et al. for the National Tumor Institute of Milan (158). Over 700 women with tumors under 2 cm were randomized to mastectomy versus quadrantectomy with axillary dissection followed by radiotherapy. Adjuvant chemotherapy using cyclophosphamide, methotrexate, and 5-fluorouracil (CMF) was administered to all patients with node-positive disease. With 20 years of follow-up, the actuarial disease-free and overall survivals were similar in both groups. The Danish Cooperative Group conducted a similar study of 895 patients and once more showed that with 6 years of follow-up, equivalent rates of local recurrence and overall survival were achieved (159). Finally, Arriagada et al. reported the results of a randomized trial involving 179 patients treated at the Institut Gustave-Roussy and once more demonstrated an equivalent disease-free and overall survival (160). Notable studies from the NCI and European Organization for Research and Treatment of Cancer (EORTC) showed a higher risk for local recurrences with breast conservation compared to mastectomy, but these studies were flawed for either inadequate margin assessment or frank margin involvement, respectively (161,162).

In the final analysis, the weight of evidence supports equivalence of breast conservation therapy versus radical or modified radical mastectomy for early-stage breast cancer. The NSABP trials rigorously and systematically both challenged and advanced breast cancer surgical technique and systemic therapy. Ongoing debate about which patients were candidates for BCT continued for decades, ultimately landing at the determination based on the breast-to-tumor volume ratio, absence of multicentric disease, and eligibility for postlumpectomy radiation (163).

The NSABP applied similar methodology in evaluating the benefit of surgery and radiation in the management of ductal carcinoma *in situ* (DCIS). From the NSABP B-17 and B-24 trials we learned that lumpectomy with radiation achieved the lowest rate of local recurrence but did not affect overall survival, and that tamoxifen could decrease not only ipsilateral recurrence but also contralateral new disease (164). NSABP B-32 compared axillary dissection to sentinel node biopsy in the management of the clinically negative axilla and demonstrated the success of sentinel node mapping in predicting the axilla (165). Most recently, the results of the second prevention trial from the NSABP, P-2 (*S*tudy of *T*amoxifen *A*nd *R*aloxifine trial), demonstrated the equivalent efficacy of raloxifine for risk reduction of a new primary in postmenopausal women, but with a reduction in untoward side effects such as thromboembolic events, cataracts, and endometrial carcinoma, the latter not achieving statistical significance (166).

In Situ Disease

In the past DCIS was managed, like any breast cancer, by mastectomy. This was effective from a cancer point of view and resulted in a local recurrence rate of only 1% (167). Interestingly, at a time when breast conservation surgery was being advocated for invasive breast cancer, total mastectomy was still the standard of care for DCIS. Current therapies have since evolved based on extrapolation of the trials of breast conservation therapy with total mastectomy in invasive breast cancer, although there are no phase 3 studies comparing breast conservation therapy with total mastectomy in DCIS.

Currently, DCIS is treated by wide local excision which is now the standard of care. Margin status and size of the lesion appear to be significant factors related to risk of recurrence (168,169). Silverstein et al. created the Van Nuys Prognostic Index (VNPI) by combining pathologic classification (non–high-grade nuclei without necrosis; non–high-grade nuclei with necrosis; high-grade nuclei), tumor size, and closest margin width (170). The VNPI score ranges from 4 to12 and has been shown to stratify the risk of local recurrence after breast-conserving surgery. However, with respect to lesion size, accuracy is often problematic at pathologic evaluation because most DCIS is not grossly evident, yet it is not practical to submit all tissue from an excisional biopsy for microscopic evaluation. Most pathologists rectify this by sectioning of the biopsy specimen guided by the type of lesion and radiographic findings. Of note, mammography can often give a more accurate size of the lesion, though only in tumors that are entirely marked by calcifications. Margin width is most easily measured microscopically in perpendicular sections, which is only possible if the margins are inked in color, which is a prerequisite for identification of each margin.

The indications for mastectomy for DCIS are (a) persistent positive margins; (b) multicentric disease, i.e., DCIS involving more than one quadrant; (c) cosmetically unacceptable breast conservation surgery due to a large DCIS process in a comparatively small breast. For these cases a total or skin-sparing mastectomy with sentinel lymph node biopsy is most clearly recommended, to ensure that the opportunity for lymphatic mapping will not have been sacrificed should occult invasive disease be identified on final pathology.

The role of sentinel node biopsy in DCIS treated with lumpectomy is less clear. Some have advocated for sentinel node biopsy in DCIS treated by lumpectomy when the diagnosis is based on a core needle biopsy since the risk of an invasive cancer at definitive excision ranges between 10% and 20%. In the largest series of sentinel node biopsy for pure DCIS, a 5% rate of nodal metastasis was described; however, 70% of these metastases were detected only by immunohistochemical (IHC) staining (171). Others have suggested stratifying the risk of invasion based on retrospective studies, acknowledging that the implications of IHC-positive nodes are unclear, especially in the context of known disease-specific survival from DCIS of 99% (172). Taking into account the published literature, consideration of lymphatic mapping is reasonable for a span of DCIS greater than 4 cm or a mass on mammography, palpable DCIS, high-grade DCIS, and in the presence or question of microinvasion (173).

Early Invasive Disease

Early invasive breast cancer is almost uniformly diagnosed by imaging modalities. Although breast MRI has emerged as a valuable adjunct in the diagnostic evaluation of breast cancer, its widespread use as a screening tool has yet to be largely realized. Therefore, the majority of patients will present with lesions that have been identified by mammography.

Once the diagnosis of invasive cancer is established in early-stage disease, surgical planning starts. A thorough history and physical examination are essential to establish both the patient's presentation and extent of clinically apparent disease, and to screen for contraindications to breast conservation therapy or to adjuvant radiation therapy, such as connective tissue disorders or prior irradiation. Particular attention to the location of the tumor, its palpability, fixation to the skin or underlying chest wall, cutaneous changes, nipple irregularities, and regional nodal assessment are paramount.

Breast conservation surgery should aim to resect the primary tumor with clear margins. This can be achieved either with the needle localization technique, or one of the other many techniques that have been described in the literature to localize the lesion, such as intraoperative ultrasound localization or radioisotope-guided resection (174,175). The ideal margin for breast cancer in a wide local excision has been a well-published challenge; after all, an acceptable margin for one pathology may not be appropriate for another. In an exhaustive review of the technique and significance of the surgical margin for invasive breast cancer, Singletary analyzed 38 representative studies examining the impact of surgical margin on local recurrence (176). Although it is difficult to discern a distinction between the significance of 1-, 2-, 3-, or greater than 5-mm margins in patients with invasive breast cancer treated with whole breast irradiation with tumor bed boost, she demonstrated an increased local recurrence rate in patients with positive margins. Young age, large tumor size, postive lymph nodes, and the absence of systemic chemotherapy or endocrine therapy were identified as significant independent predictors of locoregional recurrence. The time-dependent nature of recurrence is further elaborated by Neuschatz et al., who showed that graded tumor bed escalation in breast irradiation may establish equivalence in local recurrence for involved margins initially, but that after 5 years of follow-up, the local failure in the close/positive margin groups becomes apparent (177).

Intraoperative margin analysis to ensure adequacy has been explored primarily using frozen section analysis, touch prep, or intraoperative imaging. A promising technique of treating potential positive margins is the use of intraoperative radiofrequency ablation, where a multipronged probe is deployed into the surrounding breast tissue at the completion of the lumpectomy before wound closure (178). Ablation is performed under ultrasound visualization for 15 minutes. Twenty-five percent of patients avoided returning for re-excision due to close margins evident on final pathologic analysis. However, longer follow-up is needed to ensure that the local recurrence remains low.

Locally Advanced Breast Cancer

Locally advanced breast cancer is variously defined as primary tumor size greater than 3 to 5 cm, involvement of the chest wall, skin ulceration or satellitosis, and/or positive axillary nodes (179,180). Approximately 6% of breast cancers in the United States present as locally advanced breast cancer (LABC). These patients are candidates for neoadjuvant chemotherapy or endocrine therapy, which results in a higher rate of breast conservation, without a reduction in either disease-free or overall survival (181). Additionally, neoadjuvant therapy has not been shown to increase the complication rate of surgery or delay the onset of further postoperative treatment. From a biologic standpoint, neoadjuvant therapy provides the opportunity to assess the chemosensivity of breast tumors *in vivo*. The use of neoadjuvant chemotherapy does result in a 30% to 40% decrease in the incidence of axillary nodal involvement, and up to a 20% complete response in responding patients (182–184). Although neoadjuvant chemotherapy has not been shown to improve survival in locally advanced breast cancer, it has demonstrated that up to 80% of patients have significant breast tumor shrinkage and only 2% to 3% will have progression of disease (180,181).

Approximately 25% of patients who were not candidates for breast conservation before treatment were able to conserve their breast after the administration of neoadjuvant chemotherapy. Data from the NSABP B-18 trial demonstrated that patients who achieved a pathologic complete response (pCR) have better survival than those who were partial responders (182). Kuerer et al. also demonstrated that the presence of residual disease in the axillary lymph nodes was a predicator of poor outcome and was associated with a higher incidence of locoregional (14% vs. 5% in patients achieving a pCR in the nodes) and distant metastases (41 vs. 15%) (184). In this study the eradication of nodal metastases was associated with improved survival. In addition, a pathologic complete response to neoadjuvant therapy has been more commonly noted in younger patients and in tumors that are estrogen receptor–negative cancer, high grade, and ductal. Cancers with a high proportion of intraductal cancer are also less likely to shrink significantly. Neoadjuvant endocrine therapy has been used mainly in older women with estrogen receptor–positive disease; aromatase inhibitors are more effective than tamoxifen in inducing a local response, but pCR is rare with endocrine therapy alone.

A core biopsy of the breast is used to establish diagnosis and to obtain prognostic histologic features of the primary tumor. Multiple cores allow for staining for receptors and HER2/neu. A negative biopsy in the setting of a clinically suspicious or dominant breast mass should prompt additional workup with open biopsy. If the patient could be a candidate for breast conservation with appropriate down staging of tumor size, a microclip should be placed in the breast. This facilitates later identification of the cancer site in case of complete response to neoadjuvant therapy. Additionally, axillary evaluation is also required to establish the nodal stage. For palpable disease a needle biopsy can be performed, with sentinel node biopsy being reserved for nonpalpable disease.

However, clinical examination of the axilla remains unreliable, with reported false-negative examination in 21% to 42% of cases (182,185,186). Hence, it is important to identify other methods of accurately staging the axilla before initiation of treatment. Ultrasound combined with physical examination has been shown to increase the reliability of axillary evaluation (187). Further, fine-needle aspiration cytology of suspicious nodes, defined as size greater than 1 cm, loss of fatty hilum, cortical hypertrophy, and hypoechogenic parenchyma, has a reported sensitivity and specificity of 36% to 92% and 69% to 100%, respectively (86,87,188). In a study of 103 cases of indeterminate or suspicious-appearing lymph nodes from the M. D. Anderson Cancer Center, only 11% of node-positive patients were missed by ultrasound-guided cytology (86). All cases with three or more positive nodes, and 93% of cases where the size of the metastatic deposit was greater than 5 mm, could be identified by this technique. In this study, the overall sensitivity of US-FNA was 86%, specificity was 100%, positive predictive value was 100%, and the negative predictive value was 67%. Despite this, the false-negative rate of US-FNA remains 15% to 20% in the reported literature and a major limitation of ultrasound remains the inability to detect metastases less than 5 mm in size. While the identification of node-positive disease by US-FNA can reduce the number of sentinel lymph node biopsy (SLNB) procedures by up to 15% and identify those patients who would not otherwise be candidates for neoadjuvant chemotherapy, sentinel node biopsy is still required in those patients who are node negative based on US-FNA (87,88). Re-evaluation of the axilla after neoadjuvant therapy has also been reported in small studies to be predictive of axillary downstaging (187).

The timing of sentinel node biopsy in the US-FNA node-negative patient relative to chemotherapy remains controversial. Small single-institution studies demonstrate the feasibility of lymphatic mapping subsequent to neoadjuvant chemotherapy, and described a false-negative rate of 9%, which is comparable to the NSABP B-32 trial results for sentinel node biopsy in patients undergoing primary surgery. However, given the potential downstaging of the axilla, there remain concerns about establishing the extent of nodal involvement as patients with greater than four positive nodes will have alteration in radiation therapy field distribution. Chagpar et al. have attempted to develop a nomogram to assist in identifying those patients more likely to require extended field radiotherapy (189).

All patients with locally advanced breast cancer should undergo a baseline bone scan and CT scans of the chest, abdomen, and pelvis since 30% of these patients have metastatic disease (190). Patients are clinically assessed for response after two to three cycles, and radiologic response can also be recorded at this time. If no response is present, a decision is made to continue with surgery if possible, or to change systemic therapy. Prior to surgical decisions being made, reimaging of the breast should be performed as clinical examination alone is unreliable (191–194). Occasional patients will have residual microcalcifications or DCIS while the invasive cancer has a complete pathologic response (195). The contraindications for breast conservation after neoadjuvant chemotherapy are similar to those for primary breast conservation therapy and include residual tumor >5 cm, skin edema or involvement, chest wall fixation, diffuse calcifications on postchemotherapy mammogram, multicentric disease, and contraindications to radiation therapy. As the risk of local recurrence after breast conservation in patients undergoing neoadjuvant therapy is slightly higher, the use of postmastectomy radiation in patients with larger cancers is recommended (181,196). Neoadjuvant endocrine therapy in hormone receptor–positive patients has also been shown to be effective.

Immediate reconstruction in patients with locally advanced breast cancer undergoing mastectomy has been shown to have a slightly higher rate of complications and results in a delay in treatment, as well as problems with cosmesis when postmastectomy radiation therapy is required. Given the multiple issues that are at play in the patient desiring immediate reconstruction, early consultations with both plastic surgeon and radiation oncologist should be performed, preferably before any surgery takes place.

Management of the Axilla

Although the clinical implications of axillary lymph node involvement has taken a varied course over the years, it still remains a major prognostic indicator of survival in breast cancer (197). Additionally, an axillary dissection remains of value in improving local control in patients with clinically positive axillae, though this has not translated into improved survival.

The largest prospective, randomized trial evaluating the role of axillary lymphadenectomy was the NSABP B-04 trial (197). In this trial, 1,079 women underwent radical mastectomy including an axillary dissection, total mastectomy with axillary radiation, or total mastectomy alone. Of note, patients did not receive systemic therapy on study. The results showed an axillary recurrence rate of 5% in clinically node-negative patients treated with surgery or irradiation compared to 20% when the axilla was observed. However, there was no difference in the rate of distant metastases or in survival in clinically node-negative breast cancer patients after 25 years. Most patients with axillary recurrence were salvaged by the performance of a delayed axillary dissection, whereas one patient had inoperable regional disease. This study thus demonstrated that leaving behind axillary nodes with metastatic disease had no significant impact on the overall outcome of the disease.

Cabanes et al. reported the results of a randomized trial of breast conservation therapy with breast irradiation, with or without axillary dissection in clinically node-negative patients, and showed a survival benefit for axillary dissection (198). However, this could be explained by the greater use of adjuvant chemotherapy and radiation in patients with positive nodes discovered at axillary dissection, whereas patients who were observed did not undergo these treatments. The rate of axillary recurrence without axillary dissection was only 7 of 332 (2%), compared to 3 of 326 (1%), even when an axillary dissection had been performed. In another study of 401 patients with T1 breast cancer (<2 cm) treated only with tangential breast radiation ports without an axillary dissection or sampling, Greco et al. reported that only 25 patients (7.5%) subsequently developed clinically suspicious axillary nodes, although at biopsy only 19 of the 25 patients had a histologic confirmed axillary relapse (199).

A Danish randomized trial compared an extended radical mastectomy with nodal resection to total mastectomy with postoperative radiation, showing similar survival and suggesting that axillary radiation might be an acceptable alternative to surgical dissection of the axilla (200). Similarly, the 30-year results of a randomized trial of 737 patients treated with a radical mastectomy versus an extended radical mastectomy with internal mammary lymphadenectomy and with no adjuvant therapy demonstrated that the involvement of the internal mammary nodes was a predictor of poor outcome, but did not demonstrate a survival benefit (201).

In contrast, a meta-analysis reported a 5% survival advantage with axillary dissection versus observation (202). This has been questioned since the trials on which this meta-analyis were based have since been updated, reflecting no survival advantage with axillary dissection, though maintaining a lower axillary recurrence rate with axillary dissection (203). Few women in the era when the trials included in this meta-analysis were performed had mammographically identified or nonpalpable tumors, and few received chemotherapy. Thus, extrapolation of these data to contemporary breast cancer management is quite difficult, given the changes in presentation of breast cancer.

A complete axillary dissection involves removal of the level I-II nodal tissue from the axilla. This is defined as the space bounded by the pectoral muscles anteriorly, the latissimus dorsi muscle posteriorly, and superiorly by the axillary vein. The nerves to the latissimus dorsi and serratus anterior are preserved. If possible, the intercostobrachial nerve is also preserved to decrease the risk of arm paresthesias. Level III nodes, which can be accessed only by dividing the pectoral tendon, are usually not removed. These are included in the radiation field, which is recommended if multiple nodes are involved.

Sentinel Node Biopsy

The concept of sentinel lymph node biopsy was designed to evaluate the stage of the disease in lieu of lymphadenectomy. It has revolutionized the surgical management of the axilla, and largely replaced axillary dissection in the node-negative axilla. In a recent meta-analysis involving 69 trials run between 1970 and 2003 and over 8,000 patients, the false-negative rate averaged 7.3% across studies (ranging from 0% to 29%) (204).

Donald Morton et al. pioneered lymphatic mapping in the surgical management of melanoma (205). The simplicity and elegance of this technique were overwhelming and led to its adoption in several malignancies, but none as robustly as breast cancer. Armando Guiliano championed the blue-dye-only technique using lymphazurin dye to identify the sentinel nodes, and the radioisotopic technique followed 1 year later, which is credited to Krag (165,206). Currently, a combination of these techniques has become most widely employed, although continued controversy persists on the different techniques of injection, whether it be peritumoral or subareolar or subdermal (207,208). Although all are likely successful in the majority of patients, the peritumoral technique may be important for posteriorly situated lesions. The subareolar technique may not drain to the internal mammary nodes (209).

Following injection of isotope, the dissection begins with a separate axillary incision. Dissection is taken down to the clavipectoral fascia, which is opened. The axilla is interrogated with a handheld receiving device, and further exploration for the "hot" node is performed. The node is carefully dissected from the surrounding tissue, paying attention to close dissection, as the critical motor nerves have not been identified. Each node is subsequently removed and counted over 10 seconds; if more than one node comes out together they should be separated. The node with the highest count becomes the benchmark and all nodes with greater than 10% activity are considered sentinel nodes. If blue dye is used, any blue node or node with a blue-stained lymphatic adjacent is a sentinel node. The sentinel nodes may be hot, blue, or hot and blue. Each technique used independently gives a 90% identification rate, and 95% when combined. Each agent's benefits are inherently obvious: the visualization of the blue dye, and the audibility of the isotope. Before completion of the procedure, the axilla must be digitally evaluated for any palpable nodes, as false negativity is common with nodes replaced by tumor. Furthermore, care to try to identify low-lying nodes in the axillary tail of the breast is useful. While lymphatic mapping to the internal mammary chain has been performed, its impact on outcome remains unclear.

It has now been demonstrated that sentinel lymph node evaluation is feasible, and accurately predicts the regional nodal status (205,206,210). The analysis of the few removed sentinel lymph nodes enabled pathologists to do multiple sections and a far more careful analysis of a few nodes, rather than a single section of the 10 to 20 nodes usually obtained from an axillary dissection. This detailed examination has sharply increased (by 20% to 30%) the proportion of "positive" nodes.

Intraoperative assessment of sentinel lymph nodes using touch imprints and routine IHC staining is used by some to enable an immediate therapeutic lymphadenectomy if the nodes were positive, thus sparing the patient from a second procedure. However, intraoperative assessment may have unacceptable rates of false-negative results, ranging from 36% to 71% (211). The increased yield of small macrometastases and micrometastases from regional lymph nodes by use of multiple thin sections and immunohistochemistry had been well demonstrated even in the presentinel lymph node era, and led to the recommendation for the current careful pathologic analysis of sentinel lymph nodes (212–215). With the technique of sentinel lymph node biopsy and the pathologic analysis now relatively standardized, the more recent focus is on the clinical significance of "positive" sentinel nodes. The most recent sixth edition of the AJCC *Staging Manual* defines nodal metastases less than 0.2 mm in extent and detected by IHC only as $N_{0(ITC)}$, indicating the uncertain prognostic implication of these minor cancer cell discoveries. Not all "positive" sentinel lymph nodes require a subsequent therapeutic lymphadenectomy since studies have shown low risk of regional nodal recurrence after observation only for patients with a positive sentinel lymph node (216). This thesis formed the hypothesis of the American College of Surgeons Oncology Group (ACOSOG) Z-11 trial, which randomized women with sentinel node positive breast cancer to observation only or completion axillary dissection. Unfortunately, this study closed early due to poor accrual, but results are expected in the near future.

Yet even now we strive to ascertain which of the patients with a positive sentinel node need to return for axillary node dissection. Nomograms have been developed to assist in this decision-making process, and the rate of completion axillary dissection has fallen off as these data have matured, likely recognizing that the extent of nodal involvement will not affect chemotherapeutic recommendations (217,218). Furthermore, in an appropriately performed sentinel node biopsy, bulky disease should not be left behind.

Current data suggest that with smaller tumor size in the era of mammographic screening, only 30% of breast cancers are node positive at presentation. In approximately 50% to 60%, the only positive node is the sentinel node. Data from the NSABP B-04 and other trials performed before the routine use of systemic chemotherapy demonstrated no survival benefit in removing the axillary lymph nodes for occult disease.

The use of axillary dissection comes at a cost to the patient. The incidence of lymphedema after axillary dissection and after axillary radiation is similar (15% to 25%) and is higher when the two are combined. Overall, 50% to 70% of patients have some complaint after axillary dissection, including restricted shoulder motion (17%), intercosto-brachial nerve numbness (78%), and pain (25%) (186). Though these problems are not life threatening, their effect on the quality of life is significant (219).

Oncoplastic Surgery

Subsequent to the revolutionary advances taking surgeons from radical mastectomy to lumpectomy and axillary dissection, there remained a cohort of patients who required mastectomy to either resect their disease adequately or had significant risk of future breast carcinoma such that breast conservation was deemed inappropriate. For these patients, continuing with the standard simple mastectomy, and nodal evaluation lagged behind advances already achieved. But over the past 15 years, immediate reconstruction after mastectomy has been documented to be both safe, from an oncological perspective, and psychologically beneficial to the patient's well-being (220). Simmon et al. have championed a more ideal technique of complete resection of the breast while preserving unaffected structures (221). Her landmark article compared recurrence patterns in women treated by skin-sparing mastectomy (SSM) versus non–skin-sparing mastectomy and demonstrated local recurrence rates of 3.90% and 3.25%, respectively, with an equivalent distant recurrence rate of 3.9% at 5 years.

SSM involves resection of the nipple areolar complex and nodal evaluation, but preservation of the entire overlying skin. Although initially reserved for early-stage breast cancer, Foster et al. have shown that SSM can be used in locally advanced breast cancer stages IIB and III with comparable local recurrence (222). A recent analysis of recurrence patterns revealed that local recurrence is usually in the same quadrant as the disease and is more common with high-grade DCIS or grade 3 invasive tumors (223).

Further analysis led Simmons to advance the concept of areola-sparing mastectomy, advocating that the perserved areola would enhance nipple reconstruction (224). Although retrospective, it suggested that malignant involvement of the areola was uncommon (0.9%), whereas involvement of the nipple was present in 11% of patients. Ultimately, the idea of nipple preservation has been pursued. While long-term results available in the European literature suggest comparable rates of success in appropriately selected patients, i.e., small peripheral tumors, the local recurrence rates remain higher (25%) than in the U.S. experience (225,226). The Milan group has used intraoperative radiotherapy to reduce recurrence, but the risk of nipple necrosis is approximately 10% in most series (227). Intraoperative frozen section analysis of the subareolar ductal system to exclude occult disease is reported at 98.5%, but this is likely to be dependent on local expertise. The sensitivity of the perserved nipple areolar complex ranges widely in the literature.

While the reconstructed breast proved to appear more natural, the desire for improved breast conservation has remained paramount, where we can provide not only the greatest assurance of nipple/areolar function, but, to a lesser extent, minimize the sense of "violation" by the patient. Taking techniques from breast reduction, breast surgeons have now expanded their armamentarium in achieving cosmetically desirable lumpectomy. Incorporation of mastopexy with lumpectomy has yielded successful results that translate to improved cosmesis for patients with lesions in ptotic breasts, as well as techniques of local tissue transfer that diminish skin retraction post lumpectomy (228).

CHEMOTHERAPY

Adjuvant Therapy

An important principle in the adjuvant use of chemotherapy is the concept of dose intensity. This issue governs the treatment in breast cancer following evidence suggesting that reductions in planned dosing may have an adverse impact on survival outcomes that are often quoted to our patients. In 1995, Bonadonna et al. reported the effect of dose intensity as part of an analysis on the effectiveness of adjuvant cyclophosphamide, methotrexate, and 5-fluorouracil (CMF) following radical mastectomy for women with node-positive breast cancer (229). Groups were stratified by the percentage of planned dose actually received (also known as relative dose intensity today). If patients received at least 85% of the planned dose, estimated relapse-free and overall survival at 20 years was over 50%. However, below this, 20-year survival dropped to approximately 30%. Of even more concern was the determination that patients receiving less than or equal to 65% of the planned dose experienced similar survival outcomes to those women who did not receive chemotherapy. Similar data have been reported by Lyman et al. (230).

Early Breast Cancer Trialists' Collaborative Group Meta-analyses

Ever since the effectiveness of treating metastatic disease with systemic therapy was established, the role of chemotherapy in the treatment of breast cancer has been evaluated in numerous clinical trials. To place this into a proper perspective, the Early Breast Cancer Trialists' Collaborative Group (EBCTCG) has performed meta-analyses of all randomized trials performed evaluating the adjuvant treatment of breast cancer, provided that at least 5 years of follow-up is provided. These analyses are performed every 5 years with the first performed in 1985. In the EBCTCG, all trials evaluating a similar intervention (doxorubicin-based therapy) are grouped for subsequent analysis. Baseline risks are defined by the "control" group, which may or may not be a placebo.

In 1998, the meta-analysis included 23,000 women from randomized trials looking into the role of chemotherapy (231). In 47 trials randomization was to polychemotherapy versus no chemotherapy (n = 18,000); in 11 trials it was longer versus short-duration treatments (n = 6,000); and in 11 randomization was to anthracycline-based versus cyclophosphamide (C), methotrexate (M), and 5-fluorouracil (F), collectively referred to as CMF (n = 6,000). The use of multiagent chemotherapy was found to reduce the annual risk of relapse by 35% in women under 50 and 20% in women aged 50 to 69. For mortality, the reduction was 27% for women under 50 and 11% for women aged 50 to 69.

In 2005, the overview on the use of chemotherapy reported the endpoints of risk reduction at 10 and 15 years (232). The analysis included 8,000 women treated on an anthracycline-containing treatment (CAF, cyclophosphamide, doxorubicin, 5-fluorouracil or FEC, 5-fluorouracil, epirubicin, cyclophosphamide) versus placebo; 14,000 women on trials of CMF versus placebo; and an additional 14,000 women on athracycline-based versus CMF-type treatment. Again, no trial was included that used taxanes or trastuzumab. The meta-analysis showed that women under 50 benefited from the use of an anthracycline-containing regimen, which resulted in a reduction in the annual breast cancer death rate by 38%. Women 50 to 60 years old also benefited, with a risk reduction of 20%. These results support the gains made for adjuvant chemotherapy in not only reducing 5-year recurrence rates, but also affecting 15-year survival.

Treatment of Node-Positive Breast Cancer: Taxanes

Among the most important agents for breast cancer, and not considered in the published meta-analyses, is the role of taxanes in the treatment for breast cancer. Paclitaxel was first used in metastatic breast cancer in a study conducted by the NCI (233). In that trial of 25 patients, a 56% response rate was obtained including 12% who had a complete response. Since that time it has been utilized in numerous schedules and doses, confirming its activity in node-positive breast cancers. The first reported trial in the adjuvant setting was by Hudis et al. at Memorial Sloan-Kettering Cancer Center (234). In that study, patients with breast cancer with four or more positive nodes were treated at 14-day intervals. The drugs administered were doxorubicin (A) 90 mg/m^2 for three cycles, paclitaxel (T) 250 mg/m^2 over 24 hours for three cycles, followed by cyclophosphamide (C) 3,000 mg/m^2 for three cycles. Forty-two patients were treated on this regimen with over 90% dose-intensity given. At 4 years, the actuarial disease-free survival was 78%, suggesting this as a feasible and active regimen.

The role of paclitaxel in the adjuvant treatment for all women with node-positive breast cancer has been studied. Hayes et al. recently reported findings from a retrospective analysis of Cancer and Leukemia Group B (CALGB) 9344/INT0148, which evaluated the benefit of four cycles of paclitaxel after four cycles of AC (235). With 10 years of follow-up, paclitaxel continued to show overall improvements in both disease-free (HR 0.81; 95% CI, 0.73 to 0.91) and overall survival (HR 0.81; 95% CI, 0.72 to 0.92). Of more interest was their analysis evaluating interactions between paclitaxel response, HER2/neu status, and ER status. Their analysis showed that HER2/neu positivity (by either IHC or FISH) predicted improvements in disease-free and overall survival from the AC followed by paclitaxel. However, no benefit of paclitaxel was suggested in women with tumors that were positive for ER but negative for HER2/neu.

The concept of dose-dense therapy was tested against standard every-3-week treatment using paclitaxel in the Cancer and Leukemia Group B Trial, CALGB 9741 (236). Over 2,000 women with node-positive invasive breast cancer were enrolled in this two-by-two randomized trial evaluating chemotherapy delivered every 2 (dose-dense) versus every 3 weeks with the second randomization to sequential single-agent therapy of A 60 mg/m^2, followed by C 600 mg/m^2, followed by T 175 mg/m^2, with each given for four cycles, or combination AC for four cycles followed by T for four cycles (AC → T). Women randomized to the every-2-week treatments were given growth factors to support hematopoietic recovery. At a median of 36 months follow-up, dose-dense therapy was associated with improvements in both disease-free (risk ratio [RR], 0.74) and overall survival (RR, 0.69). Four-year disease-free survival (DFS) was 82% with dose-dense therapy compared to 75% for treatment every 3 weeks. Survival outcomes were similar by drug sequence (AC → T or sequence A, C, T).

Another trial evaluating taxane versus no-taxane adjuvant treatment was conducted by the Breast Cancer International Research Group, the BCIRG 001 trial (237). In this study almost 1,500 women were randomized to docetaxel 75 mg/m^2, A 50 mg/m^2, and C 500 mg/m^2 (TAC) versus F 400 mg/m^2, A 50 mg/m^2, and C 500 mg/m^2 (FAC). Compared to FAC, treatment with TAC resulted in improved 5-year DFS, 75% versus 68%, respectively ($p = 0.001$), and overall survival, 87% versus 81%, respectively, $p = 0.008$. The prophylactic utilization of myeloid growth factors has enabled treatment on time with both of these schedules, which are in and of themselves significantly myelosuppressive.

Given the activity of taxanes in the adjuvant therapy in node-positive disease, studies now seek to address whether anthracyclines are required. One of the first to address this question was conducted by U.S. Oncology and evaluated AC versus a nonanthracycline regimen of TC (docetaxel 75 mg/m^2 and cyclophosphamide 600 mg/m^2) (238). This trial enrolled over 1,000 women with stage I-III breast cancer following definitive excision. At a median follow-up of 5 years, TC was associated with a significant increase in DFS over AC (86% vs. 80%, respectively, $p = 0.015$) with similar overall survival (OS) (90% vs. 87%, respectively, $p = 0.13$). TC treatment was associated with increased myalgias, athralgias, edema, and episodes of febrile neutropenia over AC treatment.

Considering emerging data, there is no clear standard of care for women with node-positive breast cancer. In addition, recent data support the contention that treatment recommendations should be tailored to the features of the individual patient's breast cancer. This has been most evidently demonstrated when it comes to hormone receptor expression. In a recent meta-analysis involving over 6,000 women treated on adjuvant node-positive breast cancer trials conducted by CALGB, Berry et al. reported that the benefits of chemotherapy were larger in women with ER-negative disease, where the risk reduction in both recurrence and death was 55%, translating into a 16.7% absolute improvement in overall survival at 10 years. This contrasts to the estimates for women with ER-positive disease where the reduction in the relative risk of recurrence was estimated at 26% and in the risk of death was 23%. This translated into an approximate 4% absolute benefit in overall survival (138).

Adjuvant Treatment of Node-Negative Breast Cancer

Adjuvant therapy clinical trials have often sought to include patients with node-negative disease on the basis of poor prognostic factors (large tumor size, ER-negative disease, HER2/neu positivity, and high-grade features). Thus, there have been few trials defining the appropriate chemotherapy management specifically in women with node-negative breast cancer. A large rationale for this approach is that the prognosis for women with small tumors (defined as under 1 cm) without node involvement remains favorable such that the benefits of chemotherapy are likely minimal. For those with tumors above 1 cm, receptor positivity has played a role, especially given the profound effect of endocrine therapy in both reducing risk of relapse and improving overall survival. In this group, women at high risk or with receptor-negative disease are often considered for adjuvant chemotherapy and several important trials bear mentioning.

The NSABP recently reported an update on trials where women with node-negative ER-negative tumors were enrolled (239). The trials included B-13 (n = 760 assigned to observation vs. MF), B-19 (n = 1,095 assigned to MF vs. CMF), and B-23 (n = 2,008 assigned to CMF vs. AC). The analysis showed steady gains in overall survival with the use of MF versus observation (HR = 0.75; 95% CI, 0.58 to 0.98) and then CMF versus MF (HR = 0.71; 95% CI, 0.55 to 0.92). However, with 8 years median follow-up, the use of AC did not demonstrate continued gains in overall survival compared to CMF (HR = 0.92; 95% CI, 0.79 to 1.27), nor did it show improvements in relapse-free survival (HR = 1.0).

Linden et al. reported the results of a Southwest Oncology Group (SWOG) trial, which tested single-agent sequential A then C versus combination AC in women with high-risk node-negative or low-risk node-positive breast cancer (240). The study enrolled 3,176 patients between 1994 and 1997 and no difference in OS at 5 years was seen: 88% AC versus 89% A then C. However, sequenced therapy showed much higher grade 4 hemotoxicity.

Recommendations for the adjuvant treatment in this population often require an individualized approach based on risk of recurrence, and several tools are currently available to aid the clinician in decision making. Among them is Adjuvant! Online (241). Developed by Peter Ravdin et al., this computer-based program takes into account multiple clinical factors including age, presence of comorbidities, ER status, tumor grade, and nodal involvement in calculating a baseline 10-year risk for both recurrence and death (242). Using Surveillance, Epidemiology, and End Results (SEER) data, overview results on the use of chemotherapy and endocrine therapy, and results of contemporary clinical trials, the relative benefits of endocrine therapy, chemotherapy, or a sequential approach of the two are calculated. To make it more understandable, a graphic depiction is included which gives estimates of lives saved out of 100 women treated with each strategy.

For women with node-negative disease, the FDA has approved a genomic microarray for clinical use. Commercially marketed as the MammaPrint assay, it stratifies patients based on an expression signature into those with a good versus bad prognosis. It was validated in a study using 295 women with stage I-II breast cancers that were node negative (n = 151) or positive (n = 144) and under 53 years old (243). In this series, 180 women fell into the poor prognosis category. Their 10-year survival rate was 54.6% ± 4.4% with a 10-year relapse-free survival rate of 50.6 ± 4.4%. For the 115 with a good prognosis, the corresponding figures were 94.5% ± 2.6% and 85.2 ± 4.3%. It is currently approved for T1-2, node-negative patients regardless of ER status. However, rigorous specimen processing is required including at least a 5 mm biopsy obtained within 1 hour of surgery, which must be placed in the provided preservative overnight and up to 1 month in a −20° freezer.

An additional option for risk stratification is the Oncotype DX. Unlike the MammaPrint, it can be performed on representative archived tissue of the primary breast cancer. The assay uses a risk algorithm based on the expression of 21 genes (16 cancer genes representing groups of proliferative, invasion, HER2, and estrogen-receptor–associated genes and five reference genes). Scoring in these groups is then used to assign a recurrence score (RS) (244). In testing Oncotype DX, data from the prospective trial NSABP B-14, which enrolled 658 women with T1-2, node-negative, ER-positive tumors on tamoxifen for 5 years followed by randomization to further tamoxifen therapy versus placebo, was used. Using tumor specimens from this trial, 51% of patients were assigned to a low-risk category (RS <18) and had less than a 7% rate of distant recurrence at 10 years. Twenty-two percent were placed into an intermediate risk category and had a 14.3% rate of distant disease, and 27% were assigned the high-risk category (RS=31) and had a 30.5% rate of distant recurrence. Although such information may help guide discussion of who may *not* need chemotherapy, there are obvious limitations of the Oncotype DX assay as it cannot predict chemotherapeutic benefits, nor does the RS predict breast cancer–specific mortality.

Adjuvant Treatment: HER2/neu-Positive Breast Cancers

Among the biggest findings in the last 5 years is the use of trastuzumab in adjuvant therapy for women with HER2/neu-positive breast cancer, now considered the standard of care in women with high-risk node-negative breast cancer (defined as tumor size >2 cm if ER positive or >1 cm if ER negative) and those with node-positive breast cancer. The trials that have helped establish this standard are summarized in Table 29.9. The NSABP B-31 trial enrolled 2,043 women to AC/T every 3 weeks or AC every 3 weeks for four cycles followed by T for 12 weeks with trastuzumab followed by trastuzumab consolidation to complete 1 year. During this same period, the NCCTG 98311 trial enrolled 3,000 women to every-3-week AC for four cycles followed by weekly T as a control arm versus the same followed by 1 year of trastuzumab or T given with trastuzumab followed by trastuzumab consolidation to a total of 1 year. The results were reported in a combined analysis and showed that adjuvant trastuzumab resulted in improvements in both 4-year disease-free survival (HR = 0.48, $p < 0.0001$) and overall survival (HR = 0.67, $p = 0.015$) (245). Several studies have also confirmed the benefits of trastuzumab in the adjuvant setting (246–248).

The duration of consolidation required continues to be an area of evaluation. Although the majority of trials have compared observation to 1 year of trastuzumab, the FinHER evaluated the benefits of 9 weeks of chemotherapy with or without trastuzumab (248). In that trial, those women who were HER2/neu positive were randomized to chemotherapy (vinorelbine or docetaxel) with or without trastuzumab, followed by FEC. Two-hundred and thirty-two women were enrolled and they reported that adding trastuzumab to chemotherapy improved disease-free survival (89.6% vs. 76.8% without trastuzumab, $p = 0.01$) and showed a trend toward improved overall survival (94.8% vs. 88%, $p = 0.07$).

In addition, although the standard of care has been set for women with high-risk node-negative disease, another issue yet to be determined is whether all women with HER2/neu-positive invasive breast cancer warrant trastuzumab, regardless of tumor size. The consideration of the benefits, particularly in those with tumors less than 1 cm in size, must be weighed against the risks of trastuzumab therapy, especially if it follows anthracycline-based treatment.

Neoadjuvant Chemotherapy: Considerations and Outcomes

Neoadjuvant, or primary, therapy has become a standard option in the management of locally advanced breast cancer. The rationale for its use is historically based on the use of primary chemotherapy in inflammatory and advanced breast cancer, where chemotherapy was shown to be an effective treatment with the potential to provide a long-lasting remission in otherwise poor-prognosis patients. Currently neoadjuvant therapy allows patients facing a mastectomy the option of breast conservation by downstaging the primary tumor while not adversely impacting survival endpoints. In addition, it provides a measure of chemotherapy effectiveness to the intact cancer, which may guide prognosis, particularly in the patient experiencing a pathologic complete remission.

NSABP B-18 was a large randomized trial evaluating neoadjuvant therapy. The primary endpoint of the study was surgical and was measured by the proportion achieving breast conservation surgery (249). In this trial, 1,523 women with operable breast cancer were randomly assigned to AC every 3 weeks for four cycles preoperatively or postoperatively. In women treated with neoadjuvant AC, 81% underwent breast conservation surgery, compared to 57% treated with adjuvant therapy. For women with tumors ≥5 cm, preoperative chemotherapy increased the rate of breast conservation by 175%. Neither overall survival nor disease-free survival was affected by primary or adjuvant AC therapy, suggesting that the timing of systemic chemotherapy will not affect breast cancer outcome. However, this trial also suggested that among those who are treated with primary chemotherapy, final pathologic findings predict survival, and those who achieve a pathologic complete response (pCR) have the best prognosis. Among the factors that were associated with a pCR were being ER negative, ductal histology, being HER2/neu positive, and a high histologic grade. These factors have been used to construct nomograms to predict the likelihood of achieving a pCR for women being considered for this approach (250).

TABLE 29.9

SEMINAL TRIALS OF TRASTUZUMAB IN THE ADJUVANT THERAPY OF BREAST CANCER

Trial	N	Arms	Disease-free survival (%)	*p* value	Overall survival (%)	*p* value
NSABP B-31 (245)	2,043	AC→T	67.1		86.6	
				<0.0001		0.015[a]
NCCTG 98311 (245)	3,000	AC→T + Tr	85.3		91.4	
HERA (246)	5,081	Observation	74		89.2	
		Tr	80.6	<0.0001	92.4	<0.0051
		Tr × 24 mo	NR		NR	
BCIRG 006 (247)	3,222	AC → Doc	77		86	
		AC → Doc + Tr	83	<0.00001	92	0.004[b]
		Carbo + Doc + Tr	82		91	
FinHER (248)	210	Chemo × 9 wk → FEC	76.8		88	
				0.01		0.07[c]
		Chemo + Tr × 9 wk → FEC	89.6		94.8	

Notes: A, doxorubicin; BCIRG, Breast Cancer International Research Group; C, cyclophosphamide; Carbo, carboplatin; Doc, docetaxel; FEC, 5-fluorouracil, epirubicin, cyclophosphamide; FinHER, ; HERA, ; NCCTG, North Central Cancer Treatment Group; NSABP, National Surgical Breast and Bowel Project; T, paclitaxel; Tr, trastuzumab. Unless otherwise stated, trastuzumab treatment was for a total duration of 1 year.
[a]Joint analysis of 3,351 women (1,679 receiving AC → T; 1,672 receiving trastuzumab) reported survival analysis at 4 years.
[b]The second interim analysis reported survival endpoints at 4 years.
[c]One thousand and ten women were randomized in the FinHER trial to vinorelbine versus docetaxel, followed by FEC. The subgroup with HER2/neu-positive disease underwent additional randomization to trastuzumab or no trastuzumab.

Although women with a pCR after neoadjuvant chemotherapy have a very good prognosis, the opposite is also true. Women who do not achieve complete pathologic response tend to be at highest risk for relapse, but there is no clear consensus on the best treatment approach following surgery. While women with ER-positive tumors are candidates for endocrine therapy and those with HER2/neu-positive tumors are candidates for extended trastuzumab therapy, the use of further chemotherapy is of unclear benefit, and no randomized trials to date have addressed this issue. Considering the paucity of data on "adjuvant treatment" after neoadjuvant therapy, referral to appropriate clinical trials is encouraged. Completed randomized trials of primary chemotherapy are summarized at the end of this chapter. At this time, primary chemotherapy should be reserved for patients where the results of neoadjuvant treatment might positively impact cosmetic results or facilitate breast and/or axillary surgery.

Metastatic Breast Cancer

Patients who recur or develop metastatic breast cancer do not comprise a homogenous group and prognosis is guided by the sites of cancer involvement. Women with bone-only metastatic disease may survive for years following their diagnosis, while those who recur in the visceral organs (liver or lungs most commonly) face a more guarded prognosis. Current national practice guidelines stratify treatment options based on biologic factors and recommend first-, second-, and even third-line endocrine therapies for women with ER-positive disease; trastuzumab-based therapies are recommended for women whose tumors are HER2/neu positive. Women with visceral disease, are otherwise symptomatic, have hormone receptor–negative cancers, and/or are HER2/neu negative are treated with chemotherapy. In addition, the palliative intent of treatment in this context reinforces the importance of considering the patient's wishes when choosing treatments. A young mother may be willing to undergo significant toxicity if there is a chance for a second remission, while an older woman may not want agressive therapy, opting instead to maintain her quality of life as much as possible.

Multiple agents are active in metastatic breast cancer, and both single-agent and combination therapies are reasonable choices. Perhaps one of the biggest controversies is whether to use single-agent sequential therapies or combination treatment for metastatic breast cancer. A meta-anlysis by Fossati et al. evaluated the role of polychemotherapy versus single-agent therapy in this population (251). The meta-analysis incorporated 12 trials and over 1,900 women and showed that polychemotherapy afforded an 18% proportional reduction in mortality (HR 0.82; 95% CI, 0.75 to 0.90). However, it has been criticized because none of the trials included taxane therapies, nor did the meta-analysis evaluate *sequential* single-agent treatments.

In the intergroup trial sponsored by the Eastern Cooperative Oncology Group, ECOG 1193, over 670 women with metastatic breast cancer were randomized to doxorubicin and paclitaxel (AT) in combination or as single agents (252). It showed that the overall response rates were significantly improved with AT, compared to either single-agent doxorubicin or paclitaxel (47% vs. 36%, $p < 0.007$, and 34%, $p < 0.004$, respectively). In addition, median time to treatment failure was improved with the combination to 8 months, compared to 5.8 months with doxorubicin ($p < 0.003$) and 6 months with paclitaxel ($p < 0.009$). However, there was no difference in overall survival in any of these arms (22.4 months with AT, 19.1 months with doxorubicin, 22.5 months with paclitaxel). Sequential therapy was also shown to be beneficial in this trial where approximately 56% of patients randomized to doxorubicin crossed over to paclitaxel and vice versa, and in each case 20% of patients experienced a response. The median time to treatment failure following crossover was 4 months in both single-agent arms. Given the higher response rate seen in this trial, combination therapy continues to be an acceptable choice for some patients. Recently, two combinations have received FDA approval for metastatic breast cancer: capecitabine/docetaxel and gemcitabine/paclitaxel (253,254). A newer taxane that utilizes nanotechnology to package paclitaxel into albumin, nAb-paclitaxel, has also been approved recently as single-agent therapy (255). Another drug, ixabepilone, an epothilone B analog that stabilizes microtubules and therefore works similarly to paclitaxel, received approval in the treatment of metastatic breast cancer, in combination with capecitabine or as a single agent. Most notably, however, it has been approved in women whose tumors are resistant or refractory to standard agents including anthracyclines, taxanes, and capecitabine. In the latter approval, 126 patients were treated on a single-arm trial using a dose of ixabepilone 40 mg/m^2 as a 3-hour infusion on day 1 of a 21-day cycle. Eighty-eight percent of patients had received more than two lines of prior therapy (256). The overall response rate was 18% with an additional 50% achieving stable disease. Median progression-free survival was 3 months and overall survival in this heavily treated cohort was almost 9 months. The major toxicity included grade 3-4 sensory neuropathy in 14% of patients, fatigue/asthenia in 13%, myalgia in 8%, and stomatitis in 6%.

Biologic therapies are another area of active investigation. The most recent FDA approval was for the combination of capecitabine and the dual tyrosine kinase inhibitor lapatinib for the treatment of HER2/neu-positive breast cancer following progression on trastuzumab-based therapy. The approval was based on an interim analysis of a multicenter randomized trial comparing capecitabine monotherapy (2,500 mg/m^2 per day) versus capecitabine (2,000 mg/m^2 per day) with lapatinib (1,250 mg/day) for 14 days of a 21-day cycle (257). Combination therapy increased time to progression (HR 0.49; 95% CI, 0.34 to 0.71) with a median time to progression reported of 8.4 months, compared to 4.4 months in those randomized to capecitabine alone. Antiangiogenesis agents such as bevacizumab continue to be evaluated in clinical trials in the neoadjuvant, adjuvant, and metastatic settings.

ENDOCRINE THERAPY

The role of endocrine therapy has grown significantly over the past several years as both our understanding of breast cancer has matured and new therapeutic options have developed. It has become increasingly clear that endocrine therapy is the backbone of treatment for hormonally responsive breast cancer, independent of stage.

Adjuvant Endocrine Therapy

Perhaps no data set has been more instructive in helping to define the benefit of adjuvant hormonal therapy than the meta-analysis generated by the Early Breast Cancer Trialists' Collaborative Group (232). One of the principles appreciated through this overview analysis is that the proportional benefit of a given treatment is constant through risk groups (e.g., stage) and that the absolute benefit changes based on the estimated risk of systemic recurrence. For instance, if hormonal therapy decreases the risk of cancer recurrence by 30% in a given individual, the absolute benefit would be 3% if the 10-year risk of relapse were 10%, but 18% if the 10-year risk of relapse were 60%. This concept of proportional and absolute benefit from adjuvant therapy is a guiding principle when women are counseled regarding treatment options in the adjuvant setting.

Expression of the estrogen receptor or the progesterone receptor is predictive of response to hormonal therapy. Therefore, essentially any woman with invasive breast cancer should receive adjuvant hormonal therapy if her tumor is estrogen receptor positive (ER+) and/or progesterone receptor positive (PR+). Conversely, hormonal therapy is inappropriate in the ER−/PR− setting. The choices for treatment and duration of therapy continue to be the subject of active investigation.

Tamoxifen was the first hormonal agent used in the adjuvant setting for breast cancer (258,259). As a selective estrogen receptor modulator (SERM), tamoxifen has differential effects on various tissues. While tamoxifen may achieve its beneficial effect in the treatment of breast cancer through multiple means, the principal mode of action appears to be through competitive binding to the estrogen receptor. By preventing estrogen binding, translocation and nuclear binding of the estrogen receptor are inhibited, altering transcriptional and posttranscriptional events mediated by the receptor. The antagonistic properties of tamoxifen toward breast cancer are contrasted with its agonistic effects on other tissues, such as bone and uterus. Tamoxifen, like estrogen, improves bone mineral density in postmenopausal women and is a risk factor for endometrial cancer. Tamoxifen may negatively affect bone density in premenopausal women. The risk of endometrial cancer with the use of tamoxifen is estimated at three- to fourfold over the general population risk, though the risk is likely lower in premenopausal women and perhaps close to the general population risk as demonstrated in the NSABP P-1 trial (260). It is recommended that women on tamoxifen follow general guidelines for gynecologic screening and follow-up but, importantly, report any menstrual changes, dysfunctional uterine bleeding, or other symptoms to their gynecologist (261). Women should discuss the use of tamoxifen with their gynecologist to ensure that they are being properly evaluated.

Another important risk associated with tamoxifen is that of venous thrombosis. While perhaps less so in premenopausal women, as demonstrated by the NSABP P-1 trial, tamoxifen has an approximate fourfold increase in risk for deep venous thrombosis (DVT) over the general population risk (260). This risk is sometimes described as similar to that associated with the use of oral contraceptives and may influence choice of hormonal therapy in the postmenopausal setting. Other potential side effects of tamoxifen include hot flashes, weight gain, mood changes, increased vaginal discharge, cataracts, and rarely retinal abnormalities. Several studies have suggested an increase in risk of stroke with tamoxifen. Tamoxifen can increase fertility by increasing ovarian stimulation and is a teratogen and is therefore contraindicated during pregnancy. Moreover, premenopausal women on tamoxifen need to ensure appropriate contraception as it is possible to become pregnant while on this medication.

Benefit from the use of tamoxifen in the adjuvant setting has been demonstrated in multiple clinical trials. The Scottish tamoxifen trial published in *The Lancet* in 1987 evaluated the use of tamoxifen 20 mg daily for 5 years in 1,312 premenopausal node-negative or postmenopausal women with any nodal status (258). This trial defined tamoxifen as an effective adjuvant in node-negative and node-positive patients as well as in the pre- and postmenopausal setting and is considered a landmark trial. NSABP B-14 evaluated the use of tamoxifen versus placebo for 5 years in 869 premenopausal and 1,949 postmenopausal women with node-negative breast cancer, demonstrating statistically significant improvement in disease-free and overall survival with the use of tamoxifen (259). Although multiple dosing strategies have been tried, there is no demonstrated dose-response curve between 20 and 40 mg. Thus, 20 mg per day is the recommended dose currently. Five years of tamoxifen appears to have equal efficacy to 10 years of therapy with less toxicity and is more effective than 2 years of therapy (262,263). Therefore, 5 years of treatment is recommended. We generally estimate that the proportional benefit of tamoxifen in the adjuvant setting ranges from 30% to 50% in reducing the odds of systemic cancer recurrence (138).

Another decision-making tool in women who have an option of endocrine therapy or chemotherapy is the Oncotype DX assay. Using 668 available paraffin blocks from the B-14 trial, Paik et al. evaluated 16 cancer-related genes to define an algorithm to assess risk of recurrence at 10 years (244). By creating a continuum of recurrence score based on gene expression analysis, three risk groups were broken out: low risk, intermediate risk, and high risk. Looking at this group of node-negative hormone receptor–positive women, all of whom received tamoxifen, individuals in the low-risk category did not appear to benefit from the addition of chemotherapy to tamoxifen and are likely best served by hormonal therapy alone. Women in the high-risk group likely benefit from the addition of chemotherapy to hormonal therapy. Whether hormonal therapy alone is adequate in the intermediate risk group is less clear and is currently being studied in a prospective, randomized trial. Gene- and protein-expression prognostic and predictive models will continue to be developed to aid in defining appropriate therapy across risk groups and will complement established prognostic and predictive factors such as tumor size, grade, receptor status, nodal involvement, and Her2 overexpression.

While tamoxifen remains the only established hormonal agent in premenopausal women, choices in the postmenopausal setting have increased through the study and development of aromatase inhibitors. Initially, through the study of first-generation aromatase inhibitors such as aminoglutethimide, these agents were found to be effective therapy for postmenopausal women. Aromatase inhibitors block estrogen production by preventing conversion of androgens produced by the adrenal gland, such as androstenedione, to estrogens, such as estrone, which is later converted to estradiol. This block occurs in the breast as well as in peripheral tissues such as adipose tissue. The resulting decrease in circulating estrogen has been demonstrated through multiple clinical trials to be effective treatment for receptor-positive breast cancer. Of the three commercially available aromatase inhibitors, anastrozole and letrozole are nonsteroidal while exemestane is a steroidal aromatase inhibitor. There are currently no demonstrable differences in efficacy or toxicity among these three products. Toxicities of aromatase inhibitors commonly include hot flashes and joint or muscle aches. Unlike tamoxifen, aromatase inhibitors can contribute to osteopenia and osteoporosis, and therefore bone density should be followed carefully in women receiving these medicines. Other possible side effects include hypertension, gastrointestinal disturbance, depression, urovaginal symptoms, and possibly cardiac events. Aromatase inhibitors are not associated with an increased risk of endometrial cancer and have a lower risk for DVT compared to tamoxifen.

Several studies have demonstrated the efficacy of aromatase inhibitors in the adjuvant setting. The ATAC trial is the largest prospective adjuvant trial in breast cancer, randomizing 9,300 postmenopausal women to tamoxifen, anastrozole, or the combination (264). With a median follow-up of 47 months, there was a statistically significant benefit in disease-free survival of anastrozole over tamoxifen with a hazards ratio of 0.82 in estrogen receptor–positive patients. There was no benefit with the combination. The Coombes trial randomized 4,700 postmenopausal women to tamoxifen for 2 to 3 years followed by either tamoxifen or exemestane to complete 5 years of adjuvant therapy (265). With a median follow-up of 55.7 months, there was a statistically significant benefit in disease-free survival for the inclusion of the aromatase inhibitor with a hazard ratio of 0.76 and a modest benefit to overall survival with a hazard ratio of 0.83. Lastly, the Goss trial studied the addition of letrozole after 5 years of tamoxifen and showed a statistically significant benefit to the inclusion of an aromatase inhibitor with a median follow-up of 30 months and a hazard ratio of 0.58 (266). The Breast International Group (BIG) 1-98 study prospectively randomized 8,010 postmenopausal women with hormone receptor–positive breast cancer to either tamoxifen for 5 years, letrozole for 5 years, tamoxifen for 2 years switching to letrozole for 3 years, or letrozole for 2 years switching to tamoxifen for 3 years. After a median follow-up of 26 months, the two groups that were assigned letrozole initially had a statistically significant improvement in disease-free survival with a hazard ratio of 0.81 (267). A follow-up analysis of this trial published in 2007 focused on the groups receiving either continuous tamoxifen or letrozole for 5 years (268). At a median follow-up of 51 months, there was an 18% improvement in disease-free survival with a hazard ratio of 0.82 favoring letrozole.

Based on these four trials, it is recommended that all postmenopausal women receiving adjuvant hormonal therapy receive at least 2 to 3 years of an aromatase inhibitor (AI) unless contraindicated, and treatment with an AI beyond 5 years is the subject of current investigation. We await further data from the BIG 1-98 trial to assess the benefit of sequential versus continuous therapy.

The degree of benefit and choice of hormonal therapy may be further influenced by primary tumor characteristics. The level of expression and potentially the relative expression of estrogen- and progesterone-receptor positivity on the surface of breast cancer cells are predictive of the responsiveness of the tumor to hormonal manipulation (265). It is therefore important to incorporate the degree of ER and PR positivity into adjuvant therapy decisions. The differential expression of ER and PR may also be important in defining response to specific hormonal agents and this remains an area of active investigation. The differential benefit to tamoxifen and aromatase inhibitors in the postmenopausal ER+/Her2+ setting also requires further study.

Ovarian Ablation

Ovarian ablation (OA) has long been explored as a therapeutic option for women with breast cancer. As the ovaries are the major source for estrogen, silencing the ovaries via surgical oophorectomy, radiotherapy, or the use of gonadotropin-releasing hormone (GnRH) analogues may provide a benefit, although controversy continues as to its role in modern breast cancer management. The EBCTCG overview on ovarian ablation included 12 trials that compared OA by surgery or radiation to control and encompassed 2,012 women with early breast cancer (269). The meta-analysis concluded that OA was associated with both disease-free and overall survival advantages when compared to observation. At 15 years, 52% were alive of those who underwent OA, compared to 46% who did not ($p = 0.001$) and 45% were disease-free, compared to 39% ($p = 0.0007$). When trials using OA versus chemotherapy following breast surgery were analyzed, however, the benefits of OA were more modest and did not achieve statistical significance. Still, among women who do not receive chemotherapy, OA may play a role in management.

Since the meta-analysis, several results have been published in this area. The International Breast Cancer Study Group (IBCSG) Trial VIII randomized 1,063 women with node-negative breast cancer to chemotherapy (CMF) versus goserelin (G) versus CMF followed by G (270). Of note, 30% of women in this study had ER-negative disease. Restricting the analysis to women with ER-positive disease, the 5-year disease-free survival (DFS) in those treated with either chemotherapy or goserelin alone was 81%; for those receiving sequential therapy there was a trend toward improved 5-year DFS at 86%. Arriagada et al. randomized 926 women with node-positive or grade 2-3 tumors who had completed surgery and chemotherapy to ovarian ablation (by surgery or with triptorelin) or observation (271). Of the cohort, 63% were ER positive. Estimated 10-year disease-free and overall survivals were similar in both groups, though subgroup analysis suggested that women under 40 who had ER-positive disease benefited significantly. Finally, the TABLE study (Takeda Adjuvant Breast cancer study with Leuprolide Acetate) published their results with 5.8 years of follow-up (272). Six-hundred ninety-nine women with ER-positive node-positive disease enrolled in this trial comparing CMF to leuprolide acetate (LA). Disease-free survival at 5 years was similar (63.9% with CMF vs. 63.4% with LA, $p = 0.83$) but overall survival favored LA over CMF (81% vs. 71.9%, $p = 0.05$).

Contemporary trials will hopefully provide more guidance as to the role of ovarian ablation in women with hormone-positive breast cancer. This is an especially important issue given the marginal benefits of chemotherapy in women with ER-positive breast cancer and the availability of antiestrogen endocrine therapy. Whether ovarian ablation adds an additional benefit to endocrine therapy remains a question not sufficiently addressed.

Endocrine Therapy in Metastatic Breast Cancer

Hormonal therapy is optimal initial therapy in the setting of stage IV hormone receptor–positive breast cancer unless aggressive recurrence mandates chemotherapy to maximize time to response (e.g., significant hepatic metastasis). Options include ovarian suppression in the premenopausal setting with or without the addition of tamoxifen or an aromatase inhibitor, or even tamoxifen alone. In the postmenopausal setting, tamoxifen or aromatase inhibitors are initial appropriate options, with data suggesting that aromatase inhibitors might be more effective as first-line therapy when compared to tamoxifen and have more favorable toxicity profiles (273). Fulvestrant is a pure anti-estrogen approved for use in the postmenopausal setting and is given by monthly intramuscular injection. Data from the EFFECT trial demonstrate equivalence to exemestane as second-line therapy after use of a nonsteroidal aromatase inhibitor (274). The goal of treating recurrent disease is palliative, trying to prolong survival while maximizing quality of life and minimizing treatment-related toxicities. Response to initial hormonal therapy can be predictive of response to subsequent hormonal treatments, which can be achieved with serial enodcrine agents over many years (273,275). Hormonal resistance can evolve over time, necessitating the use of chemotherapy for cancer control. The mechanisms behind the evolution of hormonal resistance and strategies to reinduce hormonal sensitivity in stage IV breast cancer are actively being investigated.

Neoadjuvant Endocrine Therapy

As in the adjuvant and metastatic setting, hormonal therapy can also be beneficial for women presenting with locally advanced breast cancer. If chemotherapy is not being employed, neoadjuvant (preoperative) hormonal therapy in the hormonally positive setting can be important in increasing the ability to surgically resect the primary tumor as well as to increase the ability for breast-conserving surgery. Studies suggest that neoadjuvant aromatase inhibitors are superior to tamoxifen in the postmenopausal setting.

Endocrine Therapy for Prevention

The use of tamoxifen in early adjuvant trials appeared to have the benefit of decreasing the risk of second primary breast tumors. As well, tamoxifen in the NSABP B-24 trial has demonstrated a decreased risk of invasive and *in situ* disease in women with a history of ductal carcinoma *in situ* (DCIS) (164). Based on these findings, the NSABP has studied the use of tamoxifen in high-risk women. Requiring a Gail model risk for developing breast cancer over 5 years of at least 1.66%, the NSABP randomized over 13,000 high-risk women 35 years of age or older to receive tamoxifen or placebo (260). After a median follow-up of 69 months, tamoxifen decreased the risk of breast cancer by approximately 50%. Women with atypical ductal hyperplasia (ADH), which, like lobular carcinoma *in situ* (LCIS), is a risk factor for subsequent breast cancer, had the greatest benefit for breast cancer risk reduction of 86%. The incorporation of tamoxifen as a risk reduction strategy has been limited, however, based on potential toxicity and on the modest absolute benefits it likely provides. For example, if a woman has a risk for developing breast cancer of 1% per year, the absolute benefit of tamoxifen as risk reduction would be 0.5% per year.

To maintain efficacy and decrease toxicity, the NSABP P-2 trial (STAR trial) studied the use of tamoxifen or another SERM, raloxifine, as prevention for high-risk postmenopausal women (166). Published in 2006, raloxifine appeared similar to tamoxifen in decreasing the risk of invasive breast cancer but was less effective in decreasing the risk of DCIS, which appears counterintuitive and requires further study. Raloxifine was associated with a reduced incidence of endometrial cancer compared to tamoxifen, though this was not a statistically significant finding. Overall, it did provide a more favorable toxicity profile.

Still, based on these two trials, both raloxifine and tamoxifen are FDA approved for cancer prevention. While tamoxifen can be used in both pre- and postmenopausal women, raloxifine is reserved as a risk-reducing agent only in postmenopausal women who would have met risk eligibility for the NSABP P-2 trial. Further efforts to study risk reduction, such as the benefit of aromatase inhibitors compared to raloxifine, have been thwarted by the lack of NCI funding.

RADIATION THERAPY

Radiation therapy is a well-established treatment modality in breast cancer, and for women with localized, operable breast cancer, breast conservation surgery followed by radiation provides as effective treatment as mastectomy. It is noteworthy, however, that one of the first studies to compare radical mastectomy with breast conservation surgery and radiation was negative (276). The study, reported by Atkins et al., showed a high degree of unacceptable local recurrences and inferior survival rates with the use of radiation. Further examination of the trial design, however, showed that the dose of radiation was insufficient compared to modern standards; most patients received only 35 to 38 Gy. In addition, the radical mastectomy group ultimately received adjuvant nodal radiation, including to the internal mammary nodes. Fortunately, this did not deter other investigators.

The NSABP B-04 trial was one of the first to evaluate nodal irradiation and total mastectomy to radical mastectomy in lymph node–positive patients (277). It was followed by the EORTC 10801 trial, which compared breast conservation (with radiotherapy) versus mastectomy, and this trial also showed equivalent survival (both disease-free and overall survival) endpoints (162). However, the rate of locoregional recurrence was significantly different, with a rate of 20% in those treated with breast conservation and 12% in those treated with mastectomy ($p = 0.01$). Examination of results was noteworthy in that 50% of the lumpectomy specimens had positive margins. With adoption of the "negative margin," however, the subsequent trial, NSABP B-06, showed a decrease in local recurrence with lumpectomy and axillary lymph node dissection from 39.2% in those not receiving radiation compared with 14.3% for those treated with adjuvant radiation (197). These results were confirmed by the Milan III trial of quadrantectomy plus axillary lymph node dissection with and without radiation therapy (278).

In 1989 the NSABP initiated the B-21 trial for all age women with tumors up to 1 cm, estrogen receptor–positive, lymph node–negative invasive breast cancer (279). Women were randomized to adjuvant treatment with tamoxifen alone versus radiation plus placebo versus tamoxifen plus radiation with primary endpoints of in-breast tumor recurrence (IBTR) and incidence of contralateral breast cancer (CBC). This study enrolled over 1,000 women and showed that tamoxifen was not as effective in preventing IBTR as radiation when given as single therapies, and that both were less effective then tamoxifen plus radiation; the incidence of IBTR at 8 years was 16.5%, 9.3%, and 2.8%, respectively. However, the rates of distant recurrences were similar between the groups and, in fact, no overall survival advantage was seen with any of the modalities used; 8-year overall survival was 93% in the tamoxifen group, 94% in the radiation group, and 93% in those receiving both ($p = 0.93$).

Besides work evaluating the role of radiation in small breast tumors, research into the role of radiation therapy among older cohorts of women has been evaluated recently. A Canadian trial examined the possibility of omitting radiation for women 50 years and older with node-negative tumors less than or equal to 5 cm. Participants ($n = 769$) were randomized following lumpectomy to tamoxifen alone or with radiation, though it is notable that the majority of patients were over 60 with tumors less than 3 cm (280). At 5 years the addition of radiation led to a significant decrease in local recurrence in the breast and axilla, 7.7% without versus 0.6% with radiation. However, there was no difference noted in the rate of distant recurrence or overall survival. A subsequent trial by CALGB evaluated the additional benefit of radiotherapy in women over 70 years old treated by lumpectomy and tamoxifen and showed similar results (281). While the rate of local recurrence was higher among women who did not receive radiation (4% vs. 1% in those who received breast radiation, $p < 0.001$), there were no other differences in distant disease or 5-year overall survival.

Although individual trials failed to show an improvement in overall survival with the use of adjuvant radiotherapy, the Early Breast Cancer Trialists' Collaborative Group meta-analysis of radiation after both breast-conserving surgery and mastectomy demonstrated a small but significant overall survival benefit for radiation therapy, with a gain at 15 years of 5.3% and 4.4%, respectively (282). Radiation produced a 70% reduction in the risk of local recurrence irrespective of age, tumor grade/size/estrogen receptor status, or amount of nodal disease, which corresponded to a 17% to 19% absolute reduction in 5-year local recurrence. This was demonstrated despite an excess of mortality in the radiation arms from causes other than breast cancer—namely, lung cancer and cardiac disease. Most local recurrences (~75%) were discovered within the first 5 years and appeared nearby the primary tumor. These should be considered "true recurrences," whereas those occurring beyond 5 years were more likely to represent new primary breast cancers (282).

The value of including the nodal areas in the radiation field for patients with positive lymph nodes remains controversial and we await the results of currently enrolling trials including EORTC 22922, which is evaluating the role of radiotherapy to the internal mammary and supraclavicular regions in stage I-III patients. A similar trial by the National Cancer Institute of Canada is ongoing. In the absence of randomized data, radiation is considered for patients with multiple positive lymph nodes.

The standard radiation therapy field after breast conservation surgery encompasses the entire breast tissue plus or minus some or all the regional lymph nodes (axillary/supraclavicular/internal mammary) depending on the extent of the axillary-node dissection as well as the pathologic findings in those nodes dissected. In those patients requiring chemotherapy it is usual for it to precede radiation therapy, and a recent update on a study from the Joint Center for Radiation Therapy found no difference in local control, site of first failure, time to any event, distant metastasis–free survival, or overall survival when chemotherapy was given before or after radiation therapy (283). In this study, the delivery of chemotherapy before radiation was notably beneficial for patients with greater than or equal to four positive lymph nodes, and the delivery of radiation prior to chemotherapy appeared to benefit patients with close but not positive margins.

For women who undergo a mastectomy and are deemed to be at high risk for local failure, postchemotherapy irradiation to the chest wall and regional lymphatics is indicated. Criteria that are used to consider one "high risk" has been reconsidered on the basis of randomized trials published in the late 1990s. The Danish Breast Cancer Cooperative Group (DBCCG) conducted a randomized trial involving 1,708 premenopausal women with pathologic stage II or III breast cancer who were randomized to CMF with or without irradiation of the chest wall and regional nodes (284). Radiation therapy was associated with a reduction in locoregional recurrence (alone or with evidence of distant disease) over those who received chemotherapy only, 9% versus 32%, respectively ($p < 0.001$). It was also associated with a survival benefit at 10 years where 54% who received radiation were alive, compared to 45% who had received CMF only ($p < 0.001$). Ragaz et al. reported on a similar trial comparing CMF with or without radiation therapy, but in 318 postmenopausal women with node-positive disease (285). In this group of women, the addition of radiation therapy was associated with a significant reduction in the rate of recurrence (relative risk, 0.67; 99% CI, 0.50 to 0.90) and in mortality (relative risk, 0.71; 95% CI, 0.51 to 0.99). In 1999, the results of DBCCG trial 82c, which randomized stage II-III postmenopausal women to tamoxifen with or without radiation, was published (286). Over 1,300 women were enrolled, but tamoxifen in this trial was prescribed as 30 mg daily for only 1 year. With a median follow-up of over 10 years, radiation therapy was associated with a significant reduction in locoregional recurrence, 8% versus 35% with 1 year of tamoxifen ($p < 0.001$). Overall survival was 45% and 36%, respectively ($p = 0.03$).

In Situ Breast Disease

Approximately 20% of patients treated with local excision alone for DCIS have a recurrence, with about half of these recurrences being invasive cancer. Given this, radiation is often delivered as a means of risk reduction. To date, three randomized trials have compared excision alone with excision followed by whole breast radiation therapy and all demonstrated that radiation therapy reduces the risk of a subsequent breast event by 38% to 62% (287–289).

The NSABP B-17 trial enrolled over 800 women with localized DCIS to lumpectomy with or without radiation and showed a statistically significant reduction in both noninvasive in-breast tumor recurrence (IBTR, 13.4% without radiation vs. 8.2% with radiation, $p = 0.007$) and invasive IBTR (13.4% vs. 3.9%, respectively, $p < 0.0001$) (289). EORTC 10853 enrolled over 1,000 women with surgically excised DCIS up to 5 cm in widest diameter to observation or radiation (288). The reported 4-year local relapse rate was 84% and 91%, respectively ($p = 0.005$) with similar reductions seen in both invasive and noninvasive recurrences. Finally, Houghton et al. reported on a 2 × 2 randomized trial in this population where over 1,700 women were randomized to both radiation and tamoxifen, either as a single agent, or to no further therapy (287). Although reported follow-up was only 1 year, recurrent DCIS was already shown to be reduced with tamoxifen treatment (HR 0.68; 95% CI, 0.49 to 0.96). Radiation was shown to reduce the incidence of both ipsilateral invasive (HR 0.45; 95% CI, 0.24 to 0.85) and noninvasive disease (HR 0.36; 95% CI, 0.19 to 0.66). The issue of tamoxifen therapy and radiation therapy has been further addressed by the NSABP. Unlike the prior study, the B24 trial showed that the addition of tamoxifen further reduced the number of invasive breast cancer events by 50% and did so in both breasts, but had a nonsignificant effect on reducing the DCIS recurrences (290).

Finally, a recent meta-analysis of the role of radiation in breast conservation therapy for DCIS demonstrated an approximate 60% reduction in local recurrence (291). The greatest benefit was seen with high-grade lesions and/or positive margins, but all age groups benefited, and as expected there was no difference in distant metastases or survival rates.

Radiation Therapy in Recurrent Disease

Palliative radiation for painful or recurrent locoregional disease in the chest wall or regional lymphatics is quite effective and has also been used to treat lesions involving the bone, brain, spinal cord, liver, and lung among other areas. Many of these lesions are now being treated on stereotactic body radiotherapy (SBRT) trials whereby a limited number of large fractions are delivered to a well-localized site (292). Palliative radiation courses usually last from a one-time 8 Gy 1-day treatment to a 2- to 3-week course of 2.5 to 3 Gy per fraction for a total dose of 30 to 37.5 Gy. There is less concern about the late effects associated with these large fractions given that most of these patients may not survive long enough to experience them. This stands in contrast to the 6- to 8-week course of low-dose-per-fraction radiation usually used to treat localized disease where the focus is on both cure and minimizing long-term/late side effects of radiation therapy.

Radiation Therapy Techniques for the Intact Breast

Following breast conservation surgery, the entire residual breast tissue, along with a small portion of the underlying chest wall and lung, is included in the irradiated volume, although careful attention to these areas is given to limit their exposure. Before treatment, patients undergo a planning session or simulation to ensure the radiation field has been mapped out. It is essential that the plan be consistently applied on a day-to-day basis to ensure the uniformity of treatment. Small tattoos are placed to ensure proper localization on a daily basis. In women who require retreatment for chest wall disease, they also serve to define the original field to avoid overlapping fields (Fig. 29.30).

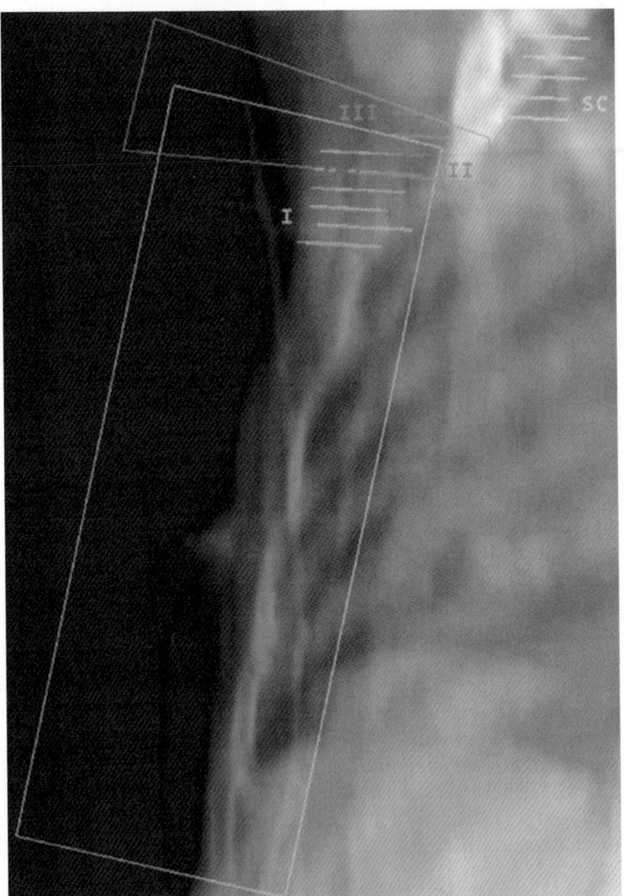

FIGURE 29.30. Medial breast/chest wall tangential field with axillary lymph node levels I, II, III and supraclavicular nodes outlined. *Source:* Reprinted with permission from Goodman RL, Grann A, Saracco P, et al. The relationship between radiation fields and regional lymph nodes in carcinoma of the breast. *Int J Radiat Oncol Biol Phys* 2001;50(1):101.

Photon energies of 4 to 6 MV are preferred to treat the breast. Energies greater than 6 MV may underdose superficial tissue beneath the skin surface, but may be helpful in large breasts to decrease the integral breast dose, and wedges are used to achieve uniform dose distributions. It is usually unnecessary to apply bolus (tissue equivalent material) to the skin as it is not at risk for recurrence, unlike in the postmastectomy setting where the bolus is applied to the mastectomy scar to increase dose superficially.

As the excised tumor bed may also harbor microscopic foci of disease, a radiation boost to the tumor bed is often given and consists of a series of an additional five to eight treatments directed to the tumor bed plus a 1.5- to 2-cm margin. However, the need for a boost if the surgical margins at breast excision are clear is controversial. The EORTC 22881-10882 trial involved over 5,500 women with stage I or II breast cancer who were randomly assigned to whole breast treatment with or without a "boost" dose of 16 Gy (293). At 10 years, the rate of local relapse was 10.2% in the no-boost group and was 6.2 % in the boost group ($p < 0.0001$), but there was no difference in overall survival noted (82% in both arms). A subsequent trial from France was also conducted with similar reduction in local relapse with a 10 Gy boost dose (294).

Irradiation of Regional Lymphatics

Most tangential breast fields include at least level I axillary lymph nodes inadvertently. The low axilla (levels I and II) is

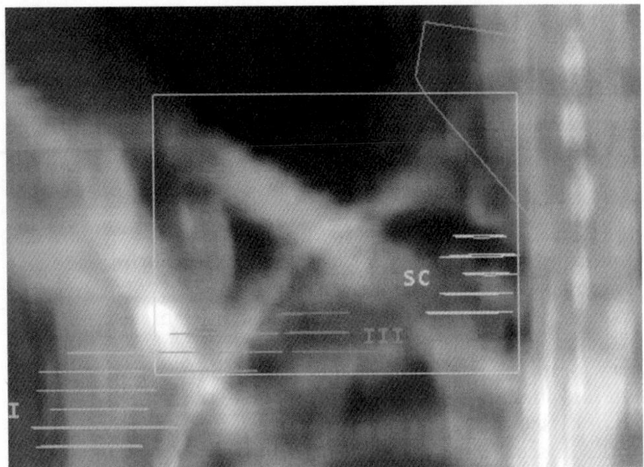

FIGURE 29.31. A right-sided supraclavicular field including the supraclavicular nodes as well as the axillary lymph node levels II and III as outlined. *Source:* Reprinted with permission from Goodman RL, Grann A, Saracco P, Needham MF. The relationship between radiation fields and regional lymph nodes in carcinoma of the breast. *Int J Radiat Oncol Biol Phys* 50(1):102.

treated along with the supraclavicular field when there is extranodal/capular invasion, when greater than 50% of the lymph nodes removed are involved with carcinoma, or in the absence of an adequate axillary dissection. The supraclavicular field is extended inferiorly to the second rib or angle of Louie to cover the axilla while the lateral border falls off the anterior axillary fold of skin (Fig. 29.31). A supplemental dose delivered by a posterior axillary boost (PAB) ensures complete radiation therapy has been accomplished (Fig. 29.32). An EORTC trial is ongoing whereby patients with a positive sentinel lymph node are randomized to axillary radiation without axillary lymph node dissection or to axillary lymph node dissection in an attempt to avoid extra surgery in these patients.

Irradiation of the supraclavicular area is indicated in women with three or more axillary nodes involved. For purposes of radiation planning, surgical clips in the area of axillary dissection provide a useful guide to the design of this radiation field. Ideally, the humeral head is shielded without compromising coverage of the high axillary lymph nodes (level III).

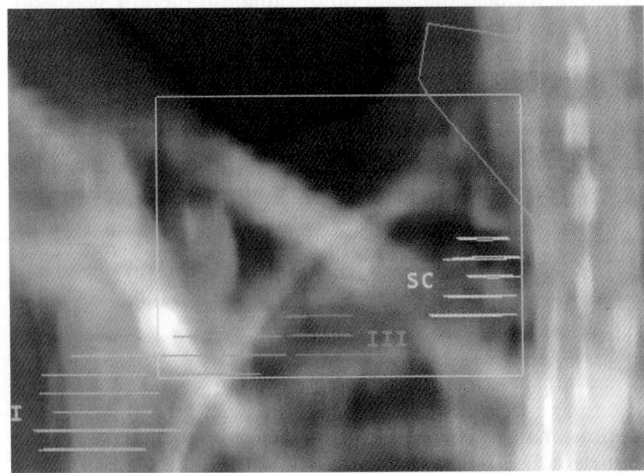

FIGURE 29.32. A left-sided posterior axillary boost (PAB) field showing the nearby levels I, II, and III axillary lymph nodes as well as the supraclavicular nodes as outlined. *Source:* Reprinted with permission from Goodman RL, Grann A, Saracco P, et al. The relationship between radiation fields and regional lymph nodes in carcinoma of the breast. *Int J Radiat Oncol Biol Phys* 50(1):103.

The total dose delivered to the supraclavicular field is 46 to 50.8 Gy. If supraclavicular node involvement is documented on biopsy, this area may be treated with a "boost" as well.

Radiotherapy to the internal mammary lymph nodes remains unresolved, although the internal mammary nodes (IMNs) are not considered to be a necessity in most patients since most patients who would be "at risk" are usually candidates for adjuvant endocrine or chemotherapy. Still, it may be an appropriate consideration in women with medial breast tumors, those with tumors larger than 2 to 3 cm, those with multiple involved axillary nodes, or those with biopsy-proven or radiographically suspected IMN involvement. If treatment is recommended, the lymph nodes should be outlined using the CT obtained at simulation by covering the first three intercostal spaces medially while limiting the heart dose as much as possible on the left side (295). Active breathing control devices have been used to spare the heart dose, whereby radiation is delivered during maximum inspiration when the heart is pushed out of the radiation field by the expanded lung (296).

Irradiation Dose to the Contralateral Breast

A dose of 0.5 to 2 Gy to the contralateral breast has been reported in women receiving a dose of 50 Gy to the intact breast with the use of tangential fields (297). As expected, radiation fields encompassing the regional lymph nodes increase the dose to the contralateral breast significantly. A detailed dosimetric study demonstrated that most of the scatter dose received by the opposite breast originates in the collimator and accessories of the accelerator and can be significantly decreased by increasing the distance between the source and the patient's skin (298). The use of independent jaws combined with beam splitters following the contour of the chest wall of the patient can be very helpful in decreasing the dose to the contralateral breast. Most breast radiation plans include a lateral and medial wedge. The medial wedge, however, contributes most to the contralateral breast dose, and attempts at treatment without this wedge have been successful with a resultant decrease in contralateral breast dose without a significant decrease in dose homogeneity in the treated breast (299). The clinical significance of the inadvertent radiation dose to the opposite breast is uncertain, with various studies failing to show an increased risk of contralateral breast cancer (300–302).

Irradiation Techniques to the Chest Wall

For women undergoing chest wall radiation following mastectomy, the technique in large part is determined by their anatomy, and the area treated includes the chest wall and supraclavicular fossa. If a patient has undergone an immediate reconstruction, a three-field technique is used, with two tangent fields directed at the chest wall and reconstruction with a third, carefully matched field encompassing the supraclavicular nodal area and the apex of the axilla. Photon beams are in the 4 to 6 MV range, and doses of 50 Gy over 5 weeks are appropriate, with a boost dose of 10 Gy to the mastectomy scar itself. For patients undergoing mastectomy in whom adjuvant radiation is being considered, simultaneous consultations involving plastic surgery and radiation oncology are recommended before surgery to discuss the timing and appropriateness of reconstruction and radiotherapy. In most cases, the reconstruction should occur after the radiation is completed to increase the probability of implant viability and cosmesis of the reconstructed breast (303).

For women who recur in the chest wall or regional nodes, treatment should be approached with curative intent. If possible, surgical resection remains the best option for long-term disease control and adjuvant radiotherapy may increase this likelihood. The radiation fields are similar to the approach for the postmastectomy patient in terms of field design and dose. If palpable disease remains following resection, a boost is used to increase the total dose over 50 Gy in the affected field.

FOLLOW-UP CARE

Women treated for a diagnosis of breast cancer should be examined every 3 to 4 months for the first 2 to 3 years, then every 4 to 6 months to year 5, and then annually. Ideally, visits should be split among a woman's multiple providers, including her surgeon, medical oncologist, radiation oncologist, and her primary care providers. Cancer follow-up requires history and physical with careful attention to new or increasing symptoms. For example, new bone pain that wakes one up from sleep may be a sign of new onset bone metastases and would require a bone scan. For the asymptomatic patient, there is no role for surveillance lab work, tumor markers such as CEA, CA 15-3, and CA 27-29, or radiographic testing and they are not recommended (304). Although they may lead to an earlier diagnosis of metastatic disease, there is no evidence that they impact survival (305). Attention to screening should be emphasized annually, and this includes tracking dates of mammography, breast MRI in high-risk patients, and screening colonoscopy (if over the age of 50 or earlier in the presence of a family history of colon cancer). Addressing health risks should be a part of routine follow-up, including smoking cessation and discussion of alcohol use. Finally, screening for issues such as sexual dysfunction, depression, and anxiety is important, as they are known to be issues in cancer survivors and can profoundly affect long-term quality of life.

SEQUELAE OF TREATMENT

The multidisciplinary treatment program can be difficult for women. Each modality has its own set of side effects and the duration of treatment (up to or more than 1 year in some cases) can exert a psychological and emotional toll.

Women who have received chemotherapy report difficulties with short-term memory ("chemo-brain") which may or may not resolve with time, and if severe, can even have an impact on a woman's ability to work. Unfortunately, the magnitude of the problem remains poorly characterized. Both doxorubicin and trastuzumab can affect cardiac function, which may not be reversed with the passage of time. In a recent review of trials that evaluated trastuzumab into anthracyline-containing adjuvant treatment, as much as 4% of patients experienced congestive heart failure, going as high as 14% in the NSABP B-31 trial, which in some cases was not reversed (306). Fatigue is an almost universal consequence of chemotherapy, worsens with each successive cycle, and may take a year or more to resolve. Severe menopausal symptoms and accelerated bone loss are potential issues for the premenopausal woman who experiences chemotherapy-induced amenorrhea. Treatments for hot flashes are readily available and include use of antidepressants, gabapentin, and vaginal estrogen preparations. Caution is required with the use of vaginal estrogen tablets, particularly in women with hormone-positive breast cancers, as the impact of even low subclinical rises in estrogen levels on effectiveness of antiestrogen agents (especially the aromatase inhibitors) and consequently on tumor relapse is unknown. Recently the empiric use of the bisphosphonate residronate was evaluated in this population in a randomized, placebo-controlled trial and demonstrated that treatment significantly increased bone mineral density at both the hip (by 1.3%) and the spine (by 1.2%), compared to placebo where decreases of 0.9% at the spine and 0.8% at the hip were seen ($p < 0.01$) (307). The Cancer and Leukemia

Group B has recently completed a similar trial (CALGB 79809) evaluating the use of zoledronic acid compared to placebo and results are awaited. Finally, a recently described arthralgia syndrome can accompany treatment with the aromatase inhibitors, and may lead to cessation of this therapy in some patients (308). The incidence and etiology of this have yet to be elucidated.

Besides the side effects of chemotherapy, there are sequelae from radiation treatment that may occur acutely or follow the end of treatment, taking months to years after treatment to manifest. The most common acute effects of radiation therapy include fatigue, skin irritation, breast swelling, and general breast discomfort; other side effects include muscle pain (in motion), incision-site pain, and rib pain. In one series, 31% of patients complained of breast swelling and approximately 20% complained of breast pain following radiation therapy after breast-conserving surgery (309). In another, approximately 10% to 15% of patients developed moist desquamation during their treatment (310). Generally, this occurs in the inframammary fold and can be treated conservatively. Very rarely, a patient will need a break for any of the above conditions. Almost all patients experience some form of fatigue, which is generally mild and manageable and improves over time. Most patients recover to baseline within 2 months after completion of the radiation treatment.

Of the late effects of radiation treatment in a woman who has undergone breast conservation, perhaps one of the most disturbing can be impaired cosmesis secondary to fibrosis and atrophy (311). Cosmetic outcome has been directly related to adjuvant chemotherapy, the dose of radiation, fraction size, and the degree of surgery (311,312). Whole breast radiotherapy doses greater than 50 Gy as well as total dose to the tumor site greater than 65 Gy have been shown to adversely affect cosmesis (313). Abner et al. reported on the cosmesis outcomes in 1,625 patients receiving BCT and chemotherapy, showing that long-term cosmesis was remarkably worse for those receiving concurrent and sequential chemoradiation as compared to radiation alone (314). Excellent cosmesis was seen in 56% of patients receiving sequential therapy versus 32% for concurrent chemoradiation and 75% for no adjuvant chemotherapy.

Arm edema is also one of the most feared late-term complications of radiation treatment, and the incidence of this complication is related to the extent of axillary surgery and regional radiation (315–320). Arm edema is found in only a few percent of women who undergo sentinel lymph node biopsy, level I-II dissection, or radiation alone, and adding nonaxillary radiation to a more limited surgery does not substantially increase the risk of arm edema (321,322). However, women who experience axillary node dissection and axillary radiation have a significantly higher risk of arm edema (323,324). In one report that included 200 women treated for early-stage breast cancer, arm edema developed in 38% of those treated with axillary node dissection plus axillary radiation compared to 7% to 9% of those undergoing either axillary node dissection or axillary radiotherapy (323).

Symptomatic pneumonitis is an infrequent occurrence after breast conservation surgery and is noted 1 to several months after irradiation (325). Patients present with dry cough (88%), shortness of breath (35%), or fever (53%). On radiographic studies a pulmonary infiltrate is observed in the irradiated volume (326). The risk of radiation pneumonitis is directly related to the volume of irradiated lung and is approximately 5% when treating the chest wall where there is minimal lung volume in the field (326,327). The risk increases when a supraclavicular field is added or the internal mammary nodes are treated (328,329). Concurrent chemotherapy has also been shown to increase the risk of pneumonitis. One study showed that when patients treated with the three-field technique received chemotherapy concurrently with irradiation, the incidence of radiation pneumonitis was 8.8% (8 of 92) compared with 1.3% (3 of 236) for those who received sequential chemotherapy (329). Of note, when radiation was given to the breast alone without chemotherapy the incidence was 0.5% (6 of 1,296, $p = 0.002$). There have been conflicting data involving increased risk of pneumonitis when taking tamoxifen concurrently with radiation. Two studies found an increased risk of pulmonary fibrosis, while a series from Fox Chase Cancer Center did not show an increase in clinical radiation pneumonitis (330–332).

Another concern related to breast radiation is cardiac toxicity. The most significant risk factors for this side effect include older radiation techniques, the addition of chemotherapy, and treatment of left-sided breast cancer. Fortunately, improvement in radiation technique has substantially decreased late-term cardiac complications, and most recent trials utilizing modern radiation techniques have found no increase in cardiovascular toxicity (333–336). Valagussa et al. reported on cardiac effects after adjuvant chemotherapy and breast irradiation for operable breast cancer (333). They retrospectively evaluated 825 women in prospective trials with respect to irradiation, with or without administration of doxorubicin; 360 patients had breast conservation therapy. With a median follow-up of 80 months, the overall incidence of congestive heart failure in all patients was 0.5%. Patients receiving doxorubicin chemotherapy without irradiation had a 0.8% incidence of congestive heart failure. Patients receiving both doxorubicin and left-breast irradiation had an incidence of 2.6%, and two fatalities secondary to congestive heart failure occurred in this group.

Brachial plexus dysfunction is another possible complication of regional nodal radiation therapy and must be distinguished from neuropathies caused by axillary dissection or recurrence. Pierce et al., in a review of 1,624 patients, reported brachial plexus involvement in 1.8% of patients, though other investigators have found the incidence to be less than 1% (321,332,337).

Pregnancy and Fertility in the Breast Cancer Survivor

It has been reported that approximately 5% to 15% of young breast cancer survivors will become pregnant following treatment (338). Currently, there are no prospective studies evaluating the safety of a subsequent pregnancy after a diagnosis of breast cancer, but several retrospective studies have demonstrated no worsening of survival or increased risk of recurrence (339–342). Of interest, a number of studies report that pregnancy is associated with an improved survival, though the issue of the "healthy mother effect" as a potential confounder has been reported (339). That is, only women who feel physically and emotionally healthy will attempt pregnancy while those who continue to be affected by the disease do not. Alternatively, it is possible that the high hormonal levels of pregnancy have a beneficial effect given the documented antitumor effects seen both *in vitro* and in animal models of high-dose estrogens and progestins (338).

Those women who become pregnant following breast cancer treatment may be able to breast-feed, though this has only been reported in case series. Higgins and Haffty reported on 11 patients who subsequently experienced 13 pregnancies (343). Lactation was possible in the treated breast in four of ten women; in three, lactation was pharmacologically suppressed. The time interval from initial treatment to delivery did not appear to affect successful lactation. Still, this issue will need to be studied in larger series.

It may seem helpful to wait before attempting pregnancy since this is the time of highest risk of recurrence, but the available data have not clearly shown a worse prognosis if pregnancy is achieved sooner. Discussing fertility options after receiving treatment for breast cancer may be too late. Several investigators have reported that women prefer to discuss these issues at the time of treatment planning and early follow-up, suggesting that options for preserving fertility should be addressed early, including a referral to a fertility specialist as needed (344,345). Recently, the American Society of Clinical Oncology (ASCO) convened an expert panel to develop guidelines for fertility preservation and made similar recommendations (346). Still, concerns that embryo banking will inappropriately delay necessary treatment for newly diagnosed patients have been raised. A recent report by Madriagno et al. compared time intervals between egg retrieval and treatment in 23 newly diagnosed women with breast cancer. He reported that there was no delay, with average time from first consult to egg retrieval of 33 days, and time from definitive surgery to start of chemotherapy at 47 days. This suggests that embryo banking could be incorporated into the workup and surgical management of new breast cancer patients, again emphasizing the importance of early referral to reproductive specialists (347).

SPECIAL CONSIDERATIONS

Breast Cancer in Pregnancy

Pregnancy-associated breast cancer is defined as cancer diagnosed during pregnancy, lactation, or up to 12 months postpartum (348). Among women of child-bearing potential, approximately 13% of breast cancers will occur in this group, and among women younger than 40 years an estimated 10% will be pregnant (349,350). As increasing numbers of women delay pregnancy, many speculate that the incidence of pregnancy-associated breast cancer will increase.

Most women diagnosed with pregnancy-associated breast cancer present with a painless breast mass. While the differential diagnosis of a palpable mass during pregnancy involves a majority of benign masses, including lactating adenomas, fibroadenomas, and galactoceles, evaluation is warranted if palpable findings persist. Clinical breast examination is limited in a pregnant patient due to hormonally induced breast engorgement. Similarly, the usefulness of mammography during pregnancy has been questioned; however, recent studies show that with proper abdominal shielding, the irradiation dose to the fetus from a standard two-view mammography is less than 50.5 μGy, which is within the limits considered acceptable during pregnancy and well below the threshold exposure of 10 rad (100 mGy), where the estimated risk of fetal malformation and central nervous system (CNS) problems is 1% (351).

Studies on the effectiveness of imaging in pregnant cancer patients are limited. Yang et al. performed a retrospective study of 23 women with 24 cancers diagnosed during pregnancy (352). Of those who underwent preoperative mammography, radiographic findings were "positive" in 18 out of 20 cancers (90%) despite dense breast parenchymal patterns; the addition of ultrasonography was noted to be 100% sensitive. Although MRI has been used during pregnancy, the gadolinium required for a meaningful breast study crosses the placenta and is associated with fetal abnormalities in animals (category C), and thus contrast-enhanced breast MRI cannot be recommended (348).

As happens for nonpregnant women, negative findings on breast imaging should not delay obtaining definitive diagnosis in a persistently palpable mass. Currently ultrasound-guided core biopsies can be performed safely and this is the preferred method for diagnosis. Despite concerns to the contrary, reports of milk fistulae are rare (353).

Historically, studies reported that pregnancy-associated breast cancer had a dismal prognosis with survival rates of less than 20% at 5 years (354–356). These statistics may have reflected the later diagnosis of these lesions, as pregnancy-associated cancers are typically larger and more often node positive (56% to 89%) compared to nonpregnant women (38% to 54%) (357,358). In addition, patients diagnosed in pregnancy frequently have high-grade tumors, are hormone negative, and are HER2/neu positive (358–360). Therefore, after controlling for these factors, patient age and stage of diagnosis at presentation, the overall prognosis of patients appears similar to nonpregnant women, and the 5- and 10-year survival for node-negative and node-positive pregnancy-associated breast cancer ranges from 60% to 100% and 31% to 52%, respectively (348,351).

There is no role for termination to improve prognosis, and it is not considered a therapeutic option. The safety of surgical intervention during pregnancy is well established, and modified radical mastectomy is considered the standard of care. This approach virtually eliminates the need for irradiation and allows optimal control of disease within the axilla. However, breast conservation is increasingly seen as a reasonable alternative to pregnant women, particularly if diagnosis is made in the latter second and third trimesters, when breast irradiation can be safely delayed until the postpartum period. In addition, for the patient presenting with locally advanced disease, the increased use of neoadjuvant chemotherapy allows a delay in definitive surgical management and a concomitant delay in postoperative radiotherapy (348). While full axillary dissection remains the most common approach to lymph node evaluation in pregnant patients, increasing reports have documented the efficacy and safety of sentinel lymph node biopsy despite the numerous concerns raised regarding the risk of fetal irradiation with use of radiocolloid in pregnancy (361–363). Still, sentinel node biopsy in pregnant women has not been systematically evaluated. Currently, it is considered *reasonable* to offer to pregnant patients but only after appropriate counseling. It is important to remember that both isosulfan blue dye and methylene blue dye are classified as pregnancy category C drugs, and intra-amniotic injection of methylene blue has been associated with hemolytic anemia, hyperbilirubinemia, methemoglobinemia, duodenal atresia, deep blue staining of the newborn, and even fetal death (364–367). Whether subareolar injections of dye would result in a similar outcome is unclear; however, its use is generally not recommended.

Most experts consider postoperative therapeutic irradiation during pregnancy to be contraindicated. If breast conservation is chosen, adjuvant radiotherapy is typically delayed until the postpartum period. However, this perspective has recently been challenged by some who feel that the risks of radiation to the fetus are overestimated (368). Kal et al. argue that fetal exposure to radiotherapy can be sufficiently reduced by proper shielding, resulting in fetal exposure doses that fall below accepted threshold doses. Unfortunately, the lack of prospective data continues to make the use of radiotherapy during pregnancy contraindicated.

Given the high prevalence of node-positive disease among women diagnosed with breast cancer during pregnancy, chemotherapy plays a crucial role in both the adjuvant and neoadjuvant treatment of these women. The effects of chemotherapy on fetal development and growth vary depending on gestational age. When administered during the first trimester, chemotherapy can result in high rates of miscarriages and malformations (369). As a result, chemotherapy is generally contraindicated during this period of organogenesis. Outside of the first trimester, chemotherapy has proven to be safe, although all chemotherapy agents are still considered category D agents. The overall incidence of major fetal malformations following administration of chemotherapy in the second and third trimesters is reported to be ~3%, which is similar to the estimated baseline population risk of major congenital malformations (2% to 3%) (370). The most commonly reported side effects are fetal growth restriction, low birth weight, preterm delivery, and transient leukopenia of the newborn.

Several prospective case series have reported on the use of anthracycline-based chemotherapy administered every 3 to 4 weeks during the second and third trimesters (371,372). Hahn et al. reported that among 57 women treated with FAC in the second and third trimesters, there were no stillbirths reported, and no miscarriages or perinatal deaths (371). The most common neonatal complication was respiratory distress and 10% required ventilatory support; one child developed a subarachnoid hemorrhage in association with thrombocytopenia and neutropenia. The potential risk of anthracycline-associated fetal cardiotoxicity later in life during childhood or adulthood remains a concern for those fetuses exposed to chemotherapy *in utero*. Despite this, Meyer-Wittkopf et al. were not able to identify any abnormalities on echocardiograms performed *in utero* and up to 2 years of age in infants exposed to doxorubicin and cyclophosphamide starting at 24 weeks gestation (373). Aviles and Neri reported on a cohort of 84 children born to mothers who received combination chemotherapy during pregnancy for hematologic malignancies (374). Physical, neurologic, and psychologic development was normal for all children and there were no malignancies diagnosed in this group of children. At present, the dosing recommendations for chemotherapy during pregnancy are weight based. Current recommendations are to avoid the administration of chemotherapy approximately 1 month before delivery to minimize the possibility of infectious complications or hemorrhage from pancytopenia to either the mother or the fetus. The use of trastuzumab is limited to case reports and currently is considered a category B drug in pregnancy. There are no long-term data available of children following exposure to endocrine agents, such as tamoxifen, *in utero*. However, tamoxifen remains contraindicated in pregnancy and the use of nonhormonal contraception is recommended during tamoxifen treatment and for 2 months after stopping, due to its extended half-life (375).

Breast Cancer in the Elderly

Age is a well-characterized risk factor for the development of breast cancer. Yet despite the high prevalence of breast cancer in older women, there is substantial evidence that they are less likely to receive standard care (376,377). Defining the optimal treatment strategies for these women is complicated by the relatively few numbers of women over 65 enrolled in multi-instititional trials. Barriers to recruitment of older women to multi-institutional trials likely include "physician bias" and/or "patient and family bias," based on the fear that patients may not tolerate treatment or that the potential toxicity does not outweigh the potential benefits of the treatment (378).

Studies indicate that the survival from breast cancer appears to be worse among older women, though the factors underlying this finding remain unclear (379,380). Although breast cancer presentation in older women may be more advanced at diagnosis, they also tend to be more indolent with a more favorable biologic profile and overall less aggressive disease than in younger women. Multiple studies have shown that breast cancer in older women is typically well- or moderately differentiated, node negative, estrogen and progesterone receptor positive, and HER2/neu negative (115,381,382).

Older patients tolerate surgery, including breast-conserving surgery or mastectomy, as well as their younger counterparts, and the operative mortality of patients who are in reasonable health with a reasonable functional status is negligible (383). Careful preoperative screening will identify the small group of women who would suffer significant morbidity and/or mortality from surgery.

Some have questioned the benefit of axillary evaluation in elderly women, particularly in the presence of endocrine-responsive disease, but several studies have shown not only that it is feasible, but that treatment decisions are still made on the basis of the nodal status. The International Breast Cancer Study Group compared the outcome of axillary clearance versus no clearance in women older than 60 years (median age, 74 years) with clinically negative, operable breast cancer (384). All women with endocrine-responsive breast cancer received 5 years of tamoxifen. Although axillary relapse was not the primary endpoint, the results were reassuring and showed a low local relapse rate of 2% after 5 years of follow-up. McMahon et al. reviewed the outcomes of 261 women who were 70 years of age or older who underwent a sentinel lymph node (SLN) biopsy (385). The overall SLN identification rate was 97.1% and sentinel node status was associated with significantly different rates of systemic therapy for tumors less than 2 cm, but not with larger tumors. Finally, despite earlier studies suggesting that primary medical treatment with tamoxifen was as effective as surgery for the treatment of operable breast cancer in elderly patients, more recent randomized studies have demonstrated a more favorable outcome following surgical management of these patients. In one, women treated with surgery plus tamoxifen had a 70% relapse-free survival as compared to 47% for those treated with tamoxifen alone (386). Subsequent studies have yielded similar results, and have been confirmed by a recent Cochrane group meta-analysis (387–389).

The role of radiotherapy in older women has also been subjected to trials. In a Canadian trial patients 50 years of age or older with tumors up to 5 cm who had been treated with surgery and tamoxifen were randomized to adjuvant radiotherapy or observation (280). The local recurrence rate among women who underwent radiation and those who did not was 0.6% and 7.7%, respectively. Similarly, CALGB conducted a trial in women 70 years or older and found no significant differences between those who did not and those who did undergo radiation therapy regarding subsequent mastectomy rates, distant metastases, or overall survival. However, the rate of locoregional recurrences was significantly different (1% in those who underwent radiotherapy vs. 4% in those who did not, $p < 0.001$) (281). Based on this, radiotherapy might be reasonably with held in the older patient who takes endocrine therapy following surgery.

The confirmed benefit of adjuvant hormonal therapy and the associated risk profiles of the available agents must be considered in the older patient. Tamoxifen may cause endometrial cancer, though rarely, and is associated with an increased risk of thromboembolic disease. As such, it is generally not recommended in patients with small (<1 cm) node-negative tumors in the presence of other serious comorbid conditions, particularly if their life expectancy is less than 10 years, as the benefits of endocrine manipulation are not likely to be realized (390). Although the aromatase inhibitors have been shown to be less of a risk in causing endometrial cancer or thromboembolic disease, they did statistically increase the risk of bone fractures compared to tamoxifen (264,268). In addition to bony disease, letrozole demonstrated significant increases in cardiac events compared to tamoxifen, including grade 3-5 ischemic disease (0.6% vs. 1.1%, respectively, $p = 0.013$), and in congestive heart failure (0.1% vs. 0.5%, respectively, $p = 0.006$) (268). For the estimated 30% of older patients with tumors negative for ER/PR receptor expression, decisions about chemotherapy must take into account tumor characteristics, the ensuing risk of relapse, and one's competing comorbidities. Still, chemotherapy may be an option especially in healthy elderly women with hormone receptor–negative tumors considered at high risk, particularly if their estimated life expectancy would otherwise exceed 5 years (391). Still, the optimal chemotherapy regimens, doses, and schedules for elderly patients remain undefined.

Disparities in Breast Cancer

There is a relative paucity of data regarding outcomes among other ethnic groups, such as Latinas, and hence much of what we have learned about disparities among ethnic minority women we have learned from work done with the African American (AA) community. The impact of racial disparities on breast cancer survival has been the subject of multiple studies. Specifically, it has been well documented that despite a consistently higher incidence of breast cancer among white women when compared to AA women, AA women still suffer the greater mortality from breast cancer (350).

Many attribute the widening racial disparity to the fact that racial and ethnic minorities in the United States often receive less than adequate health care. Health insurance coverage and socioeconomic status have been described as important factors associated with general medical outcomes, but do not entirely explain the disparities in breast cancer in ethnic minority women. Newman and Martin conducted a meta-analysis of studies reporting on survival of AA versus white patients with breast cancer (392). After adjusting for socioeconomic status, age, and stage of diagnosis, they found that AA women still experienced a higher risk of mortality, with a mortality hazard ratio of 1.27 (95% CI, 1.18 to 1.38) Similarly, Field et al. evaluated survival among AA and white breast cancer patients receiving care through the Cancer Research Network, which covers patients using managed care health plans (393). Despite similar health coverage and access to care, 5-year survival was lower for AA women (74% vs. 82%). They concluded that among women with invasive breast cancer, being insured and having access to medical care does not eliminate the survival disparity for AA women. More recently, Jatoi et al. evaluated the medical records of 23,612 women diagnosed and treated for primary breast carcinoma through the Department of Defense health care system (394). They reported that when AA women were compared to white women, the hazard ratio for survival was 1.27 in those diagnosed between 1980 and 1984, but it had increased to 1.85 between 1995 and 1999. Therefore, it appears that inequalities in access to health care, while a reality for many AA women in the United States, are not solely responsible for the racial disparities evident among women diagnosed with breast cancer.

Some argue that differences in tumor biology or other extrinsic factors account for a significant proportion of the disparity evidenced (395,396). It is documented that AA women are diagnosed at a younger age compared to white women and that, compared to white women, AA women experience a higher incidence of disease before 45 years and declining rates after 50 years of age. Reproductive history–related risk factors have been suggested as an explanation for the younger age distribution noted among AA women (397). In addition, reports suggest that a higher frequency of aggressive subtypes of infiltrating ductal carcinoma are present among AA women, such as medullary, basaloid, and inflammatory breast cancer (398,399). Finally, studies have also demonstrated a higher prevalence of high-grade, hormone receptor–negative, and triple-negative breast cancer among AA women with more advanced stages of disease at diagnosis (400,401).

Disparities in the delivery of adjuvant chemotherapy to eligible patients also may account for disparities among AA women, and studies continue to demonstrate this disturbing trend. For example, White et al. reported that among 1,263 patients with node-positive breast cancer eligible for chemotherapy, 85.3% of white women received the indicated treatment, compared to 78.7% of AA and Latina patients (402). More recently, Bickell et al. reported data from six New York City hospitals and found that AA patients were twice as likely to be under-treated with regard to chemotherapy, radiation therapy, and/or endocrine therapy compared with white patients (403). Similar data suggest that surgical therapies, such as sentinel node biopsies and breast reconstruction, are impacted as well (403–406).

Effective evaluation of the determinants of racial disparities in breast cancer treatment will require adequate participation in randomized clinical trials, which means that efforts to increase the proportion of patients offered trials and addressing eligibility so more women qualify for trials are needed. In one study, only 21% of AA patients were offered a clinical trial, compared to 42% of white patients (404). In another, evaluating barriers to enrollment of minorities into clinical trials, Adams-Campbell et al. reported that among 235 AA patients with breast cancer, only 8.5% were deemed eligible for trial participation; most were excluded due to comorbid disease (407).

Documented racial disparities exist in the incidence, treatment, and outcomes of women with breast cancer. Of great concern, the mortality among AA women diagnosed with breast cancer exceeds that of white women, despite a lower prevalence of disease overall. The determinants of these disparities are likely multifactorial, and despite numerous studies evaluating breast cancer treatment among AA women, they remain incompletely understood. Data evaluating other ethnic groups are limited, and emphasizes the need for continued studies into this area of breast cancer research.

FUTURE DIRECTIONS

The evolution in breast therapy continues to move at a very fast pace, with new technologies under development that may transform the landscape of breast surgical practice, medical care, and radiation techniques. These will be briefly summarized.

Surgery: Contemporary Strategies

The literature is replete with reports of the successful use of thermal ablation of lung, liver, bone, adrenal, kidney, and prostate in both the metastatic and primary setting. Advances in the understanding of thermal biology, and advances in both the delivery systems and tumor imaging systems have extended this therapeutic option to other tumor sites, including breast cancer. The initial reports of ablative techniques in breast cancer therapy focused on radiofrequency ablation (RFA) (408). However, this technique suffered from two serious flaws. First, thermal heating is associated with intense discomfort for the patient; second, visualization of the treatment zone is severely compromised when RFA is administered with ultrasound guidance.

Cryoablation represents an alternative to radiofrequency ablation and may be ideally suited to breast cancer therapy (409). First, the majority of invasive breast cancers are identified by mammography, and characterized and biopsied under ultrasound guidance, making the small handheld ultrasound probe an ideal modality to guide breast therapeutic interventions. In addition, cryoablation produces a ball of frozen tissue that is imminently visible under ultrasound, in direct contradistinction to thermally heated tissue. The cryoablative process involves a freeze-thaw-freeze cycle that results in tissue destruction through intracellular ice formation, causing cellular wall disruption, subsequent osmotic injury, and delayed microvascular disruption leading to tissue ischemia. The usual treatment time for sub 4 cm lesions is 30 minutes. In a prospective, randomized trial, 310 patients undergoing lumpectomy for a diagnosis of breast cancer were randomized to cryoassisted localization (CAL) or needle-wire localization (NWL) (410). Comparisons between the CAL and NWL groups showed no differences in positive margins (for invasive tumor) (28% vs. 31%, respectively) or in re-excision rates. The volume of tissue removed was significantly less with CAL (49 mL) compared to NWL (66 mL, $p = 0.002$). Of note, there was a trend for a higher positive margin rate for *in situ* disease with CAL (30%) versus NWL (18%, $p = 0.052$). The American College of Surgeons Oncology Group is preparing a study evaluating the sensitivity of MRI to detect residual disease after a course of therapeutic cryoablation for infiltrating ductal carcinomas less than 1.5 cm. As we have abandoned axillary dissection for sentinel nodes, so we may in a select group of patients abandon wide local excision for *in situ* ablation.

Medical Therapy: Redefining Standard of Care and Incorporating New Technology

Currently there is no one standard of care in the treatment of breast cancer. Multiple options exist at every stage along the continuum of care for the breast cancer patient. However, ongoing clinical trials will help define appropriate therapies for our patients. The NSABP B-38 trial is a node-positive randomized trial directly comparing dose-dense AC/T to the TAC regimen given every 3 weeks, and compares them to a novel regimen of dose-dense AC followed by paclitaxel and gemcitabine. This trial will help to establish the standard of care in this population. For women with node-negative disease, there is the NSABP B-36 trial, which randomizes women to four cycles of AC versus six cycles of 5-FU, cyclophosphamide, and the novel anthracycline, epirubicin (FEC). Other trials continue to explore drug sequence, such as the Hellenic Oncology Research group trial of epirubicin and docetaxel, as combination or sequential therapy. The NSABP B-42 trial will address the question of extended endocrine therapy by randomizing women completing 5 years of endocrine therapy (in at least 2 of which they must have used an aromatase inhibitor) to letrozole or placebo.

Novel regimens also continue to be explored. In the BCIRG-006 trial, women with HER2/neu-positive breast cancers are being randomized to anthracycline-containing and non-anthracycline–containing regimens. In arm I patients receive AC followed by docetaxel; in arm 2, patients will receive AC followed by docetaxel and trastuzumab followed by 1 year of consolidation trastuzumab; and arm 3 patients receive a platinum (carboplatin or cisplatin) and docetaxel followed by trastuzumab consolidation. Along with evaluation of survival endpoints, this novel trial will also explore the comparative toxicity (including cardiotoxicity) of these regimens.

PACCT-1 is the first trial from the NCI Program for the Assessment of Clinical Cancer Tests. It is also known as the TAILOR-Rx trial. Women with node-negative hormone-positive breast cancers will undergo an Oncotype DX test for treatment stratification. Patients who have a low recurrence score will undergo endocrine therapy, while those with a high recurrence score will undergo chemotherapy. Those with an indeterminate recurrence score (RS 11-25) will be the subjects for randomization to chemotherapy or endocrine therapy. This trial will be the pivotal validation study for the Oncotype DX assay and, if positive, will likely lead to its more widespread use in tailoring cancer therapy in this population.

The role of biologics will also be further examined. Most notable in this area will be the role of bevacizumab in the treatment of breast cancer. Contemporary trials are already under way incorporating this agent in the neoadjuvant, adjuvant, and recurrent disease setting. Already, important trials have been reported on the use of bevacizumab in metastatic breast cancer. One trial compared capecitabine with or without bevacizumab as a second-line therapy for metastatic disease (411). Four hundred sixty-two women were enrolled in this trial with a study endpoint of prolongation of progression-free survival. While the addition of bevacizumab improved response rates (20% with combination vs. 9% with capecitabine alone, $p = 0.001$), there was no difference in either progression-free or overall survival seen. However, in a first-line metastatic disease study, the combination of bevacizumab and paclitaxel was associated with an increased response rate (30% vs. 14%, $p < 0.0001$) over paclitaxel alone, and in improved progression-free survival (HR 0.48; 95% CI, 0.387 to 0.594) (412).

The incorporation of new technology will continue to be a challenge. An example is the use of a recently developed assay to detect circulating tumor cells (CTCs) in the plasma of breast cancer patients. In the seminal paper published in the *New England Journal of Medicine,* Cristofanilli et al. demonstrated that the number of CTCs at baseline and then at first follow-up were independent predictors of both progression-free (PFS) and overall survival (OS) in women with breast cancer (413). At baseline, CTCs of five or more were associated with a shorter median PFS (2 vs. 7 months, $p < 0.001$) and median OS (10 vs. >18 months, $p < 0.001$). At first follow-up, similar findings emerged. Since then, Budd et al. showed that enumerating CTCs was an earlier indication of disease status than radiologic imaging (414). In that trial, 138 patients on a new treatment regimen underwent pretreatment and repeat imaging (at a median of 10 weeks). CTC counts were also determined at 4 weeks following treatment initiation. He showed that among patients who did not demonstrate radiologic evidence of progression, a CTC of five or more was associated with a median overall survival of 15 months, which was significantly shorter than for those with a CTC of less than five who had a median OS of 27 months ($p = 0.04$). The exact role of this assay in the clinic and its use in determining future treatment plans remain an area of active investigation.

Finally, we continue to explore the role of ovarian suppression or ablation in the treatment of breast cancer. Two studies currently ongoing include the SOFT (Suppression of Ovarian Function) trial (BIG 2-02) and the TEXT (Tamoxifen and Exemestane trial). In the SOFT trial, premenopausal women who are ER and/or PR positive will undergo ovarian suppression medically (using triptorelin), surgically, or by way of ovarian radiation therapy. Subsequently, they will be randomized to tamoxifen or exemestane for 5 years. In the TEXT trial, premenopausal patients will be randomized to a combination of triptorelin and exemestane or tamoxifen alone. In both trials, patients may have undergone chemotherapy, but must continue to menstruate to meet eligibility. These results are eagerly awaited.

Evolving Techniques in Radiation Therapy

Accelerated Partial Breast Irradiation

Accelerated partial breast irradiation (APBI) generally entails 5 days of treatment twice a day, and is quickly becoming a treatment of choice for many patients and physicians. Unlike traditional whole breast radiation, this method of radiation treats only the part of the breast where the tumor was located. This localized treatment can be theoretically validated by many pathologic and clinical studies which demonstrate that the majority of local recurrences in breast cancer are located in the same quadrant as the original cancer (415,416). Patients

TABLE 29.10

SELECTION CRITERIA FOR ACCELERATED PARTIAL BREAST IRRADIATION

Criteria	ABS	ASBS
Age	=45	=45
Histology	IDC	IDC or DCIS
Size	=3 cm	=3 cm
Margin	Negative	Negative microscopic margin
Axillary node status	Negative	Negative

Note: ABS, American Brachytherapy Society; ASBS American Society of Breast Surgeons; DCIS, ductal carcinoma *in situ;* IDC, invasive ductal carcinoma.

at a higher risk of recurrence, including recurrences away from the original tumor, should not be considered candidates for APBI. However, there is no consensus about who belongs to this group. The American Brachytherapy Society and the American Society of Breast Surgeons have established separate, but similar, criteria for administering APBI (Table 29.10) (417).

There have been no completed phase 3 trials comparing recent methods of APBI to conventional whole breast radiation. However, institutional and phase 2 multicenter trials investigating APBI have shown excellent local control rates with low morbidity (418,419). The largest study compared women who had APBI to equally matched, low-risk women who received whole breast radiation, and APBI was associated with similar local recurrence rates. However, the trial suffers from limited follow-up and inclusion of highly selected patients (420). Currently, there are four principal methods of administering APBI: (a) multicatheter interstitial brachytherapy (interstitial), (b) balloon-based brachytherapy, (c) external beam three-dimensional conformal radiotherapy (3D-CRT), and (d) intraoperative radiotherapy (IORT).

Interstitial Brachytherapy

Interstitial brachytherapy, the oldest APBI technique, involves placing catheters surrounding the lumpectomy or seroma cavity. Generally, the catheters will be placed postoperatively 1.0 to 1.5 cm apart, extending 1.5 to 2.0 cm beyond the lumpectomy cavity. A typical implant will require between 14 and 20 catheters. Most commonly, high-dose-rate (HDR) is used with a total of 34 Gy given in ten fractions over 5 days. Although this form of APBI requires the highest level of skill, it is the most adaptable and flexible technique. Any lumpectomy cavity, regardless of size, shape, or location, can be assessed. Because it is the oldest technique, it has the most mature data (316,421). RTOG 95-17 enrolled 99 patients between 1997 and 2000 (316). The selection criteria was very broad, excluding greater than three involved lymph nodes, greater than 3 cm tumors, positive margins, DCIS, and invasive lobular carcinoma. At 3.7 years of median follow-up, the ipsilateral breast tumor recurrence rate (IBTRR) was 3%. Grade 3 or 4 toxicity was seen in 4% of the patients.

Intracavitary Balloon-Based Brachytherapy

Intracavitary balloon-based brachytherapy uses a balloon with a central catheter where an HDR source dwells. The balloon comes in different sizes and shapes to accommodate various lumpectomy cavities. The insertion of the balloon into the lumpectomy cavity is most often done after surgery, when final pathology has been performed. An imaging device, usually either ultrasound or CT, is utilized in the placement of the balloon. Generally, the physician prescribes 3.4 Gy per fraction to 1 cm away from the center of the balloon. The total dose is 34 Gy in ten fractions over 5 days. In contrast to the multicatheter method of APBI, the MammoSite is very easy to use. Neither the insertion nor the dosimetry requires as much skill or experience, hence its popularity. However, the ability to use the MammoSite is highly dependent upon the geometry and location of the lumpectomy cavity. The radiation oncologist must work closely with the surgeon to ensure that the cavity conforms to the balloon surface while maximizing the balloon-to-skin distance. Often the surgeon must close the cavity subcutaneously to improve the depth to the balloon surface. The balloon occasionally ruptures, requiring replacement of the balloon, reimaging, and replanning. Several acute side effects are common with the MammoSite including erythema, hyperpigmentation of the skin overlying the implant, seroma formation, and breast tenderness. Other, less common side effects include moist desquamation, delayed healing, and infection. Chronic toxicity includes fat necrosis, skin atrophy, telangiectasia, and fibrosis. Intracavitary ballon therapy is fairly new; therefore, long-term data are limited. The longest follow-up is 48 months, in which there have been no local failures and good/excellent cosmesis in 82.5% of the patients (422).

Three-Dimensional Conformal Radiation

3D-CRT is a newer technique in which multiple external radiation beams are used to treat the lumpectomy cavity with a margin. The lumpectomy cavity is identified by surgical clips at the time of the CT planning session. The clinical target volume is expanded 5 mm to include movement secondary to normal breathing and 10 mm for random and systematic components of setup error (423). The planning tumor volume (PTV) excludes the chest wall and 5 mm of skin. Patients are treated with 3.85 Gy per fraction for a total of 38.5 Gy in ten fractions over 5 days. This technique has become very popular primarily because it does not involve a surgical procedure or special equipment. Additionally, it has more homogeneity of dose than the brachytherapy options. The primary disadvantage is that larger volumes of normal breast tissue are irradiated, restricting the number of candidates for this treatment. It is recommended that 50% of the ipsilateral breast volume receive <50% of the prescribed dose. The heart and lung volumes must be below those for whole breast tangents. Additionally, the patient's setup must be reproducible. There are no studies with long-term follow-up using modern fractionation and techniques. However, a William Beaumont retrospective study with 10 months median follow-up reported 61% of patients with grade 1 toxicity, 10% with grade 2, and 0% with grade 3 toxicity. The cosmetic results were rated as good/excellent in all patients (420).

Intraoperative Accelerated Partial Breast Irradiation

IORT is utilized in a limited number of institutions that have an adequate knowledge base, technology, and facilities. Currently, there are three main devices available for IORT. The intrabeam uses soft x-rays at 50 kv, while the Mobitron and Novac7 use electrons at 4 to 12 MeV. The intrabeam machine delivers a dose of 20 to 22 Gy to the tumor bed and about 5 to 7 Gy 1 cm from the tumor bed. An applicator of varying sizes is placed in the tumor bed and, if necessary, the chest wall and skin can be protected by a tungsten-filled material. The advantage of the IORT is one of convenience to the patient, who completes all local treatment at one time. Early and late side effects are minimal secondary to the small volume of tissue irradiation. Unfortunately, long-term data are lacking on the safety and effectiveness of using IORT as the sole method of radiation treatment.

SUMMARY OF CONTEMPORARY CLINICAL TRIALS

Surgical

NSABP B-32

NSABP B-32 (165) examined whether sentinel node biopsy was equivalent to axillary dissection but with less toxicity among women with a clinically node-negative breast cancer. This trial enrolled 5,611 women who were randomly assigned to sentinel node biopsy followed by full axillary dissection (group 1) or sentinel node biopsy alone (group 2), provided it was negative. All women with a positive sentinel node biopsy underwent an axillary dissection in this trial. Among group 1, the overall accuracy of sentinel node biopsy was 97% with a false-negative rate of 9.8%. Allergic reactions to blue dye were seen in less than 1% of patients.

CALGB 9343/RTOG 9702

The CALGB trial (281) was opened to women over the age of 70 with early estrogen receptor–positive breast cancer (T1N0) treated by lumpectomy. It enrolled 636 women who were randomized to tamoxifen with or without adjuvant breast radiotherapy. The primary endpoints were time to local, regional, or distant recurrence, breast cancer–specific and overall survival. After 5 years of follow-up, overall survival was 87% with radiotherapy compared to 86% in those who did not undergo radiation ($p = 0.94$). The incidence of local failure was 1% versus 5%, respectively. Both groups experienced a 2% incidence of breast cancer–specific mortality. These data support the treatment of women over 70 without adjuvant radiation therapy, provided they are candidates for endocrine treatment following surgery.

Prevention

NSABP P-2 (STAR Trial): Study of Tamoxifen and Raloxifine

This was a prospective randomized double-blind trial comparing raloxifine 60 mg/day to tamoxifen 20 mg/day as primary prevention of invasive breast cancer (166). Eligible patients were 35 and over and in general good health. Postmenopausal women with a be at high risk for breast cancer based on the Gail model risk score. Patients with ALH or ADH were eligible, but those with DCIS were excluded. This trial enrolled 19,747 postmenopausal women with a mean risk of 4.03% based on the Gail model. There was no difference in diagnoses of invasive breast cancer with raloxifine or tamoxifen (relative risk [RR], 1.02; 95% CI, 0.82 to 1.28), but there was an increase in the diagnosis of noninvasive breast cancers with raloxifine compared with tamoxifen (RR 1.40; 95% CI, 0.98 to 2.00). Uterine cancer was less frequently diagnosed with raloxifine (RR 0.62; 95% CI, 0.35 to 1.08).

Early Breast Cancer

ATAC: Anastrozole Versus Tamoxifen, Alone or in Combination

This was a trial involving 6,241 postmenopausal women with early invasive breast cancer who were randomized to anastrozole 1 mg daily versus tamoxifen 20 mg daily versus anastrozole and tamoxifen (264). Anastrozole was shown to improve disease-free survival compared to tamoxifen (HR 0.87; 95% CI, 0.78 to 0.97), as well as time to recurrence (HR 0.79; 95% CI, 0.70 to 0.90) and time to distant disease (HR 0.86; 95% CI, 0.74 to 0.99). Five-year overall survival was similar between the two arms (84.3% with anastrozole vs. 83.8% with tamoxifen, $p = 0.7$). Comparing anastrozole to tamoxifen, anastrozole was associated with an increased risk of bone fractures (11% vs. 7.7%, $p < 0.0001$) and musculoskeletal complaints (35.6% vs. 29.4%, $p < 0.0001$). However, anastrozole had a lower incidence of hot flashes (35.7% vs. 40.9%, $p < 0.0001$), vaginal bleeding (5.4% vs. 10.2%, $p < 0.0001$), thromboembolic events (2.8% vs. 4.5%, $p = 0.0006$), and ischemic cerebrovascular events (2.0% vs. 2.8%, $p = 0.0006$). The incidence of uterine cancer was 0.2% with anastrozole, compared to 0.8% with tamoxifen ($p = 0.02$).

BIG 1-98: Breast International Group 1-98 Study

This was a four-arm trial involving 8,028 postmenopausal women with hormone receptor–positive early breast cancer (268). Arms in this trial were letrozole 2.5 mg daily versus tamoxifen 20 mg daily versus letrozole followed by tamoxifen versus tamoxifen followed by letrozole, with each arm treated for 5 years. To date, data involving the 4,922 women randomized to letrozole or tamoxifen have been reported. At 51 months, letrozole is associated with improvement in disease-free survival over tamoxifen (HR 0.82; 95% CI, 0.71 to 0.95) but there is no difference in overall survival noted (HR 0.91; 95% CI, 0.75 to 1.11).

MA-17

This trial enrolled 5,187 postmenopausal women who had completed 5 years of tamoxifen and randomized them to placebo or letrozole 2.5 mg daily (424). At 4 years, disease-free survival was 94.4% in those receiving letrozole and 89.8% in those receiving placebo ($p < 0.001$). Overall survival was similar (95.4% vs. 95%, respectively).

IES: Intergroup Exemestane Study

This was a randomized trial whereby 4,742 women completing 2 to 3 years of adjuvant tamoxifen therapy were randomized to tamoxifen or exemestane 25 mg daily to complete 5 years of total treatment (265). At 2.5 years, disease-free survival favored switching to exemestane over continuing on tamoxifen (HR 0.76; 95% CI, 0.66 to 0.88). At the time of report, there was no difference in overall survival was seen.

ARNO-95

In this trial 3,200 postmenopausal women on tamoxifen for 2 years were randomized to continuation of tamoxifen or switching to anastrozole for 3 years (275). Disease-free survival was prolonged with a switch to anastrozole (HR 0.66; 95% CI, 0.44 to 1.00). Unlike other trials, however, this showed that sequencing treatment from tamoxifen to anastrozole was also associated with a significant improvement in overall survival (HR 0.53; 95% CI, 0.28 to 0.99).

BCIRG 001

This trial enrolled 1,491 women with invasive breast cancer with axillary node involvement to docetaxel 75 mg/m^2, doxorubicin 50 mg/m^2, and cyclophosphamide 500 mg/m^2 (TAC) or 5-fluorouracil 500 mg/m^2, doxorubicin 50 mg/m^2, and cyclophosphamide 500 mg/m^2 (FAC) (237). All patients received six cycles of chemotherapy at 3-week intervals. At 55 months median follow-up, 5-year disease-free survival was 75% versus

68%, respectively ($p = 0.001$); 5-year overall survival was 87% versus 81%, respectively ($p = 0.008$). TAC was associated with increased grade 3/4 neutropenia (65.5% vs. 49.3%, respectively; $p < 0.001$), febrile neutropenia (24.7% vs. 2.5%, respectively; $p < 0.001$), and grade 3/4 anemia (4.3% vs. 1.6%, respectively; $p < 0.001$).

CALGB 9741

This adjuvant chemotherapy trial evaluated the frequency and sequencing of doxorubicin 60 mg/m^2 (A), cyclophosphamide 600 mg/m^2 (C), and paclitaxel 175 mg/m^2 (T) over 3 hours in a 2 × 2 factorial design (236). Patients were randomized to either every-2-week (dose-dense) or every-3-week treatment and to treatment using AC followed by T or to A then C then T. Women randomized to dose-dense treatment were also given prophylactic G-CSF. Results showed that dose-dense therapy significantly improved disease-free (risk ratio [RR] 0.74, $p = 0.01$) and overall survival (RR 0.69, $p = 0.013$). At 4 years, dose-dense therapy was associated with an 82% survival, compared to 75% if treatment was administered every 3 weeks. No differences were observed in the sequence of treatment used.

NSABP B-31/NCCTG 98311

These two trials explored the role of adjuvant trastuzumab in combination with chemotherapy in women with high-risk node-negative (defined as tumor >1 cm if ER negative or tumor >2 cm if ER positive) or node-positive HER2/neu-positive breast cancer (245). The NSABP B-31 tested doxorubicin and cylophosphamide followed by paclitaxel (AC/T) every 3 weeks versus the same followed by 52 weeks of trastuzumab initiated with the first dose of paclitaxel. The NCCTG trial compared three arms consisting of AC followed by 12 weeks of paclitaxel versus AC/weekly paclitaxel and 52 weeks of trastuzumab (to start with paclitaxel) versus AC/weekly paclitaxel followed by 52 weeks of trastuzumab. In the combined analysis, adjuvant trastuzumab improved disease-free (HR 0.48, $p < 0.0001$) and overall survival (HR 0.67, $p = 0.015$).

Locally Advanced Breast Cancer

NSABP B-18

NSABP B-18 was a neoadjuvant trial that enrolled 1,523 women with T1-3, N0M0 invasive breast cancers (249). Patients were randomized to preoperative AC versus postoperative AC. The rate of breast conservation was 67% versus 60%, respectively. The pathologic complete response (pCR) rate to preoperative AC was 13%. At 9 years of follow-up, survival is 69% and 70%, respectively ($p = 0.80$). Disease-free survival is 55% and 53%, respectively ($p = 0.50$). The rate of in-breast tumor recurrence was 10.7% versus 7.6% (not significant).

NSABP B-27

NSABP B-27 evaluated the role of docetaxel in patients with operable breast cancer (425). In this trial 2,411 women were randomized to preoperative AC versus preoperative AC/docetaxel versus preoperative AC followed by postoperative docetaxel. The pCR in those receiving AC was 13.7%; in those receiving preoperative docetaxel it was 26.1%, $p < 0.001$. However, the frequency of breast conservation was similar between those receiving AC (61%) and AC/docetaxel (63%) as preoperative treatment ($p = 0.70$). The addition of docetaxel did not improve overall survival.

Aberdeen Tax-301

The Tax-301 trial was designed with two phases of treatment and 145 patients completed the planned eight cycles of treatment (426). In the first phase, patients with locally advanced breast cancer received a combination of cyclophosphamide, vincristine, doxorubicin, and prednisolone (CVAP). Following four cycles patients underwent clinical re-evaluation for response. In the second stage, responding patients were randomized to four cycles of docetaxel or continued with CVAP. In those not responding, treatment was switched to docetaxel for four cycles. The pCR rate was 31% in those receiving docetaxel and 15% in those completing treatment with CVAP ($p = 0.06$). Of note, the pCR rate on docetaxel in patients who did not respond to the initial treatment of CVAP was only 2%. At surgery, the rate of breast conservation was significantly higher in those women who sequenced to docetaxel (67%) as opposed to continuing with CVAP (48%), $p < 0.01$. Additionally, at 5 years of follow-up, overall survival was 97% in patients who received docetaxel, compared to 78% of those who had completed eight cycles of CVAP.

SUMMARY

The field of breast oncology has evolved significantly, with gains made in prevention, screening, diagnosis, and management. All of this has led to a reduction in the mortality rate from breast cancer with a resultant increase in the population who are considered breast cancer survivors. Despite this, multiple questions remain: How should new radiologic technologies, such as tomosynthesis, be incorporated into routine screening practice? Should breast MRI utilization be expanded to all women with a new diagnosis of breast cancer? How can we maximize the use of neoadjuvant chemotherapy in women with invasive disease? How should we treat patients who have persistent disease following primary chemotherapy? Is partial breast radiation as safe as whole breast radiation? These are only a few of the issues that oncology will need to address as we look forward into the future.

Unlike the gynecologic malignancies, there is no one standard of care in the management of the patient with breast cancer. The indications for the use of chemotherapy continue to evolve as evidence mounts that women with breast cancer cannot be considered one and the same. Hormone receptor status can predict who will benefit from endocrine therapy, and appears to also predict who has little to gain from chemotherapy. Our current understanding of the treatment landscape in breast cancer has reinforced one point, that treatment must be individualized, especially since multiple options are considered reasonable. The evolution of breast cancer management will undoubtedly continue as reasearchers seek to define more targets for treatment and refine the appropriate therapies for the patient with breast cancer, tailored to hormone and HER2/neu status. Utilization of new technologies for treatment and follow-up will be better characterized, such as the use of accelerated partial breast irradiation or the use of circulating tumor cells. Hopefully, we will continue to improve the outcomes for our patients with breast cancer, and increase the chances more women will be cured.

References

1. American Cancer Society. *Cancer Facts & Figures 2007*. Atlanta: American Cancer Society, Inc.; 2007.
2. Chlebowski RT, Hendrix SL, Langer RD, et al. Influence of estrogen plus progestin on breast cancer and mammography in healthy postmenopausal women: the Women's Health Initiative Randomized Trial. *JAMA* 2003;289(24):3243–3253.

3. Stefanick ML, Anderson GL, Margolis KL, et al. Effects of conjugated equine estrogens on breast cancer and mammography screening in postmenopausal women with hysterectomy. *JAMA* 2006;295(14):1647–1657.
4. Marchbanks PA, McDonald JA, Wilson HG, et al. Oral contraceptives and the risk of breast cancer. *N Engl J Med* 2002;346(26):2025–2032.
5. Gail MH, Brinton LA, Byar DP, et al. Projecting individualized probabilities of developing breast cancer for white females who are being examined annually. *J Natl Cancer Inst* 1989;81(24):1879–1886.
6. Claus EB, Risch N, Thompson WD. Autosomal dominant inheritance of early-onset breast cancer. Implications for risk prediction. *Cancer* 1994;73(3):643–651.
7. Miki Y, Swensen J, Shattuck-Eidens D, et al. A strong candidate for the breast and ovarian cancer susceptibility gene *BRCA1*. *Science* 1994;266 (5182):66–71.
8. Wooster R, Neuhausen SL, Mangion J, et al. Localization of a breast cancer susceptibility gene, *BRCA2*, to chromosome 13q12-13. *Science* 1994;265(5181):2088–2090.
9. Tokunaga M, Land CE, Yamamoto T, et al. Incidence of female breast cancer among atomic bomb survivors, Hiroshima and Nagasaki, 1950-1980. *Radiat Res* 1987;112(2):243–272.
10. Aisenberg AC, Finkelstein DM, Doppke KP, et al. High risk of breast carcinoma after irradiation of young women with Hodgkin's disease. *Cancer* 1997;79(6):1203–1210.
11. Michels KB, Mohllajee AP, Roset-Bahmanyar E, et al. Diet and breast cancer: a review of the prospective observational studies. *Cancer* 2007;109(12 Suppl): 2712–2749.
12. Hartmann LC, Sellers TA, Frost MH, et al. Benign breast disease and the risk of breast cancer. *N Engl J Med* 2005;353(3):229–237.
13. Worsham MJ, Abrams J, Raju U, et al. Breast cancer incidence in a cohort of women with benign breast disease from a multiethnic, primary health care population. *Breast J* 2007;13(2):115–121.
14. Boyd NF, Guo H, Martin LJ, et al. Mammographic density and the risk and detection of breast cancer. *N Engl J Med* 2007;356(3):227–236.
15. Wellings SR, Jensen HM, Marcum RG. An atlas of subgross pathology of the human breast with special reference to possible precancerous lesions. *J Natl Cancer Inst* 1975;55(2):231–273.
16. Faverly DR, Burgers L, Bult P, et al. Three dimensional imaging of mammary ductal carcinoma *in situ*: clinical implications. *Semin Diagn Pathol* 1994;11(3):193–198.
17. Gaffney DK, Tsodikov A, Wiggins CL. Diminished survival in patients with inner versus outer quadrant breast cancers. *J Clin Oncol* 2003;21(3): 467–472.
18. Tulinius H, Sigvaldason H, Olafsdottir G. Left and right sided breast cancer. *Pathol Res Pract* 1990;186(1):92–94.
19. Lee YT. Breast carcinoma: pattern of metastasis at autopsy. *J Surg Oncol* 1983;23(3):175–180.
20. Bloom HJ. The natural history of untreated breast cancer *Ann NY Acad Sci* 1964;114:747–754.
21. Valagussa P, Bonadonna G, Veronesi U. Patterns of relapse and survival in operable breast carcinoma with positive and negative axillary nodes. *Tumori* 1978;64(3):241–258.
22. Fisher B. Laboratory and clinical research in breast cancer—a personal adventure: the David A. Karnofsky memorial lecture. *Cancer Res* 1980;40(11):3863–3874.
23. Early Breast Cancer Trialists' Collaborative Group. Favourable and unfavourable effects on long-term survival of radiotherapy for early breast cancer: an overview of the randomised trials. *Lancet* 2000;355(9217): 1757–1770.
24. Hellman S. Karnofsky Memorial Lecture. Natural history of small breast cancers. *J Clin Oncol* 1994;12(10):2229–2234.
25. Perry S. Recommendations of the Consensus Development Panel on breast cancer screening. *Cancer Res* 1978;38(2):476–477.
26. Hendrick RE, Smith RA, Rutledge JH 3rd, et al. Benefit of screening mammography in women aged 40–49: a new meta-analysis of randomized controlled trials. *J Natl Cancer Inst Monogr* 1997(22):87–92.
27. Nystrom L, Rutqvist LE, Wall S, et al. Breast cancer screening with mammography: overview of Swedish randomised trials. *Lancet* 17 1993; 341(8851):973–978.
28. Duffy SW, Tabar L, Chen HH, et al. The impact of organized mammography service screening on breast carcinoma mortality in seven Swedish counties. *Cancer* 2002;95(3):458–469.
29. Smith RA, Saslow D, Sawyer KA, et al. American Cancer Society guidelines for breast cancer screening: update 2003. *CA Cancer J Clin* 2003;53(3): 141–169.
30. Rosenquist CJ, Lindfors KK. Screening mammography beginning at age 40 years: a reappraisal of cost-effectiveness. *Cancer* 1998;82(11): 2235–2240.
31. Hollingsworth AB, Taylor LD, Rhodes DC. Establishing a histologic basis for false-negative mammograms. *Am J Surg* 1993;166(6):643–647; discussion 647–648.
32. Burrell HC, Sibbering DM, Wilson AR, et al. Screening interval breast cancers: mammographic features and prognosis factors. *Radiology* 1996;199(3):811–817.
33. Laya MB, Larson EB, Taplin SH, et al. Effect of estrogen replacement therapy on the specificity and sensitivity of screening mammography. *J Natl Cancer Inst* 1996;88(10):643–649.
34. Congress, U. Mammography Quality Standard Act of 1992. In: Session SN, ed. 1992:102–448.
35. Liberman L, Abramson AF, Squires FB, et al. The breast imaging reporting and data system: positive predictive value of mammographic features and final assessment categories. *AJR Am J Roentgenol* 1998;171(1):35–40.
36. Pisano ED, Yaffe MJ. Digital mammography. *Radiology* 2005;234(2): 353–362.
37. Pisano ED, Yaffe MJ, Hemminger BM, et al. Current status of full-field digital mammography. *Acad Radiol* 2000;7(4):266–280.
38. Pisano ED, Gatsonis C, Hendrick E, et al. Diagnostic performance of digital versus film mammography for breast-cancer screening. *N Engl J Med* 27 2005;353(17):1773–1783.
39. Skaane P, Young K, Skjennald A. Population-based mammography screening: comparison of screen-film and full-field digital mammography with soft-copy reading—Oslo I study. *Radiology* 2003;229(3):877–884.
40. Lewin JM, Hendrick RE, D'Orsi CJ, et al. Comparison of full-field digital mammography with screen-film mammography for cancer detection: results of 4,945 paired examinations. *Radiology* 2001;218(3):873–880.
41. Lewin JM, D'Orsi CJ, Hendrick RE, et al. Clinical comparison of full-field digital mammography and screen-film mammography for detection of breast cancer. *AJR Am J Roentgenol* 2002;179(3):671–677.
42. Cole E, Pisano ED, Brown M, et al. Diagnostic accuracy of Fischer Senoscan Digital Mammography versus screen-film mammography in a diagnostic mammography population. *Acad Radiol* 2004;11(8): 879–886.
43. Hendrick RE, Lewin JM, D'Orsi CJ, et al. Non-inferiority study of FFDM in an enriched diagnostic cohort: comparison with screen-film mammography in 625 women. In: Yaffe MJ, ed. *IWDM 2000: 5th International Workshop on Digital Mammography*. Madison, WI: Medical Physics; 2001:475–481.
44. Kerlikowske K, Grady D, Barclay J, et al. Effect of age, breast density, and family history on the sensitivity of first screening mammography. *JAMA* 1996;276(1):33–38.
45. Boyd NF, Dite GS, Stone J, et al. Heritability of mammographic density, a risk factor for breast cancer. *N Engl J Med* 2002;347(12):886–894.
46. Byrne C, Schairer C, Wolfe J, et al. Mammographic features and breast cancer risk: effects with time, age, and menopause status. *J Natl Cancer Inst* 1995;87(21):1622–1629.
47. Carney PA, Miglioretti DL, Yankaskas BC, et al. Individual and combined effects of age, breast density, and hormone replacement therapy use on the accuracy of screening mammography. *Ann Intern Med* 2003;138(3): 168–175.
48. Wolfe JN. Risk for breast cancer development determined by mammographic parenchymal pattern. *Cancer* 1976;37(5):2486–2492.
49. Cupples TE, Cunningham JE, Reynolds JC. Impact of computer-aided detection in a regional screening mammography program. *AJR Am J Roentgenol* 2005;185(4):944–950.
50. Morton MJ, Whaley DH, Brandt KR, et al. Screening mammograms: interpretation with computer-aided detection—prospective evaluation. *Radiology* 2006;239(2):375–383.
51. Birdwell RL, Bandodkar P, Ikeda DM. Computer-aided detection with screening mammography in a university hospital setting. *Radiology* 2005;236(2):451–457.
52. Freer TW, Ulissey MJ. Screening mammography with computer-aided detection: prospective study of 12,860 patients in a community breast center. *Radiology* 2001;220(3):781–786.
53. Birdwell RL, Ikeda DM, O'Shaughnessy KF, et al. Mammographic characteristics of 115 missed cancers later detected with screening mammography and the potential utility of computer-aided detection. *Radiology* 2001;219(1):192–202.
54. Warren Burhenne LJ, Wood SA, D'Orsi CJ, et al. Potential contribution of computer-aided detection to the sensitivity of screening mammography. *Radiology* 2000;215(2):554–562.
55. Brem RF, Baum J, Lechner M, et al. Improvement in sensitivity of screening mammography with computer-aided detection: a multiinstitutional trial. *AJR Am J Roentgenol* 2003;181(3):687–693.
56. Fenton JJ, Taplin SH, Carney PA, et al. Influence of computer-aided detection on performance of screening mammography. *N Engl J Med* 2007; 356(14):1399–1409.
57. Stavros AT, Thickman D, Rapp CL, et al. Solid breast nodules: use of sonography to distinguish between benign and malignant lesions. *Radiology* 1995;196(1):123–134.
58. Kolb TM, Lichy J, Newhouse JH. Comparison of the performance of screening mammography, physical examination, and breast US and evaluation of factors that influence them: an analysis of 27,825 patient evaluations. *Radiology* 2002;225(1):165–175.
59. Buchberger W, DeKoekkoek-Doll P, Springer P, et al. Incidental findings on sonography of the breast: clinical significance and diagnostic workup. *AJR Am J Roentgenol* 1999;173(4):921–927.
60. Kolb TM, Lichy J, Newhouse JH. Occult cancer in women with dense breasts: detection with screening US—diagnostic yield and tumor characteristics. *Radiology* 1998;207(1):191–199.
61. Gordon PB, Goldenberg SL. Malignant breast masses detected only by ultrasound. A retrospective review. *Cancer* 1995;76(4):626–630.
62. Gordon PB. Ultrasound for breast cancer screening and staging. *Radiol Clin North Am* 2002;40(3):431–441.

63. Poplack SP, Tosteson TD, Kogel CA, et al. Digital breast tomosynthesis: initial experience in 98 women with abnormal digital screening mammography. *AJR Am J Roentgenol* 2007;189(3):616–623.
64. Rafferty E, Niklason L, Jameson-Meehan L. Breast tomosynthesis: one view or two? *RSNA 2006*. Chicago, IL; 2006.
65. Kuhl C. The current status of breast MR imaging. Part I. Choice of technique, image interpretation, diagnostic accuracy, and transfer to clinical practice. *Radiology* 2007;244(2):356–378.
66. Heywang SH, Hahn D, Schmidt H, et al. MR imaging of the breast using gadolinium-DTPA. *J Comput Assist Tomogr* 1986;10(2):199–204.
67. Heywang-Kobrunner SH. Contrast-enhanced magnetic resonance imaging of the breast. *Invest Radiol* 1994;29(1):94–104.
68. Liberman L, Morris EA, Lee MJ, et al. Breast lesions detected on MR imaging: features and positive predictive value. *AJR Am J Roentgenol* 2002;179(1):171–178.
69. Brinck U, Fischer U, Korabiowska M, et al. The variability of fibroadenoma in contrast-enhanced dynamic MR mammography. *AJR Am J Roentgenol* 1997;168(5):1331–1334.
70. Orel SG, Schnall MD, LiVolsi VA, et al. Suspicious breast lesions: MR imaging with radiologic-pathologic correlation. *Radiology* 1994;190(2): 485–493.
71. Harms SE, Flamig DP, Hesley KL, et al. MR imaging of the breast with rotating delivery of excitation off resonance: clinical experience with pathologic correlation. *Radiology* 1993;187(2):493–501.
72. Kaiser WA, Zeitler E. MR imaging of the breast: fast imaging sequences with and without Gd-DTPA. Preliminary observations. *Radiology* 1989; 170(3 Pt 1):681–686.
73. Menell JH, Morris EA, Dershaw DD, et al. Determination of the presence and extent of pure ductal carcinoma *in situ* by mammography and magnetic resonance imaging. *Breast J* 2005;11(6):382–390.
74. Berg WA, Gutierrez L, NessAiver MS, et al. Diagnostic accuracy of mammography, clinical examination, US, and MR imaging in preoperative assessment of breast cancer. *Radiology* 2004;233(3):830–849.
75. Hwang ES, Kinkel K, Esserman LJ, et al. Magnetic resonance imaging in patients diagnosed with ductal carcinoma-*in-situ*: value in the diagnosis of residual disease, occult invasion, and multicentricity. *Ann Surg Oncol* 2003;10(4):381–388.
76. Williams TC, DeMartini WB, Partridge SC, et al. Breast MR imaging: computer-aided evaluation program for discriminating benign from malignant lesions. *Radiology* 2007;244(1):94–103.
77. Morris EA, Liberman L, Ballon DJ, et al. MRI of occult breast carcinoma in a high-risk population. *AJR Am J Roentgenol* 2003;181(3):619–626.
78. Liberman L. The high risk woman and magnetic resonance imaging. In: Morris E, Liberman L, eds. *Breast MRI: Diagnosis and Intervention.* New York: Springer; 2005:184–199.
79. Sardanelli F, Podo F, D'Agnolo G, et al. Multicenter comparative multimodality surveillance of women at genetic-familial high risk for breast cancer (HIBCRIT study): interim results. *Radiology* 2007;242(3): 698–715.
80. Saslow D, Boetes C, Burke W, et al. American Cancer Society guidelines for breast screening with MRI as an adjunct to mammography. *CA Cancer J Clin* 2007;57(2):75–89.
81. Lehman CD, Gatsonis C, Kuhl CK, et al. MRI evaluation of the contralateral breast in women with recently diagnosed breast cancer. *N Engl J Med* 2007;356(13):1295–1303.
82. Liberman L, Morris EA, Dershaw DD, et al. MR imaging of the ipsilateral breast in women with percutaneously proven breast cancer. *AJR Am J Roentgenol* 2003;180(4):901–910.
83. Fischer U, Kopka L, Grabbe E. Breast carcinoma: effect of preoperative contrast-enhanced MR imaging on the therapeutic approach. *Radiology* 1999;213(3):881–888.
84. Yeh E, Slanetz P, Kopans DB, et al. Prospective comparison of mammography, sonography, and MRI in patients undergoing neoadjuvant chemotherapy for palpable breast cancer. *AJR Am J Roentgenol* 2005; 184(3):868–877.
85. Parker SH, Burbank F, Jackman RJ, et al. Percutaneous large-core breast biopsy: a multi-institutional study. *Radiology* 1994;193(2):359–364.
86. Krishnamurthy S, Sneige N, Bedi DG, et al. Role of ultrasound-guided fine-needle aspiration of indeterminate and suspicious axillary lymph nodes in the initial staging of breast carcinoma. *Cancer* 2002;95(5): 982–988.
87. Somasundar P, Gass J, Steinhoff M, et al. Role of ultrasound-guided axillary fine-needle aspiration in the management of invasive breast cancer. *Am J Surg* 2006;192(4):458–461.
88. van Rijk MC, Deurloo EE, Nieweg OE, et al. Ultrasonography and fine-needle aspiration cytology can spare breast cancer patients unnecessary sentinel lymph node biopsy. *Ann Surg Oncol* 2006;13(1):31–35.
89. American Joint Committee on Cancer. Breast. In: *AJCC Cancer Staging Manual.* 6th ed. New York, Springer; 2002.
90. Dupont WD, Page DL. Risk factors for breast cancer in women with proliferative breast disease. *N Engl J Med* 17 1985;312(3):146–151.
91. Santen RJ, Mansel R. Benign breast disorders. *N Engl J Med* 2005;353(3): 275–285.
92. Schnitt SJ, Connolly JL, Tavassoli FA, et al. Interobserver reproducibility in the diagnosis of ductal proliferative breast lesions using standardized criteria. *Am J Surg Pathol* 1992;16(12):1133–1143.
93. Margenthaler JA, Duke D, Monsees BS, et al. Correlation between core biopsy and excisional biopsy in breast high-risk lesions. *Am J Surg* 2006;192(4):534–537.
94. Schnitt SJ, Vincent-Salomon A. Columnar cell lesions of the breast. *Adv Anat Pathol* 2003;10(3):113–124.
95. Azzopardi JG. Problems in breast pathology. In: Bennington JL, ed. *Major Problems in Pathology.* Vol 11. London: Saunders; 1979.
96. Fraser JL, Raza S, Chorny K, et al. Columnar alteration with prominent apical snouts and secretions: a spectrum of changes frequently present in breast biopsies performed for microcalcifications. *Am J Surg Pathol* 1998;22(12):1521–1527.
97. Collins LC, Achacoso NA, Nekhlyudov L, et al. Clinical and pathologic features of ductal carcinoma *in situ* associated with the presence of flat epithelial atypia: an analysis of 543 patients. *Mod Pathol* 2007;20(11): 1149–1155.
98. Fernandez-Aguilar S, Simon P, Buxant F, et al. Tubular carcinoma of the breast and associated intra-epithelial lesions: a comparative study with invasive low-grade ductal carcinomas. *Virchows Arch* 2005;447(4):683–687.
99. Abdel-Fatah TM, Powe DG, Hodi Z, et al. High frequency of coexistence of columnar cell lesions, lobular neoplasia, and low grade ductal carcinoma *in situ* with invasive tubular carcinoma and invasive lobular carcinoma. *Am J Surg Pathol* 2007;31(3):417–426.
100. Page DL, Dupont WD, Rogers LW, et al. Continued local recurrence of carcinoma 15-25 years after a diagnosis of low grade ductal carcinoma *in situ* of the breast treated only by biopsy. *Cancer* 1995;76(7): 1197–1200.
101. Rosai J. Breast: *in situ* carcinoma. In: Rosai J, ed. *Ackerman's Surgical Pathology, 9th edition.* Vol 2. St. Louis: Mosby; 2004.
102. Holland R, Connolly JL, Gelman R, et al. The presence of an extensive intraductal component following a limited excision correlates with prominent residual disease in the remainder of the breast. *J Clin Oncol* 1990;8:113–118.
103. Wells WA, Carney PA, Eliassen MS, et al. Pathologists' agreement with experts and reproducibility of breast ductal carcinoma-in-situ classification schemes. *Am J Surg Pathol* 2000;24(5):651–659.
104. de Mascarel I, MacGrogan G, Mathoulin-Pelissier S, et al. Breast ductal carcinoma *in situ* with microinvasion: a definition supported by a long-term study of 1248 serially sectioned ductal carcinomas. *Cancer* 15 2002;94(8): 2134–2142.
105. Silverstein MJ, Waisman JR, Gamagami P, et al. Intraductal carcinoma of the breast (208 cases). Clinical factors influencing treatment choice. *Cancer* 1990;66(1):102–108.
106. Frykberg ER. Lobular carcinoma *in situ* of the breast. *Breast J* 1999;5(5): 296–303.
107. Fisher ER, Land SR, Fisher B, et al. Pathologic findings from the National Surgical Adjuvant Breast and Bowel Project: twelve-year observations concerning lobular carcinoma *in situ. Cancer* 15 2004;100(2):238–244.
108. Li CI, Malone KE, Saltzman BS, et al. Risk of invasive breast carcinoma among women diagnosed with ductal carcinoma *in situ* and lobular carcinoma *in situ,* 1988–2001. *Cancer* 15 2006;106(10):2104–2112.
109. Hutter RV. The management of patients with lobular carcinoma *in situ* of the breast. *Cancer* 1984;53(3 Suppl):798–802.
110. Arpino G, Allred DC, Mohsin SK, et al. Lobular neoplasia on core-needle biopsy—clinical significance. *Cancer* 2004;101(2):242–250.
111. Elsheikh TM, Silverman JF. Follow-up surgical excision is indicated when breast core needle biopsies show atypical lobular hyperplasia or lobular carcinoma *in situ:* a correlative study of 33 patients with review of the literature. *Am J Surg Pathol* 2005;29(4):534–543.
112. Simpson PT, Gale T, Fulford LG, et al. The diagnosis and management of pre-invasive breast disease: pathology of atypical lobular hyperplasia and lobular carcinoma *in situ. Breast Cancer Res* 2003;5(5):258–262.
113. Elston CW, Ellis IO. Pathological prognostic factors in breast cancer. I. The value of histological grade in breast cancer: experience from a large study with long-term follow-up. *Histopathology* 1991;19(5):403–410.
114. Bane AL, Tjan S, Parkes RK, et al. Invasive lobular carcinoma: to grade or not to grade. *Mod Pathol* 2005;18(5):621–628.
115. Diab SG, Clark GM, Osborne CK, et al. Tumor characteristics and clinical outcome of tubular and mucinous breast carcinomas. *J Clin Oncol* 1999; 17(5):1442–1448.
116. Goldstein NS, Kestin LL, Vicini FA. Refined morphologic criteria for tubular carcinoma to retain its favorable outcome status in contemporary breast carcinoma patients. *Am J Clin Pathol* 2004;122(5):728–739.
117. Walsh MM, Bleiweiss IJ. Invasive micropapillary carcinoma of the breast: eighty cases of an underrecognized entity. *Hum Pathol* 2001;32(6):583–589.
118. Pettinato G, Manivel CJ, Panico L, et al. Invasive micropapillary carcinoma of the breast: clinicopathologic study of 62 cases of a poorly recognized variant with highly aggressive behavior. *Am J Clin Pathol* 2004; 121(6):857–866.
119. Collins LC, Carlo VP, Hwang H, et al. Intracystic papillary carcinomas of the breast: a reevaluation using a panel of myoepithelial cell markers. *Am J Surg Pathol* 2006;30(8):1002–1007.
120. Solorzano CC, Middleton LP, Hunt KK, et al. Treatment and outcome of patients with intracystic papillary carcinoma of the breast. *Am J Surg* 2002;184(4):364–368.
121. Moatamed NA, Apple SK. Extensive sampling changes T-staging of infiltrating lobular carcinoma of breast: a comparative study of gross versus microscopic tumor sizes. *Breast J* 2006;12(6):511–517.

122. Wheeler DT, Tai LH, Bratthauer GL, et al. Tubulolobular carcinoma of the breast: an analysis of 27 cases of a tumor with a hybrid morphology and immunoprofile. *Am J Surg Pathol* 2004;28(12):1587–1593.
123. Carter MR, Hornick JL, Lester S, et al. Spindle cell (sarcomatoid) carcinoma of the breast: a clinicopathologic and immunohistochemical analysis of 29 cases. *Am J Surg Pathol* 2006;30(3):300–309.
124. Beatty JD, Atwood M, Tickman R, et al. Metaplastic breast cancer: clinical significance. *Am J Surg* 2006;191(5):657–664.
125. Chaney AW, Pollack A, McNeese MD, et al. Primary treatment of cystosarcoma phyllodes of the breast. *Cancer* 2000;89(7):1502–1511.
126. Telli ML, Horst KC, Guardino AE, et al. Phyllodes tumors of the breast: natural history, diagnosis, and treatment. *J Natl Compr Canc Netw* 2007; 5(3):324–330.
127. Sher T, Hennessy BT, Valero V, et al. Primary angiosarcomas of the breast. *Cancer* 2007;110(1):173–178.
128. Vorburger SA, Xing Y, Hunt KK, et al. Angiosarcoma of the breast. *Cancer* 2005;104(12):2682–2688.
129. Perou CM, Sorlie T, Eisen MB, et al. Molecular portraits of human breast tumours. *Nature* 2000;406(6797):747–752.
130. Sorlie T, Perou CM, Tibshirani R, et al. Gene expression patterns of breast carcinomas distinguish tumor subclasses with clinical implications. *Proc Natl Acad Sci USA* 2001;98(19):10869–10874.
131. Sorlie T, Tibshirani R, Parker J, et al. Repeated observation of breast tumor subtypes in independent gene expression data sets. *Proc Natl Acad Sci USA* 2003;100(14):8418–8423.
132. Bertucci F, Finetti P, Rougemont J, et al. Gene expression profiling identifies molecular subtypes of inflammatory breast cancer. *Cancer Res* 2005;65(6):2170–2178.
133. Carey LA, Perou CM, Livasy CA, et al. Race, breast cancer subtypes, and survival in the Carolina Breast Cancer Study. *JAMA* 2006;295(21): 2492–2502.
134. Lakhani SR, Reis-Filho JS, Fulford L, et al. Prediction of *BRCA1* status in patients with breast cancer using estrogen receptor and basal phenotype. *Clin Cancer Res* 2005;11(14):5175–5180.
135. Bane AL, Beck JC, Bleiweiss I, et al. *BRCA2* mutation-associated breast cancers exhibit a distinguishing phenotype based on morphology and molecular profiles from tissue microarrays. *Am J Surg Pathol* 2007;31(1):121–128.
136. Allred DC, Bustamante MA, Daniel CO, et al. Immunocytochemical analysis of estrogen receptors in human breast carcinomas. Evaluation of 130 cases and review of the literature regarding concordance with biochemical assay and clinical relevance. *Arch Surg* 1990;125(1):107–113.
137. Layfield LJ, Gupta D, Mooney EE. Assessment of tissue estrogen and progesterone receptor levels: a survey of current practice, techniques, and quantitation methods. *Breast J* 2000;6(3):189–196.
138. Berry DA, Cirrincione C, Henderson IC, et al. Estrogen-receptor status and outcomes of modern chemotherapy for patients with node-positive breast cancer. *JAMA* 2006;295(14):1658–1667.
139. Kennedy SM, O'Driscoll L, Purcell R, et al. Prognostic importance of survivin in breast cancer. *Br J Cancer* 2003;88(7):1077–1083.
140. Fitzgibbons PL, Page DL, Weaver D, et al. Prognostic factors in breast cancer. College of American Pathologists Consensus Statement 1999. *Arch Pathol Lab Med* 2000;124(7):966–978.
141. Gusterson BA, Gelber RD, Goldhirsch A, et al. Prognostic importance of c-erbB-2 expression in breast cancer. International (Ludwig) Breast Cancer Study Group. *J Clin Oncol* 1992;10(7):1049–1056.
142. Muss HB, Thor AD, Berry DA, et al. c-erbB-2 expression and response to adjuvant therapy in women with node-positive early breast cancer. *N Engl J Med* 1994;330(18):1260–1266.
143. Paik S, Bryant J, Park C, et al. erbB-2 and response to doxorubicin in patients with axillary lymph node-positive, hormone receptor-negative breast cancer. *J Natl Cancer Inst* 1998;90(18):1361–1370.
144. Slamon DJ, Leyland-Jones B, Shak S, et al. Use of chemotherapy plus a monoclonal antibody against HER2 for metastatic breast cancer that overexpresses HER2. *N Engl J Med* 2001;344(11):783–792.
145. Wolff AC, Hammond ME, Schwartz JN, et al. American Society of Clinical Oncology/College of American Pathologists guideline recommendations for human epidermal growth factor receptor 2 testing in breast cancer. *J Clin Oncol* 2007;25(1):118–145.
146. Livasy CA, Karaca G, Nanda R, et al. Phenotypic evaluation of the basal-like subtype of invasive breast carcinoma. *Mod Pathol* 2006;19(2): 264–271.
147. Rakha EA, El-Sayed ME, Green AR, et al. Prognostic markers in triple-negative breast cancer. *Cancer* 2007;109(1): 25–32.
148. Fulford LG, Easton DF, Reis-Filho JS, et al. Specific morphological features predictive for the basal phenotype in grade 3 invasive ductal carcinoma of breast. *Histopathology* 2006;49(1):22–34.
149. Bauer KR, Brown M, Cress RD, et al. Descriptive analysis of estrogen receptor (ER)-negative, progesterone receptor (PR)-negative, and HER2-negative invasive breast cancer, the so-called triple-negative phenotype: a population-based study from the California Cancer Registry. *Cancer* 2007; 109(9):1721–1728.
150. Halsted WS. The results of operations for the cure of cancer of the breast performed at the Johns Hopkins Hospital from June 1889 to January 1894. *Johns Hopkins Hosp Rep* 1894;4:297.
151. Meyer W. An improved method of the radical operation for carcinoma of the breast. *Med Rec* 1894;46:746.
152. Halsted WS. The results of radical operations for the cure of carcinoma of the breast. *Ann Surg* 1907;46:1.
153. Urban JA. Radical excision of the chest wall for mammary cancer. *Cancer* 1951;4(6):1263–1285.
154. Halsted WS. Parasternal invasion of the thorax in breast cancer and its suppression by the use of radium tubes as an operative precaution. *Surg Gynecol Obstet* 1927;45:721–782.
155. McWhirter R. The value of simple mastectomy and radiotherapy in the treatment of cancer of the breast. *Br J Radiol* 1948;21:599.
156. Patey DH, Dyson WH. The prognosis of carcinoma of the breast in relation to the type of operation performed. *Br J Cancer* 1948;2:7–13.
157. Fisher B, Anderson S, Bryant J, et al. Twenty-year follow-up of a randomized trial comparing total mastectomy, lumpectomy, and lumpectomy plus irradiation for the treatment of invasive breast cancer. *N Engl J Med* 2002;347(16):1233–1241.
158. Veronesi U, Cascinelli N, Mariani L, et al. Twenty-year follow-up of a randomized study comparing breast-conserving surgery with radical mastectomy for early breast cancer. *N Engl J Med* 2002;347(16):1227–1232.
159. Blichert-Toft M, Rose C, Andersen JA, et al. Danish randomized trial comparing breast conservation therapy with mastectomy: six years of life-table analysis. Danish Breast Cancer Cooperative Group. *J Natl Cancer Inst Monogr* 1992(11):19–25.
160. Arriagada R, Le MG, Rochard F, et al. Conservative treatment versus mastectomy in early breast cancer: patterns of failure with 15 years of follow-up data. Institut Gustave-Roussy Breast Cancer Group. *J Clin Oncol* 1996;14(5):1558–1564.
161. Poggi MM, Danforth DN, Sciuto LC, et al. Eighteen-year results in the treatment of early breast carcinoma with mastectomy versus breast conservation therapy: the National Cancer Institute Randomized Trial. *Cancer* 2003;98(4):697–702.
162. van Dongen JA, Voogd AC, Fentiman IS, et al. Long-term results of a randomized trial comparing breast-conserving therapy with mastectomy: European Organization for Research and Treatment of Cancer 10801 trial. *J Natl Cancer Inst* 2000;92(14):1143–1150.
163. Veronesi U, Zurrida S. Optimal surgical treatment of breast cancer. *Oncologist* 1996;1(6):340–346.
164. Fisher B, Land S, Mamounas E, et al. Prevention of invasive breast cancer in women with ductal carcinoma *in situ:* an update of the national surgical adjuvant breast and bowel project experience. *Semin Oncol* 2001;28(4): 400–418.
165. Krag DN, Anderson SJ, Julian TB, et al. Technical outcomes of sentinel-lymph-node resection and conventional axillary-lymph-node dissection in patients with clinically node-negative breast cancer: results from the NSABP B-32 randomised phase III trial. *Lancet Oncol* 2007;8(10):881–888.
166. Vogel VG, Costantino JP, Wickerham DL, et al. Effects of tamoxifen vs raloxifene on the risk of developing invasive breast cancer and other disease outcomes: the NSABP Study of Tamoxifen and Raloxifene (STAR) P-2 trial. *JAMA* 2006;295(23):2727–2741.
167. Boyages J, Delaney G, Taylor R. Predictors of local recurrence after treatment of ductal carcinoma *in situ:* a meta-analysis. *Cancer* 1999;85(3):616–628.
168. Neuschatz AC, DiPetrillo T, Steinhoff M, et al. The value of breast lumpectomy margin assessment as a predictor of residual tumor burden in ductal carcinoma *in situ* of the breast. *Cancer* 2002;94(7):1917–1924.
169. Douglas-Jones AG, Logan J, Morgan JM, et al. Effect of margins of excision on recurrence after local excision of ductal carcinoma *in situ* of the breast. *J Clin Pathol* 2002;55(8):581–586.
170. Silverstein MJ, Lagios MD, Craig PH, et al. A prognostic index for ductal carcinoma *in situ* of the breast. *Cancer* 1996;77(11):2267–2274.
171. Wilkie C, White L, Dupont E, et al. An update of sentinel lymph node mapping in patients with ductal carcinoma *in situ. Am J Surg* 2005;190(4): 563–566.
172. Yen TW, Hunt KK, Ross MI, et al. Predictors of invasive breast cancer in patients with an initial diagnosis of ductal carcinoma *in situ:* a guide to selective use of sentinel lymph node biopsy in management of ductal carcinoma *in situ. J Am Coll Surg* 2005;200(4):516–526.
173. Klauber-DeMore N, Tan LK, Liberman L, et al. Sentinel lymph node biopsy: Is it indicated in patients with high-risk ductal carcinoma-*in-situ* and ductal carcinoma-*in-situ* with microinvasion? *Ann Surg Oncol* 2000;7(9):636–642.
174. Haid A, Knauer M, Dunzinger S, et al. Intra-operative sonography: a valuable aid during breast-conserving surgery for occult breast cancer. *Ann Surg Oncol* 2007;14(11):3090–3101.
175. Duarte GM, Cabello C, Torresan RZ, et al. Radioguided Intraoperative Margins Evaluation (RIME): Preliminary results of a new technique to aid breast cancer resection. *Eur J Surg Oncol* 2007;33(10):1150–1157.
176. Singletary SE. Surgical margins in patients with early-stage breast cancer treated with breast conservation therapy. *Am J Surg* 2002;184(5):383–393.
177. Neuschatz AC, DiPetrillo T, Safaii H, et al. Long-term follow-up of a prospective policy of margin-directed radiation dose escalation in breast-conserving therapy. *Cancer* 2003;97(1):30–39.
178. Klimberg VS, Kepple J, Shafirstein G, et al. eRFA: excision followed by RFA—a new technique to improve local control in breast cancer. *Ann Surg Oncol* 2006;13(11):1422–1433.
179. Oruwari JU, Chung MA, Koelliker S, et al. Axillary staging using ultrasound-guided fine needle aspiration biopsy in locally advanced breast cancer. *Am J Surg* 2002;184(4):307–309.

180. Lee MC, Newman LA. Management of patients with locally advanced breast cancer. *Surg Clin North Am* 2007;87(2):379–398, ix.
181. Fisher B, Brown A, Mamounas E, et al. Effect of preoperative chemotherapy on local-regional disease in women with operable breast cancer: findings from National Surgical Adjuvant Breast and Bowel Project B-18. *J Clin Oncol* 1997;15(7):2483–2493.
182. Mansour EG, Gray R, Shatila AH, et al. Survival advantage of adjuvant chemotherapy in high-risk node-negative breast cancer: ten-year analysis—an intergroup study. *J Clin Oncol* 1998;16(11):3486–3492.
183. Khan A, Sabel MS, Nees A, et al. Comprehensive axillary evaluation in neoadjuvant chemotherapy patients with ultrasonography and sentinel lymph node biopsy. *Ann Surg Oncol* 2005;12(9):697–704.
184. Kuerer HM, Sahin AA, Hunt KK, et al. Incidence and impact of documented eradication of breast cancer axillary lymph node metastases before surgery in patients treated with neoadjuvant chemotherapy. *Ann Surg* 1999;230(1):72–78.
185. Davies GC, Millis RR, Hayward JL. Assessment of axillary lymph node status. *Ann Surg* 1980;192(2):148–151.
186. Petrek JA, Blackwood MM. Axillary dissection: current practice and technique. *Curr Probl Surg* 1995;32(4):257–323.
187. Vlastos G, Fornage BD, Mirza NQ, et al. The correlation of axillary ultrasonography with histologic breast cancer downstaging after induction chemotherapy. *Am J Surg* 2000;179(6):446–452.
188. Bonnema J, van Geel AN, van Ooijen B, et al. Ultrasound-guided aspiration biopsy for detection of nonpalpable axillary node metastases in breast cancer patients: new diagnostic method. *World J Surg* 1997;21(3): 270–274.
189. Chagpar AB, Scoggins CR, Martin RC 2nd, et al. Prediction of sentinel lymph node-only disease in women with invasive breast cancer. *Am J Surg* 2006;192(6):882–887.
190. Samant R, Ganguly P. Staging investigations in patients with breast cancer: the role of bone scans and liver imaging. *Arch Surg* 1999;134(5): 551–553; discussion 554.
191. Newman LA, Buzdar AU, Singletary SE, et al. A prospective trial of preoperative chemotherapy in resectable breast cancer: predictors of breast-conservation therapy feasibility. *Ann Surg Oncol* 2002;9(3):228–234.
192. Helvie MA, Joynt LK, Cody RL, et al. Locally advanced breast carcinoma: accuracy of mammography versus clinical examination in the prediction of residual disease after chemotherapy. *Radiology* 1996; 198(2):327–332.
193. Delille JP, Slanetz PJ, Yeh ED, et al. Invasive ductal breast carcinoma response to neoadjuvant chemotherapy: noninvasive monitoring with functional MR imaging pilot study. *Radiology* 2003;228(1):63–69.
194. Chagpar AB, Middleton LP, Sahin AA, et al. Accuracy of physical examination, ultrasonography, and mammography in predicting residual pathologic tumor size in patients treated with neoadjuvant chemotherapy. *Ann Surg* 2006;243(2):257–264.
195. Mazouni C, Peintinger F, Wan-Kau S, et al. Residual ductal carcinoma *in situ* in patients with complete eradication of invasive breast cancer after neoadjuvant chemotherapy does not adversely affect patient outcome. *J Clin Oncol* 2007;25(19):2650–2655.
196. Chung CS, Harris JR. Post-mastectomy radiation therapy: Translating local benefits into improved survival. *Breast* 2007;16(Suppl 2):578–583.
197. Fisher B, Jeong JH, Anderson S, et al. Twenty-five-year follow-up of a randomized trial comparing radical mastectomy, total mastectomy, and total mastectomy followed by irradiation. *N Engl J Med* 2002;347(8):567–575.
198. Cabanes PA, Salmon RJ, Vilcoq JR, et al. Value of axillary dissection in addition to lumpectomy and radiotherapy in early breast cancer. The Breast Carcinoma Collaborative Group of the Institut Curie. *Lancet* 1992;339(8804):1245–1248.
199. Greco M, Agresti R, Cascinelli N, et al. Breast cancer patients treated without axillary surgery: clinical implications and biologic analysis. *Ann Surg* 2000;232(1):1–7.
200. Johansen H, Kaae S, Schiodt T. Simple mastectomy with postoperative irradiation versus extended radical mastectomy in breast cancer. A twenty-five-year follow-up of a randomized trial. *Acta Oncol* 1990;29(6): 709–715.
201. Veronesi U, Marubini E, Mariani L, et al. The dissection of internal mammary nodes does not improve the survival of breast cancer patients. 30-year results of a randomised trial. *Eur J Cancer* 1999;35(9):1320–1325.
202. Orr RK. The impact of prophylactic axillary node dissection on breast cancer survival—a Bayesian meta-analysis. *Ann Surg Oncol* 1999;6(1): 109–116.
203. Louis-Sylvestre C, Clough K, Asselain B, et al. Axillary treatment in conservative management of operable breast cancer: dissection or radiotherapy? Results of a randomized study with 15 years of follow-up. *J Clin Oncol* 2004;22(1):97–101.
204. Kim T, Giuliano AE, Lyman GH. Lymphatic mapping and sentinel lymph node biopsy in early-stage breast carcinoma: a metaanalysis. *Cancer* 2006;106(1):4–16.
205. Morton DL, Wen DR, Wong JH, et al. Technical details of intraoperative lymphatic mapping for early stage melanoma. *Arch Surg* 1992;127(4): 392–399.
206. Giuliano AE, Kirgan DM, Guenther JM, et al. Lymphatic mapping and sentinel lymphadenectomy for breast cancer. *Ann Surg* 1994;220(3): 391–398; discussion 398–401.
207. Chagpar AB, Martin RC, Scoggins CR, et al. Factors predicting failure to identify a sentinel lymph node in breast cancer. *Surgery* 2005;138(1): 56–63.
208. Tuttle TM. Technical advances in sentinel lymph node biopsy for breast cancer. *Am Surg* 2004;70(5):407–413.
209. Ting AC, Cumarasingam B, Szeto ER. Successful internal mammary visualization with periareolar injections of Tc-99m antimony sulfur colloid in sentinel node breast lymphoscintigraphy. *Clin Nucl Med* 2006;31(10): 593–597.
210. Krag DN, Weaver DL, Alex JC, et al. Surgical resection and radiolocalization of the sentinel lymph node in breast cancer using a gamma probe. *Surg Oncol* 1993;2(6):335–339; discussion 340.
211. Van Diest PJ, Torrenga H, Borgstein PJ, et al. Reliability of intraoperative frozen section and imprint cytological investigation of sentinel lymph nodes in breast cancer. *Histopathology* 1999;35(1):14–18.
212. Cibull ML. Handling sentinel lymph node biopsy specimens. A work in progress. *Arch Pathol Lab Med* 1999;123(7):620–621.
213. Prognostic importance of occult axillary lymph node micrometastases from breast cancers. International (Ludwig) Breast Cancer Study Group. *Lancet* 1990;335(8705):1565–1568.
214. Dowlatshahi K, Fan M, Bloom KJ, et al. Occult metastases in the sentinel lymph nodes of patients with early stage breast carcinoma: a preliminary study. *Cancer* 1999;86(6):990–996.
215. Fisher ER, Swamidoss S, Lee CH, et al. Detection and significance of occult axillary node metastases in patients with invasive breast cancer. *Cancer* 1978;42(4):2025–2031.
216. Naik AM, Fey J, Gemignani M, et al. The risk of axillary relapse after sentinel lymph node biopsy for breast cancer is comparable with that of axillary lymph node dissection: a follow-up study of 4008 procedures. *Ann Surg* 2004;240(3):462–468; discussion 468–471.
217. Park J, Fey JV, Naik AM, et al. A declining rate of completion axillary dissection in sentinel lymph node-positive breast cancer patients is associated with the use of a multivariate nomogram. *Ann Surg* 2007;245(3): 462–468.
218. Van Zee KJ, Manasseh DM, Bevilacqua JL, et al. A nomogram for predicting the likelihood of additional nodal metastases in breast cancer patients with a positive sentinel node biopsy. *Ann Surg Oncol* 2003; 10(10):1140–1151.
219. Pyszel A, Malyszczak K, Pyszel K, et al. Disability, psychological distress and quality of life in breast cancer survivors with arm lymphedema. *Lymphology* 2006;39(4):185–192.
220. Noone RB, Frazier TG, Noone GC, et al. Recurrence of breast carcinoma following immediate reconstruction: a 13-year review. *Plast Reconstr Surg* 1994;93(1):96–106; discussion 107–108.
221. Simmons RM, Fish SK, Gayle L, et al. Local and distant recurrence rates in skin-sparing mastectomies compared with non-skin-sparing mastectomies. *Ann Surg Oncol* 1999;6(7):676–681.
222. Foster RD, Esserman LJ, Anthony JP, et al. Skin-sparing mastectomy and immediate breast reconstruction: a prospective cohort study for the treatment of advanced stages of breast carcinoma. *Ann Surg Oncol* 2002;9(5): 462–466.
223. Vaughan A, Dietz JR, Aft R, et al. Scientific Presentation Award. Patterns of local breast cancer recurrence after skin-sparing mastectomy and immediate breast reconstruction. *Am J Surg* 2007;194(4):438–443.
224. Simmons RM, Brennan M, Christos P, et al. Analysis of nipple/areolar involvement with mastectomy: can the areola be preserved? *Ann Surg Oncol* 2002;9(2):165–168.
225. Sacchini V, Pinotti JA, Barros AC, et al. Nipple-sparing mastectomy for breast cancer and risk reduction: oncologic or technical problem? *J Am Coll Surg* 2006;203(5):704–714.
226. Benediktsson KP, Perbeck L. Survival in breast cancer after nipple-sparing subcutaneous mastectomy and immediate reconstruction with implants: a prospective trial with 13 years median follow-up in 216 patients. *Eur J Surg Oncol* 2008;34(2):143–148.
227. Petit JY, Veronesi U, Orecchia R, et al. Nipple-sparing mastectomy in association with intra operative radiotherapy (ELIOT): a new type of mastectomy for breast cancer treatment. *Breast Cancer Res Treat* 2006; 96(1):47–51.
228. Chen CY, Calhoun KE, Masetti R, et al. Oncoplastic breast conserving surgery: a renaissance of anatomically-based surgical technique. *Minerva Chir* 2006;61(5):421–434.
229. Bonadonna G, Valagussa P, Moliterni A, et al. Adjuvant cyclophosphamide, methotrexate, and fluorouracil in node-positive breast cancer: the results of 20 years of follow-up. *N Engl J Med* 1995;332(14):901–906.
230. Lyman GH, Dale DC, Crawford J. Incidence and predictors of low dose-intensity in adjuvant breast cancer chemotherapy: a nationwide study of community practices. *J Clin Oncol* 2003;21(24):4524–4531.
231. Polychemotherapy for early breast cancer: an overview of the randomised trials. Early Breast Cancer Trialists' Collaborative Group. *Lancet* 1998;352(9132):930–942.
232. Effects of chemotherapy and hormonal therapy for early breast cancer on recurrence and 15-year survival: an overview of the randomised trials. *Lancet* 2005;365(9472):1687–1717.
233. Holmes FA, Walters RS, Theriault RL, et al. Phase II trial of taxol, an active drug in the treatment of metastatic breast cancer. *J Natl Cancer Inst* 1991;83(24):1797–1805.

234. Hudis C, Seidman A, Baselga J, et al. Sequential dose-dense doxorubicin, paclitaxel, and cyclophosphamide for resectable high-risk breast cancer: feasibility and efficacy. *J Clin Oncol* 1999;17(1):93–100.
235. Hayes DF, Thor AD, Dressler LG, et al. HER2 and response to paclitaxel in node-positive breast cancer. *N Engl J Med* 2007;357(15):1496–1506.
236. Citron ML, Berry DA, Cirrincione C, et al. Randomized trial of dose-dense versus conventionally scheduled and sequential versus concurrent combination chemotherapy as postoperative adjuvant treatment of node-positive primary breast cancer: first report of Intergroup Trial C9741/Cancer and Leukemia Group B Trial 9741. *J Clin Oncol* 2003;21(8):1431–1439.
237. Martin M, Pienkowski T, Mackey J, et al. Adjuvant docetaxel for node-positive breast cancer. *N Engl J Med* 2005;352(22):2302–2313.
238. Jones SE, Savin MA, Holmes FA, et al. Phase III trial comparing doxorubicin plus cyclophosphamide with docetaxel plus cyclophosphamide as adjuvant therapy for operable breast cancer. *J Clin Oncol* 2006;24(34):5381–5387.
239. Fisher B, Jeong JH, Anderson S, et al. Treatment of axillary lymph node-negative, estrogen receptor-negative breast cancer: updated findings from National Surgical Adjuvant Breast and Bowel Project clinical trials. *J Natl Cancer Inst* 2004;96(24):1823–1831.
240. Linden HM, Haskell CM, Green SJ, et al. Sequenced compared with simultaneous anthracycline and cyclophosphamide in high-risk stage I and II breast cancer: final analysis from INT-0137 (S9313). *J Clin Oncol* 2007;25(6):656–661.
241. Ravdin PM, Siminoff LA, Davis GJ, et al. Computer program to assist in making decisions about adjuvant therapy for women with early breast cancer. *J Clin Oncol* 2001;19(4):980–991.
242. www.adjuvantonline.com. Accessed October 4, 2007.
243. van de Vijver M, He YD, van't Veer LJ, et al. A gene expression signature as a predictor of survival in breast cancer. *N Engl J Med* 2002;347:1999–2009.
244. Paik S, Shak S, Tang G, et al. A multigene assay to predict recurrence of tamoxifen-treated, node-negative breast cancer. *N Engl J Med* 2004;351(27):2817–2826.
245. Romond EH, Perez EA, Bryant J, et al. Trastuzumab plus adjuvant chemotherapy for operable HER2-positive breast cancer. *N Engl J Med* 2005;353(16):1673–1684.
246. Piccart-Gebhart MJ, Procter M, Leyland-Jones B, et al. Trastuzumab after adjuvant chemotherapy in HER2-positive breast cancer. *N Engl J Med* 2005;353(16):1659–1672.
247. Slamon D, Eiermann W, Robert N, et al. BCIRG 006: 2nd interim analysis phase III randomized trial comparing doxorubicin and cyclophosphamide followed by docetaxel (AC→T) with doxorubicin and cyclophosphamide followed by docetaxel and trastuzumab (AC→TH) with docetaxel, carboplatin and trastuzumab (TCH) in Her2neu positive early breast cancer patients. Abstr 52. Paper presented at the 19th Annual San Antonio Breast Cancer Symposium, 2006; San Antonio, TX.
248. Joensuu H, Kellokumpu-Lehtinen PL, Bono P, et al. Adjuvant docetaxel or vinorelbine with or without trastuzumab for breast cancer. *N Engl J Med* 2006;354(8):809–820.
249. Wolmark N, Wang J, Mamounas E, et al. Preoperative chemotherapy in patients with operable breast cancer: nine-year results from National Surgical Adjuvant Breast and Bowel Project B-18. *J Natl Cancer Inst Monogr* 2001(30):96–102.
250. Rouzier R, Pusztai L, Delaloge S, et al. Nomograms to predict pathologic complete response and metastasis-free survival after preoperative chemotherapy for breast cancer. *J Clin Oncol* 2005;23(33):8331–8339.
251. Fossati R, Confalonieri C, Torri V, et al. Cytotoxic and hormonal treatment for metastatic breast cancer: a systematic review of published randomized trials involving 31,510 women. *J Clin Oncol* 1998;16(10):3439–3460.
252. Sledge GW, Neuberg D, Bernardo P, et al. Phase III trial of doxorubicin, paclitaxel, and the combination of doxorubicin and paclitaxel as front-line chemotherapy for metastatic breast cancer: an intergroup trial (E1193). *J Clin Oncol* 2003;21(4):588–592.
253. O'Shaughnessy J, Miles D, Vukelja S, et al. Superior survival with capecitabine plus docetaxel combination therapy in anthracycline-pretreated patients with advanced breast cancer: phase III trial results. *J Clin Oncol* 2002;20(12):2812–2823.
254. Albain KS, Nag S, Calderillo-Ruiz G, et al. Global phase III study of gemcitabine plus paclitaxel (GT) vs. paclitaxel (T) as frontline therapy for metastatic breast cancer (MBC): first report of overall survival. *Journal of Clinical Oncology, 2004 ASCO Annual Meeting Proceedings (Post-Meeting Edition).* 2004;22(14 Suppl):510.
255. Gradishar WJ, Tjulandin S, Davidson N, et al. Phase III trial of nanoparticle albumin-bound paclitaxel compared with polyethylated castor oil-based paclitaxel in women with breast cancer. *J Clin Oncol* 2005;23(31):7794–7803.
256. Perez EA, Lerzo G, Pivot X, et al. Efficacy and safety of ixabepilone (BMS-247550) in a phase II study of patients with advanced breast cancer resistant to anthracycline, a taxane, and capecitabine. *J Clin Oncol* 2007;25(23):3407–3414.
257. Geyer CE, Forster J, Lindquist D, et al. Lapatinib plus capecitabine for HER2-positive advanced breast cancer. *N Engl J Med* 2006;355(26):2733–2743.
258. Adjuvant tamoxifen in the management of operable breast cancer: the Scottish Trial. Report from the Breast Cancer Trials Committee, Scottish Cancer Trials Office (MRC), Edinburgh. *Lancet* 1987;2(8552): 171–175.
259. Fisher B, Costantino J, Redmond C, et al. A randomized clinical trial evaluating tamoxifen in the treatment of patients with node-negative breast cancer who have estrogen-receptor-positive tumors. *N Engl J Med* 1989;320(8):479–484.
260. Fisher B, Costantino JP, Wickerham DL, et al. Tamoxifen for prevention of breast cancer: report of the National Surgical Adjuvant Breast and Bowel Project P-1 Study. *J Natl Cancer Inst* 1998;90(18):1371–1388.
261. Sonoda Y, Barakat RR. Screening and the prevention of gynecologic cancer: endometrial cancer. *Best Pract Res Clin Obstet Gynaecol* 2006;20(2):363–377.
262. Benson JR. Re: Five versus more than five years of tamoxifen for lymph node-negative breast cancer: updated findings from the National Surgical Adjuvant Breast and Bowel Project B-14 Randomized Trial. *J Natl Cancer Inst* 2001;93(19):1493–1494.
263. Fisher B, Dignam J, Bryant J, et al. Five versus more than five years of tamoxifen therapy for breast cancer patients with negative lymph nodes and estrogen receptor-positive tumors. *J Natl Cancer Inst* 1996;88(21):1529–1542.
264. Baum M, Buzdar A, Cuzick J, et al. Anastrozole alone or in combination with tamoxifen versus tamoxifen alone for adjuvant treatment of postmenopausal women with early-stage breast cancer: results of the ATAC (Arimidex, Tamoxifen Alone or in Combination) trial efficacy and safety update analyses. *Cancer* 2003;98(9):1802–1810.
265. Coombes RC, Kilburn LS, Snowdon CF, et al. Survival and safety of exemestane versus tamoxifen after 2-3 years' tamoxifen treatment (Intergroup Exemestane Study): a randomised controlled trial. *Lancet* 2007;369(9561):559–570.
266. Goss PE, Ingle JN, Martino S, et al. A randomized trial of letrozole in postmenopausal women after five years of tamoxifen therapy for early-stage breast cancer. *N Engl J Med* 2003;349(19):1793–1802.
267. Thurlimann B, Keshaviah A, Coates AS, et al. A comparison of letrozole and tamoxifen in postmenopausal women with early breast cancer. *N Engl J Med* 2005;353(26):2747–2757.
268. Coates AS, Keshaviah A, Thurlimann B, et al. Five years of letrozole compared with tamoxifen as initial adjuvant therapy for postmenopausal women with endocrine-responsive early breast cancer: update of study BIG 1-98. *J Clin Oncol* 2007;25(5):486–492.
269. Ovarian ablation for early breast cancer. *Cochrane Database Syst Rev.* 2000(3):CD000485.
270. Castiglione-Gertsch M, O'Neill A, Price KN, et al. Adjuvant chemotherapy followed by goserelin versus either modality alone for premenopausal lymph node-negative breast cancer: a randomized trial. *J Natl Cancer Inst* 2003;95(24):1833–1846.
271. Arriagada R, Le MG, Spielmann M, et al. Randomized trial of adjuvant ovarian suppression in 926 premenopausal patients with early breast cancer treated with adjuvant chemotherapy. *Ann Oncol* 2005;16(3):389–396.
272. Schmid P, Untch M, Kosse V, et al. Leuprorelin acetate every-3-months depot versus cyclophosphamide, methotrexate, and fluorouracil as adjuvant treatment in premenopausal patients with node-positive breast cancer: the TABLE study. *J Clin Oncol* 2007;25(18):2509–2515.
273. Buzdar A, Jonat W, Howell A, et al. Anastrozole, a potent and selective aromatase inhibitor, versus megestrol acetate in postmenopausal women with advanced breast cancer: results of overview analysis of two phase III trials. Arimidex Study Group. *J Clin Oncol* 1996;14(7):2000–2011.
274. Howell A, Robertson JF, Quaresma Albano J, et al. Fulvestrant, formerly ICI 182,780, is as effective as anastrozole in postmenopausal women with advanced breast cancer progressing after prior endocrine treatment. *J Clin Oncol* 2002;20(16):3396–3403.
275. Kaufmann M, Bajetta E, Dirix LY, et al. Exemestane improves survival compared with megoestrol acetate in postmenopausal patients with advanced breast cancer who have failed on tamoxifen. Results of a double-blind randomised phase III trial. *Eur J Cancer* 2000;36(Suppl 4):S86–87.
276. Atkins H, Hayward JL, Klugman DJ, et al. Treatment of early breast cancer: a report after ten years of a clinical trial. *Br Med J* 1972;2(5811):423–429.
277. Fisher B, Redmond C, Fisher ER, et al. Ten-year results of a randomized clinical trial comparing radical mastectomy and total mastectomy with or without radiation. *N Engl J Med* 1985;312(11):674–681.
278. Veronesi U, Marubini E, Mariani L, et al. Radiotherapy after breast-conserving surgery in small breast carcinoma: long-term results of a randomized trial. *Ann Oncol* 2001;12(7):997–1003.
279. Fisher B, Bryant J, Dignam JJ, et al. Tamoxifen, radiation therapy, or both for prevention of ipsilateral breast tumor recurrence after lumpectomy in women with invasive breast cancers of one centimeter or less. *J Clin Oncol* 2002;20(20):4141–4149.
280. Fyles AW, McCready DR, Manchul LA, et al. Tamoxifen with or without breast irradiation in women 50 years of age or older with early breast cancer. *N Engl J Med* 2004;351(10):963–970.
281. Hughes KS, Schnaper LA, Berry D, et al. Lumpectomy plus tamoxifen with or without irradiation in women 70 years of age or older with early breast cancer. *N Engl J Med* 2004;351(10):971–977.
282. Clarke M, Collins R, Darby S, et al. Effects of radiotherapy and of differences in the extent of surgery for early breast cancer on local recurrence and 15-year survival: an overview of the randomised trials. *Lancet* 2005;366(9503):2087–2106.

283. Bellon JR, Come SE, Gelman RS, et al. Sequencing of chemotherapy and radiation therapy in early-stage breast cancer: updated results of a prospective randomized trial. *J Clin Oncol* 2005;23(9):1934–1940.
284. Overgaard M, Hansen PS, Overgaard J, et al. Postoperative radiotherapy in high-risk premenopausal women with breast cancer who receive adjuvant chemotherapy. Danish Breast Cancer Cooperative Group 82b Trial. *N Engl J Med* 1997;337(14):949–955.
285. Ragaz J, Jackson SM, Le N, et al. Adjuvant radiotherapy and chemotherapy in node-positive premenopausal women with breast cancer. *N Engl J Med* 1997;337(14):956–962.
286. Overgaard M, Jensen MB, Overgaard J, et al. Postoperative radiotherapy in high-risk postmenopausal breast-cancer patients given adjuvant tamoxifen: Danish Breast Cancer Cooperative Group DBCG 82c randomised trial. *Lancet* 1999;353(9165):1641–1648.
287. Houghton J, George WD, Cuzick J, et al. Radiotherapy and tamoxifen in women with completely excised ductal carcinoma *in situ* of the breast in the UK, Australia, and New Zealand: randomised controlled trial. *Lancet* 2003;362(9378):95–102.
288. Julien JP, Bijker N, Fentiman IS, et al. Radiotherapy in breast-conserving treatment for ductal carcinoma *in situ:* first results of the EORTC randomised phase III trial 10853. EORTC Breast Cancer Cooperative Group and EORTC Radiotherapy Group. *Lancet* 2000;355(9203):528–533.
289. Fisher B, Dignam J, Wolmark N, et al. Lumpectomy and radiation therapy for the treatment of intraductal breast cancer: findings from National Surgical Adjuvant Breast and Bowel Project B-17. *J Clin Oncol* 1998;16(2): 441–452.
290. Fisher B, Dignam J, Wolmark N, et al. Tamoxifen in treatment of intraductal breast cancer: National Surgical Adjuvant Breast and Bowel Project B-24 randomised controlled trial. *Lancet* 1999;353(9169):1993–2000.
291. Viani GA, Stefano EJ, Afonso SL, et al. Breast-conserving surgery with or without radiotherapy in women with ductal carcinoma *in situ:* a meta-analysis of randomized trials. *Radiat Oncol* 2007;2:28.
292. Kavanagh BD, Scheftera TE, Wersall PJ. Liver, renal, and retroperitoneal tumors: stereotactic radiotherapy. *Front Radiat Ther Oncol* 2007;40: 415–426.
293. Bartelink H, Horiot JC, Poortmans PM, et al. Impact of a higher radiation dose on local control and survival in breast-conserving therapy of early breast cancer: 10-year results of the randomized boost versus no boost EORTC 22881-10882 trial. *J Clin Oncol* 2007;25(22):3259–3265.
294. Romestaing P, Lehingue Y, Carrie C, et al. Role of a 10-Gy boost in the conservative treatment of early breast cancer: results of a randomized clinical trial in Lyon, France. *J Clin Oncol* 1997;15(3):963–968.
295. Kirova YM, Servois V, Campana F, et al. CT-scan based localization of the internal mammary chain and supra clavicular nodes for breast cancer radiation therapy planning. *Radiother Oncol* 2006;79(3):310–315.
296. Jagsi R, Moran JM, Kessler ML, et al. Respiratory motion of the heart and positional reproducibility under active breathing control. *Int J Radiat Oncol Biol Phys* 2007;68(1):253–258.
297. Fraass BA, Roberson PL, Lichter AS. Dose to the contralateral breast due to primary breast irradiation. *Int J Radiat Oncol Biol Phys* 1985;11(3): 485–497.
298. Muller-Runkel R, Kalokhe UP. Scatter dose from tangential breast irradiation to the uninvolved breast. *Radiology* 1990;175(3):873–876.
299. Ikner CL, Russo R, Podgorsak MB, et al. Comparison of the homogeneity of breast dose distributions with and without the medial wedge. *Med Dosim* 1998;23(2):89–94.
300. Dewar JA, Arriagada R, Benhamou S, et al. Local relapse and contralateral tumor rates in patients with breast cancer treated with conservative surgery and radiotherapy (Institut Gustave Roussy 1970-1982). IGR Breast Cancer Group. *Cancer* 1995;76(11):2260–2265.
301. Veronesi U, Salvadori B, Luini A, et al. Conservative treatment of early breast cancer. Long-term results of 1232 cases treated with quadrantectomy, axillary dissection, and radiotherapy. *Ann Surg* 1990;211(3): 250–259.
302. Hill-Kayser CE, Harris EE, Hwang WT, et al. Twenty-year incidence and patterns of contralateral breast cancer after breast conservation treatment with radiation. *Int J Radiat Oncol Biol Phys* 2006;66(5):1313–1319.
303. Javaid M, Song F, Leinster S, et al. Radiation effects on the cosmetic outcomes of immediate and delayed autologous breast reconstruction: an argument about timing. *J Plast Reconstr Aesthet Surg* 2006;59(1):16–26.
304. Hurria A, Hudis C. Follow-up care of breast cancer survivors. *Crit Rev Oncol Hematol* 2003;48(1):89–99.
305. Kattlove H, Winn RJ. Ongoing care of patients after primary treatment for their cancer. *CA Cancer J Clin* 2003;53(3):172–196.
306. Telli ML, Hunt SA, Carlson RW, et al. Trastuzumab-related cardiotoxicity: calling into question the concept of reversibility. *J Clin Oncol* 2007;25(23): 3525–3533.
307. Greenspan SL, Bhattacharya RK, Sereika SM, et al. Prevention of bone loss in survivors of breast cancer: a randomized, double-blind, placebo-controlled clinical trial. *J Clin Endocrinol Metab* 2007;92(1):131–136.
308. Burstein HJ. Aromatase inhibitor-associated arthralgia syndrome. *Breast* 2007;16(3):223–234.
309. McCormick B, Yahalom J, Cox L, et al. The patients perception of her breast following radiation and limited surgery. *Int J Radiat Oncol Biol Phys* 1989;17(6):1299–1302.
310. Recht A, Come SE, Henderson IC, et al. The sequencing of chemotherapy and radiation therapy after conservative surgery for early-stage breast cancer. *N Engl J Med* 1996;334(21):1356–1361.
311. Harris JR, Levene MB, Svensson G, et al. Analysis of cosmetic results following primary radiation therapy for stages I and II carcinoma of the breast. *Int J Radiat Oncol Biol Phys* 1979;5(2):257–261.
312. Veronesi U, Luini A, Galimberti V, et al. Conservation approaches for the management of stage I/II carcinoma of the breast: Milan Cancer Institute trials. *World J Surg* 1994;18(1):70–75.
313. Wazer DE, DiPetrillo T, Schmidt-Ullrich R, et al. Factors influencing cosmetic outcome and complication risk after conservative surgery and radiotherapy for early-stage breast carcinoma. *J Clin Oncol* 1992;10(3):356–363.
314. Abner AL, Recht A, Vicini FA, et al. Cosmetic results after surgery, chemotherapy, and radiation therapy for early breast cancer. *Int J Radiat Oncol Biol Phys* 1991;21(2):331–338.
315. Pezner RD, Patterson MP, Hill LR, et al. Breast edema in patients treated conservatively for stage I and II breast cancer. *Int J Radiat Oncol Biol Phys* 1985;11(10):1765–1768.
316. Kuske RR. Breast conservation therapy: the radiation oncologist's perspective. *Clin Obstet Gynecol* 1989;32(4):819–829.
317. Beadle GF, Come S, Henderson IC, et al. The effect of adjuvant chemotherapy on the cosmetic results after primary radiation treatment for early stage breast cancer. *Int J Radiat Oncol Biol Phys* 1984;10(11):2131–2137.
318. Ray GR, Fish VJ. Biopsy and definitive radiation therapy in stage I and II adenocarcinoma of the female breast: analysis of cosmesis and the role of electron beam supplementation. *Int J Radiat Oncol Biol Phys* 1983; 9(6):813–818.
319. Clarke D, Martinez A, Cox RS, et al. Breast edema following staging axillary node dissection in patients with breast carcinoma treated by radical radiotherapy. *Cancer* 1982;49(11):2295–2299.
320. Montague ED, Paulus DD, Schell SR. Selection and follow-up of patients for conservation surgery and irradiation. *Front Radiat Ther Oncol* 1983;17:124–130.
321. Delouche G, Bachelot F, Premont M, et al. Conservation treatment of early breast cancer: long term results and complications. *Int J Radiat Oncol Biol Phys* 1987;13(1):29–34.
322. Larson D, Weinstein M, Goldberg I, et al. Edema of the arm as a function of the extent of axillary surgery in patients with stage I-II carcinoma of the breast treated with primary radiotherapy. *Int J Radiat Oncol Biol Phys* 1986;12(9):1575–1582.
323. Kissin MW, Querci della Rovere G, Easton D, et al. Risk of lymphoedema following the treatment of breast cancer. *Br J Surg* 1986;73(7):580–584.
324. Borup Christensen S, Lundgren E. Sequelae of axillary dissection vs. axillary sampling with or without irradiation for breast cancer. A randomized trial. *Acta Chir Scand* 1989;155(10):515–519.
325. Kaufman J, Gunn W, Hartz AJ, et al. The pathophysiologic and roentgenologic effects of chest irradiation in breast carcinoma. *Int J Radiat Oncol Biol Phys* 1986;12(6):887–893.
326. Lingos TI, Recht A, Vicini F, et al. Radiation pneumonitis in breast cancer patients treated with conservative surgery and radiation therapy. *Int J Radiat Oncol Biol Phys* 1991;21(2):355–360.
327. Jackson A, Kutcher GJ, Yorke ED. Probability of radiation-induced complications for normal tissues with parallel architecture subject to non-uniform irradiation. *Med Phys* 1993;20(3):613–625.
328. Neal AJ, Yarnold JR. Estimating the volume of lung irradiated during tangential breast irradiation using the central lung distance. *Br J Radiol* 1995;68(813):1004–1008.
329. Bornstein BA, Cheng CW, Rhodes LM, et al. Can simulation measurements be used to predict the irradiated lung volume in the tangential fields in patients treated for breast cancer? *Int J Radiat Oncol Biol Phys* 1990;18(1):181–187.
330. Koc M, Polat P, Suma S. Effects of tamoxifen on pulmonary fibrosis after cobalt-60 radiotherapy in breast cancer patients. *Radiother Oncol* 2002;64(2):171–175.
331. Bentzen SM, Skoczylas JZ, Overgaard M, et al. Radiotherapy-related lung fibrosis enhanced by tamoxifen. *J Natl Cancer Inst* 1996;88(13):918–922.
332. Fowble B, Fein DA, Hanlon AL, et al. The impact of tamoxifen on breast recurrence, cosmesis, complications, and survival in estrogen receptor-positive early-stage breast cancer. *Int J Radiat Oncol Biol Phys* 1996;35(4):669–677.
333. Valagussa P, Zambetti M, Biasi S, et al. Cardiac effects following adjuvant chemotherapy and breast irradiation in operable breast cancer. *Ann Oncol* 1994;5(3):209–216.
334. Rutqvist LE, Johansson H. Long-term follow-up of the randomized Stockholm trial on adjuvant tamoxifen among postmenopausal patients with early stage breast cancer. *Acta Oncol* 2007;46(2):133–145.
335. Nixon AJ, Manola J, Gelman R, et al. No long-term increase in cardiac-related mortality after breast-conserving surgery and radiation therapy using modern techniques. *J Clin Oncol* 1998;16(4):1374–1379.
336. Gyenes G, Rutqvist LE, Liedberg A, et al. Long-term cardiac morbidity and mortality in a randomized trial of pre- and postoperative radiation therapy versus surgery alone in primary breast cancer. *Radiother Oncol* 1998;48(2):185–190.
337. Pierce SM, Recht A, Lingos TI, et al. Long-term radiation complications following conservative surgery (CS) and radiation therapy (RT) in patients

with early stage breast cancer. *Int J Radiat Oncol Biol Phys* 1992; 23(5):915–923.
338. Partridge AH, Ruddy KJ. Fertility and adjuvant treatment in young women with breast cancer. *Breast* 2007;16(Suppl 2):S175–S181.
339. Sankila R, Heinavaara S, Hakulinen T. Survival of breast cancer patients after subsequent term pregnancy: "healthy mother effect." *Am J Obstet Gynecol* 1994;170(3):818–823.
340. von Schoultz E, Johansson H, Wilking N, et al. Influence of prior and subsequent pregnancy on breast cancer prognosis. *J Clin Oncol* 1995;13(2): 430–434.
341. Petrek JA. Pregnancy safety after breast cancer. *Cancer* 1994;74(1 Suppl): 528–531.
342. Gemignani ML, Petrek JA. Pregnancy after breast cancer. *Cancer Control* 1999;6(3):272–276.
343. Higgins S, Haffty BG. Pregnancy and lactation after breast-conserving therapy for early stage breast cancer. *Cancer* 1994;73(8):2175–2180.
344. Thewes B, Meiser B, Taylor A, et al. Fertility- and menopause-related information needs of younger women with a diagnosis of early breast cancer. *J Clin Oncol* 2005;23(22):5155–5165.
345. Duffy CM, Allen SM, Clark MA. Discussions regarding reproductive health for young women with breast cancer undergoing chemotherapy. *J Clin Oncol* 2005;23(4):766–773.
346. Lee SJ, Schover LR, Partridge AH, et al. American Society of Clinical Oncology recommendations on fertility preservation in cancer patients. *J Clin Oncol* 2006;24(18):2917–2931.
347. Madrigrano A, Westphal L, Wapnir I. Egg retrieval with cryopreservation does not delay breast cancer treatment. *Am J Surg* 2007;194(4):477–481.
348. Loibl S, von Minckwitz G, Gwyn K, et al. Breast carcinoma during pregnancy. International recommendations from an expert meeting. *Cancer* 2006;106(2):237–246.
349. Merkel DE. Pregnancy and breast cancer. *Semin Surg Oncol* 1996;12(5): 370–375.
350. Ries L, Eisner M, Kosary C, et al. SEER Cancer Statistics Review, 1975–2002. NCI; 2005.
351. Streffer C, Shore R, Konermann G, et al. Biological effects after prenatal irradiation (embryo and fetus). A report of the International Commission on Radiological Protection. *Ann ICRP* 2003;33(1–2):5–206.
352. Yang WT, Dryden MJ, Gwyn K, et al. Imaging of breast cancer diagnosed and treated with chemotherapy during pregnancy. *Radiology* 2006;239(1): 52–60.
353. Schackmuth E, Harlow C, Norton L. Milk fistula: a complication after core breast biopsy. *AJR Am J Roentgenol* 1993;161:961–962.
354. White TT. Carcinoma of the breast and pregnancy. *Ann Surg* 1923; 1954(139):9.
355. Kilgore AR, Bloodgood IC. Tumors and tumor-like lesions of the breast in association with pregnancy. *Arch Surg* 1929;18:2079.
356. Haagensen C, Stout A. Carcinoma of the breast. *Ann Surg* 1943;118: 859–870.
357. Ishida T, Yokoe T, Kasumi F, et al. Clinicopathologic characteristics and prognosis of breast cancer patients associated with pregnancy and lactation: analysis of case-control study in Japan. *Jpn J Cancer Res* 1992;83(11): 1143–1149.
358. Middleton LP, Amin M, Gwyn K, et al. Breast carcinoma in pregnant women: assessment of clinicopathologic and immunohistochemical features. *Cancer* 2003;98(5):1055–1060.
359. Reed W, Sandstad B, Holm R, et al. The prognostic impact of hormone receptors and c-erbB-2 in pregnancy-associated breast cancer and their correlation with *BRCA1* and cell cycle modulators. *Int J Surg Pathol* 2003;11(2):65–74.
360. Elledge RM, Ciocca DR, Langone G, et al. Estrogen receptor, progesterone receptor, and HER-2/neu protein in breast cancers from pregnant patients. *Cancer* 1993;71(8):2499–2506.
361. Pandit-Taskar N, Dauer LT, Montgomery L, et al. Organ and fetal absorbed dose estimates from 99mTc-sulfur colloid lymphoscintigraphy and sentinel node localization in breast cancer patients. *J Nucl Med* 2006;47(7): 1202–1208.
362. Keleher A, Wendt R 3rd, Delpassand E, et al. The safety of lymphatic mapping in pregnant breast cancer patients using Tc-99m sulfur colloid. *Breast J* 2004;10(6):492–495.
363. Nicklas AH, Baker ME. Imaging strategies in the pregnant cancer patient. *Semin Oncol* 2000;27(6):623–632.
364. Kidd SA, Lancaster PA, Anderson JC, et al. Fetal death after exposure to methylene blue dye during mid-trimester amniocentesis in twin pregnancy. *Prenat Diagn* 1996;16(1):39–47.
365. Gluer S. Intestinal atresia following intraamniotic use of dyes. *Eur J Pediatr Surg* 1995;5(4):240–242.
366. McEnerney JK, McEnerney LN. Unfavorable neonatal outcome after intraamniotic injection of methylene blue. *Obstet Gynecol* 1983;61 (3 Suppl):35S–37S.
367. Cragan JD. Teratogen update: methylene blue. *Teratology* 1999;60(1): 42–48.
368. Kal HB, Struikmans H. Radiotherapy during pregnancy: fact and fiction. *Lancet Oncol* 2005;6(5):328–333.
369. Ring AE, Smith IE, Jones A, et al. Chemotherapy for breast cancer during pregnancy: an 18-year experience from five London teaching hospitals. *J Clin Oncol* 2005;23(18):4192–4197.
370. Kalter H, Warkany J. Medical progress. Congenital malformations: etiologic factors and their role in prevention (first of two parts). *N Engl J Med* 1983;308(8):424–431.
371. Hahn KM, Johnson PH, Gordon N, et al. Treatment of pregnant breast cancer patients and outcomes of children exposed to chemotherapy *in utero*. *Cancer* 2006;107(6):1219–1226.
372. Berry DL, Theriault RL, Holmes FA, et al. Management of breast cancer during pregnancy using a standardized protocol. *J Clin Oncol* 1999;17(3):855–861.
373. Meyer-Wittkopf M, Barth H, Emons G, et al. Fetal cardiac effects of doxorubicin therapy for carcinoma of the breast during pregnancy: case report and review of the literature. *Ultrasound Obstet Gynecol* 2001; 18(1):62–66.
374. Aviles A, Neri N. Hematological malignancies and pregnancy: a final report of 84 children who received chemotherapy *in utero*. *Clin Lymphoma* 2001;2(3):173–177.
375. Barthelmes L, Gateley CA. Tamoxifen and pregnancy. *Breast* 2004;13(6):446–451.
376. Lavelle K, Todd C, Moran A, et al. Non-standard management of breast cancer increases with age in the UK: a population based cohort of women > or =65 years. *Br J Cancer* 2007; 96(8):1197–1203.
377. Hebert-Croteau N, Brisson J, Latreille J, et al. Compliance with consensus recommendations for the treatment of early stage breast carcinoma in elderly women. *Cancer* 1999;85(5):1104–1113.
378. Kemeny MM, Peterson BL, Kornblith AB, et al. Barriers to clinical trial participation by older women with breast cancer. *J Clin Oncol* 2003;21(12): 2268–2275.
379. Host H, Lund E. Age as a prognostic factor in breast cancer. *Cancer* 1986;57(11):2217–2221.
380. Holli K, Isola J. Effect of age on the survival of breast cancer patients. *Eur J Cancer* 1997;33(3):425–428.
381. Daidone MG, Silvestrini R. Prognostic and predictive role of proliferation indices in adjuvant therapy of breast cancer. *J Natl Cancer Inst Monogr* 2001(30):27–35.
382. Molino A, Giovannini M, Auriemma A, et al. Pathological, biological and clinical characteristics, and surgical management, of elderly women with breast cancer. *Crit Rev Oncol Hematol* 2006;59(3):226–233.
383. Ramesh HS, Pope D, Gennari R, et al. Optimising surgical management of elderly cancer patients. *World J Surg Oncol* 2005;3(1):17.
384. Rudenstam CM, Zahrieh D, Forbes JF, et al. Randomized trial comparing axillary clearance versus no axillary clearance in older patients with breast cancer: first results of International Breast Cancer Study Group Trial 10-93. *J Clin Oncol* 2006;24(3):337–344.
385. McMahon LE, Gray RJ, Pockaj BA. Is breast cancer sentinel lymph node mapping valuable for patients in their seventies and beyond? *Am J Surg* 2005;190(3):366–370.
386. Gazet JC, Ford HT, Coombes RC, et al. Prospective randomized trial of tamoxifen vs surgery in elderly patients with breast cancer. *Eur J Surg Oncol* 1994;20(3):207–214.
387. Bates T, Riley DL, Houghton J, et al. Breast cancer in elderly women: a Cancer Research Campaign trial comparing treatment with tamoxifen and optimal surgery with tamoxifen alone. The Elderly Breast Cancer Working Party. *Br J Surg* 1991;78(5):591–594.
388. Mustacchi G, Ceccherini R, Milani S, et al. Tamoxifen alone versus adjuvant tamoxifen for operable breast cancer of the elderly: long-term results of the phase III randomized controlled multicenter GRETA trial. *Ann Oncol* 2003;14(3):414–420.
389. Hind D, Wyld L, Beverley CB, et al. Surgery versus primary endocrine therapy for operable breast cancer in elderly women (70 years plus). The Cochrane Collaboration, Cochrane reviews, 2007. http://www.cochrane.org/reviews/en/ab004272.html. Accessed October 3, 2007.
390. Crivellari D, Aapro M, Leonard R, et al. Breast cancer in the elderly. *J Clin Oncol* 2007;25(14):1882–1890.
391. Muss HB. Adjuvant treatment of elderly breast cancer patients. *Breast* 2007;16(Suppl 2):S159–S165.
392. Newman LA, Martin IK. Disparities in breast cancer. *Curr Probl Cancer* 2007;31(3):134–156.
393. Field TS, Buist DS, Doubeni C, et al. Disparities and survival among breast cancer patients. *J Natl Cancer Inst Monogr* 2005(35):88–95.
394. Jatoi I, Becher H, Leake CR. Widening disparity in survival between white and African-American patients with breast carcinoma treated in the U.S. Department of Defense Healthcare system. *Cancer* 2003;98(5): 894–899.
395. Elledge RM, Clark GM, Chamness GC, et al. Tumor biologic factors and breast cancer prognosis among white, Hispanic, and black women in the United States. *J Natl Cancer Inst* 1994;86(9):705–712.
396. Eley JW, Hill HA, Chen VW, et al. Racial differences in survival from breast cancer. Results of the National Cancer Institute Black/White Cancer Survival Study. *JAMA* 1994;272(12):947–954.
397. Pathak DR, Osuch JR, He J. Breast carcinoma etiology: current knowledge and new insights into the effects of reproductive and hormonal risk factors in black and white populations. *Cancer* 2000;88(5 Suppl):1230–1238.
398. Li CI, Malone KE, Daling JR. Differences in breast cancer hormone receptor status and histology by race and ethnicity among women 50 years of age and older. *Cancer Epidemiol Biomarkers Prev* 2002;11(7): 601–607.

399. Middleton LP, Chen V, Perkins GH, et al. Histopathology of breast cancer among African-American women. *Cancer* 2003;97(1 Suppl):253–257.
400. Joslyn SA, Foote ML, Nasseri K, et al. Racial and ethnic disparities in breast cancer rates by age: NAACCR Breast Cancer Project. *Breast Cancer Res Treat* 2005;92(2):97–105.
401. Carey LA, Dees EC, Sawyer L, et al. The triple negative paradox: primary tumor chemosensitivity of breast cancer subtypes. *Clin Cancer Res* 2007;13(8):2329–2334.
402. White J, Morrow M, Moughan J, et al. Compliance with breast-conservation standards for patients with early-stage breast carcinoma. *Cancer* 2003;97(4):893–904.
403. Bickell NA, Wang JJ, Oluwole S, et al. Missed opportunities: racial disparities in adjuvant breast cancer treatment. *J Clin Oncol* 2006;24(9):1357–1362.
404. Tseng JF, Kronowitz SJ, Sun CC, et al. The effect of ethnicity on immediate reconstruction rates after mastectomy for breast cancer. *Cancer* 2004;101(7):1514–1523.
405. Morrow M, Scott SK, Menck HR, et al. Factors influencing the use of breast reconstruction postmastectomy: a National Cancer Database study. *J Am Coll Surg* 2001;192(1):1–8.
406. Maggard MA, Lane KE, O'Connell JB, et al. Beyond the clinical trials: How often is sentinel lymph node dissection performed for breast cancer? *Ann Surg Oncol* 2005;12(1):41–47.
407. Adams-Campbell LL, Ahaghotu C, Gaskins M, et al. Enrollment of African Americans onto clinical treatment trials: study design barriers. *J Clin Oncol* 2004;22(4):730–734.
408. van der Ploeg IM, van Esser S, van den Bosch MA, et al. Radiofrequency ablation for breast cancer: a review of the literature. *Eur J Surg Oncol* 2007;33(6):673–677.
409. Gass JS. Future of breast surgery. *Med Health R I* 2005;88(10):357–358.
410. Tafra L, Fine R, Whitworth P, et al. Prospective randomized study comparing cryo-assisted and needle-wire localization of ultrasound-visible breast tumors. *Am J Surg* 2006;192(4):462–470.
411. Miller KD, Chap LI, Holmes FA, et al. Randomized phase III trial of capecitabine compared with bevacizumab plus capecitabine in patients with previously treated metastatic breast cancer. *J Clin Oncol* 2005;23(4):792–799.
412. Sledge GW, Rugo HS, Burstein HJ. The role of angiogenesis inhibition in the treatment of breast cancer. *Clin Adv Hematol Oncol* 2006;4 Suppl 21(10):1–12.
413. Cristofanilli M, Budd GT, Ellis MJ, et al. Circulating tumor cells, disease progression, and survival in metastatic breast cancer. *N Engl J Med* 2004;351(8):781–791.
414. Budd GT, Cristofanilli M, Ellis MJ, et al. Circulating tumor cells versus imaging—predicting overall survival in metastatic breast cancer. *Clin Cancer Res* 2006;12(21):6403–6409.
415. Liljegren G, Holmberg L, Bergh J, et al. 10-Year results after sector resection with or without postoperative radiotherapy for stage I breast cancer: a randomized trial. *J Clin Oncol* 1999;17(8):2326–2333.
416. Clark RM, McCulloch PB, Levine MN, et al. Randomized clinical trial to assess the effectiveness of breast irradiation following lumpectomy and axillary dissection for node-negative breast cancer. *J Natl Cancer Inst* 1992;84(9):683–689.
417. Consensus statement for accelerated partial breast irradiation. http://www.breastsurgeons.org/officialstmts/officialstmt3.shtml. Accessed October 10, 2007.
418. Perera F, Engel J, Holliday R, et al. Local resection and brachytherapy confined to the lumpectomy site for early breast cancer: a pilot study. *J Surg Oncol* 1997;65(4):263–267; discussion 267–268.
419. King TA, Bolton JS, Kuske RR, et al. Long-term results of wide-field brachytherapy as the sole method of radiation therapy after segmental mastectomy for T(is,1,2) breast cancer. *Am J Surg* 2000;180(4):299–304.
420. Vicini FA, Remouchamps V, Wallace M, et al. Ongoing clinical experience utilizing 3D conformal external beam radiotherapy to deliver partial-breast irradiation in patients with early-stage breast cancer treated with breast-conserving therapy. *Int J Radiat Oncol Biol Phys* 2003;57(5):1247–1253.
421. Arthur DW, Vicini FA. Accelerated partial breast irradiation as a part of breast conservation therapy. *J Clin Oncol* 2005;23(8):1726–1735.
422. Keisch M, Vicini F, Kuske RR, et al. Initial clinical experience with the MammoSite breast brachytherapy applicator in women with early-stage breast cancer treated with breast-conserving therapy. *Int J Radiat Oncol Biol Phys* 2003;55(2):289–293.
423. Baglan KL, Sharpe MB, Jaffray D, et al. Accelerated partial breast irradiation using 3D conformal radiation therapy (3D-CRT). *Int J Radiat Oncol Biol Phys* 2003;55(2):302–311.
424. Goss PE, Ingle JN, Martino S, et al. Efficacy of letrozole extended adjuvant therapy according to estrogen receptor and progesterone receptor status of the primary tumor: National Cancer Institute of Canada Clinical Trials Group MA.17. *J Clin Oncol* 2007;25(15):2006–2011.
425. Bear HD, Anderson S, Smith RE, et al. Sequential preoperative or postoperative docetaxel added to preoperative doxorubicin plus cyclophosphamide for operable breast cancer: National Surgical Adjuvant Breast and Bowel Project Protocol B-27. *J Clin Oncol* 2006;24(13):2019–2027.
426. Smith IC, Heys SD, Hutcheon AW, et al. Neoadjuvant chemotherapy in breast cancer: significantly enhanced response with docetaxel. *J Clin Oncol* 2002;20(6):1456–1466.

SPECIAL MANAGEMENT TOPICS

CHAPTER 30 ■ MANAGEMENT OF INFECTIONS IN PATIENTS WITH GYNECOLOGIC MALIGNANCY

AMAR SAFDAR AND ISSAM I. RAAD

Patients with gynecologic cancer are susceptible to local and systemic infection. The risk of developing an infection can arise from a number of factors such as (a) tumor encroachment and invasion of adjacent structures; (b) tumor necrosis; (c) complications arising from antineoplastic chemotherapy; (d) early and late effects of abdominopelvic radiation therapy; (e) surgical tumor excision and removal of internal organs; (f) structural abnormalities resulting from surgical diversion procedures; and (g) other causes that disrupt protective barriers in the lower and upper female reproductive tract (1,2).

The spectrum of causative organisms most frequently arises from patients' endogenous microflora. The vagina, lower urinary tract, and intestinal tract colonization with bacteria and yeast serve as important sources for infection. The normal aerobic and anaerobic vaginal bacterial flora may be altered in patients undergoing antineoplastic therapy. Among factors that influence changes in colonization are hormonal dysfunction, frequent exposure to broad-spectrum antimicrobial agents, antineoplastic therapy, hospitalization, and instrumentization. In a recent report, however, patients receiving external-beam radiotherapy for gynecologic malignancy did not experience changes in aerobic microflora in the vagina, cervix, or rectum (3,4). Whereas a significant growth in vaginal yeasts occurred during the first 2 weeks of radiation therapy mostly due to *Candida albicans* and *Candida tropicalis*, the increase of growth in *Candida* species returned to preradiation levels after 4 weeks (5). Exposure to health care facilities, especially centers that care for immunosuppressed cancer patients, has been recognized as a major influence in promoting change in cutaneous, orointestinal, and genitourinary microflora. The changes in vaginal and lower urinary tract microflora occur less commonly, even in patients following repeat exposure to the hospital environment, and are often limited to patients who undergo instrumentization. The health care–associated organisms are often less susceptible to commonly prescribed antibiotics and may lead to severe disease. It is, however, important to appreciate that changes in a host's microflora are in most cases transient and restitution of normal intestinal and vaginal flora occurs once factors promoting the change have been removed.

The female genital tract is rich in anaerobic microflora. Bacteria belonging to *Peptococcaceae* are the most prominent organisms in the normal vaginal flora. Quantitative vaginal cultures in recent studies showed that anaerobic bacteria outnumbered aerobic bacteria by nearly 10:1; peptococci, *Lactobacillus*, *Corynebacterium*, *Eubacterium*, and *Bacteroides* species are common organisms isolated (6). *Escherichia coli*, *Klebsiella* species, and *Enterobacter* species are the aerobic gram negatives and streptococci, enterococci, and coagulase-negative staphylococcus are gram-positive bacteria isolated from the lower female genital tract. These organisms provide an important reference to local and invasive infections seen in patients undergoing treatment for gynecologic malignancy.

In this chapter we provide an overview of infections encountered in patients receiving treatment for cancers involving the female reproductive system. A detailed review of specific diseases such as postsurgical abdominopelvic infections, febrile neutropenia, and bacteremia is presented. A focused discussion regarding the changing epidemiology of causative organisms, the increasing rate of infection due to drug-resistant organisms, and an update on new antimicrobial agents is briefly discussed.

PATIENTS WITH FEVER

The factors that increase the risk for infection are shown in Table 30.1. Knowledge of underlying predisposing factor(s) is necessary in the selection of appropriate empiric therapy. Antibiotic prophylaxis and/or recent treatment with broad-spectrum antimicrobials increase the risk of breakthrough infection due to less-drug-susceptible organisms and systemic candidiasis. Awareness of specific cancer-therapy associated risks and the host's underlying immune dysfunction may allow for proper selection of empiric antibiotic therapy in critically ill patients prior to the results of microbiologic culture and radiographic studies becoming available. It is important to note that patients with gynecologic cancer may have a high risk of polymicrobial infections due to the anatomic proximity to the lower intestinal and urinary tracts. In certain infections, such as deep-tissue abscess, cellulitis in patients with chronic fistula tract, presence of large necrotic tumor, and history of multiple instrumentization, the probability of polymicrobial infection remains high (7). Furthermore, patients with a known anaerobic bloodstream infection have a high probability of concurrent bacteremia due to aerobic organism(s) (7). Patients with advanced cancer and history of radiation therapy may develop obstruction to the pelvic venous and lymphatic flow, which increases the risk for cellulitis, abscess formation, and septic thrombophlebitis.

TUMOR RELATED

The tumor-associated infections are dependent on the site and extent of tumor involvement. In patients with an early stage of locally involved cancer such as stage I cervical cancer, most

TABLE 30.1

PREDISPOSING RISK FACTORS AND INFECTIONS IN PATIENTS WITH GYNECOLOGIC TUMOR

TUMOR RELATED	Septic deep thrombophelibitis
Obstruction of gastrointestinal or urinary tract	Fasciitis, myositis, and gas gangrene are rare complications
Erosion into bowel, urinary tract, peritoneum, or retroperitoneal	
Necrosis of rapidly growing cancer promotes abscess formation	**CHEMOTHERAPY**
Lymphatic obstruction	Febrile neutropenia
	Pneumonia
SURGERY	Neutropenic enterocolitis
Aspiration pneumonia	
Hospital-acquired pneumonia, including ventilator-associated pneumonia	**RADIATION THERAPY**
Wound infection; skin, and skin structure infection	Enteritis
Tissue necrosis due to disruption of blood supply	Urinary tract infection
Infected hematoma	Poor wound healing
Fistula tract communication between intestinal and urinary tracts	
Complicated peritonitis	**CATHETER AND IMPLANTABLE DEVICES**
	Device infection
	Peritonitis
	Bloodstream infection
	Urinary tract infection

infections remain localized to the vagina. Whereas in patients with advanced cervical cancer infections may involve the fallopian tubes or ovaries, leading to tubo-ovarian abscess, uterine involvement may cause less frequently seen pyometra. Extension of these infections to adjacent structures such as the urinary tract presents as ascending pyelonephritis, rectal abscess, and complicated peritonitis, which are serious and difficult-to-treat infections (8,9). It is also important to note that an infection may be the primary presentation of an undiagnosed malignancy involving the female reproductive tract. In a study of postmenopausal women who presented with tubo-ovarian abscess, nearly half of these patients were subsequently diagnosed with a gynecologic malignancy (10). Therefore, a thorough investigation for possible underlying cancer should be considered in postmenopausal women or those with no risk factors for sexually transmitted diseases who present with tubo-ovarian abscess or pyometra.

In a large study conducted at the M. D. Anderson Cancer Center, septicemia, pneumonia, and peritonitis in patients with gynecologic cancer were associated with high infection-associated mortality (11). In the last 2 decades, with early diagnosis, identification of factors associated with poor prognosis, empiric antimicrobial therapy in patients at high risk of infection, advances in antineoplastic and radiation therapy, and surgical techniques have substantially improved outcomes in these patients. The advances in improved outcomes for serious systemic bacterial and yeast infections are in most part due to the availability of well-tolerated broad-spectrum antimicrobial agents. The recent emergence and spread of multidrug-resistant (MDR) organisms, however, may abrogate these advances, and even patients with solid-organ cancer with limited immune suppression may develop life-threatening septicemia, pneumonia, and peritonitis as was noted during the 1970s (11).

SURGERY RELATED

Patients undergoing surgery for cervical cancer have a higher rate of infectious complications, while patients with endometrial cancer tolerate surgery better and have fewer infections during the early and late postoperative period (12). Pelvic exenteration is performed in patients with advanced and/or treatment refractory cervical and upper reproductive tract malignancy. Infections remain as serious morbidity following pelvic exenteration; early postsurgical wound infection and wound dehiscence are not uncommon (13,14). Urinary tract infections are also frequently seen in patients with urinary fistula and/or those who develop urethral obstruction. Studies show that greater than 40% of patients undergoing pelvic exenteration for gynecologic and rectal cancer had urinary tract infection and wound dehiscence (13). Late infections such as ascending pyelonephritis may be serious, as these infections are often recurrent and seen in patients with usually irreparable structural damage to the urinary reservoir, urethral stenosis, and anastomosis obstruction. Ureterointestinal fistula, stones in the urinary reservoir, and stenosis all contribute to increased risk of infections, and unless the anatomical abnormality is corrected, these patients remain at increased risk for recurrent urinary tract infections and complications arising from prolonged systemic antibiotic therapy and hospitalization. Empiric therapy includes adequate coverage for possible polymicrobial infection, and the choice should include drugs that provide adequate coverage for enteric coliforms, enterococci, including vancomycin-resistant *Enterococcus* species, especially in patients with known prior intestinal or genitourinary tract colonization due to these drug-resistant bacteria (15). As most infections in this setting may also have an anaerobe as a co-pathogen, even in patients with negative microbiologic evidence of anaerobic infection, antibiotic selection should entertain non-representational negative anaerobic culture results. We recommend secondary suppressive antimicrobial therapy in patients with recurrent deep pelvic infection to reduce morbidity and subsequent hospitalization and surgeries. It is critical to select high-risk patients judiciously so patients are not given prolonged courses of broad-spectrum antibiotics, which is the single most important factor in promoting drug resistance in health care–associated infections.

Infections remain the main concern in patients following radical vulvar resection and inguinal lymphadenectomy. Early postoperative cellulitis is noted in nearly one third of patients undergoing inguinal lymphadenectomy, and in over 20% early surgical wound breakdown also occurred (16). Late surgery-site cellulitis was noted in patients with chronic lymphedema, and in most patients the surgical wound was not compromised (16).

Wound Infection

Infected surgical wounds in patients following female genital tract surgery include *Staphylococcus aureus*, including multidrug-resistant strains (MRSA) obtained from health care microflora (health care associated; HA) or community acquired (CA)-MRSA, which has now become the leading source of MRSA in the United States. *Streptococcus* species (group A, B, C, and G) are also common pathogens in this population and nearly one third of infections, especially those with involvement of the lower intestinal tract and urinary tract, are less likely to be monomicrobial.

In certain subpopulations of patients who have been receiving systemic corticosteroids for extended periods, patients with morbid obesity, and those with poorly controlled diabetes mellitus have a higher risk of developing postoperative wound infections. Coagulase-negative *Staphylococcus*, *Streptococcus* species, *S. aureus*, enteric gram-negative bacteria, and *Bacteroides* species are potential pathogens.

Patients who have a complicated hospital course following surgery may develop infections due to organisms acquired from the health care microenvironment. In critically ill patients infections are treated empirically, and the spectrum of causative organism(s) may not be available at the time of medical decision making. Knowledge of regional and institutional prevalence of drug-resistant organisms is required in prescribing an appropriate treatment regimen. The empiric therapy in patients with prolonged hospitalization and anatomic abnormalities such as enterouretheral, entero- or rectovaginal, or enterovesicular fistula increases the probability of recurrent infection due to resistant HA–gram-negative bacteria such as *Pseudomonas* species, extended-spectrum beta-lactamases-producing *Enterobacteriaceae*, including *E. coli*. Other nonfermentative gram-negative bacteria like *Acinetobacter* spp. and *Stenotrophomonas maltophilia* are often resistant to a wide spectrum of commonly used antibiotics, and treatment for these MDR bacteria remains a daunting task (17,18).

Intra-abdominal and Pelvic Abscess

An infected collection within the peritoneal cavity may develop as a consequence of instrumentization, and breach in the physical barriers may also occur in patients with necrotizing tumors. The secondary seeding of the intraperitoneal tumor mass in patients with bloodstream infection arising from a different primary source, such as the urinary tract, or antineoplastic therapy–induced orointestinal mucositis may also occur. The spectrum of causative organisms includes enteric bacteria such as *E. coli*, *Enterococcus*, *Staphylococcus* species, *Bacteroides*, and other anaerobes. *Candida* species infection is less frequent in non-neutropenic patients, although patients with high yeast counts in multiple body sites, exposure to prolonged broad-spectrum antibiotics, poorly controlled diabetes mellitus, systemic corticosteroid use, as well as stay in critical care units and presence of foreign devices may increase the risk for invasive candidiasis.

Hematogenous or direct seeding of the retroperitoneal space may lead to paraspinal and psoas abscess; these infections escape early detection as patients may not have high-grade fever, and increase in chronic low back pain remains subject to interpretation. In the absence of a direct extension from the intestinal or urinary tract, these retroperitoneal infections are usually monomicrobial, and diagnosis requires prompt aspiration of the infected collection. In tuberculosis endemic regions, *Mycobacterium tuberculosis* must be considered in determining the etiology of these infections, especially in patients in whom the vertebral column is involved.

Pelvic abscesses that develop after instrumentization or following surgery are often polymicrobial and treatment is directed toward normal intestinal tract and cutaneous microflora.

Peritoneal infections following bowel perforation, anastomotic leaks, or fistula tracts may present with fever, abdominal pain, and fistula drainage and/or surgical wound dehiscence. Most infections, as expected, are polymicrobial and *Enterobacteriaceae*, *S. aureus*, *Streptococcus*, and *Enterococcus* species including vancomycin-resistant strains are frequently encountered. *Bacteroides fragilis* and *Clostridium* species are common anaerobes; *Fusobacterium*, *Peptostreptococcus*, and *Eubacterium* occur less frequently. Patients with peritoneal infections following surgery involving the nonsterile bowel and lower genitourinary tract may also have an increased risk for *Pseudomonas* species infection.

CHEMOTHERAPY AND RADIATION RELATED

Patients receiving chemotherapy may have an increased risk of infection; neutropenia for less than a week increases risk for systemic bacterial infections due to *S. aureus* and *Pseudomonas* species. Patients who remain neutropenic for longer than 5 days are also at an increased risk for developing systemic *Candida* species infection (1,2). Disruption of orointestinal and genitourinary tract mucosa compromises an important barrier in the prevention of bacterial and yeast invasion. In patients with severe treatment-induced mucositis, alpha hemolytic streptococcal and anaerobic septicemia may lead to devastating consequences (19).

Radiation therapy in patients with vulvar, vaginal, and cervical cancer causes microvascular damage to the tissue and may lead to difficult-to-treat intestinal, vaginal, and urologic complications.

Increased doses of radiation for gynecologic cancer have been associated with improved cancer-free survival (20). However, with increased radiation dose, the rate of complications has also risen (21). Noninfectious complications arising from high-dose radiotherapy include tissue and bone necrosis, fistula formation, enteritis, and fibrosis that may lead to vaginal, rectal, and ureteric stenosis, and increased risk for secondary infection due to stagnation and inadequate physiologic drainage (22). In rare cases, patients with radiation-induced necrosis of pelvic bones may present with osteomyelitis; for these patients, a challenging and multifaceted treatment approach may be needed for successful outcomes (23). A patient with osteomyelitis in the setting of radiation-induced bone necrosis may need surgical debridement and an appropriate selection of antibiotics for a prolonged period. A high clinical suspicion remains critical in the timely diagnosis of radiation-related infectious and noninfectious complications.

Bacteremia

Most hematogenous bloodstream infections in adult neutropenic cancer patients are due to coagulase-negative *Staphylococcus*, viridans streptococci, *E. coli*, *Pseudomonas aeruginosa*, and *S. aureus* (24). In patients with solid-organ cancer, *E. coli* and coagulase-negative *Staphylococcus* account for nearly 40% of bacteremia, whereas *Pseudomonas*, *S. aureus*, and enterococcal bloodstream infections account for 10% or less, each (25). *Klebsiella* species, other *Enterobacteriaceae*, and *S. maltophilia* are a serious concern and may become prominent bloodstream infections in certain geographic regions.

Cancer patients with bacteremia who present with extensive tissue involvement/infection are significantly less likely to respond to antimicrobial therapy (26). Other factors associated with poor prognosis in bacteremic patients with an underlying malignancy include shock, infection due to multidrug-resistant bacteria, and *Pseudomonas* and *Clostridium* species infection (26).

Bacteroides and *Clostridium* species are the most frequent cause of anaerobic bacteremia, which is most frequently seen in patients with abdominal and pelvic malignancy (26,27). Cancer patients with nonsporulating anaerobes bacteremia, *B. fragilis*, and *Fusobacterium* may be isolated more frequently compared with *Peptostreptococcus* and *Eubacterium* species (28). Polymicrobial infections are more frequent in patients with anaerobic bacteremia compared with aerobic bacterial infections. *E. coli*, *Pseudomonas*, *Klebsiella* species, and among gram-positive cocci, *Streptococcus*, *Enterococcus*, and *Staphylococcus epidermidis* may accompany anaerobic bloodstream infection (28). Concurrent candidemia is rarely seen in patients with anaerobic bacteremia. Over 90% of patients with nonsporulating anaerobic bacteremia may also have a deep tissue abscess (28). The authors suggest that all patients with gynecologic malignancy who present with anaerobic bacteremia be thoroughly evaluated for an infected abdominopelvic pelvic collection, which may not be clinically apparent at the time of initial presentation.

Clostridial bacteremia is often seen in patients with gastrointestinal or genitourinary cancer, and acute leukemia (29). Nearly one third of patients with bacteremia with *Clostridium* species alone and nearly half with polymicrobial infection present with septic shock (29). *Clostridium perfringens* is a common species, and *Clostridium septicum* is a rare, albeit serious infection seen mostly in patients with an intra-abdominal cancer (29,30). Diffuse, rapidly spreading cellulitis involving the abdominal wall, groin, and upper thigh area, gas gangrene, and acute intravascular hemolysis indicate the possibility of clostridial infection (29). Early appropriate therapy remains critical in improved response and outcome for patients with systemic anaerobic infection.

Febrile Neutropenia

The organisms associated with infections in patients with neutropenia are shown in Table 30.2. *Pseudomonas* spp. is a well-recognized cause of serious systemic infections in febrile neutropenic patients. The other nonfermentative gram-negative bacteria such as *S. maltophilia* have emerged and present as life-threatening pneumonia, bacteremia, or deep-tissue infection; these infections are commonly resistant to standard broad-spectrum antipseudomonal antibiotics, and despite appropriate therapy response may remain suboptimum (17). Patients with peripheral blood neutrophil counts of less than 500 have significantly higher risk of serious infection, especially if the duration of neutropenia is more than 7 days (1,2). During the first 5 days of neutropenia, bacterial infections are prominent; if neutropenia extends beyond a week, invasive candidiasis becomes a concern; and in patients with greater than 2 weeks of profound neutropenia invasive mold infections such as aspergillosis may be occasionally encountered. In most patients with gynecologic malignancy, isolation of a mold even from sterile samples does not indicate invasive fungal disease; in patients with no known established predisposing factors (31), these saprophytic molds usually represent colonization or laboratory contamination (32).

Catheter-Related Bloodstream Infection

In patients with solid-organ cancer, nearly 70% of gram-positive bacteremia is associated with an infected catheter; similarly, 60% of gram-negative bacteria is also related to an infected catheter, whereas only 19% of gram-negative bacteremia in patients with hematologic cancer is due to an infected catheter (33). Coagulase-negative *Staphylococcus* remains the most commonly isolated organism in blood cultures drawn from an indwelling central venous catheter and is frequently regarded as catheter-related infection. Similarly, *S. aureus*, including MRSA bacteremia, may result from an infected indwelling catheter and successful therapy requires selection of antimicrobial agents that penetrate the biofilm and are effective against the nonplanktonic, stationary phase of the bacteria (34). *S. aureus* bloodstream infections are associated with high rates of complications (35). Patients with solid-organ cancer with catheter-related *S. aureus* bacteremia have a fivefold higher probability of developing intravascular complications such as septic thrombosis and infective endocarditis (35).

Patients with gynecologic malignancy have a higher rate of postoperative infection, catheter malfunction, and unplanned catheter removal following external intravascular catheter compared with subcutaneous/implantable venous access devices (36,37). Nearly one third of all intravascular catheters were associated with delayed complications in this cancer population; bacteremia was significantly more common in patients with nonimplantable (Hickman catheters) versus implantable (infusaport or peripheral access system ports) indwelling intravenous devices (38).

TABLE 30.2

MICROORGANISMS COMMONLY ASSOCIATED WITH INFECTION IN NEUTROPENIC PATIENTS

GRAM-NEGATIVE ORGANISMS	Coagulase-negative *Staphylococcus* such as *S. epidermidis* and *S. saprophyticus*
Escherichia coli	Beta-hemolytic streptococci, group A, B, G
Klebsiella spp.	Alpha-hemolytic streptococci (viridans streptococcus spp.)
Pseudomonas aeruginosa	*Enterococcus* spp. including vancomycin-resistant strains
Stenotrophomonas maltophilia	
Enterobacter spp.	FUNGI[a]
GRAM-POSITIVE ORGANISMS	*Candida* spp. including *C. albicans, C. glabrata, C. tropicalis,* and *C. parapsilosis*
Staphylococcus spp. including vancomycin-tolerant organisms	
Staphylococcus aureus	

[a]Patients receiving multiple courses of fluconazole therapy or prolonged antifungal supression or prophylaxis are at higher risk for infections due to drug-resistant *C. glabrata* and *C. krusei*.

IMPLANTABLE DEVICE INFECTIONS

Peritoneal, hepatic, and pleural implantable devices for delivering chemotherapy or drainage of recurring malignant effusions have been successfully used in the last decade. These devices are well tolerated; major complications including bowel perforation are uncommon, and serious infections are seen in less than 5% of cases (39–44). Overall, infections are seen in less than 20% of cases. While serious infections including pocket infections are seldom noticed, when infections such as these do occur, they should be treated aggressively, requiring prompt removal of the infected reservoir and appropriate systemic antimicrobial therapy (39). Abdominal pain and chemotherapy-related discomfort remain the main problems with these chemotherapy infusion devices.

Urinary Tract Infection

Patients with gynecologic cancer have an increased risk for urinary tract infection. The factors that promote infections are listed in Table 30.3. Nearly one third of patients, while undergoing pelvic radiotherapy for gynecologic cancer, may have symptoms of urinary tract infection at the onset of therapy or develop infection during the course of radiation therapy (45). Despite appropriate therapy, infections may recur and require several courses of antibiotic therapy (45). Patients who have undergone pelvic exenteration remain at increased risk for ascending urinary tract infection (14); recurrent pyelonephritis in these patients may lead to permanent renal damage. Older patients with advanced gynecologic cancer are also being considered for pelvic exenteration surgery (46). In these and other patients with lower renal reserves, a severe episode of pyelonephritis may precipitate irreversible dysfunction and renal failure. We suggest that in selected high-risk patients, preemptive antimicrobial therapy or even secondary antibiotic prophylaxis be considered after an episode of urinary tract infection.

ANTIMICROBIAL AGENTS

It is important to refer to the spectrum of local and regional drug resistance among commonly encountered pathogens in selecting appropriate antimicrobials, especially when treatment is initiated empirically or in patients awaiting microbiologic results.

SURGICAL ANTIMICROBIAL PROPHYLAXIS

Operative Site

Guidelines for the administration of antibiotics to uninfected patients undergoing pelvic surgical procedures were first proposed by Ledger et al. in 1975 (47). Prophylactic antibiotics are indicated for women undergoing pelvic surgery for malignancy. There have been few studies evaluating this prophylaxis in such cases. Recently, cefazolin was showed to be inferior to cefotetan as a single-dose prophylaxis in women undergoing elective abdominal hysterectomy (48). A placebo-controlled trail showed that using a broad-spectrum cephalosporin plus beta-lactamase inhibitor significantly reduced the risk of major operation-site infection from 27% in patients not given antimicrobial prophylaxis, whereas none given antibiotic developed operative-site infection (49).

The overall postoperative infection rate has been as high as 46% and surgical-site infection is seen in nearly one fourth of patients (50). The risk of postoperative infection is adversely affected by prolonged duration of surgery for >5 hours, presence of remote infection at the time of surgery, and duration of hospitalization for longer than 3 weeks; in patients with all three risk factors the relative risk of infections increases to 7.3 compared to 3 in patients who have only one of these risk factors (50). Risk factors that have been associated with an increased incidence of infection in patients undergoing surgery for reproductive tract carcinoma include lower socioeconomic status, preoperative colonization, failure to administer perioperative heparin, obesity, older patient age, a longer operative

TABLE 30.3

FACTORS PROMOTING URINARY TRACT INFECTIONS

TUMOR OBSTRUCTION	SURGERY
Retrograde urine flow leading to ascending pyelonephritis	Urinary diversions
Stagnation in patients with outlet obstruction and abscess formation	Organ resection
	Lymph node dissection
	Anastomotic leak
INSTRUMENTIZATION	Chronic surgical wound breakdown
Cystoscopy-related introduction of pathogens	
Dilatation of strictures	CHEMOTHERAPY
	Neutropenia
FOREIGN BODY	Suppression of local immune surveillance and response to bacterial invasion
Urethral stent	Mucosal damage and disruption
Percutaneous nephrostomy tube placement/replacement[a]	
Surgical drains for extended duration	
RADIOTHERAPY	
Inflammation of bladder mucosa	
Suppression of local innate cellular and acellular immune response	

[a]Patients undergoing routine replacement of percutaneous nephrostomy tubes may develop transient bacteremia in the event of prior colonization.

period, and a longer hospital stay before surgery (51,52). Extent of surgery plays a central role in predicting probability and severity of postoperative infections (12–14,52). However, these risk factors were not uniform among investigators' evaluations.

Clinical Investigation

The overall operative-site infection rate ranges from 6.7% to 44%. Interestingly, patients with preoperative cervical colonization did not have an increase in postoperative complications including duration of hospitalization, operative time, or febrile episodes compared with patients in whom no cervical colonization was demonstrated (53). An overall decrease in significant postoperative infections was reported in retrospective studies among patients undergoing radical hysterectomy (54,55). The benefit, however, was thought to be associated only with reduced local wound infections (56).

Prospective data have not resolved this issue. Numbers of patients in comparative arms have been small, and the data may be, therefore, inadequate for detecting a statistically significant infection rate. No significant difference in overall operative-site infection was observed after preoperative prophylaxis by the research groups Rosenshein et al. (57) and Marsden et al. (58), but significantly lower incidences of infection were reported by Sevin et al. (59) and Micha et al. (60). Sevin et al. reported that a short course (three doses) of prophylaxis was as effective as a long course (12 doses) in preventing major infection after radical hysterectomy (61). If separate operative-site data from prospective studies are combined, the overall incidence of pelvic infection and wound infection was significantly reduced by the administration of prophylactic antimicrobials.

A cost-benefit analysis of three doses of cefazolin antimicrobial prophylaxis showed a 29% reduction in infectious morbidity following vaginal hysterectomy and an 18% reduction in postoperative infections in patients following abdominal hysterectomy (62).

One patient population that has a significant surgical incision breakdown is that of women undergoing radical vulvectomy. Anecdotal experience indicates the principal pathogens to be *S. aureus* and *S. epidermidis*. The administration of broad-spectrum medications, such as piperacillin or mezlocillin, did not significantly reduce the incidence of postoperative wound infection; 8 of 12 women undergoing radical vulvectomy for vulvar carcinoma who were given single-dose piperacillin or mezlocillin developed postoperative infections (63). Drain sites fall into the same category. The foreign body undoubtedly contributes to the infections; local attention, rather than parenteral or oral antibiotics, is the appropriate preventive approach.

AGENT ADMINISTRATION

Intravenous administration of antibiotics is recommended to achieve high serum and tissue drug concentration and should be given before anesthesia. Antiobiotics administered to women undergoing hysterectomy for benign indications by suppository, by spray, and orally, with significant reduction in operative-site infection (64–66). There are no similar data for women undergoing hysterectomy for gynecologic cancer, and these routes of administration are presently not advised.

Timing of Drug Administration

The first dose of an antibiotic should be given intravenously in the operating room. Combination regimens and prolonged administration did not appear to offer superior infection prevention when compared with that provided by a single agent given once. If the interval between the first dose and opening the vagina exceeds 2.5 to 3 hours, a second intravenous dose should be given 15 to 30 minutes before the anticipated vaginal entry. This conclusion is based on data provided by Shapiro et al. (67). This has not been clinically studied, but administration at longer fixed intervals has not enhanced protection at hysterectomy for benign indications. In patients who are expected to undergo a prolonged surgical procedure (>4 hours), the dose may be repeated after 4 to 6 hours.

Recommendations

Intravenous administration of 2 g cefazolin should be given in the operating room. Cefazolin provides activity against gram-negative and gram-positive aerobic and anaerobic bacteria; it is an uncommon therapeutic agent and is comparatively inexpensive—beneficial attributes for a prophylactic antibiotic. A single dose of a prophylactic agent did not result in the selection of a resistant species, as did three doses of antibiotics at hysterectomy for benign disease (68). A 1-g dose may suffice, but 2 g was superior to 1 g for vaginal hysterectomy, and three 1-g doses over 16 hours were statistically inferior to a single 2-g dose for cesarean delivery (69). A single dose (1 g) of cefotetan was significantly ($p < 0.05$) superior to 1 g of cefazolin in preventing operative-site infection after elective abdominal hysterectomy for benign diagnoses. Although the cost per vial was higher, there was an overall reduction in hospital costs owing to fewer infections and shorter hospital stays (70). Kobamatsu et al. also found superior protection for women undergoing radical hysterectomy when using expanded-spectrum cephalosporins compared with first-generation agents (71). Other alternatives include ampicillin-sulbactam, although there is little evidence to support this practice; similarly, using metronidazole as a single agent may be less effective at preventing infection compared with broad-spectrum cephalosporin agents (72). More prospective data are necessary in patients with gynecologic malignancy undergoing surgery.

If the patient is allergic to cephalosporins, or if she has a history of a type I immediate hypersensitivity reaction to a penicillin, and if she is not allergic to a tetracycline, the recommendation is 100 mg doxycycline orally at bedtime the night before surgery and again the day of surgery about 3 hours before departure for the operating room. This regimen has been evaluated prospectively in Parkland Memorial Hospital, but in a nonrandomized study using very few patients and no control regimen. If the woman is allergic to tetracycline, the recommendation is intravenous administration of 900 mg of clindamycin given preoperatively, as for cefazolin. The new generation of fluoroquinolones such as moxifloxacin may be particularly suited for the gynecologic cancer patient scheduled for pelvic surgery because of its spectrum of activity and half-life. Further studies are needed.

BOWEL PREPARATION

Unobstructed Bowel

There are approximately 10^{11} bacteria in a gram of feces, making sepsis a major hazard if the colon is opened. It is desirable to reduce the patient's normal colonic microflora to diminish the postoperative infection rate in case it is necessary to perform colonic resection and reanastomosis. Preparation for colonoscopy is a regimen of clear liquids the day before surgery and 3 tablespoons of Fleet Phospho-Soda in one-half cup of cool water at 4:00 PM and 6:00 PM the day before surgery. Patients should be cautioned to drink eight to ten 8-fluid ounce glasses of clear liquids the day before surgery. Additional clear fluid is acceptable. Some surgeons prefer to add a Fleet enema 2 hours before surgery. An alternative mechanical preparation is whole gut irrigation with chilled polyethylene glycol and electrolyte therapy or a similar lavage solution given orally at a rate of approximately 1 L/h until the rectal effluent is clear, but for not more than 4 hours. A recent multicenter, randomized trial has placed routine mechanical bowel preparation practice into serious question; in patients who underwent elective colorectal surgery, no difference in anastomotic leak or other septic complications such as fascia dehiscence were noted in the group who had preoperative bowel preparation (73).

In the antimicrobial approach, 1 g each of erythromycin and neomycin is given orally at 1:00 PM, 2:00 PM, and 11:00 PM the day before surgery. This regimen was initially proposed in 1971 by Nichols and Condon (74). An alternative is 1 g each of metronidazole and neomycin at 2:00 PM and at 11:00 PM the day before surgery. There should be no need to add further antimicrobial prophylaxis to 2 g of cefazolin or other agents. Because this may alter hydration status and serum electrolytes, many administer intravenous fluids to patients undergoing mechanical bowel preparation (75).

Obstructed Bowel

There can be no mechanical prophylaxis for preoperative management of the obstructed bowel. Treatment principles include fluid and electrolyte therapy with mechanical decompression of the bowel from above and timed surgical intervention. Women with mechanical intestinal obstruction immediately after surgery may be able to be treated conservatively with decompression only. If necessary, surgery should be performed within 24 hours of the mechanical obstruction; these patients have the lowest mortality rate. A dose of intravenous antibiotic should be given in the operating room before the procedure, with a second dose given in the recovery room, and a third 8 hours later if it is necessary to enter the bowel lumen. The single-agent or combination regimen should provide broad coverage of both gram-positive and gram-negative aerobic and anaerobic bacterial species with a broader spectrum of antibacterial activity than with cefazolin. Evaluation has produced no evidence for a superior regimen. A single agent usually suffices unless the patient is septic, in which case triple antibiotics are appropriate because therapy, not prophylaxis, is necessary.

CLINICAL SYNDROMES

Peritonitis and Intra-abdominal Abscess

Etiology

Infection in the patient with pelvic cancer most commonly involves the pelvis and abdomen. The potential causes of infection include complications of the primary tumor, surgery, and radiation therapy. The tumor can compromise the integrity of the vaginal wall and allow seeding of endogenous vaginal flora into the pelvic and peritoneal cavities. Previous antibiotics, radiation therapy, and the tumor itself may alter the normal genital flora. The tumor can also erode into the bowel and allow entry of fecal material into the peritoneal cavity. Rare cases of several other syndromes arising from untreated pelvic tumor, including spontaneous clostridial gas gangrene and pneumoperitoneum, have been reported (76,77). Peritonitis, with or without abscess formation, may occur postoperatively after hysterectomy or with bowel injury. Radiation therapy to the pelvis can cause radiation enteritis, leading to a chronic diarrheal syndrome, which may develop years after radiation therapy is completed. These patients are also at higher risk for bowel adhesions and subsequent obstruction, and subclinical perforation may present as late insidious intra-abdominal or deep pelvic abscess.

Signs and Symptoms

In the patient with pelvic cancer, peritonitis may develop at any time, including at initial diagnosis (e.g., tumor infiltration of bowel), immediately postoperatively, or days or weeks after surgery (e.g., tumor infiltration or radiation therapy). The signs are generally dramatic and familiar: abdominal pain, fever, and signs of peritoneal irritation. However, among postoperative patients or patients who have received radiation or corticosteroid therapy, the physical findings may resemble those of a routine postoperative patient, making the diagnosis more difficult. To ensure proper diagnosis, frequent examinations and close observation are required.

Abscess formation can also occur in several settings. In some patients, a subclinical microperforation of the bowel is successfully walled off by the body's immune system, forming a pericolic or intraperitoneal abscess. This has been shown to occur 7 to 10 days after microperforation (78). Fever or mechanical obstruction may be the only presenting sign. Subphrenic, psoas, or liver abscesses may present as a fever of unknown origin and may require a methodical, diligent evaluation for diagnosis. A fistula, usually caused by tumor but also occurring postoperatively, may form between any two organ systems, including the bladder, vagina, bowel, or skin. Persistent suppuration despite therapy or the presence of a feculent discharge from the skin, bladder, or vagina may suggest the development of a fistula.

Diagnosis

The diagnosis of peritonitis is usually made on clinical grounds. In patients who have clinical evidence of peritonitis but are unable to undergo surgery because of bulky tumor, multiple prior surgeries, or general debility, paracentesis with appropriate cultures may be useful in guiding antibiotic therapy. Radiologic investigation is generally required to diagnose an abscess. Regular plain x-ray films of the abdomen are seldom revealing. A sonogram, computed tomographic (CT) scan, or magnetic resonance image (MRI) of the abdomen may show the collection. A gallium scan may also be helpful. In a particularly confusing case in which abnormalities of scans can represent an abscess, metastatic tumor, or postoperative changes, a labeled leukocyte scan may be required to diagnose the abscess with certainty.

The diagnosis of a fistula requires demonstration of abnormal drainage from one organ system to another. This can be shown by intravenous or intravesical injection of dye for fistulae arising from the bladder, oral or rectal instillation of dye for those arising from the gastrointestinal tract, or a fistulogram for a fistula involving the skin.

In all cases, laboratory abnormalities, including an elevated leukocyte count, an elevated erythrocyte sedimentation rate, and abnormal liver function tests, may suggest the diagnosis and direct the workup. The microbiologic diagnosis in each of these syndromes requires culture for aerobes and anaerobes. Blood cultures are only rarely positive. Some patients may have an unexplained bacteremia of enteric gram-negative rods or anaerobes. This is probably from a microperforation of the bowel. Any patient with pelvic tumor and enteric gram-negative rods or anaerobic bacteremia should be radiologically evaluated for evidence of perforation.

Therapy

Acute, generalized peritonitis where gastrointestinal perforation is suspected usually requires urgent surgery to irrigate the peritoneum and repair any perforation. Broad-spectrum antibiotic coverage with agents such as cefoxitin, ticarcillin–clavulanic acid, metronidazole, clindamycin with ampicillin, and an aminoglycoside such as gentamicin is generally effective for the polymicrobial infection. Addition of the aminoglycoside is particularly important for patients who have been recently or frequently hospitalized or who have had past courses of antibiotics. These situations predispose the patient to the development of resistant organisms.

Effective treatment of an abscess requires drainage. Percutaneous drainage is adequate in many cases, but laparotomy is occasionally required. Large or persistent abscesses may require placement of a suction drain. Patients with fistulae generally require resection of the involved tissue.

For intra-abdominal infection, intravenous antibiotics directed at the recovered bacteria should continue for at least 7 to 10 days after drainage. Some patients who have been on antibiotics may have evidence of pus but no growth on cultures. In this situation, broad-spectrum antibiotics directed at enteric gram-negative rods and anaerobes should be administered. Laboratory parameters such as leukocyte counts should be followed to determine the exact duration.

Patients who are inoperable can be treated with chronic suppressive therapy, intravenously or orally. Oral agents such as amoxicillin–clavulanic acid (875 mg bid) or clindamycin (450 mg q 6 to 8 hours) may be effective. Ciprofloxacin, moxifloxacin, or levofloxacin alone should not be used in this situation because they provide limited enterococcal coverage.

Patients with infections due to vancomycin-resistant enterococci and/or vancomycin-tolerant (79) *Streptococcus* or *Staphylococcus* infections may be treated with daptomycin (6 mg/kg daily) or linezolid (600 mg twice daily), usually in combination with drugs with gram-negative and anaerobic activity. The recently approved tigecycline has a broad spectrum of antimicrobials, including multidrug-resistant gram-negative bacteria such as extended-spectrum beta-lactamase positive *E. coli*, multidrug-resistant *Acinetobacter*, *S. maltophilia*, vancomycin-resistant enterococci, and multidrug-resistant *S. aureus*. There is limited clinical data for its use in patients with gynecologic malignancy, and due to poor activity against *Pseudomonas* species it should be used cautiously. Furthermore, emergence of drug-resistant bacteria or selection of less-susceptible organisms remains a concern for widespread use of drugs with broad-spectrum antimicrobial coverage. Similarly, antipseudomonal carbapenems such as imipenem-cilastatin and meropenem should also be reserved for seriously ill patients with polymicrobial infection, as emergence and spread of multidrug-resistant gram-negative bacteria are increasing in immunosuppressed cancer patients (80). Ertapenem, a carbapenem without antipseudomonal activity, was as effective as piperacillin-tazobactam for the treatment of acute pelvic infection (81), and can be administered as a single daily dose, albeit due to lack of enterococcal coverage it is important to select patients carefully.

Urinary Tract Infection

Etiology

Many clinical situations predispose a patient to urinary tract infection. Urinary tract infection continues to be the leading cause of infectious morbidity in this population. One study showed that half of the patients with pelvic cancer admitted to the hospital because of infection had a urinary tract infection; *E. coli* was the most common organism isolated (82). Another report found that the frequency of urinary tract infections is increased as much as threefold in patients undergoing pelvic irradiation (20–22). Many patients who undergo pelvic surgery require prolonged bladder catheterization, usually with a Foley catheter. These patients may develop the well-recognized infectious complications of chronic bladder catheterization, the most common of which is recurrent infection. In addition, tumor can cause urinary obstruction and subsequent infection. The role of silver- or antibiotic-impregnated Foley catheters has not yet been defined.

Signs and Symptoms

Some patients with gynecologic malignancy and urinary tract infection have the familiar clinical picture of dysuria, fever, flank or suprapubic tenderness, elevated leukocyte count, and abnormal urinalysis. In many others, these signs and symptoms are obscured by the rest of the clinical picture. For instance, a postoperative patient may be expected to have abdominal tenderness, an elevated leukocyte count, and fever. The physician should consider the entire clinical setting before embarking on a course of therapy.

Diagnosis

Diagnosis is generally made on the basis of a urine culture, from a "clean catch" or through a catheter, but the initial urinalysis is extremely helpful. Pyuria is expected in any nongranulocytopenic patient with a urinary tract infection. Gram stain of urinary sediment can direct antibiotic therapy in advance of the culture results. A common problem confronting the physician is when patients, especially those with indwelling catheters or nephrostomy tubes, have positive urine cultures but do not appear to be ill. Differentiating colonization from invasive infection is never simple and requires clinical judgment. Any patient who is not granulocytopenic should also have pyuria along with positive urine cultures. The absence of pyuria in a patient with a positive urine culture suggests the likelihood of contamination/colonization. From a practical standpoint, in a clinically stable patient, it is reasonable to withhold antibiotics pending repeated urinalysis and urine culture. If an organism persists, therapy should be considered.

Therapy

Therapy should be based on the sensitivity pattern of the recovered organism, and intravenous antibiotics are reserved for patients with drug-resistant bacteria and those with systemic infection, ascending infection, or pyelonephritis. Optimum duration of therapy in a patient with a urethral stent or a permanent indwelling catheter is often difficult to determine. It is virtually impossible to eradicate an infection in the presence of a foreign body, and removal of the foreign object is the obvious therapy. However, removal is not always feasible. A patient with a urinary tract infection and a foreign body in the urinary collecting system should be considered for chronic suppressive therapy if she has recurrent infection. In general, among patients with gram-negative rods, chronic suppressive therapy may include ampicillin, trimethoprim-sulfamethoxazole, doxycycline, or an oral fluoroquinolone such as ciprofloxacin. Patients with a chronic enterococcal infection may benefit from chronic suppressive therapy with amoxicillin–clavulanic acid (Augmentin) or amoxicillin alone or doxycycline.

In patients with pyuria and fever in whom a urinary tract infection is suspected, empiric antibiotic therapy should be given pending urine culture results. Gram stain of urinary sediment may be helpful in directing treatment. However, for those cases in which Gram stain is not helpful, broad-spectrum coverage should be given. For a patient who has had frequent or prolonged hospitalizations, effective coverage of potentially resistant gram-negative rods dictates that two drugs be given, preferably a beta-lactam and an aminoglycoside. Cefazolin (1 to 2 g IV, q 8 hours) and gentamicin (4 to 5 mg/kg per day IV in three divided doses) is a good empiric combination for many patients. For more debilitated patients or those with prolonged hospitalizations and frequent past courses of antibiotics, a third-generation cephalosporin, such as ceftazidime (1 to 2 g IV, q 8 hours), should be substituted for cefazolin. After culture results are known, antibiotics can be adjusted and the spectrum narrowed. For any gynecologic cancer patient with an unexplained predisposition to recurrent urinary tract infection, a full investigation should be undertaken to exclude obstruction from tumor as the cause.

Wound Infections

There are important variables that influence the development of wound infection after surgery. These include hospital flora, patient flora, operative technique and variables, patient nutrition, and immunocompetency. Women being treated for reproductive tract cancer may be at risk because of specific problems with immunocompetency, possible prior chemotherapy or radiotherapy, poor nutritional status, hypoproteinemia, or low socioeconomic status. Additional risk factors for incisional infection include obesity and diabetes. Surgical variables include operative procedures in excess of 4 hours, breaks in surgical technique, excessive inoculum at the operative site, excessive cautery, passive drains, shaving of the area in which the incision is made immediately before surgery, and placement and types of sutures. Infections may range from a mild cellulitis to a devastating fasciitis, deep infection with myonecrosis, and mixed anaerobic–aerobic synergistic abdominopelvic gangrene (83).

Cellulitis

Etiology. Cellulitis is a relatively frequent occurrence. The presence of a foreign body in a wound is an unavoidable risk factor in many cases, but this variable should be removed or reduced as much as possible. Devitalized tissue, especially fat, can also act as a foreign body. Excess cautery causes thermal injury; the charred tissue may act as a foreign body. The presence of significant amounts of devitalized tissue usually produces a wound defect. A mechanical wound retractor can cause fat necrosis, and there appears to be only minimal ability to resorb these areas during wound healing. These areas should be carefully identified and excised before closing the wound. If drains are used, they should be closed, and drains should be vacuumed. Drains should not exit through the wound but rather through an adjacent puncture site, and they should be removed as early as possible. *S. aureus* is recovered from 50% or more of wound infections. If the operative procedure involves transection of the vagina, the infections may harbor other species of normal flora of the lower reproductive tract, such as gram-positive and gram-negative anaerobes and *Enterobacteriaceae*. Cellulitis of the leg occurs with increased frequency in patients after vulvectomy (84). The affected leg is not always edematous. Group B beta-hemolytic streptococci are frequently recovered. Prophylactic therapy with oral penicillin may reduce recurrences in some patients (84).

Signs and Symptoms. Cellulitis is almost uniformly associated with pain and erythema in the incisional margins, with an increase in local skin and tissue temperature, and many times with fever. Incisions are usually tender at examination. Incisional cellulitis may not become evident until the 4th postoperative day or later.

Diagnosis. The infected surgical incision should be explored. This can frequently be performed at the bedside. Opposing skin edges in such incisions are usually separated without difficulty and may expose underlying purulent material, seromas, hematomas, or any combination of these. The wound should be explored thoroughly, and if the wound shows unusual features, aerobic and anaerobic cultures should be obtained. Foreign bodies such as sutures or drains should be removed, and obviously necrotic areas should be removed after the patient has been given parenteral pain medication. It is important to document deep fascial integrity. If this cannot be done at the bedside, it should be performed in the operating room.

Therapy. The wound should be packed open with fine-mesh gauze approximated to the incisional margins. Gauze is used to fill the intervening spaces after each dressing change. The dressing is changed two to four times daily, with chemical and mechanical debridement of necrotic areas. Commonly used solutions are hydrogen peroxide, acetic acid, and Dakin's solution (0.25% sodium hypochlorite). In general, these debriding solutions should be removed from the wound with sterile normal saline before packing because they may impede healing. Except in unusual instances, it is unnecessary to administer parenteral antimicrobials. These incisions may be left open to heal by secondary intent, or they may be closed before discharge from the hospital after the margins are completely granulated. The optimal time for secondary closure is about the 4th day after institution of wound therapy. Studies have shown that normal wound healing occurs as long as the hematocrit exceeds 17%, but that a lower level will impede healing (85).

Necrotizing Fasciitis

Necrotizing fasciitis is a potentially life-threatening infection of the soft tissues above deep fascia that can involve the abdominal wall or vulva with extension to the proximal thighs and buttocks (85). There are several descriptive names for this infection, such as beta-hemolytic streptococcal gangrene, hospital gangrene, gram-negative anaerobic cutaneous gangrene, nonclostridial gas gangrene, gangrenous erysipelas, or synergistic necrotizing cellulitis, but the name used by most is that coined by Wilson in 1952, that is, necrotizing fasciitis (86). This significant infection has been reported in patients with endometrial cancer following irradiation and hysterectomy (87–89). It has also been found in endopelvic fascia, in a suprapubic catheter site during chemotherapy, in the vulva in diabetes, and after diagnostic laparoscopy (90–95).

Etiology. Bacteria recovered from necrotizing fasciitis infectious sites include anaerobes, particularly *Peptostreptococcus*, *Prevotella*, and *Bacteroides* species, as well as *E. faecalis*, *S. aureus*, and *Enterobacteriaceae*. These bacteria produce large quantities of proteolytic and other enzymes and toxins that allow rapid spread to contiguous tissues. Superficial vessels are occluded, depriving the affected areas of oxygen, other nutrients, and antibiotics. This deprivation interferes with bacterial eradication. Patients at particularly high risk of developing this infection include women older than 50 years of age and those with arteriosclerotic heart disease, diabetes, or other chronic diseases.

Signs and Symptoms. Early in the course of necrotizing fasciitis, the signs and symptoms are those of any wound cellulitis. Because there is no response to the usual methods of therapy, antibiotic therapy will frequently be initiated. The infection, however, seems to smolder initially, then rapidly progresses to involve the wound and to produce clinical sepsis. Mortality rates for this infection have been as high as 76%. The degree of disease evident on the skin is only a small fraction of the total amount of tissue that is involved because the skin is not the primary area of infection. Hallmarks of this infection include excessive pain, edema that is unusual for the apparently minimal degree of infection, and superficial tissue crepitance. The skin overlying the affected area becomes blue or brown as the disease progresses, and there may be formation of bullae. Edema progresses, and there may be seepage of grayish fluid from the skin, which slips over underlying tissue and does not bleed if cut. Lack of familiarity with this infection and failure to recognize its signs may delay diagnosis. Even when recognized and treated early, there is a high mortality rate.

Diagnosis. Diagnostic criteria as first outlined by Fisher et al. include (96):

1. Extensive necrosis of the superficial fascia with widespread undermining of surrounding tissue
2. A moderate to severe systemic toxic reaction
3. Absence of muscle involvement
4. Failure to demonstrate *Clostridium* species in the wound or blood cultures
5. Absence of major vascular occlusion
6. Histologic demonstration of intense leukocytic infiltration, focal necrosis of the superficial fascia and surrounding tissues, and microvascular thrombosis

Early diagnosis followed as soon as possible by appropriate treatment produces the highest cure rate. Radiologic evaluation, particularly with MRI, may confirm the diagnosis rapidly, and should be ordered whenever the disease is suspected. The average interval between diagnosis and initiation of treatment is approximately 5 days. If the interval is 4 days or less, survival rates are high, but an interval of 7 days or more is more likely to result in patient death because even intense antimicrobial therapy is rarely successful at this late stage.

Therapy. Although the administration of broad-spectrum antimicrobials is important, wide and often disfiguring surgical debridement is the treatment required for preservation of life. The excision must extend to areas that bleed. The areas of debridement should be treated as are areas of burns. Adjunctive therapy with whirlpool baths and perhaps hyperbaric oxygen may be of use.

Clostridial Myonecrosis

Clostridial myonecrosis (gas gangrene) was described by Altmeier (97). It is an infection that occurs in muscle and adjacent tissues beneath the deep fascia and is seen most commonly after trauma. However, it can be seen after intra-abdominal surgery or surgery in an area that has been contaminated by feces. Mortality rates are about 25%, and poor-prognosis factors are leukopenia, advanced age, renal failure, and intravascular hemolysis.

Etiology. Clostridial myonecrosis is caused by *C. perfringens* (80% to 95%), *C. novyi* (10% to 40%), or *C. septicum* (5% to 20%). It is usually seen in association with gastrointestinal mucosal ulceration or perforation because *Clostridium* species are normal inhabitants of the gastrointestinal tract. *C. perfringens* may be isolated from as many as 20% of the women with upper genital tract infections not involving sexually transmitted diseases. The mere presence of *C. perfringens* in a wound does not mean that the patient will develop gas gangrene; it develops in only 1% to 2% of wounds in which that species can be isolated.

Signs and Symptoms. Early signs and symptoms of clostridial myonecrosis are tense edema in tissue that is extremely tender and pain that rapidly intensifies. If an incision is open, it is not uncommon to see a swollen, herniated muscle. There is frequently a serosanguinous, dirty discharge that has many gram-positive or gram-variable rods but few leukocytes. There may also be gas bubbles, and the secretions have a particularly sweet, offensive odor. The surrounding tissue frequently has crepitus. The skin becomes red to green-purple and then turns yellow before becoming a characteristic bronze color. The usual incubation period is about 2 to 3 days, but it can be as short as 6 hours after the bacterial inoculation. With progression of the infection, the patient becomes obviously ill, pale, and sweaty, with increased pulse rate and decreased blood pressure. Temperature is usually elevated, but hypothermia may occur with shock.

Diagnosis. A positive wound culture may accompany the characteristic signs and symptoms of clostridial myonecrosis. X-ray films of the affected area frequently show gas deep in the tissues. Blood cultures grow clostridia in approximately 15% of the cases. It is common to find a decrease in hemoglobin and an increase in circulating leukocytes. Involved muscle is pale and edematous, with loss of elasticity, and it does not bleed or contract with stimulation. Histologic findings demonstrate coagulation necrosis of muscle fibers.

Therapy. Clostridial myonecrosis is another infection that requires prompt and extensive debridement in the operating room. Cultures must be performed, and because clostridia may develop plasmid-mediated antibiotic resistance, repeated cultures with sensitivity testing may be required if a patient is slow to respond. In addition to wide debridement, the treatment of choice is penicillin G at a dose of 1 to 2 million units every 2 to 3 hours. Gram stain also may indicate the presence of gram-negative bacteria, in which case coverage should be provided for those bacteria as well. Chloramphenicol is as effective against *Clostridium* species as it is against many gram-negative species, although seldom used. Metronidazole, imipenem, or clindamycin, all of which have good *in vitro* activity against *C. perfringens*, may be considered. Other antibiotics with good *in vitro* activity include tetracycline, erythromycin, and rifampin. Hyperbaric oxygen may be adjunctive, but its efficacy is uncertain.

Intraperitoneal Catheter Infections

Etiology

Delivery of chemotherapeutic agents through an intraperitoneal catheter has enabled physicians to deliver high concentrations of drug locally while decreasing systemic side effects (42,98). However, intraperitoneal catheters can become infected at the exit site, along the catheter tunnel, or secondary peritonitis may occur in rare cases. *S. epidermidis* is the most common organism followed by *S. aureus* and *Streptococcus* species. Gram-negative bacilli and anaerobes, presumably from the bowel, are also found, especially in patients with polymicrobial infections. Patients who have been treated for bacterial peritonitis in the past may develop peritonitis due to *Candida* species.

Signs and Symptoms

With exit-site or tunnel infections, patients report discomfort at the site. Patients with peritonitis may complain of diffuse abdominal pain, with or without a change in bowel pattern. Fever may be absent in peritonitis, making the diagnosis more difficult because many patients with pelvic tumor have abdominal pain. On examination, patients with exit-site or tunnel infections have redness and sometimes have discharge where the catheter has been inserted. Patients with peritonitis have tenderness and frequently have abdominal rebound.

Diagnosis

Diagnosis of exit-site and tunnel infections is made clinically, with support from a Gram stain and culture of any discharge. Patients with suspected peritonitis should have withdrawal of peritoneal fluid for cell count and microbiologic evaluation. A rough guideline, derived from experience among patients receiving continuous ambulatory peritoneal dialysis, is that any leukocyte count in peritoneal fluid >100 cells/mm^3 suggests infection. Gram stain and culture should reveal the specific organism. Chemical peritonitis after instillation of chemotherapy can mimic infectious peritonitis. Peritoneal fluid cultures are often helpful in distinguishing between infectious versus chemical peritonitis, although occasionally peritoneal fluid cultures may not yield an organism, especially in infections due to a fastidious organism.

Therapy

For patients with peritonitis, systemic therapy is advised according to the recovered organisms. Treatment should be continued 10 days or longer, with serial peritoneal fluid cell counts guiding therapy. The peritoneum provides a large absorptive surface, and antibiotics delivered intraperitoneally readily enter the intravascular space; however, we suggest that intraperitoneal antibiotic therapy should be reserved for patients with serious, treatment-refractory infection. Treatment of fungal peritonitis is a unique problem. Amphotericin B can cause adhesions if delivered intraperitoneally. Caspofungin appears to be the treatment of choice for patients with intra-abdominal and peritoneal candidiasis (99). Fluconazole, which can be administered orally or intravenously, was shown in one study of patients receiving continuous ambulatory peritoneal dialysis to effectively treat *C. albicans* peritonitis and should be avoided in patients with *Candida glabrata* and *Candida krusei* infection (100). Fluconazole may be used for long-term therapy in patients with *Candida* peritonitis who have responded to initial aggressive therapy with amphotericin B or caspofungin therapy.

Septic Pelvic Thrombophlebitis

Septic pelvic thrombophlebitis, also known as suppurative pelvic thrombophlebitis, is a disorder that has been diagnosed most frequently after antimicrobial therapy for pelvic infection after cesarean section or septic abortion, but it can be seen as a complication of infection after any type of pelvic surgery. The mortality rate observed in 1917 was 52% after surgical therapy (101). Fortunately, this complication of pelvic infection is now very rare. The use of antimicrobial prophylaxis and the enhanced antibacterial activity of current therapeutic regimens are presumed to be paramount in the disappearance of this potentially lethal infection.

Etiology

Septic pelvic thrombophlebitis is clot formation in the pelvic veins as a result of infection. It can be seen after hysterectomy, other pelvic operative procedures including brachytherapy, and in association with pelvic trauma or perirectal abscess. Classically, there is relative venous stasis before phlebitis that develops adjacent to pelvic infection. The intimal lining of the veins is invaded by bacteria, including *Enterobacteriaceae*, especially *E. coli*, aerobic and anaerobic streptococci, and *Bacteroides*. The veins involved may be the ovarian, hypogastric, or uterine, with essentially equal involvement in the right and left sides. If common iliac veins are involved, clot formation is more frequently seen on the left for unknown reasons. Infected clot may embolize to the lungs, kidneys, liver, brain, and spleen.

Signs and Symptoms

A clinical diagnosis may not be readily evident. Presentation is essentially that of a fever of unknown cause, and the physician must rule out infections such as pyelonephritis, pneumonia, and pelvic or abdominal abscess. The most frequent presentation currently seen is persistence of fever associated with tachycardia after clinical response to antimicrobial therapy for a pelvic infection. Physical examination is normal in most instances, but it may be possible to palpate tender cords in the vaginal fornices. In patients with bacteremia and septic emboli, chills are observed in as many as 67% of the patients, pyrexia may be elevated to 41°C, and the variations in temperature may be quite hectic. Dyspnea, tachypnea, pleuritic pain, cough, hemoptysis, restlessness, anxiety, and perhaps angina may all be seen with septic embolization.

Diagnosis

Compatible clinical presentation and CT or MRI scan are used for diagnosis (102). Criteria for diagnosis of venous thrombosis using CT studies include enlargement of the involved vein(s), sharply defined vessel walls enhanced by contrast media, and a low-density intraluminal mass (103). Diagnosis using MRI is based on intense intraluminal signals from clot in involved veins and a lack of signal with normal blood flow in uninvolved vessels; no contrast agent is needed. Blood culture should be performed if there is suspicion of septicemia. Tests for blood gases, a chest radiograph, and a ventilation-perfusion scan should be performed if there is suspicion of embolization. A gallium scintiscan may be necessary to identify very small septic embolic foci in the lungs.

Therapy

Early treatment of venous thrombosis was surgical (101). The first to advocate the use of anticoagulants in addition to antibiotics were Schulman and Zatuchni (104). In some cases antibiotics alone may be adequate and can be used in patients in whom anticoagulation can be detrimental (105). In the largest published study of heparin therapy, the mean time to become afebrile was 2.5 days, and the average duration of heparin therapy was 8 days (106,107). It is unnecessary to initiate warfarin sodium (Coumadin) therapy in patients without evidence of emboli. Thromboembolism during or after treatment with heparin has not been reported. Antibiotic therapy must be continued. If there is significant improvement in the pulse rate and temperature pattern within 12 to 48 hours after addition of heparin, reassessment is mandatory eatment with low-molecular-weight heparin has not been studied or standardized for this condition (108). Heparin therapy is not without complications. Between 2% and 5% of patients may have an allergic reaction; bleeding occurs in 7% to 10% of patients; and the most devastating effect is the development of the "white clot syndrome" (109). This occurs in <1% of patients, but it may be associated with major limb amputation in 20% of those suffering from it, and death has been reported for 50%. This phenomenon is a paradoxical arterial platelet aggregation associated with thrombocytopenia, and it should be suspected in patients with decreasing platelet counts or an increasing requirement of heparin to maintain adequate anticoagulation. The only current indications for surgical intervention are embolization during heparin therapy or lack of response. The usual intervention is placement of a vena cava filter, which is a procedure usually performed by an interventional radiologist.

Neutropenia and Fever

Etiology

Patients with severe neutropenia are at particularly high risk for severe morbidity and mortality unless empiric intravenous antibiotic therapy is instituted at the first evidence of fever or clinical worsening. Most commonly, the febrile neutropenic patient does not have an obvious source of fever. Even in those with bacteremia, the source is rarely clinically evident. Bacteria often enter the bloodstream through the gastrointestinal tract because of the small chemotherapy-induced ulcerations of the intestinal mucosa and the accompanying neutropenia and thrombocytopenia. Neutropenic patients may also develop a clinically diagnosed group of infections, including pneumonia and cellulitis. Neutropenic patients with these clinically diagnosed infections may progress very rapidly, may have exceedingly subtle clinical signs and symptoms, and always require early, aggressive therapy of their infections to achieve a response.

Signs and Symptoms

Fever is often the only complaint of patients with neutropenia and bacteremia. Patients receiving chemotherapy should be instructed to take their own temperature at home twice a day (more frequently if a subjective feeling of fever develops) and to contact their treating physician for temperatures above 38.0°C or 100.4°F.

Diagnosis

Diagnosis is made by blood culture. Of all febrile, neutropenic patients from whom blood cultures are obtained, only 10% to 20% have an organism isolated. The others probably have enough organisms to cause fever and illness, but an insufficient load of organisms to be cultivated using current techniques. Coagulase-negative *Staphylococcus*, *S. aureus*, streptococci, *E. coli*, *Klebsiella* species, and *Pseudomonas* species are frequently isolated bacteria (110). In a recent report of 2,142 patients with febrile neutropenia, 499 (23%) patients developed bacteremia due to gram-positive bacteria (57%), gram-negative bacteria (34%) and polymicrobial infection was seen in 10% (111). Mortality rates were lowest (5%) in patients with gram-positive infection followed by 18% with gram-negative bacteremia, and they were 13% in patients in whom polymicrobial bloodstream infection was diagnosed (111). Polymicrobial infections are often under-reported and neutropenic patients with intestinal and genitourinary tract mucosal damage have a higher risk of systemic infection due to multiple organisms (7).

Therapy

The Infectious Disease Society of America (IDSA) updates guidelines for management of the patient with fever and neutropenia. Full consideration of this complex topic is beyond the scope of this chapter (112). In general, a febrile neutropenic patient should receive antibiotics with activity against *P. aeruginosa* pending results of blood cultures. Numerous regimens are effective, and their use should be determined according to sensitivity patterns for *P. aeruginosa* at a given hospital. In general, good results have been achieved with a beta-lactam antibiotic (e.g., semisynthetic penicillin such as ticarcillin–clavulanic acid or a third/fourth-generation cephalosporin such as ceftazidime or cefipime) or a carbapenem (imipenem or meropenem) with or without an aminoglycoside. Monitoring peak and trough levels of aminoglycosides is recommended to limit ototoxicity and nephrotoxicity. The choice of the specific aminoglycoside (e.g., gentamicin, tobramycin, amikacin) is dictated by the sensitivity patterns in a given hospital. Once-daily dosing of aminoglycosides is not recommended for the neutropenic patient but can be given in other settings. The length of therapy for neutropenic patients is determined by many factors and must be individualized. Patients with prolonged neutropenia and fever should be followed by an infectious disease specialist.

Fungal Infections

Etiology

Patients with pelvic cancer may be at risk for the development of fungal infections, particularly those caused by *Candida* species, including *C. albicans, C. tropicalis, C. parapsilosis*, and *C. glabrata* (113). Infection may include fungemia, pelvic abscess, or infected urinary stent in patients with extensive pelvic disease and urinary outflow obstruction. Risk factors for the development of invasive candidiasis include prolonged courses (7 to 10 days) of intravenous broad-spectrum antibiotics; an intravenous catheter, particularly a central venous catheter; major abdominal surgery; prolonged neutrocytopenia, usually related to chemotherapy; and immunosuppressive therapy, especially with corticosteroids (114).

Signs and Symptoms

Patients with the appropriate risk factors who have unexplained fevers may be fungemic. Other than fevers, which can include rigors and hypotension and closely resemble bacteremia, there may be no other symptoms. Blood cultures are positive in only 50% of the patients with autopsy-proven disseminated candidiasis. Any blood culture positive for yeast should be considered to be significant. A full evaluation for a hidden source should be completed, including a thorough re-evaluation with history and physical examination, and appropriate laboratory tests that include repeat blood cultures. An ophthalmoscopic examination to exclude endophthalmitis should be performed since this complication may occur in up to 5% to 15% of patients with fungemia.

Much has been written suggesting that any patient with *Candida* species cultured from three sites (i.e., sputum, urine, wound) should be considered to have invasive disease and treated accordingly. Although somewhat helpful, antifungal therapy in all patients meeting this criterion should not be initiated until a full evaluation is performed. In many cases, no antifungal therapy will be required.

Candida species may cause urinary tract infection in a patient with such indwelling devices as a Foley catheter, internal stents, or percutaneous nephrostomies. Rarely a "fungus ball," consisting of a matted mass of yeast, may cause urinary obstruction.

Candida species almost never cause pneumonia except as a preterminal event in a critically ill intensive care unit patient or patients with refractory relapsed acute myelogenous leukemia and prolonged severe neutropenia. Thus, recovery of any yeast from a respiratory specimen should be considered to be most likely due to oral thrush contaminating the culture. Unlike patients with leukemia and recipients of allogeneic hematopoietic stem cell transplantation, in patients with gynecologic malignancy invasive mold disease is exceedingly rare. Identification of filamentous fungi, such as *Aspergillus*, should be approached with great caution and mold-active drug therapy reserved for highly immunosuppressed patients with clinical and radiographic evidence of invasive aspergillosis. Rarely, patients with solid-organ cancer may present with non-*Aspergillus* locally invasive disease due to drug-resistant organisms (115).

Diagnosis

The diagnosis of a fungal infection is often quite difficult. The physician must differentiate between invasive disease, which must be treated, and colonization, which does not require therapy. The recovery of fungi from a urine, sputum, or wound culture does not necessarily mean that the fungus is pathogenic, and clinical judgment must be used to determine if a patient requires therapy. In general, cultures from sterile sites (e.g., blood, cerebrospinal fluid, pleural or peritoneal fluid) should be considered to represent invasive infection until a full evaluation is done. Also, fungi recovered from the initial specimen of drainage from an obstructed biliary or urinary tract should be considered to be pathogenic.

With most specimens however, the distinction between colonization and infection is not so simple. For urine, the presence or absence of pyuria is the simplest and most reliable means of differentiation: Those without pyuria are very likely only colonized and need no therapy. In such patients, a repeat urinalysis and culture may clarify the situation.

Therapy

Treatment options for invasive candidiasis have expanded in recent years. Amphotericin B and associated amphotericin B products (AmBisome and Abelcet) have the longest record for treatment of invasive fungal infections (113). The optimal duration of therapy for candidemia is not well defined and should be determined by individual responses. However, a 7- to 14-day course of therapy is probably adequate for most episodes (113).

In addition to amphotericin B products, both intravenous fluconazole therapy (400 mg daily) alone or in combination with amphotericin B and caspofungin (70-mg load and then 50 daily IV) are highly effective for non-neutropenic patients with fungemia (99,116,117). These agents offer comparable effectiveness but have fewer side effects than the amphotericin B products.

Patients who have *Candida* species consistently cultured from urine but no evidence of systemic fungal infection may benefit from bladder irrigation with amphotericin B, which reduces or eradicates bladder yeast colonization, and may prevent invasive fungal infection. Fluconazole is increasingly being given for this indication and appears to be effective.

Pneumonia

Etiology

Postoperative pneumonia remains a common cause of fever in any surgical patient, including those with gynecologic cancer. Infection may occur from aspiration during intubation or extubation or from hypoaeration due to "splinting" in patients with severe postoperative pain. Postobstructive pneumonia may occur in patients with tumor metastatic to the lungs. In addition, pneumonia may occur in patients with chemotherapy-induced neutropenia (see above).

Signs and Symptoms

The familiar signs and symptoms of pneumonia are cough, fever, chest discomfort, and dyspnea and evidence of pulmonary consolidation on lung examination.

Diagnosis

The diagnosis is usually suggested by the clinical situation and by the findings on physical examination. These are further supported by chest radiographs and sputum examination and culture. Chest radiography may show consolidation. Gram-negative organisms predominate in the mouth flora of hospitalized patients, so an aspiration pneumonia occurring in a hospitalized patient is typically due to gram-negative rods. Although thought by many to be a substantial contributor, anaerobes seldom cause aspiration pneumonia in the hospital.

Therapy

Empiric, rather than pathogen-based, coverage of a postoperative patient with clinical pneumonia is usually necessary and varies according to the setting (118). For a patient who has been hospitalized less than 3 days and has had no other recent hospitalizations or recent courses of oral or intravenous antibiotics, single-drug therapy with levofloxacin or moxifloxacin is adequate (118). For the patient who has been hospitalized for a longer period or who has received recent antibiotics (increasing the likelihood of infection due to resistant organisms), *P. aeruginosa* should be covered by the addition of an aminoglycoside such as gentamicin or tobramycin (3 to 5 mg/kg per day in three divided doses), and a beta-lactam should be selected to cover the usual isolates in that hospital. *S. maltophilia* is now increasingly seen in cancer patients without traditional risk factors such as severe neutropenia, prolonged stay in critical care units, or mechanical ventilation (119). Treatment includes high-dose trimethoprim-sulfamethoxazole (15 mg/kg in three to four divided doses) in combination with a second drug to which the bacteria are susceptible (17). Patients with drug-resistant *S. aureus* pulmonary infection may present with rapidly progressive, necrotizing pneumonia in a substantial number of cases during influenza season; these infections are especially serious postviral superinfections and require urgent, appropriate antibiotic therapy. Vancomycin (1 g twice daily), or linezolid (600 mg every 12 hours) may be given in patients with severe pneumonia and history of recent influenza-like illness. Therapy for patients with pneumonia should extend up to 10 to 14 days depending on clinical response. Various professional societies have codified recommendations for pneumonia management (120).

Gastroenterologic Sources of Infection

Diarrhea Associated With Antibiotics or Chemotherapy

Etiology. Diarrhea is a common finding in patients undergoing treatment of gynecologic malignancy. In a study of 351 hospitalized women with gynecologic cancer, 12% developed diarrhea during the course of their hospital stay; 10% had diarrhea due to *Clostridium difficile* (121). In cancer patients *C. difficile* diarrhea may be due to exposure to broad-spectrum antibiotics or chemotherapy alone (121,122).

Signs and Symptoms. Antibiotic-associated diarrhea can occur at any time during an antibiotic course and for at least a month after discontinuation. Patients typically develop abdominal pain, fever, and frequent watery diarrhea defined as ≥5 bowel movements per day lasting for more than 48 hours; however, *C. difficile* colitis may sometimes cause abdominal pain and fever without diarrhea.

Diagnosis. Any patient with antibiotic- or chemotherapy-associated diarrhea should have a full evaluation of stool, including routine cultures and a test for evidence of *C. difficile* toxin (123). In patients with a highly suspicious clinical presentation but no evidence of *C. difficile* toxin in stool, sigmoidoscopy or colonoscopy may reveal the pathognomonic mucosal pseudomembranes. One study has suggested that evaluation of stool for *C. difficile* toxin is the only cost-effective test (121). A markedly elevated white blood cell count may also be a clue to diagnosis (124).

Therapy. Oral therapy with metronidazole (250 mg to 500 mg four times daily for 2 to 4 weeks) is adequate to treat most cases of antibiotic-associated diarrhea (122–124). Because of continued reports of vancomycin-resistant bacteria (125), the use of oral vancomycin is restricted in many hospitals. Oral vancomycin should be given only to patients with proven *C. difficile* diarrhea who have not responded to metronidazole. Some patients may require repeated or prolonged courses of metronidazole, particularly if their clinical course necessitates continuation of the provocative agent (i.e., continued antibiotics or chemotherapy). Antidiarrheal compounds such as Lomotil or Imodium should not be given routinely. If, however, diarrhea persists after appropriate tests and cultures, symptomatic therapy should be considered. Nitazoxanide is a nitrothiazolide and effectively treats intestinal infestation of *Cryptosporidium* and *Giardia* species; at low concentrations nitazoxanide also inhibits *C. difficile*. A recent trial showed that nitazoxanide 500 mg twice daily was as effective in eradicating *C. difficile* as metronidazole given 250 mg four times daily (126). Nitazoxanide may be used for patients with metronidazole-refractory or recurrent *C. difficile* colitis.

Noninfectious Causes of Fever

Not all patients with gynecologic malignancy and fever have an infection. Pulmonary embolus, drug-related fever, and tumor-related fever represent the main noninfectious sources of fever, but others, such as factitious fever and underlying collagen vascular disorder, must also be considered. The use of procalcitonin and neopterin levels has been suggested to help distinguish between infected and noninfected patients, although further studies are needed to validate these tests (127).

Pulmonary embolus should be considered in a bed-bound or postoperative patient with any combination of fever, chest pain, dyspnea, or an abnormal chest radiograph. Patients with bulky pelvic tumors are also at risk. A high level of suspicion is important and spiral chest CT scans or ventilation-perfusion scans may establish the diagnosis; in rare instances a more definite pulmonary angiogram may be performed. Therapy remains anticoagulation with low-molecular-weight heparin. For patients who are unable to tolerate these drugs or who continue to have pulmonary emboli despite therapy, inferior vena caval filters are required.

Any antibiotic may cause fever (128). Patients typically develop fever and a diffuse maculopapular rash after several days of therapy. Eosinophilia, although a helpful sign, is usually lacking. Mild elevations in liver function tests may be present though nonspecific. Atypical presentations of drug fever, including patients without rash or those who develop fever weeks into therapy or after completion of therapy, can also occur. The diagnosis is usually made by discontinuing the antibiotic and observing the patient. It is important to remember that some drug fevers may take as long as a week to resolve. Supportive measures, such as antipyretics and antipruritics, may decrease symptoms.

The diagnosis of tumor fever can be made only after systematic exclusion of all other potential causes of fever. Most patients with tumor fever have metastatic disease involving the liver or lung. In these patients, the fever may be as high as 40°C, and chills may be absent; when not febrile, these patients often feel relatively well. In patients suspected of having tumor fever, a clinical trial of broad-spectrum antibiotics is given. If the fever does not abate and no other clear infection source is evident, the likelihood of tumor fever increases.

References

1. Safdar A, Armstrong D. Infections in patients with neoplastic diseases. In: Grenvik M, Ayers SM, Holbrook PR, et al., eds. *Textbook of Critical Care*, 4th ed. Philadelphia: W.B. Saunders; 2000:715–726.
2. Safdar A, Armstrong D. Infectious morbidty in critically ill patients with cancer. *Crit Care Clin* 2001;17:531–570.
3. Gilstrap LC, Gibbs RS, Michel TJ, et al. Genital aerobic bacterial flora of women receiving radiotherapy for gynecologic malignancy. *Gynecol Oncol* 1986;23:35–39.
4. Gordon AN, Martens M, LaPread Y, et al. Response of lower genital tract flora to external pelvic irradiation. *Gynecol Oncol* 1989;35:233–235.
5. Talwar P, Chakrabarti A, Patel F, et al. Yeasts at different mucosal sites in patients with carcinoma cervix before and following radiotherapy. *J Hyg Epidemiol Microbiol Immunol* 1992;36:311–316.
6. Evaldson G, Heimdahl A, Kager L, et al. The normal human anaerobic microflora. *Scand J Infect Dis* 1982;35:9–15.
7. Rolston KVI, Bodey GP, Safdar A. Polymicrobial infection in patients with cancer: an underappreciated and underreported entity. *Clin Infect Dis* 2007;45:228–233.
8. Barton DPJ, Fiorica JV, Hoffman MS, et al. Cervical cancer and tubo-ovarian abscesses: a report of three cases. *J Reprod Med* 1993;38: 561–564.
9. Imachi M, Tanaka S, Ishikawa S, et al. Spontaneous perforation of pyometra presenting as generalized peritonitis in a patient with cervical cancer. *Gynecol Oncol* 1993;50:384–388.
10. Protopappas AG, Diakomanolis ES, Milingos SD, et al. Tubo-ovarian abscess in postmenopausal women: gynecologic malignancy until proven otherwise. *Eur J Obstet Gynecol Reprod Biol* 2004;114:203–209.
11. Inagaki J, Rodriguez V, Bodey GP. Causes of death in cancer patients. *Cancer* 1974;33:568–573.
12. Iatrakis G, Sakellaropoulos G, Georgoulias N, et al. Gynecologic cancer and surgical infectious morbidity. *Clin Exp Obstet Gynecol* 1998;25:36–37.
13. Chang HK, Lo KY, Chiang HS. Complications of urinary diversion after pelvic exenteration for gynecologic malignancy. *Int Urogynecol J* 2000; 11:358–360.
14. Wydra D, Emerich J, Sawicki S, et al. Major complications following exenteration in cases of pelvic malignancies: a 10-year experience. *World J Gastroenterol* 2006;12:1115–1119.
15. Matar MJ, Safdar A, Rolston KV. Relationship of colonization with vancomycin-resistant enterococci and risk of systemic infection in patients with cancer. *Clin Infect Dis* 2006;42:1506–1507.
16. Gould N, Kamelle S, Tillmanns T, et al. Predictors of complications after inguinal lymphadenopathy. *Gynecol Oncol* 2001;82:329–332.
17. Safdar A, Rolston KV. *Stenotrophomonas maltophilia*: changing spectrum of a serious bacterial pathogen in patients with cancer. *Clin Infect Dis* 2007;45:1602–1609.
18. Safdar A, Rodriguez GH, Balakrishnan M, et al. Changing trends in etiology of bacteremia in patients with cancer. *Eur J Clin Microbiol Infect Dis* 2006;25:522–526.
19. Han XY, Kamana M, Rolston KV. Viridans streptococci isolated by culture from blood of cancer patients: clinical and microbiologic analysis of 50 cases. *J Clin Microbiol* 2006;44:160–165.
20. Green JA, Kirwan JM, Tierney JF. Survival and recurrence after concomitant chemotherapy and radiotherapy for cancer of the uterine cervix. *Lancet* 2001;385:781–786.
21. Yessaian A, Magistris A, Burger RA, et al. Radical hysterectomy followed by tailored postoperative therapy in the treatment of stage 1B2 cervical cancer: feasibility and indications for adjuvant therapy. *Gynecol Oncol* 2004;94:61–66.
22. Jurado M, Martinez-Monge R, Garcia-Foncillas J, et al. Pilot study of concurrent cisplatin, 5-fluorouracil, and external beam radiotherapy prior to radical surgery +/− intraoperative electron beam radiotherapy in locally advanced cervical cancer. *Gynecol Oncol* 1999;74:30–37.
23. Micha JP, Goldstein BH, Rettenmaier MA, et al. Pelvic radiation necrosis and osteomyelitis following chemoradiation for advanced stage vulvar and cervical carcinoma. *Gynecol Oncol* 2006;101:349–352.
24. Wisplinghoff H, Cornely OA, Moser S, et al. Outcomes of nosocomial bloodstream infections in adult neutropenic patients: a prospective cohort and matched case-control study. *Infect Control Hosp Epidemiol* 2003; 24:905–911.
25. Anatoliotaki A, Valatas V, Mantadakis E, et al. Bloodstream infections in patients with solid tumors: associated factors, microbial spectrum and outcome. *Infection* 2004;32:65–71.
26. Elting LS, Rubenstein EB, Rolston KV, et al. Outcomes of bacteremia in patients with cancer and neutropenia: observations from two decades of epidemiological and clinical trials. *Clin Infect Dis* 1997;25:247–259.
27. Zahar JR, Farhat H, Chachaty E, et al. Incidence and clinical significance of anaerobic bacteremia in cancer patients: a 6-year retrospective study. *Clin Microbiol Infect* 2005;11:724–729.
28. Fainstein V, Elting LS, Bodey GP. Bacteremia caused by non-sporulating anaerobes in cancer patients—a 12-year experience. *Medicine (Baltimore)* 1989;68:151–162.
29. Bodey GP, Rodriguez S, Fainstein V, et al. Clostridial bacteremia in cancer patients—a 12-year experience. *Cancer* 1991;67:1928–1942.
30. Pelletier JP, Plumbley JA, Rouse EA, et al. The role of *Clostridium septicum* in paraneoplastic sepsis. *Arch Pathol Lab Med* 2000;124:353–356.
31. Safdar A. Strategies to enhance immune function in hematopoietic transplantation recipients who have fungal infections. *Bone Marrow Transplant* 2006;38:327–337.
32. Safdar A, Singhal S, Mehta J. Clinical significance of non-*Candida* fungal blood isolation in patients undergoing high-risk allogeneic hematopoietic stem cell transplantation (1993–2001). *Cancer* 2004;100:2456–2461.
33. Raad I, Hachem R, Hanna H, et al. Sources and outcome of bloodstream infections in cancer patients: the role of central venous catheters. *Eur J Clin Microbiol Infect Dis* 2007;26:549–556.
34. Raad I, Hanna H, Jiang Y, et al. Comparative activities of daptomycin, Linezolid, and tigecycline against catheter-related methicillin-resistant *Staphylococcus* bacteremic isolates embedded in biofilm. *Antimicrob Agents Chemother* 2007;51:1656–1660.
35. Ghanem GA, Boktour M, Warneke C, et al. Catheter-related *Staphylococcus aureus* bacteremia in cancer patients: high rate of complications with therapeutic implications. *Medicine (Baltimore)* 2007;86:54–60.
36. Estes JM, Rocconi R, Straughn JM, et al. Complications of indwelling venous access devices in patients with gynecologic malignancies. *Gynecol Oncol* 2003;91:591–595.

37. Silver DF, Hempling RE, Recio FO, et al. Complications related to indwelling caval catheters on a gynecologic oncology service. *Gynecol Oncol* 1998;70:329–333.
38. Minassian VA, Sood AK, Lowe P, et al. Long-term central venous access in gynecologic cancer patients. *J Am Coll Surg* 2000;191:403–409.
39. Roybal JJ, Feliberti EC, Rouse L, et al. Pump removal in infected patients with hepatic chemotherapy pumps: when is it necessary? *Am Surg* 2006; 72:880–884.
40. Strecker EP, Heber R, Boos I, et al. Preliminary experience with locoregional intraarterial chemotherapy of uterine cervical or endometrial cancer using the peripheral implantable port system (PIPS): a feasibility study. *Cardiovasc Intervent Radiol* 2003;26:118–122.
41. Shoji T, Tanaka F, Yanagihara K, et al. Phase II study of repeated intrapleural chemotherapy using implantable access system for management of malignant pleural effusion. *Chest* 2002;121:821–824.
42. Sakuragi N, Nakajima A, Nomura E, et al. Complications related to intraperitoneal administration of cisplatin or carboplatin for ovarian carcinoma. *Gynecol Oncol* 2000;79:420–423.
43. Driesen P, Boutin C, Viallat JR, et al. Implantable access system for prolonged intrapleural immunotherapy. *Eur Respir J* 1994;7:1889–1892.
44. Adachi S, Noda T, Ito K, et al. Complications associated with CDDP intraperitoneal chemotherapy. *Asia Oceania J Obstet Gynaecol* 1994;20: 7–12.
45. Prasad KN, Pradhan S, Datta NR. Urinary tract infection in patients of gynecologic malignancies undergoing external pelvic radiotherapy. *Gynecol Oncol* 1995;57:380–382.
46. Roos EJ, Van Eijkeren MA, Boon TA, et al. Pelvic exenteration as treatment of recurrent or advanced gynecologic and urologic cancer. *Int J Gynecol Cancer* 2005;15:624–629.
47. Ledger WJ, Gee C, Lewis WP. Guidelines for antibiotic prophylaxis in gynecology. *Am J Obstet Gynecol* 1975;121:1038–1045.
48. Hemsell DL, Johnson ER, Hemsell PG, et al. Cefazolin is inferior to cefotetan as single-dose prophylaxis for women undergoing elective total abdominal hysterectomy. *Clin Infect Dis* 1995;20:677–684.
49. Hemsell DL, Bernstein SG, Bawdon RE, et al. Preventing major operative site infection after radical abdominal hysterectomy and pelvic lymphadenectomy. *Gynecol Oncol* 1989;35:55–60.
50. Velasco E, Thuler LC, Martins CA, et al. Risk factors for infectious complications after abdominal surgery for malignant disease. *Am J Infect Control* 1996;24:1–6.
51. Brooker DC, Savage JE, Twiggs LB, et al. Infectious morbidity in gynecologic cancer. *Am J Obstet Gynecol* 1987;156:513–520.
52. Morgan LS, Daly JW, Monif GR. Infectious morbidity associated with pelvic exenteration. *Gynecol Oncol* 1980;10:318–328.
53. Orr JW Jr, Shingleton HM, Hatch KD, et al. Correlation of perioperative morbidity and conization to radical hysterectomy interval. *Obstet Gynecol* 1982;59:726–731.
54. Berkeley AS, Orr JW, Cavanagh D, et al. Comparative effectiveness and safety of cefotetan and cefoxitin as prophylactic agents in patients undergoing abdominal or vaginal hysterectomy. *Am J Surg* 1988;155: 81–85.
55. Mann WJ Jr, Orr JW, Shingleton HM, et al. Perioperative influences on infectious morbidity in radical hysterectomy. *Gynecol Oncol* 1981;11: 207–212.
56. Gussman D, RJ Carlson JA Jr. Prophylaxis for radical hysterectomy. *Infect Surg* 1987;6:55.
57. Rosenshein NB, Ruth JC, Villar J, et al. A prospective randomized study of doxycycline as a prophylactic antibiotic in patients undergoing radical hysterectomy. *Gynecol Oncol* 1983;15:201–206.
58. Marsden DE, Cavanagh D, Wisniewski BJ, et al. Factors affecting the incidence of infectious morbidity after radical hysterectomy. *Am J Obstet Gynecol* 1985;152:817–821.
59. Sevin BU, Ramos R, Lichtinger M, et al. Antibiotic prevention of infections complicating radical abdominal hysterectomy. *Obstet Gynecol* 1984;64:539–545.
60. Micha JP, Kucera PR, Birkett JP, et al. Prophylactic mezlocillin in radical hysterectomy. *Obstet Gynecol* 1987;69:251–254.
61. Sevin BU, Ramos R, Gerhardt RT, et al. Comparative efficacy of short-term versus long-term cefoxitin prophylaxis against postoperative infection after radical hysterectomy: a prospective study. *Obstet Gynecol* 1991;77:729–734.
62. Shapiro M, Schoenbaum SC, Tager IB, et al. Benefit-cost analysis of antimicrobial prophylaxis in abdominal and vaginal hysterectomy. *JAMA* 1983;249:1290–1294.
63. van Lindert AC, Giltaij AR, Derksen MD, et al. Single-dose prophylaxis with broad-spectrum penicillins (piperacillin and mezlocillin) in gynecologic oncological surgery, with observation on serum and tissue concentrations. *Eur J Obstet Gynecol Reprod Biol* 1990;36: 137–145.
64. Smith CV, GD, Gibbs RL, et al. Oral doxycycline vs. parenteral cefazolin: prophylaxis for vaginal hysterectomy. *Infect Surg* 1989;99:64.
65. Turner S. The effect of penicillin vaginal suppositories on morbidity in vaginal hysterectomy and on the vaginal flora. *Am J Obstet Gynecol* 1950;60:806–812.
66. Wright VC, Lanning MN, Natale R. Use of a topical antibiotic spray in vaginal surgery. *Can Med Assoc J* 1978;118:1395–1398.
67. Shapiro M, Munoz A, Tager IB, et al. Risk factors for infection at the operative site after abdominal or vaginal hysterectomy. *N Engl J Med* 1982;307:1661–1666.
68. Hemsell DL, Heard MC, Hemsell PG, et al. Alterations in lower reproductive tract flora after single-dose piperacillin and triple-dose cefoxitin at vaginal and abdominal hysterectomy. *Obstet Gynecol* 1988;72:875–880.
69. Hemsell DL, Bawdon RE, Hemsell PG, et al. Single-dose cephalosporin for prevention of major pelvic infection after vaginal hysterectomy: cefazolin versus cefoxitin versus cefotaxime. *Am J Obstet Gynecol* 1987;156: 1201–1205.
70. Hemsell DL, Johnson ER, Hemsell PG, et al. Cefazolin inferior to cefotetan for single-dose prophylaxis in women undergoing hysterectomy. *Clin Infect Dis* 1995;20:677.
71. Kobamatsu Y, Makinoda S, Yamada T, et al. Evaluation of the improvement of cephems on the prophylaxis of pelvic infection after radical hysterectomy. *Gynecol Obstet Invest* 1991;32:102–106.
72. Bratzler DW, Hunt DR. The surgical infection prevention and surgical care improvement projects: national initiatives to improve outcomes for patients having surgery. *Clin Infect Dis* 2006;43:322–330.
73. Contant CM, Hop WC, van't Sant HP, et al. Mechanical bowel preparation for elective colorectal surgery: a multicenter randomized trial. *Lancet* 2008;370:2112–2117.
74. Nichols RL, Condon RE. Preoperative preparation of the colon. *Surg Gynecol Obstet* 1971;132:323–337.
75. Lichtenstein GR, Cohen LB, Uribarri J. Review article: bowel preparation for colonoscopy—the importance of adequate hydration. *Aliment Pharmacol Ther* 2007;26:633–641.
76. Braverman J, Adachi A, Lev-Gur M, et al. Spontaneous clostridia gas gangrene of uterus associated with endometrial malignancy. *Am J Obstet Gynecol* 1987;156:1205–1207.
77. Douvier S, Nabholtz JM, Friedman S, et al. Infectious pneumoperitoneum as an uncommon presentation of endometrial carcinoma: report of two cases. *Gynecol Oncol* 1989;33:392–394.
78. Weinstein WM, Onderdonk AB, Bartlett JG, et al. Experimental intra-abdominal abscesses in rats: development of an experimental model. *Infect Immun* 1974;10:1250–1255.
79. Safdar A, Rolston KV. Vancomycin tolerance, a potential mechanism for refractory gram-positive bacteremia observational study in patients with cancer. *Cancer* 2006;106:1815–1820.
80. Ohmagari N, Hanna H, Graviss L, et al. Risk factors for infections with multidrug-resisatnt *Pseudomonas aeruginosa* in patients with cancer. *Cancer* 2005;104:205–212.
81. Roy S, Higareda I, Angel-Muller E, et al. Ertapenem once a day versus piperacillin-tazobactam every 6 hours for treatment of acute pelvic infections: a prospective, multicenter, randomized, double-blind study. *Infect Dis Obstet Gynecol* 2003;11:27–37.
82. McNeeley SG Jr, Hopkins MP, Ehlerova B, et al. Infection on a gynecologic oncology service. *Gynecol Oncol* 1990;37:183–187.
83. Henderson W. Synergistic bacterial gangrene abdominal hysterectomy. *Obstet Gynecol* 1977:49(1 suppl):24–27.
84. Bouma J, Dankert J. Recurrent acute leg cellulitis in patients after radical vulvectomy. *Gynecol Oncol* 1988;29:50–57.
85. Hunt TK, Rabkin J, von Smitten K. Effects of edema and anemia on wound healing and infection. *Curr Stud Hematol Blood Transfus* 1986;53:101–113.
86. Bahary CM, Joel-Cohen SJ, Neri A. Necrotizing fasciitis. *Obstet Gynecol* 1977;50:633–637.
87. Wilson B. Necrotizing fasciitis. *Am Surg* 1952;18:416–431.
88. Daly JW, King CR, Monif GR. Progressive necrotizing wound infections in postirradiated patients. *Obstet Gynecol* 1978;52(Suppl):5S–8S.
89. Husseinzadeh N, Nahhas WA, Manders EK, et al. Spontaneous occurrence of synergistic bacterial gangrene following external pelvic irradiation. *Obstet Gynecol* 1984;63:859–862.
90. Bearman DM, Livengood CH 3rd, Addison WA. Necrotizing fasciitis arising from a suprapubic catheter site. A case report. *J Reprod Med* 1988;33:411–413.
91. Hoffman MS, Turnquist D. Necrotizing fasciitis of the vulva during chemotherapy. *Obstet Gynecol* 1989;74:483–484.
92. Roberts DB. Necrotizing fasciitis of the vulva. *Am J Obstet Gynecol* 1987;157:568–571.
93. Pruyn SC. Acute necrotizing fasciitis of the endopelvic fascia. *Obstet Gynecol* 1978;52(Suppl):25–45.
94. Sotrel G, Hirsch E, Edelin KC. Necrotizing fasciitis following diagnostic laparoscopy. *Obstet Gynecol* 1983;62(3 Suppl):67S–69S.
95. McNeeley SG Jr, Hendrix SL, Bennett SM, et al. Synthetic graft placement in the treatment of fascial dehiscence with necrosis and infection. *Am J Obstet Gynecol* 1998;179:1430–1434.
96. Fisher JR, Conway MJ, Takeshita RT, et al. Necrotizing fasciitis. Importance of roentgenographic studies for soft-tissue gas. *JAMA* 1979;241:803–806.
97. Altmeier WA. Gas gangrene. *Surg Gynecol Obstet* 1947;84:504.
98. Fujiwara K, Sakuragi N, Suzuki S, et al. First-line intraperitoneal carboplatin-based chemotherapy for 165 patients with epithelial ovarian carcinoma: results of long-term follow-up. *Gynecol Oncol* 2003;90:637–643.
99. Mora-Duarte J, Betts R, Rotstein C, et al. Comparison of caspofungin and amphotericin B for invasive candidiasis. *N Engl J Med* 2002;347: 2020–2029.

100. Blot SI, Vandewoude KH, Waele JJ. *Candida* peritonitis. *Curr Opin Crit Care* 2007;13:195–199.
101. Miller C. Ligation or excision of the pelvic veins in the treatment of puerperal pyaemia. *Surg Gynecol Obstet* 1917;25:431.
102. Twickler DM, et al. Imaging of puerperal septic thrombophlebitis: prospective comparison of MR imaging, CT, and sonography. *AJR Am J Roentgenol* 1997;169:1039–1043.
103. Zerhouni EA, Barth KH, Siegelman SS. Demonstration of venous thrombosis by computed tomography. *AJR Am J Roentgenol* 1980;134:753–758.
104. Schulman H, Zatuchni G. Pelvic thrombophlebitis in the puerperal and postoperative gynecology patient. Obscure fever as an indication for anticoagulant therapy. *Am J Obstet Gynecol* 1964;90:1293–1296.
105. Twickler DM, Setiawan AT, Evans RS, et al. Imaging of puerperal septic thrombophlebitis: prospective comparison of MR imaging, CT, and sonography. *AJR Am J Roentgenol* 1997;169:1039–1043.
106. Josey WE, Staggers SR Jr. Heparin therapy in septic pelvic thrombophlebitis: a study of 46 cases. *Am J Obstet Gynecol* 1974;120:228–233.
107. Brown CE, Stettler RW, Twickler D, et al. Puerperal septic pelvic thrombophlebitis: incidence and response to heparin therapy. *Am J Obstet Gynecol* 1999;181:143–148.
108. Lee AY, et al. Low-molecular-weight heparin versus a coumadin for the prevention of recurrent venous thromboembolism in patients with cancer. *N Engl J Med* 2003;349:146–153.
109. Stanton PE Jr, Evans JR, Lefemine AA, et al. White clot syndrome. *South Med J* 1988;81:616–620.
110. Raad II, Escalante C, Hachem RY, et al. Treatment of febrile neutropenic patients with cancer who require hospitalization. A prospective randomized study comparing imipenem and cefepime. *Cancer* 2003;98:1039–1047.
111. Klastersky J, Ameye L, Maertens J, et al. Bacteremia in febrile neutropenic cancer patients. *Int J Antimicrob Agents* 2007;30(Suppl 1):51–59.
112. Hughes WT, Armstrong D, Bodey GP, et al. 2002 guidelines for the use of antimicrobial agents in neutropenic patients with cancer. *Clin Infect Dis* 2002;34:730–751.
113. Rex JH, Walsh TJ, Sobel JD, et al. Practice guidelines for the treatment of candidiasis. Infectious Diseases Society of America. *Clin Infect Dis* 2000;30:662–678.
114. Marsh PK, Tally FP, Kellum J, et al. Candida infections in surgical patients. *Ann Surg* 1983;198:42–47.
115. Safdar A. Progress cutaneous hyalohyphomycosis due to *Paecilomyces lilacinus*: rapid response to treatment with caspofungin and itraconazole. *Clin Infect Dis* 2002;34:1415–1417.
116. Rex JH, Bennett JE, Sugar AM, et al. A randomized trial comparing fluconazole with amphotericin B for the treatment of candidemia in patients without neutropenia. Candidemia Study Group and the National Institute. *N Engl J Med* 1994;331:1325–1230.
117. Rex JH, Pappas PG, Karchmer AW, et al. A randomized and blinded multicenter trial of high-dose fluconazole plus placebo versus fluconazole plus amphotericin B as therapy for candidemia and its consequences in nonneutropenic subjects. *Clin Infect Dis* 2003;36:1221–1228.
118. Marik PE. Aspiration pneumonitis and aspiration pneumonia. *N Engl J Med* 2001;344: 665–671.
119. Aisenberg G, Rolston KV, Dickey BF, et al. *Stenotrophomonas maltophilia* pneumonia in cancer patients without traditional risk factors for infection, 1997–2004. *Eur J Clin Microbiol Infect Dis* 2007;26:13–20.
120. Mandell LA, Wunderrink RG, Anzueto A, et al. Infectious Diseases Society of America/American Thoracic Society consensus guidelines on the management of community-acquired pneumonia in adults. *Clin Infect Dis* 2007;44(Suppl 2):S27–S72.
121. Cirisano FD, Greenspoon JS, Stenson R, et al. The etiology and management of diarrhea in the gynecologic oncology patient. *Gynecol Oncol* 1993;50:45–48.
122. Satin AJ, Harrison CR, Hancock KC, et al. Relapsing *Clostridium difficile* toxin-associated colitis in ovarian cancer patients treated with chemotherapy. *Obstet Gynecol* 1989;74:487–489.
123. Turgeon DK, Novicki TJ, Ouick J, et al. Six rapid tests for direct detection of *Clostridium difficile* and its toxins in fecal samples compared with the fibroblast cytotoxicity assay. *J Clin Microbiol* 2003;41:667–670.
124. Wanahita A, Goldsmith EA, Marino BJ, et al. *Clostridium difficile* infection in patients with unexplained leukocytosis. *Am J Med* 2003;115: 543–546.
125. Low DE, Keller N, Barth A, et al. Clinical prevalence, antimicrobial susceptibility, and geographic resistance patterns of enterococci: results from the SENTRY Antimicrobial Surveillance Program, 1997–1999. *Clin Infect Dis* 2001;32(Suppl 2):S133–S145.
126. Musher DM, Logan N, Hamill RJ, et al. Nitazoxanide for the treatment of *Clostridium difficile* colitis. *Clin Infect Dis* 2006;43:421–427.
127. Ruokonen E, Ilkka L, Niskanen M, et al. Procalcitonin and neopterin as indicators of infection in critically ill patients. *Acta Anaesthesiol Scand* 2002;46:398–404.
128. Hirschmann JV. Fever of unknown origin in adults. *Clin Infect Dis* 1997;24:291–300; Quiz 301–302.

CHAPTER 31 ■ MANAGEMENT OF COMPLICATIONS OF GYNECOLOGIC CANCER TREATMENT

DAVID G. MUTCH, CATHERYN YASHAR, MAURIE MARKMAN, AND STEPHEN C. RUBIN

The treatment of a serious illness such as cancer always involves the judicious search for a proper balance between efficacy and toxicity. Although we strive to maximize cure and minimize side effects, a certain acceptable level of treatment-related complications is unavoidable. This chapter reviews the management of the late complications of the major therapeutic modalities used in cancer treatment: chemotherapy, radiation therapy, and surgery. The distinction between the acute and late complications of therapy is arbitrary; we consider late toxic effects to be those that initially become clinically evident more than several months after the initiation of therapy.

CHEMOTHERAPY

Anemia, myelosuppression, and thrombocytopenia, which are among the most common acute complications of chemotherapy, may persist for months after the completion of treatment. In general, a delay in return of marrow function to normal does not imply that the patient will experience any long-term hematopoietic effects of treatment. However, if the patient requires future treatment with marrow-toxic drugs, it is likely that the marrow reserve will be limited.

Myelodysplastic Syndrome and Acute Nonlymphocytic Leukemia

Perhaps the most feared long-term complication of the administration of chemotherapeutic agents is the potential for the development of myelodysplasia and acute leukemia. Although first recognized more than a decade ago in patients with ovarian cancer treated with alkylating agents, it is now clearly documented that the *chronic* administration of this class of antineoplastic agents is associated with roughly a tenfold increased risk for the development of acute nonlymphocytic leukemia (1,2). Granulocytic leukemia is not a common disease; only approximately 12,000 cases are diagnosed in the United States each year. The peak incidence of secondary leukemia occurs 4 to 5 years after chemotherapy administration; an increased risk is noted for at least 8 years after the cessation of cytotoxic drug treatment.

Survival after the diagnosis of treatment-related acute nonlymphocytic leukemia is generally measured in months. Specific antileukemia therapy, although occasionally of clinical benefit, is usually unsuccessful in producing complete or long-lasting remission. In many patients with this clinical syndrome, it is most appropriate that the management plan involves supportive and comfort measures only (i.e., transfusions, antibiotic therapy, pain medications).

Current chemotherapy for gynecologic or other malignancies is quite different from the prolonged alkylating agent therapy reported to result in an unacceptably high incidence of acute leukemia. In ovarian cancer, studies have demonstrated that five or six treatment cycles or more prolonged treatment regimens produce equivalent therapeutic results (response rates and survival) (3,4). With fewer courses, both short-term (marrow suppression, emesis) and chronic side effects, including the risk of acute leukemia, should be reduced.

Because the majority of reports that estimated the risk of secondary leukemia after cytotoxic drug therapy in ovarian cancer were from the pre-cisplatin chemotherapy era, an association between cisplatin and leukemia remains unsettled (5–10). One report has suggested that the use of cisplatin in ovarian cancer may increase the risk for the development of acute leukemia by approximately fourfold (11). However, it is important to note that essentially all patients who received cisplatin in the pre-paclitaxel era also received an alkylating agent (generally cyclophosphamide), a class of drugs known to be leukemogenic (2,12). Based on all available data, it is appropriate to state that even this small increase in the risk of developing acute leukemia is an acceptable price to pay for the substantial improvement in overall survival associated with the use of platinum agents in ovarian cancer.

In view of the documented risk of acute leukemia associated with the long-term use of alkylating agents in ovarian cancer and the known low response rate of the disease to this class of drugs (delivered at standard dose levels) in individuals who fail an initial cisplatin-based regimen (13), the administration of chronic oral alkylating agent therapy (chlorambucil, melphalan) as a second- or third-line treatment is strongly discouraged. Several studies have confirmed that the use of etoposide is strongly associated with the development of acute leukemia (14–17). This risk appears to be highly correlated with the total cumulative dose of the drug administered over time. Therefore, for diseases in which etoposide is an appropriate or required component of treatment (e.g., germ cell tumors), management of the malignancy should include the use of optimal doses/schedules of the agent delivered for the minimal acceptable number of cycles.

Cardiac Toxicity

Doxorubicin, which has demonstrated activity in several gynecologic malignancies, is an important component of a number of commonly used treatment regimens (18). Its most serious potential side effect is cardiac toxicity (19). Whereas acute cardiac dysfunction (e.g., arrhythmias, pericarditis) may occasionally be observed, chronic heart failure is much more common. The incidence of subclinical and clinical congestive heart failure is directly related to the cumulative dose of doxorubicin administered (20). Cardiac abnormalities are rarely observed with a total doxorubicin dose <350 mg. With a cumulative dose of >550 mg/m^2, the incidence of cardiac dysfunction is 1% to 10%.

Risk factors for cardiac toxicity necessitating a lowering of the doxorubicin dose that can be safely administered include a history of significant hypertension or pre-existing cardiac disease, prior cardiac or mediastinal irradiation, and age >70 years (19). Patients who have received cardiac irradiation are at a particularly high risk for developing cardiac complications even when the "safe" dose level of doxorubicin is reduced by 50% (250 mg/m^2) compared with those without such a history.

Doxorubicin-induced heart injury is unique, and specific histologic features are observed in tissue obtained through a cardiac biopsy during a right-heart catheterization (21). When morphologic abnormalities are graded, an objective scoring system appears to correlate well with the severity of the underlying pathologic process. However, although the results of a cardiac biopsy are predictive of future clinical symptoms, it is not a practical procedure to use in routine clinical practice.

Evaluation of serial echocardiogram (ECG)-gated blood-pool scans allows for a reasonably accurate assessment of the effect of doxorubicin on cardiac function (22,23). In most patients, a major drop in the cardiac ejection fraction is observed *before* the onset of clinical symptoms, allowing for discontinuation of the antineoplastic agent before more serious damage results.

Treatment of doxorubicin-induced heart failure focuses on improving myocardial contractility with afterload reduction and diuresis. Many patients improve symptomatically. Continued improvement in cardiac function has been noted more than a year after initial symptoms are observed.

Several methods have been used in standard clinical practice and experimentally to reduce the risk of the development of chronic cardiac dysfunction associated with doxorubicin, including administration by continuous infusion for several days (rather than by bolus instillation) (24) and the use of dexrazoxane, the first drug demonstrated to reduce anthracycline-induced cardiac injury (25). Neither technique appears to decrease the antineoplastic activity of doxorubicin compared with standard bolus administration.

The combination of doxorubicin and paclitaxel can result in an increased risk for cardiac toxicity compared with the use of doxorubicin alone (12). The appropriate sequencing of the drugs appears to reduce the risk of cardiac effects.

The combination of doxorubicin and herceptin (anti–HER2/neu monoclonal antibody) also appears to potentiate the cardiac toxicity of doxorubicin and to a lesser extent that of paclitaxel (26). There is currently inadequate information available to recommend specific management strategies to reduce the risk of toxicity when either chemotherapeutic agent is combined with this novel monoclonal antibody.

Although paclitaxel itself has been considered to be an agent with potential cardiac toxicity, particularly in individuals with pre-existing cardiac abnormalities, available data have suggested that most individuals can safely receive the drug without concern for the development of either acute (arrhythmias) or chronic (congestive heart failure) cardiac toxicities (27).

Pulmonary Toxicity

Bleomycin, an antitumor antibiotic, is a common component of the treatment regimen for patients with carcinoma of the cervix and malignant germ cell tumors (18). The most serious toxic effect of bleomycin is subacute or chronic interstitial pneumonitis (28). This inflammatory process may progress to a fibrotic stage, with subsequent significant impairment of pulmonary function.

The most common early symptoms of bleomycin-induced pulmonary toxicity are cough and dyspnea. Bibasilar pulmonary infiltrates have been reported in as many as 5% of patients who receive total cumulative doses of bleomycin <450 mg. The incidence rises to 10% with higher cumulative doses. However, it should be noted that severe pulmonary toxicity has been observed at total bleomycin doses <100 mg.

In addition to the cumulative dose received, other risk factors for bleomycin-induced pulmonary dysfunction include pre-existing emphysema, age >70 years, single doses >25 mg/m^2, and prior chest irradiation.

An interesting, potentially serious complication of bleomycin is the development of postoperative respiratory failure in patients previously treated with this agent (29). It has been postulated that bleomycin makes the lung more susceptible to oxygen toxicity. Lowering the inspired oxygen concentration during surgery to an FIO_2 of 0.24 and avoiding fluid overload during surgery appear to substantially reduce the risk of postoperative respiratory insufficiency.

The pathogenesis of bleomycin-induced pulmonary dysfunction is not completely understood. The agent produces an inflammatory intra-alveolar infiltrate with edema, followed by a proliferation of alveolar macrophages and subsequent interstitial fibrosis. In experimental systems, high concentrations achieved after bolus administration of bleomycin produced more pulmonary damage than either continuous infusion or delivery of low doses on a frequent dosing schedule. These data provide strong support for the clinical use of the agent either as a continuous intravenous infusion or on a low-dose weekly bolus schedule.

No specific treatment exists for bleomycin pulmonary toxicity except discontinuing the agent if pulmonary function tests, particularly the carbon monoxide–diffusing capacity, demonstrate a significant deterioration compared with baseline. Mild worsening in pulmonary function (10% to 15%) is common in patients treated with >240 mg of bleomycin. A more substantial worsening observed in pulmonary function tests should lead to the discontinuation of the antineoplastic drug. Steroid therapy may help reduce inflammation and improve symptoms, but it has little or no impact on established fibrotic lesions. Fortunately, most patients with subclinical disease or mild symptoms demonstrate improvement in symptoms, radiographic findings, and pulmonary function tests.

Mitomycin C, an antineoplastic agent used in patients with several gynecologic malignancies, can produce a syndrome similar to bleomycin-induced pulmonary insufficiency (17). Higher cumulative doses of the agent (20 mg/m^2) appear to increase the risk of mitomycin C–induced pulmonary dysfunction (30). Symptoms include cough and progressive dyspnea. Corticosteroids may be helpful, but patients can develop progressive pulmonary insufficiency. As many as 5% to 7% of patients treated with mitomycin C have been reported to have clinical or subclinical evidence of pulmonary toxicity (30).

Neurotoxicity

The dose-limiting side effect of cisplatin, one of the most important drugs in the management of gynecologic malignancies, is neurotoxicity (31–33). The neurologic effects of cisplatin include peripheral sensory neuropathy, ototoxicity, retinal toxicity, seizures, and autonomic dysfunction.

It is difficult to know the precise incidence of cisplatin-induced neurotoxicity because most early reports only occasionally noted this form of toxicity. In the past, the dose-limiting toxicity of cisplatin was acute renal dysfunction, and in most patients, it was not possible to administer high enough cumulative doses of cisplatin to observe nervous system toxicity (34). With the development of intensive hydration regimens, it has become possible to significantly increase the amount of cisplatin administered to individual patients.

Although cisplatin-induced neurotoxicity may occur after a single dose, most reports suggest that the incidence of this class of side effects increases with higher cumulative doses (31). A summary of the oncologic literature reveals that the incidence of cisplatin neurotoxicity is approximately 15% with a total cumulative dose <300 mg/m^2, but it rises to 85% with doses of >300 mg/m^2 (31).

The most common cisplatin-induced neurologic side effects result from toxicity to the peripheral sensory nerves. Patients complain of numbness, tingling, and paresthesia that involve the feet, legs, hands, and arms. Symptoms generally begin in the feet or hands and proceed proximally. Reflexes (ankle, knee) are lost, and vibratory sensation is greatly diminished. With continued treatment, patients may lose the ability to sense touch or pinprick. Ultimately, patients have difficulty walking and using their hands for fine motion (e.g., writing, picking up a fork).

Fortunately, recovery after cisplatin-induced peripheral neuropathy is common, although frequently not complete. Improvement in symptoms has been noted more than 2 years after the discontinuation of therapy, although most patients begin to note improvement within several months of stopping the antineoplastic drug.

Another important feature of cisplatin-induced neuropathy is that the initial symptoms may develop months after the last dose, and symptoms commonly worsen when the drug is stopped, only to improve several months later. This factor makes it difficult for the clinician to know whether a patient who experiences a mild neuropathy should continue to receive the agent because the ultimate severity of the current symptoms may not be known until after the next dose is scheduled to be given.

Cisplatin administration may also cause tinnitus and hearing loss in the high-frequency range (35). High-dose cisplatin regimens (100 mg/m^2 per dose) that achieve very high peak plasma levels appear to result in a greater incidence of ototoxicity than lower-dose regimens (35,36). Paclitaxel (Taxol) can also produce a peripheral neuropathy, which is a dose-limiting toxicity of the agent (37). The neuropathy has been noted to worsen with higher cumulative dosing in some patients and to persist for considerable periods of time (>6 months) (37).

The combination of paclitaxel and cisplatin has been shown to have the potential to produce a higher incidence of peripheral neuropathy than either agent used alone. Of particular concern is the combination of cisplatin (75 mg/m^2) and 3-hour infusion of paclitaxel (175 mg/m^2), where several studies have demonstrated a 20% to 25% incidence of severe (grade 3) peripheral neuropathy (38,39).

Although less neurotoxic than cisplatin plus paclitaxel, combination chemotherapy with carboplatin and paclitaxel, a commonly employed regimen in several gynecologic malignancies, also has the potential to produce distressing symptoms associated with the development of a peripheral neuropathy (40).

Renal Insufficiency

Cisplatin is the chemotherapeutic agent most commonly associated with renal compromise (34). Although the damage to the kidney is reversible in most patients, persistent abnormalities in renal function are common in patients who experience acute toxicity. In addition, severe irreversible renal toxicity secondary to cisplatin has been reported; fortunately, however, it is rare.

Cisplatin produces its nephrotoxic effects by damaging the renal tubules. Vigorous saline diuresis has been shown to prevent the development of major renal impairment in most patients who receive this agent, although significant decreases in creatinine clearance are common after standard cisplatin treatment programs for ovarian cancer (400 to 600 mg/m^2 cumulative dose).

In addition to abnormalities in renal function tests, hypomagnesemia secondary to renal magnesium wasting is common after cisplatin administration. Although this defect generally does not result in clinical symptoms of hypomagnesemia, renal magnesium wasting can be demonstrated in many patients more than a year after discontinuation of cisplatin.

Mitomycin may also be associated with renal damage and kidney failure of such severity that chronic dialysis is required (41).

Infertility and Mutagenic Potential

One of the greatest concerns of younger female patients who receive chemotherapy is its effect on fertility. The data that directly address the influence of antineoplastic agents on fertility are limited because accurate figures on the incidence of subsequent pregnancies are not available.

The development of amenorrhea during chemotherapy is influenced by patient age, as well as the specific drug used. Younger patients appear to be able to receive higher cumulative doses of cytotoxic drugs than older women before amenorrhea occurs (42). Existing data reveal that the majority of young women treated with standard chemotherapy for gynecologic malignancies, including the intensive regimens employed in ovarian germ cell tumors, have an excellent chance to maintain fertility (43–45).

One summary of the literature on the influence of chemotherapy on ovarian function concludes that, if a woman continues to menstruate after administration of cytotoxic antineoplastic therapy, no therapy-related impairment in her ability to become pregnant should exist (42). However, it remains uncertain whether such women will experience premature menopause; therefore, a woman must consider this factor in any decisions about family planning.

An additional important question about fertility is the risk of an increase in congenital abnormalities in the children of women treated with cytotoxic drug therapy. Again, although the available data in the medical literature that address this point are limited and conflicting, the consensus is that no significant increase of spontaneous abortions or fetal abnormalities in pregnancies occurs in this setting, and fetal development (including intellectual function) appears to be normal (46,47).

It is noteworthy that the administration of specific chemotherapeutic agents, most notably the antimetabolites (e.g., methotrexate), during early pregnancy is associated with the development of fetal abnormalities (46). In addition, follow-up of children exposed to antineoplastic agents *in utero* is of limited duration, and the ultimate impact of such therapy will be known only when long-term follow-up is available (47).

RADIATION THERAPY

Radiation therapy is used in the primary treatment of cervical, vulvar, uterine, and vaginal carcinomas as well as in the adjuvant setting and is often used as a palliative measure. Recent advances such as chemoradiation have improved outcomes

TABLE 31.1

RADIATION THERAPY ONCOLOGY GROUP MORBIDITY GRADING SYSTEM

Grade	Morbidity
1	Minor symptoms requiring no treatment
2	Symptoms responding to simple outpatient management; lifestyle (performance status) not affected
3	Distressing symptoms altering patient's lifestyle (performance status); hospitalization for diagnosis or minor surgical intervention (e.g., urethral dilatation) may be required
4	Major surgical intervention (e.g., laparotomy, colostomy, cystectomy) or prolonged hospitalization is required
5	Fatal complications

Source: Reprinted with permission from Pilepich MV, Pajak T, George FW, et al. Preliminary report on phase III RTOG studies of extended-field irradiation in carcinoma of the prostate. *Am J Clin Oncol* 1983;6:485–491.

but toxicity and overall control for locoregionally advanced tumors remain a concern (48–53). To combat toxicity, new treatment modalities such as intensity-modulated radiation therapy (IMRT), image-guided radiation therapy (IGRT), and 3D-based brachytherapy are under investigation as are radioprotectors such as amifostine (Ethyol).

Despite advances, radiation inevitably leads to effects on normal tissues that can be divided into two categories: acute effects and late effects. Acute effects begin during a radiation course at approximately 2,000 cGy with symptoms gradually increasing during treatment and typically resolving completely in 4 to 6 weeks. Late effects initially are manifest as early as 1 month following the completion of therapy and can last a lifetime. These effects can be seen in the skin, urinary tract, gastrointestinal tract, and reproductive tract. A significant correlation between the severity of acute effects and the development of late effects has been controversial with some studies finding a relationship (54–58).

Multiple grading systems have been used in the past to quantify normal tissue reactions and complications. In 1983, the Radiation Therapy Oncology Group (RTOG) published a meaningful grading system for radiation complications (Table 31.1). By 2007, most cooperative groups adopted a unified system to make communication easier and more complete. The reporting systems used by both the Gynecologic Oncology Group and the Radiation Therapy Oncology Group are the National Cancer Institute Common Terminology Criteria for Adverse Events and the Common Toxicity Criteria (found at the NCI website address http://ctep.cancer.gov/reporting/ctc.html).

Normal tissue effects are influenced by dose fractionation, field arrangement, total dose, volume irradiated, and inherent tissue sensitivity. Some reports in the literature have demonstrated a correlation between increased total external beam doses and higher complication rates (Table 31.2). Radiobiologists estimate that in the case of injury to the normal tissues, only 5% to 20% of the damage is repaired. The radiation-induced late tissue effects are usually attributed to progressive obliterative endarteritis that leads to decreased blood flow and subsequent hypoxia and scarring (59). Further injury from surgery, biopsy, or recurrent tumor will leave the tissues at even greater risk for poor healing, ulceration, fistulization, and necrosis. Table 31.3 lists tolerance of normal tissue to therapeutic irradiation.

Bone Injury

The bony pelvis is weakened by radiotherapy due to progressive microvascular obliteration leading to decreased osteoblast/osteoclast function. The subsequent changes can lead to increased fragility with subsequent stress fracture or outright necrosis

TABLE 31.2

INCIDENCE OF GRADE 2 AND 3 GASTROINTESTINAL COMPLICATIONS (RTOG SCALE) IN RELATION TO EXTERNAL PELVIC IRRADIATION DOSE

Reference	No. of patients	Whole pelvic dose (Gy)	Complications (%)
Hamberger et al. (196)	192	40	3.1
	111	50	10
	15	60	20
Strockbine et al. (224)	11	30	0
	341	40	3
	85	50	8.5
	331	60	12
	63	70	26 (all grades 3–5 complications)
Logsdon (225)	260	60	40
	301	70	17
	184	most >52 Gy	40
	162	most <51 Gy	17

Note: RTOG, Radiation Therapy Oncology Group.
Source: Reprinted with permission from Logsdon MD, Eifel PJ. FIGO IIIB squamous cell carcinoma of the cervix: an analysis of prognostic factors emphasizing the balance between external beam and intracavitary radiation therapy. *Int J Radiat Oncol Biol Phys* 1999;43(4):763–775.

TABLE 31.3

NORMAL TISSUE TOLERANCE TO THERAPEUTIC IRRADIATION

	TD 5/5 volume			TD 5/50 volume			
Organ	1/3	2/3	3/3	1/3	2/3	3/3	Selected endpoints
Kidney	5,000	3,000[a]	2,300	—	4,000[a]	2,800	Clinical nephritis
Bladder	N/A	8,000	6,500	N/A	8,500	8,000	Symptomatic bladder contracture and volume loss
Bone: femoral head	—	—	5,200	—	—	6,500	Necrosis
Skin	10 cm²	30 cm²	100 cm²	10 cm²	30 cm²	100 cm²	Telangiectasia, necrosis, ulceration
	—	—	5,000	—	—	6,500	—
	7,000	6,000	5,500	—	—	7,000	—
Stomach	6,000	5,500	5,000	7,000	6,700	6,500	Ulceration/perforation
Small intestine	5,000	—	4,000[a]	6,000	—	5,500	Obstruction, perforation/fistula
Colon	5,500	—	4,500	6,500	—	5,500	Obstruction/perforation
Rectum	Volume 100 cm²	No volume effect	6,000	Volume 100 cm²	No volume effect	8,000	Severe proctitis/ necrosis/fistula, stenosis
Liver	5,000	3,500	3,000	5,500	4,500	4,000	Liver failure
Bone marrow	4,000	1,000	400	4,500	1,000	650	—
Spinal cord	5,000	5,000	4,700	7,000	7,000	—	—

Note: N/A, not available; TD, total dose.
[a]<50% of volume does not make a significant change.
Source: Reprinted with permission from Emami B, Lyman J, Brown A, et al. Tolerance of normal tissue to therapeutic irradiation. *Int J Radiat Oncol Biol Phys* 1991;21:109–113.

affecting the pelvis and femoral bones (60,61). In addition, the radiation profoundly affects the bone marrow both acutely and permanently.

The incidence of asymptomatic insufficiency fractures following pelvic radiation for uterine cancer was found to range from 34% to 89% but symptomatic fracture is lower at 13%. (62–64). Diagnosis can be made with magnetic resonance imaging (MRI) or bone scan. Presenting symptoms include pelvic pain on average 1 year following completion of radiotherapy. Expectant management or treatment with nonsteroidal anti-inflammatories can provide relief until recovery, but multiple fractures are not infrequent.

The quoted tolerance dose for the femoral head for a 5% incidence of fracture at 5 years is 45 Gy and every effort should be made to minimize the irradiation of the femoral head (65). However, a review from Washington University found a 15% incidence of femoral neck fracture at 15 years when doses exceeded 42 Gy, especially in those women with pre-existing osteoporosis or tobacco use (66). Postmenopausal women with low estrogen are at particular risk and women should be screened and treated for osteoporosis before and after radiotherapy and treated with estrogens, calcium, and bisphosphonates as appropriate.

Finally, since approximately 40% of the bone marrow volume lies within the pelvis, large volume irradiation may lead to subsequent changes in hematopoietic tissues with symptoms and signs manifested from 2 weeks to 2 months after the completion of radiotherapy. Permanent bone marrow changes can affect subsequent chemotherapeutic tolerance, necessitating the use of hematopoietic growth factors such as filgrastim and erythropoietin (67). Use of IMRT has been shown to decrease this effect (68–71).

Gastrointestinal Tract

The gastrointestinal tract is more susceptible to radiation injury than other pelvic organs. This includes both acute and late effects. In addition to pre-existing conditions such as diverticulitis, pelvic inflammatory disease, age, body mass index, tobacco use, and prior surgery may increase the likelihood of radiation bowel damage (72,73). The tolerance quoted for large bowel or rectum is 70 to 75 Gy and includes patients who are treated with a combination of external radiation and brachytherapy. The small bowel tolerance is quoted as 45 Gy, but small bowel is relatively spared secondary to episodic motion in and out of the radiation field. If the loops of small bowel are immobilized secondary to adhesions from tumor or prior surgery they are more susceptible to injury. Anal tolerance is somewhat lower at 60 to 65 Gy with higher doses potentially causing damage to the myenteric plexus and subsequent dysfunction (74,75). Inclusion of the para-aortic nodal chain also increases the likelihood of bowel injury as more volume is included in the radiation field. One the most common areas of injured bowel is the terminal ileum, especially when fixed in the right lower quadrant.

Radiation for intact cervical carcinoma usually includes both external beam and brachytherapy. Historically a rectal point was chosen to represent dose, but studies have demonstrated this point to inadequately represent the full dose spectrum to the rectum and sigmoid (76). In addition, intestinal injury has not always correlated with dose to this point. With the advent of computed tomography and magnetic resonance imaging in planning of radiation, dose-volume histograms have been used to better assess dose to intestinal structures (51,52,77,78).

The increased sensitivity of the gastrointestinal tract to radiation is secondary to physiologic superficial cell turnover and high cell division rates, with a cycle time of 12 to 15 hours (79). As these cells die, rapid loss leads to initial thinning of the mucosa followed by denuded epithelium, loss of fluids, malabsorption, and diarrhea (80–82). These injuries usually resolve at the completion of radiotherapy with the robust regenerative capacity of these cells, but vascular endothelial damage may lead to small vessel obliteration, fibrosis, tissue hypoxia, and late damage (82–84).

Symptoms of acute radiation enteritis range from loose, frequent stools and tenesmus to abdominal pain with severe bloody diarrhea at times necessitating a treatment break and fluid resuscitation. Symptoms usually start at about 20 Gy of conventionally fractionated radiation. Early symptoms can be managed with a low residue diet and oral loperamide or diphenoxylate. Oral intake stimulates the bowels so it is best to take the antidiarrheal prior to meals and bedtime. One to two tablets before meals and bedtime with a maximum of eight tablets a day, titrated to bowel activity, will manage most patients. If the patient has had a recent course of antibiotics or complains of bloody diarrhea, *Clostridium difficile* colitis should be eliminated as an aggravating factor. If the diarrhea is persistent despite loperamide or diphenoxylate, Kaopectate, paregoric, or in extreme cases somatostatin and bowel rest may be used. One should pay particular attention to hydration status and electrolytes with frequent, watery diarrhea and correct abnormalities as needed. Proctitis and tenesmus can usually be managed with Proctofoam HC or Cortifoam HC per rectum twice a day for 14 days or with anti-inflammatory suppositories such as Anusol. Oral and rectal sucralfate has been used, but data demonstrating its efficacy is lacking (85–87).

Long-term complications include tenesmus, urgency, hematochezia, chronic intermittent diarrhea, bowel stricture, obstruction, incontinence, and fistulas. Late toxicity to the gastrointestinal tract is estimated to be 1% per year for the first 2 years and then decreasing to 0.06% per year thereafter. Prior surgery increases the risk of subsequent injury. Radiographically a smooth, narrowed bowel with proximal dilatation suggests injury, and direct visualization demonstrates pale mucosa with superficial telangiectasias. Management includes intake of a low residue diet, daily Metamucil, and loperamide or diphenoxylate as needed. Telangiectasias can be locally but gingerly treated with laser, and extreme cases of hematochezia may necessitate sucralfate enema, intraluminal formalin, or surgical diversion (88–90).

Genetic and Fetal Effects

Irradiation causes random damage to the DNA so generalizations are difficult. Differences in cell stage and type, dose rate, sex, oxygenation, and species all affect the mutation rate and repair. Data in models are difficult to extrapolate to humans and direct evidence is scarce. There are certainly examples of radiation-induced tumors such as an excess of skin cancers with x-rays, lung cancer in pitchblende miners, bone tumors in radium dial painters, and liver tumors in those given Thorotrast. The Japanese survivors of the atomic bombs have been the largest human group studied and results indicate an increase in death from cancer (91). There are also reports of radiation-induced increases in other diseases (92). Other studied populations including the Oak Ridge National Laboratory have also contributed to the body of knowledge regarding increased death rates and relationship to radiation exposure (93).

Radiation is thought to increase the spontaneous mutation rate, not create unique mutations. The doubling dose (doubling dose is the dose of radiation that will double the rate of spontaneous mutations) was initially based on animal data but the atomic bomb data suggests that the doubling rate may be higher than originally predicted from 1 to 2 Gy for acute exposure and 4 Gy for chronic exposure (94). There is no known threshold dose for the genetic effects of radiation. In females permanent sterility is affected by age of exposure. The published threshold is thought to be 2.5 to 6 Gy for acute exposure in females.

Effects on the fetus are varied and depend on dose, dose rate, and gestational age at exposure. After radiation one can see embryonic, fetal, or neonatal death; growth retardation; and/or malformations. The recommendation is to limit dose for the entire gestational period to ≤0.5 rem (~0.5 cGy), with monthly exposures limited to 0.05 rem. A therapeutic abortion should be discussed with any woman exposed to ≥10 cGy between 1 and 26 weeks gestation. Radiation for cervical carcinoma will result in fetal demise and spontaneous abortion usually follows this. The peak in congenital malformations occurs during major organogenesis (10 to 40 days). Later exposure can lead to microcephaly and mental retardation, especially from 8 to 15 weeks of gestation. In general it is believed that high doses in the first 2 weeks primarily lead to resorption. Irradiation from 4 to 16 weeks may precipitate severe abnormalities such as deformity, stunted growth, microcephaly, and mental retardation. With irradiation from 16 to 20 weeks mild microcephaly is seen but mental retardation and growth abnormalities are most common. Irradiation after 30 weeks is unlikely to cause gross malformations (59).

Genitourinary Tract

The quoted tolerance of the whole bladder is 65 Gy with an increase in tolerance to 75 to 80 Gy when the high dose volume is limited (65). In gynecologic carcinoma external radiation is often combined with brachytherapy that concentrates dose in a specified area close to the tissue at risk. Historically, low-dose-rate (LDR) radiation (dose rate 50 to 100 cGy/h) has been used for brachytherapy, but high-dose-rate (HDR, dose rate 100 to 300 Gy/min) is becoming more common. The recommendation for HDR is to keep the bladder dose below 70% of the dose to point A, as toxicity correlates with total dose to the bladder (95,96). With the adoption of dose-volume histograms and experience with image-guided radiotherapy, a more complete characterization of the tolerance of the bladder may be achieved (97–99).

Acute radiation effects in the genitourinary tract may cause symptoms such as frequency, urgency, dysuria, hematuria, and/or bladder spasms. Histologically, the bladder wall demonstrates submucosal edema with an inflammatory infiltrate. As most patients are relatively or overtly immunocompromised from cancer, radiotherapy, and chemotherapy, it is prudent to check a urinalysis and culture in symptomatic patients. Pyridium may be successfully used for dysuria while an antispasmodic such as oxybutynin chloride will help with urinary spasms. Antibiotics should be prescribed to treat any noted infection.

Long-term bladder complications include ulceration, fistula formation, ureteral stenosis, contracted bladder, and hematuria. For curative early-stage cervical cancer the actuarial rate of major urinary complications is estimated at 0.7% per year for the initial 3 years and decreases to 0.25% per year thereafter (100). Cystoscopy demonstrates areas of pallor or intense erythema and petechiae with occasional ulceration. With progressive small-vessel fibrosis from radiation, ulcers may form. Biopsies should be avoided if the appearance is typical as further stress can precipitate fistulization (101). Fistulas are most commonly seen in patients who have bladder invasion by tumor, but can certainly be seen in its absence and likelihood is increased with prior surgery or brachytherapy.

Fistulas are often surgically corrected, many times with urinary diversion as radiated tissue exhibits a decreased healing capacity. Ureteral stricture is an uncommon but well described late radiation complication. The possibility of stricture is increased when radical surgery is combined with radiation as both modalities compromise blood supply (102,103). The incidence of stricture has been estimated retrospectively to be 2.5% at 20 years and unilateral injury is more common than bilateral. Recurrent disease should always be entertained in the differential diagnosis of late ureteral stricture (104). For hematuria, treatment can range from cystoscopic cauterization of bleeding to cautious intravesical instillation of formalin (105,106). Hyperbaric oxygen treatment has also been used successfully for hemorrhagic cystitis following pelvic radiation (107,108).

Lymphatics

Surgery or radiation alone in the pelvis or groin can lead to lymphedema, but when combined the incidence of lymphedema increases (109,110). The prevalence of lymphedema is quoted from 11% to 18% and is greater in those treated for vulvar carcinoma with inguinofemoral lymphadenectomy and adjuvant radiation (109,110). Symptoms may be unilateral or bilateral and range from mild, soft, pitting edema to severe, indurated, brawny edema placing the woman at risk for cellulitis. Treatment includes compression stockings, massage, elevation, and good skin and nail care to avoid infection.

Nerve Injury

Although rare, reports of sacral neuropathy with doses commonly used in cervical carcinoma have been reported (111). Symptoms vary along a spectrum ranging from sensory changes to muscle weakness and paralysis. An electromyogram (EMG) will show injury similar to that seen in diabetes, and recurrent tumor as a cause must be eliminated.

Reproductive Tract

Radiation has demonstrable effects on all the reproductive organs but with varying sensitivities. The cervix and uterus can tolerate an unusually high radiotherapy dose that translates into a high locoregional control rate compared to other similarly sized solid tumors. In fact, frank necrosis is uncommon despite doses to point A exceeding 90 Gy (112). In addition, the vaginal mucosa is relatively radioresistant, tolerating a mucosal dose of 140 Gy prior to severe complications or necrosis. In fact, more recent reports suggest this may be an underestimate, and the tolerance may be closer to 175 Gy (113). The distal vagina is more radiosensitive than the proximal vagina and surface doses should be limited to 98 Gy (114). As an end organ, the vulva is more radiosensitive than other gynecologic tissues and doses should be limited to 50 to 70 Gy (70 Gy only with gross disease and shrinking, limited fields). Ovarian function after radiation is highly dependent on patient age and radiation dose, but therapeutic radiation that includes the ovaries will invariably lead to premature menopause. The supporting cells of the meiotic oocytes are more radiosensitive than the oocytes themselves, but without these cells estrogen production ceases, and the follicles fail to develop. A dose of 24 Gy leads to granulosa cell death, sterilization, and menopause, but the precipitating dose may be much lower in women over 40 years of age. Permanent sterility and menopause have been reported with doses as low as 4 Gy (115,116). Those women who desire fertility or preservation of ovarian function should have options such as cryopreservation or ovarian transposition discussed (117–120).

Acutely the patient may have symptoms of vaginitis or vulvitis with pruritus, discharge, or denuded mucosa. Most patients will experience at least patchy wet desquamation of the vulva with therapeutic doses. Vulvar reactions are exacerbated by friction and the moisture typically present in this area of the body. Acute vulvar symptoms may be managed by two to three daily sitz baths with complete perineal drying by either patting or using cool air as with a fan or hair dryer set on cool. Undergarments should be cotton to allow "breathing" and ointments should be avoided. Vaginal mucositis may respond to gentle douching twice a day with a 1:10 mixture of hydrogen peroxide in water.

After radiotherapy, the vagina may become dry, contracted, and shortened with thinning of the mucosa, especially if the patient is naturally or iatrogenically postmenopausal (121,122). The effects on the vagina are long lasting and commonly interfere with normal sexual functioning (123). If the patient is not sexually active vaginal dilators should be prescribed to maintain a patent vagina. Other vaginal symptoms such as dryness or pruritus may be alleviated by lubrication, and local and/or systemic estrogen therapy (124,125). Examination will demonstrate pale mucosa, telangiectasias, fibrosis, and/or ulceration. Biopsies of abnormalities should be undertaken cautiously as fistulas can form. Pap smears after radiotherapy may show abnormal cells attributable to the radiation and consultation with the pathologist and colposcopy should always precede biopsy. If recognized early, most superficial ulceration will heal with gentle use of douches. In cases of pernicious or deep ulceration, debridement and possibly hyperbaric oxygen may be required with flap coverage once granulation tissue has started. Late vulvar effects may include atrophy and fibrosis, hypo- or hyperpigmentation, permanent epilation, and telangiectasias.

Long-term effects on the uterus and cervix are usually less symptomatic, but atrophy and cervical stenosis are common. Preservation of partial uterine function has been reported despite the high doses used in curative radiotherapy and this should be taken into account if hormone therapy is prescribed (126).

Women may or may not complain of sexual dysfunction after treatment, but active investigation should remain the responsibility of the treating physician as permanent changes are inevitable. Dysfunction is often characterized by lack of lubrication, dyspareunia, and loss of libido and orgasm. This aspect of radiation has unfortunately been poorly prospectively evaluated. In completed studies to date, some degree of dysfunction after pelvic radiotherapy commonly exists and improves with intervention (127,128). Studies have demonstrated increased compliance with interventions if counseling is included as part of the recovery process (129,130). The EROS device has been shown to correct sexual dysfunction in patients post radiotherapy by increasing the blood flow to the clitoris with gentle suction (131,132). Subsequent vascular engorgement then leads to increased vaginal lubrication and a decrease in physiologic dysfunction (133).

Strategies to Minimize Normal Tissue Injury

Strategies have developed over the years to help minimize normal tissue damage including treatment of all fields each day, use of a four-field technique, 3D conformal therapy with blocking of normal structures, shrinking-field techniques, prone position, and the use of belly boards to exclude bowel

(134,135). Newer techniques such as IMRT and IGRT hold promise to decrease acute and long-term toxicity. With the introduction of high-dose-rate brachytherapy, fears were raised that the increased dose rate would lead to higher complications, but prospective studies have not demonstrated this to be the case (136–139).

Intensity-Modulated Radiation Therapy

Intensity-modulated radiation therapy is becoming rapidly adopted as the treatment of choice in many cancers. IMRT uses highly sophisticated computer software and hardware to shape the form and intensity of the radiation beam to conform more precisely to a patient's tumor and to avoid the normal tissues. It is standardly used in many centers for the treatment of head and neck and prostate cancers and interest is increasing in gynecologic cancer as well. A survey of IMRT use in 2002 and repeated in 2004 demonstrated an increase in any use from 32% to 73% of radiation oncologists and is likely far higher today (140). The first American national trial allowing the use of IMRT for gynecologic cancers for postoperative endometrial and cervical cancers was opened by the RTOG in March 2006. Interest in IMRT as a future standard for gynecologic cancers has grown as several studies have demonstrated a decrease in hematologic, gastrointestinal, and genitourinary side effects (70,141–143). While these early reports demonstrate success in an institutional setting, national adoption will require standards and trials demonstrating superiority, reproducibility, safety, and efficacy (144–146).

Image-Guided Radiation Therapy

Image-guided radiation therapy is in its infancy but holds promise for more accurately targeting IMRT. Many linear accelerators can now be equipped with on-board imaging that includes conventional x-rays and computed tomography (CT) scanners. With this technology, daily imaging of tumors or normal tissues holds promise in allowing more accurate tissue sparing and adaptation of treatment plans to organ motion or tumor shrinkage (147,148).

3D Brachytherapy

Brachytherapy as an integral part of the successful treatment of gynecologic cancers is undisputed as it allows for higher control rates as well as decreased normal tissue toxicity (149,150). Traditional low-dose-rate brachytherapy was based on clinical experience and empirical rules established with two-dimensional imaging. Doses are prescribed in two systems, mg-hrs and dose to a point, point A. Both systems have evolved over time and have clear limitations (151–153). As imaging modalities improve with the advent of CT scanners and MRI, brachytherapy equipment is adapted to include systems designed to eliminate artifact and allow more accurate evaluation. The three-dimensional view afforded by new imaging has led clinicians and researchers in gynecologic radiotherapy to investigate the actual doses received by target and normal tissues. A standard nomenclature is being adopted worldwide and data is being collected in a unified drive toward volume-directed therapy. Hopefully, this new examination of the relationship of brachytherapy implants to external radiotherapy, normal tissues, and tumor may also allow increased control and decreased normal tissue toxicity (89,99,100).

Radioprotectors

Over the years many therapies have been studied as radioprotectors and sensitizers. One of the most promising is amifostine (WR-2721; Ethyol). Amifostine is a compound extensively studied by the Walter Reed Army Institute of Research for radioprotection and has noted protective effects on the salivary glands, bone marrow, oral mucosa, esophagus, intestinal mucosa, and bladder mucosa (154,155).

The compound is an organic thiophosphate dephosphorylated to the active metabolite (WR-1065) in the tissue. The differential protection of normal versus tumor tissue is due to a differential concentration of tissue alkaline phosphatase and pH differences that allow variable metabolite uptake (156). The compound is rapidly absorbed into normal tissues with a prolonged retention time and a differential concentration of normal tissue:tumor of 100:1. After cellular uptake WR-1065 scavenges oxygen free radicals and by this mechanism affords normal tissue radioprotection.

Several published studies have demonstrated the efficacy of amifostine for normal tissue protection without sacrificing tumoricidal effects. A phase 3 trial in head and neck cancers demonstrated a statistically superior decrease in permanent salivary gland damage (157). Two randomized trials in pelvic radiation demonstrated a significant decrease in bladder and gastrointestinal toxicity without compromising median survival or therapeutic response (158,159). The rectal cancer trial of Liu et al. demonstrated a 50% reduction in toxicity in the genitourinary and the gastrointestinal tract. Grade 3 and 4 toxicity was seen in 14% of those treated without daily amifostine compared to 0% treated with amifostine. The RTOG has recently completed a phase 1/2 trial using amifostine as a radioprotector for chemoradiotherapy for cervical carcinoma when treating the pelvis and para-aortics. The results of this trial are still forthcoming. Toxicities of amifostine include hypotension and nausea. Subcutaneous administration has decreased the incidence of hypotension, but nausea must be actively managed, especially when combined with cisplatin (160). Skin toxicity has also been seen with subcutaneous administration.

SURGERY

The complications of surgery per se occur almost exclusively in the perioperative period; therefore, a discussion of the role of surgery as it pertains to the late effects of therapy of gynecologic cancer is principally a discussion of the surgical management of irradiation injury to the intestinal and lower urinary tracts. The management of intraoperative and early postoperative complications, such as bleeding and surgical damage to the urinary and intestinal tracts, is covered only briefly in this chapter. Readers interested in detailed discussions of these topics are referred to excellent texts on the subject (161,162).

Intraoperative Urinary Tract Injuries

Intraoperative injury to the urinary tract is a relatively uncommon occurrence during surgery for gynecologic cancer. Recognized intraoperative injury to the ureter occurs in approximately 1% of nonirradiated patients undergoing radical hysterectomy for cervical cancer (163). This represents a significant improvement in the injury rate from series reported before 1980. Injuries can occur by a variety of mechanisms, but usually involve crushing or laceration of the ureter. Crushing injuries typically involve clamping and/or ligation of the ureter. When identified intraoperatively, the clamp or ligature should be removed immediately and the ureter mobilized sufficiently from surrounding tissue so that it can be carefully inspected. Observation over a period of time may be necessary to assess the blood supply and extent of damage. Intravenous indigo carmine can be administered if there is concern about urinary leakage. If the ureter appears viable and there is no extravasation, the site of injury can be stented with a self-retaining stent (single or double pigtail) passed through either a ureterotomy or a cystotomy over a wire. The retroperitoneum near the site of injury should also be drained with a closed suction drain. Lesser degrees of injury such as those resulting from mass ligation of the ureter may not require stenting; simply removing the suture may suffice. Severe crushing injuries may require resection of the damaged segment of ureter and, depending on the site of the injury and the anatomy, either primary anastomosis or reimplantation into the bladder. Stenting should also be performed in these cases.

Ureteral lacerations that do not compromise the blood supply of the ureter can be closed primarily with absorbable suture over a stent. Larger injuries or complete transections will require primary repair or ureteroneocystostomy. Injuries below the pelvic brim can generally be managed by ureteroneocystostomy, with bladder mobilization and psoas muscle hitch if required. Those above the pelvic brim are often best managed by anastomosis, or intestinal interposition. Generally, a ureteroneocystostomy should be performed when possible, as the complication rate of this procedure is significantly lower than with other types of anastomosis. Permanent suture should never be used when suturing the uroendothelium.

Injuries above the pelvic brim can be managed with a variety of techniques, including ureteroureteral anastomosis, transureteroureteral anastomosis, Boari flap, Demel technique, or intestinal interposition. Intestinal interposition uses a portion of the ilium as a ureteral extender and interposes a segment between distal ureter and bladder. The two flaps described must be raised carefully from medial to lateral, taking care to keep the superior vesicle artery intact. This will help keep the flap well vascularized. Transureteroureterostomy is potentially dangerous, because the function of both kidneys can be compromised if there is a technical problem with the anastomosis and, in the authors' opinion, should be avoided.

Intraoperative bladder injuries occur in approximately 1% to 2% of radical hysterectomy patients or other cases of radical surgery. They are generally easily repaired with a two-layer closure using absorbable suture, followed by bladder drainage for 5 to 14 days. Irradiated bladders generally should be drained longer than nonirradiated bladders.

Postoperative Urinary Tract Complications

With modern surgical techniques, the incidence of ureterovaginal fistula following radical hysterectomy has fallen to 1% to 2% from a rate of 10% to 20% several decades ago. Most become apparent from the 5th to the 14th day postoperatively. Placement of a vaginal tampon and instillation of intravesical methylene blue can allow discrimination of a bladder fistula from a ureteral fistula. Intravenous indigo carmine intravenous pyelography, cystoscopy, and retrograde pyelography may be useful to define the site of the problem. Initial therapy of ureterovaginal fistula is directed toward elimination of infection and maintenance of renal function. Retrograde stenting should be attempted and, if successful, the stent should be left in place for several months. This will often allow spontaneous healing of the fistula. If a retrograde stent cannot be passed, percutaneous nephrostomy and antegrade stenting should be performed. If antegrade stenting cannot be accomplished, nephrostomy drainage should be established, and a decision made about the timing of surgical repair. If an active intraperitoneal urine leak is present, immediate repair is indicated. In the absence of this, many authorities prefer to wait 6 to 8 weeks before surgical repair, although there are also proponents of routine immediate repair.

Postoperative vesicovaginal fistulas are less common following radical hysterectomy and often heal spontaneously after prolonged bladder drainage. If surgical repair is necessary, many of these can be approached by the vaginal route. One of the most troubling complications after radical hysterectomy for cervical cancer is bladder dysfunction, a result of the necessary disruption of the nerve supply to the bladder that occurs during the radical pelvic dissection (164). Minor degrees of sensory and motor dysfunction, detectable by cystometrogram, are seen in essentially all patients, and approximately 2% to 3% of patients will have long-term clinically significant difficulties with bladder function that may require chronic intermittent self-catheterization. Almost all patients have some element of bladder dysfunction after radical hysterectomy, and their bladder function should be monitored carefully.

Fistulas that occur after the patient has received a combination of radiation therapy and surgery are less likely to heal spontaneously and often require surgical intervention. Vesicovaginal fistulas resulting from radiation injury almost always require surgical correction. The repair can be achieved vaginally or abdominally. Vaginal repair often uses a portion of the bulbocavernosus muscle (Martius flap) (165,166). This allows new blood supply to be brought into the radiated field. Alternatively, abdominal repair may require using a flap of nonirradiated tissue such as the omentum between the bladder and vagina to improve the success of repair by including additional blood supply.

Urinary diversion is often required to divert the urinary stream in patients in whom it is felt a primary repair of the area cannot be achieved. The type of diversion can be continent or incontinent, depending on the clinical situation at the time that the repair is needed. Also, it will depend on the patient's willingness to care for an extraneous device. If the patient already has a colostomy, she may be more willing to care for such a device. Early complications of urinary diversion include urine leak and vascular complications. Urine leak that is clinically important is seen approximately 5% of the time (167,168). This may present as urine leaking from the perineum, incision, or stoma or through a cutaneous drain. Evidence of leakage may also manifest itself by fever with abscess formation, ileus, or decreased urine output with a contemporaneous rise in BUN or creatinine. Initial management should always be conservative. Percutaneous drains or nephrostomies can be placed by interventional radiology for drainage of the urine or abscess. The tracts will often close under appropriate conservative management. Surgical intervention should be avoided, as the operative mortality is exceedingly high. In the case of urinary diversion, one can occasionally consider an "undiversion." In this situation, the urinary conduit is attached to the dome of the bladder, reconnecting the urinary stream.

Penalever et al. (169) reported on the complications of continent urinary diversions. They observed a complication rate of over 53% and a postoperative mortality of 9%. Early complications included stricture or obstruction, anastomotic leak, pyelonephritis, sepsis, and reservoir cutaneous fistula. Late complications included stricture or obstruction, incontinence, difficulty with catheterization, and urinary stones. All complications should be treated initially with drainage and nonoperative intervention until the complication is stabilized, then appropriate surgical management can be considered.

Intraoperative Intestinal Injuries

Intraoperative injury to the intestinal tract may occur from time to time in patients undergoing surgery for gynecologic cancers. Predisposing factors include prior extensive surgery, irradiation, inflammatory disease, and perhaps intraperitoneal chemotherapy. Intraoperative intestinal injuries generally lead to no serious sequelae, provided that the bowel has been adequately prepared and the injuries are recognized and repaired appropriately. The extent of the bowel preparation should be tailored to the surgical procedure being performed and the likelihood of intestinal injury. For high-risk patients or for those in whom intestinal resection is contemplated, a complete antibiotic and mechanical bowel preparation is indicated (see Bowel Preparation section in Chapter 11). All bowel preparations can cause dehydration, and special attention should be given to the elderly patient to prevent dehydration with associated postoperative acute tubular necrosis; this may mean administering intravenous fluids during the bowel preparation.

Small injuries to the intestinal serosa usually do not require repair. Larger injuries or those occurring in irradiated bowel should be oversewn. Injuries that transgress both the serosa and the muscular layers of the bowel wall can be recognized by a bulging of the mucosa when gentle pressure is applied. These should be repaired, generally with a single layer of interrupted sutures. Injuries that enter the intestinal lumen must be dealt with according to their site and severity, as well as the condition of the intestine. Uncomplicated injuries to the small intestine and to the well-prepared large intestine can usually be closed primarily. A common technique uses a first layer of continuous or interrupted absorbable suture, followed by an interrupted layer of permanent suture, such as 3-0 silk or Vicryl. In the presence of more extensive injury, vascular compromise, tumor, or obstruction, a more extensive procedure, such as resection and anastomosis, may be required. In the case of injury to the unprepared large bowel, diverting colostomy should be considered.

Postoperative Intestinal Complications

The spectrum of postoperative intestinal complications includes obstruction and leakage of intestinal contents. Postoperative mechanical obstruction generally results from adhesions forming in the early postoperative period. Initial management should be conservative, including gastric decompression and, possibly, intravenous nutritional support, as many postoperative obstructions will resolve spontaneously. Those that do not resolve with conservative management may require surgical correction (170).

Leakage of intestinal contents can be a devastating complication. It may occur at the site of intestinal injury or anastomosis or may develop spontaneously in unmanipulated bowel. Predisposing factors include the presence of tumor and distal obstruction. Prior radiation therapy not only increases the risk of intestinal complications, but also makes their management more difficult (discussed later in this chapter). Management must be individualized, but basic principles include cessation of oral intake, establishing a route of drainage for the leaking intestinal contents, and treatment of infection. Emergency operation and intestinal diversion may be required in the case of gross intraperitoneal leakage of intestinal contents. In less acute cases, such as enterocutaneous fistulas following surgery, supportive management with gastric suction, total parenteral nutrition, and the use of somatostatin may allow spontaneous healing.

The use of automatic-stapling devices to perform low-rectal anastomoses has greatly facilitated the avoidance of permanent colostomy in gynecologic cancer patients. The technical feasibility of the anastomosis, however, must be weighed against the risk of immediate and long-term complications. In patients at risk for poor healing of the anastomosis, a diverting colostomy should be considered. If a leak does occur postoperatively, simple diversion of the fecal stream usually prevents serious complications. The protective colostomy or ileostomy should be well out of the irradiated field if possible. A small proportion of patients undergoing low-rectal anastomosis with circular stapling devices will experience problems with long-term stenosis of the stapled anastomosis. It is important to use the largest staple cartridge that can be accommodated by the patient's intestinal lumen. Dilatation of the anastomosis under anesthesia may be effective in relieving symptomatic stenosis. Digital inspection of the anastomosis at regular office visits can help prevent progressive or recurrent stenosis. Very low anastomoses may also produce some degree of fecal urgency and incontinence, probably related to loss of the reservoir function of the rectal ampulla and denervation of the sphincter itself during the procedure. Radical pelvic resections as described above may also result in loss of bladder function and lead to atonic bladder; therefore, postvoid residuals should be checked during the postoperative period.

The reported frequency of anastomotic leaks varies significantly, depending on the type of anastomosis and site. The rate of clinical leak varies from 0% to 30%. This rate has been shown to be even higher when integrity of the anastomosis is investigated prospectively with water-soluble contrast material. Rectal anastomoses have a higher complication rate than all other anastomoses. The complication rate may also be related to the distance from the anal verge. Authors from the Mayo Clinic reported a 1% clinical leak rate in 402 patients undergoing hand-sewn colon anastomosis. Almost 6% (5 of 107) of the patients' colorectal anastomoses developed a leak (171,172). Pelvic abscess following an anastomosis may occur and is often heralded by high spiking fevers. The diagnosis is usually confirmed by CT scan and is usually best treated by percutaneous drainage under radiographic guidance (173).

A major long-term complication of colorectal anastomoses is stricture. This may occur in as many as 3% of very low anastomoses, particularly if the EEA stapler is used. The EEA stapler allows lower anastomoses than hand-sewn, but at a cost of increased risk of stricture, particularly if the area has been irradiated (172,174). It is unusual in anastomoses of the proximal rectum. The lower anastomoses, particularly those below the peritoneal reflection, can be dilated. Other more proximal strictures, including those of the small bowel, may require surgical correction (175).

Another common complication in gynecologic cancer patients is small bowel obstruction. Unfortunately, there is little information on management of this problem in our patients. Most of the management techniques are extrapolated from the general surgery literature. Small bowel obstruction presents with dilated loops of small bowel, air fluid levels, and associated nausea and vomiting. If there is air in the rectum on abdominal x-ray, the diagnosis of obstruction secondary to ileus is made. This usually resolves with conservative management and nasogastric suction over 1 to 7 days. Any surgical procedure, whether peritoneal or extraperitoneal, may result in an ileus. Treatment for adynamic ileus is bowel rest with nasogastric (NG) suction. Some have advocated agents to increase bowel motility, but this has not been shown to be effective in any peer-reviewed publications.

Mechanical small bowel obstruction occurs in a significant portion of patients with gynecologic malignancies. The differential diagnosis is ileus, fecal impaction ischemia, and, of course, gastroenteritis. Treatment is immediate NG suction. This problem requires immediate medical attention, but may no longer require immediate surgical attention. It is now generally accepted that a trial of conservative management is warranted in cases of small bowel obstruction, provided that there is no evidence of ischemic bowel or evidence of strangulation. The majority of cases of partial small bowel obstruction resolve with NG suction and electrolyte replacement, whereas fewer than 50% of cases of complete obstruction resolve with this treatment and ultimately require surgical intervention (176–179). The use of contrasted bowel studies is often helpful in distinguishing high-grade from low-grade obstruction and may be helpful in determining the site of obstruction. The type of contrast used is controversial. Barium often yields a better study, but can complicate subsequent operative procedures, as barium is quite caustic if spilled in the peritoneal cavity. Soluble contrast is safer, but often is diluted to such a degree that the study is not helpful (179). If one believes that there could be a large bowel obstruction, an enema with contrast should be performed before an upper GI study. If the obstruction is in the distal small bowel, evaluation by enema can also be helpful if the patient has an incompetent ileocecal valve.

The timing and advisability of surgery on a patient who has end-stage ovarian cancer are controversial and require experience and associated judgment. If the physician feels that the patient's life expectancy is greater than 3 to 4 months and that the surgery is technically feasible, it is reasonable to proceed. Patients with disseminated carcinomatosis often have large segments of dysfunctional bowel, making resection necessary if the obstruction is to be relieved, and the risk of fistula is high. A gastrostomy tube and prolonged bowel rest should be used in this setting.

Large bowel obstructions often present with progressive symptoms of constipation and difficulty defecating. Once the obstruction is complete, surgical intervention is mandatory to avoid perforation at the cecum. The risk of cecal perforation increases when the cecum acutely dilates to more than 10 cm. Management is almost always a colostomy in the form of a loop or end, depending on the clinical situation (180). A more proximal obstruction may necessitate ileostomy with mucous fistula formation.

Late medical complications of intestinal surgery include those that follow extensive resection of the ileum and right colon, which may produce chronic diarrhea from impaired absorption of water, fat, and bile salts, and problems related to poor absorption of nutrients, including the fat-soluble vitamins and vitamin B_{12}.

Postoperative Incisional Complications

Incisional complications after surgery include varying degrees of wound separation in the early postoperative period, as well as incisional hernias that become apparent in the later postoperative period. Superficial wound separations, involving only the skin and subcutaneous tissues, are generally minor problems. They may be managed by reclosure, if the tissues are in good condition, or allowed to heal by secondary intention. Wound separations involving the deep fascia are more serious. Fortunately, the use of single-layer bulk closure of the abdominal wall, a kind of "internal retention" suture, has made fascial dehiscence quite uncommon, even in high-risk patients. Fascial dehiscence must, of course, be repaired emergently.

Wound infection occurs in approximately 4% of patients undergoing a surgical procedure. The infection rate varies with the type of patient, her medical characteristics, and the type of wound. It is important to follow appropriate preoperative measures to minimize the wound infection rate (161,162).

Incisional hernia is a long-term complication that is also quite uncommon after single-layer bulk closure of the abdominal wall. However, the reported rate of hernias in the gynecologic oncology population is approximately 5% (181,182). Incisional hernia occurs more often in patients who have factors that adversely affect healing, such as advanced malignancy, poor nutrition, and the use of radiation therapy and chemotherapy. It is also more common in patients who have had multiple prior operations and in those who have postoperative incisional complications, such as infection. The need for elective repair should be determined on an individual basis. Extensive hernias may require the use of a prosthetic material to bridge the fascial gap.

Surgical Management of Radiation Injury

The Patterns of Care Outcome Study of cervical cancer published in 1983 analyzed data on 706 patients treated with radiation therapy at 163 institutions across the United States (183). Major complications (those that required hospitalization) occurred in 86 patients (12%). Fewer than half of these complications required surgery for management.

Perez et al. (184), reporting on 811 patients with cervical cancer treated at the Mallinckrodt Institute of Radiology (St. Louis, Missouri, USA), found that complications requiring surgery occurred in approximately 5% of patients. The most common intestinal complications included rectovaginal fistula, sigmoid stricture, small bowel obstruction, and sigmoid perforation. The most common urinary tract complications were bladder ulcer, vesicovaginal fistula, and ureteral stricture. In this report, irradiation dose and technique were the primary clinical features related to risk of complications. No relationship was demonstrated between complications and age or a history of previous pelvic disease. As mentioned previously, additional risk factors cited by other investigators include conditions that predispose to atherosclerosis, such as diabetes and hypertension (185). It is reasonable to estimate that approximately 5% to 7% of patients who undergo radiation therapy for cervical cancer will experience major treatment complications including fistulas that require surgery. The incidence of complications is significantly lower in women who receive irradiation for endometrial cancer, because of the lower central doses used. On the other hand, patients who undergo whole-abdominal irradiation as salvage treatment of ovarian cancer after chemotherapy failure have a risk of major complications reported in the range of 40% to 50% (186,187). Because of the high morbidity and low efficacy, this treatment has gained only limited acceptance.

Intestinal Tract

Radiation injury to the intestinal tract severe enough to require surgery generally becomes manifest in the first 2 years after treatment. In a series of 71 patients from the M. D. Anderson Cancer Center who required surgery for radiation injury to the small intestine, Smith et al. (188) reported that 48% of the injuries developed within 1 year after completion of treatment and 74% developed within 2 years. Occasionally, however, complications may develop much later, perhaps as a result of the natural development of atherosclerosis that accompanies aging.

The most common sites of intestinal injury in patients who undergo pelvic irradiation are areas of the intestinal tract that typically lie in the pelvic field. The ileum is the most frequent site of injury, because of the greater radiosensitivity of the small intestine compared with the colon. In a series from the Mayo Clinic, Schmitt and Symmonds (189) reported that, among 93 patients who underwent surgery for radiation injury to the intestine, 78 (84%) had involvement of the ileum. The rectosigmoid colon and the cecum are also frequent sites of involvement.

The decision to operate on patients with radiation injury must never be made lightly. Surgery may be required in the management of radiation injury to the intestinal tract for palliation of severe symptoms that fail to respond to the previously outlined conservative management, as well as for relief of life-threatening complications, such as obstruction or perforation. In a review of all intestinal surgeries performed during a 3-year interval on the Gynecology Service at Memorial Sloan-Kettering Cancer Center, Rubin et al. (190) reported that 79 (46%) of the 171 operations that involved intestinal surgery were performed in previously irradiated patients. The most common indications for these operations were intestinal obstruction (44%) and intestinal fistula or perforation (32%) that occurred in patients treated for cervical or corpus cancer.

Smith and DeCosse (15), in a review on radiation damage to the small intestine, emphasized three phases that can be applied to the management of radiation injury in all areas of the intestinal tract: stabilization, evaluation, and surgery. The patient's fluid, electrolyte, and nutritional status should be assessed and optimized before surgery; total parenteral nutrition is often required. Some investigators have suggested that the use of somatostatin to decrease gastrointestinal secretions may promote the healing of enteric fistulas (191). As mentioned previously, in contrast to fistulas in the nonirradiated intestine, those involving irradiated bowel only rarely heal with a program of intestinal rest and parenteral alimentation. In cases of bowel obstruction, intestinal intubation and decompression should be performed preoperatively. If infection is present, preoperative antibiotic therapy should be given.

Except in emergency situations, a careful evaluation of the entire intestinal tract should be made before any contemplated surgery. One should always bear in mind that recurrent cancer may, in part, be responsible for the intestinal problems; if cancer is present, the appropriate management may be altered. Radiographic studies of the large and small intestine should be performed. Cutaneous fistulas can be studied by injection of contrast medium, and stomas can be explored endoscopically. Evaluation of the ureters and bladder by intravenous pyelogram and cystoscopy may also provide useful information. As Marks and Mohiudden (192) pointed out, the extent of radiation injury may be greater than anticipated, and the patient must understand the possible need for intestinal or urinary diversion.

At operation, it is generally advisable to explore the entire abdominal cavity. Intestinal adhesions are frequently encountered, making exploration a difficult undertaking. Irradiated intestine must be handled with great care, and meticulous dissection must be used to lyse adhesions. Injuries to the intestinal wall that may be trivial in the nonirradiated patient may lead to fistulization of irradiated intestine. Frequently, in patients with gynecologic cancer, the surgeon encounters a matted mass of distal ileum densely fixed in the pelvis that is the site of obstruction or fistula. It is often not possible to release such a mass without damage to the involved intestine and risk of injury to adjacent structures, such as the urinary bladder and ureters, rectosigmoid colon, and major pelvic blood vessels. The decision whether to resect or bypass such an agglutinated mass of bowel may tax the judgment of even the most experienced surgeon. In general, such masses are best resected, particularly in the presence of intestinal necrosis, perforation, abscess formation, and fistulization, if resection can be accomplished without undue risk of gross contamination of the peritoneal cavity or damage to adjacent structures. Bypass procedures may be more likely to lead to the development of the blind-loop syndrome or to result in subsequent spontaneous perforation or fistulization of diseased defunctionalized intestine left *in situ*. In a series of 77 patients who underwent surgery for radiation injury to the small intestine, no difference in short-term complications was noted whether patients underwent resection or bypass, although it is likely that the two groups were not comparable in clinical features (188). The authors did believe that the long-term complications of fistula formation and continued small bowel necrosis could be avoided by primary resection. In patients with peritonitis caused by perforation, Swan et al. (193) emphasized the option of ileostomy to avoid the risk of a failed intestinal anastomosis under these circumstances. In most cases, however, anastomosis can be performed. As pointed out by Hoskins et al. (194), anastomosis in the irradiated terminal ileum should be avoided by wide resection of the terminal ileum and ascending colon with ileocolonic anastomosis.

Decisions about bypass or resection of irradiated small intestine must also take into account the presence of enteric fistulas that are draining via the vagina, bladder, or skin. Smith et al. (195), reporting on 68 enteric fistulas managed on the Gynecology Service at Memorial Sloan-Kettering Cancer Center, emphasized that if fistulized loops cannot be resected, they should be totally excluded from the intestinal stream to minimize continued fistulous drainage. For example, in the common case of a terminal ileal fistula, this exclusion may be accomplished by dividing the ileum proximal to the fistula, performing an ileocolonic anastomosis, bringing out the ileal stump as a mucous fistula, and placing a staple line across the ascending colon to prevent reflux of intestinal contents through an incompetent ileocecal valve. The ultimate decisions as to the operative management of patients with radiation injury to the small intestine must be in the hands of the operating surgeon. Under appropriate circumstances, satisfactory results may be obtained with either the resection or bypass procedure.

The surgical management of radiation injury to the large intestine presents a different set of considerations. Usually, the injury is to the rectosigmoid, where it may be manifested as proctitis, ulceration, stricture, perforation with abscess formation, or rectovaginal fistula (196). Lesser degrees of bleeding may be controllable by dietary modifications, hydrocortisone-containing enemas (Cortifoam, Proctofoam), or the use of the endoscopic YAG laser (197). Surgery is required for bleeding that fails to respond to conservative measures or is massive, recurrent, or associated with perforation. Colostomy alone, without resection of the involved intestinal segment, may be sufficient in some cases to control the bleeding, presumably by decreasing mechanical irritation and infection of the diseased area of the colon. In more severe cases, excision of the rectosigmoid is required, although this procedure may be technically difficult as a result of radiation fibrosis of the pelvic soft tissues. Under favorable circumstances, restoration of intestinal continuity by coloanal anastomosis may be feasible (198). The refinement of surgical stapling instruments over the last decade has extended the ability of the surgeon to perform such low anastomoses successfully.

Patients with rectal perforation and abscess formation may require urgent surgery after correction of fluid and electrolyte imbalance. The extent of the surgical procedure depends on the degree of radiation injury, the severity of the infection, and the general condition of the patient. Often, a diverting colostomy and drainage of the abscess control infection without the increased morbidity that may result from attempts at resection of the involved rectum. In chronic situations without active severe infection, resection and low anastomosis with a protective colostomy that can be closed several months after satisfactory healing has been demonstrated to be efficacious and may be considered.

Fistulization of the large intestine after pelvic radiation therapy usually occurs between the rectum and the vagina. Occasionally, the sigmoid colon or cecum may fistulize to the vagina, cervix, uterine fundus, or urinary bladder. Because these fistulas result from radiation necrosis of the intestinal wall, simple closure is doomed to failure. After a radiographic evaluation of the intestinal tract, generous biopsy specimens of the fistulous tract should be taken. If recurrent cancer is documented, a diverting colostomy is generally indicated for relief of symptoms, and attention should be given to further treatment of the cancer. If no evidence of recurrence is found,

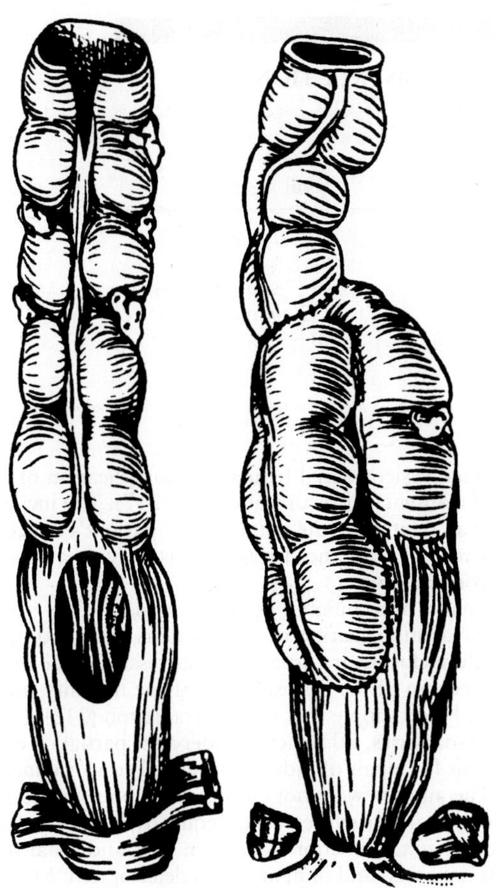

FIGURE 31.1. Bricker's technique for repair of postirradiation rectovaginal fistula. The proximal end of the colon is anastomosed end-on to the fistula, or it can be increased by an antimesenteric slit to fit a larger fistulous defect. *Source:* Reprinted with permission from Bricker EM, Johnston WD. Repair of postirradiation rectovaginal fistula and stricture. *Surg Gynecol Obstet* 1979;148:499–506.

closure of the fistula can be attempted after fecal diversion. Successful fistula repair requires the delivery of a new vascular supply to the damaged area. Perhaps the simplest means of accomplishing this task is to develop the bulbocavernosus fat pad from the labium major for use as a vascular pedicle graft between the rectum and vagina, as described by Martius (199). Although short-term results appear satisfactory with this technique (200), late breakdown can occur (201). Graham (202) has described the use of the gracilis and rectus muscles in the closure of large rectovaginal fistulas after irradiation with good success. More recently, Bricker and Johnston (203) have described an innovative technique that uses a folded piece of normal colon as a patch over the fistula, with restoration of intestinal continuity above the level of the fistula (Fig. 31.1).

Urinary Tract

Serious urinary tract complications after irradiation are somewhat less common than intestinal complications, presumably because of the greater resistance of the urinary tract to the damaging effects of ionizing radiation. Ureteral and bladder injuries that result from irradiation most often become manifest 1 to 3 years after therapy. In the series of Cushing et al. (204), 12.3 months was the mean interval for major radiation-related urinary tract complications to develop in patients treated for carcinoma of the cervix. Ureteral injury occurred at a median time of 18 months in the report by Muram et al. (205), whereas the peak time of development of bladder injuries was 2 to 3 years in Kottmeier's (206) series. Occasionally, complications occur much later. Ureteral fistula as a complication of radiation therapy alone in the absence of surgery or recurrent cancer is extremely rare.

The incidence of ureteral stricture after pelvic radiation therapy has markedly diminished with the refinement of irradiation techniques in recent years. Everett (207), writing in 1939, noted a 15% incidence of severe ureteral obstruction in a small group of patients treated for carcinoma of the cervix. Kaplan (208) noted a 1% incidence of postirradiation ureteral obstruction in his patient population, but pointed out that this figure was probably an underestimate because patients were not routinely investigated. In the series of Underwood et al. (209), symptomatic ureteral stricture occurred in only 0.33% of 2,393 patients who underwent radiation therapy for carcinoma of the cervix; however, pyelographic evidence of stricture was noted in 4% of 100 asymptomatic patients studied 5 or more years after treatment. Villasanta (210) has pointed out that ureteral stenosis generally occurs after cervicovaginal necrosis and parametritis and must be considered at least in part a complication of infection in irradiated patients. The most common site of ureteral stricture after pelvic irradiation appears to be 4 to 6 cm above the ureterovesical junction at the point at which the ureter passes through the parametrium (208), although obstruction may also occur at the ureterovesical junction (20) or may involve a long segment of ureter from the pelvic brim downward (211).

Because most patients who develop ureteral obstruction after irradiation for cancer of the cervix have recurrent cancer as the cause of obstruction, a thorough evaluation for recurrence must be undertaken before appropriate management can be determined. In addition to a complete physical examination and routine laboratory tests, patients should generally undergo an intravenous pyelogram. Creatinine clearance and isotope renography can be performed to determine precisely the degree of impairment of renal function. Computed tomography or magnetic resonance imaging of the abdomen and pelvis should be done to look for evidence of recurrent cancer, with needle biopsies of suspicious areas performed under radiologic guidance. All patients should undergo pelvic examination under anesthesia, with cystoscopy. Biopsies of the cervix, parametrium, and bladder may help detect recurrence. Antegrade or retrograde pyelography may be needed to determine the site of obstruction or the anatomy of the involved urinary tract. In some cases, exploratory laparotomy may be needed to document recurrent cancer; however, as Boronow (212) pointed out, given the lack of effective therapy for recurrent cervical cancer after radiation therapy, unless pelvic exenteration is contemplated, laparotomy for diagnosis of recurrence is seldom indicated. However, one must be wary of making a clinical diagnosis of recurrent cancer in the absence of histologic confirmation. In an autopsy series of 68 patients with fatal hydronephrosis and uremia, Kirchoff (213) found radiation fibrosis only as the cause of urinary obstruction in 18 patients.

Once recurrent cancer has been excluded, the site and length of the ureteral stricture have been determined, and differential renal function has been assessed, a plan of management may be developed. If infection is present in an obstructed renal unit, antibiotic treatment and decompression, usually by percutaneous nephrostomy, should be undertaken. In general, the goal of intervention is to eliminate infection and preserve renal function. A patient with a mild degree of hydronephrosis may be followed with serial evaluations. If significant impairment of renal function is present or develops under observation, intervention is indicated. Temporary relief of obstruction may be achieved by stenting of the ureter, either retrograde or antegrade, with an internal self-retaining stent. Although

TABLE 31.4

LATERALITY OF IRRADIATION-RELATED URETERAL OBSTRUCTION

	No. of obstructions		
Reference	Unilateral	Bilateral	Total
Muram et al. (205)	9	3	12
Kaplan (208)	10	1	11
Kirkinen et al. (219)	9	10	19 (7 simultaneous)
Underwood et al. (209)	3	5	8 (2 simultaneous)
Total	31 (62%)	19 (38%)	50

mechanical dilatation of radiation-related ureteral strictures has been attempted, it usually does not produce lasting relief of obstruction, probably owing to the intense degree of periureteral fibrosis present in these patients. Despite the common assumption that ureteral stricture resulting from irradiation should be a bilateral process, a summary of reports providing information on laterality of involvement shows that, in approximately 60% of patients, involvement was unilateral (Table 31.4). Temporization does have the advantage of allowing one to observe the patient for the development of stricture on the opposite side, because bilateral involvement may not always develop simultaneously.

If surgery is required, the specific operative intervention depends on the site and extent of the damage and the remaining renal function on the affected side. As reported by a number of authors, simple lysis of the ureter from its fibrotic bed in the retroperitoneum is rarely successful in eliminating the obstruction (190,214). In general, it is necessary to resect the strictured segment of ureter and reconstruct the urinary tract using healthy tissue. Patients who have been heavily irradiated may have extensive fibrosis of the bladder, which makes direct reimplantation of the ureter difficult, particularly if a procedure such as bladder flap formation or psoas hitch is required to bridge the gap between the bladder and the ureter. In selected cases with minimal bladder fibrosis, satisfactory results may be obtained by ureteroneocystostomy, implanting the ureter into the lateral dome of the bladder, which usually has received a lesser dose of radiation. Often, the most prudent procedure is to interpose an isolated segment of intestine between the healthy ureter and the bladder (215,216). This bowel segment can also be used to increase bladder capacity if it has been significantly diminished as a result of irradiation. When considering how to reestablish intestinal continuity, one must remember that the ileum generally is heavily irradiated. Occasionally, a transureteroureterostomy above the irradiated field is appropriate, although one is naturally hesitant about the possibility of a complication that involves the opposite, relatively normal ureter. In extreme cases with bilateral ureteral injury or a bladder that can no longer function, urinary diversion may be required. This procedure is discussed fully in the section on pelvic exenteration, but may include continent urinary diversion, transverse or sigmoid colon conduit, or a Bricker-type conduit.

The bladder is subject to a spectrum of injuries from irradiation, which may produce sequelae including cystitis, hematuria, contracture, and occasionally severe necrosis and fistula formation. Bladder fistulas after irradiation for cancer of the cervix usually occur between the anterior vaginal wall and the posterior bladder wall because this area of the bladder receives the highest dose of radiation. In a series of 2,729 patients who underwent radiation therapy for cervical cancer at the M. D. Anderson Cancer Center, 34 patients (1.2%) experienced vesicovaginal fistula as a complication of irradiation in the absence of recurrent cancer (217). The incidence of fistula was related to the stage of the patient's cancer, with patients who had advanced-stage disease having a greater risk of this complication.

Conventional techniques of vesicovaginal fistula repair that involve wide mobilization of the fistulous tract and a layered direct suture closure are usually not successful in the irradiated patient because of the fibrosis, poor tissue mobility, and compromised blood supply that follow irradiation (212). In the M. D. Anderson series, 20 patients underwent partial or complete colpocleisis for repair of radiation-induced vesicovaginal fistula (217). The authors were not enthusiastic about this technique, because several procedures were frequently required to achieve continence, coital function was often lost, and renal function was not improved and in many cases deteriorated. More often, once recurrent tumor has been ruled out and enough time has elapsed to allow for maturation of the fistula margins, closure may be attempted by a variety of techniques that involve the mobilization of well-vascularized tissue into the area. Boronow (212), who has contributed much to the subject, advises waiting 12 months between fistula formation and attempted closure. Gracilis muscle, omentum, and bulbocavernosus muscle have been used successfully (203,205,218,219).

Often, permanent urinary diversion is necessary. If one can subsequently repair the bladder, it is possible to attach the urinary conduit to the bladder dome in a procedure described by Boronow as the "undiversion."

In cases of bladder contracture that produces intolerable symptoms unresponsive to conservative measures, such as anticholinergic medications and bladder dilatation, augmentation cystoplasty may be indicated. Although some authors have suggested that bladder excision and replacement is preferable in radiation bladder disease (220), in the experience of others augmentation generally suffices if the bladder mucosa is not grossly abnormal (221). Techniques of augmentation cystoplasty have been described using ileum, cecum, or colon (222). In general, a nonirradiated segment of intestine should be selected and detubularized to allow it to hold a larger volume and ensure better healing (223).

References

1. Green MH, Boice JD, Greer BE, et al. Acute nonlymphocytic leukemia after therapy with alkylating agents for ovarian cancer: a study of five randomized clinical trials. *N Engl J Med* 1982;307:1416.
2. Kaldor JM, Day NE, Petterson F, et al. Leukemia following chemotherapy for ovarian cancer. *N Engl J Med* 1990;322:1.
3. Bertelsen K, Jakobsen A, Stroyer I, et al. A prospective randomized comparison of 6 and 12 cycles of cyclophosphamide, Adriamycin, and cisplatin in advanced epithelial ovarian cancer: a Danish Ovarian Study Group Trial (DACOVA). *Gynecol Oncol* 1993;49:30.

4. Hakes TB, Chalas E, Hoskins WJ, et al. Randomized prospective trial of 5 versus 10 cycles of cyclophosphamide, doxorubicin, and cisplatin in advanced ovarian carcinoma. *Gynecol Oncol* 1992;45:284.
5. Bassett WB, Weiss RB. Acute leukemia following cisplatin for bladder cancer. *J Clin Oncol* 1986;4:614.
6. Chambers SK, Chopyk RL, Chambers JT, et al. Development of leukemia after doxorubicin and cisplatin treatment for ovarian cancer. *Cancer* 1989;64:2459.
7. Ratain MJ, Kaminer KS, Bitran JD, et al. Acute nonlymphocytic leukemia following etoposide and cisplatin combination chemotherapy for advanced non–small-cell carcinoma of the lung. *Blood* 1987;70:1412.
8. Reed E, Evans MK. Acute leukemia following cisplatin-based chemotherapy in a patient with ovarian cancer. *J Natl Cancer Inst* 1990;82:431.
9. Travis LB, Curtis RE, Boice JD Jr, et al. Second malignant neoplasms among long-term survivors of ovarian cancer. *Cancer Res* 1996;56:1564.
10. Winick NJ, McKenna RW, Shuster JJ, et al. Secondary acute myeloid leukemia in children with acute lymphoblastic leukemia treated with etoposide. *J Clin Oncol* 1993;11:209.
11. Slater JM, Fletcher GH. Ureteral strictures after radiation therapy for carcinoma of the uterine cervix. *Am J Roentgenol Radium Ther Nucl Med* 1971;111:269.
12. Gianni L, Munzone E. Capri G, et al. Paclitaxel by 3-hour infusion in combination with bolus doxorubicin in women with untreated metastatic breast cancer: high antitumor efficacy and cardiac effects in a dose-finding and sequence-finding study. *J Clin Oncol* 1995;13:2688.
13. Pater JL, Carmichael JA, Krepart GV, et al. Second-line chemotherapy of stage III-IV ovarian carcinoma: a randomized comparison of melphalan to melphalan and hexamethylmelamine in patients with persistent disease after doxorubicin and cisplatin. *Cancer Treat Rep* 1987;71:277.
14. Bajorin DF, Motzer RJ, Rodriguez E, et al. Acute non-lymphocytic leukemia in germ cell tumor patients treated with etoposide-containing chemotherapy. *J Natl Cancer Inst* 1993;85:60.
15. Smith DH, DeCosse JJ. Radiation damage to the small intestine. *World J Surg* 1986;10:189.
16. Stine KC, Saylors RL, Sawyer JR, et al. Secondary acute myelogenous leukemia following safe exposure to etoposide. *J Clin Oncol* 1995;13:2688.
17. Verweij J, van der Burg MEL, Pinedo HM. Mitomycin C-induced hemolytic uremic syndrome: six case reports and review of the literature on renal, pulmonary and cardiac side effects of the drug. *Radiother Oncol* 1987;8:33.
18. Thigpen T, Vance R, Lambuth B, et al. Chemotherapy for advanced or recurrent gynecologic cancer. *Cancer* 1987;60:2104.
19. Von Hoff DD, Layard MW, Basa P, et al. Risk factors for doxorubicin-induced congestive heart failure. *Ann Intern Med* 1979;91:710.
20. Unal A, Hamberger AD, Seski JC, et al. An analysis of the severe complications of irradiation of carcinoma of the uterine cervix: treatment with intracavitary radium and parametrial irradiation. *Int J Radiat Oncol Biol Phys* 1981;7:999.
21. Bristow MR, Mason JW, Billingham ME, et al. Doxorubicin cardiomyopathy: evaluation by phonocardiography, endomyocardial biopsy, and cardiac catheterization. *Ann Intern Med* 1978;88:168.
22. Alexander J, Dainiak N, Berger HJ, et al. Serial assessment of doxorubicin cardiotoxicity with quantitative radionuclide angiocardiography. *N Engl J Med* 1979;300:278.
23. Schwartz RG, McKenzie WB, Alexander J, et al. Congestive heart failure and left ventricular dysfunction complicating doxorubicin therapy: seven-year experience using serial radionuclide angiocardiography. *Am J Med* 1987;82:1109.
24. Legha SS, Benjamin RS, Mackay B, et al. Reduction of doxorubicin cardiotoxicity by prolonged continuous intravenous infusion. *Ann Intern Med* 1982;96:133.
25. Speyer JL, Green MD, Kramer E, et al. Protective effect of the bispiperazinedione, ICRF187, against doxorubicin-induced cardiac toxicity in women with advanced breast cancer. *N Engl J Med* 1988;319:745.
26. Slamon D, Leyland-Jones B, Shak S, et al. Addition of herceptin (humanized anti-HER2 antibody) to first line chemotherapy for HER2 overexpressing metastatic breast cancer (HER2+?MBC) markedly increases anticancer activity: a randomized multinational controlled phase III trial. *Proc Am Soc Clin Oncol* 1998;17:98a.
27. Markman M, Kennedy A, Webster K, et al. Paclitaxel administration to gynecologic cancer patients with major cardiac risk factors. *J Clin Oncol* 1998;16:3483.
28. Blum RH, Carter SK, Agre K. A clinical review of bleomycin—a new antineoplastic agent. *Cancer* 1973;31:903.
29. Goldiner PL, Carlon GC, Critkovic E, et al. Factors influencing postoperative morbidity and mortality in patients treated with bleomycin. *BMJ* 1978;1:1664.
30. Verweij J, van Zanten T, Souren T, et al. Prospective study on the dose relationship of mitomycin C-induced interstitial pneumonitis. *Cancer* 1987;60:756.
31. Cersosima RJ. Cisplatin neurotoxicity. *Cancer Treat Rev* 1989;16:195.
32. Hall DJ, Diasio R, Goplerud DR. Cisplatinum in gynecologic cancer. III. Toxicity. *Am J Obstet Gynecol* 1981;141:309.
33. Thompson SW, Davis LE, Kornfeld M, et al. Cisplatin neuropathy: clinical, electrophysiologic, morphologic, and toxicologic studies. *Cancer* 1984;54:1269.
34. Blachley JD, Hill JB. Renal and electrolyte disturbances associated with cisplatin. *Ann Intern Med* 1981;85:628.
35. Kopelman J, Budnick AS, Sessions RB, et al. Ototoxicity of high-dose cisplatin by bolus administration in patients with advanced cancers and normal hearing. *Laryngoscope* 1988;98:858.
36. Pollera CF, Marolla P, Nardi M, et al. Very high-dose cisplatin-induced ototoxicity: a preliminary report on early and long-term effects. *Cancer Chemother Pharmacol* 1988;21:61.
37. Donehower RC, Rowinsky EK, Grochow LB, et al. Phase I trial of Taxol in patients with advanced cancer. *Cancer Treat Rep* 1987;71:1171.
38. Connelly E, Markman M, Kennedy A, et al. Paclitaxel delivered as a 3-hour infusion with cisplatin in patients with gynecologic cancers: unexpected incidence of neurotoxicity. *Gynecol Oncol* 1996;62:166.
39. Piccart MJ, Bertelsen K, James K, et al. Randomized intergroup trial of cisplatin-paclitaxel versus cisplatin-cyclophosphamide in women with advanced epithelial ovarian cancer: Three-year results. *J Natl Cancer Inst* 2000;92:669.
40. Neijt J, Engelholm S, Tuxen M, et al. Exploratory phase III study of paclitaxel and cisplatin versus paclitaxel and carboplatin in advanced ovarian cancer. *J Clin Oncol* 2000;18:3084.
41. Hamner RW, Verani R, Weinman EJ. Mitomycin-associated renal failure: case report and review. *Arch Intern Med* 1983;143:803.
42. Gradishar WJ, Schilsky RL. Ovarian function following radiation and chemotherapy for cancer. *Semin Oncol* 1989;16:425.
43. Tangir J, Zelterman D, Wenging M, et al. Reproductive function after conservative surgery and chemotherapy for malignant germ cell tumors of the ovary. *Am Coll Obstet Gynecol* 2003;101:251.
44. Bower M, Newlands E, Holden L, et al. EMA/CO for high-risk gestational trophoblastic tumors: results from a cohort of 272 patients. *J Clin Oncol* 1997;15:2636.
45. Brewer M, Gershenson D, Herzog C, et al. Outcome and reproductive function after chemotherapy for ovarian dysgerminoma. *J Clin Oncol* 1999; 17:2670.
46. Doll DC, Ringenberg QS, Yarbo JW. Antineoplastic agents and pregnancy. *Semin Oncol* 1989;16:337.
47. Garber JE. Long-term follow-up of children exposed *in utero* to antineoplastic agents. *Semin Oncol* 1989;16:427.
48. Whitney CW. Randomized comparison of fluorouracil plus cisplatin versus hydroxyurea as an adjunct to radiation therapy in stages IIB-IVA carcinoma of the cervix with negative para-aortic lymph nodes. A Gynecologic Oncology Group and Southwest Oncology Group study. *J Clin Oncol* 1999;17:1339.
49. Morris M. Pelvic radiation with concurrent chemotherapy versus pelvic and para-aortic radiation for high-risk cervical cancer: a randomized Radiation Therapy Oncology Group clinical trial. *N Engl J Med* 1999;340: 1137.
50. Rose PG. Concurrent cisplatin-based chemoradiation improves progression-free and overall survival in advanced cervical cancer: results of a randomized Gynecologic Oncology Group study. *N Engl J Med* 1999;340:1144.
51. Keys HM. A comparison of weekly cisplatin during radiation therapy versus irradiation alone, each followed by adjuvant hysterectomy in bulky stage IB cervical carcinoma: A randomized trial of the Gynecologic Oncology Group. *N Engl J Med* 1999;340:1154.
52. Peters WA. Cisplatin and 5-fluorouracil plus radiation therapy are superior to radiation therapy as adjunctive in high-risk early-stage carcinoma of the cervix after radical hysterectomy and pelvic lymphadenectomy: report of a phase II intergroup study. *Soc Gynecol Oncol Abstracts*, 1999.
53. Montana GS, Thomas GM, Moore DH, et al. Preoperative chemo-radiation for carcinoma of the vulva with N2/N3 nodes: a Gynecologic Oncology Group study. *Int J Radiat Oncol Biol Phys* 2000;48:1007.
54. Jereczek-Fossa BA, Jassem J, Badzio A. Relationship between acute and late normal tissue injury after postoperative radiotherapy in endometrial cancer. *Int J Radiat Oncol Biol Phys* 2002;52:476.
55. Wang CJ, Leung SW, Chen HC, et al. The correlation of acute toxicity and late rectal injury in radiotherapy for cervical carcinoma: evidence suggestive of consequential late effect (CQLE). *Int J Radiat Oncol Biol Phys* 1998;40:85.
56. Budach W, Classen J, Belka C, et al. Clinical impact of predictive assays for acute and late radiation morbidity. *Strahlenther Onkol* 1998;174 (Suppl 3):20.
57. Weiss E, Hirnle P, Arnold-Bofinger H, et al. Therapeutic outcome and relation of acute and late side effects in the adjuvant radiotherapy of endometrial carcinoma stage I and II. *Radiother Oncol* 1999;53:37.
58. O'Brien PC, Franklin CI, Poulsen MG, et al. Acute symptoms, not rectally administered sucralfate, predict for late radiation proctitis: longer term follow-up of a phase III trial—Trans-Tasman Radiation Oncology Group. *Int J Radiat Oncol Biol Phys* 2002;54:442.
59. Hall EJ. *Radiobiology for the Radiologist*, 5th ed. Philadelphia: Lippincott Williams & Wilkins; 2000.
60. Iyer RB, Jhingran A, Sawaf H, et al. Imaging findings after radiotherapy to the pelvis. *Am J Roentgenol* 2001;177:1083.
61. Libshitz HI. Radiation changes in bone. *Semin Roentgenol* 1994;29:15.
62. Abe H, Nakamura M, Takahashi S, et al. Radiation-induced insufficiency fractures of the pelvis: evaluation with 99mTc-methylene diphosphonate scintigraphy. *Am J Roentgenol* 1992;158:599.

63. Blomlie V, Rofstad EK, Talle K, et al. Incidence of radiation-induced insufficiency fractures of the female pelvis: evaluation with MR imaging. *Am J Roentgenol* 1996;167:1205.
64. Ikushima H, Osaki K, Furutani S, et al. Pelvic bone complications following radiation therapy of gynecologic malignancies: clinical evaluation of radiation-induced pelvic insufficiency fractures. *Gynecol Oncol* 2006;103: 1100.
65. Emami B, Lyman J, Brown A, et al. Tolerance of normal tissue to therapeutic irradiation. *Int J Radiat Oncol Biol Phys* 1991;21:109.
66. Grigsby PW, Roberts HL, Perez CA. Femoral neck fracture following groin irradiation. *Int J Radiat Oncol Biol Phys* 1995;32:63.
67. Parmentier C, Morardet N, Tubiana M. Late effects on human bone marrow after extended field radiotherapy. *Int J Radiat Oncol Biol Phys* 1983;9:1303.
68. Mell LK, Kochanski JD, Roeske JC, et al. Dosimetric predictors of acute hematologic toxicity in cervical cancer patients treated with concurrent cisplatin and intensity-modulated pelvic radiotherapy. *Int J Radiat Oncol Biol Phys* 2001;66:1356.
69. Brixey CJ, Roeske JC, Lujan AE, et al. Impact of intensity-modulated radiotherapy on acute hematologic toxicity in women with gynecologic malignancies. *Int J Radiat Oncol Biol Phys* 2002;54:1388.
70. Salama JK, Mundt AJ, Roeske J, et al. Preliminary outcome and toxicity report of extended-field, intensity-modulated radiation therapy for gynecologic malignancies. *Int J Radiat Oncol Biol Phys* 2006;65:1170.
71. Lujan AE, Mundt AJ, Yamada SD, et al. Intensity-modulated radiotherapy as a means of reducing dose to bone marrow in gynecologic patients receiving whole pelvic radiotherapy. *Int J Radiat Oncol Biol Phys* 2003;57:516.
72. Jereczek-Fossa BA, Badzio A, Jassem J. Factors determining acute normal tissue reactions during postoperative radiotherapy in endometrial cancer: analysis of 317 consecutive cases. *Radiother Oncol* 2003;68:33.
73. Eifel PJ, Jhingran A, Bodurka DC, et al. Correlation of smoking history and other patient characteristics with major complications of pelvic radiation therapy for cervical cancer. *J Clin Oncol* 2002;20:3651.
74. Cummings BJ, Keane TJ, O'Sullivan B, et al. Epidermoid anal cancer: treatment by radiation alone or by radiation and 5-fluorouracil with and without mitomycin C. *Int J Radiat Oncol Biol Phys* 1991;21:1115.
75. Abbasakoor F, Vaizey CJ, Boulos PB. Improving the morbidity of anorectal injury from pelvic radiotherapy. *Colorectal Dis* 2006;8:2.
76. International Commission on Radiation Units and Measurements. *Report 38: Dose and Volume Specification for Reporting Intracavitary Therapy in Gynecology*. Bethesda, MD: International Commission on Radiation Units and Measurements; 1985.
77. Fellner C, Potter R, Knocke TH, et al. Comparison of radiography- and computed tomography-based treatment planning in cervix cancer in brachytherapy with specific attention to some quality assurance aspects. *Radiother Oncol* 2001;58:53.
78. Kirisits C, Potter R, Lang S, et al. Dose and volume parameters for MRI-based treatment planning in intracavitary brachytherapy for cervical cancer. *Int J Radiat Oncol Biol Phys* 2005;62:901.
79. Williamson RC. Intestinal adaptation (first of two parts). Structural, functional and cytokinetic changes. *N Engl J Med* 1978;298:1393.
80. Haboubi NY, Schofield PF, Rowland PL. The light and electron microscopic features of early and late phase radiation-induced proctitis. *Am J Gastroenterol* 1988;83:1140.
81. Sedgwick DM, Howard GC, Ferguson A. Pathogenesis of acute radiation injury to the rectum. A prospective study in patients. *Int J Colorectal Dis* 1994;9:23.
82. Fajardo LF, Berthrong M, Anderson RE. *Radiation Pathology*. New York: Oxford University Press, Inc.; 2001.
83. Anseline PF, Lavery IC, Fazio VW, et al. Radiation injury of the rectum: evaluation of surgical treatment. *Ann Surg* 1981;194:71.
84. Hasleton PS, Carr N, Schofield PF. Vascular changes in radiation bowel disease. *Histopathol* 1985;9:517.
85. Kochhar R, Sriram PV, Sharma SC, et al. Natural history of late radiation proctosigmoiditis treated with topical sucralfate suspension. *Dig Dis Sci* 1999;44:973.
86. Kochhar R, Patel F, Dhar A, et al. Radiation-induced proctosigmoiditis. Prospective, randomized, double-blind controlled trial of oral sulfasalazine plus rectal steroids versus rectal sucralfate. *Dig Dis Sci* 1991;36:103.
87. Kneebone A, Mameghan H, Bolin T, et al. Effect of oral sucralfate on late rectal injury associated with radiotherapy for prostate cancer: a double-blind, randomized trial. *Int J Radiat Oncol Biol Phys* 2004;60:1088.
88. Biswal BM, Lal P, Rath GK, et al. Intrarectal formalin application, an effective treatment for grade III haemorrhagic radiation proctitis. *Radiother Oncol* 1995;35:212.
89. Chun M, Kang S, Kil HJ, et al. Rectal bleeding and its management after irradiation for uterine cervical cancer. *Int J Radiat Oncol Biol Phys* 2004;58:98.
90. Donner CS. Pathophysiology and therapy of chronic radiation-induced injury to the colon. *Dig Dis Sci* 1998;16:253.
91. Preston DL, Shimizu Y, Pierce DA, et al. Studies of mortality of atomic bomb survivors. Report 13: Solid cancer and noncancer disease mortality: 1950–1997. *Radiat Res* 2003;160:381.
92. Yamada M, Wong FL, Fujiwara S, et al. Noncancer disease incidence in atomic bomb survivors, 1958–1998. *Radiat Res* 2004;161:622.
93. Wing S, Shy CM, Wood JL, et al. Mortality among workers at Oak Ridge National Laboratory. Evidence of radiation effects in follow-up through 1984. *JAMA* 1991;265:1397.
94. Schull WJ. The children of atomic bomb survivors: a synopsis. *J Radiol Prot* 2003;23:369.
95. Nag S, Erickson B, Thomadsen B, et al. The American Brachytherapy Society recommendations for high-dose-rate brachytherapy for carcinoma of the cervix. *Int J Radiat Oncol Biol Phys* 2000;48:201.
96. Perez CA, Grigsby PW, Lockett MA, et al. Radiation therapy morbidity in carcinoma of the uterine cervix: dosimetric and clinical correlation. *Int J Radiat Oncol Biol Phys* 1999;44:855.
97. Potter R, Haie-Meder C, Van Limbergen E, et al. GEC ESTRO Working Group. Recommendations from gynaecological (GYN) GEC ESTRO working group (II): concepts and terms in 3D image-based treatment planning in cervix cancer brachytherapy—3D dose volume parameters and aspects of 3D image-based anatomy, radiation physics, radiobiology. *Radiother Oncol* 2006;78:67.
98. Wachter-Gerstner N, Wachter S, Reinstadler E, et al. Bladder and rectum dose defined from MRI based treatment planning for cervix cancer brachytherapy: comparison of dose-volume histograms for organ contours and organ wall, comparison with ICRU rectum and bladder reference point. *Radiother Oncol* 2003;68:269.
99. Pelloski CE, Palmer M, Chronowski GM, et al. Comparison between CT-based volumetric calculations and ICRU reference-point estimates of radiation doses delivered to bladder and rectum during intracavitary radiotherapy for cervical cancer. *Int J Radiat Oncol Biol Phys* 2005;62:131.
100. Eifel PJ, Levenback C, Wharton JT, et al. Time course and incidence of late complications in patients treated with radiation therapy for FIGO stage IB carcinoma of the uterine cervix. *Int J Radiat Oncol Biol Phys* 1995; 32:1289.
101. Herbst AL. Cancer of the vagina. In: Gusberg SB, Frick HC, eds. *Corscaden's Gynecologic Cancer*, 5th ed. Baltimore: Williams & Wilkins; 1978:120.
102. Gellrich J, Hakenberg OW, Oehlschlager S, et al. Manifestation, latency and management of late urological complications after curative radiotherapy for cervical carcinoma. *Onkologie* 2003;26:334.
103. Rotman M, John M, Roussis K, et al. The intracavitary applicator in relation to complications of pelvic radiation: the Ernst system. *Int J Radiat Oncol Biol Phys* 1978;4:951.
104. McIntyre JF, Eifel PJ, Levenback C, et al. Ureteral stricture as a late complication of radiotherapy for stage IB carcinoma of the uterine cervix. *Cancer* 1995;75:836.
105. Dewan AK, Mohan GM, Ravi R. Intravesical formalin for hemorrhagic cystitis following irradiation of cancer of the cervix. *Int J Gynaecol Obstet* 1993;42:131.
106. Lojanapiwat B, Sripralakrit S, Soonthornphan S, et al. Intravesicle formalin instillation with a modified technique for controlling haemorrhage secondary to radiation cystitis. *Asian J Surg* 2002;25:232.
107. Corman JM, McClure D, Pritchett R, et al. Treatment of radiation induced hemorrhagic cystitis with hyperbaric oxygen. *J Urol* 2003;169:2200.
108. Chong KT, Hampson NB, Corman JM. Early hyperbaric oxygen therapy improves outcome for radiation-induced hemorrhagic cystitis. *Urology* 2005;65:649.
109. Snijders-Keilholz A, Hellebrekers BW, Zwinderman AH, et al. Adjuvant radiotherapy following radical hysterectomy for patients with early-stage cervical carcinoma (1984–1996). *Radiother Oncol* 1999;51:161.
110. Ryan M, Stainton MC, Slaytor EK, et al. Aetiology and prevalence of lower limb lymphoedema following treatment for gynaecological cancer. *Aust N Z J Obstet Gynaecol* 2003;43:148.
111. Georgiou A, Grigsby PW, Perez CA. Radiation induced lumbosacral plexopathy in gynecologic tumors: clinical findings and dosimetric analysis. *Int J Radiat Oncol Biol Phys* 1993;26:479.
112. Perez CA, Fox S, Lockett MA, et al. Definitive irradiation in carcinoma of the vagina: long-term evaluation of results. *Int J Radiat Oncol Biol Phys* 1988;15:1283.
113. Au SP, Grigsby PW. The irradiation tolerance dose of the proximal vagina. *Radiother Oncol* 2003;67:77.
114. Hintz BL, Kagan AR, Chan P, et al. Radiation tolerance of the vaginal mucosa. *Int J Radiat Oncol Biol Phys* 1980;6:711.
115. Grigsby PW, Russell A, Bruner D, et al. Late injury of cancer therapy on the female reproductive tract. *Int J Radiat Oncol Biol Phys* 1995;31:1281.
116. Ogilvy-Stuart AL, Shalet SM. Effect of radiation on the human reproductive system. *Environ Health Perspec* 1993;101(Suppl 2):10.
117. Gershenson DM. Fertility-sparing surgery for malignancies in women. *J Natl Cancer Inst Monogr* 2005;(34):43.
118. Huang KG, Lee CL, Tsai CS, et al. A new approach for laparoscopic ovarian transposition before pelvic irradiation. *Gynecol Oncol* 2007;105:234.
119. Martin JR, Kodaman P, Oktay K, et al. Ovarian cryopreservation with transposition of a contralateral ovary: a combined approach for fertility preservation in women receiving pelvic radiation. *Fertil Steril* 2007;87:189.
120. Chambers SK, Chambers JT, Holm C, et al. Sequelae of lateral ovarian transposition in unirradiated cervical cancer patients. *Gynecol Oncol* 1990;39:155.
121. Bruner DW, Lanciano R, Keegan M, et al. Vaginal stenosis and sexual function following intracavitary radiation for the treatment of cervical and endometrial carcinoma. *Int J Radiat Oncol Biol Phys* 1993;27:825.

122. Jensen PT, Groenvold M, Klee MC, et al. Longitudinal study of sexual function and vaginal changes after radiotherapy for cervical cancer. *Int J Radiat Oncol Biol Phys* 2003;56:937.
123. Bergmark K, Avall-Lundqvist E, Dickman PW, et al. Vaginal changes and sexuality in women with a history of cervical cancer. *N Engl J Med* 1999;340:1383.
124. Pitkin RM, Bradbury JT. The effect of topical estrogen on irradiated vaginal epithelium. *Am J Obstet Gynecol* 1965;92:175.
125. Fraunholz IB, Schopohl B, Bottcher HD. Management of radiation injuries of vulva and vagina. *Strahlenther Onkol* 1998;174(Suppl 3):90.
126. de Hullu JA, Pras E, Hollema H, et al. Presentations of endometrial activity after curative radiotherapy for cervical cancer. *Maturitas* 2005;51:172.
127. Leenhouts GH, Kylstra WA, Everaerd W, et al. Sexual outcomes following treatment for early-stage gynecologic cancer: a prospective and cross-sectional multi-center study. *J Psychosom Obstet Gynaecol* 2002;23:123.
128. Amsterdam A, Krychman ML. Sexual dysfunction in patients with gynecologic neoplasms: a retrospective pilot study. *J Sex Med* 2006;3:646.
129. Robinson JW, Faris PD, Scott CB. Psychoeducational group increases vaginal dilation for younger women and reduces sexual fears for women of all ages with gynecologic carcinoma treated with radiotherapy. *Int J Radiat Oncol Biol Phys* 1999;44:497.
130. Jeffries SA, Robinson JW, Craighead PS, et al. An effective group psychoeducational intervention for improving compliance with vaginal dilation: a randomized controlled trial. *Int J Radiat Oncol Biol Phys* 2006;65:404.
131. Schroder M, Mell LK, Hurteau JA, et al. Clitoral therapy device for treatment of sexual dysfunction in irradiated cervical cancer patients. *Int J Radiat Oncol Biol Phys* 2005;61:1078.
132. Wilson SK, Delk JR, Billups KL. Treating symptoms of female sexual arousal disorder with the Eros-Clitoral Therapy Device. *J Gend Specif Med* 2001;4:54.
133. Munarriz R, Maitland S, Garcia SP, et al. A prospective duplex Doppler ultrasonographic study in women with sexual arousal disorder to objectively assess genital engorgement induced by EROS therapy. *J Sex Marital Ther* 2003;29(Suppl 1):85.
134. Weiss E, Richter S, Hess CF. Radiation therapy of the pelvic and paraaortic lymph nodes in cervical carcinoma: a prospective three-dimensional analysis of patient positioning and treatment technique. *Radiother Oncol* 2003;68:41.
135. Shanahan TG, Mehta MP, Bertelrud KL, et al. Minimization of small bowel volume within treatment fields utilizing customized "belly boards." *Int J Radiat Oncol Biol Phys* 1990;19:469.
136. Patel FD, Sharma SC, Negi PS, et al. Low dose rate vs. high dose rate brachytherapy in the treatment of carcinoma of the uterine cervix: a clinical trial. *Int J Radiat Oncol Biol Phys* 1994;28:335.
137. Teshima T, Inoue T, Ikeda H, et al. High-dose rate and low-dose rate intracavitary therapy for carcinoma of the uterine cervix. Final results of Osaka University Hospital. *Cancer* 1993;72:2409.
138. Hareyama M, Sakata K, Oouchi A, et al. High-dose-rate versus low-dose-rate intracavitary therapy for carcinoma of the uterine cervix: a randomized trial. *Cancer* 2002;94:117.
139. Lertsanguansinchai P, Lertbutsayanukul C, Shotelersuk K, et al. Phase III randomized trial comparing LDR and HDR brachytherapy in treatment of cervical carcinoma. *Int J Radiat Oncol Biol Phys* 2004;59:1424.
140. Mell LK, Mehrotra AK, Mundt AJ. Intensity-modulated radiation therapy use in the U.S., 2004. *Cancer* 2005;104:1296.
141. Mundt AJ, Lujan AE, Rotmensch J, et al. Intensity-modulated whole pelvic radiotherapy in women with gynecologic malignancies. *Int J Radiat Oncol Biol Phys* 2002;52:1330.
142. Mundt AJ, Mell LK, Roeske JC. Preliminary analysis of chronic gastrointestinal toxicity in gynecology patients treated with intensity-modulated whole pelvic radiation therapy. *Int J Radiat Oncol Biol Phys* 2003;56:1354.
143. Salama JK, Mundt AJ, Roeske J, et al. Preliminary outcome and toxicity report of extended-field, intensity-modulated radiation therapy for gynecologic malignancies. *Int J Radiat Oncol Biol Phys* 2006;65:1170.
144. Randall ME, Ibbott GS. Intensity-modulated radiation therapy for gynecologic cancers: pitfalls, hazards, and cautions to be considered. *Semin Radiat Oncol* 2006;16:138.
145. Georg P, Georg D, Hillbrand M, et al. Factors influencing bowel sparing in intensity modulated whole pelvic radiotherapy for gynaecological malignancies. *Radiother Oncol* 2006;80:19.
146. Varlotto JM, Gerszten K, Heron DE, et al. The potential nephrotoxic effects of intensity modulated radiotherapy delivered to the para-aortic area of women with gynecologic malignancies: preliminary results. *Am J Clin Oncol* 2006;29:281.
147. Dawson LA, Jaffray DA. Advances in image-guided radiation therapy. *J Clin Oncol* 2007;25:938.
148. Perkins CL, Fox T, Elder E, et al. Image-guided radiation therapy (IGRT) in gastrointestinal tumors. *JOP* 2006;7:372.
149. Lanciano RM, Martz K, Coia LR, et al. Tumor and treatment factors improving outcome in stage III-B cervix cancer. *Int J Radiat Oncol Biol Phys* 1991;20:95.
150. Montana GS, Fowler WC, Varia MA, et al. Carcinoma of the cervix, stage III. Results of radiation therapy. *Cancer* 1986;57:148.
151. Tod MC, Meredith WJ. A dosage system for use in the treatment of cancer of the uterine cervix. *Br J Radiol* 1938;11;809.
152. Tod M, Meredith WJ. Treatment of cancer of the cervix uteri: a revised Manchester method. *Br J Radiol* 1953;26:252.
153. Potish RA, Gerbi BJ. Role of point A in the era of computerized dosimetry. *Radiology* 1986;158:827.
154. Utley JF, Marlowe C, Waddell WJ. Distribution of 35S-labeled WR-2721 in normal and malignant tissues of the mouse. *Radiat Res* 1976;68:284.
155. Yuhas JM, Spellman JM, Culo F. The role of WR-2721 in radiotherapy and/or chemotherapy. *Cancer Clin Trials* 1980;3:211.
156. Calabro-Jones PM, Fahey RC, Smoluk GD, et al. Alkaline phosphatase promotes radioprotection and accumulation of WR-1065 in V79-171 cells incubated in medium containing WR-2721. *Int J Radiat Biol Relat Stud Phys Chem Med* 1985;47:23.
157. Brizel DM, Wasserman TH, Henke M, et al. Phase II randomized trial of amifostine as a radioprotector in head and neck cancer. *J Clin Oncol* 2000;18:3339.
158. Athanassiou H, Antonadou D, Coliarakis N, et al. Protective effect of amifostine during fractionated radiotherapy in patients with pelvic carcinomas: results of a randomized trial. *Int J Radiat Oncol Biol Phys* 2003;56:1154.
159. Liu T, Liu Y, He S, et al. Use of radiation with or without WR-2721 in advanced rectal cancer. *Cancer* 1992;69:2820.
160. Koukourakis MI, Kyrias G, Kakolyris S, et al. Subcutaneous administration of amifostine during fractionated radiotherapy: a randomized phase II study. *J Clin Oncol* 2000;18:2226.
161. Morrow CP, Curtin JP, eds. *Gynecologic Cancer Surgery*. New York: Churchill Livingstone; 1996:141.
162. Orr JW, Shingleton HM. *Complications in Gynecologic Surgery*. Philadelphia: JB Lippincott Co.; 1994.
163. Underwood PB, Wilson WC, Kreutner A, et al. Radical hysterectomy: a critical review of twenty-two years' experience. *Am J Obstet Gynecol* 1979;134:889.
164. Gellrich J, Hakenberg OW, Oehlschlager S, et al. Manifestation, latency and management of late urological complications after curative radiotherapy for cervical carcinoma. *Onkologie* 2003;26:334.
165. Carmody E, Thurston W, Yueng E, et al. Transrectal drainage of deep pelvic collections under fluoroscopic guidance. *Can Assoc Radiol J* 1993;44:429.
166. Hoskins WJ, Park RC, Long R, et al. Repair of urinary tract fistulas with bulbocavernous myocutaneous flaps. *Obstet Gynecol* 1984;63:588.
167. Hancock KC, Copeland LJ, Gershenson DM, et al. Urinary conduits in gynecologic oncology. *Obstet Gynecol* 1986;67:680.
168. Regan JB, Barrett DM. Stented versus non-stented ureteroileal anastomoses: is there a difference with regard to leak and stricture? *J Urol* 1985;134:1101.
169. Penalever MA, Angioli R, Mirhashimi R, et al. Management of early and late complications of ileocolonic continent urinary reservoir (Miami pouch). *Gynecol Oncol* 1998;69:185.
170. Montz FJ, Holschneider CH, Solh S, et al. Small bowel obstruction following radical hysterectomy: risk factors, incidence, and operative findings. *Gynecol Oncol* 1994;53:114.
171. Beard RW, Kelly KA. Randomized prospective evaluation of the EEA stapler for colorectal anastomosis. *Am J Surg* 1981;141:143.
172. Jex RK, Van Heersen JA, Wolf BG, et al. Gastrointestinal anastomoses: factors affecting early complications. *Ann Surg* 1987;206:138.
173. Castro JR, Issa P, Fletcher GH. Carcinoma of the cervix treated by external irradiation alone. *Radiology* 1970;95:163.
174. Dziki AJ, Duncan JD, Harmon JW, et al. Advantages of hand-sewn over stapled anastomoses. *Dis Colon Rectum* 1991;34:44.
175. Max E, Sweeney WB, Bailey HR, et al. Results of 1,000 single layer continuous polyprolene intestinal anastomosis. *Am J Surg* 1991;162:461.
176. Brolin RE, Krasna MJ, Mast BA. Use of tubes and radiographs in the management of small bowel obstruction. *Ann Surg* 1987;206:126.
177. Snyder CL, Ferrel KL, Goodale RL, et al. Nonoperative management of small bowel obstruction with endoscopic long tube placement. *Ann Surg* 1990;56:587.
178. Sosa J, Gardner B. Management of patients diagnosed as acute intestinal obstruction secondary to adhesions. *Ann Surg* 1993;59:125.
179. Joyce WP, Delaney PV, Gorey TF, et al. The value of water soluble contrast radiology in the management of acute small bowel obstruction. *Ann R Coll Surg Engl* 1992;74:422.
180. Farmer KCR, Phillips RKS. True and false large bowel obstruction. *Baillieres Clin Gastroenterol* 1991;5:563.
181. Hoffman MS, Villa A, Roberts WS, et al. Mass closure of the abdominal wound with absorbable suture in surgery for gynecologic cancer. *J Reprod Med* 1991;36:356.
182. Shepard JH, Cavanaugh D, Riggs D, et al. Abdominal wound closure using a nonabsorbable single-layer technique. *Obstet Gynecol* 1983;61:248.
183. Hanks GE, Herring DF, Kramer S. Patterns of Care Outcome Studies: results of the national practice in cancer of the cervix. *Cancer* 1983;51:959.
184. Perez CA, Breaux S, Bedwinek JM, et al. Radiation therapy alone in the treatment of carcinoma of the uterine cervix. II. Analysis of complications. *Cancer* 1984;54:235.
185. van Nagell JR, Maruyuma Y, Parker JC, et al. Small bowel injury following radiation therapy for cervical cancer. *Am J Obstet Gynecol* 1974;118:163.

186. Kucera PR, Berman ML, Treadwell P, et al. Whole-abdominal radiotherapy for patients with minimal residual epithelial ovarian cancer. *Gynecol Oncol* 1990;36:338.
187. Linstadt DE, Stern JL, Quivey JM, et al. Salvage whole abdominal irradiation following chemotherapy failure in epithelial ovarian cancer. *Gynecol Oncol* 1990;36:327.
188. Smith ST, Seski JC, Copeland LJ, et al. Surgical management of irradiation-induced small bowel damage. *Obstet Gynecol* 1985;65:563.
189. Schmitt EH, Symmonds RE. Surgical treatment of radiation induced injuries of the intestine. *Surg Gynecol Obstet* 1981;153:896.
190. Rubin SC, Benjamin I, Hoskins WJ, et al. Intestinal surgery in gynecologic oncology. *Gynecol Oncol* 1989;34:30.
191. Curtin JP, Burt LL. Successful treatment of small intestinal fistula with somatostatin analog. *Gynecol Oncol* 1990;39:225.
192. Marks G, Mohiudden M. The surgical management of the radiation-injured intestine. *Surg Clin North Am* 1983;63:81.
193. Swan RW, Fowler WC Jr, Boronow RC. Surgical management of radiation injury to the small intestine. *Surg Gynecol Obstet* 1976;142:325.
194. Hoskins WJ, Burke TW, Weiser EB, et al. Right hemicolectomy and ileal resection with primary anastomosis for irradiation injury of the terminal ileum. *Gynecol Oncol* 1987;26:215.
195. Smith DH, Pierce VK, Lewis JL Jr. Enteric fistulas encountered on a gynecologic oncology service from 1969 through 1980. *Surg Gynecol Obstet* 1984;158:71.
196. Hamberger AD, Unal A, Gershenson DM. Analysis of the severe complications of irradiation of carcinoma of the cervix: whole pelvis irradiation and intracavitary radium. *Int J Radiat Oncol Biol Phys* 1983;9:367.
197. Ahlquist DA, Gostout CJ, Viggiano TR, et al. Laser therapy for severe radiation induced rectal bleeding. *Mayo Clin Proc* 1986;61:927.
198. Schofield PF, Car ND, Holden D. The pathogenesis and treatment of radiation bowel disease. *J R Soc Med* 1986;79:30.
199. Martius H. Sphincter und Harnrohrenplastik aus dem M. bulbocavernosis. *Chirurgie* 1929;17:49.
200. Boronow RC. Repair of the radiation-induced vaginal fistula using the Martius technique. *World J Surg* 1986;10:237.
201. Aartsen EJ, Sindram IS. Repair of the radiation induced rectovaginal fistula without or with interposition of the bulbocavernosus muscle (Martius procedure). *Eur J Surg Oncol* 1988;14:171.
202. Graham JB. Vaginal fistulas following radiotherapy. *Surg Gynecol Obstet* 1965;120:1019.
203. Bricker EM, Johnston WD. Repair of postirradiation rectovaginal fistula and stricture. *Surg Gynecol Obstet* 1979;148:499.
204. Cushing RM, Towell HM, Liegner LM. Major urological complications following radium and x-ray therapy for carcinoma of the cervix. *Am J Obstet Gynecol* 1968;101:750.
205. Muram B, Oxorn H, Currie RJ, et al. Postradiation ureteral obstruction: a reappraisal. *Am J Obstet Gynecol* 1981;139:289.
206. Kottmeier HL. Complications following radiation therapy in carcinoma of the cervix and their treatment. *Am J Obstet Gynecol* 1964;88:854.
207. Everett HS. The effect of carcinoma of the cervix uteri and its treatment upon the urinary tract. *Am J Obstet Gynecol* 1939;38:889.
208. Kaplan AL. Postradiation ureteral obstruction. *Obstet Gynecol Surv* 1977;32:1.
209. Underwood PB, Lutz MH, Smoak DL. Ureteral injury following irradiation therapy for carcinoma of the cervix. *Obstet Gynecol* 1977;49:663.
210. Villasanta U. Complications of radiotherapy for carcinoma of the uterine cervix. *Am J Obstet Gynecol* 1972;114:717.
211. Altvater G, Imholz G. Ureteral stenosis in carcinoma of the cervix uteri: prognostic significance and surgical treatment. *Geburtshilfe Frauenheilkd* 1960;20:1214.
212. Boronow RC. Urologic complications secondary to radiation alone or radiation and surgery. In: Delgado G, Smith JP, eds. *Management of Complications in Gynecologic Oncology.* New York: John Wiley & Sons; 1982:163.
213. Kirchoff H. *Geburtshilfe Frauenheilkd* [The place of gynecologic radiotherapy in radiology.] 1960;920:34.
214. Burns BC, Upton RT. *Cancer of the Uterus and Ovary*. Chicago: Year Book Medical Publishers; 1969.
215. Krupp P, Hoffman M, Roeling W. Terminal ileum as ureteral substitute. *Obstet Gynecol* 1970;35:416.
216. Perry CP, Massey FM, Moore TN, et al. Treatment of irradiation injury to the ureter by ileal substitution. *Obstet Gynecol* 1975;46:517.
217. Boronow RC, Rutledge F. Vesicovaginal fistula, radiation, and gynecologic cancer. *Am J Obstet Gynecol* 1971;111:85.
218. Bastiaanse M. Bastiaanse's method for surgical closure of very large radiation fistulae of the bladder and rectum. In: Youssef AF, ed. *Gynecologic Oncology*. Springfield, IL: Charles C Thomas Publishers; 1960:280.
219. Kirkinen P, Kauppila A, Kontturi M. Treatment of ureteral strictures after therapy for carcinoma of the uterus. *Surg Gynecol Obstet* 1980;151:487.
220. Mundy AR. Cystoplasty. In: Mundy AR, ed. *Current Operative Surgery: Urology*. Eastbourne, UK: Bailliere; 1986:140.
221. Barnard RJ, Lupton EW. Treatment of radiation urinary tract disease. In: Schofield PF, Lupton EW, eds. *The Causation and Clinical Management of Pelvic Radiation Disease*. London: Springer-Verlag; 1989:123.
222. Goodwin WE. Experiences with intestine as a substitute for the urinary tract. In: King LR, Stone AR, Webster GD, eds. *Bladder Reconstruction and Continent Urinary Diversion*. Chicago: Year Book Medical Publishers; 1987:9.
223. Concepcion RS, Koch MO, McDougal S, et al. Detubularized intestinal segments in urinary tract reconstruction: why do they work? *J Urol* 1988;139:310a.
224. Strockbine MD, Hancock JE, Fletcher GH. Complications in 831 patients with squamous cell carcinoma of the intact uterine cervix treated with 3,000 rads or more whole pelvis irradiation. *Am J Roentgenol Radium Ther Nucl Med* 1970;108:293–304.
225. Logsdon MD, Eifel PJ. Figo IIIB squamous cell carcinoma of the cervix: an analysis of prognostic factors emphasizing the balance between external beam and intracavitary radiation therapy. *Int J Radiat Oncol Biol Phys* 1999;43:763–775.

CHAPTER 32 ■ MANAGEMENT OF PAIN

RUSSELL K. PORTENOY, DAMEAN FREAS, AND PAULINE LESAGE

The heterogeneous patient population managed by gynecologic oncologists presents a broad range of problems in pain management. The incidence of cancer pain varies, depending on the type of neoplasm, stage, and extent of spread. Acute pains are highly prevalent, including the rather straightforward incisional pain that follows surgical procedures. Chronic pain occurs in the context of numerous other physical and psychosocial symptoms, often in the population with advanced disease. Effective relief of pain may improve mood, coping, function, and other aspects of quality of life. Gynecologic oncologists have the opportunity and obligation to effectively treat pain.

SCOPE OF THE PROBLEM

Pain is highly prevalent in the cancer population. Overall, 30% to 50% of patients undergoing active antineoplastic therapy and 75% to 90% of those with advanced disease experience chronic pain severe enough to warrant therapy (1–3). Although data specific to gynecologic tumors are meager, those extant suggest that the overall prevalence rates mirror these averages (1,4–6).

A survey of patients with ovarian cancer illustrates the prevalence and characteristics of chronic pain in this population (6). The sample included 111 inpatients and 40 outpatients. The median age was 55 years (range 23 to 86 years), and most patients (82%) had stage III or IV disease at presentation and active disease (69%) at the time of the survey. Forty-two percent (n = 63) reported "persistent or frequent pain" during the preceding 2 weeks. This pain had a median duration of 2 weeks (range <1 to 756 weeks) and was usually abdominal/pelvic (80%), frequent or almost constant (66%), and moderate to severe. Most patients reported that pain caused moderate or greater interference with various aspects of function, particularly activity (68%), mood (62%), work (62%), and overall enjoyment of life (61%). In a study of 97 outpatients with breast cancer (54% metastatic disease), 47% of patients experienced cancer-related pain substantially interfering with their mood, quality of life, and functional status. The most prevalent underlying pathology was postmastectomy syndrome (56%), followed by pain from bone metastasis (26%).

Tissue injury related to the neoplasm itself is the most common cause of chronic cancer pain. Pain prevalence increases with the extent of disease and can be as high as 80% among populations with advanced illness (7). Chronic pain also may be related to an antineoplastic treatment, such as surgery (8–10), and in a small minority of patients, pain is unrelated to either the malignancy or its treatment.

Observational studies suggest that satisfactory relief of chronic pain is possible in 70% to 90% of patients with cancer (11–14). Undertreatment remains a serious problem, however (15–19), despite the availability of well-accepted guidelines for pain management (20).

Although the prevalence of severe acute pain in patients with gynecologic cancers has not been determined, and is likely changing with the increasing use of minimally invasive procedures, it is nonetheless presumed to be common and potentially controllable in a very large majority of cases. As more cancer surgeries are performed in the ambulatory setting, the ability to provide adequate treatment in unmonitored settings has become a greater challenge.

Patients with cancer, and particularly those with advanced disease, also experience numerous symptoms other than pain. The most common of these symptoms are fatigue and anxiety or depression. Acute treatment-related symptoms, such as chemotherapy-induced nausea and vomiting, also are prevalent. In the aforementioned survey of patients with ovarian cancer, the median number of symptoms per patient was nine (range 0 to 25) (Table 32.1) (6). In addition to pain, the most prevalent symptoms were fatigue ("lack of energy"), psychologic distress ("worrying," "feeling sad," and "feeling nervous"), and insomnia ("difficulty sleeping"). All of these symptoms had a prevalence of >50%. Compared to norms, approximately one third of the patients in this survey recorded heightened psychologic distress. The most important predictor of heightened distress was progressive impairment in physical functioning.

Fatigue is one of the most common complications of cancer and its treatment, and exemplifies the problem of concurrent symptoms in the patient with significant pain. In a recent analysis, patients perceived fatigue to be the most distressing symptom adversely affecting quality of life (21). A definition proposed for the International Classification of Diseases 10th Revision–Clinical Modification (ICD-10-CM) stresses the multidimensional nature of the phenomenon (22) and the National Comprehensive Cancer Network 2007 guidelines identified seven factors that should be assessed as potential causes of prolonged fatigue, one of which is pain (others include emotional distress, sleep disturbance, anemia, nutrition, activity level, and other comorbidities) (23). Patients with pain should be evaluated for meaningful concomitant symptoms, and the assessment of other symptoms should prompt an assessment of pain.

ASSESSMENT OF CANCER PAIN

The assessment of chronic pain in patients with gynecologic cancer requires an understanding of its phenomenology, pathophysiology, and syndromes. Optimally, this assessment must also consider the broad range of physical, psychologic, and social disturbances concurrently experienced by these patients. Patients with acute pain, particularly acute postoperative pain, pose less complex management problems, but could still potentially benefit from an ongoing comprehensive assessment.

TABLE 32.1

PREVALENCE AND CHARACTERISTICS OF SYMPTOMS ASSOCIATED WITH OVARIAN CANCER (N = 151)

Symptom	Overall prevalence (%)	Intensity[a] (%)	Frequency[b] (%)	Distress[c] (%)
Worrying	71.7	55.4	33.5	25.0
Lack of energy	68.6	52.6	37.3	28.0
Feeling sad	63.8	46.4	22.8	22.2
Pain	61.8	50.4	32.9	24.1
Feeling nervous	61.5	39.9	25.0	19.6
Difficulty sleeping	57.3	44.0	30.7	20.7
Dry mouth	45.6	30.2	18.8	8.7
Feeling drowsy	45.3	32.7	15.9	9.3
Feeling irritable	45.9	33.8	12.2	10.8
Numbness/tingling in hands/feet	42.7	24.0	26.0	9.3
"I don't look like myself"	35.8	25.0	—	12.8
Nausea	35.6	18.8	9.4	8.1
Difficulty concentrating	34.7	16.0	7.3	11.3
Feeling bloated	34.7	26.0	17.3	8.7
Constipation	28.6	20.4	—	11.6
Lack of appetite	28.4	20.4	14.2	8.2
Change in the way food tastes	25.7	16.2	—	8.1
Hair loss	26.4	15.0	—	9.5
Cough	25.3	11.3	6.0	4.0
Itching	22.3	11.5	8.1	3.4
Diarrhea	20.8	10.1	6.0	4.0
Swelling of arms or legs	18.9	12.2	—	8.8
Shortness of breath	18.7	10.0	7.3	6.0
Weight loss	18.5	4.8	—	3.4
Problems with sexual interest or activity	17.6	14.9	10.9	6.8
Dizziness	16.2	5.4	2.7	2.7
Vomiting	13.3	8.7	3.3	6.0
Mouth sores	8.1	4.7	1.4	2.0
Nightmares	8.0	5.3	2.0	2.0
Problems with urination	7.3	5.3	4.0	3.3
Urinary accidents	7.4	4.1	0.7	1.4
Difficulty swallowing	5.4	3.4	2.7	2.0

[a]Percentage of sample describing the symptom as "moderate," "severe," or "very severe."
[b]Percentage of sample describing the frequency of the symptom as "frequently" or "almost constantly."
[c]Percentage of sample describing the distress associated with the symptom as "quite a bit" or "very much."
Source: Reprinted with permission from Portenoy RK, Kornblith AB, Wong G, et al. Pain in ovarian cancer: prevalence, characteristics, and associated symptoms. *Cancer* 1994;74:907–915.

National medical organizations have developed guidelines in an effort to more effectively detect and monitor pain. The Joint Commission on Accreditation of Healthcare Organizations developed a standard requiring that pain be assessed initially and periodically in all hospitalized patients. The National Comprehensive Cancer Network 2007 Adult Cancer Pain Guidelines require a formal pain assessment, measurement of pain intensity, reassessment of pain intensity at specific intervals, psychosocial support, and specific educational material (23).

Definition of Pain

According to the International Association for the Study of Pain, pain is "an unpleasant sensory and emotional experience associated with actual or potential tissue damage, or described in terms of such damage" (24). Reported pain may be perceived by the clinician to be greater than or less than the observable degree of tissue injury. In the cancer population, a physical process capable of explaining the pain can usually be identified, but this does not obviate the need for a careful assessment of other factors, including psychologic disturbances, that could be influencing the intensity of the pain or contributing to pain-related distress.

The definition of pain can be further clarified by the distinctions among nociception, pain, and suffering (Fig. 32.1) (25). Nociception is the activity produced in the afferent nervous system by potentially tissue-damaging stimuli. Clinically, nociception is inferred to exist whenever tissue damage is identified. Pain is the perception of nociception and, like other perceptions, can be determined by more than the activity in the sensorineural apparatus alone. Although tissue damage related to the tumor or its treatment is common in those with cancer pain, a careful assessment is needed to infer the degree to which the pain report is consistent with the nociception presumed by the clinician on the basis of the physical findings. In all cases, factors other than nociception, including neuropathic processes that can sustain pain in the absence of ongoing

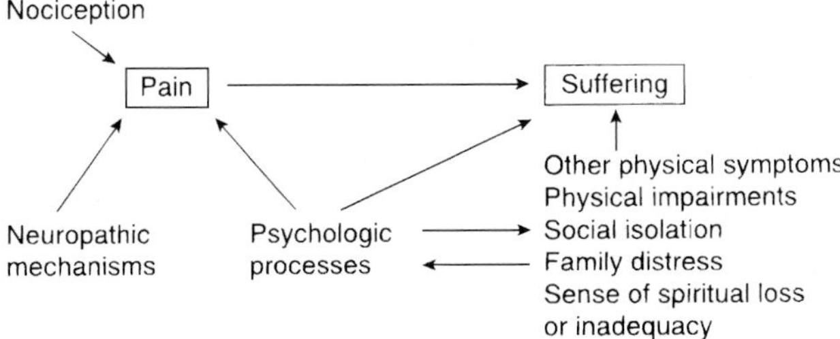

FIGURE 32.1. Distinctions and interactions between nociception, pain, and suffering. *Source:* Reproduced with permission from Portenoy RK. Cancer pain: pathophysiology and syndromes. *Lancet* 1992;339:1026–1031.

tissue injury (see below) and psychologic disturbances, must be evaluated as other potential determinants of the pain. The failure to address these other factors while targeting therapy at the sources of nociception can lead to a poor outcome in which the focus of tissue damage is ameliorated but the pain continues.

Suffering, or "total pain," can be defined as a more global aversive experience determined by numerous perceptions, one of which may be pain (see below). Among the many other factors that may contribute to suffering are the perception of physical deterioration, the experience of symptoms other than pain, psychologic disturbances (e.g., depression or anxiety), disruption in the family, social isolation, and fear of death. Just as an inordinate focus on nociception, rather than pain, can lead to interventions that reduce tissue damage without alleviating symptoms, an emphasis on pain management alone in patients with profound suffering determined by other factors can fail to influence favorably the overall quality of life even if physical comfort is enhanced (26,27).

Evaluation of the Pain Complaint

The comprehensive assessment of pain should include information about temporal characteristics (onset and duration), course (stable or changing since onset, relatively constant or widely fluctuating), severity (both average and worst), location, quality, and provocative and palliative factors. This evaluation is complemented by information about the patient's extent of disease, related medical and psychosocial conditions, present and past pain management strategies and their outcomes, the impact of the pain on the patient's daily life and functioning, as well as the patient's and family's knowledge of, expectations about, and goals for pain management. Risk factors for the undertreatment of the patient's cancer pain and risk factors for serious physical or psychiatric comorbidities (such as drug abuse) should also be examined.

Characteristics of Pain

Intensity. The measurement and recording of pain intensity is an essential element in the comprehensive assessment of pain. Although more information than intensity alone is needed to understand and manage cancer pain, a systematic method for assessing intensity is foundational. The most common approaches are a verbal rating scale (none, mild, moderate, severe, excruciating) and/or an 11-point numeric scale (where 0 is no pain and 10 is the worst pain imaginable). A visual analog scale (VAS) that uses a 10-cm line anchored at one end by the words "no pain" or "least possible pain" and at the other end by "worst possible pain" is another simple and valid approach to pain measurement. The choice of scale is less important than consistency in its use over time. Brief assessment tools modeled on this approach also can be applied to the intensity measurement of nonpain symptoms, such as depression and fatigue.

Multidimensional scales are available, but usually are utilized in research settings. These scales provide a more comprehensive measure of the pain experience, often encompassing such factors as function and quality of life.

Temporal. Acute pain usually has a well-defined onset and a readily identifiable cause (e.g., surgical incision). It may be associated with anxiety, overt pain behaviors (moaning or grimacing), and signs of sympathetic hyperactivity (including tachycardia, hypertension, and diaphoresis). In contrast, chronic pain is characterized by an ill-defined onset and a prolonged, fluctuating course. Overt pain behaviors and sympathetic hyperactivity are typically absent, and vegetative signs, including lassitude, sleep disturbance, and anorexia, may be present. A clinical depression evolves in some patients. Most patients with chronic cancer pain also experience periodic flares of pain, or "breakthrough pain," an observation with important therapeutic implications (see below).

Topographic. The distinctions among focal, multifocal, and generalized pains may influence both the assessment and treatment of the patient. Some therapies, such as nerve blocks and cordotomy, depend on the specific location and extent of the pain.

The distinction between focal and referred pain is similarly important. Focal pains are experienced superficial to the underlying nociceptive lesion, whereas referred pains are experienced at a site distant from the nociceptive lesion.

Pain may be referred from a lesion involving any of a large group of structures, including nerve, bone, muscle, or other soft tissue, and viscera (28–30). Various subtypes can be distinguished: (a) pain referred anywhere along the course of an injured peripheral nerve (such as pain in the thigh or knee from a lumbar plexus lesion); (b) pain referred along a course of the nerve supplied by a damaged nerve root (known as radicular pain); (c) pain referred to the lower part of the body, usually the feet and legs, from a lesion involving the spinal cord (called funicular pain); and (d) pain referred to a site remote from the nociceptive lesion and outside the dermatome affected by the lesion (e.g., shoulder pain from diaphragmatic irritation).

Knowledge of pain referral patterns is needed in order to target appropriate assessment procedures. For example, a patient with recurrent cervical cancer who reports progressive pain in the inguinal region may require evaluation of numerous structures to identify the underlying nociceptive lesion, including the subjacent pelvic bones and hip joint, pelvic sidewall, paraspinal gutter at an upper lumbar spinal level, and intraspinal region at the upper lumbar level.

Etiology

The etiology of acute pain is usually clear-cut. Further evaluation to determine the underlying lesion or pathophysiology of the pain is not indicated unless the course varies from the expected. In contrast, the etiology of chronic cancer-related pain may be more difficult to characterize. In most cases, pain is due to direct invasion of pain-sensitive structures by the neoplasm (24,25,31). The structures most often involved are bone and neural tissue, but pain can also occur when there is an obstruction of hollow viscus, distention of organ capsules, distortion or occlusion of blood vessels, and infiltration of soft tissues. The etiology of pain in less than a quarter of patients relates to an antineoplastic treatment, and less than 10% have pain unrelated to the neoplasm or its treatment (31).

These data suggest that a careful evaluation of cancer patients with pain is likely to identify an underlying nociceptive lesion, which will usually be neoplastic. A survey of patients referred to a pain service in a major cancer hospital noted that previously unsuspected lesions were identified in 63% of patients (32). This outcome altered the known extent of disease in virtually all patients, changed the prognosis for some, and provided an opportunity for a primary antineoplastic therapy in approximately 15%.

Pathophysiology

Pain is labeled nociceptive if it is inferred that the sustaining mechanisms involve ongoing tissue injury. This injury can involve either somatic or visceral structures. The quality of somatic nociceptive pain is typically described as aching, stabbing, throbbing, or pressure-like. The quality of visceral nociceptive pain is largely determined by the structures involved. Obstruction of hollow viscus is usually associated with complaints of gnawing or crampy pain, whereas injury to organ capsules or mesentery is associated with an aching or stabbing discomfort.

Pain is labeled neuropathic if the evaluation suggests that it is sustained by abnormal somatosensory processing in the peripheral or the central nervous system (CNS). Neuropathic mechanisms are involved in approximately 40% of cancer pain syndromes and can be disease related (e.g., tumor invasion of nerve plexus) or treatment related (e.g., postmastectomy syndrome, chemotherapy-induced painful polyneuropathy) (31). Among those with metastatic disease, neuropathic pain usually results from neoplastic injury to peripheral nerves (peripheral neuropathic pain). Other, less common subtypes include (a) those in which the focus of activity is in the CNS (sometimes generically termed deafferentation pain); and (b) those in which the pain is believed to be maintained by efferent activity in the sympathetic nervous system (so-called sympathetically maintained pain). Identification of a neuropathic mechanism is extremely important in clinical management because several specific therapies may be useful for these conditions (see below).

Neuropathic pain is diagnosed on the basis of the patient's verbal description of the pain and typically supported by evidence of nerve injury. Patients may use any of a variety of verbal descriptors but some, such as "burning," "shock-like," or "electrical," are particularly suggestive of neuropathic pain (33,34). Areas of abnormal sensations are often found on physical examination. These may include hypesthesia (a numbness or lessening of feeling), paresthesias (abnormal nonpainful sensations such as tingling, cold, or itching), hyperalgesia (increased perception of painful stimuli), hyperpathia (exaggerated pain response), and allodynia (pain induced by nonpainful stimuli such as a light touch or cool air).

Although pain can occur as a primary outcome of psychologic processes, a somatoform disorder, this appears to be rare in the cancer population. Nonetheless, psychologic factors may augment or alter the pain complaint, and not surprisingly, pain may be associated with fluctuations in psychologic distress. In one series of 203 inpatients with cancer, for example, depression was independently associated with pain intensity after controlling for performance status, disease status, and perceived treatment effect (35).

To assess the complex relationship between pain and psychiatric disease, it is useful to have familiarity with the common disorders that are present in gynecologic malignancies. One study observed major depression in nearly one quarter of women hospitalized with cervical, endometrial, and vaginal cancer (36), and another reported more severe depression and poorer body image among gynecologic patients than those with breast cancer undergoing mastectomy (37).

If the assessment of the pain does not provide enough information to categorize it as primarily nociceptive or neuropathic, or mixed, or yield a sufficient understanding of the psychologic factors that may be influencing the pain, it is important to acknowledge this lack of certainty and avoid labeling the patient with a term that may inappropriately direct care. The greatest concern in this regard is the labeling of pain as psychogenic when the assessment does not yield positive evidence of a psychiatric disorder but an alternative answer is lacking. In this case, it is best to label the pain idiopathic than to speculate about underlying factors that are not clearly demonstrable from the evaluation.

Pain Syndromes

Efforts to improve the assessment of cancer pain have been greatly encouraged by the description of numerous pain syndromes, each of which is defined by a cluster of symptoms and signs (Table 32.2) (24,25,31,38). Syndrome identification can help direct the diagnostic evaluation, clarify the prognosis, and target therapeutic interventions. Recognition of pain syndromes that occur commonly among patients with gynecologic

TABLE 32.2

CANCER PAIN SYNDROMES

- I. Pain associated with direct tumor involvement
  - A. Due to invasion of bone
    1. Base of skull
    2. Vertebral body
    3. Generalized bone pain
  - B. Due to invasion of nerves
    1. Peripheral nerve syndromes
    2. Painful polyneuropathy
    3. Brachial, lumbar, sacral plexopathies
    4. Leptomeningeal metastases
    5. Epidural spinal cord compression
  - C. Due to invasion of viscera
  - D. Due to invasion of blood vessels
  - E. Due to invasion of mucous membranes
- II. Pain associated with cancer therapy
  - A. Postoperative pain syndromes
    1. Post-thoracotomy syndrome
    2. Postmastectomy syndrome
    3. Postradical neck dissection
    4. Postamputation syndromes
  - B. Postchemotherapy pain syndromes
    1. Painful polyneuropathy
    2. Aseptic necrosis of bone
    3. Steroid pseudorheumatism
    4. Mucositis
  - C. Postirradiation pain syndromes
    1. Radiation fibrosis of brachial or lumbosacral plexus
    2. Radiation myelopathy
    3. Radiation-induced peripheral nerve tumors
    4. Mucositis
- III. Pain indirectly related or unrelated to cancer
  - A. Myofascial pains
  - B. Postherpetic neuralgia
  - C. Chronic headache syndromes

TABLE 32.3

PAIN SYNDROMES COMMONLY ENCOUNTERED AMONG PATIENTS WITH GYNECOLOGIC CANCER

ACUTE PAIN SYNDROMES
At any stage of disease:
- Postoperative pain
- Mucositis

In advanced stages of disease:
- Recurrent bowel obstruction
- Ureteral obstruction
- Movement-related pain in brachial/lumbosacral plexopathy
- Movement-related pain from bony lesions

CANCER-RELATED CHRONIC PAIN SYNDROMES
- Brachial/lumbosacral plexopathy
- Chronic abdominal pain: bowel obstruction, ascites, hepatomegaly
- Tenesmoid pain
- Bone pain from metastases

TREATMENT-RELATED CHRONIC PAIN SYNDROMES
- Postmastectomy syndrome
- Radiation-induced plexopathy
- Chemotherapy-induced peripheral neuropathy (paclitaxel, cisplatin)

cancers (Table 32.3) can also facilitate the assessment of these patients.

Comprehensive Assessment

A comprehensive assessment that incorporates this pain-related information can be used to elaborate a problem list that guides the priorities and direction of therapy. In many situations, such as acute postoperative pain or chronic pain related to a well-characterized lesion (e.g., pathologic fracture), the assessment issues are simple and the problem list is brief and straightforward. In other cases, most often in populations with advanced disease, a complex group of symptoms, medical disorders, and psychosocial disturbances greatly complicate the assessment process. In these cases, a comprehensive assessment encourages efficient selection of an appropriate multimodal therapy.

The biopsychosocial model implied by this clinical reality also has provided a framework for pain research. Reflecting this, a consensus has been reached that the core outcome domains for studies of chronic pain are pain intensity, physical functioning, emotional functioning, participant ratings of improvement and satisfaction with treatment, and other symptoms and adverse events (39).

Patients whose pain had been responsive to pain medication but experience an increase in pain intensity or a change in pain characteristics should be comprehensively reassessed as the initial step in management. The goal is to determine whether specific contributing factors can be identified. Relapse or disease progression, for example, may be amenable to primary therapeutic strategies, such as chemotherapy to address disease progression associated with loss of analgesic effectiveness. Other factors such as cord compression, systemic or local infection, and psychologic distress (e.g., depression) also may be treatable.

MANAGEMENT OF ACUTE PAIN

Although the treatment of patients with acute pain, particularly postoperative pain, is typically less challenging than the long-term management of chronic pain, the outcomes achieved in routine practice settings are often inadequate. Given the potential efficacy of widely used strategies such as patient-controlled analgesia (PCA), problematic outcomes may be more related to systems issues, such as access to a pain service, prolonged pharmacy preparation times, or other factors, rather than purely clinical issues. Cancer patients may have concurrent medical problems, psychologic disturbances, and prior drug exposure that increase the heterogeneity of the population and diminish the likelihood that routine measures will provide adequate relief of pain. The need for clinicians and administrators to attend to the problem of acute pain and provide the resources and systems for expert management is therefore particularly important in this population.

"Routine" Approach to Postoperative Pain

Despite great variability in the pharmacokinetics and pharmacodynamics of single opioid doses (40), and the large proportion of patients who fail to attain adequate analgesia with routine postoperative care, many patients do respond adequately to an opioid, traditionally morphine or meperidine, administered "as needed." In the cancer population, the starting dose must take into account the prior opioid exposure of the patient. A reasonable starting dose is the equivalent of 5% to 10% of the total opioid consumption during the previous 24 hours. If the drug or route of administration is changed, an equianalgesic dose table must be consulted to calculate the equivalent total daily dose of the new drug. Once a dose is selected, it can be initially administered every 2 to 3 hours as needed.

As-needed dosing of this type may be considered when a procedure is likely to yield no more than moderate pain for a short while. In these cases, the use of an opioid with a short half-life, such as morphine or hydromorphone, is preferred and use of the intravenous route through slow injection or brief infusion will reduce distress associated with painful injections. Meperidine, although likely to be safe during brief therapy, is generally not preferred because of the availability of safer drugs (see below).

The proportion of cancer patients with postoperative pain who will be undertreated by an as-needed dosing schedule can be diminished if several factors are recognized. The variability in analgesic requirements may require changes in the starting dose, adjustment in the dosing interval during the immediate postoperative period, or both. Some patients require several dose adjustments. Similarly, variability in pain duration after any particular operation is great and the duration of opioid treatment must be flexible and be determined solely by patient response. Some patients have concerns about opioid-induced side effects and addiction, which may augment distress and diminish patient compliance with therapy unless strong reassurance is provided by the physician and other staff.

In some populations, the routine approach to postoperative pain management can be enhanced by the use of a nonopioid analgesic, specifically a nonsteroidal anti-inflammatory drug (NSAID). In the United States, ketorolac has been approved for short-term parenteral use. In opioid-naïve patients, a standard dose of ketorolac can provide analgesia equivalent to a parenteral dose of morphine of 10 mg (41). The addition of intravenous ketoprofen (not approved in the United States) to intravenous PCA with tramadol after major gynecologic cancer surgery also significantly reduced opioid consumption (42). At the present time in the United States, patients who are highly predisposed to opioid side effects or toxicity, such as those with severe preexisting lung disease, may benefit from a trial of ketorolac either in lieu of opioid therapy or in combination with an opioid. Ketorolac should not be used when NSAID treatment is contraindicated.

Patient-Controlled Analgesia

PCA has achieved great popularity in the management of postoperative pain and there is strong evidence that it improves analgesia, decreases the risk of pulmonary complications, and increases patient satisfaction when compared with conventional opioid analgesia (43). Theoretically, the self-administration of small doses on a frequent basis allows the patient to tailor the dose to the pain and enhance a sense of personal control while achieving a more stable plasma drug concentration. However, not all studies of this modality have been positive. For example, a randomized, controlled trial of 227 gynecologic cancer patients undergoing intra-abdominal surgery found that patients who were switched from parenteral to oral morphine on the first postoperative day experienced the same degree of pain control as those who received parenteral morphine via PCA pump (44). The latter studies suggest that careful attention to dosing rather than the availability of a pump per se is the key factor in achieving adequate pain control.

Other Approaches to Acute Pain Management

Numerous alternative approaches to postoperative pain management have been explored. Some require the expertise of pain specialists.

Preemptive Analgesia

The administration of an analgesic prior to surgical tissue injury may reduce postoperative pain and opioid requirements, and possibly have longer-term benefits (45). There are conflicting data, however, and the influence of type of analgesia, timing, and range of outcomes has not been elucidated. The role of this strategy in gynecologic surgery is unclear and it is not generally pursued.

Oral Pretreatment and Postoperative Combination Therapy

Pretreatment with sustained-release morphine reduces postoperative pain and analgesia requirements (46,47). This technique is seldom used but may be an option in patients whose postoperative pain management is expected to be problematic.

Presurgical or postsurgical addition of an NSAID in combination with an opioid can augment analgesia and reduce the use of opioids, potentially leading to reduction of opioid side effects. A recent controlled trial, for example, demonstrated that postoperative celecoxib improved outcomes and was well tolerated in patients undergoing laparascopic surgery (48). Equally important, there is now substantial data demonstrating that the combination of gabapentin, a neuronal calcium channel modulator widely used for the treatment of chronic neuropathic pain, with an opioid improves a range of outcomes in diverse surgeries, including hysterectomy (49).

Intraspinal Analgesia

Epidural analgesia is now common practice in many hospitals. There is strong evidence that analgesia is better with this approach than with parenteral opioids (50–53). There may also be a lower risk of some postoperative complications (54,55). Some studies suggest benefits that are prolonged into the recovery phase after surgery, but the extant data are insufficient to judge these benefits adequately (51). Some side effects are more likely with this technique than with conventional systemic opioid therapy, including pruritus and hypotension, and resources, including staff with special competencies, are needed to implement the approach safely.

Given the abundant evidence of better analgesia and related outcomes, patients undergoing major gynecologic surgery should be considered for epidural analgesia if the resources exist to provide it. Although there is less clinical experience in the use of subarachnoid opioid administration for postoperative pain, the technique can also provide excellent relief (56–58).

Regional Anesthetic Techniques

There are numerous regional anesthetic techniques that may be useful for the management of acute pain. The simplest is the application of local anesthetic at the surgical site. Topical anesthetics that are longer acting are in development and may offer substantial benefits in the future.

Neural blockade capable of denervating the painful site is a potential approach in most cases. Catheters that deliver local anesthetic at a dose high enough to produce a sensory block can be placed in the epidural space or along peripheral nerves or plexus. Regional anesthesia can be used during an operation and then continued into the postoperative setting for pain control. For example, a recent study demonstrated that subarachnoid block for vaginal hysterectomy yielded significantly better immediate postoperative analgesia versus standard general anesthesia (59).

Other Approaches

Transcutaneous electrical nerve stimulation (TENS) has been suggested to be a useful modality for incisional pain after abdominal surgery (60). Despite the evident simplicity and safety of the approach, there has been little application of its potential.

Cognitive approaches, including stress reduction, relaxation, hypnosis, and distraction techniques, have also reduced postoperative pain and analgesic requirements (61,62). These techniques are labor intensive and are almost never sufficient as the sole means of analgesia. Nonetheless, studies have established that higher levels of anxiety and depression can negatively influence postoperative pain and analgesic requirements (63), and efforts to reduce anxiety through preoperative education and postoperative psychologic interventions are likely to have salutary effects.

MANAGEMENT OF CHRONIC CANCER PAIN

The successful management of acute postoperative pain is an important concern of the gynecologic oncologist, and satisfactory pain relief should be considered a norm of practice. The treatment of chronic pain is a far more challenging problem, particularly among those with advanced illness.

Cancer Pain, Symptom Distress, and Palliative Care

Most cancer patients who experience chronic pain also develop other physical and psychologic symptoms. Pain, fatigue, and psychologic distress are the most prevalent symptoms across populations (64,65). A broad assessment of symptom distress, followed by concurrent therapy of the most problematic symptoms other than pain, is a fundamental aspect of pain management.

Symptom distress, in turn, is only one aspect of the multifaceted problem of suffering (26,27,66). The assessment of suffering requires an evaluation in multiple domains, including the physical, psychologic, social, and spiritual. This in turn requires open and ongoing communication between the clinician and the patient.

The assessment and management of problems that relate to the broad constructs of suffering and quality of life are part of the therapeutic model of palliative care, which focuses on patients with progressive incurable illness and their families. This therapeutic approach aims to enhance the quality of life of the patient and family throughout the course of the disease. In the United States, palliative care is rapidly evolving. Specialist care now has a well-defined purview, as codified in a consensus document published by the National Consensus Project for Quality Palliative Care (67). The American Board of Medical Specialties approved Hospice and Palliative Medicine as a formal subspecialty, and in an unprecedented event, ten separate primary boards are co-sponsoring, including the American Board of Obstetrics and Gynecology. Specialist care is now being provided by institution-based palliative care programs, which now exist in approximately 40% of U.S. hospitals, and through hospice programs.

The evolution of specialist-level palliative care highlights the paradigm of generalist-level palliative care. The effort to provide optimal palliative care should be considered to be one aspect of oncology best practice. Physicians who are caring for patients with serious illness such as cancer must understand the necessity of palliative care from the time of diagnosis onward. They must acknowledge the multidimensional nature of this endeavor, including a focus on communicating well, setting goals, coordinating care, sharing decision making, promoting advance care planning, managing symptoms, providing psychosocial and spiritual support, addressing practical needs in the home, assisting the family as needed, and dealing with the challenges of end-of-life care when this is necessary. Referral to specialist services to address complex needs, or provide hospice home care services, is central to the role of the generalist.

General Principles of Pain Management

The development of a successful strategy for pain management must consider the etiology and pathophysiology of pain, the patient's medical status, and the goals of care. Although the main approach for the management of cancer pain is opioid-based pharmacotherapy, other interventions, including disease-oriented treatments (e.g., surgery, chemotherapy, or radiation) or other analgesic techniques, may be appropriate in selected cases.

Role of Primary Therapies

Effective treatment of the pathology underlying the pain can be analgesic (68,69). Primary treatment includes antineoplastic therapies and interventions directed at specific structural pathologies (e.g., lysis of adhesions). There is evidence in a limited number of cancers that specific chemotherapy regimens yield analgesic effects and it is a common observation that patients who attain a partial or complete response also experience improved symptoms. In a study of patients with metastatic breast cancer, for example, palliative chemotherapy with doxorubicin with or without vinorelbine resulted in an improvement of pain in 60.4% of the 111 patients who suffered from pain at baseline (70); although patients with an objective tumor response were more likely to have an improvement in pain (84.9%), fully 61% of patients with stable disease also benefited. In a small study of patients with advanced ovarian cancer, palliative chemotherapy was associated with improvement in symptom control, emotional well-being, and global quality of life (71). In a study of patients with recurrent/advanced cervical cancer, 67% of patients experienced improvement of pain after alternating treatment with PBM (platinum, bleomycin, and methotrexate) and PFU (platinum and 5-fluorouracil [5-FU]) (72).

TABLE 32.4

APPROACHES USED IN THE MANAGEMENT OF CHRONIC CANCER PAIN

Primary therapies
Radiation therapy
Chemotherapy
Surgery
Antibiotics
Primary analgesic therapies
Pharmacologic approaches
Interventional approaches
Physiatric approaches
Neurostimulatory approaches
Psychologic approaches
Complementary and alternative medicine approaches

Radiation therapy commonly is used to manage pain and there is evidence that it can provide effective and durable palliation of pain and other symptoms in chemotherapy-refractory patients with ovarian cancer (73,74) and cervical cancer (75). Radiation therapy can also provide analgesia to as many as 80% of those treated for bone metastases (76). Patients with widespread bone metastasis or bone pain refractory to local field radiotherapy may benefit from treatment with radiopharmaceuticals, such as strontium 89 or samarium-153 (77). In addition, analgesia may be an expected result when radiation is used to treat epidural disease, tumor ulceration, cerebral metastases, superior vena cava obstruction, and bronchial obstruction.

Unfortunately, many patients with chronic cancer pain have no option for primary antineoplastic therapy or did not achieve symptomatic relief from these interventions. The approach to these patients involves a diverse group of primary analgesic treatments (Table 32.4). Several concurrent interventions are often required to manage the pain. The benefits of analgesic therapies must be balanced against the side effects they produce in a way that optimizes the outcome for the patient. Repeated assessments, performed as part of a broader approach to palliative care, are essential in this process and often lead to adjustments in the therapy.

THERAPEUTIC APPROACHES: PHARMACOLOGIC MANAGEMENT

Prospective trials indicate that more than 70% of patients can achieve adequate relief of cancer pain using a pharmacologic approach (3,12–14). Effective pain management requires

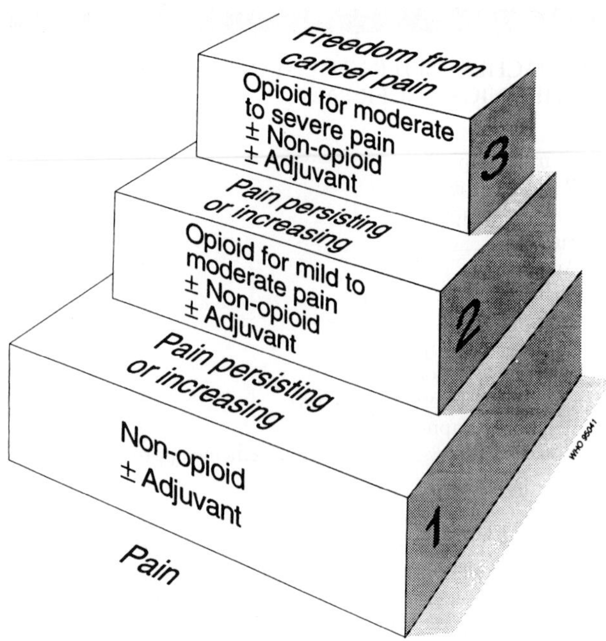

FIGURE 32.2. The three-step "analgesic ladder" proposed by an expert committee of the Cancer Unit of the World Health Organization. *Source:* Reproduced with permission from the World Health Organization. *Cancer Pain Relief.* 2nd ed. Geneva: World Health Organization; 1996.

expertise in the administration of three groups of analgesic medications: NSAIDs, opioid analgesics, and adjuvant analgesics. The term *adjuvant analgesic* is applied to a diverse group of drugs that have primary indications other than pain but can be effective analgesics in specific circumstances, such as in the treatment of neuropathic pain.

A model approach to the selection of these drugs, known as the "analgesic ladder," has been developed by the World Health Organization (WHO) (Fig. 32.2) (3). According to this approach, patients with mild to moderate cancer-related pain are first treated with acetaminophen (paracetamol) or an NSAID. This drug is combined with an adjuvant drug that can be selected either to provide additional analgesia (i.e., an adjuvant analgesic) or to treat a side effect of the analgesic or a coexisting symptom. Patients who present with moderate to severe pain, or who do not achieve adequate relief after a trial of an NSAID, should be treated with an opioid conventionally used to treat pain of this intensity (previously designated a "weak" opioid), which is typically combined with an NSAID and may be administered with an adjuvant if there is an indication for one. Those who present with severe pain or who do not achieve adequate relief following appropriate administration of drugs on the second rung of the analgesic ladder should receive an opioid conventionally used for severe pain (previously called a "strong" opioid), which may be combined with an NSAID or an adjuvant drug as indicated.

The analgesic ladder is important historically and is still widely cited in the developing world in an effort to encourage policy makers to expand medical access to opioid drugs. It is a limited clinical guideline in most developed countries, where access to numerous opioid formulations and other analgesic modalities has influenced clinical practice. Nonetheless, the concept promoted by the analgesic ladder model—opioid therapy on a long-term basis should be considered the mainstay for the therapy of chronic moderate to severe cancer-related pain—remains widely accepted and a very important message of the original paradigm.

Nonsteroidal Anti-inflammatory Drugs

In the United States, the nonopioid analgesics comprise acetaminophen and the NSAIDs (Table 32.5). These drugs have a well-established role in the treatment of cancer pain (78–81). Based on clinical observations, NSAIDs appear to be especially useful in patients with bone pain or pain related to grossly inflammatory lesions, and relatively less useful in patients with neuropathic pain (82). In addition, NSAIDs have an opioid-sparing effect that may be helpful to prevent the occurrence of dose-related side effects (83,84).

NSAIDs inhibit the enzyme cyclo-oxygenase (COX) to reduce production of peripheral and central prostaglandins, and this action presumably underlies their analgesic effects. There are two forms of COX, a constitutive form (COX-1) and an inducible form (COX-2). Compounds that are relatively more selective for COX-2 than COX-1 have a lower risk of inducing gastrointestinal adverse effects (85,86), and some drugs that are relatively COX-2 selective have been labeled in this way and promoted for their enhanced gastrointestinal safety. In the United States, the only drug of the latter type now on the market is celecoxib. Rofecoxib and valdecoxib were previously available, but were taken off the market due to concerns related to cardiovascular safety.

The cardiovascular safety of the NSAIDs, including the newer COX-2 selective drugs, has been under intense review. Based on numerous studies, it is most reasonable to conclude that an increased risk of peripheral vascular disease, myocardial infarction, transient ischemic attacks, and stroke occurs during treatment with any of the NSAIDs (87,88). Mechanistically, this risk is associated with COX-2 inhibition, whether produced by the nonselective COX-1 and COX-2 inhibitors or by the COX-2 selective drugs. Although the risk varies across drugs, large comparative studies have been retrospective and results have been conflicting.

NSAIDs should be administered with caution to patients with significant risk factors for peptic ulcer disease, renal disease, cardiovascular disease, or bleeding diathesis. For patients who are predisposed to ulcer disease or would have difficulty tolerating a gastrointestinal hemorrhage, the increased safety of the COX-2 selective drugs—celecoxib in the United States—is likely to be an advantage. Coadministration of a proton pump inhibitor, such as omeprazole or misoprostol, also should be considered to reduce the risk of gastrointestinal damage induced by NSAIDs (89).

Selective COX-2 inhibitors and nonselective NSAIDs seem to be equally nephrotoxic and, therefore, should be used with the same caution. The safest nonopioid to use in patients with existing renal disease is acetaminophen, notwithstanding some data that suggest that this drug can also produce renal toxicity (90).

Other factors may also be important in the selection of an NSAID. First, there is substantial variability in the response of individual patients to different agents, and the response to an NSAID in the past should guide drug selection in the present. Second, it may be useful to consider the drug's duration of effect when selecting an NSAID. The need to improve treatment adherence or provide a simpler dosing regimen encourages the use of a drug that can be administered once daily (e.g., nabumetone) or twice daily (e.g., celecoxib and many others), whereas the desire for as-needed dosing suggests the use of a short-duration drug (e.g., ibuprofen). Finally, drug selection may be influenced by cost, which varies greatly among both drugs and pharmacies.

The toxicities associated with the use of NSAIDs are dose-related and often occult until severe morbidity occurs. Although patients with cancer pain are commonly treated with standard doses, it is reasonable to explore the dose range and seek the minimal effective dose for long-term therapy. Dose escalation in poor responders is limited by dose-related

TABLE 32.5

NONSTEROIDAL ANTI-INFLAMMATORY DRUGS (NSAIDS)

Class and generic name	Trade name	Approx. half-life (h)	Dosing schedule	Recommended starting dose[a]	Comment[b]
P-AMINOPHENOL DERIVATIVES					
Acetaminophen[c]	Tylenol, Datril, Panadol	3–4	q 4–6 h	650 mg q 4 h (5 doses daily)	Overdosage produces hepatic toxicity. Not anti-inflammatory and therefore not preferred as first-line analgesic or coanalgesic in patients with bone pain. Lack of GI or platelet toxicity; however, may be important in some cancer patients. At high doses, liver function tests should be monitored.
NAPTHYLALKANONES					
Nabumetone	Relafen	22–30	q 24 h	500–1,000 mg q 12 h	Appears to have a relatively low risk of GI toxicity; once-daily dosing can be useful.
SALICYLATES					
Acetylsalicylic acid[c]	Aspirin	3–12[d]	q 4–6 h	650 mg q 4 h (5 doses daily)	Standard for comparison. May not be tolerated as well as some of the newer NSAIDs.
Diflunisal[c]	Dolobid, Dolobis	8–12	q 12 h	1,000 mg × 1, then 500 mg q 12 h	Less GI toxicity than aspirin
Choline magnesium trisalicylate[c]	Trilisate	8–12	q 12 h	500–1,000 mg q 12 h	Choline magnesium trisalicylate and salsalate have minimal GI toxicity and no effect on platelet aggregation despite anti-inflammatory effects. May therefore be particularly useful in some cancer patients.
Salsalate	Disalacid	8–12	q 12 h	500–1,000 mg q 12 h	
PROPRIONIC ACIDS					
Ibuprofen[c]	Motrin, Advil, Nuprin	3–4	q 4–8 h	400–600 mg q 8 h	Available over-the-counter.
Naproxen[c]	Naprosyn	13	q 12 h	250–500 mg q 12 h	Available as a suspension.
Naproxen sodium[c]	Aleve, Anaprox, Naprelan	13	q 12 h	275–550 mg q 12 h	—
Fenoprofen	Nalfon, Fenopron, Progesic	2–3	q 6 h	200 mg q 6 h	—
Ketoprofen	Orudis, Oruvail	2–3	q 6–8 h	25–50 mg q 8 h	—
Flurbiprofen[c]	Ansaid	5–6	q 8–12 h	100 mg q 12 h	—
Oxaprozin	Daypro	40	q 24 h	600 mg q 24 h	Once-daily dosing may be useful.
ACETIC ACIDS					
Indomethacin	Indocin, Indocid	4–5	q 8–12 h	25 mg q 8 h	Available in sustained-release and rectal formulations. Higher incidence of side effects, particularly GI and CNS, than proprionic acids.
Tolmetin	Tolectin	1	q 6–8 h	200 mg q 8 h	
Sulindac	Clinoril	14	q 12 h	150 mg q 12 h	Less renal toxicity than other NSAIDs.
Diclofenac	Voltaren	2	q 6–8 h	25 mg q 8 h	
Ketorolac[c]	Toradol	4–7	q 4–6 h	30–60 mg load, then 15–30 mg q 6 h (parenteral); 10 mg q 6 h (oral)	Only parenteral formulation available. Approved for postoperative use. Experience too limited to evaluate higher doses.

(continued)

TABLE 32.5

NONSTEROIDAL ANTI-INFLAMMATORY DRUGS (NSAIDS) (CONTINUED)

Class and generic name	Trade name	Approx. half-life (h)	Dosing schedule	Recommended starting dose[a]	Comment[b]
OXICAMS					
Piroxicam	Feldene	45	q 24 h	20 mg q 24 h	Administration of 40 mg for over 3 weeks is associated with a high incidence of peptic ulcer, particularly in the elderly.
FENAMATES					
Mefenamic acid[c]	Ponstel, Ponstan	2	q 6 h	250 mg q 6 h	Not recommended for use longer than 1 week and, therefore, not indicated in cancer pain therapy.
PYRAZOLES					
Phenylbutazone	Antadol, Butazolidin	50–100	q 68 h	100 mg q 8 h	Not a first-line drug owing to risk of serious bone marrow toxicity. Not preferred for cancer pain therapy.
COX-2 INHIBITORS					
Celecoxib	Celebrex	11	q 12 h	100–200 mg q 12 h	Fewer GI side effects; no effect on platelet function.

Note: CNS, central nervous system; GI, gastrointestinal.
[a]Starting dose should be one-half to two-thirds of the recommended dose for the elderly, those on multiple drugs, and those with renal insufficiency. Doses must be individualized. Low initial doses should be titrated upward if tolerated and clinical effect is inadequate. Doses can be incremented weekly. Studies of NSAIDs in the cancer population are meager; dosing guidelines are thus empiric.
[b]With all NSAIDs, stool guaiac and liver function tests, BUN, creatinine, and urinalysis should be monitored; frequency of monitoring should be increased for those on relatively high doses.
[c]Pain is approved indication.
[d]Half-life of aspirin increases with dose.

toxicities and a ceiling dose for analgesia above which additional dose increments fail to produce more relief. If an increase in dose maintains the therapy in the conventionally accepted safe range and provides more analgesia, it should be continued. The lack of additional pain relief following a dose increase, however, suggests that the ceiling has been reached, and the dose can then be lowered to the previously effective dose or the drug can be discontinued. All patients receiving an NSAID should be evaluated periodically for occult fecal blood, changes in blood pressure, and effects on renal or hepatic function.

Opioid Analgesics

Expertise in the administration of opioid analgesics (Table 32.6) is the foundation of cancer pain management. The clinician should have knowledge of opioid pharmacology and a clear grasp of practical guidelines for dosing (91,92).

Opioid Classes

Based on receptor interactions, the opioid analgesics can be divided broadly into pure agonists and agonist-antagonists. The pure agonist drugs used in the management of chronic cancer pain are agonists at the μ-receptor subtype. The agonist-antagonist drugs comprise a mixed agonist-antagonist subclass, which includes drugs that are weak antagonists at the μ receptor and agonists at another receptor subtype, and a partial agonist subclass, which includes drugs that are partial agonists at the μ receptor. In the United States, the mixed agonist-antagonist drugs include pentazocine, nalbuphine, dezocine, and butorphanol, and the partial agonists include buprenorphine.

All the agonist-antagonist drugs share properties that together suggest a limited role in the management of chronic cancer pain. These drugs have a ceiling dose for analgesia, and all have the potential to produce an abstinence syndrome in patients already physically dependent on an agonist drug. Some of the mixed agonist-antagonists, particularly pentazocine, are also more likely to produce psychotomimetic effects than the pure agonist drugs. In patients with chronic pain, the lack of oral formulations for all but pentazocine and buprenorphine (sublingual formulation) also limits the utility of these drugs.

Agonist drugs, the prototype of which is morphine, are preferred in the management of chronic cancer pain (Table 32.6). To optimize the administration of these drugs, widely accepted dosing guidelines must be applied systematically.

"Weak" Versus "Strong" Opioids. Unlike the division of the opioids into agonist and agonist-antagonist classes, the distinction between "weak" opioids and "strong" opioids, which was originally incorporated into the WHO analgesic ladder approach (3), is more operational than pharmacologic. The so-called weak opioids are now designated as those that are conventionally administered orally for moderate pain in patients with no or limited prior opioid exposure (second rung of the analgesic ladder), and the so-called strong opioids are those that are conventionally used to treat severe pain or moderate to severe pain in patients already using an opioid (third rung of the analgesic ladder). In the United States, the former group comprises codeine, hydrocodone, dihydrocodeine, oxycodone, propoxyphene, and occasionally meperidine. Tramadol, a unique centrally-acting analgesic with a mechanism of action that is partly opioid, also is generally included with this group. The other opioids used conventionally on the third rung of the

TABLE 32.6

OPIOID ANALGESICS

Drug	Dose (mg) equianalgesic to morphine 10 mg IM[a] PO	IM	Half-life (h)	Peak effect (h)	Duration (h)	Comment[b]
Morphine	20–30[c]	10	2–3	0.5–1.0	36	Standard for comparison
Morphine CR	20–30	10	2–3	3–4	8–12	Various formulations are not bioequivalent
Morphine SR	20–30	10	2–3	2–3	12–24	—
Codeine	200	130	2–3	1.5–2.0	3–6	Combined with aspirin or acetaminophen. Usually for moderate pain. Also available without coanalgesic
Hydromorphone	7.5	1.5	2–3	0.5–1.0	2–4	Potency may be greater, i.e., hydromorphone: morphine = 3:1 rather than 6.7:1 during prolonged use
Oxycodone	20	—	2–3	1	3–4	Combined with aspirin or acetaminophen, for moderate pain; available orally without coanalgesic and useful for severe pain
Oxycodone CR	20	—	2–3	2–3	8–12	—
Oxymorphone	10 (rectal)	1	2–3	1.5–3.0	2–4	—
Oxymorphone CR	20 (oral)	—	2–3	1.5–3.0	2–4	—
Methadone	20	10	12–190	0.5–1.5	4–12	Although 1:1 ratio with morphine was in single-dose study, there is a change with chronic dosing and large dose reduction (75%–90%) is needed when switching to methadone. Risk of delayed toxicity
Levorphanol	4	2	12–15	0.5–1	4–6	Usage limited because only 2 mg tablets are available
Fentanyl	—	—	7–12	—	—	Can be administered as a continuous IV infusion or SC infusion; based on clinical experience, 100 μg/h is roughly equianalgesic to morphine 4 mg/h
Fentanyl TTS	—	—	16–24	—	48–72	Based on clinical experience, 100 μg is roughly equianalgesic to morphine 4 mg
Meperidine	300	75	2–3	0.5–1.0	3–4	Not preferred for cancer patients owing to potential toxicity

Note: IM, intramuscular; IV, intravenous; SC, subcutaneous.
[a]Dose that provides analgesia equivalent to 10 mg intramuscular morphine.
[b]All opioids may produce various common side effects, (e.g., constipation, nausea, sedation). Respiratory depression is rare in cancer patients.
[c]Extensive survey data suggest that the relative potency of IM:PO morphine of 1:16 changes to 1:23 with chronic dosing.

analgesic ladder include morphine, hydromorphone, oxymorphone, levorphanol, fentanyl, and methadone.

Among those opioids conventionally used for moderate pain in the United States, codeine and propoxyphene are usually, but not always, combined with a coanalgesic (aspirin or acetaminophen); hydrocodone and dihydrocodeine are only available in combination products; tramadol is available as a single entity and combined with acetaminophen. Oxycodone, which is available both as a single entity and as a combination tablet combined with aspirin or acetaminophen, can be considered to be a drug for the second step of the ladder when used in combination with a coanalgesic and a drug for severe pain when used alone.

The designation of the drugs conventionally used to treat moderate pain as "weak" was a misnomer because none of these drugs is characterized by a ceiling effect that would limit its use. Rather, other considerations have led to the customary use of these opioids at doses limited to those capable of treating moderate pain in the relatively nontolerant patient. For example, the dose of any opioid combined in a single tablet with acetaminophen or aspirin can only be escalated until the dose of the nonopioid coanalgesic reaches a level associated with toxicity. As noted, hydrocodone and dihydrocodeine are available only in such combinations, and most of the other drugs in this group are typically administered in this form.

Propoxyphene and meperidine should not be used at higher doses because of the risk of enhanced toxicity due to accumulation of a metabolite. The metabolite of propoxyphene, norpropoxyphene, has not been a problem at the doses at which the parent compound is used clinically. However, this drug is associated with serious cardiac toxicity in overdose, and for this reason and its limited efficacy in the doses marketed, it is not preferred and rarely used. The metabolite of meperidine, normeperidine, has been observed to produce clinically relevant side effects in the cancer population, including tremulousness, hyperreflexia, myoclonus, and even seizures (93). This risk suggests that meperidine should not be used in the management of cancer pain.

As suggested by the analgesic ladder, the simplest approach to the management of moderate pain in the cancer patient with limited or no prior exposure to opioids begins with a combination product containing a nonopioid drug and an opioid, usually codeine, oxycodone, or hydrocodone. The dose can be increased to maximally safe levels of the coanalgesic; in products containing acetaminophen, this is usually 4 g per day.

Selection of an Opioid

The selection of an opioid for severe cancer pain is similarly empirical. Traditionally, morphine often was considered to be the preferred first-line drug based on worldwide experience, ease of dosing, and the availability of numerous formulations. The intraindividual variability in the response to the different opioids is very substantial, however, and any of the other drugs may yield a better response in the individual patient. This variability also suggests that therapeutic failure with one drug may be followed by remarkable success with another (94).

The predominant metabolic pathway for morphine is glucuronidation to morphine-3-glucuronide (M3G) and morphine-6-glucuronide (M6G), and the accumulation of morphine metabolites may be associated with side effects, such as myoclonus and chronic nausea (95). Renal insufficiency results in accumulation of M3G and M6G (96,97). For this reason, morphine should be administered cautiously to patients with renal insufficiency. The occurrence of morphine toxicity in these patients should be followed by a trial of an alternative opioid, such as hydromorphone or fentanyl. Although the supporting data are limited, morphine is often viewed unfavorably when patients have very poor renal function or are on dialysis or have renal function that is expected to change. In the latter situations, studies are inadequate to generate guidelines that are evidence based, but hydromorphone and fentanyl are often preferred (98). Given concern about the theoretical accumulation of hydromorphone metabolites, some authors recommend against this drug as well (99).

The selection of an opioid for the treatment of severe cancer pain is also influenced by pharmacokinetic factors, the most salient of which is duration of effect. In an effort to improve adherence and convenience, numerous long-acting extended-release formulations of short half-life opioids have been developed. Oral once-daily or twice-daily formulations of morphine, oxycodone, oxymorphone, and hydromorphone are available in the United States or other countries. Transdermal fentanyl provides a dosing interval of 2 to 3 days and is preferred by some patients.

Although both levorphanol and methadone have relatively long half-lives (Table 32.6), patients typically require doses at least every 6 hours to maintain stable effects. Methadone has become an increasingly popular drug for chronic pain, presumably because of its low cost, potential for unexpectedly high potency, and relatively low abuse potential and low likelihood of diversion by individuals with a history of substance use disorder. Clinical experience suggests that rotation to methadone after inadequate treatment with another opioid can indeed produce surprisingly good results, an outcome that has been speculated to be related to the d-isomer in the formulation that is commercially available in most countries; this isomer is not an opioid, but rather blocks another receptor (the N-methyl-D-aspartate receptor, or NMDA) and in this way may potentiate analgesia or reverse some degree of opioid tolerance (100,101).

Methadone is a challenging drug to use, however, and clinicians must understand its unique pharmacology to administer it in a safe manner. Methadone's half-life ranges between 12 and 190 hours, and substantial delayed toxicity has been observed many days after methadone treatment was begun or altered (102). Its potential to have an unexpectedly high potency when substituting for another opioid increases the challenge of dose selection when starting the drug. Finally, observational studies indicate that methadone can prolong the QTc interval (103,104). Although the risk of cardiac toxicity appears very low and there is no consensus concerning electrocardiographic (ECG) monitoring, this risk suggests that a baseline ECG is reasonable in patients with heart disease or concurrent treatment with other cardioactive drugs, and in those whose methadone dose reaches relatively high levels (e.g., above 200 mg per day). Given the increased potential for serious toxicity and the need for prolonged monitoring with methadone, it is reasonable to view this drug as a second-line agent for patients predisposed to opioid side effects, including the elderly and those with major organ dysfunction.

The patient's previous favorable experience with opioid drugs should also be considered when choosing an opioid. The exception to this is meperidine, the toxic metabolite of which may accumulate with repeated dosing. A favorable experience with this drug during short-term administration should not be viewed as predictive of the response to chronic dosing.

Routes of Administration

The oral and transdermal routes are preferred in the management of chronic cancer pain. Alternative routes may be required, however, and the clinician must recognize their indications and be familiar with the accepted approaches. In a survey of patients with advanced cancer, more than half required two or more routes of administration prior to death and almost a quarter required three or more (105).

Transdermal Delivery. The transdermal route of administration is available for the highly lipophilic opioid fentanyl (106). This formulation, which offers a 48- to 72-hour dosing interval, is preferred by some patients and may be associated with relatively less constipation (107). The transdermal route may be very useful for the patient who is unable to swallow or absorb an orally administered opioid; this is particularly appropriate when the underlying pain syndrome is relatively stable. Pains that are rapidly fluctuating and require multiple supplemental doses may be more easily managed using an ambulatory infusion device with a PCA option. Transdermal fentanyl is relatively contraindicated in patients with anticipated episodes of fever; increased ambient temperature changes the delivery characteristics of the patch and fever may be associated with overdose.

Transdermal buprenorphine is efficacious and available in some countries. Although buprenorphine is a partial agonist and has a ceiling dose, and a capacity to induce abstinence if administered to a patient who is already physically dependent on another opioid, a recent observational study suggests that some patients with severe cancer can benefit and make use of this formulation until death (108).

Rectal. Rectal formulations of oxymorphone, hydromorphone, and morphine are available in the United States. There also is anecdotal experience with rectal administration of controlled-release morphine or oxycodone tablets. The rectal route usually is considered for patients who are relatively opioid nontolerant and become temporarily unable to take oral medications. The potency of opioids administered rectally is believed to approximate oral dosing (109), absorption is variable, and relative potency may be higher or lower than expected, depending on a variety of factors, including location of the suppository (low in the rectum, where the blood supply is systemic, or high in the rectum, where blood flows through the portal circulation) and contents of the rectum at the time of dosing.

Transmucosal, Buccal, and Sublingual. Absorption through the oral cavity potentially can occur with any opioid, and those that are lipophilic and relatively potent may be absorbed sufficiently to have clinical use (110). Two different types of oral transmucosal formulations of fentanyl were approved in the United States after having been shown to be safe and efficacious when used as a "rescue" dose for the treatment of breakthrough pain in cancer patients receiving a fixed-schedule opioid (111,112). These formulations appear to have an onset of action faster than orally administered drugs. They were developed for breakthrough pain on this basis. Given the perception that rapid-onset formulations address an unmet clinical need, other formulations are in development. These will deliver fentanyl, or some other opioid, intranasally, sublingually, transbuccally, and via the intrapulmonary route.

In some clinical situations, a trial of an injectable formulation placed under the tongue is reasonable. Although there is considerable experience in the use of sublingual administration of concentrated oral morphine solution during the care of patients at the end of life, this drug is relatively hydrophilic, and is poorly absorbed by this route; it is likely that most of the effects obtained occur following enteral absorption after swallowing.

Intranasal butorphanol is available, but as noted, this opioid is an agonist-antagonist and has characteristics that make it unfavorable for long-term administration to cancer patients. It is rarely used in this setting. A sublingual preparation of buprenorphine is indicated in the United States for the office-based treatment of addiction. Experience in the treatment of pain is very limited.

Continuous Infusion. Patients who are unable to swallow or absorb opioid drugs are candidates for long-term parenteral dosing. Repetitive intramuscular or subcutaneous injections are painful and should be rarely considered. Repetitive intravenous injections may be effective, but they usually require skilled nursing and may be associated with prominent "bolus" effects (toxicity at peak concentration, pain breakthrough at the trough, or both). Repetitive dosing through a "butterfly" needle placed under the skin has been used effectively in end-of-life care and experience suggests that the needle can be in place for a week without the development of local pain or other problems.

Continuous infusion. Eliminates the fluctuations in plasma concentration associated with repetitive bolus injections. Any opioid available in an injectable formulation can be used for continuous infusion. The availability of continuous subcutaneous infusion using ambulatory infusion devices has markedly enhanced the clinical utility of infusion techniques, allowing long-term administration of opioids and other drugs in the home environment (113). A diverse group of pumps that range considerably in features, complexity, and cost are now available, and the clinician often has the option of selecting a pump based on the needs and resources of the patient. PCA can be combined with continuous infusion to address episodic pains. In most cities, skilled nursing organizations can assist in the management of therapy at home.

Intraspinal Opioids. The discovery of opioid receptors in the spinal cord provided the foundation for the development of techniques to deliver opioid analgesics intraspinally. Intraspinal administration can provide selective analgesia (i.e., without the sensory or motor blockade produced by local anesthetics) at doses lower than those required systemically. The strongest indication for a trial of intraspinal opioid administration is the occurrence of intolerable somnolence or confusion in patients who are not experiencing adequate analgesia during systemic opioid treatment of pain.

Many methods of intraspinal opioid administration are now in use (114). The most commonly used include a percutaneous epidural catheter, which is usually tunneled to the anterior abdominal wall and there connected to an ambulatory infusion pump; a totally implanted epidural catheter connected to a subcutaneous portal, which in turn is connected to an ambulatory pump; and an intrathecal catheter connected to a totally implanted continuous infusion device. The preferred drugs for chronic intraspinal infusion are morphine and hydromorphone, but many others are used empirically, and admixtures (e.g., opioid plus local anesthetic or clonidine, or both) are now commonplace.

The use of intraspinal infusion in the management of cancer pain is likely to increase with further evidence of favorable outcomes in the oncology population (115). Implantable pump systems, which are refilled percutaneously, are often chosen for patients with life expectancies of 3 or more months. A controlled trial that compared neuraxial infusion to comprehensive medical management demonstrated that the spinal opioid treatment improved pain, side effects, quality of life, and even survival (116). The potential utility of neuraxial analgesia is also likely to change with the advent of more choices in drug selection.

Based on a systematic review of the literature (117), an expert panel created an algorithm for the progressive use of an array of drugs during intrathecal therapy (118). Therapy is initiated with a single-agent opioid (either morphine or hydromorphone). If adequate pain relief cannot be achieved, a second agent is added, either bupivacaine or clonidine. Clonidine, an $alpha_2$-adrenergic agonist that was shown in a controlled trial to be effective in neuraxial analgesia (119), is one of several classes of nonopioid and nonanesthetic drugs now being used. Ziconotide, a unique calcium-channel blocker, is now available in the United States and has been shown to be effective for cancer pain in controlled trials (120). A 2007 update of the evidence-based algorithm for drug selection during neuraxial infusion is pending publication and incorporates these and other agents. Intraspinal therapy is now often initiated with a combination of drugs in an effort to reduce side effects, such as sensory and motor block, urinary retention, pruritus, and nausea, and potentiate analgesia (121).

Guidelines for the Administration of Opioid Drugs

As noted, all patients who develop moderate to severe persistent pain should be considered for an opioid-based regimen. The opioid-naïve patient usually is offered a short-acting combination product (conventionally used on the analgesic ladder's second rung). It is acceptable, however, to initiate therapy with a long-acting formulation, as long as the dose is appropriate (122). For example, long-acting morphine can be started at a dose of 15 mg twice daily, or 20 to 30 mg once daily, depending on the formulation. Long-acting oxycodone or oxymorphone can be started at doses of 10 mg twice daily or 5 mg twice daily, respectively. Transdermal fentanyl can be initiated at 12 μg/h in opioid-naïve patients. Given the availability of these long-acting formulations in doses appropriate for the opioid-naïve, the decision to start a short-acting or long-acting drug in a patient with new-onset persistent pain is a clinical judgment based on patient preference, convenience, cost and availability, and experience.

If a patient is receiving a short-acting drug, but pain is not controlled, it is conventional practice to switch to a single-entity pure μ agonist (third-rung drug), typically in a long-acting formulation. Starting doses may be slightly higher if the patient has been requiring regular administration of the short-acting drug. On a daily basis, the milligram dose of a long-acting drug is the same as the short-acting formulation of the same drug.

Following selection of a starting dose, dose adjustment is almost always required. Once a favorable balance between analgesia and side effects is obtained, this is usually maintained for a prolonged time unless there is progression in the pain-producing pathology. Although several large surveys have established that patients with stable disease usually demonstrate stable dosing patterns, most patients with cancer pain do not have stable disease. Recurrent pain or the new occurrence of side effects necessitates another period of dose titration. Inadequate adjustment of the dose is probably the most common reason for unsuccessful long-term management of cancer pain.

In all cases, the dose of an opioid should be increased until acceptable analgesia is produced or intolerable and unmanageable side effects supervene. Ceiling doses for the pure agonist opioids have not been identified clinically, and doses can, therefore, become extremely high—equivalent to grams of morphine per day—as upward dose titration proceeds. The absolute dose of the opioid is immaterial as long as the balance between analgesia and side effects remains acceptable for the patient.

In many countries, it is common to coadminister a short-acting opioid on an "as-needed" basis in combination with the fixed schedule regimen of the long-acting drug. Surveys have demonstrated that one-half to two-thirds of patients with cancer pain will experience clinically significant breakthrough pain (123,124), and this approach—known as "rescue" dosing—has become widely accepted as a means to treat it. As described previously, rapid-onset transmucosal formulations have been developed specifically in an effort to improve the management of breakthrough pain, most of which have a time course that is more rapid than the typical time-action profile of an orally administered opioid.

Treatment of common side effects is an essential element in the successful management of opioid therapy (see below). Patients who experience intolerable toxicity despite treatment should be designated as poorly responsive to the specific drug and route, and an alternative strategy for pain control should be implemented (125–127). This may include more sophisticated management of the treatment-limiting side effect, the addition of a pharmacologic or nonpharmacologic analgesic approach that could reduce the opioid requirement, or opioid rotation.

Opioid rotation, or the switching from one drug to another in an effort to improve the outcomes of an opioid regimen, is now widely used, despite guidelines that remain based on experience rather than research (128). Switching requires an appreciation of relative potency, as codified on the equianalgesic dose table (Table 32.6). To switch to another opioid drug or route, the equianalgesic dose table is used to calculate a dose of the new drug that would be theoretically equianalgesic with the old drug or route. With few exceptions, the dosing regimen based on this calculated dose should be reduced by 25% to 50% to account for incomplete cross-tolerance between drugs. A larger reduction, 75% to 90%, is prudent if the new drug is methadone (because of a unique pharmacology in this agent). In contrast, no reduction in the equianalgesic dose is needed if the switch is to transdermal fentanyl (because a reduction is already built into the recommended equianalgesic ratios).

Management of Common Opioid Side Effects

Although there is no maximum dose or ceiling dose for the μ-agonist opioids, the appearance of side effects imposes a practical limit on dose escalation. Given the importance of side effects in determining the response to an opioid, the successful management of common adverse side effects is a fundamental aspect of therapy (129). The most common side effects are related to gastrointestinal and neuropsychologic function (Table 32.7).

TABLE 32.7

COMMONLY USED PHARMACOLOGIC APPROACHES IN THE MANAGEMENT OF OPIOID SIDE EFFECTS

Opioid side effect	Treatment
Constipation	Approaches for all patients: Increase fluid intake and dietary fiber Ensure comfort and convenience, etc. Discuss approaches with patient and select one or more: Daily contact laxative plus stool softener (e.g., senna plus docusate) Daily osmotic laxative or lavage agent Intermittent use of laxative Consider alternative approaches in refractory cases: Enema Prokinetic agent (metoclopramide) Oral naloxone
Nausea	Several approaches: If associated with vertigo or if markedly exacerbated by movement, antivertiginous drug (e.g., scopolamine, meclizine, dimenhydrinate) If associated with early satiety, prokinetic agent (metoclopramide) In other cases, dopamine antagonist drugs (e.g., prochlorperazine, chlorpromazine, haloperidol, metoclopramide)
Somnolence, mental clouding	If analgesia is satisfactory, reduce opioid dose by 25% to 50% If analgesia is satisfactory and the toxicity involves confusion, consider a trial of a neuroleptic (e.g., haloperidol) If analgesia is satisfactory and the toxicity is somnolence, consider a trial of a psychostimulant (e.g., methylphenidate) Consider pharmacologic approaches to reduce the opioid requirement (addition of a coanalgesic or adjuvant) Consider trial of an alternative opioid If appropriate, consider nonpharmacologic analgesic approaches

Constipation is a highly prevalent side effect of opioid therapy. It may contribute to abdominal pain, distension, nausea, and worsening anorexia, and occasionally may progress to obstipation and bowel obstruction. The management of drug-induced constipation should begin with the elimination of nonessential constipatory drugs and, if possible, an increase in both fluid and fiber intake. Fiber should not be increased in those with likely partial bowel obstruction or marked debility because of the potential for worsening obstruction.

Laxative therapy should be considered whenever constipation cannot be controlled through nutritional measures. Routine laxative therapy should not be administered, however, if there is reason to believe that obstruction or impaction is present. These problems should be addressed before laxative therapy is initiated. Patients who are starting opioid therapy and have other predisposing factors for constipation should be considered for prophylactic laxative therapy.

There are numerous types of laxatives, including bulk-forming agents, osmotic agents, lubricants, surfactants, contact cathartics, prokinetic drugs, agents for colonic lavage, and oral opioid antagonists (129,130). The conventional first-line approach is a combination of a stool softener, usually docusate, and a cathartic agent, such as senna. Most patients respond to this therapy. The oral lavage agent, propylethylene glycol, in a powdered formulation offers another well-tolerated and usually effective approach. Osmotic agents, such as lactulose, are often tried in more refractory cases. Lubiprostone, a chloride channel opener, is available in the United States and also may be considered. A variety of other strategies are used seldomly, for challenging cases. These include trials of metoclopramide, misoprostol, colchicine, or donezepil.

Oral opioid antagonist therapy also can be tried for refractory constipation and is likely to become more common with the availability of new drugs. Opioid antagonists that can reverse opioid-induced constipation through local action on opioid receptors in the gut without causing systemic opioid withdrawal may be useful laxatives. At the present time, this treatment is implemented using oral naloxone, which is typically administered at a dose of 0.8 mg twice daily; the dose is doubled every 2 to 3 days until favorable effects occur or side effects are experienced (131,132). The daily dose needed to reverse constipation usually is 12 to 18 mg per day. Quarternary opioid antagonists, such as methylnaltrexone and alvimopan, are undergoing development as peripherally acting antagonists and may expand the utility of this approach in the future (132–134).

Nausea or vomiting constitutes a problem for some 10% to 30% of cancer patients receiving opioid therapy (135). Potential contributing etiologies should be evaluated and the treatment adjusted accordingly. If the assessment suggests that factors other than opioids are contributing to the nausea, antiemetic therapy may be combined with specific interventions to reverse or minimize these factors. The usual first-line drugs are the dopamine antagonists, including prochlorperazine, metoclopramide, and haloperidol. Patients with refractory nausea may need other pharmacologic approaches. Although the antiemetic efficacy of corticosteroids is unexplained, these drugs are clearly beneficial for some patients. Others respond to a commercially available cannabinoid. Although a 5HT antagonist, such as ondansetron, can be beneficial for patients with refractory symptoms, they are very costly and should be considered only after other therapies have failed. In difficult cases, combinations of drugs from unrelated classes often are tried.

Sedation or mental clouding is very common when an opioid regimen is begun or the dose increased. Most patients develop tolerance to this effect relatively quickly, but some do not, and some have other factors that cause cognitive impairment and compound the effect of the opioid. If these side effects are mild, reassurance and education are usually sufficient interventions. When toxicity is severe or persistent enough to compromise the benefits of therapy, other interventions are needed. Treatment of potential etiologies other than the opioid (e.g., elimination of another nonessential drug or treatment of a metabolic disturbance), when feasible and indicated, is the first step in the management of neuropsychologic symptoms. If pain is well controlled, it is reasonable to try an opioid dose reduction of 25% to 50%.

Symptomatic therapies for opioid-induced sedation or mental clouding also should be considered (Table 32.7), but few have been well studied in clinical trials. Methylphenidate has been shown to decrease opioid-induced sedation in cancer patients (136–138). The starting dose is 5 mg at breakfast and at lunchtime. Other psychostimulants that have been used empirically for this indication include dextroamphetamine, amphetamine, and modafinil. A role for modafinil in cancer has been suggested by a positive controlled study that demonstrated improvement across cognitive, mood, and fatigue outcome measures, with the maximum benefit at 8 weeks after initiation of treatment (139). A new stimulant drug, atomoxetine, has a pharmacology that may indicate its utility for fatigue but experience is lacking and it has not yet been studied.

Tolerance, Physical Dependence, and Addiction

The clinical implications of tolerance, physical dependence, and addiction are commonly misunderstood by patients and clinicians. These misapprehensions may lead to concern about adverse events and, possibly, undertreatment of pain.

Tolerance is a pharmacologic property of opioid drugs defined by the need for escalating doses in order to maintain effects (140,141). Patients may have other reasons for declining analgesic effects, however, among which are progressive nociception and increasing psychologic distress. Abundant survey data suggest that the most common reason for dose increase is worsening pain due to progression of a nociceptive lesion. Most patients with stable disease continue to require the same opioid dose for extremely long periods of time (141,142). Fear of analgesic tolerance should never delay the implementation of opioid therapy, and tolerance should not be invoked to explain the need for higher opioid doses unless a comprehensive reassessment has failed to identify an alternative explanation.

Physical dependence also is a pharmacologic property of opioid drugs, which is defined by the occurrence of an abstinence syndrome following abrupt dose reduction or administration of an antagonist (140). Neither the dose nor the duration of dosing required to produce physical dependence is known, and it is prudent to assume that all patients who have received an opioid drug for more than a few days have the potential for withdrawal. This implies that dosing should not be discontinued suddenly and that antagonist drugs, including the agonist-antagonist opioids, should be avoided.

Patients who become physically dependent on opioids appear to develop increased sensitivity to the effects of antagonist drugs. Very small doses of naloxone may produce a severe abstinence syndrome. For this reason, the use of naloxone should be limited to patients with symptomatic respiratory depression. When naloxone must be used in patients receiving chronic opioid therapy, only a dilute solution (e.g., 0.4 mg in 10 mL saline) should be administered and incremental doses should be given only until respiration improves. The goal of this intervention is improved respiration and not a return of consciousness, which may be associated with recurrent pain and withdrawal phenomena.

Both tolerance and physical dependence are distinct from addiction. Because the labels applied to patients can determine the attitudes and behaviors of caregivers, it is extremely important that appropriate terms are used to describe these phenomena. Patients who are perceived to have the capacity for withdrawal should be labeled physically dependent and not "addicted."

Addiction is a genetic, psychologic, and behavioral syndrome characterized by craving, loss of control over drug use, compulsive use, and continued use despite harm to the patient or others (140). Although abusable drugs, including opioids, can be shown to have reinforcing effects in animals, the capacity to produce addiction should not be considered an inherent property of the drug. Addiction presumably results from an interaction between the drug and a variety of factors that predispose the individual to compulsive use. These factors probably encompass genetic vulnerability, situational factors, and psychologic disturbances, as well as access to the drug.

Cancer patients who engage in aberrant drug-taking behaviors, such as hoarding or selling, unsanctioned dose escalation, or manipulation of the medical system to obtain additional drugs, may or may not meet criteria for the diagnosis of addiction. If such aberrant behaviors are identified, measures should be taken to eliminate them while a detailed assessment is performed to clarify their meaning. In some cases, aberrant drug-related behaviors appear to be driven by uncontrolled pain. This has been termed pseudoaddiction and is managed by improved efforts to provide pain relief. Occasionally, aberrant behaviors are related to a psychiatric disorder other than addiction or to the development of a mild encephalopathy, which leads to confusion about drug taking. These explanations for problematic drug use are not mutually exclusive and the complexity of the clinical situation requires careful assessment, and often referral of the patient to a pain specialist or an addiction medicine specialist. The clinician must avoid the stigmatizing label of addiction for patients who have reasonable alternative explanations for aberrant behaviors, but be willing to render the diagnosis of addiction in those who actually have this disease.

The risk of true iatrogenic addiction is clearly relevant in judging the overall utility of opioid therapy for chronic cancer pain. There is substantial evidence that this risk is extremely low among those with no prior history of abuse or addiction (143). It is now widely accepted that all patients who are being considered for a trial of an opioid should be evaluated for risk factors that may predict aberrant drug-related behavior, such as a history of substance abuse, a family history of substance abuse, and major psychiatric disorder, but that fear of addiction should not be considered a contraindication to opioid therapy of severe cancer pain. Rather, patients should be stratified by risk before therapy begins, and monitored for aberrant drug-related behavior during the course of therapy. Should concerns arise, the clinician may structure therapy in a way to reduce risk, or refer appropriately.

TABLE 32.8

ADJUVANT ANALGESICS

Indication	Drugs
Neuropathic pain	Antidepressants
	Tricyclic antidepressants
	Amitriptyline
	Desipramine
	"Newer" antidepressants
	Duloxetine
	Anticonvulsants
	Gabapentin
	Pregabalin
	Carbamazepine
	Phenytoin
	Valproate
	Clonazepam
	Lamotrigine
	Sodium channel blockers
	Mexiletine
	Tocainide
	Alpha$_2$-adrenergic agonists
	Clonidine
	Tizanidine
	NMDA receptor antagonists
	Ketamine
	Dextromethorphan
	Cannabinoids
	Tetrahydrocannabinol (THC)
	Topical anesthetics
	Capsaicin
	Lidocaine
	Miscellaneous
	Baclofen
	Calcitonin
Bone pain	Bisphosphonates (e.g., pamidronate)
	Calcitonin
	Radiopharmaceuticals (e.g., strontium 89 and samarium 153)
Bowel obstruction	Scopolamine
	Glycopyrrolate
	Octreotide
Multipurpose	Corticosteroids
	Dexamethasone
	Prednisone

Adjuvant Drugs

Most patients with cancer pain require multiple drugs for symptom management. Some of these adjuvant drugs are used to treat symptoms other than pain, particularly those that occur as side effects of the opioid (Table 32.7). Other drugs are used in an effort to provide additive analgesia. The latter drugs comprise the NSAIDs and the so-called adjuvant analgesics. Adjuvant analgesics may be defined as drugs that are commercially available for indications other than pain but may be analgesic in selected circumstances (144). In recent years, the number of these drugs has increased substantially, and several have become approved for primary pain indications due to the abundance of evidence for analgesic efficacy.

The adjuvant analgesics are particularly helpful in the treatment of pain syndromes that are often relatively less responsive to opioids, such as neuropathic pains (Table 32.8). Although neuropathic pains, such as postmastectomy syndrome, painful polyneuropathy, and painful plexopathy, can respond well to an opioid regimen, they are relatively more likely to be poorly responsive and represent the most common target of the adjuvant analgesics.

Corticosteroids are among the adjuvant analgesics commonly used to treat neuropathic pain. These drugs also may improve anorexia, nausea, and fatigue, and are often used in open-ended therapy when cancer is relatively advanced. Anticonvulsants and antidepressants are the most commonly used adjuvant analgesics for neuropathic pain. Evidence for analgesic efficacy is best for specific anticonvulsants, such as gabapentin and pregabalin (145–149); for the tricyclic antidepressants, such as amitriptyline and desipramine (150,151); and for the serotonin and norepinephrine reuptake inhibitors, specifically duloxetine (152). Gabapentin or pregabalin usually is tried first, given their lack of drug-drug interactions, but sequential trials of various drugs often are required before a well-tolerated and effective adjuvant analgesic is identified.

If the drugs with relatively good evidence of analgesic efficacy in neuropathic pain are not tolerated or are ineffective, trial of other anticonvulsants or antidepressants may be undertaken empirically. Other second-line agents for neuropathic pain also are considered in refractory cases. Sodium channel blockers may be given orally (e.g., mexiletine) or tried via brief infusion of lidocaine (153,154). NMDA antagonists have limited evidence of efficacy, with the exception of ketamine, and this drug is sometimes tried at subanesthetic doses (155,156). Cannabinoids are analgesic (157–159), and a marijuana derivative is available in some countries, with approval for pain due to multiple sclerosis and to cancer. This drug is under development in the United States, where tetrahydrocannabinol and nabilone are the commercially available cannabinoids. Experience with the latter drugs as analgesics is very limited. In contrast, there is a larger experience with the gamma-aminobutyric acid (GABA) agonist baclofen and with the alpha$_2$-adrenergic drugs tizanidine and clonidine; these drugs also are tried in selected patients with refractory neuropathic pain.

The use of topical agents represents another adjuvant analgesic strategy. A lidocaine patch (Lidoderm)® (160,161) is now available and has been shown to be effective in postherpetic neuralgia. This formulation is commonly tried for all types of neuropathic and musculoskeletal pains. Topical creams also are used empirically in patients with cancer pain, including compounds containing other local anesthetics, capsaicin, an NSAID, a tricyclic antidepressant, or an opioid.

Opioid-refractory malignant bone pain is another syndrome for which adjuvant analgesics often are considered. The preferred drugs include bisphosphonates, radiopharmaceuticals, and calcitonin. Although the bisphosphonates carry the risks of renal insufficiency and osteonecrosis of the jaw, there is evidence that they can improve overall morbidity associated with bone metastases, and a trial of one of these agents is typically considered in the setting of significant bone pain (162).

Adjuvant analgesics also are commonly employed in the setting of bowel obstruction that is not surgically correctable. Aggressive pharmacotherapy, particularly in those with advanced disease, may control symptoms and obviate the need for drainage procedures. Treatment usually involves the combination of anticholinergic drugs (e.g., scopolamine or glycopyrrolate), octreotide, corticosteroids, and opioids (163).

THERAPEUTIC APPROACHES: OTHER APPROACHES IN CHRONIC PAIN MANAGEMENT

Although most patients with cancer pain can achieve adequate relief with pharmacologic approaches alone, a multimodality strategy always should be considered in an effort to optimize the balance between analgesia and side effects, promote better function, or concurrently manage other problems. Multiple therapies commonly are needed to address the broader palliative care concerns of the patient and family, which derive from the complex interaction between pain and suffering (Fig. 32.1).

When the focus is pain control, there are a large number of noninvasive and invasive approaches that may be considered adjunctive to opioid-based pharmacotherapy. Only a small minority of patients will require an invasive analgesic modality if the other therapies are optimally administered.

Interventional Approaches

The interventional strategies include injections, neural blockade, and implant therapies. Trigger point injections may be considered within the purview of all practitioners. Myofascial pains are extremely common in patients with chronic cancer pain, and the use of local anesthetic injections into painful trigger points may be a useful adjunctive approach in these patients.

The advances in neuraxial infusion of opioids and other drugs, as described previously, have largely supplanted the neurodestructive approaches that were employed in the past for pain syndromes refractory to systemic opioid therapy. Nonetheless, some types of neural blockade continue to be widely used (114). Sympathetic nerve blocks with local anesthetic are used to manage those cancer-related neuropathic pains that are presumed to be perpetuated at least in part by sympathetic efferent function. Other temporary somatic nerve blocks may be diagnostic, prognostic, or therapeutic. Diagnostic blocks elucidate the afferent pathways involved in the experience of pain. Prognostic blocks are implemented prior to a neurolytic procedure, and although extensive clinical experience indicates that a favorable response does not predict permanent relief following neurolysis, the failure to achieve pain relief with local anesthetic is commonly viewed as a contraindication to a destructive procedure. Repeated therapeutic blocks with local anesthetic are occasionally used in cancer patients who obtain substantial and fairly prolonged relief after such a temporary block. Recently, local anesthetics have been used to provide more prolonged neural blockade through techniques of perineural or epidural infusion.

Neural blockade with neurolytic solutions, usually alcohol or phenol, have been developed to denervate virtually any area of the body (114). Their use is very limited, however, because of the short-term risks associated with the injection of these substances, such as damage to soft tissues and local hemorrhage or infection, and the longer-term risks of neuritis and deafferentation pain. The one generally accepted exception is celiac plexus blockade for the management of epigastric pain due to neoplastic invasion of the celiac axis. The response to neurolytic celiac plexus blockade in pain due to pancreatic cancer has been observed to be so satisfactory that earlier use is warranted whenever the typical pain syndrome occurs (164).

Intermittent nitrous oxide inhalation is an anesthetic technique that has been proven to be useful in the management of severe breakthrough pain in patients with advanced cancer (165). Although the availability of masks that reduce ambient leakage of the gas has increased the potential usefulness of this approach, it continues to be applied rarely.

Neurostimulatory Approaches

It has been appreciated for some time that stimulation of afferent neural pathways may result in analgesia. The best-known application of this principle is TENS. Other approaches include counterirritation (i.e., systematic rubbing of the painful part), percutaneous electrical nerve stimulation, dorsal column stimulation, and brain stimulation. Published experience in the use of these modalities for the management of cancer pain is meager. Surveys of the techniques that have been used most extensively in nonmalignant pain (TENS and dorsal column stimulation) suggest that the majority of patients will achieve analgesia soon after the approach is implemented but only a few can obtain prolonged relief. A trial of TENS is usually considered in patients with neuropathic pain that has been proven to be difficult to manage with opioids.

Physiatric Approaches

Although evidence from clinical trials is lacking, the potential for analgesic effects from physiatric therapies, including the use of orthoses or prostheses, occupational therapy and physical therapy, and modalities such as heat, cold, vibration, and ultrasound, is well accepted. For example, refractory movement–induced pains may be partially relieved by bracing the painful part, such as in patients with back pain due to metastatic lesions of the spine and those with arm pain related to a malignant brachial plexopathy, and a well-fitting prosthesis can reduce stump pain. In addition to the potential for salutary effects on symptoms, physical therapy and occupational therapy can potentially forestall painful complications, such as contractures, and generally increase well-being.

Neurosurgical Approaches

Procedures designed to denervate the painful area surgically have been developed for every level of the nervous system from peripheral nerves to cortex. Historically, the most useful approach has been cordotomy. Like neurolytic blocks, however, these procedures are rarely considered now, largely due to the advent of more sophisticated, nonneurodestructive interventions such as neuraxial infusion.

Psychologic Approaches

Some patients or families who present with severe psychologic distress may benefit from a multidisciplinary approach in which psychologic interventions are emphasized within a program designed to palliate symptoms and provide family support. These goals may be accomplished in some cases through referral to a hospice or palliative care program. Occasionally, patients with psychiatric disorders are identified, indicating the need for further assessment and treatment by an appropriate specialist (166).

Specific cognitive and behavioral approaches also have been applied in the management of pain and related symptoms (167,168). Cognitive approaches include relaxation training, distraction techniques, hypnosis, and biofeedback, all of which may enhance a patient's sense of personal control and reduce pain. Although many of these approaches require experienced personnel to implement, several forms of relaxation training can be taught by the nonspecialist. Behavioral therapy, which has achieved wide acceptance in the management of nonmalignant pain, is occasionally considered in patients with limited disease whose level of functional impairment is perceived to be out of proportion to the effects of the neoplasm. Cognitive and behavioral psychologic approaches can focus the patient's attention on issues related to function and quality of life and reduce rumination about the disease.

Complementary and Alternative Medicine Approaches

Therapies that are typically considered to be complementary or alternative have had a growing role in pain management (169). These approaches often are very attractive to patients because they endorse a holistic strategy that is perceived as providing hope and self-control. Some interventions that are termed "complementary" are actually used routinely by specialists in pain medicine or palliative care. These include mind-body therapies (e.g., relaxation, meditation, and others), nutritional support, acupuncture, and massage. Other interventions, such as homeopathy, naturopathy, and many others, are considered to be far outside the mainstream and are rarely suggested (170). Health care professionals have the difficult task of expressing concerns about some of the latter therapies, while respecting patients' pursuit of complementary treatments that may be beneficial or, at least, offer no significant chance of harm.

CONCLUSION

Pain is highly prevalent among patients with gynecologic tumors. The clinicians involved in the care of these patients have a challenging task in being able to provide state-of-the-art management approaches for both acute pain and chronic pain. Fortunately, the most effective strategy for both acute and chronic pain, namely, opioid-based pharmacotherapy, is clearly within the purview of all practitioners. The knowledge and skills necessary to optimize this therapy, and integrate it with the broader principles of palliative care, are fundamental to the practice of gynecologic oncology.

References

1. Kanner RM. The scope of the problem. In: Portenoy RK, Kanner RM, eds. *Pain Management: Theory and Practice*. Philadelphia: FA Davis Co.; 1996:40–47.
2. Vainio A, Auvinen A. Prevalence of symptoms among patients with advanced cancer: an international collaborative study. *J Pain Symptom Manage* 1996;12:3–10.
3. World Health Organization. *Cancer Pain Relief*. 2nd ed. Geneva: World Health Organization; 1996.
4. Ferrell B, Smith S, Cullinane C, et al. Symptom concerns of women with ovarian cancer. *J Pain Symptom Manage* 2003;25:528–538.
5. Olson SH, Mignone L, Nakrasieve C, et al. Symptoms of ovarian cancer. *Obstet Gynecol* 2001;98:212–217.
6. Portenoy RK, Kornblith AB, Wong G, et al. Pain in ovarian cancer: prevalence, characteristics, and associated symptoms. *Cancer* 1994;74:907–915.
7. Twycross, RG, Fairfield, S. Pain in far-advanced cancer. *Pain* 1982;14: 303–310.
8. Miaskowski C, Dibble SL. The problem of pain in outpatients with breast cancer. *Oncol Nurs Forum* 1995;22:791–797.
9. Tasmuth, T, von Smitten, K, Hietanen, P, et al. Pain and other symptoms after different treatment modalities of breast cancer. *Ann Oncol* 1995;6:453–458.
10. Perkins FM, Kehlet H. Chronic pain as an outcome of surgery. *Anesthesiology* 2000;93:1123–1133.
11. Moulin DE, Foley KM. Review of a hospital-based pain service. In: Foley KM, Bonica JJ, Ventafridda V, eds. *Advances in Pain Research and Therapy*. Vol. 16. New York: Raven Press; 1990:413–427.
12. Schug SA, Zech D, Dorr U. Cancer pain management according to WHO analgesic guidelines. *J Pain Symptom Manage* 1990;5:27–32.
13. Ventafridda V, Tamburini M, Caraceni A, et al. A validation study of the WHO method for cancer pain relief. *Cancer* 1987;59:850–856.
14. Walker VA, Hoskin PJ, Hanks GW, et al. Evaluation of WHO analgesic guidelines for cancer pain in a hospital-based palliative care unit. *J Pain Symptom Manage* 1988;3:145–149.
15. Caraceni A, Portenoy RK, a working group of the IASP task force on cancer pain. An international survey of cancer pain characteristics and syndromes. *Pain* 1999;82:263–274.
16. Cleeland CS, Gonin R, Hatfield AK, et al. Pain and its treatment in outpatients with metastatic cancer. *N Engl J Med* 1994;330:592–596.
17. Von Roenn JH, Cleeland CS, Gonin R, et al. Physician attitudes and practice in cancer pain management. A survey from the Eastern Cooperative Oncology Group. *Arch Intern Med* 1993;119:121–126.
18. Deandrea S, Montanari M, Moja L, et al. Prevalence of undertreatment in cancer pain. A review of published literature. *Ann Oncol* 2008;19(12): 1985–1991.
19. Zenz M, Zenz T, Tryba M, et al. Severe undertreatment of cancer pain: a 3-year survey of the German situation. *J Pain Symptom Manage* 1995; 10:187–191.
20. Jacox A, Carr DB, Payne R, et al. *Management of Cancer Pain (Adults)*. Clinical practice guideline no. 9. (no. 94-0592). Rockville, MD: U.S. Department of Health and Human Services, Public Health Service; 1994.
21. Newell S, Sanson-Fisher RW, Girgis A, et al. The physical and psychosocial experiences of patients attending an outpatient medical oncology department: a cross-sectional study. *Eur J Cancer Care* 1999;8:73–82.
22. Cella D, Peterman A, Passik S, et al. Progress toward guidelines for the management of fatigue. *Oncology* 1998;12:369–377.
23. National Comprehensive Cancer Network Practice Guidelines in Oncology: Cancer-Related Fatigue; 2007.
24. Merskey H, Bogduk N, eds. *Classification of Chronic Pain: Descriptions of Chronic Pain Syndromes and Definitions of Pain Terms*. 2nd ed. Seattle: IASP Press; 1994.
25. Portenoy RK. Cancer pain: pathophysiology and syndromes. *Lancet* 1992;339:1026–1031.
26. Cherny NI, Coyle N, Foley KM. Suffering in the advanced cancer patient: a definition and taxonomy. *J Palliat Care* 1994;10:57–70.
27. Portenoy RK. Pain and quality of life: theoretical aspects. In: Osoba D, ed. *Quality of Life in Cancer Patients*. New York: CRC Press; 1991:279–292.
28. Kellgren JH. On distribution of pain arising from deep somatic structures with charts of segmental pain areas. *Clin Sci* 1939;4:35–46.
29. Ness TJ, Gebhart GF. Visceral pain: a review of experimental studies. *Pain* 1990;41:167–234.
30. Torebjork HE, Ochoa JL, Schady W. Referred pain from intraneural stimulation of muscle fascicles in the median nerve. *Pain* 1984;18:145–156.
31. Foley KM. Pain syndromes in patients with cancer. In: Portenoy RK, Kanner RM, eds. *Pain Management: Theory and Practice*. Philadelphia: FA Davis Co.; 1996:191–215.

32. Gonzales GR, Elliott KJ, Portenoy RK, et al. The impact of a comprehensive evaluation in the management of cancer pain. *Pain* 1991;47:141–144.
33. Boureau F, Doubrere JF, Luu M. Study of verbal description in neuropathic pain. *Pain* 1990;42:145–152.
34. Grond S, Radbruch L, Meuser T, et al. Assessment and treatment of neuropathic cancer pain following WHO guidelines. *Pain* 1999;79:15–20.
35. Chen ML, Chang HK, Yeh CH. Anxiety and depression in Taiwanese cancer patients with and without pain. *J Adv Nurs* 2000;32:944–951.
36. Golden RN, McCartney CF, Haggerty JJ, et al. The detection of depression by patient self-report in women with gynecologic cancer. *Int J Psychiatry Med* 1991;21:17–27.
37. Evans DL, McCartney CF, Nemeroff CB, et al. Depression in women treated for gynecologic cancer: clinical and neuroendocrine assessment. *Am J Psychiatry* 1986;143:447–452.
38. Chang VT, Janjan N, Jain S, et al. Update in cancer pain syndromes. *J Palliat Med* 2006;9(6):1414–1434.
39. Turk DC, Dworkin RH, Allen RR, et al. Core outcome domains for chronic pain clinical trials: IMMPACT recommendations. *Pain* 2003;106:337–345.
40. Austin KL, Stapleton JV, Mather LE. Multiple intramuscular injections: a major source of variability in analgesic response to meperidine. *Pain* 1980;8:47–62.
41. Stouten EM, Armbruster S, Houmes RJ, et al. Comparison of ketorolac and morphine for postoperative pain after major surgery. *Acta Anaesth Scand* 1992;36:716–721.
42. Tuncer S, Pirbudak L, Balat O, et al. Adding ketoprofen to intravenous patient-controlled analgesia with tramadol after major gynecologic cancer surgery: a double-blinded, randomized, placebo-controlled clinical trial. *Eur J Gynaecol Oncol* 2003;24:181–184.
43. Ballantyne JC, Carr DB, Chalmers TC, et al. Postoperative patient-controlled analgesia: meta-analyses of initial randomized trials. *J Clin Anesth* 1993;5:182–193.
44. Pearl ML, McCauley DL, Thompson J, et al. A randomized controlled trial of early oral analgesia in gynecologic oncology patients undergoing intra-abdominal surgery. *Obstet Gynecol* 2002;99:704–708.
45. Katz J, Cohen L. Preventive analgesia is associated with reduced pain disability 3 weeks but not 6 months after major gynecologic surgery by laparotomy. *Anesthesiology* 2004;101(1):169–174.
46. Kay B, Healy TE. Premedication by controlled-release morphine. *Anaesthesia* 1984;39:587–589.
47. Pinnock CA, Derbyshire DR, Elling AE, et al. Comparison of oral slow release morphine (MST) with intramuscular morphine for premedication. *Anaesthesia* 1985;40:1082–1085.
48. White PF, Sacan O, Tufanogullari B, et al. Effect of short-term postoperative celecoxib administration on patient outcome after outpatient laparoscopic surgery. *Can J Anaesth* 2007;54(5):342–348.
49. Mathiesen O, Moiniche S, Dahl JB. Gabapentin and postoperative pain: a qualitative and quantitative systematic review, with focus on procedure. *BMC Anesthesiol* 2007;7:6.
50. Marret E, Remy C, Bonnet F, Postoperative Pain Forum Group. Meta-analysis of epidural analgesia versus parenteral opioid analgesia after colorectal surgery. *Br J Surg* 2007;94(6):665–673.
51. Liu SS, Wu CL. The effect of analgesic technique on postoperative patient-reported outcomes including analgesia: a systematic review. *Anesth Analg* 2007;105(3):789–808.
52. Simon DA, Connor JP, Kushner DM, et al. Epidural analgesia superior to patient-controlled analgesia for postoperative pain relief in gynecologic oncology surgery. *J Pelvic Med Surg* 2007;13(4):191–196.
53. Yavuz L, Eroglu F, Ozsoy M. The efficacy of intravenous versus epidural tramadol with patient-controlled analgesia (PCA) in gynecologic cancer pain. *Eur J Gynaecol Oncol* 2004;25(2):215–218.
54. Rawal N, Sjostrand U, Christoffersson E, et al. Comparison of intramuscular and epidural morphine for postoperative analgesia in the grossly obese: influence on postoperative ambulation and pulmonary function. *Anesth Analg* 1984;63:583–592.
55. De Leon-Casasola OA, Parker BM, Lema MJ, et al. Epidural analgesia versus intravenous patient-controlled analgesia. Differences in the postoperative course of cancer patients. *Reg Anesth* 1994;19:307–315.
56. Swart M, Sewell J, Thomas D. Intrathecal morphine for caesarean section: an assessment of pain relief, satisfaction and side-effects. *Anaesthesia* 1997;52:373–377.
57. Sarma VJ, Bostrom UV. Intrathecal morphine for the relief of post-hysterectomy pain—a double-blind, dose-response study. *Acta Anaesthesiol Scand* 1993;37:223–227.
58. Fleron MH, Weiskopf RB, Bertrand M, et al. A comparison of intrathecal opioid and intravenous analgesia for the incidence of cardiovascular, respiratory, and renal complications after abdominal aortic surgery. *Anesth Analg* 2003;97:2–12.
59. Sprung J, Sanders MS, Warner ME, et al. Pain relief and functional status after vaginal hysterectomy: intrathecal versus general anesthesia. *Can J Anaesth* 2006;53(7):690–700.
60. Bjordal JM, Johnson MI, Ljunggreen AE. Transcutaneous electrical nerve stimulation (TENS) can reduce postoperative analgesic consumption. A meta-analysis with assessment of optimal treatment parameters for postoperative pain. *Eur J Pain* 2003;7:181–188.
61. Good M, Anderson GC, Stanton-Hicks M, et al. Relaxation and music reduce pain after gynecologic surgery. *Pain Manag Nurs* 2002;3:61–70.
62. Weis OF, Sriwatanakul K, Weitraus M, et al. Reduction of anxiety and postoperative analgesic requirements by audiovisual instruction. *Lancet* 1983;1:43–44.
63. Ozalp G, Sarioglu R, Tuncel G, et al. Preoperative emotional states in patients with breast cancer and postoperative pain. *Acta Anaesthesiol Scand* 2003;47:26–29.
64. Curtis EB, Krech R, Walsh TD. Common symptoms in patients with advanced cancer. *J Palliat Care* 1991;7:25–29.
65. Portenoy RK, Thaler HT, Kornblith AB, et al. Symptom prevalence, characteristics and distress in a cancer population. *Qual Life Res* 1994; 3:183–189.
66. Cassell EJ. *The Nature of Suffering and the Goals of Medicine*. New York: Oxford University Press; 1991.
67. http://www.nationalconsensusproject.org.
68. Ellison NM. Palliative chemotherapy. In: Berger A, Weissman D, Portenoy RK, eds. *Principles and Practice of Supportive Oncology*. Philadelphia: Lippincott-Raven Publishers; 2002:667–669.
69. McIllmurray M. Palliative medicine and the treatment of cancer. In: Doyle D, Hanks GWC, Cherny N, Calman K, eds. *Oxford Textbook of Palliative Medicine*. Oxford: Oxford University Press; 2004:229–239.
70. Geels P, Eisenhauer E, Bezjak A, et al. Palliative effect of chemotherapy: objective tumor response is associated with symptom improvement in patients with metastatic breast cancer. *J Clin Oncol* 2000;18:2395–2405.
71. Doyle C, Crump M, Pintilie M, et al. Does palliative chemotherapy palliate? Evaluation of expectations, outcomes, and costs in women receiving chemotherapy for advanced ovarian cancer. *J Clin Oncol* 2001;19:1266–1274.
72. Chambers SK, Lamb L, Kohorn EI, et al. Chemotherapy of recurrent/advanced cervical cancer: results of the Yale University PBM-PFU protocol. *Gynecol Oncol* 1994;53:161–169.
73. Gelblum D, Mychalczak B, Almadrones L, et al. Palliative benefit of external-beam radiation in the management of platinum refractory epithelial ovarian carcinoma. *Gynecol Oncol* 1998;69:36–41.
74. Tinger A, Waldron T, Peluso N, et al. Effective palliative radiation therapy in advanced and recurrent ovarian carcinoma. *Int J Radiation Oncology Biol Phys* 2001;51:1256–1263.
75. Spanos WJ Jr, Pajak TJ, Emami B, et al. Radiation palliation of cervical cancer. *J Natl Cancer Inst Monogr* 1996;21:127–130.
76. Falkmer U, Jarhult J, Wersall P, et al. A systematic overview of radiation therapy effects in skeletal metastases. *Acta Oncol* 2003; 42:620–633.
77. Hillegonds DJ, Franklin S, Shelton DK, et al. The management of painful bone metastases with an emphasis on radionuclide therapy. *J Natl Med Assoc* 2007;99(7):785–794.
78. Eisenberg E, Berkey CS, Carr DB, et al. Efficacy and safety of nonsteroidal antiinflammatory drugs for cancer pain: a meta-analysis. *J Clin Oncol* 1994;12:2756–2765.
79. Lomen PL, Samal BA, Lamborn KR, et al. Flurbiprofen for the treatment of bone pain in patients with metastatic breast cancer. *Am J Med* 1986; 80:83–87.
80. Mercadante S. The use of anti-inflammatory drugs in cancer pain. *Cancer Treat Rev* 2001;27:51–61.
81. Wallenstein DJ, Portenoy RK. Nonopioid and adjuvant analgesics. In: Berger AM, Portenoy RK, Weissman DE, eds. *Principles and Practice of Palliative Care and Supportive Oncology*. Philadelphia: Lippincott–Raven Publishers; 2002:84–97.
82. Mercadante S, Cassucio A, Agnello A, et al. Analgesic effects of nonsteroidal anti-inflammatory drugs in cancer pain due to somatic or visceral mechanisms. *J Pain Symptom Manage* 1999;17:351–356.
83. Mercadante S, Sapio M, Caligara M, et al. Opioid-sparing effect of diclofenac in cancer pain. *J Pain Symptom Manage* 1997;14:15–20.
84. Mercadante S, Fulfaro F, Casuccio A. A randomised controlled study on the use of anti-inflammatory drugs in patients with cancer pain on morphine therapy: effects of dose-escalation and a pharmacoeconomic analysis. *Eur J Cancer* 2002,38:1358–1363.
85. Bombardier C, Laine L, Reicin A, et al. Comparison of upper gastrointestinal toxicity of rofecoxib and naproxen in patients with rheumatoid arthritis. VIGOR Study Group. *N Engl J Med* 2000;343:1520–1528.
86. Silverstein FE, Faich G, Goldstein JL, et al. Gastrointestinal toxicity with celecoxib vs. nonsteroidal anti-inflammatory drugs for osteoarthritis and rheumatoid arthritis: the CLASS study: a randomized controlled trial. Celecoxib long-term arthritis safety study. *JAMA* 2000; 284:1247–1255.
87. Waksman JC, Brody A, Phillips SD. Nonselective nonsteroidal antiinflammatory drugs and cardiovascular risk: are they safe? *Ann Pharmacother* 2007;41:1163–1173.
88. Hinz B, Renner B, Brune K. Drug insight: cyclo-oxygenase-2 inhibitors-a critical appraisal. *Nat Clin Pract Rheumatol* 2007;3:552–560.
89. Peng S, Duggan A. Gastrointestinal adverse effects of non-steroidal anti-inflammatory drugs. *Expert Opin Drug Saf* 2005;4:157–169.
90. McLaughlin JK, Lipworth L, Chow W-H, et al. Analgesic use and chronic renal failure: a critical review of the epidemiologic literature. *Kidney Int* 1998;54:679–686.
91. Fine P, Portenoy RK. *Opioid Analgesia*. 2nd ed. New York: McGraw Hill; 2007.
92. Bruera EB, Portenoy RK, eds. *Cancer Pain*. London: Assessment and management. New York: Cambridge University Press.

93. Kaiko RF, Foley KM, Grabinski PY, et al. Central nervous system excitatory effects of meperidine in cancer patients. *Ann Neurol* 1983;13:180–185.
94. Galer BS, Coyle N, Pasternak GW, et al. Individual variability in the response to different opioids: report of five cases. *Pain* 1992;49:87–91.
95. Sjøgren P. Clinical implications of morphine metabolites. In: Portenoy RK, Bruera E, eds. *Topics in Palliative Care.* Vol 1. New York: Oxford University Press; 1997;163–175.
96. Peterson GM, Randall CT, Paterson J. Plasma levels of morphine and morphine glucuronides in the treatment of cancer pain: relationship to renal function and route of administration. *Eur J Clin Pharmacol* 1990; 38:121–124.
97. Portenoy RK, Foley KM, Stulman J, et al. Plasma morphine and morphine-6-glucuronide during chronic morphine therapy for cancer pain: plasma profiles, steady-state concentrations and consequences of renal failure. *Pain* 1991;47:13–19.
98. Dean M. Opioids in renal failure and dialysis patients. *J Pain Symptom Manage* 2004;28(5):497–504.
99. Murtagh FE, Chai MO, Donohoe P, et al. The use of opioid analgesia in end-stage renal disease patients managed without dialysis: recommendations for practice. *J Pain Palliat Care Pharmacother* 2007;21(2):5–16.
100. Bryson J, Tamber A, Seccareccia D, et al. Methadone for treatment of cancer pain. *Curr Oncol Rep* 2006;8:282–288.
101. Inturrisi CE. Pharmacology of methadone and its isomers. *Minerva Anestesiol* 2005;71:435–437.
102. Mercadante S. Morphine vs. methadone in the pain treatment of advanced-cancer patients followed-up at home. *J Clin Oncol* 1998;16:3656–3661.
103. Kornick CA, Kilborn MJ, Santiago-Palma J, et al. QTc interval prolongation associated with intravenous methadone. *Pain* 2003;105:499–506.
104. Cruciani RA, Sekine R, Homel P, et al. Measurement of QTc in patients receiving chronic methadone therapy. *J Pain Symptom Manage* 2005; 29:385–391.
105. Coyle N, Adelhardt J, Foley KM, et al. Character of terminal illness in the advanced cancer patient: pain and other symptoms in the last 4 weeks of life. *J Pain Symptom Manage* 1990;5:83–93.
106. Portenoy RK, Southam M, Gupta SK, et al. Transdermal fentanyl for cancer pain: repeated dose pharmacokinetics. *Anesthesiology* 1993;28:36–43.
107. Ahmedzai S, Brooks D. Transdermal fentanyl versus sustained-release oral morphine in cancer pain: preference, efficacy and quality of life. *J Pain Symptom Manage* 1997;13:254–261.
108. Muriel C, Failde I, Micó JA, et al. Effectiveness and tolerability of the buprenorphine transdermal system in patients with moderate to severe chronic pain: a multicenter, open-label, uncontrolled, prospective, observational clinical study. *Clin Ther* 2005;27:451–462.
109. Beaver WT, Feise GA. A comparison of the analgesic effect of oxymorphone by rectal suppository and intramuscular injection in patients with postoperative pain. *J Clin Pharmacol* 1977;17:276–291.
110. Weinberg DS, Inturrisi CE, Reidenberg B, et al. Sublingual absorption of selected opioid analgesics. *Clin Pharmacol Ther* 1988;44:335–342.
111. Coluzzi PH, Schwartzberg L, Conroy JD Jr, et al. Breakthrough cancer pain: a randomized trial comparing oral transmucosal fentanyl citrate (OTFC) and morphine sulfate immediate release (MSIR). *Pain* 2001;91: 123–130.
112. Portenoy R, Taylor D, Messina J, et al. A randomized, placebo-controlled study of fentanyl buccal tablets for breakthrough pain in opioid-treated patients with cancer. *Clin J Pain* 2006:22:805–811.
113. Wilcock A, Jacob JK, Charlesworth S, et al. Drugs given by a syringe driver: a prospective multicentre survey of palliative care services in the UK. *Palliat Med* 2006;20(7):661–664.
114. Swarm RA, Karanikolas M, Cousins MJ. Anaesthetic techniques for pain control. In: Doyle D, Hanks GWC, Cherny N, et al., eds. *Oxford Textbook of Palliative Medicine.* Oxford: Oxford University Press; 2004:390–414.
115. Du Pen SL, Du Pen AR. Intraspinal analgesic therapy in palliative care: evolving perspective. In: Portenoy RK, Bruera EB, eds. *Topics in Palliative Care.* Vol. 4. New York: Oxford University Press; 2000:217–235.
116. Smith TJ, Staats PS, Deer T, et al. Implantable Drug Delivery Systems Study Group. Randomized clinical trial of an implantable drug delivery system compared with comprehensive medical management for refractory cancer pain: impact on pain, drug-related toxicity, and survival. *J Clin Oncol* 2002;20:4040–4049.
117. Bennett G, Serafini M, Burchiel K, et al. Evidence-based review of the literature on intrathecal delivery of pain medication. *J Pain Symptom Manage* 2000;20:S12–36.
118. Hassenbusch SJ, Portenoy RK, Cousins M, et al. Polyanalgesic Consensus Conference 2003: an update on the management of pain by intraspinal drug delivery—report of an expert panel. *J Pain Symptom Manage* 2004;27:540–563.
119. Eisenach JC, DuPen S, Dubois M, et al. Epidural clonidine analgesia for intractable cancer pain. *Pain* 1995;61:391–399.
120. Staats PS, Yearwood T, Charapata SG, et al. Intrathecal ziconotide in the treatment of refractory pain in patients with cancer or AIDS: a randomized controlled trial. *JAMA* 2004;291:63–70.
121. de Leon-Casasola OA. Interventional procedures for cancer pain management: when are they indicated? *Cancer Invest* 2004;22:630–642.
122. Klepstad P, Kaasa S, Jystad A, et al. Immediate- or sustained-release morphine for dose finding during start of morphine to cancer patients: a randomized, double-blind trial. *Pain* 2003;101:193–198.
123. Portenoy RK, Payne D, Jacobsen P. Breakthrough pain: characteristics and impact in patients with cancer pain. *Pain* 1999;81:129–134.
124. Caraceni A, Martini C, Zecca E, et al., a working group of an IASP task force on cancer pain. Breakthrough pain characteristics and syndromes in patients with cancer pain. An international survey. *Palliat Med* 2004;18:177–183.
125. Mercadante S, Portenoy RK. Opioid poorly-responsive cancer pain. Part 1: Clinical considerations. *J Pain Symptom Manage* 2001;21:144–150.
126. Mercadante S, Portenoy RK. Opioid poorly responsive cancer pain. Part 2: Basic mechanisms that could shift dose-response for analgesia. *J Pain Symptom Manage* 2001;21:255–264.
127. Mercadante S, Portenoy RK. Opioid poorly responsive cancer pain. Part 3: Clinical strategies to improve opioid responsiveness. *J Pain Symptom Manage* 2001;21:338–354.
128. Indelicato RA, Portenoy RK. Opioid rotation in the management of refractory cancer pain. *J Clin Oncol* 2002;20:348–352.
129. Swegle JM, Logemann C. Management of common opioid-induced adverse effects. *Am Fam Physician* 2006;74:1347–1354.
130. Kyle G. Constipation and palliative care—where are we now? *Int J Palliat Nurs* 2007;13(1):6–16.
131. Culpepper-Morgan JA, Inturrisi CE, Portenoy RK, et al. Treatment of opioid-induced constipation with oral naloxone: a pilot study. *Clin Pharmacol* 1992;52:90–95.
132. Kurz A, Sessler DI. Opioid-induced bowel dysfunction: pathophysiology and potential new therapies. *Drugs* 2003;63:649–671.
133. Shaiova L, Rim F, Friedman D, et al. A review of methylnaltrexone, a peripheral opioid receptor antagonist, and its role in opioid-induced constipation. *Palliat Support Care* 2007;5:161–166.
134. Paulson DM, Kennedy DT, Donovick RA, et al. Alvimopan: an oral, peripherally acting, mu-opioid receptor antagonist for the treatment of opioid-induced bowel dysfunction—a 21-day treatment-randomized clinical trial. *J Pain* 2005;6:184–192.
135. Campora E, Merlini L, Pace M, et al. The incidence of narcotic-induced emesis. *J Pain Symptom Manage* 1991;6:428–430.
136. Bruera E, Miller MJ, MacMillan K, et al. Neuropsychological effects of methylphenidate in patients receiving a continuous infusion of narcotics for cancer pain. *Pain* 1992;48:163–166.
137. Bruera E, Driver L, Barnes E, et al. Patient controlled methylphenidate for cancer related fatigue: a preliminary report. *J Clin Oncol* 2003; 4439–4443.
138. Wilwerding MB, Loprinzi CL, Maillard JA, et al. A randomized, crossover evaluation of methylphenidate in cancer pateints receiving strong opioids. *Support Care Cancer* 1995;3:135–138.
139. Kaleita TA, Wellisch DK, Graham CA, et al. Pilot study of modafinil for treatment of neurobehavioral dysfunction and fatigue in adult patients with brain tumors (abstract). *J Clin Oncol* 2006;24:58s.
140. Savage SR, Joranson DE, Covington EC, et al. Definitions related to the medical use of opioids: evolution towards universal agreement. *J Pain Symptom Manage* 2003;26(1):655–667.
141. Portenoy RK. Tolerance to opioid analgesics: clinical aspects. In: Hanks GW, ed. *Palliative Medicine: Problem Areas in Pain and Symptom Management.* Plainview, NY: Cold Spring Harbor Laboratory Press; 1994:49–66.
142. Kanner RM, Foley KM. Patterns of narcotic drug use in a cancer pain clinic. *Ann N Y Acad Sci* 1981;362:161–172.
143. Portenoy RK, Payne R, Passik S. Acute and chronic pain. In: Lowinson JH, Ruiz P, Millman RB, eds. *Comprehensive Textbook of Substance Abuse.* 4th ed. Baltimore: Williams and Wilkins; 2005:863–903.
144. Lussier D, Portenoy RK. Adjuvant analgesics. In: Doyle D, Hanks G, Cherny NI, Calman K, eds. *Oxford Textbook of Palliative Medicine.* 3rd ed. Oxford: Oxford University Press; 2004:349–377.
145. Rowbotham M, Harden N, Stacey B, et al. Gabapentin for the treatment of postherpetic neuralgia: a randomized controlled trial. *JAMA* 1998;280(21):1837–1842.
146. Backonja M, Beydoun A, Edwards KR, et al. Gabapentin for the symptomatic treatment of painful neuropathy in patients with diabetes mellitus: a randomized controlled trial. *JAMA* 1998;280:1831–1836.
147. Gilron I, Flatters SJ. Gabapentin and pregabalin for the treatment of neuropathic pain: a review of laboratory and clinical evidence. *Pain Res Manag* 2006;11(Suppl A):16A–29A.
148. van Seventer R, Feister HA, Young JP Jr, et al. Efficacy and tolerability of twice-daily pregabalin for treating pain and related sleep interference in postherpetic neuralgia: a 13-week, randomized trial. *Curr Med Res Opin* 2006;22:375–384.
149. Caraceni A, Zecca E, Martini C, et al. Gabapentin as an adjuvant to opioid analgesia for neuropathic cancer pain. *J Pain Symptom Manage* 1999; 17:441–445.
150. Kalso E, Tasmuth T, Neuvonen PJ. Amitriptyline effectively relieves neuropathic pain following treatment of breast cancer. *Pain* 1996;64: 293–302.
151. Watson CPN. The treatment of neuropathic pain: antidepressants and opioids. *Clin J Pain* 2000;16:S49–55.
152. Wernicke JF, Pritchett YL, D'Souza DN, et al. A randomized controlled trial of duloxetine in diabetic peripheral neuropathic pain. *Neurology* 2006; 67(8):1411–1420.
153. Sinclair R, Westlander G, Cassuto J, et al. Postoperative pain relief by topical lidocaine in the surgical wound of hysterectomized patients. *Acta Anaesthesiol Scand* 1996;40;589.

154. Sloan P, Basta M, Storey P, et al. Mexiletine as an adjuvant analgesic for the management of neuropathic cancer pain. *Anesth Analg* 1999; 89:760–761.
155. Mercadante S, Arcuri E, Tirelli W, et al. Analgesic effect of intravenous ketamine in cancer patients on morphine therapy: a randomized, controlled, double-blind, crossover, double-dose study. *J Pain Symptom Manage* 2000;20:246–252.
156. Ogawa S, Kanamura T, Noda K, et al. Intravenous microdrip infusion of ketamine in subanaesthetic doses for intractable terminal cancer pain. *Pain Clin* 1994;7:125–129.
157. Burns TL, Ineck JR. Cannabinoid analgesia as a potential new therapeutic option in the treatment of chronic pain. *Ann Pharmacother* 2006; 40:251–260.
158. Campbell FA, Tramer MR, Carroll D, et al. Are cannabinoids an effective and safe treatment option in the management of pain? A qualitative systematic review. *BMJ* 2001;323:13–16.
159. Iskedjian M, Bereza B, Gordon A, et al. Meta-analysis of cannabis based treatments for neuropathic and multiple sclerosis-related pain. *Curr Med Res Opin* 2007;23(1):17–24.
160. Galer BS, Rowbotham MC, Perander J, et al. Topical lidocaine patch relieves postherpetic neuralgia more effectively than a vehicle topical patch: results of an enriched enrollment study. *Pain* 1999;80:533–538.
161. Gammaitoni AR, Davis MW. Pharmacokinetics and tolerability of lidocaine patch 5% with extended dosing. *Ann Pharmacother* 2002; 36:236–240.
162. Lipton A. Efficacy and safety of intravenous bisphosphonates in patients with bone metastases caused by metastatic breast cancer. *Clin Breast Cancer* 2007;7(Suppl 1):S14–20.
163. Ripamonti C. Management of bowel obstruction in advanced cancer patients. *J Pain Symptom Manage* 1994;9:193–200.
164. Brown DL, Bulley CK, Quiel EL. Neurolytic celiac plexus block for pancreatic cancer pain. *Anesth Analg* 1987;66:869–873.
165. Fosburg MT, Crone RK. Nitrous oxide analgesia for refractory pain in the terminally ill. *JAMA* 1983;250:511–513.
166. Massie MJ, Spiegel L, Lederberg MS, et al. Psychiatric complications in cancer patients. In: Lawrence W, Lenhard RE, Murphy GP, eds. *Textbook of Clinical Oncology*. 2nd ed. Atlanta: American Cancer Society; 1995: 685–698.
167. Jacobsen PB, Hann DM. Cognitive-behavioral interventions. In: Holland JC, ed. *Psycho-oncology*. New York: Oxford University Press; 1998: 717–729.
168. Meyer TJ, Mark MM. Effects of psychosocial interventions with adult cancer patients: a meta-analysis of randomized experiments. *Health Psychol* 1995;14:101–108.
169. Pan CX, Morrison S, Ness J, et al. Complementary and alternative medicine in the management of pain, dyspnea, and nausea and vomiting near the end of life: a systematic review. *J Pain Symptom Manage* 2000;20: 374–387.
170. Doan BD. Alternative and complementary therapies. In: Holland JC, ed. *Psycho-oncology*. New York: Oxford University Press; 1998:817–827.

CHAPTER 33 ■ NUTRITION SUPPORT OF PATIENTS WITH GYNECOLOGIC CANCER

MARK SCHATTNER AND MOSHE SHIKE

INTRODUCTION

Cachexia and weight loss are common manifestations of cancer and exert major impacts on quality of life and survival. Malnutrition is a complex, multifactorial phenomenon that leads to progressive weight loss and deficiency of specific nutrients. Both the cancer and its various therapeutic modalities contribute to cachexia. Advances in understanding nutritional requirements and intermediary metabolism, and major technologic progress in the ability to provide nutritional support, have made it possible to feed almost any patient with cancer. Nevertheless, the indications for and the appropriate use of the various modalities of nutritional support are still evolving, and many questions remain unanswered.

Malnutrition in most patients with cancer is usually a manifestation of general calorie-protein deficits that result in progressive weight loss and weakness; however, it is important to recognize that in some patients specific nutrient deficiencies, such as magnesium deficiency or vitamin B_{12} deficiency, can be present even in the absence of weight loss and can contribute significantly to morbidity and even mortality.

Gynecologic malignancies and their multimodal therapies may be associated with severe malnutrition. Although some nutritional problems occur in patients with cervical and endometrial cancer, they are most commonly seen in those with ovarian cancer, particularly in advanced stages when intra-abdominal metastasis severely impairs gastrointestinal function. Because of the high incidence of malnutrition and its impact on the patient with cancer, nutritional assessment and appropriate therapy should be integral parts of the overall treatment plan.

NUTRITIONAL ASSESSMENT

Nutritional assessment in cancer patients is an ongoing process. It should be a part of the patient's initial evaluation and should be updated periodically. It is especially important to determine the nutritional state prior to therapeutic interventions as well as during and after an acute illness, with the goal of identifying those patients who could benefit from a specific form of nutritional support. The nutritional assessment method used must be simple, accurate, and inexpensive. Anthropometric parameters, serum protein measurements, and immunologic tests had classically formed the basis of the nutritional evaluation; however, they all have significant deficiencies.

Anthropometric and Biochemical Markers

Anthropometric measurements such as weight, skin fold thickness, midarm muscle circumference and creatinine/height index can all provide useful information but have major limitations. Change in weight is the single most useful measurement of the nutritional status when the change does not reflect changes in total body water. The often-present edema, effusions, ascites, or intravenous hydration limit the use of weight as a nutritional parameter. In addition, inaccuracies in scales and different clothing in hospitals and at home can often be sources of misleading information on changes in weight. Measurements of skin folds and midarm muscle circumference (1) are useful tools in studies but have very limited use in clinical practice. A creatinine/height index derived by dividing the patient's 24-hour creatinine excretion by that of a healthy person of the same height offers a sensitive measure of early protein calorie malnutrition (2) but requires collection of a 24-hour urine specimen and is affected by alterations in renal function which may not be indicative of the nutritional state.

Low levels of serum proteins such as albumin, pre-albumin, transferrin, and retinol-binding protein were classically thought to represent malnutrition. However, in the malnourished, sick patient low levels of these proteins can be nonspecific. They are dependent on intact hepatic synthetic function as well as hydration status. At times they can be low as a manifestation of severe illness (infection, metastatic cancer, multisystem organ failure) without being a reflection of the nutritional state. In addition, they can function as acute phase reactants and therefore be in the normal or elevated range in a clinically malnourished patient. The role of serum protein measurements in the nutritional assessment of an ill patient with cancer is therefore very limited. Similar limitations apply to the role of immunologic parameters such as total lymphocyte count and delayed cutaneous hypersensitivity. In simple starvation both of these measures may be decreased and can return to normal with initiation of nutritional support. However, in the cancer patient undergoing chemotherapy, surgery, radiotherapy, or in the midst of an acute illness, these parameters have little determinative value in the assessment of the nutritional state (3,4).

The above parameters have been combined to create numerous nutritional assessment indices. The most extensively studied is the Prognostic Nutritional Index (PNI), which factors measurements of serum albumin, serum transferrin, triceps skin fold, and delayed cutaneous hypersensitivity (5). Buzby et al. prospectively studied the PNI in patients undergoing gastrointestinal surgery and found that it could accurately stratify patients into high, intermediate, or low risk of developing postoperative complications (6). It must be understood, however, that the index is only as good as the parameters from which it is calculated, and the same limitations outlined above are present in any of these indices.

Subjective Global Assessment

The clinical assessment of the nutritional status has always been used to some extent as part of the general medical history and physical examination. The validity of a formal clinical assessment of the nutritional status was demonstrated in a landmark study by Baker et al., who developed the Subjective Global Assessment (SGA) (7). The SGA is based on a complete history and physical examination with special emphasis on six areas: change in weight, dietary intake, gastrointestinal symptoms, functional capacity, physiologic stress, and physical signs of nutritional deficiencies. These data are used to place the patient into one of three groups. Group "A" (normal nutritional status) is made up of those patients without restriction of food intake or absorption, no change in functional status, and stable or increasing weight. Group "B" (mild malnutrition) consists of patients with evidence of decreased food intake and functional status but little or no change in body weight, while those with severe reduction in food intake, functional status, and loss of weight comprise group "C" (severe malnutrition).

The SGA has consistently been shown to be reproducible and reliable in identifying patients at risk for developing complications associated with malnutrition. In the initial study of 59 patients electively admitted to a general surgical ward, interobserver reproducibility in classification of the nutritional status was 81%, and in a later study of 202 patients it was found to be 91% (7,8). Group assignment based on the SGA had prognostic significance on the ensuing clinical course. The initial study by Baker et al. showed a significant increase in incidence of infection, use of antibiotics, and length of hospitalization in group C when compared to group A (7). In the follow-up study of 202 patients undergoing gastrointestinal surgery, the rate of septic and nonseptic complications in group C was seven times greater than in group A (8). However, it must be recognized that although nutritional parameters are used to determine the SGA, the classification may still represent severity of illness rather than specific nutritionally related complications. Only a determination that the classification predicts which patients will respond favorably to nutritional support (with a decrease in complications) can validate the specificity of this technique. Nevertheless, the SGA provides a simple, reproducible, and accurate method to identify patients who are malnourished who could possibly benefit from nutritional support. Clinical assessments similar to the SGA have been shown to be superior to immunologic testing, plasma protein measurements, and bioelectrical impedance in providing a useful evaluation of nutritional status (7,9–12).

PREVALENCE OF MALNUTRITION

The prevalence of malnutrition depends on the tumor type and stage, the organs involved, and the anticancer therapy. Concurrent nonmalignant conditions such as diabetes and intestinal diseases can be important contributing factors.

The prevalence of weight loss during the 6 months preceding diagnosis of cancer was reported from a multicenter cooperative study of patients with 12 types of cancer (13). The lowest frequency (31% to 40%) and severity of weight loss were found in patients with breast cancer, hematologic cancers, and sarcomas. Intermediate frequency of weight loss was found in patients with colon, prostate, and lung cancer (54% to 64%). Patients with cancer of the pancreas and stomach had the highest frequency (over 80%) and severity of weight loss. Approximately 35% of the patients with lung cancer lost more than 5% of their body weight. This underscores the fact that even if the tumor does not involve the gastrointestinal tract directly, there can be significant weight loss because of systemic and metabolic derangements and loss of appetite. The study did not report on patients with gynecologic malignancies, in whom weight loss can also be very frequent and severe. Other studies revealed that over 40% of patients receiving medical treatment for a variety of cancers were malnourished (14,15). Among surgical patients in a Veterans Administration hospital, 39% of those undergoing a major operation for cancer were malnourished, as judged by either a nutrition risk index or a combination of weight loss and low serum proteins (16). In a study from our institution, the majority of patients with pancreatic cancer undergoing a curative resection were malnourished, as determined by weight loss (17).

Data on the prevalence and impact of malnutrition in patients with gynecologic tumors are limited. The findings in these patients mirror the observations in patients with other cancers. A recent study of 67 consecutive patients hospitalized with gynecologic cancers at the University of Texas found that 54% of the women were malnourished as determined by the prognostic nutritional index (18). In 1983 Tunca (19) examined the nutritional state of gynecologic oncology patients at time of diagnosis using serum albumin, serum transferrin, immune response, and weight loss. Patients with advanced (stage III or IV) ovarian carcinoma had the highest incidence of severe malnutrition while those with cancer of the cervix, endometrium, or vulva reported weight loss with no indication of malnutrition from serum markers or immune response testing. Twenty of the 21 patients with advanced ovarian carcinoma were anergic to recall antigens, and the mean levels of all serum markers examined were significantly lower than those found in patients with early (stage I or II) ovarian carcinoma or cancer of the cervix, vulva, or endometrium. Orr et al. (20,21) assessed the degree of protein-calorie malnutrition and evidence of vitamin deficiency in 78 patients with untreated cervical cancer. The incidence of protein-calorie malnutrition as assessed by anthropometrics, serum markers, and immune testing was directly related to tumor stage: 4% in stage I, 20% in stage II and III, and 60% in stage IV disease (20). Two thirds of patients with untreated cervical cancer were found to have reduced blood levels of at least one vitamin. Mean serum levels of folate, beta-carotene, and vitamin C at the time of admission were all significantly below control values (21). Similar observations of significant protein-calorie malnutrition were seen in 25 patients with endometrial cancer (22).

At Memorial Sloan-Kettering Cancer Center, 49 inpatients with gynecologic malignancies were referred to the clinical nutrition service over a 2-year period (1998 to 2000). This represented a diverse group of patients with the vast majority being evaluated for support with parenteral nutrition and tended to represent the sickest population. Thirty-five of the patients had ovarian cancer, six had endometrial cancer, seven had cervical cancer, and one patient had cancer of the vulva. Twenty patients had intestinal obstruction, seven had enterocutaneous fistulas, three had intractable nausea and vomiting, eight had prolonged ileus (>5 days), and the remainder had gastric outlet obstruction, mucositis, or dysphagia. The average weight loss in this group at the time of consultation was 8 kg, which represented a loss of 9.1% of the usual body weight. The weight loss in these patients was multifactorial in origin, secondary to the effects of the tumor and therapeutic interventions on the gastrointestinal tract, decreased appetite, and possibly metabolic effects of the underlying malignancy.

These patients, representing the sickest of those with gynecologic malignancies, demonstrate the association between the frequently seen complications (fistulae, intestinal obstruction, ileus, etc.) and significant weight loss.

SIGNIFICANCE OF MALNUTRITION

The impact of malnutrition on the cancer patient was demonstrated in a report by Warren in 1932 (23). Based on data from autopsies, the conclusion was that cachexia was the leading cause of death in a group of 400 patients with various cancers. More recent studies have confirmed the significant impact of malnutrition on the quality of life and prognosis of the cancer patient. In the aforementioned multicenter cooperative study of patients receiving chemotherapy (13), those who presented with weight loss at the time of diagnosis had decreased performance status and survival as compared with those without weight loss. In a study of patients with limited, inoperable lung cancer, weight loss was a major predictive factor for survival (14). The negative impact of malnutrition was also demonstrated in surgical patients with malignant and benign diseases. Malnourished patients undergoing a major operation were at greater risk for postoperative morbidity and mortality than were well-nourished patients (16,24).

The impact of malnutrition in patients with a primary gynecologic malignancy is striking. In 1988, while examining the role of total parenteral nutrition (TPN) in their patients, Terada et al. noted that those patients who developed major complications such as a fistula, wound infection, pneumonia, renal failure, respiratory failure, or died had significantly more weight loss and lower serum transferrin levels at the time of presentation (25). They concluded that these parameters might be of value in predicting clinical outcome in patients requiring nutritional support. Undernutrition also adversely affects surgical outcome in patients with primary gynecologic malignancies. Burnett et al. (26) reported that in 92 gynecologic oncology patients requiring colonic surgery, those who were classified as malnourished on the basis of serum markers were significantly more likely to develop major perioperative complications or die. Donato et al. (27) reported that of 104 patients with ovarian carcinoma undergoing intestinal surgery those considered to be malnourished on the basis of serum protein measurements and weight loss preoperatively had significantly more infectious complications, while other variables including preoperative bowel obstruction, extent of debulking, number of intestinal procedures, or hand versus stapled anastomosis failed to correlate with the rate of infectious complications. In 1993, Massad et al. reported on 128 patients undergoing operations by the gynecologic oncology service at Barnes Hospital in St. Louis and showed that serum markers of malnutrition including decreased preoperative albumin and hemoglobin concentrations were strong indicators of increased length of hospitalization (28). Among women with gynecologic cancers who were hospitalized for any reason, malnutrition was associated with prolonged hospital stay (18).

ETIOLOGY OF MALNUTRITION

Cancer can induce a wide variety of derangements in the nutritional status, ranging from generalized malnutrition with severe weight loss and muscle wasting to a single nutrient deficiency. The etiology of malnutrition in the cancer patient is multifactorial. Nutritionally relevant derangements can be induced by the tumor locally (i.e., gastrointestinal obstruction), by malabsorption, or by humoral factors produced by the tumor itself or by reaction of the immune system to the tumor. All modalities of cancer therapy—surgery, radiation, chemotherapy, immunotherapy, and palliative treatments—may be associated with side effects and complications that can impair the nutritional status.

The etiologic factors of malnutrition in the cancer patient whether caused by the tumor or antitumor therapies can be classified into three major categories: decreased food intake, malabsorption, and metabolic derangements that result in inefficient, wasteful metabolism.

Impaired Food Intake and Absorption

Both tumor and cancer treatment modalities can lead to decreased food intake through direct effects on the gastrointestinal tract or systemic effects leading to anorexia. Obstruction of the gastrointestinal tract can be caused by any gynecologic malignancy through external compression, or more rarely, by direct invasion. Although at times localized obstructions can be relieved surgically, the obstruction due to peritoneal carcinomatosis often seen in advanced ovarian cancer is particularly difficult to manage surgically. Often, draining gastrostomy with parenteral nutrition (when appropriate) is the only option for providing nutrition and symptomatic relief (29–31).

Tumors can induce anorexia without local involvement of the gastrointestinal tract. The pathophysiology of this phenomenon is not well understood. Norton et al. (32) utilized a model of surgically coupled tumor-bearing and normal rats with parabiotic cross-circulation to show that tumor-induced anorexia is mediated by circulating substances. Tumor-induced impairment of smell and taste has been well described (24,33–36), but the mechanism has not been defined. There is growing evidence that glycoproteins, cytokines, and neuropeptides play an important role in the pathogenesis of cancer cachexia. Bernstein et al. (37,38) demonstrated in a rat model that infusion of tumor necrosis factor (TNF) mimics tumor-induced anorexia and these effects are mediated via the area postrema and the caudal medial nucleus of the solitary tract in the central nervous system.

Therapies used for gynecologic malignancies often result in complications which impair nutrient intake and absorption. Surgical interventions can lead to fistulae, short bowel syndrome, infections, and ileus, all of which impair oral intake significantly. In a review of 12 years of colonic surgery in gynecologic oncology patients, the rate for major systemic complications (myocardial infarction, pulmonary embolism, renal failure, sepsis) was 13.7%, and the rate of major bowel complications (abscess, fistulae, hemorrhage, obstruction) was 12.1% (26). Adjuvant radiation and chemotherapy have been shown to increase the incidence of major complications after pelvic exenteration (39).

Radiotherapy can lead to various derangements in the structure and function of the gastrointestinal tract. Damage to the gastrointestinal tract following radiation to the abdomen and pelvis most commonly affects the small bowel, followed by the transverse colon, sigmoid, and rectum. Predisposing risk factors include previous abdominal surgery, pelvic inflammatory disease, thin body habitus, hypertension, and diabetes mellitus (40). In general, a dose of 5,000 rads is the threshold for significant injury. In the acute phase of radiation enteritis virtually all patients experience anorexia, nausea, and vomiting, which are thought to be mediated by effects of serotonin on the gut (41) and the central nervous system (42). This is followed 2 to 3 weeks later by diarrhea caused by direct injury to the intestinal mucosa resulting in diarrhea and mild to moderate malabsorption. Most patients will have complete resolution of these acute symptoms. However, a significant minority of patients who received radiotherapy will experience chronic dysfunction of the gastrointestinal tract (43).

There is often a latent period of 1 to 2 years and possibly as long as 20 years before the symptoms of chronic radiation enteropathy surface (44,45). In a review of 102 patients with radiation enteritis after treatment for cervical or endometrial cancer, the median time to development of severe symptoms such as obstruction or perforation was 18 months (46).

Chronic radiation enteropathy is characterized pathologically by transmural injury leading to submucosal fibrosis, edema, lymphatic ectasia, and obliterative endarteritis, which can induce colicky abdominal pain, diarrhea, steatorrhea, ulceration, perforation, stricture, and fistula formation (40). Yeoh et al. (47) retrospectively studied the effects of pelvic irradiation given for the treatment of cervical cancer in 30 randomly selected women who had undergone radiotherapy 1 to 6 years earlier. Significant dysfunction of the gastrointestinal tract was detected. Nineteen of the patients had frequency of bowel movements, bile acid absorption, and vitamin B_{12} absorption outside of the control range. The authors concluded that abnormal gastrointestinal function is essentially an inevitable long-term complication of pelvic irradiation (47). Husebye et al. (48) prospectively studied the gastrointestinal motility patterns in 41 patients with chronic abdominal complaints after radiotherapy for gynecologic cancer. Impaired fasting motility was found in 29% of patients, and motor response after a meal was attenuated in 24%. Postprandial delay of the migrating motor complex was found to be an independent predictor of malnutrition as assessed by weight loss and serum albumin. Impaired motility of the small bowel, therefore, is a key factor in the symptoms experienced by patients with chronic radiation enteropathy (48). Chronic radiation enteritis predisposes to numerous secondary complications. Danielson et al. (49) studied 20 patients with chronic or intermittent diarrhea occurring in women 2 or more years after receiving radiotherapy for gynecologic tumors. Bile acid malabsorption was detected in 65% of patients while evidence of bacterial overgrowth on D-xylose or cholyl-glycine breath tests was found in 45%. Treatment with bile acid binders or antibiotics resulted in a significant decline in the number of daily bowel movements. The authors concluded that treatment of these secondary complications of radiation-induced enteropathy can offer significant symptomatic relief. In 47 patients with gynecologic malignancies who had gastrointestinal complaints lasting more than 4 months after radiotherapy, Kwitko et al. (50) found 19 partial small bowel obstructions, 11 cases of malabsorption, and five fistulae. The mortality from radiation damage to the small bowel in this report was 32%. Improved fractionation of radiotherapy and protective shielding of the intestine where possible have reduced these complication rates (51). More recent studies of patients who received radiation therapy for uterine cancer found the prevalence of significant chronic radiation enteritis to be approximately 4% (52).

Chemotherapy is often associated with decreased food intake. Odynophagia, oral ulcers, and diarrhea are commonly seen during therapy with cytotoxic agents which affect the replicating cells of the intestinal mucosa such as 5-flourouracil, methotrexate, and bleomycin. The Vinca alkaloids can cause ileus and constipation mediated by toxic effects on gastrointestinal neural pathways, while cisplatin and nitrosoureas are highly emetic (53,54). Significant nausea, vomiting, stomatitis, and diarrhea occur in 15% of patients receiving intravenous paclitaxel (Taxol) and in 55% of those receiving the drug orally (55).

The psychologic impact of a malignancy and its associated therapies can also lead to decreased nutrient intake. Depression is a frequent cause of anorexia in this population and learned food aversions are a common consequence of radiation or chemotherapy. As many as 56% of patients undergoing chemotherapy and 62% of those undergoing radiation therapy developed a learned food aversion in one study (56). This is characterized by a psychologic association between the consumption of a particular food and a temporally related unpleasant reaction to the therapy such as nausea and vomiting. This results in future avoidance of that particular food item. A recent Swedish study of patients with ovarian cancer showed that a multidisciplinary approach involving antiemetic drugs, in conjunction with anxiolytics, training in relaxation techniques, nutritional advice, and continuity of nursing care resulted in significantly less cisplatin-induced emesis than antiemetics alone (57).

Metabolic Derangements

Even with normal nutrient intake patients with cancer are at risk for malnutrition due to inefficient nutrient utilization and wasteful metabolic pathways. Compared to simple starvation, cancer cachexia is associated with altered metabolism of carbohydrates, fat, protein, vitamins, and minerals. Therefore, in order to optimize nutritional support in the cancer patient it is imperative to consider metabolic derangements along with problems of ingestion, digestion, and absorption.

Increase in basal energy expenditure has been reported in many but not all studies of patients with malignancy (58–64). In patients with newly diagnosed small cell lung cancer Russel et al. (62) showed a mean increase of 37% in basal energy expenditure, which fell substantially in those who responded to chemotherapy. Similar findings have been reported for gastric cancer (59) and sarcoma (65). Elevated basal energy expenditure will drop after tumor resection (66). There are limited data on the metabolic rate in patients with gynecologic cancers (64). Dickerson et al. (67) used indirect calorimetry to determine the resting energy expenditure in 31 patients with ovarian cancer and 30 patients with cervical cancer. Fifty-five percent of those with ovarian cancer were found to be hypermetabolic (BEE >110% predicted by the Harris-Benedict equation) while only 13% of patients with cervical cancer were hypermetabolic. These differences could not be explained by differences in the extent of disease, nutritional status, body temperature, or nutrient intake.

Abnormalities in carbohydrate metabolism in cancer patients include glucose intolerance and peripheral insulin resistance (68–71). These most often become apparent in the patient with advanced metastatic cancer found to have hyperglycemia, which is refractory to high-dose insulin infusion (71,72). In comparison, in simple starvation, patients are most often euglycemic or hypoglycemic. The hyperglycemia in cancer patients is exacerbated by increased hepatic gluconeogenesis. Shaw et al. (73) showed that this increase in glucose production is correlated with tumor burden and decreases after tumor resection. A number of energy wasting metabolic cycles involving glucose have been identified. In the Cori cycle, glucose is converted to lactate by tumor cells and by the liver. This futile cycle results in a net loss of adenosine 5′-triphosphate (ATP) and may contribute to the loss of energy and weight experienced by the cancer patient (64,74,75).

Lipid metabolism may also be abnormal in patients with a malignancy. There is often increased lipolysis with weight loss and this leads to a decrease in fat mass, which can be out of proportion to the loss of lean body mass (70,76). In addition, patients with cancer are often hyperlipidemic and this may be mediated by TNF-α (77). In contrast to normal homeostasis cancer patients fail to suppress lipolysis with glucose infusion (73). Several causes of increased lipolysis have been proposed including decreased food intake, stress response to illness with adrenal medullary stimulation and increased circulating catecholamine levels, insulin resistance, and release of lipolytic factors produced by the tumor itself or by myeloid tissue cells (78). One such factor has been well characterized (79). Lipid-mobilizing factor (LMF), a 24 kDa glycoprotein produced by tumors, has been shown to stimulate increased lipid mobilization from adipocytes (80). Lipid-mobilizing factor has recently been shown to be identical to the plasma protein zinc-α2-glycoprotein (ZAG) (81). It is thought to act through binding of β-adrenergic receptors and subsequent upregulation of mitochondrial uncoupling proteins (82,83). Animal studies demonstrate that lipid-mobilizing factor causes loss of body weight (specifically a loss of body fat), which is independent of caloric food intake (84). The activity of lipid-mobilizing factor in the urine and serum of cancer patients has been shown to correlate with the degree of weight loss (85) and tumor burden (86). In addition to its effect on lipid metabolism, there is preliminary evidence that lipid-mobilizing factor may protect tumor cells from free radical toxicity and may therefore make tumors less responsive to certain chemotherapeutic agents which induce oxidative damage (87).

High total body protein turnover, with increased synthesis and catabolism, characterizes the alterations of protein metabolism seen in cancer patients (88,89). This results in depletion of muscle mass and loss of nitrogen and contrasts with the adaptive decrease in protein turnover seen in patients with uncomplicated starvation (90). Total parenteral nutrition given to patients with cancer will result in gains of weight and body fat, net gains of total body nitrogen, but no suppression of the high protein flux (89,90). The predominant mechanism of muscle protein loss in cancer patients is a ubiquitin-associated pathway (91). In this pathway, polyubiquitin chains are attached to proteins, which are then recognized and degraded by a proteasome complex. This pathway is regulated, in part, by proteolysis-inducing factor, a 24 kDa glycoprotein produced by tumors (92). Effective treatment of the underlying cancer has been shown to reverse ubiquitin-dependent proteolysis of skeletal muscle (93). Better understanding of this process holds the promise of improving therapy to attenuate the loss of protein seen in patients with cancer (94).

Cytokines play an important role in inducing the metabolic derangements seen in the cancer patient (64). They mediate increased energy expenditure, whole body protein turnover, rise in serum triglyceride levels, and high glycerol turnover (23,95). TNF can be detected in the serum of cancer patients (96), and in animal models it causes protein wasting, depletion of body fat, and anorexia (97,98). High serum levels of interleukin-1 and interleukin-6 are also present in patients with advanced cancer and cachexia. Interventions to down-regulate these cytokines result in improved appetite, body weight, and quality of life (99).

The combined effects of these wasteful and inefficient alterations in metabolism make it difficult to restore nutritional status in the patient with cancer and cachexia despite use of specialized nutritional support. This is in contrast with what is seen in patients with uncomplicated starvation who exhibit changes in metabolism that act to conserve energy and body tissues and in whom nutritional support is highly efficacious in reversing the effects of malnutrition.

NUTRITIONAL THERAPIES

There are four types of nutritional therapies: parenteral nutrition, enteral nutrition, oral dietary therapy, and drug therapy aimed at improving appetite and food intake. Depending on the patient's condition, nutritional support in the cancer patient has two distinct objectives: (a) provision of nutrition during anticancer therapies to counteract their nutritionally related side effects and improve outcome following these therapies; (b) provide support in patients with long-term or permanent severe impairment of the gastrointestinal tract. In these patients nutritional support may be required for indefinite periods of time. Results of numerous clinical trials support the use of nutritional support only in limited situations during anticancer therapies. In the group with prolonged gastrointestinal failure, nutrition support may be a lifesaving therapy because patients could die of starvation without TPN or enteral feeding.

Total Parenteral Nutrition

TPN is an effective method for delivery of nutrients directly into the blood, and thus overcomes the major causes of cancer cachexia, including decreased food intake and dysfunction of the gastrointestinal tract. Survival for more than 20 years in patients nourished exclusively by TPN clearly demonstrates the lifesaving role of this method of nutritional support. Initially, it seemed logical that TPN would be an effective adjuvant therapy for most cancer patients undergoing radiation therapy, surgery, or chemotherapy because of the accompanying cachexia and inability to eat adequately. Randomized studies, however, have shown that TPN only benefits a select subgroup of cancer patients during anticancer therapy.

Efficacy

In patients receiving chemotherapy with or without radiation therapy TPN can lead to improvements of several nutritional parameters. Both body weight and body fat increase (90). Deficits of specific vitamins, minerals, and trace elements can be corrected and hydration status can be improved (90,100). TPN, however, does not alter many of the metabolic derangements encountered in the cancer patient. Increased glucose oxidation and turnover persist (73,101) as does muscle proteolysis (102,103) and increased lipolysis (104). Finally, TPN is does not stop the overall losses of body nitrogen (105). The relevant issue for the clinician is the effect of TPN on the morbidity and mortality associated with cancer therapy and whether TPN can allow more intense therapy as was initially hoped. Numerous randomized trials have examined this issue. Studies of patients undergoing chemotherapy for carcinoma of the ovary (29), lung (106,107), colon (105), testes (108), lymphoma (109), and other tumors (110) have been conducted. However, the patients in these studies were largely unselected. Many were not malnourished and others had adequate oral intake with intact gastrointestinal function, thus making intravenous nutrition unnecessary, futile, and potentially harmful. Numerous meta-analyses concluded that nondiscriminatory use of TPN in patients undergoing chemotherapy offers no improvement in mortality, response to chemotherapy, or reduction in treatment-associated complications (111–113). This conclusion was echoed in a recent joint consensus statement from the National Institutes of Health, the American Society for Parenteral and Enteral Nutrition, and the American Society for Clinical Nutrition (114). The improvement in nutritional parameters afforded by TPN in patients receiving chemotherapy is not necessarily translated into improved clinical outcome. Thus, the routine use of TPN in these patients is not indicated. There are circumstances, however, in which nutritional support with parenteral nutrition should be considered. These include prevention of the effects of starvation in a patient unable to tolerate oral or enteral feedings for a prolonged period of time (usually more than 7 to 10 days), maximization of performance status in a malnourished patient prior to chemotherapy or surgery, and in patients undergoing bone marrow transplantation (115).

TPN may have a stimulatory effect on tumor cell cycle kinetics (116). It was hoped that this effect would induce improved tumor response to cell cycle–specific chemotherapy. Conclusive proof of such a response remains elusive.

A few randomized studies have examined the use of TPN in patients receiving radiotherapy to the abdomen and pelvis (117–120). These studies did not show any clear benefit from the routine administration of TPN.

The role of TPN in the perioperative period has been extensively studied (16,17,121–125). In an early study by Mueller et al. (125), 10 days of preoperative TPN was associated with nutritional improvement and significant reduction in major postoperative complications and mortality. These impressive results have not been confirmed in subsequent studies. At Memorial Sloan-Kettering Cancer Center, a prospective study of 117 patients undergoing curative resection for pancreatic cancer randomized to receive TPN or intravenous fluids in the postoperative period showed no benefit from routine use of postoperative TPN (17). The group receiving TPN had a significant increase in postoperative infectious complications. The largest prospective, randomized trial investigating the role of TPN in the perioperative setting was the Veterans Administration Cooperative Study (16). In this study 395 patients were randomized to receive 7 to 15 days preoperative and 3 days postoperative TPN, or oral feeding plus intravenous fluids. TPN did not improve morbidity or 90-day mortality. However, subgroup analysis showed that patients considered to be severely malnourished had fewer infectious complications if they received TPN. The authors concluded that the routine administration of preoperative TPN should be limited to patients who are severely malnourished unless there are other specific indications.

Randomized studies specifically examining the role of perioperative TPN in patients with gynecologic malignancies are lacking. In a report by Terada et al. (25), perioperative parenteral nutritional support was given to 84 of 99 patients. There were no major complications attributed to TPN, but 27% of the patients experienced minor complications: 11% due to central line placement or catheter sepsis, 2% due to fluid overload, and 13% had metabolic complications. There was no report on overall perioperative morbidity or mortality in comparison to patients who did not receive perioperative TPN.

These data and others provide the basis for the recent joint consensus statement from the National Institutes of Health, the American Society for Parenteral and Enteral Nutrition, and the American Society for Clinical Nutrition regarding the use of perioperative TPN, which states the following: (a) 7 to 10 days of preoperative TPN in a malnourished patient with gastrointestinal cancer results in a 10% reduction in postoperative complications; (b) routine use of postoperative TPN in malnourished surgical patients who did not receive preoperative TPN results in a 10% *increase* in complications; (c) if by postoperative day 5 to 10, a patient is unable to tolerate oral or enteral feedings then TPN is indicated to prevent the adverse effects of starvation. This panel, however, cautions that in the majority of studies looking at perioperative TPN the amount and type of parenteral nutrition given was not optimal, and often patients were given excess calories. Therefore, the results may differ with the provision of relatively hypocaloric formulas (114). It is reasonable to extend these recommendations to the gynecologic oncology patient undergoing surgery (Table 33.1).

Composition of TPN Solution

Once the decision to proceed with parenteral nutritional support is made, access to a large-bore central vein should be obtained. This allows the use of calorically dense, hypertonic solutions, which are often necessary in severely ill patients who may have restriction on the amount of intravenous fluids they can receive. When possible, this line should be used exclusively for TPN infusion and should be treated with strict aseptic technique. The composition of the TPN solution should be individualized based on the patient's condition and requirements, preferably by a dedicated nutrition support team (126). The solution must provide the protein and caloric needs, fluid, minerals, trace elements, and vitamins. Although indirect calorimetry and nitrogen balance can be used to determine energy and protein requirements, they are too costly and cumbersome for routine use. There are numerous formulas, charts, and tables that can provide estimates of protein and calorie requirements. Estimates of nutrition requirements are based on weight and adjusted for the degree of physiologic stress encountered by the patient. Generally, patients require 30 Kcal/kg nonprotein calories, 1 g/kg amino acids, and about 2,000 mL of fluid. As illness severity increases and organ functions change, adjustments may be required. Thus, patients with kidney or liver failure require decreased amounts of amino acids while those with heart failure require restriction of sodium and fluids. Nonprotein calories can be provided as dextrose or lipid and the relative amounts of these should also be individualized. Lipids provide 9 Kcal/g compared to 3.4 for dextrose. (In dextrose solutions the glucose is present as glucose-monohydrate, hence a gram contains less than 4 Kcal.) Lipid calories are particularly useful in patients who have high caloric requirements but cannot

TABLE 33.1

INDICATIONS FOR TPN IN HOSPITALIZED PATIENTS WITH GYNECOLOGIC CANCERS

Perioperative	Seven to 10 days preoperatively in a malnourished patient (who cannot be fed enterally) Postoperative complications that prevent oral or enteral intake for more than 7 to 10 days Enterocutaneous fistula *No* indication for routine use
During radiation or chemotherapy	Maximization of performance status prior to therapy in a malnourished patient who cannot be fed enterally Severe persistent (more than 7 to 10 days) mucositis, diarrhea, ileus, or emesis *No* indication for routine use
General	After 7 to 10 days of inability to tolerate oral or enteral feeding due to any cause

Note: TPN, total parenteral nutrition.

tolerate a large fluid load. In addition, lipids are useful in patients with severe pulmonary or hepatic dysfunction as glucose metabolism produces more carbon dioxide, which can add to the burden of the ailing lung and can lead to fatty infiltration of the liver. Up to 60% of caloric requirements can be provided as lipid, but serum triglyceride levels must be monitored closely. Appropriate electrolyte content of TPN solutions is of critical importance. The amounts have to be tailored to the patient's requirements and organ function. Care must be taken to prevent potentially fatal hypokalemia or hypophosphatemia (particularly in the patient with severe weight loss), which can be precipitated by insulin-induced transport of the minerals to the intracellular space when inadequate amounts are given. Other electrolyte disorders such as cisplatin-induced hypomagnesemia and syndrome of inappropriate antidiuretic hormone secretion (SIADH) are common in the patient with gynecologic malignancy and must be addressed when ordering TPN. The TPN solution must also contain vitamins, minerals, and trace elements. Typically these are available as standard commercial combination products. However, certain patients require specific modifications. For example, a patient with persistent diarrhea requires zinc supplementation in excess of the amounts present in standard trace element solutions.

Complications

Complications associated with TPN can be classified as catheter related, metabolic, or infectious. Catheter complications most often occur during placement of a central venous catheter and include pneumothorax, hemothorax, arterial injury, and hematoma. These can all be minimized when the procedure is performed by an experienced physician (127). Cobb et al. (128) reported a 3% incidence of pneumothorax, arrhythmia, thrombus, or bleeding during 523 intravenous catheter placements. A more recent study of subcutaneous peripheral infusion ports in women with gynecologic malignancies demonstrated a thrombosis rate of 26% during a mean follow-up of 105 days. The authors concluded that other types of vascular access devices may be preferable in this patient population (129).

Metabolic derangements are frequently encountered during support with TPN and the prescribing physician must be well versed in the pathophysiology of these disorders. Hyperglycemia is the most common abnormality (127) and if not corrected can lead to an osmotic diuresis, dehydration, acidosis, and hyperosmolar coma. Patients receiving parenteral nutrition should have continuous monitoring for glycosuria and if the dipstick is positive, the blood sugar concentration should be determined and sliding scale insulin coverage should be provided. One metabolic complication that deserves special mention is the "refeeding syndrome." In chronically ill patients with severe malnutrition there is often a depletion of total body phosphorus and potassium. The phosphorous deficits may be masked by increased renal phosphorous absorption designed to maintain normal serum levels. When TPN is initiated the infusion of a large glucose load with subsequent surge in insulin leads to increased cellular uptake of phosphorous and potassium, which may induce severe life-threatening hypokalemia and hypophosphatemia (130,131). These disorders cause widespread tissue and organ dysfunction including muscle weakness, rhabdomyolysis, heart failure, cardiac arrhythmias, and respiratory failure and may result in death in extreme cases (131). Therefore, in patients with evidence of severe undernutrition, TPN should be initiated with small amounts of dextrose calories, supplemental phosphorous and potassium, and careful monitoring of serum phosphorous and electrolytes.

TPN has been associated with cholestatic liver disease as well as fatty infiltration of the liver and glycogen deposition. These abnormalities have been attributed to infusion of excessive glucose calories, imbalance of amino acids, and rarely fatty acid deficiency (132). Elevation of serum transaminases may occur but it is generally mild (132,133). Severe liver dysfunction in adult TPN recipients is rare and requires a search for causes other than TPN.

Infections are particularly serious complications in patients with malignancy receiving TPN. In an evaluation of seven studies comparing TPN plus chemotherapy to chemotherapy alone, Klein and Koretz found four studies that showed an increase in infectious complications in patients receiving TPN (119). A meta-analysis by the American College of Nutrition showed a fourfold increase in infections when patients receiving chemotherapy were given TPN (111). In a prospective, randomized study of TPN following pancreatic resection, recipients of TPN had significantly more infectious complications (17). Data from a Veteran's Administration randomized cooperative study showed that patients with mild to moderate malnutrition given perioperative TPN had increased rates of infections, while those with severe malnutrition developed significantly fewer infections when supported with TPN (16). Infectious complications are related to both central venous catheters and a variety of sites (wound infection, abscess, and pneumonia). While there are now promising data to show that the use of catheters impregnated with antimicrobials may provide a significant reduction of catheter-related sepsis (134), it is not clear that the use of these catheters will eliminate the increase in infections in patients receiving TPN.

Home TPN

Long-term TPN in the home can be a lifesaving treatment in an appropriately selected group of patients. It is clear that cancer patients who have had severe gastrointestinal injury, such as massive intestinal resection or severe radiation enteritis, and in whom the cancer has been cured or is well controlled, benefit from long-term TPN at home (135). Survival rates and TPN-related complications in such patients are comparable to those seen in patients with benign diseases (Crohn's disease, intestinal necrosis) who require home TPN. Among patients with widely metastatic disease and poor prognosis, home TPN offers very limited benefit (103). Only 15% of such patients survive longer than 1 year on home TPN (48). Recently developed techniques for placing feeding tubes make it possible to hydrate and feed patients enterally, even in the presence of gastrointestinal obstruction (115), and thus obviate the need for home TPN in patients with upper gastrointestinal tract dysfunction. In terminally ill patients TPN should be avoided. The concern that such patients should not be "starved to death" is not a justification for TPN. A recent uncontrolled study of terminally ill cancer patients hospitalized at a long-term care facility suggests that these patients did not experience hunger or thirst, and that in those who experienced such symptoms, small amounts of food alleviated the symptoms (136). In such patients the utilization of TPN either in the home or at health care facilities cannot be justified.

At Memorial Sloan-Kettering Cancer Center the clinical nutrition service prescribed home TPN for 20 patients with gynecologic malignancies (3 cervical, 15 ovarian, and 2 endometrial) from 1995 through 1998. This represented 9% of all cancer patients given this therapy. The indications for home TPN included bowel obstruction (ten patients), enterocutaneous fistula (seven patients), radiation enteritis (two patients), and short bowel syndrome (one patient). These patients were given home TPN because they had a good performance status or were considered candidates for further antitumor therapies. On average, they received home TPN for 163 days. Thirteen of the patients were able to resume oral or enteral feedings in amounts sufficient to sustain themselves after additional

TABLE 33.2

INDICATIONS FOR HOME TPN IN PATIENTS WITH GYNECOLOGIC CANCERS

Severe chronic radiation enteropathy
Short bowel syndrome
Persistent enterocutaneous fistula
Selected patients with obstruction due to peritoneal carcinomatosis (selection based on performance status and potential for further chemotherapy)

therapy and seven patients died while still dependent on TPN.

For patients with inoperable bowel obstruction due to metastatic ovarian cancer, predicting which patients will benefit from home TPN can be difficult (137). In a review of 9,897 days of home TPN administered to 75 patients with various cancers and intestinal obstruction it was shown that a Karnofsky performance status greater than 50 at the initiation of TPN could accurately predict which patients would have improved quality of life while on home TPN. The authors concluded that home TPN should be avoided if the performance status is below this level (138). In addition, patients with a life expectancy of less than 2 to 3 months will not benefit from home TPN (103,138). In a study from Yale-New Haven Hospital of 17 patients with inoperable bowel obstruction due to malignancy, patients with ovarian cancer had the shortest survival (39 days) compared to patients with colon cancer (90 days) and appendiceal cancer (184 days) (139). Therefore, only a highly selected minority of patients with inoperable bowel obstruction can potentially benefit from home TPN. A recent study from Brown University evaluated 55 patients with terminal ovarian cancer and found that the use of TPN conferred a median survival benefit of 4 weeks (140). Currently the best selection criteria for such patients are a fair or better performance status and the potential for further antitumor therapy (Table 33.2).

Enteral Nutrition

Enteral feeding delivers a liquid-nutrient formula into the gastrointestinal tract through tubes placed into the stomach or small intestine. As in oral feeding, an adequately functioning small intestinal mucosa is required for absorption of nutrients. Enteral feeding can overcome many difficulties encountered in patients with a wide variety of gastrointestinal tract dysfunctions. A proximal gastrointestinal obstruction can be bypassed; tubes can be placed distal to obstructions as far as the jejunum and thus circumvent obstructing lesions of the oral cavity, esophagus, stomach, duodenum, or proximal jejunum (141,142). The liquid-nutrient formula can be delivered as a slow, continuous infusion, thus maximizing absorption by a limited intestinal surface, which can be overwhelmed by the higher volume delivered during oral feeding. Such an approach may be useful in patients with radiation enteritis, short bowel syndrome (with adequate remaining short bowel, usually 3 to 4 feet), or partial obstruction of the bowel.

Route of Administration and Nutrient Formula

Short-term (<2 weeks) access to the gastrointestinal tract can be obtained through nasogastric or nasoenteric tubes. Patients requiring longer nutritional support should have a gastrostomy or jejunostomy tube placed endoscopically, radiologically, or surgically. In comparison to nasal tubes, gastrostomy or jejunostomy tubes are wider (15 to 24 French) and therefore less likely to be obstructed by medications or nutrient solutions. In addition, they are fixed in the stomach or the upper intestine and do not migrate into the esophagus. Thus, the risk of aspiration is considerably decreased (141). These tubes are more comfortable and aesthetically pleasing (143). These benefits were demonstrated in a recent randomized study of patients after an acute dysphagic stroke, which showed that patients fed with a gastrostomy tube had more optimal provision of nutrients, achieved a better nutritional state, and had less mortality than those fed with nasogastric tubes (144). Patients with gastrostomy tubes have been shown in prospective studies to receive over 90% of prescribed feedings compared to only 55% in patients fed through nasal tubes. These differences are largely attributed to nasogastric tube dislodgment (145). In a randomized study of 33 women with gynecologic malignancies, enteral feedings through a needle catheter jejunostomy maintained postoperative nutrition as measured by serum transferrin levels and was associated with few complications (146). The authors concluded that women with gynecologic cancers should have a jejunostomy placed at the time of operation if it is anticipated that long-term nutritional support will be required.

Endoscopically placed percutaneous gastrostomy tube (PEG) has become the procedure of choice for placement of enteral feeding tubes because of its ease, safety, and the ability to perform it on an outpatient basis. Percutaneous jejunostomy (PEJ) tubes can also be placed endoscopically (142). PEJs allow for continued enteral feeding in patients with gastric resection, gastric outlet obstruction, or gastroparesis. Major complications (bleeding, peritonitis, abdominal wall abscess, colonic perforation, and aspiration) from PEG and PEJ placement are rare, occurring in 0% to 2.5% of patients, while minor complications (wound infection, tube migrations, or leak) are seen in 5% to 15% (65,142,147,148). This favorably compares to the 2.5% to 16% complication rate and 1% to 6% mortality from a laparotomy required for surgical placement of feeding tubes (149–151).

More than 100 different enteral feeding formulas are currently commercially available (152). They are designed to provide either complete nutrition, single nutrients, or only fluids and electrolytes. Formulas differ in protein concentration, calories, osmolarity, and percentage of nonprotein calories delivered as carbohydrates or fats. Enteral feeding formulas that provide 1,500 to 2,000 Kcal per day normally contain all the necessary nutrients including proteins, vitamins, minerals, and trace elements. In addition, there are disease-specific formulations for patients with diabetes or hepatic, renal, or pulmonary dysfunction. The choice of formula should be individualized and often helps to minimize problems such as diarrhea, bloating, or hyperglycemia (141).

Enteral solutions may be administered by either bolus feedings or by continuous infusion (141,149,150). Bolus feeding is possible when the tip of the feeding tube is in an intact stomach. Up to 500 mL of a feeding formula can be infused over 10 to 15 minutes by a syringe or gravity into the stomach. The pyloric sphincter regulates flow into the duodenum. All bolus feedings should be done with the patient sitting upright to minimize the risk of aspiration. When the tip of the feeding tube is distal to the pylorus, continuous feeding must be employed to avoid abdominal distention and diarrhea. Rates as high as 150 mL per hour are generally well tolerated (141).

Efficacy

Data from randomized trials examining the efficacy of enteral nutrition given as an adjuvant therapy in patients receiving chemotherapy for a variety of cancers have failed to demonstrate a clear benefit in terms of survival or response to treatment (153–157). The validity of the conclusions of these studies, however, is limited by their small size and poor design. Similar difficulties plague the studies examining the role of standard enteral nutrition in the perioperative period (158–161). While recent data examining early (postoperative day 1) enteral feeding in patients following resection of an upper gastrointestinal tract tumor showed improved protein metabolism, there is no evidence that this translates into improved clinical outcome (162). In a prospective, randomized study of early enteral feeding in 195 patients after resection of upper gastrointestinal malignancy there was no proven benefit. Complication rates, mortality, and length of hospital stay were not affected by early postoperative enteral feedings (163). Therefore, routine use of enteral nutrition support in patients receiving chemotherapy or undergoing operations for cancer cannot be justified. Accepted indications for enteral nutrition in cancer patients include (a) obstruction of the upper digestive tract in those who are not candidates for an operation, (b) the presence of chronic malnutrition due to inadequate oral intake, (c) perioperative support of the malnourished patient (164).

Complications

Enteral nutrition is generally safe if careful attention is paid to the following: (a) choice of an appropriate formula, (b) infusion into an appropriate portion of the gastrointestinal tract, (c) use of the correct infusion method, and (d) an ongoing clinical and metabolic monitoring of the patient. The most serious complication of enteral feeding is aspiration, which occurs in 1% to 32% of patients (153,165,166). The risk is minimized by keeping patients upright during bolus feedings and using jejunal feedings if there is predisposition for aspiration, gastroparesis, or an impaired gag reflex. Diarrhea is reported in 5% to 30% of patients receiving enteral nutrition (167). While the diarrhea may be related to underlying disorders of the gastrointestinal tract such as radiation enteritis or short bowel syndrome, a commonly overlooked cause is medications. Patients on enteral feeding often receive magnesium-containing antacids or antibiotics, both of which may induce diarrhea. Metabolic complications include dehydration, azotemia, hyperglycemia, and hyperkalemia. These are usually due to the patients' underlying disease and can be avoided with the choice of the proper formula and careful monitoring.

Home Enteral Nutrition

Home enteral nutrition (HEN) is increasingly being used to provide nutrients and fluids outside the hospital. Cancer is the most common indication for its use and accounts for 42% of all patients receiving HEN (135,141). It is a safe therapy in patients with cancer with only a 0.4% annual rate of complications requiring hospitalization (168). The overall 1-year survival for cancer patients on HEN is 30%. However, in patients with cancer of the head and neck who have been successfully treated, HEN has provided good nutrition for periods exceeding 7 years (65,141). Regular medical follow-up is essential to ensure appropriate functioning of the feeding tube and optimization of the nutrition regimen. This form of therapy is useful in patients with gynecologic malignancies with upper gastrointestinal tract obstructions that cannot be treated surgically.

Oral Dietary Therapy

Patients who are able to eat but have impairment of the gastrointestinal tract or have special metabolic requirements may benefit from a specialized oral dietary therapy (159). Often this may obviate the need for more costly and complex interventions such as parenteral nutrition. In oral dietary therapy the regular diet is modified based on the pathophysiologic changes induced by the underlying disorder with the goal of providing the most optimal nutrition possible (159). When the main problem is inadequate food consumption, various commercial oral supplements can be used but usually for only short periods because of taste fatigue. Some preparations provide complete nutrition while others are intended to supplement deficits of specific nutrients. Problems common in patients with gynecologic malignancies such as partial small bowel obstruction, chronic radiation enteritis, and short bowel syndrome may all be amenable to dietary therapies. In partial small bowel obstruction or motility dysfunction a diet comprised of frequent, small, calorically dense meals with minimal amounts of fiber is indicated. Patients with radiation enteritis should receive a low-fat, low-fiber, and lactose-free diet. Dietary management of short bowel syndrome patients includes frequent small meals; limitation of fiber, lactose, and simple sugars; taking liquids separately from meals; and supplementation of calcium and zinc orally and magnesium and vitamin B_{12} parenterally.

Bye et al. (169) conducted a prospective, randomized trial of a low-fat, low-lactose diet in 143 women with gynecologic malignancies undergoing radiation therapy. The intervention group had significantly less diarrhea. Diarrhea in the control group correlated with increased fatigue and decreased physical function. The authors concluded that diet intervention during radiotherapy reduced the severity of diarrhea, influenced patients' ability to cope with diarrhea, and gave them more control over their situation.

The successful implementation of prescribed diets depends to a large extent on a dietitian converting the prescribed diet to a meal plan and working with the patient to implement it. In a prospective, randomized study of 57 patients undergoing chemotherapy for ovarian, breast, or lung cancer, those who received intensive dietary counseling had improved long-term food intake (170). Similar data have been demonstrated in cancer patients undergoing radiotherapy (171) and in patients with acute leukemia undergoing induction chemotherapy (172).

Pharmacologic Agents

Agents that will reverse the wasting seen in advanced cancers have long been sought to complement or replace the provision of nutrients via the oral, enteral, or parenteral route. Hormones, appetite stimulants, and most recently, cytokine antagonists have been examined. Studies of growth hormone (173,174), insulin-like growth factor (IGF)-I alone (174), or IGF-I with insulin (175) in cancer-bearing rodent models showed significant attenuation of tumor-induced weight loss. In human clinical trials, these agents provided modest gain in weight but no improvement in quality of life and no other benefits (176).

Appetite Stimulants

Anabolic steroids have no proven efficacy in treating cancer cachexia. In a murine model, administration of norandrolone propionate resulted in weight gain but this was largely due to fluid retention (177). In human trials steroids produced transient improvement of nutritional parameters and appetite, but continued use is associated with negative nitrogen balance, net calcium loss, glucose intolerance, and immunosuppression (176).

Megestrol acetate is a progestational agent that has been shown to improve appetite and ameliorate weight loss in numerous but not all studies of patients with cancer and cachexia (176). Doses in these studies ranged from 160 mg per day to 1,200 mg per day, and maximal weight gain was generally seen within 8 weeks. However, the change in weight is largely due to increased adipose tissue and edema (178). Nevertheless, improvement in quality of life has consistently been demonstrated in several large, prospective studies in patients with cancer cachexia treated with megestrol acetate (179,180). It is generally well tolerated but can exacerbate underlying diabetes mellitus and rarely lead to adrenal suppression. Dronabinol, a marijuana derivative, has shown some promise in small studies, improving appetite and causing weight gain; however, large randomized trials are lacking (176). Food and Drug Administration (FDA) approval is currently limited to treatment of nausea and vomiting during chemotherapy and for cachexia in HIV-positive patients.

Cytokine Inhibitors

Inhibitors of cytokines involved in cancer cachexia and anorexia have the potential to be potent agents in the treatment of malnutrition in cancer. Monoclonal antibodies against TNF lead to improved food intake and diminished loss of protein and fat in murine models of cancer cachexia (168). Similar data are available for anti–interleukin-6 (anti–IL-6) (181,182) and anti–interferon-γ (anti–IFN-γ) (183). Suramin, a direct IL-6 receptor antagonist, decreased several key parameters of cachexia in tumor-bearing mice (184). A recent study from Japan of a novel inhibitor of IL-1 and TNF-α showed that direct injection of the drug into tumor did not alter tumor growth but did result in attenuation of loss of body weight and epididymal fat in tumor-bearing mice (185). Human studies utilizing the anticytokine approach are limited. Pentoxifylline and thalidomide have been shown to inhibit TNF-α, but only thalidomide improved weight loss associated with AIDS and tuberculosis (186). Interestingly, recent data show that the clinical anticachexia effect of megestrol acetate is due, at least in part, to inhibition of cytokines (Table 33.3) (99).

Drugs to Relieve Symptoms

The use of medications to relieve cancer or treatment-related symptoms that impair oral intake is an important adjuvant to nutritional support in these patients. For example, optimal antiemetic therapy can now adequately control acute and delayed emesis in 70% to 90% of patients (187). Despite this the incidence of chemotherapy-induced nausea and emesis is underestimated by oncologists and nurses (188). This highlights the importance of a careful history and review of systems when completing a nutritional evaluation of a cancer patient. Many cancer patients assume that nausea and vomiting are normal during treatment and will not report it as a problem unless specifically asked.

Antidepressant medications should be considered when evaluating a patient with cancer and malnutrition. Depression occurs in 25% to 45% of cancer patients and can lead to loss of appetite and weight loss (189). Pharmacotherapy for depression utilizing selective serotonin reuptake inhibitors or tricyclic antidepressants is effective in cancer patients (189). Methylphenidate, a stimulant, has also been shown to be effective for the treatment of cancer-related depression (190). Although the relief of depression may improve appetite, it should be noted that in patients without cancer, selective serotonin reuptake inhibitors and tricyclic antidepressants are associated with weight gain that is independent of the response of the

TABLE 33.3

PHARMACOLOGIC AGENTS USED FOR THE TREATMENT OF CANCER CACHEXIA AND ANOREXIA

Class of agent	Example	Efficacy	Adverse effects
Hormones	Insulin, IGF, GH	Attenuation of tumor-induced weight loss; *no* improvement in survival or quality of life demonstrated	Hypoglycemia, hypokalemia
Anabolic steroids	Oxandrolone, nandrolone	Transient improvement in appetite	Fluid retention; net loss of calcium and nitrogen; hyperglycemia, immunosuppression
Progestational agents	Megestrol acetate	Improved appetite, weight, and quality of life	Weight gain is mostly due to fluid retention and adipose tissue; may exacerbate diabetes mellitus; rare cases of adrenal insufficiency
Cannabinoids	Dronabinol	Improved appetite and weight gain in small studies	CNS effects (slurred speech, nausea, dizziness, sedation)
Cytokine inhibitors	Pentoxifylline, thalidomide, suramin, monoclonal antibodies to IL-1, IL-6, and TNF-α	Improved food intake and attenuation of protein loss in animal models	Clinical studies pending

Note: CNS, central nervous system; GH, growth hormone; IGF, insulin-like growth factor; IL, interleukin; TNF, tumor necrosis factor.

underlying depression (191). Pilot studies suggest that these drugs may also produce weight gain in patients with cancer (192). As for methylphenidate, it is associated with anorexia in patients without cancer; however, in patients with cancer-related depression and anorexia its use is associated with relief of anorexia (193). Therefore, methylphenidate can be used to treat depression in cancer patients with depression and malnutrition.

ETHICAL CONSIDERATIONS

Prior to the advent of enteral and parenteral feedings the inability to receive nutrients through oral intake inevitably led to wasting and death. Therefore, in the majority of patients the natural history of cancer led to death because of dehydration and starvation (194). In patients with potentially curable or stable disease, nutritional support, when indicated, is an important and often critical part of the overall treatment plan. On the other hand, the role of nutritional support in the terminally ill is a subject filled with ethical and legal dilemmas. These problems come to light when the wishes of the patient or the patient's representative are not in agreement with the recommendations of the physicians. For example, a patient may wish to forego nutritional support despite recommendations that such a therapy should be given. Alternatively, patients or their representatives may want to initiate or continue TPN even after all anticancer therapies have failed and the patient is in a terminal state. Two general principles apply: in the first case, autonomy, and in the second, medical futility.

Autonomy is the right of competent patients to make decisions about their care and implies that the physician must solicit these decisions. It was not until the mid-1960s, a time of vast societal changes and challenges to authority, that autonomy began to supersede the Hippocratic tradition with its emphasis on the authoritarian role of the physician. This principle is clearly outlined in a report from the President's Commission for the Study of Ethical Problems in Medicine and Biomedical and Behavioral Research, which states, "The voluntary choice of a competent and informed patient should determine whether or not life sustaining therapy will be undertaken, while healthcare institutions and professionals should try to enhance patients' abilities to make decisions on their own and to promote understanding of the available options" (195). With regard to most treatments (operations, chemotherapy, radiation therapy), the patient's knowledge and experience may be very limited and thus the physician's recommendations may form the sole basis for the patient's decisions. This is not the case with nutrition. People understand the role of nutrition in sustaining life and it is often hard for a layperson to understand why parenteral nutrition may not be indicated or even harmful when the patient has no other source of nourishment. In such situations it is the responsibility of the physician to thoroughly explain the reasons for withholding TPN.

The principle of medical futility often surfaces in discussions of nutritional support of the cancer patient, especially if the disease is advanced and unresponsive to therapy. There are four aspects to medical futility (196): (a) lack of physiologic rationale for the proposed therapy; (b) failure of the same therapy in a previous attempt; (c) all possible treatments for the underlying disease have failed; (d) the therapy will not improve quality of life or achieve a goal of care (such as living to see a particular life event). In the case of parenteral (and rarely enteral) nutritional support of the cancer patient, aspects (c) and (d) may be specifically applicable.

It should be noted that these principles, autonomy and medical futility, should govern decisions for both initiation and withdrawal of an ongoing therapy. As stated in the report from the President's Commission, "A justification that is adequate for not commencing a treatment is also sufficient for ceasing it. Moreover, establishing a higher requirement for cessation might unjustifiably discourage vigorous initial attempts to treat seriously ill patients that sometimes succeed" (195).

Religious beliefs will often strongly influence decisions regarding nutritional support. Publicly stated opinions on the subject include (a) a statement from the Archbishop of Canterbury that removal from life support was permitted if it was better to allow the patient to die (197); (b) a report from the National Conference of U.S. Catholic Bishops, which states that Catholics are not required to use extraordinary means when recovery is hopeless and only the burden of care remains (198); and (c) a review of Orthodox Jewish rabbinical decisions, which concluded, "the imperative to preserve life supersedes, with a few exceptions, quality of life considerations" (199).

For the gynecologic oncologist, management of the patient with an inoperable bowel obstruction due to peritoneal carcinomatosis is a difficult and recurrent problem. A recent review attempts to outline the role of parenteral nutrition in this population (137). TPN should be considered in only those patients with a good performance status, and careful attention must be paid to likely medical and symptomatic outcomes as well as ethical considerations. It is interesting to note the views of patients on various life-sustaining treatments. In a study from the University of Michigan, 90% of women undergoing treatment for a gynecologic cancer could envision a time when they would refuse ventilatory support, but only 37% could foresee a time when they would refuse artificial nutrition (200). It is important for the physician and other members of the health care team to inform the patient and the family that in the terminally ill, provision of food and water by enteral or parenteral routes will not improve comfort (136,176) and, in fact, may add to discomfort (136,201–203). At Memorial Sloan-Kettering Cancer Center TPN is used infrequently in patients with gynecologic cancer and bowel obstruction due to malignant carcinomatosis who do not receive any further anticancer therapy. TPN is used under these conditions only when it is judged that it will enhance the quality of life of a patient who is not at imminent risk of dying in spite of the widely metastatic disease. When considering the chance of improving the quality of life, the burden of TPN administration and monitoring and the risk of complications have to be considered.

References

1. Trosian M, Mullen JL. Nutritional assessment. In: Kaminski M, ed. *Hyperalimentation: A Guide for Clinicians*. New York: Marcel Dekker; 1985:47.
2. Nixon DW, Heymsfield SB, Cohen AE, et al. Protein-calorie undernutrition in hospitalized cancer patients. *Am J Med* 1980;69:491.
3. Dowd PS, Heatley RV. The influence of undernutrition on immunity. *Clin Sci Mol Med* 1984;66:241
4. Meakins JL, Christou NV, Shizgal HM, et al. Therapeutic approaches to anergy in surgical patients. *Ann Surg* 1979;190:286.
5. Mullen JL, Buzby GP, Waldman MT, et al. Prediction of operative morbidity and mortality by preoperative nutritional assessment. *Surg Forum* 1979;30:80.
6. Buzby GP, Mullen JL, Matthews DC, et al. Prognostic nutritional index in gastrointestinal surgery. *Am J Surg* 1980;139:160.
7. Baker JP, Detsky AS, Wesson DE, et al. Nutritional assessment: a comparison of clinical judgment and objective measurements. *N Engl J Med* 1982;306:969.
8. Detsky AS, Baker JP, O'Rourke K, et al. Predicting nutrition associated complications for patients undergoing gastrointestinal surgery. *JPEN* 1987;11:440.
9. Detsky AS, Baker JP, Mendelson RA, et al. Evaluating the accuracy of nutritional assessment techniques applied to hospitalized patients: methodology and comparisons. *JPEN* 1984;8:153.
10. Crowe PJ, Snyman AM, Dent DM, et al. Assessing malnutrition in gastric carcinoma: bioelectrical impedance or clinical impression? *Aust N Z J Surg* 1992;62:390.

11. Ottow RT, Bruining HA, Jeekel J. Clinical judgment versus delayed hypersensitivity skin testing for the prediction of postoperative sepsis and mortality. *Surg Gynecol Obestet* 1984;159:475.
12. Pettigrew RA, Hill GL. Indicators of surgical risk and clinical judgement. *Br J Surg* 1986;73:47.
13. Dewys WD, Begg C, Lavin PT, et al. Prognostic effect of weight loss prior to chemotherapy in cancer patients. *Am J Med* 1980;69:491.
14. Lanzotti VJ, Thomas DR, Boyle LE. Survival with inoperable lung cancer. *Cancer* 1977;39:303.
15. Ollenschlager G, Viell B, Thomas W, et al. Tumor anorexia: causes, assessment, treatment. *Recent Results Cancer Res* 1991;121:249.
16. Veterans Affairs Total Parenteral Nutrition Cooperative Study Group. Perioperative total parenteral nutrition in surgical patients. *N Engl J Med* 1991;325:525.
17. Brennan MF, Pisters PWT, Posner M, et al. A prospective randomized trial of total parenteral nutrition after major pancreatic resection for malignanacy. *Ann Surg* 1994;220:436.
18. Santoso JT, Canada T, Latson B, et al. Prognostic nutritional index in relation to hospital stay with gynecologic cancer. *Obstet Gynecol* 2000;95 (6 Pt 1):844–846.
19. Tunca JC. Nutritional evaluation of gynecologic cancer patients during initial diagnosis of their disease. *Am J Obstet Gynecol* 1983;147:893.
20. Orr JW Jr, Wilson K, Bodiford C, et al. Nutritional status of patients with untreated cervical cancer. I. Biochemical and immunologic assessment. *Am J Obstet Gynecol* 1985;151:625.
21. Orr JW Jr, Wilson K, Bodiford C, et al. Nutritional status of patients with untreated cervical cancer. II. Vitamin assessment. *Am J Obstet Gynecol* 1985;151:632.
22. Orr JW Jr, Wilson K, Bodiford C, et al. Corpus and cervix cancer: a nutritional comparison. *Am J Obstet Gynecol* 1985;153:775.
23. Warren RS, Starnes HF, Gabrilove JL, et al. The acute metabolic effects of tumor necrosis factor administration. *Arch Surg* 1987;122:1396.
24. Dempsey DT, Mullen JL, Buzby GP. The link between nutritional status and clinical outcome: can nutritional intervention modify it? *Am J Clin Nutr* 1985;47(Suppl 2):352.
25. Terada KY, Christen C, Roberts JA. Parenteral nutrition in gynecology. *J Reprod Med* 1988;33:957.
26. Burnett AF, Potkul RK, Barter JF, et al. Colonic surgery in gynecologic oncology. Risk factor analysis. *J Reprod Med* 1993;38:137.
27. Donato D, Angelides A, Irani H, et al. Infectious complications after gastrointestinal surgery in patients with ovarian carcinoma and malignant ascities. *Gynecol Oncol* 1992;44:40.
28. Massad LS, Vogler G, Herzog TJ, et al. Correlates of length of stay in gynecologic oncology patients undergoing inpatient surgery. *Gynecol Oncol* 1993;51:214.
29. Abu-Rustum NR, Barakat RR, Venkatraman E, et al. Chemotherapy and total parenteral nutrition for advanced ovarian cancer with bowel obstruction. *Gynecol Oncol* 1997;64:493.
30. Jong P, Sturgeon J, Jamieson CG. Benefit of palliative surgery for bowel obstruction in advanced ovarian cancer. *Can J Surg* 1995;38:454.
31. Zoetmulder FA, Helmerhorst TJ, Van Coevorden F, et al. Management of bowel obstruction in patients with advanced ovarian cancer. *Eur J Cancer* 1994;30A:1625.
32. Norton JA, Moley JF, Green MV, et al. Parabiotic transfer of cancer anorexia/cachexia in male rats. *Cancer Res* 1985;45:5547.
33. Carson JA, Gormican A. Taste acuity and food attitudes of selected patients with cancer. *J Am Diet Assoc* 1977;70:361.
34. Dewys WD. Anorexia as a general effect of cancer. *Cancer* 1979;43:2013.
35. Dewys WD, Walters K. Abnormalities of taste sensation in cancer patients. *Cancer* 1975;36:1988.
36. Trant AS, Serin J, Douglass HO. Is taste related to anorexia in cancer patients? *Am J Clin Nutr* 1982;36:45.
37. Bernstein IL. Neural mediation of food aversions and anorexia induced by tumor necrosis factor and tumors. *Neurosci Biobehav Rev* 1996;20:177.
38. Bernstein IL, Taylor EM, Bentson KL. TNF induced anorexia and learned food aversions are attenuated by area postrema lesions. *Am J Physiol* 1991;260:906.
39. Orr JW Jr, Shingleton HM, Hatch KD, et al. Gastrointestinal complications associated with pelvic exenteration. *Am J Obstet Gynecol* 1983; 145:325.
40. Turtel PS, Shike M. Diseases of the small bowel. In: Shils ME, Olsen JA, Shike M, et al., eds. *Modern Nutrition in Health and Disease*. 9th ed. Philadelphia: Williams & Wilkins; 1999:1151.
41. Scarantino CW, Ornitz RD, Hoffman LG, et al. On the mechanism of radiation-induced emesis: the role of serotonin. *Int J Radiat Oncol Biol Phys* 1994;30:825.
42. Bodis S, Alexander E 3rd, Kooy H, et al. The prevention of radiosurgery-induced nausea and vomiting by ondansetron: evidence of a direct effect on the central nervous system chemoreceptor trigger zone. *Surg Neurol* 1994;42:249.
43. Sedgwick DM, Howard GC, Ferguson A. Pathogenesis of acute radiation injury to the rectum. A prospective study in patients. *Int J Colorect Dis* 1994;9:23.
44. Kinsella TJ, Bloomer WD. Tolerance of the intestine to radiation therapy. *Surg Gynecol Obstet* 1980;151:273.
45. Loiudice TA, Lang JA. Treatment of radiation enteritis: a comparison study. *Am J Gastroenterol* 1983;78:481.
46. Libotte F, Autier P, Delmelle M, et al. Survival of patients with radiation enteritis of the small and large intestine. *Acta Chir Belg* 1995;95:190.
47. Yeoh E, Horowitz M, Russo A, et al. A retrospective study of the effects of pelvic irradiation for carcinoma of the cervix on gastrointestinal function. *Int J Radiat Onc Bio Phys* 1993;26:229.
48. Husebye E, Hauer-Jensen M, Kjorstad K, et al. Severe late radiation enteropathy is characterized by impaired motility of the proximal small intestine. *Dig Dis Sci* 1994;39:2341.
49. Danielson A, Nhylin H, Persson H, et al. Chronic diarrhoea after radiotherapy for gynaecological cancer: occurrence and aetiology. *Gut* 1991; 32:1180.
50. Kwitko AO, Pieterse AS, Hecker R, et al. Chronic radiation injury to the intestine: a clinico-pathological study. *Aust N Z J Med* 1982;12:272.
51. Curran WJ. Radiation-induced toxicities: the role of radioprotectants. *Semin Radiat Oncol* 1998;4(Suppl 1):2.
52. Kagei K, Tokuuye K, Okumura T, et al. Long-term results of proton beam therapy for carcinoma of the uterine cervix. *Int J Radiat Oncol Biol Phys* 2003;55(5):1265–1271.
53. Bajorin D, Kelsen D. Toxicity of antineoplastic therapy. In: Turnbull ADM, ed. *Surgical Emergencies in the Cancer Patient*. Chicago: Year Book Medical Publishers; 1987:14.
54. Mitchell EP, Schein PS. Gastrointestinal toxicity of chemotherapeutic agents. *Semin Oncol* 1982;9:52.
55. Calbresi P, Chabner B. Chemotherapy of neoplastic diseases. In: Gilman AG, Rall TW, Nies AS, et al., eds. *The Pharmacologic Basis of Therapeutics*. New York: Pergamon Press; 1990:1201.
56. Mattes RD, Curran WJ Jr, Alavi J, et al. Clinical implications of learned food aversions in patients with cancer treated with chemotherapy or radiation therapy. *Cancer* 1992;70:192.
57. Fletcher JC, Spencer EM. Incompetent on the slippery slope. *Lancet* 1995;345:271.
58. Arbiet JM, Lees DE, Corsey R, et al. Resting energy expenditure in controls and cancer patients with localized and diffuse disease. *Ann Surg* 1984;199:292.
59. Dempsey DT, Furer ID, Knox LS, et al. Energy expenditure in malnourished gastrointestinal cancer patients. *Cancer* 1984;53:1265.
60. Hansell DT, Davies JWL, Burns HJG. The relationship between resting energy expenditure and weight loss in benign and malignant disease. *Ann Surg* 1986;203:240.
61. Peacock JL, Inculet RI, Corsey R, et al. Resting energy expenditure and body cell mass alterations in sarcoma patients. *Surg Forum* 1986; 90:195.
62. Russel DM, Shike M, Marliss EB, et al. Effects of total parenteral nutrition and chemotherapy on the metabolic derangements in small cell lung cancer. *Cancer Res* 1984;44:1706.
63. Warnold I, Lundholm K, Schersten T. Energy balance and body composition in cancer patients. *Cancer Res* 1978;38:1801.
64. Gadducci A, Cosio S, Fanucchi A, et al. Malnutrition and cachexia in ovarian cancer patients: pathophysiology and management. *Anticancer Res* 2001;21(4B):2941–2947.
65. Shike M, Berner YN, Gerdes H, et al. Percutaneous endoscopic gastrostomy and jejunostomy for long-term feeding in patients with cancer of the head and neck. *Otolaryngol Head Neck Surg* 1989;101:549.
66. Lutetich JD, Mullen JL, Feurer ID, et al. Ablation of abnormal energy expenditure by curative tumor resection. *Arch Surg* 1990;125:337.
67. Dickerson RN, White KG, Curiello PG, et al. Resting energy expenditure of patients with gynecologic malignancies. *J Am Coll Nutr* 1995;15:448.
68. Holroyde CP, Gabuzda TG, Putnam RC, et al. Altered glucose metabolism in metastatic carcinoma. *Cancer Res* 1975;35:3710.
69. Holroyde CP, Skutches CL, Boden G, et al. Glucose metabolism in cachectic patients with colorectal cancer. *Cancer Res* 1984;44:5910.
70. Kern KA, Norton JA. Cancer cachexia. *JPEN* 1988;12:286.
71. Lundhohm K, Holm G, Schersten T. Insulin resistance in patients with cancer. *Cancer Res* 1978;38:4665.
72. Cersosimo E, Pisters PW, Pesola G. et al. The effect of graded doses of insulin on peripheral glucose uptake and lactate release in cancer cachexia. *Surgery* 1991;109:459.
73. Shaw JH, Wolfe RR. Glucose and urea kinetics in patients with early and advanced gastrointestinal cancer: the response to glucose infusion, parenteral feeding, and surgical resection. *Surgery* 1987;101:181.
74. Holroyde CP, Reichard GA. Carbohydrate metabolism in cancer cachexia. *Cancer Treat Rep* 1981;64:55.
75. Waterhouse C. Lactate metabolism in patients with cancer. *Cancer* 1974;33:66.
76. McAndrew PF. Fat metabolism and cancer. *Surg Clin North Am* 1986; 66:1003.
77. Beutler B, Cerami A. Cachectin and tumour necrosis factor as two sides of the same biological coin. *Nature* 1986;320:584.
78. Klein S, Wolfe RR. Whole-body lipolysis and triglyceride-fatty acid cycling in cachectic patients with esophageal cancer. *J Clin Invest* 1990; 86:1403.
79. Todorov PT, McDevitt TM, Meyer DJ, et al. Purification and characterization of a tumor lipid-mobilizing factor. *Cancer Res* 1998;58:2353.

80. Hirai K, Hussey HJ, Barber MD, et al. Biological evaluation of a lipid-mobilizing factor isolated from the urine of cancer patients. *Cancer Res* 1998;58:2359.
81. Sanders PM, Tisdale MJ. Effect of zinc-alpha2-glycoprotein (ZAG) on expression of uncoupling proteins in skeletal muscle and adipose tissue. *Cancer Lett* 2004;212:71.
82. Russell ST, Hirai K, Tisdale MJ. Role of beta3-adrenergic receptors in the action of a tumour lipid mobilizing factor. *Br J Cancer* 2002;86:424.
83. Bing C, Russell ST, Beckett EE, et al. Expression of uncoupling proteins-1, -2 and -3 mRNA is induced by an adenocarcinoma-derived lipid-mobilizing factor. *Br J Cancer* 2002;86:612.
84. Russell ST, Zimmerman TP, Domin BA, et al. Induction of lipolysis *in vitro* and loss of body fat *in vivo* by zinc-alpha2-glycoprotein. *Biochim Biophys Acta* 2004;1636:59.
85. Groundwater P, Beck SA, Barton C, et al. Alteration of serum and urinary lipolytic activity with weight loss in cachectic cancer patients. *Br J Cancer* 1990;62:816.
86. Beck SA, Groundwater P, Barton C, et al. Alterations in serum lipolytic activity of cancer patients with response to therapy. *Br J Cancer* 1990; 62:822.
87. Sanders PM, Tisdale MJ. Role of lipid-mobilising factor (LMF) in protecting tumour cells from oxidative damage. *Br J Cancer* 2004;90(6):1274.
88. Eden E, Ekman L, Bennegard K, et al. Whole body tyrosine flux in relation to energy expenditure in weight losing cancer patients. *Metabolism* 1984;33:1020.
89. Norton JA, Stein TP, Brennan MF. Whole body protein synthesis and turnover in normal man and malnourished patients with and without known cancer. *Ann Surg* 1981;194:123.
90. Shike M, Russel DM, Detsky A, et al. Changes in body composition in patients with small cell lung cancer. The effect of total parenteral nutrition as an adjunct to chemotherapy. *Ann Intern Med* 1984;101:303.
91. Hasselgren PO, Wray C, Mammen J. Molecular regulation of muscle cachexia: it may be more than the proteasome. *Biochem Biophys Res Commun* 2002;290:1.
92. Lorite MJ, Smith HJ, Arnold JA, et al. Activation of ATP-ubiquitin-dependent proteolysis in skeletal muscle *in vivo* and murine myoblasts *in vitro* by a proteolysis-inducing factor (PIF). *Br J Cancer* 2001;85:297.
93. Tilignac T, Temparis S, Combaret L, et al. Chemotherapy inhibits skeletal muscle ubiquitin-proteasome-dependent proteolysis. *Cancer Res* 2002;62: 7133.
94. Attaix D, Aurousseau E, Combaret L, et al. Ubiquitin-proteasome-dependent proteolysis in skeletal muscle. *Reprod Nutr Dev* 1998;38:153.
95. Warren RS, Donner DB, Starnes HF, et al. Modulation of endogenous hormone action by recombinant human tumor necrosis factor. *Proc Natl Acad Sci USA* 1987;84:8619.
96. Balkwill F, Osborne R, Burke F, et al. Evidence for tumor necrosis factor/cachectin production in cancer. *Lancet* 1987;1:1229.
97. Fong Y, Mildawer LL, Merano M, et al. Cachectin/TNF or IL-1a induces cachexia with redistribution of body protein. *Am J Physiol* 1989;256: R659.
98. Tracey KJ, Wei H, Manoque KR, et al. Cachectin/TNF induces cachexia, anorexia and inflammation. *J Exp Med* 1987;167:1211.
99. Mantovami G, Maccio A, Lai P, et al. Cytokine activity in cancer-related anorexia/cachexia: role of megestrol acetate and medroxyprogesterone acetate. *Semin Oncol* 1998;2(Suppl 6):45.
100. Lowry SF, Smith JC, Brennan MF. Zinc and copper replacement during total parenteral nutrition. *Am J Clin Nutr* 1981;34:1853.
101. Shaw JH, Humberstone DM, Wolfe RR. Energy and protein metabolism in sarcoma patients. *Ann Surg* 1988;207:283.
102. Jeevanandam M, Horowitz GS, Lowry SF, et al. Cancer cachexia and protein metabolism. *Lancet* 1984;1:1423.
103. Sharp JW, Roncagli T. Home parenteral nutrition in advanced cancer. *Cancer Pract* 1993;1:119.
104. Shaw JH, Wolfe RR. Fatty acid and glycerol kinetics in septic patients and in patients with gastrointestinal cancer. The response to glucose infusion and parenteral feeding. *Ann Surg* 1987;205:368.
105. Nixon DW, Moffitt S, Lawson DH, et al. Total parenteral nutrition as an adjunct to chemotherapy of metastatic colorectal cancer. *Cancer Treat Rep* 1981;65(Suppl 5):121.
106. Serrou B, Cupissol D, Plagne R, et al. Parenteral intravenous nutrition (PIVN) as an adjunct to chemotherapy in small cell anaplastic lung carcinoma. *Cancer Treat Rep* 1981;65(Suppl 5):151.
107. Valdivieso M, Bodner GP, Benjamin RS, et al. Role of intravenous hyperalimentation as an adjunct to intensive chemotherapy for small cell bronchogenic carcinoma. *Cancer Treat Rep* 1981;65(Suppl 5):154.
108. Samuels ML, Selig DE, Ogden S, et al. IV hyperalimentation and chemotherapy for stage III testicular cancer: A randomized study. *Cancer Treat Rep* 1981;65:615.
109. Daly JM, Reynolds J, Thom A, et al. Immune and metabolic effects of arginine in the surgical patient. *Ann Surg* 1988;208:512.
110. Fletcher JP, Little JM. A comparison of parenteral nutrition and early postoperative enteral feeding on the nitrogen balance after major surgery. *Surgery* 1986;100:21.
111. American College of Physicians position paper. Parenteral nutrition in patients receiving cancer chemotherapy. *Ann Intern Med* 1989;110:734.
112. Klein S, Simes J, Blackburn GL. Total parenteral nutrition and cancer clinical trials. *Cancer* 1986;58:1378.
113. McGeer AJ, Detsky AS, O'Rourke K. Parenteral nutrition in cancer patients undergoing chemotherapy: a meta-analysis. *Nutrition* 1990;6:233.
114. Klein S, Kinney J, Jeejeebhoy MB, et al. Nutrition support in clinical practice: review of published data and recommendations for future research directions. *Am J Clin Nutr* 1997;66:683.
115. Weisdorf SA, Lysne J, Wind D, et al. Positive effects of prophylactic total parenteral nutrition on long-term outcome of bone marrow transplantation. *Transplantation* 1987;43:833.
116. Baron PL, Lawrence W, Chan WM, et al. Effects of parenteral nutrition on cell cycle kinetics of head and neck cancer. *Arch Surg* 1986;121:1282.
117. Ghavimi F, Shils ME, Scott BF, et al. Prospective study of nutritional support during pelvic irradiation: comparison of children requiring abdominal radiation and chemotherapy with and without total parenteral nutrition. *J Pediatr* 1982;4:530.
118. Kinsella TJ, Malcom A, Bothe A, et al. Prospective study of nutrition support during pelvic irradiation. *Int J Radiat Oncol Biol Phys* 1981;7:543.
119. Klein S, Koretz RL. Nutrition support in patients with cancer: what do the data really show? *Nutr Clin Pract* 1994;9:91.
120. Van Eys J, Copeland EM, Cangier A, et al. A clinical trial of hyperalimentation in children with metastatic malignancies. *Med Pediatr Oncol* 1980;8:63.
121. Detsky AS, Baker JP, O'Rourke K, et al. Perioperative parenteral nutrition: a metanalysis. *Ann Intern Med* 1989;107:195.
122. Fan ST, Lo M, Lai ECS, et al. Perioperative nutritional support in patients undergoing hepatectomy for hepatocellular carcinoma. *N Engl J Med* 1994;331:1547.
123. Hotler AR, Fischer JE. The effects of perioperative hyperalimentation on complications in patients with carcinoma and weight loss. *J Surg Res* 1977;23:31.
124. Hotler AR, Rosen HM, Fischer JE. The effects of hyperalimentation on major surgery in malignant disease: a prospective study. *Acta Chir Scand* 1976;86(Suppl):466.
125. Mueller JM, Brenner U, Dienst C, et al. Perioperative parenteral feeding in patients with gastrointestinal cancer. *Lancet* 1982;1:68.
126. Trager SM, Willimas GB, Milliren G, et al. Total parenteral nutrition by a nutrition support team: improved quality of care. *JPEN* 1986;10:408.
127. Weisner RL, Bacon J, Butterworth LE. Central venous alimentation: a prospective study of the frequency of metabolic abnormalities among medical and surgical patients. *JPEN* 1982;6:421.
128. Cobb DK, High KP, Sawyer RG, et al. A controlled trial of scheduled replacement of central venous and pulmonary artery catheters. *N Engl J Med* 1992;327:1062.
129. Cunningham MJ, Collins MB, Kredentser DC, et al. Peripheral infusion ports for central venous access in patients with gynecologic malignancies. *Gynecol Oncol* 1996;60:397.
130. Solomon SM, Kirby DF. The refeeding syndrome: a review. *JPEN* 1990;14:90.
131. Weisner RL, Krumdieck CL. Death resulting from overzealous total parenteral nutrition: the refeeding syndrome revisted. *Am J Clin Nutr* 1981;34:393.
132. Lowry SF, Brennan MF. Abnormal liver function during parenteral nutrition: relation to infusion excess. *J Surg Res* 1979;26:300.
133. Burt ME, Lowry SF, Gorschboth C, et al. Metabolic alterations in noncachectic animal tumor systems. *Cancer* 1981;47:2138.
134. Darouiche RO, Issam IR, Heard SO, et al. A comparison of two antimicrobial-impregnated central venous catheters. *N Engl J Med* 1999;340:1.
135. Howard L, Ament M, Fleming R, et al. Current use and clinical outcome of home parenteral and enteral nutrition therapies in the United States. *Gastroenterology* 1995;109:355.
136. McCann RM, Hall WJ, Groth-Junker A. Comfort care for terminally ill patients. *JAMA* 1994;272:1263.
137. Philip J, Depczynski B. The role of total parenteral nutrition for patients with irreversible bowel obstruction secondary to gynecologic malignancy. *J Pain Sympt Manag* 1997;13:104.
138. Cozzaglio L, Balzola F, Cosentino F, et al. Outcome of cancer patients receiving home parenteral nutrition. Italian Society of Parenteral and Enteral Nutrition (S.I.N.P.E.) *JPEN* 1997;21:339.
139. August DA, Thorn D, Fisher RL, et al. Home parenteral nutrition for patients with inoperable malignant bowel obstruction. *JPEN* 1991;15:323.
140. Brard B, Weitzen S, Strubel-Lagan S, et al. The effect of total parenteral nutrition on the survival of terminally ill ovarian cancer patients. *Gynecol Oncol* 2006;103:176.
141. Shike M. Enteral feeding. In: Shils ME, Olsen JA, Shike M, et al., eds. *Modern Nutrition in Health and Disease.* 9th ed. Philadelphia: Williams & Wilkins; 1999:1643.
142. Shike M, Latkany L. Direct percutaneous endoscopic jejunostomy. *Gastro Endo Clin NA* 1998;8:569.
143. Daly JM. Malnutrition. In: Wilmore DW, Brennan MF, Harken AH, et al., eds. *Care of the Surgical Patient. Section VII: Special Problems in Perioperative Care.* New York: Scientific American, Inc.; 1994:1.
144. Norton B, Homer-Ward M, Donnelly MT, et al. A randomised prospective comparison of percutaneous endoscopic gastrostomy and nasogastric tube feeding after acute dysphagic stroke. *BMJ* 1996;312:13.

145. Di Lorenzo C, Lachman R, Hyman PE. Intravenous erythromycin for postpyloric intubation. *J Pediatr Gastroenterol Nutr* 1990;11:45.
146. Spirtos NM, Ballon SC. Needle catheter jejunostomy: a controlled, prospective, randomized trial in patients with gynecologic malignancy. *Am J Obstet Gynecol* 1988;158:1285.
147. Safadi BY, Marks JM, Ponsky JL. Percutaneous endoscopic gastrostomy. *Gastro Endo Clin NA* 1998;8:551.
148. Ponsky JL, Gauderer MW, Stellato TA. Percutaneous endoscopic gastrostomy. Review of 150 cases. *Arch Surg* 1983;118:913.
149. Gallagher MW, Tyson KR, Ashcraft AW. Gastrostomy in pediatric patients: an analysis of complications and techniques. *Surgery* 1973;74: 536.
150. Holder TM, Leape LL, Ashcraft KW. Gastrostomy: its use and dangers in pediatric patients. *N Engl J Med* 1972;286:1345.
151. Shellito PC, Malt RA. Tube gastrostomy. Techniques and complications. *Ann Surg* 1985;201:180.
152. Shils ME, Olsen JA, Shike M, et al., eds. *Modern Nutrition in Health and Disease.* 9th ed. Philadelphia: Williams & Wilkins; 1999:A-206.
153. Strong RM, Condon SC, Solinger MR, et al. Equal aspiration rates from postpylorus and intragastric-placed small-bore nasoenteric feeding tubes: a randomized, prospective study. *JPEN* 1992;16:59.
154. Evens WK, Nixon DW, Daly JM. A randomized study of oral nutritional support versus ad lib nutritional intake during chemotherapy for advanced colorectal and non-small-cell lung cancer. *J Clin Oncol* 1987;5:113.
155. Elkort RJ, Baker FL, Vitale JJ, et al. Long-term nutritional support as an adjunct to chemotherapy. *JPEN* 1981;5:385.
156. Bozzetti F. Effects of artificial nutrition on the nutritional status of cancer patients. *JPEN* 1989;4:406.
157. Bounous G, Gentile JM, Hugon J. Elemental diet in the management of the intestinal lesion produced by 5-fluorouracil in man. *Can J Surg* 1971;14:312.
158. Smith RC, Hartemink RJ, Hollinshead JW, et al. Fine bore jejunostomy feeding following major abdominal surgery: a controlled randomised clinical trial. *Br J Surg* 1985;72:458.
159. Shils ME, Shike M. Nutritional support of the cancer patient. In: Shils ME, Olsen JA, Shike M, et al., eds. *Modern Nutrition in Health and Disease.* 9th ed. Philadelphia: Williams & Wilkins; 1999:1297.
160. Ryan JA, Page CP, Babcock L. Early postoperative jejunal feeding of elemental diet in gastrointestinal surgery. *Am Surg* 1981;47:393.
161. Flynn MB, Leightty FF. Preoperative outpatient nutritional support of patients with squamous cancer of the upper aerodigestive tract. *Am J Surg* 1987;154:359.
162. Hochwald SN, Harrison LE, Heslin MJ, et al. Early postoperative enteral feeding improves whole body protein kinetics in upper gastrointestinal cancer patients. *Am J Surg* 1997;174:325.
163. Heslin MJ, Latkany L, Leung D, et al. A prospective, randomized trial of early enteral feeding after resection of upper gastrointestinal tract malignancy. *Ann Surg* 1997;226:577.
164. Kirby DF, Teran JC. Enteral feeding in critical care, gastrointestinal diseases, and cancer. *Gastro Endo Clin NA* 1998;8:623.
165. Mullan H, Roubenhoff RA, Roubenhoff R. Risk of pulmonary aspiration among patients receiving enteral nutrition support. *JPEN* 1992;16:160.
166. Montecalvo MA, Steger KA, Farber HW, et al. Nutritional outcome and pneumonia in critical care patients randomized to gastric versus jejunal tube feedings. The Critical Care Research Team. *Crit Care Med* 1992; 20:1377.
167. Bliss DZ, Guenter PA, Settle RG. Defining and reporting diarrhea in tube-fed patients—what a mess! *Am J Clin Nutr* 1992;55:753.
168. Sherry BA, Gelin J, Fong Y, et al. Anticachectin/tumor necrosis factor-alpha antibodies attenuate development of cachexia in tumor models. *FASEB J* 1989;3:1956.
169. Bye A, Ose T, Jaasa S. Quality of life during pelvic radiotherapy. *Acta Obstet Gynecol Scand* 1995;74:147.
170. Ovensen L, Allingstrup L, Hannibal J, et al. Effects of dietary counseling on food intake, body weight, response rate, survival, and quality of life in cancer patients undergoing chemotherapy: a prospective, randomized study. *J Clin Oncol* 1993;11:2043.
171. Macia E, Moran J, Santos J, et al. Nutritional evaluation and dietetic care in cancer patients treated with radiotherapy: prospective study. *Nutrition* 1991;7:205.
172. Ollenschlager G, Thomas W, Konkol K, et al. Nutritional behaviour and quality of life during oncological polychemotherapy: results of a prospective study on the efficacy of oral nutrition therapy in patients with acute leukemia. *Eur J Clin Invest* 1992;22:546.
173. Bartlett DL, Stein TP, Torosian MH. Effect of growth hormone and protein intake on tumor growth and host cachexia. *Surgery* 1995;117:260.
174. Ng EH, Rock CS, Lazarus DD, et al. Insulin-like growth factor preserves hast lean tissue mass in cancer cachexia. *Am J Physiol* 1992;262:R426.
175. Tomas FM, Chandler CS, Coyle P, et al. Effects of insulin and insulin-like growth factors on protein and energy metabolism in tumour-bearing rats. *Biochem J* 1994;301:769.
176. Ottery FD, Walsh D, Strwford A. Pharmacologic management of anorexia/cachexia. *Semin Oncol* 1998;25(2 Suppl 6):35.
177. Lyden E, Cvetkovska E, Westin T. Effects of nandrolone propionate on experimental tumor growth and cancer cachexia. *Metabolism* 1995; 44:445.
178. Strang P. The effect of megestrol acetate on anorexia, weight loss and cachexia in cancer and AIDS patients. *Anticancer Res* 1997;17:657.
179. Beller E, Tattersall M, Lumley T, et al. Improved quality of life with megestrol acetate in patients with endocrine-insensitive advanced cancer; a randomised placebo-controlled trial. Australasian Megestrol Acetate Cooperative Study Group. *Ann Oncol* 1997;8:277.
180. Skarlos DV, Fountzilas G, Pavlidis N, et al. Megestrol acetate in cancer patients with anorexia and weight loss. A Hellenic Co-operative Oncology Group (HeCOG) study. *Acta Oncol* 1993;32:37.
181. Fujimoto-Ouchi K, Tamura S, Mori K, et al. Establishment and characterization of cachexia-inducing and non-inducing clones of murine colon 26 carcinoma. *Int J Cancer* 1995;61:522.
182. Gelin J, Moldawer LL, Lonnroth C, et al. Role of endogenous tumor necrosis factor alpha and interleukin 1 for experimental tumor growth and the development of cancer cachexia. *Cancer Res* 1991;51:415.
183. Matthys P, Dijkmans R, Proost P, et al. Severe cachexia in mice inoculated with interferon-gamma-producing tumor cells. *Int J Cancer* 1991;49:77.
184. Strassmann G, Kambayashi T. Inhibition of experimental cancer cachexia by anti-cytokine and anti-cytokine receptor therapy. *Cytokines Mol Ther* 1995;1:107.
185. Yamamoto N, Kawamura I, Nishigaki F, et al. Effect of FR143430, a novel cytokine suppressive agent, on adenocarcinoma colon26-induced cachexia in mice. *Anticancer Res* 1998;18:139.
186. Haslett PA, Anticytokine approaches to the treatment of anorexia and cachexia. *Semin Oncol* 1998;2(Suppl 6):53.
187. Licitra L, Spinazze S, Roila F. Antiemetic therapy. *Crit Rev Oncol Hematol* 2002;43:93.
188. Grunberg SM, Deuson RR, Mavros P, et al. Incidence of chemotherapy-induced nausea and emesis after modern antiemetics. *Cancer* 2004;100: 2261.
189. Fisch M. Treatment of depression in cancer. *Natl Cancer Inst Monogr* 2004;(32):105.
190. Homsi J, Nelson KA, Sarhill N, et al. A phase II study of methylphenidate for depression in advanced cancer. *Am J Hosp Palliat Care* 2001;18:403.
191. Kulkarni SK, Kaur G. Pharmacodynamics of drug-induced weight gain. *Drugs Today* 2001;37:559.
192. Theobald DE, Kirsh KL, Holtsclaw E, et al. An open-label, crossover trial of mirtazapine (15 and 30 mg) in cancer patients with pain and other distressing symptoms. *J Pain Symptom Manage* 2002;23:442.
193. Fernandez F, Adams F. Methylphenidate treatment of patients with head and neck cancer. *Head Neck Surg* 1986;8:296.
194. Warren S. The immediate causes of death in cancer. *Am J Med Sci* 1932;184:610.
195. President's Commission for the Study of Ethical Problems in Medicine and Behavior Research. *Deciding to Forego Life-Sustaining Treatment. A Report on the Ethical, Medical, and Legal Issues in Treatment Decisions.* Washington, DC: United States Government Printing Office; 1983:3,61.
196. Shils ME. Nutrition and medical ethics: the interplay of medical decisions, patients' rights, and the judicial system. In: Shils ME, Olsen JA, Shike M, et al., eds. *Modern Nutrition in Health and Disease.* 9th ed. Philadelphia: Williams & Wilkins; 1999:1689.
197. Coggan HD. Edwin Stevens Lecture. On dying and dying well. Moral and spiritual aspects. *Proc R Soc Med* 1977;70:75.
198. Position of the American Dietetic Association: legal and ethical issues in feeding permanently unconscious patients. *J Am Diet Assoc* 1995;95:231.
199. Scostak RZ. Jewish ethical guidelines for resuscitation and artificial nutrition and hydration of the dying elderly. *J Med Ethics* 1994;20:93.
200. Brown D, Roberts JA, Elkins TE, et al. Hard choices: the gynecologic cancer patient's end-of-life preferences. *Gynecol Oncol* 1994;55:355.
201. Zerwekh JV. The dehydration question. *Nursing* 1983;13:47.
202. Schmitz P. The process of dying with and without feeding and fluids by tube. *Law Med Health Care* 1991;19:23.
203. Printz LA. Is withholding hydration a valid comfort measure in the terminally ill? *Geriatrics* 1988;43:84.

CHAPTER 34 ■ QUALITY OF LIFE ISSUES IN GYNECOLOGIC ONCOLOGY

LARI WENZEL, RICHARD PENSON, JEANNE CARTER, DANA CHASE, AND DAVID CELLA

INTRODUCTION

Health-related quality of life (QOL) is an increasingly important endpoint in clinical trials, and a fundamentally important issue for patients. Quality of life is a multifaceted and complex paradigm that reflects patient's experiences with disease, treatment, and accompanying long-term sequelae (1,2). While a specific definition of quality of life may require articulating the patient's status on physical, functional, emotional, and social well-being (3), it can also encompass the disparate aspects of patient demography (age, ethnicity, education, income), social circumstances (relationships and roles), and spiritual issues. It is no longer acceptable to pursue curative treatment with the hope of improving mortality without consideration of treatment morbidity, and without including patient-centered decision-making and quality of life implications. Therefore, this chapter provides an overview of state-of-the-science perspectives broadly incorporating medical interventions (e.g., recent clinical trials) which have influenced quality of life and other patient-reported outcomes, and gynecologic cancer survivorship issues, including several challenging symptoms (e.g., fatigue, neurotoxicity, lymphedema) and long-term concerns (e.g., sexual dysfunction, reproductive concerns, emotional well-being).

QUALITY OF LIFE

Quality of life is an abstract, multidimensional construct that covers the subjective perceptions of the positive and negative aspects of patients' experience. We all know good quality of life, but it is rarely simple. It integrates symptoms; physical, emotional, social, and cognitive functions; and reflects the impact of cancer and the side effects of treatment (4,5). Figure 34.1 lists elements of quality of life (6–8).

Considering well-being or quality of life is as old as Aristotle's concept of eudaimonia, or "good." The first attempt to quantitatively measure the impact of cancer was described in 1949, when Karnofsky and Burchenal reported a simple 11 (0 to 10) point scale for the clinical evaluation of chemotherapy. This was simplified into the ECOG (Eastern Cooperative Oncology Group) Zubrod scale (0 = asymptomatic, 1 = symptomatic, 2 = functional for >half the day, 3 = functional for <half the day, 4 = moribund), and performance status probably remains the single most significant bias that contributes to the big differences between the results of phase 2 studies (9). Early QOL studies rapidly revealed considerable discrepancy between observers and between the doctor's and his or her patient's evaluation of the patient's QOL, and it became clear that any method for measuring QOL, quintessentially subjective, would have to rely on patients themselves and not caregivers (10). Patient-reported outcomes (PROs) are now widely considered an excellent methodology to evaluate the utility of treatment. A simple composite measure of clinical benefit (measurements of pain [analgesic consumption and pain intensity], Karnofsky performance status, and weight) was used as the primary efficacy measure in a small but randomized study that led to Food and Drug Administration (FDA) approval of gemcitabine in advanced pancreatic cancer (11). Quality-adjusted time without symptoms of disease or toxicity of treatment (QTWIST) was an important addition as duration of symptoms, where they occur in the trajectory of the disease, and their source (disease or treatment) all influence their perception and impact (12). Recently, large randomized, controlled trials incorporating QOL endpoints have reported that docetaxel is associated with less neurotoxicity than paclitaxel (13), and erythropoietin (rHuEpo) significantly impacts anemia and fatigue (14). As physical functioning deteriorates, relational, spiritual, and psychologic issues become relatively more important (15,16).

Quality of life has been shown to predict survival in numerous disease settings (17,18). In the Heart and Soul Study, a study of outcomes in 1,024 patients with coronary artery disease, depressive symptoms were more predictive of overall health than conventional measures of cardiac function such as ejection fraction and ischemia (19). Recent work conducted within the Gynecologic Oncology Group (GOG) suggests that baseline QOL scores predict survival and may serve as an early barometer of patients who may or may not respond to aggressive treatment (20,21).

Quantitative measure of patient outcomes is dependent on the use of validated instruments of psychometric data. Such questionnaires, or scales, list items (questions about particular constructs) in related domains (dimension or focus of behavior or experience). Retesting between subjects and over time establishes reliability (test-retest, interobserver variation, and correlation with related instruments), responsiveness, and applicability (generalizability or external validity). Good scales have to be (a) internally consistent (similar domains report agreement—Cronbach's alpha ≥ 0.7), (b) stable (reliability coefficient), (c) equivalent or superior to other scales purporting to measure the same thing (kappa statistics), and (d) accepted by patients and experts. Approximately 500 instruments have been developed (22). Commonly used tools include the Functional Assessment of Cancer Therapy (FACT—with gynecologic and

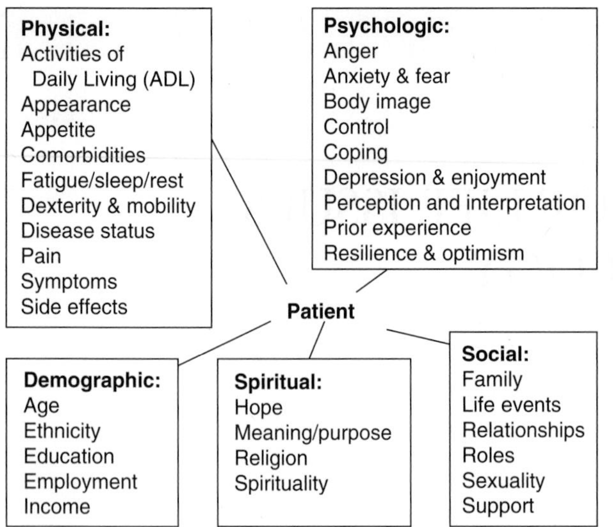

FIGURE 34.1. Elements of quality of life. *Note:* ADL, activities of daily living. *Source:* Modified from Ferrell B, Smith SL, Cullinane CA, et al. Psychological well being and quality of life in ovarian cancer survivors. *Cancer* 2003;98:1061–1071; Gralla RJ. Silk purse in Atlanta: a commentary on SWOG 9509, an advanced non-small cell lung cancer trial. *Oncologist* 1999;4:188–190; Kornblith AB, Thaler HT, Wong G, et al. Quality of life of women with ovarian cancer. *Gynecol Oncol* 1995;59:231–242.

symptom subscales), the European Organization for the Research and Treatment of Cancer QLQ-C30 (EORTC QLQ-C30), Hospital and Anxiety Depression Scale (HADS), Profile of Mood States (POMS), Rotterdam Symptom Checklist(RSCL), MOS-Short Form 36 (SF-36), and Visual Analogue Scale (VAS).

The Functional Assessment of Cancer Therapy (FACT) instrument (scale) is a 27- (generic core) to 50-item compilation of specific subscales, comprising physical, social/family, emotional, functional, and disease-specific well-being/concerns (http://www.facit.org/) (23,24). The EORTC also developed a similar QOL instrument consisting of a core component applicable to all cancer patients and modules developed for specific cancer sites (25). EuroQol-5Dimension (EQ5D) utilizes a brief five-item questionnaire covering mobility, self-care, usual activities, pain/discomfort, and anxiety/depression, and a thermometer visual analogue scale ranging from 0 (worst imaginable health state) to 100 (best imaginable health state) (26).

For much of the last decade the research agenda has been dominated by the comparison of instruments that evaluate the harder to measure aspects of clinical care (Fig. 34.2) (27,28). These studies have helped develop tools that have allowed important randomized clinical trials to now report QOL data (13,29). Formalizing the evaluation of health-related QOL is becoming established, with ongoing debate over methodology and the distillation of a minimum set of criteria for assessing outcomes in cancer clinical trials that inform decisions in clinical practice (30). New modeling approaches that account for nonrandom omission of data are beginning to be accepted (31). Evaluating QOL helps describe populations, predict outcomes, and guide decisions (trade-offs and gambles), and can screen for dysfunction, help allocate resources, and improve awareness as patients approach end-of-life issues (32).

A novel approach to patient-reported outcomes is now funded by the National Institutes of Health (NIH). The Patient-Reported Outcomes Measurement Information System (PROMIS) network, which is part of the NIH Roadmap Initiative, aims to improve how PROs are selected and assessed in clinical research. PROMIS is establishing a publicly available resource of self-reported health domain measures, including those specifically targeted to cancer. More information can be found at http://www.nihpromis.org/ (23). Additional useful resources for quality of life measurement include http://www.facit.org/, http://www.isoqol.org/, http://www.euroqol.org/, http://www.cancer.gov, and http://www.ql-recorder.com/.

QOL OUTCOMES AND CLINICAL TRIAL UPDATES FOR ENDOMETRIAL, CERVICAL, AND OVARIAN CANCER

Integrated multidisciplinary care has appropriately become the necessary standard of the complex care of patients frequently in specialist centers, with goals of care changing over the course of the disease (Fig. 34.3).

Endometrial Cancer

Recent literature has identified quality of life data that may inform therapeutic choices for women with endometrial cancer. In a recent study, advanced endometrial cancer patients were randomized to whole abdominal irradiation (WAI) versus doxorubicin-cisplatin (AP) chemotherapy. Although overall QOL did not differ between the two treatment groups, there were symptom-related differences (33). Specifically, WAI patients reported significantly higher fatigue than those who received

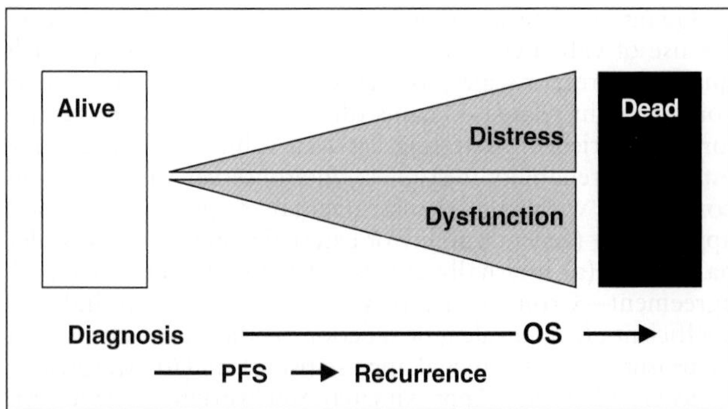

FIGURE 34.2. Health-related quality of life—measuring the grey outcomes. Black and white outcomes: PFS, progression-free survival; OS, overall survival.

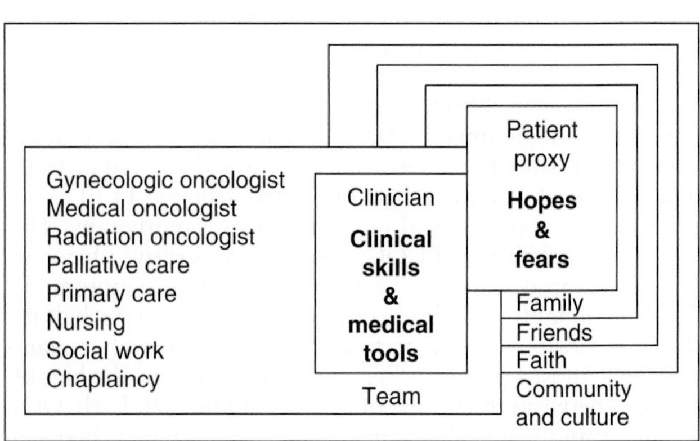

FIGURE 34.3. Holistic care.

AP chemotherapy for seven cycles plus an additional cycle of cisplatin alone. Significant differences in functional alterations due to changes in bowel function were identified at the end of treatment ($P < 0.01$), and at 3 months ($P < 0.01$), with radiation associated with poorer scores. However, the AP group showed significantly higher peripheral neuropathy scores at the end of treatment and at 3 and 6 months posttreatment compared to the WAI group ($p < 0.01$). Therefore, although doxorubicin-cisplatin showed increased survival, the authors emphasize that the patients should be counseled regarding significant peripheral neuropathy that may have a significant impact on QOL.

Notably, quality of life has also recently been evaluated in comparisons of laparoscopy versus laparotomy (34,35). In both studies, QOL was superior in the laparoscopy group. In the GOG LAP2 trial, which compared differences in quality of life between those endometrial cancer patients who underwent comprehensive surgical staging via laparoscopic technique versus traditional laparotomy, patients treated by laparoscopy had a superior quality of life through 6 weeks postsurgery compared to those treated by laparotomy, likely due to it being a less invasive procedure resulting in less pain, faster recovery, and a small but significant reduced length of hospital stay. However, except for a significantly better body image in the laparoscopy than the laparotomy group, these differences were not sustained at 6 months.

Cervical Cancer

In treatment of advanced cervical cancer, quality of life considerations are primary. Several recent studies have demonstrated important QOL results which have influenced clinical trial paradigms. For example, a randomized phase 3 trial demonstrated that although there was greater toxicity in the cisplatin/paclitaxel (CP) regimen, there was no statistically significant difference in overall QOL scores between this treatment arm and the cisplatin (C) single-agent regimen. This finding, combined with the improved response rate and progression-free survival (PFS) in the CP arm and a higher dropout rate in the C arm, suggests a worse outcome for the single-agent regimen. In this case QOL measurement contributed to the conclusion that CP is superior to C alone with respect to response rate, progression-free interval, and sustained or improved QOL for patients treated with cisplatin versus cisplatin plus paclitaxel (20,36).

Several other trials have reported quality of life as a secondary endpoint to use in addition to survival data when choosing chemotherapeutic regimens to treat advanced cervical cancer (37,38). These authors effectively argue that when determining if certain chemotherapy combinations may improve survival, it is critical to consider quality of life, as toxicity may worsen. One such study prospectively assessed the impact of treatment with cisplatin alone (C), versus C in combination with topotecan (C+T) on QOL in patients with advanced or recurrent cervical cancer, and explored the prognostic value of baseline QOL scores. Importantly, results from this study employing the FACT-Cx measure indicated there were no statistically significant differences in QOL up to 9 months postrandomization, despite more hematologic toxicity in the C+T arm. The baseline FACT-Cx was also associated with predicting survival (38). This was the first advanced cervical cancer study to note that patient-reported QOL measures may be an important prognostic tool in advanced cervix cancer. These phase 3 trials have challenged a traditional study design for chemotherapeutic agents by incorporating patient-reported outcomes into the interpretations and implications of the relative value of these regimens. Clearly, quality of life is a critical factor in palliative chemotherapy for recurrent and/or persistent advanced cervical cancer, where life expectancy is likely to be brief (36).

Ovarian Cancer

Several recent phase 3 clinical trials have included longitudinal assessment of quality of life as a secondary study endpoint. This information continues to influence a comprehensive interpretation of results, clinical trial design, and clinical decision making. For example, in a study of suboptimally debulked advanced ovarian cancer, although the addition of interval secondary cytoreduction to postoperative chemotherapy resulted in no notable long-term difference, a clinically significant QOL improvement was seen in both arms at 6 and 12 months after starting therapy. Of interest, fewer complaints of neurotoxicity at 6 months were reported among patients who did versus did not undergo interval secondary cytoreduction, likely due to the break in chemotherapy (39). In this study it was also shown for the first time in ovarian cancer that baseline QOL scores could predict survival, attributed primarily to the lowest scoring quartile on the FACT-O. QOL has also predicted survival for patients participating in a phase 3 trial comparing gemcitabine with pegylated liposomal doxorubicin (40).

A controversial randomized phase 3 trial in optimal stage III epithelial ovarian cancer showed that intravenous paclitaxel plus intraperitoneal cisplatin and paclitaxel significantly lengthened progression-free survival and overall survival compared to intravenous paclitaxel and cisplatin (41). During active treatment, patients on the intraperitoneal arm experienced more health-related quality of life disruption, abdominal discomfort, and neurotoxicity compared to those receiving conventional intravenous therapy. However, only neurotoxicity remained significantly greater for intraperitoneal patients 12 months posttreatment, and generally for both groups QOL improved over time (42). Given the continued controversy regarding intraperitoneal therapy, QOL information will continue to provide clinically meaningful information from which to guide treatment decisions.

Several additional recent phase 3 trials have incorporated quality of life endpoints into advanced ovarian cancer clinical trials (e.g., 43–48). For example, du Bois et al. compared paclitaxel plus cisplatin (PT) with paclitaxel plus carboplatin (TC) in patients with advanced ovarian cancer, evaluating QOL utilizing the EORTC QLQ-C30 questionnaire (45). There were significant QOL differences in favor of the TC arm, therefore leading to the conclusion that paclitaxel plus carboplatin is a more reasonable and better-tolerated treatment overall. In a subsequent study, Greimel et al. (47) examined hematologic and nonhematologic toxicity of the paclitaxel/carboplatin (TC) versus paclitaxel/cisplatin (PT) regimens, and the effects of toxicity on QOL. Again, quality of life was better in the TC regimen, resulting in confirmation that where two regimens have equal progression-free and overall survival, paclitaxel/carboplatin is preferable. A similar recommendation can be made from QOL data where it was demonstrated that gemcitabine plus carboplatin significantly improved progression-free survival and response rate without worsening QOL (44). The relationship between cancer treatment efficacy, benefit, and quality of life for elderly patients is also being studied. In one phase 3 trial comparing cisplatin and paclitaxel to carboplatin and paclitaxel, although quality of life scores did not differ between elderly and younger patients, the elderly patients showed a higher rate of early treatment discontinuation. The authors speculate that this may be due to provider and/or patient unwillingness to continue treatment in the setting of toxicities which might otherwise be managed differently in a younger population (49).

CHALLENGES IN GYNECOLOGIC CANCER SURVIVORSHIP

As noted previously, treatment side effects can influence short-term quality of life for many women, and longer if sequelae persist or worsen over time. Recognition of and management for these issues can vary from simple strategies to improve quality of life (i.e., managing nausea and vomiting), to complex psychosocial issues (e.g., reproductive concerns), for which clear guidelines may not exist. This section illustrates some of the current, potentially unique, and more complicated aspects of gynecologic cancer survivorship.

Pretreatment factors may influence a patient's quality of life both during and posttreatment. Several authors have noted that quality of life is affected by preoperative factors such as education, lifestyle, general health, and obesity (50–52), all of which in turn may affect a patient's ability to tolerate therapy. The interplay between cancer or cancer treatment symptoms and quality of life is well documented in the gynecologic cancer literature (e.g., 53,54). Several recent and/or prominent investigations deserve mention.

Although a considerable and growing body of literature exists specific to cognitive impairment and fatigue during and after chemotherapy, only recently has this been considered within the gynecologic cancer cohort. For example, Hensley et al. were the first to study cognitive functioning prospectively in an ovarian cancer trial (55). Although they did not find significant decreases in cognitive functioning in women receiving paclitaxel, gemcitabine, and carboplatin in a phase 2 trial, they did note that highly educated women might suffer greater impairments and thus future trials should include cognitive functioning measures in their quality of life assessments. Fatigue, during and subsequent to cancer treatment, is a related, prevalent, and understudied issue for gynecologic cancer patients.

Fatigue occurs in 70% to 100% of patients with cancer, and is often underdiagnosed, inadequately treated, and hard to disentangle from other symptoms of physical compromise and psychologic distress (56). Treatable causes of fatigue include anemia, malnutrition, medications, infections, pain, depression, insomnia, muscle dysfunction, and anticancer therapy (57,58). In a notably important QOL investigation, in 2,370 anemic cancer patients undergoing chemotherapy, recombinant human erythropoietin significantly improved patient-reported functional capacity and quality of life independent of tumor response (14). Many authorities also advocate either energy conservation or pushing apparent boundaries with graded exercise and cognitive-behavioral therapy (59). Psychostimulants, such as short- and long-acting methylphenidate, have been initially positive, but more rigorous studies have suggested that there is questionable benefit over placebo or daily telephone calls from a research nurse (60).

Neurotoxicity, an increasingly documented long-term problem, can cause sensory loss, pain, loss of function, loss of mobility, and for some women loss of professional and recreational activity. Platinum compounds, the mainstay of treatment for most gynecologic malignancies (61), are associated with cumulative myelosuppression (particularly thrombocytopenia), neurotoxicity, and nephrotoxicity, as well as severe nausea and vomiting (62,63). Neurotoxicity, anemia, and nausea/vomiting all have well-known adverse effects on QOL. Paclitaxel in combination with a platinum compound is now considered the standard of care as first-line chemotherapy for advanced ovarian cancer (64,65). However, paclitaxel has a number of toxicities (e.g., granulocytopenia, neurotoxicity) that synergistically overlap those of the platins, and the coadministration of paclitaxel and a platinum compound can increase the frequency and/or severity of shared toxicities, especially neurotoxicity. Docetaxel is associated with significantly less neurotoxicity (66).

Administration of glutamine or the antidepressant venlafaxine may be helpful in cases of paclitaxel-induced neuropathy, and amifostine may provide protection from cisplatin-induced neuropathy (67,68). However, at present there appears to be no drug available to reliably prevent or treat chemotherapy-induced neuropathy (67,69). Therapeutic interventions for neurotoxicity remain controversial with vitamins B_6 and E possibly reducing the efficacy of alkylator chemotherapy. Nonpharmacologic approaches to treatment of chemotherapy-induced neuropathy are based on patient education about potential neuropathic side effects, and the impact of these side effects on performance of daily activities and related safety issues (e.g., tripping in the dark, driving).

It is worth noting that a new, reliable, and valid patient-reported measure is now available to document symptoms of neurotoxicity. The FACT/GOG-NTX measure consists of 11 items assessing sensory, motor, and hearing symptoms as well as possible functional impact, and was administered to 263 advanced endometrial cancer patients prior to each of seven cycles of chemotherapy. Results of this study indicated that the patient-reported sensory symptom scores (sum of four item scores) increased significantly over the treatment duration ($p < 0.001$) in the paclitaxel/doxorubicin/cisplatin (TAP) arm compared to the doxorubicin/cisplatin (AP) arm. It was also noted that as few as four sensory symptoms in the FACT/GOG-NTX subscale can be used to reliably and sensitively assess chemotherapy-induced neurologic symptoms in clinical oncology without compromising the psychometric properties of the overall scale (70).

Lymphedema is a chronic, progressive condition in which protein-rich fluid accumulates in the superficial tissues of the body, ranging from a mild and reversible condition (stage 1) to chronic edema (stage 2), or a persistent condition with moderate to severe edema (stage 3) (71). The specific incidence of lower extremity lymphedema following treatment for gynecologic cancer as well as risk factors for development of lymphedema are not well documented in the literature, in contrast to research on upper extremity lymphedema (72). Several studies have estimated that lymphedema occurs in approximately one third of gynecologic patients treated for vulvar cancer (73,74). Recent findings from a retrospective study demonstrate that women treated with radical hysterectomy for cervical cancer were at an eightfold increased risk of developing lymphedema (75). Lymphedema in patients undergoing lymphadenectomy for endometrial cancer has been reported in the 5% to 10% range (76,77), although prospective data are sparse. Nodal sampling has also been documented as a factor in the development of symptomatic lymphedema (73,78), with an increased risk after removal of greater than ten or more regional nodes during surgical staging (79).

Studies examining the psychologic ramifications of lymphedema in other cancer cohorts (i.e., breast cancer) note that signs and symptoms may come as a shock if adequate information is not provided (80). Feelings of distress, anger, and helplessness emerge from limited and conflicting information (81,82). Many women are unaware of the risk factors, symptoms, and management of lymphedema (83). Furthermore, significant psychologic ramifications (i.e., anxiety, depression, and adjustment problems), as well as physical and sexual difficulties have been described in the literature (84). Untreated cluster symptoms (i.e., heaviness, swelling, and numbness) of lymphedema may contribute to poorer QOL (85,86). Additional issues of financial burdens (i.e., compression garments, medications, and bandages), limited clothing options, decreased activities due to restrictions from swollen legs, recurrent infection, and loss of work can also be problematic (87,88). Lymphedema may also be socially embarrassing or undermine confidence in appearance or body image (88). The chronicity of this condition also serves as a reminder of ones' cancer history, possibly heightening fear of recurrence or advancing disease (89).

Manual decompression therapy (massage and bandaging, or compression stockings) appears to help, but is an ongoing commitment. Other therapies are unproven. Lymphedema requires long-term management, and the psychomorbidity of lower extremity edema on a patient's quality of life can be significant. Future research should focus on prospective studies assessing the prevalence of lower extremity lymphedema following surgical staging and adjuvant therapy for gynecologic malignancy, which is a significant limitation in gynecologic oncology. This deficit prevents us from understanding not only the risk factors for lymphedema, but also the implications of this chronic condition on the emotional well-being and overall quality of life of cancer survivors.

Sexual dysfunction—all of the therapies associated with the treatment of gynecologic malignancies have been shown to interfere with multiple aspects of sexuality including body image, desire, frequency, satisfaction, vaginal dryness, dyspareunia, and a decrease in vaginal length. Intimacy can be disrupted and altered in the setting of a cancer diagnosis and treatment. The most common changes in sexual function for female cancer survivors include decreased libido or sexual interest and dyspareunia (90,91). Various surgical procedures can directly affect sexual functioning (92), depending on the anatomy involved. For women diagnosed with gynecologic cancer, surgery could involve the removal of the ovaries, uterus, cervix, vulva, and/or vagina. Surgical procedures may lead to damage to nerves as well as the possibility of scarring or adhesions in the pelvic area as part of the healing process. When ovaries are removed hormonal deprivation occurs, resulting in abrupt menopause for many women. Research on surgical treatment and sexual function demonstrates that hysterectomy for benign conditions does not appear to impair sexual function (93). Recent studies investigating sexual function after treatment for cervical cancer noted changes in lubrication, vaginal elasticity, pain, or arousal difficulties, much of which resolves by 1 year (94–96). However, vaginal dryness and decreased sexual satisfaction/interest have been shown to persist up to 2 years or more (95,96).

Abdominal and sexual sequelae have been reported in long-term survivors (97–99), since survivors may face the reality of surgical scarring and loss of body parts on a daily basis. Individuals receiving treatment for advanced disease or bowel obstruction may require the placement of temporary or permanent ostomy(ies) for urine or stool. Management of these appliances requires practice and support from medical specialists and often other patients (100). Radiation therapy can also have long-term adverse effects on sexual functioning. Issues of dyspareunia, vaginal stenosis, scarring, and fibrosis can emerge (101,102). Some authors note that chronic fibrotic changes to the pelvis may worsen vaginal atrophy over time, in some cases up to 5 or more years post radiation therapy (103).

Simple strategies have been shown to be helpful in rehabilitating sexual function with cancer survivors (104–106). The first step in restoring vaginal health should address using water-based vaginal lubricants, nonhormonal vaginal moisturizers, and pelvic floor exercises. For women with persistent vaginal dryness interfering with quality of life, a low-dose vaginal estrogen may be considered for a short time span, but many questions exist about hormone replacement in the setting of cancer. Low-dose vaginal estrogens may initially show a temporary increase in serum hormone levels, creating a complex and controversial issue for patients and medical professionals (107); however, these levels return to the normal postmenopausal range. This is not the case for systemic absorption of oral or transdermal administration of estrogen and testosterone (106,108). More safety data and long-term studies are needed in cancer populations.

For treatment of dyspareunia, vaginal dilators can be beneficial in treating vaginal stenosis and adhesions (104,109). Dilator therapy has been recommended as the only modality meeting reasonable standards for evidence-based medicine in the treatment of pelvic radiation–induced sexual dysfunction (110). The theory behind vaginal dilator therapy is that it mechanically stretches the vaginal tissues, allowing for the secondary remodeling of fibrotic tissue, thus improving elasticity. However, some authors question whether stimulation of the vaginal walls improves blood flow to the affected area (106). More research is warranted, but a combination of dilator therapy with pelvic floor exercises to get both potential benefits is not unreasonable. A recent study evaluated the reliability of an instrument (the Vaginal Sound) which was designed to measure vaginal length. The Vaginal Sound is a simple, inexpensive, reproducible instrument that has demonstrated acceptable reliability and appears to be able to detect hypothesized changes in vaginal length (33). This instrument can be used to document the degree of vaginal stenosis associated with radical hysterectomy and radiation therapy plus or minus chemotherapy in women treated for cervical carcinoma. The ability to measure vaginal length and correlate vaginal stenosis with sexual function will provide a rationale for much needed interventional studies to maintain vaginal length and sexual function.

Embarrassment and fear have been shown to decrease compliance with dilator therapy, but in most cases, education and support can enhance compliance (104). Unfortunately, for many hospitals and office settings, it is not feasible or practical to have a sexual health program or professional on staff. Therefore, it is important to identify a referral network of local professionals with experience in treating sexual difficulties, which may include mental health professionals as well as gynecologists with expertise in treating patients with changes in sexual function (i.e., menopause) related to medical illness. Educational resources are also available to help patients achieve greater comfort with these issues.

Reproductive concerns of female cancer survivors have been shown to negatively impact quality of life (39). Gynecologic cancer can present before childbearing has been started or completed, during pregnancy, or can even arise out of pregnancy (gestational trophoblastic disease). Reproductive concerns can vary by site of disease, and some women may have the option of conservative surgical management. For example, radical surgery was previously recommended for early-stage operable patients up to stage IIA. More recently, however, cone biopsy alone has become a therapeutic option for young patients with stage IA1 cervical cancer who wish to preserve fertility (111,112), and radical trachelectomy, initially received with skepticism because of the small but definite increase in risk of recurrence, is gradually gaining recognition and acceptance (113) (see Chapter 22).

However, many women will be medically unable to have fertility-preserving treatment, leaving the meaning and emotional ramifications of infertility to be dealt with as a cancer survivorship issue (114). Gynecologic cancer survivors have reported feelings of sadness and grief lasting more than a year posttreatment (115), with some feeling deprived of choices or misunderstood (116) in the setting of cancer-related infertility. Others have voiced feelings of stigma or being "less than a woman" due to loss of reproductive organs (109,117). A woman's reaction will be contingent on her personal desire for a biologic child, the degree of fertility impairment, and willingness to use and access to reproductive assistance or family building options. It is heartening to note that a recent study of women treated for malignant ovarian germ cell tumors found that reproductive and sexual functioning was encouraging, although emphasizing the importance of a stable relationship at the time of diagnosis (118).

A recent study investigating the emotional impact of fertility-preserving surgical treatment for early-stage cervical cancer (radical trachelectomy) found that distress about future conception, pregnancy, childbirth, and cancer recurrence persisted postoperatively over time (119). Recent guidelines published by the American Society of Clinical Oncology highlight the lack of research on the reproductive concerns of cancer survivors as well as the need for more information (120). Despite the availability of reproductive technology, little is known about whether patients are utilizing reproductive assistance or have knowledge about resources, or the emotional impact of fertility/family building issues in survivorship.

Psychologic well-being—patients with gynecologic malignancies face an array of emotional challenges, many of which persist 5 to 10 years after diagnosis (99). Psychologic sequelae can include distress, depression, anxiety, fear, and social disruption. Distress extends along a continuum, ranging from common normal feelings of vulnerability, sadness, and fear, to problems that can become disabling, such as depression, anxiety, panic, social isolation, and spiritual crisis. Recently the National Comprehensive Cancer Network (NCCN) has advocated recording distress as the sixth vital sign using a simple thermometer (10 cm) VAS (121), given that 20% to 40% of patients have significant distress, and only 10% of them are identified and referred for psychosocial evaluation (122). Depression is the least recognized and least effectively treated psychologic problem in patients with cancer (123). In the context of life-threatening illness, diagnostic criteria for depression typically include a significant change in mood on most days for more than 2 weeks. Clinically significant levels of distress and depression, greater than what would be expected in the general population, have been documented in gynecologic cancer patients (97). Specifically, higher levels of distress have been identified in the newly diagnosed, in those undergoing intracavitary brachytherapy (124), in patients with advanced or recurrent disease (6,125), or younger patients (97,114,125), perhaps due to the loss and adjustment many experience about issues of sexuality, fertility, and premature menopause (98,115).

Psychologic shifts have also been observed in women following completion of cancer treatment. In a prospective study with ovarian cancer patients, depression levels were found to decrease 3 months after completion of chemotherapy; however, levels of anxiety were shown to increase (126), perhaps reflective of the uncertainty that many women face about possible recurrence and concerns of future prognosis. However, studies with long-term survivors (5 to 10 years) show that disease-free early-stage survivors have resilience and adjustment over time with an overall good quality of life (99). Despite the identification of many psychologic difficulties within the gynecologic cancer experience, the literature also reveals that many women are not using psychologic services (125), but specify a need for cancer-specific support (127). It has been noted that patients may not be aware of or have access to supportive resources, but would utilize them if offered (99).

Psychologic care considerations—outcomes are improved by an integrative approach, only possible through a proactive collaboration with surgical, radiation, medical, and nurse oncologists working together with psychosocial support. Psychosocial support should include services such as emotional, spiritual, nutritional, genetic, and financial counseling, and general cancer information and support, as needed. At the core of a compassionate response there has to be both acknowledging and responding to physical, psychologic, and spiritual issues. An empathic response occurs when the clinician explicitly makes the connection between the clinical situation and how the patient is feeling. A compassionate response requires action, mobilizing the whole medical team to challenge fear and isolation (128). The medical interaction should be therapeutic on every level. Building a relationship takes more than asking questions. Courteous introductions and a genuine effort to establish rapport pay huge dividends. Consultations should have clear, explicit objectives. Avoid assumptions and be flexible, using focused but open-ended questions, frequently summarizing and screening for concerns. Find out how the illness affects the person. Information should be simple and clear and tailored to the patient's understanding, with the goal of reinforcing realistic hopefulness and supporting shared decision making.

The very process of exploring a patient's emotional symptoms can be therapeutic, but many patients may benefit from professional counseling, support groups, and/or medication. Meta-analyses indicate that preventive psychologic interventions in cancer patients may have a moderate clinical effect upon anxiety but less on depression, and that group therapy is perhaps at least as effective as individual psychotherapy (129). Treatment of anxiety can include antidepressant and antianxiety medication (e.g., buspirone, clonazepam), counseling, and behavioral therapies (130). A wide variety of antidepressant medications with different mechanisms of action and adverse effects are available. Selective serotonin reuptake inhibitors (e.g., fluoxetine, paroxetine, sertraline, and citalopram) are usually well tolerated and can improve depression within 2 to 4 weeks in 60% of patients. The tricyclics (amitriptyline and nortriptyline) have a slightly longer onset of action but can be useful for patients with significant sleep disturbances. "Atypical antidepressants" (bupropion, venlafaxine, and mirtazapine) have a relatively rapid onset of action and paucity of adverse effects. Stimulants (methylphenidate and pemoline) provide the most rapid onset (hours to days). With respect to novel counseling methodologies, a recent psychosocial telephone counseling intervention was shown to improve quality of life for cervical cancer survivors, compared to controls (131). This type of intervention has promise for people unlikely to access traditional services. However, counseling information and resources should be routinely provided to all patients.

CONCLUSION

Quality of life research activity in gynecologic cancer has increased substantially over the past decade. This has included key findings developed within and disseminated through national and international cooperative groups. These contributions have become more robust and influential as the study and science of QOL and other patient-reported outcomes have advanced. Consequently, future directions in gynecologic cancer quality of life research are likely to include a continued focus on measurement science and trial interpretation to aid in treatment decision making, as well as provision of interventions to enhance quality of life. For example, in endometrial cancer we may see areas of active investigation which include the role of obesity as a comorbid factor in the development of this cancer, as well as the role of obesity on potential response to treatment and survival. Cervical cancer investigations may emphasize identifying behavioral or social factors that influence uptake of the human papillomavirus (HPV) vaccine. With respect to this disease, additional QOL studies specific to outcomes and morbidity from multimodality therapy are anticipated. Areas of active investigation in ovarian cancer will continue to focus on evolving paradigms of care such as intraperitoneal therapy, treatment for an asymptomatic rising CA-125, and continual or intermittent therapy for recurrent disease versus therapy only for symptomatic progression. The quality of life implications in each of these treatment considerations are paramount and should be systematically studied within well-designed trials. Further investigation is also needed in palliative care strategies for women with gynecologic cancer. This may include careful examination of the role of chemotherapy in the elderly, as well as interventions to reduce significant issues associated with advanced or advancing disease (e.g., bowel obstructions, neurotoxicities). In each case, evaluation of quality of life and other patient-reported outcomes will serve a significant role in advancing gynecologic cancer care and survivorship.

References

1. Cella D. What do global quality-of-life questions really measure? Insights from Hobday et al. and the "do something" rule. *J Clin Oncol* 2003;21(16): 3178–3179; author reply 3179.
2. WHO. Study protocol for the World Health Organization project to develop a quality of life assessment instrument (WHOQOL). *Qual Life Res* 1993;2(2):153–159.
3. Cella DF. Measuring quality of life in palliative care. *Semin Oncol* 1995; 22(2 Suppl 3):73–81.
4. Bottomley A. The cancer patient and quality of life. *Oncologist* 2002; 7(2):120–125.
5. Velikova G, Stark D, Selby P. Quality of life instruments in oncology. *Eur J Cancer* 1999;35(11):1571–1580.
6. Ferrell B, Smith SL, Cullinane CA, et al. Psychological well being and quality of life in ovarian cancer survivors. *Cancer* 2003;98(5):1061–1071.
7. Gralla RJ. Silk purse in Atlanta: a commentary on SWOG 9509, an advanced non-small cell lung cancer trial. *Oncologist* 1999;4(3):188–190.
8. Kornblith AB, Thaler HT, Wong G, et al. Quality of life of women with ovarian cancer. *Gynecol Oncol* 1995;59(2):231–242.
9. Karnofsky D, Burchenal JH. The clinical evaluation of chemotherapeutic agents in cancer. In: MacLeod C, ed. *Evaluation of Chemotherapeutic Agents*. New York: Columbia University Press; 1949:199–205.
10. Slevin ML, Plant H, Lynch D, et al. Who should measure quality of life, the doctor or the patient? *Br J Cancer* 1988;57(1):109–112.
11. Burris HA 3rd, Moore MJ, Andersen J, et al. Improvements in survival and clinical benefit with gemcitabine as first-line therapy for patients with advanced pancreas cancer: a randomized trial. *J Clin Oncol* 1997;15(6): 2403–2413.
12. Gelber RD, Goldhirsch A, Cavalli F. Quality-of-life-adjusted evaluation of adjuvant therapies for operable breast cancer. The International Breast Cancer Study Group. *Ann Intern Med* 1991;114(8):621–628.
13. Kaye SB, Vasey PA. Docetaxel in ovarian cancer: phase III perspectives and future development. *Semin Oncol* 2002;29(3 Suppl 12):22–27.
14. Demetri GD, Kris M, Wade J, et al. Quality-of-life benefit in chemotherapy patients treated with epoetin alfa is independent of disease response or tumor type: results from a prospective community oncology study. Procrit Study Group. *J Clin Oncol* 1998;16(10):3412–3425.
15. Groenvold M. Methodological issues in the assessment of health-related quality of life in palliative care trials. *Acta Anaesthesiol Scand* 1999;43(9): 948–953.
16. Cohen SR, Mount BM. Living with cancer: "good" days and "bad" days—what produces them? Can the McGill quality of life questionnaire distinguish between them? *Cancer* 2000;89(8):1854–1865.
17. Coates A, Gebski V, Signorini D, et al. Prognostic value of quality-of-life scores during chemotherapy for advanced breast cancer. Australian New Zealand Breast Cancer Trials Group. *J Clin Oncol* 1992;10(12):1833–1838.
18. Spiegel D. Mind matters—group therapy and survival in breast cancer. *N Engl J Med* 2001;345(24):1767–1768.
19. Ruo B, Rumsfeld JS, Hlatky MA, et al. Depressive symptoms and health-related quality of life: the Heart and Soul Study. *JAMA* 2003;290(2): 215–221.
20. McQuellon RP, Thaler HT, Cella D, et al. Quality of life (QOL) outcomes from a randomized trial of cisplatin versus cisplatin plus paclitaxel in advanced cervical cancer: a Gynecologic Oncology Group study. *Gynecol Oncol* 2006;101(2):296–304.
21. Wenzel L, Monk B, Huang H, et al. Clinically meaningful quality-of-life changes in ovarian cancer: results from Gynecologic Oncology Group clinical trial 152. In: Quality of Life III: Translating the Science of Quality-of-Life Assessment Into Clinical Practice—An Example-Driven Approach for Practicing Clinicians and Clinical Researchers. Scottsdale, Arizona: Clinical Therapeutics: The International Peer-Reviewed Journal of Drug Therapy; 2003.
22. Carr D, Goudas L, Lawrence D, et al. Management of cancer symptoms: pain, depression and fatigue: evidence report/technology assessment No. 61. AHRQ publication No. 02-E032. Rockville, MD: Agency for Healthcare Research and Quality; 2002.
23. Garcia S, Cella D, Clauser SB, et al. Standardizing patient-reported outcomes assessment in cancer clinical trials: a patient-reported outcomes measurement information system initiative. *J Clin Oncol* 2007;25(32): 5106–5112.
24. Cella DF, Tulsky DS, Gray G, et al. The Functional Assessment of Cancer Therapy scale: development and validation of the general measure. *J Clin Oncol* 1993;11(3):570–579.
25. Aaronson NK, Ahmedzai S, Bergman B, et al. The European Organization for Research and Treatment of Cancer QLQ-C30: a quality-of-life instrument for use in international clinical trials in oncology. *J Natl Cancer Inst* 1993;85(5):365–376.
26. Schulz MW, Chen J, Woo HH, et al. A comparison of techniques for eliciting patient preferences in patients with benign prostatic hyperplasia. *J Urol* 2002;168(1):155–159.
27. Levine MN, Ganz PA. Beyond the development of quality-of-life instruments: where do we go from here? *J Clin Oncol* 2002;20(9): 2215–2216.
28. Browman GP. Science, language, intuition, and the many meanings of quality of life. *J Clin Oncol* 1999;17(6):1651–1653.
29. Parmar MK, Ledermann JA, Colombo N, et al. Paclitaxel plus platinum-based chemotherapy versus conventional platinum-based chemotherapy in women with relapsed ovarian cancer: the ICON4/AGO-OVAR-2.2 trial. *Lancet* 2003;361(9375):2099–2106.
30. Efficace F, Bottomley A, Osoba D, et al. Beyond the development of health-related quality-of-life (HRQOL) measures: a checklist for evaluating HRQOL outcomes in cancer clinical trials—does HRQOL evaluation in prostate cancer research inform clinical decision making? *J Clin Oncol* 2003;21(18):3502–3511.
31. Curran D, Molenberghs G, Aaronson NK, et al. Analysing longitudinal continuous quality of life data with dropout. *Stat Methods Med Res* 2002; 11(1):5–23.
32. Dalrymple JL, Levenback C, Wolf JK, et al. Trends among gynecologic oncology inpatient deaths: is end-of-life care improving? *Gynecol Oncol* 2002;85(2):356–361.
33. Bruner DW, Barsevick A, Tian C, et al. Randomized trial results of quality of life comparing whole abdominal irradiation and combination chemotherapy in advanced endometrial carcinoma: a Gynecologic Oncology Group study. *Qual Life Res* 2007;16(1):89–100.
34. Zullo F, Palomba S, Russo T, et al. A prospective randomized comparison between laparoscopic and laparotomic approaches in women with early stage endometrial cancer: a focus on the quality of life. *Am J Obstet Gynecol* 2005;193(4):1344–1352.
35. Kornblith AW, J Huang H, Cella D. Quality of life of patients in a randomized clinical trial of laparoscopy (scope) vs open laparotomy (open) for the surgical resection and staging of uterine cancer: a Gynecologic Oncology Group study GOG-2222. In: Society of Gynecologic Oncologists. 2006.
36. Moore DH, Blessing JA, McQuellon RP, et al. Phase III study of cisplatin with or without paclitaxel in stage IVB, recurrent, or persistent squamous cell carcinoma of the cervix: a Gynecologic Oncology Group study. *J Clin Oncol* 2004;22(15):3113–3119.
37. Long HJ 3rd, Monk BJ, Huang HQ, et al. Clinical results and quality of life analysis for the MVAC combination (methotrexate, vinblastine, doxorubicin, and cisplatin) in carcinoma of the uterine cervix: a Gynecologic Oncology Group study. *Gynecol Oncol* 2006;100(3):537–543.
38. Monk BJ, Huang HQ, Cella D, et al. Gynecologic Oncology Group. Quality of life outcomes from a randomized phase III trial of cisplatin with or without topotecan in advanced carcinoma of the cervix: a Gynecologic Oncology Group study. *J Clin Oncol* 2005;23(21):4617–4625.
39. Wenzel L, Huang HQ, Monk BJ, et al. Quality-of-life comparisons in a randomized trial of interval secondary cytoreduction in advanced ovarian carcinoma: a Gynecologic Oncology Group study. *J Clin Oncol* 2005;23(24): 5605–5612.
40. Mutch DG, Orlando M, Goss T, et al. Randomized phase III trial of gemcitabine compared with pegylated liposomal doxorubicin in patients with platinum-resistant ovarian cancer. *J Clin Oncol* 2007;25(19):2811–2818.
41. Armstrong DK, Bundy B, Wenzel L, et al. Intraperitoneal cisplatin and paclitaxel in ovarian cancer. *N Engl J Med* 2006;354(1):34–43.
42. Wenzel LB, Huang HQ, Armstrong DK, et al. Gynecologic Oncology Group. Health-related quality of life during and after intraperitoneal versus intravenous chemotherapy for optimally debulked ovarian cancer: a Gynecologic Oncology Group study. *J Clin Oncol* 2007;25(4):437–443.
43. Pfisterer J, Vergote I, Du Bois A, et al. Combination therapy with gemcitabine and carboplatin in recurrent ovarian cancer. *Int J Gynecol Cancer* 2005;15(Suppl 1):36–41.
44. Pfisterer J, Weber B, Reuss A, et al. Randomized phase III trial of topotecan following carboplatin and paclitaxel in first-line treatment of advanced ovarian cancer: a Gynecologic Cancer Intergroup trial of the AGO-OVAR and GINECO. *J Natl Cancer Inst* 2006;98(15):1036–1045.
45. du Bois A, Lück HJ, Meier W, et al. A randomized clinical trial of cisplatin/paclitaxel versus carboplatin/paclitaxel as first-line treatment of ovarian cancer. *J Natl Cancer Inst* 2003;95(17):1320–1329.
46. du Bois A, Weber B, Rochon J, et al. Addition of epirubicin as a third drug to carboplatin-paclitaxel in first-line treatment of advanced ovarian cancer: a prospectively randomized Gynecologic Cancer Intergroup trial by the Arbeitsgemeinschaft Gynaekologische Onkologie Ovarian Cancer Study Group and the Groupe d'Investigateurs Nationaux pour l'Etude des Cancers Ovariens. *J Clin Oncol* 2006;24(7):1127–1135.
47. Greimel ER, Bjelic-Radisic V, Pfisterer J, et al. Randomized study of the Arbeitsgemeinschaft Gynaekologische Onkologie Ovarian Cancer Study Group comparing quality of life in patients with ovarian cancer treated with cisplatin/paclitaxel versus carboplatin/paclitaxel. *J Clin Oncol* 2006;24(4):579–586.
48. ten Bokkel Huinink W, Lane SR, Ross GA. Long-term survival in a phase III, randomised study of topotecan versus paclitaxel in advanced epithelial ovarian carcinoma. *Ann Oncol* 2004;15(1):100–103.
49. Hilpert F, du Bois A, Greimel ER, et al. Feasibility, toxicity and quality of life of first-line chemotherapy with platinum/paclitaxel in elderly patients

aged >or=70 years with advanced ovarian cancer—a study by the AGO OVAR Germany. *Ann Oncol* 2007;18(2):282–287.
50. Gil KM, Gibbons HE, Jenison EL, et al. Baseline characteristics influencing quality of life in women undergoing gynecologic oncology surgery. *Health Qual Life Outcomes* 2007;5:25.
51. Courneya KS, Karvinen KH, Campbell KL, et al. Associations among exercise, body weight, and quality of life in a population-based sample of endometrial cancer survivors. *Gynecol Oncol* 2005;97(2):422–430.
52. von Gruenigen VE, Gil KM, Frasure HE, et al. The impact of obesity and age on quality of life in gynecologic surgery. *Am J Obstet Gynecol* 2005; 193(4):1369–1375.
53. Le T, Hopkins L, Kee Fung MF. Quality of life assessment during adjuvant and salvage chemotherapy for advance stage epithelial ovarian cancer. *Gynecol Oncol* 2005;98(1):39–44.
54. Vaz AF, Pinto-Neto AM, Conde DM, et al. Quality of life of women with gynecologic cancer: associated factors. *Arch Gynecol Obstet* 2007;276(6): 583–589.
55. Hensley ML, Correa DD, Thaler H, et al. Phase I/II study of weekly paclitaxel plus carboplatin and gemcitabine as first-line treatment of advanced-stage ovarian cancer: pathologic complete response and longitudinal assessment of impact on cognitive functioning. *Gynecol Oncol* 2006;102(2):270–277.
56. Servaes P, Prins J, Verhagen S, et al. Fatigue after breast cancer and in chronic fatigue syndrome: similarities and differences. *J Psychosom Res* 2002;52(6):453–459.
57. Cella D, Davis K, Breitbart W, et al. Fatigue Coalition. Cancer-related fatigue: prevalence of proposed diagnostic criteria in a United States sample of cancer survivors. *J Clin Oncol* 2001;19(14):3385–3391.
58. Wilkinson PM, Antonopoulos M, Lahousen M, et al. EPO-INT-45 Study Group. Epoetin alfa in platinum-treated ovarian cancer patients: results of a multinational, multicentre, randomised trial. *Br J Cancer* 2006;94(7): 947–954.
59. Gielissen MF, Verhagen S, Witjes F, et al. Effects of cognitive behavior therapy in severely fatigued disease-free cancer patients compared with patients waiting for cognitive behavior therapy: a randomized controlled trial. *J Clin Oncol* 2006;24(30):4882–4887.
60. Bruera E, Valero V, Driver L, et al. Patient-controlled methylphenidate for cancer fatigue: a double-blind, randomized, placebo-controlled trial. *J Clin Oncol* 2006;24(13):2073–2078.
61. Pignata S, De Placido S, Biamonte R, et al. Residual neurotoxicity in ovarian cancer patients in clinical remission after first-line chemotherapy with carboplatin and paclitaxel: the Multicenter Italian Trial in Ovarian Cancer (MITO-4) retrospective study. *BMC Cancer* 2006;6:5.
62. Armstrong DK. Relapsed ovarian cancer: challenges and management strategies for a chronic disease. *Oncologist* 2002;7(Suppl 5):20–28.
63. Dunton CJ. Management of treatment-related toxicity in advanced ovarian cancer. *Oncologist* 2002;7(Suppl 5):11–19.
64. McGuire WP, Hoskins WJ, Brady MF, et al. Cyclophosphamide and cisplatin compared with paclitaxel and cisplatin in patients with stage III and stage IV ovarian cancer. *N Engl J Med* 1996;334(1):1–6.
65. Ozols RF, Bundy BN, Greer BE, et al. Phase III trial of carboplatin and paclitaxel compared with cisplatin and paclitaxel in patients with optimally resected stage III ovarian cancer: a Gynecologic Oncology Group study. *J Clin Oncol* 2003;21(17):3194–3200.
66. Vasey PA, Jayson GC, Gordon A, et al. Phase III randomized trial of docetaxel-carboplatin versus paclitaxel-carboplatin as first-line chemotherapy for ovarian carcinoma. *J Natl Cancer Inst* 2004;96(22):1682–1691.
67. Hilpert F, Stähle A, Tomé O, et al. Neuroprotection with amifostine in the first-line treatment of advanced ovarian cancer with carboplatin/paclitaxel-based chemotherapy—a double-blind, placebo-controlled, randomized phase II study from the Arbeitsgemeinschaft Gynakologische Onkologoie (AGO) Ovarian Cancer Study Group. *Support Care Cancer* 2005;13(10): 797–805.
68. Lorusso D, Ferrandina G, Greggi S, et al. Phase III multicenter randomized trial of amifostine as cytoprotectant in first-line chemotherapy in ovarian cancer patients. *Ann Oncol* 2003;14(7):1086–1093.
69. Annas GJ. Informed consent, cancer, and truth in prognosis. *N Engl J Med* 1994;330(3):223–225.
70. Huang HQ, Brady MF, Cella D, et al. Validation and reduction of FACT/GOG-Ntx subscale for platinum/paclitaxel-induced neurologic symptoms: a Gynecologic Oncology Group study. *Int J Gynecol Cancer* 2007;17(2): 387–393.
71. Badger C, Preston N, Seers K, et al. Physical therapies for reducing and controlling lymphoedema of the limbs. *Cochrane Database Syst Rev* 2004;(4):CD003141.
72. Petrek JA, Senie RT, Peters M, et al. Lymphedema in a cohort of breast carcinoma survivors 20 years after diagnosis. *Cancer* 2001;92(6):1368–1377.
73. Judson PL, Jonson AL, Paley PJ, et al. A prospective, randomized study analyzing sartorius transposition following inguinal-femoral lymphadenectomy. *Gynecol Oncol* 2004;95(1):226–230.
74. Ryan M, Stainton MC, Jaconelli C, et al. The experience of lower limb lymphedema for women after treatment for gynecologic cancer. *Oncol Nurs Forum* 2003;30(3):417–423.
75. Bergmark K, Avall-Lundqvist E, Dickman PW, et al. Lymphedema and bladder-emptying difficulties after radical hysterectomy for early cervical cancer and among population controls. *Int J Gynecol Cancer* 2006;16(3): 1130–1139.
76. Nunns D, Williamson K, Swaney L, et al. The morbidity of surgery and adjuvant radiotherapy in the management of endometrial carcinoma. *Int J Gynecol Cancer* 2000;10(3):233–238.
77. Fujiwara K, Kigawa J, Hasegawa K, et al. Effect of simple omentoplasty and omentopexy in the prevention of complications after pelvic lymphadenectomy. *Int J Gynecol Cancer* 2003;13(1):61–66.
78. Ohara K, Tsunoda H, Satoh T, et al. Use of the small pelvic field instead of the classic whole pelvic field in postoperative radiotherapy for cervical cancer: reduction of adverse events. *Int J Radiat Oncol Biol Phys* 2004; 60(1):258–264.
79. Abu-Rustum NR, Alektiar K, Iasonos A, et al. The incidence of symptomatic lower-extremity lymphedema following treatment of uterine corpus malignancies: a 12-year experience at Memorial Sloan-Kettering Cancer Center. *Gynecol Oncol* 2006;103(2):714–718.
80. Woods M. Patients' perceptions of breast-cancer-related lymphoedema. *Eur J Cancer Care (Engl)* 1993;2(3):125–128.
81. Carter BJ. Women's experiences of lymphedema. *Oncol Nurs Forum* 1997; 24(5):875–882.
82. Hare M. The lived experience of breast cancer-related lymphoedema. *Cancer Nurse Practice* 2001:12–19.
83. Radina ME, Armer JM, Culbertson SD, et al. Post-breast cancer lymphedema: understanding women's knowledge of their condition. *Oncol Nurs Forum* 2004;31(1):97–104.
84. Passik SD, McDonald MV. Psychosocial aspects of upper extremity lymphedema in women treated for breast carcinoma. *Cancer* 1998;83 (12 Suppl American):2817–2820.
85. Armer JM, Radina ME, Porock D, et al. Predicting breast cancer-related lymphedema using self-reported symptoms. *Nurs Res* 2003;52(6):370–379.
86. Armer JM. The problem of post-breast cancer lymphedema: impact and measurement issues. *Cancer Invest* 2005;23(1):76–83.
87. Pereira de Godoy JM, Braile DM, de Fátima Godoy M, et al. Quality of life and peripheral lymphedema. *Lymphology* 2002;35(2):72–75.
88. Janda M, Obermair A, Cella D, et al. Vulvar cancer patients' quality of life: a qualitative assessment. *Int J Gynecol Cancer* 2004;14(5):875–881.
89. Ridner SH. Quality of life and a symptom cluster associated with breast cancer treatment-related lymphedema. *Support Care Cancer* 2005;13(11): 904–911.
90. Schover LR. Sexuality and fertility after cancer. *Hematol Am Soc Hematol Educ Program* 2005:523–527.
91. Andersen BL, Woods XA, Copeland LJ. Sexual self-schema and sexual morbidity among gynecologic cancer survivors. *J Consult Clin Psychol* 1997;65(2):221–229.
92. Wilmoth MC, Spinelli A. Sexual implications of gynecologic cancer treatments. *J Obstet Gynecol Neonatal Nurs* 2000;29(4):413–421.
93. Thakar R, Ayers S, Georgakapolou A, et al. Hysterectomy improves quality of life and decreases psychiatric symptoms: a prospective and randomised comparison of total versus subtotal hysterectomy. *BJOG* 2004;111(10): 1115–1120.
94. Grumann M, Robertson R, Hacker NF, et al. Sexual functioning in patients following radical hysterectomy for stage IB cancer of the cervix. *Int J Gynecol Cancer* 2001;11(5):372–380.
95. Jensen PT, Groenvold M, Klee MC, et al. Early-stage cervical carcinoma, radical hysterectomy, and sexual function. A longitudinal study. *Cancer* 2004;100(1):97–106.
96. Pieterse QD, Maas CP, ter Kuile MM, et al. An observational longitudinal study to evaluate miction, defecation, and sexual function after radical hysterectomy with pelvic lymphadenectomy for early-stage cervical cancer. *Int J Gynecol Cancer* 2006;16(3):1119–1129.
97. Bodurka-Bevers D, Basen-Engquist K, Carmack CL, et al. Depression, anxiety, and quality of life in patients with epithelial ovarian cancer. *Gynecol Oncol* 2000;78(3 Pt 1):302–308.
98. Stewart DE, Wong F, Duff S, et al. "What doesn't kill you makes you stronger": an ovarian cancer survivor survey. *Gynecol Oncol* 2001;83(3): 537–542.
99. Wenzel LB, Donnelly JP, Fowler JM, et al. Resilience, reflection, and residual stress in ovarian cancer survivorship: a Gynecologic Oncology Group study. *Psychooncology* 2002;11(2):142–153.
100. Schover LR. Counseling cancer patients about changes in sexual function. *Oncology (Williston Park)* 1999;13(11):1585–1591; discussion 1591–1592, 1595–1596.
101. Jensen PT, Groenvold M, Klee MC, et al. Longitudinal study of sexual function and vaginal changes after radiotherapy for cervical cancer. *Int J Radiat Oncol Biol Phys* 2003;56(4):937–949.
102. Bergmark K, Avall-Lundqvist E, Dickman PW, et al. Vaginal changes and sexuality in women with a history of cervical cancer. *N Engl J Med* 1999; 340(18):1383–1389.
103. Frumovitz M, Sun CC, Schover LR, et al. Quality of life and sexual functioning in cervical cancer survivors. *J Clin Oncol* 2005;23(30):7428–7436.
104. Robinson JW, Faris PD, Scott CB. Psychoeducational group increases vaginal dilation for younger women and reduces sexual fears for women of all ages with gynecologic carcinoma treated with radiotherapy. *Int J Radiat Oncol Biol Phys* 1999;44(3):497–506.
105. Ganz PA, Greendale GA, Petersen L, et al. Managing menopausal symptoms in breast cancer survivors: results of a randomized controlled trial. *J Natl Cancer Inst* 2000;92(13):1054–1064.

106. Schover LR, Jenkins R, Sui D, et al. Randomized trial of peer counseling on reproductive health in African American breast cancer survivors. *J Clin Oncol* 2006;24(10):1620–1626.
107. Kendall A, Dowsett M, Folkerd E, et al. Caution: vaginal estradiol appears to be contraindicated in postmenopausal women on adjuvant aromatase inhibitors. *Ann Oncol* 2006;17(4):584–587.
108. Cardozo L, Bachmann G, McClish D, et al. Meta-analysis of estrogen therapy in the management of urogenital atrophy in postmenopausal women: second report of the Hormones and Urogenital Therapy Committee. *Obstet Gynecol* 1998;92(4 Pt 2):722–727.
109. Juraskova I, Butow P, Robertson R, et al. Post-treatment sexual adjustment following cervical and endometrial cancer: a qualitative insight. *Psychooncology* 2003;12(3):267–279.
110. Denton AS, Maher EJ. Interventions for the physical aspects of sexual dysfunction in women following pelvic radiotherapy. *Cochrane Database Syst Rev* 2003;(1):CD003750.
111. Morris M. Management of stage IA cervical carcinoma. *J Natl Cancer Inst Monogr* 1996;(21):47–52.
112. Rose PG. Type II radical hysterectomy: evaluating its role in cervical cancer. *Gynecol Oncol* 2001;80(1):1–2.
113. Roy M, Plante M. Radical vaginal trachelectomy for invasive cervical cancer. *J Gynecol Obstet Biol Reprod (Paris)* 2000;29(3):279–281.
114. Wenzel L, Dogan-Ates A, Habbal R, et al. Defining and measuring reproductive concerns of female cancer survivors. *J Natl Cancer Inst Monogr* 2005;(34):94–98.
115. Carter J, Rowland K, Chi D, et al. Gynecologic cancer treatment and the impact of cancer-related infertility. *Gynecol Oncol* 2005;97(1): 90–95.
116. Corney R, Everett H, Howells A, et al. The care of patients undergoing surgery for gynaecological cancer: the need for information, emotional support and counselling. *J Adv Nurs* 1992;17(6):667–671.
117. Schover L. *Sexuality and Fertility After Cancer*. New York: John Wiley & Sons; 1997.
118. Gershenson DM, Miller AM, Champion VL, et al. Reproductive and sexual function after platinum-based chemotherapy in long-term ovarian germ cell tumor survivors: a Gynecologic Oncology Group study. *J Clin Oncol* 2007;25(19):2792–2797.
119. Carter J, Sonoda Y, Abu-Rustum NR. Reproductive concerns of women treated with radical trachelectomy for cervical cancer. *Gynecol Oncol* 2007;105(1):13–16.
120. Lee SJ, Schover LR, Partridge AH, et al. American Society of Clinical Oncology recommendations on fertility preservation in cancer patients. *J Clin Oncol* 2006;24(18):2917–2931.
121. Holland JC, Bultz BD. The NCCN guideline for distress management: a case for making distress the sixth vital sign. *J Natl Compr Canc Netw* 2007;5(1):3–7.
122. Kadan-Lottick NS, Vanderwerker LC, Block SD, et al. Psychiatric disorders and mental health service use in patients with advanced cancer: a report from the Coping with Cancer Study. *Cancer* 2005;104(12):2872–2881.
123. Pirl WF. Evidence report on the occurrence, assessment, and treatment of depression in cancer patients. *J Natl Cancer Inst Monogr* 2004;(32):32–39.
124. Kamer S, Ozsaran Z, Celik O, et al. Evaluation of anxiety levels during intracavitary brachytherapy applications in women with gynecologic malignancies. *Eur J Gynaecol Oncol* 2007;28(2):121–124.
125. Norton TR, Manne SL, Rubin S, et al. Prevalence and predictors of psychological distress among women with ovarian cancer. *J Clin Oncol* 2004;22(5):919–926.
126. Hipkins J, Whitworth M, Tarrier N, et al. Social support, anxiety and depression after chemotherapy for ovarian cancer: a prospective study. *Br J Health Psychol* 2004;9(Pt 4):569–581.
127. Ferrell BR, Smith SL, Ervin KS, et al. A qualitative analysis of social concerns of women with ovarian cancer. *Psychooncology* 2003;12(7):647–663.
128. Baile WF, Buckman R, Lenzi R, et al. SPIKES—a six-step protocol for delivering bad news: application to the patient with cancer. *Oncologist* 2000;5(4):302–311.
129. Sheard T, Maguire P. The effect of psychological interventions on anxiety and depression in cancer patients: results of two meta-analyses. *Br J Cancer* 1999;80(11):1770–1780.
130. Fricchione G. Clinical practice. Generalized anxiety disorder. *N Engl J Med* 2004;351(7):675–682.
131. Wenzel L. *Psychological, Social, and Employment Impacts on Breast and Cervical Cancer Survivors: Biobehavioral Outcomes of a Telephone Counseling Intervention for Cervical Cancer Survivors*. London: International PsychoOncology Society; 2007.

CHAPTER 35 ■ END OF LIFE CARE

JOANNA M. CAIN AND SUSAN TOLLE

The goal of end of life care is to provide, in the continuum of oncology care, maximal palliation of symptoms and maximal psychologic support at the end of life. Ensuring that our patients get the best care as the goal of medicine shifts from curing disease to relief of suffering is one of the obligations of health professionals. To do so effectively requires engaging not only the physicians and nurses who have been part of the oncology treatment, but also the skilled assistance of palliative care and hospice professionals with the patient and their caregiving network of family and friends.

THE END OF LIFE TRANSITION

Discussions about the nature of disease, the status of treatment, and the expectation and side effects of treatment are an ongoing conversation in oncology care. With the lengthening of survival for even the most deadly gynecologic cancer, ovarian cancer, and the multiplicity of options for ongoing chemotherapy, the decision to limit chemotherapy or other interventions may come out of any of the multiple conversations over time aimed at balancing the potential side effects of new chemotherapies or other treatments against the expected benefit and impact on quality of life for the patient. In this setting of continuing conversation between the health care team and the patient with or without her significant support individuals, there is often a point at which the ongoing therapy aimed at disease control or cure has a harm to quality of life that is greater than any benefit—a point in which the transition to comfort-focused end of life care is more clear, although palliative care may well have been initiated for some symptoms prior to this point (Table 35.1).

The balance can be difficult, as Callahan points out: "The most fundamental problem with technological medicine is two-fold: that it can give us a longer life and a slower dying and that it can keep us alive when we might be better off dead" (1). Patient perspectives on what constitutes high-quality end of life care reinforces the importance of interactions most physicians would identify such as communication, accessibility, continuity, and emotional support, but surprisingly oncology patients compared to terminal patients with other diagnoses more often hold on to a desire to maintain hope (2). Keeping this door open while realistically portraying prognosis and options, and pursuing palliative care can be the hardest balance of all.

The timing and expectation of death for cancer patients continues to change. Thirty years ago survival from high-grade ovarian cancer longer than 2 years was very unlikely and now is routine. As a backdrop to this advance, the age of death in the developed world has steadily increased, as the major cause of death has changed over the past hundred years from sudden death from infection, trauma, and childbirth in the young to a slower decline from chronic illnesses usually in advanced age. Cancers that previously caused a rapid death now follow a more chronic recurring course, which changes not only patient and family perceptions about the length of time until they need to deal with the issue of death, but offers a longer time to work through the phases of dying and the opportunity to bring to closure key goals for an individual. Even the gender and role of caregivers at the end of life are changing, and the role of men as caregivers for women with gynecologic cancers deserves special attention (3). The development of palliative care teams, usually in hospital settings, has added significant expertise to symptom management, discharge planning, and accomplishing improved end of life care (4). Given this prolonged course, the advance planning for end of life care has both more time for consideration and can evolve as the patient's prognosis changes.

ADVANCE PLANNING FOR END OF LIFE CARE: REDUCING THE EMOTIONAL BURDEN ON SURROGATE DECISION MAKERS

Along with improved symptom management at end of life have come improved vehicles for ensuring that patients have their wishes represented in their care, in terms of legal documents, but also ensuring that surrogate decision makers adequately represent patient wishes.

Serving as a surrogate for a woman with advanced cancer who can no longer make her own treatment decisions places a profound burden on the surrogate. Nothing can completely lift this burden, but advance planning can make the burden lighter. Health care professionals often underestimate the burden of serving as a decision maker. Formal measures of stress document that months after serving as a surrogate in a decision to withdraw life-sustaining treatment the surrogate's emotional stress levels remain remarkably high. One study found that the stress of serving as a health care decision maker was twice as high as the stress levels on households who had lost their homes to fire in the Berkeley-Oakland fire storm (5). Decision makers commonly report waking up at two in the morning and wondering if they made the right decision. They make statements such as, "It was the hardest thing I have ever done in my life."

Some surrogates experience far more distress than others. When patients have not previously documented their wishes about life-sustaining treatment, the stress levels of their surrogate decision makers tend to be even higher. When surrogates are guided by the patient's written advance directive, their stress levels are about 30% lower, when measured 2 months after a decision to stop life support (5).

TABLE 35.1

KEY ISSUES TO ADDRESS WHEN THE THERAPEUTIC FOCUS SHIFTS FROM CURE TO CARE

Issue	Examples
Communication about terminal nature of cancer should occur in the course of ONGOING communication.	"We are not achieving the goals we set together with this chemotherapy." "The cancer is continuing to grow despite our efforts with this new agent."
Assess what the patient WANTS to know.	"I would not continue any further chemotherapy at this point, but feel we should focus on relieving your symptoms of . . . What do you think?" "Do you have questions about what we just discussed?"
Identify that, in fact, the patient's condition is terminal, and particularly if asked directly.	"Am I going to die of this?" "Yes, but our attention now needs to be focused on making whatever time you have as pain-free and active as it possibly can be."
Identify the goals that the patient wants to achieve.	"Are there any special events or things that are on your agenda that we need to know about as we plan your treatment?"
Identify what resources the patient is planning to access (e.g., support systems as well as insurance coverage/hospice coverage).	"Have you talked to your . . . spouse/partner/children/friends about your plans to be at home, and do they have ideas about how that will work?"
Make sure that the priority items for the patient are dealt with immediately.	"What is the number one issue for you right now?"

Surrogates who "stand by" and affirm the patient's prior written instructions worry less about whether they made the right decision. Those who had never talked with the patient ahead of time feel the anguish of "deciding for" a woman they love. An important message to women with cancer who are reluctant to engage in advance care planning is, "Lift a burden from those you love: complete an advance directive."

THE ROLE OF TRADITIONAL ADVANCE DIRECTIVES

Advance directives provide a woman with a means to legally document her preferences about medical treatments in the event she is no longer able to make her own decisions. The legal details and breadth of clinical context vary substantially by state within the United States, and by country of the world. In many jurisdictions, these documents allow the formal appointment of a surrogate who becomes the woman's legally authorized medical decision maker in the event of future incapacity. Being asked to document one's preferences for treatment in conditions like "imminent death regardless of treatment" and "persistent vegetative state" can be anxiety-provoking for anyone. The context of a new diagnosis of cancer often makes completing an advance directive seem very real, and perhaps overwhelming. It is difficult to combine conversations about advance care planning with initial discussions of curative treatment. It is tempting to put off these discussions until they have no further treatment options to offer or the patient declines further curative treatment.

Waiting until the patient is near death to have these important conversations risks that the patient may become too ill to be able to make her wishes known. If the patient has not given any instruction, the burden of decision making often weighs more heavily on surrogates. Without prior planning, the patient will not have appointed the surrogate of her choice. Sometimes, family and friends disagree on treatment decisions, which adds further to family distress. In addition, patients and their loved ones often benefit from having advance planning be more of a process than an event. Having discussions with the patient about who should and should not be given medical information can naturally lead into who would be the most appropriate decision maker should the patient temporarily be unable to make decisions for herself. When the patient reveals strongly held value differences within her social network, or when she indicates that her most trusted surrogate is not her legal next of kin, the patient should be strongly encouraged to complete a written advance directive.

Advance directives are remarkably effective in allowing the patient to designate her choice of a surrogate decision maker. These legal instruments are also effective in silencing those whose wishes and values diverge from the patient's. Advance directives are also helpful to focus end of life treatment decisions on what the patient would have wanted. Advance directives are effective in designating a surrogate but are less effective in turning values into action, which require medical orders. Increasingly, we have learned that advance directives alone are not enough to ensure that patients' wishes regarding life-sustaining treatment will be followed (6).

MEETING THE NEED FOR MEDICAL ORDERS: THE POLST PARADIGM PROGRAM

In technologically developed countries, decisions about whether to use cardiopulmonary resuscitation, ventilators, antibiotics, and feeding tubes are an integral part of the care of women with advanced gynecologic cancers. Most persons with advanced stages of cancer and other chronic diseases ultimately make a decision to forego some forms of life-sustaining treatment. Interviews with over 1,000 next of kin reveal that in the months prior to death, a majority of patients or their surrogates make a decision to withhold or withdraw a medical treatment (7).

When a thoughtful decision has been made to forego attempts at resuscitation, it is most distressing to family members to have the patient receive unwanted cardiopulmonary resuscitation (CPR). Surrogates sometimes anguish over having "let Mom down." Family members express surprise to learn that emergency medical personnel cannot follow the patient's traditional advance directive. Emergency medical personnel need written medical orders indicating not to provide specific treatments like CPR. Without such medical orders, emergency medical services (EMS) must attempt all possible life-sustaining treatments.

Because traditional advance directives have vague language that requires further interpretation, they have proven inadequate in ensuring that a woman's wishes to limit life-sustaining treatment will be respected. As patients move from one place to another, a uniform set of medical orders is needed to be sure the patient's wishes will be followed no matter what their setting of care.

One of the best-studied systems of medical orders to document advance care planning is the Physician Orders for Life-Sustaining Treatment paradigm. The POLST program is designed primarily for patients with advanced disease who the physician would not be surprised if they died in the coming year. The POLST document is a brightly colored medical order form that converts patient treatment preferences into written medical orders based on a conversation among health care professionals, the patient, and/or surrogates about treatment goals. The form transfers with the patient across care settings, to ensure that her wishes are honored no matter whether she is cared for at home, in an ambulance, in a nursing home, or in an acute care hospital. A 1-year prospective study of nursing home residents with advanced chronic illness followed residents whose POLST forms included a Do Not Resuscitate order and an order for comfort measures only. None of these patients received unwanted intensive care, ventilator support, or cardiopulmonary resuscitation (8).

In summary, women beginning cancer treatment often benefit from the first stage of advance care planning, which is formally appointing a surrogate decision maker who shares their wishes and values. Women with advanced cancer who wish to forego one or more forms of life-sustaining treatment are more likely to have their wishes respected if the POLST or other standardized medical orders are written to provide guidance to all other health care personnel who currently are, or in the future may, provide care in life's last chapter (www.polst.org).

ROLE OF FAMILY IN DECISION MAKING

Given the sequential and repetitive conversations described above, the inclusion of family and other support persons is almost universal and clearly preferable. For many patients, they are the ones with whom they have shared their lives and their dearest and deepest emotions. They are also the ones by whom the patient wants to be surrounded during the last phase of life. However, patients have the right to exclude or include whomever they wish in conversations, and occasionally medical events are so acute that they trigger discussions with family members, without clarity, about what the patient herself would have wished or about which family member truly speaks for the patient. Expert communication with the family then becomes the most critical means of ensuring that the patient's best interests are served. Unfortunately, research suggests that communication is not as effective as it needs to be in these circumstances. Fifty-four percent of families did not understand basic information (diagnosis, prognosis, treatments) after physician-family meetings in an intensive care setting (9), a finding that could lead to potential conflict with families that could impede an appropriate transition to palliative care in any setting. Well-structured discussions that focus on the disease process, the goals of palliative therapy, and understanding the concerns of family members may help the family formulate decisions that support the dignity and choices that the patient herself would have chosen.

To prevent problems, it is wise to respect several rules:

- Always ask the patient if she has preferences in her contacts with friends and relatives. Often, she wants special persons to be more involved than others.
- Ask the patient for one or two contact persons to organize the communication with family and friends. Communicate essential information always in the presence of them or of other relatives or friends chosen by the patient. In this way, the family and friends are well informed and they share the same information with the patient. They can also help the patient with the evaluation of the information afterward.
- Never talk about the patient "behind her back." If the physician does, and the patient finds out, the relationship of trust may be upset and will take quite some time and work to be restored. This also prevents the patient from thinking that the family knows more than she does, which can also put pressure on family relationships.
- In countries where health care is a financial burden to the family, it is the responsibility of the physician to ensure that decision making concerning continuation of treatment or starting a treatment is based on the ethical principles of autonomy, beneficence, and nonmalfeasance. It is not acceptable that this decision making is driven by financial pressures alone.

At the end of life, we can expect emotional reactions by patients and their significant others, including family, to the inevitable lifestyle changes and impending death. It is the task of the physician to try to understand the thoughts and behavior of the patient regarding death and dying as well as her worries and unfinished emotional and personal business. Information on the patient's values and beliefs should be sought—even information about very personal matters like relationships and sexuality might be needed for a proper assessment of her situation. Also, it is important to respect the balance, and the patient has to know that she has the choice to what extent she wants to participate in this assessment and what information she is comfortable to share both with the physician or care team and with her family and friends. In normal life, family and friends often meet the spiritual and emotional needs of a patient, and the role of the health team is to support these relationships.

UNIQUE CIRCUMSTANCES FOR DECISION MAKING: PREGNANT PATIENTS

A rare but particularly poignant context of end of life decision making is that of the pregnant woman with terminal, metastatic cancer where survival even to the end of a normal pregnancy is unlikely. The choices for palliative therapy (e.g., pelvic radiation for control of local bleeding and pressure) may directly impact the likelihood of fetal survival. The possibility of delivery of a newborn—particularly prematurely with all the known consequences—without surviving to mother the child make the choices even more complex for the woman and for her family. The primary objective of care for the mother is alleviation of symptoms, and choices to decrease the level of palliative care in order to facilitate fetal development are considered only if strongly desired and pursued by the patient herself. Maternal autonomy in making such decisions has been supported by both ethical and legal reviews, and these confirm that the patient's wishes must guide decisions regarding fetal well-being, including accepting or not accepting caesarian section in the terminal phase of disease (10). There is no role for withholding appropriate and maximal pain and symptom management simply because the woman has a concurrent pregnancy (11). The health care team carries a special burden in this circumstance to ensure that the patient has all relevant and unbiased information regarding harms and benefits of all potential options for her and for her pregnancy, to maximize her ability to make choices.

In the absence of the ability of the patient to speak for herself, the surrogate decision makers must weigh not only her wishes regarding a premature timing of delivery of the child and invasion with a surgical procedure such as a caesarian section, but also the likelihood of viability of the fetus and the supporting family's ability and choices about caring for a significantly premature child. End of life directives for pregnant patients that specifically address these issues may be helpful in discussion and documentation of patient wishes (12). Some states and countries have special restrictions regarding decision making about limiting life-sustaining treatment in terminally ill pregnant women. In fact, 27 states have statutes that prohibit an out of hospital Do Not Resuscitate order being written on a pregnant woman or otherwise have a "pregnancy limitation." The role of the woman in fixing the parameters for balancing fetal well-being against her own needs for alleviation of pain and suffering is central, both if she can speak for herself or in representing those wishes by surrogate decision makers, and it is her health care team's obligation to make sure that these are well defined, described, and that the patient's wishes about her health care (autonomy) are respected in the terminal phase of her disease.

MAXIMIZING PALLIATION: MANAGING SYMPTOMS AT THE END OF LIFE

Pain Control

The mainstay of pain management at any time, and even more critically at the end of life, is a careful assessment of the type of pain (nociceptive [somatic or visceral], or neuropathic), the level of pain, the location and referral of pain, and the actions that increase or decrease the pain. This assessment will need multiple repetitions as the kind of pain and level are likely to shift with disease progression. The management strategy is to focus on not only the type and level of pain but also the level of consciousness and the level of activity that a woman would like to achieve, and to vary the strategies accordingly (13).

The World Health Organization's three-tier pain ladder starts with low to increasing levels of pain and increasing strategies from acetaminophen and nonsteroidal anti-inflammatory drugs to opioid analgesics for more severe pain. Using usually a 1 to 10 (10 being the worst) pain scale with patients fixes their position on the tier and suggests management strategy, although combinations from other levels or even within a level may be required for maximal comfort. Given that many gynecologic oncology patients are in the severe category (7 to 10) at the end of life, this might even include combining two opioids, particularly during pain syndrome escalation, to control the pain (14). In the course of adequate pain or symptom management, the anticipated side effects may shorten the time to death (principle of double effect), which is a well-recognized consequence of ensuring maximal palliative care. The ethical obligation is to alleviate the pain and suffering first and foremost, and the side effects that cannot be avoided (which rarely impact time to death simply because most patients already have substantial tolerance for narcotic pain medications) are accepted in this setting.

Pharmacologic measures to address severe nociceptive pain usually require narcotic medications. The options for administration are broad and can be tailored to the patient's circumstances. As a principle that supports patient and family control, a means such as dermal, oral (pill, sublinqual, and liquid), buccal, or rectal can make administration easier. With long-term sustained-release formulations, the goal is to establish adequate base pain coverage with every 8- to 12-hour dosing and adequate breakthrough pain coverage with an immediate-release form of the agents. Having the patient or caregiver track the amount and timing of breakthrough dosing can help adjust both the base and rescue dosing and timing. Sustained-release formulations are available for morphine, oxycodone, and hydromorphone (15).

Methadone is another option that has been utilized and can be particularly helpful when morphine is not adequate or is problematic for individual patients. It has a variable conversion ratio and pharmacokinetics in individuals and is much more difficult to titrate and manage with other medications. Methadone may be particularly helpful in patients where neuropathic pain resistant to opiods is a significant part of the pain complex. The final option to avoid intravenous pain management is the transdermal fentanyl patch. This is particularly helpful, when stabilized dosing is reached, for individuals who require continuous baseline coverage but are unreliable about taking doses of pain medications. The downside is the long time to peak concentrations, which renders initial evaluation and titration of dosages difficult and requires significant use of short-term release opioids to cover (16).

The use of intravenous forms of opioids with patient-controlled analgesia pumps can be accomplished in the home setting if needed. The use of a basal intravenous infusion with patient-controlled boluses is the preferred method. Subcutaneous infusion of opioids can also be used, with near equivalent efficacy, and it can be more easily managed in some home settings (17). For all methods, titration to comfort is the goal, with management of secondary symptoms such as nausea or sleepiness as needed by the patient and within the context of her goals. The last few hours of life can be marked by both increased or decreased pain, and a strategy to address this needs to be in place as part of the pain control program.

The multiplicity of tumor-related and therapy-related pain syndromes that result in neuropathies from invasion, radiation, or other therapy often require additional therapies (18). Anticonvulsants are helpful adjuncts. The most commonly used would be gabapentin, which is routinely used for postherpetic, chemotherapy-related, and diabetic neuropathies. Clonazepam and lamotrigine also may be effective. Additionally, tricyclic antidepressants (e.g., amitriptyline, desipramine, nortriptyline) may be helpful for neuropathic pain as they also treat underlying depression, have their own direct analgesic effect, and potentiate opioid analgesia (19). Alpha 2 adrenergic agonists, usually clonidine, have also been effective adjuvant analgesics for neuropathic pain as they work through a different receptor from opioids and decrease sympathetic outflow related to neuropathic pain. Corticosteroids such as dexamethasone can provide additional relief, particularly for inflammation irritating nerve endings. For the extensive pelvic tumor invading the nerves in the pelvic floor, the use of sacral or regional nerve blocks, epidural pumps, or ablation of nerve roots may have an important role (20).

Nausea, Vomiting, and Bowel Obstruction

The etiology of nausea and vomiting at the end of life can be related to medications, but more often for gynecologic cancer patients it is related to malignant bowel obstruction. Ovarian and endometrial cancers have a higher likelihood of developing obstruction. It is critical to distinguish the obstructed bowel from constipation/obstipation for obvious reasons in terms of management. Since the majority of patients are already at risk for constipation from medications (opioids as well as serotonin antagonist antiemetics) as well as low motility of the bowel, initiation of a bowel program or extension of one is part of palliative care. Initial efforts with fiber in the diet and fluid intake can assist in management. Both peristalsis stimulants and fecal softeners may be required for an adequate bowel program with rectal laxatives added as needed. Usually the use of propulsive agents such as the anthranoid laxatives (senna) or polyphenolic compounds rather than stool softeners will better manage the constipation related to opiate and other drug use, and may require higher doses of these to resolve constipation (21).

If obstruction is diagnosed, the consideration for surgery should be limited to those in whom their overall condition is otherwise good. Various studies have shown that advanced age, poor general health or nutritional status, diffuse peritoneal carcinomatosis, ascites, palpable masses, prior radiation, and multiple obstructed sites carry a higher mortality and morbidity (22). Careful selection of patients has been shown to not only achieve symptom relief but extend survival (23,24). Evaluation to ascertain the likelihood of benefit for individual patients should include imaging procedures (Gastrografin enemas, carefully chosen use of computed tomographic, and limited upper gastrointestinal evaluations) that target the identification of multiple sites of obstruction. Failure to identify the presence of multiple sites of obstruction can lead to failure of the procedure and add to the pain and discomfort of the patient during the dying phase.

Symptom management is usually the path taken in the treatment of bowel obstruction. Nasogastric tubes provide quick relief, but are uncomfortable, and some reports suggest that they are ineffective in longer-term management of symptoms. Gastrostomy tubes are generally more comfortable, but require surgical or radiology intervention that may not be desired by patients. For individuals with partial and complete bowel obstruction and carcinomatous ileus, gastrostomy tubes can provide significant symptom management with just dependent drainage or suction. Distal rectal obstruction can sometimes be relieved through the use of stent placement (25,26) if that is available, and is worth consideration.

Additionally, there are pharmacologic options to consider, with haloperidol being an additional choice for antiemetics in the setting of bowel obstruction (27). Additionally, hysocine hydrobromide and hysocine butyl bromide are helpful with patients experiencing colicky pain and nausea. Corticosteroids have been used to reduce inflammation, and potentially reduce the obstruction in some patients, and are worth a trial as part of conservative management. Dexamethasone in a dose of 4 to 8 mg per day for 3 to 5 days is generally used for this (28). Finally, somatostatin analogues such as octreotide can limit the secretions and motility and diminish the symptoms of bowel obstruction overall (29). Octreotide has the option of a long-acting formulation, which only requires monthly injections and has been shown to assist in the setting of advanced ovarian cancer (30).

Nutritional Management at End of Life

The value of end of life nutritional maintenance must be firmly set in the context of what the goal of the intervention is. Giving artificial nutrition in the dying phase of life has generally not been shown to prolong survival, adds risk, and may not enhance comfort (31). Families and patients can have culturally and religious-based concerns about not providing "nutrition" in the dying phase, often framed as "starving" the patient, which need to be addressed. It is very important to explain to patients and families that hunger and thirst are symptoms that are experienced differently in healthy people from those who are seriously ill. Those who are near death are often comfortable even though they are no longer eating.

At times, earlier in the trajectory of the patient's illness, management of nutrition as a trial to achieve another palliative or quality of life goal, for example to maximize stamina for a special event with a limited time line for treatment, may be an appropriate strategy. In this context, nutritional support might be started as a trial to evaluate whether this can achieve greater palliation of symptoms or to reach a clearly defined goal of the patient, such as attending a specific event, and defined time lines need to be discussed with patients ahead of time to assess the efficacy of this strategy in meeting these goals. In a sense, it allows patients to try to meet the energy needs for the energy expenditure they have set as a goal that they are otherwise unable to accomplish.

The options for artificial nutrition are enteral if feasible and parenteral if not. Most patients at the end of life have tried increased oral feeding, but owing to low transit times with associated nausea and lack of appetite, have ceased trying to eat. If a time-limited option to increase appetite is desired, then corticosteroids such as dexamethasone can be considered, although their efficacy is limited. Additional appetite stimulants include progesterones such as Megace. Both can have a limited impact on oral intake. Diet supplements then form the basis for increasing nutritional input, including simple formulations such as instant breakfast or intact protein formulations with low lactose.

Other enteral feeding approaches generally focus on feeding tubes either placed under fluoroscopy via a nasogastric approach or surgically placed in the jejunum or the stomach. These use protein hydrolysates with timed feedings or continuous infusions (32,33). The discomfort of nasogastric feeding tubes sometimes prevents this means of enteral feeding from being effective, but does allow for easy removal. J tubes require surgical intervention in abdomens where landmarks are possibly obscured by tumor, and placement must be evaluated in light of the potential issues with the type of tumor and the likelihood of surgical difficulty. In patients with low motility and partial obstruction, the use of enteral feeding formulations may allow the patient to meet her goals without requiring the cumbersome and more difficult to adjust total parenteral nutrition (TPN).

TPN remains the final option for attempting to improve nutritional status transiently in end of life care. Undertaking TPN ties a patient to an intravenous line as well as incurring increased expense and potential for morbidity that could add to the burden of symptoms such as dyspnea at the end of life. It is often more than a support person can manage at home, and may obligate the individual to undesired nursing home or hospital care settings. Furthermore, intravenous access with ports in the face of terminal disease and often-compromised immune surveillance can result in infections that diminish access not only for TPN, but also access for needed pain control or other intravenous medications (34). This, therefore, must be understood in a framework that defines clear stopping parameters (failure to meet goals of symptom relief or improved stamina for an event) and a clear overall time line. In general, TPN is not of benefit in the end of life for patients with cachexia from metastatic cancer (31).

Ascites Management

For women with ovarian cancer, ascites (and associated pleural effusions) create continual pressure, pain, and diminished pulmonary capacity that significantly impact activities of daily life and their quality of life in the dying process. Management relies on elements of constriction of influx and increasing efflux. The pathophysiology of malignant ascites is not only obstructed efflux through lymphatics in the diaphragm (35), but also increased production of fluid. The fact that the protein content of the fluid is 85% of plasma levels versus 25% of plasma levels for transudates suggests that the vessel walls are compromised. An emerging culprit is vascular endothelial growth factor (VEGF) (36). This suggests that VEGF receptor inhibitors might have a role in palliative management of this problem.

The mainstay of ascites management, however, remains paracentesis, and this has been improved through ultrasound guidance. The use of pleuracentesis kits and vacuum bottles allows this to be done in outpatient settings or even at the bedside at home with ease, and many patients are managed simply with once or twice weekly removal of 1 to 4 L in an office setting, often without fluid replacement (37). Use of the closed drainage system developed for pleural drainage (Pleur-X; Denver Biomedical, Golden, Colorado, USA) has been successful with malignant ascites as well and offers a method that can be managed by the patient and family (38). Large volumes of fluid (10 L) can be removed (39), but this must be balanced with colloid infusions and risks further diminishing of the intravascular albumin and protein concentrations (40), leading to worsening anasarca and associated symptoms.

Another common strategy in the management of ascites is the use of diuretics to diminish vascular volume and loss through the vascular tree. Spironolactone is the mainstay of managing ascites associated with cirrhosis and is worth considering for malignant ascites (41). Other diuretics can be considered as well, particularly furosemide, but their primary benefit may be the peripheral edema associated with hypoproteinemia. There have been no clear head-to-head studies of diuretics versus paracentesis and quality of life outcomes in these patients to guide therapy.

In the presence of a slow-growing malignancy, but a palliative stage of disease that requires frequent paracentesis, peritoneovenous shunts as well as the tunneled catheter described above can be considered. Both Denver and Le Veen shunts have been used, with a complication rate of 25% being quoted in a review of multiple series by Helzberg and Greenberger (42). More radical means such as laparoscopically guided intraperitoneal hyperthermic chemotherapy have a role in earlier palliative care, but would rarely be applicable in the end of life setting (43).

Pulmonary Management

Among the most frightening symptoms for women and their families at the end of life are the symptoms of dyspnea and chest pain. Three etiologies stand out in metastatic gynecologic cancers: malignant pleural effusions, parenchymal metastases, and nodal/mediastinal metastases with airway compromise. Although quite different in etiology, some basic principles form the basis of symptom management. These include the use of oxygen, relief of brochospasm, control of secretions, and measures to promote relaxation, which are helpful with all these etiologies.

Probably the most difficult issue to treat is pleural effusions, particularly as they compound the pulmonary constriction caused by ascites in ovarian cancer patients. Thoracentesis (with ultrasound guidance) gives immediate relief, but reaccumulations are common. Repeated thoracentesis may be a strategy appropriate to short-term management or if only needed every few weeks, with the 4% or greater risk of pneumothorax with each procedure as well as the concurrent discomfort (44). Alternatives are restricted to those who have recurrent symptomatic pleural fluid, where this is the primary source of symptomatology and survival is expected to be more than a few weeks. One option is a tunneled closed system pleural catheter which can provide considerable relief without requiring more major surgery and is successful in over 80% of patients (45). Another option for these patients is chemical pleuradesis, now virtually always done with talc by direct application with video-assisted thoracoscopic surgery (VATS) or through a chest tube (46,47). Success is more limited in the setting of repeated prior thoracentesis with scarring that can make the procedure less effective. Any suggestion of a trapped lung or an endobronchial obstruction further diminishes success to the point that pleuradesis would not be a useful choice (48). Most individuals will have a fever and moderate to severe pain around the time of instillation, and complications include arrhythmias, pneumonitis, empyema, and respiratory failure. Such a procedure requires the patient to be in the hospital, occasionally in the intensive care unit for observation overnight if a VATS plus talc procedure is done, and creates costs and side effects that must be weighed carefully against the benefits. Pleuradesis should be restricted to individuals in whom this intervention has a significant chance of alleviating the primary symptoms to avoid exposing women unnecessarily to pain and side effects that further burden their dying phase of life.

Management of pulmonary metastases in the end of life setting, even if solitary, is focused on symptom relief. Many parenchymal lesions are asymptomatic, but pleural irritation can be problematic with coughing as well as hypoxemia. Lymphangitic carcinomatosis is less common in gynecologic malignancies than in others, such as breast or lung cancer, but dyspnea and hypoxemia with the thickened septa and interstitial edema are the primary symptoms to be managed. The dyspnea associated with lymphangitic spread is often symptomatically greater than the actual pulmonary disease present (49). Strategies to treat these symptoms are attention to environment, and diminishing walking or activity requires doing simple activities of daily living by changing the environment. The use of a fan for air circulation, nasal oxygen (with portable units), and trials of pursed lip breathing may all help. Certainly, consideration should be given to diuretic therapy if there is any component of fluid overload, and opiates, particularly morphine, are helpful. Morphine, often in use for pain control, also has a role in decreasing air hunger and dyspnea and should be tried in this setting if not already in use. Anxiolytics, although helpful for the anxiety component and commonly used as an adjuvant, can occasionally worsen symptoms by causing respiratory depression and more air hunger and should be used judiciously in addressing pulmonary symptoms.

Airway obstruction and cough have similar symptoms, and some of the therapy is similar. Cough may be due to multiple issues including conditions unrelated to malignancy such as asthma or sinusitis and from gastroesophageal reflux, which is more common with ascites. Therapies tailored specifically to these issues such as the use of inhaled or intranasal steroids, antihistamines, and proton pump inhibitors for reflux are appropriate. Cough due to airway obstruction responds to narcotic suppression with morphine or codeine. Occasionally, steroid inhalers add additional relief from bronchial irritation induced by metastatic disease. Even humidifiers may be helpful for some patients, particularly for coughs from irritated mucosal linings from prior mediastinal chest radiation. In some cases, radiation therapy targeted to specific areas of obstructing disease in the mediastinum, with an obviously longer survival estimate, may be of value in managing symptoms. In sum, the therapies for pulmonary symptoms rely on supplemental oxygen, local suppression of inflammation, suppression of cough and air hunger through opiates, and removal of fluid compression as needed.

Central Nervous System Involvement: Management of Seizures, Brain Metastases, and Mental Status Changes

Mental status changes are usually present at the end of life and management of this symptom is often the key toward patients achieving their personal goals at the end of life, many of which center around being awake and conversant to bring closure with family and friends. Delirium is particularly distressing to family members who also are seeking closure with the dying patient. For both, the decline in function from a prior baseline heralds more losses to come and creates even greater anxiety. Etiologies can be metabolic abnormalities (sepsis, renal failure), innumerable drugs, and structural brain lesions with obvious differences in approach to treatment. There are clear predisposing factors, including age, multisensory impairment, medical illness, depression, dehydration, and abnormal serum electrolyte levels, pertinent to the end stage of malignancies (50–52).

Understanding the nature of the delirium is important in addressing what may be more than one contributing factor. Assessing alertness, distractibility, the patient's ability to concentrate and talk easily, and simple cognitive disturbances of memory, reasoning, or perception all contribute to the delirium, along with specific neurologic deficits or neuromuscular activity that can point to central nervous system metastases. Laboratory and physical evaluation with infection, hypercalcemia, renal failure, hypoglycemia, hypomagnesemia, and hypoxemia being key conditions to look for (53–55). Tuma and DeAngelis (56) noted that with appropriate workup, a significant number of patients can improve their symptoms (68%) even when terminal.

Addressing electrolytic abnormalities and treating infection have value when the goal of a clearer sensorum at the end of life can be achieved. If opioid-induced delirium is the diagnosis, then rotation of types of opioids used can be helpful in restoring function (57). If there are hallucinations and agitation, particularly in elderly dying patients, consideration of haloperidol or droperidol if more sedation is desired is appropriate (58,59). Given intravenously, haloperidol can be effective within 30 minutes and generally lasts for at least 4 hours. Given by mouth, the half-life of haloperidol is considerably longer, and could be used in mild delirium states. It is important to remember that these drugs have the potential of lowering the seizure threshold, as the more common electrolytic abnormalities associated with prior chemotherapy such as magnesium deficiency also may be present and compound the risk. Finally, some patients may benefit from combining drugs and including a benzodiazepine to decrease associated agitation. Some studies have noted that delirium in patients with advanced cancer more commonly requires more than one medication (60). The most commonly used are lorazepam (up to 2 mg) or midazolam, which is preferred if a subcutaneous route is to be used (61).

Another source of delirium or abnormalities in central nervous system function is brain metastasis. Initial therapy after diagnosis is the immediate use of corticosteroids to decrease local edema and also headache associated with this. This may, in fact, be all that is needed if the patient has a very short time to live as median survival with brain metastasis with steroids alone is about 2 months. However, if a patient is otherwise functional and treatment could improve her overall quality of life, then targeted radiation therapy should be considered. For this use, generally 300 Gy total dose given in 30-Gy fractions is administered (62). For care at the end of life, more aggressive resection and radiation is generally not appropriate.

Control of seizures depends on the etiology of the seizures. The more common causes in gynecologic oncology patients would be electrolyte induced, often hypomagnesemia or hyponatremia. Primary brain etiologies range from brain metastases to brain hemorrhage and stroke. Virtually all will be able to be controlled initially with lorazepam either intravenously or by mouth. Electrolyte repletion should be undertaken (63). Seizures associated with brain metastasis may be controlled with simply the decrease in inflammation with corticosteroids.

Local Comfort Measures

Many of the measures for comfort at the end of life are related to simple things that can escape notice but create comfort for the dying woman (64). The environment itself gives comfort if familiar things are around, including sounds, smells, and pictures that hold meaning for the woman. Assuring that the issues of access and fall prevention are addressed by a care team is important to the success of home care. Skin protection through rotation if the patient is bed bound and early identification and treatment of skin breakdown prevents unnecessary sources of pain and infection. Many patients derive great comfort from gentle massage and virtually all benefit from human touch and presence. Developing a plan for passive (or active) movement during the day alleviates pain and discomfort from decreased mobility. Eye care with artificial tears or even hydrogel eye patches may be needed. Perineal care and the use of urinary catheters to eliminate skin breakdown in the perineum are commonly used when the patient is no longer mobile. Families and patients sometimes need "permission" from their health care team to make the environment home rather than a hospital at home. Yet it is the breeze from the window, the smells of home, the sights of loved ones rocking in a chair beside them that bring the most comfort—and the physician must actively support choices that make this possible at the end of life.

Management of Fistulas in the Terminal Care Setting

The fistulas encountered at the end of life from both the urinary system and the gastrointestinal (GI) system are often the most difficult for family and caregivers to deal with. The principles of management are simple but difficult to achieve. The options are diversion, containment, and closure regardless of the site of the fistula.

Enterocutaneous fistulae can occur from every part of the bowel, but those from the small bowel have high output and are irritating to the skin. Diversion is rarely an option in the setting of terminal cancer, primarily because the intra-abdominal spread of disease is frequently the etiology of the fistula itself in association with prior therapies such as radiation. Surgical diversion, if the patient is medically stable and surgery could be limited, has benefits solely to provide better control and better fit of pouches over the ostomy site than over a fistula site. As noted by Marsden et al., this does not remove the problem as there may still be a discharge from the site of tumor-related necrotic material that must be managed (65). If this is not possible, the only recourse—similar to bowel obstruction—is to attempt to diminish flow through the GI tract with octreotide and then to minimize and manage skin irritation actively. Large bowel fistula, most commonly to the vagina, can be more easily diverted and this is the first choice if the patient is medically stable. Even a simple loop colostomy can provide relief from the volume of vaginal discharge. However, some discharge usually remains. The use of metronidazole for tumor necrosis and discharge in the vaginal area relieves some of the anaerobic odors, and sitz baths and douches as needed to control odor are also helpful.

Vesicovaginal and ureterovaginal fistulae are primarily handled by diversion, if appropriate. The primary problem with diversion is the discomfort and management of new percutaneous nephrostomies, and the additional factor that for some patients there may be a component of renal failure that there is no desire to reverse. Additionally, nephrostomies alone may not be adequate for resolution, and the use of ureteral occlusion with coils and sponge pledgets may also be helpful (66). Local measures, including scrupulous management of pelvic and perineal hygiene, the use of adult diapers, and the use of creams such as 1% silver sulfasalazine or skin barriers are primary measures. There are no vaginal means to control or contain the output that have so far been effective. Various measures such as the use of diaphragms glued to catheters or local tissue glues have generally been ineffective in this setting.

Bleeding related to the pelvic/vaginal fistula or to vaginal recurrence can potentially be controlled by single fraction pelvic radiation (67) or if severe and causing significant distress with embolization. Local measures such as Monsel's solution have only limited efficacy and packing can add considerably to patient discomfort. So, try to pick an approach that fits both the overall status of the patient (if only a few days are likely, then the value of any intervention would be negligible) and the comfort and decrease in anxiety she might gain from addressing the bleeding.

Management of Bone Metastases

Bone metastases are rare in terminal gynecologic cancers, being primarily confined to unusually high-grade cell types such as glassy cell malignancies, neuroendocrine tumors, melanomas, small cell malignancies, or clear cell malignancies. When they occur, however, the pain associated with bone metastases can be the most excruciating of all the symptoms to be managed at the end of life. Corticosteroids and nonsteroidal anti-inflammatory drugs may have a significant role in managing the inflammatory pain from bone metastases and should be considered as part of initial management. If the metastases are localized, radiation therapy on a palliative basis may supply additional pain relief with a success rate of 24% to 50% total pain relief and 80% to 90% of patients noting relief of pain (68). Relief of pain may be immediate or it may require several months, and the use of anti-inflammatory pain medications during treatment may aid in symptom relief until the effects of radiation become evident.

Key aspects of treatment include ensuring that radiation fields encompass the entire area of bone involvement (69) and also the prevention of overlap with prior radiation fields. Multiple schemes have been used depending on the urgency and the overall expected survival time of the patient. There does not seem to be a difference between single-fraction versus multiple-fraction approaches, except for the need for retreatment with single fraction (70). Also, if there is a longer life expectancy, consideration should be given to prophylactic surgical fixation of weight-bearing bones with >50% cortical destruction or size >2.5 cm prior to radiation therapy (71,72).

Another option for consideration is the use of osteoblast-affinic agents such as strontium 89 or samarium 153 that deliver localized radiation to osteoblastic bony metastases. The primary problem in their use is bone marrow suppression, which often limits their use in patients with ongoing residual suppression from their prior therapies. These agents are not appropriate for use in hypercalcemic patients, and the pain relief is slower in onset with a duration of about 12 weeks. This option may require multiple doses to increase efficacy (73,74).

Psychologic Needs in Terminally Ill Cancer Patients

An important aspect of palliative care in terminally ill cancer patients is the recognition and treatment of psychologic symptoms to improve quality of life at the end of life. The understanding of suffering requires not just addressing physical needs, but also distress, existential concerns, and social relational worries which contribute to overall suffering in terminal cancer patients (75). Health care professionals often ignore the role that religion and spirituality play in coping with terminal illness. Most patients consider religion or spiritual aspects to be at least somewhat important and the majority report that their spiritual needs were supported minimally or not at all by the medical system (76). Referral to chaplaincy services or other integrative medicine services is seen as having value to our patients and assessing their desire for this should be part of psychologic assessment and treatment (77). This is an area where little training and modeling exist in medical education, and the ability to address spirituality comfortably with patients is limited but important for health professionals to improve in discussing and addressing (78,79).

Depression and anxiety occur in a high percentage of cancer patients, particularly as disease advances and curative cancer treatment fails (80). The prevalence of depression in cancer patients has been the subject of numerous studies, and the reported rates have ranged from as high as 58.0% to as low as 4.5% with age, lower performance status, smaller social networks, and less participation in organized religious services all significant in predicting depression and anxiety (81).

Anxiety in terminally ill cancer patients has received less attention than depression. Anxiety commonly increases as patients become aware of both the relative ineffectiveness of medical treatments in halting the progress of their disease and, consequently, their limited life expectancy (82). The awareness of the inevitable death is likely to cause anxiety in terminally ill cancer patients. Breitbart et al. suggest that the incidence of both anxiety and depression in cancer patients increases with higher levels of disability, advanced illness, and pain (83). The closer the patient is to dying, the higher the score on depression and the lower the score on physical performance.

Although depression and anxiety are important to continually assess in terminally ill patients prior to death, data show that a relatively high percentage of terminally ill cancer patients suffer from psychologic distress a few weeks before death, which appears to be related to physical symptoms. Treating the physical symptoms maximally is the first task in addressing depression and anxiety. Standard treatment for depression and anxiety is effective in this population, and tricyclic antidepressants which additionally address neuropathic pain are reasonable choices. Lorazepam is often used for assisting in managing other symptoms but also provides relief for anxiety. Some integrative medicine solutions such as aromatherapy massage can be shown to assist in decreasing anxiety and depression (84). In sum, psychologic symptoms in terminally ill cancer patients need to be systematically assessed and considered by the care team in the overall decision-making and treatment plan at the end of life. Treatment of anxiety and depression clearly also improves overall management of pain as well as making the process of closure more possible for dying women. If patients can reconcile their concerns with psychologic and pharmacologic support, this will substantially remove the suffering from emotional distress for the patient and her family.

REQUESTS FOR HELP IN DYING

Sometimes, patients ask to end their life because of fear of an inability to control suffering at the end of life or inadequately managed pain or suffering. In most countries in the world, the law forbids assisted suicide. In the Netherlands, Belgium, and the United States (State of Oregon), individuals have access to laws that make assisted suicide available for those experiencing unbearable suffering and this access is highly regulated. Data from the Oregon experience (85) show that most patients do not follow through even with an expressed intent for assisted suicide.

Regardless of where health providers are in the world, this is a question that will come up directly or indirectly if actively caring for dying patients—and challenges our communication skills as few have been educated specifically for end of life discussions (86). Additionally, having such a discussion requires physicians to address for themselves their own understanding and barriers to discussing dying, futility, and assisted suicide (87).

Dying patients expect and need at least a minimal level of emotional support defined by them as compassion and treating the whole person and not just the disease (88). Set in this context, this conversation is an opportunity to embrace the compassion and acknowledgment of the whole person that is expected by the patient and to enhance understanding of the fears and the needs of the patient in the present. Patients who state that they would like "extra" prescriptions for pain medicine or anxiolytics, or who blatantly state that they are thinking of ending it all themselves or would like help in doing so are asking for an exploratory conversation about how "unbearable" dying will be.

Even in the middle of a busy clinic, time has to be made for this discussion. Confirming that the patient's request has been heard and confirming the patient's importance to her health professionals is part of the therapeutic relationship. A consult room with the inclusion of whomever the patient wants to include (or not) is a better setting than an examination room if available. Exploration with more open-ended questions such as, "Why do you feel you need this extra prescription right now?" "What do you think will happen that might make you think of (whatever phrasing the patient used)?" is a way to begin the dialog. Remembering that suffering is not only physical, but also psychologic and spiritual is important to be sure that all dimensions of fear and questions are answered, or if unanswerable, acknowledged as important. Follow-up questions that explore the patient's motivation are outlined in Bascom and Tolle's article (85). Then exploring each fear and, more importantly, assuring that with maximal effort at palliative care this can be addressed (and how), and that the patient is not viewed as a burden and is valued will open critical communication and provides an opportunity to address the underlying concern of the patient. In addition, this is an optimal time to introduce or reintroduce the importance of advance directives and to implement specific written orders regarding life-sustaining treatments (89). If this is an area of communication that is uncomfortable to the physician, then having another member of the team lead this discussion with the patient would be valuable, but with the specific assurance that respecting her wishes and continuing to care for the patient are still of importance to the physician who has been a critical member of that patient's care.

BEREAVED FAMILY AND FRIENDS

Medicine focuses on the individual care of patients, and the needs and issues of the social network that supports patients are often ignored. End of life care, however, engages that entire social network of family and friends and requires understanding their needs and roles as the patient nears the end of life. Families define high-quality end of life care as first achieving good palliation of symptoms for the patient, but they also weigh quality on how well the dying person was able to control decisions and whether the family members felt that they had to be constant advocates for the wishes of the dying person. In addition, education and emotional support for the family and friends caring for the patient were seen as important (90). All the members of this network of care for the patient experience high levels of stress, burden, and diminished quality of life that can be helped with specific coping skills training (91). Caregivers who are able to accept and reframe the patient's illness feel less strain and feel more capable of solving illness-related problems, all of which will directly improve the care of the dying woman (92).

While the care and comfort of the families and friends of dying patients are not a direct responsibility of the oncologic physician, advocating for the development of support for this network for patients and providing access to such support are. In addition, regardless of whether the physician and primary oncology team are directly involved in the end of life care of the patient, acknowledging the patient's death and the team's concern for her family with a card or phone call to the family is important in closing the circle for the family as well as the primary oncology team.

CARE FOR THE CAREGIVERS

Within palliative care in general and end of life care in particular, there is a tendency for patients and relatives to demand and benefit from a more personal care and personal approach. Because of this contact-intensive nature of end of life care, it can be expected that physicians and nurses run a serious risk of depleting their emotional resources, especially when they cross the border between their professional and personal involvement. This can result in burnout. Physicians and nurses should be aware of the risk factors in order to prevent this serious threat to their health. In oncology, and especially in end of life care, the stressors appear to be strongly related to the social and interpersonal aspects of the job, including relationships with patients and co-workers on the team (93–96).

To understand and prevent emotional exhaustion and burnout, physicians and nurses should be able to share their responses and feelings with others at work. This can be done by the organization of support groups at work where they can discuss what moved them and how they dealt with the situation (97–99). Improvement in physician communication skills around these stressful issues actually diminishes physician stress since the doctor-patient relationship plays an important role in this regard (100). The participants get the opportunity to discuss the emotional aspects of the care of the terminal patient. This can include revisiting conversations that were held about death with patients and their families. The team listens and discusses how these emotional events affected the person involved. Especially for younger and inexperienced personnel, this type of guidance by "peers" is very important. For the more experienced members, the team meetings can work as control. Much experience can result in diminished emotional involvement and distancing the relationships to a routine. Comments, advice, and help of colleagues are important factors in staying mentally fit—again, a message for all health professionals, at all parts of end of life care.

CONCLUSIONS

End of life care is a very important part of caring for women with cancer. It requires total commitment of the entire health care team. It includes medical interventions to relieve suffering, but also psychosocial care. Communication skills are very important to ensure optimal end of life care. In this communication, the autonomy of the patient has to be respected. The caregivers must respect the delicate balance between professional and personal involvement. Communication not only involves the patient, but also her relatives and friends. It is important that this communication take place in the presence of the patient as much as possible to avoid misunderstandings. Psychologic symptoms need to be routinely assessed and considered by physicians in the overall decision making concerning the end of life. Special attention must focus on anxiety and depression to be sure that all domains of suffering are addressed.

End of life care in oncology does not mean that the physician has to postpone the inevitable as long as possible. The goal is quite simply to continue the expert and compassionate care the patient has received throughout her treatment into the maximal alleviation of symptoms and suffering at the end of life.

References

1. Callahan D. Living and dying with medical technology. *Crit Care Med* 2003;31:S344–S346.
2. Curtis JR, Wenrich MD, Carline JD, et al. Patients' perspectives on physician skill in end-of-life care: differences between patients with COPD, cancer, and AIDS. *Chest* 2002;122:356–362.
3. Fromme EK, Drach LL, Tolle SW, et al. Men as caregivers at the end of life. *J Pall Med* 2005;8:1167–1175.
4. Fromme EK, Bascom PB, Mith MD, et al. Survival, mortality and location of death for patients seen by a hospital-based palliative care team. *J Pall Med* 2006;9:903–911.
5. Tilden VP, Tolle SW, Nelson CA, et al. Family decision-making to withdraw life-sustaining treatments from hospitalized patients. *Nurs Res* 2001; 50(2):105–115.
6. Hickman SE, Hammes BJ, Moss AH, et al. Hope for the future: achieving the original intent of advance directives. *Hastings Center Special Report* 2005;35(6):S26–S30.
7. Tilden VP, Tolle SW, Drach LL, et al. Out-of-hospital death: advance care planning, decedent symptoms, and caregiver burden. *JAGS* 2004;52: 532–539.
8. Tolle SW, Tilden VP, Dunn P, et al. A prospective study of the efficacy of the Physician Orders for Life Sustaining Treatment. *JAGS* 1998;46(9): 1097–1102.
9. Evans N, Walsh H. The organization of death and dying in today's society. *Nurs Stand* 2002;16:33–38.
10. Finnerty JJ, Chisholm CA. Patient refusal of treatment in obstetrics. *Semin Perinatol* 2003;27:435–445.
11. Milliez J, Veronique C. Palliative care with pregnant women. *Best Pract Res Clin Obstet Gynecol* 2001;15:323–331.
12. Finnerty JF, Fuerst CW, Karns LB, et al. End-of-life discussions for the primary care obstetrician/gynecologist. *Am J Obstet Gynecol* 2002;187: 296–301.
13. Thomas JR, vonGunten CF. Pain in terminally ill patients: guidelines for pharmacologic management. *CNS Drugs* 2003;17:621–631.
14. Mercadante S, Villari P, Ferrera P, et al. Addition of a second opioid may improve opioid response in cancer pain: preliminary data. *Support Care Cancer* 2004;12:762–766.
15. Bercovitch M, Adunsky A. High dose controlled-release oxycodone in hospice care. *J Pain Pall Care Pharm* 2006;20:33–39.
16. Ellershaw JE, Kinder C, Aldridge J, et al. Care of the dying: is pain control compromised or enhanced by continuation of the fentanyl transdermal patch in the dying phase? *J Pain Symptom Manage* 2003;26:589–590.
17. Anderson SL, Shreve ST. Continuous subcutaneous infusion of opiates at end of life. *Ann Pharmacother* 2004;38:1015–1023.
18. Gordin V, Weaver MA, Hahn MB. Acute and chronic pain management in palliative care. *Best Pract Res Clin Obstet Gynecol* 2001;15:203–234.
19. Hammond DL. Pharmacology of central pain-modulating networks (biogenic amines and non-opioid analgesics). *Adv Pain Res Ther* 1985:9;499–512.
20. Harrison GR. The use of epidural ropivacaine in high doses for the management of pain from invasive carcinoma of the cervix. *Anesthesia* 1999; 54:459–465.
21. Solomon R, Cherny NI. Constipation and diarrhea in patients with cancer. *Cancer J* 2006;12:355–364.
22. Baines MJ. The pathophysiology and management of malignant intestinal obstruction. In: Doyle D, Hanks GWC, MacDonald N, eds. *Oxford Textbook of Palliative Medicine*. Oxford, UK: Oxford University Press; 1998:526–534.
23. Sartori E, Chiudinelli F, Pasinetti B, et al. Palliative care in advanced ovarian cancer patients with bowel obstruction. *Gynecol Oncol* 2005;99:S215–S216.
24. Rubin SC, Hoskins WJ, Benjamin I, et al. Palliative surgery for intestinal obstruction in advanced ovarian cancer. *Gynecol Oncol* 1989:34:16–19.
25. Diaz PL, Pinto PI, Fernandex LR, et al. Palliative treatment of malignant colorectal strictures with metallic stents. *Cardiovasc Intervent Radiol* 1999;22:29–36.
26. Tack J, Gevener AM, Rutgeerts P. Self-expandable metallic stents in the palliation of rectosigmoid carcinoma: a follow up study. *Gastrointest Endosc* 1998;48:267–271.
27. Baines MJ. Nausea, vomiting, and intestinal obstruction. In: Fallon M, O'Neill B, eds. *ABC of Palliative Care*. London: BMJ Books; 1998:16–18.
28. Phillip J, Lickiss N, Grant PT, et al. Corticosteroids in the management of bowel obstruction in advanced ovarian cancer. *Gynecol Oncol* 1999;74: 68–73.
29. Mangili G, Franchi M, Mariani A, et al. Octreotide in the management of bowel obstruction in terminal ovarian cancer. *Gynecol Oncol* 1996;61: 345–348.
30. Matulonis UA, Seiden MV, Roche M, et al. Long acting octreotide for the treatment and symptomatic relief of bowel obstruction in advanced ovarian cancer. *J Pain Symptom Manage* 2005;30:563–569.
31. Casarett D, Kapo J, Caplan A. Appropriate use of artificial nutrition and hydration—fundamental principles and recommendations. *N Engl J Med* 2005;353:2607–2611.
32. Gore DC, DeLegge M, Gervin A, et al. Surgically placed gastrojejunostomy tubes have fewer complications compared to feeding jejunostomy tubes. *J Am C Nutrit* 1996;15:144–146.
33. Jabbar A, McClave SA. Prepyloric versus post pyloric feeding. *Clin Nutrit* 2005;24:719–726.
34. Chang L, Tsai JS, Huang SJ, et al. Evaluation of infectious complications of the implantable venous access system in a general oncologic population. *Am J Infect Control* 2003;31:34–39.
35. Nagy JA, Herzberg KT, Dvorak JM, et al. Pathogenesis of malignant ascites formation: initiating events that lead to fluid accumulation. *Cancer Res* 1993;53:2631–2643.
36. Kraft A, Weindel K, Ochs A, et al. Vascular endothelial growth factor in the sera and effusions of patients with malignant and nonmalignant disease. *Cancer* 1999;85:178–187.
37. Macdonald R, Kirwan J, Roberts S, et al. Ovarian cancer and ascites: a questionnaire on current management in the United Kingdom. *J Pall Med* 2006;9:1264–1270.
38. Richard HM 3rd, Coldwell DM, Boyd-Kranis RL, et al. Pleurx tunneled catheter in the management of malignant ascites. *J Vasc Interv Radiol* 2001;12:373–375.
39. Arroyo V, Gines P, Planas R. Treatment of ascites in cirrhosis. Diuretics, peritoneovenous shunt, and large-volume paracentesis. *Gastroenterol Clin North Am* 1992;21:237–256.
40. Gough IR, Balderson GA. Malignant ascites: a comparison of peritoneovenous shunting and nonoperative management. *Cancer* 1993;71: 2377–2382.
41. Greenway B, Johnson PJ, William R. Control of malignant ascites with spironolactone. *Br J Surg* 1982;69:441–442.
42. Helzberg JH, Greenberger NJ. Peritoneovenous shunts in malignant ascites. *Dig Dis Sci* 1985;30:1104–1107.
43. Garafalo A, Valle M, Garcia J, et al. Laparoscopic intraperitoneal hyperthermic chemotherapy for palliation of debilitating malignant ascites. *EJSO* 2006;32:682–685.
44. Bartter T, Mayo PD, Pratter MR, et al. Lower risk and higher yield for thoracentesis when performed by experienced operators. *Chest* 1993; 103:1873–1876.
45. vandenToorn LM, Schaap E, Surmont VF, et al. Management of recurrent malignant pleural effusions with a chronic indwelling pleural catheter. *Lung Cancer* 2005;50:123–127.
46. Luh SP, Chen CY, Tzao CY. Malignant pleural effusion treatment outcomes: pleurodesis via video assisted thoracic surgery (VATS) versus tube thoracostomy. *Thorac Cardiovasc Surg* 2006;54:332–336.
47. Arapis K, Caliandro R, Stern JB, et al. Thorascopic palliative treatment of malignant pleural effusions: results in 273 patients. *Surg Endosc* 2006;20: 919–923.
48. Sahn SA. Malignancy metastatic to the pleura. *Clin Chest Med* 1998; 19:351–356.
49. Tucakovic M, Bascom R, Bascom PB. Pulmonary medicine and palliative care. *Best Pract Res Clin Obstet Gynecol* 2001;15:291–304.
50. Schor JD, Levkoff SE, Lipsitz LA, et al. Risk factors for delirium in hospitalized elderly. *JAMA* 1992;267:827–831.
51. Bruera E, Miller L, McCallion J, et al. Cognitive failure in patients with terminal cancer: a prospective study. *J Pain Symptom Manage* 1992;7: 192–195.
52. Minagawa H, Yosuke U, Yamawaki S, et al. Psychiatric morbidity in terminally ill cancer patients: a prospective study. *Cancer* 1996;78: 1131–1137.
53. deStoutz ND, Tapper M, Faisinger RL. Reversible delirium in terminally ill patients. *J Pain Symptom Manage* 1995;10:249–253.
54. Seymour DG, Henschke PJ, Cape RDT, et al. Acute confusional states and dementia in the elderly: the role of dehydration volume depletion, physical illness and age. *Age Ageing* 1980;9:137–146.
55. Bruera E. Severe organic brain syndrome. *J Palliat Care* 1991;7:36–38.
56. Tuma R, DeAngelis L. Altered mental status in patients with cancer. *Arch Neur* 2000;57:1727–1731.
57. Morita T, Takigawa C, Hideki O, et al. Opioid rotation from morphine to fentanyl in delirious cancer patients: an open label trial. *J Pain Symptom Manage* 2005;30:96–103.
58. Breitbart W, Marotta R, Platt MM, et al. A double-blind trial of haloperidol, chlorpromazine, and lorazepan—the treatment of delirium in hospitalized AIDS patients. *Am J Psychiatry* 1996;153:231–237.
59. Resnick M, Burton B. Droperidol vs haloperidol in the initial management of acutely agitated patients. *J Clin Psychiatry* 1984;45:298–299.
60. Stiefel F, Fainsinger R, Bruera E. Acute confusional states in patients with advanced cancer. *J Pain Symptom Manage* 1992;7:94–98.
61. Bottomley D, Hanks G. Subcutaneous midazolam infusion in palliative care. *J Pain Symptom Manage* 1990;5:259–261.
62. Gaspar L, Scott C, Rotman M, et al. Recursive partitioning analysis (RPA) of prognostic factors in three Radiation Therapy Oncology Group (RTOG) brain metastases trials. *Int J Radiat Oncol Biol and Phys* 1997;37:745–751.
63. Singh G, Rees JH, Sander JW. Seizures and epilepsy in oncological practice: causes, course, mechanisms, and treatment. *J Neurol Neurosurg Psychiatry* 2007;78:342–349.
64. Cain JM. Practical aspects of hospice care at home. *Best Pract Res Clin Obstet Gynecol* 2001;15:305–311.
65. Marsden DE, Lickiss JN, Hacker NF. Gastrointestinal problems in patients with advanced gynecologic malignancy. *Best Pract Res Clin Obstet Gynecol* 2001;15:253–263.

66. Farrell T, Wallace M, Hichs M. Long term results of transrenal occlusion with use of gianturco coils and gelatin sponge pledgets. *J Vasc Interv Radiol* 1997;24:449–452.
67. Onsrud M, Hagen B, Stickert T. 10 Gy single fraction pelvic irradiation for palliation and life prolongation in patients with cancer of the cervix and corpus uteri. *Gynecol Oncol* 2001;82:167–171.
68. Carstens D. Palliative radiation therapy in female genital cancers. In: Vahrson HW, Brady LW, Heilmann HP, eds. *Radiation Oncology of Gynecologic Cancers*. New York: Springer; 1997:55–65.
69. Smith SC, Koh W. Palliative radiation therapy for gynecologic malignancies. *Best Pract Res Clin Obstet Gynecol* 2001;15:265–278.
70. Chow E, Harris K, Fan G, et al. Palliative radiotherapy trials for bone metastases: a systematic review. *J Clin Oncol* 2007;25:1423–1436.
71. Fidler M. Incidence of fracture through metastasis in long bones. *Acta Orthop Scand* 1981;52:623–627.
72. Townsend PW, Smalley SR, Cozad SC, et al. Role of postoperative radiation therapy after stabilization of fractures caused by metastatic disease. *Int J Radiat Oncol Biol Phys* 1995;31:43–49.
73. Lin A, Ray ME. Targeted and systemic radiotherapy in the treatment of bone metastasis. *Cancer Metastasis Rev* 2006;25:669–675.
74. Bauman G, Charette M, Reid R, et al. Radiopharmaceuticals for the palliation of painful bone metastasis: a systemic review. *Radiother Oncol* 2005;75:258–270.
75. Wilson KG, Chochinov M, McPherson CJ, et al. Suffering with advanced cancer. *J Clin Oncol* 2007;25:1691–1697.
76. Balboni TA, Vanderwerker LC, Block SD, et al. Religiousness and spiritual support among advanced cancer patients and associations with end of life treatment preferences and quality of life. *J Clin Oncol* 2007;25: 467–468.
77. Skalla K, McCoy JP. Spiritual assessment of patients with cancer: the moral authority, vocational, aesthetic, social and transcendent model. *Oncol Nurs Forum* 2006;33:745–751.
78. Daaleman TP, VandeCreek L. Placing religion and spirituality in end of life care. *JAMA* 2000;284:2514–2517.
79. McCord G, Ghilchrist VJ, Grossman SD, et al. Discussing spirituality with patients: a rational and ethical approach. *Ann Fam Med* 2004;2: 356–361.
80. Breitbart W. Identifying patients at risk for, and treatment of major psychiatric complications of cancer. *Support Care Cancer* 1995;3:45–60.
81. Wilson KG, Chochinov HM, Skirko MG, et al. Depression and anxiety disorders in palliative cancer care. *J Pain Symptom Manage* 2007;33: 118–129, 67, 68.
82. Shuster JL, Jones GR. Approach to the patient receiving palliative care. In: Stem TA, Herman JB, Slavin PL, eds. *The MGH Guide to Psychiatry in Primary Care*. New York: McGraw-Hill; 1998:147–165.
83. Breitbart W, Bruera E, Chochinov HM, et al. Neuropsychiatric syndromes and psychological symptoms in patients with advanced cancer. *J Pain Symptom Manage* 1995;9:412–415.
84. Wilkinson SM, Love SB, Westcombe AM, et al. Effectiveness of aromatherapy massage in the management of anxiety and depression in patients with cancer: a multicenter randomized controlled trial. *J Clin Oncol* 2007;25:532–539.
85. Bascom PB, Tolle SW. Responding to requests for physician-assisted suicide: "These are uncharted waters for both of us. . ." *JAMA* 2002; 288(1): 91–98.
86. Ramondetta LM, Tortolero-Luna G, Bodurka DC, et al. Approaches for end of life care in the field of gynecologic oncology: an exploratory study. *Int J Gynecol Cancer* 2004;14:5380–5388.
87. von Gruenigen VE, Daly BJ. Futility: clinical decisions at the end of life in women with ovarian cancer. *Gynecol Oncol* 2005;97:638–644.
88. Wenrich MD, Curtis JR, Amrozy DA, et al. Dying patients' need for emotional support and personalized care from physicians: perspectives of patients with terminal illness, families, and health care providers. *J Pain Symptom Manage* 2003:25:236–246.
89. Teno JM, Bruneir A, Schwartz Z, et al. Association between advance directives and quality of end of life care: a national study. *J Am Gerontol Soc* 2007;55:189–194.
90. Teno JM, Casey VA, Welch LC, et al. Patient focused, family centered end of life medical care: views of the guidelines and bereaved family members. *J Pain Symptom Manage* 2001;22:738–751.
91. McMillian SC, Small BJ, Weitzner M, et al. Impact of coping skills intervention with family caregivers of hospice patients with cancer: a randomized clinical trial. *Cancer* 2006;106:214–222.
92. Redinbaugh EM, Baum A, Tarbell S, et al. End of life caregiving: what helps family caregivers cope? *J Palliat Med* 2003;6:901–909.
93. Physician stress and burnout course. Texas Medical Association; 1999.
94. Penson RT, Dignan FC, Canellos GP, et al. Burnout: caring for the caregivers. *Oncologist* 2000;5:425–434.
95. Whippen D, Canellos GP. Burnout syndrome in the practice of oncology: results of a random survey of 1000 oncologists. *J Clin Oncol* 1991;9:1916–1920.
96. Halperin JD, Zabora JR, Brintzenhofe S. The emotional health of oncologists. *Oncol Issues* 1997;21:20–22.
97. Ramirez A, Graham J, Richards M, et al. Mental health of hospital consultants: the effects of stress and satisfaction at work. *Lancet* 1996;347:724–728.
98. Ramirez A, Graham J, Richards M, et al. Burnout and psychiatric disorder among cancer clinicians. *Br J Cancer* 1995;71:1263–1269.
99. Creagan ET. Stress among medical oncologists: the phenomenon of burnout and a call to action. *Mayo Clin Proc* 1993;68:614–615.
100. Armstrong J, Holland J. Surviving the stresses of clinical oncology by improving communication. *Oncology* 2004;18:363–368.

INDEX

Note: Page numbers referencing figures are italicized and followed by an "*f*." Page numbers referencing tables are italicized and followed by a "*t*."

C

D

E

F

G

H

I

J

K

L

M

N

P

Q

R

S

T

U

W

X

Y

Z

CCS0409